DIVISION OF RADIATION ONCOLOGY
UNIVERSITY HOSPITALS
410 WEST 10TH AVENUE
COLUMBUS, OHIO

DIVISION OF RADIATION ONCOLOGY
UNIVERSITY HOSPITALS
410 WEST 10TH AVENUE
COLUMBUS, OHIO

CANCER
Principles & Practice of Oncology

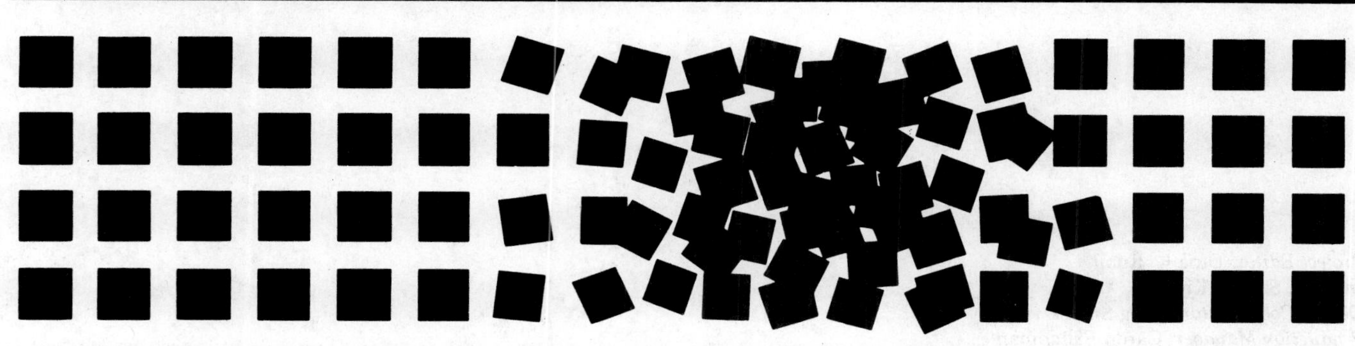

4th Edition

Volume 2

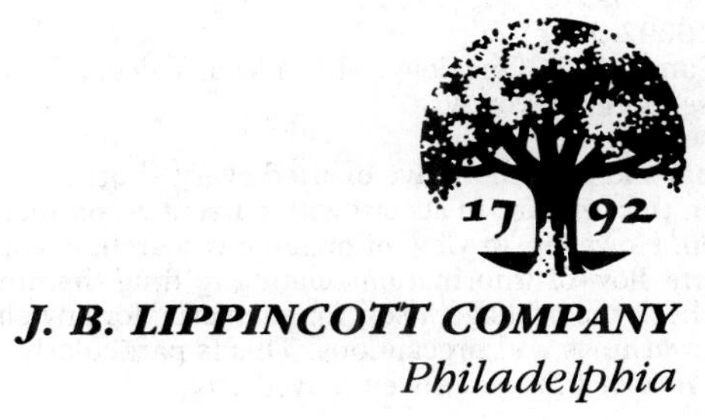

J. B. LIPPINCOTT COMPANY
Philadelphia

Project Editor: Dina K. Rubin
Indexer: Sandra King
Design Coordinator: Doug Smock
Production Manager: Caren Erlichman
Production Coordinator: Sharon McCarthy
Compositor: Tapsco Incorporated
Printer/Binder: Courier Book Company/Westford
Color Insert Printer: Village Craftsmen/Princeton Polychrome Press

4th Edition

Printed in the United States of America. For information write J. B. Lippincott Company, 227 East Washington Square, Philadelphia, Pennsylvania 19106.

6 5 4 3 2 1

Library of Congress Cataloging in Publications Data

Cancer: principles and practice of oncology/[edited by] Vincent T. DeVita, Jr., Samuel Hellman, Steven A. Rosenberg; 214 contributors.—4th ed.
p. cm.
Includes bibliographical references.
Includes index.
ISBN 0-397-51214-7 (one-vol. ed.)
ISBN 0-397-51321-6 (two-vol. set)
ISBN 0-397-51322-4 (vol. 1)
ISBN 0-397-51323-2 (vol. 2)
ISSN 0892-0567
1. Cancer. 2. Oncology. I. DeVita, Vincent T., Jr. II. Hellman, Samuel. III. Rosenberg, Steven A.

The authors and publisher have exerted every effort to ensure that drug selection and dosage set forth in this text are in accord with current recommendations and practice at the time of publication. However, in view of ongoing research, changes in government regulations, and the constant flow of information relating to drug therapy and drug reactions, the reader is urged to check the package insert for each drug for any change in indications and dosage and for added warnings and precautions. This is particularly important when the recommended agent is a new or infrequently employed drug.

Dedicated to

Mary Kay
Rusty
Alice

PUBLISHER'S FOREWORD

The physicians and surgeons who edit textbooks all have the same objective—the writing and publication of a textbook which, although edited by several and written by many, will nonetheless seem to reflect the knowledge and clinical wisdom of one mind. As every student and practitioner knows, the realization usually falls short of intention. What was to have been a divisible whole turns out to be a confusing, perplexing mosaic of contradiction, with some of the pieces missing. Such are the characteristics of most multiauthored textbooks in medicine and in surgery. There are few exceptions.

Cancer: Principles and Practice of Oncology is an exception, as thousands of oncologists, surgeons, and internists throughout the world have recognized since the publication of the first edition in January 1982. That the book *seems* to reflect one mind is no accident. As described in the Publisher's Foreword to the first edition, before the text was written the editors had exhaustive sessions with their contributors, sessions which, in many cases, lasted far into the night. Chapters were drafted and redrafted. The three editors and I (representing the publisher) met together for 1 week, and all editors reviewed all chapters—together. The chapters were then returned to the contributors with suggestions for amplification or clarification, or the deletion or addition of illustrations, drawings, and tables. The revised chapters were once again reviewed before being delivered to the publisher.

As with the first edition, so with the second, the third, and now the fourth. After the initial changes were decided on, the chapters were assigned, written, reviewed collectively, revised, and then reviewed again. The result of such effort you hold in your hands, and I am convinced that this is now the most rigorously edited and the most comprehensive textbook to have been written in oncology.

There are many rewards in medical publishing, but the most gratifying reward is to be associated with a textbook that is the best, that really works, and that has made a positive difference in the lives of cancer patients throughout the world, including me.

J. Stuart Freeman, Jr

CONTENTS

Volume One

PART 2

Volume Two

43

44

45

48

49

* *Deceased.*

CANCER
Principles & Practice of Oncology

Volume 2

Cancer: Principles & Practice of Oncology, Fourth Edition,
edited by Vincent T. DeVita, Jr., Samuel Hellman, Steven A. Rosenberg.
J.B. Lippincott Co., Philadelphia © 1993.

Jeffrey A. Norton
Bernard Levin
Robert T. Jensen

CHAPTER **41**

Cancer of the Endocrine System

THE THYROID GLAND

Malignant disease of the thyroid gland is a heterogenous disorder that affects all age groups but is more serious in the elderly. No single treatment plan is preferred because of the high long-term survival in most patients with differentiated thyroid cancers regardless of the type of treatment and even with no treatment.[1] The thyroid gland is the most common site of endocrine tumor. Occult thyroid cancer is found in 3% of individuals who die from other causes and microscopic cancer in 10% of individuals who die from other causes.[2] Because some thyroid cancers are malignant and potentially lethal, a thorough attempt to provide definitive diagnosis of all lesions of the thyroid gland is indicated and will suggest the appropriate therapy. Mortality from thyroid cancer equals or exceeds mortality from all other endocrine glands combined excluding the ovary.[2]

EPIDEMIOLOGY

The estimated number of new cases of thyroid cancer in the United States during 1990 was 12,100, with 8900 of these cases in women (Table 41–1).[3] The estimated number of deaths from thyroid cancer in 1990 was 1025, about 9% of the total number of new cases (see Table 41–1). The incidence of thyroid cancer in females was 5.8 persons per 100,000 in 1986, whereas the incidence in males was only 2.4 persons per 100,000 population.[4] Thyroid neoplasms are the most common endocrine cancers, accounting for 89% of endocrine malignancies and for 59% of deaths related to endocrine cancer (see Table 41–1).

Between 1973 and 1987, the estimated incidence of thyroid cancer increased by 14.6%, whereas the estimated death rate caused by thyroid cancer decreased by 20.6%.[4] Most cases occur in patients between 25 and 65 years of age, but thyroid cancer also occurs in the very young and the elderly. For well-differentiated thyroid cancers, age at diagnosis is an important prognostic variable[5–13] and some reports indicate that it is the most important prognostic variable.[6,7,13] The recurrence and survival rates of patients in the low-risk group (men younger than 40 years and women younger than 50 years) are strikingly different from patients in the high-risk group (all older patients). The high-risk age for well-differentiated thyroid cancer is the fourth or fifth decade.[5–14]

Since the report in 1969 by Sampson and associates on the prevalence of thyroid carcinoma in the autopsy population of Hiroshima and Nagasaki, there have been similar studies of the prevalence of thyroid cancer at autopsy in patients dying of other diseases.[15,16] The more carefully the gland is examined, the more occult and minute cancers are found. Most series report a prevalence of thyroid cancer at autopsy between 5% and 10%,[17] except in Japan and Hawaii, where the incidence can be as high as 28%.[18] These small, occult (almost always papillary) cancers are of minimal clinical significance even if lymph node spread is present.[19] However, other investigators suggest that some occult, small papillary carcinomas of the thyroid may be locally invasive and have a propensity for local recurrence and spread to cervical nodes.[20] The prevalence of thyroid cancer in autopsy series does not correlate with increased clinical incidence, recurrence, or mortality from thyroid cancer.[21]

The prevalence of clinical thyroid cancer increases with solitary nodular or multinodular thyroid disease. The evaluation of nodular thyroid disease is an integral part of the clinical evaluation of thyroid cancer. The prevalence of thyroid nodules depends on the population studied. In children not exposed to radiation, the prevalence is between 0.22% and 1.5%.[22] Prevalence increases linearly with age, with sponta-

TABLE 41–1. Estimated New Cases of and Deaths From Thyroid Cancer in the United States in 1990

	Estimated New Cases			*Estimate Deaths*		
Gland	*Both Sexes (%)*	*Male (%)*	*Female (%)*	*Both Sexes (%)*	*Male (%)*	*Female (%)*
Thyroid	12,100 (89)	3200 (80)	8900 (93)	1025 (59)	375 (48)	650 (67)
Other*	1500 (11)	800 (20)	700 (7)	725 (41)	400 (52)	325 (33)
Total	13,600	4000	9600	1750	775	975

* Other sites include the endocrine glands except the thyroid but exclude the reproductive organs. (Data from Silverberg E, Boring CC, Squires TS. Cancer statistics. CA 1990;40:9)

neous nodules occurring at a rate of 0.08% per year through the eighth decade. In the United States, clinical nodules are present in 4% to 7% of the adult population and are more common in women than men.[23] The absolute prevalence of thyroid cancer in solitary and multinodular glands is about 10% to 20%.[24–27] Thyroid irradiation increases the incidence of thyroid nodules and the likelihood that a thyroid nodule will be malignant, and after radiation exposure as many as 30% of thyroid nodules are found to be malignant.[28]

PATHOLOGY

Most malignant tumors of the thyroid gland are of glandular epithelial origin and are carcinomas (Table 41–2). Some well-differentiated thyroid cancers grow slowly,[1] so that the diagnosis of malignancy depends on blood vessel or capsular invasion rather than on histopathologic appearance.[21] Because lesions with vascular invasion and distant spread may have a benign clinical course, some investigators argue that aggressive therapy is not warranted.[1]

TABLE 41–2. Incidence and Classification of Malignant Tumors of the Thyroid Glands

Incidence (%)	*Tumor Type*
	I. Well-Differentiated Thyroid Carcinoma
	A. Papillary or Mixed Papillary-Follicular Carcinoma
70	1. Good-prognosis variants of papillary
	Micropapillary
	Encapsulated
	Solid
	Follicular
5	2. Poor-prognosis variants of papillary
	Tall cell
	Columnar
	Diffuse sclerosing
	Insular
15	B. Follicular Carcinoma
	Hürthle cell
5	II. Carcinoma of the Parafollicular C Cells (Medullary)
<5	III. Undifferentiated (Anaplastic)
Rare	IV. Other
	A. Sarcoma
	B. Lymphoma
	C. Metastatic Tumor

Primary tissue given to the pathologist must be adequate and include the thyroid nodule and the adjacent ipsilateral thyroid lobe. This resection allows the pathologist to evaluate carefully the margin of the nodule or tumor and the thyroid. Examination of the junction of the neoplasm and the thyroid allows determination of capsular invasion. Malignant papillary neoplasms of the thyroid may be multifocal, a finding with adverse prognostic importance.[29] Multifocality has been documented in up to 80% of patients with papillary cancer.[30] A recent prospective analysis of the totally resected thyroid gland from 44 patients with papillary thyroid carcinoma found an incidence of bilateral disease (both lobes involved) of 32% and an incidence of multicentric disease (multiple tumor loci in one lobe) of 50%.[31] An important prognostic feature is the age of the patient at diagnosis,[6–14] which is also an important criterion in staging.[29] An important clinicopathologic observation is the presence or absence of direct extension into contiguous structures in the neck or of extracapsular invasion which affect subsequent recurrence rates.[2,29,32] There is controversy about the prognostic significance of lymph node metastases in patients with papillary thyroid cancer. Some investigators suggest that lymph node metastases are associated with a favorable prognosis,[13,33] whereas others suggest that they are linked to a less favorable prognosis.[7,9,10] In patients with medullary thyroid cancer, lymph node metastasis is associated with a poorer prognosis.

The diagnosis of undifferentiated or anaplastic thyroid cancer has a uniformly poor prognosis regardless of stage at presentation or method of treatment.[34] Because of the problems posed by staging of thyroid carcinoma, a uniform staging system has not been applied routinely. An acceptable staging system based on the TNM classification has been developed recently by the American Joint Committee on Cancer (Table 41–3).[29] Prognosis depends on the type of thyroid cancer, the extent of disease, and, for papillary or follicular histologies, the age of the patient.

Papillary Adenocarcinoma

In the United States, papillary cancer of the thyroid represents the most common type of thyroid malignancy (about 75%). It is the most common thyroid cancer in patients older than 45 years.[35,36] Papillary cancer is characterized by an infiltrative pattern of growth, multicentricity, and spread to regional lymph nodes.[36] The nuclear membrane of the papillary cancer cells is delicate and has an opaque, ground-glass appearance

TABLE 41–3. Staging Malignant Tumors of the Thyroid Gland

Definition of TNM

Primary Tumor (T)

TX	Primary tumor cannot be assessed
T0	No evidence of primary tumor
T1	Tumor 1 cm or less
T2	Tumor > 1 cm and < 4 cm
T3	Tumor > 4 cm
T4	Tumor extending beyond thyroid capsule

Lymph Nodes (N)

NX	Regional nodes cannot be assessed
N0	No metastasis
N1	Regional nodal metastasis
N1a	ipsilateral node
N1b	contralateral or bilateral or mediastinal node(s)

Distant Metastasis (M)

MX	Distant metastasis cannot be assessed
M0	No distant metastasis
M1	Distant metastasis

Staging

Papillary or Follicular

	Patients Under 45 Years	*Patients Older Than 45 Years*
Stage I	Any T, any N, M0	T1, N0, M0
Stage II	Any T, any N, M1	T2, N0, M0
Stage III		T4, N0, M0
Stage IV		Any T, any N, M1

Medullary

Stage I	T1	N0	M0
Stage II	T2	N0	M0
	T3	N0	M0
	T4	N0	M0
Stage III	Any T	N1	M0
Stage IV	Any T	Any N	M1
Undifferentiated	All cases stage IV		

(Data from American Joint Committee on Cancer. Manual for staging of cancer. Philadelphia: JB Lippincott, 1988)

(the so-called Orphan Annie appearance).[36] Mixed papillary and follicular carcinomas are classified as papillary carcinomas because they have similar biologic behaviors and prognoses. Most papillary cancers are slow growing, and few prognostic differences have been detected.

The variants of papillary thyroid cancer associated with a good prognosis include the micropapillary, encapsulated, solid, and follicular variants.[36] Micropapillary tumors may be called *occult* or *small* and usually are less than 1.5 cm in diameter and detected incidentally. Encapsulated tumors have a well-defined fibrous demarcation between the neoplastic cells and the adjacent thyroid tissue, although capsular infiltration without vascular invasion is often found. Solid variants of papillary thyroid cancer consist primarily (at least 50% or more) of solid elements. The follicular variant is composed of follicles lined by the characteristic clear or ground-glass nuclei.[36]

Papillary thyroid carcinoma varies in necrosis and gross appearance depending on size. Occult thyroid papillary cancers usually are small (less than 1.0 or 1.5 cm in diameter) and often are minute. They are sometimes multiple and have no clinical significance. There is a high incidence of occult thyroid cancer in autopsy studies, but most patients (517 of 518 in one study)[37] reach the end of normal lifespan without clinical manifestations or awareness of a tumor. Even if occult papillary cancers metastasize to lymph nodes, the prognosis is still excellent and it is important not to overtreat these occult tumors. Only a rare case of a metastasis to bone from an occult cancer has been reported.[38] The larger tumors usually are poorly defined, although some may show attempts at encapsulation. Associated fibrosis is common, and calcium may be deposited in fibrotic areas. The classic appearance is one of papillary projections formed by a fibrovascular pedicle with its covering epithelium. Mitoses are uncommon. Squamous metaplasia, psammoma bodies, multifocality (30–40%), and lymphatic invasion are common. Whether the multifocality is multicentricity of primary papillary tumors or lymphatic spread through the thyroid has been debated. Extension of the tumor into adjacent neck structures worsens the prognosis, as does the presence of distant metastasis.

Just as there are types of papillary thyroid cancer associated with good prognosis (about 90%), there are types that appear to be associated with poor prognosis. These include the tall cell, columnar cell, and diffuse sclerosing types.[36] The tall cell variant is composed of tall columnar cells lining the glandular and papillary structures. These tumors tend to occur in older patients, to have extrathyroidal and vascular invasion, and to be associated with distant metastases to lung and bone.[39,40] The columnar cell variant is associated with poor prognosis, and patients may die of the disease. Histologically, it is similar to the tall cell variant.[41] Each of these tumor types appears to be more aggressive than typical papillary thyroid cancer.

Follicular Carcinoma

Follicular carcinoma of the thyroid gland occurs less frequently than does papillary carcinoma of the thyroid gland.[2,35,42] Although the incidence of papillary thyroid cancer is nearly seven times the incidence of follicular cancer, patients with follicular cancer account for more deaths from disease than do patients with papillary thyroid cancer (Table 41–4). Follicular adenomas and carcinomas usually have a uniform, microfollicular pattern. The detection of papillae or

TABLE 41–4. The Incidence and Deaths From Papillary and Follicular Thyroid Cancer Among 961 Cases of Differentiated Thyroid Cancer*

	No. of Patients (%)	*Deaths From Thyroid Cancer No. (% of Cases) (% of Deaths)*
Papillary thyroid cancer	842 (87)	17 (2) (35)
Follicular thyroid cancer	119 (13)	31 (26) (65)

* Data are a tabulation of three recently reported series.[2,35,42]

cytologic characteristics of papillary carcinoma (*e.g.*, Orphan Annie nucleus, psammoma bodies) are not consistent with follicular carcinoma. The distinction between follicular adenomas and carcinomas is based on the presence or absence of invasion of vessels or the tumor capsule. The term *atypical adenoma* denotes a follicular tumor without invasion but with sufficient cellular and nuclear atypia to suggest cancer. *Encapsulated follicular carcinoma* is a follicular tumor that appears encapsulated but has microscopic invasion of the capsule or vessels or both. Nineteen patients with this diagnosis treated with surgical resection and thyroid replacement had a 10-year survival rate of 78%. Primary lesions larger than 3.5 cm were associated with recurrent or metastatic disease.[43]

Multivariate analyses of populations of patients with follicular thyroid cancer emphasize the slow growth and good prognosis of these tumors if the tumor is small (≤4.0 cm), occurs in a person younger than 50 years, and is localized without marked vascular invasion.[42] Compared with papillary thyroid carcinoma, lymph node metastases are infrequent. The prognosis is poorer in patients older than 50 years, in males, in cancer that extends into contiguous neck structures, and in cancer that develops distant metastases.[42] The most important diagnostic distinction with regard to prognosis is between minimally invasive (encapsulated) and extensively invasive carcinomas.[42,44] The growth rate of distant metastases may be slow and they may respond, at least temporarily, to radioiodine therapy if the thyroid gland has been ablated.

Hürthle cell (or oxyphil cell) tumors, when studied by electron microscopy or biochemistry, have been shown to be derived from the follicular cell. Tumors show occasional formation of colloid and thyroglobulin and may have enzymes to synthesize thyroid hormone. Hürthle cell neoplasms usually are composed of sheets of Hürthle cells and not just an occasional Hürthle cell. Malignant criteria for these tumors are similar to those for other follicular neoplasms, namely capsular or vascular invasion. Thompson and colleagues started a controversy in 1974 when they described 25 patients with Hürthle cell tumor, most of whom died, including 3 of 4 in whom the diagnosis of adenoma had been made.[45] They concluded that the diagnosis of oxyphil or Hürthle cell adenoma should not be used. A follow-up study from the same institution indicated that total thyroidectomy for malignant Hürthle cell neoplasms or benign neoplasms larger than 2 cm resulted in a lower recurrence rate than in historical controls (21% versus 59%).[46] However, studies done at other institutions disagree and the pathologist can reliably distinguish a benign from a malignant Hürthle cell neoplasm based on capsular or vascular invasion. The chance of a benign Hürthle cell adenoma demonstrating malignant behavior is low (1.5–2.5%).[47,48] In general, the pathologist's diagnosis of Hürthle cell adenoma or carcinoma corresponds to the clinical behavior of the tumor.

Medullary Thyroid Carcinoma

Medullary thyroid carcinoma (MTC) makes up about 5% of all thyroid cancers (see Table 41–2). MTC is slightly more common in women. It may occur at any age with the highest incidence in the fifth and sixth decades. MTC is a tumor of calcitonin-secreting cells (C cells) of the thyroid gland. These tumors secrete a variety of other hormone products, and plasma levels of calcitonin gene-related peptide recently have been used to identify patients with MTC.[49–51] Although plasma levels of calcitonin remain the circulating marker of choice, plasma levels of calcitonin gene-related peptide may help predict more malignant tumors and the presence of metastases.[49] MTC can serve as an important model for the study of human epithelial cell transformation. About 20% of patients acquire this neoplasm through an autosomal dominant inheritance pattern, and considerable progress has been made in identifying chromosomal abnormalities associated with MTC. Investigators first proposed that a constitutional deletion of part of the short arm of chromosome 20 was a predisposing factor in some families with hereditary MTC.[52] Other investigators have not been able to detect this deletion in most families with the tumor or in MTC cells grown in tissue culture.[53] Germ line abnormalities on chromosome 10 are linked to three different familial forms of MTC: multiple endocrine neoplasia type IIa (MEN-IIa), MEN-IIb, and familial non-MEN MTC.[54–58] The genetic abnormality associated with each of the familial forms of MTC maps to the pericentromeric region of chromosome 10. This finding suggests that each abnormality is an allelic mutation at the same locus or represents a cluster of genes involved in the regulation of neuroendocrine tissue development.[54–58]

In patients with MEN-IIa, the earliest thyroid abnormality is referred to as C-cell hyperplasia and is characterized by multicentric patches of C cells. These lesions progress to become foci of microscopic carcinoma as cells break out of the C cell hyperplasia cluster and grow. Ultimately, macroscopic foci of MTC are evident. In the future, hybridization histochemistry by Northern gel analysis of mRNA for calcitonin and calcitonin gene-related peptide may help differentiate C-cell hyperplasia from MTC in situ.[59] This diagnosis has been difficult to make pathologically and some investigators have relied on sensitive preoperative elevations in plasma levels of calcitonin in response to calcium or pentagastrin stimulation.[60] These agents are especially useful in establishing the diagnosis of MTC at an early stage. Two recent studies demonstrated that of 41 patients who were from kindreds with MEN-IIa and had MTC diagnosed by an abnormal plasma calcitonin response to pentagastrin or calcium, each had MTC within the resected thyroid gland and 38 (93%) were biochemically cured.[51,61] Furthermore, because familial MTC is inherited most commonly as an autosomal dominant trait in patients from families with MEN-IIa, it is possible to determine who is at risk for the development of MTC and who is not. Using specific genetic markers linked to the pericentromeric region of chromosome 10, it is possible to predict individuals from kindreds with MEN-IIa who are at risk for developing clinical evidence of the disease (MTC) and who, therefore, should be screened periodically for pentagastrin-stimulated or calcium-stimulated plasma levels of calcitonin. Conversely, it is possible to determine who does not need to be screened.[62,63]

In patients with familial MTC or MEN-II, the neoplasm is present in both thyroid lobes.[64] In sporadic (nonfamilial) MTC, the neoplasm occurs unilaterally.[65] The solid, firm tumor is usually gray-white, and the cut surface shows areas of hemorrhage, necrosis, fibrosis, and calcification. The tumors usually are located at the junction of the upper and middle portion of each lobe, the area with the highest concentration of C cells. The tumor cells commonly are arranged in solid, irregular cords and clusters. The anaplastic variant can be recognized only by argyrophilic and calcitonin immunoreactivity. The tumor stroma is hyaline and variable in amount, and amyloid is almost always demonstrated by amyloid stains such as congo red or by electron microscopy. Calcitonin determination in tumor tissue by immunoperoxidase technique has been diagnostic.

The tumor metastasizes by way of the lymphatics and the blood stream. The growth rate of MTC compared with anaplastic carcinoma is slow and variable, yet the ultimate prognosis is not good, with about 50% 10-year survival. With earlier diagnosis and treatment, that is, with needle aspiration of thyroid mass lesions for sporadic patients and provocative testing of plasma calcitonin levels for familial patients, the survival appears to be better than 50%. In recent analyses, the 10-year survival of patients with sporadic MTC is 80%.[51] With MTC in the setting of MEN-IIa, survival is about 90%.[51,66] The prognosis is worse for older patients, patients with MEN-IIb,[67] and patients with large tumor size, lymph node metastases, or distant metastases.[66,68] There is considerable evidence that hyperplasia of the C cells precedes neoplasia. Basal and pentagastrin stimulated plasma levels of calcitonin are elevated in hyperplasia, and thyroidectomy is recommended. In familial settings, the cure rate is high (nearly 100%) if calcitonin levels are elevated and the tumor is not palpable but low if the tumor is palpable (17%).[69]

Anaplastic Thyroid Cancer

The relative frequency of undifferentiated or anaplastic thyroid cancer has been decreasing steadily for several decades to about 5% or less of all thyroid cancers (see Table 41–2).[70,71] The decreasing incidence of anaplastic thyroid tumors may mean that newer diagnostic techniques are better able to differentiate two confusing diagnoses, MTC and lymphoma. In one study, 9 of 14 undifferentiated thyroid cancers were reviewed with immunoperoxidase staining for calcitonin and electron microscopy and found to be MTC.[72] Newer monoclonal antibody methods specific for lymphoma can detect lymphomas masquerading as small cell anaplastic thyroid carcinoma.[73] Electron microscopy studies have shown that anaplastic cancers have cells with features such as lysosomal bodies and microvilli that resemble normal follicular cells.[74] Studies to determine the frequency of hormonal, epithelial, and sarcoma markers in anaplastic thyroid carcinoma indicate that 27% stain for thyroglobulin, 48% for α-antichymotrypsin, and 47% for vimentin. Thirty percent were not positive for any marker, indicating a total lack of differentiation.[70] Keratin and vimentin antibodies are generally found in anaplastic thyroid tumors. Of 32 different anaplastic thyroid cancers, between 70% and 80% stained positive with antibodies to keratin and 94% were positive for vimentin.[34] These findings are nonspecific and markers are of limited value in differentiating anaplastic from other thyroid tumors.

The prognosis of anaplastic thyroid cancer is dismal. All tumors of this type are placed in stage IV (see Table 41–3), regardless of extent of disease. Most studies show almost no 2-year survival. The mean survival in a recent series from the M. D. Anderson Hospital was only 7 months.[71] Aldinger found a 7% 5-year survival in 84 patients treated with combination therapy.[75] About 35% of anaplastic thyroid cancer arises in preexisting differentiated thyroid cancer in the elderly. There may be a greater incidence in countries with endemic goiter.[21]

ETIOLOGY

Radiation

The treatment of thymic enlargement in infancy with external irradiation was first reported in 1907. Subsequently, x-irradiation was used to treat enlarged tonsils and adenoids, mastoiditis, sinusitis, hemangiomas, lymphadenopathy, and acne. Thousands of patients in this country have received neck irradiation for these indications. In 1950, thyroid carcinoma was reported in 9 of 28 children who had previously received thymic irradiation.[76] Many subsequent studies have confirmed the association between therapeutic irradiation of the head and neck region and the development of thyroid carcinoma, salivary, neural, and parathyroid tumors 20 to 35 years later.[77] The risk for developing thyroid cancer is dose-dependent and the risk increases with doses as small as 6.5 to 80 cGy. At more than 2000 cGy, the risk declines. Risk is inversely related to age at the time of irradiation and is highest among children exposed before the age of 10.[78] The incidence of radiation-induced thyroid cancer has been increasing but appears to be reaching a plateau. The incidence of death from radiation-induced thyroid cancer appears to be decreasing.[79]

Marshall Islanders, who received about 1200 cGy from the atomic bomb fallout, showed an increased incidence of thyroid neoplasia, especially among children. There was a linear dose-response relation between distance from bomb blast site and chance of development of thyroid nodules.[80] Treatment of Graves' disease with radioactive iodine does not cause thyroid cancer because the gland receives a dose in excess of 5000 cGy.[81] It seems likely that lower doses of irradiation damage thyroid tissue and lead to mutational changes. However, lower doses of ^{131}I exposure have not been linked to increased cancer rates.[79] These studies of ^{131}I exposure are relevant to nuclear accidents, such as the Chernobyl incident in 1986, which appear likely to increase the rate of thyroid cancer.[82] Studies of people in China exposed to continuous chronic low-dose background radiation for years (330 mR/year, which is three times the normal background radiation) found no evidence of increased risk for thyroid cancer.[83] The incidence of thyroid neoplasia appears to be a function of the radiation dose, with the dose-response curve being linear, initially at 3 per 200 person-years at risk per 1000 cGy. Risk factors include sex (women have increased risk), age (the younger the patient at the time of radiation the greater the risk for subsequent cancer), interval (the more years since radiation the greater chance of cancer), and dose (risk is linear from 300–1200 cGy). Radiation increases the risk for thyroid cancer and thyroid nodules.[80,84] Furthermore, increased secretion of thyroid-stimulating hormone (TSH) as a result of impaired thyroid hormone secretion may play a cancer-promoting role in this condition.[85]

Iodine

Papillary carcinoma of the thyroid may be more common in areas with iodination of salt (United States) or a high-iodine diet (Sweden).[86] In contrast to papillary carcinoma, follicular carcinoma is much more common in iodine-deficient goitrous areas (Switzerland). The high incidence of follicular neoplasia in goitrous areas may be related to the prolonged stimulatory effect of TSH.[87]

Goiters

In the rat, prolonged exposure of the thyroid gland to TSH stimulation induced by antithyroid drugs causes a high yield of malignant tumors including rat MTC. Some series have indicated that a higher proportion of anaplastic and follicular carcinomas of the thyroid gland occur in endemic goiter regions.[21,88] Many studies suggest that anaplastic carcinoma may originate within long-standing abnormal thyroid glands. A history of nodular goiter is obtained in a high proportion of patients affected with anaplastic carcinoma.[70] The preexisting abnormality may represent an adenomatous goiter, an adenoma, or a well-differentiated carcinoma. This striking association and its frequency by history and histology has led several investigators to infer transformation of a low-grade or benign lesion into a highly malignant one.[21,70,89] Some researchers suggest that external radiation may enhance the potential for this transformation.[89] However, most radiation-induced thyroid cancers are well differentiated and behave biologically exactly like excellent prognosis papillary cancer.[90,91]

Familial

The carcinoma of the thyroid that is most influenced by genetic factors is MTC. Although the exact genetic abnormality remains unclear, recent research has pinpointed it to the centromere of chromosome 10.[54–58] This tumor is inherited as an autosomal dominant trait in 20% of cases.[64,92] It occurs in three distinct familial settings: familial MTC,[93] MEN-IIa,[65] and MEN-IIb.[51,67] Papillary thyroid carcinoma usually does not show a familial disposition, but two groups have suggested that it occurs in families and one group has suggested an association with familial polyposis of the colon and Gardner's syndrome (benign adenomatous colonic polyps, lipomas, fibromas, and mandibular osteomas).[94,95]

Oncogenes

Models for tumorigenesis suggest that a series of genetic alterations occur during progression from the normal cell to the malignant phenotype. Mutations in each of the 3 *RAS* genes (K-*RAS*, H-*RAS*, and N-*RAS*) have been identified in many human tumors including thyroid cancer. In one recent study, normal thyroid tissue did not contain point mutations in codons 12, 13, and 61 of these *RAS* oncogenes. However, 4 of 19 nodules from benign goiter (21%), 6 of 24 from benign tumors (25%), and 3 of 14 papillary carcinomas (21%) contained *RAS* point mutations, whereas none of 3 follicular carcinomas had these changes.[96] Similarly, another study demonstrated that *RAS* gene activation was found in a similar proportion of benign and malignant tumors of the thyroid.[97] Together, these two studies suggest that *RAS* gene activation is equally prevalent in benign and malignant thyroid neoplasms. The mutation of these oncogenes may be an early event in the tumoral process.

Thyroid tumors, benign and malignant, have been screened for a variety of gene rearrangements of the protooncogenes, including C-*MYC*, C-*MYB*, C-*FOS*, c-*ERBB1*, c-*ERBB2*, c-*ERBA*, N-*RAS*, K-*RAS*, and H-*RAS*. Only mutations of H-*RAS* were observed. Of 18 malignant thyroid tumors studied, 4 (22%) had H-*RAS* gene rearrangement.[98] Some suggest that *RAS* gene activation correlates with the metastatic potential of thyroid tumors, because 80% of follicular cancers in one study had activated *RAS* oncogenes, whereas only 20% of papillary tumors had this finding.[99] This finding was confirmed in a more recent study in which 2 of 14 patients with follicular carcinomas had N-*RAS* oncogene mutations and both of these patients had bone metastases.[100] In animal studies, H-*RAS* activation has been associated with chemically induced thyroid tumors, whereas K-*RAS* activation has been associated with ionizing radiation-induced tumors. Another recent study found a significantly greater rate (10-fold) of K-*RAS* mutation in radiation-associated follicular carcinomas than in nonradiation-associated follicular carcinomas. These findings suggest that radiation may preferentially activate K-*RAS* gene expression in human tumors as it does in animal tumors.[101]

Using DNA transfection analysis on NIH 3T3 cells, a new oncogene was identified from 5 separate papillary thyroid cancer specimens and 2 of the respective human lymph node metastases.[102] That the same oncogene is active in 5 thyroid papillary carcinomas suggests a tissue-specific activation for the oncogene. The transforming oncogene was called *PTC* for papillary thyroid cancer and was detected in about 15% of papillary thyroid carcinoma specimens.[103] Later it was determined that *PTC* is a novel rearrangement of the *RET* protooncogene and displays tyrosine protein kinase activity.[103] The gene has been cloned.[104] The gene appears to be specific for papillary thyroid carcinoma and has been detected in 19% of a large number of papillary thyroid cancer specimens. It has not been detected in other benign and malignant thyroid tumors including follicular, anaplastic, and medullary thyroid cancers.

Summary of Etiologic Factors

Chronic TSH stimulation appears to play a permissive but not initiative role in the etiology of well-differentiated thyroid cancer. Iodine deficiency may lead to follicular cancer, and iodine abundance is associated with papillary thyroid cancer. Low-dose radiation leads to thyroid nodules and papillary thyroid cancer. Preliminary experimental data suggest that the K-*RAS* oncogene is associated with radiation-induced thyroid cancer.[101] The *RAS* and *PTC* oncogenes appear to play a role in the pathogenesis, with the former activated in various well-differentiated forms (especially follicular forms) and the latter primarily in papillary carcinomas.[54–57,105] Genetic factors are most important in the genesis of MTC and related syndromes. The defect in familial MTC appears to be near the centromere of chromosome 10.[54–58] Thyroiditis does not appear to predispose patients to carcinoma; however, the prevalence of lymphoma of the thyroid gland may increase in patients with severe Hashimoto thyroiditis.[106]

DIAGNOSIS

Clinical Presentation

The manner of evaluating and treating a thyroid nodule is evolving. The incidence of thyroid nodules is relatively high (4–7% of the adult population and 20–30% of the radiation-exposed adult population).[28] Cancer occurs relatively infrequently, however, with a 10% to 20% incidence of cancer in nodules without radiation exposure[23] and a 30% to 50% incidence of cancer in radiation-exposed nodules.[28] For these reasons, the workup of a thyroid nodule should suggest surgical resection for nodules that are malignant and should avoid unnecessary surgery for nodules that are benign. The problem is that no preoperative test can perfectly differentiate malignant from benign nodular disease.

History and Physical Examination

The history may suggest the likelihood of cancer in a thyroid nodule. Exposure to ionizing radiation is a well-documented risk factor for the later development of thyroid cancer.[107] Whether patient age affects the likelihood of a nodule being cancerous is not clear. Local symptoms such as airway obstruction, hoarseness, and dysphagia may be associated with extensive thyroid cancer or goiter. The appearance of a new nodule or rapid growth of a nodule are associated with malignancy but are nonspecific. Because thyroid cancer is usually slow growing, a dominant nodule of long duration needs the same diagnostic attention as a new nodule. The risk for malignant disease in a multinodular goiter is significantly lower than the risk in a solitary nodule.[23] The neck must be examined for jugular or central lymph nodes, which increase the likelihood of a thyroid nodule being malignant; however, physical examination characteristics of the nodule are poor predictors of a malignant lesion. It is important to be able to palpate the thyroid nodule, because workup and evaluation of a nodule are based on the presence of the nodule on physical examination.

Laboratory Tests

Laboratory tests are minimally helpful in the evaluation of a patient with a thyroid nodule. Thyroid function studies, including measurement of serum levels of TSH, triiodothyronine (T_3), thyroxine (T_4), and free T_4, are done first. Most patients with malignant thyroid nodules have normal serum levels of these hormones. If the patient has elevated serum levels of T_3 and T_4 with low TSH levels, a thyroid scan is indicated to determine if the palpable thyroid nodule is hot (*i.e.*, hyperfunctional compared with the remainder of the thyroid). Hot nodules should be removed surgically but are seldom malignant.

Serum levels of thyroglobulin may be of use in the management of patients with well-differentiated thyroid cancer and nodular disease of the thyroid secondary to previous neck irradiation. Serum levels of thyroglobulin are elevated in patients with differentiated thyroid tumors that arise from follicular epithelium and are normal or low in patients with anaplastic or medullary tumors. The levels of thyroglobulin cannot predict whether a given nodule is benign or malignant, nor can they predict whether a cancer is present in a multinodular goiter. After total thyroidectomy for differentiated thyroid cancer with follicular elements, serum thyroglobulin levels return to normal and may become elevated with recurrent or metastatic disease.[108] Serum thyroglobulin levels have been used to follow patient populations at risk for developing thyroid cancer after radiation treatment in childhood. Increasing levels of serial serum thyroglobulin determinations in this patient population were associated with individuals who subsequently developed thyroid nodules and cancer.[109] An increment of serum level of thyroglobulin greater than 18 ng/ml in this specific patient population was predictive for the development of cancer.[109] Thyroglobulin levels are elevated in noncancerous thyroid diseases such as Graves' disease, nontoxic goiter, and thyroiditis. Because of lack of specificity and sensitivity, only sequential thyroglobulin determinations are useful in an individual patient (*e.g.*, follow-up of patients with metastatic or recurrent thyroid cancer and serial evaluation of patients with a history of radiation).

Serum levels of carcinoembryonic antigen (CEA) are elevated in many patients with MTC,[110] but serum calcitonin elevations are specific for MTC and are the most specific marker available in oncology. Combined with provocative agents such as calcium or pentagastrin, calcitonin levels become the most sensitive marker available in clinical oncology.[111] Although MTC is a rare form of thyroid cancer, these tests are useful if there is a family history of the cancer.

Thyroid Gland Suppression

A thyroid nodule is suppressed by administering thyroid hormone exogenously for several months. Supposedly, benign nodules will suppress in size but malignant nodules will not. TSH receptors are present and binding occurs on normal and malignant thyroid tissue.[112,113] Indirect evidence for the TSH dependence of thyroid cancer includes lower recurrence rates for patients receiving thyroid hormone postoperatively than for those who do not receive it.[107] The success rate of suppression therapy for solitary nodules has ranged from 0 to 60%, with 0 to 38% of patients having a complete response and 10 to 60% a partial response.[23] A prospective double-blind placebo-controlled study of the ability to suppress solitary nodules of the thyroid demonstrated that none of 28 patients randomized to receive TSH-suppressive doses of synthroid had evidence of a decrease in nodule size by repetitive ultrasonography.[114] This study failed to demonstrate any efficacy of levothyroxine sodium (Synthroid) therapy for thyroid nodules. Furthermore, the incidence of malignant disease that suppresses is completely unknown. Successful suppression of thyroid nodules does not exclude malignant disease, and confirmed carcinomas have been reported that responded to suppression.[115,116] The lack of suppression to thyroid hormone is not specific for malignant disease; most benign nodules will not suppress.[114] In two small studies in which nonresponders to suppression underwent thyroid resection, the incidence of thyroid cancer was 20% and 40%.[117,118] We use suppression for selected small nodules that have a benign cellular appearance on aspiration cytology. If an aspiration indicates malignant cytology, we proceed to surgery without suppression. When trying to suppress a nodule, measure TSH levels and make certain that circulating levels are actually suppressed on a given dose of levothyroxine sodium. If the nodule increases on suppression, a surgical resection should be done. At the end of 6 months of suppression, reevaluate the nodule with another aspiration if it is smaller but has not disappeared. If it remains unchanged, surgical resection may be necessary. With careful follow-up, delay in definitive treatment of well-differentiated thyroid cancer does not appear to translate into morbidity or mortality.

Radionuclide Imaging

The three common isotopes used in thyroid scanning are iodine 123, iodine 131, and sodium pertechnetate Tc 99m. These isotopes image nodules and thyroid tissue because these tissues trap iodine. ^{123}I has advantages over ^{131}I for imaging studies because ^{123}I does not have the high β-emission of ^{131}I. Although the β-emission is useful therapeutically, it does not contribute diagnostic information and adds to the patient's dose of radiation.[119] A survey indicated that ^{99m}Tc and ^{123}I accounted for 54% and 35%, respectively, of the thyroid imaging done in the United States.[120] ^{131}I remains indicated for uptake studies, for evaluation of metastatic thyroid carcinoma, and for treatment. Malignant thyroid tissue either does not incorporate iodine or incorporates less iodine than normal thyroid tissue, so that a malignant lesion appears as a cold area on the scan.[121]

Thyroid scanning cannot differentiate benign from malignant nodules and can be used only to assign a probability of malignancy based on the functional status of a nodule. Ashcraft and Van Herle reviewed 22 series in which radioiodine scans were obtained and all patients underwent operation regardless of the functional status of a nodule. They reported that 84% of nodules were cold, 10.5% were warm (same as normal thyroid), and 5.5% were hot.[122,123] Malignant thyroid disease was documented in 16% of cold nodules, 9% of warm nodules, and 4% of hot nodules. These results indicate that thyroid scanning does not successfully differentiate benign from malignant thyroid nodules. Cold nodules are more likely to be malignant, but hot and warm nodules also may be malignant.[123] Another group takes strong exception to the claim that hot nodules may be malignant because they have found no evidence for any malignant hot nodules.[124,125] Whether hot thyroid nodules can be malignant is not crucial because hot nodules comprise only 5.5% of all nodules and only 4% are malignant. The problem is that the likelihood of cold nodules (85% of all nodules) being malignant is also small (10–20%), so that the nuclide scan cannot reliably differentiate benign from malignant thyroid nodules. Therefore, we have not used thyroid scanning as part of the initial workup of a thyroid nodule unless the patient has serum levels of thyroid hormones that suggest hyperthyroidism.

MTC that recurs locally in the neck after thyroidectomy and in metastatic locations has been imaged using thallium ^{99m}Tc scintigraphy.[126] This study may help image recurrent or metastatic disease in patients who develop elevation of plasma calcitonin levels after thyroid resection.[126] Thallium is a blood pool marker. Because MTC and thyroid are vascular,[126] thallium is concentrated in the tumor and thyroid, whereas ^{99m}Tc is concentrated only in thyroid. A computer is used to subtract the technetium scan from the thallium scan to image MTC. This technique has been used to image parathyroid adenomas and is not specific for MTC.[127]

Meta-iodobenzylguanidine (MIBG) labeled with ^{131}I has imaged primary[128] and metastatic[129] MTC successfully. ^{131}I-MIBG also has been used to image pheochromocytomas. In one patient with MEN-IIa who had pheochromocytomas and MTC, it also imaged the MTC.[128] Subsequently, it has been used to image metastatic MTC to bone and liver. Because the isotope is taken up and incorporated into the MTC cell, it has been suggested that metastatic MTC can be treated with doses of ^{131}I-MIBG. In our experience, locally recurrent or metastatic MTC generally is not imaged by labeled MIBG and has not been useful for this tumor type. Two recent approaches appear to have developed a more efficacious method. First, anti-CEA monoclonal antibodies labeled with indium or iodine may image metastatic MTC in selected patients (2 have been reported).[130,131] Imaging by this method may have treatment implications, but treatment efficacy has not been demonstrated. Second, pentavalent ^{99m}Tc dimercaptosuccinic acid (DMSA) scintigraphy has been used to image 10 patients with suspected primary, recurrent, or metastatic MTC. It was helpful in 9 of 10 patients, including 7 of 8 asymptomatic patients with elevated peak plasma levels of calcitonin.[132,133] These findings are by a single group and are preliminary; however, if the findings are confirmed by others, noninvasive DMSA scintigraphy may be the method of choice to localize recurrent and metastatic disease in patients with MTC and hypercalcitonemia.

Ultrasonography

Ultrasound examination of the thyroid gland accurately measures the size of a given nodule, determines whether it is solid or cystic, and detects the exact number of nodules. Conventional B-mode ultrasound classifies nodules as solid, cystic, or mixed solid-cystic, with more than 90% accuracy. In one large review of 16 series in which conventional techniques were used, 21% of the solid lesions, 12% of the mixed lesions, and only 7% of the cystic lesions were malignant.[122] A solid mass within the thyroid most often is benign, but it has the highest chance of being malignant. Conversely, a cystic mass is not always benign, but it has a higher likelihood of being benign than a solid mass.

In patients with previous radiation exposure who are at risk for developing radiation-induced thyroid carcinoma, the results of two different groups support conservative management (close observation or aspiration and not surgical resection) of small nodules that are not palpable or are barely palpable and are detected by ultrasonography. The chance of this type of nodule becoming clinically significant thyroid cancer, even in patients with previous radiation, is low.[134]

Ultrasound cannot differentiate benign from malignant lesions. High-resolution real-time scanning depicts most malignant thyroid tumors as sonolucent compared with the surrounding echogenic thyroid. No ultrasound appearance is unequivocal for malignant or benign tumors. The *halo sign* is a thin sonolucent rim that supposedly occurs around a benign tumor[135] and has been observed around papillary and follicular carcinomas.[136] Lymph node metastases from a thyroid neoplasm can be detected and have the sonolucent characteristics of the primary. Nonspecific lymph node enlargement also may appear sonolucent. Ultrasound is observer-dependent and requires a dedicated ultrasonographer. It is noninvasive and sensitive but not specific. It is the most accurate method to measure and follow the exact size of a lesion in a patient on thyroid suppression. It can be used to guide aspiration or biopsy of large lesions (1–3 cm) in the posterior part of the thyroid, which may be clinically significant but not readily palpable. In patients from kindreds with MEN-II and in patients with elevated calcitonin levels, it can detect small foci of MTC that appear sonolucent with calcification.[137] It is more sensitive than physical examination in detecting locally recurrent thyroid carcinoma in high-risk individuals after thyroidectomy.[136] Because of its safety, flexibility, and sensitivity as a real-time extension of the physical examination, high-resolution ultrasound has a role in the evaluation and follow-up of thyroid neoplasms.

Biopsy

Fine-needle aspiration biopsy has emerged as the most valuable aid in the diagnosis and management of thyroid nodular disease because it is safe and inexpensive and has resulted in better selection of patients for operation.[23] The diagnostic accuracy of cytologic analysis with aspiration biopsy has been low in some centers (71%) and high in other centers (96%; Table 41–5).[123,138] The experience and technique of physicians performing the biopsy and of cytopathologists reading the slides appear to be the major reasons why one institution has excellent results and another poor results. We use local anesthesia, a syringe holder, and a 21- or 22-gauge needle in most instances. The lesion should be fixed between two fingers and the needle placed in the center of the nodule for small lesions (1–2 cm) and at the periphery for larger lesions (2–4 cm). We advise taking at least 6 good samples because most false-negative results are caused by inadequate sampling. For a detailed description of the preferred method for aspiration cytology, the reader is referred to the discussion by Hamburger and Hamburger.[139] The difficulty of obtaining adequate cytologic specimens decreases with physician experience and number of aspirations,[138] so that satisfactory specimens can be obtained in about 95% of nodules.[118,140] Large rapidly growing lesions (greater than 4 cm) in which there is a concern about lymphoma or anaplastic thyroid carcinoma may be better assessed by cutting-needle biopsy.[141,142] In lymphoma of the thyroid, fine-needle aspiration may give a diagnosis of thyroiditis, whereas cutting-needle biopsy usually provides the correct diagnosis.[142] This differentiation is important because surgery is not part of the usual treatment for lymphoma. The fine-needle aspiration cytology and the large-needle biopsy are complementary. In studies analyzing both in the same patient,[141] biopsy has given fewer false-negative diagnoses than aspiration.[143] Reported false-negative rates for fine-needle aspiration range from 2.2% to 10%.[144] The sensitivity and specificity of fine-needle aspiration is about 80% (see Table 41–5).[145] The addition of large-needle biopsy can decrease the false-negative rate to 1% and increase the sensitivity and specificity.[146] The problem with large-needle cutting biopsy is that small nodules (<4 cm) are not easily amenable to this technique. Large-needle cutting biopsy has more side effects than fine-needle aspiration[134] and, in general, has similar or better accuracy rates.[141] Nevertheless, large-needle cutting biopsy of lesions that are indeterminant on fine-needle aspiration may occasionally provide a definitive diagnosis.[141,147] We reserve fine-needle aspiration cytology for most thyroid nodules, but we use cutting-needle biopsy for larger nodules (>4 cm) that are more consistent with anaplastic carcinoma or lymphoma.

When a satisfactory fine-needle aspirate has been obtained, three cytologic results are possible: benign, suspicious, or malignant.[145] Reviewing results from four series with a total of 848 patients, 78% of the patients had benign aspirates, 20% had suspicious aspirates, and 12% had malignant aspirates.[148–151] These data indicate improvement in fine-needle aspiration results with more experience, because previous studies included about 35% of patients in the suspicious or indeterminant group.[147,152,153] In studies in which all patients with suspicious lesions underwent operation, the incidence of thyroid cancer ranged from 11% to 71%, with an overall rate of 36% (Table 41–6). If a fine-needle aspiration indicates a benign diagnosis, the probability of a malignant lesion is low (3%). Conversely, if the aspirate is diagnostic for cancer, there is a high probability that the lesion is malignant (85%; see Table 41–6). The predictive value of fine-needle aspiration biopsy is affected by whether suspicious lesions are considered positive. If a suspicious nodule is not included in the positive group, the procedure has few false-positive results but is not sensitive enough and misses too many cancers in the suspicious group (overall 36% chance of a suspicious aspirate having cancer). If the suspicious aspirate is included in the positive group, the aspiration cytology can diagnose about 97% of thyroid cancers but the specificity decreases to about 70% (see Table 41–6).

The difficulty in evaluating suspicious lesions reflects the inability to differentiate benign Hürthle cell and follicular tu-

TABLE 41–5. Analysis of Accuracy of Fine-Needle Aspiration in the Evaluation of Patients With Nodular Thyroid Disease

No. of Studies	*Total No. of Patients*	*Mean Sensitivity % (Range)*	*Mean Specificity % (Range)*	*Mean Accuracy % (Range)*	*Mean Negative Predictive Value % (Range)*	*Mean Positive Predictive Value % (Range)*
10	1553	79 (46–93)	78 (44–94)	80 (71–96)	72 (50–96)	86 (72–91)

(Data from Cusick EL, MacIntosh CA, Krukowski VMM, et al. Management of isolated thyroid swellings: a prospective six year study of fine needle aspiration cytology in diagnosis. Br Med J 1990;301:318)

TABLE 41–6. Accuracy of Preoperative Fine-Needle Aspiration (FNA) Cytology

			Pathology		
Investigations	*Group*	*FNA (No.)*	*Benign (No.)*	*Malignant (No.)*	*Malignant (%)*
Hawkins et al, 1987[153]	Benign	336	326	10	3
	Suspicious	28	13	15	54
	Malignant	51	3	47	92
Harsoulis et al, 1986[1094]	Benign	150	146	4	3
	Suspicious	14	4	10	71
	Malignant	26	3	23	88
Abu-Nema et al, 1987[1095]	Benign	89	88	1	1
	Suspicious	28	28	0	0
	Malignant	7	0	7	100
Ramacciotti et al, 1984[1096]	Benign	87	79	8	9
	Suspicious	15	12	3	20
	Malignant	17	4	13	76
Hamburger and Hamburger, 1986[139]	Benign	—	—	—	—
	Suspicious	149	133	16	11
	Malignant	284	66	218	77
Mayo[139]	Benign	—	—	—	—
	Suspicious	233	173	60	26
	Malignant	98	0	98	100
Cusick et al, 1990[145]	Benign	115	115	0	0
	Suspicious	165	39	126	76
	Malignant	21	0	21	100
Cumulative Experience	Benign	777	754	23	3
	Suspicious	632	402	230	36
	Malignant	504	76	427	85

mors from their malignant counterparts.[154] Papillary carcinoma is less of a cytologic problem except when the cellularity of a sample is poor or diagnostic features of cancer such as psammoma bodies are not present. Repeat aspiration or cutting-needle biopsy may be helpful. However, with follicular neoplasms no preoperative evaluation has been able to differentiate benign from malignant tumors consistently. The diagnosis does not depend on cell features but on invasion of the capsule or blood vessels. This distinction is poorly evaluated on frozen section tissue examination and may require permanent histologic examination. Attempts have been made to use DNA content, nuclear size, and nuclear ploidy to differentiate malignant from benign follicular neoplasms, but conflicting results have been reported.[155–157] In general, the potential value of DNA aneuploidy in differentiating benign from malignant follicular thyroid neoplasms is limited, and definitive diagnosis requires histologic examination.[158] Surgical excision of all suspicious thyroid nodules is recommended, because the complications of surgery are infrequent (≤1%), the chance of malignancy is 20% to 40%, and there is no way to identify only malignant nodules.

The real benefit of fine-needle aspiration cytology is for the benign aspiration group and the malignant aspiration group. Benign aspiration results may be present in about 78% of patients.[148–151] Only about 3% of patients with benign aspiration results have thyroid cancer, and the development of thyroid cancer can be detected by repeat aspiration cytology.[148] When 246 patients who initially had a benign aspirate were followed for 6 months, and underwent repeat fine-needle aspiration, changes in diagnosis from benign to suspicious occurred in 12 patients. Changes in diagnosis from benign to malignant occurred in 6 patients, and only 6 cancers were detected (2%).[159] Another recent study demonstrated that the risk of cancer developing in 641 patients with a benign fine-needle aspiration diagnosis was only 0.7% with a median follow-up of 6.1 years.[160] Therefore, surgical resection is not necessary for patients with benign aspirations. These patients can undergo suppression and careful follow-up evaluations with repeat aspiration cytology. Patients with malignant aspiration cytologies should undergo immediate surgical resection, and they have about an 85% chance of a true malignant lesion. Some investigators advocate definitive surgical resection based on aspiration cytology rather than on frozen section.[149] Most studies demonstrate that this strategy results in occasional incorrect diagnoses and that operative frozen section determination or postoperative permanent section determination is necessary before proceeding with a definitive cancer-type operation.[161,162]

Fine-needle aspiration cytology has had a substantial impact on the management of thyroid nodules and provides far more diagnostic information than any other diagnostic technique. Workup of nodules with history, physical examination, thyroid scan, and ultrasound yielded only 10% to 20% malignancy rates in surgically resected nodules. Fine-needle aspiration cytology has halved the number of patients who undergo operations and has doubled the incidence (40%) of malignant disease found at surgical resection.[23] This effect has been estimated to eliminate significant health care costs in the management of patients with a thyroid nodule.[150,151]

Standard Workup

The initial step in patient evaluation is a careful history of childhood irradiation, including the dose and the interval from treatment to presentation with a thyroid nodule. Physical examination determines the size and location of the nodule or nodules. Careful palpation is required to detect jugular, supraclavicular, and submandibular lymph nodes. Hoarseness, difficulty swallowing liquids, or dyspnea with exertion may necessitate indirect laryngoscopy. Fine-needle aspiration cytology is the primary diagnostic procedure for smaller lesions ($\leq$4 cm). Ultrasound is used to measure exact lesion size before suppression and to ensure that no larger thyroid masses or suspicious lymph nodes have been missed. If the lesion appears totally cystic on ultrasound, aspiration may completely eliminate it. If the thyroid mass is large (>4 cm), cutting-needle biopsy is the preferred diagnostic maneuver. Therapeutic intervention is based on biopsy results.

If the fine-needle aspiration cytology or biopsy is benign, ultrasound is used to measure the mass and thyroid suppression is started. It the results are suspicious or malignant, surgical resection is indicated. During TSH suppression therapy for benign tumors, the responsible physician must be certain that TSH levels are actually suppressed by the dose of levothyroxine sodium. If the nodule remains unchanged or decreases without resolution after 6 months, repeat aspiration cytology is indicated. If the nodule increases in size, surgical resection is indicated. Nodule size can be accurately reevaluated by physical examination and ultrasound as necessary. The entire scheme is outlined in Figure 41–1.

TREATMENT

Thyroid Nodules: Surgical Approach

Once the decision is made to operate, surgical resection is performed on the assumption that the nodule represents a carcinoma. Nodule excision is not performed. Thyroid lobectomy of the ipsilateral thyroid lobe is the procedure of choice. For isthmus lesions, the isthmus is resected along with the lobe in closer propinquity to the nodule. The pathologist needs the relation of the nodule to the adjacent normal thyroid to make the diagnosis. In addition, in the event that a given nodule is malignant and a simple nodulectomy is performed, any reoperation in the same lobe is technically difficult and increases the risk for recurrent laryngeal nerve injury sixfold. The local recurrence rate of a simple nodulectomy compared with a lobectomy may be higher because some well-differentiated carcinomas are multifocal or multicentric (about 20–40%).[152]

Most studies that have considered the extent of thyroid resection for primary well-differential thyroid carcinoma (*i.e.*, total thyroidectomy versus subtotal or partial thyroidectomy) have concluded that subtotal resection is preferred, especially in patients with small tumors (about 1 cm) and younger than 45 years.[163,164] The reasons are that there is no difference in survival or recurrence rates between the two groups and that total thyroidectomy is associated with greater morbidity. In older patients with larger, locally aggressive, or metastatic well-differentiated tumors, near-total

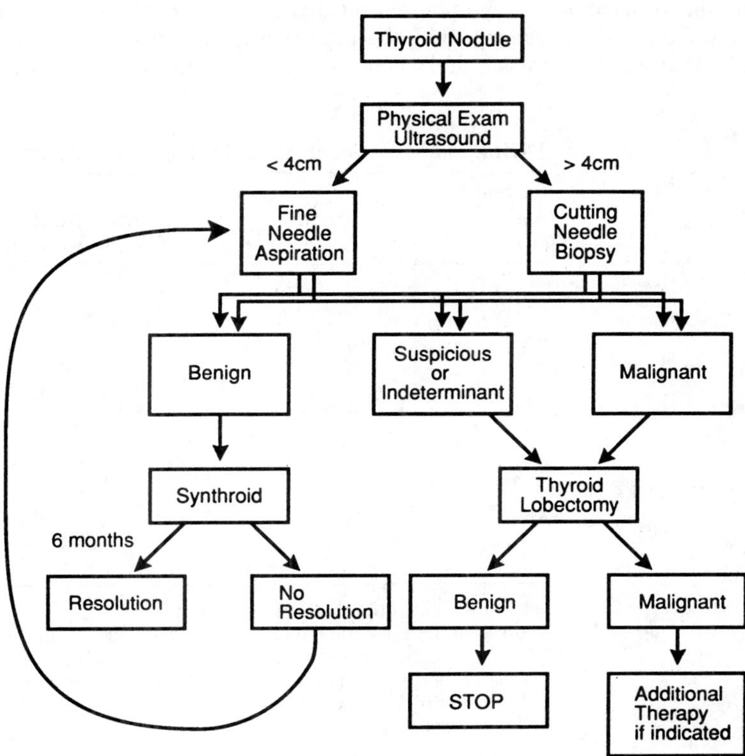

FIGURE 41–1. Flow diagram for evaluation of a thyroid nodule.

or total thyroidectomy is preferred because the tumors may be bilateral or multifocal, and tumor treatment with ^{131}I is facilitated. Prospective randomized trials regarding the extent of resection for thyroid carcinoma have not been done and may be impossible because of the slow-growing benign nature of the neoplasm in most patients. Thyroid carcinoma can behave like cancer in older patients with large tumors and extracapsular invasion.[5–13,32,165,166]

If the nodule is benign on frozen section, malignant, and small, or if the pathologist cannot be certain of malignancy, the operative procedure may be terminated with one lobe removed. The contralateral lobe is exposed and carefully palpated to make certain that no obvious tumors or suspicious nodules are present in it. If permanent pathology results indicate that the removed nodule is malignant, we use the same criteria used intraoperatively to remove the contralateral lobe. Indications for completion of near-total thyroidectomy include large lesions (>2 cm), older patients, and poor-prognosis variants of papillary thyroid cancer including tall cell, columnar, diffuse sclerosing, and follicular cancers. This point is controversial and some surgeons would not reoperate.[167] The risk of a reoperation on the contralateral lobe done before 1 week postoperatively is no greater than the same procedure performed at the initial operation. The risk would increase if the lobe was extensively dissected and about 1 month had passed.

Management of Well-Differentiated Thyroid Cancer

Surgery

Surgical resection is the method of choice for exact diagnosis and initial treatment of well-differentiated thyroid carcinoma and MTC. Large-needle biopsy is the preferred method for diagnosis of thyroid lymphoma and anaplastic thyroid carcinoma. Surgical resection may be indicated for small (<3 cm) thyroid lymphomas[168] and small anaplastic carcinomas,[169] but most of these malignancies present with large bulky lesions and surgery has no role in treatment. The extent of surgical resection and adjuvant treatment for well-differentiated thyroid carcinoma is given in Table 41–7. In general, the use of near-total or total thyroidectomy is advocated except in younger patients with tumors less than 2 cm and no evidence of lymph nodes or extrathyroidal disease. In patients undergoing near-total or total thyroidectomy for well-differentiated thyroid carcinoma, the incidence of disease in the contralateral lobe ranges from 20% to 87%.[152,170]

Tumors recur in the neck more than twice as often in patients who have had subtotal thyroidectomy than in patients who have had total thyroidectomy, although these recurrences are not associated with decreased survival. Another argument for total thyroidectomy is the ease of subsequent documentation of recurrent or metastatic disease by serum thyroglobulin determination and ^{131}I uptake. ^{131}I ablation doses are reduced so that treatment doses can be administered within a safer range. Studies report no postoperative mortality after total thyroidectomy for differentiated thyroid carcinomas. The incidence of permanent recurrent laryngeal nerve damage is 2% to 2.5%, and there is a 1% to 2.7% incidence of permanent hypoparathyroidism.[171] Experienced thyroid surgeons can perform total thyroidectomy safely. In patients with papillary and follicular thyroid carcinoma, TSH-suppressive doses of thyroid hormone and ^{131}I ablation after thyroidectomy have been demonstrated to decrease recurrence rates, but neither treatment has been shown to improve survival.[107,172] The presence of lymph node metastases at diagnosis is not associated with decreased survival rates but is associated with increased local recurrence rates. The correlation of younger age with frequent nodal metastases and older age with less frequent nodal metastases suggests a biologic difference between risk groups with thyroid cancer. Even in poor-prognosis older patients with thyroid cancer, lymph node involvement does not appear to influence survival as seen in other types of cancer.[6]

TABLE 41–7. Recommended Therapeutic Approach to Well-Differentiated Thyroid

Patient Age (y)	*Size of Lesion*	*Extrathyroidal Disease*	*Recommended Therapy*
<45	<2 cm	Absent	Thyroid lobectomy or NTT with suppression
<45	2–4 cm	Absent	NTT/TT with suppression ^{131}I ablation and treatment†
≥45	2–4 cm	Absent	NTT/TT with suppression ^{131}I ablation and treatment
Any	>4 cm*	Present with direct invasion†	NTT/TT with suppression ^{131}I ablation and treatment
Any	Any	Distant metastasis‡ (bone on lung)	NTT/TT with suppression ^{131}I ablation and treatment

NTT/TT, near total/total thyroidectomy.
Suppression, thyroxine (Synthroid) to decrease serum levels of TSH.
* One may consider additional local radiation therapy (see text).
† Treatment doses dependent on uptake during diagnostic whole-body scan.
‡ Resection of localized, solitary distant, or recurrent local well-differentiated thyroid cancer may be considered.

In general, the prognosis of well-differentiated thyroid cancer is excellent as long as some type of thyroid resection is performed. In certain risk groups, ^{131}I is added, along with levothyroxine sodium (Synthroid) to suppress serum levels of TSH. A suggested treatment strategy is outlined in Table 41–7. Certain factors indicate more aggressive disease and may dictate more aggressive treatment. The higher risk factors include distant metastases at presentation, older age (>45 years), males, direct invasion into adjacent structures from large primary lesions, and poor-prognosis variants of papillary including those with tall cell, columnar, diffuse sclerosing, and follicular histology.[5,7,10,32,44,162,165,173] Contrary to previous reports, radiation-induced thyroid carcinoma does not worsen prognosis[91] but behaves exactly like well-differentiated thyroid carcinoma. Regardless of the type of treatment, the survival of patients with papillary or follicular thyroid carcinoma is excellent as long as surgical resection is performed with or without levothyroxine sodium or ^{131}I (Table 41–8). The major morbidity and mortality appear to occur in elderly patients (5%) who present with locally advanced or distant disease. The use of more aggressive treatment strategies may be indicated in this subgroup.

Management of Hürthle Cell Neoplasia

Hürthle cell neoplasms of the thyroid, also called *oxyphil cell tumors,* are really a subgroup of follicular carcinomas of the thyroid gland.[21,174] The histologic appearance is not merely an occasional oxyphil or Hürthle cell, but rather sheets of uniform Hürthle cells. The controversy regarding these tumors comes from a single institution's experience in which the authors describe Hürthle cell neoplasms larger than 2 cm that resulted in metastatic or locally recurrent disease and death of the patient, even in the absence of vascular or capsular invasion.[45,46] This study indicates that total thyroidectomy for all histologically malignant tumors and for tumors greater than 2 cm in size results in a lower recurrence rate (21% versus 59%) than a historical control group.[46] Rosen and colleagues reported that 9% of patients with Hürthle cell malignancies had carcinoma in the contralateral lobe after total thyroidectomy and that 12% of patients developed contralateral lobe tumors after lobectomy.[175] Therefore, the incidence of bilateral malignant Hürthle cell neoplasms was about 10%.[175]

The first question that must be answered about Hürthle cell neoplasms of the thyroid gland is whether they usually appear benign or malignant. A review of nine series indicates that most of these neoplasms appear benign pathologically; that is, they do not have vascular or capsular invasion (Table 41–9). The recurrence rate in tumors that are diagnosed as malignant pathologically ranges from 25% to 53%. Malignant Hürthle cell carcinomas have been found to have a greater proportion of aneuploidy on flow cytometry studies, but the hallmark pathologic finding of malignancy remains capsular or vascular invasion.[176,177] The 10-year survival for malignant Hürthle cell carcinoma ranges from 65% to 95%, with a median survival of 80%.[176] The recurrence rate in tumors that are diagnosed as benign ranges from no recurrence to 12%, with a mean rate of 2% (see Table 41–9). This review indicates that most Hürthle cell neoplasms are benign and act benign after thyroid lobectomy. If the pathologist diagnoses a malignant Hürthle cell carcinoma, there is a higher incidence of recurrent disease. Total or near-total thyroidectomy is advocated for Hürthle cell carcinomas proved pathologically. Total thyroidectomy should not be performed for all Hürthle cell neoplasms. Recent updated reviews corroborate this approach.[174,176–178]

TABLE 41–8. Survival of Well-Differentiated Thyroid Carcinoma After Treatment

Investigations	*No. of Patients*	*5-Year Survival (%)*	*10-Year Survival (%)*	*20-Year Survival (%)*
Papillary				
Schroder et al, 1986[1097]	104	97	—	—
McConahey et al, 1986[152]	859	—	—	93
Mazzaferri et al, 1977[107]	576	—	92.4	—
Joensuu et al, 1986[5]	121	92	74	—
Akslen et al, 1991[7]	1528	93	—	—
Simpson et al, 1987[10]	1074	90	87	
Radiation-Induced Papillary Carcinoma				
Schneider et al, 1985[77]	296	—	99	—
Follicular Carcinoma				
Schroder et al, 1986[1097]	23	96	—	—
Lang et al, 1986[44]	170	—	94	—
Harness et al, 1984[173]	37	—	84	—
Crile et al, 1985[1098]	84	73	43	—
Joensuu et al, 1986[5]	46	87	66	—
Akslen et al, 1991[7]	459	83	—	—
Simpson et al, 1987[10]	504	75	65	—

TABLE 41–9. Incidence of Hürthle Cell Carcinoma, Recurrence Rates, and Late Metastases in Patients With Hürthle Cell Neoplasm of the Thyroid Gland

Investigations	*No. of Patients With Hürthle Cell Tumors (Benign and Malignant)*	*No. of Patients With Benign Tumors (%)*	*Recurrence Rate in Malignant Tumors (%)*	*Recurrence Rate in Benign Tumors (%)*
Thompson et al, 1974[45]	62	26 (42)	29	12
Heppe et al, 1985[47]	20	10 (50)	—	0
Savino et al, 1981[1099]	42	27 (64)	53	0
Rosen et al, 1985[175]	34	25 (73)	—	0
Bondeson et al, 1981[183]	42	34 (81)	25	0
Arganini et al, 1986[48]	47	40 (85)	43	2.5
Caplan et al, 1984[1100]	27	24 (88)	33	0
Gosain and Clark, 1984[1101]	75	71 (95)	25	0
Bronner and LiVolis, 1988[174]	50	34 (68)	31	0
Total	399	291 (73)	34	2

(Modified from Arganini M, Behar R, Wu C, et al. Hürthle cell tumors: a twenty-five year experience. Surgery 1986;100:1108)

Management of Radiation-Induced Thyroid Carcinoma

There is considerable evidence that clinically inapparent thyroid cancer, even radiation-induced occult thyroid cancer, runs an indolent course and does not result in morbidity or mortality. Autopsy studies demonstrate that there is increased papillary cancer in patients exposed to previous radiation, that the clinical course of that cancer was benign, and that the patients died of other causes.[2,15,17] Experience with radiation-induced thyroid carcinoma compared with thyroid carcinoma in patients with no history of head and neck irradiation demonstrates that patients with previous thyroid irradiation more often present with cancer not limited to the thyroid gland and bilateral thyroid lobe involvement.[179] The prognosis of well-differentiated thyroid cancer in patients with a history of irradiation was similar to the prognosis of patients with the same disease extent but without such a history.[179] These data underline the importance of careful follow-up with physical examination and serial serum thyroglobulin levels as a predictor of new malignancy.[109] If a patient has a history of head and neck irradiation, other risk factors can make the patient likely to develop cancer, including higher doses, being female, and younger age at the time of irradiation. Some groups recommend total thyroidectomy for all radiation-induced thyroid carcinomas because the incidence of bilaterality is high (54–75%).[180] However, a prospective study indicated that although thyroid lobectomy may leave occult malignancies in unresected thyroid tissue, there was no significant difference in outcome between patients with limited resection and total thyroidectomy after a 12-year follow-up.[181]

The administration of thyroid hormone to suppress TSH levels has reduced the number of postresection recurrences in radiation-induced papillary and follicular carcinoma.[91] No reduction in recurrence rate could be demonstrated with a greater extent of surgical resection or with the administration of postoperative radioactive iodine,[91] which has been advocated in all radiation-induced carcinomas by some researchers.[182] The clinical course of radiation-induced thyroid carcinoma appears to be similar to neoplasms without a history of radiation (Table 41–8), and therapy should be similar to that of other well-differentiated thyroid carcinomas (see Table 41–7). Furthermore, some investigators estimate that the incidence of radiation-induced thyroid cancer is decreasing.[178]

Postoperative Therapy and Follow-up of Well-Differentiated Thyroid Cancers

There is good evidence that all patients with well-differentiated thyroid cancer should take thyroid hormone (Synthroid) postoperatively to suppress TSH levels.[107,172] This treatment can decrease the recurrence rate of radiation-induced thyroid carcinoma,[91] although reduced recurrence rates do not appear to translate into any difference in survival with the use of levothyroxine sodium postoperatively.[10,107,172] We recommend the postoperative administration of levothyroxine sodium to suppress TSH levels in all patients with thyroid carcinoma (see Table 41–7). The use of postoperative ^{131}I therapy has provided similar data; that is, decreased recurrence rates but no prolongation of survival.[10,112,183] Ablative doses of ^{131}I (30 mCi) should be administered postoperatively to the following patients with primary well-differentiated thyroid cancers: patients older than 45 years, patients with multiple or locally invasive tumors or tumors larger than 2.5 cm, and patients with local or distant metastases, provided adequate uptake of the radionuclide can be demonstrated on scan (see Table 41–7).[182]

Locally recurrent disease in the neck that is detected by physical examination or ultrasound should be surgically excised if the procedure can be performed with low morbidity. Radical neck dissections are not indicated for differentiated thyroid carcinoma. Localized distant metastases that do not take up radioiodine may be resected.[2] External-beam irradiation may be of benefit for less differentiated recurrent or locally advanced lesions (see the section on treatment of anaplastic carcinoma). Metastatic thyroid carcinoma confined to lung has been treated successfully by radioactive iodine, and 54% of patients were alive and without disease 20 years after ^{131}I treatment.[184] In contrast, patients with bony involvement treated by radioactive iodine seldom survive 10 years after treatment.[184] Some patients who have localized bony metastases that take up iodine on whole-body scan and who are treated with radioactive iodine plus aggressive surgery may be rendered disease free, and 30% of patients are still alive at 86 months.[185] After a successful ablative dose of ^{131}I and failure to find extrathyroidal uptake, a patient should be given thyroid hormone replacement (levothyroxine sodium) and TSH levels should be measured to ensure suppression. If the ablation is successful, the patient is not scanned again unless serum thyroglobulin levels are persistently elevated or become elevated, suggesting recurrent or persistent disease.[186]

In a recent study of 98 patients, a serum thyroglobulin level of more than 23 ng/ml correlated 100% with recurrent disease in patients with well-differentiated thyroid cancer who had undergone a total thyroidectomy and received an ablative dose of ^{131}I. The converse was also true; if the serum thyroglobulin level was less than 23 ng/ml, the patient did not have recurrent tumor.[187] Some patients with thyroid cancer may develop antithyroglobulin antibodies that interfere with the ability to measure serum levels of thyroglobulin. This appears to be more common in patients with progressive metastatic disease.[188] As useful and sensitive as serum levels of thyroglobulin are in the follow-up of patients with well-differentiated thyroid cancer, they are inadequate alone and should be coupled with diagnostic whole-body scan for maximal determination of recurrent disease.[189]

Although the use of radioactive iodine to treat metastatic or persistent well-differentiated thyroid cancer is efficacious and generally safe, it can be associated with complications. The side effects of ^{131}I therapy in order of frequency include temporary bone marrow suppression, nausea, sialoadenitis, pain in metastatic deposits, vomiting, pulmonary fibrosis, and leukemia.[186] Patients who have had less extensive surgery (*e.g.*, lobectomy) for the primary tumor often have more neck pain with radioactive iodine.[190] Most authorities use a therapeutic dose of 100 to 200 mCi to treat recurrent or metastatic disease and may repeat the dose several times.[2] A reasonable limiting factor is 200 cGy to blood. One mCi of ^{131}I gives 0.67 cGy to blood, so 300 mCi would be the maximum tolerable dose. If bulk disease or distant metastatic disease exists, dosimetry is required to allow maximal dose with minimal risk. Hematologic complications such as hypoplasia and leukemia may occur when the total dose exceeds 800 mCi.[184,191] Women have had normal pregnancies and deliveries after a total dose of 500 to 600 mCi.

Survival rates from time of discovery of lung and bone metastases from differentiated thyroid carcinoma are less favorable than rates for localized disease. One analysis of 283 patients indicates that 53% were alive at 5 years, 38% at 10 years, and 30% at 15 years.[191] A more recent analysis suggests that the 1-year survival is 50%.[8] Survival after the development of pulmonary metastases from well-differentiated thyroid cancer depends on whether the tumor takes up radioactive iodine. Fortunately, 63% to 80% of metastases from well-differentiated thyroid cancer avidly take up ^{131}I. Metastases that take up ^{131}I are usually treatable with ^{131}I therapy.[192] Six variables have an independent prognostic significance for survival in these patients: extensive metastases, older age at discovery of metastases, advanced local disease, male sex, absence of radioactive iodine uptake by metastases, and follicular cell type.[8,191] These variables were documented in another study, in which pulmonary metastases occurred less often in patients treated initially by total thyroidectomy than in those treated with less than total thyroidectomy.[193]

The aim of management of patients with differentiated thyroid carcinoma after surgery should be to detect and treat metastases with radioactive iodine as early as possible. The incidence of pulmonary metastases is lowest in patients with papillary carcinoma (9%), intermediate with follicular carcinoma (13%), and highest with Hürthle cell carcinoma (25%).[176,178,193] Surgical resection of distant metastases from differentiated thyroid carcinoma has been advocated by some researchers.[2] Indications for resection include reduced administration of radioiodine, pain, and pathologic fracture. Estimated cumulative survival rates from the time of resection of distant disease were 45% for 5 years and 33% for 20 years after removal of a solitary metastasis.[2] This heroic treatment may be indicated for solitary metastases to bone or lung that do not take up radioiodine.

Chemotherapy for metastatic well-differentiated thyroid cancer has not been effective. The best regimen has been high-dose single-drug therapy with doxorubicin. Doses in the range of 60 to 150 mg/m^2 given every 3 weeks have resulted in a 33% to 39% partial response rate. Combination regimens have not had better results than monotherapy doxorubicin (see the section on chemotherapy in the treatment of anaplastic thyroid cancer).[194]

Management of Medullary Thyroid Carcinoma

In 1959, Hazard and colleagues described MTC as a distinct clinical and pathologic entity. This neoplasm presents in sporadic form (nonfamilial) and is associated with three clinical syndromes: MEN-IIa, MEN-IIb, and familial non-MEN MTC, a disease characterized by hereditary MTC without associated endocrinopathies.[51,65,93,178] In the three familial presentations of MTC, the disease is almost always bilateral and requires a total thyroidectomy combined with central lymph node dissection.[51,178,195] MTC that presents sporadically is usually unilateral, but it still requires the same operation because the familial disease cannot be ruled out by history alone. In MEN-IIa and MEN-IIb, MTC is associated with pheochromocytoma, a potentially life-threatening situation if an unprepared patient undergoes anesthetic stress for thyroidectomy. For this reason, if the diagnosis of MTC is known preoperatively by abnormal plasma level of calcitonin or by needle biopsy, pheochromocytoma must be ruled out by measurement of 24-hour urine for vanillylmandelic acid (VMA), metanephrines, and catecholamines or by measurement of serum levels of norepinephrine and epinephrine.[51,65] In the familial setting, individuals from kindreds who are at risk for the development of MTC can be identified accurately by specific genetic probes.[62,63] These individuals can then be screened at yearly intervals for the early diagnosis of MTC (Fig. 41–2). The early diagnosis of C-cell hyperplasia, C-cell carcinoma in situ, or MTC confined to the thyroid gland can be made by provocative testing with calcium and pentagastrin. An abnormal response is a rise in plasma calcitonin levels after use of these agents (see Fig. 41–2). This abnormal response to pentagastrin or calcium is diagnostic for MTC or MTC in situ or premalignant C-cell hyperplasia (see Fig. 41–2). Individuals

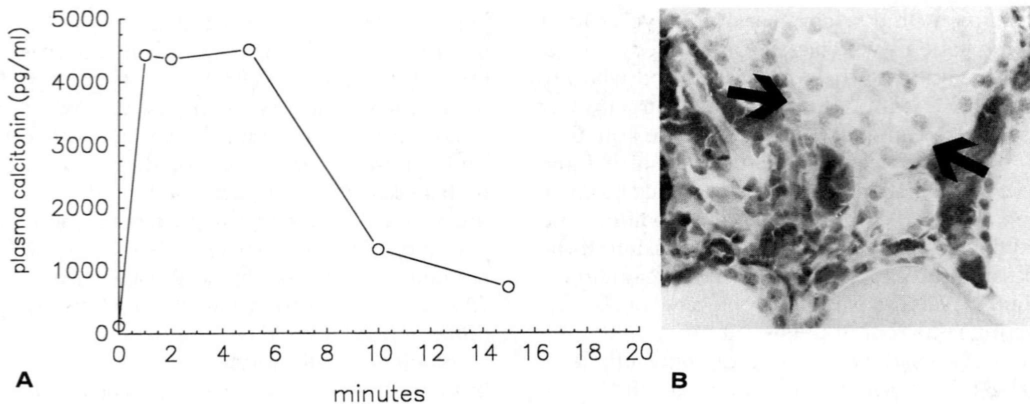

FIGURE 41–2. The results of a screening pentagastrin stimulation test and a photomicrograph from a 21-year-old man whose family has multiple endocrine neoplasia. **(A)** Although the patient's basal calcitonin level was normal (<200 pg/ml), his peripheral plasma level was abnormally elevated at 1, 2, 5, 10, and 20 minutes after the intravenous administration of pentagastrin (0.5 μg/kg body weight). **(B)** A thyroidectomy specimen showing C-cell hyperplasia (*arrows*). A similar focus was found in both thyroid lobes. The patient had no evidence of extrathyroidal metastases and was cured by total thyroidectomy (H & E, original magnification × 250). (Alexander HR, Norton JA. Biology and management of medullary thyroid carcinoma of the parafollicular cells. Ann Intern Med 1991;115:133)

diagnosed in this fashion have a high probability of cure (Table 41–10).

Plasma calcitonin levels (basal and stimulated) increase with an increase in the extent of disease. In a study of patients from kindreds with MTC who had undetectable basal calcitonin levels and who had levels less than 100 pg/ml after pentagastrin-calcium stimulation, 24 of 25 patients had MTC localized to the thyroid gland and were cured after total thyroidectomy.[111] Telander and colleagues demonstrated that MTC is present in children from kindreds at a mean age of 7 years (range, 1.5–12 years).[196] A total thyroidectomy cured 14 of 17 children at this early age, and the 3 children with persistent disease had MEN-IIb. Provocative testing helps in the management of patients from kindreds with MEN-IIa and familial non-MEN MTC. Furthermore, recent reports contradict past dogma[67] and suggest that children with MTC in the setting of MEN-IIb may be cured. Investigators at Washington University School of Medicine performed total thyroidectomy and central node dissection in 7 children (age 3–10 years) with a family history of MEN-IIb based on increased plasma concentrations of calcitonin (either basal or pentagastrin stimulated). Five of 7 children treated in this manner had no evidence of MTC 3 to 10 years after thyroidectomy.[197] In older studies, most patients with MEN-IIb had spread of MTC outside the thyroid gland at presentation. These patients were not cured by thyroid surgery.[67]

Sporadic MTC usually presents with a neck mass, and the diagnosis can be obtained by aspiration cytology, cutting-needle biopsy, or measurement of serum calcitonin levels. Serum calcitonin is a specific, sensitive circulating marker for MTC but usually is not measured as part of the workup of a thyroid nodule. Patients with sporadic MTC may present with lymph node metastases or extrathyroidal disease, and surgery may not be curable in this setting. However, in a study of 12 patients with sporadic MTC who were treated at the National Institutes of Health, 5 were cured after total thyroidectomy and central lymph node dissection (see Table 41–10).[51] High-resolution real-time ultrasound can be used to stage accurately the extent of disease in the neck. MTC appears bright and echogenic and may be detected in the thyroid or lymph nodes.[198] The only significant predictor of survival after resection of primary MTC is tumor invasion beyond the

TABLE 41–10. Outcome of Patients With Medullary Thyroid Carcinoma According to Method of Diagnosis

Investigations	*Disease and Method of Diagnosis*	*No. of Patients*	*Follow-Up (y)*	*No. of Cured Patients (%)*	*No. of Patients Dead From Disease (%)*
Alexander and Norton, 1991[51]	MEN-IIa* by screening	19	13	19 (100)	0
Gagel et al, 1988[61]	MEN-IIa by screening	22	11	19 (86)	0
Alexander and Norton, 1991[51]	MEN-IIa by palpation of mass	17	19	5 (29)†	2 (12)
Alexander and Norton, 1991[51]	Sporadic MTC by palpation of mass	12	12	5 (42)†	2 (17)

* MEN-IIa, multiple endocrine neoplasia type IIa.
† Significantly less than MEN-IIa by screening ($p < 0.01$, Fisher's exact test).

thyroid capsule or metastases to cervical lymph nodes. The overall survival after surgical resection of sporadic MTC varies; the historical 10-year survival was 40% to 60%.[21,199] With meticulous surgery and earlier diagnosis, the 10-year survival may be better (about 80%).[51]

Several studies have attempted to localize and resect lymph nodes containing microscopic or macroscopic MTC after thyroidectomy. One study used selective venous catheterization and pentagastrin stimulation to detect regions draining calcitonin in patients with recurrent and MTC.[200] Another study used additional extensive neck dissections after thyroidectomy to remove tumor in lymph nodes.[201] Both studies were able to remove MTC in clinically normal-appearing lymph nodes, and both were able to normalize postoperative basal calcitonin levels in some patients. The impact of these techniques on survival has not been demonstrated.[200,201] Most recent analyses of larger groups of patients with MTC suggest that this strategy can normalize plasma levels of calcitonin in 50% of patients and may render some patients free of disease.[202] Several groups have used thallium and technetium scanning or pentavalent ^{99m}Tc-DMSA to detect recurrent MTC and advocate resection of recurrent or persistent macroscopic disease.[126,132,133,203] Surgery alone seldom has been able to cure patients with MTC spread outside the thyroid gland. Whether resection of local or distant metastases from MTC impacts on survival is not clear because of the indolent course of this neoplasm.

The tragedy of not detecting MTC confined to the thyroid gland when it is surgically curable can be appreciated if one considers the ineffectiveness of nonoperative treatment of recurrent or metastatic disease.[65] Chemotherapy has been of little use for metastatic MTC. Gottlieb and Hill reported remissions in 3 of 5 patients with metastatic MTC,[204] but these results have not been confirmed by others.[205] Cisplatin, streptozocin, carmustine (BCNU), methotrexate, and 5-fluorouracil (5-FU) have been used without benefit.[65] One recent case report demonstrated some efficacy of low-dose doxorubicin at 15 mg/m^2 intravenously each week for 20 weeks for a total dose of 300 mg/m^2. The patient had a complete response that has lasted 18 months.[206] Another patient had a partial response to a combination of dacarbazine and 5-FU that lasted 10 months.[207] Because ^{131}I-MIBG is taken up by metastatic and recurrent MTC,[128,129] it may be of use in the treatment of metastatic MTC, although no studies have been reported. We have attempted to image several patients with metastatic MTC with iodinated MIBG without success. This strategy does not appear useful. Monoclonal antibodies to CEA have been used to image metastatic MTC and may have potential in experimental treatment of metastatic MTC.[130,131]

Radiation therapy for localized inaccessible tumor deposits may be useful in patients with MTC.[208] Work with sensitizers may increase radiation efficacy in MTC, but the data are limited (see the section on anaplastic thyroid carcinoma). In general, MTC is not very sensitive to radiation. Potential benefits from radiation therapy must be weighed against complications.

Patients with metastatic MTC may be asymptomatic even with substantial tumor burdens. The most troubling symptom is severe voluminous secretory diarrhea, which generally develops when plasma calcitonin levels exceed 20 ng/ml. The etiology of this diarrhea is unknown. It may be due to calcitonin[209] or to other tumor hormone products, because C cells in MTC can secrete many different hormones.[65] This symptom is especially bothersome because it is not well controlled by medical regimens. In some cases, debulking of grossly evident tumor ameliorates the diarrhea. One patient with metastatic MTC, elevated pancreatic polypeptide levels, and severe refractory diarrhea has been reported to respond with complete resolution of diarrhea to the long-acting somatostatin analog octreotide.[210] Three other patients with metastatic MTC have had their diarrhea controlled with octreotide in a similar protocol, in which octreotide was administered by continuous pump at a dose of 0.6 to 1.0 mg/day.[211] Octreotide does not appear to have antitumor effects in these studies. It does lower circulating levels of calcitonin and other hormones and appears to derive its beneficial effects on the diarrhea by inhibiting secretion of diarrhea-producing peptides. Tachyphylaxis may develop and requires increasing the administered dose.[211] Low-dose use of interferon-α (3 million units) three times per week subcutaneously ameliorated the diarrhea in 2 patients with metastatic MTC.[212] This immune stimulatory agent appears to decrease plasma levels of calcitonin without any change in tumor size.[212]

Management of Anaplastic Thyroid Carcinoma

Treatment of anaplastic thyroid carcinoma is poor, and most patients with this diagnosis are dead within 1 year with a median survival of 4 months.[213] The clinical manifestations of thyroid carcinoma present a true paradox; it is a cancer that in its differentiated form may be one of the most benign types of cancer[1] and in its undifferentiated form may be one of the most malignant forms.[213] Surgical resection is indicated for small tumors or tumors in which it is technically feasible;[169] however, most tumors are unresectable at presentation. If the tumor is large and apparently unresectable, cutting-needle biopsy is recommended to establish the diagnosis. Radiation therapy alone has not been useful for anaplastic thyroid carcinoma; however, the combination of doxorubicin as a sensitizer and 5760 cGy delivered over 40 days has had dramatic local control rates for anaplastic giant and spindle cell carcinoma of the thyroid gland.[214] The regimen consists of once weekly low-dose doxorubicin (10 mg/m^2) and hyperfractionated radiation therapy. The radiation therapy is carried out with fractional doses of 160 cGy per treatment twice a day for 3 days each week to a total dose of 5760 cGy in 40 days. Using this protocol, 16 of 19 patients (84%) achieved complete tumor regression in the primary area and 13 (68%) remained disease free in the neck until death.[214,215] The same group has treated 22 patients with locally advanced differentiated thyroid carcinoma with a similar treatment regimen, and 91% of patients achieved complete tumor regression in the neck.[215,216] The regimen did not disproportionately enhance normal tissue morbidity and appears to be a breakthrough for the treatment of locally advanced anaplastic or differentiated thyroid carcinoma. External-beam irradiation has been shown to reduce massive mediastinal disease from follicular thyroid carcinoma, resolving superior vena caval syndrome.[217] Most patients with anaplastic cancer develop distant metastases and die within 1 year, and systemic therapies need to be developed.

Drug therapies for advanced thyroid carcinoma and anaplastic thyroid carcinoma have been disappointing. Regimens with doxorubicin have shown the highest response rates, and doxorubicin itself is the best single agent (Table 41–11). Some researchers suggest that doxorubicin-only therapy is better than multidrug therapy.[194] Cisplatin and bleomycin have had some activity, although two trials using these active agents in advanced thyroid carcinoma had conflicting results. The combination of doxorubicin (60 mg/m^2) and cisplatin (60 mg/m^2) had only 2 (9%) partial remissions in 22 evaluable patients with advanced thyroid cancer.[218] These results were inconsistent with a previous study that showed that doxorubicin plus cisplatin was significantly better than doxorubicin alone in a similar group of patients with advanced thyroid carcinoma.[219] Eighty-four evaluable patients were stratified by histologic type and randomized to doxorubicin alone (60 mg/m^2 intravenously every 3 weeks) or to a combination of doxorubicin (60 mg/m^2) and cisplatin (40 mg/m^2) intravenously every 3 weeks. The total dose of doxorubicin was 550 mg/m^2. Forty-one patients received doxorubicin alone and 7 had partial responses (17%). Forty-three patients received the combination of drugs, and there were 5 complete and 6 partial responses (26%). The finding of 5 complete responses in the combination group was significantly better than no complete responses in the doxorubicin alone group. The 5 CRs in the combination group included 3 complete responders of 18 with anaplastic carcinoma, and an overall response rate in anaplastic carcinoma of 33%. Four of 5 complete responders survived for more than 2 years. The toxicity was similar in the two-drug regimens and indicated that doxorubicin plus cisplatin had a better response rate than doxorubicin alone.[219] Bukowski and colleagues treated 11 patients with advanced thyroid carcinoma with a combination of doxorubicin, bleomycin, vincristine and melphalan.[220] They reported a response in 4 of 11 patients (36%), with one durable complete response in a patient with anaplastic carcinoma.[220]

The findings of durable complete response in patients with anaplastic carcinoma are provocative. One potential diagnostic error is thyroid lymphoma, which may mimic anaplastic carcinoma. However, there may be subsets of patients with advanced or anaplastic thyroid carcinoma that will respond to combination chemotherapy. A recent phase II study of 15 patients in Germany with anaplastic thyroid carcinoma showed more potential efficacy with a different regimen. Drugs included cisplatin (100 mg/m^2), mitoxantrone (20 mg/m^2), and vincristine (1.5 mg/m^2). Ten of 15 patients (67%) responded to chemotherapy, with 4 patients (27%) having a compete response. Responders demonstrated a longer survival than nonresponders (mean 21 months versus 4 months).[105] Patients with anaplastic thyroid carcinoma are rare, and it will take cooperative trials to answer questions about certain regimens. The treatment of anaplastic thyroid carcinoma should include doxorubicin, fractionated radiation therapy to control primary tumors, and combination chemotherapy using either doxorubicin with cisplatin or the combination of Bukowski and colleagues.[214,219,220]

THE PARATHYROID GLAND

Primary hyperparathyroidism is a common disease, with an incidence between 1 and 5 persons per 1000. An increased incidence of hyperparathyroidism has been reported in persons who have been exposed previously to irradiation of the head and neck.[221] The parathyroid tumor associated with previous radiation has been adenoma and not carcinoma. Patients usually present with symptoms related to increased urinary excretion of calcium (urinary calculi and nephrocalcinosis) or demineralization of bony skeleton (bone pain and elevated serum alkaline phosphatase) or both. The diagnosis of primary hyperparathyroidism is established biochemically by concomitant serial elevations of serum calcium levels and inappropriately elevated serum parathyroid hormone levels. Elevated urinary cyclic adenosine monophosphate (UcAMP) levels are present in 92% of patients with primary hyperparathyroidism.[222] Once the diagnosis is established, surgical exploration generally is recommended. The extent of surgery depends on the etiology of the hyperparathyroidism. The three possible etiologies of primary hyperparathyroidism and incidences are adenoma (83%), hyperplasia (15%), and car-

TABLE 41–11. Chemotherapy for Thyroid Carcinoma

Investigations	*Drugs*	*No. of Evaluable Patients*	*No. of Responders (%)*	*No. of Complete Responders (%)*
Gottlieb and Hill, 1974[204]	Doxorubicin alone	43	15 (35)	0
Shimaoka et al, 1985[219]	Doxorubicin alone	41	7 (17)	0
Ahuja and Ernst, 1987[194]	Doxorubicin alone	248	95 (38)	8 (3)
Shimaoka et al, 1985[219]	Doxorubicin + cisplatin	43	11 (26)	5 (12)
Williams et al, 1986[218]	Doxorubicin + cisplatin	22	2 (9)	0
Bukowski et al, 1983[220]	Doxorubicin + bleomycin + vincristine + melphalan	11	4 (36)	1 (19)
Sokal and Harmar, 1978[1102]	Doxorubicin + vincristine + bleomycin	14	9 (64)	0
Kober et al, 1990[105]	Cisplatin, mitoxantrone, vincristine	15	10 (67)	4 (27)

cinoma (1–2%; Table 41–12). Parathyroid hyperplasia means multiple gland involvement and can be inherited as part of two familial syndromes (MEN-I and MEN-IIa). Parathyroid adenomas are the most common cause of primary hyperparathyroidism and require identification and simple excision of the tumor. Parathyroid carcinomas are rare and require identification and resection of the tumor along with the ipsilateral lobe of the thyroid and abnormal central nodal tissue. The diagnosis of parathyroid carcinoma can be confusing and it is the purpose of this section to help the clinician and the pathologist differentiate parathyroid carcinoma from parathyroid adenoma.

The diagnosis of parathyroid carcinoma may be suspected at the time of clinical presentation. Parathyroid carcinoma has been reported in 3 patients from different families with familial hyperparathyroidism. This finding is rare and implies transformation of hyperplastic parathyroid tissue into carcinoma.[223,224] Parathyroid carcinoma usually presents in the fourth decade. The hallmark preoperative signs are severe hypercalcemia (serum calcium >15 mg/dl), palpable neck mass, and bone and renal disease.[225] Parathyroid adenomas rarely present with palpable tumors, and serum levels of calcium are usually significantly lower, although similar hypercalcemia can be seen with parathyroid adenomas.[226] The principal histologic features of parathyroid carcinoma that distinguish it from adenoma include a trabecular pattern, mitotic figures, thick fibrous bands, and capsular and blood vessel invasion.[225] The major problem with parathyroid carcinoma

TABLE 41–12. Differential Causes of Primary Hyperparathyroidism: Etiology, Incidence, Diagnostic Features, and Long-Term Results

Diagnosis	*Etiology*	*Relative Frequency*	*Palpable Neck Mass or Vocal Cord Paralysis*	*Serum Calcium Level (mg/dl)*	*Parathyroid Hormone*	*Gross Pathology*	*Surgical Procedure*	*Microscopic Pathology*	*Recurrent Hyperparathyroidism**
Hyperplasia	Familial pattern	14%	Absent	12	Elevated	Multiple gland enlargement; soft reddish brown appearance	Either 3½ gland resection or 4 gland resection with autograft	Decreased fat content and increased gland cellularity in multiple glands	Intermediate (10–30%)
Adenoma	Associated with previous irradiation	85%	Absent	12	Elevated	Single gland enlargement; soft reddish brown appearance	Excision of abnormal gland	Decreased fat content and increased cellularity; occasionally attached normal parathyroid gland	Low (<1%)
Carcinoma	? Familial pattern	1%	Usually	>14	Markedly elevated	Single enlarged gland that is firm, whitish gray	Resection of abnormal gland in continuity with ipsilateral thyroid lobe and suspicious central lymph nodes	Trabecular pattern; mitotic figures; thick fibrous bands; capsular and blood vessel invasion	High (>50%)

* Recurrent means that patient initially has normal serum levels of calcium postoperatively and more than 6 months later develops recurrent hypercalcemia.

is intraoperative recognition of the malignancy and performance of an appropriate resection procedure including ipsilateral thyroid lobectomy and dissection of the central lymph node region.[227] In two large series of patients, the 5-year survival rates were 44% and 29% and the 10-year survival rates were 22% and 15%, respectively.[228,229] This is in marked contrast to a more recent series in which 8 of 9 patients were alive with a median follow-up of 6 years.[227] Distant metastases develop to lung, bone, and liver in order of highest frequency.[229,230] Radiation therapy has been unsuccessful at controlling primary and metastatic lesions.[229,230] Bukowski and colleagues reported a single patient with metastatic lesions who had a complete remission of 5 months' duration with a combination of 5-fluorouracil (500 mg/m^2), cyclophosphamide (500 mg/m^2), and dacarbazine (200 mg/m^2).[231] Another group also documented a dramatic response of metastatic parathyroid cancer to dacarbazine.[232] Based on these two reports, dacarbazine appears active and may be useful in the treatment of parathyroid carcinoma.

The major morbidity of recurrent or metastatic parathyroid carcinoma is due to severe hypercalcemia, which is difficult to control medically and results in death. Aggressive surgical resection of bulk recurrent or metastatic disease has been advocated by some surgeons because of the indolent, slow-growing nature of the tumor and the potential to control hypercalcemia.[233] Unfortunately, surgery is not always possible or successful, especially if the carcinoma has metastasized widely. Attempts to inhibit the actions of parathyroid hormone with calcitonin, mithramycin, or diphosphonates have been disappointing. Recent evidence suggests that gallium nitrate is effective for cancer-related hypercalcemia and may be useful to manage the hypercalcemia of patients with parathyroid cancer.[234] Intravenous etidronate may be helpful in the acute setting with severe hypercalcemia.[235] Unfortunately, the hypercalcemia associated with parathyroid cancer is a chronic problem and needs better antitumor therapy to control. Proper intraoperative identification of malignancy and appropriate initial surgery is crucial to therapy of parathyroid carcinoma. The characteristics that distinguish patients at risk preoperatively and the intraoperative malignant tumor characteristics that allow the surgeon and pathologist to make the correct diagnosis are listed in Table 41–12. If malignant parathyroid neoplasms are recognized and proper initial resections performed, a greater number of patients will be cured.

THE ADRENAL GLAND

PATHOLOGY OF THE ADRENAL CORTEX

Hyperplasia

The term hyperplasia is defined as an increased number of cells in an organ.[236] It is a pathologic change associated with increased function or compensatory change. In pituitary-based hypercortisolism (Cushing's disease), which is the most common endogenous form of hypercortisolism, the gross adrenal enlargement is not impressive. The adrenal gland is about twice the normal size. The weight of each adrenal ranges from 6 to 8 g, although occasionally the adrenal weighs 12 g (a normal adrenal weighs from 3–6 g). Microscopically, there is a widened inner zone of the compact zona reticularis and a sharply demarcated outer zone of clear cells. The appearance of adrenal glands in ectopic ACTH syndrome is similar except that the glands are usually larger, weighing at least 12 g and as much as 30 g. Macronodular adrenal hyperplasia (3-cm nodules of adrenal cortex weighing 30–50 g and as much as 100 g) usually is a secondary response of the adrenal gland to adrenocorticotropic hormone (ACTH), whereas pigmented micronodular adrenal hyperplasia (1- to 5-mm nodules with pigmented appearance and normal glandular weight) is more likely to be autonomous and to occur in children including infants.[237] ACTH levels are low or undetectable. This histology is rare and can occur in a familial pattern.[238]

Adrenocortical Adenoma

Adrenal adenoma is a benign neoplasm of adrenocortical cells that resembles normal adrenal cells histologically but may possess functional autonomy.[236] An adenoma usually does not exceed 5 cm, although benign tumors exceeding 10 cm have been reported. One suggested cut-off for benign adenomas is a weight of 100 g. Cellular pleomorphism and tumor necrosis may be present but are rare. The exact functional type of neoplasm cannot be described based solely on histology, although there are consistent differences. Adenomas produce syndromes of hypercortisolism and hyperaldosteronism but seldom produce adrenogenital syndromes. Larger tumors producing adrenogenital syndromes are consistent with carcinoma,[239] as are pleomorphism, tumor necrosis, and mitotic activity.[239] The prognosis of adrenocortical adenomas producing Cushing's syndrome is excellent, and successful resection invariably produces cure. The prognosis of adrenocortical adenomas producing hyperaldosteronism may not be as favorable. Resection is followed by a response in blood pressure and correction of hypokalemia; however, 30% of patients with resected aldosteronomas develop recurrent hypertension but not recurrent hypokalemia. If the preoperative diagnosis was incorrect and the patient had hyperaldosteronism secondary to hyperplasia, unilateral adrenalectomy does not improve the syndrome. Adenomas that produce the adrenogenital syndrome have the least favorable outcome. Many of these tumors are really misdiagnosed carcinomas that develop local recurrence or metastases.[239]

Adrenocortical Carcinoma

Adrenocortical carcinoma is a malignant neoplasm of adrenocortical cells demonstrating partial or complete histologic and functional differentiation. Adrenocortical carcinomas are rare neoplasms and comprise only 0.05% to 0.2% of all cancers.[240] This incidence translates to a rate of only 2 persons per million in the world population.[241] Women appear to develop functional adrenocortical carcinomas more commonly than men, and men develop nonfunctioning malignant adrenal tumors more commonly than women. There is a bimodal occurrence by age with a peak incidence at less than 5 years of age and a second peak in the fourth and fifth decade. Adrenocortical carcinoma has been described as part of a complex hereditary syndrome including sarcoma and breast and lung cancer.[242] Cytogenetic analysis of primary adrenocortical carcinoma revealed clonal rearrangements of several autosomes and sex chromosomes. In all metaphases, the following marker chromosomes were present: 4 pt, t(3;12) (p14;p3), 14q+,t(15;20)(p11;q11), t(5;18)(p13.3;p11.2), psu dic (18) t(18;3) (p11.39;p12), and psu dic (20)t(20;9) (q11.2;p11).[243] Two recent studies suggest that loss of heterozygosity at loci on the short arm of chromosome 11 (11p) may be important in the pathogenesis of malignant adrenocortical tumors.[244,245]

Adrenocortical carcinomas weigh between 100 and 5000 g. Areas of necrosis and hemorrhage are common and are consistent with malignancy. Invasion and metastases are common. Microscopically, their appearance varies with the functional syndrome but also varies within the same tumor. The presence of cells with big nuclei, hyperchromatism, and enlarged nucleoli are all consistent with malignancy.[236] Nuclear changes are more common in tumors larger than 500 g. Vascular invasion and mitoses are diagnostic of adrenocortical malignancy. Broad desmoplastic bands are associated with metastatic potential of tumors.

The diagnosis of malignancy in adrenocortical neoplasms is difficult, especially in tumors that weigh between 50 and 100 g. Differentiating between adrenal carcinoma and renal carcinoma also may be difficult. Immunostaining for vimentin, epithelial membrane antigen, cytokeratin, and blood group antigens can separate the two diagnoses. Adrenal carcinoma and adenoma stain positive for vimentin, whereas renal carcinoma is negative for vimentin but positive for the others.[246] Table 41–13 attempts to differentiate benign from malignant adrenal tumors based on criteria suggested by Page and colleagues.[236] Immunostaining profiles of adrenocortical carcinoma and adenoma are similar, so that the pathologist must rely on clinical and morphologic criteria.[246] Although the difference in natural history between benign and malignant adrenocortical neoplasms is clear, it is not always possible to histologically separate one from the other. The only reliable criterion is the presence of nodal or distant metastases. The data used to differentiate benign from malignant adrenocortical neoplasms include whether hormone is produced and what type, the amount of tumor necrosis, fibrosis, vascular invasion, number of mitoses, and tumor weight. In a series that analyzed 43 adrenocortical tumors histologically, mitotic activity and venous invasion correlated best with metastasizing or recurring tumors (*i.e,* carcinoma).[247] Another more recent analysis demonstrated that number of mitoses is the most important predictor of outcome. Patients who had more than 20 mitoses per 50 high-power fields had a median survival of 14 months, whereas patients with fewer than 20 had a median survival of 58 months.[248] Nuclear DNA ploidy may predict survival because patients with aneuploid tumors appear to have shortened survival.[249] A final criterion is based on the observation that cells from carcinomas produce abnormal amounts of androgens and 11-deoxysteroids.[250] Only 10% of malignant tumors are associated with masculinization and only 12% with feminization; the rest usually produce a combination of hormones including aldosterone.

CLINICAL PRESENTATIONS OF ADRENOCORTICAL NEOPLASMS

Cushing's Syndrome or Hypercortisolism

Signs

Hypercortisolism results in the signs and symptoms of Cushing's syndrome. The signs and symptoms are widespread and diverse, affecting nearly every organ in the body.[251,252] However, no single symptom or sign is common to every patient with endogenous hypercortisolism. Although hypercortisolism is the most common presentation for adrenocortical neoplasms, Cushing's syndrome is rare with an estimated incidence of only 10 persons per million population.[251] The most common cause of hypercortisolism is iatrogenic administration of steroids to treat other diseases. Hypercortisolism usually is not associated with MEN-I, although it can be present in this familial syndrome.[253] It has been reported in 5% of patients with sporadic Zollinger-Ellison syndrome (ZES) and in 19% of patients with both ZES and MEN-I.[251,254]

Progressive weight gain is the most universal symptom of patients with hypercortisolism. Obesity is usually truncal, and patients demonstrate thin extremities due to muscle wasting. Increased fat in the dorsal neck region combined with dorsal kyphosis secondary to osteoporosis gives the appearance of a buffalo hump. Serial photographs demonstrate a rounding of the face. Increased blood pressure in Cushing's syndrome is usually mild and is caused primarily by excess mineralocorticoid secretion. Hypertension is less frequent in iatrogenic Cushing's syndrome because physicians prescribe pure glucocorticoids. Striae are reliable clinical signs of Cushing's. Hirsutism consists of excessive fine hair on the face, upper

TABLE 41–13. Diagnosis of Malignancy in Adrenocortical Neoplasms

Reliability	*Clinical Criteria*	*Pathologic Criteria*
Diagnostic of malignancy	Weight loss, feminization, nodal or distant metastases	Tumor weight >100 g, tumor necrosis, fibrous bands, vascular invasion, mitosis
Consistent with malignancy	Virilism, Cushing's virilism, no hormone production	Nuclear pleomorphism
Suggestive of malignancy	Elevated urinary 17-ketosteroids	Capsular invasion
Unreliable	Hypercortisolism, hyperaldosteronism	Tumor giant cells, cytoplasmic size variation, ratio between compact and clear cells

(Adapted from Page DL, DeLillis RA, Hough AJ. Tumors of the adrenal. In: Atlas of tumor pathology. Washington DC: Armed Forces Institute of Pathology, 1986)

back, and arms. Virilization including clitoromegaly, deep voice, and balding suggest adrenocortical carcinoma. Glucose intolerance with hyperglycemia is common, and patients may present with diabetes mellitus. Weakness secondary to muscle atrophy is a common complaint and is especially common in ectopic ACTH syndrome with hypokalemia. Menstrual irregularity or amenorrhea is common in women with Cushing's syndrome, whereas men with Cushing's syndrome have loss of libido or impotency. Dilatation of blood vessels and thinning of the subcutaneous tissue give the face a ruddy appearance. Mental changes in Cushing's syndrome vary from mild depression to severe psychosis and appear to correlate directly with serum levels of cortisol and ACTH. Hypokalemia worsens the weakness associated with Cushing's syndrome and suggests the etiology of adrenocortical carcinoma or ectopic ACTH syndrome. Impaired immune surveillance is an important part of the morbidity associated with Cushing's syndrome. Opportunistic infections including cryptococcosis, aspergillosis, nocardiosis, and *Pneumocystis carinii* pneumonia are more common in patients with Cushing's syndrome and may be lethal.[255–257] In children with Cushing's syndrome, the most common presenting sign is obesity or an arrest of normal growth with short stature.[258] The early diagnosis of Cushing's syndrome depends primarily on a knowledge of the many different signs and symptoms of the disorder and a high clinical index of suspicion.

Workup and Diagnosis of Cushing's Syndrome

The initial step in the workup of a patient with presumptive hypercortisolism is to establish biochemically whether hypercortisolism is present. The second step is to determine whether the hypercortisolism is considered pituitary-dependent or pituitary-independent, and the final step is to determine the exact etiology of the hypercortisolism (Fig. 41–3). Laboratory testing allows the correct diagnosis of the presence and the cause of the hypercortisolism in nearly every case.[251]

Establish Hypercortisolism. Urinary excretion of unmetabolized (free) cortisol is directly proportional to the amount of free cortisol in the plasma. As the cortisol-binding globulin becomes saturated (at plasma cortisol levels of 20 μg/dl), small increases in cortisol secretion produce exponential increases in urinary free cortisol. This amplification effect makes 24-hour urinary free cortisol the single best measurement to dif-

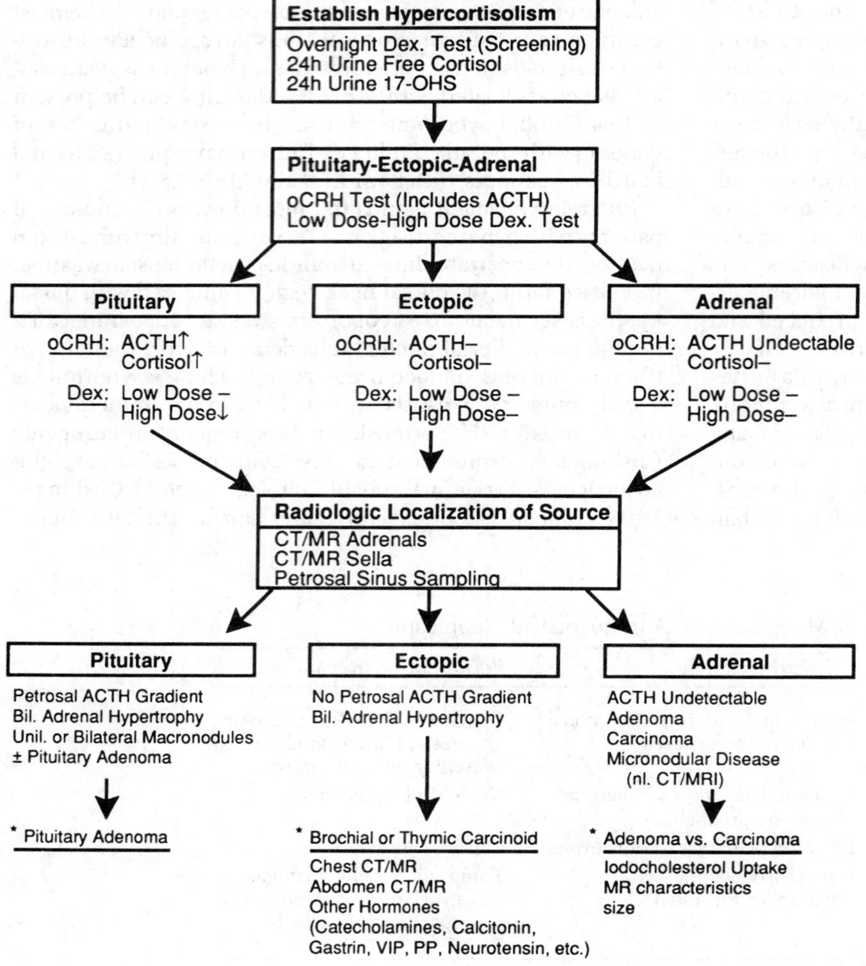

FIGURE 41–3. Flow diagram for evaluation of a patient with suspected hypercortisolism or Cushing's syndrome.

ferentiate normal from hypercortisolemic states (see Fig. 41–3). The overnight single-dose dexamethasone test works because of the lack of normal feedback that occurs in all forms of hypercortisolism (Fig. 41–4).[259] Normal subjects given 1 mg of dexamethasone orally at 11:00 P.M. have plasma cortisol levels less than 5 μg/dl at 8:00 A.M. the next day. Patients with endogenous hypercortisolism do not suppress and have cortisol levels greater than 5 μg/dl. The major advantage of this test is a 3% incidence of false-negative results (patients with Cushing's syndrome whose cortisol levels suppress). This test may have false-positive results (30%) including depression, alcoholism, stress, and primary cortisol resistance.[260–262] A normal-single dose dexamethasone test and urinary free cortisol (less than 100 μg/day in most laboratories) virtually exclude the diagnosis of hypercortisolism.[251] Another study that can be used to discriminate hypercortisolism is the 24-hour urine test for 17-hydroxysteroids corrected for gram creatinine. This study is older but has results similar to urinary measurement of free cortisol levels.

Etiology of Hypercortisolism. Patients with pituitary Cushing's syndrome respond to 1 μg/kg of corticotropin-releasing hormone (CRH) by increasing plasma ACTH and cortisol levels, and patients with depression have a blunted ACTH response to CRH.[263] A CRH test can differentiate pituitary Cushing's syndrome (Cushing's disease) from ectopic secretion of ACTH. Twenty-nine of 33 patients with Cushing's disease had increased plasma ACTH and cortisol levels after CRH, whereas none of 8 patients with ectopic ACTH responded. The CRH test worked as well as the standard dexamethasone test, and the diagnostic power was enhanced when the two tests were combined.[264] Patients with Cushing's syndrome have abnormalities in the diurnal rhythm of plasma cortisol and ACTH levels. Serial samples taken over several days are necessary because patients with Cushing's disease can have episodic secretion of cortisol. Nevertheless, a low midnight cortisol level (<2 μg/dl) excludes the diagnosis of endogenous hypercortisolism. Determination of simultaneous plasma ACTH levels are helpful. Primary adrenal tumors or hyperplasia cause very low plasma ACTH levels. Pituitary-dependent hypercortisolism causes intermediate levels of plasma ACTH, and ectopic ACTH-producing tumors have very high levels of plasma ACTH (about 60% of these patients have ACTH levels of more than 300 pg/ml). Radioimmunoassays for ACTH in plasma have been difficult to perform reliably and to interpret because of platelet-associated proteases that degrade ACTH. Samples must be collected using recommended procedures including pre-chilled tubes on ice. Urinary 17-ketosteroids can help the differential diagnosis of hypercortisolism. Low levels (<10 mg/day) suggest an adrenal adenoma and very high levels (>60 mg/day) occur more commonly in patients with adrenal cancer and ectopic ACTH. Hypokalemia is seen in most patients with ectopic ACTH (16/16 in one series) and in only 10% of patients with Cushing's disease.[265]

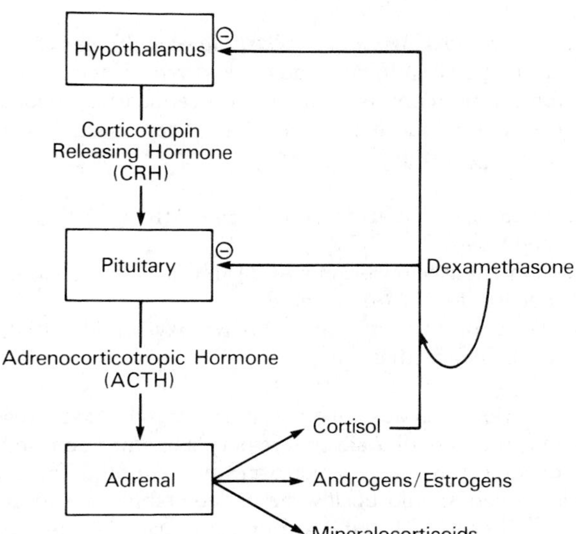

FIGURE 41–4. Model of cortisol secretion indicates the mechanism of dexamethasone suppression and CRH stimulation of normal cortisol secretion.

The standard dexamethasone suppression test remains one of the most useful tests in establishing the cause of hypercortisolism (see Fig. 41–3). The expected results are that urinary 17-hydroxysteroid levels will be less than 2.5 mg/day when normal subjects receive 2 mg of dexamethasone per day, but this dose has no effect on patients with endogenous hypercortisolism. High-dose dexamethasone (8 mg/day) suppresses urinary 17-hydroxysteroids to less than 50% of baseline levels in patients with pituitary-dependent hypercortisolism (Cushing's disease), but has no effect on hypercortisolism from other causes. This single test differentiates hypercortisolism from normal and pituitary-dependent hypercortisolism, the most common cause, from all other causes with about 95% accuracy.[266]

Radiologic Evaluation of Hypercortisolism. Sellar computed tomography (CT) scans detect abnormal sellar enlargement in up to 15% of patients with pituitary-dependent Cushing's disease and can detect more subtle abnormalities in 23% to 60% of these patients.[267] Sellar CT scans may detect ACTH-secreting tumors whose greatest diameter is between 5 and 10 mm, but this study cannot reliably detect the more common microadenoma (less than 5 mm). Pituitary magnetic resonance imaging (MRI) studies have similar resolution capabilities, even those done with gadolinium.[268] In patients with pituitary-dependent hypercortisolism, CT and MRI may be normal, but simultaneous bilateral petrosal sinus sampling for ACTH concentrations produces a hormone gradient in most cases. Resection of the ipsilateral half of the pituitary with the ACTH gradient is followed by biochemical and clinical remission, and pathologic analysis demonstrates microadenomas in most patients.[269] Recent data in 281 patients indicate that petrosal sinus sampling is the single best method to differentiate a pituitary source of hypercortisolism (Cushing's disease) from an ectopic ACTH-producing tumor.[268] Petrosal sinus sampling worked best when combined with the administration of ovine corticotropin-releasing hormone and requires bilateral sampling of the inferior petrosal sinus and peripheral sampling for plasma ACTH levels before and after CRH. A peak inferior petrosal sinus to peripheral plasma ACTH level greater than 3.0 after CRH administration correctly identified all 203 patients with Cushing's disease (sensitivity, 100%) with no false-positive results (specificity,

100%). Furthermore, petrosal sinus sampling predicted correct localization of the ACTH-producing microadenoma in about 70% of patients.[268] Although this new study is invasive and requires a significant degree of experience and expertise by the radiologist, it is the study of choice to diagnose and localize pituitary tumors in patients with Cushing's disease, the most common form of endogenous hypercortisolism.

Adrenal CT and MRI have been able to detect small adrenal abnormalities with certainty (Fig. 41–5). CT scans can detect normal adrenal glands in about 97% of patients.[270] CT scans can differentiate cortical hyperplasia from tumor.[271–274] Although CT scanning has great sensitivity (>95%), it lacks specificity. In a patient with Cushing's syndrome, early detection of an adrenal neoplasm by CT scan simplifies the workup. About 15% of patients with Cushing's syndrome have a primary adrenal neoplasm as the source of the hypercortisolism. Unilateral adrenal tumors require the detection of a normal adrenal gland on the contralateral side (Figure 41–5A). Adrenal hyperplasia may be detected if both glands appear enlarged. MRI may be able to add specificity to the sensitivity of CT scanning and to differentiate adrenal adenoma (Fig. 41–5B) from carcinoma or from a pheochromocytoma by the brightness of the lesion on the T2-weighted image.[272,275] Functional adenoma and nonfunctional adenoma appear darker than the liver on the T2-weighted MRI. Carcinomas, whether primary adrenocortical or metastatic, appear as bright as or slightly brighter than the liver on T2-weighted image (Fig. 41–6). Pheochromocytomas appear about three times brighter than the liver on T2-weighted MRI.[275]

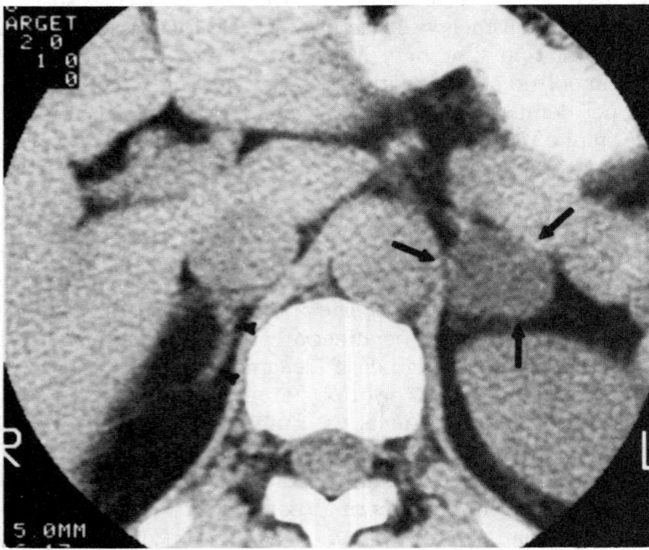

A

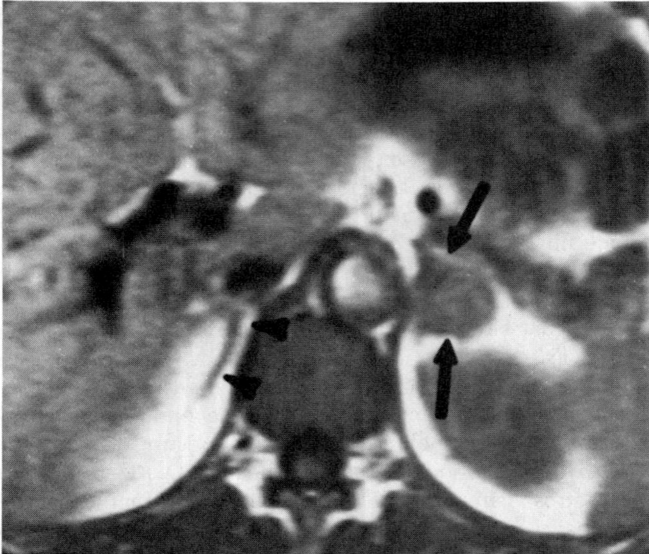
B

FIGURE 41–5. Left adrenal adenoma in a patient with Cushing's syndrome. **(A)** CT scan of the left adrenal (*arrows*) shows a mass and a normal contralateral adrenal gland (*arrowheads*). **(B)** T2-weighted MRI of the same tumor (*arrows*) and normal contralateral adrenal gland (*arrowheads*). Because the tumor has less density than the liver (darker) on T2 image, the image suggested a benign adrenal adenoma, which was removed subsequently for resolution of the hypercortisolism.

Radioisotope imaging of adrenals using labeled iodocholesterol such as ^{131}I-6-β-iodomethyl norcholesterol can be useful in differentiating unilateral adrenal adenoma with suppression of the contralateral gland from bilateral hyperplasia.[276] It can help differentiate a benign cortical neoplasm (adenoma), which usually takes up iodocholesterol (images), from a malignant cortical neoplasm (carcinoma), which usually does not take up the tracer.[277] A recent study demonstrated that labeled iodocholesterol correctly imaged 14 of 14 benign functional adenomas, only 1 of 4 carcinomas, and 4 of 4 adrenal pairs in primary nodular adrenocortical hyperplasia.[278] Radioisotope imaging is helpful in micronodular hyperplasia, in which uptake in both adrenal glands confirms the diagnosis, and can be useful in instances of recurrent hypercortisolism after bilateral adrenalectomy, in which ectopic rests of tissue enlarge with chronic ACTH stimulation. The limitations of radioiodocholesterol scans are the magnitude of the radiation dose, limited availability of the scan and isotope, and poor imaging of malignant adrenal neoplasms.

Interpretation of Workup for Cushing's Syndrome. Once the laboratory tests confirm endogenous hypercortisolism, the workup can pinpoint its cause. If an adrenocortical neoplasm is the source of the hypercortisolism, the workup produces the following results:

1. Imaging of the tumor on CT and MRI (see Figs. 41–5 and 41–6)
2. Consistently low plasma ACTH levels when concomitant cortisol levels are elevated
3. No suppression of urinary 17-hydroxysteroids with high-dose dexamethasone.

If criterion 1 is absent but criteria 2 and 3 are present, primary micronodular adrenal hyperplasia must be ruled out by iodocholesterol scan or petrosal sinus sampling for ACTH levels, which should be low or undetectable (see Fig. 41–3).[279,280] If criteria 1 and 3 are present but ACTH levels are consistently elevated, urinary catecholamines, VMA, and metanephrines should be measured because the patient may have an ACTH-producing pheochromocytoma.[281]

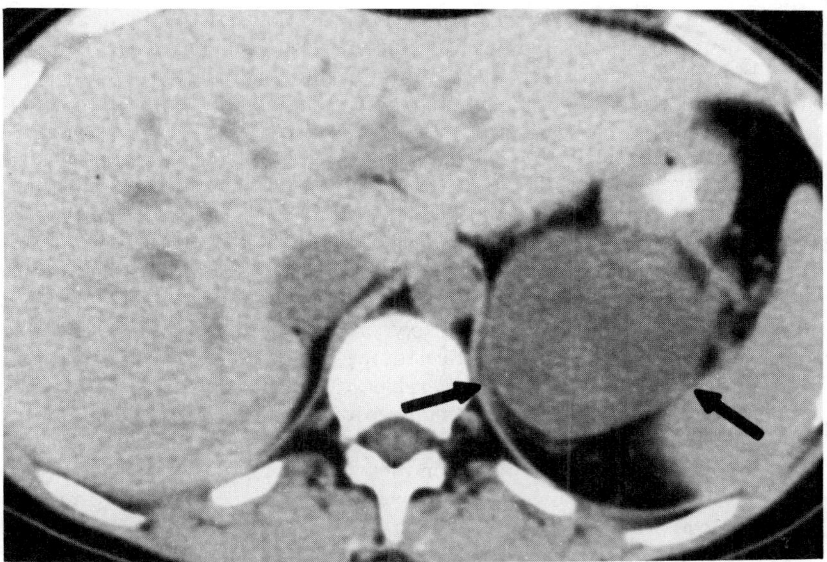

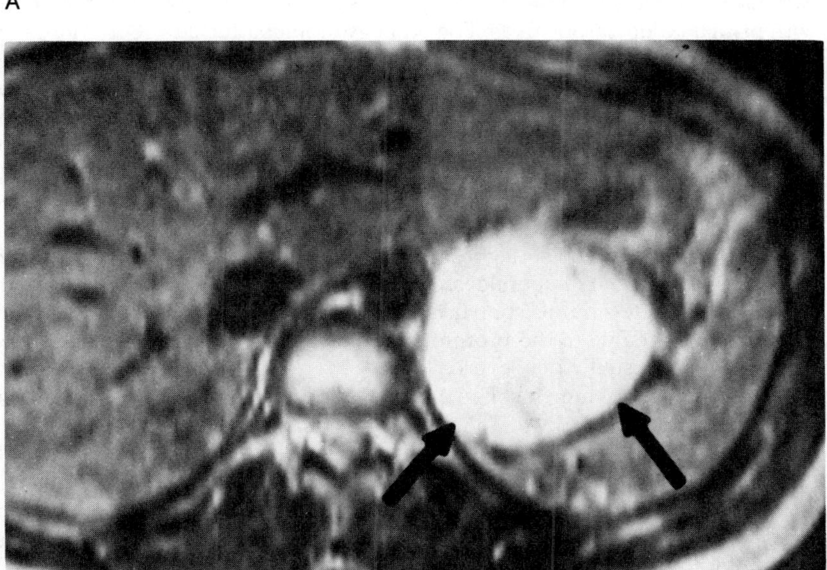

FIGURE 41–6. Adrenocortical carcinoma of the left adrenal. **(A)** CT scan of mass in left adrenal gland (*arrows*) in a patient with Cushing's syndrome. **(B)** T2-weighted MRI demonstrates that the mass (*arrows*) is brighter than the liver, consistent with adrenal cortical carcinoma. After surgical resection, pathologic analysis diagnosed adrenocortical carcinoma.

In patients with ectopic ACTH syndrome, one would expect to find the following:

1. Normal or bilateral hyperplasia of adrenals on CT
2. Normal or greatly elevated ACTH levels in plasma
3. No suppression with high-dose dexamethasone
4. No evidence of lateralization of ACTH plasma levels on petrosal sinus sampling with CRH.

Some bronchial ACTH-producing carcinoid tumors may suppress with dexamethasone, but the false suppression of ectopic ACTH-producing tumors is rare.[251] If the results are inconsistent, rely on petrosal sinus sampling for ACTH levels[268,269] and on CRH test results. More than 95% of patients with ectopic ACTH have no ACTH or cortisol increase after CRH.[264]

If the patient has pituitary-dependent hypercortisolism or Cushing's disease, the most common cause of endogenous hypercortisolism, one expects to find the following:

1. Normal or bilateral hyperplasia of the adrenal glands
2. Normal or mildly elevated plasma ACTH levels
3. No suppression with low-dose dexamethasone but greater than 50% suppression with high-dose dexamethasone
4. Lateralization with petrosal sinus sampling and a petrosal sinus to peripheral gradient of 3 or more after CRH.

More than 90% of patients with Cushing's disease have increased plasma levels of ACTH and cortisol after CRH,[264] and all patients have a gradient on petrosal sinus sampling with CRH.[268,269] In less than 5% of instances, results may be confusing and ectopic ACTH syndrome may not be distinguishable from Cushing's disease. This problem fortunately is not common,[282] and new data with petrosal sinus sampling with CRH suggest that diagnostic ambiguity may be eliminated.[268]

Conn's Syndrome (Primary Aldosteronism)

Diagnosis

Aldosterone overproduction with elevated plasma levels is the cause of hypertension in patients with primary aldosteronism or Conn's syndrome. Elevated urinary or serum levels of deoxycorticosterone, 18-hydroxycorticosterone, 18-hydroxydeoxycorticosterone, corticosterone, 18-hydroxycortisol, 18-oxocortisol, and other mineralocorticoids have been detected in patients with primary aldosteronism.[283,284] These mineralocorticoid metabolites contribute to the hypertension detected clinically.[285] The most common cause of primary aldosteronism is an aldosterone-producing adenoma, and the second most common cause is idiopathic hyperaldosteronism.[286,287] The third most common cause is adrenocortical carcinoma, but it is rare for adrenal cancers to present solely with primary aldosteronism.[288] The etiology of idiopathic adrenal hyperplasia is not clear, but some studies have suggested that a pituitary factor stimulates proliferation of the adrenal cortex.[289]

Hypertension, hypokalemia, hyperaldosteronism, and decreased plasma renin levels are essential for the diagnosis of primary aldosteronism. Secondary aldosteronism that occurs with renal artery stenosis, cirrhosis, and conditions of decreased kidney perfusion is diagnosed by an increase in plasma renin activity. Primary hyperaldosteronism is associated with weakness, muscle cramps, polyuria, and polydipsia. These clinical signs are due to the prominent hypokalemia.[285] The hypertension is usually not severe.

The serum potassium level in primary aldosteronism is usually less than 3.9 mEq/L.[290] Another possible diagnosis is essential hypertension that has been treated with diurectics. Although patients with the later diagnosis seldom have potassium levels of less than 3.9 mEq/L, the diuretic should be stopped and 24-hour urinary potassium excretion should be measured. In most patients with primary aldosteronism, 24-hour urinary excretion of potassium is greater than 30 mEq. Patients who are taking antihypertensive medications including diuretics and spironolactone should have all medications stopped for 1 month before measurement of plasma aldosterone levels and concomitant plasma renin activity. Patients with primary hyperaldosteronism are expected to have elevated plasma aldosterone levels and low renin activity. The plasma aldosterone to renin ratio is usually greater than 30. The final proof of the diagnosis of primary hyperaldosteronism relies on an inability to lower plasma aldosterone levels and a similar inability to raise plasma renin activity. A suppression test that simplifies the evaluation of primary aldosteronism uses captopril.[291] The patient takes 25 mg of captopril orally in the morning. Two hours later, plasma levels of aldosterone and renin activity are obtained. In normal subjects and in patients with essential hypertension, plasma aldosterone levels decrease and plasma renin activity increases after captopril administration. In patients with primary aldosteronism, plasma levels of aldosterone and renin activity do not change. A postcaptopril plasma aldosterone level greater than 15 ng/dl and an aldosterone to renin ratio greater than 50 are diagnostic of primary aldosteronism (Table 41–14).

Etiology: Adenoma Versus Hyperplasia

Once the diagnosis of primary aldosteronism is established, the next important consideration is whether the patient has idiopathic adrenocortical hyperplasia (IAH) or a tumor that produces aldosterone (see Table 41–14). Determining the exact cause of primary aldosteronism is crucial because treatment is primarily medical for IAH and primarily surgical for a neoplasm. Patients with neoplasm generally have serum 18-hydroxycorticosterone levels greater than 100 ng/dl, whereas patients with IAH have levels less than 90 ng/dl; however, there is some overlap and these measurements do not always discriminate between the two diagnoses.[283]

About 75% to 90% of aldosteronomas can be imaged preoperatively on CT scans; however, tumors smaller than 7 to 10 mm may not be imaged.[292–294] CT scanning does not accurately identify IAH because these glands appear normal and small tumors may be missed. CT scan evidence of a tumor does not predict the functional significance of the tumor.[292–294]

Iodocholesterol scans are able to image 64% of aldosteronomas, and the agent ^{131}I-β-iodomethyl-19-norcholesterol combined with adrenal suppression with dexamethasone can image 88% of tumors.[292] The advantage of these nuclear studies over CT scans is that they provide functional information about the neoplasm. Generally, CT scanning is more sensitive, more available, and uses less radiation per study than iodocholesterol scans. However, in some patients with equivocal studies, iodocholesterol scans may be helpful. In patients with IAH as a cause of hyperaldosteronism, the adrenal scan shows symmetrical uptake in both adrenal glands; and in patients with adrenal carcinoma causing hyperaldosteronism, the study may show no uptake by the tumor, whereas in adenomas tumor uptake is usually evident.[292]

The study of choice for determining whether hyperaldosteronism is caused by a tumor or by hyperplasia is sampling of the adrenal veins for aldosterone.[294] The procedure is performed by simultaneous selective catheterization of the veins and a peripheral vein. Serum levels of aldosterone and cortisol are measured at each site. A unilateral elevation of the aldosterone level or of the aldosterone to cortisol ratio indicates the presence of an aldosterone-secreting adenoma. Bilateral levels of aldosterone that are similar and are greater than peripheral levels are consistent with IAH. Adrenal venous sampling for aldosterone (96%) has been more sensitive than CT scans (75%) and adrenal venography (78%) in prospective comparisons.[287,294] Venous sampling is invasive and expensive, but it is the best study to confirm a functioning aldosteronoma.

The clinical response to spironolactone appears to be useful in predicting the subsequent outcome of surgical resection of an aldosteronoma. In one series before a trial of spironolactone, only 66% of patients were cured after surgical resection. When the guideline of a good response to the preoperative administration of spironolactone was used, the cure rate was increased to 92%.[295]

Treatment of Hyperaldosteronism

The treatment of primary aldosteronism depends on the diagnosis. IAH is best managed medically with spironolactone

TABLE 41–14. Evaluation of Patient With Hyperaldosteronism

Diagnosis of Primary Aldosteronism

Measure	*Result*
Blood pressure	Hypertension
Serum potassium levels	Hypokalemia (serum $K^+ < 3.9$ mEq/L)
Urinary potassium levels	Elevated urinary K^+ excretion (>25–30 mEq/day)
Plasma aldosterone and plasma renin activity	Ratio > 30 (elevated aldosterone and low renin)
Captopril suppression test (25 mg orally)	After captopril aldosterone > 15 ng/ml Aldosterone/renin ratio > 50

Etiology of Primary Aldosteronism: Idiopathic Adrenal Hyperplasia (IAH) Versus Neoplasm

Measurement	*IAH*	*Neoplasm*
Serum 18-hydroxycorticosterone	<90 ng/dl	>100 ng/dl
High-resolution CT scan	Normal adrenals	Tumor (tumors < 7–10 mm may be missed)
Iodocholesterol scan	Symmetric uptake bilaterally	Uptake or tracer by benign adenoma (malignant tumors may not take up tracer)
Spironolactone	Fair response	Good repsonse
Adrenal vein sampling	Aldosterone levels elevated from both adrenal veins and greater than simultaneous peripheral sample	Aldosterone levels elevated on side with tumor, contralateral side equal to simultaneous peripheral samples

or amiloride, in conjunction with other antihypertensive drugs. Another drug with potential for managing the hypokalemia and hypertension associated with primary aldosteronism (IAH and adenoma) is the calcium-channel blocker nifedipine. In a 4-week study of 10 patients (5 with aldosteronoma and 5 with IAH), nifedipine controlled blood pressure and normalized potassium and aldosterone levels in every patient.[296] These drugs usually allow effective blood pressure control.[285,297] There may be subsets of patients with primary adrenal hyperplasia who respond favorably to subtotal (75%) adrenalectomy.[298] However, most patients with hyperplasia (IAH) should be treated medically. Because of adrenal venous aldosterone levels and the ability to localize a small aldosteronoma to one adrenal gland, it is preferable to use a posterior approach for unilateral adrenalectomy in patients with a localized adrenocortical adenoma.

Results for resection of an aldosteronoma have not been entirely satisfactory. A high percentage of patients become normotensive and normokalemic postoperatively (about 95%, dependent on accurate diagnosis), and 20% to 30% of patients develop recurrent hypertension within 2 to 3 years.[297] This hypertension may not be associated with recurrent hypokalemia. Prolonged preoperative hypertension from an aldosteronoma may alter renal function and lead to renal impairment and persistent postoperative hypertension despite successful resection of the tumor.[299] Aldosterone-producing adrenocortical carcinomas are rare (2% of all carcinomas).[300] Patients with primary aldosteronism due to adrenocortical carcinoma usually have higher levels of deoxycorticosterone and aldosterone than patients with benign adenomas.[301] In addition, their hypokalemia and weakness are usually more severe than in the typical patient with Conn's syndrome.[301] Treatment is similar to that for other patients with adrenal carcinoma and is discussed later in this chapter.

Asymptomatic Adrenal Mass

With the availability of high-resolution CT scanners, a new diagnostic problem has arisen—the evaluation of a patient with an asymptomatic adrenal mass seen or detected by CT scan. Unexpected adrenal masses have been detected on 0.6% of abdominal CT scans.[302,303] Most adrenal masses detected in this manner are benign, silent adrenocortical adenomas, which occur in 8.7% of autopsy series (incidentalomas may appear similar to the tumors shown in Fig. 41–5).[304] Adrenal carcinomas are rare. Metastases to the adrenal gland from a known or occult primary tumor, a pheochromocytoma, or an early adrenal carcinoma cannot be diagnosed based on CT scan morphology. When managing these masses, one must remember that most are benign and nonfunctional. Percutaneous aspiration biopsy of occult unsuspected pheochromocytomas identified in this manner has resulted in severe morbidity including hypertensive crises, hemorrhage, and even sudden death.[305] The suggested procedure for evaluating an incidental adrenal mass (incidentaloma) is given in Figure 41–7.

In the evaluation of an adrenal incidentaloma, two questions arise: is the tumor functional, and is it cancer?[304] Attempting to answer these questions is the basis for the diagnostic evaluation. One difficulty is that nonfunctioning adrenocortical carcinomas may occur.[306,307] With earlier diagnosis and measurement of urinary 17-ketosteroids, most nonfunctional adrenocortical carcinomas are secreting increased amounts of some steroid.[308]

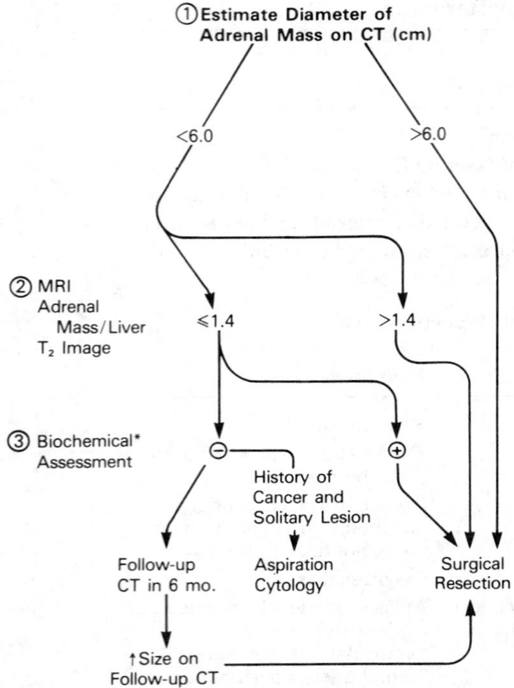

FIGURE 41–7. Flow diagram for evaluation of an incidentally discovered adrenal mass. All three studies are performed on each patient. *Biochemical assessment includes 24-hour urine for VMA, metanephrine, catecholamines, and serum levels of potassium. Biochemical assessment for hypercortisolism or virilization is reserved for patients with clinical signs of the disease.

The first step in evaluation of an asymptomatic adrenal mass is a careful history and physical examination including blood pressure. The clinician should examine for evidence of the following: weight change, weakness, or hypokalemia; Cushing's syndrome; hypertension; virilization or feminization; change in menstruation; and evidence of occult malignancy (stool guaiac, pap smear, anemia).

The laboratory evaluation of an asymptomatic adrenal mass should consist of measurement of a 24-hour urine for VMA, metanephrines, and catecholamines. If urinary levels of catecholamines are elevated, see the section on management of pheochromocytoma. If the patient is hypertensive, the serum potassium concentration should be measured. Hormonal screening for an excess of glucocorticoids or androgens to detect functional adrenocortical tumors that have a low prevalence, such as glucocorticoid-producing adenoma, should be limited to patients with clinical features suggestive of these disorders.[309] Therefore, plasma testosterone levels should be measured if a woman or child has clinical evidence of hirsutism or virilization. Elevated serum testosterone levels are usually associated with elevated urinary levels of 17-ketosteroids, but serum testosterone levels may be elevated in some patients with normal urinary levels of 17-ketosteroids.[310] Serum estrogen levels should be measured if there is a clinical suspicion of feminization. Although urinary levels of 17-ketosteroids are usually elevated in patients with feminization, levels may be normal, so that measurement of serum estrogen levels may be indicated.[304] Serum levels of aldosterone should be measured in any patient with an adrenal mass accompanied by hypertension or hypokalemia.

The size of the adrenal mass on CT scan is probably the most helpful determinant of the nature of a biochemically silent lesion.[304] Most adrenocortical carcinomas are greater than 6 cm in diameter, and most benign lesions are less than 6 cm. A smaller lesion should not be ignored. Early diagnosis may lead to discovery of smaller adrenocortical carcinomas, which may lead to better prognosis and survival. In three series, all 5 patients with nonmetastatic adrenocortical carcinoma and primary tumors less than 5 cm were alive 5 years postoperatively, whereas only about 10% of patients with larger tumors or metastases survived longer than 5 years.[311–313] CT scans can accurately image normal glands, hyperplastic adrenal glands, and neoplasms but cannot differentiate benign from malignant neoplasms by criteria other than size, direct invasion, or distant metastases. More recent studies confirm earlier reports that CT scanning cannot differentiate benign from malignant adrenal masses.[314] MRI of the adrenal gland is a new modality but already has resolution similar to that of CT. Small tumors (<1 cm) can be imaged accurately by MRI.[315] Some studies suggest that MRI can reliably differentiate adrenal cancer or metastases from pheochromocytoma and adenoma based on appearance on T2-weighted spin echo scans.[275,315] Adenomas appear dark, carcinomas intermediate (1.4 times as bright as liver), and pheochromocytomas bright (3 times as bright as liver) when T2-weighted images are compared with the adjacent liver.[316–318]

Fine-needle aspiration biopsy of an adrenal mass is of limited use in differentiating benign from malignant adrenal lesions. Because fine-needle aspiration cytology may be catastrophic if the patient has an unsuspected pheochromocytoma, MRI or measurement of urinary catecholamine levels is indicated before needle biopsy.[305,319] In patients with suspected metastatic disease to the adrenal gland and inconclusive MRI, needle aspiration may be helpful. In a study of 16 patients with known primary cancers, 7 patients had adrenal metastases confirmed by aspiration cytology.[320] Because aspiration cytology usually cannot differentiate benign from malignant adrenal neoplasms and may be life-threatening if the patient has an unsuspected pheochromocytoma, it should not be performed routinely in the evaluation of asymptomatic adrenal masses.

The suggested approach to an asymptomatic adrenal mass is outlined in Figure 41–7. All three suggested tests—CT, MRI, and biochemical assessment—should be performed on each patient because each provides information important to management. Initially, the adrenal mass diameter is carefully measured by CT scans, with a size greater than 6 cm an indication for surgical resection. Because the incidence of cancer in solid adrenal masses larger than 6 cm ranges from about 35% to 98%, most experts recommend excision of these adrenal mass lesions.[309] Ultrasound may be useful in the evaluation of large masses to determine if the mass is solid or cystic. Cystic masses are rare but should be aspirated with ultrasound guidance. Lesions smaller than 3.5 to 4 cm on CT scan are usually benign adenomas,[318] but aldosteronoma, pheochromocytoma, and early carcinomas must be considered. MRI and measurement of urinary catecholamine levels can rule out the presence of pheochromocytoma. Density of fat as determined by CT scan may raise the diagnostic possibility of myolipoma. An increase in MRI signal intensity (>1.4 compared with liver) on T2-weighted image for an intermediate-size adrenal lesion may suggest surgical resection for possible cancer. If a surgical resection is not done, a follow-up CT scan examination in 3 months is indicated to determine whether the mass has enlarged. If it has increased in size, surgical excision is recommended.[309] Finally, clinical evidence of hypercortisolism or Conn's syndrome and a positive biochemical assessment also mandate surgical resection. This schema provides early surgical intervention for functional and malignant adrenal masses, and it is hoped that it will limit surgical resection of nonfunctional benign adrenal adenomas.

Sex Hormone Excess

The final way adrenocortical carcinoma may present is with excessive sex hormone secretion. This presentation may consist primarily of excessive levels of estrogen or testosterone or may be combined with excessive levels of cortisol or aldosterone or both. In children, the clinical signs of increased androgen production include increased growth, premature development of pubic and facial hair and acne, genital enlargement, increased muscle mass, and deepening voice. In women, the clinical signs of excess androgen production include hirsutism, acne, amenorrhea, infertility, increased muscle mass, deep voice, and temporal balding. In children, the clinical signs of increased estrogen production include gynecomastia in boys and precocious breast enlargement or vaginal bleeding in girls. In men, hyperestrogenism presents with gynecomastia, decreased sexual drive, impotence, and infertility. In women, hyperestrogenism presents primarily with irregular menses in premenopausal women and dysfunctional uterine bleeding or vaginal bleeding in postmenopausal women.[251] The workup requires measurement of 24-hour urinary 17-ketosteroids, 17-hydroxysteroids, and urinary free cortisol levels and, depending on virilization or feminization, serum levels of testosterone or estrogen.

Virilization secondary to an adrenal neoplasm may accompany Cushing's syndrome and usually indicates adrenocortical carcinoma. Adrenal-induced virilization in the absence of Cushing's syndrome may occur due to adrenocortical adenoma[310] or carcinoma.[321] Although many other disorders can cause virilization in women and children, in working up a patient with virilization, an imaging study of both adrenals (either CT or MRI) is indicated to rule out an adrenal neoplasm. Hyperestrogenism of adrenal origin is usually caused by an adrenal adenoma or carcinoma and may be associated with hypercortisolism. An imaging study of both adrenal glands (either CT or MRI) is indicated to rule out a neoplasm before proceeding with the differential diagnosis of hyperestrogenism.

TREATMENT OF ADRENOCORTICAL NEOPLASM

Adenomas of the Adrenal Cortex

The definitive treatment of benign adenomas is surgical resection of the adrenal gland with the adenoma. MRI can help characterize the biology of a tumor, and if the tumor appears malignant on MRI (adrenal mass to liver ratio of >0.4:<3.0 on T2-weighted image), the anterior approach is preferred.[275] Baker and colleagues reported 2 patients who had benign adrenal adenomas with increased adrenal mass to liver ratio on T2-weighted MRI, but they agree with the general ability of the MRI signal intensity to differentiate malignant neoplasms from pheochromocytomas.[322] In patients who are undergoing resection of an adrenal tumor that causes Cushing's syndrome, steroid replacement during and after surgery is necessary. Mineralocorticoid replacement is not required. Postoperative glucocorticoid replacement is necessary until the patient has complete recovery of the hypothalamic-pituitary-adrenal axis. In most cases, glucocorticoid replacement is necessary for about 2 years.[323] Surgical resection of an adenoma is curative.[323] Larger lesions that weigh between 50 to 100 g and appear benign histologically (no mitoses and no vascular invasion) may need careful follow-up including detection of hormonal abnormalities and CT or MRI.

Carcinoma of the Adrenal Cortex

The mainstay of treatment of adrenocortical carcinoma is complete resection of all gross tumor. If the carcinoma is intimately associated with the kidney, liver, or diaphragm on the right, or with the pancreas on the left, it may be necessary to resect part or all of the contiguous structures at the time of definitive resection. The best time for potentially curative surgery is at the initial surgery. The surgeon needs adequate imaging of the mass including CT and MRI.[275,322] CT and MRI should include the chest to rule out metastatic disease above the diaphragm. If the right adrenal is involved and the inferior vena cava is compressed, an inferior vena caval contrast study or caval ultrasound is useful to assess blood flow through the cava. If resection of one kidney is planned along with resection of the primary tumor, an intravenous pyelogram or an intravenous contrast CT scan is indicated to be sure that the contralateral kidney is functioning. A bone scan is necessary to rule out bony metastases. A complete bowel preparation is helpful in case the tumor invades bowel.

In children, adrenocortical carcinoma usually occurs before age 6, with a higher incidence in girls than in boys. Twice as many girls as boys develop childhood adrenal cancer. The median age in children with adrenal cancer is 4 years. Virilization is the most common presenting feature (93%), although children may present with precocious puberty or Cushing's syndrome.[324–328] Some children with adrenal cancer can be cured primarily by complete surgical resection. In one recent report, 17 of 26 (65%) children with completely resected adrenal cancer remained in continuous complete remissions.[327] In a multivariate analysis of predictors of outcome, only primary tumor size greater than 200 cm^3 independently identified a poor-prognosis group of children who may require more aggressive adjuvant therapy after surgery.[327]

The second peak age of occurrence of adrenal cancer is between 40 and 50 years, and about 70% of these patients present with hormonal syndromes.[300] The surgical staging of adrenal carcinoma is outlined as follows (Table 41–15):

Stage I	Tumor less than 5 cm without local invasion of nodal or distant metastases
Stage II	Same as stage I except the tumor is greater than 5 cm

TABLE 41–15. Staging Criteria for Adrenocortical Carcinoma*

Stage	*Criteria*
	Tumor ≤ 5 cm, invasion absent
T1	Tumor > 5 cm, invasion absent
T2	Tumor outside adrenal in fat
T3	Tumor invading adjacent organs
T4	
N0	No positive lymph nodes
N1	Positive lymph nodes
M0	No distant metastases
M1	Distant metastases
	TNM Criteria
I	T1, N0, M0
II	T2, N0, M0
III	T1 or T2N1M0, T3N0M0
IV	Any T, any NM1, T3T4N1

* Staging criteria from references 312, 329, and 1103.

Stage III Tumor with local invasion or positive lymph nodes

Stage IV Tumor with local invasion and lymph nodes or distant metastases

Most patients (70%) present with stage III or IV disease.[300,329]

The definitive initial treatment for all stage disease including locally aggressive stage III disease is en bloc resection, which may include the adjacent kidney. This procedure usually requires a combined thoracoabdominal approach. Surgical resection of localized disease can be curative.[300,312,329] However, in a recent analysis of 105 patients with adrenal cancer, only 80 patients were able to undergo surgery for possible cure and the median disease-free interval postoperatively was 12 months.[330] The overall 5-year survival was 22%.[330] Age of more than 40 years and the presence of metastases at the time of diagnosis were predictive of a poor prognosis.[330]

If complete resection of tumor cannot be achieved, remove as much of the primary tumor as possible to decrease the amount of cortisol-secreting tissue and to minimize complications due to tumor mass. Patients who undergo definitive resection should be monitored for appropriate steroid hormone levels postoperatively. The steroid levels depend on the secretion of the neoplasm before resection and at the time of diagnosis. If hypercortisolism was present, urinary free cortisol levels should be measured. If levels of urinary 17-ketosteroids were elevated preoperatively, postoperative levels are most helpful. Plasma measurements of 11-deoxycortisol, dehydroepiandrosterone, deoxycorticosterone, or other steroids may help detect recurrences in an individual patient.[251] CT and MRI can help detect local recurrences and pulmonary metastases. If a solitary recurrence is detected, it should be removed surgically if possible with acceptable morbidity. Prolonged remissions have been reported after resection of hepatic, pulmonary, and cerebral metastases from adrenocortical carcinoma.[331–335] If complete resection of tumor metastases is not possible, near-total resection may still be helpful in some hormonally productive, slow-growing adrenocortical cancers.[306,335] A recent nonrandomized retrospective study of patients with locally recurrent or metastatic adrenal cancer compared treatment by surgery plus mitotane chemotherapy with treatment by mitotane alone.[335] The benefit of aggressive re-resection of adrenal cancer appeared greatest in one third of patients who were able to survive more than 5 years from the time of first recurrence with an improvement in the symptoms and signs of hypercortisolism. However, aggressive surgical therapy was not able to cure any patient with recurrent adrenal cancer.[335] Palliation of bony metastases may be achieved by radiation therapy.[300] Percapto and Knowlton reported that abdominal radiation therapy was palliative in two thirds of patients with local recurrences and that it even relieved one bowel obstruction.[334] However, it did not improve the length of survival.[300,334]

Chemotherapy of Adrenocortical Carcinoma

Once a patient has recurrent or metastatic adrenocortical carcinoma, chemotherapy with o,p-DDD (mitotane) is usually started.[336] Therapy is initiated at a dose of 2 to 6 g daily in two or three divided doses and increased until adverse reactions occur. Adverse reactions include gastrointestinal toxicity (anorexia, nausea, vomiting, and diarrhea), neuromuscular toxicity (depression, dizziness, tremors, headache, confusion, and weakness) and skin rash. Of patients treated with mitotane, 79% suffer from gastrointestinal toxicity, 50% from neuromuscular toxicity, and 15% from skin rash.[336] Mitotane is associated with prolonged bleeding time and abnormal platelet aggregation responses consistent with an aspirin-like defect. It may cause a significant defect in platelet function.[337] A decrease in levels of urinary 17-hydroxysteroids and 17-ketosteroids occurs in 67% of patients treated with mitotane, due to its direct effect on steroid metabolism,[338,339] and a partial response occurs in about 33% of patients. It is important to measure blood levels of o,p-DDD and to achieve serum levels higher than 14 μg/ml. In one study, patients who had blood levels less than 10 μg/ml had no demonstrable therapeutic effects, whereas 7 of 8 patients who had levels greater than 14 μg/ml had objective responses and significantly longer survival rates.[340] Unfortunately, the difference between efficacy and toxicity is small, and levels greater than 20 μg/ml are associated with symptoms of neuromuscular toxicity.[340]

Tumor responses usually occur in the first 6 weeks after the initiation of mitotane treatment. Although most patients who demonstrate an objective response to o,p-DDD subsequently relapse, there have been a few long-term survivors with metastatic adrenocortical carcinoma.[341] Mitotane can be an unpleasant drug, and if clinical toxicity is present, the dose must be adjusted to minimize side effects. Because patients with adrenocortical carcinoma are rare, there have been no controlled studies to establish that mitotane can significantly alter the natural course of adrenocortical carcinoma. Some suggest that adjuvant o,p-DDD improves survival after initial surgery for adrenocortical carcinoma.[342] although most experts do not recommend it as an adjuvant drug after total resection of primary adrenocortical cancer. In a recent report of 59 patients with adrenal cancer who received mitotane therapy at a dose between 7 and 10 g/day, 37 patients were evaluable for tumor response.[330] Of the 37 patients, only 8 (22%) had a documented partial response. These findings are similar to three other recent reports, none of which recommends mitotane for the management of patients with adrenocortical cancer.[335,343–345] Other researchers argue that the dose of mitotane is critical and must be pushed to toxicity to see the higher response rates described in some studies.[346] At best, the response rate with mitotane alone is 60%, and few complete responses have been seen. Mitotane appears to be of use in controlling hypercortisolism but of limited use as an antitumor agent. We do not recommend mitotane because the dose of drug must be pushed to toxicity to see modest efficacy. A potential use of mitotane in patients with adrenal cancer is to block the decreased chemotherapy drug accumulation mediated by the multidrug resistance gene (*MDR1*/p-glycoprotein). It appears that adrenocortical cancers have high levels of expression of this gene and that treatment with mitotane blocks gene expression and increases chemotherapeutic drug accumulation within the cancer.[347] This in vitro finding suggests a rationale for combining chemotherapy and mitotane in the treatment of adrenocortical cancer, but human trials have not been done.

Chemotherapy regimens besides o,p-DDD have been ineffective against adrenocortical carcinoma. Partial responses have been reported with regimens based on doxorubicin[345,348,349] and alkylating agents.[349] Promising regimens include cisplatin and etoposide. In two different studies using cisplatin and etoposide in patients with metastatic adrenocortical carcinomas for whom mitotane therapy had not been effective, there were 5 responses in 6 patients, including 1 patient with a complete response that lasted only 1 year.[350,351] In another study, an active regimen that included 5-FU, doxorubicin, and cisplatin produced a response in all 3 patients treated, and 1 patient had a complete response that lasted for 42 months.[352,353] Suramin is known to inhibit the binding of growth factors (*e.g.,* epidermal growth factor, platelet-derived growth factor, and transforming growth factor-β) to tumor receptors and may reduce tumor growth by antagonizing the ability of these factors to stimulate tumor growth.[354] Suramin was used as a phase I agent in 21 patients with metastatic adrenocortical cancer in whom other therapy had failed. It produced 3 partial responses (14%) but no complete responses.[354–356] It has toxicity related to blood coagulation, and some patients have had thrombocytopenia and hemorrhage.[357] In one recent retrospective review, 2 inoperable patients were treated preoperatively with mitotane and streptozocin and each had a 50% reduction in primary tumor size. One patient also had complete regression of pulmonary metastases. Tumor was resected in both patients and both were treated with more chemotherapy postoperatively. Both patients have remained completely free of disease for 9 and 5 years postoperatively.[358] Gossypol has been shown to inhibit adrenal cancer growth and prolong survival in in vitro studies with adrenocortical carcinoma cells and in nude mice studies.[359] In phase I human studies with metastatic cancer, it has only had a partial response rate of about 20%. There is no consistently active cytotoxic drug or drug combination in the treatment of adrenocortical carcinoma. Steroid hormone receptors have been detected in vitro in adrenocortical carcinomas, indicating a dependence on progesterone and glucocorticoid.[360] In vivo studies of therapy related to manipulation of receptors have not been done. The available chemotherapy agents and results are summarized in Table 41–16.

Survival of Patients With Adrenocortical Carcinoma

Adrenocortical carcinoma is a rare but very malignant tumor. Some have categorized it into two subpopulations, anaplastic and differentiated, with different prognoses and survival. The anaplastic variant of adrenocortical carcinoma occurred more commonly in males, produced more frequent cutaneous metastases, and was associated with a lack of clinical or laboratory evidence of hormone production. Median survival of patients with anaplastic adrenocortical cancer was only 5 months. Differentiated adrenocortical cancer usually occurred in women, produced clinical or laboratory evidence of hormonal excess, and had a median survival of 40 months.[306]

Most patients present with stage III and stage IV tumors (see Table 41–15). The metastatic sites of adrenal cancer are lymph nodes (68%), lung (71%), liver (42%), and bone (26%).[307] Surgical cure is possible only in stage I or II tumors (tumors confined to the adrenal gland).[361]

In patients with invasion of contiguous structures at presentation, median survival was 2.3 years.[300] In one large series from the Mayo Clinic, 39% of patients presented with stage I or stage II adrenocortical carcinoma.[329] Mean survival for patients presenting with stage I and stage II tumors was only 25 and 24 months, respectively, compared with 28 and 12 months for stages III and IV. Only patients with stage IV tumors had a significantly shortened survival.[329] In a recent study from the Cleveland Clinic, patients who presented with stage I disease had a 50% 5-year survival, whereas patients who presented with stage II or III disease had a 10% 5-year survival.[343] In another study, most patients presented with functional tumors, abdominal mass, and distant or nodal metastases (stage IV). In those patients with tumors confined to the adrenal gland, the mean duration of survival was 5 years.[300] For all patients, the 6-year survival is only about 10% to 20%, indicating that most patients present with locally advanced or distant disease.[330] Most clinicians recommend aggressive surgical resection of locally recurrent or metastatic cancer in these patients, but a recent study demonstrates that even with this aggressive intervention the 5-year survival is about 10% to 20%.[335] These data indicate the poor prognosis of all patients with adrenocortical carcinoma and support the use of adjuvant systemic chemotherapy for resectable lesions (stages I, II, and III). However, chemotherapy is not recommended except as part of a study because effective regimens have not been developed.

Future challenges for the treatment of adrenocortical carcinoma include facilitating earlier diagnosis and finding better adjuvants than o,p-DDD. Earlier diagnosis can be facilitated by an index of suspicion for hormonal excess during history and physical examinations. Changes in body appearance and menstrual history are important clues to earlier diagnosis. The use of MRI to differentiate benign from malignant incidentalomas of the adrenal may help clinicians find early resectable adrenocortical cancers. Drugs such as cisplatin and etoposide or mitotane combined with mitotane[347] may be useful in the management of this difficult disease.

TABLE 41–16. Chemotherapy Agents Used to Treat Adrenocortical Carcinoma

Investigations	*Drug*	*Dose*	*Frequency*	*No. of Patients*	*Efficacy*
Gutierrez and Crooke, 1980[336] Fukishima et al., 1971[338] Hellman et al, 1973[339] Luton et al, 1990[330] Van Slooten et al, 1984[340] Jarabak and Rice, 1981[341]	o,p-DDD (mitotane)	1–12 g/d	bid or tid	37	22–33% PR 0 CR
Venkatesh et al, 1989[344]		7–10 g/d not given	bid	72	29% PR 0 CR
Decker et al, 1991[345]		6 g/d	—	36	22% PR
Stein et al, 1989[354] Allolio et al, 1989[355] LaRocca et al, 1990[356]	Suramin	1–1.5 mg/m²	q wk	21	3 PR
Stein et al, 1989[345] Hag et al, 1980[349]	Doxorubicin	60 mg/m² 40 mg/m²	q 3 wk q 4 wk	16 8	19% PR 1 PR
Chun et al, 1983[1104]	Cisplatin	120 mg/m²	q 4 wk	5	0 PR 0 CR
Johnson and Creco, 1986[350]	Cisplatin + etoposide (VP-16)	40 mg/m²/d 100 mg/m²/d	Daily for 3 d	2	2 PR 0 CR
Van Slooten and van Oosterom[348]	Cyclophosphamide + doxorubicin + cisplatin	600 mg/m² 40 mg/m² 50 mg/²	q 3 wk	11	2 PR 0 CR
Hag et al, 1980[349]	Cyclophosphamide + vincristine + methyl-CCNU + bleomycin	Not given	Not stated	2	1 PR 0 CR
Hag et al, 1980[349]	Cyclophosphamide + melphalan or peptichermio	Not given		12	2 PR 0 CR
Heskel et al, 1987[351]	Cisplatin + etoposide + bleomycin	40 mg/m² 100 mg/m² 30 U	q 4 wk	4	1 CR 2 PR
Schlumberger et al, 1991[352]	5-Fluorouracil + doxorubicin + cisplatin	500 mg/m² on days 1, 2, 3 60 mg/m² on day 2 120 mg/m² on day 2	q 4 wk	13	1 CR 2 PR

PR, partial remission; CR, complete remission.

Ectopic ACTH Syndrome

The first report of a patient who exhibited features of Cushing's syndrome described an oat cell carcinoma of the bronchus secreting a peptide now called corticotropin or ACTH.[362] Similar patients who had adrenal hyperplasia without pituitary tumors were reported over the next 30 years, but it was Christy[363] and Liddle[364] who established the presence of ACTH-like material in tumors other than pituitary tumors and in the blood, and the presence of subnormal quantities in the pituitary itself.[363,364] The term *ectopic ACTH syndrome* was introduced in 1962.[364]

The diagnosis of ectopic ACTH syndrome is based on the metabolic evaluation of the patient who presents with hypercortisolism. An early clue to the diagnosis is the presence of Cushing's syndrome and severe hypokalemia (potassium <3.3 mEq/L). The diagnosis is based primarily on high plasma ACTH and cortisol levels, which do not change with high-dose dexamethasone or administration of CRH,[264] and on results of petrosal sinus sampling, which demonstrate low levels of ACTH draining the pituitary gland that do not change with CRH.[252,268,269] The simultaneous bilateral inferior petrosal sinus venous and peripheral determination of ACTH levels with and without CRH stimulation always differentiates ectopic ACTH syndrome from pituitary Cushing's disease.[268] Once the diagnosis is established, the primary therapeutic goal is to find and eradicate the neoplasm that is secreting ACTH. When this is accomplished by surgery, chemotherapy, or radiation therapy, long-term cures can be achieved.[251] The main clinical problems have been finding the source of ectopic ACTH in some patients and treating the aggressive, underlying tumor in others.

The causative tumors, in approximate order of frequency, are as follows:

1. Oat cell carcinoma of the bronchus
2. Carcinoid tumor of the bronchus
3. Epithelial carcinoma of the thymus or thymic carcinoids
4. Pancreatic endocrine tumor
5. Medullary carcinoma of the thyroid gland
6. Pheochromocytoma

7. Gut carcinoids
8. Ovarian adenocarcinoma
9. Pancreatic cystadenoma
10. Adenocarcinoma of unknown site[365–367]

Other than small cell carcinoma of the lung, the most common cause of ectopic ACTH syndrome is a bronchial or thymic carcinoid tumor that secretes ACTH. The recommended radiographic procedures to localize ACTH producing tumors include the following:

Chest and abdominal CT
Chest and abdominal MRI
Urinary catecholamines to screen for pheochromocytomas
Plasma level of calcitonin to rule out MTC
Inferior petrosal sinus sampling with CRH in any patients in whom the differential diagnosis of Cushing's disease (pituitary) is unclear

Any suspicious finding in chest or abdomen can be unequivocally confirmed by fine-needle aspiration and radioimmunoassay for ACTH in the aspirate.[368]

The goal of therapy for patients with ectopic ACTH production is to find and treat (usually by resection except in oat cell carcinoma) the neoplasm that is the source of ACTH. Cancer resection is indicated for patients with bronchial carcinoid tumors (lobectomy with lymph nodes) because 50% have positive lymph node metastases. Despite this malignant potential, about 75% of patients are cured by surgical resection.[369] The proper therapy for ACTH-producing neoplasms depends on the diagnosis (exact tumor that produces ACTH) and extent of disease.

Any of these tumors may be malignant and may metastasize. Therefore, in some patients with ectopic ACTH production the primary disease cannot be eradicated and therapy must be directed toward correcting the life-threatening metabolic and hormonal abnormalities. Hypokalemia and excess mineralocorticoid activity may be managed with potassium supplementation and spironolactone. Hypercortisolism may be managed with metyrapone,[370] aminoglutethimide,[371] or mitotane. Bilateral adrenalectomy is recommended for patients who have ectopic ACTH secondary to tumors that cannot be localized despite diligent radiographic efforts and for patients who have stable but unresectable metastatic disease.[367]

Pheochromocytoma

Pheochromocytomas are rare tumors that rise from chromaffin cells in the adrenal medulla and elsewhere. Pheochromocytomas secrete catecholamines and cause intermittent, episodic, or sustained hypertension. In autopsy series, only 0.005% to 0.1% of persons have unsuspected pheochromocytomas.[236] When urinary catecholamines are measured as a screening test for pheochromocytoma in hypertensive patient populations, the tumor is present in only 0.1% of the patients.[372] Although these tumors are rare, it is important to diagnose and localize pheochromocytomas for several reasons.[373] Sustained hypertension caused by a pheochromocytoma may be curable with tumor resection. Sudden death has been described in patients with pheochromocytoma secondary to paroxysmal hypertensive crisis. Pheochromocytomas can be malignant. Earlier diagnosis and therapy may lessen the probability of death from malignancy and improve the prognosis. Incidence of malignancy in pheochromocytomas has been reported to be as low as 5%[373] and as high as 46%.[374] Extraadrenal tumors are more commonly cancerous.[375] The presence of pheochromocytomas can be part of associated endocrine or nonendocrine inherited disorders.

Bilateral adrenal medullary pheochromocytomas are components of MEN-IIa and MEN-IIb. MEN-IIa includes MTC, parathyroid hyperplasia, and pheochromocytomas. MEN-IIb includes a characteristic body and facial appearance, bony abnormalities, MTC, and pheochromocytomas. The presence of pheochromocytomas must be excluded before operating on patients with MTC because an unexpected pheochromocytoma can result in hypertensive crisis and death during general anesthesia. Familial pheochromocytoma also has been described. Affected individuals have bilateral adrenal pheochromocytomas and no other manifestation of MEN syndromes.[376] In other families without evidence of MEN, extraadrenal pheochromocytomas have been reported usually in the same extraadrenal location (*e.g.*, bladder) in all affected individuals from one kindred.[377] Pheochromocytomas occur in about 25% of patients with von Hippel-Lindau disease[378] and have been reported in less than 1% of patients with neurofibromatosis and von Recklinghausen's disease.[379]

Pheochromocytomas produce catecholamines, which can cause the clinical symptoms of anxiety attacks and marked or sustained hypertension. Pheochromocytomas produce other hormones, including ACTH, and patients may have concomitant Cushing's syndrome.[252,281] Pheochromocytomas contain other peptide hormones, including somatostatin,[380] calcitonin,[381] oxytocin, and vasopressin,[382] that are seldom of clinical significance.

Oncogene

Pheochromocytomas originate from the neural crest and may develop by arrest at various points during normal differentiation.[383] The *RAS* oncogene does not appear to be involved in the tumoral process of pheochromocytoma because one recent study failed to detect any abnormality of *RAS* gene sequence in 10 pheochromocytomas.[384] Loss of heterozygosity at specific loci may help localize tumor suppressor genes involved in the formation of various familial and sporadic pheochromocytomas. Of 41 tumors tested, significant allelic losses were found on chromosome 1p (42%), 3p (16%), 17p (24%) and 22q (31%). Furthermore, there appeared to be a correlation between loss of heterozygosity on chromosome 1p with urinary excretion of metanephrine and loss of heterozygosity on chromosomes 1p, 3p, and 17p with tumor volume.[385]

Pathology

Pheochromocytomas arise from chromaffin cells,[373] which are widespread and are associated with sympathetic ganglia during fetal life. After birth, most chromaffin cells degenerate but many remain in the adrenal medulla.[373] This may explain why about 90% of pheochromocytomas are in the adrenal medulla. Extraadrenal pheochromocytomas may arise anywhere including in the carotid body, within the heart,[386] along the aorta (thoracic and abdominal), and within the urinary bladder. The most common extraadrenal location is the organ of Zuckerkandl, which is near the origin of the inferior mesenteric artery to the left of the aortic bifurcation. Bilateral adrenal pheochromocytomas occur in familial syndromes including MEN-IIa and MEN-IIb. Some researchers believe that unilateral adrenal medullary tumors can occur in these patients, but with resection both adrenals usually have neoplasms or medullary hyperplasia. In patients with MEN-IIa who undergo unilateral adrenalectomy for pheochromocytoma, recurrent biochemical disease and imageable pheochromocytomas may develop in the contralateral adrenal gland with a long follow-up period.[387] Sturge-Weber syndrome is associated with cavernous hemangiomas of the trigeminal nerve and pheochromocytoma.

Data from series of patients with sporadic pheochromocytomas indicate that the right adrenal gland harbors a tumor more commonly than the left gland does.[372,388] Pheochromocytomas resected from hypertensive patients usually measure between 3 and 5 cm in diameter and weigh about 100 g.[389] These tumors appear tan or gray and have a soft, smooth consistency. Larger tumors may be cystic or have necrotic areas and often have calcification. Microscopically, pheochromocytomas resemble the cell of origin. Tumors are usually arranged in cords or alveolar patterns[236] and may be composed of cords of cells lining vascular structures and having an angiomatous appearance.[390] Tumors generally are separated clearly from the adrenal cortex by a thin band of fibrous tissue. Extension of the pheochromocytoma into the cortex or vascular invasion may occur in benign neoplasms.[236]

The pathologic distinction between benign and malignant pheochromocytomas is not clear, and pathologists have relied on the reported benign natural history of most pheochromocytomas. However, pheochromocytomas may be malignant more often than expected.[374] In one large series, the tumor recurrence rate was 10% and most recurrences occurred within 5 years.[388] In another series, tumors recurred in 16 of 69 (23%).[391] In another experience, tumors recurred in 46% of 176 patients studied.[374] These results partly reflect the referral pattern of tertiary institutions, but they may also reflect a higher malignancy rate than originally predicted. Malignant tumors tend to be larger and weigh more than benign pheochromocytomas, although this is not an absolute criterion.[236] The only absolute criteria for malignancy are secondary tumors in sites where chromaffin cells are not usually present and visceral metastases.[392] Paradoxically, benign pheochromocytomas may demonstrate marked nuclear pleomorphism, whereas malignant ones may demonstrate less.[236] Malignant pheochromocytomas usually have many more mitoses than benign tumors, but capsular and vascular invasion occurs with equal frequency in both.[236] Nuclear DNA ploidy may indicate malignant potential.[393–395] Flow cytometry has been used to define a subgroup of patients with pheochromocytoma who have malignant tumor. Tumors in which DNA ploidy studies demonstrated tetraploidy, polyploidy, or aneuploidy had a significantly higher chance of a malignant course compared with most other tumors, which were normally diploid.[394] It has been suggested that neuropeptide Y gene expression by tumors may be used to differentiate benign from malignant pheochromocytomas. In one study, neuropeptide Y mRNA was expressed in 9 of 9 benign tumors and in only 4 of 11 malignant tumors, suggesting that expression of this gene is seen more often in benign pheochromocytomas.[396] Other investigators have attempted to differentiate benign pheochromocytomas from malignant pheochromocytomas by measuring serum levels of neuron-specific enolase and neuropeptide Y, but observed differences were not significantly different.[397] Finally, a study by Medeiros and colleagues indicates that the malignant potential of a tumor correlates best with tumor weight and amount of necrosis (Table 41–17).[398] The prospective distinction between benign and malignant pheochromocytoma based on pathologic criteria remains a chal-

TABLE 41–17. Differentiation of Benign Versus Malignant Pheochromocytomas

Investigations	*Characteristic*	*Benign*	*Malignant*
Sherwin, 1964[392]	Metastases	–	+
Medeiros et al, 1985[398]	Weight (g)	156	759
Beierwaltes et al, 1986[374] Remine et al, 1974[388]	Occurrence (%)	50–90	10–50
Page et al, 1986[236]	Vascular invasion	+	+
Page et al, 1986[236]	Capsular invasion	+	+
Page et al, 1986[236]	Mitoses	±	++++
Page et al, 1986[236]	Nuclear pleomorphism	+	–
Sherwin, 1964[392] Lewis, 1971[393] Hosaka et al, 1986[394] Sheps et al, 1990[395]	Ploidy	Diploid	Hyperdiploid, triploid
Medeiros et al, 1985[398]	Necrosis	±	++
Helman et al, 1989[396]	Tumors with neuropeptide Y gene expression (%)	100	36
Grouzmann et al, 1990[397]	Proportion of patients with elevated serum levels of neuron-specific enolase (%)	0	50

+, extent present; –, extent absent.

lenge. This distinction is increasingly important because recent studies indicate that more patients have malignant recurrent tumors than originally believed.

Clinical Manifestations and Diagnosis

Patients with pheochromocytomas may present with symptoms such as mild labile hypertension or may experience sudden death secondary to a hypertensive crisis, myocardial infarction, or cerebral vascular accident. The classic symptoms described by patients are spells of paroxysmal headaches, pallor, palpitations, hypertension and diaphoresis. In 50% of patients, the hypertension is intermittent, whereas in the other 50% it is sustained. In 90% of children with pheochromocytomas, the hypertension is sustained.[399] Patients may have signs of chronic hypovolemia such as orthostatic hypotension secondary to excessive α-catecholaminergic stimulation and vasoconstriction. Most patients have mild weight loss, but obesity does not rule out pheochromocytoma.

The diagnosis of pheochromocytoma is based on measuring catecholamines in the urine and blood and on the clonidine suppression test (Fig. 41–8). There is no single best screening test for pheochromocytoma. Some clinicians prefer measurement of a spot urine for metanephrines. The false-negative rate is about 5%. Another recommended screening method is the separate measurement of norepinephrine and epinephrine and their metabolites in the urine or serum.[400] Measuring urinary free catecholamines by ion-pair high pressure liquid chromatography (HPLC) is another sensitive screening test.[401]

If a pheochromocytoma is suspected clinically or if a patient has a family history of MEN-IIa or MEN-IIb, the best study is

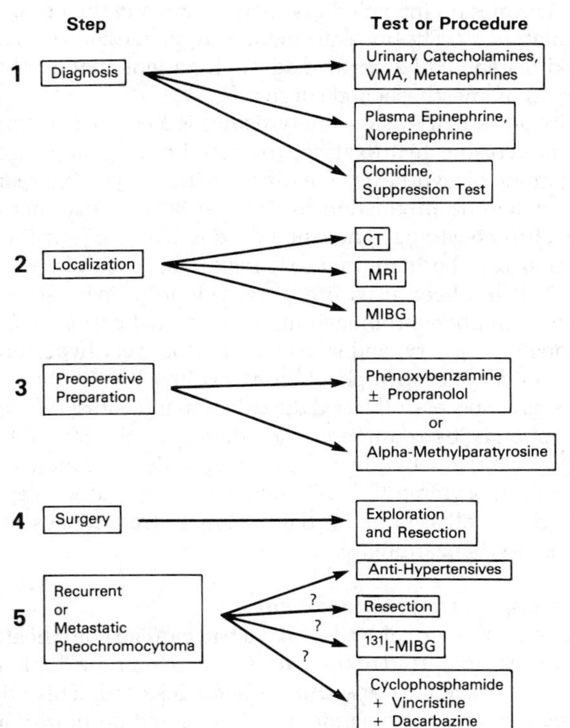

FIGURE 41–8. Flow diagram for diagnosis, localization, preoperative preparation, treatment, and follow-up of a patient with a pheochromocytoma.

a measurement of 24-hour urine for catecholamine, metanephrine, and VMA. In a recent report testing 64 patients, 30 of whom had pheochromocytomas, 24-hour urine collections for VMA, dopamine, epinephrine, and norepinephrine were analyzed. The measurement of 24-hour urine for levels of VMA and norepinephrine had the greatest sensitivity (97%), whereas the measurement for levels of VMA had the best specificity (91%).[402] Another recent study reports that urinary measurement of catecholamine, VMA, and metanephrine levels was the most sensitive screening test.[403] When patients with MTC are screened for pheochromocytomas by these urinary studies in the MEN-II setting, false-negative results can occur. Radioenzymatic assays for plasma catcholamines can provide a more direct measurement of catecholamine excess, but there have been conflicting reports comparing the value of urinary or plasma catecholamines in the diagnosis of pheochromocytoma. As the plasma assay becomes more reliable, it may be a more sensitive and specific method than the urinary assay, especially when combined with the clonidine suppression test.[400] This depends on the laboratory and the method, because recent studies still report that 24-hour urinary measurement of levels of free norepinephrine are more sensitive (sensitivity 100%) than plasma assays (sensitivity 82%). Urinary assay may be more specific if 24-hour levels of 3,4-dihydroxyphenyl glycol are also measured (specificity, 99%).[404]

Plasma levels of chromogranin A may be used as a confirmatory but not diagnostic circulating marker for pheochromocytomas. Levels are not specific for patients with pheochromocytoma but are elevated in any condition in which excessive catecholamine secretion occurs (*e.g.*, cardiac arrest).[405] The clonidine suppression test has become the test of choice to determine whether a patient with borderline urinary or plasma catecholamine level has a pheochromocytoma.[406–410] It may be the most definitive test for pheochromocytoma. In this test, the patient rests supine in a quiet room while a venous catheter for blood drawing is inserted. Blood samples are obtained for plasma epinephrine, norepinephrine, and total catecholamines after a 30-minute period. Clonidine (300 μg) is then administered orally, and 3 hours later another blood sample is obtained. In normal subjects and in patients with idiopathic hypertension, clonidine suppresses plasma levels of epinephrine and norepinephrine into the normal or less than normal range. In patients with pheochromocytomas, clonidine did not suppress these plasma levels. Combing two studies from different groups, plasma levels of epinephrine and norepinephrine after clonidine were found to be suppressed in 14 normal subjects and in 51 essential hypertensive patients without pheochromocytomas but were not suppressed in the 16 patients with proved pheochromocytomas.[408,409] Only 2 patients were diagnosed incorrectly using the clonidine suppression test; 1 patient had a false-positive result and 1 patient had a false-negative result.[411]

The clonidine suppression test remains the study of choice to diagnose pheochromocytomas in patients with plasma catecholamine concentrations between 500 and 2000 pg/ml.[412] An overnight method of this test is based on the measurement of urinary levels of norepinephrine and epinephrine that do not suppress in patients with pheochromocytoma but do suppress in other forms of hypertension.[410] This test may be more valuable because urinary determinations of catecholamines may be more sensitive and specific than plasma determinations.[404]

Localization Studies

CT and MRI are the two radiologic (non-nuclear medicine) procedures of choice to localize pheochromocytomas preoperatively (see Fig. 41–8).[318,413] Both are noninvasive and sensitive, being able to detect tumors about 1 cm in diameter. MRI is specific because of the signal intensity on the T2-weighted image. Pheochromocytomas appear more than three times as bright as liver and few if any other adrenal tumors have a similar MRI appearance.[316] CT has a greater resolution and availability than MRI does, but MRI is rapidly improving in both areas. In a Mayo Clinic study of 52 patients with pheochromocytoma, CT scans detected 51 of 52 tumors, including 9 of 10 bilateral tumors.[414] In another study, unenhanced high-resolution CT scans detected pheochromocytomas in 6 of 6 patients who had tumors found at surgery, including 2 extraadrenal retroperitoneal tumors.[415] MRI of pheochromocytomas has remarkable resolution without any radiation. In 7 patients with pheochromocytomas demonstrated on CT, MRI imaged all primary lesions and metastases to the chest, retroperitoneum, and liver.[316] Because it has no radiation exposure, it has been used to image successfully a life-threatening pheochromocytoma during pregnancy in a patient with severe hypertension.[416] In a recent study, CT scans imaged 16 of 19 pheochromocytomas (84%), whereas MRI imaged 12 of 15 (75%) for comparable sensitivity.[417] In addition, MRI successfully imaged an intrapericardial pheochromocytoma and differentiated it from the cardiac chambers and surrounding great vessels, which could not be determined by CT.[418] Adrenal arteriography and venography, formerly the best studies to localize pheochromocytomas, are no longer indicated.

Another important technique for the localization of pheochromocytomas is nuclear scanning after the administration of labeled MIBG. The compound is similar to norepinephrine and is taken up and concentrated in adrenergic tissue. ^{131}I-MIBG has been studied in 400 patients to localize suspected pheochromocytoma.[419] The results were rated as true positive, false positive, true negative, and false negative based on a combination of other imaging studies, venous sampling, and surgical pathologic results after exploration. The sensitivity of MIBG scanning was 78% in sporadic pheochromocytoma, 91% in malignant pheochromocytoma, and 94% in familial pheochromocytoma. The overall sensitivity was 87%. The specificity was nearly 100% in each category and overall. ^{131}I-MIBG used in 48 patients at another institution demonstrated a sensitivity of 77% and a specificity of 96%,[420] and two other institutions reported similar findings.[421,422] Recent data confirm previous studies and demonstrate that labeled MIBG is a useful diagnostic and imaging study for the detection and localization of pheochromocytoma.[402] In three recent studies from different institutions, it had a sensitivity of 86% and correctly diagnosed and imaged tumor in 71 of 83 patients.[402,417] It appears that MIBG scanning is safe, noninvasive, and efficacious for the localization of pheochromocytomas, including those that arise in nonadrenal sites, and malignant disease. Metastatic bone involvement of pheochromocytoma can be imaged by ^{131}I-MIBG, but standard bone scintigraphy may be more sensitive.[423,424] In summary, MIBG scanning images catecholamine-producing tumors with a high specificity and sensitivity. Whereas CT scans and MRI reflect changes in morphology, scintigraphic imaging relies on tissue function.[422] False-positive results with MIBG scintigraphy are rare, although tumors such as MTC and neuroblastoma can image, accounting for the high specificity (98% to 100%) of the study. False-negative results can occur and have an incidence of about 13% to 20%, which lowers sensitivity.[402,417,425,426] It appears that these false-negative results may be more common with multiple tumors and with metastatic disease in the same patient.[427]

Preoperative Preparation

Once the diagnosis is established and the tumor localized, preoperative preparation includes α-adrenergic blockade. Patients are started on phenoxybenzamine 10 mg orally two or three times daily (see Fig. 41–8). If tachycardia develops (heart rate of more than 100 beats/minute), β-adrenergic blocking agents (*e.g.*, propranolol) are added 1 week before surgery. Propranolol should never be started before α-blockade because unopposed vasoconstriction may worsen hypertension. One problem with intraoperative management of patients with pheochromocytomas is decreased blood volume and plasma volume secondary to tumor production of excess α-adrenergic hormones. Phenoxybenzamine blocks this excessive α-adrenergic activity and after 14 days increases the total blood volume and plasma volume to normal levels in patients with pheochromocytoma.[428] This standard regimen has been used by many and has been a marked improvement over historical unprepared patients with pheochromocytoma.[402,403,429] In addition, lactic acidosis is often present in patients with pheochromocytoma related to the effect of catecholamines on intermediary metabolism and the peripheral circulation.[430] The measurement and correction of arterial blood pH should be performed in all patients before the induction of anesthesia and surgery.[430]

Alpha-methyltyrosine (metyrosine) is a competitive inhibitor of tyrosine hydroxylase, the rate-limiting step in catecholamine biosynthesis. Treatment with metyrosine reduces catecholamine production by 50% to 80% in patients with pheochromocytoma. The usual dose is 250 mg four times a day and may be increased to a maximum dose of 3 to 4 g/day.[431] It has been used preoperatively to prepare some patients with pheochromocytoma and unusual cardiac complications for surgery, and it may be used to treat hypertensive crisis in patients with pheochromocytoma.[431,432] Other clinicians have successfully used the calcium-antagonist nifedipine with phenoxybenzamine or nicardipine alone (60–120 mg/day) to control labile hypertensive episodes in patients with pheochromocytoma.[433,434] These newer drug strategies appear to work as well as or better than the more traditional strategy of phenoxybenzamine.

Intraoperative Management

Patients who are elderly or have had cardiac complications should be transferred to the intensive care unit the day before surgery to have a Swan-Ganz catheter inserted. This allows correction of hemodynamic imbalances and optimization of cardiac performance. The morning of the operation, an arterial catheter and peripheral intravenous catheters should be inserted. Arterial blood gas should be measured to rule out acidosis. During surgery, especially during manipulation of the tumor, marked increased in blood pressure may occur, and hypertensive episodes should be controlled with α-adrenergic blocking agents such as regitine or with agents that directly relax arterial and venous smooth muscle such as sodium nitroprusside. Nitroprusside is the preferred drug because of its rapid onset and short duration. It is administered by continuous intravenous infusion with a pump, and the blood pressure is continuously titrated to acceptable levels. The use of preoperative preparation with oral α-adrenergic blocking agents and intraoperative adjustment and regulation of blood pressure with nitroprusside has greatly facilitated the surgical resection of pheochromocytomas and has reduced operative morbidity and mortality.

The operation is performed using a transabdominal incision that is either a bilateral subcostal or long midline incision. Preoperative localization studies such as CT, MRI, and ^{131}I-MIBG guide the exploration, but the entire abdomen must be carefully visualized and palpated. Others argue that localization procedures are so sensitive and specific that more direct approaches may be preferred.[435] Most pheochromocytomas can be well localized. In instances of malignant pheochromocytomas or multiple pheochromocytomas in known or unsuspected MEN syndromes, some tumors may be missed. Extraadrenal pheochromocytomas may be difficult to find. The most common locations of intraabdominal extraadrenal pheochromocytoma are the hilar region of the kidneys and the chromaffin tissue along the aorta from the celiac axis to the aortic bifurcation. The organ of Zuckerkandl at the aortic bifurcation is the most common extraadrenal location for a pheochromocytoma. Pheochromocytomas have even been described within the bladder.[436] Multiple locations, metastatic potential, and multiple tumors all support the necessity for a complete exploration of the entire abdominal cavity, which includes Kocherization of the duodenum and exploration of the lesser sac. The *rule of ten* may be of value in the management of pheochromocytomas and states that 10% are malignant, 10% are extraadrenal, and 10% are bilateral in the adrenal medulla.[407] Some researchers suggest that nearly 100% of patients with MEN-II have or will develop bilateral benign adrenal medullary pheochromocytomas,[437] whereas others suggest that the incidence of bilaterality, although high, may be significantly less (70%).[65]

Malignant Pheochromocytomas

It is generally believed that malignant pheochromocytomas do not occur in MEN syndromes and are present in about 10% of patients with pheochromocytoma.[407] However, two reports indicate that substantially more than 10% of sporadic pheochromocytoma may be malignant.[374,391] In one study, 25 of 69 patients (36%) had malignant pheochromocytomas diagnosed by recurrent or metastatic disease.[391] In another study using the same criteria, 81 of 176 patients (46%) with pheochromocytomas had malignant disease.[374] In the latter study, original histologic review by blinded pathologists failed to discriminate malignant versus benign neoplasms with accuracy. Pathologic analysis was not helpful in predicting which tumors were malignant.[374] Patients who developed metastases did not develop them until 0.2 to 28.7 years after their initial surgery. Incidence of detection for the first 9 years was 5% per year. Males were more likely to develop metastatic pheochromocytoma. Imaging with ^{131}I-MIBG was usually able to detect recurrent or metastatic pheochromocytoma. Some surgeons recommend yearly ^{131}I-MIBG scans to detect recurrent disease in all patients after resection of pheochromocytoma.[374] Others recommend lifetime follow-up with measurement of blood pressure and urinary levels of catecholamines.[391] The detection of recurrent or metastatic pheochromocytoma should be based on the same methods as detection of primary or initial pheochromocytoma. These methods include measurement of urinary and serum catecholamines, clonidine suppression test, CT, MRI, and ^{131}I-MIBG scan. Careful follow-up requires some of these studies on a yearly basis (see Fig. 41–8). With careful follow-up, the incidence of malignant pheochromocytoma may be more than 10% and may approach 30% to 50%.

Treatment of Malignant Pheochromocytoma. The basic principles in the treatment of malignant pheochromocytomas have been surgical resection of recurrences or metastases if possible and treatment of hypertensive symptoms by catecholamine blockade.[438,439] Painful bony metastases, which may be diagnosed by ^{131}I-MIBG scans or by standard bone nuclide scans,[424] respond well to radiation therapy.[440] Soft tissue masses or bony masses generally respond well to radiation therapy, if doses of 4000 cGy or more can be administered.[395] Localized or solitary soft tissue masses may be successfully resected surgically, even when metastatic to the liver or lung.[441] Standard chemotherapy regimens including doxorubicin plus streptozocin[438] and BCNU plus doxorubicin have not been effective in the treatment of malignant pheochromocytomas.

Survival data of patients with malignant pheochromocytoma are difficult to obtain because of the rarity and indolence of the tumor.[441] In a large series from the Mayo clinic, the 5-year survival rate was 36%.[439] Other investigators reported a 5-year survival rate of 60% in 15 patients with malignant pheochromocytoma.[442] In this study, patients were treated primarily by aggressive surgery and medical blood pressure control. In a final series, patients who succumbed from malignant pheochromocytoma did so within 3 years of the appearance of metastases.[443]

The early success with streptozocin in the treatment of neuroendocrine tumors of the gastrointestinal tract[444] suggested that it might be useful in the treatment of malignant pheochromocytomas. Streptozocin has had mixed responses in patients with malignant pheochromocytoma. Initial work with streptozocin was disappointing and suggested no role for it in the treatment of malignant pheochromocytoma.[438,443] However, Feldman treated one patient with a good response and suggested that the dosage schedule might be important in obtaining a beneficial result.[445] Three-year follow-up data on that patient showed that the patient maintained an 85% reduction in urinary homovanillic acid levels and a 73% reduction in urinary VMA levels with normal renal function despite 66 g of streptozocin.[446] Other investigators have tried this regimen and found no response and deterioration of renal function.[447] Some patients with malignant pheochromocytoma may respond to streptozocin chemotherapy, but many do not and it does not appear to play a major role in the treatment of patients with these rare tumors.

Because of the high sensitivity (85%) and specificity (100%) of ^{131}I-MIBG in the imaging of pheochromocytomas, its use in higher doses to treat recurrent or metastatic pheochromocytomas is a logical progression. Imaging of pheochromocytoma permits accurate dosimetry to the tumor on the basis of the diagnostic dose of ^{131}I-MIBG administered. If uptake by the primary tumor or metastases is high, it is possible to deliver radiation doses on the order of several thousand cGy by increasing the administered activity. Specific activity of ^{131}I-MIBG of 200 mCi in 5 mg has been achieved.[448] With the remarkable ability of MIBG to image tumors, one would expect its ability to treat metastatic or recurrent tumors to be equally effective; unfortunately, it has not been dramatic. Treatment response in patients with pheochromocytomas can be measured by catecholamine secretion and standard tumor size measurements. Blood pressure control of a few patients with malignant pheochromocytoma has been facilitated by ^{131}I-MIBG therapy.[442] A recent trial reports the use of ^{131}I-MIBG therapy in 15 patients with malignant pheochromocytoma. Patients were treated with ^{131}I-MIBG (specific activity 740 MBq/mg) every 3 months. The typical patients received 3 doses, with an absorbed cumulative tumor dose of 1200 to 15,500 cGy. A beneficial response to treatment was observed in 9 of the 15 patients (60%). Four patients did not respond, and the others had a slight response. No complete responses were observed. Five patients had measurable partial responses to treatment and 7 had hormonal responses. Toxicity included pancytopenia in 1 patient that resolved after discontinuation of therapy.[449] In another study of 12 patients treated with ^{131}I-MIBG, 5 (42%) had reduced catecholamine levels and 2 had decreased tumor size (17%).[450] Vetter and colleagues reported that 2 patients with malignant pheochromocytomas treated with ^{131}I-MIBG had minor reductions in tumor size but no change in catecholamine secretion.[451] There have been no complete responses.[448–451]

For a malignant pheochromocytoma to concentrate and retain ^{131}I-MIBG, the tumor must have an active neuronal pump mechanism.[451] Keiser and colleagues found that only 1 of 5 patients with metastatic pheochromocytoma had an appreciable uptake of ^{131}I-MIBG into the tumor.[452] When ^{131}I-MIBG was administered to 9 patients with metastatic pheochromocytoma, 40% to 55% of the administered radioactivity appeared in the urine as ^{131}I-MIBG in 24 hours and 70% to 90% appeared in the urine within 4 days.[453] This study suggests that the agent is stable and rapidly excreted by the kidneys and that malignant pheochromocytomas do not take up much of the administered dose. This inability of malignant pheochromocytoma to absorb ^{131}I-MIBG may be partially explained by a study in which plasma levels of dopa and catecholamines from patients with benign pheochromocytoma were compared with levels from patients with malignant pheochromocytomas and neuroblastoma.[454] Neuroblastomas are aggressive tumors of neural-crest origin that occur in children and have no association with hypertension. All the patients with neuroblastoma had high plasma levels of dopa. Patients with benign pheochromocytomas had elevated plasma levels of norepinephrine or epinephrine, and none had elevated plasma levels of dopa. In contrast, 60% of patients with malignant pheochromocytomas had elevated plasma levels of dopa. These observations suggest that patients with benign pheochromocytomas have well-differentiated tumor cells that function as normal chromaffin tissue. These cells synthesize and store norepinephrine and epinephrine, leading to hypertension. Malignant pheochromocytomas that are composed of less differentiated cells grow more rapidly and have deficient mechanisms for catecholamine synthesis or storage, explaining why malignant tumors do not take up as much ^{131}I-MIBG and why dopa is detected in the plasma of 60% of patients with malignant pheochromocytoma and in no patients with benign pheochromocytoma.[454] The similarity between malignant pheochromocytoma and neuroblastoma is further supported by the astonishing responsiveness of malignant pheochromocytomas to therapy effective in treating neuroblastomas.[452,455,456]

There are many similarities between pheochromocytoma and neuroblastoma. Both tumors arise from neuroectoderm, for example, and both contain neuron-specific enolase. Dopa is found to circulate in the plasma of patients who have either of these tumors.[452,454] Because of these similarities and because a combination of cyclophosphamide, vincristine, and dacarbazine has an 80% response rate for metastatic neuroblastoma,[457] this regimen has been used in patients with metastatic pheochromocytoma.[452] The chemotherapy regimen consisted of cyclophosphamide 750 mg/m^2 given intravenously on day 1, vincristine 1.4 mg/m^2 intravenously on day 1, and dacarbazine 600 mg/m^2 intravenously on days 1 and 2, repeated every 21 days. Doses of cyclophosphamide and dacarbazine were increased or decreased on the basis of neurotoxicity. Each of the 3 patients treated had decreased levels of catecholamines, decreased blood pressure, and a documented partial response on imaging studies. Each patient had either progressed on ^{131}I-MIBG therapy or failed to image tumor on ^{131}I-MIBG scan.[452] In a study of this regimen in 14 patients with metastatic pheochromocytoma, the ability to respond to the chemotherapy regimen correlated with plasma norepinephrine level before therapy.[456] One patient had a complete response (biochemical and imageable) that lasted for 9 months. One other patient had a biochemically complete response, and a total of 8 patients (57%) had decreases in 24-hour levels of urinary catecholamines. Seven patients (50%) had at least a 50% decrease in measurable size of tumor. Biochemical response (urinary catecholamines) correlated well with response evaluated on imaging studies. The median duration of response was more than 18 months. All responding patients have had dramatic improvement in hypertension control and performance status. The regimen has been well tolerated and toxicity has been mild.[456] Malaise, nausea, and vomiting have been limited to the 48 hours after chemotherapy. Reversible granulocytopenia has been controlled by dose reductions of cyclophosphamide and dacarbazine. Hypertensive crisis after cytotoxic drug therapy in patients with unsuspected pheochromocytomas has been reported,[458] but this potentially life-threatening complication is not a problem as long as the patients are treated with adequate α-adrenergic blockade.[452] Table 41–18 lists possible treatment regimens for metastatic pheochromocytoma.

In summary, malignant pheochromocytomas are difficult to diagnose accurately based on pathology alone. They are indolent tumors, and the overall 5-year survival rates are between 34% and 60%. These malignant tumors may be more common than previously reported, mandating diligent lifelong follow-up of all patients who undergo resection of a primary pheochromocytoma. In patients with malignant pheochro-

TABLE 41–18. Treatment of Metastatic Malignant Pheochromocytoma

Investigations	*Compound*	*No. of Patients*	*No. With Change in Catecholamine Secretion*	*Result of Imaging in Urine Levels of Catecholamine*
McEwan et al, 1985[448]	^{131}I-MIBG	12	5 partial decrease (40%)	2 decrease (16%)
Feldman et al, 1984[450]	^{131}I-MIBG	3	No change	Questionable decrease
Krempf et al, 1991[449]	^{131}I-MIBG	15	7 partial decrease (47%) 4 normal	5 decrease (33%)
Feldman, 1983[445]	High-dose streptozocin	1	Marked decrease	Marked decrease
Gross et al, 1985[447]	High-dose streptozocin	1	No change	No change
Keiser et al, 1985[452]	Cyclophosphamide + vincristine + darcarbazine	3	3 Marked decrease	3 Marked decrease
Averbuch et al, 1988[456]	Cyclophosphamide + vincristine + darcarbazine	14	2 normal 6 partial decrease (57%)	1 CR 6 PR (50%)

CR, complete remission; PR, partial remission.

mocytoma, hypertension should be controlled medically with α-adrenergic blocking agents or other antihypertensive agents. Recurrent or metastatic tumors that are solitary and well localized should be resected surgically. Bony metastases that are painful should be treated with radiation therapy. ^{131}I-MIBG scans can localize recurrent or metastatic tumor and may be used to treat malignant disease if the isotope localizes to the tumor on scan. Treatment with combination chemotherapy cyclophosphamide, vincristine, and dacarbazine may be more efficacious than ^{131}I-MIBG.

CARCINOID TUMORS

Carcinoid tumors are believed to arise from enterochromaffin (EC) cells, which are scattered throughout the body but occur primarily in the submucosa of the intestine and main bronchi. In the intestine, these cells are present at the base of the crypts and are sometimes called Kultchitzky's cells.[459,460] Some EC cells can take up and reduce silver and are called argentaffin cells. Others take up silver but do not reduce it and are called argyrophilic cells.

PATHOLOGY AND TUMOR HISTOLOGY

Carcinoids are neuroendocrine tumors and have been proposed to derive from the diffuse neuroendocrine cell system.[461,462] They have been classified as APUDomas (amine precursor uptake and decarboxylation) and share cytochemical features with melanomas, pheochromocytomas, MTC, and pancreatic endocrine tumors.[461,462] The APUDomas all share histologic, ultrastructural, and biochemical features. Histologically, they are similar to pancreatic endocrine tumors.[463,464] Both are composed of monotonous sheets of small round cells with uniform nuclei and cytoplasm. Mitotic figures are rare.[463,464] Pathologists cannot differentiate benign from malignant carcinoids based on histology, nor can they differentiate pancreatic endocrine tumors from carcinoids histologically. Malignancy can be determined unequivocally only if there is lymph node invasion or distant metastases. Ultrastructurally, carcinoid tumors possess electron-dense neurosecretory granules.[465] Studies using immunoperoxidase staining have shown that carcinoid tumors synthesize numerous bioactive amines, peptides such as neuron-specific enolase, 5-hydroxytryptamine, 5-hydroxytryptophan, synaptophysin, and chromogranin A and C, other peptides such as insulin, growth hormone, neurotensin, ACTH, melanocyte stimulating hormone (B-MSH), gastrin, pancreatic polypeptide, calcitonin, substance P and other tachykinins (*e.g.*, neuropeptide K), growth hormone-releasing hormone, and bombesin.[466–472] Shared biochemical characteristics include increased activity of tissue enzymes such as diamine oxidase, L-dopa decarboxylase, cholinesterase, and nonspecific esterase.[462] APUDomas originally were proposed to be of neural crest origin.[461,462] Later studies suggest that some of these tumors are of endodermal origin.[468] The numerous similarities of these tumors to carcinoid tumors make the concept of the APUDoma useful.

Most carcinoid tumors can be identified tentatively on routine histology.[469,472] Diagnostic problems can arise because adenocarcinomas occasionally have carcinoid-like features, in that both produce mucus, express carcinoembryonic antigen, and produce various cytokeratins.[473–476] For this reason, general endocrine tumor markers such as the argyrophil reaction of Grimelius and the immunocytochemical localization of chromogranin, synaptophysin, and neuron-specific enolase generally have been used.[469,472] The chromogranins (A, B, and C) are a family of acidic polypeptides that are the major components of the secretory granules of many neuroendocrine cell types.[469,471,472] There usually is a close correspondence between neuroendocrine cells sharing chromogranin A immunoreactivity and an argyrophil reaction, which may be partially explained by argyrophilic nature of pure chromogranin A.[472] Generally, chromogranin A immunoreactivity is more specific than the argyrophil reaction because the latter identifies other intracellular proteins such as melanin.[472] Neuron-specific enolase is a glycolytic enzyme that occurs in the cytoplasm of most neuroendocrine cells and is positive in most carcinoid tumors and other APUDomas.[469,472,477] NSE occasionally can be misleading because some tumors not considered to be neuroendocrine (*e.g.*, breast tumors) may show considerable neuron-specific enolase activity.[472] Synaptophysin is a calcium-binding vesicle membrane glycoprotein that is synthesized independently of other neuroendocrine proteins.[478] In a recent study of 12 patients with carcinoid tumors, special staining for neuron-specific enolase was positive in 100%, chromogranin A in 92%, synaptophysin in 50%, and the Grimelius reaction in 75%.[479]

In addition to the general histologic neuroendocrine tumor markers discussed above, specific markers for carcinoid tumors may help identify the tumor as a carcinoid tumor. Serotonin can be identified by various methods including the argentaffin reaction of Masson or the use of antibodies to serotonin.[469,472,480] In midgut carcinoids, the argentaffin reaction of Masson generally is positive and the serotonin antibody localization weak or negative, whereas in foregut and hindgut carcinoids, serotonin immunoreactivity is detected more often than is the argentaffin reaction.[472,480]

Numerous biogenic amines and peptide hormones are secreted by carcinoid tumors and can be detected in the plasma (Table 41–19). Many of these cause symptomatic syndromes such as the carcinoid syndrome, Cushing's syndrome, and the classic syndromes caused by pancreatic endocrine tumors (*e.g.*, ZES, acromegaly due to release of growth-hormone releasing factors [GRFoma], and somatostatinoma syndrome). Measurement of the plasma levels of these secreted products (*e.g.*, biogenic amines, serotonin and its precursors or metabolites, chromogranins, or subunits of human chorionic gonadotropin [HCG]) are used to diagnosis and assess malignancy and are discussed in later sections.

Williams and Sanders originally proposed a classification of carcinoids by their site of origin. This classification is useful because carcinoid tumors from different areas have different functional manifestations, histochemistry, and secretory products (see Table 41–19).[481] Foregut carcinoids generally have a low serotonin (5-HT) content, are argentaffin negative but argyrophilic, occasionally secrete 5-hydroxytryptophan (5-HTP) and ACTH, are associated with the typical carcinoid syndrome, are often multihormonal, and may metastasize to bone (see Table 41–19). Although many foregut carcinoids contain peptides, clinical syndromes rarely are produced, and elevated levels of hormones in the plasma generally are not detected. Midgut carcinoids are argentaffin positive, have a high serotonin content, have smaller number of endocrine cells than foregut tumors, cause the classical carcinoid syndrome when they metastasize, release serotonin and tachykinins (substance P, neuropeptide K, substance K), rarely secrete 5-HTP or ACTH, and rarely metastasize to bone. Hindgut carcinoid tumors are argentaffin negative, often argyrophilic, rarely contain 5-HT, rarely cause carcinoid syndrome, contain numerous gastrointestinal hormones, rarely secrete 5-HTP or ACTH, and may metastasize to bone.

Carcinoid tumors can be ubiquitous, but most arise from four sites: the bronchus, appendix, rectum, and jejunoileum.[482] Carcinoid tumors most frequently occur in the appendix (about 40%; Table 41–20). The most common extraappendiceal sites are the small intestine (27%), rectum (13%), and bronchus (11.5%). The distribution of carcinoid tumors found

TABLE 41–19. Classification of Carcinoid Tumors

	Origin		
	Foregut (Respiratory Tract, Pancreas, Stomach, Proximal Duodenum)	*Midgut (Jejunum, Ileum, Appendix, Meckel's Diverticulum, Ascending Colon)*	*Hindgut (Transverse and Descending Colon, Rectum)*
Histochemistry			
Silver staining	Argentaffin negative, argyrophilic or negative	Argentaffin positive	Argentaffin negative (75%) or occasional argyrophilic (55%)
Neuron-specific enolase	Positive	Positive	Positive
Chromogranin A staining	Positive	Positive	Positive (42%)
Cytoplasmic granules (Electron microscopy)	Round, variable density, 180 nm in size	Pleomorphilic, uniform density 230 nm in size	Round, variable density, about 190 nm in size
Products			
Tumor	Low 5-HT content, multihormonal*	High 5-HT content, multihormonal*	Rarely 5-HT multihormonal*
Blood	5-HTP, histamine, multihormonal,* occ ACTH	5-HT, multihormonal,* rarely secrete ACTH	Rarely release 5-HTP or ACTH
Urine	5-HTP, 5-HT, 5-HIAA, histamine and others	5-HT, 5-HIAA	Negative
Carcinoid syndrome	Occurs but is atypical	Occurs frequently (with metastases)	Rarely occurs
Metastasize to bone	Common	Rarely	Common

* Multihormonal tumors include tachykinins (substance P, substance K, neuropeptide K), neurotensin, insulin, glucagon, pastrin, glicentin, VIP, somatostatin, pancreatic polypeptide, ACTH, and α subunit of human chorionic gonadotropin.
(Data from references 467, 472, 481, 483, 521–524, 532, and 554)

TABLE 41–20. Carcinoid Tumors: Location, Incidence of Metastases, and Incidence of Carcinoid Syndrome by Location

	Location of Tumors (%)	*Incidence of Metastases by Site (%)*	*Incidence of Carcinoid Syndrome by Site (%)*
Foregut			
Esophagus	<1	—	—
Stomach	2	22	9.5
Duodenum	2.6	20	3.4
Pancreas	<1	20	20
Gallbladder	<1	33	5
Bile duct	<1	—	—
Ampulla	<1	14	—
Larynx	<1	50	—
Bronchus	11.5	20	13
Thymus	2	25	—
Midgut			
Jejunum	1.3	35	9
Ileum	23	35	9
Meckel's diverticulum	1	18	13
Appendix	38	2	<1
Colon	2	60	5
Liver	<1	—	—
Ovary	<1	6	50
Testis	<1	—	50
Cervix	<1	24	3
Hindgut			
Rectum	13	3	—

Percentages from review of 4349 carcinoid tumors.
(Godwin JD. Carcinoid tumors: an analysis of 2837 cases. Cancer 1975;36:560)

in surgical or clinical series differs markedly from that found at autopsy.[483,484] At autopsy, as many as 76% of all carcinoid tumors are found in the jejunoileum, whereas these make up about 25% of tumors found in clinical and surgical series, demonstrating that most small intestinal carcinoid tumors are clinically silent. The anatomic origin of carcinoid tumors has presented a changing clinical pattern over the last 10 years.[483] There has been an approximate doubling in the percentage of all carcinoid tumors of foregut origin, primarily due to an increase in occurrence of carcinoids of the bronchus from 10% (1961–1980) to 30% (1981–1989). There was a marked decrease from 65% to 25% in the occurrence of tumors of the jejunoileum, and the occurrence of tumors of the rectum decreased from 15% to 6%.[483] The percentage of tumors in the colon, stomach, liver, pancreas, and lymph nodes remained about the same. Although the reasons for this change in distribution are not clear, the authors speculate that it is due to improved diagnostic histologic methods such as the increased use of staining with neuron-specific enolase and chromogranin, which have identified some cases originally thought to be small cell lung cancer or adenocarcinoma as carcinoid tumors.[483] The exact clinical incidence of carcinoid tumors varies in different studies. In Ireland between 1920 and 1985, they were reported to occur at an annual incidence of 13 per million population per year and were 11 times as common as insulinomas and 26 times as common as gastrinomas.[485] In a series from Scandinavia, the annual incidence of clinically significant tumors was 7 per million population per year, a rate twice that for all pancreatic endocrine tumors, 7 times that of gastrinomas, and 8 times that of insulinomas.[486–489] The clinical presentation of carcinoids underestimates their occurrence, because many are asymptomatic. This is demonstrated by recent data from the Surveillance, Epidemiology, and End Results program reporting an annual incidence of 2.8 per million population for small intestinal carcinoids.[490] An autopsy study at the Mayo Clinic found 6500 cases per million.[463] In another study, the annual incidence of malignant carcinoid tumors at autopsy was 21 per million population per year.[491]

About 1 in every 200 to 300 appendectomies has a carcinoid tumor in the resected appendix.[463] Most tumors occur in the tip of the appendix and most (about 90%) are less than 1 cm in diameter without metastases.[463,492] About 50% of those tumors between 1 and 2 cm metastasize to lymph nodes.[493]

Small intestinal carcinoids may be multiple; 87% present within the ileum and 40% present within 2 feet of the ileocecal valve.[463] Primary tumors tend to remain small. If they spread to local lymph nodes, a marked fibrotic reaction can distort the gut or mesentery and present clinically as a small bowel obstruction or mesenteric infarction. Further spread generally occurs to the liver and possibly bone. Only about 20% to 35% of small intestinal carcinoids are malignant and metastasize (see Table 41–20). About 20% to 30% of patients with ileal carcinoid have one or more additional ileal primary carcinoid tumors.[494] The incidence of metastases from small intestinal carcinoid tumors depends on the size of the primary lesion. If the tumor is less than 1 cm, metastases occur in less than 15% of cases.[463] If the tumor is between 1 and 2 cm in size, metastases occur in 60% to 80% of cases.[463] If the tumor is larger than 2 cm, metastases nearly always occur.[463] In contrast to jejunoileal carcinoids, duodenal carcinoids often are discovered by endoscopy.[495] In a recent study of 99 patients with duodenal carcinoid tumors, 21% had metastases.[495] Invasion into the muscularis propria, size, and mitotic activity all correlated with metastatic spread, with invasion being the strongest predictor. No duodenal carcinoid smaller than 1 cm metastasized, whereas 33% of the tumors larger than 2 cm or 35% of tumors invading the muscularis mucosa metastasized. In this series, 25% of the tumors stained positively for somatostatin, 20% for gastrin, and 3% for both.[495] Only 5% of patients had clinical ZES, and no patient had the somatostatinoma syndrome.

In about 1 in every 2500 proctoscopies, a small gray-yellow nodule is seen and is diagnosed as a carcinoid tumor on pathologic examination.[463] Nearly all rectal carcinoids occur submucosally on the anterior or lateral walls between 4 and 13 cm above the dentate line.[463] About 80% are smaller than 1 cm in diameter and never metastasize. Tumors between 1 and 2 cm can metastasize, and tumors larger than 2 cm (which are rare) almost always metastasize.[463,493] Colorectal carcinoids not detected at autopsy are almost entirely limited to the sigmoid colon and rectum, with most occurring in the rectum.[496] Metastatic disease occurs in about 10% of colorectal carcinoids, and in all patients with metastatic disease the tumor was larger than 2 cm in diameter and invaded the muscularis propria. Greater invasiveness correlates with increased numbers of mitoses.[496] The frequency or intensity of immunohistochemical or silver positivity does not differ between metastasizing and nonmetastasizing colorectal carcinoid tumors.[496]

As recently as 1981, bronchial carcinoids were reported to be rare, accounting for only 1% to 6% of primary lung tumors.[497] However, in a study for the years 1981 to 1989, they accounted for 30% of all carcinoid tumors.[483] Pathologic features indicating a poor prognosis for bronchial carcinoid tumors include increased mitotic count, nuclear pleomorphism, vascular invasion, undifferentiated growth pattern, and lymphatic invasion. The bronchus is the site of the primary carcinoid tumor in about 2% of cases.[497,498]

Gastric carcinoids account for 3 of every 1000 gastric neoplasms, and all gastric carcinoid tumors may not be similar.[499,500] In older studies, these tumors frequently were reported to be multifocal and metastatic (36–55% of cases) and were associated with a high mortality rate of 80%.[501,502] Muscularis propria invasion was associated with tumors larger than 2 cm. Recently, gastrin-producing argyrophil carcinoids have been found with increased frequency in patients with various causes of hypergastrinemia such as pernicious anemia, atrophic gastritis, and ZES.[466,500,503] These carcinoids have been shown to be tumors of the gastric enterochromaffin-like (ECL) cell.[499,504,505] These tumors characteristically react with argyrophil stains and chromogranin A antibodies and are negative for staining with gastrin, somatostatin, or chromogranin B.[499] Only 9% of these tumors show metastases, mostly to local lymph nodes, and only 2% show distant metastases.[499] These tumors appear to have a markedly different growth behavior from gastric carcinoids, which arise independently from hypergastrinemic states and are usually solitary.[499]

Carcinoid tumors are classified by their histologic growth patterns: insular, trabecular, glandular, undifferentiated, or mixed.[472,473] The midgut carcinoid tumors frequently possess the most typical morphology, with an insular formation of regular tumor cells, surrounded by fibrotic stroma.[472] Most foregut carcinoids show a more mixed growth pattern, with a solid, ribbon-like, trabecular, or acinar pattern. Hindgut carcinoids frequently are solid or trabecular.[472,473] The histologic types have prognostic significance.[506,507] Glandular and undifferentiated carcinoids have a worse prognosis, whereas midgut carcinoids have a better prognosis than foregut or hindgut carcinoids.[506] One study demonstrated that 27% of midgut carcinoids, which have the best prognosis, were in the favorable histologic group (insular structure), whereas there were no foregut or hindgut carcinoids, which have a worse prognosis, in the insular histologic group.[507] Multivariate analysis demonstrated that histologic type and primary site have independent prognostic significance.[507]

Neither the stimulus for malignant growth nor the factors that promote the growth of carcinoid tumors are known. For some gastric carcinoids, recent data have led most[503–505] but not all[508] investigators to conclude that gastrin may be an important growth factor. Studies have shown an increased occurrence of gastric carcinoids in disease states that result in high fasting gastrin concentrations.[499,503] In pernicious anemia and atrophic gastritis, basal hypergastrinemia develops as achlorhydria develops, and the development of endocrine cell hyperplasia, nodules of mucosal argyrophilic cells and carcinoid tumors have been reported.[466,503,505,509,510] Gastric carcinoids have been reported in some patients with ZES.[466,499,503] Rats treated for prolonged periods with omeprazole, a potent long-acting inhibitor of the gastric H^+-K^+-ATPase, or rats and other animals treated by other patent gastric antisecretory agents or by partial fundectomy, develop prolonged achlorhydria and basal hypergastrinemia that result in EC hyperplasia and gastric carcinoids.[499,503,505,511] These experimental changes occur more frequently in female rats, suggesting other hormonal factors may be involved in the development of gastric carcinoids.[499,505]

CLINICAL FEATURES

The age of patients with carcinoid tumors ranges from 10 to 93 years, with a mean of 55 years and a median age of 57.[484] In most series, the most frequent age is between 50 and 70 years.[483,484] However, in one series, 17% of patients were younger than 40 years at the time of diagnosis.[484]

Carcinoid Tumors Without Systemic Features

The presentation of carcinoid tumors that do not cause the carcinoid syndrome is diverse and related to the site of origin of the tumor and the malignant spread of the tumor. In the most common site of occurrence, the appendix, carcinoid tumors are almost always found incidentally during surgery for suspected appendicitis.[492] Small intestinal carcinoids in the jejunoileum are the most common location for carcinoid tumors of clinical significance.[463,483,484,494] Most small intestinal carcinoids do not cause symptoms, but these tumors can cause fibrosis of the mesentery, which results in kinking of the bowel, intestinal obstruction, obstruction of blood supply, and gut infarction or intussusception either secondary to the tumor itself or to direct spread of the tumor. The most common clinical presentation for small intestinal carcinoid is periodic abdominal pain that is consistent with a diagnosis of intermittent small bowel obstruction.[463,484,494] Gastrointestinal bleeding is uncommon, and small intestinal carcinoids rarely ulcerate.[463] Only 24 patients with small intestinal carcinoids have been described as presenting with bleeding.[512] Because of the vagueness of the symptoms, the diagnosis of small intestinal carcinoid is frequently delayed, with the median time of onset from symptoms to diagnosis being 2 years in one study,[463,494] with a range up to 20 years. Except for an abdominal mass with or without hepatomegaly, there are no physical signs to suggest small intestinal carcinoid tumors.[463] Duodenal and gastric carcinoids are usually found incidentally during endoscopy.[484,495,500] Rectal carcinoids are usually found incidentally during endoscopy but can occasionally be large and cause obstruction.[459,496] Rectal carcinoid tumors seldom cause bleeding. Bronchial carcinoids are usually discovered as a lesion on chest x-ray films (43% in one series).[484] Patients may present with pneumonitis (11%) or cough (7%).[484] Thymic carcinoids usually present as anterior mediastinal masses on chest x-ray films or CT scans. Ovarian and testicular carcinoids may present as masses that can be reliably detected by physical examination or ultrasound. Most carcinoids present as an isolated disease; however, foregut carcinoids are associated with MEN-I,[499,513–515] gastric carcinoids with diseases causing hypergastrinemia,[466,499,503,509,510,514–517] ampullary somatostatin-rich carcinoids with von Recklinghausen's disease,[518–520] and duodenal carcinoids with tumors causing ZES.[484,503] Metastatic carcinoid tumors frequently present in fully active and productive patients with a grossly enlarged liver, minimal symptoms, and normal or near-normal liver function test results.[463]

Carcinoid Tumors With Systemic Features

The most common systemic syndrome caused by carcinoids is the malignant carcinoid syndrome, which is discussed in the following section. Carcinoid tumors have been demonstrated to contain and occasionally secrete gastrointestinal peptides. Immunocytochemical studies have identified ACTH, gastrin, somatostatin, insulin, motilin, growth hormone, calcitonin, neurotensin, B-MSH, pancreatic polypeptide (PP), vasoactive intestinal peptide (VIP), and other peptides thought to be involved in the pathogenesis of the carcinoid syndrome.[467,470,471,521–525] Because all APUDomas are carcinoid tumors and it cannot be determined which of the gastrointestinal hormones demonstrated by immunocytochemistry or histology are released in amounts sufficient to cause symptoms, carcinoids that are found in a patient with a given clinical syndrome due to excess release of a peptide are classified by that clinical syndrome (*e.g.*, carcinoid syndrome, gastrinoma, insulinoma, somatostatinoma, GRFoma, and so forth). In studies of patients with carcinoid tumors, elevated serum concentrations of PP have been reported in 43%,[467,486] motilin in 14%,[467] and subunits of HCG in 12%.[486] A slightly elevated level of gastrin was reported in 15% of these patients,[486] and no patient had an elevated level of VIP[467] or plasma gastrin-releasing peptide.[467] Even though these gastrointestinal peptides were present in the serum, they did not appear to contribute to any clinical symptoms.

Foregut carcinoids have been reported to be more likely to produce gastrointestinal peptides than midgut carcinoids.[521] Ectopic ACTH production with Cushing's syndrome is increasingly seen with carcinoid tumors.[484] In one recent study, carcinoid tumors were the most common cause of the ectopic ACTH syndrome and accounted for 54% of all patients.[526] Foregut carcinoids are reported to be more likely than midgut carcinoids to release ACTH and cause Cushing's syndrome, whereas hindgut carcinoids are not reported to cause Cushing's syndrome.[483,521,527] Acromegaly due to growth-hormone releasing factors (GRFoma) has been reported with carcinoid tumors.[520,527,528]

The Carcinoid Syndrome

Clinical Features

Even though carcinoid tumors have been known for more than 80 years, the endocrine manifestations of these tumors were not described until 1954.[529,530] The principal clinical endocrine manifestations are cutaneous flushing, diarrhea, valvular heart disease, asthma or wheezing, and facial telangiectasia. The relative percentages of patients who have these clinical features are summarized in Table 41–21.

The cardinal feature of the carcinoid syndrome is flushing attacks, which occur in 25% to 73% of patients initially and in 63% to 94% at some time during the course of the disease (see Table 41–21). The typical flush appears as a sudden deep-

TABLE 41–21. Clinical Characteristics in Patients With Malignant Carcinoid Syndrome

	At Presentation		*During Course of Disease*		
	Davis et al, 1973[531]	*Norheim et al, 1987*[486]	*Thornson, 1958*[540]	*Feldman, 1987*[538]	*Norheim et al, 1987*[486]
No. of patients	91	91	79	111	91
Symptom (%)					
Diarrhea	73	32	68	73	84
Flushing	65	23	74	63	75
Pain	NR	10	NR	NR	NR
Asthma/wheezing	8	4	18	3	15
Pellagra	2	NR	5	NR	NR
None	12	NR	NR	22	NR
Carcinoid heart disease present	11	NR	41	14	33
Sex (% males)	59	46	61	NR	46
Mean age (y)	57	59	52	NR	NR
(Range)	(25–79)	(ND)	(18–80)		
Tumor Location (%)					
Foregut	5	9	2	NR	9
Midgut	78	87	75	NR	87
Hindgut	5	1	8	NR	1
Unknown	11	2	15	NR	2

NR, not reported.

red or violaceous erythema of the upper part of the body, primarily the face and neck. Flushes often are associated with an unpleasant feeling of warmth, occasionally with lacrimation, itching, palpitations, facial or conjunctival edema, and diarrhea. Flushes may be spontaneous or precipitated by stress, alcohol, foods such as cheese, exercise, or pharmacologically by injections of agents such as catecholamines (adrenaline, noradrenaline, isoproterenol), calcium, pentagastrin, or the COOH-terminal octapeptide of cholecystokinin.[483,484,531–537] Initially, flushing attacks may be brief, lasting only 2 to 5 minutes, although they may be prolonged for hours, especially later in syndrome. These flushes usually are seen with carcinoid tumors of midgut origin but can occur in some patients with foregut tumors.[484] Although flushing has been classified into four characteristic types,[532] the most distinctive types are those associated with bronchial carcinoids or gastric carcinoids. With bronchial carcinoids, the flushes are more frequently prolonged, last for hours to days, are reddish in color, and are associated with salivation, lacrimation, diaphoresis, facial swelling, palpitations, deep furrowing of the forehead, diarrhea, and hypotension.[484,532] The flushing with bronchial carcinoids has a greater tendency to cause diffuse body involvement, and after repeated flushing of this type, patients may develop a constant red or cyanotic coloration.[463] The flush associated with gastric carcinoids is reddish and distributed in patches over the neck and face. It is frequently provoked by food intake or pentagastrin, with erythema associated with blotches and wheals with central clearing. It frequently occurs around the root of the neck and on the arms, and the lesions frequently are associated with pruritus.[463,484,532,533,537]

Diarrhea initially is present in 32% to 78% of patients with the carcinoid syndrome and in 68% to 84% at some time during the course of the disease (see Table 41–21). If diarrhea is present, it usually occurs with flushing (85% of cases) but may occur alone (15% of cases).[484,538] Typically, the patient describes the stools as watery and less commonly as frothy or as the pale bulky stool of steatorrhea, with the stool number ranging from 2 to 30 per day.[484,531,532] Steatorrhea can occur but is unusual and much less common than diarrhea.[532,539] Abdominal pain may be present with the diarrhea or independently, and the frequency of its occurrence in carcinoid syndrome ranges from 10% to 50% in different series (see Table 41–21). In one series, 55% of patients with diarrhea had abdominal cramps at the time of the diarrhea.[540]

Cardiac manifestations have been reported in 11% to 53% of patients (see Table 41–21). The cardiac disease is due to a unique form of fibrosis involving the endocardium, primarily of the right side of the heart, although left-side lesions can occur.[532,541,542] The fibrous deposits are diffuse and are found most commonly on the ventricular aspect of the tricuspid valve and the associated chordae and less commonly on the pulmonary valve cusps. These fibrous deposits tend to constrict the tricuspid and pulmonic valves. At the pulmonic valve, stenosis is usually predominant, whereas at the tricuspid valve, where the constriction results in the valve being fixed open, tricuspid regurgitation is usually predominant, although some degree of clinical tricuspid stenosis can occur.[532,541–543] In two studies, 80% of patients with cardiac lesions had evidence of heart failure.[531,540] Simultaneous appearance of the lesions on the right and left sides of the heart occurs in 30% of autopsy cases.[542] Lesions on the left side are much less extensive than those on the right side and most frequently occur on the mitral valve.[542]

Other clinical manifestations of carcinoid syndrome are wheezing or asthma-like symptoms in 8% to 25% of patients and pellagra-like skin lesions with hyperkeratosis and pigmentation in 2% to 6% of patients (see Table 41–21). Symptoms rarely reported to occur in carcinoid syndrome are rheumatoid arthritis,[540] arthralgias,[540] changes in mental state or confusion, and ophthalmic changes during flushing leading to vessel occlusion.[540,544] Noncardiac problems secondary to increased fibrous tissue have been reported, including retroperitoneal fibrosis leading to ureteral obstruction, Peyronie's disease of the penis, intraabdominal fibrosis, and occlusion of mesenteric arteries or veins.[484,532] Sexual dysfunction is a common complaint of men with carcinoid syndrome and may be related to the vascular effects of serotonin on pelvic blood vessels.[484]

Pathobiology

The carcinoid syndrome occurs only when sufficient concentrations of the hormonal products released by the tumor reach the systemic circulation. The occurrence and severity of the carcinoid syndrome are related directly to tumor size in an area that drains into the systemic circulation.[463] In almost all cases, especially with midgut carcinoids, this only occurs after distant metastases (especially to the liver). In one study, the carcinoid syndrome was associated with the presence of hepatic metastases in 95% of patients with gastrointestinal carcinoids,[545] and with distant metastases in 100% of these patients in another study.[531] In rare cases, primary gut tumors with nodal metastases, with peritoneal metastases that are extensively invasive retroperitoneally or into the ovarian veins, or with direct access to the systemic circulation can produce the carcinoid syndrome without hepatic metastases.[531,546] Ovarian carcinoids in the absence of hepatic metastases have produced the carcinoid syndrome due to the direct venous drainage of these tumors into the systemic circulation.[546] Bronchial tumors can give rise to the carcinoid syndrome without metastatic disease; however, metastases are present in most cases.[547–549] Tumors of thyroid C cells and oat cell tumors rarely have been reported to cause the carcinoid syndrome.[532,548] All carcinoid tumors do not have the same propensity to metastasize and to produce the carcinoid syndrome (see Table 41–20). Because midgut tumors are the most common tumors and frequently metastasize, they account for 75% to 87% of the carcinoids causing the carcinoid syndrome. In most series, foregut tumors account for 2% to 9% of these carcinoids, hindgut tumors for 1% to 8%, and unknown primary locations for 2% to 15% (see Table 41–21).

In the original description of the complete carcinoid syndrome, symptoms were attributed to secretion of serotonin by the tumor.[529,530] In three reports, the carcinoid syndrome with overproduction of serotonin was estimated to occur in 6%, 10%, and 18% of patients with carcinoid tumors.[494,531,550] However, it was assumed in these reports that patients with carcinoid syndrome had overproduction of serotonin, so that serotonin production was not systematically examined in all patients with carcinoid tumors.[538] In one study of 380 patients with carcinoid tumors, 56% had evidence of serotonin overproduction.[484] Eighteen percent of 500 patients in a second study[531] and 88% of 103 patients with carcinoid tumors in a third study had elevated levels of urinary 5-hydroxyindolacetic acid (5-HIAA), the major metabolite of serotonin (Fig. 41–9).[486] In one of the above series, many patients were assessed only for serotonin overproduction after resection of the tumor, so the incidence of serotonin overproduction may be underestimated.[484] When 44 consecutive cases were studied before any resection, 84% of the patients had serotonin overproduction.[484] In two of these studies, 12% to 22% of all patients with evidence of serotonin overproduction had no symptoms, and in one study only 44% of the patients with serotonin overproduction had flushing and diarrhea.[484] Serotonin overproduction was associated with 70% of carcinoid tumors arising from the cecum, jejunum, pancreas, ileum, or an unknown site, with 25% to 40% of tumors arising from the stomach, bronchus, or thymus, with 10% to 16% of tumors arising from the duodenum and rectum, with 8% of tumors arising from the appendix, and with no tumors arising from the left colon.[484]

Patients may develop typical or atypical carcinoid syndromes (see Fig. 41–9). In patients with the typical carcinoid syndrome, the conversion of tryptophan to 5-HTP is the rate-limiting step. Once formed, the 5-HTP is rapidly converted to 5-HT in the tumor by L-dopa decarboxylase and stored in the neurosecretory tumor granules or released into vascular compartments. Most 5-HT is taken up and stored in the granules of platelets. A small amount remains in the plasma, but

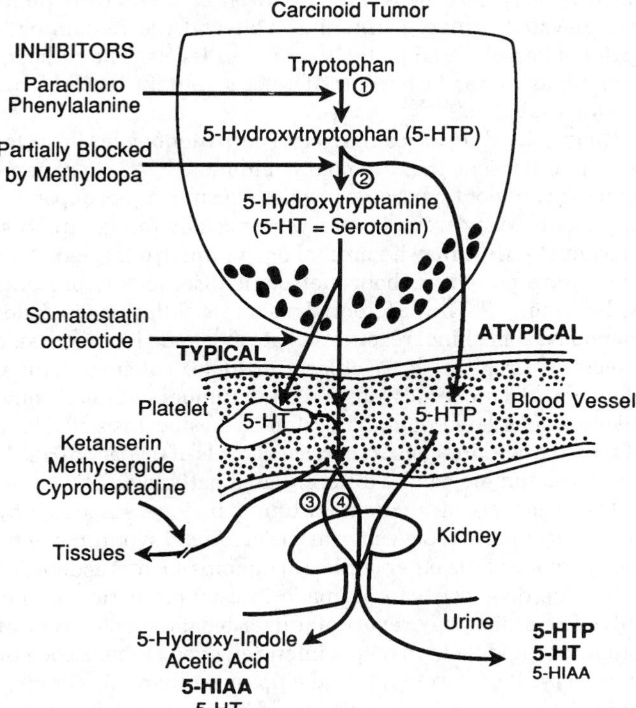

FIGURE 41–9. Synthesis, secretion, and metabolism of serotonin (5-HT) and 5-hydroxytryptophan (5-HTP) in patients with typical and atypical carcinoid syndrome. (1) Tryptophan hydroxylase; (2) Aromatic 1-amino acid decarboxylase (dopa decarboxylase); (3) Monoamine oxidase; and (4) Aldehyde dehydrogenase. Arrows indicate the sites of action of therapeutic agents used in the treatment of the carcinoid syndrome.

most 5-HT in the circulation is converted by monoamine oxidase and aldehyde dehydrogenase to 5-HIAA, which appears in large amounts in the urine (see Fig. 41–9).[538,551] Characteristically, patients with carcinoid syndrome have expansion of the serotonin pool size, increase in blood and platelet concentrations of serotonin, and elevated levels of 5-HIAA in the urine.[551] This is the typical pattern in argentaffin-positive and argyrophil-positive tumors such as midgut carcinoids, which characteristically secrete large amounts of serotonin and make up to 75% to 87% of all cases of carcinoid syndrome (see Table 41–21). Some carcinoid tumors cause an atypical carcinoid syndrome[484,521,543,552,553] and are thought to be deficient in the enzyme L-dopa decarboxylase; therefore, they cannot convert 5-HTP to 5-HT, and 5-HTP is secreted into the blood stream (see Fig. 41–9). Serotonin plasma levels are normal in these patients, but urinary levels usually are elevated because some of the 5-HTP is decarboxylated at the kidney and excreted as 5-HT. Patients with this type of carcinoid tumor may have a marked increase in urinary 5-HT and 5-HTP levels but normal or only slightly elevated 5-HIAA levels (see Fig. 41–9).[484,538] Foregut carcinoid tumors are more likely to excrete high levels of 5-HT and 5-HTP in the urine and give the atypical carcinoid syndrome.[484]

Flushing is not thought to be due to serotonin overproduction, because serotonin antagonists such as methysergide, cyproheptadine, and ketanserin generally have no effect on the flushing.[554–557] It has been proposed that serotonin has a role in provoking flushing attacks.[484,538] Early studies demonstrated that kinins, which are vasoactive substances, are released from carcinoids. Carcinoids contain kallikrein, an enzyme capable of converting plasma kininogen to lysylbradykinin, which is converted to bradykinin.[558–560] Not all patients have increased levels of bradykinin during flushing.[536,558] Moreover, a study demonstrated that plasma kallikrein levels were no different in patients with carcinoids than in normal patients and did not increase after alcohol administration, despite the fact that some patients developed a flush; these findings suggest that kallikrein levels did not cause the flush in these patients.[561] The exact etiology of the flushing in patients with carcinoid syndrome may differ depending on the tumor type. In patients with gastric carcinoids, the red, patchy, pruritic flush is thought to be caused by histamine, because this type of flushing can be prevented by the use of histamine 1 and 2 (H_1 and H_2) receptor antagonists.[534,562] Candidates for mediators of flushing seen with midgut carcinoids, which comprise 75% to 87% of all tumors causing the carcinoid syndrome (see Table 41–21), include the tachykinins (substance P, neuropeptide K) and gastrointestinal peptides or prostaglandins.[538,556,557,563] Prostaglandins E and F and other unidentified prostaglandins have been extracted from carcinoid tumors.[564] In one study, plasma prostaglandin concentrations have been shown to correlate with the severity of flushing in 1 patient, whereas in other studies there no correlation between clinical symptoms and prostaglandin blood levels.[564–566] In a review of numerous reports of prostaglandin measurements in the carcinoid syndrome and of studies generally showing a lack of effect of prostaglandin synthesis inhibitors on flushing or diarrhea in the carcinoid syndrome, the investigators concluded that prostaglandins are unlikely to be major mediators of the flushing or diarrhea in carcinoid syndrome.[567] A more recent study reached the same conclusion.[538] Studies demonstrate that numerous tachykinins are stored in carcinoid tumor and released during flushing.[467,486,557,563,568–571] One study reported that plasma levels of neuropeptide K increased during spontaneous and pentagastrin-stimulated flush.[572] Although flushing can be produced by infusion of substance P,[573] some researchers found that changes in plasma levels of substance P or neuropeptide K did not correlate with the occurrence of flushing, leading them to conclude that circulating tachykinins have a minor role or no role in flushing.[538,556,563] A recent study demonstrated that 8 of 8 patients with midgut carcinoids had elevated plasma substance P levels (*i.e.*, >10 pg/ml).[557] In addition, 88% of patients with pancreatic endocrine tumors and 71% of patients with idiopathic flushing had elevated plasma levels of substance P. With pentagastrin stimulation, plasma levels of substance P increased to more than 150 pg/ml in 50% of patients with carcinoid tumors and in 38% of patients with pancreatic endocrine tumors.[557] In this study, octreotide acutely relieved pentagastrin-induced flushing in all patients without necessarily altering the substance P response. Furthermore, pentagastrin caused flushing in some patients without rises in plasma levels of substance P, suggesting that mediators other than substance P must be important in inducing the flushing.[557] Although gastrointestinal peptides have been proposed to be involved in the flush, no changes in gastric inhibitory peptide, neurotensin, VIP, PP, motilin, insulin, glucagon, or enteroglucagon occurred with provocation of the flush.[561] The exact etiology of flushing in the carcinoid syndrome remains unexplained.

Serotonin is thought to be responsible for the diarrhea by means of its effects on gut motility.[538,574,575] It may cause fat malabsorption and probably induces a secretory state in the small intestine.[538,575,576] Furthermore, serotonin receptor antagonists (methysergide, cyproheptadine, and ketanserin) have been shown to relieve diarrhea but not flushing.[554–556,577,578] In combination with histamine, serotonin may be responsible for producing asthma[579] and may be involved in the fibrotic reactions that contribute to heart disease, Peyronie's disease, and ureteral obstruction.[521,532,556] The pathogenetic link between the carcinoid tumor and the characteristic heart disease remains a subject of debate.[484] No correlation has been established between the severity of the heart disease and other common manifestations such as flushing, diarrhea, or duration of disease.[484,580] Patients with heart disease have higher levels of urinary 5-HIAA excretion and higher plasma levels of neurokinin A and substance P than those without heart disease.[580]

Diagnosis

Diagnosis of the carcinoid syndrome relies on the measurement of levels of serotonin or its metabolites in the urine. The most commonly used test is measurement of 5-HIAA levels in a 24-hour urine sample. False-positive results may occur if the patient is eating serotonin-rich foods such as bananas, plantains, pineapple, kiwi fruit, walnuts, hickory nuts, pecans, and avocados, which elevate urinary levels of 5-HIAA.[581] Medications that contain guaifenesin, acetaminophen, salicylates, and L-dopa (*e.g.*, cough medicine) should be avoided because they may affect urinary 5-HIAA levels.[483,582]

Although a simple and inexpensive qualitative test can be used to measure increased excretion of 5-HIAA in the urine, the test is only positive if patients excrete more than 30 mg of 5-HIAA daily.[484,583] If the urine collection bottle is not refrigerated, the addition of acid before the urine collection is necessary to prevent oxidation.[484] With properly controlled dietary and medicinal intake, the normal range for urinary 5-HIAA excretion is between 2 and 8 mg every 24 hours.[484] Many patients with serotonin-secreting carcinoid tumors have an increase in urinary 5-HIAA excretion in the range of 8 to 30 mg/24 hours, making the quantitative test measuring urinary 5-HIAA levels the preferred method for diagnosing carcinoid syndrome.[584] Determination of 5-HIAA levels alone has a 73% sensitivity and a 100% specificity for the carcinoid syndrome.[538]

Most physicians rely on the measurement of urinary 5-HIAA for diagnosis; however, urinary and platelet measurement of serotonin levels may give additional information and it has been recommended recently that serotonin levels should be measured.[484,538,584] Elevated levels of 5-HIAA can occur in malabsorption states.[532,577] Foregut carcinoids tend to produce an atypical carcinoid syndrome with increases in plasma 5-HTP levels but not in serotonin levels because they lack the appropriate decarboxylase (see Fig. 41–9), with the result that urinary 5-HIAA is usually not markedly increased.[484] Patients with a normal or minimally elevated 5-HIAA should be screened for other urinary metabolites of tryptophan if there is a strong suspicion of the carcinoid syndrome.[584] Usually this is not necessary because some of the 5-HTP is decarboxylated in the intestine and other tissues and many of these patients have elevated levels of urinary 5-HT or 5-HIAA (see Fig. 41–9).[537,584] In an evaluation of 75 patients with known carcinoid tumors, 15 patients had normal or borderline elevated urinary 5-HIAA levels.[584] Eleven of these 15 patients had elevated urinary serotonin levels and the remaining 4 patients had elevated platelet serotonin levels. The radioenzymatic assay for urinary or platelet serotonin levels is not readily available.[584–586]

Diagnostic difficulties may arise in patients who flush for reasons other than the carcinoid syndrome,[483,484,587] in patients with the carcinoid syndrome in whom flushing is not apparent, in patients with carcinoid tumors, especially foregut tumors, in whom 5-HIAA may be normal or minimally elevated,[584] or in the rare patient without metastatic disease who presents with flushing.[546] The differential diagnosis of flushing includes menopausal flushing, reactions to alcohol and glutamate, side effects of drugs such as chlorpropamide, calcium-channel blockers, and nicotinic acid, and other tumors such as chronic myelogenous leukemia and systemic mastocytosis.[587] None of these conditions causes increased levels of urinary 5-HIAA, and these tumors can be differentiated pathologically.

The diagnosis of a carcinoid tumor may be suspected by clinical symptoms suggestive of the carcinoid syndrome or by the presence of the other clinical symptoms such as abdominal pain. The diagnosis can be made in asymptomatic patients only after a histology report of a liver biopsy specimen or of a tumor or nodule biopsy specimen removed at endoscopy or at surgery. Ileal carcinoids make up more than 25% of clinically detected carcinoids and should be suspected if a patient presents with bowel obstruction, abdominal pain, flushing, or diarrhea.[484] In a study of 154 consecutive patients with gastrointestinal carcinoid tumors, 60% of those tumors found at surgery were asymptomatic and 40% were symptomatic.[493] In patients with symptomatic carcinoid tumors, the time from the onset of symptoms until the diagnosis is frequently delayed, varying from 1 to 2 years in different studies.[463,486] Attempts are being made to identify specific and sensitive serum markers for carcinoid tumors that allow earlier diagnosis.[467,470,471,484,486,538,557] In one study, measurement of levels of urinary 5-HIAA had a sensitivity of 73% and a specificity of 100%, levels of plasma substance P had a sensitivity of 32% and a specificity of 85%, and levels of plasma neurotensin had a sensitivity of 41% and a specificity of 60%.[467] In another study, 88% of patients with carcinoid tumors (93% with hepatic metastases) had elevated levels of 5-HIAA, 66% has elevated levels of plasma neuropeptide K, and 43% has elevated plasma PP concentrations.[486] In a recent study, plasma levels of substance P were reported to be elevated in 100% of patients with carcinoid tumors, and in 88% of patients with pancreatic endocrine tumors, demonstrating a low specificity.[557] When a value of 50 pg/ml was used as the cutoff (normal <10 pg/ml), 63% of patients with carcinoid tumors were positive, whereas none of the noncarcinoid tumors was positive.[557] Plasma elevations of substance P were reported in 100% of 47 patients with carcinoid tumors, of whom 13 patients had midgut carcinoids and 3 had foregut carcinoids.[557] In another study of 30 patients with limited disease carcinoid tumors, all patients had an elevated plasma chromogranin levels using an antibody that recognizes chromogranin A and B, whereas only 3 patients had increased urinary 5-HIAA levels.[470] These results suggest that plasma chromogranin A and B levels may be useful in recognizing carcinoid tumors. The α-HCG or β-HCG subunits of human chorionic gonadotropin are reported to be present in carcinoid tumors as determined by immunocytochemistry,[588] and elevated plasma levels of HCG are reported in 28% of carcinoid tumors.[540,589] In a review of an ongoing prospective study, it was pointed out that HCG levels are elevated in the plasma in a much lower percentage of cases than the literature suggests; therefore, it is unlikely to be useful in diagnosis.[484] Although CEA antigen is elevated in some neuroendocrine tumors, it is usually normal or minimally elevated in patients with metastatic carcinoid tumors.[590] Markedly elevated levels suggest the presence of a second tumor.[484]

Because measurements of urinary 5-HIAA levels and plasma assays of amines or peptides are unable to identify all patients with carcinoid tumors, various provocative tests have been proposed. Adrenergic agents[535,591] and pentagastrin can stimulate flushing attacks.[533,557] Pentagastrin has been used as a provocative test in patients with carcinoid tumors,[533,538,557] and caused flushing in 100% of patients in two series.[555,557] In one study, more than 75% of patients demonstrated enhanced release of substance P after pentagastrin stimulation,[557] whereas in another study none of the patients demonstrated increased levels after pentagastrin.[555] In one study, 50% of patients demonstrated an increase of more than 150 pg/ml in plasma levels of substance P; however, 38% of patients with pancreatic endocrine tumors also demonstrated an increase, suggesting this test may be of limited usefulness.[557] Provocative tests have been used in too few patients to assess their potential usefulness.

Localization

Many techniques have been used to determine the location of the primary tumor and the tumor extent, including gastrointestinal endoscopy, gastrointestinal barium x-ray films, chest x-ray films, imaging studies (ultrasound, CT scan, MRI, angiography), selective venous sampling for hormones, and radionuclide scanning (radiolabeled octreotide, iodinated MIBG).[483,484]

Bronchial carcinoids usually are detected by chest x-ray film, MRI, and CT and occasionally are detected by bronchoscopy.[484,526,549] The bronchial carcinoid tumors appear most frequently (37%) as opacities with sharp or notched margins.[592] They were slow growing and often induced airway compression with resultant atelectasis, and enlarged hilar lymph nodes from metastasis were rare.[592] Rectal, colonic, and gastric carcinoids almost always are detected by gastrointestinal endoscopy, with barium x-ray films generally having negative results.[493,500] In one study, positive barium x-ray studies showed dilated loops of small bowel or extrinsic filling defects but rarely detected a mucosal lesion,[493] whereas ileal, cecal, and right colon tumors were diagnosed or suggested on x-ray studies by others.[483,593,594]

The main problem is in localizing small bowel carcinoids, which may be small and frequently are missed by barium studies,[594] and small carcinoids in other gastrointestinal tissues.[483] Some of these tumors can be localized by angiography[595,596] or CT scanning[596–598] but many are not seen with these modalities. Liver metastases usually are detected by CT scanning, however, and angiography remains the most sensitive method for detecting liver metastases.[484,596,597,599,600] CT scanning is the primary diagnostic modality for tumor staging. Liver lesions appear as focal hypodense lesions on nonenhanced CT scans.[600]

Recently, scanning with ^{123}I-MIBG or ^{131}I-MIBG either alone or with CT scanning has been recommended for carcinoid tumors.[483,484,601,602] ^{125}I-MIBG, which is concentrated by a sodium-dependent neuronal pump in pheochromocytomas, is also concentrated by carcinoid tumors. In a recent review of a number of series, the overall sensitivity was reported as 55% with a specificity of 95%.[483] In a study of 82 patients with carcinoid tumors, ^{131}I-MIBG identified 59% of the primary or distant metastatic sites, localized 68% of ileal carcinoids, and localized 64% of patients with an unknown carcinoid site. In only 38% of patients did ^{131}I-MIBG localize foregut tumors.[601] ^{131}I-MIBG was more likely to accumulate in patients with elevated urinary 5-HIAA levels (70%), elevated urinary serotonin levels (70%), and elevated serum serotonin levels (80%), than in patients with normal 5-HIAA levels (23%), urinary serotonin levels (44%), or plasma serotonin levels (12%).[601] However, the likelihood of the ^{131}I-MIBG scan being positive did not correlate with the presence of absence of the carcinoid syndrome (68% versus 44%).[601] In general, ^{131}I-MIBG was more useful for visualizing metastatic tumors than for identifying the primary tumor.[484,601] Because the liver concentrates a small amount of ^{131}I-MIBG, the combination of a ^{99m}Tc-liver-spleen scan and ^{131}I-MIBG scan is recommended to detect liver involvement.[484]

Carcinoid tumors possess high-affinity receptors for the hormone somatostatin in 87% of cases.[603] The somatostatin receptors were present in the primary tumor and in the metastases.[603] Recently, ^{123}I-labeled octreotide, a synthetic somatostatin analog that has a high affinity for somatostatin receptors and is only slowly degraded, has been used to localize carcinoid tumors and pancreatic endocrine tumors.[604–606] In one study, primary tumors or metastases, often previously unrecognized, were identified in 12 of 13 patients with carcinoid tumors.[606] Metastatic tumor in the liver was detected in 85% of cases, and primary tumor in the ileum was detected in all 6 cases.[606] In more than 50% of patients, extensive metastatic disease that had not been appreciated by other modalities was detected.[606] However, only a small number of patients have been assessed with iodinated MIBG or octreotide and compared with patients assessed by widely used imaging modalities such as CT with or without contrast or MRI. Therefore, the roles of these two new methods have not been defined clearly.

Bone metastases are increasingly being recognized in patients with metastatic carcinoid and pancreatic endocrine tumors.[606–608] In one recent study of 12 patients with carcinoid tumors, of which 11 had liver metastases, bony metastases were found in 8 patients (75%) using ^{125}I-radiolabeled octreotide.[606] In general, ^{99m}Tc bone scanning is more sensitive than conventional radiographs for detecting metastases to bone.[484,607]

Prognosis

The carcinoid syndrome is generally a manifestation of advanced disease. Two of every 3 patients with the carcinoid syndrome have physical signs of cancer such as an abdominal mass or hepatomegaly.[463] In the remaining patients, the disease is easy to identify on imaging studies. A positive correlation between tumor mass and urinary 5-HIAA levels makes this laboratory test a good marker for extent of disease.[463,506,531] Flushing alone does not indicate an extremely poor prognosis or the need for immediate aggressive intervention. Patients with elevated levels of urinary 5-HIAA may have only minimal symptoms such as occasional flushing or mild diarrhea for many years.

Survival rates depend on the site and the extent of the carcinoid tumors.[482] For patients with local disease only, the 5-year survival was found to be 94%, ranging from 75% for carcinoids of the small intestine and ileum to 99% for carcinoids of the appendix (Table 41–22). In patients with regional involvement, 5-year survival was 64% overall, ranging from 23% for the stomach to 100% for the appendix. For patients with distant metastases, the overall 5-year survival was 18%, ranging from no survival with carcinoids of the stomach to 19% for carcinoids of the small intestine. Five-year survival rates were highest for carcinoids of the appendix (92%–99%),[463,482] followed by lung (87%),[482] rectum (76%–100%),[482,493,609,610] small intestine (42%–71%),[463,482,494,611,612] and colon and stomach (52%; see Table 41–22).[482] The chance of finding regional invasion or metastatic disease is directly proportional to the size of the primary tumors.[463,612–615] If carcinoid tumors are smaller than 1 cm in diameter, less than 15% to 18% of patients with small bowel primaries have metastases, up to 20% with rectal primaries have metastases, and up to 2% with appendiceal primaries have metastases.[463,486,492,610] Of patients with carcinoid tumors larger than 2 cm in diameter, 86% to 95% with small bowel primaries have metastases, almost all with rectal primaries have metastases, and 33% with appendiceal primaries have metastases.[463,494,610] For all patients with carcinoid tumors, the reported 5-year survivals range from 65% to 82%.[482,486] Race, age, and sex have no influence on survival.[482]

The histologic stage of the carcinoid tumor has been shown to correlate with disease-specific survival and the risk of metastases.[493,495,496,612,613] In one recent study, carcinoid tumors were staged according to Dukes' classification and demonstrated a 10-year disease-specific survival of 100% for Dukes' A (n=3 patients), 80% for Dukes' B (n=12 patients), 55% for Dukes' C (n=22 patients), and 10% for Dukes' D classification.[612] Recently, flow cytometry has been used to define the malignant potential for gastrointestinal and bronchial carcinoids.[616–621] In two studies of gastrointestinal carcinoids, aneuploidy was found in 5% and 45% of patients and tetraploidy in 5% and 6% of patients.[616,619] The presence of metastases or decreased survival correlated with the presence of aneuploidy. In bronchial carcinoids, aneuploidy was reported to occur in 50% to 79% in two studies.[621,622] In some studies[621–623] but not others,[624] flow cytometry was able to predict the presence of metastasis or decreased survival. In one study, aneuploidy was seen significantly more frequently in atypical tumors (74% of cases) than in typical bronchial carcinoid tumors (18%; $p<0.001$).[622]

The median survivals reported for patients with carcinoid syndrome from the time of the onset of symptoms range from 3.5 to 8.5 years, and the presence of the carcinoid syndrome is associated with decreased survival.[486,531] The mean survival

TABLE 41–22. Prognosis of Carcinoid Tumors

Site	No. of Patients	Patients With Metastases (%)	5-Year Survival (%) Local	Regional Metastasis	Distant Metastasis	All Stages
Appendix	820	5	99	100	27	99
Rectum	295	15	92	44	7	83
Lung and bronchus	190	21	96	71	11	87
Small intestine and ileocecum	366	60	75	59	19	54
Colon	112	71	77	65	17	52
Stomach	41	54	93	23	0	52
All sites	1824	23	94	64	18	82

(Modified from Godwin JD. Carcinoid tumors: an analysis of 2837 cases. Cancer 1975;36:560)

after recognition of abnormal excretion of 5-HIAA was 23 months,[531] and the 5-year survivals after onset of symptoms in two studies were 30% and 67%.[486,531] Although an occasional patient lives for 30 years with carcinoid syndrome,[463] and some may live for many years excreting 300 to 400 mg of 5-HIAA per day,[531] the level of urinary 5-HIAA excretion generally correlates with survival.[531] In one study, patients who excreted 10 to 49 mg of 5-HIAA daily had a mean survival of 29 months; those with daily 5-HIAA excretions of 50 to 149 mg had a mean survival of 24 months; and those excreting more than 150 mg of 5-HIAA daily had a mean survival of 13 months.[531]

The most immediate life-threatening complication of the carcinoid syndrome, the carcinoid crisis, is observed more frequently in patients who have intense symptoms from foregut carcinoids or who have greatly elevated urinary 5-HIAA levels (>200 mg/day).[625] The carcinoid crisis may occur spontaneously or may be associated with stress, anesthesia, chemotherapy, or even biopsy of hepatic metastases.[463,626–629] Patients usually develop an intense flush, diarrhea, and abdominal pain. Mentation is altered, ranging from lightheadedness to coma. Cardiac abnormalities may occur, including tachycardia, hypertension, or profound hypotension. This crisis can be treated successfully but in many patients may be a terminal event.[463,625,626] Recent treatment strategies using the somatostatin analog octreotide have improved the treatment of carcinoid crises greatly, and these methods are discussed in the next section.

Treatment of the Carcinoid Syndrome

Many patients can have hepatic metastases from carcinoid tumor and remain active and well except for occasional episodes of flushing or diarrhea. Management of these patients includes avoiding stress and conditions or substances that precipitate flushing and dietary supplementation with nicotinamide (Fig. 41–10).[521] Heart failure may require diuretics, wheezing may require oral bronchodilators (*e.g.*, salbutamol, a bronchodilator that interacts with β-adrenergic receptors and does not induce flushing, or aminophylline), and mild diarrhea may respond to antidiarrheal agents (*e.g.*, loperamide or diphenoxylate; see Fig. 41–10). If patients still have carcinoid syndrome symptoms, agents that may help relieve the flushing, diarrhea, or wheezing should be used on a trial-and-error basis. These agents act in various ways: they inhibit the synthesis of serotonin, act as serotonin receptor antagonists, block the action of serotonin on target tissues, or inhibit the release of vasoactive substances. Parachlorophenylalanine blocks the hydroxylase enzyme that converts tryptophan to 5-HTP (see Fig. 41–9) and has been shown to relieve diarrhea and improve flushing in some patients and to reduce urinary levels of 5-HIAA.[625,630] The side effects of this agent, including hypersensitivity reactions and psychiatric disturbances, make it intolerable for long-term clinical use.[625,630] Alpha-methyldopa partially blocks the conversion of 5-HTP to serotonin (see Fig. 41–9), but its effect is partial.[537] It occasionally relieves flushing, which may be secondary to inhibiting catecholamine-stimulated release of vasoactive substances, and has little effect on gastrointestinal symptoms.[521,532] Phenoxybenzamine, an α-adrenergic antagonist, and phenothiazines, possibly acting as α-adrenergic antagonists, may block flushing provoked by alcohol or other agents, although patients frequently become refractory.[521,532,554,577] The serotonin receptor antagonists methylsergide,[554] cyproheptadine,[577,578,631–633] and,

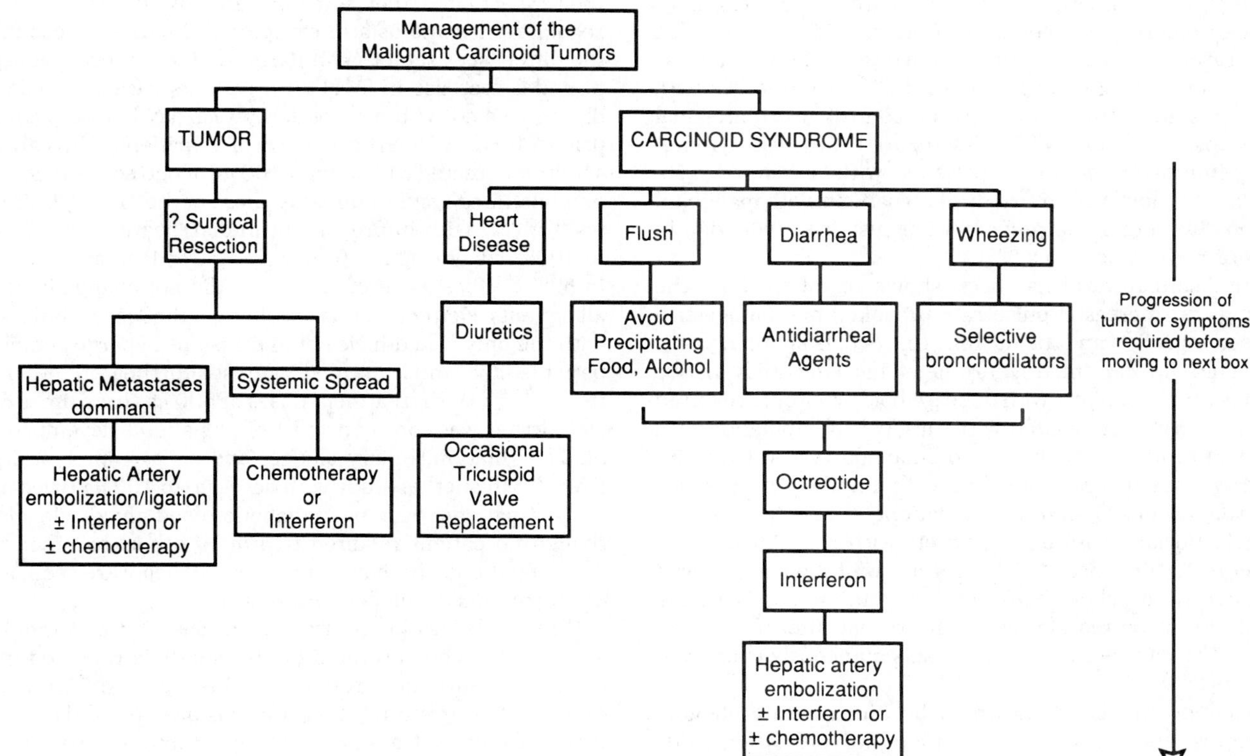

FIGURE 41–10. Flow diagram for the treatment of malignant carcinoid tumors.

more recently, ketanserin[634,635] have been used with success to treat gastrointestinal symptoms such as diarrhea but usually do not decrease flushing. In one study, cyproheptadine used at a dose of 3 to 8 mg three times daily reduced diarrhea in 50% of patients, with minimal or no effect on flushing or excretion of 5-HIAA.[463] In a study of 16 patients with carcinoid syndrome who were given up to 48 mg of cyproheptadine daily, diarrhea decreased by 50% or more in 58%, flushing decreased more than 50% in 17%, and levels of 5-HIAA did not decrease more than 50% in any patient.[578] Cyproheptadine was discontinued in 19% of patients because of side effects.[578] The recommended starting dose is 0.4 mg/kg/day given in divided portions and then reduced to a level that produces only minimal side effects.[578] If no benefit is seen in 1 week, the drug should be discontinued. Cyproheptadine is reported to have antitumor activity.[578,633] The use of methysergide is limited because it can cause or enhance retroperitoneal fibrosis. Ketanserin, like cyproheptadine, is a selective serotonin type II (S_2) receptor antagonist and has weak α-blocking and H_1 receptor blocking properties.[635] In one placebo-controlled study, a daily dose of 40 to 160 mg of ketanserin diminished the frequency and severity of flushing in 70% of patients and of diarrhea in 30% of patients.[635] In another study, ketanserin controlled pentagastrin-provoked flushing, dyspnea, and diarrhea in all patients (n=6).[634] Ketanserin decreased pentagastrin-provoked gastrointestinal symptoms in 93% of patients in another study, whereas flushing was controlled in only 6% of patients.[655] In open trials, ketanserin decreased the severity and frequency of flushing in 68% of 31 patients and lessened diarrhea in 75% of 29 patients.[634,636] An antagonist of the S_3 receptor recently has been reported to decrease diarrhea in patients with the carcinoid syndrome.[637] A combination of H_1- and H_2-receptor antagonists has been reported to be effective in carcinoid syndrome due to gastric carcinoids.[534] Prednisone in doses of 20 mg/day has been reported to give occasional relief in some cases with severe flushing, although it does not control gastrointestinal symptoms.[521,532] Tamoxifen was reported to cause symptomatic improvement in 2 patients with carcinoid syndrome.[638,639] However, in a study of 16 patients with malignant carcinoid tumors, no improvement or sustained reduction in levels of 5-HIAA occurred.[640]

Native somatostatin has been shown to inhibit both the flushing and increased pulse rate provoked by pentagastrin and food ingestion and the flushing that occurs spontaneously in patients with carcinoid syndrome.[533] In a later study, native somatostatin in patients with the carcinoid syndrome reversed the hypotension associated with surgical manipulation of a carcinoid tumor,[641] inhibited the cutaneous vasodilation induced by ethanol or norepinephrine,[642] inhibited the diarrhea and bronchoconstriction in one patient,[643] and reversed intestinal chloride secretion in a patient with a carcinoid tumor and secretory diarrhea.[644] The usefulness of the natural form is limited by its short half-life (2.5–3 minutes). With the availability of octreotide, which has a half-life of 90 minutes,[645,646] treatment can be given subcutaneously every 6 to 12 hours.[645–647]

Octreotide has been shown to be effective at relieving symptoms and decreasing hormone levels when self-administered every 6 to 12 hours subcutaneously in patients with carcinoid syndrome[463,648–652] and pancreatic endocrine tumors, which are discussed in a later section (see Pancreatic Endocrine Tumors). Octreotide recently has been shown to decrease serotonin and neuropeptide K release from midgut carcinoids by a direct action on tumor cells.[653] Octreotide inhibited release of serotonin and neuropeptide K from tumor cell cultures prepared from 4 midgut carcinoids and the synthesis of these substances by the tumor cells.[653] In Mayo Clinic studies of 53 patients with carcinoid syndrome, octreotide caused complete improvement in flushing in 53% and a 50% or more decrease in an additional 32%.[463,650,654] Diarrhea was completely improved in 25% of patients and partially improved in an additional 49%.[463,650] Levels of 5-HIAA excretion decreased by 50% or more in 68% of all patients and were reduced to normal in 5%.[463,650,654] Only 7% failed to respond in any way.[463] Forty percent of patients escaped from control after a median time of 4 months, with the remaining patients having sustained control for up to 2.5 years with all responding for more than 1 year and 33% for more than 2 years.[463] The recommended starting dose is 150 μg subcutaneously three times a day.[655] Results with octreotide vary. In one study of 23 patients, in which an objective response was defined as more than a 50% decrease in 5-HIAA levels, plasma neuropeptide K levels or tumor size were reported to decrease significantly in only 28% of patients,[652] whereas in the earlier studies,[463,650,654] 68% of patients showed such a response. In the recent study, 50% of patients showed a subjective response with less diarrhea or flushing.[652] The octreotide dose had to be increased to maintain this response in all patients. The difference between these two studies is that in the latter study patients were started on a low dose (50 μg twice daily ×6 months) then increased, whereas in the earlier study patients were treated with 150 μg three times daily.[463,650,654] The authors speculated that starting with low doses may down-regulate the somatostatin receptor and partially account for the differences seen.[652] Similarly, Richter and colleagues reported a decrease in 5-HT in 8 patients with carcinoid syndrome treated with octreotide 150 μg/day but no change in urinary 5-HIAA.[656] A recent study of 14 patients with carcinoid syndrome treated with at least 100 μg of octreotide twice daily demonstrated results similar to those of the Mayo Clinic studies,[463,650,654] with improvement in diarrhea in 83%, flushing in 100%, wheezing in 100%, and a 50% decrease in 5-HIAA in 62%.[651] Plasma serotonin levels did not change in almost all patients. Octreotide was excellent in the Mayo Clinic study, with the only side effects being transient hyperglycemia in 2 patients and mild to moderate steatorrhea in other patients.[463,650] With treatment doses of 500 μg three times daily, steatorrhea was common and 1 of 28 patients developed gallbladder dilation, biliary sludge, and an asymptomatic gallstone.[655] In another study with doses up to 100 μg twice daily, 36% of patients developed diabetic blood glucose levels, although no patient required treatment other than diet.[652] In 43% of patients, borborygmus and diarrhea were seen, and 1 of 23 patients developed bradycardia.

Octreotide has been effective in cases of carcinoid crisis.[629,655,657] The carcinoid crisis usually is reported in patients with foregut carcinoids and more than 250 mg/day of 5-HIAA excretion. It frequently is precipitated by stressful situations such as chemotherapy, tumor biopsy, or anesthesia and may result in death. The use of octreotide may be life-saving.[463,626–629,655,657]

Interferon-α is reported to be effective in the carcinoid syndrome either alone[658–662] or with hepatic artery embolization.[662,663] In one study, patients improved significantly and there was a reduction in 5-HIAA excretion in 12 of 36 patients (42%).[658] In another study, flushing and diarrhea improved in 75% of patients, but the positive effect for diarrhea disappeared by 1 year of treatment.[661] In a study in which 24 patients with malignant carcinoid syndrome were treated with 24 million units/m^2 body surface area (24 mU/m^2), 39% had a decrease in 5-HIAA excretion, flushing improved in 65%, and diarrhea improved in 33%.[662] These responses were transient, lasting a median of only 7 weeks. Human interferon-2b has been combined with hepatic embolization in 7 patients and compared with interferon given alone in 12 patients (5 mU/daily) with the carcinoid syndrome.[663] Evaluation after 1 year of treatment showed that a 50% decrease in urinary levels of 5-HIAA with interferon alone in 50% of patients; when combined with embolization, 71% of patients had such a decrease. With interferon alone, 58% of patients had decreased flushing and 67% had decreased diarrhea, whereas with embolization 86% had decreased flushing and 43% decreased diarrhea.[663]

For a patient with severe carcinoid syndrome who does not respond to other measures, hepatic artery embolization or ligation either alone or combined with interferon or chemotherapy may be effective (see Fig. 41–10).[463,662–669] In two recent studies involving 32 patients with metastatic liver disease and the carcinoid syndrome, hepatic artery embolization or ligation resulted in 50% decrease in urinary 5-HIAA levels in 63% of patients.[668,669] In the largest study, diarrhea and flushing disappeared in all patients immediately after the procedure, and 61% were free of symptoms at 1 year later.[669] Chemoembolization with gelfoam embolization and simultaneous chemotherapy (doxorubicin, mitomycin, cisplatin) was reported to result in symptomatic improvement in a significant number of patients with carcinoid syndrome.[463,666,667] Hepatic artery occlusion can have significant side effects, however, including septicemia. In one study, 5% of patients died of a complication of hepatic artery occlusion.[666] The mortality is reported as less than 3%, pain occurs in 100%, pyrexia and leukocytosis occur in 50%, and there can be occasional acute gangrenous cholecystitis from obstruction of the cystic artery, hepatic abscess, paralytic ileus, and renal failure.[668]

The approach to treatment of the carcinoid syndrome is summarized in Figure 41–10. After symptomatic treatment, patients should avoid precipitating food and alcohol. Oral antidiarrheal agents are given for mild diarrhea and oral selective bronchodilators for wheezing. Octreotide in a dose of 100 to 150 μg three times daily subcutaneously is the drug of choice, self-administered by the patient. If tachyphylaxis develops, the dose can be increased. If symptoms recur, are severe, and do not respond to an increased octreotide dose, serotonin receptor antogonists such as cyproheptadine or ketanserin should be considered. If these agents are ineffective, interferon should be considered.

TREATMENT OF THE CARCINOID TUMOR

Surgery should be considered as the only potentially curative therapy in patients with carcinoids (see Fig. 41–10). Resection of local disease or resection of local and regional nodal metastatic disease can result in cure in some patients. Because the probability of metastatic disease is directly related to primary tumor size in most carcinoid tumors, the extent of surgical resection for possible cure should be determined accordingly. In the case of appendiceal tumors smaller than 1 cm in diameter without gross metastases (more than 98% of cases encountered in the appendix), a simple appendectomy is sufficient.[463] Of 103 such patients treated with simple appendectomy, of whom 103 were followed for 5 years and 83 for 10 to 35 years, no patient developed a local recurrence or metastatic disease.[463,492] With rectal carcinoids smaller than 1 cm, local resection is adequate and results in cure.[463,496,670,671] There is no agreement about treatment of intestinal carcinoids smaller than 1 cm. In two series, 15% and 18% of tumors less than 1 cm had metastases; in other series, 69% of tumors smaller than 0.5 cm had metastases.[672] One group concluded that with midgut carcinoids malignancy is independent of size.[672] This had led one group to recommend a wide resection with en bloc resection of the adjacent lymph node-bearing mesentery for all small intestinal carcinoids.[493] If the carcinoid tumor is 2 cm or larger, which is uncommon in the case of carcinoids of the rectum or appendix but occurs in 40% of small bowel carcinoids, a full-scale cancer operation should be done.[463] In the case of a carcinoid tumor of the appendix that is 2 cm or larger, a right hemicolectomy is the operation of choice.[463,492,493] In such a tumor in the rectum, an abdominoperineal resection or a low anterior resection with primary anastomosis is recommended.[493] In one recent study, all 13 cases of patients with rectal carcinoid tumors greater than 2 cm died of metastatic complications with a median survival of 10 months after abdominal perineal or low anterior resection.[671] The investigators concluded that radical surgery is inappropriate if anorectal carcinoids can be removed by local excision. In the case of a small intestinal carcinoid 2 cm or larger, a wide resection is recommended with en bloc resection of the adjacent lymph node-bearing mesentery.[493] For carcinoids of the appendix between 1 and 2 cm, some surgeons recommend simple appendectomy,[463,492] whereas others favor partial cecectomy for those lesions located at the base of the appendix to ensure clear margins[493] or formal right hemicolectomy. For carcinoids of the rectum between 1 and 2 cm, it is estimated that only 11% have metastases.[673] It is recommended that these tumors be locally resected with a wide local full-thickness excision[671] and that tumors found to invade the muscularis propria undergo abdominoperineal or low anterior resection.[463,493,674] For gastric and duodenal carcinoids, lesions smaller than 1 cm can be locally excised[493,674] or removed endoscopically.[500,675] With larger gastric tumors, there is no agreement about the best course of treatment. If the tumor is greater than 2 cm or there is local invasion, some recommend total gastrectomy.[493,674] Another study recommends that larger tumors (2 cm or more in diameter) without muscle invasion be resected locally.[500] It is not clear whether gastric carcinoids arising in patients with atrophic gastritis or pernicious anemia should be treated differently.[675] Of 137 cases arising in patients with hypergastrinemic states, only 9% developed metastases, whereas of those arising outside of these hypergastrinemia states, 55% had metastases.[499]

Resection of isolated hepatic metastases may be markedly beneficial or curative in selected patients.[625] In one series, 10 patients who apparently had isolated areas of hepatic metastases in a surgically accessible region of the liver were chosen for possible resection.[463,625] All patients with carcinoid syndrome had symptomatic relief, and 5-HIAA levels were reduced to normal. Although only one patient was cured, the mean survival was 5 years and extended to 13.5 years in 1 patient.[463] In the presence of extensive metastases, partial hepatic resection is not indicated. One study has recommended debulking mesenteric metastases and removal of compromised intestinal segments even in the presence of liver metastases.[672] In this study of 138 patients with midgut carcinoids of whom 51 patients were subjected to surgery with the principal aim of removing the primary and debulking mesenteric metastases, the researchers concluded that surgery provided considerable symptomatic relief.[672] A similar approach involving a aggressive surgical debulking combined with transarterial embolization of hepatic arteries has been used recently in patients with carcinoid syndrome.[676]

Although a study reported that radiation therapy induced a prolonged disease-free remission for carcinoid tumors with metastases,[677] a follow-up study from the same group showed no benefit.[678] In general, radiation therapy has not been useful in the treatment of metastatic carcinoid tumors, except for treatment of symptomatic bone and skin metastases.[521] In one recent study, radiation therapy was used in 44 patients with symptomatic metastatic carcinoid tumors.[679] Survival was not prolonged, although substantial palliation was achieved in most cases. Of 8 patients with intracranial lesions, none demonstrated progression of these lesions (median dose of 3300 cGy). Local control of osseus or epidural metastases was achieved in 78% and 77% of sites respectively, and local control was obtained in 62% of patients with intraabdominal disease.[679] It is recommended that nonhepatic sites be treated with 4500 to 5000 cGy over 4 to 5 weeks.[679]

Because MIBG frequently is taken up by carcinoid tumors and concentrated, the possibility of using radiolabeled MIBG therapeutically has been evaluated recently in a small number of patients.[483,680–683] In three studies involving 10 patients with metastatic carcinoid tumors, 3 patients had decreased urinary excretion of 5-HIAA.[680–683] In one study, 20% of patients had a decrease of 50% or more.[680]

There is no general agreement on when, or even if, chemotherapy should be started in patients with malignant carcinoid tumors. One group with considerable experience suggests that only patients suffering from significant symptoms or disability due to malignant disease or syndromes or those who have a poor prognosis should undergo chemotherapy.[463] The signs of poor prognosis include impaired liver function, high levels of 5-HIAA (150 mg/day or more), or clinical evidence of carcinoid heart disease.[463] Chemotherapy for metastatic carcinoid tumors has, in general, been disappointing. With single agents such as 5-FU, doxorubicin, actinomycin, cisplatin, etoposide, cyclophosphamide, or streptozocin, responses ranged from no response to a 30% response rate (Table 41–23).[521,625,655,684–686] Combination chemotherapy for metastatic carcinoid has not been shown to have any advantage compared with single-agent chemotherapy.[687] For streptozocin with 5-FU,[506,655,688] with cyclophosphamide,[506] or with doxorubicin,[689,690] response rates varied from 11% to 40%. There was no response to the combination of ectoposide and cisplatin (see Table 41–23).[691] A three-drug regimen of streptozocin, doxorubicin, and cyclophosphamide,[692] or a four-drug regimen of streptozocin, doxorubicin, cyclophosphamide, and 5-FU, offered no additional therapeutic advantage (see Table 41–23).[655,692,693] Remissions have been short-lived with an average duration of 4 to 7 months.[463,625,655,694] Given the indolent nature of the tumor, poor efficacy, undisputed toxicity of chemotherapy, and availability of excellent symptomatic therapy (octreotide), chemotherapy usually is reserved for advanced tumors with radiologic evidence of progression.

The long-acting somatostatin analog octreotide has an antitumor effect in addition to controlling symptoms and reducing secretion of 5-HIAA or various peptides (see Table 41–23).[632,695,696] In 25 patients with carcinoid syndrome who underwent octreotide treatment (150 μg three times daily), tumor size increased in 3, remained unchanged in 22, and was reduced in 4 (a 16% response rate).[650] To determine whether an increased dose of octreotide was more effective, the effect of octreotide (500 μg three times daily) on tumor size was evaluated in 23 patients with metastatic carcinoid syndrome.[696] Of the 23 patients, 4 (17%) demonstrated a decrease of more than 50% in the diameter of the tumor, a response similar to that seen with the lower dose.[650] In more recent studies of patients with metastatic carcinoid tumors, octreotide decreased tumor size in 0 to 9% of patients (see Table 41–23).[652,695] The antitumor effects of octreotide have not been impressive in all studies.

Human leukocyte interferon or recombinant interferon-α can decrease tumor size in a significant number of patients with metastatic tumors (see Table 41–23). In early studies with human leukocyte interferon in 36 patients with malignant carcinoid tumors treated with doses of 3 to 6 million units/day, decreases in tumor size were seen in 11%.[658,697] Nineteen patients previously had failed standard chemotherapy. The median duration of response was 34 months. Adverse side effects were surmountable and less severe than with cytotoxic chemotherapy.[658,698] In a recent study using 24 million units of recombinant interferon-α three times weekly, 4 of 20 patients (20%) with metastatic carcinoid tumors had measurable regression of tumor metastases (20%); the regression was always partial.[699] The mean duration of the regression was 7 weeks from the onset of therapy, with a range of 4 to 26 weeks.[699] In a large prospective study of 111 patients with metastatic disease, 16 patients (14%) demonstrated more than a 50% reduction in tumor size, with 66% demonstrating a stabilization of the disease, and only 19% a progressive disease.[660] In this study, the mean survival of patients treated with interferon was prolonged compared with the median survival with chemotherapy with streptozocin plus 5-FU. In patients treated with interferon alone, the mean survival was more than 80 months; with chemotherapy first and then interferon, it was 64 months.[660] In this large study, interferon treatment (3–9 million units three times weekly) was associated with tolerable but significant side effects including flu-like symptoms (89% of patients), fatigue (70%), weight loss (57%), reduction of blood counts or anemia (31%), leukopenia (3%), thrombocytopenia (14%), and increased serum levels of tryglycerides (32%), liver enzymes (31%), and antibodies (5%).[660] Clinical thyroid disease developed in 76% of patients with thyroid antibodies.[700] In 22 patients, induction of the enzyme 2′,5′-oligoadenylate synthetase with interferon treatment was correlated with the development of a clinical re-

TABLE 41–23. Drug Therapy of Carcinoid Tumors

Investigations	*Agent*	*No. of Patients*	*Objective Response* Number (%)*
Single Drug			
Moertel, 1983[625]	DOX	33	7 (21)
Moertel, 1983[625]	5-FU	19	5 (26)
Kvols, 1989[655]	DTIC	18	3 (17)
Van Hazel et al, 1983[684]			
Van Hazel et al, 1983[684]	Dactinomycin	17	1 (6)
Moertel et al, 1986[685]	Cisplatin	15	1 (6)
Maton and Hodgson, 1984[521]	Alkylating agents	39	9 (23)
Kelsen et al, 1987[686]	ETOP	17	0 (0)
Maton and Hodgson, 1984[521]	STZ	23	7 (30)
	Interferon		
Oberg et al, 1986[658]	Human leukocyte	36	4 (11)
Norbin et al, 1989[661]		13	2 (15)
Valimaki et al, 1991[1106]		7	1 (14)
Moertel et al, 1989[699]	Interferon-α	20	4 (20)
Norbin et al, 1989[661]		10	1 (10)
Doberanr et al, 1987[690]		7	0 (0)
Creutzfeldt et al, 1991[695]		10	0 (0)
Kvols et al, 1986[650]	Octreotide	25	4 (16)
Creutzfeldt et al, 1991[695]		10	0 (0)
Oberg et al, 1991[652]		23	2 (9)
Kvols et al, 1987[696]		23	4 (17)
Norbin et al, 1989[669]	Hepatic artery occlusion or embolization	27	10 (37)
Marlink et al, 1991[668]		4	3 (75)
Combination			
Oberg and Erickson, 1991[660]	STZ + 5-FU	19	2 (11)
Moertel and Hanley, 1979[506]		42	14 (33)
Kvols, 1989[655]			
Engstrom et al, 1984[688]		80	18 (22)
Moertel and Hanley, 1979[506]	STZ + CTX	47	12 (26)
Kelsen et al, 1982[689]	STZ + DOX	10	4 (40)
Doberaur et al, 1987[690]		9	2 (22)
Moertel et al, 1991[1024]	ETOP + Cisplatin	13	0 (0)
Bukowski et al, 1987[692]	STZ + CTX + 5-FU	9	2 (21)
Bukowski et al, 1987[692]	STZ + DOX + CTX + 5-FU	56	17 (31)
Bukowski et al, 1983[1107]			
Moertel, 1987[463]	Hepatic artery occlusion + DTIC + DOX + 5-FU + STZ	21	18 (86)
		10	9 (90)
Hanssen, 1989[663]	Hepatic artery occlusion + inteferon-α, 2β	7	5 (71)

DOX, doxorubicin; 5-FU, 5-fluorouracil; ETOP, etoposide; STZ, streptozocin; DTIC, dacarbazine; CTX, cyclophosphamide.
* Objective response is defined as a decrease in tumor size using the investigator's criteria. Changes in tumor markers or functional improvement was not included as an objective response.

sponse.[701] It is not known whether it is predictive of changes in tumor size with interferon treatment.

Selective hepatic artery infusion of 5-FU had a response rate similar to that reported for systemic 5-FU.[521] Hepatic artery ligation surgically or embolization by interventional radiology has been reported to reduce hepatic tumor bulk.[463,662,663,665,667,669] In one series of 14 patients with metastatic carcinoid to the liver after hepatic artery occlusion either surgically or percutaneously, 7% showed complete improvement, 43% showed 75% to 100% improvement, and 43% showed a 50% to 75%[463] improvement in endocrine responses and in regression of hepatic metastases. The duration of response was short, with a mean of 5 months.[463] In two recent studies involving 31 patients, 19 patients had temporary liver dearterialization and 12 patients were treated by liver embolization.[668,669] After temporary liver dearterialization, 41% had a decrease in metastatic hepatic tumor size, whereas with embolization 50% showed a decrease and in almost all cases the reduction lasted more than 12 months. The combination of hepatic artery ligation and combination chemotherapy with dacarbazine, doxorubicin, 5-FU, and streptozocin has led to dramatic response rates in patients with carcinoid and hepatic metastases.[463,649,666,667] Of 21 patients with carcinoid tumors treated with sequential hepatic artery occlusion and cytotoxic drugs (doxorubicin, dacarbazine, streptozocin, and 5-FU), 19% had complete improvement, 57% had 75% to 100% improvement, and 10% a 50% to 75% improvement, for an 80% overall response rate that lasted a median of 24 months.[463] In a recent study of 15 patients with liver metastases from carcinoid (n=7) or pancreatic endocrine tumors (n=8) who were treated with chemoembolization (gelfoam occlusion with doxorubicin, mitomycin, and cisplatin), 4 patients (33%) demonstrated a 75% decrease in tumor size, 17% (2 patients) stable disease, and 4 patients (33%) progressive disease.[667] The median survival was 6 months (range, 0–55 months). Hepatic artery embolization has been combined with treatment with human interferon 2b (see Table 41–23).[662,663] One year after the chemoembolization, 5 of 7 patients (71%) continued to demonstrate a decrease in tumor size within the liver, whereas with interferon alone (n=10) only 10% demonstrated a decrease in tumor size.

The therapeutic potential of the uptake of MIBG by carcinoid tumors has been investigated recently.[680] In 5 patients with progressive metastatic disease who were given 5.2 to 29.5 GBq of ^{131}I-MIBG cumulatively, no decrease in tumor size was seen in any patient even though symptomatic improvement was seen.

PANCREATIC ENDOCRINE TUMORS

Pancreatic endocrine tumors share a number of features with carcinoid tumors, and their histologic features cannot be differentiated from those of carcinoid tumors.[702] Both carcinoid and pancreatic endocrine tumors can be classified as an APUDomas by histologic criteria (see the earlier section on pathology) and, except for insulinoma, both are malignant in most cases (more than 60%; Table 41–24). Both are vascular tumors with similar radiographic appearances and metastatic patterns (primarily to regional lymph nodes and the liver).

Pancreatic endocrine tumors are classified as functional if they are associated with a clinical syndrome due to ectopic hormone release of a functional tumor. They are considered nonfunctional if they are not associated with a clinical symptom due to hormone release. This latter category includes tumors releasing PP (PPomas) or neurotensin (neurotensinomas) and tumors are not associated with elevated plasma hormone levels, even though they are histologically indistinguishable from functional tumors.[702] Despite elevated plasma levels of PP or neurotensin, these tumors are classified as nonfunctional because no specific symptoms occur in most studies due to elevated plasma levels of these hormones.[702,703]

TABLE 41–24. Characteristics of Gastropancreatic and Endocrine Tumors

Tumor Name	*Syndrome Name*	*Hormone Producing Symptoms*	*Malignant (%)*	*Location (%)*
Symptoms Not Due to Released Hormones				
PPoma	PPoma	None	>60	Pancreas
Nonfunctioning	Nonfunctioning Pancreatic Endocrine Tumor	None	>60	Pancreas
Symptoms Due to Released Hormones				
Gastrinoma	Zollinger-Ellison syndrome	Gastrin	60–90	Pancreas (30–60%) Duodenum (30–43%) Other (10–20%)
Insulinoma	Insulinoma	Insulin	10–15	Pancreas (>99%)
VIPoma	Pancreatic cholera Verner-Morrison syndrome WDHA	Vasoactive intestinal peptide	80	Pancreas (90%) Adrenal (10%)
Glucagonoma	Glucagonoma	Glucagon	60	Pancreas (>99%)
Somatostatinoma	Somatostatinoma	Somatostatin		Pancreas (56%) Upper small intestine (44%)
GRFoma	GRFoma	Growth hormone-releasing peptide	30	Pancreas (33%) Lung (53%) Small intestine (10%) Other (7%)

PPoma, pancreatic endocrine tumor releasing pancreatic polypeptide; VIPoma, vasoactive intestinal peptide; GRFoma, growth hormone-releasing factor tumor; WDHA, watery diarrhea hypokalemia achlorhydria.

In general, these tumors are uncommon. Functional pancreatic endocrine tumors are reported to have a prevalence of 10 persons per million population.[704] The prevalence in unselected autopsy studies is 0.5% to 1.5%.[704–707] It is not apparent why the autopsy detection rate is so much higher than the clinical detection rate.[520] It may be because most tumors are nonfunctional, symptoms frequently are missed, or peptides are released in quantities too small to cause symptoms. The incidence of clinically significant pancreatic endocrine tumors is 3.6 to 4 persons per million population per year.[488,708] Nonfunctional pancreatic endocrine tumors or PPomas are reported to account for 15% to 30% of all pancreatic endocrine tumors.[488,709–711] Gastrinomas and PPomas are the most common malignant pancreatic endocrine tumors. Gastrinomas due to ZES usually are clinically recognized and have been studied extensively; they are discussed in detail.[712] The localization, surgical approach, and the approach to advanced disease are similar to approaches used for the more rare pancreatic tumors. Other syndromes are discussed in separate sections. The treatment of metastatic disease is similar for all metastatic pancreatic endocrine tumors and is discussed at the end of this chapter.

ZOLLINGER-ELLISON SYNDROME

In 1955, Zollinger and Ellison described 2 patients with severe peptic ulcer disease treatable only by total gastrectomy. The disease was characterized by extreme hypersecretion of gastric acid and a non-β islet cell tumor of the pancreas.[713] Extracts of tumors from patients with ZES were demonstrated to contain a potent acid secretagogue that was gastrin-like.[714] Amino acid analysis and enzymatic degradation of purified tumor extracts demonstrated that the secretagogue in the tumor was identical to human antral gastrin.[715,716] Because these tumors synthesize and release large amounts of gastrin, they have been called gastrinomas.

Recent studies estimate that ZES occurs in 1 person per 100,000 population in Denmark,[717] in 0.5 persons per million population in Ireland,[708] and in 1 to 3 persons per million per year in Sweden.[488] The prevalence of ZES varies from half as common[708] to 1.2 times as common as insulinomas.[488] Gastrinomas occur less frequently than the original estimate of 0.1% of all persons in the United States with duodenal ulcer disease.[718] In one series, gastrinomas were the most common pancreatic endocrine tumor, making up 30% of all such tumors.[488]

Pathogenesis, Pathology, and Tumor Biology

Almost all clinical manifestations, except for those late in the course of the disease, are due to gastric acid hypersecretion secondary to hypergastrinemia.[691] Effective control of the gastric hypersecretion medically or surgically abolishes all clinical manifestations, including peptic ulcer disease and diarrhea (Table 41–25).[691,719–722] In patients late in the course of their disease with metastatic gastrinoma or large primaries, symptoms such as pain or cachexia can arise due to the tumor itself. Besides basal gastric acid hypersecretion, hypergastrinemia causes trophic changes in the gastric mucosa,[723] with the result that patients with ZES have increased numbers of parietal cells and an increased maximal acid secretory capacity.[719,724,725]

Many patients with ZES have diarrhea and in some patients it is the sole presenting manifestation (see Table 41–25). The diarrhea is due to the consequences of gastric acid hypersecretion including direct injury to the small intestinal mucosa, inactivation of pancreatic lipase at low pH, and precipitation of bile acids at low pH.[719] Hypergastrinemia itself has been proposed to contribute to the diarrhea by increasing intestinal secretion.[726] This hypothesis is not supportable because diarrhea disappears and patients remain asymptomatic when the gastric acid hypersecretion is controlled, even though the hypergastrinemia remains unchanged.[503,719]

Gastrin in normal subjects and in patients with ZES has been found in different molecular sizes. In gastrinomas, gastrin-17 (G-17) is the major gastrin component, comprising 74% to 80% of the total immunoreactivity, with so-called big gastrin or gastrin-34 (G-34) comprising most of the remainder.[719,727,728] In contrast, in sera from normal subjects and patients with gastrinoma, G-34 comprises more than 60% of

TABLE 41–25. Clinical Features of Patients With Zollinger-Ellison Syndrome

Characteristic	*Ellison et al, 1964*[757]	*Regan et al, 1978*[791]	*Stage et al, 1979*[717]	*Mignon et al, 1986*[822]	*Jensen et al, 1991*[712]
No. of patients	260	40	34	144	165
MEN-I (%)	21	23	24	24	18
Mean duration of symptoms before diagnosis (y)	ND (53% = 1–4) (27% = >4)	6.5	6.4	ND	6.4
First symptoms (%)					
Abdominal pain	93	98	85	26	24
Pain and diarrhea	30	28	56	49	55
Diarrhea only	7	2	9	15	18
Dysphagia/pyrosis	0	0	6	ND	31
Mean age at onset (y)	ND	50.5	50.4	47	45
Sex (% male)	60	60	62	68	58

MEN-I, multiple endocrine neoplasia type I; ND, no data.

the total gastrin immunoreactivity.[702,719,727] In addition to G-17 and G-34, smaller and larger forms of gastrin have been described in sera and in gastrinomas from patients with ZES. Each of the gastrins can exist in two different forms (sulfated or nonsulfated), which are reported to be equipotent.[719] Early studies reported that G-17 was five times more potent than G-34,[729] but a recent study using synthetic peptides found G-34 and G-17 to be equally potent.[730] In ZES, plasma gastrin immunoreactivity includes a high-molecular-weight gastrin (big, big gastrin), an uncategorized gastrin slightly larger than G-34 (component I gastrin), and small amounts of amino-terminal, carboxyl-terminal, and carboxyl-terminal-extended fragments of gastrin.[728,731–737] Altered posttranslational processing of gastrin may occur in gastrinoma, leading to altered ratios of various fragments of gastrin and precursors.[734,738,739] In a recent study, less than 50% of the total progastrin in tumors was processed to α-amidated gastrins, whereas in normal subjects only small amounts of unprocessed, nonamidated gastrins were found.[738] In patients with ZES, large amounts of glycine-extended forms of G-17, G-34, and component I have been described in the plasma.[735,738] In addition, a high-molecular-weight progastrin has been described in plasma and tumors of patients with gastrinomas.[734,737,738,740] Elevated levels of progastrin have been found in patients with gastrinoma metastatic to liver, whereas the smaller glycine-extended gastrins predominated in benign disease.[738] Furthermore, a significantly lower percentage of α-amidated gastrin was found in patients with metastatic disease to the liver compared with patients without metastases.[738] These results suggest that a low degree of processing of progastrin predicts a malignant clinical course.[738] Some researchers reported that the relative amounts of G-17 and amino-terminal fragments and the ratio of G-17 amino-terminal immunoreactivity to G-17 carboxyl-terminal immunoreactivity was predictive of the extent of gastrinoma.[733,734,741] Others did not confirm these findings.[738] These results are preliminary and appear to vary considerably from patient to patient. It is unclear whether analysis of gastrin fragments and precursors will provide useful clinical information to help establish the presence of malignancy.

Initially, gastrinomas were thought to occur most commonly in the pancreas (Table 41–26). In early studies, gastrinomas were reported to occur in a frequency of 4:1:4 for the pancreatic head:body:tail, and 14% of all gastrinomas were found in the duodenum.[720,742] Gastrinomas in the duodenum and in lymph nodes in the pancreatic head area have been reported increasingly[741,743–745] and have been found recently in 60% of all patients in whom a tumor is found at surgery (Table 41–27).[745] Of all gastrinomas found at surgery, 65% to 90% are in the pancreatic head and duodenal area (see Table 41–27).[741,743,745,746] Occasionally, gastrinomas have been found in the liver, stomach, jejunum, mesentery, and spleen. In women, there are numerous reports of ovarian gastrinomas that are functionally indistinguishable from other gastrinomas.[747–751]

Because gastrin-containing cells (G cells) normally are not present in the adult pancreas, it has been proposed that pancreatic gastrinomas be considered ectopic, whereas gastrinomas in areas that normally contain G cells (*e.g.*, duodenum, stomach, jejunum) be considered entopic.[510,752–754] Earlier studies found a lower incidence of malignant change (38%) for gastrinomas in entopic locations and a higher incidence for ectopic gastrinomas (60–70%).[752] In recent prospective studies, duodenal gastrinomas have been found to be malignant with metastatic spread in 54% to 75% of patients.[745,755,756] The disease-free interval was shortest in patients who had resected duodenal gastrinomas and normal serum levels of gastrin and provocative tests immediately postoperatively, suggesting the presence of metastases (Fig. 41–11).[745] These data suggest that the malignant potential of ectopic and entopic gastrinomas does not differ as suggested originally and that both groups are malignant in more than 60% of cases. In early studies, 60% to more than 90% of patients with ZES had metastatic gastrinoma at the time of diagnosis.[727,757–759] In recent studies, only 34% have had metastatic disease at the time of diagnosis (see Table 41–26). Metastases usually are to the peripancreatic lymph nodes and the liver.[712] Recently, bony metastases have been reported in 12% of patients with metastatic gastrinoma in the liver.[608]

The cell of origin of gastrinomas remains obscure. Duodenal gastrinoma usually contains many well-differentiated antral G cells, in contrast to pancreatic gastrinoma, and is believed to originate from gastrin cells in the duodenal crypts and

TABLE 41–26. Pathology, Tumor Location, and Extent in Patients With Zollinger-Ellison Syndrome in Various Series

*Extent of Tumor** *(% of All Patients)*	*Tumor Location** *(% of All Patients)*	*Pathology Found*
No tumor found in 30% (8–48%)	Pancreatic in 42% (21–65%)	Gastrinoma in 90% (87–94%)†
Tumor present in 70% (52–92%)	Duodenal in 15% (6–31%)	Malignant in 61–90%‡
Metastatic in 34% (13–52%)	Other, 11% (1–26%)	Benign in 10–39%‡
Localized in 36% (23–51%)	Metastases only in 2% (0–11%)	Islet cell hyperplasia only in 10% (6–13%)†

* Mean percentages and ranges are calculated from references 722, 741–743, 745, 746, 757–759, 762, 766, 767, 799, and 823.
† Percentages from references 722, 741, 745, 757, 758, and 822.
‡ Percentages from references 727, 757, 759, and 822.

TABLE 41–27. Location of Primary Gastrinomas in a Recent Prospective 10-Year Surgical Study

	Location of Primary Gastrinoma Number (%)				
*Surgical Group**	*Duodenum*	*Pancreatic*	*Lymph Nodes Only*	*Other†*	*No Tumor Found*
Group 1 (n = 36)	4 (11)	12§ (33)	6 (17)	1 (3)	13 (36)
Group 2 (n = 37)	16‡ (43)	11 (30)	7 (19)	—	3 (8)
Both groups (n = 73)	20 (27)	23 (32)	13 (18)	1 (1)	16 (22)

* Group 1 and Group 2 differed in that patients in Group 2 underwent additional procedures to search for duodenal gastrinomas (duodenotomy, endoscopy at surgery).
† One patient had an ovarian gastrinoma.
‡ Proportion of duodenal gastrinomas found was significantly greater in group 2 versus group 1 patients ($p < 0.01$).
§ Proportion of pancreatic gastrinomas found in group 1 was greater than that of duodenal gastrinomas found in group 1 ($p < 0.05$).
(Data from Norton JA, Doppman JL, Jensen RT. Curative resection in Zollinger-Ellison syndrome: Results of a ten year prospective study. Ann Surg 1992;215:8)

Brunner's glands.[510,754] Because G cells are not seen in human pancreas and because pancreatic gastrinomas are pleomorphic with heterogenous cell types, they have been proposed to originate from a multipotential, endocrine-programmed stem cell that undergoes somewhat inappropriate and incomplete differentiation toward the G cell.[510,754] An argyrophilic cell with atypical granules has been described in islet cell tumors and may well be the precursor or stem cell for these tumors.[727]

In early studies, in which patients presented late in the course of their disease, gastrinomas were found at surgery in most patients with ZES (81–94%).[727,757,758] In subsequent studies, gastrinomas were found in only 70% of the patients with ZES (see Table 41–26).[712] In one-half of the patients, the tumor is nonmetastatic (36% of all patients), and in about one-half of these patients the tumors are multiple.[715,758] Therefore, in only 20% of all patients with ZES was a single, nonmetastatic gastrinoma found. In a recent large prospective study, when attention was directed to finding duodenal gastrinomas, tumors were found in 93% of patients.[745] Forty-three percent were duodenal, 30% were pancreatic, and 20% were in the lymph nodes (see Table 41–27). Islet cell hyperplasia and nesidioblastosis have been suggested as causes of

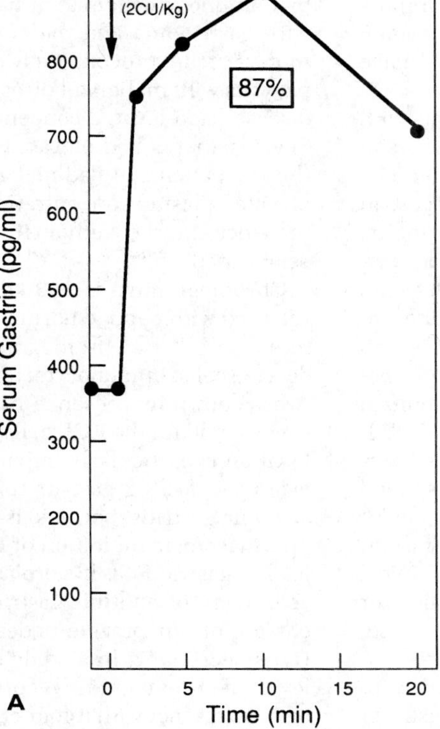

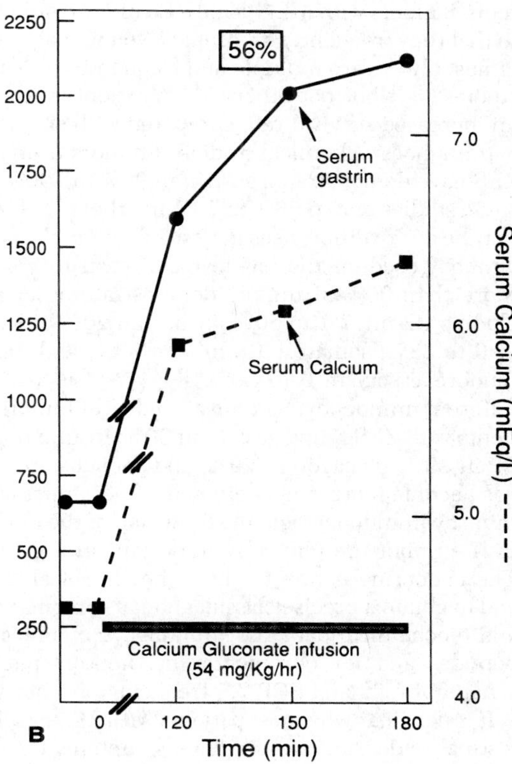

FIGURE 41-11. **(A)** Typical secretin and **(B)** calcium provocative test results in a patient with Zollinger-Ellison syndrome (ZES). Secretin (2 U/kg intravenous bolus) was given (*arrow*), and serum levels of gastrin increased more than 200 pg/ml consistent with ZES. This response is seen in 87% of patients with ZES. Calcium gluconate (54 mg/kg/h) is infused over 3 hours and serum levels of gastrin increase greater than 395 pg/ml. This response is seen in 56% of patients with ZES. Percentage data is based on responses in 96 patients with ZES.

ZES in some cases in which no gastrinoma is found.[757,758,760] Most authorities do not accept islet cell hyperplasia or nesidioblastosis as a cause of ZES for three reasons. First, islet cell hyperplasia or nesidioblastosis is common in patients with ZES who have a gastrinoma located. Second, the hyperplastic islets do not contain gastrin. Third, the possibility of a small gastrinoma that was not detected at surgery cannot be excluded. Islet cell hyperplasia or nesidioblastosis is regarded not as a cause but as a consequence of the disease.[707,727,754,761]

The percentage of gastrinomas that are actually malignant is unclear. In early studies, 60% to more than 90% of patients with ZES had a malignant gastrinoma.[727,757–759] In recent studies, only 50% of patients have had a malignant gastrinoma at the time of diagnosis (see Table 41–26). Whether this change represents earlier diagnosis or inclusion of a spectrum of the disease not previously appreciated is unclear. The diagnosis of malignancy is complicated by the fact that no histologic criteria predicts malignancy; therefore, malignancy can be established only by the presence of metastases. Even metastatic disease can be difficult to establish, because a number of extrapancreatic gastrinomas localized in lymph nodes have been described with no evidence of primary tumor. Some of these patients apparently have been cured by excision of lymph nodes, which suggests that the gastrinoma was not metastatic but originated in the lymph node.[707,746,762–764]

About 20% of patients with ZES (see Table 41–25) have a familial form of the disease with evidence of MEN-I (Wermer's syndrome). MEN-I is an autosomal dominant trait characterized by hyperplasia or tumors of multiple endocrine organs, with hyperparathyroidism the most common abnormality.[513,514] Islet cell tumors of the pancreas are the second most common characteristic, occurring in 82% of MEN-I patients, with 57% having ZES and 25% having insulinomas.[513] Pituitary and adrenal adenomas are less common. Patients with MEN-I and ZES differ from sporadic cases in that they frequently present at a younger age. Their tumors almost always are multiple and frequently are small. In some studies[762,765] but not others,[766,767] patients with MEN-I have an increased survival rate compared with sporadic cases.

Immunocytochemical studies of tumors from patients with ZES have demonstrated gastrin in 90% to 100% of tumors in some studies and in 56% to 78% in others.[691] This difference may be due to differences in tissue fixation, the type of gastrin antibody used, or the low levels of gastrin in small tumors. More than 50% of tumors demonstrate other peptides, including PP in 17% to 50%, insulin in 20% to 33%, glucagon in 0 to 33%, somatostatin in 0 to 33%, and ACTH-like immunoreactivity in 0 to 30%.[691,727,768–770] A review of seven different immunocytochemical studies of tumors from 75 patients with ZES found gastrin in 80%, insulin in 30%, human PP in 35%, glucagon in 29%, and somatostatin in 21%.[703] It has become increasingly difficult, if not impossible, to determine by immunocytochemistry which of the hormones found in the tumor are clinically important in a given patient.[691] The endocrine nature of the tumor is not always apparent, and to obtain a precise classification, a combination of clinical and biochemical data and immunocytochemical studies for peptides and for chromogranins, neuron-specific enolase, synaptophysin, and PCP 7.5 frequently are needed.[712,768]

It is not clear why most patients with ZES or other gastrointestinal endocrine tumors have symptoms characteristic of hypersecretion of only one peptide, even though their tumors contain multiple peptide hormones. It may be that only one of the peptides is released in quantities sufficient to cause symptoms, that only one of the peptides is biologically active, or that all the peptides are released and biologically active but have antagonistic physiologic actions. Early studies involving small numbers of cases reported elevated plasma concentrations of various gastrointestinal peptides in patients with ZES.[691,718,771–775] A recent prospective study of 45 consecutive cases of patients with ZES demonstrated increased plasma concentrations of a peptide besides gastrin in 62% of patients.[703] Forty-four percent had one additional peptide in abnormal amounts and 18% had two additional peptides. No patient had abnormal levels of three additional peptides. Motilin was the peptide most often present at abnormally high levels (29%). Human PP plasma levels were elevated in 27% of patients, compared with plasma PP elevations of 10% to 60% described previously.[772,773,776] Some investigators[774] but not others[777] have proposed that elevations in plasma PP levels might be a useful marker for identifying patients with ZES and metastatic liver disease. Elevated levels of neurotensin occurred in 20% of patients in one study[703] and in no patients in another study.[771] Plasma levels of gastrin-releasing peptide were elevated in 10% of patients in one study.[703] Although there have been frequent reports of finding insulin, glucagon, or somatostatin by immunocytochemical studies, and of occasional patients having ZES with a concomitant insulinoma[778] or glucagonoma,[712] the prospective study of 45 patients with ZES found no patient with increased plasma levels of these peptides.[703] The presence or absence of abnormal plasma levels of a particular peptide or extent of elevation did not correlate with location of tumor, extent of tumor, or the presence or absence of a particular symptom.[703]

Elevated concentrations of HCG subunits (α or β chains) in sera, or the presence of HCG in the tumor as determined by immunocytochemistry, have been found in some patients with gastrinoma and may be predictive of a malignant tumor.[779–782] In a recent study of 30 patients with ZES, 57% of patients with malignant disease and 45% of those with benign disease had elevated concentrations of α-HCG in plasma.[781] Seven patients had elevated levels of β-HCG in plasma. Of these 7 patients, 4 had malignant disease. The usefulness of elevated plasma concentrations of α-HCG or β-HCG or their presence in the tumor in predicting malignancy is not established.[712,764,783]

Chromogranin A is a 48-kd protein that is co-stored and co-released with peptide hormones from gut endocrine cells and tumors.[782,784–787] Chromogranin A is not produced by nonendocrine cells. Immunocytochemical staining for chromogranin A has shown its presence in gastrinomas, carcinoids, antral G cells, and fundic ECL cells of the stomach.[784–788] The latter location is particularly important because conditions that elevate the fasting gastrin concentration (*e.g.,* ZES, chronic atrophic gastritis, pernicious anemia, and antral exclusion or pharmacologic inhibition of gastric acid hypersecretion) can lead to gastric ECL hyperplasia and in some cases to the development of multiple gastric carcinoid tumors (see the discussion of omeprazole under Medical Treatment of Gastric Hypersecretion). In a study of patients with ZES, abnormal levels of chromogranin A correlated best with plasma pepsinogen levels, not with tumor characteristics.[789] The researchers speculated that the chromogranin A-producing cells in the stomach, not the gastrinoma, could be the principal source of plasma chromogranin A due to long-term hypergastrinemia with resultant hyperplasia of ECL cells.[789] This study measured plasma chromogranin A levels in 10 patients with ZES and found that the mean value was 5 times that in normal patients.[789] There was no correlation between the plasma level of chromogranin A and the amount of tumor, presence or absence of metastatic disease, or presence or absence of MEN-I.[789]

Histologic studies have demonstrated that tumors from patients with ZES are similar to other carcinoid tumors.[691,770] Different histologic classifications have been proposed based on growth patterns, including classifying tumors into a glandular pattern, solid nests of cells (solid pattern), a trabecular or ribbon-like structure (gyriform pattern), and an unclassified pattern.[691,712,754,768,770,790] Similar patterns have been demonstrated in tumors from patients with other endocrine tumors, and the type of histologic pattern does not correlate with the type of hormone produced, clinical symptoms, or malignancy. Ultrastructural classifications have been based on the type of granules seen, but this does not correlate with malignancy or clinical features.[510,691,727,754,768,783]

Clinical Features

The clinical features of ZES as reported in several studies are summarized in Table 41–25. ZES is slightly more common in males (60%) than in females (40%); the mean age is 45 to 50 years old, and about 20% have MEN-I. Abdominal pain remains the most common initial symptom, with 90% to 95% of patients developing peptic ulcer disease at some time during the course of the disease. The abdominal pain cannot be differentiated from that which occurs in patients with idiopathic peptic esophagitis or peptic ulcer disease. Diarrhea and esophageal disease are increasingly the first symptoms (see Table 41–25). Esophageal symptoms were only reported in 3% of 355 patients with ZES in early studies.[757,787,791] However, in two later small series in which esophageal disease was specifically sought, 33% of 32 patients had symptoms or endoscopic evidence of esophagitis.[792,793] In a study of 122 patients with ZES, esophageal symptoms, endoscopic abnormalities, or both were present in 61%.[794]

The change in presenting symptoms is reflected in changes in radiologic and endoscopic findings. In early studies, up to 93% of patients had a peptic ulcer, and in 36% of patients the ulcers were multiple or in unusual locations.[719,757] Although atypical ulcers, when present, strongly suggest the diagnosis, most patients with ZES have typical duodenal ulcers, and 18% to 25% of patients have no ulcer at the time of diagnosis.[719] This change in presenting symptoms and severity of peptic disease suggests that patients with ZES are being diagnosed earlier. Nevertheless, in almost all series there is a delay of 3 to 6 years between the onset of symptoms and diagnosis (see Table 41–25). Intestinal perforation, especially of the jejunum, is a presenting event, even today, in as many as 7% of patients with ZES.[795]

Diagnosis

None of the original triad of symptoms described by Zollinger and Ellison is required for the diagnosis of ZES. At time of diagnosis, 38% to 68% of patients have a solitary peptic ulcer and 14% to 25% have no peptic ulcer.[719] Although gastric acid hypersecretion remains an essential criterion of ZES, it may not be extreme, and in 8% to 48% of patients, gastrinomas are not located at the time of diagnosis (see Table 41–26). ZES is suspected on the basis of the clinical presentation and established in almost all patients by demonstrating elevated basal gastric acid secretion (basal acid output [BAO]) and fasting hypergastrinemia.

ZES should be suspected clinically in any of the clinical settings of ulcer with diarrhea, familial ulcer, ulcer in unusual locations, and recurrent or resistant ulcer. One of the most common clinical presentations is a patient whose peptic ulcer fails to heal on conventional doses of H_2 receptor antagonists.[712] Most patients present with symptoms that are similar to those in patients with idiopathic peptic disease.[717,719] Therefore, at least one preoperative fasting serum gastrin should be done for all patients who have peptic ulcer disease severe enough to require gastric surgery.

To make the diagnosis of ZES it is necessary to demonstrate fasting hypergastrinemia and an elevated BAO.[796] The fasting gastrin concentration is usually done first, and although occasional normal values have been reported in patients with ZES, this is a rare occurrence.[707,796] Disorders other than ZES are known to elevate the fasting serum level of gastrin.[719] These disorders fit into two categories—those associated with gastric acid hypersecretion (Table 41–28) and those associated with hypochlorhydria or achlorhydria including chronic gastritis, gastric cancer, pernicious anemia, or postvagotomy.[719] No absolute level of elevation of serum gastrin concentration distinguishes these two categories causing hypergastrinemias, and they can be differentiated only by measuring the BAO. If facilities are not available to measure the basal output, the pH of the gastric contents should be determined while the patient is not taking antisecretory medications. A pH of 3 or higher virtually excludes the diagnosis of ZES.[796]

The most commonly used secretory criteria for diagnosing ZES are a BAO of 15 mEq/hour or more in patients without previous acid-reducing operations and 5 mEq/hour or more in patients with previous acid-reducing operations.[712,719,798] The mean BAO in five series ranged from 34 to 53 mEq/hour in patients without previous gastric surgery and from 6 to 20 mEq/hour for patients with previous acid-reducing surgery.[691,721,791,798,799] In early studies, 33% of patients with ZES without previous gastric surgery were reported to have a BAO of less than 15 mEq/hour.[721,791,798] In recent studies, only 1 of 77 patients without previous gastric surgery had a BAO of less than 15 mEq/hour.[691,799,800] Requiring a BAO of at least 15 mEq/hour will include 66% to 99% of all patients with ZES and exclude 90% of patients with routine duodenal ulcer.[719] In patients with previous acid-reducing surgery, the mean BAO exceeded 5 mEq/hour in most studies, but in three studies, 6%, 33%, and 45% of patients had a BAO of less than 5 mEq/hour.[503,773,801] Patients with ZES have an elevated maximal acid output (MAO) and an elevated BAO/MAO ratio that often exceeds 0.6.[802] In some series, the BAO/MAO ratio is less than 0.6 in a significant proportion of patients.[721,791,798,799] Criteria based on the MAO or BAO/MAO ratio have not been shown to offer an advantage over the BAO alone.[712,719]

TABLE 41–28. Differential Diagnosis of Increased Fasting Gastrin Level and Basal Acid Output

Diagnosis	*Secretion Injection*	*Calcium Infusion*	*Meal Test*	*Other Discriminating Features*
Zollinger-Ellison syndrome	Increase > 200 pg/ml over basal	Increase > 395 pg/ml over basal	NC or increase < 100% over basal (70%)	About 50% of patients have tumor on imaging studies
Retained gastric antrum	NC or increase < 200 pg/ml	NC or small increase	NC, decrease or increase < 50% over basal	History of Billroth II operation. Positive ^{99m}Tc scan
Chronic gastric outlet obstruction	NC or increase < 200 pg/ml	NC or small increase	ND	Decreased gastric empyting; with nasogastric suction serum gastrin levels return to normal
Antral G-cell hyperplasia	NC or decrease or increase < 200 pg/ml	NC or small increase	Increase > 100% over basal	Increased numbers of G cells may be seen by immunocytochemical staining
Antral G-cell hyperfunction	NC or decrease or increase < 200 pg/ml	NC or small increase	Increase > 100% over basal	Normal number of G cells; frequently familial; may be associated with hyperpepsinogenemia I
After small bowel resection	NC or increase < 200 pg/ml	NC or small increase	ND	History of extensive small bowel resection

NC, no change; ND, not determined.

If a patient has a fasting gastrin concentration of 1000 pg/ml or more with basal acid hypersecretion, the diagnosis of ZES generally is established.[691,796] The only other disorder that can mimic ZES and cause similar elevations of acid secretion and fasting gastrin concentration is the retained gastric antrum syndrome, a rare condition that occurs in patients who underwent a Billroth II gastroenterostomy in which part of the antrum was left attached to the excluded proximal duodenal stump.[803,804] This diagnosis can be excluded if there is no history of gastric surgery. If there is such a history, the diagnosis can be excluded using the secretin test and gastric ^{99m}Tc scanning as outlined in Table 41–28.[804,805]

In a recent study, 32% of patients with ZES had a fasting gastrin concentration of 1000 pg/ml or greater.[806] In the remaining 68%, the fasting gastrin concentration was elevated but less than 1000 pg/ml, a range that overlaps with other conditions that can cause similar elevations of fasting gastrin and BAO.[719,806] These conditions are listed in Table 41–28. To differentiate them from ZES, various gastrin provocative tests frequently are necessary (Table 41–29). Provocative tests including the secretin test,[712,729,800,806–809] calcium infusion test,[800,806,807,809] and meal test[809] have been developed, and each measures the serum gastrin response. Recently, the secretin, calcium, and meal provocative tests were evaluated prospectively.[806,810] In terms of sensitivity to the three proposed criteria of positivity, gastrin levels increased by 110 pg/ml in 93%, 200 pg/ml or more in 87%,[808] and more than 50% in 85% of patients with ZES (see Table 41–29).[809] There was no significant difference in results in patients with or without MEN-I, and fasting serum gastrin levels above or below 1000 pg/ml did not correlate with extent, size, or location of tumor. The study concluded that an increase of 200 pg/ml after injection of secretin is the diagnostic criteria of choice.[806] This study analyzed different gastrin sampling times and found that 6% of patients had a positive secretin test only at 2 minutes and that no secretin test was positive at more than 20 minutes that was not positive previously. It was therefore recommended that serum gastrin levels be sampled at −15, 0, +2, +5, +10, and +20 minutes only. A typical result is shown in Figure 41–11.

During the calcium infusion test, calcium gluconate is infused at a rate of 54 mg/kg/hour for 3 hours, and serum levels of calcium and gastrin are measured.[800,806] It has been suggested that serum samples be obtained at −15, 0, +120, and +180 minutes.[806] A typical result is shown in Figure 41–11. The calcium infusion test was evaluated using the proposed criteria of at least a 395 pg/ml[800] or 50% increase[806] and compared with the secretin test results. The 395 pg/ml criteria was less sensitive (see Table 41–29). Although the 50% increase criteria had equal sensitivity to secretin, it can be seen in patients with ordinary peptic ulcer disease without ZES.[503,806]

Because of its ease, lack of side effects, high sensitivity, and low number of false-positive results, the secretin test is the provocative test of choice.[719,806,808] The calcium infusion test should be reserved for the rare patient in whom ZES is strongly suspected but the secretin test is negative.[796,808] In 33% of such patients, the calcium test is positive.[806]

To separate ZES from antral G-cell hyperfunction or hyperplasia, serum gastrin response as determined after a standard meal is reported to be useful.[809,810] After a standard meal, serum gastrin is measured at -15, 0, +30, +60, and +90 minutes.[809,810] Patients with ZES are reported to have less than 50% increase over basal values (see Fig. 41–11), whereas patients with antral G-cell hyperfunction or hyperplasia have an exaggerated response (Table 41–28).[809,810] In a recent re-

TABLE 41–29. Results of Provocative Tests Using Secretin, Calcium, and a Standard Meal Test in Patients With Zollinger-Ellison Syndrome: Proposed Criteria for a Positive Test

	*Serum Gastrin Increase**								
	After Secretin			*After Calcium*		*After Meal*			
	≥110 pg/ml	≥200 pg/ml	≥50%	≥395 pg/ml	≥50%	<50%	50–99%	≥100%	≥150%
Tumor demonstrated	93%	84%	78%	43%	74%	46%	36%	18%	9%
Tumor not demonstrated	93%	89%	93%	70%	100%	43%	14%	43%	10%

* Results are the percentage of patients with the indicated tumor status who demonstrated the indicated change in serum gastrin after receiving a secretin bolus (2 U/kg), calcium infusion (54 mg calcium gluconate/h for 3 h) or a standard meal.[809] Results are for patients with Zollinger-Ellison syndrome with fasting serum gastrin concentration < 1000 pg/ml (secretin, 54 patients; calcium 46 patients; meal, 53 patients).

(Data from Lamers CBH, van Tongeren JHM. Comparative study of the value of calcium, secretin, and meal stimulated increase in serum gastrin in the diagnosis of Zollinger-Ellison syndrome. Gut 1979;18:128; and from Frucht HJ, Howard JM, Stark HA, et al. Prospective study of meal provocative gastrin testing in patients with Zollinger-Ellison syndrome. Am J Med 1989;87:528)

view of 52 patients with antral G-cell disease, 98% of patients had an increase of 100% or more and 92% had an increase of 150% or more postmeal.[810] In a recent prospective study of patients with ZES, only 46% of patients had an increase of 50% or less, 26% had an increase of 50% to 99%, 30% had an increase of less than 100%, and 10% had a greater than 150% increase (see Table 41–28).[810] It was therefore concluded that the meal test frequently is positive in patients with ZES and does not reliably differentiate ZES from antral syndromes.[810] Antral G-cell hyperplasia is reported to mimic ZES clinically with elevated fasting serum levels of gastrin and BAO, to occur frequently in patients postvagotomy, to be due to increased numbers of antral G cells, to be curable by antrectomy, and to be differentiated from ZES by a negative secretin test and a postmeal increase of 100% or more in serum gastrin levels (see Table 41–28).[712,719,811–814] Antral G-cell hyperfunction is similar to antral G-cell hyperplasia except that normal numbers of G cells are found, the syndrome frequently is familial with autosomal dominant inheritance, and the syndrome is associated with hyperpepsinogenemia I.[712,815,816] This syndrome also was reported to be differentiated from ZES by having a negative secretin test and exaggerated increase in serum gastrin postmeal.[719,815,816] Thirty percent of patients with ZES have a positive meal test (see Tables 41–28 and 41–29).[810]

Chronic gastric outlet obstruction can be difficult to differentiate from ZES because the obstruction can be caused by ZES or can mimic ZES and be secondary to other causes of duodenal obstruction (see Table 41–28).[719,817] ZES can be differentiated from the other causes of obstruction by a secretin test and prolonged gastric suction.[719,818] In ZES, the secretin test is positive (more than 200 pg/ml increase) and prolonged nasogastric suction does not change the serum gastrin concentrations. In the other conditions, the secretin test is negative and serum gastrins decrease with nasogastric suction.[817] Massive small bowel resection has been reported to cause a transient hypergastrinemia and an elevation of BAO that can be differentiated from ZES by the history and the secretin test (see Table 41–28).[719]

Tumor Localization

Precise localization of the gastrinoma has become an increasingly important factor in evaluating patients with ZES.[764,796,819] With the increased ability to control gastric acid hypersecretion with H_2 receptor antagonists, emergency total gastrectomy is rarely necessary, allowing time to determine the location and extent of the gastrinoma.[719,820] With the increased ability to control gastric acid hypersecretion long-term medically or surgically, the growth and possible metastatic spread of the gastrinoma has become an increasingly important determinant of long-term survival.[691,712,720,759,821] In previous studies, 13% to 52% of all patients at surgery had metastatic disease (usually to the liver), and identification of these patients preoperatively can prevent unnecessary surgery (see Table 41–26).[746,762,822] Gastrinomas frequently are multiple and extrapancreatic (see Tables 41–26 and 41–27).[757,762,823,824] In as many as 40% to 60% of patients in some series (see Table 41–26), no gastrinoma is found at surgery.[823–825] Therefore, careful imaging studies should be used to assist the surgeon in localizing the tumor. A recent study using careful imaging studies was able to identify 15% of patients with metastatic disease to the liver in whom the gastrinoma was resectable.[826]

A number of techniques are helpful in localizing gastrinomas, including abdominal ultrasound, CT scans, selective abdominal angiography, MRI, selective venous sampling for gastrin from portal venous tributaries, intraarterial secretin with hepatic venous gastrin sampling, intraoperative ultrasonography (IOUS), and transillumination of the duodenum at surgery (Table 41–30). Although ultrasound has a low sensitivity for localizing primary and metastatic tumors, a recent prospective study recommended that it continue to be used because it is highly specific, noninvasive, and on occasion localizes gastrinomas not found by other modalities.[827] The CT scan detects on average 50% of all primaries and patients with metastatic liver disease (see Table 41–30). Its ability to detect primary tumors has been shown to be directly related to tumor size, detecting no tumor smaller than 1 cm, 30% of

TABLE 41–30. Ability of Various Modalities to Localize Primary and Metastatic Gastrinoma in Patients With Zollinger-Ellison Syndrome

	Sensitivity (%) Mean (Range)	*Specificity (%) Mean (Range)*
Primary Tumor		
Ultrasound	23 (21–28)	92 (92–92)
CT scan	50 (35–59)	90 (83–100)
Angiography	68 (35–68)	89 (84–94)
IOUS	83	NE
MRI	21	33
PVS	73	33
Intraarterial secretin test	78 (55–100)	100
Transillumination of duodenum*	83	88
Metastatic Tumor		
Ultrasound	14 (14–63)	100
CT scan	54 (35–72)	99 (98–100)
Angiography	62 (33–86)	98 (96–100)
IOUS	NE	NE
MRI	67	100
PVS	NE	NE

IOUS, intraoperative ultrasound; PVS, selective gastrin sampling from portal venous tributaries; NE, not evaluated.
* Data are for duodenal gastrinomas only.
(Data from Jensen RT, Gardner JD. Zollinger-Ellison syndrome: Clinical presentation, pathology, diagnosis, and treatment. In: Dannenberg A, Zakim D, eds. Peptic ulcer and other acid-related diseases. New York: Academic Research Association, 1991:117)

tumors between 1 and 3 cm, and 95% of tumors larger than 3 cm.[828] Primary tumors smaller than 1 cm, which increasingly are being found in the duodenum, usually are missed by CT.[743,745,783,829] Furthermore, CT is less sensitive for detecting extrahepatic and extrapancreatic tumors than pancreatic gastrinomas.[828] A typical CT scan showing gastrinoma metastatic to the liver is shown in Figure 41–12. Selective angiography was able to detect 68% of primary tumors and 86% of hepatic metastases in a recent large prospective study (see Table 41–30).[830] The ability to detect tumors depended on their location, with the study finding 90% of gastrinomas in the pancreatic head, 80% in the body, 45% in the tail, 34% in the duodenum, and 50% in extrapancreatic, extrahepatic, and extraduodenal locations.[830] A typical angiogram of a primary gastrinoma in the pancreatic head area is shown in Figure 41–13. In a comparative study, angiography detected 68% of hepatic metastases, 17% more than CT scans did, and the combination detected 98% of all patients with liver metastases.[830]

MRI was reported in early studies to be useful in localizing gastrinoma in a small number of cases (see Table 41–30).[831,832] A typical positive imaging study identifying metastatic disease in the liver is shown in Figure 41–13. A prospective study from 1986 to 1987 reported that MRI was less sensitive than CT or angiography.[833] A recent preliminary study suggests that contrast agents such as gadolinium may increase the sensitivity of MRI.[834] In this study, in which gadolinium was given by continuous intravenous infusion, MRI was found to be as sensitive as CT for detecting hepatic metastases in 4 of 15 patients with metastatic gastrinomas. In another recent study of 16 patients with ZES, gadolinium did not enhance the ability to find the primary or metastatic tumor.[835] MRI is rapidly improving, and in a study using MRI that corrects for motion by respiratory gating, signal averaging, and fast image analysis, MRI was more sensitive than angiography or CT for metastatic disease.[835] MRI may be the initial imaging study of choice for metastatic disease, although MRI studies remain less sensitive than angiography for primary tumor.[835]

Even though gastrinomas frequently occur in the duodenum (see Tables 41–26 and 41–27), they rarely are seen by routine upper gastrointestinal endoscopy because they are small and submucosal.[712] Endoscopic transillumination of the duodenum at surgery has been attempted and was useful in localizing small gastrinomas not found by other modalities (see Table 41–30).[836] In a recent prospective study of 26 patients, 12

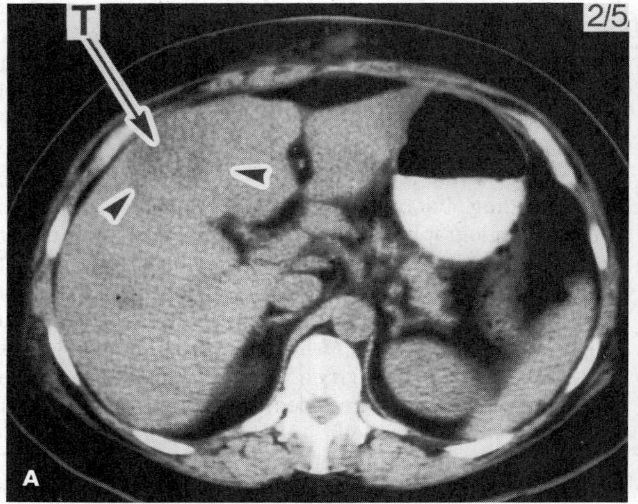

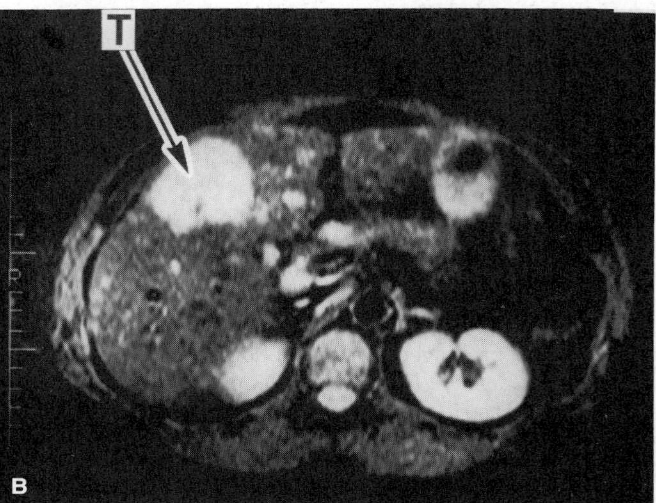

FIGURE 41–12. CT and MRI scans in a patient with metastatic gastrinoma. **(A)** The CT scan shows a large metastatic tumor (T) deposit in the left lobe of the liver (*arrowheads*). **(B)** The MRI STIR sequence more clearly demonstrates the metastatic tumor (T).

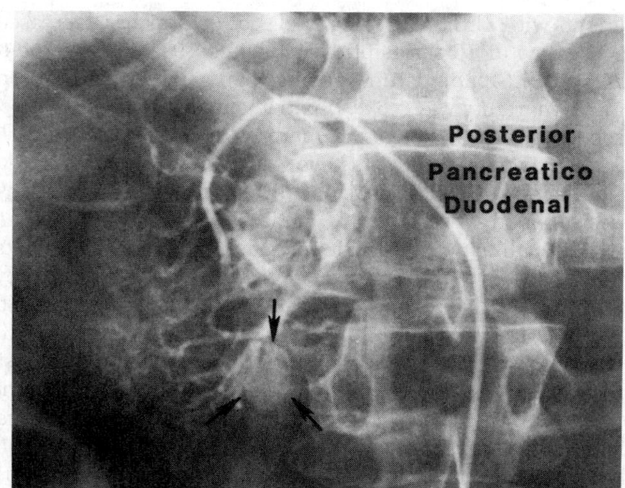

FIGURE 41–13. Selective injection of the posterior pancreaticoduodenal artery shows a small gastrinoma (*arrows*) in the posteroinferior portion of the pancreatic head in a patient with Zollinger-Ellison syndrome.

duodenal gastrinomas were found at surgery in 10 patients.[836] Operative endoscopic transillumination detected 10 of the 12 (83% sensitivity), a sensitivity significantly greater than that of preoperative imaging, which detected 3 duodenal gastrinomas (25% sensitivity), or of IOUS and palpation, which detected 5 (42% sensitivity). It is not known whether this procedure is as sensitive as duodenotomy or has less morbidity. A preliminary report suggests that endoscopic ultrasound should be helpful for preoperatively localizing duodenal tumors.[837] In this study, endoscopic ultrasound localized tumor in 8 of 13 patients (61%), including a primary pancreatic gastrinoma or gastrinoma in lymph nodes not seen on CT scan; however, it failed to localize 3 duodenal gastrinomas. Future prospective studies are needed to evaluate its potential fully.

Early studies in a small number of patients with ZES suggested that selective venous sampling for gastrin from portal venous tributaries (PVS) would be helpful (see Table 41–30).[838–840] In a recent prospective study, a combination of PVS and imaging yielded results only marginally better than imaging alone in identifying gastrinomas.[808] In this study, neither the magnitude of the gastrin gradient nor its presence or absence correlated with finding a gastrinoma at surgery. A typical result localizing a gastrinoma to the pancreatic head area is shown in Figure 41–14. A gradient of more than 50% is reported to occur in 74% of all patients with ZES.[808,841] PVS requires expertise, is time consuming, and has some morbidity, primarily abdominal pain at the catheter insertion site.[808,841] These drawbacks, combined with its limited availability and the fact that 70% to 80% of gastrinomas are in the pancreatic head, have led most investigators[796,808] but not all[842] to conclude that this procedure has limited usefulness in ZES. PVS, although occasionally helpful, is not recommended for gastrinomas. PVS has proved valuable in localizing insulinomas, which can occur throughout the pancreas.[843,844]

Most gastrinomas (91%) demonstrate a paradoxical release of gastrin with intravenous injection of secretin (see Fig. 41–11).[806–808] This characteristic has been used to localize gas-

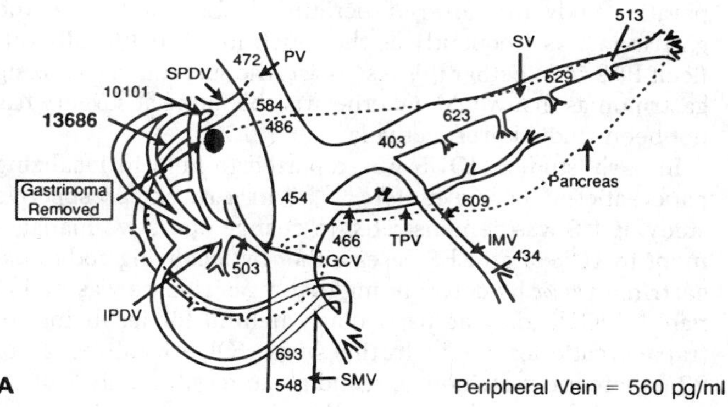

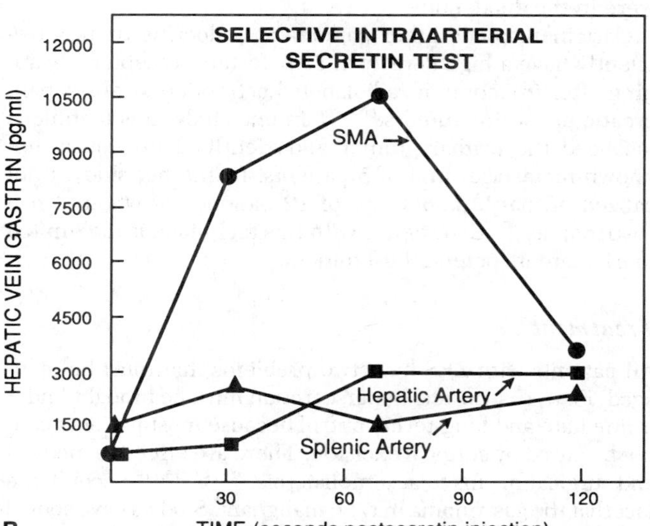

FIGURE 41–14. Selective portal venous sampling and intraarterial secretin injection to localize gastrinoma in a patient with ZES. **(A)** The selective venous gastrin concentration at different locations with a simultaneous peripheral gastrin of 560 pg/ml. This patient had a marked gradient of 2343% in the pancreatic head. The solid dot indicates the location of the 1-cm gastrinoma found subsequently in the pancreatic head at surgery. **(B)** The serum gastrin concentration (from the same patient) in the hepatic vein after secretin injection (30 units) sequentially into the hepatic, superior or mesenteric (SMA), and splenic arteries. Hepatic venous samples were collected before injection and at 0.5, 1 and 2 minutes after injection. A rapid rise from 520 pg/ml to 10,500 pg/ml at 30 seconds occurred with the SMA injection, whereas the increase with injection in the other arteries occurred later and was of less magnitude. These results localized the gastrinoma to the pancreatic head area supplied by the SMA, which was the area in which a 1-cm gastrinoma was found subsequently **(A)**. GCV, gastrocolic vein; TPA, tranverse pancreatic vein; IMV, inferior mesenteric vein; SMV, superior mesenteric vein; SPDV, superior pancreaticoduodenal vein; IPDV, inferior pancreaticoduodenal vein; PV, portal vein.

trinomas selectively by injecting secretin intraarterially into various abdominal arteries and collecting venous samples from the hepatic veins for assays of gastrin.[843,845,846] Figure 41–14 (lower panel) demonstrates a rapid increase in hepatic vein gastrin concentration after injection of secretin into the superior mesenteric artery. The other vessels demonstrated smaller increases that occurred at later times. A gastrinoma was found in this patient in the pancreatic head, which is supplied by the superior mesenteric artery. In a recent comparative study, intraarterial secretin was found to localize the gastrinoma as frequently as the much more technically difficult PVS.[846] Whether this test assists the surgeon in localizing gastrinomas that would not otherwise be found at surgery has not been studied prospectively.

In early studies, IOUS was reported to help in localizing pancreatic endocrine tumors.[847–849] In a recent prospective study, IOUS was demonstrated to change operative management in 10% of all ZES cases either by localizing additional gastrinomas or by determining that a gastrinoma was malignant.[850] IOUS may be particularly helpful for localizing intrapancreatic lesions.[850] In this study, IOUS localized 22 of 23 pancreatic gastrinomas found at surgery but only 7 of 12 extrapancreatic gastrinomas. All 5 of the gastrinomas missed were in the duodenum.[850]

Gastrinomas and other pancreatic endocrine tumors frequently have a high density of somatostatin receptors. Scanning after injection of radiolabeled octreotide localizes pancreatic endocrine tumors.[604–606] In one study, this technique localized the primary tumor and identified previously unknown metastases in 4 of 5 patients. In another study, it localized primary tumors in 7 of 12 patients, of whom 3 had gastrinomas.[606] Experience with this technique is too limited to evaluate its potential usefulness.

Treatment

All patients with ZES have two problems that must be managed. First, gastric acid hypersecretion must be brought under immediate and long-term control because most patients cannot be cured by surgical excision. There are effective medical and surgical means to accomplish this.[691,712,715,719] Second, the fact that the gastrinoma may be malignant. Studies have shown that if acid hypersecretion is controlled, these patients have an excellent quality of life. Long-term prognosis increasingly is being determined by the malignant nature of the gastrinoma.[712] Although in recent studies only about 30% patients at diagnosis have metastatic disease, in previous studies 60% to 90% of patients had metastatic disease (see Table 41–26). The exact percentage of gastrinomas that are malignant is not clear. However, in contrast to insulinomas, of which only 15% are malignant, as many as 60% to 90% of gastrinomas may be malignant (see Table 41–26).[520,702,851] Therefore, it is important to consider therapy directed at the gastrinoma itself, including therapies for metastatic disease and surgical excision of nonmetastatic gastrinoma.

Treatment of Acid Secretion

Surgical Treatment of Gastric Hypersecretion. Until recently, all patients with ZES required total gastrectomy to control gastric acid hypersecretion. In early studies, patients at the time of surgery were debilitated with complicated ulcer disease, had electrolyte abnormalities, and were malnourished. The operation frequently had to be done as an emergency, leading to a mortality rate of 15% in the postoperative period.[757,758] Operative results were unsatisfactory for patients who had less than total gastrectomy, with most patients developing recurrent ulcer disease, often with lethal complications, within days of surgery.[757,758] With the development of increasingly effective medical therapy, the mortality for patients with ZES undergoing total gastrectomy has decreased. In a review of 10 series published since 1978 involving 248 cases of ZES patients undergoing total gastrectomy, the operative mortality was 5.6%. If patients undergoing emergency procedures are excluded, the operative mortality was 2.4%.[762] Although some researchers have stated that the morbidity rate is low, adequate follow-up is not always apparent.[762] In at least one well-studied series of 18 patients undergoing total gastrectomy, all patients experienced one or several side effects, including symptoms of esophageal reflux, early satiety, cramping, or diarrhea.[766] These side effects were moderate to severe in 50% of the patients, and in 3 patients (27%) serious additional complications developed, including stenosis of the esophageal anastomosis in 2 patients, and recurrent, severe vomiting in the third patient.[766] The morbidity associated with total gastrectomy may be significant and is probably underestimated in many series.[691] Furthermore, a nutritional morbidity is associated with total gastrectomy that includes weight loss and anemia. Although one early study claimed that total gastrectomy could lead to regression of the gastrinoma in some patients,[852] recent studies have failed to substantiate this claim.[759,799,821] There is no evidence that medical therapy of gastric hypersecretion or total gastrectomy affects the growth rate of the gastrinoma.[503]

The development of increasingly effective medical therapy has led to a considerable debate over the role of total gastrectomy in controlling gastric acid hypersecretion.[691,719,762,853] Some groups continue to advocate total gastrectomy, citing high failure rates with medical therapy and improved morbidity and mortality now that total gastrectomy can be performed electively after correcting malnutrition.[722,762,853] Gastric acid hypersecretion can be controlled medically long-term in every patient who takes oral medication, using the H^+-K^+-ATPase inhibitor omeprazole.[854–861] The availability of omeprazole and its long duration of action has greatly simplified management because it can be taken once or twice per day. Therefore, most authorities recommend that total gastrectomy be reserved for patients who do not have access to routine medical follow-up or who cannot or will not take oral medication.[764,796] In all other patients, medical therapy is the treatment of choice.

A combination of anticholinergic agents and H_2 receptor antagonists has a greater effect than either drug alone.[862–864] The use of anticholinergic agents frequently is associated with side effects that limit patient acceptance.[865] Richardson and colleagues reported that parietal cell vagotomy in patients with ZES in whom no tumor was found at surgery decreased the BAO by 66% and decreased the antisecretory drug requirement by 95% in all patients.[825] Even though it is likely that the antisecretory drug dose requirement will increase slowly as the gastrinoma progresses, use of a parietal cell vagotomy will delay high-dose requirements for years in most patients.[825] Because of the availability of potent antisecretory agents such as omeprazole, parietal cell vagotomy should not be performed routinely.[796] Rather, it should be reserved for the occasional patient who has a high-dose antisecretory medication requirement and an unresectable tumor or tumor not found (Fig. 41–15).

In patients with ZES and the MEN-I syndrome, medical control of gastric hypersecretion can be facilitated greatly by correction of the hyperparathyroidism, which almost always

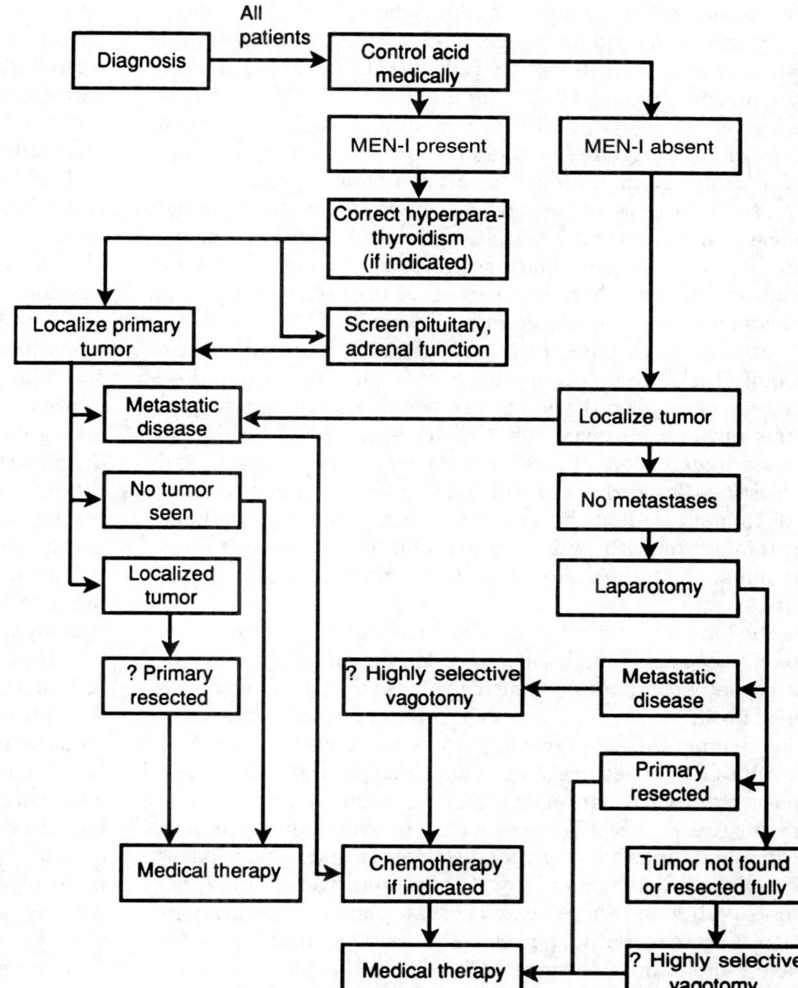

FIGURE 41–15. Flow diagram for the management of patients with Zollinger-Ellison syndrome. It is unclear whether a highly selective vagotomy should be performed in a patient in whom metastatic disease is found at the time of surgery. With the availability of omeprazole, gastric acid hypersecretion can be controlled in all such patients so that parietal cell vagotomy is indicated less frequently. If a primary tumor is seen on imaging studies in patients with MEN-I, there is no general agreement as to whether patients should undergo surgery because resection of a pancreatic tumor does not result in cure.

is present by the time ZES develops.[514] Correction of hyperparathyroidism may reduce the fasting serum gastrin concentration, increase the responsiveness to a given dose of antisecretory medication, and decrease the BAO.[866–868] Therefore, in patients with MEN-I and hyperparathyroidism, parathyroidectomy should be performed before any other surgical procedure to control acid hypersecretion.

Medical Treatment of Gastric Hypersecretion. The results of medical treatment of gastric acid hypersecretion have been reviewed extensively.[691,764,796,820,856,865,869] H_2 antagonists (*e.g.*, cimetidine, ranitidine, famotidine) alone or in combination with anticholinergic agents probanthine (*e.g.*, propantheline bromide and isopropamide) and more recently omeprazole, the substituted benzimidazole that functions as a H^+-K^+-ATPase inhibitor, have been used successfully in the long-term treatment of gastric hypersecretion in ZES. The number of patients failing medical therapy varies greatly in different series,[691,719,796,869] with failure rates ranging from 0 to 65% for cimetidine,[691,704,766,870–872] from 0 to 40% for ranitidine,[691,757,873] no reported failure for famotidine,[862,874] and from 0 to 7.5% for omeprazole.[854–861] An analysis of these series concluded that the principal factors contributing to failure of H_2 receptor antagonists to control acid hypersecretion were inadequate doses of antisecretory medication and the failure to use reliable criteria for assessing the ability of these agents to suppress BAO.[869] In general, relief of symptoms does not reflect adequately the effectiveness of antisecretory therapy.[871,872,875] To assess the adequacy of antisecretory therapy, gastric acid secretion must be measured while the patient is taking medication.[691,719,876]

The amount of antisecretory medication required varies widely from patient to patient and increases slowly with time. The optimal dose of medication must be determined for each patient initially and periodically reevaluated.[691,764,820,856] If enough antisecretory drug is used to decrease gastric acid secretion to less than 10 mEq/hour for the hour before the next dose of medications in patients without previous gastric surgery and to less than 5 mEq/hour in patients with previous acid-reducing procedures or severe esophageal disease, peptic ulcers will heal and complications of peptic ulcer disease will be prevented.[721,764,794,854,873,875] To reduce acid output to these levels before the next dose of medication, patients usually require more than twice the usual dose of H_2 antagonist or three times the usual dose of omeprazole recommended for idiopathic peptic ulcer disease. In recent studies, the median doses were 3.6 g/day for cimetidine (range, 1.2–12.6 g/day), 1.2 g/day for ranitidine (range, 0.45–6 g/day), 0.25 g/day for famotidine (range, 0.05–0.8 g/day), and 60 to 80 mg for omeprazole (range, 20–360 mg/day).[764,796,856,862,873,874] It is not clear why patients with ZES require more than the usual dose of H_2 antagonist or omeprazole to inhibit acid output adequately. Some patients have been shown to have a decreased sensitivity of the acid secretory process to H_2 antagonists or impaired or delayed absorption, but in 25% of patients no alteration in drug pharmacokinetics is found.[877,878] One study reported no alterations in absorptive or pharmacokinetic parameters for omeprazole in patients with ZES.[879]

Although high doses of H_2 antagonist or omeprazole are required initially and patients may require up to one dose increase per year, the long-term use of H_2 antagonists and omeprazole has proved effective and safe.[764,796,856] Although antiandrogen side effects (impotence, gynecomastia, and breast tenderness) occur with high-dose cimetidine in up to 60% of male patients,[880] long-term treatment with cimetidine in females or with ranitidine, famotidine, or omeprazole in patients of either sex has been demonstrated to be safe.[691,764,796,865]

The long-term use of omeprazole has caused concern about toxicity because female rats given long-term omeprazole (or other potent inhibitors of gastric acid secretion) have developed proliferation of gastric ECL cells and in some cases carcinoid tumors of the stomach.[505,856] Results have led most[505,856] but not all[508] investigators to conclude that the ECL hyperplasia and gastric carcinoid tumor formation in these animal models were most likely secondary to drug-induced achlorhydria and the resultant hypergastrinemia, and not secondary directly to a toxic action of the antisecretory drug. First, patients with long-term elevated serum gastrin concentrations such as those with ZES, pernicious anemia, or chronic gastritis have increased numbers of ECL cells in the gastric mucosa and have been reported to develop gastric carcinoid tumors.[505,856] Second, gastrin has been shown to be trophic to the gastric mucosa in animals and to cause ECL hyperplasia.[503,505,723,856] Third, ECL hyperplasia is caused not only by omeprazole or unsurmountable inhibitors of gastric acid secretion but also by large doses of H_2 receptor antagonists such as ranitidine, loxtidine, SKF9378, BL-6431, ICI 162,846, or sodium bicarbonate.[503,505,508,856] Fourth, in animal studies, hyperplasia of the ECL cells was proportional to the hypergastrinemia produced by various means and was prevented by antrectomy.[503,505,856] Fifth, other means of inducing hypergastrinemia such as gastric antral exclusion and fundectomy can increase the number of ECL cells and in some cases cause the development of carcinoid tumors.[511,881]

Hyperplasia of gastric endocrine cells occurs in patients with ZES. Quantitative studies indicate that gastric ECL cells are increased about twofold, independent of administration of antisecretory agents.[499,503,856,882–884] Of the six types of gastric endocrine cells, only the ECL cells were increased and underwent neoplastic changes in patients with ZES.[884] In two studies in which omeprazole treatment was prolonged for up to 4 years, there was no statistical increase in gastric ECL cells due to this drug.[882,883] The lack of effect of omeprazole on ECL-cell hyperplasia in patients with ZES appears to conflict with reports of gastric carcinoids in patients with ZES, some of whom were taking omeprazole.[503,856,884] Recent reports have described patients with ZES who developed carcinoid tumors of the stomach, some of whom were being treated with omeprazole.[503,856,884] In 15 of 16 patients reported with gastric carcinoids and ZES in whom the presence or absence of MEN-I could be determined, 14 had MEN-I.[503,856] In one well-studied series of 170 patients, 24% of the patients had ZES with MEN-I.[822] Both patients who developed gastric carcinoid tumors had MEN-I.[883] Therefore, about 2 of 41 patients with MEN-I and ZES developed gastric carcinoids, but of 129 patients with the sporadic form of ZES, no patient developed gastric carcinoids. Two of the 16 cases of gastric carcinoids occurred in patients with ZES who were taking omeprazole when the gastric carcinoid tumors were diagnosed and who had ZES with MEN-I.[856] Therefore, 14 of the patients with ZES reported to have gastric carcinoids were not taking omeprazole when the gastric carcinoid tumors were diagnosed, and almost all had MEN-I. These data suggest that the presence of MEN-I may be an important factor predisposing patients with ZES to the development of gastric carcinoids.[499,856]

Most patients with ZES require H_2 antagonists every 4 to 8 hours to inhibit gastric secretion adequately.[796,820,865] In contrast to optimally effective doses of cimetidine or ranitidine, which each have a duration of action of 6 to 8 hours,[862] and of famotidine, which has a duration of action of 10 hours,[720] the optimal dose of omeprazole has a long duration of action (>48 hours),[854–856,879] allowing most patients to require omeprazole only once or twice a day. Anticholinergic agents that were used extensively in the past[865] are rarely used. H_2 antagonists continue to be useful, although omeprazole is the drug of choice.[503,820,856] The usual starting dose of omeprazole is 60 mg/day, although some patients are better controlled with two doses daily.[856] Patients with ZES who have had previous gastric surgery, have moderate to severe esophageal disease, or have MEN-I usually require a higher dose and are best treated by starting with 40 mg twice a day.[794,856,885]

If the patient presents with a complication and cannot take oral antisecretory medication, or if during surgery it is important to control secretion, continuous infusions of cimetidine (median dose 3 mg/kg/hour) or ranitidine (median dose 1 mg/kg/hour) or bolus doses of omeprazole (injectable, 60 mg every 12 hours; not available in the United States) are all effective.[876,886–889] These drugs should be continued until oral antisecretory agents can be restarted.[503,876,888,889]

Treatment of Gastrinoma

The 5-year survival rate for patients with ZES ranges from 62% to 75%, and the 10-year survival ranges from 47% to 53% (Table 41–31). Although the growth of a gastrinoma generally is slow, long-term studies of patients originally treated by total gastrectomy found that in 57% of patients, death was due to tumor progression.[758,759] Therefore, with the ability to control gastric acid hypersecretion, the malignant potential of the tumor is an increasingly important determinant of long-term prognosis. Various factors that contribute to long-term survival have been identified. The extent of the tumor and whether MEN-I is present or absent have been reported to determine survival rates (see Table 41–31). In patients with no tumor found at laparotomy or in whom tumor is completely resectable, 5-year and 10-year survival rates are 90% to 100% (see Table 41–31).

TABLE 41–31. Prognosis in Patients With Zollinger-Ellison Syndrome

Investigations	*No. of Patients*	*5-Year Survival (%)*	*10-Year Survival (%)*
All Patients			
Thompson et al, 1983[762]	27	75	52
Zollinger et al, 1984[765]	40	62	47
Mignon et al, 1986[822]	144	62	53
Ellison et al, 1987[891]	60	63	52
Related to Tumor Resectability			
No tumor found			
Malagelada et al, 1983[766]	13	100	100
Zollinger et al, 1984[765]	6	100	—
Stabile and Passaro, 1984[767]	10	90	90
Zollinger, 1985[890]	8	ND	63
Norton et al, 1992[745]	16	90	ND
Tumor resected			
Malagelada et al, 1983[766]	7	100	100
Zollinger et al, 1984[765]	22	76	—
Stabile and Passaro, 1984[767]	10	90	90
Ellison et al, 1987[891]	33	69	62
Norton et al, 1992[745]	42	95	ND
Tumor incompletely resected or recurrence			
Malagelada et al, 1983[766]	10	75	20
Zollinger et al, 1984[765]	7	14	—
Norton et al, 1992[745]	15	95	ND
Unresectable			
Malagelada et al, 1983[766]	13	80	—
Zollinger et al, 1984[765]	7	30	—
Stabile and Passaro, 1984[767]	14	40	30
Hancke, 1979[1108]	15	20	—
Norton et al, 1992[745]	18	18	ND
Related to MEN-I Status			
MEN-I present			
Malagelada et al, 1983[766]	14	—	80
Thompson et al, 1983[762]	11	85	85
Zollinger et al, 1984[765]	13	85	62
Stabile and Passaro, 1984[767]	23	80	75
Zollinger, 1985[890]	7	ND	71
Ellison et al, 1987[891]	16	75	70
Podevin et al, 1990[892]	45	70	63
MEN-I absent			
Malagelada et al, 1983[766]	36	—	64
Thompson et al, 1983[762]	26	70	50
Zollinger et al, 1984[765]	27	52	40
Stabile and Passaro, 1984[767]	42	70	65
Zollinger, 1985[890]	7	ND	71
Ellison et al, 1987[891]	44	70	65
Podevin et al, 1990[892]	135	66	55

MEN-I, multiple endocrine neoplasia type I; ND, not determined.

Survival curves from a recent large prospective study of curative resection in ZES are shown in Figure 41–16, demonstrating excellent long-term survival in patients with resected disease or tumors so small they cannot be detected at surgery, whereas patients who develop advanced metastatic disease have a poor survival.[745] In contrast, patients with tumor incompletely resected or unresectable have 5-year survival averaging 50% and an average 10-year survival of 25%. In two studies, patients with MEN-I are reported to have a better 5-year and 10-year survival than patients without MEN-I,[762,765] whereas in other studies[766,767,890–892] the difference was not significant (see Table 41–31). The presence of Cushing's syndrome is associated with a poor prognosis.[893] It has not been proved a poor prognostic factor, because it usually occurs in patients with ZES without MEN-I when extensive metastases are present, a condition that already has a poor prognosis.[893]

Because of the excellent prognosis of patients with gastrinoma who are resected and the increased importance of the malignancy in determining survival, surgical resection of the gastrinoma should be considered in all patients with ZES. The general approach to the gastrinoma is summarized in the flow diagram in Figure 41–15. The first step is to control gastric acid hypersecretion medically. It must then be determined whether the patient has sporadic ZES (ZES without MEN-I) or whether ZES is present with MEN-I.[691] The role of surgery is controversial in patients with MEN-I (see the sections on MEN-I and on pancreatic endocrine tumors in MEN-I).

Treatment of Nonmetastatic Gastrinoma. The role of surgery in the treatment of the gastrinoma is becoming better defined.[745,783] All physicians agree that the ideal treatment of ZES is the surgical excision of the gastrinoma, but in early studies this was possible in only 8 of 157 patients.[717,719–721,799] Even this figure was probably an overestimation of the cure rate because in many cases follow-up was less than 1 year and in no cases were multiple secretin provocative tests performed postoperatively.[503,691] In series reported since 1986, the cure rate is higher, averaging about 40% and ranging from 17% to 100% (Table 41–32).

Surgical cure rates may continue to increase. With the development of effective antisecretory agents, all patients can undergo extensive preoperative investigational studies, surgery can be done electively, and the surgery can emphasize gastrinoma localization and removal rather than control of gastric acid hypersecretion.[503,745,783] The preoperative localization and clinical distinction between patients with and without MEN-I identifies groups of patients with different potential for cure. More than 90% of patients with gastrinoma metastatic to the liver can be identified with imaging studies, obviating unnecessary attempts at curative surgery in these patients.[745,783,828,830] Because gastrinomas occur more frequently in the duodenum than previously thought (see Tables 41–26 and 41–27), preoperative localization studies frequently do not identify extrapancreatic gastrinomas.[691,741,745,783,828–830] Even when the gastrinoma is localized, potential resectability cannot be predicted if hepatic metastases are not present.

In a recent large prospective study, the overall percentage of patients with no evidence of disease immediately postoperatively was 58%.[745] At 5 years, 30% of all patients remained

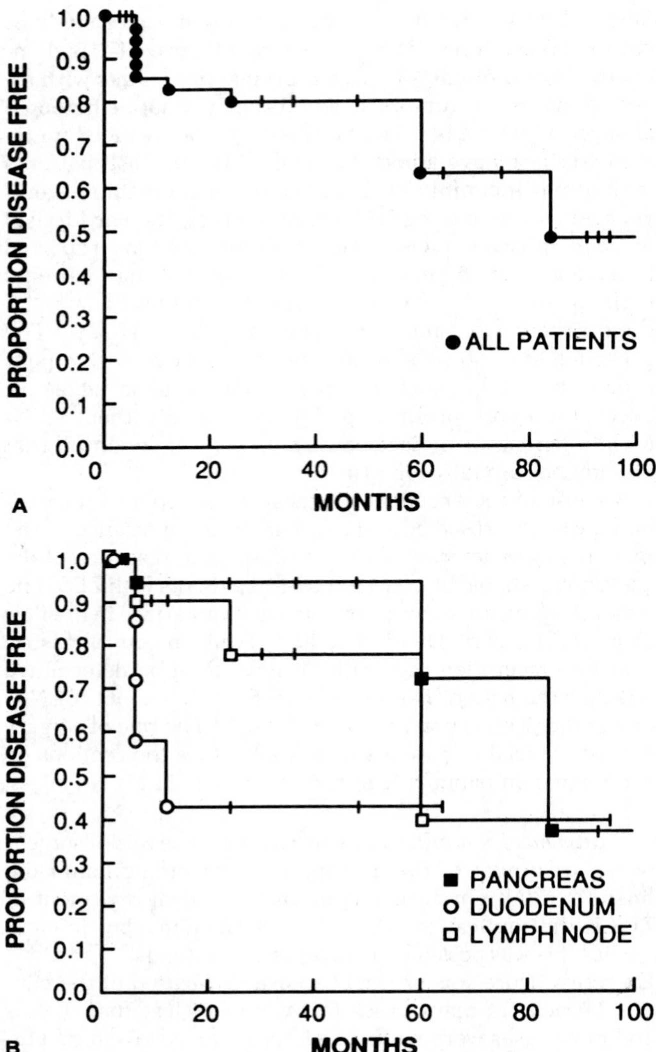

FIGURE 41–16. Time to recurrence of Zollinger-Ellison syndrome in patients initially disease-free by surgery. **(A)** The Kaplan-Meier plot of the time to recurrence for all patients (n = 42) who were disease free of Zollinger-Ellison syndrome at the initial (3- or 6-month) postoperative follow-up. *Disease-free* is defined as no evidence of gastrinoma on imaging studies, normal fasting gastrin concentration, and negative secretin and calcium provocative tests. **(B)** Kaplan-Meier plot of the time to recurrence of Zollinger-Ellison syndrome of patients who were rendered disease-free of Zollinger-Ellison syndrome at the initial postoperative follow-up divided by primary disease site: duodenum (n = 12), pancreas (n = 19), and lymph node (n = 10). One patient with the primary ovarian gastrinoma is excluded. Patients with primary duodenal gastrinomas had a significantly shorter disease-free interval than patients with pancreatic gastrinomas ($p < 0.01$). The difference between patients with duodenal gastrinomas and those with lymph node only gastrinomas was not significant ($p = 0.1$). The median disease-free survival for patients with duodenal, pancreatic, or lymph node primary gastrinomas was 12, 84, and 60 months, respectively. (Modified from Norton JA, Doppman JL, Jensen RT. Curative resection in Zollinger-Ellison syndrome: results of a 10 year prospective study. Ann Surg 1992;215:8)

TABLE 41–32. Long-Term Results of Attempts at Complete Surgical Resection of Gastrinoma

Investigations	*No. of Patients Operated**	*Patients With Normal Gastrin Postresection Number (%)*
Stage and Stadil, 1979[717]	25	1 (4)
Zollinger et al, 1980[720] †	42	2 (5)
Bonfils et al, 1981[722] †	32	6 (6.5)
Friesen, 1982[853] †	23	9 (39)
Wilson, 1982[1109] †	28	6 (22)
Wolfe et al, 1982[744] †	18	4 (22)
Thompson et al, 1983[762] †	26	3 (12)
Deveney et al, 1983[823] †	52	6 (12)
Malagelada et al, 1983[766]	44	7 (16)
Stabile et al, 1984[746] †	45	5 (11)
Richardson et al, 1985[825]	22	4 (18)
Norton et al, 1986[743]	29	12 (43 postop) (30; 6 mo–4 y)
Mignon et al, 1986[822]	125	32 (26)
Vogel et al, 1987[1110] †	20	5 (25)
Ellison et al, 1987[891]	60	10 (17)
Howard et al, 1990[748]	11	8 (73)
Delcore et al, 1989[1111]	43	12 (27)
Thompson et al, 1989[829]	5	5 (100)
Norton et al, 1992[745]	73	42 (58; 3 mo) 22 (30; 5 y)

* The total number of patients reported to have undergone exploratory laparotomy in each series.
† Series in which total gastrectomy was performed in most cases.

cured (see Fig. 41–16). The recurrence rate varied markedly for different groups of patients at different times, depending on where the primary tumor was found (see Fig. 41–16). The recurrence rate was significantly greater in patients with duodenal primaries.[745] Furthermore, 55% of duodenal tumors and only 25% of pancreatic tumors were associated with metastases, suggesting that duodenal primaries are much more malignant than previously believed.[503,755,894] The long-term survival in this study for all patients was excellent, with more than 90% surviving for all the nonmetastatic groups (Fig. 41–17).[745] Survival was similar for patients cured, patients resected but not cured, and patients in whom a small gastrinoma was not found. It might be concluded that surgery is not helpful because patients with no gastrinoma found or those cured had equal 5-year survival rates (see Fig. 41–17). It is known that if patients have a gastrinoma so small it cannot be found on a detailed exploratory laparotomy, they have an excellent prognosis.[766] Preliminary evidence suggests this group is not representative of patients with gastrinomas, including the patients who had gastrinomas found and resected. In preliminary long-term studies at the National Institutes of Health, a number of patients who did not undergo surgical resection developed metastatic disease to the liver. There is no way to predict which patients will develop metastatic disease. Therefore, all patients with sporadic gastrinoma (*i.e.*, ZES that is not associated with MEN-I) and with no serious contraindication to surgery should undergo localization studies (selective hepatic and pancreatic angiography, CT, MRI, ultrasound), preferably

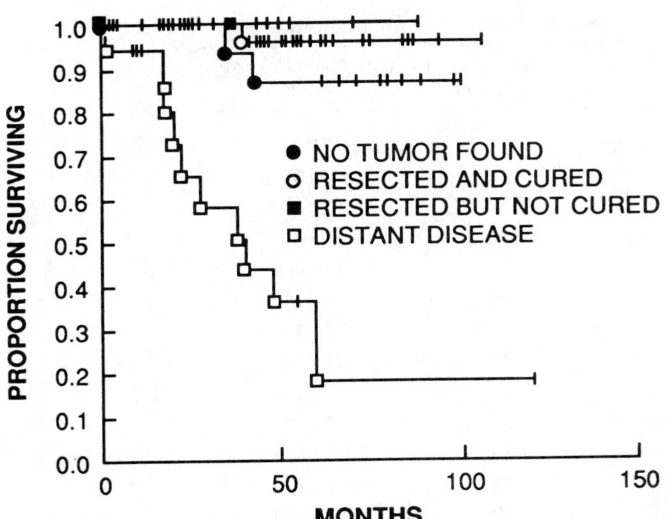

FIGURE 41–17. Survival of patients with Zollinger-Ellison syndrome from the day of diagnosis. Patients were divided into four groups based on preoperative evaluation, operative findings, and initial postoperative evaluation: (1) patients who had biopsy confirmation of bulky metastatic gastrinoma on initial evaluation (n = 18, open squares); (2) patients who had all tumor resected and were functionally disease-free (cured) at initial postoperative evaluation (n = 42, open circles); (3) patients who had all tumor resected but were functionally not disease-free (cured) (n = 15, closed squares); and (4) patients with no tumor found (closed circles). There were no significant differences seen among the three groups who did not have metastatic gastrinoma. However, the group with distant disease survived for a significantly shorter time than all other patient groups ($p < 0.001$). (Modified from Norton JA, Doppman JL, Jensen RT. Curative resection in Zollinger-Ellison syndrome: results of a 10 year prospective study. Ann Surg 1992; 215:8)

in a center with considerable experience with these patients.[691,764,796,843] If no metastases are found, the patient should undergo surgical exploration (Fig. 41–15).

In our experience, the single most important factor in achieving good surgical results is the expertise of the surgeon. Even very experienced pancreatic surgeons have almost no experience with islet cell tumors and no appreciation of the difficulty in identifying the extrapancreatic gastrinomas or the technique of enucleating lesions within the pancreas. A gastrinoma found at laparotomy as a solitary lesion in the liver should be removed, provided the resection can be performed safely. If gastrinoma is found in the pancreatic head, it should be enucleated.[743,745,796,895] If unresectable gastrinoma is found in the pancreatic head area, a pancreaticoduodenectomy (Whipple's operation) is not indicated. No studies have demonstrated an increased survival overall in patients with ZES after pancreaticoduodenectomy. Furthermore, because of the marked morbidity and mortality associated with this operation (up to 37% in one study)[783,838] and the excellent long-term prognosis of these patients, it is not established that the adverse consequences of a pancreaticoduodenectomy might not outweigh the adverse consequences of an unresected solitary gastrinoma. If no gastrinoma is found at surgery, as occurs in 7% to 30% of cases overall but in 60% of cases in one series,[825] a blind distal pancreatectomy should not be performed, because 65% to 90% of gastrinomas are found in the pancreatic head or duodenum (gastrinoma triangle[743,745,746,783] and because such an approach has not improved cure rates.[796] The use of IOUS to localize additional lesions and to confirm the significance of a palpated mass is recommended.[847–850] This allows identification of some masses as malignant and can help determine the extent of resection that may be needed.[850]

Special attention needs to be paid to finding duodenal gastrinomas. In a recent prospective study, gastrinomas were found in 64% of patients using the above described procedures, of which 11% were in the duodenum and 33% in the pancreas (see Table 41–27).[745] When transillumination of the duodenum at surgery[836] and a duodenotomy were used, gastrinomas were found in 92% of patients,[745] 43% in the pancreas and 30% in the duodenum (see Table 41–27). The increase was entirely due to the detection of additional duodenal gastrinomas, which frequently are small. A 3-cm duodenotomy is recommended along the antimesenteric aspect of the duodenum and entering on the second portion of the duodenum with the option to extend in either direction.[745] The duodenal wall should be palpated carefully, with the index finger inside the duodenum and the thumb on the outside, and the distal third and fourth parts of the duodenum examined by everting them into the incision. If no tumor is found at laparotomy, or if the gastrinoma is unresectable or metastatic to the liver and the patient had a high antisecretory drug requirement before surgery (>4.8 g/day cimetidine), a highly selective vagotomy may be considered (see Fig. 41–15).

The role of surgery in the treatment of patients with ZES with MEN-I is unclear (see Fig. 41–15).[712,719,783,896] Surgery is discussed later in this chapter in the section on pancreatic endocrine tumors in MEN-I.

Treatment of Metastatic Gastrinoma. Because patients with metastatic gastrinomas have a markedly decreased survival (Table 41–31 and Fig. 41–17) and because the malignant nature of the gastrinoma is becoming an increasingly important determinant of survival, there is an increasing need for effective treatment of metastatic gastrinoma and other metastatic pancreatic endocrine tumors. Chemotherapy, hepatic embolization, systematic removal of all resectable tumor, hormonal therapy with a somatostatin analog, and treatment with interferon (Table 41–33) have been advocated, but the role of each remains unclear.

Chemotherapy using streptozocin alone or in combination with 5-FU or 5-FU plus doxorubicin has been reported to be effective at reducing tumor size in 5% to 63% of patients with islet cell tumors (see Table 41–33). In one study, the combination of streptozocin plus 5-FU was more effective than streptozocin alone.[897] Dacarbazine and doxorubicin have given poor response rates alone (9–20%), and chlorozotocin has given about the same response rate (50%; see Table 41–33) as streptozocin alone. Almost all single studies that include significant numbers of patients and investigate the effects of chemotherapeutic agents on pancreatic endocrine tumors have been combined series that include all pancreatic endocrine tumors often compared with carcinoids. Whether these results can be extrapolated to include metastatic gastrinoma is not clear. Two studies have demonstrated no difference in response rates of various islet cell tumors to streptozocin;[897,898] however, there were only small numbers of patients with the

TABLE 41–33. Drug Therapy of Pancreatic Endocrine Tumor and Gastrinomas

Investigations	*Agent*	*No. of Patients*	*Objective Response Number (%)*
All Pancreatic Endocrine Tumors			
Broder and Carter 1973[444]	STZ	52	26 (50%)
Kvols and Buck, 1987[1019]		17	7 (41%)
Buchanan et al, 1986[898]		16	10 (62%)
Moertel et al, 1980[897]		42	14 (36%)
Moertel et al, 1982[1112]	DOX	20	4 (20%)
Bukowski et al, 1983[1113]	CZT	13	7 (53%)
Manger et al, 1986[463]	DTIC	11	1 (9%)
Manger et al, 1986[463]	Tubercidin	6	2 (33%)
Moertel et al, 1991[1024]	Etoposide + cisplatin	14	2 (14%)
Moertel et al, 1982[897]	STZ + 5-FU	40	25 (63%)
Maton, 1989[905]		22	1 (5%)
Oberg and Erikson, 1989[489]		30	19 (68%)
Kelsen et al, 1982[689]	STZ + DOX	5	1 (20%)
Frame et al, 1988[1114]		14	3 (21%)
Bonfils et al, 1986[1115]	STZ or STZ + 5-FU	45	19 (42%)
Von Schrenk et al, 1988[899]	STZ + 5-FU + DOX	10	4 (40%)
Maton et al, 1989[903]	Octreotide	46	8 (17%)
Maton 1989[905]		66	8 (11%)
Erikson et al, 1986[909]	Interferon	22	6 (27%)
Gastrinomas Only			
Jensen et al, 1983[719]	STZ	24	12 (50%)
Moertel et al, 1980[897]			
NIH 1987 (unpub. data)	DTIC	5	0 (0%)
Moertel et al, 1980[897]	STZ + 5-FU	3	1 (33%)
Mignon et al, 1986[822]		10	8 (80%)
Hofman et al, 1973[742]		5	1 (20%)
Ruszniewski et al, 1989[900]		22	1 (5%)
Bonfils et al, 1986[1115]	STZ + 5-FU	28	(42%)
Bonfils et al, 1986[1115]	STZ	17	(42%)
Von Schrenk et al, 1988[899]	STZ + 5-FU + DOX	10	4 (40%)
Kvols et al, 1987[1116]	Octreotide	9	1 (11%)
Maton et al, 1989[903]		16	3 (19%)
Maton, 1989[905]		22	3 (14%)
Erikson et al, 1986[909]	Interferon	4	2 (50%)
Slimak et al, 1991[910]		9	3 (33%)

STZ, streptozotocin; DOX, doxorubicin; CZT, chlorozotocin; 5-FU, 5-fluorouracil; DTIC, dacarbazine.

different type of pancreatic endocrine tumor. Other studies have suggested differential responses of gastrinomas, glucagonomas, and VIPomas to chemotherapeutic agents such as dacarbazine or streptozocin. When results from a number of small series are combined, streptozocin alone appears to cause an objective response in 50% of patients with metastatic gastrinoma (see Table 41–33). Streptozocin combined with 5-FU or 5-FU plus doxorubicin causes an objective response in 5% to 80% of patients with metastatic gastrinoma (see Table 41–33). For all pancreatic endocrine tumors, the combination of streptozocin and 5-FU gave a response rate of 63%, which was significantly better than the 40% response rate with streptozocin alone.[897] In a prospective study of 10 patients with metastatic gastrinoma to the liver that had increased in size over the 6 months before the patient entered the study, chemotherapy with streptozocin, 5-FU, and doxorubicin resulted in only a 40% objective response rate, no complete remissions, and no statistical difference in survival in responders versus nonresponders.[899] In another recent study of a similar group of 22 patients, only 5% of patients demonstrated an objective decrease in tumor size.[900] Therefore, the precise role and efficacy of chemotherapy in patients with metastatic gastrinoma has not been established, and it is not clear when chemotherapy should be considered in a given patient. Some patients have been followed for 20 years with stable metastatic disease,[759] whereas most die within 5 years, with a mean survival of 3 to 5 years.[720,722,762,799,826] Of the two groups with considerable experience with metastatic gastrinoma, one group proposed that patients be treated with chemotherapy when they become symptomatic.[897] If gastric acid hypersecretion is controlled adequately, symptoms due to the tumor will arise only late in the course of the disease. The other group proposed that after the initial evaluation patients be reassessed in 3 to 6 months and that those patients with evidence of increasing size of hepatic metastases should be treated with chemotherapy.[719,899] No studies have recommended chemotherapy in patients with metastases only to regional lymph nodes.

For tumors metastatic to the liver, hepatic arterial embolization has been recommended in patients with gastrinoma and other gastrointestinal endocrine tumors.[665,668,901,902] Only small numbers of gastrinomas have been treated by this technique and its effect on long-term survival is not known. Furthermore, distant metastases to bone recently have been reported to occur in 12% of all patients with hepatic metastases,[608] suggesting that procedures directed only at the disease in the liver, such as embolization, may be of limited value in many patients with extensive disease.

The data of Zollinger and colleagues suggest that removal of all resectable tumor or *debulking surgery* prolongs life expectancy.[720] There are no studies that have systematically evaluated debulking surgery. Norton and colleagues reported the successful resection of all metastatic disease in 5 of 20 patients with extensive disease, 2 of whom have maintained normal gastrin levels postoperatively.[826] Although debulking surgery requires systematic evaluation before it can be routinely recommended, these results raise the possibility that a small percentage of patients with extensive disease can be identified in whom removal of all resectable tumor may provide prolonged remission.

Hormonal therapy with octreotide is effective in controlling the symptoms of pancreatic endocrine or carcinoid-like tumors, including VIPomas, glucagonomas, GRFomas, insulinomas, gastrinomas, and carcinoids (see Table 41–33).[903–905] Octreotide has been reported to decrease the size of metastases or tumor growth of pancreatic endocrine tumors in animals[906] and humans.[905] Studies have reported a decrease in hepatic metastases in 3 patients of 22 with gastrinoma (see Table 41–33).[903,905,907,908] Another recent study of 9 patients with metastatic gastrinoma who were treated with octreotide for 1 to 11 months reported no effect.[904] Until controlled trials are done, treatment with octreotide cannot be recommended for routine use in patients with metastatic gastrinoma.

Human leukocyte interferon may be helpful in patients with metastatic pancreatic endocrine tumors including gastrinoma (see Table 41–33). In one study using interferon, 17 of 22 patients, most of whom had previously failed chemotherapy, demonstrated an objective response (defined as a decrease of more than 50% in tumor size or in tumor markers).[909] In a more recent study of 9 patients with metastatic gastrinoma to the liver that was increasing in size, interferon-α (5 million units/day) did not decrease tumor bulk but did slow tumor growth in 3 patients.[910] Because of the small numbers of cases and limited follow-up, it is unclear whether interferon can provide long-term benefit for patients with metastatic gastrinoma.

INSULINOMA

Insulin-secreting islet cell tumors encompass a broad range of diagnostic and therapeutic features. Insulinomas were first recognized by Whipple, who had seen 30 patients with hypoglycemia and pancreatic adenomas by 1935.[911] Whipple's triad, which consisted of the characteristic symptoms of hypoglycemia, blood sugars below 50 mg/dl, and immediate relief after ingestion of glucose, remained for many years the major diagnostic criteria for insulinoma.[911]

Insulinomas usually occur in patients between the ages of 20 and 75 years. The average age of presentation is between 44 and 46 years.[702,851,912,913] There is a preponderance of women in most series (60%),[702,851,914] and the reported incidence of insulinomas ranges from 0.8 to 0.9 persons per million population per year.[488,708] In these studies, the prevalence of insulinomas varied from twice as common as gastrinomas[708] to slightly less common than gastrinomas,[488] and insulinomas made up 27% of the pancreatic endocrine tumors in one series.[488]

Symptoms

The clinical symptoms of insulinomas are due to hypoglycemia in almost all instances. Most symptoms are neuroglycopenic, that is, provoked by insufficient availability to the CNS of glucose, which is the main source of energy to the brain.[482,914–917] The most common symptoms are visual disturbances (59%), confusion (51%), altered consciousness (38%), and weakness (32%). Seizures occur but are less common (23%).[482,914–917] Symptoms can occur due to catecholamine release (adrenergic symptoms)[482,915,916] such as sweating (43%) and tremulousness (23%). In one study of the initial presenting symptoms, 49% of patients had both neuroglycopenic symptoms and adrenergic symptoms, 38% had neuroglycopenic symptoms only, and 12% had adrenergic symptoms only.[915] Symptoms characteristically are associated with fasting, as when a meal is delayed or missed or with exercise.[482,851,914–916] There are numerous reports of erroneous psychiatric or neurologic diagnoses for patients with insulinomas.[918] These reports highlight the need for blood glucose measurements during any transient neuropsychiatric incident, particularly if it is recurrent. The duration of neuroglycopenic symptoms before diagnosis is usually longer than 3 years. Some patients present with a history of self-treatment by consuming frequent small meals.[919] Most patients with insulinomas are overweight and many are obese.

Diagnosis

Although there are useful clues to diagnosis of insulinoma, such as symptoms after a fast, symptoms often are nonspecific and the diagnosis can only be established by fasting with concomitant laboratory examination.[702,914,915] Investigation of patients with neuroglycopenic episodes begins with the documentation of hypoglycemia during these symptoms provoked by a fast. Organic hypoglycemia is usually defined as a blood sugar level of less than 40 mg/dl in the fasting state.[482,851,915] In healthy individuals, the blood glucose value usually does not decrease to less than 70 mg/dl after an overnight fast.[915]

In a study of patients with insulinomas, blood glucose levels after an overnight fast were less than 60 mg/dl in 53% of patients and less than 50 mg/dl in 39% of patients.[482] If this test is combined with measurement of plasma insulin levels, plasma insulin levels will be inappropriately elevated in 65% of people.[482,915] Because a single overnight fast, even when combined with a measurement of plasma insulin levels, does not establish the diagnosis of insulinoma in more than 55% of patients, a 72-hour fast usually is done with measurement of blood glucose and insulin levels at 2- to 4-hour intervals and more frequently if blood glucose levels decrease to less than 50 mg/dl.[851,914,915,917] If at any point the patient becomes symptomatic during the fast, plasma insulin and glucose values should be obtained before intravenous glucose is given and the test stopped. Within 24 hours of starting the fast, 75% of patients with an insulinoma have symptoms and a blood sugar level of less than 40 mg/dl. By 48 hours, 92% to 98% are hypoglycemic, and by 72 hours virtually all patients with insulinomas are hypoglycemic.[482,915,917,920] The test is considered positive for insulinoma if the plasma insulin to glucose ratio is greater than 0.3.[851] In some normal obese subjects, the fasting plasma insulin to glucose ratio may be elevated because hyperinsulinemia due to insulin resistance mimics the pattern in insulinoma.[915] In these patients, the fasting glucose is normal, and even with prolonged fasting blood glucose levels do not decrease to less than 55 mg/dl; therefore, during fasting they can be easily differentiated.[915]

The presence of hypoglycemia or an elevated fasting blood insulin to blood glucose ratio during fasting is consistent with but may not be caused by insulinoma. Other conditions can cause a similar result, including organic hyperinsulinism due to pancreatic islet diseases, factitious use of insulin or hypoglycemic agents, or autoantibodies against the insulin receptor or insulin.[851,920–922] To differentiate insulinoma from these other conditions, additional tests are required, including plasma determinations of proinsulin, C peptide, antibodies to insulin, and plasma sulfonylurea levels.[482,851,922] Plasma proinsulin levels are elevated in 80% to 90% of patients with insulinoma to more than 22% of the plasma insulin level.[851,915,922] In patients with surreptitious use of insulin or oral hypoglycemic agents, the proinsulin level is normal or decreased.[922] The measurement of C peptide has proved useful in differentiating organic hypersecretion of insulin such as in patients with insulinoma from patients surreptitiously using insulin, because commercial insulin preparations contain no C peptide.[922] In insulinoma, the characteristic finding is an elevated or normal C peptide plasma concentration,[922] whereas in patients surreptitiously using insulin the plasma insulin level is high and the C peptide level low.[920,922] The C peptide level does not differentiate patients surreptitiously taking oral hypoglycemic agents from patients with insulinomas in that both have low blood sugars and elevated levels of insulin and C peptide,[702,920,922] but most oral hypoglycemia drugs do produce elevated plasma levels of sulfonylurea.

Pathology

As with other APUDomas, malignancy is only defined by the presence of metastases at the time of surgery or metastases documented by other investigations.[923] Insulinomas are the opposite of gastrinomas in that 60% to 90% of gastrinomas are malignant but only 5% to 16% of insulinomas are malignant.[482,851,915,916] The pattern of metastatic spread of insulinomas is local invasion followed by spread to peripancreatic and portal nodes and then to the liver. Most insulinomas are found to be solitary benign pancreatic nodules, often encapsulated; only 2% to 10% of patients have multiple tumors.[482,920] In patients with multiple insulinomas, MEN-I should be suspected.[513] Insulinomas are uniformly distributed throughout the entire pancreas, and most are smaller than 1.5 cm in diameter.[482,915,916]

Localization

After a firm diagnosis of insulinoma is established, an attempt should be made to localize the tumor (Table 41–34 and Fig. 41–18). Radiographic investigations are concentrated on the pancreas because most insulinomas (unlike gastrinomas) are within the pancreas.[851,915,924] Preoperative localization is essential because insulinomas frequently are small (90% are less than 2 cm in diameter) and unnecessary surgery may be prevented if metastatic spread is present. CT scanning local-

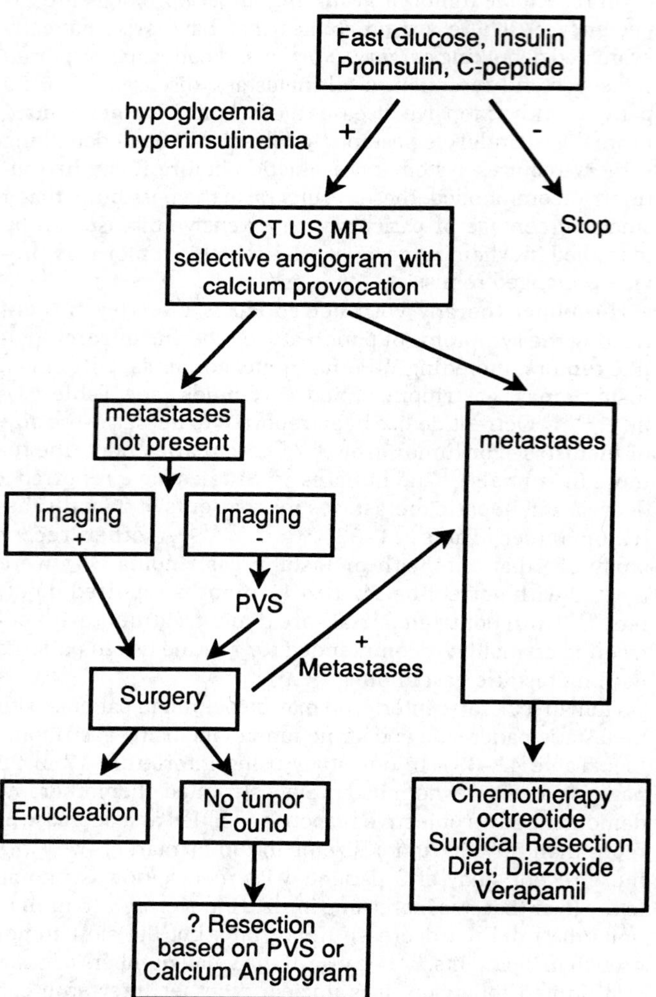

FIGURE 41–18. Flow diagram for the evaluation and management of patients with hypoglycemia.

TABLE 41–34. Localization Procedures for Insulinoma

Procedure	*Successful Localization Mean (Range)*	*References*
Ultrasound	33% (0–66%)	482, 927, 928, 1117
CT scan	35% (11–50%)	482, 927, 928, 1117
Dynamic CT scan	66%	925
Selective arteriography	63% (17–100%)	482, 927, 928, 1117
All imaging studies	80% (50–90%)	482, 927
Transhepatic portal venous sampling	92% (89–96%)	844, 926, 927, 929, 1117–1119
Operative ultrasound	83–90%	844, 850, 930

izes 35% of cases. Dynamic CT scanning is reported to be more sensitive, localizing 66% of insulinomas.[925] Selective arteriography localizes the greatest proportion of insulinomas (see Table 41–34). An average of 40% of patients do not have insulinomas localized by these imaging procedures (see Table 41–34).[482,844,926–928] Most large series report an even distribution of insulinomas within the pancreas,[915,924,928] so that a blind distal pancreatectomy has only a one in three chance of finding tumor. Therefore, additional localization procedures may be needed in some patients. PVS for insulin can localize an insulinoma to the exact region of the pancreas (head, body, or tail) in nearly all patients (see Table 41–34). A typical result localizing tumor in the pancreatic tail is shown in Figure 41–19. Four groups have reported successful localizations by PVS in the subgroup of patients not visualized by angiography, identifying 10 of 10 in one series and 6 of 7 in another.[844,851,926,928,929] In a recent study of 12 patients with insulinomas with negative imaging studies, selective venous sampling correctly localized the tumor in 75% of cases.[844] In another recent study of 35 patients with insulinoma in whom imaging studies localized the tumors in 46%, PVS localized the tumor in 100%.[926] Because PVS only localizes tumors to

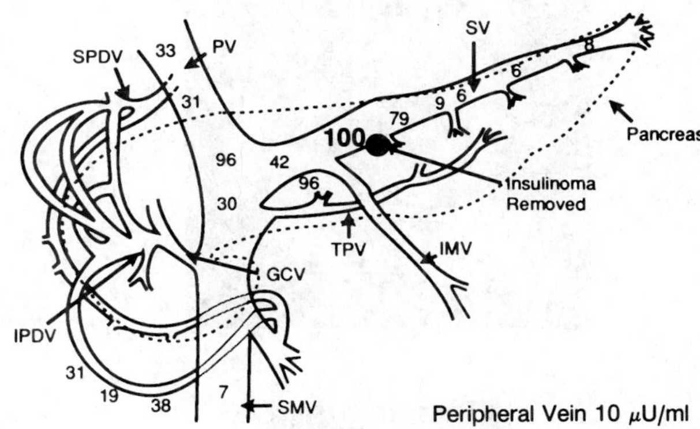

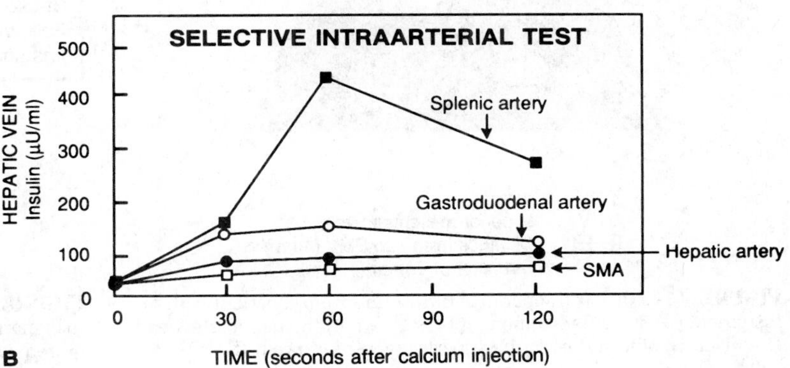

FIGURE 41–19. Selective venous sampling for insulin from portal venous tributaries **(A)** and a selective intraarterial calcium provocative test in a patient with insulinoma **(B)**. **(A)** Numbers are the plasma insulin concentrations at different locations. The simultaneous peripheral value was 10 μU/ml. A significant gradient of 900% (increase to 100 μU/ml) is seen in the proximal splenic vein. The closed circle indicates the location of a 1-cm insulioma found at surgery. **(B)** Results of calcium (0.01–0.25 mEq/kg) injected into the splenic, gastroduodenal hepatic, and superior mesenteric arteries (SMA) and of venous blood obtained from the hepatic veins. A rapid increase in plasma insulin levels was seen with injection of the splenic artery, which supplies the area where the tumor was found.

a general area of the pancreas and insulinomas may be so small that they cannot be localized by palpation at surgery within this area, IOUS has been useful in localizing insulinomas.[844,848,850,930] A typical IOUS result is shown in Figure 41–20, in which a 1.1-cm insulinoma is localized in the pancreatic head area. In one recent study of 12 patients with negative imaging studies of which 75% had a PVS gradient localizing the insulinoma to the appropriate pancreatic area, insulinomas could be localized by palpation at surgery in only 41%.[844] IOUS identified insulinomas in 5 additional patients and was the single best modality in locating the insulinoma at surgery.[844]

A new study that may be helpful in the future and may replace selective sampling for insulin from portal venous tributaries is the use of selective intraarterial injection of calcium with hepatic venous insulin sampling.[927] Small amounts of calcium (0.01–0.25 mEq Ca^{2+}/kg) are infused directly into the branches of the celiac plexus (gastroduodenal, splenic, hepatic) and superior mesenteric artery, and simultaneous blood samples are taken from the right and left hepatic artery for measurement of plasma insulin concentrations (see Fig. 41–19B). In all 4 patients, insulin increased in one of the hepatic veins after the calcium injection into one of the arteries, correctly localizing the insulinoma.[927] A typical result is shown in Figure 41–19 and compared with the PVS. In this patient, PVS demonstrated a positive gradient (900% increase; Fig. 41–19A) in the proximal pancreatic tail, and intraarterial calcium into the splenic artery demonstrated an increase in plasma insulin (Fig. 41–19B). A 1-cm insulinoma was resected from the proximal pancreatic tail. If the usefulness of this test is confirmed, it will likely obviate the need for PVS because it can be done in most centers and requires less expertise.

Many pancreatic endocrine tumors possess somatostatin receptors,[604–606,850,931] and radiolabeled somatostatin is reported to localize some tumors not localized by other modalities. The experience with this technique in patients with insulinomas is limited, with too few patients with insulinoma studied to determine whether this technique will localize tumors not found by any other modalities.

In our experience, more than 70% of insulinomas are visualized by arteriography, and 75% of the unidentified lesions are localized by PVS.[844,851] If all preoperative localization studies are negative, the patient should undergo surgical exploration by a group with experience in the use of IOUS (Fig. 41–21). Previously, the decision for surgical exploration patients with negative localization studies rested on whether the patient's symptoms could be effectively controlled medically.[932] The recent results with IOUS in these patients indicate that the insulinoma can be found and resected successfully at surgery.

Surgery

All insulinomas without evidence of metastases should be surgically removed, regardless of the severity of symptoms. Of

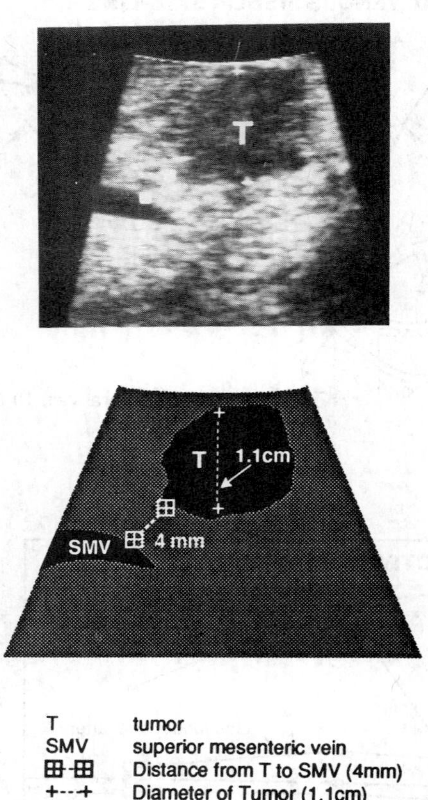

FIGURE 41–20. Intraoperative ultrasound from a patient with an insulinoma. A 1.1-cm insulinoma (T) is shown in the pancreatic head at a distance of 4 mm from the superior mesenteric vein (SMV).

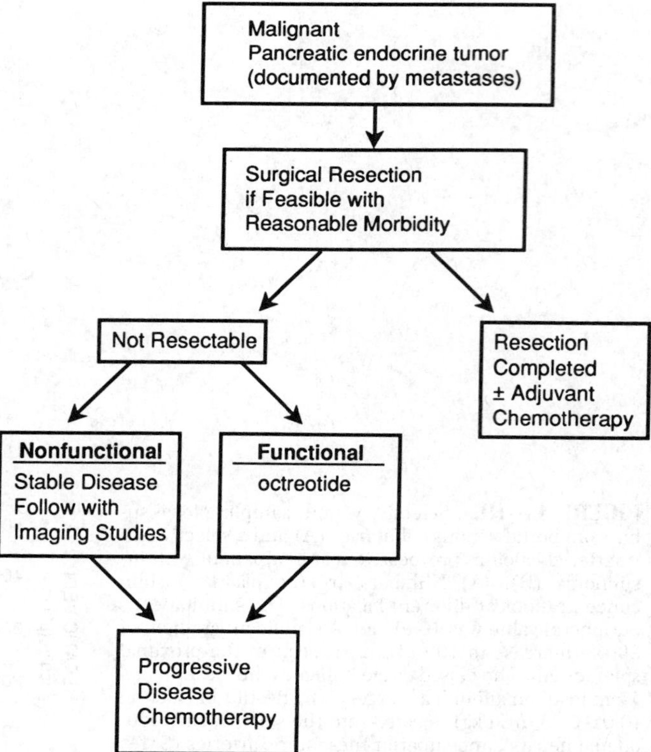

FIGURE 41–21. Flow diagram for management of patients with malignant pancreatic endocrine tumors. Chemotherapy may be required with progressive disease.

all insulinomas, 80% are benign isolated lesions whose surgical removal is curative.[915,921] The liver always must be explored for evidence of metastatic disease and the entire abdomen explored to rule out rare extrapancreatic tumors. The entire pancreas must be explored for other tumors, because multifocal tumors occur in at least 10% of patients.[844,851] Isolated lesions of the tail may be enucleated or removed en bloc by distal pancreatectomy. Body and head lesions require enucleation with careful dissection to avoid damage to the main pancreatic duct and its attendant morbidity. Division of the peritoneum lateral to the duodenum (Kocher's maneuver) is necessary to palpate the pancreatic head, and division of the peritoneum along the inferior border of the pancreas is required to palpate the body and the tail adequately. Distal pancreatectomy usually requires concomitant splenectomy. Pneumococcal vaccine (Pneumovax) should be administered preoperatively to lower the risk of catastrophic postsplenectomy sepsis.

Anecdotal reports of hypoglycemia during manipulation of the pancreas have focused attention on glucose monitoring during surgery. Use of the artificial pancreas (Biostator) has documented an increased glucose requirement during removal of insulinomas.[851] A number of centers have used the artificial pancreas or frequent glucose measurements to monitor patients for hypoglycemia and to document successful removal of the tumor by noting a *rebound hyperglycemia* or sudden decreased glucose requirement. A large retrospective study at the Mayo Clinic showed that the rebound hyperglycemia did not occur in 23% of patients who had successful extirpation of insulinoma.[933] This technique may be of more limited use in aiding the localization of insulinomas occult to preoperative studies. Kudlow and colleagues showed sensitive detection of an unlocalized tumor using a noncrushing clamp to isolate regions of the pancreas from the circulation while monitoring blood glucose with an artificial pancreas programmed to amplify small increases in blood glucose concentrations.[934] We do not use intraoperative monitoring of insulin or glucose to guide tumor localization or removal.

Even in cases of documented metastatic disease, refractory debilitating symptoms may be an indication for debulking the pancreatic lesion. Metastases are not always secretory. Removal of peripancreatic lymph nodes may be curative for malignant insulinoma if no liver metastases are present.[851,914]

Medical Therapy

The simplest form of nonsurgical treatment for insulinoma is dietary management.[851,915] Many insulinoma patients begin frequent small meals to alleviate symptoms before seeking medical evaluation, and a significant percentage report weight gain in the year before diagnosis. Slowly absorbed oral nutrients such as cornstarch, bread, potatoes, and rice are recommended.[851,926] In unusually severe cases, intravenous glucose may be required to prevent neuroglycopenic attacks. Hypertonic solutions, such as 10% dextrose, should be avoided because of electrolyte imbalances generated by combining high levels of glucose and hyperinsulinemia simultaneously. During a hypoglycemia episode, rapidly absorbable forms of carbohydrates such as fruit juice with glucose or sucrose are preferable.

A number of drugs have been reported to control the hyperinsulinemia. Diazoxide, a benzothiazide analog, directly inhibits insulin release from β cells through stimulation of α-adrenergic receptors. It has an extrapancreatic, hyperglycemic effect, possibly by inhibiting cyclic AMP phosphodiesterase, which enhances glycogenolysis.[915,920] The major side effects of diazoxide are sodium retention, gastrointestinal symptoms such as nausea, and occasional hirsutism.[851,915,920] Edema can result from the sodium retention and the addition of a diuretic such as trichlormethiazide, a benzothiadiazine derivative, can correct the edema and augment the hyperglycemia effect.[702,851,915,920] Diazoxide should be initiated with 150 to 200 mg given in two to three divided doses a day and, if not effective, increased to a maximum of 600 to 800 mg/day.[851,920] About 60% of patients respond to the diazoxide.[851,914] The calcium-channel inhibitor verapamil has been used alone and in combination with other drugs to help control hypoglycemia in a small number of patients,[935–937] as has propanolol.[915,938] Phenytoin (Dilantin) inhibits the release of insulin from β cells and has been used successfully to treat a small number of patients with refractory hypoglycemia.[915,939] Maintenance doses of 300 to 600 mg/day are used, and only in less than 33% of patients is the hypoglycemia effect of phenytoin of any clinical significance.[915] Glucocorticoids (prednisone, 1 mg/kg) and glucagon either alone or with diazoxide have been used in a few patients.[915]

The most promising results are with octreotide, which has been reported to control symptoms and hypoglycemia in 40% to 60% of patients.[903,905,940–942] Octreotide generally is well tolerated and usually is given in starting doses of 50 μg two or three times daily, which can be increased to 1500 μg/day.[905] The main side effects are gastrointestinal (*e.g.,* bloating and abdominal cramping), and long-term side effects include malabsorption and cholelithiasis.[713,905,940–942] Besides improving symptoms, octreotide decreases plasma insulin levels in 65% of patients.[905] Most patients were treated for less than 1 week before surgery, so that the long-term efficacy is not known in a significant number of patients.

Malignant Insulinoma

The documentation of metastatic disease, either at the time of surgery or by imaging studies, is the only accurate means of diagnosing malignant insulinoma. Unlike all other islet cell tumors, malignant insulinomas are uncommon, occurring in only 10% to 15% of cases (see Table 41–24). Malignant primary insulinomas usually are not occult and have a mean size of 6 cm, which is more than twice the mean size of benign insulinomas.[702,914,915,923] The median disease-free survival after curative resection of malignant insulinomas was 5 years in one recent series.[923] The recurrence rate was 63%, with the median interval to recurrence 2.8 years. The median survival with recurrent tumor was 19 months. Palliative re-resection was associated with a median survival of 4 years, and biopsy only with a survival of 11 months.[923] Surgical resection of primary and metastatic insulinomas is preferred when possible (see Fig. 41–21).[923] Malignant insulinomas, like other pancreatic endocrine tumors, may respond to chemotherapy and treatment with octreotide.[905,940–942] The use of these agents for all malignant pancreatic endocrine neoplasms is described at the end of this section (see Chemotherapy).

NONFUNCTIONAL PANCREATIC ENDOCRINE TUMORS AND PPOMAS

Nonfunctional pancreatic endocrine tumors and PPomas present in the fourth and fifth decade of life.[943–945] PPomas release the hormone PP.[702,944,945] Nonfunctioning pancreatic endocrine tumors are not associated with elevated plasma levels of any peptide.[520,943] Because no active hormone is secreted by these tumors, symptoms arise from mechanical or mass effects of the neoplasm; therefore, they present late and the tumors are usually large and locally invasive at diagnosis. In one series, 72% were greater than 5 cm in diameter.[943]

These tumors usually are solitary except in patients with MEN-I, in whom multiple microadenomata can be seen.[711,770] The tumors are distributed throughout the pancreas with a ratio of 14:2:3 for pancreatic head:body:tail in one study.[943] The malignancy rate varied from 64% to 92% in different series (see Table 41–24).[488,711,943–945] Histologically, PPomas and nonfunctioning tumors are similar and cannot be differentiated from other pancreatic endocrine tumors even by immunocytochemistry. Nonfunctioning tumors are only differentiated from PPomas by the detection of an elevated level of plasma PP.[702] Increasingly, what in the past were thought to be nonfunctioning pancreatic endocrine tumors are found to have elevated plasma PP levels.[945] In one study of those pancreatic endocrine tumors not associated with any clinical syndrome and classified as nonfunctioning in the past, 50% to 75% were PPomas.[944] That elevated plasma PP levels are specific for endocrine pancreatic tumors is suggested by a study of 53 patients with adenocarcinoma of the pancreas, in which no patient had an elevated plasma PP level.[944] There are no data to suggest that nonfunctioning pancreatic endocrine tumors and PPomas differ in biologic behavior or presentation.[702] Immunocytochemically, nonfunctioning tumors and PPomas can contain numerous other gastrointestinal peptides. In one series of 30 nonfunctioning tumors, 50% had insulin-like immunoreactivity, 30% had glucagon immunoreactivity, 43% had PP immunoreactivity, 13% had somatostatin immunoreactivity, and only 13% produced none of these peptides.[770]

Infusions of PP into animals and humans have shown this peptide to have numerous biologic effects including the following: a net secretory effect on water and electrolytes in the small intestine; inhibitory effects of fluid, electrolyte, and enzyme secretion by the pancreas; effects on esophageal, gastric, intestinal, and gallbladder motility; and metabolic effects such as decreasing somatostatin or insulin release.[946] Patients with PPomas have been reported to have symptoms that were attributed to elevated plasma levels of PP,[944] although most patients have no such symptoms.[702,947] In one study, 36% of patients presented with abdominal pain and 28% with jaundice.[948] In 16% of patients, the tumors were found incidentally at surgery, and the remaining patients had a variety of symptoms due to the tumor mass. In this series, no patient was diagnosed preoperatively. In the future, it is likely that the histologic diagnosis will be established by cytologic analysis after fine-needle aspiration. This technique has been used extensively to diagnose pancreatic cancer and increasingly is being used to diagnose pancreatic endocrine tumors.[949–952] In a recent study of 10 patients with pancreatic endocrine tumors using fine-needle aspiration combined with immunocytochemical analysis, cytologic studies showed the typical pattern of monotonous cytologic features with few mitoses.[949] Positive staining for chromogranin was seen in 5 patients, with a 78% concordance between cytochemical studies and final histology studies.

Elevated plasma levels of PP do not establish the diagnosis of a PPoma, even when a pancreatic mass is present. Plasma PP levels are reported to be elevated in 22% to 71% of patients with functional pancreatic endocrine tumors and nonpancreatic carcinoid tumors.[702,776,945,947] Furthermore, elevated plasma levels of PP can occur in other situations such as old age, bowel resection, alcohol abuse, infection, chronic noninfective inflammatory disorders, acute diarrhea, chronic renal failure, diabetes, chronic relapsing pancreatitis, hypoglycemia, or even after eating.[947] Therefore, an elevated plasma level of PP is not diagnostic of a PPoma. To increase the specificity of an elevated plasma level for a pancreatic tumor, an atropine suppression test has been proposed.[776,953] In one study of 48 patients with elevated plasma PP levels, atropine (1 mg intramuscularly) did not suppress the levels in any of the 18 patients with pancreatic endocrine tumors but did suppress the level by 50% in all patients without tumors.[776] Others have proposed a secretin provocative test.[947] A response of more than a 5000 pg/ml/minute increase is more than two standard deviations greater than seen in normal subjects. The usefulness of the atropine suppression or secretin provocative test for PP has not been investigated extensively and cannot be recommended as a routine procedure.[520]

The treatment of these tumors is surgical if possible. In more than 60% of patients, metastases are present at the time of diagnosis. Of 25 patients in one series, a Whipple procedure was done in 20%, a partial or total pancreatectomy in 25%, and a tumor excision in 10%.[948] The remaining patients had a biopsy only. The survival rates were 60% at 3 years and 44% at 5 years in this series. The cure rate of these tumors is low because of their late recognition.

LESS FREQUENT PANCREATIC ENDOCRINE TUMORS

Other pancreatic endocrine tumors occur less frequently and include VIPomas, glucagonomas, ACTHomas, somatostatinomas, and GRFomas (see Table 41–24). Each of these pancreatic endocrine tumors is usually malignant.

VIPomas

The VIPoma syndrome was first described by Verner and Morrison in 1958 and is commonly called the Verner-Morrison syndrome (see Table 41–24).[954] Because of the resemblance of the diarrheal fluid to that seen in patients with cholera, the term pancreatic cholera was proposed in 1967[955] and the acronym WDHA (watery diarrhea, hypokalemic, and achlorhydric) proposed in 1967.[954,956,957]

In adults, more than 80% to 90% of VIPomas are pancreatic in location,[958,959] with rare cases caused by VIP-producing intestinal carcinoids or pheochromocytomas.[959] VIPomas are usually large solitary tumors.[711,958,959] In one series, only 2% of tumors were multiple.[959] Seventy-five percent were reported in the pancreatic tail in one review.[941] In various series,

37% to 68% of the VIPomas have metastases at the time of diagnosis or surgery.[944,956,958–960] In one detailed pathology study, 61% of VIPomas were identified as malignant by the occurrence of metastases.[958] Characteristically in children younger than 10 years and rarely in adults (5% of cases), the VIPoma syndrome is due to a ganglioneuroma or ganglioneuroblastoma.[959] In one series, 16% of all cases were due to this tumor.[959] These tumors are extrapancreatic and are less often malignant than pancreatic VIPomas, being malignant in only 10% of cases.[959]

By immunocytochemistry, VIP was detected in 86%[958] and 57%[770] of VIPomas. Using immunocytochemical studies, 34% to 38% of VIPomas possess PP, 19% glucagon, 10% somatostatin, 5% insulin, and none gastrin.[770,958] VIPomas elaborate the peptide histidine methionine (PHM-27), a 27 amino acid peptide that shares with VIP a common precursor peptide (prepro VIP/PHM-27), and PHM-27-like immunoreactivity has been found in the plasma and tumors of patients with VIPomas.[702,957,961] On conventional microscopy, VIPomas show the typical microscopic features of endocrine tumors.[958] Mitoses were uncommon, seen in only 12%.[958] On electron microscopy, a mixture of cells were seen, usually in the same tumor.[958] The secretory granules were small (120–180 nm) and resembled those of the so-called D cells of normal gut.[958] The histologic and electron microscopic studies do not allow VIPomas to be differentiated clearly from some other pancreatic endocrine tumors; however, the presence of immunoreactive VIP is strongly suggestive for VIPoma because it is found uncommonly in other pancreatic endocrine tumors (10 of 104 pancreatic endocrine tumors in one study).[946,958]

The pathophysiology of the VIPoma syndrome is clear in that VIP is the major mediator.[958,962] For a number of years there was considerable controversy about the mediator.[962,963] In early studies, levels of substances other than VIP were reported to be elevated in the plasma of patients.[702,957,962] In early studies, plasma VIP infusions in humans did not produce the syndrome.[702,962,963] Plasma levels of VIP are consistently elevated in patients with the VIPoma syndrome.[702,957,959,962] A continuous infusion of VIP for 10 hours in normal human subjects to achieve plasma levels similar to that seen in patients with the VIPoma syndrome produced watery diarrhea in 6 to 7 hours.[964] The ability of VIP to produce diarrhea is consistent with its known actions in the intestine.[965] Receptors for VIP have been identified on intestinal epithelial cells. VIP stimulates intestinal electrolyte and fluid secretion in animals, stimulates chloride secretion with increased short circuit current, and activates adenylate cyclase and cyclic AMP in intestinal cells, which leads to intestinal secretion.[965] PHM-27-like immunoreactivity was found in 92% of VIPomas.[961] PHM was 32-fold less potent than VIP at causing intestinal secretion.[702,966] Because VIP is always present, it is likely to be the important peptide in most cases.

In two large series, the mean age for adults at the time of diagnosis was 49 and 50 years, with a range of 32 to 81 years.[959,967] There was a slight female predominance. The mean age in children was 4 years[959] and 2 years[967] in these studies, with a range from 10 months to 9 years.

The principal features of the VIPoma syndrome are the presence of severe, secretory diarrhea (100%) associated with hypokalemia (100%) and dehydration (100%).[702,957,959,967] The diarrhea is large volume with all patients with VIPomas, having more than 1 L in a number of studies and in most more than 3 L/day.[959,962] A volume of less than 700 g/day has been proposed to rule out the diagnosis of VIPoma.[962] The diarrhea fluid is described as having the appearance of weak tea and persisting during fasting.[955,962] Although abdominal cramping pain and colic were reported to be absent in earlier studies, more recent studies report these characteristics in 63% of patients.[959,968] Gross steatorrhea usually is not present, and in one study none of 52 patients with VIPomas had 24-hour fecal fat of more than 15 g/day.[959] Weight loss is almost universally present.[959] Flushing is reported in 21% of patients, is usually present in the head or trunk area, and is characteristically erythematous.[957] The clinical laboratory studies invariably demonstrate hypokalemia (100%) and, to a lesser degree, hypercalcemia (41%), hypochlorhydria (70%), and hyperglycemia (18%).[702,957,959,967] The hypokalemia is often severe, being less than 2.5 mmol/L. At some time, 93% of patients will have serum levels of potassium less than 3 mmol/L (normal 3.5-5 mmol/L).[959] The hyperglycemia is mild.[959]

The diagnosis of a VIPoma requires the demonstration of an elevated plasma concentration of VIP and the establishment of the presence of a large volume secretory diarrhea. The possibility that VIPoma is responsible for the secretory diarrhea is strongly suggested by the volume of the diarrhea.[702,956,957] In 80% to 85% of patients, the diarrhea volume is more than 3 L/day and never less than 700 ml/day.[959,962] Many possible causes for the diarrhea can be excluded by fasting the patient, because in patients with VIPomas the diarrhea persists during fasting.[702,957,962] The diarrheal fluid should be characteristic of a secretory diarrhea,[962] in which the stool electrolytes can account for all the stool water osmolality ([sodium+potassium]×2=measured osmolality]).[962] Other diseases can give a chronic secretory diarrhea with large volume and be confused with a possible VIPoma; one such syndrome is called the pseudoVIPoma syndrome.[962] Other causes include ZES[712,962] and chronic laxative abuse.[969] In some cases, the secretory diarrhea is of unknown origin.[969–971] The diagnosis of ZES can be excluded by measuring fasting serum gastrin and gastric acid secretory rate.[712,764]

To differentiate VIPomas from these other conditions, a reliable measurement of plasma VIP concentrations is required. The fasting plasma VIP level ranges in most laboratories is 0 to 170 pg/ml.[959,962,967] In one study of patients with VIPomas, the mean value was 965 pg/ml, with the lowest value at 225 pg/ml (normal less than 170 pg/ml).[967] In another large study, the mean value in patients with VIPomas was 675 pg/ml, with the highest normal value (being 53 pg/ml) seen in normal patients and the lowest value seen in a VIPoma patient was 160 pg/ml.[959] Originally, plasma VIP levels were not found to increase in some patients with VIPomas or were increased in patients without VIPomas, including patients with laxative abuse. In most recent studies, this is not the case if a reliable assay is used.[702,957,959,962]

The first objective in these patients even before considering the diagnosis is the replenishment of fluid and electrolyte losses to correct the profound hypokalemia, dehydration, and acidosis that is usually present. The patients may require 5 L/day or more of fluid[957] and more than 350 mEq/day of potassium.[957,972] In the past, numerous drugs have been used in small numbers of VIPoma patients to control, to varying degrees, the diarrheal output. These drugs include prednisone

(60 to 100 mg/day), clonidine, indomethacin, phenothiazines, lithium carbonate, propranolol, metoclopramide, loperamide, lidamidine, angiotensin II, and norepinephrine.[702,957,967] Octreotide provides short-term and long-term control of the diarrhea in 87% of patients with VIPoma and is the agent of choice.[903,905,940–942,957] In two recent reviews of 20 and 25 patients with VIPomas treated with octreotide, the drug completely abolished diarrhea in 10% of patients in one study and in 65% in the other; diarrhea improved in 90% of patients in one study and in 95% in the other.[903,905,941] In one study, octreotide continued to be effective for all patients (n=13) at 6 months.[941] Some patients have short-lived responses or may respond initially to a low dose (50–100 μg three times daily) but subsequently require a larger dose to control the diarrhea, and some symptoms may become refractory even with doses up to 1200 μg/day.[905] In a small number of nonresponsive patients or patients whose symptoms recur, the administration of glucocorticoids concomitant with octreotide has proved effective.[905] With octreotide, plasma VIP concentrations decreased in 80% to 88% of patients.[905,941]

After imaging studies to localize the primary VIPoma and determine the extent of the tumor, possible surgical cure should be considered for all patients without metastatic disease. In one series, surgical resection of a pancreatic VIPoma relieved all symptoms in 17 patients (33% of patients).[959] In another series, 30% were cured.[960] Surgical removal with complete control of all symptoms was possible in 78% of all patients with VIP-producing ganglioneuroblastomas.[959]

Glucagonoma

In 1974, Mallinson and colleagues established the association of a cutaneous rash with glucagon-producing tumors of the pancreas when they reported 9 patients with the full clinical syndrome and a glucagon-releasing tumor of the pancreas.[973] The disease was described earlier by others, but the association with elevated plasma levels of glucagon had not been established.[702,914] In 1942, the association of a pancreatic tumor with a skin rash was first described.[974] In 1966, McGavran and colleagues reported a patient with an elevated fasting glucagon level, dermatitis, diabetes, and a pancreatic endocrine tumor.[975] Wilkinson and associates in 1973 described the rash associated with endocrine tumor as necrolytic migratory erythema.[976]

Most glucagonomas are large at the time of diagnosis, with the average size between 5 and 10 cm and a range from 0.4 to 35 cm.[977] Fifty percent of glucagonomas occurred in the tail in one study[978] and 80% in another study,[979] whereas in the largest study 22% were in the head, 14% in the body, and 51% in the pancreatic tail.[977] Between 50% and 80% had evidence of metastatic spread or invasion establishing malignancy.[977–979] The most common site of metastatic spread was to the liver (43% to 82%), with metastasis to lymph nodes, bone, and mesentery less common. In most cases, glucagonomas are within the pancreas; however, a glucagonoma associated with the typical clinical syndrome was found in the proximal duodenum.[979] Glucagonomas usually occur as a single tumor, although in one series multiple tumors or diffuse involvement by a single mass were found in 10% of patients.[979]

The pathophysiology of the glucagonoma syndrome is related to the known actions of glucagon.[980] Glucagon stimulates glycogenolysis, gluconeogenesis, ketogenesis, lipolysis, and insulin secretion. Glucagon affects gut secretion, inhibits pancreatic and gastric secretion, inhibits gut motility, and increases heart rate and force of contraction. Hyperglycemia in the glucagonoma syndrome results from the increased hepatic glycogenolysis and glyconeogenesis. The weight loss has been attributed to the known catabolic effects of glucagon.[974] It is not clearly established that the skin rash is due to the hyperglucagonemia per se, because numerous patients have been given large doses of glucagon over extended periods and the skin rash did not develop.[702,974] The glucagon-induced hypoaminoacidemia that develops in 80% to 90% of patients[977–979] may be involved in causing the skin rash, because correction of the hypoaminoacidemia has been shown to correct the dermatitis without changing plasma glucagon concentrations in some patients.[702,822,974,981] The similarity of the lesions to those seen in patients with zinc deficiencies have resulted in trials of zinc in some patients with some responses.[974]

Immunocytochemical and histologic studies of glucagonomas show results typical of pancreatic endocrine tumors. Glucagon is one of the most frequently seen peptides in immunocytochemical studies of pancreatic endocrine tumors, although in many cases it is not associated with any syndrome. In one series of 1366 autopsy cases, a 0.8% frequency of adenomas was reported, and all contained glucagon-producing cells.[711,770,974] The morphology of most glucagon-producing tumors demonstrate no general features that distinguish them from other pancreatic endocrine tumors.[702,770,974,979]

Glucagonomas usually occur in middle to late age with only 16% occurring in persons younger than 40 years and most occurring in persons between 50 and 70 years.[977–979] The typical dermatitis, called necrolytic migratory erythema, occurs in 64% to 90% of patients. Diabetes mellitus or glucose intolerance occurs in 83% to 90% of patients, weight loss in 56% to 90%, diarrhea in 14% to 15%, abdominal pain in 12%, thromboembolic disease with venous thrombosis in 24%, pulmonary emboli in 11%, and psychiatric disturbances in a few patients.[520,974,977–979] Laboratory abnormalities include anemia in 44% to 85% of patients, hypoaminoacidemia in 26% to 100%, hypocholesterolemia in 80%, and renal glycosuria.[520,974,977,978]

The presence of cutaneous lesions often precedes the diagnosis of the syndrome for long periods, with a mean of 6 to 8 years in one study and a maximum of 18 years.[977] The skin lesions may wax and wane, and because of their variable nature have been misdiagnosed in various studies as pemphigus foliaceus, pemphigoid, vasculitis, acrodermatitis enteropathica, psoriasis, herpes, seborrheic or contact dermatitis, eczema, pellagra, or even a chemical burn.[979] Numerous excellent descriptions of necrolytic migratory erythema associated with glucagonoma have been published.[973,974,977–979] Typically, the rash starts as an erythematous area, usually at periorifacial or intertriginous areas such as the groin, buttocks, thighs, or perineum, and then spreads laterally. The lesions later become raised with superficial central blistering. The top of the bullae frequently detach or rupture, leaving eroded areas that crust. The lesions tend to heal in the center, while the edges continue to spread with a well-defined crusting edge. Lesions may become confluent. Healing is associated with hyperpigmentation. This entire sequence characteristically takes 1 to 2 weeks. While some new lesions are developing, others are healing; therefore, a mixed pattern of erythema, bullous formation with epidermal separation, crusting, and hyperpigmentation can occur together with normal skin. The histopathology can be as varied as the clinical presentation.[979] In their classical form, early lesions demonstrate a superficial spongiosis and necrosis with subcorneal and midepidermal bullae.[973,974,976] Fusiform keratinocytes with pyknotic nuclei are often seen, as are mononuclear inflammatory infiltrates.[973,974,976] This characteristic histologic pattern is best seen in an early lesion. Glossitis or angular stomatitis is reported to occur in 34% to 68% of patients.[977,978]

Once the diagnosis is suspected, it can be confirmed by establishing the presence of a marked elevation in plasma glucagon concentration. In most laboratories, the upper limit of normal for fasting glucagon concentration is 150 to 200 pg/ml.[977] In one large review of glucagonomas, only 2 patients had a plasma glucagon level of 200 to 500 pg/ml, 4 patients had levels between 500 and 1000 pg/ml, and 52 patients had levels of more than 1000 pg/ml.[977] These results agree with another study, in which the mean plasma glucagon concentration in 73 patients with glucagonoma was 2110±334 pg/ml, with a range of 550 to 6600 pg/ml.[979] In this study, no patient had a level less than 500 pg/ml, 30% of patients had levels between 500 and 1000 pg/ml, and the remaining patients had levels of more than 1000 pg/ml. Hyperglucagonemia is reported to occur in chronic renal insufficiency, diabetic ketoacidosis, prolonged starvation, acute pancreatitis, acromegaly, hypercortisolism, septicemia, severe burns, severe stress (trauma, exercise), familial hyperglucagonemia, and hepatic insufficiency.[974,977–979] Plasma glucagon levels in these conditions have not been reported to exceed 500 pg/ml.[974,977]

In terms of medical therapy, the rash improved with octreotide in 54% to 90% of patients and disappeared completely in up to 30%.[903,905,941] In 5 patients in whom the time course was described, the rash disappeared in 2 patients within 1 week, and within 1 month in three other patients.[905] In one study, diarrhea improved in 4 of 6 patients and resolved in the other 2 patients.[941] Diabetes mellitus was not improved with octreotide treatment.[905,941] The diabetes mellitus was severe enough to require oral hypoglycemic agents in 42% of patients and insulin in 27%.[977] With octreotide treatment, plasma glucagon levels decreased in 80% to 90% of patients but only decreased in the normal range in 10% to 20% of patients.[903,905,941]

In 50% to 80% of patients, metastases are present at the time of diagnosis.[974,977,979] In patients with resectable disease, surgical resection has been successful in many cases.[702,974,977] The exact percentage of cases that can be cured is not known. In one large review involving 92 cases of glucagonoma, only 16 of the malignant cases were treated by surgical resection only.[977] Only 7 patients had normal plasma glucagon levels after resection, and of the 5 patients that had no evidence of metastatic spread, plasma glucagon levels postoperatively were normal in 2. Even if a patient eventually develops a recurrence, an extended disease-free interval may be attained.[974] Some studies have reported a benefit to patients even if only surgical debulking is done.[974,977–979] In patients with widely metastatic disease in which surgical debulking is not possible, chemotherapeutic agents frequently are used and are described later in this chapter (see Chemotherapy).

Somatostatinoma

Somatostatin is a hormone that inhibits numerous endocrine and exocrine functions.[982] Somatostatin inhibits the release of almost all gut hormones, including insulin, glucagon, gastrin, secretin, cholecystokinin, and motilin. Somatostatin has direct effects on target organs (*e.g.,* inhibition of gastric acid secretion), increases intestinal motility, and reduces the absorption of fat.[982]

The first two cases of somatostatinoma were described in 1977 by Ganda and colleagues[983] and Larsson and colleagues.[984] Somatostatinomas are the least common of the pancreatic endocrine tumors, and fewer than 50 cases have been described.[947] Patients characteristically have diabetes mellitus, gallbladder disease, diarrhea, weight loss, steatorrhea, and hypochlorhydria.[702,944,947,983,985,986]

Somatostatinomas occur in the pancreas in 56% to 75% of cases, and the remainder occur in the upper small intestine.[944,986] The distribution of the tumors within the pancreatic head:body:tail was 11:0:3.[986] and 14:2:5.[944] In 90% of patients, the tumors were solitary and varied from 1.5 to 10 cm in diameter (mean 4.9 cm).[986] In one series, 84% of all tumors had evidence of metastatic spread.[986] However, in another study, 92% of pancreatic tumors were associated with metastases, whereas metastases were seen in only 69% of those originating in the intestine.[944] Metastases occur to the liver in about 75% of patients with metastases and less frequently to the regional lymph nodes (31%) and to bone.[944,986]

With light microscopic studies, most tumors appear as well-differentiated tumors within varying degrees of fibrous septa. In 89% of the tumors examined, the secretory granules are typical of those in D cells.[944,986] Immunocytochemical analysis of 15 cases demonstrated somatostatin-like immunoreactive material in all tumors, and 33% contained insulin, 27% calcitonin, and 13% gastrin.[986] The mean age of patients was 51 to 53 years.[944,986] Of patients with intestinal somatostatinomas, 43% were females and 66% had with pancreatic tumors.[986] Diabetes mellitus was present in 95% of patients with pancreatic tumors and in 21% of those with intestinal tumors.[944,947] Gallbladder disease was seen in 94% of pancreatic tumors and in 36% of intestinal tumors, whereas weight loss was seen in 90% of pancreatic and in 44% of intestinal cases.[944,947] Steatorrhea and hypochlorhydria occurred in 83% to 86% of pancreatic cases but in only 12% to 17% of intestinal tumors.[520,944,947] Somatostatinomas generally are found by accident.[944,986] The symptoms produced by somatostatinomas are less pronounced than those seen with other pancreatic endocrine tumors and often are not detected until patients develop high somatostatin blood levels, usually late in the course of the disease when the tumor is large. In most cases, somatostatinomas are found at the time of laparotomy for cholecystectomy or during gastrointestinal imaging studies for various nonspecific complaints such as abdominal pain or diarrhea.[944,986]

Surgery was performed in 83% of patients in one series[987] and in 60% of patients in another series.[986] In one study, 65% of patients were reported to have successful resection, but the percentage actually cured was not stated.[987] Although an occasional patient might be cured,[987] this is not possible in most series because of the late diagnosis. In patients in whom a combination of surgical resection and cytotoxic therapy was used, 60% were alive 6 months to 5 years after diagnosis.[944,986,988] Because of the malignant nature of these tumors, patients benefit from surgical resection if imaging studies demonstrate possible resectable tumor.

GRFomas

GRFomas are the most recently described pancreatic endocrine tumor syndrome and are due to excessive release of growth hormone-releasing factor (GRF).[989–991] In one recent review of 30 cases of GRFomas,[528] 30% originated in the pancreas, 53% in the lung, 10% from small intestinal tumors, and 1 case from the adrenal gland.

Multiple pancreatic tumors have been reported,[992,993] occurring in 30% of the pancreatic GRFomas in one series.[528] All occurred in patients with MEN-I. Tumors were generally large (>6 cm), varying from 1 to 25 cm in diameter.[528] Metastases were present in 30% of patients with pancreatic GRFomas and in 2 of the 3 patients with intestinal GRFomas.[528] Metastases were to regional lymph nodes and less frequently to the liver. In one series, there were no relations among tumor size, GRF levels, and the presence of metastases, and the three largest tumors were not associated with metastatic disease or invasion.[528] About 40% of all GRFomas occur in patients with ZES, and in 40% of patients Cushing's syndrome was also present.[528,702]

On light microscopic studies, the typical features of a pancreatic endocrine tumor are seen: trabecular or solid nests and sheets of uniform tumor cells.[528] In electron microscopic studies, tumor cells containing 100- to 250-nm secretory granules are seen.[528,992,994,995] Immunochemical studies demonstrated GRF-immunoreactive material in all tumors examined, with 10% to 80% of cells possessing GRF.[528] GRF-immunoreactive material was seen in 31% of all pancreatic endocrine tumors in one study[996] and in 0 to 100% in other pathology studies,[528,997,998] although few of these patients had acromegaly. The known actions of GRF as a stimulant of growth hormone release account for the clinical presentation with acromegaly.[528,989,990,999]

Patients are from 15 to 63 years old with an average age of 38.[528] The patients with intestinal GRFomas were younger, with 2 of the 3 patients younger than 20 years.[528] A female predominance (73%) is seen for all GRFomas and for patients with pancreatic GRFomas (78%). Acromegalic features were indistinguishable from patients with classical acromegaly and included enlargement of hands and feet, facial changes, skin changes, headache, and peripheral nerve entrapment.[528,999] The average time from the onset of the acromegalic changes to diagnosis was 5.3 years in patients with pancreatic GRFomas.[528] The syndromes due to other hormones were due to the presence of ZES, Cushing's syndrome, or to hyperinsulinemia and hypoglycemia.[528,702]

Patients without metastatic disease should undergo surgical resection of the GRFoma. Before surgery and in those patients with nonresectable lesions, various agents may reduce plasma growth hormone (GH) levels. Dopamine agonists such as bromocriptine are widely used in patients with classical acromegaly, having more than a 50% response rate in some series.[999] However, they rarely are able to normalize plasma GH levels in patients with GRFomas.[991] Octreotide is the agent of choice because it always significantly suppresses or normalizes growth hormone levels[905,999–1002] and in some cases is associated with pituitary shrinkage.[1000,1002] The suppression of GH secretion is mainly due to suppression at the pituitary level.[999] Surgical resection resulted in regression of the GRFoma syndrome in a small number of cases.[528,989,993,1003] The actual number of patients with long-term cure is unknown.

Other Pancreatic Endocrine Tumors

In a few studies in patients with pancreatic endocrine tumors secreting the peptide neurotensin, a neurotensinoma syndrome has been proposed.[771,944,1004–1009] Neurotensin is a 13 amino acid peptide originally isolated from bovine brain[1010] and later from human intestine and has biologic effects including tachycardia, hypotension, and cyanosis. It affects intestinal motility, stimulates jejunal and ileal fluid and electrolyte secretion, and stimulates pancreatic protein and bicarbonate secretion.[1010] Clinical features of patients with possible neurotensinomas include hypokalemia, weight loss, diabetes mellitus, cyanosis, hypotension, and flushing in a patient with a pancreatic endocrine tumor.[944] In a review of 6 patients, 50% were cured by resection of the pancreatic endocrine tumor and the remaining 50% improved with chemotherapy.[771,944,1004–1009] Recent studies question the existence of a specific neurotensinoma syndrome.[702,703,771] Of 180 patients with functional pancreatic endocrine tumors, elevated plasma neurotensin levels were found in 6 patients with VIPomas and their symptoms did not differ from patients with normal levels.[771] In another study, a similar result was found in patients with gastrinomas.[703]

Patients with pancreatic endocrine tumors with Cushing's syndrome (ACTHoma) have been reported.[893,947] In a recent study, Cushing's syndrome was reported in 19% of patients with both ZES and MEN-I.[893] In these patients, the disease was of pituitary origin and was mild. Cushing's syndrome occurs in sporadic cases of ZES[893] and in one recent prospective study was found in 5% of all cases.[702,893,1011] In these patients, the Cushing's syndrome was severe, due to ectopic ACTH production, occurred with metastatic pancreatic endocrine tumors that responded poorly to chemotherapy, and was associated with a poor prognosis.[893] Cushing's syndrome as the only manifestation of pancreatic endocrine tumors occurs and may precede any other hormonal syndrome.[1011]

Hypercalcemia has been reported to be due to a pancreatic endocrine tumor secreting a peptide similar to parathyroid hormone (PTH) or to an unknown substance that mimics the action of PTH and causes hyperparathyroidism.[1012–1017] The tumor generally has been metastatic to the liver by the time of diagnosis,[1012–1014] although in one recent case, radical resection of a pancreatic tail tumor with subsequent treatment with chemotherapy resulted in a total remission for 5 years.[1017]

Treatment

Most pancreatic endocrine tumors including VIPomas, glucagonomas, nonfunctional tumors or PPomas, somatostatinomas, and GRFomas resemble gastrinomas and are malignant with diligent follow-up. The exception is insulinoma, which has a low incidence of malignancy (10–15%; see Table 41–24). The malignant nature of these tumors cannot be detected accurately by pathology, so they require careful follow-up with imaging studies and appropriate plasma markers. The principles and treatment of malignant insulinomas, VIPomas, glucagonomas, somatostatinomas, nonfunctioning islet cell tumors, PPomas, and GRFomas are similar to that discussed previously in detail for gastrinomas. Although these tumors frequently may metastasize, many patients live comfortably and productively for many years with metastatic disease if symptoms can be controlled.

Chemotherapy alone has yielded few, if any, complete remissions in patients with metastatic disease.[520,563,702,1018,1019] Chemotherapy combined with aggressive surgical resection of all visible disease may be helpful, especially in patients with functional tumors in which medical therapy is not controlling the symptoms.[702,947,957,974] Because of the indolent growth pattern of these tumors and the fact that chemotherapy has not cured any patients with metastatic disease, chemotherapy has usually been withheld until a patient demonstrates progression of disease during follow-up or demonstrates refractory symptoms due either to the tumor or to the secreted hormone. Progression usually means increase in size or number of metastatic lesions on an imaging study. In some studies, an increase in plasma hormone marker for a given tumor has been used to assess disease activity. The former documentation is more reliable. A recent study has shown no relation between tumor growth and plasma levels of gastrin in patients with ZES treated with chemotherapy.[899]

Treatment of metastatic and primary tumors requires control of bulk disease and control of symptoms secondary to the hormonal excess in patients with functional tumors. The initial consideration and the only potentially curative treatment of malignant pancreatic endocrine tumors is surgical resection (see Fig. 41–21). This should be considered (if feasible with a reasonable operative risk) for any patient with a pancreatic endocrine tumor whether primary or metastatic. The goal of surgery is to locate and remove all gross disease. Resection must be performed with acceptable morbidity and mortality because often the disease is slow-growing and some patients may live for years with documented metastases.

Therapy for malignant pancreatic endocrine tumors consists of controlling the symptoms with octreotide or other medical therapies in patients with functional tumors. This therapy is used alone or coupled with debulking surgery in some cases and various cytotoxic therapies in others (see Table 41–33). Treatment with octreotide, with other medical therapies, and with surgical resection is discussed under the functional tumor syndromes. The remainder of this section considers cytotoxic therapies directed at the tumor itself in patients with metastatic disease.

MANAGEMENT OF METASTATIC DISEASE

The treatment of all metastatic pancreatic endocrine tumors is considered together because in most aspects it is similar for each tumor. Cytotoxic protocols and surgical approaches generally are the same. The long-term natural history of most functional pancreatic endocrine tumors (malignant insulinomas, VIPomas, glucagonomas, GRFomas, somatostatinomas) is not known because, until recently, effective treatment for the functional syndrome did not exist. Patients died of complications of the hormonal excess rather than of the tumor itself.[702] This may change with the recent availability of agents such as octreotide. In contrast to PPomas, nonfunctional pancreatic endocrine tumors, and gastrinomas, for which effective therapy for the gastric hypersecretion has existed for more than 30 years, the natural history of the malignant tumor itself can be assessed. Because of the similar biologic behavior of all endocrine tumors, the assessment of the latter tumors will likely provide insights into the natural history of all malignant pancreatic endocrine tumors.[702,948,1018] As shown in Table 41–31, the overall 5-year survival rate with gastrinomas is 63% to 75%, and survival is influenced primarily by the extent of the tumor. If the tumor is thought to be completely resected at the time of surgery, 5-year survival is 69% to 100%. If the tumor is resected incompletely or recurs, 5-year survival rates are 14% to 95%. If the tumor is unresectable, 5-year survival rates are 18% to 75%. There are no data to suggest that other pancreatic endocrine tumors differ in behavior. Limited data from PPomas, of which most were metastatic, report a 5-year survival rate of 44%, which is similar to that with metastatic gastrinomas.[948] Most authorities would therefore agree that treatment directed at the metastatic disease is indicated. There is no agreement about what type of therapy is most appropriate, when therapy should be started, and even the efficacy of various therapies because of the small numbers of patients treated with various protocols. Chemotherapy either alone or with debulking surgery, hepatic arterial embolization either alone or with chemotherapy, hormonal therapy with octreotide, and interferon all have been reported useful in small numbers of cases (see Table 41–33).

CHEMOTHERAPY

Chemotherapy for insulinomas and the less common islet cell tumors is similar to that discussed previously for gastrinomas and summarized in Table 41–33. Because of the rarity of these tumors, in most studies of chemotherapy for pancreatic endocrine tumors, chemotherapy of all pancreatic endocrine tumors is considered together. Although two series reported no difference in responsiveness to chemotherapeutic agents in different tumors, the numbers of individual tumors studied were small and it is not established that each tumor responds equally to chemotherapy.[702,897] As with gastrinomas, chemotherapy is reserved for patients with metastatic disease that is increasing in size on imaging studies or with refractory symptoms. The recommended choice for metastatic pancreatic endocrine tumors is the combination of streptozocin and 5-FU.[702,1019] Streptozocin is a glycocyamine nitrosourea compound originally derived from a *Streptomyces* species and has been in clinical use since 1967.[1020,1021] In preclinical studies, it was found to have cytotoxic effects on pancreatic islets.[1022] In 1968, streptozocin was found to have clinical effectiveness against a pancreatic endocrine tumor[1023] and since then has been used as the initial agent either alone or in combination with other agents for treating metastatic pancreatic endocrine tumors (see Table 41–33). Streptozocin alone gives an objective tumor response in 36% to 62% of patients. In contrast, other single agents such as doxorubicin, dacarbazine, or tubercidin have had a lower response rate of 6% to 33% (see Table 41–33). In various series, streptozocin treatment has caused nausea and vomiting in almost all patients

(100%),[899] transient dose-related renal dysfunction including proteinuria (40% to 50%),[899,1018] decreased creatinine clearance (26%),[1018] abnormalities in hepatic function (27%),[1018] and leukopenia and thrombocytopenia (6%).[1018] In one study, 5 patients died of renal failure, and the use of streptozocin must be carefully monitored.[444]

Etoposide, dactinomycin, or cisplatin alone have been used in a few cases but generally are not effective.[1019] Recently, a combination of etoposide and cisplatin was evaluated in 14 patients with metastatic pancreatic endocrine tumors and the results compared with metastatic carcinoid tumors (13 patients) or anaplastic neuroendocrine tumors (18 patients: 6 with tumors in the pancreas, 8 with tumors in the stomach and intestine, 1 with tumor of the lung, and 3 with tumors in unknown locations).[1024] This study was performed because recent studies demonstrate that these two agents are effective in small cell lung cancer, which has neuroendocrine features histologically similar to those seen in pancreatic endocrine tumors.[1024] Sixty-seven percent of the anaplastic neuroendocrine tumors, 14% of the pancreatic endocrine tumors, and none of the metastatic carcinoid tumors demonstrated partial to complete regression.[1024]

The combination of streptozocin and 5-FU was found to be more effective than streptozocin alone.[897] In this study, streptozocin gave a 36% response rate with 12% showing a complete response, whereas with streptozocin plus 5-FU, 63% demonstrated a response with 33% having a complete response. Response rates for different functional tumors or between functional and nonfunctional tumors did not differ.[897] In two more recent prospective studies, the response rate with streptozocin plus 5-FU was significantly lower in patients with metastatic gastrinomas to the liver (5% and 40%).[899,900] In neither study did any patient have a complete response, and in one study there was no difference in survival for responders and nonresponders.[899] The difference in response rate in the early study and the more recent ones remains unexplained. Streptozocin has been used in combination with other agents such as doxorubicin or tubercidin in small numbers of patients with response rates ranging from 20% to 100% (see Table 41–33).

Glucagonomas are reported to respond to dacarbazine.[694,1025–1031] Some patients have complete remissions with dacarbazine, whereas in other pancreatic endocrine tumors the response rate is low. In one study, 90% of VIPomas were reported to respond to streptozocin, a percentage higher than that seen in series of all pancreatic endocrine tumors (see Table 41–33).[967] Only small numbers of patients are reported with the different pancreatic endocrine tumors, and these possible differences have not been established.

SURGICAL TREATMENT

If possible, systematic removal of all resectable tumor (debulking surgery) is recommended for VIPomas,[957,967] glucagonomas,[920,974] and somatostatinomas.[1032] The survival of patients with gastrinomas was reported to improve with this approach.[720,759] Whether such an approach actually increases survival is not clear. This approach may be required in patients with symptomatic tumors in whom octreotide or the use of chemotherapy alone is not reducing plasma hormone levels and symptoms are not controlled sufficiently.

HEPATIC ARTERY EMBOLIZATION

Hepatic artery embolization with or without postocclusion chemotherapy has been used successfully in small numbers of patients with metastatic pancreatic endocrine tumors to the liver.[463,666,668,901,902,1033] Because the liver derives only 20% to 25% of its blood supply from the hepatic artery and 75% to 80% from the portal vein,[1033] and because most pancreatic islet cell tumors are vascular with an arterial supply, hepatic artery embolization has been used if the portal vein is patent. In some studies, 80% to 90% of patients demonstrate symptomatic improvement.[1033] In one study, only 14% had symptomatic improvement.[901] In a study combining hepatic arterial occlusion with chemotherapy, 64% of patients had complete symptomatic remission, 18% had a 75% to 100% improvement, and 9% had a 50% to 75% improvement.[463,666] The symptomatic improvement lasts longer with the addition of chemotherapy than without it.[463,666] This procedure is not without side effects, and almost all patients report abdominal pain, nausea, vomiting, and fever, usually lasting 3 to 10 days.[1033] Severe complications occur in 10% to 15%, including hepatic failure, infection, and death.[901,1033] Even more important than the possible side effects is the recent report that metastases to bone occur in 12% of patients with gastrinoma metastatic to liver.[608] This raises the likelihood in some cases that treatment directed only at the liver may be of limited value. Hepatic artery embolization should be considered in a patient with a symptomatic pancreatic endocrine tumor who has diffusely metastatic disease to the liver, minimal or no bone metastases, and hormone symptoms that cannot be controlled by octreotide, chemotherapy, or other medical treatment.

HORMONAL THERAPY WITH SOMATOSTATIN ANALOGS

In animal studies, somatostatin analogs can inhibit tumor growth[1034] and the growth of transplantable insulinomas and chondrosarcomas.[906] Pancreatic endocrine tumors frequently possess somatostatin receptors, which may mediate the action of somatostatin on these tumors.[605,931,1035] In one recent study, all 15 pancreatic endocrine tumors examined had somatostatin receptors.[603] Hormonal treatment with octreotide was reported to decrease tumor size in 8 of 66 patients (see Table 41–33). This included 3 of 29 patients with gastrinomas, 4 of 10 patients with VIPomas, 1 of 3 patients with GRFomas, and none of 5 patients with insulinomas, 10 patients with glucagonomas, 4 with Cushing's syndrome secondary to a pancreatic endocrine tumor, and 5 with nonfunctioning tumors. In no case did the metastases disappear.[905] Therefore, the antitumor effects of octreotide are small, at least at the doses of less than 1000 μg/day used in most of these studies.

INTERFERON

Interferon has been reported to effective at controlling symptoms in many patients with pancreatic endocrine tumors.[489,698,909,1036,1037] In one study of 22 patients with advanced pancreatic endocrine tumors, treatment with 3 to 6 million U/day of human leukocyte interferon resulted in responses in 77% of patients, with a mean duration of 8.5 months (2–

36 months).[909] In this study, 7 of 7 patients (100%) with VIPomas and 6 of 9 patients (66%) with PPomas or nonfunctioning tumors responded, whereas patients with somatostatinoma and insulinoma did not. Only 6 of 22 patients (27%) demonstrated an actual decrease in tumor size, although each patient had failed chemotherapy. One study demonstrated no effect of recombinant interferon-α in 2 patients with VIPomas.[1037] In another study of 16 patients with neuroendocrine tumors treated with doxorubicin plus interferon, 3 (18%) partial responses were reported.[1018] The exact percentage of patients who will respond with tumor reduction is unknown but appears to be low.[1038]

MULTIPLE ENDOCRINE NEOPLASIA TYPE I

In 1954, Wermer described the familial occurrence of tumors involving the pituitary gland, parathyroid glands, and the endocrine pancreas.[1039] Of the 5 affected patients, 4 had pituitary tumors, 3 had hyperparathyroidism, and 3 had pancreatic tumors. The syndrome was initially called Wermer's syndrome and then multiple endocrine adenomatosis type I. It is now termed multiple endocrine neoplasia type I (MEN-I) because the parathyroid disease is hyperplasia and some of the pancreatic endocrine tumors in affected individuals can be malignant.[513,514,1040]

MEN-I is inherited as an autosomal dominant trait.[514,1040,1041] Recent chromosomal linkage studies have localized the genetic defect to the long arm of chromosome 11 (q12,q13 locus), which is closely linked to the skeletal muscle glycogen phosphorylase locus that is altered in McArdle's disease (Table 41–35).[1041–1044] In 2 insulinomas from patients with MEN-I, there was a loss of one constitutional allele on chromosome 11 and hyperplastic pancreatic tissue showed a similar alteration.[1043] This suggests that the oncogenesis of MEN-I follows the two-hit theory of neoplasia of Knudsen,[1045] in which an inherited mutation in one chromosome is unmasked by a somatic deletion or mutation on the other normal chromosome, thereby removing the suppressor effect of the normal gene. These results are in contrast to patients without MEN-I who develop pancreatic endocrine tumors, in whom the pancreatic neoplasms even when malignant do not develop homozygous inactivation of the MEN-I gene.[1046] Recent work concerning the etiology of primary hyperparathyroidism in patients with MEN-I suggests that a circulating factor in the serum stimulates bovine parathyroid cells to proliferate.[1047,1048] Subsequent analyses of the mitogenic activity in the plasma of MEN-I patients demonstrated that basic fibroblast growth or a closely related growth factor was present in this plasma.[1048,1049] A monoclonal abnormality has been found in the hyperplastic parathyroid glands of patients with MEN-I, suggesting that the hyperplastic process in these glands may develop by inactivation of the MEN-I gene in a precursor cell.[1050]

CLINICAL PRESENTATION

The peak incidence of symptoms in women with MEN-I is during the third decade of life, whereas the peak incidence in men is during the fourth decade. More than half of patients

TABLE 41–35. Multiple Endocrine Neoplasia Syndromes and Familial Medullary Thyroid Cancer

Characterstic	*MEN-II*	*MEN-IIa*	*MEN-IIb*	*Familial Non-MEN MTC*
Genetic defect location	Chromosome 11q 12–13 near PYGM locus	Chromosome 10 near centrosome	Chromosome 10 near centrosome	—
MTC present	No	Bilateral	Bilateral	Bilateral
Pheochromocytoma present	No	70% bilateral	70% bilateral	No
Parathyroid disease	Hyperplasia	Hyperplasia	Rare	No
Specific phenotype	No	No	Bony abnormalities, multiple mucosal neuromas, marfanoid habitus, bumpy lips	No
Familial, autosomal dominant trait	Yes	Yes	Yes, but may be nonfamilial	Yes
Course of MTC	No MTC	Variable, frequently indolent	Generally more virulent	Indolent
Pancreatic endocrine tumors	PPomas (80–100%) Gastrinomas (54%) Insulinomas (21%) Glucagonomas (3%) GRFomas, VIPomas (uncommon)	No	No	No

MEN, multiple endocrine neoplasia; MTC, medullary thyroid carcinoma; PYGM locus, skeletal muscle glycogen phosphorylase locus; PPoma, pancreatic endocrine tumor releasing pancreatic polypeptide; VIPoma, vasoactive intestinal peptide; GRFoma, growth hormone-releasing factor tumor.

with MEN-I have adenomas of more than one gland, and about 20% have 3 affected glands. The frequency of glandular involvement, in descending order, is parathyroid, pancreas, pituitary, adrenal cortex, and thyroid. The frequency of clinical symptoms, in descending order, is hypercalcemia, nephrolithiasis, peptic ulcer disease, hypoglycemia, headache, visual-field loss, hypopituitarism, acromegaly, galactorrhea-amenorrhea, and Cushing's syndrome.[514,1040,1051]

PARATHYROID GLAND INVOLVEMENT

Hyperparathyroidism is the most common clinically detected abnormality in patients with MEN-I, occurring in 88% to 97% of all patients in different series.[513,514,1042,1052] The pathology associated with primary hyperparathyroidism is always hyperplasia or multiple gland disease (see Table 41–35).[513,1052] The surgical management requires removal of 3½ or 4 parathyroid glands to control the hypercalcemia. If 4 glands are removed, immediate autograft of some of the parathyroid tissue into the musculature of the nondominant forearm is recommended.[1053] Unfortunately, the incidence of recurrent or persistent hyperparathyroidism after surgery for hyperparathyroidism in MEN-I patients varies from 16% to 54% and the incidence of hypoparathyroidism from 10% to 25%.[1054,1055] Primary hyperparathyroidism adversely affects the medical management of the gastric acid hypersecretion in MEN-I patients with hyperparathyroidism and ZES. A recent study indicates that successful parathyroidectomy in these patients greatly facilitates the management of the gastric acid hypersecretion.[868]

PANCREATIC ENDOCRINE TUMORS

Pathologic examination of the resected pancreas in patients with MEN-I demonstrated multiple tumors producing multiple different hormones.[1056,1057] These pathologic studies suggest that PPomas are the most common pancreatic endocrine tumor, occurring in 80% to 100% of these patients.[520] These tumors cause symptoms only due to the tumor itself and often present when tumor growth is advanced. Furthermore, because patients with MEN-I have not been able to survive until late adulthood, the frequency with which this tumor will be clinically significant is unknown. In two large series, 81% to 82% of patients with MEN-I developed functional pancreatic endocrine tumors—54% had gastrinomas, 21% insulinomas, 3% glucagonomas, and 1% VIPomas (see Table 41–35).[513,514] Up to 33% of patients with GRFomas have MEN-I, and this tumor may occur much more frequently in patients with MEN-I than previously suspected.[702] The diagnosis and management of each of these syndromes are described earlier in this chapter.

The ideal treatment of ZES is surgical excision of the gastrinoma; however, in patients with MEN-I, excision of gastrinomas rarely results in normal serum gastrin levels.[712,719,896] In early studies in six different surgical series, no patient with MEN-I was cured by resection of gastrinoma, indicating that the probability of curing these patients in this manner is remote.[719] Therefore, the role of pancreatic surgery in the treatment of the gastrinoma in patients with ZES with MEN-I is unclear.[712,719,783,896] The possibility of surgical cure is much lower in patients with ZES and MEN-I than in patients with sporadic disease.[712,783,796,1058] Because of the low possibility of cure and the recent suggestion that the gastrinoma may be less malignant in MEN-I, some groups recommend that patients with MEN-I do not undergo explorative laparotomy.[758,766] Others recommend laparotomy only if a localized lesion is predicted by a localized gastrin gradient from selective venous sampling for gastrin,[1058] if the fasting serum PP concentration is more than three times normal,[1059] or if a localized tumor is identified by imaging studies and there is a family history suggesting early metastatic disease.[712,778] The best approach is unclear because all the above criteria are flawed. It is not established clearly that familial gastrinoma has a less malignant course.[712] In a recent study, an elevated or normal level of PP had no predictive value.[778] Selective gastrin sampling from portal venous tributaries in patients with MEN-I with ZES was not helpful.[777]

Many gastrinomas in patients with ZES with MEN-I are reported to appear in the duodenum[756,783] and not in the pancreas, as earlier studies suggested.[1056] No study has examined prospectively whether such tumors can be found routinely at surgery and what the long-term cure rate will be. These patients often have multiple duodenal nodularities with more than one endocrine tumor in the duodenum. It is not clear how the gastrinoma can be identified without radical surgery. Therefore, it is not known whether these patients will benefit by routine exploration with duodenotomy to the same extent as patients with sporadic disease.[783] In particular kindreds in which patients' parents died of metastatic gastrinoma and presentation occurs at a relatively young age with a large pancreatic tumor, a surgical approach similar to the one used in patients with sporadic disease may be warranted.[712,764,778,783] Therefore, we recommend that all patients with ZES and MEN-I have extensive localization studies but that only patients with unequivocally positive imaging studies undergo surgical exploration (see Fig. 41–15). At surgery, tumors identified in the pancreatic head are enucleated, the duodenum is carefully explored and any identified tumor is resected, and tumors in the pancreatic body or tail are resected. In a recent study, almost 50% of the patients treated in this manner had evidence of lymph nodes metastases.[778] Using this approach, cure of ZES is almost never seen; however, it is hoped that such surgery reduces the risk of later metastatic disease. No data demonstrate that this approach increases survival.

MEN-I is reported to be present in 20% of all patients with ZES and in 4% of patients with insulinomas.[520,764] The exact percentage of patients with VIPoma, glucagonomas, or somatostatinoma with MEN-I is not known but is estimated to be low (<5%).[520] The management of insulinomas and VIPomas is different from gastrinoma in patients with MEN-I.[702] Medical management of VIPomas and insulinomas is not as reliable as medical management of gastric acid hypersecretion in ZES patients. Diazoxide and octreotide are available and may be useful for short-term treatment, but they are not as reliable as surgical resection for long-term treatment (see the sections on these tumors). Unlike gastrinomas, insulinomas or VIPomas in patients with MEN-I frequently are solitary tumors, and resection may prove helpful in symptomatic management and may result in cure.[778,1056,1058,1060] Preoperative PVS for insulin or VIP can help identify the tumor or region of the pancreas from which the abnormal hormone source originates.[778,1058]

PITUITARY TUMORS

Pituitary tumors occur in 54% to 80% of patients with MEN-I.[513,514,1051] Symptoms caused by pituitary adenomas in MEN-I are usually due to local encroachment of tumor including headache and visual-field defects. In early studies, most tumors were described as nonfunctioning chromophobe adenomas, with 15% of patients having eosinophilic tumors often with acromegaly and 5% having basophilic tumors with Cushing's disease.[1051] It is likely that many of these nonfunctioning tumors are prolactinomas because serum prolactin levels were not routinely measured in these early cases.[1051] Prolactinomas are now thought to have a prevalence of 15%.[1051] Of the functional tumors, prolactinomas comprise 70%. The second most common hormone secreted is GH (25%), with resulting acromegaly.[1051] Cushing's syndrome may be more common in some patients with MEN-I than previously thought. In one recent study of patients with MEN-I and gastrinoma, 20% of patients had Cushing's syndrome.[893] In this series, Cushing's syndrome was always of pituitary origin and was mild.[893] Cushing's syndrome can result from release of ACTH-like material from the pancreatic tumor itself,[520,893,1061] although in patients with MEN-I this appears to be much less common than in patients with sporadic pancreatic endocrine tumors such as gastrinomas.[893] Transsphenoidal pituitary surgery is indicated to control any detectable pituitary mass lesion in patients with MEN-I. Incompletely resected patients can be managed with bromocriptine.

ADRENAL AND THYROID TUMORS

Adrenal abnormalities occur in 27% to 36% of patients with MEN-I.[513,514] The most common abnormality is a benign, nonfunctional cortical adenoma, although adrenocortical carcinomas and hyperplasia may occur.[513,514] Adrenocortical hyperfunction may be found secondary to a pituitary tumor[893] or rarely to a pancreatic endocrine tumor.[1061] Adrenocortical neoplasms usually are nonfunctional in patients with MEN-I. Thyroid adenomas occur in about 5% to 30% of patients with MEN-I involving diffuse or nodular hyperplasia and have little clinical significance.[513]

FAMILIAL MEDULLARY THYROID CARCINOMA AND MULTIPLE ENDOCRINE NEOPLASIA TYPES IIa AND IIb

HISTORY AND PATHOLOGY

The coexistence of thyroid cancer and pheochromocytoma was first described in 1932 by Eisenberg and Wallerstein.[1062] In 1959, Hazard and colleagues first described MTC and its striking histologic characteristics of cellular argentaffin staining and amyloid production.[1063] MTC is associated with three distinct familial syndromes: MEN-IIa, MEN-IIb, and familial non-MEN MTC, a disease characterized by hereditary MTC without associated endocrinopathies (see Table 41–35).[1064] In 1970, a radioimmunoassay was developed for calcitonin and a kindred with MEN-IIa was described with elevated serum calcitonin levels.[1065] Subsequently, patients with increased serum calcitonin levels were identified whose resected thyroid glands were normal macroscopically but on microscopic examination showed C-cell hyperplasia.[1066,1067]

In 1961, Sipple reported the unusually high incidence of bilateral pheochromocytomas in patients with thyroid malignancy.[1068] These patients were later found to have MTC, and the familial disease was inherited as a mendelian autosomal dominant trait with high gene penetrance (see Table 41–35).[1069,1070] Hyperparathyroidism later was identified as part of the syndrome.[1071] In 1968, this syndrome of MTC, pheochromocytomas, and hyperparathyroidism was termed MEN-II. It is now called MEN-IIa (see Table 41–35).

In 1966, Williams and Pollock called attention to the finding that some patients with MTC and pheochromocytomas had multiple mucosal neuromas, with or without marfanoid habitus, puffy lips, prominent jaw, pes cavus, and medullated corneal nerves (Fig. 41–22).[1072] For this group of patients, the terms MEN-IIb and MEN-II were suggested.[92] Patients with MEN-IIb do not have parathyroid disease (see Table 41–35). Recent chromosomal linkage studies have localized the genetic defects of MEN-IIa and MEN-IIb to chromosome 10 (see

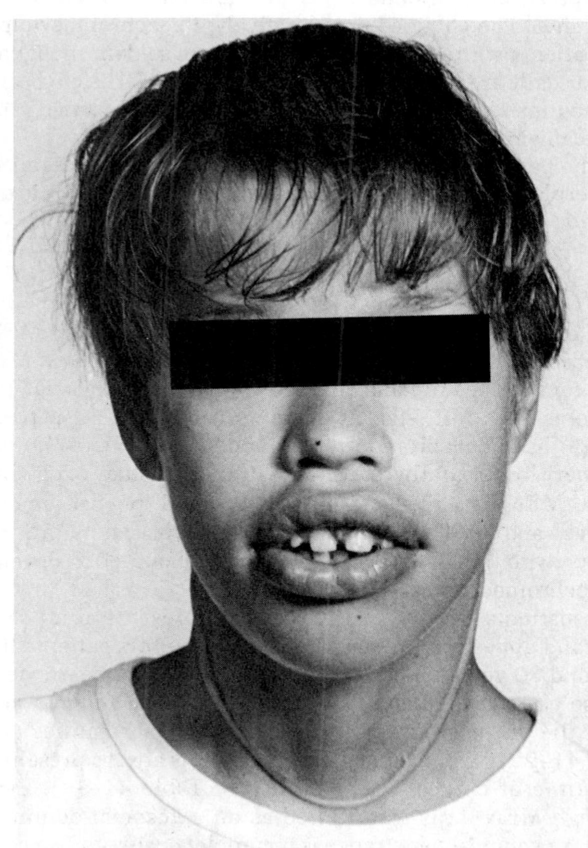

FIGURE 41–22. Characteristic appearance of a patient with multiple endocrine neoplasia type IIb. Note the mucosal neuromas, pronounced lips, poor dentition, and prominent jaw. (Norton JA, Fromme LC, Farrell RE, Wells SA Jr. Multiple endocrine neoplasia type IIb: the most aggressive form of medullary thyroid carcinoma. Surg Clin North Am 1979;59:109)

Table 41–35).[1073] In MEN-IIa, the defect has been localized to near *RBP3,* D10S5, *FNRB,* D10S15, and D10ZI near the centrosome of chromosome 10.[1074–1077] Recent linkage studies have localized the defect in MEN-IIb to chromosome 10 near *FNRB,* D10Z1.[1077–1079]

Histologically, MTC in patients with familial MTC, MEN-IIa and MEN-IIb appears identical to the MTC occurring sporadically. In each syndrome, there is bilateral involvement and the MTC usually occupies a position in the superior-lateral part of the thyroid lobe and may be multicentric, whereas in the sporadic setting it is usually unilateral. MTC is a malignant tumor of the parafollicular cells or the calcitonin-secreting cells (C cells). MTC comprises 5% to 12% of all thyroid cancers, and only 10% of all MTC is familial.[1080]

The pheochromocytomas in patients with MEN-IIa or MEN-IIb usually present in the second or third decades of life and are usually bilateral (70%).[437,1080] Tumors in patients with MEN-IIa usually are smaller than 2 to 3 cm and usually are larger in patients with MEN-IIb. Even in MEN-IIa patients with apparent unilateral pheochromocytomas, the contralateral adrenal gland almost always demonstrates medullary hyperplasia on pathologic analysis.[437] Patients with medullary hyperplasia rarely have symptoms of pheochromocytoma. ^{131}I-MIBG scans in patients with MEN-IIa may be useful to predict the presence of a clinically significant pheochromocytoma and should be obtained preoperatively. Pheochromocytomas in patients with MEN-IIa or MEN-IIb are seldom malignant and usually are found within the adrenal gland. Histologically, these tumors are indistinguishable from those occurring sporadically in a nonfamilial setting.

The parathyroid lesions in MEN-IIa consist of generalized hyperplasia[1052] and must be managed like the parathyroid disease in MEN-I (see Table 41–35).[1053]

CLINICAL PRESENTATION

Any of the neoplasms that make up the syndromes of MEN-IIa or MEN-IIb may be the presenting problem; however, MTC is a constant feature and affects 100% of individuals. Of 164 patients with MEN-IIa, all patients had MTC, 35 patients (21%) had pheochromocytomas, and 28 patients (17%) had primary hyperparathyroidism.[1080] In another study of patients with MEN-IIa, all had MTC, 40% had pheochromocytomas, and 60% had parathyroid hyperplasia.[1081] All patients with MEN-IIb have MTC and about 60% develop pheochromocytomas.[1082]

In patients with MEN-IIb, the MTC presents at an early age and appears more aggressive because few patients live beyond 30 years of age.[67] The characteristic appearance of these patients is often the first sign of disease and may suggest the diagnosis before other clinical abnormalities (see Fig. 41–22). On investigation, the MTC is always present at the time of clinical recognition (see Table 41–33). Even though MEN-IIa is transmitted as an autosomal dominant trait, the clinical penetrance is incomplete, with 40% of gene carriers not presenting with symptoms even by the age of 70 years.[1083]

Patients initially may seek medical advance because of episodic spells with headache, dizziness, or symptoms suggestive of hypertension. It is unusual for patients with MEN-IIa to present with symptoms related to parathyroid disease.[1064]

PREOPERATIVE EVALUATION AND SCREENING

When the presence of MEN-IIa or MEN-IIb is suspected, precise diagnosis depends on hormonal changes consistent with MTC, hyperparathyroidism, and pheochromocytoma. For MTC, the production of calcitonin by the tumor cells holds the key for diagnosis. Most investigators believe that the upper normal limit of plasma calcitonin levels is 300 pg/ml. Virtually all patients with MTC have elevated basal levels or stimulated plasma levels of calcitonin. Patients who present with clinically apparent disease usually have basal plasma calcitonin levels exceeding 1 ng/ml.[1084] Generally, there is a direct correlation between the tumoral mass of MTC and plasma calcitonin levels.[1084]

Minimal plasma elevations of plasma calcitonin are indicative of MTC in patients who have no other clinical evidence of the neoplasm.[1085] Some patients with normal basal plasma calcitonin levels have an increase to abnormal levels after calcium infusion (15 mg/kg over 4 hours), or pentagastrin injection (see Fig. 41–2). Short bolus calcium injection (2 mg calcium gluconate/kg over 1 minute) provokes elevated plasma calcitonin levels in MTC patients. The peak plasma calcitonin levels in patients with MTC were higher with the combination test of calcium and pentagastrin injection than with calcium chloride alone, calcium gluconate alone, or pentagastrin alone.[1086] Patients with MTC and undetectable basal calcitonin levels (<300 pg/ml) all had peak calcitonin responses above 300 pg/ml after pentagastrin and calcium injection. Three of 12 patients with MTC had peak calcitonin levels below 300 pg/ml with pentagastrin alone and with calcium gluconate alone, and would not have been diagnosed if these two provocative agents had been used separately. The combination test provides a higher diagnostic accuracy than any other provocative test and may be the most efficacious method of screening for MTC.[1086] The pentagastrin test alone is usually diagnostic (see Fig. 41–2), and patients diagnosed with MTC using this test almost always have been cured (see Table 41–12). In kindred members at risk who have borderline elevated plasma calcitonin levels (200–600 pg/ml), selective inferior thyroid venous catheterization and sampling during provocative testing is recommended.[1087] Patients with MTC have strikingly increased plasma calcitonin levels in the inferior thyroid vein effluent after provocative testing, whereas normal subjects do not. Furthermore, such subjects with MTC and minimally elevated plasma CT levels after stimulation have minimal MTC and are usually cured by thyroidectomy.[1084]

Patients and members of kindreds with MEN-IIa or MEN-IIb have been screened using various DNA markers from the pericentromeric region of chromosome 10.[1074,1077,1078] In one study,[1078] family members with a negative pentagastrin-stimulated calcitonin test were screened and the linkage study resulted in substantial changes in carrier risk for various family members. In another study of a 5-year-old child, the pentagastrin provocative test was negative but DNA linkage studies suggested a 96% chance of carrying the MEN-IIa gene.[1074] A repeat provocative test at a later time was positive for MTC. Studies combining calcitonin and restriction fragment length polymorphrism tests have identified up to 99% of MEN-IIa carriers age 25.[1076] This is an apparent improvement over pentagastrin-stimulated calcitonin screening, which detects

90% by age 30.[1078] Patients with MEN-IIa or MEN-IIb must have a pheochromocytoma excluded before undergoing surgery for MTC. Pheochromocytomas usually can be excluded by measuring normal urinary levels of epinephrine, norepinephrine, VMA, and metanephrines. If levels are elevated, tumor localization studies should be done. Abdominal CT and MRI are helpful in localizing the pheochromocytoma, but more sensitive studies may be needed.[1088,1089] MIBG is concentrated into pheochromocytoma cells and provides a means to localize these tumors functionally using scintigraphy.[1089] The sensitivity of this method varies from 79% to 91%, with a specificity of 94% to 99%.[1089]

SURGICAL MANAGEMENT

The ability to diagnose MTC in patients at risk for familial MTC allows the physician to diagnose and treat this malignancy in an early preclinical stage. If MTC is diagnosed in a patient from a MEN-IIa kindred, it is essential to screen the remainder of the family members at risk. It is in this situation that calcium gluconate and pentagastrin provocative test and DNA linkage studies are of greatest use. Most patients diagnosed with only biochemically evident MTC have surgically curable C-cell hyperplasia or carcinoma confined to the thyroid gland (see Fig. 41–3).[1090] Provocative testing is usually done in family members at risk beginning at 5 years of age and continuing at yearly intervals through the fifth decade. DNA linkage studies require only a blood sample and can be done even earlier with ease.

MEN-II patients with pheochromocytoma merit abdominal exploration and evaluation of both adrenal glands. Before surgical exploration, all patients need effective α-adrenergic receptor blockade.[1082,1089] Phenoxybenzamine should be administered 1 to 2 weeks before surgery, starting with a dose of 10 mg twice daily and increasing every second day to a usual dose of 20 to 30 mg three times daily.[1089] The end point is normotension with mild to moderate asymptomatic posterial hypotension (15 mm Hg) accompanied by symptoms of blockade including nasal stuffiness. β-Adrenergic blockade is not required[1091] except in patients with persistent sinus tachycardia.[1082,1089] The β blocker should never be administered before the institution of α-adrenergic blockage because this may result in unopposed agonism with hypertensive crises.[1089]

If a solitary pheochromocytoma is present at surgery, it should be resected. Some advocate resecting only abnormal adrenal glands confirmed by palpation,[1092] whereas others recommend routinely resecting both adrenal glands because bilateral pathology is present in most patients.[437] However, some patients have undergone only unilateral adrenalectomy and remained asymptomatic with normal urinary catecholamines for a mean follow-up of 8 years.[1092] A preoperative MIBG scan can determine unilateral versus bilateral adrenalectomy in these patients. Patients with MEN-IIa undergoing unilateral adrenalectomy should be followed carefully at 6-month or 1-year intervals because a second adrenal tumor may be diagnosed biochemically before it is clinically apparent.

The surgical management of familial MTC is total thyroidectomy with a central lymph node dissection. A total thyroidectomy must be performed because the MTC is always bilateral.

POSTOPERATIVE FOLLOW-UP

In patients with MEN-IIa and MEN-IIb, the disease that is most frequently lethal is MTC. The MTC in patients with MEN-IIb seems to be more virulent than in patients with MEN-IIa.[67] However, a recent group of children with MTC in the setting of MEN-IIb have been reported, some of whom appear to be cured of MTC.[197] Survival of patients with MTC and MEN-IIa is difficult to predict because some patients die at a young age, whereas others live a normal life expectancy. However, survival of patients with MEN-IIa depends on the extent of MTC at initial surgical resection (see Table 41-10).[1084] The survival of patients with MTC in the presence of MEN-IIa is excellent.

In a familial setting, MTC must be diagnosed at an early stage when it is confined to the thyroid gland.[1090] The prognostic significance of the stimulated plasma calcitonin level was demonstrated in a study of 92 patients with hereditary MTC.[1090] The patients were divided into four groups according to their preoperative stimulated plasma calcitonin level (group 1, 1000–1250 pg/ml; group 2, 1000–5000 pg/ml; group 3, 5000–10,000 pg/ml; and group 4, more than 10,000 pg/ml). In the 25 patients in group 1, the MTC was clinically occult and evident only on biochemical testing. Only 1 of these patients had regional lymph node metastases and only 1 patient had an elevated stimulated plasma calcitonin level postoperatively, indicating residual disease. None of the patients had distant metastases and none died during the period of observation. In the group 4 patients, 13 of the 23 had metastases to regional lymph nodes and 14 had biochemical evidence of residual disease.[1090] The only patients who had distant metastatic disease and succumbed to disease were in group 4.[1090]

With the widespread availability of reliable radioimmunoassays for calcitonin, a patient can be easily followed postoperatively. Detection of an elevated basal plasma calcitonin level, or the finding of an abnormal response to calcium and pentagastrin, indicates recurrent or persistent disease. The best strategy for patients with metastatic MTC is unclear. Radioactive iodine ablation, thyroid suppression, and radiation therapy have not been helpful. MTC is relatively insensitive to chemotherapy. Because of the indolent nature of the tumor, most physicians do not treat metastatic disease aggressively.

The 10-year survival of MTC is about 80% to 90%. Aggressive surgical resection has been used to control recurrent MTC locally because it is the only known effective therapy. In patients with MEN-IIa, the MTC may be well tolerated. The average life expectancy of patients with MTC and MEN-IIa is more than 50 years.[1093] The best therapy for familial MTC is early diagnosis and complete resection of intrathyroidal disease at initial surgery. Ablation of extrathyroidal disease when detected as persistent or current elevations of plasma calcitonin levels after total thyroidectomy requires the development of effective systemic adjuvant treatment (see Management of Medullary Thyroid Carcinoma).

REFERENCES

1. Schwartz TB. Benign metastases from thyroid malignancies. Lancet 1986;733.
2. Robbins J, Merino MJ, Boice JD Jr, et al. Thyroid cancer: A lethal endocrine neoplasm. Ann Intern Med 1991;115:133.
3. Silverberg E, Boring CC, Squires TS. Cancer Statistics. CA 1990;40:9.

4. Cancer Statistics Review. A report on the status of cancer control: 1973–1986. Cancer Statistics Review I-45, 1989.
5. Joensuu H, Klemi PJ, Paul R, Tuominen J. Survival and prognostic factors in thyroid carcinoma. Acta Radiol Oncol 1986;25:243.
6. Cady B, Rossi R, Silverman M, Wool M. Further evidence of the validity of risk group definition in differentiated thyroid carcinoma. Surgery 1985;98:1171.
7. Akslen LA, Haldorsen T, Thoresen SO, Glattre A. Survival and causes of death in thyroid cancer: A population-based study of 2479 cases from Norway. Cancer Res 1991;51:1234.
8. Hoie J, Stenwig AE, Kullmann G, Lindegaard N. Distant metastases in papillary thyroid cancer. Cancer 1988;61:1.
9. Schelfhont LJDM, Creutzberg CL, Hamming JF, et al. Multivariate analysis of survival in differentiated thyroid cancer: The prognostic significance of the age factor. Eur J Cancer Clin Oncol 1988;24:331.
10. Simpson WJ, McKinney SE, Carruthers JS, Gospodarowicz MK, Sutcliffe SB, Panzarella T. Papillary and follicular thyroid cancer. Am J Med 1987;83:479.
11. Rossi RL, Cady B, Silverman ML, et al. Surgically incurable well-differentiated thyroid carcinoma. Arch Surg 1988;123:569.
12. Schindler AM, van Melle G, Evequoz B, Scazziga B. Prognostic factors in papillary carcinoma of the thyroid. Cancer 1991;68:324.
13. Cady B. Papillary carcinoma of the thyroid. Semin Surg Oncol 1991;7:81.
14. Mueller-Gaertner HW, Grzac HT, Rehpenning W. Prognostic indices for tumor relapse and tumor mortality in follicular thyroid carcinoma. Cancer 1991;67:1903.
15. Sampson RJ, Key CF, Buncher CR, Lijima S. Thyroid carcinoma in Hiroshima and Nagasaki: Prevalence of thyhroid carcinoma at autopsy. JAMA 1969;209:65.
16. Bondeson L, Ljungberg O. Occult thyroid carcinoma at autopsy in Malmo, Sweden. Cancer 1981;47:319.
17. Sampson RJ, Woolner LB, Bahn RC, et al. Occult thyroid carcinoma in Olmsted County, Minnesota: Prevalence at autopsy compared with that in Hiroshima and Nagasaki. Cancer 1975;36:1095.
18. Fukunaga FH, Yatani R. Geographic pathology of occult thyroid carcinoma. Cancer 1975;366:1095.
19. McConahey WM, Hay ID, Woolner LB, van Heerden JA, Taylor WF. Papillary thyroid cancer treated at the Mayo Clinic 1946 through 1970: Initial manifestations, pathologic findings, therapy and outcome. Mayo Clin Proc 1986;61:968.
20. Allo MD, Christianson W, Koivunen D. Not all "occult" papillary carcinomas are "minimal." Surgery 1988;104:971.
21. Meisner WA. Tumors of the thyroid gland. In: Atlas of tumor pathology. Washington, DC: Armed Forces Institute of Pathology, 1984 (monograph).
22. Rallison ML, Dobyns BM, Keating FR, et al. Thyroid nodularity in children. JAMA 1975;233:1069.
23. Rojeski MT, Gharib H. Nodular thyroid disease. N Engl J Med 1985;313:428.
24. Shimaoka K, Sokal JE. Differentiation of benign and malignant thyroid nodules by scintiscan. Arch Intern Med 1974;114:36.
25. Groesbeck HP. Evaluation of routine scintiscanning of nontoxic thyroid nodules 1: The preoperative diagnosis of thyroid carcinoma. Cancer 1959;12:1.
26. Liechty RD, Stoffel PT, Zimmerman DE, Silverberg SG. Solitary thyroid nodules. Arch Surg 1977;112:59.
27. Messaris G, Kyriakou K, Vasilopoulos P, Tountas C. The single thyroid nodule and carcinoma. Br J Surg 1974;661:943.
28. DeGroot LJ, Reilly M, Pinnameneni K, Refetoff S. Retrospective and prospective study of radiation-induced thyroid disease. Am J Med 1983;74:852.
29. American Joint Committee on Cancer. Manual for staging of cancer. Philadelphia: JB Lippincott, 1988.
30. Clark RL, White EC, Russell WO. Total thyroidectomy for cancer of the thyroid: Significance of intraglandular dissemination. Ann Surg 1959;149:858.
31. LoGerfo P, Chabot J, Gazetas P. The intraoperative incidence of detectable bilateral and multicentric disease in papillary cancer of the thyroid. Surgery 1990;108:958.
32. Torres J, Volpato RD, Power EG, et al. Thyroid cancer survival in 148 cases followed for 10 years or more. Cancer 1985;566:2298.
33. Cady B, Sedgwick E, Meisner WA, et al. Changing clinical pathologic therapeutic and surgical patterns in differentiated thyroid carcinoma. Ann Surg 1980;192:701.
34. Ordonez NG, El-Naggar AK, Hickey RC, Samaan NA. Anaplastic thyroid carcinoma. Am J Clin Pathol 1991;96:15.
35. Mazzaferi FL. Papillary thyroid carcinoma: Factors influencing prognosis and current therapy. Semin Oncol 1987;14:315.
36. Merino MJ. Variant forms of thyroid carcinoma. In: Robbins J, moderator. Thyroid cancer: A lethal endocrine neoplasm. Ann Intern Med 1991;115:133.
37. Sampson RJ. Thyroid carcinoma. Arch Pathol Lab Med 1978;102:270.
38. Patchefsky AS, Keller IB, Mansfield CM. Solitary vertebral column metastasis from occult sclerosing carcinoma of the thyroid gland. Am J Clin Path 1970;53:596.
39. Merino MJ, Kennedy SM, Norton JA, Robbins J. Pleural involvement by metastatic thyroid carcinoma "tall cell variant": An unusual occurrence. Surg Pathol 1990;3:59.
40. Johnson TL, Lloyd RV, Thompson NW, Beierwaltes WH, Sisson JC. Prognostic implications of the tall cell variant of papillary thyroid carcinoma. Am J Surg Pathol 1988;12:22.
41. Sobrinho-Simoes MA, Nesland JM, Johannessen JV. Columnar-cell carcinoma: Another variant of poorly differentiated carcinoma of the thyroid. Am J Clin Pathol 1988;89:264.
42. Brennan MD, Bergstralh EJ, van Heerden JA, McConahey WM. Follicular thyroid cancer treated at the Mayo Clinic: 1946 through 1970. Initial manifestations, pathologic findings, therapy and outcome. Mayo Clin Proc 1991;66:11.
43. Schmidt RJ, Wang CA. Encapsulated follicular carcinoma of the thyroid: Diagnosis, treatment and results. Surgery 1986;100:1068.
44. Lang W, Choritz H, Hundeshagen H. Risk factors in follicular thyroid carcinoma. Am J Surg Pathol 1986;10:246.
45. Thompson NW, Dunn EL, Batsakis JG, Nishiyama RH. Hurthle cell lesions of the thyroid gland. Surg Gynecol Obstet 1974;139:555.
46. Gundry SR, Burney RE, Thompson NW, Lloyd R. Total thyroidectomy for Hurthle Cell Neoplasm of the thyroid. Arch Surg 1983;118:529.
47. Heppe H, Armin A, Calandra DB, et al. Hurthle cell tumors of the thyroid gland. Surgery 1985;98:1162.
48. Arganini M, Behar R, Wu TC, et al. Hurthle cell tumors: A twenty-five year experience. Surgery 1986;100:1108.
49. Carter WB, Taylor RL, Kao PC, Heath H. Determination of plasma calcitonin-gene related peptide concentrations by a new immunochemiluminometric assay in normal persons and patients with medullary thyroid carcinoma and other neuroendocrine tumors. J Clin Endocrinol Met 1991;72:327.
50. Poston GJ, Seitz PK, Townsend CM Jr, et al. Calcitonin gene-related peptide: Possible tumor marker for medullary thyroid cancer. Surgery 1987;102:1–49.
51. Alexander HR, Norton JA. Biology and management of medullary thyroid carcinoma of the parafollicular cells. In: Robbins J, moderator. Thyroid cancer: A lethal endocrine neoplasm. Ann Intern Med 1991;115:133.
52. Babu VR, Van Dyke DL, Jackson CE. Chromosome 20 deletion in human multiple endocrine neoplasias types 2A and 2B: A double blind study. Proc Natl Acad Sci USA 1985;84:2525.
53. Tanaka K, Baylin SB, Nelkin BD, Testa JR. Cytogenetic studies of a human medullary thyroid carcinoma cell line. Cancer Genet Cytogenet 1987;25:27.
54. Nelkin BD, deBustros AC, Mabry M, Baylin SB. The molecular biology of medullary thyroid carcinoma. JAMA 1989;261:3130.
55. Lairmore TC, Howe JR, Korte JA, et al. Familial medullary thyroid carcinoma and multiple endocrine neoplasia type 2B map to the same region of chromosome 10 as multiple endocrine neoplasia type 2A. Genomics 1991;9:181.
56. Mathew GGP, Chin KS, Easton DF, et al. A linked genetic marker for multiple endocrine neoplasia type 2A on chromosome 10. Nature 1987;328:527.
57. Simpson NE, Kidd KK, Goodfellow PJ, et al. Assignment of multiple endocrine neoplasia type 2A to chromosome 10 by linkage. Nature 1987;328:528.
58. Jackson CE, Norum RA, O'Neal LW, Nikolai TF, DeLaney JP. Linkage between MEN 2B and chromosome 10 markers linked to MEN 2A. Am J Hum Genet [Abstract] 1988;43:147.
59. Zajac JD, Penschow J, Mason T, et al. Identification of calcitonin and calcitonin gene-related peptide messenger ribonucleic acid in medullary thyroid carcinomas by hybridization histochemistry. J Clin Endocrinol Metab 1986;62:1037.
60. Wells SA Jr, Ontjes DA, Cooper CW, et al. The early diagnosis of medullary carcinoma of the thyroid gland in patients with multiple endocrine neoplasia type II. Ann Surg 1975;182:362.
61. Gagel RF, Tashjian AH Jr, Cummings T, et al. The clinical outcome of prospective screening for multiple endocrine neoplasia type 2a. N Engl J Med 1988;318:478.
62. Matthew CGP, Easton DF, Nakamura Y, Ponder BAJ. MEN2a International Collaborative Group. Presymptomatic screening for multiple endocrine neoplasia type 2A with linked DNA markers. Lancet 1991;337:7.
63. Sobol H, Narod SA, Assouline D, Lenon GM (GETC). Genetic screening of endocrine tumour syndromes with DNA probes: The example of medullary thyroid carcinoma. Horm Res 1989;32:34.
64. Wells SA Jr. Multiple endocrine neoplasia type II. Recent Results Cancer Res 1990;118:70.
65. Cance WG, Wells SA Jr. Multiple endocrine neoplasia type IIa. Curr Probl Surg 1985;22:1.
66. Van Heerden JA, Grant CS, Gharib H, Hay ID, Ilstrup DM. Long-term course of patients with persistent hypercalcitonemia after apparent curative primary surgery for medullary thyroid carcinoma. Ann Surg 1990;212:395.
67. Norton JA, Fromme LC, Farrell RE, Wells SA Jr. Multiple endocrine neoplasia type 2b: The most aggressive form of medullary thyroid carcinoma. Surg Clin North Am 1979;59:109.
68. Rossi R, Cady B, Meissner WA, et al. Nonfamilial medullary thyroid carcinoma. Am J Surg 1980;139:554.
69. Block MA, Jackson CE, Greenawald KA, et al. Clinical characteristics distinguishing hereditary from sporadic medullary thyroid carcinoma. Arch Surg 1980;115:142.
70. LiVolsi VA, Brooks JJ, Arendash-Durand B. Anaplastic thyroid tumors immunohistology. Am J Clin Pathol 1987;87:434.
71. Venkatesh YSS, Ordonez NG, Schultz PN, Hickey RC, Goepfert H, Samoan NA. Anaplastic carcinoma of the thyroid. Cancer 1990;66:321.
72. Kruseman ACN, Bosman FT, Henegouw JCV, et al. Medullary differentiation of anaplastic thyroid carcinoma. Am J Clin Pathol 1982;77:541.
73. Carcangiu ML, Steeper T, Zampi G, Rosai J. Anaplastic thyroid carcinoma. Am J Clin Pathol 1985;83:135.
74. Krisch K, Holzner JH, Kokoschkar J. Hemangioendothelioma of the thyroid gland: True endothelioma or anaplastic carcinoma? Pathol Res Pract 1980;170:230.
75. Aldinger KA, Samaan NA, Ibanez M, Hill CS. Anaplastic carcinoma of the thyroid. Cancer 1978;41:2267.
76. Duffy BJ Jr, Fitzgerald PJ. Cancer of the thyroid in children: A report of 28 cases. J Clin Endocrinol Metab 1950;10:1296.
77. Schneider AB, Shore-Freedman E, Ryo UY, et al. Radiation-induced tumors of the head and neck following childhood irradiation. Medicine 1985;64:1.
78. Ron E, Kleinerman RA, Boice JD Jr, LiVolsi VA, Flannery JT, Fraumeni JF Jr. A population-based case-control study of thyroid cancer. JNCI 1987;79:1.

79. Boice JD Jr, Ron E. Epidemiology of radiation-induced thyroid cancer. Ann Intern Med 1991;115:135.
80. Hamilton TE, van Belle G, LoGerfo JP. Thyroid neoplasia in Marshall islanders exposed to nuclear fallout. JAMA 1987;258:629.
81. Holm LE, Dahlquist I, Israelsson A, et al. Malignant thyroid tumors after ^{131}iodine therapy. N Engl J Med 1980;303:188.
82. Anspaugh LR, Catlin RJ, Goldman M. The global impact of Chernobyl Reactor Accident. Science 1988;242:1513.
83. Wang Z, Boice JD Jr, Wei L, et al. Thyroid nodularity and chromosome aberrations among women in areas of high background radiation in China. JNCI 1990;82:478.
84. Pottern LM, Kaplan MM, Larsen PR, et al. Thyroid nodularity after childhood irradiation for lymphoid hyperplasia: A comparison of questionnaire and clinical findings. J Clin Epidemiol 1990;43:449.
85. Larsen PR, Conrad RA, Knudsen KD, et al. Thyroid hypofunction after exposure to fallout from a hydrogen bomb explosion. JAMA 1982;247:1571.
86. Harach HR, Escalant DA, Onatavia A, et al. Thyroid cancer and thyroiditis in an endemic goiter region before and after iodine prophylaxis. Acta Endocrinol 1985;108:55.
87. William ED. The aetiology of thyroid tumours. Clin Endocrinol Metab 1979;8:193.
88. Heitz P, Moser H, Staub JJ. Thyroid cancer. Cancer 1976;37:2329.
89. Kapp DS, Li Volsi VA, Sanders MM. Anaplastic carcinoma following well-differentiated thyroid cancer: Etiological considerations. Yale J Biol Med 1982;55:521.
90. Deaconson TF, Wilson SD, Cerletty JM, Komorowski RA. Total or near total thyroidectomy versus limited resection for radiation-associated thyroid nodules: A twelve-year follow-up of patients in a thyroid screening program. Surgery 1986;100:1116.
91. Schneider AB, Recant W, Pinsky SM, et al. Radiation-induced thyroid cancer. Ann Intern Med 1986;105:405.
92. Chong GC, Beahrs OH, Sizemore GW, Woolner LH. Medullary carcinoma of the thyroid gland. Cancer 1975;35:695.
93. Farndon JR, Leight GS, Dilley WG, et al. Familial medullary thyroid carcinoma without associated endocrinopathies: A distinct clinical entity. Br J Surg 1986;73:278.
94. Phade V. R, Lawrence WR, Max MH. Familial papillary carcinoma of the thyroid. Arch Surg 1981;116:836.
95. Lote K, Andersen K, Nordal E, Brennhovd IO. Familial occurrence of papillary thyroid carcinoma. Cancer 1980;46:1291.
96. Namba H, Rubin SA, Fagis JA. Point mutations of ras oncogenes are an early event in thyroid tumorigenesis. Mol Endocrinol 1990;4:1474.
97. Lemoine NR, Mayall ES, Wyllie FS, et al. High frequency of ras oncogene activation in all stages of human thyroid tumorigenesis. Oncogene 1989;4:159.
98. Namba H, Gutman RA, Matsuo K, Alvarez A, Fagin JA. H-ras protooncogene mutations in human thyroid neoplasms. J Clin Endocrinol Metab 1988;48:4459.
99. Lemoine NR, Mayall ES, Wyllie FS, et al. Activated ras oncogenes in human thyroid cancers. Cancer Res 1988;48:4459.
100. Karga H, Lee JK, Vickery AL Jr, Thor A, Guz RD, Jameson JL. Ras oncogene mutations in benign and malignant thyroid neoplasms. J Clin Endocrinol Metab 1991;73:832.
101. Wright PA, Williams ED, Lemoine NR, Wynford-Thomas D. Radiation-associated and spontaneous human thyroid carcinomas show a different pattern of ras oncogene mutation. Oncogene 1991;6:471.
102. Fusco A, Grieco M, Santoro M, et al. A new oncogene in human thyroid papillary carcinomas and their lymph-nodal metastases. Nature 1987;328:170.
103. Bongarzone I, Pierotti MA, Monzini N, et al. High frequency of activation of tyrosine kinase oncogenes in human papillary thyroid carcinoma. Oncogene 1989;4:1457.
104. Grieco M, Santoro M, Berlingieri MT, et al. PTC is a novel rearranged form of the ret proto-oncogene and is frequently detected in vivo in human papillary thyroid carcinoids. Cell 1990;60:557.
105. Kober F, Heiss A, Keminger K, Depisch D. Chemotherapy of highly malignant thyroid tumors. Wien Klin Wochenschr 1990;102:274.
106. Jackson IMD, Cobb WE. Disorders of the thyroid. In: Kohler PO, ed. Clinical endocrinology. New York: John Wiley, 1986:73–165.
107. Mazzaferri EL, Young RL, Oertel JE. Papillary thyroid carcinoma: The impact of therapy in 576 patients. Medicine 1977;56:171.
108. Van Herle AJ, Uller RP. Elevated serum thyroglobulin: A marker of metastases in differentiated thyroid carcinoma. J Clin Invest 1975;56:272.
109. Schneider AB, Shore-Freedman E, Ryo UY, et al. Prospective serum thyroglobulin measurements in assessing the risk of developing thyroid nodules in patients exposed to childhood neck irradiation. J Clin Endocrinol Metab 1985;661:547.
110. Wells SA Jr, Haagensen DE Jr, Linehan WM, et al. The detection of elevated plasma levels of carcinoembryonic antigen in patients with suspected or established medullary thyroid carcinoma. Cancer 1978;42:1498.
111. Wells SA Jr, Dilley WG, Farndon JA, et al. Early diagnosis and treatment of medullary thyroid carcinoma. Arch Intern Med 1985;145:1248.
112. Clark OH. TSH suppression in the management of thyroid nodules and thyroid cancer. World J Surg 1981;5:39.
113. Field JB, Bloom G, Chou MCY, et al. Effects of thyroid-stimulating hormone on human thyroid carcinoma and adjacent normal tissue. J Clin Endocrinol Metab 1978;47:1052.
114. Gharib H, James FM, Charkmeau JW, Naessens JM, Offord KP, Gorman CA. Suppressive therapy with levothyroxine for solitary thyroid nodules. N Engl J Med 1987;317:70.
115. Getaz EP, Shimaoka K, Razack M, et al. Suppressive therapy for post-irradiation thyroid nodules. Can J Surg 1980;23:558.
116. Hill LD, Beebe HG, Hipp R, Jones HW. Thyroid suppression. Arch Surg 1974;108:403.
117. Blum M, Rothschild M. Improved nonoperative diagnosis of the solitary "cold" thyroid nodule: Surgical selection based on risk fastors and three months of suppression. JAMA 1980;243:242.
118. Gershengorn MC, McClung MR, Chu EW, et al. Fine needle aspiration cytology in the preoperative diagnosis of thyroid nodules. Ann Intern Med 1977;87:265.
119. Schick RM. Thyroid nodules. N Engl J Med [Letter] 1986;314:452.
120. Parker TW, Mettler FA Jr, Christie JH, Williams AG. Radionuclide thyroid studies: A survey of practice in the United States in 1981. Radiology 1984;150:547.
121. Dobyns BM, Maloof F. The study and treatment of 119 cases of carcinoma of thyroid with radioactive iodine. J Clin Endocrinol Metab 1951;11:1323.
122. Ashcraft MW, Van Herle AJ. Management of thyroid nodules I. History, physical examination, blood tests, x-ray tests and ultrasonograph. Head Neck Surg 1981;3:216.
123. Ashcraft MW, Van Herle AJ. Management of thyroid nodules II. Scanning techniques, thyroid suppressive therapy, and fine needle aspiration. Head Neck Surg 1981;3:297.
124. Hamburger JI. Thyroid nodules. N Engl J Med [Letter] 1986;314:452.
125. Miller JM, Hamburger JI. The thyroid scintigram. One hot nodule. Radiology 1965;84:66.
126. Arnstein NB, Juni JE, Sisson JC, et al. Recurrent medullary carcinoma of the thyroid demonstrated by thallium-201 scintigraphy. J Nucl Med 1986;27:1564.
127. Skibber JM, Reynolds JC, Spiegel AM, et al. Computerized technetium/thallium scan and parathyroid reoperation. Surgery 1985;98:1077.
128. Asari AN, Siegel ME, DeQuattro V, Gazarian LH. Imaging of medullary thyroid carcinoma and hyperfunctioning adrenal medulla using Iodine-131 metaiodobenzylguanidine. J Nucl Med 1986;27:1858.
129. Sone T, Fukunaga M, Otsuka N, et al. Metastatic medullary thyroid cancer: Localization with iodine-131 metaiodobenzylguanidine. J Nucl Med 1985;26:604.
130. Zanin DFA, van Dongen A, Hoefnagel CA, Bruning PF. Radioimmunoscintigraphy using iodine-131-anti-CEA monoclonal antibodies and thallium-201 scintigraphy in medullary thyroid carcinoma: A case report. J Nucl Med 1990;31:1854.
131. Edington HD, Watson CG, Levine G, Tauxe WN, Yousem SA, Unger M, Kowal CD. Radioimmunoimaging of metastatic medullary carcinoma of the thyroid gland using an indium-111-labelled monoclonal antibody to CEA. Surgery 1988;104:1004.
132. Mojiminyi OA, Udelsman R, Soper ND, Shepstone BJ, Dudley NE. Pentavalent Tc99m DMSA scintigraphy: Prospective evaluation of its role in the management of patients with medullary carcinoma of the thyroid. Clin Nucl Med 1991;16:259.
133. Udelsman R, Mojiminyi OA, Soper ND, Buley ID, et al. Medullary carcinoma of the thyroid: Management of persistent hypercalcitonemia utilizing ^{99m}Tc dimercaptosuccinic acid scintigraphy. Br J Surg 1989;76:1278.
134. Stockwell R, Davidoff F. Radiation-induced thyroid carcinoma. Ann Intern Med [Letter] 1987;106:637.
135. Nassani SN, Bard R. Evaluation of solid thyroid neoplasms by gray scale and real-time ultrasonography: The halo sign. Ultrasound Med Biol 1978;4:323.
136. Simeone JF, Daniels GH, Hall DA, et al. Sonography in the follow-up of 100 patients with thyroid carcinoma. AJR 1987;148:45.
137. Schwerk WB, Grun R, Wahl R. Ultrasound diagnosis of c-cell carcinoma of the thyroid. Cancer 1985;55:624.
138. Van Herle AJ, Rich P, Ljung BME, et al. The thyroid nodule. Ann Intern Med 1982;966:221.
139. Hamburger JI, Hamburger SW. Fine needle biopsy of thyroid nodules: Avoiding the pitfalls. New York State J Med 1986;86:241.
140. Walfish PG, Hazani E, Strawbridge HTG, et al. Combined ultrasound and needle aspiration cytology in the assessment and management of hypofunctioning thyroid nodule. Ann Intern Med 1977;87:270.
141. Nishiyama RH, Bigos ST, Goldfarb WB, et al. The efficacy of simultaneous fine-needle aspiration and large-needle biopsy of the thyroid gland. Surgery 1986;100:1133.
142. Hamburger JI, Miller JM, Kini SR. Lymphoma of the thyroid. Ann Intern Med 1983;99:685.
143. Broughan TA, Esselstyn CB. Large-needle biopsy: Still necessary. Surgery 1986;100:1138.
144. Schwartz AE, Nieburgs HE, Davies TF, et al. The place of fine needle biopsy in the diagnosis of nodules of the thyroid. Surg Gynecol Obstet 1982;155:54.
145. Cusick EL, MacIntosh CA, Krukowski Z, Williams VMM, Ewen SWB, Matheson NA. Management of isolated thyroid swellings: A prospective six year study of fine needle aspiration cytology in diagnosis. Br Med J 1990;301:318.
146. Boey J, Hsu C, Collins RJ. False-negative errors in fine-needle biopsy of dominant thyroid nodules: A prospective follow-up study. World J Surg 1986;10:623.
147. Block M. A, Dailey GE, Robb JA. Thyroid nodules indeterminant by needle biopsy. Am J Surg 1983;146:72.
148. Hamburger JI. Consistency of sequential needle biopsy findings for thyroid nodules, management implications. Arch Intern Med 1987;147:97.
149. Hamburger JI, Hamburger SW. Declining role of frozen section in surgical planning for thyroid nodules. Surgery 1985;98:307.
150. Miller JM, Hamburger JI, Kini SR. The impact of needle biopsy on the preoperative diagnosis of thyroid nodules. Henry Ford Hosp Med J 1980;28:145.
151. Hamburger B, Gharib H, Melton LJ III. Fine needle aspiration biopsy of thyroid nodules: Impact on thyroid practice and cost of care. Am J Med 1982;73:381.
152. McConahey WM, Hay ID, Woolner LB, et al. Papillary thyroid cancer treated at the Mayo Clinic, 1946 through 1970: Initial manifestations, pathologic findings, therapy and outcome. Mayo Clin Proc 1986;61:978.
153. Hawkins F, Bellido D, Bernal C, et al. Fine needle aspiration biopsy in the diagnosis of thyroid cancer and thyroid disease. Cancer 1987;59:1206.
154. Gharib H, Boellner JR, Zinsmeister AR, et al. Fine needle aspiration biopsy of the thyroid: The problem of suspicious cytologic findings. Ann Intern Med 1984;101:25.

155. Boon ME, Lowhagen T, Cardozo PL, et al. Computation of preoperative diagnosis probability for follicular adenoma and carcinoma of the thyroid on aspiration smears. Anal Quant Cytol 1982;4:1.
156. Luck JB, Mumaw VR, Frable WJ. Fine needle aspiration biopsy of the thyroid: Differential diagnosis by videoplan image analysis. Acta Cytol 1982;26:793.
157. Sprenger E, Lawhagen T, Vogt-Schaden M. Differential diagnosis between follicular adenoma and follicular carcinoma of the thyroid by nuclear DNA determination. Acta Cytol 1977;21:528.
158. Cusick EL, Ewen SWB, Krukowski ZH, Matheson NA. DNA aneuploidy in follicular thyroid neoplasia. Br J Surg 1991;78:94.
159. Hamburger JI. Consistency of sequential needle biopsy findings for thyroid nodules. Arch Intern Med 1987;147:97.
160. Grant CS, Hay ID, Gough IR, McCarthy PM, Goellner JR. Long-term follow-up of patients with benign thyroid fine-needle aspiration cytologic diagnoses. Surgery 1989;106:980.
161. Layfield LJ, Mohrmann RL, Kopald KH, Guiliano AE. Use of aspiration cytology and frozen section examination for management of benign and malignant thyroid nodules. Cancer 1991;68:130.
162. Shaha AR, DiMaio T, Webber C, Jaffe BMJ. Intraoperative decision making during thyroid surgery based on the results of preoperative needle biopsy and frozen section. Surgery 1990;108:964.
163. Rossi R, Cady B, Silverman ML, et al. Current results of conservative surgery for differentiated thyroid carcinoma. World J Surg 1986;10:612.
164. Cohn KH, Backdahl M, Forsslund G, et al. Biologic considerations and operative strategy in papillary thyroid carcinoma: Arguments against the routine performance of total thyroidectomy. Surgery 1984;96:957.
165. Tubiana M, Schlumberger M, Rougier P, et al. Long-term results and prognostic factors in patients with differentiated thyroid carcinoma. Cancer 1985;55;794.
166. Hannequin P, Liehn JC, Delisle MJ. Multifactorial analysis of survival in thyroid cancer. Cancer 1986;58:1749.
167. Brennan MF. Cancer of the endocrine system. In: DeVita VT, Hellman S, Rosenberg SA, eds. Cancer principles and practice of oncology. Philadelphia: JB Lippincott, 1985:1179–1241.
168. Tupchong L, Phil D, Hughes F, Harmer CL. Primary lymphoma of the thyroid: Clinical features, prognostic factors and results of treatment. Int J Radiat Oncol Biol Phys 1986;12:1813.
169. Goldman JM, Goren EN, Cohen MH, et al. Anaplastic thyroid carcinoma: Long-term survival after radical surgery. J Surg Oncol 1980;14:389.
170. Tollefson HR, DeCosse JJ. Papillary carcinoma of the thyroid: Recurrence in the thyroid gland after initial treatment. Am J Surg 1983;1066:728.
171. Van Heerden JA, Groh MA, Grant CS. Early postoperative morbidity after surgical treatment of thyroid carcinoma. Surgery 1986;101:224.
172. Young RL, Mazzaferri EL, Rahe AJ, et al. Pure follicular thyroid carcinoma: Impact of therapy in 214 patients. J Nucl Med 1980;21:735.
173. Harness JK, Thompson NW, McLeod MK, et al. Follicular carcinoma of the thyroid gland: Trends and treatment. Surgery 1984;966:972.
174. Bronner MP, LiVolsi VA. Oxyphilic (Askanazy/Hurthle cell) tumors of the thyroid: Microscopic features predict biologic behavior. Surg Pathol 1988;1:137.
175. Rosen IB, Luk S, Katz I. Hurthle cell tumor behavior: Dilemma and resolution. Surgery 1985;98:777.
176. Cooper DS, Schneyer CR. Follicular and Hurthle cell carcinoma of the thyroid. Endocrinol. Metab Clin North Am 1990;19:577.
177. Flint A, Lloyd RV. Hurthle-cell neoplasms of the thyroid gland. Pathol Annu 1990;577.
178. Kramer JB, Wells SA Jr. Thyroid carcinoma. Adv Surg 1989;22:195.
179. Schneider AB, Shore-Freedman E, Weinstein RA. Radiation-induced thyroid and other head and neck tumors: Occurrence of multiple tumors and analysis of risk factors. J Clin Endocrinol Metab 1986;63:107.
180. Calandra DB, Shah KH, Lawrence A, Paloyan E. Total-thyroidectomy in irradiated patients. Ann Surg 1985;202:356.
181. Deaconess TF, Wilson SD, Cerletty JM, Komorowski RA. Total or near total thyroidectomy versus limited resection for radiation-associated thyroid nodules: A twelve-year follow-up of patients in a thyroid screening program. Surgery 1986;100:1116.
182. DeGroot LJ, Reilly M. Comparison of 30- and 50- mCi doses of Iodine-131 for thyroid ablation. Ann Intern Med 1982;96:51.
183. Bondeson L, Bondeson AG, Ljungberg O, Tibblin S. Oxyphil tumors of the thyroid. Follow-up of 42 cases. Ann Surg 1981;194:677.
184. Brown AP, Greening WP, McCready VR, et al. Radioiodine treatment of metastatic thyroid carcinoma: The Royal Marsden experience. Br J Radiol 1984;57:323.
185. Marocci C, Pacini F, Elisei R, et al. Clinical and biological behavior of bone metastases from differentiated thyroid carcinoma. Surgery 1989;106:960.
186. Leeper RD. Thyroid cancer. Med Clin North Am 1985;669:1079.
187. Ruiz-Garcia J, Ruiz de Almodovar JM, Olea N, Pedraza V. Thyroglobulin as a predictive factor of tumoral recurrence in differentiated thyroid cancer. J Nucl Med 1991;32: 395.
188. Rubello D, Girelli ME, Casara D, Piccolo M, Perin A, Busnardo B. Usefulness of the combined antithyroglobulin antibodies and thyroglobulin assay in the follow-up of patients with differentiated thyroid cancer. J Endocrinol Invest 1990;13:737.
189. Robnga G, Fiorentino A, Paserio E, Signore A, Todino V, Tummarello MA, Filesi M, Baschierri I. Can iodine-131 whole-body scan be replaced by thyroglobulin measurement in the post-surgical follow-up of differentiated thyroid carcinoma? J Nucl Med 1990;31:1766.
190. Burmeister LA, deCret RP, Mariash CN. Local reactions to radioiodine in the treatment of thyroid cancer. Am J Med 1991;906:217.
191. Schlumberger M, Tubiana M, De Vathaire F, et al. Long-term results of treatment of 283 patients with lung and bone metastases from differentiated thyroid carcinoma. J Clin Endocrinol Metab 1986;63:9660.
192. Maxon MR, Smith HS. Radioactive ^{131}I in the diagnosis and treatment of metastatic well differentiated thyroid cancer. Endocrinol Metab Clin North Am 1990;19:685.
193. Samaan NA, Schultz PN, Haynie TP, Ordonez NG. Pulmonary metastasis of differentiated thyroid carcinoma: Treatment results in 101 patients. J Clin Endocrinol Metab 1985;665:376.
194. Ahuja S, Ernst H. Chemotherapy of thyroid cancer. J Endocrinol Invest 1987;10: 303.
195. Duh QY, Sancho JJ, Greenspan FS, et al. Medullary thyroid carcinoma. Arch Surg 1989;124:1206.
196. Telander RL, Zimmerman D, van Heerden JA, Sizemore GW. Results of early thyroidectomy for medullary thyroid carcinoma in children with multiple endocrine neoplasia type 2. J Pediatr Surg 1986;21:1190.
197. Decker RA, Toyama WM, O'Neal LW, Telander RL, Wells SA Jr. Evaluation of children with multiple endocrine neoplasia type IIb following thyroidectomy. J Pediatr Surg 1990;25:939.
198. Gorman B, Charboneau JW, James EM, et al. Medullary thyroid carcinoma: Role of high-resolution. Ultrasound Radiology 1987;162:147.
199. Tennvall J, Biorklund A, Moller T, et al. Prognostic factors of papillary, follicular and medullary carcinoma of the thyroid gland. Acta Radiologica Oncol 1985;24:17.
200. Norton JA, Doppman JL, Brennan MF. Localization and resection of clinically inapparent medullary carcinoma of the thyroid. Surgery 1980;87:616.
201. Tisell LE, Hansson G, Jansson S, Salander H. Reoperation in the treatment of asymptomatic metastasizing medullary thyroid carcinoma. Surgery 1986;99:60.
202. Tisell LE, Hansson S. Recent results of reoperative surgery in medullary carcinoma of the thyroid. Wien Klin Wochenschr 1988;100:347.
203. Talpos GB, Jackson CB, Froelich JW, et al. Localization of residual medullary thyroid cancer by thallium/technetium scintigraphy. Surgery 1985;98:1189.
204. Gottlieb JA, Hill CS Jr. Chemotherapy of thyroid cancer with adriamycin: Experience with 30 patients. N Engl J Med 1974;290:193.
205. Stepanas AV, Samaan NA, Hill CS Jr, Hickey RC. Medullary thyroid carinoma: Importance of serial serum calcitonin measurement. Cancer 1979;43:825.
206. Porter AT, Ostrowski MJ. Medullary carcinoma of the thyroid treated by low-dose adriamycin. Brit J of Clin Pract 1990;44:517.
207. Petursson SR. Metastatic medullary thyroid carcinoma, complete response to combination chemotherapy with dacarbazine and 5-fluorouracil. Cancer 1988;62:1899.
208. Tubiana M, Haddad E, Schlumberger M, et al. External radiotherapy in thyroid cancers. Cancer 1985;55:2062.
209. Cox TM, Fagan EA, Hillward CJ, et al. Role of calcitonin in diarrhea associated with medullary carcinoma of the thyroid. Gut 1979;20:629.
210. Jerkins TW, Sacks HS, O'Dorisio TM, et al. Medullary carcinoma of the thyroid, pancreatic nesidioblastosis and microadenosis, and pancreatic polypeptide hypersecretion: A new association and clinical and hormonal responses to long-acting somatostatin analog SMS 201-995. J Clin Endocrinol Metab 1987;64:1313.
211. Mahler C, Verhelst J, DeLonueville M, Harris A. Long-term treatment of metastatic medullary thyroid carcinoma with the somatostatin analogue octreotide. Clin Endocrinol 1990;33:261.
212. Gröhn P, Kumpulainen E, Jakobsson M. Response of medullary thyroid cancer to low-dose alpha-interferon therapy. Acta Oncol 1990;29:950.
213. Nel CJC, van Heerden JA, Goellner JR, et al. Anaplastic carcinoma of the thyroid: A clinicopathologic study of 82 cases. Mayo Clin Proc 1985;60:51.
214. Kim JH, Leeper RD. Treatment of anaplastic giant and spindle cell carcinoma of the thyroid gland with combination adriamycin and radiation therapy a new approach. Cancer 1983;52:954.
215. Kim JH, Leeper RD. Treatment of locally advanced thyroid carcinoma with combination doxorubicin and radiation therapy. Cancer 1987;60:2372.
216. Kim JH, Leeper RD. Combination adriamycin and radiation therapy for locally advanced carcinoma of the thyroid gland. Int J Radiat Oncol Biol Phys 1983;9:565.
217. Wilford MR, Chertow BS, Lepanto PB, Leidy JW Jr. Dramatic response of follicular thyroid carcinoma with superior vena cava syndrome and tracheal obstruction to external beam radiotherapy. Am J Med 1991;90:753.
218. Williams SD, Birch R, Einhorn D. Phase II evaluation of doxorubicin plus cisplatin in advanced thyroid cancer: A Southeastern Cancer Study Group trial. Cancer Treat Rep 1986;70:405.
219. Shimaoka K, Schoenfeld DA, DeWys WD, et al. A randomized trial of doxorubicin versus doxorubicin plus cisplatin in patients with advanced thyroid carcinoma. Cancer 1985;566:2155.
220. Bukowski RM, Brown L, Weick JK, et al. Combination chemotherapy of metastatic thyroid cancer. Am J Clin Oncol 1983;6:579.
221. Christensson T. Hyperparathyroidism and radiation therapy. Ann Intern Med 1978;89: 216.
222. Norton JA, Brennan MF, Saxe AW, et al. Intraoperative urinary cyclic adenosine monophosphate as a guide to successful reoperative parathyroidectomy. Ann Surg 1984;200:389.
223. Mallette LE, Bilizikian JP, Ketcham AS, Aurbach GD. Parathyroid carcinoma in familial hyperparathyroidism. Am J Med 1974;57:642.
224. Dinnen JS, Greenwood RH, Jones JH, et al. Parathyroid carcinoma in familial hyperparathyroidism. J Clin Pathol 1977;30:966.
225. Schantz A, Castleman B. Parathyroid carcinoma a study of 70 cases. Cancer 1973;31: 6600.
226. Levin KE, Galante M, Clark OH. Parathyroid carcinoma versus parathyroid adenoma in patients with profound hypercalcemia. Surgery 1987;101:649.

227. Cohn K, Silverman M, Corrado J, Sedgewick C. Parathyroid carcinoma: The Lahey Clinic experience. Surgery 1985;98:1095.
228. Wang C, Gaz RD. Natural history of parathyroid carcinoma. Diagnosis, treatment, and results. Am J Surg 1985;149:522.
229. Shane E, Bilezikian JP. Parathyroid carcinoma: A review of 62 patients. Endocr Rev 1982;3:218.
230. Gutter RD, Maier H. Carcinoma of the parathyroid. Arch Intern Med 1972;130:413.
231. Bukowski RM, Sheeler L, Cunningham J, Esselstyn C. Successful combination chemotherapy for metastatic parathyroid carcinoma. Arch Intern Med 1984;144:399.
232. Calandra DB, Chejfec G, Foy BK, et al. Parathyroid carcinoma: Biochemical and pathologic response to DTIC. Surgery 1984;96:1132.
233. Flye MW, Brennan MF. Surgical resection of metastatic parathyroid carcinoma. Ann Surg 1981;193:425.
234. Warrell RP Jr, Israel R, Frisone M, Snyder T, Gaynor JJ, Bockman RS. Gallium nitrate for acute treatment of cancer-related hypercalcemia a randomized, double-blind comparison to calcitonin. Ann Intern Med 1988;108:669.
235. Singer FR, Ritch PS, Lad TE, Ringenberg QS, et al. Treatment of hypercalcemia of malignancy with intravenous etidronate. Arch Intern Med 1991;151:471.
236. Page DL, DeLellis RA, Hough AJ. Tumors of the adrenal. In: Atlas of tumor pathology. Washington, DC: Armed Forces Institute of Pathology, 1986 (monograph).
237. Travis WD, Tsokos M, Doppman JL, et al. Primary pigmented nodular adrenocortical disease. Am J Surg Pathol 1989;13:921.
238. Schweizer-Cagrianut M, Salomon F, Hedinger E. Primary adrenocortical nodular dysplasia with cardiac myxomas. Virchows Arch [A] 1982;397:183.
239. Hough AJ, Hollifield JW, Page DL, Hartmann WH. Diagnostic factors in adrenal cortical tumors. Am J Clin Pathol 1979;72:390.
240. Hutter AM Jr, Kayhoe DE. Adrenal cortical carcinoma. Am J Med 1966;4:572.
241. National Cancer Institute Monograph. Third national cancer surgery: incidence data (DHEW publication NIH75-787). Bethesda, MD: National Cancer Institute, 1975: 41.
242. Lynch HT, Katz DA, Bogard PJ, Lynch JF. The sarcoma, breast cancer, lung cancer, and adrenocortical carcinoma syndrome revisited. Am J Dis Child 1985;139:134.
243. Limon J, Dal Cin P, Kakati S, et al. Cytogenetic findings in a primary adrenocortical carcinoma. Cancer Genet Cytogenet 1987;266:271.
244. Yano T, Linehan M, Anglard P, et al. Genetic changes in human adrenocortical carcinomas. JNCI 1989;81:518.
245. Henry I, Grandjovans S, Couillin P, et al. Tumor-specific loss of 11 p 15.5 alleles in del 11 p 13 Wilms tumor and in familial adrenocortical carcinoma. Proc Natl Acad Sci USA 1989;86:3247.
246. Wick MR, Cherwitz DL, McGlennen RC, Dehner LP. Adrenocortical carcinoma, an immunohistochemical comparison with renal cell carcinoma. Am J Pathol 1986;122: 343.
247. Weiss LM. Comparative histologic study of 43 metastasizing and nonmetastasizing adrenocortical tumors. Am J Surg Pathol 1984;8:163.
248. Weiss LM, Medeiros LJ, Vickery AL. Pathologic features of prognostic significance in adrenocortical carcinoma. Am J Surg Pathol 1989;13:202.
249. Hosaka Y, Rainwater LM, Grant CS, et al. Adrenocortical carcinoma: Nuclear deoxyribonucleic acid ploidy studied by flow cytometry. Surgery 1987;102:1027.
250. O'Hare MJ, Monaghan P, Neville AM. The pathology of adrenocortical neoplasia: A correlated structural and functional approach to the diagnosis of malignant disease. Hum Pathol 1979;10:137.
251. Loriaux DL, Cutler GB. Diseases of the adrenal glands. In: Kohler PO, ed. Clinical endocrinology. New York: John Wiley and Sons, 1986:167–238.
252. Perry RR, Nieman LK, Cutler GB, et al. Primary adrenal causes of Cushing's syndrome: Diagnosis and surgical management. Ann Surg 1989;210:59.
253. Raker JW, Henneman PH, Graf WS. Coexisting primary hyperparathyroidism and Cushing's syndrome. J Clin Endocrinol Metab 1962;22:273.
254. Maton PN, Gardner JD, Jensen RT. Cushing's syndrome in patients with the Zollinger-Ellison Syndrome. N Engl J Med 1986;315:1.
255. Kramer M, Corrado ML, Bacci V, et al. Pulmonary cryptococcosis and Cushing's syndrome. Arch Intern Med 1983;143:2179.
256. Fulkerson WJ, Newman JH. Endogenous Cushing's syndrome complicated by pneumocystis carinii pneumonia. Am Rev Respir Dis 1984;129:188.
257. Graham BS, Tucker WS Jr. Opportunistic infections in endogenous Cushing's syndrome. Ann Intern Med 1984;101:334.
258. Thomas CG Jr, Smith AT, Griffith JM, et al. Hyperadrenalism in childhood and adolescence. Ann Surg 1984;199:538.
259. Pavlatos FC, Smilo RP, Forsham PH. A rapid screening test for Cushing's syndrome. JAMA 1965;193:720.
260. Willenbring M. L, Morley JE, Niewoeher CB, et al. Adrenocortical hyperactivity in newly admitted alcoholics: Prevalence, course and associated variables. Psychoneuroendocrinology 1984;9:415.
261. Chrousos GP, Vingerhoeds A, Brandon D, et al. Primary cortisol resistance in man: A glucocorticoid receptor-mediated disease. J Clin Invest 1982;69:1261.
262. Chrousos GP, Schuermeyer TH, Doppman J, et al. Primary cortisol resistance: A family study. J Clin Endocrinol Metab 1983;56:1243.
263. Chrousos GP, Schuermeyer TH, Doppman J, et al. Clinical applications of corticotropin-releasing factor. Ann Intern Med 1985;102:344.
264. Nieman LK, Chrousos GP, Oldfield EH, et al. The ovine corticotropin-releasing hormone stimulation test and the dexamethesone suppression test in the differential diagnosis of Cushing's syndrome. Ann Intern Med 1986;105:862.
265. Howlett TA, Drury PL, Perry L, et al. Diagnosis and management of ACTH-dependent Cushing's syndrome: Comparison of the features in ectopic and pituitary ACTH production. Clin Endocrinol 1986;24:699.
266. Weiss E. R, Rayjis SS, Nelson DH, et al. Evaluation of stimulation and suppression tests in the etiological diagnosis of Cushing's syndrome. Ann Intern Med 1969;71: 941.
267. Tyrrell JB, Brooks RM, Fitzgerald PA, et al. Cushing's disease: Selective transphenoidal resection of pituitary microadenomas. N Engl J Med 1978;298:753.
268. Oldfield EH, Doppman JL, Nieman LK, et al. Petrosal sinus sampling with and without corticotropin-releasing hormone for the differential diagnosis of Cushing's syndrome. N Engl J Med 1991;325:897.
269. Oldfield EH, Chrousos GP, Shulte HM. Preoperative lateralization of ACTH-secreting pituitary microadenomas by bilateral and simultaneous inferior petrosal sinus sampling. N Engl J Med 1985;312:100.
270. Epstein AJ, Patel SK, Petasnick JP. Computerized tomography of the adrenal gland. JAMA 1979;242:2791.
271. Doppman JL, Nieman LK, Travis WD, et al. CT or MR imaging of massive macronodular adrenocortical disease: A rare cause of autonomous primary adrenal hypercortisolism. J Comput Assist Tomogr 1991;15:773.
272. Roubidoux M, Dunnick NR. Adrenal cortical tumors. Bull N Y Acad Med 1991;67: 119.
273. Remer EM, Weinfeld RM, Glazer GM, Quint LE, Francis IR, Gross MD, Bookstein FL. Hyperfunctioning and nonhyperfunctioning benign adrenal cortical lesions: Characterization and comparison with MR imaging. Radiology 1989;171:681.
274. Doppman JL, Travis WD, Nieman L, et al. Cushing syndrome due to primary pigmented nodular adrenocortical disease: Findings at CR and MR imaging. Radiology 1989;172: 415.
275. Doppman JL, Reinig JW, Dwyer AJ, et al. Differentiation of adrenal masses by magnetic resonance imaging. Surgery 1987;102:1018.
276. Bierwaltes WH, Sisson JC, Shapiro JC, Shapiro B. Diagnosis of adrenal tumors with radionuclide imaging. Spec Top Endocrinol Metab 1984;6:1.
277. Schteingart DE, Seabold JE, Gross MD, Swanson DP. Iodocholesterol adrenal tissue uptake and imaging in adrenal neoplasms. J Clin Endocrinol Metab 1981;52:1156.
278. Fig LM, Gross MD, Shapiro B, Ehrmann DA, Freitas JE, Schteingart DE, Galzer GM, Francis IR. Adrenal localization in the adrenocorticotropic hormone-independent Cushing syndrome. Ann Intern Med 1988;109:547.
279. McArthur RB, Bahn RC, Hayles AB. Primary adrenocortical nodular dysplasia as a cause of Cushing's syndrome in infants and children. Mayo Clin Proc 1982;57:58.
280. Donaldson MDC, Grant DB, O'hare MJ, et al. Familial congenital Cushing's syndrome due to bilateral nodular adrenal hyperplasia. Clin Endocrinol 1981;14:519.
281. Spark RF, Connolly PB, Gluckin DS, et al. ACTH secretion from a functioning pheochromocytoma. N Engl J Med 1979;301:416.
282. Boggan JE, Tyrrell JB, Wilson CB. Transsphenoidal microsurgical management of Cushing's disease: Report of 100 cases. J Neurosurg 1983;59:195.
283. Kern DC, Tang K, Hanson CS, et al. The prediction of anatomical morphology of primary aldosteronism using serum 18-hydroxycorticosterone levels. J Clin Endocrinol Metab 1985;60:67.
284. Gomez-Sanchez CE, Montgomery M, Ganguly A, et al. Elevated urinary excretion of 18-oxocortisol in glucocorticoid-suppressible aldosteronism. J Clin Endocrinol Metab 1984;59:1022.
285. Brown RD, Hollifield JW. Endocrine hypertension. In: Kohler PO, ed. Clinical endocrinology. New York: John Wiley & Sons, 1986:239–262.
286. Conn JW. Presidential address. Part I. Painting background. II. Primary aldosteronism, a new clinical syndrome. J Lab Clin Med 1972;264:9.
287. McLeod MK, Thompson NW, Gross MD, Grekin RJ. Idiopathic aldosteronism masquerading as discrete aldosterone-secreting adrenal cortical neoplasms among patients with primary aldosteronism. Surgery 1989;106:1161.
288. Tenschert W, Maurer R, Vetter H, Vetter W. Primary aldosteronism by carcinoma of the adrenal cortex. Klin Wochenschr 1987;65:428.
289. Carey RM, Sen S, Dolan LM, et al. Idiopathic hyperaldosteronism: A possible role for aldosterone-stimulating factor. N Engl J Med 1984;311:94.
290. Weinberger MH, Grim CE, Hollifield JW, et al. Primary aldosteronism: Diagnosis, localization and treatment. Ann Intern Med 1979;90:386.
291. Lyons DG, Kern DC, Brown RD, et al. Single dose captopril as a diagnostic test for primary aldosteronism. J Clin Endocrinol Metab 1983;57:892.
292. Guerin CK, Wahner HW, Gorman CA, et al. Computed tomographic scanning versus radioisotope imaging in adrenocortical diagnosis. Am J Med 1983;75:653.
293. Falke THM, Strake L, Shaff MI, et al. MR imaging of the adrenals: Correlation with computed tomography. J Comput Assist Tomogr 1986;10:242.
294. Geisinger MA, Zelch M, Bravo E, et al. Primary hyperaldosteronism: Comparison of CT, adrenal venography, and venous sampling. AJR 1983;141:299.
295. Auda SP, Brennan MF, Gill JR. Evolution of the surgical management of primary aldosteronism. Ann Surg 1980;191:1.
296. Nadler JL, Hsueh W, Horton R. Therapeutic effect of calcium channel blockade in primary aldosteronism. J Clin Endocrinol Metab 1985;60:896.
297. Alder GK, Williams GH. Primary aldosteronism. In: Krieger DT, Bardin CW, eds. Current therapy in endocrinology and metabolism. Toronto: BC Decker, 1985:116–121.
298. Banks WA, Kastin AJ, Biglieri EG, Ruiz AE. Primary adrenal hyperplasia: A new subset of primary hyperaldosteronism. J Clin Endocrinol Metab 1984;58:783.
299. Biglieri EG, Schambelan M, Slaton PE, et al. The intercurrent hypertension of primary aldosteronism. Circ Res 1970;26:1.
300. Cohn K, Gottesman L, Brennan M. Adrenocortical carcinoma. Surgery 1986;100: 1170.
301. Arteaga E, Biglieri EG, Kater C, et al. Aldosterone-producing adrenocortical carcinoma, preoperative recognition and course in three cases. Ann Intern Med 1984;101:316.

302. Glazer HS, Weyman PJ, Sagel SS, et al. Nonfunctioning adrenal masses: Incidental discovery on computed tomography. AJR 1982;139:81.
303. Prinz RA, Brooks MH, Churchill R, et al. Incidental asymptomatic adrenal masses detected by computed tomographic scanning: Is operation required? JAMA 1982;248: 701.
304. Copeland PM. The incidentally discovered adrenal mass, diagnosis and treatment. Ann Intern Med 1983;98:940.
305. McCorkell SJ, Miles NL. Fine-needle aspiration of catecholamine-producing adrenal masses: A possibly fatal mistake. AJR 1985;145:113.
306. Hogan TF, Gilchrist KW, Westring DW, Citrin DL. A clinical and pathological study of adrenocortical carcinoma. Cancer 1980;45:2880.
307. Didolkar MS, Bescher RA, Elias EG, Moore RH. Natural history of adrenal cortical carcinoma: A clinicopathologic study of 42 patients. Cancer 1981;47:2153.
308. Bertagna C, Orth DN. Clinical and laboratory findings and results of therapy in 58 patients with adrenocortical tumors admitted to a single medical center 1951 to 1978;. Am J Med 1981;71:855.
309. Ross NS, Aron DC. Hormonal evaluation of the patient with an incidentally discovered adrenal mass. N Engl J Med 1990;323:1401.
310. Gabrilove JL, Seman AT, Sabet R, et al. Virilizing adrenal adenoma with studies on the steroid content of the adrenal venous effluent and a review of the literature. Endocr Rev 1981;2:462.
311. Tang CK, Gray GF. Adrenocortical neoplasms: Prognosis and morphology. Urology 1975;5:691.
312. Sullivan M, Boileau M, Hodges CV. Adrenal cortical carcinoma. J Urol 1978;120: 660.
313. Bradley EL. Primary and adjunctive therapy in carcinoma of the adrenal cortex. Surg Gynecol Obstet 1975;141:507.
314. Hussain S, Belldegrun A, Seltzer SE, et al. Differentiation of malignant from benign adrenal masses: Predictive indices on computed tomography. AJR 1985;144:61.
315. Reinig JW, Doppman JL, Dwyer AJ, et al. Distinction between adrenal adenomas and metastases using MR imaging. J Comput Assist Tomogr 1985;9:898.
316. Fink IJ, Reinig JW, Dwyer AJ, et al. MR imaging of pheochromocytomas. J Comput Assist Tomogr 1985;9:454.
317. Reinig JW, Doppman JL, Dwyer AJ, Frank J. MRI of indeterminate adrenal masses. AJR 1986;147:493.
318. Reinig JW, Doppman JL. Magnetic resonance imaging of the adrenal. Radiologe 1986;26:186.
319. Casola G, Nicolet V, Van Sonnenberg E, et al. Unsuspected pheochromocytomas: Risk of blood pressure alterations during percutaneous adrenal biopsy. Radiology 1986;159:733.
320. Katz RL, Shirkhoda A. Diagnostic approach to incidental adrenal nodules in the cancer patient. Cancer 1985;55:1995.
321. Gabrilove JL, Frieberg EK, Nicolis GL. Peripheral blood steroid levels in Cushing's syndrome due to adrenocortical carcinoma or adenoma. Urology 1983;22:576.
322. Baker ME, Spritzer C, Blinder R, et al. Benign adrenal lesions mimicking malignancy on MR imaging: Report of two cases. Radiology 1987;163:669.
323. Doherty GM, Nieman LK, Cutler GB Jr, Chrousos GP, Norton JA. Time to recovery of the hypothalamic-pituitary-adrenal axis after curative resection of adrenal tumors in patients with Cushing's syndrome. Surgery 1990;108:1085.
324. Jones GS, Shah KJ, Mann JR. Adreno-cortical carcinoma in infancy and childhood: A radiological report of ten cases. Clin Radiol 1985;36:257.
325. Daneman A, Chan HSL, Martin J. Adrenal carcinoma and adenoma in children: A review of 17 patients. Pediatr Radiol 1983;13:11.
326. Neblett W, Frexes-Steed M, Scott HW. Experience with adrenocortical neoplasia in childhood. Am J Surg 1987;53:117.
327. Ribeiro RC, Sandrini NR, Schell MJ, Lacerda L, Sambaio GA, Cat I. Adrenocortical carcinoma in children: A study of 40 cases. J Clin Oncol 1990;8:67.
328. Chudler RM, Kay R. Adrenocortical carcinoma in children. Urol Clin North Am 1989;16:469.
329. Henley DJ, van Heerden JA, Grant CS, Carney JA, Carpenter PC. Adrenal cortical carcinoma—A continuing challenge. Surgery 1983;94:226.
330. Luton JP, Cerdas S, Billaud L, et al. Clinical features of adrenocortical carcinoma, prognostic factors and the effect of mitotane therapy. N Engl J Med 1990;322:1195.
331. Hajjar RA, Hickey RC, Samaan NA. Adrenal cortical carcinoma: A study of 32 patients. Cancer 1975;35:549.
332. Appelqvist P, Kostiainen S. Multiple thoracotomy combined with chemotherapy in metastatic adrenal cortical carcinoma: A case report and review of the literature. J Surg Oncol 1983;24:1.
333. Potter DA, Strott CA, Javadpour N, Roth JA. Prolonged survival following six pulmonary resections for metastatic adrenal cortical carcinoma: A case report. J Surg Oncol 1984;25:273.
334. Percarpio B, Knowlton AH. Radiation therapy of adrenal cortical carcinoma. Acta Rad Ther Phys Biol 1976;15:288.
335. Jensen JC, Pass HI, Sindelar WF, Norton JA. Recurrent or metastatic disease in select patients with adrenocortical carcinoma. Arch Surg 1991;126:457.
336. Gutierrez ML, Crooke ST. Mitotane (o,p-DDD). Cancer Treat Rev 1980;7:49.
337. Haak HR, Caekibcke-Peerlinck KMH, Van Seters AP, Briet E. Prolonged bleeding time due to mitotane therapy. Eur J Cancer 1991;27:638.
338. Fukushima DK, Bradlow HL, Hellman L. Effects of o, p-DDD on cortisol and 66-B-hydroxycortisol secretion and metabolism in man. J Clin Endocrinol Metab 1971;32: 192.
339. Hellman L, Bradlow HL, Zumoff B. Decreased conversion of androgens to normal 17-ketosteroid metabolites as a result of treatment with o,p-DDD. J Clin Endocrinol Metab 1973;366:801.
340. Van Slooten H, Moolenaar AJ, Van Seters AP, Smeek D. The treatment of adrenocortical carcinoma with o,p-DDD: Prognostic implications of serum levels monitoring. Eur J Clin Oncol 1984;20:47.
341. Jarabak J, Rice K. Metastatic adrenal cortical carcinoma, prolonged regression with mitotane therapy. JAMA 1981;246:1706.
342. Thompson NW. Adrenocortical carcinoma. In: Thompson NW, Vinik AI, eds. Endocrine surgery update. New York: Grune & Stratton, 1983:119–128.
343. Bodie B, Novick AC, Pontes JE, Straffon RA, et al. The Cleveland Clinic experience with adrenal cortical carcinoma. J Urol 1989;141:257.
344. Venkatesh S, Hickey RC, Sellin RV, Fernandez JF, Samoan NA. Adrenal cortical carcinoma. Cancer 1989;64:765.
345. Decker RA, Elson P, Hogan TF, et al. Eastern Cooperative Oncology Group Study 1989: Mitotane and adriamycin in patients with advanced adrenocortical carcinoma. Surgery 1991;110:1006.
346. Haak HR, Van Seters AP, Moolenaar AJ. Mitotane therapy of adrenocortical carcinoma. N Engl J Med 1990;322:758.
347. Bates SE, Shieh CY, Mickley LA, Dichek HL, Gazdar A, Loriaux DL, Fojo AT. Mitotane enhances cytotoxicity of chemotherapy in cell lines expressing a multidrug resistance gene (mdr-1/P-glycoprotein) which is also expressed by adrenocortical carcinomas. J Clin Endocrinol Metab 1991;73:18.
348. Van Slooten H, van Oosterom AT. CAP (cyclophosphamide, doxorubicin and cisplatin) regimen in adrenal cortical carcinoma. Cancer Treat Rep 1983;67:377.
349. Hag MM, Legha SS, Samaan NA, et al. Cytotoxic chemotherapy in adrenal cortical carcinoma. Cancer Treat Rep 1980;64:909.
350. Johnson DH, Creco A. Treatment of metastatic adrenal cortical carcinoma with cisplatin and etoposide (VP-16). Cancer 1986;58:2198.
351. Hesketh PJ, McCaffrey RP, Finkel HE, et al. Cisplatin-based treatment of adrenocortical carcinoma. Cancer Treat Rep 1987;71:222.
352. Schlumberger M, Brugieres L, Gicquel C, Travagli JP, Droz JP, Parmentier C. 5-fluorouracil, doxorubicin, and cisplatin as treatment for adrenal cortical carcinoma. Cancer 1991;67:2997.
353. Schlumberger M, Ostronoff M, Bellaiche M, Rougier P, Driz JP, Parmentier C. 5-fluorouracil, doxorubicin and cisplatin regimen in adrenal cortical carcinoma. Cancer 1988;61:1492.
354. Stein CA, LaRocca RV, Thomas R, McAtee N, Myers CE. Suramin: An anticancer drug with a unique mechanism of action. J Clin Oncol 1989;7:499.
355. Allolio B, Reincke M, Arlt W, Deuss U, Winkelmann W, Siekmann L. Suramin for treatment of adrenocortical carcinoma. Lancet 1989;1:277.
356. LaRocca RV, Stein CA, Danesi R, Jamis Dow CA, Weiss GH, Myers CE. Suramin in adrenal cancer: Modulation of steroid hormone production, cytotoxicity in vitro and clinical antitumor effect. J Clin Endocrinol Metab 1990;71:497.
357. Stein CA, LaRocca R, Myers CE. A phase II trial of suramin in metastatic adrenocortical cancer, 1991 (personal communication).
358. Grondal S, Cedermark B, Eriksson B, Grimelius L, Harach R, Kristoffersson A, Rastad J, Uden P, Akerstrom G. Adrenocortical carcinoma. A retrospective study of a rare tumor with a poor prognosis. Eur J Surg Oncol 1990;16:500.
359. Wu YW, Chek CL, Knazck RA. An in vitro study of antitumor effects of gossypol in human SW-13 adrenocortical carcinoma. Cancer Res 1989;49:3754.
360. Sanfilippo JS, Wittliff JL. Steroid hormone receptors in adrenal cortical carcinoma. Am J Obstet Gynecol 1984;150:326.
361. Richie JP, Gittes RF. Carcinoma of the adrenal cortex. Cancer 1980;45:1957.
362. Brown WH. A case of pluriglandular syndrome. Lancet 1928;2:1022.
363. Christy NP. Adrenocorticotrophic activity in plasma of patients with Cushing's syndrome associated with pulmonary neoplasms. Lancet 1961;1:85.
364. Liddle GW, Island D, Meador CK. Normal and abnormal regulation of corticotropin secretion in man. Recent Prog Horm Res 1962;18:125.
365. Imura H. Ectopic hormone syndrome. Clin Endocrinol Metab 1980;9:235.
366. Davies CJ, Hoplin GF, Welbourn RB. Surgical management of the ectopic ACTH syndrome. Ann Surg 1982;196:246.
367. Jex RK, van Heerden JA, Carpenter PC, Grant CS. Ectopic ACTH syndrome. Am J Surg 1985;149:276.
368. Doppman JL, Loughlin T, Miller DL, et al. Identification of ACTH-producing intrathoracic tumors by measuring ACTH levels in aspirated specimens. Radiology 1987;163:501.
369. Pass HI, Doppman JL, Nieman L, et al. Management of the ectopic ACTH syndrome due to thoracic carcinoids. Ann Thorac Surg 1990;50:52.
370. Liddle GW, Nicholson WE, Island DP, et al. Clinical and laboratory studies of ectopic humoral syndromes. Recent Prog Horm Res 1969;25:283.
371. Misbin RI, Canary J, Williard D. Aminoglutethimide in the treatment of Cushing's syndrome. J Clin Pharmacol 1976;16:645.
372. Beard CM, Sheps SG, Kurland L. T, et al. Occurrence of pheochromocytoma in Rochester, Minnesota, 1950 through 1979. Mayo Clin Proc 1983;58:802.
373. Cryer PE. Phaeochromocytoma. Clin Endocrinol Metab 1985;14:203.
374. Beierwaltes WH, Sisson JC, Shapiro B, et al. Malignant potential of pheochromocytoma. Proc Am Assoc Cancer Res 1986;27:617.
375. Melicow MM. One hundred cases of pheochromocytoma (107 tumors) at the Columbia Presbyterian Medical Center, 1926–1976. Cancer 1977;40:1987.
376. Irvin GL, Fishman LM, Sher JA. Familial pheochromocytoma. Surgery 1983;94:938.
377. Glowniak JV, Shapiro B, Sisson JC, et al. Familial extra-adrenal pheochromocytoma. Arch Intern Med 1985;145:257.
378. Loughlin KR, Gittes RF. Urological management of patients with von Hippel-Lindau's disease. J Urol 1986;136:789.
379. Nakagawara A. Malignant pheochromocytoma with ganglioneuroblastomatous elements in a patient with von Ricklinghausen's disease. Cancer 1985;55:2794.

380. Berelowitz M, Szabo M, Barowsky HW, et al. Somatostatin-like immunoactivity and biological activity is present in human pheochromocytoma. J Clin Endocrinol Metab 1983;56:134.
381. Weinstein RS, Ide LF. Immunoreactive calcitonin in pheochromocytomas. Proc Soc Exp Biol Med 1980;165:215.
382. Ang VTY, Jenkins JS. Neurohypophysical hormones in the adrenal medulla. J Clin Endocrinol Metab 1984;58:688.
383. Cooper MJ, Helman LJ, Israel MA. Molecular biology and the pathogenesis of neuroblastoma and pheochromocytoma. Cancer Cells 1989;7:95.
384. Moley JF, Brother MB, Wells SA, Spengler BA, Bredler JL, Brodeur GM. Low frequency of ras gene mutations in neuroblastomas, pheochromocytomas and medullary thyroid cancers. Cancer Res 1991;51:1596.
385. Khosia S, Patel VM, Hay ID, Schaid DJ, Grant CS, van Heerden JA, Thibodeau SN. Loss of heterozygosity suggests multiple genetic alterations in pheochromocytomas and medullary thyroid carcinomas. J Clin Invest 1991;87:1691.
386. Orringer MB, Sisson JC, Glazer G, et al. Surgical treatment of cardiac pheochromocytomas. J Thorac Cardiovasc Surg 1985;89:753.
387. Lips KJM, Veer JVDS, Struyvenberg A, et al. Bilateral occurrence of pheochromocytoma in patients with multiple endocrine neoplasia syndrome type 2a (Sipple's syndrome). Am J Med 1981;70:1051.
388. Remine WH, Chang GC, van Heerden JA, et al. Current management of pheochromocytoma. Ann Surg 1974;179:740.
389. Sutton MGS, Sheps SG, Lie JT. Prevalence of clinically unsuspected pheochromocytoma: Review of a 50 year autopsy series. Mayo Clin Proc 1981;56:354.
390. Shin WY, Groman CS, Berkman JI. Pheochromocytoma with angiomatous features. Cancer 1977;40:275.
391. Scott HW, Halter SA. Oncologic aspects of pheochromocytoma: The importance of follow-up. Surgery 1984;96:1061.
392. Sherwin RP. Present status of the pathology of the adrenal gland in hypertension. Am J Surg 1964;107:136.
393. Lewis PD. A cytophotometric study of benign and malignant pheochromocytomas. Virchows Arch 1971;9:371.
394. Hosaka Y, Rainwater LM, Grant CS, et al. Pheochromocytoma: Nuclear deoxyribonucleic acid patterns studied by flow cytometry. Surgery 1986;100:1003.
395. Sheps SG, Jiang NS, Klec GG, van Heerden JA. Recent developments in the diagnosis and management of pheochromocytoma. Mayo Clin Proc 1990;65:88.
396. Helman LJ, Cohen PS, Averbuch SD, Cooper MJ, Keiser HR, Israel MA. Neuropeptide y expression distinguishes malignant from benign pheochromocytoma. J Clin Oncol 1989;7:1720.
397. Grouzmann E, Gicquel C, Pluin PF, Schlumberger M, Conroy E, Bohuon C. Neuropeptide Y and neuron specific enolase levels in benign and malignant pheochromocytomas. Cancer 1990;66:1833.
398. Medeiros LJ, Wolf BC, Balogh K, Federman M. Adrenal pheochromocytoma: A clinicopathologic review of 60 cases. Hum Pathol 1985;16:580.
399. Manger WM, Gifford RW. Pheochromocytoma. New York: Springer-Verlag, 1977.
400. Hengstmann JH. Evaluation of screening tests for pheochromocytoma. Cardiology 1985;72:153.
401. Kremer R, Crawhall JC, Kolanitch R. Rapid and reliable estimation of urinary free catecholamines in patients with pheochromocytomas. J Chromatogr 1985;344:313.
402. Hanson MW, Feldman JM, Beam CA, Leight GS, Coleman E. Iodine ^{131}-labelled metaiodobenzylguanidine scintigraphy and biochemical analyses in suspected pheochromocytoma. Arch Intern Med 1991;151:1397.
403. Samaan NA, Hickey RC, Shutts PE. Diagnosis, localization and management of pheochromocytoma. Cancer 1988;62:2451.
404. Duncan MW, Compton P, Lazarus L, Smythe GA. Measurement of norepinephrine and 3,4-dihydroxyphenylglycol in urine and plasma for the diagnosis of pheochromocytoma. N Engl J Med 1988;319:136.
405. Cryer PE, Wortsman J, Shah SD, Nowak RM, Deftos LJ. Plasma chromogranin A as a marker of sympathochromaffin activity in humans. Am J Physiol 1991;260:E243.
406. Karlberg BE, Hedman L. Value of the clonidine suppression test in the diagnosis of pheochromocytoma. Acta Med Scand 1986;714:15.
407. Gifford RW, Bravo EL, Manger WM. Diagnosis and management of pheochromocytoma. Cardiology 1985;72:186.
408. Brandstetter K, Krause U, Beyer W. Preliminary results with the clonidine suppression test in the diagnosis of pheochromocytoma. Cardiology 1985;72:157.
409. Karlberg BE, Hedman L, Lennquist S, Pollace T. The value of the clonidine-suppression test in the diagnosis of pheochromocytoma. World J Surg 1986;10:753.
410. MacDougall IC, Isles CG, Stewart H, et al. Overnight clonidine suppression test in the diagnosis and exclusion of pheochromocytoma. Am J Med 1988;84:993.
411. Taylor HC, Mayes D, Anton AH. Clonidine suppression test for pheochromocytoma: Examples of misleading results. J Clin Endocrinol Metab 1986;63:238.
412. Bravo EL, Tarazi RC, Fouad FM, et al. Clonidine suppression test: A useful aid in the diagnosis of pheochromocytoma. N Engl J Med 1981;305:623.
413. Dunnick NR, Doppman JL, Gill JR, et al. Localization of functional adrenal tumors by computed tomography and venous sampling. Radiology 1982;142:429.
414. Welch TJ, Sheedy PF, van Heerden JA, et al. Pheochromocytoma: Value of computed tomography. Radiology 1983;148:501.
415. Radin DR, Ralls PW, Boswell WD, et al. Pheochromocytoma: Detection by unenhanced CT. AJR 1986;146:741.
416. Greenberg M, Moawad AH, Wieties BM, et al. Extraadrenal pheochromocytoma: Detection during pregnancy using MR imaging. Radiology 1986;161:475.
417. Velchik MG, Alavi A, Kressel HY, Engelman K. Localization of pheochromocytoma: MIBG, CT and MRI correlation. J Nucl Med 1989;30:328.
418. Fisher MR, Higgins CB, Andereck W. MR imaging of an intrapericardial pheochromocytoma. J Comput Assist Tomogr 1985;9:1103.
419. Shapiro B, Copp JE, Sisson JC, et al. Iodine-131 metaiodobenzylguanidine for the locating of suspected pheochromocytoma: Experience in 400 cases. J Nucl Med 1985;26:576.
420. Swenson SJ, Brown MJ, Sheps SG, et al. Use of ^{131}I-MIBG scintigraphy in the evaluation of suspected pheochromocytoma. Mayo Clin Proc 1985;60:299.
421. Koizumi M, Endo K, Sakahara H, et al. Computed tomography and ^{131}I-MIBG scintigraphy in the diagnosis of pheochromocytoma. Acta Radiologica Diagn 1986;27: 305.
422. Fischer M, Galanski M, Winterberg B, Vetter H. Localization procedures in pheochromocytoma and neuroblastoma. Cardiology 1985;72:143.
423. Shulkin B. L, Shen SW, Sisson JC, Shapiro B. Iodine 131 MIBG scintigraphy of the extremities in metastatic pheochromocytoma and neuroblastoma. J Nucl Med 1987;28: 315.
424. Lynn MD, Braunstein EM, Wohl RL, et al. Bone metastases in pheochromocytoma: Comparative studies of efficacy of imaging. Radiology 1986;160:701.
425. Lynn MD, Shapiro B, Sisson JC, et al. Pheochromocytoma and the normal adrenal medulla: Improved visualization with I-123 MIBG scintigraphy. Radiology 1985;156: 851.
426. Cheung PSY, Thompson NW, Dmuchowski CF, Sisson JC. Spectrum of pheochromocytoma in the ^{131}I-MIBG era. World J Surg 1988;12:546.
427. Gouch IR, Thompson NW, Shapiro B, Sisson JC. Limitations of ^{131}I-MIBG scintigraphy in locating pheochromocytomas. Surgery 1985;98:115.
428. Stenstrom G, Kutti J. The blood volume in pheochromocytoma patients before and during treatment with phenoxybenzamine. Acta Med Scand 1985;218:381.
429. Stenstrom G, Haljamae H, Tisell LE. Influence of pre-operative treatment with phenoxybenzamine on the incidence of adverse cardiovascular reactions during anaesthesia and surgery for phaeochromocytoma. Acta Anaesthesiol Scand 1985;29:797.
430. Bornemann M, Hill SC, Kidd GS. Lactic acidosis in pheochromocytoma. Ann Intern Med 1986;105:880.
431. Perry RR, Keiser HR, Norton JA, et al, Surgical management of pheochromocytoma with the use of metyrosine. Ann Surg 1990;212:621.
432. Imperato-McGinley J, Gautier T, Ehlers K, et al. Reversibility of catecholamine-induced dilated cardiomyopathy in a child with a pheochromocytoma. N Engl J Med 1987;316:793.
433. Chimori K, Miyazaki S, Nakajima T, Muira D. Preoperative management of pheochromocytoma with the calcium-antagonist nifedipine. Clin Ther 1985;7:372.
434. Proye C, Thevenin D, Cecat P, et al. Exclusive use of calcium channel blockers in preoperative and intraoperative control of pheochromocytomas: Hemodynamics and free catecholamine assays in ten consecutive patients. Surgery 1989;106:1149.
435. Irvin GL, Fishman LM, Sher JA, Yeung LK, Irane H. Pheochromocytoma lateral vs anterior operative approach. Ann Surg 1989;209:774.
436. Zimmerman ID, Biron RE, MacMahon HE. Pheochromocytoma of the urinary bladder. N Engl J Med 1953;249:25.
437. Carney JA, Sizemore GW, Sheps SG. Adrenal medullary disease in multiple endocrine neoplasia, type 2. Am J Clin Pathol 1976;66:279.
438. Brennan MF, Keiser HR. Persistent and recurrent pheochromocytoma: The role of surgery. World J Surg 1982;6:397.
439. Van Heerden JA, Sheps SG, Hamberger B, et al. Pheochromocytoma: Current status and changing trends. Surgery 1982;91:367.
440. James RE, Baker HL, Scanlon PW. The roentgenological aspects of metastatic pheochromocytoma. AJR 1972;115:783.
441. Lewi HJE, Reid R, Mucci B, et al. Malignant phaeochromocytoma. Br J Urol 1985;57: 394.
442. Guo JZ, Gong LS, Chen SX, Luo BY, Xu MY. Malignant pheochromocytoma: Diagnosis and treatment in fifteen cases. J Hypertens 1989;7:261.
443. Scott WH, Reynolds V, Green N, et al. Clinical experience with malignant pheochromocytoma. Surg Gynecol Obstet 1982;154:801.
444. Broder LE, Carter SK. Pancreatic islet cell carcinoma II Results of therapy with streptozotocin in 52 patients. Ann Intern Med 1973;79:108.
445. Feldman JM. Treatment of metastatic pheochromocytoma with streptozotocin. Arch Intern Med 1983;143:1799.
446. Feldman JM. In reply to a letter to the editor by Gross DJ, Schlank E, Ipp E. Arch Intern Med 1985;145:368.
447. Gross DJ, Schlank E, Ipp E. Streptozotocin therapy for malignant pheochromocytoma. Arch Intern Med [Letter] 1985;145:368.
448. McEwan A, Shapiro B, Sisson JC, et al. Radio-iodobenzylguanidine for the scintigraphic location and therapy of adrenergic tumors. Semin Nucl Med 1985;15:132.
449. Krempf M, Lumbroso J, Mornex R, et al. Use of ^{131}Im iodobenzylguanidine in the treatment of malignant pheochromocytoma. J Clin Endocrinol Metab 1991;72:455.
450. Feldman JM, Frankel N, Coleman RE. Platelet uptake of the pheochromocytoma-scanning agent ^{131}I-meta-iodobenzylguanidine. Metabolism 1984;33:397.
451. Vetter H, Fischer M, Muller-Rensing R, et al. [^{131}I]-meta-iodobenzylguanidine in treatment of malignant pheochromocytomas. Lancet 1983;2(8341):107.
452. Keiser H. R, Goldstein DS, Wade JL, et al. Treatment of malignant pheochromocytoma with combination chemotherapy. Hypertension 1985;7:1-18.
453. Manger TJ, Tobes MC, Wieland DW, et al. Metabolism of Iodine-131 metaiodobenzylguanidine in patients with metastatic pheochromocytoma. J Nucl Med 1986;27:37.
454. Goldstein DS, Stull R, Eisenhofer G, et al. Plasma 3,4-dihydroxyphenylalanine (Dopa) and catecholamines in neuroblastoma or pheochromocytoma. Ann Intern Med 1986;105:887.
455. Averbuch S, Steakley C, Gelmann E, et al. Malignant pheochromocytoma: Treatment

with a combination of cyclophosphamide, vincristine and darcarbazine. Proc American Society of Clinical Oncology 1987;6:241.

456. Averbuch SD, Steakley CS, Young RC, et al. Malignant pheochromocytoma: Effective treatment with a combination of cyclophosphamide, vincristine and dacarbazine. Ann Intern Med 1988;109:267.
457. Finklestein JZ, Klemperer MR, Evans A, et al. Multiagent chemotherapy for children with metaststic neuroblastoma: A report from children's cancer study group. Med Pediatr Oncol 1979;6:179.
458. Taub MA, Osburne RC, Georges LP, Sode J. Malignant pheochromocytoma: Severe clinical exacerbation and release of stored catecholamines during lymphoma chemotherapy. Cancer 1982;50:1739.
459. Masson P. Carcinoid (argentaffin-cell tumours) and nerve hyperplasia of appendicular mucosa. Am J Pathol 1982;4:181.
460. Kultschitzky N. Zur frage ueber den bau des darmkanals. Arch Mikrosk Anat 1987;49:7.
461. Bolande RP. The neurocrestopathies: A unifying concept of disease arising from neural crest maldevelopment. Hum Pathol 1974;5:409.
462. Pearse HGE. The APUD concept and hormone production. Clin Endocrinol Metab 1980;9:211.
463. Moertel CG. An odyssey in the land of small tumors. J Clin Oncol 1987;5:1502.
464. Kloppel G, Heitz PU. Pancreatic endocrine tumors. Pathol Res Pract 1988;183:155.
465. Black WC III. Enterochromaffin cell types and corresponding carcinoid tumors. Lab Invest 1968;19:473.
466. Carney JA, Go VLW, Fairbanks JF, Moore SB, Alport EC, Nora EE. The syndrome of gastric argyrophil carcinoid tumors and nonantral gastric atrophy. Ann Intern Med 1983;99:761.
467. Feldman JM, O'Dorisio TM. The role of neuropeptides and serotonin in the diagnosis of carcinoid tumors. Am J Med 1986;81:41.
468. Pearse AGE, Tabor TT. Embryology of the diffuse neuroendocrine system and its relationship to the common peptides. Fed Proc 1979;38:2288.
469. Wilander E, Scheibenpflug L, Eriksson B, Oberg K. Diagnostic criteria of classical carcinoids. Acta Oncol 1991;30:469.
470. Eriksson B, Oberg K. Peptide hormones as tumor markers in neuroendocrine gastrointestinal tumors. Acta Oncol 1991;30:477.
471. Eriksson B, Arnberg H, Oberg K, et al. Chromogranins: A new sensitive marker for neuroendocrine tumors. Acta Oncol 1989;28:325.
472. Wilander E. Diagnostic pathology of gastrointestinal and pancreatic neuroendocrine tumors. Acta Oncol 1989;28:363.
473. Soga J, Tazawa K. Pathologic analysis of carcinoids. Histologic reevaluation of 62 cases. Cancer 1971;28:990.
474. Nash SV, Said JW. Gastroenteropancreatic neuroendocrine tumors. A histochemical and immunohistochemical study of epithelial (keratin proteins, carcinoembryonic antigen) and neuroendocrine (neuron-specific enolase, bombesin and chromogranin) markers in foregut, midgut and hindgut tumors. J Clin Pathol 1986;86:415.
475. Moll R, Franke WW. Cytoskeletal differences between human neuroendocrine tumors: A cytoskeletal protein of molecular weight 46,000 distinguishes cutaneous from pulmonary neuroendocrine neoplasms. Differentiation 1985;30:165.
476. Pinkus GS, Etheridge CL, O'Connor EM. Are keratin proteins a better tumor marker than epithelial membrane antigen? A comparative immunohistochemical study of various paraffin-embedded neoplasms using monoclonal and polyclonal antibodies. Am J Clin Pathol 1986;85:269.
477. Marangos PJ, Polak JM, Pearse AGE. Neuron-specific enolase. A prove for neurons and neuroendocrine cells. TINS 1982;5:193.
478. Wiedenmann B, Franke WW, Kuhn C, Moll R, Gould VE. Synaptophysin: A marker protein for neuroendocrine cells and neoplasms. Proc Natl Acad Sci USA 1986;83: 3500.
479. Vyberg M, Horn T, Francis D, Askaa J. Immunohistochemical identification of neuron-specific enolase, synaptophysin, chromogranin and endocrine granule constituent in neuroendocrine tumors. Acta Histochem 1990;38:S179.
480. Wilander E, Lundquist M, El-Salhy M. Serotonin in foregut carcinoids: A survey of 60 cases with regard to silver stains, formalin-induced fluorescence and serotonin immunocytochemistry. J Pathol 1985;145:251.
481. Williams ED, Sanders M. The classification of carcinoid tumors. Lancet 1963;1:238.
482. Godwin JD. Carcinoid tumors: An analysis of 2837 cases. Cancer 1975;36:560.
483. Vinik AI, McLeod MK, Fig LM, Shapiro B, Lloyd RV, Cho K. Clinical features, diagnosis, and localization of carcinoid tumors and their management. Gastroenterol Clin North Am 1989;18:865.
484. Feldman JM. Carcinoid tumors and the carcinoid syndrome. Curr Probl Surg 1989;26: 835.
485. Watson RGP, Johnston CF, et al. The frequency of gastrointestinal endocrine tumors in a well-defined population: Northern Ireland 1970–1985. Q J Med 1989;72:647.
486. Norheim I, Oberg K, Theodorsson-Norheim E, et al. Malignant carcinoid tumors. Ann Surg 1987;206:115.
487. Eriksson B. Recent advances in the diagnosis and management of endocrine pancreatic tumors. Acta Universitatis Upsaliensis 1988:160:28.
488. Eriksson B, Oberg K, Skogseid B. Neuroendocrine pancreatic tumors. Acta Oncol 1989;28:373.
489. Oberg K, Eriksson B. Medical treatment of neuroendocrine gut and pancreatic tumors. Acta Oncol 1989;28:425.
490. Weiss NS, Yang CP. Incidence of histologic types of cancer of the small intestine. JNCI 1987;78:653.
491. Berge T, Linell F. Carcinoid tumors. Acta Pathol Microbiol Immunol Scand 1976;84: 322.
492. Moertel CG, Dockerty MB, Judd ES. Carcinoid tumors of the vermiform appendix. Cancer 1968;21:270.
493. Thompson GB, van Heerden JA, Martin JK, et al. Carcinoid tumors of the gastrointestinal tract: Presentation, management and prognosis. Surgery 1985;98:1054.
494. Moertel CG, Suer WG, Doherty MG, et al. Life history of the carcinoid tumor of the small intestine. Cancer 1961;14:901.
495. Burke AO, Sobin LH, Federspiel BH, Shekitka KM, Helwig EB. Carcinoid tumors of the duodenum. Arch Pathol Lab Med 1990;114:700.
496. Federspiel BH, Burke AP, Sokin LH, Shekitka KM. Rectal and colonic carcinoids. Cancer 1990;65:135.
497. Bronchial adenomas. Br Med J [Editorial] 1981;282:252.
498. Hasleton PS, Gomm S, Blair V, Thatcher N. Pulmonary carcinoid tumours: A clinicopathological study of 35 cases. Br J Cancer 1986;54:963.
499. Solcia E, Capella C, Fiocca R, Cornaggia M, Bosi F. The gastroenteropancreatic endocrine system and related tumors. Gastroenterol Clin North Am 1989;18:671.
500. Davies MG, O'Dowd GO, McEntree GP, Hennessey TPJ. Primary gastric carcinoid tumors: A view on management. Br J Surg 1990;77:1013.
501. Hasdu SI, Winawer SJ, Myer WP. Surgical management of carcinoid tumors of the gastrointestinal tract. Ann Surg 1980;41:429.
502. Sanders RJ. Carcinoids of the gastrointestinal tract. Springfield, IL: Charles L. Thomas, 1973.
503. Jensen RT, Gardner JD. Gastrinoma. In: Go VLW, Brooks FA, DiMagno EP, Gardner JD, Lebenthal E, Scheele GA, eds. The exocrine pancreas: Biology, pathobiology and disease. New York: Raven Press, 1992 (in press).
504. Solcia E, Capella C, Sessa F, et al. Gastric carcinoids and related endocrine growths. Digestion 1986;35:3.
505. Ekman L, Hansson E, Havu N, et al. Toxicological studies on omeprazole. Scand J Gastroenterol 1985;20:53.
506. Moertel CG, Hanley JA. Combination chemotherapy trials in metastatic carcinoid and malignant carcinoid syndrome. Cancer Clin Trials 1979;2:327.
507. Johnson LA, Lavin PT, Moertel CG, et al. Carcinoids: The prognostic effect of primary site histologic type variations. J Surg Oncol 1986;33:81.
508. Penston J, Wormsley KG. Achlorhydria-hypergastrinaemia: Carcinoids—a flawed hypothesis. Gut 1987;28:488.
509. Borch K, Renvall H, Liedberg G. Gastric endocrine cell hyperplasia and carcinoid tumors in pernicious anemia. Gastroenterology 1985;88:638.
510. Solcia E, Capella C, Buffa R, et al. Endocrine cells of the gastrointestinal tract and related tumors. Pathol Annu 1979;9:163.
511. Mattson H, Havu N, Brautigam J, Carlsson K, Lundell L, Carlsson E. Partial fundectomy results in hypergastrinemia and development of gastric enterochromaffin-like cell carcinoids in rats. Gastroenterology 1991;100:311.
512. Krets DJ, Guerra JJ, Saltz M, et al. Gastrointestinal hemorrhage due to carcinoid tumors of the small intestine. JAMA 1986;255:234.
513. Eberle F, Grun R. Multiple endocrine neoplasia type I. Adv Intern Med Pediatr 1981;5:76.
514. Ballard HS, Frame B, Hartsock RT. Familial multiple endocrine adenoma: Peptic ulcer complex. Medicine 1964;43:481.
515. Creutzfeldt W. The achlorhydria—carcinoid sequence: Role of gastrin. Digestion 1988;39:61.
516. Wilander E. Achylia and the development of gastric carcinoids. Virchows Arch Anat Pathol 1981;394:151.
517. Hodges JR, Isaacson P, Wright R. Diffuse enterochromaffin-like (ECL) cell hyperplasia and multiple gastric carcinoids: A complication of pernicious anemia. Gut 1981;22: 237.
518. Johnson L, Weaver M. Von Recklinghausen's disease and gastrointestinal carcinoids. JAMA 1981;245:2496.
519. Wheeler MH, Curley IR, Williams ED. The association of neurofibrometasis, pheochromocytoma, and somatostatin rich duodenal carcinoid tumor. Surgery 1986;100: 1163.
520. Jensen RT, Norton JA. Pancreatic endocrine tumors. In: Fordtran JS, Sleisinger MH, Feldman M, Scharschmidt B, eds. Gastrointestinal diseases: Pathophysiology, diagnosis and management. Philadelphia: WB Saunders, 1992 (in press).
521. Maton PN, Hodgson HJF. Carcinoid tumors and the carcinoid syndrome. In: Bouchier IAD, Allan RN, Hodgson HJF, Keighly MRB, eds. Textbook of gastroenterology. London: Bailliere-Tindall, 1984:620.
522. Falkner S, Martensson H, Nobin A, Sundler F. Peptide hormones in various types of gastro-entero-pancreatic tumors: immunohistochemical patterns and evolutionary background. In: Bresciani F, King RJB, Lippman ME, Namers M, Raynaud JP, eds. Progress in cancer research and therapy. New York: Raven Press, 1984:597.
523. Dayal Y. Endocrine cells in the gut and their neoplasms. In: Norris HT, ed. Contemporary issues in surgical pathology. New York: Churchill Livingstone, 1983:267.
524. Dayal Y, Wolfe HJ. Regulatory substances in clinically nonfunctioning gastrointestinal carcinoids. In: Falkmers W, Hakanson R, Sundler F, eds. Evolution and tumor pathology of the neuroendocrine system. Amsterdam: Elsevier Science Publishers, 1984:497.
525. Wilander E, Ed-Salhy M, Lundquist M. Argyrophilic reaction in rectal carcinoids. Path Microbiol Scand 1983;91:84.
526. Doppman JL, Nieman L, Miller DL, et al. Ectopic adreno-corticotropic hormone syndrome: Localization studies in 28 patients. Radiology 1989;172:115.
527. Leveston SA, McKeel DW Jr, Buckley PG, et al. Acromegaly and Cushing's syndrome associated with a foregut carcinoid. J Clin Endocrinol Met 1981;53:682.
528. Sano T, Asa SL, Kovacs K. Growth hormone releasing-producing tumors: Clinical, biochemical and morphological manifestations. Endocr Rev 1988;9:357.
529. Thorson A, Bjork G, Bjorkman G, Waldenstrom J. Malignant carcinoid of the small intestine with metastases to the liver, valvular disease of the right heart (pulmonary stenosis and tricuspid regurgitation without septal defect), peripheral vasomotor symptoms, bronchoconstriction and an unusual type of cyanosis. Am Heart J 1954;47: 795.

530. Pernow B, Waldenstrom J. Paroxysmal flushing and other symptoms caused by 5-hydroxytryptamine and histamine in patients with malignant tumors. Lancet 1954;2: 951.
531. Davis Z, Moertel CG, McIlrath DC. The malignant carcinoid syndrome. Surg Gynecol Obstet 1973;137:637.
532. Grahame-Smith DG. The carcinoid syndrome. London: William Heineman Medical Books, 1972.
533. Frolich JC, Bloomgarden ZT, Oates JA, et al. The carcinoid flush: Provocation by pentagastrin and inhibition by somatostatin. N Engl J Med 1978;19:1055.
534. Roberts LJ, Marney SR, Oates JA. Blockade of the flush associated with metastatic gastric carcinoid by combined H_1 and H_2 receptor antagonists: Evidence for an important role of H_2 receptors in human vasculature. N Engl J Med 1979;300:236.
535. Peart WS, Robertson JS, Andrews TM. Facial flushing produced in patients with carcinoid syndrome by intravenous adrenaline and noradrenaline. Lancet 1959;2: 715.
536. Adamson AR, Grahame-Smith DG, Peart WS, et al. Pharmacological blockade of carcinoid flushing provoked by catecholamines and alcohol. Lancet 1967;2:293.
537. Oates JA, Sjoerdsma A. A unique syndrome associated with secretion of 5-hydroxytryptophan by metastatic gastric carcinoids. Am J Med 1962;32:333.
538. Feldman JM. Carcinoid tumors and syndrome. Semin Oncol 1987;14:237.
539. Knowlessar OD, Law DH, Sleisenger MH. Malabsorption syndrome associated with carcinoid tumors. Am J Med 1959;27:673.
540. Thorson AH. Studies on carcinoid disease. Acta Med Scand 1958;334:81.
541. Roberts WC, Sjoerdsma A. The cardiac disease associated with carcinoid syndrome (carcinoid heart disease). Am J Med 1964;36:5.
542. Lundin L. Carcinoid heart disease. Acta Oncol 1991;30:499.
543. Schiller VL, Fishbein MC, Siegel RJ. Unusual cardiac involvement in carcinoid syndrome. Am Heart J 1986;112:1322.
544. Wong VW, Melman KL. Ophthalmic manifestations of the carcinoid flush. N Engl J Med 1967;277:406.
545. Waldenstrom J. Clinical picture of carcinoidosis. Gastroenterology 1958;35:565.
546. Feldman JM, Jones RS. Carcinoid syndrome from gastrointestinal carcinoids without liver metastases. Ann Surg 1982;196:33.
547. Ricci C, Patrassi N, Massa R, et al. Carcinoid syndrome in bronchial adenoma. Am J Surg 1973;126:671.
548. Moertel CG, Beahrs O, Woolmer LB, Tyce GM. Malignant carcinoid syndrome associated with noncarcinoid tumors. N Engl J Med 1965;273:244.
549. McCaughan BC, Martini H, Bains MS. Bronchial carcinoids: review of 124 cases. J Thorac Cardiovasc Surg 1985;89:8.
550. Cheek RC, Wilson H. Carcinoid tumors. Curr Probl Surg 1970;11:4.
551. Sjoerdsma A. Serotonin. N Engl J Med 1959;261:181.
552. Campbell ACP, Gowenlock AH, Platt DS, et al. A 5-hydroxytryptophan-secreting carcinoid tumor. Gut 1963;4:61.
553. Feldman JM. Serotonin metabolism in carcinoid tumors: Incidence of 5-hydroxytryptophan secreting tumors. Gastroenterology 1978;75:1109.
554. Grahame-Smith DG. Natural history and diagnosis of the carcinoid syndrome. Clin Gastroenterol 1974;3:575.
555. Ahlman H, Dahlstrom A, Gronstadt K, et al. The pentagastrin test in the diagnosis of carcinoid syndrome: Blockage of gastrointestinal symptoms by ketanserin. Ann Surg 1985;201:81.
556. Creutzfeldt W, Stockman F. The carcinoid syndrome. Am J Med 1987;82(Suppl 5B):4.
557. Vinik AI, Gonin J, England BG, Jackson T, McLeod MK, Cho K. Plasma substance-P in neuroendocrine tumors and idiopathic flushing: The value of pentagastrin stimulation tests and the effects of the somatostatin analog. J Clin Endocrinol Metab 1990;70:1702.
558. Oates JA, Melman K, Sjoerdsma M, Gillespie L, Mason DT. Release of a kinin peptide in the carcinoid syndrome. Lancet 1964;2:514.
559. Oates JA, Pettinger WA, Doctor RB. Evidence for the release of bradykinin in the carcinoid syndrome. J Clin Invest1966;45:173.
560. Melman K, Lovenberg W, Sjoerdsma A. Identification of lysylbradykinin as the peptide formed in vitro by carcinoid tumor kallikrein. Clin Chim Acta 1965;12:292.
561. Lucas KJ, Feldman JM. Flushing in the carcinoid syndrome and plasma kallikrein. Cancer 1986;58:2290.
562. Wilkin JK, Roundtree CB. Blockade of the carcinoid flush with cimetidine and clonidine. Arch Dermatol 1982;118:109.
563. Oates JA. The carcinoid syndrome. N Engl J Med 1986;315:702.
564. Sandler M, Karim SM, Williams ED. Prostaglandins in amine-peptide-secreting tumors. Lancet 1968;2:1053.
565. Smith AG, Greaves MW. Blood prostaglandin activity associated with noradrenaline-provoked flush in the carcinoid syndrome. Br J Dermatol 1974;90:547.
566. Jaffe BM, Landon C. Prostaglandin E and F in endocrine diarrheagenic syndromes. Ann Surg 1976;84:516.
567. Metz SA, McRae JR, Robertson PR. Prostaglandins as mediators of paraneoplastic syndromes: Review and update. Metabolism 1981;30:299.
568. Hakanson R, Bengmark S, Brondin E, et al. Substance P like immunoreactivity in intestinal carcinoid tumors. In: Van Euler US (Pernow B, ed). New York: Raven Press, 1977:55.
569. Theodorsson-Norheim E, Norheim I, Oberg K, et al. Neuropeptide K: A major tachykinin in plasma and tumor tissues from carcinoid patients. Biochem Biophys Res Comm 1985;131:77.
570. Conlon JM, Deacon CF, Richter G, Schmidt WE, Stockmann F, Creutzfeldt W. Measurement and partial characterization of the multiple forms of neurokinin A-like immunoreactivity in carcinoid tumors. Regul Pept 1985;131:77.
571. Emson PC, Gilbert RFT, Martensson H, Nobin A. Elevated concentrations of substance P and 5-HT in patients with carcinoid tumors. Cancer 1984;54:715.
572. Norheim I, Theodorsson-Norheim E, Brondin E, Oberg K. Tachykinins in carcinoid tumors: Their use as a tumor marker and possible role in carcinoid flush. J Clin Endocrinol Metab 1986;63:605.
573. Schaffalitsky de Muckadell OB, Aggestrup S, Stentoft P. Flushing and plasma substance P concentration during infusion of synthetic substance P in normal man. Scand J Gastroenterol 1986;21:498.
574. Hendrix TR, Arkinson M, Clifton JA, Ingelfinger FJ. The effect of 5-hydroxytryptamine on intestinal motor function in man. Am J Med 1957;23:886.
575. Feldman JM, Plank JW. Gastrointestinal and metabolic function in patients with the carcinoid syndrome. Am J Med Sci 1977;273:43.
576. Donowitz M, Binder JH. Jejunal fluid and electrolyte secretion in carcinoid syndrome. Am J Dig Dis 1975;20:1115.
577. Warner RRP. Carcinoid tumor. In: Berk JE, Haubrich WS, Kalser MH, Roth JLA, Schnaffner F, eds. Bockus: Gastroenterology. Philadelphia: WB Saunders, 1985:1074.
578. Moertel CG, Kvols LK, Rubin J. A study of cyproheptadine in the treatment of metastatic carcinoid tumor and the malignant carcinoid syndrome. Cancer 1991;67:33.
579. Herxheimer H. Influence of 5-hydroxytryptamine on bronchial function. J Physiol (Lond) 1953;122:49.
580. Lundin L, Norheim I, Landelius J, Oberg K, Theodorsson-Norheim E. Carcinoid heart disease: relationship of circulating vasoactive substances to ultrasound detectable cardiac abnormalities. Circulation 1988;77:264.
581. Feldman JM, Lee EM. Serotonin content of foods: Effect on urinary excretion of 5-hydroxyindoleacetic acid. Am J Clin Nutr 1985;42:639.
582. Feldman JM, Butler SS, Chapman BA. Interference with measurement of 3-methoxy-4-hydroxymandelic acid and 5-hydroxyindoleacetic acid by reducing metabolites. Clin Chem 1974;20:607.
583. Sjoerdsma A, Weissbach H, Udenfriend H. Simple test for diagnosis of metastatic carcinoid (argentaffinoma). JAMA 1955;159:397.
584. Feldman JM. Urinary serotonin in the diagnosis of carcinoid tumors. Clin Chem 1986;32:840.
585. Hussain MN, Sole MJ. A simple, specific radioenzymatic assay for picogram quantities of serotonin or acetylserotonin in biological fluids of tissues. Anal Biochem 1981;111: 105.
586. Feldman JM, Davis JA. Radioenzymatic assay of platelet serotonin, dopamine and norepinephrine in subjects with normal and increased serotonin production. Clin Chim Acta 1981;109:275.
587. Wilkin JK. Flushing reactions: Consequences and mechanisms. Ann Intern Med 1981;95:468.
588. Fukayama M, Hayashi Y, Shiozawa Y, Okabe S, Koike M. Human chorionic gonadotropin alpha subunit in rectal carcinoids. Am J Pathol 1989;135:1065.
589. Oberg K, Wide L. HLG and HCG subunits as tumor markers in patients with endocrine pancreatic tumors and carcinoid tumors. Acta Endocrinol 1981;98:256.
590. Feldman JM, Plonk JW. Carcinoembryonic antigen and carcinoid tumors. Ann Intern Med 1975;83:82.
591. Robertson JIS, Peart WS, Andrews TM. The mechanism of facial flushes in the carcinoid syndrome. Q J Med 1961;31:103.
592. Nessi R, Ricci D, Ricci SB, Bosco M, Blanc M. Bronchial carcinoid tumors: Radiologic observations in 49 cases. J Thorac Imaging 1991;6:47.
593. Jeffree MA, Barter SJ, Hemingway AP, Nolan DJ. Primary carcinoid tumors of the ileum: The radiological appearances. Clin Radiol 1985;35:451.
594. Banks NH, Goldstein MH, Dodd G. The roentgenologic spectrum of small intestinal carcinoid tumors. AJR 1975;123:274.
595. Goldstein HM, Miller M. Angiographic evaluation of carcinoid tumors in the small intestine: The value of epinephrine. Radiology 1975;115:23.
596. Sako M, Lunderquist A, Owman T, Martensson H, Norbin A. Angiographic and computed tomographic appearance of secondary carcinoid tumor of the liver. Cardiovasc Intervent Radiol 1982;5:90.
597. McCarthy SM, Stark DD, Moss AA, Goldberg HI. Computed tomography of malignant carcinoid disease. J Comput Assist Tomogr 1984;8:846.
598. Lackey BM, Fishman EK, Jones B, Siegelman SS. Computed tomography of abdominal carcinoid tumors. J Comput Assist Tomogr 1985;9:38.
599. Collatz L, Stage JG, Henriksen FW. Angiography in the diagnosis of carcinoid syndrome. Scand J Gastroenterol 1979;53:111.
600. Gould M, Johnson RJ. Computed tomography of abdominal carcinoid tumour. Br J Radiol 1986;59:881.
601. Hanson MW, Feldman JM, Blinder RH, Moore JO, Coleman RE. Carcinoid tumors: Iodine ^{131}I MIBG scintigraphy. Radiology 1989;172:699.
602. Adolph JMG, Kimmig BN, Georgi P, et al. Carcinoid tumors: CT and ^{131}I-metaiodobenzylguanidine scintigraphy. Radiology 1976;164:199.
603. Reubi JC, Kvols LK, Waser B, et al. Detection of somatostatin receptors in surgical and percutaneous needle biopsy samples of carcinoids and islet cell tumors. Cancer Res 1990;50:5969.
604. Bakker WH, Krenning EP, Breeman WA, et al. Receptor scintigraphy with radiolabelled somatostatin analogue: Radiolabelling, purification, biologic activity and in vivo application. J Nucl Med 1990;31:501.
605. Lamberts SW, Hofland LJ, van Koetsveld PM, et al. Parallel in vivo and in vitro detection of functional somatostatin receptors in human endocrine tumors: Consequences with regard to diagnosis, localization and therapy. J Clin Endocrinol Metab 1990;31:566.
606. Lamberts SW, Bakker WH, Reubi JC, Krenning EP. Somatostatin receptor imaging in the localization of endocrine tumors. N Engl J Med 1990;323:1246.

607. Feldman JM, Plunk JW. ^{99m}Tc-pyrophosphate bone scans in patients with metastatic carcinoid tumors. J Med 1977;8:71.
608. Barton JC, Hirschowitz BI, Maton PN, Jensen RT. Bone metastases in malignant gastrinoma. Gastroenterology 1986;91:915.
609. Orloff MJ. Carcinoid tumors of the rectum. Cancer 1971;28:175.
610. Caldarola VT, Jackman RJ, Moertel CG, et al. Carcinoid tumors of the rectum. Am J Surg 1964;107:844.
611. Brookes VS, Waterhouse JAH, Pawel DJ. Malignant carcinoids of the small intestine: A ten year survey. Br J Surg 1968;55:405.
612. Agranovich AL, Anderson GH, Manji M, Acker BD, MacDonald WC, Threlfall WJ. Carcinoid tumor of the gastrointestinal tract: Prognostic factors and disease outcome. J Surg. Oncol 1991;47:45.
613. Eller R, Frazee R, Roberts J. Gastrointestinal carcinoid tumors. Am Surg 1991;57: 434.
614. MacGillivary DG, Snyder DA, Druker W, Remine SR. Carcinoid tumors: The relationship between clinical presentation and the extent of disease. Surgery 1991;110:68.
615. Martensson H, Norbin A, Sundler F. Carcinoid tumors in the gastrointestinal tract: An analysis of 156 cases. Acta Chir Scand 1983;149:607.
616. Tsushima K, Nagorney DM, Weiland LH, Lieber MM. The relationship of low cytometry DNA analysis and clinicopathology in small-intestinal carcinoids. Surgery 1989;105: 366.
617. Tsioulias G, Muto T, Kubota Y, et al. DNA ploidy pattern of rectal carcinoid tumors. Dis Colon Rectum 1991;34:31.
618. Von Herbay A, Sieg B, Schurmann G, Betzler M, Otto HF. Proliferative activity of neuroendocrine tumors of the gastroenteropancreatic endocrine system: DNA flow cytometric and immunohistochemical investigations. Gut 1991;32:949.
619. Kujari H, Joensuu H, Klemi P, Asola R, Nordman E. A flow cytometric analysis of 23 carcinoid tumors. Cancer 1988;61:2517.
620. Wilander E, Bjelkenkrantz K, Risberg B. Nuclear DNA recordings in gastric carcinoids. A cytofluorometric study in single tumor cells. Pathol Res Pract 1987;182:331.
621. Jones DJ, Hasleton PS, Moore PN. DNA ploidy in bronchopulmonary carcinoid tumors. Thorax 1988;43:195.
622. El Nugger AK, Pallance W, Karim FW, et al. Typical and atypical bronchopulmonary carcinoids. A clinicopathologic and flow cytometry study. Am J Clin Pathol 1991;95: 828.
623. Thunnissen FB, Van Eijk J, Book JP, et al. Bronchopulmonary carcinoids and regional lymph node metastases: A quantitative pathologic investigation. Am J Pathol 1988;132: 119.
624. Travis WD, Linnoila RI, Tsokos MG, et al. Neuroendocrine tumors of the lung with proposed criteria for large-cell neuroendocrine carcinoma: An ultrastructural immunohistochemical and flow cytometry study of 35 bases. Am J Surg Pathol 1991;15: 529.
625. Moertel CG. Treatment of the carcinoid tumor and the malignant carcinoid syndrome. J Clin Oncol 1983;1:727.
626. Bissonette RT, Gibney RG, Berry BR, Buckley AR. Fatal carcinoid crisis after percutaneous fine-needle biopsy of hepatic metastasis: Case report and literature review. Radiology 1990;174:751.
627. Sukamaran M, Wilkinson ZS, Christainson L. Acute carcinoid syndrome: A complication of flexible fiberoptic bronchoscopy. Ann Thorac Surg 1982;34:702.
628. Miller R, Patel AV, Warner RPR, Parres IH. Anaesthesia for the carcinoid syndrome: A report of nine cases. Can Anaesth Soc J 1978;25:240.
629. Kvols LK, Martin JK, Marsh HM, Moertel CG. Rapid reversal of carcinoid crises with a somatostatin analogue. N Engl J Med 1985;313:1229.
630. Sjoerdsma H, Loyenberg W, Engelman K, Carpenter WT Jr, Wyatt RJ, Gessa GL. Serotonin now: Clinical implications of inhibiting its synthesis with parachlorophenylalanine. Ann Intern Med 1970;73:607.
631. Berry EM, Maunder C, Wilson M. Carcinoid myopathy and treatment with cyproheptadine (Periactin). Gut 1974;15:34.
632. Ureles AL, Murray M, Wolf R. Results of pharmacologic treatment in the malignant carcinoid syndrome. N Engl J Med 1962;267:435.
633. Harris AL, Smith IL. Regression of carcinoid tumor with cyproheptadine. Br Med J 1982;285:475.
634. Robertson JIS. Carcinoid syndrome and serotonin: Therapeutic effects of ketanserin. Cardiovasc Drug Therapy 1990;4:53.
635. Gustafsen J, Lendorf A, Raskov H, Boesby S. Ketanserin versus placebo in carcinoid syndrome. Scand J Gastroenterol 1985;21:816.
636. Sullivan PA, O'Donovan M. Ketanserin as the antagonist in symptomatic treatment of carcinoid syndrome. Irish J Med Sci 1985;155:436.
637. Coupe MO, Anderson JV, Morris JH, Alstead EM, Bloom SR, Hodgson HJF. The effect of the 5-hydroxytryptamine (5HT) receptor antagonist ICS 205-930 in the carcinoid syndrome. Aliment Pharmacol Ther 1988;2:167.
638. Stathopoulous GB, Karvountzis GG, Yiotis J. Tamoxifen in carcinoid syndrome. N J Med 1981;305:52.
639. Myers CF, Ershler WB, Tannenbaum MA, et al. Tamoxifen and carcinoid tumor. Ann Intern Med 1982;96:383.
640. Moertel CG, Engstrom PF, Schutt AJ. Tamoxifen therapy for metastatic carcinoid tumor: A negative study. Ann Intern Med 1984;100:531.
641. Thulin L, Samnegard H, Tyden G, Long DH, Efendic S. Efficacy of somatostatin in a patient with carcinoid tumor. Lancet 1978;2:43.
642. Long RG, Peters JR, Bloom SR, et al. Somatostatin, gastrointestinal peptides and the carcinoid syndrome. Gut 1981;22:549.
643. Dharmsathaphorn K, Sherwin RS, Calaland S, Jaffe B, Dobbins J. Somatostatin inhibits diarrhea in the carcinoid syndrome. Ann Intern Med 1980;92:68.
644. Davis GR, Camp RG, Raskin P, Krejs GJ. Effect of somatostatin infusion on jejunal water and electrolyte transport in a patient with secretory diarrhea due to malignant carcinoid syndrome. Gastroenterology 1980;78:346.
645. Bauer W, Briner U, Doefner W, et al. SMS-201-995 a very potent and selective octapeptide of somatostatin with prolonged actions. Life Sci 1982;31:1183.
646. Pless J, Bauer W, Briner U, et al. Chemistry and pharmacology of SMS-201-995, a long-acting octapeptide of somatostatin. Scand J Gastroenterol 1986;21(Suppl 119):54.
647. Kutz K, Nuesch J, Rosenthaler J. Pharmacokinetics of SMS-201-995 in healthy subjects. Scand J Gastroenterol 1986;21:65.
648. Vinik AI, Tsai ST, Moattari AR, Cheung P, Eckhauser FE, Cho K. Somatostatin analogue (SMS-201-995) in the management of gastroentero-pancreatic tumors and diarrhea syndromes. Am J Med 1986;81:23.
649. Kvols LK. Metastatic carcinoid tumors and the carcinoid syndrome. Am J Med 1986;81:49.
650. Kvols LK, Moertel CG, O'Connell MJ, Schutt AJ, Rubin J, Hahn RG. Treatment of the malignant carcinoid syndrome: Evaluation of a long-acting somatostatin analogue. N Engl J Med 1986;315:663.
651. Vinik AI, Moattari AR. Use of somatostatin analogue in management of carcinoid syndrome. Dig Dis Sci 1989;34:14S.
652. Oberg K, Norheim I, Theodorsson E. Treatment of malignant carcinoid tumors with a long-acting somatostatin analogue octreotide. Acta Oncol 1991;30:503.
653. Wangberg B, Nilsson O, Theodorsson E, Dahlstrom A, Ahlman H. The effect of somatostatin analogue on the release of hormones from human midgut carcinoid tumor cells. Br J Cancer 1991;64:23.
654. Kvols LK. Therapeutic considerations for the malignant carcinoid syndrome. Acta Oncol 1989;28:433.
655. Kvols LK. Therapy of malignant carcinoid syndrome. Endocrinol Metab Clin North Am 1989;18:557.
656. Richter G, Stockmann F, Lembeke B, Conlon JM, Creutzfeldt W. Short-term administration of somatostatin analogue SMS-201-995 in patients with carcinoid tumor. Scand J Gastroenterol 1986;21:193.
657. Roy RC, Carter RF, Wright KD. Somatostatin, anesthesia and the carcinoid syndrome: Perioperative administration of a somatostatin analogue to suppress carcinoid tumor activity. Anaesthesia 1987;42:627.
658. Oberg K, Norheim I, Lind E, et al. Treatment of malignant carcinoid tumors with human leukocyte interferon: Long term results. Cancer Treat Rev 1986;70:1297.
659. Oberg IL, Funa K, Alma GV. Effects of leukocyte interferon on clinical symptoms and hormone levels in patients with mid gut carcinoid tumors and carcinoid syndrome. N Engl J Med 1983;309:129.
660. Oberg K, Erickson B. The role of interferons in the management of carcinoid tumors. Acta Oncol 1991;30:519.
661. Norbin A, Lindblom A, Mansson B, Sundberg M. Interferon treatment in patients with malignant carcinoids. Acta Oncol 1989;28:445.
662. Hanssen LE, Schrompf E, Jacobsen MB, Kolbenstredt AN, Kolmannskug F, Bergan A, Dulva LO. Extended experience with recombinant 2b interferon with or without hepatic artery embolization in the treatment of midcut carcinoid tumors: A preliminary report. Acta Oncol 1991;30:523.
663. Hanssen LE, Schrumpt E, Kalbenstvedt AN, Tausjo J, Dowa LO. treatment of malignant metastatic midgut carcinoid tumors with recombinant human 2b interferon with or without prior hepatic artery embolization. Scand J Gastroenterol 1989;24:787.
664. Stockman F, von Tomatowski HJ, Reimold WV, Schuster R, Creutzfeldt W. Hepatic artery embolization for treatment of endocrine gastrointestinal tumors with liver metastases. Z Gastroenterol 1984;22:652.
665. Maton PN, Camilleri M, Friggin G, et al. The role of hepatic arterial embolization in the carcinoid syndrome. Br Med J 1983;287:932.
666. Moertel CG, May GR, Martin JK, et al. Sequential hepatic artery occlusion and chemotherapy for metastatic carcinoid tumor and islet cell carcinoma. Proc Amer Soc Clin Oncol 1985;4:80.
667. Venook A, Stagg R, Frye J, Gorden R, Ring E. Chemoembolization of patients with liver metastases from carcinoid and islet cell tumors. Proc Amer Soc Clin Oncol [Abstract] 1991;10:386.
668. Marlink RG, Lakich JJ, Robins JR, Clouse ME. Hepatic arterial embolization for metastatic hormone secreting tumors. Cancer 1991;65:2227.
669. Norbin A, Mansson B, Lunderquist A. Evaluation of temporary liver dearterialization and embolization in patients with metastatic carcinoid tumors. Acta Oncol 1989;28: 419.
670. Andaker L, Lamke LO, Smeds S. Follow-up of 102 patients operated for gastrointestinal carcinoid. Acta Chir Scand 1985;151:469.
671. Sauven P, Ridge JE, Quan SH, Siguardson ER. Anorectal carcinoid tumors: Is aggressive surgery warranted? Ann Surg 1990;211:67.
672. Makridis C, Oberg K, Juhlin C, et al. Surgical treatment of midgut carcinoid tumors. World J Surg 1990;14:377.
673. Naunheim KS, Zeitel J, Kaplan EL, et al. Rectal carcinoid tumors - treatment and prognosis. Surgery 1983;94:670.
674. Arunha G. U, Greenlee HB. Surgical management of carcinoid tumors of the gastrointestinal tract. Ann Surg 1980;41:429.
675. Stuart RC. Primary gastric carcinoids. Br J Surg 1991;78:122.
676. Ahlman H, Schensten T, Tisell L-E. Surgical treatment of patients with carcinoid syndrome. Acta Oncol 1989;28:403.
677. Gaitan-Gaitan A, Riden WD, Rush RS. Carcinoid tumor: Cured by radiation. Int J Radiat Oncol Biol Phys 1975;1:9.
678. Keane TS, Rider WP, Harwood HR, et al. Whole body radiation in the management of the metastatic carcinoid tumor. Int J Radiat Oncol Biol Phys 1981;7:1519.
679. Shupak KP, Wallner KE. The role of radiation therapy in the treatment of locally unresectable or metastatic carcinoid tumors. Int J Radiat Oncol Biol Phys 1991;20: 489.

680. Shapiro B, Fig LM. Management of pheochromocytomas. Endocrinol Metab Clin North Am 1989;18:443.
681. Bauer P, van de Fierdt E, Stettmeier H, Langhammer HR, Pabst HW. ^{125}I-MIBG therapy of carcinoid tumor of intestinal origin. Eur J Nucl Med 1988;14:234.
682. Hoefnagel LA, der van Hartog Jaeger FC, Tool GB, Abeling NG, Engelsman EE. The role of ^{125}I-MIBG in the diagnosis and therapy of carcinoids. Eur J Nucl Med 1987;13:187.
683. Hoefnagel CA, der van Hartog Jaeger FC, van Gennig AM, et al. Diagnosis and therapy of carcinoid tumor using ^{131}I metaiodobenzylguanidine. Clin Nucl Med 1986;11:150.
684. Van Hazel GA, Rubin J, Moertel CG. Treatment of metastatic carcinoid tumor with dactinomycin or dacarbazine. Cancer Treat Rep 1983;67:583.
685. Moertel CG, Rubin J, O'Connell MJ. Phase II study of cisplatin therapy in patients with metastatic carcinoid tumor and the malignant carcinoid syndrome. Cancer Treat Rep 1986;70:1459.
686. Kelsen D, Fiore J, Heelar R, et al. Phase II trial of ectoposide in APUD tumors. Cancer Treat Rep 1987;71:305.
687. Kvols LK, Buck M. Chemotherapy of endocrine malignancies. Semin Oncol 1987;14:343.
688. Engstrom PF, Lavin PT, Folsch E, Moertel CG, Douglas HO. Streptozotocin plus fluorouracil versus doxorubicin therapy for metastatic carcinoid tumors. J Clin Oncol 1984;2:1255.
689. Kelsen DG, Cheng E, Kemeny N, Magill GB, Yagoda A. Streptozotocin and adriamycin in the treatment of APUD tumors (carcinoid, islet cell and medullary thyroid). Proc Amer Assoc Cancer Res 1982;23:433.
690. Doberaur C, Niecterle N, Klobe O, Kurschel E, Schmidt GS. Zur behandlung des metastatasserten karzoids van ileum and cecum mit arkombinatem interferon alpha-2b. Oncologie 1987;10:340.
691. Jensen RT, Doppman JL, Gardner JD. Gastrinoma. In: Go VLW, Brooks FA, DiMagno EP, Gardner JD, Lebenthal E, Scheele GA, eds. The exocrine pancreas: Biology, pathobiology and disease. New York: Raven Press, 1986:727–744.
692. Bukowski RM, Johnson KG, Peterson RF, et al. A Phase II trial combination chemotherapy in patients with metastatic carcinoid tumors: A Southwest Oncology Group study. Cancer 1987;60:2891.
693. Boddie AW Jr, McMurtrey MJ, Diacco GG, McBride CM. Palliative total gastrectomy and esophagogastrectomy. Cancer 1983;51:1195.
694. Kvols LK, Buck M. Chemotherapy of endocrine malignancies: A review. Semin Oncol 1987;14:343.
695. Creutzfeldt W, Bartsch HH, Jacubaschke U, Stockmann F. Treatment of gastrointestinal endocrine tumors with interferon-α and octreotide. Acta Oncol 1991;30:529.
696. Kvols LK, Moertel CG, Schutt AJ, Rubin J. Treatment of the malignant carcinoid syndrome with a long acting somatostatin analogue (SMS 201-995): Preliminary evidence that more is not better. Proc Amer Soc Clin Oncol 1987;6:95.
697. Oberg K, Norheim I, Alm G, et al. Long-term treatment of malignant carcinoid tumors with human leukocyte interferon. In: Stewart WE, et al, eds. Biology of the interferon system. New York: Elsevier Science Publisher, 1985:433.
698. Oberg K, Eriksson B, Norheim I. Interferon treatment of neuroendocrine gut tumors. J Clin Oncol 1987;6:80.
699. Moertel CG, Rubin J, Kvols LK. Therapy of metastatic carcinoid tumor and the malignant carcinoid syndrome with recombinant leukocyte A interferon. J Clin Oncol 1989;7:865.
700. Ronnblom LE, Alm GV, Oberg KE. Autoimmunity after alpha-interferon therapy for malignant carcinoid tumors. Ann Intern Med 1991;115:178.
701. Grander D, Oberg K, Lundquist M-L, Jansun ET, Eriksson B, Einhorn S. Interferon-induced enhancement of 2′,5′-oligoadenylate synthetase in mid-gut carcinoid tumors. Lancet 1990;336:337.
702. Jensen RT, Norton JA. Pancreatic endocrine tumors. In: Yamada T, Alpers DH, Owyang C, Powell DW, Silvenstein FE, eds. Textbook of gastroenterology. Philadelphia: JB Lippincott, 1991:1912.
703. Chiang HC, O'Dorisio TM, Huang SC, et al. Multiple hormone elevations in patients with Zollinger-Ellison syndrome: Prospective study of clinical significance and of development of a second symptomatic pancreatic endocrine tumor syndrome. Gastroenterology 1990;99:1565.
704. Schein PS, DeLellis RA, Kahn CR, Gorden P, Kraft AR. Islet cell tumors: Current concepts and management. Ann Intern Med 1973;79:239.
705. Becker V. Pathologisch-anatomische aspekte bei endokrin wirksamon. Tumoren Langenbecks Arch 1971;88:426.
706. Grimelius L, Hultquist D, Stenkvist B. Cytological differentiation of asymptomatic pancreatic endocrine tumors in autopsy material. Virchows Arch A Pathol Anat Histopathol 1975;365:275.
707. Weil C. Gastroenteropancreatic endocrine tumors. Klin Wochenschr 1985;63:433.
708. Buchanan KD, Johnston CF, O'Hare MMT, et al. Neuroendocrine tumors: A European view. Am J Med 1986;81(Suppl 68):14.
709. Dent RB, van Heerden JA, Weiland LH. Nonfunctioning islet cell tumors. Ann Surg 1981;193:185.
710. Broder LE, Carter SK. Pancreatic islet cell carcinoma: Clinical features of 52 patients. Ann Intern Med 1973;79:101.
711. Koppel G, Heitz PU. Pancreatic endocrine tumors. Pathol Res Pract 1988;183:155.
712. Jensen RT, Gardner JD. Zollinger-Ellison syndrome: Clinical presentation, pathology, diagnosis and treatment. In: Dannenberg A, Zakim D, eds. Peptic ulcer and other acid-related diseases. New York: Academic Research Association, 1991:117.
713. Zollinger RM, Ellison EH. Primary peptic ulceration of the jejunum associated with islet cell tumors of the pancreas. Ann Surg 1955;142:709.
714. Gregory RA, Tracy HJ, French JM, Sircus W. Extraction of a gastrin-like substance from a pancreatic tumor in a case of Zollinger-Ellison syndrome. Lancet 1960;1:1045.
715. Gregory RA, Grossman MI, Tracy HJ, Bentley PH. Nature of the gastric secretagogue in Zollinger-Ellison tumors. Lancet 1967;2:543.
716. Gregory RA, Tracy JH, Agarwal KL. Amino acid constitution of two gastrins isolated from Zollinger-Ellison tumor tissue. Gut 1969;10:603.
717. Stage JG, Stadil F. The clinical diagnosis of the Zollinger-Ellison syndrome. Scand J Gastroenterol 1979;14:79.
718. Grossman MI, ed. Peptic ulcer. Chicago: Yearbook Medical Publishers, 1981:141–151.
719. Jensen RT, Gardner JD, Raufman JP. Zollinger-Ellison syndrome. NIH combined clinical staff conference. Ann Intern Med 1983;98:59.
720. Zollinger RM, Ellison EC, Fabri PJ, et al. Primary peptic ulceration of the jejunum associated with islet cell tumors: Twenty-five year appraisal. Ann Surg 1980;192:422.
721. Thompson JC, Reeder DD, Villar HV, et al. Natural history and experience with diagnosis and treatment of the Zollinger-Ellison syndrome. Surg Gynecol Obstet 1975;140:721.
722. Bonfils S, Landor SH, Mignon M, Hervoir P, et al. Results of surgical management in 92 consecutive patients with Zollinger-Ellison syndrome. Ann Surg 1981;194:692.
723. Johnson LR. Gut hormones on growth of gastrointestinal mucosa. In: Chey WY, Brooks FP, eds. Endocrinology of the gut. Thorofare, NJ: Charles B. Slack, 1974:163.
724. Neurburger PH, Lewin M, Bonfils S. Parietal and chief cell populations in 4 cases of the Zollinger-Ellison syndrome. Gastroenterology 1972;937.
725. Sum P, Perey BJ. Parietal cell mass (PCM) in a man with Zollinger-Ellison syndrome. Can J Surg 1969;12:285.
726. Wright HK, Hersh T, Floch MH, Weinstein LD. Impaired intestinal absorption in the Zollinger-Ellison syndrome independent of gastric hypersecretion. Am J Surg 1970;119:150.
727. Creutzfeldt W, Arnold R, Creutzfeld C, et al. Pathomorphological, biochemical and diagnostic aspects of gastrinomas (Zollinger-Ellison syndrome). Hum Pathol 1975;6:47.
728. Dockray GJ, Walsh JH, Passaro E Jr. Relative abundance of big and little gastrins in the tumors and blood of patients with Zollinger-Ellison syndrome. Gut 1975;16:353.
729. Walsh JH, Grossman MI. Gastrin. N Engl J Med 1975;292:1324.
730. Eysselein VE, Maxwell V, Peedy T, Wunsch E, Walsh JH. Similar and stimulatory potencies of synthetic human big and little gastrins in man. JNCI 1984;73:1284.
731. Dockray GJ, Walsh JH. Amino terminal gastrin fragment in serum of Zollinger-Ellison syndrome patients. Gastroenterology 1975;68:222.
732. Rehfeld JF, Stadil F. Gel filtration studies on immunoreactive gastrin in serum from Zollinger-Ellison patients. Gut 1973;14:369.
733. Kothary PC, Fabri PJ, Gower W, O'Dorisio TM, Ellis J, Vinik A. Evaluation of NH2-terminus gastrins in gastrinoma syndrome. J Endocrinol Metab 1986;62:970.
734. Kothary PC, Mahoney WC, Vinik AI. Identification of gastrin molecular variants in gastrinoma syndrome. Regul Pept 1987;17:71.
735. Hilsted L, Bardram LC. Terminally glycine extended gastrins in serum and tumors from patients with Zollinger-Ellison syndrome. Can J Physiol Pharmacol 1986:136.
736. Desmond H, Parcevelo S, Varro A, Gregory H, Yaund J, Dockray GJ. Isolation and characterization of the intact gastrin precursor from a gastrinoma. FEBS Lett 1987;210:185.
737. Pauwels S, Desmond H, Dimaline R, Dockray GJ. Identification of progastrin in gastrinoma, antrum and duodenum by a novel radioimmunoassay. J Clin Invest 1986;77:376.
738. Bardram L. Progastrin in serum from Zollinger-Ellison patients: An indicator of malignancy? Gastroenterology 1990;98:1420.
739. Del Valle G, Sugano K, Yamada T. Progastrin and its glycine-extended posttranslational processing intermediates in human gastrointestinal tissues. Gastroenterology 1987;87:1908.
740. Dockray GJ, Varro A, Desmond H, Young J, Gregory H, Gregory RA. Posttransitional processing of the porcine gastrin precursor by phosphorylation of the COOH-terminal fragment. J Biol Chem 1987;262:8643.
741. Johnson JA, Fabri PJ, Lott JA. Serum gastrins in Zollinger-Ellison syndrome: Identification of localized disease. Clin Chem 1980;26:867.
742. Hofman JW, Fox PS, Wilson SD. Duodenal wall tumors and the Zollinger-Ellison syndrome. Arch Surg 1973;107:334.
743. Norton JA, Doppman JL, Collen MJ, Harmon JW, Maton PN, Gardner JD, Jensen RT. Prospective study of gastrinoma localization and resection in patients with Zollinger-Ellison syndrome. Ann Surg 1986;204:468.
744. Wolfe MM, Alexander RW, McGuigan JE. Extrapancreatic, extraintestinal gastrinoma: Effective treatment by surgery. N Engl J Med 1982;306:1533.
745. Norton JA, Doppman JL, Jensen RT. Curative resection in Zollinger-Ellison syndrome: Results of a 10 year prospective study. Ann Surg 1992;215:8.
746. Stabile BE, Morrow DJ, Passaro E. The gastrinoma triangle: Operative implications. Am J Surg 1984;147:25.
747. Maton PN, Macken SM, Norton JA, Gardner JD, O'Dorisio TM, Jensen RT. Ovarian carcinoma as a cause of Zollinger-Ellison syndrome. Gastroenterology 1989;97:464.
748. Howard TJ, Zinner MJ, Stabile BE, Passaro E Jr. Gastrinoma excision for cure. Ann Surg 1990;211:9.
749. Primrose JN, Maloney M, Wells M, Bulgin O, Johnston D. Gastrin-producing ovarian mucinous cystadenomas: A cause of Zollinger-Ellison syndrome. Surgery 1988;104:830.
750. Bollen ECM, Lamers CBHW, Jansen JBMJ, Larsson LI, Joosten HJ. Zollinger-Ellison syndrome due to a gastrin-producing ovarian cystadenoma. Br J Surg 1981;68:776.

751. Cocco AE, Conway SJ. Zollinger-Ellison syndrome associated with ovarian mucinous cystadenocarcinomas. N Engl J Med 1975;293:485.
752. Friesen SR. Tumors of the endocrine pancreas. N Engl J Med 1982;306:580.
753. Larsson LI, Rehfeld JR, Goltermann N. Gastrin in the human fetus. Distribution and molecular forms of gastrin in the antro-pyloric gland area, duodenum, and pancreas. Scand J Gastroenterol 1977;12:869.
754. Solcia E, Capella C, Buffa R, Frigerio G, Fiocca R. Pathology of the Zollinger-Ellison syndrome. In: Fengolio LM, Wolff M, eds. Progress in surgical pathology. 1980;119.
755. Thom AK, Norton JA, Axiotix CA, Jensen RT. Location, incidence and malignant potential of duodenal gastrinomas. Surgery 1991;110:1086.
756. Pipeleers-Marichal M, Somers G, Willems G, Foulis A, Imrie C, Bishop AE, et al. Gastrinomas in the duodenums of patients with multiple endocrine neoplasic type 1 and the Zollinger-Ellison syndrome. N Engl J Med 1990;322:723.
757. Ellison EC, Wilson SD. The Zollinger-Ellison syndrome: Re-appraisal and evaluation of 260 registered cases. Ann Surg 1964;160:512.
758. Fox PS, Hofmann JW, Wilson SD, DeCosse JJ. Surgical management of the Zollinger-Ellison syndrome. Surg Clin North Am 1974;54:394.
759. Zollinger RM, Martin EW, Carey LC. Observations on the post-operative tumor growth of certain islet cell tumors. Ann Surg 1976;184:525.
760. Friesen SR. The development of endocrinopathies in the prospective screening of two families with MEN-1. World J Surg 1979;3:753.
761. Larsson LI, Ljungberg O, Sundler F, et al. Antropyloric gastrinoma associated with pancreatic nesidioblastosis and proliferation of islets. Virchows Arch [A] 1973;360: 305.
762. Thompson JC, Lewis BG, Wiener I, Townsend CM Jr. The role of surgery in the Zollinger-Ellison Syndrome. Ann Surg 1983;197:594.
763. Harmon JW, Norton JA, Collen MJ. Removal of gastrinomas for control of Zollinger-Ellison syndrome. Ann Surg 1984;200:396.
764. Jensen RT, Maton PN. Zollinger-Ellison syndrome. In: Gustavsson S, Kumar D, Graham DY, eds. The stomach. London: Churchill Livingstone, 1991:341.
765. Zollinger RM, Ellison EC, O'Dorisio T, Sparks J. Thirty years' experience with gastrinoma. World J Surg 1984;8:427.
766. Malagelada JR, Edis AJ, Adson MA, van Heerden JA, Go VLW. Medical and surgical options in the management of patients with gastrinoma. Gastroenterology 1983;84: 1524.
767. Stabile BE, Passaro E. Benign and malignant gastrinoma. Am J Surg 1984;149:144.
768. Mukai K, Greider MH, Grotting JC, Rosai J. Retrospective study of 77 pancreatic endocrine tumors using the immunoperoxidase method. Am J Surg Pathol 1982;6: 387.
769. Larsson LI. Classification of pancreatic endocrine tumors. Scand J Gastroenterol 1978;14:15.
770. Heitz PU, Kasper M, Polak JM, Kloppel G. Pancreatic endocrine tumors. Hum Pathol 1982;13:263.
771. Blackburn AM, Bryant MG, Adrian TE, Bloom SR. Pancreatic tumors produce neurotensin. J Clin Endocrinol Metab 1981;52:820.
772. Bloom SR, Adrian TE, Bryant MG, Polak JM. Pancreatic polypeptide: A marker for Zollinger-Ellison syndrome. Lancet 1978;1:1155.
773. Lamers CBH, Diemel JM, Roeffen W. Serum levels of pancreatic polypeptide in Zollinger-Ellison syndrome and hyperparathyroidism from families with multiple endocrine adenamotosis type I. Digestion 1978;18:297.
774. Taylor IL, Rotter J, Walsh JH, Passaro E Jr. Is pancreatic polypeptide a marker for Zollinger-Ellison syndrome? Lancet 1978;1:845.
775. Yamaguchi K, Abe A, Miyakawa S, Ohnami S. Multiple hormone production in endocrine tumors in the pancreas. In: Miyoshi H, ed. Gut hormones. Amsterdam: Elsevier North-Holland Biomedical Press, 1979:343.
776. Adrian TE, Uttenthal LD, Williams SJ, Bloom SR. Secretion of pancreatic polypeptide in patients with pancreatic endocrine tumors. N Engl J Med 1986;315:287.
777. Langstein HN, Norton JA, Chiang HC. V, et al. The utility of circulating levels of human pancreatic polypeptide as a marker of islet cell tumors. Surgery 1990;108: 1109.
778. Sheppard BC, Norton JA, Doppman JL, Maton PN, Gardner JD, Jensen RT. Management of islet cell tumors in patients with multiple endocrine neoplasia: A prospective study. Surgery 1989;106:1108.
779. McCarthy DM, Weintraub B. Subunits of human chorionic gonadotropin in the Zollinger-Ellison syndrome. Gastroenterology 1979;76:1198.
780. Stabile BE, Braunstein GD, Passaro E Jr. Serum gastrin and human chorionic gonadotropin in the Zollinger-Ellison syndrome. Arch Surg 1980;115:1090.
781. Bardram L, Agner T, Hagen C. Levels of alpha subunits of gonadotropin can be increased in Zollinger-Ellison syndrome, both in patients with malignant tumors and apparently benign disease. Acta Endocrinol 1988;118:135.
782. Kloppel G, Girard J, Polak JW, Vaitukaitis JL, Kasper M, Heitz PU. Alpha human chorionic gonadotropin and neuron specific enolase as markers for malignancy and neuroendocrine nature of pancreatic endocrine tumors. Cancer Detect Prev 1983;6: 161.
783. Norton JA, Jensen RT. Unresolved surgical issues in the management of patients with Zollinger-Ellison syndrome. World J Surg 1991;15:151.
784. Hagn C, Schmid KW, Rischer-Calibrie R, Winkler H. Chromogranin A, B and C in human adrenal medulla and endocrine tissues. Lab Invest 1986;55:405.
785. Lloyd RV, Mervak T, Schmidt K, Warner TGCS, Wilson BS. Immunohistochemical detection of chromogranin and neurospecific enolase in pancreatic endocrine tumors. Am J Surg Pathol 1984;8:607.
786. O'Connor DT, Deftos LJ. Secretion of chromogranin A by peptide-producing endocrine neoplasms. N Engl J Med 1986;314:1145.
787. Sobol RE, Memoli V, Deftos LJ. Hormone-negative, chromogranin A-positive endocrine tumors. N Engl J Med 1989;320:444.
788. Wiedenmann B, Waldherr R, Buhr H, Hille A, Russa P, Huttner WB. Identification of gastroenteropancreatic neuroendocrine cells in normal and neoplastic human tissue with antibodies against synaptophysin, chromogranin A, secretogranin I (chromogranin B), and secretogranin II. Gastroenterology 1988;95:1364.
789. Stabile BE, Howard TJ, Passaro EJ Jr, O'Connor DJ. Source of plasma chromogranin A elevation in gastrinoma. Arch Surg 1990;125:451.
790. Niewenhuijzen-Knuseman AC, Knijnenburg G, Ribiere GB, Bosman FT. Morphology and immunohistochemically-defined endocrine function of pancreatic islet cell tumors. Histopathology 1978;2:389.
791. Regan PT, Malagelada JR. A reappraisal of clinical, roentgenographic, and endoscopic features of the Zollinger-Ellison syndrome. Mayo Clin Proc 1978;53:19.
792. Jensen RT, Gardner JD. Zollinger-Ellison syndrome: Clinical presentation, pathology, diagnosis, and treatment. In: Zakim D, Dannenberg AJ, eds. Peptic ulcer disease and other acid-related disorders. Armonk, NY: Academic Research Associates, 1991;117–211.
793. Richter JF, Pandol SI, Castell DO, McCarthy DM. Gastroesophageal reflux disease in the Zollinger-Ellison syndrome. Ann Intern Med 1981;95:37.
794. Miller LS, Vinayek R, Frucht H, Gardner JD, Jensen RT, Maton PN. Reflux esophagitis in patients with Zollinger-Ellison syndrome. Gastroenterology 1990;98:341.
795. Waxsman I, Gardner JD, Jensen RT, Maton PN. Peptic ulcer perforation as the presentation of Zollinger-Ellison syndrome. Dig Dis Sci 1991;36:19.
796. Wolfe MM, Jensen RT. Zollinger-Ellison syndrome, Current concepts in diagnosis and management. N Engl J Med 1987;317:1200.
797. Wolfe MM, Jain DK, Edgerton JR. Zollinger-Ellison syndrome associated with persistent normal fasting serum gastrin concentrations. Ann Intern Med 1985;103:215.
798. Aoyagi T, Summerskill SHJ. Gastric secretion with ulcerogenic islet cell tumor. Arch Intern Med 1966;117:667.
799. Deveney CW, Deveney KS, Way LW. The Zollinger-Ellison syndrome: 23 years later. Ann Surg 1978;188:384.
800. Deveney CW, Deveney KS, Jaffe BM, Janes RS, Way LW. Use of calcium and secretin in the diagnosis of gastrinoma (Zollinger-Ellison syndrome). Ann Intern Med 1979;87: 680.
801. Malagelada JR, Davis CS, O'Fallon WM, Go VLW. Laboratory diagnosis of gastrinoma. Mayo Clin Proc 1982;57:211.
802. Isenberg JI, Walsh JH, Grossman MI. Zollinger-Ellison syndrome. Gastroenterology 1973;65:140.
803. Van Heerden JA, Bernatz PE, Rovelstad RA. The retained antrum-clinical considerations. Mayo Clin Proc 1971;46:25.
804. Korman MG, Scott DG, Hansky J, Wilson H. Hypergastrinemia due to excluded gastric antrum: A proposed method for differentiation from Zollinger-Ellison syndrome. Aust N Z J Med 1972;3:266.
805. Chaudhuri TK, Shirazi SS, Condon RE. Radioisotope scan: A possible aid in differentiating retained gastric antrum from Zollinger-Ellison syndrome in patients with recurrent peptic ulcer. Gastroenterology 1973;65:697.
806. Frucht H, Howard JM, Slaff JE, et al. Secretin and calcium provocative tests in patients with Zollinger-Ellison syndrome: A prospective study. Ann Intern Med 1989;111: 713.
807. Isenberg JI, Walsh JH, Passaro E Jr, Moore EW, Grossman MI. Unusual effect of secretin on serum gastrin, serum calcium, and gastric acid secretion in a patient with suspected Zollinger-Ellison syndrome. Gastroenterology 1972;62:626.
808. Cherner JA, Doppman JL, Norton JA, et al. Prospective assessment of selective venous sampling for gastrin to localize gastrinomas. Ann Intern Med 1986;105:841.
809. Lamers CBH, van Tongeren JHM. Comparative study of the value of calcium, secretin, and meal stimulated increase in serum gastrin in the diagnosis of the Zollinger-Ellison syndrome. Gut 1979;18:128.
810. Frucht H, Howard JM, Stark HA, et al. Prospective study of meal provocative gastrin testing in patients with Zollinger-Ellison syndrome. Am J Med 1989;87:528.
811. Ganguli PC, Elder JB, Polak MJ, Pearse AGE. Antral gastrin cell hyperplasia in peptic ulcer disease. Lancet 1974;1:288.
812. Polak JM, Stagg B, Pearse AGE. Two types of Zollinger-Ellison syndrome: Immunofluorescent, cytochemical, and ultrastructural studies of the antral and pancreatic gastric cells in different clinical states. Gut 1972;13:501.
813. Friesen SR, Schimke RN, Pearse AGE. Genetic aspects of Z-E syndrome: Prospective studies in two kindreds—Antral gastrin cell hyperplasia. Ann Surg 1972;176:370.
814. Friesen SR, Tomita T. Pseudo-Zollinger-Ellison syndrome: Hypergastrinemia, hyperchlorohydria without tumor. Ann Surg 1981;194:481.
815. Lamers CBH, Ruland CM, Joosten HJM, Verkooyen HCM, Tongeren JHM, Rehfeld JF. Hypergastrinemia of antral origin in duodenal ulcer. Dig Dis Sci 1978;23:998.
816. Taylor IL, Calam JK, Roth JI, et al. Family studies of hypergastrinemic hyperpepsinogenemic I duodenal ulcer. Ann Intern Med 1981;95:421.
817. Hangen D, Maltz GS, Anderson CM. Marked hypergastrinemia in gastric outlet obstruction. J Clin Gastroenterol 1989;11:442.
818. Fuerle G, Ketterer H, Becker HD, Creutzfeldt W. Circadian serum gastrin concentrations in control persons and in patients with ulcer disease. Scand J Gastroenterol 1972;7:177.
819. Saeed ZA, Doppman JL, Norton J, Maton PN, Gardner JD, Jensen RT. Gastrinoma localization in Zollinger-Ellison syndrome. Intern Med Specialist 1988;9:79.
820. Maton PN, Gardner JD, Jensen RT. Recent advances in the management of gastric hypersecretion in patients with Zollinger-Ellison syndrome. Med Clin North Am 1989;18:847.
821. Fox PS, Hofmann JW, DeCosse JJ, Wilson SD. The influence of total gastrectomy on survival in malignant Zollinger-Ellison tumors. Ann Surg 1974;180:558.

822. Mignon M, Ruszniewski P, Haffar S, Rigaud D, Rene E, Bonfils S. Current approach to the management of the tumoral process in patients with gastrinoma. World J Surg 1986;10:703.
823. Deveney CW, Deveney KE, Stark D, Moss A, Stein S, Way LW. Resection of gastrinomas. Ann Surg 1983;198:546.
824. McCarthy DM. The place of surgery in the Zollinger-Ellison syndrome. N Engl J Med 1980;302:1344.
825. Richardson CT, Peters MN, Feldman M. Treatment of Zollinger-Ellison syndrome with exploratory laparotomy, proximal gastric vagotomy, and H2-receptor antagonists. Gastroenterology 1985;89:357.
826. Norton JA, Sugarbaker PH, Doppman JL, et al. Aggressive resection of metastatic disease in select patients with malignant gastrinoma. Ann Surg 1986;203:352.
827. London JF, Shawker TH, Doppman JL, et al. Prospective assessment of abdominal ultrasound in patients with Zollinger-Ellison syndrome. Radiology 1991;178:763.
828. Wank SA, Doppman HL, Miller DL, et al. Prospective study of the ability of computerized axial tomography to localize gastrinomas in patients with Zollinger-Ellison syndrome. Gastroenterology 1987;92:905.
829. Thompson NW, Vinik AI, Eckhauser FE. Microgastrinomas of the duodenum. Ann Surg 1989;209:396.
830. Maton PN, Miller DL, Doppman HL, et al. Role of selective angiography in the management of Zollinger-Ellison syndrome. Gastroenterology 1987;92:913.
831. Tjon Tham RTO, Falke TAM, et al. CT and MR imaging in advanced Zollinger-Ellison syndrome. Comput Assist Tomogr 1989;13:821.
832. Stark DD, Moss AA, Goldberg HI, et al. Computed tomography and nuclear magnetic resonance imaging of pancreatic islet cell tumors. Surgery 1983;94:1024.
833. Frucht H, Doppman JL, Norton JA, et al. MR imaging of gastrinomas: Comparison with computed tomography, angiography and ultrasound. Radiology 1989;171:713.
834. Legman P, Ruszniewski P, Sibert A, et al. Computed tomograph (CT) and magnetic imaging (MRI) in liver metastases (LM) of digestive endocrinology tumors (DET): A prospective study in 24 patients. Gastroenterology 1989;96:294.
835. Pisegna J, Doppman JL, Metz D, Slimak GG, Gardner JD, Jensen RT. Prospective study of the ability of magnetic resonance (MRI) to detect gastrinomas in patients with Zollinger-Ellison syndrome. Program of American College of Gastroenterology Meeting, 1991.
836. Frucht H, Norton JA, London JF, et al. Detection of duodenal gastrinomas by operative endoscopic transillumination: A prospective study. Gastroenterology 1990;99:1622.
837. Ruszniewski P, Mouyal PA, Combes R, et al. Endoscopic ultrasonography (EUS) is useful for localization of primary gastrinomas. Gastroenterology [Abstract] 1991;100: 297.
838. Roche A, Raisonnier A, Gillon-Savouret MC. Pancreatic venous sampling and arteriography in localizing insulinomas and gastrinomas: Procedure and results in 55 cases. Radiology 1982;145:621.
839. Burcharth F, Stage JG, Stadil F, et al. Localization of gastrinoma by transhepatic portal catheterization and gastrin assay. Gastroenterology 1979;77:44.
840. Glowniak JV, Shapiro B, Vinik AI, Glaser B, Thompson NW, Cho KJ. Percutaneous transhepatic venous sampling of gastrin: Value in sporadic and familial islet-cell tumors and G-cell hyperfunction. N Engl J Med 1982;307:293.
841. Miller DL, Doppman JL, Metz D, Maton PN, Jensen RT. Portal venous sampling in Zollinger-Ellison syndrome: Technique, results and complications in 95 procedures. Radiology 1991 (in press).
842. Vinik A, Moattari R, Cho K, Thompson N. Transhepatic portal venous catherization for localization for sporadic and MEN gastrinomas. Surgery 1990;107:246.
843. Doppman JL, Shawker TH, Miller DC. Localization of islet cell tumors. Med Clin North Am 1989;18:793.
844. Norton JA, Shawker TH, Doppman JL, et al. Localization and surgical treatment of occult insulinomas. Ann Surg 1990;212:615.
845. Imamura M, Takashi MP, Isobe Y, Hattori Y, Satomura K, Tobe T. Curative resection of multiple gastrinomas aided by selective arterial secretin injection and intraoperative secretin test. Ann Surg 1989;210:710.
846. Doppman JL, Miller DL, Chang R, et al. Gastrinomas: Localization by means of selective intraarterial injection of secretin. Radiology 1990;174:25.
847. Sigel B, Coelho MCU, Nyhus LM, et al. Detection of pancreatic tumors by ultrasound during surgery. Arch Radiol 1982;117:1058.
848. Charboneau WJ, James EM, van Heerden JA, et al. Intraoperative realtime ultrasonographic localization of pancreatic insulinomas. J Ultrasound Med 1983;2:251.
849. Cromack DT, Norton JA, Sigel et al. The use of high-resolution intraoperative ultrasound to localize gastrinomas: An initial report of a prospective study. World J Surg 1987;11:648.
850. Norton JA, Cromack DT, Shawker TH, et al. Intraoperative ultrasonographic localization of islet cell tumors. Ann Surg 1988;207:160.
851. Comi RJ, Gorden P, Doppman HL, Norton JA. Insulinoma. In: Go VLW, Gardner JD, Brooks FP, et al, eds. The exocrine pancreas: Biology, pathology and diseases. New York: Raven Press, 1986:745–761.
852. Friesen SR. Effect of total gastrectomy on the Zollinger-Ellison tumor: Observation by second-look operations. Surgery 1967;62:609.
853. Friesen SR. Treatment of the Zollinger-Ellison syndrome. Am J Surg 1982;143:331.
854. McArthur KE, Collen MJ, Maton PN. Omeprazole: Effective convenient therapy for Zollinger-Ellison syndrome. Gastroenterology 1985;88:939.
855. Lamers CDHW, Lind T, Moberg S, Jansen JBMJ, Olbe L. Omeprazole in Zollinger-Ellison syndrome: Effects of a single dose and of long term treatment in patients resistant to histamine H2-receptor antagonists. N Engl J Med 1984;310:758.
856. Frucht H, Maton P, Jensen RT. The use of omeprazole in patients with Zollinger-Ellison syndrome. Dig Dis Sci 1991;36:405.
857. Hirschowitz BI, Denen J, Raufman JP, LaMont B, Berman R, Humphries T. A multicenter U.S. study of omeprazole treatment of Zollinger-Ellison syndrome. Gastroenterology [Abstract] 1988;94:188.
858. Delcher JC, Soule JC, Mignon M, et al. Effectiveness of omeprazole in seven patients with Zollinger-Ellison syndrome resistant to histamine H_2-receptor antagonists. Dig Dis Sci 1986;31:693.
859. Lloyd-Davis KA, Rutgerssan K, Solvell L. Omeprazole in Zollinger-Ellison syndrome: Four year international study. Gastroenterology 1986;90:1523.
860. Meijer JL, Jansen JB, Lamers CB. Omeprazole in the treatment of Zollinger-Ellison syndrome and histamine H2-antagonist refractory ulcers. Digestion 1989;44:31.
861. Maton PN, McArthur KE, Wank SA, et al. Long-term efficacy and safety of omeprazole in patients with Zollinger-Ellison syndrome. Gastroenterology 1986;90:1537.
862. Vinayek R, Howard JM, Maton PN, et al. Famotidine in the therapy of gastric hypersecretory states. Am J Med 1986;81:49.
863. Collen MJ, Howard JM, McArthur KE, et al. Comparison of ranitidine and cimetidine in the treatment of gastric hypersecretion. Ann Intern Med 1984;100:52.
864. McCarthy DM, Hyman PE. Effect of isopropamide on response to oral cimetidine in patients with Zollinger-Ellison syndrome. Dig Dis Sci 1982;27:353.
865. Miller LS, Doppman JD, Maton PN, Gardner JD, Jensen RT. Zollinger-Ellison syndrome. In: Collen MJ, Benjamin SB, eds. Pharmacology of peptic ulcer disease. Handbook of experimental pharmacology, 1991 (in press).
866. McCarthy DM, Peikin SR, Lopatin RN. Hyperparathyroidism: A reversible cause of cimetidine-resistant gastric hypersecretion. Br Med J 1979;1:765.
867. Gogel HK, Buckman MT, Cadieux D, McCarthy DM. Gastric secretion and hormonal interactions in multiple endocrine neoplasms type I. Arch Intern Med 1985;145:855.
868. Norton JA, Cornelius MJ, Doppman JL, Maton PN, Gardner JD, Jensen RT. Effect of parathyroidectomy in patients with hyperparathyroidism and Zollinger-Ellison syndrome and multiple endocrine neoplasia type 1: A prospective study. Surgery 1987;102:958.
869. Jensen RT. Basis for failure of cimetidine in patients with Zollinger-Ellison syndrome. Dig Dis Sci 1984;29:363.
870. Stadil F, Stage JG. Cimetidine and the Zollinger-Ellison (ZE) syndrome. In: Wastell C, Lance P, eds. Cimetidine. London: Churchill Livingstone, 1978:91–104.
871. Deveney CW, Stein S, Way LW. Cimetidine in the treatment of Zollinger-Ellison syndrome. Am J Surg 1983;146:116.
872. Stabile BE, Ippoliti AF, Walsh JH, Passaro E Jr. Failure of histamine H2-receptor antagonist therapy in Zollinger-Ellison syndrome. Am J Surg 1983;145:17.
873. Jensen RT, Collen MJ, McArthur KE, et al. Comparison of the effectiveness of ranitidine and cimetidine in inhibiting acid secretion in patients with gastric hypersecretory states. Am J Med 1984;77:90.
874. Howard JM, Chremos AN, Collen MJ, et al. Famotidine, a new potent long-acting histamine H2-receptor antagonist: Comparison with cimetidine and ranitidine in the treatment of Zollinger-Ellison syndrome. Gastroenterology 1985;88:1026.
875. Raufman J-P, Collins SM, Pandol SJ, et al. Reliability of symptoms in assessing control of gastrin and secretin in patients with Zollinger-Ellison syndrome. Gastroenterology 1983;84:108.
876. Metz D, Pisegna JR, Fishbeyn VA, Benya RV, Jensen RT. Control of gastric and hypersecretion in the management of Zollinger-Ellison syndrome. World J Surg 1991 (in press).
877. McArthur KE, Raufman JP, Seaman JJ, et al. Cimetidine pharmacokinetics in patients with Zollinger-Ellison syndrome. Gastroenterology 1987;93:69.
878. Ziemniak JA, Madura M, Adamonis AJ, et al. Failure of cimetidine in Zollinger-Ellison syndrome. Dig Dis Sci 1983;28:976.
879. Vinayek R, Amantea MA, Maton PN, Frucht H, Gardner JD, Jensen RT. Pharmacokinetics of oral and intravenous omeprazole in patients with Zollinger-Ellison syndrome. Gastroenterology 1991;101:138.
880. Jensen RT, Collen MJ, Allende HD, et al. Cimetidine induced impotence and breast changes in patients with gastric hypersecretory states. N Engl J Med 1983;308:883.
881. Alumets J, El Munshid HA, Hakanson R, et al. Effect of antrum exclusion on endocrine cells of rat stomach. J Physiol (Lond) 1979;286:145.
882. Maton PN, Lack EE, Collen MJ, et al. The effect of Zollinger-Ellison syndrome and omeprazole therapy on gastric endocrine cells. Gastroenterology 1990;99:943.
883. Lehy T, Mignon M, Cadiot G, et al. Gastric endocrine cell behavior in Zollinger-Ellison patients upon long-term patient antisecretory treatment. Gastroenterology 1989;96:1029.
884. D'Adda T, Corletto V, Pilato FD, et al. Quantitative ultrastructure of endocrine cells of oxyntic mucosa in Zollinger-Ellison syndrome. Gastroenterology 1990;99:17.
885. Maton PN, Frucht H, Vinayek R, Wank SA, Gardner JD, Jensen RT. Medical management of patients with Zollinger-Ellison syndrome. Gastroenterology 1988;94:294.
886. Fraker D, Norton JA, Saeed Z, Maton P, Gardner JD, Jensen RT. A prospective study of pre- and postoperative control of acid secretion in patients with Zollinger-Ellison syndrome. Surgery 1988;104:1054.
887. Saeed ZA, Norton JA, Frank W, et al. Parenteral antisecretory drug therapy in patients with Zollinger-Ellison syndrome. Gastroenterology 1989;96:1393.
888. Vinayek R, Frucht H, London JF, et al. Intravenous omeprazole in patients with Zollinger-Ellison syndrome undergoing surgery. Gastroenterology 1990;99:10.
889. London J, Frucht H, Doppman JL, Maton PN, Gardner JD, Jensen RT. Zollinger-Ellison syndrome in the acute care setting. J Intens Care Med 1989;4:272.
890. Zollinger RM. Gastrinoma: Factors influencing prognosis. Surgery 1985;97:49.
891. Ellison EC, Carey LC, Sparks J, et al. Early surgical treatment of gastrinoma. Am J Med 1987;82:17.
892. Podevin P, Ruszniewski P, Mignon M, et al. Management of multiple endocrine neoplasia type I (MEN I) in Zollinger-Ellison syndrome. Gastroenterology [Abstract] 1990;98:230.

893. Maton PN, Gardner JD, Jensen RT. The incidence and etiology of Cushing's syndrome in patients with Zollinger-Ellison syndrome. N Engl J Med 1986;315:1.
894. Delcore R Jr, Cheung LY, Friesen SR. Characteristics of duodenal wall gastrinomas. Am J Surg 1990;160:621.
895. Norton JA, Doherty GM, Fraker DL. Surgery for endocrine tumors. In: Go VLW, Gardner JD, Brooks FP, Lebenthal E, Diangano EP, Scheele G, eds. Exocrine pancreas. New York: Raven Press, 1991 (in press).
896. Norton JA. Invited commentary. World J Surg 1984;8:572.
897. Moertel CG, Hanley JA, Johnson LA. Streptozotocin alone compared with streptozotocin plus fluorouracil in the treatment of advanced islet-cell carcinoma. N Engl J Med 1980;303:1189.
898. Buchanan KD, O'Hare MMT, Russel CJF, Kennedy TL, Hadden DR. Factors involved in the responsiveness of gastrointestinal apudomas to streptozotocin. Dig Dis Sci 1986;31:511S.
899. Von Schrenck T, Howard JM, Doppman JL, et al. Prospective study of chemotherapy in patients with metastatic gastrinoma. Gastroenterology 1988;94:1326.
900. Ruszniewski PH, Rougier P, Andre-David F, et al. Prospective multicentric study chemotherapy with streptozotocin (STZ) and 5-fluorouracil (5FU) for liver metastases (LM) in Zollinger-Ellison syndrome (ZES). Gastroenterology [Abstract] 1989;96:431.
901. Carrasco CH, Chuang VP, Wallace S. Apudoma metastatic to the liver: Treatment by hepatic artery embolization. Radiology 1983;149:79.
902. Ajani JA, Carrasco CH, Charnsangavej C, et al. Islet cell tumors metastatic to the liver: Effective palliation by sequential hepatic artery embolization. Ann Intern Med 1988;108:340.
903. Maton PN, Gardner JD, Jensen RT. The use of the long acting somatostatin analogue 201-995 in patients with pancreatic endocrine tumors. Dig Dis Sci 1989;34:29.
904. Kvols HM, Buck M, Moertel LG, et al. Treatment of metastatic islet cell carcinoma with a somatostatin analogue (SMS-201-995). Ann. Intern Med 1987;107:162.
905. Maton PN. The use of the long-acting somatostatin analogue, octreotide in patients with islet cell tumors. Gastroenterol Clin North Am 1989;18:897.
906. Reubi JC. Somatostatin analogue inhibits chondrosarcoma and insulinoma tumor growth. Acta Endocrinol 1985;109:108.
907. Shepherd JJ, Senator GB. Regression of liver metastases in patients with gastrin secreting tumor treated with SMS 201-995. Lancet 1986;2:274.
908. Bonfils S, Ruszniewski P, Laucouret H, Castil J, Rene W, Mignon M. Long-term management of Zollinger-Ellison syndrome with SMS 201-995, a long-acting somatostatin analog. Can J Physiol Pharmacol 1986;63:6.
909. Erickson B, Oberg K, Alm G, et al. Treatment of malignant endocrine pancreatic tumors with human leukocyte interferon. Lancet 1986;2:1307.
910. Slimak GG, Pisegna J, Metz DL, Gardner JD, Jensen RT, Maton PN. Use of alpha interferon in patients with metastatic gastrinoma. Gastroenterology [Abstract] 1991;100:299.
911. Whipple AO. The surgical therapy of hyperinsulinism. J Int Chir 1938;3:237.
912. Galbut DL, Markowitz AM. Insulinoma: Diagnosis, surgical management and long-term followup. Am J Surg 1980;139:682.
913. Giercksky KE, Halse J, Mathisen W, et al. Endocrine tumors of the pancreas. Scand J Gastroenterol 1980;15:129.
914. Boden G. Insulinoma and glucagonoma. Semin Oncol 1987;14:253.
915. Fajans SS, Vinik AI. Insulin-producing islet cell tumors. Endocrinol Metab Clin North Am 1989;18:45.
916. Stefanini P, Carboni M, Patrassi N, Basoli A. Beta-islet cell tumor of the pancreas: Results of a study on 1,067 cases. Surgery 1974;75:597.
917. Service FJ, Dale AJ, Elveback LR, Jiang N. Insulinoma: Clinical and diagnostic features of 60 consecutive cases. Mayo Clin Proc 1976;51:417.
918. Glickman MH, Hart MJ, White TT. Insulinoma in Seattle: 39 cases in 30 years. Am J Surg 1980;140:119.
919. Nelson RL, Rizza RA, Service FJ. Documented hypoglycemia for 23 years in a patient with insulinoma. JAMA 1978;240:1891.
920. Boden G. Glucagonomas and insulinomas. Gastroenterol Clin North Am 1989;18:831.
921. Moller DE, Flier JS. Insulin resistance: Mechanisms, syndromes and implications. N Engl J Med 1991;325:938.
922. Grunberger G, Weiner JL, Silverman R, Taylor S, Gorden P. Factitious hypoglycemia due to surreptitious administration of insulin: Diagnosis, treatment and long-term follow-up. Ann Intern Med 1988;108:252.
923. Danforth DN, Gorden P, Brennan MF. Metastatic insulin secreting carcinoma of the pancreas: Clinical course and the role of surgery. Surgery 1984;96:1027.
924. Jensen RT, Norton JA. Pancreatic endocrine tumors. In: Sleisinger MH, Fordtran JS, Scharschmidt BF, Feldman M, eds. Gastrointestinal disease: Pathophysiology, diagnosis, management. Philadelphia: WB Saunders, 1992 (in press).
925. Dunnick NJ, Schaner JL, Doppman JL, et al. Computed tomography in adrenal tumors. AJR 1979;132:43.
926. Vinik AI, Delbridge L, Moattari R, Cho K, Thompson N. Transhepatic portal vein catheterization for localization of insulinomas: A ten-year experience. Surgery 1991;109:1.
927. Doppman JL, Miller DL, Chang R, Gorden P, Norton JA. Insulinomas localization with selective intraarterial injection of calcium. Radiology 1991;178:237.
928. Dunnick NR, Long JA, Krudy A, et al. Localizing insulinomas with combined radiographic methods. AJR 1980;135:747.
929. Doppman JL, Brennan MF, Dunnick NR, Kahn CR, Gorden P. The role of pancreatic venous sampling in the localization of occult insulinoma. Radiology 1981;138:557.
930. Norton JA, Sigel B, Baker AR, et al. Localization of an occult insulinoma by intraoperative ultrasonography. Surgery 1985;97:381.
931. Reubi JC, Lamberts SW, Maurer R. Somatostatin receptors in normal and tumoral tissues. Horm Res 1988;29:65.
932. Norton JA, Doppman JL, Jensen RT. Cancer of the endocrine system. In: DeVita VT, Hellman S, Rosenberg SA, eds. Cancer: Principles and practice of oncology. Philadelphia: JB Lippincott, 1989:1269–1344.
933. Tutt GO Jr, Edis AJ, Servie FJ, van Heerden JA. Plasma glucose monitoring during operation for insulinoma: A critical reappraisal. Surgery 1980;88:351.
934. Kudlow JE, Albisser AM, Angel A, et al. Insulinoma resection facilitated by the artificial endocrine pancreas. Diabetes 1978;27:774.
935. DeMarinis L, Barbarino A. Calcium antagonists and hormone release. I. Effects of verapamil on insulin release in normal subjects and patients with islet-cell tumor. Metabolism 1980;29:599.
936. Murakami K, Taniguchi H, Kobayshi T, Seki M, Olmon M, Baba S. Suppression of insulin release by calcium antagonist in human insulinoma in vivo and in vitro: Its possible role for clinical use. Kobe J Med Sci 1979;25:237.
937. Stehouwer CD, Lems WF, Fischer HR, Hackeng WH. Malignant insulinoma: Is combined treatment with verapamil and the long-acting somatostatin analogue octreotide (SMS 201-995) more effective than single therapy with either drug? Neth J Med 1989;35:86.
938. Blum I, Doron M, Laron Z, et al. Prevention of hypoglycemia attacks by propanolol in a patient suffering from insulinoma. Diabetes 1975;24:535.
939. Hofeldt FD, Dippe SE, Levin SR, Karam JH, Blum MR, Forsham PH. Effects of diphenylhydantoin upon glucose-induced insulin secretion in three patients with insulinoma. Diabetes 1974;23:192.
940. Gorden P, Comi RJ, Maton PN, Go VLW. Somatostatin and somatostatin analogue (SMS 201-995) in treatment of hormone-secreting tumors of the pituitary and gastrointestinal tract and non-neoplastic diseases of the gut. Ann Intern Med 1989;110:35.
941. Dunne MJ, Elton R, Fletcher T, Hofker PH, Shiu J. Somatostatin and gastroenteropancreatic endocrine tumors: Therapeutic characteristics. In: O'Dorisio TM, ed. Somatostatin in the treatment of GEP endocrine tumors. Berlin: Springer-Verlag, 1987:93.
942. Mozell E, Stenzel P, Woltering EA, Rosch J, O'Dorisio TM. Functional endocrine tumors of the pancreas clinical presentation, diagnosis, and treatment. Curr Probl Surg 1990;27:303.
943. Eckhauser FE, Cheung PS, Vinik AI, et al. Nonfunctioning malignant neuroendocrine tumors of the pancreas. Surgery 1986;100:978.
944. Vinik AI, Strodel WE, Eckhauser FE, et al. Somatostatinomas, PPomas, neurotensinomas. Semin Oncol 1987;14:263.
945. O'Dorisio TM, Vinik AI. Pancreatic polypeptide and mixed peptide-producing tumors of the gastrointestinal tract. In: Cohen S, Soloway RD, eds. Hormone-producing tumors of the gastrointestinal tract. London: Churchill Livingstone, 1985:117.
946. Walsh JH. Gastrointestinal hormones. In: Johnson LR, ed. Physiology of the gastrointestinal tract. New York: Raven Press, 1987:1981.
947. Vinik AI, Moattari AR. Treatment of endocrine tumors. Endocrinol Metab Clin North Am 1989;18:483.
948. Kent RB, van Heerden JA, Weiland LH. Nonfunctioning islet cell tumors. Ann Surg 1981;193:185.
949. Shaw JA, Vance RP, Geisinger KR, Marshall RB. Islet cell neoplasms: A fine needle aspiration cytology study with immunocytochemical correlations. Am J Clin Pathol 1990;94:142.
950. Hsiu J-G, D'Amato NA, Sperling MH, et al. Malignant islet-cell tumors of the pancreas diagnosed by fine needle aspiration biopsy: A case report. Acta Cytol 1985;29:556.
951. Lin TH, Tseng HC, Zhu Y, Zhong SX, Chen J, Cui QC. Insulinoma: An immunocytochemical and morphologic analysis of 95 cases. Cancer 1985;56:1420.
952. Sneige N, Ordonez NG, Vaenattukathil S, Samaan NA. Fine needle aspiration cytology in pancreatic endocrine tumors. Diagn Cytopathol 1987;3:35.
953. Schwartz TM. Atropine suppression test for pancreatic polypeptide. Lancet 1978;2:43.
954. Verner JV, Morrison AB. Islet cell tumor and a syndrome of refractory watery diarrhea and hypokalemia. Am J Med 1958;29:529.
955. Matsumoto KK, Peter JB, Schultze RG, et al. Watery diarrhea and hypokalemia associated with pancreatic islet cell adenoma. Gastroenterology 1967;52:695.
956. Verner JV, Morrison AB. Non-B islet tumors and the syndrome of watery diarrhea, hypokalemia and hypochlorhydria. Clin Gastroenterol 1974;3:595.
957. O'Dorisio TM, Mekhjian H, Gaginella TS. Medical therapy of VIPoma. Endocrinol Metab Clin North Am 1989;18:545.
958. Capella C, Polak JM, Butta R, et al. Morphologic patterns and diagnostic criteria of VIP-producing endocrine tumors: A histologic, histochemical, ultrastructural and biochemical study of 32 cases. Cancer 1983;52:1860.
959. Long RG, Bryant MG, Mitchell SJ, Adrian TE, Polak JM, Bloom SR. Clinicopathological study of pancreatic and ganglioneuroblastoma tumors secreting vasoactive intestinal polypeptide (VIPomas). Br Med J 1981;282:1767.
960. Verner JV, Morrison AB. Endocrine pancreatic islet disease with diarrhea: Report of a case due to diffuse hyperplasia of no beta islet tissue with a review of 54 additional cases. Arch Intern Med 1974;1974;133.
961. Bloom SR, Christofides ND, Yiengan T, et al. Peptide histidine isoleucine (PHI) and Verner-Morrison syndrome. Gut 1983;24:473.
962. Krejs GJ. VIPomas syndrome. Am J Med 1987;82:37.
963. Ginsberg AL. The VIP controversy: Stephen R. Bloom vs. Jerry D. Gardner. Dig Dis Sci 1978;23:30.
964. Kane MG, O'Dorisio TM, Krejs GJ. Production of secretory diarrhea by intravenous infusion of vasoactive intestinal peptide. N Engl J Med 1983;309:1482.

965. Laburthe M, Amiranoff B. Peptide receptors in intestinal epithelium. In: Makhlouf GM, ed. The gastrointestinal system: Handbook of physiology. Bethesda: American Physiological Society, 1989:215.
966. Krejs GJ. Comparison of the effect of VIP and PHI on water and ion movement in the canine jejunum in vivo. Gastroenterol Clin Biol 1984;8:868.
967. Mekhjian HS, O'Dorisio TM. VIPoma syndrome. Semin Oncol 1987;14:282.
968. Bloom SR, Long RG, Bryant MG, et al. Clinical, biochemical and pathological studies on 62 VIPomas. Gastroenterology 1980;78:1143.
969. Morris AI, Turnberg LA. Surreptitious laxative abuse. Gastroenterology 1979;77:780.
970. Read NW, Read MG, Krejs GJ, et al. A report of five patients with large volume secretory diarrhea but no evidence of endocrine tumor or laxative abuse. Dig Dis Sci 1982;27:193.
971. Read WN, Krejs G, Read MG, et al. Chronic diarrhea of unknown origin. Gastroenterology 1980;78:264.
972. Maton PN, O'Dorisio TM, Howe BA, et al. Effect of a long-acting somatostatin analogue (SMS 201-995) in a patient with pancreatic cholera. N Engl J Med 1985;312:17.
973. Mallinson CN, Bloom SR, Warin AP, et al. A glucagonoma syndrome. Lancet 1974;2:1.
974. Holst JJ. Glucagon-producing tumors. In: Cohen S, Soloway D, eds. Hormone producing tumors of the gastrointestinal tract. New York: Churchill Livingstone, 1985:57.
975. McGavran M. H, Unger RH, Recant L, et al. A glucagon-secreting alpha-cell carcinoma of the pancreas. N Engl J Med 1966;274:1408.
976. Wilkinson DS. Necrolytic migratory erythema with carcinoma of the pancreas. Trans St. John's Hosp Dermatol Soc 1973;59:244.
977. Guillausseau PJ, Gauillausseau C, Villet R, et al. Les glucagonomas: Aspect cliniques, biologiques, anatomo-pathologiques et therapeutiques (Revue general de 130 cas). Gastroenterol Clin Biol 1982;6:1029.
978. Leichter SB. Clinical and metabolic aspects of glucagonoma. Medicine 1980;59:100.
979. Stacpoole PW. The glucagonoma syndrome: Clinical features, diagnosis, and treatment. Endocr Rev 1981;2:347.
980. Bataille D. The gastrointestinal system. In: Makhlouf GN, ed. Handbook of physiology. Bethesda: American Physiological Society, 1989:455.
981. Abravia C, De Bartolo M, Katzen R, Lawrence AM. Disappearance of glucagonoma rash after surgical resection, but not during dietary normalization of serum amino acids. Am J Clin Nutr 1984;39:351.
982. Yamada T, Chiha T. Somatostatin. In: Makhlouf GN, ed. The gastrointestinal system: Handbook of physiology. Bethesda: American Physiological Society, 1979:431.
983. Ganda PO, Weir GC, Soeldner JS, et al. Somatostatinoma: A somatostatin-containing tumor of the endocrine pancreas. N Engl J Med 1977;296:963.
984. Larsson LI, Hirsch MA, Holst J, et al. Pancreatic somatostatinoma clinical features and physiologic implications. Lancet 1977;1:1666.
985. Krejs GJ, Orci L, Conlon M, et al. Somatostatinoma syndrome (biochemical, morphological, and clinical features). N Engl J Med 1979;301:285.
986. Boden G, Shimoyama R. Somatostatinoma. In: Cohen S, Soloway RD, eds. Hormone-producing tumors of the gastrointestinal tract. New York: Churchill Livingstone, 1985:85.
987. Konomi K, Chijiiwa K, Katsuta T, Yamaguchi K. Pancreatic somatostatinoma: A case report and review of the literature. J Surg Oncol 1990;43:259.
988. Soldati TK, Delnoce G, Garino M, Farin EC, De Paolis P, Balba G. Pancreatic somatostatinoma. Pan Minerva Med 1990;32:141.
989. Rivier J, Spress J, Thorner M, Vale W. Characterization of a growth-hormone releasing factor from a human pancreatic islet cell tumor. Nature 1982;300:276.
990. Thorner MO, Perryman RL, Cronin MJ, et al. Somatotroph hyperplasia. J Clin Invest 1982;70:965.
991. Guillemin R, Brazeau P, Bohlen P, Esch F, Ling N, Wehrenberg W. Growth hormone-releasing factor from a human pancreatic tumor that caused acromegaly. Science 1982;27:774.
992. Berger C, Trouillas J, Bloch B, et al. Multihormonal carcinoid tumors of the pancreas: Secreting growth hormone-releasing factor as a cause of acromegaly. Cancer 1984;54:2097.
993. Sano T, Yamasaki R, Saito H, et al. Growth hormone-releasing hormone (GHRH) secreting pancreatic tumor in a patient with multiple endocrine neoplasia type 1. Surg Pathol 1987;11:810.
994. Moller DE, Moses AC, Jones K, Thorner MO, Vance ML. Octreotide suppresses both growth hormone (GH) and GH-releasing hormone (GHRH) in acromegaly due to ectopic GHRH secretion. J Clin Endocrinol Metab 1989;68:499.
995. Von Werder K, Losa M, Stalla FK, et al. Long-term treatment of a metastasizing GRFoma with a somatostatin analogue (SMS 201-995) in a girl with gigantism. Scand J Gastroenterol 1986;21:238.
996. Christofides ND, Stephanou A, Suzuki H, Yianigou Y, Bloom SR. Distribution of immunoreactive growth hormone-releasing hormone in the human brain and intestine and its production by tumors. J Clin Endocrinol Metab 1984;59:747.
997. Bostwick DG, Quan R, Hoffman AR, Webber RJ, Chang J-R, Bensch KG. Growth-hormone-releasing factor immunoreactivity in human endocrine tumors. Am J Pathol 1984;117;167.
998. Dayal Y, Lin HD, Tallberg K, Reichlin BAS, DeLellis RA, Wolfe JH. Immunocytochemical demonstration of growth hormone-releasing factor in gastrointestinal and pancreatic endocrine tumors. Am J Clin Pathol 1986;85:13.
999. Barkan AL. Acromegaly: Diagnosis and therapy. Endocrinol Metab Clin North Am 1989;18:277.
1000. Barkan AL, Shenker Y, Grekin RJ, et al. Acromegaly from ectopic GHRH secretion by a malignant carcinoid tumor: Successful treatment with long-acting somatostatin analogue SMS Cancer 1986;61:221.
1001. Melmed S, Ziel FH, Braustein GD, et al. Medical management of acromegaly due to ectopic production of GHRH by a carcinoid tumor. J Clin Endocrinol Met 1988;67:395.
1002. Wilson DM, Hoffman AR. Reduction of pituitary size by the somatostatin analogue SMS 201-995 in a patient with an islet cell tumour secreting growth hormone releasing factor. Acta Endocrinol 1986;113:23.
1003. Caplan PH, Koob L, Abellera RM, et al. Cure of acromegaly by operative removal of an islet cell tumor of the pancreas. Am J Med 1978;64:874.
1004. Fuerle GE, Helmstaedter V, Tischbirek K, et al. A multihormonal tumor of the pancreas producing neurotensin. Dig Dis Sci 1981;26:1125.
1005. Gutniak M, Rosenqvist U, Grimelius L. Report on a patient with watery diarrhea syndrome caused by a pancreatic tumour containing neurotensin, enkephalin and calcitonin. Acta Med Scand 1980;208:95.
1006. Bloom SR, Lee YC, Lacroute JM. Two patients with pancreatic apudomas secreting neurotensin and VIP. Gut 1983;24:448.
1007. Wood JR, Wood SM, Lee YC. Neurotensin-secreting carcinoma of the bronchus. Postgrad Med J 1983;59:46.
1008. Shulkes A, Boden R, Cook I, et al. Characterization of a pancreatic tumor containing vasoactive intestinal peptide, neurotensin and pancreatic polypeptide. J Clin Endocrinol Metab 1984;58:41.
1009. Maier W, Schumacher A, Etzrodt H, et al. A neurotensinoma of the head of the pancreas: Demonstration by ultrasound and computed tomography. Eur J Radiol 1982;2:125.
1010. Ferris CF. Neurotensin. In: Makhlouf GN, ed. The gastrointestinal tract: Handbook of physiology. Bethesda: American Physiological Society, 1989:559.
1011. Clark ES, Carney JA. Pancreatic islet cell tumor associated with Cushing's syndrome. Am J Surg Pathol 1984;8:917.
1012. Deftos LJ, McMillan PJ, Sartinano GP, Abuid J, Robinson AG. Simultaneous ectopic production of parathyroid hormone and calcitonin. Metabolism 1976;25:543.
1013. Arps H, Dietel M, Schulz A, Janzarik H, Kloppel G. Pancreatic endocrine carcinoma with ectopic PTH-production and paraneoplastic hypercalcaemia. Virchows Arch [A] 1986;408:497.
1014. Cryer PE, Hill GJ. Pancreatic islet cell carcinoma with hypercalcemia and hypergastrinemia. Cancer 1976;38:2217.
1015. Palmieri GMA, Nordquist RE, Omenn GS. Immunochemical localization of parathyroid hormone in cancer tissue from patients with ectopic hyperparathyroidism. J Clin Invest 1974;53:1726.
1016. Rasbach DA, Hammond JM. Pancreatic islet cell carcinoma with hypercalcemia: Primary hyperparathyroidism or hormonal hypercalcemia of malignancy. Am J Med 1985;78:337.
1017. Bresler L, Boissel P, Conroy T, Grosdidier J. Pancreatic islet cell carcinoma with hypercalcemia: Complete remission 5 years after surgical excision and chemotherapy. Am J Gastroenterol 1991;86:635.
1018. Ajani JA, Levin B, Wallace S. Systemic and regional therapy of advanced islet cell tumors. Gastroenterol Clin North Am 1989;18:923.
1019. Kvols LK, Buck M. Chemotherapy of the metastatic carcinoid and islet cell tumors: A review. Am J Med 1987;82:77.
1020. Herr RR, Jahnke HK, Argoudelis AD. The structure of streptozotocin. J Am Chem Soc 1967;98:4808.
1021. Weiss RB. Streptozotocin: A review of its pharmacology, efficacy, and toxicity. Cancer Treat Rep 1982;66:427.
1022. Rakieten N, Rakieten ML, Nadkani MV. Studies of the diabetogenic action of streptozotocin (NSC-37917). Cancer Chemother Rep 1969;29:91.
1023. Murray-Lyon IM, Eddelsteon ALWF, Williams R, et al. Treatment of multiple hormone producing malignant islet cell tumor with streptozotocin. Lancet 1968;2:895.
1024. Moertel CG, Kvols LK, O'Connell MJ, Rubin J. Treatment of neuroendocrine carcinomas with combined etoposide and cisplatin. Cancer 1991;68:227.
1025. Duncan LA, Marynick SP. Glucagonoma and Dacarbazine. Ann Intern Med 1982;97:930.
1026. Kessinger A, Lemon HM, Foley JF. The glucagonoma syndrome and its management. J Surg Oncol 1977;9:419.
1027. Strauss GM, Weitzman SA, Aoki TT. Dimethyltriazenoimidazole carboxamide therapy of malignant glucagonomas. Ann Intern Med 1979;90:57.
1028. Marynick SP, Fagadau WR, Duncan LA. Malignant glucagonoma syndrome. Response to chemotherapy. Ann Intern Med 1980;93:453.
1029. Prinz RA, Budrinath K, Banerji M, et al. Operations and chemotherapeutic management of malignant glucagon producing tumors. Surgery 1981;90:713.
1030. Awrich AE, Peetz M, Fletcher WS. Dimethyltriazenoimidazole carboxamide therapy of islet cell carcinomas of the pancreas. J Surg Oncol 1981;17:321.
1031. Kurose T, Seino Y, Ishida LT, et al. Successful treatment of metastatic glucagonoma with dacarbazine. Lancet 1984;1:621.
1032. McFadden D, Jaffe BN. Surgical approaches to endocrine-producing tumors of the gastrointestinal tract. In: Cohen S, Soloway RD, eds. Hormone producing tumors of the gastrointestinal tract. New York: Churchill Livingstone, 1985:139.
1033. Valette PJ, Souquet JC. Pnacreatic islet cell tumors metastatic to the liver: Treatment by hepatic artery chemo-embolization. Horm Res 1989;32:77.
1034. Redding TW, Schally AV. Inhibition of growth of pancreatic carcinomas in animal models by analogs of hypothalamic hormones. Proc Natl Acad Sci USA 1984;84:248.
1035. Lamberts SW, Hofland LJ, van Koetsveld PM, et al. Parallel in vivo and in vitro detection of functional somatostatin receptors in human endocrine tumors: Consequences with regard to diagnosis, localization and therapy. J Clin Endocrinol Metab 1990;31:566.

1036. Oberg K, Lindstrom H, Alm G, Lundquist G. Successful treatment of therapy-resistant pancreatic cholera with human leukocyte interferon. Lancet 1985;1:725.
1037. Anderson JV, Bloom SR. Treatment of malignant endocrine tumors with human leukocyte interferon. Lancet 1987;1:97.
1038. Balentine JD. Pathology of oxygen toxicity. New York: Academic Press, 1982.
1039. Wermer P. Endocrine adenomatosis: Peptic ulcer in a large kindred. Am J Med 1963;35:205.
1040. Loeb JN. Polyglandular disorders. In: Wyngaarden JB, Smith LH, eds. Cecil textbook of medicine. Philadelphia: WB Saunders, 1982:1304.
1041. Oberg K, Skogseid B, Eriksson N. Multiple endocrine neoplasia type I. Acta Oncol 1989;28:383.
1042. Radford DM, Ashley SW, Wells SA Jr, Gerhard DS. Loss of heterozygosity of markers on chromosome 11 in tumors with patients with multiple endocrine neoplasia syndrome I. Cancer Res 1991;50:1154.
1043. Larsson C, Skogseid B, Oberg K, et al. Multiple endocrine neoplasia type I gene maps to chromosome 11 and is lost in insulinoma. Nature 1988;332:85.
1044. Bystrom C, Larsson C, Blomberg C, et al. Localization of the MEN-1 gene to a small region within chromosome 11 q 13 by deletion mapping in tumors. Proc Natl Acad Sci USA 1990;87:1968.
1045. Knudson AG. Mutation and cancer: Statistical study of retinoblastoma. Proc Natl Acad Sci USA 1971;68:820.
1046. Bale A. E, Norton JA, Wong EL, et al. Allelic loss on chromosome 11 in hereditary and sporadic tumors related to familial multiple endocrine neoplasia type 1. Cancer Res 1991;51:1154.
1047. Brandi ML, Aurbach GD, Fitzpatrick LA, et al. Parathyroid mitogenic activity in plasma from patients with familial multiple endocrine neoplasia type I. N Engl J Med 1986;314:1287.
1048. Brandi ML. Multiple endocrine neoplasia type I: General features and new insights into etiology. J Endocrinol Invest 1991;14:61.
1049. Zimmering MB, Brandi ML, de Grange DA, et al. Circulating fibroblast growth factor-like substance in familial multiple endocrine neoplasia-type I. J Clin Endocrinol Metab 1990;70:149.
1050. Thakker RV, Bonloux P, Wooding C, et al. Association of parathyroid tumors in multiple endocrine neoplasia type 1 with loss of alleles on chromosome 11. N Engl J Med 1989;321:60.
1051. Bone HG. Diagnosis of multiglandular endocrine neoplasias. Clin Chem 1990;36:711.
1052. Leight GS, Hensley MI. Management of familial hyperparathyroidism. Prog Surg 1987;184:106.
1053. Wells SA Jr, Farndon JR, Dale JK, et al. Long-term evaluation of patients with primary parathyroid hyperplasia managed by total parathyroidectomy and heterotopic autotransplantation. Ann Surg 1980;192:451.
1054. Prinz RA, Gamvros OI, Seller D, Lynn JA. Subtotal parathyroidectomy for primary chief cell hyperplasia of the multiple endocrine neoplasia type I syndrome. Ann Surg 1981;193:26.
1055. Rizzoli R, Green J, Marx SJ. Primary hyperparathyroidism in familial multiple endocrine neoplasia type I. Long-term follow-up of serum calcium levels after parathyroidectomy. Am J Med 1985;78:467.
1056. Thompson NW, Lloyd RV, Nishiyama RH, et al. MEN-1 pancreas:a histological and immuno-histochemical study. World J Surg 1984;8:561.
1057. Kloppel G, Willemar S, Stamm B, et al. Pancreatic lesions and hormonal profile in pancreatic tumors in multiple endocrine neoplasia type I. Cancer 1986;57:1820.
1058. Thompson NW. Surgical considerations in the MEN-1 syndrome. In: Johnston IDA, Thompson NW, eds. Endocrine surgery. Butterworths, London: 1983:144–163.
1059. Friesen SR, Tomita T, Kimmel JR. Pancreatic polypeptide update: Its role in detection of the trait for multiple endocrine adenopathy syndrome, type I and pancreatic polypeptide-secreting tumors. Surgery 1983;94:1028.
1060. Rasbach DA, van Heerden JA, Telandar RL, et al. Surgical management of hyperinsulinism in the multiple endocrine neoplasia, type I syndrome. Arch Surg 1985;120:584.
1061. Lamers CB, Stadil F, Tongeren JMH. Prevalence of endocrine abnormalities in patients with the Zollinger-Ellison syndrome and their families. Am J Med 1981;64:687.
1062. Eisenberg AA, Wallerstein H. Pheochromocytoma of the suprarenal medulla (paraglioma): A clinicopathological study. Arch Pathol 1932;14:818.
1063. Hazard JB, Hawk WH, Creile G Jr. Medullary (solid) carcinoma of the thyroid-clinicopathologic entity. J Clin Endocrinol Metab 1979;19:704.
1064. Norton JA, Wells SA Jr. Medullary thyroid carcinoma and multiple endocrine neoplasia type-II syndromes. In: Friesen S, ed. Surgical endocrinology. Philadelphia: JB Lippincott, 1988.
1065. Tashjian AH Jr, Howland BG, Melvin KEW, Hill CS Jr. Immunoassay of human calcitonin: Clinical measurement, relation to serum calcium and studies in patients with medullary carcinoma. N Engl J Med 1970;283:890.
1066. Jackson CE, Block MA, Greenawald KA, et al. The two-mutational event theory in medullary thyroid cancer. Am J Hum Genet 1979;31:704.
1067. Wolfe HJ, Melvin KEW, Cervi-Skinner SJ, et al. C-cell hyperplasia preceding medullary thyroid carcinoma. N Engl J Med 1973;189:437.
1068. Sipple JH. The association of pheochromocytoma with carcinoma of the thyroid gland. Am J Med 1961;31:163.
1069. Williams ED. A review of 17 cases of carcinoma of the thyroid and pheochromocytoma. J Clin Pathol 1965;18:288.
1070. Schimke RN, Hartmann WH. Familial amyloid-producing medullary thyroid carcinoma and pheochromocytoma: A distinct genetic entity. Ann Intern Med 1965;63:1027.
1071. Manning PC, Molnar GD, Black BM, Priestly JT, Woolner LB. Pheochromocytoma, hyperparathyroidism and thyroid carcinoma occurring coincidentally. N Engl J Med 1963;268:68.
1072. Williams ED, Pollock DJ. Multiple mucosal neuromata with endocrine tumors: A syndrome alluded to von Recklinghausen's disease. J Path Bacteriol 1989;91:71.
1073. Simpson NE, Kidd KK, Goodfellow PJ, et al. Assignment of multiple endocrine neoplasia type 2a to chromosome 10 by linkage. Nature 1987;328:528.
1074. Sobol H, Narod SA, Nakamura Y, et al. Screening for multiple endocrine neoplasia 2a with DNA polymorphism analysis. N Engl J Med 1989;312:996.
1075. Telenius H, Mathew CGP, Nakamura Y, et al. Application of DNA markers to screening families with multiple endocrine neoplasia 2A. Eur J Surg Oncol 1990;16:134.
1076. Wu JS, Larson NL, Myers S, et al. The genetic defect in multiple endocrine neoplasia type 2A maps next to the centrosome of chromosome 10. Am J Hum Genet 1990;46:624.
1077. Mathew GCP, Easton DF, Nakamura Y, et al. Presymptomatic screening for multiple endocrine neoplasia type 2A with linked DNA markers. Lancet 1991;337:7.
1078. Norum RA, Lafreniere R, O'Neal LW, et al. Linkage of multiple endocrine neoplasia type 2B gene (MEN2B) to chromosome 10 markers linked to MEN2A. Genomics 1990;8:313.
1079. Jackson CE, Norum RH, O'Neal LW, Nikolai TF, DeLaney JP. Linkage between MEN 2B and chromosome 10 markers linked to MEN 2A. Am J Hum Genet [Abstract] 1988;45:154.
1080. Grun R, Eberle F. Ergebn Inner Mediz Kinderheildk 1981;46:151.
1081. Keiser HR, Beaven MA, Doppman J, et al. Sipple's syndrome: Medullary thyroid carcinoma, pheochromocytoma and parathyroid disease. Ann Intern Med 1973;78:561.
1082. Wells SA Jr. Multiple endocrine neoplasia type II: Recent results. Cancer Res 1990;18:71.
1083. Easton DF, Ponder MA, Cummings TA, et al. The clinical and screening-age-at-onset distribution for the MEN-2 syndrome. Am J Hum Genet 1989;44:208.
1084. Wells SA Jr, Baylin SG, Leight GS, et al. The importance of early diagnosis in patients with hereditary medullary thyroid carcinoma. Ann Surg 1982;195:505.
1085. Wells SA Jr, Baylin SB, Gann DW, et al. Medullary thyroid carcinoma: Relationship of method of diagnosis to pathological staging. Ann Surg 1978;188:377.
1086. Melvin KEW, Miller HH, Tashjian AH Jr. Early diagnosis of medullary carcinoma of the thyroid by means of calcitonin assay. N Engl J Med 1971;285:1115.
1087. Wells SA Jr, Baylin SG, Linehan WM, et al. Provocative agents and the diagnosis of medullary carcinoma of the thyroid gland. Ann Surg 1978;188:139.
1088. Valk TW, Frager MW, Gross MD, et al. Spectrum of pheochromocytoma in multiple endocrine neoplasia: A scintigraphic portrayal using ^{131}I-metaiodobenzylguanidine. Ann Intern Med 1981;94:762.
1089. Shapiro B, Fig LM. Management of pheochromocytoma. Endocrinol Metab Clin North Am 1989;18:443.
1090. Wells SA Jr, Baylin SG, Johnsrude IS, et al. Thyroid venous catheterization in the early diagnosis of familial medullary thyroid carcinoma. Ann Surg 1982;196:505.
1091. Hull CJ. Pheochromocytoma: Diagnosis, preoperative preparation and anesthetic management. Br J Aneaesth 1986;58:1453.
1092. Farndon JR, Fagraeus L, Wells SA Jr. Recent developments in the management of phaechromocytoma. In: Johnston IDA, Thompson NW, eds. Endocrine surgery. London: Butterworths, 1983:189–201.
1093. Jackson CE, Talpos GB, Kanbouris A, et al. The clinical course after definitive operation for medullary thyroid carcinoma. Surgery 1983;94:995.
1094. Harsoulis P, Leontsini M, Economou A, et al. Fine needle aspiration biopsy cytology in the diagnosis of thyroid cancer: Comparative study of 213 operated patients. Br J Surg 1986;73:461.
1095. Abu-Nema T, Ayyash K, Tibblin S. Role of aspiration biopsy cytology in the diagnosis of cold solitary nodules. Br J Surg 1987;74:203.
1096. Ramacciotti CE, Pretorius HT, Chu EW, et al. Diagnostic accuracy and use of aspiration biopsy in the management of thyroid nodules. Arch Intern Med 1984;144:11669.
1097. Schroder DM, Chambous A, France CJ. Operative strategy for thyroid cancer: Is total thyroidectomy worth the price? Cancer 1986;58:2320.
1098. Crile G, Pontius KI, Hawk WA. Factors influencing the survival of patients with follicular carcinoma of the thyroid gland. Surg Gynecol Obstet 1985;160:409.
1099. Savino D, Sibley RK, Sumner H. Significance of Hurthle cell in thyroid neoplasms: Reexamination of an old but persistent problem. Lab Invest [Abstract] 1981;44:59.
1100. Caplan RH, Abellera RM, Kisken WA. Hurthle cell tumors of the thyroid gland: A clinicopathologic review and long-term follow-up. JAMA 1984;251:3114.
1101. Gosain AK, Clark OH. Hurthle cell neoplasms. Arch Surg 1984;119:515.
1102. Sokal M, Harmar GI. Chemotherapy for anaplastic carcinoma of the thyroid. Clin Oncol 1978;4:3.
1103. Macfarlane DA. Cancer of the adrenal cortex. Ann R Coll Surg 1958;23:155.
1104. Chun HG, Yagoda A, Kemeny N. Cisplatin for adrenal cortical carcinoma. Cancer Treat Rep 1983;67:513.
1105. Kahler HJ, Heilmeyer L. Klinikund pathophysiologie des karzinoids und karzinoid-syndroms unter besonderer beruck sichtigung der pharmacologie des 5-hydroxyptamins. Ergeb Inn Med Kinderheildk 1961;16:291.
1106. Valimaki M, Harvinen H, Salmela P, Sane T, Sjoblom S-J, Pelkenon R. Is the treatment of metastatic carcinoid tumor with interferon not as successful as suggested? Cancer 1991;67:547.
1107. Bukowski RM, Stephens R, Oishi N, Pedersen R, Chen T. Phase II trials of 5-FU, adriamycin, cyclophosphamide and streptozotocin in metastatic carcinoid. Proc Amer Soc Clin Oncol 1983;2:130.

1108. Hancke S. Localization of hormone-producing gastrointestinal tumors by ultrasonic scanning. Scand J Gastroenterol 1979;53:115.

1109. Wilson SD. The role of surgery in children with Zollinger-Ellison syndrome. Surgery 1982;92:682.

1110. Vogel SB, Wolfe MM, McGuigan JE. Localization and resection of gastrinomas in Zollinger-Ellison syndrome. Ann Surg 1987;205:550.

1111. Delcore R, Hermeck AS, Friesen SR. Selective surgical management of correctable hypergastrinemia. Surgery 1989;106:1094.

1112. Moertel CG, Lavin PT, Hahn RG. Phase II trial of doxorubicin for advanced islet cell carcinoma. Cancer Treat Rep 1982;66:1567.

1113. Bukowski RM, McCracken JD, Balcerzek SP, et al. Phase II study of chlorozotocin in islet cell carcinoma. Cancer Chemother Pharmacol 1983;11:48.

1114. Frame J, Kelsen D, Kemeny N, et al. A Phase II trial of streptozotocin and adriamycin in advanced APUD tumors. Am J Oncol 1988;11:490.

1115. Bonfils S, Ruszniewski P, Haffar S, Laucouret H. Chemotherapy of hepatic metastases (HM) in Zollinger-Ellison syndrome (ZES): Report of a multicenteric analysis. Dig Dis Sci 1986;31:51.

1116. Kvols LK, Buck M, Moertel CG, et al. Treatment of metastatic islet cell tumors with a somatostatin analogue. Ann Intern Med 1987;107:162.

1117. Rothmund M, Angelini L, Brunt M, et al. Treatment of metastatic islet cell tumors with a somatostatin analogue. Ann Intern Med 1990;14:393.

1118. Rayfield EJ, Goldberg IJ, Gregerich EW, et al. Transportal blood sampling for preoperative localization of insulinoma. Mt Sinai J Med 1983;50:258.

1119. Cho KJ, Vinik AI, Thompson NHD, et al. Localization of the source of hyperinsulinism. AJR 1982;139:237.

Cancer: Principles & Practice of Oncology, Fourth Edition,
edited by Vincent T. DeVita, Jr., Samuel Hellman, Steven A. Rosenberg.
J.B. Lippincott Co., Philadelphia © 1993.

James C. Yang
Steven A. Rosenberg
Eli J. Glatstein
Karen H. Antman

CHAPTER **42**

Sarcomas of Soft Tissues

Soft tissues refer to the extraskeletal connective tissues of the body that connect, support, and surround other discrete anatomic structures. This portion of the body mass lying between the epidermis and parenchymal organs includes the organs of locomotion, such as muscles and tendons, and supportive tissue structures, such as fibrous tissue, fat, and synovial tissue. The soft somatic tissues are ubiquitous and comprise more than 50% of body weight. The more than 400 muscles in the human body comprise about 40% of adult body weight.

Soft tissue sarcomas refer to malignant tumors arising in the soft tissues, and they are grouped together because of similarities in pathologic appearance, clinical presentation, and behavior. A combination of embryologic, functional, and morphologic characterizations define this tumor group.

The Greek word *sarkoma* means a fleshy growth, and virtually all tumors included in the soft tissue sarcomas arise from a common embryonic ancestry, the primitive mesoderm (Table 42–1). Nine to 13 days after fertilization of the ovum, the human embryo undergoes a transition from a phase of increasing cell number to a phase of morphologic organization into the endoderm, ectoderm, and mesoderm, the three primary germ layers of the embryo.[1] Within these layers are established commitments to developmental potentials that far precede morphologic differentiation of the cells.

The primitive mesoderm gives rise to organs such as the kidney, ureter, oviducts, uterus, gonads, and heart and a wide range of hematopoietic, lymphatic, and reticuloendothelial tissues. The primitive mesenchyme, a loose network of cells and intercellular matrix within the mesoderm, is largely responsible for the development of the common connective tissues of the body listed in Table 42–1. Tumors of these connective tissues are referred to as soft tissue sarcomas. Because of similarities in anatomic sites of origin, clinical presentation, and clinical behavior, tumors arising in Schwann cells, a class of cells surrounding peripheral nerves that arise from the neural tube of the primitive ectoderm, are also included in the category of soft tissue sarcomas.

Malignant tumors are categorized as sarcomas or carcinomas based on whether they arise from connective tissue (*i.e.*, sarcomas) or epithelial tissue (*i.e.*, carcinomas). This differentiation is imprecise, and many sarcomas arise from tissues that fit the morphologic criteria of epithelium. Epithelium is a morphologic, not embryologic, term that is used to designate cellular structures that cover or line surfaces on or in the body and may arise from ectoderm, endoderm, or mesoderm. The endothelium lining the vascular and lymphatic channels and the mesothelium lining the body cavities and visceral organs are two types of epithelium that arise from the mesoderm. These epithelial structures give rise to malignant tumors that resemble and behave like tumors that develop from connective tissue cells. Tumors arising from the endothelium and the mesothelium are included in the category of sarcomas. Sarcomas arise mostly from mesodermal structures and from connective tissue cells. Some sarcomas arise from ectodermal structures, and some arise from epithelium.

This chapter describes the natural history and treatment of the soft tissue sarcomas. All visceral organs contain connective tissue stroma that can undergo malignant transformation. These visceral sarcomas are discussed in the chapters dealing with individual organ systems.

INCIDENCE

Approximately 5800 new cases of soft tissue sarcoma and 3300 deaths from this disease occurred in the United States in 1991.[2]

TABLE 42-1. Embryonic Derivation of the Soft Tissue and Bony Sarcomas

Fertilized ovum
↓
Blastoderm (day 9–13)

- Endoderm
  - GI tract
  - Lungs, and so on
- Mesoderm
  - Hematopoietic system
  - Genitourinary system
  - Heart
  - Connective tissue and smooth muscle of viscera → Visceral sarcomas
  - Pleura, Peritoneum, Pericardium, Blood vessels (wall, endothelium), Bone, Cartilage, Muscle, Soft connective tissues (fibrous, synovial, and so on) → Soft tissue and bony sarcomas
- Ectoderm
  - Skin
    - Mammary gland, and so on
  - Nervous system
    - Brain
    - Spinal cord
    - Adrenal medulla
    - Schwann cells → Soft tissue and bony sarcomas

The annual age-adjusted incidence was 2 per 100,000 persons. Data from New Zealand suggest that the incidence and mortality from soft tissue sarcomas have been increasing (from 1.3 per 100,000 men in 1955 to 2.2 per 100,000 men in 1977) in that country, although no change in incidence was seen in Denmark during the same period.[3,4] There appears to be no sex or racial pattern for these cancers in the United States.

Soft tissue sarcomas comprise 0.7% of all cancers, although these tumors comprise 6.5% of all cancers in children younger than 15 years of age.[2] Soft tissue sarcomas rank fifth in cancer incidence among children younger than 15, behind leukemia, central nervous system cancers, lymphomas, and sympathetic nervous system cancers. Soft tissue sarcomas rank fifth as a cause of cancer death in this age group behind leukemia, nervous system cancers, renal cancer, and bone cancer.

EPIDEMIOLOGY

Little is known about epidemiologic or etiologic factors of importance in patients with soft tissue sarcomas. There is no proven genetic predisposition to the development of soft tissue sarcomas, although Li and Fraumeni reported four kindreds with pairs of young children (*i.e.,* three sets of siblings and one set of cousins) with soft tissue sarcomas.[5] This incidence exceeded that expected on a chance basis ($p = 0.06$).

This familial cancer syndrome is associated with an increased incidence of soft tissue sarcoma and with breast cancer, osteosarcoma, brain tumors, leukemia, and adrenal carcinoma. Although these kindreds have germline abnormalities of the tumor suppressor gene p53, somatic mutations of p53 are found in only a portion of sporadic, nonfamilial sarcomas.[6,7]

There have been several reports of childhood sarcomas associated with a small increase in incidence of other familial cancers (especially breast cancer) that tended to occur in mothers younger than 30 years of age.[5,8–14] Lymphangiosarcoma of the arm in women after mastectomy and axillary lymph node ablation (Stewart-Treves syndrome) almost certainly does not represent evidence of an etiologic correlation between mammary cancer and sarcoma of soft tissue, but rather is the development of lymphangiosarcoma in lymphedematous arms.[15]

Although Sloane and Hubbel reported an increased incidence of congenital defects in children with soft tissue sarcomas, this association was not seen by Li and Fraumeni.[8,16]

Soft tissue sarcomas are thought to occur with slightly increased frequency in patients with a variety of genetically transmitted diseases, such as the basal cell nevus syndrome, tuberous sclerosis, Werner's syndrome, intestinal polyposis, and Gardner's syndrome.[14,17–21] Patients with multiple neurofibromatosis (von Recklinghausen's disease) have approximately a 15% chance of developing a neurofibrosarcoma.[18]

Although many patients with soft tissue sarcomas present with a recent history of trauma, it is likely that minor trauma merely calls a preexisting lesion to the patient's attention.

Chemical carcinogens, such as 3-methylcholanthrene, and viruses can cause soft tissue sarcomas in experimental animals, but there is no convincing link between these factors and sarcomas in humans. Studies in Sweden in 1979 and 1981 linked environmental exposure to phenoxyacetic acids (a class of herbicides) and chlorophenols (wood preservatives) to a sixfold increase in the risk of developing soft tissue sarcoma.[22,23] These studies were based on small numbers of patients, and a later analysis of more than 350,000 Swedish agricultural and forestry workers potentially exposed to these chemicals failed to confirm this association.[24] A case-control study from New Zealand failed to find an association between exposure to phenoxyherbicides and the incidence of soft tissue sarcomas, and an analysis of data from Denmark also cast doubt on this association.[3,4] Because of the early Swedish reports, there was concern that Vietnam veterans exposed to Agent Orange, a mixture of two commercial phenoxyacetic acid herbicides containing trace amounts of dioxins, might have an increased incidence of soft tissue sarcomas, but two studies failed to show a significant correlation.[25,26]

Sarcomas have a tendency to occur in areas previously exposed to ionizing radiation, although sarcomas in radiation therapy fields are uncommon. In 1977, Adam and Reif could find only 7 cases in the world literature of fibrosarcoma of the chest wall in women undergoing radiation therapy after mastectomy for breast cancer.[27] The latent period of these lesions averaged 15 years after radiation exposure. An additional 7 cases were described by Kuten and colleagues in 1985.[28] Sixteen cases of radiation-induced sarcomas of the chest wall occurred at the M.D. Anderson Cancer Center in Houston between 1944 and 1984, representing 5% of the 331 sarcomas of the chest wall that were seen during that period.[29] Similar findings were reported by O'Neil and colleagues, who reviewed 11 patients with soft tissue fibrosarcomas after irradiation of the chest wall for breast cancer.[30]

Halperin and colleagues reported 5 cases of bone or soft tissue sarcomas occurring more than 5 years after treatment of Hodgkin's disease.[31] Two of these patients had received radiation therapy alone, 2 were treated with a combination of radiation and chemotherapy, and 1 received chemotherapy alone. Four cases of soft tissue sarcoma and 1 case of osteosarcoma occurred, with latent periods of 6 to 11 years. These investigators calculated the risk of developing a sarcoma in 5-year survivors of Hodgkin's disease to be 0.9%.

Osteosarcomas appear to be the most common sarcomas induced by radiation. Arlen and associates summarized 50 cases of postirradiation osteosarcoma, and Martland described osteosarcoma developing after ingestion of radium and mesothorium during the painting of luminous watch dials.[32,33]

Sarcomas are associated with foreign-body implantations in rodents, and sporadic reports of this phenomenon in humans have appeared.[34] Ott tabulated all cases published before 1966.[35] The responsible foreign bodies were mainly metal implants, bullets, shrapnel pieces, and bone transplants, with latent periods of as long as 40 years. The true incidence of foreign-body-induced sarcomas is probably minimal, because no sarcomas were seen among 11,000 women who underwent augmentation mammoplasty with a variety of materials or in 281 patients who underwent prosthetic replacement for facial defects.[36,37]

SITES OF SOFT TISSUE SARCOMAS

Because of the ubiquitous nature of the connective tissues, soft tissue sarcomas can arise anywhere in the body. Visceral sarcomas arise from the connective stroma found in all organs and are rarer than sarcomas originating in somatic sites. Visceral sarcomas are not considered in this chapter. Sites of somatic soft tissue sarcomas from nine reported series are presented in Table 42–2.[38–46] Approximately 60% of sarcomas occur in the extremities. The ratio of lower-extremity to upper-extremity tumors is 3 to 1. About 75% of lower-extremity sarcomas originate at or above the knee. Other sites include the head and neck regions (9%) and the trunk (31%). Within the trunk, approximately 40% of tumors are located in the retroperitoneum, and the remaining tumors are located in the abdominal wall, chest wall, mediastinum, and breast. Treatment approaches for patients with soft tissue sarcomas must consider the site of the origin of the tumor.

PATHOLOGIC CLASSIFICATION

PRINCIPLES OF CLASSIFICATION

Each of the soft tissues can give rise to benign and malignant groups of tumors. The transformation of a benign soft tissue tumor into a malignant sarcoma is rare. Because of the many different soft tissues, a variety of histologically distinct, but often grossly similar, sarcomas have been identified.[47–50] The pathologic classification presented in Table 42–3, based on the putative cell of origin of each tumor, was suggested by

TABLE 42-2. Sites of Soft Tissue Sarcomas

	Sites				
Investigations	*Head and Neck*	*Trunk/ Retroperitoneum*	*Upper Extremity*	*Lower Extremity*	*Total*
Shieber et al, 1961[38]	16	39	20	50	125
Hare et al, 1963[39]	42	34/5	32	48	161
Ferrell et al, 1972[40]	8	19	15	36	78
Sears et al, 1980[41]	12	16	6	26	60
Abbas et al, 1981[42]	24	66/38	42	81	251
Lindberg et al, 1981[43]	26	74	63	137	300
Potter et al, 1985[44]	12	48/36	59	152	307
Torosian et al, 1987[45]	21	92/90	81	208	492
ACS Survey, 1987[46]	406	872/568	594	2110	4550
Total	567	1997	912	2848	6324
(%)	(9)	(32)	(14)	(45)	(100)

TABLE 42-3. Histologic Classification of Soft Tissue Tumors

I. *Tumors and Tumor-like Lesions of Fibrous Tissue*
 A. Benign
  1. Fibroma
  2. Nodular fasciitis (including intravascular and cranial types)
  3. Proliferative fasciitis
  4. Proliferative myositis
  5. Fibroma of tendon sheath
  6. Elastofibroma
  7. Nuchal fibroma
  8. Nasopharyngeal fibroma
  9. Keloid
 B. Fibrous tumors of infancy and childhood
  1. Fibrous hamartoma of infancy
  2. Myofibromatosis (solitary, multicentric)
  3. Fibromatosis colli
  4. Infantile digital fibromatosis
  5. Infantile fibromatosis (desmoid type)
  6. Giant cell fibroblastoma
  7. Gingival fibromatosis
  8. Calcifying aponeurotic fibroma
  9. Hyalin fibromatosis
 C. Fibromatoses
  1. Superficial fibromatoses
   a. Palmar and plantar fibromatosis
   b. Penile (Peyronie's) fibromatosis
   c. Knuckle pads
  2. Deep fibromatoses
   a. Abdominal fibromatosis
   b. Extra-abdominal fibromatosis
   c. Intra-abdominal fibromatosis
   d. Mesenteric fibromatosis (Gardner's syndrome)
   e. Postradiation fibromatosis
   f. Cicatricial fibromatosis
 D. Malignant
  1. Adult fibrosarcoma
  2. Congenital and infantile fibrosarcoma
  3. Inflammatory fibrosarcoma
  4. Postradiation fibrosarcoma
  5. Cicatricial fibrosarcoma

II. *Fibrohistiocytic Tumors*
 A. Benign
  1. Fibrous histiocytoma
   a. Cutaneous (dermatofibroma)
   b. Deep
  2. Atypical fibroxanthoma
  3. Juvenile xanthogranuloma
  4. Reticulohistiocytoma
  5. Xanthoma
 B. Intermediate
  1. Dermatofibrosarcoma protuberans
  2. Bednar tumor
 C. Malignant
  1. Malignant fibrous histiocytoma
   a. Storiform-pleomorphic
   b. Myxoid (myxofibrosarcoma)
   c. Giant cell (malignant giant cell tumor of soft parts)
   d. Inflammatory (malignant xanthogranuloma, xanthosarcoma)
   e. Angiomatoid

III. *Tumors and Tumor-like Lesions of Adipose Tissue*
 A. Benign
  1. Lipoma (cutaneous, deep, and multiple)
  2. Angiolipoma
  3. Spindle cell and pleomorphic lipoma
  4. Lipoblastoma and lipoblastomatosis
  5. Angiomyolipoma
  6. Myelolipoma
  7. Intramuscular and intermuscular lipoma
  8. Lipoma of tendon sheath
  9. Lumbosacral lipoma
  10. Interneural and perineural fibrolipoma
  11. Diffuse lipomatosis
  12. Cervical symmetrical lipomatosis (Madelung's disease)
  13. Pelvic lipomatosis
  14. Hibernoma
 B. Malignant
  1. Liposarcoma, predominantly
   a. Well-differentiated
    (1) Lipoma-like
    (2) Sclerosing
    (3) Inflammatory
   b. Myxoid
   c. Round cell (poorly differentiated myxoid)
   d. Pleomorphic
   e. Dedifferentiated

IV. *Tumors of Muscle Tissue*
 A. Smooth muscle
  1. Benign
   a. Leiomyoma (cutaneous and deep)
   b. Angiomyoma (vascular leiomyoma)
   c. Epithelioid leiomyoma (benign leiomyoblastoma)
   d. Intravenous leiomyomatosis
   e. Leiomyomatosis peritonealis disseminata
  2. Malignant
   a. Leiomyosarcoma
   b. Epithelioid leiomyosarcoma (malignant leiomyoblastoma)
 B. Striated muscle
  1. Benign
   a. Adult rhabdomyoma
   b. Genital rhabdomyoma
   c. Fetal rhabdomyoma
  2. Malignant
   a. Rhabdomyosarcoma, predominantly
    (1) Embryonal (including botryoid)
    (2) Alveolar
    (3) Pelomorphic
    (4) Mixed
   b. Ectomesenchymoma (rhabdomyosarcoma with ganglion cell differentiation)

V. *Tumors and Tumor-like Lesions of Blood Vessels*
 A. Benign
  1. Hemangioma
   a. Capillary (including juvenile)
   b. Cavernous
   c. Arteriovenous
   d. Venous
   e. Epithelioid (angiolymphoid hyperplasia, Kimura's disease)
   f. Granulation tissue type (pyogenic granuloma)
  2. Deep hemangioma (intramuscular, synovial, perineural)
  3. Hemangiomatosis
  4. Glomus tumor
  5. Hemangiopericytoma
  6. Papillary endothelial hyperplasia (intravascular vegetant hemangioendothelioma of Masson)
 B. Intermediate
  1. Hemangioendothelioma
   a. Epithelioid
   b. Spindle cell
   c. Malignant endovascular papillary angioendothelioma
 C. Malignant
  1. Hemangiosarcoma
  2. Kaposi's sarcoma
  3. Malignant glomus tumor
  4. Malignant hemangiopericytoma

(continued)

TABLE 42-3. *(Continued)*

VI. Tumors of Lymph Vessels
- A. Benign
  - 1. Lymphangioma
    - a. Cavernous
    - b. Cystic (cystic hygroma)
  - 2. Lymphangiomatosis
  - 3. Lymphangiomyoma and lymphangiomyomatosis
- B. Malignant
  - 1. Angiosarcoma

VII. Tumors and Tumor-like Lesions of Synovial Tissue
- A. Benign
  - 1. Giant cell tumor of tendon sheath
    - a. Localized (nodular tenosynovitis)
    - b. Diffuse (florid synovitis)
- B. Malignant
  - 1. Synovial sarcoma (malignant synovioma), predominantly
    - a. Biphasic (fibrous and epithelial)
    - b. Monophasic (fibrous or epithelial)
  - 2. Malignant giant cell tumor of tendon sheath

VIII. Tumors of Mesothelial Tissue
- A. Benign
  - 1. Localized fibrous mesothelioma (subserosal fibroma)
  - 2. Multicystic peritoneal mesothelioma
  - 3. Mesothelioma of the genital tract (adenomatoid tumor)
- B. Malignant
  - 1. Diffuse and localized mesothelioma, predominantly
    - a. Epithelial
    - b. Fibrous
    - c. Biphasic

IX. Tumors and Tumor-like Lesions of Peripheral Nerves
- A. Benign
  - 1. Traumatic neuroma
  - 2. Morton's neuroma
  - 3. Neuromuscular hamartoma
  - 5. Nerve sheath ganglion
  - 5. Neurilemoma (benign schwannoma)
  - 6. Neurofibroma, solitary
    - a. Localized
    - b. Diffuse
    - c. Pacinian
    - d. Pigmented
  - 7. Granular cell tumor
  - 8. Neurofibromatosis (von Recklinghausen's disease)
    - a. Localized
    - b. Plexiform
    - c. Diffuse
  - 9. Pigmented neuroectodermal tumor of infancy (retinal anlage tumor)
  - 10. Ectopic meningioma
  - 11. Nasal glioma
  - 12. Neurothekeoma
- B. Malignant
  - 1. Malignant schwannoma, including malignant schwannoma with rhabdomyoblastic differentiation (malignant Triton tumor), glandular malignant schwannoma, and epithelioid malignant schwannoma
  - 2. Peripheral tumors of primitive neuroectodermal tissues (Neuroepithelioma)
  - 3. Malignant pigmented neuroectodermal tumor of infancy (retinal anlage tumor)
  - 4. Malignant granular cell tumor

X. Tumors of Autonomic Ganglia
- A. Benign
  - 1. Ganglioneuroma
  - 2. Melanocytic schwannoma
- B. Malignant
  - 1. Neuroblastoma
  - 2. Ganglioneuroblastoma
  - 3. Malignant melanocytic schwannoma

XI. Tumors of Paraganglionic Structures
- A. Benign
  - 1. Paraganglioma (solitary, multiple, familial)
- B. Malignant
  - 1. Malignant paraganglioma

XII. Tumors and Tumor-like Lesions of Cartilage and Bone-Forming Tissues
- A. Benign
  - 1. Panniculitis ossificans
  - 2. Myositis ossificans
  - 3. Fibrodysplasia (myositis) ossificans progressiva
  - 4. Extraskeletal chondroma
  - 4. Extraskeletal osteoma
- B. Malignant
  - 1. Extraskeletal chondrosarcoma
    - a. Well-differentiated
    - b. Myxoid (chordoid sarcoma)
    - c. Mesenchymal
  - 2. Extraskeletal osteosarcoma

XIII. Tumors and Tumor-like Lesions of Pluripotential Mesenchyme
- A. Benign
  - 1. Mesenchymoma
- B. Malignant
  - 1. Malignant mesenchymoma

XIV. Tumors and Tumor-like Lesions of Disputed or Uncertain Histogenesis
- A. Benign
  - 1. Congenital granular cell tumor
  - 2. Tumoral calcinosis
  - 3. Myxoma (cutaneous and intramuscular)
  - 4. Aggressive angiomyxoma
  - 5. Amyloid tumor
  - 6. Parachordoma
- B. Malignant
  - 1. Alveolar soft part sarcoma
  - 2. Epithelioid sarcoma
  - 3. Clear cell sarcoma of tendons and aponeuroses (malignant melanoma of soft parts)
  - 4. Extraskeletal Ewing's sarcoma

XV. Unclassified Soft Tissue Tumors and Tumor-like Lesions

(Enzinger FM, Weiss SW. Soft tissue tumors. 2nd ed. St. Louis: CV Mosby, 1988)

Enzinger and Weiss.[50] Pathologic classifications based on the appearance of the predominant cell in the lesion (*i.e.*, round cell or spindle cell sarcomas) are less useful and should not be employed. Each of the sarcomas tends to reflect the morphologic appearance of the cell of origin, and the tendency of these tumors to dedifferentiate results in a variety of overlapping patterns that can make them difficult to classify. Competent pathologists often disagree on the cell of origin of an individual tumor.[51,52] The great variation in the reported incidence of various subtypes of soft tissue sarcomas probably reflects differences of opinion among pathologists.

There are tumors arising from the soft tissues that are grossly similar to sarcomas but rarely metastasize. Many of these tumors (*e.g.*, desmoid tumors, dermatofibrosarcoma protuberans) are capable of aggressively invading local tissues in a fashion characteristic of true sarcomas. It is important to differentiate these locally aggressive, nonmetastasizing lesions from those that are truly benign or malignant because of the therapeutic implications. Injury may provoke proliferative lesions in soft tissues. These can mimic soft tissue tumors, and because of their high mitotic rate, they are often difficult to differentiate from malignant lesions. An example is myositis ossificans.

For each histologically distinct malignant sarcoma, the tendency to metastasize depends on the grade of the tumor. Low-grade sarcomas are capable of aggressive, invasive local growth but tend not to disseminate. High-grade tumors are more likely to metastasize. In a survey of 4550 sarcoma patients, Lawrence and colleagues found approximately 33% of the tumors had low-grade classifications, and the others were high-grade lesions.[46] Assigning a pathologic grade to an individual tumor as a means of predicting clinical behavior has not been easy. The general criteria for grading—mitotic rate, nuclear morphology, degree of cellularity, cellular anaplasia or pleomorphism, and the presence of necrosis—are not readily quantifiable. However, sarcomas of the various histologic types can be assigned a numeric grade. The range of grades attributed to the more common types of sarcoma is presented in Figure 42–1.[50]

Costa and colleagues at the National Cancer Institute (NCI) correlated histologic features, such as histologic type, number of mitoses, degrees of necrosis, pleomorphism, cellularity, and matrix of the primary lesion, with the overall prognoses of these patients.[53] Stratified analyses revealed that the degree of necrosis was the single best histopathologic parameter that

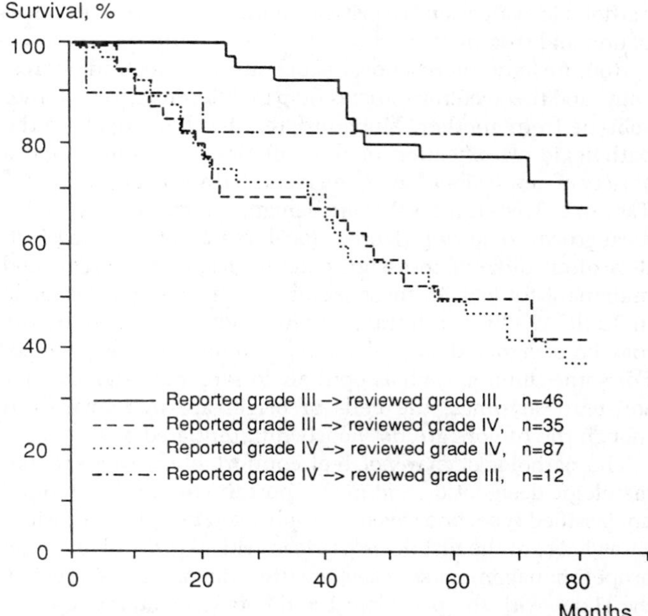

FIGURE 42–2. Comparison of overall survival of patients with high grade sarcomas based on tumor grading by individual referring pathologists and central pathology review by the Scandinavian Sarcoma Group. When compared with the prognosis of patients with agreement on tumor grading (——, grade III; and ··· grade IV), the prognosis of those with disagreement on tumor grade (---, III versus IV; -·-, IV versus III) was best predicted by the central review group. Such review of equivocal cases by pathologists with extensive experience in sarcoma grading can be crucial in estimating prognosis and planning appropriate therapy.

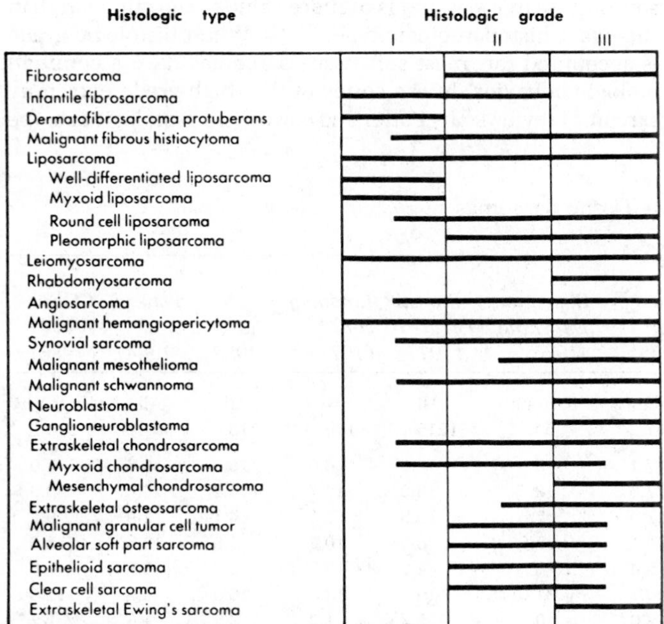

FIGURE 42–1. Soft tissue sarcomas. Estimated range of degree of malignancy based on histologic type and grade. Grade within the overall range depends on specific histologic features such as cellularity, cellular pleomorphism, mitotic activity, amount of stroma, infiltrative or expansive growth, and necrosis. (Enzinger FM, Weiss SW. Soft tissue tumors. 2nd ed. St. Louis: CV Mosby, 1988)

predicted the time to recurrence and the overall survival of patients ($p = 0.025$ and $p = 0.002$, respectively). The investigators proposed a grading system using the degree of necrosis to differentiate aggressive lesions. Grade 2 lesions were high-grade tumors with no or minimal necrosis, and grade 3 lesions were high-grade lesions with moderate or marked necrosis.[53] When using this criterion alone, a significant difference was seen between the prognoses of patients with grades 2 or 3 lesions. This system was independently confirmed by Lack and coworkers, who reviewed 300 extremity sarcomas and found the degree of necrosis to be the most significant determinant in predicting time to recurrence and overall survival.[54] However, there was only a 64% concordance rate in assigning a grade to 87 extremity soft tissue sarcomas that were previously reviewed by Costa and colleagues.[54]

A somewhat more elaborate grading system was proposed by Trojani and associates, using tumor differentiation, mitosis count, and the degree of tumor necrosis to predict the prognoses of patients with high-grade sarcomas.[55] Using this grading system, Coindre and coworkers reported a 75% concordance in grading 25 soft tissue sarcomas between an experienced panel of pathologists and a study group of 15 pathologists who had not been involved in the development of the grading system.[51]

Alvegard and Berg demonstrated that the grading of tumors by pathologists experienced in evaluating sarcomas correlated better with patient prognosis than grading assigned by referring pathologists (Fig. 42–2). This emphasizes that expert pathologic evaluation is a critical component in sarcoma evaluation and treatment.[56]

Routine light microscopy, histochemistry, electron microscopy, and tissue culture studies help to differentiate one tumor subtype from another. Much progress has been made in the pathologic classification of the soft tissue sarcomas, and a variety of new lesions have been identified and characterized.[50] Table 42–3 lists tumors that are benign, benign with aggressive local growth requiring vigorous local treatment, or malignant. It is often difficult to assign cells of origin for benign and malignant tumors. In these instances, the assignment made in Table 42–3 was arbitrary. Highly undifferentiated tumors may be designated as soft tissue sarcoma, type unspecified. For some tumors, such as epithelioid sarcomas and alveolar soft-part sarcomas, the cells of origin are unknown even though the tumors are not poorly differentiated.

The pathologist may not feel comfortable with a specific histologic designation and may report the tumor as sarcoma, unclassified type, and this may apply even to a grade 1 lesion. Knowledge of the histologic grade is critical to developing the proper management strategy, and the clinician should review the slides with the pathologist and obtain a statement about grade, even if the pathologist does not wish to specify cell type.

HISTOPATHOLOGIC CLASSIFICATION OF MALIGNANT TUMORS

Competent pathologists differ in attaching a histiogenic label to types of soft tissue sarcomas. These disagreements confound attempts to compare reports from different institutions about the incidence of histologic subtypes, frequency of tumors at different anatomic sites, stage of disease at presentation, frequency of local failure with different treatment modalities, and frequency of distant metastasis. This is particularly evident in Table 42–4, which collates the relative frequency of the various histopathologic types in several series.[38–40,44,57–65] The large differences in the incidence of different histopathologic types almost certainly reflect the differences in diagnostic criteria used by the pathologists. For example, in the series reported by Shieber and Graham and by Ferrell and Frable, there are no lesions that are considered as unclassifiable sarcomas.[38,40] In contrast, Hare and Cerny had 28.5%, Pack and Ariel had 36.4%, and Potter and coworkers had 9.5% unclassifiable sarcomas.[39,44,57] Another example of these disparities is illustrated by the 5.4% incidence of fibrosarcomas in the series by Pack and Ariel, compared with the 37% to 44% incidence of fibrosarcomas in the series reported by Simon and Enneking, Hare and Cerny, and Shieber and Graham.[38,39,57,60]

Changes in histologic classification of lesions, such as the recognition of a separate category of malignant fibrous histiocytomas, generated wide variations in the reported incidence of soft tissue sarcomas. For example, in the five series listed in Table 42–4 published before 1972, no cases of malignant fibrous histiocytomas were reported. Since 1972, this lesion has gained increasing recognition, and the 20.4% incidence reported in the series by Simon and Enneking in 1976 is comparable to the 17.5% incidence reported by Lindberg and associates, 22.8% reported by Potter and coworkers, 15.6% reported by Suit, 14.6% reported by Collin and colleagues, and 25.9% reported by Lawrence and colleagues.[44,47,60,63–65]

Presant and colleagues reviewed 216 consecutive sarcoma patients in the Southeastern Cancer Study Group experience and found concordance in histopathologic diagnoses in only 66% of cases.[52] The diagnoses of the primary member institution and a pathology review panel were compared. Coindre and coworkers reported a 61% concordance among pathologists in assigning histologic type in 25 soft tissue sarcomas.[51] The available evidence indicates that the histopathologic grade is the most important indicator of the biologic behavior of soft tissue sarcomas and is of more value to the clinician than the exact histopathologic type.[50,53–55] When histologic grade is accounted for, most soft tissue sarcomas have a common biologic behavior. In the series of 211 high-grade extremity sarcomas reviewed by Potter and coworkers, histologic subtype

TABLE 42-4. Relative Incidence (%) of Histologic Types of Soft Tissue Sarcomas in Various Studies

Soft Tissue Sarcomas	*Shieber and Graham*[38] *(1962)*	*Hare and Cerny*[39] *(1963)*	*Pack and Ariel*[57] *(1964)*	*Martin et al*[58] *(1965)*	*Ferrell and Frable*[40] *(1972)*	*Shiu et al*[59] *(1975)*	*Simon and Enneking*[60] *(1976)*	*Russell et al*[61] *(1977)*	*Lindberg et al*[63] *(1977)*	*Suit*[64] *(1983)*	*Potter et al*[44] *(1984)*	*Collins et al*[65] *(1986)*
Sites	All	All	All	All	All	Extremity	Extremity	All	All	All	All	Extremity
Total no. of cases	125	200	717	398	117	297	54	1215	166	315	307	315
Unclassified	0	28.5	36.4	14.8	0	7.1	5.6	10.0	6.0	16.5	9.5	1.0
Liposarcoma	16.0	11.5	14.6	26.9	17.0	27.6	18.5	18.2	12.7	15.2	18.3	33.9
Rhabdomyosarcoma	16.0	5.0	13.9	20.6	30.0	17.5	5.6	19.3	9.6	4.1	2.9	9.2
Synoviosarcoma	0.8	2.5	8.4	3.0	2.5	14.1	5.6	6.9	10.2	3.8	19.5	12.6
Neurofibrosarcoma	3.2	0	6.4	0	0	5.4	0	4.9	19.3	6.0	6.8	7.6
Fibrosarcoma	44.0	43.0	5.4	24.1	33.0	20.2	37.0	19.0	13.3	16.8	3.6	12.3
Angiosarcoma	4.8	0	2.6	0.3	0	2.0	0	2.7	1.2	3.2	1.6	1.2
Leiomyosarcoma	6.4	6.5	0	6.3	4.0	2.4	0	6.5	4.2	7.6	11.4	3.8
Mesenchymoma	0	0	0	0	0	0.3	0	0.3	0	0.9	0	0
Malignant fibrous histiocytoma	0	0	0	0	0	1.0	20.4	10.5	17.5	15.6	22.8	14.6
Other	8.8	3.0	12.1	4.0	13.5	2.4	7.4	1.7	6.0	10.2	3.6	3.4

was not a significant determinant of disease-free or overall survival (Fig. 42–3).[66] The difficulties in pathologic classification and its negligible importance in arbitrating therapy compel the treatment of soft tissue sarcomas as a group.

BENIGN TUMORS OF SOFT TISSUE

BENIGN TUMORS OF FIBROUS ORIGIN

There are many variants of fibrous tumors that are nonmalignant and do not metastasize. Most are successfully treated by simple excision and do not recur. Some tumors in this category, such as nodular fasciitis, can be mistaken for true fibrosarcomas. Others, such as extraabdominal desmoid tumors, require special attention because aggressive local therapy is necessary to prevent recurrence.

Fibroma

"Fibroma" has been applied to any benign fibrous growth. Many congenital malformations and reparative tissue growths fall into this category. With increased understanding of the variants of fibrous tissue neoplasms, fewer tumors are called fibromas, and the term is now restricted to benign, encapsulated, fibrous nodules that seldom grow larger than a few centimeters in diameter. A subcutaneous or soft fibroma (*i.e.*, fibroma molle) is a pedunculated subcutaneous growth composed of fibrous tissue and fat covered by epidermis. Fibroma durum is a pedunculated lesion, often arising in the oral mucosa, that may result from malocclusion or malfitting dentures. All of these lesions should be treated by simple excision. They rarely recur.

Elastofibroma

Elastofibroma is a rare lesion that usually occurs under the scapular muscles and frequently attaches to the rib cage.[67–70] Many are not noticed, and one series found them in 10% of 235 autopsy cases.[68] The lesions are benign and do not recur after simple enucleation.

Palmar and Plantar Fibromatosis

Tumor-like proliferations of the palmar and plantar aponeuroses can give rise to tumor-like nodules.[71–74] Only the palmar fibromatosis (Dupuytren's contracture) is associated with flexion contractures. Heredity affects incidence, and lesions occur six times as often in men as in women. The lesions grow slowly as localized nodular enlargements that can infiltrate the fascia and involve overlying skin and subcutaneous tissue. The lesions are benign, although they have a tendency to recur after simple excision. Consequently, small nodules should be left untouched. If excision is necessary, attempts should be made to widely excise the palmar or plantar fascia.

Juvenile Aponeurotic Fibroma

Juvenile aponeurotic fibroma (*i.e.*, Keasby's tumor) is a form of fibromatosis that affects the palms or soles of children and young adults.[75–77] The lesion can infiltrate and overgrow subcutaneous fat and muscle, but metastases never occur. The lesions invade locally and have a tendency to recur after limited excision. Attempts to achieve negative microscopic margins should be made.

Congenital Generalized Fibromatosis

Generalized fibromatosis, usually present at birth, is characterized by multiple, widely scattered, nodular and infiltrating fibroblastic lesions, diffusely present in the superficial and deep tissues, viscera, and bone.[78–80] The disease is often fatal because of vital organ involvement, but it represents a congenital rather than neoplastic condition.

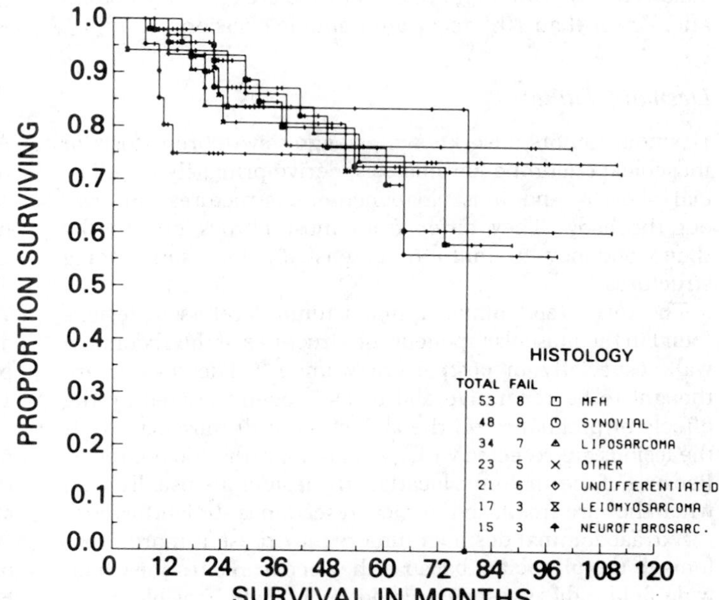

FIGURE 42–3. Actuarial analysis of overall survival for 211 patients with high-grade extremity sarcomas categorized by histologic subtype. There are no significant differences between the groups. (Potter DA, Kinsella T, Glatstein E, et al. High grade soft tissue sarcomas or the extremities. Cancer 1986;58:190–205)

Fibrous Hamartoma of Infancy

Fibrous hamartoma occurs predominantly in boys and presents in the first year of life with a solitary mass in the axilla, upper extremity, head, or neck.[81] These lesions are situated almost exclusively in the dermis or subcutaneous fat and can become large. Local excision is almost always curative, because this lesion does not metastasize.

Fibromatosis Colli

This distinctive form of fibromatosis develops in the sternocleidomastoid muscle of newborn or very young children. In many cases, a small lump in the sternocleidomastoid muscle noticed in the newborn disappears spontaneously.[82,83] If the lesion persists for several months after birth, it can grow and produce neck contractures. Lack of treatment can result in large growths, with subsequent spread to the trachea and surrounding organs. These lesions should be excised and often require removal of the entire sternocleidomastoid muscle.

Penile Fibromatosis

Also called Peyronie's disease, penile fibromatosis involves a circumscribed fibrous thickening arising in the connective tissue sheath that separates the corpus cavernosum from the tunic albuginea.[84] It causes pain and curvature of the penis on penile erection. Surgical excision of the fibrous tissue is the preferred treatment.

Nodular Fasciitis

Nodular fasciitis, also called pseudosarcomatous or proliferative fasciitis, should be treated by simple excision. Its morphologic appearance causes it to be confused with fibrosarcoma.[85–88] These lesions generally arise in the subcutaneous fascia or the superficial portions of the deep fascia. The growth of these lesions is frequently rapid. Maximal size is usually achieved within a few weeks, and then growth stops. These lesions rarely grow larger than 5 cm and are often asymptomatic. Fewer than 10% recur after simple excision.

Desmoid Tumors

Desmoid tumors, also known as aggressive fibromatosis or musculoaponeurotic fibromatosis, derive primarily from fascial sheaths and musculoaponeurotic structures throughout the body. They differ from most fibrous growths by their tendency to infiltrate extensively into surrounding structures.[89–105]

The term "abdominal desmoid tumor" refers to lesions found in the muscular aponeurotic structures of the abdominal wall, especially in postpartum women.[92] The lesions are thought to be reparative and to have been initiated by the effects of pregnancy on the abdominal wall musculature. If the lesions are resected with good margins, they do not recur. Because of the anatomic location, the lesions are usually seen when they are small, and surgical resection is straightforward.

Extraabdominal desmoid tumors may present more problems to the physician, because they occur in sites for which wide-field radical resection is not technically feasible; if attempted, irradiation may be associated with appreciable morbidity. These lesions occur around the shoulder girdle, inguinal region, and lower extremities. They are not encapsulated, infiltrate locally, and are destructive but do not metastasize. Histopathologically, these lesions are primarily fibroblastic with elongated, thin, delicate nuclei, which appear virtually normal. Mitotic figures are uncommon, usually less than 1 per 50 high-power fields.

The preferred treatment for extraabdominal desmoid is wide-field resection with negative margins in all dimensions.[106] The local recurrence rate is 50% to 75% of the cases for which margins were close or positive.

In a review of 138 patients at Memorial Sloan-Kettering Cancer Center, Posner found that inadequate surgical resection and presentation with recurrent disease were independent predictive factors for recurrence after surgery. The overall survival rate for these patients was 92% at 5 years, with 11 patients succumbing to tumor-related complications. All 11 patients had lesions in nonextremity sites, leading to obstruction, fistula, sepsis, and malnutrition.[105]

If wide resection is not feasible, radiation therapy may be an effective treatment. James Ewing, in 1928, commented that desmoid tumors slowly responded to irradiation and that this treatment could be considered for lesions not amenable to surgical resection.[93] Successful treatment by irradiation has been reported in an incidental way in describing results of large surgical series.[94]

Benninghoff and Robbins described the treatment of 4 patients with desmoid tumors, 3 of whom were treated after incomplete surgery and 1 for frank recurrent tumor.[95] Radiation doses were modest, but good responses were obtained in 3 of 4 patients. Greenberg and coworkers reported long-term control in 8 of 9 patients with desmoid tumors treated by irradiation alone or in combination with surgery.[96] Wara and associates reported a series of 16 patients with desmoid tumors, 12 of whom were treated for gross tumor (>5 cm).[98] Two died from disease, but the remaining 10 were alive without tumor 2 to 6 years after treatment. Among the 4 patients treated after incomplete surgical resection (no palpable tumor), there was 1 local recurrence at 2 years; the other 3 patients were free of evident disease at 2 to 4 years.

Suit and Russell described the results of treatment of 4 patients with desmoid tumor, 2 of whom had massive local disease and 2 of whom were treated after incomplete surgery.[99] All 4 remained disease free for 5 years. Seventeen patients treated by radiation therapy for desmoid tumors at the Massachusetts General Hospital and followed for more than 12 months were reported by Kiel and Suit.[100] Ten patients were treated by irradiation alone and 7 by irradiation and surgery. There were 3 local failures: 2 of 10 after irradiation and 1 of 7 after irradiation and surgery. However, 2 of the failures developed after doses of only 2200 and 2400 cGy. Among 15 patients who received doses greater than 5000 cGy, there was 1 local failure (follow-up, 12–96 months).

For the patient who has uncertain or minimally positive margins at the first resection, and re-resection is not feasible, the patient should be observed and treatment implemented at the first sign of regrowth. In these circumstances, local failure is not universal; some patients may be able to avoid high-dose radiation treatment. At the Massachusetts General Hospital, 8 patients with uncertain or minimally positive margins after resection were followed, and only one recurred; after re-resection, this patient is free of disease.[100]

There are reports that hormonal or antihormonal medication may achieve long-term remission of desmoid tumors. Kinzbrunner and colleagues described a patient with a 16-kg desmoid tumor of the back that regressed to a $5 \times 5 \times 2$ cm mass in 2 weeks after treatment with tamoxifen (20 mg four times daily).[101] Lanari described a small series of patients with desmoid tumors treated successfully with progesterone.[102] Using another approach, Waddell and Gerner reported that administration of indomethacin and ascorbic acid could cause regression of desmoid tumors.[103] Because of the limited toxicity of these approaches, the use of these agents in the treatment of desmoid tumors deserves further clinical study.

BENIGN TUMORS OF STRIATED MUSCLE

Rhabdomyoma

These are extremely rare benign tumors of skeletal muscle, generally occurring in the tongue, neck muscles, larynx, uvula, nasal cavity, axilla, vulva, and heart.[107,108] These tumors are treated by simple excision.

BENIGN TUMORS OF SMOOTH MUSCLE

Leiomyoma

Leiomyomas rarely occur outside of the uterus and the gastrointestinal tract.[109,110] They can occur in the skin and subcutaneous tissues and probably arise from the smooth muscle of small blood vessels in these tissues. These lesions are treated by simple excision.

Epithelioid Leiomyoma

Epithelioid leiomyoma (*i.e.*, leiomyoblastoma) are most frequently found in the wall of the gastrointestinal tract, especially in the stomach. They are similar to other smooth muscle tumors but may become large and hemorrhagic and exhibit small cystic areas. Simple excision is usually curative.

BENIGN TUMORS OF ADIPOSE TISSUE

Lipomas

Lipomas are among the most common of all benign neoplasms and arise in any location where fat is normally present. These lesions may occur in deep tissue, although they usually arise subcutaneously. They are characteristically multilobulated masses of fatty tissue that vary from small nodules to large masses weighing several kilograms.

Multiple lipomatosis is a condition of diffuse overgrowths that may occur throughout the body. These are not true tumors and are probably a result of fat metabolism disorders.

Spindle cell lipomas are rare benign tumors that occur almost exclusively in the neck and shoulders of males.[111] The major importance of these tumors is their tendency to be confused with liposarcomas.

Angiolipomas are lipomas containing a network of many small capillaries and are usually quite painful.[112] Some angiolipomas are infiltrative and require a wider margin of resection than most lipomas.

The treatment for lipomas is simple enucleation. Recurrence is uncommon after this limited treatment.

Lipoblastomatosis

Lipoblastomatosis, also called adipose hamartomatosis, is found in infants. It consists of lobular soft tissue growths separated by partitions of loose fibrous tissue.[93,113,114] About 10% of these lesions recur after simple local excision, but they have no tendency to metastasize.

Atypical Lipoma

The designation of atypical lipoma is applied to subcutaneous lipomatous neoplasms that display cytologic atypia not seen in most lipomas.[115–118] These lesions occur in the subcutaneous or deep muscular layers. Simple excision cures virtually all subcutaneous lesions, although simple excision of deep muscular lesions often results in local recurrence that may require reexcision. These lesions have no tendency to metastasize and can be controlled by reexcision.

Hibernoma

Hibernomas are unusual lipomas that are thought to arise from vestiges of brown fat, similar to the glandular, brown adipose tissue occurring in certain hibernating animal species.[119] These are benign tumors and should be treated by simple excision.

BENIGN TUMORS OF SYNOVIAL TISSUE

Giant Cell Tumor of Tendon Sheath

Giant cell tumors of tendon sheath, also called localized nodular tenosynovitis, are usually solitary and arise from the tendon sheath, joints or bursae of the hand, palm, or wrist.[120,121] These soft tissue lesions can produce atrophy of the bony cortex or actual erosion into adjacent bone. Simple excision is the treatment of choice. Villonodular synovitis is probably related to giant cell tumor of tendon sheath but almost always occurs in joints and presents with pain and swelling. This benign tumor-like growth erodes the bone and appears to be a primary bone tumor. The synovium of the affected joint is usually diffusely involved, and total synovectomy is the treatment of choice.

Ganglion

Ganglions are multilocular, fibrous-walled cysts, usually occurring on the dorsal aspect of the wrist. These lesions form as a result of synovial tissue that has become pinched off and undergoes degeneration. Simple excision is almost always curative.

BENIGN TUMORS OF NEURAL TISSUE

Neurilemoma

Neurilemomas are benign, encapsulated tumors, also called schwannomas, that almost always occur as solitary lesions.[50,122] The most common site of origin is the eighth cranial nerve (*i.e.*, acoustic neuroma), although cranial peripheral nerves are often affected. This is also the most common benign neoplasm of the spinal canal. These lesions often grow with an easily demonstrable flattened nerve seen along its capsule. These lesions rarely recur if resected locally. Every effort should be made to preserve the nerve involved if this nerve is of clinical significance (*e.g.*, the facial nerve). These lesions arise from Schwann cells, although they are different from neurofibromas.

Neurofibroma

Neurofibromas are thought to arise from Schwann cells, although they differ from neurilemomas in that they tend not to be encapsulated and have a much softer consistency. They may also occur at many different sites. These lesions may be locally infiltrative, although simple excision is almost always curative.

Multiple neurofibromas are a feature of von Recklinghausen's disease, which is an autosomal dominant disorder that affects 1 of 3000 live births.[123–132] In this condition, neurofibromas may occur in virtually all sites of the body and be associated with any peripheral or intraspinal nerves. Plexiform neurofibromas may cause massive enlargement of an extremity. About 10% to 15% of patients with von Recklinghausen's disease develop malignant schwannoma, and these malignant tumors can arise in benign, superficial neurofibromas. Neurofibromas in von Recklinghausen's disease should be removed for cosmetic reasons or if they become painful or undergo rapid enlargement. In a long-term study of 212 patients with neurofibromatosis, 57 developed malignant tumors; 21 patients developed cancers of the central nervous system, 6 developed cancers of the peripheral nervous system, and the remainder developed cancers at other sites.[132]

BENIGN TUMORS OF VASCULAR TISSUE

Hemangioma

Hemangiomas are vascular neoplasms that can occur anywhere in the body.[133–135] About 75% are present at birth, and about 60% occur in the head and neck area. Most hemangiomas of infancy spontaneously regress. Some lesions grow rapidly during the early months of life and may be a source of some concern, although most disappear by about 5 years of age. These lesions may be primarily composed of capillaries or widely dilated veins (*i.e.*, cavernous hemangioma). These lesions do not metastasize, and simple excision is often curative, although it is not necessary except for cosmetic reasons. In some instances, the hemangioma may exhibit rapid growth and abut or compromise vital structures. In these instances, low-dose radiation confined to the hemangioma may be used. Efforts should be made to use techniques that limit the dose to the vascular process itself. Radiation treatment for these lesions is rarely indicated, and even large medical centers probably do not see more than 3 or 4 patients each decade for whom radiation treatment is warranted.

Lymphangioma

Lymphangiomas are similar to hemangiomas, although the vascular spaces do not contain blood cells. These lesions can occur virtually anywhere in the body. Cystic hygromas are lymphangiomas of the neck. The lesions require surgical excision. The extent of the procedure should be dictated by the location and the desire to achieve a reasonable cosmetic result.

Glomus Tumors

The normal glomus is a 1-mm end organ arteriovenous anastomosis.[136–139] This organ enlarges into a painful and tender mass. About 15% occur in the subungual regions, although any location in the skin and soft tissue is possible. Local excision is usually curative, and metastases do not occur. Glomus tumors may be located along the larger vessels. A common syndrome is that of the glomus tumor near the jugular foramen, designated as a glomus jugulare. These lesions are not resectable and are effectively treated by radiation therapy (5000 cGy delivered over about 5 weeks). Lesions regress slowly, but permanent control of the process is regularly achieved.

Infantile Hemangiopericytomas

Although hemangiopericytomas in the adult are more benign in their behavior than most soft tissue sarcomas, these tumors can metastasize and are therefore be considered with malignant lesions.[139,140] However, hemangiopericytomas that occur in infancy appear to be benign lesions without significant metastatic potential. These tumors occur almost exclusively in the skin and may have evidence of infiltrative growth outside the main tumor mass. These lesions generally do not recur after wide local excision.

BENIGN TUMORS OF HISTIOCYTIC TISSUE

The work of Stout and colleagues has significantly improved our understanding and recognition of tumors of presumed histiocytic origin.[49,50] Variants of these tumors have received more than 30 different names in a variety of nomenclature systems. The tumors are composed wholly or in part of cells with the morphologic characteristics of histiocytes and with various fibroblastic components. It is thought that these tumors are of purely histiocytic origin, but histiocytes in these lesions can differentiate toward fibroblastic morphology.

Dermatofibroma

Dermatofibromas, also called sclerosing hemangioma or fibrous xanthoma of skin, are common soft tissue lesions that are usually about 1 cm in diameter and occur in the dermis. Simple excision is always curative.

Fibrous Histiocytoma

Many variants of histiocytoma, also called fibrous xanthoma, exist.[49,50,141] Superficially located histiocytic lesions behave in a benign manner, although deep, benign histiocytomas may invade locally into surrounding tissue. These lesions can occur anywhere in the body. Superficial lesions are always cured by simple excision, but a wider margin of normal tissue should be obtained for deep, benign fibrous histiocytomas. Local recurrence is uncommon.

Atypical Fibrous Histiocytomas

Although superficial fibrous histiocytomas are always totally benign and cured by simple excision, deep fibrous histiocytomas may have a more atypical morphologic appearance and are more ominous in their tendency to recur locally.[142–144] Although superficial lesions may occasionally fit the criteria for atypical histiocytoma (*e.g.*, 3 of 18 atypical fibrous histiocytomas reported by Soule and coworkers), almost all are located deep in soft tissue or muscle.[142] Despite the absence of obvious anaplasia, a rapidly growing, deeply occurring fibrous histiocytoma may achieve a diameter of 6 cm or larger; more than half of these lesions recur after simple excision. These lesions usually do not metastasize, although rare reports of metastases after many local recurrences for lesions with this histology have been reported. Recommended therapy includes wide local excision, with negative microscopic margins in all directions. As a result of inadequate local treatment at first resection, recurrent local extension of these tumors, especially in the retroperitoneal area, can lead to death.

Dermatofibrosarcoma Protuberans

Dermatofibrosarcoma protuberans can occur in any part of the body.[145–150] The exact histogenesis is not known, although a histiocytic origin is likely. These lesions most often begin as indurated nodules in the skin that grow slowly and are often ignored until they are large. They show an extremely aggressive tendency to invade surrounding local tissue; they should be regarded as malignant neoplasms. They do not metastasize, even after multiple recurrences. About 50% recur after simple excision, and a wide excision including a wide margin of surrounding tissue should be achieved in therapy.[150] The first resection is important, because tumor spread at the inadequate first resection may lead to uncontrollable local growth. These benign lesions may ultimately lead to amputation of extremities or even death because of extensive invasion of vital organs.

Many of the comments regarding use of radiation therapy discussed under the treatment of desmoid tumors may apply to these lesions.[96–100] In a review of the NCI experience with locally aggressive but nonmetastasizing soft tissue tumors seen between 1975 and 1982, Glenn and coworkers identified 35 cases that were completely resected. Twenty patients received radiation therapy postoperatively, and one tumor recurred. One recurrence was seen among 15 patients treated by surgery alone. Follow-up in this study ranged from 12 to 97 months, with a median of 36 months.

If surgical treatment of dermatofibrosarcoma protuberans is not feasible or requires a radical procedure, consideration should be given to radiation therapy in combination with conservative surgery or to radiation therapy alone in special circumstances.[151]

BENIGN TUMORS OF MESOTHELIAL TISSUE

Mesothelioma

The cells lining the pleura, peritoneum, and pericardium are mesothelial cells. Although most tumors of mesothelial tissue are malignant, benign tumors can occur, usually in the pleura. These lesions project outwardly from the viscera or parietal pleura into the adjacent cavity but do not infiltrate aggressively into local tissue. They may grow to be quite large, and simple excision is usually curative.

BENIGN TUMORS OF UNCERTAIN TISSUE ORIGIN

Granular Cell Myoblastoma

Granular cell myoblastomas rarely grow larger than 6 cm and can be cured by local excision.[152] If these lesions develop beneath the epidermis or mucous membranes, they can lead to squamous tissue proliferation, possibly mimicking a squamous cell carcinoma.

Mesenchymoma

Mesenchymomas, also referred to as hamartoma or mixed mesodermal tumor, are composed of at least two different mesenchymal elements.[153] Lesions often contain smooth muscle, skeletal muscle, fat, and angiomatous and osseous tissue in various combinations. Although most lesions are malignant, rare benign forms have been described. Benign tumors are generally small, and none of the individual elements contain cells with atypical or anaplastic appearance. Local excision is adequate therapy.

Myxoma

Myxoma is thought to arise from embryonic rests and is composed of spindle cells imbedded in a mucinous intercellular matrix.[154,155] It can occur in any of the soft tissues, bone, or occasionally in the heart and genitourinary tract. When these lesions develop in the soft tissues, they are generally close to a large muscle or aponeurosis. They are cured by local excision. Deep tumors can sometimes infiltrate contiguous structures, but local resection is usually curative.

There are many other less common benign tumors of soft tissue.[50]

DIAGNOSIS

Soft tissue sarcomas most often present as asymptomatic soft tissue masses. Because these lesions arise in compressible tissues and are often far from vital organs, symptoms are few until the lesions are quite large compared with the anatomic part. For example, a sarcoma often presents at 8 to 15 cm in the thigh or buttock, 3 to 4 cm in the wrist, but only 0.5 to 1 cm around the digits. Symptoms generally result from pressure or traction on adjacent nerves or muscles. There are no reliable physical signs to differentiate benign from malignant soft tissue lesions; consequently, all soft tissue lumps that persist or grow should be biopsied. Even soft and pliable subcutaneous lumps thought to be lipomas occasionally prove surprising. Leaving soft tissue lumps in place without biopsy is justified only if they have been present and unchanged for many years before being observed by the physician.

The nature of the biopsy of soft tissue sarcomas is an important aspect of the overall management of these patients. Because the biopsy site must be removed in any definitive resection, care should be taken to place the biopsy incision at a location and orientation that does not compromise subsequent surgical excision.

Adequate and representative tissue must be obtained in any biopsy of a soft tissue mass, and this typically requires an incisional or excisional biopsy. Although in centers with extensive experience with sarcoma, multiple core-needle biopsies can provide adequate pathologic material, aspiration cytology is typically not sufficient.[156] Immunohistochemistry or electron microscopy often is necessary, and these efforts are hampered by insufficient tissue. Inhomogeneity within large tumors can also lead to critical sampling errors, particularly in assigning tumor grade. If uncertainty remains after initial biopsy, do not hesitate to obtain additional tissue. The decision between excisional and incision biopsy is based on tumor size and location.

Soft tissue sarcomas grow in the path of least resistance and push surrounding tissue before them. This surrounding tissue forms a pseudocapsule and always contains invasive prongs of malignant tissue. For this reason, shelling out soft tissue sarcomas is never curative. Excision through the pseudocapsule often spreads tumor into surrounding tissue and can greatly complicate further surgical treatment. Excisional biopsy is an appropriate means of establishing a diagnosis only for soft tissue sarcomas smaller than 3 cm in diameter.

Tumors larger than 3 cm in diameter require an incisional biopsy. This technique allows acquisition of a generous wedge of tissue from the lesion and minimally disrupts the surrounding tissue planes. The incisional biopsy should be performed through a carefully placed small incision that does not compromise subsequent radical excision of the lesion. Impeccable hemostasis is essential, because hematomas resulting from biopsies of soft tissue sarcomas can spread tumor along their paths.

Although most experienced surgeons consider an incisional biopsy preferable to a limited excisional biopsy for the diagnosis of soft tissue sarcomas, a survey of surgical practices in the United States conducted by The American College of Surgeons showed that roughly half of the sarcomas were biopsied by excision.[46] This practice did not change during two intervals surveyed, 1977 to 1978 and 1983 to 1984 (Table 42–5). Only 20% of patients had a diagnosis established by incisional biopsy during these same periods.

TABLE 42-5. Biopsy Techniques for Sarcoma Diagnosis

Type of Biopsy	*1977–1978*		*1983–1984*	
	No.	*%*	*No.*	*%*
None	319	13.5	380	11.0
Needle	114	4.8	311	9.0
Incisional	466	19.8	753	21.8
Excisional	1210	51.4	1644	47.6
Other	139	5.9	278	8.0
Unknown	107	4.5	91	2.6
Total	2355	100.0	3457	100.0

(Lawrence W Jr, Donegan WL, Natarajan N, et al. Adult soft tissue sarcomas. A pattern of care survey of the American College of Surgeons. Ann Surg 1987;205:349–359)

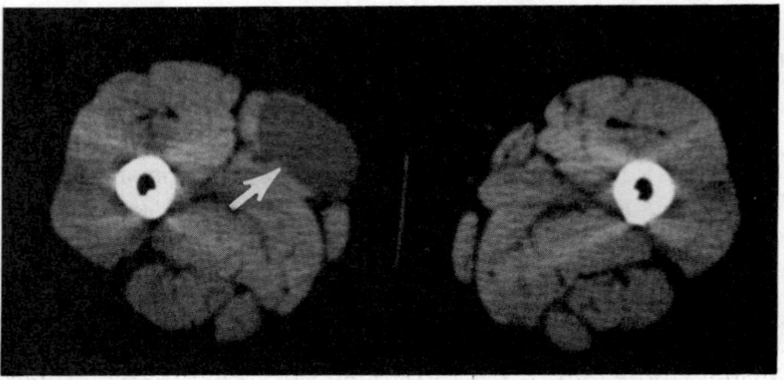

FIGURE 42–4. Computed tomography scan of midthigh region in patient with a myxoid liposarcoma (*white arrow*). Transaxial orientation demonstrates relation to underlying muscle groups.

The importance of the adequate placement of the biopsy incision cannot be overemphasized. Improper placement may preclude proper radical resection of the lesion and may lead to large increases in the radiation fields necessary to encompass all areas of possible spread. Incisions on the extremities should be placed longitudinally to prevent compromise of the muscle group excisions that may subsequently be necessary. At other sites, the incision should be parallel to the long axis of the underlying principal muscle. Biopsies of lesions in the buttocks should be placed as inferiorly as possible to allow subsequent development of skin flaps if hemipelvectomy is necessary.

Planning surgical resection or radiation therapy requires a careful and detailed determination of the pattern of local spread and assessment of the tissues probably involved by microscopic disease. The physical examination determines the approximate size of the lesion, attachment to deep or superficial structures, relation of the tumor to prior biopsy sites, functional status of the part, and presence of prior injury or concurrent medical disease that would confound the execution of the desired surgery or radiation. The radiographic evaluation of the patient with soft tissue sarcoma should include these procedures[157–165]:

1. Xerogram or soft tissue radiograph of the affected part
2. Computed tomography (CT), magnetic resonance imaging (MRI), or ultrasound through the affected region
3. CT or full-chest tomogram
4. Arteriogram in certain instances
5. Radionuclide bone scan

The most important diagnostic procedures in assessing the pattern of involvement of the primary lesion are CT (Fig. 42–4) or MR scans (Fig. 4-5). High-quality CT or MR scans are essential because these techniques permit accurate delineation of the muscle compartment or anatomic structures involved by gross disease.

Chang and colleagues performed a prospective evaluation of preoperative CT and MR scans of patients with extremity sarcomas.[164] Operative findings were correlated with the scans. CT and MRI were found comparable in evaluating the tumor's relation to major neurovascular and skeletal structures. However, MRI demonstrated better visual contrast between tumor and muscle. MRI has the advantage of displaying anatomy in coronal and sagittal views, but CT is restricted to transaxial views. Bland and colleagues reported that MRI was

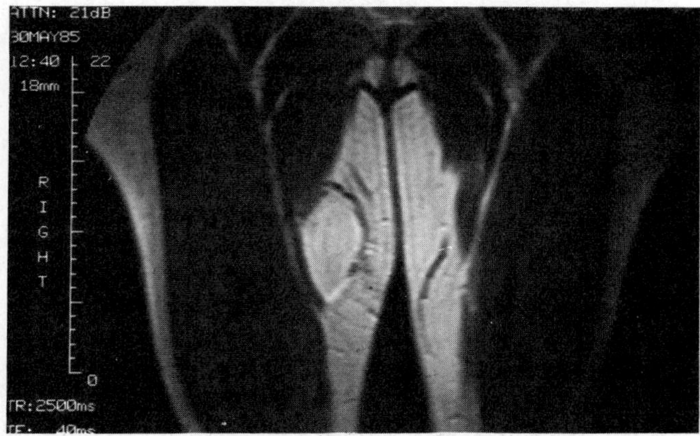

FIGURE 42–5. T1-weighted MRI scan of the same patient shown in Figure 42–3. This scan demonstrates excellent tumor to muscle contrast for this myxoid liposarcoma. The coronal image is helpful in defining the longitudinal extent of the tumor in the thigh.

significantly better than CT in predicting resectability of 53 soft tissue sarcomas in various sites.[165] This was a result of the multiplanar imaging and improved visual contrast afforded by MRI.[165]

Arteriography can also delineate the position and status of major vessels and the local extent of disease, and it is particularly useful for estimating the proximity of tumor to major vessels, for determining the pattern of displacement or deviation of vessels, and for determining the encasement of a vessel by tumor, resulting in abrupt, irregular change in the caliber of the vessel, which is characteristic of neoplastic involvement.[161–163] The late venous phase can show the venous drainage, which should be controlled intraoperatively early in the course of surgery to prevent major embolization of tumor cells. An arteriogram is of minimal benefit in planning the treatment of recurrent tumors or the reoperation of incompletely excised lesions.

Although sarcomas rarely invade bone, assessment of soft tissue reaction in the periosteum and at the margin of soft tissues may be estimated by bone scan.[46,166] A positive scan does not mean that the tumor has invaded bone or periosteum. A positive scan may simply be the consequence of periosteal reaction to the increased blood flow of a nearby tumor. This could serve as a guide to wide resection near the bone or to removing periosteum or a portion of the bone in the area that is positive on scan in the patients treated by surgery alone. Patients with positive bone scans and no radiographic periosteal reactions who are being treated by irradiation and surgery should not have stripping of periosteum unless operative findings reveal fixation of the lesion to the bone.

Sarcomas of soft tissue infrequently metastasizes to regional lymph nodes, and lymphangiography is rarely indicated.[170]

STAGING

The single most important prognostic factor in patients with soft tissue sarcomas is the histologic grade of the primary lesion.[50,53–55,61] Grades are assigned from grade 1 (well-differentiated) to grade 3 (poorly differentiated).

In the staging system for soft tissue sarcomas proposed by the American Joint Committee for Cancer Staging and End Results, the histologic grade is the most important determinant of stage.[61,62] The system is based on four parameters: G or histopathologic grade, T, N, and M. Details of the staging system, which was revised in 1987, are presented in Table 42–6. G1, G2, and G3 lesions are sarcomas that are well-differentiated, moderately differentiated, or poorly differentiated, respectively. T1 lesions are smaller than 5 cm; T2 lesions are equal to or larger than 5 cm. N1 lesions have metastatic disease in regional lymph nodes, and M1 lesions show clinical evidence of distant metastasis. All lesions that are G1 and T1 or T2 and are N0M0 are stage 1. All lesions that are G2 and T1 or T2 and are N0M0 are stage II, and all lesions that are G3 and T1 or T2 and are N0M0 are stage III. All lesions that are N1 become stage IVA, without regard to grade or size. The correlation of this staging system with prognosis

TABLE 42-6. American Joint Committee Staging System for Soft Tissue Sarcomas

T	Primary tumor
	T1 Tumor less than 5 cm
	T2 Tumor 5 cm or greater
G	Histologic grade of malignancy
	G1 Low
	G2 Moderate
	G3 High
N	Regional lymph nodes
	N0 No histologically verified metastases to regional lymph nodes
	N1 Histologically verified regional lymph node metastasis
M	Distant metastasis
	M0 No distant metastasis
	M1 Distant metastasis

Stage I	
Stage IA GIT1N0M0	Grade 1 tumor less than 5 cm in diameter with no regional lymph node or distant metastases
Stage IB G1T2N0M0	Grade 1 tumor 5 cm or greater in diameter with no regional lymph node or distant metastases
Stage II	
Stage IIA G2T1N0M0	Grade 2 tumor less than 5 cm in diameter with no regional lymph node or distant metastases
Stage IIB G2T2N0M0	Grade 2 tumor 5 cm or greater in diameter with no regional lymph node or distant metastases
Stage III	
Stage IIIA G3T1N0M0	Grade 3 tumor less than 5 cm in diameter with no regional lymph node or distant metastases
Stage IIIB G3T2N0M0	Grade 3 tumor 5 cm or greater in diameter with no regional lymph node or distant metastases
Stage IV	
Stage IVA G1–3T1–2N1M0	Tumor of any grade or size with histologically verified metastasis to regional lymph nodes, but no distant metastases
Stage IVB G1–3T1–2N0–1M1	Clinically diagnosed distant metastases

(Bears OH, Henson DE, Hutter RVP, Kennedy BJ, eds. Manual for staging cancer, American Joint Committee on Cancer. 4th ed. Philadelphia: JB Lippincott, 1992)

TABLE 42-7. Local Control and Disease-free Survival for 220 Patients with Soft Tissue Sarcoma Treated at MGH by Radiation and Surgery According to AJC Stage

		5-Year Actuarial Results	
*AJC Stage**	*No. of Patients*	*Local Control*	*Disease-free Survival*
IA	17	1.00	1.00
IB	30	0.93	0.88
IIA	40	0.88	0.83
IIB	66	0.85	0.52
IIIA	33	0.93	0.87
IIIB	69	0.79	0.39
IVA	3	1.00	1.00
Total	258	0.88	0.66

* Excludes patients with distant metastases (stage IVB) and patients with sarcomas arising from thoracic, abdominal, pelvic, and retroperitoneal sites.
(Suit HD, Mankin HJ, Willett G, et al. Limited surgery and external irradiation in soft tissue sarcomas. In: Recent Concepts in Sarcoma Treatment. Proceedings of the International Symposium on Sarcomas. Tarpon Springs, FL, October 8–10, 1987. The Netherlands: Kluwer Academic Publishers, 1988)

in 220 patients with soft tissue sarcomas of all sites, excluding retroperitoneum, treated at the Massachusetts General Hospital is presented in Table 42–7.[62]

The survivals for adults with soft tissue sarcomas by clinical and pathologic stage are shown in Fig. 42–6. For clinical stages I, II, III, and IV, the 5-year estimated survival rates are 79%, 65%, 45%, and 10%, respectively.[46]

An alternate staging system has been proposed by Enneking and colleagues (Table 42–8).[167] In this system, patients are categorized as stage I (low-grade, no metastases), stage II (high-grade, no metastases), or stage III (either grade with regional or distant metastases). Tumors are designated "A" if they are contained within an anatomic compartment and are designated "B" if they extend across fascial planes. The correlation of survival with stage of disease using this scheme in 397 patients with sarcomas of the extremity is shown in Table 42–9.[167] This staging system is practical only for extremity sarcomas.

Factors thought to be of prognostic importance in patients with soft tissue sarcomas are listed in Table 42–10.[44,61,64,16] The site of a soft tissue sarcoma often influences resectability and local control and cure. Lesions in the trunk, especially those in the retroperitoneum, mediastinum, head, and neck, often involve vital structures before they become clinically apparent. They are usually large, and local control by any approach is less likely for these tumors than for tumors on the extremity or torso. In the extremity, the exact site of the lesion has prognostic importance. Proximal lesions are less curable than distal lesions. In the series reported by Simon and Enneking, local recurrences after surgery alone in the buttock, groin, thigh, and areas below the knee were 38%, 14%, 15%, and 0%, respectively (Table 42–11).[60]

Size is an important parameter for freedom from distant metastases and for local control. Among subjects whose treatment controlled the primary lesion, distant control decreased

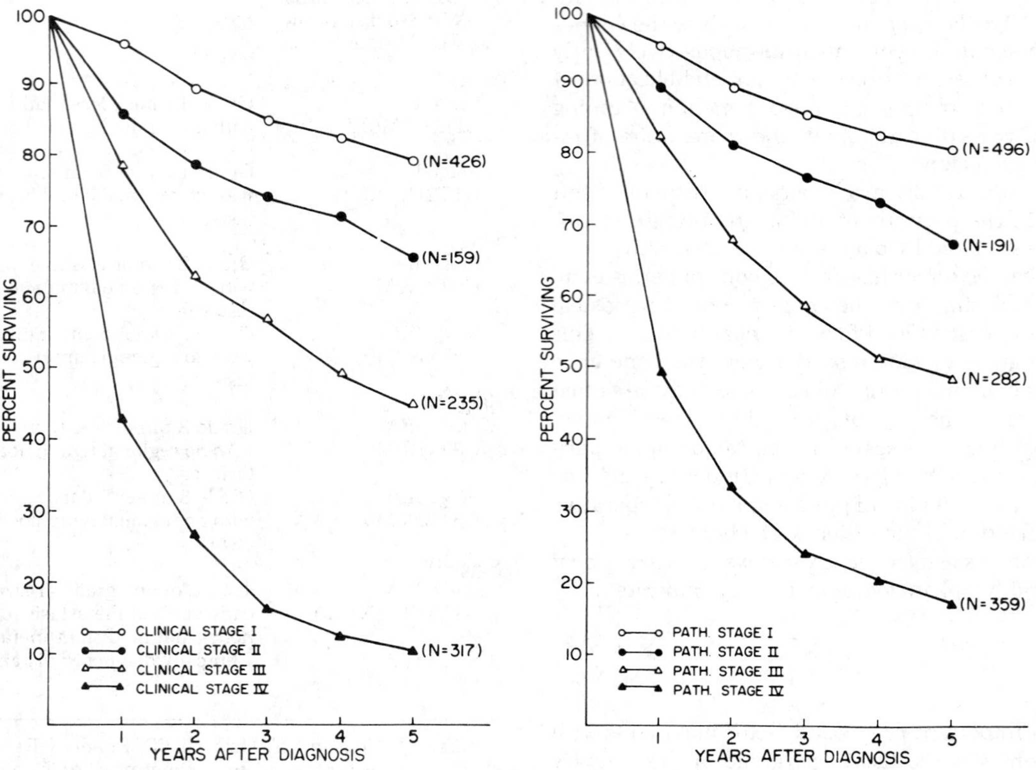

FIGURE 42–6. Overall survival of patients with soft tissue sarcomas according to AJCC clinical and pathologic grading of tumors. There is a strong correlation of survival with each stage of disease.

TABLE 42-8. Enneking System for Staging of Sarcomas of Soft Tissues or Bone

Stage	*Characteristic*
I	Low grade
IA	Intracompartmental
IB	Extracompartmental
II	High grade
IIA	Intracompartmental
IIB	Extracompartmental
III	Any grade
	N1 or M1

(Enneking WF, Spanier SS, Goodman MA. The surgical staging of musculoskeletal sarcoma. J Bone Joint Surg [Am] 1980;62:1027–1030)

rapidly with tumor size (Table 42–12).[44,61,64,169] Size is a major factor in achieving local control by surgery alone for tumors in some anatomic sites (*e.g.*, head, neck, retroperitoneum), and it is a dominant factor in the results of radiation therapy alone. For irradiation combined with surgery, local control did not depend on size for lesions up to 150 mm.

Soft tissue sarcomas rarely spread to regional lymph nodes. In a review of 374 patients referred to the NCI during 24 years, only 3 patients (2.6%) of 113 who had lymph nodes evaluated had evidence of metastases to draining lymph nodes before gross dissemination of disease.[170] In a review of more than 2500 patients in the world literature, Weingrad and Rosenberg analyzed the incidence of lymph node metastases from each of the major histologic types of soft tissue sarcomas (Table 42–13).[170] Approximately 5% of patients with soft tissue sarcomas developed nodal metastases at any point in the course of their disease, although for patients with synovial cell sarcoma and rhabdomyosarcoma the, incidence was higher. Patients with involvement of draining lymph nodes had a substantially poorer prognosis than did those whose lymph nodes were not involved. Mazeron and Suit reported an incidence of regional lymph node involvement of 5.9% for 323 patients with stage M0 soft tissue sarcoma.[171] There was no regional node involvement in patients with grade 1 sarcomas compared with 2% and 12% for grades 2 and 3, respectively. In their series, the 19 patients who had nodal involvement had a 5-year survival rate of 32%.

Rosenberg and coworkers reported an inverse correlation between prognosis and the number of perioperative blood transfusions administered to patients who underwent resections of localized high-grade sarcomas of the extremities.[172] The number of transfusions represented a prognostic variable independent of tumor size. This observation requires confirmation by others.

The histologic cell of origin of soft tissue sarcomas is not of major prognostic importance if lesions of equivalent grade are compared. There appears to be no prognostic importance attached to the age or sex of patients with soft tissue sarcomas, except that fibrosarcomas occurring in children tend to have a better prognosis than those in adult patients, even if allowances are made for grade and size.[173] Liposarcomas may be less aggressive in children.[174]

TABLE 42-9. Predicted Survival According to Stages, Based on 397 Extremity Sarcoma Patients

	Probability of Survival	
Stage	*2 Years*	*5 Years*
IA	0.99	0.97
IB	0.95	0.89
IIA	0.88	0.73
IIB	0.73	0.45
III	0.37	0.08

(Enneking WF, Spanier SS, Goodman MA. The surgical staging of musculoskeletal sarcoma. J Bone Joint Surg [Am] 1980;62:1027–1030)

NATURAL HISTORY OF SOFT TISSUE SARCOMAS

COMMON FEATURES

The poor prognosis of most patients with soft tissue sarcomas is due to the tendency of these lesions to invade aggressively into surrounding tissues and for early hematogenous dissemination, usually to the lungs. Soft tissue sarcomas invade locally along anatomic planes, such as nerve fibers, muscle bundles, fascial planes, and blood vessels. Most patients with soft tissue sarcomas present without obvious clinical metastases. Of 565 soft tissue sarcoma patients admitted to Memorial Sloan-Kettering Cancer Center between 1983 and 1985, 128 (22.7%) had evidence of metastases at presentation.[175] At the Massachusetts General Hospital between 1971 and 1981, 28 (10.3%) of 272 patients who presented with a primary sarcoma were found to have distant metastases.[176] In the American College of Surgeons survey, 1365 (23.5%) of 5812 patients who presented with soft tissue sarcoma had evidence of distant metastases.[46] The lung was the most frequent site of distant metastases, accounting for 33% of the metastatic lesions, followed by bone and liver (Table 42–14).[46]

Because the appropriate diagnosis is often not appreciated or suspected before biopsy, many soft tissue sarcomas are initially treated by shelling out the lesion through the pseudocapsule. In the American College of Surgeons survey, approximately half of sarcomas were biopsied by this procedure or by excision (see Table 42–5). Only 20% of the sarcomas were diagnosed by incisional biopsy. Excisional biopsy is inadequate as sole therapy, and more than 90% of these patients have local recurrences.

In a review of 87 patients with low-grade sarcomas with a median follow-up of 7 years, Marcus found that 14 patients

TABLE 42-10. Prognostic Factors for Patients With Primary Soft Tissue Sarcomas

Histologic grade
Site (proximal vs distal; extremity vs trunk)
Size
Lymph node involvement

TABLE 42-11. Anatomic Site Correlated With Local Recurrence Rate of Soft Tissue Sarcomas of the Extremities

Anatomic Site	*No. of Patients*	*% Total*	*No. With Recurrence*	*No. Without Recurrence*	*% Recurrence*
Lower extremity	(53)				
Intrapelvic	2	3	2	0	100
Buttock	8	11	3	5	38
Groin	7	10	1	6	14
Thigh	26	37	4	22	15
Knee	3	4	0	3	0
Below knee	7	10	0	7	0
Upper extremity	(17)				
Shoulder girdle	4	6	2	2	50
Arm	7	10	0	7	0
Below elbow	6	9	1	5	17

(Simon MA, Enneking WF. The management of soft-tissue sarcomas of the extremities. J Bone Joint Surg [Am] 1976;58:317)

had local recurrences, 3 developed distant metastases, and the estimated tumor-related mortality rate at 10 years was 7%.[177] Factors retrospectively associated with poorer disease-free survival were retroperitoneal location, no postoperative radiation therapy, and positive surgical margins. Overall survival was most affected by tumor location, with 50% of the tumor-related deaths occurring in the 8% of patients with retroperitoneal lesions. Even these deaths occurred 7.0 to 9.5 years after diagnosis. Although these results are somewhat better than those from large national surveys, this difference may be due to a low proportion of retroperitoneal tumors and pathologic tumor grading by an institution with extensive sarcoma experience.

The pattern of recurrence in patients with high-grade soft tissue sarcoma is a function of the primary site of the lesion. Potter and associates analyzed 307 patients referred to the NCI between 1975 and 1982 who underwent complete surgical resection of high-grade soft tissue sarcomas, often in combination with chemotherapy and radiation therapy.[44] The pattern of recurrence in the 107 patients is shown in Table 42–15. Patients with retroperitoneal sarcomas had a greater tendency to recur with disseminated disease throughout the abdomen, and patients with truncal sarcomas had a higher local recurrence rate than was seen in patients with primary lesions in the extremities. Among the entire group with recurrences, the lung was the predominant site (52%) of the first isolated recurrence; isolated local recurrence was seen in 20% of patients. In the American College of Surgeons survey, treatment failures in patients without metastases at initial diagnoses and with total gross resections of the soft tissue sarcomas occurred in 452 (37%) of 1209 patients.[46] Isolated locoregional recurrence occurred in 236 (52.2%) of these patients. This high rate may reflect inadequate surgical resection or inadequate adjunctive treatments. At least 25% of the patients had limited local excisions of the primary tumor if no distant disease was documented.

TABLE 42-12. Actuarial Distant Control Rates at 5 Years Among 159 Patients With G2–3 Sarcoma of Soft Tissue With Control of Primary Lesion After Treatment by Radiation and Surgery

Tumor Size (mm)	*No. of Patients*	*Actuarial Distant Control (5 y)*
<25	17	0.94
26–49	48	0.77
50–100	55	0.62
101–150	24	0.51
151–200	9	0.42
>200	6	0.17
Total	159	0.65

(Suit HD, Mankin HJ, Wood WC, et al. Treatment of the patient with stage M_0 soft tissue sarcoma. J Clin Oncol 1988;6:854–862)

TABLE 42-13. Incidence of Lymph Node Metastases in Patients With Soft Tissue Sarcomas

Histology	*No. of Series*	*No. of Patients*	*Incidence of Lymph Node Metastases* No.	*%*
Liposarcoma	7	288	15	5.7
Fibrosarcoma	14	1083	55	5.1
Rhabdomyosarcoma	13	888	108	12.2
Synoviosarcoma	13	535	91	17.0
Unclassifiable	5	125	11	8.8
Neurofibrosarcoma	2	60	0	0

(Weingrad DW, Rosenberg SA. Early lymphatic spread of osteogenic and soft-tissue sarcomas. Surgery 1978;84:231–240)

TABLE 42-14. Clinically Involved Distant Metastatic Sites at Time of Diagnosis of Sarcoma

Metastatic Sites	*1977–1978* No.	*1977–1978* %	*1983–1984* No.	*1983–1984* %
Bone	126	22.6	191	23.7
Lung	186	33.3	275	34.1
Liver	83	14.9	126	15.7
Brain	19	3.4	22	2.7
Other	144	25.8	193	23.9
Total	558	100.0	807	100.0

(Lawrence W, Donegan WL, Natarajan N, et al. Adult soft tissue sarcomas. A pattern of care survey of The American College of Surgeons. Ann Surg 1987;205:349–359)

The time until local recurrence is fairly constant in most reported series. Cantin and coworkers demonstrated that approximately 80% of all lesions that recur after surgery do so within 2 years.[178] In 54 patients treated surgically by Simon and Enneking, all local recurrences occurred by 30 months after definitive resection.[60] Lindberg and associates also reported that 80% of local recurrences occurred in the first 2 years and 100% by 3 years.[179] Shiu and associates reported 87% of local recurrences within the first 2 years.[59] Gerner and associates reported that 82% of local recurrences were evident by 2 years at Roswell Park Memorial Institute.[180]

Patients undergoing amputation or radical local excision have local recurrence rates of about 20%.[59,60] In older series from Memorial Sloan-Kettering Cancer Center, local recurrences were seen in 59% of patients undergoing conservative excision, compared with 25% for those undergoing radical excision.[178] At the M.D. Anderson Cancer Center, patients undergoing conservative excision had a 77% local recurrence rate, compared with 28% for those undergoing radical excision.[58] These series were not randomized, and these figures are highly influenced by patient selection factors. In general, however, the larger the surgical excisions in all directions from the tumors, the lower are the local recurrence rates.

Spread to draining lymph nodes is an uncommon finding. In a review by Weingrad and Rosenberg of more than 30 series, 5.8% of almost 3000 patients developed lymph node metastases some time during their course (see Table 42–13). These figures reflect the incidence of lymph node metastases at any time during the course of the disease; spread to lymph nodes in the early stages is less frequent. There was a 3.2% incidence of nodal spread in almost 6000 patients analyzed in the American College of Surgeons survey.[46] Mazeron and Suit reported a 5.9% incidence of regional nodal involvement in 323 patients with stage M0 sarcoma.[171] The incidence of lymph node metastases is somewhat higher for epithelioid sarcomas (20–40%), in synovial cell sarcoma (17%), and in rhabdomyosarcoma (12%) than for other histologic types.

Before 1977, when surgery was the primary modality of treatment, the overall 5-year survival rate in most reported series of patients with soft tissue sarcoma was approximately 50% (Table 42–16).[38,39,57–61,168,180–182]

UNIQUE FEATURES OF HISTOLOGIC SUBTYPES

Despite the common biologic behavior of equivalent-grade soft tissue sarcomas, there are some features that are unique to individual histologic types.

Fibrosarcoma

Before 1965, fibrosarcoma was the most common diagnosis of soft tissue sarcoma.[183,184] Since that time, the recognition of a larger variety of subtypes of soft tissue sarcoma has significantly decreased this diagnosis. As stated by Stout and Lattes, "One should try to restrict the term 'fibrosarcoma' to growths that are composed of cells and fibers derived from fibrocytes and exclude all the fibrous growths derived from other types of cells acting as facultative fibroblasts."[49] Although some pathologists differentiate fibroblastic fibrosarcoma from pleomorphic fibrosarcoma largely by the uniformity of the herringbone pattern of the tumor and the number of mitotic figures, this is mainly a reflection of grading.[47] Because of the changing definition of fibrosarcoma, earlier series undoubtedly contain sarcomas that would now be identified as other histologic types.[183–186] Infantile fibrosarcomas are extremely rare. There have been 3 cases of inoperable infantile fibrosarcoma that completely responded to chemotherapy.[187,188]

TABLE 42-15. Frequency of Initial Recurrence Pattern by Site of Primary Sarcoma

Primary Site	*Extremity* *No. (%)*	*Retroperitoneal* *No. (%)*	*Trunk* *No. (%)*	*Breast* *No. (%)*	*Head and Neck* *No. (%)*	*Total* *No. (%)*
Isolated lung	43 (70)	3 (17)	5 (29)	3 (75)	2 (50)	56 (52)
Isolated local	7 (10)	5 (30)	7 (41)	0	2 (50)	21 (20)
Isolated other	11 (15)	1 (6)	2 (12)	1 (25)	0	15 (14)
Multiple	4 (5)	8 (47)	3 (18)	0	0	15 (14)
Total	65 (100)	17 (100)	17 (100)	4 (100)	4 (100)	107 (100)

(Potter DA, Glenn J, Kinsella T, et al. Patterns of recurrence in patients with high-grade soft tissue sarcoma. J Clin Oncol 1985;3:353–366)

TABLE 42-16. Soft Tissue Sarcomas: Results of Surgical Excision Alone

Investigations	*No. of Patients*	*Survival Before 1977 (%)*	
		5 Years	*10 Years*
Task Force, AJC[61]	1215	41	30
Surgery Branch, NCI (before 1975)[181]	66	48	44
Gerner et al[180]	155	50	26
Shieber and Graham[38]	125	27	22
Martin and Ariel[58]	183	40	
Pack and Cerny[57]	717	39	
Hare[39]	200	39	
Shiu et al[59]	297	55	41
Suit et al[168]	100	52	
Simon and Enneking[60]	54	62	
Markhede et al[160]	97	59	

Rhabdomyosarcoma

Rhabdomyosarcoma accounts for about 15% of all sarcomas.[189–194] Because the skeletal muscle accounts for approximately 40% of adult body weight, this tumor, on a per weight basis, is one of the rarest of all tumors. Striated muscle cells are highly differentiated cells that rarely undergo mitosis in the postnatal period, which probably accounts for the low incidence of these malignancies.

The three categories of rhabdomyosarcoma are pleomorphic, alveolar, and embryonal. Many tumors contain several histologic patterns, and the assignment of a specific subtype is often nebulous. Because the alveolar and embryonal types usually occur in childhood, they are often referred to as juvenile-type rhabdomyosarcomas. "Botryoid" indicates the gross appearance of a subset of embryonal rhabdomyosarcomas that have a polypoid or grape-like appearance. Embryonal rhabdomyosarcomas with botryoid features are commonly found in the urogenital tract of infants and children, although these tumors have occurred in the oral and nasal pharynx. Embryonal tumors occasionally are found in adult and elderly patients. Lloyd and associates reported a series of 54 cases of embryonal rhabdomyosarcomas in patients 20 years or older.[194] Embryonal rhabdomyosarcomas are the most common soft tissue sarcomas of children. Discussion of these tumors is presented elsewhere in the text.

Alveolar rhabdomyosarcomas are distinguished by slit-like alveolar spaces in the tumor.

Pleomorphic rhabdomyosarcomas generally present in adulthood, although they can appear in childhood. They are rare adult sarcomas that arise within skeletal muscles. The most common sites of pleomorphic rhabdomyosarcomas are the extremities. These are often highly anaplastic lesions, having small and large cells with one or many bizarre nuclei. Their diagnosis has changed dramatically in recent years. A review by Hajdu of 214 sarcomas originally diagnosed as pleomorphic rhabdomyosarcoma led to a reclassification of 93 of these lesions as other histologic subtypes, mainly malignant fibrous histiocytoma.[47] Differentiation of pleomorphic rhabdomyosarcoma from other pleomorphic sarcomas can be aided by immunohistochemical staining using antibodies specific for constituent proteins of sarcomeric muscle.[195–197]

Leiomyosarcoma

Leiomyosarcomas are malignant neoplasms that arise from smooth muscle. Because these tumors can arise from the walls of small and large blood vessels, they can occur anywhere in the body.[198–201] Leiomyosarcomas also occur in the viscera, arising from smooth muscle (*e.g.*, the uterus) or from vessels in these organs. Leiomyosarcomas commonly arise in the retroperitoneum, where they are highly aggressive neoplasms.

Liposarcoma

Liposarcomas are malignant lesions of adipose tissue.[202–207] The incidence in men exceeds that in women by about 1.5 to 1. Multicentric liposarcomas have been described. In a series of 97 patients with liposarcomas reported by Kindbloom and coworkers, 11 patients had second liposarcomas that developed at sites remote from their first tumors.

Four subtypes of liposarcomas are recognized: well-differentiated, myxoid, lipoblastic (*i.e.*, round cell), and pleomorphic tumors. Some investigators refer to fibroblastic liposarcomas as a fifth subtype. Well-differentiated liposarcomas can exhibit aggressive local invasion and can infrequently metastasize late in their course. Lipoblastic or epithelioid sarcomas are composed of uniform round cells and are highly vascular. These are highly malignant lesions, and like the pleomorphic liposarcomas, they have only a 20% to 30% 5-year survival rate in most reported series.

Synovial Sarcoma

Synovial sarcomas are malignant neoplasms that arise from tendosynovial tissue and occur most commonly in the second through fourth decades.[208–212] The lower extremities are the most common sites of synovial sarcomas. They can occur in any muscle, although not usually close to joints. Although extremities are the most common sites, lesions can occur in the abdominal wall and in other skeletal muscles of the trunk. The two synovial sarcomas generally recognized are the monophasic and biphasic types. Monophasic synovial sarcomas are characterized by sheaths of monotonous spindle cells; the biphasic variety has slit-like spaces or clefts present within the tumor. These clefts are lined by cuboidal or tall columnar epithelial cells and sometimes resemble carcinomas. Calcified areas often appear within the synovial sarcomas and lead to a characteristic x-ray appearance of this type of soft tissue sarcoma. Some investigators consider epithelioid and clear cell sarcomas to be variants of synovial cell sarcoma, although these types are considered separately in this chapter.

Cagle and colleagues reviewed 45 synovial cell sarcoma patients and were able to identify high-risk and low-risk patients based on percent of glandularity and mitotic rates.[213] Low-risk patients, identified as having more than 50% glandular features and less than 15 mitoses per 10 high-power fields, had a 100% survival rate. High-risk patients, with less than 50% glandular features and more than 15 mitoses per 10 high-power fields, had a 37% survival rate.

Neurofibrosarcomas

Neurofibrosarcomas are malignant tumors of neural sheath origin. They have also been referred to as neurogenic sarcomas, malignant schwannomas, and malignant neurilemomas.[131,214] These tumors can occur anywhere in the body.

Neurofibrosarcomas are frequently associated with von Recklinghausen's disease, a chronic, progressive disease inherited as a mendelian-dominant trait and associated with multiple neurofibromas and skin pigment changes, which are characterized as café-au-lait spots.[123–131] About 10% of patients with neurofibromatosis develop sarcomatous changes during their lifetimes, often in preexisting, benign masses.

Angiosarcomas

Hemangiosarcomas and lymphangiosarcomas arise from blood and lymphatic vessels, respectively.[215–221] These are almost uniformly high-grade lesions, but they are uncommon, comprising only 2% of all soft tissue sarcomas. In 1948, Stuart and Treves reported 6 cases of lymphangiosarcoma in lymphedematous arms after radical mastectomy.[15,222–224] In 1972, Woodward and colleagues reported 23 cases of lymphangiosarcoma associated with chronic lymphedema seen at the Mayo Clinic and reviewed the world literature of 163 cases reported up to that time.[222] The cases of postmastectomy lymphangiosarcoma occurred at an average age of 63.9 years and at an average of 10 years and 3 months after mastectomy. Because of the diffuse nature of these tumors, most physicians recommend radical amputation (*i.e.*, shoulder disarticulation, forequarter amputation) for patients who develop lymphangiosarcoma in the upper extremity after mastectomy.[222–224]

Hemangiosarcomas may occur anywhere in the body but often arise in skin and superficial soft tissue, which contrasts sharply with the deep location of most soft tissue sarcomas.[50] Of 366 hemangiosarcomas, 33% arose in the skin and 25% in the soft tissues. Fifty percent of cutaneous hemangiosarcomas are localized in the head and neck region. These are extremely aggressive tumors despite multimodality therapy, and one series of 72 patients reported by Holden and coworkers had a 12% 5-year survival rate.[225]

Hemangiopericytoma

Malignant hemangiopericytoma is a malignant sarcoma thought to arise from the pericyte cells of smooth muscle origin that lie around small vessels.[139,140,226–228] Benign and malignant hemangiopericytomas exist, and the rarity of these lesions has led to considerable confusion in differentiating benign and malignant variants. Hemangiopericytomas should be treated as other sarcomas. In most series, 5-year survival rates of approximately 50% are recorded.

Kaposi's Sarcoma

In 1872, Kaposi described "multiple idiopathic pigmented sarcomas of the skin" that "arise in the skin, without any known local or systemic cause."[229,230] These tumors are thought to arise from endothelial cells and present as raised pigmented lesions of the skin. Four clinical types of Kaposi's sarcoma have been recognized (Table 42–17).[231] The classic Kaposi's sarcoma occurs in elderly men of Mediterranean or Jewish extraction living in the United States or Europe.[232–235] This is a rare tumor, and in 1965, Reynolds and colleagues reported a series of only 70 patients collected during 38 years.[232] These lesions usually start as a reddish nodule on the lower extremity. The disease is generally indolent and can be palliated with radiation therapy if necessary. Approximately 20% of these patients die as a direct result of Kaposi's sarcoma, usually because of gastrointestinal or pulmonary involvement.[229] Many of these patients developed second malignancies (*e.g.*, lymphomas), and in one series, death from secondary primaries, often lymphoreticular neoplasms, was as great a threat to life as was mortality from the Kaposi's sarcoma itself.[230,236]

In 1950, interest in Kaposi's sarcoma was renewed after a second form of the disease was described by Kaminer and

TABLE 42–17. Comparison of Clinical Manifestations of Kaposi's Sarcoma

Type	*Population*	*Male to Female Ratio*	*Clinical Characteristics*	*Course*
Classic	Jewish, Italian heritage (age 50–80 y)	15:1	Lower extremity cutaneous lesions	Indolent: 10–15-year survival
African	Young adult (age 25–40 y)	13:1	Lower-extremity nodular cutaneous lesions	Indolent, locally aggressive disease
	Children (age 2–13 y)	3:1	Generalized lymphadenopathy, cutaneous lesions rare	Rapidly progressive: 2–3-year survival
Renal transplant	Iatrogenic immunosuppressed patient	2.3:1	Localized cutaneous or disseminated	Indolent or progressive: fatal in 30%
Epidemic	AIDS patients	20:1	Disseminated mucocutaneous lesion and visceral involvement	Fulminant: <20% 2-year survival

(Adapted from Krigel RL, Friedman-Kien AE. Kaposi's sarcoma in AIDS. In: DeVita VT, Hellman S, Rosenberg, SA, eds. AIDS. Etiology, diagnosis, treatment, and prevention. Philadelphia: JB Lippincott, 1985:185–211)

Murray, who compiled 43 cases of Kaposi's sarcoma in Bantu men in Africa.[237] In some areas of Africa, Kaposi's sarcoma is a common neoplasm, representing between 3% and 9% of all reported malignancies.[235,238] This disease can be more aggressive than the American or European Kaposi's sarcoma. These lesions can respond to chemotherapy with dactinomycin, vincristine, and dacarbazine (DTIC).[230]

Another type of Kaposi's sarcoma is associated with renal transplantation, and the first case was reported in 1969.[239] Since then, a number of renal allograft recipients have been reported to develop Kaposi's sarcoma after the onset of immunosuppressive therapy. The incidence of Kaposi's sarcoma in patients undergoing renal transplantation appears to be 0.4%, which represents between 150 to 200 times the expected incidence of this tumor in the general population. The average time to development of Kaposi's sarcoma after transplantation is about 16 months. The extent of the tumor correlates with the degree of depression of cellular immunity. In some cases the tumors have regressed because of reduction or changes in immunosuppressive therapy.[240–243]

The Kaposi's sarcoma associated with acquired immunodeficiency syndrome (AIDS) has been called epidemic Kaposi's sarcoma. The initial reports of epidemic Kaposi's sarcoma appeared in 1981.[244] The clinical features of these patients are reminiscent of Kaposi's sarcoma of immunosuppressed renal transplant patients, underscoring the opportunistic nature of this tumor. Approximately 48% of homosexual males with AIDS present with or eventually develop Kaposi's sarcoma. Approximately 4% of all heterosexual intravenous drug users with AIDS and about 12% of Haitian AIDS patients develop epidemic Kaposi's sarcoma.[231] None of the hemophiliac patients with AIDS have developed Kaposi's sarcoma. This form of the disease can be extremely virulent, and death from the disease or related complications of immunodeficiency occurs in most patients. Kaposi's sarcoma in AIDS is reviewed in Chapter 59.

Malignant Fibrous Histiocytoma

Malignant fibrous histiocytoma was characterized by O'Brien and Stout as a group of tumors having a common origin from tissue histiocytes.[141,245–250] This diagnosis has achieved great popularity in recent years, and many cases previously diagnosed as pleomorphic rhabdomyosarcoma or undifferentiated fibrosarcoma are now categorized as malignant fibrous histiocytoma. A wide spectrum of fibrous histiocytomas exists, from those that are benign to those that are highly atypical to those that are frankly malignant. In many series, malignant fibrous histiocytoma is the most common diagnosis attached to soft tissue sarcomas.

These tumors are more common in adults, with 40% occurring in the sixth and seventh decades of life and with fewer than 5% occurring in patients younger than 20 years of age.[251–253]

Alveolar Soft Part Sarcoma

Alveolar soft part sarcomas were described by Christopherson in 1952.[254–256] These tumors have a unique histologic appearance, but the cell of origin is unknown. These are true malignant sarcomas with no benign counterpart, although they tend to have a more protracted course than most other sarcomas. Although most patients ultimately die from the disease, 5-year survival rates of 60% are common. Many patients develop metastatic disease that progresses slowly over the course of 5 to 15 years before death.

The tumor commonly arises in the thigh in adults and in the head and neck region in children.[50] In 143 patients reviewed by the Armed Forces Institute of Pathology, 44% of the tumors arose in the lower extremities, 27% in the head and neck area, 17% in the upper extremities, and 11% in the trunk.[50]

Epithelioid Sarcoma

Epithelioid sarcomas are of unknown origin and occur almost exclusively in the extremities, usually in the hand or foot, associated with aponeurotic structures.[257–262] These tumors differ in their natural history from most other sarcomas in that they have a greater tendency to spread to noncontiguous areas of skin, subcutaneous tissue, fat, and bone. The tumors have a high propensity to spread to draining lymph nodes. Chase and Enzinger reviewed 241 cases of epithelioid sarcoma in which the most common initial sites of metastases were the lymph nodes (48%) and lungs (24%).[262] A more aggressive course was associated with a proximal or axial tumor location, increased tumor size or depth, hemorrhage, mitotic figures, necrosis, or vascular invasion. More favorable behavior was observed if the tumor arose in distal extremities in younger patients or in female patients between the ages of 10 and 49. Long-term survival is similar to or slightly better than for most other soft tissue sarcomas. Recommended therapy for these patients is wide excision, often involving amputation of the extremity and regional lymph node dissection.

TREATMENT

Surgery alone, surgery combined with radiation, surgery combined with radiation and intraarterial chemotherapy, or radiation alone have been used for the treatment of soft tissue sarcomas. There has been an intense and sustained interest in evaluating treatment strategies that preserve limbs of patients with sarcomas of soft tissue of the extremities and reduce the extent of resection for patients who have lesions on the torso or in the head and neck region by combining less than radical surgery with radiation and chemotherapy.

A National Institutes of Health consensus conference in 1984 reviewed a variety of limb-sparing approaches, which included surgery plus adjunctive radiation therapy or chemotherapy, for the treatment of high-grade extremity sarcomas.[263] They concluded that limb-sparing treatment for some of these sarcoma patients was an effective treatment option. The available data indicate that the results of these conservative approaches were equivalent to those obtained by more radical surgical procedures in selected subgroups of patients.

In discussing the rationale for combining these modalities, the results are presented in terms of frequency of local control, survival, and complications. Important technical aspects are delineated for currently employed strategies.

TABLE 42–18. Local Recurrence Rate After Surgery Alone

	Local Failures/Total No. of Patients (%)		
Investigations	*Marginal Excision*	*Wide Excision*	*Radical Excision*
Simon et al[60]	3/6 (50)	7/20 (35)	3/43 (7)
Markehede et al[182] *	16/21 (76)		5/76 (7)
Gerner et al[180]	54/58 (93)	15/25 (60)	3/38 (8)
Shiu et al[59] †			54/297 (18)
Total	73/85 (86)	22/45 (49)	65/454 (14)

* Two patients received preoperative radiation therapy.
† Eighteen patients had adjunctive radiation therapy.

SURGERY

The essential ingredient in any surgical approach designed to maximize local control is to achieve adequate negative surgical margins. Until the late 1940s and the early 1950s, the surgical approach to the patient with sarcoma of a soft tissue was a local excision, which removed the grossly evident tumor mass with little or no margin of adjacent normal tissue. This is a "marginal excision." The local failure rate for this procedure is approximately 86% (range, 50–93%), as indicated in Table 42–18.[59,60,180,182] Improvement to reduce local failure rates emphasized the use of more extensive surgical procedures to obtain wider margins of normal tissue. Wide local excisions, which usually entail only soft tissue resections, are associated with local recurrences of 49% if surgery alone is performed (see Table 42–18). More radical procedures, such as amputation or muscle compartmental excisions, are associated with an even lower local failure rate of 14% (range, 7–18%), as documented in four separate series (see Table 42–18).

Resection of a soft tissue sarcoma requires that the tumor be located so that an acceptably wide margin of normal tissue can be obtained between the edge of the tumor and the adjacent critical, nonresectable structures, such as major nerves, vessels, bone, and important tendons. This guideline does not apply to many anatomic sites, such as the groin, knee, popliteal space, most portions of the leg, the ankle, many sites within the head and neck area, supraclavicular area, some axillary sites, the elbow region, and most of the forearm, wrist, and hand. Because of the inability to obtain a clear margin at those sites and still retain acceptable function, approximately half of patients with extremity sarcomas were subjected to amputation at institutions with a large experience in sarcoma surgery. Table 42–19 shows the proportion of patients with extremity sarcomas treated by radical resection or amputation at the University of Florida in Gainesville or at Memorial Sloan-Kettering Cancer Center in New York City.[59,60]

The combined results of amputation for the treatment of sarcoma of soft tissue from four centers showed that local control was obtained in 40 of 40 patients with lesions of the leg or foot.[59,60,182,264] In these patients, the level of amputation was well above the lesion and, in most instances, above the level of the proximal joint. These results can be taken as the benchmark for local control results for sarcomas of the distal extremities. If the level of amputation is closer to the tumor (*e.g.*, thigh lesions), about 10% of patients fail locally. In the University of Florida and Goteborg series, 5% and 89% local failure rates were documented after surgery obtaining adequate and inadequate margins, respectively (Table 42–20).[60,182]

TABLE 42–19. Local Control of Soft Tissue Sarcomas of the Extremities by Radical Surgery

Series Factors	*Simon and Enneking*[59]	*Shiu et al*[60]
Total number of patients	54	297
Radical local resection	25 (46%)	158 (53%)
Amputation	29 (54%)	139 (47%)
Local control		
Radical local resection	88%	72%
Amputation	79%	93%
Overall	83%	82%

Sites of failure among 464 patients treated by surgery alone at three institutions are shown in Table 40–21.[59,182,265] The total local failure rate was 19%; 35% developed distant metastases. These figures are a fair indication of the best that can be accomplished by surgery alone for soft tissue sarcoma in extremities, although patient selection can influence these results. The proportion of patients amputated in the three centers shown in Table 42–21 were 47%, 16%, and 50%, respectively; which was 41% in the combined study.[59,182,264] An average local control rate of 81% was achieved but only with a high rate of amputation.

The more conservative procedures have been employed in combined-modality treatments to reduce local recurrences but perform limb-sparing surgery. These treatments have been adopted by many institutions with extensive experience in sarcoma surgery. For example, the percentage of limb-sparing procedures being performed at Memorial Sloan-Kettering Cancer Center has increased since 1975, when approximately 50% of all extremity sarcoma patients received amputations. Between 1982 and 1984, 83% of patients had limb-sparing operations, and only 17% had amputations.[266] In recommending a limb-sparing procedure, the physician must inform the patient that the risk of local failure may be higher than for amputation.

Although a local recurrence should be avoided if possible, its true impact is not yet known.[267,268] Any association between local recurrence and distant metastases could be causally re-

TABLE 42–20. Adequacy of Margins of Radical Surgery Related to Local Failure Rate

	No. Local Failures/ Total Failures (%)	
Investigations	*Negative Margins*	*Positive Margins*
Simon and Enneking[60]	1/46 (2)	8/8 (100)
Markhede et al[182]	5/76 (7)	16/19 (84)
Total	6/122 (5)	25/27 (89)

TABLE 42–21. Patterns of Failure in Patients With Extremity Sarcomas Treated by Surgery Alone

Investigations	*No. of Patients*	*Follow-up (y)*	*Amputation (%)*	*Local Failure ± Distant Metastases (%)*	*Distant Metastases (%)*
Memorial Sloan-Kettering Cancer Center[59] *	297	5–24	139 (47)	54 (18)	88 (30)
University of Goteborg[182] †	97	3–23	17 (16)	20 (21)	46 (27)
University of Florida at Gainesville[265]	70	2–19	35 (50)	14 (20)	27 (39)
Total	464	2–24	191 (41)	88 (19)	161 (35)

* Eighteen patients received adjunctive radiation therapy.
† Series includes four patients with truncal sarcomas; two patients received preoperative radiation therapy.

lated or merely a reflection of more aggressive tumor biology. Resolution of such issues would clarify the risk of conservative surgery in marginal cases.

Technical Aspects of Surgery

Extremity Sarcomas

The categorization of surgical procedures by Enneking is useful in carefully defining the nature of the surgical procedure performed (Table 42–22).[269] There are four types of surgical procedures for soft tissue sarcomas.

Intracapsular excision involves removal of the tumor by directly incising the tumor capsule. This procedure leaves gross tumor behind and is of diagnostic value only.

In *marginal excision,* all gross tumor, including the pseudocapsule, is excised locally. Soft tissue sarcomas tend to grow by radial expansion and compress normal structures around them. This pseudocapsule gives the gross appearance of compartmentalization of the tumor from surrounding structures, but invasion of local tissues occurs through the pseudocapsule. The local recurrence rate after treatment by marginal excision alone is close to 90% (see Table 42–18).

In *wide excision,* the tumor is removed with a margin of normal surrounding tissue in continuity with the tumor. This procedure does not imply removal of entire structures within which the tumor may be found. The local recurrence rate after treatment by wide resection alone is approximately 50%.

In *radical resection,* tumor is removed with all tissue in the anatomic compartment occupied by the tumor. The excision takes place by dissecting along planes that are separated from the tumor and its tissues of origin by at least one uninvolved anatomic plane in all directions. The resected specimen includes the origin and insertion of all muscles and any bones or joints that are contained within the anatomic compartment of resection. This procedure may involve amputation, although nonablative procedures can fulfill the criteria for radical resection (Fig. 42–7). The local recurrence rate after these procedures is approximately 14%.

Amputative Procedures. In the treatment of soft tissue sarcomas of the extremities, a variety of amputative procedures can be employed.

For *amputations of the foot,* amputations of digits, ray amputations, transmetatarsal amputation, and Syme amputations at the level of the ankle joint are accepted procedures for ischemic lesions of the foot, but they infrequently give an adequate margin for soft tissue sarcomas in the foot and should be combined with adjuvant radiation therapy to maximize the changes for obtaining local control.

TABLE 42–22. Surgical Procedures for Soft Tissue Extremity Sarcomas

Margin	*How Margin Was Achieved*		*Plane of Dissection*	*Microscopic Appearance*
	Limb Salvage	*Amputation*		
Intracapsular	Intracapsular piecemeal excision	Intracapsular amputation	Within lesion	Tumor at margin
Marginal	Marginal en bloc excision	Marginal amputation	Within reactive zone, extracapsular	Reactive tissue ± microsatellites
Wide	Wide en bloc excision	Wide through-bone amputation	Beyond reactive zone through normal tissue within compartment	Normal tissue ± "skips"
Radical	Radical en bloc resection	Radical disarticulation	Normal tissue, extracompartmental	Normal tissue

(Adapted from Enneking, WF. Staging of musculoskeletal neoplasms. In: Current concepts of diagnosis and treatment of bone and soft tissue tumors. Heidelberg: Springer-Verlag, 1984)

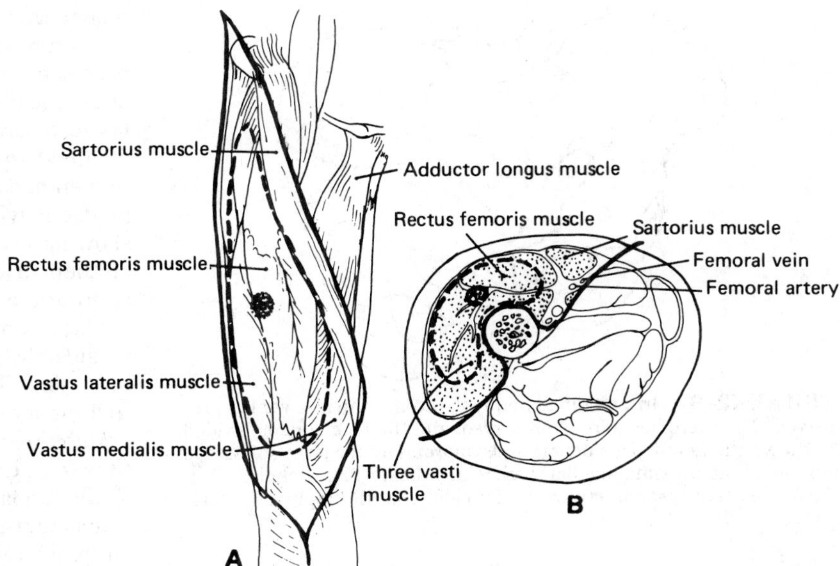

FIGURE 42–7. **(A)** Schematic drawing of the anterior thigh and **(B)** transverse section through the thigh, illustrating the anatomic extent of a radical resection, without amputation, of a soft tissue sarcoma lying within the rectus femoris muscle. (Courtesy of Dr. Martin Malawer)

Below-knee amputation is usually performed about a third the distance between the knee and the ankle and involves division of the tibia and fibula. Muscles to the ankle or foot are transected. This amputation is the treatment of choice for any substantive soft tissue sarcoma of the foot. Because the weight-bearing portions of the foot tolerate radiation therapy poorly, amputation is often the best treatment for these lesions.

Above-knee amputation through the thigh can be performed at any level distal to the lesser trochanter. Major muscle groups of the thigh are transected. This amputation is of little value for tumors occurring above the knee and is often indicated for tumors of the leg.

Hip disarticulation is a form of amputation involving disarticulation of the hip joint with complete removal of the femur. Most muscles attached to the lower extremity are removed entirely. It is often suitable for patients with lesions of the middle and distal thigh.

Hemipelvectomy involves removal of the entire lower extremity and hemipelvis with disarticulation of the sacroiliac joint and pubic symphysis (Fig. 42–8). All major muscles that attach to the lower extremity, except the iliopsoas, are removed. This operation is often applied to the treatment of proximal thigh and buttock lesions. A conventional hemipelvectomy uses a posterior flap of skin and subcutaneous tissue overlying the buttock. For lesions of the buttock, it is possible to construct an anterior flap that includes part of the quadriceps muscles and the femoral vessels. The use of anterior-flap hemipelvectomies has greatly extended the application of this procedure.

Modified hemipelvectomy allows preservation of the iliac wing and improves patient rehabilitation. This procedure is similar to the standard hemipelvectomy, except that the sacroiliac joint is preserved and the iliac bone is excised from an area below the level of the sciatic notch (Fig. 42–9). This operation does involve transection of muscles in the buttock and is not suitable for lesions in this area. Internal hemipelvectomy can be performed with removal of the innominate bone and adjacent muscles but with preservation of the ipsilateral lower extremity.[270]

Extended hemipelvectomy is used if lesions of the iliac wing are too close to the sacroiliac joint to permit its disarticulation. Extension of the standard hemipelvectomy to include excision of the sacral ala at the level of the lateral vertebral bodies adds little in morbidity to this procedure and often adds several centimeters of margin from the tumor.

Amputations of the upper extremities follow the principles enunciated for those of the lower extremities. Below-elbow amputations are often used for the treatment of tumors of the hand and wrist. Above-elbow amputations are used for tumors of the forearm. Disarticulation of the shoulder joint is an operation reserved for distal arm and elbow lesions. Forequarter amputation is applied to the treatment of lesions of the shoulder girdle or the proximal arm. This operation includes removal of the entire upper extremity, including the scapula and clavicle.

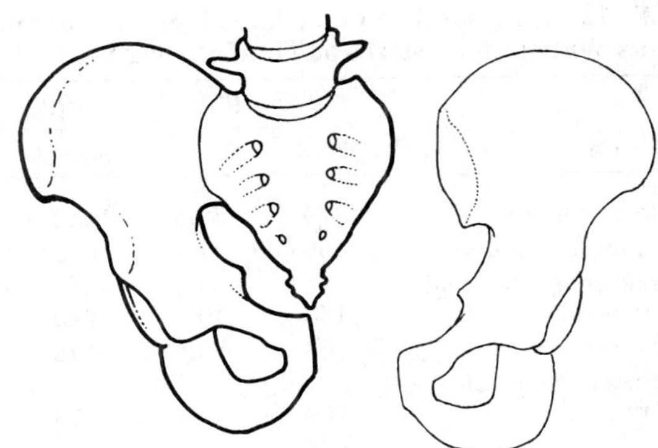

FIGURE 42–8. In a hemipelvectomy, removal of the entire lower extremity including the hemipelvis is performed by disarticulation of the sacroiliac joint and symphysis pubis. This approach may be required for large soft tissue tumors of the buttock and anterior or lateral proximal thigh. (Sugarbaker PH, Nicholson TH. Atlas of extremity sarcoma surgery. Philadelphia: JB Lippincott, 1984)

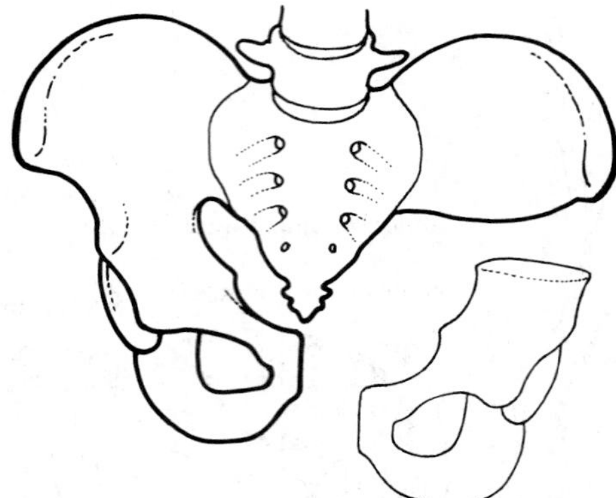

FIGURE 42–9. In a modified hemipelvectomy, the iliac wing is preserved. The sacroiliac joint is preserved, and the iliac bone is divided at the sciatic notch. This operation is appropriate for large soft tissue tumors of the proximal medial thigh. (Sugarbaker PH, Nicholson TH. Atlas of extremity sarcoma surgery. Philadelphia: JB Lippincott, 1984)

Nonamputative Procedures. Nonamputative surgical procedures used in the treatment of patients with soft tissue sarcomas of the extremities should also be known to the surgical oncologist.

Wide excision is one of the most common surgical procedures performed for extremity sarcomas. In the American College of Surgeons survey, approximately half of all sarcomas were treated with this surgical procedure (Table 42–23).[46] As indicated in Table 42–18, this procedure results in a local control rate of 50% if used alone, and wide excision is often employed with adjunctive radiation therapy.

Sound surgical principles must be adhered to (Fig. 42–10). Surgery should include wide excision of all normal tissue in the tumor area, including several centimeters of normal tissue in all directions and excision of all skin and subcutaneous tissue near the tumor. All previous scars, biopsy areas, and areas containing hematoma from previous biopsies should be resected. Surgical excision of the sarcoma should be completed without spilling of tumor, which can severely compromise the ability to deliver effective radiation therapy. A tourniquet can be placed on the extremity above the lesion before ligation of the venous outflow, as a first part of the surgical procedure, but there is no convincing evidence that this reduces the distant spread. Because these tumors rarely metastasize to draining nodes, lymph node dissection should be confined to patients with clinically suspicious and biopsy-proven nodal involvement. Current data do not support prophylactic lymph node dissection for sarcoma. For histologies showing a significant incidence of lymphatic metastases (*e.g.*, epithelioid sarcoma), an increased level of suspicion is appropriate.

TABLE 42–23. Surgical Procedures Used in Sarcoma Patients Without Metastases at Time of Diagnosis

	1977–1978		*1983–1984*	
Procedures	*No.*	*%*	*No.*	*%*
Wide local resection	879	52.4	1412	56.7
Limited local resection	455	27.1	583	23.4
Anatomic compartmental resection	168	10.0	249	14.8
Amputation	108	6.4	138	8.2
More than one type of surgery	69	4.1	108	6.4
Total	1679	100.0	2490	100.0

(Lawrence W, Donegan WL, Natarajan N, et al. Adult soft tissue sarcomas. A pattern of care survey of the American College of Surgeons. Ann Surg 1987;205:349–359)

Placement of metallic clips as a guide to the limits of the surgical dissection is essential in all nonamputative sarcoma resections. The clips identify the entire dissected area in the treatment field for construction of the radiation portals.

Muscle compartmental excision is useful for some anatomic sites (*e.g.*, thigh) containing compartments that are bounded by the fascia and its extensions. Because it is unusual for sarcomas to transgress these fascial boundaries, excision of the entire anatomic compartment containing the tumor is often successful in eradicating all local tumor. These procedures are classified as radical nonamputative excisions (see Table 42–22), and according to the American College of Surgeons survey, they were performed in approximately 10% to 15% of patients (see Table 42–23).[46]

In the thigh, there are three major compartments bounded by the fascia lata and its extensions: the anterior compartment, including the quadriceps muscle (see Fig. 42–8); the medial compartment, including the adductor muscles; the posterior compartment, including the hamstring muscles. The anterior thigh compartment consists of the quadriceps and sartorius muscles and the femoral artery, vein, and nerve. Excision of the anterior compartment leads to significant loss of motion and stability of the knee. In these situations, hamstring transfers can be performed to provide needed muscular movement at the knee. The medial thigh compartment consists of the gracilis, adductor brevis, adductor longus, adductor magnus, and the pectineus muscles. The obturator nerve supplies this compartment. In addition, the profunda femoris artery must be sacrificed when this compartment is resected. The posterior compartment consists of the semimembranosus, semitendinosus, and biceps femoris muscles and the posterior portion of the adductor magnus muscle and the sciatic nerve.

Several atlases of extremity surgery for patients with soft tissue sarcomas detail the performance of these surgical procedures.[160,271]

Truncal Sarcomas

The principles guiding the surgical therapy of extremity lesions apply to truncal sarcomas.[272–277] However, there are unique therapeutic features of these lesions that require special consideration. The anatomic location of most truncal sarcomas precludes surgical excision with margins wide enough to ensure local control, especially for sarcomas in the head and neck region and for mediastinal and retroperitoneal tumors. Surgical excision should be aimed at removing all gross tumor with as much marginal tissue in the expected areas of local spread as is compatible with reasonable morbidity. Radiation therapy should be used in the treatment of virtually all high-grade truncal sarcomas, and the surgeon should outline the margins of resection with metallic clips. For tumors

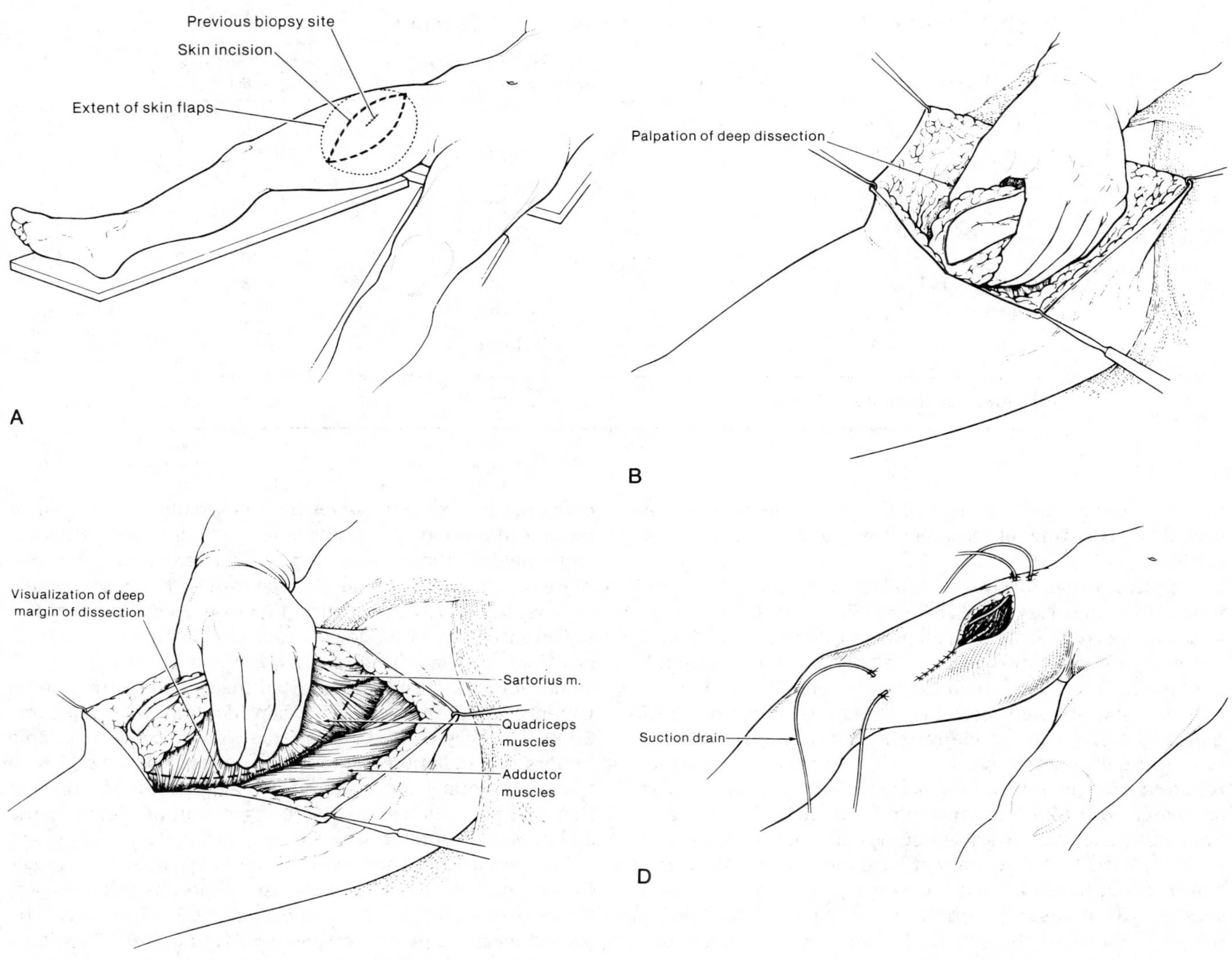

FIGURE 42–10. Wide excision of an anterior thigh sarcoma. **(A)** Elliptical skin incision encompassing previous biopsy incision(s) or drain site(s) is made. Subcutaneous skin flaps are developed to the lateral extent of the muscle margins. **(B)** Palpation of the tumor within the muscle is constantly needed to localize the mass and achieve a margin of at least 2 cm in all directions. Removal of the tumor without visualization of the mass is important. **(C)** Visualization of the deep margin is obtained and the muscle divided. **(D)** The extent of the dissection is marked with clips for subsequent planning of radiation fields. The skin flaps are closed over suction drains to allow apposition of the flaps to the surgical bed.

of the thoracic or abdominal walls, full-thickness excisions, except for skin, are indicated.[275,276,278,279] Replacement of the abdominal wall with synthetic materials does not preclude subsequent radiation therapy.

Sarcomas of the retroperitoneum present a unique surgical challenge.[280–286] These tumors tend not to cause symptoms until they are quite large, with extensive local invasion. Delamater reported a patient with an abdominal liposarcoma that reached 125 kg, and reports of tumors reaching 27 kg are not rare.[287,288] Most retroperitoneal sarcomas weigh several pounds when diagnosed and extensively invade local tissues. The most common diagnoses in the retroperitoneum are liposarcoma and leiomyosarcoma.

Evaluation of patients with retroperitoneal sarcomas should include ultrasound studies, CT, intravenous pyelogram, and if necessary, gastrointestinal contrast studies. Arteriography can delineate the blood supply of the tumor. Venacavography should be employed if invasion of the vena cava is suspected.

It is rarely possible to achieve negative microscopic margins in the excision of retroperitoneal sarcomas. An attempt should be made to remove all gross tumor, even if this involves resection of a kidney or other intraabdominal structures. In a 20-year retrospective review of 78 patients with retroperitoneal sarcomas treated between 1951 and 1971, Fortner and colleagues reported the necessity of en bloc excision of adjacent organs in 75% of patients.[289] The colon or kidney were the organs most often resected. This was similar to the experience reported by McGrath and coworkers from the Medical College of Virginia, where complete resection of tumors required en bloc excision of adjacent organs in 68% of the

TABLE 42–24. Treatment Results for Retroperitoneal Sarcomas

Investigations	*No. of Patients*	*No. With Complete Resection (%)*	*5-Year Overall Survival (%)*
Braasch and Mon[280]	37	13 (35)	16
Cody et al[281]	68	45 (66)	25
Storm et al[282]	54	28 (52)	33
Glenn et al[277]	48	37 (77)	43*
Karakousis et al[283]	68	27 (39)	30
Bose[284]	29	6 (21)	20
McGrath et al[285]	47	18 (38)	33
Jaques et al[286]	114	67 (59)	64
Total	465	241 (52)	

* Three-year overall survival rate.

patients; kidney and colon were the organs most often resected.[285] The role of postoperative radiation therapy is unclear.

Reported 5-year survival rates after treatment of retroperitoneal sarcomas vary from 16% to 37% (Table 42–24). Most series included patients with all grades of sarcoma. Although low-grade tumors can have an indolent course, the retroperitoneum is one site in which they can eventually lead to significant tumor-related mortality.[286] Marcus reported a 43% mortality rate for low-grade retroperitoneal tumors, but the median time to death was 7 years.[177] Storm and colleagues reported a 5-year survival rate of 54% for low-grade tumors compared with a 23% survival rate for high-grade tumors.[282] For high-grade and low-grade lesions in this location, a major problem is the high frequency of local recurrence. Abbas and coworkers reported a local recurrence rate of 63%.[290] In a series of 37 patients reported by the NCI, 16 had recurrences.[277] Of these 16 patients, 12 had locally recurrent disease, alone or in conjunction with recurrence in other sites.[277]

The ability to achieve complete resection of all gross disease may improve cure rates. McGrath reported a 70% 5-year survival rate after complete resections, compared with an 8% survival rate for patients undergoing partial excisions or biopsies only.[285] Complete resection of all gross disease was possible in only 49% of the patients in a combined series (see Table 42–24).

The roles of adjuvant radiation therapy and chemotherapy have not been established, and although widely used, there is no evidence that results are better than after surgical resection alone. A prospective randomized trial at the NCI comparing intraoperative radiation therapy with postoperative external-beam irradiation in 35 patients with resectable retroperitoneal soft tissue sarcomas revealed no difference in therapeutic effectiveness.[291] Innovative combined-modality approaches are needed for retroperitoneal sarcomas.

RADIATION THERAPY

Radiation Therapy Alone

Radiation therapy alone in the management of soft tissue sarcomas has been limited to patients who have locally advanced, inoperable, recurrent, or metastatic disease. The radiation doses used have been somewhat low by modern standards, and the intention of therapy was predominantly palliative. Nonetheless, there were reports documenting objective regression and occasional local control of large, inoperable tumors. In 1951, Cade reported that unresectable sarcomas in 6 of 22 patients were locally controlled with radiation therapy alone; they survived from 5 to 26 years after treatment.[292] Windeyer and coworkers reported the results of treating 58 patients with fibrosarcomas.[293] Using doses between 6000 and 8000 cGy, they treated 11 patients with large, unresectable tumors with radiation therapy alone and an additional 11 with radiation therapy for postsurgical recurrences. Fourteen of these 22 patients had complete regression of their tumors, and 27% of the tumors were locally controlled for many years.

In a series of 35 patients from the M.D. Anderson Cancer Center, high-dose radiation therapy alone was given for soft tissue sarcomas.[294] Doses ranged from 7000 to 7500 cGy. The overall local recurrence rate was 66%, and 7 of 10 patients with extremity sarcomas had recurrences. In a series from the Massachusetts General Hospital, 54 patients were treated with primary radiation therapy for soft tissue sarcomas.[295] Of the 26 patients who were treated with doses greater than 6500 cGy, 61% were locally controlled at 4 years. Most lesions smaller than 5 cm were controlled. However, of the 28 patients treated with doses less than 6500 cGy, only 2 patients were alive and free of disease for more than 2 years. An analysis of the experience with radiation therapy alone (≥6500 cGy) reported by Tepper and Suit showed an inverse association between tumor size and ability to obtain local control (Table 42–25).[296] For tumors smaller than 5 cm, 5 to 10 cm, and more than 10 cm, the local control rates with radiation therapy alone were 88%, 53%, and 33%, respectively.

Data demonstrate that the dose required to inactivate a tumor increases with the number of viable tumor cells, and radiation therapy given to microscopic disease is much more effective than treatment of gross disease.[297]

Local control can be achieved by radiation therapy alone, but it usually requires aggressive treatment with very high doses of radiation, which carries significant risks of adverse sequelae. The local control rates achieved with radiation therapy alone appear to be inferior to those obtained with surgery. Radiation therapy should be used as a primary modality only

TABLE 42–25. Relation of Size of Lesion to Local Control Achieved by Radiation Therapy Alone

Size of Lesion	*No. of Patients*	*No. Locally Controlled (%)* *
<5 cm	8	7 (88)
5–10 cm	17	9 (53)
>10 cm	10	3 (33)
Total	35	19 (54)

* Tumor dose of ≥6500 rad.
(Tepper JE, Suit HD. Radiation therapy of soft tissue sarcomas. Cancer 1985;55:2273–2277)

for patients who have lesions that are not amenable to standard treatments because of tumor size, anatomic location, medical inoperability, or refusal of a patient to agree to conventional treatment. An exception may be desmoid tumors that cannot be resected; several series have shown that excellent local control was achieved with radiation therapy alone.[298–300]

The contribution of radiation therapy for some sarcomas remains uncertain. Mirabell and colleagues reported 26 patients with positive surgical margins after resection of primary fibromatoses.[301] Without further therapy, only 9 patients had recurrences during a 5-year period. Because the risk of metastasis is negligible for this lesion, close observation is a reasonable policy if patients are reliable and wider resection would result in major functional deficits. Mirabell also reported that 10 patients treated with irradiation for primary control of desmoid tumors achieved local control. Similar data for aggressive fibromatoses were reported by McCollough and associates.[302]

Combining Radiation Therapy and Surgery

The rationale for combining surgery with adjuvant radiation therapy is to employ conservative surgery and moderate-dose radiation therapy to preserve the function of the area involved, especially limbs. Radiation therapy is used to treat microscopic tumor extending into the adjacent tissues beyond the primary tumor mass, achieving the same results as a more radical resection. An advantage of this approach is that the treatment volume for radiation therapy is designed to encompass the surrounding tissues at risk for tumor involvement, such as nerves, vessels, tendons, and bone, which would otherwise limit the ability to perform an adequate local resection. Theoretically, combined therapy offers a high degree of local control and improved functional and cosmetic results, especially in the extremities. This expectation has been realized in clinical practice in several different series.[43,44,303,304]

In 1951, Cade reported a survival rate of 61% in a series of 80 patients treated with wide excision followed by radiation therapy, compared with 27% (6 of 22) with amputation.[292] He championed the use of radiation therapy in combination with wide local excision. Results of combined-modality treatment from recent literature are shown in Tables 42–26 and 42–27. Although several reports show excellent results from combining limb-sparing surgery with radiation therapy for high-grade sarcomas of the extremities, it is still unclear if radiation therapy should be administered before, during, or after the surgical procedure. It is obvious that combining radiation therapy with conservative surgery has avoided ablative surgical procedures and maintained local control in most patients (85%), and by eliminating the need for generous surgical margins, the functional results are excellent. Additional research is needed to define the contribution of each modality and to relate results to grade, histologic type, tumor size, and anatomic site.

For low-grade sarcomas, local control is the predominant issue, but any potential enhancement of local control by radiation therapy must be weighed against functional deficits and impairment in quality of life caused by radiation therapy. The issues can only be resolved by a randomized prospective study that considers quality of life factors.

PREOPERATIVE RADIATION THERAPY. There are several theoretical advantages of preoperative radiation therapy combined with conservative surgery in the management of soft tissue sarcomas. First, inactivation of tumor cells by radiation therapy may decrease the risks of tumor implantation in the surgical wound and decrease metastatic spread from any tumor cells that enter vascular spaces during surgery. Second, the volume to be treated can be limited to clinically and radiologically evident tumor and the adjacent tissues at risk for microscopic extension, without encompassing all the tissues that are manipulated during the surgical procedure itself. Third, the mass is often smaller at the time of surgery after responding to radiation therapy, which facilitates conservative resection. Fourth, an inoperable sarcoma may be made resectable by regression with radiation therapy.

The major disadvantages of preoperative radiation therapy

TABLE 42–26. Local Control and Survival After Preoperative Radiation Therapy for Extremity Soft Tissue Sarcomas

Investigations	*No. of Patients*	*Follow-up (y)*	*Local Failure ± Distant Metastases (%)*	*5-Year Disease-Free Survival (%)*
Massachusetts General Hospital[305]	90	1–18	15 (17)	67 (74)
M.D. Anderson[306]	27	≥5	2 (7)	15 (56)
University of Florida[307]	19	1–5	1 (5)	11 (58)
Pooled data	136		18 (13)	93 (68)

TABLE 42–27. Local Recurrence Rate With Conservative Surgery and Postoperative Radiation Therapy

Investigations	*No. of Patients*	*Follow-up (y)*	*Dose (Gy)*	*Patients With Local Recurrence (%)*	*5-Year Disease-Free Survival (%)*
University California San Francisco[303]	29	>2	50–75	3 (10)	68
M.D. Anderson[43]	300	2–7	60–75	67 (22)	68
National Cancer Institute[44] *	129	1–8	63	10 (8)	60
Massachusetts General Hospital[304] *	123	1–12	60–68	16 (12)	65
Pooled data	581			96 (17)	

* Extremity sites only.

are the delay in surgical resection (a psychological disadvantage for some patients), a risk of compromising wound healing, and the necessity for the radiation therapist to have planned and executed radiation therapy before surgical resection. Often, an initial excision is carried out by a surgeon who is removing a piece of tissue for diagnosis. In some instances, the diagnosis of a sarcoma comes as a surprise and many of the potential benefits of preoperative radiation therapy cannot be realized because of a suboptimal biopsy procedure. Nonetheless, several series demonstrated that planned preoperative radiation therapy in patients with high-grade sarcomas can yield excellent results (see Table 42–26).[305–307] Radiation-induced shrinkage of an inoperable tumor resulted in some tumors becoming resectable.[294,308,309]

POSTOPERATIVE RADIATION THERAPY. Radiation therapy in combination with surgery is most commonly employed in the postoperative period. For patients for whom postoperative radiation therapy is planned, the amount of surgical resection itself remains a matter of some controversy. Although all gross tumor should be removed, some physicians advocate minimal excision of surrounding normal tissue, and others advocate the widest excision possible that is compatible with reasonable limb function. The crucial issue is that larger surgical excisions remove more normal tissue and require the use of wider radiation fields; wide excisions may ultimately reduce the functional result that can be achieved. For lesions in the groin, popliteal space, ankle, elbow, forearm, wrist, hand, or foot, the margins are necessarily close at some point in the dissection. For lesions that occur in fleshy parts of the body, the margins can be more generous. Expansion of local operations to include vascular reconstruction or bone replacement procedures has been advocated in recent years.[310–314]

The advantages of postoperative radiation therapy include immediate surgery, which can be a psychological advantage for some patients; no radiation-induced delay in wound healing; and an entire specimen available for histopathologic investigation. Moreover, the exact size and pattern of extension of the tumor are interpreted definitively.

The conservative surgical procedure itself has a moderate probability of achieving local control if the surgeon is able to get around the tumor with a negative margin. Adjuvant radiation therapy can minimize the necessity of wide margins, optimizing function, and maximize the probability of local control. However, in encompassing all tissues manipulated by the surgeon, the postoperative treatment volume is usually larger than that used for preoperative radiation. Moreover, if there is a delay in starting radiation therapy, as for wound healing, there may be a larger number of residual tumor cells. A prolonged delay in wound healing may allow residual microscopic tumor to become palpable.

There are several published series demonstrating the results of surgery with postoperative radiation therapy (see Table 42–27).[43,44,303,304] One of the earliest and largest came from the M.D. Anderson Cancer Center, where more than 300 patients with soft tissue sarcomas were treated.[43] The surgery consisted of conservative excision, usually shelling out, with removal of the gross tumor and a limited amount of normal tissue. Patients received a dose between 6000 and 7000 cGy during 6 to 7 weeks. No attempt was made to include the entire muscle or anatomic compartment in the treatment field. The local recurrence rate for all patients treated with combined conservative surgery and postoperative radiation therapy was 22% and 20% for those with extremity sarcomas. In the patients who had extremity sarcomas, most of the recurrences occurred in the fleshy portions of the extremity, where lesions typically were large and extended for significant distances along fascial planes. The disease-free survival rate at 5 years was 61% for all primary sites. For the extremities, it was 69%; for head and neck sarcomas, it was 63%; but for retroperitoneal disease, the 5-year survival rate was only 33%. Local failure rates ranged from 10% for stage I to 28% for stage III tumors. Distant metastases developed in 5% of patients with stage I, in 29% with stage II, and in 43% with stage III tumors. The investigators reported significant complications in 7% of the patients, including soft tissue necrosis, traumatic fractures of bone within the radiation field, fibrosis with limitation of motion, nerve and vascular injuries, and moderate edema. Nonetheless, of those with extremity tumors undergoing such treatment, 85% of the patients maintained functional limbs.

In a smaller series from the University of California at San

Francisco, 29 patients with extremity sarcomas were treated with surgery and postoperative radiation therapy.[303] Most had grade 3 tumors. The dose usually ranged between 5500 and 7000 cGy. Radiation fields were designed to cover the surgical bed with a generous margin; no effort was made to treat the entire involved muscle group from origin to insertion. The 5-year determinant survival rate was 81%, and the 5-year relapse-free survival rate was 68%. The local control rate was 90%. No patient required amputation due to radiation sequelae. It was demonstrated that radiation can sterilize microscopic disease and reduce the local recurrence rate in patients undergoing simple excision of soft tissue sarcomas. Of the patients undergoing conservative excision and postoperative radiation therapy, 22 had microscopically positive margins of resection, but only 3 of these 22 patients developed local recurrences after postoperative radiation therapy. Of 14 nonirradiated patients treated with conservative surgery alone in whom margins were positive, 11 developed local recurrences.

It is difficult to assess the influences of size, grade, histology, and anatomic site in comparing patients from different series. To overcome some of these potential biases, Rosenberg and colleagues conducted a randomized prospective clinical trial evaluating limb-sparing surgery plus postoperative radiation therapy compared with amputation in patients with high-grade extremity sarcomas at the NCI.[264] The dose of radiation therapy employed for the patients undergoing limb-sparing surgery was usually 6300 cGy. All patients received postoperative adjuvant chemotherapy. Forty-three patients were entered into the trial with an (updated) median follow-up of 11 years. There were 17 patients randomized to amputation and 27 to limb-sparing surgery plus postoperative radiation therapy (1:2 randomization). There were five local recurrences in the group receiving limb-sparing surgery and one (a protocol violator) in the group randomized to radical surgery (Fig. 42–11). Despite this finding, the 10-year overall survival rate for the two groups was approximately equal at 75%.

A randomized, prospective study demonstrated the benefit of radiation therapy for local control of high-grade extremity sarcoma. Yang and colleagues randomized 90 patients to receive surgery and chemotherapy or to receive surgery, chemotherapy, and radiation therapy.[315] With a median follow-up of 5 years, no patient receiving radiation therapy had a local recurrence, but 9 of 46 treated with only surgery and chemotherapy had local recurrences. The low local recurrence rate in patients not receiving radiation therapy may be attributable to their receiving chemotherapy, because several studies have indicated an effect of adjuvant chemotherapy on local recurrence.[316,317] Despite the significant difference in local recurrences, overall survival of the two groups was identical, again raising the question of the impact of local recurrence on survival (Fig. 42–12). A concurrent, prospective quality of life study of these patients indicated that radiation therapy impaired quality of life and limb function, but the magnitude of impairment was small. This confirms that radiation therapy can control local disease in sarcoma patients undergoing limb-sparing surgery, but it suggests that local recurrences may have minimal influence on overall survival. Highly selected patients who have optimal surgery for favorable tumors (and who may receive adjuvant chemotherapy) may be able to safely avoid adjuvant radiation therapy.

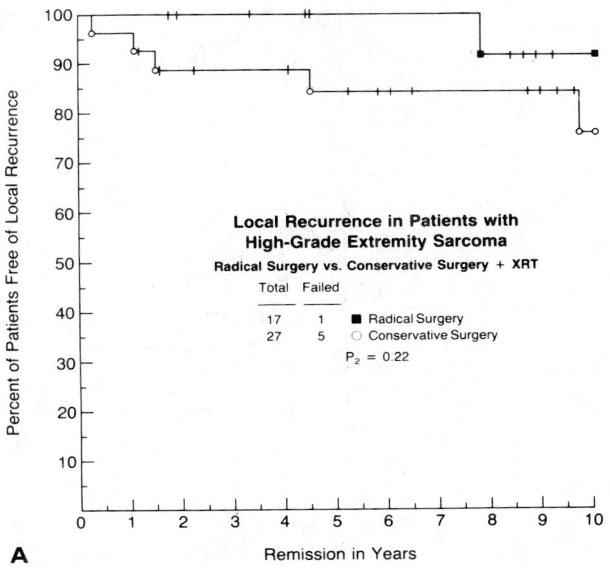

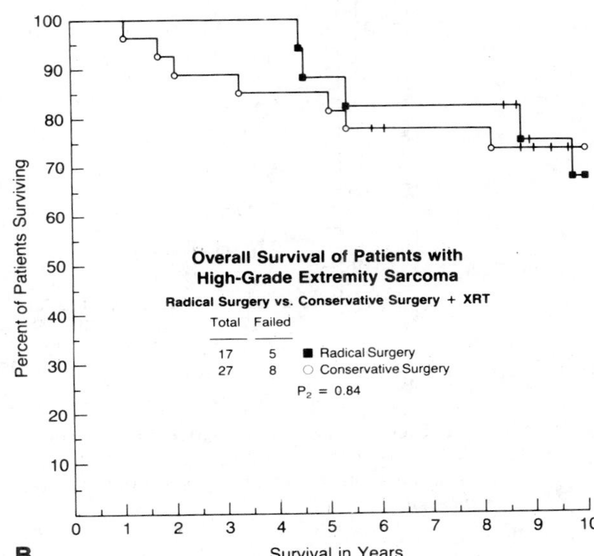

FIGURE 42–11. **(A)** Local recurrence in patients with high-grade extremity sarcoma and a limb-sparing surgical option, who were randomized to receive a limb-sparing resection with radiation therapy rather than amputation (standard therapy at the time). All patients in this trial received postoperative adjuvant chemotherapy. With few patients, there was a small, statistically insignificant difference in local recurrence. **(B)** Updated overall survival of patients in the same study. Long-term survival of patients randomized to limb-sparing surgery versus amputation appears to be similar. This represents the only prospective randomized study of this issue.

Rydholm and associates and the Scandinavian Sarcoma Group have already applied these concepts in a series of 70 patients with high-grade and low-grade sarcomas confined to the subcutaneous space or totally within a deep muscular fascia.[318] These fascial planes had not been violated by previous biopsy; many preoperative diagnoses were made on the grounds of radiographs and fine-needle aspirate. In 56 of the 70 patients, widely negative surgical margins including fascia or wide muscular cuffs were obtained and no adjuvant radia-

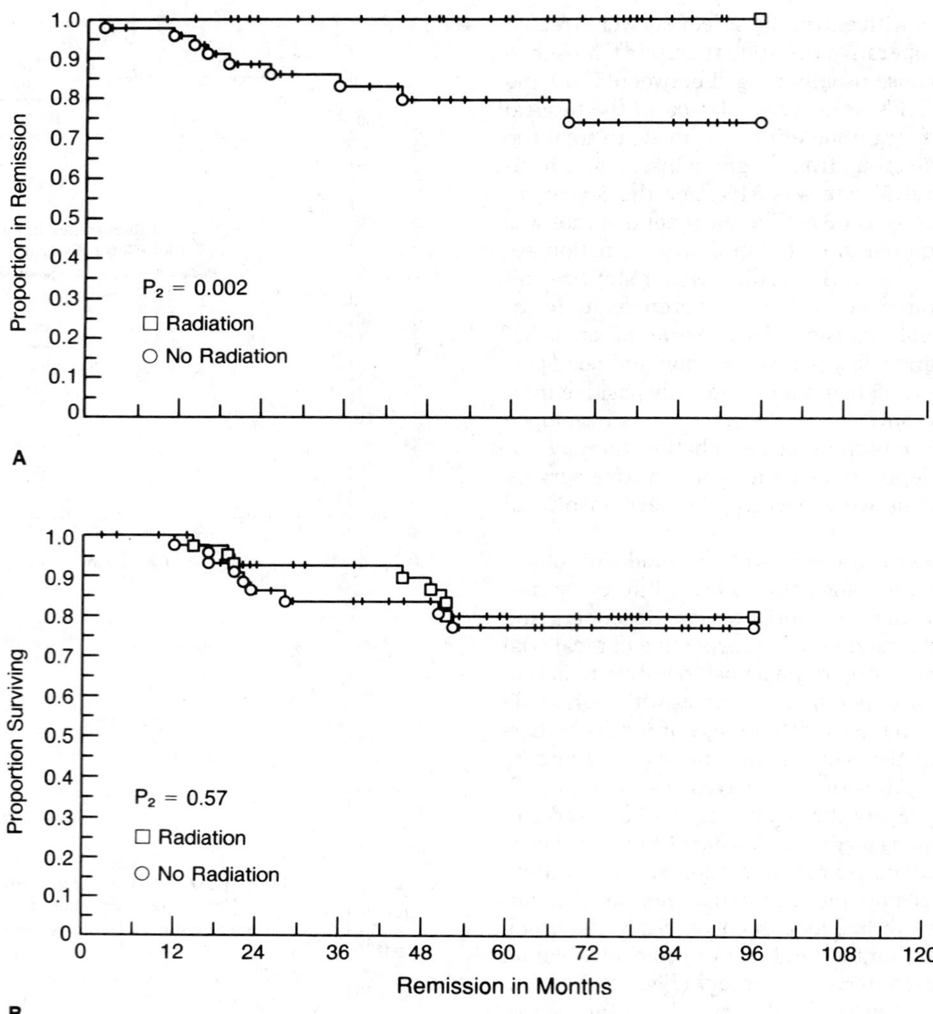

FIGURE 42–12. **(A)** Local recurrence and **(B)** overall survival of patients with high-grade extremity sarcomas treated with surgery and chemotherapy (no radiation therapy) or with surgery, chemotherapy, and radiation therapy. Despite a difference in local recurrence rate, no difference in overall survival is seen.

tion therapy was given. With a median follow-up of 5 years, only 4 (7%) of these patients had local recurrences. Despite the excellent results from this highly experienced group of investigators, the approach remains experimental and controversial and does not represent a recommendation for therapy of patients undergoing limb-sparing procedures.

INTRAOPERATIVE BRACHYTHERAPY. A less commonly employed approach combining surgery and radiation therapy is the use of intraoperative brachytherapy.[319] This approach requires a surgery and radiation therapy team with expertise in this technique. Brennan and colleagues reported a trial evaluating the efficacy of intraoperative brachytherapy in adult patients with operable soft tissue sarcomas of the extremities or superficial trunk at Memorial Sloan-Kettering Cancer Center.[320] Temporary implants of iridium 192 were employed using after-loading techniques. Usually, this consisted of a single-plane implant. A total of 117 patients were prospectively randomized to receive or not receive intraoperative brachytherapy. With median follow-up of only 16 months, 2 of 52 patients receiving brachytherapy developed local recurrences, compared with 9 of 65 in the group not receiving brachytherapy ($p = 0.06$). No survival differences were seen between the two groups during the short follow-up period. Similar data have been reported by others.[321,322]

The advantages and disadvantages of brachytherapy are somewhat similar to those for preoperative radiation therapy; however, an additional advantage is that the complete treatment is considerably shorter, because the radiation is given during the time of surgery and the immediate week or so thereafter. The treatment necessitates detailed planning and exceptionally close cooperation between the surgeon and the radiation therapist, but the results achieved with brachytherapy in this study are comparable to the best reports of treatment using external-beam radiation therapy.

Technical Aspects of Radiation Therapy

The most commonly employed technique in the treatment of soft tissue sarcomas is the combined use of surgery and postoperative radiation therapy. This approach mandates an adequate resection of all gross disease. A shell-out procedure, which involves the excision of the tumor around its pseudocapsule, is suboptimal. Giuliano and Eilber documented persistent macroscopic tumor in approximately 50% of the patients at the time of reexcision of previous shell-out operative sites.[323] A planned reexcision of the operative sites should always be performed if the initial excision is deemed inadequate.

Radiation portals should be designed to treat muscle groups from origin to insertion to encompass the entire fascial plane, which may be potentially contaminated by tumor cells within postoperative hematomas.[324] Whether this is better than a 5- to 10-cm margin around the tumor bed is unknown. For the occasional tumor involving a subcutaneous primary location without muscle involvement, an 8- to 10-cm margin around the initial tumor volume should be employed. If preoperative radiation therapy is used, an 8- to 10-cm margin around the tumor mass in all dimensions should be obtained.

For primary tumors of the extremities, the only contraindications to limb-sparing surgery and radiation therapy are lesions that are so extensive that negative margins cannot be obtained; gross invasion of a joint; extensive involvement of several compartments of the extremity; or invasion of major neurovascular or bony structures beyond the scope of grafting or reconstruction.

Radiation therapy is often planned postoperatively after wound healing. It is essential to establish the extent of disease as seen by the surgeons who carried out the surgery and the apparent site of origin, possible residual tumor, tumor spillage, or hemorrhage. Ideally, the radiation therapist should directly observe the surgery.

In planning radiation therapy, it is essential to simulate the patient in a treatment position. The extremity is immobilized in a reproducible position at the time of simulation. A cast is usually necessary to immobilize the extremity in the same position each day with respect to the table top (Fig. 42–13). If large fields are needed, the patient should not be turned, because rotation of an extremity around a major joint may occur in more than one plane. If very long fields are required, treat isocentrically with pairs of matching fields, using a shifting match-line technique or the match-line wedge technique.[325] The match-line wedge technique allows shifting the angle of obliquity in such a way that matching may occur in different planes, and this can be an advantage in designing radiation fields that correspond to an anatomic compartment. The match-line wedge technique has some theoretical advantage over shifting the match line 1 cm every 1000 cGy, as is commonly done.

Every attempt is made to define the tumor volume to optimize the radiation portals (Figs. 42–14 and 42–15). Customized, individually shaped blocks are cut out for each patient to optimize the tumor volume, and the process adds secondary collimation beyond what a linear accelerator itself can offer. Generous use of clips placed at the time of surgery to define the extent of resection allow the therapist to see at simulation where the surgeon has been, and in many instances, the clips enable planning of oblique fields, which spare unmanipulated tissues but incorporate tissues that were handled at surgery. It is often surprising to see how far beyond the surgical scar some of the clips may appear. At the time of simulation, the scar is marked with wire to visualize on simulator films how the scar will be treated within the radiation field. If the radiation port strikes the scar perpendicularly, rather than tangentially, tissue-equivalent bolus material should be applied superficially to increase the dose to the scar. This ensures that the skin-sparing effects of high-energy x-rays, applied perpendicularly to the skin, do not work to the patient's disadvantage by underdosing the scar itself.

An attempt is made to spare at least 33% of the circumference of the extremity from the direct radiation field to optimize function and minimize lymphedema. Every effort is made to exclude joints from the radiation field if the surgery permits. If the scar crosses the joint, at least some of the joint is blocked out, unless the joint was entered surgically. Active involvement of the physical therapist with the patient is essential from the beginning to motivate the patient. This is essential to maximize the function of the extremity, muscles, and joints.

Postoperative tumor doses of 6300 cGy at 180 cGy per day are recommended. If there is gross residual disease, an increase in the total dose to approximately 7000 to 7500 cGy can be achieved using shrinking-field techniques to minimize the volume receiving the highest dose. The first volume reduction is made at 4500 cGy, and if a second volume reduction is needed, it can be made at 6300 cGy.

Lesions of the hand and foot are frequently able to be treated with conservative surgery and radiation therapy with excellent functional results.[326] The radiation therapy must be planned carefully, and it frequently necessitates high-energy electrons for at least part of the treatment. Similar principles apply to sarcomas of the head and neck region.

Lesions of the chest or abdominal wall can frequently be treated with high doses of radiation therapy postoperatively using a combination of x-rays and electrons. Doses range from 6000 to 7000 cGy or even higher, depending on the volume and location of the tumor. For retroperitoneal sarcomas, dose limitations usually reflect the tolerance of the small bowel and kidney. Doses in excess of 5500 cGy carry a considerable risk of small bowel injury.

For patients who receive preoperative radiation therapy, a dose of 4500 to 5000 cGy is recommended, at the rate of 180 cGy each day. Additional boosts may be given, intraoperatively or postoperatively, depending on the surgical findings and pathologic margins. The total dose for these patients can reach 7000 cGy.

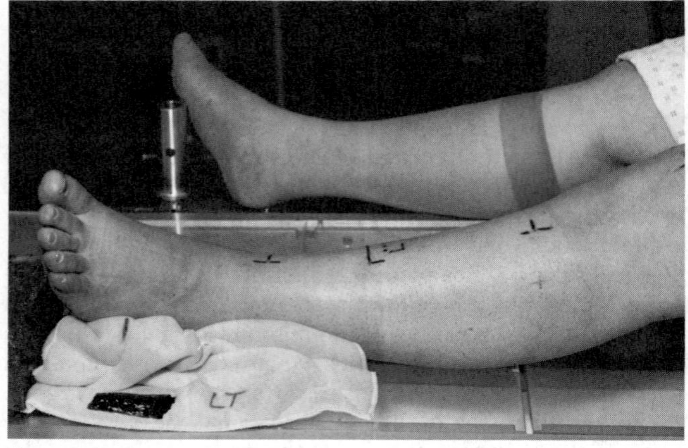

A

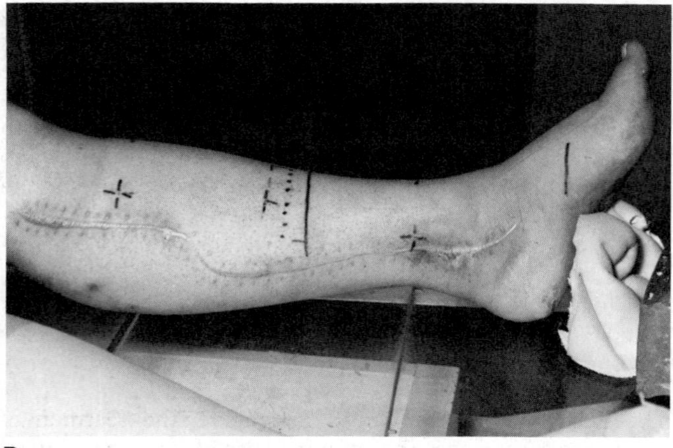

B

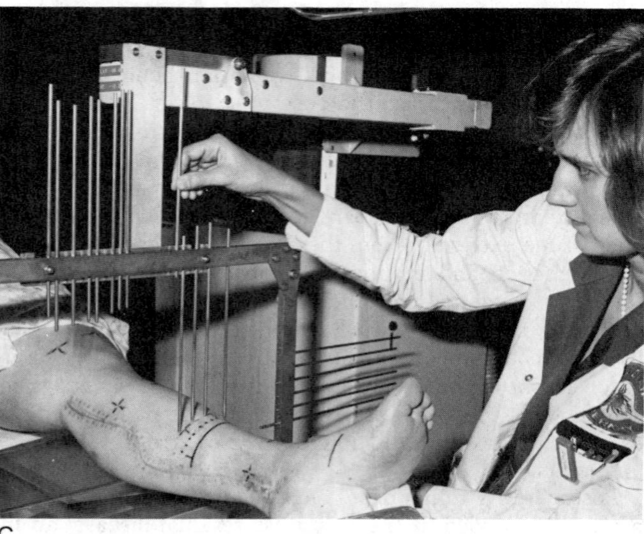

C

FIGURE 42–13. **(A)** Patient with a sarcoma of the left leg. A cast was individually molded to surround her foot and ankle such that the foot will always be in exactly the same position for each day's treatment. This is done at the time of simulation, which is a mock-up procedure during which the positioning and measurements required for treatment are determined, although treatment is not actually carried out. Diagnostic x-ray films are taken that mimic exactly what will be done with the megavoltage x-ray beam. **(B)** Medial view of the left leg. The scar can be seen, and several reference points have been marked on the skin. The cast and its relation to supporting the foot can be seen. **(C)** After positioning, it is important to determine the contour of what is being irradiated. Because the tissues vary in their thickness at any one level and because radiation is continuously attenuating as it transverses tissue, the thickness of the tissue at different levels in the radiation field will result in differing doses. To know what the discrepancies are, contours are taken at various levels. In this view, a mechanical device is being used to outline the contour at various levels in differing directions. After the contours have been determined, dose calculations can be made for the various levels that have been determined.

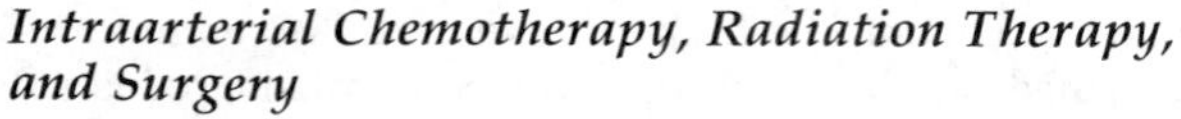

Intraarterial Chemotherapy, Radiation Therapy, and Surgery

Eilber and associates reported their extensive experience with preoperative intraarterial doxorubicin (Adriamycin) and radiation therapy for sarcomas of the extremity.[327] The rationale for this approach is to deliver regionally an active chemotherapeutic agent that has direct cytotoxic and potentially radiosensitizing effects on the tumor. In their early experience, intraarterial doxorubicin was given at 30 mg/day over 24 hours for 3 consecutive days. On the following day, radiation therapy was started, and 350-cGy fractions were administered daily for 10 days for a total dose of 3500 cGy. At 1 to 2 weeks after completion of irradiation, an en bloc resection of all gross disease was performed.

A total of 77 patients with high-grade extremity sarcomas were treated, and 74 (96%) were able to have limb-salvage surgery. Local tumor recurrence was noticed in only 3 (4%) patients. However, complications occurred in 25 (35%), with 14 (17%) requiring a second operative procedure. These complications consisted mainly of bone fractures and wound slough. Because of this high complication rate, the preoperative radiation therapy regimen was reduced to 1750 cGy in five fractions. An additional 105 patients were treated with this regimen, and 102 (97%) were able to undergo limb-salvage surgery. Complications were reduced, with reoperation required in 6 (6%) patients. Local recurrences were seen in 9 (8%) patients. With this combined preoperative regimen, more than 96% of the patients with high-grade extremity tumors were able to have nonamputative surgery with acceptable local control.

Denton and colleagues at the University of Alabama reported a local recurrence rate of 3% for 30 patients with soft tissue and bony extremity sarcomas using a similar regimen. The mean follow-up was only 22 months.[328] Results achieved with this approach are comparable to standard multimodality approaches; however, no comparative randomized trials have been performed. Lokich reported the use of preoperative systemic chemotherapy in combination with radiation therapy in 3 patients with bulky soft tissue sarcomas and noticed marked tumor regression in 2 patients.[329]

Other investigators used regional arterial chemotherapy alone or in conjunction with hyperthermic perfusion as a preoperative adjunct or as primary therapy for unresectable tumors.[330–332] The advantages of regional chemotherapy in these approaches have not been definitively demonstrated. Didolkar

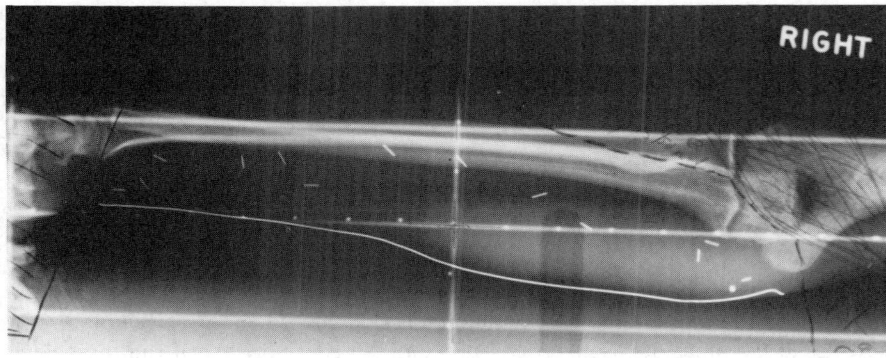

A

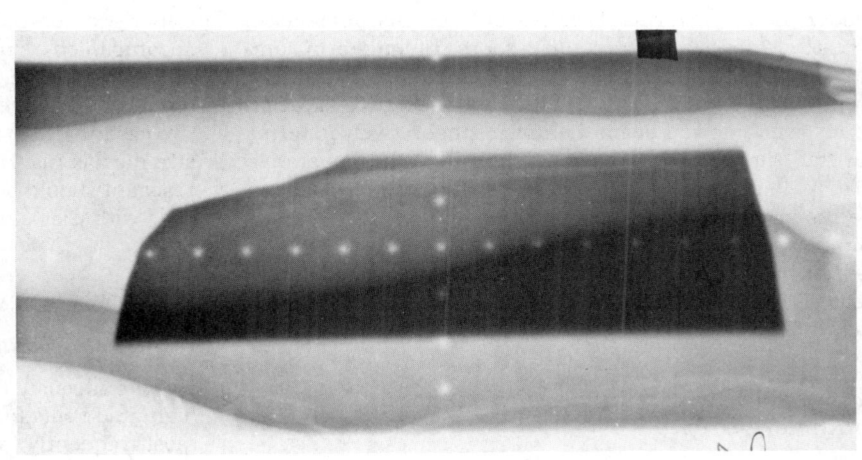

B

FIGURE 42–14. **(A)** On a different patient, a simulation process is demonstrated. Metallic clips have been placed throughout the course of the surgeon's exploration to show exactly where the surgeon has been. A piece of wire corresponds to the forearm of this particular patient, showing where the scar is in relation to the treatment field. It occurs right at the edge of the tissue being treated. The cross-mark represents the center of the radiation field, which is situated in the middle of the soft tissue of the forearm itself. The forearm has been positioned carefully in such a way that the radius and ulna superimpose on the same plane. One edge of the radiation field corresponds to the bony structures themselves, leaving soft tissue above that line which is outside the radiation field. A dotted line represents a customized block that is cut to protect approximately half of the elbow joint, keeping it outside the high-dose radiation volume. **(B)** Port film on the same patient taken with 4 MeV x-rays in the treatment position. This image matches the simulator film seen in **A.**

and colleagues reported that intraarterial doxorubicin achieved similar regional tissue levels as intravenously administered drug in animals.[333] It is difficult to assess the efficacy of preoperative intraarterial chemotherapy from any of these studies.

Fast-Neutron Therapy

At least two reports have emerged on the treatment of locally advanced sarcomas treated with fast-neutron therapy. Salinas and coworkers from the M.D. Anderson Cancer Center reported 20 (69%) of 29 patients with advanced soft tissue sarcomas who achieved local control of their tumors with fast-neutron therapy.[334] Four patients developed complications. Pelton and colleagues from the University of Washington reported that 16 patients with unresectable soft tissue sarcomas were treated with fast neutrons, including 11 who had no evidence of metastatic disease and who were treated with curative intent.[335] These patients received a mixture of neutrons and photons. Local control was achieved in approximately 60%, with no relapses seen after 30 months. Only 4 patients, however, were alive without evidence of disease. A common complication of treatment was severe subcutaneous fibrosis, which in 2 patients necessitated skin grafts. One patient who received abdominal radiation for retroperitoneal sarcomas developed a small bowel obstruction thought to be related to radiation enteritis and fibrosis.

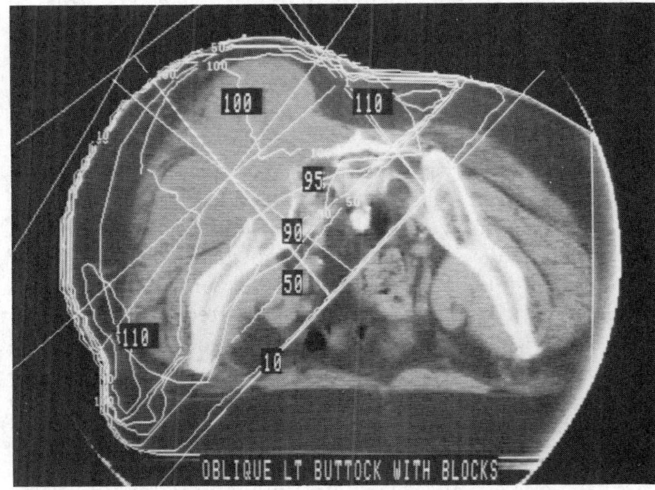

FIGURE 42–15. CT cut for a patient with a large buttock sarcoma. The patient is prone, and the extensive soft tissue mass, which could not be resected, is seen. The patient is being treated with oblique fields designed to treat the entire ilium on the right and as the soft tissue mass. The fields are wedged to account for the contour of the buttock itself, and the fields are slightly offset, so that the 50% isodose lines from each field direction coincide within the pelvis. The numbers represent different isodose curves on this particular slice (one of many sequential cuts), and they relate closely to the soft tissue mass itself. The intention is to take this entire volume to a dose of approximately 7500 cGy. In this case, treatment was carried out twice daily.

Although neutron therapy is still investigational in this country, fast-neutron therapy for patients with inoperable soft tissue sarcomas appears to offer a reasonable chance of local control and potential long-term survival, but its precise role must still be defined.

Intraoperative Radiation Therapy

Intraoperative radiation therapy is used at the time of surgery and permits a high single dose of electron-beam therapy to be delivered directly to the tumor bed, after moving as many incidental structures out of the radiation field as possible. For soft tissue sarcomas, its use has been predominantly for primary tumors in the retroperitoneum; it has not shown any significant benefit over conventional surgery and postoperative radiation therapy in terms of survival or freedom from relapse. Large single doses are potentially a source of long-term complications for ureters and nerves. In a randomized study, the NCI was unable to show the benefit of intraoperative radiation therapy over external-beam therapy postoperatively in terms of overall survival or disease-free survival.[291] Intraoperative radiation therapy was able to reduce the frequency of radiation enteritis in these patients.

Similar data were reported from Massachusetts General Hospital.[336] Because many of these patients developed sarcomatosis of the peritoneum, intraoperative radiation therapy remains investigational.

Radiation Sensitizers, Radiosensitivity, and Radioresistance

For most sarcomas, complete surgical resection is recommended if it can be accomplished without excessive morbidity. If a patient has a sarcoma that is not amenable to resection, it is still possible that radiation therapy alone can control the local disease.

Although radiation therapy may be rejected for treating soft tissue or bony sarcomas because the tumor is thought to be "radioresistant," data demonstrate that this concept is fallacious. Tepper and Suit reported a series of 35 patients who had soft tissue sarcomas that were treated with doses of 6500 cGy or more (see Table 42–25).[296] For lesions smaller than 5 cm, 7 of 8 achieved local control. For lesions between 5 and 10 cm, 9 of 17 achieved local control. For lesions larger than 10 cm, only 3 of 10 achieved local control.

Kinsella and Glatstein from NCI reported a series using a variety of intravenous radiosensitizers in the management of unresectable soft tissue and bony sarcomas.[337] Most tumors were larger than 10 cm; the median size was 14 × 14 cm. Local control (*i.e.*, freedom from all symptoms and no further growth) was achieved for at least a year in 22 of 29 patients who had extensive disease. Many tumors were radiosensitive but not radioresponsive. Radiosensitive refers to specific parameters (*e.g.*, D_o, D_q, or n) that are obtained from in vitro cell survival curves. Whether the tumor is sensitive or resistant depends on the exact quantitative parameters derived from such studies. Often a tumor is called radioresistant, but the tumor is really radio-unresponsive, because the tumor does not demonstrate any decrease in size (exactly how much is unspecified) seen relatively quickly (also unspecified) after some modest doses of radiation therapy (also unspecified). The concept of radioresponsiveness of tumors is 40 years old and was useful for differentiating tumors that shrank quickly, such as lymphomas or seminomas, from those that did not. In their review of 29 patients with massive sarcomas treated with hypoxic cell sensitizers or halogenated pyrimidines, the NCI reported patients in whom all the cells were destroyed pathologically, but in whom the mass never regressed. In some instances, the patients survived more than 5 years without any growth of tumor after irradiation.

The role of radiation sensitizers in the management of these tumors is an area of active investigation. The important point is that all the tumor cells can apparently be destroyed, even if the mass does not necessarily regress. A significant component of a sarcomatous mass may be represented by the matrix of stroma of the tumor. Depending on the extent of a tumor's composition, the death of tumor cells is not necessarily accompanied by measurable regression. Some sarcomas can be radiosensitive, but not necessarily radioresponsive. Examples of this phenomenon have been seen in other tumors, such as testicular cancer treated with chemotherapy or massive mediastinal Hodgkin's disease. Radiosensitive and radioresistant should be defined carefully, and the words must be used with precision.

CHEMOTHERAPY

Adjuvant Chemotherapy

Despite adequate local treatment, almost half of patients with high-grade soft tissue sarcomas develop metastatic disease, most frequently in the lungs. This led to intensive efforts to identify adjuvant chemotherapy regimens that can prevent metastatic spread. The studies must be carefully designed to address sarcomas of a specific grade and location and to balance factors such as size and margin status. Due to the scarcity of these tumors, studies of adequate size to detect or exclude a significant benefit of adjuvant chemotherapy are few and somewhat conflicting.

Several nonrandomized trials suggesting an improved outcome with adjuvant chemotherapy used similar agents, including doxorubicin, DTIC, vinca alkaloids, and high-dose methotrexate. Cyclophosphamide was shown to have activity against metastatic sarcoma. The results of combinations of these agents have been reported from prospective, randomized trials of adjuvant therapy for high-grade soft tissue sarcomas of the extremities, head, neck, and trunk. Due to the low risk of metastatic disease in patients with grade 1 lesions, the trials should be confined to lesions of higher grade. Because the prognosis (and possibly the efficacy of adjuvant chemotherapy) for lesions of the extremities differs from that of sarcomas in nonextremity locations, clinical trials should consider these groups separately.

There have been 11 reported prospective, randomized trials of adjuvant chemotherapy for soft-tissue sarcoma.[316,317,338–354] Five combined extremity and nonextremity tumors, but they included data analysis by tumor location.[316,317,342,349,350] Four included only patients with extremity tumors, and two studied only nonextremity tumors.[345,351–355] Data on extremity sarcomas could be obtained from nine trials, and nonextremity tumors were analyzed in seven trials as shown in Table 42–28. Of the results confined to extremity tumors, three studies

TABLE 42–28. Adjuvant Chemotherapy for Sarcoma: Randomized Studies

*Investigations**	*No. of Patients*	*Tumor Grades*	*Chemotherapy Agents†*	*Median Follow-up (mo)*	*Disease-free Survival (%)‡*		*Overall Survival (%)‡*	
					No CTX	*+CTX*	*No CTX*	*+CTX*
Extremity								
Alvegard[349] (SSG 1989)	155	2, 3	Dx	40	NR	NR	NR	NR
Antman[350] (DFCI/MGH, ECOG, ISSG 1990)	101	1–3	Dx	54	64	78	67	79
Benjamin[351] (MDA 1987)	46	2, 3	DxVCA	>120	35	(55)§	57	65§
Bramwell[316] (EORTC 1988)	223	1–3	DxVCDt	36	66	77‖	74	81‖
Chang[355] (NCI 1988)	67	2, 3	DxC	85	54	(75)	60	82
Edmunson[342] (Mayo 1984)	48	1–3	DxVCDtA	64	67	86	82	88
Eilber[352] (UCLA 1987)	119	3	Dx	36	58	58‖	75	78‖
Picci[345] (Rizzoli 1988)	77	2, 3	Dx	42	42	(68)¶	68	(88)¶
Ravaud[317] (Bergonie 1990)	36	2, 3	DxVCDt	52	NR	(NR)	NR	(NR)
Nonextremity								
Alvegard[349] (SSG 1989)	26	2, 3	Dx	40	NR	NR	NR	NR
Antman[350] (DFCI/MGH, ECOG, ISSG 1990)	67	1–3	Dx	54	47	53	52	54
Bramwell[316] (EORTC 1988)	125	1–3	DxVCDt	36	50	63‖	71	81‖
Edmunson[342] (Mayo 1984)	13	1–3	DxVCDtA	64	NR	NR	NR	NR
Omura[353] (GOG 1985)	156	NR	Dx	60	45	60	47	60
Ravaud[317] (Bergonie 1990)	23	2, 3	DxVCDt	52	NR	NR	NR	NR
Yang[354] (NCI 1992)	81	2, 3	DxC	59	57	59	65	63

* SSG, Scandinavian Sarcoma Group; DFCI, Dana-Farber Cancer Institute; MGH, Massachusetts General Hospital; ECOG, Eastern Cooperative Oncology Group; ISSG, Intergroup Sarcoma Study Group; MDA, M.D. Anderson Cancer Center; EORTC, European Organization for Research on Treatment of Cancer; NCI, National Cancer Institute; Mayo, Mayo Clinic; UCLA, University of California, Los Angeles; Rizzoli, Istituto Ortopedico Rizzoli, Bologna; Bergonie, Fondation Bergonie, Bordeaux; GOG, Gynecologic Oncology Group. Year of last update is in parnetheses.
† Dx, doxorubicin; V, vincristine; C, cyclophosphamide; A, dactinomycin; Dt, DTIC.
‡ Survival values are estimated 5-year actuarial values (taken from text or published survival curves) unless otherwise noted. Parenthetic values are significantly greater than randomized comparison group, $p \leq 0.05$. All other differences are not significant. CTX, chemotherapy; NR, not reported.
§ Estimated 10-year actuarial survival rates.
‖ Survival rates at last available patient follow-up.
¶ Estimated 4-year actuarial survival rates.

showed a significant survival advantage for doxorubicin-based chemotherapy.[317,345,346] A third study of 67 patients with extremity lesions at the NCI showed a significant overall survival benefit at 5-year follow-up, but due to a few late deaths, the difference was not significant with 9-year median follow-up.[355] The other six studies did not show significant survival differences with the use of adjuvant chemotherapy. Of eight studies with disease-free survival values presented, seven showed superior results with chemotherapy, but only four were statistically significant. Several studies showed a significant impact of chemotherapy on the incidence of local recurrence.[316,317,339,351]

Many of these studies have limited power to detect a difference, and several are open to criticism on methodologic grounds. In two studies, patients received some preoperative chemotherapy before randomization and then were randomized to stop or continue this chemotherapy.[345–347,352] In one trial that showed no effect of chemotherapy, only 75% of randomized patients were eligible, and of those eligible and randomized to chemotherapy, approximately two thirds received 85% or less of the planned chemotherapy dose.[349] Many trials included patients with low-grade tumors that are unlikely to be chemotherapy responsive.

In some studies, clinically evident doxorubicin cardiotoxicity occurred in as many as 10% of patients (with subclinical or clinical findings in as many as half of patients), and this may have offset any overall survival benefit of adjuvant chemotherapy.[356] In one NCI study, a lower-dose, less toxic doxorubicin regimen was compared with the NCI regimen with demonstrated benefit and was shown to be equally effective.[355,357]

Studies confined to lesions of the head, neck, trunk, and retroperitoneum have uniformly failed to show any statistically significant benefit from a variety of adjuvant regimens, although many are limited by small patient numbers. In the most recent NCI study, the estimated 5-year survival of 88 patients with high-grade tumors randomized to receive or not receive postoperative doxorubicin and cyclophosphamide were 63% and 65%, respectively. Disease-free survival was also similar (59% and 57%).[354]

The use of adjuvant chemotherapy for primary high-grade

adult soft tissue sarcomas remains experimental. Although existing data suggest that there may be an improvement in disease-free survival, this difference is only significant in a few studies and seems confined to sarcomas of the extremities. Many studies continue to include low-grade lesions with high-grade tumors, a practice that can only obfuscate any possible benefit of chemotherapy. Studies showing a survival benefit to adjuvant chemotherapy for node-positive breast cancer and Dukes' stage C colon cancer required many hundreds of randomized patients to attain statistical significance. The existing literature on soft tissue sarcomas can neither prove or exclude a benefit from adjuvant chemotherapy.

TREATMENT OF RECURRENT OR METASTATIC SARCOMAS

Potter and associates reviewed the initial sites of tumor recurrence after primary treatment of soft tissue sarcomas in 307 patients referred to the NCI.[44] These patients underwent complete surgical resection, often in combination with postoperative chemotherapy and radiation therapy. A total of 107 (35%) patients had local recurrences or developed distant metastases; the sites of disease are identified in Table 42–14. The lung was the predominant site of first recurrence in 52% of these patients, followed by isolated local recurrences (20%). The pattern of recurrence depended on the primary site of the sarcoma. Patients with sarcomas of the head and neck, retroperitoneum, and chest or abdominal wall had a higher local recurrence rate than those with extremity sites. In the American College of Surgeons survey, there were 452 (37%) of 1209 treatment failures in patients without metastases at the initial diagnoses who had total gross resections of their soft tissue sarcomas.[46] Among patients with recurrent disease, 236 (52%) had isolated locoregional recurrences, and 83 (18%) had isolated lung recurrences. Approximately 80% of all recurrences became evident within 5 years.

Aggressive surgical management of isolated local recurrences should be attempted. A thorough evaluation for evidence of disseminated disease must be performed before contemplating resection of a local recurrence. In the NCI experience, 20 (96%) of 21 isolated local recurrences were surgically resectable. Figure 42–16 shows the actuarial continuous disease-free and overall survival of patients who were rendered free of disease after resection of a local recurrence. The 3-year survival was 69%. Shiu and associates were able to resect 35 (81%) of 43 isolated locally recurrent extremity sarcomas, with a subsequent 5-year survival rate of 45%.[59] Giuliano and coworkers reported that 35 (92%) of 38 patients surgically rendered free of a local recurrence of an extremity or truncal (excluding retroperitoneal) sarcoma had a 5-year actuarial survival rate of 87%.[358] In the American College of Surgeons survey, the 5-year survival rate after salvage therapy of isolated local failures was 61%.[46]

Metastasectomy for isolated pulmonary recurrences is clearly warranted. Patients who are found to have pulmonary metastases by plain chest x-ray film or chest CT scans should have a thorough evaluation for extrapulmonary tumor, particularly in the primary site, to determine operability. For extremity and truncal sarcoma patients, this can be accomplished by physical examination and CT or MR scans of the

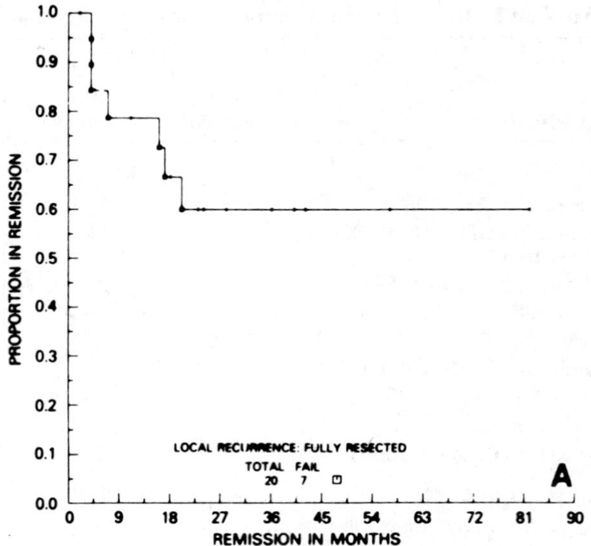

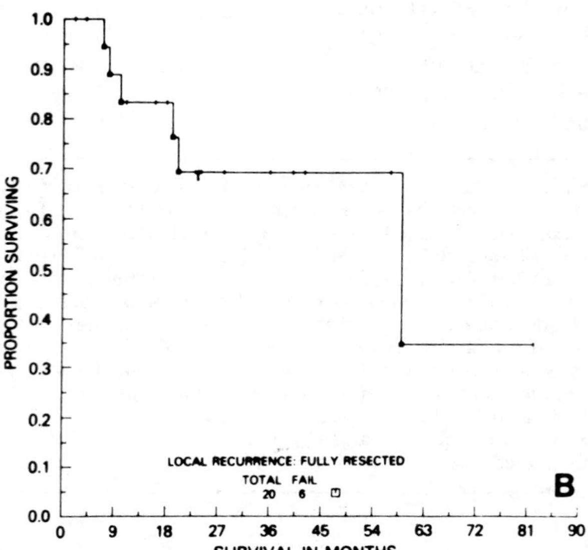

FIGURE 42–16. **(A)** Disease-free survival and **(B)** overall survival in patients with high-grade sarcomas who underwent resection of isolated locally recurrent disease. (Potter DA, Glenn J, Kinsella T, et al. Patterns of recurrence in patients with high-grade soft tissue sarcomas. J Clin Oncol 1985;3:353–366)

primary site. For patients with retroperitoneal sarcomas, an evaluation of the liver should be performed to detect metastases. Patients with extrapulmonary tumors are not candidates for pulmonary resection. In Potter's analysis of NCI patients, 40 (72%) of 56 patients with isolated pulmonary metastases were rendered free of disease after surgery, which resulted in an actuarial 3-year survival rate of 38% (Fig. 42–17).

Pass, Roth, and colleagues reported that the number of metastatic nodules (≤6) seen on preoperative CT scan, the disease-free interval (>1 year), and tumor doubling time (≥20 days) significantly correlated with survival in soft tissue sarcoma patients undergoing their first pulmonary metastasectomy.[359,360] Nevertheless, there were long-term survivors with

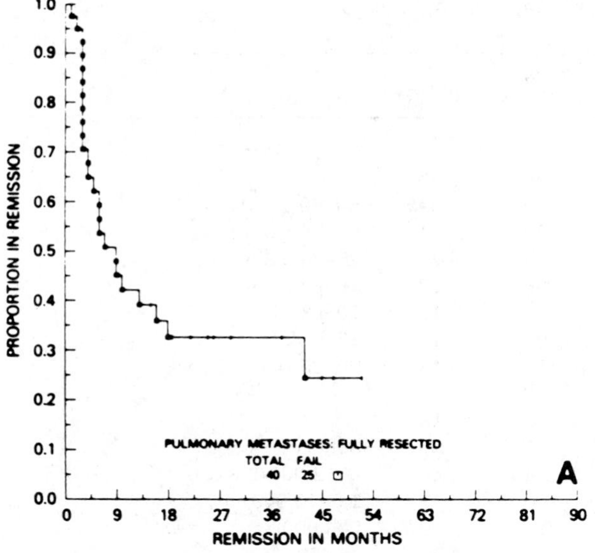

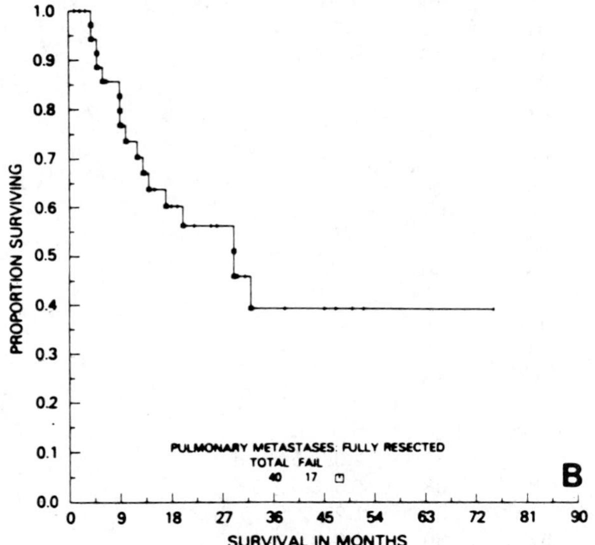

FIGURE 42–17. **(A)** Disease-free survival and **(B)** overall survival in patients with high-grade sarcomas who underwent resection of isolated pulmonary metastases. (Potter DA, Glenn J, Kinsella T, et al. Patterns of recurrence in patients with high-grade soft tissue sarcomas. J Clin Oncol 1985;3:353–366)

poor prognostic parameters, and no single criterion was sufficient to exclude attempted resection. In the American College of Surgeons survey, the 5-year survival rate after pulmonary metastasectomy was 21%.[46] Resection of recurrent pulmonary metastases can result in survival benefit. In the NCI experience, 29 patients had two or more resections for pulmonary metastases, resulting in a 22% 3-year actuarial survival rate after the second thoracotomy.[361] There have been no operative deaths after 254 pulmonary resections for metastases at the NCI since 1978. Because of the minimal morbidity and potential survival benefit of pulmonary metastasectomy, patients treated for primary soft tissue sarcomas should be closely monitored for development of pulmonary metastases at least every 6 months with lung tomograms or chest CT for 3 years after resection of the primary tumor.[362]

CHEMOTHERAPY FOR DISSEMINATED SOFT TISSUE SARCOMAS

Soft tissue sarcomas constitute a heterogenous class of neoplasms with divergent response rates to available chemotherapy. Regimens including vincristine, dactinomycin, and cyclophosphamide result in response rates of 80% or more in previously untreated embryonal and alveolar rhabdomyosarcoma, and combination chemotherapy is now established in the primary treatment of these lesions. Of the classic adult soft tissue sarcomas, malignant fibrous histiocytoma and synovial sarcomas have the highest response rates to doxorubicin-based combination chemotherapy. The lowest response rates are observed in angiosarcomas, extraskeletal chondrosarcomas, and leiomyosarcomas of gastrointestinal origin. Mesotheliomas and Kaposi's sarcoma differ from the classic soft tissue sarcomas and are not discussed in this section.

Widely divergent response rates for a given drug or combination reflect the mix of histologies included on the trial, dose and schedule of administration, prior therapy, and biases introduced by the small numbers of patients in some studies. Publication bias (*i.e.*, negative studies are rarely reported) probably also plays a role, particularly in nonrandomized studies.

Single-Agent Chemotherapy

Commercially Available Agents

Table 42–29 summarizes the activity of various single agents in soft tissue sarcoma. Single-agent doxorubicin, the most active commercially available single agent, had a response rate of 15% to 35% in various studies.[363–368] A dose-response association has been observed in nonrandomized trials and in combination with other agents in randomized trials, with dose rates of 60 to 70 mg/m² every 3 weeks superior to dose rates of 50 mg/m² or less every 3 weeks.[364–366,404] Doxorubicin administered by continuous infusion over 4 days in combination regimens has been reported to be less cardiotoxic and equally effective as bolus dosing in some studies.[405–408]

Ifosfamide is a cyclophosphamide analog with one chloroethyl group shifted to the ring nitrogen atom. Preclinical and human phase I and II trials for sarcomas, lymphoma, and small cell lung cancer have shown an apparent lack of cross-resistance with cyclophosphamide.[409–412] Ifosfamide has activity in patients with sarcoma who have failed doxorubicin-containing regimens.[385,391–393,413–415] A European Organization for Research and Treatment of Cancer (EORTC) study showed ifosfamide at 5 g/m² to be somewhat superior to cyclophosphamide at 1.5 g/m² as single-agent treatment of advanced sarcoma and resulted in less myelotoxicity.[393] The production of acrolein from ifosfamide and the resulting cystitis requires the use of the urothelial protective agent mesna (sodium-2-mecapto-ethane-sulfonate). Mesna has been shown to be superior to *N*-acetylcystein in preventing hematuria in a randomized trial of sarcoma patients receiving ifosfamide.[416]

DTIC has a single-agent response rate of 18% and is particularly active in leiomyosarcomas. Nausea associated with its administration may be decreased by administration as a continuous infusion.[394]

TABLE 42–29. Commercially Available Chemotherapeutic Agents for Soft Tissue Sarcoma by Class

Investigations	*Drug*	*No. of Patients*	*% RR**	*Dose (mg/m²)*
	Anthracyclines			
Total	Doxorubicin	356	26	
Blum[363]		130	34	60–90 q 3 wk
O'Bryan et al[364]		49	31	60–75 q 3 wk
O'Bryan et al[365]		82	28	25–70 q 3 wk
Schoenfeld[366]		66	27	70 q 3 wk
Borden et al[367]		93	19	70 q 3 wk
Borden et al[367]		92	16	15 q wk
Cruz et al[368]		15	13	20–25/day × 3 q wk
	Antimetabolites			
Total	Methotrexate, high-dose	76	13	
Rosen et al[369]		1	1/1	8000/wk
Vaughan et al[370]		14	14	5–12,000/2 wk
Isacoff and Eilber[371]		6	17	1.5–10,000
Karakousis et al[372]		18	5	2–4,000/wk
Von Hoff et al[373]		26	20	>1000
Frei et al[374]		9	0/9	2–10,000/1–4 wk
Total	Methotrexate, standard-dose	81	21	
Andrews[375]		19	10	
Subramanian[376]		41	37	
Buesa[377]		21	0	
Amato[378]	Bleomycin	32	6	
Golbey[379]	Dactinomycin	30	17	
Gold[380]	5-Fluorouracil	8	12	
	Vincas			
Total	Vincristine	103	12	
Selawry[381]		15	40	
Korbitz[382]		7	0	
Total	Etoposide	40	8	
Radice[383]		34	6	
Bleyer[384]		6	16	
	Alkylating agents			
	Ifosfamide†			
Elias[385,386]	High dose	20	35	2.0–4.5 × 4 d
Klein[387]		8	38	2.5–3.5 × 5 d
Czownicki[389]		13	38	1.25–2.5 × 5 d
Niederle[390]		57	30	1.6–3.0 × 5 d
Antman[391]		124	23	2.0–2.5 × 4 d
Wiltshaw[392]	Standard dose	42	38	5.0–8.0 × 1 d
Bramwell[393]		68	18	5.0 × 1 d
Buesa[394]	Dacarbazine (DTIC)	44	18	
Total	Cisplatin	103	12	
Bramwell[395]		17	0	
Karakousis[396]		13	23	
Samson[397]		42	7	
Thigpen[398]		19	5	
Budd[399]		40	15	200 mg/m²
Gershenson[400]		12	42	GYN only
Goldstein[401]	Carboplatin	50	12	
Total	Cyclophosphamide	82	8	
Bergsagel[402]		12	16	
Korst[403]		3	0	
Bramwell[393]		67	8	

* % RR percent response when the denominator includes at least 10 cases.
† In adults by dose per course.

TABLE 42–30. Investigational Chemotherapeutic Agents for Soft Tissue Sarcomas by Class

Drug	*References*	*No. of Patients Evaluable*	*% Responding*
Anthracyclines			
Carminomycin	417	48	27
Azotomycin	418, 419	28	18
AMSA	420–423	9	11
Iclarubicin	424	23	4
Diaziquone (AZQ)	425, 427	108	2
Mitoxantrone	428, 429	115	1
Menogaril	430	21	5
Esorubicin	431	14	7
Epirubicin	432	32	19
Echinomycin	433	34	0
Antimetabolites			
Trimetrexate	434, 435	36	8
Cycloleucine	436–438	118	11
Chlorozotocin	439–445	160	4
Cytembena	446, 447	24	4
PALA/5 fluorouracil	448, 449	23	0
PALA/dipyridamole	450, 451	46	11
Baker's Antifol	452, 453	30	0
Alkylating Agents			
Methyl-CCNU	454, 455	85	6
Hexamethylmelamine	456–458	88	5
Dibromodulcitol	459, 460	34	3
Dianhydrogalacitol	461	28	0
Gallium nitrate	462	31	0
Vinca & Related Compounds			
VM-26	463	33	3
Vindesine	464, 465	3	0
Miscellaneous			
DDMP	466	15	7
Piperazinedione	467–469	22	5
ICRF 159	460	29	5
MGBG	378, 470	54	2
Pyazofurin	470–472	47	0
Maytansine	460, 473	44	0
Bruceantin	460, 473	34	0
Homoharingtonin	474	16	0
Biologicals			
Tumor necrosis factor	475	16	0
Tumor necrosis factor	476	1	0
Interferon-α	477	16	0
Interferon-β	478	20	1
Interleukin-2	479	6	0

Investigational Agents

The studies of single investigational agents in the treatment of advanced sarcoma are shown in Table 42–30. Currently, there are no consistent data to recommend a particular agent without further study.[417–479]

Combination Chemotherapy

Randomized Studies

Most large randomized cooperative group studies have reported response rates of 17% to 30% (Table 42–31). The median survival in these trials is in the range of 12 months, with no significant differences in survival observed. This lack of effect on survival despite differences in response rates probably results from several factors: high response rates (often >50%) are required to impact on survival in patients with advanced disease, many patients not responding to one treatment subsequently receive the other agent or regimen, and the 0.5 to 2 log decrease in tumor cell number represented by many partial or complete responses is often not significant in a patient with an advanced tumor burden of 10^9 to 10^{12} cells. Other endpoints for chemotherapy such as its ability to improve the results of surgery or radiation therapy given preoperatively in patients with bulky disease deserve further study.

The addition of DTIC to doxorubicin has been evaluated in three randomized trials. The Gynecologic Oncology Group (GOG) and the Eastern Cooperative Oncology Group (ECOG) evaluated doxorubicin as a single agent and with DTIC.[367,480–481] The response rate was higher for the combination in both studies, significantly in the ECOG study. In the third Southwest Oncology Group (SWOG) study patients received doxorubicin, cyclophosphamide, and vincristine with DTIC or dactinomycin. The DTIC-containing arm was significantly more active.[482]

SWOG, ECOG, and GOG studies evaluating the addition of cyclophosphamide to an doxorubicin-containing regimen showed no advantage for the addition of cyclophosphamide.[366,483,484] In the ECOG trial, after the dose of doxorubicin was decreased from 70 mg/m^2 to 50 mg/m^2 to avoid myelosuppression from cyclophosphamide, the response rate for doxorubicin at 70 mg/m^2 as a single agent was significantly higher than for the combination with the lower doxorubicin dose.[366]

The EORTC evaluated doxorubicin alone, doxorubicin with ifosfamide, and doxorubicin, cyclophosphamide, DTIC, and vincristine (CYVADIC regimen).[485] There was significantly more myelosuppression and a trend but no significant advantage in response rate or survival for the two combinations. An ECOG study comparing doxorubicin with or without ifosfamide observed a significant difference in response for the ifosfamide arm with a trend for longer survival in the ifosfamide arm.[486]

The SWOG/CALGB study of doxorubicin and DTIC alone compared with the addition of ifosfamide demonstrated response rates of 17% and 32%, respectively.[487] Although the response rate and duration of response were significantly improved for the three-drug arm, myelosuppression (including fatal sepsis) was also significantly worse. Median survival times were 13 and 12 months, respectively.

M.D. Anderson Cancer Center compared CYVADIC at high and intermediate doses, and the EORTC compared full-dose with alternating half-dose therapy.[488] Both studies correlated dose with response.[404]

Two studies randomized patients between different schedules of similar regimens. An adjuvant trial at Memorial Sloan-Kettering Cancer Center corroborated the decreased cardio-

TABLE 42–31. Randomized Chemotherapy Trials for Measurable Soft Tissue Sarcoma

Investigations	*Group**	*Regimen†*	*No. of Patients*	*% CR‡*	*% RR‡*	*Comments*
Studies Comparing the Addition of DTIC						
Omura et al[480]	GOG	A	80	6	16	Uterine sarcoma only
		AD	66	11	24	
Lerner[481]	ECOG	A	34	3	18	
		AD	32	3	44	Leiomyosarcomas only
Borden et al[367]	ECOG	A q 3 wk	93	6	19	A 15 mg/m²/wk
		A q wk	92	4	16	A 70 mg/2 q 3 wk
		AD	95	6	30	
Benjamin et al[482]	SWOG	ACVD	221	14	52	
		ACVAd	224	12	40	
Studies Evaluating the Addition of Cyclophosphamide						
Schoenfeld et al[366]	ECOG	A	66	6	27	A 70 mg/m²
		ACV	70	4	19	A 50 mg/m²
		CVAd	64	2	11	A none
Baker et al[483]	SWOG	AD	79	14	32	
		ADC	95	13	35	
		ADAd	98	9	24	
Muss et al[484]	GOG	A	50	1	19	
		AC	54	2	20	
Studies Evaluating Vindesine						
Bordon et al[491]	ECOG	A Vindesine	149	4	17	
		A	149	6	18	
Studies Evaluating Dose and Schedule						
Zalupski et al[490]	SWOG	AD	135	7	19	Bolus
		AD	143	10	18	Continuous infusion
Casper et al[489]	MSKCC	A	32			Bolus
		A	39			Continuous infusion
Bodey et al[488]	SWOG	ADCV	27	15	67	A 50 mg/m² C 500 mg/m²
		ADCV	24	33	71	A 80 mg/m² C 800 mg/m²
Pinedo et al[404]	EORTC	ADC	71	20	38	Full dose rate
		AD-CV	74	5	14	Half dose rate
Studies Evaluating Ifosfamide						
Bramwell[393]	EORTC	I	68	2	18	5 g/m²
		C	67	1	8	1.5 g/m²
Antman[487]	ISSG	AD	170	2	17	
		ADI	166	4	32	Myelosuppression more severe
Santoro[485]	EORTC	A	212	4	24	
		AI	202	6	27	Myelosuppression more severe
		ACDV	135	8	28	Nausea vomiting more severe
Blum[486]	ECOG	A	87		20	
		AI	87		35	

* GOG, Gynecologic Oncology Group; ECOG, Eastern Cooperative Oncology Group; SWOG, Southwest Oncology Group; MSKCC, Memorial Sloan Kettering Cancer Center; EORTC, European Organization for Research and Treatment of Cancer; ISSG, Intergroup Sarcoma Study Group.
† A, doxorubicin; Ad, dactinomycin; C, cyclophosphamide; D, DTIC; I, ifosfamide; V, vincristine.
‡ CR, complete response; RR, response rate.

toxicity of continuous-infusion doxorubicin, but patients receiving the continuous infusion had a higher incidence of relapse.[489] A SWOG study compared bolus with continuous-infusion doxorubicin and DTIC. The response rate was identical, but the toxicity (particularly doxorubicin-associated cardiotoxicity and nausea and vomiting from DTIC) was substantially reduced with continuous infusion.[490]

The combination resulting in the highest response rates in soft tissue sarcomas is doxorubicin (60 mg/m^2) and ifosfamide (7.5 g/m^2) with or without DTIC (1 g/m^2). The doses of doxorubicin and DTIC should be given by continuous infusion over 4 days to decrease the risk of cardiotoxicity and the severity of nausea and vomiting. Ifosfamide should be divided and given daily over 3 days and with mesna for bladder protection. Physicians may choose single-agent doxorubicin or doxorubicin and DTIC for palliation for patients who may not tolerate the combination. Ifosfamide is currently the most active salvage agent for patients who have failed a doxorubicin-containing regimen.

Nonrandomized Studies

Nonrandomized, phase II combination chemotherapy trials are described in Table 42–32. Response rates in single-institution phase II trials are superior to similar regimens tested in randomized trials by cooperative groups. This may be due to smaller patient numbers, better patient selection, and higher dose delivery by single institutions. Small single-institution studies with poor results may be less reported. Nevertheless, these trials are helpful in estimating the range of responses for a regimen and in designing randomized trials.

Dose-Intensive Therapy

In laboratory models of sarcomas and other malignancies, the delivery of the highest possible doses of chemotherapy is essential to achieving curative therapy. Theory and experimental and clinical data suggest that sarcoma recurs despite an initial response to chemotherapy because of resistance to the chemotherapy drugs. In the laboratory, resistance to alkylating agents can often be overcome by using a five-fold to ten-fold higher dose.[544] There is ample evidence of a correlation between doxorubicin dose and tumor response from three randomized trials.[366,404,488]

Because the limiting toxicity of higher chemotherapy doses is myelosuppression, several investigators have used hematopoietic growth factors to allow delivery of the full dose on schedule.[517,545,546] Autotransplants have been used to ensure prompt marrow recovery after high doses of chemotherapy. Ewing's sarcoma, rhabdomyosarcoma, and osteosarcoma are optimal tumors for studies of the role of high-dose therapy based on their sensitivity at conventional chemotherapy doses.

Forty-three children with malignant soft tissue sarcomas were treated at the Royal Marsden Hospital in Sutton, England, with a rapid-dose-delivery schedule consisting six courses of vincristine, doxorubicin, and cyclophosphamide followed in 36 patients by high-dose melphalan with autologous bone marrow support. There was one toxic death due to infection and possible cardiomyopathy. Using International Society of Pediatric Oncology (SIOP) staging, there were 11 stage I patients, 13 stage II patients, 7 stage III patients, and 12 stage IV patients. The actuarial survival rate at 5 years was 57%, and the event-free survival rate was 44% for all stages. For patients with nonmetastatic diseases, the rates were 62% and 53%, respectively. This treatment strategy enables completion of all chemotherapy by 4 months. Radiation and surgery were conservative to minimize late sequelae.[547]

Of 95 patients with sarcoma collected in a review by Pinkerton for the European Bone Marrow Transplant Registry, 64 received high-dose therapy as consolidation after the first complete or partial response. About 20% maintained durable complete responses at more than 40 months. However, 35% of the 40 patients transplanted during complete remission were disease free.[548] At the Dana-Farber Cancer Institute, a high-dose ifosfamide, carboplatin, and etoposide regimen is being studied as consolidation therapy for patients with sarcomas responding to conventional-dose therapy.[385,386]

HORMONE THERAPY

Observing that a higher percentage of premenopausal than postmenopausal patients who developed uterine sarcomas survived for 5 years, some investigators have suggested that estrogen replacement may be efficacious in the treatment of postmenopausal women with sarcomas. Lantta and colleagues documented estradiol and progesterone receptors in two endometrial stromal sarcomas.[549] One of the patients responded to hormone treatment for 2 years. One endometrial stromal sarcoma responded to progesterone, and a second case of endometrial stromal sarcoma responded to medroxyprogesterone after failure of tamoxifen and combination chemotherapy.[550,551] However, of 29 patients with uterine sarcomas treated with 40 mg/day of tamoxifen in a Clinical Oncology Society of Australia study, 0 of 19 patients with leiomyosarcomas, none of 3 with endometrial stromal sarcomas, and 1 of 7 with malignant mixed müllerian tumors had objective responses.[552] Of 60 patients with uterine sarcomas, 48% and 30% were estrogen and progesterone receptor positive, respectively. Only 1 of 28 patients with recurrent disease had a response to hormonal therapy. Receptor status did not affect prognosis.[553]

THERAPY FOR BORDERLINE AND LOW-GRADE SARCOMAS

Desmoids are low-grade fibrosarcomas of the abdominal or chest wall, usually occurring in sites of prior trauma most frequently in women. Optimal treatment remains wide excision and radiation therapy. For recurrent and unresectable disease, tamoxifen has been used with some success.[554–556] Responses have been reported to chemotherapy regimens such as vinblastine (10 mg/week) and methotrexate (50 mg/week).[557] This regimen has produced responses in 2 of 2 patients with disabling fibromatosis and in 2 of 4 patients with neurofibromatosis.[557]

A 12-year-old boy with hemangiomatosis was reported to have normalization of his exercise tolerance, clubbing, pulmonary pressure-volume curve, and of the abnormal vascular pattern on pulmonary angiogram in response to interferon-2α.[558]

(text continues on page 1480)

TABLE 42–32. Nonrandomized Combination Chemotherapy in Untreated Sarcomas

*Combination**	*Investigations*	*Institute†*	*No. of Patients Evaluable*	*% CR‡*
Doxorubicin-based Combinations				
AD	Total		732	9
	Gottlieb[492]	SWOG	100	5
	Baker[483]	SWOG	79	15
	Borden[367]	ECOG	95	6
	Omura[480]	GOG	66	11
	Saiki[493]	SWOG	114	9
	Weh[494]	Hamburg	38	
	Baker[407]	SWOG	278	9
ADC	Total		200	14
	Benjamin[406]	MDAH	46	15
	Blum[495]	DFCI	23	17
	Baker[483]	SWOG	97	11
	Handman[496]	Minneapolis	18	28
	Ikeda[497]	Japan	16	6
ADV	Total		161	7
	Gottlieb[498]	SWOG	107	10
ADVC	Total		399	15
	Yap[499,500]	SWOG	125	17
	Benjamin[482]	MDAH	60	13
	Bui[501]	France	60	7
	Pfeffer[502]	Hadassah	31	13
	Pinedo[404]	EORTC	60	13
	Choi[503]	Hong Kong	12	17
	Bodey[488]	MDAH	51	23
ADVC-AD	Lopez[504]	Rome	40	10
ACV	Schoenfeld[366]	ECOG	70	4
ACVAd	Benjamin[482]	MDAH	224	12
ADAd	Baker[483]	SWOG	98	10
A + methyl-CCNU	Rivkin[505]	SWOG	41	7
A + streptozotocin	Chang[506]	UNCC	14	0
Epirubicin-based Combinations				
ED	Lopez[507]	Rome	52	17
EDI	Casali[508]	Milano	26	8
EP	Jelic[509]	Belgrade	35	20
EI	Elli[510]	Argentina	12	17
Ifosfamide-based Combinations				
IA	Cantwell[511]	Newcastle	16	6
IA	Dombernowshy[512]			
IA	Edmonson[513]	Mayo Clinic	44	2
IA	Loehrer[514]	Indiana	42	7
IA	Mansi[515]	Royal Marsden	54	6
IA	Schutte[516]	EORTC	175	9
IA	Steward[517]	EORTC	51	8
IA	Weh[494]	Hamburg	45	
IA	Wiltshaw[518]	Royal Marsden	60	
IAD	Bramwell[519]	London, Ontario	43	5
IAD	Elias[520]	DFCI	108	10
IC	Elias[386]	DFCI	8	12
IEtoposide	Wellens[521,522]	Duisburg	13	15
IEtoposide, hyperthermia	Issels[523]	Munich	38	16

(continued)

TABLE 42–32. *(Continued)*

*Combination**	*Investigations*	*Institute†*	*No. of Patients Evaluable*	*% CR‡*
Ifosfamide-based Combinations *(continued)*				
IE	Elli[510]	Argentina	12	17
IE	Hoffmann[524]	Leverksen, FRG	55	
IE	Toma[525]	Genoa	38	11
IDE	Casali[508]	Milano	52	10
IP	Biernbaum[526]	Essen	12	17
IP	Budd[527]	SWOG	28	4
IP	Hartlapp[528]			
IP/WLRT	Zamboglou[529]	Dusseldorf	8	75
Cisplatin-based Combinations				
	Total		219	6
AP	Klippenstein[530]	Frankfurt	18	21
APC	Edmonson[531]	Mayo Clinic	20	0
APC	Cormier[532]	Mayo Clinic	20	0
APC	Edmonson[533]	Mayo Clinic	63	0
AP Mitc	Edmonson[533]	Mayo Clinic	63	0
APV	Biernbaum[526]	Essen	16	19
APC/Hmm	Jansen (mixed mesodermal sarcoma)[534]	Rotterdam	6	33
PI	Biernbaum[526]	Essen	12	17
P/D	Piver[535]	RPMI	20	20
Methotrexate Combinations				
	Total		463	5
AM	Presgrave[536]	Austria	36	0
AMV	Kaufman[537]	RPMI	14	7
AMVD	Kaufman[537]	RPMI	5	0
AMVDAd	Shiu[538]	MSKCC	41	0
AMVAd	Shiu[538]	MSKCC	32	0
AM Mustard	Subramanian[376]	Marsen	22	15
AMC	Presant[539]	C. of Hope	105	6
AMC/ADV	Presant[539]	C. of Hope	32	16
AMCDV	Lynch, Shiu[538,540]	MSKCC	36	11
AMCDV	Pfeffer[541]	Jerusalem	24	13
AMC	Lowenbraun[542]		140	3
Dactinomycin-based Combinations				
	Total		298	1
AdVC	Jacobs[543]	UCSF	17	6
AdVC	Schoenfeld[366]	ECOG	64	2
AdVC		Mayo Clinic	61	2
AdL	Cruz[368]	MDAH	25	0
AdLV	Cruz[368]	MDAH	26	0
AdL + cycloleucine	Golbey[379]	RPMI	25	0
AdL = cycloleucine	Golbey[379]	RPMI	40	0
AdM = chlorambucil	Golbey[379]	RPMI	40	0

* A, doxorubicin; Ad, dactinomycin; C, cyclophosphamide; D, DTIC; E, Epirubicin; Hmm, hexamethylmelamine; M, high-dose methotrexate; I, ifosfamide; L, (L-PAM) melphalan; P, cisplatin; V, vincristine; Mitc, mitomycin C; WLRT, whole lung radiation therapy.

† UCSF, University of California, San Francisco; ECOG, Eastern Cooperative Oncology Group; GOG, Gynecologic Oncology Group; SIOP, International Society of Pediatric Oncology; SWOG, Southwest Oncology Group; MDAH, M.D. Anderson Cancer Center; EORTC, European Organization for Research and Treatment of Cancer; MSKCC, Memorial Sloan Kettering Cancer Center; RPMI, Roswell Park Memorial Institute, Rochester, NY.

‡ CR, complete response.

QUALITY OF LIFE ISSUES

Medical decisions should be predicated on an understanding of the influence of treatments on survival. If different treatments result in equivalent survival outcomes, the effects of these treatments on the quality of life may help in choosing the most appropriate treatment for a patient.[559] One example is the treatment of patients with high-grade extremity soft tissue sarcomas in which there is a choice between limb-sparing surgery combined with adjuvant therapy or amputation. In a prospective, randomized NCI study, Rosenberg and colleagues demonstrated that the overall survival rates of these two treatment modalities were equivalent.[264] Although intuition predicts that the limb-sparing approach should result in improved quality of life over amputation and should therefore be offered to a patient, there are few data available to determine the functional capacity and quality of life for patients who have had either treatment.

Sugarbaker and coworkers assessed quality of life for 26 patients undergoing limb-sparing surgery or amputation for soft tissue sarcomas of the extremity.[560] Psychosocial and clinical assessments were used to measure the impact of treatment on psychosocial adjustment, daily activities, economic status, mobility, pain, sexual relationships, and treatment trauma. Analysis of this study revealed no evidence of improved quality of life in patients undergoing limb-sparing surgery plus irradiation compared with amputation.

In a study reported by Weddington and colleagues, the psychological outcome of 33 patients with extremity sarcoma who underwent amputation or limb-sparing surgery were evaluated.[561] A battery of standard psychosocial assessment tests were employed and revealed no psychological advantage of limb-sparing surgery to amputation. These studies appear to indicate that the impact of amputation or limb-sparing surgery are equivalent, an idea that is contrary to intuition. This may be a result of insensitive tools in the assessment of quality of life, which is a difficult concept to measure, or these studies may reflect the ability of an amputee to compensate and adjust to a lost limb. It appears that there is no compelling reason to attempt a limb-sparing approach instead of an amputation for every patient with a high-grade sarcoma, because the impact of these treatments on survival and quality of life are equivalent. If there is concern about obtaining adequate tumor margins with a limb-sparing procedure, amputation should be performed.

Multimodality treatment of soft tissue sarcomas significantly improved patient survival. The optimal combination of surgery, radiation therapy, and chemotherapy has not been defined. Evaluation of the impact of various combined modality treatments on the quality of life of patients becomes an important determinant in optimizing therapy if survival results are not affected.[562]

In an NCI study, the role of adjuvant, postoperative radiation therapy was studied in patients with high-grade extremity sarcomas treated with limb-sparing surgery and adjuvant chemotherapy.[563] A concurrent prospective study of the quality of life evaluated economic status, sexual activity, functional parameters, and indicators of global well-being. There were significantly more local recurrences in patients treated with only surgery and chemotherapy, but the overall survival of the two groups was virtually identical. In this study, quality of life parameters helped to weigh the detriment of those few local recurrences against the detriment of administering high-dose radiation therapy in all cases. Radiation therapy was found to result in a significantly greater degree of pain, edema, and joint stiffness, which tended to abate with time. Because the magnitude of these effects was modest, no difference in activities of daily living was seen. Psychosocial parameters were not consistently influenced by irradiation, and the Functional Living Index (Cancer), a global parameter of quality of life, showed no differences beyond 6 months from surgery. Such studies should not be construed to prescribe one therapy over another, but they define and quantitate the differences between two treatments, allowing some patients to choose a therapy based on personal priorities.

REFERENCES

1. Patten BM. Human Embryology. New York: McGraw-Hill, 1968.
2. Boring CC, Squires TS, Tong T. Cancer statistics, 1991. CA 1991;41:19–39.
3. Smith AH, Pearce NE, Fisher DO, et al. Soft tissue sarcoma and exposure to phenoxyherbicides and chlorophenols in New Zealand. JNCI 1984;73:1111–1117.
4. Lynge E, Storm HH, Jensen OM. The evaluation of trends in soft tissue sarcoma according to diagnostic criteria and consumption of phenoxyherbicides. Cancer 1987;60:1896–1901.
5. Li FP, Fraumeni JF Jr. Soft-tissue sarcomas, breast cancer, and other neoplasms. A familial syndrome? Ann Intern Med 1969;71:747–752.
6. Malkin D, Li FP, Strong LC, et al. Germ line p53 mutations in a familial syndrome of breast cancer, sarcomas and other neoplasms. Science 1990;250:1233–1238.
7. Mulligan LM, Matlashewski GJ, Scrable HJ, et al. Mechanisms of p53 loss in human sarcomas. PNAS 1990;87:5863–5867.
8. Li FP, Fraumeni JF Jr. Rhabdomyosarcoma in children: Epidemiologic study and identification of a familial cancer syndrome. JNCI 1969;43:1365–1373.
9. Li FP, Tucker MA, Fraumeni JF Jr. Childhood cancer in sibs. J Pediatr 1976;88:419–423.
10. Miller RW. Deaths from childhood leukemia and solid tumors among twins and other sibs in the United States, 1960–1967. JNCI 1971;45:203.
11. Chabalko JJ, Creagon ET, Fraumeni JF Jr. Epidemiology of selected sarcomas in children. JNCI 1974;53:675.
12. Remzi D, Kendi S. Rhabdomyosarcoma of the prostate in childhood. Turk J Pediatr 1966;8:143–149.
13. Bottomley RH, Condit PT. Cancer families. Cancer Bull 1968;20:22–24.
14. Fraumeni JF Jr, Vogel CL, Easton JM. Sarcomas and multiple polyposis in a kindred. A genetic variety of hereditary polyposis? Arch Intern Med 1968;121:57–61.
15. Stewart FW, Treves NP. Lymphangiosarcoma in postmastectomy lyphedema: A report of six cases in elephantiasis chirurgica. Cancer 1948;1:64–81.
16. Sloane JA, Hubbel MM. Soft tissue sarcomas in children associated with congenital anomalies. Cancer 1969;23:175–182.
17. Schjweisguth O, Gerard-Marchant R, Lemerle J. Naevomatose baso-cellulaire association a un rhabdomyosarcome congenital. Arch Fr Pediatr 1968;25:1083–1093.
18. Heard G. Malignant disease in von Recklinghausen's neurofibromatosis. Proc R Soc Med 1963;56:502–503.
19. Reed WB, Nickel WR, Campion G. Internal manifestations of tuberous sclerosis. Arch Dermatol 1963;87:715–728.
20. Epstein CJ, Martin GM, Schultz AL, et al. Werner's syndrome. A review of its symptomatology, natural history, pathologic features, genetics and relationship to the natural aging process. Medicine (Baltimore) 1966;45:177–221.
21. Usui M, Ishii S, Yamawaki S, et al. The occurrence of soft tissue sarcomas in three siblings with Werner's syndrome. Cancer 1984;54:2580–2586.
22. Hardell L, Sandstrom A. Case-control study: Soft-tissue sarcomas and exposure to phenoxyacetic acids or chlorophenols. Br J Cancer 1979;39:711–717.
23. Eriksson M, Hardell L, Berg NO, et al. Soft tissue sarcomas and exposure to chemical substances: A case-referent study. Br J Ind Med 1981;38:27–33.
24. Wiklund K, Holm LE. Soft tissue sarcoma risk in Swedish agricultural and forestry workers. JNCI 1986;76:229–234.
25. Greenwald P, Kovasznay B, Collins DN, et al. Sarcomas of soft tissue after Vietnam service. JNCI 1984;73:1107–1109.
26. Kang H, Enzinger F, Breslin P, et al. Soft tissue sarcomas and military service in Vietnam: A case-control study. JNCI 1987;79:693–699.
27. Adam YG, Reif R. Radiation-induced fibrosarcoma following treatment for breast cancer. Surgery 1977;81:421–425.
28. Kuten A, Sapir D, Cohen Y, et al. Postirradiation soft tissue sarcoma occurring in breast cancer patients: Report of seven cases and results of combination chemotherapy. J Surg Oncol 1985;28:168–171.
29. Souba WW, McKenna RJ, Meis J, et al. Radiation-induced sarcomas of the chest wall. Cancer 1986;57:610–615.
30. O'Neil NB, Cocke W, Mason D, et al. Radiation-induced soft tissue fibrosarcoma: Surgical therapy and salvage. Ann Thorac Surg 1982;33:625–628.

31. Halperin EC, Greenberg MS, Suit HD. Sarcoma of bone and soft tissue following treatment of Hodgkin's disease. Cancer 1984;53:232–236.
32. Arlen M, Higinbotham NL, Huvos AG, et al. Radiation-induced sarcoma of bone. Cancer 1971;28:1087–1099.
33. Martland HS, Humphries RE. Osteogenic sarcoma in dial painters using luminous paint. Arch Pathol 1929;7:406–417.
34. Brand KG. Foreign body induced sarcomas. In: Becker FF, ed. Cancer. New York: Plenum Press, 1975:485–511.
35. Ott G. Fremd Körpersarkome. Exp Med Pathol Klin 1970;32:1.
36. De Cholnky T. Augmentation mammaplasty: Survey of complications in 10,941 patients by 265 surgeons. Plast Reconstr Surg 1970;45:573.
37. Rubin LR, Bromberg BE, Walden RH. Long-term human reaction to synthetic plastics. Surg Gynecol Obstet 1971;132:603.
38. Shieber W, Graham P. An experience with sarcomas of the soft tissues in adults. Surgery 1962;52:295.
39. Hare HF, Cerny MF. Soft tissue sarcoma: A review of 200 cases. Cancer 1963;16: 1332.
40. Ferrell HW, Frable WJ. Soft part sarcomas revisited. Review and comparison of a second series. Cancer 1972;30:475–480.
41. Sears HF, Hopson R, Inouye W, et al. Analysis of staging and management of patients with sarcoma. Ann Surg 1980;191:488–493.
42. Abbas JS, Holyoke ED, Moore, et al. The surgical treatment and outcome of soft tissue sarcoma. Arch Surg 1981;116:765–769.
43. Lindberg RD, Martin RG, Romsdahl MM, et al. Conservative surgery and postoperative radiotherapy in 300 adults with soft-tissue sarcomas. Cancer 1981;47:2391–2397.
44. Potter DA, Glenn J, Kinsella T, et al. Patterns of recurrence in patients with high-grade soft tissue sarcomas. J Clin Oncol 1985;3:353–366.
45. Torosian MH, Friedrich C, Godbold J, et al. Soft tissue sarcomas: Initial characteristics and prognostic factors in patients with and without metastic disease. Semin Surg Oncol 1988;4:13–19.
46. Lawrence W Jr, Donegan WL, Nachimuth N, et al. Adult soft tissue sarcomas. A pattern of care survey of the American College of Surgeons. Ann Surg 1987;205:349–359.
47. Hajdu SI. Pathology of soft tissue tumors. Philadelphia: Lea & Febiger, 1979.
48. Mirr JM. The soft tissues. In: Coulson WF, ed. Surgical pathology. Philadelphia: JB Lippincott, 1978.
49. Stout AP, Lattes R. Tumors of the soft tissue. In: Atlas of tumor pathology. 2nd series. Washington, DC: Armed Forces Institute of Pathology, 1967.
50. Enzinger FM, Weiss SW. Soft tissue tumors. St. Louis: CV Mosby, 1988.
51. Coindre JM, Trojani M, Contesso G, et al. Reproducibility of a histopathologic grading system for adult soft tissue sarcoma. Cancer 1986;58:306–309.
52. Presant CA, Russell WO, Alexander RW, et al. Soft-tissue and bone sarcoma histopathology peer review: The frequency of disagreement in diagnosis and the need for second pathology opinions. The Southeastern Cancer Study Group experience. J Clin Oncol 1986;4:1658–1661.
53. Costa J, Wesley RA, Glatstein E, et al. The grading of soft tissue sarcomas. Results of a clinicohistopathologic correlation in a series of 163 cases. Cancer 1984;53:530–541.
54. Lack EE, Steinberg SM, White DE, et al. Extremity soft tissue sarcomas: Analysis of prognostic variables in 300 cases and evaluation of tumor necrosis as a factor in stratifying higher-grade sarcomas. J Surg Oncol 1989;41:263–273.
55. Trojani M, Contesso G, Coindre JM, et al. Soft tissue sarcomas of adults. Study of pathological prognostic variables and definition of a histopathological grading system. Int J Cancer 1984;33:37–42.
56. Alvegard TA, Berg NO, et al. Histopathological peer review of high-grade soft tissue sarcoma: The Scandinavian Sarcoma Group experience. J Clin Oncol 1989;7:1845–1951.
57. Pack GI, Ariel IM. Treatment of cancer and allied diseases. In: Tumors of the soft somatic tissues and bone. Vol VIII. New York: Harper & Row, 1964.
58. Martin RG, Butler JJ, Albores-Saavedra J. Soft tissue tumors: Surgical treatment and results. In: Tumors of bone and soft tissue. Chicago: Year Book Medical Publishers, 1965.
59. Shiu MH, Castro EB, Hajdu SI, et al. Surgical treatment of 297 soft tissue sarcomas of the lower extremity. Ann Surg 1975;182:597.
60. Simon MA, Enneking WF. The management of soft tissue sarcomas of the extremities. J Bone Joint Surg [Am] 1976;58:317.
61. Bears OH, Henson DE, Hutter RVP, Kennedy BJ, eds. Manual for staging of cancer, American Joint Committee on Cancer. 4th ed. Philadelphia: JB Lippincott, 1992.
62. Suit HD, Mankin JH, Willett G, et al. Limited surgery and external irradiation in soft tissue sarcomas. In: Recent concepts in sarcoma treatment. Proceedings of the International Symposium on Sarcomas, Tarpon Springs, FL, October 8–10, 1987. The Netherlands: Kluwer Academic Publishers, 1988.
63. Lindberg RD, Martin RG, Romsdahl MM, et al. Conservation surgery and radiation therapy for soft tissue sarcomas. In: Martin RG, Ayala AG, eds. Management of primary bone and soft tissue tumors. Chicago: Year Book Medical Publishers, 1977.
64. Suit HD. Patterns of failure after treatment of sarcoma of soft tissue by radical surgery or by conservative surgery and radiation. Cancer Treat Symp 1983;2:241–246.
65. Collins C, Hadju SI, Godbold J, et al. Localized, operable soft tissue sarcoma of the lower extremity. Arch Surg 1986;121:1425–1433.
66. Potter DA, Kinsella T, Glatstein E, et al. High grade soft tissue sarcomas of the extremities. Cancer 1986;58:190–205.
67. Jarvi OH, Saxen E. Elastofibroma dorsi. Acta Pathol Microbiol Immunol Scand 1961;144: S83–S84.
68. Jarvi OH, Lansimies PH. Subclinical elastofibromas in the scapular region in an autopsy series. Acta Pathol Microbiol Immunol Scand [A] 1975;83:87–108.
69. Jarvi OH, Saxen AE, Hopsu-Havu VK, et al. Elastofibroma: A degenerative pseudotumor. Cancer 1969;23:42–63.
70. Stemmermann GN, Stout AP. Elastofibroma dorsi. Am J Clin Pathol 1962;37:490–506.
71. Conway H. Dupuytren's contracture. Am J Surg 1954;87:10.
72. Luck JV. Dupuytren's contracture. J Bone Joint Surg [Am] 1959;41:635.
73. Skoog T. Dupuytren's contracture: Pathogenesis and surgical treatment. Surg Clin North Am 1967;47:433–444.
74. Allen RA, Woolner LB, Ghormley RK. Soft-tissue tumors of the sole: With special reference to plantar fibromatosis. J Bone Joint Surg [Am] 1955;37:14–26.
75. Allen PM, Enzinger FM. Juvenile aponeurotic fibroma. Cancer 1970;26:857–867.
76. Goldman RL. The cartilage analogue of fibromatosis (aponeurotic fibroma): Further observations based on 7 new cases. Cancer 1970;26:1325–1331.
77. Keasbey LE. Juvenile aponeurotic fibroma (calcifying fibroma). Cancer 1953;6:338–346.
78. Bartlett RC, Otis RD, Haakso AO. Multiple congenital neoplasms of soft tissues. Report of 4 cases in 1 family. Cancer 1961;14:913–920.
79. Beatty EC. Congenital generalized fibromatosis in infancy. Am J Dis Child 1962;103: 620.
80. Teng P, Warden MJ, Cohn WL. Congenital generalized fibromatosis (renal and skeletal) with complete spontaneous regression. J Pediatr 1963;62:748–753.
81. Enzinger FM. Fibrous hamartoma of infancy. Cancer 1965;18:241–251.
82. Chandler A. Muscular torticollis. J Bone Joint Surg [Am] 1948;30:566.
83. Brown JB, McDowell F. Wry-neck facial distortion prevented by resection of fibrosed sternomastoid muscle in infancy and childhood. Ann Surg 1950;131:721–733.
84. Smoth BH. Peyronie's disease. Am J Clin Pathol 1966;45:670.
85. Allen PW. Nodular fascitis. Pathology 1972;4:9–26.
86. Bernstein KE, Lattes R. Nodular (pseudosarcomatous) fasciitis; a nonrecurrent lesion: Clinicopathologic study of 134 cases. Cancer 1982;49:1668–1679.
87. Soule EH. Proliferative (nodular) fasciitis. Arch Pathol 1962;73:437.
88. Hutter RVP, Stewart FW, Foote FW Jr. Fasciitis: A report of 70 cases with follow-up proving the benignity of the lesion. Cancer 1962;15:992–1003.
89. MacKenzie DH. The differential diagnosis of fibroblastic disorders. Oxford: Blackwell Scientific, 1970.
90. Das Gupta TK, Brasfield RD, O'Hara J. Extra-abdominal desmoids. Ann Surg 1969;170: 109.
91. Enzinger FM, Shiraki M. Musculoaponeurotic fibromatosis of the shoulder girdle. Cancer 1967;20:113.
92. Brasfield RD, Das Gupta TK. Desmoid tumors of the anterior abdominal wall. Surgery 1969;65:241.
93. Ewing J. Neoplastic disease. Philadelphia: WB Saunders, 1928.
94. Musgrove JE, McDonald JR. Extra-abdominal desmoid tumors: A differential diagnosis and treatment. Arch Pathol 1948;45:513–540.
95. Benninghoff D, Robbins R. The nature and treatment of desmoid tumors. Am J Roentgenol Radium Ther Nucl Med 1964;91:132–137.
96. Greenberg HM, Goebel R, Weichselbaum RR, et al. Radiation therapy in the treatment of aggressive fibromatoses. Int J Radiat Oncol Biol Phys 1981;7:305–310.
97. Kirchmer JT Jr, Woma FJ Jr. Desmoid tumors of the abdominal wall. South Med J 1977;70:1136.
98. Wara WM, Phillips TL, Hill DR, et al. Desmoid tumors—treatment and prognosis. Radiology 1977;124:225–226.
99. Suit HD, Russell WO. Radiation therapy of soft tissue sarcomas. Cancer 1975;36:759–764.
100. Kiel KD, Suit HD. Radiation therapy in the treatment of aggressive fibromatoses (desmoid tumors). Cancer 1984;54:2051–2055.
101. Kinsbrunner B, Ritter S, Domingo J, et al. Remission of rapidly growing desmoid tumors after tamoxifen therapy. Cancer 1983;52:2201–2204.
102. Lanari A. Effect of progesterone on desmoid tumors (aggressive fibromatosis). N Engl J Med 1983;309:1523.
103. Waddell WR, Gerner RE. Indomethacin and ascorbate inhibit desmoid tumors. J Surg Oncol 1980;15:85–90.
104. Khorsand J, Karakousis CP. Desmoid tumors and their management. Am J Surg 1985;149:215–218.
105. Posner MC, Shiu MH, Newsome JL, et al. The desmoid tumor: Not a benign disease. Arch Surg 1989;124:191–196.
106. Kofoed H, Kamby C, Anagnostaki L. Aggressive fibromatosis. Surg Gynecol Obstet 1985;160:124–127.
107. Czernobilsky B, Cornog JL, Enterline HT. Rhabdomyoma: Report of a case with ultrastructural and histochemical studies. Am J Clin Pathol 1968;49:782–789.
108. Morgan JJ, Enterline HT. Benign rhabdomyoma of the pharynx: A case report, review of the literature, and comparison with cardiac rhabdomyoma. Am J Clin Pathol 1964;42: 174–181.
109. Lendrum AC. Painful tumors of the skin. Ann R Coll Surg Engl 1947;1:62–67.
110. Stout AP. Solitary cutaneous and subcutaneous leiomyoma. Am J Cancer 1937;29: 435–469.
111. Enzinger FM, Harvey DA. Spindle cell lipoma. Cancer 1975;36:1852–1859.
112. Lin JJ, Lin F. Two entities in angiolipoma. A study of 459 cases of lipoma with review of infiltrating angiolipoma. Cancer 1974;34:720–727.
113. Chung EB, Enzinger FM. Benign lipoblastomatosis. An analysis of 35 cases. Cancer 1973;32:482–491.
114. Alba-Greco M, Garcia RL, Vuletin JC. Benign lipoblastomatosis. Ultrastructure and histogenesis. Cancer 1980;45:511.
115. Evans HL, Soule EH, Winkelmann RK. Atypical lipoma, atypical intramuscular lipoma,

and well-differentiated retroperitoneal liposarcoma. A reappraisal of 30 cases formerly classified as well-differentiated liposarcoma. Cancer 1979;43:574–584.
116. Dionne GP, Seemayer TA. Infiltrating lipomas and angiolipomas revisited. Cancer 1974;33:732–738.
117. Enzinger FM. Benign lipomatous tumors simulating a sarcoma. In: Martin RG, Ayala AG, eds. Management of primary bone and soft tissue tumors. Chicago: Year Book Medical Publishers, 1977:11–24.
118. Kindblom LG, Angervall L, Stener B, et al. Intermuscular and intramuscular lipomas and hibernomas: A clinical, roentgenologic, histologic, and prognostic study of 46 cases. Cancer 1974;33:754–762.
119. Mesara BW, Batsakis JC. Hibernoma of the neck. Arch Otolaryngol 1967;85:95.
120. Jones FE, Soule EH, Coventry MB. Fibrous xanthoma of synovium (giant cell tumor of tender sheath, pigmented nodular synovitis). J Bone Joint Surg [Am] 1969;51:76.
121. Gehweiler JA, Wilson VW. Diffuse biarticular pigmented villonodular synovitis. Radiology 1969;93:137.
122. Slooff JL, Kernohan JW, MacCarty CS. Primary intramedullary tumors of the spinal cord and filum terminale. Philadelphia: WB Saunders, 1964.
123. D'Agostino A. Sarcomas of the peripheral nerves and somatic soft tissues associated with multiple neurofibromatosis. Cancer 1963;16:1015.
124. Buck BE. Congenital neurogenous sarcoma with rhabdomyosarcomatous differentiation. J Pediatr Surg 1977;12:581–582.
125. Hammond JA. Detection of malignant change in neurofibromatosis by gallium-67 scanning. Can Med Assoc J 1978;119:352–353.
126. Herman J. Sarcomatous transformation in multiple neurofibromatosis. Ann Surg 1950;131:206.
127. Hunt K. Neurofibrosarcoma complicating von Recklinghausen's disease. J Ky Med Assoc 1976;74:346–349.
128. Lee C. Malignant degeneration of thoracic neurofibromata. NY State J Med 1972;75: 347–352.
129. Wander JW, Das Gupta TK. Neurofibromatosis. Curr Probl Surg 1977;14:1–81.
130. Riccardi VM. Medical progress. von Recklinghausen neurofibromatosis. N Engl J Med 1981;305:1617–1626.
131. Nambisan RN, Rao U, Moore R, et al. Malignant soft tissue tumors of nerve sheath origin. J Surg Oncol 1984;25:268–272.
132. Sorensen SA, Mulvihill JJ, Nielsen A. Long-term follow-up of von Recklinghausen neurofibromatosis survival and malignant neoplasms. N Engl J Med 1986;314:1010–1015.
133. Allen PW, Enzinger FM. Heamangioma of skeletal muscle: An analoysis of 89 cases. Cancer 1972;29:8–22.
134. Lister WA. The natural history of strawberry nevi. Lancet 1938;1:1429–1434.
135. Modlin JJ. Capillary hemangiomas of the skin. Surgery 1955;38:169–180.
136. Riveros M, Pack GT. The glomus tumors—report of 20 cases. Ann Surg 1951;133: 394.
137. Carroll RE, Berman AT. Glomus tumors of the hand: Review of the literature and report of 28 cases. J Bone Joint Surg [Am] 1972;54:691–703.
138. Shugart RR, Soule EH, Johnson EW. Glomus tumor. Surg Gynecol Obstet 1963;117: 334–340.
139. Stout AP. Tumors featuring pericytes: Glomus tumor and hemangiopericytoma. Lab Invest 1965;5:217–223.
140. Enzinger FM, Smith BH. Hemangiopericytoma. An analysis of 106 cases. Hum Pathol 1976;7:61–82.
141. Soule EH, Enriquez P. Atypical fibrous histiocytoma, malignant fibrous histiocytoma, malignant histiocytoma, and epithelioid sarcoma. A comparative study of 65 tumors. Cancer 1972;30:128.
142. Kempson RL, McGavran MH. Atypical fibroxanthomas of the skin. Cancer 1964;17: 1463–1471.
143. Kauffman SL, Stout AP. Histiocytic tumors (fibrous xanthoma and histiocytoma) in children. Cancer 1961;14:469–482.
144. O'Brien JE, Stout AP. Malignant fibrous xanthomas. Cancer 1964;17:1445–1458.
145. Brenner W, Schaefler K, Habrans C, et al. Dermatofibrosarcoma protuberans metastatic to a regional lymph node. Report of a case and review. Cancer 1975;36:1897–1902.
146. Burkhardt BR, Soule EH, Winkelman RK, et al. Dermatofibrosarcoma protuberans: Study of 56 cases. Am J Surg 1966;111:638–644.
147. Taylor HB, Helwig EB. Dermatofibrosarcoma protuberans: A study of 115 cases. Cancer 1962;15:717–725.
148. McPeak CJ, Druz T, Nicastri AD. Dermatofibrosarcoma protuberans: An analysis of 86 cases—five with metastasis. Ann Surg 1967;166:803.
149. Glenn J, Potter D, Kinsella T, et al. Unpublished results, 1985.
150. Roses DF, Valensi Q, LaTrenta G, et al. Surgical treatment of dermatofibrosarcoma protuberans. Surg Gynecol Obstet 1986;162:449–452.
151. Rinck PA, Habermalz HJ, Loceck H. Effective radiotherapy in one case of dermatofibrosarcoma protuberans. Strahlentherapie 1982;158:681–685.
152. Strong EW, McDivitt RW, Brasfield RD. Granular cell myoblastoma. Cancer 1970;25: 415–422.
153. Le Ber MS, Stout AP. Benign mesenchymomas in children. Cancer 1962;15:598–605.
154. Stout AP. Myxoma, the tumor of primitive mesenchyme. Ann Surg 1948;127:706–719.
155. Enzinger FM. Intramuscular myxoma. Am J Clin Pathol 1965;43:104.
156. Barth RJ, Merino MJ, Solomon D, et al. A prospective study of the value of core needle biopsy and fine needle aspiration in the diagnosis of soft tissue sarcoma. Surgery 1992;112:536–543.
157. Martel W, Abell MR. Radiologic evaluation of soft tissue tumors. A retrospective study. Cancer 1973;32:352–366.
158. Berger PE, Kuhn JP. Computed tomography of tumors of the musculoskeletal system in children. Clinical applications. Radiology 1978;127:171–175.
159. Neifeld JP, Walsh JW, Lawrence W Jr. Computed tomography in the management of soft tissue tumors. Surg Gynecol Obstet 1982;155:535–540.
160. Lawrence W Jr, Neifeld JP, Terz JJ. Manual of soft tissue tumor surgery. New York: Springer-Verlag, 1983.
161. Levin DC, Watson RC, Baltaxe HA. Arteriography in diagnosis and management of acquired peripheral soft-tissue masses. Radiology 1972;103:53–58.
162. Hudson TM, Haas G, Enneking WF, et al. Angiography in the management of musculoskeletal tumors. Surg Gynecol Obstet 1975;141:11–21.
163. De Santos LA, Wallace S, Finklestein JB. Angiography and lymphangiography in peripheral soft tissue sarcomas. In: Martin RG, Ayala AG, eds. Management of primary bone and soft tissue tumors. Chicago: Year Book Medical Publishers, 1977.
164. Chang AE, Matory YL, Dwyer AJ, et al. Magnetic resonance imaging versus computed tomography in the evaluation of soft tissue tumors of the extremities. Ann Surg 1987;205: 340–348.
165. Bland KI, McCoy DM, Kinard RE, et al. Application of magnetic resonance imaging and computerized tomography as an adjunct to the surgical management of soft tissue sarcomas. Ann Surg 1987;205:473–481.
166. Enneking WF. Preoperative staging of sarcomas. Cancer Treat Symp 1985;3:67–70.
167. Enneking WF, Spanier SS, Goodman MA. The surgical staging of musculoskeletal sarcoma. J Bone Joint Surg [Am] 1980;62:1027–1030.
168. Suit HD, Russell WO, Martin RG. Sarcoma of soft tissue: Clinical and histopathologic parameters and response to treatment. Cancer 1975;35:1478–1483.
169. Suit HD, Mankin HJ, Wood WC, et al. Treatment of the patient with stage M_0 soft tissue sarcoma. J Clin Oncol 1988;6:854–862.
170. Weingrad DW, Rosenberg SA. Early lymphatic spread of osteogenic and soft-tissue sarcomas. Surgery 1978;84:231–240.
171. Mazeron JJ, Suit HD. Lymph nodes as sites of metastases from sarcomas of soft tissue. Cancer 1987;60:1800–1808.
172. Rosenberg SA, Seipp CA, White DE, et al. Perioperative blood transfusions are associated with increased rates of recurrence and decreased survival in patients with high-grade soft-tissue sarcomas of the extremities. J Clin Oncol 1985;3:698–709.
173. Soule EH, Pritchard DJ. Fibrosarcoma in infants and children: A review of 110 cases. Cancer 1977;40:1711–1721.
174. Shmahler BM, Enzinger FM. Liposarcoma occurring in children. An analysis of 17 cases and review of the literature. Cancer 1983;52:567–574.
175. Brennan MF. Presentation, demographics and prognostic factors of soft tissue sarcoma. In: Shiu MH, Brennan MF, eds. Surgical management of soft tissue sarcoma. Philadelphia: Lea & Febiger, 1989.
176. Suit HD. Patterns of failure after treatment of sarcoma of soft tissue by radical surgery or by conservative surgery and radiation. Cancer Treat Symp 1983;2:241–246.
177. Marcus SG, Merino MJ, Steinberg SM, et al. Long-term outcome of patients with low grade soft tissue sarcomas. Arch Surg 1993 (in press).
178. Cantin J, McNeer GP, Chu FC, et al. The problem of local recurrence after treatment of soft tissue sarcoma. Ann Surg 1968;168:47–53.
179. Lindberg RD, Martin RG, Romsdahl MM. Surgery and postoperative radiotherapy in the treatment of soft tissue sarcomas in adults. Am J Roentgenol Radium Ther Nucl Med 1975;123:123–129.
180. Gerner RE, Moore GE, Pickren JW. Soft tissue sarcomas. Ann Surg 1975;181:803–808.
181. Rosenberg SA, Kent H, Costa J, et al. Prospective randomized evaluation of the role of limb-sparing surgery, radiation therapy, and adjuvant chemoimmunotherapy in the treatment of adult soft-tissue sarcomas. Surgery 1978;84:62–69.
182. Markhede G, Angervall L, Stener B. A multivariate analysis of the prognosis after surgical treatment of malignant soft tissue tumors. Cancer 1982;49:1721–1733.
183. Pritchard DJ, Soule EH, Taylor WF, et al. Fibrosarcoma: Clinicopathologic and statistical study of 199 tumors of soft tissues of extremities and trunk. Cancer 1974;33:888–897.
184. Stout AP. Fibrosarcoma: The malignant tumor of fibroblasts. Cancer 1948;1:30–63.
185. Pritchard DJ, Soule EH, Taylor WF, et al. Fibrosarcoma: Clinicopathological and statistical study of 199 tumors of soft tissues of extremities and trunk. Cancer 1974;33: 880.
186. Castro EB, Hajdu SI, Fortner JG. Surgical therapy of fibrosarcoma of extremities. Arch Surg 1973;107:284.
187. Grier HE, Perez-Atayde AR, Weinstein JH. Chemotherapy for inoperable infantile fibrosarcoma. Cancer 1985;56:1507–1510.
188. Delepine N, Cornille H, Desbois JC, et al. Complete response of congenital fibrosarcoma to chemotherapy. Lancet 1986;1:1453–1454.
189. Soule EH, Geitz M, Henderson EH. Embryonal rhabdomyosarcoma of the limbs and limb girdles. A clinico-pathologic study of 61 cases. Cancer 1969;23:1338–1346.
190. Maurer HM, Moon T, Donaldson M, et al. The intergroup rhabdomyosarcoma study. Cancer 1977;40:2015.
191. Ariel IM, Briceno M. Rhabdomyosarcoma of the extremities and trunk: Analysis of 150 patients treated by surgical resection. J Surg Oncol 1975;7:269–287.
192. Linscheid RL, Soule EH, Henderson ED. Pleomorphic rhabdomyosarcoma of the extremities and limb girdles: A clinico-pathologic study. J Bone Joint Surg [Am] 1965;47: 715–725.
193. Albores-Saavedra J, Martin RG, Smith JL. Rhabdomyosarcoma: A study of 35 cases. Ann Surg 1963;157:186–197.
194. Lloyd RV, Hajdu SI, Knapper WH. Embryonal rhabdomyosarcoma in adults. Cancer 1983;51:557–565.
195. Agamanolis DP, Dasu S, Krill CE. Tumors of skeletal muscle. Hum Pathol 1986;17: 778–795.

196. Osborn M, Hill C, Altmannsberger M, et al. Monoclonal antibodies to titin in conjunction with antibodies to desmin separate rhabdomyosarcomas from other tumor types. Lab Invest 1986;55:101–108.
197. De Jong Ash, Van Kessel-Van Vark M, Alsus-Lutter Che: Hum Pathol 1987;18:298–303.
198. Stout AP, Hill WT. Leiomyosarcoma of the superficial soft tissues. Cancer 11:844–854, 1958.
199. Abwasi OE, Dozois RR, Weiland LH, et al. Leiomyosarcoma of the small and large bowel. Cancer 1978;42:1375.
200. Kevorkian J, Cento DP. Leiomyosarcoma of large arteries and veins. Surgery 1973;73:390.
201. Wile AG, Evans HL, Romsdahl MM. Leiomyosarcoma of soft tissue: A clinicopathologic study. Cancer 1981;48:1022–1032.
202. Enterline HT, Culberson JD, Rochlin DB, et al. Liposarcoma. A clinicopathologic study of 53 cases. Cancer 1960;11:932–950.
203. Spittle MF, Newton KA, Mackenzie DH. Liposarcoma. A review of 60 cases. Br J Cancer 1971;24:696.
204. Kindblom L, Angervall L, Svendsen P. Liposarcoma. A clinicopathologic, radiographic and prognostic study. Acta Pathol Microbiol Immunol Scand 1975;253:1.
205. Ackerman LV. Multiple primary liposarcomas. Am J Pathol 1944;20:789–793.
206. Enzinger FM, Winslow DJ. Liposarcoma. A study of 30 cases. Virchows Arch [A] 1962;335:367–388.
207. Reszel PA, Soule EH, Coventry MB. Liposarcoma of the extremities and limb girdles. A study of 222 cases. J Bone Joint Surg [Am] 1966;48:229.
208. Cadman NL, Soule EH, Kelly PJ. Synovial sarcoma: An analysis of 134 cases. Cancer 1965;18:613–627.
209. Gerner RE, Moore GE. Synovial sarcoma. Ann Surg 1975;181:22–25.
210. Hajdu SI, Shiu MH, Fortner JG. Tendosynovial sarcoma. A clinicopathological study of 136 cases. Cancer 1977;39:1201–1217.
211. Crocker DW, Stout AP. Synovial sarcoma in children. Cancer 1959;12:1123–1133.
212. Mobergen G. Nilsonne U, Friberg S. Synovial sarcoma. Acta Orthop Scand Suppl 1968;11:3.
213. Cagle LA, Mirra JM, Storm FK, et al. Histologic features relating to prognosis in synovial sarcoma. Cancer 1987;59:1810–1814.
214. Storm FK, Eilber FR, Mirra J, et al. Neurofibrosarcoma. Cancer 1980;45:126–129.
215. Girard C, Johnson WC, Graham JH. Cutaneous angiosarcoma. Cancer 1970;26:868–883.
216. Gulesserian HP, Lawton RL. Angiosarcoma of the breast. Cancer 1969;24:1021–1026.
217. Dunegan LJ, Tobon H, Watson CG. Angiosarcoma of the breast: A report of two cases and a review of the literature. Surgery 1976;79:57–59.
218. Woodward AH, Ivins JC, Soule EH. Lymphangiosarcoma arising in chronic lymphedematous extremities. Cancer 1972;30:562–572.
219. Rosai J, Sumner HW, Kostianovsky M, et al. Angiosarcoma of the skin. A clinicopathologic and fine structural study. Hum Pathol 1976;7:83.
220. Maddox JC, Evans L. Angiosarcoma of skin and soft tissue: A study of forty-four cases. Cancer 1981;48:1907–1921.
221. Morales PH, Lindberg RD, Barkley HT. Soft tissue angiosarcomas. Int J Radiat Oncol Biol Phys 1981;7:1655–1659.
222. Woodward AH, Ivins JC, Soule EH. Lymphangiosarcoma arising in chronic lymphadematous extremities. Cancer 1972;30:562–572.
223. Silverberg SG, Kay S, Koss LG. Postmastectomy lymphangiosarcoma: Ultrastructural observations. Cancer 1971;27:100–108.
224. Nemoto T, Stubbe N, Gaeta J, et al. Pathogenesis of lymphangiosarcoma following mastectomy and irradiation. Surg Gynecol Obstet 1969;128:489–494.
225. Holden CA, Spittle MF, Jones EW. Angiosarcoma of the face and scalp, prognosis and treatment. Cancer 1987;59:1046–1057.
226. Mira JG, Chu FCH, Fortner JG. The role of radiotherapy in the management of malignant hemangiopericytoma. Report of eleven new cases and review of the literature. Cancer 1977;39:1254–1259.
227. Stout AP. Hemangiopericytoma (a study of 25 new cases). Cancer 1949;2:1027–1954.
228. O'Brien PH, Brasfield RD. Hemangiopericytoma. Cancer 1965;14:249–252.
229. Hood AF, Farmer ER, Weiss RA. Kaposi's sarcoma. Johns Hopkins Med J 1982;151:222–239.
230. Steis RG, Broder S. The clinical relationship between immunodeficiency diseases and cancer with special emphasis on acquired immunodeficiency syndrome (AIDS) and Kaposi's sarcoma. In: DeVita VT Jr, Hellman S, Rosenberg SA, eds. Important advances in oncology 1985. Philadelphia: JB Lippincott, 1985.
231. Krigel RL, Friedman-Kien AE. Kaposi's sarcoma in AIDS. In: DeVita VT Jr, Hellman S, Rosenberg SA, eds. AIDS: Etiology, diagnosis, treatment and prevention. Philadelphia: JB Lippincott, 1985:185–211.
232. Reynolds WA, Winkelmann RK, Soule EH. Kaposi's sarcoma: A clinicopathologic study with particular reference to its relationship to the reticuloendothelial system. Medicine (Baltimore) 1965;44:419–443.
233. Rothman S. Remarks on sex, age and racial distribution of Kaposi's sarcoma and on possible pathogenetic factors. Acta Union Int Contra Cancrum 1962;18:326–329.
234. Dorffel J. Histogenesis of multiple idiopathic hemorrhagic sarcoma of Kaposi. Arch Dermatol Syph 1932;26:608–634.
235. Oettle AG. Geographical and racial differences in the frequency of Kaposi's sarcoma as evidence of environmental or genetic causes. Acta Unio Int Contra Cancrum 1962;18:330–363.
236. O'Brien PH, Brasfield RD. Kaposi's sarcoma. Cancer 1966;19:1497.
237. Kaminer B, Murray JF. Sarcoma idiopathicum multiplex haemorrhagicum of Kaposi, with special reference to its incidence in the South African Negro, and two case reports. South Afr J Clin Sci 1950;1:1–25.
238. Loethe F. Kaposi's sarcoma in Uganda Africans. Acta Pathol Microbiol Immunol Scand Suppl 1963;161:1–71.
239. Siegel JH, Janic R, Alper JC, et al. Disseminated visceral Kaposi's sarcoma. JAMA 1969;207:1493.
240. Stribling J, Wertzner S, Smith GV. Kaposi's sarcoma in renal allograft recipients. Cancer 1978;42:442.
241. Zisbrod A, Hairnov M, Schanzer H, et al. Kopsi's sarcoma after kidney transplantation. Transplantation 1980;30:383.
242. Penn I. Kaposi's sarcoma in organ transplant recipients. Transplantation 1979;27:8.
243. Myers BD, Kessle E, Levi D, et al. Kaposi's sarcoma in kidney transplant recipients. Arch Intern Med 1974;133:387.
244. Hymes K, Cheung T, Greene JB, et al. Kaposi's sarcoma in homosexual men: A report of eight cases. Lancet 1981;2:598–600.
245. O'Brien JE, Stout AP. Malignant fibrous xanthomas. Cancer 1964;17:1445–1458.
246. Wasserman TH, Stuart ID. Malignant fibrous histiocytoma with widespread metastases. Autopsy study. Cancer 1974;33:141–146.
247. Kearney MM, Soule EH, Ivins JC. Malignant fibrous histiocytoma. A retrospective study of 167 cases. Cancer 1980;45:167–178.
248. Weiss SW, Enzinger FM. Malignant fibrous histiocytoma. An analysis of 200 cases. Cancer 1978;41:2250–2266.
249. Leite C, Goodwin JW, Sinkovics JG, et al. Chemotherapy of malignant fibrous histiocytoma: A Southwest Oncology Group report. Cancer 1977;40:2010–2014.
250. Reagan MT, Clowry LJ, Cox JD, et al. Radiation therapy in the treatment of malignant fibrous histiocytoma. Int J Radiat Oncol Biol Phys 1981;7:311–315.
251. Weiss SW. Malignant fibrous histiocytoma. A reaffirmation. Am J Surg Pathol 1982;6:773–784.
252. Bertoni F, Capanna R, Biagini R, et al. Malignant fibrous histiocytoma. An analysis of 78 cases located and deeply seated in extremities. Cancer 1985;56:356–367.
253. Raney RB, Allen A, O'Neill J, et al. Malignant fibrous histiocytoma of soft tissue in childhood. Cancer 1986;57:2198–2201.
254. Christopherson WM, Foote FW, Stewart FW. Alveolar soft part sarcomas: Structurally characteristic tumors of uncertain histogenesis. Cancer 1952;5:100.
255. Lieberman PH, Foote FW, Stewart FW, et al. Alveolar soft-part sarcoma. JAMA 1966;198:1047–1051.
256. Unni KK, Soule EH. Alveolar soft part sarcoma. An electron microscopic study. Mayo Clin Proc 1975;50:592–598.
257. Bryan RS, Soule EH, Dobyns JH, et al. Primary epithelioid sarcoma of the hand and forearm. A review of thirteen cases. J Bone Joint Surg [Am] 1974;56:458–465.
258. Peimer AC, Smith RJ, Sirota RL, et al. Epithelioid sarcoma of the hand and wrist: Patterns of extension. J Hand Surg [Am] 1977;2:275–282.
259. Prat J, Woodruff JM, Marcove RC. Epithelioid sarcoma. An analysis of 22 cases indicating the prognostic significance of vascular invasion and regional lymph node metastasis. Cancer 1978;41:1472–1487.
260. Enzinger FM. Epithelioid sarcoma. A sarcoma simulating a granuloma or a carcinoma. Cancer 1970;26:1029–1041.
261. Shimm DS, Suit HD. Radiation therapy of epithelioid sarcoma. Cancer 1983;52:1022–1025.
262. Chase DR, Enzinger FM. Epithelioid sarcoma. Am J Surg Pathol 1985;9:241–263.
263. National Institutes of Health Consensus Development Panel on Limb-Sparing Treatment of Adult Soft Tissue Sarcomas and Osteosarcomas. Introduction and conclusions. Cancer Treat Symp 1985;3:1–5.
264. Rosenberg SA, Tepper J, Glatstein E, et al. The treatment of soft tissue sarcomas of the extremities. Prospective randomized evaluations of (1) limb-sparing surgery plus radiation therapy compared with amputation and (2) the role of adjuvant chemotherapy. Ann Surg 1982;196:305–315.
265. Simon MA, Spainer SS, Enneking WF. Management of adult soft-tissue sarcomas of the extremities. Surg Annu 1979;1:363–402.
266. Brennan MF, Shiu MH, Collin C, et al. Extremity soft tissue sarcomas. Cancer Treat Symp 1985;3:71–81.
267. Rooser B, Gustafson P, Rydholm A. Is there no influence of local control on the rate of metastases in high-grade soft tissue sarcoma? Cancer 1990;65:1727–1729.
268. Gustafson P, Rooser B, Rydholm A. Is local recurrence of minor importance for metastases in soft tissue sarcoma? Cancer 1991;67:2083–2086.
269. Enneking WF. Staging of musculoskeletal neoplasms. In: Current concepts of diagnosis and treatment of bone and soft tissue tumors. Heidelberg: Springer-Verlag, 1984.
270. Karakousis CP. Internal hemipelvectomy. Surg Gynecol Obstet 1984;158:279–282.
271. Sugarbaker P. Atlas of extremity surgery. Philadelphia: JB Lippincott, 1985.
272. Greager JA, Das Gupta TK. Adult head and neck soft-tissue sarcomas. Otolaryngol Clin North Am 1986;19:565–572.
273. McKenna WG, Barnes MM, Kinsella TJ, et al. Combined modality treatment of adult soft tissue sarcomas of the head and neck. Int J Radiat Oncol Biol Phys 1987;13:1127–1133.
274. Weber RS, Benjamin RS, Peters LJ, et al. Soft tissue sarcomas of the head and neck in adolescents and adults. Am J Surg 1986;152:386–392.
275. King RM, Pairolero PC, Trastek VF, et al. Primary chest wall tumors: Factors affecting survival. Ann Thorac Surg 1986;41:597–601.
276. Greager JA, Patel MK, Briele HA, et al. Soft tissue sarcomas of the adult thoracic wall. Cancer 1987;59:370–373.
277. Glenn J, Sindelar WF, Kinsella T, et al. Results of multimodality therapy of resectable soft-tissue sarcomas of the retroperitoneum. Surgery 1985;97:316–324.
278. Shiu MH, Flanebaum L, Hajdu SI, et al. Malignant soft tissue tumors of the anterior abdominal wall. Arch Surg 1980;115:152–155.
279. Graeber GM, Snyder RJ, Fleming AW, et al. Initial and long-term results in the management of primary chest wall neoplasms. Ann Thorac Surg 1982;34:664–673.

280. Braasch JW, Mon AB. Primary retroperitoneal tumors. Surg Clin North Am 1967;47: 663.
281. Cody HS, Turnbull AD, Fortner JG, et al. The continuing challenge of retroperitoneal sarcomas. Cancer 1981;47:2147–2152.
282. Storm FK, Sondak VK, Economou JS. Sarcomas of the retroperitoneum. In: Eilber FR, Morton DL, Sondak VK, et al, eds. The soft tissue sarcomas. New York: Grune & Stratton, 1987:239–248.
283. Karakousis CP, Velez AF, Emrich LJ. Management of retroperitoneal sarcomas and patient survival. Am J Surg 1985;150:376–380.
284. Bose B. Primary malignant retroperitoneal tumors: Analysis of 30 cases. Can J Surg 1979;22:215–220.
285. McGrath PC, Neifield JP, Lawrence W, et al. Improved survival following complete excision of retroperitoneal sarcomas. Ann Surg 1984;200:200–204.
286. Jaques DP, Coit DG, Hajdu SI, et al. Management of primary and recurrent soft-tissue sarcoma of the retroperitoneum. Ann Surg 1990;212:51–59.
287. Delamater J. Mammoth tumor. Cleve Med Gazette 1859;1:31.
288. Enzinger FM, Winslow DJ. Liposarcoma. A study of 30 cases. Virchows Arch [A] 1962;335:367–388.
289. Fortner JG, Martin S, Hajdu S, et al. Primary sarcoma of the retroperitoneum. Semin Oncol 1981;8:180–184.
290. Abbas S, Holyoke ED, Moore R, et al. The surgical treatment and outcome of soft-tissue sarcoma. Arch Surg 1981;116:765–769.
291. Kinsella TJ, Sindelar WF, Lack E, et al. Preliminary results of a randomized study of adjuvant radiation therapy in resectable adult retroperitoneal soft tissue sarcomas. J Clin Oncol 1988;6:18–25.
292. Cade SS. Soft tissue tumors: Their natural history and treatment. Proc R Soc Med 1951;19:19–36.
293. Windeyer SB, Dische S, Mansfield CM. The place of radio-therapy in the management of fibrosarcoma of the soft tissues. Clin Radiol 1966;17:32–40.
294. Lindberg RD. Soft tissue sarcoma. In: Fletcher GH, ed. Textbook of radiotherapy. Philadelphia: Lea & Febiger, 1980:922–942.
295. Suit HD. Sarcomas of soft tissue. In: The third annual current approaches to radiation oncology, biology, and physics. San Francisco: University of California, 1983:138–141.
296. Tepper JE, Suite HD. Radiation therapy of soft tissue sarcomas. Cancer 1985;55: 2273–2277.
297. Todoroki T, Suit HD. Effect of fractionated irradiation prior to conservation and radical surgery on therapeutic gain in spontaneous fibrosarcoma of the C3H mouse. J Surg Oncol 1986;31:279–286.
298. Leibel SA, Ware WM, Hill DR, et al. Desmoid tumors: Local control and patterns of relapse following radiation therapy. Int J Radiat Oncol Biol Phys 1983;9:1167–1171.
299. Greenberg HM, Goebel R, Weichselbaum RR, et al. Radiation therapy in the treatment of aggressive fibromatoses. Int J Radiat Oncol Biol Phys 1981;7:309–319.
300. Kiel KD, Suit HD. Radiation therapy in the treatment of aggressive fibromatoses (desmoid tumors). Cancer 1984;54:2051–2055.
301. Mirabell R, Suit HD, Mankin HJ, et al. Fibromatoses: From post-surgical surveillance to combined surgery and radiation therapy. Int J Radiat Oncol Biol Phys 1990;18:535–540.
302. McCollough WM, Parons JT, van der Griend R, et al. Radiation therapy for aggressive fibromatoses. J Bone Joint Surg [Am] 1991;73:717–725.
303. Leibel SA, Transbaugh RF, Wara WM, et al. Soft tissue sarcomas of the extremities. Survival patterns of failure with conservative surgery and post-operative irradiation compared to surgery alone. Cancer 1982;50:1076–1083.
304. Suit HD, Mankin HJ, Wood WC, et al. Pre-operative, intra-operative, and post-operative radiation in the treatment of primary soft tissue sarcoma. Cancer 1985;55:2659–2667.
305. Suit HD, Mankin HJ, Schiller AL, et al. Results of treatment of sarcoma of soft tissue by radiation and surgery at Massachusetts General Hospital. Cancer Treat Symp 1985;3: 43–47.
306. Lindberg R. Treatment of localized soft tissue sarcomas in adults at M.D. Anderson Hospital and Tumor Institute (1960–1981). Cancer Treat Symp 1985;3:59–65.
307. Enneking WF, McAuliffe JA. Adjunctive preoperative radiation therapy in treatment of soft tissue sarcomas: A preliminary report. Cancer Treat Symp 1985;3:37–42.
308. Atkinson L, Garvan JM, Newton NC. Behavior and management of soft tissue sarcomas. Cancer 1963;16:1552–1562.
309. Suit HD, Proppe KH, Mankin HJ, et al. Pre-operative radiation therapy for sarcoma of soft tissue. Cancer 1981;47:2269–2274.
310. Fortner JG, Kim DK, Shiu MH. Limb-preserving vascular surgery for malignant tumors of the lower extremity. Arch Surg 1977;112:391–394.
311. Imparato AM, Roses DF, Francis KC, et al. Major vascular reconstruction for limb salvage in patients with soft tissue and skeletal sarcomas of the extremity. Surg Gynecol Obstet 1978;147:891–896.
312. Morton DL, Eilber FR, Townsend CM Jr, et al. Limb salvage from a multidisciplinary treatment approach for skeletal and soft tissue sarcomas of the extremity. Ann Surg 1976;184:268–278.
313. Steed DL, Peitzman AB, Webster MW, et al. Limb sparing operations for sarcomas of the extremities involving critical arterial circulation. Surg Gynecol Obstet 1987;164: 493–498.
314. Nambisan RN, Karakousis CP. Vascular reconstruction for limb salvage in soft tissue sarcomas. Surgery 1987;101:668–677.
315. Yang JC. Unpublished data, 1992.
316. Bramwell V, Rouesse J, Steward W, et al. European experience of adjuvant chemotherapy for soft tissue sarcoma: Interim report of a randomized trial of CYVADIC versus control. In: Ryan JR, Baker LH, eds. Recent concepts in sarcoma treatment. Dordrecht: Kluwer Academic Publishers, 1988.
317. Ravaud A, Bui NB, Coindre JM, et al. Adjuvant chemotherapy with CYVADIC in high risk soft tissue sarcoma: A randomized prospective trial. In: Salmon SE, ed. Adjuvant therapy of cancer. Vol 6. Philadelphia: WB Saunders, 1990.
318. Rydholm A, Gustafson P, Rooser B, et al. Limb-sparing surgery without radiotherapy based on anatomic location of soft tissue sarcoma. J Clin Oncol 1991;10:1757–1765.
319. Shiu MH, Turnbull AD, Nori D, et al. Control of locally advanced extremity soft tissue sarcomas by function-saving resection and brachytherapy. Cancer 1984;53:1385–1392.
320. Brennan MF, Hilaris B, Shiu MH, et al. Local recurrence in adult soft-tissue sarcoma. Arch Surg 1987;122:1289–1293.
321. Habrand JL, Gerbaulet A, Pejovic MH, et al. Twenty years experience of interstitial iridium brachytherapy in the management of soft tissue sarcomas. Int J Radiat Oncol Biol Phys 1991;20:405–411.
322. Gemer LS, Trowbridge DR, Neff J, et al. Local recurrence of soft tissue sarcoma following brachytherapy. Int J Radiat Oncol Biol Phys 1991;20:587–592.
323. Giuliano AE, Eilber FR. The rationale for planned reoperation after unplanned total excision of soft-tissue sarcomas. J Clin Oncol 1985;3:1344–1348.
324. Tepper JE, Rosenberg SA, Glatstein E. Radiation therapy technique in soft tissue sarcomas of the extremity—policies at the National Cancer Institute. Int J Radiat Oncol Biol Phys 1982;8:263–273.
325. Fraass BA, Tepper JE, Glatstein E, et al. Clinical use of a match-line wedge for adjacent megavoltage radiation field matching. Int J Radiat Oncol Biol Phys 1983;9:209–216.
326. Kinsella TJ, Loefler JS, Fraass BA, et al. Extremity preservation by combined modality therapy in sarcomas of the hand and foot: An analysis of local control, disease-free survival and function result. Int J Radiat Oncol Biol Phys 1983;9:1115–1119.
327. Eilber FR, Guiliano AE, Huth J, et al. Limb salvage for high grade soft tissue sarcomas of the extremity: Experience at The University of California, Los Angeles. Cancer Treat Symp 1985;3:49–57.
328. Denton JW, Dunham WK, Salter M, et al. Preoperative regional chemotherapy and rapid-fraction irradiation for sarcomas of the soft tissue and bone. Surg Gynecol Obstet 1984;158:545–551.
329. Lokich JJ. Preoperative chemotherapy in soft tissue sarcoma. Surg Gynecol Obstet 1979;148:512–516.
330. Stehlin JS, de Ipolyi PD, Giovanella BC, et al. Soft tissue sarcomas of the extremity. Multidisciplinary therapy employing hyperthermic perfusion. Am J Surg 1975;130: 643–646.
331. Krementz ET, Carter RD, Sutherland CM, et al. Chemotherapy of sarcomas of the limbs by regional perfusion. Ann Surg 1977;185:555–564.
332. Karakousis CP, Lopez R, Catane R, et al. Intraarterial Adriamycin in the treatment of soft tissue sarcomas. J Surg Oncol 1980;13:21–27.
333. Didolkar MS, Kanter PM, Baffi RR, et al. Comparison of regional versus systemic chemotherapy with Adriamycin. Ann Surg 1978;187:332–336.
334. Salinas R, Hussey DH, Fletcher GH, et al. Experience with fast neutron therapy for locally advanced sarcomas. Int J Radiat Oncol Biol Phys 1980;6:267–272.
335. Pelton JG, Del Rowe JD, Bolen JW, et al. Fast neutron radiotherapy for soft tissue sarcomas: University of Washington experience and review of the world's literature. Am J Clin Oncol 1986;9:397–400.
336. Willet CG, Suit HD, Tepper JE, et al. Intraoperative electron beam radiation therapy for sarcoma of retroperitoneal soft tissue sarcoma. Cancer 1991;68:278–283.
337. Kinsella TJ, Glatstein E. Clinical experience with intravenous radiosensitizers in unresectable sarcomas. Cancer 1987;59:908–915.
338. Rosenberg SA, Tepper J, Glatstein E, et al. Prospective randomized evaluation of adjuvant chemotherapy in adults with soft tissue sarcomas of the extremities. Cancer 1983;52: 424–434.
339. Rosenberg SA. Prospective randomized trials demonstrating the efficacy of adjuvant chemotherapy in adult patients with soft tissue sarcomas. Cancer Treat Rep 1984;68: 1067–1078.
340. Rosenberg SA, Chang AE, Glatstein E. Adjuvant chemotherapy for treatment of extremity soft tissue sarcomas: Review of National Cancer Institute experience. Cancer Treat Symp 1985;3:83–88.
341. Antman K, Suit H, Amato D, et al. Preliminary results of a randomized trial of adjuvant doxorubicin for sarcomas: Lack of apparent difference between treatment groups. J Clin Oncol 1984;2:601–608.
342. Edmonson JH, Felming TR, Ivins JC, et al. Randomized study of systemic chemotherapy following complete excision of nonosseous sarcomas. J Clin Oncol 1984;2:1390–1396.
343. Baker LH. Adjuvant therapy for soft tissue sarcomas. In: Ryan JR, Baker LO, eds. Recent concepts in sarcoma treatment. Dordrecht: Kluwer Academic Publishers, 1988.
344. Antman K, Amato D, Lerner H, et al. Adjuvant doxorubicin for sarcoma: Data from The Eastern Cooperative Oncology Group and Dana-Farber Cancer Institute/Massachusetts General Hospital studies. Cancer Treat Symp 1985;3:109–115.
345. Picci P, Bacci G, Gherlinzoni F, et al. Results of a randomized trial for the treatment of localized soft tissue tumors of the extremities in adult patients. In: Ryan JR, Baker LO, eds. Recent concepts in sarcoma treatment. Dordrecht: Kluwer Academic Publishers, 1988.
346. Gherlinzoni F, Bacci G, Picci P, et al. A randomized trial for the treatment of high-grade soft-tissue sarcomas of the extremities: Preliminary observations. J Clin Oncol 1986;4:552–558.
347. Eilber FR, Giuliano AE, Huth JF, et al. Adjuvant Adriamycin in high-grade extremity soft-tissue sarcoma—a randomized prospective trial. Proc Am Soc Clin Oncol 1986;5: 125.
348. Lerner HJ, Amato DA, Savlov ED, et al. Eastern Cooperative Oncology Group: A comparison of adjuvant doxorubicin and observation for patients with localized soft tissue sarcoma. J Clin Oncol 1987;5:613–617.
349. Alvegard TA, Sigurdsson H, Mouridsen H, et al. Adjuvant chemotherapy with doxorubicin

for high-grade soft tissue sarcoma: A randomized trial of the Scandinavian Sarcoma Group. J Clin Oncol 1989;7:1504–1513.

350. Antman K, Ryan L, Borden E, et al. Pooled result from three randomized adjuvant studies of doxorubicin versus observation in soft tissue sarcoma: 10-year results and review of the literature. In: Salmon SE, eds. Adjuvant therapy of cancer. Vol VI. Philadelphia: WB Saunders, 1990.
351. Benjamin TO, Terjanian TO, Fenoglio CJ, et al. The importance of combination chemotherapy for adjuvant treatment of high-risk patients with soft-tissue sarcomas of the extremities. In: Salmon SE, ed. Adjuvant therapy of cancer. Vol VI. Philadelphia: WB Saunders, 1990.
352. Eilber FR, Giuliano AE, Huth JF, et al. Postoperative adjuvant chemotherapy (Adriamycin) in high-grade extremity soft tissue sarcomas—a randomized prospective trial. In: Salmon SE, ed. Adjuvant therapy of cancer. Vol V. Orlando: Grune & Stratton, 1987.
353. Omura GA, Major FJ, Blessing JA, et al. A randomized clinical trial of adjuvant Adriamycin in uterine sarcomas: A Gynecologic Oncology Group study. J Clin Oncol 1985;3: 1240–1245.
354. Yang JC. Unpublished data.
355. Chang AE, Kinsella T, Glatstein E, et al. Adjuvant chemotherapy for patients with high-grade soft-tissue sarcomas of the extremities. J Clin Oncol 1988;6:1491–1500.
356. Dresdale A, Bonow RO, Wesley R, et al. Prospective evaluation of doxorubicin-induced cardiomyopathy resulting from postsurgical adjuvant treatment of patients with soft tissue sarcomas. Cancer 1983;52:51–60.
357. Ettinghausen SE, Bonow RO, Palmeri ST, et al. Prospective study of cardiomyopathy induced by adjuvant doxorubicin therapy in patients with soft-tissue sarcomas. Arch Surg 1986;121:1445–1451.
358. Giuliano AE, Eilber FR, Morton DL. The management of locally recurrent soft-tissue sarcoma. Ann Surg 1982;196:87–91.
359. Roth JA, Putnam JB, Wesley MN, et al. Differing determinants of prognosis following resection of pulmonary metastases from osteogenic and soft tissue sarcoma patients. Cancer 1985;55:1361–1366.
360. Jablons D, Steinberg SM, Roth J, et al. Metastasectomy for soft tissue sarcoma; Further evidence for efficacy and prognostic factors. J Thorac Cardiovasc Surg 1989;97:695–705.
361. Rizzoni WE, Pass HI, Wesley MN, et al. Resection of recurrent pulmonary metastases in patients with soft-tissue sarcomas. Arch Surg 1986;121:1248–1252.
362. Pass HI, Dwyer A, Makuch R, et al. Detection of pulmonary metastases in patients with osteogenic and soft-tissue sarcomas: The superiority of CT scans compared with conventional linear tomograms using dynamic analysis. J Clin Oncol 1985;3:1261–1265.
363. Blum RH. An overview of studies of Adriamycin (NSC-123127) in the United States. Cancer Chemother Rep 1975;6:247–251.
364. O'Bryan RM, Luce JK, Talley RW, et al. Phase II evaluation of Adriamycin in human neoplasia. Cancer 1973;32:1–8.
365. O'Bryan RM, Baker LH, Gottlieb JE, et al. Dose response evaluation of Adriamycin in human neoplasia. Cancer 1977;39:1940–1948.
366. Schoenfeld D, Rosenbaum C, Horton J, et al. A comparison of Adriamycin versus vincristine and Adriamycin and cyclophosphamide for advanced sarcoma. Cancer 1982;50:2757–2762.
367. Borden EC, Amato D, Enterline HT, et al. Randomized comparison of Adriamycin regimens for treatment of metastatic soft tissue sarcomas. J Clin Oncol 1987;5:840–850.
368. Cruz AB Jr, Thames EA Jr, Aust JB, et al. Combination chemotherapy for soft tissue sarcomas: A phase III study. J Surg Oncol 1979;11:313–323.
369. Rosen G, Caparros B, Nirenberg A, et al. High-dose methotrexate (HDMTX) with citrovorum factor rescue (CFR) in the treatment of radiation-induced sarcomas. Proc Am Assoc Clin Radiol 1981;1983:194.
370. Vaughn C, McKelvey E, Balcerzak S, et al. High-dose methotrexate with leucovorin rescue plus vincristine in advanced sarcoma: A Southwest Oncology Group study. Cancer Treat Rep 1984;68:409–410.
371. Isacoff WH, Eilber F, Tabbarah H, et al. Phase II clinical trial with high-dose methotrexate therapy and citrovorum factor rescue. Cancer Treat Rep 1978;62:1295–1304.
372. Karakousis CP, Rao U, Carlson M. High-dose methotrexate as secondary chemotherapy in metastatic soft-tissue sarcomas. Cancer 1980;46:1345–1348.
373. Von Hoff DD, Rozencweig M, Louie AC, et al. "Single"-agent activity of high-dose methotrexate therapy with citrovorum factor rescue. Cancer Treat Rep 1978;62:233–235.
374. Frie E, Blum R, Pitman S, et al. High-dose methotrexate with leucovorin rescue: Rationale and spectrum of antitumor activity. Am J Med 1979;68:370–375.
375. Andrews N, Wilson W. Phase II study of methotrexate (NSC 740) in solid tumors. Cancer Chemother Rep 1967;51:471–474.
376. Subramanian S, Wiltshaw E. Chemotherapy of sarcoma—a comparison of three regimes. Lancet 1978;1:683–686.
377. Buesa JM, Mouridsen HT, Santoro A. Treatment of advanced soft tissue sarcomas with low-dose methotrexate: A phase II trial by the European Organization for Research on Treatment of Cancer (EORTC) Soft Tissue and Bone Sarcoma Group. Cancer Treat Rep 1984;68:683–694.
378. Amato DA, Borden EC, Shiraki M, et al. Evaluation of bleomycin, chlorozotocin, MGBG, and bruceantin in patients with advanced soft tissue sarcoma, bone sarcoma, or mesothelioma. Invest New Drugs 1985;3:397–401.
379. Golbey R, Li MC, Kaufman RF. Actinomycin in the treatment of soft part sarcomas. [Abstract] James Ewing Society Scientific Program, 1968.
380. Gold G, Hall T, Shnider B, et al. A clinical study of 5-fluorouracil. Cancer 1959;19: 935–939.
381. Selawry OS, Holland JF, Wolman IJ. Effect of vincristine (NSC-67574) on malignant solid tumors in children. Cancer Chemother Rep 1968;52:497–499.
382. Korbitzs BC, Davis HL Jr, Ramirez G, et al. Low doses of vincristine (NSC-67574) for malignant disease. Cancer Chemother Rep 1969;53:249–254.
383. Radice PA, Bunn PA Jr, Ihde DC. Therapeutic trials with VP-16 and VM-26. Cancer Treat Rep 1979;63:1231–1239.
384. Bleyer WA, Chard RL, Krivit W, et al. Epipodophyllotoxin therapy of childhood neoplasia. A comparative phase II analysis of VM26 and VP16-213. Proc Am Assoc Clin Radiol 1978;19:373.
385. Elias AD, Eder JP, Shea T, Begg CB, Frei III E, Antman KH. High dose ifosfamide with mesna uroprotection: A phase I study. J Clin Oncol 1990;8:170–178.
386. Elias AD, Ayash LJ, Eder JP, et al. A phase I study of high-dose ifosfamide and escalating doses of carboplatin with autologous bone marrow support. J Clin Oncol 1991;9:320–327.
387. Klein HO, Wickramanayake PD, Coerper CL, Christian E, Pohl J, Brock N. High-dose ifosfamide and mesna as continuous infusion over five days-a phase I/II trial. Cancer Treat Rev 1983;10(suppl A):167–173.
388. Chawla SP, Rosen G, Lowenbraun S, Morton D, Eilber F. Role of high dose ifosfamide (HDI) in recurrent osteosarcoma. Proc Am Soc Clin Oncol 1990;9:310.
389. Czownicki Z, Utracka-Hutka B. Clinical studies with uromitexan-an antidote against urotoxicity of holoxan. Preliminary results. Nowotwory(Pol) 1981;30:377–383.
390. Niederle N, Scheulen ME, Cremer M, Schutte J, Schmidt CG, Seeber S. Ifosfamide in combination chemotherapy for sarcomas and testicular carcinomas. Cancer Treat Rev 1983;10(suppl A):129–135.
391. Antman KH, Ryan L, Elias A, Sherman D, Grier E. Response to ifosfamide and mesna: 124 previously treated patients with metastatic or unresectable sarcoma. J Clin Oncol 1989;7:126–131.
392. Stuart-Harris R, Harper PG, Kaye SB, Wiltshaw E. High-dose ifosfamide by infusion with mesna in advanced soft tissue sarcoma. Cancer Treat Rev 1983;10(suppl A): 163–164.
393. Bramwell V, Mouridsen HT, Santoro A, et al. Cyclophosphamide vs ifosfamide: Final report of a randomized phase II trial in adult soft tissue sarcoma. Eur J Cancer Clin Oncol 1987;23:311–321.
394. Buesa JM, Mouridsen HT, Oosterom ATV, et al. High-dose DTIC in advanced soft-tissue sarcomas in the adult. A phase II study of the EORTC soft tissue and bone sarcoma group. Ann Oncol 1991;2:307–309.
395. Bramwell VHC, Brugarols A, Mouridsen HT, et al. EORTC. Phase II study of cisplatinum in CYVADIC-resistant soft tissue sarcoma. Eur J Cancer 1979;15:1511–1513.
396. Karakousis CP, Holterman OA, Holyoke E. Cisdichlorodiamineplatinum (II) in metastatic soft tissue sarcomas. Cancer Treat Rep 1979;63:2071–2075.
397. Samson MK, Baker LH, Benjamin RS, Lane M, Plager C. Cisdichlorodiamineplatinum (II) in advanced soft tissue and bony sarcomas. A Southwest Oncology Group study. Cancer Treat Rep 1979;63:2027–2028.
398. Thigpen JT, Blessing JA, Wilbanks GD. Cisplatin as second-line chemotherapy in the treatment of advanced or recurrent leiomyosarcoma of the uterus. Am J Clin Oncol 1986;9:18–20.
399. Budd GT, Metch B, Balcerzak SP, Fletcher WS, Baker LH, Mortimer JE. High-dose cisplatin for metastatic soft tissue sarcoma. Cancer 1990;65:866–869.
400. Gershenson DM, Kavanagh JJ, Copeland LJ, Edwards CL, Stringer CA, Wharton JT. Cisplatin therapy for disseminated mixed mesodermal sarcoma of the uterus. J Clin Oncol 1987;5:618–621.
401. Goldstein D, Cheuvart B, Trump DL, et al. Phase II trial of carboplatin in soft-tissue sarcoma. Am J Clin Oncol 1990;13:420–423.
402. Bergsagel DE, Levin WC. A prelusive clinical trial of cyclophosphamide. Cancer Chemother Rep 1960;8:120–134.
403. Korst DR, Johnson D, Frenkel EP, Challener WL III. Preliminary evaluation of the effect of cyclophosphamide on the course of human neoplasms. Cancer Chemother Rep 1960;7:1–12.
404. Pinedo HM, Branwell VHC, Mouridson MD, et al. CYVADIC in advanced soft tissue sarcoma: A randomized study comparing two schedules. A study of the EORTC Soft Tissue and Bone Sarcoma Group. Cancer 1984;53:1825–1832.
405. Legha S, Benjamin RS, Mackay B, et al. Reduction of doxorubicin cardiotoxicity by prolonged continuous intravenous infusion. Ann Intern Med 1982;96:133–139.
406. Benjamin R, Yap B, Frazier O Jr, et al. Combination chemotherapy for sarcomas with cyclophosphamide and continuous infusion Adriamycin and dacarbazine (CI-CYA-DIC) with surgical intensification. Proc Am Assoc Clin Radiol Am Soc Clin Oncol [Abstract] 1981;22:526.
407. Baker LK, Green S, Ryan J, et al. Combined modality therapy for disseminated soft tissue sarcoma, phase III. Proc Am Soc Clin Oncol 1987;6:138.
408. Brennan MF, Friedrich C, Almadrones L, et al. Prospective randomized trial examining the cardiac toxicity of adjuvant doxorubicin in high grade extremity sarcomas. In: Sydney Salmon, ed. Adjuvant therapy of cancer V. Orlando: Grune & Stratton, 1987: 745–754.
409. Brock N. Pharmacological studies with ifosfamide—a new oxazaphosphorine compound. In: Semonsky M, Hejzler M, Masak S, eds. Advances in antimicrobial and antineoplastic chemotherapy. Proceedings of the Seventh International Congress of Chemotherapy, Prague, 1971. Berlin: Urban & Schwarzenberg, 1972:2:749–756.
410. Cabanillas F, Hagemeister FB, Bodey GP, Freireich EJ. IMVP-16: An effective regimen for patients with lymphoma who have relapsed after initial combination chemotherapy. Blood 1982;60:693–697.
411. Antman KH, Montella D, Rosenbaum C, Schwen M. Phase II trial of ifosfamide with mesna in previously treated metastatic sarcoma. Cancer Treat Rep 1985;69:499–502.
412. Morgan LR, Posey LE, Rainey J, et al. Ifosfamide: A weekly dose fractionated schedule in bronchogenic carcinoma. Cancer Treat Rep 1981;65:693–695.

413. Czownicki Z, Utracka-Hutka B. Contributions to the treatment of malignant tumors with ifosfamide. In: Burkeret H, Voight HC, eds. Proceedings of the International Holoxan Symposium. Dusseldorf: Asta-Werke, 1977:109–111.
414. De Kraker J, Voute PA. Ifosfamide and vincristine in pediatric tumors. A phase II study. Eur Paediatr Haematol Oncol 1984;1:47–50.
415. Magrath I, Sandlund J, Raynor A, Rosenberg S, Arasi V, Miser J. A phase II study of ifosfamide in the treatment of recurrent sarcomas in young people. Cancer Chemother Pharmacol 1986;18(suppl 2):S25–S28.
416. Legha S, Papadopoulos N, Plager C, et al. A comparative evaluation of the uroprotective effect of mercaptoethane sulfonate (mesna) and *N*-acetylcysteine in sarcoma patients treated with ifosfamide. Proc Am Soc Clin Oncol [Abstract] 1990;9:1205.
417. Perevodchikova NI, Lichinister MR, Gorbunova VA. Phase II clinical study of carminomycin: Its activity against soft tissue sarcomas. Cancer Treat Rep 1977;61:1705–1707.
418. Weiss AJ, Ramirez G, Grage T, Strawitz J, Goldman L, Downing V. Phase II study of azotomycin (NSC-56654). Cancer Chemother Rep 1968;52:611–614.
419. Chang P, Wiernik PHP. Phase II study of azotomycin in sarcomas. Cancer Treat Rep 1979;61:1719.
420. De Jager R, Body JJ, Dupong D, Klastersky J, Kenis Y. Phase I study of oral 4′-(9-acrindylamino-methanseulfonanidide) m-AMSA (C-574). Proc Am Soc Clin Oncol 1979;20:429.
421. Legha SS, Gutterman JU, Hall SW, et al. Phase I clinical investigation of 4′-(9-acridinylamino) methanesulfon-manisiside (NSC 249992), a new acridine derivative. Cancer Res 1978;38:3712–3716.
422. Von Hoff DD, Howser D, Gormley P, et al. Phase I study of methanesulfonamide, *N*-(4–9-acridinylamino)-3-methoxyphenyl-m-AMSA using a single-dose schedule. Cancer Treat Rep 1978;62:1421–1426.
423. Schneider R, Sklanoff R, Ochoa M. Phase I trial of AMSA (4′-acrindylamino)-methansulfon-manisidide). Proc Am Assoc Cancer Res 1979;20:114.
424. Bertrand M, Multhauf P, Bartolucci A, Ellison D, Gockerman J. Phase II study of aclarubicin in previously untreated patients with advanced soft tissue sarcoma. Cancer Treat Rep 1985;69:725–726.
425. Zidar B, Baker L, Rivkin S, Balcerzak SP, Stephens RL. A phase II study of diaziquone in advanced soft tissue and bony sarcoma. A Southwest Oncology Group Study. Cancer Treat Rep 1985;69:1035–1036.
426. Chan C, Bartolucci A, Brenner D, et al. Phase II trial of diaziquone in anthracycline-resistant adult soft tissue bone sarcoma patients: A Southeastern Cancer Study Group trial. Cancer Teat Rep 1986;70:427–428.
427. Slayton RE, Blessing JA, Clarke-Pearson D. A Phase II trials of Diaziquone (AZQ) in mixed mesodermal sarcomas uterus. A gynecologic oncology group study. Invest New Drugs 1991;9:93–94.
428. Presant C, Gams R, Bartolucci A. Treatment of metastatic sarcomas with mitroxantrone. Cancer Treat Rep 1984;68:813–814.
429. Bull FE, Von Hoff DD, Balcerzak SP, Stephens RL, Panettiere FJ. Phase II trial of mitoxantrone in advanced sarcomas. A Southwest Oncology Group study. Cancer Treat Rep 1985;69:231–233.
430. Buckner JC, Edmonson JH, Ingle JN, Schaid DJ. Evaluation of menogaril in patients with metastatic sarcomas and no prior chemotherapy exposure. Am J Clin Oncol 1989;12:384–386.
431. Giaccone G, Donadio M, Calciati A. Phase II study of esorubicin in the treatment of patients with advanced sarcoma. Oncology 1989;46:285–287.
432. Chevallier B, Montcuquet P, Fachini T, et al. Phase II study of epirubicin in advanced soft tissue sarcoma. Bull Cancer 1990;77:991–995.
433. Taylor SA, Metch B, Balcerzak SP, Hanson KH. Phase II trial of Echinomycin in advanced soft tissue sarcomas. A Southwest Oncology Group study. Invest New Drugs 1990;8: 381–383.
434. Quirt I, Eisenhauer E, Knowling M, et al. A phase 2 study of trimetrexate in metastatic soft tissue sarcoma. Proc Am Soc Clin Oncol 1988;7:275.
435. Licht JD, Gonin R, Antman KH. Phase II trial of trimetrexate in patients with advanced soft tissue sarcoma. Cancer Chemother Pharmacol 1991;28:223–225.
436. Johnson R. Preliminary phase II trials with 1-aminocyclopentane carboxylic acid (NSC-1026) (cycloleucine). Cancer Chemother Rep 1963;32:67–71.
437. Aust J, Andrews N, Shcroeder J, Lawton RL. Phase II study of 1-aminocyclopentane-carboxylic acid (NSC 1026) in patients with cancer. Cancer Chemother Rep 1970;54: 237–241.
438. Savlov ED, MacIntyre JM, Knight E, Woller J. Comparison of doxorubicin with cycloleucine in the treatment of sarcomas. Cancer Treat Rep 1981;65:21–27.
439. Amato DA, Borden EC, Shiraki M, et al. Evaluation of bleomycin, chlorozotocin, MGBG, and bruceantin in patients with advanced soft tissue sarcoma, bone sarcoma, or mesothelioma. Invest New Drugs 1985;3:397–401.
440. Mouridsen HT, Bramwell VH, Lacave J, et al. Treatment of advanced soft tissue sarcomas with chlorozotocin: A phase II trial of the EORTC soft tissue and bone sarcoma group. Cancer Treat Rep 1981;65:509–511.
441. Kovach JS, Moertel CG, Schutt AF. A phase I study of chlorozotocin (NSC 178248). Cancer 1979;43:2189–2196.
442. Gralla RJ, Tan CTC, Young CW. Phase I trial of chlorozotocin. Cancer Treat Rep 1979;63:17–20.
443. Presant CA, Bartolucci AA. Phase II evaluation of chlorozotocin in metastatic sarcomas. Med Pediatr Oncol 1984;12:25–27.
444. Sordillo PP, Magill GB, Gralla RJ. Chlorozotocin: Phase II evaluation in patients with advanced sarcomas. Cancer Treat Rep 1981;65:513–514.
445. Talley RW, Samson MK, Brownlee RW, Samhouri AM, Fraile RJ, Baker LH. Phase II evaluation of chlorozotocin in advanced human cancers. Eur J Cancer 1981;17:337–343.
446. Baker LH, Samson MK, Izbicki RM. Phase I and II evaluation of cytembena in disseminated epithelial ovarian cancer and sarcomas. Cancer Treat Rep 1976;60:1389–1391.
447. Matejovsky Z. Effects of cytembena in the treatment of malignant musculoskeletal tumors. Neoplasma 1971;18:473–480.
448. Kurzrock R, Yap BS, Plager C, et al. Phase II evaluation of PALA in patients with refractory metastatic sarcomas. Am J Clin Oncol 1984;7:305–307.
449. Presant CA, Ardalan B, Multhauf P. Continuous five-day infusion of PALA and 5-FU. A pilot phase II trial. Med Pediatr Oncol 1983;11:162–163.
450. Baselga J, Magill GB, Curley T, Casper ES. Phase II trial of pala + dipyridamole in patients with metastatic soft tissue sarcoma. Proc Am Assoc Cancer Res [Abstract] 1990;31:1187.
451. Casper ES, Baselga J, Smart TB, Magill GB, Markman M, Ranhosky A. A phase II trial of PALA + dipyridamole in patients with advanced soft-tissue sarcoma. Cancer Chemother Pharmacol 1991;28:51–54.
452. Rodriquez V, Gottlieb J, Burgess MA, et al. Phase I studies with Baker's antifol (NSC 139105). Cancer 1976;38:690–694.
453. Thigpen JT, O'Bryan RM, Benjamin RS, Coltman CA Jr. Phase II trial of Baker's antifol in metastatic sarcoma. Cancer Treat Rep 1977;61:1485–1487.
454. Tranum BP, Haut A, Rivkin SE, et al. A phase II study of methyl-CCNU in the treatment of solid tumors and lymphomas in the Southwest Oncology Group. Cancer 1974;35: 1148–1153.
455. Creagan ET, Hahn JH, Ahmann DL, Edmonson JH, Bisel HF, Eagan RT. A comparative clinical trial evaluating the combination of actinomycin D, cyclophosphamide, and vincristine, and a single agent, methyl-CCNU, in advanced sarcomas. Cancer Treat Rep 1976;60:1385–1386.
456. Borden EC, Larson P, Ansfield FJ, et al. Hexamethylmelamine: Treatment of sarcomas and lymphomas. Med Pediatr Oncol 1977;3:401–406.
457. Blum RH, Livingston RB, Carter SK. Hexamethylmelamine: A new drug with activity in solid tumors. Eur J Cancer 1973;9:195–202.
458. Sooriyaarachchi GS, Ramirez G, Roley EL. Hemangiopericytoma of the uterus. J Surg Oncol 1978;10:399–406.
459. Conroy JF, Roda PI, Prasavinichai S. Dibromodulcitol in the treatment of metastic hemangiopericytoma. Am J Clin Oncol 1982;5:453–456.
460. Borden EC, Ash A, Enterline HT, et al. Phase II evaluation of dibromodulcitol, ICRF-159, and maytansine for sarcomas. Am J Clin Oncol 1982;5:417–420.
461. Kimball JC, Cangir A. A phase II trial of dianhydrogalactitol in advanced soft tissue and bony sarcomas, a Southwest Oncology Group Study. Cancer Treat Rep 1979;63: 553–554.
462. Saiki J, Stephens R, Fabian C, Kraut E, Fletcher W. Phase II evaluation of gallium nitrate (NSC-15200) in soft tissue and bone sarcomas. Proc Am Assoc Cancer Res 1981;22:525.
463. Bleyer WA, Krivit W, Chard RL, Hammond D. Phase II study of VM-26 in acute leukemia, neuroblastoma, and other refractory childhood malignancies: A report from the Children's Cancer Study Group. Cancer Treat Rep 1979;63:977–981.
464. Currie VE, Wong PP, Krakoff IH, Young CW. Phase I trial of vindesine in patients with advanced cancer. Cancer Treat Rep 1978;62:1333–1336.
465. Rossof AH, Chandra G, Walter J, et al. Phase II trial of vindesine (desacetyl vinblastine amide sulfate) in advanced metastatic cancer. Proc Am Assoc Cancer Res 1979;20: 146.
466. Alberto P, De Jager RL, Brugarlas A, Hansen H, Cavalli F, Host H. Phase II study of diamino-dichlorophenyl-methylpyrimidine with folinic acid protection and rescue. Proc Am Assoc Cancer Res 1979;20:323.
467. Benjamin RS, Keating MJ, Valdivieso M, et al. Phase I–II study of piperazinedione in adults with solid tumors and acute leukemia. Cancer Treat Rep 1979;63:939–943.
468. LaGasse L, Thigpen T, Morrison F. Phase II trial of piperazinedione in treatment of advanced endometrial carcinoma, uterine sarcoma, and vulvar carcinoma. Proc Am Soc Clin Oncol 1979;20:388.
469. Thigpen T, Blessing JA, Homesley HD, Hacker N, Curry SL. Phase II trial of piperazinedione in treatment of advanced or recurrent uterine sarcoma, a GOG study. Am J Clin Oncol 1985;8:350–352.
470. Sordillo PP, Magill GB. Phase II evaluation of pyrazofurin in patients with soft-tissue sarcomas. Am J Clin Oncol 1985;8:316–318.
471. Salem PA, Bodey GP, Burgess MA, Murphy WK, Freireich EJ. A phase I study of pyrazofurin. Cancer 1977;40:2806–2809.
472. Gralla RJ, Sordillo PP, Magill GB. Phase II evaluation of pyrazofurin in patients with metastatic sarcoma. Cancer Treat Rep 1978;62:1573.
473. Blum R, Kahlert T. Maytansine: A phase I study of an ansamacrolide with antitumor activity. Cancer Treat Rep 1978;62:435–438.
474. Ajani JA, Dimery I, Chawla SP, et al. Phase II studies of homoharringtonine in patients with advanced malignant melanoma; sarcoma; and head and neck, breast, and colorectal carcinomas. Cancer Treat Rep 1986;70:375–379.
475. Rinehart J, Balcerzak SP, Hersh E. Phase II trial of tumor necrosis factor in human sarcoma: A Southwest Oncology Group study. Proc Am Soc Clin Oncol [Abstract] 1990;9: 1229.
476. Robertson PA, Ross HJ, Figlin RA. Tumor necrosis factor induces hemorrhagic necrosis of a sarcoma. Ann Intern Med 1989;111:682–684.
477. Schuff-Werner P, Bartsch H, Schreml W, Nagel GA. Treatment of soft tissue sarcoma with recombinant alpha-interferon. Antiviral Res [Abstract 1] 1984;3:93.
478. Harris JE, Das Gupta T, Vogelzang M, et al. Treatment of soft tissue sarcoma with fibroblast interferon—an American Cancer Society/Illinois Cancer Council study. Cancer Treat Rep 1986;70:293–294.
479. Rosenberg SA, Lotze MT, Muul LM, et al. A progress report on the treatment of 157 patients with advanced cancer using lymphokine-activated killer cells and interleukin-2 or high-dose interleukin-2 alone. N Engl J Med 1987;316:890–897.

480. Omura GA, Major FJ, Blessing JA, et al. A randomized study of Adriamycin with and without dimethyl trazenoimidazole carboxamide in advanced uterine sarcomas. Cancer 1983;52:626–632.
481. Lerner H, Amato D, Stevens C, Borden E, Enterline H. Leiomyosarcoma: The Eastern Cooperative Oncology Group experience with 222 patients. Proc Am Assoc Cancer Res [Abstract C-561] 1983;24:142.
482. Benjamin RS, Gottlieb JA, Baker LH. CYVADIC vs CYVADACT—a randomized trial of cyclophosphamide, vincristine and Adriamycin, plus either dacarbazine or actinomycin D in metastatic sarcomas. Proc Am Assoc Cancer Res 1976;17:256.
483. Baker LH, Frank J, Fine G, et al. Combination chemotherapy using Adriamycin, DTIC, cyclophosphamide, and actinomycin D for advanced soft tissue sarcomas: A randomized comparative trial. J Clin Onc 1987;5:851–861.
484. Muss HB, Bundy B, Di Saia PJ, et al. Treatment of recurrent advanced uterine sarcoma—a randomized trial of doxorubicin vs doxorubicin and cyclophosphamide. Cancer 1985;55:1648–1653.
485. Santoro A, Rouesse J, Steward W, et al. A randomized EORTC study in advanced soft tissue sarcomas (STS): ADM vs. ADM + IFX vs. CYVADIC. Proc Am Soc Clin Oncol [Abstract 1196] 1990;9:309.
486. Blum RH, Edmonson JH. Investigations of ifosphamide (IF) for adult soft tissue sarcomas in ECOG. Eur J Cancer 1991;27:S350.
487. Antman K, Baker L, Balcerzak S, Crowley J, for CALGB and SWOG. A randomized study of doxorubicin and dacarbazine ± ifosfamide and mesna in advanced sarcomas. Proc ECCO 1991.
488. Bodey GP, Rodriquez V, Murphy WK, Burgess A, Benjamin RS. Protected environment-prophylactic antibiotic program for malignant sarcoma: Randomized trial during remission induction chemotherapy. Cancer 1981;47:2422–2429.
489. Casper ES, Gaynor JJ, Hajdu SI, et al. A prospective randomized trial of adjuvant chemotherapy with bolus versus continuous infusion of doxorubicin in patients with high-grade extremity soft tissue sarcoma and an analysis of prognostic factors. Cancer 1991;68:1221–1229.
490. Zalupski M, Metch B, Balcerzak S, et al. Phase III comparison of doxorubicin and dacarbazine given by bolus versus infusion in patients with soft-tissue sarcomas: A Southwest Oncology Group study. JNCI 1991;83:926–932.
491. Borden EC, Amato DA, Edmonson JH, Ritch PS, Shiraki M. Randomized comparison of doxorubicin and vindesine to doxorubicin for patients with metastatic soft-tissue sarcomas. Cancer 1990;66:862–867.
492. Gottlieb JA, Baker LH, Quagliana JM, et al. Chemotherapy of sarcomas with a combination of Adriamycin and dimethyltrazeno-carboxamide. Cancer 1972;30:1632–1638.
493. Saiki J, Baker LH, Rivkin SE, et al. A useful high-dose intermittent schedule of Adriamycin and DTIC in the treatment of advanced sarcomas. Cancer 1986;58:2196–2197.
494. Weh HJ, Zugel M, Wingberg D, et al. Chemotherapy of metastatic soft tissue sarcoma with a combination of Adriamycin and DTIC or Adriamycin and ifosfamide. Onkologie 1990;13:448–452.
495. Blum R, Corson J, Wilson R, et al.: Successful treatment of metastatic sarcomas with cyclophosphamide, Adriamycin and DTIC. Cancer 1980;46:1722–1726.
496. Hamdan H, Savage P, Skubitz K. A pilot study of continuous infusion chemotherapy for soft tissue sarcomas. Proc Am Soc Clin Oncol 1990;9:316.
497. Ikeda K, Ogawa M, Inagaki J, et al. A combination chemotherapy with Adriamycin, cyclophosphamide and DTIC (ACD) for advanced adult soft part sarcoma. Gan To Kagaku Ryoho 1984;11:235–239.
498. Gottlieb JA, Baker LH, O'Brian RM, et al. Adriamycin (NSC 123127) used alone and in combination for soft tissue and bony sarcomas. Cancer Chemother Rep 1975;6: 271–282.
499. Yap B, Baker LH, Sinkovics JG, et al. Cyclophosphamide, vincristine, Adriamycin, and DTIC (CYVADIC) combination chemotherapy for the treatment of advanced sarcomas. Cancer Treat Rep 1980;64:93–98.
500. Yap BS, Sinkovics JG, Benjamin RS, et al. Survival and relapse patterns of complete responders in adults with advanced soft tissue sarcomas. Proc Am Soc Clin Oncol [Abstract] 1979;20:352.
501. Bui NB, Chauvergne J, Hocke C, et al. Analysis of a series of sixty soft tissue sarcomas in adults treated with a cyclophosphamide-vincristine-Adriamycin-dacarbazine (CY-VADIC) combination. Cancer Chemother Pharmacol 1985;15:82–85.
502. Pfeffer MR, Sulkes A, Biran S. Treatment of advanced soft tissue sarcomas with a modified CYVADIC protocol. Oncology 1984;41:308–313.
503. Choi TK, NG A, Wong J. Doxorubicin, dacarbazine, vincristine, and cyclophosphamide in the treatment of advanced gastrointestinal leiomyosarcoma. Cancer Treat Rep 1985;69:443–444.
504. Lopez M, Di Lauro L, Papaldo P, et al. Alternating combination chemotherapy of advanced soft tissue sarcomas in adults. Am J Clin Oncol 1984;7:539–542.
505. Rivkin SE, Gottlieb JA, Thigpen T, et al. Methyl-CCNU and Adriamycin for patients with metastatic sarcomas. A Southwest Oncology Group study. Cancer 1980;46:446–451.
506. Chang P, Wiernik PH. Combination chemotherapy with Adriamycin and streptozotocin. Clin Pharmacol Ther 1976;20:606–610.
507. Lopez M, Carpano S, DiLauro L, Vici P, Conti EMS. Epirubicin and DTIC for advanced soft tissue sarcomas. Oncology 1991;48:230–233.
508. Casali P, Pastorino U, Zucchinelli, P, et al. Epidoxorubicin plus ifosfamide and decarbazine (EID) in advanced soft tissue sarcomas. Ann Oncology 1992;3(Suppl 2):S125–S126.
509. Jelic S, Vuletic L, Milanovic N, Tomasevic Z, Kovcin V. High-dose epirubicin-cisplatin chemotherapy for advanced soft tissue sarcoma. Tumori 1990;76:467–471.
510. Elli A, Botto G, Mendez A, et al. Ifosfamide plus epidoxorubicin for advanced soft tissue sarcomas. Preliminary report. Proc Am Soc Clin Oncol [Abstract 1227] 1990;9: 317.
511. Cantwell BM, Carmichael J, Ghani S, Harris AL. A phase II study of ifosfamide/mesna with doxorubicin for adult soft tissue sarcoma. Cancer Chemother Pharmacol 1988;21: 49–52.
512. Dombernowsky P, Mouridsen H, Schutte J, et al. Phase II study of ifosfamide + Adriamycin in advanced soft tissue sarcoma in adults. A preliminary analysis. Cancer Chemother Pharmacol 1986;18(suppl 2):S17.
513. Edmonson JH, Buckner JC, Long HJ, Loprinzi CL, Schaid DJ. Phase II study of ifosfamide-etoposide-mesna in adults with advanced nonosseous sarcomas. JNCI 1989;81:863–866.
514. Loehrer PS, Sledge GJ, Nicaise C, et al. Ifosfamide plus doxorubicin in metastatic adult sarcomas: A multi-institutional phase II trial. J Clin Oncol 1989;7:1655–1659.
515. Mansi JL, Fisher C, Wiltshaw E, MacMillan S, King M, Stuart-Harris R. A phase I–II study of ifosfamide in combination with Adriamycin in the treatment of adult soft tissue sarcoma. Eur J Cancer Clin Oncol 1988;24:1439–1443.
516. Schutte J, Mouridsen HT, Stewart W, et al. Ifosfamide plus doxorubicin in previously untreated patients with advanced soft tissue sarcoma. The EORTC soft tissue and bone sarcoma group. Eur J Cancer 1990;26:558–561.
517. Steward WP, Verweij J, Somers R, et al. Doxorubicin plus ifosfamide with rhGM-CSF in the treatment of advanced adult soft tissue sarcomas—preliminary results of a phase II study from the EORTC soft tissue and bone sarcoma group.
518. Wiltshaw E, Westbury G, Harmer C, McKinna A, Fisher C. Ifosfamide plus mesna with and without Adriamycin in soft tissue sarcoma. Cancer Chemother Pharmacol 1986;18(suppl 2):S10–S12.
519. Bramwell V, Quirt I, Warr D, et al. Combination chemotherapy with doxorubicin, dacarbazine, and ifosfamide in advanced adult soft tissue sarcoma. JNCI 1989;81: 1496–1499.
520. Elias A, Ryan L, Sulkes A, Collins J, Aisner J, Antman K. Response to mesna, doxorubicin, ifosfamide, and dacarbazine in 108 patients with metastatic or unresectable sarcoma and no prior chemotherapy. J Clin Oncol 1989;7:1208–1216.
521. Wellens W, Donhuijsen-Ant R, Habets L, et al. Therapie progredienter Sarkome mit Etoposid und Ifosfamide. Aktuel Onkol 1981;4:159–164.
522. Wellens W, Mussgnug G, Havets L, Schafer E, Westerhausen M. The combination ifosfamide/VP 16–213 in therapy of small cell bronchogenic carcinoma and other malignant tumors. In: Burkert H, Nagel G, eds. New experience with the oxazaphosphorines with special reference to the uroprotector uromitexan. Basel: Karger, 1980: 81–87.
523. Issels RD, Prenninger SW, Nagele A, et al. Ifosfamide plus etoposide combined with regional hyperthermia in patients with locally advanced sarcomas: A phase II study. J Clin Oncol 1990;8:1818–1829.
524. Hoffmann W, Weidmann B, Migeod F, Konner J, Seeber S. Epirubicin and ifosfamide in patients with refractory breast cancer and other metastatic solid tumours. Cancer Chemother Pharmacol 1990;26(suppl 1):S69–70.
525. Toma S, Palumbo R, Songo G, et al. Doxorubicin (or epidoxorubicin) combined with ifosfamide in the treatment of adult advanced soft tissue sarcomas. Ann Oncol 1992;3(Suppl 2):S119–S123.
526. Bierbaum W, Bremer K, Firusian N, High M, et al. Chemotherapeutische behandlungsmoglichkeiten bei forgeschrittenen sarkomen. Dtsch Med Wochenschr 1981;106: 1181–1185.
527. Budd GT, Metch B, Weiss S, et al. SWOG 8641: Ifosfamide and cisplatin in the treatment of metastatic soft tissue sarcoma. Proc Am Soc Clin Oncol [Abstract 1222] 1990;9: 316.
528. Hartlapp JH, Munch HJ, Illiger HJ, Wolter H, Jensen JC. Alternatives to CYVADIC combination therapy of soft tissue sarcomas. Cancer Chemother Pharmacol 1986;18(suppl 2):S20–S22.
529. Zamboglou N, Furst G, Pape H, Bannach B, Molls M, Schmitt G. [Results of whole lung irradiation and chemotherapy in comparison with partial lung irradiation in metastasizing, undifferentiated soft tissue sarcomas]. Strahlenther Onkol 1988;164:386–392.
530. Klippenstein TH, Mitrou PS, Kochendorfer KJ, Bergmann L. High-dose Adriamycin (ADM) and cisplatin (DDP) in advanced soft-tissue sarcomas and invasive thymomas: A pilot study. Cancer Chemother Pharmacol 1984;13:78–81.
531. Edmonson JH, Hahn RG, Schutt AJ, Bisel HF, Ingle JN. Cyclophosphamide, doxorubicin, and cisplatin combined in the treatment of advanced sarcomas. Med Pediatr Oncol 1983;11:319–321.
532. Cormier WJ, Hahn RG, Edmonson JH, Eagan RT. Phase II study in advanced sarcoma: Randomized trial of pyrazofurin versus combination cyclophosphamide, doxorubicin and dichlorodiammineplatinum (CAP). Cancer Treat Rep 1980;64:655.
533. Edmonson JH, Long HJ, Richardson RL, et al. Phase II study of a combination of mitomycin, doxorubicin and cisplatin in advanced sarcomas. Cancer Chemother Pharmacol 1985;15:181–182.
534. Jansen RLH, Van der Burg MEL, Verweij J, Stoter G. Cyclophosphamide, hexamethylmelamine, Adriamycin and cisplatin combination chemotherapy in mixed mesodermal sarcoma of the female genital tract. Eur J Cancer Clin Oncol 1987;23:1131–1133.
535. Piver MS, Shashikant BL, Patsner B. *Cis*-dichlorodiammineplatinum plus dimethyltriazenoimidazole carboxamide as second- and third-line chemotherapy for sarcomas of the female pelvis. Gynecol Oncol 1986;23:371–375.
536. Presgrave P, Woods RL, Tatteresall MH, et al. Combination chemotherapy of adult soft tissue sarcomas with a combination of doxorubicin and methotrexate. Cancer Treat Rep 1987;71:1087–1088.
537. Kaufman JH, Catane R, Douglass HO. Combined Adriamycin, vincristine, and methotrexate in advanced adult soft tissue sarcoma. NY State J Med 1977;77:742–743.
538. Shiu MH, Magill GB, Hopfan S. Recent trends in treatment of soft tissue sarcomas. In: Hajdu SI, ed. Philadelphia: Lea & Febiger, 1979:537–542.

539. Lynch G, Magill GB, Sordillo PP, et al. Combination chemotherapy of advanced sarcomas in adults with cyomad. Cancer 1982;50:1724–1727.
540. Presant CA, Lowenbraun S, Bartolucci AA, et al. Metastatic sarcomas: Chemotherapy with Adriamycin, cyclophosphamide, and methotrexate alternating with actinomycin D, DTIC, and vincristine. Cancer 1981;47:457–465.
541. Pfeffer MR, Sulkes A, Biran S. Cyclophosphamide, Adriamycin, DTIC and vincristine with methotrexate in the treatment of advanced soft tissue sarcomas. Isr J Med Sci 1988;24:599–603.
542. Lowenbraun S, Moffitt JS, Smalley R, et al. Combination chemotherapy with Adriamycin, cyclophosphamide and methotrexate in metastatic sarcomas. Proc Am Soc Clin Oncol 1977;18:289.
543. Jacobs EM. Combination chemotherapy of metastatic testicular germinal cell tumors and soft part sarcomas. Cancer 1970;25:324–332.
544. Frei III E, Antman K, Teicher B, Eder P, Schnipper L. Bone marrow autotransplantation for solid tumors—prospects. J Clin Oncol 1989;7:515–526.
545. Antman KS, Griffin JD, Elias A, et al. Effect of recombinant human granulocyte-macrophage colony-stimulating factor on chemotherapy-induced myelosuppression. N Engl J Med 1988;319:593–598.
546. Steward WP, Verweij J, Somers R, et al. High dose chemotherapy with two schedules of recombinant human granulocyte-macrophage colony-stimulating factor in the treatment of advanced adult soft tissue sarcomas. Proc Am Soc Clin Oncol [Abstract 1240] 1991;10:349.
547. Pinkerton CR, Groot LJ, Barrett A, et al. Rapid VAC high dose melphalan regimen, a novel chemotherapy approach in childhood soft tissue sarcomas. Br J Cancer 1991;64: 381–385.
548. Pinkerton CR. Megatherapy for soft tissue sarcomas. EBMT experience. Bone Marrow Transplant 1991;3:120–122.
549. Lantta M, Kahanp K, Karkkainen J, Lehtovirta P, Wahlstrom T, Widholm O. Estradiol and progresterone receptors in two cases of endometrial stromal sarcoma. Gynecol Oncol 1984;18:233–239.
550. Keen CE, Philip G. Progestogen-induced regression in low-grade endometrial stromal sarcoma. Case report and literature review. Br J Obstet Gynaecol 1989;96:1435–1439.
551. O'Brien AA, O'Briain DS, Daly PA. Aggressive endometrial stromal sarcoma responding to medroxyprogesterone following failure of tamoxifen and combination chemotherapy. Br J Obstet Gynaecol 1985;92:862–866.
552. Rome RM, Campbell JJ, Cope TI, et al. Tamoxifen in advanced and recurrent uterine sarcomas: A phase II study. Cancer Treat Rep 1986;70:811–812.
553. Wade K, Quinn MA, Hammond I, Williams K, Cauchi M. Uterine sarcoma: Steroid receptors and response to hormonal therapy. Gynecol Oncol 1990;39:364–367.
554. Posner MC, Shiu MH, Newsome J, Hajdu SI, Gaynor JJ, Brennan MF. The desmoid tumor—not a benign disease. Arch Surg 1989;124:191–196.
555. Mckinnon JG, Neifeld JP, Kay S, Parker GA, Foster WC, W Lawrence Jr. Management of desmoid tumors. Surg Gynecol Obstet 1989;169:104–106.
556. Biron P, Meckenstock R, Bobin JY, et al. Presence of hormone receptors in desmoid tumors. Proc Am Soc Clin Oncol 1990;9:285.
557. Weiss AJ, Lackman RD. Response of various low grade neoplasms of mesothelial origin to chemotherapy. Proc Am Soc Clin Oncol 1990;9:315.
558. White CW, Sondheimer HM, Crouch EC, Wilson H, Fan LL. Treatment of pulmonary hemangiomatosis with recombinant interferon alfa-2a. N Engl J Med 1989;320:1197–1212.
559. Moskowitz AJ, Pauker SG. A decision analytic approach to limb-sparing treatment for adult soft tissue and osteogenic sarcoma. Cancer Treat Symp 1985;3:11–26.
560. Sugarbaker PH, Barofsky I, Rosenberg SA, et al. Quality of life assessment of patients in extremity sarcoma clinical trials. Surgery 1982;91:17–23.
561. Weddington WW, Segraves KB, Simon MA. Psychological outcome of extremity sarcoma survivors undergoing amputation or limb salvage. J Clin Oncol 1985;3:1393–1399.
562. Chang A, Culnane M, Lampert M, et al. Quality of life changes in soft tissue sarcoma patients undergoing multimodality treatment. Proc Am Soc Clin Oncol 1987;6:254.
563. Yang JC. Unpublished data, 1992.

Cancer: Principles & Practice of Oncology, Fourth Edition,
edited by Vincent T. DeVita, Jr., Samuel Hellman, Steven A. Rosenberg.
J.B. Lippincott Co., Philadelphia © 1993.

Karen H. Antman
Harvey I. Pass
Thomas DeLaney
Frederick P. Li
Joseph Corson

CHAPTER 43

Benign and Malignant Mesothelioma

EPIDEMIOLOGY

The annual incidence of malignant mesothelioma in the United States is approximately 2200 cases or about 12.1 per million white men, and the rate appears to be increasing.[1] Asbestos is the predominant cause of pleural, peritoneal, and probably epididymal mesothelioma in humans. As many as 8 million living persons in the United States have been occupationally exposed to asbestos over the last 50 years during mining and milling of asbestos and diverse manufacturing processes that use the material.[2] Many public and private buildings contain asbestos, including 10% to 15% of U.S. schools that were insulated or sprayed on interior surfaces with asbestos between 1946 and 1972.[3] The public health significance of exposure in these buildings and the cost effectiveness of asbestos removal are controversial.[4]

HISTORY OF ASBESTOS USAGE

The resistance of asbestos to heat and combustion was recognized by ancient civilizations.[5] The Industrial Revolution greatly expanded demand for asbestos as insulating and packing material for machines and power generators. Two world wars further increased the demand for asbestos in ships and other equipment of combat and transport. The availability, durability, and low cost of asbestos additionally expanded its range of uses in industrial and consumer products.[6]

Although Pliny had observed that asbestos mine slaves were less healthy than other slaves, the health hazards of asbestos exposure were generally not recognized until this century.[5] In 1898, pulmonary scarring and eventual death from respiratory failure was observed in asbestos workers from French and English asbestos textile mills.[7] However, the cause of the pulmonary fibrosis remained uncertain, because tuberculosis and other respiratory infections were often epidemic among poor laborers. In 1930, the causal association between asbestos and asbestosis was firmly established by Merewether and Price at the London Chest Hospital.[8] After limits were set on allowable industrial levels of asbestos exposure in England, many thought the asbestos problem had been solved.[5] However, case reports of lung cancer in patients with asbestosis appeared as early as 1935.[9,10] In 1955, Doll reported a case-control study that established the association between asbestos and lung cancer.[11]

MECHANISMS OF CARCINOGENICITY

Two major forms of asbestos exist: curly, pliable, serpentine asbestos (*i.e.*, chrysotile) and rod-like amphiboles (*i.e.*, crocidolite, amosite, anthophyllite, tremolite, actinolyte).[12] Chrysotile, crocidolite, and amosite are mined for their commercial utility; anthophyllite, tremolite, and actinolyte are usually contaminants. Asbestos fibers tend to separate readily and form numerous individual strands, which often are less than 1 μm in diameter. The carcinogenic effects of asbestos appear to result from its physical properties, rather than chemical structure.[13] Long, rod-like fibers of narrow diameter are more likely to induce tumors in laboratory animals.[14] After inhalation, most asbestos is expectorated or swallowed and subsequently excreted in the feces.[6] The remainder can be cleared from the tracheobronchial tree by several mechanisms, including ciliary action in the trachea, ingestion by macrophages, or penetration through the endothelial lining into interstitial tissues.[6,15,16] Short fibers are cleared more readily than long fibers. Fibers that remain preferentially accumulate in the lower third of the lungs adjacent to the visceral pleura.

Although there appears to be a consensus that serpentine asbestos is less carcinogenic than the rod-like amphiboles, debate continues over whether cases associated with chrysotile asbestos are actually caused by amphibole contamination or are due to chrysotile itself.[17,18]

Asbestos initiates an inflammatory and fibrotic process, mediated in part by cytokines released by activated alveolar macrophages.[19] At a molecular level, protooncogenes such as *PDGFB* (formerly *SIS*), which codes for the platelet-derived growth factor β-chain) are upregulated in alveolar macrophages from fibrotic lungs a factor that enhances mesothelial cell proliferation. Asbestos can transfect DNA into cells.[19] Epidermal growth factor-positive cells have been found in 68% of mesotheliomas examined and correlate with improved survival.[20]

ASBESTOS-ASSOCIATED MESOTHELIOMA

The existence of mesothelioma as a distinct pathologic entity was debated by pathologists before 1960.[21] In the late 1940s, case reports of mesotheliomas in patients with asbestosis began to appear. In 1960, Wagner and colleagues in South Africa reported 33 cases of mesothelioma diagnosed in patients between 31 and 68 years of age in a South African crocidolite mining community.[22] An additional 14 cases appeared in an addendum to the paper. Most of these patients were exposed in childhood through living in the vicinity of asbestos mills and mines; a few had occupational contacts. This study was followed by reports of mesotheliomas in asbestos workers in other parts of the world.

INCIDENCE

The actual annual incidence of mesothelioma is unknown because the neoplasm is difficult to diagnose, even by expert pathologists.[1] Data from death certificates are unreliable for estimating disease frequency despite the usually rapidly fatal outcome of malignant mesothelioma. Cancer deaths are not coded by morphology (*e.g.*, mesothelioma); the cause of mortality is assigned by primary site of the neoplasm (*e.g.*, primary neoplasms of pleural and peritoneum). In a recent study by the Surveillance, Epidemiology and the End Results (SEER) Program of the National Cancer Institute (NCI), only 274 of 1130 white decedents with mesothelioma (approximately 95% diagnosed by microscopy) were recorded as having died of a primary neoplasm of pleura or peritoneum.[23] Most mesothelioma cases were coded as having malignant neoplasm of the lung or unknown site. A reasonable estimate is that 2200 new cases (range, 1000–3000+) of mesothelioma occur annually in the United States.[23-25] Reported rates have increased in the last decade by as much as 50%.[23] Projections suggest that the number of cases will rise moderately into the next century and then decline as a result of recent legislation to reduce asbestos exposure in the workplace and the ambient environment.[25]

In the United States, mesothelioma is approximately three-fold more common in men than in women.[1,23,24] Incidence rises steadily with age, and is approximately ten-fold higher in men between the ages of 60 and 64 years than among those between 30 and 34.

PERSONS AT HIGH RISK

Persons at high risk of developing mesothelioma can be identified by tracing the processing and commercial uses of asbestos. The mineral is mined, milled, and incorporated into a wide range of industrial and commercial products, including insulation, textiles, heat protectors, filters, and construction materials (*e.g.*, spackling, roofing, siding, floor and ceiling tiles).[1,5,6] Workers with high levels of asbestos exposure are miners, millers, producers of asbestos products, and laborers who install plumbing, boilers, and heating equipment in ships, factories, and homes. The risk extends to workers who may not handle asbestos directly but are in proximity to the material, such as carpenters, electricians, and welders in shipyards.

The risk of mesothelioma associated with occupational exposure to asbestos has been examined in case-control studies and cohort studies. In case-control studies, as many as 75% of the cases had asbestos exposure, compared with a small fraction of controls.[1] In cohort studies, the proportion of asbestos workers who died of mesothelioma exceeded 10% in several studies.[26,27] However, mesothelioma risk is difficult to quantitate for several reasons. First, ambient levels of asbestos in most workplaces have not been measured. A "high" level in one study may be called "moderate" or "low" in another. Duration of employment has been used as another surrogate measure of exposure. Second, the time from exposure to the development of mesothelioma is long, usually 3 to 4 decades in most reported studies. Mathematical modeling suggests that risk of mesothelioma increases exponentially by the third to fourth power of time from first exposure, but few cohorts have been followed to the end of life. Third, the composition of the inspired asbestos differed among exposed workers. Evidence suggests that the amphiboles are more carcinogenic, perhaps because of the physical characteristics of these fibers. The long, needle-like fibers appear to lodge more readily in the distal respiratory area, where they persist longer and are transported to the pleura and peritoneum.[14,28]

Despite the obstacles to quantifying risk of mesothelioma, several consistent observations have emerged from studies worldwide. Crocidolite is associated with the high risk of mesothelioma in miners, manufacturers, and workers who install asbestos products.[29] Another amphibole, amosite, appears to carry an intermediate risk. Chrysotile, currently the major form of asbestos in production, shows the weakest association with mesothelioma.[14,30] Occupations with highest risk appear to be insulators, asbestos producers and manufacturers, and the heating and construction tradespeople. The projected lifetime risk among these workers exposed from early adulthood is as high as 20%. Working in proximity to these occupational groups in construction sites confers a relatively lower risk. Some patients with mesothelioma have reported only isolated or brief occupational exposures to asbestos.

Malignant mesothelioma is rarely curable, and screening of asbestos workers for mesothelioma is therefore inappropriate.[31] However, smoking greatly increases the risk of lung cancer (but not mesothelioma) in asbestos workers, and smoking cessation efforts are needed in this high-risk group.[31,32] Clinicians considering the diagnosis of malignant mesothelioma should take a detailed exposure history, emphasizing the period between 20 and 50 years before diagnosis and including possible household contact exposure.[33] Brief exposures may be long forgotten.[34,35]

Exposure in the Home

Mesothelioma in wives and children of asbestos workers has prompted studies that show increased asbestos levels in their homes.[30,36–38] Presumably, asbestos was brought into the home on hair and on clothing to be washed in the family laundry. Asbestos workers were required to shower and change clothing before leaving the work place only after 1972. Asbestos-related neoplasms have been reported in multiple members of some families, but genetic predisposition to the neoplasm remains to be shown.[39,40] The risk of mesothelioma in household contacts of asbestos workers may be as high as 0.4% to 1%, but the rate varies with the level of household contamination and may be overestimated in the reported data.[32]

MESOTHELIOMAS WITHOUT A HISTORY OF ASBESTOS EXPOSURE

No asbestos exposure can be documented in about 30 to 50% of cases of mesothelioma. Quantitation of asbestos fibers in some of these patients has documented background pulmonary fiber levels consistent with the absence of a substantial asbestos exposure.[41]

About 25 published cases of pleural and peritoneal mesothelioma have developed after therapeutic irradiation, and in 2 patients, tumors arose adjacent to deposits of thorium dioxide (thorotrast) still visible on chest radiographs after extravasation during diagnostic procedures years earlier.[42–45] A median of 16 years (range, 7–36 years) elapsed between irradiation and detection of mesothelioma.

A high incidence of mesothelioma (*i.e.*, 22 per 10,000 persons >25 years) observed in the Anatoli region of Turkey has been attributed to zeolite, a silicate ubiquitous in the soil and sometimes sprayed onto homes.[46,47] Erionite is associated with a high incidence of mesothelioma.[48]

MALIGNANT PLEURAL MESOTHELIOMA

PRESENTATION

Malignant pleural mesothelioma most commonly develops in the fifth to seventh decade (median age, 60). A significant proportion of patients with mesothelioma diagnosed between the ages of 20 and 40 report household or neighborhood exposure during childhood.[22,49,50] Children who present with the disease frequently have no apparent asbestos exposure.[51–56]

Men are affected five times as often as women. Dyspnea, nonpleuritic chest wall pain, or both bring patients to medical attention. Examination is remarkable for dullness at one base, and a chest radiograph reveals a large freely movable unilateral pleural effusion. Some patients are asymptomatic, with effusions found incidentally on chest radiographs. Sixty percent have right-sided lesions, and fewer than 5% have bilateral involvement at the time of diagnosis.

A computed tomography (CT) scan or magnetic resonance image (MRI) of the chest to assess the extent of disease is indicated if any treatment is contemplated.[57] Loss of lung volume is evident early on CT scan.[57,58] Scoliosis with contracture of the ipsilateral hemithorax is visible even on a chest radiograph with advanced disease. Despite a history of asbestos contact in 50% to 70% of patients, pleural plaques or interstitial fibrosis are apparent on chest radiographs in approximately 20%, but pleural calcifications are evident on almost half of CT scans and in as many as 87% at autopsy.[57,59]

DIAGNOSIS

Initial misdiagnosis is common. Pathologic opinion appears particularly diverse if litigation is involved. Because a substantial percentage of mesotheliomas develop in patients with no known asbestos exposure and because other malignancies are common in asbestos workers, asbestos exposure should not influence the diagnosis of mesothelioma. Because of the poor prognosis of pleural mesothelioma, a major role of establishing the diagnosis is to exclude the possibility of a more treatable illness. Accurate diagnosis is important in the event of subsequent litigation and for epidemiologic and therapeutic studies.

Diagnostic Surgery

It is sometimes difficult to obtain an accurate histologic confirmation of mesothelioma from pleural fluid cytology or needle biopsy specimens, but the diagnosis of mesothelioma has such a poor prognosis that an unequivocal tissue diagnosis is mandatory. This usually requires surgical intervention with thoracoscopy or thoracotomy, despite the risk of seeding the biopsy site or surgical scar with tumor.[60] For patients who are not candidates for radical surgery, thoracoscopy usually obtains sufficient tissue for histochemical analysis.[61] Later development of chest wall masses from seeding of the biopsy site or surgical scar is an uncommon complication (about 10%) of any diagnostic procedure, but it can usually be avoided by radiotherapy to the scar if appropriate.[60]

If preoperative studies suggest stage I mesothelioma in a good-risk patient with asbestos exposure, most surgeons combine the diagnostic and therapeutic surgical interventions.[62] Generous biopsies can be performed at the inception of the exploration, using frozen sections to differentiate mesothelioma from adenocarcinoma. A sample of uninvaded lung should be obtained for counting asbestos fibers.[34,63]

Bronchoscopy should be performed in all patients with suspected mesothelioma to rule out endobronchial disease, which is rare in mesothelioma.[64] The role of mediastinoscopy in patients with suspected mesothelioma is undefined. Some surgeons think it is unnecessary, because nodes can be removed with the lung. Others think that, because positive nodes indicate stage III disease, surgery is contraindicated. Nevertheless, if radical extrapleural pneumonectomy is contemplated, mediastinoscopy is recommended, because 20% of patients with mesothelioma have mediastinal lymph node involvement.[64]

Cytology, Needle Biopsies, and Sections From Cell Blocks

The results of repeated cytologic examination or biopsy may be negative despite active tumor. If tumor tissue is obtained, light microscopy often provides documentation of malignancy, but it usually does not differentiate adenocarcinoma from mesothelioma. Electron microscopy of needle biopsy or cytocentrifuge specimens from pleural fluid may establish the mesothelial origin of the malignant tumor. Sputum cytology and bronchoscopy may be helpful in documenting an occult bronchogenic adenocarcinoma.

PATHOLOGY

Gross and Microscopic Appearance

Discrete nodules and plaques of firm, grayish tumor coalesce, eventually obliterating the parietal and visceral surfaces. A rind of up to 5 cm thick may encase and constrict the lung with only superficial invasion. The chest wall, pericardium, diaphragm, and interlobar fissures are involved relatively early.[65] At autopsy, tumor invades thoracic lymph nodes in as many as 70% of patients, with occasional extension to cervical nodes.[66] Small hematogenous metastases are documented to liver and lung and less commonly to kidney, adrenal, and bone in 33% to 67% of cases.[66,67] Without careful postmortem examination, hematogenous metastases may be missed.

Extensive sampling of biopsy, pleurectomy, or pneumonectomy specimens is required. A small piece should be fixed in glutaraldehyde for electron microscopy and the remainder promptly fixed in neutral buffered formalin. There are three histologic variants: epithelial, sarcomatoid, and mixed.[65,68] Fifty percent to 60% are epithelial, characterized by tubular, papillary, solid, or vacuolated patterns. The sarcomatoid variant is composed of ovoid or spindle-shaped cells with cellularity and hyperchromatism similar to that of a fibrosarcoma. A biphasic pattern with mixed epithelial and sarcomatoid elements is virtually pathognomonic of malignant mesothelioma, although extensive sampling may be required to demonstrate the minor component.

Differential Diagnosis

Benign inflammatory and reactive processes producing mesothelial hyperplasia or other malignant tumors may mimic mesothelioma but do not invade normal tissues and lack cytologic atypia and hyperchromatism.[66] Adenocarcinomas from primary lung, breast, ovary, stomach, kidney, or prostate cancer frequently metastasize to the pleura and can be extremely difficult to differentiate from epithelial mesothelioma cytologically or histologically. Metastatic adenocarcinoma with extensive pleural involvement may grossly resemble mesothelioma (*i.e.*, pseudomesothelioma).[69] Sarcomatous mesothelioma must be differentiated from fibrosarcoma, malignant fibrous histiocytoma, malignant schwannoma, and hemangiopericytoma. Synovial sarcoma and carcinosarcoma, which may have mixed sarcomatous and epithelial components, usually present as localized masses in the lung.

Autopsy requires skilled performance and experienced interpretation to exclude other occult primary carcinomas. Advanced malignant mesothelioma tends to form peripheral visceral masses, mimicking primary carcinomas.[65] Asbestos counts and postmortem examinations may have legal and epidemiologic value.

HISTOCHEMICAL METHODS. Three methods are in common use to differentiate metastatic adenocarcinomas from epithelial mesotheliomas. The periodic acid-Schiff stain (PAS) used before and after diastase digestion is the single most reliable histochemical method available.[65] Strongly PAS-diastase-positive *neutral* mucopolysaccharides are found in intracellular secretory vacuoles and in intraacinar vacuoles in most adenocarcinomas, but they are rarely found in most mesotheliomas. Their presence is strong but not unequivocal evidence for a diagnosis of adenocarcinoma. Appropriate controls for diastase activity and to differentiate staining of vacuoles from stroma and other structures are essential. Alcian blue at pH 2.5 and colloidal-iron stain *acid* mucopolysaccharides present in mesothelioma and many adenocarcinomas.[66] Disappearance after digestion with hyaluronidase that removes hyaluronic acid in intracellular and secretory vacuoles and intercellular lumens is characteristic of mesothelioma. However, *stromal* hyaluronic acid is a nonspecific finding in many tumors. Under most staining conditions, Mayer's mucicarmine method (*i.e.*, stains neutral and weakly acidic mucopolysaccharides in intracellular and intercellular secretory vacuoles pink or red) is strongly positive in many adenocarcinomas. Mesotheliomas are usually negative but occasionally may stain strongly in some laboratories possibly due to fixation or technical conditions. The method is not completely reliable.

IMMUNOHISTOCHEMISTRY. Immunoperoxidase stains using various antibodies may be effectively applied to paraffin-embedded tumor tissue. Monoclonal antibodies against keratin proteins are strongly reactive in mesothelioma with diffuse cytoplasmic staining and perinuclear accentuation with ring formation.[70] Epithelial and spindle-shaped tumor cells of mixed and sarcomatoid variants are often stained, reflecting the transitional patterns of differentiation observed on electron microscopy.[71] This reactivity is helpful in differentiating mesothelioma from fibrosarcoma, malignant fibrous histiocytoma, and schwannoma, but carcinosarcomas and synovial sarcomas, which have biphasic histology, also express keratin proteins. Adenocarcinomas stain positively, usually with localization to the periphery of the tumor cell. Immunoperoxidase staining for Leu-M1 is usually absent in mesotheliomas but positive in most adenocarcinomas. Staining for carcinoembryonic antigen is usually weak or absent in mesotheliomas and renal, prostate, and some ovarian and endometrial carcinomas, but it is moderate to strong in most other adenocarcinomas.[72,73]

ELECTRON MICROSCOPY. The epithelial variant is composed of polygonal cells with numerous long, slender, branching surface microvilli, desmosomes, abundant tonofilaments, and intracellular lumen formation.[71,74] Primary lung, breast, and upper gastrointestinal tract adenocarcinomas have short stubby surface microvilli, fewer tonofilaments, and microvillus rootlets or lamellar bodies.[75,76] Ovarian and endometrial carcinomas lack intracytoplasmic lumens, but have few tonofilaments and may express features of intestinal metaplasia (*e.g.*, abundant mucin droplets, numerous cilia, dense core granules).[75,76] Elongated nuclei and abundant rough endoplasmic reticulin are found in the sarcomatoid variant. Stromal cells separated by matrix-containing collagen fibers appear spindled or ovoid with sarcomatoid and epithelial features, characteristic of the biphasic nature of mesothelioma.[71,74]

STAGING

Butchart and others have proposed various staging systems that predict survival with statistical significance in some series.[77] The Butchart classification (Table 43–1) suffers from an absence of TNM descriptions and vague statements about lymph node involvement and degrees of chest wall invasion. The International Union Against Cancer (UICC) proposed a TNM staging system that probably is as good an attempt to unify future reporting of mesothelioma as any other system.[78] The weighting system of the individual descriptions as they translate into stage I through IV disease is handled in a similar manner to the new International Staging System used for non-small cell lung cancer, but the impact of nodal disease and long-term survival as a function of organ of invasion or depth of invasion with confined hemothorax disease remains problematic.

Probably the major role of noninvasive procedures is to determine isolated hemithorax disease. A CT or MR scan of the primary tumor to assess the extent of disease is indicated if treatment is contemplated. Characteristic CT findings in almost 100 patients are pleural thickening in 92% (intralobar fissures in 86%), effusions in 74%, and pleural calcifications in 20% to 50%.[44,57,79] A CT scan is helpful in differentiating benign from malignant pleural thickening but does not reliably differentiate primary from metastatic malignancy. Fewer patients have been evaluated by MRI, but the extent of tumor and its invasion of adjacent structures are well documented. Coronal MRI was particularly helpful for evaluating the diaphragm.[80] Although brain, bone, and liver metastases or extension into other serosal surfaces are found in more than half of patients at autopsy, they are sufficiently uncommon at presentation to obviate the need for extensive baseline studies in the absence of symptoms or laboratory abnormalities. However, these studies may identify an occult adenocarcinoma of the lung, a pattern of widespread metastases or a markedly elevated serum or pleural fluid carcinoembryonic antigen (CEA), suggesting a diagnosis other than mesothelioma.[66,81] Although there are no definitive biomarkers for mesothelioma, future studies investigating serial serum levels of tissue polypeptide antigen or thrombomodulin may be of interest.[82,83] Mesotheliomas take up gallium 67.[84]

Pulmonary function tests may document restrictive lung disease resulting from encasement of the lung and assess the potential tolerance for pneumonectomy. Obstructive spirometric changes are unrelated to mesothelioma or asbestosis.[85] Laboratory evaluation is otherwise generally unremarkable except for an elevated platelet count and erythrocyte sedimentation rate.

TABLE 43–1. Staging Systems for Malignant Mesothelioma

Butchart Staging Classification		
I	Tumor confined within the capsule of the parietal pleura, involving only ipsilateral pleura, lung, pericardium, and diaphragm	
II	Tumor invading chest wall or involving mediastinal structures, such as esophagus, heart, opposite pleura	
III	Tumor penetrating diaphragm to involve peritoneum; involvement of opposite pleura	
	Lymph node involvement outside the chest	
IV	Distant blood-borne metastases	
UICC Staging Proposal*		
I	T1, N0, M0	
	T2, N0, M0	
II	T1, N1, M0	
	T2, N1, M0	
III	T3, N0, M0	
	T3, N1, M0	
	T1, N2, M0	
	T2, N2, M0	
	T3, N2, M0	
IV	Any T, N3, M0	
	T4, any N, M0	
	Any T, and N, M1	
	T	(Primary Tumor And Extent)
	TX	Primary tumor cannot be assessed
	T0	No evidence of primary tumor
	T1	Primary tumor limited to ipsilateral parietal or visceral pleura
	T2	Tumor invades any of the following: ipsilateral lung, endothoracic fascia, diaphragm, pericardium
	T3	Tumor invades any of the following: ipsilateral chest wall muscle, ribs, mediastinal organs or tissues
	T4	Tumor extends to any of the following: contralateral pleura or lung by direct extension, peritoneum or intraabdominal organs by direct extension, cervical tissues
	N	(Lymph Nodes)
	NX	Regional lymph nodes cannot be assessed
	N0	No regional lymph nodes metastases
	N1	Metastases in ipsilateral bronchopulmonary of hilar lymph nodes
	N2	Metastases in ipsilateral mediastinal lymph nodes
	N3	Metastases in contralateral mediastinal internal mammary, supraclavicular, or scalene lymph nodes
	M	(Metastases)
	MX	Presence of distant metastases cannot be assessed
	M0	No known distant metastases
	M1	Distant metastasis present

* Staging solely on clinical measures is designated cTNM. Staging that can be done on clinical pathologic information is designated as pTNM. Clinical and pathologic groups are identical.

NATURAL HISTORY

Prognostic variables at presentation significantly associated with a longer survival include age under 55 to 65, 0 to 1 performance status, stage I disease, epithelial histology, lack of chest pain at diagnosis, and a normal platelet count.[86–90]

Shortness of breath and chest pain can be controlled initially by repeated thoracenteses and minor narcotics. Although chest tube drainage and sclerosis are usually unsuccessful, pleural fluid eventually becomes loculated as the tumor obliterates the pleural space.[67] With advanced disease, fatigue and dyspnea increase out of proportion to x-ray findings or pulmonary function values. Because hypoxia results from shunting of desaturated blood through a poorly aerated lung, therapeutic oxygen provides little symptomatic relief.

Mesothelioma tends to be locally invasive. Chest wall masses develop in about 10% of patients over thoracentesis, chest tube drainage, or thoracotomy tracts.[67,91] Direct involvement of esophagus, ribs, vertebrae, nerves, and the superior vena cava cause dysphagia, pain, cord compression, brachial plexopathy, Horner's syndrome, or superior vena cava syndromes, respectively.[92] Fevers and sweats with no documented source of infection are common and often accompanied by significant weight loss, poor performance status, and an early death. Thrombocytosis and other clotting abnormalities occur in 10% to 20% (more frequently in peritoneal mesothelioma).[93,94] Disseminated intravascular coagulation, thrombophlebitis, pulmonary emboli, Coombs-positive hemolytic anemia, and hypercalcemia associated with elevated levels of a parathyroid hormone-like peptide have been reported.[95,96]

The median survival is 4 to 18 months in various series (range, weeks to 16 years). Patients usually die of respiratory failure or pneumonia. Small bowel obstruction from direct extension through the diaphragm develops in about one third, and 10% die of pericardial or myocardial involvement.[50,92]

Localized malignant fibrous tumors of the pleura may resemble sarcomatous mesotheliomas histologically. Of 82 malignant localized tumors, 45% were cured by simple excision.[97] If the nature of the lesion is ambiguous, involvement of the pleura on random biopsy would establish a diagnosis of diffuse, malignant disease.

CYTOGENETICS

Asbestos, a poor mutagen, can be cytotoxic and is associated with chromosomal abnormalities in exposed cells.[39,40,98] Asbestos induces mesothelial proliferation, but in vitro malignant transformation has not been demonstrated.

Ploidy status and the percentage of cells actively synthesizing DNA have been analyzed by flow cytometry in almost 200 malignant mesotheliomas.[99–102] Ploidy and S-phase fraction seem to be consistent in different sections from the same tumor and were not associated with histologic subtype.[100] In the various studies, 60% to 65% were diploid and 27% were near diploid. In contrast, 85% of lung cancers are aneuploid.[99] Significantly shorter survival is associated with a high percentage of S-phase cells but not aneuploidy.[100,101] The number of copies of 7p correlated inversely with survival.[103] Recurring chromosomal changes, including partial deletions of 1p, 3p, 9p and monosomy 4 and 22, suggest a cascade of events involving alterations of genes on more than one chromosome. These regions should be targeted for molecular investigation into the possibility of suppressor genes in mesothelioma.[104–108] Mesotheliomas displayed little genetic instability (heterogeneity) within tumor populations, unlike lung cancers.[105]

HUMORAL FACTORS

Hyaluronic acid has been useful in diagnosis or for following response but is relatively nonspecific.[109] A markedly elevated serum or pleural fluid CEA suggests a diagnosis other than mesothelioma. Hematopoietic growth factors and blood group antigens have been produced by normal and malignant mesothelial cell lines.[110–114]

TREATMENT

Surgery

Although some physicians feel strongly that mesothelioma patients should be referred to institutions with research programs, others advocate supportive care alone after definitive biopsy because reported cures with any treatment remain anecdotal. In 68 patients in Glasgow with mesothelioma managed supportively, the median survival was 30 weeks (*i.e.*, 22 weeks for patients with pain and 44 weeks for patients with dyspnea).[90] A similar median survival of 7 months was recorded by Ruffie and colleagues for 176 patients with mesothelioma treated supportively in Canada.[115] Harvey reported a 6-month median survival for 76 nonsurgically treated patients; 33 had had pleurodesis, chemotherapy, or radiation.[116]

Diffuse malignant mesothelioma is usually associated with chest wall pain and recurrent effusions.[117] Pleurectomy successfully controls recurrent effusions in 88% of patients. Surgery probably has no role in the palliation of the pain associated with chest wall invasion, which is better treated with nonnarcotic analgesics, antiinflammatory agents, or opiates.[117]

Although the staging of mesothelioma has been inconsistent, it is reasonable to consider surgical therapy in patients with stage I disease, defined by Butchart as a tumor confined within the capsule of the parietal pleura, involving only the ipsilateral lung, pericardium, and diaphragm.[77] Stage I disease, however heterogenous, is associated with a longer survival, although this may be solely associated with lead-time bias. Cases in which tumor extends beyond the confines of the parietal pleural capsule, with diffuse invasion of neighboring structures, are probably not amenable to radical surgery.

Preoperative Evaluation

Any patient considered for radical surgical therapy must be able to withstand pneumonectomy and prolonged anesthesia. Cardiac status should be screened by an electrocardiogram, and the patient should be questioned for signs of acquired heart disease that may need further noninvasive investigation. Adequate pulmonary reserve is crucial. The forced expiratory volume (FEV_1) of more than 2 L per second is desirable; if the FEV_1 is less than this, quantitative ventilation-perfusion scanning should be performed to document that residual FEV_1 after pneumonectomy will be greater than 1 L per second. As with primary lung cancer, good-risk patients usually have good nutritional status. Some surgeons think that age over 65 years is a contraindication to surgery.[62]

Surgical Technique

Pleurectomy. Pleurectomy has been strongly advocated by the Memorial Sloan-Kettering Cancer Center (MSKCC) group.[64] Da Valle uses pleurectomy in patients with minimal invasion of the visceral pleura (*i.e.*, free pleural space without tissue invasion) for attempted cure.[62] Extrapleural dissection of the parietal pleura is begun after a generous posterolateral thoracotomy. The pleura is stripped from the apex of the lung to the diaphragm, along with the pericardium, as necessary (Fig. 43–1). Most of the mediastinum and chest wall pleura can be removed, but the diaphragmatic pleura usually cannot be completely resected. Hemostasis is controlled as the procedure is performed, and blood replacement is frequently necessary. Two large intercostal catheters are used to drain blood and to manage peripheral bronchopleural fistulas. Large fistulas are suture ligated to allow maximal expansion of the underlying lung with underwater seal drainage. Operative mortality is low (1–2%), but complications include bronchopleural fistulas, hemorrhage, and subcutaneous emphysema.

Extrapleural Pneumonectomy. Extrapleural pneumonectomy is a more radical procedure, which includes en bloc removal of the parietal pleura, lung, pericardium, and diaphragm (Fig. 43–2 and Table 43–2). The approach can be by posterolateral thoracotomy (in the sixth interspace) or by thoracoabdominal incision (in the sixth or seventh interspace) with subdiaphragmatic blunt dissection of the peritoneum. The latter approach allows easier resection of the diaphragm and avoids the lower thoracotomy counter-incision needed if the posterolateral incision is used. Extrapleural dissection to the hilum, early entry into the pericardium retrosternally to accomplish intrapericardial pneumonectomy, and use of double-lumen anesthesia were described by Da Valle.[62] Diaphragmatic resection is followed by reconstruction using Dacron or Gortex material to prevent abdominal content herniation. Right-sided pericardial resections are usually reconstructed to prevent cardiac herniation. Intercostal tube drainage after pneumonectomy is optional. Operative mortality, earlier reported to be as high as 27% to 31%, is now 5% to 9%. Serious complications have been seen in 25% of the patients, including bronchopleural fistulas and empyema, vocal cord paralysis, chylothorax, arrhythmia, and respiratory insufficiency.[62]

Results of Surgical Treatment

Palliation. There is poor documentation of the results of palliative surgical intervention for mesothelioma. Law controlled 22 of 25 recurrent effusions by pleurectomy and reported objective relief of pain and dyspnea lasting weeks to months.[117,127] In a report by Ruffie, 63 patients had partial decortication and debulking for mesothelioma, which prevented recurrence of pleural effusion in 86% of cases.[115] Brancatisano has verified the efficacy of effusion control in 44 of 45 patients having subtotal parietal pleurectomy.[128]

Survival. Survival figures after pleurectomy or extrapleural pneumonectomy are difficult to interpret due to the different treatment philosophies and ways in which patients are selected for these operations. They should be considered separately. The MSKCC series investigated the use of pleurectomy with selective brachytherapy and postoperative radiation therapy from 1976to 1988. Forty-one patients received only external-beam irradiation after decortication and pleurectomy, and 54 patients received an implant and external-beam therapy. Median survival for the entire group was 12.6 months, with a 2-year survival rate of 35%. A select group of 27 patients who had pure epithelial histology and who did not require an implant had a median survival of 22.5 months and a 2-year survival rate of 41%.[64] Ruffie reported a median survival of 9.8 months in this group of decorticated patients and Brancatisano's patients survived a median of 16 months.[115,128] Law, in a series of 28 patients, reported a 2-year survival rate of 32% after pleurectomy alone, with a median survival of 20 months.[117,127] The median survival for 23 patients after pleurectomy performed by Da Valle was 11.2 months.[62] Lewis reported an older series of patients with a median survival of 6.7 months after pleurectomy.[129]

Because the degree of tumor debulking varied in the pleurectomy series, the potential impact of radical surgery is

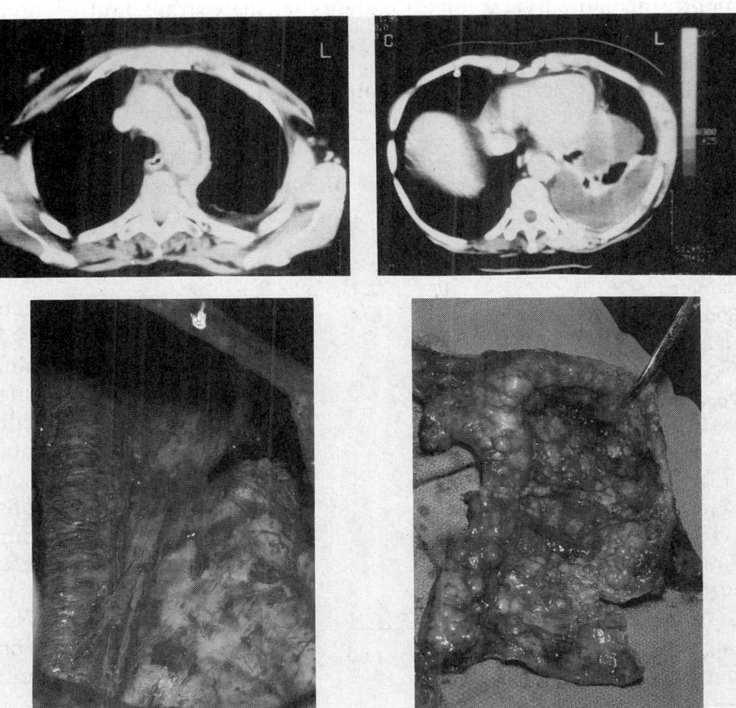

FIGURE 43–1. Pleurectomy for diffuse pleural mesothelioma. Preoperative tomograms demonstrate thickened pleura and fluid; the operative photograph and specimen are depicted below.

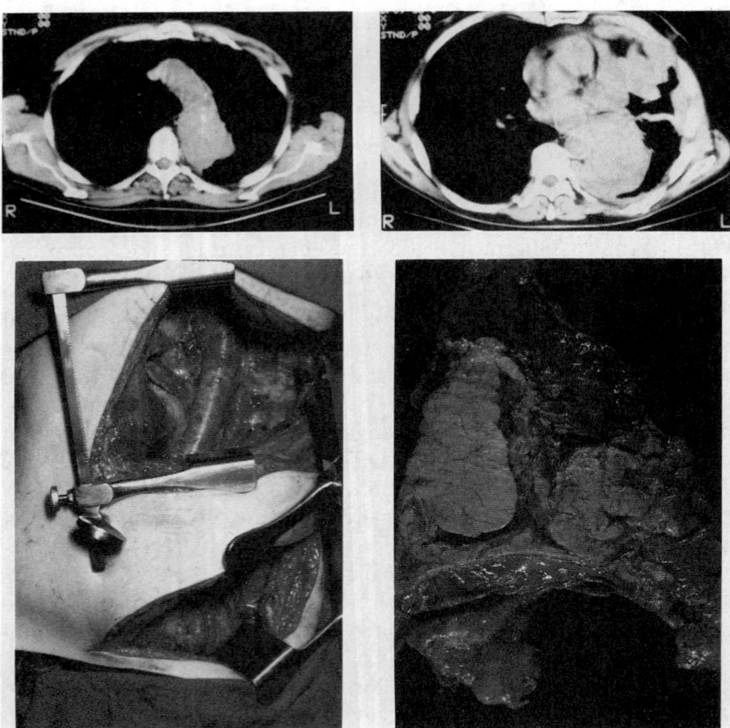

FIGURE 43–2. Left-sided diffuse mesothelioma. Two CT cuts show chest wall, fissure involvement, and aortic arch abutment. The surgical photograph demonstrates the skeletonized aorta, partial pericardectomy, and partial diaphragmatic removal through a counter incision. The surgical specimen is demonstrated in the lower right.

probably more accurately assessed by long-term survival after extrapleural pneumonectomy. Butchart reported a 9% 2-year survival after extrapleural pneumonectomy compared with a 24% 2-year survival and 15% 3-year survival for Da Valle's 33 patients. The Ontario and Quebec group of 23 patients with extrapleural pneumonectomy had a 2-year survival of 17%, and Rusch reported a 2-year survival of 33% with a 10-month median survival for 20 patients having extrapleural pneumonectomy.[125] This last series is probably one of the most representative of the modern surgical management of mesothelioma; although it is not randomized, it represents a detailed analysis of recurrence patterns after pleurectomy and extrapleural pneumonectomy. The implication from the study was that extrapleural pneumonectomy may alter the natural history of pleural mesothelioma in that relapse occurred predominantly in systemic sites, but lesser operations were characterized predominantly by local and progressive pleural relapses.

TABLE 43–2. Extrapleural Pneumonectomy for Diffuse Pleural Mesothelioma

Investigations	*No. of Patients*	*Mortality (%)*	*Median Survival (mo)*
Woern (1974)[118]	62	Unspecified	19
Bamler (1976)[119]	17	23	
Butchart (1978)[77]	29	31	4
DeLaria (1985)[120]	11	0	
DaValle (1986)[62]	33		
Vogt-Moykopf (1987)[121]	55	5.5	10.2
Faber (1988)[122]	33	9	13.5
Probst (1989)[123]	111*	6.3	9
Geroulenos (1990)[124]	18	7	20
Rusch (1991)[125]	20	15	10
Sugarbaker (1991)[126]	31	6	21

* Includes patients with pleurectomy and extrapleural pneumonectomy.

Conclusions and Recommendations. To consider any surgical management for patients with pleural mesothelioma, the diagnosis must be certain with immunohistochemical techniques or electron microscopic confirmation. Thoracoscopic techniques will probably be used with greater frequency and earlier to define patients with earlier-stage disease. If repeated semiinvasive attempts do not secure the diagnosis, open biopsy is indicated. In patients with minimal disease or persistent pleural effusion, pleurectomy and decortication usually clinch the definitive diagnosis and palliate the effusion. If the lung and pleura cannot be mobilized easily from the chest wall due to invasion, a generous biopsy specimen should be obtained and the procedure terminated. Extrapleural pneumonectomy, especially with diaphragmatic removal, may be appropriate for selected patients. If the patient has had concomitant diagnosis and pleurectomy, most of the disease is debulked, and baseline computerized tomography after the pleurectomy does not reveal disease that could be scored in response to therapy, it is reasonable to defer further treatment. When local or systemic recurrences can be documented, referral to or participation in a defined treatment protocol should be initiated.

Radiation Therapy

PRINCIPLES. The efficacy of irradiation, like that of other treatment modalities, remains uncertain in the definitive treatment of patients with pleural mesothelioma. Its use has not been subjected to randomized clinical trials. Although several series suggest benefit, the variable clinical course of the disease and the frequent use of radiation in conjunction with surgery or chemotherapy make it difficult to assess its contribution to an overall treatment program.

Mesothelioma cells are more sensitive to radiation (*i.e.*, assessed by the surviving fraction after 200 cGy) than non-small cell lung cancer cells, but they are less sensitive than small cell lung cancer cells.[130] The use of irradiation for mesothelioma differs considerably from its use in lung cancer because of the extensive pleural involvement seen in mesothelioma. If irradiation is used for definitive treatment of malignant mesothelioma, treatment of the entire pleura is indicated. This treatment volume is extremely difficult to irradiate to tumoricidal doses without causing significant injury to the normal tissues of adjacent lung, heart, and liver.[131]

Most recent series document occasional regressions of gross disease with modest doses of radiation but do not indicate that survival is significantly altered by irradiation compared with supportive care (Table 43–3). Between 1971 and 1980, 116 patients in good general condition and without evidence of extrathoracic disease were seen at the Brompton and Royal Marsden Hospitals in London.[117,127] Fifty-two patients underwent active treatment, and the other 64 received supportive care, with the choice determined by physician preference. No difference in survival was seen between the two groups, with a 2-year survival rate of about 33% and 4-year survival rates of 0% to 11%. Active treatment consisted of parietal pleurectomy and decortication of the lung for 28 patients, radiation therapy for 12 patients (after surgery in 8), and chemotherapy for the remaining 12 patients (8 of whom had surgery). Radiation consisted of 5000 to 5500 cGy using rotating arc fields designed to treat the pleura and spare underlying lung. One patient showed a dramatic response to radiotherapy with resolution of effusion, pain, and dyspnea. She was well and active 4 years after completion of treatment. Two other patients experienced sustained regression of recurrent pleural effusions after radiotherapy. Although the treatment volume and normal tissue tolerance limit radiation dose, radiation therapy to these large bulky tumors can occasionally produce significant regression and worthwhile palliation.

Another large series from South Africa failed to demonstrate any convincing evidence that currently employed therapies significantly affected the course of the disease. Alberts and colleagues compiled the treatment outcome for 262 patients treated between 1965 and 1985 with chemotherapy, radiotherapy, chemotherapy plus radiotherapy, or decortication plus radiotherapy and chemotherapy.[135] The median survival of 9.6 months was similar for all groups. Only a small group of patients treated with doxorubicin and irradiation with 1000 cGy every 6 weeks for four courses appeared to show prolonged survival, with a median survival of 23 months.

Because of the variable course of the disease, the different radiation treatment techniques used (*e.g.*, anteroposterior-posteroanterior rotational arc, combined photon-electron radiotherapy), and normal tissue constraints on radiation dose, the relation between radiation dose and treatment response is not well established. The series from the Joint Center for Radiation Therapy in Boston included 29 treatment courses for palliation between 1968 and 1980.[91] Relief of pain, dyspnea, and other symptoms was seen in 4 of 6 patients treated with doses of 4000 cGy or more, but only 1 of 23 treatment courses at lower doses achieved successful palliation. Doses of 1500 to 2000 cGy (*i.e.*, the normal tissue tolerance dose of whole lung irradiation) were ineffective in controlling disease in patients with diffuse involvement of the visceral pleura with 1- to 2-mm nodules.

A report from the Peter MacCallum Cancer Institute in Australia described successful palliation in 17 (65%) of 26 evaluable palliative radiation courses.[136] Short-course treatment with 2000 cGy in five fractions appeared to give comparable palliation to that seen with more protracted courses (*i.e.*, 3000–4000 cGy in 10–15 fractions). Fifteen patients were given high-dose radiotherapy with radical therapeutic intent. Twelve completed treatment to 5000 cGy. The median survival of the 12 patients completing treatment was 17 months, with an estimated 2-year survival of 17%.[136] In a series from Thomas Jefferson Medical School in Philadelphia, 2 of 9 patients had local control for 20 and 40 months, respectively,

TABLE 43–3. Radiation Series

Investigations	*No. of Patients*	*Dose (cGy)*	*Outcome*
University of Iowa[132]	3	2000–2500	Symptomatic improvement
Brompton/Royal Marsden[117,127]	12	5000–5500	1 asymptomatic for 4 y
			2 with effusions controlled until demise
Joint Center for Radiation Therapy[91]	6	>4000	4 with significant symptomatic relief
	23	<4000	1 with significant symptomatic relief
Institut Gustave-Roussy[133]	14	3500–5000	4 alive at 1–41 mo
			10 dead at 1–37 (median, 15) mo
Thomas Jefferson Medical School[134]	9	6000	2 with local control at 20 and 40 mo

after 6000 cGy to the entire ipsilateral pleura, mediastinum, and involved areas of lung.[134] Radiation was given in three courses of 2000 cGy over a total of 10 weeks by a split-course technique.

Although information is limited, histologic subtype does not appear to have a major impact on the outcome of irradiated patients. In the early MSKCC series of patients from 1939 to 1972 with disease confined to the hemithorax treated primarily with radiotherapy, 15 patients with the epithelial subtype of mesothelioma had a median survival of 8 months, compared with 9 months in patients with the fibrosarcomatous subtype.[137] Although the volume of disease influences radiotherapeutic outcome in many other sites, its impact on the radiation response of pleural mesothelioma is not well characterized.

The combination of irradiation with debulking surgery can be rationalized if the patient can be rendered with only microscopic residual disease on most pleural surfaces after surgery. Irradiation is more effective at a given dose level for treating microscopic than for gross disease.[138] Higher doses of boost irradiation with brachytherapy or localized external-beam irradiation can be used to sites of residual gross disease. This strategy can maximize local control while minimizing the normal tissue complications from irradiation.

Irradiation has been used to prevent seeding of biopsy tracts and surgical wounds. In one series from Marseilles, irradiation consisting of 2100 cGy in three fractions prevented the development of wound seeding after thoracoscopy or thoracotomy in 24 patients.[139] Before initiation of prophylactic irradiation, wound seeding occurred in 17 (61%) of 33 biopsied patients. None of the patients who had developed growth of nodules in an incision responded to subsequent irradiation.

In considering the use of irradiation in this disease, the potential complications of high-dose irradiation to a large volume should be weighed in the treatment decision. The frequency, type, and severity of radiation complications depend on technique, volume, dose, fractionation, and normal tissue in the field and type and timing of any other treatment, such as chemotherapy. Remarkably, some earlier series reported no acute or chronic complications from the use of radiotherapy alone.[91,133] This may have been a function of limited-volume treatment or short survival. One series reported few complications with radiotherapy after 5000 to 5500 cGy were delivered with an off-axis rotational technique. Among 12 patients, complications included nausea and malaise in 6, transient radiation hepatitis in 1, and mild esophagitis in 1.[117,127] No case of radiation pneumonitis was seen. However, if no attempt has been made to shield lung or if the organ tolerance of other tissues such as the liver has been exceeded, significant complications have occurred. Ball and Cruikshank reported a case of fatal radiation hepatitis in a patient treated for a right pleural mesothelioma and a case of radiation myelitis (after 4000 cGy) in their series of 12 radically irradiated patients.[136] Maasilta reported deterioration in lung function after high-dose irradiation (5500–7100 cGy) given with chemotherapy.[140,141] Forced vital capacity and diffusing capacity showed significant declines at 1.5 to 2 months after radiotherapy and continued to decline over the year after radiation therapy. By radiologic assessment, treatment essentially obliterated lung function on the affected side. Hypoxemia and pathologic physiologic shunting increased in 2 of 6 patients monitored. Lung function should be evaluated to assess potential tolerance before undertaking hemithorax irradiation. Liver position should be determined and adequate hepatic shielding should be used after 3000 cGy. Maasilta and Hallman reported the association of bronchoalveolar lavage plasmin and surfactant in mesothelioma patients with radiation pulmonary injury.[141,142]

The use of radioactive colloids (*i.e.*, ^{198}Au or ^{32}P in chromic phosphate) instilled into the pleural space has been studied. Pleural effusions have disappeared for as long as 3.5 years.[143] The exact response rate and duration to this approach is unknown. In a series from Hahnemann Medical College, all 6 patients were alive at 12 months or longer after instillation of isotopes.[144] The extent of other treatment and exact length of survival were not reported. Because of the physical characteristics of these isotopes (especially ^{32}P), their effect on bulky disease is limited. ^{32}P is a pure beta (electron) emitter with maximal tissue penetration of 8 mm and the bulk of energy deposited in the first 2 mm. ^{198}Au emits 90% of its energy as beta particles with an energy of 0.96 MeV. These have tissue penetrations of less than 5 mm, although the emitted photons have energies of 0.412 to 1.099 MeV and can penetrate several centimeters. An equally important limitation on the use of radiocolloids is the problem of obtaining optimal distribution of isotope throughout the pleural space. Gordon and colleagues attempted radioisotope instillation in 3 patients, but fluoroscopy or gamma camera measurements indicated that the distribution was suboptimal.[91] Both agents may have limited roles in patients with low-volume disease or in conjunction with surgery in patients with an adequate pleural distribution. The distribution of a radiotracer or contrast material should be tested before the therapeutic administration of these agents.

RADIATION THERAPY TECHNIQUES. Several different radiation therapy techniques have been used to irradiate the pleura to high doses. Because of the diffuse pleural involvement, the target volume is large and includes the pleural surface, diaphragm, and mediastinum. Attempts at radical irradiation must be limited to patients with disease confined to one hemithorax. Field borders must extend above the first rib superiorly; below the diaphragmatic reflection of the pleura inferiorly, which is usually at about the lower border of the twelfth thoracic vertebra; laterally to clear the bony rib cage; and include the full width of the mediastinum. The field size can be increased to include masses extending through the chest wall or diaphragm or to include the whole heart when the pericardium is involved. The demarcation of sites of residual gross disease with surgical clips placed at thoracotomy greatly facilitates planning by allowing accurate, high-dose boost irradiation and lessens the likelihood of normal tissue injury. CT scans can delineate sites of gross disease, but they may miss invasion of tumor into the mediastinum or through the diaphragm and areas of miliary seeding of the pleura.[57,145,146] MRI can delineate mediastinal invasion by mesothelioma and may have an increasing role in radiologic assessment and treatment planning.[80,147]

Radical irradiation has delivered 4000 to 5500 cGy to the entire pleural surface (with the exception of the reflections extending into the fissures in the lung) and the mediastinum. Other structures such as the heart have been included as clinically indicated. This dose has been followed by boost treatment to 5500 to 7100 cGy to focal areas of gross disease through reduced portals. Although some have chosen to irradiate the entire hemithorax with opposed anterior and posterior photon fields to doses of 4000 to 5000 cGy without lung shielding followed by conning down to smaller fields, such techniques can cause irreversible pulmonary injury.[131,136]

Techniques have been developed to spare the lung. One involves the use of an off-axis beam rotational technique to irradiate a maximal area of the pleural space to high dose while shielding underlying lung.[117,127] Several others involve matching photon and electron beams.[134,145,148,149] These involve the use of large, opposed anterior and posterior external-beam portals with central lung blocking. The pleural areas underneath the blocks are treated with electron beams of appropriate energy (10–15 MeV). CT scans are used to define the thickness of the chest wall, delineate patient contour, and plan treatment. Tissue compensators may improve dose distribution. Currently no completely satisfactory technique for high-dose irradiation of the pleura exists. Even careful photon and electron techniques deliver substantial doses to the lung because of the penetrating ability of the electron beams in the lung and contribution from side scattered electrons set in motion during photon irradiation.[149] Advances in sophisticated conformal radiotherapy may improve the available dose distribution.[150]

With fractions of 180 to 200 cGy given five times weekly, reasonable treatment precautions limit the spinal cord dose to 4000 cGy, the esophagus to 4500 to 5000 cGy, the whole lung to 2000 cGy, a functional portion of the liver to 3000 cGy, and 50% of the heart to 4000 cGy. Radiation tolerances may be lowered if irradiation is given in conjunction with chemotherapy, especially doxorubicin, despite separation of the two modalities by weeks or months.

A single report on the use of fast neutrons describes a complete regression of bulk disease without evidence of recurrence 78 months after treatment.[151] In this report, a portion of the disease was treated with cobalt 60 radiation with similar response. Because of the poor depth-dose characteristics of the available neutron beams, only very thin patients could be treated with a pure neutron technique. However, these or other particles may have a role in selected patients in delivering boost treatment to sites of gross disease.

Chemotherapy

SINGLE-AGENT STUDIES. Before the wide availability of CT scans, most mesotheliomas were not strictly measurable. Measurable masses on chest radiographs were frequently obscured by effusions, producing data that are totally unreliable in determining response to therapy. Response rates to standard agents remain difficult to define. Relatively small positive studies are reported promptly, but larger series with lower response rates may never be published. Nevertheless, data from single-agent studies are shown in Table 43–4. Response rates are included in the table if the number of evaluable patients exceeded 10. Doxorubicin appears to have some activity against mesothelioma, although response rates vary considerably. Methotrexate with rescue, 5-azacytidine, and 5-fluorouracil may also have single-agent activity. Cisplatin as a single agent does not appear to be significantly active, with 5 of 49 patients responding in several phase II studies.

COMBINATION CHEMOTHERAPY. Response rates for combination regimens range from 30% to 40% of 10 to 20 patients in single-institution series to 0% to 14% for cooperative group trials of the same combinations (Table 43–5). Response rates for combinations with and without doxorubicin are similar to the 18% response rate of single-agent doxorubicin (see Table 43–4). Doxorubicin and cyclophosphamide with or without dacarbazine yielded response rates of 7% in both arms of a large randomized trial that accrued advanced-disease patients concurrently with a second study for stage I and II mesothelioma.[229] The response rates may be artificially low in this study because good prognosis patients were treated on a competing study. The Cancer and Leukemia Group B randomized patients with measurable mesothelioma to cisplatin and doxorubicin or to cisplatin and mitomycin C. The objective response rates (24%) in patients with measurable disease were similar.[230] Based on the activity of intraperitoneal cisplatin, the Lung Cancer Study Group completed a trial of 47 patients treated with intrapleural cisplatin and cytarabine. Of the 37 patients evaluated, 49% had at least 75% decrease in the size of their effusions.[125]

Surgery With Intraoperative and Postoperative Adjuvant Therapy

Most patients with mesothelioma cannot be rendered free of disease with surgical therapy alone, and local and systemic recurrences lead to ultimate failure. In a MSKCC report of 41 patients who underwent parietal pleurectomy between 1976 and 1982, disease at the completion of surgery remained on the diaphragm (49%), visceral pleura (51%), mediastinum (49%), chest wall (27%), and lung (5%).[245] Seventy-eight percent had residual gross disease after surgery. Radical pleuropneumonectomy can remove more disease in selected patients but may still have residual microscopic or gross tumor after even the most aggressive surgical resection.

In a Dana-Farber Cancer Institute and Brigham and Women's Hospital select series of 44 patients treated from 1980 to 1991, extrapleural pneumonectomy followed by cisplatin, doxorubicin, and cyclophosphamide chemotherapy and external-beam irradiation resulted in a 48% 2-year survival rate.[126] The operative mortality rate was 5%.[126] Those with lymph node involvement or sarcomatous histology had a significantly poorer survival. In a multivariate analysis of their mesothelioma registry, survival was significantly prolonged for patients who underwent pleuropneumonectomy and chemotherapy and radiotherapy.[86]

Rusch at MSKCC has been investigating the combination of pleurectomy and intraoperative intracavitary administration of cisplatin, followed by postoperative systemic therapy with cisplatin and mitomycin C. The results of this study are forthcoming. At the M.D. Anderson Cancer Center, 20 patients initially received cyclophosphamide, doxorubicin, and DTIC. Five whose disease responded partially underwent surgical resection. Follow-up was short at the time of publication.[238]

A completely different approach has been studied in at the NCI. Recognizing the magnitude of the problem of local control, patients undergo debulking of the disease to a minimum of 5 mm by modified extrapleural pneumonectomy or pleurectomy decortication and intraoperative photodynamic therapy. Before surgery, patients receive the photosensitizer di-

TABLE 43–4. Single-Agent Response Rates in Malignant Mesothelioma Studies With More Than 5 Patients

Agent	*No. of Patients Evaluable*	*No. of Patients Responding*	*Response (%)*	*References*
Anthracyclines				
Doxorubicin	164	29	18	134, 152–162
THP-doxorubicin	15	0		163
Pirarubicin	85	11	14	164–166
Epirubicin	69	8	12	167, 168
Detorubicin	21	9	43	169
Aclacinomycin A	10	1	10	170
Alkylating Agents				
Cyclophosphamide	14	4	28	154, 171–174
Ifosfamide	43	7	16	175, 176
Mechlorethamine	6	2		177–182
Thiotepa	7	1		152, 171, 180, 181, 183
Melphalan	3	2		174, 183
Procarbazine	6	2		184
Mitomycin C	12	2	17	50, 185
Cisplatin	56	8	14	186–192
Cisplatin (weekly)	9	4	44	193
Carboplatin	97	11 (2 CR)	11	194–200
Iproplatin	7	0		198, 199
Vincas				
Vincristine	23	0		201
Etoposide	51	3	6	202–205
Vindesine	37	1	3	206, 207
Antimetabolites				
5-Fluorouracil	28	4	14	154, 156, 208, 209
Methotrexate, high dose	9	4		171
Dideazafolic acid (CB3717)	18	1	6	198, 210
5-Azacytidine	7	0		211, 212
Dihydro-5-azacytadine	55	4 (1 CR)	7	213, 214
Bleomycin	6	1		215, 216
Miscellaneous				
AMSA	19	1	5	217
Cycloleucine	7	2		215
AZQ	20	0	0	218
Biologicals				
BCG (after surgery)	30		Inevaluable	219
RNA (intrapleural)	10	8	80	220
Interferon				
α	13	2	15	221
β	14	0		222
γ (intrapleural)	99	24 (7 CR)	24	223–226
γ (intrapleural)	10	0		225
Interleukin-2 (intrapleural)	24	10	42	225, 227, 228

CR, complete response.

TABLE 43–5. Reported Therapeutic Combinations in Series With More Than 15 Patients

Agents Used	*No. of Patients Evaluable*	*No. of Patients Responding*	*Response (%)*	*References*
Doxorubicin-containing Combinations				
5-Azacytadine	36	8	27	87, 216, 231
Ifosfamide	27	5	19	232, 233
Cisplatin	54	14	26	230, 234–236
Cisplatin, bleomycin, mitomycin	25	(1 CR) 11	44	237
Cyclophosphamide ± DTIC	81	6	7	229, 238
Cyclophosphamide, DTIC, vincristine	30	8	21	181, 239, 240
Radiotherapy	24	4	16	87, 161
Nondoxorubicin-containing Combinations				
Cisplatin, etoposide	26	3	12	241
Cisplatin, pirarubicin	39	6	15	166, 242
Cisplatin, mitomycin C	32	10	31	230, 243
Rubidizone, decarbazine	23	0	0	244

hematoporphyrin ether. Theoretically, when the sensitizer that is retained by residual tumor tissue is activated by 630-mm light from two argon pump dye lasers, the resulting photochemical reaction results in cytotoxicity. First-generation light dosimetry has been developed for this technique, and total hemothorax illumination uses light-dispersing media. These trials may lead to the use of water-soluble chemoluminescent compounds as a source of photon delivery.

The use of intraoperative brachytherapy to give a boost dose of radiation to residual areas of gross disease after surgical resection has theoretical appeal because of the opportunity to deliver higher doses to residual disease while sparing normal tissue.[64,245] Forty-one patients were treated between 1976 and 1982 with aggressive surgical exploration, permanent ^{125}I implantation if the volume of residual disease was small (4 patients), or temporary ^{192}Ir implantation if disease was more diffuse (11 patients). Nine patients underwent complete resection of all gross disease, and boost was not attempted. Seven patients also had installation of ^{32}P 5 to 7 days postoperatively. All patients received 4500 cGy of external-beam irradiation to the entire hemithorax 4 to 6 weeks postoperatively with a mixed photon-electron technique to minimize the dose to the lung parenchyma. Some patients also received chemotherapy. The median survival for all patients was 21 months (range, 6–32 months), with 2-year survival of 40%. Disease-free survival was only 13% at 2 years. Isolated local failures occurred in 7 (17%), and 22 patients had distant failures. Four patients developed complications of radiotherapy (*e.g.*, pneumonitis, pulmonary fibrosis, pericardial effusion, esophagitis). In principle, intraoperative electron-beam or brachytherapy boosts may improve local control; in practice, little advantage has been demonstrated. The median time to appearance of a local recurrence in this series was 9 months.

A large nonrandomized series from Hamburg has shown some prolongation of life expectancy with multimodal treatment compared with best supportive care.[246] Ninety-three patients younger than 71 years of age with malignant pleural mesothelioma, a Karnofsky performance status greater than 60, and no other major medical problems underwent aggressive multimodal treatment or best supportive care according to patient preference. Aggressive treatment included surgery (*i.e.*, parietal pleurectomy or extrapleural pneumonectomy) if possible, followed by doxorubicin, vindesine, and cyclophosphamide. Of the 57 patients in the aggressive treatment group who were in partial or complete remission without progression at the completion of the chemotherapy, 16 received 4500 to 6000 cGy using rotating tangential technique to areas of original extension of tumor. The median survival in the treated patients was 13 months, compared with 7 for those receiving best supportive care. The treated patients, however, were younger, had a better performance status at presentation, and were more amenable to surgery.

Combined radiotherapy and chemotherapy may be more effective than radiotherapy or chemotherapy alone. Theoretically, cisplatin or doxorubicin can be used as a radiosensitizer. A small group of South African patients treated with doxorubicin and radiation of 1000 cGy every 6 weeks for four courses survived a median of 23 months.

MALIGNANT PERITONEAL MESOTHELIOMA

PRESENTATION AND DIAGNOSIS

Patients usually present with symptoms and signs of advanced disease, including pain, ascites, weight loss, or an abdominal mass.[247–249] A tumor in the omentum may be palpable as an epigastric mass.

No satisfactory staging system has been proposed for peritoneal mesothelioma, which is usually confined to the abdomen at diagnosis. Chest radiographs reveal pleural plaques in about 50% of patients with peritoneal primaries, compared with 20% in patients with pleural mesothelioma, reflecting the higher level of asbestos exposure in patients with peritoneal disease. Classic findings on CT scan include mesenteric thickening, peritoneal studding, hemorrhage within the tumor mass, and ascites, but patients may have advanced disease with relatively normal CT scans.[250–252] MRI offers the possibility of improved resolution. Given the low incidence of bone, brain, or liver metastasis at presentation, extensive evaluation for metastatic disease is inappropriate without laboratory test abnormalities. Adrenal, intrapulmonary, or bony metastases should raise the possibility of an alternative diagnosis.

Peritoneal fluid from malignant ascites may be a watery transudate or a viscous fluid rich in mucopolysaccharides. No diagnostic significance has been attached to the character of the fluid, although a viscous ascites with high fluid hyaluronidase levels may suggest the diagnosis. Massive ascites may result in confusion of mesothelioma with severe cirrhosis. Cytologic analysis establishes the diagnosis for only 5% to 10% of patients.[249] Definitive diagnosis requires adequate tissue sampling, preferably from peritinoscopy or an open, visually directed biopsy. A generous biopsy specimen is required to perform immunohistochemical stains and electron microscopy. Open biopsy permits inspection of the abdominal cavity for extent of disease with particular attention to the bowel and ovaries to differentiate mesothelioma from more common causes of peritoneal carcinomatosis. Peritoneal mesotheliomas can be confused with adenocarcinomas arising from any abdominal organ, but the pattern of spread and tendency to accumulate in the pelvis readily leads to confusion with adenocarcinoma of the ovary or carcinoma arising from mullerian duct remnants in the peritoneum.

The tumor usually remains confined to the abdomen until late in the course, and even then, it is more likely to spread to one or both pleural cavities than to disseminate hematogenously. Thrombocytosis is common and associated with a poor prognosis. Other common clotting abnormalities include phlebitis, emboli, hemolytic anemia, and disseminated intravascular coagulation. Most patients die without metastases or involvement of the chest.[249] Esophageal achalasia, secondary amyloidosis, and dermatomyositis have been reported.[253–255] The median survival of untreated patients in most series is 4 to 12 months.[95,247,248,256]

PATHOLOGY

Rare, well-differentiated papillary variants found in younger woman and a syndrome of recurrent peritoneal mesothelial cysts have been associated with a prolonged survival despite bulky disease.[257,258] The disease rarely progresses over time to a typical malignant mesothelioma.[259] Treatment should be provided only with clearly documented progression.[259–261]

Multilocular peritoneal inclusion cysts (*i.e.,* cystic mesotheliomas) are associated with prior surgery, endometriosis, or pelvic inflammatory disease.[262] Although predominantly affecting women, men have been affected.[263–267] Local recurrences develop in about half of the patients. Neither lesion size nor proliferation correlate with outcome.[262] Some investigators advocated classifying this lesion as reactive proliferation rather than as malignant.[262]

THERAPY

Surgery

Surgical and autopsy series have shown that peritoneal mesothelioma involves all peritoneal surfaces, often with masses of 5 cm or more.[268,269] Sites of local invasion included the liver, abdominal wall, diaphragm, retroperitoneum, gastrointestinal tract, and bladder. Seeding of laparotomy scars and biopsy tracts has been observed. The tumor is usually confined to the peritoneal cavity at the time of initial diagnosis and remains there for much or all of the subsequent clinical course.[95] Effective local therapy may have a substantial impact on the survival of patients with this disease. Complete surgical resection is rarely feasible and has not been shown to afford survival benefit without additional therapy. Nevertheless, surgical intervention can provide palliation for small bowel obstruction and relief of massive ascites by peritovenous shunting or paracentesis with a Tenckhoff catheter.[270]

Radiation Therapy

Despite its use in the few reported survivors in this disease, the role of radiation therapy remains unclear. Megavoltage external radiotherapy can deliver a homogeneous dose to the entire abdominal cavity and its contents, although critical organ tolerance limits dose in several areas. Several techniques have been described and used predominantly for the therapy of ovarian carcinoma.[271] The first report was the moving-strip technique, which was necessary because of limited field size and dose rate with ^{60}Co units but which was shown to have a higher morbidity than the open-field techniques.[272] The technique reported from the Joint Center for Radiation Therapy (JCRT) uses open fields with a 67% transmission block to attenuate the dose given to the abdomen superior to the L5–S1 interspace.[273] The superior border of the field is placed above the maximal excursion of the diaphragm by 1 to 2 cm as observed by fluoroscopy. The inferior border is placed at the ischial tuberosities. Laterally, the field extends 1 to 2 cm beyond the properitoneal fat stripe. Daily fractions of 120 cGy in the upper abdomen and 180 cGy in the pelvis are given 5 times weekly to opposed anterior and posterior fields, with both fields treated daily. Doses are prescribed to midplane on the central axis. Total doses of 3000 cGy in the upper abdomen and 4500 cGy in the pelvis are given in 5 weeks. Full-thickness kidney blocks are added to anterior and posterior fields after 1800 cGy. When intraperitoneal chemotherapy is used, the transmission block is omitted and a uniform daily dose of 120 cGy is given to a total dose of 3000 cGy. Blocks are also placed over a portion of the heart and the inferior pelvis lateral to the abdominal cavity to protect the femoral heads and soft tissue. Treatment breaks are given when the total leukocyte count drops to 1500 to 2000/μl or the platelet count drops below 75 to 100,000/μl.

Intraperitoneal instillation of radioactive colloidal gold (^{198}Au) was first reported to improve the symptoms of peritoneal mesothelioma in 1955.[274] Nine other patients treated by the administration of colloidal ^{198}Au have been reported.[182] Two of nine were disease free for 3.5 and 5 years, respectively. Four other patients had clinical improvement of symptoms. The concentration of radiocolloid is generally greatest in the pelvis and lateral gutters, but adhesions from prior surgery and tumor can cause adherence of loops of bowel that may result in inhomogenous spread of the radiocolloid.[181,275] Neither ^{198}Au nor ^{32}P give substantial dose to tumor cells within gross tumor masses. The estimated dose from 20 mCi of ^{32}P is 18,000 cGy at 0.04 mm but only 4300 cGy at 1 mm and 1700 cGy at 2 mm.[276] The distribution of a radiotracer or contrast material should be tested before the therapeutic administration of these agents. The major complication associated with intraperitoneal instillation of radiocolloids is small bowel obstruction, which occurs in 2% to 10% of patients.[277,278] If external-beam irradiation is also given to the pelvis, as many as 33% of patients may develop bowel complications.[273,279]

Chemotherapy

Because the results of intravenous chemotherapy in patients with malignant mesothelioma have been disappointing and because there is a tendency for the disease to remain confined to the peritoneum, interest has focused on the use of intraperitoneal chemotherapy. The primary theoretical obstacle to this form of treatment is the shallow depth of drug penetration into tumor nodules. Advantages include greatly enhanced drug concentrations in the peritoneal cavity and decreased systemic toxicity. Substantial intravenous drug concentrations are obtained from peritoneal absorption of some drugs like cisplatin. The combination of free-surface diffusion and intracapillary drug flow may be more effective than intravenous treatment alone. Intraperitoneal cisplatin and intravenous thiosulfate protection resulted in a 59% complete response rate, but many patients relapsed quickly after treatment, implying incomplete eradication of tumor using cisplatin alone. Mitomycin C, doxorubicin, and epidoxorubicin have been used intraperitoneally.[248,280,281]

Combined-Modality Approaches

Because surgery or radiotherapy alone have resulted in only a few anecdotal long-term mesothelioma survivors, intensive combined-modality approaches are being studied at several institutions. One of four patients treated at Seattle with surgery, radiotherapy, and chemotherapy had no tumor as assessed by follow-up CT scan at the time of publication.[282]

Three sequential series of patients were treated at the Dana-Farber Cancer Institute and JCRT with surgery, radiotherapy, and chemotherapy. One of 3 patients treated with surgery, intravenous cyclophosphamide, doxorubicin, and DTIC (before and after whole-abdominal radiotherapy) remains alive and well 10 years after diagnosis.[248] Patients treated on a phase I trial between 1982 and 1985 were initially evaluated by computerized tomography. The protocol surgeon was unwilling to attempt resection in 7 of 13 patients with bulky tumors. The remaining 6 patients underwent resection of all lesions larger than 1 cm in diameter and placement of a Tenchkoff catheter or a Portacath intraperitoneal access device. Two of the 6 patients had received prior debulking surgery and intravenous chemotherapy. They then received doxorubicin (20–50 mg) total dose and cisplatin (20–100 mg/m^2) separately administered intraperitoneally for a total of 8 to 12 treatments. At the time of second laparotomy for removal of the access device, all 6 patients had at least an objective 50% decrease in the size of the tumor. (None of the seven patients who presented with inoperable tumor had more than a minimal response to intravenous or intraperitoneal chemotherapy.) Chemotherapy was followed by whole-abdominal irradiation in 5 patients. One patient did not receive irradiation because of prior limited-field irradiation for Hodgkin's disease. Currently, 4 of the 6 patients (including 3 of 5 who received irradiation) remain disease-free 8 to 10 years after diagnosis.[248,256] One patient currently requires chronic intravenous hyperalimentation due to malabsorption, but the remaining 3 patients have normal performance status.

A phase II trial began in 1986.[256] Twenty patients have completed therapy. The median survival for the entire treated group is 16.4 months. Intensive multimodality therapy produces a high response rate and may ultimately prolong survival for this otherwise rapidly fatal disease.

MALIGNANT MESOTHELIOMA OF THE TUNICA VAGINALIS TESTIS

There are about 37 cases of malignant mesothelioma of the tunical vaginalis testis reported in the literature.[283,284] Asbestos exposure was documented in about half of the more recently reported cases. Patients usually present with a hydrocele or "hernia." There may be diffuse peritoneal or abdominal lymph node involvement at diagnosis. Mesotheliomas arising in the tunica vaginalis testes appear to have a more indolent disease course.[283,285–287]

MALIGNANT MESOTHELIOMA OF THE PERICARDIUM

There are just over 100 cases of malignant mesothelioma of the pericardium reported in the literature.[288] Asbestos exposure has not been documented in most patients. Children with pericardial mesothelioma have been reported.[289] Patients usually present with a pericardial effusion, congestive heart failure, an anterior mediastinal mass, or tamponade.[288–292] Diffuse pericardial involvement is found at surgery. The diagnosis is often unsuspected before surgery or autopsy.[293–295]

BENIGN MESOTHELIOMA

Benign tumors involving mesothelium arise with some frequency in the pleura and peritoneum, the tunica vaginalis testis, the atrioventricular node of the heart, and rarely in the mediastinum, liver, and adrenal.[296–301] Those of peritoneum, including tunica vaginalis testis and adrenal, are mesothelial derived, but the others are of disputed histogenesis (*e.g.*, atrioventricular node) or appear to arise from submesothelial mesenchymal cells that do not exhibit mesothelial differentiation.

BENIGN FIBROUS TUMORS OF THE PLEURA

Benign fibrous tumors of the pleura are approximately one third as common as diffuse malignant mesotheliomas and are most common in patients between 40 and 70 years of age.[302] Because they appear to arise from subsurface fibrous tissue, rather than from the mesothelial lining, they have also been called submesothelial fibromas, localized fibrous mesothelioma, or solitary fibrous tumor of the pleura.[302–304] Few patients have been exposed to asbestos, approximating the incidence of exposure in the general population. CT scan and MR imaging are useful but non specific. The differential diagnosis between benign and malignant lesions is based on histologic study.[305] Lesions have ranged in diameter from 1 to 36 cm. Associated effusions can be serosanguineous. Hypertrophic pulmonary osteoarthropathy has occurred in about one third of patients, particularly associated with lesions larger than 10 cm. Hypoglycemia has also been associated with large lesions, associated in some cases with tumor production of insulin-like growth factor.[306,307]

Mesotheliomas are often pedunculated, and 80% arise from but usually do not invade the visceral pleura.[97] Benign pleural mesotheliomas usually have a sharp separation between tumor and compressed lung, and resection can be performed without pulmonary resection. Others may require a limited chest wall resection. Although usually cured if completely resected, recurrences have been reported after several decades, and 12% of patients eventually die of extensive local tumor.[59,120,302]

Localized malignant fibrous tumors of the pleura have also been described. Of 82 malignant localized tumors, 45% were cured by simple excision.[97] If the nature of the lesion is ambiguous, involvement of the pleura on random biopsy can establish a diagnosis of diffuse, malignant disease.

BENIGN FIBROUS MESOTHELIOMAS OF THE GENITAL TRACTS

Called benign mesotheliomas in the past, these neoplasms are probably more accurately designated adenomatoid tumors.[308,309] They usually arise in the scrotum and epididymis. Similar tumors histologically also are occasionally described in women. Talc granulomas have been described in proximity to the tumor in one case.[310]

BENIGN MESOTHELIOMA OF THE CARDIAC ATRIOVENTRICULAR NODE

Patients with benign mesotheliomas of the atrioventricular node present most frequently with heart block.[311] Sudden death has been reported despite the implantation of a pacemaker. The diagnosis is often made at autopsy.[312] Patients have ranged newborn to elderly.[313] The histologic origin of the tumor is disputed.[314]

REFERENCES

1. McDonald AD, McDonald JC. Epidemiology of malignant mesothelioma. In: Antman K, Aisner J, eds. Asbestos-related malignancy. Orlando: Grune & Stratton, 1987:31–55.
2. Hogan MD, Hoel DG. Estimated cancer risk associated with occupational asbestos exposure. Risk Analysis 1981;1:67–76.
3. Irving KF, Alexander RG, Bavley H. Asbestos exposures in Massachusetts public schools. Am Ind Hyg Assoc J 1980;41:270.
4. Mossman BT, Bignon J, Corn M, Seaton A, Gee JB. Asbestos: Scientific developments and implications for public policy. Science 1990;247:294–301.
5. Lee DHK, Selikoff IJ. Historical background to the asbestos problem. Environ Res 1979;18:300.
6. Editorial. A physician's guide to asbestos-related diseases. JAMA 1984;252(18):2593–2597.
7. Women Inspectors of Factories. Annual Report for 1898. London: Her Majesty's Stationery Office, 1899.
8. Merewether ERA, Price CV. Report on effects of asbestos dust in the lungs and dust suppression in the asbestos industry. London: Her Majesty's Stationery Office, 1930.
9. Lynch KM, Smith WA. Pulmonary asbestosis. III. Carcinoma of lung in abestosilicosis. Am J Cancer 1935;14:56–64.
10. Gloyne SR. Two cases of squamous carcinoma of the lung occurring in asbestosis. Tubercle 1935;17:5.
11. Doll R. Morality from lung cancer in asbestos workers. Br J Med 1955;12:81.
12. Craighead JE, Mossman BT. The pathogenesis of asbestos-associated disease. N Engl J Med 1982;306:1446.
13. Timbrell V. Physical Factors as etiological mechanisms. In: Biological effects of asbestos. Lyon: International Agency of Research on Cancer, 1973.
14. Stanton MF, Layard M, Tegeris A, EM, May M, Kent E. Carcinogenicity of fibrous glass: Pleural response in relation to fiber dimension. JNCI 1977;58:589–603.
15. Editorial. Asbestos in water. Lancet 1981;2:132.
16. Lee KP, Barras CE, Griffith FD, Waritz RD. Pulmonary response and transmigration of inorganic fibers by inhalation exposure. Am J Pathol 1981;102:314–323.
17. Gibbs AR, Griffiths DM, Pooley FD, Jones JS. Comparison of fibre types and size distributions in lung tissues of paraoccupational and occupational cases of malignant mesothelioma. Br J Ind Med 1990;47:621–626.
18. Rogers AJ, Leigh J, Berry G, Ferguson DA, Mulder HB, Ackad M. Relationship between lung asbestos fiber type and concentration and relative risk of mesothelioma. A case-control study. Cancer 1991;67:1912–1920.
19. Rom WN, Travis WD, Brody AR. Cellular and molecular basis of the asbestos-related diseases. Am Rev Respir Dis 1991;143:408–422.
20. Dazzi H, Hasleton PS, Thatcher N, Wilkes S, Swindell R, Chatterjee AK. Malignant pleural mesothelioma and epidermal growth factor receptor (EGF-R). Relationship of EGF-R with histology and survival using fixed paraffin embedded tissue and the F4, monoclonal antibody. Br J Cancer 1990;61:924–926.
21. Robertson HE. Endothelioma of the pleura. Cancer Res 1924;8:317.
22. Wagner JC, Sleggs EA, Marchand P. Diffuse pleural mesothelioma and asbestos in the North Western Cape Province. Br J Ind Med 1960;17:260.
23. Connelly RR, Spirtas R, Myers MH, Percy CL, Fraumeni JF. Demographic patterns for mesothelioma in the United States. JNCI 1987;78:1053.
24. Enterline PE, Henderson VL. Geographic Patterns for female pleural mesothelioma deaths for 50 states. JNCI 1987;79:1.
25. Walker AM, Loughlin JE, Freidlander ER, Rothman KJ, Dreyer NA. Projections of asbestos-related disease 1980–2009. J Occup Med 1983;25:409–425.
26. Selikoff IJ, Hammonds EC, Seidman H. Mortality experience of insulation workers in the United States and Canada, 1943–76. Ann N Y Acad Sci 1979;330:195–203.
27. Selikoff IJ, Hammond EC, Seidman H. Latency of asbestos disease among insulation workers in the United States and Canada. Cancer 1980;46:2736–2740.
28. Wagner JC, Sleggs EA, Marchand P. The effects of the inhalation of asbestos in rats. Br J Cancer 1974;29:252–269.
29. Wagner JC, Berry G, Polley FD. Mesotheliomas and asbestos type in asbestos textile workers: A study of lung contents. Br Med J 1982;285:603–606.
30. Anderson HA, Lilis R, Daum SM, Fischbein AS, Selikoff IJ. Household-contact asbestos neoplastic risk. Ann N Y Acad Sci 1976;271:311–323.
31. McNeil BJ, Eddy DM. The costs and effects of screening for cancer among asbestos-exposed workers. J Chron Dis 1982;35:351.
32. Selikoff IJ, Churg J, Hammond EC. Asbestos exposure and neoplasia. JAMA 1964;188:142.
33. Carey TS, Hadler NM. The role of the primary physician in disability determination for social security insurance and workers' compensation. Ann Intern Med 1986;104:706–710.
34. Churg A. Fiber counting and analysis in the diagnosis of asbestos-related disease. Hum Pathol 1982;13:381.
35. Thomson JG, Kaschula ROC, MacDonald RR. Asbestos as a modern urban hazard. Afr Med J 1963;37:77.
36. Li FP, Lokich J. Familial mesothelioma after intense asbestos exposure at home. JAMA 1978;240:467.
37. Risberg B, Nickels J, Wagermark J. Familial clustering of malignant mesothelioma. Cancer 1980;45:2422.
38. Vianna NJ, Polan AK. Non-occupational exposure to asbestos and malignant mesothelioma in females. Lancet 1978;1:1061–1063.
39. Lechner D. Effects of asbestos on cultured human lung epithelial and mesothelioma cells. Proc Am Assoc Cancer Res [Abstract 228] 1983;24:58.
40. Mossman BT, Craighead JE. Asbestos-induced epithelial changes in organ cultures of hamster trachea: Inhibition by retinyl methyl ether. Science 1980;207:311.
41. Gibbs AR, Jones JS, Pooley FD, Griffiths DM, Wagner JC. Non-occupational malignant mesotheliomas. IARC Sci Publ 1989;90:219–228.
42. Antman KH, Corson JM, Li FP, et al. Malignant mesothelioma following radiation exposure. J Clin Oncol 1983;1:695–700.
43. Horie A, Hiraoka K, Yamamoto O, et al. An autopsy case of peritoneal malignant mesothelioma in a radiation technologist. Acta Pathol Jpn 1990;40:57–62.
44. Kawashima A, Libshitz HI, Lukeman JM. Radiation-induced malignant pleural mesothelioma. Can Assoc Radiol J 1990;41:384–386.
45. Lerman Y, Learman Y, Schachter P, et al. Radiation associated malignant pleural mesothelioma. Thorax 1991;46:463–464.
46. Artvinli M, Baris YI. Malignant mesothelioma in a small village in the Anatolian region of Turkey: An epidemiologic study. JNCI 1979;63:17.
47. Suzuki Y. Malignant mesothelioma induced by asbestos and zeolite in the mouse peritoneum. Proc Am Assoc Cancer Res 1983;24:240.

48. Gardner MJ, Saracci R. Effects on health of non-occupational exposure to airborne mineral fibres. IARC Sci Publ 1989;90:375–397.
49. Kane MJ, Chahinian AP, Holland JF. Malignant mesothelioma in young adults. Cancer 1990;65:1449–1455.
50. Antman K, Blum R, Greenberger J, et al. Multimodality therapy for mesothelioma based on a study of natural history. Am J Med 1980;68:356–362.
51. Bellocq JP, Chenard NM, Marcellin L, et al. [Malignant peritoneal mesothelioma in a child. Diagnostic difficulties in a locally "non tumoral" form, revealed by cervical lymph node metastasis.] Arch Anat Cytol Pathol 1989;37:240–247.
52. Bento L, Martinez MA, Conde J, Bardaji C, Montes M, Gonzalez A. Mesothelial cysts of the peritoneum in children. Cir Pediatr 1989;2:140–142.
53. Cooper SP, Fraire AE, Buffler PA, Greenberg SD, Langston C. Epidemiologic aspects of childhood mesothelioma. Pathol Immunopathol Res 1989;8:276–286.
54. Geary WA, Mills SE, Frierson HJ, Pope TL. Malignant peritoneal mesothelioma in childhood with long-term survival. Am J Clin Pathol 1991;95:493–498.
55. Lin CM, Lee Y, Ho MY. Malignant mesothelioma in infancy. Arch Pathol Lab Med 1989;113:409–411.
56. Tewari SC, Kurian G, Jayaswal R, Chakravorty S, Chadha SK, Chauhan MS. Malignant mesothelioma in the young (with prosthetic aortic valve an unusual association). J Assoc Physicians India 1989;37:187–189.
57. Grant DC, Seltzer SE, Antman KH, et al. Computer tomography of malignant pleural mesothelioma. J Comput Assist Tomogr 1983;7:626.
58. Mirvis S, Dutcher JP, Haney PJ, et al. CT of malignant pleural mesothelioma. AJR 1983;140:665.
59. Antman KH. Clinical presentation and natural history of benign and malignant mesothelioma. Semin Oncol 1981;8:313–320.
60. Shearn JC, Jackson D. Malignant pleural mesothelioma: Report of 19 cases. J Thorac Cardiovasc Surg 1981;31:53.
61. Menzies R, Charbonneau M. Thoracoscopy for the diagnosis of pleural disease. Ann Intern Med 1991;114:271–276.
62. DaValle MJ, Faber LP, Kittle CF. Extrapleural pneumonectomy for diffuse, malignant mesothelioma. Ann Thorac Surg 1986;42:612.
63. Roggli VL, Greenberg SD, McLarty JL, et al. Asbestos body content of the larynx in asbestos workers: A study of five cases. Arch Otolaryngol 1980;106:533.
64. Martini N, McCormach PM, Baines MS, et al. Pleural mesothelioma. Ann Thorac Surg 1987;43:113.
65. Kannerstein M, Churg C, McCaughery WTE, eds. Asbestos and mesothelioma: A review. New York: Appleton-Century-Crofts, 1978:81.
66. Kannerstein M, Churg J. A critique of the criteria for the diagnosis of diffuse malignant mesothelioma. Mt. Sinai J Med 1977;44:485.
67. Elmes PC, Simpson M. The clinical aspects of mesothelioma. Q J Med 1976;45:427.
68. Winslow DJ, Taylor HB. Malignant peritoneal mesotheliomas. 1960;13:127.
69. Harwood TR, Grecey DR, Yokoo H. Pseudomesotheliomatous carcinoma of the lung. A variant of peripheral lung carcinoma. Am J Clin Pathol 1976;65:159.
70. Corson J, Pinkus G. Cellular localization patterns of keratin proteins in pleural mesothelioma and metastatic adenocarcinomas a diagnostic discriminant. Lab Invest 1991;64:114A.
71. Suzuki Y, Churg C, Kannerstein M. Ultrastructure of human malignant diffuse mesothelioma. Am J Pathol 1976;85:241.
72. Corson JM, Pinkus GSS. Mesothelioma: Profile of keratin proteins and carcinoembryonic antigen; and immunoperoxidase study of 20 cases and comparison with pulmonary adenocarcinomas. Am J Pathol 1982;108:80.
73. Said J, Nash G, Lee M. Immunoperoxidase localization of keratin, proteins, carcinoembryonic antigen, and factor VIII in adenomatoid tumors: Evidence for a mesothelial derivation. Hum Pathol 1982;13:1106.
74. Bolen JW, Thorning D. Mesotheliomas: A light and electron microscopical study concerning the histogenic relationships between the epithelial and the mesenchymal variants. Am J Surg Pathol 1980;4:451.
75. Warhol WJ, Hickey WF, Corson J. Malignant mesothelioma: Ultrastructural distinction from adenocarcinoma. Am J Surg Pathol 1982;6:307.
76. Warhol MJ, Hunter NJ, Corson JM. An ultrastructural comparison of mesotheliomas and adenocarcinomas of the ovary and endometrium. Int J Gynecol Pathol 1982;1: 125.
77. Butchart EG, Ashcroft T, Barnsley WC, et al. Pleuropneumonectomy in the management of diffuse malignant mesothelioma of the pleura: Experience with 29 patients. Thorax 1976;31:15.
78. Rusch VS, Ginsberg RJ. New concepts in the staging of mesotheliomas. In: Deslauriers J, Lacquet LK, ed. International trends in general thoracic surgery. Vol. 6. St. Louis: CV Mosby, 1990:336–343.
79. Leung AN, Muller NL, Miller RR. CT in differential diagnosis of diffuse pleural disease. AJR 1990;154:487–492.
80. Lorigan JG, Libshitz HI. MR imaging of malignant pleural mesothelioma. J Comput Assist Tomogr 1989;13:617–620.
81. McDonald AD, Magner D, Eyssen G. Primary malignant mesothelial tumors in Canada, 1960–1968. Cancer 1973;31:869.
82. Pluygers E, Badewyns P, Minette P, Beandoin M, Gourdin P. Biomarker assessments in asbestos-exposed workers as indicators for selective prevention of mesothelioma or bronchogenic carcinoma: Rationale and practical implications. Eur J Canc Prev 1991;1.
83. Collins CL, Ordonez NG, Schaefer R, et al. Thrombomodulin expression in malignant pleural mesothelioma and pulmonary adenocarcinoma. Am J Pathol 1992;141(4): 827–833.
84. Nakano T, Maeda J, Iwahashi N, Tamura S, Hada T, Higashino K. Gallium-67 scanning in patients with malignant pleural mesothelioma. Jpn J Med 1990;29:255–260.
85. Weill H. Asbestos-associated diseases. Science, public policy and litigation. Chest 1983;84:601–608.
86. Antman K, Shemin R, Ryan L, et al. Malignant mesothelioma: Prognostic variables in a registry of 180 patients, the Dana-Farber Cancer Institute and Brigham and Women's Hospital experience over two decades 1965–1985. J Clin Oncol 1988;6:147–153.
87. Chahinian AP, Pajak T, Holland J, et al. Diffuse malignant mesothelioma: Prospective evaluation of 69 patients. Ann Intern Med 1982;96:746.
88. Ruffie P, Feld R, Minkin S, et al. Diffuse malignant mesothelioma of the pleura in Ontario and Quebec: A retrospective study of 332 patients. J Clin Oncol 1989;7:1157–1168.
89. Schildge J, Kaiser D, Henss H, Fiebig H, Ortlieb H. [Prognostic factors in diffuse malignant mesothelioma of the pleura.] Pneumologie 1989;43:660–664.
90. Hulks G, Thomas JS, Waclawski E. Malignant pleural mesothelioma in Western Glasgow 1980–86. Thorax 1989;44:496–500.
91. Gordon W, Antman K, Breenberger J, Weichselbaum R, Chaffey J. Radiation therapy in the management of patients with mesothelioma. Int J Radiat Oncol Biol Phys 1982;8: 19.
92. Antman KH. Malignant mesothelioma. N Engl J Med 1980;303:200–202.
93. Wojtukiewicz MZ, Zacharski RL, Memoli VA, et al. Absence of components of coagulation and fibrinolysis pathways in situ in mesothelioma. Thromb Res 1989;55:279–284.
94. De Pangher, Manzini V, Brollo A, Bianchi C. Thrombocytosis in malignant pleural mesothelioma. Tumori 1990;76:576–578.
95. Antman K, Pomfret E, Aisner J, McIntyre J, Osteen RT, Greenberger JS. Peritoneal mesothelioma: Natural history and response to chemotherapy. J Clin Oncol 1983;1: 386–391.
96. McAuley P, Asa SL, Chiu B, Henderson J, Goltzman D, Drucker DJ. Parathyroid hormone-like peptide in normal and neoplastic mesothelial cells. Cancer 1990;66:1975–1979.
97. England DM, Hochholzer L, McCarthy MJ. Localized benign and malignant fibrous tumors of the pleura. A clinicopathologic review of 223 cases. Am J Surg Pathol 1989;13: 640–658.
98. Olofsson K, Mark J. Specificity of asbestos-induced chromosomal aberrations in short-term cultured human mesothelial cells. Cancer Genet Cytogenet 1989;41:33–39.
99. Burmer GC, Rabinovitch PS, Kulander BG, Rusch V, McNutt MA. Flow cytometric analysis of malignant pleural mesotheliomas. Hum Pathol 1989;20:777–783.
100. Dazzi H, Thatcher N, Hasleton PS, Chatterjee AK, Lawson RA. DNA analysis by flow cytometry in malignant pleural mesothelioma: Relationship to histology and survival. J Pathol 1990;162:51–55.
101. Pyrhonen S, Laasonen A, Tammilehto L, et al. Diploid predominance and prognostic significance of S-phase cells in malignant mesothelioma. Eur J Cancer 1991;27:197–200.
102. Tierney G, Wilkinson MJ, Jones JS. The malignancy grading method is not a reliable assessment of malignancy in mesothelioma. J Pathol 1990;160:209–211.
103. Tiainen M, Tammilehto L, Rautonen J, Tuomi T, Mattson K, Knuutila S. Chromosomal abnormalities and their correlations with asbestos exposure and survival in patients with mesothelioma. Br J Cancer 1989;60:618–626.
104. Fletcher JA, Weidner N, Corson JM. Laboratory investigation and genetics in sarcomas. Curr Opin Oncol 1990;2:467–473.
105. Fletcher J, Cibas E, Granados R, et al. Consistent chromosome aberrations and genetic stability in malignant mesotheliomas: Diagnostic relevance. Proc US Can Acad Pathol [Abstract]1991;64:114.
106. Decker HJ, Li FP, Bixenman HA, Sandberg AA. Chromosome 3 and 12p rearranged in a well-differentiated peritoneal mesothelioma. Cancer Genet Cytogenet [Letter] 1990;46:135–137.
107. Flejter WL, Li FP, Antman KH, Testa JR. Recurring loss involving chromosomes 1, 3, and 22 in malignant mesothelioma: Possible sites of tumor suppressor genes. Genes Chromosom Cancer 1989;1:148–154.
108. Hagemeijer A, Versnel MA, Van DE, et al. Cytogenetic analysis of malignant mesothelioma. Cancer Genet Cytogenet 1990;47:1–28.
109. Hillerdal G, Lindqvist U, Engstrom AL. Hyaluronan in pleural effusions and in serum. Cancer 1991;67:2410–2414.
110. Demetri GD, Zenzie BW, Rheinwald JG, Griffin JD. Expression of colony-stimulating factor genes by normal human mesothelial cells and human malignant mesothelioma cells lines in vitro. Blood 1989;74:940–946.
111. Nakamura Y, Ozaki T, Yanagawa H, Yasuoka S, Ogura T. Eosinophil colony-stimulating factor induced by administration of interleukin-2 into the pleural cavity of patients with malignant pleurisy. Am J Respir Cell Mol Biol 1990;3:291–300.
112. Okazaki H, Kano S, Hatake K, et al. [A case of malignant pleural mesothelioma producing colony-stimulating factor (CSF).] Nippon Naika Gakkai Zasshi 1989;78:506–511.
113. Jordon D, Jagirdar J, Kaneko M. Blood group antigens, Lewisx and Lewisy in the diagnostic discrimination of malignant mesothelioma versus adenocarcinoma. Am J Pathol 1989;135:931–937.
114. Kawai T, Suzuki M, Torikata C, Suzuki Y. Expression of blood group-related antigens and *Helix pomatia* agglutinin in malignant pleural mesothelioma and pulmonary adenocarcinoma. Hum Pathol 1991;22:118–124.
115. Ruffie P, Feld R, Minkin S, et al. Diffuse malignant mesothelioma of the pleura in Ontario and Quebec: A retrospective study of 331 patients. J Clin Oncol 1990;45:40–42.
116. Harvey JC, Fleischman EH, Kagan R, Streeter OE. Malignant pleural mesothelioma: A survival study. J Surg Oncol 1990;45:40–42.
117. Law MR, Hodson ME, Turner-Warurch M. Malignant mesothelioma of the pleura: Clinical aspects and symptomatic treatment. Eur J Respir Dis 1984;65:162.

118. Woern H. Mopeglichkeiten und Ergebnisse der chirurgischen Behandlung des malignen Pleuramesotheliomas. Thoraxchirurgie 1974;22:339–356.
119. Bamler KJ, Maassen W. Malignant pleura mesotheliomas. Thoraxchirurgie 1974;22: 386.
120. DeLaria G, Jensik R, Faber LP, Kittle CF. Surgical management of malignant mesothelioma. Ann Thorac Surg 1978;26:375.
121. Voyt-Moykopf I, Etspule W, Bulzebruck H. Das diffuse meligne pleuramesotheliom: Diagnostik, therapie and prognose. Z Herz Thorac Gefabchir 1987;1:67–77.
122. Faber LP. Surgical treatment of asbestos related disease of the chest. Surg Clin North Am 1988;68:525–530.
123. Probst G, Buelzebruck H, Bauer H, Branscheld HG, Vogt-Moykopf I. The role of pleuropneumonectomy in the treatment of diffuse malignant mesothelioma of the pleura. In: Deslauriers J, Lacquet LK, eds. Thoracic surgery: Surgical management of pleural diseases. St. Louis: CV Mosby, 1990:344–350.
124. Geroulanos S, Lampe P, Hafner F, Buchmann P, Largiader F. Malignant pleural mesothelioma: Diagnosis, therapy and prognosis. Schweiz Rundsch Med Prax 1990;79: 361–367.
125. Rusch VW, Piantadose S, Holmes EC. The role of extrapleural pneumonectomy in malignant pleural mesothelioma. A Lung Cancer Study Group trial. J Thorac Cardiovsc Surg 1991;102:1–9.
126. Sugarbaker DJ, Lee TH, Coupe G, et al. Extrapelural pneumonectomy, chemotherapy and radiotherapy in the treatment of diffuse malignant pleural mesothelioma. J Thorac Cardiovasc Surg 1991;102:10–15.
127. Law MR, Gregor A, Hodson ME, Bloom HJG, Turner-Warwick M. Malignant mesothelioma of the pleura: A study of 52 untreated patients. Thorax 1984;39:255–259.
128. Brancatisano RR, Joseph MG, McCaughan BC. Pleurectomy for mesothelioma. Med J Aust 1991;154:455–457.
129. Lewis RJ, Sisler GE, Mackenzie JW. Diffuse mixed malignant pleural mesothelioma. Ann Thoracic Surg 1981;3:153–160.
130. Carmichael J, Degraff WG, Gamson J, et al. Radiation sensitivity of human lung cancer cell lines. Eur J Cancer Clin Oncol 1989;25:527–534.
131. Maasilta P. Deterioration in lung function following hemithorax irradiation for pleural mesothelioma. Int J Radiat Oncol Biol Phys 1991;20:433–438.
132. Ehrenhaft JL, Sensenig DM, Lawrence MS. Mesotheliomas of the pleura. J Thorac Cardiovasc Surg 1960;40:393–409.
133. Eschwege F, Schlienger M. La Radiotherapie des mesotheliomes pleuraux malins: A propos de 14 cas irradies a dose elevees. J Radiol Electrol 1973;54:255–259.
134. Dobelbower RR, Strubler KA, Vaisman I. Clinical applications of high energy electron beams: The pancreas, pleura, and spine. In: High energy electrons in radiation therapy. Berlin: Springer-Verlag, 1980:91–97.
135. Alberts AS, Falkson G, Goedhals L, et al. Malignant pleural mesothelioma: A disease unaffected by current therapeutic maneuvers. J Clin Oncol 1988;6:527–535.
136. Ball DL, Cruickshank DG. The treatment of malignant mesothelioma of the pleura: Review of a 5-year experience, with special reference to radiotherapy. Am J Clin Oncol 1990;13:4–9.
137. Wanebo HJ, Martini N, Melamed MR, Hilaris B, Beattie EJ. Pleural mesothelioma. Cancer 1986;38:2481–2488.
138. Todoroki T, Suit HD. Effect of fractionated irradiation prior to conservative and radical surgery on therapeutic gain in a spontaneous fibrosarcoma of the C3H mouse. J Surg Oncol 1986;31:279–286.
139. Boutin C, Irrisson M, Rathelot P, Petite JM. L'extension parietale des mesotheliomas pleu raux malins diffus apres biopsies: Prevention par radiotherapie locale. Presse Med 1983;12:1823.
140. Maasilta P, Kivisaari L, Holsti LR, Tammilehto L, Mattson K. Radiographic chest assessment of lung injury following hemithorax irradiation for pleural mesothelioma. Eur Respir J 1991;4:76–83.
141. Maasilta P, Salonen EM, Vaheri A, Kivisaari L, Holsti LR, Mattson K. Procollagen-III in serum, plasminogen activation and fibronectin in bronchoalveolar lavage fluid during and following irradiation of human lung. Int J Radiat Oncol Biol Phys 1991;20:973–980.
142. Hallman M, Maasilta P, Kivisaari L, Mattson K. Changes in surfactant in bronchoalveolar lavage fluid after hemithorax irradiation in patients with mesothelioma. Am Rev Respir Dis 1990;141:998–1005.
143. Richart R, Sherman CD. Prolonged survival in diffuse pleural mesothelioma treated with Au198. Cancer 1959;12:799–805.
144. Brady LW. Mesothelioma the role for radiation therapy. Semin Oncol 1981;8:329–334.
145. Bricout PB, Engler MJ. Computerized tomography scanning and the planning of high-dose radiotherapy for pleural mesothelioma: A report of five patients. Int J Radiat Oncol Biol Phys 1981;7:821–826.
146. Rusch VW, Godwin JD, Shuman WP. The role of computed tomography scanning in the initial assessment and the follow-up of the malignant pleural mesothelioma. J Thorac Cardiovasc Surg 1988;96:171–177.
147. Shimojo M, Tsuda N, Kamihata H, et al. [Magnetic resonance imaging for cardiovascular masses.] J Cardiol 1989;19:583–592.
148. Kutcher GJ, Kestler C, Greenblatt D, et al. Technique for external beam treatment for mesothelioma. Int J Radiat Oncol Biol Phys 1987;13:1747–1752.
149. Soubra M, Dunscombe PB, Hodson DI, et al. Physical aspects of external beam radiotherapy for the treatment of malignant pleural mesothelioma. Int J Radiat Oncol Biol Phys 1990;18:1521–1527.
150. Takahashi K, Purdy J, Liu YY. Work in progress: Treatment planning system for conformation radiotherapy. Radiology 1983;147:567–573.
151. Blake PR, Catterall M, Emerson PA. Pleural mesothelioma treated by fast neutron therapy. Thorax 1985;40:72–73.
152. Bonadonna G, Beretta G, Tancini G, et al. Adriamycin studies at the Instituto Nazionale Tumori, Milan. Cancer Chemother Rep 1975;6:231–245.
153. Benjamin RS, Wiernik PH, Bachur NR. Adriamycin: A new effective agent in the therapy of disseminated sarcomas. Med Pediatr Oncol 1975;1:63–67.
154. Gerner RE, Moore GE. Chemotherapy of malignant mesothelioma. Oncology 1974;30: 152–1555.
155. Gottlieb JA, Baker LH, O'Bryan RM, et al. Adriamycin (NSC 123127) used alone and in combination for soft tissue and bony sarcomas. Cancer Chemother Rep 1975;6: 271–282.
156. Harvey VJ, Slevin ML, Ponder BA, et al. Chemotherapy of diffuse malignant mesothelioma: Phase II trials of single-agent 5-fluorouracil and Adriamycin. Cancer 1984;54: 961–964.
157. Kucuksu N, Thomas W, Ezdinli E. Chemotherapy of malignant diffuse mesothelioma. Cancer 1976;37:1265–1274.
158. Lerner H, Amato D, Shiraki M, et al. A prospective study of Adriamycin programs in malignant mesothelioma. Proc Am Soc Clin Oncol [Abstract C-901] 1983;2:230.
159. Mischler NE, Chuprevich T, Johnson RO, et al. Malignant mesothelioma presenting in the pleura and peritoneum. J Surg Oncol 1979;11:185–191.
160. O'Bryan RM, Luce JK, Talley RW, et al. Phase II evaluation of adriamycin in human neoplasia. Cancer 1973;32:1–8.
161. Stock RJ, Fu YS, Carter JR. Malignant peritoneal mesothelioma following radiotherapy for seminoma of the testis. Cancer 1979;44:914–919.
162. Van Dyk JJ, VanDer AM. Adriamycin in the treatment of cancer. S Afr Med J 1976;50: 61–66.
163. Ruffie P, Salomon C, Herait P, et al. Phase II study of THP-Adriamycin (THP-A) in malignant pleural mesothelioma (MPM). Presented at the First International Mesothelioma Conference. Paris, 1991:40.
164. Kaukel E, Koschel G, Gatzemeyer U, Salewski E. A phase II study of pirarubicin in malignant pleural mesothelioma. Cancer 1990;66:651–654.
165. Sridhar KS, Hussein AM, Feun LG, Zubrod CG. Activity of pirarubicin (4'-0-tetrahydropyranyladriamycin) in malignant mesothelioma. Cancer 1989;63:1084–1091.
166. Koschel G, Calavrezos A, Kaukel E, et al. Phase III randomized comparison of pirarubicin vs. pirarubicin and cisplatin for treatment of pleural mesotheliomas. Proceedings of the Sixth European Congress Against Cancer. 1991;6.
167. Magri MD, Veronesi A, Foladore S, et al. Epirubicin in the treatment of malignant mesothelioma: A phase II cooperative study. The North-Eastern Italian Oncology Group—Mesothelioma Committee. Tumori 1991;77:49–51.
168. Mattson K, Giaccone G, Kirkpatrick A, et al. Epirubicin in malignant mesothelioma: A phase II study of the EORTC lung cancer cooperative group. J Clin Oncol 1992; 10: 824–828.
169. Colbert N, Izrael V, Vannetzel JM, et al. A prospective study of detorubicin in malignant mesothelioma. Am Soc Clin Oncol 1985;4:127.
170. Earhart RH, Amato DJ, Chang AY, et al. Phase II trial of 6-diazo-5-oxo-L-norleucine versus aclacinomycin-A in advanced sarcomas and mesotheliomas. Invest New Drugs 1990;8:113–119.
171. Butt WO. Mesothelioma of the pleura. J Can Assoc Radiol 1962;13:40–49.
172. Di Pietro S, Gennari L. Successful cyclophosphamide treatment in a case of diffuse pleural mesothelioma. Tumori 1963;49:69–73.
173. Hichock HT. Mesothelioma of the pleura. Irish J Med Sci 1970;3:453–456.
174. Yap BS, Benjamin RS, Burgess MA, et al. The value of Adriamycin in the treatment of diffuse malignant pleural mesothelioma. Cancer 1978;42:1692–1696.
175. Alberts AS, Falkson G, Zyl LV. Malignant pleural msothelioma: Phase II pilot study of ifosfamide and mesna. JNCI 1988;80:698–700.
176. Zidar BL, Metch B, Balcerzak SP, et al. A phase II evaluation of ifosfamide and mesna in unresectable diffuse malignant mesothelioma: A Southwest Oncology Group study. Cancer 1992;70:2547–2551.
177. Champion P. Two cases of malignant mesothelioma after exposure to asbestos. Am Rev Respir Dis 1971;103:821–826.
178. Cafrey PF, Lucido JL. The clinical and pathologic aspects of pleural mesotheliomas. Surgery 1961;49:690–695.
179. Gray FW, Tom BCK. Diffuse pleural mesothelioma: A survival of one year following nitrogen mustard therapy. J Thorac Cardiovasc Surg 1962;44:73–77.
180. Jara F, Takita H, Rao UN. Malignant mesothelioma: Clinicopathologic observation. N Y State J Med 1977;77:1885–1888.
181. Kaplan WD, Zimmerman RE, Bloomer WD, Knapp RC. Therapeutic intraperitoneal ^{32}P: A clinical assessment of the dynamics of distribution. 1981;138:683–688.
182. Legha SS, Muggia FM. Pleural mesothelioma: Clinical features and therapeutic implications. Ann Intern Med 1977;87:613–621.
183. McGowan L, Bunnag B, Arias LF. Mesothelioma of the abdomen in women; monitoring of therapy by peritoneal fluid study. Gynecol Oncol 1975;3:10–14.
184. Falkson G, DeVilliers PC, Falkson HC. *N*-isopropyl-L-2-methylhydrazino)-*p*-toluamide hydrochloride (NSC 77213) for the treatment of cancer patients. Cancer Chemother Rep 1965;46:7–16.
185. Kelsen D, Bajorin D, Mintzer D. Phase II trial of mitomycin C in malignant mesothelioma. Am Soc Clin Oncol [Abstract] 1985;4:146.
186. Dabouis G, Le Mevel B, Coroller J. Treatment of diffuse pleural malignant mesothelioma by cisdichlorodiammine platinum in nine patients. Cancer Chemother Pharmacol 1981;5:209–210.
187. Daboys G, Delajartre MB, Le Mevel BP. Treatment of diffuse pleural malignant mesothelioma by *cis*-diaminedichloroplatinum: Preliminary results in eleven patients. Med Oncol Soc Nice France 1979;52:98.
188. Glatstein E, Fuks Z, Bagshaw M. Diaphragmatic treatment in ovarian carcinoma: A new radiotherapeutic technique. Int J Radiat Oncol Biol Phys 1977;2:357–362.

189. Hayes DM, Cvitkovic E, Golbey RB, et al. High dose cisplatinum diaminedichloride. Cancer 1977;39:1372–1381.
190. Mintzer D, Kelson D, Frimmer D, et al. Phase II trial of high dose cisplatin in patients with malignant mesothelioma. Proc Am Soc Clin Oncol 1984;3:258.
191. Rossoff AH, Slayton RE, Perlia CP. Preliminary clinical experience with cisdiamine dichloroplatinum (II) (NSC 119875 CACO). Cancer 1972;30:1451–1456.
192. Samson MK, Baker LH, Benjamin RS, et al. *Cis*-dichlorodiammineplatinnum III in advanced soft tissue and bony sarcomas: A Southwest Oncology Group study. Cancer Treat Rep 1979;63:11–12.
193. Planting A, Goey H, Verweij J. Phase II study of six weekly courses of high dose cisplatin in mesothelioma. Proc Am Assoc Cancer Res [Abstract 1158] 1991;32:194.
194. Raghavan D, Gianoutsos P, Bishop J, et al. Phase II trial of carboplatin in the management of malignant mesothelioma. J Clin Oncol 1990;8:151–154.
195. Vogelzang NJ, Goutsou M, Corson JM, et al. Carboplatin in malignant mesothelioma: A phase II study of the Cancer and Leukemia Group B. Cancer Chemother Pharmacol 1990;27:239–242.
196. Mbidde EK, Harland SJ, Calvert AH, Smith IE. Phase II trial of carboplatin (JM8) in treatment of patients with malignant mesothelioma. Cancer Chemother Pharmacol 1986;18:284–285.
197. Mbidde EK, Smith IE, Harland S. Phase II trial of carboplatin (JM8) in the treatment of patients with mesothelioma (M). Br J Cancer 1986;54:215.
198. Cantwell BMJ, Harris AL, Ghani S. Phase II studies of a novel antifolate CB3717, and the platinum analogues JM8 and JM9, in mesothelioma of pleura and peritoneum. Br J Cancer 1986;54:216.
199. Cantwell BMJ, Franks CR, Harris AL. A phase II study of the platinum analogues JM8 and JM9. Cancer Chemother Pharmacol 1986;18:286–288.
200. Rebattu P, Riou R, Pacheco Y, Clavel M, Perrin-Fayolle M. Phase II study of very high dose cisplatin in the treatment of malignant mesothelioma. Presented at the First International Mesothelioma Conference. Paris, 1991:36.
201. Martensson G, Sorenson S. A phase II study of vincristine in malignant mesothelioma: a negative report. Cancer Chemother Pharmacol 1989;24:133–134.
202. Falkson G, Falkson H. Clinical trial of the oral form 4′-dimethylepipodophyllotoxin-*p*-D-ethylidene glucoside (NSC 141540) and VP-16-213. Am Assoc Cancer Res 1978;1: 160.
203. Nissen NI, Larsen V, Pederson H, et al. Phase I clinical trial of a new antitumor agent, 4′dimethylepipodophyllotoxin-9-(4,6-*O*-ethylidene-beta-D-glucopyranoside) (NSC 141540). Cancer Chemother Rep 1972;56:769–777.
204. Nissen NI, Dombernowsky P, Hansen HH, et al. Phase I clinical trial of an oral solution of VP16-213. Cancer Treat Rep 1976;60:943–945.
205. Smit EF, Berendsen HH, Postmus PE. Etoposide and mesothelioma. J Clin Oncol [Letter] 1990;8:1281.
206. Boutin C, Irisson M, Guerin J, et al. Phase II trial of vindesin on malignant pleural mesothelioma. Cancer Treat Rep 1987;71:205–206.
207. Kelsen D, Gralla R, Chang E. Vindesine in the treatment of malignant mesothelioma: A phase II study. Cancer Treat Rep 1983;67:821–822.
208. Porter JM, Cheek JM. Pleural mesothelioma: Review of tumor histogenesis and report of 12 cases. J Thorac Cardiovasc Surg 1968;55:882–890.
209. Riddell RJ. Three cases of mesothelioma. Med J Aust 1966;2:554–559.
210. Cantwell MJ, Earnshaw M, Harris AL. Phase II study of a novel antifolate, *N*-10-propargyl-5,8-dideazafolic acid (CB3717) in malignant mesothelioma. Cancer Treat Rep 1986;70: 1335–1336.
211. Vogler WR, Arkun S, Valez-Garcia E. Phase I study of twice weekly-azacytidine. Cancer Chemother Rep 1974;58:895–899.
212. Vogler WR, Miller DS, Keller JW. 5-Azacytidine: A new drug for the treatment of myeloblastic leukemia. Blood 1976;48:331–337.
213. Harmon D, Vogelzang N, Roboz J, et al. Dihydro-5-azacytidine (DHAC) in malignant mesothelioma (Meso) using serum hyalluronic acide (SHA) as a tumor marker: A phase II trial of the CALGB. Proc Am Soc Clin Oncol [Abstract 1248] 1991;10:351.
214. Dhingra HM, Murphy WK, Winn RJ, Raber MN, Hong WK. Phase II trial of 5,6-dihydro-5-azacytidine in pleural malignant mesothelioma. Invest New Drugs 1991;9: 69–72.
215. Lerner H, Schoenfeld D, Martin A, Falkson G, Borden E. Malignant mesothelioma: The Eastern Cooperative Oncology Group Experience. Cancer 1983;52:1981–1985.
216. Chahinian AP, Pajak T, Holland J, et al. Evaluation of 63 patients with diffuse malignant mesothelioma. Proc Am Assoc Cancer Res/Am Soc Clin Oncol 1980;21:360.
217. Falkson G, Vorobiof DA, Lerner JH. A phase II study of M-AMSA in patients with malignant mesothelioma with cyclophosphamide, Adriamycin and vincristine. Cancer Chemother Pharmacol 1980;4:135.
218. Eagan R, Frytak S, Richardson R, et al. Phase II trial of diaziquone in malignant mesothelioma. Cancer Treat Rep 1986;70:429.
219. Webster I, Cochrane JWC, Burkhardt KR. Immunotherapy with BCG vaccine in 30 cases of mesothelioma. S Afr Med J 1982;81:277–278.
220. Esposito S. RNA Therapy for pleural mesothelioma. Lancet 1969;2:1203–1204.
221. Christmas TI, Musk AW, Robinson BW. Phase II study of recombinant human alpha interferon therapy in malignant pleural mesothelioma. Proc Am Assoc Cancer Res 1990;31:A1678.
222. Von Hoff DD, Metch B, Lucas JG, Balcerzak SP, Grunberg SM, Rivkin SE. Phase II evaluation of recombinant interferon-beta (IFN-beta ser) in patients with diffuse mesothelioma: A Southwest Oncology Group study. J Interferon Res 1990;10:531–534.
223. Brandely M, Sousell Sante R. A Phase II multicentre study of recombinant interferon (r-IFN-γ) in malignant mesothelioma. Presented at the First International Mesothelioma Conference. [Abstract] Paris, 1991:5.
224. Boutin C, Viallat JR, Astoul P. Treatment of mesothelioma with interferon gamma and interleukin 2. Rev Pneumol Clin 1990;46:211–215.
225. Boutin C. Treatment of malignant mesothelioma using intrapleural gamma interferon. Bull Acad Natl Med [Discussion 427] 1990;174:421–426.
226. Boutin C, Viallat JR, Zandwijk NV, et al. Activity of intrapleural recombinant gamma-interferon in malignant mesothelioma. Cancer 1991;67:2033–2037.
227. Stoter G, Goey SH, Slingerland R, Bolhuis RL, Eggermont AM. Intrapleural interleukin-2 (IL-2) in malignant pleural mesothelioma: A phase I–II study. Proc Am Assoc Cancer Res [Abstract] 1990;31:275.
228. Robinson BWS, Bowman RV, Christmas TI, Manning LS, Musk AW. Clinical experience using immunotherapy (IL-2/LAK cells or interferon alpha 2a) in malignant mesothelioma. Presented at the First International Mesothelioma Conference. Paris, 1991:38.
229. Samson M, Baker L, Wasser L, et al. Randomized comparison of cyclophosphamide, DTIC and adriamycin vs. cyclophosphamide and adriamycin in patients with advanced malignant mesothelioma: A sarcoma intergroup study. Proc Am Soc Clin Oncol 1985;4: 128.
230. Chahinian AP, Antman K, Aisner J, et al. Cisplatin with Adriamycin or mitomycin for malignant mesothelioma: A randomized phase II trial. Proc Am Assoc Clin Oncol [Abstract] 1987;6:183.
231. Chahinian AP, Holland JF. Treatment of diffuse malignant mesothelioma: A review. Mt Sinai J Med 1978;45:54–67.
232. Carmichael J, Cantwell BM, Harris AL. A phase II trial of ifosfamide/mesna with doxorubicin for malignant mesothelioma. Eur J Cancer Clin Oncol 1989;25:911–912.
233. Alberts AS, Falkson G, van ZL. Ifosfamide and mesna with doxorubicin have activity in malignant mesothelioma. Eur J Cancer [Letter; comment] 1990;26:1002.
234. Zidar B, Pugh R, Schiffer L, et al. Treatment of six cases of mesothelioma with doxorubicin and *cis*-platinum. Cancer 1983;52:1788–1791.
235. Ardizzoni A, Rosso R, Salvati F, et al. Activity of doxorubicin and cisplatin combination chemotherapy in patients with diffuse malignant pleural mesothelioma. An Italian Lung Cancer Task Force Phase II study. Cancer 1991;67:2984–2987.
236. Niki Y, Nakayama S, Soga T, et al. [A case of remission induced in diffuse pleural malignant mesothelioma by the treatment with cisplatin and doxorubicin.] Gan To Kagaku Ryoho 1989;16:3635–3638.
237. Breau JL, Boaziz C, Morere JJF, Sadoun D, Israel L. Combination chemotherapy with cisplatinum, Adriamycin, bleomycin and mitomycin C, plus systemic and intrapleural hyaluronidase in 25 consecutive cases of stages II, III pleural mesothelioma. Presented at the First International Mesothelioma Conference. Paris, 1991:5.
238. Dhingra H, Valdivieso M, Tannir N, et al. Combined modality treatment for mesothelioma with Cytoxan, Adriamycin, and DTIC (CYADIC) and adjuvant surgery. Am Soc Clin Oncol [Abstract] 1983;2:205.
239. Spremulli E, Wampler G, Regelson E, et al. Chemotherapy of malignant mesothelioma. Cancer1977;40:2038–2045.
240. Gottlieb JA, Bodney GP, Sinkovics JG, et al. An effective new four-drug combination regimen (CY-VA-DIC) for metastatic sarcomas. Proc Am Assoc Cancer Res/Am Soc Clin Oncol 1974;15:162.
241. Eisenhauer EA, Evans WK, Murray N, Kocha W, Wierzbicki R, Wilson K. A Phase II study of VP-16 and cisplatin in patients with unresectable malignant mesothelioma. An NCI Canada clinical trials group study. Invest New Drugs 1988;6:327–329.
242. Niki Y, Soga T, Nishimura A, et al. [A diffuse, pleural, malignant mesothelioma kept in long remission by chemotherapy combining pirarubicin and cisplatin.] Gan No Rinsho 1990;36:2463–2467.
243. Chahinian AP, Norton L, Szrajer L, et al. Mitomycin C and cisplatin in human malignant mesothelioma xenografts in nude mice: Clinical correlation. Proc Am Assoc Cancer Res [Abstract 597] 1983;24:151.
244. Zidar BL, Benjamin RS, Frank J, et al. Combination chemotherapy for advanced sarcomas of bone and mesothelioma utilizing rubidazone and DTIC: A Southwest Oncology Group Study. Am J Clin Oncol 1983;6:71–74.
245. Hilaris BS, Dattatreyudu NK, Wong E, Kutcher GJ, Martini N. Pleurectomy and intraoperative brachytherapy and postoperative radiation in the management of malignant pleural mesothelioma. Int J Radiat Oncol Biol Phys 1984;10:325–331.
246. Calavrezos A, Koschel G, Husselmann H, et al. Malignant mesothelioma of the pleura. Klin Wochenschr 1988;66:607–635.
247. Moertel C. Peritoneal mesothelioma. Gastroenterology 1972;63:346.
248. Antman K, Osteen R, Klegar K, et al. Early peritoneal mesothelioma: A treatable malignancy. Lancet 1985;2:977–982.
249. van Gelder T, Hoogsteden HC, Versnel MA, de Beer P, Vandenbroucke JP, Planteydt HT. Malignant peritoneal mesothelioma: A series of 19 cases. Digestion 1989;43:222–227.
250. Whitley NO, Brenner DE, Antman KH, Grant K, Aisner J. Computed tomographic evaluation of peritoneal mesotheliomas: An analysis of eight cases. AJR 1982;138: 531–535.
251. Cozzi G, Bellomi M, Frigerio LF, et al. Double contrast barium enema combined with non-invasive imaging in peritoneal mesothelioma. Acta Radiol 1989;30:21–24.
252. Fukuda T, Hayashi K, Mori M, et al. [Radiologic manifestations of peritoneal mesothelioma.] Nippon Igaku Hoshasen Gakkai Zasshi 1991;51:643–648.
253. Nensey YM, Ibrahim MA, Zonca MA, Ma CK. Peritoneal mesothelioma: An unusual cause of esophageal achalasia. Am J Gastroenterol 1990;85:1617–1620.
254. Rashchupkina ZP, Karmilov VA, Iudina LI, Burtsev VI. [Malignant mesothelioma of the peritoneum with secondary amyloidosis of the internal organs.] Klin Med (Mosk) 1990;68:99–101.
255. von Hirschhausen R, Clemens M. [Paraneoplastic dermatomyositis in peritoneal mesothelioma.] Med Klin 1990;1:113–115.
256. Weissmann L, Osteen R, Corson J, Herman T, Antman K. Combined modality therapy for intraperitoneal mesothelioma. Proc Am Soc Clin Oncol 1988;7:274:1063.
257. Foyle A, Al-Jabi M, McCaughey WTE. Papillary peritoneal tumors in women. Am J Surg Pathol 1981;5:241.

258. Katsube Y, Mukai K, Silverberg SG. Cystic mesothelioma of the peritoneum: A report of five cases and review of the literature. Cancer 1982;50:1615.
259. Burrig KF, Pfitzer P, Hort W. Well-differentiated papillary mesothelioma of the peritoneum: A borderline mesothelioma. Report of two cases and review of literature. Virchows Arch [A] 1990;417:443–447.
260. Daya D, McCaughey WT. Well-differentiated papillary mesothelioma of the peritoneum. A clinicopathologic study of 22 cases. Cancer 1990;65:292–296.
261. Lammer F, Scherrer C, Hacki WH. [Well-differentiated papillary mesothelioma of the peritoneum. Rare, but prognostically important differential diagnosis.] Schweiz Med Wochenschr 1991;121:954–946.
262. Ross MJ, Welch WR, Scully RE. Multilocular peritoneal inclusion cysts (so-called cystic mesotheliomas). Cancer 1989;64:1336–1346.
263. O'Neil JD, Ros PR, Storm BL, Buck JL, Wilkinson EJ. Cystic mesothelioma of the peritoneum. Radiology 1989;170:333–337.
264. Villaschi S, Autelitano F, Santeusanio G, Balistreri P. Cystic mesothelioma of the peritoneum. A report of three cases. Am J Clin Pathol 1990;94:758–761.
265. Baddoura FK, Varma VA. Cytologic findings in multicystic peritoneal mesothelioma. Acta Cytol 1990;34:524–528.
266. Canty MD, Williams J, Volpe RJ, Yunan E. Benign cystic mesothelioma in a male. Am J Gastroenterol 1990;85:311–315.
267. Kristensen KA, Ostergaard E. Cystic mesothelioma of peritoneum: Occurrence in a man. J Clin Gastroenterol 1990;12:702–704.
268. McCaughey WTE. Criteria for diagnosis of diffuse mesothelial tumors. Ann N Y Acad Sci 1965;132:603.
269. Kannerstein M, Churg J. Peritoneal mesothelioma. Hum Pathol 1977;8:83.
270. Lomas DA, Wallis PJ, Stockley RA. Palliation of malignant ascites with a Tenckhoff catheter. Thorax 1989;44:828.
271. Einhorn N, Hamos KV, Hindmarsh T, et al. Radiation therapy of ovarian carcinoma: Presentation of a six-field technique. Radiother Oncol 1986;7:125–131.
272. Fazekas J, Maier JG. Irradiation of ovarian carcinomas: A prospective comparison of the open-field and moving strip techniques. AJR 1974;120:118–123.
273. Lederman GS, Recht A, Herman T, Osteen R, Corson J, Antman KH. Long-term survival in peritoneal mesothelioma. The role of radiotherapy and combined modality treatment. Cancer 1987;59:1882–1886.
274. Rose RG, Palmer JD, Lougheed MN. Treatment of peritoneal mesothelioma with radioactive colloidal gold. Cancer 1955;8:478–481.
275. Leichner PK, Rosenshein N, Leibel SA, Order SE. Distribution and tissue dose of intraperitoneal administered radioactive chromic phosphate (^{32}P) in New Zealand white rabbits. Radiology 1980;134:729–734.
276. Cross WG. Table of beta dose distributions. In: Chalk River, Ontario, 1967.
277. Piver SM. Radioactive colloids in the treatment of stage IA ovarian cancer. Obstet Gynecol 1972;40:42–44.
278. Pezner RD, Stevens KR, Tong D, Allen CV. Limited epithelial carcinoma of the ovary treated with curative intent by the intraperitoneal installation of radiocolloids. Cancer 1978;42:2563–2571.
279. Klaassen D, Starreveld A, Shelly W, et al. Levitt M. External beam pelvic radiotherapy plus intraperitoneal radioactive chromic phosphate in early stage ovarian cancer: A toxic combination. Int J Radiat Oncol Biol Phys 1985;11:1801–1804.
280. Hayashi T, Nasu Y, Aramaki K, Johnsen T, Matsuura H. [A case of peritoneal malignant mesothelioma with disappearance of ascites result of intraperitoneal instillation of mitomycin C and oral administration of UFT.] Gan To Kagaku Ryoho 1989;16:2449–2452.
281. Sugarbaker PH, Cunliffe WJ, Graves T, et al. Phase I and pharmacologic studies with early postoperative intraperitoneal epiadriamycin. Fourth International Conference on Advances in Regional Cancer Therapy. Berchtesgaden, Germany, 1989.
282. Taylor RA, Johnson LP. Mesothelioma: Current perspectives. West J Med 1981;134: 379–383.
283. Antman K, Cohn S, Green M. Malignant mesothelioma of the tunica vaginalis testis. J Clin Oncol 1984;2:447–451.
284. Carp NZ, Petersen RO, Kusiak JF, Greenberg RE. Malignant mesothelioma of the tunica vaginalis testis. J Urol 1990;144:1475–1478.
285. Kamiya M, Eimoto T. Malignant mesothelioma of the tunica vaginalis. Pathol Res Pract 1990;186:680–684.
286. Rodriguez AJ, Garmendia LJ, Hernandez LI, et al. [Diffuse malignant mesothelioma of the testicular tunica vaginalis. Report of a new case.] Arch Esp Urol 1990;43:897–899.
287. Smith AH, Handley MA, Wood R. Epidemiological evidence indicates asbestos causes laryngeal cancer. J Occup Med 1990;32:499–507.
288. Asoh Y, Nakamura M, Maeda T, et al. [Brain metastasis from primary pericardial mesothelioma. Case report.] Neurol Med Chir (Tokyo) 1990;30:884–887.
289. Eker R, Cantez T, Dogan O, Demiryent M, Celik A, Karabocuoglu M. Pericardial mesothelioma. A pediatric case report. Turk J Pediatr 1989;31:305–309.
290. Taguchi T, Fujiwara Y, Ichiki H, Kohno N, Hiwada K. [A case of malignant pericardial mesothelioma detected by gallium-67 scintigraphy.] Kaku Igaku 1991;28:281–284.
291. Aggarwal P, Wali JP, Agarwal J. Pericardial mesothelioma presenting as a mediastinal mass. Singapore Med J 1991;32:185–186.
292. Pascual MA, Povar J, Munoz J, et al. [Pericardial mesothelioma: Apropos of a case.] Rev Esp Cardiol 1989;42:559–561.
293. Dai RP. [Primary pericardial mesothelioma: A report of four cases.] Chung Hua Fang She Hsueh Tsa Chih 1989;23:90–92.
294. Gurevich MA, Odinokova VA, Smirnov VB, Iankovskaia MO. [Clinico-morphological characteristics of pericardial mesothelioma.] Sov Med 1991;1991:8–11.
295. Torii T, Takasuga H, Mizushima M, Ito J, Kanaya T, Matsushima T. [Primary malignant mesothelioma of the pericardium masquerading as malignant pleural mesothelioma: Report of an autopsy case and review of the reported cases in Japan as to its invasion to neighboring organs.] Kokyu To Junkan 1989;37:1027–1032.
296. De Klerk DP, Nime F. Adenomatoid tumors (mesothelioma) of testicular and paratestic ular tissue. Urology 1975;6:635.
297. Fenoglio JJ, Jacobs DW. Ultrastructure of the mesothelioma of the atrioventricular node. 1977;40:721.
298. Scully R, Mark EJ, McNeeley BU. Case record of the Massachusetts General Hospital. N Engl J Med 1982;306:32.
299. Balassiano M, Reichert N, Rosenman Y, Hertcheg E, Lieberman Y, Yellin A. Localized fibrous mesothelioma of the mediastinum devoid of pleural connections. Postgrad Med J 1989;65:788–790.
300. Kottke MK, Hart WR, Broughan T. Localized fibrous tumor (localized fibrous mesothelioma) of the liver. Cancer 1989;64:1096–1102.
301. Simpson PR. Adenomatoid tumor of the adrenal gland. Arch Pathol Lab Med 1990;114: 725–727.
302. Briselli M, Mark EJ, Dickersin GR. Solitary fibrous tumors of the pleura: Eight new cases and review of 360 cases in the literature. Cancer 1981;47:2678.
303. Scharifker D, Kaneko M. Localized fibrous "mesothelioma" of pleura (sub-mesothelial fibroma). A clinicopathologic study of 18 cases. Cancer 1979;43:627.
304. Dalton WT, Zolliker AS, McCaughey WTE, et al. Localized primary tumors of the pleura. An analysis of 40 cases. Cancer 1979;44:1465.
305. Majoulet JF, Millant P, Bouillet P, Le BA, Gaillard S. [Radiologic aspect of benign pleural fibrous mesothelioma. Reports of 4 cases.] Ann Radiol (Paris) 1990;33:229–236.
306. Strom EH, Skjorten F, Aarseth LB, Haug E. Solitary fibrous tumor of the pleura. An immunohistochemical, electron microscopic and tissue culture study of a tumor producing insulin-like growth factor I in a patient with hypoglycemia. Pathol Res Pract 1991;187:109–113.
307. Scotte M, Bessou JP, Andro JF, et al. [Hypoglycemic pleural mesothelioma. A case report.] Ann Chir 1990;44:688–691.
308. Davies JH, Notley RG. Adenomatoid tumours of the male genital tract. Review of 5 men presenting with an intrascrotal swelling subsequently diagnosed as an adenomatoid tumor. Eur Urol 1989;16:393–394.
309. Lopez JI, Aranda FI. Absence of estrogen immunoreactivity in adenomatoid tumors of male reproductive system. Pathol Res Pract 1990;186:395–396.
310. Kupryjanczyk J. Adenomatoid tumor of the ovary and uterus in the same patient. Zentralbl Allg Pathol 1989;135:437–444.
311. Corbi P, Jebara V, Fabiani JN, et al. [Benign tumors of the heart (excluding myxoma). Experience with 9 surgically treated cases.] Ann Cardiol Angeiol (Paris) 1990;39:433–436.
312. Subramanian R, Flygenring B. Mesothelioma of the atrioventricular node and congenital complete heart block. Clin Cardiol 1989;12:469–472.
313. Fontaliran F, Guillois B, Colin A, et al. Congenital atrioventricular block and maternal lupus erythematosus. Histologic discovery of tumor of the artrioventricular node. Arch Mal Coeur 1989;82:609–613.
314. Monma N, Satodate R, Tashiro A, Segawa I. Origin of so-called mesothelioma of the atrioventricular node. An immunohistochemical study. Arch Pathol Lab Med 1991;115: 1026–1029.

Cancer: Principles & Practice of Oncology, Fourth Edition,
edited by Vincent T. DeVita, Jr., Samuel Hellman, Steven A. Rosenberg.
J.B. Lippincott Co., Philadelphia © 1993.

Martin M. Malawer
Michael P. Link
Sarah S. Donaldson

CHAPTER **44**

Sarcomas of Bone

Malignant tumors arising from the skeletal system are rare, representing only 0.2% of all new cancers. Approximately 2100 new cases in the United States occur annually.[1] Osteosarcoma and Ewing's sarcoma are the two most common bone tumors; they occur mainly during childhood and adolescence.[2-4] Other mesenchymal (spindle cell) neoplasms—fibrosarcoma, chondrosarcoma, and malignant fibrous histiocytoma—that characteristically arise after skeletal maturity are less common.[5-18] These are sometimes associated with underlying benign bony tumors, previous irradiation, or primary bone disease.[5-16]

The surgical, chemotherapeutic, and radiotherapeutic principles developed in the treatment of osteosarcomas form the basis of the management strategy for most of the spindle cell neoplasms. Within the past decade, there has been an explosion of clinical knowledge and experience in the management of bony neoplasms.[18-28] The development of centers with specific interest in these tumors has played an important role in the advancement of biologic understanding, surgical management, and multimodality treatment of these tumors.[24-27] A surgical staging system that permits standardized preoperative evaluation, analysis, and end-result reporting has been developed.[28]

Amputation was once the standard method of treating bony sarcomas, but the past decade has witnessed the development of limb-sparing surgery for most malignant and aggressive benign tumors.[29-39] Advances in orthopedics, bioengineering, radiographic imaging, radiation therapy, and chemotherapy have contributed to safer, more reliable surgical procedures.[40-80] Axial computerized tomography (CT) and magnetic resonance imaging (MRI) permit extremely accurate evaluation of the local anatomy and enhance the possibility of safe resection.[81-88] Limb-sparing surgery is considered safe and routine for a large number of carefully selected patients. An evaluation system to determine a patient's functional status has been developed.[28] This system has enabled evaluation and comparison of the various limb-sparing procedures and types of surgical reconstructions.

Paralleling these advances has been the demonstrated effectiveness of adjuvant chemotherapy in dramatically increasing overall survival, and the bleak 15% to 20% survival rate with surgery alone before the 1970s rose to 55% to 80% with various adjuvant treatment regimens during the 1980s.[49-52,89-91] Multidrug regimens are now considered essential treatment. The timing, mode of delivery, and different combinations of these agents are being investigated at many centers. Preoperative chemotherapy regimens, administered by the intravenous or intraarterial route, and postoperative regimens are being evaluated to determine their effect on the tumor and their impact on the choice of operative procedure and on overall survival.[92-99]

This chapter focuses on malignant spindle cell tumors; Ewing's sarcoma is presented elsewhere. Benign tumors are described briefly, and their significance for the oncologist is explained.[2,3] We emphasize natural history, surgical staging, criteria of patient selection for amputation or limb-sparing surgery, and the technique of limb-sparing procedures. The development, role, timing, and mode of delivery of adjuvant chemotherapy and its relation to stage of disease is discussed. The role of radiation therapy in specific clinical situations is presented.

CLASSIFICATION AND TYPES OF BONE TUMORS

Bone consists of cartilaginous, osteoid, and fibrous tissue and of bone marrow elements. Each tissue can give rise to benign or malignant spindle cell tumors.[2-4] The classification of bone tumors is based on cell type and recognized products of proliferating cells. The classification, described by Lichtenstein in 1954 and modified by Dahlin is presented in Table 44–1.[3,55] Jaffe recommends that each tumor be considered a separate clinical-pathologic entity.[4] Radiographic, histologic, and clinical data are necessary to form an accurate diagnosis and to determine the degree of activity and malignancy of each lesion.

Cartilage tumors are lesions in which cartilage is produced. They are the most common bone tumors. Osteochondroma is the most common benign cartilage tumor; 1% to 2% of solitary osteochondromas become malignant.[56–57] Enchondroma is a benign cartilage tumor that occurs centrally; in an adult, malignant transformation may occur. Chondrosarcoma, the most common malignant cartilage tumor, occurs intramedullarly or peripherally. Ten percent are secondary, arising from an underlying benign lesion.[2] Most chondrosarcomas are low grade, although 10% differentiate into a high-grade spindle cell sarcoma or a rare mesenchymal chondrosarcoma.[2,56]

Osteoid tumors are lesions in which the stroma produces osteoid. The benign forms are osteoid and osteoblastoma. Osteoid osteomas are never malignant. Osteoblastomas rarely metastasize; if they do, it is only after multiple local recurrences.[58] Osteosarcomas are the most common primary malignant tumors of the bone. Histologically, they are composed of malignant spindle cells and osteoblasts that produce osteoid or immature bone. Several variants are now recognized.[59] Parosteal, periosteal, and low-grade intraosseous osteosarcoma are histologically and radiographically distinct from the classic central medullary osteosarcomas and have more favorable prognoses.[60–62]

Fibrous tumors of bone are rare. Desmoplastic fibroma is a locally aggressive, nonmetastasizing tumor, analogous to fibromatosis of soft tissue.[5,6] Fibrosarcoma of bone appears histologically as its soft tissue counterpart. Multiple sections must be obtained to demonstrate the lack of osteoid production. If osteoid is present, the lesion is classified as an osteosarcoma. Malignant fibrous histiocytoma (MFH), the counterpart of soft tissue MFH, has been described in bone.[7–9] It rarely occurs. The pathology of bone and soft tissue MFH is similar, consisting of a storiform pattern with a histiocytic component. Giant cell tumors are of unknown origin; originally called benign, they are now considered to be low-grade sarcomas. They have a high rate of local recurrence and malignant transformation.[63,64]

Tumors presumably arising from bone marrow elements are the round cell sarcomas. The two most common are Ewing's sarcoma and non-Hodgkin's lymphoma, which are discussed in other chapters.

RADIOGRAPHIC EVALUATION AND DIAGNOSIS

Radiographic evaluation, combined with the clinical history and histology, is necessary for accurate diagnosis. Bone scans, angiography, CT scans, and MRI generally are not helpful in determining a diagnosis but are important in delineating the extent of local involvement.

A systematic approach to the radiographic evaluation of skeletal lesions was described by Madewell and colleagues, who studied and correlated several hundred radiographic and pathologic specimens.[65] They considered the radiograph as

TABLE 44–1. General Classification of Bone Tumors

*Histologic Type**	*Benign*	*Malignant*
Hematopoietic (41.4%)		Myeloma Reticulum cell sarcoma
Chondrogenic (20.9%)	Osteochondroma Chondroma Chondroblastoma Chondromyxoid fibroma	Primary chondrosarcoma Secondary chondrosarcoma Dedifferentiated chondrosarcoma Mesenchymal chondrosarcoma
Osteogenic (19.3%)	Osteoid osteoma Benign osteoblastoma	Osteosarcoma Parosteal osteogenic sarcoma
Unknown origin (9.8%)	Giant cell tumor (Fibrous) histiocytoma	Ewing's tumor Malignant giant cell tumor Adamantinoma (Fibrous) histiocytoma
Fibrogenic (3.8%)	Fibroma Desmoplastic fibroma	Fibrosarcoma
Notochordal (3.1%)		Chordoma
Vascular (1.6%)	Hemangioma	Hemangioendothelioma Hemangiopericytoma
Lipogenic (<0.5%)	Lipoma	
Neurogenic (<0.5%)	Neurilemmoma	

* Distribution based on Mayo Clinic experience.
(Adapted from Dahlin DC. Bone tumors: General aspects and data on 6,221 cases. 3rd ed. Springfield, IL, Charles C. Thomas, 1978; classification based on Lichtenstein: Classification of primary tumors of bone. Cancer 1951;4:335–351)

the gross specimen from which a detailed histologic interpretation could be made and biologic activity accurately diagnosed. According to their system, a bone tumor is evaluated by five radiographic parameters: anatomic site, borders, bone destruction, matrix formation, and periosteal reaction.

Specific anatomic sites of the bone give rise to specific groups of lesions. Johnson explained this by a field theory, which hypothesizes that the most active cells of a certain area of bone give rise to tumors that are characteristic of that area.[66] Figure 44–1 summarizes the anatomic sites of common bone tumors. In general, spindle cell sarcomas are metaphyseal, and round cell sarcomas tend to be diaphyseal.

The border reflects the growth rate and the response of the adjacent normal bone to the tumor. Most tumors have characteristic borders. Benign lesions (*e.g.*, nonossifying fibromas, unicameral bone cysts) have well-defined borders and a narrow transition area that is often associated with a reactive sclerosis. Aggressive or benign tumors (*e.g.*, chondroblastoma, giant cell tumors) tend to have faint borders and wide zones of transition with little sclerosis, reflecting a more rapidly growing lesion. Poorly delineated or absent margins indicate an aggressive or malignant lesion.

Bone destruction is the hallmark of a bone tumor. Bone destruction is described as a geographic, moth-eaten, or permeative pattern.[67] In general, these patterns are found in the tubular bone rather than in the flat bone and represent a combination of cortical and cancellous destruction. These patterns reflect the progressively increasing growth rate of the underlying tumor.

Calcification of the matrix or new bone formation can produce an area of increased density within the lesion. Calcification typically appears as flocculent or stippled rings or clusters. The appearance of the new bone varies from dense sclerosis that obliterates all evidence of normal trabeculae to small, irregular, circumscribed masses described as "wool" or "clouds." Calcification and ossification may appear in the same lesion. Neither type of matrix formation is diagnostic of malignancy.

Periosteal reaction indicates malignancy but is not pathognomonic of a particular tumor. A combination of periosteal changes is often found. In malignant tumors, periosteal reaction is noncontinuous and thin, with multiple laminations. A parallel or a perpendicular pattern may be present.

The radiographic parameters of benign and malignant tumors are quite different. Benign tumors have round, smooth, well-circumscribed borders. There is no cortical destruction and generally no periosteal reaction. Malignant lesions have irregular, poorly defined margins. There is evidence of bone destruction and a wide area of transition with periosteal reaction. Soft tissue extension is common.

NATURAL HISTORY

Tumors arising in bone have characteristic patterns of behavior and growth that differentiate them from other malignant lesions.[68,88] These patterns form the basis of a staging system and current treatment strategies. These principles and their relation to management, as formulated by Enneking, are described here.[68,88]

BIOLOGY AND GROWTH

A spindle cell sarcomas form a solid lesion that grows centrifugally. The periphery of this lesion is the least mature. Unlike a true capsule that surrounds a benign lesion and is

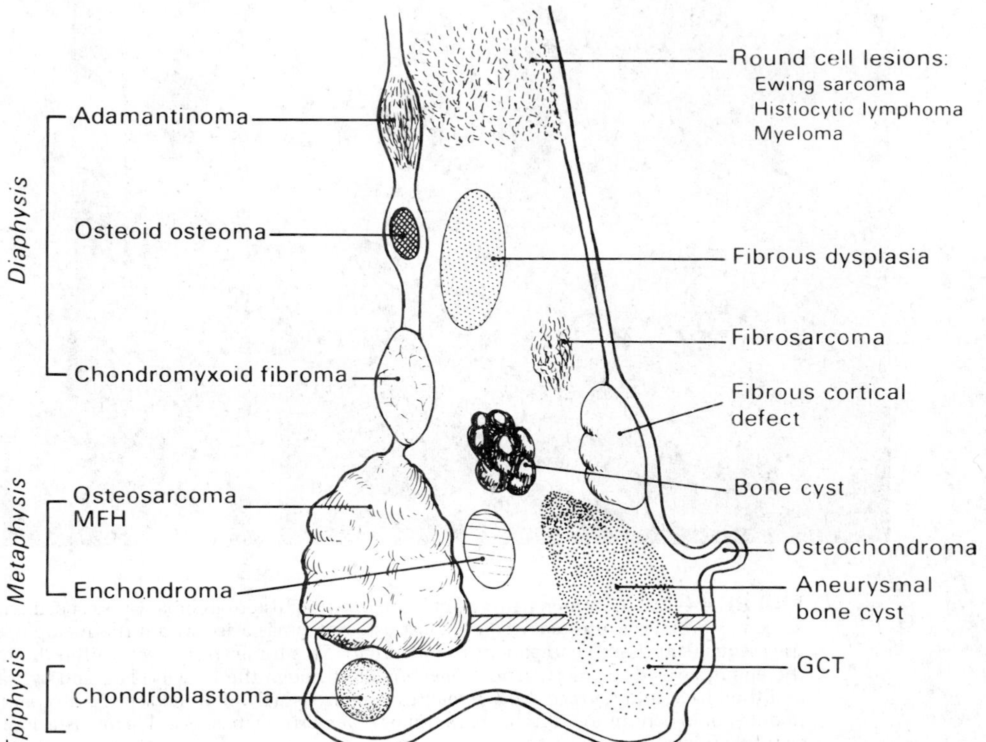

FIGURE 44–1. Common anatomic sites of bone tumors. (Modified from Madewell JE, Ragsdale ED, Sweet DE. Radiographic and pathologic analysis of solitary bone lesions. Radiol Clin North Am 1981;19:715–814)

composed of compressed normal cells, the malignant tumor is generally enclosed by a pseudocapsule and consists of compressed tumor cells and a fibrovascular zone of reactive tissue with a inflammatory component that interdigitates with the normal tissue adjacent to and beyond the lesion. The thickness of the reactive zone varies with the degree of malignancy and histiogenic type. The histologic hallmark of sarcomas is their potential to break through the pseudocapsule to form satellite lesions of tumor cells. This characteristic differentiates a nonmalignant from a malignant mesenchymal tumor.

High-grade sarcomas have a poorly defined reactive zone that may be invaded and destroyed by the tumor (Fig. 44–2). There may be tumor nodules in tissue that appear to be normal and not contiguous with the main tumor. These are called skip metastases. Although low-grade sarcomas regularly demonstrate tumor interdigitation into the reactive zone, they rarely form tumor nodules beyond this area.

The three mechanisms of growth and extension of bone tumors are compression of normal tissue, resorption of bone by reactive osteoclasts, and direct destruction of normal tissue. Benign tumors grow and expand by the first two mechanisms, and direct tissue destruction is characteristic of malignant bone tumors. Sarcomas respect anatomic borders and remain within one compartment. Local anatomy influences tumor growth by setting the natural barriers to extension. Bone sarcomas usually take the path of least resistance. Most benign bone tumors are unicompartmental; they remain confined and may expand the bone in which they arose. Malignant bone tumors are bicompartmental; they destroy the overlying cortex and go directly into the adjacent soft tissue. The determination of anatomic compartment involvement has become more important with the advent of limb-preservation surgery.

PATTERNS OF SPREAD AND CLASSIFICATION

Based on biologic considerations and natural history, Enneking classified bone tumors into five categories, each of which shares certain clinical characteristics and radiographic patterns and requires similar surgical procedures.[68,118]

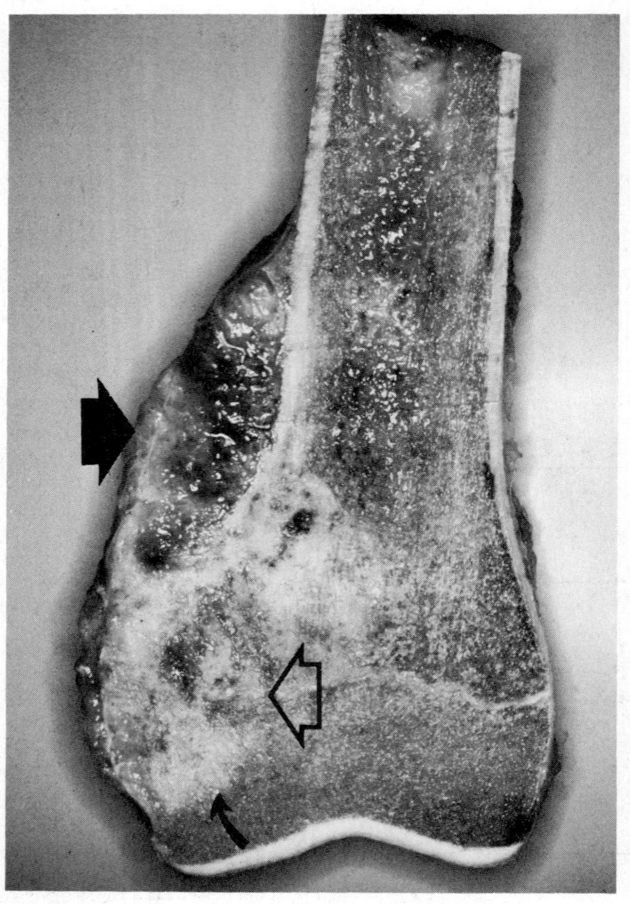

A

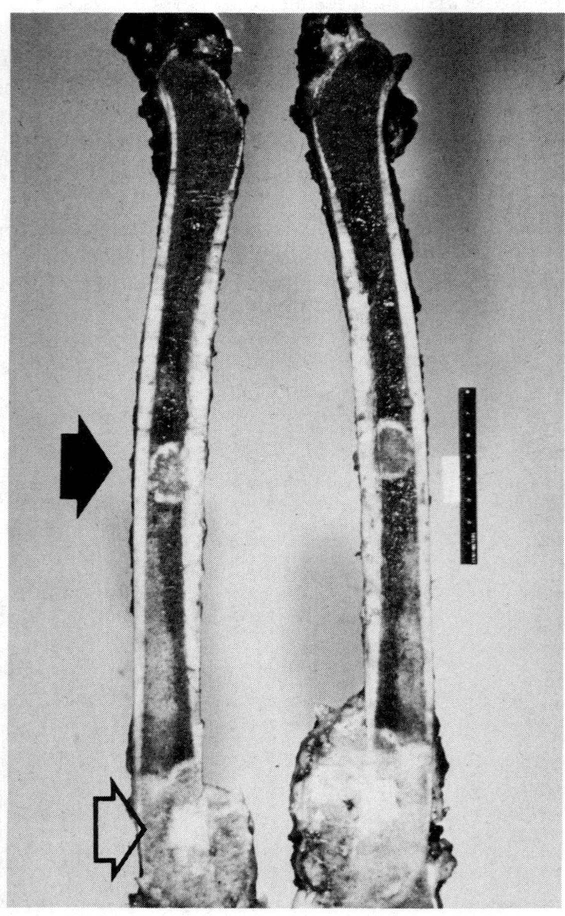

B

FIGURE 44–2. Common patterns of local growth of osteosarcoma. Gross specimens of two femoral osteosarcomas. **(A)** Typical osteosarcoma. Most osteosarcomas arise within the metaphysis and have a large extraosseous (soft tissue) component (*solid arrow*). This tumor has arisen within the metaphysis and involves the epiphysis by direct destruction (*open arrow*) through the growth plate and by tracking along the cortex and then back into (*curved solid arrow*) the epiphysis. **(B)** Skip metastasis. A separate tumor (*solid arrow*) nodule not in continuity with the main tumor (*open arrow*) mass is a skip metastasis. This is a poor prognostic sign for survival.

Benign and latent: lesions whose natural history is to grow slowly during normal growth of the person and then stop, with a tendency to heal spontaneously. They never become malignant and, if treated by simple curettage, they heal rapidly. Surgery is not indicated unless they become symptomatic.

Benign and active: lesions whose natural history is one of progressive growth. Simple curettage leaves a reactive rim with some tumor. Curettage has a high recurrence rate. Wide excision through normal bone results in local control in approximately 95% of patients.

Benign and aggressive: lesions that are locally aggressive but do not metastasize. The tumor extends through the capsule into the reactive zone. Local control can be obtained only by removing the lesion with a margin of normal bone beyond the reactive zone.

Low-grade malignant: lesions that have a low potential to metastasize. Histologically there is no true capsule but a pseudocapsule. Tumor nodules exist within the reactive zone but rarely beyond. Local control can be accomplished only by removal of all tumor and reactive tissue with a margin of normal bone. These lesions can be treated successfully by surgery alone.

High-grade malignant: lesions whose natural history is to grow rapidly and to metastasize early. Tumor nodules are often found within and beyond the reactive zone and at some distance in the normal tissue. Surgery is necessary for local control, and systemic therapy is warranted to prevent metastasis.

METASTASES

Bone tumors, unlike carcinomas, disseminate almost exclusively through the blood; bones lack a lymphatic system. There have been rare reports of early lymphatic spread to regional nodes.[18,100] Lymphatic involvement, which has been found in 10% of cases at autopsy, is a poor prognostic sign.[69] McKenna observed that 6 (3%) of 194 patients with osteosarcoma who underwent amputation demonstrated lymph node involvement. None of these patients survived 5 years.[70] Hematogenous spread is manifested by pulmonary involvement in its early stages and secondarily by bony involvement.[70–75] Bone metastasis is occasionally the first sign of dissemination. With the use of adjuvant chemotherapy, the skeletal system has become a more common site of initial relapse.[45,101,102]

SKIP METASTASIS

A skip metastasis is a tumor nodule that is located within the same bone as the main tumor but not in continuity with it. Transarticular skip metastases are located in the joint adjacent to the main tumor.[76] Skip metastases are most often seen with high-grade sarcomas. A skip lesion develops by the embolization of tumor cells within the marrow sinusoids; in effect, they are local micrometastases that have not passed through the circulation (see Fig. 44–2). Transarticular skips are believed to occur through periarticular venous anastomosis. The clinical incidence of skip metastases is less than 1%.[77] These lesions connote a poor prognosis.[76,77]

Wuisman and Enneking reported the natural history of 23 osteosarcomas with skip metastases evaluated at the University of Florida.[102a] Twenty-three patients with documented skip metastases were compared with 224 patients with stage II osteosarcoma without skip metastases. Seventeen skip metastases were in the same bone and six were transarticular. There was no difference in the mean age, sex ratio, or distribution of patients. Only 10 skip metastases were picked up on preoperative staging studies. The remaining 13 were detected only on examination of whole mount macrosections. Skip metastasis has a significant impact on local recurrence (30% versus 10%) and metastatic disease (95% versus 50%). Neither prognosis nor incidence of skip metastasis differed by age for groups older or younger than 21 years. The researchers reported an overall incidence of 6%. They concluded that adjuvant chemotherapy had no effect on patients with skip metastasis.

LOCAL RECURRENCE

Local recurrence of a benign or malignant lesion is due to inadequate removal. The aggressiveness of the tumor determines which surgical procedure is required for local control. Ninety-five percent of all local recurrences, regardless of histology, develop within 24 months of attempted removal.[68,78,79] Local recurrence of a high-grade sarcoma decreases overall survival prospects substantially. Local recurrence in patients who have undergone therapy may be associated with an even poorer prognosis.[74]

JOINT INVOLVEMENT

The articular cartilage is thought to be a natural barrier to direct articular extension by tumor. In a careful study of 45 macrosections of primary bone sarcomas, Simon reported 17 (38%) with articular extension.[80] He described three mechanisms: pericapsular, direct extension along intraarticular structures, and direct extension through the articular cartilage. Pathologic fracture, which opens a direct communication from tumor bone to joint cartilage, is a fourth mechanism (Fig. 44–3).

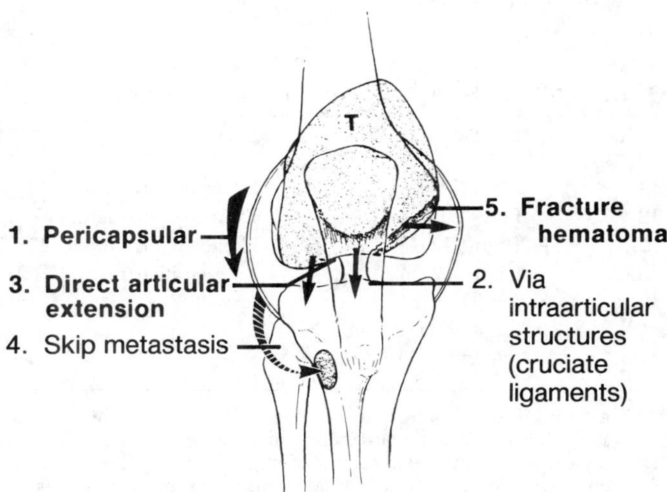

FIGURE 44–3. Mechanisms of articular involvement by high-grade bone sarcomas.

STAGING BONE TUMORS

In 1980, the Musculoskeletal Tumor Society adopted a surgical staging system for bone sarcomas (Table 44–2).[118] The system is based on the fact that mesenchymal sarcomas of bone behave similarly, regardless of histiogenic type. The surgical staging system described by Enneking and colleagues is based on GTM classification: grade (G), location (T), and lymph node involvement and metastases (M) (see Table 44–2).

SURGICAL GRADE

In the staging system, G represents the histologic grade of a lesion and other clinical data. These factors are used to make a surgical determination of low grade (G1) or high grade (G2) (Fig. 44–4).

SURGICAL SITE

T represents the site of the lesion, which may be intracompartmental (T1) or extracompartmental (T2). Compartment is defined as an anatomic structure or space bounded by natural barriers of tumor extension. The significance of T1 lesions is easier to define clinically, surgically, and radiographically than that of T2 lesions, and there is a higher chance of adequate removal of the former by a nonamputative procedure. Low-grade bone sarcomas are usually intracompartmental (T1), and high-grade sarcomas are extracompartmental (T2).

LYMPH NODES AND METASTASES

Lymphatic spread is a sign of wide dissemination (M). Regional lymphatic involvement is equated with distal metastases.

The surgical staging system developed by Enneking and colleagues for surgical planning and assessment of bone sarcomas is summarized:

Stage IA (G1,T1,M0): low-grade intracompartmental lesion, without metastasis
Stage IB (G1,T2,M0): low-grade extracompartmental lesion, without metastasis

TABLE 44–2. Surgical Staging of Bone Sarcomas

Stage	*Grade**	*Site*
IA	Low (G1)	Intracompartmental (T1)
IB	Low (G1)	Extracompartmental (T2)
IIA	High (G2)	Intracompartmental (T1)
IIB	High (G2)	Extracompartmental (T2)
III	Any G	Any (T)
	Regional or distant metastasis (M1)	

* G, grade; G1 is any low-grade tumor, and G2 is any high-grade tumor. T, site; T1 intracompartmental location of tumor, and T2 extracompartmental location of tumor. M, regional or distal metastases; M0 represents no metastases, and M1 represents any metastases. (Enneking WF, Spanier SS, Goodman MA. A system for the surgical staging of musculoskeletal sarcoma. Clin Orthop 1980;153:106–120)

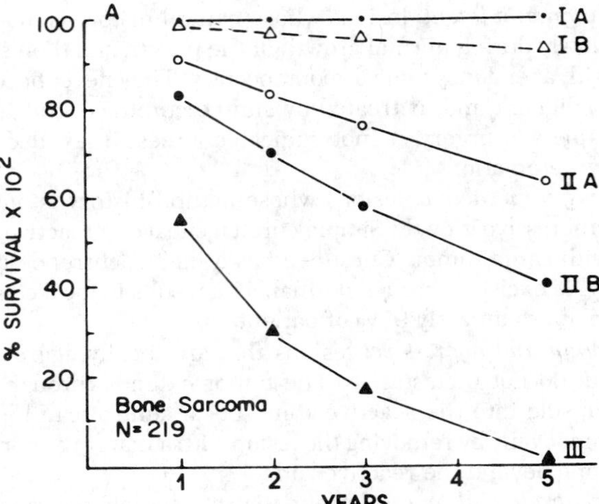

FIGURE 44–4. Survival rates of patients over a 5-year period with bone sarcoma according to stage of disease. (Enneking WF, Spanier SS, Goodman MA. A system for the surgical staging of musculoskeletal sarcoma. Clin Orthop 1980;153:106–120)

Stage IIA (G2,T1,M0): high-grade intracompartmental lesion, without metastasis
Stage IIB (G2,T2,M0): high-grade extracompartmental lesion, without metastasis
Stage IIIA (G1 or G2,T1,M1): intracompartmental lesion, any grade, with metastasis
Stage IIIB (G1 or G2,T2,M1): extracompartmental lesion, any grade, with metastasis

Spanier and coworkers further evaluated and refined stage IIB osteosarcoma and divided them into six categories (E1 to E6) depending on their local growth patterns (Table 44–3)

TABLE 44–3. Definitions of Anatomic Extent for Stage IIB Tumors

Maximal Extent	*Definition*
E1	Tumor touches but does not elevate or penetrate the periosteum
E2	Tumor elevates but does not penetrate the periosteum
E3	Tumor penetrates into but not through the periosteum
E4	Minimal extraperiosteal extension, not into a defined structure or space, seen as a nodule of tumor of one centimeter or less in fat just outside the periosteum, where muscle does not insert onto bone; the nodule often lies next to a small artery and may represent a small venous embolus that has destroyed the wall of the vein
E5	Tumor invades any one of the following: tendon; ligament; periarticular structures (tumor is covered by synovial tissue); joint (tumor is intraarticular); muscle; bone; or space, such as the popliteal fossa or the axilla
E6	Tumor invades two structures or more

(Spanier SS, Schuster JJ, Vander Griend RA. The effect of local extent of the tumor on prognosis in osteosarcoma. J Bone Joint Surg [Am] 1990;72:643–652)

and correlated it with prognosis (*i.e.*, disease-free interval) in 51 patients who had osteosarcoma.[102b] E6 was the worse prognostic factor for stage IIB osteosarcoma (*i.e.*, if the tumor invades two or more structures adjacent to the bone, the risk of failure was 5.9 times greater than if the tumor was smaller and more circumscribed). They did not determine any relation to sex, age, or size. They agreed that the most important factor determining prognosis was the initial extent of local disease and that it must be given primary consideration in evaluating and comparing different therapeutic regimens.

PREOPERATIVE EVALUATION

If the plain radiographs suggest an aggressive or malignant tumor, staging studies should be performed before biopsy. All radiographic studies are influenced by surgical manipulation of the lesion, making interpretation more difficult.[39,68] The biopsy site may be in a location that is not optimal for subsequent en bloc removal or radiation therapy.[24,103,104] Bone scintigraphy, MRI, CT, or angiography are required to delineate local tumor extent, vascular displacement, and compartmental localization.[42–46,68,78,82–88]

BONE SCANS

Bone scintigraphy assists in determining polyostotic involvement, metastatic disease, and intraosseous extension of tumor.[42,43,45] Malignant bone tumors, although solitary, may in rare cases present with skeletal metastasis.[46] Skip metastases are rarely detected by bone scans because they are small and localized to the fatty marrow and do not excite cortical response.[76,77]

Appreciation of the intraosseous extension of a bone tumor is important in surgical planning. Watts recommended removal of bone 6 to 7 cm beyond the area of scintigraphic abnormality.[32] This has been accepted as a safe margin for limb-sparing procedures.

COMPUTED TOMOGRAPHY

CT allows accurate determination of intraosseous and extraosseous extension of skeletal neoplasms.[40–44] It accurately depicts the transverse relation of a tumor. By varying window settings, the examiner can study cortical bone, intramedullary space, adjacent muscles, and extraosseous soft tissue extension. CT should include the entire bone and the adjacent joint. Infusion of intravenous contrast material permits identification of the adjacent large vascular structures. CT evaluation must be individualized. To obtain the maximal benefit of image reconstruction, the surgeon should discuss the information desired with the radiologist. Three dimensional reconstruction may be useful.

MAGNETIC RESONANCE IMAGING AND STAGING

MRI has several advantages in the diagnoses of bone sarcomas.[81–88] It has better contrast discrimination than any other modality, and imaging can be performed in any plane (Fig. 44–5). MRI is ideal for imaging the medullary marrow and for the detection of tumor and the extraosseous component. It has proven especially helpful in several difficult clinical situations, such as detecting small lesions, evaluating a positive bone scan if the corresponding plain radiograph is negative, determining the extent of infiltrative tumors, and detecting skip metastases. MRI has become invaluable in the planning of limb-sparing procedures.[86,88]

ANGIOGRAPHY

The technique of arteriography for bone lesions differs from that used for arterial disease. A minimum of two views (biplane) is necessary to determine the relation of the major vessels to the tumor.[105] Experience with limb-sparing procedures has increased, and it has become essential to determine individual vascular patterns before resection. This is especially crucial for tumors of the proximal tibia, where vascular anomalies are common.[106] Angiography is the most reliable means of determining vascular anatomy and displacement, but MRI and CT better demonstrate extraosseous extension.

CHOOSING A RADIOGRAPHIC METHOD FOR EVALUATION

One or all of the described studies are required in the preoperative evaluation of a bone sarcoma. There are unique benefits to each study. Bloem performed a prospective study comparing results of CT, MRI, scintigraphy, and angiography with 56 resected specimens to determine the appropriate choice of procedures.[106a] MRI was the best single modality to use. It was the most accurate for determining intraosseous extent of tumor, and scintigraphy and CT were often misleading. Angiography was performed only if the primary tumor was in the vicinity of the primary tumor. They also reported CT and MRI were as accurate in evaluation of cortical changes. MRI was superior in detection of muscular involvement in the knee, pelvis, and shoulder compared with CT.

MRI and CT (transverse data), combined with bone scans and angiography, allow the physician to develop a three-dimensional construct of the local tumor area before surgery and formulate a detailed surgical approach.

BIOPSY TECHNIQUE AND TIMING

The biopsy of a suspected bone tumor must be performed with great care and skill.[103,104] This principle cannot be overemphasized. The consequences of a poorly executed biopsy are often the deciding factor in the choice between a limb-salvage procedure or an amputation. Murray and colleagues from M.D. Anderson Cancer Center (MDACC) judged that only 19% of patients referred to that institution for treatment of primary bone sarcomas had properly placed biopsies.[24] All of these patients had open (incisional) biopsies, although 92% of such procedures performed at MDACC over the same period were needle biopsies. Similarly, Mankin compared the results of biopsies performed at the referring institution with those performed at the treatment center.[104] In this study, which involved 329 patients, a major error in diagnosis occurred for 60% of patients from referring hospitals, and 18.2% of the referred patients had to have less than optimal treatment due

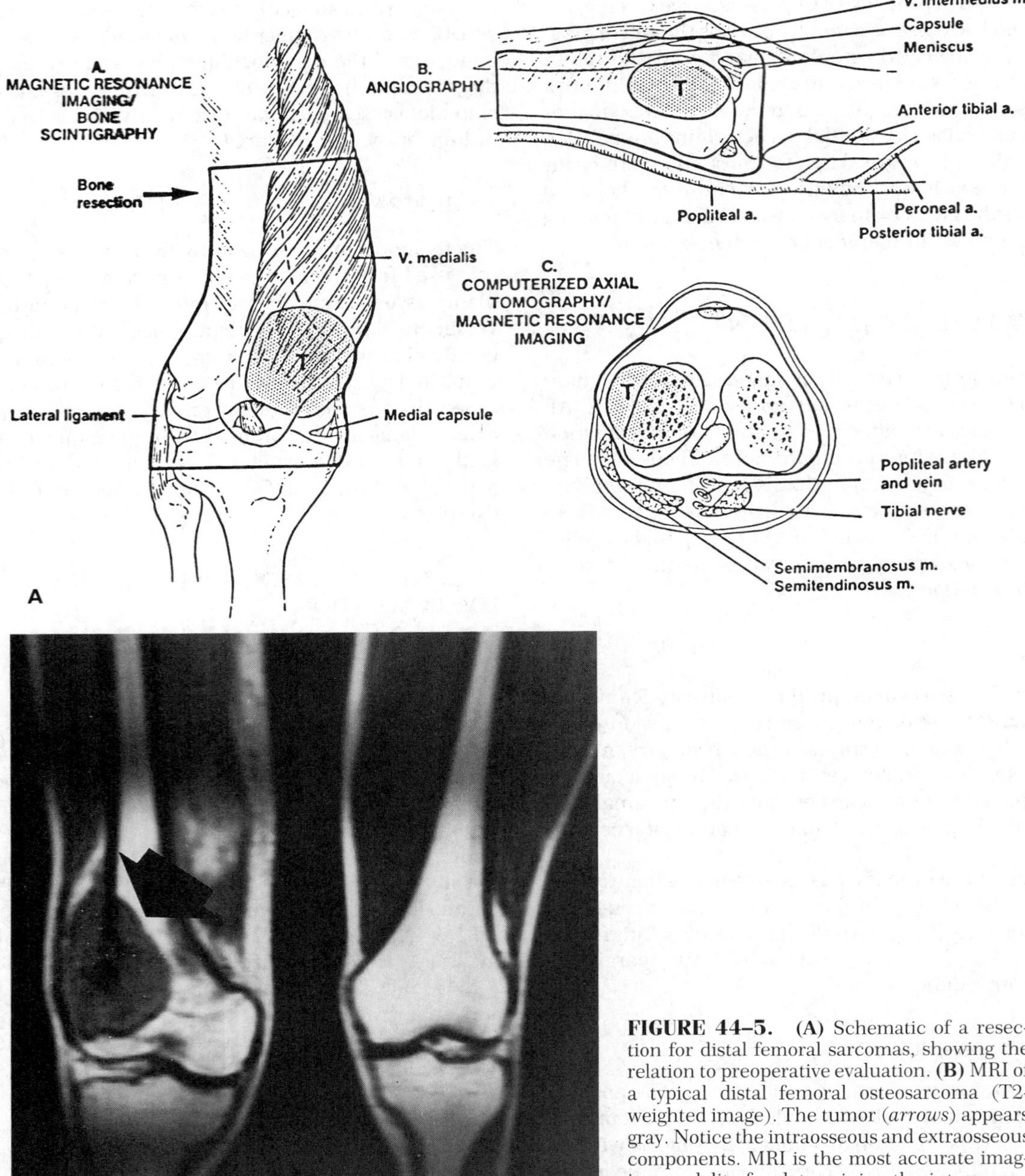

FIGURE 44–5. **(A)** Schematic of a resection for distal femoral sarcomas, showing the relation to preoperative evaluation. **(B)** MRI of a typical distal femoral osteosarcoma (T2-weighted image). The tumor (*arrows*) appears gray. Notice the intraosseous and extraosseous components. MRI is the most accurate imaging modality for determining the intraoseous extent of tumor.

to problems related to the biopsy, and for 8.5% of the total, the prognosis and outcome were adversely affected by the biopsy.

The biopsy should be performed by the surgeon who makes the ultimate decision about the operative procedure. This entails the referral of some patients who are strongly suspected of having primary bony malignancies to a regional cancer center for biopsy.

Trephine or core biopsy is recommended and often obtains an adequate specimen for diagnosis.[107–109] Multiple samples can be obtained from the same puncture site by slightly changing the angle of approach. Radiographs should be obtained to document the position of the trocar. Core biopsy is preferred if limb-sparing is an option, because it entails less local contamination than open biopsy. Core biopsy is especially helpful in difficult areas, such as the spine, pelvis, and hips. If a core biopsy proves to be inadequate, a small incisional biopsy is performed.

Every precaution should be taken to avoid contamination in performing an open biopsy. A tourniquet is used if feasible. If there is a soft tissue component, there is no need to biopsy the underlying bone. To decrease subsequent hemorrhage, polymethylmethacrylate (PMMA) is used to plug a cortical window; Gelfoam is used for hemostasis in the soft tissue. The overlying pseudocapsule is carefully closed to ensure maximal hemostasis. If it is necessary to biopsy the underlying bone, it is essential to use a small, rounded cortical window. This is especially true for a tumor that requires primary radiation therapy. Large segments do not reossify, often leading to fracture and the need for amputation. Regardless of the technique used, tumor cells contaminate all tissue planes and compartments transversed. All biopsy sites must be removed en bloc if the tumor is resected or irradiated.

Frozen-section analyses are obtained for all biopsy specimens. Many bone tumors can be adequately sectioned with a microtome. The purpose of the initial frozen section is to determine whether enough viable tumor has been obtained to yield satisfactory paraffin sections for interpretation. If not, additional specimens must be obtained. Frozen-section studies may suggest that additional material is necessary for electron microscopy studies or special staining techniques.

Interest has been renewed in frozen-section diagnosis and immediate surgery. Although the idea is attractive, there is no evidence that this procedure increases survival. Its major advantage is to decrease the risk of tumor microextension and contamination in a bloodless field, if a tourniquet has been used.[68,109]

RESTAGING AFTER PREOPERATIVE CHEMOTHERAPY

With the advent of preoperative (*i.e.*, neoadjuvant) chemotherapy for osteosarcoma, a need has developed to serially evaluate the clinical and radiographic response of the tumor before surgery. The staging and preoperative clinical studies previously described are used in evaluating tumor response. These studies are summarized in other reports.[110–114]

CLINICAL EVALUATION

Pain often decreases after the induction of chemotherapy. Alkaline phosphatase levels also decrease. The tumor becomes smaller, especially if significant matrix is not present. Conversely, increase of pain, elevation of alkaline phosphatase, or increasing tumor size are obvious signs of tumor progression.

PLAIN RADIOGRAPHY

There is a good correlation between radiographic response and the amount of necrosis.[112,113] Smith described the radiographic responses seen on serial radiographs: increased ossification of tumor osteoid, marked thickening and new bone formation of the periosteum and tumor border (giving the tumor a more benign appearance), and decrease in soft tissue mass (Fig. 44–6A,B).[113] The healing ossification is usually solid, homogenous, and regular and is easily differentiated from tumor osteoid.[112] There are less significant changes within the intramedullary component, including increased sclerosis and lysis, presumably due to necrosis and hemorrhage.

ANGIOGRAPHY

After chemotherapy, there is a marked decrease in vascularity.[111,112] Chuang evaluated 53 patients and reported that those with a complete angiographic response had more than 90% necrosis; among those with a partial response, necrosis ranged from 40% to 78%.[112] He concluded that angiographic evaluation was as reliable as pathologic evaluation and that the angiographic features were the best clinical criteria for the evaluation of tumor response.

Carrasco and coworkers from MDACC reported their extensive experience with intraarterial chemotherapy for osteosarcoma (81 patients) and evaluated the angiographic appearance and changes after two and four cycles of preoperative chemotherapy.[112a] They developed a simple radiographic system for angiographic changes. They evaluated the midarterial and parenchymal (capillary) phase:

1. Angiographic response with complete disappearance of tumor vascularity and stain
2. Total disappearance of tumor vascularity with slight persistence of tumor stain (capillary phase)
3. No response and persistence of tumor vascularity and capillary stain

They reported that 40% of the histologic responders (>90% tumor necrosis) and 91% of nonresponders were identified after two cycles. After four cycles, 91% of the responders but only 50% of the nonresponders were identified. The number of courses were not different between the responders and nonresponders. They concluded the disappearance of tumor vascularity after two courses of chemotherapy was highly suggestive of a good histologic response and was unlikely to occur in the histologic nonresponders.

COMPUTED TOMOGRAPHY

The most consistent finding in patients responding to therapy is a decrease in soft tissue mass and the development of a rim-like calcification similar to that seen on plain radiographs (Fig. 44–6C,D).[110] Changes in marrow are not helpful in evaluating response.

BONE SCINTIGRAPHY

Bone scan changes are difficult to evaluate. A decrease in activity generally indicates a favorable response; however, reparative bone formation, signalled by increased activity, may be misleading. Dynamic bone scans (quantitative bone scans), which are based on tumor blood flow and regional plasma clearance by bone and soft tissue, may allow more valid evaluations.[114] Regions that show a greater than 20% decrease in ^{99m}Tc-monodiphosphate plasma clearance are reported to be associated with necrotic tumor.

MAGNETIC RESONANCE IMAGING

MRI is a promising modality for evaluating chemotherapy-induced tumor necrosis. A preliminary report by W.R. Hogeboom and coworkers evaluated 10 patients undergoing preoperative therapy.[112b] They reported variable changes associated with tumor necrosis: decreased tumor size, cystic formation, reactive calcification, and changes in the T2 signal. They emphasized that a marked increase in T2 signal intensity is the result of necrosis, but much more investigation is required to correlate MRI findings with the spectrum of tumor necrosis before it is considered a reliable technique.

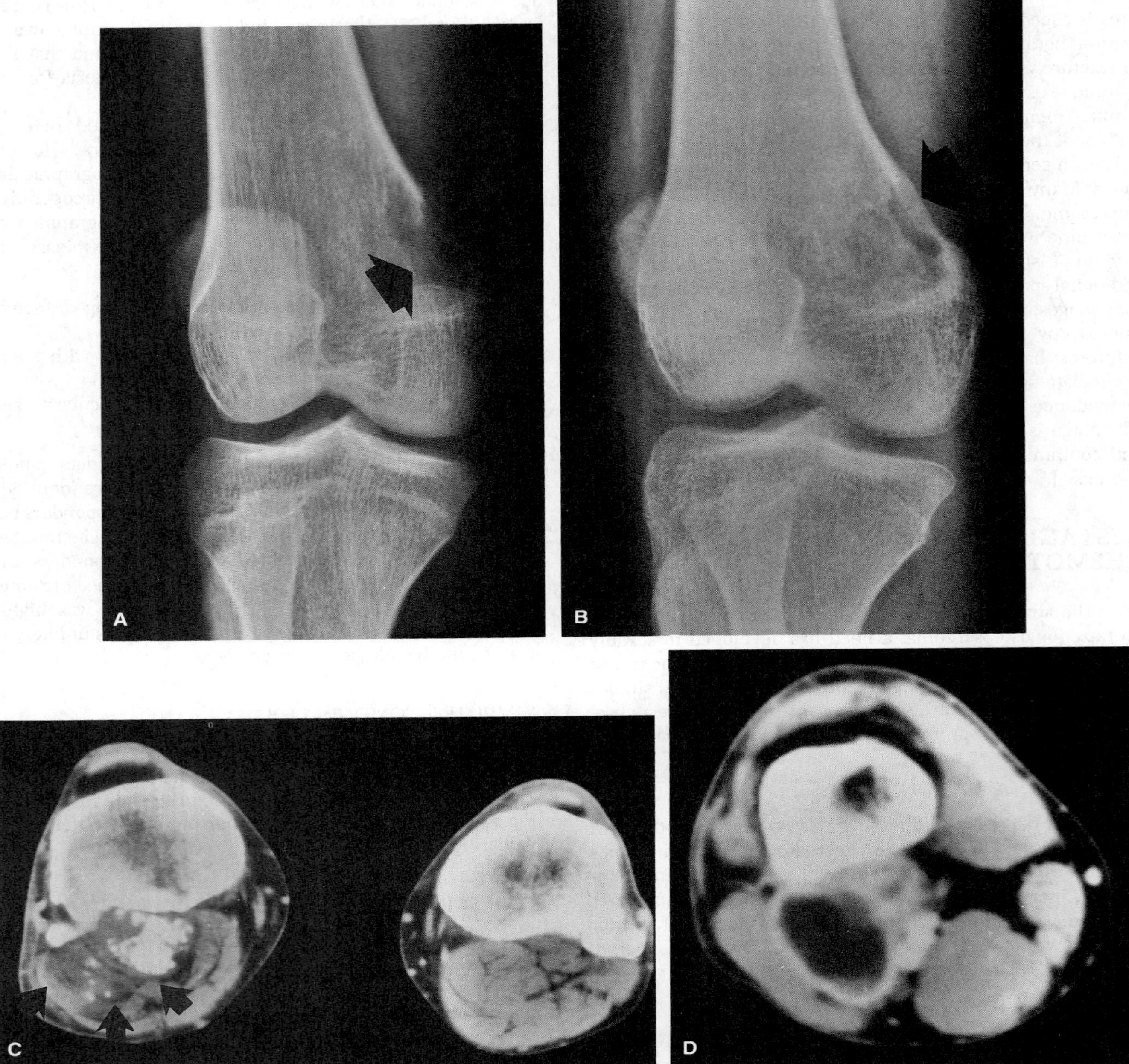

FIGURE 44–6. Response of osteosarcoma to preoperative (neoadjuvant) chemotherapy. **(A)** Plain radiograph of a small distal femoral osteolytic osteosarcoma of the medial femoral condyle. Notice the cortical destruction (*arrow*). **(B)** Plain radiograph after two cycles of intraarterial chemotherapy. Notice the reossification of the medullary space and healing of the cortical defect (*arrow*). These changes are considered typical of tumor necrosis with secondary healing response. This new bone is nontumor reparative bone and not neoplastic. **(C)** CT scan of another patient with a distal femoral osteosarcoma with a large posterior extraosseous component (*arrows*). This patient initially would have required amputation. **(D)** CT scan after two courses of neoadjuvant, intraarterial chemotherapy. There was mark necrosis (*dark center*) with new, nonneoplastic bone rimming associated with some shrinkage of the tumor mass. This patient underwent a limb-sparing procedure. Pathologic examination showed 100% tumor necrosis. The rim of reossification is typically seen on CT scans and indicates a good tumor response.

TABLE 44–4. Classification of Surgical Procedures for Bone Tumors

*Margin**	*Local*	*Amputation*
Intralesional	Curettage or debulking	Debulking amputation
Marginal	Marginal excision	Marginal amputation
Wide	Wide local excision	Wide through bone, amputation
Radical	Radical local resection	Radical disarticulation

* Tumors are classified by the type of margin achieved and whether obtained by a local or ablative procedure.
(Enneking WF, Spanier SS, Goodman MA. A system for the surgical staging of musculoskeletal sarcoma. Clin Orthop 1980;153:106–120)

HISTOLOGY

Serial needle biopsies are unreliable due to the possibility of sampling error.

SURGICAL MANAGEMENT OF SKELETAL TUMORS

Surgical removal, including curettage, resection, and amputation, is the traditional method of managing skeletal neoplasms. Limb-sparing techniques were developed during the early 1970s.[20–22,28–39] Marcove has described cryosurgery for some bony tumors.[115–117] Enneking and colleagues formulated means of classifying of surgical procedures based on the surgical plane of dissection in relation to the tumor (Table 44–4) and the method of accomplishing the removal (Table 44–5). The scheme summarized below permits meaningful comparisons of various operative procedures and gives surgeons a common language.[68,78,118]

1. *Intralesional.* An intralesional procedure passes through the pseudocapsule of the neoplasm directly into the lesion. Macroscopic tumor is left, and the entire operative field is potentially contaminated. Curettage is an intralesional procedure.
2. *Marginal.* A marginal procedure is one in which the entire lesion is removed in a single piece. The plane of dissection passes through the pseudocapsule or reactive zone around the lesion. If performed for a sarcoma, it leaves macroscopic disease.
3. *Wide* (intracompartmental). A wide excision, commonly called en bloc resection, includes the entire tumor, the reactive zone, and a cuff of normal tissue. The entire structure of origin of the tumor is not removed. In patients with high-grade sarcomas, this procedure may leave skip nodules.
4. *Radical* (extracompartmental). The entire tumor and the structure of origin of the lesion are removed. The plane of dissection is beyond the limiting fascial or bony borders.

Any of these procedures may be accomplished by a local (*i.e.*, limb-sparing) procedure or by amputation. Amputation may entail a marginal, wide, or radical excision, depending on the plane in which it passes. An amputation does not necessarily remove all cancer, but it can achieve a specific margin. The local anatomy determines how such a margin is to be obtained. The aim of preoperative staging is to assess local tumor extent and important local anatomy to enable the surgeon to decide how to achieve a desired margin and evaluate the feasibility of surgical procedures. This system allows meaningful comparisons of surgical procedures, end-results reporting, and analysis of combined data. In general, benign bone tumors may be treated adequately by an intralesional procedure (*i.e.*, curettage) or a marginal excision. Malignant tumors require a wide (*i.e.*, intracompartmental) or radical (*i.e.*, extracompartmental) removal, which may be an amputation or an en bloc procedure. Wide excision combined with adjuvant chemotherapy is the treatment of most high-grade bone sarcomas. Radical resections are rarely performed.

LIMB-SPARING SURGERY

Principles and Techniques

Limb salvage surgery is a safe operation for selected patients.[23–36,119–121] This technique may be used for all spindle cell sarcomas, regardless of histogenesis. Between 30% and 80% of patients with osteosarcoma can be treated successfully with this technique.[24,26,28,32,39,118]

The successful management of localized osteosarcomas and other sarcomas requires careful coordination and timing of staging studies, biopsy, surgery, and preoperative and postoperative chemotherapy, and radiation therapy.

TABLE 44–5. Surgical Procedure, Plane or Dissection, and Residual Disease for Musculoskeletal Tumors

Type	*Plane of Dissection*	*Result*
Intralesional	Piecemeal debulking or curettage	Leaves macroscopic disease
Marginal	Shell out en bloc through pseudocapsule or reactive zone	May leave either "satellite" or "skip" lesions
Wide	Intracompartmental en bloc with cuff of normal tissue	May leave "skip" lesions
Radical	Extracompartmental en bloc, entire compartment	No residual

(Enneking WF, Spanier SS, Goodman MA. A system for the surgical staging of musculoskeletal sarcoma. Clin Orthop 1980;153:106–120)

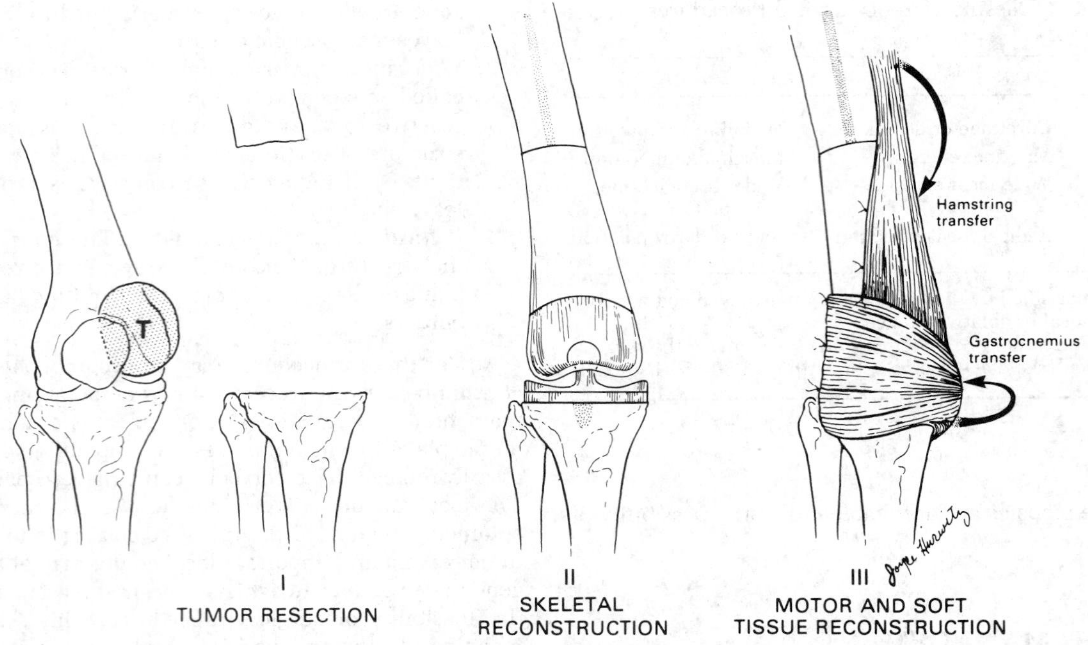

FIGURE 44–7. Schematic diagram of the three phases of a limb-sparing procedure.

Successful limb-sparing procedures consist of three surgical phases (Fig. 44–7).[120]

1. *Resection of tumor.* This strictly follows the principles of oncologic surgery. Avoiding local recurrence is the criterion of success and the main determinant of the amount of bone and soft tissue to be removed (Fig. 44–8).
2. *Skeletal reconstruction.* The average skeletal defect after adequate bone tumor resection is 15 to 20 cm. Techniques of reconstruction vary and are independent of the resection, although the degree of resection may favor one technique over the other.
3. *Soft tissue and muscle transfers.* Muscle transfers are performed to cover and close the resection site and to restore motor power. Adequate skin and muscle coverage is mandatory. Distal tissue transfers are not used because of the possibility of contamination.

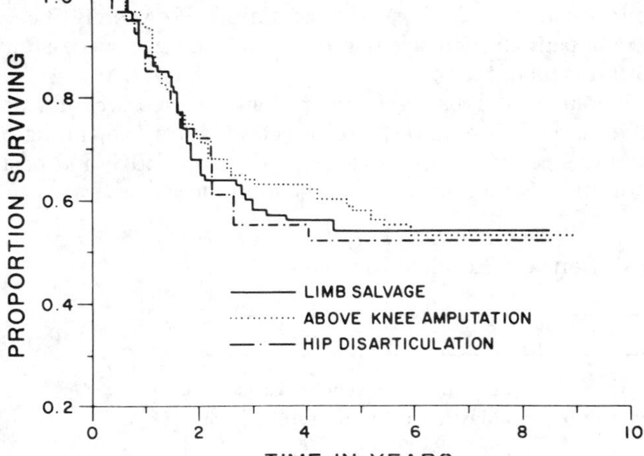

FIGURE 44–8. Length of survival versus type of operative procedure for 227 patients (pooled data) with high-grade osteosarcoma of the distal femur (Kaplan-Meier analysis). There is no survival difference for patients treated by hip disarticulation, above-knee amputation, or a limb-sparing procedure. (Simon MA, Aschliman MA, Thomas N, et al. Limb-salvage treatment versus amputation for osteosarcoma of the distal end of the femur. J Bone Joint Surg [Am] 1986;68:1331–1337)

The surgical guidelines and technique of limb-sparing surgery used by Malawer are summarized[120]:

1. No major neurovascular tumor involvement
2. Wide resection of the affected bone, with a normal muscle cuff in all directions
3. En bloc removal of all previous biopsy sites and all potentially contaminated tissue
4. Resection of bone 3 to 4 cm beyond abnormal uptake, as determined by CT or MRI and bone scan
5. Resection of the adjacent joint and capsule
6. Placement of the tourniquet proximal to the lesion, if possible
7. Adequate motor reconstruction, accomplished by regional muscle transfers
8. Adequate soft tissue coverage

Types of Skeletal Reconstruction

Large skeletal defects are reconstructed after tumor resection by several different methods. Osteoarticular defects are most often reconstructed by segmental, custom prostheses that are fixed to the remaining intramedullary bone by PMMA (Fig. 44–9). The newer knee prostheses allow some rotation and flexion and extension, and this mobility decreases the forces on the bone-cement interface and lessens the risk of loosening. There has been interest in combining porous coating to the

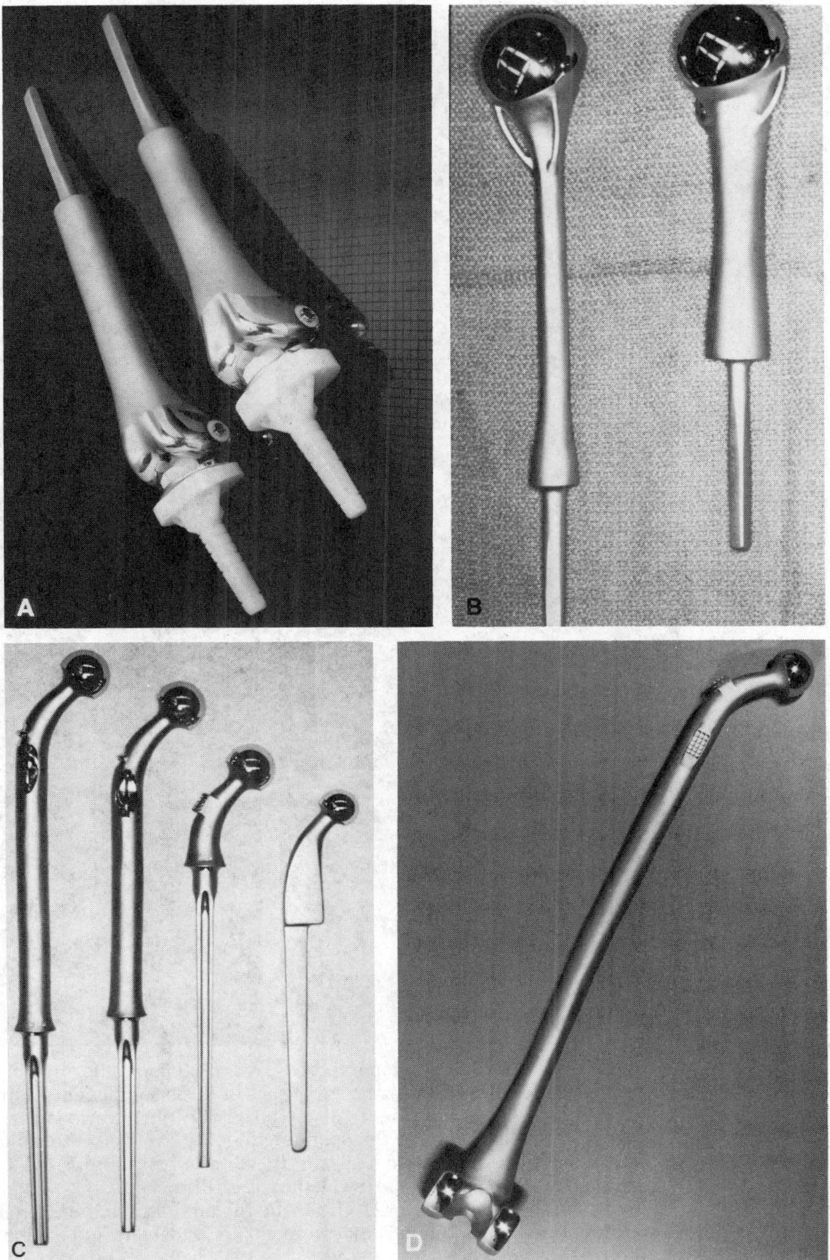

FIGURE 44–9. Prostheses used in selected patients for skeletal reconstruction using limb-sparing procedure. Different lengths are necessary to reconstruct the various resection defects. **(A)** Segmental distal femoral replacements with a total-knee component. **(B)** Segmental proximal humeral replacements. **(C)** Segmental proximal femoral replacements. **(D)** Total femoral replacement.

prosthesis to obtain biologic ingrowth, in the hope of obtaining long-term or permanent fixation.[37,122–124] Titanium, a new alloy with superior metallurgical properties, has been introduced. Most of these devices can be custom made within several weeks. In the hope of eliminating even this delay, modular systems that can be assembled in the operating room are now being evaluated (Fig. 44–10).[37,122] Alternative methods of segmental replacement include large autograft or allograft, used to obtain an arthrodesis, or osteoarticular allografts that may replace the affected joint.[33,122,124,125] Composite allograft (*i.e.*, allograft placed over a prosthesis) has been used. In general, allografts have been used successfully for low-grade sarcomas or giant cell tumors of bone that do not require chemotherapy or radiation therapy.

Contraindications

One contraindication to limb-sparing surgery is major neurovascular involvement. Although vascular grafts may be used, the adjacent nerves are usually at risk, making successful resection less likely. The magnitude of resection in combination with vascular reconstruction is often prohibitive.

Pathologic fractures contraindicate surgery. A fracture through a bone affected by a tumor spreads tumor cells by the hematoma beyond accurately determined limits. The risk of local recurrence increases under such circumstances. If a pathologic fracture heals after neoadjuvant chemotherapy, a limb-salvage procedure may be performed successfully.[125a]

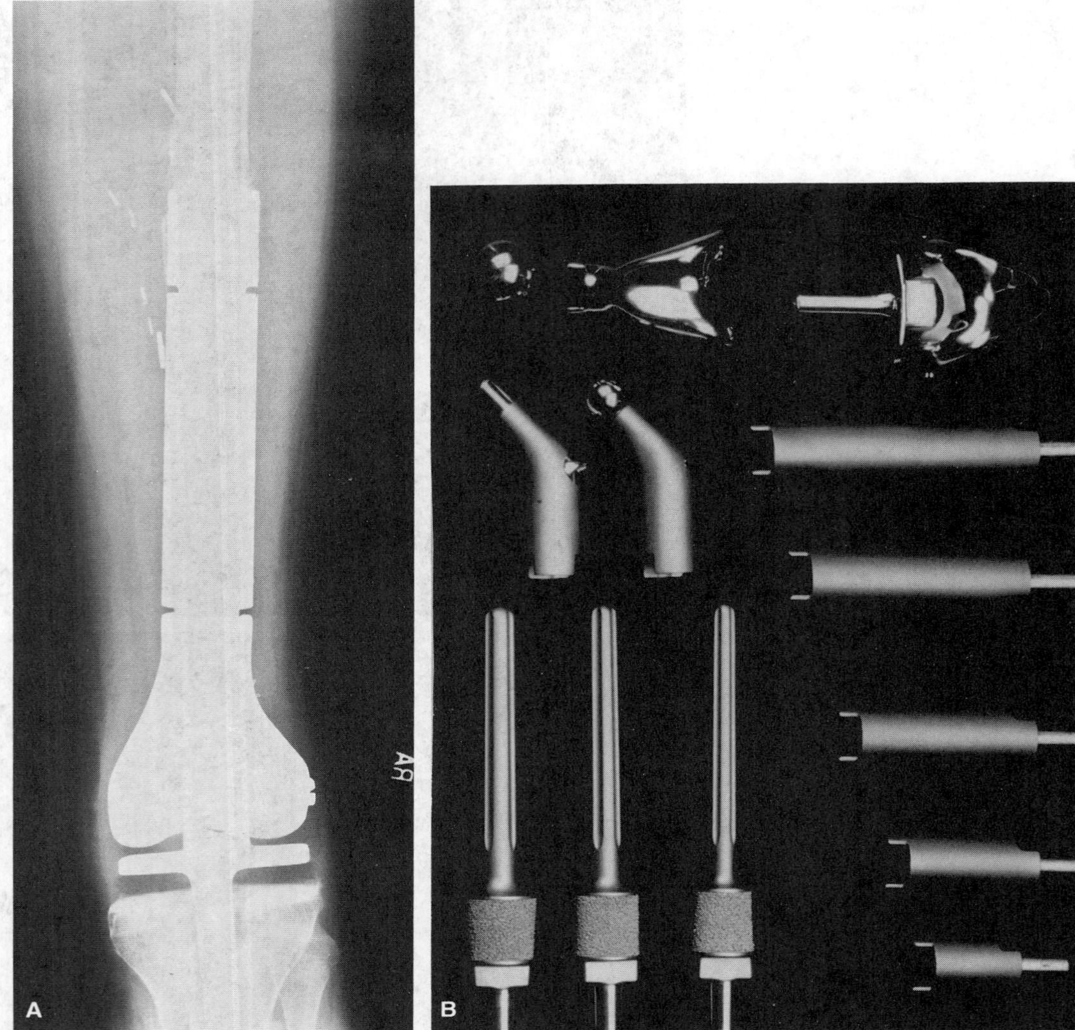

FIGURE 44–10. Distal femoral prosthesis. **(A)** Plain radiograph of a recently designed modular prosthesis of the distal femur. This prosthesis consists of three components: intramedullary stem, body segment, and a rotating-hinge knee component. All components come in various sizes. This permits immediate construction and use of the prosthesis in the operating room. It avoids the customary 4 to 6 weeks of delay in obtaining a truly custom prosthesis. Modular prostheses are available for the proximal tibia, proximal humerus, and proximal femur. (Courtesy of Howmedica, Inc., Rutherford, NJ). **(B)** Modular Segmental Replacement System (Howmedica, Inc., Rutherford, NJ) for the hip and distal femur. A modular system for large segmental prosthetic replacements permits almost immediate availability and choice of sizes without the need for customization and avoids delays in surgery.

An inappropriate or poorly planned biopsy jeopardizes local tumor control by contaminating normal tissue planes and compartments.

The risk of infection after implantation of a metallic device or allograft in an infected area is prohibitive. Sepsis jeopardizes the effectiveness of adjuvant chemotherapy.

Immature skeletal age contraindicates limb-sparing surgery. The predicted leg-length discrepancy should not be greater than 6 to 8 cm. Expandable prostheses have been used in this situation with success. Upper-extremity reconstruction is independent of skeletal maturity.

There must be enough uninvolved muscle remaining to reconstruct for a functional extremity.

Prognosis

Makley and coworkers reported from the Children's Cancer Study Group in a randomized study of 166 patients the relation of various aspects of surgical management to prognosis for disease-free survival.[125b] They found no advantage to the various aspects of surgical management: interval from first symptom to definitive surgery, interval from biopsy to definitive surgery, surgical sequence, type of surgery, or site of primary tumor.

Evaluation of Limb-Sparing Procedures

A comprehensive and reliable evaluation schema and rating system of limb-sparing procedures have been developed.[126,127]

The system sets forth six primary factors whose specific criteria depend on the unique considerations of six major functional anatomic regions. The primary factors are motion, pain, stability or deformity, strength, emotional acceptance and function, and complications. Extensive analysis using these criteria performed for 1323 patients was presented at the Third International Symposium on limb salvage. The mean follow-up of these patients was 47.8 months. The most common tumors were osteosarcoma, chondrosarcoma, and giant cell tumor; together these account for 70% of all tumors in this group of patients. The functional results are summarized:

1. *Periacetabular pelvic resections.* "Internal hemipelvectomy" had a higher recurrence rate than resection in other anatomic regions. Arthrodesis of the femur to the ilium produced the best results. Prosthetic and allograft reconstruction had an extremely high incidence of complications, especially infection.
2. *Modular versus customized devices.* There were no significant differences in the functional results of modular or customized prostheses. A significant problem with both systems was the lack of soft tissue reattachments.
3. *Resections about the knee.* There were no overall functional differences between arthrodesis, osteoarticular allografts, prosthetic arthroplasty, and rotationplasty. All were better than a prosthetic limb after an above-knee amputation. Each, however, had unique limitations that were not reflected in the overall ratings.

AMPUTATIONS

An amputation provides definitive surgical treatment in patients in whom a limb-sparing resection is not a prudent option. A significant number of patients still require amputation, despite the advent of limb-sparing surgery. Amputations for cancer, compared with those performed for other causes, tend to be at a more proximal anatomic level, to occur in younger people (reflecting the incidence of bone sarcomas), and to be technically more difficult.[128] The resultant psychological and cosmetic losses are more substantial. The amputation experience of the National Cancer Institute (NCI) during the past 30 years has been reviewed; 89% of these procedures were done for sarcomas.[128] Fifty-five percent of the lower-extremity amputations were hip disarticulations or hemipelvectomies. One half of the upper-extremity amputations were interscapulothoracic (*i.e.,* forequarter) resections. Osteosarcoma accounted for one third all amputations. Large lesions around the pelvis or proximal femur usually require amputation, but most sarcomas of the shoulder girdle and knee can now be resected.

CRYOSURGERY

Cryosurgery is the use of liquid nitrogen (−196°C) after curettage of a tumor cavity to kill the remaining tumor cells.[115–117,129–132] Necrosis occurs between −20°C and −40°C.[128] In general, a double freeze and thaw cycle is required. The aim of this technique is to enhance local tumor control after a careful curettage and avoid resection of the involved bone. Cryosurgery was initially developed by Marcove at Memorial Sloan-Kettering Cancer Center (MSKCC) for the treatment of metastatic bone tumors.[115,117] Marcove applied this technique to the treatment of aggressive benign tumors, specifically giant cell tumors and to low-grade sarcomas and chordomas.[130–132] The local recurrence rate after cryosurgery for these aggressive benign tumors decreased from 30% to 40% to between 5% and 10%.[115–117] This technique is not used for high-grade sarcomas.

CHEMOTHERAPY FOR BONE SARCOMAS

Before the advent of effective adjuvant chemotherapy, the outlook for patients with osteosarcoma was dismal. Most patients who presented without evidence of metastases and were treated only with surgery ultimately developed metastases and died.[129–133] A review of the literature published in 1972 summarized experience with 1337 patients in 11 studies conducted between 1946 and 1971.[133] Approximately half of the patients developed metastatic disease—usually in the lung—within 6 months after surgery of the primary tumor, and more than 80% developed recurrent disease. Fewer than 20% of the patients survived 5 years. The inescapable conclusion is that 80% of patients presenting without overt metastases had microscopic subclinical metastases at the time of diagnosis. The expectation that fewer than 20% of patients would survive beyond 5 years appeared to be reasonable, and this expectation served as the background for trials of adjuvant chemotherapy conducted in the 1970s and 1980s.

By the late 1970s, the prognosis for patients with osteosarcoma was improving, and this improvement was largely attributed to the beneficial effects of adjuvant chemotherapy. However, investigators from the Mayo Clinic and elsewhere challenged the apparent contribution of adjuvant chemotherapy, reporting that the prognosis of patients treated with or without adjuvant therapy had apparently improved over time.[134–140]

Two randomized, controlled trials were conducted in the mid-1980s by investigators of the Multi-institutional Osteosarcoma Study (MIOS) and investigators from the University of California in Los Angeles (UCLA) to resolve the controversy over the role of adjuvant chemotherapy in osteosarcoma. Both studies included a control group treated only with surgery of the primary tumor and no postsurgical adjuvant chemotherapy. Preliminary and mature results of these studies confirm the favorable impact of adjuvant chemotherapy in the treatment of osteosarcoma.[141–144] Life tables of event-free survival for patients in the control groups of these studies recapitulated the historic experience before 1970.

It is apparent from results of these recent trials that the natural history of osteosarcoma has not changed in the past 20 years; fewer than 20% of patients treated only with surgery of the primary tumor can be expected to survive without relapse. The bleak historic experience that served as the background for many uncontrolled adjuvant trials in the 1970s appears to be equally valid as a control for studies in the 1980s, 1990s, and beyond. Microscopic, subclinical metastatic disease can be presumed to exist in virtually all patients at the time of diagnosis. Although the more favorable results from the Mayo Clinic for patients treated without adjuvant chemotherapy remain unexplained, it is apparent from the MIOS and UCLA studies that the administration of adjuvant chemotherapy has a significant favorable influence on outcome and should be recommended for all patients with osteosarcoma.

ADJUVANT CHEMOTHERAPY

The rationale for adjuvant chemotherapy of osteosarcoma is derived from experimental evidence that microscopic metastatic disease can be eradicated if the treatment is initiated when the total body burden of metastatic tumor is sufficiently low.[145–147]

The strategy of adjuvant chemotherapy after surgical removal of the primary tumor has been applied successfully in the management of other childhood tumors. However, osteosarcoma is a relatively drug-resistant neoplasm, and results of studies of the activity of single agents and drugs in combination against macroscopic osteosarcoma have been disappointing (Table 44–6). Few drugs have produced responses in more than 15% of patients, and most responses are partial. Notable exceptions are the responses observed in trials of doxorubicin (Adriamycin), cisplatin, high-dose methotrexate with leucovorin rescue, and ifosfamide.[148–156] The effectiveness of high-dose methotrexate, however, has not been universally accepted; reported response rates have varied widely, ranging from no response to 80%.[153–155,157,158] The effectiveness of this drug may be dose dependent, because dose escalation has produced responses in patients found previously to be unresponsive to treatment.[159] A steep dose-response relation may also pertain to doxorubicin.[148,160] The combination of bleomycin, cyclophosphamide, and dactinomycin (BCD regimen) is used, although its effectiveness has been disputed.[161]

Logic dictates that the application of agents inactive against macroscopic osteosarcoma should not influence the natural history of this disease. Experimental evidence, however, suggests that eradication of microscopic metastases is possible, even with drugs that are marginally effective or ineffective against gross macroscopic tumors.[145–147,162] The hopeless prognosis for patients with osteosarcoma encouraged the enthusiastic application of the available agents, singly or in combination, as adjuvant therapy for patients with nonmetastatic osteosarcoma. Results of some of the important adjuvant chemotherapy trials of the 1970s and early 1980s are summarized in Table 44–7.

Concerns have been raised that adjuvant chemotherapy for osteosarcoma may delay but not prevent relapse. However, the results of many of the adjuvant studies reported in Table 44–7, some with follow-up beyond 10 years, suggest that life tables of event-free survival have stable plateaus beyond 4 years and that relapses after 3 years are infrequent. Most patients surviving 3 years without evidence of recurrence are probably cured.

Examination of the results of chemotherapy trials reveals a trend in the direction of improved outcome for patients treated on more intensive chemotherapy regimens. Considering that so few drugs have demonstrable activity against macroscopic osteosarcoma, the results reported in adjuvant trials are remarkable. Approximately 60% to 65% of patients with osteosarcoma treated with modern intensive adjuvant chemotherapy regimens survive without recurrence. The development of adjuvant regimens has been largely empiric, and newer, more intensive regimens have resulted in additional improvements in outcome. Further improvements in results of treatment will probably result from the development of new active agents. The activity of ifosfamide has been demonstrated, and this drug is now incorporated into newer regimens under study with promising preliminary results.[181]

TABLE 44–6. Representative Studies and Pooled Data for Single-Agent Chemotherapy Response in Overt, Primary or Metastatic Osteosarcoma

Agent	*Responders/ Evaluable Patients*	*% PR + CR**
Cyclophosphamide	4/28	15
Melphalan	5/32	15
Mitomycin C	3/23	13
Vincristine/vinblastine	0/21	0
Uracil mustard	0/10	0
Hydroxyurea	0/10	0
Procarbazine	0/10	0
DTIC	2/14	14
Doxorubicin	28/109	26
5-Fluorouracil	0/11	0
Cisplatin	8/24	33
Dactinomycin	4/26	15
Methotrexate	0/14	0
High-dose methotrexate plus vincristine and leucovorin		
Every 3 weeks	11/26	42
Every week	9/11	82†
Ifosfamide	6/18	33

* PR, partial response; CR, complete response. CR is less than 10% of total response rate in all major trials.
† May include some patients who concurrently received surgery or coned down irradiation to metastases.
(Adapted with permission from Bode U, Levine AS. The biology and management of osteosarcoma. In: Levine AS, ed. Cancer in the young. New York: Masson Publishing USA, 1982;575–602)

PRESURGICAL CHEMOTHERAPY

Presurgical chemotherapy has been used with increasing frequency during the past decade in the management of osteosarcoma. This strategy evolved concurrently with limb-sparing procedures. Initial attempts at limb salvage at the MSKCC in 1973 involved the fabrication of customized endoprostheses for selected patients undergoing en bloc resection. While the prosthesis was being made (requiring as long as 3 months), chemotherapy was administered to prevent tumor progression.[178] Retrospectively, patients treated with presurgical chemotherapy fared better than did patients treated during the same period with immediate surgery and postoperative adjuvant therapy.[179]

On histologic evaluation, the response in the primary tumor to preoperative chemotherapy was found to be a powerful prognostic factor; unfavorable responders were likely to develop distant metastases despite continued use of chemotherapy with the same agents after surgery.[182] The prognostic significance of tumor response to preoperative chemotherapy has been confirmed in studies conducted by the German So-

TABLE 44–7. Results of Representative Trials of Adjuvant Therapy for Osteosarcoma

*Investigations**	*Adjuvant Regimen**	*No. of Patients*	*Relapse Free (%)*
DFCI[163,164]	HDMTX, VCR (study I)	12	42
NCI[165]	HDMTX, VCR ± BCG†	39	38
CALGB[160,166,167]	ADRIA	88	39
CALGB[168]	ADRIA ± HDMTX†	62	50
DFCI[164]	ADRIA + VCR ± HDMTX (study II)	22	59
DFCI[164,169]	ADRIA + VCR + HDMTX (weekly) (study III)	46	60
CCSG[170]	ADRIA + VCR + (HDMTX vs IDMTX)*	166	38
SWOG[171–173]	COMPADRI I (CTX, VCR, ADRIA, PAM)	43	49
SWOG[172,173]	COMPADRI II (CTX, VCR, ADRIA, PAM, HDMTX)	53	35
SWOG[172,173]	COMPADRI III (CTX, VCR, ADRIA, PAM, HDMTX)	84	38
St. Jude[174]	ADRIA + HDMTX + CTX (OSTEO 72)	26	50
St. Jude[174]	ADRIA + HDMTX + CTX (OSTEO 77)	50	56
Roswell Park[175,176]	ADRIA + CDDP	22	61
Mayo Clinic[140]	HDMTX + VCR vs no adjuvant therapy‡	38	40 (chemotherapy) 44 (no chemotherapy)
MIOS[141,142]	BCD + HDMTX + ADRIA + CDDP vs no adjuvant therapy§	36 randomized 165 nonrandomized	63 (chemotherapy) 12 (no chemotherapy)
UCLA[144]	BCD + HDMTX + VCR + ADRIA (+intraarterial ADRIA + XRT) vs no adjuvant therapy§	59	55 (chemotherapy) 20 (no chemotherapy)
EORTC[139,177]	Whole-lung irradiation vs no adjuvant treatment‖	86	43 (with treatment) 28 (no treatment)
Mayo Clinic[138]	Whole-lung irradiation (+dactinomycin) vs no adjuvant treatment*	53	40
MSKCC[178–180]	HDMTX + VCR + ADRIA + CTX (T4 + T5 pooled)	52 (<21 years)	48

* HDMTX, high-dose methotrexate (5 g/m² or more) + leucovorin rescue; VCR, vincristine; BCG, bacillus Calmette-Guérin; ADRIA, doxorubicin (Adriamycin); IDMTX, intermediate-dose methotrexate (750 mg/m²) + leucovorin rescue; CTX, cyclophosphamide; PAM, phenylalanine mustard; CDDP, cisplatin; BCD, bleomycin, cyclophosphamide, dactinomycin combination; DFCI, Dana-Farber Cancer Institute; NCI, National Cancer Institute; CALGB, Cancer and Acute Leukemia Group B; CCSG, Children's Cancer Study Group; SWOG, Southwest Oncology Group; MIOS, Multiinstitutional Osteosarcoma Study; UCLA, University of California, Los Angeles; EORTC, European Organization for Research on Treatment of Cancer; MSKCC, Memorial Sloan-Kettering Cancer Center.
† Randomized study; no significant difference in relapse-free survival for patients on each treatment arm of study.
‡ Randomized study; no significant difference in relapse-free survival for patients receiving and not receiving adjuvant HDMTX.
§ Randomized study; difference in results of treatments highly significant ($p < 0.01$).
‖ Randomized study; difference in results of treatments significant at 6% level.

ciety for Pediatric Oncology (GPO),[183–185] and in studies from the Instituto Rizzoli,[186] the Children's Cancer Study Group,[187] and the MDACC.[180] Patients at high risk for recurrent disease can be identified early in treatment based on the poor response of the primary tumor to presurgical chemotherapy.

Although the initial impetus for presurgical chemotherapy was limb salvage, several theoretical advantages of presurgical chemotherapy apply to all patients with osteosarcoma (Table 44–8).[179] Because chemotherapy is administered soon after biopsy and diagnosis, treatment of the micrometastases known to be present in most patients can be instituted early. This offers a substantial advantage over the traditional adjuvant approach, in which the administration of systemic chemotherapy is delayed by a month or more for surgery and wound healing. Earlier administration of systemic treatment may reduce the emergence of drug-resistant cells in the micrometastases.[189–190] For the surgeon, presurgical chemotherapy has some advantages, because it allows time for fabrication of a prosthesis and may effect a reduction of bulky tumors, increasing the feasibility of limb-salvage surgery in selected patients.

ASSESSMENT OF TUMOR RESPONSE

Assessment of the response of primary tumors has been based on clinical and radiographic data, but the histologic appearance of the resected tumor specimen after presurgical chemotherapy has emerged as the standard for measuring response.[180,182,187,191] Several systems for grading the effect of preoperative chemotherapy have been proposed, all of which are based on the degree of cellularity and necrosis in the resected specimen. The grading system designed at MSKCC by Huvos has been used widely (Table 44–9).[180,182] Grade III and IV responses, indicating extensive to complete response in the primary tumor, are favorable. Grade I and II responses, indicating minimal destruction of the tumor, are unfavorable

TABLE 44–8. Considerations for Presurgical and Postsurgical Chemotherapy Regimens

Timing of Chemotherapy	*Advantages*	*Disadvantages*
Preoperative chemotherapy	Early institution of systemic therapy against micrometastases	High tumor burden (not optimal for first-order kinetics)
	Reduced chance of spontaneous emergence of drug-resistant clones in micrometastases	Increased probability of the selection of drug-resistant cells in primary tumor, which may metastasize
	Reduction in tumor size, increasing the change of limb salvage	Delay in definitive control of bulk disease; increased chance for systemic dissemination
	Provides time for fabrication of customized endoprosthesis	
	Less chance of viable tumor being spread at the time of surgery	Psychological trauma of retaining tumor
	Individual response to chemotherapy allows selection of different risk groups	Risk of local tumor progression with loss of a limb-sparing option
Postsurgical chemotherapy	Radical removal of bulk tumor decreases tumor burden and increases growth rate of residual disease, making S-phase-specific agents more active and optimizing conditions for first-order kinetics	Delay of systemic therapy for micrometastases No preoperative in vivo assay of cytotoxic response
	Decreased probability of selecting a drug-resistant clone in the primary tumor	Possible spread of viable tumor by surgical manipulation

(Fig. 44–11). In studies using the Huvos Grading System, patients with a favorable response (grade III or IV) fare extremely well, but those with an unfavorable histologic response to preoperative chemotherapy (grade I or II) are likely to develop distant metastases. An update of data from MSKCC trials suggest that modification of the Huvos system is in order. It is apparent that only grade IV response predicts an excellent outcome; patients with grade II and III responses fare equally, with an intermediate prognosis; and patients demonstrating only minimal response to chemotherapy have the worst outcome.[193] The Huvos grading system has served as a model for other systems for grading tumor response.

TABLE 44–9. Histologic Grading of the Effect of Preoperative Chemotherapy on Primary Osteosarcoma

Grade	*Effect*
I	Little or no effect identified
II	Area of acellular tumor osteoid, necrotic, or fibrotic material attributable to the effect of chemotherapy, with other areas of histologically viable tumor
III	Predominant areas of acellular tumor osteoid, necrotic, or fibrotic material attributable to the effect of chemotherapy with only scattered foci of histologically viable tumor cells identified
IV	No histologic evidence of viable tumor identified within the entire specimen

(Reproduced with permission from Rosen G, et al. Primary osteogenic sarcoma: Eight-year experience with adjuvant chemotherapy. J Cancer Res Clin Oncol [Suppl] 1983;106:55–67)

The grading system formerly used by the GPO identifies six categories of response.[191] In the COSS-80 study, favorable response was defined as greater than 50% tumor destruction after presurgical chemotherapy, but in GPO studies, 90% destruction is required. The grading system favored by investigators at the MDACC divides response into three categories: no effect or doubtful effect with less than 40% tumor destruction; partial effect with 40% to 60% tumor destruction; and definite effect, in which more than 60% of the tumor is destroyed and fibrovascular regeneration is present.[192] Grading systems are necessarily imprecise and subject to sampling errors. However, with scrupulous attention to adequate sectioning from many sites of the surgical specimen, the degree of response can be reliably and reproducibly assessed.

TAILORING OF CHEMOTHERAPY

One of the most compelling rationales for presurgical chemotherapy is its use as an in vivo drug trial to determine the drug sensitivity of an individual tumor and to customize postoperative chemotherapy. Results of studies from the MSKCC and elsewhere suggest that patients whose tumors are re-

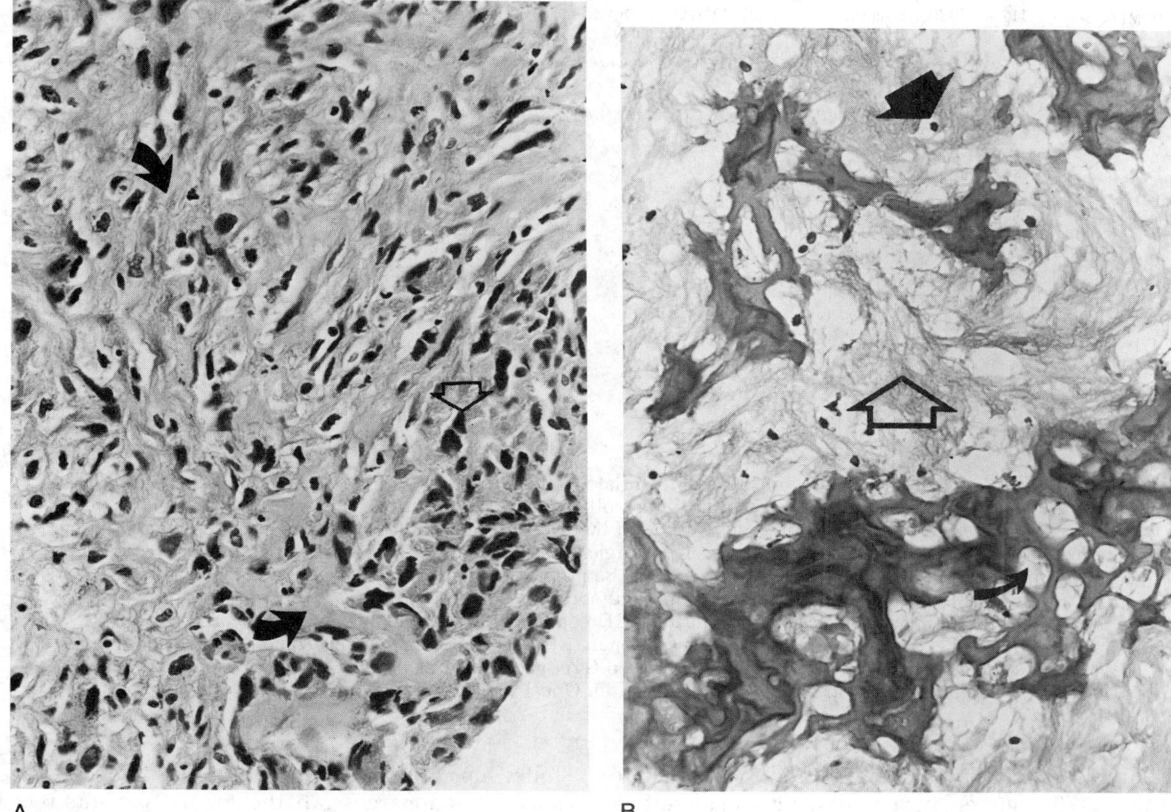

FIGURE 44–11. Two histologic effects of preoperative chemotherapy. **(A)** The section demonstrates a typical high-grade osteosarcoma (hematoxylin & eosin stain; original magnification ×200). Notice the typical osteoid (*solid curved arrows*) being made by malignant stroma cells (*open arrow*). **(B)** Photomicrograph demonstrating complete tumor cell necrosis. There are no viable cells remaining in this section; the lacunae are empty, and only the extracellular matrix (osteoid and tumor bone) remains. Osteosarcomas may not shrink much despite complete necrosis due to the persistence of their extracellular matrix.

sponsive to presurgical therapy are destined to do well when the same therapy is continued postoperatively. Patients whose tumors are unresponsive to the presurgical regimen have a much less favorable outlook and may benefit from a change in chemotherapeutic agents.

This strategy was pioneered at MSKCC in the T-10 protocol (Fig. 44–12A).[180,194] Patients were treated preoperatively with high-dose methotrexate, the BCD combination, and doxorubicin. Those with favorable (grades III and IV) histologic responses continued to receive the same agents postoperatively (T-10B regimen). Patients demonstrating unfavorable (grades I and II) histologic responses were treated on regimen T-10A, consisting of doxorubicin and cisplatin with the BCD combination (without high-dose methotrexate) postoperatively (Fig. 44–12B). Although only 39% of patients achieved a favorable histologic response to presurgical chemotherapy (51% if only patients younger than 21 were analyzed), virtually all of the favorable responders were projected to survive free of recurrence.[180,194] The patients whose primary tumors demonstrated an unfavorable histologic response were switched to the cisplatin-containing regimen, and almost 85% were initially projected to remain relapse free at 3 years. Overall, in preliminary reports, 90% of patients treated on the T-10 regimen with tailored therapy were projected to remain disease free at 3 years. Moreover, a significant difference in outcome could no longer be detected between favorable and unfavorable responders to presurgical chemotherapy, supporting the contention that poor responders were "salvaged" by the administration of alternative chemotherapy postoperatively. Because of these favorable preliminary results, the T-10 protocol served as a model for many of the osteosarcoma treatment studies launched in the 1980s, virtually all of which featured the use of presurgical chemotherapy and tailoring of treatment based on responsiveness of the primary tumor.

NEOADJUVANT CHEMOTHERAPY

Results reported from representative trials using presurgical chemotherapy are summarized in Table 44–10. Responses in the primary tumor have been variable with favorable responses observed in 30% to 85% of patients. The overall results are excellent, but comparable to adjuvant studies that used regimens of equal intensity without any preoperative chemotherapy (see Table 44–7). The importance of tailoring therapy (*i.e.*, postoperative chemotherapy is individualized based on response of the primary tumor) in this strategy remains to be defined.

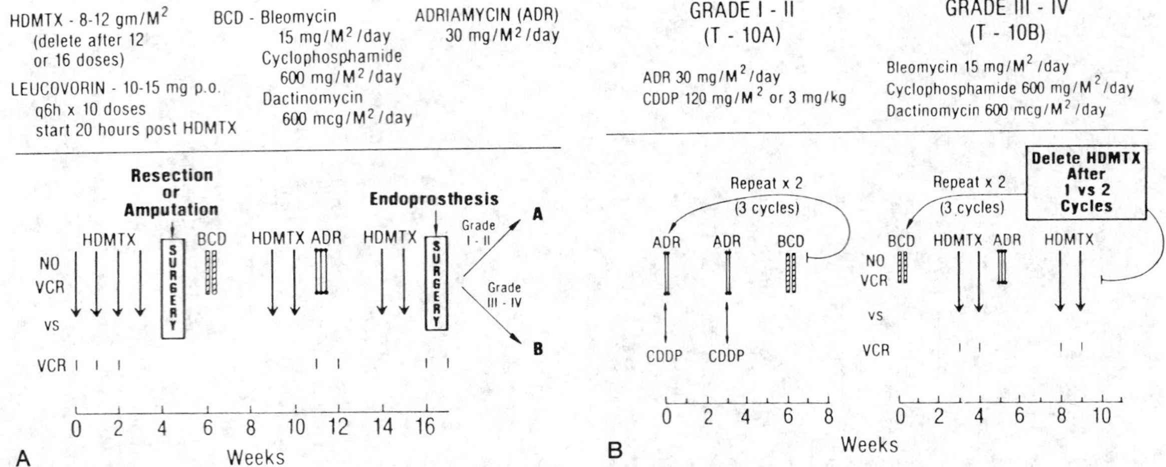

FIGURE 44–12. The T-10 regimen from Memorial Sloan-Kettering Cancer Center. **(A)** All patients receive the initial 16-week regimen. The presurgical chemotherapy regimen features four weekly courses of high-dose methotrexate and leucovorin rescue followed by resection of amputation. Patients undergoing endoprosthetic replacement receive 16 weeks of presurgical chemotherapy. **(B)** Postoperative chemotherapy is determined by the histologic grade of response of the primary tumor to presurgical chemotherapy. Patients achieving an unfavorable response in the primary tumor (grades I and II) receive T-10A regimen postoperatively, featuring doxorubicin, cisplatin, and the BCD combination. Patients achieving a favorable response (grades III and IV) receive the T-10B regimen postoperatively and continue to receive high-dose methotrexate with doxorubicin and the BCD combination. (Rosen G, et al. Primary osteogenic sarcoma: Eight-year experience with adjuvant chemotherapy. J Cancer Res Clin Oncol 1983;106[Suppl]:55–67)

The Children's Cancer Study Group (CCSG) attempted to duplicate the T-10 regimen in a multiinstitutional setting (CCSG 782).[187] Results were not as favorable as those initially reported from MSKCC; only 30% of the patients demonstrated favorable responses in the primary tumor. These patients fared extremely well, with 90% projected to remain disease free at 2 years. The remaining poor-responding patients did not benefit from a change in therapy postoperatively. Overall, 61% of patients in the CCSG study were projected to remain free of recurrent disease at 2 years—a disappointing result compared with the initial results reported from MSKCC.

The COSS-82 trial of the GPO also tested the strategy of tailoring treatment.[185] As in the CCSG trial, results suggest that patients demonstrating poor response of the primary tumor are destined to do poorly and that treatment of poor responders with salvage regimens (as in the T-10 protocol) is inadequate to improve their prognosis. Investigators of the GPO concluded that active agents should not be withheld from the initial therapy of newly diagnosed patients.

At the Instituto Rizzoli overall results have improved over time concurrent with the adoption of the strategy of presurgical chemotherapy.[186,197] However, the Rizzoli investigators conclude that the improvement in prognosis more likely reflects improved effectiveness of the agents used rather than the use of presurgical chemotherapy, because a group of patients treated concurrently at the same institution without the benefits of presurgical chemotherapy fared just as patients treated with presurgical chemotherapy.[197] As in the CCSG and COSS-82 trials, favorable responders in the Rizzoli trial had a better overall outcome; however, change in the postoperative chemotherapy for poor responders did not alter their unfavorable prognosis.

An update of results of the MSKCC studies indicates that the promising preliminary results have eroded with additional follow-up.[193] Moreover, no difference in overall disease-free survival is apparent, whether or not patients received presurgical chemotherapy as part of their management. Although histologic response to preoperative chemotherapy strongly predicted subsequent disease-free survival and overall survival, with longer follow-up, the MSKCC investigators were unable to demonstrate an improvement in disease-free survival for poor responders who received a modification of their postoperative chemotherapy compared with a similar group of patients treated without such tailoring of treatment.[193]

Whether the administration of presurgical chemotherapy (with or without tailoring of treatment based on tumor response) results in an improvement in outcome for patients with chemotherapy remains to be demonstrated conclusively. A study designed to test this question is currently being conducted by the Pediatric Oncology Group.

Although responsiveness of the primary tumor to presurgical chemotherapy is a powerful predictor of outcome, the likelihood that an individual patient will respond favorably cannot be predicted at the time of diagnosis. Because it is apparent that most poor responders relapse and that modifications of postsurgical chemotherapy fail to influence this unfavorable outcome, strategies are needed to predict favorably and poorly responding patients before the initiation of therapy so that more aggressive approaches can be used for poor-prognosis patients earlier in treatment. Analysis of tumor DNA content or expression of a multidrug resistance gene (*MDR*) in primary tumors before therapy may prove to be useful for this purpose.[198]

INTRAARTERIAL CHEMOTHERAPY

Presurgical chemotherapy may be administered directly into the arterial supply of the tumor to maximize drug delivery to

TABLE 44–10. Results of Representative Trials Incorporating Presurgical Chemotherapy for Osteosarcoma

*Investigations**	*Regimen**	*No. of Patients*	*Relapse Free (%)*
MSKCC[179,180,193]	HDMTX + VCR + ADRIA + BCD (T-7)	54 (under 21 years)	74
MSKCC[179,180,194]	HDMTX + VCR + ADRIA + BCD ± CDDP (depending on response) (T-10)	79 (under 21 years)	76
GPO[183,184]	ADRIA + HDMTX + (BCD or CDDP) ± interferon (COSS 80)†	116	68
Mount Sinai[195]	HDMTX + ADRIA + CDDP	25	77
CCSG[187]	HDMTX + VCR + ADRIA + BCD ± CDDP (depending on response) (CCSG-782)	192	61
GPO[185]	HDMTX + ADRIA + CDDP + IFOS (COSS-82)	125	58
EOIS[196]	ADRIA + CDDP ± HDMTX‡	231	63 (−HDMTX) 48 (+HDMTX)
Rizzoli[186]	IA CDDP + (HDMTX vs IDMTX) + ADRIA ± BCD (depending on response)§	127	51% (overall) (58%) (HDMTX) (42%) (IDMTX)
M.D. Anderson[188]	(IA CDDP vs HDMTX) + ADRIA (postoperative therapy determined based on response to preoperative therapy) (TIOS I)	43	60
M.D. Anderson	IA CDDP + ADRIA ± CTX (depending on response) (TIOS III)	24	

* HDMTX, high-dose methotrexate (12 g/m^2 or more) + leucovorin rescue; IDMTX, intermediate-dose methotrexate (750 mg/m^2) + leucovorin rescue; VCR, vincristine; ADRIA, doxorubicin (Adriamycin); BCD, bleomycin, cyclophosphamide, dactinomycin combination; CDDP, cisplatin; IA, intraarterial administration; CTX, cyclophosphamide.
MSKCC, Memorial Sloan-Kettering Cancer Center; GPO, German Society for Pediatric Oncology; CCSG, Children's Cancer Study Group; EOIS, First European Osteosarcoma Intergroup Study; Rizzoli, Instituto Ortopedico Rizzoli; M.D. Anderson, M.D. Anderson Cancer Center.
† Randomized study; no significant difference in relapse-free survival for patients on each treatment arm of study.
‡ Randomized study; favors treatment without HDMTX. (Some patients treated only adjuvantly).
§ Randomized study; difference in results of treatments significant at 7% level.

the tumor vasculature.[186,192,199,200] Doxorubicin and cisplatin have been delivered by prolonged intraarterial infusion to the extremities. Pharmacokinetic studies have shown that intraarterial chemotherapy produces high local drug concentrations.[199] Dramatic responses in the primary tumors have been observed in these patients, facilitating limb-salvage surgery. Significant skin and muscle necrosis, however, can occur as an inadvertent complication of intraarterial infusion.[201] The technique has appropriately been limited to centers with excellent angiographic support facilities.

The rationale for the use of intraarterial therapy is not self-evident for several reasons. Even in the prechemotherapy era, control of the primary tumor in patients with extremity primaries was rarely a problem; it was micrometastatic disease in the lung that ultimately killed the patient. Improvements in the outcome of patients with osteosarcoma have resulted directly from improvements of systemic chemotherapy for micrometastatic disease rather than from better local control measures, although the rate of limb salvage has increased dramatically.

Strategies that improve drug delivery to the primary tumor at the expense of drug delivery to micrometastatic disease are counterintuitive. Most intraarterial regimens use single-agent chemotherapy for the first 2 to 3 months of treatment, but improvements in outcome for patients with osteosarcoma have resulted from the application of multiagent chemotherapy. There is little evidence to suggest that responses observed from intraarterial administration are superior to those seen with systemic intravenous administration of the same agents. In the COSS-86 study of the GPO, responses observed in primary tumors of patients receiving intraarterial chemotherapy were not superior to responses seen in patients given the same agents intravenously.[202] Nor is it certain that the administration of intraarterial chemotherapy translates into superior overall outcome for patients as determined by improvement in relapse-free survival. An update of studies from the MDACC, where intraarterial chemotherapy was pioneered, indicates that the overall disease-free survival for pediatric patients treated with intraarterial cisplatin, definitive surgery, and postoperative adjuvant chemotherapy is projected to be 60%—a disappointing result from a single-institution trial compared with results achieved in other multiinstitutional trials with or without presurgical or intraarterial chemotherapy (see Tables 44–7 and 44–10).[188]

INFLUENCE OF REGIONAL CHEMOTHERAPY ON THE CHOICE OF SURGICAL PROCEDURE

A relatively new concept in the management of extremity sarcomas is the use of regional chemotherapy employing the intraarterial route (Fig. 44-13).[172,189,190,201,206] To improve the

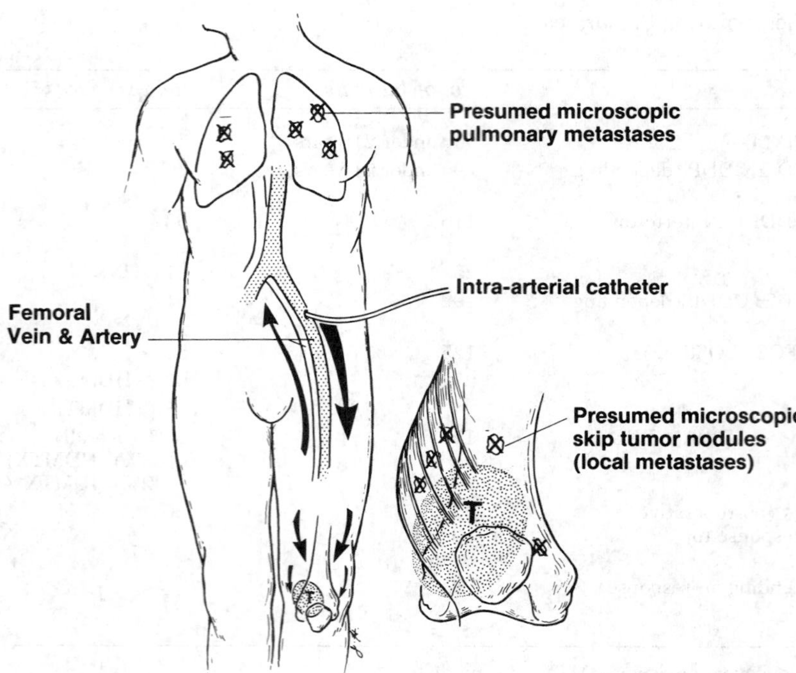

FIGURE 44–13. Postulated mechanism of the regional effect of neoadjuvant chemotherapy. The chemotherapeutic agent is delivered to the tumor at a presumed high dose and then becomes systemic to treat the probable micrometastases in the lungs. (Malawer MM, Buch R, Reaman G, et al. Impact of two cycles of preoperative chemotherapy with intraarterial cisplatin and intravenous doxorubicin on the choice of surgical procedure for high-grade bone sarcomas of the extremities. Clin Orthop Rel Res 1991;270:214–222)

results of preoperative intravenous chemotherapy, further downstage the tumor, and increase the limb-sparing procedure rate, some surgeons and oncologists began using intraarterial chemotherapy preoperatively. Presumably, this allows a higher cytotoxic concentration of chemotherapy to be directed to the primary tumor. Doxorubicin and cisplatin are the two most common drugs evaluated using this technique. A large experience has been reported from UCLA, MDACC, Children's Hospital in Washington, and the Rizzoli Institute in Italy.[138,143,155,172,187,189–191,201–206]

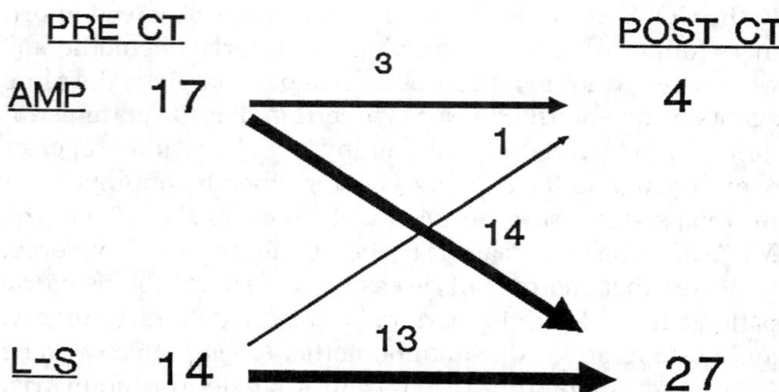

FIGURE 44–14. The impact of neoadjuvant chemotherapy on the choice of surgical procedure: surgical decisions made before receiving chemotherapy (PRE CT) compared with actual surgical procedure performed after induction with intraarterial chemotherapy (POST CT). Initially 17 (55%) of 31 patients would have required an amputation, compared with only 4 (13%) of 31 amputations actually performed (limb salvage rate of 87%). Notice that 14 (82%) of 17 patients were converted from an amputative decision to a limb-sparing procedure. (Malawer MM, Buch R, Reaman G, et al. Impact of two cycles of preoperative chemotherapy with intraarterial cisplatin and intravenous doxorubicin on the choice of surgical procedure for high-grade bone sarcomas of the extremities. Clin Orthop Rel Res 1991;270:214–222)

Malawer and colleagues reported an 82% conversion rate for patients with extremity osteosarcomas that would have required amputation (14 of 17 patients) before treatment and subsequently obtained a good clinical response to intraarterial chemotherapy, resulting in a limb-sparing procedure being performed (Fig. 44–14).[206a] Only 1 patient deemed initially resectable progressed during the preoperative (intraarterial) phase of treatment. It is the subjective impression of many surgeons that intraarterial chemotherapy results in a higher limb-sparing rate for extremity sarcomas, although no difference in overall survival has been demonstrated. We think that only rarely should a patient be treated by primary amputation without determining the patient's response to preoperative (intraarterial or intravenous) chemotherapy.

RADIATION THERAPY FOR BONE TUMORS

In keeping with the multidisciplinary, multimodality approach to the treatment of bone tumors, all patients should be evaluated by a radiation oncologist and by an orthopedic and medical (or pediatric) oncologist before decisions concerning therapy are made. Close communication between members of the care team is crucial. Tumors of the axial skeleton and facial bones are treated by a combination of limited surgery and radiation therapy. Ewing's sarcoma and peripheral primitive neuroectodermal tumors of bone may be managed by definitive radiation treatment, complete surgical excision, or combined surgical and radiation therapy approaches and are discussed elsewhere in this text. In general, radiation therapy is not used in the primary treatment of osteosarcoma. Patients who refuse definitive surgery, require palliation, or have tumors in axial locations may require radiation therapy.

TREATMENT PLANNING

Optimal radiation therapy of bone tumors requires careful planning (Table 44–11). Planning begins with tumor localization and accurate definition of the clinical and radiographic extent of tumor and of all tissue at risk for microscopic involvement. Precise, three-dimensional definition is required. This evaluation is identical to that done for surgical evaluation (see Preoperative Evaluation). These composite studies are used to establish the maximal tumor dimensions.

With the clinical physicist, decisions are made about the optimal choice of irradiation beam (*e.g.*, photon, electron), technique (*e.g.*, external-beam, brachytherapy, intraoperative therapy), beam modifiers (*e.g.*, compensators, wedge filters), and immobilization system. All patients should undergo simulation and be treated with megavoltage therapy units. There is no role for orthovoltage (low kV x-rays) in the management of primary tumors of bone.

Patient immobilization is essential to optimal radiation therapy. The patient should be placed in a comfortable position on the treatment table. The precise patient set-up should be planned using three points for reproducibility.[207] Immobilization devices such as casts, shells, vacuum pillows, and sandbags are frequently necessary.[208] Molding techniques that require a cast of the anatomic site to be treated are generally preferred if treatment fields are complex and the irradiation course is lengthy.

DOSE AND VOLUME CONSIDERATIONS

Large treatment volumes that include the entire clinical and radiographic extent of tumor plus a generous margin for microscopic or subclinical extension of disease are needed. For tumors that tend to spread along the medullary canal (*e.g.*, lymphoma, Ewing's sarcoma), the standard radiation field has included the entire bone, with a boost of radiation to the area of bulky disease. Current protocols suggest that irradiation to an involved field only may be sufficient for children with small round cell bone tumors who have responded to induction chemotherapy. If large fields are needed, it is desirable to use an extended source-to-skin distance to enable the entire radiation field to fit into one portal. If extended distances are not possible and two radiation fields must be abutted, this should be done through areas of microscopic rather than gross disease. Matchlines should be routinely moved every 1000 cGy.

TABLE 44–11. Guidelines for Optimal Radiation Therapy in the Treatment of Bone Sarcomas

Tumor localization
Simulation
Patient immobilization
Megavoltage irradiation
High radiation dose
Large treatment fields, with use of shrinking and cone-downed fields
Beam-shaping devices
Beam modifiers—compensators, wedges
Multiple fields treated each day

The irradiated field should encompass at least the same volume of tissue that would be resected plus an allowance of approximately 2 cm for patient movement and dose fall-off at the margin of the field. Extremity fields should be planned with a strip of tissue purposely out of the beam to allow lymphatic and venous return and to decrease morbidity. This nonirradiated strip should overlie the lymphatic drainage, which is located medially in the lower and upper extremities.

Because high doses are often necessary in the treatment of malignant bone tumors, a shrinking field technique is advised. This allows treatment to a large volume of subclinical disease with a moderate radiation dose, while the area of gross tumor is treated to a higher, sterilizing dose.

Additional principles involve the use of multiple beam-shaping devices so that shaped fields can be designed to conform to the individual tumor volume and patient anatomy. Multiple fields should be used to optimize the radiation dosage, and all fields must be treated every day. Beam modifiers, including compensating filters and wedge filters, should be employed to account for individual variations in patient thickness. The use of multiple small radiation fractions per day (*i.e.*, hyperfractionation) may allow the administration of higher tumor doses while simultaneously protecting sensitive nearby normal structures, such as the spinal cord, from the late effects of radiation therapy.

If chemotherapy and radiation therapy are being used, it is important to avoid the concomitant administration of drugs, such as doxorubicin and dactinomycin, that may act as radiosensitizers in normal tissues.

COMPLICATIONS OF IRRADIATION

The complications of irradiation are directly related to treatment dose and volume. Reactions occurring during the early stages of treatment are usually reversible and not of major significance. These include erythema, dry desquamation of the skin, and epilation. More serious late reactions may include fibrosis, contracture, atrophy, impaired growth, secondary fracture, and radiation-induced sarcoma. If pelvic treatment is required, it is important to consider ovarian transposition in young women whenever possible, techniques to move the small bowel out of the pelvis, and avoidance of treating the entire bladder if cyclophosphamide or ifosfamide are also being used. Fibrosis and contracture can be minimized and possibly avoided by embarking on an active physical therapy program during radiation therapy; the program should be continued after irradiation. Whenever possible, the radiologists should avoid treating across a joint space and avoid treating an open epiphysis. The risk of secondary fracture increases if there has been extensive destruction of bone such that remodeling and repair do not reconstitute the affected part. For tumors of weight-bearing bones, partial weight bearing and protective bracing are important until reossification occurs.

IRRADIATION FOR BENIGN BONE TUMORS

Some benign bone tumors are difficult to differentiate from their malignant counterparts. They have a significant rate of local recurrence and may undergo malignant transformation. The oncologist may be called to aid in establishing the correct diagnosis of a benign bone tumor or to treat local recurrence.

In general, benign tumors are managed surgically and are not considered for irradiation. However, specific indications for considering irradiation may include one or multiple recurrences and inability to completely resect.

There are several guidelines to consider in contemplating a course of irradiation for benign disease. Determine the consequences of no treatment and the natural history of the benign disease. Determine the risk-benefit ratio of radiation treatment and other therapies. Consider radiation treatment if surgical approaches have not succeeded in alleviating the condition and if the risk of other therapies is greater than the risk of radiation therapy. Determine the potential long-term risk of radiation treatment; the quality of radiation, dose, volume, time, underlying organs at risk, and any underlying disease. Obtain informed consent.[209]

Several benign tumors that deserve special consideration are discussed in the following sections.

Solitary and Multiple Osteochondromas

Osteochondromas are the most common benign bone tumor. These tumors are characteristically sessile or pedunculated, arising from the cortex of a long tubular bone adjacent to the epiphyseal plate. Osteochondromas are usually solitary, except in patients with multiple hereditary exostosis. Plain radiographs are usually diagnostic, and no additional tests are required. Sessile osteochondromas are difficult to diagnose, especially if they occur in unusual sites such as the distal posterior femur, where they must be differentiated from a parosteal osteosarcoma. Bone scintigraphy and CT scans are helpful in differentiating these two entities.

Osteochondromas "grow" with the person until skeletal maturity is reached. Growth of an osteochondroma during adolescence therefore does not signify malignancy. Pain is not a sign of malignancy in childhood or adolescence, although in adulthood, it is a significant warning sign. Pain in a child may be due to a local bursitis, mechanical irritation of adjacent muscles, or pathologic fracture.

Between 1% and 2% of solitary osteochondromas undergo malignant transformation; patients with multiple hereditary exostosis are at higher risk.[2,4,56,57] Malignant tumors arising from a benign osteochondroma are usually low-grade chondrosarcomas. Proximal osteochondromas are more likely to undergo malignant transformation than distal lesions. Surgical removal is recommended only for symptomatic osteochondromas and for those arising along the axial skeleton and pelvic or shoulder girdle.

Enchondromas

Enchondromas are composed of mature hyaline cartilage that arises within a bone (Fig. 44–15). They may be solitary or multiple (*i.e.*, Ollier's disease) and have been reported in most bones.[3,4] Their biologic potential is often overestimated or underestimated. Pathologic interpretation of cartilage tumors is more difficult than for other bone tumors; it is particularly difficult to differentiate a benign enchondroma from a grade I chondrosarcoma.[10,11,210] Malignant transformations do occur, but the rate is difficult to determine.[211] Lesions of the pelvis, femur, and ribs are generally at higher risk for malignant transformation than lesions at more distal sites.

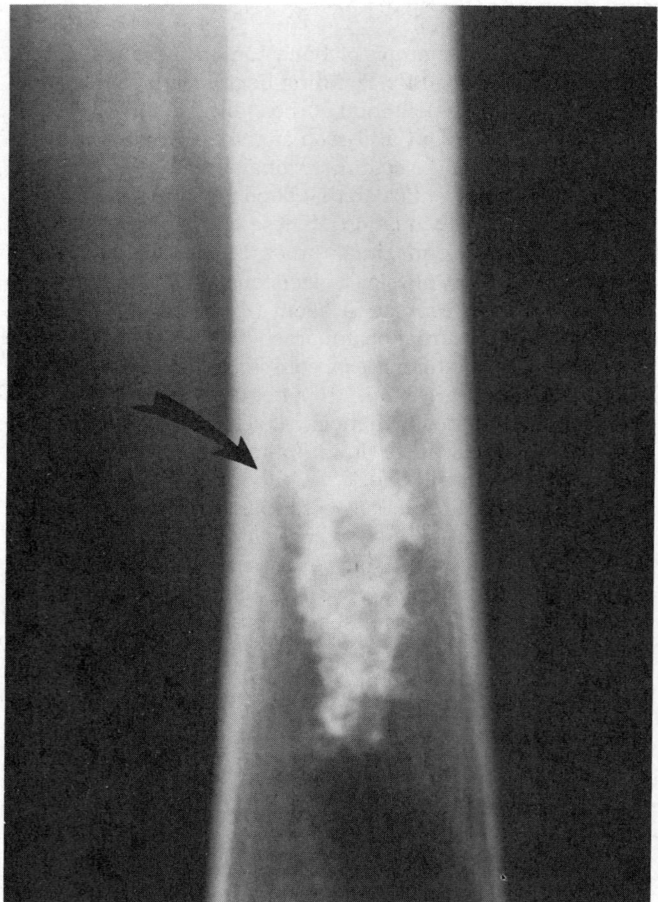

FIGURE 44–15. Enchondroma. Typical enchondroma occurring in the diaphysis of the femur. There is minimal cortical response to the tumor without evidence of bony destruction. Endosteal scalloping (*arrow*) indicates an active lesion. The differentiation from a low-grade intramedullary chondrosarcoma is based on clinical symptoms, histology, and radiographic changes.

Pain is a sign of local aggressiveness and possible malignancy. Enchondromas of the hands and feet are benign, regardless of pathology, but cartilage tumors of the pelvic or shoulder girdle are often malignant, even though the histology appears benign.[3] Plain radiographs may be helpful in this differentiation. Radiographic scalloping is a sign of local aggressiveness. Bone scintigraphy is not helpful in differentiating a low-grade chondrosarcoma from an "active" enchondroma. Patient age is an important indicator of possible malignancy; enchondromas rarely undergo malignant transformation before skeletal maturity. Painful, benign-appearing proximal enchondromas in adults are often malignant, despite their histology. The correlation of symptoms, plain radiographic findings, and histology is crucial.

Chondroblastoma, Osteoblastoma, and Osteoid Osteoma

Chondroblastoma and osteoblastoma are characterized by immature but benign chondroid and osteoid production, respectively. Both may undergo malignant transformation in rare cases.[58,211] Osteoid osteomas are small (<1 cm), painful, bone-forming tumors that are always benign (Fig. 44–16). The oncologist must be aware of these entities and be able to differentiate them from their malignant counterparts, chondrosarcoma and osteosarcoma. Chondroblastomas appear radiographically in the epiphysis of a child; conversely, primary chondrosarcomas are rarely epiphyseal and occur in adults. Although osteoblastomas may be found in any bone, the spine and skull account for 50% of all reported cases. Osteoblastomas must be differentiated from osteosarcomas and osteoid osteoma.

Chondroblastomas and osteoblastomas are considered aggressive, benign lesions with a high recurrence rate after simple curettage.[2–4,211] Local control can be obtained by primary resection; however, routine resection cannot be recommended for tumors adjacent to a joint. Marcove reports a 5% to 10% local recurrence rate if curettage is combined with cryosurgery.[211] This method has avoided the need for resection and extensive reconstruction in selected patients. Osteoid osteomas are treated by simple excision. Because surgical removal is the treatment of choice for these benign bone lesions, the role of radiation therapy is limited. For nonresectable tumors, radiation therapy has been associated with long-term control, but most radiation oncologists do not believe irradiation plays a role in the management of these conditions.[209]

Aneurysmal Bone Cyst

Aneurysmal bone cysts (ABCs) are benign tumors of childhood, occurring typically before skeletal maturity.[2–4] They never become malignant. ABCs often involve the metaphyseal regions of the long bones or the vertebrae. Radiographically, ABCs are eccentric, lytic, and expansile, characterized by cortical destruction and periosteal elevation (see Fig. 44–16). ABCs can grow rapidly and appear extremely aggressive. Differentiation from a primary malignancy may be difficult. Differential diagnosis includes giant cell tumor and telangiectatic osteosarcoma. ABCs may contain some osteoid, but careful examination reveals this to be reactive and not neoplastic. Approximately one third of ABCs arise in conjunction with another (underlying) bony neoplasm.[211,214] The classic treatment is simple curettage and bone graft, which has a recurrence rate of 20% to 35%.[4] Wide curettage may decrease the recurrence rate to approximately 10%. Marcove recommends curettage and cryosurgery as the primary treatment. Radiation therapy is recommended in surgically inaccessible sites.[3,214,215] Megavoltage doses of 2500 to 3000 cGy in 18 to 24 days have been associated with a decrease in local recurrence from 32% to 8% and are generally recommended.[180,181,209,214,215]

Desmoplastic Fibroma

Desmoplastic fibroma is an extremely rare bone tumor; only 50 cases have been reported.[211] It is characterized by abundant collagen formation and a fibrous stroma without evidence of mitosis or pleomorphism. It presents radiographically as an osteolytic lesion with well-defined margins. The basic differential diagnosis is primary fibrosarcoma of bone. Treatment is en bloc resection; curettage has a significant rate of local recurrence.

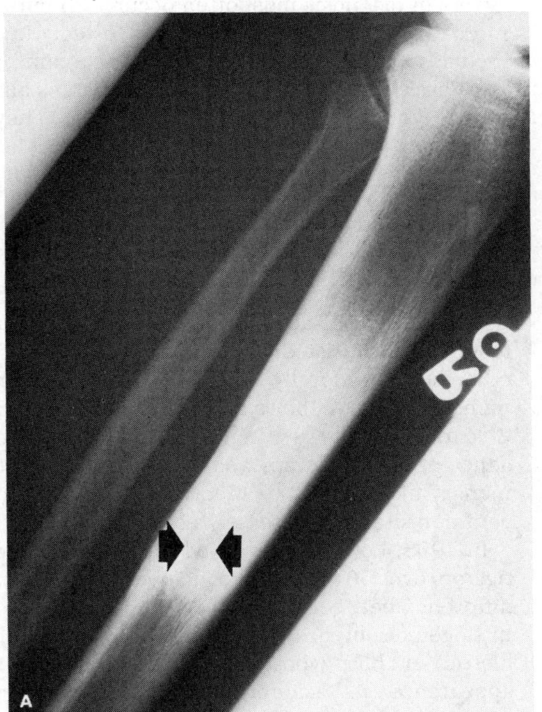

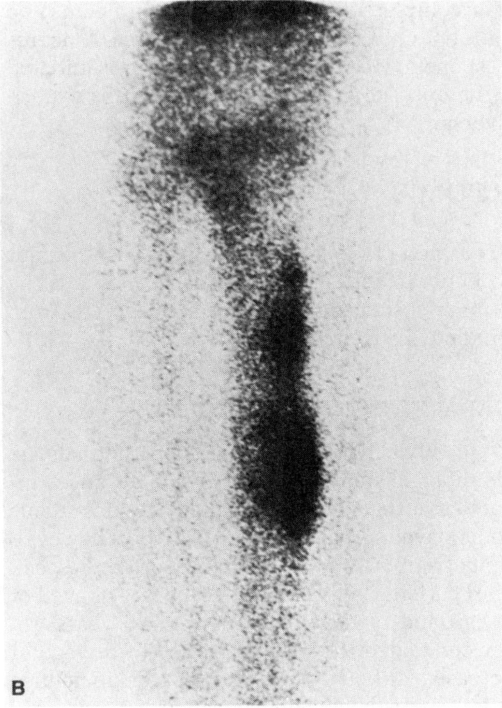

FIGURE 44–16. Osteoid osteoma. **(A)** Osteoid osteomas are characteristically a small lesion, represented radiographically as a small radiolucent nidus between 1 and 10 mm in diameter (*arrow*) surrounded by a large amount of reactive, nonneoplastic sclerotic bone. Tomograms are often necessary to demonstrate the nidus. **(B)** Bone scans will always demonstrate marked uptake that corresponds with the nidus and the reactive bone. The main radiologic differential is a sclerosing osteosarcoma.

Histiocytosis X

Langerhans' cell histiocytosis is a more descriptive and currently accepted term to describe the disease commonly referred to as histiocytosis X. The solitary or multifocal osseous lesions (Greenberger stage IA and IB) were formerly referred to as eosinophilic granuloma.[217] Histiocytosis X can be difficult to diagnose and may mimic radiographically a primary bone malignancy.

Almost any bone can be involved. Radiographically, it appears as a lytic, destructive defect, with poorly defined margins. Periosteal elevation occurs in half of all cases. This combination of characteristics strongly resembles that of Ewing's sarcoma or osteomyelitis. If arising in a flat bone, specifically the pelvis, there may be a large soft tissue component. Solitary lesions are treated by curettage.

The indications for radiation therapy include lesions of the mandible, gingiva and maxilla, where loose or painful teeth cause symptoms or reluctance to eat; lesions of weight-bearing bone at risk of fracture (*e.g.*, lytic lesion of femoral head, where curettage is not appropriate); local recurrence after surgery; local lesions showing no clinical or radiographic signs of healing after curettage or excision; expansile lesions producing symptoms or compromise of critical structures (*e.g.*, spinal cord compression or pressure on the ocular globe or optic nerve); lesions producing cosmetic deformity (*e.g.*, facial, orbital, or skull bones); painful lesions despite chemotherapy; and diabetes insipidus. Low radiation doses in the range of 600 to 1000 cGy are generally recommended and produce complete responses in approximately 90% of sites irradiated.[215–222] Local recurrences have been reported after 450 cGy, but they are rare after 600 cGy.[217] Vertebral lesions causing partial or complete collapse (*e.g.*, vertebra plana) do not require treatment unless they are symptomatic. Diabetes insipidus may respond to local irradiation if therapy is initiated promptly after the onset of symptoms, although this experience is not universal.[218,219]

OSTEOSARCOMA

Osteosarcoma is a high-grade, malignant spindle cell tumor arising within a bone. Its differentiating characteristic is the production of "tumor" osteoid or immature bone directly from a malignant spindle cell stroma.[2,3,59,220]

CLINICAL CHARACTERISTICS

Osteosarcoma typically occurs during childhood and adolescence. An epidemiologic study from the Swedish Cancer Institute documented that the mean and median ages of patients with osteosarcoma have increased since 1971.[220a] They evaluated 227 patients from 1971 to 1984 and reported the peak incidence to be in patients between 10 to 19 years of age but observed the mean and median to be 29 and 20 years, respectively. They concluded the true incidence in the age of patients had increased, although the overall annual incidence of 2.1 cases per million had not changed. When osteosarcoma occurs in patients older than 40 years, it is usually associated with a preexistent condition, such as Paget's disease, irradiated bones, multiple hereditary exostosis, or polyostotic fibrous dysplasia.[2,220–224] Bones of the knee joint and the proximal humerus are the most common sites, accounting for 50% and 25%, respectively, of all osteosarcomas.[211] Approximately 80% to 90% of osteosarcoma occur in the long tubular bones.[2,4,56,221,226–228] The axial skeleton is rarely affected. Less than 1% are found in the hands and feet.[2]

With the exception of serum alkaline phosphatase levels, which are elevated in 45% to 50% of patients, laboratory findings are usually not helpful.[226] Elevated alkaline phosphatase is not diagnostic, because it is also associated with other skeletal diseases. Pain is the most common complaint. Physical examination demonstrates a firm, soft tissue mass fixed to the underlying bone with slight tenderness. There is no effusion in the adjacent joint, and motion is normal. Incidence of pathologic fracture is less than 1%. Systemic symptoms are rare.

RADIOGRAPHIC CHARACTERISTICS

Typical radiographic findings are increased intramedullary radiodensity due to tumor bone or calcified cartilage, an area of radiolucency due to nonossified tumor, a pattern of permeative destruction with poorly defined borders, cortical destruction, periosteal elevation, and extraosseous extension with soft tissue ossification.[226–228] This combination of characteristics is not seen in other lesions. Wilner classified 600 radiographs of osteosarcoma seen at MSKCC into three broad categories: sclerotic osteosarcoma (32%), osteolytic (22%), and mixed (46%) (Fig. 44–17).[228] Although there was no statistically significant difference among overall survival rates among these types, the patterns are important to recognize. The sclerotic and mixed type offer few diagnostic problems. Errors of diagnosis most often occur with pure osteolytic tumors. The differential diagnosis of osteolytic osteosarcoma includes giant cell tumor, ABC, fibrosarcoma, and MFH.[229] In a series of 305 osteosarcomas, De Santos and Edeiken reported that 42 (13.5%) were purely lytic. They usually presented as ill-defined lesions with moderate or large soft tissue components. Nine of the lesions had benign radiographic features.

CLINICAL AND PROGNOSTIC CONSIDERATIONS

Before the era of adjuvant chemotherapy, treatment of osteosarcoma consisted of amputation. Metastasis to lungs and other bones generally occurred within 24 months. A large number of series shows an overall survival of 5% to 20% at 2 years (Fig. 44–18).[71–74] This pattern has been altered by adjuvant chemotherapy and aggressive thoracotomy for pulmonary disease.[45,101,230] Metastases may now appear at less common sites, and disease-free intervals are longer.[230]

In 1968, Lockshin reviewed the experience of 100 investigators over 50 years and concluded there was no significant difference between survival rates of patients with the three histiogenic subtypes (*i.e.*, osteoblastic, chondroblastic, fibroblastic) or those whose lesions had a different radiographic appearance (*i.e.*, sclerotic, osteolytic, or mixed).[231] Size of tumor, patient age, and degree of malignancy did not correlate with survival.[231] The most significant variable was anatomic site. Patients with pelvic and axial lesions had a lower survival rate than those with tumors of the extremities, probably due to surgical inaccessibility and incomplete removal. Patients

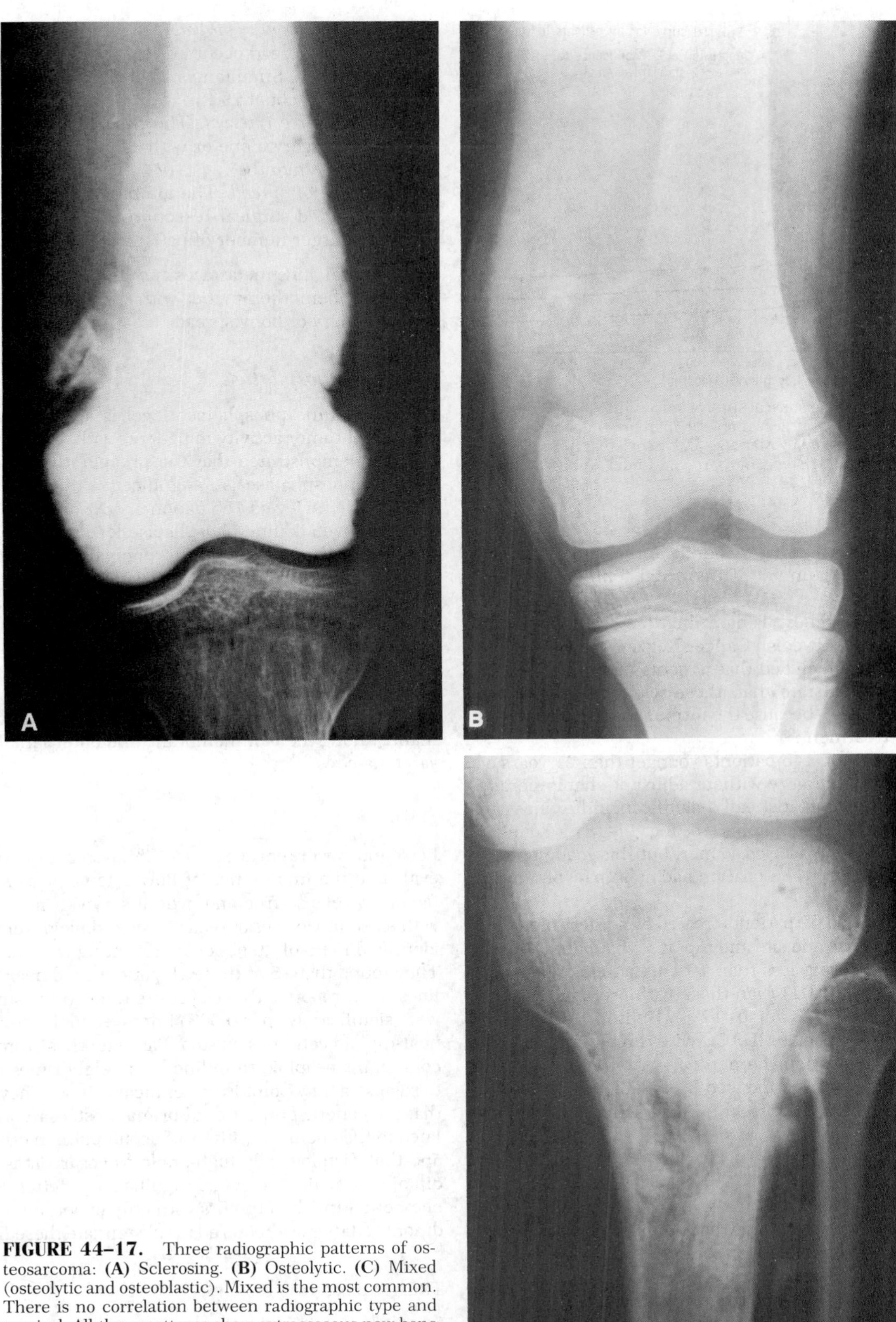

FIGURE 44–17. Three radiographic patterns of osteosarcoma: **(A)** Sclerosing. **(B)** Osteolytic. **(C)** Mixed (osteolytic and osteoblastic). Mixed is the most common. There is no correlation between radiographic type and survival. All three patterns show extraosseous new bone formation. This is pathogenomic of a bone-forming neoplasm.

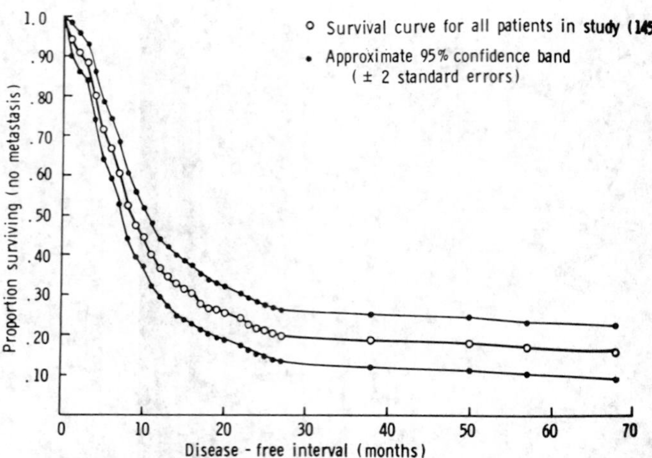

FIGURE 44–18. The historical survival curve for 145 patients with osteosarcoma treated by surgery alone at Memorial-Sloan Kettering Cancer Center, as reported by Marcove and associates. (Marcove RC, Mick V, Hajek JV, et al. Osteogenic sarcoma under the age of 21. J Bone Joint Surg [Am] 1966;48:1–26)

with tumors of the tibia had a significantly higher survival rate than those with tumors of the distal femur (35% versus 16%).

Larsson and colleagues, using a multifactorial analysis of all patients from the Swedish Cancer Registry between 1958 to 1968, similarly concluded that patients with tibial lesions had a better survival rate than those with femoral lesions (38.1% versus 15.1%), because the former were less advanced at the time of treatment.[232]

Marcove, reviewing 145 patients younger than 21 years of age who underwent surgery without adjuvant chemotherapy at MSKCC, found no statistically significant differences in race, sex, or duration of symptoms (see Fig. 44–18).[71] Younger patients developed metastases sooner, but this made no difference in overall survival. Location had no impact on 5-year survival.

Brostrom evaluated 52 patients treated by surgery alone.[233] He studied tumor size and site and reported that patients with distal lesions measuring less than 10 cm had a significantly higher survival ($p < 0.01$) than those with proximal lesions greater than 10 cm (43% versus 12%). Hudson, after evaluating 98 patients treated at MDACC with three different protocols, reported that tumor burden ($p = 0.04$) and the percentage of tumor necrosis induced by induction therapy ($p = 0.01$) were the most important prognostic factors.[233a]

Changing Pattern of Metastasis

The classic pattern and time frame of metastatic dissemination of osteosarcoma has been somewhat modified by the use of adjuvant chemotherapy and thoracotomy. Bacci and coworkers evaluated the pattern of metastatic spread of osteosarcoma in 193 patients at the Rizzoli Orthopaedic Institute.[234] Thirty patients treated with surgery alone were compared with 163 patients treated with adjuvant chemotherapy:

1. *Site of initial relapse.* No difference was found in sites of first relapse; approximately 90% of cases in both groups occurred in the lungs.
2. *Extrapulmonary spread.* After chemotherapy, extrapulmonary spread occurred in 10% of patients, usually in bony sites. Simultaneous bone and lung metastases occurred in about 2%.
3. *Disease-free interval.* The time to metastases differed with surgery alone or with adjuvant chemotherapy (13 versus 8 months).
4. *Pattern of spread.* The alteration of metastatic spread permitted surgical resection of pulmonary metastases in a larger number of patients (51% versus 29%).

In general, lung metastases appear later and are fewer after adjuvant chemotherapy but with variable difference on extrapulmonary or bony spread.

Alkaline Phosphatase

Serum alkaline phosphatase level is an important biologic marker of tumor activity in patients with osteosarcoma.[235,236] Francis demonstrated that the preoperative serum level of alkaline phosphatase is a significant prognosticator of survival.[226] He reviewed 155 patients, 46% of whom had normal preoperative alkaline phosphatase levels. Of the 2-year survivors, 85% had normal levels, compared with 12% of those dying of disease. Of the 10-year survivors, 93% had normal alkaline phosphatase levels. Scranton and coworkers found similar findings; 16 (42%) of 38 patients had elevated alkaline phosphatase levels before definitive surgery; 12 (54%) of 22 patients with normal levels survived, but only 3 (18.7%) of 16 of those with elevated levels survived.[237] Electromicroscopy has demonstrated that alkaline phosphatase is found predominantly along the cell membrane and outer lamella of osteosarcoma cells.[235,236]

DNA

Look and coworkers at St. Jude Children's Research Hospital evaluated the importance of flow cytometry as a prognostic factor on relapse-free and overall survival times in patients with extremity osteosarcoma.[238] Hyperdiploid stem lines were identified in 25 of 26 patients presenting without metastasis. They found that 15 of these 26 patients had near-diploid cell lines. They reported the relapse-free and overall survival times were significantly ($p < 0.003$) improved in the group in which near-diploid cell lines existed. Patients whose tumors did not contain near-diploid stem lines were eight times more likely to relapse at any point in the clinical course. They concluded that the genetic properties of primary osteosarcoma were related to the chemosensitivity of occult pulmonary metastases and that histologically high-grade osteosarcomas with near-diploid stem lines respond significantly better to adjuvant chemotherapy than tumors with only hyperdiploid lines. Additional studies are required to substantiate these findings.[238a]

TREATMENT

Surgical Resection of Localized Extremity Osteosarcoma

The traditional procedure for localized osteosarcoma has been amputation one joint above the tumor-containing bone or, occasionally, transmedullary amputation.[2,3,71–73] Within the past decade, parallel developments in radiology, orthopedics, and oncology have made nonamputative procedures an option for 50% to 80% of patients.[20–33] A significant impetus for these developments was the introduction of effective chemotherapeutic agents in the early 1970s.[47–52]

Springfield and coworkers from the University of Florida compared limb-sparing surgery with amputation in 53 patients with stage IIB osteosarcoma.[239] For ethical reasons, the patients were not randomized. There was no difference in survival between amputation and resection or between radical or wide surgical margins. There were three local recurrences. They recommended a wide surgical resection for adequate local control. They recommended amputation if the major neurovascular bundle was involved. They concluded that local recurrence was due to an extremely aggressive tumor or to skip metastases. The unique features of evaluation, management, and resection of tumors are described in the following sections.

SHOULDER GIRDLE. A surgical classification of shoulder girdle resections is shown schematically in Fig. 44–19.[241,242] This classification is useful for all limb-sparing procedures of the shoulder girdle. It is recommended that osteosarcomas arising from the proximal humerus be treated by a type VB resection (see Fig. 44–19). Figure 44–20 illustrates the types of local spread for a sarcoma involving the shoulder joint.

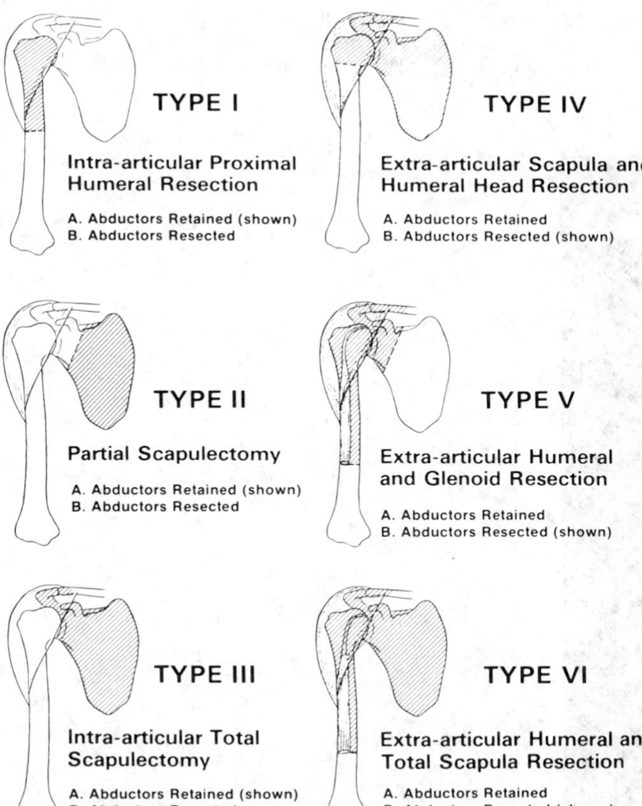

FIGURE 44–19. Schematic of proposed surgical classification of shoulder girdle resections. In general, types I–III are for benign or low-grade tumors, and types IV–VI are for high-grade tumors. A and B denote the status of the abductor mechanism: A, intact; B, partially or completely excised. Types I–III and types IV–VI are intraarticular and extraarticular resections, respectively.

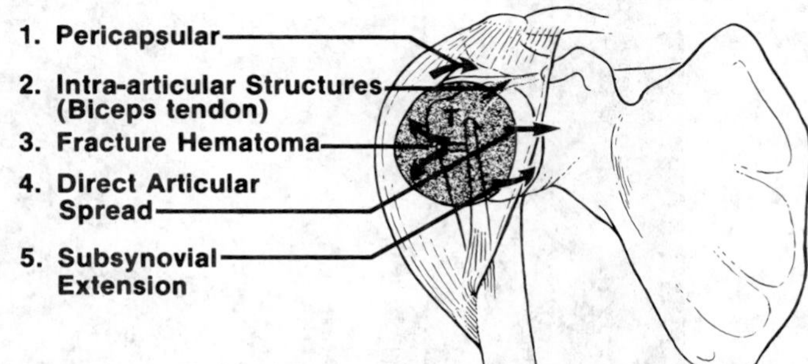

FIGURE 44–20. Mechanisms of local tumor spread for sarcomas of the shoulder. (Malawer MM, Buch R, Reaman G, et al. Impact of two cycles of preoperative chemotherapy with intraarterial cisplatin and intravenous doxorubicin on the choice of surgical procedure for high-grade bone sarcomas of the extremities. Clin Orthop Rel Res 1991;270:214–222)

PROXIMAL HUMERUS. Adequate resection of the proximal humerus requires removal of 15 to 20 cm of the humerus and shoulder joint with the deltoid, rotator cuff, and portions of the biceps and triceps muscles (Figs. 44–21 and 44–22).[240] The procedure involves suspension of the arm, motor reconstruction, and provision of adequate soft tissue coverage (Fig. 44–23).

Proximal humeral lesions should not be biopsied through the deltopectoral interval, because this contaminates the subscapularis and pectoralis muscles and the area adjacent to the axillary sheath. Biopsy under fluoroscopy through the anterior third of the deltoid by a trocar is preferred. Angiography is the most useful preoperative study. If the neurovascular bundle is clear of tumor, resection is feasible. All other structures can be removed. The major contraindications to local resection are tumor involvement of the lymph nodes or chest wall, pathologic fracture, or massive soft tissue contamination.

Resectability is determined by early exploration of the neurovascular structures by division of the pectoralis major. This approach does not jeopardize formation of an anterior flap in patients who require forequarter amputation. Preservation of the musculocutaneous nerve is important. The short biceps muscle, responsible for elbow flexion, is the most important muscle left after resection. Extraarticular resection of the glenohumeral joint by medial scapulosteotomy is safer than intraarticular resection.

A custom prosthesis is used for reconstruction. Soft tissue reconstruction and suspension are essential to avoid postoperative pain, instability, and fatigability (see Fig. 44–23). Suspension by Dacron tape and muscle transfers are effective. Hand and wrist functions are normal after resection. Shoulder motion is minimal but stable, and scapulothoracic motion provides some internal and external rotation. Cosmesis is acceptable and can be enhanced with use of a shoulder pad.

DISTAL FEMUR. Adequate en bloc resection includes 15 to 20 cm of the distal femur and proximal tibia and portions of the adjacent quadriceps (Fig. 44–24).[120] Biplane angiography is crucial to determine popliteal vessel involvement.

(text continues on page 1542)

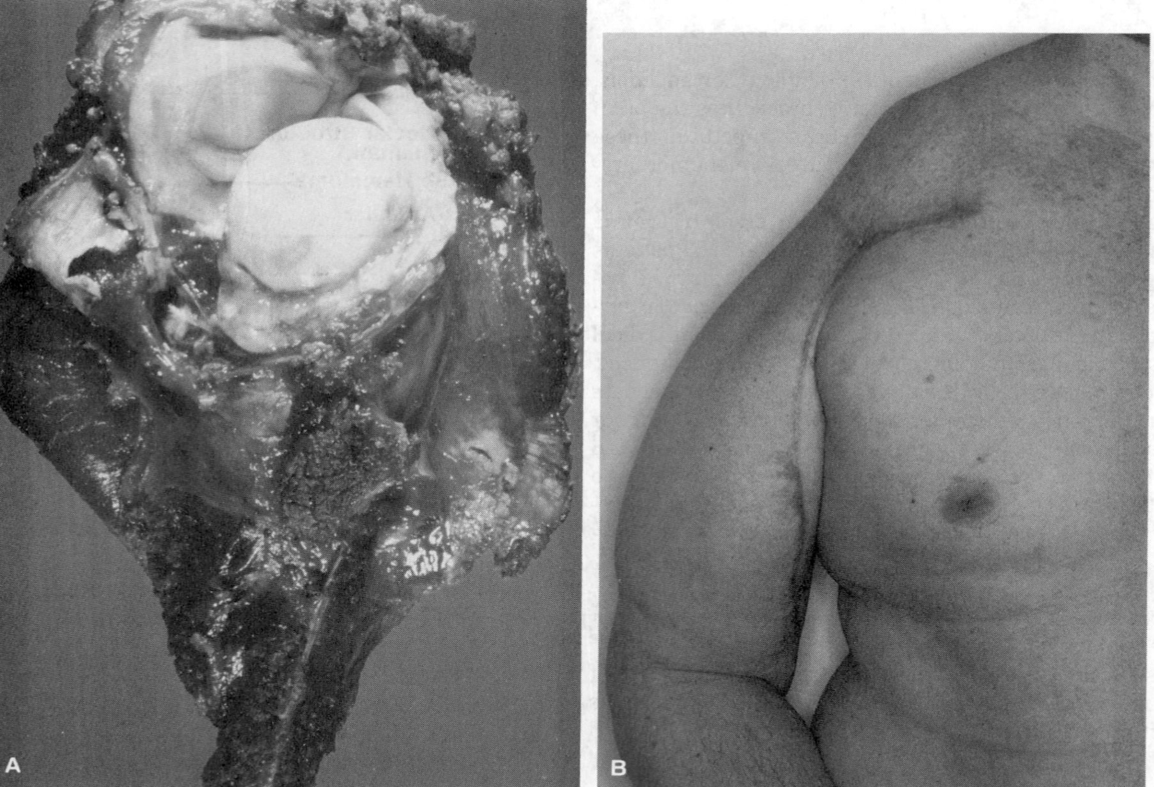

FIGURE 44–21. Osteosarcoma of the proximal humerus treated by a type V shoulder-girdle resection. **(A)** Gross specimen demonstrates the glenohumeral joint. This resection was extraarticular due to the high risk of tumor involvement of the joint. **(B)** Clinical appearance 2 years after surgery. The patient has a stable shoulder with normal elbow and hand function.

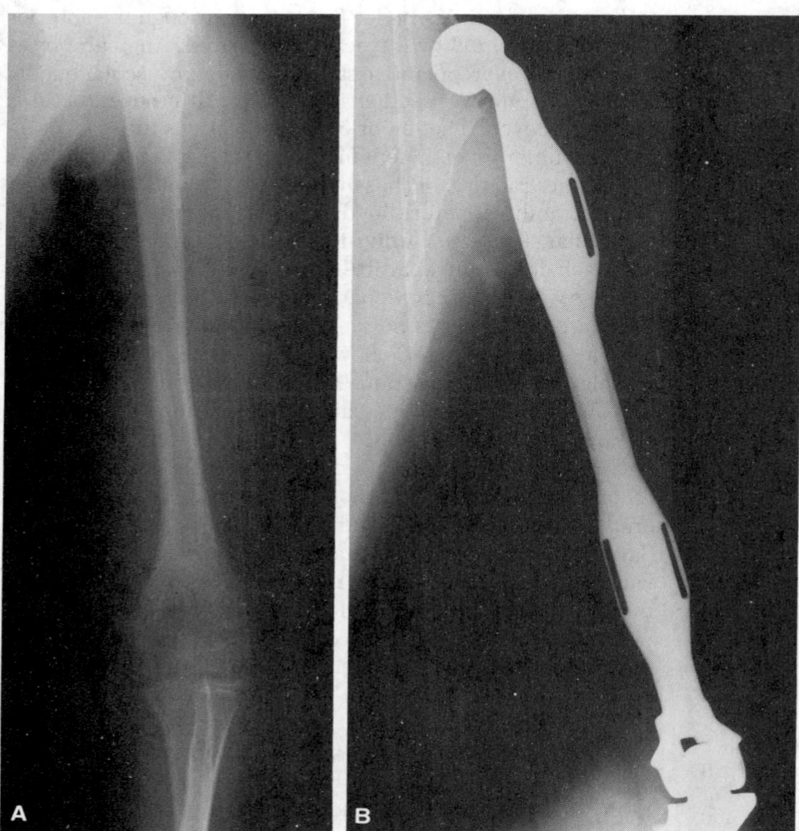

FIGURE 44–22. Osteosarcoma involving the entire humeral shaft, determined by bone scan and MRI. **(A)** Plain radiograph before chemotherapy. **(B)** This patient was treated by a custom total humeral resection and reconstruction by a custom total humeral prosthesis, including a hinge-elbow joint, showing the advancements made in design and manufacture of a custom prosthesis.

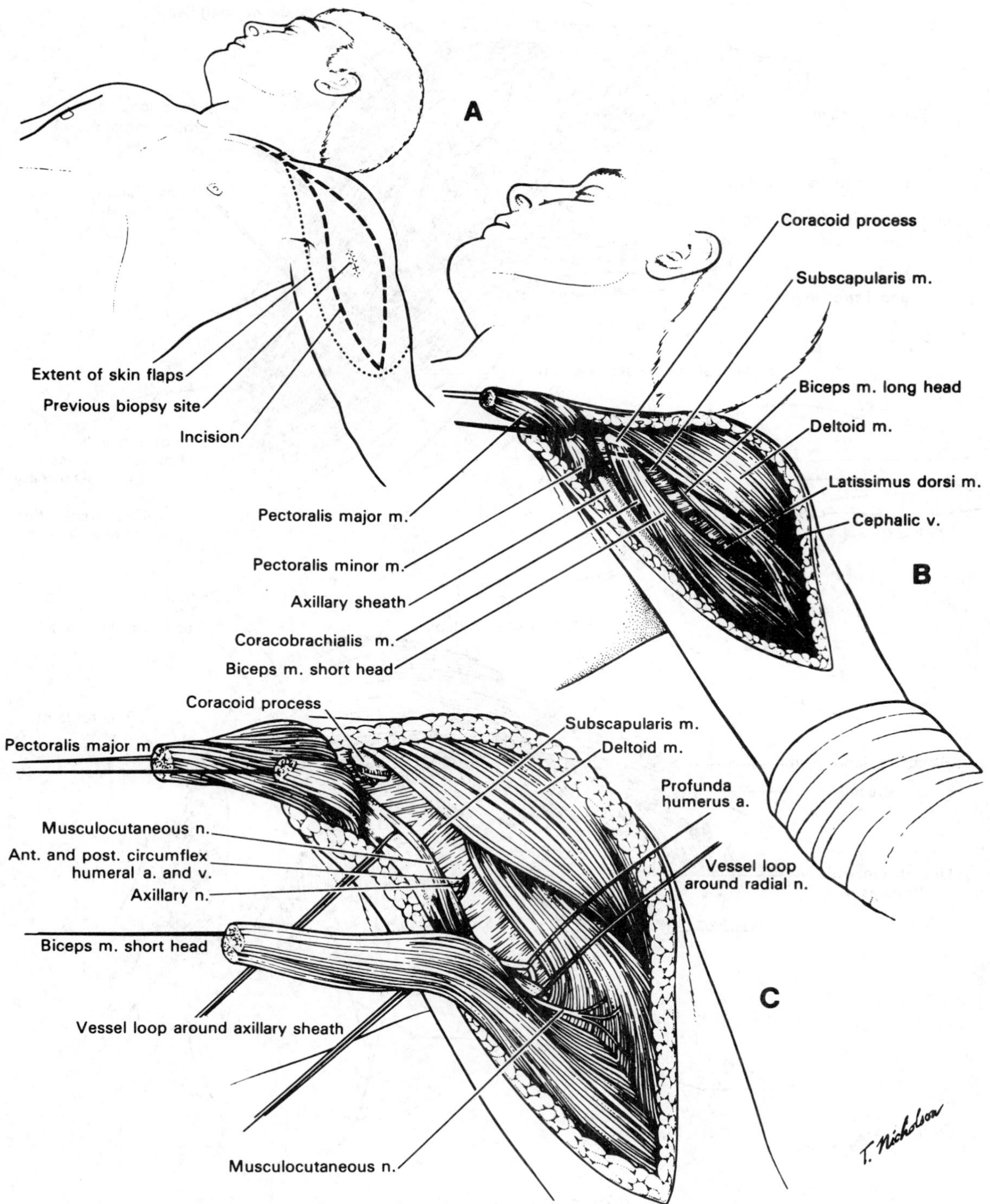

FIGURE 44–23. Technique of shoulder girdle resection for high-grade sarcomas of the proximal humerus.

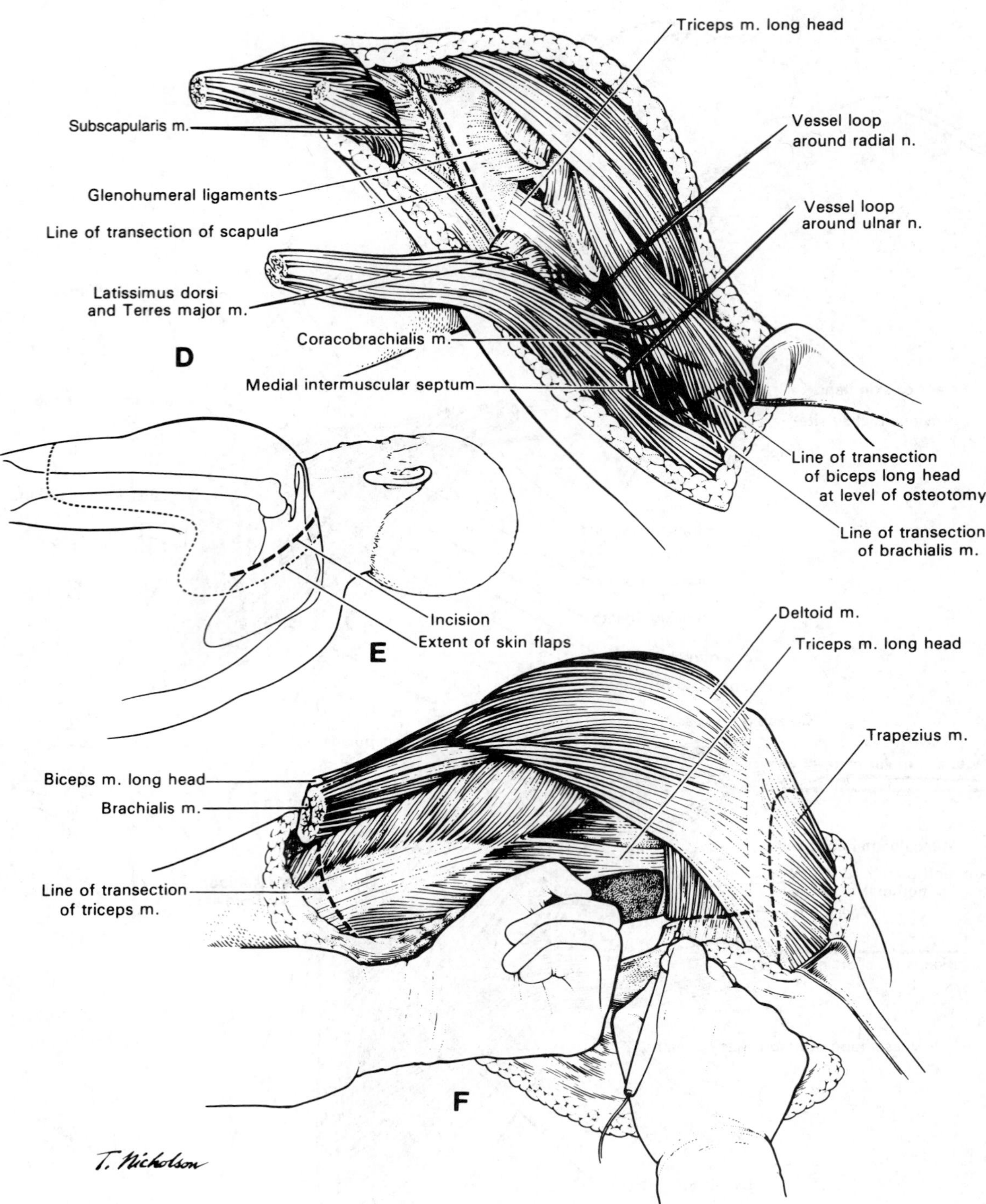
Triceps m. long head
Subscapularis m.
Vessel loop
around radial n.
Glenohumeral ligaments
Line of transection of scapula
Vessel loop
around ulnar n.
Latissimus dorsi
and Terres major m.
Coracobrachialis m.
D
Medial intermuscular septum
Line of transection
of biceps long head
at level of osteotomy
Line of transection
of brachialis m.
Incision
Extent of skin flaps
E
Deltoid m.
Triceps m. long head
Trapezius m.
Biceps m. long head
Brachialis m.
Line of transection
of triceps m.
F
T. Nicholson

FIGURE 44–23. *(Continued)*

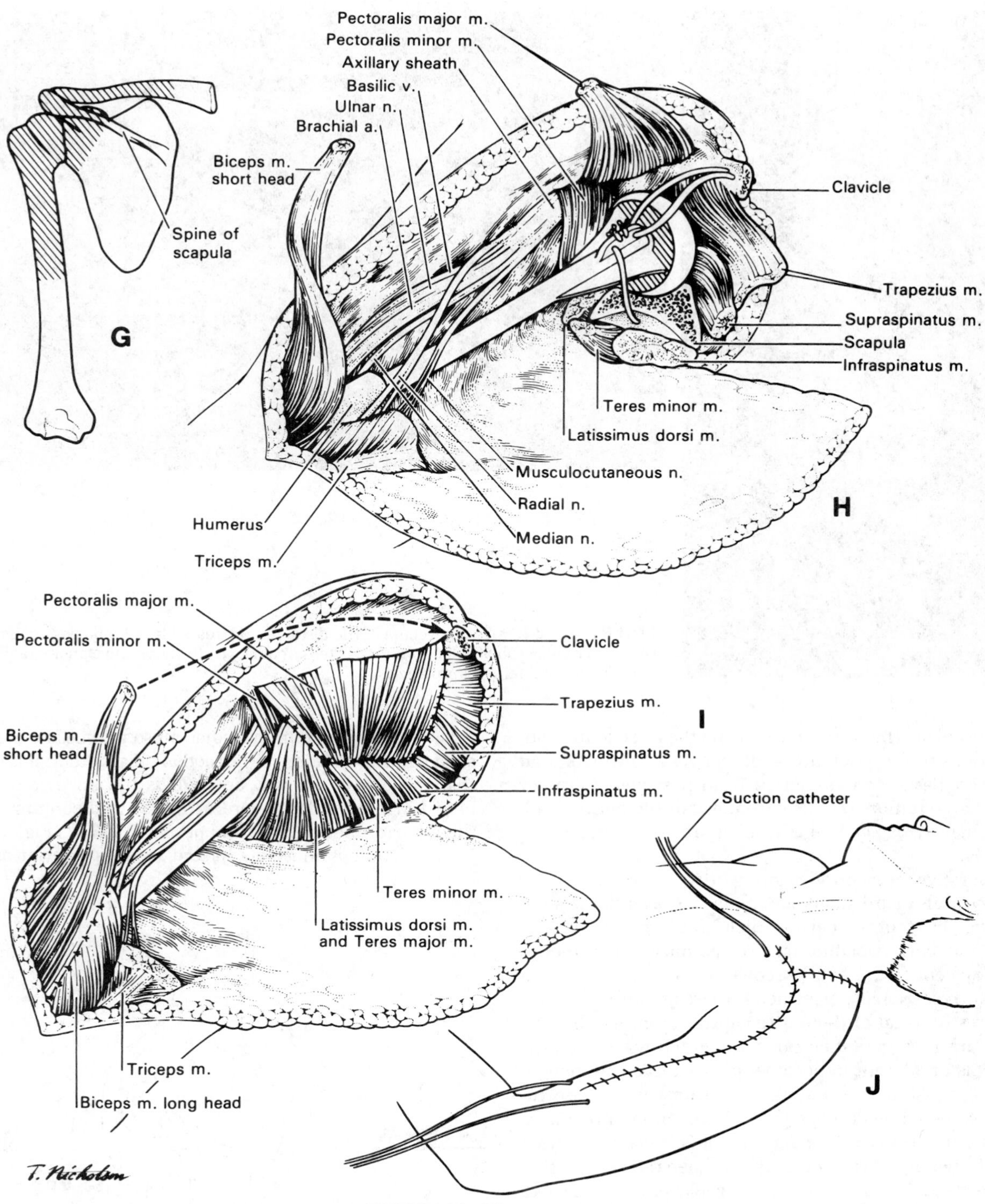
Pectoralis major m.
Pectoralis minor m.
Axillary sheath
Basilic v.
Ulnar n.
Brachial a.
Biceps m. short head
Spine of scapula
G
Clavicle
Trapezius m.
Supraspinatus m.
Scapula
Infraspinatus m.
Teres minor m.
Latissimus dorsi m.
Musculocutaneous n.
Radial n.
Median n.
Humerus
Triceps m.
H
Pectoralis major m.
Pectoralis minor m.
Clavicle
Trapezius m.
I
Biceps m. short head
Supraspinatus m.
Infraspinatus m.
Suction catheter
Teres minor m.
Latissimus dorsi m. and Teres major m.
Triceps m.
Biceps m. long head
J
T. Nicholson

FIGURE 44–23. *(Continued)*

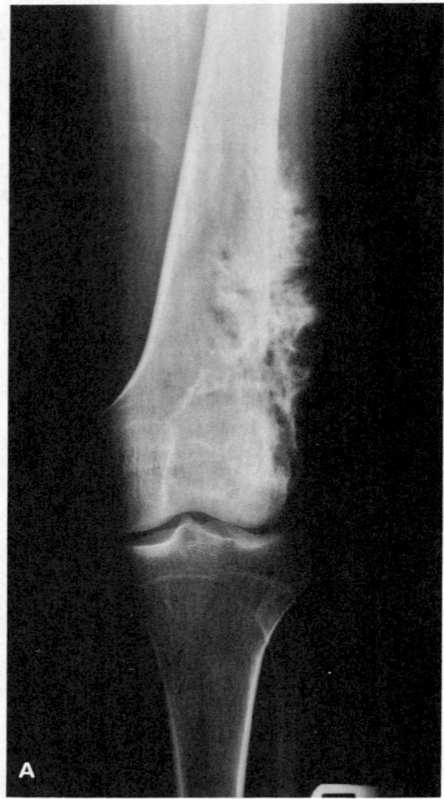

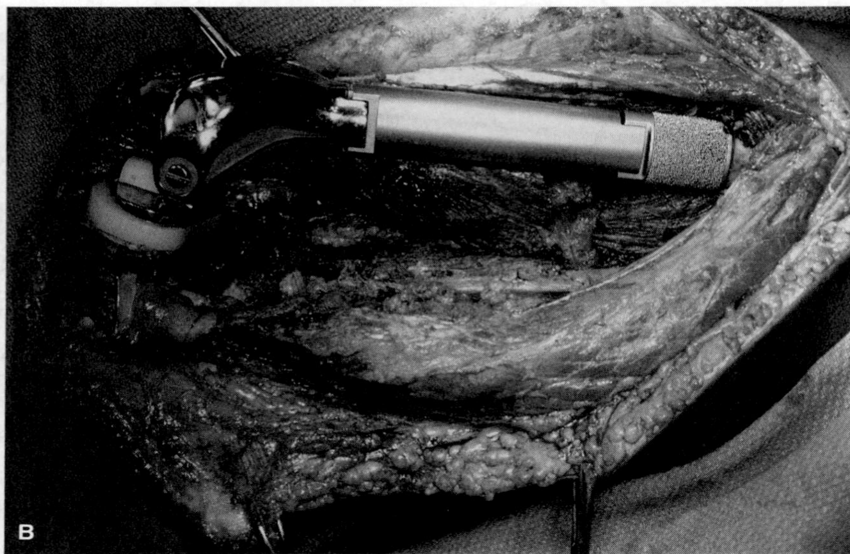

FIGURE 44–24. Osteosarcoma of the distal femur treated by a limb-sparing resection. **(A)** Plain radiograph of a distal femoral osteosarcoma. **(B)** Intraoperative photograph shows a modular distal femoral prosthesis.

Biopsy must avoid the sartorial canal and the knee joint. Contraindications to resection are popliteal vessel involvement, massive soft tissue contamination from previous biopsy, or fracture. Large tumors requiring removal of the entire quadriceps or hamstrings can be adequately reconstructed by an arthrodesis.

The operative procedure begins with exploration of the popliteal vessels. Care should be taken to preserve the sural vessels and the neurovascular pedicle to the gastrocnemius muscles. The corresponding quadriceps muscle is removed en bloc adjacent to the extraosseous tumor component. Extraarticular resection is performed if there are effusions; this necessitates removal of the entire capsule from its tibial insertion. Care must be taken not to lengthen the extremity, because this may result in postoperative arterial thrombosis. Hamstring transfers are required to reconstruct the corresponding resected quadriceps if motor function is required. A gastrocnemius transposition flap is routinely used to provide additional coverage.[243] Postoperatively, knee range of motion exercise is begun early if a prosthetic replacement was used. If an arthrodesis is performed, a long-leg cast is required until incorporation of the grafts. Hip and ankle motion are usually normal. A cane and brace are routinely recommended for 12 months.

PROXIMAL TIBIA. Limb-sparing procedures often are not feasible for tumors of the proximal tibia.[244] It is more difficult to obtain an adequate margin of resection and a good functional result with lesions of the proximal tibia, which tend to have a higher incidence of local complications than do distal femoral tumors. These problems are directly related to the anatomic constraints: minimal adjacent soft tissue and the normal subcutaneous location of the medial tibial border. It is essential that the biopsy is small and avoids the knee joint. A core biopsy of medial flare is preferred to avoid contamination of the anterior musculature and peroneal nerve (Fig. 44–25).

The popliteus muscle adjacent to the posterior aspect of

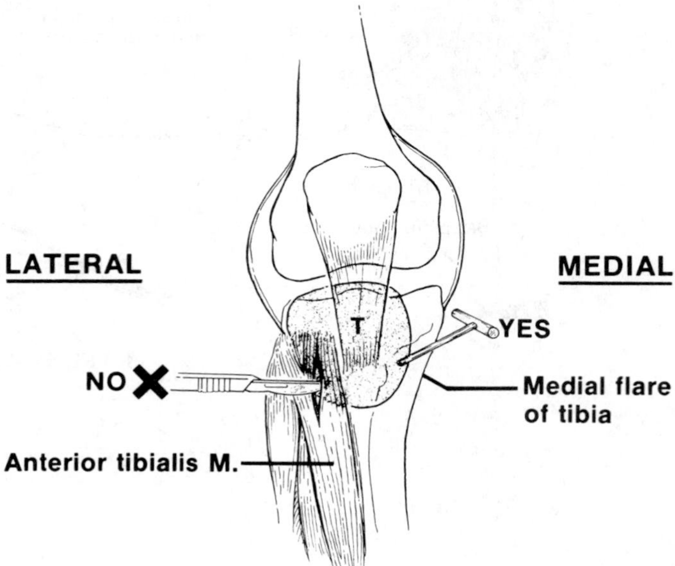

FIGURE 44–25. Biopsy technique for proximal tibial sarcomas. The biopsy should always be performed medially to avoid contamination of the anterior tibial muscles.

the tibia prevents direct tumor involvement of the neurovascular bundle.[244,245] Lateral angiography is essential to demonstrate this interval. A large posterior tumor component makes resection unadvisable. The anteroposterior projection is useful to delineate anomalous vascular patterns. Adequate resection of the proximal tibia requires ligation of the anterior tibial artery and, in most cases, the peroneal artery. The remaining posterior tibial artery leaves a viable extremity in a young person.[244] An anomalously absent posterior tibial artery, which occurs in 5% of patients, is a contraindication for resection.[246] Tumor extension often involves the tibiofibular capsule.[244] Extraarticular resection of the proximal tibiofibular joint en bloc with the tibia is required to obtain a safe margin. The average resection length is 15 to 18 cm.

Reconstruction is by prosthetic replacement, arthrodesis, or allograft (Fig. 44–26). The medial gastrocnemius is routinely transferred to provide soft tissue coverage of the reconstructed area.[243] Dacron tape is used to reattach the patella to the transferred gastrocnemius and prosthesis. Postoperative management is similar to that used for distal femoral resections.[244]

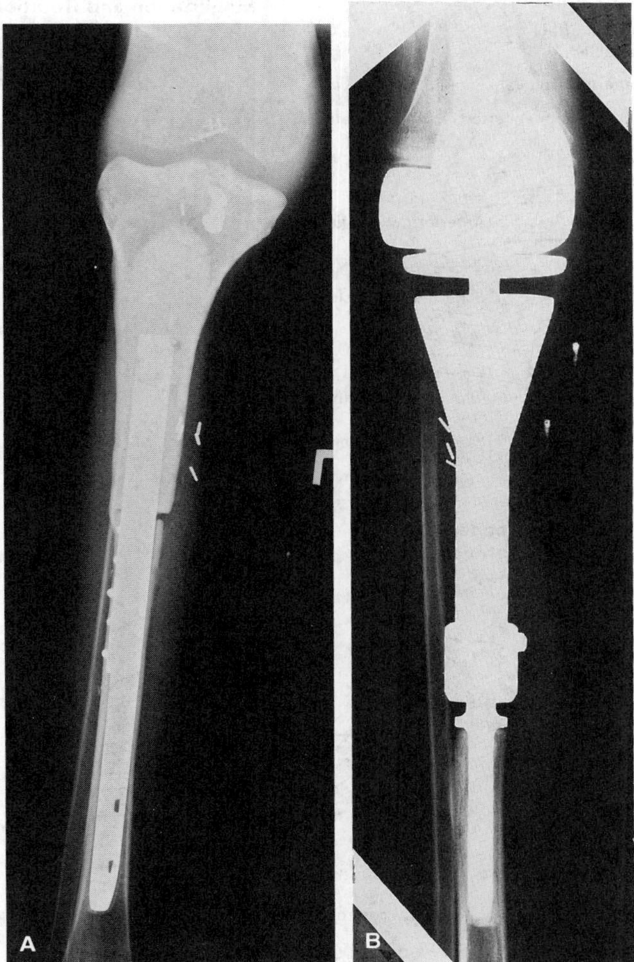

FIGURE 44–26. Two methods of reconstruction after resection of the proximal tibia. **(A)** Allograft replacement. **(B)** Expandable custom prosthesis used for the skeletal immature patient.

PROXIMAL FIBULA. Tumors of the proximal fibula require the same evaluation as proximal tibial lesions.[246] Unique considerations are early soft tissue extension, proximity to the lateral tibial condyle, necessity of ligation of the anterior and peroneal arteries, sacrifice of the peroneal nerve, and tumor infiltration of the tibiofibular joint capsule. Large tumors are often unresectable. Biplane angiography is necessary to determine anomalous vascular patterns and vascular displacement. Bone scintigraphy with multiple rotation views of the proximal tibia or MRI is essential to determine bony involvement of the adjacent tibial plateau. Contraindications to resection are direct tibial involvement, an anomalously absent posterior tibial artery, and intraarticular knee joint extension. Due to the multiple musculotendinous attachment of the proximal fibula, muscle infiltration generally occurs along muscle planes beyond visible borders.

Adequate resection includes the fibula, the tibiofibular joint, the anterior and lateral muscle compartments, and a portion of the lateral gastrocnemius, soleus, and intermuscular septum (Fig. 44–27). Wide excision of all adjacent muscle groups is mandatory (Fig. 44–28). No reconstruction of the bony defect is required. The lateral collateral ligament is reattached to the lateral joint capsule. A lateral gastrocnemius transposition flap is used to close the resultant defect.[243] After surgery, the only functional deficit is a drop foot, treated by an orthosis. Knee function is normal.[246]

Osteosarcoma of the Pelvis and Proximal Femur

Osteosarcomas of the pelvis and proximal femur (Fig. 44–29) are less common than those occurring at other anatomic areas, accounting for 10% and 5%, respectively, of all osteosarcomas.[211] Tumors arising from these structures are often large, involve important structures, and are difficult to resect. Hemipelvectomy is often required for pelvic tumors, and modified hemipelvectomy is used for tumors of the proximal femur.[128] The limb-sparing options, if feasible, are all functionally superior to amputation at this level.[126,127] A poorly planned biopsy often contaminates the extrapelvic structures, making a hemipelvectomy the only safe option. The technique of pelvic biopsy is shown in Fig. 44–30. Detailed anatomic and surgical considerations are discussed in the section on chondrosarcomas, which more commonly arise in these sites.

Limb-Sparing Surgery or Amputation

Limb-sparing surgery is now considered the preferred treatment for a significant number of patients with osteosarcomas and other high-grade bone sarcomas.[23,107,119,122,128] Amputations are reserved principally for patients in whom the primary tumor is deemed unresectable.[128] Extensive data have been obtained within the past 5 years about the crucial factors in the decision to perform a limb-sparing procedure or an amputation.[107–109,126,127] The major considerations and goals to be met in choosing a limb-salvage procedure are summarized[23]:

1. *Local recurrence.* The chance of local recurrence should not be higher than that associated with amputation.
2. *Survival.* Overall survival should not be jeopardized due to treatment delay or an ineffective (adjuvant) treatment program.

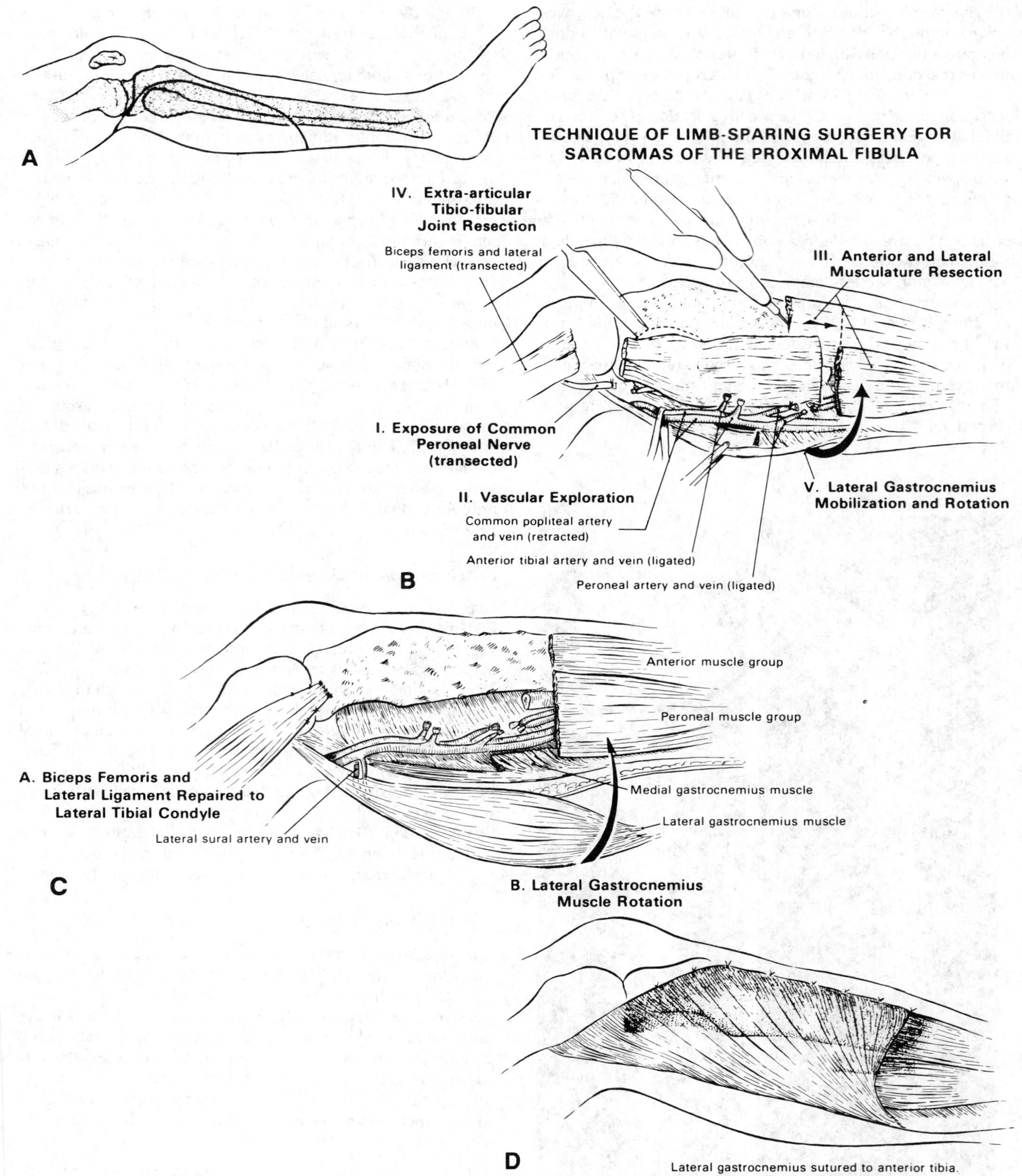

FIGURE 44–27. Technique of limb-sparing surgery for sarcomas of the proximal fibula. **(A)** Utilitarian incision. **(B)** Steps of resection of tumor. **(C)** Resection defect. Notice that both the anterior tibial and peroneal arteries have been ligated and the anterior and lateral muscle compartments removed. The defect is closed routinely by a lateral gastrocnemius muscle transfer. **(D)** Bony reconstruction is not necessary. (Malawer MM. Surgical management of aggressive and malignant tumors of the proximal fibula. Clin Orthop 1984;186:172–181)

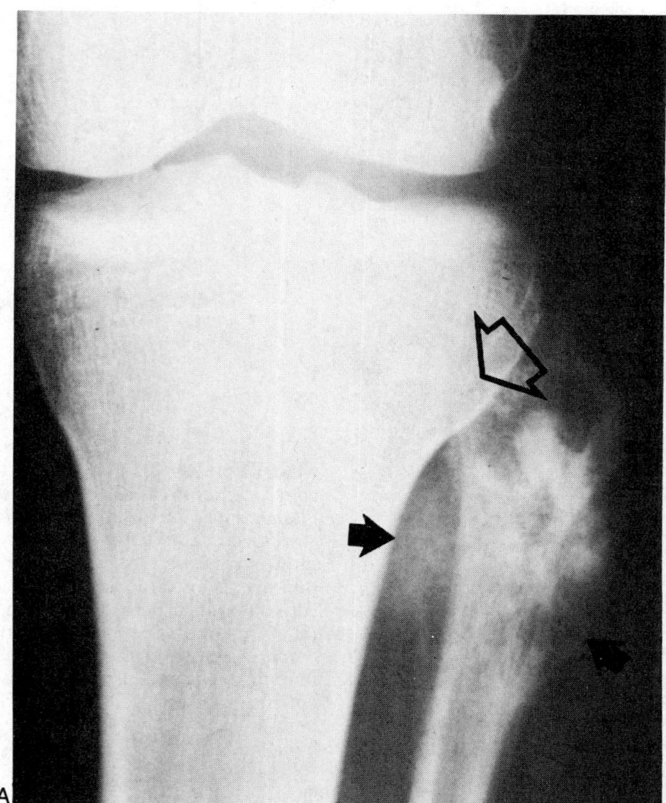

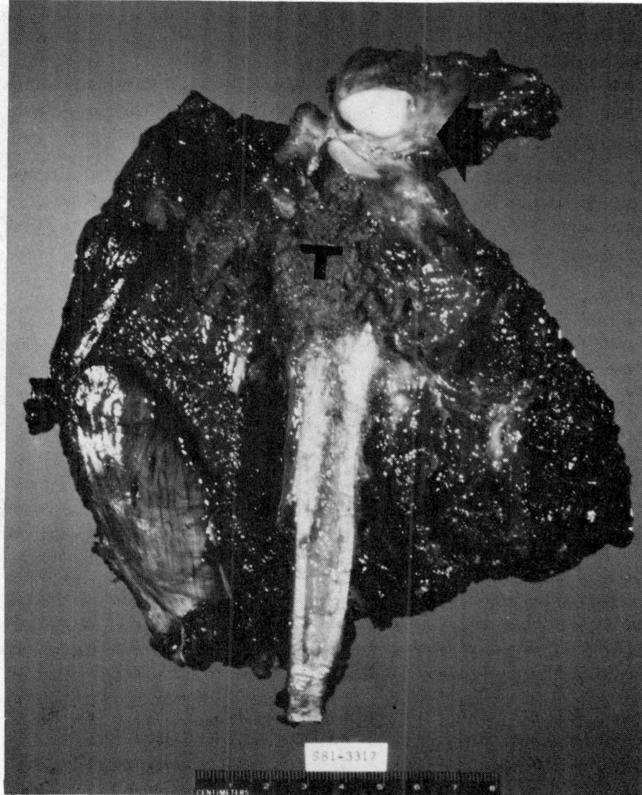

FIGURE 44–28. **(A)** Osteosarcoma of the proximal fibula. Plain radiograph of the knee demonstrates an osteosarcoma of the proximal fibula. Notice the large soft tissue component (*solid arrows*) and the intimate relation to the proximal tibiofibular joint. Tumors arising from the proximal fibula can often be treated by a limb-sparing procedure. **(B)** Gross specimen of a fibula resection for an osteosarcoma. An extraarticular resection was performed. The libiofibular joint (*solid arrow*) was opened and demonstrated pericapsular tumor extension. This is a common finding and emphasizes the need for routine extraarticular resection for sarcomas of the proximal fibula. T, tumor. (Malawer MM. Surgical management of aggressive and malignant tumors of the proximal fibula. Clin Orthop 1984;186:172–181)

3. *Function.* The means of reconstruction should be functional, with minimal long-term morbidity and need for additional surgery. The psychological impact and duration of rehabilitation must be considered.

Many studies have demonstrated that the risk (<5%) of local recurrence in patients who have undergone limb-sparing surgery is the same or less than the risk in those treated by amputation.[23,26–28,126] However, these are carefully selected patients, and the procedures have been performed in institutions whose staff is familiar with the techniques. The reported continuous disease-free survival rates are the same or better than those in large series of patients undergoing amputation alone.[26,27,30,33,36,38,52,53] If the criteria for patient selection are met, despite the variations among institutions, limb-salvage is a safe procedure. Eilber and colleagues from UCLA reported 78% (64 of 83) consecutive patients with malignant skeletal tumors who were treated by a limb-sparing resection, with no difference in overall survival compared with those treated by amputation.[26] The overall local recurrence rate was 2.7%. Eckardt and associates, from the same institution, subsequently reported their experience specifically with stage IIB osteosarcoma for the period 1972 to 1984. Seventy-eight (67%) of 116 patients were treated by a limb-sparing resection, with a local recurrence rate of 3.8%.[23]

The functional advantages of limb-sparing surgery merit careful consideration. Preservation of the upper humerus after resection of a proximal humeral sarcoma, for example, leaves a normal hand and elbow that are far superior to any prosthesis. Except for lack of shoulder motion, function is essentially normal. The advantage of such a procedure over forequarter amputation is obvious. Similarly, the functional advantages of preservation of the lower extremity after proximal femoral resection or pelvic resection are far superior to a hemipelvectomy. Initially, there was concern regarding the functional outcome of limb-sparing procedures about the knee, but Enneking reported that resections followed by reconstruction at this site by several different modalities all had a higher functional rating than an amputation in a multiinstitutional study using a standard evaluation scheme.[122]

Effect of Chemotherapy on Surgical Decisions

The initial impetus to limb-sparing surgery in the mid-1970s was the introduction of doxorubicin and methotrexate. Surgeons decided that adjuvant therapy might allow something

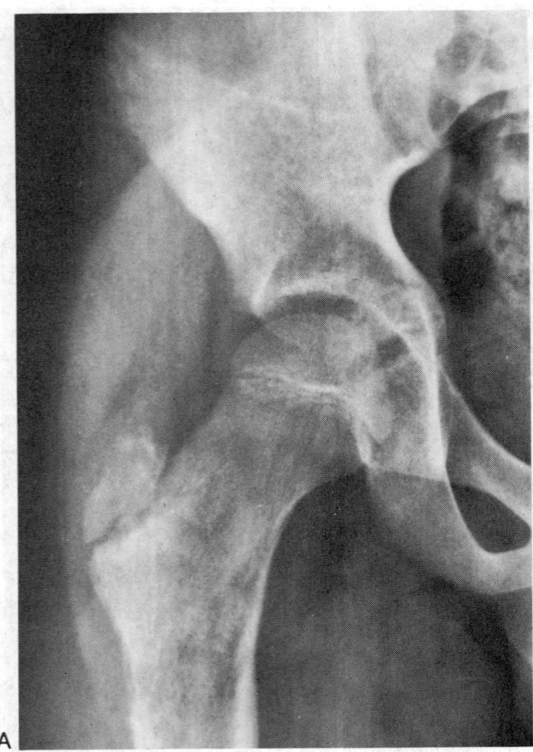

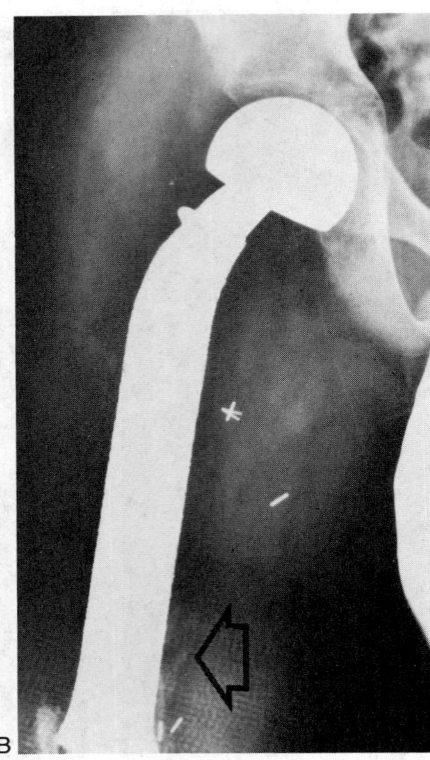

FIGURE 44–29. Osteosarcoma of the proximal femur. **(A)** Plain radiograph of an osteolytic osteosarcoma of the proximal femur. Notice the mottled destruction of the intertrochanteric area with lateral cortical destruction. **(B)** Postoperative radiograph demonstrates a custom proximal femoral replacement with porous coating to permit soft tissue and bony incorporation (*open arrow*, bone graft).

less than radical surgery. Most surgeons now think that adjuvant chemotherapy permits limb-sparing surgery to be performed more safely, with a lower local recurrence rate. Can a narrower surgical margin be a safe one with adjuvant chemotherapy? Although many surgeons believe this is possible, some evidence suggests that adjuvant chemotherapy has a beneficial effect, and other data suggest that it does not.[26,74]

Eilber and colleagues reported an encouragingly low 2.6% (5 of 183 patients) local recurrence rate for high-grade bone and soft tissue tumors and concluded that it was due to multimodal therapy (*i.e.*, preoperative irradiation and intraarterial and postoperative chemotherapy) that destroys microscopic disease at the periphery of the primary tumor.[26] The exact modality responsible for the favorable outcome was undetermined, but these researchers doubted that it was related to more accurate surgery. Conversely, Picci and associates evaluated by detailed mapping 50 osteosarcoma (Fig. 44–31) specimens from patients who had followed two different intravenous preoperative regimens. They reported a high incidence (63%) of viable tumor within the extraosseous soft tissue.[248] They concluded that a wide surgical margin is required because viable tumor is often at the periphery.

Because all preoperative chemotherapeutic agents entail the risk of increased local morbidity, skin breakdown, infection, and possible tumor progression and the possibility of losing a nonamputative option, additional studies are needed to determine the relation of preoperative chemotherapy to the choice of surgical margin.

Clinical Presentations of Osteosarcoma and Treatment Considerations

LOCALIZED EXTREMITY DISEASE. Management requires the expertise of a multidisciplinary team familiar with

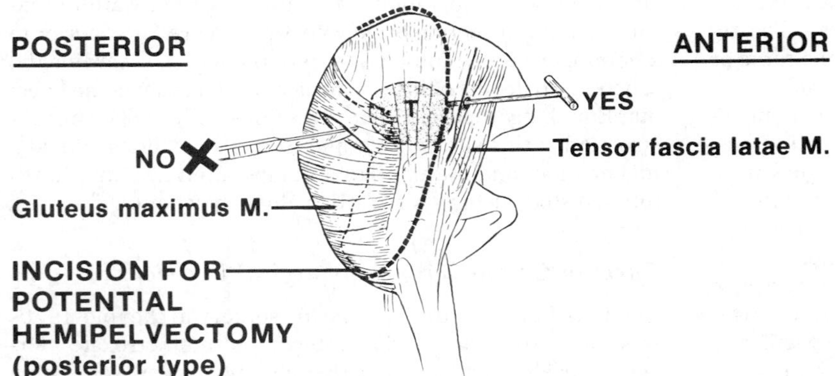

FIGURE 44–30. Biopsy technique for buttock and iliac tumors. The potential posterior hemipelvectomy flap (*dotted line*) should never be violated. A small biopsy from the lateral aspect is recommended.

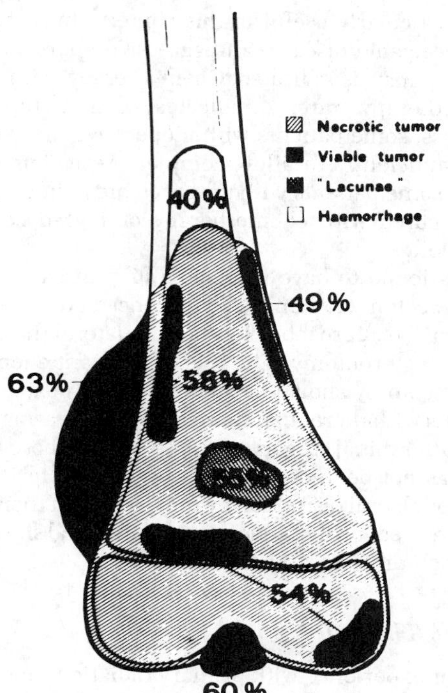

FIGURE 44–31. The percentage of viable tumor in each preferential site found in patients with viable tumor after preoperative treatment for osteosarcoma as for 50 patients. (Picci P, Bacci G, Companacci M, et al. Histological evaluation of necrosis in osteosarcoma induced by chemotherapy, regional mapping of viable and nonviable tumor. Cancer 1985;56:1515–1521)

the various management options. Patients with a suspected diagnosis of osteosarcoma (based on radiographic findings) should be referred to centers with treatment programs before biopsy.

The patient with a primary tumor of the extremity without evidence of metastases requires surgery to control the primary tumor and chemotherapy to control micrometastatic disease. The choice between amputation and limb-sparing resection must be made by an experienced orthopedic oncologist. Most distal femoral, proximal tibial, and proximal humerus osteosarcomas can be treated by limb-sparing resection. Routine amputations are no longer performed, and all patients should be evaluated for limb-sparing options. Intensive, multiagent chemotherapeutic regimens have provided the best results to date (see Tables 44–7 and 44–10). Patients who are judged unsuitable for limb-sparing options may become suitable candidates for limb-sparing operations after neoadjuvant chemotherapy. The management of these patients mandates close cooperation between chemotherapist and surgeon. Malawer recommends all patients be treated with neoadjuvant chemotherapy before making a surgical decision.

PELVIC TUMORS AND VERTEBRAL BODY TUMORS. In some pelvic and most vertebral primary tumors, complete resection is often not possible. Most pelvic osteosarcomas can be treated by hemipelvectomy; more centrally located pelvic tumors, especially those involving the sacrum, are unresectable. Only a few pelvic osteosarcomas can be treated by limb-sparing resection (internal hemipelvectomy). Contraindications to resection are unusually large extraosseous extensions with sacral plexus or major vascular involvement. Rarely, vertebral and sacral resections have been attempted.[203–205] In general, these tumors cannot be resected with negative margins and are best treated by radiation therapy and chemotherapy. Some success has been achieved with systemic or intraarterial chemotherapy, which is administered to convert apparently inoperable tumors into lesions that can be ablated surgically.[206,247a] In 1991, Tienghi and coworkers reported their results of 26 patients with pelvic osteosarcoma treated with infusional and postoperative intravenous chemotherapy. Only 1 patient remained disease free.[248a] This emphasizes the difficulty of treatment for pelvic osteosarcoma.

Patients with primary tumors of the axial skeleton have had poor outcomes because local control was rarely achieved. The prognosis for these patients may improve with a more aggressive surgical approach and more effective chemotherapy. Patients whose tumors can be completely resected should be approached with curative intent; radiation therapy provides significant palliation in patients with unresectable primary tumors.

Sundaresan and coworkers from MSKCC reviewed their experience of 35 years with vertebral osteosarcomas and reported their results of 24 patients.[248b] All lesions were stage IIB. They concluded that surgical resection should be part of the treatment strategy and not simple decompression and irradiation. Otherwise, local recurrence and dissemination is almost certain to occur. They observed the initial presentation was usually pain associated with neurologic deficit. The plain radiograph usually showed a mixed osteoblastic and osteolytic involvement of the anterior vertebral structures. CT and MRI is required and almost always demonstrates an extraosseous component. The researchers strongly recommended a two-stage surgical procedure after the diagnosis was established. The first stage should be a partial anterior spondylectomy followed by combination chemotherapy while monitoring the patient's tumor response. If the tumor remains under control, the remainder of the tumor should be resected by a posterior approach (*i.e.*, total spondylectomy) with additional stabilization by instrumentation, bone graft, or cementation. External-beam irradiation is given postoperatively.

METASTATIC PULMONARY DISEASE AT DIAGNOSIS. Metastatic disease detected at initial diagnosis does not preclude a curative treatment strategy, although the presence of extrathoracic metastases makes it extremely unlikely. In general, the surgical principles outlined for the treatment of relapsing patients apply equally to the patient presenting with macroscopic metastases. Newly diagnosed patients have not been exposed to chemotherapy and are likely to have drug-resistant tumors, and several options are therefore available for them.

For the patient presenting with resectable disease (*i.e.*, usually fewer than 15 pulmonary nodules and a primary tumor of the extremity), the traditional approach has been resection of all evidence of macroscopic disease by median sternotomy and limb amputation or resection, followed by intensive adjuvant chemotherapy. The tumor burden is reduced to a minimum before the application of adjuvant therapy. Some investigators favor treatment with chemotherapy, followed weeks or months later by definitive surgery for residual macroscopic disease in primary and metastatic sites.[249,250] Arguments advanced to justify this approach are similar to those used to support the strategy of preoperative chemotherapy in general, and the theoretical advantages and disadvantages of this strategy as discussed for patients with nonmetastatic osteosarcoma apply here as well. The risk for the patient with metastases is that growth of tumor nodules in the face of chemotherapy may render small, operable metastases unresectable and prevent cure. Primary treatment with chemotherapy may be appropriate, however, in patients with inoperable metastases, which may respond sufficiently to allow complete resection. Patients with widespread unresectable metastases are also best treated first with chemotherapy, with definitive surgery reserved for those achieving a satisfactory response. Because these patients usually require surgery for the primary tumor as a palliative procedure, early surgery may be recommended despite unresectable pulmonary disease.

RECURRENT DISEASE AFTER CURATIVE ATTEMPT. Historically, patients developing recurrent disease had a poor prognosis and were treated palliatively; most patients died within 1 year of the development of metastatic disease. Because more than 85% of metastases occur in the lung, surgical resection of tumor nodules can be readily accomplished. With the advent of thoracic CT scanning, metastatic nodules can be detected when quite small and more easily resectable, although the surgeon usually discovers more lesions at thoracotomy than anticipated from the CT scan.[251] In many patients, the lungs are likely to be the only site of metastases, especially in cases in which recurrences appear more than 1 year after diagnosis and in which the metastatic lesion is solitary. These recurrent tumors are likely to behave more indolently and may not further metastasize. These patients have been cured by thoracotomy alone.

Complete surgical resection of all overt metastatic disease is a prerequisite for long-term salvage after relapse.[252–255] Patients not treated by thoracotomy have little hope for cure, because complete responses of macroscopic metastases to chemotherapy are rare.[253,254] The completeness of surgical resection is an important determinant of outcome, because patients left with measurable or microscopic disease at the resection margins are unlikely to be cured.[253]

CHEMOTHERAPY AND METASTATIC DISEASE. Many investigators have recommended adjuvant chemotherapy after thoracotomy for the management of metastatic osteosarcoma to destroy residual microscopic tumor deposits after surgical treatment of overt metastases.[249,256–258] For patients who develop recurrent disease within 1 year of initial surgery, the possibility of microscopic metastatic disease is quite high, and additional chemotherapy is indicated. Long-term survival has been reported for some patients with recurrent osteosarcoma who were treated only with surgery without further chemotherapy.[253–255] These survivors were more likely to be patients suffering late relapses with solitary pulmonary nodules.

If overt metastatic disease is discovered, a thorough search for all metastatic lesions is essential. The discovery of unresectable extrathoracic metastases or unresectable pulmonary disease is a contraindication to aggressive thoracotomy, and the patient should be treated palliatively. Radiation therapy may be particularly useful in this context. In some patients with unresectable disease, an aggressive approach with curative intent may be indicated. Chemotherapy, with or without radiation therapy, rarely eradicates all metastatic disease; nonetheless, some patients with inoperative metastases may respond sufficiently to allow complete resection of disease later, and some patients with unresectable pulmonary metastases are cured with chemotherapy or high-dose radiation therapy alone.

Patients found to have resectable lung disease should undergo thoracotomy to remove all evidence of disease. Bilateral disease may be approached by staged bilateral thoracotomies or a median sternotomy. The role of adjuvant chemotherapy after thoracotomy should be studied; it is probably indicated for patients with more than three lesions appearing 6 months to 1 year after initial surgery and for patients whose metastatic disease has not been completely resected or for those with evidence of pleural disruption by tumor. Repeat thoracotomies may be required for subsequent recurrence and should be performed if all disease can be resected.

Radiation Therapy

Significant experience with primary radiation therapy for osteosarcomas was obtained in the 1950s and early 1960s. Primary radiation therapy with delayed amputation gained acceptance in 1955, when Cade advocated initial therapy with irradiation and delayed amputation for patients in whom there was no evidence of metastasis 4 to 6 months after radiation therapy.[259] This approach was designed to circumvent amputation in most patients who were destined to suffer an early relapse. Radiation doses were 7000 to 8000 cGy in 7 to 9 weeks at 1000 cGy each week. There were a few patients in Cade's series who were not subjected to delayed amputation who were controlled with irradiation alone, and amputation was eventually performed. The 5-year survival rate was 21.8%. Other investigators followed a similar regimen, using various radiation doses and schedules (Table 44–12). Subsequent surgical specimens of many of the patients managed in this fashion were found to have no histologic evidence of their tumor.[260–265] The ability of high radiation doses to sterilize some tumors was associated with significant necrosis of normal tissue.

Results of preoperative irradiation were subsequently evaluated. Overall success with preoperative irradiation followed by ablative surgery was suboptimal; most patients relapsed shortly after treatment. This led Jenkin and colleagues at Princess Margaret Hospital to recommend limiting irradiation to patients who had unresectable tumors or those being treated for palliation only.[266–267] Beck and coworkers observed no survival advantage for preoperative irradiation followed by surgery over surgery alone; only 43% of their patients obtained any palliative benefit from radiation therapy.[268] Disappointingly, no benefit has been observed from irradiation delivered under conditions of local tissue hypoxia, split-course radiation therapy, or with hydrogen peroxide or cytotoxic drug therapy.[269–271]

Radiation therapy has been successful in several clinical situations: facial lesions, palliation, and as a postoperative adjuvant.

TABLE 44–12. Series of Primary Radiation Followed by Delayed Surgery for Osteosarcoma

No. of Patients	*Dose*	*Machine*	*Survival (%)*	*References*
133	7000–8000 cGy/7–9 wk, 1000 cGy/wk	2 MV	21.8	243
10	10,000 cGy, 180 cGy/fraction	^{60}Co	60	245
92	6000–8000 cGy in 230-cGy fractions	or 2 MV	21.8	244a
16	1600–10,500 cGy in 200-cGy fractions	Orthovoltage and 2 MV	75 (1–16 y) Follow-up	244b
54	Variable	Variable	27.5	244c
23	1800–12,000 cGy/2–29 wk	Orthovoltage and 2 MV	26	244d
27	5000–6000 cGy in 25–30-cGy fractions		0	247
27	5000–6000 cGy/5–6 wk repeated × 1 7000–8000 cGy/8–9 wk	Orthovoltage or 1–4 Mv	23	249

OSTEOSARCOMA OF THE MAXILLA OR MANDIBLE. Osteosarcoma arising from facial bones, specifically the maxilla or mandible, have a different biology and natural history from those located elsewhere in the body. There is a lower risk of dissemination. Tumors arising in these sites have a high rate of local recurrence if treated by surgery alone. Clark and associates reported 66 patients with maxillary or mandibular primary tumors; 43 died, most with primary local recurrences.[272] Chambers and Mahoney suggested preoperative radiation therapy for such patients.[273] They reported a 73% survival rate at 5 years among 33 patients treated with high-dose radiation therapy (*i.e.*, interstitial technique or external-beam) followed immediately by wide surgical excision (*i.e.*, hemimandibulectomy and resection of surrounding soft tissues). Long-term survival after surgery alone ranged between 35% to 45%.[274] Surgical excisions associated with a high local recurrence rate are explained by difficulties in achieving adequate surgical margins. The increased survival after combined-modality treatment supports the fact that high radiation doses can eradicate microscopic disease. De Fries and colleagues and Abbiyik reported similar improved survival rates using a combination of preoperative irradiation, resection, and chemotherapy.[275,276] Conversely, Livolsi reported 5 patients irradiated in the postoperative period for osteosarcoma of the maxilla, all of whom died.[277] The long delay between the completion of surgery and the start of postoperative radiation therapy may have contributed to the poor results.

PALLIATION. Radiation therapy is extremely beneficial for patients requiring palliation of metastatic bony sarcomas, tumors at axial sites (which are unresectable), and advanced, inoperable lesions of the pelvis or extremities. A novel approach using high-dose-per-fraction irradiation and intraarterial 5′-bromodeoxyuridine (BUDR) as a radiosensitizer was undertaken by the Stanford Group.[278] Pulsed 48-hour BUDR infusions were performed before each 600-cGy radiation fraction, with a total radiation dose to the primary site of 4200 to 4800 cGy in 5 weeks in seven or eight fractions. Infusions of methotrexate-leucovorin were administered simultaneously. Local control was achieved in 7 (78%) of the 9 patients treated.[279] However, local tissue toxicity was excessive and included subcutaneous fibrosis, nonhealing traumatic fractures, peroneal neuropathy, and atrophy. Because the patients were treated with an unusual fractionation scheme using large fractions and intravenous chemotherapy, the specific role of BUDR in local control with its excessive toxicity was not established.

Kinsella used intravenous radiosensitizers of BUDR, iododeoxyuridine (IUDR), or misonidazole with high-dose radiation therapy, with various fractionation schemes and usually with chemotherapy, in patients with large, unresectable primary or metastatic sarcomas.[280] Twenty-one (75%) of 29 patients achieved local control, defined as freedom from symptoms and absence of growth. These studies demonstrated the efficacy of radiation therapy in obtaining long-term local control and palliation. The results lend support to additional clinical investigations using radiation sensitizers with high-dose radiation therapy.

ADJUVANT PULMONARY IRRADIATION. Variable results have been achieved from the use of adjuvant pulmonary irradiation in patients with primary osteosarcoma.[281,283–287] Breur and associates performed a randomized trial comparing amputation plus adjuvant whole-lung irradiation with amputation alone in 86 patients.[240,264–266] The midplane pulmonary lung dose was 1750 cGy in 10 fractions in 12 days, which, with lung correction, equalled slightly less than 2000 cGy. They found a significant benefit in the 3-year disease-free survival in the group that received adjuvant radiation therapy among patients younger than 17 years of age. Forty-eight percent of these patients survived without disease, compared with 28% in the group receiving surgery alone. This study is now being extended to the European Organization for Research on the Treatment of Cancer (EORTC) in a trial comparing amputation and lung irradiation with surgery and adjuvant chemotherapy and with all three treatments.[283–287] Their study, EORTC-SIOP 03 trial 20781, revealed a 4-year disease-free survival rate of 24% and overall survival rate of 43%, with no difference between the treatment arms.[286] For patients who subsequently developed lung metastases, successful pulmonary surgery could be done more frequently among patients who had elective lung irradiation of 2000 cGy than the other group. In this study, elective lung irradiation had an equal effect and provided the same survival as those receiving adjuvant chemotherapy (*i.e.*, methotrexate, vincristine, doxorubicin, cyclophosphamide).[286]

The French Bone Tumor Study Group gave the combination of intensive chemotherapy (*i.e.*, mitomycin C, vincristine, methotrexate, doxorubicin, dacarbazine, cyclophosphamide) and prophylactic lung irradiation of 2000 cGy after primary local treatment of surgery or radiation therapy to patients with osteosarcoma of the extremities.[287] They reported a 5-year survival rate of 66% and disease-free survival rate of 58%, but there was impairment of pulmonary function, which had not been seen when lung irradiation was given without simultaneous chemotherapy. Conversely, Rab and colleagues used a lower midplane radiation dose of 1500 cGy with concomitant dactinomycin in a randomized study and failed to show a survival benefit over amputation alone.[288] No toxicity was seen. Similarly, Jenkin found no benefit from 1500 cGy in 14 days of pulmonary irradiation with simultaneous dactinomycin.[289] Caceres and associates found no advantage over adjuvant doxorubicin alone.[290] Today, lung irradiation is rarely performed in the United States.

VARIANTS OF CLASSIC OSTEOSARCOMA

Dahlin has identified 11 variants of the classic osteosarcoma.[59] These accounted for 268 (28%) of 1021 cases reviewed at the Mayo Clinic. Osteosarcoma arising in the jaw bones, the most common variant, is characterized by well-differentiated cells with a low metastatic potential.[59] Excluding tumors arising secondary to Paget's disease, irradiation, or dedifferentiation of a chondrosarcoma, parosteal and periosteal osteosarcomas are the most common variants of classic osteosarcoma arising in the extremities, unlike classic osteosarcoma, which arises within a bone (intramedullary), both arise on the surface of the bone (juxtacortical).

Parosteal Osteosarcoma

Parosteal osteosarcoma is a distinct variant of conventional osteosarcoma, accounting for 4% of all osteosarcoma.[60] It arises from the cortex of a bone and generally occurs in an older persons. It has a better prognosis than classical osteosarcoma.

CLINICAL CHARACTERISTICS. There is a slight predominance of parosteal osteosarcoma in women. The distal posterior femur is involved in 72% of all cases; the proximal humerus and proximal tibia are the next most frequent sites. Parosteal osteosarcoma metastasizes slowly and has an overall survival rate of 75% to 85%.[60,291] Unni and colleagues found that all patients who died of tumor lived more than 5 years. The natural history of parosteal osteosarcoma is progressive enlargement and late metastasis. Parosteal osteosarcoma presents as a mass and occasionally is associated with pain. In contrast with conventional osteosarcoma, duration of symptoms varies from months to years. Unni reported that 50 of 79 patients had complaints of greater than 1 year, and one third of this group had pain for more than 5 years.[291] Tumor size, location, and duration of symptoms did not correlate with survival.[60]

RADIOGRAPHIC FINDINGS. Radiographs characteristically show a large, dense, lobulated mass broadly attached to the underlying bone without involvement of the medullary canal (Fig. 44–32). If old enough, the tumor may encircle the entire bone. The periphery of the lesion is characteristically less mature than the base. Ahuja emphasized that intramedullary extension is difficult to determine from plain radiographs.[60] Unni emphasized that high-grade foci did not usually alter the radiographic appearance of these tumors.[291]

PATHOLOGY AND GRADING. Parosteal osteosarcoma is characterized by well-formed lamellar or woven bone with a mature spindle cell stroma with few signs of malignancy. The cellularity of the spindle cell components varies; generally, it is not anaplastic and there are few mitoses.[2–4,59,60] The dif-

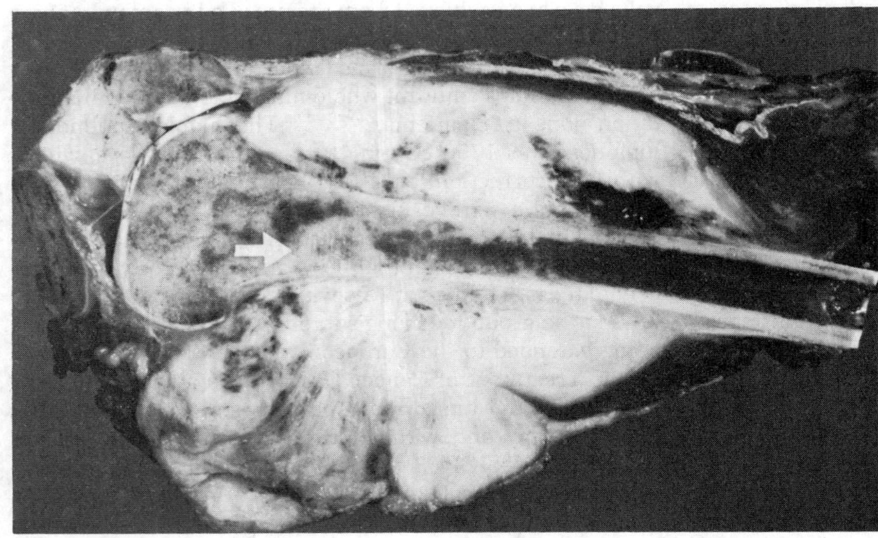

FIGURE 44–32. Parosteal osteosarcoma with intramedullary extension (*arrow*). Large parosteal osteosarcoma of the distal femur treated by an above-knee amputation. The patient refused treatment for 4 years before amputation. Intramedullary extension is a sign of advanced disease.

ferential diagnoses are osteochondroma, myositis ossificans, and conventional osteosarcoma. Cortical tumors of the posterior femur should always be suspected of malignancy; this is a rare location for a benign osteosarcoma. Unlike sarcoma, myositis ossificans is rarely attached to the underlying bone. The periphery is more mature, radiographically and histologically.

Ahuja reviewed all the parosteal osteosarcoma at MSKCC from 1934 to 1975 and described three grades: grade I (low grade), grade II (intermediate), and grade III (high grade).[60] He emphasized the importance of evaluating the fibroblastic, cartilaginous, and osseous components independently. Of the tumors of 24 patients, 8 were grade I, 10 were grade II, and 6 were grade III. Unni from the Mayo Clinic reviewed 79 patients and reported 18 (23%) were grade II and 7 (9%) had high-grade foci.[291] Neither Unni nor Ahuja could differentiate the three grades on plain radiographs. The survival rate of patients with grade III tumors is similar to that of patients with conventional osteosarcoma.

Intramedullary involvement does not necessarily imply a worse prognosis, although this may be the case in patients with high-grade lesions.[60] Eleven (46%) of 24 patients reviewed by Ahuja had medullary involvement; all patients with medullary involvement who had local resections had local recurrences.

TREATMENT. Wide excision of the tumor is the treatment of choice. This may be accomplished by an amputation or a limb-sparing procedure. There has been no experience reported of preoperative chemotherapy or radiation therapy. Parosteal osteosarcomas are often amenable to limb preservation due to their distal location, low grade, and lack of local invasiveness. If the adjacent neurovascular bundle is free of tumor, resection is feasible. Vascular displacement is not a contraindication for resection. The major surgical decision usually is whether to remove the entire end of the bone and the adjacent joint or to preserve the joint. Small lesions can be resected with joint preservation. If the medullary canal is involved, the joint usually cannot be preserved. A second factor mitigating against joint preservation is extensive cortical involvement. Techniques of resection and reconstruction are similar to those described for conventional osteosarcoma. The major difference is that only a small amount of soft tissue usually needs to be resected; consequently, a good functional result is obtained. Grade III parosteal lesions warrant systemic therapy due to the risk of metastasis.

Periosteal Osteosarcoma

Periosteal osteosarcoma is a rare cortical variant of osteosarcoma that arises superficially on the cortex, usually on the tibial shaft.[61] Radiographically, it is a small, radiolucent lesion with some evidence of bone spiculation. The cortex is characteristically intact with a scooped-out appearance and a Codman's triangle (Fig. 44–33). Histologically, periosteal osteosarcomas are relatively high-grade chondroblastic osteosarcomas composed of malignant cartilage with areas of anaplastic spindle cells and osteoid production. Unni and col-

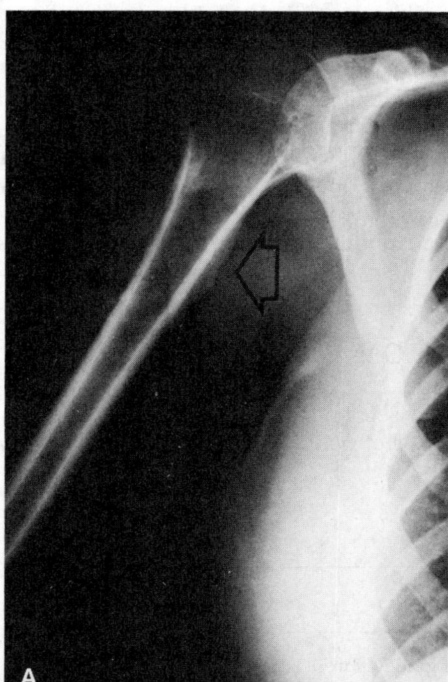

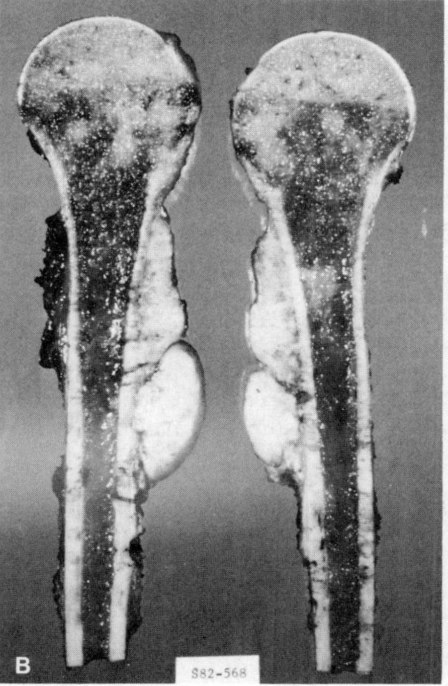

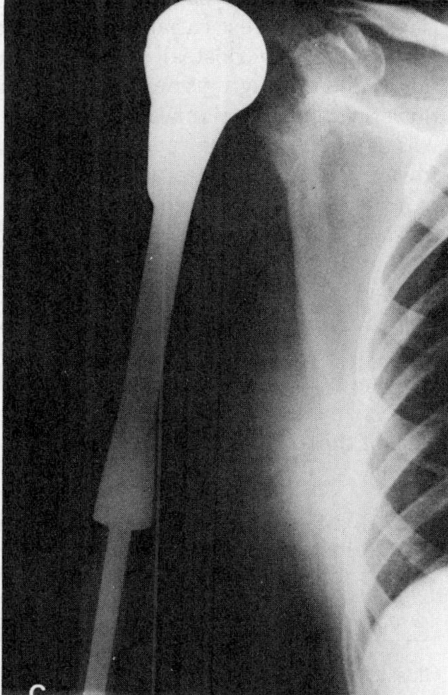

FIGURE 44–33. Periosteal osteosarcoma. **(A)** Typical radiograph of a periosteal osteosarcoma of the humerus. Notice the cortical location with a scooped-out defect of the lateral aspect of the shaft and the diaphyseal location. **(B)** Longitudinal section of the gross specimen after a limb-sparing resection. The tumor seems to arise on the outer cortex without any evidence of cortical involvement. **(C)** Postoperative radiograph. A custom prosthesis was used to reconstruct the defect. (Dunham WK, et al. Periosteal osteosarcoma. Cancer 1985;55:165–171)

leagues, in a report of 23 cases, found periosteal osteosarcomas to be one third as frequent as the parosteal variant.[61] The largest tumor measured 2.5 × 3.5 cm. Four of the 23 patients died of metastatic disease. Treatment is similar to that of other high-grade lesions. En bloc resection should be performed if feasible; otherwise, amputation is indicated. Table 44–13 compares the significant characteristics of periosteal tumors with those of conventional osteosarcoma.

Paget's Sarcoma

Approximately 1% of patients with Paget's disease develop a primary bone sarcoma.[223,224] Greditzer reported 41 sarcomas among 4415 patients with Paget's disease followed at the Mayo Clinic; 35 were osteosarcomas, and 6 were fibrosarcomas.[224] The average patient age was 64, and the most common sites were the pelvis, femur, and humerus. One half were osteolytic; the remainder had a mixed pattern. Cortical destruction and a soft tissue component were the most common signs found; periosteal elevation was rare. Most patients with this condition present with pain; a patient with known Paget's disease who complains of increasing pain, especially if it is well localized, should be evaluated radiographically. The diagnosis is usually made by plain radiography and confirmed by biopsy. Traditionally, fewer than 8% of patients survive, and most deaths occur within 2 years.[225] Treatment is similar to that recommended for adolescent patients with osteosarcoma without metastatic disease.

High-Grade Surface Osteosarcoma

High-grade surface osteosarcomas (*i.e.*, peripheral, conventional) is the rarest variant of surface osteosarcomas.[292] The parosteal and periosteal osteosarcomas have a better prognosis, and the high-grade surface variant has the same prognosis as the conventional, intramedullary lesion. This variant was previously called type III parosteal osteosarcoma. Schajowicz and coworkers studied the different surface osteosarcomas.[292] They reported that only 7 (9%) of 80 surface osteosarcomas were considered to be high-grade variants. The median age of patients was 13.5 years (younger than for other surface lesions), and most tumors were located in the diaphyseal region of the bone. The femur was the most common site. These tumors may show extensive intramedullary involvement. Radiographically, it appears as a small or moderate-sized lesion with slight to heavy calcification. The broad base of the lesion abuts the cortex. The radiographic features often are misleading and may suggest the periosteal variant. The preoperative diagnosis may be difficult. However, the young age, diaphyseal location, and highly malignant histologic features indicate the correct diagnosis. Wide excision with limb-preservation has been reported. Adjuvant chemotherapy is warranted due to its high rate of metastases.

Small Cell Osteosarcoma

Small cell osteosarcoma is a rare variant of osteosarcoma that resembles Ewing's sarcoma and is often classified as an "atypical" Ewing's sarcoma.[293,294] Characteristically, there are areas of osteoid and some chondroid formation. Differentiation from Ewing's sarcoma or the typical osteosarcoma is important, because its response to treatment is poorly defined. Sim and colleagues recommend surgery, but at the Pediatric Branch of the NCI, these tumors, like other pediatric round cell tumors, are treated by a combination of radiation therapy and chemotherapy.[293,294]

Radiation-Induced Osteosarcoma

Osteosarcomas that arise in a previously irradiated field and that meet the general criteria of a radiation-induced sarcoma (*i.e.*, latent for 5–20 years, documented secondary sarcoma, and occurring in a documented irradiated field) are rare. Amendola and coworkers from the University of Michigan reviewed 22,306 patients treated with irradiation between 1934 to 1983 and reported 23 patients with radiation-associated sarcomas.[295] The incidence was 0.1%. The median latent period was 13 years (range, 3–34 years). All sarcomas originated in previously normal tissues within the irradiated field. There were 5 bone sarcomas and 18 soft tissue sarcomas. The radiation dose ranged from 2500 to 7200 cGy. Their data suggested that intensive chemotherapy may have shortened the latency period. The treatment of radiation-induced osteosarcoma is wide resection if possible combined with adjuvant chemotherapy. The unique difficulty to the surgeon is the difficulty a previously irradiated field presents when choosing the best local treatment option. Increased local complications may be anticipated.

CHONDROSARCOMA

Chondrosarcoma is the second most common primary malignant spindle cell tumor of bone.[2] Chondrosarcomas form a

TABLE 44–13. Radiographic and Clinical Differential of Classic, Parosteal, and Periosteal Osteosarcoma

Type of Tumor	*Common Anatomic Site*	*Location*	*Radiographic Appearance*	*Histology*	*Metastases*
Classic	Distal femur, proximal tibia	Intramedullary	Destructive, osteoblastic/ osteolytic	High grade (fibroblastic, chondroblastic and osteoblastic)	Early
Parosteal	Posterior distal femur	Cortical	Dense, homogenous new bone	"Mature" bone and fibroblastic stroma, low grade	Late
Periosteal	Proximal tibia and humerus	Cortical	"Scooped-out" lesion with calcification	Chondroblastic high grade	Intermediate

heterogenous group of tumors whose basic neoplastic tissue is cartilaginous without evidence of direct osteoid formation. Occasionally, bone formation occurs from differentiation of cartilage. If there is evidence of direct osteoid or bone production, the lesion is classified as an osteosarcoma. There are five types of chondrosarcoma: central, peripheral, mesenchymal, differentiated, and clear cell.[2–4,10] The classic chondrosarcomas are central (arising within a bone) or peripheral (arising from the surface of a bone). The other three are variants and have distinct histologic and clinical characteristics.

Central and peripheral chondrosarcomas can arise as primary tumors or secondary to underlying neoplasm (Fig. 44–34). Seventy-six percent of primary chondrosarcomas arise centrally.[2,10–12,212] Secondary chondrosarcomas most often arise from benign cartilage tumors. The multiple forms of benign osteochondromas or enchondromas have a higher rate of malignant transformation than the corresponding solitary lesions.[11,12,57,210]

CENTRAL AND PERIPHERAL CHONDROSARCOMAS

Clinical Characteristics

Half of all chondrosarcomas occur in patients older than 40.[2,211] Only 3.8% occur in patients younger than 20.[2] The most common sites are the pelvis (31%), femur (21%), and shoulder girdle (13%).[11,12,210–211] Chondrosarcomas are the most common malignant tumors of the sternum and scapula. The clinical presentation varies. Peripheral chondrosarcomas may become quite large without causing pain, and local symptoms develop only because of mechanical irritation. Pelvic chondrosarcomas are often large and present with referred pain to the back or thigh, sciatica secondary to sacral plexus irritation, urinary symptoms from bladder neck involvement, or unilateral edema due to iliac vein obstruction, or as a painless abdominal mass. Conversely, central chondrosarcomas present with dull pain. A mass is rare. Pain, which indicates active growth, is an ominous sign of a central cartilage lesion. This cannot be overemphasized. An adult with a plain radiograph suggestive of a "benign" cartilage tumor but associated with pain probably has a chondrosarcoma.

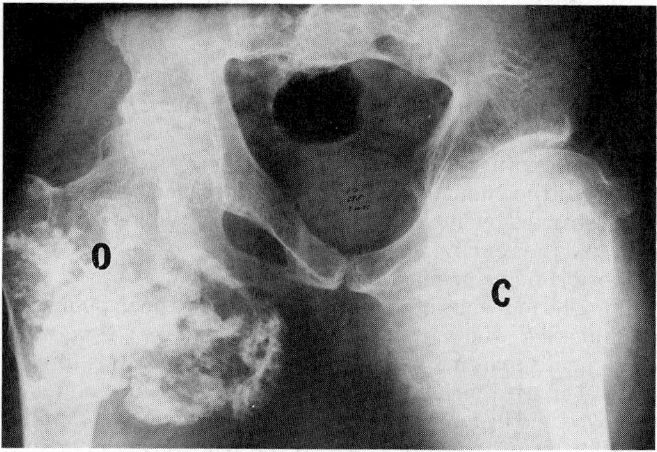

FIGURE 44–34. Radiograph of a patient with multiple hereditary osteochondromas. Notice the large sessile, lobulated osteochondroma (O) on the patient's right and a secondary (peripheral) chondrosarcoma (C) on the left. Secondary osteochondromas characteristically arise from benign underlying osteochondromas. Radiographically, they have poorly defined borders associated with a large soft tissue component with calcifications. This patient underwent a left modified hemipelvectomy.

Histology and Grading

Chondrosarcomas are graded I, II, and III. Most chondrosarcomas are grade I or II.[1,10–12,210–212] The metastatic rate of moderate grade lesions is 15% to 40%; for high-grade lesions, it is 75%.[1,10–12,85,210] Grade III lesions have the same metastatic potential as osteosarcomas.[11,212]

Because cartilage tumors are difficult to grade histologically, some investigators have attempted to apply cytologic, histochemical and biochemical analysis to evaluate these lesions.[10,210,211,296,297] Sanerkin described a combination of cytologic and histologic criteria.[210] He emphasized that cytologic analysis evaluates nuclear abnormalities better than conventional histologic sections, and histologic evaluation of the bone-tumor interface is the best predictor of local aggressiveness. Krocberg performed a retrospective study of DNA content of 45 chondrosarcomas as an indicator of malignancy by evaluating diploid (normal DNA content) and hyperploid (abnormal increase in DNA) and correlating this to 10-year survival.[298] Regardless of tumor grade, size, and location, patients with diploid content had better prognoses than those with hyperploid DNA. A preliminary report on assessing the malignancy of cartilage tumor by flow cytometry to determine the percentage of diploid, tetraploid, and aneuploid cells indicates that it may be a promising method of grading chondrosarcomas.[299]

Radiographic Diagnosis and Evaluation

Central chondrosarcomas have two distinct radiologic patterns.[300] One is a small, well-defined lytic lesion with a narrow zone of transition and surrounding sclerosis with faint calcification. This is the most common malignant bone tumor that may appear radiographically benign. The second type has no sclerotic border and is difficult to localize. The key sign of malignancy is endosteal scalloping. It is difficult to diagnose on plain radiographs and may go undetected for a long period. In contrast, peripheral chondrosarcoma is recognized easily as a large, calcified mass protruding from a bone (see Fig. 44–34). Its differential diagnosis includes large benign osteochondroma, parosteal osteosarcoma, and juxtacortical myositis ossificans. Correlation of clinical, radiographic, and histologic data is essential for accurate diagnosis and evaluation of the aggressiveness of cartilage tumor. Proximal or axial location, skeletal maturity, and pain point toward malignancy, even though the cartilage may appear "benign."

Prognosis

Metastatic potential tends to correlate with the histologic grade of the lesion.[10–12,212] Marcove reported long-term follow-up of 113 chondrosarcomas of the proximal femur and pelvis.[212] The survival rates in patients with grade I, II, and III lesions were 47%, 38%, and 15%, respectively; the overall survival rate was 52%. There was no significant difference between grades I and II; however, the mortality rate for grade III was significantly higher ($p < 0.02$) than for the other two. Eleven of 59 deaths occurred after 5 years. He emphasized that the meaningful survival interval should be considered 10 or 15 years. There was no relation between prognosis and grade, age, sex, or location. There was no statistical difference between primary and secondary chondrosarcomas. Adequacy of surgical removal was the main determinant of recurrence. In general, chondrosarcomas occurring during childhood have a worse prognosis than those occurring in adulthood.[301]

In a review of 125 chondrosarcomas at the Instituto Ortopedico Rizzoli, Gitellis reported that adequacy of treatment was the main determinant of local recurrence, length of survival, and length of disease-free interval.[13] Patients adequately treated had a 6% local recurrence rate, but the recurrence rate among those inadequately treated was 69%. The 10-year survival rates were 78% (adequately treated) and 61% (inadequately treated). There was no relation between local recurrence and grade.

Peripheral chondrosarcomas have a lower grade than central lesions. Gitellis and associates reported that 43% of peripheral lesions were grade I, compared with 13% of central lesions.[13] Ten-year survival rates among those with peripheral lesions were 77%, compared with 32% among those with central lesions. Secondary chondrosarcomas arising from osteochondromas also have a low malignant potential; 85% are grade I. Garrison reported only 3% of 75 patients with secondary chondrosarcoma from an osteochondroma developed metastases, although 12% died of local recurrence.[57]

Treatment

Treatment of chondrosarcoma is surgical removal.[10,12,212,278,279,301,302] There have been no reports of effective adjuvant chemotherapy. Resection guidelines for high-grade chondrosarcomas are similar to those for osteosarcoma. The shoulder and pelvic girdle are the most common sites for chondrosarcoma. These sites, combined with the fact that chondrosarcomas tend to be low grade, make them amenable to limb-sparing procedures. Lesions of the ribs and sternum are treated by wide excision. Cryosurgery, a technique using liquid nitrogen after thorough curettage of the lesion, has been used for central, low-grade chondrosarcomas.[116,117] There have been a few reports of effective radiation therapy for axial chondrosarcomas, and most encouraging reports used fractionated proton radiation therapy for the low-grade chondrosarcomas arising at the base of the skull.[303] The Massachusetts General Hospital group report a 5-year local control rate of 82%, and a 10-year local control rate of 58% among 28 patients with low-grade base of skull chondrosarcomas treated to approximately 69 CGE (cobalt GY equivalent) using the proton beam.[303] High-grade chondrosarcomas warrant consideration of adjuvant chemotherapy.

Limb-Sparing Procedures for Specific Anatomic Sites

The four most common sites of chondrosarcomas are the pelvis, proximal femur, shoulder girdle, and diaphyseal portions of long bones.

Pelvis. The pelvis consists of three areas: ilium, periacetabulum, and pubic rami (Fig. 44–35). Each site may be resected independent of the others.[29,279] Resections are classified type I (iliac wing), type II (acetabulum), and type III (pubic rami, pelvic floor). Bone scan most accurately determines specific bony involvement, and CT and MRI can delineate the extraosseous component (Fig. 44–36). Contraindications to resection are vascular (*e.g.,* iliac artery and vein), peritoneal, and sacroiliac joint or sarcoplexus involvement.

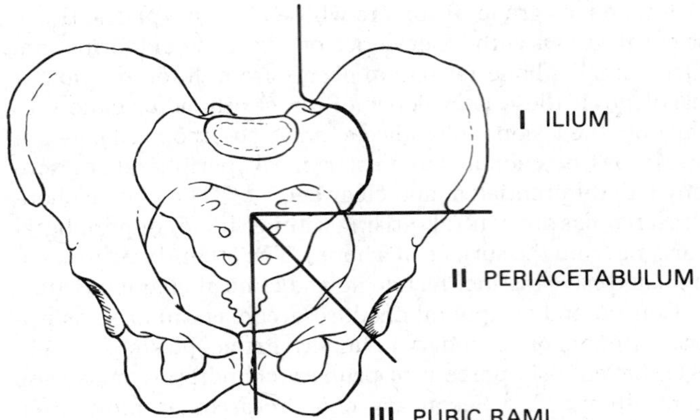

FIGURE 44–35. Segmental resection for pelvic tumors.

The retroperitoneal space is explored first to determine resectability. Type I resection is performed by a supraacetabular osteotomy and disarticulation of the sacroiliac joint. Type II resection may require removal of the femoral head; intraarticular involvement of the hip joint by tumor is evaluated by arthrotomy before finalizing the surgical plan. Types II and III resections require mobilization of the iliac vessels and femoral nerve. Care must be taken to protect these structures. The type III procedure requires mobilization of the bladder and urethra before resection. Bilateral pelvic floor resection may be used for chondrosarcomas arising from the midline of the symphysis pubis, in which case urethral resection and reconstruction may be required. Partial cystectomy may be necessary.

Despite the magnitude of resection, pelvic reconstruction is less complex than that at other anatomic sites. Type I and III resections do not require bony reconstruction. In type I, the abductor musculature is closed to the abdominal wall muscles, and in type III, the perineal muscles are approximated to the adductor muscles. The periacetabular area is reconstructed by intentionally creating a nonunion of the femur and the remaining portion of the ilium or pubic rami or by performing a primary arthrodesis.

Long-term results of these procedures have been published by Enneking, who reported that local recurrence was only 4% if adequate margins were obtained.[29] Function was almost normal if the hip joint was preserved. If the hip joint was removed and fusion was obtained, results were good. A saddle prosthesis (Fig. 44–37) permits reconstruction after periacetabular resections with minimal morbidity.[304]

Proximal Femur. Chondrosarcoma of the proximal femur can often be treated successfully by resection and prosthetic replacement. A lateral trephine biopsy is recommended. Care must be taken to avoid intraarticular contamination. A posterior approach should be avoided because of potential con-

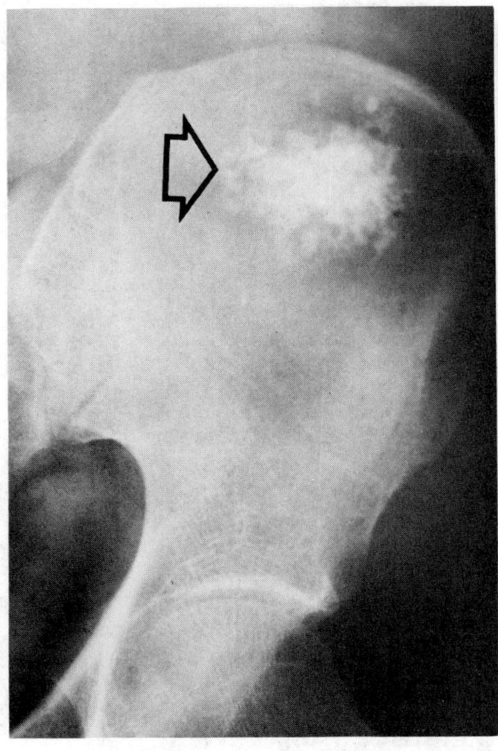

A

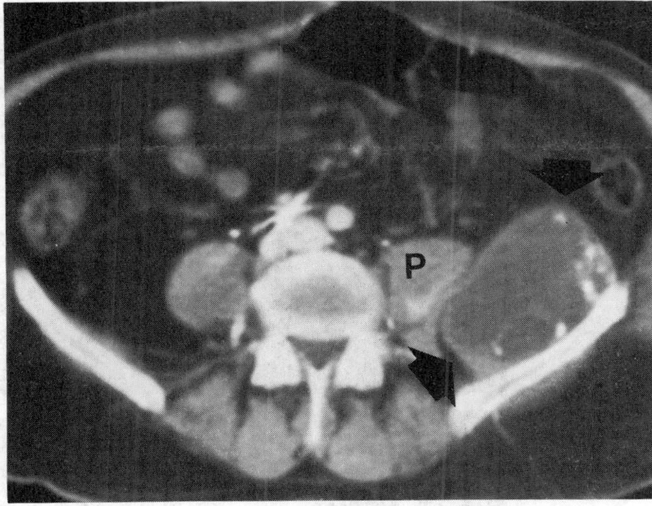

B

FIGURE 44–36. Chondrosarcoma of the pelvis. (**A** Plain radiograph demonstrates a small area of calcification within the ilium, suggesting a small intraosseous chondrosarcoma. (**B**) CT scan of the same area that surprisingly demonstrated a large chondrosarcoma (*solid arrows*) arising from the ilium, displacing the psoas muscle medially. The small area of calcification (*small solid arrow*) correlated with the plain radiograph (**A**).

tamination of the posterior flap in the event a hemipelvectomy is required.

Shoulder. The technique of resection of chondrosarcomas of the proximal humerus is similar to that described for osteosarcomas. In low-grade, intracompartmental (stage IA) tumors, preservation of the deltoid, rotator cuff musculature, and glenoid is possible, and there are several alternatives for reconstruction. Endoprosthesis, fibula autografts, and allografts have high rates of success.[34–39,125–127]

Segmental Resection for the Tibia, Femur, Humerus. Central diaphyseal chondrosarcomas can be adequately treated by segmental resection without sacrificing the adjacent joint. Because the ends of the bones are not involved, function is excellent. Reconstruction is performed by allografts or autografts combined with internal fixation.

Cryosurgery

Marcove pioneered the technique of cryosurgery for bone tumors. This method involves thorough curettage and cryotherapy of the cavity with liquid nitrogen.[115–117] With increasing experience, he expanded the indications to low-grade intramedullary cartilage tumors and to some high-grade lesions. Employing these indications, he has treated 30 chondrosarcomas with only one local recurrence. The major advantages of cryosurgery are preservation of bone stock and the avoidance of resection.

Radiation Therapy

Unresectable or inoperable chondrosarcomas arising within the axial skeleton and pelvic or shoulder girdle can be controlled and, in some cases, cured by radiation therapy. For chondrosarcomas of the facial bones and skull, a combination of radiation therapy and surgery have been successful.

Although chondrosarcomas have been considered radioresistant, data show that some are radiocurable.[309] Among 38 patients undergoing radical irradiation, with or without concurrent chemotherapy, at the Princess Margaret Hospital, 5- and 10-year actuarial survival rates of 41% and 36%, respectively, were achieved. Median survival was 46 months.[309] The best results, a 48% 5-year actuarial survival rate, were obtained in the group with favorable (well and moderately differentiated) histology. Conversely, for those with unfavorable (mesenchymal and poorly differentiated) histology the 5-year survival rate was only 22%. Radical radiation therapy was defined as a minimum of 4000 cGy in 4 or more weeks of megavoltage therapy. Of the 38 patients treated, 17 developed local recurrence. The investigators recommend 5000 cGy in 4 weeks with treatment to the whole bone if possible and, if not, at least a 5-cm margin of normal bone. They found tumor regression continued slowly for 2 to 3 years after therapy.

McNaney and colleagues from MDACC reported 20 patients with chondrosarcoma treated with photons or neutrons, with or without chemotherapy.[310] The doses of radiation administered ranged from 4000 to 7000 cGy. Thirteen (65%) of 20 patients were surviving at a median of 30 months after treatment. Among the 11 patients treated with radiation therapy alone, 6 (54%) survived. Six patients, all of whom had received photon therapy alone, developed local failures. There were no local failures among the 4 patients treated with a mixed beam of photons and neutrons.

After radical irradiation, clinical regression of tumor is slow and may take months to complete. Radiographically, the affected bone never returns to normal. The combination of ex-

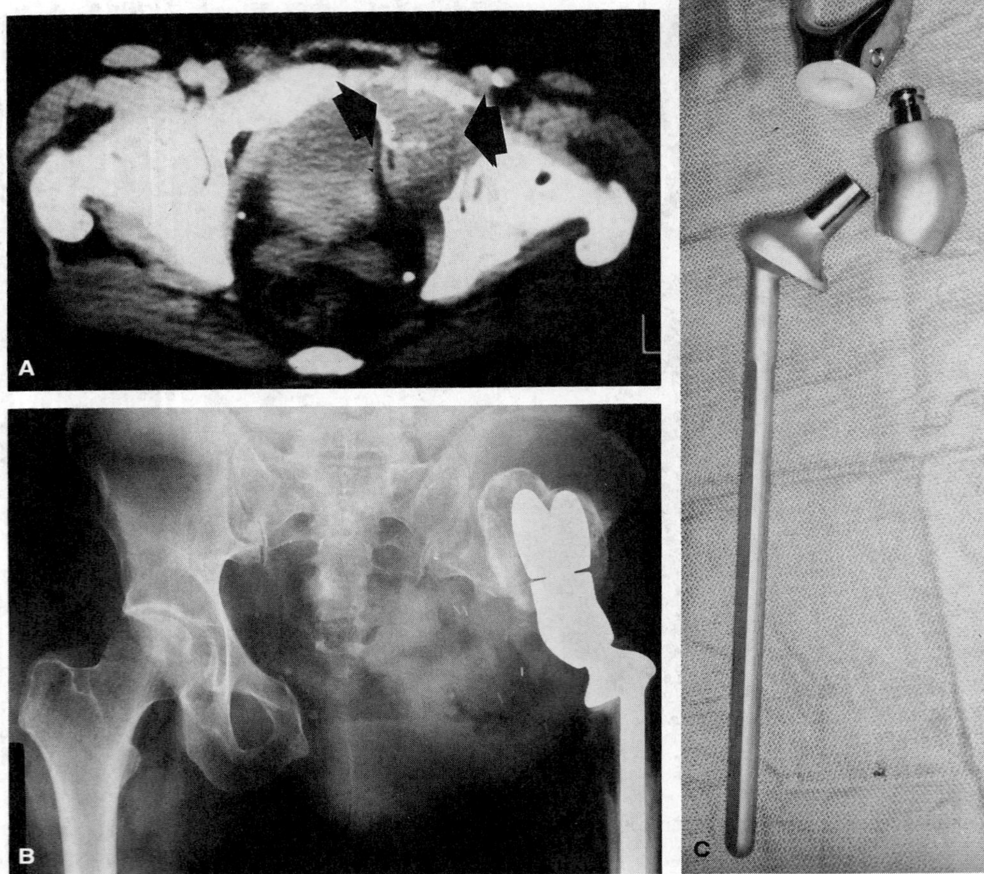

FIGURE 44–37. Limb-sparing resection for a large periacetabular chondrosarcoma involving the pelvic floor. **(A)** CT scan shows acetabular destruction by a large tumor mass (*arrows*) with involvement of the pubic rami. **(B)** The patient was treated by an internal hemipelvectomy (type II and III resection). **(C)** A custom-made saddle prosthesis was used for the reconstruction. This is a new type of pelvic prosthesis that has made pelvic reconstruction more reliable with less morbidity than other techniques.

tremely slow regression of tumor with a persistent radiologic defect makes follow-up and assessment of response difficult. Unfortunately, there are no rebiopsy data to document long-term sterilization of these tumors. Radiation therapy for chondrosarcoma can provide palliation. In such cases, high doses (approximately 5000 cGy in 4 to 5 weeks or its equivalent) are necessary; low doses for symptomatic relief are ineffective.[311]

Ryall and associates used irradiation and the radiosensitizer Razoxane (ICRF-159) in 8 patients with 12 chondrosarcomas. Seven tumors in 5 patients achieved complete or partial remission after 4500 to 6000 cGy. Two of the responders were disease free 2.5 years after treatment.[312]

Data on the relation between dose and tumor control probability are lacking; however, it seems apparent that prolonged local control requires a high radiation dose. Treatment planning requires documentation by CT of the extent of soft tissue disease.

There is some experience using radioactive ^{35}S for treatment of metastatic chondrosarcoma.[2,287] ^{35}S is selectively taken up by chondrocytes and bone marrow, causing tumor necrosis. Because of reports of associated ^{35}S-induced bone marrow suppression and severe aplastic anemia, this technique is not recommended.[2,313]

Treatment of the Maxilla, Mandible, and Skull

The treatment of chondrosarcomas of the maxilla, mandible, and skull entails irradiation and surgery, a combination that has a better potential for improving local control than surgery alone. Local recurrence rates as high as 85% have been reported for head and trunk lesions.[311,314] Among 18 patients with tumors of the head and neck, the MSKCC group reported local recurrence in 11 (61%).[315] The high local recurrence rate reflects the anatomic constraints on the surgical procedure. Austin-Seymour and associates reported an improved actuarial 5-year disease-free survival rate of 76% and local control rate of 82% for 28 patients receiving focused proton beam radiation therapy for low-grade chondrosarcomas of the base of the skull.[303]

VARIANTS OF CHONDROSARCOMA

Clear Cell Chondrosarcoma

Clear cell chondrosarcoma, the rarest form of chondrosarcoma, is a slow growing, locally recurrent tumor resembling a chondroblastoma but with some malignant potential.[305] It usually occurs in adults. The most difficult clinical problem is early recognition. It is often confused with chondroblastoma.

Metastases occur only after multiple local recurrences. Primary treatment is wide excision. Systemic therapy is not required.

Mesenchymal Chondrosarcoma

Mesenchymal chondrosarcoma is a rare, aggressive variant of chondrosarcoma characterized by a biphasic histologic pattern (*i.e.*, small, compact cells intermixed with islands of cartilaginous matrix).[306–308] These tumors have a predilection for flat bones; long, tubular bones are rarely affected.[211] They tend to occur in the younger age group and have a high rate metastatic potential. Harwood reported 8 of 17 patients died within 1 year of diagnosis.[306] The 10-year survival rate is 28%.[306] This entity responds favorably to radiation therapy. It is hypothesized that the round cell component, similar to other round cell sarcomas, is relatively radiosensitive. Treatment is surgical removal combined with adjuvant chemotherapy. Radiation therapy is recommended if the tumor cannot be completely removed.[306]

Approximately 10% of chondrosarcomas may dedifferentiate into a fibrosarcoma or osteosarcoma.[2,10,11,56] This occurs in older persons and is highly fatal. Surgical treatment is similar to that described for other high-grade sarcomas. Adjuvant therapy is warranted.

GIANT CELL TUMOR OF BONE

Giant cell tumor (GCT) of bone is an aggressive, locally recurrent tumor with a low metastatic potential.[14–16,63–64,211,313] It consists of spindle-shaped and ovoid cells uniformly interspersed with multinucleated giant cells. GCT refers to the de novo, malignant GCT, not the tumor that arises from the transformation of a giant cell tumor previously thought to be benign. These two lesions are separate clinical entities.

CLINICAL CHARACTERISTICS

GCTs occur slightly more often in female than male patients. Pain, mass, local tenderness, and decreased motion in the adjacent joint are the most common clinical symptoms. Eighty percent of GCTs in the long bones occur after skeletal maturity, and 75% of these develop around the knee joints.[2,3,63] Effusion or pathologic fracture, uncommon with other sarcomas, are common with GCT. The tumors occasionally occur in the vertebrae (2–5%) or the sacrum (10%).[2–4]

GRADING AND PATHOLOGIC CHARACTERISTICS

Jaffe attempted to grade GCTs: grade I (completely benign), grade II (borderline), and grade III (frankly sarcomatous).[4] Grades I and II do not correlate well with biologic behavior. There is also a poor correlation between the histologic pattern and the tendency for recurrence or malignant transformation.[14,15,63,211] Nineteen percent to 25% of giant cell tumors have some osteoid production.[211] If osteoid formation is found, care must be exercised in differentiating a GCT from an osteosarcoma. Conversely, an osteosarcoma with giant cells may be misinterpreted as a benign GCT. There is no correlation between osteoid formation and increased risk of recurrence or metastasis. Necrosis or hemorrhage is often found. Neither is related to malignant potential or local recurrence rate.[63]

NATURAL HISTORY

Although GCTs are rarely malignant de novo (2–8%), they may undergo transformation and demonstrate malignant potential histologically and clinically after multiple local recurrences.[14–16,177,288] Between 8.6% and 22% of known GCTs become malignant after local recurrence.[14–16,211,314] This rate decreases to less than 10% if patients who have undergone radiation therapy are excluded from the series. Hutter found that 40% of malignant GCTs were malignant at the first recurrence.[15] The remainder had become malignant by the second or third recurrence; each recurrence increases the risk of malignant transformation of typical GCT, especially if the transformation occurs after radiation therapy. Local recurrence of a GCT is determined by the adequacy of surgical removal rather than histologic grade.

RADIOGRAPHIC AND CLINICAL EVALUATION

Giant cell tumors are eccentric lytic lesions without matrix production. They have poorly defined borders with a wide area of transition. They are juxtaepiphyseal with a metaphyseal component. Although the cortex is expanded and appears destroyed at surgery, it is usually found to be attenuated but intact. Periosteal elevation is rare; soft tissue extension is common.

TREATMENT

Treatment of GCT of bone is surgical removal. Resection is curative for 90% of these tumors.[14,15,308] Curettage, with or without bone grafts, has a recurrence rate of 40% to 75%.[14–16,63,316] Johnson and Dahlin reported a recurrence rate of 29% within 1 year of curettage and of 54.1% within 5 years.[16] Although en bloc excision offers a reliable cure, routine resection is not recommended.[316] Primary resection of a joint has a significant morbidity. It is recommended for GCT of the proximal radius and fibula, distal ulna, tubular bones of hand and foot, coccyx, sacrum, and pelvic bones. Under certain situations, it is reasonable to perform a curettage. Goldenberg recommends that small tumors with an intact cortex and symptoms of less than 2 to 3 months' duration be treated by curettage.[63] If the lesion heals, resection is avoided. Curettage does not rule out a later curative resection.

The current technique of curettage is more extensive than previously performed. Curettage is accomplished through a large cortical window, equal to the length of the bony defect, using mechanical curettage and a mechanical burr. This extensive technique has been called "curettage/resection" and has significantly decreased the rate of local recurrence to approximately 15% to 25%. Bone graft and PMMA are used to reconstruct the surgical defect.

Amputation is reserved for massive recurrence, malignant transformation, or infection. Due to the biologic propensity for malignant transformation, irradiation is reserved for specific lesions, usually lesions of the spine, which cause bone destruction in a confined area and can lead to spinal cord compression and severe deformity.[107a] Treatment of GCT of the vertebrae and sacrum must be individualized. A combination of surgical excision and cryosurgery or radiation therapy is required to eradicate the tumor and prevent neurologic impairment.[106–107a]

Cryosurgery

Cryosurgery has been used more successfully for GCTs than for any other type of bone tumor.[115–117,317] Marcove developed the technique of cryosurgery because of the high recurrence rates after curettage and the significant risk of sarcomatous degeneration in tumors treated by irradiation. He found cryosurgery effective in eradicating the tumor while preserving joint motion and avoiding resection or amputation. He reported a 17-year experience of 100 GCTs treated by thorough curettage and cryosurgery.[117] He found a recurrence rate of 16% in the first 50 cases and 2% in the following 50 cases. The major complications of cryosurgery are necrosis of the adjacent bones, which may develop a late pathologic fracture, and delayed union. Rate of secondary pathologic fracture has been decreased by a combination of PMMA augmentation, bone graft, internal fixation of the cavity, and postoperative use of a long-leg brace with a quadrilateral socket.[317,318] Persson from Sweden reported curettage with PMMA augmentation of the bony defect with bony necrosis due to the heat of polymerization. This technique may provide better local control than curettage alone.[319]

Radiation Therapy

The indications for irradiation include inoperable and incompletely resected lesions and locally recurring lesions despite definitive surgery. These situations are most likely to occur in the spine.[320] Doses of 4500 to 5500 cGy in 5 to 6 weeks using megavoltage equipment are recommended.[181,215,295,321,322]

There has been a long and justified apprehension that some patients may develop a malignant and fatal neoplasm after irradiation.[324,325] This concern was supported by Dahlin from the Mayo Clinic, who reported that malignant degeneration ultimately appeared in 37 patients treated with irradiation alone or in combination with a surgical procedure.[323] The average time for malignant change was approximately 9 years. McGrath presented data from the Bristol Tumor Registry that substantiate this concern.[324] Neither of these studies break down the radiation dose to bone in patients who did or did not develop malignancies. It is known that some of these patients were treated with orthovoltage radiation, and multiple courses were given.

The Princess Margaret Hospital group reported that local tumor has been controlled in 13 of 14 patients with giant cell tumor treated with one course of megavoltage radiation. The disease of 12 patients was controlled for longer than 5 years.[321] The researchers observed no instance of malignant transformation. Larsson and colleagues reported 3 patients with giant cell tumor of the spine and sacrum treated by moderate doses of radiation therapy; all have done well.[320]

MALIGNANT FIBROUS HISTIOCYTOMA

CLINICAL CHARACTERISTICS

Malignant fibrous histiocytoma (MFH) is a high-grade bone tumor histologically similar to its soft tissue counterpart.[7–9] It is a disease of adulthood. The most common sites are the metaphyseal ends of long bones, especially around the knee. Alkaline phosphatase values are normal. Pathologic fracture is common. Huvos emphasized that a lytic metaphyseal lesion with a pathologic fracture in an adult with a normal serum alkaline phosphatase level suggests a primary MFH rather than an osteosarcoma or fibrosarcoma.[9] MFH disseminates rapidly. Spanier reported that 9 of 11 patients died of the tumor. The average disease-free survival was 6 months.[7] She reported one third of patients (3 of 9) with pulmonary metastasis had lymph node dissemination. She hypothesized that lymphatic spread was due to the histiocytic component of the tumor.

RADIOGRAPHIC CHARACTERISTICS

MFH is an osteolytic lesion associated with marked cortical disruption, minimal cortical or periosteal reaction, and no evidence of matrix formation.[9] The extent of the tumor routinely exceeds plain radiographic signs. McCarthy and associates reporting on 35 patients with MFH, found that four tumors were multicentric and four were associated with bone infarcts.[8]

TREATMENT

There have been few reports about the efficacy of chemotherapy for MFH of bone.[213,326,327] Bacci and colleagues reported 12 patients treated by surgery and chemotherapy, compared with 18 patients treated with surgery alone over the same time at the Instituto Ortopedico Rizzoli.[326] The disease-free survival rates were 59% (7 of 12) and 5% (1 of 18), respectively. Heeten reported 3 patients with MFH treated by preoperative chemotherapy; a grade IV response (100% necrosis) was obtained in all 3.[327]

Earl and coworkers from the Royal National Orthopedic Hospital evaluated the chemosensitivity of MFH of bone.[328] Eighteen patients were treated with preoperative and postoperative chemotherapy consisting of methotrexate, ifosfamide, and doxorubicin. Four patients had 100% tumor necrosis; 2 patients had more than 90%, and the remainder had between 50% and 70% tumor necrosis. Of 13 patients presenting with localized disease (median, 24 months), only 1 patient had died at the time of the report. They concluded that MFH of bone was a chemosensitive lesion and suggested long-term studies to determine if there is a survival advantage to adjuvant chemotherapy.

Due to the extremely poor prognosis of MFH, chemotherapy is thought to be justified. Although there are only limited data, there are striking similarities to the results seen with osteosarcoma. The primary approach to treatment of MFH of bone is radical surgical resection combined with adjuvant chemotherapy.

FIBROSARCOMA OF BONE

CLINICAL CHARACTERISTICS

Fibrosarcoma of bone is a rare entity characterized by interlacing bundles of collagen fibers (*i.e.*, herringbone pattern) without any evidence of tumor bone or osteoid formation.[5] Fibrosarcoma occurs in middle age. The long bones are most affected. Fifteen percent of tumors are found in the bones of the head and neck.[211] Fibrosarcomas occasionally arise in conjunction with an underlying disease, such as fibrous dysplasia, Paget's disease, bone infarcts, osteomyelitis, and postirradiation bone and giant cell tumor.[5] Fibrosarcoma may be central or cortical (*i.e.*, periosteal). The histologic grade is a good prognosticator of metastatic potential. Huvos reported overall survival rates of 27% and 52% for central and peripheral lesions, respectively.[5] Late metastases do occur, and 10- and 15-year survival rates vary. Periosteal tumors usually have a better prognosis than central lesions.

RADIOGRAPHIC DIAGNOSIS AND TREATMENT

Fibrosarcoma is a radiolucent lesion that shows minimal periosteal and cortical reaction. The radiographic appearance closely correlates with the histologic grade of the tumor.[5] Low-grade tumors are well defined, but high-grade lesions demonstrate indistinct margins and bone destruction similar to osteolytic osteosarcoma. Plain radiographs often underestimate the extent of the lesion. Pathologic fracture is common (30%) because of the lack of matrix formation. Differential diagnosis includes GCT, aneurysmal bone cyst, MFH, and osteolytic osteosarcoma.[5,6]

Fibrosarcoma of bone is primarily managed surgically. Irradiation is recommended for inoperable tumors and for patients with postsurgical residual disease and for palliation.

CHORDOMA

CLINICAL PRESENTATION AND DIAGNOSIS

Chordoma is a rare neoplasm arising from notochordal remnants in the midline of the neural axis and involving the adjacent bone. The ends of the spine are the most common sites. The sacrococcus and the base of the skull (35%) near the sphenooccipital area are most commonly involved, accounting for 50% and 35%, respectively, of all chordomas.[211] Histologically, the physaliferous cell is pathognomonic. Large areas of syncytial strands of cells lying in a mass of mucus are typically present. Myxoid chondrosarcoma and metastatic carcinoma must be differentiated. This tumor is highly fatal due to the high rate of local recurrence and local complications.[329–332] Death is most commonly due to local disease.[329] Gray and colleagues reviewed 222 cases from the literature and observed that only 2 patients were disease free at 10 years.[332] Average survival was 5.7 years. Mindell emphasized the main malignant potential of chordomas resides in their critical locations adjacent to important structures, their locally aggressive nature, and their extremely high rate of recurrence.[329] Chordomas at the base of the skull are often described as chondroid chordomas. Patients with these lesions at this site tend to survive longer than those with sacrococcygeal tumors.

The most common complaint of patients with sacrococcygeal tumors is dull pain; constipation is an occasional symptom. Bladder and sensory loss are late complaints. Clinical suspicion is the key to early diagnosis. Rectal examination characteristically reveals a large presacral mass. Sphenooccipital tumors present with signs of cranial nerve or pituitary dysfunction. CT and MRI are essential for accurate evaluation (Fig. 44–38). Myelography is used to determine intraspinal extension. A transrectal biopsy should not be performed because of potential contamination. A small midline posterior incision or trocar biopsy is recommended.

TREATMENT

Surgery

The first surgical procedure has the best chance of cure.[331,332] Inadequate surgery results in local recurrence, with little chance of subsequent surgical removal. Sacrococcygeal tumors are best removed by a combined abdominosacral approach, as described by Localio and colleagues.[302,303] They emphasized wide excision of the sacrum one level higher than the lesion. A lateral position is used. The rectum can be mobilized and the iliac vessels controlled anteriorly. The rectum may be removed with the sacrum if necessary. Guterberg and

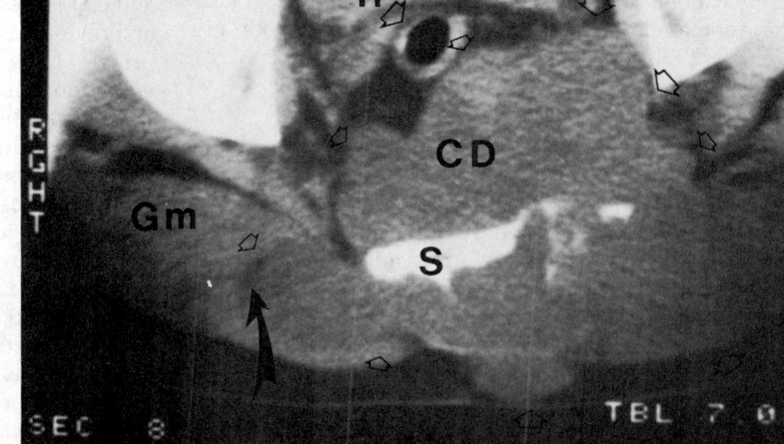

FIGURE 44–38. Computed tomography of a chordoma arising within the sacrum (s). There is destruction of the body of the sacrum with a huge soft tissue component (outlined by *small arrows*). The tumor (CD) extends to the rectum (R) and is infiltrating the gluteus maximus (Gm) muscle (*black arrow*). These are typical findings of a sacrococcygeal chordoma, which explains the difference in obtaining local control. Differential diagnosis includes metastatic carcinoma and giant cell tumor of the sacrum.

associates reported that if only half of the first sacral vertebra remains bilaterally, the pelvic girdle is still stable enough to allow immediate mobilization.[333] Recently De Vries reported 2 long-term survivors (7 and 10 years) after cryosurgery of sacral chordomas.[334]

Radiation Therapy

Because local recurrence is common with chordomas, radiation therapy is an integral treatment modality, particularly for tumors of the base of skull and sphenooccipital region. Results of conventional radiation therapy have been disappointing. Heffelfinger and colleagues reported 36 patients with nonchondroid varieties of chordomas of the base of skull, none of whom were rendered free of disease by surgery, irradiation, or a combination thereof.[335] However, the chondroid variant is more sensitive; of 19 patients with chondroid chordomas, 7 were alive, and 6 were disease free. Other investigators reported 5 patients with cervical chordomas, only one who was alive and disease free 5 years after irradiation and surgery.[336]

Amendola and associates reported 21 patients with a 5-year survival rate of 50% but a disappointing 10-year survival rate of only 20%. This is not surprising, because chordomas are relatively slow growing.[337] Long-term survival free of tumor regrowth over 10 years is relatively rare.[338] Amendola emphasized the importance of using CT in planning the radiation field, high radiation doses (*i.e.,* 5500–7000 cGy with megavoltage equipment), and use of irradiation immediately after surgery to prolong local control, rather than reserving it until recurrence. The Massachusetts General Hospital (MGH) experience of 48 patients is similar to that reported by others; 50% of the patients survived 5 years or more.[339] Radiation doses varied from 4500 to 8040 cGy, but even with high doses, there was a 45% incidence of local recurrence.

Investigators at MGH and the University of California now advocate using precision heavy-charged-particle irradiation, particularly for chordoma of the basisphenoid region and cervical spine. The MGH experience now includes 68 patients, 40 with chordomas and 28 with low-grade chondrosarcomas of the basisphenoid region and cervical spine who have been treated with proton-beam radiation therapy at a median tumor dose of 69 CGE. The actuarial 5-year disease free survival rate is 76%, and the local control rate is 82%.[340,341] There was no difference in local control between patients with low-grade chondrosarcoma and those with chondroid or nonchondroid chordoma.[303,340]

SMALL ROUND CELL SARCOMAS OF BONE

Round cell sarcomas of bone behave differently and require different therapeutic management from spindle cell sarcomas.[342,343] These tumors consist of poorly differentiated small cells without matrix production. They present radiographically as osteolytic lesions. These lesions are best treated with irradiation and chemotherapy; surgery is reserved for special situations. Non-Hodgkin's lymphoma and Ewing's sarcoma are the two most common small cell sarcomas. The differential diagnosis of all round cell sarcomas includes metastatic neuroblastoma, metastatic undifferentiated carcinoma, histocytosis, small cell osteosarcoma, osteomyelitis, and multiple myeloma.

LYMPHOMAS OF BONE

CLINICAL PRESENTATION AND DIAGNOSIS

Diffuse large cell lymphoma of bone (previously called reticulum cell sarcoma of bone) accounts for only 5% of the primary bone tumors. Lymphoma presenting in bone is usually a sign of disseminated (stage IV) disease; occasionally, it may be a true solitary lesion defined as "involvement of single extralymphatic organ or site (stage IE)."[342,343] Reimer at the NCI reported that only 1 of 12 patients presenting with bone lymphomas had a true solitary lesion.[342] Sweet and colleagues from the University of Chicago reported that 50% of so-called solitary lesions were associated with disease elsewhere.[343] Sweet presented a useful algorithm for the evaluation and treatment of bone lymphomas. He emphasized that all patients with a presumed solitary lymphoma of bone should undergo a thorough evaluation for other involvement.[343]

Treatment is based on extent of disease. Stage IE lesions have traditionally been treated with radiation therapy, with a reported 90% cure rate.[342] The role of surgery is limited to obtaining adequate tissue for diagnosis and treatment of pathologic fracture. The technique of biopsy is important to avoid secondary fracture through potentially irradiated bone. Biopsy for a suspected round cell tumor should always include a frozen section and additional material for electron microscopy, tissue culture, and immunophenotyping. Patients presenting with pathologic fractures require fixation. To prevent late fractures, all patients treated with radiation therapy should be protected with a brace until reossification occurs.

RADIATION THERAPY

Local control of the primary tumor with retention of good function of the affected part is commonly achieved after radiation therapy. Radiation therapy is administered to the entire bone and soft tissue extent with a dose of 4000 cGy and a boost to the original tumor area to 5000 cGy. Regional lymph nodes should be included in the radiation port if they are adjacent to the area treated or if clinically involved. Mendenhall and colleagues from the University of Florida, achieved local and regional control in all irradiated sites of 21 patients with primary bone lymphoma.[344] Two patients relapsed in apparently uninvolved regional lymph node sites that had not been included in the primary treatment portal.

Patients with lymphoma of the bone should be considered as having systemic disease and accordingly require chemotherapy. Investigators from Dana-Farber Cancer Center reported 11 children who had been treated with irradiation and chemotherapy consisting of APO (doxorubicin, prednisone, cyclophosphamide), with an 8-year actuarial lymphoma-free survival of 100% and a disease-free survival rate of 79%, for an overall actuarial survival rate of 90%.[345] There were no relapses. This is consistent with experience from the Bone Tumor Center, Bologna, Italy, where 23 (88%) of 26 patients survived disease free after irradiation and chemotherapy with oxorubicin, vincristine, and cyclophosphamide, with no local relapses at 7.5 years (median) of follow-up.[346] In the Dana-Farber experience, 2 patients developed second bone tumors, 5 and 7.5 years after beginning therapy. Because of the success from intensive combination chemotherapy, investigators have begun to question the need for primary radiation therapy among children responding to multiagent chemotherapy.[347,348] Current pediatric protocols using multiagent chemotherapy for non-Hodgkin's lymphoma do not routinely use radiation therapy for those with primary lymphoma of the bone.

REFERENCES

1. Silverberg E, Lubera, J. Cancer statistics, 1987. CA 1987;37:2–20.
2. Dahlin DC. Bone tumors: General aspects and data on 6,221 cases. 3rd ed. Springfield: Charles C Thomas, 1978.
3. Lichtenstein L. Bone tumors. 5th ed. St. Louis: CV Mosby, 1977.
4. Jaffe HL. Tumors and tumorous conditions of the bone and joints. Philadelphia, Lea & Febiger, 1958.
5. Huvos AG, Higinbotham NL. Primary fibrosarcoma of bone. A clinicopathologic study of 130 patients. Cancer 1975;35:837–847.
6. Wilner D. Fibrosarcoma. In: Wilner D, ed. Radiology of bone tumors and allied disorders, I. Philadelphia: WB Saunders, 1982:2291–2324.
7. Spanier SS, Enneking WF, Enriquez P. Primary malignant fibrous histiocytoma of bone. Cancer 1975;36:2084–2098.
8. McCarthy EF, Matsuno T, Dorfman HD. Malignant fibrous histiocytoma of bone: A study of 35 cases. Hum Pathol 1979;10:57–70.
9. Huvos AG. Primary malignant fibrous histiocytoma of bone. Clinicopathologic study of 18 patients. N Y State J Med 1976;76:552–559.
10. Shives TS, Wold LE, Dahlin DC, Beaubout JW. Chondrosarcoma and its variants. In: Sim FH, ed. Diagnosis and treatment of bone tumors: A team approach. Thorofare, NJ: Slack, 1983:211–217.
11. Marcove RC. Chondrosarcoma: Diagnosis and treatment. Orthop Clin North Am 1977;8:811–819.
12. Pritchard DJ, Lunke RJ, Taylor WF, et al. Chondrosarcoma: A clinicopathologic statistical analysis. Cancer 1980;45:149–157.
13. Gitellis S, Bertoni F, Chieti PP, Campanacci M. Chondrosarcoma of bone. J Bone Joint Surg [Am] 1981;1248–1256.
14. Dahlin DC, Cupps RE, Johnson EW Jr. Giant cell tumor: A study of 195 cases. Cancer 1970;25:1061–1070.
15. Hutter VP, Worcester JN Jr, Francis KC, et al. Benign and malignant giant cell tumor of bone. A clinicopathological analysis of the natural history of the disease. Cancer 1962;15:653–690.
16. Johnson EW Jr, Dahlin DC. Treatment of giant cell tumor of bone. J Bone Joint Surg [Am] 1959;41:895–904.
17. Nascimento AG, Huvos AC, Marcove RC. Primary malignant giant cell tumor of bone: A study of eight cases and review of the literature. Cancer 1979;44:1393–1402.
18. Weingard DN, Rosenberg SA. Early lymphatic spread of osteogenic and soft-tissue sarcomas. Surgery 1978;84:231–240.
19. Enneking WF, Spanier SS, Goodman MA. A system for the surgical staging of musculoskeletal sarcoma. Clin Orthop 1980;153:106–120.
20. Marcove RC, Rosen G. En bloc resection for osteogenic sarcoma. Cancer 1980;45: 3040–3044.
21. Malawer MM. Distal femoral osteogenic sarcoma, principles of soft tissue resection and reconstruction in conjunction with prosthetic replacement (adjuvant surgery). In: Chao EYS, ed. Design and application of tumor prosthesis for bone and joint reconstruction. New York: Thieme-Stratton, 1983:297–309.
22. Morton DL, Eilber FR, Townsend CM Jr, et al. Limb salvage from a multidisciplinary treatment approach for skeletal and soft tissue sarcomas of the extremity. Ann Surg 1976;184:268–278.
23. Enneking WF, Dunham WK. Resection and reconstruction for primary neoplasms involving the innominate bone. J Bone Joint Surg 1978;60:731–746.
24. Marcove RC, Lewis MM, Rosen G, et al. Total femur and total knee replacement: A preliminary report. Clin Orthop 1977;126:147–152.
25. Eilber FR, Morton DL, Eckardt J, et al. Limb-salvage for skeletal and soft tissue sarcomas: Multidisciplinary preoperative therapy. Cancer 1984;53:2579–2584.
26. Eilber FR, Eckhardt J, Morton DL. Advances in the treatment of sarcomas of the extremity: Current status of limb salvage. Cancer 1984;54:2695–2701.

26a. Weisenberg TH, Eilber FR, Grant TT, et al. Multidisciplinary "limb salvage" treatment of soft tissue and skeletal sarcomas. Int J Radiat Oncol Biol Phys 1981;7:1495.

27. Simon MA, Aschliman MA, Thomas N, et al. Limb-salvage treatment versus amputation for osteosarcoma of the distal end of the femur. J Bone Joint Surg [Am] 1986;68: 1331–1337.
28. Enneking WF. Modification of the system for functional evaluation of surgical management of musculoskeletal tumors. In: Enneking WF, ed. Limb-sparing surgery for musculoskeletal tumors. New York: Churchill Livingstone, 1987:626–639.
29. Enneking WF, Dunham WK. Resection and reconstruction for primary neoplasms involving the innominate bone. J Bone Joint Surg [Am] 1978;60:731–746.
30. Marcove RC, Lewis MM, Rosen G, et al. Total femur and total knee replacement. A preliminary report. Clin Orthop 1977;126:147–152.
31. Mankin HJ, Fogelson FS, Thrasher AZ, et al. Massive resection and allograft transplantation in the treatment of malignant bone tumors. N Engl J Med 1976;294:1247–1255.
32. Watts HG. Introduction to resection of musculoskeletal sarcomas. Clin Orthop 1980;153:31–38.
33. Enneking WF, Shirley PD. Resection-arthrodesis for malignant and potentially malignant lesions about the knee using an intramedullary rod and local bone graft. J Bone Joint Surg [Am] 1977;59:223–235.
34. Janeck CJ, Nelson CL. Enbloc resection of shoulder girdle: Technique and indications. Report of a case. J Bone Joint Surg [Am] 1972;54:1754–1758.
35. Francis KC, Worcester JN Jr. Radical resection for tumors of the shoulder with preservation of a functional extremity. J Bone Joint Surg [Am] 1962;44:1423–1429.
36. Marcove RC, Lewis MM, Huvos AG. En bloc upper humeral-interscapular resection, the Tikhoff-Linberg procedure. Clin Orthop 1977;124:219–228.
37. Chaos EYS, Ivins JC. Design and application of tumor prosthesis for bone and joint reconstruction—The design and application. New York: Thieme-Stratton, 1983.
38. Malawer MM, Sugarbaker PH, Lambert M, et al. Limb-salvage surgery for tumors of the proximal humerus and shoulder girdle. The Tikhoff-Linberg procedure and its modifications. Surgery 1955;97:518–528.
39. Sim FH, Bowman WE, Chao EYS. Limb salvage surgery and reconstructive techniques. In: Sim FH, ed. Diagnosis and treatment of bone tumors: A team approach. Thorofare, NJ: Slack, 1983:75–105.
40. De Santos LA, Bernardino ME, Murry JA. Computed tomography in the evaluation of osteosarcoma: Experience with 25 cases. AJR 1979;132:535–540.
41. Destouet JM, Gilula LA, Murphy W. Computed tomography of long bone osteosarcoma. Radiology 1979;131:439–445.
42. Mckillop JH, Etcubanas E, Goris ML. The indications for and limitations of bone scintigraphy in osteogenic sarcoma: A review of 55 patients. Cancer 1981;48:1133–1138.
43. Levine E. Computed tomography of musculoskeletal tumors. Crit Rev Diagn Imaging 1981;16:279–309.
44. Rosenthal DI. Computed tomography in bone and soft tissue neoplasms: Application and pathologic correlation. Crit Rev Diagn Imaging 1982;18:243–278.
45. Goldstein H, McNeil BJ, Zufall E, et al. Changing indications for bone scintigraphy in patients with osteosarcoma. Radiology 1980;135:177–180.
46. Bacci G, Picci P, Calderoni P, et al. Full-lung tomograms and bone scanning in the initial work-up of patients with osteogenic sarcoma. A review of 126 cases. Eur J Cancer Clin Oncol 1982;18:967–971.
47. Jaffe N, Link MP, Cohen D, et al. High-dose methotrexate in osteogenic sarcoma. NCI Monogr 1981;56:201–206.
48. Cortes EP, Holland JF, Wang JJ, et al. Amputation and Adriamycin in primary osteosarcoma. N Engl J Med 1974;291:998–1000.
49. Rosen G, Marcove RC, Caparros B, et al. Primary osteogenic sarcoma. The rationale for preoperative chemotherapy and delayed survey. Cancer 1979;43:2163–2177.
50. Rosen G, Caparros B, Huvos AC, et al. Preoperative chemotherapy for osteogenic sarcoma: Selection of postoperative adjuvant chemotherapy based upon the response of the primary tumor to preoperative chemotherapy. Cancer 1982;49:1221–1230.
51. Muggia F, Catani R, Lee YJ, et al. Factors responsible for therapeutic success in osteosarcoma. In: Jones S, Salmon S, eds. Adjuvant therapy for cancer. 2nd ed. New York: Grune & Stratton, 1979.
52. Cortes EP, Holland JP. Adjuvant chemotherapy for primary osteogenic sarcoma. Surg Clin North Am 1981;61:1391–1404.
53. Rosen G, Murphy ML, Huvos AG, et al. Chemotherapy, en bloc resection and prosthetic replacement in the treatment of osteogenic sarcoma. Cancer 1976;37:1–11.
54. Goorin AM, Frei E II, Abelson HT. Adjuvant chemotherapy for osteosarcoma: A decade of experience. Surg Clin North Am 1981;61:1379–1389.
55. Lichtenstein L. Classification of primary tumors of bone. Cancer 1951;4:335–341.
56. Spjut HJ, Dorfman HD, Fechner DE, Ackerman LV. Tumors of bone and cartilage. In: Atlas of tumor pathology, fasc. 5, 2nd series. Washington, DC: Armed Forces Institute of Pathology, 1971.
57. Garrison RC, Unni KK, Mcleod RA, et al. Chondrosarcoma arising in osteochondroma. Cancer 1982;49:1890–1897.
58. Merryweather R, Middlemiss JH, Sanerkin NG. Malignant transformation of osteoblastoma. J Bone Joint Surg [Br] 1980;62:381–384.
59. Dahlin DC, Unni KK. Osteosarcoma of bone and its important recognizable varieties.
60. Ahuja SC, Villacin AB, Smith J, et al. Juxtacortical (parosteal) osteogenic sarcoma. J Bone Joint Surg [Am] 1977;59:632–647.
61. Unni KK, Dahlin DC, Beaubout SW. Periosteal osteogenic sarcoma. Cancer 1976;37: 2476–2485.
62. Unni KK, Dahlin DC, McLeod RA, Pritchard DJ. Interosseous well-differential osteosarcoma. Cancer 1977;40:1337–1347.
63. Goldenberg RR, Campbell CJ, Bongfiglio M. Giant cell tumor of bone. An analysis of two hundred and eighteen cases. J Bone Joint Surg [Am] 1970;52:619–664.
64. Johnson EW, Dahlin DC. Treatment of giant cell tumor of bone: An evaluation of 24 cases treated at the Johns Hopkins hospital between 1925–1955. Orthopedics 1969;62: 187–191.
65. Madewell JE, Ragsdale BD, Sweet DE. Radiographic and pathologic analysis of solitary bone lesions. Radiol Clin North Am 1981;19:715–814.
66. Johnson LC. A general theory of bone tumors. Bull N Y Acad Med 1953;19:164–171.
67. Lodwick GS. The bone and joints. In: Enneking WF, ed. Atlas of tumor radiology. Chicago: Year Book Medical Publishers, 1971.
68. Enneking WF. Musculoskeletal tumor surgery, vol. I. New York: Churchill Livingstone, 1983:1–60.

69. Jeffree GM, Price CHG, Sissins HA. The metastatic spread of osteosarcoma. Br J Cancer 1975;32:87–107.
70. McKenna RJ, Schwinn CP, Soong KY, Higinbotham NL. Sarcomata of the osteogenic series (osteosarcoma, fibrosarcoma, chondrosarcoma, parosteal osteosarcoma and sarcomata arising in abnormal bone: An analysis of 552 cases. J Bone Joint Surg [Am] 1966;48:1–26.
71. Marcove RC, Mike V, Hajack JV, et al. Ostegenic sarcoma under the age of twenty-one. J Bone Joint Surg [Am] 1970;52:411–423.
72. Sweetnam R. Surgical management of primary osteosarcoma. Clin Orthop 1975;111: 57–64.
73. Campanacci M, Bacci G, Bertoni F, Picci P, Minutillo A, Franceschi C. The treatment of osteosarcoma of the extremities: Twenty years' experience at the Instituto Ortopedico Rizzoli. Cancer 1981;48:1569–1581.
74. Campanacci M, Bacci G, Bertoni F, et al. The treatment of osteosarcoma of the extremity: Twenty years' experience at the Instituto Orthopedico Rizzoli. Cancer 1981;48:1569–1581.
75. Brostrom L-A. On the natural history of osteosarcoma. Aspects of diagnosis, prognosis and endocrinology. Acta Orthop Scand Suppl 1980;183:1–38.
76. Enneking WF, Kagan A. Intramarrow spread of osteosarcoma. In: Management of primary bone and soft tissue tumors. Chicago: Yearbook Medical Publishers, 1976: 171–177.
77. Malawer MM, Dunham WF. Skip metastases in osteosarcoma: Recent experience. J Surg Oncol 1983;22:236–245.
78. Enneking WF, Spanier SS, Malawer MM. The effect of the anatomic setting on the results of surgical procedure for soft parts sarcoma of the thigh. Cancer 1981;47: 1005–1022.
79. Simon MA, Spanier SS, Enneking WF. The management of soft tissue tumors of the extremities. J Bone Joint Surg [Am] 1976;60:317.
80. Simon MA. Intra-articular extension of adult primary bone sarcomas: Implications for limb-sparing surgical procedures. In: Chao, EYS, Ivins JS, eds. Tumor prosthesis for bone and joint reconstruction. The design and application. New York: Thieme-Stratton, 1983.
81. Bohndorf, K, Reiaer M, Lochner B, et al. Magnetic resonance imaging of primary tumours and tumour-like lesions of bone. Skeletal Radiol 1986;15:511–517.
82. Cohen MD, Weetman RM, Provisor AJ, et al. Efficacy of magnetic resonance imaging in 139 children with tumors. Arch Surg 1986;121:522–529.
83. Turner DA. Nuclear magnetic resonance in oncology. Semin Nucl Med 1985;15: 210–223.
84. Zimmer WD, Berquist TH, McLeod RA, et al. Bone tumors: Magnetic resonance imaging versus computed tomography. Radiology 1985;155:709–718.
85. Powers JA. Magnetic resonance imaging in marrow diseases. Clin Orthop 1985;206: 79–85.
86. Sundaram M, McGuire MH, Herbold DR. Magnetic resonance imaging of osteosarcoma. Skeletal Radiol 1987;16:23–29.
87. Easton EJ, Powers JA. Musculoskeletal magnetic resonance imaging. Thorofare, NJ: Slack, 1986.
88. Pettersson H, Springfield DS, Enneking WF. Radiologic management of musculoskeletal tumors. New York: Springer-Verlag, 1986.
89. Link MP. Adjuvant therapy in the treatment of osteosarcoma. In: DeVita VT, Hellman S, Rosenberg SA, eds. Important advances in oncology. Philadelphia: JB Lippincott, 1986:193–207.
90. Link MP, Goorin AM, Miser AW, et al. The effect of adjuvant chemotherapy on relapse-free survival in patients with osteosarcoma of the extremity. N Engl J Med 1986;314:1600–1606.
91. Eilber F, Giliano A, Eckardt J, et al. Adjuvant chemotherapy for osteosarcoma: A randomized prospective trial. J Clin Oncol 1987;5:21–26.
92. Edmonson J, Creagan E, Gilchrist G. Phase II study of high dose methotrexate in patients with unresectable metastatic osteosarcoma. Cancer Treat Rep 1981;65:5438–5439.
93. Rosen G, Nirenberg A. Chemotherapy for osteogenic sarcoma: An investigative method, not a recipe. Cancer Treat Rep 1982;66:1687–1697.
94. Dahlin DC. The problems in assessment of new treatment regimens of osteosarcoma. Clin Orthop 1980;153:81–85.
95. Goorin A, Perez-Atayde A, Gebhardt A, et al. Weekly high-dose methotrexate and doxorubicin for osteosarcoma: The Dana Farber Cancer Institute/The Children's Hospital—study III. J Clin Oncol 1987;5:1178–1184.
96. Ettinger LJ, Douglas HO, Mindell ER, et al. Adjuvant adriamycin and cisplatin in newly diagnosed, non-metastatic osteosarcoma of the extremity. J Clin Oncol 1986;4: 353–362.
97. Rosen G, Marcove RC, Huvos AG, Caparros BI, Lane JM, Nirenberg A, Cacavio A, Groshen S. Primary osteogenic sarcoma: 8-Year experience with adjuvant chemotherapy. J Cancer Res Clin Oncol 1983;106:55–67.
98. Winkler K, Beron G, Kotz R, et al. Neoadjuvant chemotherapy for osteogenic sarcoma: Results of a Cooperative German/Austrian study. J Clin Oncol 1984;2:617–624.
99. Winkler K, Beron G, Delling G, et al. Neoadjuvant chemotherapy of osteosarcoma: Results of a randomized cooperative trial (COSS-82) with salvage chemotherapy based on histological tumor response. J Clin Oncol 1988;6:329–337.
100. Tobias JD, Pratt CB, Parham DM, et al. The significance of calcified regional lymph nodes at the time of diagnosis of osteosarcoma. Orthopedics 1985;8:49–52.
101. Giuliano AE, Feig S, Eilber F. Changing metastatic patterns of osteosarcoma. Cancer 1984;54:2160–2164.
102. Jaffee N, Smith E, Abelson H, Frei E. Osteogenic sarcoma. Alterations in the pattern of pulmonary metastases with adjuvant chemotherapy. J Clin Oncol 1983;1:251–254.
102a. Wuisman P, Enneking WF. Prognosis of patients who have osteosarcoma with skip metstasis. J Bone Joint Surg [Am] 1990;72:60–68.
102b. Spanier SS, Schuster JJ, Vander Griend RA. The effect of local extent of the tumor on prognosis in osteosarcoma. J Bone Joint Surg [Am] 1990;72:643–652.
103. Enneking WF. The issue of the biopsy. [Editorial] J Bone Joint Surg [Am] 1982;64: 1119–1120.
104. Mankin HJ, Lange TA, Spanier S. The hazards of biopsy in patients with malignant primary bone and soft-tissue tumors. J Bone Joint Surg [Am] 1982;64:1121–1127.
105. Hudson TM, Hass G, Enneking WF, Hawkins EF. Angiography in the management of musculoskeletal tumors. Surg Gynecol Obstet 1975;141:11–21.
106. Malawer MM, McHale KA. Limb-sparing surgery for high grade malignant tumors of the proximal tibia: Surgical technique and a new method of extensor mechanism reconstruction. Presented at the 4th International Symposium on Limb-salvage Surgery in Musculoskeletal Oncology, Kyoto, Japan, 1987.
106a. Bloem JL, Taminiau AHM, Eulderink F, Hermans J, Pauwels EKJ. Radiologic staging of primary bone sarcoma: MR imaging, scintigraphy, angiograhpy and CT correlated with pathologic examination. Radiology 1988;169:805–810.
107. Moore TM, Meyers MH, Patzakis MJ, et al. Closed biopsy of musculoskeletal lesions. J Bone Joint Surg [Am] 1979;61:375–380.
107a. Savino R. Gherlinzoni F, Morandi M, et al. Surgical treatment of giant-cell tumor of the spine. J Bone Joint Surg [Am] 1983;65:1283–1289.
108. Schajowicz F, Derqui JC. Puncture biopsy in lesions of the locomotor system. Review and results in 4050 cases, including 941 vertebral punctures. Cancer 1968;21:5331–5487.
109. Springfield DS, Goodman MA. Biopsy of musculoskeletal lesions. Orthopedics 1980;3: 868–870.
110. Mail JT, Cohen MD, Mirkin LD, Provisor AJ. Response of osteosarcoma to preoperative intravenous high-dose methotrexate chemotherapy: CT evaluation. AJR 1985;144: 89–93.
111. Jaffe N, Knapp J, Chuang VP, Wallace S, et al. Osteosarcoma: Intraarterial treatment of the primary tumor with *cis*-diammine-dichlorplatinum II (CDP): Angiographic, pathologic, and pharmacologic studies. Cancer 1983;51:402–407.
112. Chuang VP, Benjamin R, Jaffe N, et al. Radiographic and angiographic changes in osteosarcoma after intra-arterial chemotherapy. AJR 1982;139:1065–1069.
112a. Carrasco CH, Charnsangavel C, Raymond AK, et al. Osteosarcoma: Angiographic assessment of response to preoperative chemotherapy. Radiology 1989;170:839–842.
112b. Hogeboom WR, Hoekstra HJ, Mooyaart EL, Oosterhuis JE, Postma A, Veth RPH, Koops HS. Magnetic resonance imaging (MRI) in evaluating in vivo response to neoadjuvant chemotherapy for osteosarcomas of the extremities. Eur J Surg Oncol 1989;15:424, 430.
113. Smith J, Heelan RT, Huvos AG, et al. Radiographic changes in primary osteogenic sarcoma following intensive chemotherapy. Radiology 1982;143:355–360.
114. Sommer H-J, Knop J, Heise U, Winkler K, Delling G. Histomorphometric changes of osteosarcoma after chemotherapy, Correlation with ^{99}Tc methylene diphosphonate functional imaging.
115. Marcove RC, Lyden JP, Huvos AC, Bullough PB. Giant cell tumor treated by cryosurgery. Report of 25 cases. J Bone Joint Surg [Am] 1973;55:1633–1644.
116. Marcove RC, Stovell P, Huvos AC, Bullough P. The use of cryosurgery in the treatment of low and medium grade chondrosarcoma: A preliminary report. Clin Orthop 1977;122:147–156.
117. Marcove RC. A 17-year review of cryosurgery in the treatment of bone tumors. Clin Orthop 163:231–233.
118. Enneking WF, Spanier SS, Goodman MA. A system for the surgical staging of musculoskeletal sarcoma. Clin Orthop 1980;153:106–120.
119. Marcove RC, Rosen G. En bloc resection for osteogenic sarcoma. Cancer 1980;45: 3040–3044.
120. Malawer MM. Distal femoral osteogenic sarcoma, principles of soft tissue resection and reconstruction in conjunction with prosthetic replacement (adjuvant surgery). In, Chao EYS, ed. Design and application of tumor prosthesis for bone and joint reconstruction. New York: Thieme—Stratton, 1983:297–309.
121. Morton DL, Eilber FR, Townsend CM Jr, Grant TT, et al. Limb salvage from a multidisciplinary treatment approach for skeletal and soft tissue sarcomas of the extremity. Ann Surg 1976;184:268–278.
122. Enneking WF. Concluding material. In: Enneking WF, ed. Limb-sparing surgery for musculoskeletal tumors. New York: Churchill Liningstone, 1987:624–639.
123. Malawer MM, Meller I. Porous-coated segmental prosthesis for large tumor defects—a prosthesis based upon immediate fixation (PMA) and extracortical bone fixation: Analysis of 20 consecutive patients. Annual meeting of the Musculoskeletal Tumor Society, Toronto, 1987.
124. Heck DA, Chao EY, Sim FH, et al. Titanium fibermetal segmental replacement prostheses and radiographic analysis and review of current status. Clin Orthop 1987;204:266–285.
125. Mankin HJ, Fogelson FS, Thrasher AZ, et al. Massive resection and allograft transplantation in the treatment of malignant bone tumors. N Engl J Med 1976;294:1247–1255.
125a. Malawer MM. Unpublished data.
125b. Makley JT, Krailo M, Ertel IJ, et al. The relationship of various aspects of surgical management to outcome in childhood nonmetastatic osteosarcoma: A report from the Children's Cancer Study Group. J Pediatr Surg 1988;23:146–151.
126. Enneking WF. A system for the functional evaluation of the surgical management of musculoskeletal tumors. In Enneking WF, ed. Limb-sparing surgery for musculoskeletal tumors. New York: Churchchill Livingstone, 1987.

127. Miller G. Opening remarks. In Enneking WF, ed. Limb-sparing surgery for musculoskeletal tumors. New York: Churchill Livingstone, 1987.
128. Malawer MM, Baker A. Amputations for tumor. In: Evarts CM, ed. Surgery of the musculoskeletal system. 2nd ed. New York: Churchill Livingstone, 1989.
129. Marcove RC, Mike V, Hajek JV, Levin AG, Hutter RVP. Osteogenic sarcoma under the age of twenty-one. A review of one hundred and forty-five operative cases. J Bone Joint Surg [Am] 1970;52:411–423.
130. Mike V, Marcove RC. Osteogenic sarcoma under the age of 21: Experience at Memorial Sloan-Kettering Cancer Center. In: Terry WD, Windhorts D, eds. Immunotherapy of cancer: Present status of trials in man. New York: Raven Press, 1978.
131. Gehan EA, Sutow WW, Uribe-Botero G, Romsdahl M, Smith TL. Osteosarcoma: The M.D. Anderson experience, 1950–1974. In: Terry WD, Windhorst D, eds. Immunotherapy of cancer: Present status of trials in man. New York: Raven Press 1978.
132. Uribe-Botero G, Russell W, Sutow W, Martin R. Primary osteosarcoma of bone: A clinicopathologic investigation of 243 cases, with necropsy studies in 54. Am J Clin Pathol 1977;67:427–435.
133. Friedman MA, Carter SK. The therapy of osteogenic sarcoma: Current status and thoughts for the future. J Surg Oncol 1972;4:482–610.
134. Taylor WF, Ivins JC, Dahlin DC, Edmonson JH, Pritchard DJ. Trends and variability in survival from osteosarcoma. Mayo Clin Proc 1978;53:695–700.
135. Taylor WF, Ivins JC, Dahlin DC, Pritchard DJ. Osteogenic sarcoma experience at the Mayo Clinic, 1963–1974. In: Terry WD, Windhorts D, eds. Immunotherapy of cancer: Present status of trials in man. New York: Raven Press, 1978.
136. Taylor WF, Ivins J, Pritchard D, Dahlin DC, Gilchrist GS, Edmonson JH. Trends and variability in survival among patients with osteosarcoma: A 7-year update. Mayo Clin Proc 1985;60:91–104.
137. Strander H, Adamson U, Aparisi T, et al. Adjuvant interferon treatment of human osteosarcoma. Recent Results Cancer Res 1979;68:40–44.
138. Rab GT, Ivins JC, Childs DS, Cupps RE, Pritchard DJ. Elective whole lung irradiation in the treatment of osteogenic sarcoma. Cancer 1976;38:939–942.
139. Breur K, Cohen P, Schweisguth O, Hart A. Irradiation of the lungs as an adjuvant therapy in the treatment of osteosarcoma of the limbs: An EORTC randomized study. Eur J Cancer 1978;14:461–471.
140. Edmonson JH, Green SJ, Ivins JC, et al. A controlled pilot study of high-dose methotrexate as post surgical adjuvant treatment for primary osteosarcoma. J Clin Oncol 1984;2:152–156.
141. Link MP, Goordin AM, Miser AW, et al. The effect of adjuvant chemotherapy on relapse-free survival in patients with osteosarcoma of the extremity. N Engl J Med 1986;314:1600–1606.
142. Link MP, Shuster JJ, Goorin AM, et al. Adjuvant chemotherapy in the treatment of osteosarcoma: Results of the Multi-institutional Osteosarcoma Study. In: Ryan J, Baker LO, eds. Recent concepts in sarcoma treatment. Proceedings of the International Symposium on Sarcomas, Tarpon Springs, Florida, October 8–10, 1987. Dorecht, The Netherlands: Kluwer Academic Publishers, 1988:283–290.
143. Link MP, Goorin AM, Horowitz M, Meyer WH, Belasco J, Baker A, Ayala A, Shuster J. Adjuvant chemotherapy of high grade osteosarcoma of the extremity: Updated results of the Multi-institutional Osteosarcoma Study. Clin Orthop 1991;Sept(270): 8–14.
144. Eilber F, Giuliano A, Eckardt J, Patterson K, Moseley S, Goodnight J. Adjuvant chemotherapy for osteosarcoma: A randomized prospective trial. J Clin Oncol 1987;5: 21–26.
145. Laster WR Jr, Mayo JG, Simpson-Herren L, Griswold DP Jr, Lloyd HH, Schabel FM Jr, Skipper HE. Success and failure in the treatment of solid tumors. II. Kinetic parameters and "cell cure" of moderately advanced carcinoma 755. Cancer Chemother Rep 1969;53:169–188.
146. Schabel FM. Rationale for adjuvant chemotherapy. Cancer 1977;39:2875–2882.
147. Schabel FM Jr. The use of tumor growth kinetics in planning "curative" chemotherapy of advanced solid tumors. Cancer Res 1969;29:2384–2389.
148. Cortes EP, Holland JF, Wang JJ, Sinks LF. Doxorubicin in disseminated osteosarcoma. JAMA 1972;221:1132–1138.
149. Nitschke R, Starling KA, Vats T, Bryan H. *Cis*-diamminedichloroplatinum (NSC-119875) in childhood malignancies: A Southwest Oncology Group study. Med Pediatr Oncol 1978;4:127–132.
150. Ochs JJ, Freeman AL, Douglass HO, Higby DS, Mindell ER, Sinks LF. *Cis*-dichlorodiammineplatinum (II) in advanced osteogenic sarcoma. Cancer Treat Rep 1978;62: 239–245.
151. Baum ES, Gaynon P, Greenberg L, Krivitt W, Hammond D. Phase II study of *cis*-dichlorodiammineplatinum (II) in childhood osteosarcoma: Children's Cancer Study Group report. Cancer Treat Rep 1979;63:1621–1627.
152. Gasparini M, Rouesse J, van Oosterom A, et al. Phase II study of cisplatin in advanced osteogenic sarcoma. Cancer Treat Rep 1985;69:211–213.
153. Jaffe N, Farber S, Traggis D, et al. Favorable response of metastastic osteogenic sarcoma to pulse high-dose methotrexate with citrovorum rescue and radiation therapy. Cancer 1973;31:1367–1373.
154. Pratt C, Howarth C, Ransom J, et al. High dose methotrexate used alone and in combination for measurable primary and metastatic osteosarcoma. Cancer Treat Rep 1980;64:11–20.
155. Jaffe N, Frei E, Traggis D, Watts H. Weekly high-dose methotrexate-citrovorum factor in osteogenic sarcoma. Pre-surgical treatment of primary tumor and overt pulmonary metastases. Cancer 1977;39:45–50.
156. Marti C, Kroner T, Remagen W, Berchtold W, Cserhati M, Varini M. High-dose ifosfamide in advanced osteosarcoma. Cancer Treat Rep 1985;69:115–117.
157. Edmonson J, Creagan E, Gilchrist G. Phase II study of high dose methotrexate in patients with unresectable metastatic osteosarcoma. Cancer Treat Rep 1981;65:538–539.
158. Grem J, King S, Wittes R, Leyland-Jones B. The role of methotrexate in osteosarcoma. JNCI 1988;80:626–655.
159. Rosen G, Nirenberg A. Chemotherapy for osteogenic sarcoma: An investigative method, not a recipe. Cancer Treat Rep 1982;66:1687–1697.
160. Cortes EP, Holland JF, Wang JJ, Sinks LF, Blom J, Senn H, Bank A, Glidewell O. Amputation and Adriamycin in primary osteosarcoma. N Engl J Med 1974;291:998–1000.
161. Mosende C, Gutierrez M, Caparros B, Rosen G. Combination chemotherapy with bleomycin, cyclophosphamide and dactinomycin for the treatment of osteogenic sarcoma. Cancer 1977;40:2779–2786.
162. Frei E, Jaffe N, Skipper HE, Gero MG. Adjuvant chemotherapy of osteogenic sarcoma: Progress and perspectives. In: Salmon SE, Jones SE, eds. Adjuvant therapy of cancer. Amsterdam: Elsevier/North Holland Biomedical Press, 1977:49–64.
163. Jaffe N, Frei E, Traggis D, Bishop Y. Adjuvant methotrexate and citrovorum-factor treatment of osteogenic sarcoma. N Engl J Med 1974;291:994–997.
164. Goorin A, Delorey M, Gelber RD, Price K, Vawter G, Jaffe N, Watts H, Link M, Frei E, Abelson HT. The Dana-Farber Cancer Institute/The Children's Hospital adjuvant chemotherapy trials for osteosarcoma: Three sequential studies. Cancer Treat Rep 1986;3:155–159.
165. Rosenberg SA, Chabner BA, Young RC, et al. Treatment of osteogenic sarcoma. I. Effect of adjuvant high-dose methotrexate after amputation. Cancer Treat Rep 1979;63: 739–751.
166. Cortes EP, Holland JF, Glidewell O. Amputation and Adriamycin in primary osteosarcoma: A 5-year report. Cancer Treat Rep 1978;62:271–277.
167. Cortes EP, Holland JF, Glidewell O. Adjuvant therapy of operable primary osteosarcoma—Cancer and Leukemia Group B experience. Recent Results Cancer Res 1979;68:16–24.
168. Cortes E, Necheles TF, Holland JF, Carey RW, Blom J, Brunner K, Falkson G, Weinberg V. Adjuvant chemotherapy for primary osteosarcoma: A Cancer and Leukemia Group B experience. In: Salmon S, Jones S. eds. Adjuvant therapy of cancer, III. New York: Grune & Stratton, 1981:201–210.
169. Goorin A, Perez-Atayde A, Gebhardt M, et al. Weekly high dose methotrexate and doxorubicin for osteosarcoma: The Dana Farber Cancer Institute/The Children's Hospital—study III. J Clin Oncol 1987;5:1178–1184.
170. Krailo M, Ertel I, Makley J, et al. A randomized study comparing high-dose methotrexate with moderate-dose methotrexate as components of adjuvant chemotherapy in childhood nonmetastatic osteosarcoma: A report from the Children's Cancer Study Group. Med Pediatr Oncol 1987;15:69–77.
171. Sutow WW, Sullivan MP, Fernbach DJ, Cangir A, George SL. Adjuvant chemotherapy in primary treatment of osteogenic sarcoma. A Southwest Oncology Group study. Cancer 1975;36:1598–1602.
172. Sutow WW, Gehan EA, Dyment PG, Vietti T, Miale T. Multidrug adjuvant chemotherapy for osteosarcoma: Interim report of Southwest Oncology Group studies. Cancer Treat Rep 1978;62:265–269.
173. Herson J, Sutow WW, Elder K, Vietti TJ, Falletta JM, Crist WM, Vats TS, Miale T. Adjuvant chemotherapy in nonmetastatic osteosarcoma: A Southwest Oncology Group study. Med Pediatr Oncol 1980;8:343–352.
174. Pratt CB, Champion JE, Fleming ID, Rao B, Kumar PM, Evans WE, Green AA, George S. Adjuvant chemotherapy for osteosarcoma of the extremity. Long-term results of two consecutive prospective protocol studies. Cancer 1990;65:439–445.
175. Ettinger LJ, Douglass HO, Higby DJ, Mindell ER, Nime F, Ghoorah J, Freeman AI. Adjuvant Adriamycin and *cis*-diamminedichloroplatinum (*cis*-platinum) in primary osteosarcoma. Cancer 1981;47:248–254.
176. Ettinger LJ, Douglass HO, Mindell ER, Sinks L, Tebbi CK, Risseeuw D, Freeman AI. Adjuvant Adriamycin and cisplatin in newly diagnosed, non-metastatic osteosarcoma of the extremity. J Clin Oncol 1986;4:353–362.
177. van der Schueren E, Breur K. Role of lung irradiation in the adjuvant treatment of osteosarcoma. Recent Results Cancer Res 1982;80:98–102.
178. Rosen G, Murphy ML, Huvos AG, Gutierrez M, Marcove RC. Chemotherapy, en bloc resection, and prosthetic bone replacement in the treatment of osteogenic sarcoma. Cancer 1976;37:1–11.
179. Rosen G, Marcove RC, Caparros B, Nirenberg A, Kosloff C, Huvos AG. Primary osteogenic sarcoma. The rationale for preoperative chemotherapy and delayed surgery. Cancer 1979;43:2163–2177.
180. Rosen G, Marcove RC, Huvos AG, Caparros BI, Lane JM, Nirenberg A, Ccavio A, Groshen S. Primary osteogenic sarcoma: Eight-year experience with adjuvant chemotherapy. J Cancer Res Clin Oncol 1983;106:55–67.
181. Miser J, Arndt C, Smithson W, et al. Treatment of high grade osteosarcoma (OGS) with ifosamide (Ifos), mesna, Adriamycin (ADR), and high dose methotrexate (HDMTX). Proc Am Soc Clin Oncol 1991;10:310.
182. Huvos A, Rosen G, Marcove RC. Primary osteogenic sarcoma. Pathologic aspects in 20 patients after treatment with chemotherapy, en bloc resection and prosthetic bone replacement. Arch Pathol Lab Med 1977;101:14–18.
183. Winkler K, Beron G, Kotz R, et al. Neoadjuvant chemotherapy for osteogenic sarcoma: Results of a cooperative German/Austrian study. J Clin Oncol 1984;2:617–624.
184. Winkler K, Beron G, Kotz R, et al. Adjuvant chemotherapy in osteosarcoma—effects of cisplatinum, BCD, and fibroblast interferon in sequential combination with HD-MTX and Adriamycin. Preliminary results of the COSS 80 study. J Cancer Res Clin Oncol 1983;106:1–7.
185. Winkler K, Beron G, Delling G, et al. Neoadjuvant chemotherapy of osteosarcoma: Results of a randomized cooperative trial (COSS-82) with salvage chemotherapy based on histological tumor response. J Clin Oncol 1988;6:329–337.

186. Bacci G, Picci P, Ruggieri P, et al. Primary chemotherapy and delayed surgery (neoadjuvant chemotherapy) for osteosarcoma of the extremities. The Instituto Rizzoli experience in 127 patients treated preoperatively with intravenous methotrexate (high versus moderate doses) and intraarterial cisplatin. Cancer 1990;65:2539–2553.
187. Provisor A, Nachman J, Krailo M, Ettinger L, Hammond D. Treatment of non-metastatic osteogenic sarcoma of the extremities with pre- and post-operative chemotherapy. Proc Am Soc Clin Oncol 1987;6:217.
188. Hudson M, Jaffe MR, Jaffe N, et al. Pediatric osteosarcoma: Therapeutic strategies, results and prognostic factors derived from a 10-year experience. J Clin Oncol 1990;8: 1988–1997.
189. Goldie JH, Coldman AJ. A mathematical model for relating the drug sensitivity of tumors to their spontaneous mutation rate. Cancer Treat Rep 1979;63:1727–1733.
190. DeVita VT. The relationship between tumor mass and resistance to chemotherapy. Cancer 1983;51:1209–1220.
191. Salzer-Kuntschik M, Delling G, Beron G, Sigmund R. Morphological grades of regression in osteosarcoma after polychemotherapy. Study COSS 80. J Cancer Res Clin Oncol 1983;106:21–24.
192. Jaffe N, Prudich J, Knapp J, et al. Treatment of primary osteosarcoma with intraarterial and intravenous high-dose methotrexate. J Clin Oncol 1983;1:428–431.
193. Meyers PA, Heller G, Healey J, et al. Chemotherapy for non-metastatic osteogenic sarcoma: The Memorial-Sloan-Kettering experience. J Clin Oncol 1992;10:5–15.
194. Rosen G, Caparros B, Huvos AG, et al. Preoperative chemotherapy for osteogenic sarcoma: Selection of postoperative adjuvant chemotherapy based on the response of the primary tumor to preoperative chemotherapy. Cancer 1982;49:1221–1230.
195. Weiner M, Harris M, Lewis M, Jones R, Sherry H, Feuer EJ, Johnson J, Lahman E. Neoadjuvant high-dose methotrexate, cisplatin, and doxorubicin for the management of patients with nonmetastatic osteosarcoma. Cancer Treat Rep 1986;70:1431–1432.
196. Bramwell V, Burgers M, Sneath R, Jelliffe A, van Oosterom A, Voute T, Freedman L, van Glabbeke M. Preliminary report of the First European Osteosarcoma Intergroup study. Proc Am Soc Clin Oncol 1988;7:273.
197. Avella M, Bacci G, McDonald DJ, et al. Adjuvant chemotherapy with six drugs (Adriamycin, methotrexate, cisplatinum, bleomycin, cyclophosphamide, and dactinomycin) for non-metastatic high grade osteosarcoma of the extremities. Results of 32 patients and comparison to 127 patients concomitantly treated with the same drugs in a neoadjuvant form. Chemioterapia 1988;7:133–137.
198. Look AT, Douglass EC, Meyer WH. Clinical importance of near-diploid tumor stem lines in patients with osteosarcoma of an extremity. N Engl J Med 1988;318:1567–1572.
199. Jaffe N, Knapp J, Chuang VP, et al. Osteosarcoma: Intra-arterial treatment of the primary tumor with *cis*-diammine-dichloroplatinum II (CDP): Angiographic, pathologic and pharmacologic studies. Cancer 1983;51:402–407.
200. Jaffe N, Robertson R, Ayala A, et al. Comparison of intra-arterial *cis*-diamminedichloroplatinum II with high dose methotrexate and citrovorum factor rescue in the treatment of primary osteosarcoma. J Clin Oncol 1985;3:1101–1104.
201. Eilber FR, Eckardt J, Morton DL. Advances in the treatment of sarcomas of the extremity. Current status of limb salvage. Cancer 1984;54:2695–2701.
202. Winkler K, Bielack S, Delling G, et al. Effect of intraarterial versus intravenous cisplatin in addition to systemic doxorubicin, high-dose methotrexate, and ifosfamide on histologic tumor response in osteosarcoma (study COSS-86). Cancer 1990;66: 1703–1710.
203. Martin NS, Williamson J. The role of surgery in the treatment of malignant tumors of the spine. J Bone Joint Surg [Br] 1970;52:227–237.
204. Sterner B. Total spondylectomy in chondrosarcoma arising in the seventh thoracic vertebra. J Bone Joint Surg [Br] 1971;53:288–295.
205. Sterner BL, Johnson OE. Complete removal of three vertebra for giant cell tumor. J Bone Joint Surg [Br] 1971;53:278–287.
206. Maobiglet GM, Benjamin R, Patt YZ, et al. Intra-arterial *cis*-platinum for patients with inoperable skeletal tumors. Cancer 1981;48:1–4.
206a. Malawer MM, Buch R, Reaman G, et al. Impact of two cycles of preoperative chemotherapy with intraarterial cisplatin and intravenous doxorubicin on the choice of surgical procedure for high-grade bone sarcomas of the extremities. Clin Orthop Rel Res 1991;270:214–222.
207. Martinez A, Donaldson SS, Bagshaw MA. Special set-up and treatment techniques for the radiotherapy of pediatric malignancies. Int J Radiat Oncol Biol Phys 1977;2: 1007–1016.
208. Watkins DMB. Radiation therapy mold technology. Toronto: Pergamon Press, 1981.
209. Order SE, Donaldson SS. Radiation therapy of benign disease. Berlin: Springer-Verlag, 1990.
210. Sanerkin NG. The diagnosis and grading of chondrosarcoma of bone. A combined cytologic and histologic approach. Cancer 1980;45:582–594.
211. Huvos AG. Bone tumors. Diagnosis, treatment and prognosis. Philadelphia: WB Saunders, 1979.
212. Marcove RC, Mike V, Hutter RVP, et al. Chondrosarcoma of the pelvis and upper end of femur. J Bone Joint Surg [Am] 1972;54:561–572.
213. Bacci G, Springfield D, Picci P, et al. Adjuvant chemotherapy for malignant fibrous histiocytoma in the femur and tibia. J Bone Joint Surg [Am] 1985;67:620–625.
214. Nobler MP, Higginbotham NL, Phillips RF. The cure of aneurysmal bone cyst: Irradiation superior to surgery in an analysis of 33 cases. Radiology 1968;90:1185–1192.
215. Cassady JR. Radiation therapy in less common primary bone tumors. In: Jaffe N, ed. Solid tumors in childhood. Littleton, MA: PSG Publishing, 1979:205–214.
216. Anonsen CK, Donaldson SS. Langerhans' cell histiocytosis of the head and neck. Laryngoscope 1987;97:537–542, 1987
217. Greenberger JS, Crocker AC, Vawter G, et al. Results of treatment of 127 patients with systemic histiocytosis (Letterer-Siwe syndrome, Schuller-Christian syndrome and multifocal eosinophilic granuloma). Medicine (Baltimore) 1981;60:311–338.
218. Greenberger JS, Cassady JR, Jaffe N, et al. Radiation therapy in patients with histiocytosis: Management of diabetes insipidus and bone lesions. Int J Radiat Oncol Biol Phys 1979;5:1749–1755.
219. Gramatovici R, D'Angio GJ. Radiation therapy in soft-tissue lesions in histiocystosis X (Langerhans' cell histiocytosis). Med Pediatr Oncol 1988;16:259–262.
220. Dahlin DC, Conventry MB. Osteosarcoma, a study of 600 cases. J Bone Joint Surg [Am] 1967;49:101–110.
220a. Stark A, Kricbergs S, Nilsonne U, Silversward C. The age of osteosarcoma patients is increasing. An epidemiological study of osteosarcoma in Sweden 1971 to 1984. J Bone Joint Surg [B] 1990;72:89–93.
221. Richter MP, D'Angio GJ. The role of radiation therapy in the management of children with histiocytosis X. Am J Pediatr Hematol Oncol 1981;3:161–163.
222. Selch MT, Parker RG. Radiation therapy in the management of Langerhans cell histocytosis. Med Pediatr Oncol 1990;8:151–154.
223. Wick MR, Siegal GP, Unni KK, et al. Sarcomas of bone complicating osteitis deformas (Paget's disease), 50 years' experience. Am J Surg Pathol 1981;5:47–59.
224. Greditzer HG, McLeod RA, Unni KK, et al. Bone sarcomas in Paget's Disease. Radiology 1983;146:337–333.
225. Huvos AG, Wooard HQ, Cahan WG, et al. Postradiation osteogenic sarcoma of bone and soft tissues, a clinicopathologic study of 66 patients. Cancer 1982;55:1244–1255.
226. Francis KC, Kohn H, Malawer MM. Osteogenic sarcoma. J Bone Joint Surg [Am] 1976;55:754.
227. Enneking WF. Musculoskeletal tumor society, VII. New York: Churchill Livingstone, 1983:1021–1125.
228. Wilner D. Osteogenic sarcoma (osteosarcoma). In: Wilner D, ed. Radiology of bone tumors and allied disorders. Philadelphia: WB Saunders, 1982:1897–2095.
229. De Santos LA, Edeiken B. Purely lytic osteosarcoma. Skeletal Radiol 1982;9:1–7.
230. Jaffe N, Smith E, Abelson HT, et al. Osteogenic sarcoma: Alterations in the pattern of pulmonary metastases with adjuvant chemotherapy. J Clin Oncol 1983;1:251–254.
231. Lockshin MD, Higgins TT. Prognosis in osteogenic sarcoma. Clin Orthop 1968;58: 85–101.
232. Larsson SE, Lorentzon R, Wedron H, Boquist L. The prognosis in osteosarcoma. Int Orthop 1981;5:305–310.
233. Brostrom L, Strander H, Nisonne U. Survival in osteosarcoma in relation to tumor size and location. Clin Orthop 1982;167:250–254.
233a. Hudson M, Jaffe MR, Jaffe N, et al. Pediatric osteosarcoma: Therapeutic strategies, results, and prognostic factors derived from a 10-year experience. J Clin Oncol 1990;8: 1988–1997.
234. Bacci G, Avella M, Picci P, Briccoli A, Dallari D, Campanacci M. Metastatic patterns in osteosarcoma. Tumori 1988;74:421–427.
235. Levine AM, Rosenberg SA. Alkaline phosphatase levels in osteosarcoma tissue are related to prognosis. Cancer 1979;44:2291–2293.
236. Levine AM, Trich T, Rosenberg SA. Osteosarcoma cells in tissue culture: II. Characterization and location of alkaline phosphatase activity. Clin Orthop 1975;3:33–41.
237. Scranton PE Jr, DeCicco FA, Totten RS, Yunis EJ. Prognostic factors in osteosarcoma. A review of 20 years experience at the University of Pittsburgh Health Center Hospitals. Cancer 1975;36:2179–2191.
238. Look AT, Douglass EC, Meyer WH. Clinical importance of near-diploid tumor stem lines in patients with osteosarcoma of an extremity. N Engl J Med 1988;318:1567–1572.
238a. Bauer HCF, Kricbergs A, Silversward C. Prognostication including DNA analysis in osteosarcoma. Acta Orthop Scand 1989;60:353–360.
239. Springfield DS, Schmidt R, Grahm-Pole J, Marcus RB Jr, Spanier SS, Enneking WF. Surgical treatment for osteosarcoma. J Bone Joint Surg [Am] 1988;70:1124–1130.
240. Malawer MM, Sugarbaker, PH, et al. The Tikhoff-Linberg procedure and its modifications, In: Sugarbaker PH, ed. Atlas of sarcoma surgery. Philadelphia: JP Lippincott, 1984.
241. Malawer MM, Meller I, Dunham WK. A new surgical classification system for shoulder-girdle resections, analysis of 38 patients. Clin Orthop Rel Res 1991;267:33–43.
242. Malawar MM, Meller I, Dunham WK. Proposed surgical classification of shoulder girdle resections for bone and soft tissue tumors: Description of a new system and analysis of 38 patients. American Society of Shoulder and Elbow Surgery, New Orleans, 1987.
243. Malawer MM, Price WM. Gastrocnemius transposition flaps in conjunction with limb-sparing surgery for primary sarcomas around the knee. Plast Reconstr Surg 1984;73: 741–750.
244. Malawer MM, McHale KA. Limb-sparing surgery for high grade tumors of the proximal tibia and a new method of extensor mechanism reconstruction. 4th International Symposium on Limb-salvage in Musculoskeletal Oncology. Kyoto, Japan, 1987.
245. Hudson TM, Springfield DS, Schiebler M. Popliteus muscle as a barrier to tumor spread: Computer tomography and angiography. J Comput Assist Tomogr 1984;8: 498–501.
246. Malawer MM. Surgical management of aggressive and malignant tumors of the proximal fibula. Clin Orthop 1984;186:172–181.
247. Rosen G. Preoperative chemotherapy in osteogenic sarcoma. In: Enneking WF, ed. Limb-sparing surgery for musculoskeletal tumors. New York: Churchill Livingstone, 1987:260–267.
247a. Sundaresan N, Rosen G, Fortner JG, et al. Preoperative chemotherapy and surgical resection in the management of posterior paraspinal tumors. J Neurosurg 1983;58: 446–450.

248. Picci P, Bacci G, Companacci M, et al. Histological evaluation of necrosis in osteosarcoma induced by chemotherapy, regional mapping of viable and nonviable tumor. Cancer 1985;56:1515–1521.
248a. Tienghi A, Fiorentini G, Monti T, Graziani G, Bardella D, Margangolo M. Neo-adjuvant locoregional chemotherapy (NALC) in pelvic osteosarcoma (PO). Ann Oncol 1990;1: 97.
248b. Sundaresan N, Rosen G, Huvos AG, Krol G. Combined treatment of osteosarcoma of the spine. Neurosurgery 1988;23:714–719.
249. Rosen G, Huvos AG, Mosende C, Beattie EJ, Exelby PR, Capparos B, Marcove RC. Chemotherapy and thoracotomy for metastatic osteogenic sarcoma. A model for adjuvant chemotherapy and the rationale for timing of thoracic surgery. Cancer 1978;41: 841–849.
250. Pratt C, Champion J, Senzer N, et al. Treatment of unresectable or metastastic osteosarcoma with cisplatin or cisplatin-doxorubicin. Cancer 1985;56:1930–1933.
251. Cregan E, Frytak S, Pairolero P, Hahn RG, Muhm JR. Surgically proven pulmonary metastases not demonstrated by computed chest tomography. Cancer Treat Rep 1978;62:1404–1405.
252. Telander R, Pairolero P, Pritchard D, Sim F, Gilchrist G. Resection of pulmonary metastastic osteogenic sarcoma in children. Surgery 1978;84:335–341.
253. Putnam JB, Roth J, Wesley M, Johnston M, Rosenberg SA. Survival following aggressive resection of pulmonary metastases from osteogenic sarcoma: Analysis of prognostic factors. Ann Thorac Surg 1983;36:516–523.
254. Goorin A, Delorey M, Lack E, et al. Prognostic significance of complete surgical resection of pulmonary metastases in patients with osteogenic sarcoma: Analysis of 32 patients. J Clin Oncol 1984;2:425–431.
255. Meyer WH, Schell MJ, Kumar APM, Rao BN, Green AA, Champion J, Pratt CB. Thoracotomy for pulmonary metastatic osteosarcoma. An analysis of prognostic indicators of survival. Cancer 1987;59:374–379.
256. Weichselbaum R, Cassady J, Jaffe N, Filler R. Preliminary results of aggressive multimodality therapy for metastastic osteosarcoma. Cancer 1977;40:78–83.
257. Beattie E, Martini N, Rosen G. The management of pulmonary metastases in children with osteogenic sarcoma with surgical resection combined with chemotherapy. Cancer 1975;35:618–621.
258. Pappo A, Meyer W, Marina N, Mahmoud H, Pratt C. Chemotherapy for recurrent osteosarcoma (OS): Is it worth it? In, Proc Am Soc Clin Oncol 1992;11:368.
259. Cade S. Osteogenic sarcoma: A study based on 133 patients. J R Coll Surg Edinb 1955;1:79–111.
260. Lee ES, MacKenzie DH. Osteosacoma: A study of the value of preoperative megavoltage radiotherapy. Br J Surg 1964;51:252–274.
261. Farrell C, Reventos A. Experience in treating osteosarcoma at the Hospital of the University of Pennsylvania. Radiology 1964;83:1080–1083.
262. Sweetnan R, Knowelden J, Seedon H. Bone sarcoma: Treatment by irradiation, amputation, or a combination of the two. Br Med J 1971;2:363–367.
263. Phillips TL, Sheline GE. Radiation therapy of malignant bone tumors. Radiology 1969;92:1537–1545.
264. Allen CV, Stevens KR. Preoperative irradiation for osteogenic sarcoma. Cancer 1973;31:1365–1366.
265. Gaitan-Yanguas M. A study of the response of osteogenic sarcoma and adjacent normal tissues to radiation. Int J Radiat Oncol Biol Phys 1981;7:593–595.
266. Jenkin RD. Radiation treatment of Ewing's sarcoma and osteogenic sarcoma. Can J Surg 1977;20:530–536.
267. Jenkin RDT, Allt WEC, Fitzpatrick PJ. Osteosarcoma. An assessment of management with particular reference to primary irradiation and selective delayed amputation. Cancer 1972;30:393–400.
268. Beck JC, Wara WM, Bovill EG, et al. The role of radiation therapy in the treatment of osteosarcoma. Radiology 1976;120:163–165.
269. Suit HD. Radiation therapy given under conditions of local tissue hypoxia for bone and soft tissue sarcoma. In: M.D. Anderson Hospital: Tumors of bone and soft tissue. Chicago: Year Book Medical Publishers, 1965:143–163.
270. Scanlon PW. Split-dose radiotherapy for radioresistant bone and soft tissue sarcoma: Ten years' experience. AJR 1972;114:544–552.
271. Lee ES. Treatment of bone sarcoma. Proc R Soc Med 1971;64:1179–1180.
272. Clark JL, Unni KK, Dahlin DC, et al. Osteosarcoma of the jaw. Cancer 1983;51: 2311–2316.
273. Chambers RG, Mahoney WD. Osteogenic sarcoma of the mandible: Current management. Am Surg 1970;36:463–471.
274. Suit HD. Role of therapeutic radiology in cancer of bone. Cancer 1975;35:930–935.
275. De Fries HO, Perlin E, Leibel SA. Treatment of osteogenic sarcoma of the mandible. Arch Otolaryngol 1970;105:358–359.
276. Akbiyik N, Alexander LL. Osteosarcoma of the maxilla treated with radiation therapy and surgery. J Natl Med Assoc 1981;73:355–356.
277. Livolsi VA. Osteogenic sarcoma of the maxilla. Arch Otolaryngol 1977;103:485–488.
278. Goffinet DR, Kaplan HS, Donaldson SS, et al. Combined radiosensitizer infusion and irradiation of osteogenic sarcoma. Radiology 1975;117:211–214.
279. Martinez A, Goffinet DR, Donaldson SS, et al. Intra-arterial infusion of radiosensitizer (BUdR) combined with hypofractionated irradiation and chemotherapy for primary treatment of osteogenic sarcoma. Int J Radiat Oncol Biol Phys 1985;2:123–128.
280. Kinsella TJ, Glatstein E. Clinical experience with intravenous radiosensitizers in unresectable sarcomas. Cancer 1987;59:908–915.
281. Weichselbaum RR, Cassady JR. Radiation therapy in osteosarcoma. In: Jaffe N, ed. Solid tumors in childhood, 1979:183–190.
282. Newton KA, Barrett A. Prophylactic lung irradiation in the treatment of osteogenic sarcoma. Clin Radiol 1978;29:493–496.
283. Breur K, Cohen P, Schweisguth O, et al. Irradiation of the lungs as an adjuvant therapy in the treatment of osteosarcoma of the limbs. An E.O.R.T.C. randomized study. Eur J Cancer 1978;14:461–471.
284. Breur K, Schweisguth O, Cohen P, et al. Prophylactic irradiation of the lungs to prevent development of pulmonary metastases in patients with osteosarcoma of the limbs. NCI Monogr 1981;56:233–236.
285. Breur K, van der Schueren E. Adjuvant therapy in the management of osteosarcoma: Need for critical reassessment. Recent Results Cancer Res 1978;68:5–15.
286. Burgers JMV, van Glabbeke M, Busson A, et al. Osteosarcoma of the limbs. Report of the EORTC-SIOP 03 trial 20681 investigating the value of adjuvant treatment with chemotherapy and/or prophylactic lung irradiation. Cancer 1988;61:1024–1031.
287. French Bone Tumor Study Group. Age and dose of chemotherapy as major prognostic factors in a trial of adjuvant therapy of osteosarcoma combining two alternating drug combinations and early prophylactic lung irradiation. Cancer 1988;61:1304–1311.
288. Rab GT, Luins JC, Child DS, et al. Elective whole lung irradiation in the treatment of osteogenic sarcoma. Cancer 1976;38:949–952.
289. Jenkin RDT. The Treatment of osteosarcoma with radiation: Current indications. In: Management of primary bone and soft tissue tumors. Chicago: Year Book Medical Publishers, 1976:151–162.
290. Caceres E, Zaharia M, Moran M, et al. Adjuvant whole lung radiation with or without Adriamycin treatment in osteogenic sarcoma. Cancer Treat Rep 1978;62:297–299.
291. Unni KK, Dahlin DC, Beaubout SW, Ivins JC. Parosteal osteogenic sarcoma. Cancer 1976;37:2466–2475.
292. Schajowicz F, McGuire MH, Araujo S, Muscolo DL, Gitelis S. Osteosarcoma arising on the surfaces of long bones. J Bone Joint Surg [Am] 1988;70:555–564.
293. Martin SE, Dwyer A, Kissane JM, et al. Small-cell osteosarcoma. Cancer 1982;50: 990–996.
294. Sim FH, Unni Ku, Beaubout JW, et al. Osteosarcoma with small cells simulating Ewing's tumor. J Bone Joint Surg [Am] 1979;61:207–215.
295. Amendola BE, Amendola MA, McClatchey KD, Miller CH Jr. Radiation-associated sarcoma: A review of 23 patients with postradiation sarcoma over a 50-year period. Am J Clin Oncol 1989;12:411–415.
296. Mankin HJ, Cantley KD, Lipielo L, et al. The biology of human chondrosarcoma. I. Description of the cases, grading, and biochemical analyses. J Bone Joint Surg [Am] 1980;62:160–176.
297. Mankin HJ, Cantley KD, Schiller AL, et al. The biology of human chondrosarcoma. II. Variations in chemical composite among types and subtypes of benign and malignant cartilage tumors. J Bone Joint Surg [Am] 1980;62:176–188.
298. Krocberg A, Zelterberg A, Soderberg G. A comparative study of cellular DNA content and clinicopathologic features. Cancer 1982;50:577–583.
299. Alho A, Connor JF, Mankin HJ, Schiller AL, Campbell C. Assessment of malignancy of cartilage tumors using flow cytometry. A preliminary report. J Bone Joint Surg [Am] 1983;65:779–785.
300. Edeiken J. Bone tumors and tumor-like conditions. In: Edeiken J, ed. Roentgen diagnosis of diseases of bone. 3rd ed. Baltimore: Williams & Wilkins, 1981:30–414.
301. Aprin H, Riserborough EJ, Hall JE. Chondrosarcoma in children and adolescents. Clin Orthop 1982;166:226–232.
302. Steel HH. Partial or complete resection of the hemipelvis: An alternative to hindquarter amputation for periacetabular chondrosarcoma of the pelvis. J Bone Joint Surg [Am] 1978;60:719–730.
303. Austin-Seymour M, Munzenrider J, Goitein M, et al. Fractionated proton radiation therapy of chordoma and low-grade chondrosarcoma of the base of the skull. J Neurosurg 1989;70:13–17.
304. Aboulafia AJ, Faulks C, Li W, Buch R, Matthews J, Malawer MM. Reconstruction using the saddle prosthesis following excision of malignant periacetabular tumors. In: Brown, KLB, ed. Complications of limb salvage, prevention, management and outcome. Montreal: ISLOS, 1991.
305. Unni KK, Dahlin DC, Beaubout JW, Sim FH. Chondrosarcoma: Clear-cell variant. A report of 16 cases. J Bone Joint Surg [Am] 1976;57:676–683.
306. Harwood AR, Krajbich JI, Fornasier VL. Mesenchymal chondrosarcoma: A report of 17 cases. Clin Orthop 1981;158:144–148.
307. Huvos AG, Rosen G, Dabska M, Marcove RC. Mesenchymal chondrosarcoma: A clinicopathologic analysis of 35 patients with emphasis on treatment. Cancer 1983;51: 1230–1237.
308. Mankin HJ, Doppelt SH, Sullivan TR, Tomford WW. Osteoarticular and intercalary allograft transplantation in the management of malignant tumors of bone. Cancer 1982;50:613–630.
309. Krochak R, Harwood AR, Cummings BJ, et al. Results of radical radiation for chondrosarcoma of bone. Radiother Oncol 1983;1:109–115.
310. McNaney D, Lindberg RD, Ayala AG, et al. Fifteen year radiotherapy experience with chondrosarcoma of bone. Int J Radiat Oncol Biol Phys 1982;8:187–190.
311. Harwood AR, Krajbich JI, Fornasier VL. Radiotherapy of chondrosarcoma of bone. Cancer 1980;45:2769–2777.
312. Ryall RDH, Bates T, Newton KA, et al. Combination of radiotherapy and RA 20X and (ICRF 159) for chondrosarcoma. 1979;44:891–895.
313. Marcove RC. The surgery of tumors of bone and cartilage. 2nd ed. New York: Grune & Stratton, 1984.
314. Nascimento AG, Huvos AC, Marcove RC. Primary malignant giant cell tumor of bone study of eight cases and review of the literature. Cancer 1979;44:1393–1402.
315. Arlen M, Tollefsen HR, Huvos AS, et al. Chondrosarcoma of the head and neck. Am J Surg 1970;120:456–460.
316. Campanacci M, Giunti A, Olmi R. Giant-cell tumors of bone: A study of 209 cases with long-term follow-up in 130. Ital J Orthop Traumatol 1977;1:249–277.
317. Marcove RC, Weiss L, Vaghaiwall M, Pearson R. Cryosurgery in the treatment of

giant cell tumor of bone: A report of 52 consecutive cases. Clin Orthop 1978;134: 275–289.

318. Malawer MM, Dunham WK, Zaleski T, Zielinski CJ. The management of aggressive and low grade malignant bone tumors by cryosurgery: analysis of 40 consecutive cases. In: Enneking WF, ed. Limb-sparing surgery for musculoskeletal tumors. New York: Churchill Livingstone, 1987:498–510.
319. Persson BM, Wouters HW. Curettage and acrylic cementation in surgery of giant cell tumor of bone. J Bone Joint Surg [Am] 1976;120:125–133.
320. Larsson SE, Lorenzton R, Boquist L. Giant cell tumors of the spine and sacrum causing neurological problems. Clin Orthop 1975;111:201–211.
321. Bell RS, Harwood AR, Goodman SB, et al. Supervoltage radiotherapy in the treatment of difficult giant cell tumors of bone. Clin Orthop 1983;174:208–216.
322. Harwood AR, Fornasier VL, Rider WD. Supervoltage irradiation in the management of giant-cell tumor of bone. Radiology 1977;125:223.
323. Dahlin DC, Cupps RE, Johnson EW. Giant cell tumor: A study of 195 cases. Cancer 1970;25:1061–1070.
324. McGrath PH. Giant cell tumor of the bone: An analysis of fifty-two cases. J Bone Joint Surg [Br] 1972;54:216–229.
325. Tountas AA, Fornasier VL, Harwood AR, et al. Post-irradiation sarcoma of bone. Cancer 1979;43:182–187.
326. Bacci G, Springfield D, Picci P, et al. Adjuvant chemotherapy for malignant fibrous histiocytoma in the femur and tibia. J Bone Joint Surg [Am] 1985;67:620–625.
327. Heeten GJ, Koops HS, Kamps WA, et al. Treatment of malignant fibrous histiocytoma of bone, a plea for primary chemotherapy. Cancer 1985;56:37–40.
328. Earl HM, Morittu MD, Pringle J, Kemp H, Souhami. Sensitivity of malignant fibrous histiocytoma of bone (MFHB). Ann Oncol (in press).
329. Mindell ER. Current concept review. Chordoma. J Bone Joint Surg [Am] 1981;63: 501–505.
330. Localio AS, Eng K, Ranson JHC. Abdominosacral approach for retrorectal tumors. Am Surg 1980;179:555–560.
331. Localio AS, Francis KC, Rossano PC. Abdominosacral resection of sacrococcygeal chordoma. Ann Surg 1967;166:394–400.
332. Gray SW, Singhabhandhu B, Smith RA, Skandalakis JE. Sacrococcygeal chordoma: Report on a case and review of the literature. Surgery 1975;78:573.
333. Guterberg B, Romanus B, Sterner BL. Pelvic strength after major amputation of the sacrum. An experimental study. Acta Orthop Scand 1976;47:635–642.
334. DeVries J, Oldhoff J, Hadders, HN. Cryosurgery treatment of sacrococcyceal chordoma: Report of four cases. Cancer 1986;58:2348–2354.
335. Heffelfinger MJ, Dahlin DC, MacCarthy CS, et al. Chordomas and cartilaginous tumors of the skull base. Cancer 1973;32:410–420.
336. Sundaresian N, Galicich JH, Chu FCH, et al. Spinal chordoma. J Neurosurg 1979;50: 312–319.
337. Amendola BE, Amendola MA, Oliver E, et al. Chordoma: Role of radiation therapy. Radiology 1986;158:839–843.
338. Cummings BJ, Hodson ID, Bush RS. Chordoma: The results of megavoltage radiation therapy. Int J Radiat Oncol Biol Phys 1983;9:633–642.
339. Rich TA, Schiller A, Suit HD, et al. Clinical and pathologic review of 48 cases of chordoma. Cancer 1985;56:182–187.
340. Austin-Seymour M, Munzenrider J, Goitein M, et al. Proton radiation therapy of chordoma and low grade chondrosarcoma of the base of the skull and cervical spine. Int J Radiat Oncol Biol Phys 1986;12(suppl 1):98.
341. Raffel C, Wright DC, Gutin PH, et al. Cranial chordomas: Clinical presentation and results of operative and radiation therapy in twenty-six patients. Neurosurgery 1985;17: 703–710.
342. Reimer RR, Chabner BAC, Young RC, et al. Lymphoma presenting in bone. Results of histopathology, staging and therapy. Ann Intern Med 1977;87:50–55.
343. Sweet DL, Moss DP, Simon MA, et al. Histiocytic lymphoma (reticulum-cell sarcoma) of bone. Current strategy for orthopedic surgeons. J Bone Joint Surg [Am] 1981;63: 79–84.
344. Mendenhall NP, Jones JJ, Kramer BS, et al. The management of primary lymphoma of bone. Radiother Oncol 1987;9:137.
345. Loeffler JS, Tarbell NJ: Kozakewich H, et al. Primary lymphoma of bone in children: Analysis of treatment results with Adriamycin, prednisone, Oncovin (APO), and local radiation therapy. J Clin Oncol 1986;4:496–501.
346. Bacci G, Jaffe N, Emiliani E, et al. Therapy for primary non-Hodgkin's lymphoma of bone and a comparison of results with Ewing's sarcoma. Ten years' experience at the Instituto Orthopedico Rizzoli. Cancer 1986;57:1468–1472.
347. Coppes MJ, Patte C, Couanet D, et al. Childhood malignant lymphoma of bone. Med Pediatr Oncol 1991;19:22–27.
348. Furman WL, Fitch S, Hustu HO, et al. Primary lymphoma of bone in children. J Clin Oncol 1989;7:1275–1280.

Cancer: Principles & Practice of Oncology, Fourth Edition,
edited by Vincent T. DeVita, Jr., Samuel Hellman, Steven A. Rosenberg.
J.B. Lippincott Co., Philadelphia © 1993.

Bijan Safai

CHAPTER 45

Cancers of the Skin

The skin is the largest organ of the body and consists of three layers: epidermis, dermis, and subcutis (*i.e.*, hypodermis). It is a specialized structure with a wide range of functions that include protection from the environment, synthesis of vitamin D, production of a large number of cytokines, antigen presentation, thermoregulation, and sensation of touch and temperature. Several different cell and tissue types, originating from all three embryonic layers, participate in the formation of the three layers of the skin and its associated appendages. These cell and tissue elements can transform to produce a large number of benign and malignant growths (Tables 45–1 and 45–2). This chapter summarizes the nonmelanoma skin cancers and precancerous conditions.

EPIDEMIOLOGY

Nonmelanoma skin cancers are the most common cancers in the U.S. white population. More than 600,000 new cases are diagnosed annually, according to the data from the American Cancer Society.[1] The mortality rate for the nonmelanoma skin cancers is approximately 2100 per year.[1] Because most skin cancers are diagnosed and treated in private office settings or outpatient clinics, the available statistics are thought to grossly underestimate the actual number of nonmelanoma skin cancer cases.

Basal cell carcinoma is the most frequently diagnosed skin cancer in whites, accounting for approximately 75% to 80% of all reported cases.[2] Squamous cell carcinoma is the second most common skin cancer and is estimated to represent 20% to 25% of all reported skin cancer cases.[2]

Persons with fair skin who sunburn easily are more susceptible to developing basal cell carcinoma on the sun-exposed areas of their skin. Basal cell carcinoma occurs less often in darkly pigmented persons, in whom squamous cell carcinoma is the most common skin cancer. Basal cell carcinoma is seen more frequently in men than in women, and it mostly occurs later in life. However, recent observations indicate an increased incidence of basal cell carcinoma in younger age groups.

Other skin cancers, such as soft tissue sarcomas involving the dermis and subcutis and the adnexal carcinomas, are much less frequent and, although they are encountered in clinical practice, are not as common as basal cell carcinoma or squamous cell carcinoma.

ETIOLOGY AND PATHOGENESIS OF SKIN CANCERS

The two major factors influencing the development of skin cancers are exposure to ultraviolet radiation and type of skin (Table 45–3). Chemical carcinogens have been extensively studied, especially in laboratory animals, as etiologic factors for cutaneous malignancies. Ionizing radiation and primary chronic irritation play major roles in skin cancers. Attention has recently been focused on viruses that may cause skin cancers, specifically human papillomavirus causing skin and mucous membrane carcinomas. Host genetic makeup and host immunity also play roles in the development of skin cancers.

EXPOSURE TO ULTRAVIOLET LIGHT AND SKIN TYPE

Ample evidence supports the combined influence of ultraviolet (UV) light and skin type on the incidence of skin cancer. There is a higher incidence of skin cancer in albinos than in normally pigmented persons living in Africa. The incidence of skin cancer is higher in Australia than in Scandinavian

We acknowledge the significant contribution of Keon Menzies.

TABLE 45–1. Tumors Arising From Epidermal Cells

Keratinocytic Tumors
- Benign
  - Seborrheic keratosis
  - Epidermal nevi
  - Clear cell acanthoma
  - Kyrle's disease
  - Epidermal cyst
  - Trichilemmal cyst
  - Birt-Hogg-Dube syndrome
  - Becker's nevus
  - Warty dyskeratoma
- Premalignant
  - Actinic (solar) keratosis
  - Large cell acanthoma
  - Chondrodermatitis nodularis helicis
  - Cutaneous horn
  - Radiation dermatitis
  - Bowen's disease
  - Erythroplasia of Queyrat
  - Bowenoid papulosis
  - Epidermodysplasia verruciformis
  - Leukoplakia
  - Organoid (sebaceous) epidermal nevi
  - Porokeratosis
  - Fibroepithelioma of Pinkus
  - Keratoacanthoma
- Malignant
  - Basal cell carcinoma
  - Squamous cell carcinoma

Tumor of Merkel's Cells
- Merkel's cell carcinoma

Tumors of Langerhans Cells
- Histiocytosis X
- Letterer-Siwe disease
- Hand-Schüller-Christian disease
- Eosinophilic granuloma

Tumors of Melanocytic Origin
- Benign
  - Melanocytic nevi
- Premalignant
  - Dysplastic nevi
  - Congenital nevi
- Malignant
  - Malignant melanoma

Tumors of Epidermal Appendages
- Tumors of hair follicles
- Benign
  - Inverted follicular keratosis
  - Trichodiscoma
  - Tumors of the follicular infundibulum
  - Trichilemmoma
  - Trichofolliculoma
  - Trichoepithelioma
  - Pilomatricoma

Tumors of hair follicles (Continued)
- Malignant
  - Trichilemmocarcinoma
  - Pilomatrix carcinoma
- Tumors of sebaceous glands
- Benign
  - Fox-Fordyce anomaly
  - Organoid (sebaceous) nevi
  - Sebaceous gland hyperplasia
  - Sebaceous adenoma
  - Sebaceous epithelioma
- Malignant
  - Sebaceous carcinoma
- Tumors of apocrine glands
- Benign
  - Supernumerary nipple
  - Apocrine hidrocystoma
  - Syringocystadenoma papilliferum
  - Hidradenoma papilliferum
- Premalignant
  - Extramammary Paget's disease
- Malignant
  - Apocrine adenocarcinoma
- Tumors of eccrine glands
- Benign
  - Poroma
  - Syringoma
  - Chondroid syringoma
  - Hidrocystoma
  - Spiradenoma
  - Hidradenoma
  - Cylindroma
- Primary malignant
  - Syringoid eccrine carcinoma
  - Mucinous eccrine carcinoma
  - Clear cell carcinoma
  - Microcystic eccrine carcinoma
  - Adenoid cystic carcinoma
  - Aggressive digital papillary adenocarcinoma
  - Eccrine adenocarcinoma
- Secondary malignant
  - Porocarcinoma
  - Malignant syringoacanthoma
  - Malignant chondroid syringoma
  - Spiradenocarcinoma
  - Hidradenocarcinoma
  - Cylindrocarcinoma

TABLE 45–2. Tumors Arising in the Dermis and Subcutis

Fibrous or Connective Tissue Tumors
Benign
- Dermatofibroma
- Keloid (Hypertrophic scars)
- Angiofibroma

Malignant
- Dermatofibrosarcoma protuberans
- Atypical fibroxanthoma
- Malignant fibrous histiocytoma
- Epithelioid sarcoma

Neural Sheath Tumors
- Neurofibroma
- Neurofibromatosis
- Malignant neurofibroma
- Schwannoma (Neurilemmoma)
- Malignant schwannoma
- Granular cell tumor
- Malignant granular cell tumor

Vascular Tumors
Benign
- Angiokeratomas
- Pyogenic granuloma
- Lymphangioma
- Glomus tumors

Malignant
- Angiosarcoma
- Endovascular papillary angioendothelioma
- Spindle cell hemangioendothelioma
- Epithelioid vascular tumor
- Malignant angioendothelioma
- Kaposi's Sarcoma

Tumors Arising From Smooth Muscle
Benign
- Leiomyomas

Malignant
- Leiomyosarcomas

Tumors of Adipose Tissue Involving The Skin
Benign
- Lipoma

Malignant
- Liposarcoma
- Lipoblastoma

countries, where the population has similar skin, but UV light exposure is different. Squamous cell carcinoma usually occurs in the sun-exposed areas of head and neck. Persons with outdoor occupations, such as sailors and farmers, have a higher incidence of skin cancers than those with indoor occupations. Epidemiologic studies worldwide suggest that UV radiation is the most important etiologic agent for skin cancers.[3,4] The incidence of nonmelanoma skin cancers directly correlates with the proximity to the equator. A quantitative association has been observed between the lifetime sun exposure and the risk of developing nonmelanoma skin cancers. In outdoor workers, the most common sites for skin cancers are on the head, neck, and dorsum of the hands, which are the sites of maximal chronic sun exposure. Chronic UV exposure has changed from occupational to a more recreational pattern, and younger and younger persons are being diagnosed with skin cancers.

TABLE 45–3. Skin Type Assessment

Skin Type	Sunburn and Tanning History
I	Always burns, never tans
II	Always burns, minimal tan
III	Burns often, tans gradually (light brown)
IV	Burns minimally, tans well (moderate brown)
V	Burns rarely, tans profusely (dark brown)
VI	Never burns, deeply pigmented (black)

There is considerable environmental concern about the depletion of the ozone layer by certain chemicals. The ozone layer acts as a strong barrier in absorbing a major portion of UV radiation and preventing it from reaching the earth.[5] The chemicals responsible for the depletion of the ozone layer include chlorofluorocarbons, which are found in aerosol sprays and refrigerators. It is thought that the depletion of ozone over the next few years will rapidly increase the incidence of skin cancers.

Persons with light complexions have a higher chance of developing skin cancers than those with darker skin, who are protected from solar damage by the melanin pigment in the skin. Cutaneous malignancies are rare in dark-skinned persons, but African albinos have a high incidence of skin cancers on sun-exposed areas.

UV light may influence the development and progression of skin cancers by affecting the host immune system. The classic work of Kripke and colleagues showed that UV-induced cancers in mice are highly antigenic and that most are rejected by the host's immune system after transplantation into a normal, genetically identical animal.[6,7] However, the primary host in whom the tumor was induced by UV light becomes tolerant to the tumor and allows its rapid growth. Kripke's work indicates the development of suppressor factors and cells that suppress the host's immune system and prevent rejection of UV-induced skin cancer. These observations have not yet been confirmed in humans, but it is likely that UV light affects Langerhans cells in human skin, which may alter the host immune system, allowing the development and progression of skin cancer.

CHEMICAL CARCINOGENESIS

Most information about cutaneous carcinogenesis has been obtained from studies using laboratory animals, especially mice. After topical application of a carcinogen at regular intervals, the animals develop multiple squamous papillomas, most of which regress spontaneously. Some of the lesions develop the cytologic criteria of malignant cells, and these tumors may become locally invasive.

Three stages of progression have been identified for chemical carcinogenesis: initiation, promotion, and carcinogenesis. During the initiation phase, the DNA configuration of the cells undergoes some basic changes.[8] The process of initiation may remain unchanged for the life of the tissue, or it may progress to malignancy. The epidermal cells in psoriasis share many features with initiated cells. The initiated cells are usually terminally differentiated but may lose their pattern of differentiation and retain their ability to multiply. For the promoter to be effective and cause malignancies, the cell must have been initiated previously. Most promoters usually cause inflammation and hyperplasia, and their effects are reversible. Promoters can induce tumors only after initiation.[9] Some initiators and promoters are listed in Table 45–4.

Tar, which contains polycyclic aromatic hydrocarbons, is an initiator, and it has been used for treating psoriasis.[10] Nitrogen mustard is an accepted treatment for cutaneous T-cell lymphoma. Phorbol esters, which are found in croton oil, are known promoters. Anthralin, used in the treatment of psoriasis, and benzoyl peroxide, used in the treatment of acne, are also known promoters. Long-term use of these agents in humans has not been associated with an increased incidence of malignancy.[10,11] No chemical carcinogen has been identified that gives rise to basal cell carcinoma or malignant melanoma in animals, but experiments with cutaneous chemical carcinogenesis in laboratory animals cannot be directly applied to humans.

The well-documented cases of scrotal carcinoma in chimney sweepers offer the classic description of chemical carcinogenesis in man.[12] Arsenic is recognized as a chemical carcinogen. Increased incidence of cancers are reported in localities where there is a high level of arsenic in the drinking water.[13] Medical exposure to arsenic in the form of Fowler's solution, Donovan's solution, and Asiatic pills in the treatment of asthma and syphilis predisposes to the development of arsenical keratosis, skin cancer, and possibly lung cancer.

IONIZING RADIATION

Exposure to ionizing radiation can induce cutaneous malignancies in humans, usually basal cell carcinoma, squamous cell carcinoma, and spindle cell carcinoma.[14] Radiation-induced cancers of the skin have been reported in patients receiving ionizing radiation as therapy. In the past, acne, facial hair, and tinea capitis were treated with x-ray therapy. Patients receiving these types of therapy later developed severe radiodermatitis in the form of skin atrophy, telangiectasia, hypopigmentation, or hyperpigmentation. Some of these patients developed large, invasive, deforming skin cancers. These inappropriate uses of x-ray therapy have been discontinued, but accidental exposure to x-rays and exposure for medical reasons continues to cause radiation dermatitis. Occupational exposure and the resultant radiodermatitis and skin cancers, such as squamous cell carcinoma on the fingers of dentists, is no longer seen. The use of fractionated doses of radiation has reduced the long-term side effects of radiation therapy.

TABLE 45–4. Initiators and Promoters Used in Dermatologic Therapy

Initiators	*Promoters*
Ultraviolet light	Ultraviolet light
Tar (polycyclic aromatic hydrocarbons)	Phenol
Nitrogen mustard	Anthralin
Psoralen	Phorbol esters
	Benzoyl peroxide

CHRONIC IRRITATION OR INFLAMMATION

Skin cancers can develop in areas of chronic inflammation or irritation. Examples of such tumors include cancers developing in the area of chronic osteomyelitis sinus, lupus erythematosus, decubitus ulcers, scars of burns, and sinus formation.[15–21] Chewing tobacco or betel nuts can cause squamous cell carcinoma of the oral cavity and lip.

VIRAL ONCOGENESIS

Many malignant neoplasms are caused by viruses in animals. In humans, such associations have rarely been documented. Human papillomavirus (HPV) has been identified in lesions of verrucous carcinoma, bowenoid papulosis, and in situ epidermoid carcinoma.[22–24] Many papillomavirus subtypes have been identified, and HPV types 5, 8, 14, 16, 17, and 33 are associated with various epidermal carcinomas and carcinoma of the cervix.[25,26] It is possible that other inducing factors are needed to produce the malignant tumor from some of these papillomaviruses. These papillomaviruses appear potentially oncogenic in humans.[27] There are other viruses, such as human T-cell lymphotrophic virus-I in leukemia-lymphoma and Epstein-Barr virus in Burkitt's lymphoma and nasopharyngeal carcinoma, that may be associated with some of the human malignancies, but conclusive information is not available.

IMMUNOLOGIC FACTORS

The concept of immune surveillance suggests that many potentially fatal tumor cells are continuously being detected and destroyed by the immune system before they can form large enough tumors to permit clinical detection. Antibody-mediated and cell-mediated cytotoxic antitumor responses have been detected in animal tumors, but in humans, the detection of immunologic reactivity against malignant tumors and the value of destruction of tumor cells by immune cells are not well documented. The findings of tumor immunology are applicable to several areas of cutaneous oncology.

The work of Kripke and coworkers indicates that a suppressor T cell and suppressor factor are produced in mice, in response to the effect of UV radiation on the immune system.[6,7] Immunoregulation and carcinogenesis have been extensively investigated in murine systems, but the interaction between UV light and the human immune system is not well delineated.

Patients with primary or secondary immunodeficiencies are prone to develop de novo cutaneous malignant neoplasms.[28] Those receiving immunosuppressive therapy (*e.g.*, renal transplant recipients) also develop cutaneous malignant tumors.[29–32] Patients with lymphoreticular malignancies have a higher incidence of nonmelanoma skin cancers, and these skin cancers behave more aggressively in the immunocompromised host.[32–35] It appears that there is some association between the host's immune status and the development of skin cancer, but this relation is not well understood.

GENETIC FACTORS

Several genetically inherited syndromes increase susceptibility for the development of skin cancers. These genodermatoses include xeroderma pigmentosum, nevoid basal cell carcinoma, familial dysplastic nevus syndrome, Bazex's syndrome, and multiple self-healing epithelioma of Ferguson-Smith. Some other genodermatoses, such as Torre's syndrome, Cowden's syndrome, Gardner's syndrome, Peutz-Jeghers syndrome, dyskeratosis congenita, and Carney's syndrome, manifest with some nonmalignant skin lesions and are usually associated with internal malignancies.

CLASSIFICATION OF SKIN TUMORS

To describe the various tumors of the skin in an orderly fashion, the cellular origin and the location in the three layers are followed. Tables 45–1 and 45–2 summarize the tumor of the skin based on their cell of origin, biologic behavior, and location in the three layers of the skin.

BENIGN TUMORS ARISING FROM EPIDERMAL KERATINOCYTES

Benign tumors are commonly diagnosed. They rarely give rise to malignant tumors, but they may be confused with some of the malignant lesions. It is important for clinicians to be able to recognize and differentiate them from malignant skin tumors.

SEBORRHEIC KERATOSIS

Seborrheic keratosis or basal cell papilloma is a common benign lesion produced by the overgrowth of epidermal keratinocytes. It occurs most often on the trunk, face, and neck of middle-aged and elderly persons. Lesions may be found on the extremities but not on the palms and soles. Essential diagnostic features include multiple domed or flat-topped, round or ovoid, verrucous papules that are brown to black. These slightly raised, sharply demarcated lesions appear to be stuck on the surface of the skin. Histologic features are characteristic and consist of acanthosis, hyperkeratosis, and papillomatosis with keratin horn and pseudocysts. The lesion consists mostly of squamous and basaloid epidermal cells. Histologic types include acanthotic, hyperkeratotic, reticulated (adenoidal), clonal and irritated (inflamed) lesions. Other types include melanoacanthoma, dermatosis papulosis nigra, stucco keratosis, and seborrheic keratoses of the Leser-Trélat sign. Leser-Trélat sign is characterized by a sudden appearance of innumerable new lesions of seborrheic keratosis, which may be a sign of an internal malignancy.[36] Rare transformations of seborrheic keratosis to basal cell carcinoma and squamous cell carcinoma have been reported.[37]

Differential diagnosis consists of intraepidermal epithelioma, verruca vulgaris, dermal nevus, pigmented basal cell carcinoma, well-differentiated squamous cell carcinoma, and malignant melanoma. If histologic confirmation is necessary for differential diagnosis, shave excision is the method of choice. Because of its relatively superficial location, seborrheic keratoses may be removed by curettage and light electrodesiccation or by cryosurgery with liquid nitrogen or carbon dioxide ice.

EPIDERMAL NEVI

Epidermal nevi are benign, congenital, hyperplastic lesions with a smooth or hyperkeratotic surface. They typically appear at birth or in early childhood. Epidermal nevi are uncommon. Lesions may be solitary or multiple, or they may form a plaque covering a large area of skin, usually in an asymmetric or linear distribution. The lesions vary in color from skin color to deeply pigmented brown to black. Clinical variants include nevus verrucosus, linear epidermal nevus, systematized epidermal nevus, ichthyosis hystrix, inflammatory linear epidermal nevus, and epidermal nevus syndrome.[38] Epidermal nevus syndrome or large verrucous epidermal nevus may present with widespread involvement but predominantly on one side of the body. It frequently coexists with central nervous system and skeletal abnormalities.[39] Epidermal nevi remain benign and require treatment only if cosmetically indicated. There have been rare cases of transformation to carcinomas.[40]

CLEAR CELL ACANTHOMA

Clear cell acanthoma appears as a solitary, pink to red, scaly nodule on the lower leg.[41] The lesion is slow growing, sharply delineated, and 1 to 2 cm in diameter. Lesions appear stuck on, like seborrheic keratosis, and vascular, like granuloma pyogenicum. The growth is usually asymptomatic, but the thin, crusty cover may ooze some moisture. Multiple lesions are uncommon.[42] Histologically, the lesion consists of a proliferating population of slightly enlarged keratinocytes with abundant, clear cytoplasm, rich in glycogen. The nuclei appear normal. The lesion is usually excised for histologic diagnosis.

KYRLE'S DISEASE

Kyrle's disease (*i.e.*, hyperkeratosis follicularis et parafollicularis in cutem penetrans) appears as multiple hyperkeratotic lesions with inflammation and crusting.[43] The lesions are seen mostly on the lower extremities but appear on upper limbs, trunk, soles, and rarely on other areas of the body. It is thought that the condition is produced by the hyperkeratotic lesions penetrating from the epidermis into the dermis, forming a keratotic plug that stimulates inflammatory and foreign-body giant cell reactions. The histologic picture includes hyperkeratosis, mainly around hair follicles, lichenoid reactions, and lymphocytic infiltration.[44]

Kyrle's disease and perforating folliculitis are clinically and histologically hard to differentiate. Uremic follicular hyperkeratosis is used to describe lesions that have features of Kyrle's disease and perforating folliculitis.[45] Unlike the rarity of Kyrle's disease, this new entity is fairly common and occurs mostly in patients with diabetes and renal failure.[46] These lesions must be differentiated from actinic keratosis and squamous cell carcinoma, and they require biopsy and histologic confirmation. No effective treatment is available, but cryotherapy may be of some value.

CYSTS

Cysts are relatively common lesions occurring in young and middle-aged persons, and they are usually of great concern to patients. Two of the more common forms are epidermal cyst and trichilemmal (*i.e.*, pilar) cyst.

Epidermal cysts are single or multiple lesions, mostly found on the face, neck, chest, and back. They arise spontaneously or may form as a result of trauma. A cyst normally enlarges to about 1 to 5 cm, but remains as a firm, asymptomatic mass unless it becomes infected. Histologically, epidermal cysts are intradermal or subcutaneous cavities lined with normal surface epidermis and filled with fluid and epithelial debris. Development of basal cell carcinoma, squamous cell carcinoma, and Bowen's disease from epidermal cysts have been reported.[47–49] Effective treatment requires complete removal of the cyst and its sac.

Trichilemmal cysts are clinically indistinguishable from epidermal cysts. Trichilemmal cysts may be single or multiple lesions, frequently seen on the scalp but rarely on the face and neck. Histologically, the pilar cyst is lined by epithelium resembling hair follicle epithelium. The absence of the granular layer differentiates it from the epidermal cyst, which consists of all the layers of the epidermis.[50,51] Trichilemmal cysts may have a more hyperplastic presentation, and they are referred to as proliferating trichilemmal cysts.[52,53] Malignant degeneration with metastasis of proliferating trichilemmal cysts has been reported.[54] Treatment is surgical excision of the entire cyst.

BIRT-HOGG-DUBE SYNDROME

Birt-Hogg-Dube syndrome is inherited as an autosomal dominant trait and consists of the triad of trichodiscoma, fibrofolliculoma, and acrocordan.[55–57] The patient has multiple, asymptomatic, flesh-colored papules on the face, mainly around the nose. Histologically, the lesions may show proliferation of the superficial hair follicle (*i.e.*, trichodiscoma) or proliferation of the dermal part of the hair follicle (*i.e.*, fibrofolliculomas) or features of fibrous skin tags (*i.e.*, acrochordon). Lesions are removed only if cosmetically indicated.

BECKER'S NEVUS

Becker's pigmented hairy epidermal nevus (*i.e.*, Becker's melanosis) is a relatively common condition presenting with a patch of hyperpigmented, coalescing macules on the shoulders and upper extremities, mostly in young men.[58] Hypertrichosis is frequently associated with the tan or brown patches. This condition is usually preceded by a sunburn of the involved area. Histologically, the skin appears normal except for an increased number of melanocytes, especially in the dermis, and the increased melanin in the basal layer of the epidermis.[59] The hair follicles appear normal, but the diameter of the hair may be thicker than normal. There is no need for treatment except if cosmetically indicated.

WARTY DYSKERATOMA

Warty dyskeratoma presents in middle-aged patients as a solitary lesion on the scalp, face, or neck, but it may occur in unexposed skin and the oral mucosa.[60,61] It occurs as a slightly elevated, circumscribed papule or nodule with a raised border and keratotic umbilicated or pore-like center. The lesion typically grows to about 1 to 10 mm in diameter. Common complaints are itching, burning sensation, recurrent drainage, and bleeding due to trauma. Histologically, the lesion appears as a large, cup-shaped invagination with a keratotic and parakeratotic plug. The upper portion of the invagination shows numerous acantholytic and dyskeratotic cells. One or more pilosebaceous structures are commonly associated with warty dyskeratoma, but they are not etiologic, because lesions may also occur on the oral mucosa. In older patients, these lesions are frequently associated with premalignant and malignant lesions, such as solar keratosis, squamous cell carcinoma, basal cell carcinoma, and adnexal carcinomas. Differential diagnosis includes Darier's disease, sebaceous cyst, solar keratosis, basal cell carcinoma, verrucae, nevocellular nevus, and folliculitis. Surgical excision is the most commonly recommended treatment approach.

PREMALIGNANT TUMORS OF THE EPIDERMIS

Because of the absence of good epidemiologic data, it is difficult to determine with certainty whether a lesion is a true precancerous lesion and gives rise to a malignant condition or if the association is a coincidental finding. An example of this is keratoacanthoma, which is usually a benign, self-healing lesion, but it may predispose the patient to squamous cell carcinoma.

ACTINIC OR SOLAR KERATOSIS

Actinic or solar keratoses are common asymptotic lesions seen mostly on sun-exposed areas of light-skinned persons. The lesions are commonly multiple and appear on sun-damaged skin as skin-colored to yellow-brown, firm, raised papules with scaly, rough, keratotic surfaces and erythematous bases. Unlike seborrheic keratosis, actinic keratosis appears to arise from within the epidermis, rather than being "stuck on" the skin. Common sites for actinic keratosis are the face, dorsum of the hands, the upper chest, upper back, and lower lip. The lesions are typically a few millimeters to 1 cm in diameter. In Australia, 40% of persons over age 40 have one or more actinic keratoses.[62] Histologic features include epidermal dysplasia sparing the skin appendages, hyperkeratosis and inflammation with lymphocytic infiltration, and evidence of actinic elastosis and telangiectasia in the dermis. Abnormal keratinocytes appear less basophilic than normal keratinocytes and vary in size and shape.

Approximately 20% to 25% of actinic keratoses eventually transform into carcinoma in situ and finally into invasive squamous cell carcinoma years after their initial appearance (Fig. 45–1).[63,64] If induration, erythema, or erosion are observed, possible progression to squamous cell carcinoma should be suspected. If malignant transformation is suspected, shave excision of the lesion and histologic examination are recommended. Lesions may transform into squamous cell carcinoma more rapidly in patients who are immunosuppressed or have genetic defects of DNA repair enzymes (*e.g.*, xeroderma pigmentosum). The report from Australia indicates a much lower number, approximately 1%, developing into basal cell carcinoma.[62]

Differential diagnosis includes seborrheic keratoses, lichenoid keratoses, warts, pigmented basal cell carcinomas, lentigo maligna, malignant melanomas, and early squamous cell carcinomas. Existing lesions are treated by curettage and electrodesiccation or liquid nitrogen cryotherapy. Multiple and widespread lesions may be treated with application of a cream or solution containing 5-fluorouracil (5-FU) for approximately 3 weeks, but this treatment may produce considerable discomfort.[65] Dermatoabrasion may be an alternative. Some reports indicate spontaneous regression of lesions.[66] Protection against excessive sun exposure by the use of protective clothing and sunscreens helps to prevent actinic keratosis.

CHEMICAL AND OTHER KERATOSES

Other keratoses that may be considered as premalignant cutaneous dysplasia are arsenical keratosis (Fig. 45–2) induced by exposure to arsenic, tar keratoses induced by exposure to tars and other polycyclic aromatic hydrocarbons, thermal keratoses induced after prolonged (≤20 years) exposure to infrared radiation that causes chronic cutaneous thermal damage, chronic radiation keratoses induced by exposure to x-rays, and chronic cicatrix keratoses or scar keratoses that may degenerate to scar carcinoma with metastatic potential.

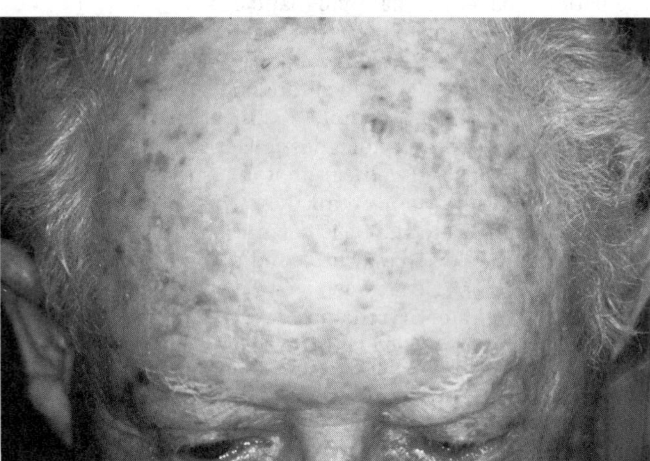

FIGURE 45–1. Severely sun-damaged skin, solar keratosis, basal cell carcinoma, and squamous cell carcinoma on sun-exposed skin of a white man.

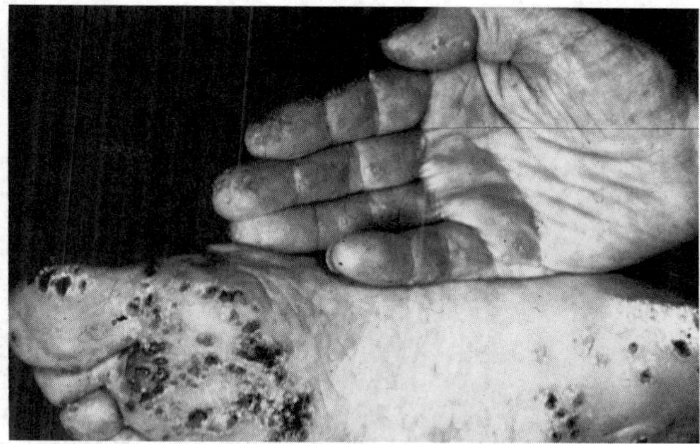

FIGURE 45–2. Arsenic keratosis on the palm and sole.

LARGE CELL ACANTHOMA

Large cell acanthoma occurs mostly on sun-exposed skin as a sharply demarcated, slightly hyperkeratotic, scaly, pigmented lesion, usually less than 1 cm in diameter.[67] Most lesions are solitary, but some multiple lesions are seen.[68] It is clinically similar to actinic keratosis, but this rare lesion is easily differentiated histologically from actinic keratosis by the presence of large keratinocytes with proportionally large nuclei scattered in a disordered arrangement of epidermal cells.[69] Another differential diagnosis is Bowen's disease. The management of large cell acanthoma is similar to actinic keratosis.

CHONDRODERMATITIS NODULARIS HELICIS

Chondrodermatitis nodularis helicis is most commonly seen in elderly men and appears as tender, painful, inflamed, scaly, erythematous papules or nodules on the apex of the ear.[70–72] Lesions are occasionally ulcerated and crusted. Advanced cases show significant cartilage destruction and distortion of the pinna. A few of these patients develop squamous cell carcinoma if left untreated. Histologic features include actinic damage in the epidermis and dermis, but the essential feature for diagnosis is inflammation and damage of underlying cartilage by a lymphocytic infiltration. Management includes use of a topical or intralesional corticosteroid and, if not effective, surgical excision.

CUTANEOUS HORN

Cutaneous horn appears as a protuberant, raised, hard, hyperkeratotic nodule with an erythematous base commonly occurring on the sun-exposed areas of white-skinned persons (Fig. 45–3). It usually develops due to the underlying dysplasia or frank neoplasm, and it is therefore considered a marker of skin cancer. The histopathology of the underlying lesion includes actinic keratosis, seborrheic keratosis, filiform verruca, trichilemmoma, basal cell carcinoma, or squamous cell carcinoma.[73–75] A histopathologic study indicates that 39% of underlying lesions were premalignant and malignant epidermal lesions, and 61% were benign lesions.[75] The lesion with a portion of the base should be removed for histologic ex-

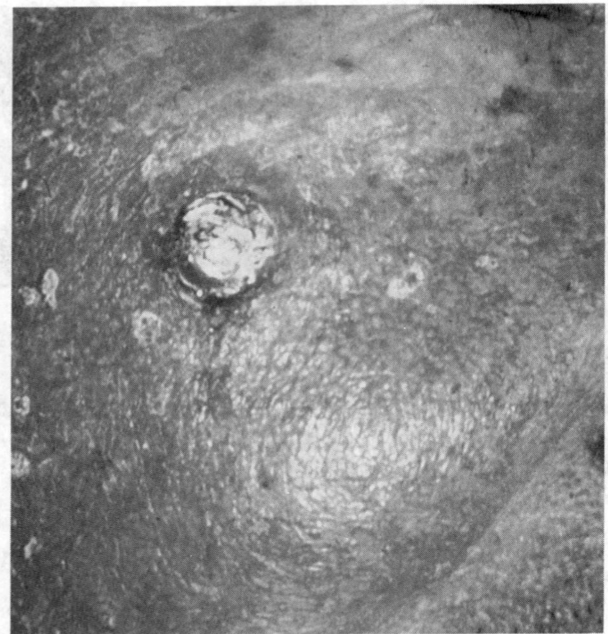

FIGURE 45–3. Cutaneous horn on severely sun-damaged facial skin.

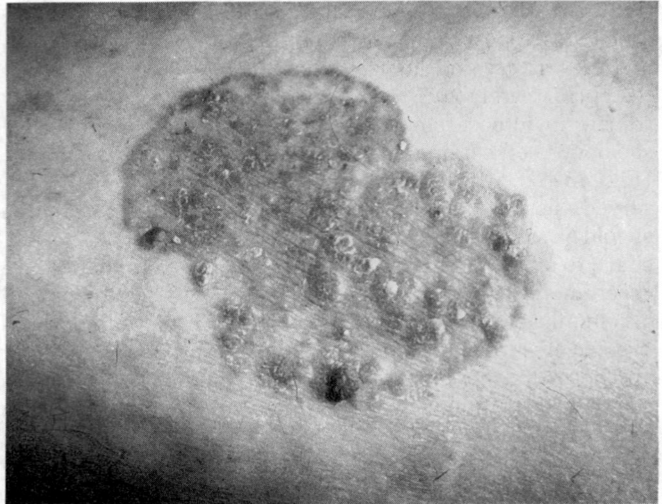

FIGURE 45–4. Bowen's disease on the trunk.

amination. Final treatment is usually determined by the pathology of the underlying tissue.

RADIATION DERMATITIS

Radiation dermatitis is the term used to describe skin damage due to x-irradiation, whether exposure occurs as a result of occupational hazard or therapeutic treatments.[76] Involved skin is dry, scaly, erythematous, thin, and discolored. Areas of telangiectasia, hyperpigmentation and hypopigmentation, and hyperkeratosis and ulceration are common. Histologically, the damaged area shows atrophy and loss of polarity of epidermal keratinocytes, changes in elastic and collagen bundles of the dermis, and destruction of hair follicles, sebaceous glands, and sweat glands. There is a potential for developing actinic keratosis, basal cell carcinoma, and squamous cell carcinoma on this kind of skin.[77,78] Management includes removal of any overlying skin lesion and continuous skin care. Soft tissue sarcomas may develop in the irradiated tissue.[79,80]

BOWEN'S DISEASE

Bowen's disease or intraepidermal carcinoma in situ is an intraepidermal squamous cell carcinoma that may involve any area of the skin but tends to favor sun-exposed areas of the face, neck, and extremities (Fig. 45–4). In one third of the patients, the lesions may be multiple. Bowen's disease is papulosquamous and appears as a slowly enlarging, sharply defined, round to irregular plaque with a rough, scaly, hyperkeratotic, erythematous surface. Other surface characteristics include pigmentation, fissures, erosion, and ulceration. Similar to in situ epidermoid carcinoma, Bowen's lesions may progress to invasive squamous cell carcinoma. This transformation to squamous cell carcinoma is reported in 3% to 5% of the cases, with most cases remaining as carcinoma in situ.[81,82]

The cause of Bowen's disease is unknown, but UV radiation, HPV-induced epidermodysplasia verruciformis, and history of ingestion of inorganic arsenic (*e.g.*, water or medication) are considered etiologic factors.[23,83,84] Bowen's disease has been seen on nonexposed areas of the skin in younger persons without a history of arsenic ingestion and without HPV infections.

Histologic features of Bowen's disease include gross dysplasia of the upper layers of epidermal cells with the basal cell layer relatively normal, individual cell keratinization, and giant keratinocytes with atypical mitoses. It has been suggested that patients with Bowen's disease are more likely to develop other cancers, including basal cell carcinoma, adnexal carcinoma, melanoma, or cancers of the lung, gastrointestinal tract, genitourinary tract, and the reticuloendothelial system, but the role of Bowen's disease as a marker of internal malignancies is unclear. A report from the Armed Forces Institute of Pathology indicates that as many as 80% of the cases of Bowen's disease have other cutaneous and noncutaneous malignancies.[85] Another report suggests that as many as 29% of the patients have internal malignancies.[86]

Many of the published reports contain major deficiencies, such as lack of sufficient control groups.[87] In view of the existing controversies, it is recommended that patients with Bowen's disease have a complete clinical examination combined with the necessary diagnostic workup. Differential diagnosis includes basal cell carcinoma, psoriasis, extramammary Paget's disease, and actinic keratosis. Excisional biopsy of the most indurated area is recommended for histologic confirmation of Bowen's disease and detection of squamous cell carcinoma. Surgical excision of the entire lesion provides the highest cure rate. Cryotherapy or curettage and desiccation have been recommended, but there is a higher chance of recurrence.

ERYTHROPLASIA OF QUEYRAT

Erythroplasia of Queyrat is a clinicopathologic variant of Bowen's disease, occurring almost exclusively on the glans penis of uncircumcised, middle-aged and older men (Fig. 45–

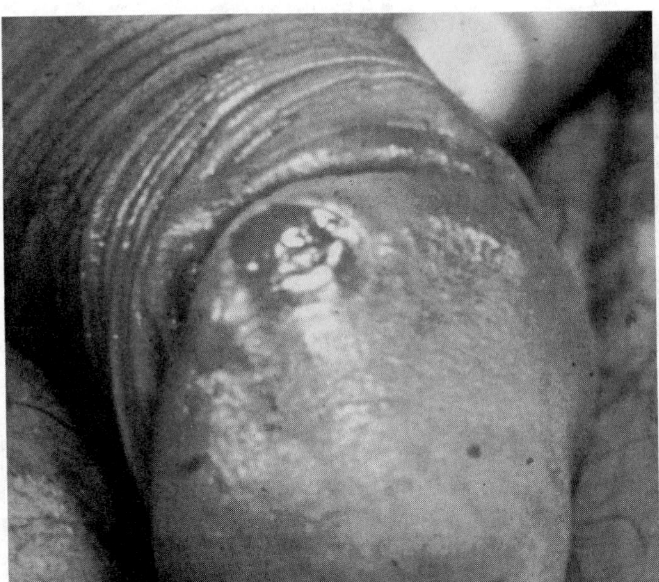

FIGURE 45–5. Erythroplasia of Queyrat occurring as in situ epidermoid carcinoma on the penis.

5). It may occur on the penile shaft, scrotum, and the vulva, but it is questionable whether these presentations are Bowen's disease of the anogenital region. The lesion appears as an asymptomatic, sharply demarcated, bright red, shiny plaque with a smooth, velvety surface.[88,89] The histologic features are identical to Bowen's disease, especially of the anogenital region. However, the rate of transformation into invasive squamous cell carcinoma is much higher for Bowen's disease, and the resultant squamous cell carcinoma tends to be more aggressive.[88,90] Cryotherapy and curettage and electrodesiccation have been used. It is advisable to use surgical excision of the tumor with microscopic control of the margin (Mohs' micrographic surgery) and to circumcise the penis.

BOWENOID PAPULOSIS

Bowenoid papulosis is a multicentric anogenital dysplasia that presents as verrucous or lichenoid pink to reddish-brown papules, erythematous macules, or leukoplakia-like lesions in young men and women.[23,91–94] Lesions of the oral mucosa have been reported.[95] Although pruritus and inflammation with tenderness and pain are occasionally reported, most patients with bowenoid papulosis have no symptoms. The lesions typically present as inconspicuous, noncondylomatous papules with mostly smooth and only slightly papillomatous surfaces. The lesions are 0.2 to 3.3 cm in diameter, with small papules coalescing into large pigmented plaques.[94,96] Bowenoid papulosis is a cutaneous manifestation of the sexually transmitted HPV. It is mostly linked with HPV type 16, but types 18, 34, and 39 have also been linked to its pathogenesis. This condition normally follows a benign but persistent course over many years. Occasional spontaneous regression, particularly in pregnant women, and progression to anogenital carcinoma has been reported.[91,97–101] These lesions are frequently confused with genital warts.

The histology is similar to Bowen's disease. Bowenoid papulosis does not show the full-thickness epidermal involvement and disorderly keratinocyte maturation characteristic of Bowen's disease and in situ squamous cell carcinoma. It has dysplastic keratinocytes scattered throughout the epidermis in a background of orderly keratinocyte maturation. These atypical keratinocytes have crowded nuclei that appear large, hyperchromatic, and pleomorphic, and are often in metaphase. The epidermis exhibits papillated hyperplasia with focally prominent, hypergranular areas. There are atypical mitotic figures, individual cell necrosis, dyskeratosis, and multinucleated keratinocytes scattered in the epidermis. If podophyllin has been used topically for the treatment of these lesions, histologic sections may exhibit a pattern of pseudoepitheliomatous hyperplasia with bizarre keratinocytic forms, because podophyllin causes metaphase arrest.

The clinical features usually differentiate bowenoid papulosis from Bowen's disease. Bowenoid papulosis usually presents in young, sexually active men and women between 20 and 40 years of age, and the lesions appear as multiple, small papules.[23,91–94,96] Bowen's disease occurs in patients older than 50 years of age and is usually a single plaque.[81,82] The lesions respond well to local destructive therapy, such as electrodesiccation, laser surgery, cryosurgery, and ablation.[102] Topical treatment with 5-FU and intramuscular or intralesional interferons have also been used in the treatment of bowenoid papulosis.[103] Recurrences after treatment are common, due to the life-long nature of HPV infections. Patients with this condition, especially women, and their sexual partners are at high risk for anogenital carcinomas and should have frequent evaluations.

EPIDERMODYSPLASIA VERRUCIFORMIS

Epidermodysplasia verruciformis is a rare, chronic, and often hereditary disease characterized by widespread eruption of flat, wart-like lesions and reddish-brown plaques with slightly scaly surfaces and irregular borders.[104–106] The wart-like lesions are mainly distributed on the hands, feet, and face, sometimes in a linear arrangement, and the pigmented plaques preferentially involve the trunk, neck, and proximal parts of the extremities. These premalignant lesions have many characteristics of actinic keratoses. Malignant transformation to squamous cell carcinoma in predominantly sun-exposed areas occurs in 30% of patients. Most patients show defects in cell-mediated immunity characterized by anergy to dinitrochlorobenzene and common skin antigens, depressed lymphocyte blastogenic reactivity to mitogens, abnormal T-lymphocyte populations, and decreased number of T lymphocytes.[83,107–109] However, the humoral immune system is left intact.[110]

The cause is attributed to rare types of human papillomavirus (HPV), mostly type 5, 8, 12, and 14. HPV appears to take advantage of the immunologic state to induce epidermodysplasia verruciformis.[107–112] The occurrence of HPV infections and epidermodysplasia verruciformis in immunosuppressed renal allograft recipients, in an immunosuppressed patient with systemic lupus erythematous, and in a patient with Hodgkin's disease provides support for this hypothesis.[111–114] Another line of evidence comes from the family members of patients with epidermodysplasia verruciformis, in whom the wart-like lesions started to appear but eventually regressed.[106] However, there are patients with epidermodys-

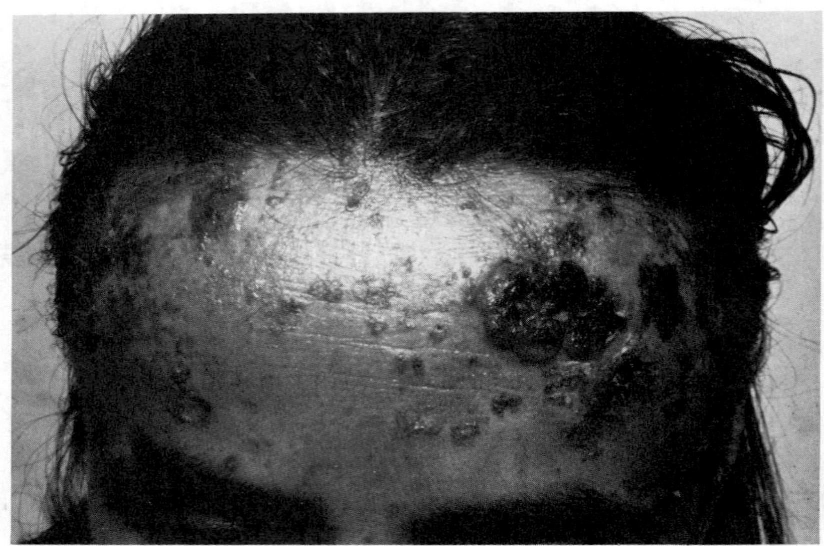

FIGURE 45–6. Multiple lesions of in situ superficial squamous cell carcinoma on the face of a woman with epidermodysplasia verruciformis.

plasia verruciformis without immune dysfunction.[115,116] Some investigators believe that the impaired cellular immunity could be a result of the HPV infection. The etiologic factors associated with the development of epidermodysplasia verruciformis are HPV infection, impaired cellular immunity, and the genetic makeup of the host. It is important for HPV-infected, immunosuppressed patients to have regular dermatologic examinations.

Epidermodysplasia verruciformis is an extremely protracted disease that usually begins in infancy or early childhood (5–11 years) with various types of warts and plaques. Later, it may progress to form verrucous plaques and nodules or transform to in situ squamous cell carcinoma. The rate of appearance of new lesions varies considerably, with some lesions disappearing in some areas as more appear in other areas. Malignant tumors typically develop in the third or fourth decade of life in approximately one third of the patients. These patients are not inconvenienced by these transformations, which are neither painful nor itchy. Malignant lesions are numerous and continue to progress as noninvasive in situ carcinoma without metastasis (Fig. 45–6). They are locally destructive if not treated. There is no effective therapy for epidermodysplasia verruciformis, but aromatic retinoids, such as etretinate and etretin, may have some beneficial effects.[83] Interferons produce only partial responses during therapy, with lesions returning in the same locations after therapy is discontinued.[116] Surgical removal, electrosurgical approaches, and cryotherapy are used.

LEUKOPLAKIA

Leukoplakia appears as white patches on the mucous membranes of the oral mucosa and vulva.[117] Leukoplakia is a clinical description. About 20% of the patients have histologies that consist of epithelial dysplasia and hyperkeratosis of the mucosa. Approximately 15% of the dysplastic cases develop carcinoma in situ, and 3% to 6% develop invasive squamous cell carcinoma within the involved area.[117,118] Differential diagnosis includes lichen planus, candidiasis, hairy leukoplakia, white sponge nevus, pachyonychia congenita, and dyskeratosis congenita.

ORGANOID OR SEBACEOUS NEVI

Organoid or sebaceous nevi are skin lesions composed of abnormal numbers of pilosebaceous structures and apocrine glands. These congenital lesions appear as raised, yellowish papules that grow gradually to develop a papillomatous surface.[119,120] They usually occur on the scalp and are present at birth. Basal cell carcinoma has been reported in as many as 10% of patients, and squamous cell carcinoma occurs rarely.[121] Syringocystadenoma papilliferum derived from the apocrine gland and basal cell carcinomas may be associated with organoid nevus (Fig. 45–7). Histologically, the lesion consists

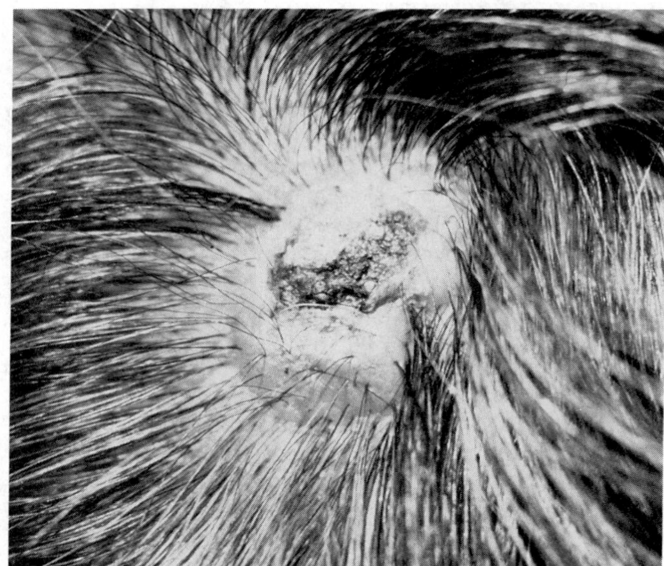

FIGURE 45–7. Basal cell carcinoma at a previous site of a sebaceous nevus.

of large numbers of skin appendages, including sebaceous, eccrine, and apocrine glands, hair follicles, and smooth muscle. Because of these structures, the term organoid nevus appears more appropriate. In syringocystadenoma papilliferum, cystic lesions of the epidermis are lined by a double layer of columnar epithelium showing decapitation secretion, suggesting apocrine gland origin.[119] After histologic confirmation of the diagnosis, the lesion is usually removed by surgical excision.

POROKERATOSIS

Porokeratosis describes a variety of epidermal disorders that share a dyskeratotic histologic pattern.[122] Except for the punctate type, porokeratosis is characterized by a distinct peripheral, raised, hyperkeratotic ridge that corresponds histologically to a parakeratotic column, called the coronoid lamella, which is a keratin-filled invagination of the epidermis. The central portion is typically flattened or of normal thickness but rarely acanthotic. The disseminated superficial actinic type is the most common and is reported in some instances to be inherited as an autosomal dominant trait.[123] The skin lesions are small, multiple, circular patches with slightly raised borders, usually on sun-exposed areas.[124] This type has been reported in renal transplant recipients and after chemotherapy for other malignancies, suggesting that immunosuppression may be involved in the development of porokeratosis.[125–127] The plaque type was originally described by Mibelli and typically begins in childhood. The lesions have atrophic centers and raised rims, and they tend to expand peripherally. This clinical picture and the lack of sweating in the center is characteristic of this condition.[125,128]

The linear nevoid variant may be widely distributed or may be localized to a segment of the body.[129] Clinically, the lesions resemble those of linear verrucous epidermal nevus. The disseminated palmoplantar variety typically presents on the palms and soles of adolescents and young adults and later may involve other areas of the body.[130] This type lacks the history of sun exposure. The punctate type is confined to the palms and soles and presents as numerous, moderately tender, 1- to 2-mm keratotic plugs.[131] Various types of malignancies, including squamous cell carcinoma, basal cell carcinoma, and Bowen's disease, have been reported to develop within porokeratotic lesions.[128,132–134] Differential diagnosis includes verruca vulgaris and solar keratosis, which may also have the coronoid lamella structure. The punctate type may be impossible to differentiate from plantar and palmar warts. Specimens for histologic diagnosis must include the peripheral raised ridge. Porokeratosis of Mibelli (plaque type) and disseminated superficial actinic porokeratosis should be treated with surgical excisions and close observation because of the possibility of progression to malignancy. The other types may be controlled with cryotherapy.

FIBROEPITHELIOMA OF PINKUS

Fibroepithelioma of Pinkus is usually seen on the back and appears as flesh-colored skin tags. Characteristic histologic features consist of a network of anastomosing epithelial strands connected to the overlying epidermis and admixed with a fibrous stroma. The network may be a few layers thick. Acanthosis of the epidermis and horn cysts make the lesion resemble seborrheic keratosis. Basal cell carcinomas are reported to develop in a small percentage of these fibroepithelial tumors.[78,135] Management is by surgical excision for histologic diagnosis.

KERATOACANTHOMA

Keratoacanthoma is a rapidly growing hyperkeratotic papule that presents on sun-exposed skin of middle-aged and elderly persons.[136] Clinically and histologically, this lesion resembles squamous cell carcinoma and is sometimes associated with actinic keratosis. They usually spontaneously regress or involute in about 6 months, but some may show atypical features and behave more aggressively. It is difficult to differentiate between keratoacanthoma and squamous cell carcinoma.[137–140] Keratoacanthoma behaves more aggressively in immunosuppressed hosts.

The lesion initially appears as a rapidly growing, reddish papule and reaches full size in 1 to 3 months. Most lesions remain between 1 to 2 cm, are firm, and have a raised rolled border and a central keratin plug (Fig. 45–8). At the end of the growth phase, the lesion becomes quiescent for a while, and then slowly undergoes spontaneous regression, leaving an ugly scar. Keratoacanthoma usually appears as an isolated lesion, although multiple eruptive and multiple self-healing lesions have been reported.[141,142] The most common sites for lesions are sun-exposed skin of the face, head and neck, and the dorsum of the hands in persons older than 40 years of age.

Histologically, keratoacanthoma is diagnosed by a central keratin plug with a surrounding proliferation of squamous epithelium extending down into the dermis. Histologic confirmation is only possible if the biopsy of the lesion includes the lateral border and the central crater. A wedge resection of the lesion from one side to the other, deep into the subcutaneous

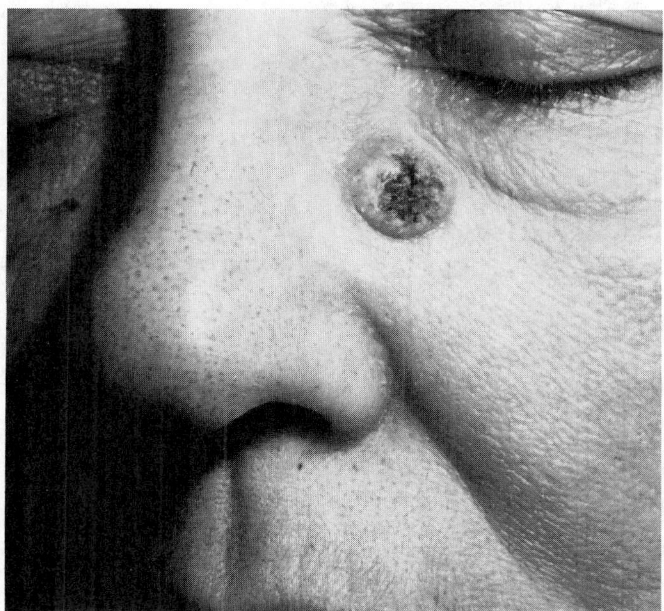

FIGURE 45–8. Keratoacanthoma. Notice the central crater.

fat, should be forwarded for histologic examination. This biopsy procedure may result in regression of the lesion. If the lesion persists longer or if more acceptable cosmetic results are required, it is best to surgically excise the lesion. Shave excision down to the deep dermis is effective for the treatment of keratoacanthoma. In cases of aggressive keratoacanthoma or if squamous cell carcinoma cannot be ruled out, complete surgical excision with appropriate margins is recommended.

MALIGNANT EPIDERMAL TUMORS

BASAL CELL CARCINOMA

Basal cell carcinoma is the most common cancer among whites, accounting for most of the 600,000 new cases of nonmelanoma skin cancer in the United States each year.[1] Basal cell carcinoma rarely metastasizes and is easily treated and cured.[143] It appears on sun-exposed areas in fair-skinned persons who have had long-standing sun exposure. It is usually seen in elderly persons and those suffering from xeroderma pigmentosum, Bazex's syndrome, basal cell nevus syndrome, and linear basal cell nevi.[78,121,144–147] Its incidence increases with age, but because of easy access to the sunbelt areas and outdoor recreational activities and because it has become fashionable to be suntanned, basal cell carcinoma is now seen more often in younger persons. It is no longer surprising to see basal cell carcinoma in patients in their third or fourth decade of life.

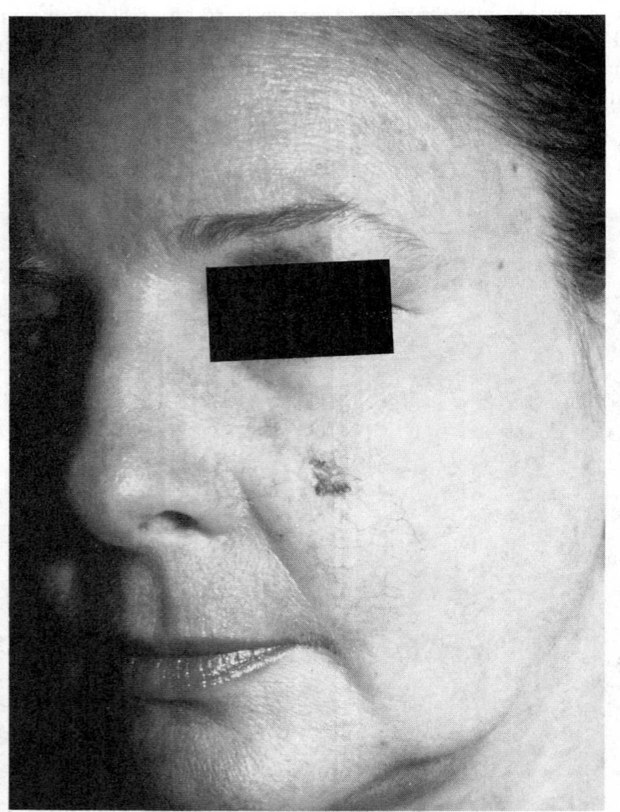

FIGURE 45–9. Basal cell carcinoma on the face of a white woman.

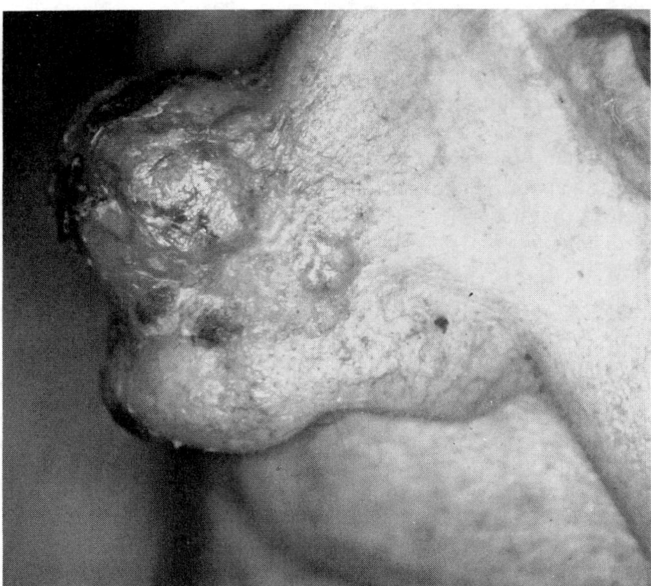

FIGURE 45–10. Large, tumorous basal cell carcinoma on the nose. Notice the concomitant sun-damaged skin.

Most basal cell carcinomas occur on sun-exposed areas such as the face (Figs. 45–9 and 45–10), especially the nose, the nasolabial fold, and the inner canthus areas. Solitary basal cell carcinomas are seen in the geographic areas with temperate climate. Multiple tumors and tumors on areas other than the face are seen usually in tropical and equatorial regions. Basal cell carcinoma occurs more commonly in men than in women, with the incidence increasing with age and with the latitude.[62,148]

Clinical Presentation

Basal cell carcinoma appears as a slowly growing, shiny, skin-colored to pink, translucent, raised papule. Telangiectasia is seen on the surface of the lesion. As the lesion enlarges, it may ulcerate and develop a rolled border and crusted center. The lesion may then regress to a smaller and less visible size.

Several clinicopathologic variants of basal cell carcinoma have been described.[78,149–152] They are nodular, multiple superficial, cystic, adenoid, pigmented, and morphea types. Pigmented basal cell carcinoma may be confused with malignant melanoma. Some basal cell carcinomas may have a hyperkeratotic surface and scaly appearance and may be confused with actinic keratosis, sebaceous keratosis, squamous cell carcinoma, and Bowen's disease. The morphea-type basal cell carcinoma has a scar-like sclerotic appearance and lacks telangiectasia and translucency, and the usual distinct border is not seen. The lesion is larger and more indurated in palpation than on inspection. Another form of basal cell carcinoma is the so-called basosquamous cell carcinoma.[153] This lesion has biologic behavior and pathologic features intermediate between basal cell and squamous cell carcinomas.

Most basal cell carcinomas are diagnosed when the tumors are a few millimeters to 1 to 2 cm in diameter (Figs. 45–11 and 45–12). However, much larger, ulcerated tumors may be

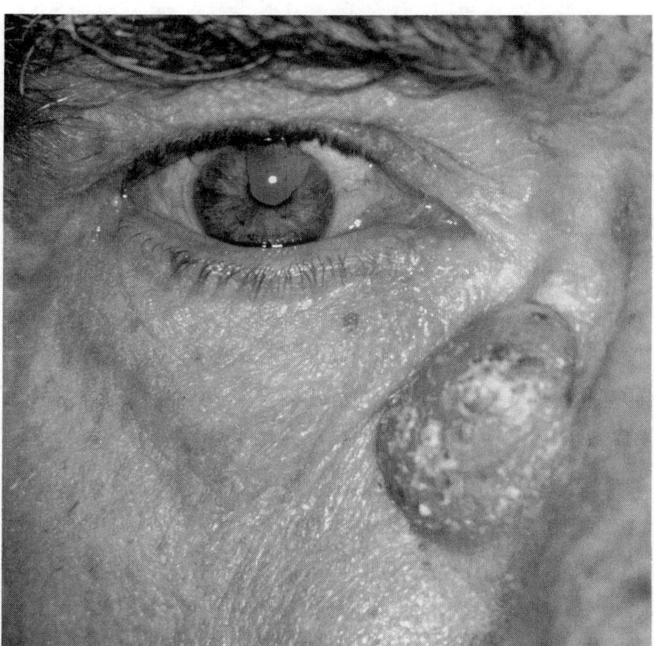

FIGURE 45–11. Nodular basal cell carcinoma.

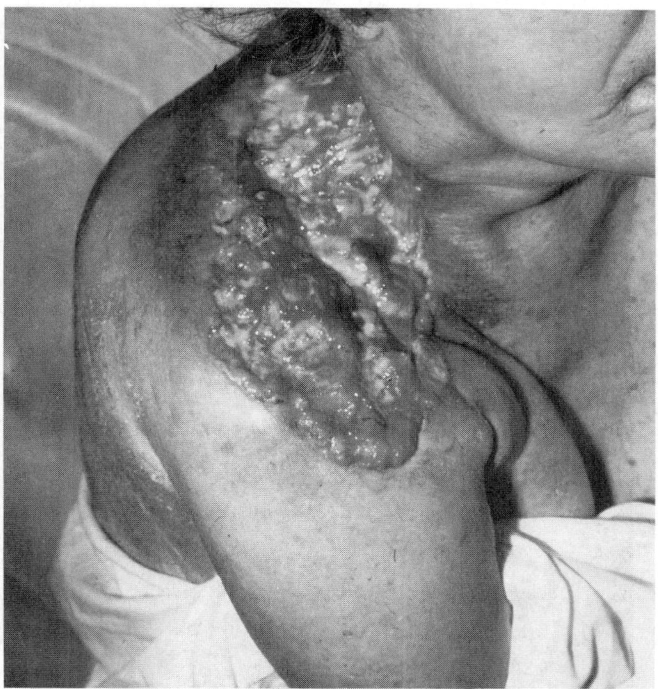

FIGURE 45–13. Large, invasive, ulcerative basal cell carcinoma.

seen (Fig. 45–13). Basal cell carcinoma does not usually metastasize, but it can invade underlying tissues and organs slowly and cause destruction of skin, cartilage, soft tissue, and bone.[154,155] Rarely, if basal cell carcinoma reaches the bone or blood circulation, it may metastasize.[143] The world literature indicates fewer than 300 cases of metastatic basal cell carcinoma. After it reaches metastatic levels, it behaves as aggressively as other types of cancers and can spread to vital organs such as lymph nodes and lung.

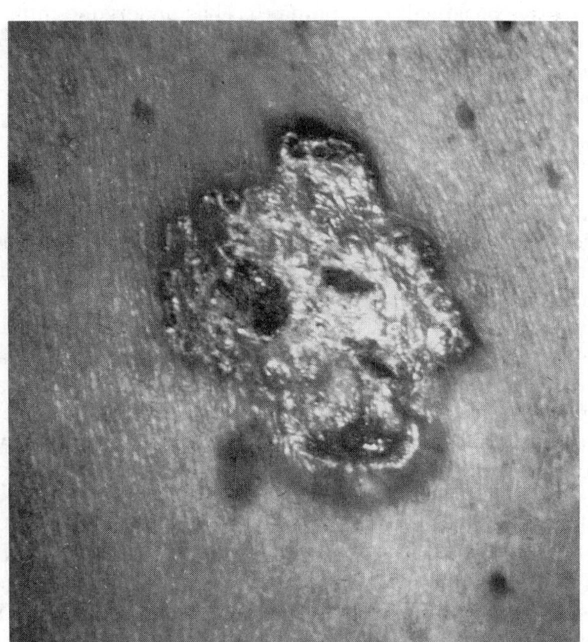

FIGURE 45–12. Ulcerated basal cell carcinoma.

Pathogenesis

Most reports indicate the importance of fair complexion, blue eyes, and fair hair in the development of basal cell carcinoma. This is especially true if the people have fair complexions and live in a sunny region, such as Scandinavians who live in Australia.[62,148,156,157] The role of genetic susceptibility to the development of basal cell carcinoma has been suggested and is well documented in cases of xeroderma pigmentosum (Fig. 45–14) and basal cell nevus syndrome.[78,144,146,147] The proven role of genetic markers is that of inheritance of the fair complexion. Although few recent reports indicate a possible role for the major histocompatibility complex, there are no confirmed data proving the role of HLA antigens (*e.g.*, DR-5) in the development of basal cell carcinoma.[158]

The association of chronic UV light exposure and development of basal cell carcinoma is well accepted.[62,148,156,157] It is the cumulative effect of UV light over many years that causes the development of basal cell carcinoma. After the necessary level of sun exposure (threshold) is reached, the exposed person continues to develop basal cell carcinomas; the process appears to be irreversible. The chance of developing basal cell carcinoma directly relates to the number of previous basal cell carcinomas.[159] For example, a person who has had 10 basal cell carcinomas has the chance to develop one new tumor each year thereafter. Other conditions that may predispose to the development of basal cell carcinoma include other primary malignancies, especially lymphoreticular types, immunodeficiency states, and trauma, such as traumatic injuries or small pox vaccination.[78,158,160–162] Although basal cell carcinomas are most commonly seen on the sun-exposed areas of the skin, many basal cell carcinomas are seen in less exposed areas, such as the nasolabial fold and the inner canthus,

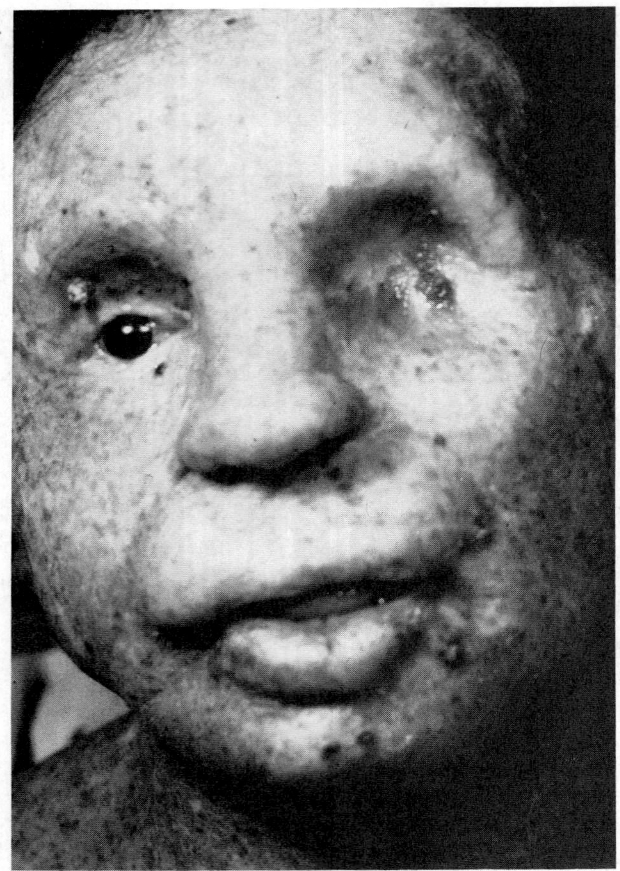

FIGURE 45–14. Severe solar damage, basal cell carcinoma, and squamous cell carcinoma developed in a man with xeroderma pigmentosum who lost one of his eyes.

suggesting that other factors (*e.g.*, embryologic closure lines) may contribute to the development of the tumor.

Basal cell carcinomas are reported only on hair-bearing skin, but in cases of basal cell nevus syndrome and linear basal cell nevi, basal cell carcinomas may be seen on the soles and palms.[146] These observations suggest that the tumors may originate from epithelial cells of hair follicles. Ionizing radiation, whether received from the environment or as part of therapeutic modalities, can promote the development of basal cell carcinoma. X-irradiated skin shows evidence of chronic dermatitis several years later and may give rise to basal cell or squamous cell carcinomas.[76–78,163,164] In the 1950s and 1960s, x-irradiation was used for the treatment of acne and hypertrichosis. Many patients who received therapeutic x-rays developed radiation dermatitis and multiple skin cancers of the face 20 to 30 years later.

Histopathology

In all forms of basal cell carcinomas, the histologic features include masses of compactly arranged basaloid cells resembling cells in the basal layer of epidermis extending down from the epidermis into the dermis (Fig. 45–15).[152,165,166] There is usually a variable dermal stroma reaction. In the sclerosing type of basal cell carcinoma, the cells are more fusiform and are admixed with a more pronounced stromal

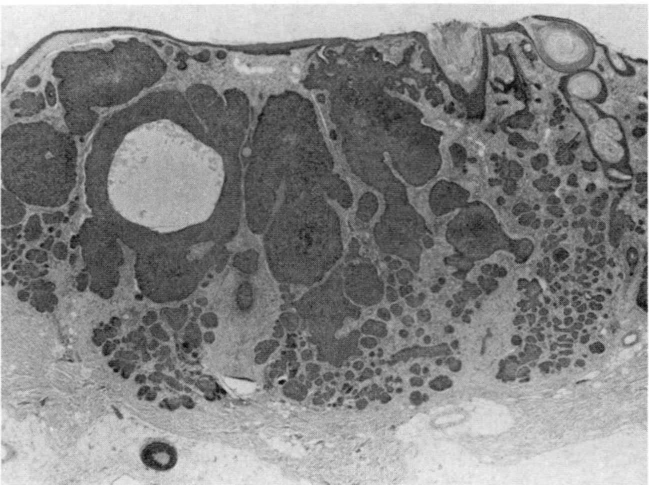

FIGURE 45–15. Histologic section of basal cell carcinoma.

reaction. In most cases, especially in the nodular, cystic, and adenoid types, there is a clear peripheral palisading of the dark epithelial cells that is characteristic of basal cell carcinoma. The differential diagnosis includes trichoepithelioma, which may also show some palisading of the cells.[167] Pigmented basal cell carcinoma is due to aggregation of melanin within the tumor. Basosquamous cell carcinoma consists of a fibrous stroma admixed with a downward proliferation of epithelial cells that lack palisading and have some of the features of squamous cell carcinoma and more frequent mitosis.[149,153]

Metastasizing Basal Cell Carcinoma

Basal cell carcinoma usually spreads by direct extensions from the primary tumor site and has little tendency to metastasize.[143,168] Fewer than 300 cases have been reported in the world literature. Metastatic disease usually arises from a more aggressive basal cell carcinoma that has undergone multiple recurrences after treatment. The tumor invades and destroys the underlying tissues, and when metastases reach vital organs, they behave aggressively.[154,155]

Management of Basal Cell Carcinoma

Several methods are available for the treatment of basal cell carcinoma (Table 45–5).[167,169,170] The choice is usually based on the location, type of lesion, and experience of the physician. Smaller lesions can be treated with surgical excision or curettage and desiccation.[171,172] Radiation therapy, although used less frequently, is the most appropriate treatment for basal cell carcinoma of the eyelid, nose, and lips. Cryosurgery and topical use of 5-FU have also been suggested, but the cure rate is not as high as with other techniques. Tumors with poorly defined margins and recurrent basal cell carcinomas are best treated by microscopically controlled excisional surgery that is known as Mohs' micrographic surgery.[173–175] This technique allows the removed tissue to be mapped in relation to the underlying site. Additional tissue removal is carried out at sites where tumor cells are present microscopically. The treatment is considered complete when there is no tumor found in removed tissue. Cure rates of 90% to 95% are

TABLE 45–5. Management of Nonmelanoma Skin Cancer

Type of Cancer	*Therapy*
Basal Cell Carcinomas	
Superficial	Topical chemotherapy, cryotherapy, curettage and electrodesiccation, excision, laser vaporization, irradiation, Mohs' micrographic surgery (for multicentric or >2–3 cm)
Nodular-ulcerative	Cryotherapy, curettage and electrodesiccation, excision, irradiation, Mohs' micrographic surgery (high-risk anatomic site, aggressive clinical or histologic pattern, or >2–3 cm)
Morphea	Excision, Mohs' micrographic surgery
Basosquamous	Excision, Mohs' micrographic surgery
Recurrent	Irradiation, Mohs' micrographic surgery
Squamous Cell Carcinoma	
In situ epidermoid cancer	Cryotherapy, laser vaporization, curettage and electrodesiccation, excision, irradiation, Mohs' micrographic surgery
Invasive cancer	Excision, irradiation, Mohs' micrographic surgery
Verrucous carcinoma	Excision, Mohs' micrographic surgery
Adnexal Cancer	
Eccrine, apocrine, and sebaceous carcinomas	Excision, Mohs' micrographic surgery
Extramammary Paget's disease	
Merkel's cell tumor	

achieved with most methods of treating primary basal cell carcinoma. Mohs' surgery has a cure rate of 96% to 99%.[173–175]

Recurrent lesions are larger than 1 to 2 cm, are located over embryologic cleavage planes, or are the sclerosing type. Some lesions are more aggressive and have multiple recurrences, and Mohs' surgery is the treatment of choice. The superficial spreading type of basal cell carcinoma usually recurs, no matter what method of treatment is chosen, because there are small nests of basaloid cells away from the visible margin of the tumor.

Intralesional injection of interferon has been used for treating basal cell carcinoma.[176] The available data are not convincing, and this approach is still experimental. Systemic retinoids have also been used in the treatment of multiple skin cancers and basal cell carcinomas, but the results are not promising. Avoidance of excessive and long periods of sun exposure are effective in the prevention of this cancer.

SQUAMOUS CELL CARCINOMA

Squamous cell carcinoma is a malignant skin cancer arising from epidermal keratinocytes with the potential for metastasis. Squamous cell carcinomas are usually seen in fair-skinned persons who have had excessive sun exposure and developed actinic keratosis (see Fig. 45–1).[62,78,148,156,157] It is more common in men than women. The incidence is estimated to be 20% to 25% of that of basal cell carcinoma. The true incidence of basal cell and squamous cell carcinomas is not available because many practitioners remove and treat these forms of skin cancer without reporting them to the appropriate cancer registry. Any figure is likely to be an underestimation. In Australia, where data are perhaps more accurate, the incidence of squamous cell carcinoma is 166 per 100,000 people, 652 per 100,000 for basal cell carcinoma, and 19 per 100,000 for melanoma.[62,148] In blacks and whites who are treated with PUVA, the incidence of basal cell and squamous cell carcinoma is approximately the same.[177,178]

Pathogenesis

As in basal cell carcinoma, it is the cumulative amount of lifetime UV exposure that influences the development of squamous cell carcinoma.[179–181] Albinos are at especially high risk for developing squamous cell carcinoma early in life if they are exposed to excessive amounts of UV light, indicating the protective value of pigmentation.[182] Occupational and nonoccupational exposure to sunlight are significant risk factors. It is reported that there is an increased incidence of squamous cell carcinoma in persons who have been treated with PUVA.[183] PUVA treatment has been available in the United States for the past 17 years and consists of the systemic intake of psoralen, which is a photosensitizing drug, and exposure to long-wave UV radiation (UVA of 320–360 nm).[177,178] In Europe, however, the use of this photochemotherapy has not been associated with increased squamous cell carcinoma.[184]

The incidence of squamous cell carcinoma is increased among patients who are on immunosuppressive therapy for organ transplantation.[111,185] In these patients, the ratio of basal cell carcinoma to squamous cell carcinoma is reversed, suggesting that the immune system may influence the control of early squamous cell carcinoma. Chronic ulceration, chronic sinus disease, chronic inflammation, and scar tissues increase the chance of developing squamous cell carcinoma. Exposure to ionizing radiation can result in the development of squamous cell carcinoma several years later.

Certain topical agents used for the treatment of chronic skin conditions are carcinogenic and perhaps cause squamous cell carcinoma. Tar causes skin cancer in laboratory animals, but there is no evidence for tar causing skin cancer in humans.[11] Squamous cell carcinoma was considered an occupational hazard among cotton spinners due to contact with the cotton oil. Industrial exposure to chemicals (*e.g.*, cutting oils) is now recognized as a risk factor for squamous cell carcinoma. The historic reports of scrotal malignancies in chimney sweeps was assumed to be due to contact with carcinogenic soot.[12] Arsenic was also recognized to be a carcinogen producing skin cancer and cancers of other organs. In the presteroid era, arsenic was used in the treatment of many diseases.[84,186]

Human papillomavirus has been found in some squamous cell carcinomas.[97,98,185,187–189] HPV types 16 and 18 were found in cancers of the cervix.[91] HPV infections are normally found in patients who are not immunosuppressed.

Clinical Presentation

Squamous cell carcinoma usually appears on the areas of the skin that are damaged by sun exposure. The most common sites of squamous cell carcinoma are the face, neck, back, forearm, and dorsum of the hand of an elderly, white patient with sun-damaged skin (Figs. 45–1 and 45–16 through 45–19). The primary lesion manifests as a red, indurated papule that appears de novo or on an actinic keratosis and expands rapidly, producing a large nodule that eventually ulcerates and metastasizes to a local draining lymph node. Bowen's disease, cutaneous horn (Fig. 45–20), chondrodermatitis nodularis helicis, chronic ulcers, scar tissues, and radiodermatitis may be precursor sites of squamous cell carcinomas (Figs. 45–21 and 45–22) and basal cell carcinomas.[62–64,77,78] The patient may have several primary lesions developing at the same time or in a rapid succession. Tumors arising from sun-damaged skin have relatively lower rates of metastasis, but tumors arising on the mucocutaneous surface or those arising from skin with previous tissue changes (*e.g.*, scars of burns, sites of trauma) tend to be more aggressive, invade locally, and metastasize rapidly.

Squamous cell carcinoma of mucocutaneous sites usually occurs in patients with a history of heavy smoking and heavy alcohol intake.[190] These lesions may arise from an area of leukoplakia or an indurated or ulcerated plaque and metastasize rapidly. Chewing tobacco and betel nuts can influence the development of oral squamous cell carcinoma. Verrucous carcinoma may occur in the oral cavity or sole of the foot and may present as a persistent, firm or vegetating plaque on these areas.

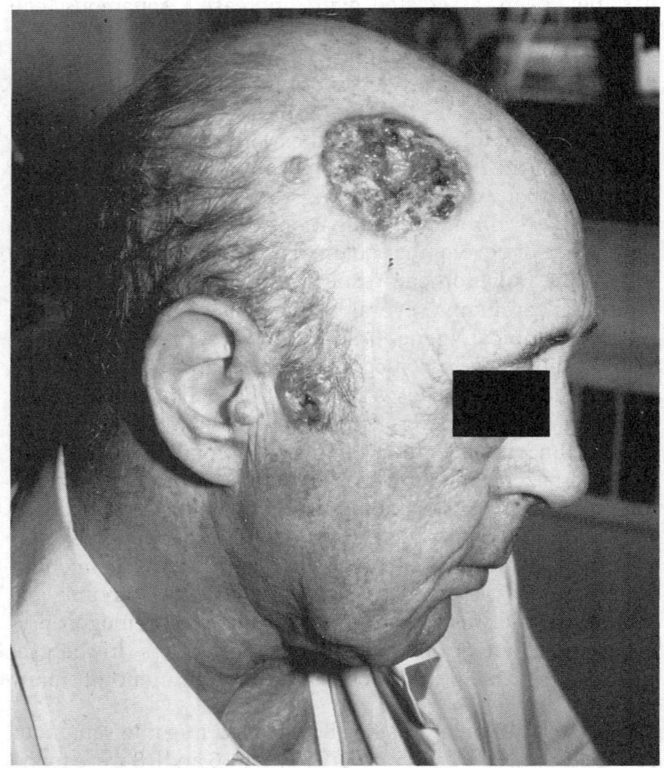

FIGURE 45–16. Large, ulcerated squamous cell carcinoma on the face and scalp.

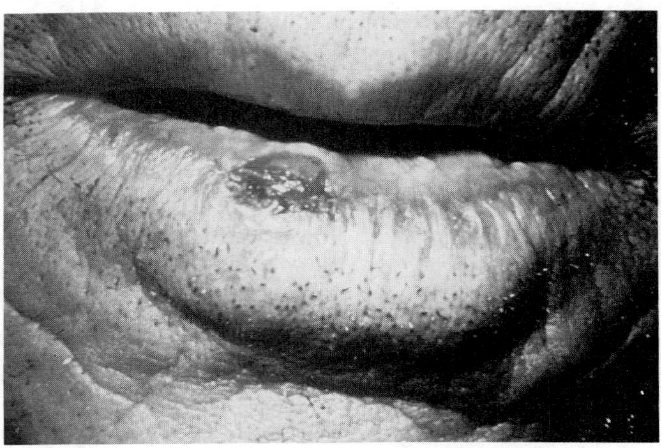

FIGURE 45–17. Squamous cell carcinoma on the lower lip.

Giant condylomata of Buschke-Lowenstein usually presents as warty lesions on male genitalia. This condition is associated with HPV.[191] Squamous cell carcinoma may develop in a preexisting condition of Buschke-Lowenstein condylomata. Epithelioma cuniculatum usually presents as a small ulcer with peripheral hyperkeratosis on the soles of the feet.[192] This lesion is difficult to eradicate.

Squamous cell carcinoma arising in patients receiving photochemotherapy appears similar to those seen in normal persons and occurs on normal-appearing skin as small crusted nodules.[183] In immunosuppressed patients, it is important to perform skin biopsies on suspected lesions of basal cell carcinoma, squamous cell carcinoma, or actinic keratosis.

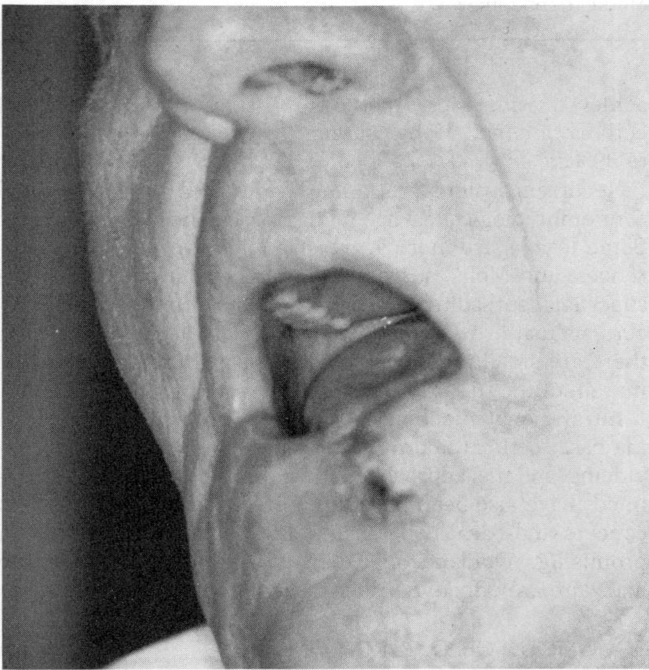

FIGURE 45–18. Large, invasive squamous cell carcinoma on the lower lip.

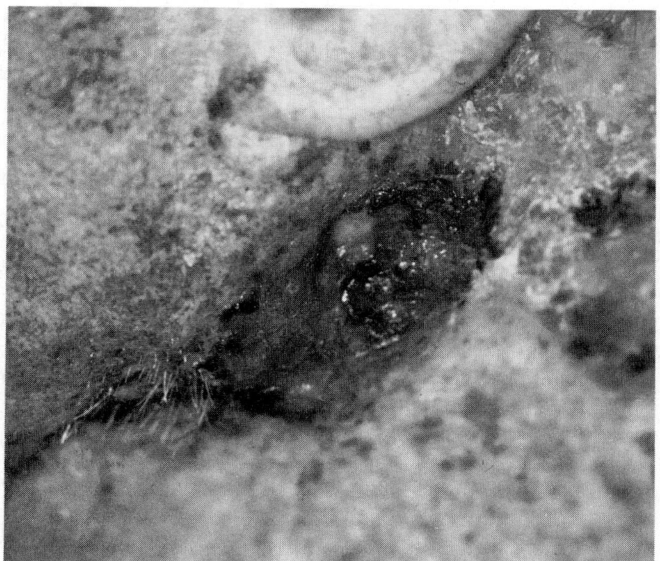

FIGURE 45–19. Large, ulcerated, invasive squamous cell carcinoma on the neck and face.

Classification and Prognosis

The characteristic features of squamous cell carcinoma include proliferation of atypical squamous cells invading the underlying dermis producing an irregular, disorganized architecture. Individually keratinized cells and horn cysts are present. In verrucous carcinoma, giant condyloma of Buschke-Lowenstein, and epithelioma cuniculatum, there is hyperplasia of the mucous membrane epidermis but no evidence of invasion into the dermis.[190–192] Mitotic figures are infrequent.

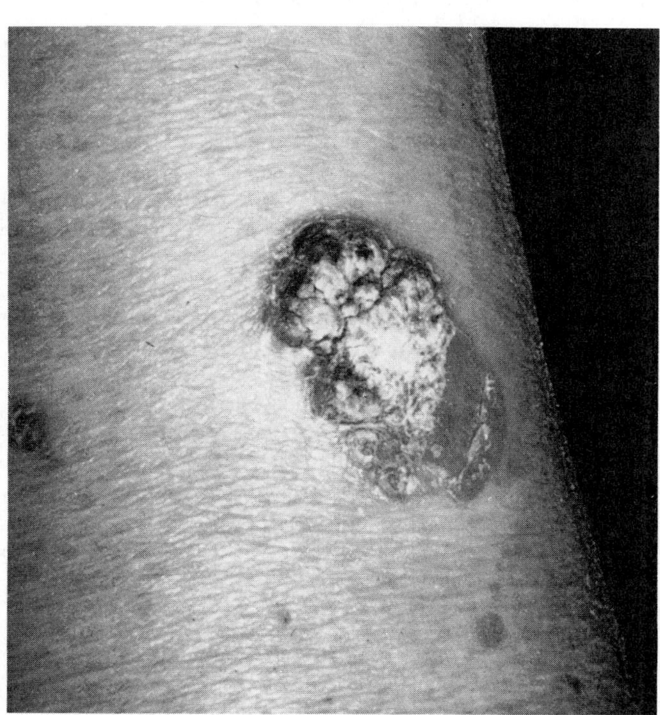

FIGURE 45–20. Squamous cell carcinoma manifesting with a cutaneous horn.

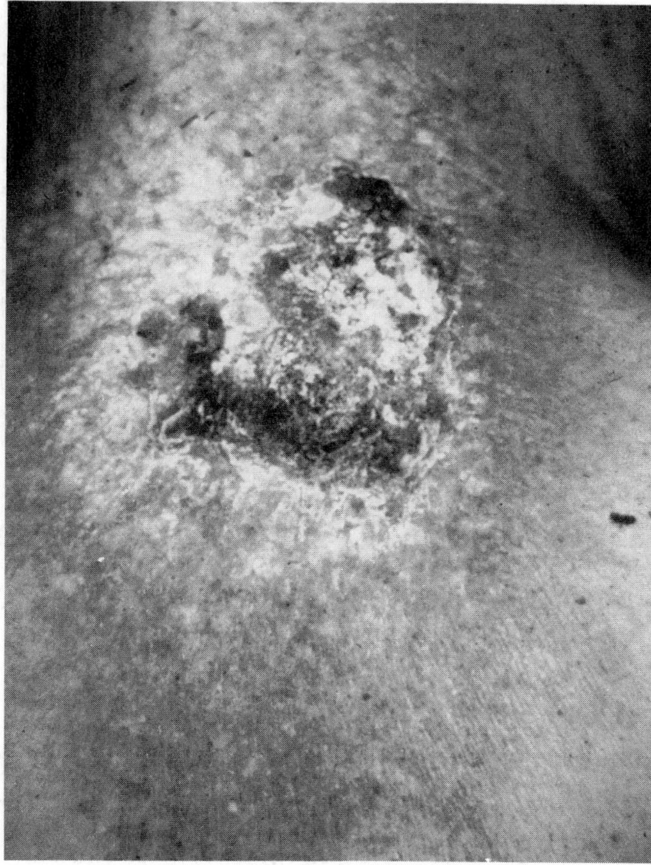

FIGURE 45–21. Squamous cell carcinoma at the site of radiation dermatitis.

Attempts have been made to classify squamous cell carcinoma based on the percentage of the undifferentiated cells and to relate this to the prognosis. There are four grades (1–4) of squamous cell carcinoma.[193] Grade 1 has fewer than 25% undifferentiated cells, and grade 4 has more than 75%. The higher the number of undifferentiated cells, the worse is the prognosis. Differential diagnosis of squamous cell carcinoma includes keratoacanthoma, spindle cell melanoma, and soft tissue sarcoma with spindle cells. Antikeratin antibodies can be used to identify and confirm the keratinocyte origin of a given tumor.[194] This is even possible in formalin-fixed, paraffin-embedded specimens. Antibodies against S-100 proteins or NKIC3 indicate a possible melanoma.

Management

Most practitioners use similar treatment modalities for basal cell carcinoma and squamous cell carcinoma (see Table 45–5).[195] Squamous cell carcinoma requires a more aggressive approach, such as wider excision. Tumors on the mucous membranes must be excised with good margins; Mohs' micrographic surgery may be used.[173,196] Close follow-up for recurrences and metastatic spread is highly recommended. In most cases, surgery is preferred to radiation therapy.

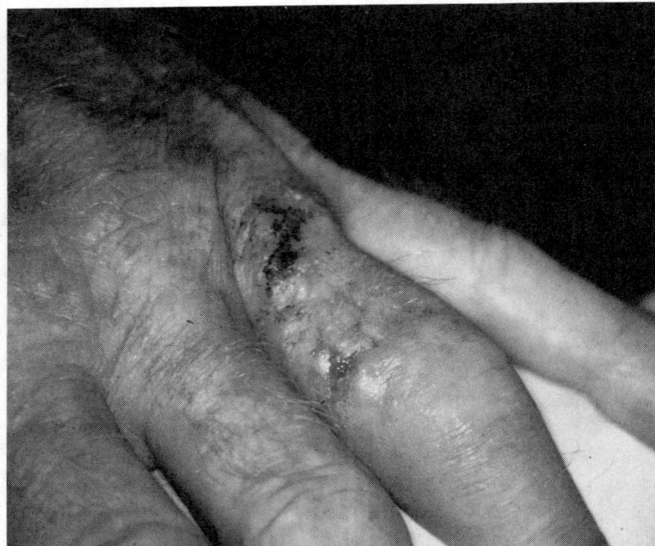

FIGURE 45–22. Squamous cell carcinoma on the finger secondary to radiation exposure.

CANCER-ASSOCIATED GENODERMATOSES

Several inherited dermatoses are associated with the development of cutaneous malignancies. These include xeroderma pigmentosum, nevoid basal cell carcinoma, familial dysplastic nevus syndrome, and multiple self-healing epithelioma of Ferguson-Smith.

XERODERMA PIGMENTOSUM

Xeroderma pigmentosum is a rare disease that occurs in approximately 1 in 250,000 persons in the general population. It is inherited as an autosomal recessive trait and is characterized by severe sun sensitivity, photophobia, cutaneous pigmentary changes, advanced solar damage, multiple skin cancers (*e.g.,* basal cell carcinoma, squamous cell carcinomas, malignant melanoma), and ocular or neurologic changes.[147]

The defect in these patients includes the inability of mast cell strains to excise UV-induced pyrimidine dimers, which results in unrepaired UV-damaged DNA and the development of skin cancers. The remaining repair capability is expressed as unscheduled DNA synthesis and is confirmed by complementary methods of DNA-incising capacity and post-UVL-exposed colony-forming ability. There are nine complementation groups that vary greatly in the degree of defect of unscheduled DNA repair.

The severity of the disease correlates closely with the residual repair capacity. Avoidance of the sun and use of total sunblocks as early in life as possible should be initiated. With the use of sunscreens and other protection mechanisms, these patients live much longer, and they usually die of neurologic involvement and infection rather than UV-induced cancer. Neurologic involvement and progressive mental dysfunction are seen in more than 50% of those who live longer.

Diagnosis of xeroderma pigmentosum is confirmed by a DNA repair study of a fibroblast culture. The best treatment is protection from UV exposure. Actinic keratosis and various skin cancers should be treated appropriately. The use of topical 5-FU or cryotherapy for multiple lesions is helpful. Radiation therapy is not recommended, although the fibroblasts are not sensitive to x-ray damage. Oral retinoid therapy has been used, but the value of this approach requires proof.

BASAL CELL NEVUS SYNDROME

Basal cell nevus syndrome is inherited as an autosomal dominant gene with complete penetrance and variable expression.[146] It is a relatively common genodermatosis, but almost 67% of the patients have no family history, suggesting a high rate of spontaneous mutation. Clinical features are seen in skin, bone, optic tissue, and in the central nervous system. Skin lesions consist of basal cell carcinoma that have atypical features resembling skin tags or pink or flesh-colored, small papules and palmar and plantar pits. Bone cysts are seen in the mandible, and abnormalities of the ribs occur. The ophthalmic evidence includes coloboma or cataracts. Other manifestations include intracranial calcification, ocular hypertelorism, enlarged occipitofrontal head circumference, and increased risk of medulloblastoma and meningioma.

It is thought that the expression of the autosomal dominant gene requires solar radiation. Skin lesions usually develop in large numbers between puberty and age 35. They may become nodular or ulcerative and aggressive. After basal cell carcinoma appears, various modes of therapy should be used to remove the tumors completely. Radiation therapy is not recommended.

FAMILIAL DYSPLASTIC NEVUS SYNDROME

Familial dysplastic nevus syndrome is described elsewhere in this book. The syndrome has an autosomal dominant pattern and consists of large numbers of nevi in the family members of patients with malignant melanoma.

MULTIPLE SELF-HEALING EPITHELIOMA OF FERGUSON-SMITH

Multiple self-healing epithelioma of Ferguson-Smith is an autosomal dominant condition in which affected patients develop crops of raised nodules, most of which regress spontaneously and leave depressed scars. Two large families have been carefully studied. Sporadic cases are also seen. Lesions are seen in early adult life on sun-exposed areas. The histologic features are indistinguishable from squamous cell carcinoma, but the clinical history resembles keratoacanthoma.

TORRE'S SYNDROME

Torre's syndrome includes cutaneous lesions of sebaceous adenoma, sebaceous carcinoma, and basal cell carcinoma in association with carcinoma of the gastrointestinal tract, especially the colon. Multiple keratoacanthomas may also exist. Full colonoscopy and careful long-term follow-up is recommended.

COWDEN'S SYNDROME

Cowden's syndrome presents as multiple hair follicle tumors, mainly tricholemmomas. Oral papillomas are associated with breast carcinoma. The syndrome is thought to be inherited as an autosomal dominant condition. Thyroid carcinoma, ocular and neurologic abnormalities, gastrointestinal problems, and skeletal abnormalities are reported.

GARDNER'S SYNDROME

Gardner's syndrome is an autosomal dominant condition manifesting with cutaneous cysts, bony abnormalities, and colonic polyps that may progress to carcinoma. Adrenal, thyroid, and ovarian carcinomas and carcinoids are also associated with Gardner's syndrome.

CARNEY'S SYNDROME

Carney's syndrome consists of myxomas, endocrine dysfunction, pigmentary abnormalities and breast and endocrine cancers. The exact mode of this rare syndrome is not as yet well established.

TUMORS ARISING FROM EPIDERMAL MERKEL'S CELL

MERKEL'S CELL CARCINOMA

Merkel's cell carcinoma, formerly called trabecular carcinoma, is an uncommon, highly malignant, primary cutaneous neuroendocrine carcinoma arising from Merkel's cells located in the basal layer of the epidermis and in the hair follicles.[197,198] Merkel's cells are associated with sensory neurites in the dermal papillae, forming mechanoreceptor in the skin. The neoplastic Merkel's cells are characteristically small, round to polygonal, undifferentiated tumor cells with scanty cytoplasm. These tumor cells exhibit different histologic patterns.[199] The most common pattern is the solid type, which is composed of irregular groups of tumor cells interconnected by strands of connective tissue. The trabecular type is characterized by well-defined cords of cells that form invading columns or cords between collagen bundles. The diffuse type exhibits poor cohesion and a lymphoma-like diffuse type of growth.

This lesion occurs mostly in white, elderly persons, with an equal incidence in men and women. It is usually localized to the sun-exposed areas of the head and neck but does occur on the extremities, trunk, and genitalia in a random distribution. The clinical presentation is a rapidly growing, painless, firm, nontender, shiny, bluish-red, intracutaneous nodule 0.5 to 5 cm in diameter. The tumor arises in the dermis and extends into the subcutis. The epidermis is infrequently involved, and the overlying skin is intact and rarely ulcerated. There is a high incidence of distant metastases, regional lymph node involvement, and locoregional recurrences, resulting in poor prognosis even after treatment.[199–202] The prognosis of Merkel's cell carcinoma shows a sex differentiation, with 3-year survival rates of 35.6% for men and 67.6% for women.[201] The three reported instances of spontaneous regression occurred in women.[203,204] The recommended treatment is wide surgical excision of the tumor and prophylactic regional node dissection. Postoperative radiation therapy to the local site and regional lymph nodes is helpful.[205,206] Chemotherapy is considered effective in some reports.[207]

TUMORS ARISING FROM EPIDERMAL LANGERHANS CELLS

HISTIOCYTOSIS X

Langerhans cells are bone marrow-derived dendritic cells that reside in the upper layer of the epidermis. Proliferation of Langerhans cells results in development of a clinically heterogenous group of diseases commonly called histiocytosis X. Three distinct variants have been described: Letterer-Siwe disease, Hand-Schüller-Christian disease, and eosinophilic granuloma.

Letterer-Siwe Disease

Letterer-Siwe disease is seen in children younger than 2 years of age and manifests with fever, lymphadenopathy, hepatosplenomegaly, pulmonary involvement, cutaneous eruption, and thrombocytopenia. Skin eruptions are in the form of seborrheic dermatitis or purpuric red-brown papules.

Hand-Schüller-Christian Disease

Hand-Schüller-Christian disease occurs in children between the ages of 2 and 6 years with the triad of exophthalmos, diabetes insipidus, and bony involvement of the skull. This is a more chronic progressive form of histiocytosis X than Letterer-Siwe disease, which is acute, fulminant, rapidly progressive, and usually fatal.

Eosinophilic Granuloma

Eosinophilic granuloma is commonly seen in children and young adults with solitary bone lesions or involvement of other organs.

Overlap of these three diseases makes classification difficult. Staging according to the extent of disease and the type of organ(s) involved is reported to have prognostic value. More detailed descriptions of these conditions can be found in other chapters of this book.

TUMORS ARISING FROM SKIN APPENDAGES

Skin appendages or adnexa include eccrine and apocrine sweat glands, hair follicles, sebaceous glands, and nail beds. Many adnexal tumors have been described, but these tumors are rare and often are difficult to diagnose clinically because of lack of distinguishable features.[208,209] Histologically, most of these tumors present a diagnostic dilemma to the pathologist. To identify the origin of these tumors, histochemical staining, ultrastructural studies, antikeratin antibodies, antibodies to epithelial membrane antigen (EMA), and carcinoembryonic antigen (CEA) have been used. The antigen tests are positive in sweat glands and negative in hair follicles. Most of the skin appendage tumors are slow growing and benign. Those considered malignant are mostly locally invasive. There are rare cases of metastasizing and highly malignant tumors. Morphologic criteria may not correlate with biologic behavior of the tumors.

TUMORS OF HAIR FOLLICLES

Many tumors may arise from various segments of the hair follicle (see Table 45–1 and Fig. 45–23).[210] These tumors proliferate but do not metastasize. Some of the more frequent types are summarized here.

INVERTED FOLLICULAR KERATOSIS

Inverted follicular keratosis usually appears as a firm, gray, flat plaque on the face that is indistinguishable from seborrheic keratosis and may sometimes be similar to verruca vulgaris.[211] It is suspected to be a virally induced lesion, but no HPV has been found in this tumor. Histologically, it is thought to be a proliferation of the keratinocytes of the follicular infundibulum or the intraepidermal part of the hair follicle. Under low-power light microscopy, a papillomatous mass of keratinocytes is seen. Squamous eddies and keratin cyst within a hair follicle sometimes gives a true pattern of inverted follicular keratosis.

TRICHODISCOMA

Trichodiscoma usually appears as multiple, skin-colored papules on the face. It is sometimes seen in family members.[55–57,212] It is thought that the lesion arises from the dermal component of the hair disk, giving a regular dome-shaped fibrovascular histology in the papillary dermis with a hair follicle at the margin.

TUMORS OF THE FOLLICULAR INFUNDIBULUM

Tumors of the follicular infundibulum appear as smooth, raised, skin-colored papules on the face. They are thought to arise from the infundibulum of the hair follicle, which is the area above the entry point of the sebaceous duct into the hair canal.[213] Histologically, the tumor is composed of pale epithelial cells rich in glycogen.

TRICHILEMMOMA

Trichilemmoma (*i.e.,* trichilemmocarcinoma) appears as single or multiple small nodules on the face and is usually asymptomatic. Hair may be seen in these lesions. The lesions resemble common warts. In women with multiple lesions of this type, Cowden's syndrome must be considered. Tumors originate from the outer part of the hair root sheath. Histologically, tumors contain large, lobulated, palisading epithelial cells with pale cytoplasm high in glycogen content.[73] These tumors are CEA and EMA negative and can be differentiated from tumors of eccrine origin that may have similar histology but are CEA and EMA positive. Malignant trichilemmoma (*i.e.,* trichilemmocarcinoma) has been reported with local lymph node metastasis.[214,215]

TRICHOFOLLICULOMA

Trichofolliculoma presents as multiple, skin-colored papules with tufts of hair emerging from some of the lesions. The lesions may coalesce to form plaques several centimeters in diameter. The histology consists of poorly formed hair follicles that are easily diagnosable from other hair follicles in these tumors.[216] A variant called sebaceous trichofolliculoma is composed of lobules of sebaceous epithelium with acini and duct formations.[217]

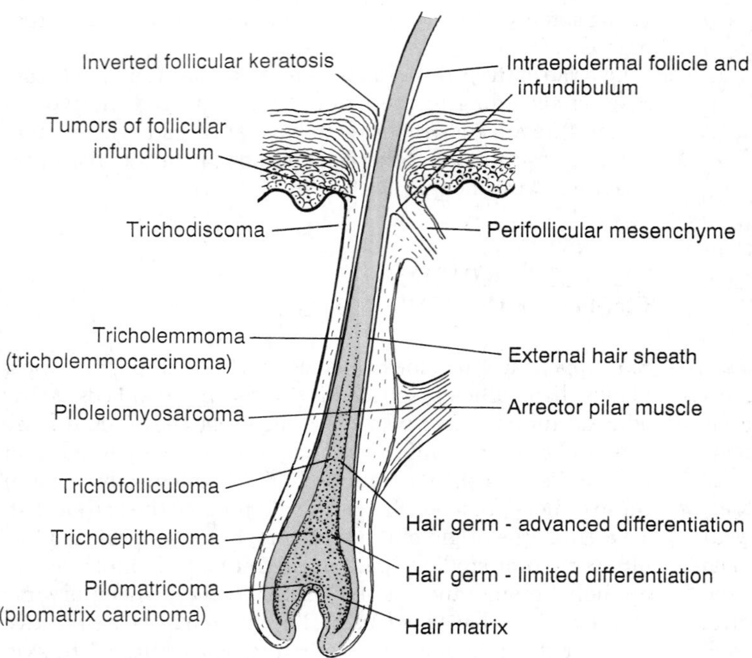

FIGURE 45–23. Schematic diagram of tumors arising from the hair follicle.

TRICHOEPITHELIOMA

Trichoepithelioma may be single or multiple and appears as nondescript skin-colored papules on the face, especially the nasolabial fold, eyelids, and central face. The tumors are inherited as an autosomal dominant trait. The tumor arises from the hair shaft deep in the sebaceous gland attachment. Histologically, this tumor has some of the features of morphea-type basal cell carcinoma and should be differentiated from it.[218]

PILOMATRICOMA

Pilomatricoma (*i.e.*, calcifying epithelioma of Malherbe) arises from the hair matrix.[219] The tumor may be single or multiple and appears mostly during the first decades of life and are occasionally familial. The tumor manifests as a solid, hard nodule a few centimeters in diameter. The histologic picture is fairly specific; darkly stained basaloid cells are seen in some areas, and in other areas, the cells have changed and developed configurations of shadow or ghost cells. Around these ghost cells, calcification usually usually makes the nodule firm. A fibrous stroma is seen around both cell types and calcification. Giant cells are frequent. Malignant transformation to pilomatrix carcinoma is rare.[219–221] Malignant tumors may invade locally but do not metastasize.

TUMORS OF SEBACEOUS GLANDS

Tumors of sebaceous glands are rare and mostly benign, but they may progress to malignancy.

FOX-FORDYCE ANOMALY

Fox-Fordyce anomaly is a condition in which sebaceous glands are found on mucosal surfaces, mostly in the oral mucosa.[222] Sebaceous glands are usually present on skin and not on mucous membranes. These mucosal sebaceous glands appear as yellowish papules. Histologically, they consist of collections of sebaceous glands.

ORGANOID OR SEBACEOUS NEVI

Organoid or sebaceous nevi are skin lesions composed of abnormal numbers of skin appendages with a high tendency of basal cell carcinoma developing secondarily to this lesion (see Fig. 45–7).[119–121] The term organoid nevus is more accurate because skin appendages other than sebaceous gland, such as eccrine gland and smooth muscle, may be present. However, because of its appearance and the presence of sebaceous glands in this tumor, it may still be referred to as sebaceous epidermoid nevus.

SEBACEOUS GLAND HYPERPLASIA

Sebaceous gland hyperplasia is a common skin lesion of the face of most elderly persons. The lesion appears as multiple, raised, yellowish papules with depressed centers and some telangiectasia.[223] Differential diagnosis includes basal cell carcinoma. Histopathologic features include collections of layers of sebaceous gland shadows.

SEBACEOUS ADENOMAS AND EPITHELIOMAS

Sebaceous adenomas and epitheliomas are two conditions that present as yellow or white raised papules on the face. Collections of sebaceous gland cells with foamy cytoplasm are seen in the sebaceous gland adenoma.[224] In sebaceous gland epithelioma, the histopathology consists of masses of compact sebaceous cells, some of which are the small, dark, basaloid type.[225] Differential diagnosis includes hair follicle tumors and basal cell carcinoma. The possibility of Muir-Torre syndrome should be considered.

SEBACEOUS CARCINOMA

Sebaceous carcinoma occurs most frequently on the upper eyelids of women in their sixties, but it may also be seen on the scalp and face.[225,226] On the eyelid, it may appear as a chronic conjunctivitis or chalazion.[227–229] On the face, it may have the appearance of a yellowish, raised papule or plaque that is translucent with a greasy surface.[230,231] Pathologic features include lobules of cells with foamy cytoplasm and basaloid cells with large numbers of mitotic figures. The tumors may extend to subcutaneous tissue and may perforate through the fascia and muscles and then rapidly metastasize. The histologic differential diagnosis includes squamous cell carcinoma, Paget's disease, and malignant melanoma. Special stains for fat, anticytokeratins, and EMA are helpful in the histologic diagnosis. Radiation therapy and chemotherapy have been used, but surgical excision with microscopic control of the margin is the best approach.[232–234]

TUMORS OF APOCRINE GLANDS

SUPERNUMERARY NIPPLE

Supernumerary nipple appears as a firm nodule on the area near the nipple. It is similar to an intraepidermal nevus or skin tag. Pathologic features consist of ectopic breast tissue, dilated mammary glands, hair follicles, and isolated smooth muscles.[235]

APOCRINE HIDROCYSTOMA

Apocrine hidrocystoma or cystadenoma appears as translucent bluish papules occurring most commonly on the face.[236] Differential diagnosis is pigmented basal cell carcinoma or nevus. Pathologic features include cystic structures lined with a row of tall columnar cells and a layer of myoepithelial cells in the periphery.

SYRINGOCYSTADENOMA PAPILLIFERUM

Syringocystadenoma papilliferum or papillary syringoadenoma presents as highly verrucous lesions appearing mostly on the scalp and face. The lesion may develop on an organoid nevus.[119] More than 50% are reported at birth and 25% at puberty. Histopathology consists of invaginated cystic structures lined with two layers of columnar epithelial cells and a plasma cell-rich stroma. Rare cases of transformation into adenocarcinoma with regional lymph node metastases have been reported.[237]

HIDRADENOMA PAPILLIFERUM

Hidradenoma papilliferum is found exclusively in women on the vulvar area and appears as a palpable lesion on the labia majora. It may also be found in the perineal and perianal regions. Histopathology is similar to syringocystadenoma papilliferum, except that there is no plasma cell infiltration. One case of malignant transformation has been reported. It developed into a fatal, metastasizing squamous cell carcinoma.[238]

PAGET'S DISEASE

Paget's disease of the skin is identified as atypical cells present within the epidermis. It may clinically and pathologically be confused with Bowen's disease.[239] Paget's disease may occur frequently on the areola and nipple (*i.e.*, mammary Paget's disease) or less commonly on the vulva, scrotum, or perineal and perianal areas (*i.e.*, extramammary Paget's disease). Characteristic histologic features of Paget's disease are large epithelioid (Paget's) cells with dark hyperchromatic nuclei, cytologic atypia, and frequent mitotic figures within the epidermis.

After confirmation of the diagnosis by skin biopsy for histologic examination, the extramammary Paget's disease is usually treated with wide excision of the involved area. In cases of Paget's disease of the breast, surgical approach of the skin and underlying carcinoma is recommended.

Extramammary Paget's disease is a rare form of adenocarcinoma observed mostly in the skin of the anogenital and axillary regions, and less frequently in the esophagus, oral mucosa, tongue, bronchial epithelium, urethra, buttocks, thighs, chest, external auditory canal, and eyelid. The lesions appear as a solitary, well-defined patch with an eczematous surface. Differential diagnosis includes psoriasis and eczematous dermatosis. It shares histologic resemblances to mammary Paget's disease, showing characteristic large anaplastic Paget's cells with round or ovoid nucleus and clear cytoplasm, occurring singly or in small groups within the epidermis.[240] Although mammary Paget's disease is an epidermal manifestation of an underlying mammary duct adenocarcinoma, extramammary Paget's disease arises from an underlying adenocarcinoma or from intraepithelial precursors, and it occurs in areas with a high density of apocrine or eccrine glands. There is controversy about whether Paget's cells originate from the ductal carcinoma or from the epidermis. Extramammary and mammary Paget's disease are presumed to be variants of epithelial carcinoma, possessing the potential to develop from or to be the cause of an underlying adenocarcinoma.

Treatment of extramammary Paget's disease depends on the area of involvement, but it is usually by wide local excision or Mohs' micrographic surgery with or without subsequent radiation therapy.[241] Depending on the area involved, a split skin graft may be necessary.

APOCRINE ADENOCARCINOMAS

Apocrine adenocarcinoma is a rare tumor that usually occurs in the areas with apocrine glands, such as the axillae and the anogenital region. It has developed in other sites, such as the auditory meatus, where ceruminal glands are found. Apocrine gland carcinoma may locally invade or metastasize to regional lymph nodes. The histopathology is that of adenocarcinoma with various degrees of differentiation. Even in poorly differentiated tumors, recognition of an apocrine structure is usually possible in some sections. The tumor shows high activity for apocrine enzymes such as acid phosphatase, β-glucuronidase, and indoxyl acetate esterase, but there is no activity of eccrine enzymes such as phosphorylase and succinic dehydrogenase.

TUMORS OF ECCRINE GLANDS

Eccrine sweat glands can be the source of many benign or malignant tumors (Fig. 45–24). Secondary eccrine gland carcinomas arise directly from eccrine glands through a malignant transformation. These malignant tumors are rare and usually develop from a preexisting eccrine appendage tumor of lesser maturity.[209] There is at least one recognizable tumor for each morphologic region. The diagram simplifies the locations where various tumors originate (see Fig. 45–24 and Table 45–1).

BENIGN TUMORS

Poroma

Poromas are benign neoplasms arising from the outer cells of the intraepidermal duct and the uppermost region of the straight intradermal duct. Variants of poromas or poroid neoplasms include hidroacanthoma simplex, eccrine poroma, dermal duct tumor, and poroid hidradenoma.[242–250] Hidro-

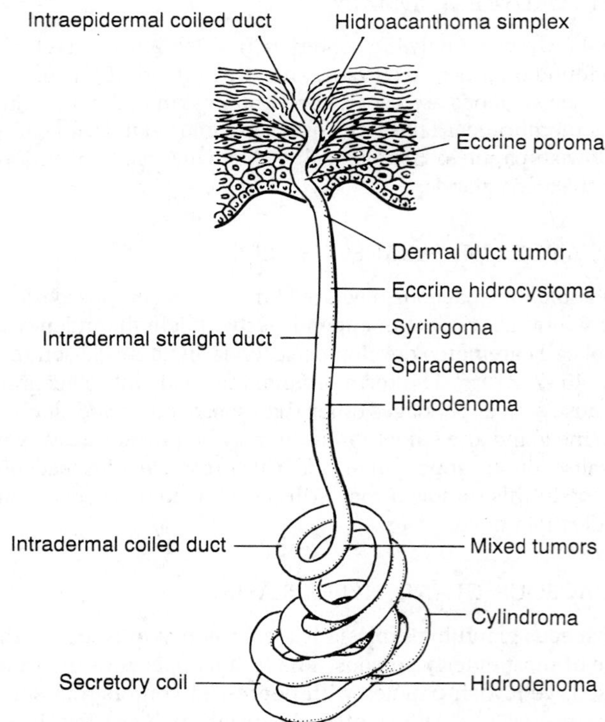

FIGURE 45–24. Schematic diagram of tumors arising from the eccrine gland.

acanthoma simplex and eccrine poroma are confined within the epidermis. Dermal duct tumor is detached from the epidermis and occurs as an intradermal nodule.[248] Poroid hidradenoma has features of poroma and hidradenoma. This variant is a wholly intradermal neoplasm with solid and cystic components of a typical hidradenoma, but on closer examination, the same cells as those in hidroacanthoma simplex, eccrine poroma, and dermal duct tumor are observed. The four poroid neoplasms have similar architectural aspects and identical cytologic features, and a sharp demarcation among types of poromas is not always possible.

The poroid cells are slightly smaller than keratinocytes and have plump, oval to round nuclei, inconspicuous nucleoli, and scant cytoplasm. There is little variation in size and shape of cells seen within poromas. Poromas also contain cuticular cells, which are larger than poroid cells, having slightly larger nuclei with more pronounced chromatin. They are situated around the lumen of eccrine ducts. One of these two cell types tends to predominate in poromas, giving these neoplasms a monomorphous appearance.

Hidroacanthoma simplex appears as a small plaque on the face and is benign.[242] Malignant hidroacanthoma simplex has been reported, but it is controversial if these are truly malignant because hidroacanthoma simplex has some histologic features of carcinoma in situ.[196,243,251] Eccrine poroma appears as raised, pink to red nodules most often on the soles of the feet. Malignant transformation of this tumor to porocarcinoma is rarely reported.[246,249–251] Porocarcinomas are mostly located on the lower extremities and may metastasize. In the malignant form, mitotic figures, duct formation, and atypical cells in the vascular slit-like spaces are seen. The malignant form should be differentiated from Paget's disease, squamous cell carcinoma, and other carcinomas. Management is surgical excision. The behavior of malignant poromas is relatively unpredictable, and microscopically checked surgical excision is advised for this malignant neoplasm.

Syringoma

Syringomas or eccrine mixed tumors are benign tumors of the luminal cells of the intradermal portion of the eccrine duct. The disease presents as multiple, smooth, firm, dome-shaped, slightly yellow or skin-colored papules that are 1 to 5 mm in diameter. Lesions are usually found on the lower eyelids and upper parts of the cheeks. They occur with much less frequency on the neck, chest, axillae, pubic area, scalp, and periumbilical region. Histologically, the tumor consists of well-circumscribed nodules in the upper dermis containing small solid nests, cords, and tubules of neoplastic epithelial cells randomly distributed throughout a prominent stroma of markedly thickened, closely packed bundles of collagen.[252] Epithelial cells have dark-staining nuclei with scanty cytoplasm or with abundant pale-staining cytoplasm. A variant called clear cell syringoma consists mostly of solid aggregates of the epithelial cell with abundant cytoplasm.[253]

Syringomas are usually diagnosed in middle-aged or older persons. This tumor often make its first appearance at puberty or in adolescence. Women are affected twice as often as men. Japanese women have an unusually high incidence that is sixfold greater than white or black women.[254] Patients with Down's syndrome also have a high incidence, with females affected more often than male patients.[255]

Another form of syringomas, an eruptive type, presents as numerous widespread crops of syringomas and is found most often in pubescent girls, almost exclusively on the anterior aspects of the neck, trunk, axillae, and inner aspects of extremities.[255,256] The crops of syringomas appear episodically and erupt over 2 to 3 years, after which the neoplasms persist without further growth. During this growth period, papules may be so numerous that they become confluent to form plaques. These lesions have identical histology to those of conventional syringoma.

The differential diagnosis is desmoplastic trichoepithelioma. In rare cases, syringomas may transform to syringomatous carcinoma.[257–261]

Chondroid Syringoma

Chondroid syringoma presents as well-encapsulated, spherical or lobulated, dermal or subcutaneous nodules on the head and neck areas, and the lesions may reach large sizes.[262,263] Twice as many men as women are affected. The lesions are also called mixed tumors because they have epithelial components that may differentiate into eccrine, apocrine, and follicular structures. Pathologic features include a mixed collection of cells in an ill-defined peripheral border. Some lesions contain more tubular structures, and others are more solid. The tubular structures are embedded in a dense fibrous stroma. The tubular structures are lined by eccrine secretory cells. Rarely, areas suggestive of apocrine glands are seen. Malignant chondroid syringomas have been reported rarely.[264–270] The tumor occurs on the extremities and may arise from a preexisting benign mixed tumor or may be malignant from the onset. It can recur locally and metastasize.

Eccrine Hidrocystoma

Eccrine hidrocystoma appears mostly on the face as solitary or multiple small translucent nodules with some bluish to dark brown-black pigmentation.[271] Histologic examination reveals a single cyst lined by two layers of cuboidal rather than columnar (as in apocrine) cells and does not show evidence of decapitation secretion. The lesions are usually located within the papillary dermis.

Eccrine Spiradenoma

Eccrine spiradenoma presents as deeply seated nodules on any part of the skin but most frequently on the face, scalp, neck, trunk, and arms, and it often causes spontaneous pain.[272–274] This lesion occurs with equal distribution among men and women. Tumors may be solitary, or multiple nodules may be grouped together and confined to a circumscribed region where they may become confluent or remain discrete. The epidermis overlying these dermal or subcutaneous nodules may show no change in color or may be pink or bluish, but it is rarely ulcerated.

Malignant forms (*e.g.*, spiradenocarcinoma) are rare.[275–278] This carcinoma occurs within a preexisting spiradenoma or may appear as a satellite nodule. The rapidly expanding nodule may cause inflammation and ulceration of the lesion. One patient died of widespread metastasis and local recurrence.[277] Spiradenomas arises from intradermal straight duct of eccrine glands. The histology consists of cords of epithelial cells in an edematous stroma. The cords contain two cell types: small basaloid cells with dark-staining nuclei lying at the periphery of slit-like tubular lumens and larger cells with pale nuclei lying within the cords. The cords and stroma form encapsulated lobules with the dermis and with no interconnection to the epidermis. The cells show high levels of phosphorylase activity, indicating their eccrine origin. In malignant tumors, some areas with typical spiradenoma structures are replaced with broad, confluent sheets of cells without intervening cords and tubular structures. These solid areas have many mitotic figures and show patterns similar to squamous metaplasia, spindle cell sarcoma, and poorly differentiated adenocarcinoma.[275–277] Large cyst formations are also found in malignant areas of spiradenoma.

The differential diagnosis includes cylindroma, lymphangioma, and other vascular neoplasms. Management consists of surgical excision.

Eccrine Hidradenoma

Eccrine hidradenoma manifests clinically as reddish-blue nodules on any area of skin but mostly on the face. This tumor arises from the secretory coil of the eccrine duct as a well-circumscribed tumor within the dermis and with no epidermal connection. It may show differentiation that is reminiscent of the lower portion of the intradermal straight duct.

Histopathologic examination reveals two main cell types: small cuboidal cells with basophilic cytoplasm and round nucleus (*i.e.*, duct lining cells) and larger cells with clear cytoplasm and small, dark nuclei (*i.e.*, secretory coil cells). The proportions of these cell types vary among lesions. These cells form a well-defined tumor mass with occasional cystic or duct-like formations. The clear cells in hidradenoma are similar to the cells seen in tricholemmoma or clear cell carcinoma of the kidney. However, the presence of tubular lumens and cystic spaces is characteristic of hidradenomas and may be used for differential diagnosis. The clear cells are derived form the secretory coil that is active in secretion and resorption. These clear cells are more prone to malignant transformations.[279–286] Clear cell hidradenocarcinomas are discussed later. Hidradenomas mostly contain cells of eccrine origin, but cells with apocrine secretory features may be seen in some areas. Surgical excision is the treatment of choice.

Cylindroma

Cylindroma (*i.e.*, turban tumor) is postulated to have eccrine, apocrine, and pilar differentiation, but new information indicates that it is a benign neoplasm arising from the intradermal coiled duct of eccrine glands.[287,288] This lesion may be solitary, but most often it presents as multiple, firm, smooth, dome-shaped, movable, pink to red papules or nodules that are 3 to 30 mm in diameter. Ulceration is uncommon and is usually a consequence of trauma. Women are affected four times more frequently than men. About 10% of all cylindromas are hereditary in an autosomal dominant fashion with variable penetrance; carriers of the trait may not necessarily manifest the disease.

Lesions usually appear in early adult life, but the onset may be as early as childhood or adolescence. Papules, nodules, and tumors occur mainly on the scalp, but they may be found on the face and upper part of the trunk. If tumors are widespread in the skin, the clinical picture, at first glance, may resemble neurofibromatosis. The neoplasm grows slowly but persistently, with new tumors continuously appearing and becoming confluent in some areas. If nodules of cylindromas cover the entire scalp and are heaped up, they resemble a turban.

The nonhereditary expression of cylindroma (90% of patients) usually appears as a solitary lesion arising on a hair-bearing area. If cylindromas occur on extremities, the patients also tend to have lesions on the scalp.

Histologically, cylindromas are composed of islands of epithelial cells surrounded by prominent thick rims of hyalinized basement membrane material. Globules of the same material are found within islands of neoplastic cells. Nodules are well circumscribed but not encapsulated, are situated in the dermis and subcutis, and lack foci of necrosis. Aggregations of epithelial cells vary considerably in size and shape, but cells are close to one another in a pattern resembling a jigsaw puzzle. These aggregates are composed of a centrally located population of neoplastic epithelial cells with large nuclei and abundant cytoplasm surrounded by a peripheral population of cells with smaller nuclei and scanty cytoplasm. Tubules may be found in some of these islands of epithelial cells. The lumen of these tubules are lined by cells with cuticular features like those of normal eccrine or apocrine ducts. Scalp tumors may extend to the fascia and the periosteum. The epidermis is not involved, but it is usually thinned due to the pressure of the underlying tumor. Cylindromas may contain zones that are almost indistinguishable from spiradenomas, giving further evidence for its eccrine origin.[288]

Cylindromas have rarely progressed to cylindrocarcinoma.[289–291] Most of the cases have developed from long-standing tumors of cylindroma. Histologically, the tumors are similar to cylindromas but are marked by large numbers of mitotic figures and atypical mitoses. Cylindrocarcinomas are aggressive, with metastases to lymph nodes, bone, and visceral organs.

PRIMARY ECCRINE GLAND CARCINOMAS

Primary eccrine gland carcinomas may arise from preexisting, less mature eccrine gland tumors or may develop de novo from eccrine glands within the skin. Primary eccrine gland carcinomas include syringoid eccrine carcinoma, mucinous eccrine carcinoma, clear cell carcinoma, microcystic eccrine carcinoma, adenoid cystic carcinoma, aggressive digital papillary adenocarcinoma, and eccrine adenocarcinoma.

The clinical features of these tumors are nonspecific, and the final diagnosis is always based on histology. The tumors usually are located on the head, neck, or extremities and manifest as slow-growing nodules or infiltrated plaques.[292] These are rare tumors, with only about 200 cases reported in the world literature. Several different subtypes have been described (see Fig. 45–24 and Table 45–1).

Syringoid Eccrine Carcinoma

Syringoid eccrine carcinoma appears as a solitary, firm, plaque-like, verrucous tumor on the head or face of elderly persons. The lesion may secrete fluid and resemble syringocystadenoma papilliferum. Scalp lesions may cause alopecia. The common benign lesions of syringoma are multiple papules distributed on the lower eyelids, and the benign lesions of eruptive syringoma are located on the neck, chest, umbilicus, or genitalia. Syringoma may be associated with Down's syndrome, Marfan's syndrome, or Ehlers-Danlos syndrome. Histology consists of tubulocystic proliferations with epithelial cord, the so-called tadpole picture, which is also seen in benign syringoma and hence the name syringoid eccrine carcinoma. Slight cellular atypia, nuclear hyperchromatism, deep invasion, and numerous crowded tubulocystic structures signify that the tumor is not benign syringoma. Syringoid eccrine carcinomas may be locally destructive or metastasize widely.[257–261]

Mucinous Eccrine Carcinoma

Mucinous eccrine carcinoma appears as a solitary, slow-growing, painless nodule, most frequently on the eyelids, but it may appear on the head, neck, or elsewhere on the body.[293–299] Local recurrences are reported, but metastasis is rare. Small cystic structures and tubular cords formed by basaloid cells are common. These structures resemble eccrine ducts. The cells show features of low-grade malignant tumors. There is a mucinous degeneration of the stroma that stains with Alcian blue.

Clear Cell Carcinoma

Clear cell carcinoma (*i.e.*, malignant clear cell hidradenoma, clear cell hidradenocarcinoma, or malignant clear cell acrospiroma) is a solitary tumor of the face, head, hand, or foot.[282–285] Widespread metastases are common.[282,286] These tumors may appear de novo as malignant tumors or develop as a malignant transformation of benign clear cell hidradenoma (*i.e.*, acrospiroma). The histology is similar to the benign condition except for cellular atypia and invasive borders. Clear cells, produced by large amounts of glycogen, are admixed with large oval or spindle-shaped cells. Large cystic spaces, lined with these clear cells, may be found in some tumors.

Microcystic Eccrine Carcinoma

Microcystic eccrine carcinoma manifests as an indurated, ill-defined, slow-growing, solitary nodule or plaque on the upper lip and cheek of middle-aged women.[300–304] The surface may appear smooth or crusted. Local recurrence is common, but metastasis is rare. Histologic examination reveals small cystic spaces, eccrine duct-like structures, and keratinous cysts in a fibrous stroma. The best sign of malignancy in these tumors is the deep infiltration with perivascular, perineural, and muscular invasions. The lesions may look like morphea-type basal cell carcinoma. Lesions are CEA positive, indicating the sweat gland origin. Differential diagnosis includes syringoma, desmoplastic trichoepithelioma, and papillary eccrine adenoma.

Adenoid Cystic Carcinoma

Adenoid cystic carcinoma is an extremely rare, indolent tumor that preferentially occurs on the scalp but may occur elsewhere.[305–308] Alopecia may be associated with this condition. It presents as crusted verrucous plaques or deep-seated nodules. Metastasis was reported in only 1 patient.[309] The histologic features of this tumor are similar with those of adenoid cystic carcinoma of the salivary gland.[310] The microscopic picture shows dermal nodules with no epidermal contact. As the name implies, there are many cystic spaces with areas of solid tissue. Small basaloid cells with scanty cytoplasm are the prominent cell type, but numerous fibroblasts and lymphocytic infiltrates can be found. These are in a fibrous stroma. The tumor shows an infiltrative growth pattern extending into the dermis or the subcutis. The adenoid cystic variant of basal cell carcinoma may present a diagnostic problem for this adnexal carcinoma.[310]

Aggressive Digital Papillary Adenocarcinoma

Aggressive digital papillary adenocarcinoma is a rare eccrine tumor with an acral location. These tumors present most often in older persons as a solitary, asymptomatic, slowly enlarging mass, most frequently on a digit or adjacent tissue.[311,312] The lesion is freely movable. Some patients may experience pain or tenderness, and the surface of the lesion may be ulcerated and bleeding. Deep infiltration of the underlying soft tissue results in a high local recurrence rate with a possibility of metastases to lymph nodes, bone, and visceral organs. Locally aggressive tumors are hard to differentiate from those that may metastasize. The histologic picture shows poor glandular differentiation, presence of necrosis, prominent cellular atypia, and invasion of the underlying tissue and bone. Lesions show a tubuloalveolar pattern with cystic spaces and atypical cells forming glandular structures. The epidermis is usually intact, except if ulceration and bleeding occur. Cells stain positive for CEA and S-100, showing their eccrine origin.

Differential diagnosis includes giant tumor of the tendon sheath, inclusion cyst, glomus tumor, metastatic tumor, pyogenic granuloma, and cavernous hemangioma. Treatment is wide excision or amputation of the digit. Chemotherapy is ineffective. After metastasis occurs, the prognosis is poor.

Eccrine Adenocarcinoma

Eccrine adenocarcinomas manifest as enlarging ulcerated nodules with no distinct clinical features.[261,313–319] Histologic examination reveals solid masses with various glandular differentiations resembling normal eccrine glands and ducts in a well-differentiated tumor. The poorly differentiated form of eccrine adenocarcinoma is highly malignant and may metastasize rapidly. Differentiation from metastatic adenocarcinoma may be impossible, but after visceral carcinomas are ruled out, the diagnosis of eccrine adenocarcinoma should be considered.

SECONDARY ECCRINE CARCINOMAS

Some of the benign eccrine gland tumors may transform and become malignant. Rapid enlargement, change in color, pain, or ulceration are usually signs of malignant transformation. In some instances, a benign-appearing lesion is removed but histologically is proven to consist of a small area of malignant degeneration.

Several secondary eccrine carcinomas arising from benign eccrine tumors are described (see Fig. 45–24 and Table 45–1). These include spiradenocarcinoma, cylindrocarcinoma, porocarcinoma, malignant chondroid syringoma, malignant syringoacanthoma, and hidradenocarcinoma. These malignant degenerations are discussed in the sections describing their benign counterparts. The bulk of tumor cells in all these tumors (*e.g.*, poromas, spiradenomas, cylindromas) are CEA negative, but in the malignant phenotype in which the tumor has undergone ductal differentiation, the cells are CEA positive.

TUMORS ARISING FROM THE DERMIS

Various cellular elements existing within the dermis may give rise to a variety of benign and malignant tumors. Because of their localization, these lesions clinically appear as subcutaneous nodules with a normal overlying epidermis. Accurate diagnosis is only possible after surgical excision and histologic evaluation. The most common of these lesions are summarized in Table 45–2. Detailed descriptions of these conditions can be found in other chapters in this book.

LYMPHORETICULAR TUMORS AND RELATED CONDITIONS

Skin is an immunologic organ and as such participates in the traffic and housing of immune cells. It is not surprising to see that malignant transformation of some of these cells may take place within the skin. The group of diseases classified under the cutaneous T-cell lymphomas appears to have special tropism for the epidermal tissues (*i.e.*, epidermotropism), and they originate and remain within the skin for a long period. The nonepidermotropic cutaneous T-cell lymphomas and the cutaneous B-cell lymphomas are other lymphoreticular malignancies involving skin. Other forms of lymphomas and leukemias may spread to skin and produce skin infiltrates.

TUMORS METASTATIC TO SKIN

Skin metastasis is rare, discovered in 0.2% to 9% of autopsies of cancer patients. The incidence of skin metastasis is associated with the type of primary cancer and with the sex of the patient. The site of metastasis to skin varies, and an increased frequency of metastasis to certain sites of skin is reported for some cancers.[244,320,321] Skin metastasis usually occurs if the disease is widespread with metastasis to multiple sites. Skin metastasis is usually a poor prognostic sign, but sometimes it is seen before the primary malignancy is recognized.

The frequency of skin metastasis in women is 69% for breast cancer, 9% for large intestine cancer, 5% for melanoma, 4% for lung cancer, 4% for ovarian cancer, 2% for sarcoma, 2% for uterine cervical cancer, 2% for pancreatic cancer, 1% for squamous cell carcinoma of oral cavity, and 1% for bladder cancer. In men, the frequency of cutaneous metastasis is 24% for lung, 19% for large intestine, 13% for melanoma, 12% for squamous cell carcinoma of oral cavity, 6% for kidney cancer, 6% for stomach cancer, 3% for esophageal cancer, 3% for sarcoma, 2% for pancreatic cancer, 2% for urinary bladder cancer, 2% for salivary gland tumors, 2% for breast cancer, and 1% each for prostate, thyroid, liver, and squamous cell carcinoma of skin.

Some skin metastases have certain morphologic and clinical features that differentiate them from other lesions. Neuroblastoma may appear as multiple, firm, nontender, mobile, bluish, subcutaneous nodules, described by the term "blueberry muffin." In breast cancer, the metastasis may present as inflammatory carcinoma, or it may appear in several other forms. Hypernephroma may clinically resemble Kaposi's sarcoma pyogenic granuloma. The primary sources of skin metastasis in women younger than 40 are, in descending order, breast cancer, melanoma, colon cancer, and ovarian cancer; in women older than 40, they are breast, colon cancer, lung cancer, ovarian cancer, and melanoma; for men younger than 40, the primary sources are melanoma, colon cancer, and lung cancer; for men older than 40, the sources are lung cancer, colon cancer, oral squamous cell carcinoma, and melanoma.

PRINCIPLES OF DIAGNOSIS AND TREATMENT

In many skin tumors, the clinical diagnosis is obvious and most dermatologists feel reasonably confident about the clinical impression. However, surveys of prehistologic diagnoses of basal cell carcinoma and malignant melanoma indicate that even among trained dermatologists there can be a wide margin of error in clinical diagnosis.

There are instances for which a definitive clinical diagnosis cannot be easily entertained, and a series of differential diagnoses are usually considered. The problem is much greater for skin appendage tumors and tumors arising from soft tissues of the skin. It is essential to develop a systematic approach in the diagnosis and management of skin tumors and use all the available resources to reduce the margin of error and select the appropriate treatment.

As part of the evaluation of patients with a malignant skin tumor the following input should be obtained: duration of the lesion, associated symptoms (*e.g.*, pain, itching), and recent changes; occupational and recreational history and history of prior sun exposure; type of skin and ethnic background; medical history including radiation exposure, history of arsenic ingestion, chronic ulcer, burn scars, osteomyelitis, and the presence of other coexisting diseases (*e.g.*, carcinomas, organ transplantation, immunodeficiency); and family history of skin and other cancers.

A complete skin examination, including examination of the scalp, ears, palms, soles, interdigital areas, and mucous membranes, should be undertaken. The extent of sun damage to skin should be assessed, evaluating the level of solar elastosis, scaling, erythema, telangiectasia, and solar lentigines. The size, location, shape, color, and other morphologic characteristics of the tumor should be recorded and marked on an anatomic chart. Regional and distant lymph nodes should be assessed. Clinical photographs are valuable in the field of skin cancers. Photographs should be taken whenever possible with a centimeter scale and date adjacent to the lesion before any procedure. This should become part of the routine procedures in all dermatology clinics. Biopsy specimens are processed for routine histologic studies. Special stains, antibodies for cell markers using immunoperoxidase, and ultrastructural studies are used for confirming certain diagnoses.

Other tests, such as blood screening for anemia, lymphoreticular disorders, anergy panel, immunosuppression, coagulation disorders, and markers of malignancies, may be necessary in some cases. Chest radiography, lymphangiography, computed tomography, liver and spleen scans, and magnetic resonance imaging should only be performed if indicated. After completion of these evaluations, a final diagnosis can be entertained and treatment can be planned.

BIOPSY AND TREATMENT PLANNING

Biopsy of a skin tumor allows microscopic examination of the tissue specimen and usually results in an accurate histologic diagnosis. The histologic diagnosis permits the physician to choose the appropriate therapy.

Biopsy

Four different biopsy techniques are used for skin lesions suspected for malignant tumors. Shave biopsy uses a scalpel to slice a superficial portion of the tumor. Punch biopsy uses a cylindrical instrument with an internal diameter of 2 to 8 mm to remove a deeper portion of the tumor down to the level of dermis or subcutaneous tissue. In incisional biopsy, a portion of the tumor is removed with a scalpel. In excisional biopsy, the entire lesion with a small border of normal skin is excised with a scalpel.

The selected technique should yield the primary specimen for an accurate diagnosis. For example, superficial specimens using a skin biopsy is adequate for the diagnosis of noduloulcerative, cystic, or superficial basal cell carcinoma. However, the diagnosis of squamous cell carcinoma may be missed in a superficial shave biopsy, because squamous cell carcinoma extends into the papillary dermis. A punch biopsy, incisional biopsy, or excisional biopsy are more appropriate in such cases. For pigmented skin lesions for which the differential diagnoses includes pigmented basal cell carcinoma and malignant melanoma, incisional or excisional biopsies are recommended. Punch biopsy should not be performed on possible melanomas, because tumor cells can be driven deeper into the dermis. In the case of morphea basal cell carcinoma, it is best to perform a punch or incisional biopsy. Shave biopsy does not provide sufficient tissue for differentiation of this entity from benign processes such as scar lesions or trichoepithelioma.

Keratoacanthomas are considered to be benign neoplasms, but the histologic picture of keratoacanthomas can be confused with squamous cell carcinoma. The diagnosis of keratoacanthoma can only be differentiated from squamous cell carcinoma based on the gross architectural pattern. Therefore biopsy of any lesion suspected for keratoacanthoma must include both opposite edges plus the central portion of the lesion. A wedge-shaped incision of the lesion from the center of the lesion to both opposite edges provides a sufficient specimen. For adnexal tumor or subcutaneous tumors, incisional or excisional biopsies are recommended. Biopsies are usually performed in an outpatient setting with the use of local anesthetic such as 1% or 2% lidocaine. These are usually uncomplicated procedures with little morbidity.

Treatment Planning

There are several acceptable choices for the treatment of cutaneous malignancies. These include curettage and electrodesiccation, excision, Mohs' micrographic surgery, cryotherapy, radiation therapy, topical chemotherapy, and laser vaporization. After the histologic diagnosis has been confirmed, several factors must be considered to determine the appropriate therapeutic approach. The size of the lesion, the anatomic location, the clinical nature, histologic characteristics, general health and age of the patient, and whether the lesion is primary, recurrent, or metastatic should be considered.

The size of the tumor is important in deciding the treatment plan and assessing the final outcome. In the case of basal cell carcinoma, the larger the tumor, the greater is the chance of recurrence. This is even true when Mohs' micrographic surgery is used.[173,322] Lesions larger than 2 to 3 cm have a much lower rate of cure than those smaller than 1 cm.

The location of the tumor also plays an important role in the final outcome of the treatment. Skin areas located along the embryonal fusion planes have the potential for deep invasion and higher rates of recurrences. These areas include the midface under the eyes, periauricular and postauricular areas, the paranasal, nasolabial, and inner canthal areas. For these high-risk areas, select the type of treatment that gives the highest cure rate and least chance of recurrence, such as Mohs' micrographic surgery. The anatomic function of the area and the final cosmetic appearance of the wound are also important in selecting the method of treatment.

The longer the tumor has been present, the greater is the chance for deeper invasion. The duration of the tumor correlates with the biologic behavior of the tumor. Tumors with well-defined borders and slow growth pattern have less chance of recurrence than tumors with ill-defined borders and multicentric, aggressive natures.

Tumors with histologic patterns of basosquamous or morphea types have a higher rate of recurrence and should be treated with modalities with higher cure rates. Another factor that should be considered in selecting a treatment modality is the pattern of spread of the tumor. The inadequacy of the standard histopathologic methods should be kept in mind when interpreting the reports about the margins of the tumor. Routine histopathologic methods allow pathologists to evaluate selected portions of the surgical specimen, and they are therefore offering an incomplete analysis of all the surgical margins.

The general health of the patient must be carefully considered. For patients with coagulopathy, a less invasive procedure should be selected and, if necessary, the problem should be temporarily corrected before surgery (*e.g.*, infusion of platelets before surgery in cases of thrombocytopenia). In elderly, debilitated patients, procedures requiring one or two office visits are preferred to those needing 10 to 15 visits. In patients with immunodeficiency states, the chance of infection is increased and the tumor may be more aggressive.

If tissue preservation is important (*e.g.*, eyelids, vermilion border of the lip, the tip of the nose), less destructive methods are usually recommended. These include radiation therapy or Mohs' micrographic surgery.

CURETTAGE AND ELECTRODESICCATION

Curettage and electrodesiccation are commonly used to treat basal cell carcinoma, superficial squamous cell carcinoma, and precancerous and benign lesions. Treatment is based on the difference in the consistency between the tumor and the normal surrounding tissues.

Curettage is performed with the use of a curet, which is a pencil-like instrument with a round or oval tip, sharpened on one side. Using the curet, the tumor is debulked down to the normal tissue, which is indicated by the sound and texture. Normal skin is firm and has a gritty sound on curettage. Electrodesiccation is used to destroy any residual tumor cells and produce hemostasis. A biopsy is recommended before the use of curettage and electrodesiccation. If possible, a shave biopsy is preferred, because it is easier to perform curettage after shave biopsy than after a punch or incisional biopsy. This technique is frequently used for the treatment of basal cell carcinoma, superficial squamous cell carcinoma, selected cases of Bowen's disease, keratoacanthomas, and hypertrophic actinic keratoses.

The cure rate with this approach is 77% to 97%. Immediately after the procedure, 12% to 30% of patients have nests of basal cell carcinoma in the treated areas. The inflammatory reaction after the procedure or possibly an immunologic reaction may be responsible for the destruction of these tumors after curettage and electrodesiccation. The cure rate for this technique also depends on patient selection. It is important to avoid high-risk patients who have more aggressive histology, larger tumors, longer duration of disease, or tumors located in high-risk anatomic areas. Morphea-like basal cell carcinomas are not suitable for treatment with this technique. Lesions larger than 1 cm, especially on the face, have an increased tendency to recur.[323] Tumors that are present longer have a tendency to become more infiltrative and break down into smaller more invasive cords with a more fibrotic stromal reaction. This type of histology is more resistant to curettage and electrodesiccation and causes more recurrences. It is also likely that older tumors may invade deeply across a broad front until they reach a tissue barrier of skin. In these cases, tumors extend deceptively beyond the reach of the curet.

Curettage and electrodesiccation is best used in superficial and nodular basal cell carcinoma of low recurrence areas. It is not effective for morphea basal cell carcinoma, recurrent basal cell carcinoma, or squamous cell carcinoma. This technique should not be used in certain areas because of cosmetic considerations, such as wound contracture around eyes and mouth. In the hands of skilled experienced practitioners, the cure rate can be as high as 95% to 97%.[324–327] A high recurrence rate is reported if less experienced dermatology residents performed the procedure.

In the current technique, the curet is used to define the size, shape, and extent of the tumor and then excise the area with a 2- to 3-mm margin.[328] Electrodesiccation is used to destroy tiny pockets of tumor cells and an extra rim of tissue at the base and periphery of the defect produced by curettage and to produce hemostasis. A high-frequency (500,000–1,000,000 Hz), highly damped alternating current of high voltage (>2000 V) and low amperage (100–1000 mA) is used for electrodesiccation. The electrical resistance of the skin generates sufficient heat to produce tissue injury at the point of contact. The heat causes dehydration of the cells and instantaneous cell death. Because of the low amperage, there is sharp delineation between normal and destroyed tissue. Increasing the current (amperage) causes more heat, deeper penetration, and excessive tissue destruction and scarring. Hemostasis results from thrombosis of affected vessels.

CRYOTHERAPY

The first report of cryotherapy in the treatment of malignant tumors of the skin appeared in 1963 by Cooper.[329] Although Cooper is recognized as the father of cryosurgery, the use of this technique began after the turn of the century.[330]

Cryotherapy takes advantage of the cryonecrosis that is achieved by cellular and microvascular response to subzero temperatures. Using liquid nitrogen (−195.5°C), freezing temperatures are achieved in viable tissues, transforming water into ice. Some changes in cells in subzero temperatures include the formation of extracellular and intracellular ice, abnormal concentration and crystallization of electrolytes, and denaturation of lipoprotein complexes that are lethal to the cells.[331] The more severe effect of cryotherapy is thought to be on the microvasculature of the skin and the tumor tissues. With proper selection of the tumor size and location, it is possible to achieve a high cure rate, excellent would healing, and cosmetically acceptable results (Fig. 45–25).

This technique is especially useful for patients with pacemakers, those with adverse reactions to local anesthetic, and those who are poor surgical risks. It can be used for the treatment of lesions smaller than 2 cm that are located on the eyelid, nose, ear, chest, back, or tip of the nose. It is recommended for the treatment of recurrent tumors and tumors with definable margins. A 3- to 5-mm tumor-free margin is used to increase the cure rate. The involved region is anesthetized with local anesthetic, and the freezing time is decided based on the size of the tumor. Open spray takes a longer period than spray through a plastic cone. The freeze-thaw time is usually 1:2 for direct spray or 1:4 for spray through plastic cone. The temperature of the tissue is controlled by a thermocoupler inserted under the tumor. A temperature of −50°C is thought to be sufficient for cryotherapy. A double freeze-thaw cycle is recommended for safe and accurate treatment.

Cryotherapy is not an option for the treatment of morphea-type basal cell carcinoma. It cannot be used in patients with abnormal cold intolerance (*e.g.*, cryoglobulinemia, Raynaud's disease) or on tumors located in certain anatomic areas such as free margin of eyelid, vermilion border of the lip, ala nasi, anterior and posterior ear, or scalp and for tumors larger than 3 cm. Tumors located on the nasolabial fold or inner canthi require wider margins of freezing to increase the cure rate. The morbidity of cryotherapy is moderate and includes edema, oozing, erosions, hemorrhaging, and secondary infections. The cosmetic result is good except for hypopigmentation or hyperpigmentation. The latter condition usually fades within a few months after therapy.

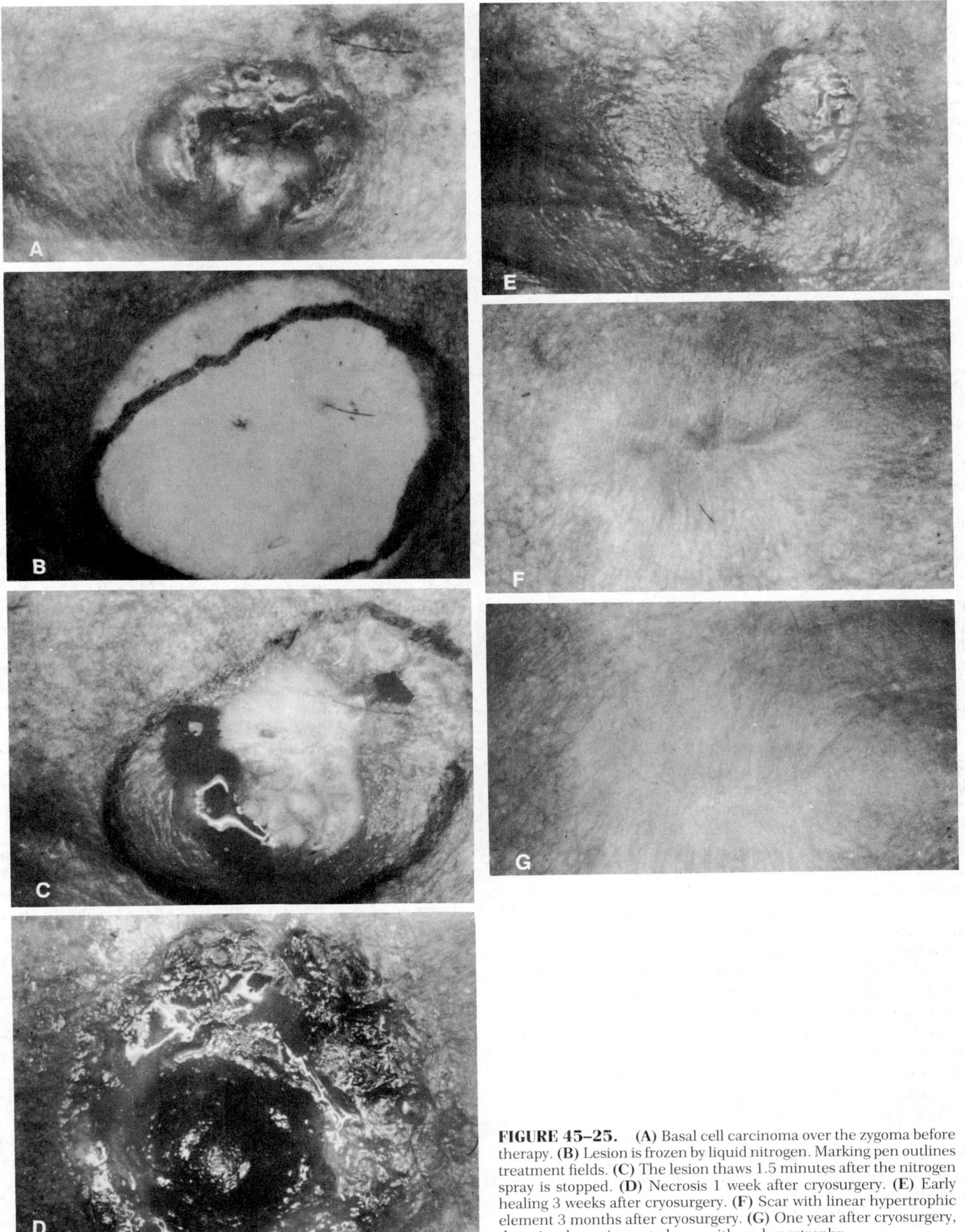

FIGURE 45–25. **(A)** Basal cell carcinoma over the zygoma before therapy. **(B)** Lesion is frozen by liquid nitrogen. Marking pen outlines treatment fields. **(C)** The lesion thaws 1.5 minutes after the nitrogen spray is stopped. **(D)** Necrosis 1 week after cryosurgery. **(E)** Early healing 3 weeks after cryosurgery. **(F)** Scar with linear hypertrophic element 3 months after cryosurgery. **(G)** One year after cryosurgery, there is a hypopigmented scar with no hypertrophy.

CHEMOTHERAPY

Topical chemotherapy has been used for the treatment of precancerous (*e.g.*, actinic keratoses) and cancerous (*e.g.*, basal cell carcinoma) lesions of the skin.[332–334] Many chemicals have been tried, including salicylic acid, pyrogallic acid, podophyllin, thiotepa, BCNU, 5-FU, and retinoids. With the exception of 5-FU, which has been effective, these agents have been unsatisfactory. BCNU is effective in the treatment of cutaneous T-cell lymphoma, and retinoids are still in clinical trials.

5-FU blocks the action of the enzyme thymidylate synthetase, which catalyzes the methylation of 2-dioxyuridylic acid to thymidylic acid. 5-FU prevents DNA synthesis and cellular reproduction by inhibition of the production of thymidylic acid. The inhibition of nucleic acid synthesis is most notable in rapidly proliferating neoplastic cells, compared with normal cells with a normal rate of metabolism.

5-FU is used topically as a cream or lotion once or twice per day for several weeks and produces a severe inflammatory response in the precancerous and malignant areas. 5-FU is available in concentrates of 1%, 2%, and 5% and can be used to achieve desired levels of inflammation. The lotion is best applied by a soft brush and the cream with fingertip. Topical steroid cream can be used to alleviate the inflammation without lessening the efficacy of 5-FU. It is not necessary to induce extreme discomfort in patients' skin to obtain results. Mild to moderate erythema is sufficient. If no erythema occurs with the 1% 5-FU cream, the concentration should be increased to 2% or 5%. Facial areas, the dorsum of the hand, and lower extremities are often treated with 5-FU. Concomitant use of topical 13-all-*trans*-retinoic acid (*i.e.*, tretinoin cream) enhances the effect of topical 5-FU.[335] Sun exposure may induce more severe reactions and photosensitivity. After the completion of the treatment with 5-FU, a careful examination of the skin is recommended to identify and biopsy any persistent or newly developed lesions.

Complications of treatment with 5-FU includes allergic reaction to the vehicle, erythema, and pigmentary changes. 5-FU is quite effective in the treatment of actinic keratoses and superficial basal cell carcinoma. It has been shown to be ineffective in other forms of cancer, including other types of basal cell carcinoma.

5-FU has been tried in combination with topical immune therapy with agents such as 2,4-dinitrochlorobenzene (DNCB). This combination has been used in a few cases of in situ epidermal cancer and Bowen's disease.[336]

Systemic chemotherapy, such as the use of 5-FU and cisplatin, has not been effective in the treatment of nonmelanoma skin cancer. Chemotherapy for squamous cell carcinoma and adnexal tumors of the skin has been unsuccessful.[337,338] This approach may be helpful for treating metastatic tumors. Isotretinoin, a vitamin A derivative, has been used in the treatment of advanced primary squamous cell carcinoma, but not enough data are available.[339]

Topical use of tretinoin cream has been effective in reducing sun damage to the skin.[340] Use of this agent for over a year results in thickened epidermis and new collagen formation in the dermis.[341] This work has not yet been confirmed by other investigators.

Many believe that 5-FU is not a good modality for the treatment of basal cell carcinoma because it may result in a tumor-free surface while the tumor underneath continues to grow. Other investigators have reported the use of 5-FU in the treatment of in situ epidermal carcinoma, but this approach is not accepted by other clinicians.[342–344]

Nitrogen mustard is an accepted modality in the treatment of cutaneous T-cell lymphomas.[345] Topical application of BCNU has been used occasionally in the treatment of cutaneous T-cell lymphoma.[346] Methotrexate was used to treat basal cell carcinoma alone or in combination with demecolcine and thiocolchicine but was not effective.[335,347,348] Dactinomycin, cytosine arabinoside, and spiramycin were ineffective in treating basal cell carcinoma.[347,348]

SURGICAL EXCISION

Surgical excision is an effective treatment approach for all forms of skin tumors in most anatomic locations (Fig. 45–26). Surgical excision is performed in an elliptical shape along the Langer's cleavage lines, and in most instances, primary closure of the wound is possible and results in good cosmetic healing. The procedure is usually performed under local anesthesia with the use of scalpel and curved scissors. Surgical margins of excision vary according to the type of tumor; a 3- to 5-mm margin is acceptable for basal cell carcinomas that do not metastasize, but a margin of several centimeters is considered sufficient for Merkel cell carcinoma and squamous cell carcinoma. For recurrent basal cell carcinoma or morphea basal cell carcinoma, a wider margin (*e.g.*, 1 cm) is used. Although specific guidelines about the margin of resection for tumors such as squamous cell carcinoma, Merkel's cell carcinoma, or eccrine carcinoma have not been developed, it is accepted that wider margins should be taken with tumors that are larger or extend deeper into the skin and underlying tissue. Local draining lymph nodes are examined and removed only if they are clinically palpable.

Split-thickness or full-thickness skin grafts are sometimes necessary for the closure of wounds if the tumor is large and primary closure is not possible or if primary closure may result in undesirable cosmetic appearance (*e.g.*, excision of tumors from the lip, nose, or eyelid).

Split-thickness grafts are usually obtained with a mechanical dermatome and are used to cover large surgical defects with minimal vascularity, such as periosteum.[349] Split-thickness skin grafts are well accepted by noninfected recipient sites. However, the color of split-thickness graft is not matched, and it creates a donor site that heals slowly by secondary intention. Full-thickness grafts are used when a good color match is important, and the donor sites require primary closure.

Split- and full-thickness grafts are immobilized after surgery to prevent movement and bleeding. It usually takes 5 to 7 days to accept the graft and 2 to 3 months for the tissue to mature and become cosmetically acceptable skin (Fig. 45–27).

A skin flap is another choice for the closure of surgical excision site. Skin flaps are attached on one side to the donor area and carry their own blood supplies. While attached to the base by a pedicle, the separated skin is advanced or rotated to cover the surgical defect. Rotation flaps are simple and are

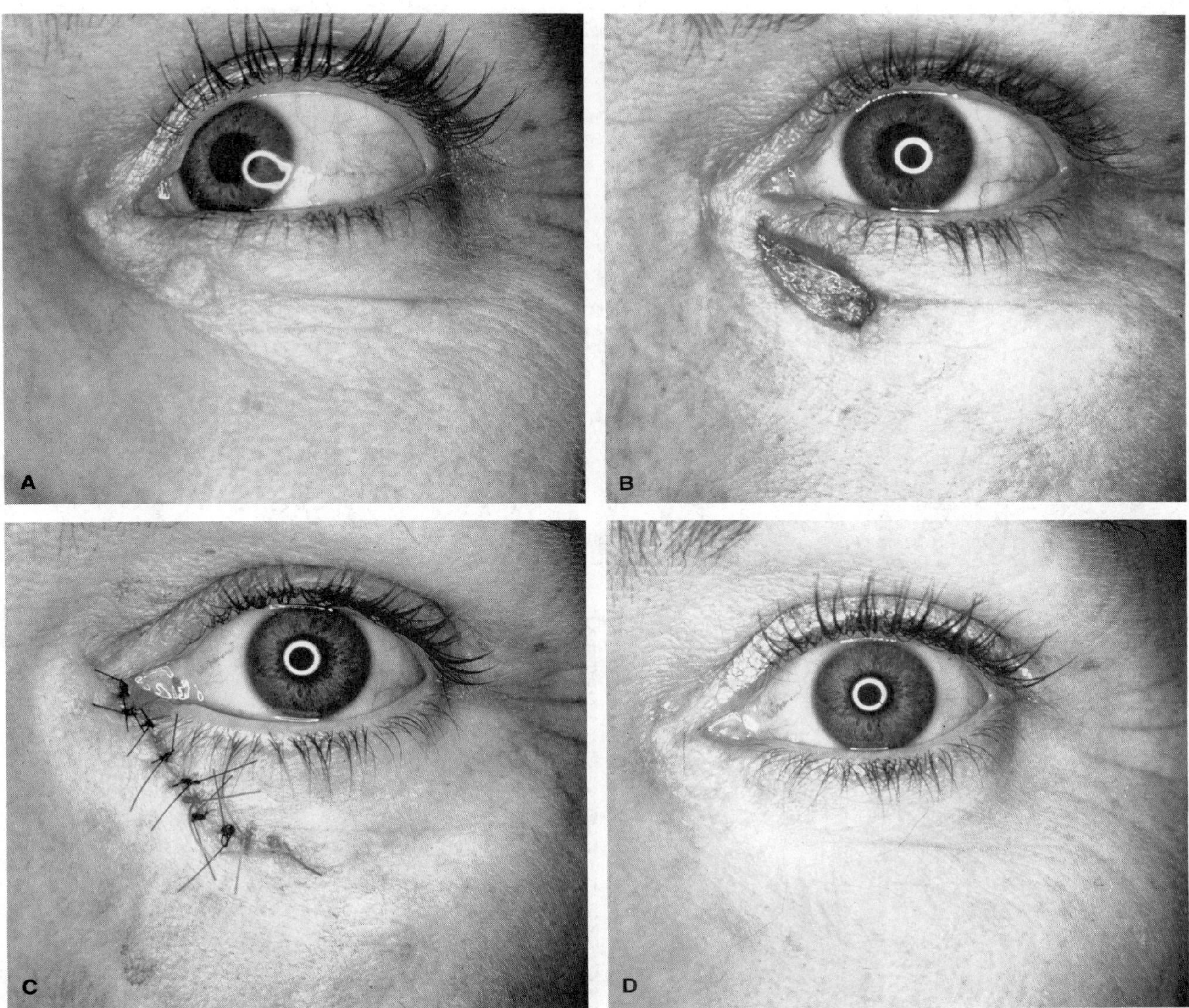

FIGURE 45–26. **(A)** Primary basal cell carcinoma in an infraorbital site close to the inner canthus. **(B)** Surgical excision of the tumor. **(C)** Primary closure. **(D)** Same patient 9 months after surgery.

commonly used to cover surgical defects. They can be designed to fit the desired anatomic site.

With advancement of microvascular surgery, the tissue transfer from one part of the body to another can be achieved by anastomosing the donor artery and vein to the recipient artery and vein. The technique of surgical excision allows microscopic evaluation of the entire tumor and its margins. The technique can be performed with minimal discomfort and complications and with good cosmetic results. It can be performed on the trunk, extremities, cheeks, forehead, chin, and scalp. For important anatomic sites, such as lesions located on the alar rim of the nose, lip, or eyelids, special care should be taken to prevent distortion if the tissue and poor cosmetic results.

The decision to preform surgical excision should be made only after consideration of all other therapeutic modalities available.

RADIATION THERAPY

Indications and Applications

Most skin cancers are radiosensitive, and this method of treatment is one of the most effective therapies for selected skin tumors. This approach is usually recommended for patients who are poor surgical risks or are elderly debilitated or when the tumor is large. The advantages of radiation therapy include acceptability by most patients, because there is no pain involved, no hospitalization required, and patients can continue to function normally in their own environment during the course of therapy. Radiation therapy does not cause keloid formation, contracture, or ectropion. Radiation therapy allows the uninvolved tissue to be preserved and produces a much lesser degree of defect. Among the disadvantages of this method are multiple patient visits and loss of hair follicles and sweat glands at the site of therapy. The decision about

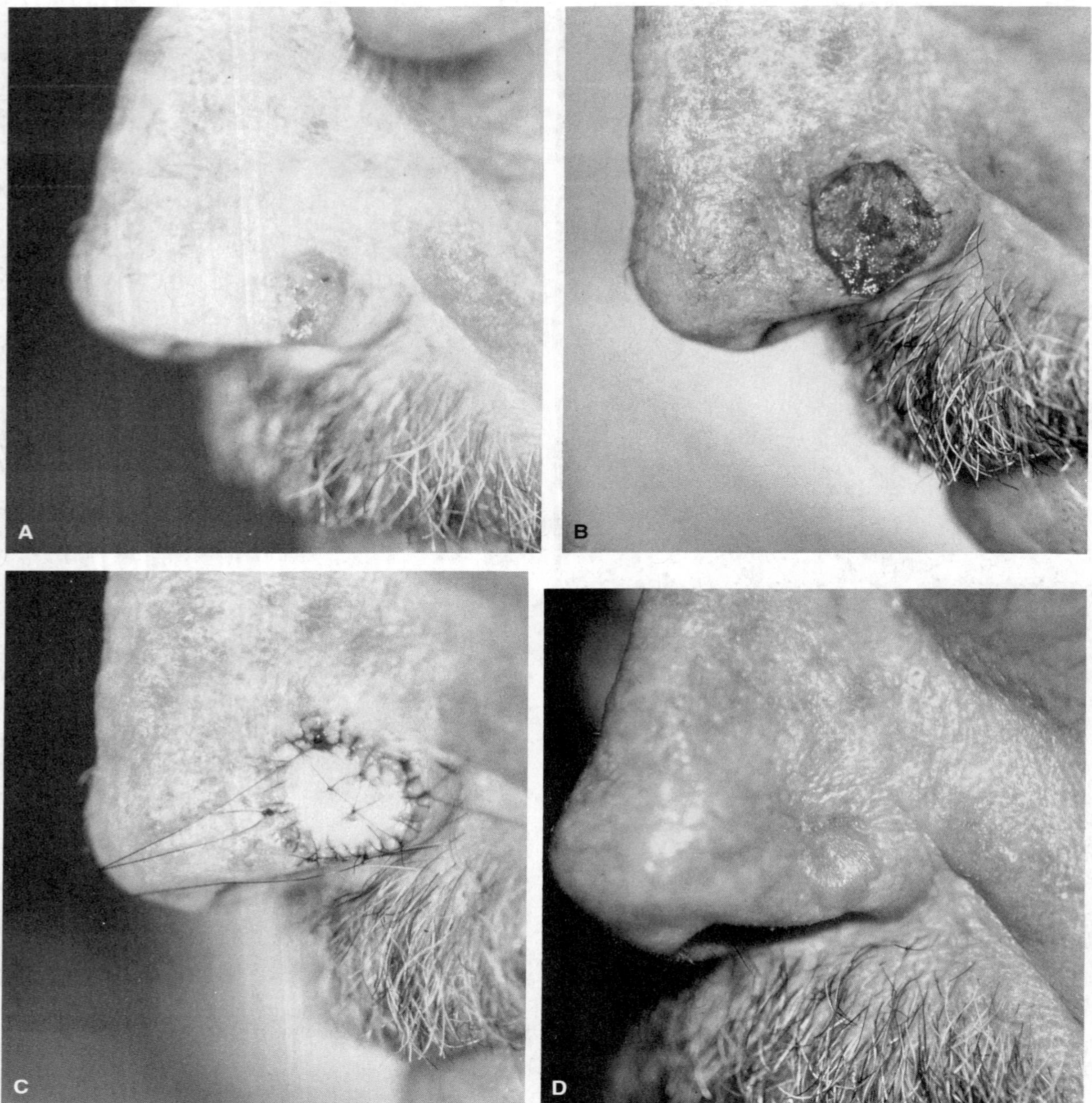

FIGURE 45–27. **(A)** Basal cell carcinoma of the ala nasi. **(B)** The site after surgery. **(C)** Full-thickness graft. **(D)** The same patient 6 months after surgery.

whether to use radiation therapy or other modalities is based on the size and anatomic location of tumor, histology of the neoplasm, age of the patient, recurrence rates, and the anticipated cosmetic results.

Radiation therapy is usually the best choice of treatment for skin cancers located on the nose, eye, lip, eyelid, and inner and outer canthi (Figs. 45–28 through 45–31). Skin tumors along the embryonal fusion planes can also be treated and cured with this modality. Radiation therapy is usually recommended for primary basal cell carcinoma and squamous cell carcinoma, but it can be used for recurrent lesions as well (Fig. 45–32). It is not appropriate to treat recurrent skin cancers with radiation therapy if the tumor was initially treated with this approach. Morphea basal cell carcinoma is ill defined in depth and borders and not suitable for radiation treatment, but it is radiosensitive.

The cure rate for radiation therapy is 96.4% for basal cell carcinoma and 91.9% for squamous cell carcinoma, if therapy is performed by an experienced specialist.[350] Similar results were reported by another group.[351] The selection of appropriate treatment modality for a given tumor and the experience of the physician administrating the treatment are important in the final outcome.

The cosmetic results of radiation therapy is good and acceptable to the patients. However, as time passes, chronic radiation dermatitis may take place in the form of atrophy,

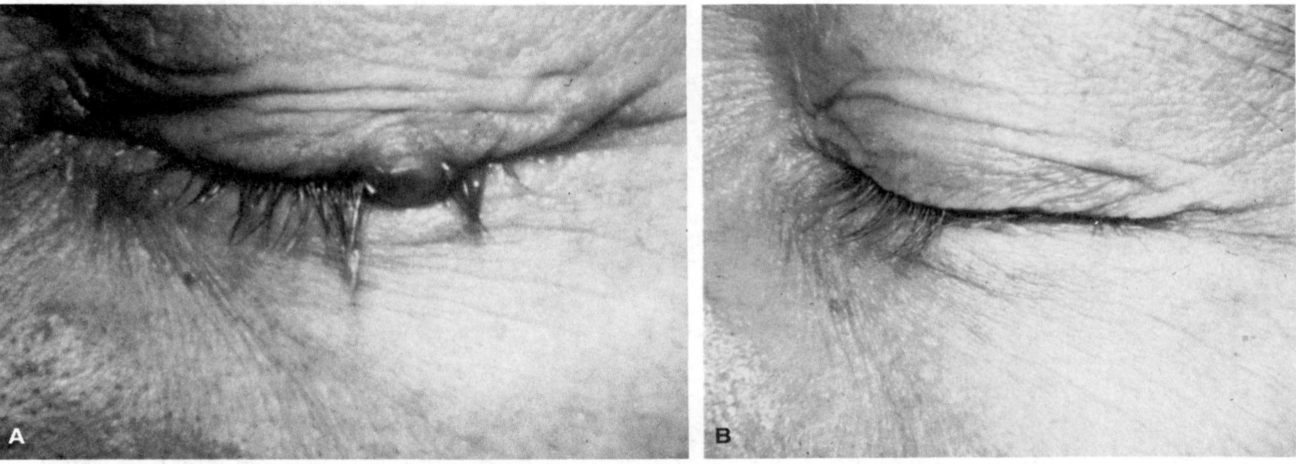

FIGURE 45–28. **(A)** Basal cell carcinoma on the margin of the upper eyelid. **(B)** Same patient 1 year after treatment with x-ray therapy.

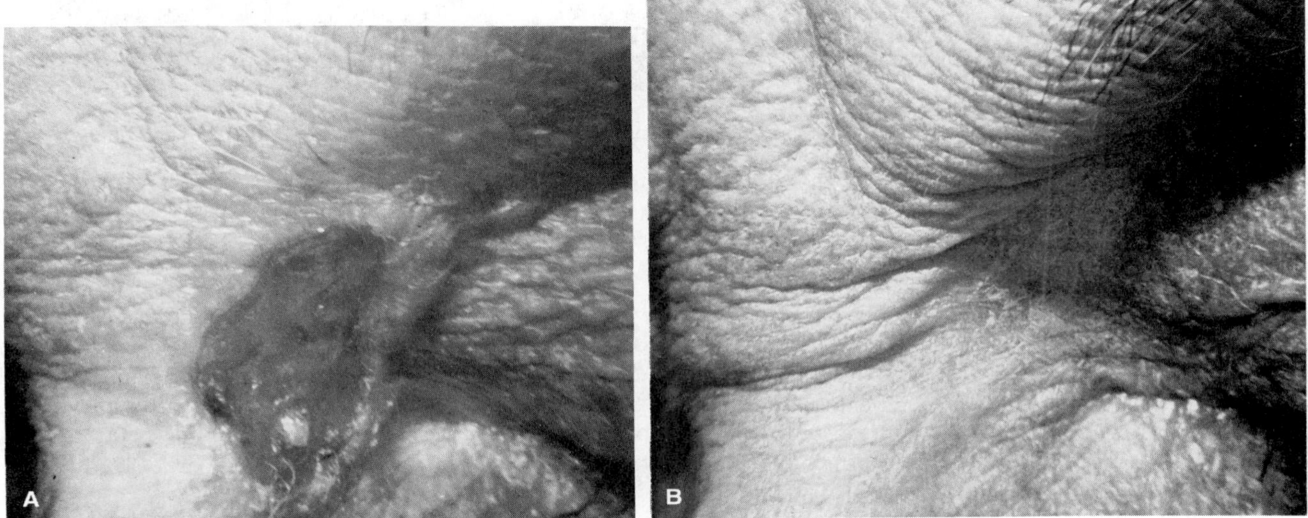

FIGURE 45–29. **(A)** Basal cell carcinoma of the left inner canthus. **(B)** After using 10 x-ray treatments of 400 cGy each for a total dose of 4000 cGy and an HVL of 0.5 mm of aluminum.

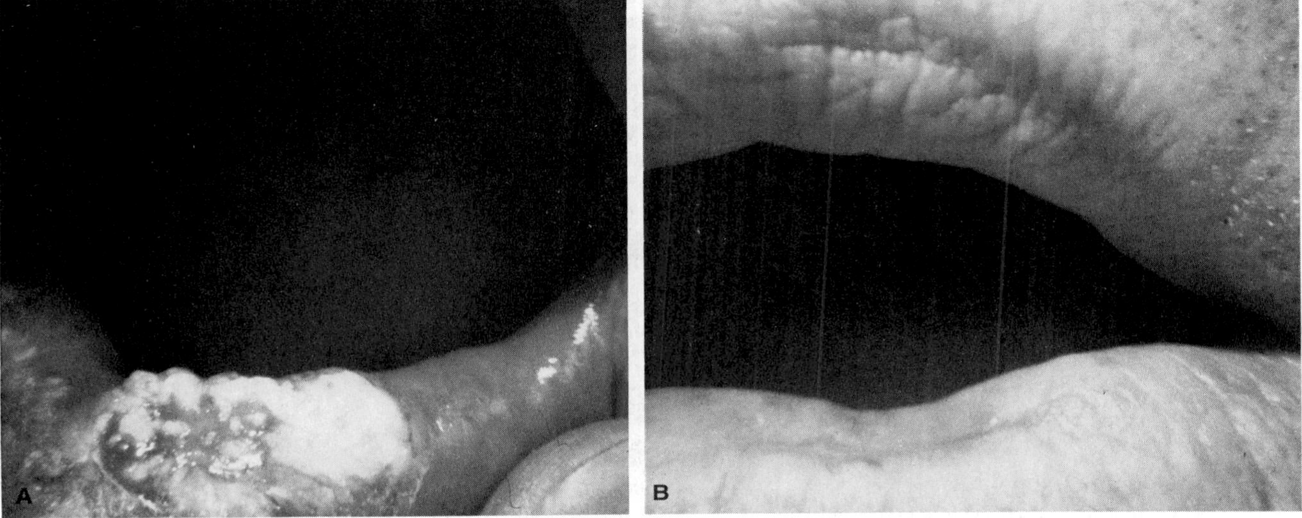

FIGURE 45–30. **(A)** Squamous cell carcinoma on the lower lip of a smoker. **(B)** The same patient after using 10 radiation treatments of 450 cGy each for a total dose of 4500 cGy and an HVL of 1 mm of aluminum.

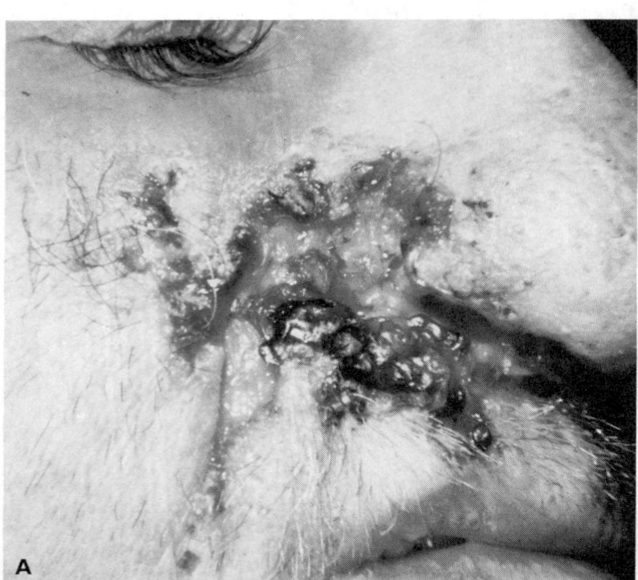
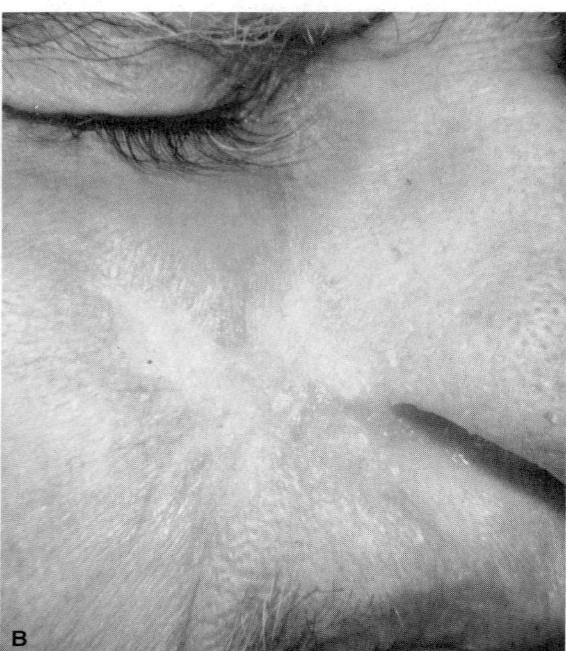

FIGURE 45–31. **(A)** Recurrent basal cell carcinoma of right nosolabial fold. **(B)** The same patient after using 10 treatments of 360 cGy each for a total of 3600 cGy and an HVL of 2 mm of aluminum.

telangiectasia, hyperpigmentation, or hypopigmentation, and radiation-induced precancerous lesions may appear. Radiation therapy is therefore recommended for selected cases, and only for patients 50 years of age or older.

A biopsy should always be performed for histologic diagnosis before initiation of radiation therapy. History of prior treatment, specifically the use of x-ray therapy, should be obtained for skin cancers or for other skin conditions such as acne, removal of hair, tinea capitis. The tumor is evaluated, and a lead shield with a portal exposure to fit the tumor and at least a 0.5 cm of normal tissue is produced. Wider margins are necessary for recurrent lesions and for lesions located at the embryonal fusion plane. The clinical margin for the tumor should be well defined, even if multiple biopsies are necessary. The tumor is exposed to x-rays through the port in the lead shield by touching the lead glass cone of the x-ray machine to the lead shield, reducing the scattered radiation. Specially sensitive areas, such as thyroid glands, gonads, and eyes, are covered with lead shields before each treatment. Protection from the exit dose of radiation is also recommended. An in-

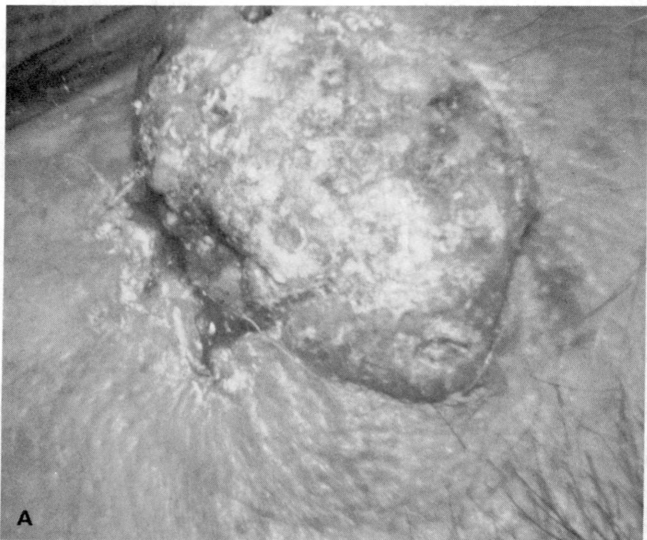
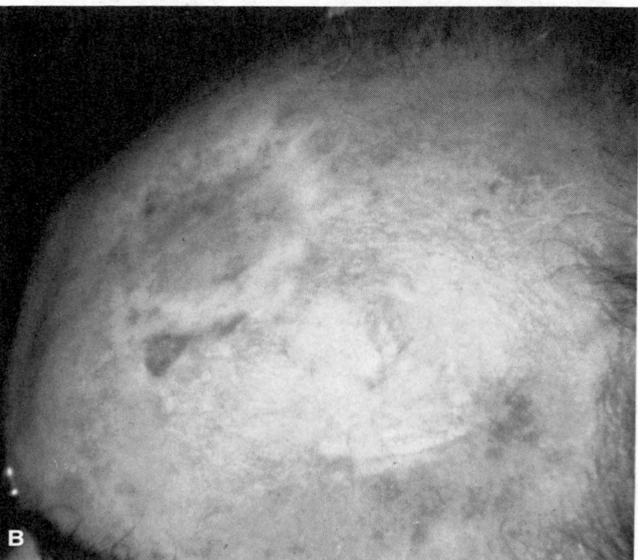

FIGURE 45–32. **(A)** The 5-cm fungating tumor is a recurrent basal cell carcinoma at the site of an old surgical graft. **(B)** The same patient after using 10 treatments of 400 cGy each for a total dose of 4000 cGy and an HVL of 2 mm of aluminum. The surgical graft scar is adjacent to the lesion.

ternal nasal shield, gum shield, and eye shield are used when treating these organs.

Immediate side effects include erythema and exudative reaction at treatment sites, loss of eyelashes when treating eyelids, and mucositis when treating the nose. The treatment is repeated until the appropriate amount of radiation is administered to the skin tumor.

Radiation Technology

The goal of radiation is to selectively destroy the tumor tissue and spare the normal surrounding area. Modern radiologic technology has made it possible to select the quality, dose, and fractionation of the radiation so that only the neoplastic tissue is destroyed.

The quality of radiation is determined by the amount of kilovoltage and by the type of filter used. The half-value layer (HVL) is the thickness of a given filter material that reduces the intensity of a beam of photons to 50% of the original exposure. The thickness of tissue or tissue depth measured in millimeters that absorbs 50% of the surface dose is called half-value depth ($D_{1/2}$). In the treatment of each skin cancer, the amount of kilovoltage and the thickness and type of the filter is selected so that the $D_{1/2}$ is equal to the thickness of the tumor, and the tissue underlying the tumor is minimized. Softer radiation reaching normal tissue causes a less chronic radiation reaction.

$D_{1/2}$ is determined by kilovoltage, the HVL, the distance between the anode (target) of the x-ray tube and the target-to-skin distance, and by the size of the field. Based on the available calculation, the intensity or dose rate of radiation at a given point is inversely proportional to the square of its distance from the target. The dose to the base of the lesion is equal to one half of the surface dose. If the depth (thickness) of the tumor is known, the appropriate quality of radiation can be selected from precalibrated table available for each x-ray machine. An x-ray machine producing superficial x-rays with a $D_{1/2}$ of 7 to 10 mm is sufficient for most skin tumors. Most basal cell carcinomas and squamous cell carcinomas infiltrate to the depth of 2 to 5 mm.[352] A total dose of 2000 to 3000 cGy for the depth of the tumor is recommended for the treatment of most skin cancers that correspond to 4000 to 6000 cGy on the surface. To prevent radiation sequela of short or long term, the entire dose of x-rays is fractionated into smaller doses and is administered over 3 to 4 weeks. For example, to achieve a good cosmetic result and high cure rate, a 4000-cGy dose could be divided into 10 fractions of 400 cGy each. Fractionation of the dose can be achieved in many different ways, but all approaches give a high cure rate and low recurrence rate. For smaller lesions (*e.g.*, eyelids), the physician can use the so-called contact x-ray, which could be produced by 50 to 60 kV, an HVL of 2 to 4 mm of aluminum, and a short distance from target to skin (1.5–3 cm).[353] This approach allows most x-rays to be absorbed by the tumor and a rapid drop down of radiation to normal tissue.

Another x-ray machine that is now commonly used is a soft x-ray unit with beryllium windows. These machines range from 10 to 100 kV and have lower inherent filtration that allows higher dose rates. Modern units have predetermined and fixed kV-filter combinations and special mechanisms to prevent errors of delivery.

Another effective approach is the use of electron-beam irradiation in the treatment of superficial skin tumors. The depth of penetration of electrons depends on the amount of the voltage used to produce them (2–15 MeV).[354,355] Because of limited depth of penetration electron-beam irradiation does not affect deep tissues and produces excellent cosmetic results. Electrons are more precise than x-rays, give better cosmetic results, and are useful in treating certain skin cancers like large carcinomas located on the scalp or lesions overlying cartilage or in elderly persons, for whom there is a risk of bone and cartilage necrosis if low-energy photons are used.[354] However, the electron beam is not widely available, is more costly, and requires a lengthy recalibration for each patient.

Radium molds and implants have been used in the past for the treatment of skin cancers, but because of the hazards, they are no longer in use.

CHEMOSURGERY AND MOHS' MICROGRAPHIC SURGERY

The combination of surgical and microscopic approaches to eradicate skin tumors was initially formulated by Frederick Mohs. When he was a medical student, he observed that injection of 20% zinc chloride into tissues resulted in fixation and preservation of histologic structure when later viewed under a microscope. This observation led him to develop the technique of chemosurgery for the treatment of skin cancers.[173–175,356] Zinc chloride paste is used to fix the tumor in situ. The tumor is then serially removed, and a careful map of the area and the specimen are developed and color coded. The excised tumor is divided into several segments, and horizontal sections are prepared by the frozen-tissue technique and evaluated for the presence of tumors by light microscopy. The lateral and deep margins of resected tumors are examined, and the areas with tumor involvement are marked on the color-coded maps of the removed tissue. These steps are repeated for the areas identified as involved with tumor until all the margins are free of the tumor, and the entire neoplastic mass is removed (Figs. 45–33 and 45–34). The fixed-tissue technique, which is effective but time consuming, has been eliminated and replaced by the frozen-section technique of cryosectioning. This technique has recently been renamed as Mohs' micrographic surgery.[173–175]

Mohs' micrographic surgery is indicated for tumors of skin that are difficult to treat using other methods. The technique's greatest success has been in the treatment of difficult basal cell carcinomas and squamous cell carcinomas (Fig. 45–35). This technique has been used to treat other cancers that have a high recurrence rate using conventional surgery and other therapeutic modalities (Fig. 45–36). In these cases, it is sensible to combine the step-wise surgical removal with precise microscopic control of removed tumor tissue to achieve a more complete removal and higher cure rate.

Mohs' micrographic surgery is currently used to treat some of the more difficult skin cancers, including basal cell carcinoma, squamous cell carcinoma, erythroplasia of Queyrat, bowenoid papulosis, Bowen's disease, verrucous carcinoma, keratoacanthoma, microcytic adnexal carcinoma, sebaceous carcinoma, extramammary Paget's disease, malignant melanoma, Merkel's cell carcinoma, dermatofibrosarcoma protuberans, atypical fibroxanthoma, leiomyosarcoma, and an-

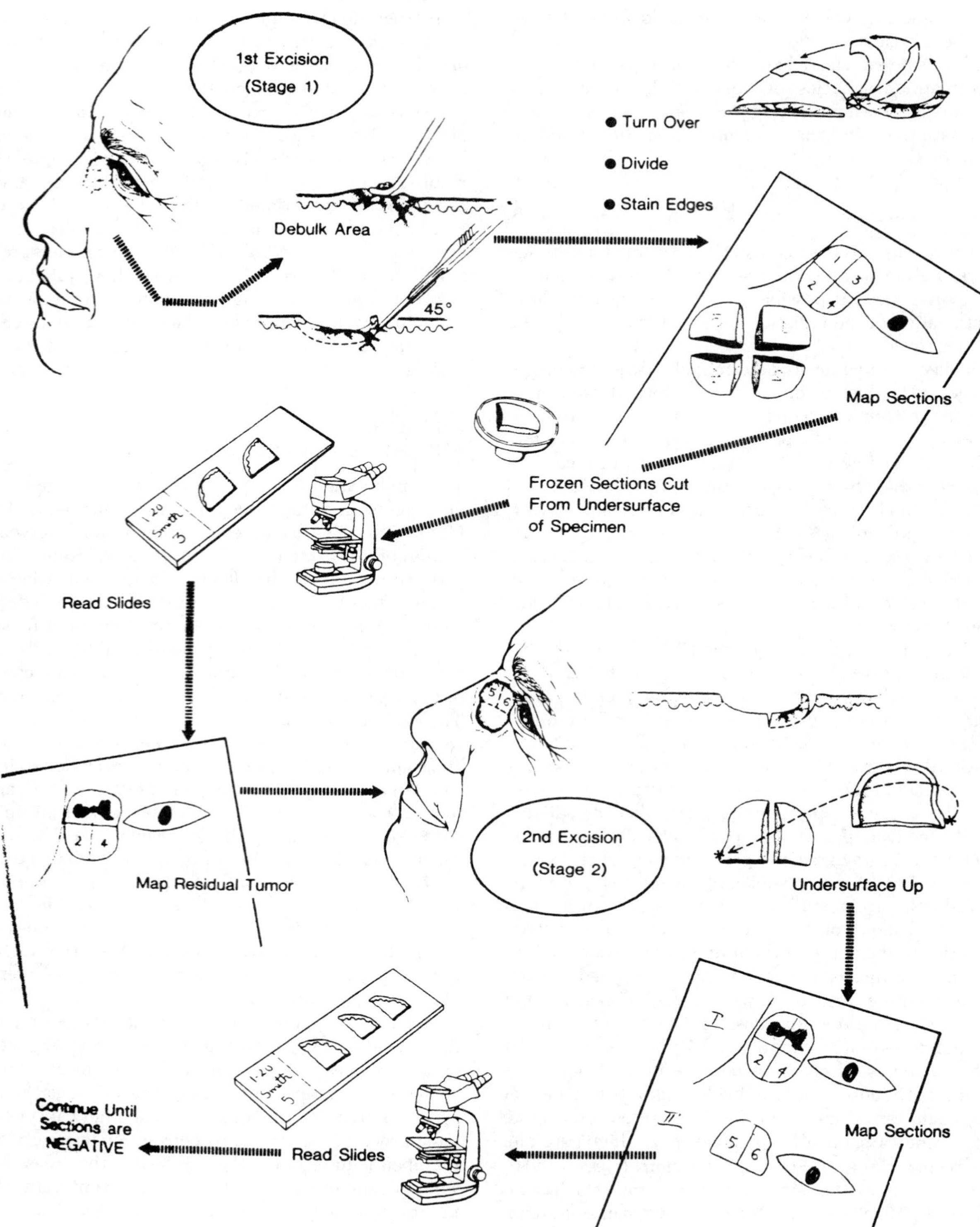

FIGURE 45–33. Schematic representation of the technique of Mohs' surgery.

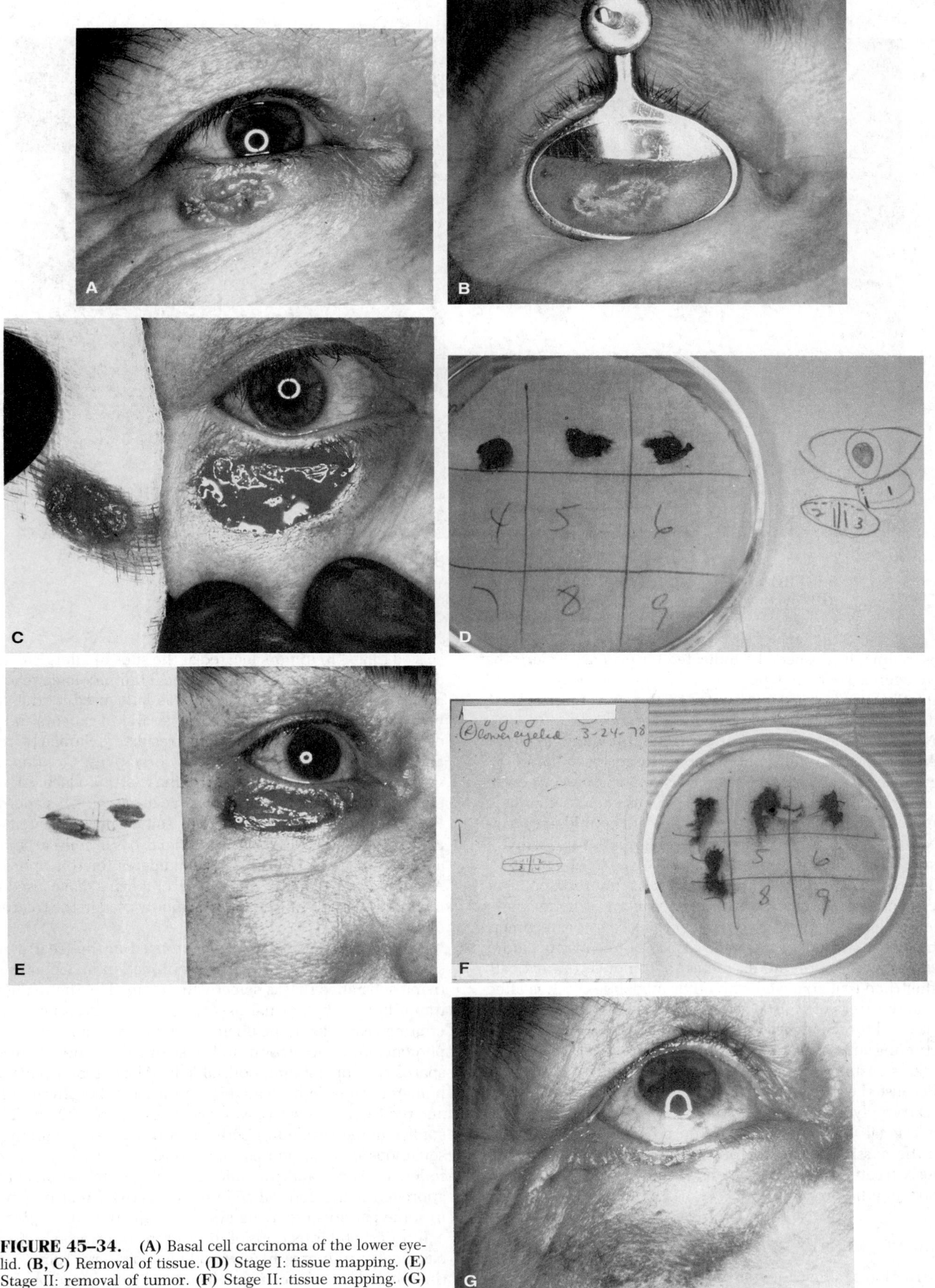

FIGURE 45–34. **(A)** Basal cell carcinoma of the lower eyelid. **(B, C)** Removal of tissue. **(D)** Stage I: tissue mapping. **(E)** Stage II: removal of tumor. **(F)** Stage II: tissue mapping. **(G)** Seven months after surgery.

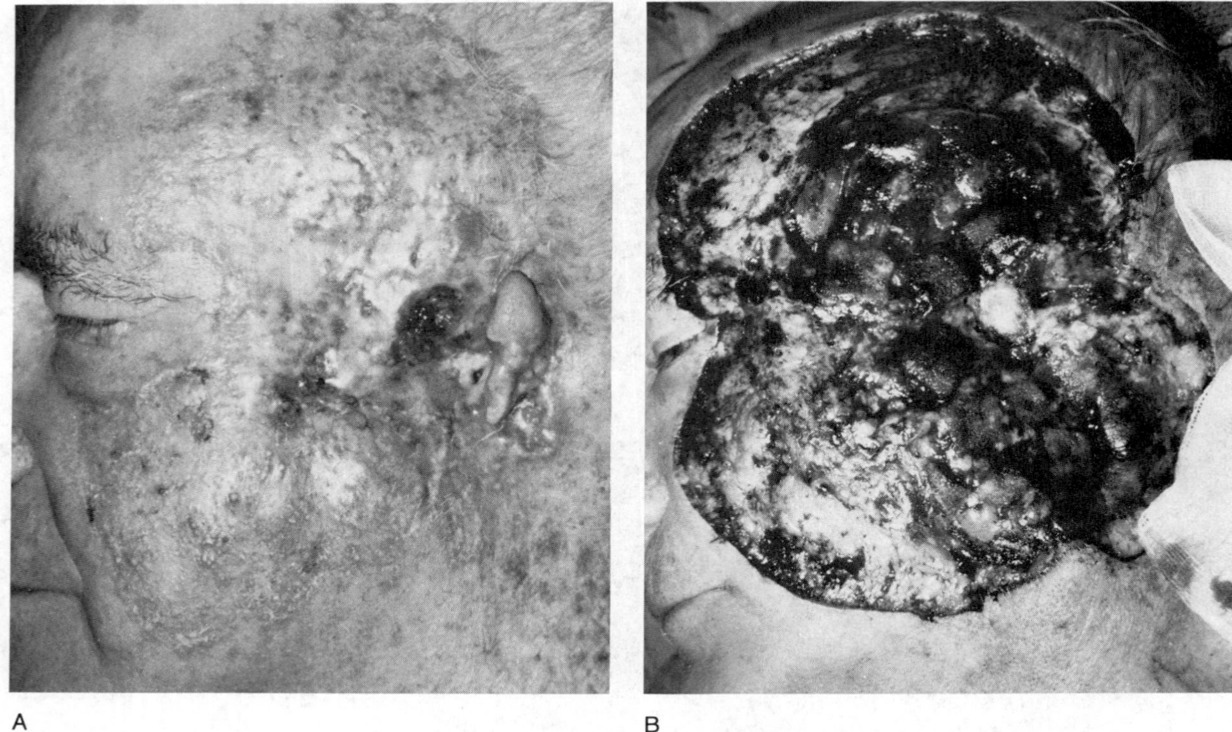

FIGURE 45–35. **(A)** Extensive infiltrating, destructive morpheaform basal cell carcinoma of the left cheek. **(B)** The tumor extends far beyond the clinical margins defined by Mohs' micrographic surgery.

giosarcoma. It is especially indicated for primary lesions that have aggressive histologic patterns (*e.g.*, morphea-like, infiltrative) or primary lesions located on the areas that are likely to have subclinical spread or high recurrence rate.

Normal tissue preservation is essential for functional and cosmetic reasons. Mohs' micrographic surgery is the preferred technique if tissue-sparing surgery is important, as when removing basal cell carcinoma or squamous cell carcinoma located on the embryonal fusion planes of the midface, nasal area, or periauricular areas that are high risk for deeply invasive tumors.

There are several advantages for Mohs' micrographic surgery. The procedure is performed within a few hours and in an outpatient setting, and the defect produced by the technique can heal by secondary intention or can be reconstructed immediately. The cure rate for recurrent tumors is dramatically higher than that achieved with other modalities.[357] It is effective in the areas of high recurrence, in cosmetically important areas, and for deeply invasive tumors, because the horizontal sectioning and examination of the entire lateral and deep margins ensures complete removal of the tumor.

Because the defect of removing a large invasive tumor could be extremely large and potentially devastating to the patient, it is crucial to discuss the procedure, the expected defects, and the possibilities for reconstruction. Photographs of previously treated cases and the end results are helpful in demonstrating the procedure.

IMMUNOTHERAPY AND EXPERIMENTAL MODALITIES

Destruction of skin cancer by the local cell-mediated reaction was initially described by Klein.[358] He and his associates observed that skin tumors located at the sites of allergic contact dermatitis were destroyed by the local immunologic reaction, and DNCB, a sensitizing agent, was later used by the same investigators in the treatment of several skin cancers and precancerous lesions with acceptable results.[358] Similarly, recall antigens, such as purified protein derivatives, *Candida,* pertussis, *Trichophyton,* and streptokinase-streptodornase, were used in the treatment of some skin cancers.[359] This approach was effective in the treatment of some uncomplicated skin cancers. Actinic keratosis, superficial basal cell carcinoma, and Bowen's disease are good candidates for this approach. Although other investigators and clinicians have used this technique, it has not become commonly used in the treatment of skin cancers.

Photodynamic therapy has been used in the treatment of skin cancers.[360] It is based on the injection of a photosensitizing substance that is selectively retained by the malignant tumor but not by normal tissue.[361,362] After exposure to penetrating visible light, the photosensitizing substance undergoes photodynamic activation and destroys the tumor cells and spares the surrounding normal skin. Most studies have used hematoporphyrin derivative (*i.e.*, dihematoporphyrin ether) and red laser light with a wavelength of 600 to 700 nm. These studies demonstrated effectiveness in basal cell carcinoma, squamous cell carcinoma, and Bowen's disease. Long-term follow-up is not yet available. One of the limitations of this approach is the generalized photosensitivity that may occur in some patients receiving systemic injection of porphyrin.

Intralesional injections of interferon (interferon α-2a) into basal cell carcinoma may provide a short-term remission of the tumor.[176] Long-term results are not yet known. Although there has been limited morbidity, the repeated injections

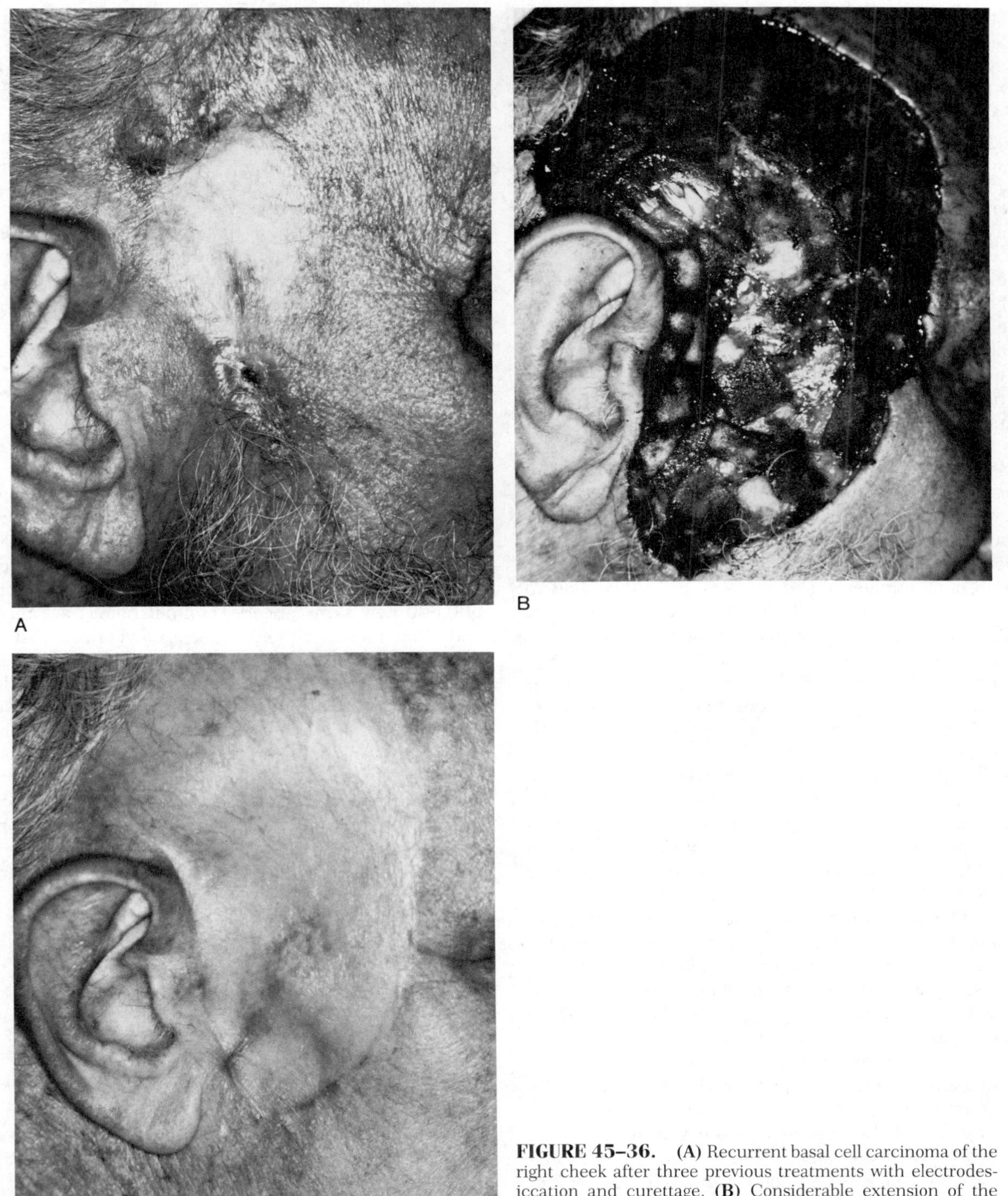

FIGURE 45–36. **(A)** Recurrent basal cell carcinoma of the right cheek after three previous treatments with electrodesiccation and curettage. **(B)** Considerable extension of the wound after six stages of Mohs' micrographic surgery. **(C)** Four months postoperatively. The defect was covered by a full-thickness skin graft after surgery.

needed to eradicate the tumor could be a limiting factor and increase the cost of the therapy. Newer developments in this field may allow the use of biologic factors to become a standard therapy for skin cancers in the future.

TRENDS IN DIAGNOSIS AND TREATMENT

Basal cell carcinoma and squamous cell carcinoma are the most common cancers in the white population. Although the mortality rate from these cancers is low, they exert a heavy burden on the health care system in developed countries. All indicators point to a continued increase in the incidence of skin cancers and their heavy burden on the health care system because of the availability of outdoor recreational activities and sunbathing all year round and because of the cultural norms of our society.

Severe sun exposure and UV damage to the skin continues for years. The problem is compounded by the rapid and continuous depletion of the ozone layer due to the release of ozone-damaging chemicals in the industrialized world. Although the government has placed a ban on production and release of these chemicals, the depletion of ozone will continue for many years. Another important factor is the continuous increase in the aging population, which is accompanied by an increasing number of skin cancers. Even if we find an effective way to protect all children from excessive exposure to UV light starting today, it would take several generations to eliminate those who have been severely damaged. Most likely, in most of these cases the initiation and promotion has occurred in the sun exposed persons and it will continue to cause skin cancers in a significant proportion of the aging population.

Currently, the most logical and effective approach is to identify the risk population for skin cancer, provide early diagnosis guidelines, and educate the public about preventing additional sun exposure. Early diagnosis of skin cancers can only be achieved with public educational programs indicating the importance of early diagnosis and treatment. In the past 6 years, public education and awareness has been increased by free skin cancer screening offered to the public every May or June in the United States. Considerable experience has been gained about the optimal means of public education, and awareness has increased greatly, but a significant workload is generated due to the large numbers of normal persons who have to be seen and reassured.

Excessive sun damage can be prevented with commercially available sunscreens. Sunscreens have protected against further development of UV-induced papillomas in hairless mice, and it is possible that the same is true for humans, but some questions remain unanswered about sunscreen use for humans.[363] Increased pigmentation in persons with white skin could be an alternative approach. Several laboratories are experimenting with a melanocyte-stimulating hormone analog, which produces greater melanization of the skin after topical or systemic application.[364]

Another possible approach is the reversal of actinic damage before the development of skin cancers. It is thought that UV-induced photoaging is a precursor of actinic keratosis, which is a precursor of nonmelanoma skin cancers. By reversing photoaging, it may be possible to prevent development of nonmelanoma skin cancers. Even delay in progression to the malignant stage could be valuable. It is reported that after 1 year of using UV protection measures, approximately 25% of actinic keratoses are reversed.[66] Daily topical use of retinoic acid (0.1%) has reversed the aging process of facial skin over a period of 4 to 5 months.[365]

Work is in progress to develop more effective modes of therapy for skin cancers, including the development of newer types of lasers for the management of precancerous and cancerous skin lesions and the use of newer biologic agents, such as interferon. It is certain that over the next few years other biologic agents will be used in the treatment of skin cancers. Further development is needed of photodynamic therapy, specifically the use of hematoporphyrin derivative and UV light. The use of gene therapy is in the preclinical stages and may soon become available for clinical trails. Culturing of basal cell carcinoma opens a new avenue for the study of the biochemistry and molecular biology of the disease.[366] Drugs can be tested on these cell lines before going into clinical trials.

FINANCIAL CONSIDERATIONS OF TREATMENT

The cost of management and care of precancerous and malignant cutaneous diseases caused by UV light accounts for a significant portion of the health care budget. More than 600,000 new skin cancers (nonmelanoma) are recognized and treated in the United States each year at a cost of more than 1 billion dollars. Because the aging population is increasing in size, because of uncertainties about the biologic effect of depletion of the ozone, and because of the continued cultural and habitual exposure to sunlight, we will continue to be faced with increasing numbers of skin cancers and associated expenses.

The prudent approach is to develop new measures to prevent further depletion of the ozone, increase public and medical practitioners' awareness about skin cancers and the importance of early diagnosis, and continue investigations into prevention, control, and care of more advanced disease.

REFERENCES

1. Boring CC, Squires TS, Tong T. Cancer Statistics, 1992. CA 1992;42:19–38.
2. Yiannias JA, Goldberg LH, Carter-Campbell S, et al. The ratio of basal cell carcinoma to squamous cell carcinoma in Houston, Texas. J Dermatol Surg Oncol 1988;14:886–889.
3. MacKie RM, Elwood JM, Hawk JLM. Links between exposure to ultraviolet radiation and skin cancer. J R Coll Physicians Lond 1987;21:91–96.
4. Council on Scientific Affairs. Harmful effects of ultraviolet radiation. JAMA 1989;262:380–384.
5. National Institutes of Health. Summary of the consensus development conference on sunlight, ultraviolet radiation, and the skin. J Am Acad Dermatol 1991;24:608–612.
6. Kripke ML, Sass ER, eds. Anitgenicity of murine skin tumors induced by UV light. JNCI 1974;53:1333–1336.
7. Kripke ML. Immunology and photocarcinogenesis. J Am Acad Dermatol 1986;14:149–155.
8. Brookes P, Lawley PD. Evidence for binding of polynuclear aromatic hydrocarbons to the nucleic acids of mouse skin: Relation between carcinogenic hydrocarbons and their binding to DNA. Nature 1964;202:781–784.
9. Marks F, Furstenberger G. Experimental evidence that skin carcinogenesis is a multistep phenomenon. Br J Dermatol 1986;115:1.
10. Jones SK, MacKie RM, Hole DJ, et al. Further evidence for the safety of tar in psoriasis. Br J Dermatol 1985;113:97–101.
11. Yuspa SH. Chemical carcinogenesis related to the skin. Prog Dermatol 1981;15:1.
12. Potter M. Percivall Pott's contribution to cancer research. NCI Monogr 1963;10:1.
13. Yeh S. Relative incidence of skin cancer in Chinese in Taiwan with special reference to arsenical cancer. NCI Monogr 1963;10:81.
14. Traenkle HL. X-ray induced cancer in man. NCI Monogr 1963;10:423–440.

15. Bowers RF, Young JM. Carcinoma arising in scars, osteomyelitis and fistulae. Arch Surg 1960;80:564.
16. Cruickshank AH, McConnell EM, Miller DG. Malignant degeneration in burn scars, chronic ulcers and sinuses. J Clin Pathol 1963;16:573.
17. Giblin T, Pickrell K, Pitts W, et al. Malignant degeneration in burn scars: Marjolin's ulcer. Ann Surg 1965;162:291.
18. Sedlin ED, Fleming JL. Epidermoid carcinoma arising in chronic osteomyelitic foci. J Bone Joint Surg [Am] 1963;45:827.
19. Hejna WF. Squamous cell carcinoma developing in the chronic draining sinuses of osteomyelitis. Cancer 1965;18:128.
20. Mustoe T, Upton J, Marcellino V, et al. Carcinoma in chronic pressure sores: A fulminant disease process. Plast Reconstr Surg 1986;77:116.
21. Rattner H, Bluefarb SM, Johnson HJ. Squamous cell epithelioma superimposed on a patch of chronic discoid lupus erythematosus. Arch Dermatol 1956;73:601.
22. Lutzner MA. The human papillomaviruses. Arch Dermatol 1983;119:631.
23. Ikengerg H, Gissmann L, Gross G, et al. Human papillomavirus type 16-related DNA in genital Bowen's disease and in bowenoid papulosis. Int J Cancer 1983;32:563–565.
24. Oblek S, Jablonska S, Orth G. HPV-associated intraepithelial neoplasia of external genitalia. Clin Dermatol 1985;3:104.
25. Meanswell CA, Cox MF, Blackledge G, et al. HPV 16 DNA in normal and malignant cervical epithelium: Implications for the aetiology and behavior of cervical neoplasia. Lancet 1987;1:703–707.
26. . Human papillomaviruses and cervical cancer: A fresh look at the evidence. Lancet 1987;1:725–726.
27. Ostrow RS, Bender M, Niimura M, et al. Human papillomavirus DNA in cutaneous primary and metastasized squamous cell carcinomas from patients with epidermodysplasia verruciformis. Proc Natl Acad Sci USA 1982;79:1634.
28. Walder BK, Robertson MR, Jeremy D. Skin cancer and immunosuppression. Lancet 1971;2:1282.
29. Hoxtell EO, Mandel JS, Murray SS, et al. Incidence of skin carcinoma after renal transplantation. Arch Dermatol 1977;113:436.
30. Koranda FC, Dehmel EM, Kahn G, et al. Cutaneous complications in immunosuppressed renal homograft recipients. JAMA 1974;229:419.
31. Penn I, Halgrimson CG, Starzl TE. De novo malignant tumors in organ transplant recipients. Transplant Proc 1971;3:773.
32. Westburg SP, Stone OJ. Multiple cutaneous squamous cell carcinomas during immunosuppressive therapy. Arch Dermatol 1973;107:893.
33. Berg JW. The incidence of multiple primary cancers: 1. Development of further cancers in patients with lymphoma, leukemias and myeloma. JNCI 1967;38:741.
34. Turner JE, Callen JP. Aggressive behavior of squamous cell carcinoma in a patient with preceding lymphocytic lymphoma. J Am Acad Dermatol 1981;4:446.
35. Weimar VM, Ceilley RI, Goeken JA. Aggressive behavior of basal and squamous cell cancers in patients with chronic lymphocytic lymphoma or chronic lymphocytic leukemia. J Dermatol Surg Oncol 1979;5:609.
36. Gitlin MC, Pirozzi DJ. The sign of Leser-Trelat. Arch Dermatol 1975;111:792–793.
37. Gallimore AP. Malignant transformation of a clonal seborrhoeic keratosis. Br J Dermatol 1991;124:287–290.
38. Su WPD. Histopathologic varieties of epidermal nevus. Am J Dermatopathol 1982;4: 161–170.
39. Solomon LM, Fretzin DF, Dewald RL. The epidermal nevus syndrome. Arch Dermatol 1977;113:767–769.
40. Levin A, Amazon K, Rywlin AM. A squamous cell carcinoma that developed in an epidermal nevus: Report of a case and review of the literature. Am J Dermatopathol 1984;6:51–55.
41. Degos R, Civatte J. Clear cell acanthoma. Experience of 8 years. Br J Dermatol 1970;83: 248–254.
42. Trau H, Fisher BK, Schewach-Millet M. Multiple clear cell acanthoma. Arch Dermatol 1980;116:433–434.
43. Carter VH, Constantine VS. Kryle's disease: I. Clinical findings in five cases and review of the literature. Arch Dermatol 1968;97:624–632.
44. Constantine VS, Carter VH. Kryle's disease: II. Histopathologic findings in five cases and review of the literature. Arch Dermatol 1968;97:633–639.
45. Gracia-Bravo B, Rodriguez-Pichardo A, Camacho F. Uraemic follicular hyperkeratosis. Clin Exp Dermatol 1985;10:448–454.
46. Hood AF, Hardegen GL, Zarate AR, et al. Kyrle's disease in patients with chronic renal failure. Arch Dermatol 1982;118:85–88.
47. Delacretaz J. Keratotic basal cell carcinoma arising from an epidermoid cyst. J Dermatol Surg Oncol 1977;3:310–311.
48. McDonald LW. Carcinomatous change in cysts of skin. Arch Dermatol 1963;87:208–211.
49. Shelly WB, Wood MG. Occult Bowen's disease in keratinous cysts. Br J Dermatol 1981;105:105–108.
50. Cotton DWK, Kirkham N, Young BJJ. Immunoperoxidase antikeratin staining of epidermal and pilar cysts. Br J Dermatol 1984;111:63–68.
51. McGavran MN, Binnington B. Keratinous cysts of the skin: Identification and differentiation of pilar cysts from epidermal cysts. Arch Dermatol 1966;94:499–508.
52. Baptista AP, Silva LGE, Born MC. Proliferating trichilemmal cyst. J Cutan Pathol 1983;10:178–187.
53. Brownstein MN, Arluk DK. Proliferating trichilemmal cyst: A simulant of squamous cell carcinoma. Cancer 1981;48:1207–1214.
54. Saida T, Oohara K, Hori Y, et al. Development of a malignant proliferating trichilemmal cyst in a patient with multiple trichilemmal cysts. Dermatologica 1983;166:203–208.
55. Birt AR, Hogg GR, Dube WJ. Herediatry multiple fibrofolliculomas with trichodiscomas and acrochorodons. Arch Dermatol 1977;113:1674–1677.
56. Fujita WH, Barr RJ, Headley JL. Multiple fibrofolliculmas with trichodiscomas and acrochordons. Arch Dermatol 1981;117:32–35.
57. Ubogy-Rainey Z, James WD, Lupton GP, et al. Fibrofolliculomas, trichodiscomas, and acrochordons the Birt-Hogg-Dube syndrome. J Am Acad Dermatol 1987;16:452–457.
58. Copeman PWM, Wilson JE. Pigmented hairy epidermal nevus (Becker). Arch Dermatol 1965;92:249–251.
59. Tate PR, Hadge SJ, Owen LG. A quantitative study of melanocytes in Becker's nevus. J Cutan Pathol 1980;7:404–409.
60. Tanay A, Mehregan AH. Warty dyskeratoma. Dermatologica 1969;138:155–164.
61. Harriest TJ, Murphy GF, Mihm MC Jr. Oral warty dyskeratoma. Arch Dermatol 1980;116:929–931.
62. Marks R. Non-melanoma skin cancer and solar keratoses in Australia. Eur J Epidemiol 1985;1:319–322.
63. Montgomery H. Precancerous dermatosis and epithelioma in situ. Arch Dermatol Syphilol 1939;39:387.
64. Brownstein MH, Rabinowitz AD. The precursors of cutaneous squamous cell carcinoma. Int J Dermatol 1979;18:1–16.
65. Bercovitch L. Topical chemotherapy of actinic keratoses of the upper extremity with tretinoin and 5-fluorouracil: A double-blind controlled study. Br J Dermatol 1987;116: 549–552.
66. Marks R, Foley P, Goodman G, et al. Spontaneous remission of solar keratoses. The case for conservative management. Br J Dermatol 1986;115:649–655.
67. Rahbari H, Pinkus H. Large cell acanthoma: One of the actinic keratoses. Arch Dermatol 1978;114:49–52.
68. Rabinowitz AD. Multiple large cell acanthoma. J Am Acad Dermatol 1983;8:840–845.
69. Sanchez Yus E, De Diego V, Urrutia S. Large cell acanthoma. Am J Dermatopathol 1988;10:197–208.
70. Santa Cruz DJ. Chondrodermatitis nodularis helicis: A transepidermal perforating disorder. J Cutan Pathol 1980;7:70–76.
71. Goette DK. Chondrodermatitis nodularis chronica helicis: A perforating necrotic granuloma. J Am Acad Dermatol 1980;2:148–154.
72. Bard JW. Chondrodermatitis nodularis chronica helicis. Dermatologica 1981;163:376.
73. Brownstein MH, Shapiro EE. Trichilemmal horn: Cutaneous horn overlying trichilemmoma. Clin Exp Dermatol 1979;4:59–63.
74. Sandbank M. Basal cell carcinoma at the base of cutaneous horn (cornu cutaneum). Arch Dermatol 1971;104:97–98.
75. Yu RCH, Pryce DW, Macfarlane AW, et al. A histopathological study of 643 cutaneous horns. Br J Dermatol 1991;124:449–452.
76. Goldschmidt H, Sherwin WK. Reactions to ionizing radiation. J Am Acad Dermatol 1980;3:551–579.
77. Lazar P, Cullen SI. Basal cell epithelioma and chronic radiodermatitis. Arch Dermatol 1963;88:172–175.
78. McGibbon DH. Malignant epidermal tumors. J Cutan Pathol 1985;12:224–238.
79. Seo IS, Warner TFCS, Warren JS, et al. Cutaneous postirradiation sarcoma. Ultrastructural evidence of pluripotential mesenchymal cell derivation. Cancer 1985;56: 761–767.
80. Souba WW, McKenna RJ Jr, Meis J, et al. Radiation-induced sarcomas of th chest wall. Cancer 1986;57:610–615.
81. Kao GF. Carcinoma arising in Bowen's disease. Arch Dermatol 1986;122:1124–1126.
82. Ackerman AB. Bowenoid papulosis. J Am Acad Dermatol 1981;4:608.
83. Lutzner MA, Blanchet-Bradon C, Orth G. Clinical observations, virologic studies, and treatment trials in patients with epidermodysplasia verruciformis, a disease induced by specific human papillomaviruses. J Invest Dermatol 1984;83:18–25S.
84. Bettley FR, O'Shea JA. The absorption of arsenic and its relation to carcinoma. Br J Dermatol 1975;92:563–568.
85. Graham JH, Helwig EB. Bowen's disease and its relationship to systemic cancer. Arch Dermatol 1959;80:133–159.
86. Callen JP, Headington J. Bowen's amd non-Bowen's squamous intraepidermal neoplasia of the skin. Arch Dermatol 1980;116:422–426.
87. Arbesman H, Ransohoff DF. Is Bowen's disease a predictor for the development of internal malignancy? JAMA 1987;257:516–518.
88. Graham JH, Helwig EB. Erythroplasia of Queyrat. Cancer 1973;32:1396–1414.
89. Goette DK. Erythroplasia of Queyrat. Arch Dermatol 1974;110:271–273.
90. Mikail GR. Cancers, precancers, and pseudocancers on the male genetalia. J Dermatol Surg Oncology 1980;6:1027–1035.
91. Obalek SJ, Jablonska S, Beaudenon MB, et al. Bowenoid papulosis of the male and female genitalia: Risk of cervical neoplasia. J Am Acad Dermatol 1986;14:433–444.
92. Wade TR, Kopf AW, Ackermann AB. Bowenoid papulosis of the penis. Cancer 1978;42: 1890–1903.
93. Wade TR, Kopf AW, Ackermann AB. Bowenoid papulosis of the genitalia. Arch Dermatol 1979;115:306–308.
94. Schwartz RA, Janniger CK. Bowenoid papulosis. J Am Acad Dermatol 1991;24:261–264.
95. Karatochvil FJ, Cioffi GA, Auclair PL, et al. Virus-associated dysplasia (bowenoid papulosis?) of the oral cavity. Oral Surg Oral Med Oral Pathol 1989;68:312–316.
96. Patterson JW, Kao GF, Graham JH, et al. Bowenoid papulosis: A clinicopathologic study with ultrastructural observations. Cancer 1986;57:823–836.
97. Rudlinger R, Buchmann P. HPV 16-positive bowenoid papulosis and squamous cell carcinoma of the anus in an HIV-positive man. Dis Colon Rectum 1989;32:1042–1045.
98. Bonnekoh B, Mahrle G, Steigleder GK. Transition of bowenoid papulosis (HPV-16) into cutaneous squamous cell carcinoma in two patients. Z Hautkr 1987;62:773–784.
99. Skinner MS, Sternberg WH, Ichinose H, et al. Spontaneous regression of bowenoid atypia of the vulva. Obstet Gynecol 1973;42:40–46.

100. Friedrich EG. Reversible vulvar atypia: A case report. Obstet Gynecol 1972;39:173–181.
101. Berger BW, Hori Y. Multicentric Bowen's disease of the genitalia: Spontaneous regression of lesions. Arch Dermatol 1978;114:1698–1699.
102. Landthaler M, Haina D, Brunner R, et al. Laser therapy of bowenoid papulosis and Bowen's disease. J Dermatol Surg Oncol 1986;12:1253–1257.
103. Gross G, Roussaki A, Papendick U. Efficacy of interferons on bowenoid papulosis and other precancerous lesions. J Invest Dermatol 1990;95:152S–157S.
104. Lutzner M. Epidermodysplasia verruciformis: An autosomal recessive disease characterized by viral warts and skin cancer. Bull Cancer 1978;65:169–182.
105. Androphy E, Dvoretzky I, Lowry D. X-linked inheritance of epidermodysplasia verruciformis. Arch Dermatol 1981;121:864–868.
106. Jablonska S, Orth G, Jarzabek-Chorzelska M. Twenty-one years of follow-up studies of familial epidermodysplasia verruciformis. Dermatologica 1979;158:309.
107. Glinski W, Obalek S, Jablonska S, et al. T cell defect in patients with epidermodysplasia verruciformis due to human papilomavirus type 3 and 5. Dermatologica 1981;162: 141–147.
108. Majewski S, Skopinska-Rozewska E, Jablonska S, et al. Partial defect of cell mediated immunity in patients with epidermodysplasia verruciformis. J Am Acad Dermatol 1986;15:996.
109. Majewski S, Malejczyk J, Jablonska S, et al. Natural cell-mediated cytotoxicity against various target cells in patients with epidermodysplasia verruciformis. J Am Acad Dermatol 1990;22:423–427.
110. Obalek S, Glinski W, Hagtek M, et al. Comparative studies on cell-mediated immunity in patients with different warts. Dermatologica 1980;161:73–83.
111. Pfister H, Iftner TH, Fuchs PG. Papillomaviruses from epidermodysplasia verruciformis patients and renal allograft recients. Papillomaviruses: Molecular and clinical aspects. UCLA Symp Mol Cell Biol 1985;32:85–100.
112. Rudlinger R, Smith JW, Bunney MH, et al. Human papillomavirus infections in a group of renal transplant recipients. Br J Dermatol 1986;115:681–692.
113. Tanigaki T, Kanda R, Sato K. Epidermodysplasia verruciformis (L-L, 1922) in a patient with systemic lupus erythematous. Arch Dermatol Res 1986;278:247–248.
114. Gross G, Ellinger K, Roussaki A, et al. Epidermodysplasia verruciformis in a patient with Hodgkin's disease: Characterization of a new papillomavirus type and interferon treatment. J Invest Dermatol 1988;91:957–962.
115. Claudy A, Touraine J, Mitanne D. Epidermodysplasia verruciformis induced by a new human papillomavirus (HPV-8): Report of a case without immune dysfunction. Effects of treatment with an aromatic retinoid. Arch Dermatol Res 1982;27:213–219.
116. Androphy E, Dvoretzky I, Maluish A, et al. Response of warts in epidermodysplasia verruciformis to treatment with systemic and intralesional alpha interferon. J Am Acad Dermatol 1984;11:197–202.
117. Waldron CA, Shafer WG. Leukoplakia revisited. A clinicopathologic study of 3256 oral leukoplakias. Cancer 1975;36:1386–1392.
118. Silverman S Jr, Gorsky M, Lozada F. Oral leukoplakia and malignant transformation. A follow-up study of 257 patients. Cancer 1984;53:563–568.
119. Wilson JE. Naevus sebaceous. Br J Dermatol 1970;82:99–117.
120. Morioka S. The natural history of nevus sebaceous. J Cutan Pathol 1985;12:200–213.
121. Domingo J, Helwig EB. Malignant neoplasms associated with the nevus sebaceous of Jadassohn. J Am Acad Dermatol 1979;1:545–556.
122. Chernosky ME. Porokeratosis. Arch Dermatol 1986;122:869–870.
123. Chernosky ME, Anderson DE. Disseminated superficial actinic porokeratosis. Genetic aspects. Arch Dermatol 1969;99:408–412.
124. Schwarz T, Seiser A, Gschnait F. Disseminated superficial "actinic" porokeratosis. J Am Acad Dermatol 1984;11:724–730.
125. MacMillian AL, Roberts SOB. Porokeratosis of Mibelli after renal transplantation. Br J Dermatol 1974;90:45–54.
126. Lederman JS, Sober AJ, Lederman GS. Immunosuppression: A cause of porokeratosis? J Am Acad Dermatol 1985;13:75–79.
127. Neumann RA, Knobler RM, Metze, et al. Disseminated superficial porokeratosis and immunosuppression. Br J Dermatol 1988;119:375–380.
128. Brodkin RH, Ricket RR, Fuller FW, et al. Malignant disseminated porokeratosis (DSAP). Arch Dermatol 1987;123:1521–1526.
129. Rahbari H, Cordero AA, Mehregan AH. Linear porokeratosis. Arch Dermatol 1974;109: 526–528.
130. Shaw JC, White CR Jr. Porokeratosis plantaris, plamaris et disseminata. J Am Acad Dermatol 1984;11:454–460.
131. Himmelstein R, Lynnfield YL. Punctate porokeratosis. Arch Dermatol 1984;120:263–264.
132. Coskey RJ, Mehregan A. Bowen disease associated with porokeratosis of Mibelli. Arch Dermatol 1975;111:1480–1481.
133. Lozinski AZ, Fisher BK, Walter JB, et al. Metastatic squamous cell carcinoma in linear porokeratosis of Mibelli. J Am Acad Dermatol 1987;16:448–451.
134. Shrum JR, Cooper PH, Greer KE, et al. Squamous cell carcinoma in disseminated superficial actinic porokeratosis. J Am Acad Dermatol 1982;6:58–62.
135. Pinkus H. Premalignant fibroepithelial tumors of the skin. Arch Dermatol 1953;67: 598–615.
136. Rook A, Whimster I. Keratoacanthoma. A 30-year retrospect. Br J Dermatol 1979;100: 41–47.
137. Walinsky S, Silvers DV, et al. Spontaneous regression of a giant keratoacanthoma. Cancer 1978;41:12–16.
138. Golddenhersh MA, Olsen TG. Invasive squamous cell carcinoma initially diagnosed as giant keratoacanthoma. J Am Acad Dermatol 1984;10:372–378.
139. Chalet MD, Connors RC, Ackerman AB. Squamous cell carcinoma vs. keratoacanthoma: Criteria for histologic differentiation. J Dermatol Surg 1975;1:16–17.
140. Kern WH, McCray MK. The histopathologic differentiation of keratoacanthoma and squamous cell carcinoma of the skin. J Cutan Pathol 1980;7:318–325.
141. Sullivan JJ, Donoghue MF, Kynaston B, et al. Multiple keratoacanthomas. Aust J Dermatol 1980;21:16–24.
142. Winkelmann RK, Brown J. Generalized eruptive keratoacanthoma. Arch Dermatol 1968;97:615–623.
143. Domarus HV, Stevens PJ. Metastatic basal cell carcinoma: Report of five cases and review of 170 cases in the literature. J Am Acad Dermatol 1984;10:1043–1060.
144. Rahbari H, Mehregan AH. Basal cell epithelioma (carcinoma) in childern and adolescents. Cancer 1982;49:350–353.
145. Plosila M, Kiistala R, Niemi KM. The Bazex syndrome: Follicular atrophoderma with multiple basal cell carcinomas, hypotrichosis, and hypohidrosis. Clin Exp Dermatol 1981;6:31–37.
146. Gorlin RJ. Nevoid basal cell carcinoma syndrome. J Med 1992;66:98–113.
147. Khatri ML, Shafi M, Mashina A. Xeroderma pigmentosum. J Am Acad Dermatol 1992;26: 75–78.
148. Giles G, Marks R, Foley P. The incidence of non-melanocytic skin cancer in Australia. Br Med J 1988;296:13–17.
149. Kuflik EG. Clinical variants of basal cell carcinoma. Cutis 1981;28:403–408.
150. Miller SJ. Biology of basal cell carcinoma (part I). J Am Acad Dermatol 1991;24:1–13.
151. Miller SJ. Biology of basal cell carcinoma (part II). J Am Acad Dermatol 1991;24: 161–175.
152. Sexton M, Jones DB, Maloney ME. Histologic pattern analysis of basal cell carcinoma. J Am Acad Dermatol 1990;23:1118–1126.
153. Borel DM. Cutaneous basosquamous carcinoma. Review of the literature and report of 35 cases. Arch Pathol 1973;95:293–297.
154. Gormley DE, Hirsch P. Aggresive basal cell carcinoma of the scalp. Arch Dermatol 1978;114:782–783.
155. Jacobs GH, Rippey JJ, Altini M. Prediction of aggressive behavior in basal cell carcinoma. Cancer 1982;49:533–537.
156. Urbach F. Geographic distribution of skin cancer. J Surg Oncol 1971;3:219.
157. Hall AF. Relationship of sunlight, complexion and heredity to skin carcinogenesis. Arch Dermatol Syphilol 1950;61:589.
158. Myskowski PL, Pollack MS,, Schorr E, et al. Human leukocyte antigen associations in basal cell carcinoma. J Am Acad Dermatol 1985;12:997–1000.
159. Robinson JK. Risk of developing another basal cell carcinoma: A 5-year prospective study. Cancer 1987;60:118.
160. Abram H, Barsky S. Pigmented basal cell epithelioma arising in the scar of an onchocerciasis nodule. Int J Dermatol 1984;23:658–660.
161. Rich JD, Shesol BF, Horne DW. Basal cell carcinoma arising in a smallpox vaccination site. J Clin Pathol 1980;33:134–135.
162. Korula R, Hughes CF. Squamous cell carcinoma arising in a sternotomy scar. Ann Thorac Surg 1991;51:667–669.
163. Schwartz RA, Burgess GH, Milgrom H. Breast carcinoma and basal cell epitheliomaa after x-ray therapy for hirsutism. Cancer 1979;44:1601–1605.
164. Anderson NP, Anderson HE. Development of basal cell epitheliomas as a consequence of radiodermatitis. Arch Dermatol Syphilol 1951;63:586–596.
165. Sexton M, Jones DB, Maloney ME. Histologic pattern analysis of basal cell carcinoma. Study of a series of 1039 consecutive neoplasms. J Am Acad Dermatol 1990;23:1118–1126.
166. Pollack SW, Goslen JB, Sheretz, et al. The biology of basal cell carcinoma. A review. J Am Acad Dermatol 1982;7:569–577.
167. Brooke JD, Fitzpatrick JE, Golitz LE. Papillary mesenchymal bodies: A histologic finding useful in differentiating trichoepitheliomas from basal cell carcinomas. J Am Acad Dermatol 1989;21:523–528.
168. Lo JS, Snow SN, Reizner GT, et al. Metastatic basal cell carcinoma: Report of twelve cases with a review of the literature. J Am Acad Dermatol 1991;24:715–719.
169. Drake LA, Ceilley RI, Cornelison RL, et al. Guidelines of care for basal cell carcinoma. J Am Acad Dermatol 1992;26:117–120.
170. McGrouther DAM. Treatment of basal cell carcinoma. A plastic surgeon's view. Br J Dermatol 1987;117:399.
171. Spiller WF, Spiller RF. Treatment of basal cell carcinoma by curettage and electrodesiccation. J Am Acad Dermatol 1984;11:808.
172. Cott RE, Wood MG, Johnson BL. Use of curettage and shave excision in office practice. J Am Acad Dermatol 1987;16:1243–1251.
173. Swanson N. Mohs' surgery. Arch Dermatol 1983;119:761–773.
174. Hruza GJ. Mohs' micrographic surgery. Otolaryngol Clin North Am 1990;23:845–864.
175. Mikhail GR. Mohs' micrographic surgery. Philadelphia: WB Saunders, 1991.
176. Greenway HT, Cornell RC, Tanner DJ, et al. Treatment of basal cell carcinoma with intralesional interferon. J Am Acad Dermatol 1986;15:437–443.
177. Lindelof B, Sigurgeirsson B, Tegner E, et al. PUVA and cancer: A large-scale epidemiological study. Lancet 1991;338:91–93.
178. Chaung TY, Heinrich LA, Schultz MD, et al. PUVA and skin cancer. J Am Acad Dermatol 1992;26:173–177.
179. Aubry F, McGibbon B. Risk factors of squamous cell carcinoma of the skin: A case-control study in the Montreal region. Cancer 1985;55:907–911.
180. Kwa RE, Campana K, Moy RL. Biology of cutaneous squamous cell carcinoma. J Am Acad Dermatol 1992;26:1–26.
181. Johnson TM, Rowe DE, Nelson BR, et al. Squamous cell carcinoma of the skin (excluding lip and oral mucosa). J Am Acad Dermatol 1992;26:467–484.
182. Luande J, Henschke CI, Mohammed N. The Tanzanian human albino skin: Natural history. Cancer 1985;55:1823.

183. Stern RS, Laird N, Melski J, et al. Cutaneous squamous cell carcinoma in patients treated with PUVA. N Engl J Med 1984;310:1156–1161.
184. Henseler T, Christophers E, Honigsmann H, et al. Skin tumors in the European PUVA study. J Am Acad Dermatol 1987;16:108–116.
185. Benton EC, Bunney MH, Barr BB, et al. Skin cancers and their relationship to human papilloma virus infection in a group of renal allograft recipients. Br J Dermatol [Abstract] 1988;118:270.
186. Arhelger SW, Kremem AJ. Arsenical epitheliomas of medicinal origin. Surgery 1951;30: 977.
187. Eliezri YD, Silverstein SJ, Nuovo GJ. Occurrence of human papillomavirus type 16 DNA in cutaneous squamous and basal cell neoplasms. J Am Acad Dermatol 1990;23: 836–842.
188. Obalek S, Favre M, Jablonska S, et al. Human papillomavirus type 2-associated basal cell carcinoma in two immunosuppressed patients. Arch Dermatol 1988;124:930–934.
189. Eliezri YD, Silverstein SJ, Nuovo GJ. Occurrence of human papillomavirus type 16 DNA in cutaneous squamous and basal cell neoplasms. J Am Acad Dermatol 1990;23: 836–842.
190. Headington JT. Verrucous carcinoma. Cutis 1978;21:207–211.
191. Okagaki T, Clark BA, Zachow KR, et al. Presence of human papillomavirus in verrucous carcinoma (Ackerman) of the vagina. Immunocytochemical, ultrastructural and DNA hybridization studies. Arch Pathol Lab Med 1984;108:567–570.
192. Kao G, Graham JH, Helwig EB. Carcinoma cuniculatum. Cancer 1982;49:2395–2403.
193. Broders S. Practical points in the microsurgic grading of carcinoma. N Y State J Med 1932;32:667–680.
194. Kahn H, Baumal R, From L. Role of immunohistochemistry in the diagnosis of undifferentiated tumors involving the skin. J Am Acad Dermatol 1986;14:1063.
195. Robbinson JK. What are adequate treatment and follow-up care for nonmelanoma cutaneous cancer? Arch Dermatol 1987;123:331–332.
196. Mohs FE, Sahl W. Chemosurgery for verrucous carcinoma. J Dermatol Surg Oncol 1979;5:302.
197. Toker C. Trabecular carcinoma of the skin. Arch Dermatol 1972;105:107–110.
198. Bayrou O, Avril MF, Charpentier P, et al. Primary neuroendocrine carcinoma of the skin. J Am Acad Dermatol 1991;24:198–207.
199. Pilloti S, Rilke F, Bartoli C, et al. Clinicopathologic correlations of cutaneous neuroendocrine Merkel cell carcinoma. J Clin Oncol 1988;6:1863–1873.
200. Goepfert H, Rammler D, Silva E, et al. Merkel cell carcinoma (endocrine carcinoma of the skin) of the head and neck. Arch Otolaryngol Head Neck Surg 1984;110:707–712.
201. Meland NB, Jackson IT. Merkel cell tumor diagnosis, prognosis, and management. Plast Reconstr Surg 1986;77:632–638.
202. Hitchcock CL, Bland KI, Laney RG,III, et al. Neuroendocrine (Merkel cell) carcinoma of the skin: Its natural history, diagnosis, and treatment. Ann Surg 1988;207:201–207.
203. Kayashima K, Ono T, Johno M, et al. Spontaneous regression in Merkel cell (neuroendocrine) carcinoma of the skin. Arch Dermatol 1991;127:550–553.
204. O'Rourke MGE, Bell JR. Merkel cell tumor with spontaneous regression. J Dermatol Surg Oncol 1986;12:994–997.
205. Cotlar AM, Gate JO, Gibbs FA. Merkel cell carcinoma: Combined surgery and radiation therapy. Am Surg 1986;52:159–164.
206. Shaw JHF, Rumball E. Merkel cell tumor: Clinical behavior and treatment. Br J Surg 1991;78:138–142.
207. Crown J, Lipzstein R, Cohen S, et al. Chemotherapy of metastatic Merkel cell cancer. Cancer Invest 1991;9:129–132.
208. Cotton D. Troublesome tumors: I. Adnexal tumors of the skin. J Clin Pathol 1991;44: 543–548.
209. Hashimoto K, Mehregan AH, Kumakiri M. Tumors of skin apendages. Boston: Butterworths, 1987.
210. Headington JT. Tumors of the hair follicle. Am J Pathol 1976;85:480–505.
211. Spielogel RL, Austin C, Ackerman AB. Inverted follicular keratosis is not a specific keratosis but a verruca vulgaris (or seborrheic keratosis) with squamous eddies. Am J Dermatol 1983;5:427–442.
212. Starink TM, Kisch LS, Meijer CJ. Familial multiple trichodiscomas. Arch Dermatol 1985;121:888–891.
213. Mehregan AH. Tumor of follicular infundibulum. Dermatologica 1971;142:177–183.
214. Arico M, LaRocca E, Noto G, et al. Proliferating trichilemmal tumor with lymph node metastases. Br J Dermatol 1989;121:793–797.
215. Ten Seldam REJ. Tricholemmocarcinoma. Aust J Dermatol 1977;18:62–67.
216. Gray FHR, Helwig EB. Trichofolliculoma. Arch Dermatol 1962;86:619–625.
217. Pelwig G. Sebaceous trichofolliculoma. J Cutan Pathol 1980;7:395–403.
218. Takei Y, Fukushiro S, Ackerman AB. Criteria for histologic differentiation of desmoplastic trichoepithelioma (sclerosing epithelial hamartoma) from morphea-like basal cell carcinoma. Am J Dermatopathol 1985;7:207–221.
219. Wick MR, Coffin CM. Sweat gland and pilar carcinomas. In: Wick MR, ed. Pathology of unusual malignant cutaneous tumors. New York: Marcel Dekker, 1985.
220. Manivel C, Wick MR, Muka K. Pilomatrix carcinoma: An immunohistochemical comparison with benign pilomatrixoma and other benign cutaneous lesions of pilar origin. J Cutan Pathol 1986;13:22–29.
221. Tateyama H, Eimoto T, Tada T, et al. Malignant pilomatricoma. Cancer 1992;69:127–132.
222. Chambers SO. The structure of Fordyce's disease as demonstrated by wax reconstruction. Arch Dermatol Syphilol 1928;18:666–672.
223. Banse-Kupin L, Morales A, Barlow M. Torre's syndrome: Report of two cases and review of the literature. J Am Acad Dermatol 1984;10:803–817.
224. Troy JL, Ackerman AB. Sebaceoma: A distinctive benign neoplasm of adnexal epithelium differentiating toward sebaceous cells. Am J Dermatopathol 1984;6:7–13.
225. Wolfe JT, Wick MR, Campbell RJ. Sebaceous carcinoma of the oculocutaneous adnexa and extraocular skin In: Wick MR, ed. Pathology of unusual malignant cutaneous tumors. New York: Marcel Dekker, 1985:77–106.
226. Wick MR, Goellner JR, Wolfe JT, et al. Adnexal carcinomas of the skin. II. Extraocular sebaceous carcinomas. Cancer 1985;56:1163–1172.
227. Dixon RS, Mikhail GR, Slater HC. Sebaceous carcinoma of the eyelid. J Am Acad Dermatol 1980;3:241–243.
228. Rao NA, Hidayat AA, McLean IW, et al. Sebaceous carcinomas of the ocular adnexa: A clinicopathologic study of 104 cases, with five-year follow-up data. Hum Pathol 1982;13:113–122.
229. Wolfe JT, Yeatts RP, Wick MR, et al. Sebaceous carcinoma of the eyelid. Am J Surg Pathol 1984;8:597–606.
230. King DT, Hirose FM, Gurevitch AW. Sebaceous carcinoma of the skin with visceral metastases. Arch Dermatol 1979;115:862.
231. Pricolo VE, Rodil JV, Vezeridis MP. Extraorbital sebaceous carcinoma. Arch Surg 1985;120:853–855.
232. Pardo FS, Wang CC, Albert D, et al. Sebaceous carcinoma of the ocular adnexa: Radiotherapeutic management. Int J Radiat Oncol Biol Phys 1989;17:643–647.
233. Whittington R, Browning ME, Farrell GR, et al. Radiation therapy and chemotherapy in malignant sweat gland tumors. J Am Acad Dermatol 1986;15:1093–1097.
234. Tan KC, Cheah ST. Surgical treatment of sebaceous carcinoma of eyelids with clinicopathological correlation. Br J Plast Surg 1991;44:117–121.
235. Mehregan AH. Supernumerary nipple. A histologic study. J Cutan Pathol 1981;8:96–104.
236. Hassan MO, Khan MA, Kruse TV. Apocrine cystadenoma. Arch Dermatol 1979;115: 194–200.
237. Numata M, Hosoe S, Itoh N, et al. Syringadenocarcinoma papilliferum. J Cutan Pathol 1985;12:3–7.
238. Shenoy YMV. Malignant perianal papillary hidradenoma. Arch Dermatol 1961;83: 965–967.
239. Guldhammer B, Norgaard T. The differential diagnosis of intraepidermal malignant lesions using immunohistochemistry. Am J Dermatopathol 1986;8:295–301.
240. Ordóñez NG, Awalt H, MacKay B. Mammary and extramammary Paget's disease: An immunochemical and ultrastructural study. Cancer 1987;59:1173–1183.
241. Coldiron BM, Goldsmith BA, Robinson JK. Surgical treatment of extramammary Paget's disease: A report of six cases and a reexamination of Mohs' micrographic surgery compared with conventional surgical excision. Cancer 1991;67:933–938.
242. Rahbari H. Hidroacanthoma simplex: A review of 15 cases. Br J Dermatol 1983;109: 219–225.
243. Ishikawa K. Malignant hidroacanthoma simplex. Arch Dermatol 1971;114:529–532.
244. Strayer DS, Santa Cruz DJ. Carcinoma in situ of the skin: A review of histopathology. J Cutan Pathol 1981;7:244–259.
245. Bottles K, Sagebiel RW, McNutt NS, et al. Malignant eccrine poroma: Case report and review of the literature. Cancer 1984;53:1579–1585.
246. Shaw M, McKee PH, Lowe D, et al. Malignant eccrine poroma. A study of 27 cases. Br J Dermatol 1982;107:675–680.
247. Gschnait F, Horn F, Lindlbauer R, et al. Malignant eccrine poroma. J Cutan Pathol 1980;7:349–353.
248. Hu CH, Marques AS, Winkelmann RK. Dermal duct tumor: A histochemical and electron microscopic study. Arch Dermatol 1978;114:1659–1664.
249. Mishima Y, Marioka S. Oncogenic differentiation of the intraepidermal eccrine sweat duct: Eccrine poroma, poroepithelioma, and porocarcinoma. Dermatologica 1969;138: 238.
250. Pinkus H, Mehregan A. Epidermotropic eccrine carcinoma. Arch Dermatol 1963;88: 597.
251. Bardach H. Hidroacanthoma simplex with in situ porocarcinoma. J Cutan Pathol 1978;5: 236.
252. Hashimoto K, Gross B, Lever W. Syringoma: Histochemical and electron microspic studies. J Invest Dermatol 1966;46:150.
253. Feibelman CE, Maize JC. Clear cell syringoma. A study by conventional and electron microscopy. Am J Dermatopathol 1984;6:139–150.
254. Butterworth T, Strean LP, Beerman H, et al. Syringoma and mongolism. Arch Dermatol 1964;91:483–487.
255. Urban C, Cannon J, Cole R. Eruptive syringomas in Down's syndrome. Arch Dermatol 1981;117:374.
256. Hashimoto K, DiBella RJ, Borsuk GM, et al. Eruptive hidradenoma and syringoma: Histological, histochemical, and electron microspic studies. Arch Dermatol 1967;96: 511–519.
257. Cooper PH, Mills SE, Leonard DD. Sclerosing sweat duct (syringomatous) carcinoma. Am J Surg Pathol 1985;9:422–433.
258. Weber P, Gretzula J, Garland L, et al. Syringoid eccrine carcinoma. J Dermatol Surg Oncol 1987;13:1.
259. Moy RL, Rivkin JE, Lee H, et al. Syringoid eccrine carcinoma. J Am Acad Dermatol 1991;24:864–867.
260. Lipper S, Peiper SC. Sweat gland carcinoma with syringomatous features: A light microscopic and ultrastructural study. Cancer 1979;44:157–163.
261. Mehregan AH, Hashimoto K, Rahbari H. Eccrine adenocarcinoma. A clinico-pathologic study of 35 cases. Arch Dermatol 1983;119:104–114.
262. Headington J. Mixed tumors of skin: Eccrine and apocrine types. Arch Dermatol 1961;84: 989.
263. Hirch P, Helwig EG. Chondroid syringoma. Mixed tumor of the skin salivary gland type. Arch Dermatol 1961;84:835–847.

264. Botha JBC, Kahn LB. Aggressive chondroid syringoma. Report of a case in an unusual location and with local recurrence. Arch Dermatol 1978;114:954–955.
265. Harrist TJ, Aretz TH, Mihm MC Jr, et al. Cutaneous malignant mixed tumor. Arch Dermatol 1981;117:719–724.
266. Hilton JMN, Blackwell JB. Metastasizing chondroid syringoma. J Pathol 1973;109: 167–170.
267. Webb JN, Stott WG. Malignant chondroid syringoma of the thigh. Report of a case with electron microscopy of the tumour. J Pahtol 1975;116:43–46.
268. Redono C, Rocamora A, Villoria F, et al. Malignant mixed tumor of the skin. Malignant chondroid syringoma. Cancer 1982;49:1690–1696.
269. Matz LR, McCully DJ, Stokes BAR. Metastasizing chondroid syringoma: Case report. Pathology 1969;1:77.
270. Ishimura E, Iwamoto H, Kobashi Y, et al. Malignant chondroid syringoma. Report of a case with widespread metastasis and review of the pertinenet literature. Cancer 1983;52:1966–1973.
271. Cordero AA, Montes LF. Eccrine hidrocystoma. J Cutan Pathol 1976;3:292–293.
272. Mambo NC. Eccrine spiradenoma: Clinical and pathologic study of 49 tumors. J Cutan Pathol 1983;10:312–320.
273. Tsur H, Lipskier E, Fisher BK. Multiple linear spiradenomas. Plast Reconstruct Surg 1981;68:100–102.
274. Schmoeckel C, Burg G. Congenital spiradenoma. Am J Dermatopathol 1992;10:541–545.
275. Evans HL, Daniel Su WP, Smith L, et al. Carcinoma arising in eccrine spiradenoma. Cancer 1979;43:1881–1884.
276. Cooper PH, Frierson HF Jr, Morrison G. Malignant transformation of eccrine spiradenoma. Arch Dermatol 1985;121:1445.
277. Dabska M. Malignant transformation of eccrine spiradenoma. Pol Med J 1972;11:388.
278. Yaremchuck MJ, Elias LS, Graham RR, et al. Sweat gland carcinoma of the hand: Two cases od malignant eccrine spiradenoma. J Hand Surg 1984;9A:910–914.
279. Keasbey LE, Hadley GC. Clear cell hidradenoma. Three cases with widespread metastases. Cancer 1954;7:934–952.
280. Kersting DW. Clear cell hidradenoma and hidradenocarcinoma. Arch Dermatol 1963;87: 323–333.
281. Hernandez-Perez E, Cruz FA. Clear cell hidradenocarcinoma. Dermatologica 1976;153: 249–252.
282. Headington JT, Neiderhuber JE, Beals TF. Malignant clear cell acrospiroma. Cancer 1978;41:641.
283. Hernandez-Perez E, Cruz FA. Clear cell hidroadenocarcinoma: Report of an unsual case. Dermatologic 1976;153:249.
284. Czarnecki DB, Aarons I, Dowling JP, et al. Malignant clear cell hidradenoma: A case report. Acta Dermatovenereol 1982;62:173–176.
285. MacKenzie DH. A clear-cell hidradenocarcinoma with metastases. Cancer 1957;10: 1021–1023.
286. Keasbey LE, Hadley GG. Clear-cell hidradenoma. Report of three cases with widespread metastases. Cancer 1954;7:934–952.
287. Cotton DNK, Braye SG. Dermal cylindromas originate from the eccrine sweat gland. Br J Dermatol 1984;111:53–61.
288. Goette DK, McConnell MA, Fowler VR. Cylindroma and eccrine spiradenoma coexistent in the same lesion. Arch Dermatol 1982;118:273–274.
289. Urbanski SJ, From L, Abramowicz A, et al. Metamorphosis of dermal cylindroma: Possible relation to malignant transformation. J Am Acad Dermatol 1985;12:188–195.
290. Lyons JB, Rouillard LM. Malignant degeneration of turban tumour of scalp. Trans St John's Hosp Dermatol Soc 1961;46:74–77.
291. Bondeson L. Malignant dermal eccrine cylindroma. Acta Derm Venereol (Stockh) 1979;59:92–94.
292. Glatt HJ, Proia AD, Tsoy EA, et al. Malignant syringoma of the eyelid. Ophthalmology 1984;91:987–990.
293. Headington JT. Primary mucinous carcinoma of skin. Cancer 1977;39:1055.
294. Santa Cruz D, et al. Primary mucinous carcinoma of the skin. Br J Dermatol 1978;98: 645.
295. Wright J, Font R. Mucinous sweat gland adenocarcinoma of eyelid. Cancer 1979;44: 1757.
296. Gardner T, O'Grady R. Mucinous adenocarcinoma of the eyelid: A case report. Arch Ophthalmol 1984;102:912.
297. Yeung K, Stinson J. Mucinous (adenocystic) carcinoma of sweat glands with widespread metastases. Cancer 1977;39:2556.
298. Mendoza S, Helwig E. Mucinous (adenocystic) carcinoma of the skin. Arch Dermatol 1971;103:68.
299. Baandrup U, Sogaard H. Mucinous (adenocystic) carcinoma of the skin. Dermatologica 1982;164:338.
300. Cooper PH, Dahl M. Sclerosing carcinomas of sweat ducts (microstic adnexal carcinoma). Arch Dermatol 1986;122:261–264.
301. Glodstein DJ, Barr RJ, Santa Cruz DJ. Microscystic adnexal carcinoma. A distinct clinicopathologic entity. Cancer 1982;50:566–572.
302. Lupton GP, McMarlin SL. Microscystic adnexal carcinoma. Report of a case with 30-year follow-up. Arch Dermatol 1986;122:286–289.
303. Nickoloff BJ, Fleischmann HE, Carmel J, et al. Microcystic adnexal carcinoma. Immunohistologic observations suggesting dual (pilar and eccrine) differentiation. Arch Dermatol 1986;122:290–294.
304. Fleischmann HE, Rath RJ, Wood C, et al. Microscystic adnexal carcinoma treated by microscopically controlled excision. J Dermatol Surg Oncol 1984;10:873–875.
305. Salzman MJ, Eades E. Primary cutaneous adenoid cystic carcinoma: A case report and reveiw of the literature. Plast Reconstr Surg 1991;88:140–144.
306. Cooper PH, Adelson G, Holthaus W. Primary cutaneous adenoid cystic carcinoma. Arch Dermatol 1984;120:774–777.
307. Seab JA, Graham JH. Primary cutaneous adenoid cystic carcinoma. J Am Acad Dermatol 1987;17:113–118.
308. Perzin K, Gullane P, Conley J. Adenoid cystic carcinoma involving the external auditory canal: A clinicopahtologic study of 16 cases. Cancer 1982;50:2873.
309. Sanderson KV, Batten JC. Adenoid cystic carcinoma of the scalp with pulmonary metastasis. Proc R Soc Med 1975;68:649–650.
310. Wick MR, Swanson PE. Primary adenoid cystic carcinoma of the skin. A clinical, histological, and immunocytochemical comparison with adenoid cystic carcinoma of salivary glands and adenoid basal cell carcinoma. Am J Surg Pathol 1986;8:2–13.
311. Kao GF, Helwig EB, Graham JH. Aggressive digital papillary adenoma and adenocarcinoma. A clinicopathological study of 57 patients, with histochemical, immunopathological, and ultrastructural observations. J Cutan Pathol 1987;14:129.
312. Ceballos PI, Penneys NS, Acosta R. Aggressive digital papillary adenocarcinoma. J Am Acad Dermatol 1990;23:331–334.
313. Teloh H, Balkin R, Grier J. Metastasizing sweat-gland carcinoma: Report of a case. Arch Dermatol 1957;76:80.
314. Grant R. Sweat gland carcinoma with metastases. JAMA 1960;173:490.
315. Miller W. Sweat gland carcinoma. Am J Clin Pathol 1967;47:767.
316. Dave V. Eccrine sweat gland carcinoma with metastases. Br J Dermatol 1972;86:95.
317. Chow C, Campbell P, Burry A. Sweat gland carcinoma in children. Cancer 1984;53: 1222.
318. Wick M, et al. Adnexal carcinomas of the skin. I. Eccrine carcinoma. Cancer 1985;56: 1147.
319. Cruz DJS. Sweat gland carcinomas: A comprehensive review. Semin Diagn Pathol 1987;4:38–74.
320. Brownstein MH, Helwig EB. Pattern of cutaneous metastases. Arch Dermatol 1972;105: 862–868.
321. Reingold IM. Cutaneous metastases from internal carcinoma. Cancer 1966;19:162–168.
322. Mohs FE. Chemosurgery, microscopically controlled surgery for skin cancer. Springfield: Charles C Thomas, 1978.
323. Dubin N, Kopf AW. Multivariate risk score for recurrence of cutaneous basal cell carcinoma. Arch Dermatol 1983;119:373.
324. Chernosky ME. Squamous cell and basal cell carcinoma: Preliminary study of 3816 primary skin cancers. South Med J 1978;71:802.
325. Freeman RG, Knox JM, Heaton CL. The treatment of skin cancer: A statistical study of 1341 skin tumors comparing results obtained with irradiation, surgery, and curettage followed by electrodesiccation. Cancer 1964;17:535.
326. Spiller WF, Spiller RF. Treatment of basal cell epithelioma by curettage and electrodesiccation. J Am Acad Dermatol 1984;11:808.
327. Knox J, Lyles TW, Shapiro EM, et al. Curettage and electrodesiccation in the treatment of skin cancer. Arch Dermatol 1960;82:197.
328. Johnson TM, Tromovitch TA, Swanson NA. Combined curettage and excision: A treatment method for primary basal cell carcinoma. J Am Acad Dermatol 1991;24:613–617.
329. Cooper IS. Cryogenic surgery: New method of destruction or extirpation of benign and malignant tumors. N Engl J Med 1963;268:743.
330. Whitehouse HH. Liquid air in dermatology: Its indications and limitations. JAMA 1907;49:371.
331. Zacarian SA. Cryosurgery for skin cancer and cutaneous disorders. St. Louis: CV Mosby, 1985.
332. Belisario JC. Topical cytotoxic therapy for cutaneous cancer and precancer. Arch Dermatol 1965;92:293.
333. Street ML, White JW, Gibson LE. Multiple keratoacanthomas treated with oral retinoids. J Am Acad Dermatol 1990;23:862–866.
334. Dillaha CJ, Jansen GT, Honeycutt WM, et al. Selective cytotoxic effects of topical 5-fluorouracil. Arch Dermatol 1983;119:774.
335. Peck GL. Topical tretinoin in actinic keratosis and basal cell carcinoma. J Am Acad Dermatol 1986;15:829–835.
336. Raat JH, Krown SE, Pinske CM, et al. Treatment of Bowen's disease with topical dinitrochlorobenzene and 5-fluorouracil. Cancer 1976;37:1633.
337. Coker DD, Elias EG, Virvathana T, et al. Chemotherapy for metastatic basal cell carcinoma. Arch Dermatol 1983;119:44.
338. Woods RL, Stewart JF. Metastic basal cell carcinoma: Report of a case responding to chemotherapy. Cancer 1983;52:1583.
339. Lippman S, Meyskens F. Treatment of advanced squamous cell carcinoma of the skin with isotretinoin. Ann Intern Med 1987;107:499.
340. Weiss JS, Ellis CN, Headington JT, et al. Topical tretionin improves photoaged skin: A double-blind vehicle-controlled study. JAMA 1988;259:527–532.
341. Kligman AM, Grove GL, Hirose R, et al. Topical tretinoin for photoaged skin. J Am Acad Dermatol 1986;15:836–859.
342. Dillaha CJ, Jansen GT, Honeycutt WM, et al. Selective cytotoxic effect of topical 5-fluorouracil. Arch Dermatol 1963;88:247.
343. Fulton JE, Carter DM, Hurley HJ. Treatment of Bowen's disease with topical 5-fluorouracil under occlusion. Arch Dermatol 1968;97:178.
344. Jansen GT, Honeycutt WM, Dillaha CJ. Bowenoid condition of the skin: Treatment with topical 5-fluorouracil. South Med J 1967;60:185.
345. Waldrof DS. Mycosis fungoides—response with topical nitrogen mustard. Arch Dermatol 1968;97:608.
346. Zackheim H, Epstein EH Jr, McNutt NS, et al. Topical carmustine (BCNU) for mycosis fungoides and related disorders: Ten-year experience. J Am Acad Dermatol 1983;9: 363.

347. Klein E, Stoll H, Milgrom H, et al. Tumors of the skin. IV. Double blind study of effects of local administration of anti-tumor agents in basal cell carcinoma. J Invest Dermatol 1965;44:351–353.
348. Klein E, Stoll H, Milgrom H, et al. Tumors of the skin V. Local administration of anti-tumor agents to multiple superficial basal cell carcinoma. J Invest Dermatol 1965;45: 489–495.
349. Stegman S, Tromovitch T, Glogau R. Grafts. In: Stegman S, ed. Basics of dermatologic surgery. Chicago: Year Book Medical Publishers, 1982.
350. Knox JM, Freeman RG, Duncan WC, et al. Treatment of skin Cancer. South Med J 1967;60:241.
351. Kopf AW. Computer analysis of 3531 basal cell carcinomas of the skin. J Dermatol 1979;6:267.
352. Atkinson HR. Skin carcinoma depth and dose homogeneity in dermatological x-ray therapy. Aust J Dearmatol 1962;6:208.
353. Domonkos AN. Treatment of eyelid carcinoma. Arch Dermatol 1965;91:364.
354. Grosch E, Lambert HE. The treatment of difficult cutaneous basal and squamous cell carcinomata with electrons. Br J Radiol 1979;52:472.
355. Viravathana T, Prempree T, Sewchand W, et al. Technique and dosimetry in the management of extensive basal cell carcinomas od the head and neck region by irradiation with electron beams. J Dermatol Surg Oncol 1980;6:290.
356. Mohs FE. Chemosurgery for skin cancer: Fixed and fresh tissue technique. Arch Dermatol 1976;11:211.
357. Menn H, Robins P, Kopf A, et al. The recurrent basal cell epithelioma. Arch Dermatol 1971;103:628.
358. Klein E, Holterman OA, Helm F, et al. Immunologic approaches to the management of primary and secondary tumors involving the skin and soft tissues: Reviews of a ten-year program. Transplant Proc 1975;7:297.
359. Holterman OA, Papermaster BW, Walker MJ, et al. Regression of cutaneous neoplasms following delayed-type hypersensitivity challenge reactions to microbial antigens or lymphokines. J Med 1975;6:157.
360. Pennington DG, Waner M, Knox A. Photodynamic therapy for multiple skin cancers. Plast Reconstr Surg 1988;82:1067–1071.
361. Dougherty TJ, Weishaupt KR, Boyle DG. Photoradiation therapy of human tumors. In: Regan JD, Parrish JA, eds. The science of photomedicine. New York: Plenum Press, 1982:625.
362. Dougherty TJ. Photodynamic therapy (PDT) of malignant tumors. Crit Rev Oncol Hematol 1984;2:83.
363. Klingman LH, Akin FJ, Kligman AM. Sunscreens prevent ultraviolet photocarcinogenesis. J Am Acad Dermatol 1980;3:30–35.
364. Kolata G. Futuristic treatments for the hair and skin. N Y Times Med Sci 1987;15:24.
365. Weiss JS, Ellis CN, Headington JT, et al. Topical tretinoin improved photoaged skin. JAMA 1988;259:527–531.
366. Brusk MM, Santschi CH, Bell T, et al. Culture of basal cell carcinoma. J Invest Dermatol 1992;98:45–49.

Cancer: Principles & Practice of Oncology, Fourth Edition,
edited by Vincent T. DeVita, Jr., Samuel Hellman, Steven A. Rosenberg.
J.B. Lippincott Co., Philadelphia © 1993.

Charles M. Balch
Alan N. Houghton
Lester J. Peters

CHAPTER 46

Cutaneous Melanoma

Cutaneous melanoma is becoming a more common disease. In 1991, an estimated 32,000 persons developed melanoma, and almost 6500 died. The incidence of melanoma has increased during the past decade at a rate faster than that for any other cancer except lung cancer in women. The reasons for this increase are unclear, but factors may include increased recreational exposure to sunlight, an increased amount of ultraviolet irradiation from the midrange sunbeam spectrum (UVB) that reaches the earth's surface, and earlier detection of melanoma. This disease is largely confined to whites, in whom the age-adjusted incidence rate in the United States is about 12 per 100,000 persons and is threefold higher (30 per 100,000) in some geographic areas.[1–3] In 1935, only 1 in 1500 persons developed melanoma. The incidence dropped dramatically to 1 in 250 in 1980 and to 1 in 135 in 1987. Assuming present trends, the incidence will be 1 in 90 persons by the year 2000 (Fig. 46–1).[4]

Fortunately, most new patients are diagnosed early in the disease's clinical course, when it can be cured with simple surgical treatment. More than 90% of melanomas can be recognized as malignant by experienced observers; therefore, it behooves each physician to know the clinical characteristics of melanoma so that biopsies can be performed on suspicious moles or skin lesions as early as possible. Histologic verification and microstaging are essential before embarking on treatment. The options for therapy range from very conservative surgical treatment for early lesions to more radical approaches for biologically aggressive melanomas. Judgment, experience, and knowledge of the prognostic factors are essential for choosing the most appropriate treatment for individual patients.

CLINICAL CHARACTERISTICS

HIGH-RISK POPULATIONS

The typical melanoma patient has a fair complexion and a tendency to sunburn rather than tan, even after a brief exposure to sunlight.[5,6] The importance of these features was delineated in a case-control study in which 287 women with melanoma were compared with 574 age-matched controls.[5] Red hair was associated with a tripling of relative risk, blond hair with a 60% risk increase, and fair skin with a doubling of risk. There was a more than threefold increase in risk for those patients with more than 20 nevi.

A patient with a melanoma has a higher risk for developing a second primary melanoma than an individual in the general population has for developing a melanoma.[7] This risk varies from 3% to 5% in different series,[8–10] a risk 900-fold that of the general population.[11] A patient who has multiple dysplastic nevi or has a familial form of melanoma has an even greater risk for developing multiple primary melanomas.[8,12,13]

Familial melanomas are uncommon but have been well documented, and individuals in such families constitute an identifiable high-risk group.[9,13–18] Between 4% and 10% of patients describe a history of melanoma among their first-degree relatives.[14] Clark and colleagues described an autosomal dominant hereditary occurrence of melanoma,[19] originally termed the B-K mole syndrome and now referred to as the dysplastic nevus syndrome, familial type.[20] Patients with this syndrome typically have between 10 and 100 pigmented lesions located predominantly on the trunk, buttocks, or lower extremities. Genetic factors may play an important role

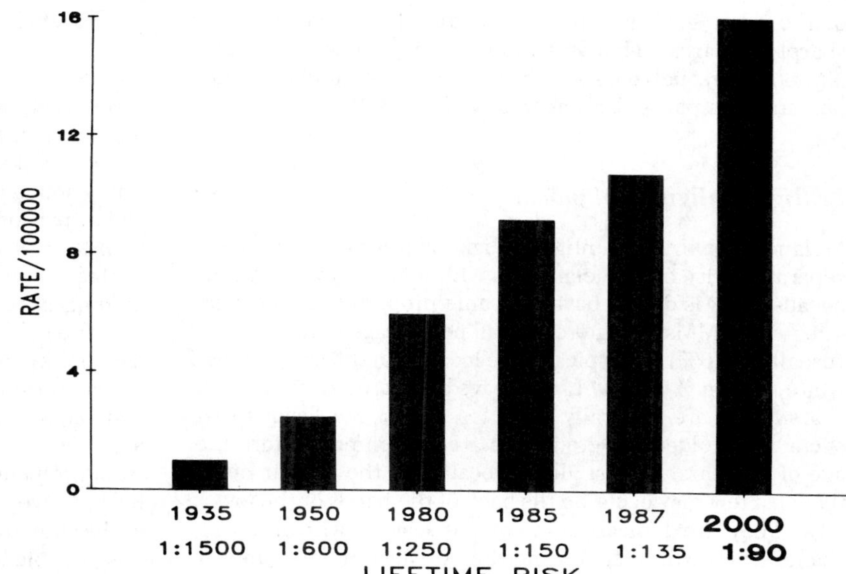

FIGURE 46–1. Past, current, and projected lifetime risk of a person in the United States developing malignant melanoma. (Rigel DS, Kopf AW, Friedman RJ. The rate of malignant melanoma in the US: Are we making an impact? J Am Acad Dermatol 1987;17:1050)

in the predisposition to melanoma, perhaps by genes controlling some aspect of immune response to melanoma antigens.[14,21,22] Melanoma-prone patients appear to have increased frequencies of certain blood, complement, and HLA phenotypes.[14,21,23–26]

SIGNS AND SYMPTOMS

Melanomas can be located anywhere on the body, but they occur most commonly on the lower extremities in women and on the back in men. Some of the clinical characteristics of melanoma are illustrated in Color Figure 46–2.[27–30] Typical features of cutaneous melanoma include variegation, an irregular raised surface, an irregular perimeter with indentations, and ulceration of the surface epithelium. Although melanomas may have a variety of clinical appearances, the common denominator is their changing nature. Any pigmented lesion that undergoes a change in size, configuration, or color should be considered a melanoma, and an excisional biopsy should be performed.

GROWTH PATTERNS

A convenient way to categorize melanomas is by their growth patterns.[27,31,32] These growth patterns represent distinct pathologic entities and have unique clinical features that can be recognized by the experienced clinician. The different categories of melanoma are all distinct from benign lesions, and each category portends a different prognosis. Histologic confirmation is essential before making any definitive treatment plans. The four major growth patterns are superficial spreading melanoma (SSM), nodular melanoma (NM), lentigo maligna melanoma (LMM), and acral lentiginous melanoma (ALM).

Superficial Spreading Melanoma

About 70% of melanomas are SSMs.[27,31–33] The lesions generally arise in a preexisting nevus. A history of slowly evolving change of the precursor lesion for more than 1 to 5 years is not uncommon, with more rapid growth developing months before diagnosis. SSMs can occur at any age after puberty. A typical SSM first appears as a deeply pigmented area in a brown junctional nevus. The lesion may take on a lacy appearance. Often, patches of regression are recognizable by an amelanotic area. Early in its evolution, an SSM is generally a flat lesion. It may develop an irregular surface, usually asymmetrically, depending on the vertical growth phase that develops as it enlarges. As the lesion grows, the surface may become glossy. Characteristically, there is notching or indentation of the perimeter, especially as the SSM enlarges.

Nodular Melanoma

The nodular growth pattern is the second most common growth pattern in most series (15–30% of patients).[27,31–33] NMs are more aggressive tumors and usually develop more rapidly than SSMs. They can occur at any age (but usually in middle age) and are most common on the trunk or head and neck. Men tend to have more NMs than women, whereas the opposite is true for SSMs. NMs are usually 1 to 2 cm in diameter but can be much larger. They begin more commonly in uninvolved skin than in preexisting nevi.

NMs are generally darker than SSMs, more uniform in coloration, and more raised or dome-shaped. The typical NM is a blue-black lesion that often resembles a blood blister or hemangioma. It may have other shadings of red, gray, or purple. About 5% of NMs lack pigment altogether (*i.e.*, are amelanotic) and have a fleshy appearance. NMs are often symmetrical but sometimes appear as irregularly shaped plaques. They lack the radial (horizontal) growth phase that is typical of the other growth patterns and therefore have discrete, sharply demarcated borders, often with irregular perimeters. NMs that are polypoid and have a stalk or cauliflower appearance are particularly aggressive lesions.[34]

Lentigo Maligna Melanoma

Melanomas with the lentigo maligna pattern appear to be a separate entity from melanomas with other growth patterns because LMMs do not have the same propensity to metastasize.[32,35,36] LMMs constitute a small percentage of melanomas (usually 4–10%) and typically are located on the face in older white women.[37] Usually LMMs have been present for 5 to 15 years. They are generally large (> 3 cm), flat lesions that occur in an older age group and are uncommon before the age of 50 years. Almost all are located on the face or neck, though a few may occur on the back of the hands or the lower legs. They are typically tan-colored lesions with differing shades of brown. Irregular mottling or flecking may appear as the lesions enlarge, with areas of dark brown or black in some parts and areas of regression in others. LMMs can have convoluted borders with prominent notching and indentation, which generally represent areas of regression. The diagnosis of LMM requires the presence of sun-related changes in both the epidermis and dermis.[32,36,37]

Acral Lentiginous Melanoma

Melanomas with the acral lentiginous growth pattern characteristically occur on the palms or soles or beneath the nail beds.[28,38–42] Not all plantar or volar melanomas are ALMs; a minority are SSMs or NMs.[43–46] ALMs occur in only 2% to 8% of white patients with melanoma[47] but in a substantially higher proportion (35–60%) of dark-skinned patients, including black, Asian, and Hispanic patients.[41,48–51]

Most ALMs are located on the sole of the foot.[40] They are generally large, with an average diameter of about 3 cm.[39] ALMs generally occur in older people, with the average patient's age in the 60s. Their evolution is short, ranging from a few months to several years, with an average of 2.5 years. Initially, these lesions appear as tan or brown flat stains on the palm or sole and often resemble LMMs. The haphazard array of color is characteristic. A minority of such lesions take on a flesh-colored appearance that can be misdiagnosed as granuloma. Ulceration is not uncommon, and fungating masses can result from neglected lesions. As with LMMs, these lesions often have irregular, convoluted borders. ALMs are much more aggressive than LMMs and are more likely to metastasize.

ALMs include subungual melanoma, an infrequently seen presentation of cutaneous melanoma.[43–45,52,53] It develops in only 2% to 3% of white patients but in a higher proportion of dark-skinned patients. It occurs equally in men and women and is most often diagnosed in older patients (median age of 55 to 65 years). More than three fourths of subungual melanomas involve either the great toe or the thumb. The most common sign of an early subungual melanoma is a brown to black discoloration under the nail bed.

BIOLOGY OF MELANOMA

Melanoma arises from melanocytes, which are dendritic pigmented cells found usually within epithelial surfaces. In adults, most melanocytes are located at the epidermal-dermal junction of the skin and in the choroid of the eye, but melanocytes can be found in the meninges, along mucosa of the alimentary and respiratory tracts, and even in lymph node capsules. More than 90% of melanomas arise in the skin, and a small percentage arise in the eye. Primary melanoma can occur in the meninges, respiratory tract, gallbladder, and other sites, although such incidences are rare. About 4% of melanomas have no known primary site. Although most of these melanomas presumably come from primary lesions in the skin that have completely regressed, some primary melanomas may arise from undiagnosed internal sites. Melanocytes arise from the neural crest early in the development of the fetus. By 4 to 6 weeks, they have migrated to their final destinations in the skin, uveal tract, meninges, and ectodermal mucosa.[54] It is possible that the ability of melanoma cells to metastasize rapidly and widely is determined by traits that facilitate the migration of melanocyte precursors through tissues before reaching epithelial tissues.

The melanocyte is a specialized cell type that synthesizes the pigment melanin using the enzyme tyrosinase in organelles called melanosomes. The presence of melanosomes, as detected by electron microscopy, or of pigment in an undifferentiated tumor can assist in the diagnosis of melanoma. Gene products other than tyrosinase regulate pigmentation. The techniques of molecular genetics have been used to identify the gene encoding tyrosinase and other genes specifically expressed in melanocytes.[55] Some of these gene products are potential targets for immunotherapies and chemically mediated cytotoxic therapies.[56–59] For example, some intermediates in the melanin synthetic pathway can be cytotoxic. This phenomenon has led to research into new strategies for treatment with compounds that can augment the production of toxic metabolites in the melanin pathway.[57–59]

Antigenic markers have been used to investigate the differentiation of melanocytes and the pathogenesis of melanoma.[60,61] Markers of melanocytic cells are useful to confirm the histologic diagnosis when the clinical pattern does not fit a diagnosis of melanoma or when melanoma is suspected in an undifferentiated tumor. Two widely used markers are S-100 protein and HMB-45, both of which can be detected by antibodies in paraffin-embedded tissues.[62] S-100 is expressed by almost all melanomas, but is expressed by sarcomas, nerve sheath tumors, and a subset of carcinomas. HMB-45 is more specific for melanocytic cell but is not always positive in metastatic melanomas. HMB-45 and S-100 are most effective when applied as part of a panel of markers, including cytokeratins, leukocyte common antigen, and other specialized markers.

Melanoma has emerged as an excellent paradigm to study events of malignant transformation and tumor progression. Clark and colleagues have proposed a model of tumor progression for melanoma.[63] The model defines lesions that represent putative steps in progression from normal melanocyte to melanoma. Lesions range from benign to most malignant in the following progression:

common acquired nevus → dysplastic nevus

→ primary melanoma (superficial or radial growth phase)

→ primary melanoma (deep or vertical growth phase)

→ metastatic melanoma.

The common acquired and dysplastic nevi are benign proliferative lesions, and each subsequent step displays properties of increasing malignant potential. For instance, cells in deep primary melanoma lesions (vertical growth phase) have the ability to invade into underlying tissue, and a subpopulation of these cells presumably has competence for metastasis. This model has formed a framework for identifying high-risk premalignant lesions and for characterizing specific molecules involved in the pathogenesis of melanoma.

Studies of melanoma cell growth, adhesion, and differentiation may lead to novel pharmacologic or biologic approaches for therapy. Normal melanocytes require exogenous growth factors for proliferation. Each of these growth factors bind to cell-surface receptors with tyrosine kinase activities, including basic fibroblast growth factor (bFGF), insulin or insulin-like growth factors, hepatocyte growth factor, and kit ligand.[64–66] Melanoma cells can grow in the absence of any exogenous growth supplements, suggesting that they produce their own growth factors. One of the best characterized melanoma growth factors is bFGF. Melanoma cells, but not melanocytes, produce their own bFGF, and bFGF production appears to be an early event in melanoma progression. Antisense oligodeoxynucleotides or antibodies against bFGF have been used to inhibit bFGF production by melanoma cells, leading to inhibition of melanoma cell growth.[67,68] Autocrine production of bFGF alone does not appear to be sufficient to cause malignant transformation of melanocytes.[69] Melanoma cells express a variety of cell-surface adhesion molecules that could play a role in cell invasion and metastasis. Several of these cell-surface markers might be useful in predicting prognosis (*e.g.*, propensity for distant metastases), including the intercellular adhesion molecule-1, the ganglioside GD2, and the $\beta 3$ integrin subunit.[70,71]

GENETIC ALTERATIONS IN MELANOMA

Specific genetic alterations have been implicated in the pathogenesis of melanoma. At least four distinct genes located on chromosomes 1, 6, 7, and 9 may play a role in melanoma. Genes located on different chromosomes also may contribute to melanoma progression. These findings suggest that melanoma is the result of a complex series of genetic events. Clues to the location or identity of genes involved in melanoma have come from genetic investigations of familial melanoma and from cytogenetic studies of pigmented lesions and melanomas.

Familial melanoma is a syndrome accounting for 4% to 10% of melanoma cases in the United States. Studies of heritable forms of melanoma, performed in families that have frank dysplastic nevus syndromes, have suggested that melanoma in this setting can be inherited in a highly penetrant, autosomal dominant mode.[72,73] DNA markers have been used to map a melanoma susceptibility gene to chromosome 1p in six kindreds.[74] A familial melanoma gene on chromosome 1p remains unconfirmed. Two other studies of different family groups have failed to detect a melanoma gene on chromosome 1p.[75,76] One difficulty has been the inability to define reproducible criteria for the diagnosis of the dysplastic nevus syndrome. These preliminary findings suggest that familial melanoma may be a heterogenous set of syndromes influenced by different genes.

Cytogenetic studies have shown that chromosomes in metastatic melanoma cells are highly aneuploid, whereas normal melanocytes are diploid. The occurrence of nonrandom chromosome alterations suggests that there are genes at these chromosomal locations that are necessary for malignant transformation and melanoma progression. The chromosomes most frequently involved in melanoma are 1, 6, and 7.[77–83] A review of the literature by Fountain and colleagues reported that chromosomes 1, 6, and 7 were rearranged in, respectively, 83%, 66%, and 61% of melanomas.[84] Chromosome 9 is the next most common chromosome to show rearrangements and is altered in almost half of all melanomas.[83] Alteration in chromosome 9 may be an early event in the pathogenesis of melanoma because alterations are found in some nevi, including dysplastic nevi.[85–87] Chromosomes 2, 3, 10, and 11 are involved in about one third of melanomas. In addition to nonrandom chromosomal abnormalities in melanomas, genetic analysis has shown widespread loss of genes throughout chromosomes in cultured melanomas.[88] About one fourth of genetic loci examined have shown a loss of genes. There is evidence that melanoma arises from a single transformed cell and is therefore clonally derived.[89] Genetic alterations appear to start early within the primary lesion, or even in precursor lesions, but widespread genetic alterations continue during metastasis.[89]

Sites of specific chromosomal alterations in cancer have provided clues to the location of tumor suppressor genes.[90] The most prevalent tumor suppressor locus identified in human cancer so far, p53, appears to be mutated only very infrequently in melanomas.[91] Evidence for a tumor suppressor locus on chromosome 6 has come from in vitro experiments that have introduced a normal copy of chromosome 6 into melanoma cell lines by microcell hybridization.[92] Expression of the normal chromosome 6 suppressed the malignant phenotype, reversing cell morphology, anchorage-independent growth in soft agar, and tumorigenicity in mice.

Selective chromosomal alterations may predict clinical course and prognosis. This approach has proved useful in the management of hematopoietic malignancies but has not been applied readily to solid tumors. Preliminary investigations have suggested that abnormalities in chromosomes 7 and 11 correlate with survival of patients with stage IV metastatic melanoma.[93] Although these results need to be confirmed, they suggest that cytogenetic analyses of melanoma could be useful in predicting clinical course.

EPIDEMIOLOGY

Exposure to sunlight (*i.e.*, UVB irradiation) is considered the major cause of cutaneous melanoma.[94] That the association is causal is supported by the demographic pattern of occurrence in humans, by the observation that DNA is sensitive to damage by solar radiation,[95] by sporadic induction of melanomas in animals through dual exposure to chemical carcinogens and UVB light,[96,97] and by evidence that the immune system may be depressed by UVB rays.[98]

In humans, the following patterns of melanoma occurrence suggest that sunlight is a cause of melanoma:

1. There is an inverse relation between incidence of melanoma and degree of skin pigmentation.
2. Incidence rates are higher in persons residing closer to the equator.[99,100]
3. The incidence of certain types of melanomas increases in anatomic sites exposed to sunlight.[101]
4. Migration studies suggest that risk is increased by moving to an area of more intense sun exposure.[102]
5. The risk for melanoma increases with increasing recreational exposure to the sun.

Inability to tan, higher frequency of sunburns, and younger age at first sunburn also have been associated with a predisposition to melanoma.[5] Finally, LMMs occur almost exclusively in sun-exposed parts of the body and in elderly persons, suggesting cumulative sunlight exposure as a contributing etiologic factor.

Several observations are not consistent with UVB irradiation as a sole cause of melanoma.[103] First, the incidence of melanoma does not increase consistently across geographic areas with increasing sunlight, although the relation may be skewed by the variable mix of people with different ethnic backgrounds and skin color. Second, melanoma affects white-collar, educated, urban workers more often than outdoor or blue-collar workers. Third, most melanomas occur in relatively young persons who have not had years of constant exposure to sunlight. Finally, some melanomas occur in relatively unexposed anatomic sites such as the palms, soles, bathing trunk areas, and mucous membranes. These observations are inconsistent with assigning cumulative sunlight exposure as the only etiologic factor, although it is possible that brief, intense exposure may contribute to or initiate carcinogenic events.

For SSMs and NMs, the pattern of risk suggests that susceptibility to sunburn determines the risk to the same or greater degree than the actual incidence of sunburn events does. Cumulative sunlight exposure has not been a consistent finding in many epidemiologic studies. No major environmental factors other than UVB irradiation have been identified as contributing substantially to the increasing incidence of cutaneous melanoma. The inheritable combination of light skin color and freckling suggests that genetically determined host susceptibility may play a more important role in the etiology of cutaneous melanoma than previously appreciated. The above characteristics are consistent with the two-step model of UVB-ray carcinogenesis, in which the initiation and promotion events result in melanoma in a genetically susceptible subpopulation of individuals.

The incidence of and mortality from cutaneous melanoma are rising steadily among white populations throughout the world.[48,94,104] In most studies, the incidence is doubling every 6 to 10 years. It is estimated that the incidence of melanoma among white persons in the United States will be 1 in 90 persons by the year 2000 (see Fig. 46–1).[5] In Queensland, Australia, the incidence has increased from 15 per 100,000 persons (the highest incidence in the world) in the 1963 to 1968 period to 28.4 per 100,000 in the 1979 to 1980 period.[105,106] In Sweden, the incidence has increased from 2.5 per 100,000 in 1958 to 11.6 per 100,000 in 1980.[107] Compare this high incidence in a fair-skinned population to the incidence of only 0.8 melanomas per 100,000 persons in China.[48,108,109]

CHANGES IN THE NATURAL HISTORY OF MELANOMA

The incidence of melanoma has been increasing rapidly, especially during the past two decades. A detailed analysis involving 7040 stage I melanoma patients treated over 30 years demonstrated major changes in the clinical and the pathologic features of the disease.[110] Over this period, there was a steady increase in the proportion of patients initially diagnosed as having localized disease (73% before 1960 compared with 81% by 1990). Melanomas have become thinner, less invasive, less ulcerative, and more curable. Most melanomas seen at many institutions measure less than 1 mm in thickness,[110,111] and more melanomas exhibit a radial growth phase with a superficial spreading growth pattern. The median thickness of melanomas decreased from about 3.0 mm before 1960 to less than 1.0 mm since 1985 (Fig. 46–3).[110] There was a significant increase during this period of extremity melanomas and a corresponding decrease of head and neck melanomas.[110] No significant change in site distribution was observed for trunk melanomas. The changes that have occurred probably

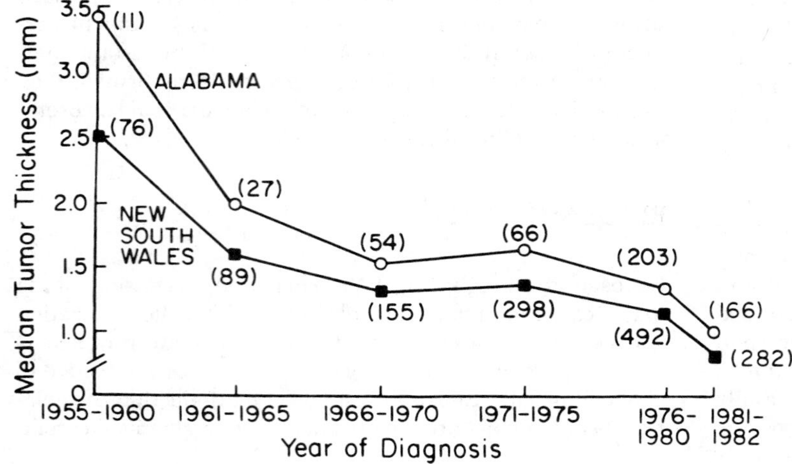

FIGURE 46–3. Changes in the median tumor thickness of melanomas treated from 1955 to 1982. The number of patients is shown in parentheses. (Balch CM, Shaw HM, Soong S-j, et al. Changing trends in the clinical and pathologic features of melanoma. In: Balch CM, Milton GW, eds. Cutaneous melanoma: Clinical management and treatment results worldwide. Philadelphia: JB Lippincott, 1985:313)

result from earlier diagnosis and changes in the biologic nature of the disease.

STAGING SYSTEMS

MICROSTAGING

Microstaging is an integral part of the staging and clinical management of melanoma. Two methods have been used. The Breslow microstaging method measures the thickness of the lesion using an ocular micrometer. The total vertical height (not just the depth) of the melanoma is measured, from the granular layer to the area of deepest penetration.[112] If the lesion is ulcerated, measurements should be made from the surface of the ulcer to the deepest part of the lesion. The Clark microstaging method categorizes levels of invasion that reflect increasing depth of penetration into the dermal layers of the subcutaneous fat (*i.e.*, levels II, III, IV, or V).[27]

Although the tumor thickness and the level of invasion can predict the risk for metastases, data from several institutions have demonstrated that tumor thickness is a more accurate and reproducible prognostic parameter than interpreting the level of invasion. Significant regression of the tumor invalidates the prognostic value of these microstaging methods.

ORIGINAL THREE-STAGE SYSTEM

The original and most widely used system involves three stages: stage I for localized melanoma, stage II for regional metastases, and stage III for distant metastases.[113,114] It is simple and easy to recall but, unfortunately, does not include important disease criteria (*e.g.*, tumor thickness) that allow for more accurate staging. A major limitation of this system is that 85% or more of melanoma patients diagnosed now have clinically localized disease (stage I). This disproportionate number of patients in one stage defeats the purpose of a classification system designed to categorize metastatic risk.

NEW STAGING SYSTEM ADOPTED BY THE AMERICAN JOINT COMMITTEE ON CANCER

The American Joint Committee on Cancer (AJCC) has worked for more than 10 years to develop uniform staging systems for all cancer types. In its extensive retrospective studies of melanoma, many factors influencing treatment results were identified. Based on these factors, a four-stage system was adopted (Table 46–1).[115,116] This system divides patients with clinically localized melanomas into two groups according to microstaging criteria, with the result that the metastatic risk categories are more evenly grouped among four stages (Fig. 46–4). It is a useful and practical classification for clinicians treating melanoma.

TABLE 46–1. New Staging System for Melanoma Adopted by the American Joint Committee on Cancer

Stage	*Criteria*
IA	Localized melanoma ≤0.75 mm or level II* (T1N0M0)
IB	Localized melanoma 0.76–1.5 mm or level III* (T2N0M0)
IIA	Localized melanoma 1.5–4 mm or level IV* (T3N0M0)
IIB	Localized melanoma >4 mm or level V* (T4N0M0)
III	Limited nodal metastases involving only one regional lymph node basin, or fewer than 5 in-transit metastases without nodal metastases (any T, N1M0)
IV	Advanced regional metastases (any T, N2M0) or any patient with distant metastases (any T, any N, M1 or M2)

* When the thickness and level of invasion criteria do not coincide within a T classification, thickness should take precedence.

(Ketcham AS, Balch CM. Classification and staging systems. In: Balch CM, Milton GW, eds. Cutaneous melanoma: Clinical management and treatment results worldwide. Philadelphia: JB Lippincott, 1985: 55)

PROGNOSTIC FEATURES OF MELANOMA

Many factors are known to predict the risk for metastatic disease in melanoma. A prognostic factors analysis of melanoma is therefore essential to identify the dominant variables that can be used for evaluating results of clinical research trials involving adjunctive systemic therapy and for making surgical decisions. In evaluating treatments, it is important to account for those prognostic variables that can categorize patients accurately into different risk groups for metastatic disease. Otherwise, differences (or lack of differences) between treatment regimens may not be due to the treatments themselves but may reflect imbalances of prognostic factors.

This section reviews a prognostic factors analysis involving more than 8500 patients with cutaneous melanoma treated at the University of Alabama in Birmingham (UAB) and the University of Sydney Melanoma Unit (SMU) over 25 years (1955–1980).[117] The median follow-up of all patients was 8 years.

CLINICALLY LOCALIZED MELANOMA (AJCC STAGES I AND II)

Characteristics of 6515 patients with localized melanoma were analyzed by single and multifactorial statistical analysis to determine which clinical and pathologic features of melanoma would predict the risk for metastases.[117]

Anatomic Location of Primary Lesion

Melanomas were divided evenly among the four major anatomic locations; 52% were on the upper and lower extremities, and 47% occurred on the trunk or head and neck. Patients with melanomas on the extremities had a better survival rate than those with melanomas of the trunk or head and neck ($p < 0.00001$), and those with melanomas on the upper extremities had a slightly better survival rate than those with melanomas on the lower extremities ($p = 0.08$). Analysis of anatomic subsites revealed some further differences in prognosis. Among those with melanomas in the head and neck region, patients with melanomas located on the scalp had worse prognoses than those with lesions on the face or neck. These differences remained even after accounting for sex and tumor thickness.[35,117] There was no sex difference in prognosis for patients with lesions on these head and neck subsites. There was no survival difference between patients with back lesions

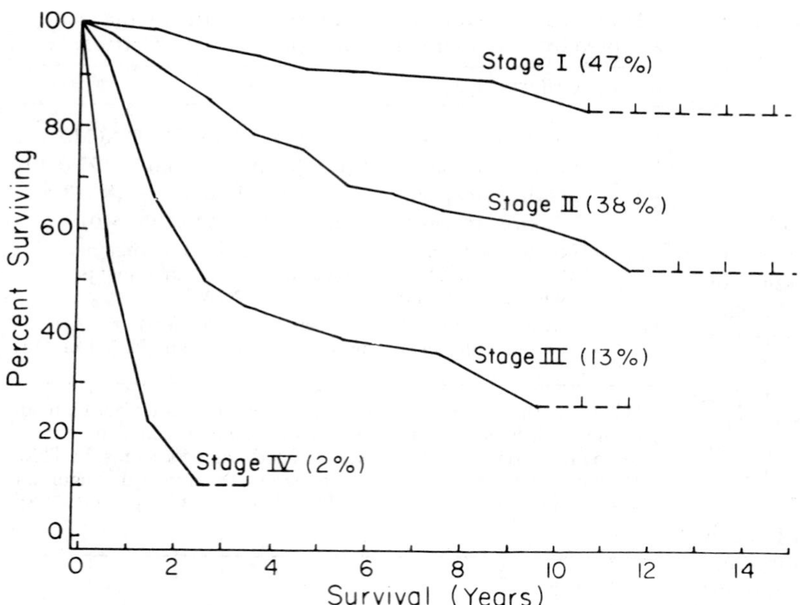

FIGURE 46–4. Fifteen-year survival results for more than 4000 melanoma patients treated at the University of Alabama in Birmingham and the University of Sydney. Patients are subgrouped according to the new four-stage system adopted by the American Joint Committee on Cancer. The distribution of patients is shown in parentheses. Patients with clinically localized melanomas (stage I by the original three-stage system) have now been divided into two stages according to tumor thickness and level of invasion (the newly designated stages I and II). (Ketcham AS, Balch CM. Classification and staging systems. In: Balch CM, Milton GW, eds. Cutaneous melanoma: Clinical management and treatment results worldwide. Philadelphia: JB Lippincott, 1985:55)

and those with chest lesions, even when subgrouped by sex. Female patients with melanomas on the back had a better survival rate than did male patients with back melanomas ($p = 0.016$). Patients with melanomas located on the hands and feet had significantly worse prognoses than those with lesions on the arms or legs.[117–119] Women with extremity melanomas had better prognoses than men did ($p < 0.00001$). Part of this sex difference in prognosis could be accounted for by the higher proportion of men with ulcerated melanomas (29% versus 19%).

Gender

Numerous studies of melanoma patients have shown that women have a better survival rate than men.[48,117–125] In the UAB-SMU analysis, women had a statistically significant survival advantage over men ($p < 0.00001$). A primary reason for better survival rates in women was that their melanomas occurred more commonly on the extremities (a more favorable prognostic site) and were less frequently ulcerated.

Tumor Thickness

The total vertical height of a melanoma is the single most important prognostic factor in stages I and II melanoma.[120,126–128] It is a quantitative parameter that can define subsets of patients with different survival rates ($p < 0.00001$). Numerous groups of thickness subsets have been analyzed for their prognostic value (*e.g.*, < 1 mm, 1 to 4 mm, > 4 mm), and only one subset was found to be more discriminating than those originally advocated by Breslow.[128] As demonstrated by actuarial survival curves, a more significant survival difference was found using the 4 mm rather than the 3 mm criterion.[117,120] There are apparently no natural breakpoints.[129] Instead, statistically defined subgroups vary from one data set to another depending on the number of patients, the duration

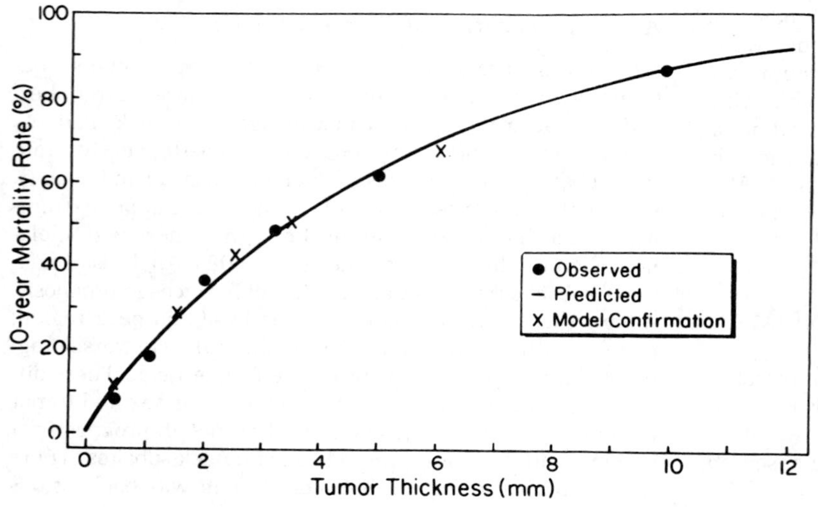

FIGURE 46–5. Observed and predicted 10-year mortality based on a mathematic model derived from tumor thickness.[117] The mathematic model is 9(T) = 1 − 0.966.e − 0.2016T and is described in more detail by Soong.[130] The solid line represents the 10-year mortality predicted by the model; the closed circles represent the actual observed mortality for 2627 patients. The accuracy of the model was confirmed by applying it to 747 AJCC stage I and II melanoma patients from the WHO Melanoma Group (data that were not used in the derivation of the model). Mortality for these patients is indicated by the Xs. The linear nature of the curve demonstrates that there are no natural breakpoints; rather, there is a continuous correlation of survival with tumor thickness. (Balch CM, Soong S-j, Shaw HM, et al. An analysis of prognostic factors in 4000 patients with cutaneous melanoma. In: Balch CM, Milton GW, eds. Cutaneous melanoma: Clinical management and treatment results worldwide. Philadelphia: JB Lippincott, 1985:321)

of follow-up, and the distribution of other factors (*e.g.*, ulceration, anatomic site of primary lesion, sex). The large number of patients in the UAB-SMU series has permitted the derivation of a simple nonlinear mathematic model that describes the relation between tumor thickness and 10-year mortality as a continuous event (Fig. 46–5).[130]

Level of Invasion

There is an inverse correlation between increasing level of melanoma invasion and survival. The level of invasion is a significant prognostic factor by single-factor analysis ($p < 0.00001$) and differentiates patients at various risks for metastases.

Comparison of Level of Invasion With Thickness as a Prognostic Indicator

A direct comparison of the level of invasion and tumor thickness microstaging methods was made by subdividing each level of invasion into thickness categories. Within levels III, IV, and V, gradations of thickness influenced survival (Fig. 46–6). Converse relations were not observed when analyzing sets of melanoma thickness subdivided by levels of invasion. For example, the 5-year survival rates for patients with level III, IV, or V lesions that measured 1.5 to 4.0 mm were not significantly different. These observations demonstrate that the measurement of tumor thickness is a more accurate prognostic factor than level of invasion.[48,118,119,120–123,126,127,131–135]

Ulceration

Ulcerated melanomas appear to be more aggressive lesions biologically because they invade through the epidermis rather than pushing it upward. The presence of ulceration in microscopic sections of melanoma was a significant adverse determinant of survival ($p < 0.00001$) in the UAB-SMU study.[117] Patients with stages I and II melanoma with ulceration had a 10-year survival rate of 50%, whereas those without ulceration had a 79% 10-year survival rate ($p < 0.0001$). Men had a higher proportion of ulcerated lesions than women (26% versus 20%). There was a positive correlation between ulceration and thickness ($p < 0.0001$). The median tumor thickness for patients with ulcerated lesions was 2.6 mm, whereas those without ulcerated lesions had a median tumor thickness of 0.8 mm. Lesions more than 1.5 mm thick were associated with a 46% incidence of ulceration.

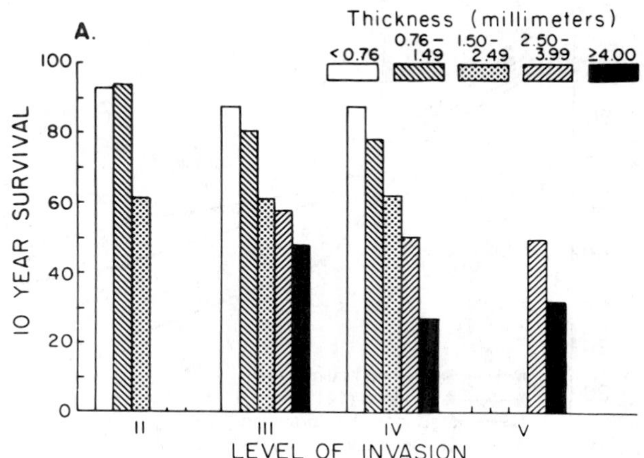

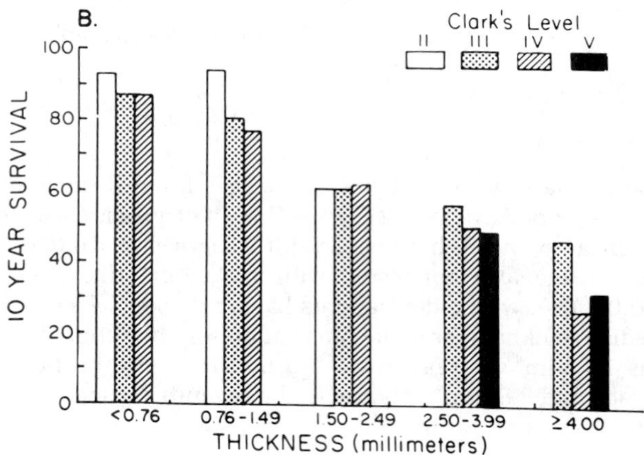

FIGURE 46–6. Comparison of two microstaging methods: tumor thickness versus level of invasion. **(A)** Ten-year survival rates for AJCC stages I and II melanoma patients according to levels of invasion and subgrouped by tumor thickness. There were statistically significant differences in survival rates for patients with lesions of various thicknesses within levels III, IV, and V. **(B)** Ten-year survival rates for AJCC stages I and II melanoma patients according to tumor thickness subgrouped by levels of invasion. There were no statistically significant differences in survival rates for patients with lesions of various levels of invasion within each thickness subgroup. (Balch CM, Soong S-j, Shaw HM, et al. An analysis of prognostic factors in 4000 patients with cutaneous melanoma. In: Balch CM, Milton GW, eds. Cutaneous melanoma: Clinical management and treatment results worldwide. Philadelphia: JB Lippincott, 1985:332)

Growth Pattern

Patients with SSM and LMM lesions had the best survival rate, whereas those with NM lesions had the worst. The most statistically significant difference among these groups was between SSM and NM ($p < 0.0001$). When patients with SSM and NM were matched for lesion thickness and their 10-year survival rates calculated, no difference was found between growth patterns as prognostic factors (Fig. 46–7). Patients with SSMs appear to have better prognoses than those with NMs only because the former are thinner lesions. Those with LMMs constituted only a small number of patients (4%). These lesions were all located on the face or neck and were generally thinner lesions. When matched thickness for thickness, patients with LMM lesions had better prognoses than the other growth pattern groups.[35,36] Even patients with LMM lesions 3 mm thick or greater had an 80% 10-year survival rate. It should be emphasized that other characteristics of LMM lesions (*e.g.*, face and neck locations, chronic skin damage, older patients) may contribute to the distinctiveness of this growth pattern as much as its histologic appearance. ALMs constituted only 2% of all cases. When matched by lesion thickness, patients with ALM lesions had worse prognoses than those of any growth pattern (see Fig. 46–7).

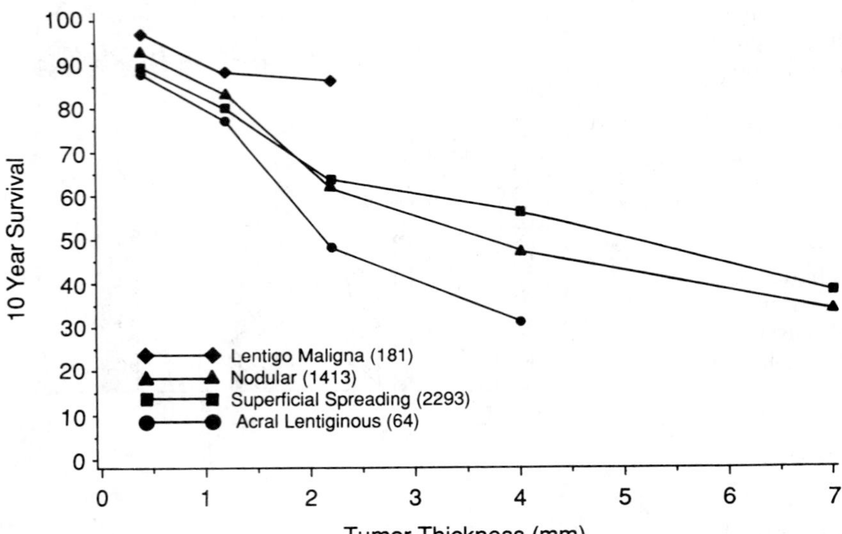

FIGURE 46–7. Ten-year survival rates for stages I and II melanoma patients according to growth pattern and tumor thickness. Among patients with melanomas of equivalent tumor thickness, those with nodular and superficial spreading melanomas had similar survival rates, those with lentigo maligna melanomas had a much more favorable prognosis, and those with acral lentiginous melanomas had the worst prognosis. The number of patients is shown in parentheses. (Balch CM, Soong S-j, Shaw HM, et al. An analysis of prognostic factors in 4000 patients with cutaneous melanoma. In: Balch CM, Houghton AN, Milton GW, Sober AJ, Soong S-j, eds. Cutaneous melanoma. 2nd ed. Philadelphia: JB Lippincott, 1992:165)

Age

The median age of patients with stages I and II melanoma was 45 years. Advanced age at the time of diagnosis correlated significantly with a shortened length of survival ($p < 0.00001$). Patient age also correlated with melanoma thickness ($p < 0.00001$), with older patients having thicker lesions. The median thickness for melanoma patients in their third decade was 1.1 mm, whereas it was 1.5 mm for those in the fifth decade and 2.8 mm for those in the seventh decade.

Multifactorial Analysis

The above clinical and pathologic parameters were simultaneously compared for their prognostic strength using multifactorial analysis. The influence of these factors on survival was examined using a cohort of 4568 patients with AJCC stages I and II melanoma for whom information was available for all prognostic factors being analyzed. The dominant factors predicting survival were thickness of the melanoma, melanoma ulceration (presence or absence), and anatomic location (upper extremity, lower extremity, trunk, or head and neck). Four other variables correlated to a lesser extent with survival in certain subgroups of patients: (1) the type of initial surgical management (primary excision alone versus excision plus elective lymph node dissection), (2) pathologic stage (I, II, or III), (3) level of invasion, and (4) sex.

Most other major studies using multifactorial analysis have established tumor thickness to be the most important prognostic factor in their series of patients with stages I and II melanoma.[48,118,119,121,123,131–137] Similarly, ulceration was found to be another strong predictor of survival in seven other patient series.[119,122,123,132,133,135,136,138] Three of these series confirmed that anatomic location of the primary lesion was another major predictor of survival.[118,119,132]

Other factors analyzed by multifactorial analysis that emerged as important variables overall or within selected subgroups in other series included sex[121,122,137] and age of the patient[132] and such tumor features as lymphocytic infiltration,[122,131] tumor diameter,[122,123,134] cell type,[122,135] microscopic satellites,[138] mitotic activity,[118,123,131–137] and level of invasion.[132] The timing of the biopsy before first definitive treatment was found to have a significant influence on survival in one series.[122] Flow cytometry analyses of DNA content (aneuploidy versus diploidy) correlated with survival in several recent studies.[138a]

METASTATIC MELANOMA IN REGIONAL LYMPH NODES

(AJCC STAGE III)

Twelve prognostic factors of melanoma were examined in a series of 1698 patients with nodal metastases who were treated at UAB and SMU during the past 30 years.[117]

Sex

Most patients with AJCC stage III melanomas were men (69%), whereas they constituted a minority of stages I and II patients (48%). There were no differences in survival rates among male and female stage III melanoma patients, even when the data were cross-analyzed by other categories.

Anatomic Location of Primary Lesion

Primary melanomas accompanied by nodal metastases occurred in anatomic locations distributed throughout the body, with 55% arising in axial locations (trunk or head and neck). Patients with melanomas on the trunk constituted the largest group (35% of the entire series). There was no statistically significant difference in survival rates for patients with stage III melanoma when subgrouped by anatomic sites. Those with melanomas of the extremities had the best survival rates.

Age

The median age of the entire stage III patient population was 46 years. Older stage III melanoma patients tended to have a worse prognosis than younger patients. For example, only 20% of patients were alive after 5 years if they were older than 50 years at the time of the initial diagnosis, compared with 38% of patients who developed melanoma when they were 50 years old or younger. This difference was statistically significant ($p = 0.0001$). Significant differences appeared when the data were subgrouped further by gender. Men 50 years or younger had a much higher survival rate than older men ($p = 0.0006$), whereas the difference between younger and older women was not as great ($p = 0.02$).

Number of Metastatic Nodes

There was a direct correlation between number of metastatic nodes and survival. Patients with one metastatic node had a better survival rate than patients with two metastatic nodes or more.[139] Data from patients with different numbers of nodal metastases were analyzed for survival differences. The greatest differences in this series were between patients with one metastatic node, patients with two to four nodes, and patients with five or more nodes (Fig. 46–8). Thirty-seven percent of patients had one metastatic node, 38% had two to four, and 25% had five or more. Their 10-year survival rates were 40%, 18%, and 9%, respectively ($p < 0.001$). Ten-year survival rates demonstrated that only patients with one positive node had a reasonable prospect of cure (40% were alive at 10 years), whereas only about 15% of patients with two or more metastatic nodes were alive at 10 years.

Ulceration

Ulceration was the most important predictor of the risk for subsequent nodal metastases in patients with AJCC stages I and II melanoma, and it continued to be an important predictive factor once nodal metastases had occurred.[139,140] The 3-year survival for patients with stage III ulcerative melanomas was only 29%, compared with 61% for nonulcerative melanomas ($p = 0.0002$). For each category of nodal metastasis, the presence of ulceration in the primary lesion implied a worse prognosis than if the melanoma had an intact overlying epithelium. Patients with one positive node and no ulceration of the primary melanoma had the most favorable prognoses of any stage III patient group, having a 50% 10-year survival rate.

Tumor Thickness

The median thickness for stage III melanomas was 3.4 mm, compared with 1.2 mm for stages I and II lesions ($p < 0.001$). Forty percent of patients with stage III disease had thick melanomas (> 4 mm thick). A significant relation was identified between thickness and ulceration. Patients with nonulcerative melanomas of 4 mm or less had a more favorable 5-year survival rate compared with patients whose lesions were greater than 4 mm thick (37% versus 24%, respectively); patients with ulcerated melanomas greater than 4 mm had only an 18% 10-year survival rate.

Multifactorial Analysis

Each of the above prognostic factors was examined for its predictive value for metastatic risk and survival in stage III melanoma patients.[117,139] By single-factor analysis, the most significant prognostic variables were (1) the number of metastatic nodes, (2) the presence or absence of ulceration of the primary melanoma, (3) tumor thickness of the primary melanoma (< or > 4 mm), and (4) the patient's age. The multifactorial analysis showed that the number of metastatic nodes ($p = 0.0001$), the anatomic site of the primary melanoma ($p < 0.0151$), and tumor ulceration ($p = 0.0661$) were the dominant prognostic variables. Tumor thickness and patient age strongly correlated with prognosis in the combined UAB and SMU data ($p = 0.0001$), but the SMU data did not include the number of metastatic nodes as a variable in the multifactorial analysis.

The number of metastatic nodes was first shown to be of prognostic significance in a multifactorial analysis by Cohen and associates.[141] Later, Day and associates[142] and Callery and associates[143] demonstrated that tumor thickness and the number of metastatic nodes were dominant and independent

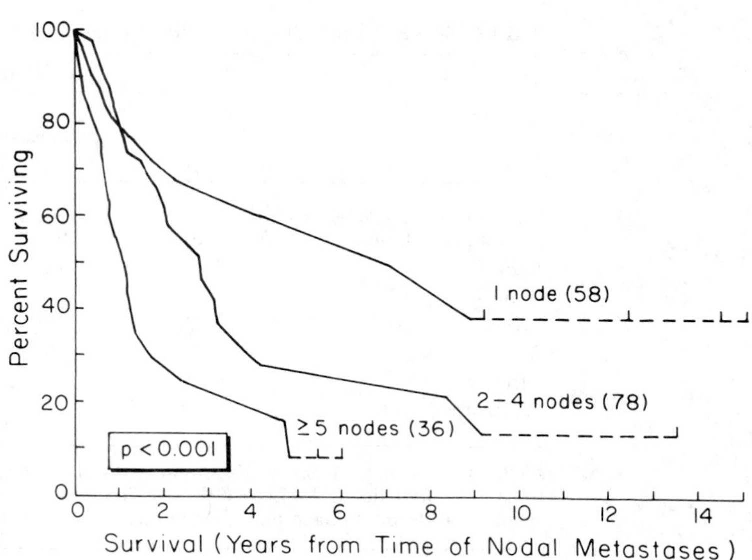

FIGURE 46–8. Survival for all stage III (AJCC) melanoma patients according to the number of metastatic nodes. (Balch CM, et al. A multifactorial analysis of melanoma patients with lymph node metastases [stage II]. Ann Surg 1981;193:377)

variables in stage III patients. Cascinelli and colleagues identified the extent of nodal metastases (*i.e.*, confined to or invading through the lymph node capsule) and the number of metastatic nodes as the most significant factors in a multifactorial analysis of 530 stage III patients.[121,144]

METASTATIC MELANOMA AT DISTANT SITES (AJCC STAGE IV)

The data for 200 patients with distant metastases treated at UAB were analyzed for predictive factors affecting survival rates.[145]

Site of Distant Metastases

The locations of distant metastases were an important prognostic factor when examined by single-factor analysis ($p = 0.0001$). The skin, subcutaneous tissues, and distant lymph nodes were the most common first sites of relapse, which occurred in 59% of patients. In 23% of patients, nonvisceral metastases at these sites were the sole manifestation of disease (14% for skin, 5% for subcutaneous sites, and 4% for distant lymph nodes). The median survival duration for the entire patient group was 7 months, with 25% alive at 1 year. There was no difference in survival among patients with metastases at any combination of these three sites. The next most common site of first relapse was the lungs (36% of patients). Patients with isolated lung metastases had the longest median survival duration (11 months) of patients with metastases at site. The brain, liver, and bone were the next most common sites of first relapse. The median duration of survival for these patients was very poor, ranging from 2 to 6 months, with a 1-year survival rate of only 8% to 10%.

The presence of visceral metastases had an overriding influence on survival, because those patients with combined visceral and nonvisceral metastases had the same poor prognoses as those with visceral metastases alone.

Number of Metastatic Sites

Patients with a single distant metastasis had longer survivals than patients with metastases at two or more sites (see Fig. 46–8). Number of metastatic sites was the most significant factor predicting survival in patients with distant metastases by single-factor analysis ($p < 0.00005$). The median survival was 7 months for patients with one metastatic site, 4 months for those with two sites, and 2 months for those with three or more metastatic sites.

Similarly, the 1-year survival rate was 36% for patients with one metastatic site and 13% for patients with two sites, with no 1-year survival for patients with three or more sites. Within the single-site group, patients with metastases in the lung, skin, subcutaneous tissue, or distant lymph nodes had a better survival rate than patients with metastases at any other single site (Table 46–2).

Sex

Once melanoma progressed to distant metastases, there was no correlation between the sex of the patient and the clinical courses ($p = 0.98$). Survival curves for male and female AJCC stage IV melanoma patients were superimposable.

Remission Duration

The length of remission was not a statistically significant factor, by single-factor analysis, in predicting the clinical course of disease when the survival rates were calculated from the onset of distant metastases ($p = 0.25$).

Multifactorial Analysis

Each of the prognostic factors was examined for its predictive value for metastatic risk and survival rate.[145] Only the number of metastatic sites and the location of the sites (visceral, nonvisceral, or both) correlated with survival rates in a single-factor analysis. When all factors were analyzed in a Cox regression analysis, the dominant factors for stage IV mela-

TABLE 46–2. First Site of Distant Metastases

		Site Alone		*Plus Other Sites*	
Site	*Overall (%)*	*Incidence (%)*	*Median Survival (mo)*	*Incidence (%)*	*Median Survival (mo)*
Skin, subcutaneous tissues, distant lymph nodes	59	23	7.2	36	5.0
Lung	36	11	11.4	25	4.0
Brain	20	8	5.0	12	1.4
Liver	20	3	2.4	17	2.0
Bone	17	3	6.0	14	4.0
Other	12	2	2.2	10	2.0
Widespread	4		2.4		2.4

(Balch CM, Soong S-j, Shaw HM. An analysis of prognostic factors in 400 patients with cutaneous melanoma. In: Balch CM, Milton GW, eds. Cutaneous melanoma: Clinical management and treatment results worldwide. Philadelphia: JB Lippincott, 1985:321)

noma patients were as follows: (1) the number of metastatic sites (one, two, or three or more; $p = 0.00001$), (2) the remission duration (< 12 months versus > 12 months; $p = 0.019$), and (3) the site of metastases (visceral versus nonvisceral; $p = 0.019$). These results were the same even after accounting for palliative chemotherapy. There were no histologic criteria of the primary melanomas that predicted the patients' clinical courses once they developed distant metastases.

Another multifactorial analysis of stage IV patients was performed by Presant and colleagues.[146] They found significant determinants of survival to include high performance (activity) status, no liver involvement, female sex, and bone involvement only.

MANAGEMENT OF THE PRIMARY MELANOMA

INDICATIONS AND TECHNIQUES OF BIOPSY

Biopsies for melanomas can be either excisional or incisional.[147] Whichever technique is used, full-thickness biopsy into the subcutaneous tissue must be performed to permit microstaging of the lesion (for thickness and level of invasion). Shave or curette biopsies should never be used for lesions suspected of being melanomas.

Excisional Biopsies

An excisional biopsy is indicated for a suspicious lesion that is not large (*i.e.*, < 1.5 cm in diameter) and is located in an area in which the amount of skin excised is not crucial (*e.g.*, on the trunk). The lesion should be excised with an elliptical incision including a narrow margin (2 mm) of normal-appearing skin. Taking slightly larger margins (*e.g.*, 1 cm) of skin may be insufficient for a malignant lesion and excessive for a benign one.

The direction of the biopsy incision is important, because a biopsy that is not oriented properly may necessitate a skin graft when an elliptical incision and primary closure might have been possible. The biopsy incision should be oriented so that it can be reexcised with optimal skin margins and minimal skin loss if the lesion proves to be malignant. The excisional biopsy technique is illustrated in Figure 46–9.

Incisional Biopsies

Incisional biopsies should be performed when the amount of skin removed is crucial (*e.g.*, face, hands, feet). They may be indicated for large lesions, for which an excisional biopsy would be a formidable procedure. An incisional biopsy can be made with a scalpel, but usually a 6-mm punch biopsy is preferred to take a full-thickness core of skin and subcutaneous tissues from the most raised or irregular area of the lesion.

The biopsy specimen should not be taken at the periphery of the lesion unless there are areas of raised nodularity at this location. No decrease in survival rates or increase in local recurrence rates has been observed in our experience with the incisional approach[147] and in the experience of others.[148,149] Moreover, an incisional biopsy is a simple, expedient office procedure and provides representative tissue if taken properly. Such an approach is more cost-effective than inpatient biopsies, especially those taken under general anesthesia.

SURGICAL MARGINS OF EXCISION

Local control of a primary melanoma requires wide excision of the tumor or biopsy site with a margin of normal-appearing skin. Until recently, the routine surgical approach was to excise all primary melanomas with a 3- to 5-cm margin and

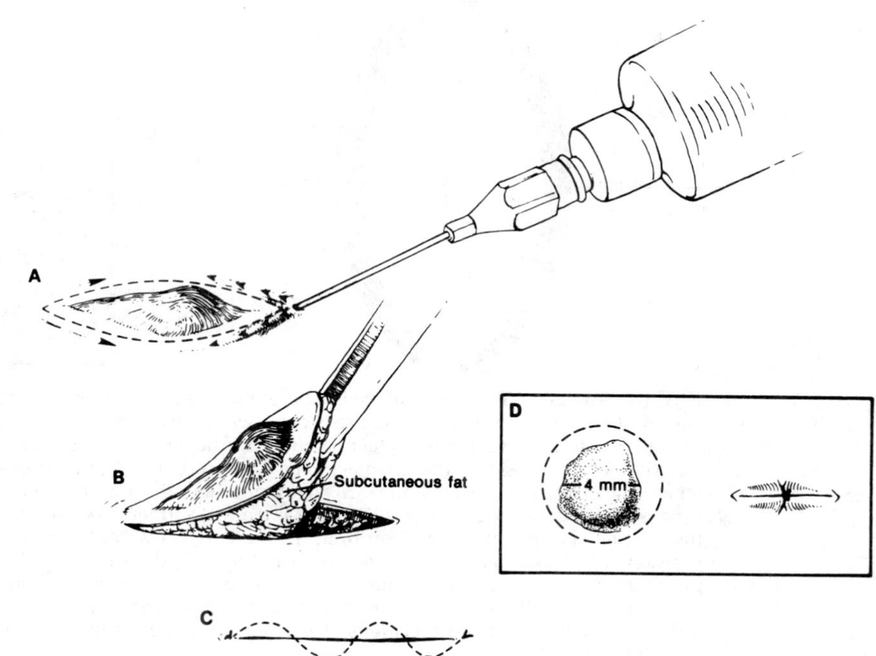

FIGURE 46–9. Technique of excisional biopsy for melanoma. **(A)** The suspicious lesion is first injected with local anesthetic around but not into the lesion itself. **(B)** The entire lesion is excised with a narrow rim (1 to 2 mm) of normal-appearing skin around it, including the underlying subcutaneous fat. Care is taken to avoid crushing the specimen with forceps. **(C)** The incision is closed after hemostasis is completed. This can be performed with a subcuticular closure using synthetic absorbable sutures or with simple interrupted nylon sutures. **(D)** An alternative approach for small lesions. An excision with a 6-mm punch is an inexpensive and expedient office procedure. The lesion is completely excised with the punch biopsy instrument, and the skin edges are closed with a single 4-0 nylon suture. (Urist MM, Balch CM, Milton GW. Surgical management of the primary melanoma. In: Balch CM, Milton GW, eds. Cutaneous melanoma: Clinical management and treatment results worldwide. Philadelphia: JB Lippincott, 1985:74)

apply a split-thickness skin graft to the defect. It has become increasingly clear that the risk for local recurrence correlates more with the tumor thickness than with the margins of surgical excision.[127,150–153] Therefore, it seems more rational to excise melanomas using surgical margins that vary according to tumor thickness and ulceration, because these factors correlate best with the risk for local recurrence.

The earliest lesion is a melanoma in situ.[154] This is a noninvasive tumor that does not metastasize but is capable of recurring locally.[155] Although the natural history of these noninvasive lesions is not completely understood, there is a risk for local recurrence as an in situ or invasive melanoma if they are not reexcised after biopsy.[155,156] It is recommended that the biopsy site of an in situ melanoma be excised, usually with a 0.5- to 1-cm margin of skin.

For thin melanomas (< 1.00 mm in thickness), there has been only minimum risk for local recurrence in all reported patient series,[127,147,148,150,152,156–158] despite wide variations in margins of excision. In other words, survival is not influenced by the size of the resection margins. This does not mean that reexcision is unnecessary, but that the minimal standards for a safe margin have not been established in any scientific study. A wide excision consisting of at least a 1-cm margin of skin is recommended by many melanoma surgeons.[127,147,152,156,157,159–161] This can be performed as a generous elliptical excision and a primary skin closure (Fig. 46–10). In a recent study of 936 patients with melanomas less than 1 mm thick, there was no local recurrence, despite the fact that 61% of patients had conservative margins (< 2 cm) of excision.[147] For intermediate and thick melanomas (> 1.0 mm thick), a margin of 2 to 3 cm is usually employed. The risk for local recurrence may exceed 10% to 20% for those melanomas more than 4 mm thick.[127,152,158,161] Because LMMs have a low risk for recurrence and generally occur on the face, they can be safely excised with a 1-cm margin of excision.

Results of the first randomized study involving surgical margins for melanomas less than 2 mm thick have been reported recently by the World Health Organization (WHO) Melanoma Group.[162] In a study of 612 evaluable patients who were randomly assigned to either a 1-cm or 3-cm surgical margin of excision, there were no local recurrences in the group with melanomas less than 1 mm thick. There were three local recurrences in the group of patients with melanomas 1.0 to 2.0 mm thick, and all 3 patients had received narrow excisions.[162a] These results demonstrate conclusively that a narrow excision for thin melanomas (< 1.0 mm) is safe, but no conclusion could be reached about the safety of excising melanomas more than 1.0 mm in thickness. A randomized prospective study conducted by the Intergroup Melanoma Committee has evaluated 2- to 4-cm radial margins of excision for intermediate thickness melanomas (1.0–4.0 mm). The trial has been closed to patient accrual, and the preliminary results indicate that a 2 cm excision margin is safe.

Special Sites

FINGERS AND TOES. A melanoma located on the skin of a digit or beneath the fingernail must be removed by a digital amputation. When such a biopsy-confirmed lesion is located on the finger (especially the thumb), it is important to save as much of the digit as possible to maximize function. The amount that can be saved depends on the extensiveness of the lesion (*i.e.*, amount of nail bed or paronychial involvement) and the location of its proximal border. In general, amputations of digits are performed proximal to the distal joint of the thumb and at the middle interphalangeal joint of

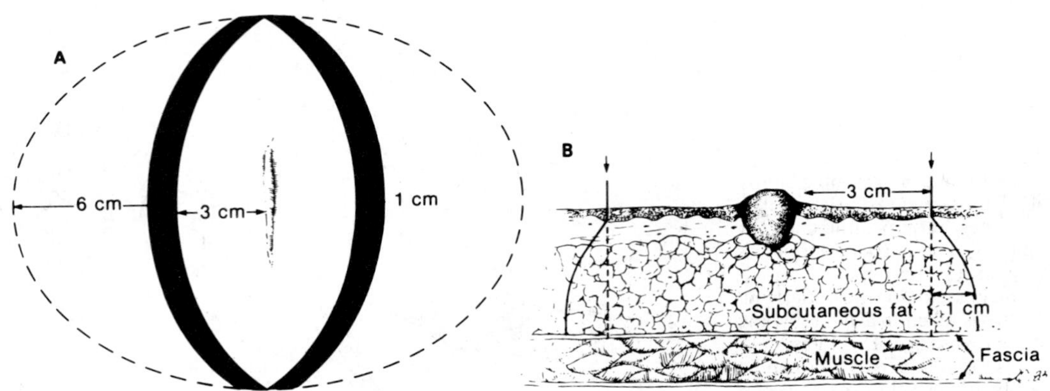

FIGURE 46–10. Technique of excising a primary melanoma with an elliptical excision and primary skin closure. **(A)** The surgical margin consists of a 3-cm radius of normal-appearing skin surrounding the biopsy site or the lateral margin of the intact melanoma. The long axis of the incision should be three to four times the width of the incision. After the melanoma is excised, skin flaps are raised in a plane above the deep fascia for a sufficient distance to close the skin edges without undue tension. The most extensive area of mobilization is near the center of the flaps, and it often is necessary to mobilize the skin flaps for a distance twice that of the excised skin margin. A suction drain in the surgical wound may be needed. **(B)** Cross-section of the excision site. A skin margin of 3 cm from the tumor is shown. Flaps of gradually increasing thickness are raised for an additional 1 to 2 cm to remove any surrounding subdermal lymphatics. Excising the fascia is optional. (Urist MM, Balch CM, Milton GW. Surgical management of the primary melanoma. In: Balch CM, Milton GW, eds. Cutaneous melanoma: Clinical management and treatment results worldwide. Philadelphia: JB Lippincott, 1985:78)

the fingers, as long as the lesions are small and confined to the nail bed. For a melanoma located on a toe, an amputation of the entire digit at the metatarsal-phalangeal joint is indicated; this generally does not cause any significant morbidity.

SOLE OF THE FOOT. A melanoma on the plantar surface often involves a sizable defect in a weight-bearing area. If possible, a portion of the heel or ball of the plantar surface should be retained to bear the greatest burden of pressure. If possible, the deep fascia over the extensor tendons should be preserved as a base for the skin coverage.

EAR. For a small suspicious lesion of the helix, the preferred initial procedure for diagnosis is excisional biopsy followed by a wedge reexcision if the diagnosis of melanoma is confirmed. A partial amputation may be necessary for larger lesions. A total amputation of the ear should be restricted to patients with widespread local disease or those with recurrence after partial amputation.

FACE. Facial lesions usually cannot be excised with more than a 1-cm margin because of adjacent vital structures. In these cases, the surgeon should use his best judgment based on the width and thickness of the melanoma and its exact location on the face. The expected local recurrence rate after surgery is 4%. Radiation therapy has been used with some success for LMMs located on the face.[163]

ROLE OF RADIATION THERAPY

Superficial contact radiation therapy has been used in Europe for more than 60 years in the treatment of cutaneous melanoma. This technique results in very high incident doses of radiation, often in excess of 10,000 cGy, with very rapid falloff (about 50% at 1 mm), and is therefore suitable only for superficial lesions. Conventional radiation therapy has little role in the initial treatment of primary melanoma, except perhaps for the LMM variety. Harwood reported in 1983 on a series of 28 patients with LMM treated definitively with conventionally fractionated radiation therapy at Princess Margaret Hospital from 1958 to 1982.[163] Only 2 patients had recurrences, although some lesions took up to 24 months to regress completely after radiation.

LOCAL RECURRENCES AND THEIR MANAGEMENT

A local recurrence is defined as any tumor that occurs within 5 cm of the scar of a previously excised melanoma. This definition is important in analyzing the risk factors involved and the influence of the surgical margins of excision of the primary melanoma. Local recurrences should be considered as retained extensions of the primary tumor. They are distinct from satellites and in-transit metastases that are intralymphatic in origin and occur between the primary tumor site and the regional lymph nodes.

Risk Factors in Local Recurrences

In general, patients with the highest risk for local recurrence have melanomas that have metastasized or melanomas with poor prognostic features. One analysis of local recurrence demonstrated that AJCC stages I and II patients with the highest risk had melanomas with any of the following features: thickness of 4 mm or more (13% of patients), ulceration (11.5%), or location on the foot, hand, scalp, or face (5–12%).[147]

The overall risk for local recurrence is very low and is about 3.2% in collected series involving 3520 patients.[147] Local recurrences usually develop within 5 years after the primary melanoma excision but sometimes occur as late as 10 years afterward.[153,164]

Management of Local Recurrences

Comparative studies of treatment alternatives have not been performed for local recurrences. There are three options: (1) surgical excision, (2) isolated limb perfusion with regional chemotherapy and hyperthermia, or (3) radiation therapy. A single local recurrence, especially in a patient with a previously excised melanoma having favorable prognostic features, can probably be excised with a generous surgical margin and no further treatment. On the other hand, a patient who has multiple recurrences (either simultaneous or sequential) or poor prognostic features of the primary melanoma (*e.g.*, tumors > 4 mm thick, especially with ulceration) might be considered for isolated limb perfusion, because the risks of additional recurrences and in-transit metastases are substantially increased.[165] In patients for whom surgical excision is not feasible, or whose lesions have recurred on multiple occasions, radiation therapy with or without adjuvant hyperthermia should be considered. Our recommendation for treatment of local recurrences is the same as that for metastatic dermal or subcutaneous metastases.

Local recurrences imply a poor prognosis and are usually the first sign that metastases will develop, because most patients with local recurrences subsequently develop metastatic disease.[147,158,166] In a study of 95 patients with local recurrences, the median survival was 3 years, with a 10-year survival rate of only 20%.[147]

REGIONAL METASTATIC MELANOMA

DIAGNOSIS AND CLINICAL EVALUATION

Regional metastases are the most common indication of metastatic melanoma. The physician managing melanoma must be vigilant in making the diagnosis and instituting prompt treatment because some patients can be cured. Moreover, effective palliation can be provided even to those who are not curable. Any adenopathy suspected of harboring metastatic disease should be investigated. If the index of suspicion for metastatic disease is low, the node may be monitored by frequent examination until a diagnosis can be made. In some instances, either fine-needle aspiration or open biopsy is warranted if the examination is equivocal or close follow-up is not possible.

Surgical excision of metastatic nodes is the only effective treatment for cure or local disease control. Some surgeons prefer to excise only clinically demonstrable metastatic nodes. This type of excision has been termed a therapeutic or delayed lymph node dissection. Other surgeons choose to excise the nodes even when they appear normal because of the risk for occult or microscopic metastases. This excision has been termed an elective lymph node dissection (ELND) (called an immediate or prophylactic lymph node dissection). Surgical treatment for established nodal metastases is best described by discussing each of the major lymph node basins where metastatic melanoma can occur. Later sections describe the management of in-transit metastases and the rationale for ELND for micrometastases in the lymph nodes.

ILIOINGUINAL NODAL METASTASES

Rationale

The surgical technique for ilioinguinal lymph node dissection has been described and illustrated.[167–170] There are two contiguous node-bearing basins in the ilioinguinal area that might contain metastatic melanoma. The first is composed of the femoral nodes located within the femoral triangle. The second nodal basin is composed of the iliac and obturator lymph nodes.

In patients with demonstrable nodal metastases, a combined dissection of the iliac and femoral lymph nodes is recommended because at least 25% of patients with femoral nodal metastases have iliac nodal involvement as well.[171,172] There is some controversy concerning the benefit of iliac lymph node dissection. Some surgeons have stated that patients with melanoma of the lower extremities cannot be cured if their nodal metastases extend above the inguinal ligament and that a combined ilioinguinal lymph node dissection is associated with a higher risk for leg edema and wound complications compared with excision of the inguinal nodes alone.[173] Other surgeons have demonstrated that some patients with iliac nodal metastases can be cured or experience prolonged survival (with a 9% to 30% 5-year survival rate) with ilioinguinal lymph node dissection, particularly those patients with microscopic metastases in the inguinal nodes.[171,172,174,175] Excision of the obturator lymph nodes is important, because they can be metastatically involved.[170,176]

Complications and Their Management

In an analysis of 58 patients who underwent inguinal groin dissections, the short-term complications were infrequent and of short duration.[177] Leg edema was a frequent long-term complication (in 26% of patients) but was largely confined to the thigh, and only 8% of patients had edema of the lower leg. Seroma occurred in 23% of patients despite the use of suction catheters, but treatment with simple incision and drainage is generally straightforward. Pain (5% of patients) and functional deficit (3%) were uncommon. Only 1 patient (2%) had persistent severe edema. A wound complication extended hospitalization by an average of 2.1 days. Increasing age was the only risk factor for the development of more wound complications. Residual edema can be a debilitating result of inguinal node dissection.

Three series using preventive measures such as perioperative antibiotics, elastic stockings, leg elevation exercises, and diuretics have shown a decreased incidence of leg edema after groin dissection.[169,177,178] Vigorous prophylactic measures are important because it is difficult to reverse the progression of edema. The patients in one series who followed this prophylactic regimen had a strikingly lower incidence of leg edema than those who did not (7% versus 46%; $p < 0.004$).[178]

AXILLARY NODAL METASTASES

Rationale

The most important feature of axillary node dissection is the completeness of the dissection, including the level III lymph nodes medial to the pectoralis minor muscle. A partial axillary node dissection is simply not in the patient's best interest; moreover, there is little additional morbidity or operative time involved in a complete axillary node dissection. The surgical technique for axillary node dissection has been described and illustrated by others.[167,179–181]

Complications and Their Management

The complication rate for axillary node dissection is low. The most frequent complication is wound seroma.[177,179,180] In a series of 98 radical axillary node dissections in melanoma patients treated at UAB,[177] wound-related complications included infections (7% of patients), seroma (27%), nerve dysfunction or pain (22%), and hemorrhage (1%). Wound-related complications extended the average hospitalization by less than 1 day. Long-term complications included arm edema (1% of patients), pain at the operative site (6%), and functional deficit (9%). Analysis of risk factors showed that increasing age was significantly associated with wound complications, whereas being female or obese only approximated statistical significance as predictive factors.

CERVICAL NODAL METASTASES

Rationale

Metastases to lymph nodes from primary melanomas in the head and neck area through the lymphatics are fairly predictable.[167] Melanomas occurring anterior to the pinna of the ear generally metastasize to the parotid, submandibular, submental, upper jugular, and posterior triangle (spinal accessory and transverse cervical) lymph nodes. Lesions occurring inferior to the lateral fissure of the lip will spread to cervical lymph nodes rather than to parotid nodes. Melanomas occurring on the scalp posterior to the pinna of the ear usually spread to occipital, postauricular, posterior triangle, or jugular chain nodes.

Radical neck dissection is recommended when nodal metastases are clinically evident. The surgical technique for this operation has been published previously.[167,182–185]

Modified Neck Dissection

Although there has never been a comparative study of modified versus radical neck dissection for melanoma, many surgeons have adopted the modified approach because of favorable results in patients with squamous cell carcinoma.[185,186] Modified neck dissection is generally reserved for patients undergoing elective neck dissection, but patients with limited metastatic disease are considered, except when it occurs in the posterior triangle near the spinal accessory nerve. Several variations of a basic technique have been described.[186–191] In comparison with the radical neck dissection discussed above, the only differences in the modified neck dissection are the sparing of the spinal accessory nerve and the sternomastoid muscle.

There are two advantages to modified neck dissection. First, there is better shoulder function and no shoulder drop. Second, the cosmetic result is better. Studies evaluating the functional results of modified neck dissection have shown a good cosmetic result; however, 30% of patients do not retain full spinal accessory nerve function.[192]

Complications and Their Management

A review of complications after radical neck dissection for melanoma revealed that short-term complications (seroma, pain, and skin slough) were common (10–19% of patients). Long-term problems such as neck pain and functional deficit occurred in only 6% to 7% of patients.[177]

A chylous leak can occur even when great care is used to detect leaks before closing the neck wound. Once the leakage rate is less than 50 ml daily, it usually stops within 7 to 10 days.

PAROTID LYMPH NODE DISSECTION

Rationale

Parotid lymph node metastases may be extraglandular or intraglandular. The most common extraglandular nodal metastases are in the preauricular nodes and the nodes located about the tail of parotid. Metastatic intraglandular nodes are generally found within the substance of the parotid gland and are usually located superficial to the seventh cranial nerve.

Melanomas arising on the scalp or face, anterior to the pinna of the ear, and superior to the commissure of the lip are at risk to metastasize to parotid lymph nodes.[193] This parotid chain of nodes is contiguous to the cervical nodes; for this reason, it is generally advisable to combine neck dissection with parotid lymph node dissection if there are metastases to the parotid nodes. The exception to this rule might be a tumor arising immediately over the parotid gland and requiring wide local excision, thereby necessitating parotid dissection to avoid injury to the seventh cranial nerve. Details of the surgical technique have been published.[167,194,195]

Complications and Their Management

Complications after parotidectomy are uncommon when the principles outlined above are followed. The incidence of facial nerve injury is proportional to the extent of dissection and the type and amount of tumor.[196–198] For elective dissection of parotid tumors in general, temporary paralysis of the facial nerve is reported in 10% to 20% of patients and permanent paralysis in 1% to 3%. When recognized during surgery, facial nerve injury should be repaired by primary anastomosis or nerve grafting from the contralateral greater auricular nerve. Seromas and salivary fistulas are uncommon and usually are self-limited. Gustatory sweating (Frey's syndrome) occurs more often than is generally reported but presents problems in only about 5% of patients.[197]

MANAGEMENT OF IN-TRANSIT METASTASES

DIAGNOSIS

In-transit metastases are located between the primary melanoma and the first major regional nodal basin. They probably originate from melanoma cells trapped in lymphatics. Although they may occur in deeper lymphatics, in-transit metastases usually are observed as subcutaneous or intracutaneous metastases (*i.e.,* satellitosis).

The number and location of in-transit metastases and the presence or absence of regional nodal metastases have implications for survival. Those patients with few in-transit metastases have better prognoses than those with multiple lesions. In the Tulane Medical Center series, patients with four or fewer lesions had better outcomes than those with five or more lesions.[199] Regional nodal metastases occur in about two thirds of patients with in-transit metastases and, if present, are associated with a lower survival rate.[200,201]

The reported incidence of in-transit metastases varies. This variation is due in part to the different definitions of in-transit metastases, the referral patterns of the reporting institution, and the proportion of patients with high-risk melanomas. The centers that practice isolated limb perfusion report a substantially higher incidence of in-transit metastases than those that do not. The actual incidence is probably 2% in most surgical practices. The reported incidence of 10% to 20% in some series reported in the 1960s and early 1970s[173,174,202,203] probably results from the fact that most melanomas diagnosed at that time were thicker, more likely to be ulcerated, and associated with a higher risk for nodal metastases than are the melanomas diagnosed in the 1980s.

TREATMENT OPTIONS

The treatment for in-transit metastases is not standardized. The treatment chosen depends primarily on the number and location of lesions in the integument, the presence of metastases elsewhere, the risk of the treatment, and whether previous metastases have been treated successfully. Aggressive local treatment is more effective than available systemic treatment.

Surgery

Surgery may be considered for one or a few lesions. Even with multiple lesions, excision of larger metastases (*i.e.,* those lesions greater than 2 cm) may prevent or relieve symptoms. A regional lymph node dissection usually is performed in patients with in-transit metastases, if it was not done previously, because there is a substantial risk of nodal metastases. Amputation of an extremity is rarely indicated, and then only when other treatments have failed and the patient is symptomatic with pain, bleeding, or odor.

Isolated Limb Perfusion

Isolated limb perfusion is probably the treatment of choice for most patients with in-transit metastases involving an extremity. Sometimes dramatic results can occur in terms of local disease control and prolongation of life.[165] One prospective controlled clinical trial provides evidence that prophylactic perfusion increases survival rates.[204]

Regional Chemotherapy Infusion

Intraarterial infusion of dacarbazine (DTIC) or cisplatin can reduce tumor burden in some patients.[205–207] It may be considered for lesions of the extremities if isolated limb perfusion has previously failed or is unavailable. Partial response rates of 40% to 50% have been reported, but the response durations were short.

Radiation Therapy

In-transit metastases too extensive for surgical excision often can be controlled effectively by radiation therapy. Wide fields and the use of an electron beam of 6 to 9 MeV with an appropriate bolus to eliminate skin sparing are recommended. Postoperative irradiation is indicated after excision of in-transit metastases that recurred after previous excision. Our recommendation for treatment for local recurrences is the same as that for dermal or subcutaneous metastases.

Intralesional Immunotherapy

Some of the first successful treatments using nonspecific immunotherapy were for in-transit metastases. Immunotherapy has been administered as intralesional injections of a variety of agents, including bacillus Calmette-Guérin (BCG), vaccinia virus, and DNCB.[208–210]

Systemic Chemotherapy

In most instances, systemic DTIC chemotherapy (alone or in combination with other agents) offers little chance of success for controlling in-transit metastases. Nevertheless, tumor growth can be temporarily arrested in a few patients but usually for only a few months. Systemic chemotherapy may be considered for multiple lesions, especially if the lesions are symptomatic and if other treatment alternatives cannot be used or have failed.

ELECTIVE LYMPH NODE DISSECTION

RATIONALE

The issue of ELND is probably one of the most important controversies in the management of patients with melanoma. Two randomized prospective studies of extremity melanomas did not demonstrate any survival advantage for ELND, whereas three nonrandomized studies involving melanomas from all anatomic sites showed a statistically significant improvement in survival for a subgroup of intermediate thickness melanomas.[211] Although surgeons are in unanimous agreement that all melanoma patients do not need ELND, there is still a continuing debate that centers around two issues. First, is it possible to identify accurately a subgroup of melanoma patients at high risk for microscopic regional nodal metastases? Second, if such a high-risk group can be identified, what is the optimal timing of dissection (immediate versus delayed)? Prospective randomized studies are in progress to resolve this issue. In the meantime, it is justified to consider ELND in selected intermediate thickness melanoma patients in whom the benefit is sufficiently high and the morbidity sufficiently low to justify in an individual patient.

Theoretically, elective lymphadenectomy has the major advantage of treating a nodal metastasis at a relatively early stage in its natural history, when the tumor burden is generally less than several million cells. The disadvantage is that some patients may be subjected to surgery when they do not have nodal metastases. Conversely, the advantage of delayed lymphadenectomy is that only patients with demonstrable metastases undergo major operations. The great disadvantage, however, is that treatment is delayed until the metastases are clinically palpable, a time when the tumor burden is much greater (*i.e.*, many billions of metastatic cells). As a consequence, the chances for cure are diminished. By the time regional nodal metastases can be detected clinically, 70% to 85% of patients have distant micrometastases of which they will eventually die.[139]

SELECTION OF PATIENTS

Lymphadenectomy

Before defining risk factors for occult metastatic disease in melanoma patients with clinically normal lymph nodes, it is important to categorize patients biologically into three groups: (1) those patients with melanoma localized to the primary lesion site, (2) those with local disease plus possible regional nodal micrometastases, and (3) those with local disease plus distant micrometastases irrespective of whether they have nodal micrometastases. The intuitive surgical strategies are wide excision of the primary lesion site as the sole procedure for patients in the first group and removal of regional nodes containing microscopic or occult metastases for patients in the second group. Regardless of the surgical treatment at the primary and regional sites, the survival of patients in the third category is dictated by the presence of micrometastases at distant sites.

Tumor thickness provides a quantitative estimate of the risk for occult metastatic melanoma at regional and distant sites (Fig. 46–11). Melanoma thickness is the most important but not the sole guide for selecting patients who might benefit from ELND.[127] The major advantage of using tumor thickness for these surgical decisions is that it can provide a quantitative estimate of the risk for occult metastatic melanoma in regional and distant sites.[112,117,120,126–128] Thin melanomas (< 0.76 mm) are associated with localized disease and a 95% or greater cure rate. ELND would provide no therapeutic benefit in such patients. Patients with intermediate thickness melanomas (0.76 mm to 4 mm) have an increased risk (up to 60%) of harboring occult regional metastases, but have a relatively low risk (< 20%) of distant metastases (see Fig. 46–11). Patients with these lesions might therefore benefit from ELND.[112,126,127,211–216] Patients with thick melanomas (> 4 mm) are at high risk for regional nodal micrometastases (> 60%) and for occult distant disease (> 70%) at the time of initial presentation.[112,120,127,140,211,214] These patients do poorly as a group, because the distant metastases in most instances negate the benefit of surgically excising the regional

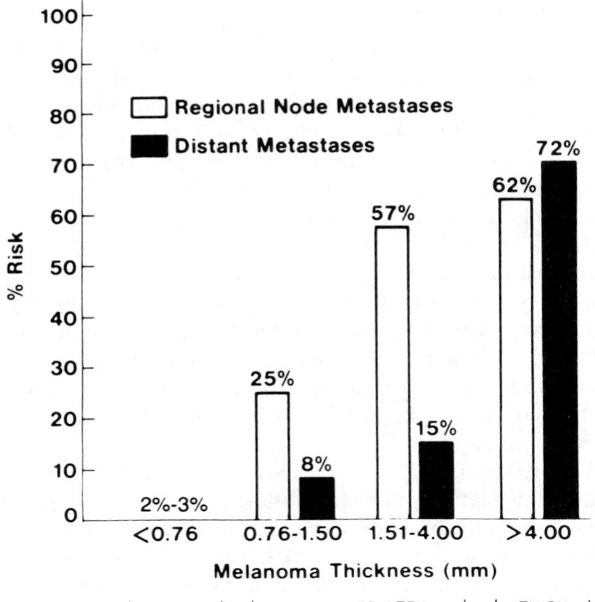

FIGURE 46–11. Estimated biologic risk that microscopic metastases become clinically evident in regional nodes (within 3 years) and at distant sites (within 5 years) for melanomas subgrouped by thickness categories. (Balch CM. Surgical management of regional lymph nodes in cutaneous melanoma. J Am Acad Dermatol 1980;3:511)

lymph nodes. The treatment goal of removing these nodes is palliative, and the operation might be deferred until nodal metastases become clinically evident. Some surgeons prefer to perform ELND as expectant palliation in patients with thick melanomas to avoid the probability (about 30%) of a second operation for lymph node metastases.[214] ELND might be justified as a staging procedure to document the pathologic status of the lymph nodes in patients with thick melanomas before entry into clinical trials involving systemic adjuvant chemotherapy or immunotherapy.

The anatomic site of the melanoma is an important criterion in predicting the risk for regional nodal micrometastases. Patients with melanomas on the extremities have more favorable prognoses, whereas those with melanoma on the trunk or head and neck area have a higher risk for microscopic metastatic disease, even with equivalent tumor thicknesses. Extremity melanomas in women have the lowest biologic potential for metastasis compared with lesions of equivalent thickness on the extremities of men, and patients with melanomas located on the trunk or head and neck area fare worse regardless of sex.[124,125,211,217] Finally, ulcerative melanomas have a higher risk for micrometastases than their nonulcerated counterparts, even when matched for other prognostic parameters such as tumor thickness.[126,213,218,219]

The growth pattern is important to consider in this decision-making process. Patients with LMMs have a low biologic risk for metastases, so ELND is not recommended.[217,220] The decision to perform ELND is made selectively based on the estimated risk for nodal metastases in regional lymph nodes and at distant sites.

ELND for extremity melanomas in women usually is not recommended unless the tumor thickness is at least 1.5 mm or more.[211] Conversely, ELND is recommended more liberally for patients at higher risk, such as men with extremity melanomas and men or women with melanomas located on the trunk or head and neck area. A recommendation for ELND might be considered in these latter patients whose tumor thickness is as low as 1.0 mm. In patients with melanomas more than 4 mm thick, the risk for distant microscopic metastases is so high that it negates any potentially curative benefit of a regional operation.

Tumor thickness should not be the sole criterion for making surgical treatment decisions. Other factors, such as the presence or absence of tumor ulceration, the patient's sex and age, the anatomic location of the melanoma, and the operative risk should all be considered when making the decision to perform ELND on any individual patient.

Identifying the Regional Lymph Nodes At Risk

Because melanomas located on the trunk and on the head and neck area have unpredictable lymphatic drainage, it is difficult to decide which nodal basin is at risk for metastatic disease. In many patients, this problem has been surmounted by performing a radionuclide cutaneous scan that can locate accurately the nodes that are the primary drainage site for a melanoma located anywhere on the trunk.[221–224] All of the regional nodes should be removed, or a policy of monitoring multiple nodal sites at risk should be followed. An ELND of two nodal basins (*e.g.,* bilateral axillary dissection) for trunk melanomas may be warranted in select cases, but removing more than two nodal basins or performing a bilateral cervical dissection as an ELND is never indicated. A bilateral inguinal dissection is usually not performed electively because of its attendant side effects, especially edema of the extremities and genitalia.

Results of Treatment

Results of a prospective but nonrandomized trial of ELND involving 1319 surgically treated patients at the SMU have demonstrated an improved survival rate for those with intermediate thickness melanomas ranging from 0.76 to 4.0 mm (Fig. 46–12).[126,211,212,215] For patients with extremity melanomas, the benefit was greater in men than women.[211,217] A similar analysis of 676 patients treated at UAB during the past 25 years also demonstrated a benefit of ELND for patients who have intermediate thickness melanomas ranging from 1.5 to 4.0 mm (see Fig. 46–12).[35,112,126,140,211,217] Men with melanomas in the 0.76 to 1.5 mm range had the same trend toward an improved survival rate, but this was not statistically significant, largely because the sample size was smaller (Table 46–3). A retrospective data analysis from the Duke Medical Center and the Memorial Sloan-Kettering Cancer Center demonstrated an improved survival rate for patients with intermediate thickness melanomas who undergo ELND,[213,216] although a similar analysis from the University of Pennsylvania did not.[220]

Patients with melanomas located on axial sites (*i.e.,* trunk and head and neck) have a higher risk for metastases than those patients with extremity melanomas.[211,212] There have been no randomized prospective trials of the benefits of ELND for axial melanomas. It is incorrect in our view to extrapolate the data from extremity melanomas and apply it to the treat-

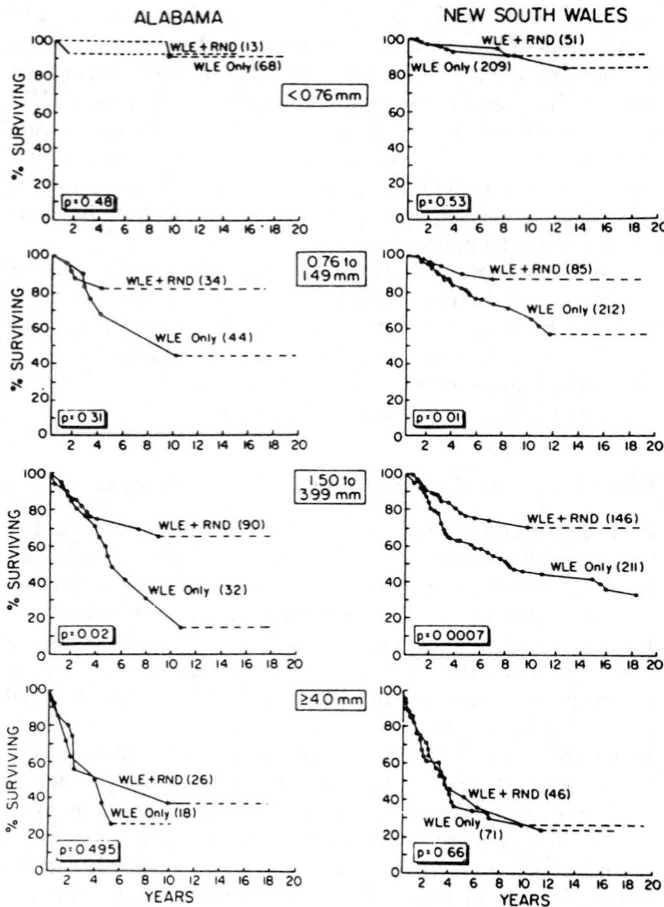

FIGURE 46–12. Actuarial survival curves calculated over 20 years for clinical AJCC stages I and II melanoma patients at the University of Alabama in Birmingham and the University of Sydney. Patients are subgrouped by tumor thickness and initial surgical management (wide local excision [WLE] + elective lymph node dissection [ELND]). The number of patients in each group is shown in parentheses. The *p* values were calculated for differences between each pair of survival curves. The benefit of ELND was greatest in patients with tumors 1.50 to 3.99 mm thick. For 0.76- to 1.49-mm melanomas, the differences were significant only for the Australian patients. The survival curves did not begin to diverge significantly until 5 to 8 years postoperatively. Patients with thin melanomas (< 0.76 mm) and thick melanomas (> 4.00 mm) did not benefit from an ELND. (Balch CM, Cascinelli N, Milton GW, et al. Elective lymph node dissection: Pros and cons. In: Balch CM, Milton GW, eds. Cutaneous melanoma: Clinical management and treatment results worldwide. Philadelphia: JB Lippincott, 1985:135)

ment of patients with axial melanomas. The results from the UAB and SMU data demonstrate an improved survival rate for patients with axial melanomas of intermediate thickness (0.76 to 4 mm) who underwent ELND. The risk for regional nodal metastases is greater and the benefit of ELND is even more apparent in this patient group than in those with extremity melanomas (see Table 46–3).[35,211,212,217] Hansen and McCarten, in a retrospective analysis of 50 patients with head and neck melanomas, also demonstrated an apparent improved survival rate with ELND for melanomas exceeding 1.5 mm in thickness.[225]

Other Considerations

Some investigators have argued that the number of metastatic lymph nodes identified by the pathologist is small after ELND. The proportion of patients with demonstrable metastatic disease in surgically excised nodes ranged from 10% to 25% in different series.[226–228] Within thickness categories, this incidence ranged from less than 5% for melanomas less than 1.5 mm thick to 40% or more for melanomas exceeding 3.0 mm in thickness.[127,214,216] One interpretation of these results is that most patients have no metastatic disease in their nodes and are being overtreated with surgical excision. These figures significantly underestimate the actual incidence of nodal metastases, because micrometastases may have been present in unsampled areas of the specimens. It would require multiple sections of each lymph node to ensure that micrometastases were not present.

A more accurate approach is to analyze the incidence of regional nodal metastases in a follow-up evaluation of patients treated initially by wide excision alone. In a retrospective analysis of patients treated at UAB, patients whose melanomas were greater than 1.5 mm thick and who had wide excision of their melanomas as their only initial surgical management had a 57% risk that nodal micrometastases would become clinically detectable within 3 years of diagnosis (see Fig. 46–11).[127] This percentage is more than double the incidence of occult nodal metastases found by examining randomly sectioned lymph nodes after ELND and is substantiated in part by the studies of Lane and colleagues[229] and Das Gupta,[230] who examined serial sections of nodes removed electively and found occult metastases in 42%.

Results of Randomized Clinical Trials Involving ELND

Two prospective trials to evaluate ELND in the treatment of stage I and stage II melanoma have been performed: an international cooperative study conducted by the WHO Melanoma Group[231–233] and a study by surgeons at the Mayo Clinic.[234] These studies demonstrated that all patients did not benefit from ELND. The question remains, however, whether any subgroup of patients might benefit. Both studies included melanomas of all thicknesses and did not specifically address the potential benefit of ELND in the subgroup of intermediate thickness melanomas described above.

The WHO Melanoma Group study involved 553 patients with stages I and II primary melanoma in the distal two thirds of the limbs. Of these patients, 286 (52%) were randomized to receive wide excision of the primary melanoma as initial treatment and node dissection only if regional node metastases became clinically detectable; 267 (48%) received wide excision plus ELND. The two groups were matched according to the major prognostic criteria. No differences in survival were noted between the two groups. Because subgroups of patients may have benefited from ELND, survival was evaluated according to prognostic criteria: sex, invasion levels III and IV, tumor thickness, and ulceration. No significant survival differences were reported in any of these subgroups. A separate analysis of the data demonstrated a 22% increase in 10-year survival in a small subgroup with intermediate-risk lesions.[211]

TABLE 46–3. Ten-Year Survival Rates of Clinical Stage I Melanoma Patients Treated at the Sydney Melanoma Unit, Australia, and the University of Alabama, Birmingham

Tumor Thickness (mm)	*Extremity Melanomas*			*Trunk and Head and Neck Melanomas*		
	WLE Only	*WLE and ELND*	*p Value*	*WLE Only*	*WLE and ELND*	*p Value*
<0.76	94% ± 5% (n = 142)	100% ± 0% (n = 26)	0.230	86% ± 6% (n = 135)	83% ± 8% (n = 38)	0.343
0.76–1.49	74% ± 8% (n = 125)	92% ± 4% (n = 66)	0.042	56% ± 10% (n = 131)	80% ± 7% (n = 51)	0.049
1.50–3.99	54% ± 7% (n = 114)	80% ± 6% (n = 107)	0.005	33% ± 6% (n = 129)	64% ± 7% (n = 129)	0.0008
≥4.0	30% ± 10% (n = 33)	44% ± 13% (n = 34)	0.400	22% ± 9% (n = 56)	26% ± 13% (n = 38)	0.806

ELND, elective (prophylactic) lymph node dissection; WLE, wide local excision.
(Balch CM, Cascinelli N, Milton GW, Sims FH. Elective lymph node dissection: Pros and cons. In: Balch CM, ed. Cutaneous melanoma. 2nd ed. Philadelphia: JB Lippincott, 1992:345)

Surgeons at the Mayo Clinic conducted a clinical study from 1972 to 1976 in which 171 stage I melanoma patients were randomized into one of three treatment groups. Sixty-two patients had their nodes left intact, 55 patients had ELND that was delayed 30 to 60 days after the primary melanoma excision, and 54 patients had elective lymphadenectomy concomitantly with the primary melanoma excision.[234] Patients with lesions of the head and neck and midline trunk were excluded. Compared with the two groups of patients who underwent ELND, patients who did not have ELND were older, more often men, and had worse prognostic features (*i.e.*, deeper invasion, thicker lesions, and more nodular lesions). The subgroup that received immediate ELND had more sites involving the trunk than did the other subgroups. None of these differences was statistically significant, although the subgroup with intact nodes was biased toward an unfavorable prognosis. Six characteristics were analyzed: initial surgical treatment, age, sex, anatomic site, tumor thickness, and growth pattern. The only factors that were significantly related to survival were tumor thickness ($p < 0.0001$) and growth pattern ($p = 0.02$).

When overall survival and disease-free survival of the three surgical treatment groups were compared, there were no significant differences.[234] The 5-year survival rate was 85% when the nodes were left intact, 85% when the nodes were removed immediately, and 91% when delayed ELND was performed. Survival and disease-free survival were significantly related to the thickness of the lesion.

The Mayo Clinic and the WHO Melanoma Group studies indicated no benefit from routine ELND for patients with stages I and II melanoma involving the extremities. There are legitimate differences in interpreting the results of the two trials.[211,217] These differences can be resolved only by continuing to perform randomized clinical trials using stratification criteria, extending these studies to all anatomic sites but confining the patient eligibility to intermediate thickness melanomas. Multiinstitutional surgical trials are being conducted in North America and Europe to assess the optimal timing of lymphadenectomy (immediate versus delayed if necessary) in a randomized prospective manner for intermediate thickness melanomas.

THE ROLE OF ADJUVANT RADIATION THERAPY

The role of radiation therapy as a surgical adjuvant after therapeutic node dissection or as an alternative to ELND in the regional treatment of patients with intermediate to thick melanomas has not been defined clearly. The rationale for its consideration in this context is that ELND, although effectively reducing regional recurrence rates, carries varying degrees of morbidity and does not offer any survival advantage in patients with thick primary tumors.[211,215] On the other hand, therapeutic dissection of pathologically involved nodes is associated with a local recurrence rate of up to 50% in patients with head and neck melanomas.[185,235]

Because of the management problems associated with uncontrolled locoregional disease and the extent of elective dissections required for scalp and facial primary sites, a study was initiated at the M.D. Anderson Cancer Center in 1983 to evaluate the role of radiation therapy in the treatment of clinically uninvolved lymph drainage areas. The study evaluated the use of radiation therapy in patients at high risk for nodal metastases and as an adjunct to surgery in patients undergoing therapeutic nodal dissections.

The preliminary results of this trial indicate an apparent advantage in terms of locoregional recurrence for adjuvant radiation therapy and were published by Ang and colleagues in 1990.[236] The following is an update of the study. Through August 1991, 153 patients were entered and divided into three groups. Group I consisted of 67 patients with primary lesions more than 1.5 mm in thickness (median 3.0 mm) or at Clark's level III or greater who had no clinically palpable lymphadenopathy. After wide local excision, these patients received radiation therapy to the tumor bed and draining lymphatics of 3000 cGy Dmax delivered in 5 fractions over 2.5 weeks with electron beams of appropriate energy. This group of patients had an overall 5-year rate of locoregional control of 87%, and 5-year survival of 63%. All patients with level III lesions less than 1.5 mm thick survived 5 years, and 82% of those whose primary lesion was 1.6 to 4 mm in thickness were 5-year survivors with adjuvant radiation therapy (Fig. 46–13). These results are similar to those obtained with elective nodal dissections for intermediate thickness melanomas (see Fig. 46–13).

Group II consisted of 29 patients with previously untreated disease who presented with clinically positive lymphadenopathy. These patients mostly received postoperative radiation therapy (3000 cGy Dmax delivered in 5 fractions over 2.5 weeks); the remainder received preoperative treatment (200 cGy Dmax delivered in 4 fractions over 2 weeks). These patients achieved a 5-year locoregional control rate of 96% and a 5-year survival of 44%. Survival was inversely proportional to the number of pathologically involved lymph nodes.

Group III consisted of 57 patients who presented with recurrent regional or local disease, but without evidence of distant metastases. These patients were treated in the same manner as group II patients. Their 5-year locoregional control rate was 88%, and the survival rate was 39%.

These results demonstrate that adjuvant radiation therapy, either alone in clinically node-negative patients or as a surgical adjuvant in pathologically node-positive patients, can achieve locoregional control in excess of 85%. This is substantially better than rates previously reported with surgery alone in comparable patients. The radiation therapy schedule used was not associated with any significant morbidity. In total, 3 of the 153 patients treated have sustained mild to moderate sequelae. There have been no severe complications. Although these data are impressive, proof of a therapeutic benefit from adjuvant radiation therapy can be obtained only from a prospective randomized trial. Such a trial, based on our pilot study, is under development by the Radiation Therapy and Oncology Group (RTOG).

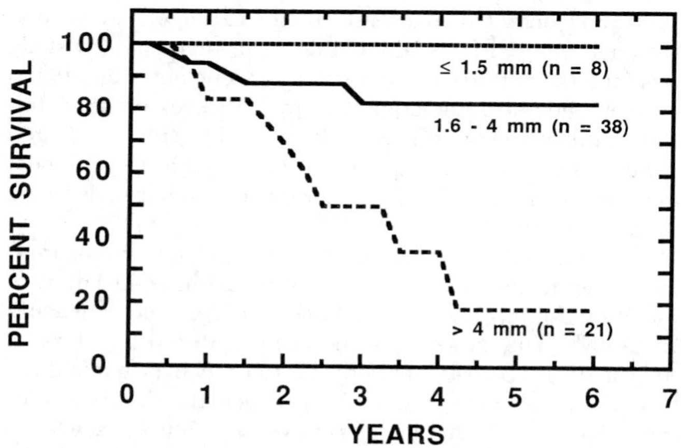

FIGURE 46–13. Survival of patients at The University of Texas M.D. Anderson Cancer Center receiving elective irradiation of the draining lymphatics of primary cutaneous melanomas of the head and neck, as a function of tumor thickness. All patients had primary lesions invading to Clark's level III or greater.

METASTATIC MELANOMA AT DISTANT SITES

SITES AND PATTERNS OF METASTASES

Melanoma can metastasize to almost every major organ and tissue. Average survival is very short when metastases are detected in multiple visceral sites. Autopsy series have revealed that the lung is involved in 70% to 87% of cases, liver in 54% to 77%, bowel in 26% to 58%, brain in 36% to 54%, heart in 40% to 45%, adrenals in 36% to 54%, kidney in 35% to 48%, and bone in 23% to 49% (Table 46–4).[236,237] Most patients die with disseminated disease involving multiple organ sites; the actual cause of death is often respiratory failure or brain complications.[238,239] In clinical series, metastases to the lung, liver, brain, and bone occur in 11% to 36% of patients, well below the frequencies detected in autopsy series.[145,238–246] Metastases to the heart, adrenals, pancreas, and kidney have been detected only infrequently in clinical series (< 1% of cases), although abdominal visceral metastases are identified at higher frequencies with the use of computed tomography (CT) scans and magnetic resonance imaging (MRI). These studies suggest that clinical evaluation of patients often underestimates the extent of metastatic disease and actual tumor burden.

The site of first distant metastasis is an important prognostic variable (see Table 46–4). After treatment for primary or regional disease, the most frequent distant sites for first recurrence are the skin, subcutaneous tissues, and distant lymph nodes (up to 59% of patients; see Table 46–4).[117,247] This pattern of recurrence confirms the importance of a careful physical examination in monitoring patients with AJCC stage I, II, or III melanoma who are free of disease. The median survival of patients with skin, subcutaneous tissue, and distant

TABLE 46–4. Common Distant Sites of Metastatic Melanoma

Site	*Clinical Series* (%)*	*Autopsy Series* (%)*
Skin, subcutaneous, lymph nodes	42–59	50–75
Lungs	18–36	70–87
Liver	14–20	54–77
Brain	12–20	36–54
Bone	11–17	23–49
GI tract	1–7	26–58
Heart	<1	40–45
Pancreas	<1	38–53
Adrenals	<1	36–54
Kidneys	<1	35–48
Thyroid	<1	25–39

* From references 145, 238, 240, 241, 242, 243, 244, 245, 246, and 250.
(Adapted from Balch CM, Milton GW. Diagnosis of metastatic melanoma at distant sites. In: Balch CM, Milton GW, eds. Cutaneous melanoma: Clinical management and treatment results worldwide. Philadelphia: JB Lippincott, 1985:221)

lymph node metastases is 7 months, but there is wide variability of survival in this group of patients. The second most frequent site for first relapse is the lung (up to 36% of patients); patients with lung involvement have a median survival of 11 months. The liver, brain, and bone comprise the next most frequent sites of recurrence (median survival for these patients ranges from only 2 to 6 months). In general, patients with visceral metastases (with or without skin, subcutaneous tissue, or lymph node involvement) do very poorly. In the UAB series, more than 80% of patients with visceral metastases were dead within 1 year and almost all died within 2 years.[117] Patients with lung metastases as their only visceral metastatic site generally fared better (median survival 11.4 months) than patients with tumors at other visceral sites. In the series from UAB, median survival of patients with a single distant metastatic site was 7 months, with two sites 4 months, and with three sites 2 months.[117,145] Disease-free intervals of 1 year[145] and 2 years[248] have been associated with longer survival.

DIAGNOSTIC EVALUATION OF METASTATIC DISEASE

The evaluation for metastatic disease in patients who are clinically free of tumors should include a careful physical examination, chest x-ray films, and liver function tests. Serum lactate dehydrogenase (LDH) is a useful marker for widespread metastases, especially for the detection of liver disease.[243,249,250] Blood in the stool and abdominal and gastrointestinal symptoms should be investigated as possible indications of metastases. Particular attention should be paid to signs or symptoms of central nervous system involvement. In all patients with systemic melanoma metastases, there should be a high index of suspicion for associated brain, spinal cord, or meningeal metastases. Extensive radiographic evaluation of patients with AJCC stage I, II, or III melanomas who are free of disease rarely reveals metastases. Chest tomography, upper gastrointestinal series, barium enema, abdominal ultrasound, intravenous pyelogram, brain CT scan, and radionuclide scans of brain, bone, and liver rarely reveal metastases in the absence of symptoms, signs, or abnormal standard test results (*e.g.*, chest x-ray films, hemogram, liver function tests including LDH).[244,251–260] The rate of false-positive tests makes extensive evaluations costly. Likewise, conventional scanning with ^{67}Ga is not a sufficiently sensitive or specific screening test, although it can detect metastatic melanoma.[261–265]

Although metastases can remain stable for months, even without treatment, progression of existing tumors or appearance of new tumors can occur rapidly, sometimes accompanied by precipitous clinical deterioration. Patients need to be evaluated at frequent intervals by medical personnel who are familiar with the patient's diagnosis and conditions. Despite the poor prognoses and the availability of prognostic indicators for patients with systemic metastases, it is often difficult to predict the course of an individual patient's disease. Periods of stability without evident tumor growth can be interrupted by a medical emergency (*e.g.*, seizure due to intracranial hemorrhage from a brain metastasis or acute gastrointestinal bleeding from a small bowel lesion).

TREATMENT MODALITIES

Patients with systemic metastases (AJCC stage IV) have poor prognoses. The mean survival is about 6 months,[117,145,248] and cure is not a realistic aim. Treatment of this group of patients should include careful evaluation for the potential role of surgery, radiation therapy, and systemic therapy.[266] General guidelines for choosing treatment modalities are presented in Table 46–5. Selection of treatment options should take into account the general medical condition of the patient, the potential for prevention or relief of symptoms, and improve-

TABLE 46–5. Treatment Options for Systemic Metastatic Melanoma

Treatment Option	*Site of Metastases*	*Comments*
Surgery	Superficial lesions Brain Symptomatic visceral Occasional lung	Best for solitary lesions, especially symptomatic; low-risk patients
Radiation therapy	Superficial lesions Brain Bone	Treatment of symptomatic lesions
Chemotherapy	Systemic metastases	Skin, subcutaneous tissue, lymph node, and lung lesions most responsive
Limb perfusion	Local recurrences	Restricted to extremity lesions; requires major surgery
Hyperthermia	Liver lesions Large superficial lesions	Experimental treatment
Intralesional therapy	Skin lesions	Experimental treatment; can be locally effective for dermal metastases
Systemic immunotherapy	Systemic metastases	Experimental treatment

(Adapted from Houghton AN, Balch CM. Treatment for advanced melanoma. In: Balch CM, ed. Cutaneous melanoma. 2nd ed. Philadelphia: JB Lippincott, 1992:468)

ment in the quality of life. The median age of patients with melanoma, about 45 years, is young compared with the age of most adult cancer patients. Careful consideration must be given to the impact of prognosis and treatment for these patients, who are frequently primary providers for their families and have full-time occupations.

NO TREATMENT

The option of no treatment is important, especially in asymptomatic patients, those who are terminally ill, or those at advanced ages. There are two groups of patients for whom no treatment is a major consideration. The first group consists of asymptomatic patients with tumors in favorable sites, such as the lung or bone (but not brain). The physician may elect to observe these lesions if they are growing slowly and are not causing symptoms. Quality of life is maintained in this instance, and treatment can be deferred until the lesions begin to progress, either by size or multiplicity, or until the patients develop symptoms. The second group consists of patients who are terminally ill or very old and for whom the benefit-to-risk ratio is small. The decision to forego treatment can be difficult; it is often best made by the patients themselves with the assistance of close relatives or medical or nursing advisors. A patient should not be denied treatment when there is a reasonable expectation that the treatment will be successful and the risk or toxicity is low.

SURGERY

Surgery is an effective palliative treatment for isolated metastases, especially because melanoma often metastasizes sequentially and effective chemotherapy is not available. Surgical excision of metastatic melanoma probably gives the patient the best, quickest, and longest lasting palliation. On some occasions, the palliative effect can last for 5 to 10 years.[242,267–269] The favorable experience with surgical resection of distant metastases in selected patients treated at four institutions is shown in Table 46–6.

The limitation of surgery is that it is a local form of treatment, and the patient will eventually die from metastatic disease elsewhere. Careful patient selection is important. Observation for several weeks may provide relevant information about the rate of tumor growth and the presence of other multiple metastases, which could emerge during the observation period. Surgery should be confined to situations involving accessible lesions that are limited in size and number and in which the operation can be safely performed. Some examples of accessible lesions include isolated visceral metastases (especially brain) and occasional lung metastases. Most amenable to this approach are gastrointestinal metastases that cause obstructions, and superficially located lesions in the skin, subcutaneous tissues, or distant lymph nodes. Liver metastases are associated with such a short survival (*i.e.*, 2–4 months) that surgical excision generally is not indicated.

The choice of surgical excision as a means of palliation depends on the site of the disease and the duration of anticipated survival. If the patient's life is likely to be measured in weeks, the surgical ablation of a large growth is not justified, whereas longer anticipated survival makes excision of gross disease worth considering. Each case has to be considered on its own merits.

RADIATION THERAPY

Over the past two decades, a large number of retrospective clinical studies on the role of radiation therapy for metastatic and recurrent melanoma have been published and are reviewed by Peters and colleagues.[270] These studies involved a variety of metastatic sites (*e.g.*, cutaneous, lymph nodes, brain, bone, lung, and other viscera), and no general conclusions can be drawn from them. In the treatment of cutaneous and lymph node metastases, most investigators observed improved response rates with higher fractional doses.[271–280] The interpretation of the role of fraction is complicated by the variability in total dose administered and by the heterogeneity of the clinical material. Bentzen and colleagues[281] recently undertook an analysis of the role of fraction size correcting for total dose and tumor volume, using the data base of Overgaard and colleagues[279] and more recently accrued cases. They found that the probability of local control increased with size of dose per fraction, at least up to 900 cGy (Fig. 46–14). However, the use of high fractional doses limits the total dose that can be administered without causing injury to many late-reacting normal tissues.[282] The optimal size of dose per fraction represents a trade-off between the probability of sterilizing the melanoma versus the probability of causing normal tissue damage. Using subcutaneous fibrosis as the normal tissue end-

TABLE 46–6. Median Survival of Melanoma Patients After Complete Surgical Resection of Distant Metastases

	Survival in Months (No. of Patients)			
Site	*M.D. Anderson Cancer Center*[242]	*Memorial Hospital*[268]	*Univ. of Alabama Hospitals*[269]	*Roswell Park Institute*[267]
Skin, subcutaneous	23 (64)	25 (12)	17 (13)	31 (25)
Lung	16 (26)	19 (17)	9 (17)	9 (13)
Brain	15 (16)	7.5 (5)	8 (17)	5 (4)
GI (excluding liver)	18 (9)	15 (12)	8 (5)	8 (3)
Overall 2-year survival	15%	21%	16%	31%

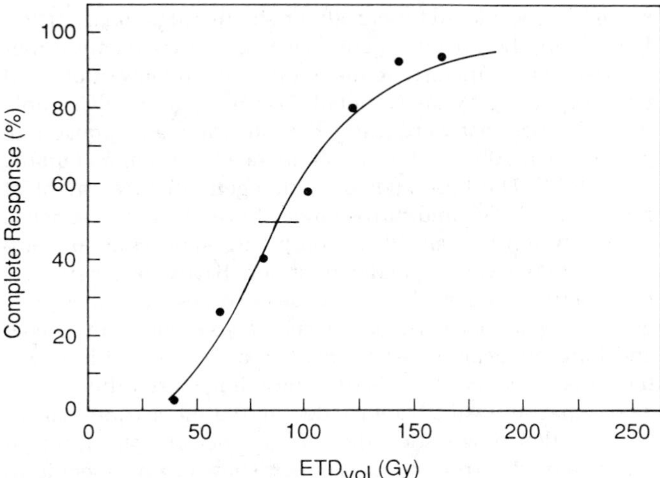

FIGURE 46–14. Dose-response relation showing the probability of achieving complete response as a function of volume-corrected extrapolated total dose (ETD_{vol}). The horizontal bar indicates the 95% confidence limits of the 50% complete response probability. (Overgaard J, et al. Some factors of importance in the radiation treatment of malignant melanoma. Radiother Oncol 1986;5:187)

point, Bentzen and colleagues calculated the therapeutic ratio as a function of dose per fraction.[281] The therapeutic ratio increased rapidly between 200 and 500 cGy and gradually thereafter. However, the lower confidence limit for the therapeutic ratio showed a peak in the range of 500 to 600 cGy which would, therefore, define the safest dose per fraction to be used when damage to connective tissue is dose limiting. Although this analysis supports the use of larger than conventional fractional doses, at least for the treatment of subcutaneous and lymph nodal metastases, a recent RTOG study failed to demonstrate any significant advantage of a treatment regimen consisting of 4 fractions of 800 cGy compared with one consisting of 20 fractions of 250 cGy.[283] A total of 137 patients were entered into this study, which included all metastatic sites other than the abdomen or brain. Most metastases were in soft tissues, skin, or lymph nodes. Tumors were stratified according to whether they were greater or less than 5 cm in largest diameter, but otherwise size was not recorded or corrected in the analysis. Total response rates were 59.7% with the 4 × 800 cGy regimen, and 57.8% with the 20 × 250 cGy regimen.

In summary, the question of optimal fraction in the treatment of melanoma remains controversial. It is certain that no single fraction size is optimal for all patients because of variability of the radiobiologic characteristics of individual tumors. Although most retrospective studies and the elegant analysis of Bentzen and colleagues[281] support the use of larger than standard dose fractions, no advantage was observed in the randomized RTOG trial.[283] We believe that the appropriate recommendation for dose fractionation should be based on considerations of normal tissue tolerance. The treatment should be convenient for the patient, at least as effective as standard treatment, and used at sites where hypofractionated treatment is well tolerated. The hypofractionated regimen is not recommended when the dose-limiting normal tissue is the central nervous system or the abdominal viscera because of the poor tolerance of these organs to large-dose fractions.

EXPERIMENTAL THERAPIES

Because the results achieved in melanoma by standard radiation therapy are less than optimal regardless of fractionation schedule, a variety of experimental therapies have been proposed and tested.

Hyperthermia

A good review of the value of hyperthermia as an adjuvant to radiation therapy in the management of malignant melanoma was published in 1987 by Overgaard and Overgaard.[284] These authors reported that in patients with subcutaneous or lymph node metastases, the response to radiation therapy was significantly improved by the addition of hyperthermia to a temperature of 43°C for 30 minutes. When the two treatments were given immediately sequentially ("simultaneously"), no improvement in therapeutic ratio was observed, because normal tissue reactions were exacerbated to the same extent as tumor response was improved. When hyperthermia was delayed until 3 to 4 hours after administration of each of three radiation therapy doses of 800 cGy, a significant improvement in therapeutic ratio was observed. Many other researchers have reported increased response rates with adjuvant hyperthermia in the treatment of malignant melanoma, and their work is reviewed by Meyer and colleagues.[285] With the exception of a study by Overgaard and Overgaard,[284] few attempts have been made to measure the therapeutic ratio, and improvement in this parameter has not been demonstrated in a randomized trial.

Clinical hyperthermia is limited by the technical difficulty associated with heating large or deep-seated tumors. Nonetheless, for accessible superficial lesions, it seems reasonable to use adjuvant hyperthermia when it is available.

High Linear Energy Transfer Irradiation

On radiobiologic grounds, fast neutron radiation therapy would be expected to achieve results equal to, or possibly better than, high dose per fraction x-ray or gamma-ray radiation therapy. The largest series of patients reported for whom such therapy has been employed is from the Hammersmith Hospital in London. In a series of 68 patients with 87 recurrent or metastatic lesions, Blake and colleagues reported a 71% complete response rate that was durable for the remainder of the patients' lives in 91% of cases.[286] A high complication rate of 22% was observed; however, most of these complications occurred in treatments of lower limb, groin, and axilla. Further studies of the value of fast neutron radiation therapy using somewhat lower biologically effective doses than those employed at Hammersmith are under way in the United States. No data from these studies are available.

Radiosensitizers

Both hypoxic and aerobic cell sensitizers are being studied as radiation therapy adjuvants for metastatic melanoma. Dische reported complete and sustained remission in 5 of 7 cases of recurrent cutaneous or lymph node disease treated with high-dose radiation therapy (5200–5600 cGy in 20 fractions) in conjunction with the hypoxic cell sensitizer Ro-03-8799 (pimonidazole).[287] Because a significant proportion of hypoxic cells has been demonstrated in autochthonous metastases of human melanoma,[288] further studies using sensitizers specific to hypoxic cells are indicated.

Another class of sensitizers is being tested by the RTOG in the treatment of brain metastases. In this study, the halogenated pyrimidine iododeoxyuridine is the sensitizer. The drug is incorporated into the DNA of cells during the S phase of the cell cycle and is therefore preferentially incorporated into brain metastases relative to the surrounding normal brain. No data on the results of this trial are available.

Photodynamic Therapy

The principle of photodynamic therapy is based on the cytotoxic effects of visible light on cells that have taken up dyes extracted from hematoporphyrin. Several such dyes are selectively retained in neoplastic tissue, affording a therapeutic advantage when these tissues can be illuminated with visible light. Photodynamic therapy is of particular interest in the treatment of dermal metastases from malignant melanoma. It is too early to assess the value of this approach in relation to other therapies. For a recent review of photodynamic therapy, see DeLaney and Glatstein.[289]

Thermal Neutron Capture Therapy

When the isotope boron 10 is irradiated with thermal neutrons, it undergoes nuclear disintegration and releases an α particle with a range of 10 to 14 μm, allowing highly selective irradiation of cells that concentrate the isotope. Mishima and associates recently reported on the first human treatment with neutron capture therapy using the melanoma-seeking drug ^{10}B1-para-boronophenylalanine HCl (^{10}B1-BPA HCl).[290] The patient had a metastatic lesion in the left occipital region. A ^{10}B tumor concentration of 24 μg/g was achieved in the tumor, and the lesion was then irradiated with thermal neutrons from a nuclear reactor. Complete regression of the lesion occurred and had been maintained for 10 months at the time the report was published. The ability to target ^{10}B selectively to melanoma by incorporating the isotope into a precursor of melanin synthesis makes this approach an attractive one for future development.

Radiolabeled Antibodies

The use of radiolabeled antibodies specific to melanoma antigens is an appealing concept, especially for adjuvant systematic therapy for a disease in which cytotoxic chemotherapy is of limited efficacy. Major problems relating to antibody specificity, stability, radionuclide specific activity, antigenic heterogeneity, and modulation of expression must be resolved before the full potential of this approach is realized. This strategy is discussed in more detail in the section on monoclonal antibodies.

Chemotherapy

Systemic therapy for melanoma, both as adjuvant therapy and for treatment of disseminated (stage IV) disease, remains unsatisfactory. Patients with high-risk or metastatic disease should be considered for enrollment in investigational studies. Few chemotherapeutic agents have demonstrated antitumor activity against metastatic melanoma. In a review of phase II trials supported by the National Cancer Institute (NCI), only 2 of 30 drugs that were tested demonstrated a response rate greater than 10% (with 80% confidence limits) in melanoma patients.[291] The best-studied single agents for treatment of melanoma, DTIC and nitrosoureas, have objective response rates between 10% and 20%. Complete responses are uncommon. Patients who respond to treatment have a longer survival than nonresponders, but responses are observed most frequently in patients with skin, subcutaneous tissue, lymph node, and lung metastases—sites that are associated with longer median survival.[292–294] It is therefore difficult to differentiate a potential survival advantage due to treatment from that related to other prognostic indicators, and no survival advantage associated with treatment has been shown to be specific to treatment and independent from other prognostic factors.

The evaluation of experimental systemic treatments for melanoma should take into account the following two prognostic factors for metastatic disease: (1) sites of tumor (skin, subcutaneous tissues, lymph nodes, and lung versus non-lung visceral sites), and (2) number of organs or tissues involved with disease (one, two, three or more). Occasionally, individual skin or subcutaneous lesions that are small (< 1 cm in diameter) can wax and wane without treatment. It is therefore important to choose sizable indicator lesions that can be confidently measured. Spontaneous regression that would fit the criterion for objective response to treatment (*i.e.*, greater than 50% decrease in the product of the greatest perpendicular diameters of measurable lesions, lasting at least 1 month) occurs infrequently when measurable indicator lesions are used.

SINGLE-AGENT CHEMOTHERAPY. DTIC remains the most active single agent for the treatment of systemic melanoma. The response rate is about 20% (Table 46–7), and patients with skin, subcutaneous tissue, and lymph node involvement respond most frequently.[292–316] Lung metastases are also responsive to DTIC, but liver, bone, and brain metastases respond infrequently. The median duration of response is 5 to 6 months. Complete responses were observed in about 5% of 580 patients entered into phase III trials, and most of these complete responses occurred in subcutaneous and lymph node metastases.[308] A minority (31%) of patients who achieved complete response survived and remained disease-free at 6 years. Overall, about 2% of patients treated with DTIC sustain long-term complete responses.

DTIC is typically well tolerated. The major side effects of DTIC used to be nausea and vomiting, but effective antiemetic regimens can control this toxicity in a high proportion of patients.[317,318] Ondansetron or a combination of lorazepam, dexamethasone, and metoclopramide appear to be effective antiemetic regimens. Other side effects of DTIC include local pain at the injection site, neutropenia, and thrombocytopenia, which are usually mild and occur between days 10 and 21, and flu-like symptoms and diarrhea. Photosensitivity reactions occur infrequently. Dose-related and life-threatening liver failure due to hepatic necrosis and venoocclusive disease has been seen in rare cases. DTIC may be given as a 1-day, 5-day, or 10-day regimen. Recommended doses are as follows: (1)

TABLE 46–7. Active Chemotherapy for Metastatic Melanoma

Agent	*No. of Evaluable Patients*	*Response*		*References*
		No. of CR + PR (%)	*95% CI (%)*	
Dacarbazine (DTIC)	1936	382 (20)	18–22	291–316
Carmustine (BCNU)	122	22 (18)	11–25	319–321
Lomustine (CCNU)	270	35 (13)	9–17	322–324, 326
Tauromustine (TCNU)	42	7 (17)	6–31	331
Fotemustine	153	37 (24)	17–31	329, 330
Cisplatin	188	43 (23)	17–29	332–339
Carboplatin	43	7 (16)	5–27	340
Vincristine	52	6 (12)	3–20	341–347
Vinblastine	62	8 (13)	5–21	348–357
Vindesine	273	39 (14)	10–18	358–369
Taxol	65	12 (18)	9–28	370–372
Dibromodulcitol	205	28 (14)	9–18	373–381
Detorubicin	42	8 (19)	7–31	382
Piritrexim	31	7 (23)	8–37	383

CR, complete response; PR, partial response; CI, 95% confidence interval for response rates.

850–1000 mg/m^2 given intravenously for 1 day every 3 to 4 weeks; (2) 250 mg/m^2/day given intravenously for 5 days every 3 weeks; or (3) 2 to 4.5 mg/kg/day given intravenously for 10 days repeated every 4 weeks. There is no evidence that response rates or duration are affected by schedule or daily dose. With the advent of effective antiemetic regimens, the 1-day schedule repeated every 3 to 4 weeks is acceptable and often is least intrusive to the patient. It is generally well tolerated and should be administered in an appropriate outpatient setting. Dose can be escalated as tolerated, depending on neutropenia and thrombocytopenia, because hematologic toxicity is not usually cumulative. Blood counts should be followed carefully during treatment.

The nitrosoureas are a second group of agents with defined activity against melanoma (see Table 46–7). Response rates are generally between 10% and 20%. Hematologic toxicity of the nitrosoureas can be more severe than with DTIC and is cumulative. Carmustine (BCNU), lomustine (CCNU), semustine (methyl-CCNU), and fotemustine are the best studied of this class.[319–331] Sites of responses are similar to those responding to DTIC (*e.g.,* skin, subcutaneous tissues, lymph nodes, lungs). Because the central nervous system is a common site for metastasis, it was hoped that the lipid-soluble nitrosoureas would induce frequent responses at brain sites. This generally has not been the case, with the possible exception of fotemustine. Fotemustine was synthesized to facilitate penetration into cells and through the blood–brain barrier by addition of an amino acid analogue 1-amino-ethyl-phosphonic acid chain onto a chlorethyl-nitrosourea to take advantage of cellular amino acid transport systems. Although response rates of fotemustine are similar to those observed with other nitrosoureas and with DTIC, fotemustine was reported to induce 9 partial responses in 36 patients with brain metastases, an observation that needs to be confirmed.[330] Recently, a new nitrosourea, tauromustine (TCNU), has demonstrated activity in melanoma.[331]

Activity against melanoma has been detected with several other classes of agents (see Table 46–7). Cisplatin and the related compound carboplatin have measurable, although generally limited, activity against melanoma.[332–340] The vinca alkaloids vindesine, vincristine, and vinblastine have marginal activity against metastatic melanoma, with response rates in the range of 12% to 14%.[341–369] Both these classes have been used widely in combination therapies for melanoma. Taxol, a plant product derived from the Western yew tree (*Taxus brevifolia*), promotes microtubule assembly. Because of limited supply, clinical trials with taxol have been restricted, but preliminary findings in melanoma are encouraging and need to be extended.[370–372] Dibromodulcitol (mitolactol), a lipid-soluble agent with alkylating properties, has been shown to have activity in melanoma.[373–381] It has been suggested that a daily dose schedule is more effective than an intermittent dose schedule. Two other agents, the semisynthetic anthracycline detorubicin and the dihydrofolate reductase inhibitor piritrexim, have been reported to have activity in single phase II trials, but these studies need to be confirmed.[382,383]

HIGH-DOSE CHEMOTHERAPY WITH OR WITHOUT AUTOLOGOUS BONE MARROW TRANSPLANTATION. Increasing dose is one strategy to overcome resistance to therapy. Because single agents have only limited activity in melanoma, dose could be a factor in establishing more respectable complete response rates in melanoma, particularly with alkylating agents. Most studies exploring high-dose chemotherapy have been phase I–II trials using autologous bone marrow rescue. Several drugs have been evaluated, including alkylating agents (*e.g.,* melphalan, thiotepa), DTIC, and nitrosoureas.[384–400]

High-dose chemotherapy trials with autologous bone marrow rescue have generally involved small numbers of patients (Table 46–8). Responses have been observed in 38% of patients treated with high-dose BCNU.[389] High-dose melphalan

TABLE 46–8. Results of High-Dose Chemotherapy Trials With Autologous Bone Marrow Transplantation

Agent	*No. of Patients*	*Response (%)*	*CR (%)*	*Median Response Duration (mo)*	*References*
Melphalan	48	58	19	3–6	390–392
Thiotepa	51	57	8	3	393
BCNU	29	38	13	6	389
DTIC + melphalan or ifosfamide	37	49	14	4	400
BCNU combinations*	38	50	8	2–4	385, 394–396, 399

CR, complete response.
* BCNU plus varying combinations of melphalan, cisplatin, and cyclophosphamide.

or thiotepa has induced responses in 50% to 60% of patients.[390–393] High-dose BCNU has been added to varying combinations of melphalan, thiotepa, cyclophosphamide, or cisplatin, with a 50% overall response rate.[385,394–396,398,399] High doses of DTIC plus melphalan or ifosfamide have produced responses in 49% of patients.[400] Although these results are encouraging, they cannot be considered a meaningful advance. Toxicity of these regimens is substantial, and they are associated with fatalities (in up to a third of cases at very high doses). Although advances in hematopoietic growth factors suggest that this approach can be extended, life-threatening toxic reactions can occur at extramedullary sites (*e.g.*, liver, lung). The least encouraging aspect of these trials has been the low rate of long-term responses. In trials with adequate follow-up, median durations of response have been short, in the range of 3 to 6 months, and meaningful remissions in non-lung visceral lesions have been infrequent.

There has been considerable interest in the past few years in the dose-response relation of cisplatin in the treatment of melanoma. The aggregate of studies has not found a dose-response relation after systemic treatment with doses of up to 200 mg/m^2 (Table 46–9). In general, response rates with high doses of cisplatin, either alone or in combination, are not discernibly improved over standard doses.[320–339] However, a regimen of cisplatin (60 to 150 mg/m^2) in combination with WR 2721 (ethiofos), a thiol derivative that protects normal host tissues, has been reported to give an objective response rate of 45% (23 of 51 patients, including patients with metastatic sites in the liver).[335,401,402] Median duration of response was only 3 months. A recent update showed a 55%

TABLE 46–9. Cisplatin-based Chemotherapy in Melanoma

Regimen	*No. of Evaluable Patients*	*No. of Responses (%)*	*Complete Response (%)*	*References*
Single-Agent Therapy				
Cisplatin (all doses)	18	43 (23)	3	332–339
<100 mg/m^2	10	1 (10)	0	333
100–149 mg/m^2	125	28 (22)	2	320, 334, 335
≥150 mg/m^2	53	14 (26)	6	335–339
Combination Chemotherapy				
Cisplatin (all doses)	1279	363 (28)	7	321, 406–409, 442–447, 449, 451, 453–469, 470–473, 476, 478, 479, 482, 484
<100 mg/m^2	764	199 (26)	5	321, 406, 407–409, 442, 447, 452, 456–462, 464, 465, 467–469, 470, 472, 473, 478, 479, 482
100–149 mg/m^2	389	126 (32)	10	443–446, 451, 453, 455, 457, 430–457
≥150 mg/m^2	126	38 (30)	10	449, 451, 454, 475, 476, 484

(Adapted from Steffens TA, Bajoin DF, Chapman PB, et al. A phase II trial of high-dose cisplatin and dacarbazine: Lack of efficacy of high-dose cisplatin-based therapy for metastatic melanoma. Cancer 1991;68:1230) response rate (5 complete and 15 partial responses) in 36 patients treated with 150 mg/m^2 cisplatin plus WR 2721; the median duration of response was 6 months.[402] This regimen is given as a rapid 30-minute infusion every 3 to 4 weeks, and it has been suggested that the schedule of treatment might be important, because most high-dose regimens of cisplatin with lower response rates have used divided dose schedules.[402] The cisplatin/WR 2721 regimen is being tested in an Eastern Cooperative Oncology Group randomized trial.

Regional administration of cisplatin has allowed very high doses to be administered. Regional perfusion of high-dose cisplatin, 100 to 200 mg/m^2, with hyperthermia (38–40.5°C) in limbs with in-transit disease produced responses in 67% of 15 patients (95% confidence interval, 43–91%).[403] Complete responses were observed in 6 patients (40%), but only 3 responses were durable (> 2 years). Toxicity was severe at doses of more than 150 mg/m^2. In this study, very high plasma levels in the isolated limb were achieved, with doses (areas under the curve) generally 10-fold higher than similar doses given systemically. Despite treatment with extraordinary doses, durable responses were achieved in a minority of patients with favorable sites of disease. Intrahepatic arterial chemoembolization using cisplatin combined with polyvinyl sponges has been reported to produce responses in 46% of 30 patients with liver metastases from ocular melanoma.[404,405] Liver metastases from ocular melanoma rarely respond to systemic therapy with cisplatin-based combination regimens or to intrahepatic infusion of cisplatin alone, suggesting that tissue injury or necrosis produced by embolization might overcome cisplatin resistance.

COMBINATION THERAPY FOR SYSTEMIC METASTATIC MELANOMA. The role of combination chemotherapy in treatment of advanced melanoma is not entirely clear. This is because the history of combination chemotherapy for melanoma is not orderly. There have been many single and unconfirmed reports of initial high response rates, followed by confirmatory trials or randomized studies that find response rates that are similar to DTIC. For example, despite an initial encouraging report of high response rates for a combination of cisplatin, vinblastine, and bleomycin (PVB), confirmatory trials and randomized studies comparing PVB with DTIC showed no advantage for the combination.[406–409] Because toxicity of DTIC is minimal when treatment is accompanied by effective antiemetic therapy, it is important to demonstrate meaningful therapeutic gains of potentially more toxic and expensive combination regimens.

Combination chemotherapy trials for melanoma can be categorized into two types. The first approach has been to develop combinations of agents that have demonstrated single-agent activity. Despite an impression that combination regimens containing cisplatin are generally superior to DTIC alone, this has not been formally established (see Table 46–9). The overall response rates in combination regimens containing either low-dose or high-dose cisplatin are not detectably greater than DTIC. Clinical trials of DTIC in combination with nitrosoureas, vinca alkaloids, interferon-α, or cisplatin have response rates of 13% to 32%, in the range of rates with these single agents used alone.[410–436] The lack of clearly additive or synergistic antitumor effects of combinations has been disappointing.[410–442] This is perhaps due to the marginal activity of most of these drugs and suggests that resistance mechanisms of melanoma cells crosses these different classes of drugs.

Three groups of combination regimens in Table 46–10 are worth noting. First, combinations of DTIC, a vinca alkaloid, and cisplatin have had an overall response rate of 32% in reported trials.[420–436] Without direct comparison with DTIC, it is not possible to affirm that these combination regimens are definitely better than DTIC, and they certainly involve more toxicity. One regimen of this sort is the CVD combination developed at the M.D. Anderson Cancer Center: cisplatin 20 mg/m^2 intravenously on days 1 to 5, vinblastine 1.6 mg/m^2 intravenously on days 1 to 5, and DTIC 800 mg/m^2 on day 1.[436] A combination regimen, often called the Dartmouth regimen, comprised of DTIC, BCNU, cisplatin and ta-

TABLE 46–10. Results of Combination Regimens Containing DTIC

Regimen	*No. of Evaluable Patients*	*% Response Rate (95% CI)*	*Complete Response (%)*	*References*
DTIC Plus:				
Nitrosourea	302	21 (16–25)	7	294, 297, 410–416
Vinca alkaloid	223	18 (13–23)	4	311, 315, 325, 410, 417–420
Interferon-α	387	27 (23–31)	9	421–430
Nitrosourea + vinca alkaloid	1114	23 (20–25)	6	307, 308, 311, 431–440
Cisplatin + vinca alkaloid	255	32 (26–38)	7	441–447
Cisplatin + tamoxifen	23	13 (0–27)	9	476
Nitrosourea + cisplatin + tamoxifen	141	46 (38–54)	11	402, 477–480

95% CI, 95% confidence interval for response rates.

moxifen, has a reported response rate of 46% (95% confidence interval, 38–54%) in 141 evaluable patients in sequential phase II studies.[439–441] The reported complete response rate was 11% (95% confidence interval, 6–17%).[402] Again, no direct comparison with DTIC has been made. Toxicity is generally greater than observed with DTIC and includes occasional severe neutropenia and thrombocytopenia, which can be related to cumulative dose (especially for BCNU). This regimen was initially published by Del Prete and colleagues, with follow-up studies from McClay and colleagues.[439–441] The doses of drugs are as follows: cisplatin 25 mg/m^2 and DTIC 220 mg/m^2 administered intravenously daily for 3 days every 4 weeks, BCNU 150 mg/m^2 intravenously once every 8 weeks, and tamoxifen 10 mg orally twice a day throughout therapy.[440] Because tamoxifen has no demonstrated activity against melanoma and might contribute to toxicity (in particular deep vein thrombosis and pulmonary embolism), it was eliminated from the combination in a follow-up study.[441–443] Responses were observed in only 10% (2 of 20) of patients.[367]

In a subsequent study by the same group, adding tamoxifen increased the response rate back to 53%.[402] This intriguing observation suggested that tamoxifen might be critical for the activity of the combination. In clonogenic assays, the combination of tamoxifen with cisplatin, but not BCNU, has been reported to be synergistic.[442] A pilot study of escalated doses of tamoxifen (160 mg daily) with DTIC, BCNU, and cisplatin produced a possible increase in hematologic toxicity, and 7 responses (including 4 complete responses) were observed in 15 patients.[402] The basis for the possible increased activity of this regimen is a mystery. If this regimen has an improved response rate, BCNU and tamoxifen may be crucial. This is suggested by a phase II trial of cisplatin, DTIC, and tamoxifen (without BCNU) in which there were responses in only 3 of 23 patients (13% response rate; 95% confidence interval, 0–27%), a result consistent with response rates observed with cisplatin plus DTIC or DTIC alone.[437–438] Results of a randomized study comparing the Dartmouth regimen with DTIC are needed to assess further the efficacy of the Dartmouth regimen. A third combination regimen uses DTIC plus interferon-α (see below for a discussion of interferon-α therapy). The mean overall response rate in these trials is 27%.[410–419] Results of randomized trials are conflicting. A small randomized trial showed a significantly higher response rate in patients treated with DTIC plus interferon-α compared with DTIC alone.[419] However, a preliminary report from a larger randomized trial showed no response rate advantage for combinations of DTIC plus interferon-α versus DTIC, but did demonstrate a significant prolongation of response duration for the combination.[418]

A second approach has been to combine defined active agents (*e.g.*, DTIC, nitrosoureas) with agents having little or no known activity against melanoma.[444,445] It is not surprising that these trials have usually shown discouraging results, particularly noticeable in confirmatory studies after preliminary reports of high response rates. Response rates with these combination regimens are not distinctly better than single-agent DTIC or the same combination of active drugs used without the inactive agent (*e.g.*, regimens containing DTIC, nitrosourea, vinca alkaloid, and bleomycin compared with the same drugs without bleomycin). For example, a regimen of CCNU, procarbazine (minimal single-agent activity), and vincristine was originally reported to have a response rate of 48% in 44 patients, with 25% of patients achieving complete responses. However, a confirmatory trial by the NCI of Canada observed only a 12% response rate (2% complete responses) with the same regimen in 65 patients.[444,445]

Biologic Therapy

There is evidence that the immune system can influence the pathogenesis of melanoma. Several biologic agents have been tested in patients with metastatic melanoma and have demonstrated antitumor activity (Table 46–11). The rapid evo-

TABLE 46–11. Clinical Trials With Recombinant Interferon-α

Interferon Type	*Dose (mU/m^2)*	*Weekly Schedule*	*No. of Evaluable Patients*	*No. of PR + CR (%)*	*CR*	*References*
α2a	12–50	tiw	96	22 (23)	4	494
α2a	18–36	qd	17	4 (24)	0	495
α2a	15–50	—	18	2 (11)	2	496
α2a	10	biw	12	1 (8)	0	497
α2a	18–36	tiw	62	5 (8)	0	498
α2b	10–50	qd × 5	23	4 (17)	2	499
α2b	10	tiw	45	10 (22)	4	501
α2b	20	qd × 5	12	0 (0)	0	502
α2b	—	—	24	7 (29)	2	503
α2b	30	qd × 5	27	1 (4)	0	504
α2b	20	qd × 5	26	3 (12)	2	505
α2c	≤30	qd	10	2 (20)	1	506
α2c	5–30	qd	8	1 (12)	1	507
Total			380	60 (16)	18	

PR, partial response; CR, complete response.

lution of recombinant DNA technology to produce cytokines such as interferons and interleukins and of hybridoma methodology to develop monoclonal antibodies has allowed purified reagents to be produced in large quantities for clinical trials. The availability of these agents and the development of assays to measure them are allowing better studies about their pharmacology, mechanisms of action, and effects on various components of the immune system. Among this class of agents, the type I interferons (specifically recombinant interferon-α) and interleukin-2 (IL-2) have been studied most extensively. Other treatments under intensive investigation are monoclonal antibodies and active immunotherapy by vaccination.

INTERFERON-α. Interferon-α is an active agent in the treatment of metastatic melanoma.[446] Initial clinical investigations of interferon-α in patients with cancer used a purified preparation obtained from virus-stimulated buffy coat leukocytes.[447] The purification of small quantities of interferon-α required huge amounts of blood products and resulted in a final product that was less than 2% pure. Production was made more complicated by the fact that the interferon-α family consists of at least 20 proteins with a high degree of identity (> 80%) in amino acid sequences. The isolation of genes coding for leukocyte interferon-α allowed clinical studies of the pure (> 95%) recombinant materials to begin in 1983.

Although responses were observed infrequently in trials using purified natural interferon-α, trials using recombinant human interferon-α have confirmed that these agents have antitumor activity against melanoma (see Table 46–11).[448–463] Toxicity is manifested mainly by flu-like symptoms, myalgia, headache, chills, fever, and anorexia, with an accompanying drop in performance status during treatment with higher doses. Neutropenia can occur, and increases in serum transaminase levels occasionally require cessation of therapy. Continued treatment generally is associated with a decrease in side effects. Objective response rates average about 15% (see Table 46–11). Trials using daily or 3 times weekly schedules generally show more activity than trials using interrupted or intermittent schedules. As with other treatments, most responses have been partial and short-lived and occur mainly in skin, subcutaneous tissue, lymph node, and lung sites. Complete responses have been observed in about 5% of treated patients. Occasional durable complete responses have been observed.[446,450] An optimal dose of interferon-α has not been established, although there is a trend in favor of higher doses, suggested by a higher proportion of complete responses and a tendency toward longer durations of response.[448,449] Another notable feature of treatment with interferon-α is delay in response after starting treatment, a pattern different from most other therapies.[446] For example, a remarkable patient reported by Kirkwood and colleagues initially progressed after starting interferon-α but then achieved a complete response at 12 months.[446] Interferon-α is being evaluated in combination with cytotoxic agents, with other immunologic agents such as IL-2 and monoclonal antibodies, and in adjuvant trials.

Interferon-β binds to the same cell surface receptor as interferon-α. Side effects of interferon-β are similar to interferon-α, but it is unclear whether there might be a difference in clinical efficacy.[464] Interferon-γ, also called immune interferon, binds to distinct receptors and has several biologic properties that are distinct from interferon-α. Little activity against melanoma has been observed in preliminary clinical studies of interferon-γ.[465–468]

INTERLEUKIN-2 AND ADOPTIVE IMMUNOTHERAPY. A large body of evidence has demonstrated that rejection of established tumors can be mediated by cellular immune responses. Observations in experimental animal models, using both immunogenic and poorly immunogenic tumors, showed that high doses of IL-2 could induce tumor regressions of established micrometastases in liver and lung.[469–474] When lymphocytes are activated by IL-2, they acquire enhanced lytic activity for tumor cells and are called lymphokine-activated killer (LAK) cells.[470] The addition of LAK cells to treatment with high doses of IL-2 has produced higher therapeutic efficacy in animal models than either treatment alone.[471–474]

These experimental studies in animal models led Rosenberg and colleagues to design phase I trials to evaluate IL-2 and activated lymphocytes individually and then in combination.[475] Clinical trials of high-dose bolus injections of IL-2, with or without the addition of LAK cells, have demonstrated reproducible responses in patients with metastatic melanoma, with response rates of 10% to 25% using several doses and schedules of administration.[475–494] Table 46–12 lists results of studies using IL-2 alone or combined with adoptive cellular therapy with LAK cells. Activity of IL-2 was first described by Rosenberg and colleagues at the NCI Surgery Branch in Maryland using bolus injection of IL-2 and subsequently was confirmed by other groups. Partial responses are typically of short duration, but durable complete responses have been observed in a small proportion of patients. The toxic effects of high-dose IL-2 can be severe and are dependent on dose and schedule. They include oliguria, pulmonary insufficiency, central nervous system changes, arrhythmias, hypotension, and, infrequently, myocardial infarction.[495–498] Toxicities generally clear rapidly with the exception of neurologic effects, which can reverse more slowly. Treatment-associated mortality has been observed in 1% to 2% of patients, usually related to myocardial infarction and central catheter sepsis.

Continuous intravenous infusion of IL-2 is biologically more active than bolus IL-2, as measured by the height of rebound lymphocytosis after treatment and the activity of circulating lymphocytes during treatment. However, response rates of IL-2 administered by continuous infusion generally have been inferior to clinical results with bolus IL-2 administration, and bolus IL-2 is the preferred schedule of administration. Response rates are similar with and without LAK cells, suggesting that any effect of LAK cells is marginal. Data from the NCI Surgery Branch show a possible advantage for durable responses in patients treated with LAK, but this observation remains to be confirmed.[478] A report from Mitchell and colleagues has suggested that the addition of low-dose cyclophosphamide to low-dose infusion IL-2 can result in a response rate greater than 20%.[493,494]

T lymphocytes may play a crucial role in tumor regression produced by treatment with IL-2. This has been demonstrated in animal models.[499,500] Cytotoxic T lymphocytes that specifically kill or proliferate in response to autologous melanoma cells can be isolated from patients with advanced melanoma.[434,512] Regressing tumors biopsied after IL-2 therapy show infiltration of T lymphocytes.[513] Animal models have

TABLE 46–12. Clinical Trials With Interleukin-2

Schedule	*No. of Evaluable Patients*	*No. of Responses (%)*	*No. of Complete Responses (%)*	*95% Confidence Interval (%)*	*References*
Bolus I.V.					
IL-2 alone	175	31 (18)	4 (2)	12–23	522, 525, 526, 532, 534, 536
IL-2/LAK	164	24 (15)	8 (5)	9–20	519–522, 525–527, 534, 536
IL-2/TIL*	20	11 (55)	1 (5)	33–77	559, 560
Continuous I.V.					
IL-2 alone	85	8 (9)	0 (0)	3–16	523, 531, 533, 535
IL-2/LAK	147	18 (12)	2 (1)	7–17	523, 528–530, 533
IL-2/TIL*	21	5 (24)	1 (5)	6–42	561
IL-2/CTX	38	9 (27)	2 (5)	11–38	537, 538
Bolus/Continuous I.V.					
IL-2/LAK	50	7 (14)	1 (2)	4–24	524

* IL-2/TIL was administered with cyclophosphamide.
LAK, lymphokine-activated killer cells; TIL, tumor-infiltrating lymphocytes; CTX, cyclophosphamide.

shown substantial antitumor activity of adoptive immunotherapy using lymphocytes isolated from tumor sites (tumor-infiltrating lymphocytes, or TILs).[514] Animals primed with either cyclophosphamide or total body irradiation were injected with IL-2-expanded TIL and treated with IL-2.[514] Much lower doses of IL-2 were needed to attain the equivalent antitumor effects seen in animals treated with high-dose IL-2 plus LAK cells. Based on these preclinical studies, clinical evaluation of adoptive immunotherapy with TIL and IL-2 were initiated.[515,516] A trial from the NCI Surgery Branch observed 11 responses in 20 patients (55%) treated with bolus IL-2 and TIL in conjunction with cyclophosphamide.[515,516] A trial using continuous infusion IL-2 and TIL plus cyclophosphamide observed a 24% response rate in 21 patients, consistent with the lower response rate of continuous infusion IL-2.[517]

MONOCLONAL ANTIBODIES. The diagnosis and treatment of melanoma with monoclonal antibodies has been treated in detail elsewhere.[518,519] Two strategies are being pursued for monoclonal antibody (MoAb) treatment of melanoma: treatment with MoAb alone to activate the host immune system, and treatment with MoAb conjugated to cytotoxic agents, either radioisotope or plant toxins (*e.g.*, ricin A chain).

Clinical trials have been performed with unconjugated MoAbs and MoAbs conjugated to radionuclides or toxins. Phase I studies of mouse MoAb alone have shown that MoAb can reach tumor sites after systemic administration.[520–525] Responses have been observed after treatment with several MoAbs against the gangliosides GD2 and GD3.[520,521,525–531] However, responses have not been observed after treatment with unconjugated MoAb against two glycoprotein antigens (p97 and the high molecular weight proteoglycan antigen).[521,523,524,532] Responses have been reported after treatment with MoAb conjugated to radionuclide or the A chain of the plant toxin ricin.[533–536]

The most intensively studied MoAbs have been anti-GD3 MoAbs, particularly MoAb R24.[520,525–528] Several other MoAbs against GD3 have been investigated, including MoAbs MG-21 and ME36.1.[529,530] These anti-GD3 MoAbs are notable because they are efficient at mediating activation of human complement and triggering killing of melanoma cells in the presence of human peripheral blood mononuclear cells (antibody-dependent cellular cytotoxicity). MoAb R24 can induce inflammatory responses specifically within tumor sites after intravenous administration.[520,525,527] Toxicity generally has been mild to moderate after treatment with low doses. The maximum tolerated doses have not been defined for most unconjugated MoAbs. However, the maximum tolerated dose of MoAb R24 resulted in malignant hypertension, associated with markedly excessive serum levels of catecholamines, at cumulative doses of more than 1200 mg/m^2 administered over 5 to 7 days.[537] This side effect is probably caused by weak reactivity of MoAb with the adrenal medulla, an organ that has a developmental origin that is similar to melanocytes. No other severe end-organ symptom has been observed, for example, to be related to reactivity of R24 with melanocytes in the skin or eye.

Trials of MoAb have been limited until recently by difficulties in production of MoAb for clinical use. However, several phase I trials have been performed. Responses have been observed with anti-GD3 MoAb in phase I trials at 5 different institutions (Table 46–13).[520,526–530,538] Most trials have been performed using systemic administration, but in one trial, isolated limb perfusion with R24 was performed.[528] Most responses have been observed at lower doses ($\leq$ 30 mg/m^2 daily). Durable responses in soft tissue or visceral lesions have been observed in a small number of patients, in some cases

TABLE 46–13. Phase I Trials of Unconjugated Monoclonal Antibodies Against GD2 and GD3 Ganglioside Antigens

MoAb	*Antigen*	*Route*	*No. of Evaluable Patients*	*Response*	*References*
R24	GD3	I.V.	21	4 PR	564, 569
R24	GD3	I.V.	5	2 PR	570
R24	GD3	I.V.	6	1 CR 1 PR	595
R24 (high-dose)	GD3	I.V.	7	NR	590
R24	GD3	ILP	12	1 PR	572
MG21	GD3	I.V.	8	1 CR	573
Me36.1	GD2/GD3	I.V.	13	1 CR	574
3F8	GD2	I.V.	9	2 PR	566
L72	GD2	IL	8	4 PR	575

CR, complete response; IL, intralesional; ILP, isolated limb perfusion; I.V., intravenous; MoAb, monoclonal antibody; NR, no response; PR, partial response.

lasting more than 2 years.[530,530a] MoAb 3F8 against the related ganglioside GD2 has shown antitumor activity against melanoma in phase I trials.[521] Anti-GD2 MoAbs but not anti-GD3 MoAbs can produce neurologic symptoms, particularly severe pain.[521] This toxicity is observed even at low doses and may be related to reactivity of anti-GD2 MoAb with peripheral nerve fibers. This side effect may limit the application of some anti-GD2 MoAbs in melanoma.

A pilot trial of MoAb fragments against the glycoprotein p97 antigen and conjugated to the radionuclide iodine 131 has been reported.[533] Up to 500 mCi of radioisotope was administered, and the primary dose-limiting toxic effects (thrombocytopenia and neutropenia) were due to marrow irradiation. Ricin, a natural product of beans from the plant *Ricinus communis,* is a potent inhibitor of protein synthesis. Ricin is composed of two chains, designated A and B, that are disulfide linked. The A chain is able to inhibit protein synthesis. The ricin A chain has been conjugated to MoAbs, and phase I trials have demonstrated generally mild toxicity (*e.g.,* flu-like symptoms, hepatic enzyme elevations).[534–536] A phase II study in 46 patients with melanoma has been completed; 1 complete response and 3 partial responses were observed.[536]

Because most antimelanoma MoAbs are of mouse origin, they have generally induced a human immunoglobulin (Ig) G response to the mouse immunoglobulin.[520,521,523,524,537–539] This immune resistance to mouse MoAb can effectively prevent the MoAb from reaching tumor sites. Two methods are being explored to bypass the human antimouse immunoglobulin response. First, genes coding for mouse MoAbs can be genetically manipulated to construct humanized MoAbs composed of mouse antigen-binding regions ligated to human immunoglobulin sequences.[540,541] These engineered humanized MoAbs should be reaching clinical trials shortly. A second approach is to derive human MoAbs from melanoma antigens. Human MoAbs to the gangliosides GD2 and GD3 have been isolated, and a pilot trial of intralesional injection of a human IgM anti-GD2 MoAb showed partial and complete regression of injected skin lesions.[531]

ACTIVE IMMUNIZATION: TUMOR VACCINES. Tumor vaccines have a long history, but the search for effective methods to induce active immunity against tumors has been difficult. Repeated attempts have been made to inhibit the outgrowth of tumors and to influence the natural history of melanoma by immunization with tumor cells or extracts of tumor cells. More recently, purified antigens, recombinant vaccines, genetically modified melanoma cells, and antiidiotype antibodies have entered into clinical trials. Evidence is mounting that vaccination can induce immune responses to melanoma. Trials have been initiated to evaluate potential efficacy of vaccines as adjuvant therapy in high-risk patients. Table 46–14 lists the strategies that are being taken to construct melanoma vaccines. At this point, there is no consensus on which approaches are most promising. Most clinical studies have been performed in patients after resection of regional

TABLE 46–14. Strategies for Immunization

- I. Whole Melanoma Cells
  - A. Autologous cells
  - B. Allogeneic cells
  - C. Neuraminidase-treated cells
  - D. Haptenized cells
- II. Melanoma Cell Lysates
  - A. Viral oncolysates
    - 1. Vaccinia virus
    - 2. Newcastle disease virus
    - 3. Vesicular stomatitis virus
  - B. Shed melanoma cell supernatant
- III. Purified Antigens
  - A. Gangliosides
- IV. Recombinant Vaccines
  - A. v-P97ny
- V. Gene Therapy
  - A. Expression of tumor necrosis factor and interleukin-2 in melanoma cells
- VI. Antiidiotype Monoclonal Antibodies
  - A. Anti-HMW-MAA
  - B. Anti-GD3 ganglioside

lymph node metastases or high-risk primary lesions and in patients with advanced metastatic disease. Responses have been observed in a few patients with advanced disease, but these appear to be infrequent. Patients who develop evidence of immune responses have improved disease-free survival and overall survival.[541–549] This does not mean that vaccines improve the clinical course (*e.g.*, patients who a priori have a better prognosis may be more likely to develop an immune response to vaccination) but is consistent with the hypothesis that an immune response induced by vaccination can prevent cancer recurrence.

Problems exist in the construction of tumor vaccines, including weak immunogenicity of tumor antigens, heterogeneity of antigen expression in tumors, and the ability of tumors to escape an immune response.[60,61,70] Most melanoma antigens on tumor cells are not tumor-specific (*i.e.*, present only on cancer cells) but are shared with certain normal cells.[60,70]

Early specific vaccination trials in melanoma (as opposed to nonspecific vaccination with BCG) used immunization with unmodified, irradiated allogeneic or autologous melanoma cells, either alone or in combination with BCG and other nonspecific immunomodulators. In these trials, it has been difficult to show that vaccination had any benefit or elicited any specific immune responses.[550–553] One exception has been immune responses to gangliosides, the major acidic glycolipid of melanoma cells, in some patients immunized with selected allogeneic melanoma cells.[543,544]

Efforts have been made to improve immunogenicity of allogeneic tumor cells by using the enzyme neuraminidase to remove sialic acid residues from the cell surface.[554,555] Strategies have been developed to augment the immune response to tumor antigens by infecting tumor cells with nonpathogenic viruses. Viral proteins presented on the cell membrane of tumors have been shown to augment the immunogenicity of tumor antigens.[546,547,549] Several centers have investigated the immunogenicity of lysates derived from tumor cells infected with Newcastle disease virus, vaccinia virus, and vesicular stomatitis virus. Prospective randomized clinical trials are under way to evaluate the potential efficacy of viral oncolysates in an adjuvant setting. Another approach to increasing immune response has been to alter tumor cells by binding haptens to autologous tumor cells.[556] Genetic alteration of melanoma cells, called gene therapy, is being investigated to augment the immune response against weakly immunogenic melanoma antigens. Cells have been altered to secrete the immunologically active molecules tumor necrosis factor and IL-2, and clinical studies of vaccination with genetically modified cells have been initiated.[557,558]

An effort is under way to immunize patients with purified or partially purified preparations of potentially immunogenic molecules from melanoma cells. The rationale for this approach comes from the identification of antigens on melanoma cells that can be recognized by antibodies in sera or lymphocytes from patients with melanoma. Gangliosides have been shown to induce antibody responses after immunization.[543,544] Of particular interest, the ganglioside GM2 can induce IgM antibody responses in up to 90% of immunized patients, and prospective randomized studies have been started to evaluate GM2 and other ganglioside vaccines. Another strategy has been to use supernatants containing a mixture of shed melanoma antigens for immunization.[544]

Other molecules that are recognized by the humoral immune response of melanoma patients, the antigens, have been isolated, and genes encoding these antigens have been cloned.[56,559] These genes are being used to construct recombinant DNA vaccines. A vaccine has been constructed by expressing the p97 melanoma antigen in vaccinia virus vector, and clinical trials have been initiated.[559] In preclinical studies, the p97 glycoprotein antigen was immunogenic in primates immunized with the recombinant vaccine. The identification of melanoma antigens recognized by T lymphocytes opens avenues for the construction of vaccines to elicit specific cellular immune responses.[560]

A final approach has been to mimic melanoma antigens using antiidiotype MoAb. Certain antiidiotype monoclonal antibodies can function as "images" of tumor antigens to elicit immune responses. Antiidiotype monoclonal antibodies have been shown to mimic the high molecular weight proteoglycan melanoma antigen and the ganglioside GD3.[561–564] Clinical trials have been initiated with antiidiotype vaccines in patients with stages III and IV melanomas.

There are several agents that might be used to augment nonspecifically the immunogenicity of vaccines. First, immune adjuvants can augment the level, duration, and quality of the immune response elicited by specific antigens. The standard adjuvant, alum, has not been shown to be very effective. BCG is an effective adjuvant for vaccines with GM2 ganglioside.[544] Detoxified endotoxin, liposomes, saponin, muramyl peptides, and other substances are being actively investigated as adjuvants. A clinical trial using allogeneic melanoma cell lysates and an adjuvant containing detoxified endotoxin (DETOX) observed 4 responses in 25 patients with metastatic melanoma.[565]

A second issue has been the phenomenon of suppressor lymphocytes. Studies in mice bearing transplantable tumors have demonstrated that a population of T lymphocytes can actively suppress specific immune responses, and suppression mediated by these T lymphocytes can be abrogated by low doses of cyclophosphamide.[566] Studies in humans suggest that low-dose cyclophosphamide can enhance humoral and cell-mediated response to tumor antigens, and some vaccine trials have incorporated pretreatment with cyclophosphamide.[566–569] Responses have been observed occasionally in patients treated with autologous melanoma cell vaccine plus low-dose cyclophosphamide.[565,570]

INTRALESIONAL THERAPY. A high proportion of skin lesions have been shown to regress after injection with nonspecific immunomodulatory agents such as BCG. The first study of this kind was done by Morton in 1971, and subsequent investigations confirmed that injection of BCG into superficial cutaneous lesions leads to responses at the injected sites (in about two thirds of lesions) and occasionally at uninjected sites (in 21% of lesions in proximity to injected lesions).[571–575] Other agents, including purified protein derivative, methanol extracted residue, and dinitrochlorobenzene, have produced similar results.[576–579] Intralesional therapy is most likely to induce regressions of small dermal lesions; the response of subcutaneous or large tumors is substantially lower.

Combinations of Biologic Agents and Chemotherapy

Exploration of combinations of biologic agents and chemotherapy for treatment of melanoma is an active area of investigation. Combinations of chemotherapy and immunologic agents have a long history. Early clinical trials of chemotherapy combined with nonspecific immunomodulators such as BCG, *Corynebacterium parvum,* or levamisole did not demonstrate any beneficial effects. Recent in vitro and preclinical studies in animals have suggested that combinations of recombinant cytokines or monoclonal antibodies (*e.g.,* IL-2 and interferon-α, monoclonal antibody and IL-2, tumor necrosis factor and interferon-γ) are additive or synergistic. Clinical trials of cytokines with and without chemotherapy have been initiated.[580–583]

Phase I–II studies have evaluated combinations of IL-2, interferon, and chemotherapy, including cisplatin, DTIC, and cyclophosphamide.[493,494,515,516,584–592] The combination of DTIC and interferon-α is discussed in the section on combination chemotherapy. Preliminary results of a series of small studies using combinations of IL-2, interferon-α, and cisplatin either alone or in combination chemotherapy regimens have reported overall response rates of 40% in 169 patients (95% confidence interval, 32–47%).[588–592] These preliminary results need to be extended in larger prospective trials. Combinations of IL-2 and interferon (interferon-α or interferon-β) have been examined in preliminary trials.[593–603] There is a suggestion that response rates to the combination may be higher than with either cytokine alone, particularly at higher dose levels, but toxicity may be additive.

Biologic agents that induce inflammation are beginning to be explored. Inflammatory monoclonal antibodies are being used in combination with IL-2, interferon-α, macrophage colony-stimulating factor, or tumor necrosis factor-α.[604] The proinflammatory cytokines tumor necrosis factor-α and interferon-γ have synergistic effects in vitro and have been studied clinically in combination in a phase I trial.[605] A preliminary report of the combination of tumor necrosis factor-α, interferon-γ, and melphalan administered as a regional limb perfusion was reported to induce complete response in 89% of patients with in-transit metastases, although substantial toxicity was observed.[606]

Endocrine Therapy

There appears to be little role for single-agent endocrine therapy in the treatment of melanoma. Clinical reports of responses to tamoxifen are mainly anecdotal, and extensive trials have demonstrated minimal or no activity for tamoxifen, the antiandrogen cyproterone acetate, or medroxyprogesterone acetate.[606] Tamoxifen has been proposed to have synergistic effects with a combination of DTIC, BCNU, and cisplatin.[441,443]

Status of Adjuvant Therapy

Advances in melanoma treatment over the past decade have evolved primarily from more detailed knowledge about prognostic factors of primary and metastatic lesions. Within the larger group of melanoma patients who undergo potentially curative treatment by surgical resection, subgroups can be identified who are at high risk for recurrence and for development of systemic metastases. Patients with thick primary melanomas (> 4.0 mm thick), in-transit lesions, and regional lymph node involvement are at particular risk. Once distant metastases develop, most patients die of their diseases. The investigation of adjuvant systemic treatment that can prevent melanoma recurrence remains a critical area of investigation. The rationale and general principles for adjuvant treatment of cancer are based on the premise that treatment, whether chemotherapy or immunotherapy, is more effective when the tumor cell population is small. Randomized trials using DTIC, nitrosoureas, a variety of combination chemotherapy regimens, BCG, *Corynebacterium parvum,* transfer factor, and combinations of immunotherapy and chemotherapy have not demonstrated any advantage for treatment.

Adjuvant treatment for melanoma should be considered within clinical research protocols. It is recommended that the option of experimental adjuvant treatment be considered for patients with AJCC stage II or III melanoma who are free of disease but are at high risk for recurrence. Investigations of adjuvant treatment include the following:

1. *Interferon.* No randomized trial has observed significant advantage for treatment with interferons. The Eastern Cooperative Oncology Group has a trial of adjuvant therapy with high-dose interferon-α2b compared with observation in stage II–III high-risk patients. Preliminary results suggest a survival advantage for the treated group, but the data have not reached maturity to support statistical significance.[607] Severe hepatic and neurologic toxicity were observed frequently in the 110 patients in the treatment arm. Two ongoing randomized intergroup trials are comparing high-dose and low-dose interferon-α with observation: a WHO randomized trial in AJCC stage III patients and a North Central Oncology Treatment Group trial in high-risk patients. A recent randomized trial of interferon-γ by the Southwest Oncology Group was closed because of possible adverse effects in the interferon-γ treatment arm.[608]
2. *Active immunization.* Various approaches to melanoma vaccination have been reviewed above. None of the randomized trials has demonstrated a survival or disease-free survival advantage in vaccinated patients. Small randomized studies of adjuvant vaccination with neuraminidase-treated allogeneic melanoma cells with BCG or with the ganglioside GM2 plus BCG have not demonstrated any benefit.[543,544,553] Survival advantage has been demonstrated in patients who develop specific immune responses to vaccination, but this observation does not establish that vaccination is causally related to improved survival.[543–549] There are several randomized trials ongoing to evaluate vaccination in an adjuvant setting, including studies using viral oncolysates and allogeneic melanoma cell lysates plus DETOX. Trials evaluating novel melanoma vaccine constructs are also under way (see Table 46–14).
3. *Levamisole.* Several randomized trials have been conducted with levamisole as an adjuvant agent. Three trials have shown no significant advantage of adjuvant therapy with levamisole over placebo.[609–615] A randomized trial of combination chemotherapy by the Southwest Oncol-

ogy Group demonstrated no advantage when levamisole was included with chemotherapy.[613] A recent randomized trial from the NCI of Canada Clinical Trials Group demonstrated a significant improvement in survival in groups treated with levamisole or levamisole plus BCG compared with an untreated control arm, providing the only evidence of adjuvant activity of levamisole.[610]

4. *Chemotherapy.* This option includes treatment with combination chemotherapy regimens that have activity against advanced metastatic melanoma. High-dose chemotherapy with autologous bone transplant has been evaluated in adjuvant trials. Agents with the best established activity against advanced melanoma, DTIC, and nitrosoureas, either alone or in combinations, have not shown any statistical advantage in survival or disease-free survival in adjuvant trials.
5. *Regional perfusion* of chemotherapy with or without hyperthermia has not shown any reduction in mortality in clinical studies to date when used as adjuvant therapy in patients at high-risk for locoregional recurrence.
6. *Other modalities.* A recent retrospective analysis of randomized trials from several centers suggested a survival advantage in patients with resected locoregional metastatic melanoma who were treated with *Corynebacterium parvum* compared with patients treated with BCG.[616] A small randomized study of megestrol acetate versus observation suggested a survival advantage for treated patients that approached significance ($p = 0.06$).[617]

MANAGEMENT OF SPECIFIC SITES OF METASTASES

Skin, Subcutaneous Tissues, and Distant Lymph Nodes

The most common sites of distant metastases are the skin and subcutaneous tissues.[145,242,243] Lesions are generally 0.5 to 2.0 cm in diameter and are readily detectable by physical examination. Occasionally, it may be clinically difficult to differentiate a cutaneous metastasis from a second primary melanoma. Distant metastases can occur in any lymph node chain and generally are asymptomatic. Superficial nodal metastases are easily diagnosed by physical examination. They usually can be detected on chest x-ray films, with CT scans or tomograms used as confirmatory tests, whereas abdominal metastatic nodes generally are detected by CT scans or ultrasonography.[255,618–621]

If distant nodal metastases are isolated (one or a few), surgical excision is the treatment of choice, providing a safe, quick, and effective treatment (see Table 46–6). They usually should be excised before they become bulky and symptomatic and require even more extensive surgery. These lesions should be excised with a rim of normal-appearing tissue (usually 0.5–1.0 cm) to minimize the risk of recurrence. Sequential metastases can be excised surgically unless they are multiple or appear in rapid succession. For multiple or recurrent lesions, radiation therapy may be considered as a second option.[270–281,283] For most dermal, subcutaneous, and lymph node metastases, we recommend treatment with 6 fractions of 600 cGy given twice weekly. The overall reported probability of a complete or partial response to radiation therapy in these sites is about 65%. This response rate is rather meaningless when tumor size is not considered. For lesions of 1 cm or less, response to radiation is almost universal, and about two-thirds of the tumors undergo complete and durable regression.[281] Conversely, a complete response was obtained in only about 20% of lesions greater than 5 cm in diameter in the RTOG study.[283] The use of radiation therapy should, therefore, be considered before metastatic deposits reach massive proportions.

Palliative radiation therapy is occasionally indicated for symptomatic nodal metastases in the mediastinum or retroperitoneum. When treating these sites, we recommend using a conventional fractionation regimen because of the poor tolerance of the thoracic spinal cord and abdominal viscera to large dose fractions. Systemic therapy, either experimental or standard, may be considered for widespread multiple lesions or symptomatic deep lymph nodes not accessible to radiation therapy. About 40% of patients with metastases localized in skin, subcutaneous tissues, or lymph nodes without visceral involvement survive more than 1 year, and 5% to 10% of these patients are alive at 5 years.

Lung, Pleura, and Mediastinum

The second most common initial sites of metastasis are the lungs and pleura (see Table 46–2). These lesions are evaluated by chest x-ray films preoperatively and during follow-up, whereas suspicious intrathoracic metastases are evaluated further by tomograms, CT scans, or bronchoscopy.

For screening purposes, standard chest x-ray films are sufficiently sensitive and cost-effective to be used for all melanoma patients. The yield of the more expensive pulmonary tomograms or CT scans is too low and the cost too high to justify when the chest x-ray films are normal.[244,619,622] Evaluation of suspicious metastases begins when one or more lesions are seen on chest x-ray films, the usual presentation of pulmonary metastases from melanoma.[145,243,623–625] Most patients have multiple pulmonary nodules; only 22% have solitary nodules.[626] Hilar and mediastinal adenopathy frequently accompany pulmonary metastases.[627]

Whole-lung tomograms or CT scans of the chest are of value in evaluating suspicious chest lesions or in determining whether the metastatic disease seen on chest x-ray films is also present elsewhere in the chest.[619,628–631] Bronchoscopy with biopsy may be considered in a few patients when the diagnosis of pulmonary lesions is in doubt. For solitary pulmonary metastases in asymptomatic patients, surgical excision may be indicated if no new lesions appear during an observation period of 3 to 4 weeks and if the tumor has a slow growth rate.[632] Whole-lung tomograms or CT scans are essential, for often a patient with a solitary lesion appearing on chest x-ray films actually has other pulmonary or intrathoracic lesions as well.[626,630,633] The operation is safe (< 1% mortality), but careful patient selection is important because only a minority of patients benefit. Surgical lesion of solitary pulmonary metastases is justified in selected patients, because truly long-term survival can be achieved.[242,267–269,633–638] The median postoperative survival ranges from 16 to 24 months, with 5-year survival rates of 12% to 21% in some large series. Not all institutions, however, have had such favorable results (see Table 46–6).[639,640]

Another justification for excising solitary pulmonary lesions is to confirm that they do not represent a second primary malignancy or a benign process. This situation can occur in up to one third of patients whose workups culminate in thoracotomies.[633,635] Patients who are not considered for surgery, such as those with multiple, slow-growing tumors, might be followed with no treatment at all while the tumors are asymptomatic. If the pulmonary metastases grow rapidly, especially if multiple visceral sites are involved or if the patient is symptomatic, an initial course of chemotherapy might be given. The response rate of DTIC chemotherapy is particularly poor for pulmonary metastases, and there is no evidence that the drug prolongs life.[250,641]

Brain and Spinal Cord

The brain is the initial site of metastases in 12% to 20% of melanoma patients and is usually associated with widespread visceral disease (Fig. 46–15).[145,240,246,250,642–646] At autopsy, cerebral metastases are present in 36% to 54% of patients.[230–240,241,250] The hemispheres generally are involved equally, with the cerebrum, usually the frontal lobe, involved most frequently, followed by the cerebellum, base of the brain, and spinal cord. Hydrocephalus is associated with about 33% of posterior fossa lesions. Cerebral metastases are solitary in only about 25% of patients.[246,645–648] An unusual feature of cerebral metastases is their propensity for hemorrhage, which occurs much more frequently than with other histologic types of metastases. Hemorrhage occurs in 33% to 50% of patients with melanoma metastases involving the brain.[645,649–651]

Headaches, alterations of mental status, and focal neurologic deficits are the most common symptoms of brain metastases.[245,646,648,649,652,653] Seizures are more common in patients with melanoma metastases in the brain than in patients with other types of brain tumors but occur in only about 25% of the melanoma patients with brain involvement.[649,652–654] It is common for these melanoma patients to present with subarachnoid or intracerebral hemorrhages.[645,649,650,655–660]

Routine brain scans are not useful for detecting occult metastases in asymptomatic patients in any disease stage. This was demonstrated in five separate series involving 504 patients with local or regional disease; not a single true-positive brain scan was obtained.[245,252,254,661,662] In patients with stage IV melanomas, cerebral metastases were detected by brain scan in 11% to 16% of patients studied, but all patients with positive scans had antecedent symptoms.[245,258,645,663]

The radiologic diagnosis of symptomatic melanoma metastases of the central nervous system has been reviewed in several published series.[510,650] The best single test for the diagnosis of intracerebral metastases is either an MRI or CT scan with contrast enhancement.[645,650,653,664–666] Compared with CT scans, MRI appears to have a better ability to distinguish hemorrhage from tumor. Leptomeningeal metastases can occur, usually in association with other distant metastases.[667,668]

Corticosteriods are the mainstay of initial treatment for brain metastases, the most effective being dexamethasone (up to 100 mg/day). This can reduce the edema around the tumor and relieve symptoms in most patients, at least temporarily.[669–671] Eighty-six percent of patients with multiple brain lesions treated with radiation therapy remained steroid dependent, whereas only 33% of patients with solitary lesions treated with surgery with or without radiation have remained steroid dependent.[654] Lack of improvement or exacerbation of symptoms during a trial of steroids can be due to intratumor hemorrhage with intracerebral hematoma.

Radiation therapy is the treatment of choice for multiple tumors. Chemotherapy generally is not effective for brain metastasis from melanoma.[250,643,652,670] Surgical excision is preferred for solitary and surgically accessible lesions. A craniotomy is a relatively safe procedure (with operative mortality of less than 5%) that alleviates symptoms in most patients and prevents further neurologic damage in patients with demonstrable metastases. It should be considered for some patients with symptomatic brain metastases, even when there is limited disease at other sites, because their estimated life span can exceed 2 to 3 months and their neurologic status usually improves. Whole-brain irradiation is generally given postoperatively.[242,269,643,644]

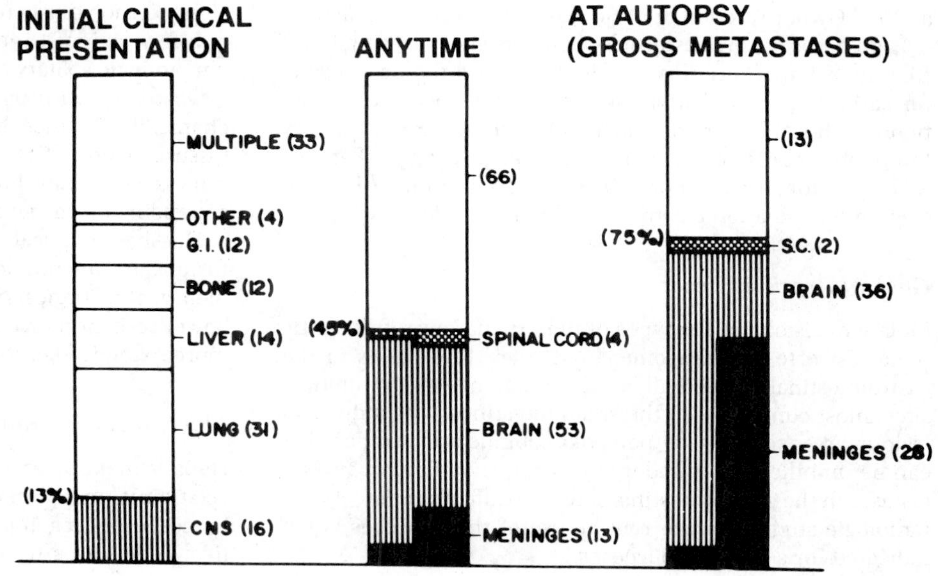

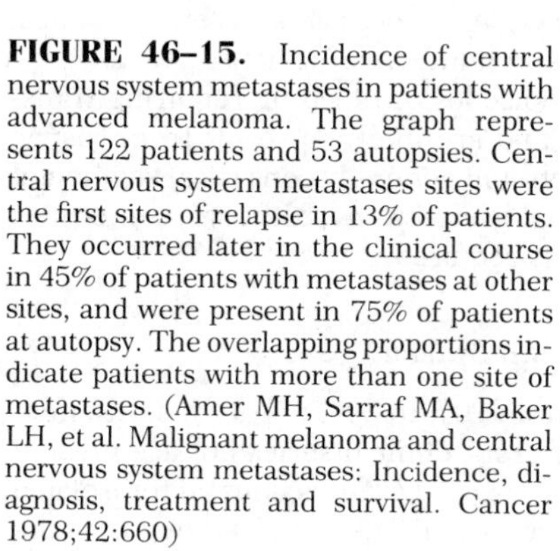

FIGURE 46–15. Incidence of central nervous system metastases in patients with advanced melanoma. The graph represents 122 patients and 53 autopsies. Central nervous system metastases sites were the first sites of relapse in 13% of patients. They occurred later in the clinical course in 45% of patients with metastases at other sites, and were present in 75% of patients at autopsy. The overlapping proportions indicate patients with more than one site of metastases. (Amer MH, Sarraf MA, Baker LH, et al. Malignant melanoma and central nervous system metastases: Incidence, diagnosis, treatment and survival. Cancer 1978;42:660)

Survival in different series averages about 7 months for surgically treated patients (see Table 46–6) and ranges from 2 to 20 months.[242,258,267–269,642–644,646–649,672–675] Satisfactory improvement in neurologic condition occurs in most patients. Survival results are influenced by remission duration, neurologic status at time of surgery, and presence of metastases at other sites.[676] Although long-term survival is uncommon, a few patients will live 3 to 5 years or more after surgery.[246,647,674,677–679]

Radiation therapy should be considered if the lesions are multiple or located in an area that would preclude a safe operation. Brain metastases present a challenging radiotherapeutic management problem. Although about 60% to 70% of patients receiving whole-brain radiation therapy experience measurable improvement in their performance status, benefit is usually of short duration and essentially all patients die with active intracranial disease. No modification of fractionation schedule[275,680,681] has been shown to be consistently superior to the reference standard of 3000 cGy in 10 fractions over 2 weeks for melanoma that is metastatic to the brain. There is a subset of good-prognosis patients treated with a high-dose accelerated fractionation regimen who may have derived a survival benefit.[682] We currently recommend 3000 cGy in 10 fractions to the whole brain as best standard treatment for patients with multiple metastases.

When surgical removal of brain metastases is possible, this should be performed and followed by whole-brain irradiation. A recent study from the M.D. Anderson Cancer Center demonstrated that combined treatment provided significantly improved survival over surgery alone.[683] If surgical margins are inadequate, a coned-down boost to the resection site to deliver a dose of 4500 cGy is justified. Patients with solitary brain metastases that are unresectable are candidates for treatment by stereotaxic radiosurgery, in which a large single ablative dose is given to a small volume encompassing the gross disease.[684]

Surgical decompression of obstructing spinal cord lesions is indicated in selected patients, although there is evidence that radiation therapy might be an effective alternative in some patients.[653,685] To maximize spinal cord tolerance in patients with a significant life expectation, we recommend treatment with conventional fractionation to a total dose of 4500 cGy at 250 cGy per fraction or 5000 cGy at 200 cGy per fraction.

High doses of corticosteroids should be given as well. Early treatment intervention is essential, because the best results for surgery and irradiation treatments have occurred in patients with mild neurologic symptoms; there have been very few treatment responses in totally paraplegic patients. Patients with symptomatic but nonobstructive disease might be considered for radiation treatment of the local area.[277]

Gastrointestinal Tract

Melanoma is one of the types of tumors that most frequently metastasize to the gastrointestinal tract. Metastases to the gastrointestinal tract usually occur simultaneously in multiple sites, most commonly in the small intestines. The individual lesions are exophytic or polypoid submucosal nodules that can be umbilicated or undergo central cavitation.[695–699] Metastases in the gastrointestinal tract are difficult to detect with radiologic studies, so the routine use of these studies is not indicated for screening purposes.

Early involvement of the gastrointestinal tract usually causes vague and subtle symptoms. The most common clinical manifestations are due to the following: chronic bleeding with anemia, anorexia, and weight loss; obstruction of the small bowel with abdominal pain, nausea, and vomiting; or acute bleeding with hematemesis or melena.[244,250,688,691–697]

Intussusception is a frequent cause of obstructive symptoms and other abdominal complaints, and numerous cases have been reported in the literature.[688,695,696,698] Intussusception usually follows a chronic or subacute course, characterized by an insidious onset. The triad of abdominal cramps, nausea without vomiting, and abdominal distention was the most consistent symptom in one series.[698]

The diagnosis of gastrointestinal metastases is usually made by barium contrast radiographs or by endoscopy. Several reviews have been written about the radiologic detection of metastatic melanoma involving the gastrointestinal tract.[688–690,699] All patients undergoing an upper gastrointestinal series for abdominal complaints should have a small bowel follow-through examination, because metastases are most likely to be present in this area. If the small bowel series is normal but there is a strong clinical suspicion of metastases, then a small bowel enteroclysis can be performed.

One of the most common symptoms of gastrointestinal metastases is chronic bleeding. In anemic patients, this can be treated with repeated blood transfusions. Systemic therapy can be considered for patients with multiple gastrointestinal lesions, and surgical excision is the treatment of choice for solitary metastases, if the patient's condition permits and there are no other visceral metastases.

Surgery is recommended for most patients with the acute complications of obstruction, massive bleeding, or perforation. These complications cannot be treated by other modalities, and the only alternative is to allow the patient to die. The final decision depends on the patient's overall condition, but symptoms can be successfully alleviated in most cases, and survival after surgical excision of the metastases averages 4 to 8 months.[240,242,244,267–269,691–696,698] In patients with multiple gastrointestinal metastases, only lesions causing immediate symptoms should be removed unless those remaining are relatively few and can be safely excised. Survival of 2 to 5 years after excision of gastrointestinal metastases has been reported in a few patients, most of whom had palliative excision for symptomatic solitary or intestinal metastases.[240,242,267–269,691–696]

Obstruction is usually due to large polypoid lesions that mechanically obstruct the bowel or act as leading points for intussusception.[693,696,698] These submucosal lesions generally are removed with bowel resections or, occasionally, enterotomies, depending on the sites and numbers of lesions.

Massive or repeated episodes of bleeding requiring transfusions are uncommon and are likely to result from gastric metastases. Surgical treatment generally consists of segmental bowel resection or partial gastrectomy, although sometimes more extended surgery is required.[242,246,267–269,691–693,695]

Liver, Biliary Tract, and Spleen

Hepatic metastases occur in 10% to 20% of patients with metastatic melanoma in different clinical series but are present in most cases at autopsy.[145,240,246,250,700] It is unusual for isolated liver metastases to occur in patients with cutaneous melanoma. Patients with liver metastases generally have widespread melanoma. The prognoses of these patients are poor (*i.e.*, median survival of 2 to 4 months), and treatment options are few.

Screening tests for liver metastases should consist only of a history, physical examination, and measurement of serum liver chemistries. These are sufficiently accurate and the most cost-effective of all available tests. There are now numerous studies that document the futility of using liver scintiscans, ultrasound studies, or CT scans to screen for occult liver metastases in melanoma patients.[244,245,252,254,661,662,701] They are neither warranted nor cost-effective as screening tests in patients with localized or regional melanoma.

The patterns of abnormal liver chemistries that suggest liver metastases are elevated LDH or alkaline phosphatase levels in the presence of normal or only slightly elevated serum glutamic-oxaloacetic transaminase or bilirubin levels.[243,250,663,702] An elevated LDH level is a clinically useful and specific indicator for metastatic melanoma.[703] When liver metastases are suspected, the confirmatory radiologic tests to be considered include ultrasound, CT scan, radionuclide liver scan, or hepatic arteriogram.[518] Most comparative studies have found that abdominal CT scans are somewhat more accurate and reliable than ultrasound and radionuclide liver scans for evaluation of liver masses.[255,704–706]

Metastatic melanoma involving the gallbladder or bile ducts is present in 4% to 20% of patients at autopsy.[246,250,251] Patients with symptoms of gallbladder metastases should be considered for cholecystectomy if metastasis is confined to the gallbladder and if they are medically fit and have life expectancies exceeding several months.[688,707–710] Short-term relief of symptoms is usually successful, but all reported patients have died within a year.[708–710]

Melanoma is one of the few tumors that metastasizes to the spleen.[240,244,246] It may rarely cause splenomegaly but is more often diagnosed as an incidental finding on a liver-spleen scan or abdominal CT scan or at laparotomy. Most patients with splenic metastases (up to 88%) have concomitant liver or pancreatic metastases.

Bone

Bone metastases occur infrequently (11% to 17%) in most clinical series but are more commonly observed in autopsy series (see Table 46–4).[240,246,711,712] Skeletal metastases generally occur in patients with widespread metastatic disease but occasionally represent the first evidence of recurrence.[711,712] The life span of these patients is short, but effective palliative treatment can be achieved in many cases, so it is worthwhile to pursue the diagnosis. In the asymptomatic melanoma patient, particularly with AJCC stage I or II disease, the yield of occult bone metastases on bone scan is too low to justify it as a screening procedure.[245,252,661–663,713]

Bone metastases from melanoma are medullary in location and destructive in nature. They generally appear osteolytic on x-ray films and provoke little if any bone formation. Patterns of bone metastases have been described previously.[711,712,714] Axial metastases account for up to 80% of bone lesions and are most common in the spine.[246,711,712] When they involve the vertebral body, there are often compression fractures that may lead to neurologic symptoms such as radicular back pain, paresthesia or paresis of the legs, or urinary retention. Only about 10% of lytic lesions occur in weight-bearing bones, which could result in pathologic fractures.[246,712]

Skeletal radionuclide scintigraphy has established itself over radiographic skeletal surveys as the initial test for evaluating suspected bone metastases. Scan abnormalities are nonspecific and must be correlated with radiographic studies and patient histories (for fractures, trauma, arthritis) to differentiate between benign and malignant causes.

The life span of melanoma patients with bone metastases is 4 to 6 months on the average and even shorter when other sites are involved.[145,711,712] The treatment chosen depends on the degree of symptoms, the location and magnitude of bone lesions, and the expected life span. Symptomatic metastases generally involve non-weight-bearing bones, particularly the spine or ribs. In these cases, radiation therapy to the lesions usually gives relief for up to 6 months; however, the fields should generally be restricted to the area of symptomatic involvement. A high-dose, short-course schedule minimizes patient travel time and hospitalization.[277,824] The available chemotherapy generally is not effective for palliation of skeletal metastases.[531]

Irradiation is effective in palliating the pain of bone metastases in most patients. A fractionation schedule of 3000 cGy in 10 fractions is usually recommended, although it has not been established as optimal in any comparative study. More abbreviated schedules, such as 2000 cGy in 5 fractions, are effective but are not recommended for spinal or pelvic bone metastases requiring large fields because of their acute gastrointestinal toxicity. Pathologic fractures in long bones should be stabilized before radiation therapy is given. In weight-bearing long bones judged radiographically to be at risk for pathologic fracture, prophylactic internal fixation is advisable. Radiation therapy should begin immediately after surgery in these patients to minimize the period of hospitalization. In this clinical situation, we recommended a radiation dose of 3600 cGy in 6 fractions. The higher biologic dose for pathologic fractures is recommended because bone healing requires more regression of metastatic tumor than does simple pain relief.

Kidneys and Urinary Tract

Although metastatic melanoma frequently appears in the kidneys and urinary tract at autopsy, metastases in these sites rarely cause clinically recognizable symptoms, and usually these symptoms are terminal manifestations of the disease. Solitary or symptomatic metastases that are amenable to treatment do occur occasionally.

Renal metastases generally occur as multiple, small (3 to 10 mm) cortical nodules that are usually asymptomatic but can cause hematuria or melanuria. Some may be large enough to cause obstructive lesions with hydronephrosis or bleeding.[717] Although patients with bladder metastases commonly have multiple subepithelial pedunculated or sessile lesions, solitary lesions can occur.[718–722]

Kidney and urinary tract metastases generally are asymptomatic until the terminal stages of disease, and death usually occurs within 1 to 4 months after the clinical diagnosis is made. Metastatic melanoma can occasionally mimic primary renal or bladder carcinomas, both endoscopically and radiographically.[729] The most common symptom prompting a urinary tract investigation is gross or microscopic hematuria.[240,246] In most patients, the diagnosis of metastases can be made by intravenous pyelogram, cystogram, cystoscopy, or imaging scans (CT or sonar). Occasionally, cytologic examination of the urine reveals melanoma cells.[723]

Bladder metastases can be treated by transurethral resection or partial cystectomy, depending on their number, sizes, and locations.[718] Symptoms usually can be relieved, but survival after treatment averages only 3 to 6 months. Patients rarely survive longer than 1 year.

Kidney and ureteral metastases causing bleeding or obstruction can be treated by ureteronephrectomy in selected patients or by a ureteral stent if the patient is not a candidate for surgery.[717,724] In most cases, survival averages only 4 months. Prostate and urethral metastases can cause hematuria, dysuria, or hesitancy.[725] Symptomatic prostate metastases rarely occur but can be treated by transurethral resection or open prostatectomy.[717,725]

METASTATIC MELANOMA FROM UNKNOWN PRIMARY SITE

A small proportion of melanoma patients present with metastatic diseased lymph nodes or distant sites but no detectable primary site. Patients presenting with occult primary melanoma comprise between 1% and 12% of patients with metastatic disease.[139,726–732] About two thirds of these patients present with tumors in lymph nodes (most frequently in the axilla) and one third with distant metastases (most frequently in the skin, subcutaneous tissues, lungs, and brain). All patients with occult primary melanoma should be examined carefully for potential sequestered primary lesions, especially in the eye and scalp. In this group of patients, it is important to get a careful history of previous treatment for nevi. About 10% to 20% of patients describe previous nevi within the lymphatic drainage areas of metastatic lymph nodes. About one third of patients have had treatment for pigmented lesions, often by nondiagnostic procedures such as curettage or diathermy.[236,733] Any biopsy specimens from previously excised pigmented lesions that are available should be reevaluated by an experienced pathologist, because occasionally these turn out to be well-differentiated primary melanomas on review. Two thirds of patients give no history of suspicious pigmented lesions.

The survival rate of patients with unknown primary lesions is no different from that of patients with metastatic cutaneous melanoma when matched for prognostic factors. When appropriate, surgical management should be considered first. Lymphadenectomy for nodal disease can be associated with long-term survival similar to the results seen in patients with cutaneous metastases to lymph nodes; survival is generally better if only one node is involved than if multiple nodes contain tumors. Two-year survival rates of 30% to 40% can be observed in patients with skin and subcutaneous metastases from cutaneous and unknown primary sites.[236,729] A small proportion of melanoma patients present with metastatic disease either in lymph nodes or at distant sites, and no primary site can be detected. Patients presenting with occult primary melanoma comprise between 1% and 12% of patients with distant metastatic disease.[139,726–732]

REFERENCES

1. McLeod GR, David NC, Little JH, et al. Melanoma in Queensland, Australia: Experience in the Queensland Melanoma Project. In: Balch CM, Milton GW, eds. Cutaneous melanoma: Clinical management and treatment results worldwide. Philadelphia: JB Lippincott, 1985:379.
2. Roush GC, Schymurs M, Holford TR. Risk for cutaneous melanoma in recent Connecticut birth cohorts. Am J Publ Health 1985;75:679.
3. Redman JC, Mora DB. Malignant melanomas of the skin diagnosed and treated in Albuquerque, New Mexico in 1980. J Dermatol Surg Oncol 1982;8:41.
4. Rigel DS, Kopf AW, Friedman RJ. The rate of malignant melanoma in the US: Are we making an impact? J Am Acad Dermatol 1987;17:1050.
5. Armstrong BK, English DR. Epidemiologic studies. In: Balch CM, Houghton AN, Milton GW, Sober AJ, Soong S-j, eds. Cutaneous melanoma. 2nd ed. Philadelphia: JB Lippincott, 1992:12–22.
6. Gellin GA, Kopf AW, Garfinkel L. Malignant melanoma: A controlled study of possibly associated factors. Arch Dermatol 1969;99:43.
7. Scheibner A, Milton GW, McCarthy WH, et al. Multiple primary melanoma: A review of 90 cases. Aust J Dermatol 1982;23:1.
8. Bellet RE, Vaisman I, Mastrangelo MJ, et al. Multiple primary malignancies in patients with cutaneous melanoma. Cancer 1977;40:1974.
9. Lynch HT, Frichot BC III, Lynch J, et al. Family studies of malignant melanoma and associated cancer. Surg Gynecol Obstet 1975;141:517.
10. Moseley HS, Giuliano AE, Storm FK, et al. Multiple primary melanoma. Cancer 1979;43:939.
11. Veronesi U, Cascinelli N, Bufalino R. Evaluation of the risk of multiple primaries in malignant cutaneous melanoma. Tumori 1976;62:127.
12. Elder DE, Goldman LI, Goldman SC, et al. Dysplastic nevus syndrome: A phenotypic association of sporadic cutaneous melanoma. Cancer 1980;46:1787.
13. Wallace DC, Exton LA, McLeod GRC. Genetic factor in malignant melanoma. Cancer 1971;27:1262.
14. Acton RT, Balch CM, Budowle B, et al. Immunogenetics of melanoma. In: Reisfeld RA, Ferrone S, eds. Melanoma antigens and antibodies. New York: Plenum, 1982:1.
15. Greene MH, Reimer RR, Clark WH Jr, et al. Precursor lesions in familial melanoma. Semin Oncol 1978;5:85.
16. Lynch HT, Frichot BC III, Lynch JF. Familial atypical multiple mole-melanoma syndrome. J Med Genet 1978;15:352.
17. Reimer RR, Clark WH Jr, Greene MH, et al. Precursor lesions in familial melanoma: A new genetic preneoplastic syndrome. JAMA 1978;239:744.
18. Wallace DC, Beardmore GL, Exton LA. Familial malignant melanoma. Ann Surg 1973;177:15.
19. Clark WH Jr, Reimer RR, Greene M, et al. Origin of familial malignant melanomas from heritable melanocytic lesions: The B-K mole syndrome. Arch Dermatol 1978;114:732.
20. Elder DE, Green MH, Guerry D, et al. The dysplastic nevus syndrome: Our definition. Am J Dermatopathol 1982;4:455.
21. Acton RT, Balch CM, Barger BO, et al. The occurrence of melanoma and its relationship with host, lifestyle and environmental factors. In: Costanzi JJ, ed. Malignant melanoma 1. The Hague: Martinus Nijhoff, 1983:151.
22. Clark DA, Necheles T, Nathanson L, et al. Apparent HL-A5 deficiency in malignant melanoma. Transplantation 1973;15:326.
23. Barger BO, Action RT, Soong S-j, et al. Increase of HLA-DR4 in melanoma patients from Alabama. Cancer Res 1982;42:4276.
24. Budowle B, Barger BO, Balch CM, et al. Associations of properdin factor B with melanoma. Cancer Genet Cytogenet 1982;5:247.
25. Pandey JP, Johnson AH, Funderberg HH, et al. HLA antigens and immunoglobulin allotypes in patients with malignant melanoma. Hum Immunol 1981;2:185.
26. Walter G, Brachtel R, Hilling M. On the incidence of blood group O and Gm phenotypes in patients with malignant melanoma. Hum Genet 1979;49:71.
27. Clark WH Jr, Ainsworth AM, Bernardino EA, et al. The developmental biology of primary human malignant melanomas. Semin Oncol 1975;2:83.
28. Fitzpatrick TB, Milton GW, Balch CM, Shaw HM, McCarthy WH, Sober AJ. Clinical characteristics. In: Balch CM, Houghton AN, Milton GW, Sober AJ, Soong S-j, eds. Cutaneous melanoma. 2nd ed. Philadelphia: JB Lippincott, 1992:223–233.
29. Mihm MC Jr, Fitzpatrick TB, Lane-Brown MM, et al. Early detection of primary cutaneous malignant melanoma: A color atlas. N Engl J Med 1973;289:989.
30. Sober AJ, Fitzpatrick TB, Mihm MC Jr, et al. Early recognition of cutaneous melanoma. JAMA 1979;242:2795.
31. Clark WH Jr, From L, Bernardino EA, et al. The histogenesis and biologic behavior of primary human malignant melanomas of the skin. Cancer Res 1969;29:705.
32. McGovern VJ, Murad TM. Pathology of melanoma: An overview. In: Cutaneous melanoma: Clinical management and treatment results worldwide. Philadelphia: JB Lippincott, 1985:29.
33. Mihm MC Jr, Clark WH Jr, Fromm L. The clinical diagnosis, classification and histogenetic concepts of the early stages of cutaneous malignant melanomas. N Engl J Med 1971;284:1078.
34. Manci EA, Balch CM, Murad TM, et al. Polypoid melanoma, a virulent variant of the nodular growth pattern. Am J Clin Pathol 1981;75:810.
35. Urist MM, Balch CM, Soong S-j, et al. Head and neck melanoma in 536 clinical stage I patients: A prognostic factors analysis and results of surgical treatment. Ann Surg 1984;200:769.
36. McGovern VJ, Shaw HM, Milton GW, et al. Is malignant melanoma arising in a Hutchinson's melanotic freckle a separate entity? Histopathology 1980;4:235.

37. Clark WH Jr, Mihm MC Jr. Lentigo maligna and lentigo-maligna melanoma. Am J Pathol 1969;55:39.
38. Arrington JH III, Reed RJ, Ichinose H. Plantar lentiginous melanoma: A distinctive variant of human cutaneous malignant melanoma. Am J Surg Pathol 1977;1:131.
39. Coleman WP III, Loria PR, Reed RJ, et al. Acral lentiginous melanoma. Arch Dermatol 1980;116:773.
40. Krementz ET, Reed RJ, Coleman WP, et al. Acral lentiginous melanoma: A clinicopathologic entity. Ann Surg 1982;195:632.
41. Seiji M, Takahashi M. Acral melanoma in Japan. Hum Pathol 1982;13:607.
42. Sondergaard K, Olsen G. Malignant melanoma of the foot: A clinicopathological study of 125 primary cutaneous malignant melanomas. Acta Pathol Microbiol Immunol Scand [Abstract] 1980;88:275.
43. Feibleman CE, Stoll H, Maize JC. Melanomas of the palm, sole and nailbed: A clinicopathologic study. Cancer 1980;46:2492.
44. Paladugu RR, Winberg CD, Yonemoto RH. Acral lentiginous melanoma: A clinicopathologic study of 36 patients. Cancer 1983;52:161.
45. Patterson RH, Helwig EB. Subungual malignant melanoma: A clinical-pathologic study. Cancer 1980;46:2074.
46. Hughes LE, Horgan I, Taylor BA, et al. Malignant melanoma of the hand and foot: Diagnosis and management. Br J Surg 1985;72:813.
47. Lopansri S, Mihm MC Jr. Clinical and pathological correlation of malignant melanoma. J Cutan Pathol 1979;6:180.
48. Balch CM, Cascinelli N, Drzewiecki KT, et al. A comparison of prognostic factors worldwide. In: Balch CM, Houghton AN, Milton GW, Sober A, Soong S-j, eds. Cutaneous melanoma. 2nd ed. Philadelphia: JB Lippincott, 1992;188.
49. Balch CM, Urist MM, Maddox WA, et al. Melanoma in the Southern United States: Experience at the University of Alabama in Birmingham. In: Balch CM, Milton GW, eds. Cutaneous melanoma: Clinical management and treatment results worldwide. Philadelphia: JB Lippincott, 1985.
50. Reintgen DS, McCarty KM Jr, Cox E, et al. Malignant melanoma in black American and white American populations: A comparative review. JAMA 1982;248:1856.
51. McCarthy WH, Shaw HM, Milton GW, et al. Melanoma in New South Wales, Australia: Experience at the Sydney Melanoma Unit. In: Balch CM, Milton GW, eds. Cutaneous melanoma: Clinical management and treatment results worldwide. Philadelphia: JB Lippincott, 1985:371.
52. Pack GT, Oropeza R. Subungual melanoma. Surg Gynecol Obstet 1967;124:571.
53. Papachristou DN, Fortner JG. Melanoma arising under the nail. J Surg Oncol 1982;21: 219.
54. Le Douarin N. Migration and differentiation of neural crest cells. Curr Top Dev Biol 1980;61:31.
55. Hearing VT. Enzymatic control of pigmentation in mammals. FASEB J 1991;5:2902.
56. Vijayasaradhi S, Bouchard B, Houghton AN. The melanoma antigen gp75 is the human homologue of the mouse *brown* locus product. J Exp Med 1990;171:1375.
57. Wick MM, Byers L, Frei E III. L-Dopa: Selective toxicity for melanoma cells in vitro. Science 1977;197:468.
58. Pawelek JM, Lerner AB. 5,6-dihydroxyindole is a melanin precursor showing potent cytotoxicity. Nature 1978;276:627.
59. Morrison ME, Yagi MJ, Cohen G. In vitro studies of 2,4-dihydroxyphenylalanine, a prodrug targeted against malignant melanoma cells. Proc Natl Acad Sci USA 1985;82: 2960.
60. Houghton AN, Eisinger M, Albino AP, et al. Surface antigens of melanocytes and melanomas: Markers of melanoma differentiation and melanoma subsets. J Exp Med 1982;156:1755.
61. Houghton AN, Real FX, Davis LJ, et al. Phenotypic heterogeneity of melanoma: Relation to the differentiation program of melanoma cells. J Exp Med 1987;164:812.
62. Barnhill RL, Mihm MC Jr. Histopathology of malignant melanoma and its precursor lesions. In: Balch CM, Houghton AN, Milton GW, Sober AJ, Soong S-j, eds. Cutaneous melanoma. 2nd ed. Philadelphia: JB Lippincott, 1992:234.
63. Clark WH Jr, Elder ED, Guerry D IV et al. The precursor lesions of superficial spreading and nodular melanoma. Hum Pathol 1984;15:1147.
64. Rodeck U, Melber K, Kath R, et al. Constitutive expression of multiple growth factor genes by melanoma cells but not normal melanocytes. J Invest Dermatol 1991;97: 20.
65. Halaban R. Growth factors and tyrosine protein kinases in normal and malignant melanocytes. Cancer Metastasis Rev 1991;10:129.
66. Herlyn M, Houghton AN. Biology of melanocytes and melanoma. In: Balch CM, Houghton AN, Milton GW, Sober AJ, Soong S-j, eds. Cutaneous melanoma. 2nd ed. Philadelphia: JB Lippincott, 1992:234.
67. Becker D, Meier CB, Herlyn M. Proliferation of human malignant melanomas is inhibited by antisense oligodeoxynucleotides targeted against basic fibroblast growth factor. EMBO J 1989;8:3685.
68. Halaban R, Kwon BS, Ghosh S, et al. bFGF as an autocrine growth factor for human melanomas. Oncogene Res 1988;3:177.
69. Dotto GP, Moellmann G, Ghosh S, et al. Transformation of murine melanocytes by basic fibroblast growth factor cDNA and oncogenes and selective suppression of the transformed phenotype in a reconstituted cutaneous environment. J Cell Biol 1989;109: 3115.
70. Houghton AN, Herlyn M, Ferrone S. Melanoma antigens. In: Balch CM, Houghton AN, Milton GW, Sober AJ, Soong S-j, eds. Cutaneous melanoma. 2nd ed. Philadelphia: JB Lippincott, 1992:234.
71. Albeda SM, Mette SP, Elder DE, et al. Integrin distribution in malignant melanoma: Association of the $\beta 3$ subunit with tumor progression. CA
72. Lynch HT, Frichot BC III, Lynch JF. Familial atypical multiple mole melanoma syndrome. J Med Genet 1978;15:352.
73. Greene MH, Goldin LR, Clark WH Jr, et al. Familial cutaneous malignant melanoma: Autosomal dominant trait possibly linked to the Rh locus. Proc Natl Acad Sci USA 1983;80:6071.
74. Bale SJ, Dracopoli NC, Tucker MA, et al. Mapping the gene for hereditary cutaneous malignant melanoma-dysplastic nevus to chromosome 1p. N Engl J Med 1989;320: 1376.
75. van Haeringen A, Bergman W, Nelen MR, et al. Exclusion of the dysplastic nevus syndrome locus from the short arm of chromosome 1 by linkage studies in Dutch families. Genomics 1989;5:61.
76. Cannon-Albright LA, Goldgar DE, Wright EC, et al. Evidence against the reported linkage of the cutaneous melanoma-dysplastic nevus syndrome locus to chromosome 1p36. Am J Hum Genet 1990;46:912.
77. Becher R, Gibas Z, Karakousis C, et al. Nonrandom chromosome changes in malignant melanoma. Cancer Res 1983;43:5010.
78. Trent JM, Rosenfeld SB, Meyskens FL. Chromosome 6q involvement in human malignant melanoma. Cancer Genet Cytogenet 1983;9:177.
79. Pathak S, Drwinga HL, Hsu TC. Involvement of chromosome 6 in rearrangements in human malignant melanoma cell lines. Cytogenet Cell Genet 1983;36:573.
80. Balaban G, Herlyn M, Guerry D, et al. Cytogenetics of human malignant melanoma and premalignant lesions. Cancer Genet Cytogenet 1984;11:429.
81. Balaban GB, Herlyn M, Clark WH Jr, et al. Karyotypic evolution in human malignant melanoma. Cancer Genet Cytogenet 1986;19:113.
82. Limon J, Dal Cin P, Sait SNJ, et al. Chromosome changes in metastatic human melanoma. Cancer Genet Cytogenet 1988;30:201.
83. Pedersen MI, Bennett JW, Wang N. Nonrandom chromosome structural aberrations and oncogene loci in human malignant melanoma. Cancer Genet Cytogenet 1986;20: 11.
84. Fountain JW, Bale SJ, Housman DE, Dracopoli NC. Genetics of melanoma. Cancer Surv 1990;9:645.
85. Richmond A, Fine R, Murray D, et al. Growth factor and cytogenetic abnormalities in cultured nevi and malignant melanomas. J Invest Dermatol 1986;86:295.
86. Cowan JM, Halaban R, Francke U. Cytogenetic analysis of melanocytes from premalignant nevi and melanomas. JNCI 1988;80:1159.
87. Parmiter AH, Balaban G, Clark WH Jr, et al. Possible involvement of the chromosome region 10q24–26 in early stages of melanocyte neoplasia. Cancer Genet Cytogenet 1988;30:313.
88. Dracopoli NC, Houghton AN, Old LJ. Loss of polymorphic restriction fragments in malignant melanoma: Implications for tumor heterogeneity. Proc Natl Acad Sci USA 1985;82:1470.
89. Dracopoli NC, Alhadeff B, Houghton AN. Loss of heterozygosity at autosomal and X-linked loci during tumor progression in a patient with melanoma. Cancer Res 1987;47: 3995.
90. Cavenee WK, Dryja TP, Phillips RA, et al. Expression of recessive alleles by chromosomal mechanisms in retinoblastoma. Nature 1983;305:779.
91. Volkenandt M, Schlegel U, Nanus DM, Albino AP. Mutational analysis of the human p53 gene in malignant melanoma. Pig Cell Res 1991;4:35.
92. Trent JM, Stanbridge EJ, McBride HL, et al. Tumorigenicity in human melanoma cell lines controlled by introduction of human chromosome 6. Science 1990;247: 568.
93. Trent JM, Meyskens FL, Salmon SE, et al. Relation of cytogenetic abnormalities and clinical outcome in metastatic melanoma. N Engl J Med 1990;22:1508.
94. Lee JAH. The causation of melanoma. In: Balch CM, Milton GW, eds. Cutaneous melanoma: Clinical management and treatment results worldwide. Philadelphia: JB Lippincott, 1985:303.
95. Lee JAH. Melanoma and exposure to sunlight. Epidemiol Rev 1982;4:110.
96. Berkelhammer J, Oxenhandler RW. Evaluation of premalignant and malignant lesions during the induction of mouse melanomas. Cancer Res 1987;47:1251.
97. Pawlowski A, Haberman HF, Menon IA. Junctional and compound pigmented nevi induced by 9,10-dimethyl-1,benzanthracene in skin of albino guinea pigs. Cancer Res 1976;36:2813.
98. Kripke ML, Fisher MS. Immunologic parameters of ultraviolet carcinogenesis. JNCI 1976;57:211.
99. Crombie IK. Variation of melanoma incidence with latitude in North America and Europe. Br J Cancer 1979;40:774.
100. Lee JAH. Melanoma in cancer epidemiology and prevention. In: Schottenfeld D, Fraumeni JF Jr, eds. Cancer, epidemiology and prevention. Philadelphia: WB Saunders, 1982:984.
101. Elwood JM, Gallagher RP. Site distribution of malignant melanoma. Can Med Assoc J 1983;128:1400.
102. Katz L, Ben-Tuvla S, Steinitz R. Malignant melanoma of the skin in Israel: Effect of migration. In: Magnus K, ed. Trends in cancer incidence. Washington, DC: Hemisphere, 1982:419.
103. Newell GR. Is ultraviolet irradiation the sole cause of melanoma? Melanoma Lett 1987;5:4.
104. Jensen OM, Bolander AM. Trends in malignant melanoma of the skin. World Health Stat Q 1980;33:2.
105. Greene A. Incidence and reporting of cutaneous melanoma in Queensland. Aust J Dermatol 1982;23:105.
106. McLeod GR, Davis NC, Little JH, et al. Melanoma in Queensland, Australia: Experience in the Queensland Melanoma Project. Personal communication, 1990.
107. Eldh J, Boeryd B, Suurkula M, et al. Melanoma in Sweden: Experience at the University of Goteborg. In: Balch CM, Milton GW, eds. Cutaneous melanoma: Clinical management and treatment results worldwide. Philadelphia: JB Lippincott, 1985:469.
108. Crombie IK. Radical differences in melanoma incidence. Br J Cancer 1979;40:185.

109. Lam K-H, Wong J. Melanoma in Hong Kong. Experience at the Queen Mary Hospital. In: Balch CM, Milton GW, eds. Cutaneous melanoma: Clinical management and treatment results worldwide. Philadelphia, JB Lippincott, 1985:495.
110. Balch CM, Soong S-j, Shaw HM, et al. Changing trends in the clinical pathological features of melanoma. In: Balch CM, Houghton AN, Milton GW, Sober A, Soong S-j, eds. Cutaneous melanoma. 2nd ed. Philadelphia: JB Lippincott, 1992:40.
111. Balch CM, Soong S-j, Milton GW, et al. A comparison of prognostic factors and surgical results in 1,786 patients with localized (stage I) melanoma treated in Alabama, USA, and New South Wales, Australia. Ann Surg 1982;196:677.
112. Breslow A. Thickness, cross-sectional areas and depth of invasion in the prognosis of cutaneous melanoma. Ann Surg 1970;172:902.
113. Goldsmith HS. Melanoma: An overview. CA 1979;29:194.
114. McNeer G, Das Gupta TK. Prognosis in malignant melanoma. Surgery 1964;56:512.
115. Beahrs OH, Myers MH. Manual for staging of cancer: American Joint Committee on Cancer. Philadelphia: JB Lippincott, 1983:117.
116. Ketcham AS. Classification and staging. In: Balch CM, Houghton AN, Milton GW, Sober A, Soong S-j, eds. Cutaneous melanoma, 2nd ed. Philadelphia: JB Lippincott, 1992:213.
117. Balch CM, Soong S-j, Shaw HM, Urist MM, McCarthy WH. An analysis of prognostic factors in 8500 patients with cutaneous melanoma. In: Balch CM, Houghton AN, Milton GW, Sober A, Soong S-j, eds. Cutaneous melanoma. 2nd ed. Philadelphia: JB Lippincott, 1992:165.
118. Day CL Jr, Sober AJ, Kopf AW. A prognostic model for clinical stage I melanoma of the lower extremity: Location on foot as independent risk factor for recurrent disease. Surgery 1981;89:599.
119. Day CL Jr, Sober AJ, Kopf AW. A prognostic model for clinical stage I melanoma of the upper extremity: The importance of anatomic subsites in predicting recurrent disease. Ann Surg 1981;193:436.
120. Balch CM, Murad TM, Soong S-j, et al. A multifactorial analysis of melanoma: Prognostic histopathological features comparing Clark's and Breslow's staging methods. Ann Surg 1978;188:732.
121. Cascinelli N, Morabito A, Bufalino R, et al. Prognosis of stage I melanoma of the skin. Int J Cancer 1980;26:733.
122. Drzewiecki KT, Andersen PK. Survival with malignant melanoma: A regression analysis of prognostic factors. Cancer 1982;49:2414.
123. Schmoeckel C, Bockelbrink A, Bockelbrink H, et al. Low-and high-risk malignant melanoma. I. Evaluation of clinical and histological prognosticators in 585 cases. Eur J Cancer Clin Oncol 1983;19:227.
124. Shaw HM, McGovern VJ, Milton GW, et al. Histologic features of tumors and the female superiority in survival from malignant melanoma. Cancer 1980;45:1604.
125. Shaw HM, McGovern VJ, Milton GW, et al. Malignant melanoma: Influence of site of lesion and age of patient in the female superiority in survival. Cancer 1980;46:2731.
126. Balch CM, Soong S-j, Milton GW, et al. A comparison of prognostic factors and surgical results in 1,786 patients with localized (stage I) melanoma treated in Alabama, USA, and New South Wales, Australia. Ann Surg 1982;196:677.
127. Balch CM, Murad TM, Soong S-j, et al. Tumor thickness as a guide to surgical management of clinical stage I melanoma patients. Cancer 1979;43:883.
128. Breslow A. Thickness, cross-sectional areas and depth of invasion in the prognosis of cutaneous melanoma. Ann Surg 1970;172:902.
129. Day CL Jr, Lew RA, Mihm MC Jr, et al. The natural break points for primary-tumor thickness in clinical stage I melanoma. N Engl J Med 1981;305:1155.
130. Soong S-j. A computerized mathematical model and scoring system for predicting outcome in patients with localized melanoma. In: Balch CM, Houghton AN, Milton GW, Sober A, Soong S-j, eds. Cutaneous melanoma. 2nd ed. Philadelphia: JB Lippincott, 1992:200.
131. Day CL Jr, Sober AJ, Kopf AW, et al. A prognostic model for clinical stage I melanoma of the trunk: Location near the midline is not an independent risk factor for recurrent disease. Am J Surg 1981;142:247.
132. Eldh J, Boeryd B, Peterson LE. Prognostic factors in cutaneous malignant melanoma in stage I: A clinical, morphological and multivariate analysis. Scand J Plast Reconstr Surg 1978;12:243.
133. Prade M, Bognel C, Charpentier P, et al. Malignant melanoma of the skin: Prognostic factors derived from a multifactorial analysis of 239 cases. Am J Dermatopathol 1982;4:411.
134. Schmoeckel C, Bockelbrink A, Bockelbrink H, et al. Low- and high-risk malignant melanoma. II. Multivariate analyses for a prognostic classification. Eur J Cancer Clin Oncol 1983;19:237.
135. Van der Esch EP, Cascinelli N, Preda F, et al. Stage I melanoma of the skin: Evaluation of prognosis according to histologic characteristics. Cancer 1981;48:1668.
136. Cox EB. Prognostic factors in malignant melanoma. In: Seigler HF, ed. Clinical management of melanoma. The Hague: Martinus Nijhoff, 1982:279.
137. Hacene K, Le Doussal V, Brunet M, et al. Prognostic index for clinical stage I cutaneous malignant melanoma. Cancer Res 1983;43:2991.
138. Day CL Jr, Sober AJ, Kopf AW, et al. A prognostic model for clinical stage I melanoma of the upper extremity: The importance of anatomic subsites in predicting recurrent disease. Ann Surg 1981;193:436.
138a. Kheir SA, Bines SD, Vonroenn JH, Soong-S-j, Urist MM, Coon JS. Prognostic significance of DNA aneuploidy in stage I cutaneous melanoma. Ann Surg 1988;207:455.
139. Balch CM, Soong S-j, Murad TM, et al. A multifactorial analysis of melanoma. III. Prognostic factors in melanoma patients with lymph node metastases (stage II). Ann Surg 1981;193:377.
140. Balch CM, Soong S-j, Murad TM, et al. A multifactorial analysis of melanoma. II. Prognostic factors in patients with stage I (localized) melanoma. Surgery 1979;86:343.
141. Cohen MH, Ketcham AS, Feix EL, et al. Prognostic factors in patients undergoing lymphadenectomy for malignant melanoma. Ann Surg 1977;186:635.
142. Day CL Jr, Sober AJ, Lew RA, et al. Malignant melanoma patients with positive nodes and relatively good prognoses: Microstaging retains prognostic significance in clinical stage I melanoma patients with metastases to regional nodes. Cancer 1981;47:955.
143. Callery C, Cochran AJ, Roe DJ. Factors prognostic for survival in patients with malignant melanoma spread to the regional lymph nodes. Ann Surg 1982;196:69.
144. Cascinelli N, Nava M, Vaglini M, et al. Melanoma in Italy. Experience at the National Cancer Institute of Milan. In: Balch CM, Milton GW, eds. Cutaneous melanoma: Clinical management and treatment results worldwide. Philadelphia: JB Lippincott, 1985:447.
145. Balch CM, Soong S-j, Murad TM, et al. A multifactorial analysis of melanoma. IV. Prognostic factors in 200 melanoma patients with distant metastases (stage III). J Clin Oncol 1983;1:126.
146. Presant CA, Bartolucci AA (for the Southeastern Cancer Study Group). Prognostic factors in metastatic malignant melanoma: The Southeastern Cancer Study Group experience. Cancer 1982;49:2192.
147. Singletary SE, Balch CM, Urist MM, McCarthy WH, Cascinelli N. Surgical treatment of primary melanoma. In: Balch CM, Houghton A, Milton GW, Sober A, Soong S-j, eds. Cutaneous melanoma. 2nd ed. Philadelphia: JB Lippincott, 1992:269.
148. Bagley FH, Cady B, Lee A, et al. Changes in clinical presentation and management of malignant melanoma. Cancer 1981;47:2126.
149. Jones WM, Williams WJ, Roberts MM, et al. Malignant melanoma of the skin: Prognostic value of clinical features and the role of treatment in 111 cases. Br J Cancer 1968;22:437.
150. Cascinelli N, van der Esch EP, Breslow A, et al. Stage I melanoma of the skin: The problem of resection margins. Eur J Cancer 1980;16:1079.
151. Day CL Jr, Mihm MC Jr, Sober AJ, et al. Narrower margins for clinical stage I malignant melanoma. N Engl J Med 1982;306:479.
152. Elder DE, Guerry D IV, Heiberger RM, et al. Optimal resection margin for cutaneous malignant melanoma. Plast Reconstr Surg 1983;71:66.
153. Milton GW, Shaw HM, Farago GA, et al. Tumour thickness and the site and time of first recurrence in cutaneous malignant melanoma (stage I). Br J Surg 1980;67:543.
154. Ackerman AB. Malignant melanoma in situ. The fat, curable stage of malignant melanoma. Pathology 1985;17:298.
155. Jones RE Jr, Cash ME, Ackerman AB. Malignant melanomas mistaken histologically for junctional nevi. In: Ackerman AB, ed. Pathology of malignant melanoma. New York: Masson, 1981:93.
156. Kelly JW, Sagebiel RW, Calderon W, et al. The frequency of local recurrence and microsatellites as a guide to re-excision margins for cutaneous malignant melanoma. Ann Surg 1984;6:759.
157. Breslow A, Macht SD. Optimal size of resection margin for thin cutaneous melanoma. Surg Gynecol Obstet 1977;145:691.
158. Roses DF, Harris MN, Rigel D, et al. Local and in-transit metastases following definitive excision for primary cutaneous malignant melanoma. Ann Surg 1983;198:65.
159. Schmoeckel C, Bockelbrink A, Bockelbrink H, et al. Low- and high-risk malignant melanoma: Prognostic significance of the resection margin. Eur J Cancer Clin Oncol 1983;19:237.
160. Cosimi AB, Sober AJ, Mihm MC. Conservative surgical management of superficially invasive cutaneous melanoma. Cancer 1984;53:1256.
161. Milton GW, Shaw HM, McCarthy WH. Resection margins of melanoma. Aust NZ J Surg 1985;55:225.
162. Veronesi U, Cascinelli N, Adamus J, et al. Primary cutaneous melanoma 2 mm less in thickness. Results of a randomized study comparing wide with narrow surgical excision: A preliminary report. N Engl J Med 1988;318:1159–1162.
162a. Veronesi U, Cascinelli N. Narrow excision (1-cm margin): A safe procedure for thin cutaneous melanoma. Arch Surg 1991;126:438–441.
163. Harwood AR. Conventional fractionated radiotherapy for 51 patients with lentigo maligna and lentigo maligna melanoma. Int J Radiat Oncol Biol Phys 1983;9:1019.
164. Briele HA, Beattie CW, Ronan SG, et al. Late recurrence of cutaneous melanoma. Arch Surg 1983;118:800.
165. Krementz ET, Ryan RF, Muchmore JH, Carter RD, Sutherland CM, Reed RJ. Hyperthermic regional perfusion for melanoma of the limbs. In: Balch CM, Houghton AN, Milton GW, Sober A, Soong S-j. Cutaneous melanoma, 2nd ed. Philadelphia: JB Lippincott, 1992:403.
166. Elias EG, Didolkar MS, Goel IP, et al. A clinicopathologic study of prognostic factors in cutaneous malignant melanoma. Surg Gynecol Obstet 1977;144:327.
167. Karakousis CP. Groin dissection. In: Balch CM, Houghton AN, A, Soong S-j, eds. Cutaneous melanoma. 2nd ed. Philadelphia: JB Lippincott, 1992:392.
168. Das Gupta TK. Radical groin dissection. Surg Gynecol Obstet 1969;129:1275.
169. Holmes EC, Moseley HS, Morton DL, et al. A rational approach to the surgical management of melanoma. Ann Surg 1977;186:481.
170. Karakousis CP. Ilioinguinal lymph node dissection. Am J Surg 1981;141:299.
171. Dasmahapatra KS, Karakousis CP. Therapeutic groin dissection in malignant melanoma. Surg Gynecol Obstet 1983;156:21.
172. Finck SJ, Giuliano AE, Mann BD, et al. Results of ilioinguinal dissection for stage II melanoma. Ann Surg 1982;196:180.
173. McCarthy JG, Haagensen CD, Herter FP. The role of groin dissection in the management of melanoma of the lower extremity. Ann Surg 1974;179:156.
174. Fortner JG, Booher RJ, Pack GT. Results of groin dissection for malignant melanoma in 220 patients. Surgery 1964;55:485.

175. Karakousis CP, Lawrence JE, Rao UR. Groin dissection in malignant melanoma. Am J Surg 1986;152:491.
176. Harris MN, Gumport SL, Berman IR, et al. Ilioinguinal lymph node dissection for melanoma. Surg Gynecol Obstet 1973;136:33.
177. Urist MM, Maddox WA, Kennedy JE, et al. Patient risk factors and surgical morbidity after regional lymphadenectomy in 204 melanoma patients. Cancer 1983;51:2152.
178. Karakousis CP, Heiser MA, Moore RH. Lymphedema after groin dissection. Am J Surg 1983;145:205.
179. Chretien PB, Ketcham AS, Hoye RC, et al. Axillary dissection with preservation of the pectoralis major muscle. Ann Surg 1971;173:554.
180. Harris MN, Gumport SL, Maiwandi H. Axillary lymph node dissection for melanoma. Surg Gynecol Obstet 1972;135:936.
181. Ames FC, Balch CM, McCarthy W. Axillary lymph node dissection. In: Balch CM, Houghton AN, Milton GW, Sober A, Soong S-j. Cutaneous melanoma. 2nd ed. Philadelphia: JB Lippincott, 1992:384.
182. Bakamjian VY, Miller SH, Poole AG. A technique for radical dissection of the neck. Surg Gynecol Obstet 1977;144:419.
183. Beahrs OH. Surgical anatomy and technique of radical neck dissection. Surg Clin North Am 1977;57:663.
184. Martin HE, Del Balle B, Ehrlich H, et al. Neck dissection. Cancer 1951;4:441.
185. Byers RM. Cervical and parotid node dissections. In: Balch CM, Houghton AN, Milton GW, Sober A, Soong S-j, eds. Cutaneous melanoma. 2nd ed. Philadelphia: JB Lippincott, 1992:376.
186. Turkula LD, Woods JE. Limited or selective nodal dissection for malignant melanoma of the head and neck. Am J Surg 1984;148:446.
187. Becker GD, Parell GJ. Technique of preserving the spinal accessory nerve during radical neck dissection. Laryngoscope 1979;89:827.
188. Bocca E, Pagnataro O. A conservative technique in radical neck dissection. Ann Otol Rhinol Laryngol 1967;76:975.
189. Calearo CV, Teatini G. Functional neck dissection: Anatomical grounds, surgical technique, clinical observations. Ann Otol Rhinol Laryngol 1983;92:215.
190. Jesse RH, Ballantyne AJ, Larson D. Radical or modified neck dissection: A therapeutic dilemma. Am J Surg 1978;136:516.
191. Lingeman RE, Helmus C, Stephens R, et al. Neck dissection: Radical or conservative. Ann Otol Rhinol Laryngol 1977;86:737.
192. Schuller DE, Reiches NA, Hamaker RC, et al. Analysis of disability resulting from treatment including radical neck dissection or modified neck dissection. Head Neck Surg 1983;6:551.
193. Storm FK, Eilber FR, Sparks FC, et al. A prospective study of parotid metastases from head and neck cancer. Am J Surg 1977;134:115.
194. Beahrs OH, Adson MA. The surgical anatomy and techniques of parotidectomy. Am J Surg 1958;95:885l.
195. Woods JE. Parotidectomy: Points of technique for brief and safe operation. Am J Surg 1983;145:678.
196. Dunn EJ, Kent T, Hines J, et al. Parotid neoplasms: A report of 250 cases and review of the literature. Ann Surg 1976;184:500.
197. Powell ME, Clairmont AA. Complications of parotidectomy. South Med J 1983;76: 1109.
198. Woods JE. The facial nerve in parotid malignancy. Am J Surg 1983;146:493.
199. Sutherland CM, Mather FJ, Krementz ET. Factors influencing survival among patients with regional melanoma treated by regional perfusion. Surg Gynecol Obstet 1987;164: 111.
200. Stehlin JS Jr, Smith JL Jr, Jing B, et al. Melanomas of the extremities complicated by in-transit metastases. Surg Gynecol Obstet 1966;122:3.
201. Treidman L, McNeer G. Prognosis with local metastasis and recurrence in malignant melanoma. Ann NY Acad Sci 1963;100:123.
202. Moore GE, Gerner RE. Malignant melanoma. Surg Gynecol Obstet 1971;132:427.
203. Stehlin JS Jr, Clark RL. Melanoma of the extremities: Experiences with conventional treatment and perfusion in 339 cases. Am J Surg 1965;110:366.
204. Ghussen F, Nagel K, Groth W, et al. A prospective randomized study of regional extremity perfusion in patients with malignant melanoma. Ann Surg 1984;200:764.
205. Calvo DB III, Patt YZ, Wallace S, et al. Phase I–II trial of percutaneous intra-arterial cis-diamminedichloroplatinum (II) for regionally confined malignancy. Cancer 1980;45:1278.
206. Einhorn LH, McBride CM, Luce JK, et al. Intra-arterial infusion therapy with 5-(3,3-dimethyl-1-triazeno) imidazole-4-carboxamide (NSC-45388) for malignant melanoma. Cancer 1973;32:749.
207. Savlov ED, Hall TC, Oberfield RA. Intra-arterial therapy of melanoma with dimethyl triazeno imidazole carboxamide (NSC-45388). Cancer 1971;28:1161.
208. Karakousis CP, Choe KJ, Holyoke ED. Biologic behavior and treatment of intransit metastasis of melanoma. Surg Gynecol Obstet 1980;150:29.
209. Morton DL, Eilber FR, Holmes EC, et al. BCG immunotherapy of malignant melanoma: Summary of a seven-year experience. Ann Surg 1974;180:634.
210. Shingleton WW, Seigler HF, Stocks LH, et al. Management of recurrent melanoma of the extremity. Cancer 1975;35:574.
211. Balch CM, Milton GW, Cascinelli N, Milton GW, Sim FH. Elective node dissection: Pros and cons. In: Balch CM, Houghton AN, Milton GW, Sober A, Soong S-j, eds. Cutaneous melanoma. 2nd ed. Philadelphia: JB Lippincott, 1992:345.
212. Milton GW, Shaw HM, McCarthy WH, et al. Prophylactic lymph node dissection in clinical stage I cutaneous malignant melanoma: Results of surgical treatment in 1319 patients. Br J Surg 1982;69:108.
213. Reintgen DS, Cox EB, McCarty KM Jr, et al. Efficacy of elective lymph node dissection in patients with intermediate thickness primary melanoma. Ann Surg 1983;198:379.
214. Schneebaum S, Briele HA, Walker MJ, et al. Cutaneous thick melanoma: Prognosis and treatment. Arch Surg 1987;122:707–711.
215. McCarthy WH, Shaw HM, Milton GW. Efficacy of elective lymph node dissection in 2,347 patients with clinical stage I malignant melanoma. Surg Gynecol Obstet 1985;161:575.
216. Wanebo HJ, Woodruff J, Fortner JG. Malignant melanoma of the extremities: A clinicopathologic study using levels of invasion (microstage). Cancer 1975;35:666.
217. Balch CM. The role of elective lymph node dissection in melanoma: Rationale, results and controversies. J Clin Oncol 1988;6:163, 392.
218. Balch CM, Wilkerson JA, Murad TM, et al. The prognostic significance of ulceration of cutaneous melanoma. Cancer 1980;45:3012.
219. McGovern VJ, Shaw HM, Milton GW, et al. Ulceration and prognosis in cutaneous malignant melanoma. Histopathology 1982;6:399.
220. Elder DE, DuPont G, VanHorn M, et al. The role of lymph node dissection for clinical stage I malignant melanoma of intermediate thickness (1.51–3.99 mm). Cancer 1985;56:413–418.
221. Fee HJ, Robinson DS, Sample WF, et al. The determination of lymph shed by colloid fold scanning in patients with malignant melanoma: Preliminary study. Surgery 1978;84:626.
222. Sullivan DC, Croker BP, Harris CC, et al. Lymphoscintigraphy in malignant melanoma: Tc-antimony sulfur colloid. AJR 1981;137:847.
223. Meyer CM, Lecklitner ML, Logic JR, et al. Technetium-99m sulfur colloid cutaneous lymphoscintigraphy in the management of truncal melanoma. Radiology 1979;131: 205.
224. Lamki LM, Logic JR. Defining lymphatic draining patterns with cutaneous lymphoscintigraphy. In: Balch CM, Houghton AN, Milton GW, Sober AJ, Soong S-j, eds. Cutaneous melanoma. 2nd ed. Philadelphia: JB Lippincott, 1992:367.
225. Hansen MG, McCarten AB. Tumor thickness and lymphocytic infiltration in malignant melanoma of the head and neck. Am J Surg 1974;128:557.
226. Goldsmith HS, Shah JP, Kim DH. Prognostic significance of lymph node dissection in the treatment of malignant melanoma. Cancer 1970;26:606.
227. Gumport SL, Harris MN. Results of regional lymph node dissection for melanoma. Ann Surg 1974;179:105.
228. Sugarbaker EV, McBride CM. Melanoma of the trunk: The results of surgical excision and anatomic guidelines for predicting nodal metastasis. Surgery 1976;80:22.
229. Lane N, Lattes R, Malm J. Clinicopathological correlations in a series of 117 malignant melanomas of the skin of adults. Cancer 1958;11:1025.
230. Das Gupta TK. Results of treatment of 269 patients with primary cutaneous melanoma: A five-year prospective study. Ann Surg 1977;186:201.
231. Veronesi U, Adamus J, Bandiera DC, et al. Inefficacy of immediate node dissection in stage I melanoma of the limbs. N Engl J Med 1977;297:627.
232. Veronesi U, Adamus J, Bandiera DC, et al. Stage I melanoma of the limbs: Immediate versus delayed node dissection. Tumori 1980;66:373.
233. Veronesi U, Adams J, Bandiera DC, et al. Delayed regional lymph node dissection in stage I melanoma of the skin of the lower extremities. Cancer 1982;49:2420.
234. Sim FH, Taylor WF, Pritchard DJ, et al. Lymphadenectomy in the management of stage I malignant melanoma: A prospective randomized study. Mayo Clin Proc 1986;61: 697.
235. Bowsher WG, Taylor BA, Hughes LE. Morbidity, mortality and local recurrence following regional node dissection for melanoma. Br J Surg 1986;73:906.
236. Ang KK, Byers RM, Peters LJ, Maor MH, Wendt CD, Morrison WH, Goepfert H. Regional radiotherapy as adjuvant treatment for head and neck malignancy melanoma. Arch Otolaryngol Head Neck Surg 1990;116:169–172.
237. Lee YT. Malignant melanoma: Patterns of metastasis. Can J Physician 1980;30:137.
238. Budman DR, Camacho E, Wittes RE. The current causes of death in patients with malignant melanoma. Eur J Cancer 1978;14:327.
239. Patel JK, Didolkar MS, Pickren JW, et al. Metastatic pattern of malignant melanoma: A study of 216 autopsy cases. Am J Surg 1978;135:807.
240. Amer MH, Al-Sarraf M, Vaitkevicius VK. Clinical presentation, natural history and prognostic factors in advanced melanoma. Surg Gynecol Obstet 1979;149:687.
241. De la Monte SM, Moore GW, Hutchins GM. Patterned distribution of metastases from malignant melanoma in humans. Cancer Res 1983;43:3427.
242. Feun LG, Gutterman J, Burgess MA, et al. The natural history of resectable metastatic melanoma (stage IVA melanoma). Cancer 1982;50:1656.
243. Finck SJ, Giuliano AE, Morton DL. LDH and melanoma. Cancer 1983;51:840.
244. Meyer JE, Stolbach L. Pretreatment radiographic evaluation of patients with malignant melanoma. Cancer 1978;42:125.
245. Roth JA, Eilber FR, Bennett LR, et al. Radionuclide photoscanning: Usefulness in preoperative evaluation of melanoma patients. Arch Surg 1975;110:1211.
246. Das Gupta T, Brasfield R. Metastatic melanoma: A clinicopathological study. Cancer 1964;17:1323.
247. Sacre R, Lejeune FJ. Patterns of metastases distribution in 173 stage I and II melanoma patients. Anticancer Res 1982;2:47.
248. Nambisan RN, Alexiou G, Reese PA, et al. Early metastatic patterns and survival in malignant melanoma. J Surg Oncol 1987;34:248.
249. Garg R, McPherson TA, Lentle B, et al. Usefulness of an elevated serum lactate dehydrogenase value as a marker for hepatic metastases in malignant melanoma. Can Med Assoc J 1979;120:1114.
250. Einhorn LH, Burgess MA, Vallejos C, et al. Prognostic correlations and response to treatment in advanced metastatic malignant melanoma. Cancer Res 1974;34:1995.
251. Muss HB, Richards F II, Barnes PL, et al. Radionuclide scanning in patients with advanced malignant melanoma. Clin Nucl Med 1979;4:516.
252. Aranha GV, Simmons RL, Gunnarsson A, et al. The value of preoperative screening procedures in stage I and II malignant melanoma. J Surg Oncol 1979;11:1.

253. Thomas JH, Panoussopoulous D, Liesmann GE, et al. Scintiscans in the evaluation of patients with malignant melanoma. Surg Gynecol Obstet 1979;149:574.
254. Evans RA, Bland KI, McMurtrey MJ, et al. Radionuclide scans not indicated for stage I melanoma. Surg Gynecol Obstet 1980;150:532.
255. Doiron MJ, Bernardino ME. A comparison of non-invasive imaging modalities in the melanoma patient. Cancer 1981;47:2581.
256. Au FC, Maier WP, Malmud LS, et al. Preoperative nuclear scans in patients with melanoma. Cancer 1984;53:2095.
257. Iscoe N, Kersey P, Gapski J, et al. Predictive value of staging investigations in patients with clinical stage I malignant melanoma. Plast Reconstr Surg 1987;80:233.
258. Lewi HJ, Roberts MM, Donaldson AA, et al. The use of cerebral computer assisted tomography as a staging investigation of patients with carcinoma of the breast and malignant melanoma. Surg Gynecol Obstet 1980;151:385.
259. Ardizzoni A, Grimaldi A, Repetto L, et al. Stage I–II melanoma: The value of metastatic workup. Oncology 1987;44:87.
260. Zartman GM, Thomas MR, Robinson WA. Metastatic disease in patients with newly diagnosed malignant melanoma. J Surg Oncol 1987;35:163.
261. Milder MS, Frankel RS, Bulkley BG, et al. Gallium-67 scintigraphy in malignant melanoma. Cancer 1973;32:1350.
262. Romolo JL, Fischer SG. Gallium-67 scanning compared with physical examination in the preoperative staging of melanoma. Cancer 1979;44:468.
263. Berkerman C, Hoffer PB, Bitran JD. The role of gallium-67 in the evaluation of cancer. Semin Nucl Med 1984;14:296.
264. Rossleigh MA, McCarthy WH, Milton GW, et al. The role of gallium-67 studies in the management of malignant melanoma. Med J Aust 1984;140:401.
265. Kirkwood JM, Meyers JE, Vlock DR, et al. Tomographic gallium-67 citrate scanning: Useful new surveillance for metastatic melanoma. Ann Surg 1983;198:102.
266. Houghton AN, Legha S, Bajorin DF. Treatment for advanced melanoma. In: Balch CM, Houghton AN, Milton GW, Sober A, Soong S-j, eds. Cutaneous melanoma. 2nd ed. Philadelphia: JB Lippincott, 1992:468.
267. Hena MA, Emrich LJ, Nambisan RN, et al. Effect of surgical treatment of stage IV melanoma. Am J Surg 1987;153:270.
268. Overett TK, Shiu MH. Surgical treatment of distant metastatic melanoma: Indications and results. Cancer 1985;56:1222.
269. Wornom IL, Smith JW, Soong S-j, et al. Surgery as palliative treatment for distant metastases of melanoma. Ann Surg 1986;204:181.
270. Peters LJ, Byers RM, Ang KK. Radiotherapy for melanoma. In: Balch CM, Houghton AN, Milton GW, Sober AJ, Soong S-j, eds. Cutaneous melanoma. 2nd ed. Philadelphia: JB Lippincott, 1992:509–521.
271. Habermalz HJ, Fischer JJ. Radiation therapy of malignant melanoma: Experience with high individual treatment doses. Cancer 1976;38:2258.
272. Hornsey S. The relationship between total dose, number of fractions and fraction size in the response of malignant melanoma in patients. Br J Radiol 1978;51:905.
273. Katz HR. The results of different fractionation schemes in the palliative irradiation of metastatic melanoma. Int J Radiat Oncol Biol Phys 1981;7:907.
274. Lobo PA, Liebner EJ, Chao JJ, et al. Radiotherapy in the management of malignant melanoma. Int J Radiat Oncol Biol Phys 1981;7:21.
275. Strauss A, Dritschilo A, Nathanson L, et al. Radiation therapy of malignant melanomas. An evaluation of clinically used fractionation schemes. Cancer 1981;47:1262.
276. Trott KR, von Lieven H, Kummermehr J, et al. The radiosensitivity of malignant melanomas. II. Clinical studies. Int J Radiat Oncol Biol Phys 1981;7:15.
277. Adam JS, Habeshaw T, Kirk J. Response rate of malignant melanoma to large fraction irradiation. Br J Radiol 1982;55:605.
278. Doss LL, Memula N. The radioresponsiveness of melanoma. Int J Radiat Oncol Biol Phys 1982;8:1131.
279. Overgaard J, von der Masse H, Overgaard MA. A randomized study comparing two high-dose per fraction radiation schedules in recurrent or metastatic melanoma. Int J Radiat Oncol Biol Phys 1985;11:1837.
280. Overgaard J, Overgaard M, Hansen V, et al. Some factors of importance in the radiation treatment of malignant melanoma. Radiother Oncol 1986;5:183.
281. Bentzen SM, Overgaard J, Thames HD, Overgaard M, Hansen PV, van der Masse H. Clinical radiobiology of malignant melanoma. Radiother Oncol 1989;16:169.
282. Thames HD, Withers HR, Peters LJ, Fletcher GH. Changes in early and late radiation responses with altered dose fractionation: Implications for dose-survival relationships. Int J Radiat Oncol Biol Phys 1982;8:219.
283. Sause WT, Cooper JS, Rush S, Ago CT Cosmatos D, Coughlin CT, et al. RTOG 83-05: A randomized trial evaluating fraction size in external beam radiation therapy in treatment of melanoma. Int J Radiat Oncol Biol Phys 1991;20:429.
284. Overgaard J, Overgaard M. Hyperthermia as an adjuvant to radiotherapy in the treatment of malignant melanoma. Int J Hyperthermia 1987;3:483.
285. Meyer JL, Kapp DS, Fessemdem P. Hahn GH. Hyperthermic oncology: Current biology, physics and clinical results. Pharmacol Ther 1989;42:251.
286. Blake PR, Catterall M, Errington RF. Treatment of malignant melanoma by fast neutrons. Br J Surg 1985;75:517.
287. Dische S. Radiotherapy using the hypoxic cell sensitizer Ro 03-8799 in malignant melanoma. Radiother Oncol 1987;10:11.
288. Chapman JD, Urtasun RC, Frank AJ, Raleigh JA, Meeker BE, McKinnon SA. The measurement oxygenation status of individual tumors. In: Paliwal BR, Fowler JF, Herbert DE, Kinsella TJ, Orton CG, eds. Prediction of response in radiation therapy: The physical and biological basis. New York: American Institute of Physics, 1989:49.
289. DeLaney TF, Glatstein E. Photodynamic therapy of cancer. Compr Ther 1988;14:43.
290. Mishima Y, Ichilhashi M, Hatta S, Honda Ch, Yamamura K, Nakagawa T, et al. First human clinical trial of melanoma neutron capture: Diagnosis and therapy. Strahlenther Onkol 1989;165:251.
291. Marsoni S, Hoth D, Simon R. Clinical drug development. An analysis of phase II trials, 1970–1985. Cancer Treat Rep 1987;71:71.
292. Comis RL. DTIC (NSC-45388) in malignant melanoma: A perspective. Cancer Treat Rep 1976;64:1123.
293. Luce JK. Chemotherapy of malignant melanoma. Cancer 1972;30:1604.
294. Costanza ME, Nathanson L, Schoenfeld D, et al. Results with methyl-CCNU and DTIC in metastatic melanoma. Cancer 1977;40:1010.
295. Wagner DE, Ramirez G, Weiss AJ. Combination phase I–II study of imidazole carboxamide (NSC-45388). Oncology 1971;26:310.
296. Nathanson L, Wolter K, Horton J. Characteristics of prognosis and response to an imidazole carboxamide in malignant melanoma. Clin Pharmacol Ther 1971;12:955.
297. Costanza ME, Nathanson L, Lenhard R, et al. Therapy of malignant melanoma with an imidazole carboxamide and bischloroethyl nitrosourea. Cancer 1972;30:1457.
298. Moon JH, Gailanai S, Cooper MR, et al. Comparison of the combination of 1,3-bis (2-chloroethyl)-1-nitrosourea (BCNU) and vincristine with two dose schedules of 5-(3,3-dimethyl-1-triazeno) imiadazole 4-carboxamide (DTIC) in the treatment of disseminated malignant melanoma. Cancer 1975;35:368.
299. Van der Merwe AM, Falkson G, Van Eden EB. Metastatic malignant melanoma. Imidazole carboxamide in its treatment. Med Proc 1971;17:399.
300. Luce JK, Thurman WG, Isaacs BL, Talley RW. Clinical trials with the antitumor agent 5-(3,3-dimethyl-1-triazeno) imidazole-4-carboxamide (NSC-45388). Cancer Chemother Rep 1970;54:119–124.
301. Gerner RE, Moore GE. Study of 5-(3,3-dimethyl-1-triazeno) imidazole-4-carboxamide (NSC-45388) in patients with disseminated melanoma. Cancer Chemother Rep 1973;57:83.
302. Gottlieb JA, Serpick AA. Clinical evaluation of 5-(3,3-dimethyl-1-triazeno) imidazole 4-carboxamide in malignant melanoma and other neoplasms: Comparison of twice weekly and daily administration schedules. Oncology 1971;25:255.
303. Burke PJ, McCarthy NWH, Milton GW. Imidazole carboxamide therapy in advanced malignant melanoma. Cancer 1971;27:744.
304. Cowan DH, Bersagel DE. Intermittent treatment of metastatic malignant melanoma with high-dose 5-(3,3-dimethyl-1-triazeno) imadazole-4-carboxamide (NSC-45388). Cancer Chemother Rep 1971;55:175.
305. Vogel CL, Comis RL, Ziegler JL, Kiryabwire JW. Study of 5-(3,3-dimethyl-1-triazeno) imadazole-4-carboxamide (NSC-45388) given intravenously in the treatment of malignant melanoma in Uganda. Cancer Chemother Rep 1973;55:143.
306. Costanza J. DTIC (NSC-45388) studies in the Southwest Oncology Group. Cancer Treat Rep 1976;60:189.
307. Pritchard KI, Quirt IC, Cowan DH et al. DTIC therapy in metastatic malignant melanoma: A simplified dose schedule. Cancer Treat Rep 1980;64:1123.
308. Hill GJ II, Krementz ET, Hill HZ. Dimethyl triazeno imidazole carboxamide and combination therapy for melanoma. IV. Late results after complete response to chemotherapy. Cancer 1984;53:1299.
309. Einhorn LH, Burgess MA, Vallejos C, et al. Prognostic correlations and response to treatment in advanced metastatic melanoma. Cancer Res 1974;34:1995.
310. Thatcher N, Anderson H, James R, et al. DTIC by 24 hour infusion for metastatic melanoma. Proceedings of the First International Conference on Skin Melanoma (Venice), 1985;1:156.
311. Carter RD, Krementz ET, Hill GJ II, et al. DTIC (NSC-45388) and combination therapy for melanoma. I. Studies with DTIC, BCNU, CCNU, vincristine, and hydroxyurea. Cancer Treat Rep 1976;60:601.
312. Bellet RE, Mastrangelo MJ, Laucius JF, et al. Randomized prospective trial of DTIC (NSC-45388) alone versus BCNU (NSC-409962) in the treatment of metastatic malignant melanoma. Cancer Treat Rep 1976;60:595.
313. Carter SK, Friedman MA. 5-(3,3-dimethyl-1-triazeno) imidazole-4-carboxamide (DTIC, DIC, NSC-45388): A new tumor agent with activity against malignant melanoma. Eur J Cancer 1972;8:85.
314. Salem PA, Sinno B, Hajj A, et al. High dose intermittent therapy with 5-(3,3-dimethyl-1-triazeno) imidazole-4-carboxamide (DTIC) in melanoma and other solid tumors. Proc Am Assoc Cancer Res 1976;17:116.
315. Ahmann DL, Hahn RG, Bisel HF, et al. Clinical evaluation of 5-(3,3-dimethyl-1-triazeno) imidazole-4-carboxamide (NSC-45388), melphalan (NSC-8806) and hydroxyurea (NSC-32065) in the treatment of disseminated malignant melanoma. Cancer Chemother Rep 1972;56:369.
316. Carbone PP, Costello W. Eastern Cooperative Oncology Group studies with DTIC (NSC-45388). Cancer Treat Rep 1976;60:193–198.
317. Tyson LB, Clark RA, Gralla RJ, et al. High-dose metoclopramide: Control of dacarbazine-induced emesis in a preliminary trial. Cancer Treat Rep 1982;66:2108.
318. Clark RA, Tyson LB, Gralla RJ, et al. Antiemetic therapy: Management of chemotherapy-induced nausea and vomiting. Semin Oncol Nurs 1989;5:53.
319. Ramirez G, Wilson W, Grage T, et al. Phase II evaluation of 1,3-bis(2-chloroethyl-nitrosourea) (BCNU; NSC-409962) in patients with solid tumors. Cancer Chemother Rep 1972;56:787.
320. DeVita VT, Carbone PP, Owens AH Jr, et al. Clinical trials with 1,3,-bis(2-chloroethyl)-1-nitrosourea, NSC-409962. Cancer Res 1965;25:1875.
321. Ahmann DL. Nitrosoureas in the management of disseminated malignant melanoma. Cancer Treat Rep 1976;60:747.
322. Beretta G, Pancera G, Locatelli C, et al. Lomustine (CCNU) and epirubicin as alternative treatments to dacarbazine (DIC) for advanced malignant melanoma. Proceedings of the First International Conference on Skin Melanoma (Venice), 1985;1:148.
323. Ahmann DL, Hahn RG, Bisel HF. A comparative study of 1-(2-chloroethyl)-3-cyclohexyl-1-nitrosourea (NSC-79037) and imidazole carboxamide (NSC-45388) with

vincristine (NSC-67574) in the palliation of disseminated malignant melanoma. Cancer Res 1972;32:2432.

324. Hoogstraten B, Gottlieb JA, Caoili E, et al. CCNU (1-(2,chloroethyl)-3-cyclohexyl-1-nitrosourea, NSC-79037) in the treatment of cancer. Cancer 1973;32:38.
325. Ahmann DL, Hahn RG, Bisel HF. Evaluation of 1-(2-chloroethyl-3-4-methyl-cyclohexyl)-1-nitrosourea (methyl-CCNU, NSC-95441) versus combined imidazole carboxamide (NSC-45388) and vincristine (NSC-67574) in palliation of disseminated melanoma. Cancer 1974;33:615.
326. Wasserman TH, Slavik M, Carter SK. Review of CCNU in clinical cancer therapy. Cancer Treat Rev 1974;1:131.
327. Young RC, Canellos GP, Chabner BA, et al. Treatment of malignant melanoma with methyl-CCNU. Cancer Pharmacol Ther 1974;15:617.
328. Wasserman TH, Slavik M, Carter SK. Methyl-CCNU in clinical cancer therapy. Cancer Treat Rev 1974;1:251.
329. Jacquillat C, Khayat D, Banzet P, et al. Final report of the French multicenter Phase II study of the nitrosourea fotemustine in 153 evaluable patients with disseminated malignant melanoma including patients with cerebral metastases. Cancer 1990;66:1873.
330. Khayat D, Lokiec F, Bizzari J-P, et al. Phase I clinical study of the new amino acid-linked nitrosourea S10036 administered on a weekly schedule. Cancer Res 1987;47:6782.
331. Nolte H, Lindgaard-Nedsen E, Bloomquist E, et al. Phase II evaluation of tauromustine in disseminated malignant melanoma. Proc Am Soc Clin Oncol 1988;7:249.
332. Al-Sarraf M, Fletcher W, Oishi N, et al. Cisplatin hydration with and without mannitol diuresis in refractory disseminated malignant melanoma: A Southwest Oncology Group study. Cancer Treat Rep 1982;66:31.
333. Goodnight JE Jr, Moseley HS, Eilber FR, et al. Cis-dichlorodiammineplatinum (II) alone and combined with DTIC for treatment of disseminated malignant melanoma. Cancer Treat Rep 1979;63:2005.
334. Schilcher RB, Wessels M, Niederle N, Seeber S, Schmidt CG. Phase II evaluation of fractionated low and single high dose cisplatin in various tumors. J Cancer Res Clin Oncol 1984;107:57.
335. Glover D, Glick J, Weiler C, Fox K, Grabelsky S, Guerry D. High dose cis-platinum (DDP) and WR-2721 in metastatic melanoma. Proc Am Soc Clin Oncol 1988;7:247.
336. Song SY, Chary KK, Higby DJ, Henderson ES, Klein E. Cisdiamminedichloride platinum (II) in the treatment of metastatic malignant melanoma. Clin Res 1977;25:411.
337. Chary KK, Higby DJ, Henderson ES, Swinerton KD. Phase I study of high-dose cis-dichlorodiammineplatinum (II) with forced diuresis. Cancer Treat Rep 1977;61:367.
338. Mortimer JE, Chestnut T, Higano CS, Goodman G. High dose cisplatin in metastatic melanoma: Comparison of two schedules. Proc Am Soc Clin Oncol 1988;7:254.
339. Kim S, McClay E, Kirmani S, et al. Biweekly intravenous (IV) cisplatin with sodium thiosulfate. Proc Am Soc Clin Oncol 1990;9:88.
340. Evans L, Casper ES, Rosenbluth R. Phase II trial of carboplatin in advanced malignant melanoma. Cancer Treat Rep 1987;71:171.
341. Rumke PH. The use of chemotherapy in the management of patients with malignant melanoma. Dev Oncol 1984;25:190.
342. Costa G, Hreshchyshyn MM, Holland JF. Initial clinical studies with vincristine. Cancer Chemother Rep 1962;24:39.
343. Holland JF, Scharlay C, Gailanai S, et al. Vincristine treatment of advanced cancer: A cooperative study of 392 cases. Cancer Res 1264;33:1258.
344. Gubisch NJ, Norena D, Perlia CP, et al. Experience with vincristine in solid tumors. Cancer Chemother Rep 1963;32:19.
345. Shaw RK, Brunner JA. Clinical evaluation of vincristine (NSC-67574). Cancer Chemother Rep 1964;42:45.
346. Reitmeier RJ, Moertel CG, Blackburn CM, et al. Vincristine (NSC-67574) therapy of adult patients with solid tumors. Cancer Chemother Rep 1964;34:21.
347. Smart CR, Ottoman RE, Rochlin DB, et al. Clinical experience with vincristine (NSC-67574) in tumors of the central nervous system and other malignant diseases. Cancer Chemother Rep 1968;52:733.
348. Frei E, Franzino A, Shnider BI, et al. Clinical studies of vinblastine. Cancer Chemother Rep 1961;12:125.
349. Armstrong JG, Dyke RW, Fouts PJ, et al. Hodgkin's disease, carcinoma of the breast and other tumors treated with vinblastine sulfate. Cancer Chemother Rep 1962;18:49.
350. Acute Leukemia Group B, Eastern Cooperative Group. Neoplastic diseases: Treatment with vinblastine. Arch Intern Med 1965;111:846.
351. Bond WH, Rohn RJ, Bates LH, et al. Treatment of neoplastic diseases with an improved oral preparation of vinblastine sulfate. Cancer 1966;19:213.
352. Hodes ME, Rohn RJ, Bond WH, Yardley JM, Corpening WS. Vincaleukoblastine. IV. A summary of two and one half years' experience in the use of vinblastine. Cancer Chemother Rep 1962;16:401.
353. Hill JM II, Loeb E. Treatment of leukemia, lymphoma, and other malignant neoplasms with vinblastine. Cancer Chemother Rep 1961;15:41.
354. Falkson G, Van Dyk JJ, Verwoerd HF. The chemotherapy of malignant melanoma. S Afr Med J 1968;42:89.
355. Wright TL, Hurley J, Korst DR, et al. Vinblastine in neoplastic disease. Cancer Res 1963;23:169.
356. Smart CR, Rochlin DB, Nahum AM, et al. Clinical experience with vinblastine sulfate (NSC-49842) in squamous cell carcinoma and other malignancies. Cancer Chemother Rep 1964;34:31.
357. Bleehan NM, Jellifee AM. Vinblastine sulfate in the treatment of malignant disease. Br J Cancer 1965;19:268.
358. Currie VE, Wong PP, Krakoff IH, et al. Phase I trial of vindesine in patients with advanced cancer. Cancer Treat Rep 1978;62:1333.
359. Camacho FJ, Young CW, Wittes RE. Phase II trial of vindesine in patients with malignant melanoma. Cancer Treat Rep 1980;64:179.
360. Retsas S, Peat I, Ashford R, et al. Updated results of vindesine as a single agent in the therapy of advanced malignant melanoma. Cancer Treat Rev 1980;7(Suppl):87.
361. Carmichael J, Atkinson RJ, Calman KC, Mackie RM, Naysmith AM, Smyth JF. A muticentre phase II trial of vindesine in malignant melanoma. Eur J Cancer Clin Oncol 1982;18:1293.
362. DiBella NJ, Berris R, Garfield D, Fink K, Speer J, Sakamoto A. Vindesine in advanced breast cancer, lymphoma and melanoma. Invest New Drugs 1984;2:323.
363. Quagliana JM, Stephens RL, Baker LH, Costanzi JJ. Vindesine in patients with metastatic malignant melanoma. J Clin Oncol 1984;2:316.
364. Smith IE, Hedley DW, Powles TJ, et al. Vindesine: A phase II study in the treatment of breast carcinoma, malignant melanoma and other solid tumors. Cancer Treat Rep 1978;62:1427.
365. Nelimark RA, Peterson BA, Vosika GJ, et al. Vindesine for metastatic malignant melanoma. Eur J Cancer Clin Oncol 1983;18:1293.
366. Rumke P, Everall JD, Mulder JH, et al. EORTC phase II trial of vindesine in advanced melanoma. Eur J Cancer Clin Oncol 1983;19:1173.
367. Arseneau JC, Mellette SJ, Kuperminc M, et al. Phase II study of vindesine in metastatic malignant melanoma. Cancer Treat Rep 1981;65:355.
368. Wagstaff J, Anderson HA, Shiu W, et al. Phase II study of vindesine infusion in visceral metastatic malignant melanoma. Cancer Treat Rep 1983;67:839.
369. Mayol XF, Beltran J, Rubio-Bazan R, et al. Multicenter phase II trial with 5-day continuous infusion of vindesine in metastatic malignant melanoma. Cancer Treat Rep 1983;68:1199.
370. Wiernik PH, Schwartz EL, Einzig A, et al. Phase I trial of taxol given as a 24-hour infusion every 2 days: Responses observed in metastatic melanoma. J Clin Oncol 1987;5:1232.
371. Einzig A, Trump DL, Sasloff J, et al. Phase II pilot study of taxol in patients with malignant melanoma. Proc Am Soc Clin Oncol 1988;7:249.
372. Legha SS, Ring S, Papadopoulos N, et al. A phase II trial of taxol in metastatic melanoma. Cancer 1990;65:2478.
373. Andrews NC, Weiss AJ, Ansfield FJ, et al. Phase I study of dibromodulcitol (NSC-104800). Cancer Chemother Rep 1971;55:61.
374. Phillips RW, Brook J. Clinical experience with dibromodulcitol (NSC-104800) in solid tumors. Cancer Chemother Rep 1971;55:567.
375. Andrews NC, Weiss AJ, Wilson W, et al. Phase II study of dibromodulcitol (NSC-104800). Cancer Chemother Rep 1974;58:653.
376. Bellet RE, Catalano RB, Mastrangelo MJ, et al. Positive phase II trial of dibromodulcitol in patients with metastatic melanoma refractory to DTIC and nitrosoureas. Cancer Treat Rep 1978;69:2095.
377. Simmonds MA, Lipton A, Harvey HA, et al. Phase II study of mitolactol in metastatic malignant melanoma. Cancer Treat Rep 198;69:65.
378. Amato DA, Bruckner H, Guerry D IV, et al. Phase II evaluation of dibromodulcitol and actinomycin D, hydroxyurea and cyclophosphamide in previously untreated patients with malignant melanoma. Invest New Drugs 1987;5:293.
379. Medina W, Kirkwood JM. Phase II trial of mitolactol in patients with metastatic melanoma. Cancer Treat Rep 1985;69:723.
380. Murray N, Silver H, Shah A, et al. Phase II study of mitolactol in advanced malignant melanoma. Cancer Treat Rep 1985;69:723.
381. Malden LT, Coates AS, Milton GW, et al. Mitolactol chemotherapy for malignant melanoma. Cancer Treat Rep 1984;68:1045.
382. Friustaci S, Gafprini G, Galligioni E, et al. Phase II trial of Esorubicin in patients with advanced melanoma. Cancer Treat Rep 1987;71:325.
383. Feun LG, Gonzalez R, Savaraj N, et al. Phase II study of piritrexim in metastatic melanoma using intermittent, low dose administration. J Clin Oncol 1991;9:464.
384. Phillips GL, Fay JW, Herzig GP, et al. Intensive 1,3-bis(2-chloroethyl)-1-nitrosourea (BCNU) with autologous bone marrow transplantation therapy of refractory cancer: A preliminary report. Exp Hematol 1979;7:372.
385. Thomas MR, Robinson WA, Glode LM, et al. Treatment of advanced malignant melanoma with high-dose chemotherapy and autologous bone marrow transplantation: Preliminary results—phase I study. Am J Clin Oncol 1982;5:611.
386. Lazarus HM, Herzig RH, Graham-Pole J, et al. Intensive melphalan chemotherapy and cryopreserved autologous bone marrow transplantation for the treatment of refractory cancer. J Clin Oncol 1983;1:359.
387. Spitzer G, Dicke K, Zander AR, et al. High-dose chemotherapy with autologous bone marrow transplantation. Cancer 1984;54:216.
388. Tchekmedyian NS, Tait N, van Echo D, et al. High-dose chemotherapy without autologous bone marrow transplantation in melanoma. J Clin Oncol 1986;4:1811.
389. Phillips GL, Fay JW, Herzig GP, et al. Intensive 1,3-bis(2-chloroethyl)-1-nitrosourea (BCNU), NSC-409962 and cryopreserved autologous marrow transplantation for refractory cancer: A phase I–II study. Cancer 1983;52:1792.
390. Lazarus HM, Herzig RH, Wolff SN, et al. Treatment of metastatic malignant melanoma with intensive melphalan and autologous bone marrow transplantation. Cancer Treat Rep 1985;69:473.
391. McElwain TJ, Hedley DW, Burton G, et al. Marrow autotransplantation accelerates hematological recovery in patients with malignant melanoma treated with high-dose melphalan. Br J Cancer 1979;40:72.
392. McElwain TJ, Hedley DW, Gordon MY, et al. High dose melphalan and non-cryopreserved autologous bone marrow treatment of malignant melanoma and neuroblastoma. Exp Hematol 1979;7(Suppl):360.
393. Wolff SN, Herzig RH, Fay JW, et al. High dose thiotepa with autologous bone marrow

transplantation for metastatic melanoma: Results of phase I–II studies of the North American Bone Marrow Transplantation Group. J Clin Oncol 1989;7:245.
394. Antman K, Eder JP, Elias A, et al. High dose combination alkylating agent preparative regimen with autologous bone marrow support: The Dana-Farber Cancer Institute/Beth Israel Hospital experience. Cancer Treat Rep 1987;71:119.
395. Ciobanu N, Dutcher J, Gucalp R, et al. High dose chemotherapy with autologous bone marrow transplantation for malignant melanoma after failure of interleukin-2 and lymphokine activated killer cells. Proc Am Soc Clin Oncol 1989;8:281.
396. Slease RB, Benear JB, Selby GB, et al. High dose combination alkylating agent therapy with autologous bone marrow rescue for refractory solid tumors. J Clin Oncol 1988;6:1314.
397. Eder JP, Antman K, Elias A, et al. Cyclophosphamide and thiotepa with autologous bone marrow transplantation in patients with solid tumors. JNCI 1988;80:1221.
398. Shea TC, Antman KH, Eder JP, et al. Malignant melanoma: Treatment with high-dose combination alkylating chemotherapy and autologous bone marrow support. Arch Dermatol 1988;124:878.
399. Moormeier JA, Williams SF, Kaminer LS, et al. High-dose tri-alkylator chemotherapy with autologous stem cell rescue in patients with refractory malignancies. JNCI 1990;82:29.
400. Thatcher N, Lind M, Morgenstern G, et al. High dose double alkylating agent chemotherapy with DTIC, melphalan or ifosphamide and marrow rescue for metastatic malignant melanoma. Cancer 1989;63:1296.
401. Glover D, Glick JH, Weiler C, et al. WR 2721 and high-dose cis-platin: An active combination in the treatment of metastatic melanoma. J Clin Oncol 1987;5:574.
402. Mastrangelo MJ, Berd D, Bellet RE. Aggressive chemotherapy for melanoma. PPO Updates 1991;5:1.
403. Coit DG, Bajorin DF, Menedez-Botet C, et al. A phase I study of hyperthermic isolation limb perfusion using cisplatin for metastatic melanoma. Proc Am Soc Clin Oncol 1991;10:294.
404. Mavligit G, Carrasco C, Papadopoulos N, et al. Regression of ocular melanoma metastatic to the liver after chemoembolization with cis-platinum and polyvinyl sponge. Proc Am Soc Clin Oncol 1987;6:830.
405. Mavligit GM, Charnsangavej C, Carrasco CH, et al. Regression of ocular melanoma metastatic to the liver after hepatic arterial chemoembolization with cisplatin and polyvinyl sponge. J Am Med Assoc 1988;260:974.
406. Nathanson L, Kaufman SD, Carey RW. Vinblastine infusion, bleomycin, and cis-dichlorodiammine-platinum chemotherapy in metastatic melanoma. Cancer 1981;48:1290.
407. Nathanson L, Wittenberg BK. Pilot study of vinblastine and bleomycin combinations in the treatment of metastatic melanoma. Cancer Treat Rep 1980;64:133.
408. National Cancer Institute of Canada Melanoma Group. Vinblastine, bleomycin, and cis-platinum for the treatment of metastatic malignant melanoma. J Clin Oncol 1984;2:131.
409. Luikart SD, Kennealey GT, Kirkwood JM. Randomized phase III trial of vinblastine, bleomycin, and cis-dichlorodiammine-platinum versus dacarbazine in malignant melanoma. J Clin Oncol 1984;2:164.
410. Kirkwood JM, Ernstoff MS, Guiliano A, et al. Interferon-α2a and dacarbazine in melanoma. JNCI 1990;82:1062.
411. McLeod GRC, Thomson DB, Hersey P. Recombinant interferon alpha-2b in advanced melanoma: A phase I–II study in combination with DTIC. Int J Cancer 1987;1(Suppl):31.
412. Breier S, Pensel R, Roffe C, et al. High dose DTIC with recombinant interferon-α2b for the treatment of metastatic malignant melanoma. Proc Am Soc Clin Oncol 1990;9:821.
413. Vorobiof DA, Falkson G, Voges CW. DTIC versus DTIC and recombinant interferon-α2b in treatment of patients with advanced malignant melanoma. Proc Am Soc Clin Oncol 1989;8:284.
414. Bajetta E, Negretta E, Giannotti B, et al. Phase II study of interferon-α2a and dacarbazine in metastatic melanoma. Proc Am Soc Clin Oncol 1989;8:286.
415. Mickiewicz E, Estevez R, Rao F, et al. Interferon-α2b for the treatment of metastatic melanoma. Proc Am Soc Clin Oncol 1990;9:281.
416. Kerr R, Pippen P, Mennel R, et al. Treatment of metastatic malignant melanoma with a combination of interferon-α2a and dacarbazine. Proc Am Soc Clin Oncol 1989;8:288.
417. Mulder NH, Schraffordt S, Koops H, et al. Dacarbazine and α-interferon for disseminated metastatic melanoma. Proc Am Soc Clin Oncol 1990;9:279.
418. Sertoli MR. DTIC with or without recombinant interferon α-2A at different dosages in the treatment of stage IV melanoma patients: Preliminary results of a randomized clinical trial. Proc Advances Biol Clin Management Melanoma 1991;34:138.
419. Falkson CI, Falkson G, Falkson HC. Improved results with the addition of interferon α-2b to dacarbazine in the treatment of 6 patients with malignant melanoma. J Clin Oncol 1991;9:1403.
420. Hill II JG, Metter GE, Krementz ET, et al. DTIC and combination therapy for melanoma. II. Escalating schedules of DTIC with BCNU, CCNU, and vincristine. Cancer Treat Rep 1979;63:1989.
421. McKelvey EM, Luce JK, Talley RW, et al. Combination chemotherapy with bis-chloroethyl nitrosourea (BCNU), vincristine and dimethyl triazeno imidazole carboxamide (DTIC) in disseminated malignant melanoma. Cancer 1977;39:1.
422. Berretta G, Bajetta E, Bonadonna G, et al. Polichemioterapia con 5 (3,3-dimetil-triazeno)-imidazole-4-carboxamide (DTIC; NSC-45388), 1,3-bis (2-chloretil)-1-nitrosourea (BCNU; NSC-409962) e vincristina (NSC-67574) nel melanoma in fase metastatizzata. Tumori 1973;59:239.
423. Berretta G, Bonadonna G, Cascinelli N, et al. Comparative evaluation of three combination regimens for advanced malignant melanoma: Results of an international cooperative study. Cancer Treat Rep 1976;60:33.
424. Cohen SM, Greenspan EM, Ratner LH, et al. Combination chemotherapy of malignant melanoma with imidazole carboxamide, BCNU, and vincristine. Cancer 1977;39:41.
425. Luce JK, Torin LB, Price H. Combination dimethyltriazeno imidazole carboxamide (NSC-45388), vincristine (NSC-67574; VCR) and 1,3-bis (2-chloroethyl)-1-nitrosourea (NSC-409962; BCNU) chemotherapy of disseminated malignant melanoma. Proc Am Assoc Cancer Res 1970;11:50.
426. Einhorn LH, Furnas B. Combination chemotherapy for disseminated malignant melanoma with DTIC, vincristine and methyl-CCNU. Cancer Treat Rep 1977;61:881.
427. Carmo-Pereira J, Costa FO, Pimentel P. Combination cytotoxic chemotherapy for metastatic cutaneous malignant melanoma with DTIC, BCNU and vincristine. Cancer Treat Rep 1976;60:1381.
428. Kleeberg UR, Schreml W. Polychemotherapie des metastasierenden melanomas. Vincristin, carmustin, dacarbazin. Deutsch Med Wochenschr 1976;101:890.
429. Berretta G, Bonadonna G, Bajetta E, et al. Combination chemotherapy (NSC-45388) in advanced malignant melanoma, soft tissue sarcomas and Hodgkin's disease. Cancer Treat Rep 1976;60:1381.
430. Gunderson S. Dacarbazine, vindesine and cisplatin combination chemotherapy in advanced malignant melanoma. Cancer Treat Rep 1987;71:997.
431. Carey RW, Anderson JR, Green M, et al. Treatment of metastatic malignant melanoma with vinblastine, dacarbazine and cisplatin: a report from the Cancer and Leukemia Group B. Cancer Treat Rep 1986;70:329.
432. Verschraegen CF, Kleeberg UR, Mulder J, et al. Combination of cisplatin, vindesine and dacarbazine in advanced malignant melanoma: A phase II study of the EORTC Malignant Melanoma Cooperative Group. Cancer 1988;62:1061.
433. Ringborg U, Jungnelius J, Hansson J, Strander H. DTIC-vindesine-cisplatin in disseminated malignant melanoma: A phase II study. Proc Am Soc Clin Oncol 1987;6:212.
434. Wussow P, Hartman F, Block B, Schmoll HJ, Deicher H, Peter HH. Treatment of advanced malignant melanoma with dacarbazine, vindesine and cisplatin (DVP). Proceedings of the Fourth European Conference on Clinical Oncology and Cancer Nursing (Paris), 1987:238.
435. Gundersen S. Dacarbazine, vindesine and cisplatin combination chemotherapy in advanced malignant melanoma: A phase II study. Cancer Treat Rep 1987;71:997.
436. Legha SS, Ring S, Papadopoulos N, Plager C, Chawla S, Benjamin R. A prospective evaluation of a triple-drug regimen containing cisplatin, vinblastine and DTIC (CVD) for metastatic melanoma. Cancer 1989;64:2024.
437. Steffens TA, Bajorin DF, Chapman PB, et al. A phase II trial of high-dose cisplatin and dacarbazine: Lack of efficacy of high-dose cisplatin-based therapy for metastatic melanoma. Cancer 1991;68:1230.
438. Buzaid AC, Murren JR, Durivage HJ. High-dose cisplatin with dacarbazine and tamoxifen in the treatment of metastatic melanoma. Cancer 1991;68:1238.
439. Del Prete SA, Maurer LH, O'Donnell J. Combination chemotherapy with cisplatin, carmustine, dacarbazine, and tamoxifen in metastatic melanoma. Cancer Treat Rep 1984;68:1403.
440. McClay EF, Mastrangelo MJ, Bellet RE. Combination chemotherapy and hormonal therapy in the treatment of malignant melanoma. Cancer Treat Rep 1987;71:465.
441. McClay EF, Mastrangelo MJ, Sprandio JD, et al. The importance of tamoxifen to a cisplatin-containing regimen in the treatment of metastatic melanoma. Cancer 1989;63:1292.
442. McClay EF, Albright K, Jones J, et al. Modulation of cisplatin resistance by tamoxifen in human malignant melanoma. Proc Advances in the Biology and Clinical Management of Melanoma 1991;43:101.
443. McClay EF, Sprandio JD, Mastrangelo MJ, et al. Importance of tamoxifen to a combination chemotherapy regimen for melanoma. Proc Am Soc Clin Oncol 1988;7:251.
444. Carmo-Pereira J, Kosta SO, Henriques E. Combination cytotoxic chemotherapy with procarbazine, vincristine and lomustine in disseminated malignant melanoma: Eight years follow-up. Cancer Treat Rep 1984;68:1211.
445. Shelley W, Quirt I, Bodurtha A, et al. Lomustine, vincristine and procarbazine in the treatment of metastatic melanoma. Cancer Treat Rep 1985;69:941.
446. Kirkwood JM, Ernstoff M. Potential application of the interferons in oncology: Lesions drawn from studies of human melanoma. Semin Oncol 1986;13:48.
447. Krown SE, Burk MW, Kirkwood JM, et al. Human leukocyte (α) interferon in metastatic malignant melanoma: The American Cancer Society phase II trial. Cancer Treat Rep 1984;68:723.
448. Creagan ET, Ahmann DL, Green SJ, et al. Phase II study of recombinant leukocyte A interferon (rIFN-αA) in disseminated malignant melanoma. Cancer 1984;54:2844.
449. Creagan ET, Ahmann DL, Green SJ, et al. Phase II study of low-dose recombinant leukocyte A interferon in disseminated malignant melanoma. J Clin Oncol 1985;2:1002.
450. Creagan ET, Ahman DL, Frytak S, et al. Recombinant leukocyte A interferon (rIFN-α2A) in the treatment of disseminated malignant melanoma: Analysis of complete and long-term responding patients. Cancer 1986;58:2576.
451. Jacquillat C, Mural J, Chelq C, et al. Treatment of metastatic malignant melanoma with Roferon A. Proceedings of the Third European Conference on Clinical Oncology and Cancer Nursing (Stockholm), 1985;3:183.
452. Hersey P, Hasic E, MacDonald M, et al. Effects of recombinant leukocyte interferon (rIFN-αA) on tumor growth and immune responses in patients with metastatic melanoma. Br J Cancer 1985;51:815.
453. Thompson DB, McLeod GR. Pilot efficacy study of recombinant leukocyte A interferon (Ro 22-8181; IFN-rA) in patients with metastatic melanoma. Proceedings of the

Third European Conference on Clinical Oncology and Cancer Nursing (Stockholm), 1984;3:47.

454. Legha SS, Papadopoulos NEJ, Plager C, et al. Clinical evaluation of recombinant interferon-α2A (Roferon-A) in metastatic melanoma using two different schedules. J Clin Oncol 1987;5:1240.

455. Kirkwood JM, Ernstoff MS, Davis CA, et al. Comparison of intramuscular and intravenous recombinant interferon in melanoma and other cancers. Ann Intern Med 1985;103:32.

456. Robinson WA, Kirkwood J, Harvey H et al. Effective use of recombinant α2a-interferon in metastatic malignant melanoma. Proc Am Soc Clin Oncol 1984;3:60.

457. Robinson WA, Mughal TI, Thomas MR, et al. Treatment of metastatic melanoma with recombinant interferon α2. Immunobiology 1986;172:275.

458. Coates A, Rallings M, Hersey P, et al. Phase II study of recombinant α-2 interferon in advanced malignant melanoma. J Interferon Res 1986;6:1.

459. Dorval T, Palangie T, Jouve M, et al. Treatment of metastatic malignant melanoma with recombinant interferon alpha-2b. Invest New Drugs 1987;5:561.

460. Hawkins MJ, McCune CS, Speyer JL, et al. Recombinant α-2 interferon (SCH 30500) in patients with metastatic malignant melanoma: An ECOG pilot study. Proc Am Soc Clin Oncol 1984;3:51.

461. Miller RL, Steis RG, Clark JW, et al. Randomized trial of recombinant α-2B-interferon with or without indomethacin in patients with metastatic malignant melanoma. Cancer Res 1989;49:1871.

462. Kokaschka EM, Micksche M, Babits R, et al. Phase I study with high dose recombinant α-2 interferon in chemotherapy-resistant malignant melanoma patients. Antiviral Res 1984;3:105.

463. Kuzmits R, Kokoschka EM, Micksche M, et al. Phase II results with recombinant interferons: Renal cell carcinoma and malignant melanoma. Oncology 1985;42:26.

464. Hawkins MJ, Horning S, Konrad MW, et al. Phase I evaluation of a synthetic mutant of β-interferon. Cancer Res 1985;45:5914.

465. Creagan ET, Ahmann DL, Long HJ, et al. Phase II study of recombinant interferon-gamma in patients with disseminated malignant melanoma. Cancer Treat Rep 1987;71: 843.

466. Ernstoff MS, Trautman T, Davis CA, et al. A randomized phase I/II study of cutaneous versus intermittent intravenous interferon gamma in patients with metastatic malignant melanoma. J Clin Oncol 1987;5:1804.

467. Gutterman JU, Rosenblum MG, Rios A, et al. Pharmacokinetic study of partially pure gamma-interferon in cancer patients. Cancer Res 1984;44:4164.

468. Kurzrock R, Quesada JR, Talpaz M, et al. Phase I study of multiple dose intramuscularly administered recombinant gamma interferon. J Clin Oncol 1986;4:1101.

469. Truitt RL, Gale RP, Bortin MM. Cellular immunotherapy of cancer. Prog Clin Biol Res 1987;244:1.

470. Grimm EA, Mazumder A, Zhang HZ, et al. Lymphokine-activated killer phenomenon: Lysis of natural killer resistant fresh solid tumor cells by interleukin-2-activated autologous human peripheral blood lymphocytes. J Exp Med 1982;155:1823.

471. Mule JJ, Shu S, Schwarz SL. Successful adoptive immunotherapy of established pulmonary metastases with LAK cells and recombinant interleukin 2. Science 1984;255: 1487.

472. Rosenberg SA, Mule JJ, Spiess PJ, et al. Regression of established pulmonary metastases and subcutaneous tumor mediated by the systemic administration of high-dose recombinant interleukin 2. J Exp Med 1985;161:1169.

473. Mule JJ, Shu S, Rosenberg SA. The antitumor efficacy of lymphokine-activated killer cells and recombinant interleukin 2 in vivo. J Immunol 1985;135:646.

474. Lafreniere R, Rosenberg SA. Successful immunotherapy of experimental hepatic metastases with lymphokine-activated killer cells and recombinant interleukin 2. Cancer Res 1985;45:3755.

475. Rosenberg SA, Lotze MT, Muul LM, et al. Special report: Observations on the systemic administration of autologous lymphokine-activated killer cells and recombinant interleukin-2 to patients with metastatic cancer. N Engl J Med 1985;313:1485.

476. Dutcher JP, Creekmore S, Weiss GR, et al. Phase II study of high dose interleukin-2 and lymphokine activated killer cells in patients with melanoma. Proc Am Soc Clin Oncol 1987;6:970.

477. Rosenberg SA, Lotze MT, Muul LM, et al. A progress report on the treatment of 157 patients with advanced cancer using lymphokine-activated killer cells and interleukin-2 or high-dose interleukin-2 alone. N Engl J Med 1987;316:889.

478. Rosenberg SA, Lotze MT, Yang JC, Aebersold PM, et al. Experience with the use of high-dose interleukin-2 in the treatment of 652 cancer patients. Ann Surg 1989;210: 474.

479. West WH, Tauer KW, Yanelli JR, et al. Constant infusion recombinant interleukin 2 adoptive immunotherapy of advanced cancer. N Engl J Med 1987;316:898.

480. Bar MH, Sznol M, Atkins MB, et al. Metastatic melanoma treated with combined bolus and continuous infusion interleukin-2 and lymphokine-activated killer cells. J Clin Oncol 1990;7:1138.

481. Dutcher JP, Creekmore S, Weiss GR, et al. A phase II study of interleukin-2 and lymphokine-activated killer cells in patients with metastatic melanoma. J Clin Oncol 1989;7:477.

482. Parkinson DR, Abrams JS, Wiernik PH, et al. Interleukin-2 therapy in patients with metastatic malignant melanoma. J Clin Oncol 1990;8:1650.

483. Mittelman A, Gafney L, Penichet K, et al. A phase I dose escalation study of recombinant interleukin-2 and lymphokine-activated killer cells in patients with advanced cancer. Proc Am Soc Clin Oncol 1987;6:237.

484. Dutcher JP, Gaynor ER, Boldt DH, et al. A Phase II study of high-dose continuous infusion interleukin-2 with lymphokine-activated killer cells in patients with metastatic melanoma. J Clin Oncol 1991;9:641.

485. Dillman RO, Barth N, Oldham RK, et al. Continuous interleukin-2 and lymphokine-activated killer cells in advanced cancer. Proc Am Soc Clin Oncol 1989;8:188.

486. Dillman RO, Oldham RK, Tauer KW, et al. Continuous interleukin-2 and lymphokine-activated killer cells for advanced cancer: A National Biotherapy Study Group Trial. J Clin Oncol 1991;9:1233.

487. Perez EA, Scudder SA, Meyers F, et al. Weekly 24 hour continuous infusion interleukin-2 for metastatic melanoma and renal carcinoma. Proc Am Soc Clin Oncol 1989;8: 190.

488. Whitehead RP, Kopecky KJ, Samson MK, et al. A phase II study of IV bolus recombinant interleukin-2 in metastatic malignant melanoma: A Southwest Oncology Group Study. Proc Am Soc Clin Oncol 1989;8:284.

489. Richards JM, Bajorin DF, Vogelzang NJ, et al. Treatment of metastatic melanoma with continuous intravenous IL-2 ± LAK cells: A randomized trial. Proc Am Soc Clin Oncol 1990;9:279.

490. McCabe MS, Stablein D, Hawkins MJ. The modified group C experience: Phase III randomized trials of IL-2 vs IL-2/LAK in advanced renal cell carcinoma and advanced melanoma. Proc Am Soc Clin Oncol 1991;10:213.

491. Dorval T, Mathiot C, Fridman WH, et al. Phase II trial of recombinant interleukin-2 in patients with metastatic melanoma. Proc Am Soc Clin Oncol 1991;10:297.

492. Blair S, Flaherty L, Valdivieso M, et al. Comparison of high dose interleukin-2 with combined chemotherapy/low dose IL-2 in metastatic malignant melanoma. Proc Am Soc Clin Oncol 1991;10:294.

493. Mitchell MS, Kempf RA, Harel W, et al. Effectiveness and tolerability of low-dose cyclophosphamide and low-dose intravenous interleukin-2 in disseminated melanoma. J Clin Oncol 1988;6:409.

494. Mitchell MS, Kempf RA, Harel W, et al. Low-dose cyclophosphamide and low-dose interleukin-2 for malignant melanoma. Bull NY Acad Med 1989;65:128.

495. Lotze MT, Matory YL, Raynor AA, et al. Clinical effects and toxicity of interleukin-2 in patients with cancer. Cancer 1986;58:2764.

496. Ognibene FP, Rosenberg SA, Lotze MT, et al. Interleukin-2 administration causes reversible hemodynamic changes and left ventricular dysfunction similar to those seen in septic shock. Chest 1988;94:750.

497. Webb DE, Austin HA, Belldegrun A, et al. Metabolic and renal effects of interleukin-2 immunotherapy for metastatic cancer. Clin Nephrology 1988;30:141.

498. Szybalski W. X-ray sensitization by halopyrimidines. Cancer Chemother Rep 1974;58: 539–557.

499. Hatanaka H, ed. Neutron capture therapy, Proceedings of the Second International Symposium on Neutron Capture Therapy, Teikyo University, Tokyo, October 1985. Niigata, Japan: Nishimura, 1986.

500. Greenberg PD, Kern DE, Cheever MA. Therapy of disseminated murine leukemia with cyclophosphamide and immune Lyt 1 + 2-T cells: Tumor eradication does not require participation of cytotoxic T cells. J Exp Med 1985;161:4303.

501. Anichini A, Fossati G, Parmiani G. Clonal analysis of cytotoxic T lymphocyte response to autologous human metastatic melanoma. Int J Cancer 1985;35:683.

502. De Vries JE, Spits H. Cloned cytolytic T lymphocyte (CTL) lines reactive with autologous melanoma cells. I. In vitro generation, isolation, and analysis of phenotype and specificity. J Immunol 1984;132:510.

503. Herin M, Lemoine C, Weynant P, et al. Production of stable cytolytic T lymphocyte (CTL) against autologous human melanoma. Int J Cancer 1987;39:390.

504. Hersey P, MacDonald M, Schibeci S, et al. Clonal analysis of cytotoxic T lymphocytes (CTL) against autologous melanoma: Classification based on phenotype, specificity, and inhibition of monoclonal antibodies to T cell structures. Cancer Immunol Immunother 1986;22:15.

505. Fossati G, Anichini A, Parmiani G. Melanoma cell lysis by human CTL clones: Differential involvement of T3, T8 and HLA antigens. Int J Cancer 1987;39:689.

506. Anichini A, Fossati G, Parmiani G. Heterogeneity of clones from a human metastatic melanoma detected by autologous cytotoxic T lymphocyte clones. J Exp Med 1986;163: 215.

507. Itoh K, Tilden AB, Balch CM. Interleukin 2 activation of cytotoxic T lymphocytes infiltrating into human metastatic melanoma. Cancer Res 1986;46:3011.

508. Itoh K, Platsoucas CD, Balch CM. Autologous tumor-specific cytotoxic T lymphocytes in the infiltrate of human metastatic melanoma. J Exp Med 1988;168:1419.

509. Muul LM, Spiess PJ, Director EP, et al. Identification of specific cytolytic immune responses against autologous tumors in humans bearing malignant melanoma. J Immunol 1987;138:989.

510. Mukherji B, MacAlister TJ. Clonal analysis of cytotoxic T cell response against human melanoma. J Exp Med 1983;158:240.

511. Knuth A, Danowski B, Oettgen HF, et al. T cell mediated cytotoxicity against autologous malignant melanoma: Analysis with interleukin 2 dependent T cell cultures. Proc Natl Acad Sci USA 1984;81:3511.

512. Topalian SL, Solomon D, Rosenberg SA. Tumor-specific cytolysis by lymphocytes infiltrating human melanoma. J Immunol 1989;142:3714.

513. Cohen PJ, Lotze MT, Roberts JR, et al. The immunopathology of sequential tumor biopsies in patients treated with interleukin-2. Correlation of response with T-cell infiltration and HLA-DR expression. Am J Pathol 1987;129:208.

514. Rosenberg SA, Spiess PJ, Lafreniere R. A new approach to adoptive immunotherapy of cancer with tumor-infiltrating lymphocytes. Science 1986;233:1318.

515. Topalian S, Solomon D, Avis FP, et al. Immunotherapy of patients with advanced cancer using tumor infiltrating lymphocytes in recombinant interleukin-2: A pilot study. J Clin Oncol 1988;6:838.

516. Rosenberg SA, Packard BS, Aebersold PM, et al. Use of tumor-infiltrating lymphocytes and interleukin-2 in the immunotherapy of patients with metastatic melanoma: A preliminary report. N Engl J Med 1988;319:1676.

517. Dillman RO, Oldham RK, Barth NM, et al. Continuous interleukin-2 and tumor-infiltrating lymphocytes as treatment of advanced melanoma: A National Biotherapy Study Group Trial. Cancer 1991;68:1.
518. Houghton AN, Chapman PB, Bajorin DF. Antibodies in cancer therapy: Clinical application. 22.3 Melanoma. In: Devita VT Jr, Hellman S, Rosenberg SA. Biologic therapy of cancer. Philadelphia: JB Lippincott, 1991:533.
519. Houghton AN, Scheinberg DA. Monoclonal antibodies: Potential applications to the treatment of cancer. Semin Oncol 1986;13:165.
520. Houghton AN, Mintzer D, Cordon-Cardo C et al. Mouse monoclonal IgG3 antibody detecting GD3 ganglioside: A phase I trial in patients with malignant melanoma. Proc Natl Acad Sci USA 1985;82:1242.
521. Goodman GE, Beaumier P, Hellstrom I, et al. Pilot trial of murine monoclonal antibodies in patients with advanced melanoma. J Clin Oncol 1985;3:340.
522. Cheung N-K, Lazarus H, Miraldi FD, et al. Ganglioside GD2 specific monoclonal antibody 3F8: A phase I study in patients with neuroblastoma and malignant melanoma. J Clin Oncol 1987;5:1430.
523. Oldham RK, Foon KA, Morgan AC, et al. Monoclonal antibody therapy of malignant melanoma: In vivo localization in cutaneous metastasis after intravenous administration. J Clin Oncol 1984;2:1235.
524. Schroff RW, Woodhouse CS, Foon KA, et al. Intratumor localization of monoclonal antibody in patients with melanoma treated with antibody to a 250,000 dalton melanoma-associated antigen. JNCI 1985;74:299.
525. Vadhan-Raj S, Cordon-Cardo C, Carswell E, et al. Phase I trial of a mouse monoclonal antibody against GD3 ganglioside in patients with melanoma: Induction of an inflammatory response at tumor sites. J Clin Oncol 1988;6:1636.
526. Dippold WG, Berhard H, Dienes HP, et al. Treatment of patients with melanoma by monoclonal ganglioside antibodies. Eur J Cancer Clin Oncol 1988;21:S65.
527. Dippold WG, Knuth A, Meyer zum Buchenfelde KH. Inflammatory tumor response to monoclonal antibody infusion. Eur J Cancer Clin Oncol 1985;21:97.
528. Coit D, Houghton AN, Cordon-Cardo C, et al. Isolation limb perfusion with monoclonal antibody R24 in patients with malignant melanoma. Proc Am Soc Clin Oncol 1988;7:962.
529. Goodman GE, Hellstrom I, Hummel D, et al. Phase I trial of monoclonal antibody MG-21 directed against a melanoma-associated GD3 ganglioside antigen. Proc Am Soc Clin Oncol 1987;6:823.
530. Lichtin A, Iliopoulos D, Guerry D, et al. Therapy of melanoma with an anti-melanoma ganglioside monoclonal antibody: A possible mechanism of a complete response. Proc Am Soc Clin Oncol 1988;7:247.
530a. Houghton, AN. Personal communication.
531. Irie RF, Morton DL. Regression of cutaneous metastatic melanoma by intralesional injection with human monoclonal antibody to ganglioside GD2. Proc Natl Acad Sci USA 1986;83:8694.
532. Schroff RW, Morgan AC Jr, Woodhouse CS, et al. Monoclonal antibody therapy in malignant melanoma: Factors effecting in vivo localization. J Biol Response Mod 1987;6:457.
533. Larson SM, Carrasquillo JA, Krohn KA, et al. Localization of 131-I labeled p97-specific Fab fragments in human melanoma as a basis for radiotherapy. J Clin Invest 1983;72:2101.
534. Vitteta ES, Fulton RJ, May RD, et al. Redesigning nature's poisons to create anti-tumor reagents. Science 1987;238:1098.
535. Spitler LE, Del Rio M, Khentigan A, et al. Therapy of patients with malignant melanoma using a monoclonal antimelanoma antibody-ricin A chain immunotoxin. Cancer Res 1987;47:1717.
536. Spitler LE. Clinical trials of immunotoxin. Second International Congress on Monoclonal Antibody 1987;1:26.
537. Bajorin DB, Chapman PB, Wong G, et al. A phase I trial of high-dose R24 mouse monoclonal antibody in patients with metastatic melanoma. Proc Am Assoc Cancer Res 1991;32:265.
538. Raymond J, Kirkwood J, Vlock D, et al. A phase IB trial of murine monoclonal antibody R24 (anti-GD3) in metastatic melanoma. Proc Am Soc Clin Oncol 1991;10:298.
539. Schroff RW, Foon KA, Beatty SM, et al. Human anti-mouse immunoglobulin response in patients receiving monoclonal antibody therapy. Cancer Res 1985;45:879.
540. Morrison SL, Oi V. Transfer and expression of immunoglobulin genes. Ann Rev Immunol 1984;2:239.
541. Reichmann L, Clark MR, Waldmann H, et al. Reshaping antibodies for therapy. Nature 1988;332:323.
542. Yamaguchi H, Furukawa K, Fortunato S, et al. Cell surface antigens of human melanoma recognized by human monoclonal antibodies. Proc Natl Acad Sci USA 1987;84:2416.
543. Morton DL, Nizze RJ, Gupta RK, et al. Active specific immunotherapy of malignant melanoma. In: Kim JP, Jim BS, Park J-G, eds. Current status of cancer control and immunobiology. Seoul, Korea, 1987:152.
544. Livingston PO, Natoli EJ, Calves MJ, et al. Vaccines containing purified GM2 ganglioside elicit GM2 antibodies in melanoma patients. Proc Natl Acad Sci USA 1987;84:2911.
545. Bystryn J-C, Oratz R, Harris MN, et al. Immunogenicity of a polyvalent melanoma antigen vaccine in humans. Cancer 1988;61:1065.
546. Hersey P, Edwards A, Coates A, et al. Evidence that treatment with vaccinia melanoma cell lysates (VMCL) may improve survival of patients with stage II melanoma. Cancer Immunol Immunother 1987;25:257.
547. Hersey P, Edwards A, Coates A, et al. Evidence that treatment with vaccinia melanoma cell lysates (VMCL) may improve survival of patients with stage II melanoma. Cancer Immunol Immunother 1987;25:257.
548. Jones PC, Sze LL, Liu PY, et al. Prolonged survival for melanoma patients with elevated IgM antibody to oncofetal antigen. JNCI 1981;66:249.
549. Wallack MK, Bash JA, Leftheriotis E, et al. The positive relationship of clinical and serologic responses to vaccinia melanoma oncolysate. Arch Surg 1987;122:1460.
550. Livingston PO, Oettgen HF, Old LJ. Specific active immunotherapy in cancer treatment. In: Mihich E, ed. Immunological approaches to cancer therapeutics. New York: John Wiley & Sons, 1982:363.
551. Livingston PO, Takeyama H, Pollack MS, et al. Serological responses of melanoma patients to vaccines derived from allogeneic cultured melanoma cells. Int J Cancer 1983;31:567.
552. Livingston PO, Kaelin K, Pinsky CM, et al. The serologic response of patients with stage II melanoma to allogeneic melanoma cell vaccines. Cancer 1985;56:2194.
553. Fisher RI, Terry WD, Hodes RJ, et al. Adjuvant immunotherapy or chemotherapy for malignant melanoma. Surg Clin North Am 1981;61:1267.
554. Seigler HF, Cox E, Mutzner F, et al. Specific active immunotherapy for melanoma. Ann Surg 1979;190:366.
555. Cox EB, Vollmer RT, Seigler HF. Melanoma in the Southeastern United States: Experience at the Duke Medical Center. In: Balch CM, Milton GW, eds. Cutaneous melanoma: Clinical management and treatment results worldwide. Philadelphia: JB Lippincott, 1985:407.
556. Berd D, Murphy G, McGuire HC Jr, Mastrangelo MJ. Immunization with haptenized, autologous tumor cells induces inflammation of human melanoma metastases. Cancer Res 1991;51:2731.
557. Gansbacher B, Gee C, Houghton AN, et al. Retroviral lymphokine gene transfer induced secretion of interleukin-2 or interferon-gamma by human melanoma cells. Proc Am Assoc Cancer Res 1991;32:255.
558. Rosenberg SA. Immunotherapy and gene therapy of cancer. Gottlieb Award lecture. Proc Adv Biol Clin Management Melanoma 1991;43:61.
559. Estin CD, Stevenson US, Plowman GD, et al. Recombinant vaccinia virus vaccine against the human melanoma antigen p97 for use in immunotherapy. Proc Natl Acad Sci USA 1987;85:1052.
560. Van der Bruggen P, Traversari C, Chomez P, et al. A gene encoding an antigen recognized by cytolytic T lymphocytes on a human melanoma. Science 1991;254:1643.
561. Kageshita T, Chen ZJ, Kim J-W, et al. Murine anti-idiotypic monoclonal antibodies to syngeneic antihuman high molecular weight-melanoma associated antigen monoclonal antibodies: Development, characterization and clinical application. Pigment Cell Res 1988;1(Suppl):185.
562. Kusama M, Kageshita T, Tsujisaki M, et al. Syngeneic antiidiotypic antisera to murine antihuman high molecular weight melanoma-associated antigen monoclonal antibodies. Cancer Res 1987;47:4312.
563. Mittelman A, Chen ZJ, Kageshita T, et al. Active specific immunotherapy in patients with melanoma: A clinical trial with mouse antiidiotypic monoclonal antibodies elicited with syngeneic anti-high-molecular weight-melanoma-associated antigen monoclonal antibodies. J Clin Invest 1990;86:2136.
564. Chapman PB, Houghton AN. Induction of IgG antibodies against GD3 ganglioside in rabbits by an anti-idiotypic monoclonal antibody. J Clin Invest 1991;88:186.
565. Mitchell MS, Harel W, Kempf RA, et al. Active-specific immunotherapy for melanoma. J Clin Oncol 1990;8:856.
566. North RJ. Cyclophosphamide-facilitated adoptive immunotherapy of an established tumor depends on elimination of tumor-induced suppressor T-cells. J Exp Med 1982;35:1063.
567. Livingston PO, Hoffman MK, Enker WE. Inhibition of suppressor cell activity in melanoma patients by cyclophosphamide. Proc Am Soc Clin Oncol 1984;3:58.
568. Berd D, Mastrangelo MJ, Engstrom PF, et al. Augmentation of the human immune response by cyclophosphamide. Cancer Res 1982;42:4862.
569. Berd D, Danna V, Maguire HC, et al. Induction of cell mediated immunity to autologous melanoma cells and regression of metastases after treatment with a melanoma cell vaccine preceded by cyclophosphamide. Cancer Res 1986;46:2572.
570. Berd D, Maguire HC Jr, McCue P, Mastrangelo MJ. Treatment of metastatic melanoma with an autologous tumor-cell vaccine: Clinical and immunologic results in 64 patients. J Clin Oncol 1990;8:1858.
571. Morton DL. Immunological studies with human neoplasms. J Reticuloendothel Soc 1971;10:137.
572. Mastrangelo MJ, Bellet RE, Berd D. Immunology and immunotherapy of human cutaneous malignant melanoma. In: Clark WH Jr, Goldman LI, Mastrangelo MJ, eds. Human malignant melanoma. New York: Grune & Stratton, 1979:355.
573. Pinsky CM, Hirshaut Y, Oettgen HF. Treatment of malignant melanoma by intratumoral injection of BCG. NCI Monogr 1973;39:255.
574. Mastrangelo MJ, Sulit HL, Prehn LM. Intralesional BCG in the treatment of metastatic malignant melanoma. Cancer 1976;37:684.
575. Klein E, Holterman OA. Immunotherapeutic approaches to the management of neoplasms. NCI Monogr 1972;35:379.
576. Klein E, Holterman OA, Helm F et al. Immunologic approaches to the management of primary and secondary tumors involving the skin and soft tissues. Review of a ten year program. Transplant Proc 1975;7:297.
577. Tisman G, Wu SJG, Safire GE. Intralesional PPD in malignant melanoma. Lancet 1975;1:161.
578. Krown SE, Hilal E, Pinsky CM. Intralesional injection of the methanol extraction residue of Bacillus Calmette-Guerin (MER) into cutaneous metastases of malignant melanoma. Cancer 1978;42:2648.
579. Cohen MH, Feliz E, Jessup J, et al. Treatment of metastatic melanoma by intralesional injection of BCG, organic chemicals and *C. parvum*. In: Crispen RG, ed. Neoplasm immunity mechanisms. Philadelphia: Franklin Institute Press, 1975:121.

580. Cameron RB, McIntosh JK, Rosenburg SA. Synergistic antitumor effects of combination immunotherapy with recombinant interleukin-2 and recombinant hybrid interferon-α in the treatment of established murine hepatic metastases. Cancer Res 1988;48:5810.
581. Rosenberg SA, Schwarz S, Spiess P. Combination immunotherapy of cancer: Synergistic antitumor interactions of interleukin-2, interferon-α and tumor-infiltrating lymphocytes. JNCI 1988;80:1392.
582. Rosenberg SA, Lotze MT, Yang JC, et al. Combination therapy with interleukin-2 and interferon-α for the treatment of patients with advanced cancer. J Clin Oncol 1989;7:1863.
583. Eisenthal A, Cameron RC, Uppenkamp I, et al. Effect of combined therapy with lymphokine activated killer cells, interleukin-2 and specific monoclonal antibody on established B16 melanoma lung metastases. Cancer Res 1988;48:7140.
584. Shiloni E, Pouillart P, Janssens J, et al. Sequential dacarbazine chemotherapy followed by recombinant interleukin-2 in metastatic melanoma: A pilot multicentre phase I-II study. Eur J Cancer Clin Oncol 1989;25(Suppl 3):45.
585. Papadopoulos NEJ, Howard J, Murray JL, et al. Phase I–II DTIC and interleukin 2 (IL2) trial for metastatic malignant melanoma. Proc Am Soc Clin Oncol 1989;8:290.
586. Shiloni E, Pouillart P, Janssens J, et al. Sequential dacarbazine chemotherapy followed by recombinant interleukin-2 in metastatic melanoma: A pilot multicentre phase I–II study. Eur J Cancer Clin Oncol 1989;25:45.
587. Stoter G, Aamdal S, Rodenhuis S, et al. Sequential administration of recombinant human interleukin-2 and dacarbazine in metastatic melanoma: A multicentric phase II study. J Clin Oncol 1991;9:1687.
588. Richards JM, Ramming K, Bitran JD, et al. Combination of chemotherapy and biologic therapy for the treatment of melanoma. Clin Res [Abstract] 1990;38:844.
589. Sznol M, Clark J, Smith J, et al. A phase II study of IL-2/LAK in combination with chemotherapy and interferon-alfa in patients with metastatic melanoma and renal cell carcinoma. Proc Am Soc Clin Oncol [Abstract] 1990;9:759.
590. Sznol M, Clark J, Smith J, et al. A pilot evaluation of interleukin-2 (IL-2) and lymphokine-activated killer (LAK) cells in combination with chemotherapy and α-interferon. Proc Am Soc Clin Oncol [Abstract] 1989;8:742.
591. Demshak PA, Mier JW, Robert NJ, et al. Interleukin-2 and high-dose cisplatin in patients with metastatic melanoma: A pilot study. J Clin Oncol 1991;1821.
592. Khayat D. Cisplatin, IL-2 and interferon. Proc Adv Biol Clin Management Melanoma, Houston, 1991:29.
593. Pichert G, Jost LM, Fierz W, et al. Clinical and immune modulatory effects of alternative weekly interleukin-2 and interferon alfa-2a in patients with advanced renal cell carcinoma and melanoma. Br J Cancer 1991;63:287.
594. Rosenberg SA, Lotze MT, Yang JC, et al. Combination therapy with interleukin-2 and α-interferon for the treatment of patients with advanced cancer. J Clin Oncol 1989;7:1863.
595. Bergmann L, Weidmann E, Mitrou PS, et al. Interleukin-2 in combination with interferon-α in disseminated malignant melanoma and advanced renal cell carcinoma: A phase II study. Onkologie 1990;13:137.
596. Sznol M, Mier JW, Sparano J, et al. A phase I study of high-dose interleukin-2 in combination with interferon-α2b. J Biol Response Modifiers 1990;9:529.
597. Mittelman A, Huberman B, Fallon S, et al. Phase I study of recombinant interleukin-2 (IL-2) and recombinant human interferon α (IFN-Roche) in patients (pts) with melanoma, renal cell carcinoma (Ca), colorectal CA and malignant B-cell disease. Proc Am Soc Clin Oncol 1989;8:179.
598. Budd GT, Osgood B, Barna B, et al. Phase I clinical trial of interleukin 2 and α-interferon: Toxicity and immunologic effects. Cancer Res 1989;49:6432.
599. Lee KH, Talpaz M, Rothberg JM, et al. Concomitant administration of recombinant human interleukin-2 and recombinant interferon α-2A in cancer patients: A phase I study. J Clin Oncol 1989;7:1726.
600. Mittelman A, Huberman M, Puccio C, et al. A phase I study of recombinant human interleukin-2 and α-interferon-2a in patients with renal cell cancer, colorectal cancer, and malignant melanoma. Cancer 1990;66:664.
601. West W, Schwartzberg L, Blumenchein G, et al. Continuous infusion interleukin-2 (IL-2) plus SC interferon α-2B (IFN) in advanced malignancy. Proc Am Soc Clin Oncol [Abstract] 1990;9:738.
602. Huberman M, Mittelman A, Fallon B, et al. Preliminary observations from a phase I study of recombinant human interleukin-2 (IL2) and roferon-a (recombinant human α-IFN) in patients with malignant b-cell disease, renal and colorectal cancer, and melanoma. Proc Am Soc Clin Oncol [Abstract] 1988;7:653.
603. Krigel R, Poiesz B, Comis R, et al. A phase I study of recombinant interleukin-2 (RIL-2) plus recombinant beta ser 17 interferon (IFN-beta ser). Proc Am Soc Clin Oncol 1986;5:225.
604. Bajorin DF, Chapman PB, Wong G, et al. Phase I evaluation of a combination of monoclonal antibody R24 and interleukin 2 in patients with metastatic melanoma. Cancer Res 1990;50:7490.
605. Urba WJ, Kopp WC, Clark JW, et al. The in vivo immunomodulatory effects of recombinant interferon gamma plus recombinant tumor necrosis factor-α. J Clin Oncol 1991;9:1831.
606. Lienard D, Ewalenko P, Delmotte J-J, Renard N, LeJeune FJ. High dose recombinant tumor necrosis factor α in combination with interferon gamma and melphalan in isolation perfusion of the limbs for melanoma and sarcoma. J Clin Oncol 1992;10:52.
607. Kirkwood JM. Rationale for use of interferon in the therapy of high risk melanoma. Eur J Cancer 1992 (in press).
608. Meyskens FL, Kopecky K, Samson M, et al. Recombinant human interferon-γ: Adverse effects in high-risk stage I and II cutaneous malignant melanoma. JNCI 1990;82:1071.
609. Spitler LE, Sagebiel R. A randomized trial of levamisole versus placebo as adjuvant therapy in malignant melanoma. N Engl J Med 1980;303:1143.
610. Quirt IC, Shelley WE, Pater JL, et al. Improved survival in patients with poor-prognosis malignant melanoma treated with adjuvant levamisole: A phase III study by the National Cancer Institute of Canada Clinical Trials Group. J Clin Oncol 1991;9:729.
611. Gonzalez RL, Spitler LE, Sagebiel RW, et al. Effect of levamisole as a surgical adjuvant therapy for malignant melanoma. Cancer Treat Rep 1978;62:1703.
612. Loutfi A, Shakr A, Jerry M, et al. Double-blind randomized prospective trial of levamisole/placebo in stage I cutaneous malignant melanoma. Clin Invest Med 1987;10:325.
613. Costanzi JJ, Fletcher WS, Balcerzak SP, et al. Combination chemotherapy plus levamisole in the treatment of disseminated malignant melanoma: A Southwest Oncology Group study. Cancer 1984;53:833.
614. Stevenson HC, Green I, Hamilton JM, et al. Levamisole: Known effects on the immune system, clinical results, and future application to the treatment of cancer. J Clin Oncol 1991;9:2052.
615. Parkinson DR. Levamisole as adjuvant therapy for melanoma: Quo vadis? J Clin Oncol 1991;9:716.
616. Lipton A, Harvey HA, Balch CM, et al. Corynebacterium parvum versus Bacille Calmette-Guerin adjuvant immunotherapy of stage III malignant melanoma. J Clin Oncol 1991;9:1151.
617. Creagan ET, Ingle JN, Schutt AJ, et al. A prospective randomized control trial of megestrol acetate among high risk patients with resected malignant melanoma. Am J Clin Oncol 1989;12:152.
618. Bernardino ME, Goldstein HM. Gray scale ultrasonography in the evaluation of metastatic melanoma. Cancer 1978;42:2529.
619. Heaston DK, Putman CE. Radiographic manifestations of thoracic malignant melanoma. In: Seigler HF, ed. Clinical management of melanoma. The Hague: Martinus Nijhoff, 1982:62.
620. Braman SS, Whitcomb ME. Endobronchial metastasis. Arch Intern Med 1975;135:543.
621. Feldman L, Kricun ME. Malignant melanoma presenting as a mediastinal mass. JAMA 1979;241:396.
622. Curtis A McB, Ravin CE, Deering TF, et al. The efficacy of full-lung tomography in the detection of early metastatic disease from melanoma. Diagn Radiol 1982;144:27.
623. Chen JTT, Dahmash NS, Ravin CE, et al. Metastatic melanoma to the thorax: Report of 130 patients. AJR 1981;137:293.
624. Gromet MA, Ominsky SH, Epstein WL, et al. The thorax as the initial site for systemic relapse in malignant melanoma: A prospective survey of 324 patients. Cancer 1979;44:776.
625. Simeone JF, Putman CE, Greenspan RH. Detection of metastatic malignant melanoma by chest roentgenography. Cancer 1977;39:1993.
626. Webb WR, Gamsu G. Thoracic metastasis in malignant melanoma: A radiographic survey of 65 patients. Chest 1977;71:176.
627. Webb WR. Hilar and mediastinal lymph node metastases in malignant melanoma. AJR 1979;133:805.
628. Chang AE, Schaner EG, Conkle DM, et al. Evaluation of computed tomography in the detection of pulmonary metastases: A prospective study. Cancer 1979;43:913.
629. Mintzer RA, Malave SR, Neiman HL, et al. Computed vs. conventional tomography in evaluation of primary and secondary pulmonary neoplasms. Radiology 1979;132:653.
630. Neifeld JP, Michaelis LL, Doppman JL. Suspected pulmonary metastases: Correlation of chest x-ray, whole lung tomograms, and operative findings. Cancer 1977;39:383.
631. Schaner EG, Chang AE, Doppman JL, et al. Comparison of computed and conventional whole lung tomography in detecting pulmonary nodules: A prospective radiologic-pathologic study. AJR 1978;131:51.
632. Morton DL, Joseph WL, Ketcham AS, et al. Surgical resection and adjunctive immunotherapy for selected patients with multiple pulmonary metastases. Ann Surg 1973;178:360.
633. Cahan WG. Excision of melanoma metastases to lung: Problems in diagnosis and management. Ann Surg 1973;178:703.
634. Cline RE, Young WG Jr. Long term results following surgical treatment of metastatic pulmonary tumors. Am Surg 1970;36:61.
635. McCormack, Martini N. The changing role of surgery for pulmonary metastases. Ann Thorac Surg 1979;28:139.
636. Thayer JO Jr, Overholt RH. Metastatic melanoma to the lung: Long-term results of surgical excision. Am J Surg 1985;149:558.
637. Vidne BA, Richter S, Levy MJ. Surgical treatment of solitary pulmonary metastasis. Cancer 1976;38:2561.
638. Morrow CE, Vassilopoulos PP, Grage TB. Surgical resection for metastatic neoplasms of the lung: Experience at the University of Minnesota Hospitals. Cancer 1980;45:2981.
639. Mathisen DJ, Flye MW, Peabody J. The role of thoracotomy in the management of pulmonary metastases from malignant melanoma. Ann Thorac Surg 1979;27:295.
640. Wilkins EW Jr, Head JM, Burke JF. Pulmonary resection for metastatic neoplasms in the lung: Experience at the Massachusetts General Hospital. Am J Surg 1978;135:480.
641. Presant CA, Bartolucci AA, Smalley RV, et al. Cyclophosphamide plus (3,3-dimethyl-l-triazeno)-imidazole-4-carboxamide (DTIC) with or without *Corynebacterium parvum* in metastatic malignant melanoma. Cancer 1979;44:899.
642. Vieth RG, Odom GL. Intracranial metastases and their neurosurgical treatment. J Neurosurg 1965;23:375.
643. Amer MH, Al-Sarraf M, Baker LH, et al. Malignant melanoma and central nervous

system metastases: Incidence, diagnosis, treatment and survival. Cancer 1978;42: 660.
644. Fell DA, Leavens ME, McBride CM. Surgical versus nonsurgical management of metastatic melanoma of the brain. Neurosurgery 1980;7:238.
645. Ginaldi S, Wallace S, Shalen P, et al. Cranial computed tomography of malignant melanoma. AJR 1981;136:145.
646. Pennington DG, Milton GW. Cerebral metastasis from melanoma. Aust NZ J Surg 1975;45:405.
647. Bullard DE, Cox EB, Seigler HF. Central nervous system metastases in malignant melanoma. Neurosurgery 1981;8:26.
648. Posner JB, Chernik NL. Intracranial metastases from systemic cancer. Adv Neurol 1978;19:579.
649. Bremer AM, West CR, Didolkar MS. An evaluation of the surgical management of melanoma of the brain. J Surg Oncol 1978;10:211.
650. Enzmann DR, Kramer R, Norman D, et al. Malignant melanoma metastatic to the central nervous system. Radiology 1978;127:177.
651. Gildersleeve N Jr, Koo AH, McDonald CJ. Metastatic tumor presenting as intracerebral hemorrhage: Report of 6 cases examined by computed tomography. Radiology 1977;124:109.
652. Carella RJ, Gelber R, Hendrickson F, et al. Value of radiation therapy in the management of patients with cerebral metastases from malignant melanoma: Radiation Therapy Oncology Group brain metastases study I and II. Cancer 1980;45:679.
653. Posner JB. Management of central nervous system metastases. Semin Oncol 1977;4: 81.
654. Byrne TN, Cascino TL, Posner JB. Brain metastases from melanoma. J Neurooncol 1983;1:313.
655. Hayward RD. Malignant melanoma and the central nervous system: A guide for classification based on the clinical findings. J Neurol Neurosurg Psychiatry 1976;39:526.
656. Hayward RD. Secondary malignant melanoma of the brain. Clin Oncol 1976;2:227.
657. McCann WP, Weir BKA, Elvidge AR. Long-term survival after removal of metastatic malignant melanoma of the brain: Report of two cases. J Neurosurg 1968;28:483.
658. McNeel DP, Leavens ME. Long-term survival with recurrent metastatic intracranial melanoma: Case report. J Neurosurg 1968;29:91.
659. Scott M. Spontaneous intracerebral hematoma caused by cerebral neoplasms: Report of eight verified cases. J Neurosurg 1975;42:338.
660. Wolpert SM, Zimmer A, Schechter MM, et al. The neuroradiology of melanomas of the central nervous system. AJR 1967;101:178.
661. Felix EL, Sindelar WF, Bagley DH, et al. The use of bone and brain scans as screening procedures in patients with malignant lesions. Surg Gynecol Obstet 1975;141:867.
662. Thomas JH, Panoussopoulous D, Liesmann GE, et al. Scintiscans in the evaluation of patients with malignant melanomas. Surg Gynecol Obstet 1979;149:574.
663. Muss HB, Richards F II, Barnes PL, et al. Radionuclide scanning in patients with advanced malignant melanoma. Clin Nucl Med 1979;4:516.
664. Bardfeld PA, Passalaqua AM, Braunstein P, et al. A comparison of radionuclide scanning and computed tomography in metastatic lesions of the brain. J Comput Assist Tomogr 1977;1:315.
665. Holtas S, Cronqvist S. Cranial computed tomography of patients with malignant melanoma. Neuroradiology 1981;22:123.
666. Solis OJ, Davis KR, Adair LB, et al. Intracerebral metastatic melanoma: CT evaluation. Comput Tomogr 1977;1:135.
667. Wasserstrom WR, Glass JP, Posner JP. Diagnosis and treatment of leptomeningeal metastases from solid tumors: Experience with 90 patients. Cancer 1982;49:759.
668. Fleisher M, Wasserstrom WR, Schold SC, et al. Lactic dehydrogenase isoenzymes in the cerebrospinal fluid of patients with systemic cancer. Cancer 1981;47:2654.
669. Fletcher JW, George EA, Henry RE, et al. Brain scans, dexamethasone therapy, and brain tumors. JAMA 1975;232:1261.
670. Gottlieb JA, Frei E III, Luce JK. An evaluation of the management of patients with cerebral metastases from malignant melanoma. Cancer 1972;29:701.
671. Ruderman NB, Hall TC. Use of glucocorticoids in the palliative treatment of metastatic brain tumors. Cancer 1965;18:298.
672. Atkinson L. Melanoma of the central nervous system. Aust NZ J Surg 1978;48:14.
673. Cooper JS, Carella R. Radiotherapy of intracerebral metastatic malignant melanoma. Radiology 1980;134:735.
674. Hafstrom L, Jonsson P-E, Stromblad L-G. Intra-cranial metastases of malignant melanoma treated by surgery. Cancer 1980;46:2088.
675. Winston KR, Walsh JW, Fischer EG. Results of operative treatment of intracranial metastatic tumors. Cancer 1980;45:2639.
676. Galicich JH, Sundearesan N, Arbit E, et al. Surgical treatment of single brain metastasis: Factors associated with survival. Cancer 1980;45:381.
677. Bauman ML, Price TR. Intracranial metastatic malignant melanoma: Long-term survival following subtotal resection. South Med J 1972;65:344.
678. Mandybur TI. Intracranial hemorrhage caused by metastatic tumors. Neurology 1977;27:650.
679. Reyes V, Horrax G. Metastatic melanoma of the brain: Report of a case with unusually long survival period following surgical removal. Ann Surg 1950;131:237.
680. Ziegler JC, Cooper JS. Brain metastases from malignant melanoma: Conventional vs. high-dose-per-fraction radiotherapy. Int J Radiat Oncol Biol Phys 1986;12:1839.
681. Vlock DR, Kirkwood JM, Leutzinger C, et al. High dose fraction radiation therapy for intracranial metastases of malignant melanoma. Cancer 1982;49:2289.
682. Choi KN, Withers R, Rotman M. Metastatic melanoma in brain: Rapid treatment or large dose fractions. Cancer 1985;56:10.
683. Skibber JM, Soong S-j, Austin L, Balch CM, Urist MM, Peters LJ, Sawaya R. Cranial irradiation after surgical excision of brain metastases in melanoma patients. 1992 (in press).
684. Loeffler JS, Alexander ED, Kooy HM, Wen PY, Fine HA, Black PM. Radiosurgery for brain metastases. PPO Updates 1991;5(2):1–12.
685. Young RF, Post EM, King GA. Treatment of spinal epidural metastases: Randomized prospective comparison of laminectomy and radiotherapy. J Neurosurg 1980;53:741.
686. Booth JB. Malignant melanoma of the stomach: Report of a case presenting as an acute perforation and review of the literature. Br J Surg 1965;52:262.
687. Das Gupta TK, Brasfield RD. Metastatic melanoma of the gastrointestinal tract. Arch Surg 1964;88:969.
688. Goldstein HM, Beydoun MT, Dood GD. Radiologic spectrum of melanoma metastatic to the gastrointestinal tract. AJR 1977;129:605.
689. Oddson TA, Rice RP, Seigler HF, et al. The spectrum of small bowel melanoma. Gastrointest Radiol 1978;3:419.
690. Thompson WH. Radiographic manifestations of metastatic melanoma to the gastrointestinal tract, hepatobiliary system, pancreas, spleen and mesentery. In: Seigler HF, ed. Clinical management of melanoma. The Hague: Martinus Nijhoff, 1982:133.
691. Fraser-Moodie A, Hughes RG, Jones SM, et al. Malignant melanoma metastases to the alimentary tract. Gut 1976;17:206.
692. Giler S, Kott I, Urca I. Malignant melanoma metastatic to the gastrointestinal tract. World J Surg 1979;3:375.
693. Goodman PL, Karakousis CP. Symptomatic gastrointestinal metastases from malignant melanoma. Cancer 1981;48:1058.
694. Harris MN. Massive gastrointestinal hemorrhage due to metastatic malignant melanoma of small intestine. Arch Surg 1964;88:1049.
695. Klausner JM, Skornick Y, Lelcuk S, et al. Acute complications of metastatic melanoma to the gastrointestinal tract. Br J Surg 1982;69:195.
696. Macbeth WAAG, Gwynne JF, Jamieson MG. Metastatic melanoma in the small bowel. Aust NZ J Surg 1969;38:309.
697. Shah SM, Smart DF, Texter EC Jr, et al. Metastatic melanoma of the stomach: The endoscopic and roentgenographic findings and review of the literature. South Med J 1977;70:379.
698. Karakousis C, Holyoke ED, Douglass HO Jr. Intussusception as a complication of malignant neoplasm. Arch Surg 1974;109:515.
699. Beckly DE. Alimentary tract metastases from malignant melanoma. Clin Radiol 1974;25:385.
700. Felix EL, Bagley DH, Sindelar WF, et al. The value of the liver scan in preoperative screening of patients with malignancies. Cancer 1976;38:1137.
701. Seigler HF, Fetter BF. Current management of melanoma. Ann Surg 1977;186:1.
702. Garg R, McPherson TA, Lentle B, et al. Usefulness of an elevated serum lactate dehydrogenase value as a marker of hepatic metastases in malignant melanoma. Can Med Assoc J 1979;120:1114.
703. Bernardino ME, Thomas JL, Barnes PA, et al. Diagnostic approaches to liver and spleen metastases. Radiol Clin North Am 1982;20:469.
704. MacCarty RL, Stephens DH, Hattery RR, et al. Hepatic imaging by computed tomography: A comparison with ^{99m}Tc-sulfur colloid, ultrasonography, and angiography. Radiol Clin North Am 1979;17:137.
705. Smith TJ, Kemeny MM, Sugarbaker PH, et al. A prospective study of hepatic imaging in the detection of metastatic disease. Ann Surg 1982;195:486.
706. Snow JH Jr, Goldstein HM, Wallace S. Comparison of scintigraphy, sonography, and computed tomography in the evaluation of hepatic neoplasms. AJR 1979;132:915.
707. Balthazar EJ, Javors B. Malignant melanoma of the gallbladder. Am J Gastroenterol 1975;64:332.
708. Bowdler DA, Leach RD. Metastatic intrabiliary melanoma. Clin Oncol 1982;8:251.
709. McFadden PM, Krementz ET, McKinnon WMP, et al. Metastatic melanoma of the gallbladder. Cancer 1979;44:1802.
710. Shimkin PM, Soloway MS, Jaffe E. Metastatic melanoma of the gallbladder. AJR 1972;116:393.
711. Fon GT, Wong WS, Gold RH, et al. Skeletal metastases of melanoma: Radiographic, scintigraphic, and clinical review. AJR 1981;137:103.
712. Stewart WR, Gelberman RH, Harrelson JM, et al. Skeletal metastases of melanoma. J Bone Joint Surg [Abstract] 1978;60:645.
713. Devereux D, Johnston G, Blei L, et al. The role of bone scans in assessing malignant melanoma in patients with stage III disease. Surg Gynecol Obstet 1980;151:45.
714. Steiner GM, MacDonald JS. Metastases to bone from malignant melanoma. Clin Radiol 1972;23:52.
715. Tong D, Gillick L, Hendrickson FR. The palliation of symptomatic osseous metastases: Final results of the study by the Radiation Therapy Oncology Group. Cancer 1982;50: 893.
716. Harrelson JM. Orthopaedic considerations in the treatment of malignant melanoma. In: Seigler HF, ed. Clinical management of melanoma. The Hague: Martinus Nijhoff, 1982:435.
717. McKenzie DJ, Bell R. Melanoma with solitary metastasis to ureter. J Urol 1968;99: 399.
718. Das Gupta T, Grabstald H. Melanoma of the genitourinary tract. J Urol 1965;93:607.
719. deKernion JB, Golub SH, Gupta RK, et al. Successful trans-urethral intralesional BCG therapy of a bladder melanoma. Cancer 1975;36:1662.
720. Goldstein HM, Kaminsky S, Wallace S, et al. Urographic manifestations of metastatic melanoma. Radiology 1974;121:801.
721. Sheehan EE, Greenberg SD, Scott R Jr. Metastatic neoplasms of the bladder. J Urol 1963;90:281.
722. Weston PAM, Smith BJ. Metastatic melanoma in the bladder and urethra. Br J Surg 1964;51:78.
723. Woodard BH, Ideker RE, Johnston WW. Cytologic detection of malignant melanoma in urine. Acta Cytol 1978;22:350.

724. Nakazono M, Iwata S, Kuribayashi N. Disseminated metastatic ureteral melanoma: A case report. J Urol 1975;114:624.
725. Lowsley OS. Melanoma of the urinary tract and prostate gland. South Med J 1951;44: 487.
726. Baab GH, McBride CM. Malignant melanoma: The patient with an unknown site of primary origin. Arch Surg 1975;110:896.
727. Chang P, Knapper WH. Metastatic melanoma of unknown primary. Cancer 1982;49: 1106.
728. Das Gupta T, Bowden L, Berg JW. Malignant melanoma of unknown primary origin. Surg Gynecol Obstet 1963;117:341.
729. Giuliano AE, Moseley HS, Morton DL. Clinical aspects of unknown primary melanoma. Ann Surg 1980;191:98.
730. Milton GW, Shaw HM, McCarthy WH. Occult primary malignant melanoma: Factors influencing survival. Br J Surg 1977;64:805.
731. Reintgen DS, McCarty KS, Woodard B, et al. Metastatic malignant melanoma with an unknown primary site. Surg Gynecol Obstet 1983;156:335.
732. Mundth ED, Guralnick EA, Raker JW. Malignant melanoma: A clinical study of 427 cases. Ann Surg 1965;162:15–28.
733. Elder DE. Metastatic melanoma. Pigment Cell 1987;8:182.

Cancer: Principles & Practice of Oncology, Fourth Edition,
edited by Vincent T. DeVita, Jr., Samuel Hellman, Steven A. Rosenberg.
J.B. Lippincott Co., Philadelphia © 1993.

Jose A. Sahel
John D. Earle
Daniel M. Albert

CHAPTER **47**

Intraocular Melanomas

Melanomas are the commonest primary intraocular malignancy in the white population. They arise from uveal melanocytes, mature melanin-producing and melanin-containing cells, residing in the uveal stroma. These cells originate from the neural crest and possess long, dendrite-like processes. Melanomas may also arise in the conjunctiva. Proliferations of cells other than uveal melanocytes can arise in the eye; the epithelia of the iris, ciliary body, and retina can undergo reactive or neoplastic proliferations, forming adenomas or adenocarcinomas.[1–5] This chapter deals exclusively with uveal melanomas, with particular emphasis on the current therapeutic issues and controversies.

EPIDEMIOLOGY

The annual age-adjusted incidence of noncutaneous melanomas as reported in the Surveillance, Epidemiology, and End Results (SEER) Program during the period of 1973 to 1977 was 0.7 per 100,000 population in the United States.[6] Similar data were reported from epidemiologic studies conducted in New England (0.65 per 100,000 residents from 1984 to 1985),[7] the Swedish West Coast (0.72 per 100,000 from 1956 to 1975),[8] and Iceland (0.7 per 100,000 in men and 0.5 per 100,000 in women from 1955 to 1979).[9]

In the Third National Cancer Survey, conducted from 1969 to 1971, the annual age-adjusted incidence of intraocular melanomas in the United States was estimated at 0.6 per 100,000.[10] The precise anatomic origin of ocular melanomas was unspecified in about 25% of cases. Seventy-three percent of the tumors arose within the globe (mainly from the choroid), and 2% developed from the conjunctiva. Melanoma accounted for 70% of all primary eye malignancies, followed in frequency by the childhood tumor retinoblastoma (13%). In persons older than 20 years of age, melanoma was the reported diagnosis for 80% of all primary ocular cancers.[10] Data from the Missouri Department of Health,[11] China,[12] the SEER Program,[6] New England,[7] Iceland,[9] Finland,[13] and the Ocular Melanoma Task Force[14] are similar to those reported by the Third National Cancer Survey.[10] (Few studies have provided reliable, long-term survival rates. The Finnish study showed that the 5-, 10-, and 15-year survival rates were 65%, 52%, and 46%, respectively.[13]) The annual age-adjusted incidence of ocular melanomas is about one eighth that of skin melanoma in the United States.[13] The recently observed increase in the incidence of cutaneous melanomas has not been observed for uveal melanomas.[15–19] Although the incidence increases steadily by decade, with a peak in the seventh decade, uveal melanoma cases can occur before the age of 20 years, as illustrated by 101 of the 6359 cases on file at the Registry of Ophthalmic Pathology at the Armed Forces Institute of Pathology (AFIP), 40 of 3706 consecutive patients seen at Wills Eye Hospital, and several other reports.[7,12,20–27] Most studies show a median age at diagnosis of about 55 years, with rates decreasing after the age of 70 years.[13,23,28,29]

White persons have an eightfold greater risk for ocular melanoma than black persons (compared with a sixfold greater risk for skin melanomas)[10,14,30–32] and a threefold greater risk than certain Asian populations.[5,15] Although Scotto and associates found that the overall risk for ocular melanomas did not vary by sex,[5] Jensen,[23] Gislason and colleagues,[9] and others[7,16,33] noted a predominance of men. Ocular and skin melanoma show similar age patterns, with more women affected at younger ages and more men affected later in life.[5] The Third National Cancer Survey indicated a left-sided excess of 18% for ocular melanomas in men and a right-sided excess in women.[10]

ETIOLOGY AND HISTOGENESIS

As for most human cancers, the specific causes of ocular melanomas are unknown. However, epidemiologic, electron microscopic, and experimental data allow the characterization of risk factors, predisposing conditions, and hypothetical genetic or oncogenic causes.

PREDISPOSING CONDITIONS

Ocular melanocytosis and oculodermal melanocytosis (nevus of Ota) predipose to the development of uveal melanomas. In 4.6% of reported cases of nevus of Ota, malignant transformation was recorded,[36–38] and except for a single anecdotal case,[35] the melanoma occurred in the affected eye. Rare cases of uveal melanomas have been reported in patients with neurofibromatosis.[38,39]

Evidence that nevi are the origin of most choroidal melanomas has been provided by Yanoff and Zimmerman and others.[3,40,41] Yet a nevus-like configuration associated with choroidal melanoma may in some instances be explained by other mechanisms, such as flattening of normal uveal melanocytes or tumor cells; a secondary proliferative effect of the malignancy; or common oncogenic stimuli.[3,42,43] The last two mechanisms have been postulated in a few cases of bilateral, diffuse melanocytic tumors of the uvea in patients with systemic carcinoma.[3,44,45] In some instances, a familial increased occurrence of uveal melanoma has been recorded.[28,46–48]

Data on the occurrence of uveal melanocytic tumors in patients with the dysplastic nevus syndrome are controversial but generally support periodic ophthalmoscopic examination of these patients.[49–53] The association between uveal melanomas and other cancers is controversial. Turner and coworkers showed that the overall prevalence of nonbasal cell cancers in uveal melanoma patients was twice the expected number based on an age- and sex-matched population.[54] A link between cutaneous and uveal melanoma was suspected based on their association in three cases of primary uveal and cutaneous melanomas among 333 patients. A family history of cutaneous or uveal melanoma was present in 14 and 2 patients, respectively.[54] Lischko and associates conducted a case-control study among 197 New England cases with 385 matched control subjects and 337 cases (from the United States) with 800 control subjects.[55] They concluded that the association of prior malignancies with uveal melanomas is weak. In a similar study of 407 uveal melanoma patients from the Western United States compared with 870 control subjects, Holly and colleagues found no excess of prior cancers.[56] Cytogenetic studies of uveal melanoma tissues from 19 patients suggest that recessive alleles at some chromosome 2 loci may be important in the oncogenesis of these tumors.[57]

ONCOGENIC STIMULI

Certain electron microscopic and biomolecular studies of ocular melanomas suggest a possible etiologic role of viruses.[58] Viruses such as the feline sarcoma virus have been used successfully in the induction of ocular melanoma in animals.[58–61] In a study of a single population of chemical workers, a statistically significant and higher than expected incidence of ocular melanomas was found.[62] Nicotine has been incriminated in the unusual incidence of uveal melanomas in men.[63] Various chemicals, including nickel bisulfamide, platinum, methylcholanthrene, ethionine, *N*-2-fluorenylacetamide, radium, and *N*-methyl-*N*-nitrosourea, have been reported to induce ocular melanocytic tumors in animals.[59–70] A possible connection between levodopa therapy in Parkinson's disease and malignant melanoma has been mentioned.[71]

The role of hormonal factors and pregnancy has been suggested in some publications. Hartge and coworkers reported a case-controlled study comparing 238 women with uveal melanoma with 223 matched control women.[72] They showed that women with a past medical history of pregnancy or hormonal substitutive treatment with estrogens had an increased risk (relative risk of 1.4),[72] whereas a past medical history of oophorectomy had a decreased influence on relative risk (0.6), and oral contraceptives had none.[72] The role of pregnancy in the growth of uveal melanoma has been documented by Seddon and associates[73] and Shields and colleagues.[74] Whether the growth observed clinically is secondary to cellular growth or other factors, such as fluid retention and vascular engorgement, is unclear.

A case-controlled study lends support to the etiologic role of sunlight exposure.[75] A study of host factors (Northern European ancestry, light skin color, ten or more cutaneous nevi), ultraviolet radiation, and the risk for uveal melanoma indicated that personal attributes are strong independent risk factors.[76] Holly and associates proved that light skin color and easily sunburned skin increased the risk for uveal melanoma twofold, whereas ultraviolet exposure increased this risk fourfold and sevenfold, if intensive.[77] These data, which contradict previous studies,[10,78] confirm the high association between light iris color and the presence of iris melanocytic lesions.[79]

HISTOPATHOLOGY, PROGNOSTIC PARAMETERS, AND NATURAL HISTORY

CHOROIDAL AND CILIARY BODY MELANOMAS: CYTOLOGIC AND HISTOLOGIC CLASSIFICATION

The accurate histologic diagnosis of uveal melanoma is, in most instances, easily made by the experienced histopathologist. Rarely, differentiation from metastatic carcinoma may be facilitated by immunohistochemical labeling of S100 protein. This technique is not helpful in differentiating other neural crest-derived tumors, such as schwannomas, neurofibromas, and leiomyomas.[3] The S100 immunophenotypes of uveal melanoma differ considerably from cutaneous melanoma.[80] HMB-45 immunostaining may be a useful adjunct in the differentiation between uveal melanomas and nevi.[81] Otherwise, immunocytochemistry has not provided reliable characterization of uveal melanoma using cutaneous melanoma antibodies or antihuman leukocyte antigen antibodies or allowed preparation of reliable monoclonal antibodies.[82–85]

In 1931, Callender recognized major cell types in the spectrum of cells composing uveal melanomas, and this finding provided a cytologic classification clearly correlated with prognosis after enucleation.[86] The different cell types are shown in Table 47-1 and discussed in the following sections.[3,86,87]

TABLE 47–1. Histopathologic Classification of Choroidal and Ciliary Body Melanocytic Tumors

Iris

Pretreatment Clinical Classification (cTNM)

Primary Tumor (T)

TX	Minimum requirements to assess the primary tumor cannot be met
T0	No evidence of primary tumor
T2	Tumor involving not more than one quadrant, with extension into the anterior chamber angle
T3	Tumor involving more than one quadrant, with extension into the anterior chamber angle
T4	Tumor with extraocular extension

Regional Lymph Nodes (N)

NX	Minimum requirements to assess the regional lymph nodes cannot be met
N0	No evidence of regional lymph node involvement
N1	Evidence of involvement of the regional lymph nodes

Distant Metastases (M)

MX	Minimum requirements to assess the presence of distant metastases cannot be met
M0	No evidence of distant metastases
M1	Evidence of distant metastases

Ciliary Body

Pretreatment Clinical Classification (cTNM)

Primary Tumor (T)

TX	Minimum requirements to assess the primary tumor cannot be met
T0	No evidence of primary tumor
T1	Tumor limited to the ciliary body
T2	Tumor with extension into the anterior chamber and/or iris
T3	Tumor with extension into the choroid
T4	Tumor with extraocular extension

Regional Lymph Nodes (N)

NX	Minimum requirements to assess the regional lymph nodes cannot be met
N0	No evidence of regional lymph node involvement
N1	Evidence of involvement of the regional lymph nodes

Distant Metastases (M)

MX	Minimum requirements to assess the presence of distant metastases cannot be met
M0	No evidence of distant metastases
M1	Evidence of distant metastases

Choroid

Pretreatment Clinical Classification (cTNM)

Primary Tumor (T)

TX	Minimum requirements to assess the primary tumor cannot be met
T0	No evidence of primary tumor
T1	Tumor not more than 10 mm in its greatest dimension, and/or with an elevation of not more than 3 mm
T1A	Tumor not more than 7 mm in its greatest dimension and with an elevation of not more than 2 mm
T1B	Tumor more than 7 mm but not more than 10 mm in its greatest dimension and with an elevation of more than 2 mm but not more than 3 mm
T2	Tumor more than 10 mm but not more than 15 mm in its greatest dimension and with an elevation of more than 3 mm but not more than 5 mm
T3	Tumor more than 15 mm in its greatest dimension or with an elevation of 5 mm or more
T4	Tumor with extraocular extension *Note:* When dimension and elevation show a difference in classification, the highest category should be used for classification.

Regional Lymph Nodes (N)

NX	Minimum requirements to assess the regional lymph nodes cannot be met
N0	No evidence of regional lymph node involvement
N1	Evidence of involvement of regional lymph nodes

Distant Metastases (M)

MX	Minimum requirements to assess the presence of distant metastases cannot be met
M0	No evidence of distant metastases
M1	Evidence of distant metastases

Spindle A cells are uniform, cohesive cells with small, slender, spindle-shaped nuclei often showing longitudinal folds in the nuclear membrane. The nucleoli are not distinct, and mitotic figures are rare. The cell borders are difficult to identify.

Spindle B cells are plumper, cohesive spindle cells with larger ovoid nuclei containing a coarse chromatin network and a conspicuous nucleolus. Mitotic figures are seen more frequently. The cell borders are difficult to discern. Spindle A and B cells may be arranged in rows or palisades, constituting the fascicular pattern, which is now regarded as having no prognostic significance.[3,88] A careful reappraisal of 90 pure spindle A melanomas by McLean and colleagues found that 15 had features of benignity, whereas the other 75 had larger, hyperchromatic nuclei with frequent mitotic activity associated with histologic features of malignancy (*e.g.*, invasiveness) and greater size.[89] In the revised AFIP classification of uveal melanomas, the spindle A and B subtypes are no longer separated.[89]

Epithelioid cells were described by Callender as larger, more pleomorphic, poorly cohesive, polygonal cells with abundant eosinophilic cytoplasm.[86] The nuclei are round and contain large single or multiple nucleoli. Mitotic figures are abundant. A subtype consisting of small cells with less cytoplasm and a smaller nucleus is now included in this category, because it has other typical features of epithelioid cells, such as large eosinophilic nucleoli and lack of cohesiveness.[90] According to Callender's cytologic characterization, uveal melanomas are divided into the following three categories:

1. Spindle cell melanomas, type A, B, or both, accounting for 30% of intraocular tumors
2. Mixed cell melanomas containing spindle and epithelioid cells
3. Epithelioid cell melanomas accounting for 5% of intraocular tumors

The major cell types described by Callender are part of a continuous spectrum, and the pathologist's identification of a particular cell type involves subjective judgment.[91,92] In the Collaborative Ocular Melanoma Study (COMS), it was found useful to include an "intermediate" category of cells that share characteristics of spindle B and epithelioid cells.[93]

This issue was also addressed by Gamel and McLean, who described a more objective method of assessing uveal melanomas histopathologically.[94] This method, which uses computerized cytomorphology, mainly entails evaluating the inverse of the standard deviation of the nucleolar area and, more recently, measurement of the mean of the ten largest nucleoli. This measure appears to be the best objective determination of a tumor's malignant potential ($p > 0.001$).[95–98] Studies by Gamel and associates and others have corroborated the well-documented prognostic value of Callender's classification, especially as to the pejorative significance of high epithelioid cell content.[30,86,88,90,95–102]

Several attempts to evaluate the growth and malignant potential of uveal melanomas have been made recently using DNA cell cycle studies, for example, bromodeoxyuridine uptake or Ki-67 antibody as a marker of cycling cells[102,103] and DNA or RNA content by flow cytometry.[103,106] The value of these methods and the usefulness of silver-stained nucleolar-organizer regions must still be prospectively compared with cytomorphometric determinations and conventional cytology by an experienced pathologist.[103–108]

Paul and coworkers reviewed 2652 cases accessioned at the AFIP by 1959 and found that 95% of patients with spindle A tumors, 85% of those with spindle B tumors, 60% of those with mixed cell tumors, and 83% of those with epithelioid tumors were alive 5 years after enucleation.[30] At 16 years after enucleation, the survival rates were 85%, 80%, 46%, and 34%, respectively.[62] McLean and colleagues, in a review of 3432 cases from the AFIP, found that the overall mortality from metastasis 15 years after enucleation was 46%.[102] The mortality of patients with mixed cell melanomas was three times that of patients with pure spindle cell lesions.

In Jensen's series of 302 reported cases from Denmark that had been observed for 25 years, 150 (50%) of the patients died from metastatic melanoma.[23,109,110] Fewer than 1% of patients with spindle A tumors died from metastatic disease; 83% with mixed cell tumors were dead; and in 71% of patients with epithelioid tumors, the cause of death was metastatic melanoma.

After the studies of Rosenberg and coworkers on the prognostic and therapeutic value of tumor-infiltrating lymphocytes, a reappraisal of the well-known lymphocytic infiltration of some uveal melanomas has been undertaken.[111–115] Analysis of tumor-infiltrating lymphocytes detected in five tumors (among 27 melanomas studied) has shown the predominance of cytotoxic T cells and the predominant expression of T-cell receptor V α7.[111,112]

The role of infiltrating lymphocytes in the regression of animals with tumors is a current avenue of investigation.[100–102]

NATURAL HISTORY

Growth Rate

Little is known about the natural history of uveal melanomas; until recently, all patients underwent enucleation immediately after the diagnosis.[3,116,117] Data on the growth pattern of small melanomas from series of patients observed by Gass and others have contributed to the knowledge of the rate of intraocular tumor growth before treatment.[110,118–121]

These findings and other selected reports[122,123] suggest a Gompertzian (expotential) growth curve, as postulated by Manschot and associates.[124] The doubling time of uveal tumors may vary from 2 months or less[119–125] to several years.[117–119] In rapidly growing tumors, a high mitotic activity and the presence of epithelioid cells have been documented.[119,123,125] Rarely, spontaneous regression of a choroidal melanoma has been reported.[126]

Intraocular Spread

Small melanomas usually grow from a discoid to a hemispheric shape. They progressively obliterate the choriocapillaris and displace Bruch's membrane and the retina inward. When Bruch's membrane is disrupted, the tumor grows in the subretinal space in a mushroom configuration.[3,127–136] The retinal pigment epithelium overlying the tumors undergoes early changes, including drusen formation and orange pigment (lipofuscin) accumulation.[3,127–133] The neurosensory retina is detached frequently and, in some instances, infiltrated by tumor cells, which can seed into the vitreous.[132]

Anterior choroidal and ciliary body tumors are more likely to affect the lens and to seed the posterior chamber. The zonule, lens, iris, anterior chamber, and angle may be involved. Secondary glaucoma may result from obstruction of the outflow pathways by tumor cells, cell debris, and phagocytic cells swollen with ingested cell debris (melanomalytic glaucoma).[133,134] The tumor may infiltrate through the scleral spur into the trabecular network.

Although the sclera is stated to be an effective barrier against extraocular extension, scleral infiltration by tumor cells along ciliary vessels and nerves and along the vortex veins is frequent (32.3% of large melanomas in a series reported by Shammas and Blodi).[135] Approximately 5% of melanomas grow diffusely in the plane of the uvea or circumferentially along the root of the iris. They induce a slight thickening of the uvea (approximately 3–5 mm) and are often unsuspected or are diagnosed late in the course of the tumor, when secondary glaucoma or extraocular spread occur. Such extraocular extension may occur adjacent to or through the optic nerve or can occur anteriorly about the limbus.[136]

Extraocular Extension

Although extrascleral extension may be observed with small tumors,[137,138] it is more likely to occur when the tumor has reached a larger size. In a study by Shammas and Blodi, extrascleral extension was observed in 18% of tumors exceeding 10 mm in diameter.[138] The overall incidence of transcleral extension was determined to about 13% among 1842 malignant melanomas studied by Starr and Zimmerman.[139] Others series have compiled similar data.[140,141] Starr and Zimmerman noted a tenfold increase in the incidence of postoperative recurrence if the tumor extended to the surgical margin. The depth of the scleral extension may have a prognostic significance.[142] Other paths of extraocular spread include the optic nerve[143,144] and the lumen of the vortex veins.[145]

Because of the absence of lymphatics in the eye, lymphatic spread has not been demonstrated; this is in contrast to cutaneous melanomas.[146] Hematogenous dissemination to the liver is a frequent form of metastatic spread.[3,15,147,148] The respective roles of nonspecific trapping and of cell-surface antigens in the invasiveness and dissemination of uveal melanomas remain poorly explored fields of investigation.[149–154]

Some clones of melanoma cells with a preferential propensity for liver metastasis mediated by cell-surface properties have been characterized.[155,156] Patients with preexisting liver damage are more likely to be affected.[157,158] Metastases to other sites (lungs, heart, gastrointestinal tract, lymph nodes, pancreas, skin, central nervous system, bones, spleen, adrenal glands, kidneys, ovaries, and thyroid gland) generally occur in association with liver metastases.[133] In a recent survey of metastases from proton beam-treated melanomas, liver involvement was documented in almost all patients[159]; the overall 1-year survival was 13%.[159]

In a series of studies, Zimmerman and McLean found that most deaths from metastatic disease occurred in the first 5 years after enucleation, with a peak mortality in the second and third years (about 8% per year), and compared these data with the natural course of untreated melanomas.[3,90,116,160] In a conclusion that remains controversial, they incriminated enucleation as a risk factor and suggested two principal mechanisms: (1) dissemination of tumor cells during traumatic operations, as demonstrated experimentally by Fraunfelder and colleagues,[161] and (2) decreased host resistance to disseminated tumor cells. This latter mechanism has been called by Niederkorn and coworkers the "loss of intraocular induced concomitant immunity" mediated by cytotoxic T lymphocytes.[115,162,163] Zimmerman's and McLean's assumptions have been challenged by several investigators. Seigel and associates concluded that the statistical data can be interpreted differently and that there was no evidence to suggest that the existing pattern of treatment be altered.[164] Manschot and Van Peperzeel,[124] Kersten and Blodi,[165] and Davidorf[166] pointed out that most melanomas are diagnosed only when they have reached a relatively large size and concomitantly have given rise to metastases, and only then are they enucleated. The clinical consequences of these controversies have been employment of less traumatic techniques for enucleation and new impetus to the search for alternative treatments.[129,167]

PROGNOSTIC ASSESSMENT OF CHOROIDAL AND CILIARY BODY MELANOMAS

In most studies, the second most important prognostic parameter after the number of epithelioid cells is the largest tumor diameter.[3,90,100,101,135,169] This is followed, according to Seddon and colleagues, by the location of the anterior margin of the tumor, the invasion of the line of transsection, and the degree of pigmentation.[100,101,135] In a study of 253 choroidal and ciliary body melanomas for which a follow-up of 5 years or more was available, Shammas and Blodi identified the following eight factors that significantly influenced prognosis:

- Age of the patient at enucleation
- Location of the tumor
- Location of the anterior border of the tumor
- Largest tumor diameter in contact with the sclera
- Height of the tumor
- Integrity of Bruch's membrane
- Cell type
- Scleral infiltration by tumor cells

Using a multivariate analysis, McLean and coworkers reached similar conclusions for small melanomas.[102] Parameters that significantly influenced prognosis were cell type, largest dimension, scleral extension, and mitotic activity. A single factor analysis identified three additional factors of significance: degree of scleral invasion, optic nerve invasion, and pigmentation. In most of the studies, increased pigmentation has been associated with increased mortality.[15,30,102,110,135] In a multivariant analysis, however, these three parameters appear statistically related to cell type and tumor size,[55,100,101,168,169] but a close interval by interval analysis of the prognostic value of size and cell type shows a decline over time after tumor excision.[170]

In summary, all studies show that the prognosis of a patient with a choroidal or ciliary body melanoma treated by enucleation is *adversely affected* if the following occur:

- The tumor contains epithelioid cells.
- The tumor involves the ciliary body.
- The largest tumor dimension exceeds 10 mm.
- The tumor extends to the sclera.
- Numerous mitotic figures are present.

Many of these prognostic parameters are lacking in patients treated conservatively (*i.e.,* by methods other than enucleation). Because of reports with a brief follow-up period, bias in patient selection and sample size, and use of different survival analysis models, the comparison of survival rates with either conservative approaches or enucleation remains a subject of intense controversy.[167,169–172] The survival rates in large series after 5 years do not differ significantly: the reported tumor-related mortality 5 years after radiation therapy ranges from 11% to 25%,[169–181] whereas preliminary assumptions based on a log normal model may indicate a poorer life prognosis after 10 years for patients treated conservatively.[172] COMS, a prospective, multicenter study, should provide answers to this crucial and controversial issue.[173]

Several studies have established a correlation between rapid tumor regression after radiation therapy and poor prognosis for life.[175–178] Rapid regression of tumor height after irradiation appears to be a risk factor for metastasis.[175] That can possibly be correlated with a less differentiated cell type found in rapidly regressing tumors. However, this hypothesis is difficult to support because (1) cytologic study of such melanomas would depend on needle biopsy, which is rarely performed before radiation therapy; (2) in those rare cases, cytologic aspiration does not provide a reliable characterization of the cell type; and (3) histologic study of enucleated eyes after irradiation may not reflect accurately the cytologic features of the tumor before irradiation, particularly in mixed cell tumors.

DISTINGUISHING FEATURES OF IRIS MELANOMAS

Malignant melanoma of the iris is rare compared with melanomas of the rest of the uvea; the estimated ratios range from 1 in 6 to 1 in 30.[15,182–187] The average age at diagnosis of iris melanocytic tumors, including nevi, is 40 to 50 years.[109,110,127–130,185–187] Many patients (17–33%) give a long history of a noticeable pigmented iris lesion before clinical diagnosis. This observation is widely interpreted as suggesting that such tumors arose from preexisting nevi.[184,185,188–192] Zimmerman and others believe that the difference in size between tumors of the iris and other uveal tumors is the most critical feature affecting tumor behavior.[161,193,196] Iris melanomas are comparatively small lesions, generally much smaller than the posterior uveal tract tumors that come to clinical attention.[166,193–196] Iris melanomas grow more slowly than posterior uveal melanomas. Kersten and colleagues,[194] applying the scheme proposed by Apple and Blodi for choroidal melanomas,[197] suggested that the slow growth rate is related to the small size of iris melanomas. This slow growth and the high proportion of spindle A cells probably account for the low number of recurrences, metastasis, or death from disease several years or decades after the onset of symptoms.[194,198] The literature has continued to stress the relatively benign behavior and good prognosis of iris melanomas compared with melanomas of the choroid and ciliary body. Those melanomas in the ciliary body and choroid are associated with a mortality tenfold higher than the mortality from iris melanomas.[90] Green, reviewing 783 cases from the literature, noted 18 (2.29%) reported deaths from metastatic disease.[4] In two recent clinicopathologic studies, 138 and 107 patients, respectively, with a previous diagnosis of iris melanomas had no tumor-related deaths.[182,188] These series emphasize that many lesions previously called melanomas are actually nevi. Jakobiec and Silbert reclassified 138 lesions with an initial histopathologic diagnosis of melanoma into a nine-part classification, including three malignant categories; on reexamination using their criteria, only 13% of lesions were judged malignant.[182] In a similar series of 107 such tumors,[188] a ten-part classification derived from Jakobiec and Silbert was applied. Only 10% of the lesions were considered melanomas. The argyrophilic-stained nucleolar organizer region-associated count may provide an accurate prediction of the malignant nature and potential or iris melanocytic lesions.[199,199a] However, the low malignant potential of iris melanocytic tumors is accepted by most authors.[192–194,198,200,201] Moreover, the prognostic assessment of iris melanoma should consider that local spread of some melanocytic tumors, even with "benign" cytology, may lead to sight-threatening complications, such as refractory secondary glaucoma, and that incomplete or inappropriate surgery may increase both local and systemic malignant potential.[182,191,192,198,202,203]

DIAGNOSIS OF UVEAL MELANOMAS

CHOROIDAL AND CILIARY BODY MELANOMAS

The diagnosis of choroidal and ciliary body melanomas has reached a high degree of accuracy at eye centers where experienced clinicians and modern ancillary testing facilities are available.[204–210] This point is well illustrated by a comparison of the misdiagnosis rates among the eyes on file at the AFIP: 19% (of 529 eyes) until 1962, 20% (of 208 eyes) between 1963 and 1970, and 6.4% (of 744 eyes) between 1970 and 1980.[204–207] During the 11-year period of the last study, the rate of misdiagnosis declined from 12.5% to 1.4%.[207] Between 1954 and 1977, the misdiagnosis rate was 2.6% (of 244 eyes) at the Mayo Clinic.[208] In this series, in addition, six clinically unsuspected melanomas were found.[208] This high rate of correct clinical diagnosis is particularly impressive, because only outpatient procedures (including clinical examination, ultrasound, and fluorescein angiography) were used. No biopsies were performed, as is done for many other tumors. A review of 395 eyes enucleated during a 50-year period, based on the pathology files of Ohio State University, revealed a misdiagnosis rate of 10.9% from 1931 to 1959, which decreased to 1.7% from 1960 to 1981. Nine percent of choroidal melanomas were unsuspected preoperatively, and all of these were in eyes with opaque media.[209] In a series of 400 consecutive patients referred to the oncology unit of the Wills Eye Hospital with an incorrect diagnosis of melanoma (*i.e.*, patients proved to have pseudomelanomas), the correct diagnosis was reached through clinical evaluation in 397 cases (99%).[210] In that series, the most commonly encountered conditions mimicking a melanoma included suspicious choroidal nevi (26.5%), peripheral disciform degeneration (11%), congenital hypertrophy of the retinal pigment epithelium (9.5%), and choroidal hemangioma (8%). Most metastatic carcinomas had been diagnosed correctly by the referring opthalmologists.[210] A high rate of accuracy was recently reported in the multicenter COMS.[211]

The cornerstone of diagnosis of posterior uveal melanoma remains clinical examination, particularly indirect ophthalmoscopy through a dilated pupil. Fundus contact lens examination and the use of a three-mirror lens can be extremely helpful.[127–130] Scleral transillumination as advocated by Reese is also a useful aid.[128] Pigmented conjunctival lesions, such as conjunctival melanoma, staphylomas, scleral ectasia, hematoma, cellular blue nevi, and ocular melanocytosis, may mimic extraocular extension of uveal melanomas.[212] Visual field studies are of little help in diagnosis or in distinguishing melanomas from choroidal nevi.[42,91,129,213,216] Although clinical examination by an experienced observer remains the most important test in establishing the presence of an ocular melanoma, ancillary diagnostic testing can be extremely valuable.[46,127–130,215]

Fluorescein angiography and monochromic photography have proved useful in differentiating subretinal or choroidal hemorrhage and hemangioma from melanoma. Although no angiographic pattern is pathognomonic for choroidal melanomas, features of value include early mottling, fluorescence, orange pigment over the margin of the tumor, progressive fluorescence of the lesion with late staining, and multiple pinpoint leaks that increase in size. Breaks in Bruch's membrane and retinal invasion can be detected from abnormalities such as a "double circulation" pattern.[44,127–130,215–218]

The combined use of A- and B-mode ultrasound techniques is valuable in confirming the clinical diagnosis of choroidal melanoma, especially in the presence of opaque media.[129,130,173,205,210,219–228] The B-mode ultrasound characteristics useful in differentiating melanomas from metastases or hemangiomas are acoustic hollowness, choroidal excavation, and orbital shadowing. Small tumors elevated less than 2 to 3 mm cannot be evaluated accurately. In large tumors, ultrasound provides valuable size data for serial measurements.[220,226] However, a difference between ultrasonographic and histopathologic measurements of tumor thickness was demonstrated, probably resulting from tumor shrinkage after laboratory preparation.[220] Extrascleral extension can be detected by contact B-mode ultrasound.[221] Ultrasound is an important follow-up tool after conservative treatment of uveal melanoma.[229] Recent reports on the usefulness of color-coded

Doppler imaging are promising in characterization and follow-up studies.[230–232]

The usefulness of radioactive phosphorus (phosphorus 32) in determining malignancy is more controversial. It probably has limited indications for use in routine cases in which adequate support for a diagnosis of ocular melanoma has been obtained with less complicated procedures.[129,130,233–236]

Radiologic examination, including computed tomography (CT), is useful in evaluating the presence and size of extraocular extension of tumor.[237–239]

Images of uveal melanoma were included in early reports of magnetic resonance imaging (MRI) studies.[240] This imaging modality has become more useful with the increase in its availability, the use of thin-section imaging, the development of surface coils, and the employment of contrast material (gadolinium).[240–246] Typically, pigmented melanomas are hyperintense on T1-weighted images with enhancement by gadolinium.[205,243–246] Therefore, this method is promising in the detection, the characterization, and the delimitation of difficult cases. Phosphorus 31 magnetic resonance spectroscopy may be helpful in this respect soon.[247,248] Nevertheless, ultrasonography is currently the main imaging modality employed in intraocular melanomas.

Immunologic testing does not yet offer reliable results.[249–255] Using the indirect immunoperoxidase method, Felberg and coworkers found that 78% of patients with uveal malignancy had tumor-associated antibodies (TAA), whereas 24% of control subjects tested positive for TAA.[249] Unfortunately, TAA assays could not be used to separate primary from secondary uveal tumors. Studies of monoclonal antibodies, as discussed earlier, are not yet convincing.[252,254] Radioimmunoscintigraphy using technetium 99m (^{99m}Tc)-labeled monoclonal antibodies are too preliminary to be considered as reliable diagnostic tools.[253,255] However, surveillance of melanoma-associated antigens and carcinoembryonic antigens may be useful for monitoring recurrence or metastatic disease.[251,256,257]

In a review of 51 consecutive patients who had undergone enucleation for a choroidal melanoma and 50 patients with simulating lesions, Char and colleagues found that the ophthalmoscopic examination was the most accurate diagnostic modality, allowing correct diagnosis of choroidal melanomas in all patients with clear media.[258] Subretinal fluid, orange pigmentation, and collar button configuration occurred more often with melanomas than with other lesions. In 63% of melanoma patients, fluorescein angiography was diagnostic, and in 82%, A- and B-mode ultrasonography was diagnostic.[258]

In some dubious cases, fine-needle aspiration biopsy has been proposed.[129,130,259] However, the interpretation of aspirates may be difficult, even in the hands of an experienced pathologist, and subsequent tumor cell seeding in the needle track has been reported.[260,261] Nevertheless, in selected cases, this technique has proved useful to differentiate benign from malignant lesions.[129,130,259,262] The lack of histologic data before conservative treatment of most uveal melanomas imposes a major limitation on an understanding of tumor response to irradiation and the accurate adaptation of conservative approaches and on the estimate of prognosis for such examinations.

Despite ancillary examinations, the differential diagnosis of small tumors may be difficult. Careful follow-up study of such patients at short intervals with photography, fluorescein angiography, and ultrasound is advocated to demonstrate tumor growth.[42,66,129,130,204,263]

Patients with suspected intraocular melanoma should undergo a physical examination and metastatic workup. Clinical laboratory studies should include routine blood studies, chest radiography, and liver enzyme measurements. CT should be performed if other tests suggest liver involvement.[127–130,147,148,157,173,205,264–266] Liver ultrasonography and liver-spleen scans may be useful.

IRIS MELANOMAS

Iris tumors are visible not only to the ophthalmologist but also to the patient, family, and friends.[127–130,193] Patients frequently are aware of a spot on the iris that has been present for many years but has only recently shown growth. The ophthalmologist can examine the lesion carefully with a slit-lamp biomicroscope and gonioscopy, and with the aid of serial iris fluorescein photography, can determine the size and vasculature of the tumor.[130,267] Iris tumors are usually small, discrete lesions replacing the normal architecture of the iris stroma, but they may be extensive (*e.g.*, diffuse or ring), infiltrative, or even multiple, such as the hypopigmented, multifocal nodules composing the picture of tapioca melanomas.[3,127–130,182] Only a few clinical findings—increased vascularity, involvement of the ciliary body, secondary glaucoma, and documented tumor growth—are helpful in distinguishing benign from malignant iris melanocytic tumors.[182,185,187,195,196,269–271] The differential diagnosis includes entities characterized by diffuse increased pigmentation, including melanosis, siderosis bulbi, heterochromia iridis, foreign bodies encapsulated by fibrous tissue, iris cysts, essential iris atrophy, peripheral anterior synechia, tumors of the retinal pigment epithelium, leiomyomas, granulomas—as seen in tuberculosis, herpes, or sarcoidosis—metastatic neoplasms, syphilitic gummas, and nevoxanthoendothelioma.[152,195,196,269–272]

TREATMENT OF UVEAL MELANOMAS

PRETREATMENT CLINICAL STAGING

It is useful to discuss the treatment of choroidal and ciliary body melanomas in terms of the following tumor sizes: (1) small 2 to 2.5 mm elevated $<$16 mm base; (2) medium $\geq$2.5 to $\leq$10.0 mm elevated $\leq$16 mm base; (3) large $>$10 mm elevated $>$16 mm base *or* at least 2 mm elevated *and* $>$16 mm base.[3,127–139,205] This division by size is referred to in the remainder of this chapter.

Comparisons of results from various series would benefit from more uniform staging of uveal tumors. The American Joint Committee on Cancer has developed a staging classification of uveal melanomas based on the tumor, node, metastasis (TNM) system (see Table 47-1).[3,273] However, this classification is not widely used for various reasons, including the rarity of detectable metastases at the time of diagnosis, particularly lymphatic lesions. Moreover, in contrast to the Reese-Ellsworth classification of retinoblastomas,[128] this classification is of marginal help in predicting the visual outcome of conservative approaches, because of such factors as the distance to the optic nerve and macula. Moreover, as mentioned earlier, the lack of histopathologic data in most patients managed conservatively has given emphasis to evaluation of the tumors based solely on patterns of tumor growth before and tumor regression after radiation therapy. Therefore, the comparison of data from most retrospective and often incomplete studies would increase the current confusion and controversies.

TREATMENT OF CHOROIDAL AND CILIARY BODY MELANOMAS

In the late nineteenth century, enucleation became the standard and almost universally accepted treatment for all choroidal or ciliary body melanomas.[276] Early enucleation continues to have its ardent advocates[124,180,275]; however, in recent years enucleation has been reassessed as a conventional means of treating malignant melanomas of the choroid and ciliary body. This reassessment has resulted from (1) the development of newer and more precise diagnostic tests for recognizing malignant melanomas and the serial documentation of their size; (2) more information about clinical and pathologic features that determine survival; (3) additional observations about the natural course of untreated ciliary body and choroidal melanomas; (4) therapeutic developments other than enucleation to treat these tumors without destroying the eye; and (5) disagreements regarding the value and risks of enucleation.[3,61,90,100,101,116,118,126,160–167,173,174,180,197,205]

Currently, most authors agree that the goals for treating a uveal melanoma should be to destroy or inactivate the neoplasm, to maintain useful vision in the involved eye, to use a treatment with few side effects, and, most important, to provide the patient with the best prognosis for life among the treatment alternatives that are available.[127–130,173,174,205] Beyond these basic statements, many controversies will continue until results from prospective, randomized treatment trials are collected.[129,167,173,205] Therefore, the treatment ultimately selected is determined currently by the specific findings in the individual patient with regard to tumor size, location, and growth rate, the preferences of the ophthalmologist, and the desires of the patient.

SMALL MELANOMAS

The choices open to the physician treating a small choroidal or ciliary body melanoma include observation; some method of local treatment, including radiation therapy, photoradiation, cryotherapy, ultrasonic hyperthermia, local resection; and enucleation.

Observation

An accumulating body of evidence indicates that the risks to these patients in observing these tumors are low (Table 47-2).[91,117–119,126,129,130,214,215,277–280] Serial examination every 3 months without intervention seems appropriate if the tumor is asymptomatic or appears dormant; if the diagnosis is equivocal; if no growth is seen on serial ophthalmoscopic, photographic, and ultrasound examinations; in elderly, seriously ill patients; or for a tumor in the patient's only useful eye when the tumor is growing slowly.[129,176,210,215,277–281]

If the tumor shows progression, particularly rapid growth or an increase in size beyond 10 mm in diameter and 3 mm in elevation, or if the lesions results in significant impairment of vision, treatment is indicated.

Photocoagulation

In this method, the xenon arc, the argon laser, photoradiation with red light after photosensitization with hematoporphyrin derivatives, or dye laser after phthalocyanine photosensitization can be used.[129,130,281–296] Some success with photocoagulation has been documented histologically in small series.[128,130,288] The following criteria for selecting patients with melanoma for photocoagulation treatment were suggested by Meyer-Schwickerath[281] and Vogel[282] and adapted by Shields and others[29,205,294]:

1. The diagnosis of melanoma and evidence of growth should be documented thoroughly.

TABLE 47–2. Observation Versus Enucleation of Small Tumors of the Choroid and Ciliary Body

Aspect Evaluated	*Char et al*[118]	*Gass*[263]*	*Shields*[222]	*Davidorf et al*[280]	*McLean et al*[90]	*Shammas et al*[135]	*Barr et al*[278]	*Thomas et al*[279]	*Seddon et al*[100]
No. of eyes	20	100	150	38	37	129	16	27	267
Management	Observation: enucleation if growth	Observation: enucleation or further follow-up if growth	Observation: enucleation if growth	Enucleation	Enucleation	Enucleation	Enucleation	Enucleation	Enucleation
Follow-up	1–19 y before enucleation; average 4.5 y after enucleation	>8 y	2–5 y	>5 y	6 y	5 y	6 y	10 y	8 y
Evidence of growth	45%	36%	10–15%						
Deaths from metastases	—	3%	—	5% 5 y 19% 10 y	25%	8% 5 y 10% 10 y	11%	10%	12% 5 y 18% 10 y

* Gass assumed that tumors exhibiting no growth over 5 years were actually nevi.

2. The tumor should not be greater than 5 diopters in elevation and 6 disk diameters at its greatest diameter.
3. The tumor must be surrounded completely without damaging the fovea or the optic disk.
4. The patient must have clear ocular media and a sufficient mydriasis to enable photocoagulation to be performed.
5. The tumor surface should not have large overlying retinal vessels.

Photocoagulation requires several outpatient treatment sessions and is carried out after mydriasis and (for xenon photocoagulation) induction of retrobulbar anesthesia. A double confluent row of heavy coagulation is repeated three times at monthly intervals to encircle the tumor and to obliterate the choroidal vasculature supplying the gray discoloration and a surrounding atrophic choroidal scar.

Long-term complications of photocoagulation include retinal vascular obstruction, visual field defect, macular pucker, cystoid macular edema, choroid neovascularization, vitreous hemorrhage, and retinal detachment.[129,205,282,294] Recurrences may appear, usually within 2 years of treatment. In a 20-year follow-up of 54 patients with uveal melanomas, Vogel reported that 63% were alive, although only 46% were considered cured by photocoagulation.[282] Twenty percent of patients subsequently underwent enucleation. Of the 20 patients (37%) who died, 8 did so as a result of metastatic disease, 3 died from other causes, and 9 died from undetermined causes.[282] Shields reported that among 35 patients treated between 1976 and 1979, 25 retained useful vision, 5 had poor vision, and 5 subsequently underwent enucleation.[129] There were no tumor-related deaths. Comparison of xenon arc and argon laser photocoagulation in 38 consecutive patients with a minimal follow-up of 58 months showed that recurrences were less frequent and appeared later after xenon photocoagulation irradiation.[286] Photocoagulation seems best suited for small posterior melanomas located within 3 mm of the optic disk or fovea. In such lesions (photocoagulation-induced) retinopathy may cause visual loss.[129,130,205] The patient's desire to avoid radiation therapy or enucleation may be the deciding factor for using this modality. Photocoagulation is also helpful in the treatment of secondary serious macular detachments.[297] Reports on hematoporphyrin and phthalocyanine phototherapy are too preliminary.[261–264,267,272,273]

Radiation

For lesions meeting the clinical criteria for choroidal melanomas that are no larger than about 10 mm in height or 16 mm in diameter, brachytherapy is an acceptable therapeutic option. Before 1930, Moore used radon 222 seed to treat choroidal melanomas.[298] In the 1960s, Stallard popularized cobalt ^{60}Co as a brachytherapy source.[299] Although dosimetry was still relatively crude, the use of standardized plaques became common because of the long half-life of ^{60}Co. Results in a large series of patients managed in similar fashion became available, demonstrating the equivalence with enucleation within the limits of balancing the prognostic factors in these retrospective analyses. Markoe and associates used the Cox proportional hazards model to compare results in 100 patients treated with ^{60}Co plaques with results in enucleated patients.[300] Survival was better for the plaque-treated patients, although the findings were not statistically significant. Vision deteriorated in a roughly linear fashion: approximately 40% had better vision than 20/200 visual acuity at 5 years.[300]

In 1976, Sealy and coworkers first reported using iodine ^{125}I for choroidal melanomas.[301] In 1979, Packer and Rotman suggested ^{125}I as the isotope of choice for brachytherapy of choroidal melanomas, based on the ease of shielding the adjacent structures and the safety of medical personnel.[302] Of 58 patients, 8 failed locally, and 45 remained alive without disease. Thirty-eight percent had deterioration of vision of two or more lines on the Snellen chart.[303] Garretson and colleagues reported results in 26 patients treated with ^{125}I plaques who were followed for a minimum of 2 years (mean, 45 months).[304] One patient died at 21 months. Visual acuity remained within two Snellen lines of preoperative levels in 54%. Of the 12 patients who lost more than two lines of acuity, 8 developed retinal changes, and 3 developed cataracts. Enucleation accounted for the loss of vision in the last patient. Enucleation was necessary in a single patient because of tumor growth.

Lommatzsch has published results comparable with those achieved with ^{125}I or ^{60}Co plaque using β-particles from ruthenium 106 and rhubidium 106.[305] He notes a 10-year survival of 67% in 309 cases.[306]

The COMS, involving some 42 clinical centers and 6 central units carefully monitoring quality, is conducting two randomized clinical trials. The first trial compares enucleation with ^{125}I brachytherapy for melanomas 2.5 to 10 mm in height and as much as 16 mm in diameter. Eligible patients randomized to irradiation receive treatment with ^{125}I sources in a gold-backed plaque shielding the posterior tissues. A dose of 100 Gy is delivered at 50 to 125 cGy/hour at the apex of the tumor (for tumors 5–10-mm high and to 5 mm for tumors 2.5–5-mm high). The second trial tests the value of preoperative external-beam irradiation (2000 cGy in five fractions) versus enucleation alone for patients with large tumors.[173]

More than 1000 patients were entered into these controlled trials through 1991. Heavy-charged particle beams are being investigated, using cyclotron-produced protons at Massachusetts General Hospital and synchrocyclotron-generated helium ions at the Lawrence Laboratory at Berkeley. These beams were selected because of their sharp penumbra and the Bragg peak, describing the greater deposition of energy at a depth. Both facilities use careful patient evaluation before treatment and sophisticated immobilization procedures that allow precise positioning of ports guided by radiographic confirmation of the tumors, the bases of which are marked by tantalum rings sutured to the sclera around the margin demonstrated by transillumination and indirect ophthalmoscopy. For treatment, generally 4000 to 10,000 cGy (^{60}Co equivalent dose corrected for relative biologic effect [RBE] with a factor of 1.1) is delivered in five fractions over 8 to 10 days at Harvard. At Berkeley, 7000 or 8000 cGy (^{60}Co equivalent dose corrected for RBE 1.3) is delivered over five fractions.

With a relatively short follow-up period, Saunders and coworkers have reported that irradiation failed locally in 5 of 75 patients, and 18% had neovascular glaucoma.[307] Twenty patients received a 70-Gy equivalent dose. Because of the high local failure rate, the dose was increased to 80-Gy equivalent for the remaining 55 patients. The mean follow-up at the time of the reporting was only 18 months. Local recurrence was detected in 4 of 20 patients treated with 70-Gy equivalent, and 1 of the 55 patients treated to 80-Gy equivalent has recurred (mean follow-up in the latter group was 14 months). Of the 42 patients followed for more than 1 year, 10 had vision worse than 20/200.[307]

Between 1975 and 1981, 128 patients were treated at the Massachusetts General Hospital cyclotron. The results are reported with a median follow-up of 5.4 years. Vision seemed to be declining linearly, with 69% of patients having at least 20/200 visual acuity at 5 years. Eight eyes were enucleated because of complications (6%), and metastases developed in 20.5% of patients.[308] Poorer outcome was seen for thicker tumors and tumors located nearer the optic disk and fovea.[309]

Other Local Nonsurgical Techniques

Preliminary reports on the experimental use of microwave, ferromagnetic, or ultrasonically induced hyperthermia described tumor regression in most patients.[310–317] This technique has been used in association with radiation in some instances, with good results in tumor control with lower doses of irradiation.[312–317]

Lincoff and coworkers obtained discouraging results with cryotherapy of ocular melanomas in 4 patients.[318] There are anecdotal reports of successful treatments for small peripheral melanomas.[129,277,319,320] Documented evidence for the efficacy of these alternative approaches is scant.

Local Resection

Peyman and coworkers developed a technique of local sclerochorioretinal resection for choroidal melanomas.[321–325] After a series of photocoagulation treatments around the tumor to create a firm chorioretinal adhesion or an area of bare sclera, the tumor is surgically removed, along with the adjacent sclera and retina. The defect is replaced by a scleral graft. Peyman and coworkers suggested that surgical candidates should have the following:

1. No evidence of metastatic disease
2. The ability to tolerate general anesthesia
3. A tumor base no larger than 12 mm and tumor location at least three disk diameters from the optic disk
4. Exudative retinal detachment no larger than one third of the fundus
5. Clear media

After local resection, one third of the eyes needed enucleation because of complications, including vitreous hemorrhage and retinal detachment.[11–35] Shields and associates advocate the use of partial lamellar sclerouvectomy in selected cases.[326] Most authors report that patients treated by local resection are also amenable to radiation therapy and that early visual loss is far more frequent after surgical resection.[129,130,205,327] The risk of leaving viable tumor cells in the eye after resection is a matter of concern. For these reasons, this technique has not been adopted widely.

Iridocyclectomy has proved useful in the treatment of ciliary body melanomas in several series.[129,130,328,329] In the series of Forrest and associates of 107 iridocyclectomies for ciliary body melanoma, 6% of the patients had subsequent enucleation; most problems related to surgical management or to the tumor area occurred within 4 years of surgery.[328] Foulds and Damato, who promoted this method, have employed the approach for many years with good results.[329,330] In contrast to resection of choroidal melanomas, iridocyclectomy is widely accepted for the treatment of ciliary body melanomas.[329,330]

Enucleation

In the case of patients with a healthy second eye, enucleation is advised if the tumor shows evidence of rapid progression and invasion of the optic nerve or extraocular extension is suspected.[119,130,205] Other complications, including loss of central vision, failure of previous conservative treatment, and the patient's desires, may make enucleation the treatment of choice.

TREATMENT OF LARGE MELANOMAS OF THE CHOROID AND CILIARY BODY

Most clinicians agree that it would be inadvisable to treat cases of large melanoma by methods other than enucleation.[125,130,331] Possible exceptions include patients with the tumor occurring in their only seeing eye, occasional patients in whom vision can be salvaged by irradiation, and patients who refuse enucleation.[337] Abramson and Ellsworth recommend local irradiation in these latter difficult cases.[331,332]

Some authors recommend external irradiation before enucleation,[333–338] but convincing evidence for the usefulness of this therapy is still lacking.[338–340] This method is being evaluated currently in the COMS.[173,341]

Zimmerman and associates have suggested that when enucleation is carried out, the "no-touch" technique of Fraunfelder should be considered.[3,342] This method was designed to minimize the possibility of seeding of tumor cells into the blood vessels during enucleation. The authors claim that this technique avoids intraocular pressure elevations higher than 15 mm before complete freezing occurs around the tumor. Subsequently, cryotherapy prevents the flow of fluid and blood to or from the tumor before the manipulation necessary for enucleation. Although most surgeons do not use the no-touch technique, it is increasingly recognized that enucleation should be carried out by a surgeon skilled and experienced in the procedure and that surgery should be done with a minimum of unnecessary manipulation.[127–130,205,343]

TREATMENT OF MEDIUM-SIZED MELANOMAS OF THE CHOROID AND CILIARY BODY

Treatment of medium-sized tumors is the subject of current controversy. Although general agreement exists that observation of small melanomas carries little risk and that large melanomas should be enucleated, there is less consensus regarding medium-sized melanomas. Good results with radiation therapy using various modalities have been reported.[119,130,176,343–350] This method is unequivocally advocated in patients in whom the tumor occurs in their only seeing eye, in patients whose eyes retain useful vision, and in patients who refuse enucleation. However, in most instances, both treatment options remain possible, and personal choice is often the deciding factor. For these reasons, a nationwide, prospective, randomized comparison of radiation versus enucleation has been undertaken under the auspices of the National

Eye Institute "in order to demonstrate that either radiation or enucleation offers a better chance for survival, or that there is no difference in survival."[173,341] In this multicenter study, tumors 2.5 to 10 mm in height and no more than 16-mm basal diameter are randomized. Immunotherapy and chemotherapy have not been established as significantly useful modalities for primary or adjuvant treatment of medium-sized melanomas of the choroid or ciliary body.[351–354] However, in view of the likelihood of subclinical metastases being present at the time of diagnosis, a systemic treatment should be tested when an effective agent becomes available.

TREATMENT OF TUMORS WITH EXTRASCLERAL EXTENSION

Patients with extrascleral extension of an intraocular tumor have a poor prognosis.[139] Affeldt and coworkers reported that two thirds of 60 patients followed up after enucleation for uveal melanoma with extrascleral extension eventually died from metastatic disease.[355] Attempts should be made to detect extraocular extension preoperatively with ultrasound, CT, and MRI. At the time of surgery, the episcleral surface should be inspected carefully. These visual and imaging findings should be confirmed subsequently by frozen-section study.[3] Excision of adjacent Tenon's capsule and orbital tissue is then performed. The indications for primary or secondary exenteration remain controversial, because no clear evidence exists for an increase in life expectancy after exenteration compared with enucleation. Of 15 patients who underwent exenteration in the series reported by Starr and Zimmerman, only 1 survived longer than 13 months.[139] Affeldt and colleagues concluded that exenteration within 2 months after enucleation is beneficial.[355] In 1977, Shammas and Blodi initially reported good results of exenteration, particularly if the operation was performed promptly after recognition of residual tumor in the orbit.[138] However, a subsequent study of long-term results at the same institution showed little improvement in survival.[356] The usefulness of exenteration remains disputed.[356–359] Hykin and coworkers advocate postenucleation orbital radiation therapy in patients with extrascleral extension.[360]

METASTATIC DISEASE

Metastatic disease is observed in about 2% of patients at the time of diagnosis.[14,147,148,361] Fournier and coworkers[362] and Gronemeyer and coworkers[363] have suggested that local resection of solitary hepatic metastases in patients with uveal melanoma may be an effective palliative treatment and possibly lead to longer survival. Other authors have reported prolonged periods of remission after hepatic artery embolization.[366] Experimental studies using immunologic approaches are in progress,[365] but these tentative treatments are still anecdotal. Currently, metastatic melanoma is incurable and usually is treated palliatively with chemotherapy and radiation therapy (see Chap. 46).[205,366–369]

TREATMENT OF IRIS MELANOMA

In the past 30 years, gradual recognition of the better prognosis of iris melanoma has led to a conservative approach. Every effort is made to avoid enucleation in most cases.[128–130,182,189,190] Different options are possible, according to the clinical situation.

OBSERVATION

If the following factors are present, surgical intervention is not necessary:

1. There is no clinical evidence that the lesion is progressing.
2. There is a lack of pronounced neovascularization.
3. The lesion is not producing any visual disturbances.
4. No significant complications, such as hemorrhage into the anterior chamber, trabecular involvement, secondary glaucoma, and an obvious extension outside the eye, are evident.
5. The lesion arises in the only seeing eye.
6. The lesion is situated near the pupil.

CONSERVATION EXCISION

The anecdotal nature of reports on photocoagulation of iris melanomas does not allow definitive conclusions to be drawn.[370,371] Surgery should be considered if there is evidence of rapid tumor growth, the tumor interferes with vision, and the tumor induces noncontrollable secondary glaucoma.[129,130,271,372]

In 1958, Reese pointed out that iris melanoma, with or without ciliary body involvement, seldom metastasizes or spreads by seeding.[128] Iris melanomas are capable of local extension and infiltration. Subsequently, interest developed in the use of iridectomy, iridocyclectomy, and corneoscleroiridocyclectomy, with grafting, as alternatives to enucleation.[128–130] Although some authors advocate diagnostic needle biopsy of the iris lesion,[182,203,372] this procedure is usually not performed because of the risk of tumor dissemination.

The object of excisional iridectomy is to remove the tumor entirely without allowing tumor cells to disseminate in the eye or in the incision. The procedure is similar to that described by Reese, in which a limbal incision is made that is large enough to allow removal of the lesion by basal iridectomy under direct observation.[128] Iridectomy of peripheral tumors should be performed before the lesion extends to the trabecular meshwork. Some authors emphasize the local and systemic risks of delaying the removal of a growing tumor.[271,373] If the trabecular meshwork is involved in the quadrant of the tumor, inducing secondary glaucoma, iridotrabeculectomy is indicated. When the iris tumor extends to the ciliary body, iridocyclectomy must be considered, as was advocated by Raubitschek[376] and Verhoeff[375] many years ago and introduced into clinical practice through the efforts of Muller and associates[376] and Stallard.[377,378] A basic technique for resecting the iris tumor together with involved ciliary body has been reported by Jones.[379] Many patients requiring more extensive surgery than iridectomy for iris tumor removal also require an operation more extensive than iridocyclectomy. Examples are patients in whom the tumor not only invades the ciliary body but also fills the chamber angle and is adjacent to the tissue in the angle or to the cornea itself. In such cases, the surgeon should consider corneoscleroiridocyclectomy with or without a corneoscleral graft.[129,130,329] Surgical complications include intraocular hemorrhage, hypotony, subluxation of the lens, cataract, late detachment of the retina, corneal edema, macular edema, and vitreous loss. If the excision is incomplete, tumor may recur. Therefore, the finding of spindle B cells should lead to frequent and extremely thorough follow-up examinations. If similar numbers of epithelioid cells are disclosed histopathologically, their lack of cohesiveness argues toward enucleation in view of a high risk for recurrence and exteriorization.[182]

ENUCLEATION

Enucleation for an iris melanoma is not exceptional but must be considered in individual cases if the following conditions exist:

1. The melanoma is clearly growing and involves more than half the iris and anterior chamber angle.
2. The tumor, growing in a blind eye, is too bulky to be removed by excision.
3. There is a secondary glaucoma refractory to medical treatment, particularly after vision is lost.
4. Histopathologic features point toward a high risk for recurrence or exteriorization, or both.
5. Extraocular extension is present.
6. The tumor has recurred after previous iridectomy or iridocyclectomy and is judged unsuitable for further treatment.

In the case of extraocular spread or metastatic disease, or both, the treatment is the same as for advanced choroidal or ciliary body melanomas.

REFERENCES

1. Rawles ME. Origin of pigment cells from neural crest in mouse embryos. Physiol Zool 1947;20:248–266.
2. Zimmerman LE. Melanocytes, melanocytic nevi, and melanocytomas. Invest Ophthalmol Vis Sci 1965;4:11–41.
3. Zimmerman LE. Malignant melanoma of the uveal tract. In: Spencer WH, ed. Ophthalmic pathology. Vol 3. Philadelphia: WB Saunders, 1986:2072–2139.
4. Green WR. The uvea. In: Spencer WH, ed. Ophthalmic pathology. Vol 3. Philadelphia: WB Saunders, 1986:1352–2072.
5. Scotto, J, Fraumeni JF, Lee JAH. Melanomas of the eye and other noncutaneous sites. JNCI 1976;56:489–491.
6. Young JL, Percy CL, Asire AJ, et al. Cancer incidence and mortality in the United States, 1973–1977. Cancer Inst Monogr 1981;57:1–187.
7. Egan KM, Seddon JM, Gradoudas ES, et al. Uveal melanoma in New England: Profile of cases diagnosed in 1984 to 1985. Invest Ophthalmol Vis Sci 1987;28(Suppl):144.
8. Abrahamson M. Malignant melanoma of the choroid and the ciliary body, 1956–1975. Acta Ophthalmol (Copenh) 1982;61:600–610.
9. Gislason I, Magnussen G, Tulinius H. Malignant melanoma of the uvea in Iceland, 1955–1979. Acta Ophthalmol (Copenh) 1985;63:385–394.
10. Cutler SJ, Young JL, eds. Third National Cancer Survey: Incidence data. NCI Monogr 1975;41:1–454.
11. Chang JC. Personal communication. St. Louis, Missouri Department of Social Services, Division of Health, October 4, 1983.
12. Kuo PK, Puliafito CA, Wang KM, et al. Uveal melanoma in China. Int Ophthalmol Clin 1982;22:57–71.
13. Teikari JM, Rairio I. Incidence of choroidal melanoma in Finland in the years 1973–1980. Acta Ophtlamol (Copenh) 1985;63:661–665.
14. Graham BJ, Duane TD. Meetings, conferences, symposia: Report of the Ocular Melanoma Task Force. Am J Ophthalmol 1981;90:728–733.
15. Haukulin T, Teppo L, Saxen F. Cancer of the eye: A review of trends and differentials. World Health Stat Q 1978;31:143–158.
16. Jensen QA, Prause JU. Malignant melanomas of the human uvea in Denmark: Incidence and a 25-year follow-up of cases diagnosed between 1943 and 1952, In: Lommatzsch PK, Blodi FC, eds. Intraocular tumors. Berlin: Springer-Verlag, 1983:85–92.
17. Strickland D, Lee JHA. Melanomas of the eye: Stability of rates. Am J Epidemiol 1981;113:700–702.
18. Swerdlow AJ. Epidemiology of eye cancer in adults in England and Wales, 1962–1977. Am J Epidemiol 1983;118:294–300.
19. Houghton, A, Flannery J, Viola MV. Malignant melanoma in Connecticut and Denmark. Int J Cancer 1980;25:95–104.
20. Rosenbaum PS, Boniuk M, Font RL. Diffuse uveal melanoma in a 5-year-old child. Am J Ophthalmol 1988;106:601–6060.
21. Barr CC, McLean IW, Zimmerman LE. Uveal melanoma in children and adolescents. Arch Ophthalmol 1981;95:2133–2134.
22. Shields CL, Shields JA, Milite J, et al. Uveal melanoma in teenagers and children. Ophthalmology 1991;98:1662–1666.
23. Jensen OA. Malignant melanoma of the uvea in Denmark, 1943–1952: A clinical, histopathological and prognostic study. Acta Ophthalmol 1963;75(Suppl):1–200.
24. Apt L. Uveal melanomas in children and adolescents. Int Ophthalmol Clin 1962;2: 403–410.
25. Fledelius H, Land A. Malignant melanoma of the choroid in an 11-month-old infant. Acta Ophthalmol 1975;53:1 160–166.
26. Jones ST. Choroidal malignant melanoma in a child. Br J Ophthalmol 1967;51:489–491.
27. Verdauger J. Prepubertal and pubertal melanomas in ophthalmology. Am J Ophthalmol 1965;60:1002–1011.
28. Raivo I. Uveal melanoma in Finland: An epidemiological, clinical, histological and prognostic study. Acta Ophthalmol 1977;133(Suppl):3–64.
29. Egan KM, Seddon JM, Glynn RJ, et al. Epidemiologic aspects of uveal melanoma. Surv Ophthalmol 1988;32:239–251.
30. Paul EV, Parnell BL, Fraker M. Prognosis of malignant melanomas of the choroid and ciliary body. Int Ophthalmol Clin 1968;5:387–402.
31. Malik MOA, El Sheikh EH. Tumors of the ey and adnexa in the Sudan. Cancer 1979;44: 293–303.
32. Miller B, Abraham C, Cole CG, et al. Ocular malignant melanoma in South African blacks. Br J Ophthalmol 1981;65:720–722.
33. Swerlow AJ. Epidemiology of melanoma of the ey in the Oxford region, 1952–78. Br J Cancer 1983;47:311–313.
34. Albert DM, Scheie HG. Nevus of Ota with malignant melanoma of the choroid. Arch Ophthalmol 1963;69:774–777.
35. Body FC. Ocular melanocytes and melanoma. Am J Ophthalmol 1975;80:389.
36. Dutton JJ, Anderson RL, Schelper RL, et al. Orbital malignant melanoma and oculodermal melanocytes: Report of two cases and review of the literature. Ophthalmology 1984;91:946–507.
37. Gonder JR, Shields JA, Albert DM, et al. Uveal malignant melanoma associated with ocular and oculodermal melanocytosis. Ophthalmology 1982;89:953–960.
38. Yanoff M, Zimmerman LE. Histogenesis of malignant melanomas of the uvea: III. The relationship of congenital ocular melanocytosis and neurofibromatosis to uveal melanomas. Arch Ophthalmol 1967;77:331–336.
39. Gartner S. Malignant melanoma of the choroid in von Recklinghausen's disease. Am J Ophthalmol 1940;23:73–78.
40. Yanoff M, Zimmerman LE. Histogenesis of malignant melanomas of the uvea: II. Relationship of uveal nevi to the malignant melanomas. Cancer 1967;20:497–507.
41. Volker HE, Naumann GO. Multicentric primary malignant melanomas of the choroid: Two separate malignant melanomas of the choroid and two uveal nevi in one eye. Br J Ophthalmol 1978;62:408–413.
42. Sahel JA, Albert DM. Choroidal nevi. In: Ryan SJ, ed: Retina. Vol 1. St Louis: CV Mosby, 1989:625–637.
43. Albert DM, Lahav M, Packer S, et al. Histogenesis of malignant melanomas of the uvea: Occurrence of nevus-like structures in experimental choroidal tumors. Arch Ophthalmol 1974;92:318–323.
44. Gass JDM. Stereoscopic atlas of macular diseases. St Louis: CV Mosby, 1987:182–195.
45. Margo CE, Paven PR, Gendelman D, et al. Bilateral melanocyte uveal tumors associated with systemic non-ocular malignancy: Malignant melanomas or benign paraneoplastic syndrome. Retina 1987;7:137–141.
46. Walker JP, Weiter JJ, Albert, DM, et al. Uveal malignant melanoma in three generations of the same family. Am J Ophthalmol 1979;88:723–726.
47. Lynch H, Anderson D, Krush A. Heredity and intraocular malignant melanoma: Study of two families and review of 45 cases. Cancer 1968;21:119–125.
48. Reese AB. Tumors of the eye. 3rd ed. Hagerstown, MD: Harper & Row, 1976: 177–178.
49. Reese AB. Association of uveal nevi with skin nevi. Arch Ophthalmol 1952;48:271–275.
50. Albert DM, Chang MA, Lamping KA, et al. The dysplastic nevus syndrome: A pedigree with primary malignant melanomas of the choroid and skin. Ophthalmology 1985;92: 1728–1734.
51. Albert DM, Searl SS, Forget B, et al. Uveal findings in patients with cutaneous melanoma. Am J Ophthalmol 1987;95:474–479.
52. Rodriquez-Sains RS. Ocular findings in patients with dysplastic nevus syndrome. Ophthalmology 1986;93:661–665.
53. Taylor MR, Guerry D IV, Dondl EE, et al. Lack of association between intraocular melanoma and cutaneous dysplastic nevi. Am J Ophthalmol 1984;98:478–482.
54. Turner BJ, Statkowski RM, Ausberger JJ, et al. Other cancers in uveal melanoma patients and their families. Am J Ophthalmol 1989;107:601–608.
55. Lischko AM, Seddon JM, Gragoudas ES, et al. Evaluation of prior primary malignancy as a determinant of uveal melanoma: A case-control study. Ophthalmology 1989;96: 1716–1721.
56. Holly EA, Ashton DA, Ahn DK, et al. No excess prior cancer in patients with uveal melanoma. Ophthalmology 1991;98:608–611.

57. Mukai S, Dryja TP. Loss of alleles at polymorphic loci on chromosome 2 in uveal melanoma. Cancer Genet Cytogenet 1986;22:45–53.
58. Albert DM. The association of viruses with uveal melanoma. Trans Am Ophthalmol Soc 1980;77:367–421.
59. Albert DM, Shadduck JA, Lin HS, et al. Animal models for the study of uveal melanomas. Int Ophthalmol Clin 1980;20:143–160.
60. Albert DM. Need for animal models of human diseases of the eye. Am J Pathol 1980;101:177–185.
61. Albert DM. Ocular melanoma: A challenge to visual science. Invest Ophthalmol Vis Sci 1982;23:550–580.
62. Albert DM, Puliafito CA, Fulton AB, et al. Increased incidence of choroidal malignant melanoma occurring in a single population of chemical workers. Am J Ophthalmol 1980;89:323–337.
63. Keeny AH, Waddell WJ, Perraut TC. Carcinogenesis and nicotine in malignant melanoma of the choroid. Trans Am Ophthalmol Soc 1987;80:131–142.
64. Albert DM, Gonder JR, Papale J, et al. Induction of ocular neoplasms in Fischer rats by introcular injection of nickle subsulfide. Invest Ophthalmol Vis Sci 1982;22:768–782.
65. Evgenyeva TP. Pigmented tumors in rats induced by introduction of platinum and cellophane films into the chamber of the eye. Buill Eksp Biol Med (Moscow) 1972;74: 76–77.
66. Patz A, Wulff LB, Rogers SW. Experimental production of ocular tumors. Am J Ophthalmol 1959;48:98–111.
67. Benson WR. Intraocular tumor after ethionine and *N*-2-fluorenyl-acetamide. Arch Pathol 1962;73:404–406.
68. Taylor GH, Dougherty TF, Mays CW, et al. Radium-induced eye melanomas in dogs. Radiat Res 1972;51:361–373.
69. Albert DM, Puliafito CA, Haluska FG, et al. Induction of ocular neoplasms in Wistar rats by *N*-methyl-*N*-nitrosourea. Exp Eye Res 1986;42:83–86.
70. Folberg R, Baron J, Reeves RD, et al. Animal model of conjunctival primary acquired melanomas. Ophthalmology 1989;96:1006–1013.
71. Van Rens GH, DeJohn P, Demols E, et al. Uveal malignant melanoma and levodopa therapy in Parkinson's disease. Ophthalmology 1982;89:1464–1466.
72. Hartge P, Tucker MA, Shields JA, et al. Case-control study of female hormones and eye melanoma. Cancer Res 1989;49:4622–2625.
73. Seddon JM, MacLaughlin DT, Albert DM, et al. Uveal melanomas presenting during pregnancy and the investigation of estrogen receptors in melanomas. Br J Ophthalmol 1982;66:695–704.
74. Shields CL, Shields JA, Eagle RC Jr, et al. Uveal melanoma and pregnancy. Ophthalmology 1991;98:1667–1673.
75. Tucker MA, Shields JA, Hartge P, et al. Sunlight exposure as risk factor for malignant melanoma. N Engl J Med 1985;313:789–792.
76. Seddon JM, Gragoudas ES, Glynn RJ, et al. Host factors, UV radiation, and risk of uveal melanoma: A case control study. Arch Ophthalmol 1990;108:1274–1280.
77. Holly EA, Aston DA, Char DH, et al. Uveal melanoma in relation to ultraviolet light exposure and host factors. Cancer Res 1990;50:5773–5777.
78. Edwood JM, Lee JA, Walter SD, et al. Relationship of melanoma and other skin cancer mortality to latitude and ultraviolet radiation in the United States and Canada. Int J Epidemiol 1972;3:325–332.
79. Kliman GH, Augsburger JJ, Shields JA. Association between iris color and iris melanocytic lesions. Am J Ophthalmol 1985;100:547–548.
80. Kan-Mitchell J, Rao N, Albert DM, et al. S-100 immunopheotypes of uveal melanomas. Invest Ophthalmol Vis Sci 1990;31:1492–1496.
81. Beckenkamp G, Schafer HJ, Von Domarus D. Immunocytochemical parameters in ocular malignant melanomas. Eur J Cancer Clin Oncol 1988;24:542–645.
82. Van Der Pol JP, Jager MJ, DeWolff-Rouendaal D, et al. Heterogeneous expression of melanoma-associated antigens in uveal melanomas.
83. Bomanji J, Garner A, Prasad J, et al. Characterization of ocular melanoma with cutaneous melanoma antibodies. Br J Ophthalmol 1987;71:647–650.
84. Natali PG, Bigotti A, Necotra MR, et al. Analysis of the antigenic profile of uveal melanoma lesions with anti-cutaneous melanoma-associated antigen and anti-HLA monoclonal antibodies. Cancer Res 1989;49:1269–1274.
85. Damato BE, Campbell AM, McGuire BJ, et al. Monoclonal antibodies to uveal melanoma. Eye 1987;1:686–690.
86. Callender GR. Malignant melanotic tumors of the eye: A study of histologic types in 111 cases. Trans Am Acad Ophthalmol Otolaryngol 1931;36:131–142.
87. Zimmerman LE, Sobin LH. International histological classification of tumors: Histological typing of tumors of the eye and its adnexa. No. 24. Geneva: World Health Organization, 1980.
88. McLean IW, Foster WD, Zimmerman LE, et al. Modification of Callender's classification of uveal melanoma at the Armed Forces Institute of Pathology. Am J Ophthalmol 1983;96:502–509.
89. McLean IW, Zimmerman LE, Evans RM. Reappraisal of Callender's spindle A type of malignant melanoma of the choroid and ciliary body. Am J Ophthalmol 1978;86: 557–564.
90. McLean IW, Foster MD, Zimmerman LE. Uveal melanoma: Location, size, cell type and enucleation as risk factors in metastasis. Hum Pathol 1981;13:123–132.
91. Gass JDM. Problems in the differential diagnosis of choroidal nevi and malignant melanomas. Am J Ophthalmol 1977;83:299–323.
92. Gamel JW, McLean IW. Quantitative analysis of the Callender classification of uveal melanoma cells. Arch Ophthalmol 1977;95:686–691.
93. Collaborative Ocular Melanoma Study manual of procedures. National Technical Information Service. NTIS PB90-115536. Springfield, VA, 1989.
94. Gamel JW, McLean IW. Modern developmenst in histopathologic assessment of uveal melanomas. Ophthalmology 1984;91:679–684.
95. Gamel JW, McLean IW, Greckey RA, et al. Objective assessment of the malignant potential of intraocular melanomas with standard microslides stained with hematoxylin-eosin. Hum Pathol 1985;16:689–692.
96. Donoso LA, Augsburger JJ, Shields JA, et al. Metastatic uveal melanoma: Correlation between survival time and cytomorphology of primary tumors. Arch Ophthalmol 1986;104:76–82.
97. Wilder HC, Callender GR. Malignant melanoma of the choroid: Further studies on prognosis by histologic type and fiber content. Am J Ophthalmol 1939;22:851–855.
98. Seddon JM, Polivogianis L, Hsieh CC, et al. Death from uveal melanoma: Number of epithelioid cells and inverse SD of nucleolar areas as prognostic factors. Arch Ophthalmol 1987;105:801–806.
99. McCurdy JB, Gamel JW, McLean IW. A simple, efficient, and reproducible method for determining the malignant potential of uveal melanoma. Invest Ophthalmol Vis Sci 1991;32(ARVO Suppl):1197.
100. Seddon JM, Albert DM, Lavin PT, et al. A prognostic factor study of disease-free interval and survival following enucleation for uveal melanoma. Arch Ophthalmol 1983;101:1894–1899.
101. Lavin PT, Albert DM, Seddon JM, et al. A deficit survival analysis to assess the history of uveal melanoma. J Clin Dis 1984;37:481–487.
102. McLean IW, Foster WD, Zimmerman LE. Prognostic factors in small malignant melanomas of the choroid and ciliary body. Arch Ophthalmol 1977;95:48–58.
103. Bardenstein DS, Char DH, Kaleta-Michaels S, et al. Ki-67 and bromodeoxyuridine labelling of human choroidal melanoma cells. Curr Eye Res 1991;10:479–484.
104. Char DH. DNA cell cycle studies in uveal melanoma. Trans Am Ophthalmol Soc 1989;86:561–580.
105. Rennie IG, Ress RC, Parsons MA, et al. Estimation of DNA content in uveal melanomas by flow cytometry. Eye 1989;3:611–617.
106. Chen TC, Char DH, Waldman F, et al. Flow cytometry measurement of nuclear RNA content in uveal melanoma. Ophthalmic Res 1990;22:187–193.
107. McLean IW, Gamel JW. Prediction of metastasis of uveal melanoma: Comparison of spectrophotometric determination of DNA. Invest Ophthalmol Vis Sci 1988;29:507–511.
108. Marcus DM, Minkovitz JB, Wardwell SD, et al. The value of nucleolar organizer regions in uveal melanoma. Am J Ophthalmol 1990;110:527–534.
109. Jensen OA. Malignant melanomas of the human uvea: Recent follow-up of cases in Denmark, 1943–1952. Acta Ophthalmol 1970;46:1113–1128.
110. Jensen OA. Malignant melanomas of the human uvea: 25-year follow-up of cases in Denmark, 1943–1952. Acta Ophthalmol 1982;60:161–182.
111. Durie FH, Campbell AM, Lee WR, et al. Analysis of lymphocytic infiltration in uveal melanoma. Invest Ophthalmol Vis Sci 1990;31:2106–2110.
112. Nitta R, Oksenberg JR, Rao NA, et al. Predominant expression of T cell receptor V alpha 7 in tumor infiltrating lymphocytes of uveal melanoma. Science 1990;248: 671–674.
113. Knisely T, Niederkorn JY. Immunologic evaluation of spontaneous regression of an intraocular murine melanoma. Invest Ophthalmol Vis Sci 1990;31:247–257.
114. Richardson JT, Burns RP, Misfeldt ML. Association of uveal melanocyte destruction in melanoma-bearing swine with large granular lymphocyte cells. Invest Ophthalmol Vis Sci 1989;30:2455–2460.
115. Niederkorn JY, Benson JL. Differential expression of tumor-specific cytotoxic T lymphocyte activity and delayed type hypersensitivity in the anterior chamber of the eye. Invest Ophthalmol Vis Sci 1991;32(ARVO Suppl):937.
116. Curtin VT, Cavender JC. Natural course of selected malignant melanomas of the choroid and ciliary body. Mod Prob Ophthalmol 1974;12:523–527.
117. McLean IW, Foster MD, Zimmerman LE, et al. Inferred natural history of uveal melanoma. Invest Ophthalmol Vis Sci 1980;19:760–770.
118. Char DH, Heilborn DL, Juster RR, et al. Choroidal melanoma growth patterns. Br J Ophthalmol 1983;67:575–578.
119. Gass JDM. Comparison of uveal melanoma growth rates with mitotic index mortality. Arch Ophthalmol 1985;103:924–931.
120. Char DH, Hogan MJ. Management of small elevated pigmented choroidal lesions. Br J Ophthalmol 1977;61:54–58.
121. Curtin VT. Choroidal and ciliary body malignant melanomas. Mod Prob Ophthalmol 1979;20:115–120.
122. Friberg TR, Finchberg E, McQuaig S. Extremely rapid growth of a primary choroidal melanoma. Arch Ophthalmol 1983;11:1376–1377.
123. Sahel JA, Pesavento R, Frederick AR Jr, et al. Uveal melanoma arising de novo over a 16-month period. Arch Ophthalmol 1988;106:381–385.
124. Manschot WA, van Peperzeel HA. Choroidal melanoma: Enucleation or observation? A new approach. Arch Ophthalmol 1980;98:71–77.
125. Augsburger JJ, Gonder JR, Amsel J, et al. Growth rates and doubling time of posterior uveal melanomas. Ophthalmology 1984;91:1709–1715.
126. Lambert JR, Char DH, Howes E Jr, et al. Spontaneous regression of a choroidal melanoma. Arch Ophthalmol 1988;104:732–734.
127. Brini A, Dhermy P, Sahel J. Oncology of the eye and adnexa: Atlas of clinical pathology. In: Monographs in Ophthalmology Series. Vol. 13. Dordrecht: Kluwer, 1990:143.
128. Reese AB. Tumors of the eye. 3rd ed. Hagerstown, MD: Harper & Row, 1976:174–262.
129. Shields JA. Diagnosis and management of intraocular tumors. St Louis: CV Mosby, 1983:75–254.
130. Char DH. Clinical ocular oncology. New York: Churhill Livingstone, 1989:91–166.
131. Font RL, Zimmerman LE, Armaly MF. The nature of the orange pigment over a

choroidal melanoma: Histochemical and electron microscopic observation. Arch Ophthalmol 1974;91:359–365.
132. Dunn WJ, Lambert HM, Kincaid MC, et al. Choroidal melanoma with early vitreous seeding. Retina 1988;8:155–192.
133. Yanoff M. Glaucoma mechanism in ocular malignant melanomas. Am J Ophthalmol 1970;70:898–904.
134. El Baba F, Hagler WS, De la Cruz A, et al. Choroidal melanoma with pigment dispersion into the vitreous and melanomalytic glaucoma. Ophthalmology 1988;956:370–376.
135. Shammas HF, Blodi FC. Prognostic factors in choroidal and ciliary body melanomas. Arch Ophthalmol 1977;95:63–69.
136. Font RL, Spaulding AG, Zimmerman LE. Diffuse malignant melanoma of the uveal tract: A clinicopathologic report of 56 cases. Trans Am Acad Ophthalmol Otolaryngol 1968;72:877–894.
137. Duffin RM, Straatsma BR, Foos RY, et al. Small malignant melanoma of the choroid with extraocular extension. Arch Ophthalmol 1981;99:1027–1020.
138. Shammas HF, Blodi FC. Orbital extension of choroidal and ciliary body melanomas. Arch Ophthalmol 1977;93:2002–2005.
139. Starr HJ, Zimmerman LE. Extrascleral extension and orbital recurrence of a malignant melanoma of the choroid and ciliary body. Int Ophthalmol Cent V 1962;2:369–385.
140. Affeldt JC, Minckler DS, Azen SP, et al. Prognosis in uvealmelanoma with extrascleral extension. Arch Ophthalmol 1980;98:1975–1979.
141. Pach JM, Robertson DM, Taney BS, et al. Prognostic factors in choroidal and ciliary body melanomas with extrascleral extension. Am J Ophthalmol 1988;101:325–331.
142. Packard RBS. Pattern of mortality in choroidal malignant melanoma. Br J Ophthalmol 1980;64:565–573.
143. Shammas HF, Blodi FC. Peripapillary choroidal melanomas: Extension along the optic nerve and its sheaths. Arch Ophthalmol 1978;96:440–444.
144. Chess J, Albert DM, Bellows AR, et al. Uveal melanoma: Case report of extension through the optic nerve to the surgical margin in the orbital apex. Br J Ophthalmol 1984;68:272–275.
145. Ruiz RS. Early treatment in malignant melanomas of the choroid. In: Brockhurst RJ, Boruchoff SA, Hutchinson BT, et al, eds. Controversy in ophthalmology. Philadelphia: WB Saunders, 1977:604–610.
146. Lock-Anderson J, Partoft S, Jensen MG. Patterns of the first lymph node metastases in patients with cutaneous malignant melanoma of axial localization. Cancer [Abstract] 1988;62:9.
147. Pack JM, Robertson DM. Matastases from untreated uveal melanomas. Arch Ophthalmol 1986;104:1624–1625.
148. Wagoner MD, Albert DM. The incidence of metastases from untreated ciliary body and choroidal melanoma. Arch Ophthalmol 1982;100:939–940.
149. Fornabio DM, Alterman AL, Stackpole CW. Matastatic dissemination of B16 melanoma: Evidence that metastases can result from non-specific trapping of disseminated cells. Invasion Metastasis 1988;8:1–16.
150. Albelda SM, Mette SP, Elder DE, et al. Integrin distribution in malignant melanoma: Association of the B3 subunit with tumor progression. Cancer Res 1990;50:6757–6764.
151. Kath R, Jambrosio J, Holland L, et al. Development of invasive and growth factor independent cell variants from primary melanoma. Cancer Res 1991;51:4853–4858.
152. Hart IR, Brich M. Cell adhesion receptors in melanoma progression and metastasis: The biology of melanoma. In: The 35th Annual Clinical Conference and 24th Annual Special Pathology Program: Advances in the biology and clinical management of melanoma. Houston, November 20–23, 1991:8.
153. Raz A. Tumor cell migration and the metastatic cascade: The biology of melanoma. In: The 35th Annual Clinical Conference and 24th Annual Special Pathology Program: Advances in the biology and clinical management of melanoma. Houston, November 20–23, 1991:9–10.
154. Price JE, Zhang RD. Melanoma brain metastasis. The biology of melanoma. In: The 35th Annual Clinical Conference and 24th Annual Special Pathology Program: Advances in the biology and clinical management of melanoma. Houston, November 20–23, 1991:10, 11.
155. Fidler IJ, Nicholson CJ. Organ selectiveity for implantation survival and growth of B16 melanoma. JNCI 1976;57:1199–1201.
156. Donoso LA, Nagy RM, McFall RC, et al. Metastatic choroidal melanoma: Hepatic binding protein reactivity toward a liver metastasizing clone. Arch Ophthalmol 1983;101:787–790.
157. Zimmerman LE. Gamma-glutamyl transpeptidase in the prognosis of patients with uveal melanomas. Am J Ophthalmol 1983;96:409–411.
158. Pascal SG, Saulenas AM, Fourner GA, et al. An investigation into the association between liver damage and metastatic uveal melanoma. Am J Ophthalmol 1985;100: 448–453.
159. Gragoudas ES, Egan KM, Seddon JM, et al. Survival of patients with metastases from uveal melanoma. Ophthalmology 1991;98:383–390.
160. Zimmerman LE. Does enucleation of the eye containing a malignant melanoma prevent or accelerate the dissemination of tumor cells? Br J Ophthalmol 1978;62:420–425.
161. Fraunfelder FT, Boozman FW, Wilson RS, et al. No-touch technique for intraocular malignant melanomas. Arch Ophthalmol 1977;95:1616–1620.
162. Niederkorn JY, Streihlen JW. Intracamerally induced concommitant immunity: Mice harboring progressively growing intraocular tumors are immune to spontaneous metastases and secondary tumor challenge. J Immunol 1983;131:2587–2594.
163. Niederkorn JY. Enucleation-induced metastasis of intraocular melanoma in mice. Ophthalmology 1984;91:692–700.
164. Seigel D, Myers M, Ferris F III, et al. Survival rates after enucleation of eyes with malignant melanomas. Am J Ophthalmol 1979;87:761–765.
165. Kersten RC, Blodi FC. Prognosis of choroidal melanomas. Ophthal Forum 1983;1: 21–27.
166. Davidorf FH. The melanoma controversy: A comparison of choroidal, cutaneous, and iris melanomas. Surv Ophthalmol 1981;25:373–377.
167. Albert DM. Towards resolving the ocular melanoma controversy. Arch Ophthalmol 1979;97:431–432.
168. Kidd MN, Cyness RW, Patterson CC, et al. Prognostic factors in malignant melanomas of the choroid: A retrospective survey of cases occurring in Northern Ireland between 1965 and 1980. Trans Ophthalmol Soc UK 1986;105:114–121.
169. Seddon JM, Egan KM, Gragoudas ES. Choroidal melanoma: Prognosis. In: Ryan SJ, ed. Retina. Vol 1. St Louis: CV Mosby, 1989:363–373.
170. Gamel JW, McLean IW, Greenberg RA. Interval by interval Cox model analysis of 3480 cases of intraocular melanoma shows a decline in the prognostic value of size and cell type over time after tumor excision. Cancer 1988;61:574–579.
171. Seddon JM, Gragnodas ES, Egan KM, et al. Relative survival rates after alternative therapy for uveal melanoma. Ophthalmology 1990;97:769–777.
172. Augsburger JJ, Gamel JW. Log normal distribution of uveal melanoma deaths following cobalt 60 plaque. Invest Ophthalmol Vis Sci 1991;32(ARVO Suppl):980.
173. COMS Group: Collaborative ocular melanoma study manual of procedures. National Technical Information Service, Springfield, VA, 1989. NTIS Accession No. PB90-115536.
174. Shields JA. Introduction to the management of posterior uveal melanomas. In: Ryan SJ, Ogden TE, Schchat AP, eds. Retina. Vol 1. St Louis: CV Mosby, 1989:683–686.
175. Augsburger JJ, Gamel JW, Shields JA, et al. Post-irradiation regression of choroidal melanomas as risk factor for death from metastatic disease. Ophthalmology 1987;94: 1173–1177.
176. Abramson DH, Servodidio CA, McCormick B, et al. Changes in height of choroidal melanomas after plaque therapy. Br J Ophthalmol 1990;74:359–362.
177. Guthoff R, Hasse J, Von Domarus D, et al. Regression behavior of choroidal melanoma after radiotherapy: A new prognosis parameter. Klin Monatsbl Augenheilkd 1990;196: 6–10.
178. Glynn RJ, Seddon JM, Gragoudas ES, et al. Evaluation of tumor regression and other prognostic factors for early and late metastasis after proton irradiation of uveal melanoma. Ophthalmology 1989;96:1566–1573.
179. Grange JD, Thacoor S, Bienvelez B, et al. Comparative study of the speed of tumor regression in 127 uveal melanomas treated with ^{106}Ru/^{106}Ru: Correlations between cytologic analysis, histopathology of enucleated eyes and tumor regression on one hand, vital prognosis on the other hand. Ophthalmologie 1990;4:221–224.
180. Manschot WA, Van Strik R. Choroidal melanoma: Analysis of published therapeutic results. Forschr Ophthalmol 1987;84:183–186.
181. Adams KS, Abramson DH, Ellsworth RM, et al. Cobalt plaques versus enucleation for uveal melanoma: Comparison of survival rates. Br J Ophthalmol 1988;72:494–497.
182. Jakobiec FA, Silbert G. Are most iris "melanomas" really nevi. Arch Ophthalmol 1981;99:2117–2132.
183. Holland G. Zur Klinik und Pathologie der Pigmenttumoren der Iris. Klin Monatsbl Augenheilkd 1967;150:359–370.
184. Rones B, Zimmerman LE. The prognosis of primary tumors of the iris treated by iridectomy. Arch Ophthalmol 1964;60:193–205.
185. Ashton N. Primary tumors of the iris. Br J Opththalmol 1964;48:65–68.
186. Heath P. Tumors of the iris: Classification and clinical follow-up. Trans Am Ophthalmol Soc 1964;62:51.
187. Duke JR, Dunn SN. Primary tumors of the iris. Arch Ophthalmol 1958;59:204.
188. Colt CA, Sahel JA, Seddon JM. unpublished data.
189. Reese AB. Tumors of the eye. 3rd ed. Hagerstown, MD: Harper & Row, 1976:229–262.
190. Cleasby GW. Malignant melanom of the iris. Arch Ophthalmol 1958;60:403–417.
191. Arentsen JJ, Green WR. Melanoma of the iris: Report of 72 cases treated surgically. Ophthalmic Surg 1975;6:23–32.
192. Green WR. The uveal tract. In: Spencer WH, ed. Ophthalmic pathology. Vol 3. Philadelphia: WB Saunders, 1986:1300–1342.
193. Zimmerman LE. Histologic considerations in the management of tumors of the iris and ciliary body. Ann Inst Barraquer 1972;10:27–56.
194. Kersten RC, Tse D, Andersen DR. Iris melanoma: Nevus or malignancy? Surv Ophthalmology 1985;29:423–433.
195. Shields JA. Melanocytic tumors of the iris. In: Shields JA, ed. Diagnosis and management of intraocular tumors. St Louis, CV Mosby, 1983:
196. Char DH. Anterior uveal tumors. In: Char DH, ed. Clinical ocular oncology. New York: Churchill Livingstone, 1989:
197. Apple D, Blodi FC. Pathologic observations and clinical approach to uveal melanomas. In: Nicholson D, ed. Ocular pathology update. New York: Masson Publishing, 1980: 213–226.
198. Sunba MN, Rahj AHS, Morgan G. Tumors of the anterior uveal tract: I. Metastasizing malignant melanoma of the iris. Arch Ophthalmol 1980;98:82–85.
199. Deuble K, McCartney A. Nucleolar organizer regions in iris melanocytic tumors: An accurate predictor? Eye 1990;4:743–750.
199a. Marcus DM, Mawn LA, Egan KM, Albert DM. Nucleolar organizer regions in iris nevi and melanoma. Am J Ophthalmol 1992;114:202–207.
200. Geisse LJ, Robertson DM. Iris melanomas. Am J Ophthalmol 1985;99:638.
201. McGalliard JN, Johnston PB. A study of iris melanoma in Northern Ireland. Br J Opthalmol 1989;73:591.
202. Planten JT. An unnecessary mistake. Ophthalmologica 1970;160:369.

203. Grossniklaus HE, Brown RH, Stulting RD, et al. Iris melanoma seeding through a trabeculectomy site. Arch Ophthalmol 1990;1287:
204. Ferry AP. Lesions mistaken for malignant melanoma of the posterior uvea: A clinicopathologic analysis of 100 cases with ophthalmoscopically visible lesions. Arch Ophthalmol 1964;72:463–469.
205. Shields JA, Zimmerman LE. Lesions simulating malignant melanoma of the posterior uvea. Arch Ophthalmol 1973;89:466–471.
206. Zimmerman LE. Problems in the diagnosis of malignant melanomas of the choroid and ciliary body. Am J Ophthalmol 1973;75:917–929.
207. Chang M, Zimmerman LE, McLean IW. The persisting pseudomelanoma problem. Arch Ophthalmol 1984;102:726–727.
208. Robertson DM, Campbell RJ. Errors in the diagnosis of malignant melanoma of the choroid. Am J Opthalmol 1979;87:269–275.
209. Daviddorf FH, Letson AD, Weiss ET, et al. Incidence of misdiagnosed and unsuspected choroidal melanomas. Arch Ophthalmol 1983;101:410–412.
210. Shields JA, Augsberger JJ, Brown GC. The differential diagnosis of posterior uveal melanoma. Ophthalmology 1980;87:518–522.
211. Collaborative Melanoma Study Group. Accuracy of diagnosis of choroidal melanoma in the Collaborative Ocular Melanoma Study: COMS Report No. 1. Arch Ophthalmol 1990;108:1268–1273.
212. Donoso LA, Shields JA, Nagy RM. Epibulbar lesions simulating extraocular extension of uveal melanoma. Am Ophthalmol 1982;14:1120–1123.
213. Flindall RJ, France SM. Visual field studies of benign choroidal melanoma. Arch Ophthalmol 1969;81:41–44.
214. Augsburger JJ, Schroeder RP, Territo C, et al. Clinical parameters predictive of enlargement of melanocytic choroidal lesions. Br J Ophthalmol 1989;73:911–917.
215. Shields JA, Shields CL, Donoso LA. Management of posterior melanoma. Surv Ophthalmol 1991;36:161–195.
216. Augsburger JJ, Golden MI, Shields JA. Fluorescein angiography of choroidal malignant melanomas with retinal invasion. Retina 1986;4:232–241.
217. Cantrill HL, Cameron JD, Ramsay, et al. Retinal vascular changes in malignant melanoma of the choroid. Am J Ophthalmol 1984;97:411–418.
218. Leff SR, Augsburger JJ, Shields JA. Focal fluorescence of choroidal melanoma. Br J Ophthalmol 1986;70:104–106.
219. Coleman DJ, Abramson DH, Jack RL, et al. Ultrasonic diagnosis of tumors of the choroid. Am J Ophthalmol 1974;91:344–364.
220. Nicholson DH, Frazier-Byrne S, Chin MT, et al. Echographic and histologic tumor height measurements in uveal melanoma. Am J Ophthalmol 1985;100:456–457.
221. Martin JA, Robertson DM. Extrascleral extension of choroidal melanoma diagnosed by ultrasound. Ophthalmology 1983;90:1334–1339.
222. Shields JA. Current approaches to the diagnosis and management of choroidal melanomas. Surv Ophthalmol 1977;21:443–463.
223. Shields JA, McDonald PR, Leonard BC, et al. The diagnosis of uveal malignant melanoma in eyes with opaque media. Am J Ophthalmol 1977;83:95–105.
224. Dixon PA, Abrams GW, Caya JG. Acoustic analysis of the cytologic structure of malignant melanomas with standardized echography. In: Ossoinig KC, ed. Ophthalmic echography. Proceedings of the 10th SIDUO Congress, St. Petersburg Beach, Florida, November 7–10, 1984. Martinus Nijhoff, Dr W Junk Publi, Dordrecht Doc Opthalmol Proc Series, 1987;48:347–356.
225. Ossoinig KC, Reshef DS, Harrie RP, Hasenfratz GC. Acoustic tissue differentiation with standardized echography in reference to melanomas and pseudomelanomas. In: Ossoinig KC, ed. Ophthalmic echography. Proceedings of the 10th SIDUO Congress, St Petersburg Beach, Florida, November 7–10, 1984. Martinus Nijhoss, Dr Junk Publ, Dordrecht Doc Ophthalmol Proc Series, 1987;48:363–364.
226. Char DH, Kroll S, Stone RD, Harrie R, Kerman B. Ultrasonographic measurement of uveal melanoma thickness: interobserver variability. Br J Ophthalmol 1990;74: 183–185.
227. Coleman DJ, Silverman RH, Rondeau MJ, Lizzi FL, McLean IW, Jakobiec FA. Correlations of acoustic tissue typing of malignant melanoma and histopathologic features as a predictor of death. Am J Ophthalmol 1990;110:380–388.
228. Gosbell AD, Barry WR, Favilla I, Burgess F. Volume measurement of intraocular tumors by cross-sectional ultrasonographic scans. Aust/NZ J Ophthalmol 1991;19: 327–333.
229. Abramson DH, Servodidio CA, McCormick B, Fass D, Zang E. Changes in height of choroidal melanomas after plaque therapy. Br J Ophthalmol 1990;74:359–362.
230. Lieb WE, Cohen SM, Marton DA, et al. Color Doppler imaging of the eye and orbit: Technique and normal vascular anatomy. Arch Ophthalmol 1991;109:527–531.
231. Lieb WE, Shields JA, Cohen SM, et al. Color Doppler imaging in the management of intraocular tumors. Ophthalmology 1990;97:1660–1664.
232. Guthoff RF, Berger RW, Winkler P, Helmke K, Chumbley LC. Doppler ultrasonography of malignant melanomas of the uvea. Arch Ophthalmol 1991;109:537–541.
233. Wollensak J, Heinrich M. In vivo and in vitro measurement of P32 untake inthe ocular tissue in cases of malignant melanoma. Graefes Arch Clin Exp Ophthalmol 1981;217:35–44.
234. McLean IW, Shields JA. Prognostic value of ^{33}P uptake in posterior uveal melanomas. Ophthalmology 1980;87:543–548.
235. Boniuk M, Ruiz RS. Viewpoints: The ^{33}P test in the diagnosis of ocular melanoma. Surv Ophthalmol 1980;24:671–678.
236. Goldberg B, Kara GB, Previtte LR. The use of radioactive phosphorus (^{32}P) in the diagnosis of ocular tumors. Am J Ophthalmol 1980;90:817–828.
237. Mafee MF, Peyman GA, McKusick MA. Malignant uveal melanoma and similar lesions studied by computed tomography. Radiology 1985;156:403–408.
238. Peyster RG, Augsburger JJ, Shields JA, et al. Choroidal melanoma: Comparison of CT, fundoscopy and ultrasound. Radiology 1985;136:675–680.
239. Augsburger JJ, Peyster RG, Markoe AM, et al. Computed tomography of posterior uveal melanomas. Arch Ophthalmol 1987;105:1512–1516.
240. Sobel DF, Kelly W, Kjos BO, et al. MR imaging of orbital and ocular disease. AJNR 1983;6:259–264.
241. Mafee MF, Peyman GA, Grisdano JF, et al. Malignant melanoma and stimulating lesions: MR imaging evaluation. Radiology 1986;160:773–780.
242. De Keiser RJ, Vielvoye GJ, de Wolff-Rouendahl D. Nuclear magnetic resonance imaging of intraocular tumors. Am J Ophthalmol 1986;102:438–441.
243. Chambers RB, Davidorf FH, McAdoo JF, Chakeres DW. Magnetic resonance imaging of uveal melanomas. Arch Ophthalmol 1987;105:917–921.
244. Bond JB, Haik BG, Mihara F, Gupta KL. Magnetic resonance imaging of choroidal melanoma with and without gadolinium contrast enhancement. Ophthalmology 1981;98:459–466.
245. Raymond WR, Char DH, Norman D, Protzko EE. Magnetic resonance imaging evaluation of uveal tumors. Am J Ophthalmol 1991;5:633–641.
246. Peyster RG, Augsburger JJ, Shields JA, Hershey BL, Eagle R Jr, Haskin ME. Intraocular tumors: Evaluation with MR imaging. Radiology 1988;168:773–779.
247. Kurhanewicz J, Winguth SD, Char DH, et al. ^{31}P magnetic resonance spectroscopy of animal uveal melanoma. Invest Ophthalmol Vis Sci 1990;31:1745–1753.
248. De Potter P, Von Weymarn C, Zografos L. In vivo phosphorus 31 magnetic resonance spectroscopy of human uveal melanomas and other intraocular tumors. Am J Ophthalmol 1991;111:276–288.
249. Felberg NT, Donoso LA, Federman JL. Tumor-associated antibodies in the serum of patients with ocular melanoma. Ophthalmology 1980;87:529–533.
250. Felberg NT, Pro-Landazuri JM, Shields JA, et al. Tumor-associated antibodies in the serum of patients with ocular melanoma. Arch Ophthalmol 1979;97:256–259.
251. Donoso LA, Felberg NT, Edelberg K, et al. Metastatic uveal melanoma: An ocular melanoma-associated entigen in the serum of patients with metastatic disease. J Immunol 1986;7:273–283.
252. Ringens PJ, Van Haperen R, Vennegoor C, et al. Monoclonal antibodies in detection of choroidal melanoma. Graefe Arch Clin Exp Ophthalmol 1989;227:287–290.
253. Schaling DF, Van Kroonenburgh MJPG, Borsje RA, et al. Radioimmuno-scintigraphy with melanoma-associated monoclonal antibody fragments in choroidal melanoma. Graefe Arch Clin Exp Ophthalmol 1989;227, 3:291–294.
254. Whitmore WG, Witkin SS, Ellsworth RM. Circulating melanoma-associated antigens in ocular melanoma. Am Ophthalmol 1988;20:212–217.
255. Schaling DF, Van Der Pol JP, Jager MJ, Van Kroonenburgh MJPG, Oosterhuis JA, Ruiter DJ. Radioimmunoscintigraphy and immunohistochemistry with melanoma-associated monoclonal antibodies in choroidal melanoma: A comparison of the clinical and immunohistochemical results. Br J Ophthalmol 1990;74:538–541.
256. Meyer E, Navon D, Zonis S. The role of carcinoembryonic antigen in surveillance of patients with choroidal malignant melanoma: A prospective study. Ann Ophthalmol 1987;19:24–25.
257. Meyer F, Navon D, Zonis S. The role of carcinoembryonic antigen in surveillance of patients with choroidal malignant melanoma: A prospective study. Ann Ophthalmol 1987;19:24–25.
258. Char DH, Stone RD, Irvine AR, et al. Diagnosis modalities in choroidal melanoma. Am J Ophthalmol 1980;89:223–230.
259. Augsburger JJ, Shields JA, Folberg R, et al. Fine needle aspiration biopsy in the diagnosis of intraocular cancer: Cytologic-histologic correlations. Ophthalmology 1985;92:39–49.
260. Karcioglu ZA, Gordon RA, Karcioglu GC. Tumor seeding in ocular fine needle aspiration biopsy. Ophthalmology 1985;92:1763–1767.
261. Glasgow BJ, Brown HH, Zargoza AM, Foos RY. Quantitation of tumor seeding from fine needle aspiration of ocular melanomas. Am J Ophthalmol 1988;105:538–546.
262. Char DH, Miller TH, Crawford JB. Cytopathologic diagnosis of benign lesions simulating choroidal melanomas. Am J Ophthalmol 1991;112:70–75.
263. Gass JDM. Observation of suspected choroidal and ciliary body melanomas for evidence of growth prior to enucleation. Ophthalmology 1980;87:523–528.
264. Felberg NT, Shields JA, Maguire J, et al. Gamma-glutamyl transpeptidase in the prognosis of patients with uveal malignant melanoma. Am J Ophthalmol 1983;95: 467–473.
265. Donoso LA, Nagy RG, Brochman RJ, et al. Metastatic uveal melanoma: Hepatic cell-surface enzymes, isoenzymes, and serum sialic acid levels in early metastatic disease. Arch Ophthalmol 1983;101:791–794.
266. Donoso LA, Bend D, Augsberger JF. Metastatic uveal melanoma: Pretherapy serum liver enzyme and liver scan abnormalities. Arch Ophthalmol 1985;103:796–798.
267. Jakobiec FA, Depot MJ, Henkind P, et al. Fluorescein angiographic patterns of iris melanocytic tumors. Arch Ophthalmol 1982;100:1288–1299.
268. Ferry AP. Lesions mistaken for malignancy of the iris. Arch Ophthalmol 1985;74:9–18.
270. Shields JA, Sanborn GE, Augsburger JJ. The differential diagnosis of malignant melanoma of the iris: A clinical study of 300 patients. Ophthalmology 1983;90:716–720.
271. Territo C, Shields CL, Shields JA, Augsburger JJ, Schroeder RP. Natural course of melanocytic tumors of the iris. Ophthalmology 1988;95:1251.
272. Gupta K, Hoepher JA, Streeten BW. Pseudomelanoma of the iris in herpes simplex keratitis. Ophthalmology 1986;93:1524–1527.
273. Beras OH, Myers MH. Manual for staging of cancer. 2nd ed. Philadelphia: JB Lippincott, 1983:197–208.
274. Fuchs E. Das sarcom des uvealtractus. Wein: Wilhelm, Braumueller, 1882.
275. Kersten RC. Management of choroidal malignant melanoma at Iowa. Ophthalmologica 1984;189:24–35.
276. Char DH. Therapeutic options in uveal melanomas. Am J Ophthalmol 1984;98:796–799.

277. Char DH. Management of choroidal melanoma and retinoblastoma. In: Kanski JJ, Morse PM, eds. Disorders of the vitreous, retina, and choroid. Butterworth international medical review in ophthalmology. London: Butterworth, 1983:122–146.
278. Barr CC, Sipperley JO, Nicholson DH. Small melanomas of the choiroid. Arch Ophthalmol 1978;96:1580–1582.
279. Thomas JV, Green WR, Waumenee AE. Small choroidal melanomas: A long-term follow-up study. Arch Ophthalmol 1979;97:861–864.
280. Davidorf FH, Lang JR. The natural history of malignant melanoma of the choroid and ciliary body: Small versus large tumors. Trans Am Acad Ophthalmol Otolaryngol 1975;79:310–320.
281. Meyer-Schwickerath G. The preservation of vision by treatment of intraocular tumors with light coagulation. Arch Ophthalmol 1961;66:458–466.
282. Vogel MH. The application of photocoagulation in the treatment of the choroid. Ophthalmic Forum 1983;1:46–47.
283. Foulds WS, Danato BF. Low-energy long-exposure laser therapy in the management of choroidal melanoma. Graefes Arch Clin Exp Ophthalmol 1986;224:26–31.
284. Lin LH, Ni C. Hematoporphyrin phototherapy for experimental intraocular malignant melanoma. Arch Ophthalmol 1983;101:301–303.
285. Gomer CJ, Doinon DR, White L, et al. Hematoporphyrin derivative photoradiation-induced damage to normal and tumor tissue of the pigmented rabbit eye. Curr Eye Res 1984;3:229–237.
286. Tse DT, Dutton JJ, Weingeist TA, et al. Hematoporphyrin photoradiation therapy for intraocular and orbital malignant melanoma. Arch Ophthalmol 1984;102:833–838.
287. Bruce RA Jr. Evaluation of hematoporphyrin photoradiation therapy to treat choroidal melanomas. Lasers Surg Med 1984;4:59–64.
288. Vogel MH. Histopathologic observations of photocoagulated malignant melanomas of the choroid. Am J Ophthalmol 1972;74:466–474.
289. Jaffe GJ, Mieler WF, Burke JM, Williams GA. Photoablation of ocular melanoma with a high-powered argon endolaser. Arch Ophthalmol 1989;107:113–118.
290. Phillips AMR, Browne BH, Allan D, Szczesny PJ, Lee WR, Foulds WS. Haematoprophyrin photosensibilization treatment of experimental choroidal melanoma: Annual Congress of the Ophthalmology Society, United Kingdom, April 1987. Eye 1987;1: 680–685.
291. Bruce RA, McCaugnan JS. Lasers in uveal melanoma. Ophthalmol Clin North Am 1989;2:597–604.
292. Shukla M, Gerke E, Bornfeld N, Meyer-Schwickerath G. Tumor regression after photocoagulation of malignant melanomas of the choroid: An ultrasonographic study. Ophthalmologica 1987;194:119–125.
293. Jalkh AE, Trempe CL, Nasrallah FP. Treatment of small choroidal melanomas with photocoagulation. Ophthalmic Surg 1988;19:738–742.
294. Shields JA, Glazer LC, Mieler WF, Shields CL, Gottlieb MS. Comparison of xenon ard and argon laser photocoagulation in the treatment of choroidal melanomas. Am J Ophthalmol 1990;109:647–655.
295. Bauman WC, Mones JM, Tritten JJ, et al. Transpupillary phthalocyanine photodynamic therapy of experimental posterior malignant melanoma. Invest Ophthalmol Vis Sci 1991;32(suppl):713.
296. Ozler SA, Nelson JS, De Queiroz JL, et al. Photodynamic therapy of experimental choroidal melanoma model using chloroaluminum sulfonated phtalocyanine. Invest Ophthalmol Vis Sci 1991;32:1196.
297. Folk JC, Weingeist TA, Coonan P, Blodi CF, Folberg R, Kimura AE. The treatment of serous macular detachment secondary to choroidal melanomas and nevi. Ophthalmology 1989;96:547–551.
298. Moore RF. Choroidal sarcoma treated by the intraocular insertion of radon seeds. Br J Ophthalmol 1930;14:14–152.
299. Stallard HB. Radiotherapy for malignant melanoma of the choroid. Br J Ophthalmol 1966;50:147–155.
300. Markoe AM, Brady LW, Shields JA, et al. Malignant melanoma of the eye: Treatment of posterior uveal lesions by Co-60 plaque radiotherapy versus enucleation. Radiology 1985;156:801–803.
301. Sealy R, Le Roux PLM, Rapley F, et al. The treatment of ophthalmic tumors with low energy sources. Br J Urol 1976;49:551–554.
302. Packer S, Rotman M. Radiotherapy of choroidal melanoma with iodine-125. Ophthalmology 1980;87:582–590.
303. Bosworth JL, Packer S, Rotman M, Ho T, Finger PT. Choroidal melanoma I-125 plaque therapy. Radiology 1988;169:249–251.
304. Garretson BR, Robertson DM, Earle JD. Choroidal melanoma treatment with iodine-125 brachytherapy. Arch Ophthalmol 1987;105:1394–1397.
305. Loammatsch PK. B-irradiation of choroidal melanoma within 106R/106Rh applicators: 16 years' experience. Arch Ophthalmol 1983;101:713–717.
306. Lommatzsch PK. Results after beta-irradiation (106 Ru/106Rh) of choroidal melanomas: 20 years' experience. Am J Clin Oncol 1987;10:146–151.
307. Saunder WH, Char DH, Quivey JM. Precision high-dose radiotherapy: Helium ion treatment of uveal melanoma. Int J Radiat Oncol Biol Phys 1985;11:227–233.
308. Gragoudas ES, Seddon JW, Eagan KM, et al. Long-term results of proton beam radiated uveal melanomas. Ophthalmology 1987;94:395–453.
309. Seddon JM, Gragoudas ES, Polivogianis L, et al. Visual outcome after proton beam irradiation of uveal melanoma. J Ophthalmol 1986;93:666–674.
310. Finger PT, Packer S, Svitra PP, et al. Hyperthermic treatment of intraocular tumors. Arch Ophthalmol 1986;102:1477, 1481.
311. Burgess JE, Chang S, Svitra PP, et al. Effects of hyperthemia on experimental choroidal melanoma. Br J Ophthalmol 1985;69:854–860.
312. Finger PT, Packer S, Sviltra PP, et al. Thermoradiotherapy for intraocular tumors. Arch Ophthalmol 1985;103:1574–1578.
313. Riedel KG, Svitra PP, Seddon JM, et al. Proton beam irradiation and hyperthermia: Effects on experimental choroidal melanoma. Arch Ophthalmol 1985;103:1862–1869.
314. Coleman DJ, Lizzi FL, Burgess SE, et al. Ultrasonic hyperthermia and radiation in the management of intraocular malignant melanoma. Am J Ophthalmol 1986;101: 635–642.
315. Finger PT, Packer S, Paglione RW, Gatz JF, Ho TK, Bosworth JL. Thermoradiotherapy of choroidal melanoma: Clinical experience. Ophthalmology 1989;96:1384–1388.
316. Mieler WF, Jaffe GJ, Steevens RA. Ferromagnetic hyperthermia and iodine 125 brachytherapy in the treatment of choroidal melanoma in a rabbit model. Arch Ophthalmol 1989;107:1524–1528.
317. Swift PS, Stauffer PR, Fries PD, et al. Microwave hypertehrmia for choroidal melanoma in rabbits. Invest Ophthalmol Vis Sci 1990;31:1754–1760.
318. Lincoff H, McLean T, Long R. The cryosurgical treatment of intraocular tumors. Am J Ophthalmol 1977;63:389–390.
319. Abramson DH, Lisman RD. Cryopexy of a choroidal melanoma. Ann Ophthalmol 1979;11:1418–1421.
320. Hidayat AA, LaPiana FG, Kramer KK, et al. The effect of rapid freezing on uveal melanomas. Am J Ophthalmol 1987;103:66–80.
321. Peyman GA, Ericson ES, Axelrod AJ, et al. Full-thickness eyewall resection in primates: An experimental approach to the treatment of choroidal melanoma. Arch Ophthalmol 1973;89:410–412.
322. Peyman GA, Apple DJ. Local excision of a choroidal malignant melanoma: Full-thickness eyewall resection. Arch Ophthalmol 1974;92:216–218.
323. Peyman GA. Eyewall resection. Ophthalmic Forum 1983;4:38–41.
324. Peyman GA, Juarez CL, Diamond FG, et al. Ten-year experience with eyewall resection for uveal malignant melanomas. Ophthalmology 1984;91:1720–1723.
325. Peyman GA, Gremillon CM. Eyewall resection in the management of uveal neoplasms. Jpn J Ophthalmol 1989;33:458–471.
326. Shields JA, Shields CL, Shah P, Sivalingram V. Partial lamellar sclerouvectomy for ciliary body and choroidal tumors. Ophthalmology 1991;98:971–983.
327. Augsbuerger DJ, Lowry JC, Eisenman R. Matched group study of surgical resection versus cobalt-60 plaque radiotherapy for primary choroidal or ciliary body melanoma. Ophthalmic Surg 1990;21:682–688.
328. Forrest AW, Keyser RB, Spencer WH. Iridocyclectomy for melanomas of the ciliary body: A follow-up study of pathology and surgical mortality. Trans Am Acad Opthalmol 1978;85:1237–1249.
329. Damato B, Foulds Ws. Ciliary body tumors and their management. Trans Ophthalmol Soc UK 1986;103:256–264.
330. Foulds WS, Damato BE. Surgical resection of choroidal melanomas. In: Ryan SJ, ed. Retina. Vol 1. St Louis: CV Mosby, 1989:713–720.
331. Blodi FC. Ophthalmology. JAMA 1980;243:2202–2203.
332. Abramson DH, Ellsworth RM. Treatment of choroidal melanomas. Bull NY Acad Med 1978;54:849–854.
333. Char DH, Phillips TL. Pre-enucleation irradiation of uveal melanoma. Br J Ophthalmol 1986;69:177–179.
334. Augsburger JJ, Eagle RC, Chiu M., Shields JA. The effect of pre-enucleation radiotherapy on mitotic activity of choroidal and ciliary body melanomas. Ophthalmology 1987;94:1627–1630.
335. Jager MJ, Van Der Pol JP, De Wolff-Rouendaal D, De Jong PTVM, Ruiter DJ. Decreased expression of HLA class II antigens on human uveal melanoma cells after in vivo x-ray irradiation. Am J Ophthalmol 1988;105, 1:78–86.
336. Rousseau AP, Deschenes J, Pelletier G, Tremblay M, Larochelle-Belland M. Effect of pre-enucleation radiotherapy on the viability of human choroidal melanoma cells. Can J Ophthalmol 1989;24:10–14.
337. Mooy CM, De Jong PTVM, Van Der Kwast TH, Mulder PGH, Jager MJ, Ruiter DJ. Ki-67 immunostaining in uveal melanoma: The effect of pre-enucleation radiotherapy. Ophthalmology 1990;97:1275–1280.
338. Krissig I, Rohrbach M, Lincoff H. Irradiation of choroidal melanomas before enucleation? Retina 1989;9:101–104.
339. Char DH, Phillips TL, Andejeski Y, Crawford JB, Kroll S. Failure of prenucleation radiation to decrease uveal melanoma mortality. Am J Ophthalmol 1988;106:21–26.
340. Kenneally CZ, Farber MG, Smith ME, Devineni R. In vitro melanoma cell growth after preenucleation radiation therapy. Arch Ophthalmol 1988;106:223–224.
341. Straatsma BR, Fine SL, Earle JD, Hawkins BS, Diener-West M, McLaughlin JA. The collaborative ocular melanoma study research group: Enucleation versus plaque irradiation for choroidal melanoma. Ophthalmology 1988;95:1000–1004.
342. Wilson RS. Ocular melanoma. Surgical experience with "no touch" enucleation. South Med J 1983;76:202–204.
343. Davidorf FH, McAdoo JF. Enucleation for choroidal melanoma. In: Ryan SJ, ed. Retina. Vol 1. St Louis: CV Mosby, 1989:687–691.
344. Augsburger JJ, Gamel JW, Lauritzen K, Brady LW. Cobalt-60, plaque radiotherapy vs enucleation for posterior uveal melanoma. Am J Ophthalmol 1990;109:585–592.
345. Egan KM, Gragoudas ES, Seddon JM, et al. The risk of enucleation after proton beam irradiation of uveal melanoma. Ophthalmology 1989;96:1377–1383.
346. Char DH, Castro JR, Kroll SM, Irvine AR, Quivey JM, Stone RD. Five-year follow-up of hemium ion therapy for uveal melanoma. Arch Ophthalmol 1990;108:209–214.
347. Gragoudas ES, Seddon JM, Egan K, et al. Ophthalmology 1987;94:349–353.
348. Zografos L, Gaillaud C, Perret C, et al. Conservative treatment of uveal melanomas at Lausanne University Eye Clinic. 80 Jahreskongr Scheiz Ophthalmol Ges, Engelberg, September 9–12, 1987. Klin Monatsbl Augenheildk 1988;192:572–578.
349. Grange JD, Gerard JP, Ragab M, et al. Place of beta-ray brachytherapy in the conservative treatment of choroidal and ciliary body melanomas. Ophthalmologie 1989;3: 175–179.

350. Lommatzch PK, Kirsch IH. 106RU/106RH plaque radiotherapy for malignant melanomas of the choroid. Doc Ophthalmol 1988;68:225–238.
351. Smith GM. Ocular melanoma and immunotherapy. Ophthalmologica (Basel) 1979;178: 111–113.
352. The TH, De Gast GC, Huiges HA, et al. Immunologic aspects of melanoma. Ophthalmologica (Basel) 1977;175:25–27.
353. Stark WJ, Rosenthal AR, Mullins GM, et al. Simultaneous bilateral uveal melanomas responding to BCNU therapy. Trans Am Acad Ophthalmol Otolaryngol 1971;75:70–83.
354. Liu HS, Refojo MF, Albert DM. Experimental combined systemic and local chemotherapy for intraocular malignancy. Arch Ophthalmol 1980;98:905–908.
355. Affeldt JC, Minckler DS, Azen SP, et al. Prognosis of malignant melanoma of the choroid and ciliary body. Int Ophthalmol Clin 1962;5:389–402.
356. Kersten RC, Tse D, Anderson RL, et al. Role of orbital exenteration in malignant melanoma with extrascleral extension. Ophthalmology 1985;92:436–443.
357. Rini FJ, Jakobiec FA, Hornblass A, Beckerman BL, Anderson RL. The treatment of advanced choroidal melanoma with massive orbital extension. Am J Ophthalmol 1987;104:634–640.
358. Shields CL, Shields JA, Yarian DL, Augsberger JJ. Intracranial extension of choroidal melanoma via the optic nerve. Br J Ophthalmol 1987;71:172–176.
359. Shields JA, Shields CL. Massive orbital extension of posterior uveal melanoma. J Ophthalmol Plast Reconstr Surg 1991;7:238–251.
360. Hykin PG, McCartney ACE, Plowman PN, Hungerford JL. Postenucleation orbital radiotherapy for the treatment of malignant melanoma of the choroid with extrascleral extension. Br J Ophthalmol 1990;74:36–39.
361. Gragoudas ES, Seddon JM, Egan KM, et al. Metastasis from uveal melanoma after proton beam irradiation. Ophthalmology 1988;95:992–999.
362. Fournier GA, Albert DM, Arrigg CA, et al. Resection of solitary metastasis: Approach to palliative treatment of hepatic involvement with choroidal melanoma. Arch Ophthalmol 1984;102:80–82.
363. Gronemeyer U, Enger Mann R, Thiede A. Erfolgreiche Entfernung siner Lebersmetastase 15 Jahre nach Enukleation wegen Aderhaut melanom. Fortschr Ophthalmol 1984;81:363–364.
364. Carrasco CH, Wallace S, Charnsangavny C, et al. Treatment of hepatic metastases in ocular melanoma: Embolization of the hepatic artery with polyvinyl spone and asplatin. JAMA 1986;255:3152–3151.
365. Harning R, Szalay J. A treatment for metastasis of murine ocular melanoma. Invest Ophthalmol Vis Sci 1988;29:1505–1510.
366. Schiller JH, Storer B, Bittner G, Willson JK, Borden EC. Phase II trial of a combination of interferon-beta and interferon-gamma in patients with advanced malignant melanoma. J Interferon Res 1988;8:581–589.
367. Creagan ET. Interferon trials in the management of malignant melanoma and other neoplasms: An overview. In: Nathanson L, ed. Basic and clinical aspects of malignant melanoma. 1987:167–194.
368. McCutcheon IE, Baranco RA, Katz DA, Saris SC. Adoptive immunotherapy of intracerebral metastases in mice. J Neurosurg 1990;72:102–109.
369. The 35th Annual Clinical Conference and 24th Annual Special Pathology Program. Advances in the biology and clinical management of melanoma. Symposium 3. Treatment for distant metastases. November 20–23, 1991.
370. Wilson RS, Fraunfelder FT, Hanna C. Recurrent tapioca melanoma of the iris and ciliary body treated with argon laser. Am J Ophthalmol 1976;82:213–217.
371. Cleasby GW, van Wertenbrugge JA. Treatment of iris melanoma by photocoagulation: A case report. Ophthalmic Surg 1987;18:42–44.
372. Char DH, Crawford JB, Gonzales J, Miller T. Iris melanoma with increased intraocular pressure: Differentiation of focal solitary tumors from diffuse or multiple tumors. Arch Ophthalmol 1989;107:548.
373. Hungerford J. Prognosis in ocular melanoma. Br J Ophthalmol [Editorial] 1989;73: 689.
374. Raubitschek E. Uber Iristumoren. Klin Monatsbl Augenheikd 1914;52:683–694.
375. Verhoeff FH. Sarcoma of the iris. Trans Am Ophthalmol Soc 1933;31:270–271.
376. Muller HK, Sollner F, Lund OE. Erfahrunger bei der operativen von Tumeren der Iris wurzel und des Ciliarkorpers. Berl Dtsch Ophthalmol Ges Heidelberg 1961;63: 194–199.
377. Stallard HB. Partial cyclectomy. Br Ophthalmol 1961;45:797–802.
378. Stallard HB. Partial iridocyclectomy and sclerectomy. Br J Ophthalmol 1966;50:656–659.
379. Jones IS. Iridocyclectomy and corneoscleroiridocyclectomy. In: Reese AB, ed. Tumors of the eye. 3rd ed. Hagerstown, MD: Harper & Row, 1976:238–239.

Cancer: Principles & Practice of Oncology, Fourth Edition,
edited by Vincent T. DeVita, Jr., Samuel Hellman, Steven A. Rosenberg.
J.B. Lippincott Co., Philadelphia © 1993.

Victor A. Levin
Philip H. Gutin
Steven Leibel

CHAPTER **48**

Neoplasms of the Central Nervous System

INCIDENCE AND CLASSIFICATION

Extrapolating available Surveillance, Epidemiology, and End Results (SEER) registry data for 1978 to 1984, the combined incidence of all recorded primary intracranial and spinal axis tumors is between 2 and 19 in 100,000 per year, depending on age.[1] There is an early peak (3.1 in 100,000) between 0 and 4 years, a trough (1.8 in 100,000) between 15 and 24 years, and then a steady rise in incidence that reaches a plateau (17.9–18.7 in 100,000) between 65 and 79 years of age.

The diversity in primary intracranial and spinal axis tumors partly results from the diversity of phenotypically distinct cells capable of transformation into tumors. Table 48–1 shows the hypothetical 15 cell types that can give rise to these tumors. The relative frequency of the seven commonest families of intracranial tumors is given in Table 48–2, and the distribution of spinal tumors is shown in Table 48–3.[2] The commonest tumors are those that are derived from glial precursors (astrocytes, ependymocytes, and oligodendrocytes). The existence of histologically mixed astrocytoma-oligodendroglioma and the less common astrocytoma-ependymoma implies that astrocytomas, oligodendrogliomas, and ependymomas may arise from common stem or progenitor cells. The facts that these tumors arise in different locales within the cranium and the spinal axis and that various types predominate at different ages suggest that differing molecular and genetic mechanisms may underly tumorigenesis at different times in the life span.

Central nervous system (CNS) tumors are the most prevalent solid neoplasms of childhood, the second leading cancer-related cause of death in children younger than 15 years of age, and the third leading cancer-related cause of death in adolescents and adults between the ages of 15 and 34 years. However, most intracranial tumors occur in people older than 45 years. Table 48–4 lists the frequency of intracranial tumors by tumor type and age at first presentation. Glioblastoma rarely occurs in people younger than 15 years but dramatically increases after the age of 45. The incidence of most glial tumors, other than glioblastoma multiforme, actually decreases with increasing age. There is some concern that the incidence of anaplastic astrocytoma and glioblastoma multiforme is increasing in the elderly population,[3] although incorrect ascertainment preceding the widespread availability of computed tomography (CT) scans in the late 1970s may account for some of the presumed increase in incidence.[4,5]

A similar age-related increase in prevalence occurs with differentiated or "benign" meningiomas that increase from 0.2% of all primary intracranial tumors in patients younger than 24 years of age to 39% of tumors in patients older than 65 years.[6] Table 48–4 shows a different pattern for malignant meningiomas, which increase from 0.2% in children to 2.4% in adults older than 60 years of age.

The overall incidence of primary spinal cord tumors is approximately 15% of that of brain tumors. For gliomas, the age-adjusted incidence is 0.11% to 0.14%; for meningiomas, 0.08% to 0.28%, depending on sex (females higher than males); and for nerve sheath tumors, 0.07% to 0.13%.[7] As shown in Table 48–3, the frequency of specific spinal cord tumors is strikingly different from that of the brain tumors. Gliomas constitute approximately 23% of spinal tumors, and most are ependymomas with a predilection for the cauda equina. Schwannomas and meningiomas account for approximately 60% of spinal tumors, with schwannomas being

TABLE 48–1. Classification of Primary Intracranial Tumors by Cell of Origin

Normal Cell	*Tumor*
Astrocyte	Astrocytomas, glioblastoma multiforme
Ependymocyte	Ependymoma, ependymoblastoma
Oligodendrocyte	Oligodendroglioma
Arachnoidal fibroblasts	Meningioma
Nerve cell or neuroblast	Ganglioneuroma, neuroblastoma, retinoblastoma
External granular cell or neuroblast	Medulloblastoma
Schwann cell	Schwannoma (neurinoma)
Melanocyte	Melanotic carcinoma
Choroid epithelial cell	Choroid plexus papilloma or carcinoma
Pituitary	Adenoma
Endothelial or "stromal" cell	Hemangioblastoma
Primitive germ cells	Germinoma, pinealoma, teratomas, cholesteatoma
Pineal parenchymal cell	Pineocytoma
Notochordal remnant	Chordoma

slightly more frequent; both types occur most often in adult life. Other less common spinal tumors are the lipomas, dermoids, and hemangioblastomas.

TUMORIGENESIS

Several cytogenetic studies have demonstrated an increased copy number of chromosomes 7 and 22 and nonrandom losses associated with chromosomes 9p, 10, and 17p in human gliomas.[8,9] The amplification of genetic material suggests the presence of a protooncogene, whereas the loss of genomic loci implies a possible tumor-suppressor gene. With respect to the increasing malignancy of gliomas, it has been shown that chromosomal loss of chromosome 17p is an early event seen in all grades of astrocytoma malignancy[10] and that the *p53* gene, which is one of the tumor-suppressor genes that maps to p13 of chromosome 17, is mutated frequently.[11] The loss of chromosome 9p appears to represent an intermediate event that occurs in most higher-grade astrocytomas,[12] whereas the loss of a portion of chromosome 10 is a late event seen primarily in glioblastoma multiforme tumors.[13] Some evidence suggests that losses on chromosome 19 may be involved in oligodendrogliomas.[14] Ependymomas are associated with a duplication of the long arm of chromosome 12 and losses on chromosome 22.[15]

TABLE 48–2. Frequency of Primary Intracranial Brain Tumors

Type	*Frequency (%)*
Gliobastoma multiforme	30
Astrocytoma	20
Other gliomas (ependymoma, oligodendroglioma, medulloblastoma)	7
Meningioma	18
Nerve sheath (*e.g.*, neurinoma)	9
Pituitary	5
Other (unspecified)	11

(Modified from the Office of Biometry and Epidemiology [Tables 3–1C, 3–5, and 3–6A], 1977)

TABLE 48–3. Distribution of Primary Spinal Tumors

Histology	*Sloff et al*[2]	*Preston-Martin*[7]
Neurilemmoma	29.0	22.0
Meningioma	25.5	42.0
Ependymoma	12.8	15.1
Sarcoma	11.9	
Astrocytoma	6.5	11.2
Other gliomas		1.9
Vascular tumors	6.2	
Chordomas	4.0	
Epidermoids	1.4	
Other	2.7*	5.6

* Lipoma and subarachnoid seeding from primary intracranial tumor.

For meningiomas, multiple deletions of chromosome 22 and constitutional heterozygosity have been observed in a high percentage of cases.[16–18] The neurofibromatosis type II (*NF*2) gene is located on chromosome 22. Recent evidence suggests that the *NF*2 gene is centromeric to break points in meningiomas, suggesting the suspected meningioma tumor-suppressor and *NF*2 genes are separate entities.[18] Interestingly, for females, alterations on chromosome 22 are much larger than any alterations seen for males with meningiomas.[18,19]

For CNS tumors of children, the commonest genomic alteration identified by karyotypic and molecular analyses is the short arm of chromosome 17 (17p).[20–22] Medulloblastomas have shown extra copies of chromosome 11 and marker chromosomes 8q+, 17p+, and 20q+,[23] and unbalanced translocations resulting in a partial 1q trisomy and 6q monosomy.[24] Nonrandom alterations were observed also in chromosomes 1, 6, 10, 11, 13, and 22. Additionally, amplification of c-*MYC* and epidermal growth factor receptor (EGF-R) has been observed to be associated with medulloblastomas and pediatric gliomas, respectively.[25,26] Although a limited number of specimens were examined in each of the studies, the results indicate that losses in genomic material or the amplification of protooncogenes occur in pediatric brain tumors, similar to those observed for adult tumors. These results strongly implicate the loss of function of tumor-suppressor genes and the possible consequences of germ line mutations.

In addition to chromosomal abnormalities, cytokine and receptor aberrations are seen in gliomas. For instance, transforming growth factor-α (TGF-α)-producing cells are seen throughout all grades of astrocytoma, but amplified EGF-R and TGF-α are seen more often in higher-grade astrocytomas.[27] The amplification of chromosome 22 may also be associated with increased expression of platelet-derived growth factor-β (PDGF-β). PDGF-α maps to chromosome 7, which

TABLE 48–4. Frequency of Intracranial Tumors as a Function of Age Range

	Age Ranges (y)						
Histology	*0–9*	*10–19*	*20–29*	*30–39*	*40–49*	*50–59*	*60–74*
Astrocytoma	60	59	76	81	86	87	91
"Low-grade"	9.8	7.1	7.1	4.9	2.5	1.5	1.8
"Astrocytoma"	28.0	31.7	40.4	41.9	38.2	31.1	28.8
Anaplastic	18.5	10.9	11.0	12.8	9.6	8.3	11.0
Mixed	2.5	2.7	2.8	3.4	2.2	2.1	0.7
Glioblastoma	1.3	7.4	14.4	18.2	32.9	44.2	51.0
Medulloblastoma	21.0	10.0	5.5	2.3	1.0	0.1	0.0
Ependymoma*	8.7	2.7	4.3	1.8	0.8	1.3	0.5
Oligodendroglioma	1.1	4.0	5.0	6.4	6.2	3.6	1.6
Embryonal/teratoid†	1.0	1.3	0.3	0.3	0.0	0.0	0.0
Meningioma‡	0.2	0.4	1.2	1.7	1.2	2.0	2.4

* Includes differentiated and anaplastic ependymoma.
† Includes germinoma, mixed embryonal pinealomas, and malignant teratomas.
‡ Underestimate, because SEER does not include many "benign" tumors in its registry; these are probably malignant meningiomas.
(Data based on unpublished SEER program search, 1978–1984)

is also amplified. Increased expression of basic FGF is seen in gliomas and may be important as an autocrine and angiogenic factor in high-grade gliomas. Pediatric glioblastomas and medulloblastomas have been shown to have amplification of EGF-R in similar proportions to that observed in adult tumors.[26] These results suggest that the activation of cytokines and their receptors, by any of several mechanisms, may play an important role in primary tumor initiation or progression, or both.

GENETIC FACTORS

For most brain tumors, a genetic predisposition is lacking. Some exceptions are NF1 and NF2, tuberous sclerosis, Li-Fraumeni syndrome, familial polyposis (Turcot's syndrome), and Osler-Weber-Rendu syndrome; the last two are rare. Li-Fraumeni syndrome is an autosomal dominant disorder characterized by the appearance of diverse tumors (malignant glioma, breast cancer, soft tissue sarcoma, osteosarcoma, leukemia, and adrenocortical carcinoma) that often occur at a young age. Noncancerous skin fibroblasts and lymphocytes derived from people with Li-Fraumeni syndrome have germ line p53 mutations.[28,29] Careful study of familial clusters of specific CNS tumors and CNS tumors with other neoplasms is stimulating careful molecular genetic analysis that leads to the elucidation of the critical cascades that underlie CNS malignancies.

NF1 is relatively common, with an incidence of 1 in 3500. Patients with NF1 develop cutaneous lesions (café-au-lait spots), subcutaneous neurofibroma, anterior optic nerve gliomas, and other brain tumors. NF1 is associated with a gene on chromosome 17q (*NF1* gene).[30,31]

NF2 is inherited as an autosomal dominant disorder with incomplete penetrance. It has an incidence of 1 in 50,000. Acoustic schwannomas, especially bilateral acoustic schwannomas; bony and mesenchymal abnormalities; and a spectrum of gliomas from well-differentiated astrocytoma to glioblastoma multiforme have been observed in NF2 families. Cytogenetic and linkage studies have implicated the *NF2* gene on chromosome 22q.[19] However, a specific transcribed gene responsible for the genesis of NF2 has not been identified.

Another phakomatosis associated with brain tumors is tuberous sclerosis, a hereditary disease with cutaneous, neurologic, cardiac, and kidney abnormalities. Tuberous sclerosis is normally obvious in children. It is characterized by acneiform skin lesions, angiofibromas, periungual fibromas, epilepsy, periventricular hamartomas composed of abnormal glia, and in some patients, mental retardation. Gliomas may be associated with tuberous sclerosis; the commonest type is an uncommon ganglioglioma. Potential genetic loci on 9q and 11q have been suggested.[32]

With greater sophistication in genetic investigations, specific abnormalities of the genome likely will be found for each specific brain tumor histology. As more is learned about oncogene function and the specific association of chromosomal alterations to structural proteins and enzymes, it is likely that the genetics of tumor development and the entire panoply of tumor growth control will be understood.

CHEMICAL INDUCTION AND EPIDEMIOLOGY

The epidemiology of primary CNS tumors has provided hints but few definitive observations with respect to environmental or occupational causes. Although brain tumors can be experimentally induced in a high proportion of rodents by the use of certain chemicals, the association of chemical exposure and brain tumors is limited to a few occupations. A higher than expected increase in the incidence of brain tumors has been observed as a result of purported exposure to pesticides, herbicides, and fertilizers,[33] various petrochemical industries,[34] and health professions.[35] Whether these statistical observations are credible is difficult to determine. Aside from a known association between vinylchloride and gliomas, there are no common chemical or environmental threads among these observations.[34]

VIRAL INFECTION AND CNS NEOPLASIA

Viruses have been implicated directly in the development of gliomas only in rats, dogs, and monkeys. In all cases, direct CNS injection of the virus is required. In rats, the avian sarcoma virus produces glial tumors[36]; in dogs, Rous sarcoma virus leads to gliosarcomas[37]; in owl monkeys, a human polyoma virus (JC virus) produces glial neoplasms[38]; and in hamsters, JC virus produces medulloblastomas.[39] Although a direct association between virus exposure and CNS tumors has not been established in humans, patients with primary CNS lymphoma have been observed to have a high incidence of infection with Epstein-Barr virus (EBV) and evidence of EBV in their tumor tissue.[40] Common viral exposure could explain the occasional glioma cluster observed in schools and communities. However, it is extremely difficult to pinpoint mutations due to a virus to validate this hypothesis.

TRAUMA AND CNS NEOPLASIA

CNS neoplasia, like most cancers, appears to be unassociated with prior trauma. It has been suggested that the incidence of meningiomas is higher in patients with a prior history of head trauma, but this hypothesis was not supported by a prospective study.[41] Trauma could be a progression event; however, this theory would be difficult to prove.

CNS NEOPLASIA AFTER RADIATION, CHEMOTHERAPY, AND IMMUNOSUPPRESSION

The incidence of CNS tumors after treatment for a prior malignancy is small. The literature contains several examples of astrocytomas occurring 3 to 7 years after craniospinal axis irradiation and chemotherapy for acute lymphocytic leukemia (ALL) and craniopharyngioma[42,43]; unfortunately, none of the reports contain sufficient information to determine risk assessment. In non-Hodgkin's lymphoma, 2% of 44 second malignancies were an astrocytoma.[44] As in the cases discussed previously, no measure of risk assessment is possible, although such infrequent reporting would suggest that these are uncommon or rare events. Meningiomas have been reported in association with scalp irradiation for tinea capitis, the risk for meningiomas being as high as 21% in one study.[45,46]

For unknown reasons, transplant recipients and patients with acquired immunodeficiency syndrome (AIDS) have substantially increased risks for primary CNS lymphoma but not gliomas.

ANATOMIC AND CLINICAL CONSIDERATIONS

The clinical presentation of the various tumors is best appreciated by considering the relation of signs and symptoms to anatomy.[47]

INTRACRANIAL TUMORS

Intracranial tumors produce symptoms primarily by two mechanisms: mass effect (and increased intracranial pressure), due entirely to the tumor or to the tumor and surrounding edema, or infiltration and destruction of normal tissue.

General Signs and Symptoms

Typical infiltrative intracerebral tumors, such as the various grades of astrocytoma and oligodendroglioma and some of the more primitive neuroectodermal tumors, can produce headache, gastrointestinal upset such as nausea and vomiting, personality changes, and slowing of psychomotor function. These may be the only clinical indications of tumor.

Because headache is a common presenting symptom in patients with intracranial tumor, clinical patterns and their localizing value must be appreciated. Brain parenchyma does not have pain-sensitive structures, and tumor pain (headache) has been attributed to local swelling and distortion of pain-sensitive nerve endings associated with blood vessels, primarily in the meninges. Tumors grow at different rates and, therefore, achieve variable size before signs and symptoms occur. But once a tumor has achieved a critical volume causing compression and displacement of brain, the onset and demise of headache seem to correlate with changes in intracranial pressure.

Headaches can vary in severity and quality; they often occur in the early morning hours or on first awakening. Patients sometimes complain of an uncomfortable feeling in the head rather than headache. Although there is not an exact relation between the location of tumor headache and the location of the tumor, some rules are worth remembering. More often than not, frontal and temporal tumors produce headache in frontal, retroorbital, or temporal regions, whereas infratentorial tumors tend to produce occipital and retroauricular headache. Occasionally, however, retroorbital headaches are observed with infratentorial tumors.

Gastrointestinal symptoms are common. Patients complain of loss of appetite, queasiness, nausea, and, occasionally, vomiting. Vomiting appears more commonly in children and in patients harboring infratentorial rather than supratentorial tumors. Although textbooks discuss projectile vomiting as an infrequent generalized symptom of brain tumors, in these authors' experience, it is common in children but rare in adults. From reports in the literature and discussions with experienced neurosurgeons, it seems as though there is a lower incidence of vomiting currently compared with past years; this may reflect the fact that patients are diagnosed earlier than in previous years and receive glucocorticoids that can modify dramatically many of the generalized signs and symptoms of brain tumors.

Sometimes the only presenting symptoms are changes in personality, mood, mental capacity, and concentration. Occasionally, merely a slowing of psychomotor activity is the antecedent symptom of intracranial tumor. Patients with brain tumors tend to sleep longer at night and nap during the day. These changes in function and activity often are apparent to the family and the examiner but not to the patient; in other instances, only the patient recognizes the changes in mental function. None of these symptoms are unique to brain tumors;

they could easily be confused with depression, neurasthenia, or other psychological problems.

Focal Cerebral Syndromes

Although fewer than 10% of patients presenting with seizures have a brain tumor as the cause of the seizure, seizures are a presenting symptom in approximately 20% of patients with supratentorial brain tumors. With rapidly growing infiltrative malignant gliomas, they are likely to take the form of focal motor or sensory seizures, although generalized seizures are also common. In patients with slowly growing astrocytomas, oligodendrogliomas, or meningiomas, generalized seizures may antedate the clinical diagnosis by months to years. The value of the focal seizure as a means of tumor localization is high, sufficiently so that tumor should be considered causative until proved otherwise.

The distribution of infiltrative parenchymal tumors in the brain is directly related to the mass of the lobe or region. Frontal tumors occur more commonly than parietal tumors, which, in turn, occur more often than temporal lobe tumors, and so forth. Anatomic or regional involvement by tumors, although not completely stereotypic as it is with CNS vascular disease, nonetheless has certain features that distinguish them and help the clinician localize the tumor or, at least, to consider the diagnosis.

The frontal lobe syndrome varies markedly from patient to patient. It can range from personality change to headache and mild slowing of contralateral hand movements and to contralateral spastic hemiplegia, marked elevation in mood, or loss of initiative and dysphasia (if it is the dominant lobe). Assuming the normal pattern of left hemisphere dominance, unilateral tumors affecting the right frontal lobe can cause left hemiplegia, slight elevation in mood, difficulty in adapting to new situations, loss of initiative, and even occasional primitive grasp and sucking reflexes. Left frontal lobe tumors can cause right hemiplegia and nonfluent dysphasia with or without some apraxia of lip, tongue, or hand movements.

Bifrontal disease, a condition usually associated with infiltrative gliomas and primary CNS lymphomas, can cause varying degrees of bilateral hemiplegia, spastic bulbar palsy, severe impairment of intellect, lability of mood, dementia, and prominent primitive grasp, suck, and snout reflexes.

Temporal lobe syndromes, like frontal lobe syndromes, can range from symptoms that are detectable only on careful testing of perception and spatial judgment to severe impairment of recent memory. Homonymous quadrantanopsia, auditory hallucinations, and even aggressive behavior can occur as a result of tumors of either temporal lobe. Involvement of the nondominant temporal lobe can also result in minor perceptual problems and spatial disorientation. Dominant temporal lobe involvement can lead to dysnomia, impaired perception of verbal commands, and even a full-blown, fluent Wernicke-like aphasia. Bilateral disease, involving both temporal lobes, is rare in comparison with the bilaterality of frontal lobe tumors that readily cross through the corpus callosum. This is fortunate, because bitemporal tumor involvement is devastating. It produces impairment of memory, especially recent memory, and can lead to dementia.

Parietal lobe syndromes affect sensory and perceptual functions more than motor modalities, although mild hemiparesis is sometimes seen with extensive parietal lobe tumors. Tumors impinging on either parietal lobe can produce a decrease in the perception of cortical sensory stimuli that may vary from mild sensory extinction, observable only by testing, to a more severe sensory loss with deep tumors that leads to hemianesthesia or other hemisensory abnormalities. Homonymous hemianopsia or visual inattention also may occur. In addition, involvement of the nondominant parietal lobe can lead to perceptual abnormalities and, in severe cases, to anosognosia and apraxia for self-dressing. Unilateral dominant parietal lobe tumors lead to alexia, dysgraphia, and certain types of apraxia.

Occipital lobe tumors can produce contralateral homonymous hemianopsia or visual aberrations that take the form of imperception of color, object size, or object location. Bilateral occipital disease can produce cortical blindness.

The classic disconnection syndromes associated with corpus callosum lesions are seen rarely in patients with brain tumors. Even though infiltrative gliomas often cross the corpus callosum in the region of the genu or the splenium, the involvement of additional structures complicates neurologic interpretation, obscuring classic disconnection syndromes. With respect to partial lesions, interruption of association fibers in the anterior part of the corpus callosum usually causes a failure of the left hand to carry out spoken commands. Lesions in the splenium of the corpus callosum interrupt visual fibers connecting the right occipital lobe and left angular gyrus, resulting in an inability of patients to read or name colors.

Symptoms related to thalamic tumors vary as a function of tumor size and whether the tumor produces secondary blockage of cerebrospinal fluid (CSF) flow and hydrocephalus. Occasionally, tumors in the thalamus and, less commonly, in the basal ganglia, can reach 3 to 4 cm in diameter before the patient has symptoms severe enough to seek medical attention. Patients typically present with headaches resulting from hydrocephalus and increased intracranial pressure secondary to trapping of the lateral horn of one of the ventricles. In addition or independently, patients can present with a mild sensory abnormality on the contralateral side, which is detected only by testing of sensory extinction or, rarely, severe neuropathic pain syndrome. Patients may complain of intermittent paresthesias on the contralateral side; because they are episodic and seizure-like, anticonvulsant drugs are used sometimes and actually may be beneficial. With more involvement of the basal ganglia, contralateral intention tremor and hemiballistic-like movement disorders can be observed. Thalamic tumors usually do not present in a manner typical of thalamic strokes, unless bleeding into the tumor has occurred.

Focal Infratentorial Syndromes

The brain stem, composed of the medulla oblongata and the pons, has both nuclear groups and traversing axons. Tumors invading or compressing the brain stem can produce dire consequences; even a small increase in size, for example, 1 to 2 mm, may lead to death or devastating signs and symptoms. Tumors can be primarily intrinsic or intrinsic with exophytic components in the fourth ventricle, peripontine cisterns, or in both locations. Cranial nerve involvement, therefore, can be at the nuclear level or of the cranial nerve as it leaves the brain stem.

The commonest tumor of the brain stem is an astrocytoma (glioma), the initial clinical manifestations of which are palsies involving cranial nerves VI and VII on one side in 90% of patients. These usually are followed by involvement of long tracts resulting in hemiplegia, unilateral limb ataxia, ataxia of gait, paraplegia, hemisensory syndromes, gaze disorders, and, occasionally, hiccups. Less commonly, long-tract signs precede the cranial nerve abnormalities; this is more likely with confined intrinsic brain stem lesions.

The midbrain, juxtaposed between the pons and the cerebral hemispheres, encompasses the tectum, the cerebral peduncles, and the cerebral aqueduct. If the midbrain is involved, obstructive hydrocephalus can occur, producing vomiting, drowsiness, and cerebellar signs. Patients with medullary tumors have a more rapidly progressive course and are more likely to have deficits in cranial nerves VI (usually late), VII, IX, and X, and dysarthria, personality change, and head tilt. Unlike the expansive posterior fossa tumors, headache, vomiting, and papilledema occur late.

Fourth ventricular tumors, because of their location, tend to produce obstructive hydrocephalus early in their development. This produces profound headache and vomiting and associated disturbances of gait and balance. With rapidly progressing lesions, cerebellar herniation may develop.

Tumors of the cerebellum have valuable localizing signs and symptoms. In slowly growing tumors, the initial symptoms may be headache and nausea, which are caused by increased intracranial pressure, and mild imbalance in gait or ataxia of a limb. In more rapidly growing cerebellar tumors, there may be prominent morning headache, vomiting, a stumbling gait with frequent falling, nystagmus and dizziness, and visual symptoms caused by papilledema. Abnormal posturing of the head is seen often in children but not in adults. In children, the head is tilted back and away from the side of the tumor. Posturing of the head is curious in that it indicates unilateral cerebellum-foramen magnum herniation. Bilateral sixth cranial nerve palsies are uncommon. Midline lesions in and around the cerebellar vermis lead to truncal and gait ataxia, whereas lesions in a cerebellar hemisphere lead to unilateral appendicular ataxia, most readily observed in upper extremity movements.

Tumors of the base of the skull, although not particularly common, nevertheless are important because many are curable by surgery. Table 48–5[48] summarizes the salient clinical features of seven of the more common clinical syndromes.

A classic base-of-skull tumor presentation is that associated with acoustic neurilemmomas (schwannoma), the most frequent cause of the cerebellopontine angle syndrome. Almost all such patients have involvement of the auditory or vestibular portions of cranial nerve VIII; more than 50% have facial weakness, disturbance of taste, and sensory loss of the face; approximately 40% have ataxia of gait; and fewer than 25% have unilateral appendicular ataxia. Deafness and vestibular dysfunction due to damage to the auditory and vestibular nerve branches are characteristic of these tumors. Finally, these tumors can attain an extremely large size before they are discovered.

Another group of tumors that present with distinct signs and symptoms is that which occurs in or near the sella turcica. Table 48–6 summarizes the location, tumors, and some of the salient features of sellar and parasellar tumors.[49]

Many patients present with defects of the visual field, less commonly with blindness and optic atrophy. The visual field abnormality is usually a partial or complete bitemporal hemianopsia associated with intrasellar tumors such as pituitary adenomas. With lesions that expand from below the optic chiasm, the upper temporal quadrants are affected first. Patients can also present with scotomata in either eye. With long-standing, slowly progressive disease, unilateral or bilateral optic atrophy can be observed. Expansion of tumor may

TABLE 48–5. Differential Diagnosis of Tumors at the Base of the Skull

Site of Lesion	*Associated Tumors*	*Clinical Findings*
Anterior parts	Carcinomas invasive from frontal and ethmoid sinuses; meningiomas	Unilateral anosmia, frontal lobe syndrome, seizures
Superior orbital	Meningiomas, carcinoma of nasopharynx	Lesions of cranial nerves III, IV, V, VI with ophthalmoplegia, pain, and hypesthesia in VI distribution
Cavernous sinus	Chondromas, meningiomas, sellar and parasellar tumors	Cranial nerves III, IV, VI, and sometimes V involvement with ophthalmoplegia
Apex of the petrous temporal bone	Cholesteatoma, chondroma, meningioma, neurinoma, sarcoma	Cranial nerves V and VI involvement with sensory and motor findings and diplopia
Sphenoid and petrous bones	Meningioma, chondroma, nasopharyngeal carcinoma, metastasis	Lesions of cranial nerves III, IV, VI resulting in ophthalmoplegia; fifth may be associated with trigeminal neuralgia syndrome
Jugular foramen	Glomus jugular tumors, neurinomas, chondromas, cholesteatoma, meningioma, nasopharyngeal carcinoma	Cranial nerves IX, X, XI producing difficulty with swallowing and speaking and weakness of neck muscles
Cerebellopontine angle	Neurinoma, meningioma, cholesteatoma, metastasis of cerebellar tumors	Cranial nerve VII lesions: loss of hearing, vertigo, and nystagmus; cerebellar: ataxia; cranial nerves V, VII, occasionally IX and XII; brain stem symptoms and signs of increased intracranial pressure

(Adapted from Bingas B. Tumours of the base of the skull. In: Vinken PJ, Bruyn GW, eds. Handbook of clinical neurology: Tumours of the brain and skull. Vol 17. Amsterdam: North Holland, 1974:136)

TABLE 48–6. Clinical Syndromes Associated With Tumors of Sellar Region

Tumor	*Disorders* — *Anterior Pituitary Gland*	*Disorders* — *Hypothalamus*	*Incidence and Degree*	*Syndromes*
In the Sella				
Adenoma				
Active	+			Cushing's disease, acromegaly, gigantism
Inactive	+	+/−		Forbes-Albright syndrome, hypopituitarism
Chondroma	+			
Metastasis	+			
Craniopharyngioma			Regular	
Intrasellar	+		Clinical	
Intrasellar and suprasellar	+	+		
Close to Sella				
Suprasellar craniopharyngioma		+	Regular Clinical	Adiposogenital dystrophy (Frohlich)
Suprasellar meningioma		+/−		
Suprasellar epidermoid				
Optic pathway glioma		+/−	Rare	Russell's syndrome
Hypothalamic glioma		+	Frequent	Precocious puberty
Hypothalamic hamartoma		+	Clinical	
Pineal tumors		+	Frequent Clinical	
Tumors with aqueductal obstruction and hydrocephalus		+		Cushingoid
Remote From Sella				
Cerebral hemispheres	+/−	+/−	Rare	
Meningioma glioma			Latent	

(Fahlbusch R, Marguth F. Endocrine disorders associated with intracranial tumors. In: Vinken PJ, Bruyn GW, eds. Handbook of clinical neurology: Tumours of the brain and skull. Part I, Vol 16. Amsterdam: North Holland, 1974:345)

involve the hypothalamus and compression of the third ventricle, leading to obstructive hydrocephalus and signs of increased intracranial pressure, such as headache and nausea and vomiting.

Some of the pituitary tumors produce secondary signs and symptoms, because they elaborate hormones that create various syndromes of endocrine hyperactivity (Table 48–7). A few pituitary tumors produce no detectable hormones or produce hormones in quantities that assume no clinical significance. Currently, it is uncommon for patients with endocrine-active tumors to present with large tumors; it is more common for patients with endocrine-inactive tumors to seek medical attention because of optic chiasmal compression-hypopituitarism as a consequence of a large mass. Compression leads to detectable hyposecretion of specific cells, with production of growth hormone being the most sensitive, followed closely by gonadotropins. Cells producing thyroid-stimulating hormone and corticotropin are much more resistant, and their function is impaired only at a later stage of growth.

Table 48–8 summarizes the differential diagnosis of tumors by location in children and adults.[50]

Acute and Life-Threatening Syndromes Caused by Intracranial Tumors

Because the brain and the spinal cord are surrounded by a rigid skull and dural membranes, expanding lesions within or abutting the brain or spinal cord can cause displacement of vital structures. This can lead, in the brain, to respiratory arrest and death and, in the spinal cord, to paraplegia or quadriplegia.

TABLE 48–7. Clinical Syndromes Produced by Endocrine-Activity Pituitary Adenomas

Hormone Produced	*Clinical Syndrome*
Prolactin	Amenorrhea and galactorrhea, impotence
Growth hormone	Gigantism and acromegaly
Corticotropin	Cushing's disease, Nelson's syndrome (after adrenalectomy)
Thyroid-stimulating hormone (rare)	Hyperthyroidism

TABLE 48–8. Differential Diagnosis of Tumors by Location and Age at Onset of Symptoms

Location	*Child*	*Adult*
Supratentorial	Astrocytoma	Metastatic
	Glioblastoma	Glioblastoma
	Oligodendroglioma	Astrocytoma
	Sarcoma	Meningioma
	Neuroblastoma	Oligodendroglioma
	Mixed glioma	Mixed glioma
Infratentorial	Astrocytoma	Metastatic
	Medulloblastoma	Astrocytoma
	Ependymoma	Glioblastoma
	Brain stem glioma	Ependymoma
		Brain stem glioma
Sellar and parasellar	Craniopharyngioma	Pituitary
	Optic glioma	Meningioma
	Epidermoid	
Base of the skull		Neurinoma
		Meningioma
		Chordoma
		Carcinoma
		Dermoid, epidermoid

To understand the sequence of events leading to temporal lobe-tentorial (uncal) herniation and cerebellar-foramen magnum herniation, a visual image of intracranial anatomy is needed. The tentorium cerebelli forms a rigid tissue partition between the cerebral hemispheres above and the cerebellum and brain stem below. Through this opening passes the midbrain centrally and cranial nerve III anterolaterally. Immediately lateral to cranial nerve III lies the medial portion of the temporal lobe called the *uncus*. An expanding mass lesion situated above the tentorium may displace the uncus medially and inferiorly beneath the tentorium. Table 48–9 summarizes the neurologic findings and pathologic causes for the events that constitute the temporal lobe-tentorial herniation syndrome.[51]

A rapid increase in the volume of the supratentorial compartment leading to herniation can be caused by many different factors. A rapidly growing glioblastoma can present in this manner, although it is more usual for it to occur as a terminal or near-terminal event after ineffective therapy for the tumor. It can also occur when there is a dramatic increase in the amount of edema associated with metastasis to the brain or with hyponatremia and hypoosmolar syndromes. The injudicious use of parenteral hypoosmolar 5% dextrose in water often is sufficient to produce an abrupt increase in brain edema and temporal lobe herniation. These authors also have seen temporal lobe herniation follow a group of shortly spaced seizures. Presumably, the seizures, which are associated with hypoventilation, produce local hypoxia around the tumor with a resultant increase in brain edema.

Mass lesions in the infratentorial compartment can displace brain tissue upward through the tentorium, but more commonly force brain tissue downward through the foramen magnum. In this situation, the cerebellar tonsils move caudally through the foramen magnum, and in doing so, wedge against the medulla, causing the findings summarized in Table 48–10.

Cerebellar-foramen magnum herniation frequently results from, or is contributed to by, obstructive hydrocephalus. In such instances, emergency removal of fluid from the more cephalad ventricular system may relieve symptoms and be life saving. Surgical intervention is indicated only if the reason

TABLE 48–9. Temporal Lobe-Tentorial (Uncal) Herniation

Neurologic Findings	*Pathologic Causes*
Pupillary dilation and ptosis	Compression of ipsilateral oculomotor nerve between herniating tissue and petroclinoid ligament
Ipsilateral hemiplegia	Compression of contralateral cerebral peduncle against tentorium (Kernohan's notch)
Contralateral hemiplegia	Compression of ipsilateral cerebral peduncle; when associated with compression of contralateral peduncle, bilateral corticospinal tract signs
Homonymous hemianopia	Compression of posterior cerebral artery against the tentorium can lead to occipital ischemia or infarction and contralateral homonymous hemianopia; occasionally bilateral field cuts
Midbrain syndrome: Cheyne-Stokes respirations, stupor and coma, bipyramidal signs, decerebrate rigidity, dilated fixed pupils, gaze paresis, altered oculocephalic reflexes	Crushing of midbrain between herniating temporal lobe and leaf of tentorium associated with vascular occlusion and perivascular hemorrhages
Coma, rising blood pressure, and bradycardia	These late signs occur from rising intracranial pressure and hydrocephalus as the aqueduct is compressed and the subarachnoid space becomes compromised

(Adapted from Adams RD, Victor M. Principles of neurology. New York: McGraw-Hill, 1977:586)

TABLE 48–10. Cerebellar-Foramen Magnum Herniation

Neurologic Findings	*Pathologic Causes*
Head tilt, stiff neck, posturing of neck, or paresthesias over the neck	Downward displacement of inferior hemispheres through the foramen magnum; may be unilateral or bilateral
Tonic extensor spasms of limbs and body (cerebellar "fits") and later coma	Compressive effects of cerebellum or hydrocephalus on the upper brain stem
Respiratory arrest	Medullary compression

(Adapted from Adams RD, Victor M. Principles of neurology. New York: McGraw-Hill, 1977:586)

for the herniation is treatable. In the instance of cerebellar-foramen magnum herniation aggravated by acute obstructive hydrocephalus, ventriculoperitoneal shunting is often necessary. Care must be taken, however, because too rapid a change in the CSF dynamics can lead to a rapid and damaging movement of the brain, which can lead to occlusion of posterior cerebral arteries and brain stem injury.

These two herniation syndromes will lead to death, unless there is prompt intervention. The immediate intravenous administration of hyperosmotic agents, such as mannitol or urea, and large doses of synthetic glucocorticoids, such as dexamethasone or methylprednisolone, should be given promptly to reduce intracranial pressure and to avert impending death.

Hemorrhage into a tumor is not as common as might be expected, although the incidence of intratumor hemorrhage may increase because of iatrogenic thrombocytopenia associated with the current use of chemotherapy in the treatment of brain tumors. Primary tumors that most commonly bleed de novo are glioblastoma and oligodendrogliomas; of the metastatic tumors, those from the lung, melanoma, hypernephroma, and choriocarcinoma are most likely to be associated with intratumoral hemorrhage. Signs and symptoms of intratumoral hemorrhage may be temporized by the use of osmotic agents and glucocorticoids, but if extensive and life threatening, operation and decompression are indicated. Under no circumstances should a lumbar puncture be performed in any of the acute herniation syndromes. In fact, lumbar puncture should never be done indiscriminately. The indications for lumbar puncture are discussed in another section of this chapter.

SPINAL AXIS

To understand the clinical presentation of tumors of the spinal axis, the local anatomy (Fig. 48–1) and how tumors might present with respect to anatomy must be appreciated. The cranial dura is firmly adherent to the skull (with the exception of dural duplications of the falx and tentorium), and no extradural space normally exists between dura and skull. An entirely different anatomic relation in the spinal canal accounts for a well-defined extradural space containing epidural fat and blood vessels. By way of the intervertebral foramina, this extradural space communicates with adjacent extraspinal compartments, for example, the mediastinum and the retroperitoneal space. With rare exceptions, extradural tumors are metastatic, reaching the extradural space through intervertebral foramina.

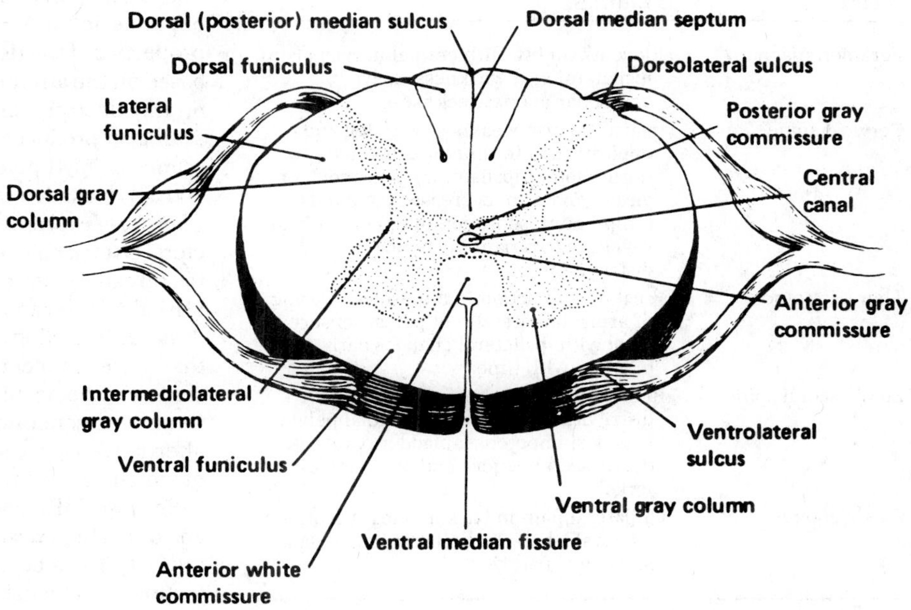

FIGURE 48–1. Cross-section of thoracic spinal cord shows relation of spinal nerves to intraspinal tracts.

Tumors arising inside of the dural tube (intradural tumors) may originate within the spinal cord (intramedullary), or they may take origin outside the spinal cord (extramedullary). The two common extramedullary intradural tumors, neurilemmoma (schwannoma) and meningioma, are attached, respectively, to sensory nerve roots and to dura and involve the spinal cord by compression.

Neurology of Spinal Cord Tumors

A spinal tumor produces two effects: local (focal) and distal (remote). Local effects indicate the tumor's location along the spinal axis, and distal effects reflect involvement of motor and sensory long tracts within the spinal cord. Table 48–11 summarizes the clinical findings useful in localizing a spinal cord tumor.

Distal effects are common to all spinal tumors sooner or later, and symptoms and signs are confined to structures innervated below the spinal cord level of involvement. Although neurologic manifestations commonly begin unilaterally, a full-blown Brown-Séquard's syndrome of cord hemisection can occur but is rare. More characteristic are motor changes: weakness and spasticity, if the tumor lies above the conus medullarus, or weakness and flaccidity, if at or below the conus. Typically, sensory impairment begins distally in the feet. Impairment of bladder function occurs later in tumors above the conus, but may be an early manifestation of tumors in or below the conus. The upper level of impaired long-tract function usually is several segments below the actual site of tumor involvement.

Local manifestations may reflect involvement of bone, with pain constituting the cardinal symptom of metastatic tumors. Involvement of spinal roots produces pain, sensory impairment, and weakness with atrophy in the appropriate radicular distribution. Less often, involvement of spinal gray matter produced by extensive pressure from extramedullary tumors or direct damage by intramedullary tumors causes segmental sensory and motor changes.

TABLE 48–11. Clinical Manifestations of Spinal Cord Tumors

Location	*Findings*
Foramen magnum	Eleventh and twelfth cranial nerve palsies; ipsilateral arm weakness early; cerebellar ataxia; neck pain
Cervical spine	Ipsilateral arm weakness with leg and opposite arm in time; wasting and fibrillation of ipsilateral neck, shoulder girdle, and arm; decreased pain and temperature sensation in upper cervical regions early; pain in cervical distribution
Thoracic spine	Weakness of abdominal muscles; sparing of arms; unilateral root pains; sensory level with ipsilateral changes early and bilateral with time
Lumbosacral spine	Root pain in groin region and sciatic distribution; weakened proximal pelvic muscles; impotence; bladder paralysis; decreased knee jerk and brisk ankle jerks
Cauda equina	Unilateral pain in back and leg, becoming bilateral when the tumor is large; bladder and bowel paralysis

Historically, tumors at or near the foramen magnum have been diagnosed incorrectly more often than have spinal tumors at any other site, because foramen magnum tumors can mimic such diverse conditions as multiple sclerosis, amyotrophic lateral sclerosis, and cervical disk disease. The frequency of delayed diagnoses of these tumors justifies the dictum that myelography or magnetic resonance imaging (MRI) is indicated as a diagnostic measure in any neurologic disease that can be accounted for by a lesion at or below the foramen magnum.

Occasionally, a cervical intramedullary tumor will mimic syringomyelia, with dissociated sensory loss, weakness, and wasting in the arms and hands and variable long-tract involvement. In most instances, the clinical presentation of a spinal tumor does not indicate if it is extradural or intradural.

The rate at which symptoms develop can be helpful in distinguishing extradural from intradural tumor, with a history of days to a few weeks characterizing metastatic extradural tumors, and a longer course, often many months, reflecting the slower growth of intradural tumors. A history of previously diagnosed cancer or other system involvement also is helpful.

NEURODIAGNOSTIC TESTS

NEUROIMAGING

The diagnosis of intracranial tumor requires radiographic confirmation. Fortunately, the great strides in radiology have yielded technologic advances best adapted for the brain and the spinal cord. Nuclear imaging, arteriography, and pneumoencephalography have been supplanted by the much more sensitive and descriptive techniques of MRI and CT. Both techniques are applicable to demonstrate intracranial and spinal lesions. Both CT and MRI produce cross-sectional digital images. In both, the depicted anatomy and pathology are based on numeric computerized representations of certain physical properties of the tissue.[52] The CT image is composed of pixels based on the attenuation of x-rays that are, in turn, dependent on the electron density of the tissue being studied. The MRI scan also produces an image based on pixels, but unlike CT scanning, MRI pixel intensity is based on proton density, T1 and T2 relaxation times, and flow (blood flow). The MRI scan, therefore, represents a complex interrelation of four parameters. Data acquisition also can be manipulated by the operator to a greater degree than can be done with CT scans. CT and MRI also differ in that MR data can be acquired in any plane desired, including oblique planes, in a primary fashion such that there is no compromise of spatial or contrast detail. CT scans can be acquired only in the axial or half-axial planes. Computer-generated reformations are required to generate alternative views, such as orthogonal and off-axis images, all of which have degradation of both spatial and contrast detail.

Because MRI scanning can generate images in any plane and offers high resolution and contrast without associated bone artifact, it has been shown to be superior to CT scan in detecting and localizing brain tumors and evaluating edema, hydrocephalus, or hemorrhage.[53] Unfortunately, MRI is not superior to CT in specificity.

Availability of modern imaging equipment varies with the economies of various communities. If MRI is unavailable, a CT scan after administration of iodinated contrast material is the imaging method of choice.

Intraaxial CNS tumors normally produce edema that is partially correlated with the rapidity of tumor growth. An exception is the benign cerebral meningioma, a slow-growing tumor that can produce profound edema. The so-called vasogenic edema associated with brain tumors is fluid that has leaked through an incompetent blood–brain barrier and is seen on the CT scan as relatively low attenuation compared with normal brain. On MRI, edema appears as an area of low-signal intensity on T1-weighted images and high-signal intensity on T2-weighted images.

Mass lesions in the brain can obstruct the ventricular system, resulting in hydrocephalus. MRI is perhaps slightly superior to CT in evaluating hydrocephalus and its causes, because more planes of view are available to the radiologist. Dilation of one or both of the lateral ventricles and not the rest of the ventricular system suggests obstruction at the foramen of Monro as is seen with colloid cysts or gliomas in this region. Dilation of a temporal horn of the ventricular system suggests a tumor in the ventricular atrium "trapping" the temporal horn. Dilation of only the lateral and third ven-

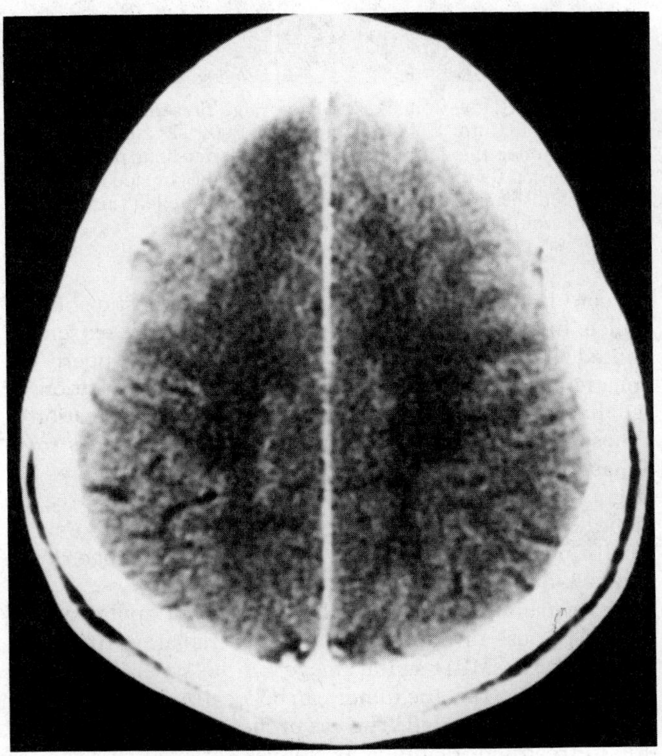

A

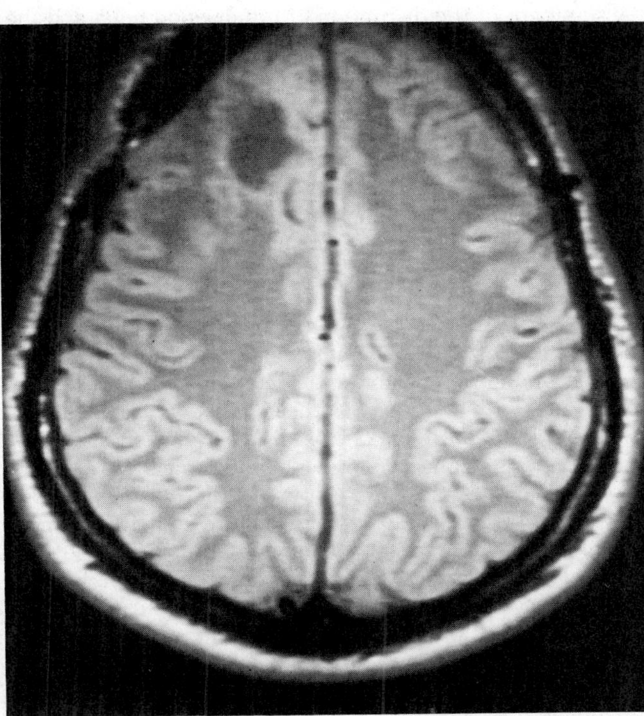

B

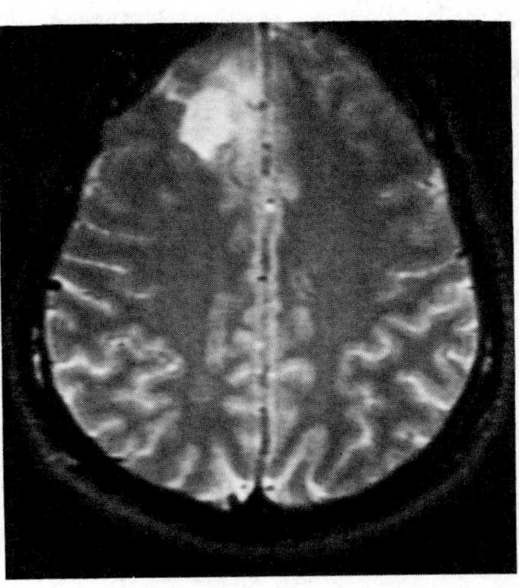

C

FIGURE 48–2. A young man presented with a single focal seizure that generalized into a major motor seizure. **(A)** A postcontrast axial CT demonstrates a poorly defined area of low density involving the most anterior portion of the corona radiata extending anteriorly to the gray matter on the right. No contrast enhancement, sulcal effacement, or mass effect is present. **(B)** After this CT scan, a T2-weighted (TR 2000, TE 20) axial MRI scan was performed that shows an area of decreased signal intensity at the gray-white junction at the most anterior medial aspect of the right frontal lobe. **(C)** On the second echo (TR 2000, TE 60), the lesion exhibits high signal intensity. On biopsy, the tumor was found to be a well-differentiated astrocytoma.

tricles points to a lesion of the aqueduct; when all the ventricles are dilated, communicating hydrocephalus caused by tumor seeding to the meninges or by the reaction to previous therapy should be considered.

Brain tumors occasionally bleed, and this bleeding can be insignificant or can cause dramatic clinical consequences. Metastatic brain tumors that tend to bleed are melanoma, renal cell carcinoma, choriocarcinoma, and thyroid carcinoma. Of the primary CNS tumors, glioblastoma and oligodendrogliomas are more commonly associated with hemorrhage than are other primary tumors. Acute hemorrhage appears as high attenuation on CT, but subacute hemorrhage may be harder to detect by CT. On MRI, acute hemorrhage is of low-signal intensity on T1 and T2; the subacute hemorrhage poorly seen on CT produces a bright signal on both T1- and T2-weighted MRI scans.

Assessment of the disruption of tumor endothelia and the passage of contrast material compared with the intact blood–brain barrier is an important step in radiologic evaluation. The use of contrast agents in CT and MRI scanning provides, in some patients, improved tumor visualization[54] and, in all patients, an improved ability to discern tumors from other pathologic entities, to discern one tumor type from another, and even to discern higher from lower grade malignancies.[55] There are few situations when administration of contrast agents should not be included in the radiologic evaluation of the patient with a brain tumor.

Approximately 50% of patients with low-grade gliomas may present with tumors that do not exhibit contrast enhancement on CT scan. Some may not be detected on CT because they are isodense with brain. It is in these patients that the differential sensitivity of MRI can be seen clearly, even in the absence of a paramagnetic contrast agent. Figure 48–2 shows an example of a CT scan on a patient with a seizure disorder that was interpreted prospectively and retrospectively as normal before and after contrast agent administration. The MRI scan is clearly abnormal. Stereotactic biopsy demonstrated a well-differentiated astrocytoma.

The possibility of obtaining high-quality coronal images without artifact associated with beam hardening through bone makes MRI particularly attractive for evaluating the base of the skull and the posterior fossa. Figure 48–3 is an example of a high-quality MRI scan on a patient with pituitary adenoma. Although this lesion would be identified readily on CT, the relation to the optic chiasm and infundibulum would certainly not be identified as clearly.

In the posterior fossa, the lack of artifact and the availability of sagittal and coronal planes make MRI uniquely suited for detecting and characterizing neoplasms. Both intraaxial and extraaxial masses are distinguished easily, and their relation to the ventricular cisternal systems is assessed easily.

In the evaluation of intracranial tumors, cerebral angiography is used much less frequently than in the past. Angiography may be used to confirm an impression on MRI or CT that the lesion in question is a vascular malformation or an aneurysm rather than a neoplasm. In certain situations, for example, with large meningiomas, angiography may be useful before surgery to determine the blood supply so that it can be embolized during the angiographic procedure or obliterated during the surgical procedure, or both.

In the evaluation of intramedullary and extramedullary spinal cord lesions, high-quality MRI is the diagnostic study of choice. Indications for myelography currently are extremely limited, because multiplanar MRI can provide superb delineation of the spinal cord contour, and the addition of gadolinium-DTPA provides enhancement and visualization of almost all intrinsic tumors (such as ependymomas, astrocytomas, meningiomas, and schwannomas) and facilitates the diagnosis of leptomeningeal disease.[56] Tumor cysts are readily identified on MRI, and currently spinal cord tumors can be distinguished much more reliably from syringomyelia (Fig. 48–4).

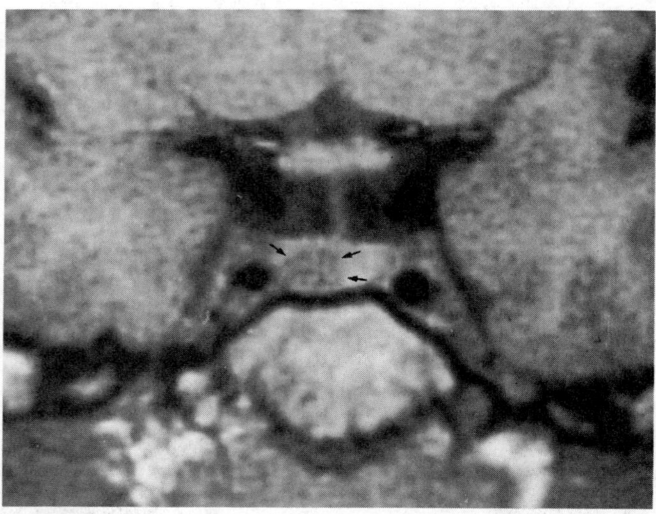

FIGURE 48–3. A woman 30 years of age presented with hyperprolactinemia. Coronal T1-weighted (TR 600, TE 20) 3-mm-thick section scan of the pituitary gland demonstrates (*arrows*) a low-intensity lesion 9 mm in diameter involving the right side of the pituitary fossa displacing the gland and the stalk to the left. Findings are typical of a pituitary microadenoma.

Another unique and particularly important application of MRI is the use of the sagittal image in radiation treatment planning. The MRI sagittal image can be superimposed on the port film so that the tumor can be localized accurately for appropriate port design. The use of the MRI scan is now routine in treatment planning of any base-of-skull or posterior fossa lesion.

TANGENT SCREEN, PERIMETRY, AUDIOMETRY, AND ELECTROENCEPHALOGRAPHY

Testing for abnormalities of the visual system is part of the neurologic examination. However, the results of confrontation visual field testing need quantitation to provide greater accuracy and to follow the effects of treatment. Formal visual field testing is done using tangent screens, and scotomas and field defects are diagnosed with perimetry. Figure 48–5 schematically represents the common visual field abnormalities and their anatomic localization.

Quantitation of deafness is performed by formal audiometric testing. This can be helpful in the diagnosis of acoustic neurinomas. The electrical equivalent of auditory signals can be observed by recording over the brain stem. These signals, called *auditory evoked responses,* correlate well with lesions in the brain stem and can be used to follow patients with brain

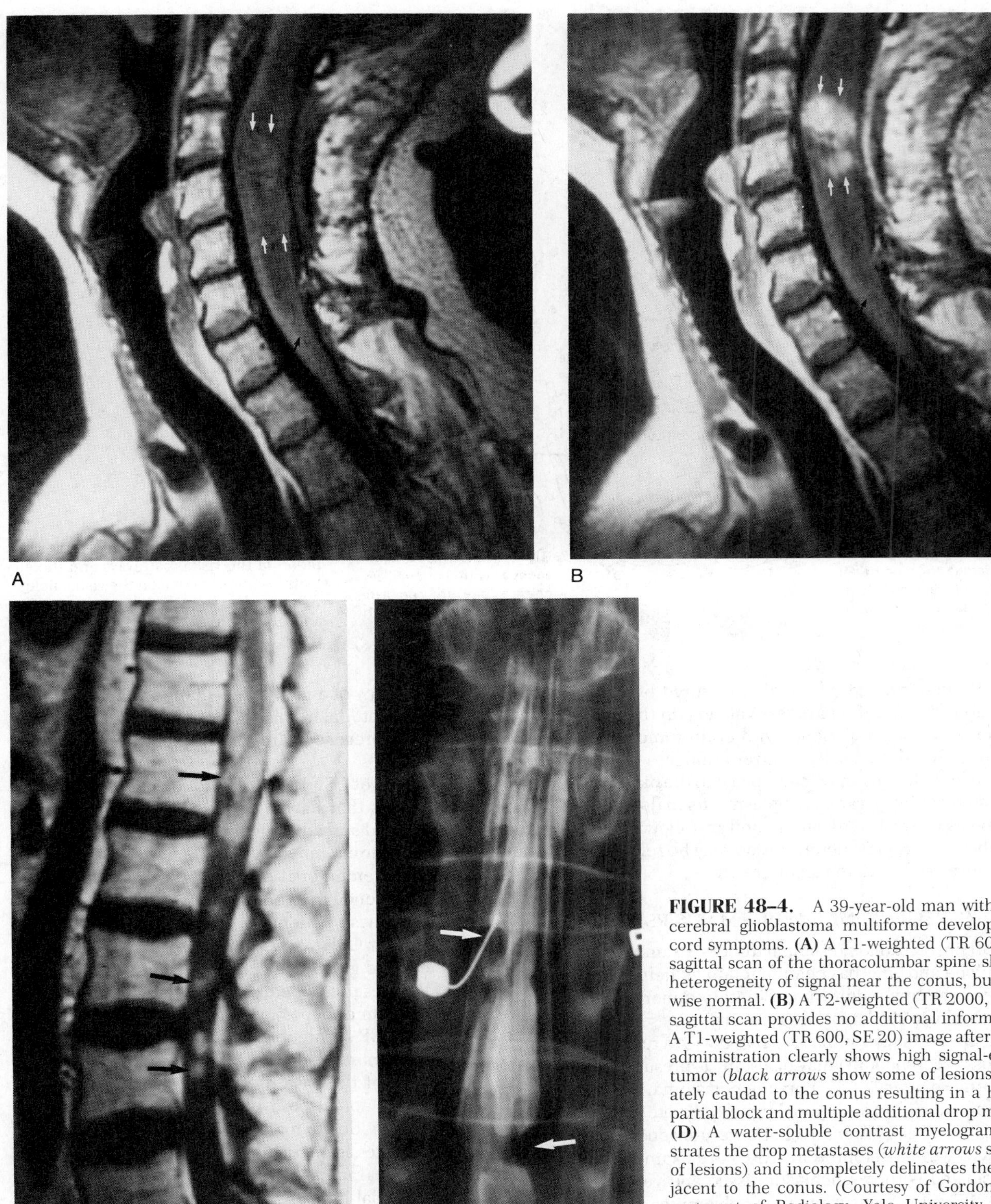

FIGURE 48–4. A 39-year-old man with a known cerebral glioblastoma multiforme developed spinal cord symptoms. **(A)** A T1-weighted (TR 600, TE 20) sagittal scan of the thoracolumbar spine shows mild heterogeneity of signal near the conus, but is otherwise normal. **(B)** A T2-weighted (TR 2000, SE 35,70) sagittal scan provides no additional information. **(C)** A T1-weighted (TR 600, SE 20) image after Gd-DTPA administration clearly shows high signal-enhancing tumor (*black arrows* show some of lesions) immediately caudad to the conus resulting in a high-grade partial block and multiple additional drop metastases. **(D)** A water-soluble contrast myelogram demonstrates the drop metastases (*white arrows* show some of lesions) and incompletely delineates the mass adjacent to the conus. (Courtesy of Gordon Sze, Department of Radiology, Yale University School of Medicine, New Haven, Connecticut)

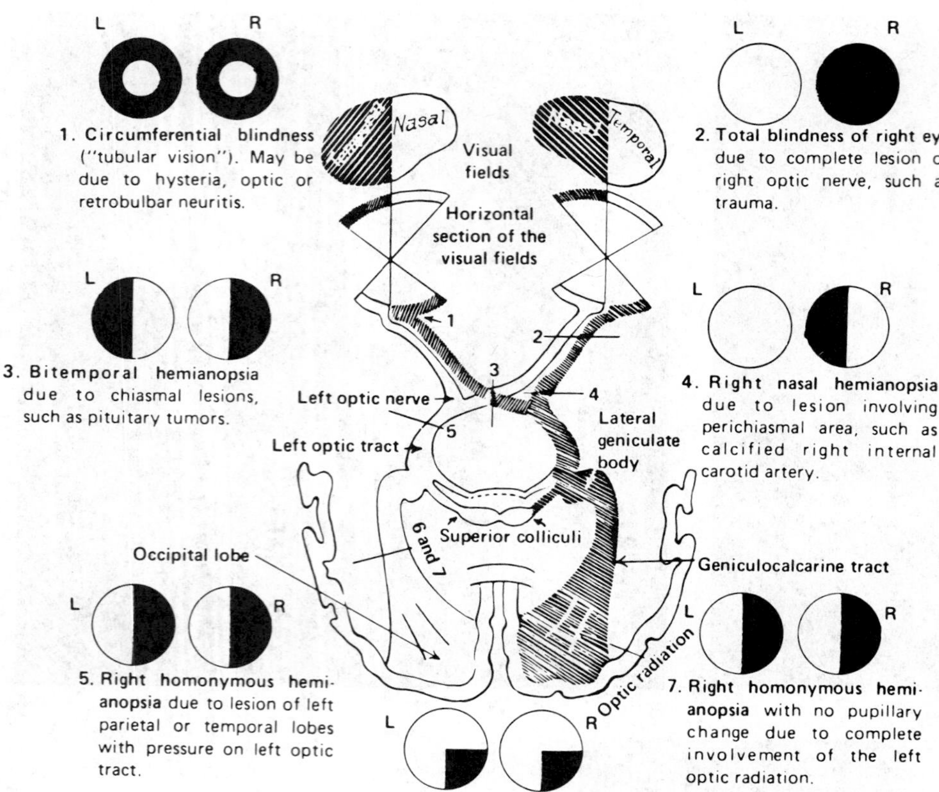

L
R
1. Circumferential blindness ("tubular vision"). May be due to hysteria, optic or retrobulbar neuritis.
Nasal
Temporal
Visual fields
Horizontal section of the visual fields
2. Total blindness of right eye due to complete lesion of right optic nerve, such as trauma.
3. Bitemporal hemianopsia due to chiasmal lesions, such as pituitary tumors.
4. Right nasal hemianopsia due to lesion involving perichiasmal area, such as calcified right internal carotid artery.
Left optic nerve
Left optic tract
Lateral geniculate body
Superior colliculi
6 and 7
Occipital lobe
Geniculocalcarine tract
Optic radiation
5. Right homonymous hemianopsia due to lesion of left parietal or temporal lobes with pressure on left optic tract.
7. Right homonymous hemianopsia with no pupillary change due to complete involvement of the left optic radiation.

FIGURE 48–5. Schematic representation of the visual pathways and the effects lesions can have on the visual fields. (Chusid JG. Correlative neuroanatomy and functional neurology. Los Altos, CA: Lange, 1973)

stem tumors. Similar evoked potentials measured over the visual cortex after visual stimuli are less valuable in the evaluation or follow-up study of patients with brain tumors, but can help distinguish multiple sclerosis from tumor.

The electroencephalogram once had a place in the diagnosis and follow-up study of intracranial neoplasms. Its major value is in the diagnosis of seizure disorders and in following the rare patient whose neurologic deterioration may be related to subclinical seizures rather than tumor growth.

TUMOR AND CEREBROSPINAL FLUID MARKERS

For patients with intracranial and spinal tumors, examination of peripheral blood and CSF has been found to be helpful for diagnosis and for therapy monitoring. Pituitary tumors often produce endocrinologic abnormalities measurable by sensitive radioimmunoassays. Polycythemia associated with a tumor of the posterior fossa (cerebellum) may be useful as presumptive evidence for the diagnosis of hemangioblastoma. Some parasellar and pineal region embryonal tumors secrete unique hormones and proteins; β-human chorionic gonadotrophic hormone (β-HCG) and α-fetoprotein (AFP) are examples of hormones associated with trophoblastic tissue and yolk sac, respectively.[57,58] Finally, measurement of polyamines such as putrescine in the CSF is helpful in following patients with tumors located near the ventricle or spinal subarachnoid space; however, it is not widely used.[59]

INDICATIONS FOR AND INTERPRETATION OF CEREBROSPINAL FLUID EXAMINATION

Lumbar puncture in a patient with headache, papilledema, and a presumed diagnosis of tumor is risky, because it increases the possibility of a fatal cerebellum-foramen magnum or temporal lobe-tentorial herniation. Lumbar puncture should follow rather than precede neuroimaging studies, such as MRI and CT scanning.

The examination of CSF is useful in following patients with intracranial tumors that have a propensity to seed the subarachnoid space and spread through the CSF pathways. Typically, medulloblastoma, ependymoma, choroid plexus carcinoma, and some embryonal pineal and suprasellar region tumors have a high enough likelihood of spread to justify CSF examinations. In these patients, it is important to obtain a lumbar puncture for CSF to examine for malignant cells (cytology), protein, and glucose and specific markers such as β-HCG and AFP. These tests determine if malignant cells are in the CSF and if tumor deposits have reached sufficient size to begin to block CSF subarachnoid pathways. A high protein concentration with normal glucose levels and normal cytology is seen in tumors of the base of the skull, such as acoustic neurinoma, and in spinal cord tumors. The appearance of xanthochromic CSF, due to high protein content, with an absence of erythrocytes is characteristic of spinal cord tumors obstructing the subarachnoid space and producing stasis of the CSF in the caudal lumbar sac.

Evaluation of Patients With Intracranial Tumors During Therapy

Critical to the evaluation of the efficacy of any therapy for brain tumors is the reliability of the measurement of tumor growth (deterioration) or tumor regression (response). Before MRI, sequential neurologic examinations, CT scans, and radionuclide scans were used to evaluate for response and regrowth.[60] Later, with improvement in CT scanners and to reduce the cost of therapy evaluations, contrast-enhanced CT scanning became the major method to evaluate patients for response and regrowth. Contrast-enhanced MRI scans are replacing CT scans in many instances. However, the extreme sensitivity of the MRI to changes in brain water content and small enhancing lesions can be confusing in the evaluation of tumor regrowth and progression. The use of magnetic resonance spectroscopy and diffusion-perfusion algorithms may improve the ability to assess tumor regrowth in the postirradiation period.

To interpret the results of therapy correctly and to improve patient care, understanding factors other than cell division is important; these are discussed in the following sections.

FACTORS THAT MAY PRODUCE CLINICAL DETERIORATION

The commonest causes of neurologic deterioration in brain tumor patients undergoing radiation therapy or chemotherapy, or both, are growth of the tumor or increased peritumoral edema. Both cause increased pressure in the cranial cavity that is transmitted primarily to the adjacent brain; in turn, hydrostatic pressure on the brain can lead to impairment of cerebral blood flow. The clinical result can be progressive impairment of functioning brain with resultant neurologic deficits. These manifestations may include signs and symptoms of increased intracranial pressure and temporal lobe or cerebellar herniation (see Tables 48–5 and 48–6).

Neurologic deterioration, without neuroimaging evidence of tumor growth, can occur for any of the following reasons:

1. Obstructive hydrocephalus can occur secondary to tumor in the ventricular system at the aqueduct of Sylvius, fourth ventricle, or foramen of Monro or communicating hydrocephalus due to infiltrative tumor (carcinomatosis, CNS leukemia, and arachnoiditis).
2. Hemorrhage into a tumor may occur.
3. Fluid imbalance, particularly hyponatremia caused by excessive administration of parenteral dextrose in water solutions, may develop.
4. Hypertension can accentuate intratumoral and peritumoral edema.
5. Reactive peritumoral edema (or demyelination) may develop early in the course of radiation therapy.
6. An "early-delayed" syndrome, observed in about 20% to 25% of patients completing a course of cranial irradiation, can be distinguished from tumor regrowth only by waiting and finding that the patient's condition improves without further treatment.[61] This encephalopathy responds to corticosteroids and resolves within several weeks without specific sequelae. This syndrome is not unique to patients with brain tumors, and is observed in leukemic children after prophylactic cranial irradiation.
7. Radiation necrosis can occur within 6 months to 10 years or longer after radiation therapy and can produce neurologic impairment that may be indistinguishable from tumor recurrence.
8. Seizures may suggest that the tumor is growing and may result in an increase in the neurologic deficit apart from any direct effect of the tumor. Recovery from any increase in weakness and mental dullness may take several hours to a week in postictal patients who are already brain injured. Even subclinical seizures can cause deterioration, persisting for hours to days, which resolves with control of the seizures. The electroencephalogram is usually diagnostic in these patients, and the treatment is better control of seizures. Patients receiving long-term chemotherapy often require higher doses of anticonvulsants or widely fluctuating dosages caused by drug-induced hepatic changes.
9. Infection and fever often exacerbate neurologic signs and symptoms, regardless of the site of infection. The more common causes of infection include pneumonia secondary to aspiration or atelectasis and urinary tract infections; meningitis and cerebral abscess are less common.
10. Metabolic disorders, anemia, fatigue, and emotional depression can cause clinical deterioration, including increase in focal deficit on testing, that is difficult to distinguish from tumor progression. Such conditions generally produce no alteration of neuroimages.

In these authors' experience, at least 10% of patients who eventually respond to therapy become significantly worse at the end of a first course of chemotherapy, and transient deterioration is observed occasionally even during the second year of continuous chemotherapy. Paradoxically, this clinical worsening early in therapy may result from an increase in tumor bulk resulting from "effective" therapy. Several factors contribute: cell mass may increase when doomed cells form giant cells or undergo one or more successful cell divisions before dying; the CNS also has an inefficient mechanism for disposing of dead cells produced by chemotherapy or irradiation; and edema, probably caused by irritative products of cell lysis, may be present within the tumor mass and in adjacent brain.

GLUCOCORTICOID USAGE

Administration of glucocorticoids is usually begun before surgery for brain tumor. If an adequate surgical decompression is achieved, the steroid dose can be tapered off rapidly and discontinued within the first week or two after the operation. Some patients require steroid maintenance because a large volume of tumor remains, because tumor occupies the brain stem or spinal cord, or because of steroid dependence resulting from long-term prior usage.

Patients who no longer require corticosteroids after surgery may need them during or after radiation therapy. Reactive edema may occur during irradiation, and there may be a transient period of drowsiness and increased deficit for 6 to 16 weeks after treatment. In both instances, signs and symptoms usually resolve within a few weeks; observation of the subsequent clinical course is often the only way to differentiate these reactions from tumor progression.

The lowest dosage of glucocorticoid that maintains patients at their maximum level of comfort and function should be sought. Ordinarily, this is determined by decreasing the dosage until symptoms increase or become apparent, then increasing the dosage until they subside. If deterioration is secondary to tumor growth or treatment-induced effects, glucocorticoids may have to be increased to keep the patient comfortable. For example, 3 mg/day of dexamethasone may have the desired effect for a patient with stabilized disease; however, a deteriorating patient may require dexamethasone doses of 64 mg/day or more.

The efficacy of chemotherapy and radiation therapy can be affected by glucocorticoid dosage. A decrease in steroid requirement suggests improvement, assuming that the previous dosage was actually required. An increase in dosage suggests deterioration. Because increased glucocorticoid dosage may improve neurologic status and reduce the image size on an MRI and CT scan, an attempt should be made to document tumor recurrence before increasing glucocorticoid dosage.

SURGERY

GENERAL CONSIDERATIONS

No other modality can reduce tumor bulk as quickly as surgery, and advances in imaging, pharmacologic agents for brain edema, neuroanesthesia, and surgical magnification, illumination, and instrumentation have made operative approaches to tumors in even the most remote corners of the CNS possible and reasonably safe. The goal of brain tumor surgery is to resect and cure the tumor completely. If surgical cure is not possible, such as in most gliomas, tumor bulk reduction and consequent decompression of the brain is the next goal and, when possible, should be the first therapeutic modality for the tumor.

An extremely important byproduct of cytoreductive surgery is the acquisition of adequate tissue for histopathologic examination. Only rarely should brain tumors be treated with irradiation or chemotherapy without a definitive tissue diagnosis. In patients with tumors that are believed to be inaccessible by open craniotomy or in patients for whom open craniotomy is deemed unhelpful, a needle biopsy should be performed with guidance from CT, MRI, or ultrasound. CT-guided stereotaxy is the easiest method for obtaining tissue with a needle.

SURGICAL PLANNING

The intrinsic characteristics of a tumor's appearance and its relative position in the brain as shown on a technically adequate MRI scan can most often narrow the diagnostic possibilities to one or two choices, and a view of the tumor in several planes simplifies surgical planning.

Cerebral angiography is important in surgical planning for tumors that may encircle critical cerebral blood vessels, such as basal meningiomas, or for tumors that can be extremely vascular, such as hemangioblastomas, meningiomas, and glomus tumors. Angiography done in temporal proximity (24–96 hours) to the planned surgical procedure can be combined with embolization of the tumor's blood supply, in many instances making the surgical procedure technically easier.

The final selection of a surgical approach is made after adequate imaging, after developing a differential diagnosis, and after assessing the patient's general condition. In the era of modern neuroanesthesia, it is rare that a craniotomy must not be done because of poor general medical status. The design of an appropriate scalp incision and bone flap is the final preoperative decision.

PREOPERATIVE AND ANESTHETIC MANAGEMENT

Patients undergoing surgery for supratentorial tumors should be placed on anticonvulsants, and corticosteroids commonly (dexamethasone) should be administered for a few days preoperatively, when possible, to reduce cerebral edema and thereby facilitate cerebral retraction for perfect exposure. Blood levels of anticonvulsants should be monitored to ensure that the therapeutic range has been achieved. Anticonvulsants should also be continued for at least 1 year. Corticosteroids should be continued into the postoperative period and then tapered, when possible. The anesthetic agents are selected for their lack of effect on intracranial pressure. In general, the head is held rigidly with pin fixation to minimize movement as the surgeon is looking through the operating microscope, where the slighest movement is dramatically amplified. As the procedure is about to commence, mannitol (1 g/kg body weight) is administered and hyperventilation to a P_{CO_2} of 25 to 30 mm Hg is accomplished for definitive reduction of the intracranial pressure in preparation for brain retraction. These authors routinely administer bromodeoxyuridine intravenously during the induction of anesthesia to obtain a labeling index of the tumor on the fixed tissue postoperatively.[62]

CRANIOTOMY FOR SUPRATENTORIAL TUMORS

The bony opening is designed so that it is generous enough to facilitate surgery. The bone flap is centered over the tumor or positioned to provide access to the route of approach. In all instances, the scalp flap is designed to accommodate the bone flap fully, and the vascular supply to the scalp is given careful consideration in the design.

After the scalp incision is made and the scalp flap reflected, burr holes are drilled and connected with a hand or power saw. The bone flap can be turned back, attached to the temporal muscle (osteoplastic flap) or its blood supply, or removed completely (free flap). The dura is opened only after the brain has been softened completely by mannitol diuresis and intraoperative hyperventilation. Sometimes a few minutes' wait is necessary to secure maximum decompression, and this brief pause can be critical to the success of the subsequent surgical approach.

The dura is reflected back, and the approach to the tumor is made. The surgeon can be confused by a field of normal-appearing cortex when seeking to expose a small subcortical lesion. In this situation, intraoperative ultrasonography is invaluable in delineating the position of a small tumor, and a cortical incision can be made directly over the lesion, thereby minimizing cortical injury. Tumor removal is usually done with grasping instruments, sponges, and suction, but removal of firm, adherent, or calcified tumor tissue can be difficult and is simplified by use of the Cavitron ultrasonic aspirator (CUSA), which ultrasonically disrupts the tumor at its tip and sucks it away. Tumor in locations where access is limited (for example, the third ventricle) and space to use graspers and other equipment is not available sometimes can be dealt with best by use of the CO_2 laser, which can vaporize tumor tissue with a "hands off" technique. Tumor removal with a laser is slow, however, and is reserved for special circumstances.

In the rare situations when brain swelling is worrisome at the time of closure, a catheter is left in the subdural space to measure the intracranial pressure. All patients are monitored in the intensive care unit for at least 1 night after surgery, and a CT scan is done within 48 hours to evaluate the success of the tumor resection. Serum electrolyte levels and osmolality are measured often in the postoperative period to ensure that the patient is relatively dehydrated through the first several days and to detect the possible onset of inappropriate secretion of antidiuretic hormone or diabetes insipidus.

CRANIOTOMY FOR POSTERIOR FOSSA TUMORS

The occiput and, commonly, the dorsal aspects of C1 and C2 are exposed. A generous craniotomy is done unilaterally or bilaterally to accommodate an approach through the vermis or through, over, or around the cerebellar hemisphere. A laminectomy of C1 and sometimes C2 is done in certain midline approaches to improve tumor exposure or extend the decompression. The CO_2 laser occasionally is more valuable than the CUSA in posterior fossa tumor resections because of the tight working space.

STEREOTACTIC TUMORS BIOPSY

For intrinsic tumors of the deep midline, for example, pontine or corpus callosum gliomas, for deep tumors of the dominant hemisphere, or for diffuse nonfocal tumors, surgical resection is not practical. In these situations, needle biopsy for diagnosis is essential. There is no longer any reason to perform a full craniotomy for the purpose of biopsy only. Tissue can be obtained through a needle directed by hand through a burr hole under CT scan guidance or a needle directed by many devices that incorporate ultrasound images. However, in these authors' opinion, nothing is as simple or accurate as CT- or MRI-directed stereotactic biopsy.

A number of image-guided stereotactic systems are available.[63,64] Figure 48–6 shows the general sequence of events using the Brown-Roberts-Wells guidance technique. Typically, the patient undergoes a CT scan with a rigid array of bars affixed tightly to the skull to minimize movement. In adults, local anesthesia usually is used; children usually require general anesthesia. The CT scan image demonstrates the lesion in which the biopsy will be performed and also the localizing rods, thereby relating the target to a volume encompassed by the rods. By digitizing the position of the target and the position of the rods, this relation is formalized, and the coordinates for a trajectory to the target are created in a way specific to the individual stereotactic system used.

The target is approached through a burr hole or a (smaller) twist drill hole. The biopsy instrument is guided to the target by use of an adjustable stereotactic arc that is placed on the head in fixed relation to the former position of the localizing rods used for the CT scan. A fragment of tissue is aspirated or grasped for removal, and a frozen section confirms the acquisition of diagnostic material and most often also suggests a working diagnosis. Experienced surgeons obtain diagnostic tissue in more than 95% of patients, and these patients stay only 1 night in the hospital.[64] The principal risk of the surgery, hemorrhage at the biopsy site, occurs in few patients.[64] Occasionally, cerebral edema is exacerbated by the procedure.

RADIATION THERAPY

GENERAL CONSIDERATIONS

Most primary CNS neoplasms are unifocal and, therefore, they are potentially curable with effective local forms of therapy. However, most of these lesions infiltrate for a considerable distance into surrounding normal CNS tissue, and their borders are poorly demarcated, even by CT scan or MRI. Therefore, it is often necessary to irradiate a substantial amount of normal tissue within the target volume to relatively high doses, and the tolerance of these tissues to irradiation becomes a limiting factor. As local treatments become more aggressive, as in the case of malignant gliomas, the incidence of radiation injury will probably increase.

TOLERANCE OF THE BRAIN

Adverse reactions associated with cranial irradiation differ in their pathogenesis and can be classified according to their time of presentation into (1) acute reactions that occur during or shortly after radiation therapy; (2) early-delayed reactions that appear within a few weeks to 2 or 3 months after irradiation; and (3) late-delayed injuries that develop several months to years after treatment.[65]

Acute reactions are thought to be caused by radiation-induced edema and to include symptoms of increased intracranial pressure if the whole brain is treated or if there is an intensification of preexisting neurologic symptoms or signs when the treatment is confined to the location of the lesion. Symptoms are generally mild and self-limited and, if necessary, can be treated effectively with corticosteroids. A dose of 60 Gy in conventional daily dose fractions of 1.8 to 2 Gy, five times per week, can be given to all or part of the brain without significant acute morbidity. Hyperfractionated irradiation schedules of 0.9 to 1.2 Gy, two or three times daily, to doses as high as 81.6 Gy, and accelerated fractionation programs of 1.6 to 2 Gy given two or three times daily to approximately 60 to 70 Gy delivered to a portion of the brain are also acutely tolerable. Individual dose fractions as much as 6 Gy to the whole brain are well tolerated, provided that the total administered dose is reduced coincident with the increase in fraction size. Severe complications, however, have been observed with higher dose fractions.[66]

The early-delayed reaction, characterized by somnolence or an exacerbation of preexisting signs and symptoms, is thought to result from temporary demyelination caused by the effects of radiation on oligodendroglial cells[61] or radiation-induced changes in capillary permeability.[67] In addition, early vascular abnormalities and tumor necrosis may induce clinical and radiographic changes that are indistinguishable from tumor progression.[68] Although signs and symptoms are usually mild, corticosteroid therapy and intensive medical support may be required. The appearance of new findings during this early posttreatment interval does not always indicate that the tumor has recurred or that a change in therapy is needed.

Late-delayed radiation injuries constitute the most serious aftereffects of therapeutic irradiation on the brain and vary in their appearance and severity from asymptomatic white matter changes to potentially fatal necrosis. The late-delayed reaction presents as a focal or as a diffuse white matter injury

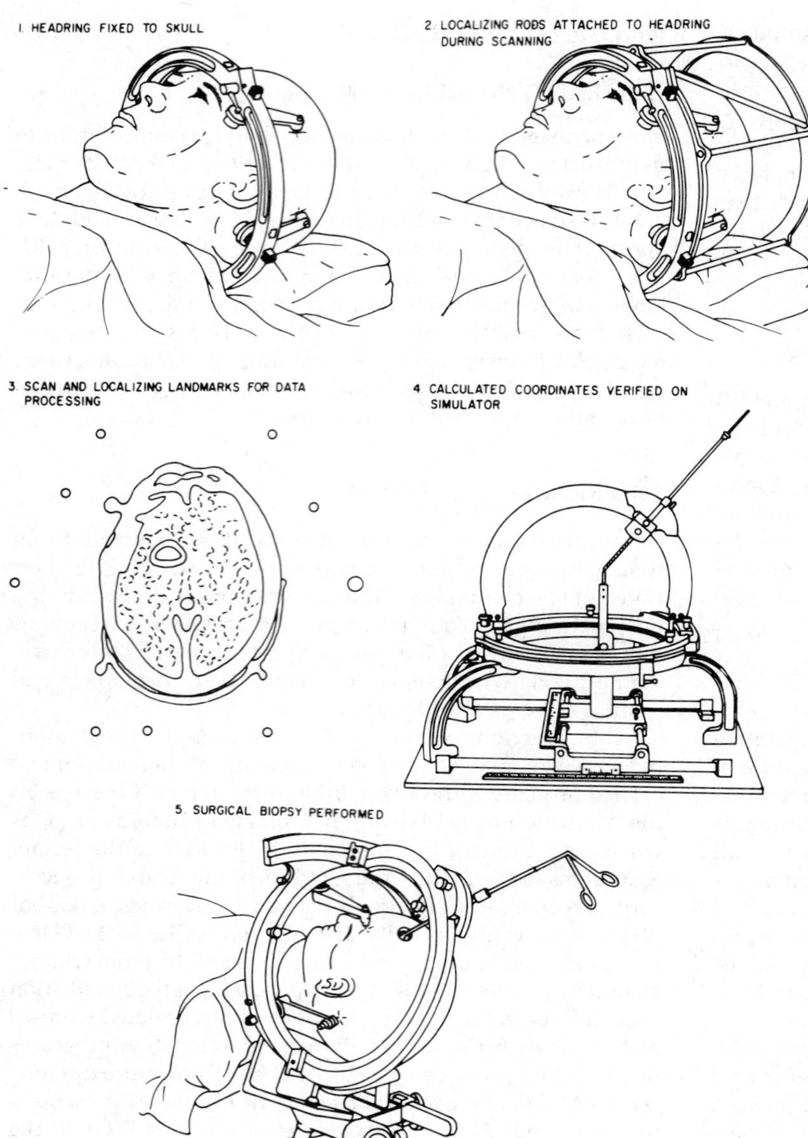
1. HEADRING FIXED TO SKULL
2. LOCALIZING RODS ATTACHED TO HEADRING DURING SCANNING
3. SCAN AND LOCALIZING LANDMARKS FOR DATA PROCESSING
4. CALCULATED COORDINATES VERIFIED ON SIMULATOR
5. SURGICAL BIOPSY PERFORMED

FIGURE 48–6. Steps and typical equipment used for CT-guided stereotactic biopsy. The equipment depicted is part of the Brown-Roberts-Wells guidance technique. (Weiss MH. Clinical neurosurgery. In: Proceedings of the Congress of Neurological Surgeons. Baltimore: Williams & Wilkins, 1983)

that may occur together in the same patient. The clinical presentation depends on the site and volume of the brain exposed. Patients with focal radiation necrosis present with localizing neurologic signs, often accompanied by symptoms of increased intracranial pressure. Focal hypodensity or a contrast-enhancing mass with surrounding vasogenic edema may be seen on CT scan. MR images show a contrast-enhancing mass with focal hyperintensity on T2-weighted images. Diffuse white matter injury typically occurs after large-volume or whole-brain irradiation. Clinical features include seizure disorders and varying degrees of neuropsychological impairment. Diffuse white matter hypodensity is seen on CT scan, often accompanied by a focal enhancing mass, whereas T2-weighted MR images show diffuse periventricular white matter hyperintensity.[69] Late radiation injury has been attributed to vascular injury or to a direct effect on glial cells, and multiple mechanisms are probably involved.[65] Rarely, therapeutic irradiation causes an intracranial vessel occlusive vasculopathy[70,71] or secondary neoplasia.[71]

The tolerance of the brain depends on the size of the dose per fraction and the total dose administered. The probability of injury increases with larger daily doses and doses in excess of 60 Gy delivered in 30 fractions over approximately 6 weeks. Sheline and associates suggested that the threshold doses for brain injury are approximately 35 Gy for 10 fractions, 60 Gy for 35 fractions, and 76 Gy for 60 fractions.[72] They further demonstrated that the isoeffective dose (termed *neuret*) formula should have an exponent of $N = -0.41$ and an exponent of $T = -0.03$ (where N is the number of fractions and T is the total time in days), but they warned that this formula may not be applicable to extremely small or large numbers of fractions or to extremely short or long overall treatment times.

Approximately 4% to 9% of patients treated for brain tumors develop clinically detectable focal radiation necrosis, and this form of injury may be found in as many as 15% to 22% of patients at autopsy. A review by Marks and colleagues of 139 patients who received irradiation for primary brain tumors with at least 45 Gy in daily dose fractions of 1.8 to 2 Gy disclosed 7 patients with brain necrosis.[73] A recalculation of their data, assuming a daily dose of 1.8 Gy given five times per week, demonstrated that the incidence of necrosis was directly related to dose. Of 51 patients who received total doses of 57.6 Gy or less, there were no cases of necrosis. Two of 60 patients (3%) who received between 57.6 and 64.8 Gy developed necrosis, and 5 of 28 patients (18%) who received 64.8 to 75.6 Gy developed necrosis.[74]

Several additional factors may affect the radiation tolerance of the brain. Children younger than 2 to 3 years of age are thought to be more susceptible to injury than are adults because of incomplete development of the CNS.[72] Vasculopathy associated with endocrine disorders,[75] CNS infection,[76] and cerebral edema[77] also appear to potentiate the effects of radiation.

The risk of injury may be amplified by some chemotherapeutic agents.[78] The most dramatic illustration of the toxicity of combined modality therapy was observed in children with acute lymphoblastic leukemia treated with prophylactic brain irradiation and methotrexate administered intravenously and intrathecally. Two delayed syndromes, necrotizing leukoencephalopathy and mineralizing microangiopathy, have been recognized in children who received 24 Gy in 1.5 to 2 Gy daily increments, which without chemotherapy are well below tolerance levels. Although necrotizing leukoencephalopathy has not been reported with a dose of 24 Gy in the absence of chemotherapy and occurs in fewer than 1% to 2% of patients receiving intrathecal and high-dose intravenous methotrexate, the incidence with all three therapies combined is as high as 45%.[79] It is currently recognized that methotrexate is most toxic when given during or after radiation therapy, and attention to this detail has reduced the frequency of this complication significantly.

Because radiation-induced changes are often indistinguishable from tumor recurrence on CT and MRI, the clinical diagnosis of radiation necrosis may be difficult to confirm. Thallium 201 single-photon emission computed tomography (SPECT)[80] and F-18 fluorodeoxyglucose positron emission tomography (PET)[81] studies may help separate patients with radiation necrosis from those with recurrent tumor. However, a biopsy may be required to confirm the diagnosis, especially when the injury occurs at or near the tumor site.

Corticosteroids may improve or stabilize the neurologic symptoms associated with the effects of radiation injury. Surgical resection is often beneficial to patients with favorably situated, focal radiation-induced lesions who deteriorate neurologically and become dependent on corticosteroids.[81]

Decreased levels of intellectual function have been observed after cranial irradiation in children and adults with acute lymphoblastic leukemia, small cell lung carcinoma, and primary brain tumors. IQ decrements and perceptual and learning disabilities seen after CNS prophylaxis in children with acute lymphoblastic leukemia have long been attributed to cranial irradiation. However, a recent study comparing the long-term cognitive outcome of children treated with 18 or 24 Gy and intrathecal methotrexate or intrathecal and intravenous methotrexate without cranial irradiation failed to demonstrate an overall decline in verbal, performance, or full-scale IQ in any of the three groups, although 22% to 30% of children in each group showed at least a 15-point decline in IQ during the study period. The authors proposed that ecologic factors or continuation-phase chemotherapy rather than radiation therapy might account for the IQ changes.[82]

Neuropsychological deterioration has been recognized in long-term surviving patients with small cell lung carcinoma who receive prophylactic cranial irradiation. These patients are treated with a variety of chemotherapeutic agents that may enhance the effects of radiation on the CNS. The risk and severity of impairment appear to be related to radiation dose and fraction size and to the type, sequence, and dose intensity of the chemotherapeutic agents used.[83]

Children irradiated for brain tumors have IQ decrements and behavioral disturbances. Most require formal psychological intervention and special education programs. Young age at treatment, supratentorial tumor sites, the use of whole-brain irradiation, poorly controlled seizure disorders, the presence of sensorimotor deficits, and the addition of chemotherapy have a negative influence on IQ.[84] The risk and severity of neuropsychological dysfunction are also affected by psychological stress, reduced school attendance, and the adequacy of rehabilitative efforts.[85]

Cranial irradiation also leads to intellectual impairment in adults. Unlike in children, however, only a limited amount of quantitative information is available, especially for patients treated with radiation therapy alone. Impairment is most pronounced in those patients who have had chemotherapy and whole-brain irradiation.[85] Decrements in tests of new learning ability, recent memory, abstraction, and problem solving have been observed,[86] and early return to work after treatment may lead to improvement or recovery of neuropsychological function.[87]

Radiation therapy may cause hypothalamic-pituitary dysfunction, and the incidence and degree of hormone suppression appear to be dose related, with a threshold of approximately 25 to 30 Gy.[88] Growth hormone deficiency is the most frequent endocrine dysfunction observed after radiation therapy. Children who undergo irradiation to the hypothalamic-pituitary axis should be evaluated for pituitary function before, and periodically after, irradiation. Early detection of a deficiency permits appropriate hormonal replacement therapy before irreversible damage has occurred.

TOLERANCE OF THE SPINAL CORD

Radiation myelopathy may present as a transient early-delayed or as a more ominous late-delayed reaction. Transient radiation myelopathy is clinically manifested by momentary, electrical shock-like paresthesias or numbness radiating from the neck to the extremities, precipitated by neck flexion (Lhermitte's sign). The syndrome develops after an average latent period of 3 to 4 months and gradually resolves over the ensuing 3 to 6 months without the need for specific therapy. These findings have been attributed to transient demyelination caused by radiation-induced inhibition of myelin-producing oligodendroglial cells in the irradiated cord segment.[89] An alternative hypothesis suggests that radiation induces a transient disruption of the blood–spinal cord barrier, resulting in vasogenic edema, which in turn leads to demyelination.[67]

Radiation myelopathy is one of the most feared complications in clinical radiotherapy. In addition to its obvious neurologic sequelae, about 50% of patients die from secondary complications.[90] The latent period between the completion of radiation therapy and the onset of symptoms is bimodal in distribution, with the first peak occurring at 12 to 14 months and the second occurring at 24 to 28 months. A dual mechanism of injury has been suggested to explain the bimodal distribution of presentation. The earlier peak is associated with demyelination and white matter necrosis due to a direct effect on oligodendroglial cells, whereas the later peak results from intramedullary microvascular injury. The signs and symptoms that accompany radiation myelopathy are irreversible. They may be partial in some patients, whereas in others there is progressive functional loss that becomes complete over several months. Less commonly, radiation myelopathy is manifested by the acute onset of paraplegia or quadriplegia that evolves over several hours or a few days, resulting from infarction of the cord. Myelopathy may also be heralded by lower motor neuron dysfunction due to selective injury to anterior horn cells.[91]

The diagnosis of radiation myelopathy requires a history of radiation therapy in doses sufficient to result in injury. The portion of the cord irradiated must be slightly above the dermatome level of expression of the lesion, and the latent period from the completion of treatment to the onset of injury must be consistent with that observed in radiation myelopathy. There are no confirmatory laboratory tests or imaging studies that distinguish radiation myelopathy from other spinal cord lesions, and the diagnosis is often one of exclusion.

The medical and legal consequences of radiation myelopathy are such that treatment with radiation therapy is often compromised to keep the spinal cord dose within a "safe" level.[92] A dose of 50 Gy in 25 fractions over 5 weeks usually is considered to be safe, the risk of myelopathy being less than 0.5%.[92] The dose of 40 to 45 Gy commonly given to the spinal cord in head and neck irradiation appears to be well below the steep portion of the dose-response curve.[92] It is estimated that with conventionally fractionated irradiation (1.8–2 Gy per fraction, five fractions per week), the incidence of myelopathy is 5% for doses in the range of 57 to 61 Gy and 50% for doses of 68 to 73 Gy.[93] At doses higher than the tolerance threshold, the risk of injury increases with the length of cord irradiated.[94] There is no convincing evidence that the cervical and thoracic cord differ in their radiosensitivity. The belief that the cervical cord is more tolerant than the thoracic cord probably arose from differences in biologic dose resulting from the practice of treating with one field per day, which was common through the mid-1970s.[93]

Various isoeffect formulas have been proposed for the spinal cord. Wara and coworkers derived an Ellis-type formula with an exponent of $N = -0.377$ and an exponent of $T = -0.058$.[95] Van der Kogel and Berendsen concluded that the isoeffect formula should have an N exponent of -0.4 and that for treatment times as long as 6 weeks, the time factor was essentially negligible.[96] These formulas suggest that in addition to the total dose given, radiation myelopathy is related to the size of the individual daily dose and predict that spinal cord tolerance will continue to increase with decreasing fraction size. However, data indicate that reducing the fraction size to lower than 2 Gy does not alter the dose response significantly,[97] and that extrapolating from a conventionally fractionated cord dose to an equivalent hyperfractionated cord dose using any isoeffect formula should be approached with caution.[93]

TUMOR TARGET VOLUME AND TREATMENT TECHNIQUES

The appropriate volume to encompass within the radiation treatment portal varies according to the specific histopathologic tumor type and, with certain histologies, is a topic of considerable controversy. Because their tendency to infiltrate beyond the lesional borders visualized by neuroimaging studies is limited, certain tumors, such as benign meningiomas, pituitary adenomas, craniopharyngiomas, and acoustic neurilemmomas, may be treated with narrow margins of surrounding normal tissue. In contrast, the astrocytic gliomas require larger margins for uncertainty because of their tendency to infiltrate beyond the identifiable tumor periphery. Improved imaging techniques and a better understanding of recurrence patterns have fostered the use of limited radiation portals rather than whole-brain irradiation for malignant gliomas. Comparisons of CT and MRI studies with clinical and pathologic findings have shown that (1) malignant gliomas are localized, and microscopic invasion of the perilesional brain is limited at the time of initial diagnosis[98]; (2) only 1.1% of patients present with multiple lesions[99]; (3) after initial treatment, most of these lesions, when they recur, do so at their original location[100]; and (4) isolated tumor cell infiltration may extend to the periphery of T2-weighted MRI abnormalities.[101] Clinical studies have failed to demonstrate that irradiating the whole brain is superior to treating more limited fields,[74] and patients surviving for extended periods after whole-brain irradiation, especially in combination with chemotherapy, may suffer considerable treatment-related morbidity.[85] Until the primary tumor can be controlled with greater frequency, and the patterns of failure in such patients suggest that local fields are unjustified, there is little rationale for treating the whole brain.

The radiation-beam energy and field arrangements are selected after consideration of the location of the tumor within the brain and the geometry of the target volume. The *tumor volume* is defined as a three-dimensional reconstruction of the tumor contour based on operative findings and data from CT and MRI studies. The *target volume* consists of the volume of tissue that must be irradiated to encompass the tumor volume with a margin of surrounding tissue considered to be at risk for microscopic tumor spread and to account for patient movement and daily set-up uncertainties. Depending on tumor size and location, treatment portals may be coaxially opposed or designed in a more complex fashion, using multiple or rotational fields with wedge filters. Three-dimensional conformal radiation therapy is a new method of treatment planning and delivery designed to enhance the conformation of the dose to the target volume, while maximally restricting the dose delivered to the normal tissue outside the treatment volume. In the future, this approach may improve the outcome of patients with brain tumors by allowing higher than traditional radiation doses to be administered safely. Megavoltage equipment with energies ranging from cobalt 60 to 15 MeV photons is used to administer radiation therapy. Treatment is generally given in daily fractions of 1.72 to 2 Gy/day five times per week. The total doses referred to in this chapter assume that this "conventional" fractionation scheme is used unless otherwise specified.

Certain neoplasms, such as medulloblastomas and primitive

neuroectodermal tumors, require treatment to the entire craniospinal axis. Patients are treated prone in an immobilization cast to ensure daily positional reproducibility. The intracranial contents, including the upper one or two segments of the cervical cord, are treated through opposed lateral fields. The spine is treated through one or two posterior fields, depending on the size of the patient. The collimator for the lateral cranial fields is angled to match the divergence of the upper border of the adjacent spinal field, and the treatment couch is angulated so that the inferior border of the cranial field is perpendicular to the superior edge of the spinal field. Individualized focused blocks protect the normal extracranial head and neck tissues from the primary radiation beam. The cranial and posterior spine fields may be abutted, but a gap of 0.5 to 1 cm is often left between the fields. When two posterior spinal fields are used, as is usually the case, a gap is calculated so that the 50% isodose lines meet at the level of the spinal cord. All junction lines are moved 0.5 to 1 cm daily or at least every 10 Gy to avoid overdosing or underdosing segments of the cord. This is accomplished by expanding the lateral cranial fields and moving the posterior spine fields caudally without changing their dimensions. A fixed block is placed at the inferior margin of the caudal spinal field to keep the lower margin of the irradiated volume at the same location. Several modifications of this approach are used in clinical practice.

CHEMOTHERAPY

GENERAL PHARMACOLOGIC CONSIDERATIONS

The use of anticancer agents in the treatment of intracranial and spinal tumors is established for many primary tumors. For parenchymal CNS tumors, however, controversy surrounds the concept of limited antitumor efficacy for agents with restricted blood–brain barrier permeability.[102] Supporting the concept is the fact that many infiltrative primary CNS tumors (*e.g.*, gliomas) have cellular regions within the brain with apparently intact normal-appearing brain capillaries. In addition, the actual extent of capillary breakdown accounting for the leakage responsible for positive-contrast CT and radionuclide brain scans is small.[103] Although drug delivery to portions of any primary tumor would be expected to occur to the same extent as with non-CNS tumors, delivery (by diffusion) to infiltrative regions distant from leaky tumor capillaries would be expected to be compromised. Diffusion, being a slow process, cannot achieve significant drug concentrations, unless plasma drug levels are sustainable for prolonged periods, and the diffusing drug is relatively stable in the tumor tissue as it diffuses.

A secondary supporting argument is that most agents with antitumor activity against CNS tumors readily cross the blood–brain barrier.[104] For example, all of the nonsugar-containing chloroethylnitrosoureas (CENUs) such as BCNU, CCNU, PCNU, and ACNU have shown efficacy as single agents, whereas sugar-containing CENUs are less effective.[47] Procarbazine, another commonly used agent, also crosses the blood–brain barrier and is active.[105] Agents such as bleomycin, doxorubicin, cisplatin, vincristine (VCR), and mithramycin have shown no activity or have activity limited to primitive childhood and embryonal tumors.

Whether ease of blood–brain barrier passage constitutes an absolute or relative advantage is somewhat academic, given the paucity of chemotypes with demonstrable antitumor activity. Even a small pharmacokinetic disadvantage takes on disproportionate importance when the selective cytotoxicity of a drug is small. This may well be the case with many of the drugs used, because they share narrow therapeutic indices because of dose-limiting systemic toxicity.

Finally, with respect to drugs for CNS tumors, many of the available anticancer drugs can be toxic to the CNS if given at extremely high doses or when given in a manner to circumvent the blood–brain barrier.[106] The blood–brain barrier exists to protect the brain from many potentially toxic compounds. If the blood–brain barrier did not exist, CNS toxicity rather than myelotoxicity or gastrointestinal toxicity would be dose limiting for most drugs.

Pharmacokinetic considerations for intracranial nonparenchymal tumors and extramedullary spinal tumors are less dependent on the ability to cross the blood–brain barrier readily, because many of these tumors gain blood supply from meningeal blood vessels that are significantly more permeable than those of the brain.

REGIONAL DRUG DELIVERY CONSIDERATIONS

Under most circumstances regional drug delivery produces greater drug exposure than does systemic intravenous or oral administration. With respect to intracranial and spinal tumors, the regional delivery takes the form of intra-CSF therapy, intraarterial infusion, and intratumoral therapy.

Therapy by the CSF route (usually by ventricular reservoir) is a form of regional drug delivery that is used to treat meningeal neoplasia resulting from primary or secondary tumor invasion of the subarachnoid space and, less commonly, one of the ventricular cavities. It is often, but not always, associated with malignant cells floating in the CSF.

The advantages of intra-CSF therapy are high local drug levels; low systemic toxicity; and the ability to increase the frequency of treatments. However, delivery of drugs through the CSF can be dangerous and is associated with a high morbidity rate. The drugs commonly used are methotrexate, cytarabine, and thiotepa. All three drugs have been reported to produce CNS damage ranging from fever and chills to leukoencephalopathy and myelitis. Efficacy is limited when gross lesions exist ($\geq$5 mm diameter) or when CSF pathways are blocked and CSF flows are diverted.

Of concern in the use of CSF therapy is that slow clearance of drug can lead to increased neurotoxicity. Normally, these authors find, after injection into a ventricular reservoir and pumping the reservoir five times, the CSF distribution and flow of radionuclide-labeled albumin in the ventricle is well distributed and the half-time from ventricle to cisterna magnum is approximately 60 minutes. In many instances, obvious hydrocephalus is not apparent by neuroimaging, but a physiologic slowing of CSF flow (and presumably CSF absorption) is present. This slowing of CSF flow can lead to poor distribution in the subarachnoid CSF for drugs with high capillary clearance, such as cytarabine, and a greater likelihood of serious CNS toxicity for a drug such as methotrexate.

Another form of regional therapy is the intraarterial administration of anticancer drugs through carotid or vertebral arteries. The advantage of this approach is an increased uptake during the first passage of drug through tumor capillaries. Increased efficacy would be expected for patients whose tumors reside within the perfusion territory of the infused artery. Contrary to what may be thought, systemic toxicity will not be reduced unless the total administered dose is reduced, because the actual amount of drug taken up into the tumor is a small fraction of the injected dose. On the other hand, focal brain and retinal morbidity are increased, as was demonstrated by the clinical trials with BCNU[107] and cisplatin.[108] Controversial results of clinical trials do not commend this form of treatment, except under controlled experimental conditions.

Intratumoral therapy is regional therapy that is applicable for cystic tumors with a narrow rim of surrounding tumor. Pharmacokinetic considerations implicate problems with maintenance of tumor cavity drug levels; diffusion distances from the cavity to the outer margin of tumor; nonspecific biodegradation and binding of drug or drug products; and the need for repeat treatments. Modern clinical trials evaluating this form of regional therapy have not been published.

CEREBRAL ASTROCYTOMAS

PATHOLOGY CLASSIFICATION

This section deals primarily with classification of astrocytomas of varying degrees of aggressiveness, ranging from juvenile pilocytic astrocytoma to glioblastoma multiforme. The slower growing or less aggressive lesions are often referred to as *low grade* or *benign,* and the more rapidly progressive neoplasms are referred to as *high grade* or *malignant.* With the exception of juvenile pilocytic astrocytomas, subependymomas, and the limited number of astrocytomas that can be completely resected, even "benign" astrocytomas are highly lethal. For low-grade astrocytomas, Bloom reported 10-year survival rates of 6% to 10%.[109] Laws and associates had 10- and 20-year survival rates of about 21% and 16% for subtotally resected low-grade cerebral astrocytomas[110]; expected survival for a comparable group of age- and sex-matched normal subjects would have been approximately 95% at 10 years. Liebel and associates had 10-year survival rates of 35% and 11%, depending on whether radiation therapy was used.[111]

Many classification systems for astrocytomas have been advanced that have advocated the presumed cell of origin or the degree of malignancy, or both. The most widely used grading system has been that of Kernohan and Sayre, in which the astrocytomas are graded from I to IV, with grade IV being the most malignant.[112] Although the grades I and II of Kernohan and Sayre have significantly longer median survival times than grades III and IV, the system is not prognostically useful for separating grades I and II from grades III and IV.[110,113] Some of the randomized trials reported during the last decade for malignant gliomas have failed to find a difference in survival for grade III compared with grade IV. In the Radiation Therapy Oncology Group (RTOG) and Eastern Cooperative Oncology Group (ECOG) prospective randomized trial of 626 patients, the median survival time for grade III astrocytoma was 10 months compared with 9 months for grade IV.[114] On the other hand, when these same patients were histologically grouped as astrocytoma with anaplastic foci versus glioblastoma multiforme, there were marked differences in both median survival time and 18-month survival rates; these were 28 months and 62%, respectively, for anaplastic astrocytoma versus 8 months and 15% for glioblastoma multiforme. Similar differences between anaplastic astrocytoma (or malignant astrocytoma) and glioblastoma multiforme have been reported in older retrospective studies from the University of California at San Francisco (UCSF),[115] Stanford,[116] and Jefferson[117] medical centers.

For most purposes, a three-tier system is satisfactory.[118] Daumas-Duport and colleagues proposed a grading system that assigned a point system to nuclear atypia, mitoses, endothelial proliferation, and necrosis.[119,120] Grade I tumors had none of these features, grade II had one feature, grade III had two features, and grade IV had three or more features. In their initial evaluation, this grouping led to distinct and separate median survival curves. A subsequent review of 251 cases at the Massachusetts General Hospital found no statistical difference in survival between grades II and III.[121] Necrosis was found to be a significant predictor of short survival, in agreement with previous studies.[122]

RATIONALE FOR SURGERY

Data from animal experiments suggest, and a large clinical experience with tumors at many sites would confirm, that maximal surgical resection improves the results of subsequent radiation therapy and chemotherapy. This principle would seem to transfer to the treatment of astrocytomas. Gross total surgical resection was among the dominant factors favoring longer survival in a large series of patients with grade I or II astrocytomas treated at the Mayo Clinic.[123] The second Brain Tumor Study Group trial of radiation therapy and chemotherapy regimens showed a correlation between the extent of surgical resection and subsequent survival in patients with the more malignant astrocytomas.[124] Salcman's review of older literature reporting on the results of treatment of more than 600 patients with such malignant gliomas who received only surgical treatment confirms this correlation.[125] Andreou and coworkers approached this problem from a different perspective, looking at the impact of the amount of tumor present on the postoperative CT scan and "useful survival" (Karnofsky performance score [KPS] $>$ 30) and demonstrating a significant inverse correlation.[126] This same inverse condition of postoperative enhancing tumor volume with survival was confirmed in a much larger group of patients studied by the Brain Tumor Cooperative Group (BTCG),[127] whereas Winger and associates showed that the extent of resection was a significant independent variable for survival in 285 consecutive patients treated for malignant gliomas.[128]

A number of factors might be responsible for the improved clinical outcome when astrocytomas are aggressively resected. An assiduous resection can remove 90% of a typical astrocytoma, thereby decompressing the brain and substantially reducing the tumor cell burden. A large tumor mass left in the brain can serve as a nidus for cerebral edema after radiation therapy because of the indolent removal of dead cells from the brain.[129,130] In addition, aggressive surgical resection reduces (1) the number of separate cell populations in these heterogenous tumors, thereby eliminating some already radioresistant and chemoresistant populations; (2) the probability of further mutation toward resistance by lowering the overall number of tumor cells; and (3) the number of cells in regions remote from blood vessels, regions where chemotherapeutic agents cannot penetrate and where hypoxia can (theoretically) confer radioresistance.[131]

SURGICAL PRINCIPLES FOR CEREBRAL ASTROCYTOMAS

The goal of every craniotomy for a cerebral astrocytoma is gross total resection, and adequate exposure should be accomplished for this purpose, although sometimes aggressive resection proves impossible at the time of the operation. Tumors are approached through an incision in the crest of an overlying gyrus, the selection of which is aided by intraoperative ultrasound images. Self-retaining retractors are placed to retract gently both sides of the cortical incision (generally about 3 cm in length), and then the operating microscope is brought in for the approach through the subcortical white matter to the tumor. The tumor is resected with suction, two-point coagulation forceps, grasping instruments, the CO_2 laser, or the CUSA, the resection proceeding from the inside out, so that surrounding normal white matter is disturbed minimally. The glistening peritumoral white matter is seen easily through the microscope as each of the tumor's margins are reached, and it is at this interface that the resection is stopped. Hemostasis is sometimes difficult but must be perfect. Hemispheric tumor cysts can be drained and, when possible, fenestrated into an adjacent ventricle to prevent reaccumulation. Tumors not amenable to resection because of their location or their diffuseness should be biopsied stereotactically. Again, there is no indication for a craniotomy when the purpose is merely to biopsy (and not resect) a tumor.

The introduction of cortical mapping procedures into brain tumor surgery has made feasible the extensive resection of tumors in functionally critical areas. By use of intraoperative cortical stimulation, motor- and speech-associated cortex can be mapped, and safe routes to deep-lying tumors and safe resection limits determined.[132] A principal disadvantage of surgery that incorporates mapping of speech is that the patient cannot be given general anesthesia, and the surgeon must, therefore, anticipate unexpected patient movement and inferior brain relaxation during the operation.

REOPERATION FOR CEREBRAL ASTROCYTOMAS

Evidence is accumulating that reoperation for resection of cerebral astrocytomas at the time of their recurrence can be efficacious.[125,133,134] The rationale cited earlier for the aggressive initial resection of cerebral astrocytomas seems to fit equally well the prospect for re-resection at recurrence. This is only true, however, if there is some treatment modality (*e.g.*, chemotherapy and brachytherapy) that the patient can receive after the reoperation, and most often there is.

Salcman proposes from experience with reoperation of all patients who were to receive further therapy for recurrence of malignant glioma that relatively nonselective approach might be rational, given that reoperation is safe and of potential benefit despite the patient's age, performance status, tumor grade, or interval between initial surgery and recurrence.[125] Salcman emphasizes that reoperation is technically more demanding than the initial surgery, because tissues are compromised by previous therapy and, consequently, the postoperative infection rate is high.

Young and coworkers argue for more rigid selection criteria when choosing candidates for reoperation on recurrent malignant gliomas.[133] They found that patients with a KPS higher than 60 and an interval between the initial surgery and recurrence of at least 6 months had the longest survival times after reoperation. Harsh and associates looked at the effect of reoperation on the subsequent high-quality survival (KPS of at least 70) of patients with recurrent malignant gliomas.[134] Age and preoperative KPS have effects on the duration of high-quality survival in this study, with relative youth and high performance scores being advantageous. Because their data suggest that reoperation can significantly enhance the effects of chemotherapy on recurrent brain tumors, Harsh and associates would not suggest confining reoperation to young patients in excellent condition, but would suggest instead simply using these factors as guidelines in the broader therapeutic picture.

RADIATION THERAPY

The differentiated or low-grade astrocytomas constitute a heterogenous group of tumors, and the variability in their behavior has led to uncertainties regarding their therapy and prognosis. Approximately 10% to 35% of astrocytomas are amenable to total surgical resection.[135] The local control rate for completely resected cystic cerebellar astrocytomas approaches 100%, and postoperative irradiation is not recommended.[111,113] Similarly, the 5- and 10-year survival rates for patients with juvenile pilocytic astrocytomas are almost 100% after complete or "radical subtotal" resection.[135,136] In contrast, patients with supratentorial nonpilocytic "ordinary" astrocytomas or mixed oligoastrocytomas who undergo total or radical subtotal resection do not do as well. In a series of 23 such patients, 14 of whom received postoperative irradiation, the 5- and 10-year survival rates were 52% and 21%, respectively.[135]

The 5- and 10-year survival rates for patients with low-grade cerebral astrocytomas treated by subtotal resection alone range from 0% to 25%.[137] For incompletely resected and irradiated juvenile pilocytic astrocytomas, Wallner and coworkers reported 10- and 20-year progression-free survival rates of 74% and 41%, respectively.[136] Unfortunately, the authors had no data relative to incompletely resected and nonirradiated lesions. Shaw and associates found that patients with supratentorial pilocytic astrocytomas who underwent subtotal resection or biopsy and irradiation survived longer than nonirradiated patients.[135] However, the number of patients treated with surgery alone was small, and, therefore, the efficacy of radiotherapy for this tumor is uncertain.

Retrospective reviews suggest that postoperative irradiation is valuable for other types of astrocytomas that are incompletely resected. Leibel and colleagues found that the 5- and 10-year recurrence-free survival rates with incomplete resection alone were 19% and 11%, respectively, whereas, with the addition of postoperative irradiation to doses of 50 to 55 Gy, the survival rates increased to 46% and 35%.[111] For adults, the 5-year survival rate was 10% after surgery alone and 32% with combined therapy. Fazekas reported a 5-year survival of 41% with postoperative irradiation compared with 13% with surgery alone, even though the nonirradiated patients represented a prognostically more favorable subgroup.[113] Shaw and coworkers found that survival was directly related to dose.[135] Patients receiving at least 53 Gy had a significantly longer survival than those receiving less than 53 Gy or surgery alone ($p = 0.04$).

Therapeutic recommendations currently are based on the results of retrospective studies. Postoperative irradiation is not indicated for pilocytic astrocytomas when a complete or near-complete resection has been performed. After subtotal resection, either immediate irradiation or close follow-up may be recommended, deferring treatment until there is disease progression. Postoperative irradiation appears to be beneficial for patients with incompletely removed, unfavorable astrocytomas. Radiation therapy has also been recommended for completely resected, unfavorable lesions.[135] A dose of 55 Gy is administered using conventional fractionation. Limited radiation fields are used that encompass the lesion defined by CT scan with a 2- to 3-cm margin of normal tissue and the T2-weighted MRI abnormality with a 1- to 2-cm margin, whichever volume is larger. A combined North Central Cancer Treatment Group, RTOG, and ECOG study is addressing the question of whether there is a relation between dose and tumor control in adult patients with supratentorial astrocytomas. Patients are randomized to receive 50.4 Gy in 28 fractions or 64.8 Gy in 36 fractions. An adequate dose in children younger than 5 years of age is likely to lead to unacceptable neurologic sequelae, and radiation therapy is delayed until there is evidence of disease progression. When radiation therapy is necessary, the dose is reduced to 50 Gy.

Although it is generally agreed that patients with neurologic impairment, tumor progression, or malignant transformation should undergo radiation therapy, it is common for some practitioners to defer treatment in asymptomatic patients or in those with seizures who are medically controlled. Proponents of this approach argue that with CT and MRI, the disease is diagnosed early in its natural history and that it is not certain whether there is an advantage of early irradiation over delayed irradiation or whether radiation therapy even alters the prognosis.[138] The effect of this policy on patient outcome is not known, but it is being prospectively tested in adults by the BTCG and the Southwest Oncology Group and in children by the Children's Cancer Study Group (CCSG) and the Pediatric Oncology Group (POG).

Retrospective studies indicate that the prognosis of patients with anaplastic astrocytomas is superior to that of patients with glioblastoma multiforme and that the addition of radiation therapy confers a significant survival improvement over surgery alone.[115,116] The BTCG conducted the first clinical trial in which patients with malignant gliomas were randomized to receive postoperative irradiation or supportive care only.[139] Ninety percent of the 222 evaluable patients had glioblastoma multiforme. The median survival time for patients receiving supportive care alone was 14 weeks, whereas those treated with radiation therapy had a median survival time of 36 weeks ($p = 0.001$). The 1-year survival rates were 24% with radiation therapy and 3% for the nonirradiated patients. Similar findings were reported by the Scandinavian Glioblastoma Study Group. In that study, nearly 30% of the irradiated patients maintained a full or partial working capacity, although none of the untreated patients maintained this level of performance.[140] Combining data from a series of BTCG trials, Walker and colleagues demonstrated a stepwise prolongation of survival with increasing dose.[141] The median survival times for patients in the 50-, 55-, and 60-Gy subgroups were 28, 36, and 42 weeks, respectively (difference in survival between the 50- and 60-Gy groups was significant, $p = 0.004$). A combined RTOG and ECOG study failed to demonstrate a further survival improvement when 60 Gy was compared with 70 Gy.[142] These data led to the practice of treating patients with anaplastic astrocytomas and glioblastoma multiforme with a dose of 60 Gy in single daily fractions of 1.72 to 2 Gy, five times per week.

The amount of tissue to include within the treatment volume is the subject of considerable discussion. The BTCG and RTOG malignant glioma trials use partial brain fields defined by the extent of tumor on neuroimaging studies. In the BTCG protocols, the target volume is defined as a 3-cm margin of tissue surrounding the perimeter of the CT- and MRI-defined contrast-enhancing lesion. The RTOG protocols use a shrinking field approach. Initially, the treatment volume includes the contrast-enhancing lesion and surrounding edema on the preoperative CT-MRI study with a 2-cm margin. Subsequently (after 46 Gy of a 60-Gy course), the target volume is reduced to include the enhancing lesion only (without edema) with a 2.5-cm margin.

The response of malignant gliomas to standard radiation therapy techniques is limited by their striking inherent radioresistance and the radiosensitivity of the surrounding normal brain tissue. In addition to pursuing more effective chemotherapy programs (see chemotherapy section), several new approaches, including the use of chemical radiation sensitizers, heavy particle irradiation, altered fractionation schemes, and interstitial brachytherapy, have been examined. Hypoxic cell radiation sensitizers, such as misonidazole[143] and high-linear-energy transfer radiations, have been used to overcome the effects of hypoxia. These approaches have not yet improved survival over that produced by conventional irradiation. Proton irradiation is being used selectively to boost malignant gliomas to higher than conventional doses.

The halogenated pyrimidine analogs are radiosensitizers that are selectively incorporated into rapidly dividing cells undergoing DNA synthesis.[144] When integrated into DNA in the place of thymidine before radiation, cells become more than three times more sensitive to radiation, depending on concentration, exposure time, and percentage of thymidine replaced by the analog. Two halogenated pyrimidines, bromodeoxyuridine (BUDR) and iododeoxyuridine (IUDR), are undergoing clinical testing currently.

In a phase I–II study conducted by the Northern California Oncology Group (NCOG), 310 patients with malignant gliomas received BUDR in weekly 96-hour infusions of 0.8 $mg/m^2/day$ during a 6-week course of irradiation. This was followed by 1 year of PCV chemotherapy consisting of lomustine (CCNU), 110 mg/m^2 orally on day 1; procarbazine, 60 mg/m^2 orally on days 8 to 21; and vincristine, 1.4 mg/m^2 intravenously on days 8 and 29. The median survival times for patients with anaplastic astrocytoma and glioblastoma multiforme were 252 and 64 weeks, respectively.[145,146] Compared with historical controls, the survival of patients with anaplastic astrocytoma using this regimen was particularly encouraging. This and other studies[147,148] suggest that halogenated pyrimidine radiosensitization in malignant gliomas is measurable, and methods to improve the degree of radiosensitization are under investigation.[149] A randomized study comparing BUDR-, IUDR-, and hydroxyurea-sensitized radiation therapy (all arms followed by PCV) in patients with anaplastic astrocytoma is being conducted at UCSF.

Hyperfractionated irradiation is the use of two or more treatments per day with fraction sizes smaller than conventional dose fractions to deliver a higher dose in the same overall treatment time as conventionally fractionated therapy. With hyperfractionation, tumor control probabilities should improve without increasing the risk of late complications. Further, with a 4- to 8-hour interval between doses, there is greater probability that rapidly proliferating tumor cells will be irradiated during more radiosensitive phases of the cell cycle and become "self-sensitized" by redistribution. Target cells for late sequelae proliferate slowly, and, therefore, for these tissues little redistribution or self-sensitization occurs.[150]

In a dose-escalation study reported by Urtasun and associates,[151] patients received 61.4, 71.2, and 80 Gy in fractions of 0.9 to 1.1 Gy three times daily. The median survival times for the three dose subgroups were 45.8, 37.2, and 60.5 weeks, respectively. The survival difference between the two highest dose levels was significant ($p = 0.003$). In an RTOG randomized phase II dose-escalation study, patients were given 64.8, 72, 76.8, or 81.6 Gy in 1.2-Gy twice-daily fractions. Patients receiving 72 Gy had the longest median survival, and no further improvement in outcome was observed at the higher dose levels.[152] Based on these data, the RTOG is conducting a randomized trial comparing hyperfractionated irradiation (72 Gy) with conventionally fractionated radiation therapy (60 Gy; BCNU is given in both arms).

Another fractionation option, accelerated fractionation, attempts to reduce the overall treatment time by giving conventional-sized dose fractions two or three times daily. This treatment schedule may improve the therapeutic ratio by reducing the opportunity for tumor cell repopulation during treatment, thereby increasing the probability of tumor control for a given dose level.[150] Several trials using accelerated regimens have been conducted, but none has shown a survival benefit over conventional irradiation.[153,154] These studies indicate that although rapid regeneration does not appear to explain the radioresistance of malignant gliomas, the overall treatment time can be shortened. This outcome may be especially appropriate in patients with relatively short survival expectancies.[153] Further, altered fractionation schedules provide an opportunity to integrate chemosensitizers and hypoxic cell sensitizers in a novel fashion.

Most gliomas are localized to a single area of the brain,[99,100] and they should be controllable if sufficiently high radiation doses can be delivered without damaging the surrounding normal brain tissue. One approach to augmenting the radiation dose is with interstitial brachytherapy. Iodine 125 and iridium 192 sources are most commonly used in clinical practice, and stereotactic techniques have been devised for the placement of afterloading catheters that are removed after the prescribed dose has been accrued. Well-circumscribed, peripheral, solitary supratentorial lesions measuring as large as 5 cm are best suited for implantation. Further, candidates must have good neurologic function and a KPS of at least 70. Based on these criteria, about one third of patients with newly diagnosed malignant gliomas are candidates for this procedure.[155]

Several studies have demonstrated survival improvements in patients with glioblastoma multiforme when external irradiation is combined with brachytherapy. Gutin and coworkers reported the results of an NCOG trial that evaluated brachytherapy as an adjunct to external irradiation and chemotherapy in patients with newly diagnosed supratentorial malignant gliomas.[156] Patients received involved field external irradiation to 60 Gy with concomitant hydroxyurea (300 mg/m^2 orally every other day) followed by an implant to deliver an additional minimum tumor dose of 50 to 60 Gy. Patients were then given PCV chemotherapy every 6 to 8 weeks for 1 year. Although the median survival time of patients with glioblastoma multiforme (88 weeks) compared favorably with that of historical controls, there was no apparent gain observed in performing implantation at diagnosis in patients with nonglioblastoma multiforme (median survival time, 157 weeks). Loeffler and associates reported the outcome of 35 patients with glioblastoma multiforme who underwent partial brain external irradiation (59.4 Gy in 33 fractions) followed by an additional 50 Gy given by interstitial implantation.[157] Survival rates at 1 and 2 years were 87% and 57%, respectively, for patients receiving brachytherapy compared with 40% and 12.5%, respectively, for a control group matched by radiographic and patient characteristics ($p < 0.001$). The BTCG is conducting a randomized study comparing interstitial implantation (60 Gy at 10 Gy per day) preceding external irradiation (60.2 Gy at 1.72 Gy per fraction) and BCNU with external irradiation and BCNU alone. Brachytherapy has also been shown to improve the survival and quality of life of patients with recurrent malignant gliomas who meet the criteria of implantation.[158]

To amplify the effects of interstitial implantation, brachytherapy is being combined with a variety of dose-modifying agents, including interstitial hyperthermia, halogenated pyrimidine analogs, hypoxic cell radiosensitizers, and cisplatin chemotherapy. A randomized trial testing the addition of interstitial microwave hyperthermia to the brachytherapy boost after external irradiation in newly diagnosed patients with glioblastoma multiforme is being conducted at UCSF.[156] However, as local control has improved with brachytherapy, peripheral and distant CNS relapses are becoming more common.[159] This observation suggests that efforts designed only to enhance the effects of brachytherapy may not lead to a significant additional survival gain.

CHEMOTHERAPY

It is unfortunate that only a few patients with astrocytoma receive chemotherapy; most patients are never offered the option. Nonetheless, astrocytomas have been the most extensively treated of primary intracranial tumors.

Controlled (randomized) clinical trials have demonstrated the efficacy of a number of drugs when combined with irradiation as adjuvant therapy. Table 48–12 summarizes the results of controlled (randomized) clinical trials of adjuvant chemotherapy.[114,160–170] Efficacy has been shown for BCNU, CCNU, PCNU, procarbazine, streptozotocin, and the combination of CCNU, procarbazine, and PCV.

The era of controlled clinical trials for malignant astrocytomas began with the inception of the Brain Tumor Study Group in 1967. The European Organization for Research on

TABLE 48–12. Survival Time for Studies That Combined Irradiation and Chemotherapy for Patients With Anaplastic Astrocytoma or Glioblastoma Multiforme With Karnofsky Performance Scores of 60 or Higher

Treatment	*Percentage of Glioma Multiforme*	*Survival Percentile in Weeks*	
		50%	*25%*
BCNU[114,160–162]	45–89	43–55	75–78
CCNU[163–166]	41–100	43–55	
MeCCNU[160]	82	42	73
STZ[168]	79	43	78
PCB[161]	89	47	83
CDDP[167]	77	53	
CCNU-PCB[164]	63	50	
BCNU-PCB[169]	79	50	
HU-BCNU-PCB-VM-26[169]	78	50	
MeCCNU-DTIC[114]	68	42	
"8-in-1-day" [170]	74	47	73

BCNU, carmustine; CCNU, lomustine; MeCCNU, methyl CCNU; STZ, streptozotocin; DTIC, dacarbazine; VM-26, teniposide; CDDP, *cis*-diaminedichloroplatinum; PCB, procarbazine; HU, hydroxyurea.

Treatment of Cancer then established a comparable group. In addition, other national and regional cooperative groups have conducted controlled chemotherapy trials. Tables 48–12 to 48–14 summarize selected data from some of these groups. Differences in reports are sometimes confusing, for instance, some groups report survival or time to tumor progression (TTP) from initiation of therapy, whereas others use the original surgery date for untreated patients. Some groups define histologic groups and separate glioblastoma multiforme from anaplastic astrocytoma, and others combine the two groups under the heading of malignant glioma.

In addition to histology, other factors influence the likelihood and duration of response. Major known factors are age, performance status, and extent of surgical resection at onset of therapy. For instance, younger patients are more likely to respond and for a longer period; better performance status patients do best; and patients who have more extensive surgical resection do better than those who do not have surgery or who have biopsy only.[125,199]

With consideration for these covariants, it is still clear that adjuvant chemotherapy after surgery and radiation therapy for glioblastoma and anaplastic astrocytomas increases both TTP and survival, more so for the patients with anaplastic gliomas than for glioblastoma. There is less precise information with respect to response because of differing criteria used by the various groups. However, most investigators agree on the definition of deterioration or tumor progression: TTP and survival are more universal measures for controlled clinical trials. TTP is a more pure measure of efficacy, because at time of initial progression, many patients receive other forms of therapy. Survival, however, is a better measure of the social usefulness of the life attained by the therapy.

Chemotherapy appears to benefit mostly the lower 50th percentile of patients, and especially those below the 25th percentile. This is reasonable, because in vitro tumor drug sensitivity assays suggest that approximately 60% of patients are resistant to a given agent.[200,201]

Nitrosourea-based drug combinations appear superior to monotherapy, although even this conclusion is based on only one controlled study by the NCOG. In that study, postradiation therapy BCNU was compared with the PCV combination.[171] The greatest benefit for chemotherapy, based on TTP and survival, was in PCV-treated anaplastic astrocytomas. For glioblastoma multiforme patients, TTP and survival at the 50th percentile were for PCV at 37 and 53 weeks and for BCNU at 34 and 57 weeks, respectively; for the 25th percentile, they were for PCV at 72 and 94 weeks and for BCNU at 43 and 71 weeks, respectively. This was more significant ($p = 0.009$) for anaplastic tumors. TTP and survival at the 50th percentile were for PCV at 126 and 157 weeks and for BCNU at 63 and 82 weeks, respectively; for the 25th percentile, they were for PCV at 6.1 years and were not attained (>7.7 years) and for BCNU at 2.7 years and 4.1 years, respectively. At the dose schedule used, substituting BUDR for hydroxyurea during radiation therapy appears to offer no advantage.[182,183a] For glioblastoma, no survival advantage is seen; for anaplastic gliomas, the mean survival is higher (4.6 versus 3 years), but because only 50% of patients have died, it is too soon to be certain of the statistical trend.

TABLE 48–13. Survival for Adequately Treated Glioblastoma Multiforme Patients With Karnofsky Performance Scores of 60 or Higher Treated on NCOG Protocols

Treatment	*Percentile in Weeks**	
	50%	*25%*
RT + HU-BCNU[171]	57 (34)	71 (43)†
RT + HU-PCV[171]	53 (37)	94 (72)
FU-CCNU-RT + HU + MISO-PCB-VCR-BCNU-FU[172]	50 (41)	NA (59)†
RT + BUDR-PCV[173]	62 (43)	88 (69)

NCOG, Northern California Oncology Group; BCNU, carmustine; HU, hydroxyurea; PCV, lomustine (CCNU), procarbazine (PCB), vincristine (VCR); FU, fluorouracil; RT, radiation therapy; MISO, misonidazole; BUDR, bromodeoxyuridine; NA, not available.
* Time to tumor progression in parentheses.
† Not significant.

TABLE 48–14. Survival for Adequately Treated Anaplastic Gliomas Other Than Glioblastoma Multiforme in Patients With Karnofsky Performance Scores of 60 or Higher Treated on NCOG Protocols

Treatment	*Percentile in Weeks**	
	50%	*25%*
RT + HU-BCNU[171]	82 (63)	214 (142)†
RT + HU-PCV[171]	157 (126)	NA (317)
RT + BUDR-PCV[171a]	252 (148)	NA (NA)‡

NCOG, Northern California Oncology Group; BCNU, carmustine; HU, hydroxyurea; PCV, lomustine (CCNU), procarbazine (PCB), vincristine (VCR); RT, radiation therapy; BUDR, bromodeoxyuridine; NA, not available.
* Time to tumor progression in parentheses.
† $p = 0.009$.
‡ Not significant.

TABLE 48–15. Chemotherapy of Recurrent and Progressive Supratentorial Astrocytomas

Treatment	*Percentage of Response and Stable Tumor (MTP, wk)**		
	GM	*AA*	*GM + AA†*
Single Agents			
BCNU[104,174]	29 (22)	64 (22)	
CCNU[175,176]			42 (23)
PCNU[177]	33 (8)	69 (28)	
PCB[105,178]	27 (30)	28 (49)	50 (26)
BIC[179]	20 (na)	23 (22)	
AZQ, 24 h[180]	50 (18)	47 (16)	
AZQ, bolus[181,182]			24 (24)
Melphalan (oral)[183]	0 (NA)	7 (NA)	
Melphalan (IV)[183a]	0 (NA)	0 (NA)	
Spiromustine[184]			27 (5)
Cisplatin[185a,186]		73 (8)	83 (12)
Carboplatin[185a,186]	43 (14)	54 (16)	
DFMO[183a]		21 (NA)	44 (48)
Betaseron[187]	51 (18)	50 (16)	
Combinations			
BCNU-VCR[188]			41 (17)
BCNU-PCB[60]		46 (17)	56 (23)
CCNU-PCB-VCR[189,190]	45 (15)	65 (27)	
BCNU-FU[191]		89 (32)	
BCNU-FU-HU-MP[192]		55 (23)	71 (46)
BCNU-FU, PCB, CCNU-PCB[183a]		95 (41)	
DFMO-BCNU[193]	30 (8)	57 (76)	
DFMO-MGBG[194]		72 (49)	
TG-PCB-DBD-CCNU-FU-HU[195]	61 (40)	92 (65)	
PCB-FU-HU-MP[183a]	33 (16)	50 (20)	
AZQ-BCNU[196,197]	0–28 (9)	80 (37)	
AZQ-PCB[196]	31 (25)	53 (42)	
Cytoxan-VCR[198]	60 (15)	78 (35)	
Carboplatin-FU-PCB[199a]	32 (20)	57 (36)	

GM, glioblastoma multifome; AA, anaplastic astrocytoma; BCNU, carmustine; CCNU, lomustine; PCB, procarbazine; TG, 6-thioguanine; DBD, dibromodulcitol; MTP, median time to progression; AZQ, diaziquone; DFMO, alpha-difloromethylornithine; VCR, vincristine; FU, fluorouracil; HU, hydroxyurea; MP, mercaptopurine; MGBG, methylbisguanylhydrazone; NA, not available.
* Time to tumor progression in parentheses.
† GM and AA were not analyzed separately, because histologies were not separated or too few patients were found in each group to separate activity by histology.

More approaches need to be considered to improve the results cited in Tables 48–12 to 48–14. As a rule, new protocols for controlled trials usually come from phase II studies of chemotherapy efficacy against recurrent or progressive astrocytomas. Table 48–15 summarizes many of the published studies and several studies completed recently but not published. In many ways, Table 48–15 is disappointing. As was the case with adjuvant therapy of previously untreated astrocytomas, the nitrosoureas, alone and in combination, are the most active for recurrent and progressive tumors. It is disappointing that drugs designed specifically for gliomas, such as diaziquone (AZQ) and spiromustine, are only mediocre agents in the clinic.[180–182,184] Table 48–15 shows that even though the number of patients benefiting from chemotherapy is high in some studies, nevertheless, among the response and stable tumor patients, the duration of benefit has shown only modest gains during the last decade. This failure of chemotherapy is probably a function of de novo and emergent resistance of tumor cell subclones.

The use of the combination of polyamine inhibitors for anaplastic astrocytomas is encouraging. Alpha-difloromethyl ornithine–methyl-bisguanylhydrazone (DFMO-MGBG),[194] DFMO,[183a] and DFMO-BCNU[193] have been used with good results. For DFMO-MGBG patients with recurrent or progressive disease who had been heavily pretreated with nitrosoureas, approximately 50% responded or stabilized on the combination for a median time to progression (MTP) of 52 weeks (the MTP for the stable group alone was 50 weeks). Since that study, additional patients have been treated; as of September 1, 1987, 21 of 29 patients with anaplastic astrocytomas have stabilized or responded, with a median duration of 49 weeks. As a single agent, DFMO appears to have similar activity to the DFMO-MGBG combination. In both instances, the MTP for recurrent anaplastic gliomas achieving response and stable disease was almost 1 year. The difference in response rates (72% versus 46%) may reflect too lenient entry requirements for the DFMO patients and a subsequent high number of patients who went off therapy before the first evaluation at 8 weeks.[194a]

DFMO-BCNU, a combination found active in cultured cells and against rodent tumors, was found active against recurrent gliomas with a median survival of 92 weeks.[193] These studies open new therapeutic opportunities, because these polyamine inhibitors can interact with other agents to improve their efficacy.

Another encouraging finding may be a recently completed study[195] conducted in an attempt to overcome tumor resistance to CCNU. In that study, 6-thioguanine, dibromodulcitol, and procarbazine were given before CCNU to enhance tumor cell kill by interfering with DNA repair. The results were dramatic for the anaplastic gliomas, when 95% of patients who had failed radiation therapy responded or stabilized for an MTP of 15 months, and 25% did not fail until 33 months; 61% of glioblastoma patients with response or stable disease had an MTP of 9.3 months.[195] Of those who failed earlier nitrosourea therapies, 38% of anaplastic glioma patients and 58% of glioblastoma patients benefited, with MTPs of 10.6 and 5.1 months, respectively.

Intravenous cisplatin and carboplatin have shown only modest activity with respect to TTP, although response and stable rates appear high.[185,186] This may reflect poor tumor and adjacent brain penetration of these drugs and their inability to kill tumor cells at a distance from the main tumor mass. Betaseron, an interferon-β, attained 50% response and stable rates in a cooperative study; however, the duration of benefit is low, with MTPs of 16 to 18 weeks.[187]

Autologous bone marrow transplantation (ABMT) has had few practitioners, generally because of a low rate of observed complete responses to any form of chemotherapy. Single-agent BCNU was used years ago with no definable gains over conventional-dose nitrosourea therapy.[202] Other researchers have used thiotepa[203] and etoposide.[204,205] Although neither thiotepa nor etoposide alone has shown remarkable activity against gliomas, various combinations of the three agents are being evaluated.[206,207] It is currently unclear whether ABMT has a place in the management of cerebral gliomas.

BRAIN STEM GLIOMAS

CLINICAL AND PATHOLOGIC CONSIDERATIONS

Tumor involvement of the brain stem is due, in order of decreasing frequency, to astrocytoma, glioblastoma, and ependymoma. These tumors can be primarily central, diffuse, and infiltrative or focally infiltrative with or without an exophytic; the latter carry a better prognosis. Cranial nerve involvement can be at the nuclear level or of the cranial nerve as it leaves the brain stem. The initial manifestations of a brain stem glioma are unilateral palsies of cranial nerves VI and VII in approximately 90% of patients. Cranial nerve involvement is usually followed by long tract signs, such as hemiplegia, unilateral limb ataxia, ataxia of gait, paraplegia, hemisensory syndromes, gaze disorders, and, occasionally, hiccups. Less commonly, long tract signs precede the cranial nerve abnormalities; this is more likely with confined central intrinsic lesions.

If the tumor is a well-differentiated or an anaplastic astrocytoma, it is likely to involve the midbrain and produce hydrocephalus, vomiting, drowsiness, and cerebellar signs; if the tumor is a glioblastoma, it more often involves the medulla. Children with glioblastoma characteristically have a rapidly progressive course and are likely to have deficits in cranial nerves VI, VII, IX, and X and dysarthria, personality change, and head tilt. Unlike expansive posterior fossa tumors, headache, vomiting, and papilledema occur late.

As a group, the prognosis is poor, with 5-year survival rates varying between 0% and 38% and a median survival of less than 1 year in most series.[208–210] Certain patients do better than others. For instance, patients with type II tumors do better than those with infiltrative type I tumors. Moderately anaplastic exophytic tumors do better than higher-grade anaplastic tumors.

SURGERY

Modern imaging of the CNS with MRI scanning has improved the capability for definitive diagnosis of brain stem tumors. Lesions previously difficult to distinguish from brain stem glioma, for example, clivus tumors, foramen magnum meningiomas, multiple sclerosis, occult arteriovenous malformations, and brain stem abscesses, usually can now be excluded. Still, biopsy of brain stem gliomas for confirmation of the diagnosis and for definite tumor grading should be performed when possible. Biopsy of brain stem gliomas accessible through the floor of the fourth ventricle or presenting on the lateral surface of the pons can be accomplished safely, and associated symptomatic cysts can be drained. Attempt at complete resection of these tumors is contraindicated. Stereotactic needle biopsy of brain stem gliomas using CT and MRI guidance seems to have a low complication rate, so this method is being used increasingly, with the consequence that fewer patients are being treated without a tissue diagnosis.[211]

RADIATION THERAPY

Radiation therapy, the primary treatment for brain stem tumors, improves survival and can stabilize or reverse neurologic dysfunction in 75% to 90% of patients.[212,213] Traditionally, brain stem gliomas have been treated with up to doses of 50 to 60 Gy (1.8 Gy/fraction/day) through parallel opposed portals with the tumor dose calculated at the midline on the central axis of the beam. Sagittal MRI offers improved target definition and allows the radiation portals to be tailored to the contour of the lesion. The irradiated volume includes a margin of normal tissue of approximately 2 cm around the tumor. According to a multiinstitutional survey by Freeman and Suissa,[209] the 1-, 2-, and 5-year survival rates of children treated with conventional radiation therapy techniques were 50%, 29%, and 23%, respectively.[214,215]

Because of the relatively poor results obtained with conventional radiation dose-fractionation schedules and the observation that these tumors recur locally, hyperfractionated irradiation, designed to deliver higher tumor doses, is being evaluated.[216] Consistent, although modest, improvements in outcome have been observed when patients treated with hyperfractionation regimens of up to doses of 70.2 to 72 Gy (1–1.17 Gy twice daily) have been compared with historical control patients treated with conventional or low-dose hyperfractionated irradiation.[217–219] In a trial reported by Edwards and coworkers, 53 patients (19 adults and 34 children) with brain stem gliomas were treated with hyperfractionated irradiation to 72 Gy using 1 Gy twice daily, 5 days per week, with an interfraction interval of 4 to 8 hours.[219] The median survival time was 74 weeks (adults, 92 weeks, and children, 64 weeks). No increase in acute or delayed radiation-induced neurotoxicity was observed with this fractionation schedule, and the dose was subsequently escalated to 78 Gy. Although the outcome of children treated with this protocol is better than that observed in studies using conventional radiation therapy alone or with chemotherapy, it cannot be determined currently whether this is due to the fractionation schedule used, patient selection, or improvements in tumor localization and treatment planning using MRI.[219] Although these questions can be addressed only in a randomized trial, the data provide further evidence that higher doses can be safely administered to brain tumors using hyperfractionation regimens.

CHEMOTHERAPY

As with cerebral astrocytomas, chemotherapy is primarily nitrosourea based.[221] The use of chemotherapy, adjuvant to irradiation, has been infrequent. The CCSG randomly compared radiation therapy with radiation therapy followed by CCNU, PCV, and prednisone.[222] The mean survival was 11 months, and there was no difference between the two groups. In another trial, 5-fluorouracil and CCNU before radiation therapy and hydroxyurea and misonidazole during radiation therapy were evaluated[223]; in that study, TTP (32 weeks) and survival (44 weeks) were not better than the initial CCSG study.

For recurrent or progressive brain stem gliomas, few therapies have been evaluated.[221] Some benefit has been demonstrated, but the extent of benefit was not well established. In a recent study, 5-fluorouracil, CCNU, hydroxyurea, and 6-mercaptopurine were used to treat children and adults with recurrent or progressive brain stem gliomas.[224] Sixty-nine percent of 13 patients had response or stabilization, with a relapse-free survival of 25 weeks; the overall survival was 27 weeks. This finding is somewhat worse than would be expected for supratentorial gliomas. These authors conducted a phase II study of recurrent malignant gliomas with a combination of BCNU and DFMO. In that study, 3 of 5 patients benefited, with the 3 continuing at 1 to 3 years.[193] Although not curative, some of these chemotherapeutic leads should be exploited.

CEREBELLAR ASTROCYTOMAS

CLINICAL AND PATHOLOGIC CONSIDERATIONS

Astrocytomas arising in the cerebellum are considered separately, because their prognosis is consistently better than astrocytomas arising in the cerebrum or brain stem. These tumors, which occur most often during the first two decades of life, arise in the vermis or more laterally in a cerebellar hemisphere. Cerebellar astrocytomas usually are well circumscribed; they can be cystic, solid, or an admixture of polycystic and solid.

Histologically, most astrocytomas are low grade and lack features commonly associated with anaplasia; many are pilocytic in appearance and, histologically, some are juvenile pilocytic astrocytomas. In a series on 451 children reported from the Hospital for Sick Children of Toronto, cerebellar astrocytomas accounted for 25% of all posterior fossa tumors; 99 of 111 (89%) of the cerebellar astrocytomas were low grade, with nearly all vermian in origin.[225]

Because most of these tumors arise in the vermis, the clinical presentation is similar to medulloblastoma, with truncal ataxia, headache, nausea and vomiting, and in the young, split cranial sutures and head enlargement from raised intracranial pressure.

SURGERY

Cystic cerebellar astrocytomas are exposed through a posterior fossa craniectomy. The cyst is located with a cannula and then exposed by an incision through the cerebellar folia. Self-retaining retractors are placed into the cyst and then, with the aid of the operating microscope, the cyst is examined and the vascular, firm mural module identified, dissected, and removed. The nonneoplastic cyst wall is not excised.

Solid cerebellar astrocytomas are separated carefully from surrounding cerebellar white matter, again using the improved visualization offered by the operating microscope. The texture and appearance of the tumor are usually distinct and the separation from white matter usually is not difficult, so the only barrier to complete resection becomes deep penetration of the tumor into the dentate nucleus, cerebellar peduncles, or brain stem.

RADIATION THERAPY

See the discussion in the section on cerebral astrocytomas; the same principles apply. Completely resected cerebellar astrocytomas do not require radiation therapy. The remainder receive total doses of 50 to 60 Gy, depending on the histologic features and the age of the patient.

CHEMOTHERAPY

Because surgery alone or surgery and irradiation is often curative, chemotherapy has been limited to cases of recurrence or if the tumor is histologically highly anaplastic. For these tumors, the authors' approach has been to use nitrosourea-based therapies.

Chemotherapy adjuvant to surgery and radiation has not been commonly advocated for these tumors. The authors' experience is anecdotal (Table 48–16), but appears consistent with chemotherapy results for cerebral gliomas.[226] All patients received a nitrosourea; however, the chemotherapy combinations varied depending on which program was being used at the time for supratentorial gliomas. For patients at recurrence, chemotherapy provided palliation, with relapse-free survivals in 50% of patients at 18 months and 25% of patients surviving longer than 32 months.[226] As with the adjuvant chemotherapy patients, all were treated on a protocol being used at the time for cerebral gliomas. Among these patients, 5 of 18 (28%) developed metastases to the leptomeninges (3 of 5) or intracranial extracerebellar parenchymal sites (2 of 5). All leptomeningeal disseminations occurred in conjunction with locoregional recurrences. In many patients, therefore, combined systemic and intraventricular therapy may be needed for tumor control.

OPTIC, CHIASMAL, AND HYPOTHALAMIC GLIOMAS

CLINICAL AND PATHOLOGIC CONSIDERATIONS

Nearly all gliomas of the optic nerve and chiasm are discovered in patients before the age of 20 years, and most before the age of 10 years.[227] In some patients there is a family kindred of neurofibromatosis. Lewis and colleagues prospectively evaluated 217 patients with neurofibromatosis and found that gliomas along the anterior visual pathway occurred in 15% and were occasionally bilateral.[228] Sixty-seven percent of these tumors were not suspected clinically or obvious on ophthalmologic examination.

TABLE 48–16. Chemotherapy for Recurrent Cerebellar Astrocytomas[226]

Age (y)	*Diagnosis*	*Treatment(s)*	*Survival in Months*
Adjuvant Chemotherapy			
25	GM	RT-BUDR-PCV	+45
8	GM	RT-8422	+22
15	GM	RT-8422	+19
13	AA	RT-PCV	22
13	AA	RT-CYCLE	+52
Chemotherapy at Progression			
19	GM	8522, ACNU, PCB	+20
29	AA	BCNU, PCV, 8422	18
38	AA	BFHM	10
25	AA	CYCLE, AraC, TEPA	32
11	AA	BCNU, CYCLE	+112
33	AA	BCNU	6
4	MG	CCNU	+152
31	MG	CYCLE	10
38	LG	PCV	5
42	JPA	CYCLE, HME	30

GM, glioblastoma multiforme; AA, anaplastic astrocytoma; MG, meningioma; LG, low grade; JPA, juvenile pilocytic astrocytoma; RT, radiation therapy; PCV, lomustine (CCNU) + procarbazine (PCB) + vincristine; CYCLE, carmustine (BCNU), 5-fluorouracil, CCNU, PCB; BTRC 8422 is 6-thioguanine, PCB, dibromodulcitol, CCNU, vincristine; BTRC 8522 is 6-thioguanine, PCB, dibromodulcitol, CCNU, 5-fluorouracil, hydroxyurea; HME, elliptinium; BUDR, bromodeoxyuridine; ACNU, intraventricular nimustine; AraC, intraventricular cytarabine; TEPA, intraventricular thiotepa; BFHM is BCNU, 5-fluorouracil, hydroxyurea, 6-mercaptopurine.

With respect to tumor location, Housepian and associates reported that 25% involved one optic nerve, 73% the chiasm, and 3% the optic tracts.[229] In another series, 25% involved the chiasm alone, 33% the chiasm and hypothalamus, and 42% the chiasm and optic nerves or tracts.[230] Clinically, these tumors produce loss of visual acuity (70%), strabismus and nystagmus (33%), visual field impairment (bitemporal hemianopsia, 8%), developmental delay, macrocephaly, ataxia, hemiparesis, proptosis, and precocious puberty. Funduscopic evaluation demonstrates a range of findings from normal optic disks through venous engorgement to disk pallor due to atrophy. Tumors involving the chiasm often grow to involve the hypothalamus, causing a diencephalic syndrome that is characterized by emaciation (especially in children between 3 months and 2 years of age), motor overactivity, and euphoria.

Pathologically, these tumors range from primarily piloid and stellate astrocytes (commonest), with or without oligodendroglia, through the gamut of malignant astrocytomas to glioblastoma multiforme (rare). Typically, optic gliomas appear as fusiform expansions of any part of the nerve; they tend to bridge through the optic foramen and expand as dumbbell-shaped tumors within the skull. The nerve can be infiltrated by tumor originating in the chiasm, the walls of the third ventricle, or the hypothalamus. The tumors found in patients with neurofibromatosis often affect a single optic nerve and are grossly normal in appearance, although infiltrated by tumor and surrounded by a fibrous stroma.

Diagnosis is best made by MRI scan and should use images in the sagittal plane. The CT scan is satisfactory for diagnosis but is not as sensitive or descriptive as the MRI scan. The MRI also shows hypothalamic involvement more clearly.

SURGERY

Unilateral tumors of the optic nerve (as opposed to the chiasm) should be resected, particularly when there is profound visual loss or when proptosis is disfiguring.[231] A transcranial approach to the orbit is preferred, permitting complete resection of the tumor-infiltrated nerve from the chiasm to the globe and sparing the globe for an optimum cosmetic effect.[231] The involved nerve is inspected through a unilateral craniotomy, and the nerve is sectioned at the chiasm. The orbit is then unroofed, and the optic nerve's attachment to the globe is exposed and divided, allowing the tumor to be removed.

Biopsy of smaller tumors of the optic nerve, chiasm, or the nerve and chiasm must sometimes be accomplished when radiographic studies cannot exclude meningioma or other diagnoses definitively. Subtotal resection of larger tumors of these structures is occasionally necessary for decompression, but resection of the chiasm with resultant blindness is never indicated.

RADIATION THERAPY

Treatment of optic nerve and chiasmal gliomas is controversial, because some patients with incomplete surgical resections have been followed for 10 to 20 years without progression.[227] The literature suggests, however, that untreated optic gliomas, especially those involving the chiasm or extending into the hypothalamus or optic tracts, progress locally or are fatal in 75% of patients. Tenny and coworkers found that only 21% of patients who were followed after biopsy or exploration survived compared with 64% of those who received radiation therapy.[232] In general, optic nerve gliomas have a better prognosis than those involving the chiasm, and tumors confined to the anterior chiasm have a better outcome than those that involve adjacent structures (posterior chiasmal tumors).[233–236]

Routine postoperative irradiation is not indicated for most gliomas confined to the optic nerve. In contrast, radiation therapy can prevent tumor progression, improve disease-free survival, and stabilize or improve vision in patients with chiasmal lesions. Wong and colleagues reported that 6 of 27 (22%) chiasmal gliomas that did not receive radiation therapy progressed locally, whereas 9 of 20 (45%) failed that received radiation therapy.[234] Three of these recurrences occurred in the adults with extremely aggressive, nonresponsive tumors. Further, 87% of the irradiated patients who received a dose of 50 to 55 Gy were controlled compared with 55% of those who received 46 Gy or less. Radiation therapy significantly improved the relapse-free survival but not the overall survival. In another series collected from the literature, local control was achieved in 154 of 189 (81%) irradiated anterior chiasmal tumors, whereas 92 of 142 (65%) posterior tumors were controlled. Vision improved in 61 of 210 (29%) evaluable patients and remained stable in 118 of 210 (56%) patients.[233]

Although some clinicians advocate deferring irradiation in asymptomatic patients until there are signs of disease progression, others recommend that radiation therapy be given early in the course of the disease to minimize the risk of visual deterioration.[234,237] The radiation portals are tailored to the tumor volume and designed to avoid irradiation of the lens of the eye. A three-field or bicoronal arc technique may be used to treat smaller lesions. A dosage of 50 to 55 Gy in daily 1.8-Gy fractions is recommended.

For hypothalamic tumors, radiation therapy produced radiographic improvement in 11 of 24 (46%) with an MTP of 70 months.[239] Those patients who did not receive radiation therapy initially had an MTP of 30 months.

CHEMOTHERAPY

There are few published chemotherapy trials in this group of patients. Chemotherapy has been used successfully to delay the initiation of radiation therapy in young children.[238] Packer and associates treated 24 children (median age 1.6 years) with a combination of dactinomycin and VCR.[230] Six of the cases involved the chiasm, 8 involved the chiasm and hypothalamus, and 10 involved the chiasm and visual pathways. At a median follow-up period of 4.3 years, 38% of patients had progressed.[230]

Petronio and coworkers reported on 19 infants or children with chiasmatic and hypothalamic gliomas treated with chemotherapy after surgical or radiologic diagnosis.[240] Of the 12 tumors in which a biopsy was obtained, there were 7 juvenile pilocytic astrocytomas, 2 astrocytomas, 2 anaplastic astrocytomas, and 1 subependymal giant cell astrocytoma. The children were between 3 months and 15 years of age when treated. The chemotherapy included one of three regimens: 1 with dactinomycin and VCR; 1 with the combination of BCNU, 5-fluorouracil, hydroxyurea, and 6-mercaptopurine; and 15 with the combination of 6-thioguanine, procarbazine, dibromodulcitol, CCNU, and VCR (BTRC 8422 protocol). Fifteen of 18 initially treated with chemotherapy responded or stabilized; the median follow-up period exceeded 1.5 years (range, 1.4 months to 5.8 years). The four patients who progressed responded to radiation therapy.

Rodriguez and colleagues reported a series of 33 hypothalamic gliomas,[239] some of whom were included in the Petronio series.[240] Chemotherapy at presentation or recurrence was beneficial in 10 of 16 (62%) patients.

OLIGODENDROGLIOMAS

CLINICAL AND PATHOLOGIC CONSIDERATIONS

Oligodendrogliomas have a relatively flat "peak" incidence between 25 and 49 years. Although they are commonest (80%) in the cerebral hemispheres, approximately 15% occur in the third or lateral ventricles or protrude into a ventricle from the thalamus.[241] Grossly, these tumors are often well demarcated, and in 20% they are cystic. They have a 10% likelihood of spreading through the CSF pathways. Like astrocytomas, they vary in malignancy. Attempts have been made to grade oligodendrogliomas on an A through D scale[241]; however, grades A through C vary little, and B and C are virtually identical with respect to survival such that these subdivisions seem unnecessary; a designation of *differentiated* or *highly anaplastic* may be sufficient. These tumors often have both astrocytic or ependymal elements seen at biopsy; such tumors are called *mixed gliomas.*

Clinically, these tumors present in the typical fashion of hemispheral astrocytomas. However, two features distinguish them from astrocytomas: the antecedent history, averaging 7 to 8 years, tends to be longer, and seizures are more common, occurring in 70% to 90% of patients by the time of diagnosis. Provisional diagnosis may be made by CT or MRI neuroimaging, but histologic confirmation is necessary and almost always possible. Approximately 50% of oligodendrogliomas have scattered calcification, usually related to intrinsic blood vessels, which are evident by CT scan.

At recurrence or autopsy, approximately 60% of oligodendroglioma and most mixed oligoastrocytoma patients demonstrate histologically an anaplastic astrocytoma or glioblastoma multiforme. This may belie a common origin of both types of tumors to the O2A progenitor cell.

SURGERY

The surgical resection of hemispheric oligodendrogliomas follows the same principles as discussed earlier for cerebral astrocytomas, with gross total removal being the goal when this is consistent with good neurologic outcome. The margins of oligodendrogliomas can appear to be more distinct than those of astrocytomas, but generally they are infiltrative, and surgical cure remains unlikely. Oligodendrogliomas often recur in the previous operative site. Under these circumstances, reoperation may be advisable, particularly when followed by chemotherapy.

RADIATION THERAPY

The role of postoperative irradiation in patients with differentiated oligodendrogliomas is controversial and contradictory. The lack of randomized trials precludes the statement of firm recommendations. Some authors recommend immediate postoperative irradiation for patients with incompletely resected lesions,[242,243] some advise that only patients with anaplastic tumors or mixed oligoastrocytomas receive radiation therapy,[244] and others advocate that radiation therapy be deferred until there is evidence of tumor progression or recurrence.[245] Data from three recent retrospective series suggest that the median survival time is increased from 23 to 60 months to 38 to 132 months by the addition of postoperative irradiation.[242,243,246,247]

Wallner and associates reviewed the outcome of 42 patients and observed 5- and 10-year survival rates of 61% and 33%, respectively; relapse-free survival rates were only 33% and 25%.[242] The 10-year survival rate for patients with pure oligodendrogliomas who received at least 45 Gy was 56% compared with 18% for nonirradiated patients ($p = 0.092$). The survival rates for patients with irradiated mixed oligoastrocytomas were virtually identical to those for the irradiated pure tumors. Wallner and coworkers concluded that adjunctive radiation therapy increased the time to tumor recurrence and the number of long-term survivors.[242] Lindegaard and colleagues found that radiation therapy prolonged the median survival time but did not influence the overall cure rate when given after subtotal resection, whereas it did not appear to be indicated after total resection.[243] On the other hand, Bullard and associates could find no evidence that postoperative radiation therapy was beneficial.[246]

Based on the poor long-term prognosis associated with these tumors and data that suggest that radiation therapy may be beneficial, these authors continue to recommend postoperative irradiation after incomplete resection. It is reasonable, however, to defer treatment in asymptomatic children until there are signs of tumor progression. Radiation therapy is given using fields that encompass the tumor volume with a 2- to 3-cm margin. A dose of 55 to 60 Gy is used in adults, and the dose is reduced to 50 Gy in children.

CHEMOTHERAPY

As with radiation trials, prospective clinical chemotherapy trials of oligodendroglioma patients have not been published. There are, however, individual patients reported within trials for malignant astrocytomas. In those reports, chemotherapy was limited to the treatment of recurrent, well-differentiated, and moderately anaplastic oligodendrogliomas and the primary treatment of the highly anaplastic oligodendrogliomas with surgery, radiation therapy, and chemotherapy.

Because many of these isolated patients came from the authors' own published reports, they reviewed their experience during the last decade. Table 48–17 summarizes TTP and survival results of treatment of oligodendrogliomas and mixed tumors that had been treated at recurrence. In their series, the median time to first recurrence for the oligodendrogliomas was 2.4 years; those treated with chemotherapy (primarily nitrosourea based) at recurrence had a median survival of an additional 1.4 years. These results are similar to those for well-differentiated (moderately anaplastic) astrocytomas. For the mixed tumors, the median time to first recurrence was 1.8 years, and the median time from recurrence to death was an additional 1.6 years for those treated with chemotherapy at recurrence. Cairncross and MacDonald have advocated the combination of CCNU, procarbazine, and VCR.[248] They believe that oligodendrogliomas are more sensitive to chemotherapy than are anaplastic astrocytomas, although survival differences are measurable in months, not years, between the two groups. Based on these results, they have initiated prospective trials.

TABLE 48–17. Patients With Oligodendroglioma and Oligoastrocytoma Tumors Treated for Recurrence With Chemotherapy* at UCSF between 1977 and 1987

	Percentiles	
Tumors	*50%*	*25%*
Oligodendroglioma (median age 37)		
Time to first tumor recurrence (n = 21)	2.4 y	3.8 y
Time from recurrence to death (n = 12)	1.4 y	2.8 y
Mixed Oligoastrocytoma (median age 35)		
Time to first tumor recurrence (n = 53)	1.8 y	4.9 y
TIme from recurrence to death (n = 20)	1.6 y	>2.0 y†

* Chemotherapy included nitrosourea-based therapies, the combination of PCV, procarbazine, DFMO-MGBG, and thiotepa. In addition, 20–25% had a reoperation after recurrence before starting chemotherapy.

† The 25% has not been reached, because 10 in 20 have not failed yet.

EPENDYMOMA

CLINICAL AND PATHOLOGIC CONSIDERATIONS

Ependymomal tumors arise from cells of ependymal lineage and, therefore, have a propensity for occurring in the obliterated central canal of the spinal cord, the filum terminale, and white matter adjacent to a ventricular surface (usually a highly angulated surface).[50] Sixty percent of intracranial ependymomas are infratentorial, and 40% are supratentorial.[249] Of infratentorial sites, the fourth ventricle is the commonest site. Extension into the subarachnoid space occurs in 50% of these cases, and encasement of the medulla and upper cervical cord can occur. Of supratentorial ependymomas, 50% are primarily intraventricular, and the remainder are parenchymal, arising from ependymal rests. Most of the intraventricular tumors arise in the lateral ventricles, and fewer (25%) occur in the third ventricle .

Ependymomas can be classified in various ways. Ependymomas are either differentiated (ependymoma or myxopapillary ependymoma) and, therefore, low grade or, less commonly, they are anaplastic and higher grade and more likely to disseminate through the CSF pathways.

Clinical presentations are dependent on the location of tumor. Intraventricular tumors often cause increased intracranial pressure and hydrocephalus. As a result, headache, nausea and vomiting, papilledema, ataxia, and vertigo are found in most patients at presentation. Focal neurologic signs and symptoms are more often seen with extraventricular supratentorial ependymomas.

Either MRI or CT scanning is sufficient to make the anatomic diagnosis before surgery. The presence of calcium in a fourth ventricular tumor is highly suggestive but not diagnostic of an ependymoma. Surgical exploration and biopsy are essential for the selection of appropriate treatment. For anaplastic ependymomas, staging myelography and examination of the CSF for cytologic evidence of malignancy are essential.

The inclusion of ependymoblastomas, which are known for their propensity to disseminate throughout the CNS, tends to overestimate the risk of seeding.[252,253] In a literature review, Vanuytsel and Brada found that the overall incidence of spinal seeding was 6.9%.[254] It was 1.6% for supratentorial tumors and 9.7% for infratentorial lesions, 8.4% for high-grade tumors, and 4.5% for low-grade lesions. No patient with high-grade supratentorial lesions developed spinal seeding, whereas 15.7% of those with high-grade infratentorial tumors developed spinal dissemination. For low-grade tumors, 2.7% of patients with supratentorial lesions developed seeding compared with 5.5% for those with infratentorial lesions. The incidence of spinal seeding was related directly to local tumor control, regardless of tumor grade. The incidence of spinal dissemination was 3.3% in locally controlled patients and 9.5% in those with uncontrolled primary lesions ($p < 0.05$).

SURGERY

Approximately half of hemispheric ependymomas arise from the wall of the lateral ventricle, and half appear to be intraparenchymal, arising perhaps from remote fetal ependymal cell rests.[250] Hemispheric ependymomas tend to be cystic and, even when not, are often well circumscribed from surrounding brain, allowing gross total resection. A wide craniotomy permits a transcortical exposure of the tumor through a cortical incision placed to avoid injury to vital brain tissue. The tumor is removed using the operating microscope, and every effort is made to minimize bleeding into the ventricular cavity. At the end of the resection, the ventricular system is gently irrigated free of blood and blood clots to prevent mechanical obstruction to CSF flow, to prevent the blockage of the CSF absorptive bed (arachnoid granulations), and to reduce the irritation of bloody CSF to the brain.

Ependymomas arising from the floor of the fourth ventricle are approached through a wide bilateral suboccipital craniectomy and laminectomy of C1. The tumor is exposed by retracting the cerebellar tonsils laterally and splitting the inferior aspect of the vermis, although often a tongue of tumor is visible over the dorsal aspect of the medulla and upper cervical spinal cord before the tonsils are retracted. The dorsal convexity of the tumor comes into view as the cerebellar vermis is divided, and its attachment to the floor of the fourth ventricle can then be exposed progressively and evaluated. Firm attachment precludes a gross total resection, as does infiltration of the tumor into the cranial nerves of the cerebellopontine angle through the foramen of Luschka. Tumor is removed to the extent possible using illumination and magnification afforded by the operating microscope.

There would appear to be a relation between residual ependymoma left by the surgeon and a poorer outcome after radiation therapy.[251] In ependymomas, as in most of the gliomas, a maximal surgical resection should be carried out when possible.

RADIATION THERAPY

It is well established that postoperative irradiation improves the survival of patients with intracranial ependymomas, and 5-year survival rates with doses of 45 Gy or more range from 40% to 87%.[74] Tumor grade has been considered to be the most important determinant of tumor behavior and prognosis. The 5-year survival for patients with low-grade tumors ranges from 60% to 80%, whereas for anaplastic ependymomas, it is only 10% to 47%.[74] Most series fail to distinguish patients with malignant ependymomas from those with ependymoblastomas that are classified as primitive neuroectodermal tumors and have an especially poor prognosis. Analyses suggested that when these lesions are excluded, tumor grade has less prognostic value.[252]

The risk of seeding, however, was independent of whether prophylactic spinal irradiation was given.[254] For high-grade lesions, spinal dissemination occurred in 9.4% of patients receiving craniospinal irradiation and in 6.7% of those treated with local radiation therapy only. Similarly, for low-grade tumors, spinal seeding occurred in 9.3% after craniospinal irradiation, whereas 2.2% developed seeding without prophylactic treatment.

The recommended treatment volumes for supratentorial low-grade ependymomas vary from generous local fields to the whole brain, whereas for low-grade infratentorial tumors they include local fields, the whole brain with cervical spine extension, and craniospinal axis irradiation. Wallner and coworkers reviewed the outcome of low-grade ependymomas treated with local irradiation after surgery; only 1 in 16 patients, who was eventually found to have a local recurrence, developed spinal dissemination.[255] The 5- and 10-year survival rates for those who received more than 45 Gy (approximately 50 Gy in most instances) were 67% and 57%, respectively. Recurrence at the primary tumor site was the most frequent pattern of failure. Based on this series and data from others and the greater precision in determining tumor extent currently available through high-quality diagnostic imaging, low-grade supratentorial ependymomas are treated using a generous target volume with a dose of at least 54 Gy. Spinal CT and MRI studies, myelography, and CSF evaluation are not obtained routinely in these patients. Patients with low-grade infratentorial lesions are treated similarly. The remainder of the craniospinal axis is treated only if pretreatment CSF cytology studies reveal malignant cells or if radiographic studies show evidence of tumor spread.

Most authors agree that in the case of anaplastic ependymomas, the entire craniospinal axis should be treated, although some recommend whole-brain irradiation with an additional boost for high-grade supratentorial lesions located away from the CSF pathways.[253] A dose of 54 Gy is given to the primary tumor site and 35 to 40 Gy to the remainder of the axis. If spread within the brain is demonstrated, the entire brain receives 54 Gy. Spinal imaging studies are routinely performed, and any area of gross involvement is boosted to 50 Gy. Despite the apparent superiority of craniospinal irradiation in some series,[256] the findings that local recurrence is the primary pattern of failure,[253,255,257,258] that subarachnoid failure is rare in the absence of local failure,[256,257] and that spinal metastases may not be prevented by prophylactic treatment[253,254] have led some investigators to question the routine use of craniospinal irradiation in anaplastic lesions. Future clinical trials probably will focus on more aggressive local therapy to improve primary tumor control in both low- and high-grade ependymomas and will address the necessity of spinal prophylaxis in high-grade lesions.

CHEMOTHERAPY

Because the need for chemotherapy for these tumors has been limited and, before the MRI era, they were hard to assess, most chemotherapeutic trials are anecdotal. For primary treatment of anaplastic ependymomas, these authors have been using craniospinal axis irradiation with oral hydroxyurea followed by six courses of polydrug chemotherapy (BTRC 8422) with 6-thioguanine, procarbazine, dibromodulcitol, CCNU, and VCR. Since 1984, they have treated 17 consecutive children and adults with this regimen. As of October 1991, they have had 9 failures, an MTP of 3.4 years, and a 5-year disease-free survival of 42%.

Table 48–18 summarizes some published and unpublished series of chemotherapy for recurrent differentiated or anaplastic ependymomas. The authors have, for many years, treated recurrent ependymomas with BCNU or dibromodulcitol as monotherapy.[259] Results were better than those achieved for anaplastic astrocytomas. Subsequent to those trials, they used the drug combination of 6-thioguanine, procarbazine, dibromodulcitol, CCNU, and VCR (BTRC 8422A); they achieved an 82% response and stable rate for an MTP of 21.3 months.

Goldwein and colleagues retrospectively analyzed 16 recurrent ependymoma patients treated with a variety of agents alone and in combination (VCR, cisplatin, CCNU, procarbazine, VP-16, and ifosfamide).[260] Approximately 20% of patient trials led to a partial response or stable disease (more common 7 to 1), for an approximate median of 6 to 10 months.

Gaynon and associates of the CCSG used carboplatin every 4 weeks and found a response and stable disease rate of 28% (4 in 14) with a duration of 6+, 17+, 12, and 15 months.[261] Those who did not receive prior cisplatin were more likely to respond to carboplatin. Bertolone and coworkers evaluated cisplatin and found 6 of 8 (75%) benefiting, with an MTP of 3.8 months.[185] Ettinger and colleagues, also of the CCSG, used AZQ on a 5-day every 3-week schedule in 12 children with recurrent or metastatic disease. One 35+ month response was reported.[262]

TABLE 48–18. Chemotherapy for Recurrent Ependymoma and Anaplastic Ependymomas

Treatment*	*Percentile of TTP (mo)* 50%	25%
BCNU (11/14)[183a]	13	24
DBD (9/12)[259]	16	20
AZQ (5/12)[262]	10	16
Carboplatin (4/14)[261]	14	NA
Cisplatin (6/8)[220]	3.8	4.3
VCR-CDDP-CCNU-PCB-VP-16-IFSO combinations (8/37)[260] †	9	10
6-TG-PCB-DBD-CCNU-VCR (9/11)[258a]	21.6	NA

TTP, time to tumor progression; BCNU, carmustine; NA, not available or attained; AZQ, diaziquone; VCR, vincristine; CDDP, cisplatin; CCNU, lomustine; PCB, procarbazine; VP-16, etoposide; 6-TG, 6-thioguanine; DBD, dibromodulcitol.
* (Responder + Stable)/All patients.
† 16 patients were treated on 37 different trials.

MENINGIOMAS

CLINICAL AND PATHOLOGIC CONSIDERATIONS

Meningiomas arise from arachnoidal cells in the meninges, especially in areas of the arachnoid villi. In some series, meningiomas constitute 39% of primary CNS tumors.[46] The most frequent locations of these tumors are along the sagittal sinus and over the cerebral convexity. Table 48–19 summarizes the frequency of these tumors according to location.[263] Meningiomas are extraaxial, intracranial (and sometimes spinal) tumors that produce symptoms and signs through compression of adjacent brain tissue and cranial nerves. They often also produce hyperostosis. Table 48–20 summarizes the symptoms and signs associated with these tumors.

Histologically, most meningiomas are differentiated, with low proliferative capacity and limited invasiveness. Less commonly, meningiomas are more anaplastic with a higher

TABLE 48–19. Sites of Predilections of Meningiomas Within the Intracranial Regions

Site	*Number*
Parasagittal	65
Convexity	54
Sphenoidal ridge	53
Olfactory groove	29
Suprasellar	28
Posterior fossa	23
Spinal	18
Periocular	12
Temporal fossa	8
Falx	7
Choroidal	6
Gasserian	5
Multiple	2
Combined with neurinomas	2
Intraorbital	1

(Cushing H, Eisenhardt L. Meningiomas. Vol 1. Their classification, regional behavior, life history and surgical end results. Springfield: Charles C. Thomas, 1938:73)

TABLE 48–20. Neurologic Findings Associated With Meningiomas as a Function of Their Location

Site	*Presentation*
Sphenoidal ridge	Nonpulsating, painless unilateral exophthalmos; unilateral visual loss; ophthalmoplegia; ICP
Cerebral convexity	Altered mentation; ICP; seizures
Intraventricular	Hydrocephalus; headache; mental changes; visual field abnormalities
Olfactory groove	Central scotoma; ipsilateral optic atrophy; contralateral papilledema; ipsilateral loss of smell; altered mentation; focal motor abnormalities
Tuberculum sellae	Loss of vision; bitemporal hemianopia; papilledema or optic atrophy
Other basilar sites	See Table 48–5
Cerebellar convexity	ICP; cerebellar findings
Cerebellopontine angle	Cerebellar findings; hearing loss
Foramen magnum	No findings; spastic paresis and sensory findings in upper extremities

ICP, increased intracranial pressure.

proliferative capacity and are invasive. Even though the difference in the 30-minute bromodeoxyuridine labeling index in situ for the differentiated meningiomas may be less than 1% versus 3% to 4% for anaplastic meningiomas,[264] biologically, the anaplastic meningiomas behave considerably differently than the more differentiated meningiomas.

SURGERY

The perception that meningiomas are surgically resectable gives these tumors an undeserved reputation of benignity. Although meningiomas usually are well circumscribed and do not invade adjacent brain, they can occur virtually anywhere in the CNS, and access is sometimes only by deep retraction. In addition, these tumors may be extremely vascular and can surround important structures such as cranial nerves and major arteries at the skull base. Such characteristics can preclude a smooth operation, and a total removal is commonly not possible. Simpson reported on a large series of surgically resected meningiomas and documented that even when there was a perceived total resection, the recurrence rate was 9%.[265] A more modern series from Massachusetts General Hospital shows that a "total resection" is followed by 7% recurrence rate at 5 years, 20% at 10 years, and 32% at 15 years.[266]

Nevertheless, in dramatic contrast to the more common cerebral gliomas, certain meningiomas are surgically resectable, and the neurosurgeon is usually more favorably disposed toward tackling a meningioma than operating on another glioma. The neurosurgeon's zeal must be tempered with an understanding of the risks of removing a particular meningioma in a particular location and an understanding of the impact of this meningioma on the well-being of the particular patient, because these tumors are often exceedingly slow-growing and the patients are often elderly. The presence of a meningioma is not an absolute indication for surgery; when surgery is undertaken in an elderly patient, partial removal is sometimes adequate.

Preoperative Planning

The preoperative preparation of the patient, the surgical planning, and the intraoperative anesthetic management are as described in the earlier surgery section. However, the planning of surgery for meningiomas must be extremely assiduous, because a detailed knowledge of surgical anatomy is necessary in these tumors. A preoperative angiogram to assess overall tumor vascularity and to identify arterial feeders is often important. In many instances, the angiography procedure is combined with embolization of the tumor's blood supply. The angiogram is done within 24 to 96 hours of the operative procedure, so that alternative vascular routes to the tumor do not have time to develop.

Surgical Principles

Those feeding arteries that could not be occluded by embolization are addressed first at the operation, if they are accessible. These arteries are meningeal and cerebral in origin. The tumor is retracted from surrounding normal brain progressively as the tumor bulk is reduced by the use of the CUSA or, for extremely vascular tumors, the cutting loop of the electrocoagulation unit or the CO_2 laser. Meningiomas at individual sites pose special surgical problems.

At the cerebral convexity, a large bone flap is made around the tumor, a dural incision circumscribes the tumor, and the dura attached to the tumor is used to retract the tumor from the brain as microdissection frees the adhesions between the tumor and surrounding brain.

Parasagittal meningiomas abut the midline; difficulties in removal are related to critical draining veins, to involvement of the sagittal sinus with tumor, and to the often massive overlying bony erosion or hyperostosis or both. A patent sagittal sinus cannot be transected for a complete tumor removal except in its anterior one third, so a careful study of the preoperative arteriogram looking for the patency of the sinus and for the position of the draining veins in the region is critical. Some clinicians advocate opening the sagittal sinus for removal of tumor that has grown through its wall, and others advocate resecting and grafting the involved sagittal sinus wall. In the authors' opinion, these dangerous maneuvers are not usually indicated, because recurrence-free survivals after subtotal resection of these lesions are extended,[266] and because the tumor may grow to occlude the sinus completely, thereby making complete resection possible later with a lesser risk to life.

Falx meningiomas do not involve the sagittal sinus but occupy the falx below the sinus, often becoming bilateral. Major complications of resection of falx meningiomas relate to interruption of draining veins and consequent cerebral edema and venous infarction.

Olfactory groove meningiomas grow extremely large before their neurologic sequelae lead to their discovery. Surgery is carried out through a large bifrontal bone flap based low on the forehead. The broad sessile base of the tumor is attacked first with its blood supply, then the tumor's bulk is reduced by internal coring and dissection, with attention to protection of the optic nerves, carotid artery, and anterior cerebral arteries on the tumor's posterior aspect.

Tuberculum sellae meningiomas are smaller at presentation because of their proximity to the optic apparatus. Attention to the safety of the optic apparatus and the anterior cerebral and carotid arteries is equally critical.

Sphenoid ridge meningiomas vary in approach, depending on whether they occupy the outer, middle, or inner third of the sphenoid bone. Outer third tumors can be a problem purely of tumor mass, purely of massive temporal hypertosis from en plaque tumor invading bone, or a combination of both. When it is present, the tumor mass insinuates itself in the sylvian tissue, and its removal through a frontotemporal craniotomy is complicated by the tumor's adherence (on its medial aspect) to sylvian veins. Surgical cure is not possible. Middle third tumors grow into both the frontal and temporal fossae in a globular fashion. The approach is through a frontotemporal craniotomy, with the base of the tumor approached first to eliminate the blood supply. Surgical cure is likely. Inner third tumors arise from the anterior clinoid process and compress the optic nerve and encase the carotid and middle cerebral arteries. In addition, medial sphenoidal meningiomas can grow diffusely into the cavernous sinus and optic canal. Only in those situations where the tumor presents early because of optic nerve compression is total removal even feasible. Most commonly, a complete resection is not possible, and the surgeon stops when the risk of the surgery exceeds potential benefits.

Tentorial meningiomas arise from the broad surface or free edge of the tentorium and are approached under the temporal lobe or under the occipital lobe, depending on their placement. In all instances, the principle of removal is incision of the tentorium around the tumor and gradual bulk reduction and separation of the tumor from surrounding brain. Venous sinuses and critical draining veins, particularly the vein of Labbé, must be protected.

Cerebellopontine angle or lateral posterior fossa meningiomas arise from the petrous bone and are exposed through a posterior fossa craniectomy by retracting the cerebellum medially. Involvement of cranial nerves VII and VIII can occur, and ventrally situated tumors may be marked by extreme adherence to the brain stem; no attempt at complete removal is justifiable in this situation.

Clival meningiomas have been approached under the temporal lobe, through the posterior fossa and temporal bone, and even transorally. Because these tumors involve cranial nerves and important arterial perforators to the brain stem, a conservative approach, internal decompression of the tumors, seems prudent sometimes. If possible, however, total removal should be attempted in the young patient at the first operation, because adhesions will preclude surgical cure at a subsequent reoperation.

RADIATION THERAPY

The need for adjunctive radiation therapy is determined by the extent of surgical resection and the histopathologic features of the tumor (benign versus malignant). The risk of recurrence for completely resected meningiomas is small, and postoperative irradiation is not usually recommended. In contrast, the risk of relapse after subtotal resection ranges from 33% to 60% at 5 years to more than 90% at 15 years.[247,266] Several reports suggest that postoperative irradiation prolongs the interval to recurrence, prevents tumor regrowth in some patients, and improves the survival of patients with incompletely resected meningiomas. Barbaro and associates compared the outcome of 54 patients who were treated with subtotal resection and radiation therapy with a group of 30 patients who underwent subtotal resection alone.[267] Sixty percent of the nonirradiated patients developed recurrence, whereas 32% of the irradiated patients recurred. The median time to recurrence was 10.4 years for the irradiated patients compared with 5.5 years for the nonirradiated group ($p < 0.05$). Taylor and coworkers found that 69% of their patients relapsed after subtotal excision alone, whereas only 15% of those treated with subtotal excision and postoperative irradiation recurred ($p = 0.01$).[268] The 10-year survival rate was 81% for patients treated with combined therapy compared with 49% for nonirradiated patients. The actuarial 5-, 10-, and 15-year relapse-free survival rates for patients undergoing subtotal resection and irradiation reported by Graholm and colleagues were 78%, 67%, and 56%, respectively.[269] These results compare favorably with the relapse-free survival rates of 63%, 45%, and 9% reported by Mirimanoff and associates for incompletely resected, nonirradiated patients.[266]

It is controversial whether patients should be treated with radiation therapy after their initial subtotal resection or when signs of disease progression appear. Some clinicians have found that patients with benign meningiomas do equally well with either approach[270]; others suggest that initial postoperative irradiation is preferable, because recurrence has an adverse influence on outcome, and many patients who recur after initial subtotal excision alone may not be salvaged by subsequent treatment.[268] Postoperative irradiation often is deferred in elderly patients and in those in poor medical condition until there is evidence of symptomatic progression.[268] When a surgical resection is not feasible, radiation therapy may relieve symptoms and substantially decrease the rate of tumor progression.[269]

Malignant meningiomas behave in a more aggressive manner than their benign counterparts. Chan and Thompson found that the mean survival of 6 patients treated with surgery alone was only 7.2 months, compared with 5.1 years for 12 patients treated with surgery and postoperative irradiation.[271] Six of the 9 patients with malignant histology reported by Graholm and coworkers died within 5 years.[269] The recurrence rate among 53 patients with malignant meningiomas collected from six series in the literature was 49%. The recurrence rates were 33% for patients treated with complete resection alone, 12% for those undergoing complete resection and radiation therapy, 55% for patients treated by subtotal resection and irradiation, and 100% for those treated by subtotal resection alone.[257] These data suggest that all patients with malignant meningiomas should be offered postoperative irradiation, regardless of the extent of resection.

The tumor volume for radiation therapy, defined by CT scan or MRI and modified by the neurosurgeon's description of the site of residual disease, is treated with a margin of 1.5 to 2 cm. Extensive base-of-skull tumors and malignant meningiomas require more generous margins. A dose of 55 Gy in daily fractions of 1.8 to 2 Gy is recommended for benign meningiomas, whereas the dose is increased to 60 Gy for malignant lesions.

CHEMOTHERAPY

There is currently no place for chemotherapy for newly diagnosed and nonirradiated meningiomas, because chemotherapy is not required except in the most intransigent recurrences. For patients who present with histologically malignant meningiomas or recurrent, surgically inaccessible, more-differentiated meningiomas, the situation is only slightly different. Because of the potentially lethal consequences of these two situations, the authors have been treating with aggressive surgery, focal irradiation, and cytotoxic chemotherapy.

The authors have evaluated the combinations of cyclophosphamide, doxorubicin, and VCR (9 patients); DTIC and doxorubicin (5 patients); and high-dose ifosfamide with mesna (2 patients). Little objective activity was noted for the first, 1 in 5 responses in the second, and 1 in 2 in the third. Grunberg and colleagues reported on the use of mifepristone, an antiprogesterone, in 14 patients with recurrent meningiomas; 5 in 14 showed objective response after 6 to 12 months of daily oral therapy.[272] A randomized trial for incompletely resected meningiomas is being advanced to better determine the relative merits of mifepristone chemotherapy.

PRIMARY CNS LYMPHOMA

CLINICAL AND PATHOLOGIC CONSIDERATIONS

Primary non-AIDS CNS lymphomas are often B-cell lymphomas of the histiocytic (large cell or large cell immunoblastic) type. In some patients, EBV has been found in biopsy material.[40] In the past, most patients with primary CNS lymphoma had no predisposing immunosuppressive disorder. However, primary CNS non-Hodgkin's lymphoma has been seen with inherited immunosuppression (ataxia-telangiectasia, Wiskott-Aldrich syndrome, and severe combined immunodeficiency disease [SCID]), acquired immunosuppression (systemic lupus erythematosus, tuberculosis, and vasculitis), drugs that are immunosuppressants (transplant patients), and EBV.[40,273–275] Unfortunately, these tumors are taking on greater importance because of their association with immunodeficiency states.

Before the AIDS era, CNS lymphomas represented only 1% of all lymphomas. In transplant recipients, CNS lymphomas accounted for 50% of lymphomas. As a result of the AIDS epidemic, primary CNS lymphoma has become more prevalent and, by some estimates, it will become the commonest primary CNS tumor during the 1990s.[276]

Clinically, these tumors are more prevalent among men. Before AIDS, they had their peak incidence in the fourth to sixth decades. Because of AIDS-associated CNS lymphomas, the age for the peak incidence is decreasing, with these tumors becoming more common in the third and fourth decades. The average time from onset of disease to diagnosis is approximately 1 to 2 months. In a recent literature review, Murray and associates found that 52% of cases were supratentorial, 34% were multiple, 12% were cerebellar, 2% were in the brain stem, and fewer than 0.5% were spinal.[277]

Because the level of clinical concern determines how quickly diagnosis is made and how long symptoms are allowed to progress, patterns of presentation vary from series to series. The following categories of symptoms have been observed: (1) those due to increased intracranial pressure, such as headache, nausea, and vomiting; (2) those associated with deficits in higher cortical function, including personality change, psychiatric manifestations, and dementia; (3) focal neurologic deficits; and (4) seizures. Most prevalent are symptoms and signs of confusion, lethargy, and memory loss followed by focal findings of hemiparesis or dysphasia.

The contrast-enhanced CT and MRI appearance of these lesions is sometimes distinctive. Multiple lesions and homogenous enhancement of signal in the paraventricular regions, basal ganglia, thalamus, or corpus callosum suggest CNS lymphoma. Sometimes, the extent of disease appears disproportionate to the neurologic deficit. Many tumors have minimal, if any, mass effect. The differential diagnosis of AIDS-associated CNS lymphoma must include the many opportunistic fungal and parasitic infections also common to AIDS, especially toxoplasmosis. However, as with gliomas, the diagnosis is made by biopsy.

CSF examination is sometimes helpful to identify specific cytoplasmic immunoglobulins. Although specific CSF abnormalities are seen in fewer than 30% of patients with primary CNS lymphomas, pleocytosis, increased protein, hypogalycorrhachia, positive cytology, and specific monoclonal antibody staining of surface markers may be helpful.

SURGERY

Because a tissue diagnosis is essential and surgery is not curative for patients with multiple lesions or with small and poorly accessible lesions in, for example, the thalamus, corpus callosum, or deep dominant hemisphere, these patients may receive only a CT-stereotactic biopsy. Large single hemispheric lesions should be surgically reduced, as should the largest of multiple lesions, when intracranial pressure cannot be controlled otherwise. CSF shunting procedures are sometimes necessary when there is diffuse meningeal tumor invasion and consequent communicating hydrocephalus.

RADIATION THERAPY

Primary CNS lymphomas are clinically aggressive tumors, and although they are limited to one "extranodal site," their behavior is comparable with that of disseminated high-grade systemic lymphomas.[278] Survival times from the onset of symptoms vary from 1 to 3.3 months with supportive care alone and 0.9 to 4.6 months after surgical resection (without adjuvant therapy).[279,280] Although radiation therapy generally results in prompt clinical and radiographic improvement, the duration of response is surprisingly short, and local recurrence usually ensues. The median survival time after treatment with radiation therapy ranges from 10 to 18 months,[281] and the 5-year disease-free survival rate is only 3%.[74] Because of the multifocal nature of CNS lymphomas, their predilection for leptomeningeal infiltration, and their tendency to be more widespread than indicated by imaging studies, the entire intracranial contents are included within the treatment fields. Several retrospective reviews suggest that there is a direct relation between radiation dose and outcome. Pollack and coworkers found that patients treated with doses of 40 to 50 Gy to the whole brain survived longer than those who received lower doses.[282] Further, Murray and colleagues observed that patients who received 50 Gy or more to the primary tumor site had a better outcome than those given less than 50 Gy.[283]

To examine the efficacy of high-dose radiation therapy, the RTOG conducted a prospective study in which patients were given 40 Gy to the whole brain followed by an additional 20 Gy to the primary lesion. The median survival time of the 41 evaluable patients was 11.6 months; the 1- and 2-year survival rates were 48% and 28%, respectively. Age and KPS were the most important predictors of outcome. Patients who were older than 60 years of age or had a KPS of less than 60 had an especially poor prognosis (median survival time 5.6–7.6 months) compared with younger and more functionally intact patients (median survival time 21–23 months).[284] These results suggest that even 60 Gy is inadequate and provide convincing evidence that more aggressive therapeutic regimens are needed.

Usually, it is recommended that patients with solitary lesions receive 40 to 50 Gy to the whole brain, supplemented by an additional 10 to 15 Gy to the primary tumor site using conventional fractionation schedules. Because of the risk of ocular involvement and the efficacy of orbital irradiation in affected patients,[285] inclusion of the posterior orbits within the whole-brain irradiation field has been recommended.[282] Although craniospinal axis irradiation may be of value in patients with primary leptomeningeal lymphoma, its efficacy in other patients is unproved.[74] In most situations, spinal irradiation has been replaced by intrathecal chemotherapy. The prognosis of AIDS patients with CNS lymphomas is much poorer than in non-AIDS-related CNS lymphoma. The median survival time may be as brief as 2 months, and patients often die from other causes.[276,286] For these patients, a dose of 40 Gy in 3 weeks to the whole brain provides satisfactory palliation.

CHEMOTHERAPY

Chemotherapy is of proved efficacy in the treatment of systemic lymphoma. A variety of agents and approaches have been used to treat primary CNS lymphoma with variable results. In some patients, glucocorticoids cause the temporary disappearance of contrast-enhancing lesions on CT. This effect may result from the direct cytolytic effect of glucocorticoids or from stabilization of the blood–brain barrier. This usually is a short-lived response. Unfortunately, chemotherapy trials have been sporadic and often have involved few patients.

Early studies used chemotherapy at the time of recurrence or progression. More recently, chemotherapy was given adjuvant to radiation therapy. Regimens used include nitrosoureas; procarbazine; mustard compounds; high-dose methotrexate; high-dose cytosine arabinoside; cytoxan, doxorubicin, VCR, and prednisone (CHOP); VCR, cytoxan, procarbazine or 6-mercaptopurine (VENP or VEMP); dexamethasone, high-dose cytosine arabinoside, and cisplatin (DHAP)[287]; PCV[288]; and osmotic blood–brain barrier opening with cytoxan, methotrexate, procarbazine, and dexamethasone.[289] Reports indicate that all regimens are capable of producing remission, although the resilence of remission in terms of duration is variable.

McLaughlin and associates reported on 10 patients treated with DHAP.[287] They found 2 in 4 had a complete response at initial treatment and 4 in 6 treated at relapse also achieved complete response. Chamberlain and Levin reported 10 patients treated with radiation therapy and concomitant hydroxyurea followed by PCV. Median and 25% survival times were 30 and 50 months.[288]

Neuwelt and colleagues reported on the use of osmotic blood–brain barrier disruption using intraarterial mannitol in association with intraarterial methotrexate (1–5 g) with leucovorin rescue and intravenous cyclophosphamide (30 mg/kg).[289] During the next 14 days, the patients received oral procarbazine (100 mg/day) and dexamethasone (24 mg/day). Of 13 patients treated at recurrence, the median survival was 17 months. For the 17 patients treated at initial presentation, the median survival was 55 months (radiation was used for tumor progression or recurrence).

Some of the best results have been obtained by DeAngelis and associates, using high-dose intravenous methotrexate and intraventricular methotrexate before radiation therapy.[281] Patients received preradiation therapy methotrexate (1 g/m^2) and intraventricular methotrexate; whole-brain and tumor-boosted radiation therapy; and postradiation therapy, two courses of cytarabine (3 g/m^2 for 2 days). Of 32 patients studied, the median survival was 42 months compared with 21 months for those receiving radiation therapy only.[290]

Given the scarcity of non-AIDS primary CNS lymphomas, it is clear that randomized cooperative trials are necessary to consolidate these observations and provide a more rational basis for future treatments.

PRIMITIVE NEUROEPITHELIAL TUMORS

CLINICAL AND PATHOLOGIC CONSIDERATIONS

The treatment of primitive neuroepithelial tumors is controversial and complex. Much of the controversy is based on the failure to understand that there are multiple entities included within this pathologic diagnosis. Controversy surrounds the classification of these tumors.[291] Primitive cells that remain undifferentiated or exhibit varying degrees of neuronal or glial differentiation, or both, are the hallmark of these tumors. Conceptually, these tumors can be viewed as developmentally aberrant brain cells. Therefore, primitive neuroepithelial tumors can be divided into the following classification schema: medulloepithelioma, neuroblastoma, spongioblastoma, ependymoblastoma, pineoblastoma, and medulloblastoma. With the exception of medulloblastoma, primitive neuroepithelial tumors are rare.

It has been proposed that all neoplasms showing primitive poorly differentiated neuroepithelial cells be called *primitive neuroectodermal tumors,* regardless of location or cell type. Because of the infrequency of these tumors and the controversy surrounding an all-inclusive classification schema currently, it is best to refer to each histiotype separately.

Clinically, however, these tumors share some common and disquieting features. Primarily, they are proliferative and malignant tumors that tend to spread throughout the neuraxis like medulloblastoma. As a result, a complete evaluation of the CNS, including contrast-enhanced CT scans of the entire brain, CSF cytology, and metrizamide myelography, must be performed before the initiation of treatment.

SURGERY

The initial therapy for primitive neuroectodermal tumors is surgical bulk reduction whenever feasible. Surgical principles are the same as those for astrocytoma described earlier.

RADIATION THERAPY

Because of their propensity to spread throughout the subarachnoid space, primitive neuroectodermal tumors are treated with craniospinal axis irradiation. The doses are similar to those given for medulloblastoma. The primary tumor should receive 54 Gy at 1.8 Gy/day, with the remainder of the axis receiving 30 to 40 Gy, depending on the age of the patient. These tumors appear to be less radiocurable than medulloblastomas. In a series of 14 patients reported by Gaffney and coworkers, the 5-year survival rate was 25%.[292] Two of the three long-term survivors received craniospinal irradiation, and all had chemotherapy. None of the patients with more than 90% primitive elements in their pathology specimen survived 5 years.

Within this category is a distinct pathologic and clinical entity that differs from other primitive neuroectodermal tumors, namely the primary cerebral neuroblastoma. Berger and colleagues found that 7 of the 11 patients treated with local irradiation to a dose of 50 Gy were alive with no evidence of tumor progression.[293] Of the 6 patients with cystic tumors, none had recurrent disease, whereas 4 of the 5 patients with solid tumors recurred. Based on this analysis, it is recommended that patients with primary cerebral neuroblastomas receive craniospinal axis irradiation only if there is evidence of tumor spread beyond the site of origin. If the tumor is localized, focal irradiation is the treatment of choice.

CHEMOTHERAPY

Because primitive neuroectodermal tumors are an uncommon type of tumor, there are no controlled chemotherapy trials. Reports of isolated cases and small series indicate that drugs active against medulloblastoma have activity in primitive neuroectodermal tumors (see medulloblastoma chemotherapy section that follows).

MEDULLOBLASTOMA

CLINICAL AND PATHOLOGIC CONSIDERATIONS

Medulloblastoma appears more similar to the primitive neuroectodermal tumors of childhood than to the gliomas. Although the cell of origin of these tumors is controversial, it is probable that medulloblastoma takes its origin from germinative neuroepithelial cells in the roof of the fourth ventricle.[50] Consistent with its embryonal nature is the fact that the peak incidence occurs in the first decade of life (see Table 48–4); 50% to 60% of medulloblastomas occur in the first decade, with a peak between 5 and 9 years. A second but lesser peak occurs between 20 and 30 years.

The typical location for childhood medulloblastoma is in the cerebellum, mostly in the midline and posterior vermis (Fig. 48–7); many encroach on the cisterna magna and the fourth ventricle. In adolescents and adults, there is an increasing tendency for tumors to be laterally placed in the cerebellar hemispheres. Regardless of where in the cerebellum they occur, the tendency for metastatic spread (within craniospinal intradural axis) of medulloblastoma is relatively high. At presentation, as many as 30% of patients have positive cytology or myelographic evidence of spinal metastasis.[294,295] Extra-CNS metastasis is less common and occurs in fewer than 5% of patients; most metastases are to long bones.[294]

Based on bromodeoxyuridine 30-minute labeling indices, medulloblastoma would be considered a highly proliferative tumor because its labeling index is approximately 14%, as opposed to gliomas, which range between less than 1% to 10%.[264]

The overall disease-free 5-year survival for medulloblastoma is approximately 50%.[222,294,296–299] However, the extent of disease at initial diagnosis defines risk. When risk factors are considered, survival is altered dramatically. Poor risk is defined as less than a 75% resection (probably >1 cc residual); invasion of the brain stem; metastasis to the spinal cord, cerebrum, and leptomeninges or seeding of the cerebellum; positive CSF cytology 2 weeks after surgery; and age younger than 4 years.[222,296,297] Of the poor-risk factors, two need explanation. Resection of less than 75% is an imprecise measure of remaining tumor—CT and MRI measurement of residual tumor volume would be better. However, in most patients, if the surgeon can remove more than 75% of tumor, the resection is usually a gross total resection. Poor risk associated with age 4 years and younger may relate more to the restricted irradiation to the developing CNS and its negative impact on tumor control. Most radiation therapists will not treat with full doses of craniospinal irradiation at 4 years.

The disease-free survival of poor-risk patients with craniospinal irradiation with or without chemotherapy is approximately 25% to 30%.[298] Good-risk patients, on the other hand, have 5-year disease-free survivals of 66% to 70%.[299,300]

At relapse, the major site of first recurrence is the posterior

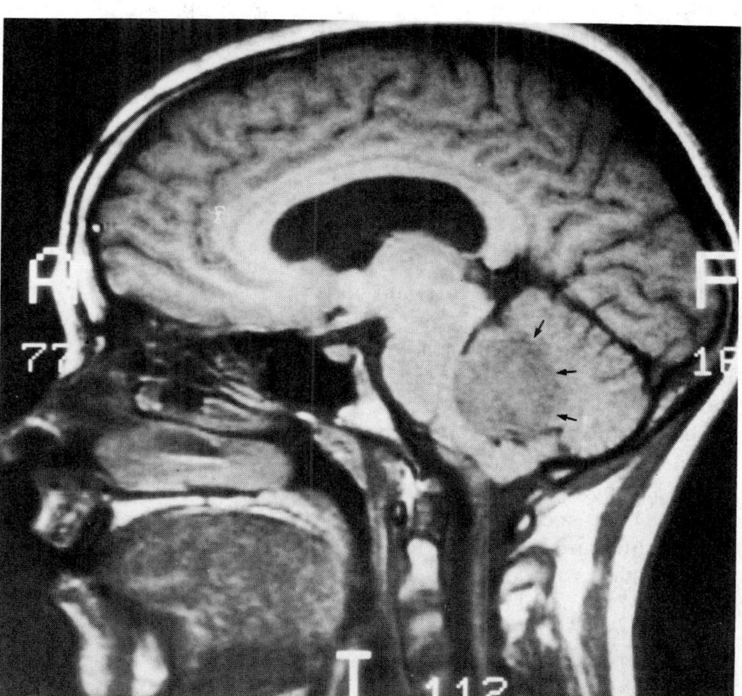

FIGURE 48–7. This young girl presented with headache and gait ataxia. A T1-weighted sagittal MRI scan (TR 600, TE 20) demonstrated a large, low-intensity mass involving the inferior aspect of the cerebellum in the midline and extending to and filling the fourth ventricle. There is arcuate stretching and displacement of the medulla and secondary hydrocephalus. The well-circumscribed nature and location of the tumor is fairly characteristic for medulloblastoma.

fossa in more than 50% of patients, the frontal lobe in nearly 20%, bone in 10% to 15%, and other cerebral and suprasellar regions in 10% to 15%.[294,300]

The incidence of systemic metastasis varies between 10% and 30%,[297,298] although the 10% incidence is most similar to the authors' experience. Most extra-CNS metastases are to long bones and ribs, with lymph nodes being a distant second site. In the series by Park and associates[297] and by Lowery and colleagues,[298] the median time to the development of extra-CNS metastasis was 10 to 12 months; in the authors' more recent study, it was 18 months.[301] In the Park study, 17% of ventriculoperitoneal-shunted patients developed systemic metastases, whereas only 4% in unshunted patients did so. In Lowery's series, 30% of patients developed systemic metastases, and none had been shunted previously. These authors' experience is that, except in patients with rampant disease, they did not find an association between ventriculoatrial or ventriculoperitoneal shunting, with or without an in-line filter, and systemic metastases. Bone metastases can occur as the only evidence of recurrence in nonshunted patients years after their initial presentation with CNS disease.

SURGERY

Although hydrocephalus associated with medulloblastoma obstructing the fourth ventricle can be relieved with a preresection CSF shunt, it is more usual to defer shunting and control increased intracranial pressure with corticosteroids. In as many as 60% of patients, aggressive resection of the tumor relieves hydrocephalus. An occipital burr hole is commonly placed at surgery, before the posterior fossa exposure is done, to allow cannulation of the ventricles for drainage of CSF to lower the increased intracranial pressure so that the dura can be opened safely.

Surgery for medulloblastoma is carried out in the prone or the sitting position. The prone position is preferred, especially in children. The incision and bony exposure are usually in the midline, but a paramedian incision and unilateral bony removal are done when the tumor is limited to one hemisphere, particularly in adults. The more commonly used midline craniectomy extends down through the foramen magnum, and a laminectomy of C1 (and rarely, C2) is performed to decompress herniated cerebellar tonsils or to remove a caudally extending tongue of tumor over the dorsum of the spinal cord.

After the dura is opened, the cerebellar tonsils are retracted laterally, and it is in the foramen of Magendie that the purplish-gray tumor usually is first seen. The floor of the fourth ventricle is separated from the tumor by a cottonoid pledget. The pledget is advanced to protect the floor of the fourth ventricle as the tumor is resected.

The thinned cerebellar vermis is progressively incised in the midline until the dorsum of the tumor is exposed. The tumor is usually soft and moderately vascular and is readily removed with suction irrigation, the CUSA, or laser, using the operating microscope for magnification and illumination. Clinical studies of cooperative groups show that an aggressive (gross total) removal is associated with an improved prognosis for the patient.[297] Dissection is continued laterally to remove tumor from the cerebellar hemispheres and ventrally to remove tumor from the fourth ventricle. When the obstructive hydrocephalus has been relieved, the CSF can be seen flowing from the aqueduct of Sylvius superiorly. It is rare for medulloblastoma to invade the floor of the fourth ventricle; when it does, careful use of the laser can be attempted to remove it. Closure is carried out in multiple layers, with particular attention to a tight dural closure to decrease the risk for pseudomeningocele (bulging wound) formation and the risk for asceptic meningitis and consequent communicating hydrocephalus from spilled blood products. Postoperative CSF shunting for hydrocephalus remains necessary in about 30% to 40% of patients.

RADIATION THERAPY

Medulloblastomas commonly infiltrate the subarachnoid space and have a striking propensity to spread throughout the CSF. As many as 25% to 30% of patients have clinically unsuspected cytologic and radiographic evidence of CNS dissemination at the time of diagnosis,[302,303] and for this reason, radiation therapy is directed to the entire craniospinal axis. Doses of 54 to 55 Gy to the primary tumor site and 35 to 36 Gy to the remainder of the craniospinal axis are generally recommended.[304] These doses usually are reduced by about 10 Gy for children younger than 2 or 3 years of age. Five-year survival rates in recent series range from 50% to 65% or higher.[74] The prognosis is affected by local tumor extent, completeness of surgical resection, presence of CSF dissemination, and age at diagnosis.[299] Although medulloblastoma is considered to be one of the most radiosensitive tumors of the CNS, local recurrence remains the primary cause of failure.[74]

Although modern radiation therapy techniques have greatly improved the prognosis for patients with medulloblastoma, the maximum benefit that can be achieved with conventional radiation therapy has probably been reached. Adjunctive chemotherapy programs are being pursued actively to further improve the outcome. Randomized trials have been conducted by the International Society of Pediatric Oncology (SIOP)[299] and the CCSG.[300] Each study compared radiation therapy plus chemotherapy with radiation therapy alone. The SIOP study used a regimen of weekly VCR during radiation therapy followed by eight courses of VCR and CCNU, cycled every 6 weeks. Patients in the CCSG study received similar chemotherapy plus prednisone. Neither trial demonstrated an overall improvement in outcome with the addition of chemotherapy. The 5-year disease-free survival rates in the CCSG and SIOP studies were 59% and 55%, respectively, for radiation therapy plus chemotherapy, and 50% and 43%, respectively, for radiation therapy alone. Chemotherapy did, however, appear to benefit certain patients with more advanced stages of disease, including those having only partial or subtotal tumor excision, those with brain stem involvement, and those with advanced T (T3 and T4) and M (M1–M3) stages. Based on these findings, patients with medulloblastoma have been separated into "low-stage" or "good-risk" and "high-stage" or "poor-risk" subgroups, and different study questions are being examined in each group.

Clinical studies in good-risk patients have been directed at decreasing treatment-related morbidity, including neuropsychological dysfunction, impaired growth of the spine, and hypothalamic-pituitary dysfunction, by reducing the dose of prophylactic irradiation to areas remote from the primary tumor site. A pilot study from the Children's Memorial Hospital and Northwestern University in Chicago found that there were no isolated spinal relapses in children given 24 Gy to the craniospinal axis.[305] However, a randomized trial conducted by CCSG and POG, which compared 23.4 Gy with the standard 36 Gy craniospinal prophylactic dose in good-risk children, was closed prematurely when an interim analysis demonstrated an excessive number of overall treatment failures and isolated neuraxis recurrences in the low-dose arm.[306]

The combination of low-dose craniospinal axis irradiation and chemotherapy also is being examined. It is expected that future studies will examine the use of more aggressive chemotherapy and seek to improve local control using approaches such as hyperfractionated irradiation. Efforts to decrease the morbidity of craniospinal axis irradiation should continue, provided that disease control is not compromised.

CHEMOTHERAPY

Medulloblastomas are responsive to a variety of antineoplastic agents, including VCR, nitrosoureas, procarbazine, dibromodulcitol, cyclophosphamide, methotrexate, platinum compounds, and various drug combinations. Table 48–21 summarizes some of the single agents and their observed response rates for CNS medulloblastoma when treated at recurrence or for progressive disease. For extra-CNS disease, these same agents have activity, although drugs such as cyclophosphamide, methotrexate, doxorubicin, and VCR may be more active than the nitrosoureas and procarbazine.

Table 48–22 summarizes some of the drug combinations that have been used for recurrent or progressive CNS medulloblastoma. It is not possible to compare the durability of these responses, because some reports pool the primitive neuroectodermal tumor patients with medulloblastoma, whereas others do not provide individual lengths of response, an MTP, or Kaplan-Meier curves. This is unfortunate, because those studies suggest an MTP range of 10 to 19 months among the better single agent and combination chemotherapy programs.[338] It is clear, however, that better treatments are needed for recurrent and progressive disease. Whether well-founded or not, current emphasis appears to be with drug combinations such as cyclophosphamide, teniposide, and cisplatin or CCNU, VCR, and cisplatin. Whether these approaches provide long-standing benefit or short-term gain awaits more careful adjuvant studies. Problems with drug delivery of these agents to the CNS may compromise long-term benefits and ultimate cure.

TABLE 48–21. Efficacy of Single-Agent Chemotherapy for Recurrent and Progressive CNS Medulloblastoma

Treatment	*Response**
Doxorubicin[308]	0/6 (0%)
PCNU[313]	0/4 (0%)
Etoposide (VP-16)[329]	0/4 (0%)
AZQ[182,208]	6/21 (28%)
BCNU[188,309]	2/6 (33%)
Carboplatin[261,317]	12/34 (35%)
Methotrexate (I.V.)[319–321]	5/13 (38%)
Cisplatin[314–316]	11/27 (40%)
Melphalan I.V.[330]	6/12 (50%)
Dibromodulcitol[259]	15/29 (51%)
Vincristine[322–327]	11/15 (73%)
Procarbazine[105]	3/4 (75%)
CCNU[174,175,310–312]	12/15 (80%)
Cyclophosphamide[318]	7/7 (100%)
Teniposide (VM-26)[328]	1/1 (100%)

VM-26, teniposide; AZQ, diaziquone; BCNU, carmustine; I.V., intravenous; CCNU, lomustine; VP-16, etoposide.
* Complete response plus partial response plus stable disease.

TABLE 48–22. Efficacy of Combination Chemotherapy for Recurrent and Progressive CNS Medulloblastoma

Treatment	*Response*
VCR-Pred-PCB(OPP)[335]	3/12 (25%)
VCR-CYT[336]	4/8 (50%)
6-TG-PCB-DBD-CCNU-VCR[258a]	6/10 (60%)
CCNU-PCB-VCR(PCV)[331]	10/16 (62%)
VM-26-CCNU-Pred[333]	2/3 (67%)
"8-in-1-day"[339]	6/9 (67%)
MOPP[334]	14/19 (73%)
VCR-MTX-BCNU[332]	8/8 (100%)
VCR-BCNU-Dex-MTX(I.V.)[337]	8/8 (100%)
CCNU-VCR-CPDD[338]	6/6 (100%)

VCR, vincristine; Pred, prednisone; PCB, procarbazine; MOPP, mustagen + Oncovin + Procarbazine + prednisone; CYT, cytoxan; 6-TG, 6-thioguanine; DBD, dibromodulcitol; CCNU, lomustine; VM-26, teniposide; MOPP, mechlorethamine, VCR, PCB, Pred; MTX, methotrexate; BCNU, carmustine; Dex, dexamethasone; CPDD, cisplatin.

As adjuvant therapy to surgery and irradiation, chemotherapy has shown inconsistent but sometimes dramatic benefit. Part of the problem resides with an agreement for the definition of good and poor risk and the tendency of some investigators to pool data from medulloblastoma with other primitive neuroectodermal tumors. Another constraint is that patients who receive craniospinal irradiation do not tolerate high-dose aggressive chemotherapy protocols well because of reduced bone marrow reserves. In an attempt to improve the tolerance to cytotoxic agents, these authors and others conducted trials to evaluate reduced craniospinal radiation therapy doses.

The authors conducted a nonrandomized trial of preradiation procarbazine and hydroxyurea during reduced craniospinal irradiation.[296] In that study they found that, after 2 weeks of oral procarbazine and irradiation with hydroxyurea, reducing the craniospinal radiation dose to 25 Gy to the spinal axis and 25 to 35 Gy to the whole brain was not detrimental with respect to disease-free survival or recurrence patterns in good- and poor-risk patients. When this group was compared with historical controls treated with conventional doses, Halberg and associates[307] found no increase in tumor recurrence in the brain or spinal axis. The 5-year disease-free survival rates for good- and poor-risk patients were 77% and 39%, respectively. In both groups, 70% of recurrences were in the posterior fossa only.

In a nonrandomized study, Packer and coworkers evaluated 108 children treated between 1975 and 1989 for medulloblastoma and other primitive neuroectodermal tumors.[340] Before 1982, children received surgery and radiation therapy, but after 1982 they also had chemotherapy with CCNU, VCR, and cisplatin. There was no difference in disease-free survival rates for children with standard risk factors; however, there was a significant difference in the 5-year survival rate for poor-risk patients treated before 1982 (35%) compared with those treated later (87%) ($p < 0.001$).

A randomized postoperative trial with postirradiation nitrogen mustard, PCV, procarbazine, and prednisone (MOPP) versus radiation therapy alone for newly diagnosed medulloblastoma found that patients treated with irradiation plus MOPP had a statistically significant increase in overall survival rate at 5 years compared with patients treated with radiation therapy alone (74% versus 56%; $p = 0.06$).[341]

The authors recently presented preliminary results of a study that opened in 1984.[342] In that study, they gave combination chemotherapy with 6-thioguanine, procarbazine, dibromodulcitol, CCNU, and VCR before and for as many as 8 cycles every 6 weeks after radiation therapy in children and adults with high-risk (more than 25% residual tumor, brain stem invasion, positive CSF cytology, positive myelogram) medulloblastoma. Radiation therapy consisted of 54 Gy to the posterior fossa and 24 Gy to the craniospinal axis. Of the 30 patients evaluable (25 children and 5 adults), there were 17 failures, a 5-year disease-free survival of 30%, and an MTP of 4.3 years. Seven pineoblastomas were also treated, with four failures to date, an MTP of 1.6 years, and 38% 5-year disease-free survival.

Hyperfractionated radiation therapy regimens, although potentially less damaging to the CNS, may lead to more bone marrow damage and less tolerance to systemic chemotherapy.

One approach that is being evaluated consists of aggressive preradiation therapy chemotherapy. The advantage of this approach is that it unequivocably defines response; the disadvantage is that some drugs may fail to achieve adequate levels in patients with poor risk due to CSF spread of tumor cells.

Kretschmar and colleagues treated 21 newly diagnosed children with poor-risk medulloblastoma on a 9-week-postoperative, preradiation therapy chemotherapy regimen of PCV and cisplatin.[343] The children older than 2 years of age then received radiation therapy. Of 13 children with measurable disease after surgery, 5 showed a definite response (1 complete response, 4 partial responses, and 5 minor responses) on CT scan. They also evaluated mustagen, Oncovin Procarbazine, and prednisone (MOP) in 6 infants until the age of 2 years, at which time they were referred for irradiation. Four of the 6 infants were disease free at 19, 32, 35, and 57 months from diagnosis.

"Eight-in-1-day" therapy has also been evaluated before radiation therapy.[339] Of 21 eligible medulloblastoma patients who received at least two courses of chemotherapy, 12 (57%) responded (including 3 complete responses and 3 partial responses). The MTP for the combined medulloblastoma-primitive neuroectodermal tumor group was 2 years.

In another study, Kovnar and associates treated 11 newly diagnosed children with measurable residual disease and characteristics indicative of poor prognosis with preradiation therapy cisplatin and etoposide.[344] There were 2 of 11 complete responses, 8 partial responses, and 1 stable disease determined radiographically in the series.

For extracranial metastases, the best results appear with aggressive combination chemotherapy. In this situation, issues of CNS drug delivery are not important, and many drugs are active. Initially, these authors evaluated the combination of cyclophosphamide, doxorubicin, and VCR; 7 patients treated responded for a median duration of 17 months, and 2 continue at 34 and 62 months without evidence of disease.[300] Other combinations with good activity are cyclophosphamide and VCR[345]; VCR, dactinomycin, and cyclophosphamide[346]; cisplatin, cyclophosphamide, and VP-16; and DTIC and doxorubicin.[183a]

PINEAL REGION TUMORS

CLINICAL AND PATHOLOGIC CONSIDERATIONS

The pineal gland is located in the posterior portion of the third ventricle. Tumors in this region are rare, accounting for fewer than 1% of intracranial tumors, although in children they constitute 3% to 8% of intracranial tumors.[347] The peak incidence of germ cell tumors is the second decade, and few present after the third decade.[348] Table 48–23 summarizes the types of tumors found in the pineal region.[349] In all series, germinomas are the commonest histology, accounting for 33% to 50% of pineal tumors (the higher frequencies are seen in Japan). Gliomas are second commonest, accounting for about 25% of pineal tumors; astrocytomas are the commonest of the glial neoplasms arising at this site.

Neurologic signs and symptoms are caused by obstructive hydrocephalus and involvement of ocular pathways. Major symptoms are headache, nausea and vomiting, lethargy, and diplopia. Signs are primarily ocular but can include ataxia and hemiparesis. The major ocular manifestation is paralysis of conjugate upward gaze (Parinaud's syndrome), although pupillary and convergence abnormalities are seen, as are skew deviation and papilledema.

Determination of tumor histology and extent of disease is

TABLE 48–23. Classification of Pineal Region Tumors

- I. Tumors of germ cell origin
  - A. Germinoma (atypical teratoma, dysgerminoma, seminoma)
  - B. Embryonal carcinoma
    - 1. Extraembryonic structures
      - a. Endodermal sinus tumors (yolk sac tumor)
      - b. Choriocarcinoma
    - 2. Embryonic endoderm, mesoderm, ectoderm
      - a. Immature teratoma
      - b. Mature teratoma
- II. Tumors of pineal parenchymal cells
  - A. Pineoblastoma
  - B. Pineocytoma
- III. Tumors of glial and other cell origin
- IV. Nonneoplastic cysts and masses

(Adapted from Herrick MK. Pathology of pineal tumors. In: Neuwelt EA, ed. Diagnosis and treatment of pineal region tumors. Baltimore: Williams & Wilkins, 1984:31) critical for optimal management of pineal region tumors. Figure 48–8 is a schema the authors use to evaluate and stage patients with pineal region tumors.

The prognosis for these tumors varies depending on the histology and size of tumor and the extent of disease at presentation. Typically, patients with mature teratomas do well with surgery alone; germinomas do best with radiation, although preradiation therapy chemotherapy may increase the cure rate and reduce the total radiation dose; gliomas respond to therapy in a manner discussed in earlier sections; and the remaining tumors respond variably to chemotherapy and radiation therapy, leading to survivals ranging from months to years before recurrence.

SURGERY

Because pineal tumors are near the center of the brain, they are among the most difficult brain tumors to remove, and it is this factor that creates some controversy in their management. Some authors promulgate decompressing the nearly invariable obstructive hydrocephalus with a shunt and then irradiating the tumor without a tissue diagnosis. However, because of an increasingly favorable experience with microsurgical approaches to the pineal region, the current recommendation is to obtain a tissue diagnosis and, when possible, to carry out a gross total resection of the tumor.[350] Resection is particularly important for pineal masses that may be relatively radioresistant or that do not require radiation therapy, such as teratomas, arachnoid cysts, and meningiomas.

Many surgical approaches to the pineal region have been described: (1) through the dilated lateral ventricle; (2) through the posterior corpus callosum; (3) under the occipital lobe; and (4) through the posterior fossa over the cerebellum.[351] The most commonly used microsurgical approaches are currently the infratentorial supracerebellar approach described first by Horsley, later by Krause, and recently resurrected and modernized by Stein, and the supratentorial approach under the occipital lobe described by Poppen and popularized recently by Clark.[351] Both have been associated with low morbidity and mortality in experienced hands.

The place of CT-guided (stereotactic) biopsy in the diagnosis of pineal region tumors is unclear. Although such biopsies have been described as relatively safe, there is a risk that tissue sampling of these heterogenous tumors may not depict accurately the correct histologic nature of the tumor.[352] Without an accurate histologic diagnosis, treatment planning may be erroneous or inadequate. In its favor is the advantage of rapid tissue diagnosis and shortened hospital stay.

RADIATION THERAPY

With certain exceptions, such as benign teratomas, radiation therapy has an established role in the treatment of pineal and suprasellar tumors of pineal parenchymal or germ cell origin. Because of their location and infiltrative nature, complete surgical extirpation often is not possible. In the past, high mortality and morbidity rates associated with biopsy or attempted resection, especially with older surgical techniques, often led to the use of radiation therapy without histologic confirmation. In such instances, response to low-dose radiation therapy, measurement of AFP and β-HCG, and CSF cytology were used to provide diagnostic information. There has been a tendency to increase the use of biopsy and attempted resection. Although surgery theoretically might be expected to increase the incidence of CSF seeding, there is no proof that this will occur. A review of older literature suggests that the incidence of spinal seeding increased from 3% for tumors in which biopsy was not obtained to 23% when biopsy was obtained from the tumors.[74] However, Linstadt and associates found no instances of failure in the spinal axis in 13 patients with biopsy-proved germinomas, only one of whom received prophylactic spinal irradiation.[353]

Five-year survival rates with radiation therapy range from 44% to 78% and vary with histology and extent of disease, age, radiation volume, and dose to the primary site.[74] Accord-

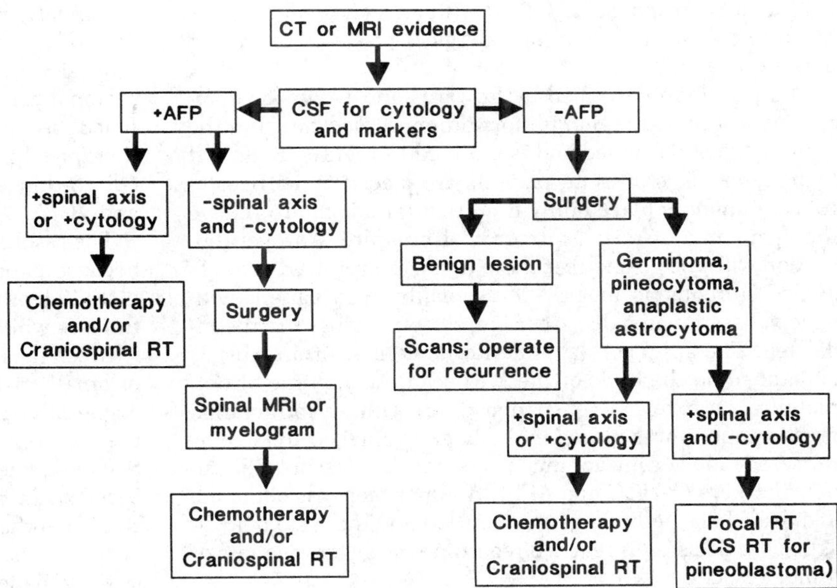

FIGURE 48–8. Treatment and evaluation schema for pineal region tumors. (Modified from Edwards MSB, Hudgins RJ, Wilson CB, et al. Pineal region tumors in children. J Neurosurg 1988;68:689)

ing to a multiinstitutional survey by Wara and coworkers, the survival of patients with pineal parenchymal cell tumors or malignant teratomas was 21% (3 of 14) compared with 72% (26 of 36) for those with germinomas.[354] This survey and the report of Jenkin and colleagues[355] indicated that patients younger than 25 to 30 years of age have survival rates of 65% to 80% compared with 35% to 40% for older patients. This finding may reflect the increased incidence of true germinomas in younger patients.

Germinomas are infiltrative tumors that tend to spread along the ventricular walls or throughout the leptomeninges. The incidence of CSF seeding ranges from 7% to 12%. Because of these features, the use of fields encompassing the entire ventricular system, the whole brain, and even the entire craniospinal axis has been recommended. In a literature review, Salazar and colleagues found a recurrence-free survival rate of 76% for patients with whole-brain irradiation compared with 61% for irradiation to the ventricular system and 51% for smaller volumes.[356] Further analysis of those data showed a 90% survival rate for patients treated with whole-brain irradiation and a tumor dose of least 50 Gy. If smaller fields were used or the dose to the primary tumor site was less than 50 Gy, the survival was 33%. With less than whole-brain irradiation, recurrences at the margin of the irradiated volume were reported in the older literature. However, the frequency of such recurrences should be reduced with the availability of CT and MRI for treatment planning. Linstadt and associates concluded that the risk for spinal metastases from germinomas was too small to justify routine prophylactic spinal irradiation, but recommended its use when there is tumor spill at surgery or in those patients with malignant CSF cytology or known subependymal or leptomeningeal metastases.[353]

At some institutions, if the histologic diagnosis is unknown and CSF cytology and myelography are negative, radiation therapy is administered at a dose of about 25 Gy at 1.8 Gy/fraction to the primary tumor site with a generous margin that includes at least the third ventricle. The CT or MRI scan is then repeated. If substantial regression has occurred, it is assumed that the lesion is a germinoma, and the whole brain is given an additional dose of approximately 25 Gy. If there is little or no response by CT or MRI, an additional 30 Gy is given to the primary field or a surgical resection is carried out, if possible.

The paradigm described by Edwards and Levin for management of pineal region tumors differs somewhat from the approach just discussed and is outlined in Figure 48–8.[350] If hydrocephalus is present, patients are placed on corticosteroids. A shunt is placed only if corticosteroids fail to relieve the symptoms of raised intracranial pressure. An open operation with the goal to resect the tumor is preferred to a CT-guided stereotactic biopsy. Occasionally, in a patient with widely disseminated disease, a stereotactic biopsy may be indicated. The approach (supratentorial versus infratentorial) is planned on the basis of the MRI scan. At the time of craniotomy, an external ventricular drain with an intracranial pressure monitor is placed in the lateral ventricle and CSF is removed to lower intracranial pressure and measure CSF tumor markers (β-HCG and AFP). A tumor biopsy is obtained, and, based on the findings at operation and the histologic diagnosis, a decision is reached regarding the aggressiveness of tumor resection.

Additional therapy is planned based on the histology, CSF markers, staging CT and MRI, and myelogram; localized germinomas (two-cell pattern) are treated with 25 Gy to the ventricular system and an additional 25 Gy to the tumor with a 1.5- to 2-cm margin. If the germinoma is disseminated, systemic chemotherapy or craniospinal irradiation is administered. Nongerminomatous malignant germ cell tumors, whether localized or disseminated, are treated with systemic chemotherapy (for six courses), followed by restaging studies. After restaging, localized tumors receive focal radiation therapy, and disseminated tumors receive craniospinal irradiation (54 Gy to the primary tumor, 45 Gy to the ventricular system, 35 Gy to the spinal cord, and 45 Gy to any localized spinal cord lesions).

Biopsy-verified tumors with little or no tendency to metastasize to the spinal cord, such as teratomas, embryonal cell carcinomas, pineocytomas, and low-grade gliomas, are treated by resection or with local radiation fields only. Craniospinal axis irradiation is reserved for tumors that have a strong tendency toward cord involvement (such as pineoblastoma), for those with positive CSF cytology, or for those with radiographic evidence of spinal cord involvement.

CHEMOTHERAPY

Chemotherapy for glial neoplasms is similar to that covered in earlier sections. The chemotherapy for germ cell tumors is in flux but is encouraging. For germinomas, complete responses before radiation therapy or at recurrence have been observed with cisplatin and bleomycin[357]; cyclophosphamide alone[358,359] or the combination of cyclophosphamide, vinblastine, and bleomycin[358]; the combination of cisplatin and etoposide[360]; and dactinomycin, methotrexate, vinblastine, and cisplatin.[348,350]

For nongerminoma malignant germ cell tumors (*e.g.*, embryonal, endodermal sinus, and mixed tumors), the benefits of chemotherapy are far less impressive, with partial rather than complete responses and recurrence within months to years being the norm. Chemotherapies with activity include combinations of cyclophosphamide, vinblastine, and bleomycin[358]; cisplatin, VCR, and bleomycin[361]; cisplatin and etoposide[362]; and cisplatin, bleomycin, and teniposide.[362a] Occasional patients with recurrent germ cell tumors who have failed the combination of cisplatin, bleomycin, and vinblastine therapies have responded to the authors' BTRC 8422 protocol (6-thioguanine, procarbazine, dibromodulcitol, CCNU, and VCR).

The results with chemotherapy have appeared paradoxical, because patients with systemic seminoma treated with cisplatin, bleomycin, and vinblastine have developed brain metastases while receiving chemotherapy.

Given the rarity of CNS germ cell tumors and the similarity of small trials reported in the literature, it is obvious that cooperative group trials are necessary to determine which of the existing chemotherapy combinations are most active. Second-generation studies could then address modifications based on a reasonable data base rather than the few anecdotal studies in the literature. Much study needs to be done to elucidate the best drug combinations and use of chemotherapy in these patients.

PITUITARY ADENOMAS

CLINICAL AND PATHOLOGIC CONSIDERATIONS

Pituitary gland tumors tend to produce neuroendocrine or neurologic symptoms and signs. Anatomically, tumors arising from the pituitary gland can compress the pituitary, grow out of the sella to compress and invade the optic chiasm, and, if growth is unabated, extend into the temporal lobe, third ventricle, and the posterior fossa. The chief finding in most patients is visual loss initially characterized by a bitemporal hemianopia. Headache occurs in about 20%. Less frequent are ocular palsies due to compression or invasion of the cavernous sinus.

Neuroendocrine abnormalities can be associated with tumor compression of the pituitary gland or hypersecretion of hormones, or both. Table 48–7 summarizes some of the more common syndromes and their endocrine abnormalities. Sexual impotence in men and amenorrhea and galactorrhea in women are commonly associated with hyperprolactinemia. Growth hormone hypersecretion is associated with acromegaly or gigantism, depending on the age of the patient. Corticotropin hypersecretion results in Cushing's disease. Elements of hypothyroidism, adrenal insufficiency, and growth hormone deficiency may follow compression of the pituitary gland by growth of an adenoma.

The diagnosis of a pituitary tumor is based on sensitive radioimmunoassays, CT scans, and, most recently, MRI. Figure 48–3 shows an MRI scan of a pituitary adenoma before surgery.

Pituitary adenomas are classified as endocrine inactive or endocrine active. Most secrete one or, occasionally, two hormones. The reported incidence of the various types of pituitary adenomas depends on the institution's referral patterns. Of 800 patients operated on at UCSF between 1970 and 1981, 630 of 800 (79%) were endocrine active; of these, 331 of 630 (52%) were prolactin secreting, 27% growth hormone secreting, 20% corticotropin secreting, and only 0.3% were thyroid-stimulating hormone secreting.[363] Undifferentiated cell adenomas are considered to be nononcocytic (null) or oncocytic (oncocytoma) tumors.

Of prognostic importance are the functional status of the tumor and how large or invasive it is. Table 48–7 is the grade and staging system used at UCSF.[363]

SURGERY

The goal of surgery for the larger (usually, but not always, endocrine inactive) pituitary tumors is to decompress the visual pathways and reduce tumor bulk, whereas the goal for hypersecreting adenomas is normalization of the hypersecretion with preservation of remaining normal pituitary function. For larger nonsecreting pituitary adenomas, surgical cure is not possible or necessary, because radiation therapy adjuvant to surgery is usually curative. In contrast, the hypersecreting adenoma should be resected in its entirety, whenever possible, because the effects of hypersecretion can be devastating, and response to radiation therapy is slow and less predictable.

The operative approach of choice for most pituitary tumors is transsphenoidal, because it is safer and better tolerated than the alternative transcranial (frontal craniotomy) approach.[364] The transsphenoidal approach is possible for tumors occupying the sella turcica and even in those with fairly large medial suprasellar extension as long as the tumor is soft (the usual case) and can drop into the sella with progressive resection. Tough, woody suprasellar tumors and those with extension laterally into the middle fossa or anteriorly beneath the frontal lobes must be resected by craniotomy.

RADIATION THERAPY

Microadenomas of the pituitary, usually diagnosed because of endocrine hypersecretion, may be totally resected. There is no indication for radiation therapy, unless there is persistent hormone elevation. Macroadenomas, particularly the endocrine inactive lesions, may invade into adjacent structures, such as the cavernous sinus, the optic chiasm, or the third ventricle. Subtotal resection and postoperative irradiation can relieve mass effect, shrink the remaining tumor, prevent regrowth, and lower hormone levels. Further, radiation therapy alone or in conjunction with medical treatment is an effective alternative to primary treatment for patients who are medically inoperable or who refuse surgery.

Radiation therapy controls tumor growth in more than 90% of patients with nonfunctioning, prolactin-secreting, and growth hormone-secreting adenomas. Sheline and Tyrrell demonstrated that patients with large, nonfunctioning adenomas or prolactin-secreting adenomas associated with visual field deficits had a 60% recurrence rate (using visual field changes as an endpoint) within 5 years after incomplete resection alone.[365] The recurrence rate was reduced to about 4% by the addition of radiation therapy, whereas 7% treated with radiation therapy alone recurred. Approximately two thirds of patients who presented with modest visual field defects, involving not more than one quadrant, who were treated by surgery or radiation therapy alone had return of normal vision in the involved eyes. With larger visual field defects, restoration of vision was better in patients who received preradiation therapy surgical decompression than in those treated by radiation therapy alone. In patients with acromegaly and visual field defects, normal vision was achieved by irradiation alone in about two thirds of patients.

Radiation therapy is less effective in controlling endocrine hypersecretion than in controlling the growth of pituitary adenomas. Radiation therapy decreases serum growth hormone concentrations to normal levels (usually defined as <10 ng/ml in the radiation therapy and surgery literature) in 80% to 85% of acromegalic patients. However, several years may be required for the levels to normalize.[364] The probability of normalization is related to the pretreatment growth hormone level. Radiation therapy is most effective in tumors with relatively small preradiation therapy growth hormone elevations (30–50 ng/ml), whereas the response is less predictable with higher growth hormone levels.[75] Radiation therapy controls hypercortisolism in 50% to 75% of adults and 80% of children with Cushing's disease. Response occurs within 6 to 9 months of treatment.[366,367]

Data on control of prolactin secretion by conventional radiation therapy are more difficult to interpret. Irradiation decreases prolactin levels by 75% to 90% on the average, and the response occurs over several years. However, normal levels are only attained in about 30% of patients when radiation therapy is used as primary treatment or after incomplete surgical resection.[368–370] Bromocriptine may be administered to reduce temporarily the prolactin level in patients with incompletely resected macroadenomas who are receiving radiation therapy. The drug is then periodically withdrawn to determine whether the prolactin level has returned to normal. Medical treatment with dopamine agonists alone does not appear to represent adequate therapy for prolactin-secreting adenomas. Bromocriptine does not produce a permanent reduction in tumor size and prolactin concentration after the course of therapy is completed and, unlike radiation therapy, does not reduce the risk of tumor expansion during pregnancy. Further, it commits the patient to a lifetime of medicinal use and its potential side effects.[371]

Pituitary adenomas may be treated using several different techniques. One approach is to use bilateral coronal arcs with moving wedge filters. The usual treatment plan includes two 110° arcs with 30° wedge filters. The field size is chosen to include the target volume in the 95% isodose line. The neck is placed in the flexed position so that the plane of rotation is behind the eyes. During simulation, markers are placed on the eyelids. Three tattoo marks are placed on the skin and used for alignment with laser beams to ensure daily positional reproducibility. For large tumors, a three-field technique with lateral opposed wedged portals and a superior or vertex field may be used. The total dose is carried to 45 Gy in 25 fractions of 1.8 Gy, calculated at the 95% isodose line. This combination of fraction size and total dose provides long-term tumor control in more than 90% of cases, and, therefore, a larger dose is not indicated.[372] Further, radiation-induced injury to optic apparatus or adjacent brain with this dose-fractionation scheme is rare, whereas larger fractions or greater total doses lead to a higher incidence of injury. The optic chiasm appears especially sensitive to radiation injury in patients with acromegaly. Bloom and Kramer reported five instances of visual complication in 40 acromegalic patients.[75] The complications were largely in patients receiving daily increments of 2 Gy and total doses of 50 Gy. Hypopituitarism, however, may develop as a late complication years after completion of radiation therapy.[364] Hypopituitarism is more likely to occur in patients who have had surgery and postoperative radiation therapy than in those who have been treated by radiation therapy or surgery alone.[373] Because hypopituitarism is largely correctable by hormone replacement therapy, patients treated for pituitary adenomas should be observed by an endocrinologist for the remainder of their lives.

CRANIOPHARYNGIOMAS

CLINICAL AND PATHOLOGIC CONSIDERATIONS

Craniopharyngiomas occur primarily in children. These tumors arise from cell rests that are remnants of Rathke's pouch at the juncture of the infundibular stalk and the pituitary gland. Most of these tumors become symptomatic only after they have attained a diameter of about 3 cm. They are usually cystic at the time of presentation. They may compress the optic chiasm or pituitary gland and extend up into the third ventricle. The cyst is high in proteinaceous material and calcium and is seen easily by CT scan or MRI.

Clinically, craniopharyngiomas produce increased intracranial pressure and hypopituitary-hypothalamic-chiasmal dysfunction. Symptoms vary and, in children, may include obesity, delayed development, decreased vision and optic atrophy, field defects, and papilledema.

SURGERY

Craniopharyngiomas usually are approached by a microsurgical procedure done through a right frontal craniotomy. Large craniopharyngioma cysts that enter and enlarge the sella turcica can be drained and resected through a transsphenoidal procedure.

The goal of most surgeons in the surgery of craniopharyngioma is total removal, but some do a more conservative operation and depend on the excellent results with radiation therapy discussed later. Aggressive removal nearly guarantees some injury to the pituitary gland and stalk, with subsequent temporary or permanent diabetes insipidus and elements of hypopituitarism. Patients injured in this manner must take replacement hormones and use inhaled desmopressin acetate spray for the control of diabetes insipidus for life. However, patients whose vision was affected by the craniopharyngioma can expect improvement after surgery. The mortality of craniopharyngioma resection should be extremely low.

In Europe, a few centers are treating craniopharyngioma cysts with stereotactic puncture and the instillation of colloidal therapeutic radioisotopes, particularly yttrium 90.[374] Such treatments are being tried in this country also with colloidal phosphorus 32. Intracystic therapy may be a good treatment for craniopharyngioma cysts recurring after conventional external-beam irradiation.

RADIATION THERAPY

Although debate exists regarding the extent to which total excision should be attempted, numerous reports demonstrate that local tumor control and survival after subtotal removal, consisting of extensive resection or of limited biopsy and cyst aspiration and irradiation, is comparable with that achieved by radical excision.[375–378] The local control rates after complete resection, subtotal resection alone, and incomplete resection and postoperative irradiation are 70%, 26%, and 75%, respectively.[379] Ten-year survival rates range from 24% to 100% for complete resection, 31% to 52% for subtotal resection, and 62% to 84% for incomplete resection and irradiation.[375–377,380,381] Patients undergoing conservative treatment including biopsy and cyst drainage and irradiation appear to enjoy a better quality of life and demonstrate less psychosocial impairment than those initially treated with more extensive resections.[377] Further, conservative therapy is associated with less hypothalamic-pituitary dysfunction[382] and a lower incidence of persistent diabetes insipidus[390] than when a total or near-total excision is attempted. More extensive resections using a subfrontal approach may be associated with frontal lobe and visual perceptual dysfunction.[383]

The radiation therapy target volume is based largely on CT scanning using relatively small margins around demonstrated tumor. The technique varies according to size and location of residual tumor, but most patients are treated by bicoronal arcs with moving wedge filters, similar to the method used for pituitary adenomas. The total dose is 55 Gy, given in daily

1.8-Gy increments. In children younger than 3 years of age, it is recommended that, if possible, irradiation be delayed until the child is older.

CEREBELLOPONTINE ANGLE NEURILEMMOMAS

CLINICAL AND PATHOLOGIC CONSIDERATIONS

The major tumors occurring in this region are the acoustic nerve tumors and meningiomas. Meningiomas have been discussed previously; therefore, the discussion that follows is limited to acoustic neurilemmomas (schwannoma and neurofibroma). These tumors originate on cranial nerve VIII, almost always on the vestibular division, at the point where the nerve acquires its reticulin and Schwann cell investment. Within the skull, this transition zone occurs in the internal auditory foramen and causes local erosion of the internal auditory meatus. Slow growth characterizes these tumors; therefore, they can grow to substantial size before clinical symptoms lead to diagnosis. They often occupy the posterior fossa at the angle between the cerebellum and the pons. By compression, they can affect cranial nerves VII, V, and, less often, IX and X alone or in various combinations. When large enough, they can compress the medulla and obstruct the CSF, leading to hydrocephalus.

Acoustic neurilemmomas are commonest in the fifth decade and can be associated with familial neurofibromatosis. In the latter instance they occur earlier, in late childhood and adolescence, and may be bilateral.

In a series from the Massachusetts General Hospital, auditory and vestibular branch involvement was found to occur in 98% of patients, facial weakness with disturbances of taste in 56%, sensory loss over the face in 56%, gait abnormality in 41%, and appendicular ataxia in 20%.[51]

Diagnosis by skull x-ray examination is suggestive, but definitive diagnosis is most effectively made with MRI or CT scan done in conjunction with the CSF administration of metrizamide contrast.

SURGERY

The aim of surgery for acoustic neurilemmomas is complete resection, with the surgical approach chosen after consideration of the patient's age and residual hearing and the size and location of the tumor.[384] When useful hearing is present, the suboccipital approach is taken because of the possibility of hearing preservation postoperatively, particularly in smaller tumors. In patients with poor hearing, the translabyrinthine approach, which produces deafness in the operated-on ear, is used for its lower overall morbidity. Occasionally, tumors that reside purely within lateral portions of the internal acoustic canal are approached through the middle cranial fossa.[384]

The translabyrinthine route requires only a small incision behind the ear through which the petrous bone is gradually removed with a high-speed drill until the facial nerve is identified and exposed to the point where it can be separated from the tumor and protected. The dura of the posterior fossa is seen easily and can be opened to gain access to the intradural component of the tumor.

The transoccipital approach requires a unilateral posterior fossa craniectomy, after which the dura is opened and the cerebellum is retracted medially to expose the cerebellopontine angle. The lower cranial nerves are protected while tumor is removed, and the porus acusticus is unroofed in an effort to identify the facial nerve, and in smaller tumors, the acoustic nerve as well. Once the facial nerve is identified, the remainder of the tumor is removed in a usually lengthy and involved operation that fully exploits the surgeon's microsurgical skill.

Complete removal of acoustic neurilemmomas through the posterior fossa can be predicted in almost every instance, and life-threatening complications are rare except in patients with extremely large tumors. As mentioned earlier, preservation of the acoustic nerve is rare in even small tumors, but the facial nerve is in continuity at the end of most acoustic tumor resections. Therefore, any postoperative paresis or paralysis tends to be temporary. When the facial nerve is divided during surgery, it is sutured together when possible, or a nerve graft is placed between the stumps. Facial paralysis with no evidence of recovery within a few months is treated by surgical reinnervation, wherein another cranial nerve, usually a branch of the accessory nerve, is joined to the facial nerve peripherally. Bilateral acoustic tumors are seen with NF2 and present difficult problems in surgical decision making.[385] In general, a conservative approach is taken, treating the largest tumor when symptoms absolutely require it. Bilateral aggressive tumor resections lead to complete deafness and confer the possibility of bilateral facial nerve paralysis, a cosmetic and functional problem.

RADIATION THERAPY

There have been few reports on the role of radiation therapy for treatment of acoustic neurilemmomas. A review by Wallner and colleagues disclosed 62 patients who were thought to have had a total resection and did not receive irradiation.[386] The recurrence rate in this group was only 3% (2 of 62). The 15-year actuarial survival and relapse-free survival rates were 98% and 94%, respectively. Thirty patients underwent subtotal resection, defined as removal of less than 90% of the tumor. Six of the 13 (46%) patients with subtotally resected lesions recurred, whereas only 1 of 17 (6%) of those treated with subtotal resection and postoperative irradiation to a dose higher than 45 Gy relapsed. The 15-year relapse-free survival rate for patients treated with subtotal resection and radiation therapy (>45 Gy) was 94% compared with 41% for nonirradiated patients ($p = 0.01$); the corresponding 15-year survival rates were 100% and 67%, respectively ($p = 0.016$). There were no recurrences among 3 patients in whom biopsy was obtained at the time of surgery that was followed by irradiation. On the other hand, 4 of 7 patients who were irradiated for disease progression after having had resection alone subsequently developed a second recurrence. Based on these data, it was concluded that postoperative irradiation should be given after subtotal resection to reduce the risk of local tumor progression. The target volume includes a narrow margin around the residual tumor. Treatment is given using a homolateral pair of angled beams with wedge filters in daily increments of 1.8 to 2 Gy to a total of 50 to 55 Gy. Stereotactic radiosurgery has been used as an alternative to surgery in selected patients with small acoustic neurilemmomas.[387]

GLOMUS JUGULARE TUMORS

CLINICAL AND PATHOLOGIC CONSIDERATIONS

Glomus jugulare tumors arise from glomus tissue in the adventitia of the jugular bulb (glomus jugulare) or along Jacobson's nerve in the temporal bone, sometimes multifocally. The tumor invades temporal bone diffusely, but growth is characteristically slow. Sometimes they are endocrine active, with a carcinoid or pheochromocytoma-like syndrome.[388]

Because glomus jugulare tumors occur in the jugular foramen, they commonly cause lower cranial nerve palsies and early symptoms of hoarseness and difficulty swallowing. Later, facial weakness, hearing loss, and atrophy of the tongue become prominent. Pulsating tinnitus also may be a presenting symptom, and a pulsating mass can sometimes be seen behind the eardrum.

A presumptive radiologic diagnosis of glomus tumor can be made by CT or MRI scanning, with jugular neurilemmoma being the main differential diagnosis. Because glomus tumors incite a tremendous blood supply, particularly by way of the ascending pharyngeal artery, cerebral angiography provides the definitive diagnosis. Because preoperative tumor embolization is essential to surgical removal of glomus tumors, the diagnostic angiogram should be performed just before surgery when possible.

Histopathologically, numerous vascular channels are distinctive. The background is composed of clear cells clumped in a fibrous matrix. A small percentage of glomus tumors are malignant.

SURGERY

The treatment of glomus jugulare tumors is controversial, with advocates for radiation,[389] surgery, and the combination.[390] Most clinicians would agree that a resection should be attempted and that in most instances gross surgical resection, if not a cure, is a realistic goal.

Surgery on glomus tumors is most often performed by a neurosurgeon and a head and neck surgeon together after preoperative embolization. The base of the skull in the region of the jugular foramen is first exposed, and neurovascular structures are identified and mobilized through a high transverse cervical incision. When the incision is extended behind the pinna and a mastoidectomy is completed, the facial nerve can be protected, and the entire tumor bulb, the jugular bulb, and the internal jugular vein can be seen passing through the base of the skull. Finally, after a suboccipital craniectomy, the sigmoid sinus above and the jugular vein below can be ligated, and the segment between them excised with the attached tumor. Complications of this procedure include CSF leak and cranial nerve (particularly facial) palsy.

RADIATION THERAPY

Even though glomus tumors are histologically benign, radiation therapy is effective and has been recommended for symptomatic lesions that cannot be totally resected or as primary treatment.[389,391–393] These tumors regress slowly after irradiation, and the success of radiation therapy is measured by the amelioration of symptoms and the absence of disease progression. The dose required for control is relatively modest. Kim and associates reported a series of 40 patients with such lesions and added a literature survey.[394] The control rate with subtotal resection and postoperative irradiation was 85%. When radiation therapy only was used for inoperable or recurrent tumors, control was achieved in 88%. Their composite data, including cases from the literature, showed a 25% recurrence rate for doses lower than 40 Gy, whereas only 1.4% recurred with doses of 40 Gy or higher.

Based on these data, a dose of 45 Gy in 5 weeks is recommended. Although a dose of 50 Gy has been advocated for more advanced tumors, there is no evidence that such lesions require higher doses.[393] Treatment is usually delivered through a homolateral pair of angled, wedged portals, depending on the precise location of the lesion.

CHORDOMAS

CLINICAL AND PATHOLOGIC CONSIDERATIONS

Chordomas occur along the pathway of the primitive notochord, which extends, in human embryos, from the tip of the dorsum sellae to the coccyx. Chordomas are extradural, multilobulated tumors, varying in consistency from extremely soft to woody and cartilaginous. They are pseudoencapsulated and may invade through the basal dura.

The typical chordoma is composed of cord-like rows of distended, vacuolated (physaliferous) cells. A variant, the chondroid chordoma, has distinctly chondroid elements and may be less aggressive.[395] None of the histopathologic characteristics of tumor aggressiveness (cellularity, pleomorphism, and mitoses) seems to be predictive in chordoma.

The diagnosis of clivus chordomas cannot be made without radiologic tests and often is delayed because symptoms are nonspecific and vague. At onset there is usually headache and intermittent diplopia. These vague symptoms often are not reported, allowing the tumor to grow to an enormous size before the diagnosis is made. Gradually, headache (upper clivus tumors) and neck pain (lower clivus tumors) worsen. Superiorly placed tumors proceed to cause diplopia and facial numbness as the cavernous sinus and Meckel's cave are invaded. Lower clivus tumors compress the lower cranial nerves and later the brain stem.

The differential diagnosis of cranial chordoma includes basal meningioma, neurilemmoma (schwannoma), nasopharyngeal carcinoma, pituitary adenoma, and craniopharyngioma. MRI scanning usually results in a working diagnosis of chordoma, but surgical biopsy (and resection) is mandatory.

SURGERY

Surgery for cranial chordomas is obligatory to obtain diagnostic tissue, to enhance the effectiveness of subsequent radiation therapy, and to improve the patient's clinical condition. With an aggressive surgical resection, a favorable effect on the severe headaches and neurologic deficits associated with chordomas can be anticipated.

Intracranial chordomas occur at the base of the skull, a region relatively remote from surgical access. Consequently, a variety of innovative approaches have been developed by neurosurgeons and head and neck surgeons, and these procedures are commonly done with both types of specialist in attendance.

For midline lesions of the upper clivus that extend into the sella or sphenoid sinus, or both, a transseptal, transsphenoidal approach (as for pituitary tumors) is best. Large, compressive, transdural extensions of these upper clivus tumors into the interpeduncular cistern must be removed through a transcranial, subtemporal, intradural approach. For the more lateralized upper clival tumor and some lateralized midclival tumors, an approach through a sphenoethmoidectomy (to which may be added a maxillectomy) is useful. For midline tumors of the midclivus and lower clivus, a transoral resection is commonly used. A combination of exposures sometimes is necessary for extremely large tumors.

A potentially serious complication of the transsphenoidal, transsphenoethmoid, and transoral approaches is CSF leakage and consequent meningitis. Therefore, every attempt must be made to keep the dura intact during these procedures. Because dural invasion by cranial chordomas may occur 50% of the time, inadvertent entry of the dura during tumor resection is sometimes unavoidable. Careful intraoperative patching of the leak with fat and muscle grafts followed by postoperative spinal CSF drainage is essential.

Cranial chordomas often recur after surgery and radiation therapy. In this situation, reoperation directed toward symptomatic improvement is the only treatment option. Reoperations are complicated by surgical scarring and tissue compromise from irradiation.

RADIATION THERAPY

Chordomas and low-grade chondrosarcomas of the base of skull, clivus, and axial skeleton are not amenable to complete surgical resection. With conventional megavoltage irradiation (median dose of 50 Gy), the local control rate for these lesions is only 27%.[396] Although higher doses appear to improve the local control rate, the proximity of dose-limiting critical structures, such as the optic nerves, the chiasm, other cranial nerves, the brain stem, the temporal lobes, and the spinal cord, limit the dose that can be delivered safely to these lesions.[397] Charged-particle beams such as protons and helium ions, which feature sharp lateral beam edges and a finite range in tissue, may be used to deliver higher doses than are possible with conventional photon irradiation while keeping the dose to neighboring critical structures at a safe level. The depth of penetration can be tailored to the clinical situation by varying the energy of the beam or by interposing bolus material in the beam path. Charged-particle beams can be made to stop in front of a critical structure, such as the spinal cord, and in combination with other lateral or oblique beams, a target volume may be "wrapped" around a critical structure. Precise tumor and normal tissue identification and beam delivery techniques, highly reproducible patient positioning, and accurate compensation for tissue inhomogeneities in the beam path are required.

Available data suggest that the higher doses that are achievable with charged-particle irradiation result in higher local control rates than have been observed with conventional radiation therapy techniques. Austin-Seymore and coworkers reported the outcome of 68 patients with chordomas or low-grade chondrosarcomas of the clivus treated postoperatively at the Harvard Cyclotron Laboratory at Massachusetts General Hospital with a 160-MeV proton beam.[396] The median dose was 69 cobalt Gy equivalent (CGE; the dose in proton Gy multiplied by 1.1, the relative biologic effectiveness [RBE] for protons compared with cobalt 60), with a range of 56.9 to 75.6 CGE. Local control was achieved in 90% of patients (61 of 68), with follow up ranging from 17 to 152 months (median of 34 months). The 5-year actuarial local control and disease-free survival rates were 82% and 76%, respectively. Treatment was complicated by unilateral or bilateral blindness in 3 patients, and 9 patients developed pituitary insufficiency requiring hormone replacement. A study comparing 66.6 CGE with 72 CGE is in progress.

Berson and colleagues reviewed the results of 45 patients with chordomas and chondrosarcomas of the base of skull and cervical spine treated at the University of California Lawrence Berkeley Laboratory with helium ion or neon beams.[398] Total doses ranged from 59.4 to 80 Gy equivalent (GyE; the physical dose multiplied by the RBE; 1.2–1.3 for helium and 2–3.3 for neon). After initial subtotal resection, 23 patients were treated with charged particles alone, and 13 were treated with photons and particles combined. Nine patients were treated for recurrent disease. The 5-year actuarial local control and survival rates were 59% and 62%, respectively. The 2-year actuarial local control rate for patients treated at initial diagnosis was 78% compared with 33% for those with recurrent tumors ($p < 0.01$). The 2-year local control rate for tumor volumes of less than 20 ml was 80%, whereas it was 33% for larger lesions ($p < 0.05$). Complications included unilateral or bilateral blindness in 5 patients, and 4 patients developed brain stem injury.

HEMANGIOBLASTOMAS AND HEMANGIOMAS

CLINICAL AND PATHOLOGIC CONSIDERATIONS

Hemangioblastoma accounts for approximately 2% of intracranial tumors, arising most often in the cerebellar hemispheres and vermis. Usually solitary, these tumors can be multiple and may also occur in the brain stem, spinal cord, and supratentorial compartment. Cerebellar hemangioblastoma can be sporadic or occur as a familial disorder as part of the von Hippel-Lindau complex that is transmitted as an autosomal dominant disorder with varying degrees of penetrance. Other entities associated with familial hemangioblastoma are hypernephroma, polycystic kidneys, pancreatic cysts, pheochromocytoma, and erythrocytosis.

Cerebellar hemangioblastomas usually are recognized in the third decade causing symptoms of increased intracranial pressure and symptoms and signs of cerebellar dysfunction. Gait disturbance and imbalance are particularly common. Clinical progression is slow, because these tumors enlarge extremely slowly.

The hemangioblastoma probably arises during embryonic life from primitive endothelial cells around the fourth ventricle. The tumor is composed of numerous capillary and sinusoidal channels lined with endothelial cells. Interspersed are nests of lipid-laden pseudoxanthoma cells. The tumor is usually cystic and contains proteinaceous, xanthochromic fluid. The cyst contains a red (vascular) firm mural nodule, the apparent source of the fluid. The cyst wall is a glial nonneoplastic reaction to the secreted fluid. Occasional hemangioblastomas (brain stem and spinal cord, particularly) are without cysts.

SURGERY

In most instances, the diagnosis can be made by CT scan or MRI. Angiography, to confirm the diagnosis, is usually done before surgery. Cerebellar hemangioblastoma tumors are readily approached and excised, with the cyst drained and the entire solid portion carefully dissected and removed. Solid hemangioblastomas of the brain stem are exceedingly vascular, and their removal is associated with high mortality; even biopsy can be associated with precipitous bleeding and significant morbidity. Such tumors are sometimes irradiated with or without a confirmatory biopsy.

RADIATION THERAPY

Radiation therapy is recommended for patients with unresectable, incompletely excised, and recurrent hemangioblastomas and for those patients who are medically inoperable. Sung and coworkers reported their experience of 23 patients treated with radiation therapy for cerebellar hemangioblastoma.[399] About half of their patients received doses of 36 Gy or lower, and the remainder (12 of 23) received 40 to 55 Gy in 4 to 6.5 weeks. The 5-, 10-, and 15-year survival rates for the lower dose group were 54.5%, 27.3%, and 8.1%, respectively, whereas the survival rates for the higher dose group were 90.5%, 56.5%, and 56.5%, respectively. These findings are similar to those reported by Smalley and associates.[400] In their series, 19 patients had gross residual disease after initial surgery or recurrent tumors, whereas 6 had only microscopic disease. The overall 5-, 10-, and 15-year survival rates were 85%, 58%, and 58%, respectively, and the recurrence-free survival rates were 76%, 52%, and 42%, respectively. Eight of the 19 patients with gross disease were locally controlled. In-field disease control rates were significantly higher in patients who received at least 50 Gy ($p = 0.06$) or a time-dose-fractionation (TDF) of more than 75 Gy (equivalent to 46–48.6 Gy at 1.8–2 Gy per fraction, 5 days per week [$p = 0.004$]) than in those who received lower doses. Five of the 6 patients treated for microscopic disease were controlled. Based on these data, doses of at least 50 to 55 Gy in 5.5 to 6 weeks appear to be warranted.

CHOROID PLEXUS PAPILLOMA AND CARCINOMA

CLINICAL AND PATHOLOGIC CONSIDERATIONS

Choroid plexus papilloma and carcinoma are rare tumors that occur most often in children younger than 12 years of age, although they can occur at any age. Nearly half of these tumors are found in patients younger than 20 years of age. The tumor is an irregularly lobulated reddish mass, which on histopathologic examination is apparently normal choroid plexus. Rarely, these tumors show malignant features and are then classified as choroid plexus carcinoma.

In children, choroid plexus papillomas most often occur in the lateral ventricles. In adults, the fourth ventricular papilloma is commonest. Third ventricle tumors are exceedingly rare. Because papillomas tend to grow slowly within ventricles, they expand to fill the ventricle and block CSF flow. In addition, papillomas are thought to secrete CSF. Choroid plexus papillomas (and carcinomas) can produce hydrocephalus secondary to obstruction of the CSF; by CSF overproduction by the tumor; or by damage to the CSF resorptive bed from recurrent hemorrhages. As a result, increased intracranial pressure without focal findings is the commonest presentation; fourth ventricular tumors can also be associated with focal findings of ataxia and nystagmus.

Although choroid plexus papillomas and carcinomas extensively seed throughout the ventricular and subarachnoid spaces, seeding from papillomas is usually subclinical, whereas that from carcinomas is frequent and dramatically symptomatic. These tumors are seen easily by CT scan and MRI. In patients with anaplastic changes, the authors advocate staging by myelography and examination of the CSF.

Therapy for anaplastic tumors should be approached in a manner similar to medulloblastoma and malignant ependymomas. Because of the aggressive nature of the more anaplastic tumors, therapy must be equally aggressive, requiring radiation therapy and, in some instances, intraventricular chemotherapy.

SURGERY

The treatment of choroid plexus papillomas is total surgical excision. Choroid plexus tumors of the lateral ventricle are approached through a high parietal cortical incision and transcortical approach to the ventricular trigone. The predilection of these tumors for the left side makes this worrisome. Hydrocephalus is the rule and simplifies the exposure when retraction into the ventricle is established. Tumor arteries and veins are identified by use of the operating microscope and then coagulated, after which smaller tumors are removed intact and larger tumors are removed piecemeal. In half of the patients, hydrocephalus is relieved by tumor resection, but persistent hydrocephalus requires shunting.

Choroid plexus papillomas of the third ventricle are exceedingly rare but can be approached through various surgical exposures of the third ventricle. The problems of removal of fourth ventricular choroid plexus tumors are similar to those associated with suboccipital removal of medulloblastomas or ependymomas, as discussed earlier.

RADIATION THERAPY

Choroid plexus papillomas usually are considered to be radioresistant, but information regarding the use and response to irradiation is anecdotal. Naguib and coworkers reported a case of an inoperable choroid plexus papilloma with extensive involvement of the mastoid bone.[401] This patient received 49.5 Gy in 32 treatments during a 33-day period. Serial CT scans showed that 16 months after completion of the radiation therapy, the mass was markedly reduced in size. Such anecdotes suggest that radiation therapy to the primary tumor site may be offered for inoperable choroid plexus papillomas and carcinomas.[402,403] With choroid plexus carcinoma, consideration must be given to treating the entire craniospinal axis, although data to support this approach are lacking. With a negative myelogram and negative CSF cytology, an alternative approach is to treat primary tumor with radiation therapy in conjunction with intrathecal and systemic chemotherapy.

CHEMOTHERAPY

Usually, chemotherapy is not used for choroid plexus papillomas. For the more anaplastic tumors, however, the authors have increasingly used chemotherapy adjuvant to surgery and irradiation to prevent the inevitable recurrence and CSF dissemination common to the choroid plexus carcinomas. As with many of the less common tumors discussed, there are no chemotherapeutic guidelines and few reports to guide the therapist.

Initially, the authors used chemotherapy only for recurrent disease. They have used combinations of cyclophosphamide, doxorubicin, and VCR and nitrosourea-based combinations. They have seen transient responses and disease control with both. They have also used intraventricular chemotherapy with low-dose methotrexate (2–3 mg/day for 5 days) or cytosine arabinoside (30 mg/day for 3 days), or both, to stave subarachnoid spread. As a result of this experience, the authors currently advocate the use of adjuvant chemotherapy with a nitrosourea-based combination after irradiation and the use of concomitant intraventricular chemotherapy. During irradiation, they have used intraventricular cytosine arabinoside and methotrexate after irradiation. Further study and additional approaches should be considered.

SPINAL AXIS TUMORS

CLINICAL AND PATHOLOGIC CONSIDERATIONS

Some of the clinical features of spinal axis tumor localization and diagnosis have been discussed previously. Most primary spinal axis tumors produce symptoms and signs as a result of spinal cord and nerve root compression rather than because of parenchymal invasion.

The reported frequency of primary spinal cord tumors is between 10% and 19% of all primary CNS tumors.[404] Although most spinal axis tumors are extradural, most *primary* spinal axis tumors are intradural. Of intradural tumors, the intradural extramedullary neurilemmomas and meningiomas are the commonest (see Table 48–3). Neurilemmomas and meningiomas are normally intradural, but occasionally they may present as extradural tumors. Other intradural extramedullary tumors are vascular tumors, chordomas, and epidermoids.

Intramedullary tumors have the same cellular origins as the other CNS tumors discussed previously. In terms of frequency, ependymomas occur in about 40% of patients with intramedullary tumors; next most common are the astrocytomas of low- and mid-anaplasia. These are followed in frequency by less common histologies such as oligodendroglioma, ganglioglioma, medulloblastoma, and various hemangiomas and hemangioblastomas.

Table 48–24 classifies spinal axis tumors by location. Although different tumor types exhibit a predilection for certain spinal regions, taken altogether, spinal tumors are distributed almost evenly along the spinal axis. Approximately 50% of spinal tumors involve the thoracic spinal canal, 30% involve the lumbosacral spine, and the remainder involve the cervical spine, including the foramen magnum. Some tumors, such as the neurilemmomas, occur with greatest frequency in the thoracic region, although they can be found throughout the spine and often extend through an intervertebral foramen to acquire a dumbbell configuration.

TABLE 48–24. Classification of Spinal Tumors by Their Location in Relation to the Spinal Cord and Dura Mater

Location	*Usual Tumor Types*
Extradural	Metastatic (carcinoma, lymphoma, melanoma, sarcoma), chordoma
Intradural	
Extramedullary	Schwannoma,* meningioma
Intramedullary	Astrocytoma, ependymoma†

* May extend along nerve root into extradural and extraspinal spaces.
† Ependymomas originating from the filum terminale and involving the cauda equina, not intramedullary in the strictest sense, are included here by custom.

Meningiomas are dural based and arise preferentially at the foramen magnum and in the thoracic spine. Astrocytomas are distributed throughout the spinal cord, and most ependymomas involve the conus medullaris and the cauda equina. Spinal chordomas are characteristically sacral.

Clinically, patients with spinal axis tumors present as a sensorimotor spinal tract syndrome; a painful radicular-spinal cord syndrome; or a central syringomyelic syndrome. In the *sensorimotor presentation,* symptoms and signs are in response to compression of the spinal cord. The onset is gradual over weeks to months, initial presentation is asymmetric, and motor weakness predominates. The level of impairment determines the muscle groups involved. Because of external compression, dorsal column involvement occurs with paresthesia and abnormalities of pain and temperature on the side contralateral to the motor weakness.

Radicular spinal cord syndromes occur because of external compression and infiltration of spinal cord roots. The main symptom is sharp, knife-like pain in the distribution of a sensory nerve root. The intense pain is often of short duration, with pain that is more aching in nature persisting for longer periods. The pain typically is exacerbated by coughing and sneezing or other maneuvers that increase intracranial pressure. Local paresthesia and impairment of sensations of pain and touch are common, as are weakness and muscle wasting. These findings commonly antedate cord compression by months.

Spinal tumors, particularly intramedullary tumors, can produce *syringomyelic dysfunction* by destruction and cavitation within the central gray matter of the cord. This produces lower motor neuron destruction and attendant segmental muscle weakness, wasting, and loss of reflexes. There is also a dissociated sensory loss of pain and temperature sensation with preservation of touch. With extension of the lesion, however, touch, vibration, and position sense are affected.

Finally, many patients with spinal axis tumors or supratentorial tumors that show a tendency toward drop metastases tend to lead to leptomeningeal neoplasia. Choucair and colleagues found that 1.2% of glioblastomas and 1.5% of anaplastic gliomas had metastatic spread of their supratentorial tumors to the spinal cord at some time during the course of their disease.[99]

SURGERY

General Considerations

The use of the operating microscope is as essential for spinal cord tumor surgery as it is for brain tumor surgery. In addition, other surgical adjuncts, such as intraoperative ultrasound, the CO_2 laser, and the CUSA, are equally valuable for the resection of spinal cord tumors. The ultrasound is particularly useful for examining the spinal cord through an intact or open dura to assess the level of maximum tumor involvement or to differentiate tumor cysts from solid tumor masses.

Surgical Planning

MRI scanning is invaluable for the diagnosis, localization, and characterization of spinal tumors (see Fig. 48–4). In all but vascular tumors (*e.g.*, hemangioblastoma), where angiography is needed, or tumors that cause extensive bony destruction (*e.g.*, metastasis), where CT scanning might be helpful, a technically excellent MRI scan is most often sufficient for preoperative planning for spinal tumors. Determination of the spinal level of the tumor and its exact relation to the spinal cord is important in localization. Corticosteroids are given before, during, and after spinal cord tumor surgery to help control spinal cord edema.

Removal of Intradural Extramedullary Tumors

Meningiomas and neurilemmomas (schwannomas) occur in the intradural extramedullary spinal compartment. Most of these tumors can be completely resected (cured), because through a laminectomy exposure they can be easily separated and rotated away from the spinal cord, which is already displaced, but not invaded, by tumor.

Neurilemmomas arise from spinal rootlets (most often dorsal rootlets), and their removal includes sections of those rootlets involved. Neurilemmomas can grow along the nerve root in a dumbbell fashion through a neural foramen; and although some of these extraspinal tumor extensions can be removed by extending the initial laminectomy exposure laterally, some must be resected at a separate operation through a thoracotomy, a costotransversectomy, or a retroperitoneal approach.

Meningiomas in most patients can be removed through a posterior (laminectomy) approach, because they are commonly lateral or anterolateral, and even the more anteriorly placed tumors cause enough lateral displacement of the spinal cord to allow access for resection without traction on the spinal cord. The uncommon tumor directly anterior to the spinal cord must sometimes be approached anteriorly, arterolaterally, or posterolaterally. Anteriorly situated meningiomas at the foramen magnum are sometimes unresectable because of their encasement of the vertebral artery.

Removal of Intramedullary Tumors

The commonest intramedullary tumors are ependymoma and astrocytoma. Hemangioblastoma is another (infrequent) tumor occurring in the spinal intramedullary compartment. Surgery is the principal treatment for all these tumors, with the exception of anaplastic astrocytomas.

Intramedullary tumors are approached through a laminectomy exposure, and after the dura is opened, a longitudinal myelotomy is made over the widened region of spinal cord and the incision deepened several millimeters to the tumor surface. Dissection planes around the tumor are sought microsurgically and, in the case of ependymomas, usually found and extended gradually around the tumor's surface, because removal of the central tumor bulk (by CO_2 laser or CUSA) causes the tumor to collapse. Usually, such tumors are completely removed. Tumors with indefinite dissection planes (usually low-grade astrocytomas) cannot be removed completely, but bulk reduction can cause long-term palliation. If frozen section shows a tumor to be malignant, surgery is aborted, and radiation therapy is the treatment.

Hemangioblastomas are extremely vascular tumors, so the tumor margins are addressed first where feeding arteries are coagulated, and the tumor is dissected and removed en bloc. The dorsal location of most of these tumors and the commonly associated cyst simplifies the removal to some extent.

RADIATION THERAPY

Radiation therapy is recommended for incompletely resected neoplasms of the spinal axis. As a rule, doses of 50 to 55 Gy are used so that the risk of radiation injury to the cord is less than that from the neoplasm itself. However, for lesions involving only the cauda equina and in situations in which irreversible and complete transverse myelopathy already has occurred, higher doses are permissible. The tumor usually is treated with a margin of 2 to 3 cm. Extension of the portals to include the thecal sac has been suggested for ependymomas that are removed piecemeal.[405] Ependymomas of the cord have a longer natural history than astrocytomas. Although most astrocytomas that recur do so within 3 years of treatment, recurrence of ependymomas may be delayed for as long as 12 years.[406]

Adjunctive radiation therapy is not necessary when ependymomas are removed completely in an en bloc fashion. However, 75% of patients (3 of 4) reported by Wen and associates recurred locally or with spread to the thecal sac after complete resection alone when the tumor was excised piecemeal.[405] All 7 nonirradiated patients with incompletely excised lesions reported by Barone and Elvidge[407] and Schuman and coworkers[408] recurred. In contrast, postoperative radiation therapy appears to improve tumor control and disease-free survival in patients with incompletely resected ependymomas. Sloof and colleagues[409] found their irradiated patients survived nearly twice as long as those who were not irradiated. Five- and 10-year survival rates in irradiated patients with localized ependymomas range from 60% to 100% and 86% to 93%, respectively, whereas 10-year relapse-free survival rates vary from 43% to 58%. Local control rates range from 60% to 100% in most reported series.[406] Myxopapillary ependymomas that arise exclusively in the conus medullaris have a better prognosis than the cellular ependymomas that arise in the cord.[405]

The 5- and 10-year survival rates for irradiated patients with low-grade astrocytomas of the spinal cord vary from 60% to 90% and 40% to 90%, respectively; the 5- and 10-year relapse-free survival rates are 66% and 53%, respectively.[406] Approximately 50% to 65% of astrocytomas are controlled locally. Patients with malignant gliomas have a much poorer prognosis; none of the patients with anaplastic astrocytoma or glioblastoma multiforme survived longer than 8 months.

CHEMOTHERAPY

There have been no reports of controlled clinical trials of chemotherapy for primary spinal axis tumors. Drugs active against intracranial astrocytomas, oligodendrogliomas, ependymomas, medulloblastoma, and germ cell tumors may logically be assumed to be equally efficacious against these same histologies in the spinal cord. Along with reports of chemotherapy activity against intracranial tumors, anecdotal patients have been included.

The authors' experience suggests that palliation is possible for astrocytomas using nitrosourea-based chemotherapy regimens. No therapy is clearly superior. For drop metastases from ependymomas, they have used BCNU and dibromodulcitol as single agents and various combinations with some benefit.[138,183a] For drop metastases from medulloblastoma, various drugs have been found to be beneficial. Specifically, cyclophosphamide, carboplatin, methotrexate, procarbazine, teniposide, and VCR have been used alone or in various combinations. These drugs would be expected to produce palliation for weeks to many months.

Although leptomeningeal spread is a common complication of primary spinal axis tumors, the use of intraventricular and intrathecal chemotherapy is limited to the treatment of microscopic deposits. Biodistribution in the subarachnoid CSF can be limited in the face of intradural extramedullary tumors. In addition, deposits of 5 mm in diameter or larger are not likely to benefit because of limitations in diffusion coupled with transcapillary loss of drug in the tumor.[410]

REFERENCES

1. SEER search performed for this chapter between 1978–1984.
2. Sloof JL, Kernohan JW, MacCary CS. Primary intramedullary tumors of the spinal cord and filum terminale. Philadelphia: WB Saunders, 1964.
3. Davis DL, Hoel D, Percy C, et al. Is brain cancer mortality increasing in industrial countries? Ann NY Acad Sci 1990;609:791.
4. Boyle P, Maisonneuve P, Saracci R, Muir CS. Is the increased incidence of primary malignant brain tumors in the elderly real? JNCI [Editorial] 1990;82:1594.
5. Greig NH, Ries LG, Yancik R, Rapoport SI. Increasing annual incidence of primary malignant brain tumors in the elderly. JNCI 1990;82:1621.
6. Percy AK, Elveback LR, Okazaki H, et al. Neoplasms of the central nervous system: Epidemiologic considerations. Neurology 1972;22:40.
7. Preston-Martin S. Descriptive epidemiology of primary tumors of the spinal cord and spinal meninges in Los Angeles County, 1972–1985. Neuroepidemiology 1990;9: 106.
8. Bigner SH, Mark J, Burger PC, et al. Specific chromosomal abnormalities in malignant human gliomas. Cancer Res 1988;48:405.
9. Jenkins RB, Kimmel DW, Moertel CA, et al. A cytogenetic study of 53 human gliomas. Cancer Genet Cytogenet 1989;39:253.
10. James CD, Carlbom E, Nordenskjold M, et al. Mitotic recombination of chromosome 17 in astrocytomas. Proc Natl Acad Sci USA 1989;86:2858.
11. Cavenee WK, Scrable HJ, James CD. Molecular genetics of human cancer predisposition and progression. Mutat Res 1991;247:199.
12. Bigner SH, Mark J, Burger PC, et al. Specific chromosomal abnormalities in malignant human gliomas. Cancer Res 1988;48:405.
13. James CD, Carlbom E, Dumanski JP, et al. Clonal genomic alterations in glioma malignancy stages. Cancer Res 1988;48:5546.
14. Ransom DT, Ritland SR, Jenkins RB, et al. Loss of heterozygosity studies in human gliomas. Cancer Res 1991;32:302.
15. Neville BG, Berry AC, Stoddart Y. A case of malignant spinal cord ependymoma in association with a duplication of part of the long arm of chromosome 12. J Med Genet 1985;22:154.
16. Collins VP. The molecular genetics of meningiomas. Brain Pathol 1990;1:19.
17. Dumanski JP, Carlbom E, Collins VP, Nordenskjold M. Deletion mapping of a locus on human chromosome 22 involved in the oncogenesis of meningiomas. Proc Natl Acad Sci USA 1987;84:9275.
18. Dumanski JP, Rouleau GA, Nordenskjold M, Collins VP. Molecular genetic analysis of chromosome 22 in 81 cases of meningioma. Cancer Res 1990;50:5863.
19. Menon AG, Ponder BAJ, Seizinger BR. The neurofibromatosis genes: Molecular cloning to cellular function. Cancer Cells 1991;3:147.
20. Griffin CA, Hawkins AL, Packer RJ, et al. Chromosome abnormalities in pediatric brain tumors. Cancer Res 1988;48:175.
21. Raffel C, Gilles FE, Weinberg KI. Reduction to homozygosity and gene amplification in central nervous system primitive neuroectodermal tumors of childhood. Cancer Res 1990;50:587.
22. James CD, He J, Carlbom E, et al. Loss of genetic information in central nervous system tumors common to children and young adults. Genes Chromosom Cancer 1990;2:94.
23. Friedman HS, Schold C Jr. Rational approaches to the chemotherapy of medulloblastoma. Neurol Clin North Am 1985;3:843.
24. Stratton MR, Darling J, Cooper CS, Reeves BR. A case of cerebellar medulloblastoma with a single chromosome abnormality. Cancer Genet Cytogenet 1991;53:101.
25. Bigner SH, Friedman HS, Vogelstein B, et al. Amplification of *c-myc* gene in human medulloblastoma cell lines and xenografts. Cancer Res 1990;50:2347.
26. Wasson JC, Saylors RL, Zeltzer P, et al. Oncogene amplification in pediatric brain tumors. Cancer Res 1990;50:2987.
27. Yung WK, Zhang X, Steck PA, Hung MC. Differential amplification of the TGF-alpha gene in human gliomas. Cancer Commun 1990;2:201.
28. Malkin D, Li FP, Strong LC, et al. Germ line p53 mutations in a familial syndrome of breast cancer, sarcomas, and other neoplasms. Science 1990;250:1233.
29. Srivastava S, Zou ZQ, Pirollo K, et al. Germ-line transmission of a mutated p53 gene in a cancer-prone family with Li-Fraumeni syndrome. Nature 1990;348:747.
30. Wallace MR, Marchuk DA, Anderson LB, et al. Type I neurofibromatosis gene: Identification of a large transcript disrupted in three NF1 patients. Science 1990;249: 181.
31. Cawthon RM, Weiss R, Xu G, et al. A major segment of the neurofibromatosis type 1 gene: cDNA sequence, genomic structure, and point mutations. Cell 1990;62:193.
32. Sampson JR, Yates JR, Pirrit LA, et al. Evidence for genetic heterogeneity in tuberous sclerosis. J Med Genet 1989;26:511.
33. Musicco M, Filippini G, Bordo BM, et al. Gliomas and (occupational) exposure to carcinogens: Case-control study. Am J Epidemiol 1982;116:782.
34. Moss AR. Occupational exposure and brain tumors. J Toxicol Environ Health 1985;16: 703.
35. McLaughlin JK, Malker HS, Blot WJ, et al. Occupational risks for intracranial gliomas in Sweden. JNCI 1987;78:253.
36. Copeland DD, Bigner DD. Glial-mesenchymal tropism of in vivo avian sarcoma virus neuro-oncogenis in rats. Acta Neuropathol (Berl) 1978;41:23.
37. Wodinski I, Kensler CJ, Rall DP. The induction and transplantation of brain tumors in neonate beagles. Proc Am Assoc Cancer Res [Abstract] 1969;99.
38. Major EO, Vacante DA, Traub RG, et al. Owl monkey astrocytoma cells in culture spontaneously produce infectious JC virus which demonstrates altered biological properties. J Virol 1987;61:1435.
39. Matsuda M, Yasui K, Nagashima K, Mori W. Origin of the medulloblastoma experimentally induced by human polyomavirus JC. JNCI 1987;79:585.
40. Hochberg RH, Miller G, Schooley RT, et al. Central nervous system lymphoma related to Epstein-Barr virus. N Engl J Med 1983;309:745.
41. Annegers JF, Laws ER Jr, Kurland LT, et al. Head trauma and subsequent brain tumors. Neurosurgery 1979;4:203.
42. Malone M, Lumley H, Erdohazi M. Astrocytoma as a second malignancy in patients with acute lymphoblastic leukemia. Cancer 1986;57:979.
43. Sogg RL, Donaldson SS, Yorke CH. Malignant astrocytoma following radiotherapy of a craniopharyngioma. J Neurosurg 1978;48:622.
44. Poster DS, Bruno S. The occurrence of second primary neoplasms in patients with non-Hodgkin's lymphomas. IRCS Med Sci Cancer 1980;8:554.
45. Rubinstein AB, Shalit MN, Cohen M, et al. Radiation-induced cerebral meningioma: A recognizable entity. J Neurosurg 1984;61:966.
46. Spallone A, Gagliardi FM, Vagnozzi R. Intracranial meningiomas related to external cranial irradiation. Surg Neurol 1979;12:153.
47. Levin VA, Wilson CB. Clinical characteristics of cancer in the brain and spinal cord. In: Crook ST, Prestayko A, eds. Cancer and chemotherapy: Introduction to neoplasia and antineoplastic chemotherapy. Vol 2. New York: Academic Press, 1981:167.
48. Bingas B. Tumours of the base of the skull. In: Vinken PJ, Bruyn GW, eds. Handbook of clinical neurology; Tumors of the brain and skull. Vol 17. Amsterdam: North Holland, 1974:136.
49. Fahlbusch R, Marguth F. Endocrine disorders associated with intracranial tumors. In: Vinken PJ, Bruyn GW, eds. Handbook of clinical neurology: Tumors of the brain and skull. Vol 16. Amsterdam: North Holland, 1974:345.
50. Russell DJ, Rubinstein LJ. Pathology of tumors of the nervous system. 4th ed. Baltimore: Williams & Wilkins, 1977.

51. Adams RD, Victor M. Principles of neurology. New York: McGraw-Hill, 1977:586.
52. Brant-Zawadzki M, Norman D, eds. Magnetic resonance imaging of the central nervous system. New York: Raven Press, 1987.
53. Brant-Zawadski M, Badami JP, Mills CM, et al. Primary intracranial tumor imaging: A comparison of magnetic resonance and CT. Radiology 1984;150:435.
54. Berry I, Brant-Zawadski M, Osaki L, et al. Gd-DPTA in clinical MR of the brain: II. Extraxial lesions and normal structures. Am J Roentgenol 1986;147:1223.
55. Butler AR, Horii SC, Kricheff I, et al. Computed tomography in astrocytomas: A statistical analysis of the parameters of malignancy and the positive contrast enhanced CT scan. Radiology 1978;129:433.
56. Dillon WP, Norman D, Newton TH, et al. Intradural spinal cord lesions: Gd-DTPA enhanced MR imaging. Radiology 1989;170:229.
57. Edwards MSB, Davis RL, Laurent JP. Tumor markers and cytologic features of cerebrospinal fluid. Cancer 1985;56:1773.
58. Inoue HK, Naganuma H, Ono N. Pathobiology of intracranial germ-cell tumors: Immunochemical, immunohistochemical, and electron microscopic investigations. J Neurooncol 1987;5:105.
59. Marton LJ, Edwards MS, Levin VA, et al. CSF polyamines: A new and important means of monitoring medulloblastoma. Cancer 1981;47:757.
60. Levin VA, Crafts D, Wilson CB, et al. BCNU and procarbazine treatment for malignant brain tumors. Cancer Treat Rep 1976;60:243.
61. Hoffman WF, Levin VA, Wilson CB. Evaluation of malignant glioma patients during the postirradiation period. J Neurosurg 1979;50:624.
62. Hoshino T, Nagashima T, Murovic J, et al. In situ cell lanetics studies on human neuroectodermal tumors with bromodeoxyuridine labeling. J Neurosurg 1986;64:453.
63. Heilbrun MP. Computed tomography-guided stereotactic systems. Clin Neurosurg 1984;31:564.
64. Apuzzo MLJ, Chandrasoma PT, Cohen D, et al. Computed imaging stereotaxy: Experience and perspective related to 500 procedures applied to brain masses. Neurosurgery 1987;20:930.
65. Leibel SA, Sheline GE. Tolerance of the brain and spinal cord to conventional irradiation. In: Gutin PH, Leibel SA, Sheline GE, eds. Radiation injury to the nervous system. New York: Raven Press, 1991:239.
66. Young DF, Posner JB, Chu F, et al. Rapid-course radiation therapy of cerebral metastases: Results and complications. Cancer 1974;34:1069.
67. Delattre JY, Rosenblum MK, Thaler HT, et al. A model of radiation myelopathy in the rat: Pathology, regional capillary permiability changes and treatment with dexamethasone. Brain 1988;111:1319.
68. Graeb DA, Steinbok P, Robertson WD. Transient early computed tomographic changes mimicking tumor progression after brain tumor irradiation. Radiology 1982;144:813.
69. Valk PE, Dillon WP. Radiation injury of the brain. AJNR 1991;12:45.
70. Brant-Zawadzki MB, Anderson M, De Armond SJ, et al. Radiation-induced large intracranial vessel occlusive vasculopathy. AJR 1980;134:51.
71. Bernstein M, Laperriere N. Radiation-induced tumors of the nervous system. In: Gutin PH, Leibel SA, Sheline GE, eds. Radiation injury to the nervous system. New York: Raven Press, 1991:455.
72. Sheline GE, Wara WM, Smith V. Therapeutic irradiation and brain injury. Int J Radiat Oncol Biol Phys 1980;6:1215.
73. Marks JE, Baglan RJ, Prassad SC, et al. Cerebral radio-necrosis: Incidence and risk in relation to dose, time, fractionation and volume. Int J Radiat Oncol Biol Phys 1981;7:243.
74. Leibel SA, Sheline GE. Radiation therapy for neoplasms of the brain. J Neurosurg 1987;66:1.
75. Bloom B, Kramer S. Conventional radiation therapy in the management of acromegaly. In: Black PM, Zervas NT, Ridgeway ED, eds. Secretory tumors of the pituitary gland. Vol 1. New York: Raven Press, 1984:179.
76. Rottenberg DA, Chernik MD, Deck MDF, et al. Cerebral necrosis following radiotherapy of extracranial neoplasms. Ann Neurol 1977;1:339.
77. Burger PC, Mahaley MS Jr, Dudka L, et al. The morphologic effects of radiation administered therapeutically for intracranial gliomas: A postmortem study of 25 cases. Cancer 1979;44:1256.
78. DeAngelis LM, Shapiro WR. Drug/radiation interactions and central nervous system injury. In: Gutin PH, Leibel SA, Sheline GE, eds. Radiation injury to the nervous system. New York: Raven Press, 1991:361.
79. Bleyer WA, Griffin TW. White matter necrosis, mineralizing microangiopathy, and intellectual abilities in survivors of childhood leukemia. In: Gilbert HA, Kagan AR, eds. Radiation damage to the nervous system. New York: Raven Press, 1980:155.
80. Kim KT, Black KL, Marciano D, et al. Thallium-201 SPECT imaging of brain tumors: Methods and results. J Nucl Med 1990;31:965.
81. Gutin PH. Treatment of radiation necrosis of the brain. In: Gutin PH, Leibel SA, Sheline GE, eds. Radiation injury to the nervous system. New York: Raven Press, 1991:271.
82. Mulhern RK, Fairclough D, Ochs J. A prospective comparison of neuropsychologic performance of children surviving leukemia who received 18-Gy, 24-Gy, or no cranial irradiation. J Clin Oncol 1991;9:1348.
83. Johnson BE, Becker B, Goff WB, et al. Neurologic, neuropsychologic, and computed cranial tomographic scan abnormalities in 2- to 10-year survivors of small-cell lung cancer. J Clin Oncol 1985;12:1657.
84. Mulhern RK, Ochs J, Kun LE. Changes in intellect associated with cranial radiation therapy. In: Gutin PH, Leibel SA, Sheline GE, eds. Radiation injury to the nervous system. New York: Raven Press, 1991:325.
85. Eiser C. Intellectual abilities among survivors of childhood leukemia as a function of CNS irradiation. Arch Dis Child 1978;53:391.
86. Hochberg FH, Slotnick B. Neuropsychologic impairment in astrocytoma survivors. Neurology 1980;30:172.
87. Maire J Ph, Coudin B, Guerin, J, et al. Neuropsychologic impairment in adults with brain tumors. Am J Clin Oncol 1987;10:156.
88. Shalet SM, Beardwell CG, Pearson D, et al. The effect of varying doses of cerebral irradiation on GH production in childhood. Clin Endocrinol 1976;5:287.
89. Jones A. A transient radiation myelopathy (with reference to Lhermitte's sign of electrical paresthesia). Br J Radiol 1964;37:727.
90. Schultheiss TE, Stephens LC, Peters LJ. Survival in radiation myelopathy. Int J Radiat Oncol Biol Phys 1986;12:1765.
91. Reagen TJ, Thomas JE, Colby MY Jr. Chronic radiation myelopathy: Its clinical aspects and differential diagnosis. JAMA 1968;203:128.
92. Marcus RB Jr, Million RR. The incidence of myelitis after irradiation of the cervical spinal cord. Int J Radiat Oncol Biol Phys 1990;19:3.
93. Schultheiss TE. Spinal cord radiation "tolerance": Doctrine versus data. Int J Radiat Oncol Biol Phys 1990;19:219.
94. Abbatucci JS, Delozier T, Quint R, et al. Radiation myelopathy of the cervical spinal cord: Time, dose and volume factors. Int J Radiat Oncol Biol Phys 1978;4:239.
95. Wara WM, Phillips TL, Sheline GE, et al. Radiation tolerance of the spinal cord. Cancer 1975;35:1558.
96. Van der Kogel AJ, Barendsen GW. Late effects of spinal cord irradiation with 300 kV x-rays and 15 MeV neutrons. Br J Radiol 1974;47:393.
97. Ang KK, Van der Kogel AJ, van der Scheuren E. Lack of evidence for increased tolerance of rat spinal cord with decreasing fraction doses below 2 Gy. Int J Radiat Oncol Biol Phys 1985;11:105.
98. Burger PC, Dubois PJ, Schold SC Jr, et al. Computerized tomographic and pathologic studies in untreated, quiescent, and recurrent glioblastoma multiforme. J Neurosurg 1983;58:159.
99. Choucair AK, Levin VA, Gutin PH, et al. Development of multiple lesions during radiation therapy and chemotherapy in patients with gliomas. J Neurosurg 1986;65:654.
100. Hochberg FH, Pruitt A. Assumptions in the radiotherapy of glioblastoma. Neurology 1980;30:907.
101. Kelly PJ, Dauman-Duport C, Kispert DB, et al. Imaging-based stereotaxic serial biopsies in untreated intracranial glial neoplasms. J Neurosurg 1987;66:865.
102. Levin VA. Pharmacokinetics and CNS chemotherapy. In: Hellmann K, Carter SK, eds. Fundamentals of cancer chemotherapy. New York: McGraw-Hill, 1986:28.
103. Levin VA, Patlak CS, Landahl HD. Heuristic modeling of drug delivery to malignant brain tumors. J Pharmacokinet Biopharm 1980;8:257.
104. Levin VA. Chemotherapy of primary brain tumors. Neurol Clin North Am 1985;3:855.
105. Kumar ARV, Renaudin J, Wilson CB, et al. Procarbazine hydrochloride in the treatment of brain tumors. J Neurosurg 1974;40:365.
106. Weiss HD, Walker MD, Wiernik PH. Neurotoxicity of commonly used antineoplastic agents. N Engl J Med 1974;291:75.
107. Feun LG, Wallace S, Yung WK, et al. Phase I trial of intracarotid BCNU and cisplatin in patients with malignant intracerebral tumors. Cancer Drug Deliv 1984;1:239.
108. Stewart DJ, Grahovac Z, Benoit B, et al. Intracarotid chemotherapy with a combination of 1,3-*bis*-(2-chloroethyl)-1-nitrosourea (BCNU), *cis*-diaminedichloroplatinum (cisplatin), and 4′-*O*-demethyl-1-*O*-(4,6-*O*-2-thenylidene-beta-*D*-glucopyranosyl) epipodophyllotoxin (VM-26) in the treatment of primary and metastatic brain tumors. Neurosurgery 1984;15:828.
109. Bloom HJG. Intracranial tumors: Response and resistance to therapeutic endeavors, 1970–1980. Int J Radiat Oncol Biol Phys 1982;8:1083.
110. Laws ER Jr, Taylor WF, Clifton MB, et al. Neurosurgical management of low-grade astrocytoma of the cerebral hemispheres. J Neurosurg 1984;61:665.
111. Leibel SA, Sheline GE, Wara WM, et al. The role of radiation therapy in the treatment of astrocytomas. Cancer 1975;35:1551.
112. Kernohan JW, Sayre GP. Tumors of the central nervous system. In: Atlas of tumor pathology. Section 10, Fascicle 35. Washington, DC: Armed Forces Institute of Pathology, 1952.
113. Fazekas JT. Treatment of grade I and II brain astrocytomas: The role of radiotherapy. Int J Radiat Oncol Biol Phys 1977;2:661.
114. Chang CH, Horton J, Schoenfeld D, et al. Comparison of postoperative radiotherapy and combined postoperative radiotherapy and chemotherapy in the multidisciplinary management of malignant gliomas. Cancer 1983;52:997.
115. Sheline GE. Radiation therapy of primary tumors. Semin Oncol 1975;2:29.
116. Marsa GW, Goffinet DR, Rubinstein LJ, et al. Megavoltage irradiation in the treatment of gliomas of the brain and spinal cord. Cancer 1975;36:1681.
117. Kramer S. Radiation therapy in the management of malignant gliomas. In: Cancer of the central nervous system. Proceedings of the Seventh National Cancer Conference. Philadelphia: JB Lippincott, 1983:823.
118. Fulling KH, Nelson JS. Cerebral astrocytic neoplasms in the adult: Contribution of histologic examination to the assessment of prognosis. Semin Diagn Pathol 1984;1:152.
119. Daumas-Duport C, Scheithauer BW, Kelly PJ. A histologic and cytologic method for the spatial definition of gliomas. Mayo Clin Proc 1987;62:435.
120. Daumas-Duport C, Scheithauer B, O'Fallon J, Kelly P. Grading of astrocytomas, a simple and reproducible method. Cancer 1988;62:2152.
121. Kim TS, Halliday AL, Hedley-Whyte ET, Convery K. Correlates of survival and the Daumas-Duport grading system for astrocytomas. J Neurosurg 1991;74:27.
122. Nelson JS, Tsukada Y, Schoenfeld D, Fulling K, Lamarche J, Peress N. Necrosis as a prognostic criterion in malignant supratentorial, astrocytic gliomas. Cancer 1983;52:550.

123. Laws ER, Taylor WF, Clifton MB, et al. Neurosurgical management of low-grade astrocytoma of the cerebral hemispheres. J Neurosurg 1984;61:665.
124. Waller MD, Alexander E Jr, Hunt WE, et al. Evaluation of BCNU and/or radiotherapy in the treatment of anaplastic gliomas: A cooperative clinical trial. J Neurosurg 1978;49: 333.
125. Salcman M. Malignant glioma management. Neurosurg Clin North Am 1990;1:49.
126. Andreou J, George AE, Wise A, et al. CT prognostic criteria of survival after malignant glioma surgery. Am J Neuroradiol 1983;4:488.
127. Wood JR, Green SB, Shapiro WR. The prognostic importance of tumor size in malignant gliomas: A computed tomographic scan study by the Brain Tumor Cooperative Group. J Clin Oncol 1988;6:338.
128. Winger MJ, MacDonald DR, Cairncross JG. Supratentorial anaplastic gliomas in adults. J Neurosurg 1989;71:487.
129. Kumar ARV, Hoshino T, Wheeler KT, et al. Comparative rates of dead tumor cell removal from brain, muscle, subcutaneous tissue, and peritoneal cavity. JNCI 1974;52: 1751.
130. Gutin PH, Leibel SA, Wara WM, et al. Recurrent malignant gliomas: Improved survival following interstitial brachytherapy with high-activity iodine-125 sources. J Neurosurg 1987;67:864.
131. DeVita VT Jr. The relationship between tumor mass and resistance to chemotherapy: Implication for surgical adjuvant treatment of cancer. Cancer 1983;51:1209.
132. Berger MS, Kincaid J, Ojemann GA, et al. Brain mapping techniques to maximize resection, safety, and seizure control in children with brain tumors. Neurosurgery 1989;25:786.
133. Young B, Oldfield EH, Markesbery WR, et al. Reoperation for glioblastoma. J Neurosurg 1981;55:917.
134. Harsh GR IV, Levin VA, Gutin PH, Seager M, Silver P, Wilson CB. Reoperation for recurrent glioblastoma and anaplastic astrocytoma. Neurosurgery 1987;21:615.
135. Shaw EG, Daumas-Duport C, Scheithauer BW, et al. Radiation therapy in the management of low-grade supratentorial astrocytomas. J Neurosurg 1989;70:853.
136. Wallner KE, Gonzales MF, Sheline GE, et al. Treatment results of juvenile pilocytic astrocytoma. Neurosurgery 1988;69:171.
137. Shaw EG, Scheithauer BW, Gilbertson DT. Postoperative radiotherapy of supratentorial low-grade gliomas. Int J Radiat Oncol Biol Phys 1989;16:663.
138. Cairncross JG, Laperriere NJ. Low-grade glioma: To treat or not to treat? Arch Neurol 1989;46:1238.
139. Walker MD, Alexander E, Hunt WE, et al. Evaluation of BCNU and/or radiotherapy in the treatment of anaplastic gliomas. J Neurosurg 1978;49:333.
140. Kristiansen K, Hagen S, Kollevold T, et al. Combined modality therapy of operated astrocytomas grade III and IV—confirmation of the value of postoperative irradiation and lack of potentiation of bleomycin on survival time: A prospective multicenter trial of the Scandinavian Glioblastoma Study Group. Cancer 1981;47:649.
141. Walker MD, Strike TA, Sheline GE. An analysis of dose-effect relationship in the radiotherapy of malignant gliomas. Int J Radiat Oncol Biol Phys 1979;5:1725.
142. Nelson DF, Diener-West M, Horton J, et al. Combined modality approach to treatment of malignant gliomas: Reevaluation of RTOG 7401/ECOG 1374 with long-term follow-up. NCI Monogr 1988;6:279.
143. Bleehen NM. Studies of high grade cerebral gliomas. Int J Radiat Oncol Biol Phys 1990;18:811.
144. Djordjevic B, Szybalski W. Genetics of human cell lines: III. Incorporation of 5-bromo- and 5-iododeoxyuridine into the deoxyribonucleic acid of human cells and its effect on radiation sensitivity. J Exp Med 1960;112:509.
145. Levin VA, Wara WM, Gutin PH, et al. Initial analysis of NCOG 6G82-1: Bromodeoxyuridine (BUdR) during irradiation followed by CCNU, procarbazine, and vincristine (PCV) chemotherapy for malignant gliomas. Proc Am Soc Clin Oncol [Abstract] 1990;9: 91.
146. Phillips TL, Levin VA, Ahn DK. Evaluation of bromodeoxyuridine in glioblastoma multiforme: A Northern California Oncology Group phase II study. Int J Radiat Oncol Biol Phys 1991;21:709.
147. Kinsella TJ, Collins J, Rowland J, et al. Pharmacology and phase I/II study of continuous intravenous infusions of iododeoxyuridine and hyperfractionated radiotherapy in patients with glioblastoma multiforme. J Clin Oncol 1988;6:871.
148. Hegarty TJ, Thornton AF, Diaz RF, et al. Intra-arterial bromodeoxyuridine radiosensitization of malignant gliomas. Int J Radiat Oncol Biol Phys 1990;19:421.
149. Rodriquez R, Kinsella TJ. Halogenated pyrimidines as radiosensitizers for high grade glioma revisited. Int J Radiat Oncol Biol Phys 1991;21:859.
150. Withers HR. Biologic basis for altered fractionation schemes. Cancer 1985;55:2086.
151. Urtasun RC, Fulton D, Huyser-Wierenga D, et al. Dose intensity in radiotherapy: "Is more better" for patient with malignant glioma? Proc Am Soc Clin Oncol [Abstract] 1989;8:84.
152. Nelson DF, Curran WJ, Nelson JS, et al. Hyperfractionation in malignant glioma report on a dose searching phase I/II protocol of the Radiation Therapy Oncology Group (RTOG). Proc Am Soc Clin Oncol [Abstract] 1990;9:90.
153. Simpson WJ, Platts ME. Fractionation study in the treatment of glioblastoma multiforme. Int J Radiat Oncol Biol Phys 1976;1:639.
154. Keim H, Potthoff PC, Schmidt K, et al. Survival and quality of life after continuous accelerated radiotherapy of glioblastomas. Radiother Oncol 1987;9:21.
155. Florell RC, MacDonald DR, Irish WD, et al. Selection bias, survival, and brachytherapy for glioma. J Neurosurg 1991;76:179.
156. Gutin PH, Prados MD, Phillips TL, et al. External irradiation followed by an interstitial high activity iodine-125 implant "boost"" in the initial treatment of malignant gliomas: NCOG Study 6G-82-2. Int J Radiat Oncol Biol Phys 1991;21:601.
157. Loeffler JS, Alexander E, Wen P, et al. Results of stereotactic brachytherapy used in the initial management of patient with glioblastoma. JNCI 1990;82:1918.
158. Leibel SA, Gutin PH, Wara WM, et al. Survival and quality of life after interstitial implantation of removable high-activity iodine-125 sources for the treatment of patients with recurrent malignant gliomas. Int J Radiat Oncol Biol Phys 1989;17:1129.
159. Loeffler JS, Alexander E, Hochberg FH, et al. Clinical patterns of failure following stereotactic interstitial irradiation for malignant gliomas. Int J Radiat Oncol Biol Phys 1990;19:1455.
160. Walker MD, Green SB, Byar DP, et al. Randomized comparison of radiotherapy and nitrosoureas for the treatment of malignant glioma after surgery. N Engl J Med 1980;303:1323.
161. Green SB, Byar DP, Walker MD, et al. Comparison of carmustine, procarbazine, and high-dose methylprednisolone as additions to surgery and radiotherapy for the treatment of malignant glioma. Cancer Treat Rep 1983;67:1.
162. Nelson DF, Schoenfeld D, Weinstein AS, et al. A randomized comparison of misonidazole sensitized radiotherapy plus BCNU and radiotherapy plus BCNU for treatment of malignant glioma after surgery: Preliminary results of an RTOG study. Int J Radiat Oncol Biol Phys 1983;9:1143.
163. Paoletti P, Cuna GRD, Knerich R, et al. Multidisciplinary treatment for central nervous system tumors with nitrosourea compounds. ACTA Neurochir 1978;41:287.
164. Eyre HJ, Quagliana JM, Eltringham JR, et al. Randomized comparisons of radiotherapy and CCNU versus radiotherapy, CCNU plus procarbazine for the treatment of malignant gliomas following surgery. J Neurooncol 1983;1:171.
165. Adinolfi D, Buoncristiani P, Casotto A, et al. Multidisciplinary treatment for brain tumors. J Neurosurg Sci 1978;22:111.
166. EORTC Brain Tumor Group. Effect of CCNU on survival rate of objective remission and duration of free interval in patients with malignant brain glioma—final evaluation. Eur J Cancer 1978;14:851.
167. Feun LG, Steward DJ, Maor M, et al. A pilot study of *cis*-diaminedichloroplatinum and radiation therapy in patients with high-grade astrocytomas. J Neurooncol 1983;1: 109.
168. Deutsch M, Green SB, Strike TA, et al. Results of a randomized trial comparing BCNU plus radiotherapy, streptozotocin plus radiotherapy, BCNU plus hyperfractionated radiotherapy, and BCNU following misonidazole plus radiotherapy in the postoperative treatment of malignant glioma. Int J Radiat Oncol Biol Phys 1989;16: 1389.
169. Shapiro WR, Green SB, Burger PC, et al. Randomized trial of three chemotherapy regimens and two radiotherapy regimens and two radiotherapy regimens in postoperative treatment of malignant glioma: Brain Tumor Cooperative Group Trial 8001. J Neurosurg 1989;71:1.
170. Rozental JM, Robins HI, Finlay J, Healy B, et al. "Eight-in-one-day" chemotherapy administered before and after radiotherapy to adult patients with malignant gliomas. Cancer 1989;63:2475.
171. Levin VA, Silver P, Hannigan J, Wara WM, Gutin PH, Davis RL, Wilson CB. Superiority of post-radiotherapy adjuvant chemotherapy with CCNU, procarbazine, and vincristine (PCV) over BCNU for anaplastic gliomas: NCOG 6G61 Final Report. Int J Radiat Oncol Phys Biol 1990;18:321.
171a. Levin VA. Unpublished observations, 1992.
172. Levin VA, Wara WM, Davis RL, et al. NCOG protocol 6G91: Seven drug chemotherapy and irradiaion for patients with glioblastoma multiforme. Cancer Treat Rep 1986;70: 739.
173. Phillips TL, Levin VA, Ahn DK, et al. Evaluation of bromodeoxyuridine in glioblastoma multiforme—a Northern California Cancer Center phase II study. Int J Radiat Oncol Biol Phys 1991;21:709.
174. Wilson CB, Gutin PH, Boldrey EB, et al. Single-agent chemotherapy of brain tumors. Arch Neurol 1976;33:739.
175. Fewer D, Wilson CB, Boldrey EB, et al. Phase II study of 1-(2-chloroethyl)-3-cyclohexyl-1-nitrosourea (CCNU) in the treatment of brain tumors. Cancer Chemother Rep 1972;56:421.
176. Rosenblum ML, Reynolds AF, Smith KA, et al. Chloroethyl-cyclohexyl-nitrosourea (CCNU) in the treatment of malignant brain tumors. J Neurosurg 1973;39:306.
177. Levin VA, Resser K, McGrath L, et al. PCNU treatment for recurrent malignant gliomas. Cancer Treat Rep 1984;68:969.
178. Rodriguez LA, Prados M, Silver P, Levin VA. Re-evaluation of procarbazine for the treatment of recurrent malignant CNS tumors. Cancer 1989;64:2420.
179. Levin VA, Crafts D, Wilson CB, et al. Imidazole carboxamides. Relationship of lipophilicity to activity against intracerebral murine glioma 26 and preliminary phase II clinical trial of 5-(3,3-bis chloroethyl)-1-triazeno)-imidazole-4-carboxamide (NSC-82196) in primary and secondary brain tumors. Cancer Chemother Rep 1975;59: 107.
180. Chamberlain MC, Prados MD, Silver P, Levin VA. A phase I/II study of 24 hour intravenous AZQ in recurrent primary brain tumors. J Neurooncol 1988;6:319.
181. Decker DA, Al-Sarraf M, Kresge C, et al. Phase II study of aziridinylbenzoquinone (AZQ NSC-182986) in the treatment of malignant gliomas recurrent after radiation: Preliminary report. J Neurooncol 1985;3:19.
182. Schold SC, Friedman HS, Bjornsson TD, et al. Treatment of patients with recurrent primary brain tumors with AZQ. Neurology 1984;34:615.
183. Chamberlain MC, Prados MD, Silver P, et al. A phase II trial of oral melphalan in recurrent primary brain tumors. Am J Clin Oncol 1988;11:52.
183a. VA Levin, et al. Unpublished observations, 1987 and 1991.
184. Prados MD, Rodriguez L, Seager M, et al. Phase II study of spirohydantoin mustard for the treatment of recurrent malignant gliomas. Cancer Treat Rep 1987;71:1105.
185. Bertolone SJ, Baum ES, Krivit W, Hammond GD. A phase II study of cisplatin therapy in recurrent childhood brain tumors. J Neurooncol 1989;7:5.
185a. Spence AM, et al. Unpublished observations, 1991.

186. Yung WKA, Mechtler L, Gleason MJ. Intravenous carboplatin for recurrent malignant gliomas: A phase II study. J Clin Oncol 1991;9:860.
187. Yung WKA, Prados MD, Levin VA, et al. Intravenous recombinant interferon-beta, betaseron, in patients with recurrent malignant gliomas: A phase I/II study. J Clin Oncol 1991;9:1945.
188. Fewer D, Wilson CB, Boldrey EB, et al. Chemotherapy of brain tumors: Clinical experience with carmustine amd vincristine. JAMA 1972;222:549.
189. Gutin PH, Wilson CB, Kumar ARV, et al. Phase II study of procarbazine, CCNU, vincristine combination chemotherapy in the treatment of malignant brain tumors. Cancer 1975;35:1398.
190. Levin VA, Edwards MS, Wright DC, et al. Modified procarbazine, CCNU, and vincristine (PCV 3) combination chemotherapy in the treatment of malignant brain tumors. Cancer Treat Rep 1980;64:237.
191. Levin VA, Hoffman WF, Pischer TL, et al. BCNU–5-fluorouracil combination in the treatment of recurrent malignant brain tumors. Cancer Treat Rep 1978;62:2071.
192. Levin VA, Phuphanich S, Liu H-C, et al. Phase II study of combined BCNU, 5-fluorouracil, hydroxyurea, and 6-mercaptopurine (BFHM) for the treatment of malignant gliomas. Cancer Treat Rep 1986;70:1271.
193. Prados M, Rodriguez L, Chamberlain M, Silver P, Levin VA. Treatment of recurrent gliomas with 1,3-*bis*(2-chloroethyl)-1-nitrosourea and α-difluoromethylornithine. Neurosurgery 1989;24:806.
194. Levin VA, Chamberlain MC, Prados MD, et al. Phase I-II study of eflornithine and mitoguazone combined in the treatment of recurrent primary brain tumors. Cancer Treat Rep 1987;71:459.
194a. Levin VA, Prados MD, Yung WK, Gleason MJ, Ictech S, Malec M. Treatment of recurrent gliomas with eflornithine. JNCI 1992;84:1432.
195. Levin VA, Prados MD, Davis RL, et al. Treatment of recurrent gliomas with a polydrug protocol designed to combat nitrosourea resistance. J Clin Oncol 1992;10:766.
196. Schold SC Jr, Mahaley MS Jr, Vick NA, et al. Phase II diaziquone-based chemotherapy trials in patients with anaplastic supratentorial astrocytic neoplasms. J Clin Oncol 1987;5:464.
197. Yung WKA, Harris MI, Bruner JM, Feun LG. Intravenous BCNU and AZQ in patients with recurrent malignant gliomas. J Neurooncol 1989;7:237.
198. Longee DC, Friedman HS, Albright RE, et al. Treatment of patients with recurrent gliomas with cyclophosphamide and vincristine. J Neurosurg 1990;72:583.
199. Byar DP, Green SB, Strike TA. Prognostic factors for malignant glioma. In: Walker MD, ed. Oncology of the nervous system. Boston: Martinus Nijhoff, 1983:379.
199a. Yung WKA, et al. Unpublished observations, 1991.
200. Rosenblum ML, Gerosa MA, Wilson CB, et al. Stem cell studies of human brain tumors. J Neurosurg 1983;58:170.
201. Thomas DGT, Darling JL, Paul EA, et al. Assay of anti-cancer drugs in tissue culture: Relationship of relapse free interval (RFI) and in vitro chemosensitivity in patients with malignant cerebral glioma. Br J Cancer 1985;51:525.
202. Goodwin W, Crowley J. A retrospective comparison of high-dose BCNU with autologous marrow rescue plus radiotherapy vs IV BCNU plus radiation therapy in high grade gliomas: A Southwest Oncology Group review. Proc Annu Meet Am Soc Clin Oncol [Abstract] 1989;8:A352.
203. Ahmed T, Feldman E, Helson L, et al. Phase I-II trial of high-dose thiotepa (HDT) with autologous bone marrow transplantation (ABMT) and localized radiotherapy (RT) for patients (pts) with astrocytoma grade III-IV. Proc Annu Meet Am Assoc Cancer Res [Abstract] 1990;31:A1023.
204. Long J, Leff R, Daly M, et al. Phase II trial of high-dose etoposide (E) and autologous bone marrow transplantation for treatment of progressive glioma. Proc Annu Meet Am Soc Clin Oncol [Abstract] 1989;8:A360.
205. Glannone L, Wolff SN. Phase II treatment of central nervous system gliomas with high-dose etoposide and autologous bone marrow transplantation. Cancer Treat Rep 1987;71:759.
206. Finlay JL, August C, Packer R, et al. High-dose multi-agent chemotherapy followed by bone marrow "rescue" for malignant astrocytomas of childhood and adolescence. J Neurooncol 1990;9:239.
207. Finlay JL. High-dose chemotherapy with bone marrow rescue in children and young adults with malignant brain tumors. Proc Annu Meet Am Assoc Cancer Res [Abstract] 1991;32:A1078.
208. Allen JC, Bloom J, Ertel I, et al. Brain tumors in children: Current cooperative and institutional chemotherapy trials in newly diagnosed and recurrent disease. Sem Oncol 1986;13:110.
209. Freeman CR, Suissa S. Brain stem tumors in children: Results of a survey of 62 patients treated with radiotherapy. Int J Radiat Oncol Biol Phys 1986;12:1823.
210. Eifel PJ, Cassady JR, Belli JA. Radiation therapy of tumors of the brainstem and midbrain in children: Experience of the Joint Center For Radiation Therapy and Children's Hospital Medical Center (1971–1981). Int J Radiat Oncol Biol Phys 1987;13: 847.
211. Coffey RJ, Lunsford LD. Stereotactic surgery for mass lesions of the midbrain and pons. Neurosurgery 1985;17:12.
212. Eifel PJ, Cassady JR, Belli JA. Radiation therapy of tumors of the brainstem and midbrain in children: Experience of the Joint Center for Radiation Therapy and Children's Hospital Medical Center. Int J Radiat Oncol Biol Phys 1987;13:847.
213. Kim TH, Chin HW, Pollan S, et al. Radiotherapy of primary brain stem tumors. Int J Radiat Oncol Biol Phys 1980;6:51.
214. Albright AL, Guthkelch AN, Packer RJ, et al. Prognostic factors in pediatric brainstem gliomas. J Neurosurg 1986;65:751.
215. Stroink AR, Hoffman HJ, Hendrick EB, et al. Diagnosis and management of pediatric gliomas. J Neurosurg 1986;65:745.
216. Halperin EC. Pediatric brain stem tumors: Patterns of treatment failure and their implications for radiotherapy. Int J Radiat Oncol Biol Phys 1985;11:1293.
217. Packer RJ, Allen JC, Goldwein JL, et al. Hyperfractionated radiotherapy for children with brainstem gliomas: A pilot study using 7,200 cGy. Ann Neurol 1990;27:167.
218. Freeman CR, Krischer J, Sanford RA, et al. Hyperfractionated radiation therapy for brain stem tumors: Results of treatment at the 7020 cGy dose level of Pediatric Oncology Group Study No. 8495. Cancer 1991;68:474.
219. Edwards MSB, Wara WM, Urtasun RC, et al. Hyperfractionated radiation therapy for brain-stem glioma: A phase I-II trial. J Neurosurg 1989;70:691.
220. Bertolone SJ, Baum ES, Krivit W, Hammond GD. A phase II study of cisplatin therapy in recurrent childhood brain tumors. J Neurooncol 1989;7:5.
221. Fulton DS, Levin VA, Wara WM, et al. Chemotherapy of pediatric brain stem tumors. J Neurosurg 1981;54:721.
222. Jenkin D. Posterior fossa tumors in childhood: Radiation treatment. Clin Neurosurg 1983;30:203.
223. Levin VA, Edwards MS, Wara WM, et al. 5-fluorouracil and CCNU followed by hydroxyurea, misonidazole and irradiation for brain stem gliomas: A pilot study of the Brain Tumor Research Center and the Children's Cancer Group. Neurosurgery 1984;14:679.
224. Rodriguez LA, Prados M, Fulton D, Edwards MSB, Silver P, Levin V. Treatment of recurrent brain stem gliomas and other CNS tumors with 5-fluorouracil, CCNU, hydroxyurea and 6-mercaptopurine. Neurosurgery 1988;22:691.
225. Humphreys RP. Posterior cranial fossa brain tumors in children. In: Youmans JR, ed. Youmans' neurological surgery. Philadelphia: WB Saunders, 1982:2747.
226. Chamberlain MC, Silver P, Levin VA. Poorly differentiated gliomas of the cerebellum—a study of 18 patients. Cancer 1990;65:337.
227. Walsh FB, Hoyt WF. Clinical neuro-opthalmology. Baltimore: Williams & Wilkins, 1969:2076.
228. Lewis RA, Gerson LP, Axelson KA, Riccardi VM, Whitford RP. von Recklinghausen neurofibromatosis: II. Incidence of optic gliomata. Ophthalmology 1984;91:929.
229. Housepian EM, Trokel SL, Jakobiec FO, et al. Tumors of the orbit. In Youmans JR, ed. Youmans' neurological surgery. Philadelphia: WB Saunders, 1982:3024.
230. Packer RJ, Sutton LN, Bilaniuk LT, et al. Treatment of chiasmatic/hypothalamic gliomas of childhood with chemotherapy: An update. Ann Neurol 1988;23:79.
231. Housepian EM. Surgical treatment of unilateral optic nerve gliomas. J Neurosurg 1969;31:604.
232. Tenny RT, Laws ER, Young BR, Rush JA. The neurosurgical management of optic gliomas: Results in 104 patients. J Neurosurg 1982;57:452.
233. Bataini JP, Delanian S, Ponvert D. Chiasmal gliomas: Results of irradiation management and review of literature. Int J Radiat Oncol Biol Phys 1991;21:615.
234. Wong JYC, Uhl V, Wara WM, Sheline GE. Optic gliomas: A re-analysis of the University of California, San Francisco experience. Cancer 1987;60:1847.
235. Danoff BF, Kramer S, Thompson N. The radiotherapeutic management of optic nerve gliomas in children. Int J Radiat Oncol Biol Phys 1980;6:45.
236. Flickinger JC, Torres C, Deutsch M. Management of low-grade gliomas of the optic nerve and chiasm. Cancer 1988;61:635.
237. Horowich A, Bloom HJG. Optic gliomas: Radiation therapy and prognosis. Int J Rad Oncol Biol Phys 1985;11:1067.
238. Rosenstock JG, Packer RJ, Bilaniuk L. Chiasmatic optic glioma treated with chemotherapy. J Neurosurg 1985;63:862.
239. Rodriguez LA, Edwards MSB, Levin VA. Management of hypothalamic gliomas in children: An analysis of 33 cases. Neurosurgery 1990;26:242.
240. Petronio J, Edwards MSB, Prados M, et al. Management of chiasmal and hypothalamic gliomas of infancy and childhood with chemotherapy. J Neurosurg 1990;74:701.
241. Ludwig CL, Smith MT, Godfrey AD, et al. A clinicopathologic study of 323 patients with oligodendrogliomas. Ann Neurol 1986;19:15.
242. Wallner KE, Gonzales M, Sheline GE. Treatment of oligodendrogliomas with or without postoperative irradiation. J Neurosurg 1988;68:684.
243. Lindegaard K-F, Mork SJ, Eide GE, et al. Statistical analysis of clinicopathological features, radiotherapy, and survival in 170 cases of oligodendroglioma. J Neurosurg 1987;67:224.
244. Halperin EC, Kun LE, Constine LS, Tarbell NJ. Pediatric radiation oncology. New York: Raven Press, 1989:58.
245. Reedy DP, Bay JW, Hahn JF. Role of radiation therapy in the treatment of cerebral oligodendroglioma: An analysis of 57 cases and a literature review. Neurosurgery 1983;13:499.
246. Bullard DE, Rawlings CE, Phillips B, et al. Oligodendroglioma: An analysis of the value of radiation therapy. Cancer 1987;60:2179.
247. Karlsson UL, Leibel SA, Wallner K, et al. Brain tumors. In: Perez CA, Brady LW, eds. Principles and practice of radiation oncology. 2nd ed. Philadelphia: JB Lippincott 1992:515.
248. Cairncross JG, MacDonald DR. Chemotherapy for oligodendroglioma: Progress report. Arch Neurol 1991;48:225.
249. Kernohan JW, Sayre GP. Tumors of the central nervous system. In: Atlas of tumor pathology. Section 10, Fascicle 35. Washington, DC: Armed Forces Institute of Pathology, 1952.
250. Svien HJ, Mabon RF, Kernohan JW, et al. Ependymoma of the brain: Pathologic aspects. Neurology 1953;3:1.
251. Healey EA, Barnes PD, Kupsky WJ, et al. The prognostic significance of post-operative residual tumor in ependymoma. Neurosurgery 1991;28:666.
252. Ross GW, Rubinstein LJ. Lack of histopathological correlation of malignant ependymomas with postoperative survival. J Neurosurg 1989;70:31.
253. Goldwein JW, Corn BW, Finlay JL, et al. Is craniospinal irradiation required to cure

children with malignant (anaplastic) intracranial ependymomas? Cancer 1991;67: 2766.
254. Vanuytsel L, Brada M. The role of prophylactic spinal irradiation in localized intracranial ependymoma. Int J Radiat Oncol Biol Phys 1991;21:825.
255. Wallner KE, Wara WM, Sheline GE, et al. Intracranial ependymomas: Results of treatment with partial or whole brain irradiation without spinal irradiation. Int J Radiat Oncol Biol Phys 1986;12:1937.
256. Salazar OM, Castro-Vita H, Van Houtte P, et al. Improved survival in cases of intracranial ependymoma after radiation therapy: Late report and recommendations. J Neurosurg 1983;59:652.
257. Marks JE, Adler SJ. A comparative study of ependymomas by site of origin. Int J Radiat Oncol Biol Phys 1982;8:3.
258. Shaw EG, Evans RG, Scheithauer BW, et al. Postoperative radiotherapy of intracranial ependymoma in pediatric and adult patients. Int J Radiat Oncol Biol Phys 1987;13: 1457.
258a. Prados M, Levin VA, Edwards MSB. Unpublished observations, 1991.
259. Levin VA, Edwards MSB, Gutin PH, et al. Phase II evaluation of dibromodulcitol in the treatment of recurrent medulloblastoma, ependymoma, and malignant astrocytoma. J Neurosurg 1984;61:1063.
260. Goldwein JW, Leahy JM, Packer RJ, et al. Intracranial ependymomas in children. Int J Radiat Oncol Biol Phys 1990;99:1497.
261. Gaynon PS, Ettinger LJ, Baum ES, et al. Carboplatin in childhood brain tumors: A Children's Cancer Study Group phase II trial. Cancer 1990;66:2465.
262. Ettinger LJ, Ru N, Krailo M, et al. A phase II study of diaziquone in children with recurrent or progressive primary brain tumors: A report from the Children's Cancer Study Group. J Neurooncol 1990;9:69.
263. Cushing H, Eisenhardt L. Meningiomas: Their classification, regional behavior, life history, and surgical end results. Springfield: Charles C Thomas, 1938:73.
264. Hoshino T, Nagashima T, Murovic J, et al. Cell kinetic studies of in situ human brain tumors with bromodeoxyuridine. Cytometry 1985;6:627.
265. Simpson D. The recurrence of intracranial meningiomas after surgical treatment. J Neurol Neurosurg Psychiatry 1957;20:22.
266. Mirimanoff RO, Dosoretz DE, Linggood RM, et al. Meningioma. Analysis of recurrence and progression following neurosurgical resection. J Neurosurg 1985;62:18.
267. Barbaro NM, Gutin PH, Wilson CB, et al. Radiation therapy in the treatment of partially resected meningiomas. Neurosurgery 1987;20:525.
268. Taylor BW, Marcus RB Jr, Friedman WA, et al. The meningioma controversy: Postoperative radiation therapy. Int J Radiat Oncol Biol Phys 1988;15:244.
269. Graholm J, Bloom HJG, Crow JH. The role of radiotherapy in the management of intracranial meningiomas: The Royal Marsden Hospital experience with 186 patients. Int J Radiat Oncol Biol Phys 1990;18:755.
270. Solan MJ, Kramer S. The role of radiation therapy in the management of intracranial meningiomas. Int J Radiat Oncol Biol Phys 1985;11:675.
271. Chan RC, Thompson GB. Morbidity, mortality, and quality of life following surgery for intracranial meningiomas. J Neurosurg 1984;60:52.
272. Grunberg SM, Weiss MH, Spitz IM, et al. Treatment of unresectable meningiomas with the antiprogesterone agent mifepristone. J Neurosurg 1991;74:861.
273. Schneck SA, Penn I. De novo brain tumors in renal transplant recipients. Lancet 1971;1:983.
274. Pitchenik AE, Fischl MA, Walls KW. Evaluation of cerebral-mass lesions in acquired immunodeficiency syndrome. N Engl J Med 1983;308:1099.
275. Payan MJ, Gambarelli D, Routy JP, et al. Primary lymphoma of the brain associated with AIDS. Acta Neuropathol 1984;64:78.
276. Rosenblum ML, Levy RM, Ziegler JL. Primary central nervous system lymphomas in patients with AIDS. Ann Neurol 1988;23(suppl):S13.
277. Murray K, Kun L, Cox J. Primary malignant lymphoma of the central nervous system. J Neurosurg 1986;65:600.
278. DeAngelis LM, Yahalom J, Rosenblum M, Posner JB. Primary CNS lymphoma: Managing patients with spontaneous and AIDS-related disease. Oncology 1987;1:52.
279. Jellinger K, Radaskiewicz TH, Slowik F. Primary malignant lymphomas of the central nervous system in man. Acta Neuropathol (Berlin) 1975;95:102.
280. Henry JM, Heffner RR Jr, Dillard SH, et al. Primary malignant lymphomas of the central nervous system. Cancer 1974;34:1293.
281. DeAngelis LM, Yahalom J, Heinemann MH, et al. Primary central nervous system lymphoma: Combined treatment with chemotherapy and radiotherapy. Neurology 1990;40:80.
282. Pollack IF, Lunsford ID, Flickinger JC, Dameshek HL. Prognostic factors in the diagnosis and treatment of primary central nervous system lymphoma. Cancer 1989;63: 939.
283. Murray K, Kun L, Cox J. Primary malignant lymphoma of the central nervous system: Results of treatment of 11 cases and review of the literature. J Neurosurg 1986;65: 600.
284. Nelson DF, Martz KL, Bonner H, et al. Definitive radiation therapy in the treatment of primary non-Hodgkin's lymphoma of the central nervous system, non-AIDS related. Report of RTOG study 8315. Int J Radiat Oncol Biol Phys 1992;23:9.
285. Margolis L, Fraser R, Lichter A, Char DH. The role of radiation therapy in the management of ocular reticulum cell sarcoma. Cancer 1980;45:688.
286. Goldstein JD, Dickson DW, Moser FG, et al. Primary central nervous system lymphoma in acquired immunodeficiency syndrome. Cancer 1991;67:2756.
287. McLaughlin P, Velasquez WS, Redman JR, et al. Chemotherapy with dexamethasone, high-dose cytarabine, and cisplatin for parenchymal brain lymphoma. JNCI 1988;80: 1408.
288. Chamberlain MC, Levin VA. Adjuvant chemotherapy for primary lymphoma of the central nervous system. Arch Neurol 1990;47:1113.
289. Neuwelt EA, Goldman D, Dahlborg SA, et al. Primary central nervous system lymphoma treated with osmotic blood-brain barrier disruption and combination chemotherapy: Prolonged survival and preservation of cognitive function. Proc Annu Meet Am Soc Clin Oncol [Abstract] 1990;9:A1047.
290. DeAngelis LM, Yahalom J. Combined modality treatment of primary central nervous system lymphoma (PCNSL). Proc Annu Meet Am Soc Clin Oncol [Abstract] 1991;10: A368.
291. McComb RD, Burger PC. Pathologic analysis of primary brain tumors. Neurol Clin North Am 1985;3:711.
292. Gaffney CC, Sloane JP, Bradley NJ, Bloom HJG. Primitive neuroectodermal tumours of the cerebrum: Pathology and treatment. J Neurooncol 1985;3:23.
293. Berger MS, Edwards MD, Wara WM, et al. Primary cerebral neuroblastoma: Long-term follow-up review and therapeutic guidelines. J Neurosurg 1983;59:418.
294. Bloom HJG. Medulloblastoma in children: Increasing survival rates and further prospects. Int J Radiat Oncol Biol Phys 1982;8:2023.
295. Deutsch M. The impact of myelography on the treatment results for medulloblastoma. Int J Radiat Oncol Biol Phys 1984;10:999.
296. Levin VA, Rodriguez LA, Edwards MSB, et al. Treatment of medulloblastoma with procarbazine hydroxyurea, and reduced radiation doses to whole brain and spine. J Neurosurg 1988;68:383.
297. Park TS, Hoffman HJ, Hendrick EB, et al. Medulloblastoma: Clinical presentation and management—experience at the Hospital For Sick Children, Toronto, 1950–1980. J Neurosurg 1983;58:543.
298. Lowery GS, Kimball JC, Patterson RB, et al. Extraneural metastases from cerebellar medulloblastoma. Am J Pediatr Hematol Oncol 1982;4:259.
299. Tait DM, Thornton-Jones H, Bloom HJG, et al. Adjuvant chemotherapy for medulloblastoma: The first multi-centre control trial of the International Society of Pediatric Oncology (SIOP I). Eur J Cancer 1990;26:464
300. Evans AE, Jenkin RD, Sposto R, et al. The treatment of medulloblastoma: Results of a prospective randomized trial of radiation therapy with and without CCNU, vincristine, and prednisone. J Neurosurg 1990;72:572.
301. Chamberlain MC, Silver P, Edwards MSB, Levin VA. Treatment of extraneural metastatic medulloblastoma with a combination of cyclophosphamide, adriamycin and vincristine (CAV). Neurosurgery 1988;23:476.
302. Deutsch M. The impact of myelography on the treatment results of medulloblastoma. Int J Radiat Oncol Biol Phys 1984;10:999.
303. Allen JC, Epstein F. Medulloblastoma and other primary CNS malignant neuroectodermal tumors: The effect of age and extent of disease on prognosis. J Neurosurg 1982;57:446.
304. Kun LE, Constine LS. Medulloblastoma-caution regarding new treatment approaches Int J Radiat Oncol Biol Phys 1991;20:897.
305. Brand WN, Schneider PH, Tokars RP. Long-term results of a pilot study of low-dose cranial-spinal irradiation for cerebellar medulloblastoma. Int J Radiat Oncol Biol Phys 1987;13:1641.
306. Deutsch M, Thomas P, Boyett J, et al. Low-stage medulloblastoma: A Children's Cancer Study Group (CCSG) and Pediatric Oncology Group (POG) randomized study of standard vs reduced neuraxis irradiation. Proc Am Soc Clin Oncol [Abstract] 1991;10: 124.
307. Halberg FE, Wara WM, Fippin LF, et al. Low-dose craniospinal radiation therapy for medulloblastoma. Int J Radiat Oncol Biol Phys 1991;20:651.
308. Benjamin RS, Wiernik PH, Bachur NR. Adriamycin chemotherapy: Efficacy, saftey, and pharmacologic basis of an intermittent single high-dose schedule. Cancer 1974;33: 19.
309. Shapiro WR. Chemotherapy of primary malignant brain tumors. Cancer Child 1975;35: 965.
310. Ward HWC. Central nervous system tumors of childhood treated with CCNU, vincristine and radiation. Med Pediatr Oncol 1978;4:315.
311. Garrett MJ, Hughs HJ, Ryall RDH. CCNU in brain tumors. Clin Radiol 1974;25:183.
312. Ward HWC. CCNU in the treatment of recurrent medulloblastoma. Br Med J 1974;1: 642.
313. Hancock C, Allen J, Tan CTC. Phase II trial of PCNU in children with recurrent brain tumors and Hodgkin's disease. Cancer Treat Rep 1984;68:441.
314. Walker RW, Allen JC. Treatment of recurrent primary intracranial childhood tumors with *cis*-diamine-dichloroplatinum. Ann Neurology 1983;14:371.
315. Bertolone SJ, Baum E, Krivit W, et al. Phase II trial of cisplatinum diamino-dichloride (CPDD) in recurrent childhood brain tumors: A CCSG trial. Proc Am Assoc Cancer Res 1983;2:72.
316. Sexauer CL, Kahn A, Burger PC, et al. *Cis*-platinum in recurrent pediatric brain tumors: A POG phase II study. Cancer 1985;56:1497.
317. Allen JC, Walker R, Luks E, et al. Carboplatin and recurrent childhood brain tumors. J Clin Oncol 1987;5:459.
318. Allen JC, Helson L. High-dose cyclophosphamide chemotherapy for recurrent CNS tumors in children. J Neurosurg 1981;55:749.
319. Rosen G, Ghavimi F, Nirenberg A, et al. High-dose methotrexate with citrovorum factor rescue for the treatment of central nervous system tumors in children. Cancer Treat Rep 1977;61:681.
320. Djerassi I, Kim JS, Shulman K. High-dose methotrexate-citrovorum factor rescue in the management of brain tumors. Cancer Treat Rep 1977;61:691.
321. Mooney C, Souhami R, Pritchard J. Recurrent medulloblastoma: Lack of response to high-dose methotrexate. Cancer Chemother Pharmacol 1983;10:135.
322. Haddy TB, Ferbach DJ, Watkins WL, et al. Vincristine in uncommon malignant disease in children. Cancer Chemother Rep 1964;41:41.
323. Lassman LP, Pearce GW, Gang J. Effect of vincristine sulfate on the intracranial gliomata of childhood. Br J Surg 1966;53:774.

324. Lampkin BC, Maurer AM, McBride BH. Response of medulloblastoma to vincristine sulfate: A case report. Pediatrics 1967;39:761.
325. Smart CR, Ottoman RE, Rochlin DB, et al. Clinical experience with vincristine in tumors of the central nervous system and other malignant diseases. Cancer Chemother Rep 1968;52:733.
326. Afra D. Vincristine therapy in malignant glioma recurrencies. Neurochirurgia 1973;16: 189.
327. Rosenstock JG, Evans AE, Schut L: Response to vincristine of recurrent brain tumors in children. J Neurosurg 1976;45:135.
328. Skylansky BD, Mann-Kaplan RS, Reynolds BF, et al. 4'-demethyl-epipodophyllotoxin-*D*-thenylidene-glucoside (PTG) in the treatment of malignant intracranial neoplasms. Cancer 1974;33:460.
329. Bleyer WA, Krivit W, Chard RL. Phase II study of VM26 in leukemia, neuroblastoma, and other refractory childhood malignancies: A report from the Children's Cancer Study Group. Cancer Treat Rep 1979;63:977.
330. Friedman HS, Schold SC Jr, Mahaley MS Jr, et al. Phase II treatment of medulloblastoma and pineoblastoma with melphalan: Clinical therapy based on experimental models of human medulloblastoma. J Clin Oncol 1989;7:904.
331. Crafts DC, Levin VA, Edwards MS, et al. Chemotherapy of recurrent medulloblastoma with combined procarbazine, CCNU, vincristine. J Neurosurg 1978;49:589.
332. Thomas P, Duffner PK, Cohen ME, et al. Multimodality therapy for medulloblastoma. Cancer 1980;45:666.
333. Seiler RW. Combination chemotherapy with VM26 and CCNU in primary malignant brain tumors of children. Helv Paediatr Acta 1980;35:51.
334. van Eys J, Baram TZ, Cangir A, et al. Salvage chemotherapy for recurrent primary brain tumors in children. J Pediatr 1988;113:601.
335. Cangir A, Ragab AH, Steubner P, et al. Combination chemotherapy with vincristine, procarbazine, prednisone with or without nitrogen mustard (MOOP vs OPP) in children with recurrent brain tumors. Med Pediatr Oncol 1984;12:1.
336. Freidman HS, Mahaley MS, Schold SC Jr, et al. The efficacy of vincristine and cyclophosphamide in the therapy of recurrent medulloblastoma. Neurosurgery 1986;18: 335.
337. Thomas PR, Duffner PK, Cohen ME, et al. Multimodality therapy for medulloblastoma. Cancer 1980;45:666.
338. Lefkowitz IB, Packer RJ, Siegel KR, et al. Results of treatment of children with recurrent medulloblastoma/primitive neuroectodermal tumors with lomustine, cisplatin, and vincristine. Cancer 1990;65:412.
339. Pendergrass TW, Milstein JM, Geyer JR, et al. Eight drugs in 1 day chemotherapy for brain tumors: Experience in 107 children and rationale for preirradiation chemotherapy. J Clin Oncol 1987;5:1221.
340. Packer RJ, Sutton LN, Goldwein JW, et al. Improved survival with the use of adjuvant chemotherapy in the treatment of medulloblastoma. J Neurosurg 1991;74:433.
341. Krischer JP, Ragab AH, Kun L, et al. Nitrogen mustard, vincristine, procarbazine, and prednisone as adjuvant chemotherapy in the treatment of medulloblastoma: A Pediatric Oncology Group Study. J Neurosurg 1991;74:905.
342. Prados M, Levin VA, Edwards MS, Wara W. Combined chemotherapy/radiotherapy for pediatric brain tumors: The UCSF experience [Abstract No. A48]. International Symposium on Pediatric Neuro-Oncology. June 1—3, 1989, Seattle, WA, 1989.
343. Kretschmar CS, Tarbell NJ, Kupsky W, et al. Pre-irradiation chemotherapy for infants and children with medulloblastoma: A preliminary report. J Neurosurg 1989;71:820.
344. Kovnar EH, Kellie SJ, Horowitz ME, et al. Preirradiation cisplatin and etoposide in the treatment of high-risk medulloblastoma and other malignant embryonal tumors of the central nervous system: A phase II study. J Clin Oncol 1990;8:330.
345. Christ WM, Ragab AH, Vietti TJ, et al. Chemotherapy of childhood medulloblastoma. Am J Dis Child 1976;13:639.
346. Nathanson L, Kovacs SG. Chemotherapeutic response in metastatic medulloblastoma: Report of two cases and a review of the literature. Med Pediatr Oncol 1978;4:105.
347. Hoffman HJ. Pineal region tumors. Prog Exp Tumor Res 1987;30:281.
348. Matsutani M, Takakura K, Sano K. Primary intracranial germ cell tumors: Pathology and treatment. Prog Exp Tumor Res 1987;30:307.
349. Herrick MK. Pathology of pineal tumors. In: Neuwelt EA, ed. Diagnosis and treatment of pineal region tumors. Baltimore: Williams & Wilkins, 1984:31.
350. Edwards MSB, Levin VA. Chemotherapy of third ventricle tumors. In: Appuzzo M, ed. Third ventricular tumors. Baltimore: Williams & Wilkins, 1987:838.
351. Schmidek HH, Waters A. Pineal masses: Clinical features and management. In: Wilkins RH, Rengachary SS, eds. Neurosurgery. New York: McGraw-Hill, 1985:688.
352. Pecker J, Scarabin J-M, Vallee B, et al. Treatment in tumours of the pineal region: Value of stereotaxic biopsy. Surg Neurol 1979;12:341.
353. Linstadt D, Wara WM, Edwards MSB, et al. Radiotherapy of primary intracranial germinomas: The case against routine craniospinal irradiation. Int J Radiat Oncol Biol Phys 1988;17:291.
354. Wara WM, Jenkin RDT, Evans A, et al. Tumors of the pineal and suprasellar region: Children's Cancer Study Group results, 1960–1975—a report from the Children's Cancer Study Group. Cancer 1979;43:698.
355. Jenkin RDT, Simpson WJK, Keen CW, et al. Pineal and suprasellar germinomas: Results of radiation treatment. J Neurosurg 1978;48:99.
356. Salazar OM, Castro-Vita H, Bakos RS, et al. Radiation therapy for tumors of the pineal region. Int J Radiat Oncol Biol Phys 1979;5:491.
357. Matsukado Y, Abe H, Tanaka R, et al. Cisplatin, vinblastine and bleomycin (PVB) combination chemotherapy in the treatment of intracranial malignant germ cell tumors—a preliminary report of a phase II study—The Japanese Intracranial Germ Cell Tumor Study Group. Gan No Rinsho 1986;32:1387.
358. Allen JC, Kim JH, Packer RJ. Neoadjuvant chemotherapy for newly diagnosed germ-cell tumors of the central nervous system. J Neurosurg 1987;67:65.
359. Jereb B, Zupancic N, Petric J. Intracranial germinoma: Report of seven cases. Pediatr Hematol Oncol 1990;7:183.
360. Mizuno M, Yoshida J, Noda S. Combined chemotherapy of CDDP and etoposide in intracranial germinomas. Gan To Kagaku Ryoho 1989;16:3457.
361. Miyamachi K, Aida T, Abe H. Five cases of primary intracranial germ cell tumor treated by combination chemotherapy with cisplatin. No Shinkei Geka 1988;16:1053.
362. Kobayashi T, Yoshida J, Sugita K, et al. Combination chemotherapy with cisplatin and etoposide for intracranial germ cell tumors [Abstract No. A5]. International Symposium on Pediatric Neuro-Oncology. June 1–3, 1989, Seattle, WA, 1989.
362a. Edwards MSB, Ablin A. Unpublished observations, 1987.
363. Wilson CB. Surgical management of endocrine-active pituitary adenomas. In: Walker MD, ed. Oncology of the nervous system. Boston: Martinus-Nijhoff, 1983:117.
364. Eastman RC, Gorden P, Roth J. Conventional supervoltage irradiation is an effective treatment for acromegaly. J Clin Endocrinol Metab 1979;48:931.
365. Sheline GE, Tyrrell JB. Pituitary tumors. In: Perez CA, Brady LW, eds. Principles and practice of radiation oncology. Philadelphia: JB Lippincott, 1987:1108.
366. Orth DN, Liddle GW. Results of treatment in 108 patients with Cushing's syndrome. N Engl J Med 1971;285:243.
367. Jennings AS, Liddle GW, Orth DN. Results of treating childhood Cushing's disease with pituitary irradiation. N Engl J Med 1977;297:957.
368. Grossman A, Besser GM. Prolactinomas. Br Med J 1985;290:182.
369. Kleinberg DL, Noel GL, Frantz AG. Galactorrhea: A study of 235 cases including 48 with pituitary tumors. N Engl J Med 1977;296:589.
370. Sheline GE, Grossman A, Jones AE, Besser GM. Radiation therapy of prolactinomas. In: Black PM, Zervas NT, Ridgway ED, Martin JB, eds. Secretory tumors of the pituitary gland. New York: Raven Press, 1984:1–35.
371. Halberg FE, Sheline GE. Radiotherapy of pituitary tumors. Endocrinol Metab Clin North Am 1987;16:667.
372. McCollough WM, Marcus RB Jr, Rhoton AL Jr, et al. Long-term follow-up of radiotherapy for pituitary adenoma: The absence of late recurrence after ≥ 4500 cGy. Int J Radiat Oncol Biol Phys 1991;21:607.
373. Feek CM, McLelland J, Seth J, et al. How effective is external pituitary irradiation for growth hormone secreting pituitary tumors? Clin Endocrinol 1984;20:401.
374. Coffey, RJ, Lunsford LD. The role of stereotactic techniques in the management of craniopharyngiomas. In: Rosanblum ML, ed. The role of surgery in brain tumor management. Philadelphia: WB Saunders, 1991:161.
375. Richmond IL, Wara WM, Wilson CB. Role of radiation therapy in the management of craniopharyngiomas in children. Neurosurgery 1980;6:513.
376. Sung DI, Chang CH, Harisiadis L, et al. Treatment results of craniopharyngiomas. Cancer 1981;47:847.
377. Fischer EG, Welch K, Belli JA, et al. Treatment of craniopharyngiomas in children, 1972–1981. J Neurosurg 1985;62:496.
378. Weiss M, Sutton L, Marcial V, et al. The role of radiation therapy in the management of childhood craniopharyngioma. Int J Radiat Oncol Biol Phys 1989;17:1313.
379. Wen B-C, Hussey DH, Staples J, et al. A comparison of the roles of surgery and radiation therapy in the management of craniopharyngiomas. Int J Radiat Oncol Biol Phys 1989;16:17.
380. Danoff BF, Cowchock FS, Kramer S. Childhood craniopharyngioma: Survival, local control, endocrine and neurologic function following radiotherapy. Int J Radiat Oncol Biol Phys 1983;9:171.
381. Carmel PW, Antunes J, Chang CH. Craniopharyngiomas in children. Neurosurgery 1982;11:382.
382. Thomsett MJ, Conte FA, Kaplan SL, Grumbach MM. Endocrine and neurologic outcome in childhood craniopharyngioma: Review of effect of treatment in 42 patients. J Pediatr 1980;97:728.
383. Cavazzuti V, Fischer EC, Welch K, et al. Neurological and psychophysiological sequelae following different treatments of craniopharyngiomas in children. J Neurosurg 1983;59: 409.
384. Jackler RK, Pitts LH. Acoustic neuroma. In: Rosenblum ML, ed. The role of surgery in brain tumor management. Neurosurg Clin North Am 1990;1:199.
385. Martuza RL, Ojemann RG. Bilateral acoustic neuromas: Clinical aspects, pathogenesis, and treatment. Neurosurgery 1982;10:1.
386. Wallner KE, Sheline GE, Pitts LH, et al. Efficacy of irradiation for incompletely excised acoustic neurilemomas. J Neurosurg 1987;67:858.
387. Flickinger JC, Lunsford LD, Coffey RJ, et al. Radiosurgery of acoustic neurinomas. Cancer 1991;67:345.
388. Farriro JB III, Hyams VL, Benke RH, et al. Carcinoid apudoma arising in glomus jugulare tumors. Laryngoscope 1980;90:110.
389. Simko TG, Griffin TW, Gerdes AJ, et al. The role of radiation therapy in the treatment of glomus jugulare tumors. Cancer 1978;42:104.
390. Gardner G, Cocke EW Jr, Robertson JT, et al. Glomus jugulare tumors: Combined treatment. I. J Laryngol Otol 1981;95:437.
391. Cummings BJ, Beale FA, Garrett PG, et al. The treatment of glomus tumors of the temporal bone by megavoltage radiation. Cancer 1984;53:2635.
392. Springate SC, Weichselbaum RR. Radiation or surgery for chemodectoma of the temporal bone: A review of local control and complications. Head Neck 1990;12: 303.
393. Million RR, Cassisi NJ. Chemodectomas (glomus body tumors). In: Million RR, Cassisi NJ, eds. Management of head and neck cancer. Philadelphia: JB Lippincott, 1984: 567.
394. Kim JA, Elkon D, Lim ML, et al. Optimum dose of radiotherapy for chemodectomas of the middle ear. Int J Radiat Oncol Biol Phys 1980;6:815.
395. Heffelfinger MJ, Dahlin DC, MacCarty CS, et al. Chordomas and cartilaginous tumors at the skull base. Cancer 1973;32:410.

396. Austin-Seymore M, Munzenrider J, Goitein M, et al. Fractionated proton radiation therapy of chordoma and low-grade chondrosarcoma of the base of the skull. J Neurosurg 1989;70:13.
397. Phillips T, Newman H. Chordomas. In: Deeley T, ed. Modern radiotherapy and oncology: Central nervous system tumors. Boston: Butterworths, 1974:184.
398. Berson AM, Castro JR, Petti P, et al. Charged particle irradiation of chordoma and chondrosarcoma of the base of skull and cervical spine: The Lawrence Berkeley Laboratory Experience. Int J Radiat Oncol Biol Phys 1988;15:559.
399. Sung DI, Chang CH, Harisiadis L. Cerebellar hemangioblastomas. Cancer 1982;49:553.
400. Smalley SR, Schomberg PJ, Earle JD, et al. Radiotherapeutic considerations in the treatment of hemangioblastomas of the central nervous system. Int J Radiat Oncol Biol Phys 1990;18:1165.
401. Naguib MG, Chou SH, Mastri A. Radiation therapy of a choroid plexus papilloma of the cerebellopontine angle with bone involvement. J Neurosurg 1981;54:245.
402. Ausman JI, Schrontz C, Chason J, et al. Aggressive choroid plexus papilloma. Surg Neurol 1984;22:472.
403. Carpenter DB, Michelsen WJ, Hays AP. Carcinoma of the choroid plexus: Case report. J Neurosurg 1982;56:722.
404. Connolly ES. Spinal cord tumors in adults. In: Youmans JR, ed. Youmans' neurological surgery. Philadelphia: WB Saunders, 1982:3196.
405. Wen B-C, Hussey DH, Hitchon PW, et al. The role of radiation therapy in the management of ependymomas of the spinal cord. Int J Radiat Oncol Biol Phys 1991;20:781.
406. Linstadt DE, Wara WM, Leibel SA, et al. Postoperative radiotherapy of primary spinal cord tumors. Int J Radiat Oncol Biol Phys 1989;16:1397.
407. Barone B, Elvidge A. Ependymomas: A clinical survey. J Neurosurg 1970;33:428.
408. Schuman R, Alvord E, Leech R. The biology of childhood ependymomas. Arch Neurol 1975;32:731.
409. Sloof J, Kernohan J, MacCarty C. Primary intramedullary tumors of the spinal cord and filum terminale. Philadelphia: WB Saunders, 1964.
410. Forman AD, Levin VA. Intraventricular therapy. In: Perry MC, ed. The chemotherapy source book. Baltimore: Williams & Wilkins, 1991:213.

Cancer: Principles & Practice of Oncology, Fourth Edition,
edited by Vincent T. DeVita, Jr., Samuel Hellman, Steven A. Rosenberg.
J.B. Lippincott Co., Philadelphia © 1993.

Philip A. Pizzo
David G. Poplack
Marc E. Horowitz
Daniel M. Hays
Larry E. Kun

CHAPTER **49**

Solid Tumors of Childhood

Despite their rarity, childhood cancers have enlightened the epidemiology, genetics, etiology, and treatment of pediatric and adult malignancies. There are, however, striking and important differences in the types of malignancies that occur in children or adults.

EPIDEMIOLOGY OF CHILDHOOD CANCER

Approximately 6500 to 7200 new cases of childhood cancer are diagnosed each year in the United States. Cancer is second only to accidents as the leading cause of death in children younger than 15 years of age. Table 49–1 lists the incidences of the most common childhood cancers. Leukemias and lymphomas comprise almost 48% of pediatric cancers, followed by tumors of the central nervous system (20%), the sympathetic nervous system, soft tissues, kidney, bone, liver, eye, and germ cells. These malignancies often have a high growth fraction and a propensity for rapid growth. Carcinomas are rare during childhood. Pediatric tumors are characterized by unique age peaks, and some have sex, genetic, race, and geographic predilections.

Age is important in pediatric cancer in at least three ways. First, as shown in Table 49–2, the predominant type of childhood cancer varies according to the age of the child. The incidence of several cancers peaks soon after birth (*e.g.*, neuroblastoma, retinoblastoma), suggesting the role of prenatal events, but the incidence of other tumors (*e.g.*, lymphomas, bone tumors) increases with age, suggesting that postnatal events are important. Second, histologically identical malignancies can behave differently at different ages. For example, neuroblastoma, the most common tumor of infancy, has an excellent prognosis if it occurs in infants younger than 1 year of age, but it has a dismal prognosis in older children. Whether these differences reflect biologic properties of the host or the tumor is an unresolved but important issue. Third, the age of the child at diagnosis may predict the tumor's malignant potential. For example, sacrococcygeal tumors rarely have malignant elements if they are diagnosed at birth. However, if diagnosis is delayed until after the child is 2 months old or older (because the mass is intrapelvic and not directly visible), 50% to 70% of these tumors are malignant.

Sex influences the incidence and outcome of certain pediatric cancers. Most pediatric neoplasms have a male predominance (see Table 49–1), although for some tumors, such as Ewing's sarcoma and rhabdomyosarcoma, this does not become apparent until after the age of 13 years. Teratomas are an exception, because almost 75% occur in girls, but their potential for malignancy is higher in boys.

Race influences the distribution and outcome of several pediatric cancers. The cancer rate for black children is approximately 20% less than that for white children. For example, Ewing's sarcoma rarely occurs in American and African blacks. Testicular cancer is unusual in black children, and the early age peak observed in white children with acute lymphocytic leukemia (ALL) is not observed in blacks. However, the prognosis for black children who do develop ALL appears to be worse than for white children, probably because of the predominance of T-cell leukemia in black patients.

During recent years, the geographic diversity of cancer has become better appreciated. For example, although Burkitt's lymphoma accounts for almost half of the childhood cancers in Uganda, it is rare outside of the "Burkitt's belt." Conversely, neuroblastoma appears to be exceedingly rare in the Burkitt's belt. Retinoblastoma accounts for only 1% of the childhood cancers in the United States but is far more common in India. Hepatic tumors, which are rare in the United States, are considerably more frequent in the Far East. The distribution of

TABLE 49–1. Incidence of Childhood Cancers

Malignancy	Rate (per million/y)	Ratio: Sex (M:F)	Ratio: Race (W:B)	Peak Age (y)
Leukemias				
Acute lymphocytic	24.7	1.3	2.4	2–5
Acute nonlymphocytic	5.0	1.2	1.0	<2
Lymphomas				
Non-Hodgkin's	9.3	2.9		6–16
Hodgkin's	7.5	3.0	1.6	>10
Central Nervous System Tumors				
Gliomas	13.4	>1.0	1.1	Constant
Medulloblastoma	4.9	1.6	0.8	5–10
Ependymoma	2.1	>1.0	2.6	<5
Solid Tumors				
Neuroblastoma	8.0	1.4	1.6	<3
Wilm's tumor	6.9	0.9	0.9	<5
Retinoblastoma	3.0	<1.0	0.8	<3
Rhabdomyosarcoma	3.7	>1.2	0.9	Bimodal: 2–6 and 14–18
Ewing's sarcoma	2.1	>1.0	>1.0	10–18
Osteosarcoma	3.1	>1.0	1.2	10–18
Primary hepatic	1.6	>1.3		Bimodal: <2 and >14
Germ cell teratoma	0.4	0.3	0.8	Bimodal: <2 and >14

Hodgkin's disease by subtype also appears to vary geographically, with the more aggressive varieties predominating in developing countries. Some of these differences reflect racial and genetic factors, whereas others are due to variations in the environment and various oncogenic cofactors, like Epstein-Barr virus (EBV), hepatitis B virus, and human T-cell lymphotropic virus (HTLV).

The most famous geographic cluster of childhood cancer was the putative concentration of childhood leukemia in a single parish in Niles, Illinois, in 1963. Several clusters have been described over the years to suggest an association of the malignancy with environmental factors (*e.g.*, viruses, chemical pollution). Most have not held up to detailed investigation, but the recent cluster of leukemia in Woburn, Massachusetts, implicating chemical water pollution is noteworthy and suggests the need for continuing vigilance and research.

Ecogenetics is the study of the interaction between environmental and genetic factors in carcinogenesis, particularly of genetic variations in response to environmental agents. Table 49–3 details environmental agents that interact with genetic traits or defects to produce a malignant phenotype. Environmental factors include chemicals, radiation, and viruses. The genetic predisposition may be created by a sporadic mutation or familial transmission.

GENETICS AND BIOLOGY

The importance of genes and inheritance is exemplified in many childhood cancers. In some families, several members are affected by the same tumor or by various types of cancers. Certain human tumors are clearly inheritable. For example, approximately 40% of retinoblastomas appear to be inherited as an autosomal dominant trait with high penetrance. Wilms' tumor and neuroblastoma may also be bilateral and inheritable. Despite this dominant pattern of transmission, it is gene loss that leads to malignancy. The genetic information in the "retinoblastoma locus" on chromosome 13q14 acts to suppress the development of retinoblastoma, and if both alleles are lost (*i.e.*, a recessive mutant), the normal suppression of this tumor is lost and retinoblastoma occurs. In familial retinoblastoma, a loss of both retinoblastoma alleles is transmitted, leading to the expression of disease. In patients who have one copy of the allele, which can effectively suppress the development of retinoblastoma, the mutation, loss, or inactivation of this allele produces retinoblastoma.

Similar modes of genetic oncogenesis appear to occur in patients with Wilms' tumor, osteosarcoma, hepatoblastoma, and rhabdomyosarcoma (Table 49–4). The Li-Fraumeni syndrome, in which there is an increased incidence of breast cancer and other malignancies in the mothers of some children with rhabdomyosarcoma or osteosarcoma, is associated with the loss of genetic material or mutation on chromosome 17 (p53 region).

Some genetic disorders are associated with an increased incidence of cancer. For example, children with trisomy 21 (Down's syndrome) have a 10-fold increase in the incidence of acute lymphocytic leukemia; those with Klinefelter's syndrome (*i.e.*, XXY) have a greater than 60-fold increase in their incidence of breast cancer. Patients with chromosome fragility and defective DNA repair (*e.g.*, xeroderma pigmentosa, Bloom's syndrome, Fanconi's anemia) have an increased risk of cancer.

TABLE 49–2. Predominant Pediatric Cancers by Age and Site

Tumors	*Newborn (<1 y)*	*Infancy (1–3 y)*	*Children (3–11 y)*	*Adolescents and Young Adults (12–21 y)*
Leukemias	Congenital leukemia AML AMMoL CML, juvenile	ALL AML CML, juvenile	ALL AML	AML ALL
Lymphomas	Very rare	Lymphoblastic	Lymphoblastic Undifferentiated	Lymphoblastic Undifferentiated (Burkitt's, Hodgkin's)
Solid Tumors				
Central nervous system	Medulloblastoma Ependymoma Astrocytoma Choroid plexus papilloma	Medulloblastoma Ependymoma Astrocytoma Choroid plexus papilloma	Cerebellar astrocytoma Medulloblastoma Astrocytoma Ependymoma Craniopharyngioma	Cerebellar astrocytoma Astrocytoma Craniopharyngioma Medulloblastoma
Head and neck	Retinoblastoma Rhabdomyosarcoma Neuroblastoma Multiple endocrine neoplasia	Retinoblastoma Rhabdomyosarcoma Neuroblastoma	Rhabdomyosarcoma Lymphoma	Lymphoma Rhabdomyosarcoma
Thoracic	Neuroblastoma Teratoma	Neuroblastoma Teratoma	Lymphoma Neuroblastoma Rhabdomyosarcoma	Lymphoma Ewing's Rhabdomyosarcoma
Abdominal	Neuroblastoma Mesoblastic nephroma Hepatoblastoma Wilms' (>6 mos)	Neuroblastoma Wilms' Hepatoblastoma Leukemia	Neuroblastoma Wilms' Lymphoma Hepatoma	Lymphoma Hepatocellular carcinoma Rhabdomyosarcoma
Gonadal	Yolk sac tumor of testis (endodermal sinus tumor) Teratoma Sarcoma Botryoides Neuroblastoma	Rhabdomyosarcoma Yolk sac tumor of testis Clear cell sarcoma kidney	Rhabdomyosarcoma	Rhabdomyosarcoma Dysgerminoma Teratocarcinoma, teratoma Embryonal carcinoma of testis Embryonal cell and endodermal sinus tumors of ovary
Extremity	Fibrosarcoma	Fibrosarcoma Rhabdomyosarcoma	Rhabdomyosarcoma Ewing's	Osteosarcoma Rhabdomyosarcoma Ewing's sarcoma

ALL, acute lymphoblastic leukemia; AML, acute myelogenous leukemia; AMMoL, acute myelomonocytic leukemia; CML, chronic myelogenous leukemia.

Many translocations specific for malignancies have been identified. Some translocations are associated with oncogenes (*MYC* and the 8:14 translocation of Burkitt's lymphoma), and some oncogenes are uniquely associated with certain tumors (*MYCN* [previously N-*myc*] in neuroblastoma). The genome of every normal cell contains at least 30 protooncogenes. Although the gene product of every oncogene is not known, it is apparent that some of their products play a role in the regulation of cell growth. The activation or mutation of oncogenes or their translocation next to sites important in growth regulation contribute to malignancy (Table 49–5). Although many of the examples in which alteration of growth factors and differentiation contribute to the expression of neoplasia have been in pediatric tumors, the genetic mechanism being elucidated has relevance for adult tumors (Table 49–6).

Certain pediatric tumors are frequently associated with congenital disorders, malformations, or syndromes (Table 49–7). Patients with these disorders should be followed with the awareness that they may be at risk for developing a cancer. Because congenital findings may be associated with an inheritable malignancy, such as retinoblastoma and multiple endocrine neoplasia syndromes, genetic counseling of the patient and family is important.

Genetic disorders that alter the immune system (*e.g.*, ataxia-telangiectasia, Wiskott-Aldrich syndrome) are associated with an increased risk of cancer. The increased occurrence of lymphoma in adult patients and leiomyomas and leiomyosarcomas in children with acquired immunodeficiency syndrome (AIDS) emphasizes the integral association between immunoregulation and cancer.

TABLE 49–3. Ecogenetics of Tumors of the Young

Environmental Agent	*Genetic Trait*	*Tumor or Outcome*
Ionizing radiation	Ataxia-telangiectasia with lymphoma	Radiation toxicity
	Retinoblastoma	Sarcoma
	Nevoid basal cell carcinoma syndrome	Basal cell carcinoma
Ultraviolet radiation	Xeroderma pigmentosum	Skin cancer, melanoma
	Cutaneous albinism	Skin cancer
	Hereditary dysplastic nevus syndrome	Melanoma
Stilbestrol	X0 Turner's syndrome	Adenosquamous endometrial carcinoma
Androgen	Fanconi's pancytopenia	Hepatoma
Iron	Hemochromatosis	Hepatocellular carcinoma
Tyrosine	Tyrosinemia	Hepatocellular carcinoma
Monosaccharides	Glycogen storage disease type I	Hepatic adenoma
Epstein-Barr virus?	Purtilo X-linked lymphoproliferative syndrome	Burkitt's and other lymphomas
Papillomavirus type 5	Epidermodysplasia verruciformis	Skin cancer

(Mulvihill JJ. Clinical genetics of pediatric cancer. In: Pizzo PA, Poplack DG, eds. Principles and practice of pediatric oncology. Philadelphia: JB Lippincott, 1993)

In addition to genetically mediated or transmitted factors, prenatal exposure to certain drugs or substances have been associated with a heightened risk for developing cancer. For example, the fetal alcohol or hydantoin syndromes have been associated with neuroblastoma, and prenatal exposure to diethylstilbestrol increases the risk for adolescent girls to develop a clear cell adenocarcinoma of the vagina.

Some pediatric tumors have the interesting biologic property of undergoing spontaneous regression. This is most common in neuroblastoma, but it has also been observed in retinoblastoma, histiocytosis, sacrococcygeal teratoma, and hepatoblastoma. Study of the genetic controls that affect this differentiation process are central to developing new treatment modalities for these neoplasms. For example, *MYCN* amplification correlates with the stage of neuroblastoma, and lowering *MYCN* expression in vitro with *cis*-retinoic acid causes differentiation of these cells into more mature neural cells. This suggests that future therapeutic strategies should focus on the differentiation of tumor cells rather than their destruction.

TABLE 49–4. Pediatric Malignancies With Recognized or Likely Recessive Genetic Alterations

Tumor	*Chromosomal Alterations*
Neuroblastoma	1p36
Embryonal tumors of Beckwith-Wiedemann syndrome	11p
Retinoblastoma	13q14
Osteosarcoma	13q14
Astrocytoma	17q12
Acoustic neuroma and meningioma	22
Meningioma	22

(Israel, MA. Cancer cell biology. In: Pizzo PA, Poplack DG, eds. Principles and practice of pediatric oncology. 2nd ed. Philadelphia: JB Lippincott, 1993)

UNUSUAL CLINICAL MANIFESTATIONS

Although most children with cancer come to medical attention because of growing masses, the signs and symptoms of cancer can sometimes be subtle, nonspecific, or confusing and can result in delays in diagnosis and treatment (see Table 49–7).

TABLE 49–5. Cancer-Associated Genes Implicated in Selected Pediatric Malignancies

Malignancy	*Genes*
Leukemia	p53, *ABL, FMS, KRAS, MYB, MYC, NRAS, SRC*
Lymphoma	*BCL, MYB, MYC, RAS*
Glioma	p53, *ERBB2, FES, MYB, MYC, NEU, NRAS, RAF, ROS, SIS*
Wilms' tumor	*WT1, MYB, MYCN*
Neuroblastoma	*MYB, MYC, MYCN, NRAS, SRC*
Retinoblastoma	*RB, MYCN, SRC*
Germ cell tumors	*HST, MYC, MYCN*
Rhabdomyosarcoma	p53, *FOS, KRAS, MYB, MYC, NRAS, REL, SRC*
Osteogenic sarcoma	*RB, MET, SIS, SRC*
Ewing's sarcoma	*DBL, ETS, MYC, RAF, SRC*
Peripheral neuroectodermal tumors	*ETS, MYC, RAF, SRC*

TABLE 49–6. Childhood Cancers Associated With Congenital Syndromes or Malformations

Syndrome or Anomaly	*Tumor*
Aniridia	Wilms' tumor
Hemihypertrophy	Wilms' tumor, hepatoblastoma, adrenocortical carcinoma
Genitourinary abnormalities (including testicle maldescent)	Wilms' tumor, Ewing's sarcoma, nephroblastoma, testicular carcinoma
Beckwith-Wiedemann syndrome	Wilms' tumor, neuroblastoma, adrenocortical carcinoma
Dysplastic nevus syndrome	Melanoma
Nevoid basal cell carcinoma syndrome	Basal cell carcinoma, medulloblastoma, rhabdomyosarcoma
Poland's syndrome	Leukemia
Trisomy 21 (Down's syndrome)	Leukemia, retinoblastoma
Blooms' syndrome	Leukemia, gastrointestinal carcinoma
Severe combined immune deficiency disease	EBV-associated B-lymphocyte lymphoma/leukemia
Wiscott-Aldridge syndrome	EBV-associated B-lymphocyte lymphoma
Ataxia-telangiectasia	EBV-associated B-lymphocyte lymphoma, gastric carcinoma
Retinoblastoma	Wilms' tumor, osteosarcoma, Ewing's sarcoma
Fanconi's anemia	Leukemia, squamous cell carcinoma
Multiple endocrine neoplasia syndromes (MEN-I, -II, -III)	Andenomas of islet cells, pituitary, parathyroid, and adrenal glands
	Submucosal neuromas of the tongue, lips, eyelids
	Pheochromocytomas, medullary carcinoma of the thyroid
	Malignant schwannoma, nonappendiceal carcinoid
Neurofibromatosis (von Recklinghausen's syndrome)	Rhabdomyosarcoma, fibrosarcoma, pheochromocytomas, optic glioma, meningioma

Several pediatric tumors are biologically active and produce a variety of oncofetal proteins and other substances that may have diagnostic or prognostic value. These indicators, listed in Table 49–8, are measured in serum or in urine. Only rarely do these substances directly affect the patient.

Some pediatric cancers may present with bilateral involvement (*e.g.,* Wilms' tumor, retinoblastoma), making thorough examination important before any surgical procedures are performed. Some nonmalignant processes can also be confused with a cancer (*e.g.,* histoplasmosis with lymphoma, osteomyelitis with bone tumors), and some cancers can mimic other malignancies (*e.g.,* neuroblastoma mimics ALL in the bone marrow or peripheral blood).

PROGNOSTIC FACTORS

Most pediatric cancers can be divided into good and poor prognostic categories. Although the stage, site, and extent of disease have provided the traditional means for classifying patients, additional refinements have been achieved using tumor histology, immunologic typing, and molecular analysis. The identification of risk groups permits therapy to be tailored so that patients likely to do well can receive less intensive and less toxic regimens, and more intensive therapies can be restricted to patients with a poorer prognosis. However, prognostic factors are dynamic and, in some cases, artificial, because improvements in therapy may modify or even nullify previously important risk factors.

Histologic variants of specific pediatric neoplasms have been recognized and correlated with prognosis. For example, Wilms' tumors can now be divided into favorable and unfavorable histologic variants, which correlate with prognosis; 57% of patients with unfavorable histology die of their tumors, compared with 7% of patients with favorable histology. Similar prognostic correlations can be achieved with immunologic classification; children with the common acute leukemia antigen, CALLA, on their lymphoblasts fare better than those lacking this antigen. Molecular analysis has determined the gene rearrangements in children with null cell leukemias, further clarifying the cell lineage and guiding treatment. Pathologic diagnosis and molecular analysis have become particularly important in defining the small, round cell tumors of childhood (*i.e.,* neuroblastoma, rhabdomyosarcoma, Ewing's sarcoma, lymphoma, peripheral neuroectodermal tumors), clarifying important prognostic features and directing new therapeutic approaches. For example, recognition that peripheral neuroepithelial tumors share a t(11;22) abnormality and an oncogene profile with Ewing's sarcoma, rather than with the histologically similar neuroblastoma, has helped to define appropriate treatment regimens.

MANAGEMENT OF PEDIATRIC TUMORS

The successful management of pediatric cancer requires a carefully orchestrated team of a pediatric oncologist; a surgeon; a radiotherapist; diagnostic specialists in radiology, nuclear medicine, pathology, and clinical laboratory data; pediatric, medical, and surgical subspecialty consultants; nurses; pharmacists; and the supportive care services of specialists in physical, respiratory, recreation, and occupational therapy. Because the child with cancer is under enormous physical and emotional stress, appropriate psychosocial resources for the patient and family are important for optimal therapy.

Therapy for certain pediatric tumors has become more specialized, raising the question of whether all children with cancer should be treated at pediatric cancer centers. The complexity of most treatment protocols and the support services necessary to deliver and monitor them has consistently demonstrated a significant survival advantage for children treated in a specialty center over those treated in a community hospital. An alternative is a shared management plan in which the daily primary care is coordinated by community physicians who work under the guidance of a specialty treatment center.

Although the major modalities of therapy—surgery, radiation, and chemotherapy—are the same for pediatric and adult neoplasms, several features distinguish their application in children.

TABLE 49–7. Nonspecific Clinical Findings Associated With or as the Sole Manifestation of a Childhood Cancer

Clinical Findings	*Tumor*
Eye or orbit	
Strabismus	Retinoblastoma
Leukokoria ("cat's eye")	Retinoblastoma
Heterochromia—anisocoria and Horner's syndrome	Neuroblastoma
Opsoclonus—myoclonus ("dancing eyes") or acute cerebellar encephalopathy	Neuroblastoma
Proptosis	Neuroblastoma, lymphoma, retinoblastoma, rhabdomyosarcoma
Chronic sinusitis or otitis media	Rhabdomyosarcoma, nasopharyngeal carcinoma
Chronic diarrhea (Verner-Morrison syndrome)	Neuroblastoma, MEN-II
Skin	
"Blueberry muffin" nodules	Neuroblastoma
Seborrheic dermatitis	Histiocytosis
Nodular "blueberry" lips	MEN-II
Hypertension	Neuroblastoma, carcinoid, APUD tumors, pheochromocytoma, Wilms'
Virilization	Hepatoblastoma, arrhenoblastoma, adrenal rest tumors, gonadoblastoma
Feminization	Chorioepithelioma, teratoma, hepatoblastoma, adrenal tumor, nongestational choriocarcinoma, embryonal cell carcinoma, granulosa thecal cell tumors

SURGERY

Two principles guide management. First, with rare exception, no child should be considered to have disease that is so far advanced that cure can be ruled out. Second, although there should be no hesitation to perform a radical procedure for cure, every attempt should be made to minimize disability and deformity. With the use of preoperative or neoadjuvant chemotherapy or radiation therapy, tumors resectable with difficulty or loss of function (*i.e.,* hepatoma, rhabdomyosarcoma) have been converted into more readily resectable lesions. Limb-sparing procedures provide important alternatives for children with extremity lesions and have become increasingly important with improvements in survival.

Attention should be given to the general principles of pediatric and cancer surgery. Care must be used to avoid excessive blood loss because the common tumors of childhood are large and vascular, originating in vascular organs (*e.g.,* hepatoma) or surrounding major blood vessels, such as the vena cava and aorta (*e.g.,* neuroblastoma, Wilms' tumor). Surgical technique must be meticulous, and presurgical planning must anticipate a vascular catastrophe. Blood replacement must be readily accomplished. If rapid transfusion is necessary, the blood should be warmed to 37°C and its pH

TABLE 49–8. Biological Markers for Pediatric Tumors

Tumors	*AFP*	*hCG*	*Ferritin*	*Catecholamines*	*NSE*	*LDH*	*Alkaline Phosphatase*	*Polyamine*	*Cystathionine*	*CEA*
Germ cell tumor	+	+				+				+
Liver tumor	+	+	+						+	+
Neuroblastoma			+	+	+	+			+	+
Ewing's sarcoma						+				
Osteosarcoma						+	+			
Medulloblastoma					+			+		
Lymphoma						+				

AFP, α_1-fetoprotein; hCG, human chorionic gonadotropin; NSE, neuron-specific enolase; LDH, lactate dehydrogenase; CEA, carcinoembryonic antigen; +, reported to be elevated in some or all patients with active disease.

buffered to 7.4 to avoid the potential for a cardiac arrest that can occur when large volumes of cold, relatively acid, bank blood (10°C, pH 7.0) are administered to the small child. The surgeon and anesthesiologist must be aware that what is considered insignificant blood loss in an adult may be life-threatening in a small child whose circulating blood volume is small. For example, the loss of 400 ml of blood in a 1-year-old child represents half of the child's blood volume.

Another important difference between children and adults is the greater heat loss that occurs when a child is anesthetized, primarily because of the proportionally large body surface area of children. Hypothermia, cardiac irritability, metabolic acidosis, and clotting abnormalities can result from excessive heat loss. To avoid this, the operating room and the child should be kept warm and monitored carefully.

RADIATION THERAPY

As with adults, the primary goal of radiation therapy in children is to deliver an effective tumoricidal dose while sparing as much normal tissue as possible. This goal is more difficult to achieve in young children because of potential growth retardation and second malignancies.

To deliver technically acceptable irradiation, careful treatment planning and simulation are essential, as is immobilization and sedation, particularly for the young or uncooperative child. Ketamine anesthesia is particularly useful in young children, especially for those who require multiple treatments.

Although children often tolerate the acute radiation reactions better than adults, late changes in skeletal and soft tissue development are important and unique consequences. Treatment planning should attempt to create symmetry wherever possible, particularly in visible areas, such as the head and neck, and in the spine. Inadequate attention to symmetric irradiation of growing bone results in abnormal development that may not become apparent until the child enters the pubertal growth phase (*e.g.*, vertebral asymmetry resulting in scoliosis). Soft tissues, teeth, and visual structures may fail to develop normally after irradiation. Decreased muscle mass can lead to imbalance and relative asymmetry. Blood vessels and other structures with the radiation field, such as the thyroid and pituitary glands, may develop imperfectly. Brain tissue is particularly susceptible to late effects, especially if radiation is combined with neurotoxic drugs like methotrexate. Similarly, radiation therapy may exacerbate chemotherapy-induced toxicities, such as doxorubicin-induced cardiomyopathy or cyclophosphamide-related hemorrhagic cystitis. The most sobering consideration is that therapeutic irradiation increases the risk of second tumors.

CHEMOTHERAPY

One of the most important differences between pediatric and adult neoplasms is their general chemosensitivity and the possibility that a cure can be attained with combination chemotherapy. Analyses confirm continued improvements during the last decade in the numbers of children with cancer who are being cured. The drugs used in children are usually the same as those used in adults. Combination chemotherapy is the rule, and for the most part, higher dosages of chemotherapeutic agents are employed in children (except newborns), because their tolerance of the acute side effects of chemotherapy is greater than that of adults. Many chemotherapeutic regimens in children consist of more intensive and frequent drug administrations, with less dose modifications for myelosuppression or infection, than in adults. However, appropriate dose adjustment and modification is necessary on a regular basis to account for the normal growth of children. Brain growth relative to body surface area is completed by the age of 3 years, and dosages of intrathecal drugs should have an upper limit based on age rather than body surface area.

Many chemotherapy regimens for children are given over prolonged periods, frequently from 1 to 3 years. Efforts are being directed at defining good-risk patients for whom shorter durations of therapy may suffice. Nonetheless, for many children extended courses of treatment are necessary. In attempting to adjust schedules so that school attendance and daily activities can be normal, many treatment protocols use oral drugs for patients who are receiving maintenance therapy. However, absorption of oral chemotherapy may result in decreased bioavailability of the chemotherapeutic agent, which can contribute to treatment failure, and children, particularly adolescents, may not take medications, necessitating careful monitoring of pediatric cancer patients.

Because long-term survival is achievable for children and because growing organs may be more susceptible to long-term damage, careful consideration must be given to the chemotherapeutic agents used in children. The magnitude of long-term complications from regimens administered a decade ago are only now being appreciated. The pediatric oncologist should anticipate the future impact of current strategies.

SUPPORTIVE CARE

The treatment program for the child with cancer cannot focus only on tumor reduction and the physical side effects of therapy. Every attempt must be made to ensure that the child survives as a functional member of the family and society, and a comprehensive support matrix must offer the child every opportunity to grow and mature as normally as possible. This requires a coordinated school program with educational monitoring and psychological counseling; psychosocial support for the patient, siblings, and family; and occupational recreational, and physical therapy.

WILMS' TUMOR

EPIDEMIOLOGY AND GENETICS

The annual incidence of Wilms' tumor is 7 per million children younger than 16 years of age, a statistic that varies little from one part of the world to another. One child in 10,000 develops Wilms' tumor. In 1991, approximately 460 new cases of Wilms' tumor occurred in the United States, accounting for 5% to 6% of childhood cancers. The tumor occurs equally in boys and girls worldwide, but a slight preponderance of girls was seen in the National Wilms' Tumor Study (NWTS). The median age at diagnosis in the NWTS experience was 39 months for patients with unilateral tumors and 26 months for those with bilateral tumor.

Congenital anomalies associated with Wilms' tumor include aniridia, hemihypertrophy, malformation of the genitalia (*e.g.*, cryptorchidism, hypospadias, pseudohermaphroditism, gonadal dysgenesis), the Beckwith-Wiedemann, Drash, and Perlman malformation syndromes, and neurofibromatosis.

Case reports and the records of the NWTS-1 document the occurrence of familial Wilms' tumor in about 1% of patients. The mode of inheritance is thought to be autosomal dominant with variable penetrance. According to the two-hit mutation model, the pathogenesis of Wilms' tumor lies in the loss of a functioning gene by mutations at homologous loci. Cytogenetic characterization of somatic and tumor cells from patients with Wilms' tumor has identified the location of this gene at band p13 of chromosome 11. Although the somatic cells of most patients are karyotypically normal, those with aniridia often have a deletion at 11p13 or half-normal levels of catalase, an enzyme mapped to that region of chromosome 11. This constitutional chromosomal abnormality, the first hit, may involve enough of the chromosome to be cytogenetically detectable, as is the case with associated aniridia, or may involve only a point mutation at the Wilms' tumor locus. A candidate recessive gene at 11p13 has been cloned and, unlike the genes in retinoblastoma, appears to be inactivated in only a subset of Wilms' tumors, especially those whose histopathology is reminiscent of intralobar nephroblastomatosis. It seems likely, based in detailed family studies, that more than a single gene is involved in the molecular pathogenesis of Wilms' tumor.

PATHOLOGY

Wilms' tumor usually presents as a large mass, the surface of which is smoother than the more irregular and nodular neuroblastoma. The tumor mass is often surrounded by a fibrous pseudocapsule composed of compressed, atrophic renal tissues and may contain cystic areas and necrosis and hemorrhage. Calcification is uncommon. The tumors are most often unicentric, but in the NWTS experience, 7% are multifocal in one kidney, and 5.4% involved both kidneys at the time of presentation or subsequently. Rarely, the tumor is extrarenal, occurring in the retroperitoneum, pelvis, or inguinal region. Local extension of tumor through the capsule and into the perinephric fat is common. Tumor invades the renal vein in 10% of patients, and tumor thrombus may extend to the right atrium. Spread to the lymph nodes of the renal hilum or the perinephric lymph nodes occurs in approximately 20% of patients and is prognostically unfavorable.

As a consequence of its derivation from the metanephric blastema, the histologic spectrum of Wilms' tumor is broad. The typical histologic pattern is triphasic, which includes blastemal, epithelial, and stromal cells, with undifferentiated spindle cells surrounding epithelial cell tubules of various sizes and shapes, sometimes forming abortive glomeruli. Biphasic patterns composed of stromal and blastemal cells and monophasic tumors consisting of one cell type are also encountered. A monophasic epithelial Wilms' tumor with papillary or tubular differentiation may be difficult to differentiate from an undifferentiated renal cell carcinoma. Because Wilms' tumor rarely poses a problem in recognition, ultrastructural and immunohistochemical studies, often essential for other childhood tumors, have little utility. Ultrastructurally, the tumor is characterized by numerous desmosomes, cilia, and distinctive flocculent densities surrounding the tumor cells.

There is a subgroup of patients with Wilms' tumor who have *anaplastic tumors*. Anaplasia is categorized as the presence of hyperdiploid mitotic figures, a threefold or greater nuclear enlargement or hyperchromasia of enlarged nuclei. Two sarcomatous variants, clear cell sarcoma and rhabdoid tumor, also confer poor prognoses. Anaplasia is recognized by hyperdiploid miotic features, threefold or greater nuclear enlargement, and hyperchromasia of enlarged nuclei. Even a single focus of anaplasia correlates with an adverse prognosis. These histologic markers of hyperploidy have been supported by flow cytoflurometric studies of DNA content in Wilms' tumors. Anaplasia occurs in approximately 5% of the tumors, is rare (2%) in children younger than 2 years, and increasingly frequent in older children, until the incidence reaches 13% in those older than 5 years. Relapses were seen in 27 (55%) of 49 NWTS-1 and NWTS-2 stage I, II, and III children with anaplastic tumors, and relapses occurred in 101 (14%) of 720 patients with nonanaplastic or "favorable histology" tumors. Stage I patients with anaplastic tumors do as well as those with histologically favorable tumors.

Clear cell sarcoma of the kidney, a distinct entity, occurs in the same age group as Wilms' tumor, but it has a poorer prognosis, with relapse common even in the stage I patients. The tumor consists of nests of polygonal to stellate cells with small nuclei, inconspicuous nucleoli, and pale vesicular cytoplasm, which form cords separated by a fine vascular network. This variant of Wilms' tumor has been associated with a high rate of skeletal metastasis and was originally called the "bone-metastasizing renal tumor of childhood."

Rhabdoid tumor of the kidney is a monomorphous tumor with cells containing prominent acidophilic cytoplasm, similar to rhabdomyoblasts, but it does not contain ultrastructural features of muscle and immunohistochemical markers. This tumor is not associated with rhabdomyosarcoma. The cell of origin is unknown, and it may occur outside the kidney. The median age at diagnosis of the cases seen in the NWTS was 13 months (range, 2 months to 5 years). Simultaneous primitive neuroectodermal tumors of the brain have developed in children with this variant. The outlook for children with rhabdoid tumor of the kidney is poor. Fewer than 20% of the patients survive, and aggressive chemotherapy has not altered this.

Nephroblastomatosis, a small cluster of blastemal cells, tubules, or stromal cells that is usually situated at the periphery of the renal lobe is thought to be the precursor lesion of Wilms' tumor. Its presence in a kidney biopsy specimen demands close follow-up to detect possible evolution of bilateral Wilms' tumor.

Congenital mesoblastic nephroma is a tumor of the newborn or young infant. It is composed of bundles of spindle cells with an interdigitating margin that extends into the renal parenchyma. Although these tumors are usually curable by surgery alone, there are subtypes that contain more cystic components and have a higher mitotic index, indicating a metastatic potential. The tumor has been diagnosed in utero by ultrasound and may be associated with polyhydramnios. This tumor is curable by a standard surgical approach that results in a histologically proven complete resection. Rarely, the tumor may infiltrate the perirenal structures, including the liver. Care must be taken in the resection of tumor infringing on the capsule of the liver, because hemostasis may be difficult to achieve and uncontrollable bleeding may result.

CLINICAL PRESENTATION AND NATURAL HISTORY

Wilms' tumor most frequently presents as an asymptomatic flank or abdominal mass, usually detected on a routine physical examination or discovered by parents when bathing the child. The differential diagnosis includes hydronephrosis, neuroblastoma, and other tumors that present with an abdominal component or organomegaly, such as leukemia, lymphoma, and hepatoma. Wilms' tumor is rare after the age of 7 years. A characteristic presentation of rapid abdominal enlargement, anemia, hypertension, and occasionally, fever with egg-shell calcification visible on plain x-ray films has been attributed to sudden subcapsular hemorrhage. Of 164 patients, 68% presented with abdominal mass, 29% with abdominal pain, 26% with hematuria, 18% with fever, and 14% with anorexia. Elevated blood pressure affects approximately 25% of patients and is caused by elevated renin.

On physical examination, the abdominal mass of Wilms' tumor is smoother in outline and usually more confined to one side of the abdomen than the irregular and nodular mass of neuroblastoma (Table 49–9). However, Wilms' tumor may be bilateral or may grow large enough that it can be felt on both sides of the abdomen. Tumor involvement can be extensive, with infiltration through the renal capsule or invasion into the renal vein (8–40%) through the vena cava to the heart.

Metastatic disease is evident at diagnosis in approximately 15% of patients with Wilms' tumor. The most common sites of hematogenous metastasis are the lung (85%) and liver (15%). Brain metastasis is a rare form of recurrence. With the exception of those with clear cell sarcoma, bone metastasis is uncommon. The regional lymph nodes are involved in 15% to 25% of patients. Positive nodes are associated with unfavorable histology (*i.e.*, anaplasia) and a relatively poor prognosis. For patients with node-positive Wilms' tumor of a favorable histologic pattern, the mortality rate is 17%, compared with a 97% survival rate for patients with negative nodes.

EVALUATION

The child with an abdominal mass should be examined thoroughly to arrive at the most likely preoperative diagnosis, assess the local and distant extent of the tumor, and prepare the patient for surgery.

Physical evaluation for evidence of concomitant congenital anomalies should be sought (see Table 49–9). Distended ab-

TABLE 49–9. Characteristic Features of Wilms' Tumor and Neuroblastoma

Characteristic Features	*Wilms' Tumor*	*Neuroblastoma*
Age at presentation	3.6 y (rare before 6 mo)	<2 y (most common tumor of infancy)
Associated congenital anomalies	Aniridia, hemihypertrophy, genitourinary abnormalities	Rare: Beckwith-Wiedemann syndrome, nisidioblastosis, von Recklinghausen's syndrome
Clinical presentation	Smooth, bulging flank mass; may enlarge rapidly; usually confined to one side	Firm and irregular flank mass frequently crossing the midline of abdomen, often fixed
Radiologic findings	Intrarenal mass with calyceal distortion and displacement but little change in axis of the kidney	Outward and downward displacement of kidney, "dropping lily," with microcalcifications
Tumor markers	None	Vanillylmandelic acid, homovanillic acid, catechols, ferritin, neuron-specific enolase
Metastases	Lungs, lymph nodes, liver, brain, bone (rare)	Liver, bone, bone marrow, lymph nodes

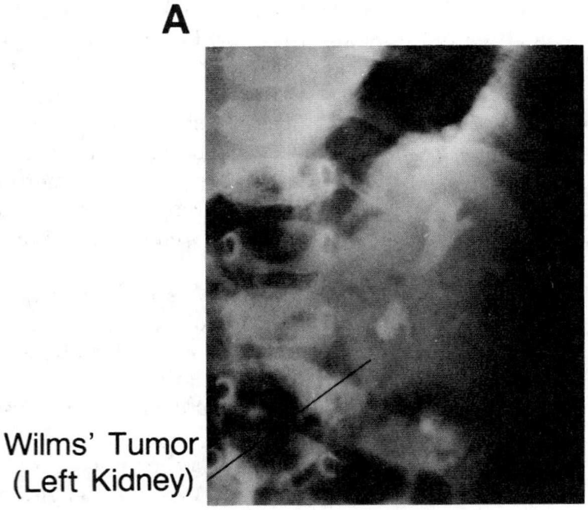

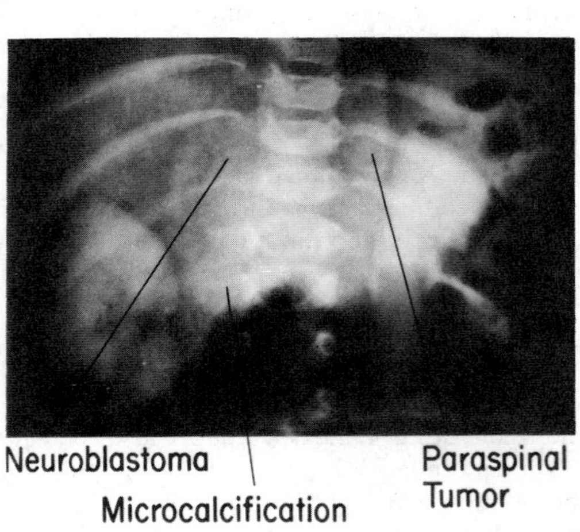

dominal veins may indicate occlusion of the inferior vena cava by tumor thrombus. Routine laboratory studies should also include tests for urine catecholamines. The most sensitive tests are not necessarily the best because the successful treatment of Wilms' tumor is founded on the chest x-ray films and intravenous pyelograms (IVP). Abdominal ultrasound can provide an accurate assessment of the mass and detect tumor thrombi in renal veins. Ultrasound can delineate tumor extension to the inferior vena cava or right atrium. Abdominal computed tomography (CT) provides the most precise means to assess the tumor. Magnetic resonance imaging (MRI) is useful for diagnosing and staging Wilms' tumor and may replace other techniques because it is noninvasive and does not employ ionizing radiation.

The metastatic workup should include four-view chest x-ray films. The use of lung CT is controversial and not advocated by the NWTS for low-risk children. Should a patient with low-stage disease whose only site of metastasis is a lung nodule, visible on CT scan but not chest x-ray films, be upstaged and treated more aggressively? There are no data to support such an approach, and most stage I and II patients assessed by chest x-ray films alone are cured. Moreover, focal atelectasis or granulomas are indistinguishable from metastatic tumor. Treatment for stage IV patients with lung disease includes irradiation of the entire thorax; whether patients with lung metastases demonstrated only by CT scan require this therapy is unknown. A decision analysis concluded that there was no advantage in routine chest CT scans and the NWTS Committee does not recommend this for low-risk children. Postoperatively, patients with a histologic diagnosis of clear cell sarcoma should be staged with bone scan and CT of the brain. This is unnecessary for other variants of Wilms' tumor. The diagnosis of rhabdoid tumor of the kidney warrants brain CT because of its association with brain metastases and primary brain tumors.

STAGING AND PROGNOSTIC FACTORS

A clinicopathologic grouping that determined the extent of tumor at diagnosis and surgery was used in NWTS-1 and NWTS-2. Analysis of these clinical trials resulted in the staging system shown in Table 49–10. Unfavorable histologic types, distant metastasis, and lymph node involvement continue to affect prognosis adversely. Conversely, analysis of NWTS-3 indicated that children younger than 2 years of age who had stage I tumors smaller than 250 g with favorable histology had the best outcome.

TREATMENT

The advances in treating Wilms' tumor reflect integration of improved methods of surgery, radiation therapy, and chemotherapy. Optimal treatment of the patient requires that the pediatric, radiation, and surgical oncologists begin to coordinate their efforts during the initial diagnostic and staging workup.

TABLE 49–10. Staging Systems for Wilms' Tumor

*Clinical Grouping (NWTS-1 and NWTS-2)**	*Clinical Staging (NWTS-3)*
I. Tumor limited to the kidney and completely resected. The surface of the renal capsule is intact. The tumor was not ruptured before or during removal. There is no residual tumor apparent beyond the margins of resection.	I. Tumor limited to the kidney and completely resected. The surface of the renal capsule is intact. The tumor was not ruptured before or during removal. There is no residual tumor apparent beyond the margins of excision.
II. Tumor extends beyond the kidney but is completely resected. There is local extension of the tumor: penetration beyond the pseudocapsule into the perirenal soft tissues or periaortic lymph node involvement. The renal vessel outside the kidney substance is infiltrated or contains tumor thrombus. There is no residual tumor apparent beyond the margins of resection.	II. Tumor extends beyond the kidney but is completely excised. There is regional extension of the tumor: penetration through the outer surface of the renal capsule into the perirenal soft tissues. Vessels outside the kidney substance are infiltrated or contain tumor thrombus. The tumor may have been biopsied or there has been local spillage of tumor confined to the flank. There is no residual tumor apparent at or beyond the margins of excision.
III. Residual nonhematogenous tumor confined to the abdomen. Any of the following may occur:	III. Residual nonhematogenous tumor confined to the abdomen. Any of the following may occur:
A. The tumor has ruptured before or during surgery, or a biopsy has been performed.	A. Lymph nodes on biopsy are found to be involved in the hilus, the periaortic chains, or beyond.
B. Implants are found on peritoneal surfaces.	B. There has been diffuse peritoneal contamination by the tumor such as by spillage of tumor beyond the flank before or during surgery, or by tumor growth that has penetrated through the peritoneal surface.
C. Lymph nodes are involved beyond the abdominal periaortic chains.	C. Implants are found on the peritoneal surfaces.
D. The tumor is completely resectable because of local infiltration into vital structures.	D. The tumor extends beyond the surgical margins either microscopically or grossly.
	E. The tumor is not completely resectable because of local infiltration into vital structures.
IV. Hematogenous metastases. Deposits beyond group III in lung, liver, bone, and brain.	IV. Hematogenous metastases. Deposits beyond stage III in lung, liver, bone, and brain.
V. Bilateral renal involvement either initially or subsequently.	V. Bilateral renal involvement at diagnosis. An attempt should be made to stage each side according to the above criteria on the basis of extent of disease before biopsy.

* The clinical group (stage) is defined by the surgeon in the operating room and is confirmed by the pathologist. In NWTS, patients are categorized by stage and histology (favorable or unfavorable).

Surgery

The goal of surgery is to remove the primary tumor, even if there are distant metastases. Two questions require consideration preoperatively. Is the mass too large for safe resection without tumor rupture? Is there any evidence for bilateral involvement?

Approximately 5% to 15% of patients have tumors that are too large for safe primary surgical resection. These tumors cross the midline, appear to be fixed to adjacent structures, or are not visualized on IVP. In the past, radiation therapy was used to achieve preoperative tumor shrinkage, and although it was effective, it frequently delayed surgery. Preoperative chemotherapy (1.0 mg/m^2 of vincristine for infants and 1.5 mg/m^2 for children, administered every 5–7 days) can substantially shrink the tumor mass in 80% of patients within 2 to 3 weeks, making subsequent surgery safe and effective.

If preoperative chemotherapy or radiation therapy is being considered, a definitive diagnosis should first be established by a needle biopsy or an open biopsy through a small retroperitoneal incision. Biopsy by one of these methods minimizes the possibility of tumor contaminating the entire abdominal cavity and eliminates the possibility of a false diagnosis and unnecessary therapy.

The possibility of bilateral Wilms' tumors (5% of cases) should be determined preoperatively. The prognosis for patients with bilateral disease is good (approximately an 87% survival rate), even if the tumors are not entirely resectable. Surgery should remove all tumor only if adequate renal parenchyma can be left on one or both sides. Treatment for bilateral Wilms' tumor should be individualized, and many different approaches have been successful. For example, in patients with a large tumor on one side and a small tumor on the other, nephrectomy is indicated for the larger lesion and partial nephrectomy for the smaller one. In patients with two large primary tumors, biopsy followed by chemotherapy and second-look surgery and, if possible, resection of the residual tumors should be considered. Bilateral nephrectomy and renal transplant has not been especially successful, and this approach is indicated only if all other measures have failed.

In patients deemed surgically resectable, good exposure should be obtained with a generous transabdominal incision that, if necessary, should extend into the thorax. The renal vein should be ligated before beginning extensive dissection, although this does not appear to affect prognosis. Avoid rupture of the tumor during surgery because operative spill, which occurs in 16% of cases, appears to increase the risk of abdominal recurrence. This liability may be overcome if the peritoneal surfaces are irradiated after the spill. Perhaps the greatest hazard in the resection of Wilms' tumor is hemorrhage due to injury to the vena cava. The vena cava should be isolated above and below the tumor so that damage to it can be quickly controlled. Tumors that invade the liver capsule usually are totally resectable, because they rarely penetrate deeply into the liver parenchyma.

After the tumor is removed with a long segment of ureter, the hilar and local paraaortic lymph nodes should be biopsied, and any enlarged or suspicious nodes should be removed. Although lymph node biopsy is important in staging, retroperitoneal lymph node dissection is not of proven value and has potential morbidity.

Tumor extending into the vena cava can usually be removed with venotomy and traction. If the tumor segment in the inferior vena cava is completely obstructed, it is best left in situ. If the tumor embolus extends into the heart, a median sternotomy and midline abdominal incision provides exposure of the right atrium and the intrapericardial portion of the inferior vena cava. Extracorporeal circulation is necessary in these cases. Intracardiac extension of Wilms' tumor of favorable histology does not impact adversely on survival. If resection is not possible, shrinkage with chemotherapy or radiation therapy should be pursued and patients managed as if stage III.

For large or hemorrhagic tumors, surgical resection may be accomplished more effectively after embolization of the renal artery with Gelfoam particles, which reduce renal vascularity and shrink tumor bulk. This procedure should be considered if the patient presents with gross hematuria but has a resectable primary tumor.

During surgery, the contralateral kidney should be carefully examined after it has been mobilized and its capsule has been opened. If, after resection of the primary tumor, an easily removable contralateral lesion is found, it should be excised if sufficient renal tissue can be left behind to maintain renal function. If this cannot be safely guaranteed, the contralateral nodule should be biopsied.

The liver and the remainder of the abdomen should be inspected for metastases, and the tumor bed or areas of extension or residual disease should be outlined with metallic clips. Although tumor resection is important, a small volume of residual tumor does not appear to adversely affect prognosis. Heroic efforts to remove the last vestiges of tumor are not indicated.

Surgical extirpation of pulmonary nodules is beneficial if the resection can be accomplished without compromising pulmonary function. Similarly, surgical resection has been successful in eradicating liver and brain metastases.

Radiation Therapy

The role of radiation therapy has become more sharply defined in recent years. Improved chemotherapy has eliminated postoperative irradiation for early-stage disease. Radiation therapy is used conservatively because of the toxic effects of large irradiation fields in very young children. There is a potential for growth disturbances, and hepatic, pulmonary, or cardiac damage can result from irradiation used in conjunction with chemotherapy. Because of the anticipated long survival of patients with Wilms' tumor, there is appropriate concern about the risk of developing second malignancies.

Radiation therapy has been effective in virtually eliminating abdominal failure because of microscopic or gross residual disease. In conjunction with chemotherapy, irradiation has achieved a high proportion of disease control in cases with pulmonary metastases. Preoperative radiation therapy had proven the value of diminishing large tumors before resection, diminishing operative spill and improving disease-free survival. The efficacy and reduced toxicity of preoperative chemotherapy has supplanted preoperative radiation.

The use of postoperative radiation therapy is dictated by operative stage and histology. The NWTS-1 and NWTS-2 trials showed that postoperative radiation therapy is not necessary for stage I patients, regardless of age, who have favorable histologic patterns, if they are treated with adjuvant vincristine and dactinomycin. Results from NWTS-3 demonstrated that stage II patients with favorable histology did not benefit from radiation therapy. Neither stage I or II patients with favorable histology require postoperative radiation therapy.

Patients with favorable stage III tumors (and some include stage II patients with intraoperative spillage), based on NWTS-3 findings, should receive limited (*e.g.*, 1080 cGy) postoperative radiation with the addition of doxorubicin (Adriamycin) to the vincristine plus dactinomycin regimen.

Postoperative radiation therapy is recommended for all patients with unfavorable histologic patterns, regardless of stage, and for patients with stage IV tumors. Abdominal treatment in stage IV presentations should be defined by the extent of abdominal disease. Radiation treatment of pulmonary metastases is independent of "abdominal stage."

Radiation therapy ports should be tailored to the extent of disease found at surgery. Whole-abdominal irradiation is used only in patients with abdominal spill (Fig. 49–1). Residual disease or documented lymph node involvement requires tumor bed irradiation, usually as hemiabdominal therapy, to encompass the initial tumor and paraaortic volume. It is important to include the full width of the vertebrae, to encompass the retroperitoneal nodes, and to avoid asymmetric closure of the vertebral epiphyses.

Radiation to extrarenal and extraabdominal sites has been integrated into treatment planning for patients with stage IV Wilms' tumor. Patients with pulmonary metastases should receive doxorubicin with 1200 cGy of whole-lung irradiation, with only the growth centers of the humeri blocked. If this treatment follows abdominal or renal fossa irradiation, care must be taken to avoid normal tissues, such as the remaining kidney or liver. Patients with hepatic, brain, or bone involvement are treated with irradiation.

Chemotherapy

Wilms' tumor was found to be responsive to dactinomycin in the 1960s. Other active agents include vincristine, doxorubicin, cyclophosphamide, and cisplatin, which have response rates of 63%, 60%, 27%, and 16%, respectively. Successive studies by single institutions, collaborative groups, and the NWTS have identified the following principles of treatment:

1. *Stage I with favorable histology or anaplastic and stage II with favorable histology:* Chemotherapy with dactinomycin and vincristine is superior to either alone. Radiation therapy is not needed.
2. *Stage III with favorable histology and stage IV with favorable histology:* Chemotherapy with dactinomycin, vincristine, and doxorubicin and postoperative irradiation.
3. *Stage II, III, and IV anaplastic tumors:* Chemotherapy with dactinomycin, vincristine, doxorubicin, and possibly cyclophosphamide (pending results from NWTS IV) and postoperative irradiation.
4. *Stage I through IV clear cell sarcoma:* Chemotherapy with doxorubicin, vincristine, and dactinomycin and irradiation.
5. *Stage V (bilateral) Wilms' tumor:* The goal is to preserve enough functioning renal parenchyma, usually by removing the kidney with the major involvement and only a portion of the less affected kidney. Bilateral nephrectomy and kidney transplantation is a last resort. Postoperative radiation therapy should be considered for both renal fossae, although lack of residual disease may make this unnecessary. The adjuvant schedules and radiation treatment should be dictated by the histology and extent of residual disease.

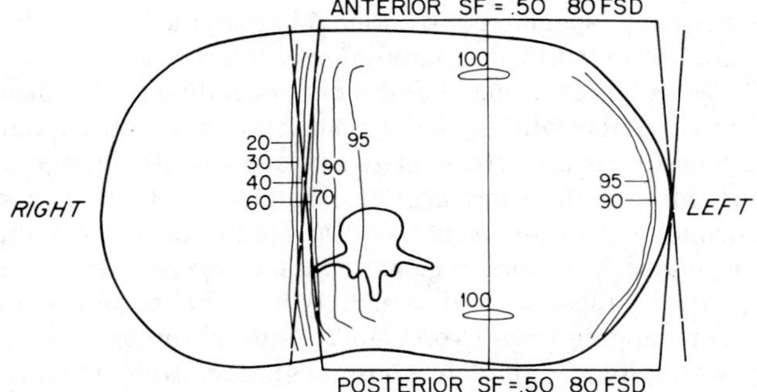

FIGURE 49–1. Dosimetry for hemiabdominal irradiation. Notice inclusion of the paraaortic lymph nodes and full width of the vertebral body within the 90% volume. Dosimetry depicts dose configuration for a field identical but contralateral to that shown.

The results of NWTS-3 are summarized in Table 49–11. Because relapse after 2 years from diagnosis is rare, most disease-free children at this point are cured. NWTS-4, now underway, will determine if there is an advantage to single-dose or divided-dose dactinomycin and doxorubicin. It will also evaluate a 6-month treatment for patients with stage II, III, or IV tumors. The International Society of Pediatric Oncology (SIOP) focused on the preoperative treatment of Wilms' tumor with radiation therapy or with chemotherapy. Results have been excellent. The group found that residual tumor at the time of surgery is a negative prognostic indicator.

The acute and long-term toxic effects of therapy have influenced treatment. Seventeen toxic deaths in NWTS-2 resulted primarily from leukopenia (7) and liver failure (41). Because 4 of 47 infants (<1 year old) died of leukopenia, chemotherapy doses have been decreased by 50% for this age group. Long-term side effects of the disease and its treatment include cardiomyopathy caused by the interaction between doxorubicin and radiation, skeletal growth disturbances after irradiation, and radiation-induced nephritis in the remaining kidney.

Most children in the United States with Wilms' tumor are treated on the NWTS. Although almost 90% of Wilms' tumor patients are curable and tolerate therapy well, the child with this disease deserves to be managed by a team experienced in pediatric cancer.

NEUROBLASTOMA

Neuroblastoma represents frustration and hope to those who treat cancer in children. Cure is elusive for most children (>1 year old) with this disease who present with disseminated tumor. Despite improved chemotherapeutic regimens that can effect complete responses, recurrence is common in older patients. However, because the molecular genetics of this tumor are better understood than most other human cancers, there is an implicit promise of more effective and less toxic treatments.

TABLE 49–11. Results in Randomized NWTS-3 Patients

Stage/ Histology	*Regimen*	*No. of Patients*	*4-Year Survival* Relapse-Free (%)		Overall (%)	
I/FH	AMD + VCR (10 wk)	306	89.0	$p = 0.19$	95.6	$p = 0.15$
I/FH	AMD + VCR (6 mo)	301	91.8		97.4	
II/FH	AMD + VCR (+RT)	70	90.0	$p = 0.89$	91.1	$p = 0.73$
II/FH	AMD + VCR (−RT)	67	87.4		94.9	
II/FH	AMD + VCR + ADR (+RT)	71	86.9		89.6	
II/FH	AMD + VCR-ADR (−RT)	70	87.9		93.6	
III/FH	AMD + VCR (1000 cGy)	71	71.4	$p = 0.22$	85.2	$p = 0.90$
III/FH	AMD + VCR (2000 cGy)	70	76.8		85.1	
III/FH	AMD + VCR-ADR (1000 cGy)	68	82.0		90.9	
III/FH	AMD + VCR-ADR (2000 cGy)	66	85.9		86.7	
IV/FH	AMD + VCR + ADR	64	71.9	$p = 0.43$	78.4	$p = 0.29$
IV/FH	AMD + VCR + ADR + CPM	56	77.9		86.6	
I-III/UH	AMD + VCR + ADR	69	67.1	$p = 0.86$	68.3	$p = 0.88$
I-III/UH	AMD + VCR + ADR + CPM	61	62.4		68.4	
IV/UH	AMD + VCR + ADR	12	58.3	$p = 0.70$	58.3	$p = 0.69$
IV/UH	AMD + VCR + ADR + CPM	17	52.9		52.9	

FH, favorable histology; UH, unfavorable histology; AMD, dactinomycin; VCR, vincristine; ADR, doxorubicin; CPM, cyclophosphamide; *p* values indicate results of test for the two or four regimens in brackets.
(Green DM, et al. Wilms' tumor [nephroblastoma, renal embryoma]. In: Pizzo PA, Poplack DG, eds. Principles and practice of pediatric oncology. 2nd ed. Philadelphia: JB Lippincott, 1993)

EPIDEMIOLOGY AND GENETICS

Neuroblastoma is the fourth most common pediatric malignancy, with an annual incidence of 10 cases per million children. In the United States, it comprises 8% to 10% of cancers diagnosed in children under 15 years of age or approximately 525 new cases annually. The incidence is significantly less in African than in American black children, raising the possibility that environmental factors are important and may be responsible for the increased incidence of neuroblastoma between 1943 and 1980. Alcohol, hair-coloring products, and certain medicines used during pregnancy may be prenatal risk factors for neuroblastoma, but none have been confirmed.

The median age at diagnosis of neuroblastoma is approximately 2 years. Half of all malignancies diagnosed in the first month of life and a third during the first year are neuroblastoma. The mortality of neuroblastoma occurring in the first year of life is far lower than that in the older child, suggesting the unique biology of this tumor. Microscopic nodules of primitive neuroblasts, usually larger than 3 mm and occasionally invading blood vessels, referred to as "neuroblastoma in situ," have been observed at autopsy in infants dying before 3 months old of other causes at 40 to 200 times the expected incidence. Autopsy examination of the adrenal glands of 92 18-week to 20-week fetuses demonstrated "neuroblastoma in situ" in all. It is clear that a normal phase in the embryogenesis of the adrenal gland, which is histologically similar to neuroblastoma, may persist into the first year of life. It is not understood how this relates to the observed spontaneous regression of neuroblastoma, especially stage IVS, or to the high rate of cure of the less than 1-year-old infant with a tumor indistinguishable from the usually fatal lesion seen in older children.

Molecular geneticists are studying neuroblastoma as a paradigm for elucidating the biology of differentiation and its relation to oncogenesis. The two-hit hypothesis, which postulates that malignancy is a function of prezygotic and postzygotic mutations, may be relevant to neuroblastomas. Neuroblastoma has been associated with the genetic diseases neurofibromatosis, Beckwith-Wiedemann syndrome (*i.e.*, omphalocele, macroglossia, visceromegaly, neonatal hypoglycemia), nisidiroblastosis, and trisomy 18 and with teratogenic syndromes caused by in utero exposure to alcohol and hydantoins. These associations are rare, indicating that they may be coincidental. Although familial neuroblastoma, characterized by multiple primaries, very young age at presentation (*i.e.*, 9 months versus 22 months for neuroblastoma in the general population), and autosomal dominant inheritance, is uncommon, its existence establishes that a germline mutation may promote tumorigenesis. Siblings and offspring of nonfamilial neuroblastoma patients are at low risk for developing the disease. A specific constitutional karyotypic abnormality has not been identified in familial neuroblastoma.

Progress has been made in the understanding of the chromosomal abnormalities of the neuroblastoma cell. Human neuroblastomas are characterized cytogenetically by partial monosomy for the short arm of chromosome 1 (1p−) and abnormality of chromosome 17. Double-minutes (DM) and homogeneously staining regions (HSR), cytogenetic evidence of gene amplification, and variability in modal chromosome number, ranging from hypodiploidy (<46 chromosomes) to hypertetraploidy (>92 chromosomes), are evident. Chromosome 1 abnormalities, specifically deletions at 1p22, are a common feature of a diverse group of pediatric solid tumors. The amplified genes identified within neuroblastoma cells as HSR and DM are designated as *MYCN* (previously designated

N-*myc* and homologous to v-*myc*). This gene is normally present in a single copy on chromosome 2. The number of copies of the *MYCN* oncogene is related to the clinical aggressiveness of the tumor and is a prognostic indicator independent of stage and age, the number of copies does correlate with the stage of the tumor and progression-free survival at 18 months from diagnosis. Amplification of *MYCN* has been detected in 30% of untreated neuroblastomas. Amplification can be detected in 5% to 10% of patients with low stages of disease or IVS and 30% to 40% of those with more advanced stages. The *MYCN* copy number is an intrinsic biologic property of each patient's tumor, remaining consistent within the tumor, in tumors at different sites, and over time, uninfluenced by treatment. The product of *MYCN* gene is yet to be identified, but it is probably related to the growth of the neuroblastoma cell.

Other oncogenes implicated in pathogenesis include *RAS*, identified initially in human neuroblastoma cell line SK-N-SH, and *SRC*, which expresses the enzyme tyrosyl kinase. Expression of *HRAS* (previously Ha-*ras*) appears to correlate with lower stage of disease and more differentiated tumors.

The DNA index of neuroblastoma cells, analyzed by flow cytometry, has been shown by investigators at St. Jude Children's Research Hospital to correlate with outcome. Tumors that are hyperdiploid are more likely to have lower stages of disease and be more chemotherapy responsive than those with a diploid DNA index.

The status of the immune system in patients with neuroblastoma has been studied. Although mild lymphopenia and leukopenia have been demonstrated at diagnosis, no general humoral or cellular immune defects have been detected. Natural killer cell activity is depressed in neuroblastoma patients. Clinical trials using the methanol-extracted residue of bacillus Calmette-Guérin (BCG), with BCG-treated and neuraminidase-treated tumor cells, to provoke an antitumor immune response in patients have not demonstrated the benefit for this immunotherapy.

Monoclonal antibodies have been raised to antigens on the surface of human neuroblastoma cells to develop reagents that have immunodiagnostic and immunotherapeutic utility. The cell-surface glycosphingolipid diganglioside GD_2 is an abundant antigen on neuroblastoma cells. Monoclonal antibodies to GD_2 recognize neuroblastoma cells relatively specifically without cross-reacting with normal marrow or lymphoid cells. With this monoclonal antibody, Cheung and coworkers were able to detect as few as 0.01% neuroblastoma cells in the marrow. They were able to identify neuroblastoma cells in the bone marrow in 74% of 35 neuroblastoma patients, and conventional histologic techniques and clonogenic assays detected 27% and 55%, respectively. Shedding of GD_2 into the plasma of patients with neuroblastoma may be useful for monitoring responses to therapy. ^{131}I-tagged monoclonal antibodies to GD_2 can ablate human neuroblastoma xenograft tumors in nude mice. Monoclonal antibodies to other neuroblastoma antigens include 5A7 to a cytoplasmic antigen and CE7, KP-NAC8, 5G3, 6–19, and UJ13A to cell-surface antigens. ^{131}I-coupled monoclonal antibodies have been administered as treatment for neuroblastoma. Responses were seen in patients with disseminated disease, but those with large tumor masses were resistant to this therapy. Substantial bone marrow toxicity was incurred, and issues of delivery and dosimetry must be addressed before the potential of this approach can be realized. Monoclonal antibodies may be useful in purging tumor cells from bone marrow for use in autologous bone marrow transplant regimens.

Neuroblastoma has a biologic characteristic unique among human cancers, the capacity to spontaneously differentiate and regress. Residual microscopic tumor left in the bed of a resected, localized neuroblastoma rarely results in recurrence of the disease. Disseminated neuroblastoma has spontaneously regressed in a subset of very young children with disease metastatic to the liver, skin, or bone marrow, but not involving bone, a condition designated as stage IVS neuroblastoma by D'Angio, Evans, and Koop. Histologic evidence of neuroblastoma having differentiated into mature ganglion cells is found in tumors removed from patients during second-look surgical procedures after induction chemotherapy and in older children with isolated mediastinal or abdominal masses, detected incidentally and found to be pure ganglioneuroma. Potential markers for determining disease may be nerve growth factor and the neurosecretory proteins chromogranin and neuropeptide Y.

This phenomenon stimulated laboratory investigation into the mechanisms of differentiation of neuroblastoma cells. In cultured neuroblastoma cells, agents such as prostaglandin E_1, 3′,5′-cyclic nucleotide phosphodiesterase inhibitors, thyroid hormone, and Bu_2cAMP that increase the intracellular cAMP levels, decrease the mitotic rate and increase the degree of differentiation. Differentiating agents, including cyclophosphamide, vincristine, the phosphodiesterase inhibitor papaverine, and the thymidylate synthetase inhibitor trifluromethyl-2-deoxyuridine, used in the treatment of neuroblastoma have resulted in good antitumor responses, but the role of the differentiating agents could not be ascertained because the patients received simultaneous high-dose chemotherapy.

Retinoic acid differentiates neuroblastoma cells in vitro. It probably interacts through a cytoplasmic protein that binds retinoic acid or by the glycosylation of cell surface constituents. Clinical studies with this agent are being initiated as a component of multimodal therapy.

PATHOLOGY AND BIOLOGIC MARKERS

Neuroblastoma is thought to be derived from the embryonic neural crest. The presumptive stem cell of the neural crest, the sympathogon, differentiates into sympathoblasts, the cells of origin of neuroblastoma, and into its more mature forms, ganglioneuroblastoma and ganglioneuroma, and the chromaffin or nonchromaffin paraganglionic cells, the progenitors of pheochromocytomas and paragangliomas. As a "small, round, blue cell" tumor, neuroblastoma consists of dense nests of cells separated by fibrovascular bundles. Hemorrhage, necrosis, and calcification are frequent. Other microscopic features include Homer-Wright neural rosettes with a central fibrillar core and a fibrillary intercellular matrix that can be shown ultrastructurally to be neural cell processes. In the more-differentiated tumor, ganglion cells are present. They are large cells with prominent nucleoli and generous cytoplasm that are scattered throughout a fibrillar matrix. Ganglioneuroblastoma contains areas of neuroblastoma and ganglion cells; ganglioneuroma has ganglion cells, Schwann cells, and nerve bundles. It is important for the pathologist to take multiple sections of a ganglioneuroma to exclude neuroblastoma.

TABLE 49–12. Immunohistochemistry in the Differential Diagnosis of Neuroblastoma

	Small Blue Round Cell Neoplasms				
Stains	*Neuroblastoma*	*Lymphoma*	*Ewing's Sarcoma*	*Rhabdomyosarcoma*	*Primitive Neuroectodermal Tumors*
Neurofilament	+	−	±	−	−
Synaptophysin	+	−	−	−	−
Neuron-specific enolase	+	−	−*	−*	+
β_2-microglobulin	−	−	−	−	+
LCA (T-200 protein)	−	+	−	−	−
Vimentin	−	±	+	+	+
Myoglobin	−	−	−	+	−
Myosin	−	−	−	+	−
Actin	−	−	−	+	−
Desmin	−	−	−	+	−

* Extraosseous Ewing's sarcoma variants of Ewing's sarcoma and rhabdomyosarcoma stain for neuron-specific enolase.
(Brodeur RM, Castleberry RP. Neuroblastoma. In: Pizzo PA, Poplack DG, eds. Principles and practice of pediatric oncology. 2nd ed. Philadelphia: JB Lippincott, 1993)

The characteristic electron microscopic finding of neuroblastoma is the dense core granule (*i.e.*, catecholamine or neurosecretory granule), which is a 50- to 200-mm membrane-bound unit found in the periphery of the cytoplasm. The ultramicroscopic appearance of the neural rosettes is that of peripherally clustered tumor nuclei surrounding a mass of neuritic processes or neuropil.

Neuroblastoma can be difficult to differentiate from other small, round cell tumors of childhood, including Ewing's sarcoma, lymphoma, rhabdomyosarcoma, and other peripheral neurally derived neoplasms, such as the peripheral neuroepithelioma or Askin's tumor. Table 49–12 lists some of the features that help to differentiate these tumors. Neuroblastoma exhibits formaldehyde-induced fluorescence as the catecholamine metabolites from isoquinolone compounds when exposed to formaldehyde, and glyoxylic acid provides a rapid and sensitive assay. Identification of specific cellular constituents, such as enzymes (*i.e.*, neuron-specific enolase) or surface antigens, by sensitive immunoperoxidase techniques, in which paraffin-embedded, formaldehyde-fixed tissues may be used with specific antisera, have become an integral part of the pathologist's workup of the small, round, blue cell tumor.

An often useful adjunct to tissue examination in the diagnosis of neuroblastoma is detection of tumor markers in the blood or urine. The most commonly used is the urinary excretion of tumor-produced catecholamines. Urinary vanillylmandelic acid (VMA) and homovanillic acid (HVA) are elevated in at least 65% of neuroblastoma patients. If both metabolites are sought, more than 90% of patients are identified. Pretreatment measurements correlate with prognosis. Higher levels of catecholamine metabolites are found in patients with more extensive disease. For stage IV patients, a ratio of VMA to HVA of more than 1.5 is associated with a better prognosis. Patients whose neuroblastomas arise from the dorsal root ganglions are nonsecretors of catecholamines. The most reliable method for detection of catecholamine metabolites is a 24-hour urine test. The LaBrosse spot test, which screens for VMA in the urine, is associated with a relatively high false-negative rate because it requires a high concentration of VMA in the samples. Dietary restrictions are not necessary for a reliable 24-hour urine catecholamine quantitation, but catecholamine medications should be avoided. In Japan, mass screening of infants 6 to 7 months old using VMA spot tests has been successful in the early detection of neuroblastoma, and studies are underway in North America and Europe.

Neuron-specific enolase is elevated in most neuroblastoma patients. Higher levels in those with more advanced disease are prognostic of a poorer outcome. Serum ferritin elevation correlates with a poorer prognosis. Cystathionine is elevated in the urine of at least 50% of neuroblastoma patients. As with the other biomarkers, lower levels were associated with a better prognosis.

CLINICAL PRESENTATION AND DIAGNOSIS

Neuroblastoma can occur anywhere along the sympathetic nervous system. The most common site of primary tumor is within the abdomen, in an adrenal gland (40%) or in a paraspinal ganglion (25%); thoracic (15%) and pelvic (5%) primaries account for the rest. Thoracic primaries are more common in children younger than 1 year old (Table 49–13). Metastatic disease is identified in half the infants and two thirds of the older children at diagnosis. (Table 49–14). The most common sites of metastases are lymph nodes, bone

TABLE 49–13. Primary Site of Neuroblastoma According to Age

Primary Site of Tumor	*Percentage of Patients by Age at Diagnosis*	
	≤12 Mo	*>13 Mo*
Head and neck	5	2–3
Thoracic	20	10–15
Abdominal	55	70–75
Pelvic	5	5
Other (or unknown)	15	2–13

TABLE 49–14. Extent of Disease at Diagnosis According to Age

Stage at Diagnosis	*No. of Patients by Age at Diagnosis*		
	≤1 Year	*>1 Year*	*Total*
Localized	93 (39)*	83 (19)	176 (26)
Regional	43 (18)	54 (13)	97 (15)
Disseminated	61 (25)	290 (68)	351 (52)
IVS	44 (18)	0 (0)	44 (7)
Total	241	427	668

* Numbers in parentheses are percentages.
(Courtesy of JJ Shuster, PhD, Pediatric Oncology Group Statistical Office. From Brodeur GM, Castleberry RP. Neuroblastoma. In: Pizzo PA, Poplack DG, eds. Principles and practice of pediatric oncology. 2nd ed. Philadelphia: JB Lippincott, 1993)

marrow, bone, liver, and subcutaneous tissue. Lung metastases are rare.

The signs and symptoms at presentation depend on the primary and metastatic sites. The most common presentation, that of a large abdominal or flank mass that is firm, irregular, and crosses the midline, must be differentiated from Wilms' tumor. Thoracic neuroblastoma presents as a posterior mediastinal mass and is usually found coincidentally when a chest radiograph is obtained for other reasons, although it occasionally causes respiratory symptoms or signs of thoracic spinal cord compression from local extension (Fig. 49–2). Neuroblastoma arising from the cervicothoracic ganglion is often confused with benign lymphadenopathy, but the presence of Horner's syndrome or heterochromia irides from sympathetic dysfunction suggests the true diagnosis. Pelvic neuroblastoma arising from the organ of Zuckerkandl may present as a palpable mass alone or with symptoms related to bladder or vascular compression.

Several unusual presentations of neuroblastoma are noteworthy. First, the firm, subcutaneous, blue-tinged nodules, reminiscent of the blueberry muffin sign associated with congenital rubella, are most often encountered in the neonate with neuroblastoma. Second is the opsoclonus-polymyoclonus syndrome of acute cerebellar and truncal ataxia and dancing eyes, which is associated with persistent neurologic sequelae but limited tumor; it indicates a favorable prognosis. A third unusual symptom is that of intractable, watery diarrhea and hypokalemia (*i.e.*, Kerner-Morrison syndrome) caused by vasoactive intestinal peptide produced by ganglioneuroblastoma and measured in the plasma of these patients. Olfactory neuroblastoma (*i.e.*, esthesioneuroblastoma) arises in the nasal cavity and presents with obstruction. It is most commonly seen in adults and is most probably a peripheral neuroepithelioma.

Neuroblastoma has an unusual predisposition to periorbital metastasis, which presents with proptosis and ecchymosis. This is secondary to sphenoid bone involvement or invasion of the retrobulbar tissues. Intracranial metastasis other than direct extension from bony lesions of the skull are rare. The so-called cerebral neuroblastoma is a supratentorial tumor of primitive neuroectoderm that is more closely related to a family of primary central nervous system (CNS) tumors.

Bone marrow involvement with neuroblastoma is common and may be difficult to differentiate from acute leukemia or other solid tumors, like rhabdomyosarcoma, metastatic to marrow. Neuroblastoma cells are more likely to be periodic acid-Schiff (PAS)-negative and form rosettes, but the clinical tests and tissue histopathology usually confirm the diagnosis.

In some neuroblastoma patients, no primary tumor site can be found. This is most common in the unique syndrome (stage IVS) that occurs in infants younger than 1 year old. It is characterized by small or undetectable tumors, usually of the adrenal, with skin, hepatic, or bone marrow (but not bone) metastases that may undergo spontaneous regression. Hepatic enlargement may be significant, causing symptoms that necessitate therapeutic intervention.

A bone marrow aspirate and a biopsy may provide tumor for diagnostic pathologic studies and adjunctive laboratory analysis such as flow cytometry for establishing the DNA index, which may be clinically useful. The international staging system calls for two aspirates and biopsies, one from each iliac crest, to enhance diagnostic sensitivity.

Evidence is accumulating that there are three genetic subsets of neuroblastoma based on chromosomal abnormalities and *MYCN*. One consists of younger patients (<1 year) who have a hyperdiploid or near-triploid karyotype with few chromosomal abnormalities and a good prognosis. A second group is older and has a near-diploid karyotype without consistent chromosomal abnormalities and more advanced, albeit slowly progressing, disease. The third group of patients, with rapidly advancing tumor that is almost always fatal (<5% survival) are older and have advanced tumor stages with near-diploid or tetraploid karyotype with deletions or LoH of 1p36, amplified *MYCN* or both.

Although other small, round, blue cell tumors metastatic to

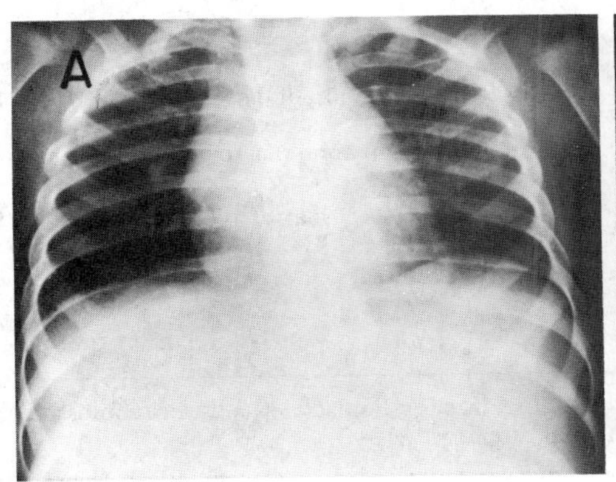

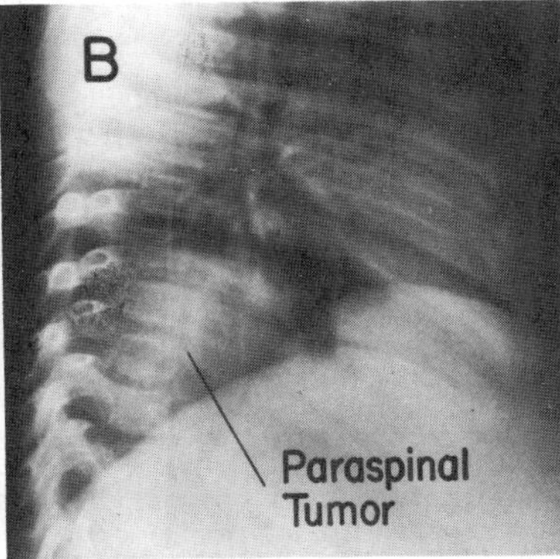

FIGURE 49–2. Chest roentgenograph in **(A)** frontal and **(B)** lateral projections, demonstrating paravertebral pleural displacement. Size of the thoracic component can be appreciated on the lateral projection.

the bone marrow may have similar histologic features, a diagnosis of neuroblastoma may be confirmed if abnormal urine catecholamine excretion is found in conjunction with the marrow findings, and this often obviates a major surgical procedure. A careful search of many slides must be undertaken before the marrow can be declared uninvolved. Examination of slides of the buffy coat made from 1 to 2 ml of heparinized marrow may increase the yield.

CT is the best imaging modality for neuroblastoma and should be performed for every patient to determine the location and extent of the primary and metastatic lesions. CT detects abdominal neuroblastoma with an extremely high sensitivity, and calcifications are seen in approximately 85% of patients. The IVP is less sensitive than a CT scan in the evaluation of an abdominal mass and should not be done routinely. Bilateral adrenal calcifications detected in an otherwise asymptomatic child with an abnormal birth history are probably due to neonatal adrenal hemorrhage. Experience with MRI of neuroblastoma visualizes the tumor in many planes, demonstrates the vascular anatomy, and improves the definition of the intraspinal extension, aiding the determination of resectability.

Nuclear medicine scans of use in evaluating neuroblastoma include the technetium 99m methylene diphosphonate bone scan, which is more sensitive than the conventional skeletal survey. Bone scanning agents are frequently taken up by extraosseous tumor, further aiding in the metastatic workup. ^{131}I-meta-iodobenzylguanidine (MIBG), which has been used in the diagnosis and treatment of pheochromocytoma because of its preferential uptake by cells with adrenergic secretory vesicles, allows the imaging of most neuroblastomas and should be performed if available.

The laboratory evaluation of neuroblastoma should include a complete blood count and coagulation studies. Coagulopathy is not uncommon in patients with disseminated disease and may be caused by intravascular coagulation. Hypocoagulability and hypercoagulability have been reported.

STAGING

There have been several staging systems for neuroblastoma (Table 49–15). Because of the prognostic influence of regional lymph node involvement and the importance of the initial surgical procedure in determining further treatment, the Pediatric Oncology Group (POG) adopted a modification of the staging system advocated by Hayes and coworkers at St. Jude Children's Research Hospital based on the surgical-pathologic staging of patients with clinically localized disease, a concept originally advocated by Pinkel in 1958. It is important that investigators working in this field be able to compare results of treatment protocols, and an international working group has been established to develop a common system. The In-

TABLE 49–15. Comparison of Staging Systems for Neuroblastoma

CCSG System[116]	*POG System*[6]	*International (INSS)*[124]
Stage I. Tumor confined to the organ or structure of origin.	Stage A. Complete gross resection of the primary tumor, with or without microscopic residual disease. Intracavitary lymph nodes not adhered to the primary tumor must be histologically free of tumor. Nodes adhered to the surface of or within the primary may be positive.	Stage 1. Localized tumor confined to the area of origin; complete gross excision, with or without microscopic residual disease; identifiable ipsilateral and contralateral lymph nodes negative microscopically.
Stage II. Tumor extending in continuity beyond the organ or structure of origin, but not crossing the midline. Regional lymph nodes on the ipsilateral side may be involved.	Stage B. Grossly unresected primary tumor. Nodes and nodules the same as in stage A.	Stage 2A. Unilateral tumor with incomplete gross excision; identifiable ipsilateral and contralateral lymph nodes negative microscopically. Stage 2B. Unilateral tumor with complete or incomplete gross excision; with positive ipsilateral regional lymph nodes; identifiable contralateral lymph nodes negative microscopically.
Stage III. Tumor extending in continuity beyond the midline. Regional lymph nodes may be involved bilaterally.	Stage C. Complete or incomplete resection of primary. Intracavitary nodes not adhered to primary must be histologically positive for tumor. Liver as in stage A.	Stage 3. Tumor infiltrating across the midline with or without regional lymph node involvement or unilateral tumor with contralateral regional lymph node involvement or midline tumor with bilateral lymph node involvement.
Stage IV. Remote disease involving the skeleton, bone marrow, soft tissue and distant lymph node groups (see stage IVS)	Stage D. Dissemination of disease beyond intracavitary nodes (*i.e.,* extracavitary nodes, liver, skin, bone marrow, bone).	Stage 4. Dissemination of tumor to distant lymph nodes, bone, bone marrow, liver, or other organs (except as defined in stage 4S).
Stage IVS. As defined in stage I or II, except for the presence of remote disease confined to the liver, skin, or marrow (without bone metastases).	Stage DS. Infants <1 year of age with stage IVS disease (see CCSG).	Stage 4S. Localized primary tumor as defined for stage 1 or 2 with dissemination limited to liver, skin, or bone marrow.

(Brodeur GM, Castleberry RP. Neuroblastoma. In: Pizzo PA, Poplack DG, eds. Principles and practice of pediatric oncology. 2nd ed. Philadelphia: JB Lippincott, 1993)

ternational Staging System is based on clinical, radiographic, and surgical assessment. Table 49–15 describes this system.

THERAPY

Successful treatment of the child with neuroblastoma requires a carefully considered multidisciplinary approach. The initial diagnostic workup establishes whether the disease is disseminated or localized. In the patient with localized disease, the operation is key to defining the local extent of tumor and to completely resecting the tumor. Radiation therapy plays a role in the treatment of the patient with localized disease and the palliative management of the patient with disseminated disease unresponsive to chemotherapy. Chemotherapy is central in the management of those with unresectable local tumor or metastatic disease.

Surgery

The surgical approach depends on tumor site, disease stage, and age of the patient. Among those with cervical, mediastinal, and to a lesser extent, pelvic tumors, complete excision is usually feasible and should be aggressively pursued. The same approach is occasionally possible for a primary abdominal tumor, particularly if it is small or laterally placed. Most localized abdominal neuroblastomas extend centrally and surround the major branches of the aorta, making the tumors unresectable by conventional surgical procedures. Every large series contains some long-surviving patients in whom these tumors were literally "carved" away from the central vessels, but there are more patients for whom this did not result in cure. In general, abdominal tumors are biopsied, and a second or third attempt is made to remove them after intensive chemotherapy or radiation therapy. If complete gross resection can be carried out during a second or third procedure, the patient will probably survive. These procedures may be instrumental in creating a favorable-prognosis group.

Among patients with metastatic disease, an early aggressive attempt to resect the primary tumor does not increase survival. In patients in whom metastatic disease can be controlled, successful secondary excisions of the primary tumors produce relatively extensive survival times.

In patients with functional neuroblastomas, early excision of the major tumor mass is essential to ameliorate symptoms. Surgery for patients with stage IVS disease should be conservative. After all disseminated disease is eliminated by chemotherapy or spontaneously, the remaining primary tumor mass is usually excised, although this has never been demonstrated to be necessary. Surgical procedures have been devised to relieve intraabdominal pressure in patients with stage IVS disease by employing plastic sheets to create an artificial ventral "hernia."

Radiation Therapy

In general, dosages of radiation for neuroblastoma range from 1500 to 3000 cGy, depending on the child's age, tumor location, and volume. Radiation therapy appears to have a clearly defined role for children with regional lymph node metastases (INSS stages 2B and 3). It has been used successfully in neonates with Evans stage IVS who developed respiratory distress secondary to hepatomegaly or for children with cord compression due to dumbbell lesions. However, fractionated radiation has not improved survival for children with metastatic disease, although local therapy can provide pain relief for children with advanced disease.

Chemotherapy

Neuroblastoma is usually chemoresponsive and sometimes curable. The complete and partial response rates vary for the most common single agents: cyclophosphamide (59%), cisplatin (46%), epipodophyllotoxins (30%), vincristine (24%), dacarbazine (14%), melphalan (24%), and ifosfamide (20%). Combination schedules are employed and, with surgery and radiation therapy, they can be combined to delineate multimodal risk-based therapy (Fig. 49–3).

Treatment of Low-Risk Patients

Infants and children with localized and resected tumors (INSS stage 1), partially resected tumors (INSS stage IIA), with regional disease (INSS 2B or 3), or INSS 4S disease are in this category of low risk.

Children with INSS stage 1 have a survival exceeding 90% with surgery alone. Neither radiation or chemotherapy are administered initially to these patients. However, postoperative chemotherapy (*i.e.*, sequential cyclophosphamide and doxorubicin) is indicated for children with INSS stage 2A, 2B, and 3 tumors and is associated with survival rates of 85%, 87%, and 89%, respectively.

Treatment of Intermediate-Risk Patients

Children with metastatic disease to regional lymph nodes only (INSS stage 2B or 3) or infants with INSS stage 4 disease are the intermediate-risk category. Children with stage 2B and 3 disease are treated with chemotherapy (*e.g.*, cyclophosphamide and doxorubicin, high-dose cisplatin and tenoposide with cyclophosphamide and doxorubicin and with radiation therapy. Similarly, infants with INSS stage 4 require intensive combination chemotherapy and radiation and may achieve survival rates ranging between 60% to 75%.

Treatment of High-Risk Patients

Most children with neuroblastoma fall into the high-risk category. They include children older than 2 years of age with disseminated (INSS stage 4) disease. Survival for this group of patients remains around 15% despite several therapeutic approaches. These children now receive intensive chemotherapy in conjunction with autologous bone marrow transplantation, and although this approach appears to improve early survival, relapses continue to occur. Most of these children are initially responsive to chemotherapy and achieve an initial remission. This suggests that drug-resistant tumor cells are present from the outset or that mutations evolve rapidly with treatment. Schedules that modulate multidrug resistance together with dose intensity may offer some hope.

New strategies are needed for children with advanced neuroblastoma, and the use of biologic agents is being studied. Included are the hematopoietic cytokines (*e.g.*, granulocyte or granulocyte-macrophage colony-stimulating factors) that can permit more timely delivery or higher doses of chemotherapy, the use of adoptive immunotherapy with tumor-

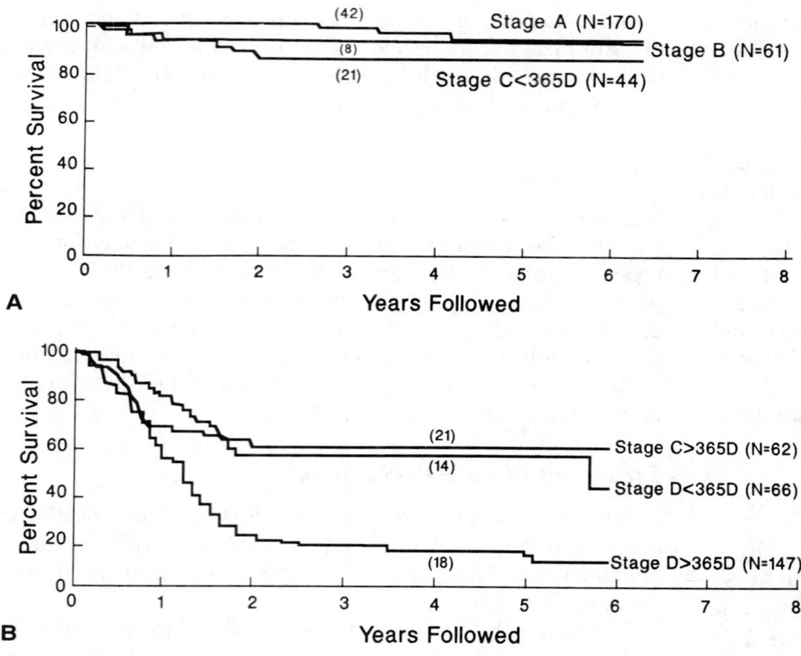

FIGURE 49–3. Survival in 550 consecutive patients with neuroblastoma treated from 1981 to 1989 on POG protocols. Based on POG stage and age (≤1 or >1 year), three prognostic groups emerged: **(A)** low risk and **(B)** intermediate and high risk.

infiltrating lymphocyte, differentiating agents, and monoclonal antibodies.

RETINOBLASTOMA

Retinoblastoma, the most common primary tumor of the eye in children, has many distinguishing features. Arising from the nuclear layer of the retina, tumors may be multifocal, bilateral, congenital, inherited, or acquired. Patients may have unique chromosomal abnormalities, and tumors can undergo spontaneous regression. Patients with the inherited form of retinoblastoma appear to be at increased risk for second, nonocular malignancies.

The estimated annual incidence of retinoblastoma is 1 in 15,000 to 34,000 live births. According to the Third National Cancer Survey and the Surveillance, Epidemiology, and End Results (SEER) group, there are approximately 11 new cases of retinoblastoma per million children younger than 5 years of age. There are approximately 200 new cases each year in the United States, 90% of which are diagnosed in children (see Table 49–1). The disease is bilateral in 40 to 60 cases. Although retinoblastoma accounts for only 1% of pediatric tumors, it serves as an important model for understanding the genetics of oncogenesis.

EPIDEMIOLOGY AND GENETICS

The mean age of presentation for retinoblastoma is 17 months, with 80% diagnosed before the age of 4 years. Although the tumor has been described in adults, it is rare in children older than 5 years. Retinoblastoma occurs in hereditary, nonhereditary, and chromosomal deletion forms. The retinoblastoma gene may be transmitted from parent to child or acquired as a new mutation. No family history of retinoblastoma is found in 90% of patients.

The hereditary form of retinoblastoma accounts for approximately 40% of cases, and it is inherited as a highly penetrant, autosomal dominant trait. A two-mutation hypothesis explains the genetics of inherited retinoblastoma. The first mutation occurs in the germinal cells, and the second occurs in the somatic cells. In the sporadic form of the disease, both mutations occur in the somatic cells. It is presumed that the timing of the mutational event in embryonic development determines whether the entire retinal anlage or only that of one eye is affected. Most patients with the hereditary form of retinoblastoma have bilateral disease, although unilateral disease occurs in almost 25% of these patients. Overall, approximately 30% of patients with retinoblastoma have bilateral disease, and 70% have unilateral involvement. Eleven patients with bilateral retinoblastoma subsequently developed pineoblastoma, suggesting that genetic susceptibility to transformation can be conferred to ectopic neuroblastic photoreceptors in the pineal gland (*i.e.*, trilateral retinoblastoma).

Most patients with retinoblastoma lack appreciable chromosomal abnormalities in most autosomal cells. A deletion on the long arm of chromosome 13 within band 13q14 has been observed in a few patients with retinoblastoma, some of whom have a syndrome that includes mental retardation, microcephaly, skeletal abnormalities, and dysmorphic features. Using recombinant DNA probes, which are homologous to unique loci on human chromosome 13, a specific retinoblastoma locus (*RB1*) has been defined, confirming that chromosome loss or loss and reduplication can lead to the expression of a recessive mutation. Dryja and coworkers examined tumor tissue obtained from 8 patients with retinoblastoma, none of whom had a family history of this disease. Four of the eight tumors demonstrated chromosome 13 homozygosity, which had no correlation with the degree of tumor differentiation or whether the tumors were multifocal or unifocal.

The tight linkage of the retinoblastoma (*RB1*) gene locus to the genetic locus of esterase D, assigned to 13q14, has demonstrated that the two independent genetic events consist of the loss or inactivation of wild-type alleles. The *RB* gene is 200,000 base pairs and encodes a 928 amino acid product that is a nuclear phosphoprotein with DNA-binding activity. Within the 13q14 band locus of the retinoblastoma gene, the loss of one *RB* allele is insufficient for tumorigenesis, but the loss of both alleles by nondisjunction or point mutation is associated with tumor production.

The genetic susceptibility for oncogenesis in patients with the inheritable form of retinoblastoma is further underscored by the fact that these patients have an increased risk for developing second malignancies that are unrelated to radiation or chemotherapy exposure. The predominant second cancers include osteosarcoma, fibrosarcoma, Ewing's sarcoma, and Wilms' tumor. Patients with bilateral retinoblastoma have a 15% to 20% chance of developing a second, nonocular neoplasm 1 to 40 years after their treatment for retinoblastoma. Fibroblasts from patients with the genetic form of retinoblastoma have increased radiation sensitivity and defective DNA repair. Fibroblasts from siblings of patients with retinoblastoma also have this radiation sensitivity pattern. The complementary sequences to the retinoblastoma gene have been cloned and demonstrate deletion at the 13q14 *RB* locus in some patients with osteosarcoma, offering an explanation for the close association of these two malignancies.

The incidence of second malignancies increases over time. For irradiated patients, the incidence of second tumor was 20% at 10 years, 50% at 20 years, and approximately 90% at 30 years. For nonirradiated patients, the incidence of second malignancies was 10% at 10 years, 30% at 20 years, and 68% at 32 years. Based on a series of 882 patients, the cumulative index of second malignancies was 2% at 12 years and 4.2% at 18 years after diagnosis. This incidence was doubled in patients with the genetic form of retinoblastoma.

Genetic counseling is important for patients with the genetic form of retinoblastoma. Assuming that the mutation is a germinal event, the risk for bearing an affected child may be as high as 50%. This is straightforward if there is a family history of the disease but more difficult for sporadic cases, because these may be heritable or nonheritable. Bilateral cases, even without a family history, are always the hereditary type, and the offspring of affected patients have a 50% risk of having retinoblastoma. Of the unilateral cases, 10% to 12% have the hereditary form, and the first child of a survivor has a 5.6% chance of having the disease (Fig. 49–4)

Parents of an affected child should always have a funduscopic examination. If a child with retinoblastoma is born to physically sound parents, the risk of a second child having retinoblastoma is 1% if the first child had unilateral retinoblastoma and 6% if the child had bilateral disease. The use of restriction fragment length polymorphism may facilitate diagnosis and permit prenatal and postnatal prediction of susceptibility to the heritable form of retinoblastoma.

Nonprogressive retinal lesions (*i.e.*, retinomas) have been described in patients presumed to carry the retinoblastoma gene. These retinomas consist of translucent, gray, elevated masses that extend from the retina into the vitreous cavity and are frequently associated with calcified foci and pigment-epithelium hyperplasia. In a recent survey of 34 patients with retinomas and 5 with phthisis bulbi, which is associated with retinoblastoma, 67% had a family history of retinoblastoma, and 23 (68%) of their offspring developed retinoblastomas. Although retinoma may represent a mutation of a more mature retinoblast, making it nonmalignant, its detection should

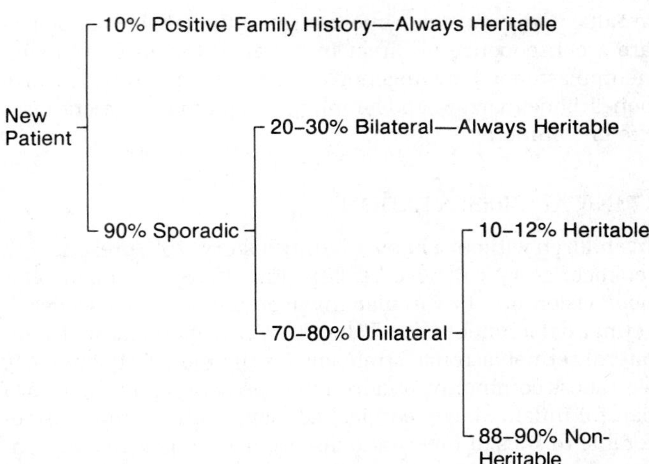

FIGURE 49–4. Flow diagram of statistical probabilities for a newly diagnosed patient with retinoblastoma. (Donaldson SS, Egbert PR. Retinoblastoma. In: Pizzo PA, Poplack DG, eds. Principles and practice of pediatric oncology. 2nd ed. Philadelphia: JB Lippincott, 1993)

prompt genetic counseling and follow-up of the affected person.

PATHOLOGIC AND ANATOMIC CONSIDERATIONS

Retinoblastoma, putatively arising from the outer layer of the retina, consists of small, round cells with scanty cytoplasm and chromatin-rich nuclei. Histologic examination shows similarity with neuroblastoma and medulloblastoma, including aggregation around blood vessels, necrosis, calcification, and Flexner-Winter stained rosettes. Tumors are often multifocal, averaging four to five lesions in as many as 84% of the patients. This multifocality and the predilection of retinoblastoma to invade the optic nerve influences treatment planning.

Endophytic and exophytic local extension of retinoblastoma are recognized. Endophytic growth is characterized by extension into the vitreous cavity, and exophytic growth invades the subretinal space, with consequent retinal detachment. With endophytic extension, tumor fragments can break away from the main tumor mass to form vitreous seeds, which is a poor prognostic finding.

Most patients with retinoblastoma have disease restricted to the eye and orbit. Local tumor growth usually involves the choroid or the sclera if subretinal seeds cross Brach's membrane. The highly vascular choroid is involved in more than 25% of patients and, although this serves as a potential site for dissemination, it is not as serious as scleral involvement. Scleral involvement usually occurs by direct extension from the choroid or by spread along emissary veins.

Glaucoma can result from tumor growth in a retinal detachment that pushes the iris forward to occlude the trabecular network. It can also result if a neovascular membrane grows on the iris and over the trabecular network, blocking the egress of aqueous fluid. Iris neovascularization may be exacerbated by radiation therapy.

Of particular concern is extension of retinoblastoma cells through the lamina cribrosa and into or along the optic nerve. If the tumor extends just 10 to 22 mm along the optic nerve, invasion into the meninges is usually a consequence, a particularly poor prognostic feature.

Slightly more than half of the deaths with retinoblastoma

are due to distant tumor metastases, although 47% of deaths are a consequence of direct intracranial extension. As with neuroblastoma, hematogenous metastases most often involve bones, bone marrow, and lymph nodes; pulmonary metastases are uncommon.

CLINICAL PRESENTATION

In children without a known family history, 75% present with leukocoria or "cat's eye" reflex (Fig. 49–5), strabismus, or poor vision due to vascular involvement, vitreous seeds, or retinal detachment (see Table 49–7). In patients with unilateral retinoblastoma, strabismus is the most frequent early sign. Less commonly, children may present with proptosis, a painful inflamed eye, cervical adenopathy, or symptoms referable to sites of metastatic disease. It is imperative that infants and children with these symptoms undergo a careful ophthalmologic evaluation. Young children do not complain of loss of vision, and intraocular tumors are not painful unless there is also glaucoma or inflammation. Any child with a known family history of retinoblastoma or retinomas should be examined at birth and at regular intervals thereafter. Of 158 infants with retinoblastoma diagnosed during the first 6 months of life (mean age, 3.6 years), 60% had leukocoria, and 68% had bilateral disease. Many of these patients had advanced disease despite their early evaluation.

In young children suspected of having retinoblastoma, examination of the retina may need to be performed under general anesthesia. This is particularly important if tumor involvement includes the ora serrata or if the tumor cannot be visualized because of retinal detachment or vitreous hemorrhage obscuring the tumor mass. The differential diagnosis includes visceral larva migrants (*i.e., Toxocara* granuloma), Coats' disease, retrolental fibroplasia, and persistent hyperplastic primary vitreous. Findings of calcification, which occurs in 50% to 75% of patients, or vitreous seedings are compatible with retinoblastoma. Orbital CT scan can detect calcification in more than 80% of patients, and in children younger than 3 years of age in whom the diagnosis is suspected, CT-detected calcification is virtually diagnostic. Two dimensional B-scan ultrasonography is of particular value in demonstrating mass lesions in the posterior segment of the fundus, because retinoblastoma has a high internal acoustic reactivity due to the pressure of calcium and the interface between necrotic and viable areas.

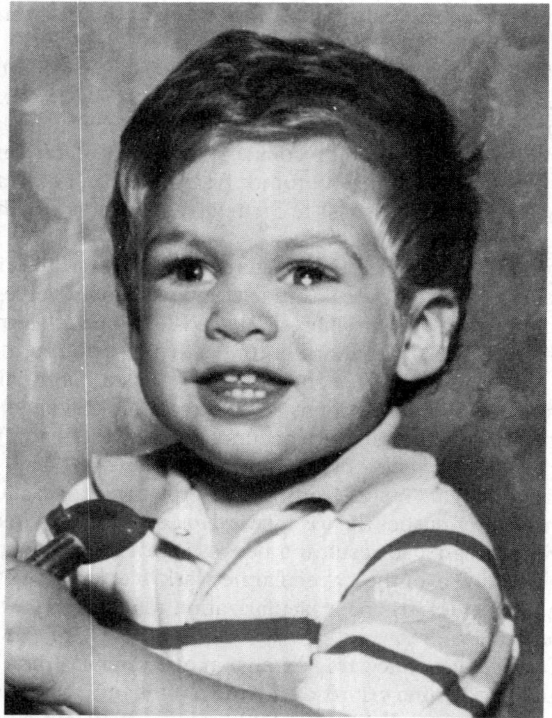

FIGURE 49–5. Child exhibiting leukokoria in the left eye, the most common presenting sign of retinoblastoma. (Donaldson SS, Egbert PR. Retinoblastoma. In: Pizzo PA, Poplack DG, eds. Principles and practice of pediatric oncology. 2nd ed. Philadelphia: JB Lippincott, 1993)

EVALUATION

Examination of the child with retinoblastoma should determine the extent of local disease and metastatic disease. Careful examination of both retinas by direct and indirect ophthalmoscopy is essential, and the extent of orbital disease and intracranial extension should be assessed by CT scan. Two-dimensional B-scan ultrasonography can help in determining whether there is a mass in the posterior segment. Because of intraocular calcifications, CT of the orbit is more sensitive than plain films of the skull. MRI can determine the extent of orbital and CNS involvement. Patients should have a lumbar puncture for cytocentrifuge CSF examination, a bone marrow aspirate, and a biopsy. Patients with extensive orbital involvement should have bone scans. Lactic acid dehydrogenase may be elevated in the aqueous humor of patients with retinoblastoma.

Because of the predominance of intraocular disease and because of improved survival, treatment planning and staging has been focused on the management of local disease and on preserving the eye and vision. The most widely used staging system for retinoblastoma assesses the likelihood of local tumor control and preservation of vision but does not predict survival. As outlined in Table 49–16, this grouping system divides patients according to the likelihood of preserving vision after radiation therapy based on tumor size, the number and location of lesions, and vitreous seeding. In this system, tumor size is expressed by comparison with the optic disk (1.5 mm diameter). Each eye should be evaluated separately to assess the most effective therapy and to determine if there is any potential for preserving or restoring useful vision. Although this system is useful in guiding management of intraocular disease, it does not predict survival for patients with advanced (group V) disease at presentation.

A histologically based staging system, which considers intraocular and extraocular tumor extension and which correlates with patient survival, has been adopted by St. Jude Children's Research Hospital (Table 49–17). This staging system permits the integration of multimodal treatment planning for patients with advanced local disease, but it is based on results of enucleation.

TREATMENT

Treatment Planning

Treatment planning must consider unilateral or bilateral involvement; the size, number, and location of local tumors;

TABLE 49–16. Reese-Ellsworth Clinical Grouping System for Retinoblastoma

Group I: Very Favorable

1. Solitary tumor, less than 4 disk diameters* in size, at or beyond equator.
2. Multiple tumors, none over 4 disk diameters in size, all at or behind equator.

Group II: Favorable

1. Solitary tumor, 4 to 10 disk diameters in size, at or behind equator.
2. Multiple tumors, 4 to 10 disk diameters in size, at or behind equator.

Group III: Doubtful

1. Any lesion anterior to equator.
2. Solitary tumors larger than 10 disk diameters behind equator.

Group IV: Unfavorable

1. Multiple tumors, some larger than 10 disk diameters.
2. Any lesion extending anteriorly to ora serrata.

Group V: Very Unfavorable

1. Massive tumors involving over half the retina.
2. Vitreous seeding.

* 1 disk diameter = 1.6 mm.

(Reese AB, Ellsworth RM. The evaluation and current concepts of retinoblastoma therapy. Trans Am Acad Ophthalmol Otolaryngol 1963;67:164–172)

TABLE 49–17. St. Jude Children's Research Hospital Staging System

I. Tumor (unifocal or multifocal) confined to retina
   A. Occupying 1 quadrant or less
   B. Occupying 2 quadrants or less
   C. Occupying more than 50% of retinal surface
II. Tumor (unifocal or multifocal) confined to globe
   A. With vitreous seeding
   B. Extending to optic nerve head
   C. Extending to choroid
   D. Extending to choroid and optic nerve head
   E. Extending to emissaries
III. Extraocular extension of tumor (regional)
   A. Extending beyond cut end of optic nerve (including subarachnoid extension)
   B. Extending through sclera into orbital contents
   C. Extending to choroid and beyond cut end of optic nerve (including subarachnoid extension)
   D. Extending through sclera into orbital contents and beyond cut end of optic nerve (including subarachnoid extension)
IV. Distant metastases
   A. Extending through optic nerve to brain
   B. Blood-borne metastases to soft tissue and bone
   C. Bone marrow metastases

(Pratt CB. Management of malignant solid tumors in children. Pediatr Clin North Am 1972;19:1141–1155)

tumor extension into the choroid, sclera, or optic nerve; and evidence of extraocular disease. The goal of therapy for patients with localized disease (Ellsworth-Reese stages I and II or St. Jude stages I, IIA, and IIB) is local control with surgery or radiation therapy. Unfortunately, most children with unilateral involvement present with far advanced disease and with little potential for preserving vision. Patients with advanced local disease may require postoperative treatment to the orbit or contiguous extension sites of the CNS. The management of patients with bilateral disease depends on the extent and group of disease in each eye. It is no longer appropriate to enucleate the most severe eye in patients with bilateral involvement. With modern radiation therapy, vision may be spared.

Surgery

ADVANCED UNILATERAL DISEASE. Most children with sporadic unilateral retinoblastoma have advanced intraocular disease at the time of presentation, often with little or no vision in the affected eye. Although the potential for visual preservation exists with irradiation, at least 50% of patients with advanced local disease subsequently require enucleation, because of irradiation-induced complications or inadequate local tumor control. Enucleation is the treatment of choice for children with advanced unilateral disease, especially if there is involvement of the optic nerve head or if the child has glaucoma. If enucleation is performed, at least 10 mm of the optic nerve should be resected to remove any disease that may have extended along the nerve. If microscopic examination detects evidence of tumor along the nerve tract, local irradiation should be administered. An artificial eye can be fitted in 6 weeks. In children younger than 3 years of age, the orbit ceases to grow normally after enucleation and, as the face grows, the orbit becomes more sunken.

LIMITED DISEASE. Patients with limited unilateral or bilateral tumors (<4 disk diameters) may be candidates for photocoagulation or cryotherapy instead of enucleation combined with radiation. Photocoagulation by the technique of Meyer-Schwicherath obliterates small tumors and destroys their blood supply. This procedure requires direct visualization of the tumor and is best restricted to posterior tumor masses. The tumor mass must be easily differentiated from the optic nerve head or macula, must not involve the choroid, and must not have a large nutrient vessel. The technique is used in cases with residual or recurrent disease after irradiation. Although successful, photocoagulation can be complicated by retinal detachment and hemorrhage.

Cryotherapy has been occasionally successfully used for primary treatment; it is more often employed for excision of residual or recurrent disease after irradiation. It is applied by a probe placed directly on the conjunctiva or sclera through a small incision in the conjunctiva. The position of the probe is guided by ophthalmoscopy, and the tumor can be observed to whiten as it freezes. Of 138 retinoblastomas treated in one study, the overall success with cryotherapy was 70%, with a 93% survival rate. Cryotherapy was useful as a primary modality in small (<4 disk diameters or <3 mm in diameter and 2 mm thick) tumors (20 of 21 cured) and for radiation failures (58 of 66). Successful cryotherapy is limited by the size, location, and elevation of the tumor. It is ineffective in the treatment of vitreous seeds. Peripheral lesions may not be effectively treated by cryotherapy.

BILATERAL DISEASE. The treatment plan for patients with bilateral disease depends on the extent of tumor involvement in each eye. If one eye has lost vision or has clearly established optic nerve head involvement, it should be enucleated, and the less involved eye should be irradiated. If vision is present and imaging studies show no obvious optic nerve involvement, both eyes may be treated by irradiation. For group I, II, and III patients with bilateral retinoblastoma treated with irradiation, tumors were controlled in 73% to 80% of the cases. If both eyes are severely affected at the time of presentation, it is preferable to administer a trial of bilateral irradiation, because the possibility for some preservation or restoration of vision exists.

Although the 5-year survival rates for patients presenting with group IV or V disease is 88%, the chance for satisfactory tumor control and preservation of vision is low (29%). Recent experience with improved radiation therapy techniques and liberal use of phototherapy or cryotherapy have resulted in disease control in almost 80%, including group IV cases. With group V disease, primary irradiation control has been reportedly anecdotally.

Radiation Therapy

The purpose of radiation therapy in retinoblastoma is the control of local disease while preserving vision. However, the advantages of this approach must be weighed against its potential short-term and long-term complications. Because most patients have multiple tumors in one or both eyes, radiation fields must include the entire anatomic extent of the retina, the anterior border of which is the ora serrata. This is important because tumor cells from the posterior retina may be channeled into the region of the ora serrata and result in local failure if not included in the radiation field.

Radiation treatment planning requires the joint efforts of the radiation therapist, ophthalmologist, and anesthesiologist. Several techniques for external-beam irradiation have been employed. Concerns about including the lacrimal gland and direct conjunctival effects limit general use of anterior fields to cases with advanced disease (including vitreous seeding). Modern techniques permit accurate lateral field arrangements, which assure adequate coverage of the retina, diminish direct irradiation of the optic lens, and limit the degree of late xerophthalmia (Fig. 49–6). Young children should be anesthetized, usually requiring ketamine to ensure immobilization and relatively fixed ocular positioning. Excellent results have been reported by using a technically precise lateral photon field or by magnetic fixation of the eye using a low-vacuum contact lens that is attached to a small iron pin. Alternatively, a Comberg lens that has a radiopaque marker on the anterior surface of the cornea can be used for the setup.

No firm radiation dose-response relation has been proved for retinoblastoma. Most clinical series report doses between 4500 to 5400 cGy delivered over 4 to 6 weeks.

The regression patterns after radiation therapy include a "cottage cheese" appearance due to calcium deposition or shrinkage and a homogenous, gray, nonvascular mass with an annulus of atrophic pigment around the bone. Determination of tumor sterilization requires experience and serial ophthalmologic examinations.

Localized radiation, using radioactive plaques or particle radiation, although useful in patients with recurrent tumors, is comparable to cryotherapy or phototherapy. Local modifications, such as addressing less than the full retinal surface, should be used for primary control only in the unusual unilateral, limited-size, unifocal tumors. Patients who have residual orbital or optic nerve tumor after surgery should receive wide-field (*i.e.*, orbit and optic nerve) irradiation after enucleation. In general, a dosage of 4500 to 5400 cGy is delivered in 1800 to 200-cGy fractions over 5 to 6 weeks. At higher doses, optic atrophy may occur. Full cranial or craniospinal irradiation is indicated for patients with brain or dural extension.

Chemotherapy

Although chemotherapy was first used in patients with retinoblastoma in 1953, its role remains undefined. Because effective local control and survival is achieved in 90% of patients with surgery and radiation, chemotherapy is best restricted to patients with locally extensive (*e.g.*, choroidal or optic nerve), regional, or distant disease. Unfortunately, responses have been unsatisfactory. Patients with CNS extension and meningeal disease may benefit from intrathecal or intraventricular methotrexate. The agents that have been most extensively used in retinoblastoma include triethanolamine (TEM), vincristine, nitrogen mustard, cyclophosphamide, doxorubicin, and methotrexate. TEM has most often been administered by an intracarotid route, usually before the start of irradiation, although without proven efficacy. Ifosfamide has produced short-term, partial responses, and combinations of cyclophosphamide and dactinomycin, cyclophosphamide and doxorubicin, and cisplatin and VM-26 have been associated with mixed or partial responses. Preirradiation chemotherapy has been used for children with extensive intraocular tumors.

PRIMARY HEPATIC TUMORS

Primary malignancies of the liver, although infrequent in childhood, pose a considerable therapeutic and diagnostic challenge. One to two hepatic tumors per million children occur annually in the United States, with hepatoblastoma predominating in children younger than 5 years of age and hepatocellular carcinoma (HCC) in older children. As with Wilms' tumor, hepatoma most often presents as an asymptomatic abdominal mass that is found in a routine physical examination or discovered coincidentally by parents. Fewer than 25% of patients experience symptoms of abdominal pain, weight loss, or malaise, but when these symptoms occur, they are usually associated with advanced disease. The primary objective is to differentiate a hepatic malignancy from benign hepatic tumors, nonneoplastic hepatomegaly, and other causes of abdominal enlargement, particularly Wilms' tumor and neuroblastoma.

From a survey of 656 hepatic tumors in children, 423 (64%) were malignant, 54% were hepatoblastomas, 35% were hepatocellular sarcomas, and 11% were sarcomas (Table 49–18). Hemangiomas and hamartomas account for approximately 75% of the benign liver tumors, and almost 90% of these lesions occur in infants younger than 6 months. Benign vascular tumors can reach considerable size in infancy and

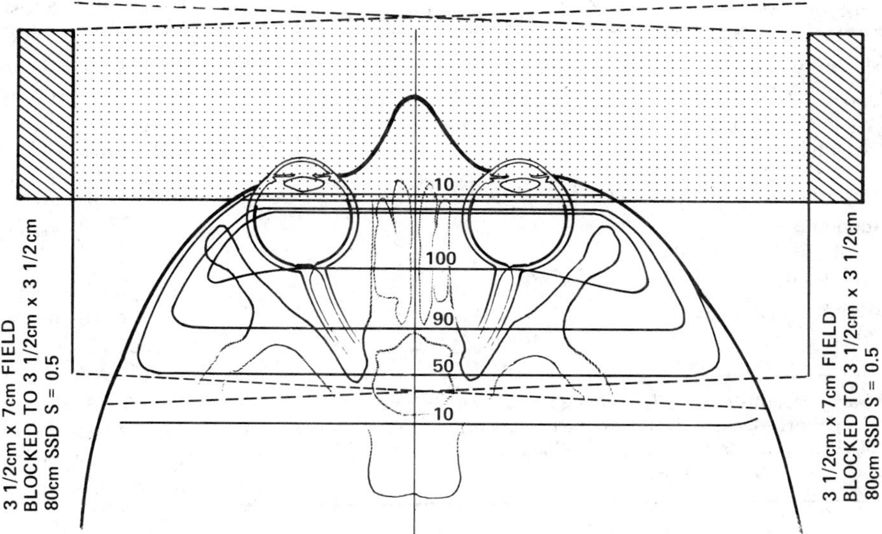

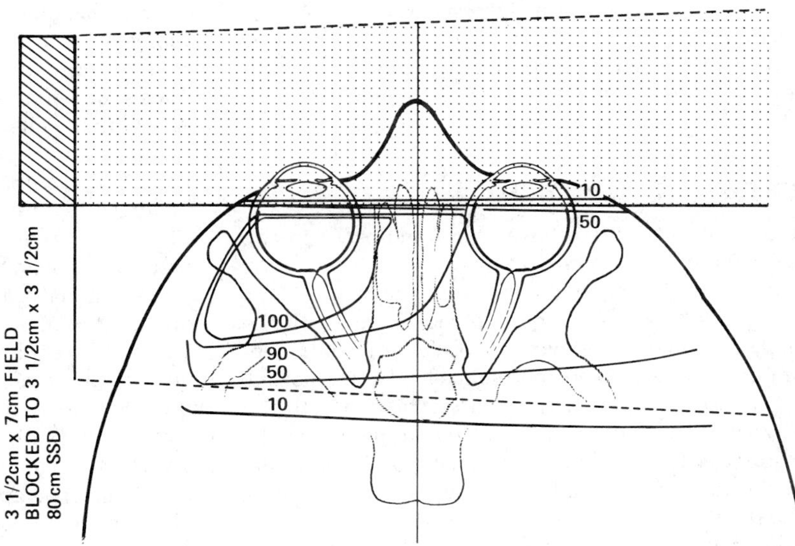

FIGURE 49–6. Isodose curves from a 4-MV linear accelerator for a 3.5 × 7 cm field blocked to an effective field of 3.5 × 3.5 cm, with the anterior border of the treatment field located at the ora serrata. Using the beam-splitting technique, the lens and pituitary receive less than 10% of the given dose. **(A)** For bilateral treatment, using equally weighted opposed lateral fields, the dose is calculated at the midplane with the retina lying within the 90% isodose curve. **(B)** For unilateral treatment, the dose is calculated to a depth of 3 cm. The retina lies within the 90% isodose curve, and the opposite eye receives 50% to 70% of the given dose.

may have an alarming clinical presentation, including high-output congestive heart failure due to arteriovenous shunting, hemorrhage, and bleeding with evidence of platelet consumption (the Kasabach-Merritt syndrome), and shock may occur after the rupture of a vascular tumor mass. Cavernous hemangioma, characterized by vascular spaces lined by a single layer of flat endothelial cells, often with evidence of old and new thrombus formation, and hemangioendotheliomas, composed of many small vascular channels lined by one or more layers of endothelial cells, are the two most important benign lesions that should be differentiated from malignant hepatic tumors. Although hemangioendotheliomas can be found at multiple sites within the liver, the metastatic potential of these tumors is exceedingly low. Benign hemangiomas can be treated with steroids and, if they fail to respond, low doses of radiation are generally successful in causing shrinkage; surgical resection is rarely necessary.

Hepatic sarcoma is a rare malignancy that constitutes approximately 10% of the primary hepatic tumors of childhood. The most common presenting symptom is abdominal pain. Evaluation should include a thorough determination of the extent of abdominal disease to guide resection and a search for metastases, especially in lung and bone. Tumors are classified as undifferentiated (*i.e.*, embryonal) sarcomas if there is no evidence of specific differentiation and the malignant elements are mesenchymal, having a myxoid background and

TABLE 49–18. Frequency of Benign and Malignant Hepatic Tumors in Children: Selected North American Series

Tumor Type	*No. of Tumors*	*Percentage of Total*
Malignant		
Hepatoblastoma	227	34.6
Hepatocellular carcinoma	148	22.5
Sarcoma*	45	6.8
Benign		
Adenoma	13	2
Focal nodular hyperplasia	12	2
Vascular tumors	118	18
Mesenchymal hamartoma	53	8
Other	40	6

* Sarcomas often arose from extrahepatic biliary tree.
(Greenberg M, Filler RM. Hepatic tumors. In: Pizzo PA, Poplack DG, eds. Principles and practice of pediatric oncology. 2nd ed. Philadelphia: JB Lippincott, 1993)

stellate cells. If there is evidence of differentiation, a more specific diagnosis may be assigned, such as rhabdomyosarcoma if striated muscle cells are present.

Treatment should begin with an aggressive attempt at complete resection. These tumors are relatively responsive to chemotherapy, and patients given therapy similar to that developed for rhabdomyosarcoma may experience long-term survival.

EPIDEMIOLOGY AND GENETICS

Hepatic tumors occur more often in boys and occur in two age peaks. Virtually all hepatoblastomas occur before 5 years of age, with 65% occurring in children younger than 2 years. Anecdotal reports have associated hepatoblastoma with the fetal alcohol syndrome or the maternal use of oral contraceptives. Four familial cases of hepatoblastoma has been reported. Hepatoblastoma has been described in association with the Beckwith-Wiedemann syndrome and its incomplete variants. Hepatoblastoma and Wilms' tumor can occur synchronously. Homozygosity for a mutant allele at the 11p locus, corresponding to the so-called WAGR locus (*i.e.*, Wilms', aniridia, genital malformation, and mental retardation) has been shown in biopsy tissue and in explants from 2 patients with hepatoblastoma.

HCC rarely occurs in infants and has its peak childhood incidence during adolescence. HCC is associated with preexisting cirrhosis and chronic hepatitis caused by the hepatitis B virus (HBV), an association that is particularly prominent in countries where there is a high prevalence of HBV infection, such as Japan. HBV sequences are integrated into the DNA of the HCC cells. Perinatal transmission of HBV has been associated with the onset of HCC 6 to 7 years later, suggesting that the latency period may be shorter in children than in adults. Epidemiologic studies suggest that control of HBV transmission and infection (*i.e.*, by vaccination) may eventually decrease the incidence of HCC in adults and children.

A variety of syndromes and congenital malformations have been associated with primary hepatic tumors, including hemihypertrophy, osteopetrosis, DeToni-Fanconi syndrome, neurofibromatosis, ataxia-telangiectasia, lipid storage disease, glycogen storage disease, hereditary tyrosinemia, biliary atremia secondary to extrahepatic biliary atresia, and the homozygous ZZ and heterozygous phenotypes of α_1-antitrypsin deficiency states. Recent studies have demonstrated an abnormality of the p53 gene at the DNA, RNA, or protein level. The relevance of this pathogenesis of HCC remains to be elucidated.

Hepatoblastoma has presented with virilization in fewer than 25 boys. Prolonged use of anabolic steroids, especially the C17 alkylated forms (*e.g.*, oxymetholone, methyltestosterone, testosterone enanthate, methandienone) have been associated with HCC. Although α-fetoprotein (AFP) is commonly detected in the serum of patients with hepatoblastoma, it is unusual to find evidence of elevated levels of choriogonadotropin (hCG). However, hCG can be detected in children with evidence of virilization, and immunoperoxidase staining has confirmed that hepatoma cells produce the hCG, although these cells may not be the same ones producing AFP. Estrogen and progesterone receptors have been found in hepatoblastoma.

PATHOLOGY

Hepatoblastoma and HCC are epithelial neoplasms. Hepatoblastomas are generally divided into tumors that consist of fetal or immature hepatic epithelial cells and tumors that consist of mixtures of epithelial and mesenchymal elements. The tumor cells have a high nuclear to cytoplasmic ratio, compact amphophilic or basophilic cytoplasm, and evidence of miotic activity. Most commonly, the tumor cells are arranged in cords two to three cells thick and have a sheet-like configuration. Acinar or pseudoglandular components can sometimes be defined, although a mixed epithelial-mesenchymal variant of hepatoblastoma, accounting for almost 30% of hepatoblastomas, can have a spindle cell component. Osteoid and extramedullary hematopoiesis are frequently observed in these mixed tumors. Although the epithelial component appears to be a prognostic determinant for patients with mixed hepatoblastomas, embryonal cells influence the malignant potential of these tumors. Less commonly, the tumor may appear more anaplastic, consisting of sheets of loosely connected cells with scant cytoplasm and a high mitotic rate.

HCC in children may be histologically identical to that seen in adults, although an important variant has been recently defined. This rare tumor, called fibrolamellar carcinoma, occurs primarily in younger patients (mean age, 25; range, 5–35 years) and is characterized by deeply eosinophilic neoplastic hepatocytes, many of which contain intracellular hyaline globules and distinct pale bodies surrounded by fibrous bands, often with a lamellar configuration. Fibrolamellar carcinoma presents as a single tumor nodule and has a much more favorable prognosis (median survival, 32 months) than other forms of HCC. Nonetheless, it is important to differentiate fibrolamellar carcinomas from benign hepatic adenomas, because survival depends on surgical resection.

HCC has a distinctive ultrastructural appearance characterized by large, round, centrally placed nuclei, prominent nucleoli, abundant large mitochondria, and microvilli on the plasma membrane.

By the time of presentation, tumor masses are usually quite large, regardless of histologic type, and frequently involve the right lobe of the liver. Spread to other parts of the liver usually occurs by direct extension, but it may take place through intrahepatic vascular or lymphatic channels. Extrahepatic tumor spread usually occurs by way of the regional lymph nodes in the porta hepatis, and the lungs are the primary sites of metastatic disease.

CLINICAL PRESENTATION

A palpable abdominal mass in the right upper quadrant is the predominant finding in more than 90% of patients with primary hepatic tumors. Usually, there are no other physical signs or symptoms. Severe osteopenia with back pain and pathologic features of weight-bearing bones can occur. Iso sexual precocity, although uncommon, can be seen in approximately 3% of the hepatoblastomas that secret β-hCG.

Abdominal pain is more frequent in patients with HCC, and the mean duration of symptoms before presentation is only 1 to 2 months. Hemoperitoneum with an acute abdominal crisis may be the primary presentation.

In patients with localized hepatic tumors, most routine laboratory tests are normal. Anemia or thrombocytopenia are important findings because they may indicate that the mass is a benign vascular tumor with associated bleeding or platelet consumption. Thrombocytosis can be seen in hepatoblastoma and HCC. Polycythemia, with hemoglobin levels higher than 16 g/100 ml may occur in patients with HCC due to the extrarenal production of erythropoietin. In patients with hepatic tumors, the SGOT and alkaline phosphatase levels may be slightly elevated, but the serum bilirubin is elevated in only 5% of patients with hepatoblastoma, compared with almost 25% of those with HCC.

An α-globulin, AFP is produced normally by embryonic hepatocytes and is present in the serum for the first few days after birth. Elevated AFP has been described in 40% of children with HCC and in 67% of children with hepatoblastomas. The protein is not specific for hepatic tumors and can be elevated in the serum of children with embryonal testicular carcinoma and teratomas. Cystanthininuria has been described in children with primary hepatic neoplasms, but it can be found in patients with neuroblastoma. Serum ferritin levels are elevated in 97% patients with HCC, but they are also elevated in 87% patients with uncomplicated cirrhosis. Although not useful diagnostically, serum ferritin levels have been observed to fall with tumor response and to rise with tumor progression. Rarely, the serum hCG levels may be elevated in patient with virilization and hepatomas. The level of unsaturated vitamin B_{12}-binding protein is elevated in the fibrolamellar variant of HCC and increases with disease progression.

Because the primary goal of the initial evaluation is to define the extent of disease and to differentiate a primary hepatic tumor from the other abdominal masses that may occur in children, a chest x-ray film, abdominal radiograph, and IVP should be obtained. Ultrasound radionuclide liver scan, CT, and to a lesser extent, arteriography are important in delineating the contour and extent of the tumor. Hepatoblastoma and HCC have diffused hyperechoic patterns, unlike benign lesions, which are usually less echogenic. CT scanning is important in defining the extent of tumor and potential operability. Characteristically, tumor masses have lower attenuation than surrounding tissue, although tumors may be isodense. CT scanning is of particular value in assessing the left lobe of the liver, a site hard to define by arteriography. MRI appears to be able to image parenchymal structure and vascular structures, making it the most accurate imaging study and a replacement for angiography.

TREATMENT PLANNING

The staging system, based on surgical resectability, correlates with outcome (Table 49–19 and Fig. 49–7). This approach is verified by the fact that cure of primary hepatic neoplasms requires complete resection. From a surgical viewpoint, the liver can be divided into lobes and segments according to its vascular supply. The right lobe of the liver contains about 70% of the total liver mass, and each segment of the left lobe represents an additional 15%. Because of the liver's remarkable ability to regenerate, it is possible to remove as much as 85% of the total liver at one time and still expect complete regeneration of liver cell mass within 3 weeks in infants and within 3 months in children after surgery. Tumors contained in one lobe of the liver and those arising in the right lobe that do not extend beyond the medial segment of the left lobe are amenable to surgical resection. Improvements in anesthesia and surgical techniques and in vigilant management before, during, and after surgery have minimized the hazards of hepatic resection.

Surgery

BIOPSY. Although excision is preferred, some tumors may be unresectable, because many liver segments are involved or because the hepatic arterial and venous inflow and outflow tracts are involved with tumors. In such cases, preoperative chemotherapy, with or without radiation, may render the tumor resectable. Before beginning such therapy, histologic di-

TABLE 49–19. Clinical Grouping of Malignant Hepatic Tumor

Designation	*Criteria*
Group I	Complete resection of tumor by wedge resection lobectomy or by extended lobectomy as initial treatment
Group IIA	Tumors rendered completely resectable by initial irradiation or chemotherapy
Group IIB	Residual disease confined to one lobe
Group III	Disease involving both lobes of the liver
Group IIIB	Regional node involvement
Group IV	Distant metastases, irrespective of the extent of liver involvement

(Greenberg M, Filler R. Hepatic tumors. In: Pizzo PA, Poplack DG, eds. Principles and practice of pediatric oncology. 2nd ed. Philadelphia: JB Lippincott, 1993)

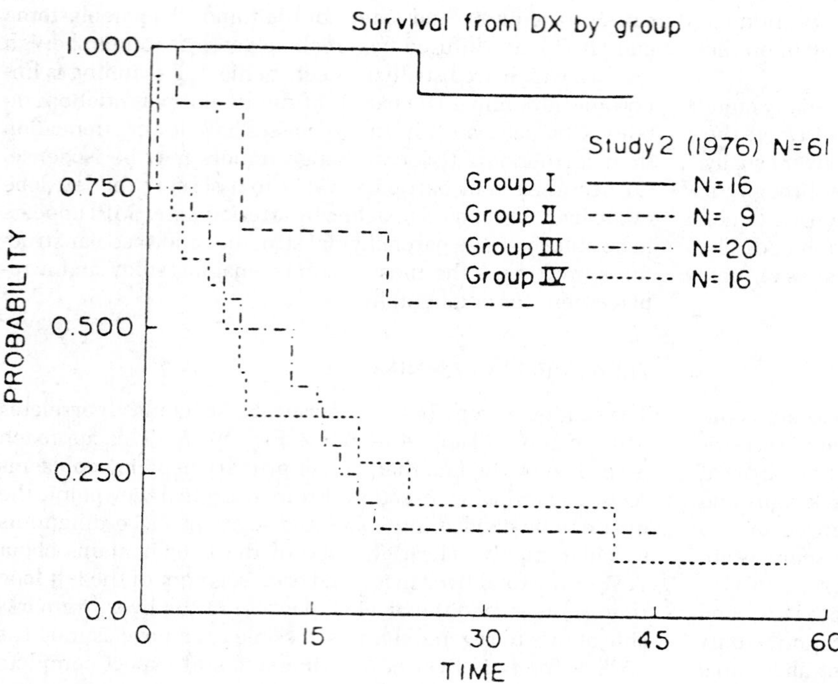

FIGURE 49–7. Life table analysis of survival in a mixed population of children with hepatoblastoma and hepatocellular carcinoma. Survival probability is correlated with clinical grouping 0 to 60 months after diagnosis and treatment. (Greenberg M, Filler RM. Hepatic tumors. In: Pizzo PA, Poplack DG, eds. Principles and practice of pediatric oncology. 2nd ed. Philadelphia: JB Lippincott, 1993)

agnosis is essential. Although an open liver biopsy has been employed, a needle biopsy is satisfactory and avoids the need for general anesthesia, although hemorrhage may occur. Some recommend preoperative chemotherapy in patients with an elevated AFP who have CT scans and anteriograms suggesting hepatoma.

OPERATIVE TECHNIQUE. The recommended procedure for hepatic resection in children is similar to that used in adults. A thoracoabdominal approach is preferred because it offers excellent exposure and precludes the development of negative intrathoracic pressure, which may cause the aspiration of air into an open venous system. This approach provides excellent visualization of the entire supradiaphragmatic inferior vena cava, into which an internal venous shunt can be placed so that liver blood flow can be isolated in the event of catastrophic hemorrhage.

After the porta hepatis is dissected, the vessels and ducts to the lobe to be excised are ligated and divided. The liver is mobilized by dividing the diaphragmatic attachments, and the diaphragm may be divided radially to the vena cava. Tapes are passed around the vena cava above and below the liver to ensure control of excessive bleeding. Before the hepatic veins are isolated, the liver capsule is incised along a lobar or segmental division, and the liver substance is divided bluntly. Bridging vessels and bile ducts are ligated as they are encountered. Because of the short extrahepatic length of the hepatic veins in children, they should be approached by dissection through the liver substance rather than at their exit from the liver. With this technique, inadvertent venous injury, which can result in difficult to control bleeding, can be minimized. Large vessels and ducts are individually ligated on the raw surface of the remnant lobe. Sump and Penrose drains are placed in the liver bed, and the incision is closed. If the gallbladder remains, it should be drained with a cholecystostomy.

Profound hypothermia with circulatory arrest has been used as an adjunct to surgery in a difficult hepatectomy. Before division of the liver, cardiopulmonary bypass is instituted and hypothermia is induced. With the child's body temperature at 20°C, the circulation can be stopped for as long as 60 minutes, and resection and repair of vascular structures can be performed in a bloodless operative field. Alternatively, a normothermic, isolated hepatic circulatory arrest in which the lower thoracic aorta, porta hepatis, and the vena cava above or below the liver are clamped to effectively stop liver circulation has been used as an adjunct to hepatic resection. Hemodilution is another procedure that produces an essentially bloodless exposure and permits the return of the patient's own erythrocytes after surgery. These techniques should be considered for children with large tumors or with tumors adjacent to the hepatic veins.

INTRAOPERATIVE MANAGEMENT. The most frequent and serious intraoperative problem is hemorrhage. Even without uncontrolled bleeding, the loss of one blood volume (up to 800 ml in a 10-kg child) is not unusual. Accurate measurement of blood lost in surgical sponges and by suction and measurement of intraarterial blood pressure, central venous pressure, and urine output is necessary to estimate replacement volumes. Because hypothermia tends to cause cardiac irritability, metabolic acidosis, and abnormal blood clotting mechanisms, blood administered during surgery should be warmed to 37°C. Unless the procedure is performed with induced hypothermia, the child's normal body temperature should be maintained by providing a warm operating room temperature and by the use of a warming blanket. Adjusting the pH 7.0 of bank blood to pH 7.4 decreases the incidence of cardiac arrest, which can be triggered by the rapid infusion of large volumes of cold, relatively acidic blood.

PREOPERATIVE CHEMOTHERAPY OR RADIATION THERAPY. Preoperative chemotherapy or radiation therapy (1200–2000 cGy) has been used to reduce the size of the primary tumors before resection. The use of continuous-infusion doxorubicin and cisplatin has shrunk tumors in 35% to 95% of patients. Ten of these patients had initially unresectable tumors, but after chemotherapy, the tumors were completely resectable. Although the experience with HCC is more limited, preoperative chemotherapy with doxorubicin and cisplatin is recommended before resection in all patients.

POSTOPERATIVE MANAGEMENT. Despite advances in surgical techniques, surgical morbidity and mortality rates are still high. Between 11% and 25% of the patients die during or after hepatic resections. Blood loss was the most common intraoperative and postoperative complication. A single blood-stained dressing may represent significant blood loss in an infant, but too vigorous volume replacement may result in pulmonary edema. Other postoperative complications include subphrenic abscess, wound infection, biliary fistula, and small bowel obstruction.

Hepatic resection may result in a variety of metabolic derangements, particularly hypoglycemia and coagulopathies. These problems can usually be avoided by the continuous intravenous infusion of 10% dextrose postoperatively, with daily infusion of albumen for the first postoperative week and the administration of vitamin K.

Radiation Therapy

The role of preoperative and postoperative radiation therapy is less defined than that for surgery and chemotherapy. When employed, doses range between 1200 and 2000 cCy. Although used for preoperative therapy in patients failing to respond to chemotherapy, radiation therapy may be better used for the treatment of microscopic residual disease after resection.

Adjuvant Chemotherapy

Approximately 50% of children with hepatoblastomas or HCC appear to be cured after complete tumor resection. In general, children with hepatoblastoma do better than those with HCC. The use of preoperative chemotherapy in patients with inoperative tumors should further improve these results. Metastatic disease is an important cause of death in patients with residual tumor. The Children's Cancer Study Group (CCSG) and POG evaluated combination chemotherapy consisting of pulses of vincristine, cyclophosphamide, and doxorubicin, alternating every 3 weeks with vincristine, cyclophosphamide, and 5-fluorouracil (5-FU) for 1 year. Of 16 patients who received adjuvant therapy after complete surgical resection, only 1 patient developed distant metastases, compared with 7 of 11 historic controls who did not receive adjuvant chemotherapy. Among the regimens recommended are cisplatin (20 mg/m^2/day) by continuous infusion for 5 days with doxorubicin (25 mg/m^2/day) for 3 days. Treatments are given every 3 to 4 weeks for six cycles, beginning 3 to 4 weeks after surgery, permitting regeneration of hepatic tissue.

GERM CELL TUMORS

The germ cell tumors of infants and children reflect the transformation of primordial cells that have failed to migrate to their predestined location. The totipotent germ cells normally arise from the yolk sac of the 4-week-old human embryo and migrate along the gonadal ridge to the gonadal anlage before their final descent into the pelvis. During embryogenesis, some of these germ cells fail to complete this migration and come to rest along the dorsal midline of the embryo. The primordial germ cells give rise to an undifferentiated cell line and a primitive, committed germ cell line. The undifferentiated germ cell undergoes differentiation into embryonic (*i.e.,* somatic cells) or the extraembryonic cells of yolk sac, chorion, and allantoin cells. Malignant transformation of these cells gives rise to tumors that reflect their embryonic features. Tumors of the embryonic germ cells are the teratomas and consist of each of the embryonic cell layers of ectoderm, mesoderm, and endoderm. However, tumors of extraembryonic cells have trophoblastic features, as in choriocarcinoma, or characteristics of the yolk sac endoderm and extraembryonic mesoderm, as in embryonal adenocarcinoma of the infantile testis (Fig. 49–8).

EPIDEMIOLOGY AND GENETICS

Germ cell tumors comprise approximately 3% of childhood neoplasms and have a bimodal age distribution. Almost 67% arise in extragonadal sites. Extragonadal teratomas and yolk sac tumors of the testis occur in infants and young children. Ovarian teratomas and dysgerminomas have their peak incidence during adolescence.

Karyotypic analysis has demonstrated several nonrandom structural changes, most commonly is chromosomes 1 and 12 but also in chromosomes 5, 7, 9, 17, 21, and 22. An isochromosome 12p[i(12p)] has been identified in various histologic subtypes of germ cell tumors. Familial inheritance of testicular and other germ cell tumors have been described. The malignant potential of histologically benign-appearing teratomas may be suggested by the DNA index, aneuploidy, and presence of the *MYC* oncogene.

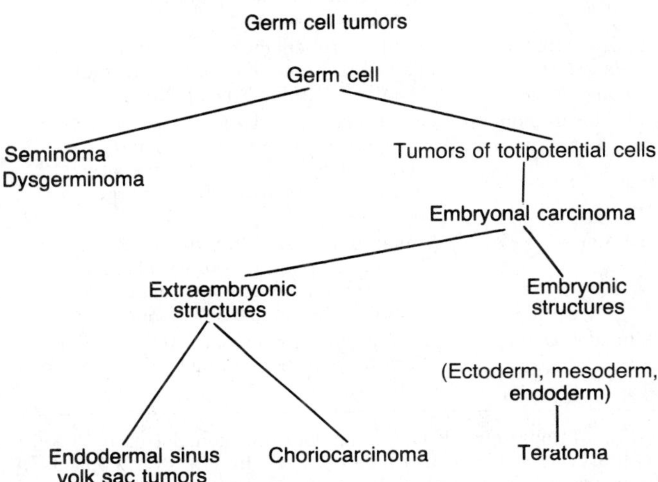

FIGURE 49–8. Histogenesis of germ cell tumors.

ANATOMIC AND PATHOLOGIC CONSIDERATIONS

The classification and comparative pathology of germ cell tumors are shown in Tables 49–20 and 49–21.

Teratomas

Teratomas are composed of tissues that are derived from three germinal layers, the endoderm, mesoderm, and ectoderm. They may be solid or cystic and are classified histologically as mature, immature, and malignant. Mature teratomas consist of well-differentiated tissues (*e.g.*, brain, skin, gastrointestinal, bone) and are benign. Immature teratomas contain embryonic tissue, usually neuroglia or neural tube-like structures, in addition to mature tumors. Teratomas with malignant potential may contain elements of germinoma, choriocarcinoma, endodermal sinus tumor, or embryonal carcinoma. There may be a mixture of mature, embryonic and unequivocally malignant elements, making examination of multiple histologic sections mandatory.

Teratomas in infants and young children are primarily extragonadal. Of 245 patients with 254 teratomas admitted to the Boston Children's Hospital Medical Center from 1928 to 1982, 49% were detected in the newborn period. Sacrococcygeal teratomas were most common (40%), followed by ovary (37%), head and neck (6%), retroperitoneum (5%), mediastinum (4%), CNS (4%), testes (3%), and liver or trunk (1%) teratomas.

Fifty percent to 75% of sacrococcygeal teratomas are diagnosed at birth, and almost 75% occur in girls. Although every teratoma has the potential to become malignant, 48% are benign, 23% have immature but nonmalignant components, and 29% are malignant. Most tumors are diagnosed within the first 2 months after birth (90% at birth) and are almost invariably benign.

Sacrococcygeal tumors can be external or internal (*i.e.*, presacral), 44% of them have an external component and an intrapelvic or intraabdominal extension. In 10% of patients, they can be entirely presacral. Tumors that are entirely or predominantly external have a lower malignant potential than presacral tumors, 8% of which are malignant, or intrapelvic or intraabdominal tumors, approximately 20% of which are malignant.

Sacrococcygeal teratomas vary in size from small localized lesions to massive tumors. Rarely, the tumor is so large in utero that a cesarean section is necessary for delivery, and death of the child due to uncontrolled hemorrhage has been reported during vaginal delivery if the tumor ruptures.

Germinoma

Germinomas are uniform in appearance, consisting of large, round cells with vesicular nuclei and clear or finely granular eosinophilic-staining cytoplasm separated by vascular fibrous septal-containing lymphocytes and focal granulomas.

The most common sites in children are the ovary, anterior mediastinum, and pineal gland, and the tumor is the predominant histologic type found in dysgenic gonads and undescended testes. Germinomas account for 10% of ovarian tumors in children and 15% of all germ cell tumors.

Embryonal Carcinoma and Endodermal Sinus Tumor

Endodermal sinus tumor (*i.e.*, yolk sac tumor) is the most common malignant germ cell tumor found in children. It is

TABLE 49–20. Comparative Characteristics of Germ Cell Tumors by Pathologic Types

Tumor Type	*Characteristic Histology*	*Frequency*	*Most Common Locations*	*Markers* AFP	HCG	PLAP
Germinoma	Large round cells, vesicular nuclei, clear eosinophilic cytoplasm; monotonous pattern	+	Ovary, anterior mediastinum, pineal, undescended testes	–	–	+
Embryonal carcinoma	Poorly differentiated, epithelial appearance; solid or glandular, anaplasia, necrosis	++	Testes, young adult	+	±	±
Yolk sac tumor (endodermal sinus tumor)	Papillary, reticular or solid pattern; papillary projections with perivascular sheaths (Schiller-Duval bodies)	+++	Testes, infant: sacrococcygeal, ovary	+	–	–
Choriocarcinoma	Cytotrophoblasts (large round cells, clear cytoplasm, vesicular nuclei) and syncytiotrophoblasts (syncytia with abundant cytoplasm); hemorrhage, necrosis	+	Mediastinal, ovary, pineal	–	+	–
Teratoma	Immature to well-differentiated tissues foreign to anatomic site with lack of organization; benign or immature may contain other malignant components	++++	Sacrococcygeal midline structures	–	–	–
Gonadoblastoma	Large germ cells surrounded by smaller Sertoli's cells containing hyaline bodies and calcium	+	Dysgenic gonads	–	–	–

AFP, α-fetoprotein; HCG, human chorionic gonadotropin; PLAP, placental alkaline phosphatase.
(Ablin A, Isaacs H Jr. Germ cell tumors. In: Pizzo PA, Poplack DG, eds. Principles and practice of pediatric oncology. 2nd ed. Philadelphia: JB Lippincott, 1993)

TABLE 49–21. Comparative Clinical Presentations of Germ Cell Tumors

Tumor	*Age*	*Relative Frequency (%)*	*Symptoms*	*Findings*	*Pathology*
Extragonadal					
Sacrococcygeal	Infants	41	Constipation, neurologic abnormalities of bladder or lower extremities	Presacral mass with or without extension to buttocks or pelvis and abdomen	65% benign 5% immature 30% malignant
Mediastinal		6	Cough, wheeze, dyspnea	Anterior mediastinal mass	Benign or malignant
Abdominal	<2 y	5	Secondary to pressure pain, GU obstruction, constipation	Often retroperitoneal; also stomach, omentum, liver	Benign or malignant
Intracranial	Children	6	Headache, paralysis of upward gaze, incoordination	Pineal or supracellular tumors; AFP or hCG in CSF	Any type germ cell tumor
Head and neck	Infants	4	Pressure-related; respiratory or swallowing difficulty	Large mass on physical examination	Usually benign
Vagina	<3 y	1	Blood-tinged vaginal discharge	Polypoid mass from vagina	Usually malignant
Gonadal					
Ovarian	10–14 y	29	Abdominal pain, nausea, vomiting, constipation, GU symptoms	Abdominal pelvic mass; calcifications in 50%; often + AFP or hCG	Any type germ cell tumor
Testicular	Infants, postpubertal	7	Painless swelling of testis or painful torsion	Testicular mass; metastases to lung in infants	Any type germ cell tumor; 82% malignant, 18% benign. Infants mostly yolk sac tumors

GU, genitourinary; AFP, α-fetoprotein; hCG, human chorionic gonadotropin.
(Ablin A, Isaacs H Jr. Germ cell tumors. In: Pizzo PA, Poplack DG, eds. Principles and practice of pediatric oncology. 2nd ed. Philadelphia: JB Lippincott, 1993)

characterized by a labyrinthine glandular pattern consisting of flat epithelial cells and rounded papillary processes with a central capillary (*i.e.,* Schiller-Duval body). The tumor represents a proliferation of yolk sac endoderm and extraembryonic mesenchyme. It was first recognized as a distinct entity by Teilum, because of its similarity to the endodermal sinus found in rat placenta. Although most yolk sac tumors present as infant testicular tumors, yolk cell tumors occurring as pure or component portions of mixed germ cell tumors are rather common in the ovaries of young girls and in several extragonadal sites, including the sacrococcygeal area, pelvis, mediastinum, liver, retroperitoneum, vagina, and CNS.

Choriocarcinoma, Gonadoblastoma, and Polyembryoma

Choriocarcinoma is an uncommon, highly malignant tumor consisting of gestational forms arising from placenta and nongestational forms arising from extraplacental tissues in a nongravid woman. In an infant, choriocarcinoma may present as a congenital tumor arising from a maternal placental primary tumor and transmitted to the fetal bloodstream; it presents as a mediastinal or ovarian tumor in young children or as a placental tumor in the pregnant adolescent. Choriocarcinomas consist of cytotrophoblasts, which are large round cells with clear cytoplasms and variable vesicular nuclei, and syncytiotrophoblasts, which are larger cells with vacuolated cytoplasm and irregular nuclei that form syncytia.

Gonadoblastoma is a rare germ cell tumor that occurs almost exclusively during the first 20 years of life in patients with dysgenic gonads, usually in association with a Y chromosome. Almost 33% of these tumors are associated with germinomas. Gonadoblastomas consist of large germ cells surrounded by smaller round, darkly staining Sertoli's cells, forming microfollicles consisting of hylanine bodies and calcium deposits.

Polyembryoma is a rare tumor that consists of embryoid bodies comparable to presomatic embryos. They stain positive for AFP and hCG, suggesting embryonic and extraembryonic differentiation.

TREATMENT

Clinical Evaluation and Treatment Planning

Depending on the anatomic site, histologic type, and stage, surgery is combined with radiation or chemotherapy in the management of children with germ cell tumors. The surgical considerations are tailored to each tumor.

Radiation Therapy

Radiation therapy, even in limited doses, can be highly curative for several germ cell tumors. However, in the more common yolk sac tumors and embryonal carcinomas or the malignant teratomas of extragonadal origin, the role of radiation therapy is less certain. Few patients with malignant sacrococcygeal teratomas have been long-term survivors. Similar data support the use of regional radiation therapy for other extragonadal tumors poorly controlled with surgery or chemotherapy.

Doses of radiation for germinomas may be limited to 2500 cGy for patients with microscopic disease or to 3500 cGy for large tumors. With endodermal sinus tumors, effective local control has only been achieved at doses of 4000 to 4500 cGy or higher.

Chemotherapy

Methotrexate was the first chemotherapeutic agent to demonstrate efficacy against germ cell tumors, producing a 47% complete response rate in gestational choriocarcinoma. Several agents have been evaluated, singly and in combination, with remarkable results in some germ cell tumors. Among the agents that have been used are vincristine, dactinomycin, cyclophosphamide, vinblastine, bleomycin, cisplatin, doxorubicin, ifosfamide, and VP-16. The most commonly employed combinations are vincristine, dactinomycin, and cyclophosphamide (VAC), vinblastine, dactinomycin, and bleomycin (VAB), or cisplatin, vinblastine, and bleomycin (PVB). For testicular tumors in adults, PVB combinations have been the standard, with complete response rates of 70% and overall response rates of 100%. Combinations of PVB plus doxorubicin have also been employed. For ovarian germ cell tumors in adults, PVB combinations have proven superior to VAC regimens for patients with endodermal sinus tumor and those with stage III or IV disease of any cell type.

Similar regimens have been employed for germ cell tumors occurring in children. Adjuvant VAC chemotherapy has been most extensively used, particularly for children with ovarian tumors and endodermal sinus tumors. Other combinations have demonstrated efficacy, particularly those with cisplatin, bleomycin, and doxorubicin in addition to vincristine, dactinomycin, and cyclophosphamide.

Vinblastine, bleomycin, cisplatin, dactinomycin, cyclophosphamide, and doxorubicin were evaluated in treating 79 children with poor-risk germ cell tumors; 39% had evidence of metastatic disease at diagnosis. Approximately 69% of these patients had complete responses and 27% attained partial responses. After 4 years, 45% of the patients are free of disease.

Epipodophyllotoxin and ifosfamide have been evaluated as salvage agents for adults and children with germ cell tumors, particularly in conjunction with high-dose cisplatin. More intensive regimens using high doses of melphalan, VP-16, and cyclophosphamide have been administered in conjunction with autologous bone marrow reconstitution. Regimens using ifosfamide and VP-16 in conjunction with cisplatin, bleomycin, cyclophosphamide, dactinomycin, doxorubicin, and vinblastine are being explored.

Specific Management Strategies

SACROCOCCYGEAL TUMORS. For infants with external masses in the sacrococcygeal area, the differential diagnosis includes meningomyelocele, chordoma, duplication of the rectum, neurogenic tumors, lipoma, vestigial tail, and hemangioma. In infants without external masses, asymmetric intergluteal folds warrant a careful rectal examination to search for a presacral lesion. The incidence of malignancy if the diagnosis is established before the infant is 2 months of age is 10% for boys and 7% for girls. If diagnosis is delayed until the infant is older than 2 months, 67% of boys and 47% of girls develop malignant tumors. A careful rectal examination is essential in the evaluation of these infants. With more advanced presacral or intrapelvic involvement, particularly if the diagnosis is delayed, infants may develop bowel or bladder dystonia as a consequence of the tumor mass. Albeit rarely, invasion of the lumbosacral plexus or spinal cord may result in lower extremity weakness and pain. Approximately 20% of infants with advanced local involvement have pulmonary metastases at the time of diagnosis.

Radiographic examination of the pelvis may demonstrate calcification in the tumor mass or the destruction of the sacrum. Barium enema, a CT scan, and an IVP should be performed to evaluate the intrapelvic extent of tumor. A chest x-ray film should always be obtained to assess the presence of metastatic disease.

The serum AFP level is elevated in malignant sacrococcygeal tumors. Of 61 infants with teratoma, the AFP level was normal in 96% with mature lesions but was elevated in 97% of those with malignant elements. It is important to monitor AFP levels, even in patients whose sacrococcygeal tumor was initially benign, because late recurrences may develop. Serum ferritin may be elevated in patients with germ cell tumors and, although not tumor specific, may serve as another biologic marker.

The operative approach depends on whether the tumor is primarily extrapelvic or there is intrapelvic or intraabdominal extension. For lesions that are predominantly external, a one-stage posterior sacral approach, in which the coccyx and possibly the lower sacrum are removed, is the treatment of choice. For lesions that extend into the pelvis, a two-stage procedure is usually necessary. An anterior approach through the abdomen is taken so that the superior extent of the tumor can be defined and removed. For the second stage, the child is positioned face downward, and a V-shaped incision is made over the upper buttocks. The lower sacrum is divided, and with the coccyx attached to the specimen, the previously mobilized intrapelvic mass is delivered. The lower part of the mass is separated from the rectum, and the skin is incised posteriorly behind the mass so that the tumor can be removed intact. The major surgical complication is massive bleeding. In most children, anal and urinary sphincter functions are not impaired.

The success of therapy correlates most closely with the histologic type and the surgical resectability of the primary tumor. With few exceptions, patients with benign, resectable tumors survive with surgery alone. If local, benign recurrence takes place, reexcision can be curative. In contrast, fewer than 10% of children whose tumors have malignant components or who have surgically unresectable tumors survive.

MEDIASTINAL GERM CELL TUMORS. Mediastinal tumors are usually located in the anterior superior mediastinum, but they rarely can be located posteriorly. Occurrence in the mediastinum is related to the fact that the urogenital ridge in the embryo extends past C6 to L4. These tumors are often asymptomatic but may result in tracheobronchial compression hemoptysis or hormone production.

In boys, most lesions are endodermal sinus tumors, but pure and malignant-element teratomas have been described. Chest CT scanning is the imaging procedure of choice, and the differential diagnosis must include thymomas, thymic cysts, lymphomas, lymphangiomas, lipomas, bronchial and enteric cysts, and neurogenic tumors.

Most mediastinal germ cell tumors can be approached by a unilateral thoracotomy or a median sternotomy. Complete excision is necessary except for immature teratomas with neuroglial elements in young children; in older children, this can be highly malignant.

ABDOMINAL GERM CELL TUMORS. The primary sites of abdominal germ cell tumors are in the retroperitoneum, but they can involve the stomach, omentum, and liver. Patients may present with vague abdominal complaints or bleeding, and abdominal germ cell tumors must be differentiated from Wilms' tumor, neuroblastoma, lymphoma, or rhabdomyosarcoma.

HEAD AND NECK TUMORS. The oral cavity is the site of almost 6% of germ cell neoplasms. They are usually found at birth, and most are benign. Intracranial germ cell tumors account for 0.5% to 2% of brain tumors in children. They arise in the pineal area and can involve the suprasellar and infrasellar regions.

TESTICULAR TUMORS. Approximately 7% of germ cell tumors and 1% of all childhood cancers arise in the testes. About 77% of testicular tumors originate from germ cells; 25% of these are benign. The most common malignant germ cell tumors of the testes have been described as infantile adenocarcinoma of the testes, embryonal carcinoma, orchioblastoma, adenocarcinoma with clear cells, and embryonal adenocarcinoma. Unifying terms for these malignancies are endodermal sinus tumor or yolk sac tumor. Choriocarcinomas and seminomas are unusual in children; the youngest patient described being 8 years old. Although testicular tumors account for less than 1% of childhood tumors, they are much less common in American and African blacks and in Asians. An increased incidence of congenital anomalies, particularly of the genitourinary tract, is associated with patients with testicular germ cell tumors.

Most infants and young boys with cancer of the testes present with a painless mass that usually has been growing slowly for months. Almost all of these children, particularly those with endodermal sinus tumors, are younger than 2 years of age. Testicular tumors rarely occur in adolescents.

Almost 25% of infants with a malignant tumor have a hydrocele, making transillumination potentially misleading. Physical examination usually reveals a hard, painless testicular mass, 2 cm in diameter or larger, not involving the scrotal wall or spermatic cord. The possibility of distant spread, particularly to lymph nodes in the inguinal and supraclavicular regions and retroperitoneum, should be carefully assessed. The scrotum should be carefully examined for evidence of direct extension to the scrotal skin and to determine if the mass is in the testis or in a paratesticular site.

Although endodermal sinus tumors tend to remain confined to the testes for a relatively long period, early diagnosis is critical. The relative rarity of these tumors and a lack of awareness that testicular cancer can occur in infants makes delays in diagnosis of as long as 3 months common.

After a testicular mass is suspected, a biopsy should be done as soon as possible. An inguinal incision should be made, and the spermatic cord should be exposed and occluded at the internal abdominal ring with a noncrushing vascular clamp before manipulation of the testis. If a gross diagnosis of neoplasm can be made when the testis is delivered into the wound, radical orchiectomy is performed by ligating and dividing the spermatic cord at the internal ring and removing the mass with the entire cord. If the testicular mass is obviously benign (*e.g.*, hydrocele), appropriate treatment is provided and the testis is returned to the scrotum. If the diagnosis is uncertain, the testis is walled off with sponges and an incisional biopsy is performed. Frozen-section diagnosis is used to determine additional treatment. It is unnecessary to excise a portion of the scrotum unless the tumor has been previously biopsied in situ or if the extragonadal tissues are grossly involved. If retroperitoneal lymph node dissection is contemplated, placement of a nonabsorbable suture on the ligated spermatic cord aids in defining the distal end of the inguinal dissection during lymphadenectomy.

The physician must determine whether the tumor is restricted to the scrotum and, if not, whether the retroperitoneal lymph nodes or distant sites are involved. This dictates retroperitoneal node dissection, radiation, or chemotherapy. The major sites of metastases for testicular germ cell cancers are the lungs, liver, lymph nodes, and CNS.

A variety of staging systems are used, and in evaluating reports from different centers, the distinction between clinical staging and pathologic staging should be recognized, although they are usually the same for boys with this neoplasm.

Virtually all patients with embryonal adenocarcinoma of the testis and 90% of patients with nonseminomatous testicular tumors have elevated serum levels of hCG and AFP. Measurement of AFP and hCG before and after surgery, and then at least monthly, can assess tumor burden or recurrence.

Ultrasonography can help in defining testicular and adnexal masses. CT scans of the chest and abdomen and a bone scan are part of the metastatic workup, and MRI of the pelvis produces optimal visualizations of pelvic structures.

Retroperitoneal node dissection has been recommended for accurate pathologic staging of testicular tumors. For example, of adults with stage I embryonal carcinoma, 53% actually had stage II disease after retroperitoneal lymphadenectomy. However, for endodermal sinus tumor, the results of node dissection have been quite different. Positive nodes were found in only 4 of 53 node dissections in clinical stage I patients. Therefore, node dissection for staging purposes is useful only for those children in whom retroperitoneal node involvement is suspected by ultrasound, MRI, or CT scan or for patients without lung metastases in whom AFP of hCG remains elevated.

After radical orchiectomy and clinical staging are completed, further therapy, possibly including retroperitoneal node dissection, chemotherapy, and irradiation, is considered. Approximately 80% of children have stage I disease, and 20% have stage II or stage III disease.

The value of node dissection in the treatment of endodermal sinus tumor is not clear cut. Current data suggest that radical orchiectomy alone is comparable to orchiectomy plus retroperitoneal node dissection for children younger than 36 months of age with stage I embryonal carcinoma or endodermal sinus tumor. However, other data describe a cure rate (84%) after orchiectomy plus node dissection that is almost twice the cure rate after orchiectomy alone (48%). These discrepancies may be due to inclusion of older patients in the early studies, histologic differences in the study populations, and the fact that less radical orchiectomies are performed than in the past. On the basis of current data, retroperitoneal lymphadenectomy is not recommended for patients with stage I disease, particularly if serum markers are positive before surgery and fall at the expected rate after inguinal orchiectomy.

If retroperitoneal lymph nodes are the site of metastatic disease (stage II), lymphadenectomy appears to increase survival. Considerable controversy surrounds the value of bilateral or unilateral lymphadenectomy. The cross-communications between the lymphatic channels of the testes support the need for bilateral retroperitoneal node dissection, but few patients have had negative ipsilateral nodes and positive contralateral nodes. Survival figures for patients with germ cell neoplasms receiving unilateral or bilateral adenectomies were comparable. Unilateral dissection is recommended if no gross tumor is discovered. When ipsilateral nodes are grossly positive, bilateral adenectomy is advised, or a modified (superior aspect only) node dissection on the contralateral side can be performed, minimizing the possibility of retrograde ejaculation, a disturbing complication of bilateral adenectomy if both second lumbar sympathetic ganglia are excised. Although some reports raise doubts about the safety of this procedure in small children, experience indicates that retroperitoneal node dissection is well tolerated. A simple midline, paramedian, or transverse abdominal incision generally gives adequate exposure in children.

Approach to the Child With an Undescended Testicle. Although the incidence of an undescended testis is 0.23%, the risk for developing testicular cancer in these cases is 20 to 40 times that in a normal testis. Almost 20% of the tumors that occur in cryptorchid patients do so in the descended testis. This suggests that there may be a genetic predisposition to develop testicular cancer in patients with an undescended testis or that a basic defect in gonadogenesis accounts for failure of the testis to descend and for subsequent oncogenesis.

Tumors of all germ cell types can arise in cryptorchid testis and can occur in adulthood (median age, 38 years). However, seminomas appear to be more common in the undescended testis than in the scrotal testis.

There is debate about orchiopexy in the child with an undescended testis. Although it is clear that orchiopexy does not prevent the development of testicular cancer, especially because it can arise in the contralateral descended testis, it does make the testis more accessible for palpation and monitoring. Because these patients have a higher risk of developing cancer, periodic evaluation is important. If the diagnosis of a cryptorchid testis is not made until after puberty, when dysgenesis and atrophy are probable, orchiectomy is recommended.

OVARIAN TUMORS. Gynecologic malignancies are extremely rare in children and adolescents and differ in their clinical presentation and histology from those occurring in adults. Ovarian tumors are the most common, but only account for 1% of cancers in girls younger than 17 years of age; nonovarian malignant tumors are even less common. The peak incidence is between 10 and 14 years of age. Unlike the pattern in adults, approximately 90% of pediatric gynecologic tumors are immature, and only 10% are differentiated carcinomas.

The ovary descends from the abdomen into the bony pelvis during puberty, and in younger children and in most adolescents, an ovarian tumor presents as an abdominal mass. The longer infundibular pedicle in the child facilitates torsion of an enlarged ovary, resulting in abdominal pain. In the adolescent, abdominal pain can be due to endometriosis, a diagnosis that is frequently overlooked. Symptoms can include constipation or genitourinary complaints. Rarely, tumors may produce hCG and can mimic signs of pregnancy. Nonneoplastic cysts comprise 25% to 35% of the ovarian masses, of which half are follicular and half are simple, parovarian, or luteal. In an infant, an adnexal mass is likely to be a nonneoplastic cyst. Mesonephric duct cysts (*e.g.,* Gartner's duct cysts) and paramesonephric duct cysts can present as abdominal or pelvic masses. If associated with symptoms or if the cystic mass is larger than 4 cm, laparoscopy or laparotomy is indicated.

The remaining 65% to 75% of ovarian tumors are true neoplasms, of which 33% are malignant. Germ cell tumors account for 60% to 89% of the ovarian tumors in children and adolescents (compared with 20% in adults) and are more likely to be malignant in younger children and infants. With increasing age, tumors of the sex cord stroma (*e.g.,* granulosa-theca cell tumor, Sertoli-Leydig cell tumors) and tumors of common epithelial origin increase in frequency; in adolescents 15 to 17 years old, almost 33% of ovarian neoplasms are epithelial tumors. Most benign tumors occur in prepubertal patients, and most malignant tumors occur after 13 years of age.

A calcified ovarian mass is found in almost half of the patients, particularly those with benign teratomas. These can be demonstrated with pelvic ultrasound, and abdominal and chest CT scans should be performed to rule out evidence of metastatic disease. Levels of hCG can be elevated with embryonal carcinoma and choriocarcinoma, and AFP increases in patients with endodermal sinus tumor.

The staging for ovarian tumors in children is modified from the International Federation of Gynecology and Obstetrics:

Stage I	Disease is limited to one or both ovaries, with the capsule intact and peritoneal fluid negative for malignant cell.
Stage II	Disease includes or is beyond the ovarian capsule with local pelvic extension. Retroperitoneal nodes and peritoneal fluid are negative for malignant cells.
Stage III	Positive retroperitoneal nodes or malignant cells are in the peritoneal fluid or abdominal extension.
Stage IV	Extraabdominal dissemination exists.

In children, the ovaries are in the abdomen, and if there are malignant ascites, they are classified as stage III disease.

Approaches to management are based on the patient's tumor type and extent.

Mature Cystic (Dermoid) or Solid Teratoma. These benign neoplasms account for approximately 40% of ovarian tumors and are the most common tumors in older adolescents. These tumors are frequently unilateral in children, but in adults, almost 25% are bilateral. Approximately 40% to 50% of mature teratomas are calcified, and diagnosis is usually suggested by a plain abdominal radiograph and ultrasonography. Malignant degeneration is rare in children. Therapy consists of oophorocystectomy with the preservation of as much ovarian tissue as possible. Oophorectomy is indicated only if there is torsion, rupture, or if the mass is so large that normal ovarian tissue cannot be reconstructed.

Immature Teratomas. Immature teratomas account for 7.4% of childhood ovarian neoplasms and most commonly occur around the age of 11 years. The tumors are composed of variable amounts of incompletely differentiated germ cell elements, most commonly of neural origin. Immature teratomas may not be clinically or grossly differentiated from benign cysts or solid teratomas, and scrupulous histologic examination is important. Teratomas containing immature elements can become malignant, and survival is closely correlated with stage. Approximately 50% of patients with immature teratomas have measurable levels of AFP. These tumors tend to be radioresistant, and treatment has included surgery (*i.e.*, salpingo-oophorectomy for unilateral lesions) and chemotherapy.

Dysgerminomas. Dysgerminomas comprise 16% of germ cell tumors. They are rare before the age of 10 and occur most frequently in prepubertal and young adolescent girls; almost 50% of these tumors occur before the age of 20. These tumors are usually surrounded by a dense capsule and may be bilateral in 5% to 10% of patients. Dysgerminomas are endocrinologically inactive; hormonal symptoms signal an undetected teratocarcinoma with chorioepitheliomatous elements. Dysgerminomas are generally considered low-grade malignancies, although spread may occur if the tumor extends through the capsule and involves lymph nodes or blood vessels.

Treatment planning should take into account that dysgerminomas are highly radiosensitive tumors. If the tumor is well encapsulated, a salpingo-oophorectomy is recommended and has been associated with a 96% survival. More advanced disease may require hysterectomy and bilateral oophorectomy. Wide-field, low-dose irradiation or chemotherapy (VAC or PVB) are indicated if the tumor has penetrated through the ovarian capsule. Better results may be attained with bleomycin, etoposide, and cisplatin (BEP). Disease has recurred 5 to 34 years after treatment.

Embryonal Cell Carcinoma. This carcinoma accounts for 6% of ovarian neoplasms, is highly malignant, and occurs primarily in girls 13 to 14 years of age. Almost 60% of these tumors are associated with endocrinologic manifestations, including precocious puberty, abnormal vaginal bleeding, and hirsutism. Both hCG and AFP are detectable in patients with this tumor. Because the survival for patients whose tumor has been completely resected, usually with salpingo-oophorectomy, is only 50%, adjuvant chemotherapy (VAC) is indicated.

Endodermal Sinus or Yolk Sac Tumors. Like embryonal cell carcinomas, yolk sac tumors are highly malignant germ cell tumors, primarily occurring in older adolescents. Elevated AFP is detectable in virtually all cases. The fact that fewer than 20% of patients with localized and completely resected tumors are curable with surgery alone is testimony to the malignant potential of these tumors. All patients, even those with completely resectable tumors, should receive adjuvant chemotherapy. Mixed germ cell tumors are infrequent and are treated according to the most malignant element present.

Mesenchymal Sex Cord Stromal Tumors. Stromal tumors account for approximately 13% of ovarian tumors in children. The granulosa-theca cell tumor is the most common type and most often presents with precocious pseudopuberty and an abdominal mass, particularly in premenarcheal girls. Postmenarcheal girls may present with menstrual abnormalities or with virilization. Unlike the typical thecal tumor in adults, the histologic picture in children consists of a diffuse or solid pattern with larger cells and prominent luteinization of cellular components; Call-Exner bodies and "coffee bean" nuclei are inconspicuous. This tumor follows a benign course in children and is usually effectively treated with a unilateral salpingo-oophorectomy. Sertoli cell tumor (*i.e.*, androblastoma) is extremely rare and is benign and effectively treated with a salpingo-oophorectomy.

Epithelial ovarian neoplasms are rarely found in premenarcheal girls, and even if they occur in adolescents, their malignant potential is less than in adults. Because of their rarity, specific therapeutic guidelines distinct from those used in adults are not defined.

CERVICAL AND VAGINAL TUMORS. Vaginal or cervical neoplasms are rare in children. In infants and young children, vaginal tumors are more likely to be rhabdomyosarcoma (botryoides variant) than carcinomas. However, with increasing age, evidence of cervical intraepithelial neoplasias has been observed with frequencies of up to 31 of 1000 female adolescents. The current recommendation is for sexually active adolescents to have PAP smears annually.

In the early 1970s, an increased frequency of clear cell adenocarcinoma was observed in young women whose mothers had received diethylstilbestrol (DES) in an attempt to prevent fetal wastage. Although the survival rate for women with clear cell adenocarcinomas is 80% to 90%, this is closely correlated with the extent and stage of disease at diagnosis, and in utero exposure to DES should be recognized as a significant risk factor. It is important to recognize that the incidence of vaginal adenosis and adenocarcinoma depends on the age of the fetus at the time of in utero exposure to DES and the dose and duration of DES treatment. As many as 20% to 90% of exposed girls can have vaginal adenosis, defined as mucinous columnar cells or metaplastic squamous cells, with or without mucinous droplets in the vaginal scrapings. Current recommendations call for all exposed girls to have pelvic examinations by an experienced gynecologist by the age of 14 or after menarche. This should include careful examination, cytologic samplings of the cervix and vagina, iodine staining of the vagina, and colposcopy and biopsy of suspicious lesions. Follow-up examinations should be performed annually. The treatment of clear cell sarcoma requires radical surgery, including vaginectomy, hysterectomy, and lymphatic resection.

RHABDOMYOSARCOMA

Rhabdomyosarcoma, arising from mesenchymal cells that initiate striated muscle differentiation, accounts for approximately 5% to 8% of all solid tumors in children. It is the most common soft tissue sarcoma in children younger than 15 years, with an annual incidence of 4.5 per million white children and 1.3 per million black children. Survival for children with rhabdomyosarcoma, like that for children with Wilms' tumor, has greatly improved since the incorporation of chemotherapy into treatment programs. With current multidisciplinary regimens, approximately two thirds of the patients are surviving 3 years from diagnosis.

Rhabdomyosarcoma can occur in infants, children, or adolescents, and because its presentations are varied, it should not be considered as a single entity. The extent of the tumor at diagnosis, its histology, and the primary site are each important factors for treatment planning and prognosis. During the last decade, many hundreds of patients have been entered into multi-institutional trials organized by the Intergroup Rhabdomyosarcoma Study (IRS), and much of our present understanding of the natural history, pathology, and treatment of rhabdomyosarcoma is derived from these studies.

EPIDEMIOLOGY AND GENETICS

Rhabdomyosarcoma appears to have two age peaks of occurrence, the first in children between 2 and 6 years of age and the second during adolescence, between 14 and 18 years. The early peak is primarily due to the occurrence of tumors in the head and neck region and the genitourinary tract. The late peak is predominately accounted for by primary tumors of the male genitourinary tract; tumors of the head and neck region, trunk, and extremity are common in this group. Orbital tumors occur at any age.

As with other pediatric malignancies, rhabdomyosarcoma has been associated with several congenital disorders, including neurofibromatosis, Gorlin's basal cell nevus syndrome, and the fetal alcohol syndrome. A few families have been described with an increased frequency of breast and other cancers in the relatives of children with rhabdomyosarcoma. This Li-Fraumeni syndrome has recently been associated with a germ line mutation in the p53 tumor suppressor gene located on chromosome 17. Other familial associations have been reported, including an excess incidence of rhabdomyosarcoma in the siblings of children with brain tumors and adrenal cortical carcinoma.

There has been work on the characterization of the molecular and cytogenetic lesions of rhabdomyosarcoma. Translocation t(2;13) (q37;q14) is a common finding in alveolar rhabdomyosarcoma, and a loss of heterogeneity on the short arm of chromosome 11 has been described. Work with human rhabdomyosarcoma cell lines led to the identification of intracellular peptides that modulate cell growth, the transforming growth factors and the insulin-like growth factor-2. The DNA content of rhabdomyosarcoma tumor cells is associated with histology; the prognosis associated with hyperdiploidy (usually found in embryonal tumors) is the best, that associated with near-tetraploid tumors (often alveolar) is intermediate, and the prognosis of diploid tumors is the worst.

Human rhabdomyosarcoma xenograft lines were grown in the flanks of immunosuppressed mice to investigate the mechanisms of resistance of rhabdomyosarcoma to cytotoxic chemotherapy. Vincristine resistance may be related to the production of an altered tubule subunit. The level of activity of a DNA repair enzyme correlates with the sensitivity of the rhabdomyosarcoma xenograft lines to the nitrosourea, methyl-CCNU. Human xenograft tumors have been invaluable for the rational development of new approaches to the treatment of rhabdomyosarcoma. The identification of melphalan as an active agent in the xenograft model has had its activity confirmed in phase II clinical studies.

PATHOLOGY

The head and neck are sites for approximately 38% of rhabdomyosarcomas, and the orbit is the most common single location. The next most common sites are the genitourinary tract (21%), extremities (18%), trunk (7%), and retroperitoneum (7%). The sites of primary involvement are related to the age of the child. Histologic subtype of rhabdomyosarcomas vary according to age and site.

Since the description in 1946 of rhabdomyosarcoma as a tumor of skeletal muscle, significant advances have been made in the histopathologic classification of this tumor and in correlating subtypes with clinical behavior and prognosis. Three major subtypes of rhabdomyosarcoma exist: embryonal, alveolar, and pleomorphic. The embryonal histologic subtype accounts for approximately 50% to 60% of childhood rhabdomyosarcoma and is characterized by variable numbers of large acidophilic myoblast cells and a large number of primitive round cells and spindle-shaped cells showing little myoblastic differentiation. The tumor stroma is usually loose and edematous. Compared with fetal tissue, the embryonal variant most closely resembles the developing muscle of a 1- to 7-week-old fetus. Although cross-striations can facilitate the diagnosis, they often are not visible by light microscopy. Sarcoma botryoides, although grossly differentiated by polypoid, edematous, and myxoid appearance, is histologically similar to embryonal rhabdomyosarcoma. The characteristic feature of the botryoides variant is the cambium layer of Nicholoson, a multilayered band of spindle cells with relatively little cytoplasm that lies parallel to and just below the mucosal surface of the tumor.

Alveolar rhabdomyosarcoma, the second most common subtype, is distinguished by a unique tissue pattern reminiscent of pulmonary alveoli. Tumor cells and giant multinucleated cells line septa and protrude into an open alveolar space. The alveolar subtype typically occurs in older children and young adults, is much more likely to occur in the extremities or perineal sites, is more likely to spread to the lymph nodes, and has a worse prognosis than the more common embryonal rhabdomyosarcoma.

Pleomorphic rhabdomyosarcoma is rarely seen in children and occurs primarily in adults 30 to 50 years old. It is a more differentiated tumor composed of haphazardly and compactly arranged spindle cells and multinucleated giant cells.

A pathologic classification was developed by the IRS. This classification divides tumors into favorable and unfavorable histologies by cytologic features rather than the tissue pattern. There are two unfavorable histologic categories. The first, called anaplastic, is similar to that described for Wilms' tumor and is characterized by the presence of enlarged, bizarre mitotic figures and diffuse nuclear hyperchromatism with pleomorphism. It can be found focally or diffusely throughout the tumor. The second, called monomorphous, is characterized by round cells of uniform size with constant cytologic features. Tumors that contain neither anaplastic nor monomorphic features are histologically favorable. Of 405 cases evaluated from the first IRS trial, 330 (81.5%) were categorized as favorable, and 75 (18.5%) were categorized as unfavorable. This histologic grading was used to evaluate the prognosis of 261 patients with localized rhabdomyosarcoma on the second IRS trial, and 89% of the 211 patients with favorable histologic subtypes survived, compared with 72% of those with unfavorable cytologic features. If the cytologic and tissue patterns are evaluated by light microscopy, a group of patients with a less favorable prognosis can be defined. Of 171 patients with completely resected rhabdomyosarcoma, 40 (23%) had unfavorable cytologic features or the alveolar subtype. The recurrence rate for these patients was 43%, compared with 15% for patients whose tumors did not have these unfavorable features. Analyses may permit the selection of patients who are at increased risk for tumor recurrence and who may profit from additional or more intensive therapy. However, the IRS criteria have not yet been fully validated.

An independent study at the National Cancer Institute (NCI) and St. Jude Children's Research Hospital evaluated the IRS cytologic criteria in conjunction with the classic histologic classification (*i.e.*, embryonal or alveolar) and other criteria (*e.g.*, solid variant of alveolar rhabdomyosarcoma) and demonstrated that the monomorphous or solid variant of alveolar rhabdomyosarcoma is associated with an aggressive clinical course, as is alveolar rhabdomyosarcoma of any cytologic type. Although various percentages of alveolar histologic features have been used by pathologists to diagnose "alveolar" rhabdomyosarcoma, it now is apparent that any amount confers a poor prognosis. Therefore, the "0% standard" is being used in IRS-III to diagnose alveolar rhabdomyosarcoma for the assignment of treatment. The current classification that is being used in IRS studies is presented in Table 49–22.

CLINICAL PRESENTATION

Rhabdomyosarcoma may occur at any body site containing striated muscle or its mesenchymal anlage. In infants, a frequent presentation is a grape-like, clustered polypoid vaginal mass, the botryoides variant of embryonal rhabdomyosarcoma. In young patients, the most common presentation is a mass in the head and neck region or genitourinary tract. In adolescence, rhabdomyosarcoma often presents as a painless extremity or truncal mass or as a nontender scrotal swelling

TABLE 49–22. IRS Staging Systems for Rhabdomyosarcoma

Clinical Grouping System		*Proposed Staging System for IRS-IV* — *Stage*	*Sites**	*Tumor Size*	*Lymph Nodes*	*Metastases*	*5-Year Progression-Free Survival (%)*
Group I	Localized disease, completely resected Regional nodes not involved A. Confined to muscle or organ of origin B. Contiguous involvement-infiltration outside the muscle or organ of origin, as through fascial planes	I	GU Non-BP, HN Non-PM, Orbits	a, b†	N0, N1	M0	73
Group II	Regional disease A. Grossly resected tumor with microscopic residual disease. No evidence of gross residual tumor. No clinical or microscopic evidence of regional node involvement B. Regional disease, completely resected (regional nodes involved completely resected with no microscopic residual) C. Regional disease with involved nodes, grossly resected, but with evidence of microscopic residual	II	All other	a	N0	M0	65
Group III	Incomplete resection or biopsy with gross residual disease	III	All other	b	N0	M0	44
				a, b	N1	M0	
Group IV	Metastatic disease present at onset	IV	Any site	a, b	N0, N1	M1	20

* GU Non-BP, genitourinary, not bladder-prostate; HN Non-PM, head and neck non-parameningeal; N0, regional nodes not involved by tumor, N1, regional nodes involved by tumor; M0, no distant metastases, M1, distant metastases.
† a, ≤5 cm; b, >5 cm.
‡ Except clinical group I paratestis, clinical group I and II orbital.

that may be separate from the testis. Intraabdominal lymph node metastases, which occur in as many as 26% of patients with paratesticular rhabdomyosarcoma, may sometimes present as an abdominal mass. The only sites not recognized by the IRS as probable primary tumors are brain, bone, and lung.

Rhabdomyosarcoma may present as a tumor mass or it may be discovered coincidentally during the evaluation of more nonspecific clinical symptoms. For example, a retroperitoneal rhabdomyosarcoma may present as an abdominal mass, with or without ascites, or it may present as an acute abdomen mimicking acute appendicitis. Rhabdomyosarcoma of the biliary tract, which is usually the botryoides type, most frequently presents with asymptomatic, direct hyperbilirubinemia due to biliary obstruction, but it may present with symptoms of acute cholecystitis or "relapsing hepatitis."

Rhabdomyosarcoma is the most common malignancy involving the bladder, prostate, or vagina in children. The clinical presentation may be as an asymptomatic abdominal or perineal mass, with tumor encroachment or obstruction. Symptoms include increased frequency of urination, urinary retention, or hematuria.

Rhabdomyosarcoma is the most common nonocular orbital tumors in children, usually presenting with proptosis, but rarely with evidence of direct extension into the CNS, perhaps because of its early diagnosis or containment by the bony orbit. Tumors of the middle ear may present as a polypoid or botryoid mass associated with ear pain and chronic otitis media, as a hemorrhagic discharge from the ear canal, or with evidence of a cranial nerve palsy. Contiguous extension into the CNS by primary parameningeal rhabdomyosarcoma may result in cranial nerve palsies, increased intracranial pressure, and meningeal symptoms. Tumors of the nasopharynx can be subtle in their presentation, including airway obstruction, sinusitis, epistaxis, local pain, and dysphagia. The rich lymphatics of the nasopharynx contribute to contiguous and distant spread. The CNS is the most common site of invasion by nasopharyngeal rhabdomyosarcoma.

Rhabdomyosarcoma spreads by direct extension to contiguous structures, such as parameningeal extension to the CNS, or by lymphatic and hematogenous metastasis. The margins of the primary tumor are often indistinct because of its pseudocapsule and are difficult to define on physical examination and at surgery. The incidence of lymph node metastases varies according to primary site in most series. There appears to be a particularly high incidence of lymph node involvement associated with primary lesions of the genitourinary tract (20%), paratesticular region (26%), extremity, and perineum (10–17%), but the incidence of lymph node metastasis from other sites appears to be lower (*e.g.*, 4% in the orbit).

The most common sites of hematogenous spread are lungs, bone, bone marrow, and liver. Because this occurs at initial diagnosis in 10% to 20% of patients, pretreatment examination should include a careful evaluation of the extent of the primary tumor and a detailed investigation of potential metastatic sites. In addition to special radiographic studies of the primary site, patients should have a bone scan, chest CT scan, bilateral bone marrow biopsies, and aspirates. Patients with head and neck primaries should have a head CT scan and spinal fluid examination. An MR scan is useful for defining the extent of the primary lesion and its resectability.

STAGING

The staging system for rhabdomyosarcoma used most commonly is the IRS clinical-pathologic grouping system, which is based on the extent of the extirpative surgery, except in cases of distant dissemination (see Table 47–22). Although this has been a useful approach to directing treatment, it obviates analysis of the local characteristics of the tumor, such as size and invasiveness, and incorporates results of therapy (*e.g.*, extent of operative resection) in outcome analysis. The IRS Committee analyzed IRS-II patients retrospectively restaged using a presurgical system. They confirmed the validity of staging by the degree of involvement of contiguous organs or structures, tumor size larger than 5 cm, and the presence of metastatic disease. IRS-IV is evaluating a prospective TNM staging system.

TREATMENT

Treatment Planning

The therapeutic plan for patients with rhabdomyosarcoma is determined by the primary site of involvement, histologic classification, and the clinical group or stage. Certain primary sites, such as the orbit, parameningeal sites, vagina, and prostate, are usually best managed by an initial biopsy followed by primary irradiation and adjuvant chemotherapy. The management of limited trunk, extremity, and paratesticular lesions usually includes the removal of all gross disease followed by adjuvant chemotherapy with irradiation as needed.

Among patients with bladder or prostate lesions, the overall bladder salvage rate on the same IRS regimens has been approximately 35%, and the mortality rate has been 20% to 30%, which is higher than the mortality associated with standard primary surgical approaches. Primary uterine tumors usually affect older patients and apparently not very responsive to chemotherapy. Primary chemotherapy has achieved its goal in eliminating anterior pelvic exenteration for patients with vaginal tumors.

Because the prognosis and approach to management vary according to the primary tumor sites, the general principles of management are considered first and then applied to specific sites of disease.

Surgery

The efficacy of radiation therapy and chemotherapy has had a major impact on the surgical procedures now recommended for rhabdomyosarcoma. Before the development of these modalities, radical operations were the only means to achieve tumor control, and even with extensive and often disabling surgery, local recurrence rates were high and cure rates were low. Some limited surgical procedures are now adequate, and the timing and extent of these procedures are important for retaining high rates of survival and improving functional results.

The exact role of surgery varies with the location, size, and extent of the tumor at presentation. Surgical extirpation is indicated if removal of the primary tumor imposes no major functional disability or if excision of the primary tumor permits the elimination of postoperative irradiation by completely excising the tumor or permits a reduction in the dose without increasing functional deficit by eliminating all but microscopic disease. This approach is especially appropriate in the treatment of rhabdomyosarcoma of the extremity, for which group I and II tumors without lymph node metastases have a much better prognosis than group III tumors. However, patients with large, invasive extremity tumors without evidence of metastatic disease do poorly even after amputation.

If only partial tumor removal is possible, particularly if removal would result in significant long-term disability, initial surgery should be limited to biopsy, preferably with sampling of regional lymph nodes. This is especially true in the treatment of orbital tumors, for which biopsy followed by irradiation and chemotherapy has resulted in excellent long-term survival. Sampling of clinically uninvolved regional nodes is recommended for tumors of the genitourinary tract, paratesticular region, extremities, and perineum. Node groups with apparent involvement are biopsied regardless of the primary site, except for patients with stage IV disease.

Preoperative chemotherapy or radiation therapy to reduce the size of the tumor, followed by removal of the residual tumor at a second operation, is currently under evaluation in the treatment of genitourinary rhabdomyosarcomas. The goals of this approach are the preservation of bladder function and achievement of long-term survival.

Radiation Therapy

Reports in the 1960s established the efficacy of high-dose, wide-field irradiation to achieve local control of rhabdomyosarcomas in children. With megavoltage equipment, orbital rhabdomyosarcoma could be controlled in 90% of patients with appropriate doses and volumes of radiation therapy.

Local control was achieved in 96% of the 27 patients treated with conservative, function-preserving surgery plus combination chemotherapy and high-dose, large-volume radiation therapy, with doses of 5500 to 6500 cGy to the primary tumor site. This approach has been confirmed in many studies.

The IRS analyzed the role of radiation therapy in the local tumor control of 524 children with rhabdomyosarcoma and showed that radiation therapy was not required for patients whose primary tumor was totally excised and who had no microscopic residual disease (group I).

For more advanced disease, radiation therapy is important for local and regional disease control. Overall local tumor control in patients with local residual disease (stages II and III) is well documented in 75% to 90% of those treated with adequate irradiation and chemotherapy.

Both principles of treatment include wide volumes, using prechemotherapy or preoperative tumor extent to determine irradiation fields. Wide margins are important; 60% local of regional failure in parameningeal tumors are due primarily to inadequate irradiation volumes. Inclusion of regional lymph nodes with documented involvement is important; irradiation of clinically uninvolved nodes is controversial.

A local control rate of more than 95% can be achieved for microscopic disease (stage II) with 4000 cGy. For patients with "gross" or "bulky" disease (stage III), doses in excess of 4500 to 5500 cGy are required. Daily fractions of 150 to 180 cGy are effective and well tolerated.

In selected patients, brachytherapy may be of value. Particularly for pelvic tumors, the use of intracavitary irradiation may facilitate disease control with less damage to surrounding normal tissues. IRS-IV is evaluating hyperfractioned radiation therapy to learn whether it can improve local control of bulky lesions without increasing morbidity.

Chemotherapy

Before the routine use of systemic chemotherapy, the long-term survival for children with rhabdomyosarcoma was poor, and cure was largely restricted to a few favorable anatomic sites, such as the orbit. The utility of adjuvant chemotherapy in patients who had been rendered disease-free with surgery or radiation therapy has been convincingly demonstrated. The survival rate for patients receiving vincristine plus dactinomycin was 82%, compared with 47% for patients not receiving chemotherapy.

Many chemotherapeutic agents have single-agent activity in rhabdomyosarcoma (Table 47–23), although the most commonly used regimens include combinations of vincristine, dactinomycin, and cyclophosphamide. Refinements of the chemotherapy regimens for rhabdomyosarcoma have been generated by the IRS studies. Data accrued from the first of these cooperative trials (IRS-I) supported the following conclusions:

1. Adjuvant chemotherapy with vincristine, dactinomycin, and oral cyclophosphamide (VAC) eliminates the need for postoperative radiation therapy in patients whose tumors were totally excised and who had no evidence of residual microscopic disease (group I).
2. A two-drug regimen (vincristine plus dactinomycin) was as effective as three drugs (VAC) for patients with grossly resected but microscopic residual disease (group II) treated with irradiation.
3. Doxorubicin did not improve the outcome when added to pulse VAC (vincristine, dactinomycin, and intravenous cyclophosphamide) for patients with gross residual

TABLE 49–23. Response of Rhabdomyosarcoma to Single Agents

Drug	*No. of Evaluable Patients*	*CR*	*PR*	*% CR + PR/ Total*
Dactinomycin	14		6	43
Cyclophosphamide	26	2	11	42
Vincristine	42	3	10	31
Doxorubicin	40	2	11	33
Cisplatin	19	1	3	21
VP-16 (etoposide)	5		1	20
DTIC	9		2	22
Methotrexate	6	1	2	50
Melphalan (newly diagnosed)	13		10	77
Melphalan (recurrent)	13		2	8
Ifosfamide	8		2	25

CR, complete response (100% disappearance); PR, partial response (50–99% disappearance).

(group III) or disseminated (group IV) disease. However, doxorubicin was given at a relatively low dose intensity.

The relapse-free survival rates at 3 years were 82% to 84% for group I, 63% to 72% for group II, 54% to 61% for group III, and 17% to 23% for group IV patients (Table 49–24). Several conclusions were drawn from the data generated in IRS-II:

1. The chemotherapy regimen for group I patients could be simplified, because a two-drug regimen (vincristine plus dactinomycin) appeared as effective (83% 2-year relapse-free survival) as the three-drug VAC regimen (87% 2-year relapse-free survival).
2. A moderately more intensive regimen of vincristine and dactinomycin was as good as or better (81% 2-year relapse-free survival) than a pulse VAC regimen of vincristine, dactinomycin, and intravenous cyclophosphamide (70% 2-year relapse-free survival) for group II patients, all of whom had postoperative irradiation.
3. Treatment of groups III and IV patients remains a problem. In this trial, the addition of doxorubicin to the VAC regimen did not result in a major improvement in survival. The preliminary results for group IV patients showed the 3-year survival in IRS-II to be 32%, compared with 17% to 23% in IRS-I.

IRS-III, which investigated the contribution of cisplatin and etoposide to the therapeutic regimen, is complete and is being analyzed. IRS-IV is comparing VAC with vincristine, dactinomycin, and ifosfamide (VAI) and vincristine, ifosfamide, and etoposide (VIE) in patients with stage II and III disease. Stage IV patients are treated with new pairs of drugs in an upfront phase II "window." The pairs include ifosfamide and doxorubicin, ifosfamide and etoposide, and vincristine and melphalan.

For patients with advanced disease, new approaches to treatment are being explored. The most prominent are new drugs, such as cisplatin, VP-16, and DTIC, added to the current chemotherapy regimen of vincristine, dactinomycin, cyclophosphamide, and doxorubicin, and the intensification of chemotherapy, particularly doxorubicin and cyclophosphamide, with or without total-body irradiation and autologous bone marrow rescue. General conclusions from the St. Jude Children's Research Hospital study of preirradiation chemotherapy in the treatment of rhabdomyosarcoma are that the approach does not jeopardize overall survival and does allow the assessment of chemotherapy response independently. Those patients with chemotherapy-resistant tumors were unlikely to be locally controlled with irradiation. This identifies subsets of patients who may be approached with experimental techniques, such as hyperfractionation or brachytherapy.

Analysis of many studies suggests that many of the patients who are disease-free at 2 years will remain in remission. However, if relapse occurs, the long-term survival rate is poor (2%), emphasizing the need to maximize primary treatment regimens and to develop better salvage protocols.

TABLE 49–24. Actuarial Survival at Three Years: Results of The Intergroup Rhabdomyosarcoma Studies I and II

Prognostic Factors	*IRS-I*	*IRS-II*
Clinical Group		
I	79	88
II	68	77
III	42	68
IV	18	32
Histologic Type		
Embryonal		69
Alveolar		56
Other		66
Primary Site		
Orbit	91	93
Genitourinary (GU)	74	
GU (mainly group III)		64
Cranial parameningeal	53	71
Other head or neck	59	69
Trunk	53	57
Extremity	53	56
Retroperitoneum-pelvis	39	46
Total	686	956

Management of Specific Tumors

HEAD AND NECK PRIMARY TUMORS. Embryonal tumors (78%) predominate in the head and neck region, including the botryoid variant in the pharynx, larynx, maxillary sinus, and middle ear. Alveolar tumors are found in 9.5% of cases; extraosseous Ewing's sarcoma is found in 2.5%; and 10% are undifferentiated.

Before the routine use of chemotherapy and adequate irradiation, the long-term survival of patients with head and neck primaries was poor (9–15%), with metastases occurring by the hematogenous and lymphatic routes. After combined modality therapy, the 3-year disease-free survival for patients with rhabdomyosarcoma of the head and neck region (groups I–III) rose to 66%.

Despite these improvements, the potential long-term complications of therapy are of concern because the mean age of children with head or neck rhabdomyosarcoma is less than 10 years. The use of high-dose local radiation therapy and prophylactic whole-brain irradiation can cause major complications for these children, and the facial, dental, mucosal, and endocrine complications of high-dose radiation therapy, especially if administered with chemotherapy, are well known.

EYE AND ORBIT TUMORS. The orbit is the most common site for rhabdomyosarcomas of the head and neck region, accounting for approximately 25% of these tumors. Since the institution of multimodality therapy for orbital rhabdomyosarcomas, 91% of patients are disease-free at 3 years. Orbital tumors are usually confined to the orbit and surrounding structures and rarely metastasize to distant sites, local nodes, or the CNS if properly irradiated. Although most orbital tumors are only biopsied and are classified as group III tumors, orbital exenteration is unnecessary because of the efficacy of radiation therapy and chemotherapy, except for local recurrence after conventional therapy.

Whether radiation should be administered before or in conjunction with systemic chemotherapy is controversial. The IRS protocols used simultaneous therapy. The total radiation dose is comparable to that prescribed for other sites, and the minimal volume usually includes the entire bony limits of the orbit. For treatment of limited disease, this field usually extends from the supraorbital ridge superiorly, to the infraoptic foramen interiorly, and across the midline to the inner canthus of the opposite eye. To avoid chronic keratoconjunctivitis, radiation therapy should be delivered with the eyelids open. Because the preauricular and upper cervical nodes appear to be negative in most cases, their inclusion in the irradiated field is unnecessary.

Adjuvant chemotherapy is necessary for all patients with orbital rhabdomyosarcoma. Treatment with radiation alone results in hematogenous metastases in approximately 33% of the patients. The most common therapy uses vincristine plus dactinomycin.

Ninety percent of the children whose orbits have been irradiated for rhabdomyosarcoma developed evidence of a cataract 1 to 4 years after completion of therapy. Enophthalmos, stenosis of the lacrimal duct, keratoconjunctivitis, photophobia, or conjunctivitis were seen in 20% of these patients. Secondary surgery was necessary in approximately 33% of these patients to improve functional results after radiation therapy; enucleation was required in 8% of patients.

PARAMENINGEAL RHABDOMYOSARCOMA. The parameningeal sites include the middle ear, auditory canal, mastoid, nasal cavity, paranasal sinuses, pharynx, pterygopalatine fossa, and the infratemporal fossa. Patients with parameningeal tumors who were enrolled in the IRS-I protocol had a significantly lower 3-year relapse-free survival rate (46%) than those with other head and neck primaries. The reason for treatment failure in 35% of these patients was tumor invasion into the CNS. None of the patients who developed this pattern of relapse survived. Detailed analysis of these patients suggested that these local treatment failures were probably a reflection of inadequate radiation dose (*i.e.*, 13 of 19 patients received <5000 cGy) and volume (*e.g.*, 11 of 19 patients had less than adequate volume). After using adequate treatment fields and doses of more than 5000 cGy, parameningeal tumor extension occurred in less than 5% of the patients. Rhabdomyosarcoma arising in a parameningeal site has a propensity for contiguous extension into the CNS, but radiation ports that include potential extension sites control the tumor in many patients. Current treatment planning includes higher radiation doses and more carefully planned radiation ports based on extensive imaging studies before chemotherapy. These modifications have produced a significant reduction in local failures and CNS extension in patients with primary parameningeal rhabdomyosarcoma. Intrathecal chemotherapy for patients with parameningeal disease is probably unnecessary if the radiation ports are adequate, and it has been eliminated from IRS-IV.

OTHER HEAD AND NECK TUMORS. Rhabdomyosarcoma can arise in the scalp, neck, parotid, oropharynx, larynx, or cheek. Surgical resection with margins that are sufficient to eliminate the need for radiation therapy are rarely possible without unacceptable functional or cosmetic consequences. Primary radiation and chemotherapy form the cornerstone of management for these patients. Of 36 patients with primaries in these areas (groups I–III), 27 (75%) have remained disease-free for 3 or more years after therapy. Four of 5 failures received no irradiation or less than 1500 cGy. Only 2 of 37 patients with nonorbital, nonparameningeal primaries of the head (excluding the neck) on IRS-I relapsed.

PRIMARY TUMORS OF THE TRUNK. The trunk is the primary site in 7% to 9% of patients. The prognosis for this group, influenced by the type, extent, and location of the tumor at diagnosis, is not as favorable as that for patients with head and neck primaries. Of 30 patients, 14 tumors occurred on the chest wall, 10 were paraspinal, and 6 were on the abdominal wall; 15 of the 30 patients remained disease free at 5+ years. The prognosis appeared to be best for patients with paraspinal tumors (7 of 10 surviving disease free) and poorest for those with chest wall tumors (5 of 15 survived disease free). Only 3 of 12 patients with alveolar tumors have remained disease free, in contrast to 12 of 18 patients with nonalveolar tumors. Of 18 patients with retroperitoneal tumors treated with multimodality therapy, 14 had a greater than 50% tumor response; however, only 4 remained alive and free of active tumor.

Patients with localized tumors of the trunk (groups I and II) fare better (9 of 14 surviving disease free) than those with extensive local or disseminated tumor at diagnosis (6 of 16 disease-free survivors). Because of the poorer prognosis for patients with gross residual disease, complete surgical removal of the tumor is recommended and should be possible in many of these patients without unacceptable consequences. Such procedures are frequently recognized as incomplete, because microscopic residual disease is found in the detailed examination of the specimen. If the tumor is completely excised with adequate margins and there is no microscopic disease, postoperative irradiation is unnecessary. Use of electron-beam irradiation and interstitial techniques and the judicious use of photon irradiation to minimize normal tissue damage are particularly important. Because the major reason for failure in this group is distant dissemination, adjuvant chemotherapy is essential.

PRIMARY TUMORS OF THE EXTREMITY. Approximately 16% of rhabdomyosarcomas occur in the extremities. In contrast to tumors of the head and neck region, rhabdomyosarcoma of the extremity is more common in adolescents, is associated with a high incidence of relapse, and has a low survival rate. Early studies suggested that upper-extremity and distal lesions had a better prognosis than lower-extremity and proximal lesions, an observation that is supported in the IRS-I study, in which 44% of patients with lower-extremity lesions relapsed, compared with 30% of those with upper-extremity disease.

Rhabdomyosarcoma of the extremity is distinct in two important ways: the high incidence of alveolar cells (44% versus 16% for all other sites) and the high incidence of lymph node metastasis (17% versus none for orbit lesions and 3% for head and neck primaries). The importance of histologic types is reflected in the higher relapse rate (65%) for patients with stage I or II disease whose extremity tumors were alveolar, compared with 33% for patients with nonalveolar tumors, although their initial response rates were similar.

Although wide surgical resection should be performed if it can be accomplished without causing a major functional defect, amputation, especially of the upper extremity, is rarely required. Delayed amputation may be necessary if significant uncorrectable growth discrepancy occurs in the lower extremity after cure of the lesion. Because of the high incidence of regional lymphatic spread, a lymph node biopsy is recommended. The radiation guidelines are similar to those for other sites, although care must be taken to avoid circumferential irradiation with its attendant risk of long-term vascular and lymphatic complications.

The major problem in the treatment of patients with alveolar rhabdomyosarcoma continues to be the failure to control systemic disease. Current regimens for patients with extremity lesions use more intensive chemotherapy schedules.

PRIMARY TUMORS OF THE GENITOURINARY SYSTEM. The genitourinary tract is the primary site of approximately 20% of rhabdomyosarcomas. The principal genitourinary sites are the prostate, bladder, vagina, and paratesticular tissues. The overall survival was 70% to 75% for patients with genitourinary primaries. The overall survival of patients with genitourinary tumors is related to stage; relapse rate is 19% for patients with localized, grossly resected bladder and prostate tumors, compared with 39% for patients with group III or IV disease at diagnosis. The most common histologic type is embryonal; the botryoid variant occurs frequently in these sites. Lymph node metastases are common but site specific. For example, 26% of patients with paratesticular primaries have paraaortic node involvement, compared with a lower incidence for vaginal primaries. The role of retroperitoneal node dissection is an area of controversy, particularly in view of its long-term complications. It is generally recommended that regional nodes be sampled, especially in patients with paratesticular primaries, and if they are positive, patients should receive radiation therapy to that region.

Although the survival of patients with tumors at these sites has improved markedly with the addition of combination chemotherapy to pelvic surgery and radiation therapy, the long-term sequelae of these therapies in young children are significant. The use of primary chemotherapy (*i.e.*, pharmacologic debulking) followed by limited surgery and irradiation has been evaluated for treatment of the primary tumors of the genitourinary tract. This sequencing has eliminated anterior pelvic exenteration for many children with vaginal tumors. Among patients with localized bladder or prostate lesions, the overall bladder salvage rate on the IRS regimens has been approximately 35%; the mortality rates of 20% to 30% with attempted bladder salvage seems higher than that associated with standard primary exenteration approaches. Primary uterine tumors are a distinct group (older age) and apparently not very responsive.

Radiation therapy seeks to include the pelvic disease with maximal sparing of the femoral heads, acetabulum, and bowel. Coordination of radiation with cyclophosphamide is important to minimize short-term and long-term bladder complications. Mesna administered with cyclophosphamide is usually successful in preventing hemorrhagic cystitis even if the bladder is irradiated. Rotational and multiple-field techniques should be used. Brachytherapy may be possible in selected cases. Dose and volume considerations are comparable to other sites. If paraaortic node biopsies and lymphangiogram are negative, irradiation of these regional nodes may be omitted. If positive, the lymph nodes should be included in the radiation fields.

EWING'S SARCOMA AND PERIPHERAL PRIMITIVE NEUROECTODERMAL TUMOR

In 1921, James Ewing described a vascular, hemorrhagic bone tumor composed of small, round cells without associated osteoid formation that usually occurred in the midshaft of the long bones or in the flat bones of the trunk. Although Ewing's sarcoma, the second most common primary bone tumor of childhood, was originally thought to arise from the endothelial cell, recent evidence suggests that it is derived from primitive neural tissue. Molecular and cytogenetic studies of this tumor produced important clues regarding the molecular pathogenesis of this disease. Multimodality therapy has increased the proportion of long-term disease-free survivors from less than 15% to more than 50% during the past 20 to 30 years.

EPIDEMIOLOGY AND BIOLOGY

Ewing's sarcoma occurs most frequently in the second decade of life and is rare before 5 or after 30 years of age (Fig. 49–9). The incidence in males is equal to that in females until age 13 years, when, as with osteosarcoma, males predominate. As with osteosarcoma, epidemiologic studies demonstrate that

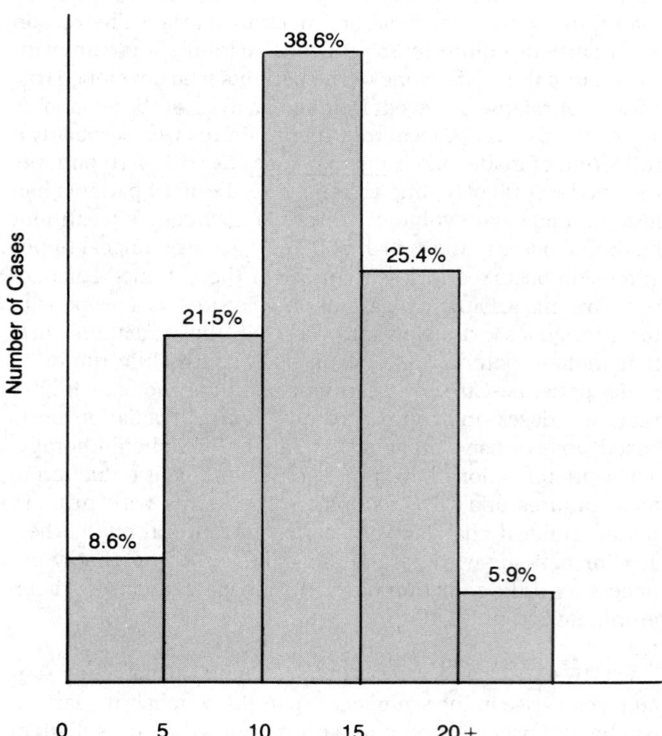

FIGURE 49–9. Age distribution of 303 patients with Ewing's bone sarcoma in the Intergroup Ewing's Sarcoma Study.

taller persons are more likely to develop Ewing's sarcoma, suggesting that its development is in some way linked to growth.

The annual incidence of Ewing's sarcoma in the United States is 1.7 cases per million white children younger than 15 years of age. A striking epidemiologic finding is the exceedingly low incidence of Ewing's sarcoma in African and American blacks and Chinese. Ewing's sarcoma has not been associated with congenital syndromes, but an association with skeletal anomalies (*i.e.*, enchondroma, aneurysmal bone cyst) and genitourinary anomalies (*i.e.*, hypospadias, duplication of the renal collecting system) has been reported. Ewing's sarcoma has been associated with retinoblastoma.

A chromosomal translocation, t(11:22), is a characteristic abnormality of Ewing's sarcoma. In a series of 13 karyotyped tumors, 9 demonstrated this translocation and two others contained a deletion on chromosome 22. The translocation is indistinguishable from that reported in peripheral neuroepithelioma by Whang-Peng and colleagues, suggesting that these entities have a common histogenesis. This is further supported by the demonstration of neuroectoderm-associated antigens on Ewing's cell lines in culture and identical patterns of protooncogene expression as seen in peripheral neuroepithelioma. Because of this realization tumors that once would have been diagnosed as Ewing's sarcoma are now often designated as peripheral neuroepithelioma or synonymously peripheral primitive neuroectodermal tumors (PPNET) based on any hint of neural differentiation at light or electron microscopic levels. For this reason, Ewing's sarcoma and PPNET are discussed together in this section. Table 49–25 compares the biologic features of Ewing's sarcoma and PPNET with neuroblastoma.

PATHOLOGY

Ewing's sarcoma is an undifferentiated round cell tumor possessing no unique morphologic markers. It is diagnosed only after the exclusion of the other small, round, blue cell tumors of childhood, which include primary sarcoma of bone (including small cell osteosarcoma and mesenchymal and myxoid chondrosarcoma), primitive sarcoma of bone, rhabdomyosarcoma, lymphoma, neuroblastoma, and peripheral neuroepithelioma. Refinements in electron microscopic, immunocytochemical, cytogenetic, and molecular genetic techniques have increased the sensitivity with which these tumors can be identified, consequently shrinking the numbers of cases left in the Ewing's "waste basket."

Biopsy should ensure that adequate tissue is obtained for these special studies. Tissue for electron microscopy is best fixed in glutaraldehyde and in alcohol for immunocytochemistry. The core-needle biopsy may compromise an accurate diagnosis, but a fine-needle aspirate is not acceptable as the sole biopsy sample.

By light microscopy, Ewing's sarcoma is a diffuse mass of homogenous tumor cells. There is often a biphasic population, with larger, clear cells and smaller, darker cells. Marked vascularity and widespread coagulative necrosis are typical features. The tumor infiltrates bone with surprisingly little destruction. Tumor margins are usually infiltrative or "pushing." A filigree pattern in which finger-like processes of compact, basophilic cells intertwine correlates with poorer survival.

The cells of Ewing's sarcoma are approximately the size of histiocytes, two to three times the size of a small lymphocyte, and have a centrally placed ellipsoid or spherical nucleus with a delicate nuclear membrane. The nuclear chromatin is usu-

TABLE 49–25. Comparison of Peripheral Neuroectodermal Tumors With Neuroblastoma and Ewing's Sarcoma

Variable	*Neuroblastoma*	*PNET*	*Ewing's Sarcoma*
Clinical Presentation			
Age	<4	Adolescence	Adolescence
Site	Abdominal	Thoracic, extremity, pelvis	Thoracic, extremity, pelvis
Biologic Markers			
Cytologic features of neural differentiation	+	±	−
EM features of neural differentiation	+	±	−
Neurotransmitters	Adrenergic	Cholinergic	Cholinergic
Surface HLA expression	−	+	+
Cytogenetic Characteristics			
Chromosomal translocation	−	t(11;22)(q24;q11–12)	t(11;22)(q24;q11–12)
Gene amplification	+	−	−
Oncogene Expression			
MYCN	+	−	−
MYC	−	+	+

(Israel MA, Miser JS, Triche TJ, et al. Neuroepithelial tumors. In: Pizzo PA, Poplack DG, eds. Principles and practice of pediatric oncology. Philadelphia: JB Lippincott, 1989:629)

ally faintly stippled, and the nucleoli are inconspicuous. The cytoplasm of Ewing's sarcoma is devoid of organelles, but cytoplasmic glycogen is usually demonstrable by electron microscopy or the PAS stain with light microscopy. A large cell variant consisting of larger, more pleomorphic cells with conspicuous nucleoli demonstrates the same clinical behavior as typical Ewing's sarcoma. An unusual pattern of intramyofiber skeletal muscle invasion by tumor cells seen in a few patients is a negative prognostic factor.

Like neuroblastoma and Ewing's sarcoma, PPNET are highly cellular and consist of a monotonous pattern of primitive-appearing round cells, most of which lack any evidence of neural differentiation. Electron microscopy may reveal evidence of dense core granules, neurites, neurotubules, and neurofilaments in prominent Golgi's apparatus. Immunocytochemical staining is often positive for neuron-specific enolase.

Ewing's sarcoma is a diagnosis of exclusion that is made with decreasing frequency by pathologists who, using electron microscopy and immunocytochemistry, diligently search for clues to a tumor's histogenesis. This can be a source of frustration for the oncologist who must determine treatment for patients with tumors that have limited "history," such as primitive sarcomas of bone and peripheral neuroepithelioma. A rational approach is to treat the Ewing's family of tumors in a uniform manner until there are data to indicate that specific subsets have biologic and clinical differences that warrant a unique approach.

NATURAL HISTORY AND EVALUATION

Although Ewing's sarcoma most commonly presents in the femur and bones of the pelvis, it can affect any bone. Unlike osteosarcoma, it often originates in the axial skeleton. Table 49–26 lists the distribution and frequency of primary sites of patients enrolled in the first Intergroup Ewing's Sarcoma Study.

TABLE 49–26. Distribution of Primary Sites in Ewing's Sarcoma

Primary Site	*Frequency (%)*	
Pelvis/sacrum	20.5	
Pelvis		17.2
Sacrum		3.3
Proximal extremity	31.4	
Humerus		10.6
Femur		20.8
Distal extremity	27.1	
Tibia		10.6
Fibula		12.2
Radius + ulna		2.0
Hands + feet		2.3
Other	14.1	
Rib		6.9
Vertebrae		4.9
Skull/face		2.8
Scapula		4.0
Clavicle		1.7
Other		0.7

Most patients with Ewing's sarcoma seek medical attention because of pain and swelling of the affected bone or region. Systemic symptoms, such as fatigue, weight loss, and intermittent fever, may be present, especially in patients with metastatic disease. The duration of symptoms before presentation may be measured in weeks or months and is often prolonged in patients who have primary sites in the axial skeleton. When intratumor hemorrhage and necrosis occur, the tumor can become fluctuant, erythematous, and warm, mimicking infection. Frequently the entire medullary cavity of the affected bone is involved with the tumor (Table 49–27).

Extension through the bony cortex and into the soft tissues often results in a large soft tissue mass that, particularly with axial lesions, may be larger than the intraosseous component (Fig. 49–10).

Less common presentations of Ewing's sarcoma include primary rib tumor associated with a pleural effusion and respiratory symptoms, mandibular lesions presenting with chin and lip parasthenias, primary vertebral tumor with symptoms of nerve root or spinal cord compression, and sacral primary with neurogenic bladder.

The chest wall is the most common site for PPNET. The trunk, abdomen, and pelvis are other primary sites. PPNET usually present as sometimes painful masses, and when invading the chest wall, they are often associated with a malignant pleural effusion. If the tumor involves the paraspinal region, extension into the spinal cord must be considered. PPNET arising in the extremities or pelvis are similar to Ewing's sarcoma, with bony involvement of a soft tissue mass and pain.

The incidence of metastatic disease at the time of presentation in patients with Ewing's sarcoma or PPNET ranges from 14% to 50%, depending on the thoroughness of the metastatic workup and the referral base of the reporting institutions. Metastasis is predominantly hematogenous, although lymph node involvement may occur. The lung is the most common site of metastatic disease at presentation and the most frequent site of initial relapse. CNS involvement is detected in fewer than 1% of patients and is the site of first relapse in fewer than 5% of patients. More commonly, the CNS is involved as a result of direct intracranial or intraspinal extension of bony metastatic disease.

The importance of the initial diagnostic biopsy in a patient with a suspected Ewing's sarcoma should be emphasized. The soft tissue component of the tumor is often viable and yields a better specimen than the frequently necrotic intramedullary component of the tumor. Electron microscopy and immunocytochemistry must be employed for an accurate diagnosis. The surgical or pediatric oncologist should tell the pathologist the suspected diagnosis before surgery. Improper placement of the initial biopsy may obviate subsequent limb-sparing surgery.

The diagnostic evaluation should include a CT scan of the primary tumor and lungs. The use of MRI complements the CT scan in defining the primary tumor. Experience with this technology suggests that it may be overly sensitive, exaggerating the size of the lesion, resulting in overly generous radiation ports. Until experience with MRI accumulates, it should not replace the CT. A radionuclide bone scan is essen-

TABLE 49–27. Typical Radiographic Characteristics of Bone Tumors

Feature	*Osteosarcoma*	*Ewing's Sarcoma*
Location in bone	Metaphyseal	Diaphyseal
Involvement of long bones	Yes	Yes
Involvement of flat bones	Rare	Yes
Diffuse medullary cavity involvement	Rare	Common ("moth-eaten" or permeative involvement)
New bone formation	Yes	No—only as secondary phenomenon
Periosteal reaction	Yes ("Codman's triangle") or spiculation	Yes ("onionskin" appearance)
	Not prominent but may be present	Yes

tial to find bony metastases. The bone marrow should be assessed with a bone aspirate and biopsy. In the event of a pelvic lesion, bone marrow distant from the primary site must be sampled to determine if there has been dissemination. Although there is no specific serum marker for Ewing's sarcoma, lactate dehydrogenase is frequently elevated in those with more advanced disease, which has negative prognostic implications.

There is no uniformly accepted staging system for Ewing's sarcoma. A system based on a TNM concept is more appropriate for this disease than a system based on the extent of disease after a surgical procedure, because the approach to the local control of this tumor is rarely surgical. Experience suggests that the size of the lesion has prognostic importance. In several studies, the prognosis of those with lesions less than 5 to 10 cm in the maximal diameter was better than for those with larger tumors. Node involvement (N) is rare. The presence of metastatic disease (M) dramatically reduces the likelihood of survival.

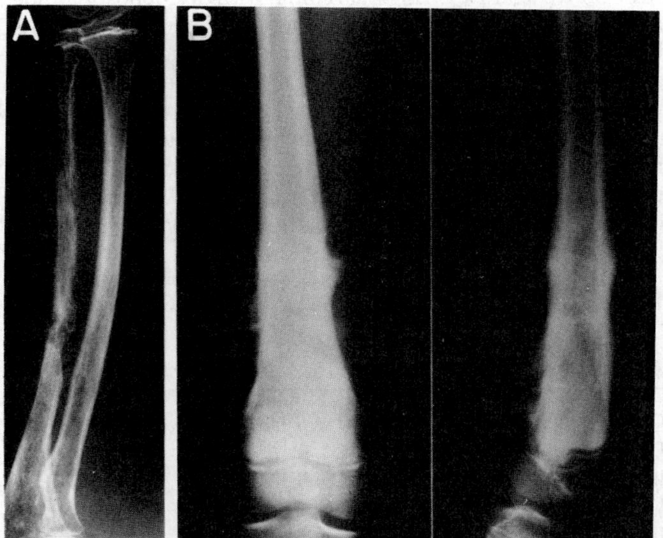

The most favorable prognostic factors are a distal primary tumor, normal serum lactate dehydrogenase, and absence of metastatic disease at presentation. Pelvic and sacral sites for primary tumors and metastatic disease are the least favorable factors. A partial or complete response to initial chemotherapy is a strong predictor of long-term disease control.

FIGURE 49–10. Radiographs of typical osteosarcoma and Ewing's tumor. **(A)** Ewing's tumor of the ulna. Notice the diaphyseal involvement with no tumor-related new bone and extensive permeative appearance. **(B)** Classic osteosarcoma of the femur in frontal and lateral projections. Typical metaphyseal location, new bone formation, lack of permeation, Codman's triangle, and spiculation are evident.

TREATMENT

Every patient with Ewing's sarcoma or PPNET should be treated with curative intent. Even patients with widely metastatic disease can, if not cured, have excellent responses to therapy, which may translate into years of disease control. Successful treatment requires close coordination among the surgeon, chemotherapist, and radiotherapist to ensure the most effective approach to controlling the primary lesion and the inevitable dissemination of the tumor.

Surgery

With surgical therapy alone, the long-term survival rates of patients in most early series were less than 10%, with failure usually caused by distant metastatic disease. The success of adjuvant chemotherapy in preventing distant failure in patients with Ewing's sarcoma and the effectiveness of radiation therapy in controlling the primary site of disease have resulted in abandoning surgery as the sole primary modality of therapy. Before improved irradiation equipment, patients whose initial treatment included surgery lived longer than patients who did not have surgery. A retrospective analysis revealed that 57 of the 334 patients had partial or complete resection of the tumor, and patients whose tumors had been resected lived longer than those who did not have surgery. Although these data must be cautiously evaluated for their potential selection bias, they do suggest that the role of surgery in the primary management of Ewing's sarcoma deserves evaluation. Balanced against this is the excellent local control attained with megavoltage irradiation and the low frequency of therapy-induced functional deficits if careful treatment planning was used. There are, however, no controlled data that compare the advantages and disadvantages of surgery and irradiation for the primary treatment of Ewing's sarcoma.

The indications for primary surgical resection of Ewing's

sarcoma used at some institutions include a lesion in an expendable bone, such as the rib, clavicle, fibula, or individual bones of the feet. Surgery usually follows initial chemotherapy, which can be expected to significantly debulk the lesion. Amputation may be indicated if there is an unmanageable pathologic fracture, but many of fractures heal during initial chemotherapy, allowing subsequent irradiation. If the tumor arises at or below the knee in a young child (<6 years) and a major uncorrectable functional deformity is expected from radiation therapy, amputation or limb-sparing surgery with an expandable prosthesis should be considered.

The two goals of therapy, local and distant tumor control and preservation of function, guide the management of an individual lesion. If a major functional loss, such as sacrifice of the peroneal nerve in resection of a fibular lesion, is likely to result from surgery, irradiation is usually preferred.

Radiation Therapy

James Ewing initially described the tumor's susceptibility to radium. It has since been recognized that this tumor is highly responsive to radiation therapy. Before the availability of chemotherapy, local control of Ewing's sarcoma was attained in 44% to 86% of patients with radiation doses greater than 4000 to 5000 cGy, even though long-term survival was low (16–25%).

With the addition of effective chemotherapy and local irradiation, local recurrence of Ewing's sarcoma is approximately 10% for distal extremity lesions and 20% to 40% for patients with proximal extremity or pelvis primaries. Coordinated therapy has increased the control of microscopic systemic disease and markedly increased survival. In a report of 193 patients treated on the first Intergroup Ewing's Sarcoma Study, the overall local control rate was 90%, and the survival had increased to 56% at 3+ years. These results have been corroborated in other studies.

Local control with primary irradiation and chemotherapy appears to depend on tumor size. Failure occurred in 2 of 20 patients with lesions less than 8 cm in diameter, compared with 9 of 30 patients with larger primary tumors. Disease-free survival rates differed even more: 72% of patients with lesions smaller than 8 cm at 5 years and 22% of patients with larger lesions. Local failures with pelvic primary tumors were only 8% for lesions less than 5 cm, compared with 17% for larger lesions. There are significant differences in local control and survival with lesions with volumes greater or smaller than 100 ml.

Radiation therapy is the primary mode of therapy for most local lesions. In conjunction with chemotherapy, doses of more than 5000 to 5500 cGy achieve tumor control in 80% to 85% of patients. Overall survival and local control have been improved by adding chemotherapy to irradiation.

To maintain function, a meticulous radiation technique is required. Necessary technical aspects include megavoltage apparatus, immobilization techniques for daily reproduction, and the use of beam-modifying devices, including compensators, wedge filters, and individually constructed blocks. Appropriate treatment of an extremity lesion includes the preservation of an unirradiated strip of skin and soft tissue to prevent late lymphedema and contractures. With the use of moderate-dose radiation therapy and systemic chemotherapy, the functional results achieved in 29 patients who survived 2 years showed that only 18% of the patients had a severe functional deficit if doses of 5000 cGy were combined with chemotherapy.

Second cancers occur in the radiation field in 3% to 18% of patients. The incidence appears to be related to total radiation dose, to radiation energy (orthovoltage), and to the use of chemotherapy.

Integrated Radiation Therapy and Chemotherapy

Current treatment protocols for Ewing's sarcoma often begin with three to five cycles of chemotherapy before irradiation. This allows for the assessment of the response to chemotherapy. Early institution of radiation therapy should be considered in a patient with progressive spinal cord compression or airway obstruction caused by the tumor. Doxorubicin and dactinomycin, commonly used chemotherapeutic agents in Ewing's sarcoma, interact with radiation, potentially exacerbating local toxicity and necessitating treatment interruptions, with negative consequences for local control. These problems may be decreased by delaying irradiation for a few days after the drugs are given and carefully planning radiation treatment.

Chemotherapy

Before the use of adjuvant chemotherapy, long-term survival of patients with Ewing's sarcoma was rare. In the largest prechemotherapy series, only 36 (9.6%) of 374 patients treated with surgery or radiation therapy survived for 5 years. As with Wilms' tumor and rhabdomyosarcoma, single-agent chemotherapy trials were initiated in the 1960s with highly encouraging results. As shown in Table 49–28, many agents appear to be active against Ewing's sarcoma, with cyclophosphamide and doxorubicin consistently the most active. Few new agents have been developed for this or other pediatric cancers, possibly because drugs are tested against tumors resistant to multiple drugs and radiation.

In 1973, a multiinstitutional randomized trial, the first Intergroup Ewing's Sarcoma Study (IESS-I), was initiated. Patients without evidence of metastatic disease were treated on one of three treatment regimens. Local tumor control was

TABLE 49–28. Phase II Studies in Ewing's Sarcoma

Agent	*Response (No. Responding/Total)*	*Response Rate (%)*
Cyclophosphamide	19/37	51
Doxorubicin	24/58	41
Ifosfamide	10/31	32
Vincristine	3/10	30
Dactinomycin	3/9	33
BCNU	6/18	33
5-Fluorouracil	5/16	31
Etoposide	3/10	30
Cisplatin	2/27	7
Melphalan (high dose)	9/11	82
Ifosfamide/etoposide	16/17	94

planned with radiation therapy to the entire involved bone in doses ranging from 4500 to 4400 cGy, depending on the patient's age, followed by a boost of 1000 cGy to gross radiographically demonstrable tumor. Daily dose fractionation was 200 cGy, delivered 5 days each week. In addition to local therapy, patients were randomly assigned to receive adjuvant VAC with doxorubicin (regimen 1); VAC without doxorubicin (regimen 2); or VAC plus bilateral pulmonary irradiation, which consisted of midplane dose of 1500 to 1800 cGy (regimen 3). The duration of chemotherapy was 1.5 to 2 years. The survival of patients on this study are listed in Table 49–29. Important results included the following:

1. The survival rate after 3 years was 56% for the entire group.
2. The addition of doxorubicin to VAC significantly improved the disease-free survival at 2 years (72% versus 36%).
3. The addition of pulmonary irradiation to VAC decreased pulmonary recurrence if compared with VAC alone, but it was less effective than the combination of VAC plus doxorubicin.
4. The local control and disease-free survival was related to treatment and to primary site. Pelvic, humeral, and femur lesions had the poorest outcome; rib lesions were intermediate; and the best results were seen in patients with primary lesions below the knee and in the skull or spine.
5. A filigree histologic pattern was associated with a poorer prognosis.

Of 44 patients with metastatic disease or advanced regional disease treated with VAC plus doxorubicin and irradiation to primary and metastatic sites, 31 (70%) responded completely. Of these, 18 (41%) remained disease free at a median of 34 months.

The second Intergroup Ewing's Sarcoma Study (IESS II) evaluated the role of a more intensive regimen, which relied heavily on the two most active agents, cyclophosphamide and doxorubicin.

The current combined POG and CCSG protocol is a randomized study to determine whether ifosfamide and etoposide can improve outcome for patients with Ewing's sarcoma or PPNET of bone. Future studies will probably incorporate the hematopoietic growth factors to learn whether increased dose intensity can improve outcome.

Single-institution studies have played a major role in the development of therapy for Ewing's sarcoma. These studies furthered the concepts of dose intensity and preirradiation chemotherapy. In one study, 79% of patients with localized disease treated with aggressive chemotherapy and local irradiation or surgery were free of disease at a median of 41 months from beginning therapy.

NCI investigators tested a strategy that maximized the use of cyclophosphamide and doxorubicin to achieve complete remission followed by irradiation to the primary and metastatic sites of disease, which was followed by total-body irradiation. Improved outcome was correlated to a higher dose intensity of doxorubicin delivered in that study and autologous bone marrow reconstitution to prevent systemic recurrence. Although most patients achieved a complete response, this has not been maintained in the patients presenting with metastatic disease. A study in progress is testing the efficacy of the intensive vincristine, doxorubicin, and cyclophosphamide regimen in combination with the noncross-resistant pair, ifosfamide and etoposide, and irradiation to the primary site.

Hayes and coinvestigators at the St. Jude Children's Research Hospital, using a cytokinetically based, sequential, moderate-dose cyclophosphamide and doxorubicin regimen based on their experience with neuroblastoma, report complete responses in patients with metastatic disease and a disease-free survival rate comparable to that achieved with more intense regimens. This approach was tested by the POG in a larger group of patients with disappointing results.

Although several groups have been successful in achieving complete responses, the actuarial disease-free survival curves have continued to drop years after diagnosis. The disheartening experience of diagnosing a relapse in a Ewing's sarcoma patient as much as 10 to 15 years after the initial treatment is all too familiar to those who treat this disease. This phenomenon is not commonly seen with the other childhood sarcomas. It is possible that the molecular abnormality that gives rise to this tumor is predisposed by a somatic defect that favors oncogenesis and that the late recurrence is, in fact, a new tumor.

TABLE 49–29. Correlation of Local Control and Disease-Free Survival With Site of Primary Disease

Site	*No. of Patients*	*Local Control (%)*	*Disease-Free Survival (%)*
Pelvis	37	31 (84)	14 (38)
Humerus	24	19 (79)	12 (50)
Femur	43	40 (93)	22 (51)
Tibia	22	20 (91)	15 (68)
Fibula	25	24 (96)	17 (68)
Ribs	10	9 (90)	6 (60)
Skull and spine	12	12 (100)	12 (100)
Others	20	18 (90)	14 (70)

LESS COMMON SARCOMAS

Approximately 25% to 45% of all soft tissue sarcomas in children have a histologic pattern other than rhabdomyosarcoma, comprising almost 3% of all tumors in children. Although these types of sarcomas are more commonly seen in adults, the prognosis may be better for children. The difference in prognosis is most pronounced for infants and younger children whose tumors often have a benign behavior and excellent prognosis with surgery alone. Soft tissue sarcomas that occur in adolescents often have a behavior similar to those in adults.

The most common sites for soft tissue sarcomas are the extremities and trunk, especially the retroperitoneum. The usual approach to the treatment of these tumors in adults is wide surgical excision. Radiation therapy is usually added postoperatively. Although debated, the role of adjuvant chemotherapy appears to be useful for adult patients with resectable, high-grade soft tissue sarcomas of the extremities.

The utility of adjuvant chemotherapy in children is being studied by POG because similar histologic patterns may have a different biologic behavior in children.

Most of the information about the treatment of children with nonrhabdomyosarcomatous soft tissue sarcomas comes from retrospective analyses of the experiences of a single institutions. Although valuable, careful prospective multiinstitutional studies are needed to determine the roles of radiation therapy and chemotherapy in the treatment of these diseases. The POG is addressing these issues in a prospective multiinstitutional trial. The ability to surgically extirpate the tumor is the most important prognostic factor. In a retrospective review of 62 cases of childhood soft tissue sarcomas other than rhabdomyosarcoma treated at St. Jude, 84% survived with no evidence of disease if the tumor could be completely removed, but only 1 of 26 patients survived if gross tumor remained after resection.

FIBROSARCOMA

Although rare, fibrosarcoma is one of the most common nonrhabdomyosarcomatous soft tissue sarcomas in children and adolescents. It occurs most frequently in the extremity, often in the distal segments. The incidence of fibrosarcoma has two age peaks, one in infants and children younger than 5 years of age, and the second in patients 10 to 15 years of age. It appears that fibrosarcoma in infants has a more benign course.

Fibrosarcoma is a spindle cell tumor with a characteristic herringbone pattern or regularly interweaving fascicles of parallel arrays of tumor cells. Important features are evidence of mitoses, nuclear pleomorphism, and increased basophilia of individual, sometimes anaplastic, tumor cells. Cells are densely packed, but reticulin stain reveals a regular pattern of stromal collagen fibers not easily appreciated by light microscopy. The differential diagnosis includes fibromatosis (which can be exceedingly aggressive locally, but which does not metastasize), nodular fasciitis, myositis ossificans, and inflammatory pseudotumor among the nonmalignant conditions and neurofibrosarcoma and poorly differentiated embryonal rhabdomyosarcoma among malignant tumors.

Of 52 cases of congenital fibrosarcoma, 37 occurred on an extremity and 15 on the trunk. Of the patients with extremity tumors, 92% were free of metastatic disease, and 95% were alive, despite a 27% local recurrence rate. Congenital fibrosarcomas of the trunk appear to be more aggressive, with 20% of patients developing metastases, and 26% dying of their disease. The standard therapy for fibrosarcoma is surgical extirpation by wide local excision, usually without additional therapy. The use of irradiation and chemotherapy in the local management of congenital fibrosarcoma is restricted to situations in which surgical removal is not possible.

There is no evidence that adjuvant chemotherapy is indicated in the treatment of congenital fibrosarcoma and nonmetastatic fibrosarcoma of young children. Several recent reports document that at least some of these tumors are sensitive to chemotherapy, and for patients who have unresectable metastatic or primary disease, chemotherapy may be useful. Several combinations of chemotherapy have been used: vincristine, doxorubicin, and cyclophosphamide; vincristine, dactinomycin, and cyclophosphamide; ifosfamide and etoposide have resulted in complete regressions of metastatic fibrosarcoma.

NEUROFIBROSARCOMA

Neurofibrosarcomas, malignant tumors of nerve sheath origin, account for approximately 5% to 10% of all nonrhabdomyosarcomatous soft tissue sarcomas in children. Neurofibrosarcoma occurs in association with a dominantly inherited syndrome, neurofibromatosis (*i.e.*, von Recklinghausen's disease) in about 50% of patients. Approximately 5% to 16% of patients with von Recklinghausen's disease develop neurofibrosarcoma.

Although superficially similar in appearance to fibrosarcoma, neurofibrosarcoma is a more aggressive tumor. The cells are usually more variable in size and shape, a herringbone pattern is absent, and typical features of adult neurofibrosarcomas often can be found in some areas of the tumor (*e.g.*, myxoid stroma, palisading of nuclei, and occasionally well-defined organoid arrays of nuclei). These features, common in benign schwannomas, are far less conspicuous in the malignant counterpart, but can be diagnostic if present. Diagnosis is best established by electron microscopy. The most common primary sites of neurofibrosarcoma appear to be the extremities (42%), retroperitoneum (25%), and trunk (21%).

As with fibrosarcoma, surgery plays a key role in the management of children with neurofibrosarcoma. Postoperative irradiation may be indicated if surgery does not attain negative margins. The role of chemotherapy in the treatment of patients with neurofibrosarcoma is unclear. Experience with extremity tumors in a few adults at the NCI suggests that a regimen of doxorubicin and cyclophosphamide may be effective in the adjuvant treatment of localized, grossly removed neurofibrosarcoma. Although chemotherapy can produce tumor regressions in patients with gross local and metastatic disease, no regimen appears to enhance disease-free survival in patients with advanced disease. The combination of ifosfamide and etoposide, a regimen highly active in the treatment of recurrent small, round cell tumors of neural origin, has produced partial tumor regressions in 2 of the 4 patients with recurrent neurofibrosarcoma who were evaluated.

MALIGNANT FIBROUS HISTIOCYTOMA

Although malignant fibrous histiocytoma (MFH) was the most common histologic diagnosis in the NCI series of adults with extremity sarcomas, accounting for 53 (25%) of 211 patients, it is much less common in children. At St. Jude, only 5 (8%) of the 62 cases of nonrhabdomyosarcomatous soft tissue sarcoma were diagnosed as MFH. The typical microscopic appearance of MFH resembles fibrosarcoma, but it is differentiated by marked cellular pleomorphism, multiple cell types (especially lipid-laden tumor cells), and a more malignant appearance. A storiform pattern of tumor cells, described as radiating fascicles of tumor cells at right angles from one another, is virtually diagnostic of this tumor.

Because of the rarity of this tumor in childhood, the approach to treatment of this malignancy is based on the adult experience. The accepted initial management is wide local excision of the tumor. Limb-sparing operations with radiation to the tumor bed have been as successful as amputations for tumors in the extremities. The role of adjuvant chemotherapy is not yet established in children with MFH. Of 7 patients with MFH, 2 had their tumor completely removed and were then treated with adjuvant chemotherapy; both were alive 1.4 and 9 years later. Comparable survivals without adjuvant chemotherapy have also been described.

Vincristine, dactinomycin, and cyclophosphamide, with or without doxorubicin, has produced objective tumor regressions in patients with advanced disease. Four of the 5 patients with group III or IV disease had complete or partial tumor regressions, and 2 remained disease free at 4.6 and 5.4 years. Responses to ifosfamide plus etoposide have been reported.

SYNOVIAL SARCOMA

Synovial sarcoma accounted for 29% of the nonrhabdomyosarcomatous soft tissue sarcomas at St. Jude Children's Research Hospital. The most common anatomic location is the lower extremity, often in the thigh and the knee; the next most common site is the upper extremity. Approximately 15% to 20% occur on the head, neck, or trunk.

Synovial cell sarcomas can have two components, a spindle cell fibrous stroma virtually indistinguishable from fibrosarcoma and a distinct glandular component with absolute epithelial differentiation.

Significant prognostic features are small tumor size (<5-cm diameter); a primary site in the hand, foot, or knee; a younger age; and a predominant epithelioid pattern. The disease-free survival rate for adult patients with localized tumors of the extremities is approximately 70%. Eight of the 18 patients treated at St. Jude were long-term survivors.

Because this tumor is relatively rare in children, the optimal treatment guidelines have not yet been established. Wide local excision is the treatment of choice to control the primary tumor. Radiation therapy may improve control with microscopically inadequate margins; treatment planning should seek to ensure normal function and normal growth by maximal sparing of bone and normal soft tissue. The effectiveness of irradiation in the control of bulky disease has not been established.

The benefit of adjuvant chemotherapy in the treatment of synovial sarcoma in children and young adults is not clear, but adjuvant cyclophosphamide and doxorubicin administered postoperatively to adult patients was beneficial. Tumor regressions in patients with advanced disease have been documented with several chemotherapy regimens. Although these treatment plans have usually included cyclophosphamide and doxorubicin, a regimen of vincristine, dactinomycin, and cyclophosphamide has been advocated. Objective tumor regressions have been seen with the combination regimen of ifosfamide and etoposide.

HEMANGIOPERICYTOMA

Hemangiopericytoma, a tumor that presumably arises from the pericyte cells that surround vascular channels, accounts for approximately 3% of all soft tissue sarcomas in children. It can be benign or malignant. The most common primary sites are the extremities, especially the lower extremities; the retroperitoneum is the second most common site of disease, followed by the head and neck region and the trunk. The most common sites of secondary disease are the lungs and bone.

The behavior of this tumor in older children is similar to that of hemangiopericytoma in adult patients. The overall 5-year survival rate for adults varies from 30% to 70%. The therapeutic approach is wide local excision. Adjuvant chemotherapy has been of value in adults with this disease. As with other soft tissue sarcomas, radiation therapy is used if complete surgical removal of the tumor cannot be accomplished.

Responses to chemotherapy have been reported with the use of vincristine, cyclophosphamide, doxorubicin, dactinomycin, methotrexate, mitoxantrone, and other alkylating agents. Although there is no randomized study confirming the role of adjuvant chemotherapy is this disease, the high incidence of metastatic disease and relative chemoresponsiveness of the tumor had led many investigators to treat these patients with chemotherapy after extirpation of the primary tumor.

Hemangiopericytoma may rarely occur in infants, and although similar in histologic appearance to the adult form, infantile hemangiopericytoma usually follows a more benign course. These tumors usually arise in the subcutis; however, occasionally they may have extensive local infiltration or metastasize. The treatment of choice for infantile hemangiopericytoma is surgery alone if the tumor is localized; however, complete regression of metastatic disease in patients with this entity has been seen with chemotherapy.

ALVEOLAR SOFT PART SARCOMA

Alveolar soft part sarcoma (ASPS) is a rare sarcoma that usually occurs in patients between the ages of 15 and 35 years. Although 6 of the 62 patients in the St. Jude series had ASPS, the actual incidence in children and adolescents is probably lower. The tumor usually occurs in the skeletal muscle of the extremities in adults, but the head and neck region is a common site in children.

The most distinctive feature of ASPS is the presence of PAS-positive, diastase-resistant inclusions in the cytoplasm, which show a regular crystalline structure. That some inclusions closely resemble neurosecretory granules provokes suspicion that the tumor may be neuroepithelial, but immunocytochemistry is inconclusive in this regard.

Alveolar soft part sarcoma usually presents as a slow-growing, painless mass. The clinical course of patients with ASPS is indolent but usually progressive. The most common sites of metastatic disease are lung, brain, bone, and lymph nodes.

The initial therapeutic approach is complete local excision alone, with radiation and chemotherapy reserved for the treatment of recurrent disease. Many patients eventually relapse and subsequently die of disease. This ominous fact strongly suggests that new approaches to the prevention of relapses are needed in the treatment of this disorder.

LEIOMYOSARCOMA

Leiomyosarcoma is rare in childhood, accounting for less than 2% of soft tissue sarcomas in children. The most common primary sites of disease are the retroperitoneum vascular tissue, peripheral soft tissue, and the gastrointestinal tract.

The tumor cells are elongate, with cigar-shaped nuclei and brightly eosinophilic cytoplasm (due to the content of myofilaments), and they are closely packed in parallel arrays. The appearance is superficially similar to fibrosarcoma, but the eosinophilic nuclei, resembling smooth muscle in normal tissues, and usual monotonous regularity of tumor cells are distinct.

The most common approach to the treatment is local excision. The role of chemotherapy and radiation therapy in children is undefined. If complete extirpation of the tumor can be achieved, the prognosis is usually good for tumors arising outside of the gastrointestinal tract; however, tumors arising in this site generally have a poor prognosis. Leiomyosarcomas of the colorectal region in children, although extremely rare, appear to have a relatively good prognosis if the tumor can be successfully excised.

LIPOSARCOMA

Although primarily a disease of adults, with a peak age of incidence between 40 and 60 years, liposarcomas may occur in children, most often in the early part of the second decade of life. The tumor rarely affects infants and young children, in whom its behavior is usually benign. The two most common primary sites are the extremities and the retroperitoneum. The tumor may be well-differentiated, myxoid, round cell, or pleomorphic (in increasing degree of malignancy and decreasing survival). Most tumor cells are fibroblastic; only rare cells show conspicuous lipoblastic differentiation. The distinction from MFH can be difficult, but the presence of a myxoid stroma, conspicuous small blood vessels, and scant mitotic activity are all typical of liposarcoma.

The treatment of choice for localized liposarcoma is wide local excision. Local recurrences may ultimately result in the death of the patient because of extension of the tumor into vital structures. The role of adjuvant chemotherapy in the treatment of liposarcomas of childhood is undefined. Radiation appears to be effective in the control of microscopic disease in adults.

HISTIOCYTOSES

The histiocytoses are an uncommon group of clinically diverse syndromes that share a histopathology characterized by granuloma formation with the infiltration and proliferation of histocytes. The classic clinical triad of the histiocytosis X syndromes includes a solitary lytic lesion of bone (*i.e.*, eosinophilic granuloma); a chronic disorder characterized by exophthalmos, diabetes insipidus, and skeletal lesions (*i.e.*, Hand-Schüller-Christian syndrome); and an acute fulminant disseminated disorder of young children manifested by skin lesions, hepatosplenomegaly, lymphadenopathy, mastoiditis, osteolytic lesions, pneumonitis, anemia, thrombocytopenia, and fever (*i.e.*, Letterer-Siwe disease). The clinical and biologic diversity has made it difficult to characterize and classify histiocytosis as a neoplastic or nonneoplastic disorder and has contributed to the controversy about its appropriate management.

BIOLOGIC CONSIDERATIONS

The infiltration and accumulation of cells in the monocyte or macrophage series into a target tissue can be a primary or secondary event, and not all diseases associated with histiocytic infiltration are classified as histiocytoses.

Histiocytes arise from the uncommitted bone marrow stem cell and differentiate along the granulocyte-macrophage axis. One of the primary functions of normal histiocytes is phagocytoses of aged erythrocytes, microbes, or tumor cells, and erythrophagocytosis is a common finding in many of the histiocytoses of childhood. The characteristic findings of histiocytoses may be the result of diverse pathogenic mechanisms. For example, in "histiocytosis-X," now known as Langerhans' cell histiocytosis, the proliferation and accumulation of histiocytes is the result of immunologic stimulation of the Langerhans' cell. It does not appear that these histiocytes are truly malignant, and improvement has been noticed with the administration of thymic extracts. In the cases of infection-associated hemophagocytic syndrome, the macrophage appears to be reacting to a foreign antigen, and this histiocytosis reverses when the infection and its antigenic stimulation abates. Other histiocytoses may represent a genetic abnormality (*e.g.*, familial erythrophagocytic lymphohistiocytosis) or a clonal neoplastic proliferation (*e.g.*, malignant histiocytosis).

PATHOLOGY

To clarify this diverse group of histiocytoses, the Histiocytosis Society has developed a classification system based on pathologic examination that divides the histiocytoses into three classes.

In class I histiocytoses, the central cell has the histopathologic feature of the Langerhans' cell and this designation replaces those syndromes previously referred to as histiocytosis X (*i.e.*, eosinophilic granuloma, Hand-Schüller-Christian syndrome, and Letterer-Siwe disease). The lesions associated with Langerhans' cell histiocytosis are granulomatous and are highlighted by the presence of Langerhans' cells with Birbeck's granules, which can be seen by electron microscopy.

Class II histiocytoses include all the other nonmalignant histiocytoses in which the mononuclear phagocyte is not a Langerhans' cell. These are reactive histiocytoses that are usually associated with a mixed lymphohistiocytic infiltrate, generally in the sinusoids, cortex, and paracortex, but without effacement of nodal architecture. The infiltrating histiocytes appear normal, and they have low nuclear to cytoplasmic ratios, mature nuclear chromatin, inconspicuous nucleoli, and abundant cytoplasm. The two disorders categorized in class II histiocytoses, the infection-associated hemophagocytic syndrome (IAHS) and familial erythrophagocytic lymphohistiocytosis (FEL), are denoted by erythrophagocytosis and the secondary accumulation of histocytes.

Class III histiocytosis is a true neoplasm, of which malignant histiocytosis is the best known disease. Lymph nodes in class III histiocytosis are characterized by nodal effacement and infiltration with cells containing reticular chromatic patterns, prominent nucleoli, and basophilic cytoplasm. Erythrophagocytosis may be observed in class III histiocytosis, but it is not a prominent as in class II.

CLINICAL PRESENTATION, DIAGNOSIS, AND TREATMENT

Class I Histiocytoses

As seen in Table 49–30, the Langerhans' cell histiocytosis has a variable presentation and clinical course and can undergo regression and exacerbation within the same patient. In acute disseminated histiocytosis, the skin is involved in 70% to 100% of patients and is characterized by a scaling, eczematoid rash over the trunk, neck, groin, and scalp. Scalp lesions are not infrequently misdiagnosed as a seborrheic dermatitis. There is often a petechial component, and in rare cases, skin lesions can antedate more widespread disease. A syndrome referred to as regressing atypical histiocytosis has been described and is characterized by noduloulcerative skin lesions composed of atypical histiocytes, monocytes, and multinucleated giant cells with erythrophagocytosis. However, these patients have cutaneous disease only, and the skin lesions are indolent and characterized by spontaneous regressions and recurrences. Recognition of this disorder is important to avoid unnecessary treatment.

Lytic bone lesions serve as the clinical hallmark of Langerhans' histiocytoses and occur with a frequency comparable to skin disease, most commonly involving the flat bones and vertebrae, frequently with pain and functional impairment. In approximately 33% of patients, there is evidence of bilateral osteomastoiditis with bilateral suppurative discharge. Skeletal survey is a more reliable diagnostic and follow-up tool in these patients than radionuclide bone scans.

Histiocytic infiltration into the reticuloendothelial system results in generalized lymphadenopathy. Enlargement of the liver and spleen, particularly if associated with functional abnormalities, carries an ominous prognosis. Although hepatosplenomegaly is infrequent in initial presentation, it develops in almost half of patients with disseminated histiocytosis, sometimes with jaundice and occasionally with the onset of cirrhosis. Similarly, pulmonary findings are infrequent at initial diagnosis, but some pulmonary manifestations, particularly a diffuse interstitial infiltrate, develop during the disease course in almost 67% of patients. Buccal and gingival infiltration occurs in about 40% of patients and is manifested as loose or floating teeth. More ominous are hematologic abnormalities, including anemia and thrombocytopenia.

Of patients with generalized disease, 25% to 50% develop diabetes insipidus during their disease course. Nonetheless, the classic Hand-Schüller-Christian syndrome, which includes diabetes insipidus, exophthalmos, and geographic skull lesions, is found in fewer than 10% of patients with disseminated histiocytosis. The presence of diabetes insipidus is rarely associated with radiographic abnormalities of the sella turcica.

TABLE 49–30. Clinical, Prognostic, and Therapeutic Aspects of the Major Childhood Histiocytoses

Variable	*LCH or Class I*	*IAHS or Class II*	*FEL or Class II*	*MH or Class III*
Clinical presentation	Wide spectrum, from mild discomfort related to lesions (lytic bone lesions, chronic otitis, diabetes insipidus) to generalized symptoms including fever and weight loss	Pancytopenia, hepatosplenomegaly, fever coagulopathy	Irritability, fever, wasting sometimes with a coagulopathy and hepatosplenomegaly	Variable, from systemic disease (*e.g.*, acute leukemia) to a localized mass lesion
Diagnostic findings	Birbeck's granules in lesional cells	Morphologically normal macrophages, documented infection, and negative family history	Morphologically normal macrophages and negative search for infection, sometimes positive family history	Malignant macrophages
Prognosis	Variable, but a self-resolving disease process in most cases	Excellent, providing underlying infection is controlled and immunosuppression can be reversed	Extremely poor; uniformly rapidly fatal	Up to 75% survival at 40 months reported with appropriate therapy for patients with MH or THL; prognosis is poor for patients with acute monocytic leukemia
Recommended treatment	None to mild radiation or chemotherapy (vinblastine or etoposide and steroids) for certain lesions	Avoidance of immunosuppressive therapy; etoposide is being explored experimentally	Experimental (etoposide); bone marrow transplantation	Doxorubicin in a combination chemotherapy regimen for MH or THL; appropriate therapy for acute monocytic leukemia

LCH, Langerhans' cell hystiocytosis; IAHS, infection-associated hemophagocytic syndrome; FEL, familial erythrophagocytic lymph histiocytosis; MH, malignant histiocytosis; THL, true histiocytic lymphoma.
(Ladisch S, Jaffe ES. The histiocytoses. In: Pizzo PA, Poplack DG, eds: Principles and practice of pediatric oncology. 2nd ed. Philadelphia: JB Lippincott, 1993)

Increasingly recognized are the delayed neurologic manifestations that include hyperreflexia, ataxia, vertigo, nystagmus, and dysarthria.

Diagnosis requires biopsy and electron microscopy to determine the presence of Birbeck's granules and to eliminate other disorders that may cause lytic bone lesions, especially metastatic neuroblastoma.

Two prognostic features stand out. First, mortality is higher for children younger than 2 years of age at the time of diagnosis. Second, organ dysfunction, especially if multiple organ systems are involved, decreases survival. Particularly ominous is hepatic involvement at the time of initial diagnosis. These factors influence approaches to therapy.

The treatment of patients with monostotic bone lesions is the most straightforward and includes surgical biopsy or curettage. Low-dose megavoltage irradiation (500–1000 cGy) is recommended only for lesions that are surgically inaccessible, including vertebral bodies or sites adjacent to major growth plates.

The treatment of patients with generalized involvement is more controversial. Which patients should be treated? If treatment is undertaken, should it be with chemotherapy or immunotherapy? What should be the intensity and duration of therapy? These questions are complicated by the clinical diversity of Langerhans' cell histiocytosis and the chance that the disease may undergo a spontaneous regression. While treating the underlying process, care should be taken to avoid iatrogenic morbidity. Symptomatic or palliative therapy should not be overlooked, because disabling problems, such as diabetes insipidus, progressive destruction of a weight-bearing bone, extensive and progressive mandibular involvement, mastoid disease, and proptosis, can often be resolved with a short course of local irradiation.

Current systemic treatment options include chemotherapy, immunotherapy, and low-dose, total-body irradiation. A variety of drugs (*e.g.*, chlorambucil, vinblastine, etoposide, methotrexate, with or without prednisone) yield complete and partial response rates of 40% to 60%. The overall response rates to combination chemotherapy do not appear to be clearly superior to single-drug schedules in most series, although one study suggested that combination therapy was preferable for children younger than 2 years of age who had extensive disease. Conversely, combination regimens are likely to be associated with more toxicity. Some investigators recommend withholding chemotherapy from patients who have multifocal disease limited to the skeleton or skin. Recent data suggest that early intervention may offset the onset of delayed, particularly neurologic, complications. Patients with more extensive disease, particularly those with evidence of hepatic dysfunction, require chemotherapy with agents such as vinblastine (for infants <1 year of age) or vinblastine or etoposide plus prednisone and 6-mercaptopurine for older children. Children who fail to respond to chemotherapy may benefit from low-dose cyclosporine alone or in combination with chemotherapy, perhaps because of its ability to affect a reduction in cytokine production.

Class II Histiocytoses

FEL is an autosomal-recessive disorder characterized by fever, irritability, leptomeningeal involvement, hepatosplenomegaly, and abnormal liver dysfunction, with bone marrow findings of histiocytic and lymphocytic infiltration and with prominent erythrophagocytosis. FEL occurs primarily in young infants, and families with several affected members have been described. Unlike histiocytosis X, FEL is differentiated by a variety of immunologic abnormalities, including depressed antibody levels, anergy, and defective lymphocyte proliferation. In one family, plasma-mediated inhibition of cellular immunity was described, which correlated with the plasma triglyceride level, raising the question of whether the immune abnormalities were primary or secondary phenomena. Clinical and immunologic improvement was observed with plasma-exchange transfusion in a patient with FEL. An increase of acidic glycosphingolipids and a decrease of α-galactosidase activity suggest that FEL may be associated with unique quantitative and qualitative abnormalities of the hepatic gangliosides.

FEL is a rapidly progressive disorder and is frequently complicated by thrombocytopenia and a disseminated intravascular coagulopathy. Progressive neurologic deterioration and brain atrophy with perivascular infiltration of the brain and meninges by lymphocytes and histiocytes can occur. An X-linked histiocytosis has been described in which there is nodal infiltration by macrophages and plasma cells with hypergammaglobulinemia.

Because of its rapidly fulminant course and lymphohistiocytic infiltration suggesting a malignant neoplasm, cytotoxic therapy has been employed for FEL. Although transient improvements have been observed with combination regimens similar to those used for acute leukemia, remissions are rarely sustained, and the patients die. Two approaches have been explored as alternatives to chemotherapy: plasma exchange and bone marrow transplantation. Plasma exchange is based on the presence of circulating immunosuppressive activity in patients with FEL. After exchange transfusion, a reduction in plasma-inhibiting activity and some reversal of the depressed cellular immunity was observed, but these responses were not sustained. Bone marrow transplantation is based on the hypothesis that FEL represents an uncontrolled proliferation of lymphocytes and histiocytes. Bone marrow transplantation has been successful for a few patients, but additional experience is necessary.

IAHS is considered a class II histiocytosis. The clinical appearance of IAHS is similar to FEL, and the diagnosis rests on presence of an infection and a negative family history for this disease. Like FEL, there is striking erythrophagocytosis in the bone marrow of children with IAHS, and with the absence of Birbeck's granules on electron microscopy, this differentiates IAHS from Langerhans' cell histiocytosis.

The keys to the successful therapy of children with IAHS are the discovery of the infectious agent and the avoidance of immunosuppressive therapy. Although cytotoxic therapy is generally contraindicated for IAHS, etoposide may be beneficial in halting disease progression. However, caution is appropriate because of the secondary leukemias observed in patients treated with etoposide.

Class III Histiocytosis

Acute monocytic leukemia and malignant histiocytosis fall into the category of class III histiocytosis. Malignant histiocytosis is a nonfamilial, rapidly fatal disorder characterized by fever, generalized tender lymphadenopathy, hepatosplenomegaly, subcutaneous inflammatory infiltration, pancytopenia, and a Coombs-positive hemolytic anemia. A characteristic finding is erythrophagocytosis in the bone marrow, liver, and spleen, along with histiocytic infiltration of the subcapsular and medullary regions of lymph nodes. Immunochemical analysis has demonstrated that malignant histiocytosis cells stain positively for the S-100 protein (a CNS-specific protein), that many contain evidence of κ or λ chains, and that many are lysosome negative, suggesting that they are derived from T-zone histiocytes rather than from the monocyte-macrophage axis. Cytogenetic analysis of malignant histiocytes from the bone marrow of an infant with malignant histiocytosis revealed a translocation [t(8:16)(p11′3)], which disappeared after clinical remission.

For patients with malignant histiocytosis and FEL, intervention is clearly necessary. However, a continuing issue is whether this should be with prednisone alone or with regimens including vincristine and cyclophosphamide. Prolonged responses have been observed in some patients with malignant histiocytosis treated with combination chemotherapy, including vincristine, prednisone, cyclophosphamide, doxorubicin, vinblastine, bleomycin, methyl-CCNU, etoposide, and cytosine arabinoside, although the overall mortality rate of these patients remains quite high (68%).

Additional insights into the immunology and classification of the histiocytoses are necessary, and continued exploration of immune replacement or its mediation are important objectives.

CARCINOMAS AND OTHER LESS COMMON TUMORS OF CHILDHOOD

Many of the tumors that are common in adults occur only rarely in children. Principles for evaluation and management are generally similar to those for adults. Some insights about the pediatric aspects of those tumors are offered here.

HEAD AND NECK TUMORS

Nasopharyngeal Carcinoma

Nasopharyngeal carcinoma is a rare neoplasm in North America. It is more common in black than white teenagers. In children, rhabdomyosarcoma and non-Hodgkin's lymphomas are much more common nasopharyngeal tumors. Nasopharyngeal carcinoma appears to be closely associated with EBV infection. Management includes irradiation (6000–7000 cGy) and chemotherapy (*e.g.,* 5-FU, methotrexate, bleomycin, cisplatin). In patients with localized involvement, a disease-free survival rate of 78% has been reported.

Oropharyngeal Tumors

Squamous cell carcinoma of the tongue and oral cavity are extremely rare in children, but the incidence is increasing because of the use of smokeless tobacco products. It has been estimated that as many as 8% to 30% of male high-school and college students regularly use smokeless tobacco, often beginning at 12 years of age. The use of these products should be discouraged by physicians caring for teenagers and young adults.

Ameloblastoma

Ameloblastoma or adamtanoma is a rare tumor that arises in the mandible, maxilla, or rarely, long bones. The primary therapeutic modalities are surgery and irradiation. The role of chemotherapy is not established.

Laryngeal Tumors

The most common childhood tumor involving the larynx is rhabdomyosarcoma, and squamous cell tumors of the larynx occur only rarely. Juvenile papillomatosis is a benign overgrowth of epithelial cells, primarily affecting the larynx and responsive to surgery or, in recurrent cases, radiation therapy or interferon.

TUMORS OF THE LUNG AND THORAX

Lung Cancer

Although rare, more that 100 cases of primary lung cancers in children have been reported, including bronchogenic carcinoma, usually of the undifferentiated or adenocarcinomatous type, occurring primarily in adolescents. Bronchial adenomas have been described, the primary treatment for which is surgical resection.

Pulmonary blastoma, a rare subpleural neoplasm has been described in children. It can metastasize and may respond to combination chemotherapy.

Thymoma

To be considered a tumor of the thymus gland, neoplastic epithelial cells must be demonstrable, because many malignant and nonmalignant processes are associated with thymomas. Included are Hodgkin's and non-Hodgkin's lymphomas, germ cell tumors, carcinoids, thymolipomas, myasthenia gravis, autoimmune diseases (*e.g.,* polymyositis, systemic lupus erythematosus, rheumatoid arthritis), and endocrine disorders (*e.g.,* hyperparathyroidism, Addison's syndromes, panhypopituitarism).

Thymomas are usually slowly growing tumors found in the anterior mediastinum. Diagnosis may be heralded by nonspecific symptoms, including cough, dyspnea, and in advanced cases, evidence of a superior vena cava syndrome. Thymomas are locally invasive, and metastases can occur in lymph nodes, bone, liver, kidney, or brain.

Thymomas are generally radiosensitive and treatment includes 3500 to 4500 cGy given over 3 to 6 weeks. Thymomas have responded to doxorubicin, cisplatin, and alkylating agents. Most authorities reserve chemotherapy for patients not responding to local therapy. Survival rates appear to be 65% to 83% for patients with locally confined tumors and 30% to 54% for invasive tumor.

Breast Cancer

Most breast tumors in pediatric patients are benign, the most common being the fibroadenomas that occur in adolescents.

Although these tumors can become quite large (*e.g.*, cystosarcoma phyllodes), they are usually benign.

Although uncommon, carcinomas of the breast have been described in boys and girls. They do not appear to be different from adult tumors, and the recommendations for therapy are the same.

ENDOCRINE TUMORS

Endocrine tumors comprise 4% to 5% of childhood neoplasms, most which are benign or low-grade malignancies. Most of these tumors do not secrete hormones, with 40% to 45% arising from gonadal origins, 30% from the thyroid, and 20% from the pituitary gland. Less commonly, tumors involve the parathyroids, adrenal gland, and the gastroenteropancreatic unit. Although most of these tumors are sporadic and of embryonic origin, a smaller percentage may be familial (*e.g.*, medullary carcinomas of the thyroid, pheochromocytoma), among which are the genetically transmitted syndromes of multiple endocrine neoplasia (MEN).

Most thyroid cancers in children are papillary or follicular, usually presenting as an asymptomatic solitary nodule or cervical adenopathy. Although a trial of thyroid suppression is recommended by some, the 14% to 40% incidence of carcinoma in children with thyroid nodules should prompt surgical resection. The 10-year survival is better for younger patients with thyroid carcinoma (83%) than for adults (60%).

Adrenal carcinomas are rare in childhood (<0.5% of pediatric tumors) and occur primarily in children younger than 8 years old. These tumors are endocrinologically active, causing Cushing's syndrome, virilization, or feminization; aldosterenomas are rare in children.

One of the primary objectives is to differentiate carcinoma from a benign adenoma. Carcinomas are usually larger and more inhomogenous by CT and ultrasound at the time of diagnosis. Tumors weighing less than 100 g have an excellent prognosis, but those weighing more than 500 g have a poor prognosis. Surgery is the treatment of choice, and awareness that tumors may be bilateral in as many as 10% of patients is important. For patients with extensive local or metastatic disease in kidney, lymph nodes, liver, lung, mesentery, brain, or bone, chemotherapy with 5-FU, dactinomycin, cyclophosphamide, and op'DDD should be administered. Inhibitors of steroid synthesis (*e.g.*, aminoglutethimide, metapyrone, ketoconazole) or glucocorticoid antagonists (*e.g.*, RU486) may be useful. If hypoaldosteronism or hypocortisolism develops, after treatment with mitolane, fludrocortisone or hydrocortisone replacement may be necessary. Studies are in progress using suramin, an antiparasitic agent that, as a side-effect, can cause the necrosis of the adrenal cortex. Preliminary results are encouraging.

MEN syndromes are exceedingly rare in pediatrics but have been described in families. MEN type I consists of tumors of the pituitary, parathyroid, and pancreas (in particular, the Zollinger-Ellison syndrome); MEN type II consists of medullary carcinoma of the thyroid and pheochromocytoma (MEN-IIa) and a familial syndrome that includes mucosal neuromas and a Marfan-like body habitus (MEN-IIb) (Table 49–31).

RENAL CELL CARCINOMA

Renal cell carcinoma (*e.g.*, clear cell carcinoma, renal cell adenocarcinoma, hypernephroma) is the most common primary kidney tumor in adults, but it is rare in children, occurring with an annual incidence of 4 per million. Renal cell carcinoma has been seen in patients with the von Hippel-Lindau syndrome, tuberous sclerosis, and a constitutional

TABLE 49–31. Comparison of Clusters of Involved Tumors in MEN Syndromes

Site of Origin	*MEN-I*	*MEN-IIa*	*MEN-IIb**
Pituitary gland	Prolactinoma Somatotropinoma Corticotropinoma		
Thyroid gland		C-cell hyperplasia Medullary carcinoma	Medullary carcinoma
Parathyroid glands	Parathyroid hyperplasia, adenoma	Parathyroid hyperplasia, adenoma	
Adrenal cortex	Adrenal adenoma, hyperplasia		
Adrenal medulla		Pheochromocytoma	Pheochromocytoma
Gastroenteropancreatic unit	Gastrinoma Insulinoma VIPoma Glucagonoma		
Other	PPoma Lipomas Carcinoids		Mucosal neuromas, ganglioneuromas

* Characterized also by marfanoid habitus.
(Chrousos GP. Endocrine tumors. In: Pizzo PA, Poplack DG, eds. Principles and practice of pediatric oncology. 2nd ed. Philadelphia: JB Lippincott, 1993)

chromosome translocation. There is a high frequency of abnormalities, t(3:8)(p14″4), of chromosome 3.

The four patterns of pathology are papillary, solid, cystic, and sarcomatous, although these have little prognostic impact. The cellular morphology includes clear cell, granular cell, and sarcomatoid types.

Unlike Wilms' tumor, in which the presenting mass is often asymptomatic, renal cell carcinoma usually presents with abdominal or flank pain and hematuria. The average age of patients with renal cell carcinoma is 11 years, but it has been described in children as young as 14 months.

The most important prognostic factor is stage. Children with stage I disease had a 100% survival rate; stage II had a 66% survival rate; stage III had 43% survival rate; and stage IV had a 12% survival rate. This is related to the therapeutic approaches. Radical nephrectomy with resection of the kidney, adrenal gland, surrounding perinephric fat, Gerota's fascia, and regional lymph nodes is the treatment for localized renal cell carcinoma. The role of radiation therapy is unclear for children, although some physicians have advocated 4000 to 4500 cGy postoperatively for children with stage II disease. Chemotherapy has not been particularly successful, but interferon and the use of interleukin-2 (IL-2) with lymphokine-activated killer (LAK) cells have been successful in adults; data for children are lacking.

GASTROINTESTINAL TRACT CARCINOMAS

Carcinomas of the stomach, colon, gallbladder, and pancreas have been described in children, although their incidence is strikingly low. These tumors are usually not suspected in children. Because the tumors are so rare in children, the treatments are similar to those used in adults.

CANCERS OF THE SKIN

Melanoma is the most common skin cancer in children, followed by basal cell and squamous cell carcinomas. Ionizing irradiation is an important risk factor and contributes to the regional distribution of these cancers.

The familial occurrence of melanoma in patients with the dysplastic nevus syndrome is recognized. These nevi are usually located on the trunk but can occur in the scalp or extremities. Approximately 10% of patients with these lesions develop melanomas.

The clinical appearance of melanomas and their local and metastatic spread is similar in children to that of adults. Biopsy is necessary for diagnosis, but whether it is incisional or excisional depends on the location and size of the lesion. If the lesion is a melanoma, a wide excision is necessary. Curettage or cryotherapy can be used for basal cell or squamous cell carcinomas. As in adults, chemotherapy has been used for patients with melanoma who have evidence of regional lymph node involvement. The use of IL-2 and LAK cells in adults with melanoma suggests therapeutic utility for children or adolescents with evidence of extensive disease.

Pediatricians should recommend decreased sun exposure, the use of sunscreens for children and teenagers, and the removal of congenital nevi.

REFERENCE

Pizzo PA, Poplack DG, eds. Principles and practice of pediatric oncology. 2nd ed. Philadelphia: JB Lippincott, 1993.

Cancer: Principles & Practice of Oncology, Fourth Edition,
edited by Vincent T. DeVita, Jr., Samuel Hellman, Steven A. Rosenberg.
J.B. Lippincott Co., Philadelphia © 1993.

David G. Poplack Ian T. Magrath
Larry E. Kun Philip A. Pizzo

CHAPTER **50**

Leukemias and Lymphomas of Childhood

There have been major advances in the treatment of children with leukemia and lymphoma during the past 30 years. The record of therapeutic achievements in these diseases constitutes one of the true success stories of modern clinical oncology. Perhaps the most dramatic example is the improvement in the outlook for children with acute lymphoblastic leukemia (ALL), a disorder that was uniformly fatal only 40 years ago. More than half of the children with this disease now are alive and free of disease more than 5 years after initial diagnosis, and most of these patients are considered cured. Forty years ago the major concern was developing better methods of inducing complete remission; today the focus has shifted to issues facing long-term survivors. The situation is somewhat different for children with acute myelogenous leukemia (AML). Although the outlook for these patients has improved, curative therapy for most of these children remains elusive. In contrast, progress in treating the childhood non-Hodgkin's lymphomas (NHL) has been particularly striking. Before the 1970s, fewer than 30% of children obtained long-term, disease-free survival. Currently, 60% to 80% of children with NHL are considered curable.[1]

Improvement in therapy for these disorders has resulted from innovative application of the principles of combination chemotherapy and the combined-modality approach. Intensive biologic, immunologic, and cytogenetic characterization has contributed significantly to our understanding of these disorders. For example, information about the differentiation status of malignant lymphoid cells, derived in part from technical advances such as immunophenotyping with monoclonal antibodies and determination of immunoglobulin and T-cell receptor gene rearrangements, has provided a more rational means of classifying these disorders. Similarly, application of the type of molecular biologic methods that led to the demonstration of oncogene expression in Burkitt's lymphoma cells is likely to help elucidate the cause of lymphoid and nonlymphoid malignancies.

EPIDEMIOLOGY AND ETIOLOGY

Acute leukemia is the most common malignancy in children. Each year in the United States, approximately 2000 cases are diagnosed. ALL accounts for three fourths of these cases; AML makes up most of the remaining cases. Chronic myelogenous leukemia (CML) is rare and comprises fewer than 5% of childhood leukemias.[2]

ALL has a peak incidence in children between 2 and 6 years of age. The increased peak incidence of ALL in whites in the United States is not observed in blacks. This difference is largely responsible for the observation that acute leukemia is almost twice as common in white than in nonwhite children.

In AML, there is no peak age of incidence in childhood. The two forms of CML in childhood tend to occur at somewhat different ages. The median age of onset for the juvenile form is approximately 2 years of age, whereas the Philadelphia chromosome-positive (Ph-positive) type more commonly appears in older children.[3] AML and CML occur with similar frequencies in whites and nonwhites.

ALL occurs more commonly in boys; this pattern is particularly striking in pubertal children. In contrast, among children younger than 5 years of age, AML occurs more commonly in girls, and between 5 to 15 years, the incidence in each sex is equal; thereafter, males are affected more frequently.

There has been considerable interest in reports of "leukemic clusters," which are a greater than expected number of leukemia cases within a given geographic area or period. Most studies have been unable to confirm this phenomenon.

A variety of possible causative factors for leukemia have been examined, including environmental and genetic factors, viruses, and immunodeficiency states. Irradiation and exposure to toxic chemicals are the most studied environmental factors. The increased incidence of leukemia observed in survivors of atomic bomb explosions in Hiroshima and Nagasaki in 1945 is well known. Persons closest to the hypocenters of these explosions had the highest incidence of leukemia. The type of leukemia that developed corresponded to the age at exposure; ALL was more common in children. There is an increased risk to children exposed to diagnostic radiation, particularly in the first trimester. A higher incidence of leukemia was found in several early studies in which irradiation was used to treat thymic enlargement in neonates, tinea capitis infection, or ankylosing spondylitis.

The use of alkylating agents to treat childhood malignancy has been associated with the development of leukemia in adulthood (*e.g.,* Hodgkin's disease). Therapy-induced leukemia is more common in those persons who also have received concomitant radiation therapy. Chronic exposure to toxic chemicals (*e.g.,* benzene) has been associated with the development of leukemia, usually AML.

There is considerable controversy about the potential risks associated with exposure to ionizing radiation from routine nuclear power plant emissions. Although an association between exposure to electromagnetic fields and the development of childhood ALL has been reported, it has not been confirmed.

There is evidence for the role of genetic factors in leukemogenesis. The incidence of leukemia is increased in children with certain constitutional chromosomal abnormalities. Children with trisomy 21 (*i.e.,* Down's syndrome) have approximately 15 times greater risk of developing leukemia than persons in the general population. ALL is most commonly observed, although AML may occur, particularly in neonatal cases. The *ETS*2 oncogene, which has been implicated in leukemogenesis may be found on chromosome 21. The development of leukemia in children with Down's syndrome is believed to reflect the presence of an unstable genome that is more susceptible to other leukemogenic factors. The observation that fibroblasts from Down's syndrome children are transformed more readily in vitro by SV40 virus supports this thesis. The same observation has been made in fibroblasts of children with Fanconi's syndrome, a rare, recessively transmitted disorder characterized by a variety of congenital abnormalities that is frequently associated with the development of AML. Patients with Bloom's syndrome, another recessively transmitted chromosomal fragility disorder, characterized by short stature and photosensitive telangiectatic erythema, also have a higher incidence of leukemia, usually AML. The development of leukemia in these patients may be a consequence of genetic recombination of somatic cell chromosomes.

Patients with ataxia-telangiectasia, an immunodeficiency disease in which abnormalities of chromosomes 14 and 7 have been observed, are at an increased risk of lymphoid malignancy, including ALL. The loci of three rearranging T-cell receptor genes, α (chromosome 14), β, and γ (chromosome 7), are at chromosomal positions susceptible to breakage and rearrangement in patients with ataxia-telangiectasia. The extent to which immune deficiency contributes to the genetic predisposition of patients to develop malignancy is unknown.

The risk of leukemia is increased in children with Klinefelter's syndrome and the trisomy G syndrome. Leukemia also has been associated with a variety of less-well-characterized chromosomal abnormalities. The increased risk of leukemia in children born to relatively older women may be related to the existence of subtle karyotypic abnormalities present in aging mothers. An increased risk of leukemia has been observed in several genetically determined congenital syndromes that are not associated with known karyotypic abnormalities, including the Rubinstein-Taybi syndrome, Schwachman's syndrome, Poland's syndrome, and neurofibromatosis.

The development of leukemia in more than one family member has been documented. The risk of leukemia is two to four times greater among siblings of leukemic children than in the general population. Those at highest risk for the development of leukemia are identical twins of children with the disease. Their risk may be as high as 25%, but it diminishes with age, and after the age of 7 years, the risk of leukemia for the unaffected twin returns to that of the general population. Although these observations strongly imply a genetic basis for the increased risk of leukemia, other factors, such as common exposure to a leukemogenic prenatal or postnatal event, cannot be excluded.

Recent attention has been focused on the p53 oncogene, a recessive tumor-suppressor gene.[4–7] Somatic p53 mutations have been reported in ALL but with a low frequency. Studies of familial ALL have identified nonhereditary p53 mutations in a few cases. It does not appear, however, that a mutant p53 gene is the cause of increased susceptibility to leukemia in most familial cases.

There has been intense interest in the possible role of viruses in the development of human leukemia. Certain retroviruses can cause leukemia in avian, murine, bovine, feline, and nonhuman primate species.[8] HTLV-I and HTLV-II, the human T-cell leukemia and lymphoma viruses, appear to play a role in the development of adult T-cell leukemia and hairy cell leukemia. No definite link has been confirmed between HTLV-I infection and children with ALL. The role of DNA viruses, particularly the Epstein-Barr virus (EBV), in lymphoid malignancy has been studied.

Infection with human immunodeficiency virus has been associated with a variety of malignancies, including lymphoma, angiogenic sarcoma, and leiomyosarcoma. Cases of B-lineage ALL have been reported.[9]

An association between immunodeficiency and the development of leukemia has been established. Children with the Wiskott-Aldrich syndrome, congenital hypogammaglobulinemia, or severe combined immunodeficiency disease have an increased incidence of lymphoid malignancy, including leukemia. Presumably, impaired immune surveillance permits the development of malignancy. The increased risk of leukemia in ataxia-telangiectasia patients probably is related to impaired immunity and genetic factors. Chronic use of immunosuppressive agents has been associated with the development of leukemia. The role that immune dysfunction plays in the development of leukemia in patients without a recognized immunodeficiency syndrome is unknown. Abnormalities in the immune system of newly diagnosed patients with ALL have been observed, but whether they precede or are a consequence of the leukemia is unclear.

ACUTE LYMPHOBLASTIC LEUKEMIA

CLINICAL PRESENTATION AND DIAGNOSIS

The presenting signs and symptoms of the child with ALL (Table 50–1) reflect the degree to which the bone marrow has been infiltrated with leukemic lymphoblasts and the extent of extramedullary spread. The most common symptoms and physical findings result from anemia, thrombocytopenia, and neutropenia and include pallor and fatigue, anorexia, petechiae, purpura, bleeding, and infection. Localized or generalized lymphadenopathy, hepatomegaly, and splenomegaly are the consequence of extramedullary leukemic spread. Overt symptoms of CNS leukemia are relatively rare at the time of initial diagnosis. Leukemic infiltration of the periosteum and bone frequently occurs, and bone pain, often manifesting as a limp or refusal to walk, is common in young children. The duration of symptoms in children presenting with ALL varies from days to months.

Because children most frequently present with relatively nonspecific symptoms, ALL clinically may mimic several childhood conditions, including infectious mononucleosis, idiopathic thrombocytopenic purpura, pertussis and parapertussis, chronic viral infections (*e.g.,* cytomegalovirus, acute infectious lymphocytosis) and rheumatoid arthritis. ALL may be confused with aplastic anemia. Rarely, it may present as the hypereosinophilic syndrome. ALL must be differentiated from other pediatric malignancies that may involve bone marrow, including non-Hodgkin's lymphoma, rhabdomyosarcoma, retinoblastoma, and neuroblastoma.

Replacement of normal bone marrow elements by leukemic cells produces an abnormal hemogram in most newly diagnosed patients (see Table 50–1). Anemia and thrombocytopenia occur in more than two thirds of patients. The peripheral leukocyte count may be normal or low, but approximately one third of patients have an initial leukocyte count of more than 20,000/mm^3. An increased leukocyte count at diagnosis connotes a poor prognosis. Leukemic cells may be seen in the peripheral blood, but morphologic assessment of these cells is often misleading. Careful examination of a bone marrow aspirate is mandatory to make a diagnosis. On rare occasions, a bone marrow biopsy may be necessary. Although the presence of greater than 5% lymphoblasts indicates leukemia, most laboratories require a minimum of 25% leukemic blast cells in the bone marrow aspirate to confirm the diagnosis.[3] A definitive diagnosis requires careful morphologic examination of marrow aspirate smears stained with Romanovsky stain and detailed cytochemistry studies using myeloperoxidase or Sudan black, periodic acid-Schiff (PAS), and nonspecific esterase stains. Immunophenotyping, biochemical analysis (*e.g.,* TdT determination), and cytogenetic analyses should also be performed (Tables 50–2 and 50–3).

In addition to a detailed history, physical examination, and hematologic evaluation, newly diagnosed leukemia patients require other laboratory studies, including uric acid and electrolyte level determinations, kidney and liver function studies,

TABLE 50–1. Symptoms, Physical Findings, and Laboratory Features in Children with ALL

Clinical or Laboratory Feature	*Patients (%)*
Symptoms and Physical Findings	
Fever	61
Bleeding (*e.g.,* petechiae or purpura)	48
Bone pain	23
Lymphadenopathy	50
Splenomegaly	62
Hepatosplenomegaly	68
Laboratory Features	
Leukocyte count (/mm^3)	
<10,000	53
10,000–49,000	30
>50,000	17
Hemoglobin (g/dl)	
<7.0	43
7.0–11.0	45
>11.0	12
Platelet count (/mm^3)	
<20,000	28
20,000 to 99,000	47
>100,000	25
Lymphoblast morphology	
L1	84
L2	15
L3	1

(Miller DR. Acute lymphoblastic leukemia. Pediatr Clin North Am 1980;27:269–291)

TABLE 50–2. Morphologic, Cytochemical, and Biochemical Characteristics Helpful in Differentiating ALL From AML

Characteristic	*ALL*	*AML*
Nuclear-cytoplasmic ratio	High	Low
Nuclear chromatin	Clumped	Spongy
Nucleoli	0–2	2–5
Granules	–	+
Auer rods	–	+/–
Cytoplasm	Blue	Blue-gray
Cytochemical reaction		
Peroxidase	–	+
Sudan Black B	–	+
Periodic acid-Schiff	+/–	–
Naphthyl ASD chloracetate esterase	–	+/–
α-Napthyl acetate esterase	–	+/–
α-Napthyl butyrate esterase	–	–
Terminal deoxynucleotidyl transferase (TdT)	+*	–

* TdT is usually negative in typical FAB L3 ALL.
(Poplack DG. Clinical manifestations of acute lymphoblastic leukemia. In: Hoffmann R, ed. Hematology, basic principles and practice. New York: Churchill Livingstone, 1990:776–784)

TABLE 50–3. Monoclonal Antibodies Commonly Used to Immunophenotype Leukemia

CD	*Antibody*	*Predominant Reactivity*
T Cell		
CD1	T6	Thymocytes
CD2	T11	Pan-T
CD3	T3	Pan-T
CD4	T4/Leu-3	T helper/inducer
CD5	T101/Leu-1	Pan-T, B-cell CLL
CD7	Leu-9	Pan-T
CD8	T8/Leu-2	T cytotoxic/suppressor
CDw29	4B4	T4+/4B4+ (helper//inducer) T4+/2H4+ (suppressor/inducer)
B Cell		
CD19	B4	Pan-B
CD20	B1	Pan-B
CD21	B2	C3dR
CD24	BA1	Pan-B
	PCA-1	Plasma cells
Myeloid		
CD11c	Leu-M5	Monocytes, hairy cell
CD13	My7	Pan-myeloid
CD14	Leu-M3/MY4/MO2	Monocytes
CD15	Leu-M1	Monocytes, granulocytes
CD33	My9	Pan-myeloid
Miscellaneous		
CD9	BA2	Hematopoietic Progenitor/leukemic blasts
CD10	CALLA/J5	ALL/Burkitt's/follicular lymphoma
CD34	My10/HPCA-1	Hematopoietic progenitor cells/HTLV-infected cells
CD41a	Plt-1	Platelets/megakaryocytes
CD45	T-200/LCA	Pan-leukocyte
	T9	Transferrin receptor/proliferating cells

(CD classification number, corresponding antibodies and their predominant reactivity are listed with permission of Jane Trepel, PhD, Medicine Branch, National Cancer Institute. Other data from Poplack DG. Clinical manifestations of acute lymphoblastic leukemia. In: Hoffmann R, ed. Hematology, basic principles and practice. New York: Churchill Livingstone, 1990:776–784)

and appropriate radiologic studies. Hyperuricemia, a consequence of increased purine metabolism in leukemia cells, often exists at diagnosis or is provoked by initiation of treatment. Adequate hydration, alkalinization, and treatment with the xanthine oxidase inhibitor allopurinol are required to prevent uric acid nephropathy. Leukemic cell lysis frequently produces elevated serum lactate dehydrogenase (LDH) levels. Liver function tests may be abnormal at diagnosis, presumably the result of leukemic infiltration of the liver. A variety of metabolic abnormalities may be seen on initial presentation, including hyperkalemia, hypomagnesemia, and hypocalcemia or hypercalcemia. Low serum levels of immunoglobulins have been reported in as many as 30% of newly diagnosed patients with ALL. Whether this represents a preexisting condition or is a consequence of the disease is not clear. Leukemic cells are capable of suppressing immunoglobulin synthesis in vitro, suggesting that in some patients this mechanism may play a role.

Chest x-ray films may reveal the presence of a mediastinal mass, particularly in high-risk patients. Leukemic infiltrates of the periosteum and bone may produce changes in the radiologic appearance of the long bones. Bone lesions may be observed radiographically even if there is no pain, and rarely, the bone lesions of ALL mimic osteomyelitis.

EXTRAMEDULLARY LEUKEMIA

Extramedullary leukemic spread may be clinically overt or detectable only by invasive diagnostic procedures. Extramedullary disease is important because it may cause local morbidity and because an extramedullary relapse frequently heralds bone marrow relapse, presumably as a result of spread to the bone marrow from the involved site. Current treatment strategies aim to prevent extramedullary relapse and to treat it aggressively if it occurs.

The two most important sites of extramedullary spread are the central nervous system (CNS) and the testes. Ovarian leukemia, perhaps because of inaccessibility to detailed physical examination, is rarely detected. Extramedullary disease can also occur in the liver, spleen, kidneys, gastrointestinal tract, and lung.

Central Nervous System Leukemia

The significance of CNS leukemia became apparent in the late 1950s and 1960s, when the CNS became the most frequent site of initial relapse because of better systemic treatment and longer survival. The incidence of CNS disease was as high as 75% to 80%. CNS disease was difficult to eradicate, and almost invariably, was rapidly followed by bone marrow relapse. The recognition of this latter phenomenon led to the development of effective CNS preventive therapy that improved the prognosis of children with this disease.

CNS leukemia is thought to develop by hematogenous seeding of circulating leukemic cells or by direct spread of leukemic cells from involved cranial bone marrow. CNS leukemia initially involves the meninges; deeper invasion of the brain parenchyma occurs in more advanced disease. Overt CNS leukemia occurs in fewer than 5% of children at diagnosis and rarely is symptomatic.[10] Symptomatic patients manifest a variety of signs and symptoms of increased intracranial pressure, including headaches, nausea, vomiting, lethargy, irritability, nuchal rigidity, and papilledema. Cranial nerve palsies may occur (most commonly of the sixth or seventh cranial nerves), often as an isolated event. More unusual presentations include the hypothalamic-obesity syndrome, diabetes insipidus, ataxia due to cerebellar involvement, and symptoms related to subdural or epidural leukemic infiltration. Any unexplained neurologic sign or symptom in a patient with ALL requires evaluation to exclude CNS leukemia.

The diagnosis of CNS disease is made by cytologic examination of cerebrospinal fluid (CSF) obtained by lumbar puncture. CSF should be examined after cytocentrifugation, a technique that concentrates the leukemic cells and increases diagnostic sensitivity tenfold. Relying solely on the demonstration of a pleocytosis in CSF is insufficient and potentially misleading. In symptomatic patients, CSF pressure is usually elevated, and hypoglycorrhachia and increased CSF protein levels are common. The heightened awareness of the possibility of CNS relapse has made surveillance lumbar punctures routine. As a result, CNS leukemia is more commonly diagnosed in the asymptomatic patient, in whom CSF pressure and chemistries may be normal and CSF leukemic cell counts relatively low. Although skull x-ray films, the computed tomography (CT) brain scan, head magnetic resonance imaging (MRI), and the electroencephalogram may occasionally be abnormal for the patient with overt CNS leukemia, none of these tests is reliable for diagnosis.

Testicular Leukemia

The incidence of testicular leukemia increased in the 1970s with improved survival of ALL patients. The testes constitute an important site of relapse, and although clinically demonstrable testicular disease is rarely evident at the initial diagnosis, occult testicular involvement has been reported in as many as 25% of newly diagnosed boys. Overt testicular recurrence, presenting as painless testicular enlargement, may occur in as many as 15% of boys undergoing chemotherapy. In one earlier study, testicular infiltration was reported in approximately 40% of boys who had successfully completed a 2.5-year to 3-year course of treatment.[11,12] Although the overall incidence of testicular disease appears to be significantly lower on current therapeutic protocols, biopsy-proven, occult testicular leukemia has been found in as many as 15% of asymptomatic boys on completion of chemotherapy, an observation consistent with relatively high incidence of late, overt relapses in these patients.

Testicular disease is more likely to occur in boys with a high initial leukocyte count (>20,000/mm^3), prominent lymphadenopathy and splenomegaly, T-cell disease, or significant thrombocytopenia (>30,000/mm^3).[13] The diagnosis of clinically suspected testicular leukemia is made by wedge biopsy. Testicular recurrence frequently is followed by systemic relapse, particularly if the testicular relapse has occurred during or immediately after maintenance chemotherapy. Isolated testicular relapse occurring 6 months or longer after cessation of therapy is associated with a relatively good prognosis if treated appropriately.

MORPHOLOGIC CLASSIFICATION

The considerable variation in the morphologic appearance of ALL cells led to numerous attempts to subclassify the disease. The system proposed by the French-American-British (FAB) cooperative working group, which divides lymphoblasts into three categories, has been most useful.[14] L1 lymphoblasts are smaller, with little cytoplasm and inconspicuous nucleoli or none at all. L2 lymphoblasts are larger, with abundant cytoplasm and prominent nucleoli. Leukemic cells of the L3 type are cytomorphologically identical to Burkitt's lymphoma cells. Approximately 85% of childhood ALL cases have L1 lymphoblasts, 14% are L2, and 1% are L3. The L2 lymphoblast is the most common type in adults. Concordance among observers using this system is high, and the FAB classification has prognostic value.[14,15] L1 lymphoblasts are associated with a higher remission induction rate and prolonged remission and survival. L2 cells convey a poor prognosis independently of other prognostic variables. Patients with the L3 variety have the least favorable prognosis. With the possible exception of L3 cells, which ordinarily possess surface immunoglobulin and other B-cell markers, there is no apparent correlation between FAB classification and immunologic cell-surface markers.[14]

DIAGNOSIS AND CLASSIFICATION

Immunophenotypes

Immunologic techniques have permitted the identification of distinct immunologic subtypes of ALL and have confirmed that ALL is a heterogenous disease in which leukemic transformation and clonal expansion may occur at different stages in lymphoid differentiation. Initially, using standard immunologic methods for surface membrane characterization, three forms of ALL were identified. Between 1% and 2% had lymphoblasts with B-cell characteristics, and most patients were found to have lymphoblasts that lacked definable T-cell or B-cell markers. Further classification using heterologous antisera and monoclonal antibodies detected a common leukemia-associated antigen (CALLA) on the leukemic cells of approximately 80% of the children with "non-T, non-B-cell" leukemia and designated these as having "common ALL" to differentiate them from the antigen-negative, non-T, non-B-cell group with "null cell" ALL.

Clinical differences were apparent among the immunologic subtypes of ALL. Children with common ALL had a relatively good prognosis, faring better than those with null cell ALL. T-cell ALL was found to have distinctive clinical features, frequently occurring in older boys presenting with a high initial leukocyte count and a mediastinal mass. T-cell ALL is associated with a poor prognosis, but it is unclear whether any immunologic subtype is a significant independent prognostic variable.

More sophisticated immunologic methods have revealed that most non-T, non-B lymphoblasts are actually early B cells. These cells are capable of differentiating in vitro into cells with B-cell markers, may possess intracytoplasmic immunoglobulin, and demonstrate immunoglobulin gene rearrangement indicative of precursor cells committed to the B-cell lineage.[16] Approximately 20% to 30% of B-cell precursor ALL cases have lymphoblasts that are cytoplasmic μ (Cμ) heavy chain positive. These pre-B-cell ALL cases represent a relatively mature stage of development and are differentiated from Cμ-negative early pre-B-cell cases of ALL.[17] Pre-B-cell ALL has a worse prognosis than the early pre-B-cell type.[17]

Using recombinant DNA technology for analysis of immunoglobulin gene rearrangement in precursor-B-cell ALL and monoclonal antibodies for immunophenotyping different B-cell antigens, investigators have defined distinct stages of differentiation for pre-B-cell ALL.[17] Monoclonal antibodies also have been used to define different subsets of normal thymocytes that correspond to different stages of intrathymic differentiation.[18] Typing with these antibodies has demonstrated that T-cell leukemias may be derived from these different stages of differentiation.

Molecular biologic analysis of the genes encoding the T-cell receptor have provided a useful marker of T-cell differentiation in an analogous fashion to immunoglobulin gene rearrangement in pre-B-cell ALL.[19] Although most ALL cells can be readily classified as B-cell or T-cell lineage, some leukemic cells coexpress cell surface marker antigens or molecular markers, suggesting that traditional views of lineage classification may be overly restrictive.[19,20] For example, immunoglobulin gene rearrangement may occur in cases of T-cell ALL, and conversely, T-cell receptor gene rearrangement occurs in some cases of B-lineage ALL (Fig. 50–1).

There are also numerous reports of ALL cases in which the leukemic cells express characteristics of more than one he-

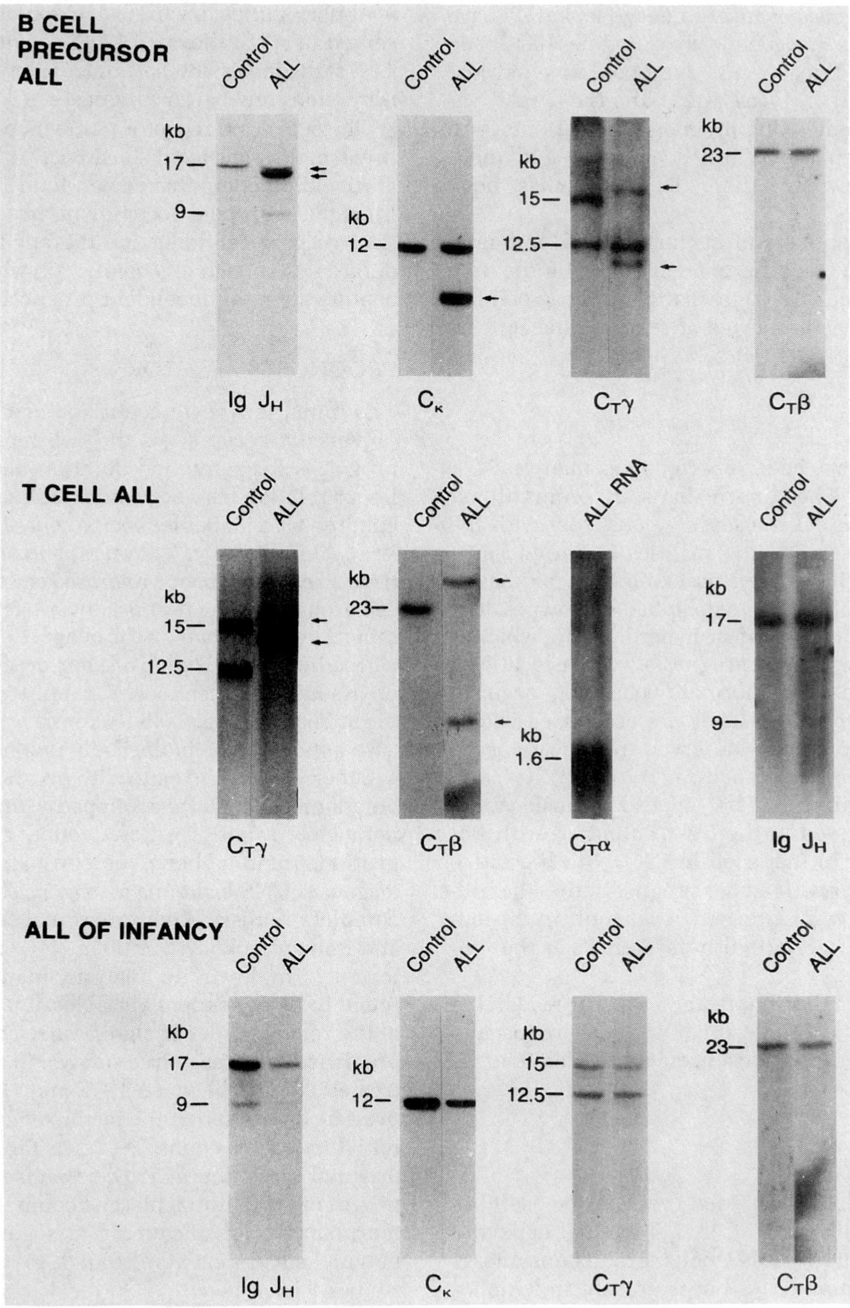

FIGURE 50–1. Examples of patterns of immunoglobulin and T-cell receptor gene rearrangement in acute lymphoblastic leukemia of childhood shown by Southern and Northern analysis. (Reproduced with permission from Carolyn Felix, MD). **(A)** B-cell precursor ALL. This case demonstrates rearrangement of both alleles of the immunoglobulin heavy chain gene, one allele of the κ light chain gene, and both alleles of the T-cell receptor γ gene. The T-cell receptor β gene remains in germline configuration. **(B)** T-cell ALL. This case illustrates rearrangement of both alleles of the T-cell receptor; γ and β line configuration of the immunoglobulin heavy chain gene is shown. **(C)** ALL of infancy (B-cell precursor). This case demonstrates the germline configuration both of immunoglobulin heavy and light chain genes and of the γ and β T-cell receptor genes. Rearrangements are indicated by arrows and germline bands by dash marks.

matopoietic lineage.[21–23] The incidence of cases that express myeloid and lymphoid markers has been reported to be as high as 25%.[24] It is not clear whether they represent leukemias that have developed from normal multilineage potential precursors or represent cases occurring from aberrant or inappropriate gene activation and thus have not been derived from a corresponding normal stage of hematopoietic development. Guidelines for the diagnosis of mixed lineage leukemia have been proposed.[25] Certain cytogenetic abnormalities have been associated with mixed lineage (*i.e.*, lymphoid-myeloid leukemias), including the t(4;11)(q21;q23) and the t(9;22) abnormalities. In most studies, the prognosis for patients with acute mixed-lineage leukemias has been poor, and more intensive chemotherapy for these leukemias has been advocated.[23]

At relapse, most patients manifest their original immunophenotypes. Expression of a different cell lineage at the time of relapse is a rare event. Although changes in blast cell immunophenotype have been reported at relapse, this appears to be the exception.

Cytogenetics

Abnormal karyotypes have been reported in as many as 90% of children with ALL.[26] The abnormalities are ordinarily restricted to the leukemia cells, a finding consistent with the clonal nature of the disease. Abnormalities in chromosome number and structure have been observed. Approximately 67% of patients have diploid or pseudodiploid karyotypes. The remaining 33% of patients manifest hyperdiploidy, which is associated with a relatively good prognosis.[27] Translocations, the most common structural abnormality observed, occur in approximately 40% of patients. They are associated with a poor prognosis. More commonly observed translocations include the t(8;14) (specific for B-cell ALL), t(9;22), t(4;11), and t(1;19) abnormalities. The typical translocation, t(9;22)(q34;q11), observed in the 5% of children with Ph-positive ALL, is similar to that seen in CML. In Ph-positive ALL, however, a disorder with a poor prognosis, the Ph chromosome is not found in remission and occurs only in the leukemic lymphoid line. There are also differences at the molecular level.[27]

Chromosomal abnormalities appear to have considerable prognostic importance. Chromosomal studies are usually normal during remission; the presence of aneuploid cells is thought to herald relapse.

Biochemistry

Study of several enzymes indicate that they may be useful in the diagnosis and classification of ALL. Terminal deoxynucleotidyl transferase (TdT), a DNA polymerizing enzyme, is not found in normal lymphocytes but is present in lymphoblasts of T-cell and non-T, non-B-cell types. TdT expression is variable in B-cell ALL. TdT determination may help to differentiate ALL from AML, in which it is rarely present. TdT activity, however, has no prognostic significance in ALL.

Several purine pathway enzymes, whose activity is abnormal in certain childhood immunodeficiency states, have specific patterns of expression that correlate with immunologic subtypes of ALL.[28] For example, T-cell lymphoblasts have elevated adenosine deaminase (ADA), but lower 5′-nucleotidase and purine nucleoside phosphorylase activity than non-T, non-B lymphoblasts.[28] These findings raised the possibility that selective therapy, aimed at taking advantage of these enzyme abnormalities, might be of value. Deoxycoformycin, an ADA inhibitor, has undergone clinical trials and has been used for in vitro marrow purging.

Abnormalities in various lysozomal enzymes have been observed in ALL. Elevated LDH activity has been observed in ALL at diagnosis; low serum LDH levels correlate with longer remissions and better prognoses.

Glucocorticoid receptor numbers have been correlated with in vitro glucocorticoid sensitivity. A lower number of glucocorticoid receptors have been found on T-cell lymphoblasts. Low glucocorticoid receptor numbers are associated with a poor response to induction therapy and a shorter remission duration, although it is not certain whether glucocorticoid receptors are an independent prognostic factor.

PROGNOSTIC FACTORS

The initial leukocyte count and age at diagnosis of ALL are universally accepted as the two most reliable indicators of prognosis for remission duration and survival.[29] There is a linear relation between initial leukocyte count and outcome; children with higher leukocyte counts have a poorer prognosis. Very young children (<2 years) and older patients (>10 years) have a relatively poor prognosis; children in the intermediate age group have the best prognosis. The worse prognosis is for infants younger than 1 year of age.[30,31] These children present with a higher incidence of poor prognostic features (*e.g.*, increased initial leukocyte count, massive organomegaly, thrombocytopenia, CNS leukemia at diagnosis) and their disease appears to be biologically unique.[30]

Other factors correlate with prognosis, including sex, race, organomegaly, lymphadenopathy, mediastinal mass, initial hemoglobin, initial platelet count, FAB morphologic classification, immunophenotype, serum immunoglobulin levels at diagnosis, CNS leukemia at diagnosis, the rapidity of attaining complete remission, chromosomal status, serum LDH level, and human leukocyte antigen (HLA) type.[27,29,32] When subjected to multivariate analysis, many of these features are found to be dependent variables.[27,29,32] A retrospective study of the relative order of significance and association of factors predictive for disease-free survival in a group of 1419 children treated for ALL between 1978 and 1982 revealed, after multivariate analysis, that the factors of greatest importance were initial leukocyte count, sex (girls fare better than boys), mediastinal mass, the marrow response on day 14 of induction treatment, age, initial platelet count, hepatomegaly, and FAB morphologic classification.[29] Cytogenetics and immunophenotypic subgroup were found to be important in other studies.[17,27]

The prognostic importance of some factors may vary somewhat from study to study, which may be caused by differences in treatment and in the patient populations.

Most current protocols use prognostic criteria (*e.g.*, initial leukocyte count, age at diagnosis) to stratify patients at diagnosis into different risk groups. Staging of this type permits selective application of treatment to different risk groups. High-risk patients are treated with more aggressive chemotherapy regimens, but low-risk patients receive less-intensive therapy, designed to be equally effective but avoid the toxicities and complications of aggressive therapy.

No single system of ALL staging has been universally accepted. An example is shown in Figure 50–2 that illustrates the event-free survival curves for patients treated on a Children's Cancer Study Group (CCSG) series of protocols that stratified patients into five risk groups: good, average, poor (primarily on the basis of initial leukocyte count, age at diagnosis, and FAB classification), infants, and patients presenting with lymphomatous features, a group at high risk of treatment failure, particularly CNS relapse.[29]

TREATMENT

As our understanding of ALL has increased, evaluation and treatment of children with this disease has become more complex. An appropriate patient workup requires sophisticated techniques (*e.g.*, immunophenotyping, cytogenetic analysis, molecular genotyping, biochemical assays) and stratification of patients into risk groups for appropriate therapy. Recognition of the biologic heterogeneity of ALL makes it inappropriate to define a standard ALL treatment regimen. Combination chemotherapy remains the primary therapeutic modality. Current treatment is divided into four phases: remission induction, CNS preventive therapy, consolidation, and maintenance.

Remission Induction

The first goal of ALL treatment is induction of complete remission, defined as the lack of any evidence of leukemia on physical examination and hematologic evaluation. The bone marrow must be normocellular, with fewer than 5% lymphoblasts, and peripheral blood counts should be within the range of normal values. There must be no detectable CNS or other extramedullary disease. It has been estimated that patients with clinically overt ALL have approximately 10^{12} leukemic cells, and patients in remission have fewer than 10^{10} blast cells. In these terms, remission induction requires a reduction in the number of leukemic cells by at least 99%. Although prednisone and vincristine traditionally have been the most widely used two-drug combination, capable of inducing remission in approximately 80% to 90% of patients, it is now clear that this combination is inadequate. The addition of a third agent, L-asparaginase or daunorubicin, raises the induction rate to 90% to 100% and significantly prolongs remission. The addition of a fourth induction agent, usually the anthracycline daunorubicin, together with intensive consolidation therapy, improves remission duration, even in patients with poor-risk factors.[33] Most induction regimens last approximately 4 weeks. There is evidence that the rapidity of cytoreduction correlates with remission duration (Fig. 50–3).

Central Nervous System Prophylaxis

The concept of CNS preventive therapy is based on the assumption that undetectable CNS leukemia is present in most patients at the time of diagnosis, residing in that "sanctuary site" protected by the blood-brain barrier from cytotoxic concentrations of most systemically administered antileukemic agents. Studies in the 1960s aimed at prevention of CNS leukemia demonstrated that administration of 2400 cGy of cranial irradiation and intrathecal methotrexate after remission induction reduced the incidence of overt CNS leukemia from more than 60% to 10% or less.

Although this approach was universally adopted in the 1970s, the adverse effects of CNS irradiation on neurologic and intellectual functions prompted a reappraisal of this strategy. There is now a large body of data documenting long-term side effects, including CT-detected brain abnormalities, impaired intellectual and psychomotor function, and neuroendocrine dysfunction, in a proportion of patients treated with 2400 cGy of cranial irradiation and intrathecal chemotherapy. This has stimulated a search for safer methods of CNS prophylaxis. Several approaches have been studied, in-

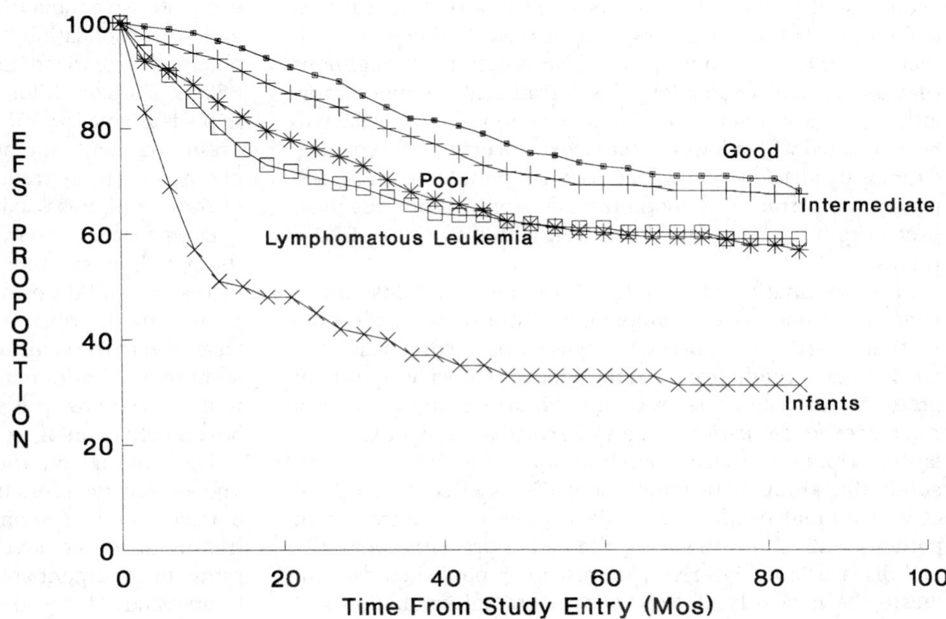

FIGURE 50–2. Event-free survival of 3507 children with ALL stratified according to prognostic groups and treated by the Children's Cancer Study Group. (Reproduced with permission of WA Bleyer, MD, and H Sather, PhD)

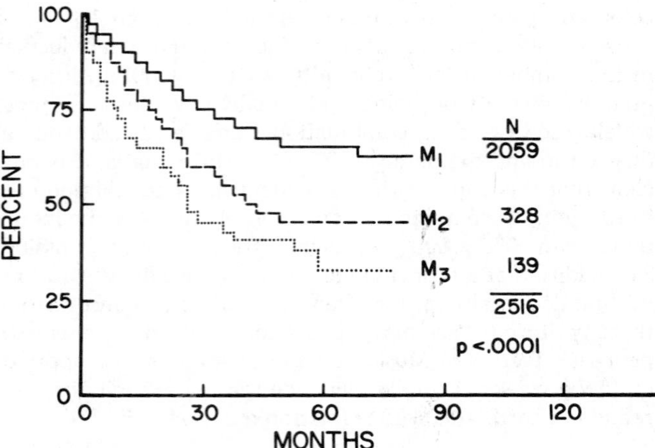

FIGURE 50–3. Disease-free survival from completion of induction treatment according to day 14 bone marrow status in 2516 children with ALL. Day 14 bone marrow status was a highly significant independent predictor of disease-free survival. (Miller D, Coccia P, Bleyer W, et al. Early response to induction therapy as a predictor of disease-free survival and late recurrence of childhood acute lymphoblastic leukemia: A report from the Childrens Cancer Study Group. J Clin Oncol 1989;7:1807–1815)

cluding using lower doses of cranial irradiation (1800 cGy) with intrathecal methotrexate; periodic intrathecal methotrexate during maintenance with intensive systemic chemotherapy; triple intrathecal chemotherapy with methotrexate, cytosine arabinoside, and hydrocortisone; intermediate-dose methotrexate alone or with concomitant intrathecal methotrexate; or high-dose systemic methotrexate alone.

The risk of developing CNS leukemia depends on certain predictive factors at presentation. Characteristics associated with an increased risk of CNS leukemia include a high initial leukocyte count, T-cell disease, thrombocytopenia, profound lymphadenopathy or hepatosplenomegaly, and patients who are very young or black.[10,30] The recognition of different risk groups led to the concept of tailoring CNS preventive therapy, using equally effective, less-intensive CNS treatment if possible. For example, it is now evident that 1800 cGy is as effective as 2400 cGy in providing CNS protection in regimens that use cranial irradiation plus intrathecal chemotherapy, although it is not yet clear if reduction in radiation dose will be associated with a lower incidence of adverse CNS sequelae. Cranial irradiation is not necessary for patients with a good prognosis; intrathecal methotrexate alone offers adequate protection for this group of children with a low risk of CNS relapse.[34]

The combination of intrathecal and moderate-dose intravenous methotrexate, maintenance intrathecal triple chemotherapy (*i.e.*, methotrexate, cytarabine, hydrocortisone), and high-dose methotrexate alone appear to provide equivalent protection to that offered by cranial irradiation and intrathecal methotrexate for patients at an intermediate risk of CNS relapse. Triple intrathecal chemotherapy given frequently and continuing throughout maintenance is as effective as 2400 cGy of cranial irradiation plus intrathecal methotrexate in patients with ALL without lymphomatous presentations or T-cell disease. For high-risk patients, most published data indicate the necessity of 1800 cGy of cranial irradiation and intrathecal methotrexate to prevent CNS relapse.[10] A study employing very-high-dose methotrexate infusions, high-dose cytarabine, and sequential intrathecal chemotherapy with methotrexate and cytarabine demonstrated effective CNS preventive therapy for high-risk patients without using cranial irradiation. Although this study requires confirmation, the results raise the possibility that the need for cranial irradiation in high-risk patients may be obviated by the use of aggressive chemotherapy.[35]

Consolidation and Maintenance Therapy

After remission induction, additional treatment is necessary. Without maintenance treatment, most patients relapse within 1 to 2 months. Methotrexate and 6-mercaptopurine are the two drugs most frequently administered during maintenance. Usually, 6-mercaptopurine is given on a daily basis; methotrexate is given intermittently (*e.g.*, once or twice weekly). The value of adding agents to standard 6-mercaptopurine and methotrexate maintenance therapy has been controversial, and the data have been somewhat contradictory. The addition of intermittent pulses of vincristine and prednisone appears to prolong remission, although the value of this approach after intensive induction therapy is unclear. The intensive, weekly use of L-asparaginase may add to the effectiveness of maintenance treatment. Other approaches include repeated pulses of an intensive combination of agents periodically during maintenance and sequential intensive multiagent therapy.[36]

The choice of an appropriate maintenance regimen may also differ for different risk groups. Although 6-mercaptopurine and methotrexate may be adequate for certain good-risk patients, more intensive maintenance therapy appears to be optimal in treating poor-risk patients.

To improve cytoreduction early in maintenance, many regimens now include a period of intensified therapy shortly after remission induction with drugs that minimize the development of cross-resistance. Intensive remission "consolidation" therapy of this type has improved treatment success even in patients with poor prognoses.[36–39] A West German study that used intensive induction and consolidation and "reinduction" and "reconsolidation" phases of therapy early in maintenance obtained prolonged disease-free survival in approximately 65% to 70% of children, with significantly improved results in poor-prognosis patients.[37] Similarly, a study employing early "reinforcement" therapy followed by a rotational combination chemotherapy approach produced an event-free survival rate of 69% in high-risk patients.[38]

Drug dosage is an important consideration in maintenance therapy. Longer remissions occurred in patients randomized to receive full-dose maintenance therapy with 6-mercaptopurine, methotrexate, and cyclophosphamide than in those treated with the same agents administered at half dose. Orally administered 6-mercaptopurine and methotrexate have profound variations in bioavailability, suggesting that this may be a mechanism of treatment failure for some patients.

The optimal duration of maintenance treatment is not known. Most centers treat patients for 2.5 to 3 years. A randomized study demonstrated that 5 years of maintenance treatment has no advantage over 3 years.[40] The optimal duration of treatment appears to be different for girls and boys; in one study, 1.5 years of therapy was sufficient for girls but inadequate for boys. It is likely that the intensity of therapy has bearing on the optimal duration of treatment. Because much of the information on which the current policy of 2.5 to 3 years of maintenance therapy is based was derived from less-intensive therapeutic regimens than many currently in use, additional study of this important question is needed.

The outlook for patients who successfully complete a full 2.5-year to 3-year course of treatment is good. Approximately 80% of these patients can expect to remain disease free. The greatest number of relapses occur in the first year after discontinuing chemotherapy. After 4 years "off" treatment, relapse is unusual.

Treatment of Relapse

BONE MARROW RELAPSE. Bone marrow relapse is the most frequent form of treatment failure in patients with ALL. Reinduction of remission is possible in most patients who suffer an initial marrow relapse, but most patients experience subsequent relapse and eventually die of the disease. Nevertheless, many patients can achieve prolonged second remissions, justifying an aggressive treatment approach to the child in relapse. Multidrug induction regimens are the most effective. The best results have been obtained with a four-drug combination, which includes vincristine, prednisone, L-asparaginase, and daunorubicin and produces remission in 90% of patients.

Other factors influence the remission induction rate for relapsed patients. Children whose relapses occur more than 6 months after completion of chemotherapy regimens have a better chance of achieving and maintaining prolonged second remission than do children who relapse while receiving maintenance therapy. Second remissions are more readily induced in patients who receive suboptimal induction or maintenance therapy as initial treatment for their disease or who had longer first remissions.

A second course of CNS preventive therapy is necessary for patients in second remission. Without additional CNS prophylaxis in these patients, almost 50% suffer CNS relapses. In previously irradiated patients, intrathecal chemotherapy is an effective form of second CNS prophylaxis.

Unfortunately, second or subsequent remissions, particularly in children relapsing on treatment, are usually short. However, it has been reported that prolonged second remissions (>2 years) can be obtained with aggressive chemotherapy in 10% to 30% of patients who relapse on therapy and in approximately one third of patients who relapse after elective cessation of therapy.[41–43]

Bone marrow transplantation is another approach used to treat relapse patients (Fig. 50–4). An early report from the Seattle transplant group on the long-term follow-up of a group of patients with ALL who received allogeneic bone marrow transplantation indicated that, with a minimum follow-up of more than 5 years, 27% of the patients transplanted in second or subsequent remissions and 15% of patients transplanted during relapse were alive and free of disease.[44] A report from Seattle confirmed other studies that have reported long-term disease-free survival for 40% or more of patients transplanted during second remission.[45–47] Allogeneic bone marrow transplantation is feasible for the approximately one third of relapsed patients who have an HLA-identical sibling. Bone marrow transplantation is considered the treatment of choice for patients in second bone marrow remission whose initial relapse occurred while undergoing chemotherapy or within 3 months of its completion.[41,48] An analysis performed by the International Bone Marrow Transplant Registry indicates that patients with late relapses (>36 months after attainment of first remission or after completion of maintenance therapy) should probably receive chemotherapy, with bone marrow transplantation reserved for subsequent relapses.[48–50]

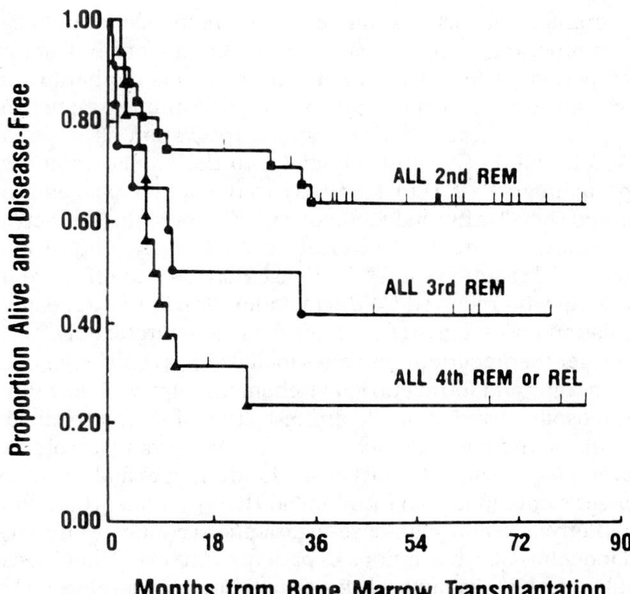

FIGURE 50–4. Disease-free survival of children receiving transplants for ALL. Patients were stratified according to their disease status at the time of transplantation. (Brochstein JA, Kernan NA, Groshen S, et al. Allogeneic bone marrow transplantation after hyperfractionated total-body irradiation and cyclophosphamide in children with acute leukemia. N Engl J Med 1987;317:1618–1624)

Methods of crossing the histocompatibility barrier are being studied in several centers and, if successful, ultimately may increase the applicability of bone marrow transplantation. Autologous transplantation with remission marrow treated in vitro with leukemia-specific monoclonal antibodies is being investigated. Relapse-free survival can be achieved in approximately 20% to 30% of relapsed patients using this approach.[51,52] Other approaches being studied for patients without a histocompatible sibling donor include the use of partially matched, related donors or unrelated matched donors identified through comprehensive bone marrow typing banks. The effectiveness of these marrow transplant approaches and their eventual role for therapy of ALL requires additional study.

CENTRAL NERVOUS SYSTEM RELAPSE. Although CNS preventive therapy has dramatically reduced its incidence, CNS relapse remains a significant cause of treatment failure in ALL. CNS relapse may occur as an isolated relapse, concomitant with bone marrow relapse or with recurrence in another extramedullary site (*e.g.*, testes). Intrathecal methotrexate, alone or together with cytosine arabinoside and hydrocortisone, produces CNS remission (*i.e.*, clearance of CSF lymphoblasts) in more than 90% of patients. Unless followed by craniospinal irradiation or by maintenance intrathecal chemotherapy, relapse ensues within 3 to 4 months. Continued periodic administration of intrathecal chemotherapy on a maintenance schedule may prolong CSF remission, but relapse usually occurs.[10] Craniospinal irradiation, at doses of 2400 to 2500 cGy (150 cGy daily) to the cranial vault and approximately 1200 to 1800 cGy to the spinal axis, administered shortly after induction of a CSF remission, is effective in achieving durable control of established meningeal leukemia.[10] Treatment of CNS disease may be less effective in patients who received CNS irradiation previously; repeat irradiation poses a greater risk for delayed neurotoxicity.[53]

Other therapeutic approaches include intraventricular chemotherapy and intraventricular chemotherapy with low-dose craniospinal irradiation.[10] Administration of methotrexate by means of an indwelling subcutaneous Ommaya reservoir has several technical and pharmacologic advantages and produces longer remissions than intralumbar therapy alone. High-dose methotrexate and high-dose cytarabine have been effective in inducing CSF remissions in patients with overt meningeal leukemia. New intrathecal agents are also being developed.[54,55] Because isolated CNS relapse often heralds a bone marrow relapse, intensification of systemic therapy at the time of isolated CNS relapse is considered essential.

TESTICULAR RELAPSE. Testicular relapse requires treatment with radiation therapy. Unilateral disease frequently has been followed by relapse in the contralateral testis, particularly in patients with early testicular relapse during therapy.[6] Bilateral testicular radiation therapy is indicated for all patients. A dosage of 2400 cGy is considered adequate, although rare cases of local recurrence have been reported. In the past, testicular recurrence frequently was followed by systemic relapse and was associated with a poor prognosis. The practice of intensifying systemic therapy or reinducing patients at the time of isolated testicular relapse has produced a dramatic improvement, and prolonged disease-free survival is now possible.[56,57]

Supportive Care

The provision of optimal supportive care is a vital element in the treatment of the child with ALL. Appropriate use of blood component therapy; an aggressive approach to detection, prevention, and management of infectious complications; maintenance of the metabolic and nutritional needs of the patient; and comprehensive, continuous psychosocial support for patient and family are mandatory.

Late Effects of Treatment

The increased survival of children with ALL has focused attention on the late effects of antileukemia therapy. Recognition of adverse sequelae is particularly important now that it is possible to define good-risk patients for whom less intensive but equally effective therapy may be designed.

The effects of CNS preventive therapy on neurologic and intellectual function have been of particular concern. The awareness of adverse sequelae has stimulated a search for equally effective alternative approaches to CNS preventive therapy. Children treated for overt CNS disease are at a higher risk for neurologic and neuropsychologic sequelae of treatment.[53] Careful monitoring of patients at risk for possible adverse CNS sequelae, with periodic neurologic examination, CT or MRI brain scans, and psychometric testing is advocated.[53]

The reproductive capacity of children exposed to prolonged antileukemic therapy has been evaluated, and most boys and girls treated with conventional chemotherapy (not including cyclophosphamide) appear to maintain gonadal function and undergo normal pubertal progression. However, boys who have received testicular irradiation have a high rate of testicular endocrine failure and may require androgen replacement therapy. As survival times increase, more patients face the prospect of parenthood. Although scarce, the available evidence suggests no increase in birth defects in the offspring of mothers or fathers previously treated for ALL.

Damage to other systems (*e.g.*, elevated liver enzymes) may occur during therapy, but long-term toxic effects after treatment are unusual. Although treatment with anthracyclines carries the possibility of cardiac toxicity, most protocols use limited cumulative doses of this agent. Some patients, however, who receive anthracyclines for ALL treatment may be at a significant risk for late-onset congestive heart failure. A study from the Dana-Farber Cancer Institute indicated that over half of a group of long-term ALL survivors had evidence of abnormal left ventricular function.[58] These results and those of other studies increased concern about late anthracycline cardiotoxicity and emphasized the need for careful cardiac monitoring and follow-up of children at risk.[59]

Second malignancies have been reported in ALL, but the incidence has been exceedingly low. There are, however, an increasing number of brain tumors (mostly secondary malignant gliomas) diagnosed in children after cranial irradiation.[60] Reports from St. Jude Children's Research Hospital indicated an unexpectedly high number of cases of secondary acute myelogenous leukemia in patients treated with intensive chemotherapy that included exposure to epipodophyllotoxins.[60a] These leukemias have been characterized by the presence of an 11q23 chromosomal abnormality. These reports and those of secondary leukemias occurring in other cancer patients treated with epipodophyllotoxins led to questions about the role of these compounds in the treatment of newly diagnosed patients with ALL.[61–63]

For many children with ALL, most therapy can be administered on an outpatient basis. Despite its length, treatment is usually compatible with a reasonably normal lifestyle. Most patients do not experience significant late sequelae and tolerate treatment well.

Treatment Obstacles

Despite the dramatic improvement in therapy, many treatment obstacles must be overcome before a cure becomes a reality for all patients.

Continued efforts must be made to define more precisely those clinical and biologic features of greatest prognostic value, permitting improved delineation of patient subgroups requiring more or less intensive therapy. The most important problem is the need for improved treatment of patients in the poor-risk category. Although efforts to intensify therapy for these patients appear promising, greater understanding of the disease that affects them is needed. The group of patients failing current therapy is known to be biologically heterogenous, manifesting differences in clinical presentation and in the cytogenetic, immunologic, and molecular features of their disease. The application of molecular biologic methods to the study of drug resistance may ultimately provide valuable information about the mechanisms of treatment failure. Studies of the role of expression of the multidrug resistance gene, *MDR1*, in patients with ALL who have experienced treatment failure are in progress.[64]

The causes of treatment failure must be identified. More than one third of children with ALL relapse, most during maintenance therapy. Recent studies, suggesting that variation and limitations in drug bioavailability may be partially responsible for treatment failure during maintenance, require confirmation.

Molecular biologic techniques are being applied to detect minimal residual disease. In the past, most methods lacked sufficient sensitivity, but studies using polymerase chain reaction technology demonstrate an enhanced ability to detect residual leukemic cells and suggest that this approach may be useful in identifying patients at risk for relapse.[65-68]

Because attention also must focus on the development of more effective treatment for the relapsed patient, the role of bone marrow transplantation in the treatment of ALL is likely to increase. Recent successes in the use of partially mismatched donors offers the possibility of totally crossing the HLA barrier. The role of autologous marrow transplantation may expand as newer methods of in vitro purging (*e.g.*, radiolabeled monoclonal antibodies or biologics) become available.

An exciting potential application for biologics in ALL treatment is in the area of molecularly cloned hematopoietic growth factors. Preclinical and early clinical studies with granulocyte-macrophage colony-stimulating factor (GM-CSF) and granulocyte colony-stimulating factor (G-CSF) confirm the potential of these agents to shorten the duration and severity of chemotherapy-induced myelosuppression. These agents may allow intensified chemotherapy for patients with ALL at high risk of treatment failure.

ACUTE MYELOGENOUS LEUKEMIA

AML represents approximately 20% of all cases of acute leukemia in children. Considerable progress has been made in the treatment of childhood AML in the past decade. The prognosis for children with this disease, although appreciably greater than that for adults, is significantly worse than for children with ALL. AML shares many features with the adult form of the disease (see Chap. 54). With some minor differences, the biology of AML is similar in children and adults, with the possible exception of neonatal leukemia.

Approximately 50% to 70% of children are classified as having AML, and 20% to 40% have acute myelomonocytic leukemia.[69] The FAB system of morphologic classification in equally applicable to childhood AML. There is some evidence that patients in the FAB M5a (acute monoblastic leukemia) and M5b (acute monocytic leukemia) subcategories have a less favorable prognosis.[70] The responses to treatment of the other FAB subtypes are similar.

Mixed-lineage leukemia has been reported in cases presenting as childhood AML. In one series, approximately 15% of cases of AML expressed lymphoid antigens. Most of these cases were FAB M1 or M2 and expressed the T-cell antigen CD7 and CD2.[71] The clinical significance of mixed lineage is not clear.[20] Acute megakaryocytic leukemia (M7), recently added to the FAB classification system, occurs more commonly in children with Down's syndrome. M7 is frequently associated with myelofibrosis.

Definable cytogenetic abnormalities are present in more than two thirds of AML cases. There are some cytogenetic differences between childhood and adult AML. The −5, 5q−, and −7 abnormalities often seen in adults are rare in children. The 11q23 translocation occurs frequently in infants and often is associated with biphenotypic leukemia. This translocation is also found in cases of secondary AML arising as a consequence of epipodophyllotoxin therapy. A t(1;22) has been associated with acute megakaryocytic leukemia in infants.

Chromosomal patterns appear to have prognostic implications. Trisomy 8, t(8;21), inv(16), and t(9;11) are associated with a high rate of complete remission; abnormalities of chromosome 7 (*e.g.*, monosomy 7) are associated with a low rate of remission induction. The t(9;11) and the t(15;17) (found in M3 disease) are associated with prolonged remission duration.

Information about the influence on prognosis of other factors such as age, sex, and leukocyte count has been somewhat conflicting. Very young age (<1 year) and high leukocyte count (>20,000/mm^3) are unfavorable prognostic factors for attaining complete remission.[69,72] Cases of M1 subtype that lack Auer rods have a low remission induction rate.[73] Remission rates are also low in cases of treatment-related secondary AML or AML that develop after a myelodysplastic syndrome. Age at diagnosis, initial leukocyte count, and FAB classification affect remission duration.[69] Children older than 2 years of age have a better prognosis than younger children, with those between 3 and 10 years of age having the best prognosis. The poor prognosis for children younger than 2 years may be related to the observation that the M4 and M5 FAB categories occur more often in these children (Table 50–4).[70]

Because AML and ALL have similar clinical presentations but quite different therapies and prognoses, it is important for the clinician to differentiate them. In addition to use of special stains (*e.g.*, myeloperoxidase, Sudan black, PAS, specific esterase), determination of TdT activity (usually lacking in AML) and immunophenotyping with myeloid-specific monoclonal antibodies are important.[74] After the diagnosis of AML is established, the FAB subtype should be determined, because this classification system has prognostic value and because certain FAB subcategories present unique clinical problems. For example, patients with the M3 (promyelocytic leukemia) subtype frequently develop a disseminated intravascular coagulation-like syndrome. Cytogenetic analysis of the initial bone marrow specimen should also be performed.

As in adults, the most effective regimens for remission induction include cytosine arabinoside plus an anthracycline (usually daunorubicin) in a two-drug combination or with additional drugs such as 6-thioguanine, prednisone, vincristine, or 5-azacytidine. To induce a complete remission, it is usually necessary to produce profound marrow aplasia. An exception may be patients with M3 (acute promyelocytic leukemia) who

TABLE 50–4. Frequencies of FAB Subtypes in Childhood Acute Nonlymphocytic Leukemia

		Incidence (%)	
FAB Type	*Common Name*	*Age <2 Years*	*Age >2 Years*
M1	Acute myeloblastic leukemia without maturation	15–20	25
M2	Acute myeloblastic leukemia with maturation		25–30
M3	Acute promyelocytic leukemia (hypergranular variant)		5
M3V	Acute promyelocytic leukemia (microgranular variant)		
M4	Acute myelomonocytic leukemia	30	25
M4Eo	Acute myelomonocytic leukemia with eosinophilia		
M5	Acute monocytic leukemia	50–55	15
M6	Erythroleukemia		≤5
M7	Acute megakaryocytic leukemia		≤5

(Adapted from Grier H, Weinstein H. Acute myelogenous leukemia. In: Pizzo PA, Poplack DG, eds. Principles and practice of pediatric oncology. 2nd ed. Philadelphia: JB Lippincott, 1993)

have a high remission induction rate if treated with all-*trans*-retinoic acid. With induction chemotherapy, the potential for morbidity and mortality from infection may be great, necessitating aggressive supportive care measures. Induction morbidity may be higher with doxorubicin (Adriamycin) than with daunomycin. In most centers, complete remission can be induced in approximately from 75% to 85% of children.

CNS leukemia appears to be more common at diagnosis in AML than in ALL, occurring in 5% to 20% of patients.[75] CNS disease appears to be more common in patients with very high initial leukocyte counts and with the monocytic and myelomonocytic subtypes.[75] Several studies have indicated benefit of CNS preventive therapy.[70,76] Most centers rely on intrathecal chemotherapy with methotrexate or with cytosine arabinoside. Cranial irradiation is not used in most frontline AML protocols.

As in ALL, maintenance chemotherapy has been employed in childhood AML to prolong the duration of the initial remission. Although a variety of strategies have been used, most regimens produced median remissions of less than 2 years. Studies using intensive treatment have demonstrated improvement, with approximately 40% of children achieving prolonged event-free survival.[70,76–79] It is not clear that, after intensive induction and consolidation therapy, maintenance therapy provides additional therapeutic benefit.[80]

Many centers perform bone marrow transplantation for patients who achieve an initial remission and have a histocompatible sibling donor (see Chap. 66). This approach is promising. The CCSG compared bone marrow transplantation with conventional AML maintenance chemotherapy in a nationwide study. The results demonstrated a statistically significant better disease-free survival rate at 3 years for transplantation (49%) than for chemotherapy (36%).[80a] Because some intensive chemotherapy programs have achieved results similar to those obtained for transplantation, there is controversy about the optimal postremission strategy. Most centers suggest marrow transplantation for patients who have an appropriately matched HLA-compatible allogeneic sibling donor.

Studies evaluating the role of autologous marrow transplantation for patients with AML suggest that this strategy may have a role in first or subsequent remission. Purging has been accomplished with chemotherapeutic agents (*e.g.*, 4-hydroperoxycyclophosphamide) or monoclonal antibodies. Autologous marrow transplantation provides a potential transplant option for patients who lack a histocompatible donor. This strategy has produced significant long-term survival of patients transplanted during second remission.[81–84] Whether autologous bone marrow transplantation offers an advantage over chemotherapy alone in children with AML in first remission is currently being assessed in a randomized study of the Pediatric Oncology Group (POG).

Recent studies have demonstrated high complete remission induction rates in patients with acute promyelocytic leukemia (M3) treated with all-*trans*-retinoic acid.[85–87] The therapeutic benefit associated with all-*trans*-retinoic acid therapy has stimulated investigation into the possible therapeutic role of other differentiation agents in the treatment of AML. In vitro studies indicate differentiation of M1 and M2 subtypes with a combination of all-*trans*-retinoic acid and other differentiating agents (*e.g.*, low-dose cytarabine, G-CSF). Clinical trials of these combinations are beginning.

NEONATAL LEUKEMIA

Neonatal leukemia occurs in the first month of life. It is a rare disorder, and most cases are AML. Neonatal or so-called congenital leukemia may be associated with Down's syndrome or other chromosomal abnormalities. Congenital leukemia frequently presents with infiltration of the skin, usually nodular, which may be ecchymotic as a result of concomitant thrombocytopenia. Leukemic infiltration of the lungs, liver, and spleen are common. The initial leukocyte count is frequently greater than 100,000/mm^3. The prognosis for neonatal leukemia has been poor. Although complete remissions have been obtained, they are usually short, and long-term survivors have not been reported. There is, however, little experience treating these children with the type of intensive combination chemotherapy regimens used to treat older children with AML.

Patients with neonatal leukemia and Down's syndrome pose a unique problem. A number of these children have had disease that resolved spontaneously over weeks or months. Some researchers have suggested that this disorder represents a defect in the regulation of granulopoiesis and should be considered a myeloproliferative syndrome. However, some patients with this transient disorder have experienced recurrences that proved fatal. The relation between these processes is unclear.

CHRONIC MYELOGENOUS LEUKEMIA

CML is relatively rare in childhood, accounting for 1% to 5% of childhood leukemias.[2] The two major forms are the adult form, which typically is seen in adolescents, and the juvenile form, which occurs mainly in infants. Adult CML is discussed in depth in Chapter 55. The juvenile form of the disease occurs less frequently and differs biologically and clinically from adult CML (Table 50–5).

Juvenile CML is a disease of infancy, rarely occurring after 5 years of age. Typically, it presents with symptoms of fatigue, pallor, and recurrent infection. An eczematoid facial rash, prominent and frequently suppurative lymphadenopathy, thrombocytopenia, and hemorrhagic manifestations at diagnosis also differentiate juvenile CML from the adult form. The Philadelphia chromosome, a hallmark of adult CML, is lacking in juvenile CML. The leukocyte count is usually less than 100,000/mm^3. These features, the presence of thrombocytopenia, and a relatively low myeloid to erythroid ratio, which reflects the hyperplasia of both lines in the bone marrow, are useful in differentiating juvenile from adult CML.[2]

In juvenile CML, in vitro bone marrow culture yields a predominance of monocytic colonies, suggesting that it is a form of myelomonocytic leukemia. Juvenile CML is also associated with several erythroid abnormalities, including a persistently high fetal hemoglobin level and other findings similar to those seen in fetal erythrocytes, suggesting that there is disordered regulation of erythropoiesis. Immunologic abnormalities have been noticed. Unlike adult CML, which has its characteristic chronic phase, the juvenile form of the disease follows a course of progressive deterioration that does not have a terminal blastic phase. In its later stages, profound erythroid hyperplasia is seen.

Treatment for juvenile CML is totally unsatisfactory; most patients survive less than 1 year after diagnosis. Chemotherapeutic intervention has not altered the natural history of this disease. Bone marrow transplantation has been attempted successfully and is appropriate to consider.

NON-HODGKIN'S LYMPHOMA

The childhood non-Hodgkin's lymphomas differ in many respects from their adult counterparts.[88] For example, pediatric lymphomas are virtually always diffuse rather than nodular,

TABLE 50–5. Features of the Adult and Juvenile Forms of Chronic Myelogenous Leukemia

Feature	*Adult Form*	*Juvenile Form*
Age at onset (median)	14.2 years	22.5 months
Sex (M:F)	6:1	2.1
Philadelphia chromosome	Present	Absent
Physical findings		
Facial rash	Absent	Present
Lymphadenopathy	Occasional	Frequent, with tendency to suppuration
Splenectomy	Marked	Mild to moderate
Hemorrhagic manifestations	Absent	Frequent
Hematologic findings		
Initial leukocyte count	Usually >100,000/mm^3	Usually <100,000/mm^3
Thrombocytopenia at diagnosis	Uncommon	Frequent
Monocytosis	Absent	Usually present
Fetal hemoglobin levels	Normal	30–70%
Erythrocyte I antigen	Normal	Reduced
Erythrocyte enzymes	?	Increased fetal enzyme systems
		Decreased carbonic anhydrase
Ineffective erythropoiesis	Absent	Present
Marrow M:E ratio	10:1–50:1	2:1–5:1
Leukocyte alkaline phosphatase	Decreased	Decreased or lower limit of normal
Serum vitamin B_{12} level	Increased	Increased
Colony-forming characterizations	Predominantly granulocytic	Almost exclusively monocytic
Urine and serum muramidase	Slightly elevated	Markedly elevated
Immunologic abnormalities	None	Increased immunoglobulin levels
		High incidence of antinuclear and anti-IgG antibodies
Response to busulfan	Good	Poor
Median survival	2.5–3 years	<9 months
Terminal phase	Blast crisis	Erythroid hyperplasia; intense normoblastemia

(Adapted from Altman AJ. Chronic leukemias of childhood. Pediatr Clin North Am 1988;35[4]:765–787)

and they are more often extranodal than nodal. Immunophenotypic studies indicate that B-cell lymphomas account for about 80% of adult NHL, but in childhood, approximately 40% of NHLs are of T-cell origin. Most childhood NHLs arise from lymphoid precursors, and almost all are included in the National Cancer Institute's (NCI) category of "high grade" lymphomas. Only a small fraction (predominantly in older children) fall into the intermediate-grade category, and essentially none are considered low grade. In contrast, high-grade lymphomas are relatively uncommon in adults, who usually have low-grade lymphomas. Childhood lymphomas are rapidly fatal if untreated, but expeditiously instituted chemotherapy results in cure of a high proportion of patients.

Childhood NHL, like adult NHL, has the propensity for early, widespread, noncontiguous dissemination. Leukemic presentation and the development of primary CNS relapse are common, and this has given rise to diagnostic confusion because in the presence of bone marrow involvement the clinical syndromes of "leukemia" and "lymphoma" are not sharply separable. Lymphoblastic lymphomas are indistinguishable cytomorphologically from acute lymphoblastic leukemias. Better definition of individual pathologic entities on the basis of their cytogenetic and molecular characteristics is likely to improve this situation. For example, it has already become clear through detailed pathobiologic characterization that the so-called B-cell ALL is the same entity as small, noncleaved cell lymphoma and should be treated as such. The separation of lymphoblastic lymphoma from ALL is more difficult. An arbitrary and widely used clinical definition is that 25% of bone marrow cells must be blasts for a diagnosis of ALL. Such a definition appears to be of little biologic or prognostic significance.

EPIDEMIOLOGY

NHL is approximately 1.5 times as common as Hodgkin's disease in children younger than 15 years; Hodgkin's disease has a higher incidence in children and young adults older than 16 years. The average annual incidence in the United States of NHL is approximately 9 cases per 1 million white children younger than 15 years old and approximately 5 per 1 million black children. There is a male preponderance, with a male to female ratio of 2.5:1 to 3:1. The peak incidence occurs between the ages of 7 to 11 years. Involvement before the age of 3 is uncommon.

Although the precise cause of NHL is unknown, it is clear that the disease results from genetic changes, the likelihood of which is influenced by environmental factors. Several inherited and acquired conditions predispose to the development of NHL. The association between inherited immunodeficiency disease and NHL is well documented; NHL accounts for more than half of all malignancies that occur in children with inherited immunodeficiency syndromes, including ataxia-telangiectasis, Wiscott-Aldrich syndrome, common variable immunodeficiency disease, severe combined immunodeficiency disease (SCID), and the X-linked lymphoproliferative syndrome.[89] In some of these immunodeficiency states, chromosomal abnormalities or the genetic instability associated with the chromosomal abnormality contribute to the increased risk of lymphoid malignancy. For example, translocations involving the long arm of chromosome 14 at band q32 are frequently encountered in ataxia-telangiectasia. Translocations that involve the immunoglobulin heavy chain locus are common in neoplasms of B-cell origin, and it seems probable that the greater activity of the enzyme system that mediates immunoglobulin gene rearrangement in ataxia-telangiectasia accounts for the increased likelihood of developing an NHL-associated chromosomal translocation. In the X-linked recessive syndrome described by Purtilo, fatal infectious mononucleosis, NHL (including immunoblastic and small, noncleaved cell lymphoma), hypogammaglobulinemia, and aplastic anemia may occur. Epstein-Barr virus EBV appears to be relevant to the pathogenesis of many of the lymphomas that develop in the inherited immunodeficiency states, because EBV genomes are frequently found in the tumor cells.

Acquired immunodeficiency is associated with the development of lymphoma. Patients undergoing chronic immunosuppressive therapy after organ allografting have an increased risk of lymphoproliferative syndromes that are almost invariably EBV associated. Patients with human immunodeficiency virus (HIV) infection have a markedly increased risk of lymphomas, some of which have the typical histologic pattern and chromosomal abnormalities of Burkitt's lymphoma. Whatever the cause of the immunosuppression, lymphomas confined to the CNS are much more common than in immunocompetent persons. In patients with HIV infection, CNS lymphomas appear to be invariably associated with EBV. This is not the case for systemic HIV-associated lymphomas, approximately 40% of which are EBV associated.

EBV and malaria have been implicated in the development of Burkitt's lymphoma in African children, and evidence suggests that the form of the disease that is endemic in equatorial Africa (with an average annual incidence of between 5 and 15 per 100,000 children younger than 15 years) represents a separate molecular subtype.[90] A retrovirus, HTLV-I, has been implicated in the pathogenesis of one form of adult T-cell leukemia-lymphoma that is prevalent in Japan, the Caribbean, and parts of the southern United States. However, retroviruses have not been linked to the pathogenesis of childhood lymphomas.

Chronic treatment with hydantoin drugs, including phenytoin (Dilantin), has been associated with development of pseudolymphomas and true malignant lymphomas, including Hodgkin's disease and NHL. NHL has developed as a second malignancy in patients treated with chemotherapy, particularly if in addition to radiation therapy, for Hodgkin's disease. Recently, epidemiologic evidence from Kansas and Nebraska has been collected that suggests that high exposure to certain herbicides is linked to lymphomagenesis. Plants containing phorbol esters have been implicated in the pathogenesis of Burkitt's lymphoma in equatorial Africa.

PATHOLOGIC AND IMMUNOLOGIC CLASSIFICATION

The histologic classification of pediatric NHL is much less complicated than the classification of adult NHL, because there are only three major categories. Unfortunately, these three categories have different names in different classification schemes.[88] In the NCI working formulation, the categories are small, noncleaved cell lymphoma, lymphoblastic lymphoma, and large cell lymphoma (Table 50–6). The corresponding categories in the older Rappaport scheme are un-

TABLE 50–6. Distribution of Histopathologic Types of Diffuse Lymphomas in Childhood

Histologic Classification	*Approximate Frequency (%)*
Lymphoblastic (convoluted and nonconvoluted)	30–40
Small non-cleaved (Burkitt's and non-Burkitt's, pleomorphic)	40–50
Large cell	15

(Magrath IT. Malignant non-Hodgkin's lymphomas. In: Pizzo PA, Poplack DG, eds. Principles and practice of pediatric oncology. Philadelphia: JB Lippincott, 1993)

differentiated lymphoma, lymphoblastic lymphoma, and histiocytic (also referred to as large cell) lymphoma. Each of these categories can be further divided on the basis of histology, immunophenotype, or both.

An indication that these histologic categories are biologically meaningful is provided by the observation that they correspond to different, although overlapping clinical syndromes. Lymphoblastic lymphomas characteristically present with supradiaphragmatic disease, particularly anterior superior mediastinal (thymic) involvement. Small, noncleaved cell lymphomas usually present with intraabdominal disease. Lymphoblastic and small noncleaved cell lymphomas are approximately equal in frequency and account for some 85% of childhood NHL. Large cell lymphomas do not have a characteristic clinical syndrome and may occur at a variety of nodal and extranodal sites, including Waldeyer's ring, lymph nodes, abdomen, chest, skin, and bone.

Immunologic classification is extremely important in childhood NHL. Lymphoblastic lymphomas are predominantly neoplasms of the precursors of functional T cells and, much less commonly, of B-cell precursors. Regardless of phenotype, lymphoblastic lymphomas almost always contain TdT. Studies using monoclonal antibodies capable of delineating the various stages of intrathymic differentiation indicate that the malignant T cells in lymphoblastic lymphoma generally bear the immunophenotypic stamp of intermediate or late thymocytes. In contrast, T-cell ALL lymphoblasts often display the characteristics of early thymocytes. A small subset of lymphoblastic lymphomas—those that present as isolated bone or lymph node involvement—have the immunophenotype of common acute lymphoblastic leukemia, a pre-B-cell phenotype. All small, noncleaved cell lymphomas, including Burkitt's and non-Burkitt's subtypes, are of B-cell origin and express various B-cell markers, including CD19, CD20, and surface immunoglobulin, predominantly IgM (associated with kappa or lambda light chains). They also express HLA-DR antigens and usually express the CALLA antigen, but they do not contain TdT. Many large cell tumors also express B-cell characteristics, but the recently described anaplastic large cell lymphomas, most of which bear T-cell surface antigens, are characterized by the uniformly high level of expression of the CD30 (Ki-1) antigen.

Pathogenesis

As is the case for all malignant tumors, NHL probably arises as a consequence of the accumulation of genetic abnormalities in a cell. The small chance that a genetic lesion able to contribute to lymphomagenesis will arise coupled to the need for multiple genetic abnormalities usually results in monoclonality of the tumor cells (although clonal evolution subsequently occurs). It is probable that dysfunction of oncogenes and antioncogenes are required, and such functional abnormalities are produced by a restricted set of changes in the genome that may include chromosomal translocation, point mutation, deletion, or amplification. Particularly characteristic of the lymphoid neoplasms is involvement of the antigen receptor genes in the molecular abnormalities.[88] An increasing number of chromosomal translocations in lymphoid malignancy have been shown to involve deregulation of "master" genes involved in the regulation of other genes (*i.e.*, transcription factors). In addition to changes in cellular genes, the expression of adventitious genes provided by viruses may contribute to the ultimate functional changes that give rise to neoplasia.

Lymphoblastic Lymphoma

The genetic changes in lymphoblastic malignancies are quite heterogenous but often result in the deregulation of master genes.[89a] Translocations sometimes produce the juxtaposition of such genes to the T-cell antigen receptor genes on chromosomes 7 (β) and 14 (α,δ), such as t(7;9), t(7;10), t(7;11), t(10;14), and t(11;14). A master gene known as *TAL1* or *SCL* is deregulated by chromosomal translocation (and juxtaposition to the T-α receptor on chromosome 14) or interstitial deletion within chromosome 1, on which *TAL1/SCL* gene is situated. These deletions have been described in some 20% of T-cell leukemias, suggesting that mechanisms other than chromosomal translocation may be more frequently employed in T-cell malignancies. Genetic abnormalities have not been described in the pre-B-cell variety of lymphoblastic lymphoma but may be similar to those reported in pre-B leukemia, such as t(1;19). There has been no clear separation of the genetic changes associated with lymphoblastic leukemias and lymphoblastic lymphomas.

Small, Noncleaved Cell Lymphoma

Small, noncleaved cell lymphoma is divided into two subtypes: Burkitt's lymphoma and non-Burkitt's lymphoma. It is not clear that this histologic distinction is meaningful in children, because most small, noncleaved cell lymphomas in this age group are Burkitt's lymphomas.[88,90] In adults, the non-Burkitt's subtype is differentiated from Burkitt's lymphoma at a molecular level. In older patients, small, noncleaved cell lymphomas may bear a quite different chromosomal abnormality, the 14;18 translocation associated with the follicular lymphomas and about 25% of large cell lymphomas. All small, noncleaved cell lymphomas are derived from B-cell lineage.

Burkitt's cells manifest a characteristic cytogenetic abnormality in which genetic material is exchanged between the q24 band of the long arm of chromosome 8, at the location of the c-*MYC* gene, and the q32 band of chromosome 14, t(8;14), the site of the immunoglobulin heavy chain genes.[90] Rarely, "variant" translocations can be demonstrated, t(8;22) or t(2;8), which involve the same band on chromosome 8 and one of the light chain immunoglobulin genes on the partner chromosome (κ on 2p12, and λ on 22q12). As a consequence of these translocations, the expression of *MYC*, a master gene involved in cell proliferation, is deregulated. In effect, *MYC* is expressed as if it were an immunoglobulin gene. Cells bearing a deregulated *MYC* gene are probably unable to enter a resting phase, and in the presence of additional genetic events, become fully malignant neoplastic clones.

Burkitt's lymphoma was originally described in equatorial Africa, and the disease there differs in several respects from the North American form of the disease and from the disease in most other parts of the world (Table 50–7). Apart from the much higher incidence rate in Africa (hence the term "endemic"), the typical presentation of African Burkitt's lymphoma, a large tumor of the maxilla or mandible, with or without orbital involvement, is rarely seen in the "sporadic" form of the disease seen in the United States. Moreover, bone marrow involvement is much more common in the American form of the disease than the African. The endemic and sporadic forms of the disease also differ biologically. EBV DNA and the EBV nuclear antigen are usually in the tumor cells in African children but are much less frequently encountered in North American patients. Although the cytogenetic findings are similar in endemic and sporadic tumors, there is a difference in the location of the breakpoint on chromosome 8. In endemic tumors, the breakpoint occurs a variable distance upstream of the gene, but in sporadic tumors, it is usually within the gene or its flanking sequences. Although genetic factors cannot be completely excluded, it seems probable that Burkitt's lymphoma is composed of a mixture of molecular subtypes and that the incidence of each type depends on the environment.

Large Cell Lymphomas

It appears that at least some large cell lymphomas have a similar pathogenesis (*i.e.*, contain the same genetic abnormalities) as the small, noncleaved cell lymphomas. However, little is known of the pathogenesis of the remaining large cell lymphomas. The anaplastic or Ki-1 subtype appears to arise from perifollicular activated lymphocytes of T-cell or B-cell lineages and frequently bears a nonrandom translocation involving chromosome band 5q35. The partner chromosome varies (*i.e.*, usually 2, but sometimes 3 or 1), and other translocations, such as t(2;13), have been described.

CLINICAL PRESENTATION

Childhood NHL can arise in almost any organ or tissue but involves peripheral lymph nodes in approximately 15% of patients.[88] Although systemic symptoms including fever, night sweats, and weight loss may be observed, these are relatively uncommon features, except in anaplastic large cell lymphomas. Symptoms usually reflect the presence of a tumor mass, except in the small number of patients with a leukemic presentation of a small, noncleaved cell lymphoma. The most frequent site of involvement at presentation is the abdomen, and most intraabdominal NHLs are small, noncleaved cell lymphomas. Pain, a palpable mass, or generalized abdominal swelling are the most common reasons for seeking medical assistance, and occult or overt bleeding from the gastrointestinal tract, with consequent anemia, is often observed. Intussusception is a frequent presentation in the younger child and is usually caused by a small intestinal tumor that often proves to be totally resectable. Involvement of the terminal ileum or ascending cecum occurs in approximately 40% of patients with small, noncleaved cell lymphomas.[88]

The chest is the next most frequently involved site, and approximately 70% of patients with lymphoblastic lymphoma have a mediastinal mass. However, large cell lymphomas, but rarely small, noncleaved cell lymphomas, may also present with a mediastinal mass.[38] Mediastinal enlargement usually presents with dyspnea, particularly if there is an associated pleural effusion, dysphagia, or superior vena cava obstruction.

Childhood NHL may present with involvement of a variety of other sites, including peripheral lymphadenopathy (frequently cervical or supraclavicular in lymphoblastic lymphoma), tonsils, nasopharynx, or other portions of Waldeyer's ring (with or without involvement of cervical lymph nodes), bone marrow, bones, skin, gonads, breast, face, or CNS. These

TABLE 50–7. Differences Between Endemic and Sporadic Burkitt's Lymphoma

Endemic	*Sporadic*
Common (100 per 1 million children)	Rare (1–2 per 1 million children)
Distribution relates to climate and geography	Distribution apparently unrelated to climate and geography
Nearly always associated with EBV (95%)	Uncommonly associated with EBV (15%)
t(8:14) common	t(8:14) common
No IgM secretion	Secretion of IgM
Chromosome 8 breakpoints upstream of c-*MYC*	Chromosome 8 breakpoints within c-*MYC*
Jaw tumors common, marrow involvement rare	Jaw tumors rare, marrow involvement common
Multiple relapses not incompatible with eventual prolonged disease-free survival	Survival uncommon after relapse

EBV, Epstein-Barr virus; CTX, cyclophosphamide; COM, cyclophosphamide, vincristsine, methotrexate.
(Magrath IT. Malignant non-Hodgkin's lymphomas. In: Pizzo PA, Poplack DG, eds. Principles and practice of pediatric oncology. Philadelphia: JB Lippincott, 1993)

tumors grow rapidly, and clinical symptoms have rarely existed for more than 6 to 8 weeks before presentation.

PRETREATMENT EVALUATION AND STAGING

The diagnosis of NHL can only be definitively established by biopsy and, wherever possible, immunophenotyping and cytogenetics. Because of the extremely rapid growth rate of the NHLs that occur in children, particularly of the small, noncleaved cell lymphomas, a rapid and expeditious assessment of disease extent is essential. In addition to a detailed history and physical examination, a complete blood count with careful examination of the peripheral smear for circulating blasts should be performed. Blood chemistries, including electrolytes, BUN, creatinine, liver function tests, and serum calcium and uric acid, should be performed routinely. In patients with the largest tumor burdens, marked abnormalities in renal function and uric acid levels may be detected. Measurement of serum LDH is a useful correlate of tumor burden. The level of soluble interleukin-2 receptor in serum appears to be a reliable prognostic factor, particularly for B-cell lymphomas.

Posterior and lateral chest x-ray films should be obtained to assess mediastinal, hilar, pericardial, or pleural involvement. The trachea and bronchi should be evaluated for patency and displacement. CT scan of the mediastinum is much more valuable in documenting the extent of chest disease than chest x-ray films, and CT scans of the abdomen are usually performed, although in very young children, ultrasound examination may be more valuable in view of the lack of retroperitoneal fat. Sometimes these studies provide complementary information. A particularly valuable whole-body screening study for the small, noncleaved cell lymphomas is the ^{67}Ga scan. Bilateral bone marrow biopsies and aspirates are advocated to maximize detection of marrow involvement. Lumbar puncture should be performed and a cytocentrifuged CSF specimen examined for malignant cells, but because intrathecal therapy is normally given to all patients, CSF examination can be performed at the same time intrathecal therapy is first administered. Mandatory and optional staging procedures for the child with NHL are shown in Table 50–8.

Because treatment consists of chemotherapy, there is no role for a staging laparotomy. However, laparotomy may be necessary for biopsy of an abdominal mass at the time of presentation, and in patients with regionally limited disease, the most common site is the terminal ileum and cecum. Complete resection of the offending tumor mass may be feasible and the safest surgical procedure. Patients who have the mass completely resected, even those with positive mesenteric nodes, have an excellent prognosis.

The Ann Arbor staging system is of limited value in childhood NHL; most pediatric lymphomas are extranodal, and unlike Hodgkin's disease, NHL in children is not orderly or predictable in its pattern of spread or relapse, and prognosis is not readily determined by the number of sites affected. The most widely used staging system in pediatric NHL is that used at St. Jude Children's Research Hospital (Table 50–9). This and similar systems differ from the Ann Arbor scheme in that they do not differentiate between primary nodal and extranodal presentations, and they recognize the poor prognosis (in American NHL) of bone marrow involvement and CNS disease. A quite widely used staging scheme, originally designed for African Burkitt's lymphoma, includes a separate stage, AR, that includes patients with more than 90% resection of intraabdominal disease.

TABLE 50–8. Staging Procedures for Non-Hodgkin's Lymphoma

Mandatory
- Complete blood count, platelet count, differential
- Chest x-ray films (posteroanterior and lateral)
- Bone marrow aspirates and biopsy
- Lumbar puncture with cytocentrifuge examination of cerebrospinal fluid
- Liver function tests
- Serum electrolytes, BUN, creatinine, and uric acid levels
- Chest and abdominal CT scan

Optional (depending on clinical circumstances)
- Bone scan and skeletal survey
- Intravenous urogram
- Barium studies on the gastrointestinal tract
- Myelography
- MRI
- Lymphangiography*
- Ultrasonography

* Rarely indicated.

Some institutions no longer use a recognized staging system. For example, the CCSG classifies children with NHL on the basis of whether they have localized or nonlocalized disease. In this definition, patients with localized disease have tumor limited to a single extranodal site, with or without positive regional nodes, or to lymph nodes in one or two adjacent lymphatic regions. All other tumors, including mediastinal disease, are classified as nonlocalized disease. Localized disease in this system corresponds to stage I and stage II disease in the St. Jude system and includes children with a particularly favorable prognoses. This system, although less elaborate, effectively separates patients with limited disease from those with extensive tumor involvement. As treatment results continue to improve, the utility of these staging systems as predictors of prognosis will diminish. Currently, they remain essential for meaningful comparison of results obtained in clinical trials and will continue to be necessary as long as treatment is predicated on the extent of disease.

TREATMENT

At the time of presentation, it is essential to recognize conditions requiring emergency treatment, such as airway or vascular obstruction, paraplegia, compression of optic nerves, cardiac tamponade, gastrointestinal perforation or bleeding, and uricosemia. Patients with extensive intraabdominal disease may have multiple causes of renal failure, including uricosemia and renal outflow tract obstruction. Before the initiation of chemotherapy in all patients with high tumor burdens, it is essential to initiate allopurinol and to establish good diuresis. If this is not possible, hemodialysis may be necessary to rectify biochemical abnormalities and to avoid severe

TABLE 50–9. Clinical Staging Systems for Childhood Lymphomas

Stage	*Memorial Sloan-Kettering (Wollner)*	*St. Jude Children's Research Hospital (Murphy)*	Stage	*National Cancer Institute (Ziegler, Magrath)*
I	One single site	A single tumor (extranodal) or single anatomic area (nodal) with the exclusion of mediastinum or abdomen	A	Single solitary extraabdominal site
II	Two or more sites on the same side of the diaphragm	A single tumor (extranodal) with regional node involvement Two or more nodal areas on the same side of the diaphragm Two single (extranodal) tumors with or without regional node involvement on the same side of the diaphragm A primary GI tract tumor, usually in the ileocecal area, with or without involvement of associated mesenteric nodes only	B	Multiple extraabdominal sites
III	Disseminated disease without marrow or CNS involvement	Two single tumors (extranodal) on opposite sides of the diaphragm Two or more nodal areas above and below the diaphragm All the primary intrathoracic tumors (mediastinal, pleural, thymic) All extensive primary intraabdominal disease All paraspinal or epidural tumors regardless of other tumor site(s)	C	Intraabdominal tumor
IV	Any of the above with bone marrow and/or CNS involvement	Any of the above with initial CNS or bone marrow involvement	D	Intraabdominal tumor with involvement of ≥ extraabdominal site
			AR	Intraabdominal tumor with >90% of tumor surgically resected

and possibly fatal worsening after rapid tumor lysis. The syndrome of rapid tumor lysis is characterized by azotemia, hyperphosphatemia, and hypocalcemia as a result of the liberation of tumor breakdown products into the bloodstream.[88] In uricosemia, alkaline diuresis is normally recommended, but after near normalization of serum uric acid levels, alkalinization should be stopped, because phosphates, which are released by lysed tumor cells and may produce renal tubular obstruction, are less soluble in alkaline urine.

Because one of the potentially most devastating consequences of rapid tumor lysis is hyperkalemia, potassium is not normally administered to patients undergoing chemotherapy. Hyperkalemia is essentially unknown in the presence of a good diuresis. Establishment and maintenance of a high urine flow is the key to the successful management of patients with massive tumor burdens and the potential for tumor lysis. Normally, 4 to 5 L/m^2 per day can be safely administered to these patients if careful monitoring is performed. This is best conducted in a critical care unit.

Chemotherapy

Before the 1970s, the overall survival of children with NHL was poor; few patients survived 5 years after diagnosis, and most survivors had limited disease. Although the use of surgery or radiation therapy was modestly effective in patients with limited disease (*e.g.*, a single extraabdominal, extrathoracic tumor site or totally resected abdominal tumor), as many as two thirds of patients experienced relapse. The pattern of relapse, with frequent recurrences at sites distant from the radiation field, including bone marrow, suggested that failure occurred because of widespread occult disease. The addition of combination chemotherapy to treat patients with limited disease raised the overall survival figures for this group to approximately 90%, making radiation therapy superfluous because it adds potential toxicity without apparent therapeutic advantage.[91] Radiation and surgery also have no role in treating patients with advanced disease. Systemic combination chemotherapy is indicated for all patients with childhood NHL. Using the most effective modern regimens, 85% to 95% of patients achieve complete remissions, and 90% of patients with limited disease and 60% to 80% of patients with extensive disease are cured. Relapse does not occur with any significant frequency beyond 2 years, and in patients with small, noncleaved cell lymphomas, relapse is rare beyond 10 months.

For purposes of treatment, childhood NHL is usually divided into lymphoblastic and nonlymphoblastic lymphomas, which includes small, noncleaved cell and large cell lymphomas. Lymphoblastic lymphomas are most often treated with regimens similar to that initially designed for the treatment of high-risk ALL. The most frequently used are modifications of the LSA$_2$-L$_2$ protocol designed at the Memorial Sloan-Kettering Cancer Center. This approach stems from a randomized trial performed by the CCSG. In this study, the LSA$_2$-L$_2$ protocol was compared with the COMP regimen, which includes cyclophosphamide, vincristine, methotrexate, and prednisone, and was modified from regimens developed for patients with Burkitt's lymphoma. Most patients in both treatment groups also received radiation therapy to sites of bulky disease. For nonlocalized lymphoblastic leukemia, 76% of patients treated with LSA_2-L_2 were disease free at 2 years, compared with 26% of patients treated with COMP. For nonlocalized nonlymphoblastic lymphoma, 57% of patients treated with COMP achieved 2-year disease-free survival, compared with 28% of children who received LSA_2-L_2 therapy. For patients with localized disease, histologic subtype did not appear to have prognostic significance. In this group, the less toxic four-drug COMP regimen was as effective as the more intensive ten-drug LSA_2-L_2 treatment (89% versus 84%). Similar results to those obtained with LSA_2-L_2 have been reported for another leukemia-type protocol, the APO regimen (Table 50–10), but patients with Burkitt's lymphoma fared badly with this regimen.

These results were originally interpreted as indicating that patients with lymphoblastic lymphoma and nonlymphoblastic lymphoma should be treated differently, but it has become clear that lymphoblastic lymphomas may be treated with lymphoma-type regimens, although patients with small, noncleaved cell lymphoma should not be treated with a leukemia-type regimen. Anthracyclines appear to be an important component of successful treatment protocols for lymphoblastic lymphomas. Regimens based on repeated alkylating agent therapy that also contain anthracyclines appear to be as successful as LSA_2-L_2. For example, an NCI regimen containing cyclophosphamide, vincristine, prednisone, and doxorubicin alternating with prolonged methotrexate infusions has been shown to be effective for lymphoblastic and nonlymphoblastic lymphomas, producing a disease-free survival at 3 years of approximately 60%, and the POG ACOP+ regimen has been shown to produce similar results to LSA_2-L_2. The results of one small series of lymphoblastic lymphoma patients treated with an ALL-like approach that omitted anthracyclines was reported. This protocol, which included cytarabine and VM-26 and was not as complicated as LSA_2-L_2, had a predicted disease-free survival rate at 4 years of 73%.[90a]

CNS prophylaxis is incorporated into all protocols, but there is no evidence that cranial irradiation is necessary, and most pediatric oncologists now use only intrathecal therapy. The optimal duration of therapy for lymphoblastic lymphoma remains unknown.

Treatment regimens for the nonlymphoblastic lymphomas, most of which are B-cell tumors, usually incorporate cyclophosphamide, vincristine, and intermediate-dose or high-dose methotrexate. Patients with limited disease are usually treated with a combination of cyclophosphamide, vincristine, prednisone, and methotrexate (COMP) or doxorubicin (*e.g.*, CHOP). In patients with extensive disease, other drugs (*e.g.*, VM-26, ifosfamide, cytarabine, BCNU) are usually employed. The most successful regimens, such as those of the French Society of Pediatric Oncology, the Berlin-Frankfurt-Münster group (BFM), and the recent NCI and Dana-Farber protocols (Fig. 50–5), include more than four drugs. The last three protocols have treatment durations of approximately 12 weeks, but produce disease-free survival rates in excess of 70% for patients with extensive disease. It seems that excellent results can be obtained with intensive, short-duration regimens containing a backbone of cyclophosphamide, high-dose methotrexate, vincristine, and high-dose cytarabine. Doxorubicin, ifosfamide, and the epipodophyllotoxins are also included in most of these regimens. A modified version of the French protocol used in a small group of patients with CNS disease at presentation proved to be highly successful. Until this report, little progress in improving survival rates had been made in treating this subgroup.

Patients with anaplastic large cell lymphomas have been treated successfully (*i.e.*, anticipated long-term survival rate of approximately 70%) with the BFM and LSA_2-L_2 protocols. There appears to be little point in treating these patients with the much longer LSA_2-L_2 regimen if intensive, short-duration therapies are equally successful.

CENTRAL NERVOUS SYSTEM PREVENTIVE THERAPY

In the past, the CNS was an initial site of relapse in almost one third of children with NHL. Some form of CNS preventive therapy is warranted for most patients. CNS spread is less common in patients with limited disease (stage I or II), and it has been suggested that CNS preventive therapy can be avoided in some patients with limited disease without producing a significant increase in subsequent CNS relapse. Included in this group are patients with totally resected abdominal disease and non-Burkitt's, nonmediastinal, limited nodal disease that is not close to the meninges. However, this policy has not been subjected to clinical trial, and for this reason, most centers treat all patients with CNS preventive therapy.

Intrathecal therapy with or without cranial irradiation has been used. Although the relative efficacy of each form of CNS preventive therapy has not been carefully studied in a randomized fashion, it is now clear that intrathecal chemotherapy alone is highly effective and cranial irradiation is unnecessary. The CCSG compared LSA_2-L_2 with COMP. The use of intrathecal chemotherapy alone was associated with an incidence of isolated CNS disease of only 6%. In the NCI study described earlier, the inclusion of intrathecal chemotherapy with methotrexate and cytosine arabinoside reduced the incidence of primary CNS relapse from approximately 20% to 2%.

Radiation Therapy

Although radiation therapy plays an important role in the treatment of adult non-Hodgkin's lymphomas, its role in pediatric NHL is limited. Specific emergency situations, including acute respiratory distress, superior vena cava syndrome, spinal cord compression, orbital proptosis, and cranial nerve palsy, may be effectively treated with radiation therapy. However, because irradiation may contribute to the development of toxicity (*e.g.*, esophagitis, cardiac failure after irradiation of a mediastinal mass), its role should be limited only to emergencies for which chemotherapy alone is not effective. In the small, noncleaved cell lymphomas, the effectiveness of chemotherapy has significantly limited the need for radiation therapy. One of the few exceptions may be the treatment of intraparenchymal brain disease. Although it has been traditional to include irradiation in the treatment of patients with localized disease, a randomized study, largely confined to patients with nonlymphoblastic lymphoma, demonstrated that irradiation added toxicity without therapeutic benefit.[91] At 4

TABLE 50–10. Chemotherapy Regimens Used for Childhood Non-Hodgkin's Lymphoma

LSA$_2$-L$_2$ (Modified)

Induction

Cyclophosphamide, 1.2 g/m^2 I.V., day 1

Vincristine, 2.0 mg/m^2 I.V. (maximum dose, 2.0 mg), days 3, 10, 17, and 24

Methotrexate, 6.25 mg/m^2 I.V., days 5, 31, and 34

Daunomycin, 60 mg/m^{2}I.V., days 12 and 13

Prednisone, 60 mg/m^2 PO (maximum dose, 60 mg), days 3–30

Consolidation

Cytosine arabinoside, 100 mg/m^2 I.V. daily for 5 days (Mon–Fri) for 2 wk

Thioguanine, 50 mg/m^2 PO 8–12 h after each cytosine arabinoside injection

Asparaginase, 6000 IU/m^2 IM daily for 14 days after completion of cytosine arabinoside and thioguanine

Methotrexate, 6.25 mg/m^2 IT twice, 3 days apart, beginning 2 to 3 days after last dose of asparaginase

Carmustine, 60 mg/m^2 I.V. single dose given 2 to 3 days after completion of methotrexate

Maintenance

1. Thioguanine, 300 mg/m^2 PO, days 1–4
2. Hydroxyurea, 2.4 g/m^2 PO, days 1–4
   Daunomycin, 45 mg/m^2 I.V., day 5
3. Methotrexate, 10 mg/m^2 I.V., days 1–4
   Carmustine, 60 mg/m^{2}I.V., day 5
4. Cytosine arabinoside, 150 mg/m^2 I.V., days 1–4
   Vincristine, 2.0 mg/m^2 I.V. (maximum dose, 2.0 mg), day 5
5. Methotrexate, 6.25 mg/m^2 IT, 2 doses given 3 days apart

Repeat maintenance cycles 1–5

COMP

Induction

Cyclophosphamide, 1.2 g/m^2 I.V., day 1

Vincristine 2.0 mg/m^2 I.V. (maximum dose, 2.0 mg), days 3, 10, 17, and 24

Methotrexate, 6.25 mg/m^2 IT, days 5, 31, 34

Methotrexate, 300 mg/m^2 I.V. (60% of dose as I.V. push, 40% as 4-h infusion) on day 12

Prednisone, 60 mg/m^2 PO (maximum dose, 60 mg), days 3–30

Maintenance

Cyclophosphamide, 1.0 g/m^2 I.V., day 1

Vincristine, 1.5 mg/m^2 I.V. (maximum dose, 2 mg), days 1 and 4

Methotrexate, 6.25 mg/m^2 IT, day 1 (excluded from first maintenance cycle)

Methotrexate, 300 mg/m^2 I.V. (60% of dose as I.V. push, 40% as 4-h infusion), day 15

Prednisone, 60 mg/m^2 PO (maximum dose, 60 mg), days 1–5 (excluded from first maintenance cycle)

Repeat maintenance cycle every 28 days

NCI 77-04

CYCLE 1

Systemic Therapy

Cyclophosphamide, 1,2 g/m^2 I.V., day 1

Methotrexate (begins on day 10), 300 mg/m^2 I.V. (over first hour), then 60 mg/m^2 I.V. hourly for next 41 h, followed by calcium leucovorin 48 mg/m^2 I.V., then 12 mg/m^2 I.V. every 6 h until plasma methotrexate levels $<5 \times 10^{-8}$ M.

Intrathecal Therapy

Cytosine arabinoside, 30 mg/m^2 IT, days 1, 2, 3, and 7

Methotrexate, 12.5 mg/m^2 IT (maximum dose, 12.5 mg), day 10, 6–8 hours after commencement of systemic methotrexate infusion

CYCLES 2 TO 6

Systemic Therapy (Begins When Granulocyte Count $\geq$ 1500/mm^3)

Cyclophosphamide, 1.2 g/m^2 I.V., day 1

Adriamycin, 40 mg/m^2 I.V., day 1

Vincristine, 1.4 mg/m^2 I.V., day 1 (maximum dose 2.0 mg)

Prednisone, 40 mg/m^2 I.V. or PO, days 1–5

Methotrexate and calcium leucovorin day 10, as in cycle 1

Intrathecal Therapy

CYCLES 2 AND 3

Cytosine arabinoside, 30 mg/m^2 IT, days 1 and 2

Methotrexate, 12.5 mg/m^2 IT (maximum dose 12.5 mg), day 3 and on day 10 6–8 h after commencement of systemic methotrexate infusion

CYCLES 4, 5, AND 6

Cytosine arabinoside, 45 mg/m^2 IT, day 1

Methotrexate 12.5 mg/m^2 IT (maximum dose 12.5 mg), day 10

Patients with Burkitt's lymphoma/ undifferentiated lymphoma, stages A, B, AR, stop therapy after 6 cycles. All other patients are treated for a total of 15 cycles.

CYCLES 7 TO 15

Cyclophosphamide, 1.2 mg/m^2 I.V., day 1

Adriamycin, 40 mg/m^2 I.V., day 1

Vincristine, 1.4 mg/m^2 I.V. (maximum dose 2.0 mg), day 1

Prednisone, 40 mg/m^2 I.V. or PO, days 1–5

Methotrexate and calcium leucovorin on day 14 as in cycle 1

Cycles are repeated on day 28 or when granulocyte count is $\geq$1500/mm^3 and platelet count $\geq$75,000/mm^3

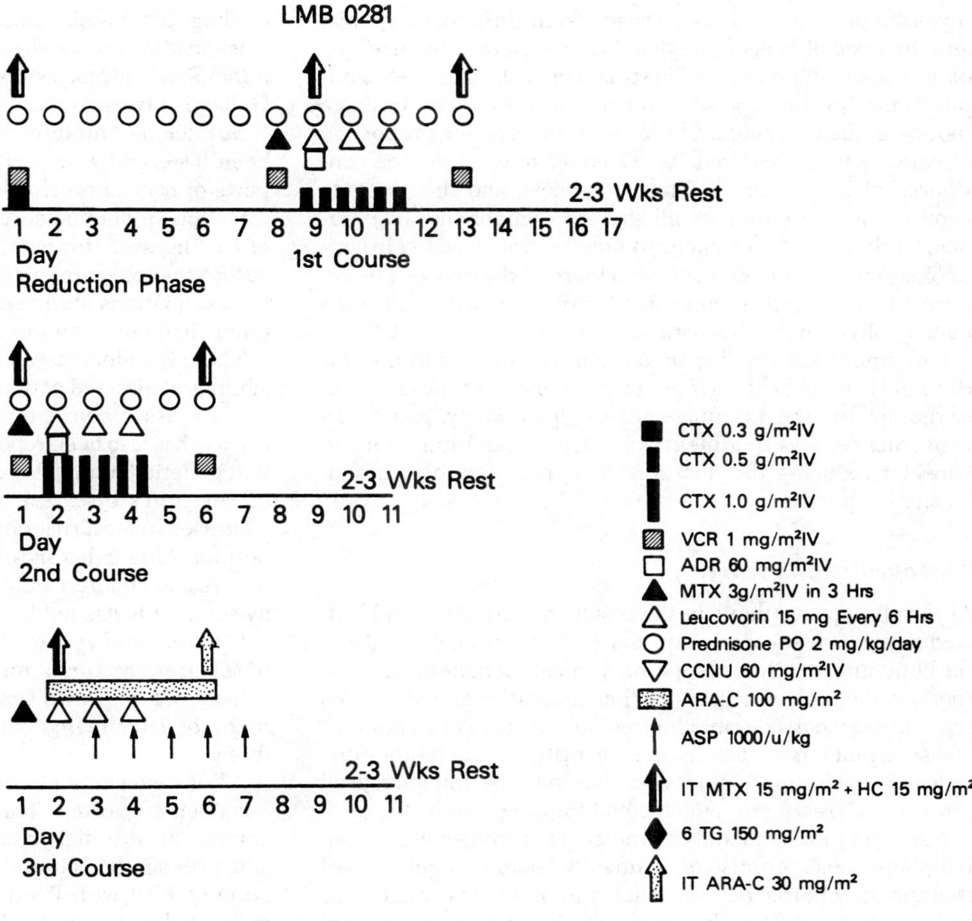

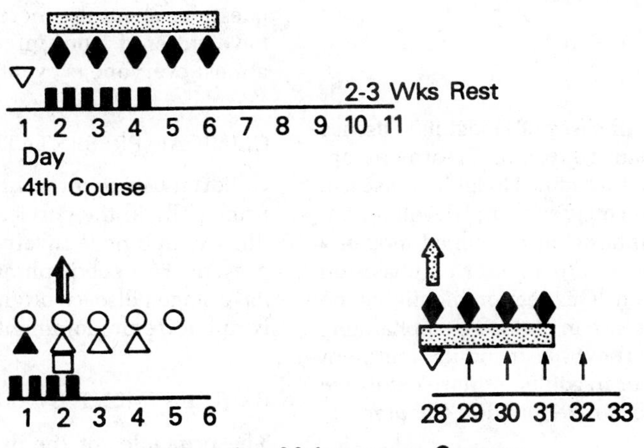

FIGURE 50–5. The LBM-02 protocol of the SFOP for B cell lymphoblastic lymphomas stages I and II (large nasopharyngeal primaries in stage II are included). Cyclophosphamide is given at the doses shown daily in two fractions. Maintenance courses are given monthly. During maintenance ara-C is given as two SC fractions; otherwise it is given as a continuous intravenous infusion. (Schema prepared from information in Patte C, Philip T, Rodary C, et al. Improved survival rate in children with stage III and IV B cell non-Hodgkin's lymphoma and leukemia using multi-agent chemotherapy: Results of a study of 114 children from the French Pediatric Oncology Society. J Clin Oncol 1986;4:1219–1226)

years, 88% of the patients in this study are projected to be disease-free survivors; no significant difference has been found in the rate of locoregional failure. Previous studies suggesting benefit using local radiation therapy in more advanced childhood NHL used less effective systemic chemotherapy.[91a] Although no randomized trial has been conducted recently using patients with advanced disease, the excellent results obtained in several treatment protocols using chemotherapy alone has led to the exclusion of radiation therapy in most current studies.

Complications of Therapy

Treatment of children with NHL may be associated with acute and chronic complications. The acute risks of multiagent systemic chemotherapy include infection as a complication of myelosuppression and hemorrhage from thrombocytopenia, and the toxic effects of individual chemotherapy include cardiomyopathy, hemorrhagic cystitis, hepatitis, and CNS complications. Sterility and second malignancies are becoming a more significant problem because of the greater proportion of patients who are cured. These issues must always be considered in the design of future protocols, and they provide good reasons to eliminate all therapy components (*e.g.*, radiation therapy, doxorubicin in small, noncleaved cell lymphomas) that do not contribute to increased survival. The report of increased second malignancies associated with epipodophyllotoxins is worrisome.

One important trend is to shorten treatment duration for the nonlymphoblastic lymphomas. Shortening the duration of therapy has the advantage of reducing toxicity, patient inconvenience, and treatment cost. It is equally important to consider reducing the duration of therapy for the lymphoblastic lymphomas.

Therapeutic Challenges

Although improvements in the results of patients with localized or extensive disease have markedly reduced enthusiasm for bone marrow transplantation as a component of primary therapy, the molecularly cloned hematopoietic growth factors have aroused considerable interest in this form of treatment. These agents may lessen the severity of chemotherapy-induced myelosuppression, and they may permit increased intensity of treatment, which could improve survival.

Attempts to understand the molecular pathogenesis of the lymphomas has promise of ultimately leading to quite novel therapeutic approaches in which tumor-specific molecular targets are identified. Unfortunately, it is likely to be many years before such approaches enter the clinic.

HODGKIN'S DISEASE

Approximately 10% to 15% of all cases of Hodgkin's disease occur in patients younger than 16 years. Treatment approaches differ from those used in adult Hodgkin's disease. The adverse effects of irradiation on growth and development in children have led to an emphasis on combined-modality therapy with limited irradiation and to a lesser emphasis on stage-specific therapy in children. This section highlights the salient features of Hodgkin's disease in children, emphasizing those aspects that differentiate the disease and its treatment in children from those that occur in adults. A more extensive discussion of Hodgkin's disease can be found in Chapter 51.

EPIDEMIOLOGY

The incidence of Hodgkin's disease increases throughout the pediatric age range. Most pediatric cases occur in children 11 years of age or older. Hodgkin's disease is rarely seen in children younger than 4.[92] Among prepubertal children, there is a striking predominance of boys. In early adolescence, the number of girls with Hodgkin's disease increases significantly.

The cause of Hodgkin's disease remains obscure. Although an increased incidence of Hodgkin's disease has been noticed in children with inherited immunodeficiency syndromes, including ataxia-telangiectasia, Chediak-Higashi syndrome, Wiskott-Aldrich syndrome, and congenital agammaglobulinemia, it is not as common in these conditions as non-Hodgkin's lymphoma.

Suspicion of an infectious cause for Hodgkin's disease has been fostered by several reported associations, including reports of case clustering, a higher incidence in patients with infectious mononucleosis, and the bimodal incidence curve of the disease. However, there is no conclusive evidence of space-time clusters in children, and it remains possible that the associations observed result from the interplay of factors other than common infections.

There is an increased incidence of Hodgkin's disease among siblings of affected patients, especially if they are of the same sex. An association between certain HLA antigens and the disease has also been reported. These two observations suggest that genetic factors play a role. A difference in the age peaks of Hodgkin's disease in industrialized and underdeveloped countries suggest that environmental factors may also be important. Although a significant association between tonsillectomies and children with Hodgkin's disease has been reported by some, this has not been confirmed.

Children and young adults receiving phenytoin for control of seizures are at risk for a lymphoma-like syndrome, which usually reverses with cessation of the drug, and the development of true malignant lymphomas, including Hodgkin's disease.

A link between socioeconomic status and Hodgkin's disease has been suggested. The incidence of Hodgkin's disease is correlated with higher family income and educational status and with smaller family size. There appears to be an association of EBV with Reed-Sternberg cells. EBV is most often associated with mixed cellular Hodgkin's disease, but its exact role in pathogenesis is unknown. The association does raise questions about the increased incidence among persons who have suffered from infectious mononucleosis, even though almost everyone is eventually infected with this virus.

CLINICAL PRESENTATION

Children usually present with disease above the diaphragm, principally in the cervical or mediastinal nodes; isolated axillary lymph node involvement is infrequent.[92] Patients who present with subdiaphragmatic involvement often prove to have stage I disease originating in inguinal lymph nodes with lymphocyte-predominant histology.

PRETREATMENT EVALUATION

The principles of the diagnostic workup for the child with Hodgkin's disease are similar to those for adults (see Chap. 51). Lymphangiography is a feasible procedure in most children, and its diagnostic accuracy in the pediatric population has been substantiated; there is a greater than 90% correlation between lymphangiographic and histopathologic results. Because the dye persists in lymph nodes, lymphangiography is also a valuable means of assessing the results of therapy. Lymphangiography may reveal disease in lymph nodes that are not enlarged, and for this reason, the yield of lymphangiography is approximately 15% above that of CT alone. In the young child, lymphangiography is understandably a more difficult procedure, but this is offset by the lesser need of lymphangiography for the detection of pathologic nodes not detectable by CT, because few patients are currently treated by irradiation alone, particularly young children.

Indications for staging laparotomy are controversial, and arguments for and against its use are considered in Chapter 51. At Stanford University, where staging laparotomy was introduced, this procedure is no longer systematically performed in children. Laparotomy can provide more information about the extent of disease. In reviews of staging laparotomies with splenectomy in pediatric populations, resultant changes in the clinical stage affected approximately 15% to 50% of patients.[93] Approximately 20% of all clinical stage I patients have occult infradiaphragmatic disease at laparotomy, and in stage II cases that are clinically supradiaphragmatic, the incidence of histologically positive disease is 30%. In lymphocyte-predominant disease limited to the neck, the yield of laparotomy is sufficiently low to obviate its use.

Although information provided by a staging laparotomy and splenectomy may be unobtainable by other means, there has been considerable concern about the morbidity of the procedure in the pediatric population. The major risk is overwhelming postsplenectomy sepsis, which in the past occurred in as many as 10% of children with Hodgkin's disease. The use of polyvalent pneumococcal vaccine or prophylactic antibiotic therapy has markedly reduced the incidence of postsplenectomy infection in children at risk, but current treatment trends and the demonstration that similarly good results can be obtained without splenectomy weigh against its use.[92]

Because laparotomy is primarily a means of identifying otherwise occult disease in the abdomen, its value is primarily as a means of guiding local or regional therapy.[94] When combined-modality therapy is to be used, it is highly questionable whether the patient should be subjected to laparotomy and splenectomy. The use of chemotherapy and extended-field, low-dose irradiation in all children with Hodgkin's disease without the use of staging laparotomy has resulted in 85% survival, and the relapse-free survival rate for clinical stages I, II, and III approaches 90%.[95] It is possible that chemotherapy alone may provide results close to those achieved with combined-modality therapy (see section on therapy).

Staging is largely used these days as a guide to the treatment approach. With the possible exception of stage IV disease, it has lost its importance as a prognostic indicator, as has histologic subtype. Few prognostic factors have retained importance in the modern era of highly effective therapy for Hodgkin's disease, although age appears to be significant. Children have a better outcome than adults, although the reasons for this may be multiple and not necessarily a consequence of the biology of the disease.

THERAPY

Because the results of the treatment of Hodgkin's disease in children have been excellent, a major consideration in current treatment approaches is to limit morbidity. Available data indicate that the use of combined-modality therapy for patients in all stages of disease, except perhaps those with stage I or certain presentations of stage IV disease, results in high survival rates and a low risk of relapse.[95,96] Gratifying results, for example, were obtained for 57 children of all stages treated at the Sick Children's Hospital, Toronto (*i.e.*, 10-year survival rate of 85%, relapse-free survival rate of 80%), in whom no staging laparotomy was performed and three cycles of MOPP were given before and three after low-dose extended-field irradiation.[97]

The universal application of this approach, however, may inappropriately expose patients to added complications from both modalities.[98] Complications of irradiation in childhood include impairment of growth and development of bones, muscles, and soft tissues; thyroid dysfunction; and an increase in the risk of second malignancies, particularly solid tumors.[92] Irradiation is responsible for a 10% to 20% increase in the late appearance of heart disease (*e.g.*, valvular, coronary). Late complications of chemotherapy include infertility and second malignancies. MOPP chemotherapy results in a high incidence of sterility in postpubertal men, although it is likely that prepubertal boys will have a lower incidence of infertility. Ovarian function may also be compromised, although younger prepubertal and pubertal girls appear to be less susceptible to these effects than older, postpubertal women.

The risk of AML after MOPP treatment alone during the first 10 years after therapy is approximately 8%, and it may be exacerbated by previous or concurrent extensive irradiation. However, in the Stanford experience with combined-modality therapy (with less use of MOPP), the risk of secondary leukemia is 3% at 10 years. Beyond 10 years, the risk of developing secondary leukemia is negligible, although the risk of other tumors, including NHL and breast cancer, which appears beyond 15 years after therapy, appears to persist indefinitely, and the overall risk of a second neoplasm may be as high as 30% at 20 years with current regimens. Chemotherapy regimens other than MOPP, such as ABVD (doxorubicin, bleomycin, vincristine, DTIC), may achieve similar disease control with less risk of secondary tumors. However, the use of ABVD carries the potential risk of severe pulmonary damage from bleomycin and anthracycline-induced cardiac failure. The latter complication is not only an acute side effect. Recent reports have indicated that cardiac failure can occur many years after the cessation of treatment, and in patients treated with mediastinal irradiation, this could prove to be an important late complication. The combined use of MOPP and ABVD may be more effective than either alone, although there are fewer data about the long-term side effects of combined regimens.

In view of the potential risks associated with chemotherapy and radiation therapy, consideration should be given to whether there are subgroups of patients for whom one or other modality may be more appropriate or even whether chemotherapy alone may produce similar results to combined-modality therapy. The possibility of developing more effective chemotherapy regimens that are associated with a lower incidence of late effects has always been a goal of medical oncologists with a special interest in Hodgkin's disease. The vinblastine, bleomycin, and methotrexate regimen used at Stanford as adjuvant (after irradiation) therapy in patients with limited disease, for example, has not been associated with infertility. A variety of approaches designed to reduce the complications of therapy have been recommended. For example, reduction in radiation volume by using high-dose involved-field techniques rather than extended-field irradiation may be sufficient for patients with favorable stage I presentations, and although relapse rates will be higher, those who relapse are likely to be salvaged by chemotherapy. A group of 28 children with stage I or II disease treated at St Bartholomew's hospital for whom clinical staging was followed by limited-volume irradiation (involved field or mantle) achieved a survival rate (96% at 10 years) at least equal to 48 patients treated at Stanford University (86% at 10 years) using pathologic staging followed primarily by extended-field irradiation. Freedom from relapse at 10 years was 90% in the Stanford series and 83% in the London series.[99] Alternatively, intermediate-dose, involved-field radiation therapy combined with chemotherapy employing MOPP, ABVD, or MOPP plus ABVD, can also reduce the radiation volume, but this approach, at least if MOPP is used as the chemotherapy regimen, is associated with a significant risk of secondary leukemia.

The use of chemotherapy alone has been studied, and as with any approach using chemotherapy, the constitution of the drug regimen was important.[42,43,45] The details of each of these strategies and the controversies surrounding them are discussed in detail in Chapter 51. No single approach is accepted by all oncologists as optimal, and the achievement of an appropriate balance between maximizing disease-free survival and minimizing treatment complications for the child with Hodgkin's disease must take into consideration the stage of disease and the age of the patient.

Most pediatric patients with Hodgkin's disease are beyond puberty. For this group, growth changes are of relatively less concern and an approach based on extended-field irradiation for patients with pathologic stage I or IIA disease, with chemotherapy reserved for children who relapse after initial irradiation, is more acceptable to those who feel strongly that irradiation should be an important component of treatment.[92] For stage I disease, local irradiation may be adequate, because it can produce a disease-free survival rate of approximately 85%, and most relapsing patients can be salvaged with chemotherapy. Older children with stage III disease have traditionally been treated with combined-modality therapy, but many consider that all stage III patients should receive chemotherapy alone.[92,96] In older patients with extensive mediastinal disease, B symptoms, or disease beyond stage IIIA, there is general agreement on the use of primary chemotherapy, although many prefer to add involved-field irradiation.[92,95,96]

Defining optimal treatment for the younger child has been more difficult. Such children with pathologic stage I lymphocyte-predominant disease limited to the neck, particularly the upper neck, have an excellent disease-free survival rate after involved-field or limited extended-field ("minimantle") treatment. Treatment of this favorable-prognosis group reduces the likelihood of significant cardiac, pulmonary, and structural effects from irradiation, and by eliminating chemotherapy, it prevents the adverse sequelae associated with combined-modality treatment.

In patients with stage II disease managed with local fields only, relapse rates of more than 30% are common, even with surgical staging. Although relapsing patients still appear to respond well to chemotherapy, the excellent overall survival must be balanced against the eventual, rather high proportion of patients who receive combined-modality therapy. In young children with extensive disease, most centers favor primary chemotherapy with involved-field or extended-field irradiation using limited radiation doses (1500–2500 cGy) to diminish the pronounced growth changes associated with large-volume, full-dose radiation therapy. This approach produces an excellent outcome with significant reduction in the risk of major deficits in growth and development.[95,96] In addition to the previously described Toronto study,[97] a series of children were treated at Stanford with 1500 to 2500 cGy of total nodal irradiation followed by six cycles of MOPP, which produced a relapse-free survival rate of 93%.[98]

In a disease in which irradiation has historically been of such importance, it is only with reluctance that this modality is abandoned. However, as doses of radiation are lowered without loss of efficacy in combined-modality approaches, the possibility that chemotherapy alone can achieve the same good results without the late complications of combined-modality therapy becomes more acceptable. Longo and coworkers reported the results of a randomized trial in adults, in which MOPP combination chemotherapy (54 evaluable patients) was compared with radiation therapy (51 patients) in patients with stages IB, IIA, IIB, or IIIA Hodgkin's disease. MOPP alone was significantly superior in patients with stages IIIA, massive mediastinal disease, patients with no B symptoms, patients with an erythrocyte sedimentation rate above 20 mm, patients with more than four sites of disease, or patients younger than 40. The overall projected 10-year disease-free survival rates were 60% for patients randomized to receive radiation therapy and 86% for patients randomized to receive MOPP chemotherapy ($p_2 = 0.009$), and the projected 10-year overall survival rates were 76% and 92%, respectively ($p_2 = 0.051$).[100]

Encouraging results with chemotherapy alone have been obtained in children. For example, an Australian group reported 92% failure-free survival (median follow-up, 45 months) for 53 children staged clinically and treated with chemotherapy alone with MOPP or ChlVPP (chlorambucil, prednisone, vinblastine, procarbazine).[101] Eighteen of 19 patients with massive mediastinal disease achieved remissions and none relapsed, and there were only four adverse events among 38 children with stage I or II disease. These data need to be complemented by long term follow-up, because knowledge of the actual survival and incidence of late effects is necessary for drawing final conclusions with respect to these divergent approaches to treatment. However, the potential avoidance of the complications associated with laparotomy and splenectomy, the obviation of radiation-induced dysmorphia, and the lower risk of second malignancies than for combined-modality therapy makes the further exploration of chemotherapy-alone approaches attractive.

In adults, some series have suggested that ABVD is more affective than MOPP alone and as effective as ABVD and MOPP combined. Whether ABVD, the MOPP plus ABVD hybrid regimen used in Vancouver, or another regimen will prove to provide optimal efficacy with the least likelihood of sterility and secondary malignancies remains to be seen, and it is one of the major issues to be resolved in the treatment of Hodgkin's disease. Few studies using ABVD for children have been conducted, but the CCSG reported a pilot study of children with stage III or IV disease treated with 12 cycles of ABVD followed by low-dose irradiation (2100 cGy). Early results are gratifying: event-free survival was 87% at 3 years, although 9% of patients developed significant pulmonary toxicity (*i.e.*, 2 of 6 patients died). It is too early to determine the incidence of second malignancies, late cardiac toxicity, or infertility. The duration of treatment in this study may be longer than is necessary, and this is likely to be an important factor in late effects. Regimens including fewer cycles must be studied. Variations in the chemotherapy regimen are not the only approach to the reduction of late effects. Alternative approaches to the prevention of infertility, such as the use of gonadotropin releasing hormone analogs in pubertal and post pubertal children, may be employed in the future, but it is difficult to envision early intervention for the prevention of secondary malignancies.

Although many issues remain to be resolved in the treatment of childhood Hodgkin's disease, the fact that there is so much focus on the late complications of therapy is a tribute to the success that has been achieved in the treatment of this disease. Overall 5- and 10-year survival rates have progressively improved, and most centers are achieving rates of approximately 90% in series including all stages of disease. It is difficult to justify staging laparotomy, and it is becoming increasingly clear that chemotherapy should be the primary modality of treatment in all stages except perhaps stage I. It will be important to establish whether even low-dose local or regional irradiation adds any therapeutic advantage to chemotherapy alone.

REFERENCES

1. Anderson JR, Wilson JF, Jenkin DJ, et al. Childhood non-Hodgkin's lymphoma: The results of a randomized therapeutic trial comparing a 4-drug regimen (COMP) with a 10-drug regimen LSA_2-L_2. N Engl J Med 1983;308:559–565.
2. Smith KL, Johnson W. Classification of chronic myelocytic leukemia in children. Cancer 1974;34:670–679.
3. Altman AJ. Chronic leukemias of childhood. Pediatr Clin North Am 1988; 35(4):765–787.
4. Malkin D, Li F, Strong L, et al. Germline p53 mutations in a familial syndrome of breast cancer, sarcomas, and other neoplasms. Science 1990;250:1233.
5. Felix C, Nau M, Takahaski T, et al. Identification of p53 gene abnormalities in acute lymphoblastic leukemia of childhood: Nonhereditary p53 mutation in the Li-Fraumeni syndrome. J Clin Invest 1992;89(2):640–647.
6. Felix CA, D'Amico D, Mitsudomi T, et al. Absence of hereditary p53 mutations in ten familial leukemia pedigrees. J Clin Invest 1992;90:653–658.
7. Till M, Rapson N, Smith P. Family studies in acute leukemia in childhood: A possible association with autoimmune disease. Br J Cancer 1979;49:62–71.
8. Kirsch I. Molecular biology of the leukemias. Pediatr Clin North Am 1988;35:693–722.
9. Rossi G, Gerla R, Cadeo G, et al. Acute lymphoblastic leukaemia of B cell origin in an anti-HIV positive intravenous drug abuser. Br J Haematol 1988;68:140–141.
10. Bleyer WA, Poplack DG. Prophylaxis and treatment of leukemia in the central nervous system and other sanctuaries. Semin Oncol 1985;12:131–1148.
11. Russo A, Schiliro G. The enigma of testicular leukemia: A critical review. Med Pediatr Oncol 1986;14:300–306.
12. Bowman WP, Aur RJA, Hustu HO, et al. Isolated testicular relapse in acute lymphocytic leukemia of childhood: Categories and influence on survival. J Clin Oncol 1984;2: 924–929.
13. Miller LP, Miller DR. Acute lymphoblastic leukemia in children: current status, controversies, and future perspective. Crit Rev Oncol Hematol 1986;1:129–197.
14. Bennett JM, Catovsky D, Daniel MT, et al. French-American-British (FAB) Cooperative Group: The morphological classification of acute leukemias-concordance among observers and clinical correlation. Br J Haematol 1981;47:553–561.
15. Miller DR, Krailo M, Bleyer WA, et al. Prognostic implications of blast cell morphology in childhood acute lymphoblastic leukemia: A report from the Children's Cancer Study Group. Cancer Treat Rep 1985;69:1211–21.
16. Korsmeyer SJ, Arnold A, Bakshi A, et al. Immunoglobulin gene rearrangement and cell surface antigen expression in acute lymphocytic leukemia of T-cell and B-cell precursor origins. J Clin Invest 1983;71:301–313.
17. Crist WM, Grosse CE, Pullen J, et al. Immunologic markers in childhood acute lymphocytic leukemia. Semin Oncol 1985;2:105–121.
18. Foon KA, Todd RF III. Immunologic classification of leukemia and lymphoma. Blood 1986;68:1–31.
19. Felix CA, Wright JJ, Poplack DG, et al. T cell receptor α-, β-, and γ-Genes in T-cell and pre-B cell acute lymphoblastic leukemia. J Clin Invest 1987;80:545–556.
20. Mirro J, Zipf TF, Pui C, et al. Acute mixed lineage leukemia: Clinicopathologic correlations and prognostic significance. Blood 1985;65:1115–1123.
21. Williams M, Innes DJ, Borowitz M, et al. Immunoglobulin and T cell receptor gene rearrangements in human lymphoma and leukemia. Blood 1987;69:79.
22. Stass S, Mirro JJ. Lineage heterogeneity in acute luekaemia: Acute mixed-lineage leukaemia and lineage switch. Clin Haematol 1986;15:811.
23. Altman A. Clinical features and biological implications of acute mixed lineage (hybrid) leukemias. Am J Pediatr Hematol Oncol 1990;12:123–133.
24. Wiersma S, Ortega J, Sobel E, et al. Clinical importance of myeloid-antigen expression in acute lymphoblastic leukemia of childhood. N Engl J Med 1991;324:800–808.
25. Hurwitz C, Loken M, Graham M, et al. Asynchronous antigen expression in B lineage acute lymphoblastic leukemia. Blood 1988;72:299–307.
26. Williams DL, Raimondi S, Rivera G, et al. Presence of clonal chromosome abnormalities in virtually all cases of acute lymphoblastic leukemia. N Engl J Med 1985;10: 640–641.
27. Look AT. The emerging genetics of acute lymphoblastic leukemia: Clinical and biologic implications. Semin Oncol 1985;12:92–104.
28. Poplack DG, Blatt J, Reaman G. Purine pathway enzyme abnormalities in acute lymphoblastic leukemia. Cancer Res 1981;41:4821–4823.
29. Hammond GD, Sather H, Bleyer WA, et al. Stratification by prognostic factors in the design and analysis of clinical trials for acute lymphoblastic leukemia. Haematology and Blood transfusion. In: Buchner T, Schellong G, Hiddemann W, Urbanitz D, Ritter J, eds. Acute leukemias. Berlin: Springer-Verlag, 1987:161–166.
30. Reaman G, Zeltzer P, Bleyer WA, et al. Acute lymphoblastic leukemia in infants less than one year of age: A cumulative experience of the Children's Cancer Study Group. J Clin Oncol 1985;3:1513–1521.
31. Crist W, Pullin J, Boyett J, et al.: Clinical and biologic features predict a poor prognosis in acute lymphoid leukemias in infants: A Pediatric Oncology Group study. Blood 1986;67:135–140.
32. Sather HN. Statistical evaluation of prognostic factors in ALL and treatment results. Med Pediatr Oncol 1986;14:158–165.
33. Steinherz PG, Gaynon P, Miller DR, et al. Improved disease-free survival of children with acute lymphoblastic leukemia at high risk for early relapse with the New York regimen—a new intensive therapy protocol: A report from the Children's Cancer Study Group. J Clin Oncol 1986;4:744–752.
34. Bleyer WA, Coccia PF, Sather HN, et al. Reduction in central nervous system leukemia with a pharmacokinetically derived intrathecal methotrexate dosage regimen. J Clin Oncol 1983;1:317–325.
35. Poplack D, Reaman G, Bleyer W, et al. Successful prevention of central nervous system (CNS) leukemia without cranial radiation in children with high risk acute lymphoblastic leukemia (ALL): A preliminary report. Proc Am Soc Clin Oncol 1989;8: 828.
36. Riehm H, Gadner H, Henze G, et al. Acute lymphoblastic leukemia: Treatment results in three BFM studies (1970–1981). In: Murphy SB, Gilbert JR, eds. Leukemia research: Advances in cell biology and treatment. New York: Elsevier Biomedical, 1983:251–263.
37. Henze G, Langermann HJ, Fengler R, et al. Acute lymphoblastic therapy study BFM 70/81 in children and adolescents: Intensified reinduction therapy for patients with different risk for relapse. Klin Pediatr 1982;194:195–203.
38. Rivera G, Raimondi S, Hancock M, et al. Improved outcome in childhood acute lymphoblastic leukaemia with reinforced early treatment and rotational combination chemotherapy. Lancet 1991;337:61–66.
39. Tubergen D, Gilchrist G, Coccia P, et al. The role of intensified chemotherapy in intermediate risk acute lymphoblastic leukemia (ALL) of childhood. CCG-105. Proc Am Soc Clin Oncol 1990;9:835.
40. Nesbit ME, Sather HN, Robison LL, et al. Randomized study of 3 years versus 5 years of chemotherapy in childhood acute lymphoblastic leukemia. J Clin Oncol 1983;1: 308–316.
41. Butturine A, Rivera GK, Bortin MM, et al. Which treatment for childhood acute lymphoblastic leukaemia in second remission? Lancet 1987;1:429–432.
42. Henze G, Fengler R, Hartmann R, et al. Chemotherapy for bone marrow relapse of childhood acute lymphoblastic leukemia. Cancer Chemother Pharmacol 1989;24: S16–19.
43. Henze G, Fengler R, Hartman R, et al. BFM group treatment results in relapsed childhood acute lymphoblastic leukemia. In: Buchner S, Hiddemann W, Ritter J, eds. Haematology and blood transfusion, acute leukemias II. Berlin: Springer-Verlag 1990: 619–626.
44. Thomas ED, Sanders JE, Flowinoy N, et al. Marrow transplantation for patients with acute lymphoblastic leukemia: A long-term follow-up. Blood 1983;62:1139–1141.
45. Sanders JE, Thomas ED, Buckner CD, et al. Marrow transplantation for children with acute lymphoblastic leukemia in second remission. Blood 1987;70:324–326.
46. Sanders J, Thomas E, Buckner C, et al. Marrow transplantation for children with acute lymphoblastic leukemia in second remission. Blood 1987;70:324–326.
47. Barrett A, Horowitz M, Gale R, et al. Marrow transplantation for acute lymphoblastic leukemia: Factors affecting relapse and survival. Blood 1989;74:862–871.
48. Gale R, Butturini A. Bone marrow transplantation in acute lymphoblastic leukemia. In: Champlin R, ed. Bone marrow transplantation. Boston: Kluwer Academic Publishers, 1990:223–233.
49. Champlin R, Gale R. Acute lymphoblastic leukemia: Recent advances in biology and therapy. Blood 1989;73:2051–2066.
50. Rivera G, Santana V, Mahmoud H, et al. Acute lymphoblastic leukemia of childhood: The problem of relapses. Bone Marrow Transplant 1989;4:80–85.
51. Kersey J, Weisdorf D, Nesbit M, et al. Comparison of autologous and allogeneic bone marrow transplantation for treatment of high-risk refractory acute lymphoblastic leukemia. N Engl J Med 1987;317:461–467.

52. Sallan S, Niemeyer C, Billett A, et al. Autologous bone marrow transplantation for acute lymphoblastic leukemia. J Clin Oncol 1989;7:1594–11601.
53. Poplack DG, Brouwers, P. Adverse sequelae of central nervous system therapy. Clin Oncol 1985;4:263–285.
54. Berg SL, Balis FM, Zimm S, et al. Phase I/II trial and pharmacokinetics of intrathecal diaziquone in refractory meningeal malignancies. J Clin Oncol 1992;10:143–148.
55. Adamson PC, Balis FM, Arndt CA, et al. Intrathecal 6-mercaptopurine: Preclinical pharmacology, phase I/II trial, and pharmacokinetic study. Cancer Res 1991;51:6079–6083.
56. Smith S, Wofford M, Shuster J, et al. Treatment of testicular leukemia in children with acute lymphoblastic leukemia (ALL): A Pediatric Oncology Group study. Proc Am Soc Clin Oncol 1990;9:841.
57. Uderzo C, Zurlo M, Adamoli L, et al. Treatment of isolated testicular relapse in childhood acute lymphoblastic leukemia: An Italian multicenter study. J Clin Oncol 1990;8: 672–677.
58. Lipshultz S, Colan S, Gelber R, et al. Late cardiac effects of doxorubicin therapy for acute lymphoblastic leukemia in childhood. N Engl J Med 1991;324:808–815.
59. Yeung S, Yoong C, Spink J, et al. Functional myocardial impairment in children treated with anthracyclines for cancer. Lancet 1991;337:816–818.
60. Shapiro S, Mealey JJ. Late anaplastic gliomas in children previously treated for acute lymphoblastic leukemia. Pediatr Neurosci 1989;15:176–180.
60a. Pui C-H, Behm F, Raimondi S, et al. Secondary acute myeloid leukemia in children treated for acute lymphoblastic leukemia. N Engl J Med 1989;321:136–142.
61. Pui C-H, Behm F, Raimondi S, et al. Secondary acute myeloid leukemia in children treated for acute lymphoid leukemia. N Engl J Med 1989;321:136–142.
62. Kreissman S, Gelber F, Sallan S, et al. Secondary acute myeloid leukemia (AML) in children treated for acute lymphoblastic leukemia (ALL). Proc Am Soc Clin Oncol 1990;9:846.
63. Ratain M, Kaminer L, Bitran J, et al. Acute nonlymphocytic leukemia following etoposide and cisplatin combination chemotherapy for advanced non-small cell carcinoma of the lung. Blood 1987;70:1412–1417.
64. Rothenberg M, Mickley L, Cole D, et al. Expression of the mdr-1/P-170 gene in patients with acute lymphoblastic leukemia. Blood 1989;74:1388–1395.
65. Yamada M, Wasserman R, Lange B, et al. Minimal residual disease in childhood B-lineage lymphoblastic leukemia. Persistence of leukemic cells during the first 18 months of treatment. N Engl J Med 1990;323:448–455.
66. Yokota S, Hansen-Hagge T, Ludwig W-D, et al. Use of polymerase chain reactions to monitor minimal residual disease in acute lymphoblastic leukemia patients. Blood 1991;77:331–339.
67. Neale G, Menaarguez J, Kitchingman G, et al. Detection of minimal residual disease in T-cell acute lymphoblastic leukemia using polymerase chain reaction predicts impending relapse. Blood 1991;78:739–747.
68. Wright JJ, Poplack DG, Bakhski A, Reaman G, Cole D, Jensen JP, Korsmeyer SJ. Gene rearrangements as markers of clonal variation and minimal residual disease in acute lymphoblastic leukemia. J Clin Oncol 1987;5:735–741.
69. Lampkin BC, Woods W, Strauss R, et al. Current status of the biology and treatment of acute non-lymphocytic leukemia in children (Report from the ANLL Strategy Group of Children's Cancer Study Group). Blood 1983;61:215–228.
70. Weinstein HJ, Mayer RJ, Rosenthal DS, et al. Chemotherapy for acute myelogenous leukemia in children and adults: VAPA update. Blood 1983;62:315–319.
71. Pui CH, Raimondi S, Head D, et al. Characterization of childhood acute leukemia with multiple myeloid and lymphoid markers at diagnosis and relapse. Blood 1991;78: 1327.
72. Creutzig U, Ritter J, Riehm H, et al. Improved treatment results in childhood acute myelogenous leukemia: A report of the German cooperative study AML-BFM-78. Blood 1985;65:298.
73. Creutzig U, Ritter J, Schellong G. Identification of two risk groups in childhood acute myelogenous leukemia after therapy intensification in study AML-BFM-83 as compared with study AML—AML-BFM-78. Blood 1991;75:1932.
74. Griffin JD, Mayer RJ, Weinstin HJ, et al. Surface marker analysis of acute myeloblastic leukemia: Identification of differentiation-associated phenotypes. Blood 1983;62:557–563.
75. Pui CH, Dahl GV, Kalwinsky DK, et al. Central nervous system leukemia in children with acute nonlymphoblastic leukemia. Blood 1985;66:1062–1067.
76. Grier HE, Gelber RD, Camitta BM, et al. Prognostic factors in childhood acute myelogenous leukemia. J Clin Oncol 1987;5:1026.
77. Grier HE, Gelber RD, Camitta BM, et al. Prognostic factors in childhood acute myelogenous leukemia. J Clin Oncol 1987;5:1026.
78. Woods WG, Ruyman FB, Lampkin B, et al. The role of timing of high-dose cytosine arabinoside intensification and of maintenance therapy in the treatment of children with acute nonlymphocytic leukemia. Cancer 1990;66:1106.
79. Ravindranath U, Steuber CP, Krischer J, et al. High dose cytarabine for intensification of early therapy of childhood acute myeloid leukemia: A Pediatric Oncology Group study. J Clin Oncol 1991;9:572.
80. Champlin R, Gale RP. Acute myelogenous leukemia: Recent advances in therapy. Prolonged survival in acute myelogenous leukemia without maintenance chemotherapy. Blood 1987;69:1551.
80a. Nesbit M, Buckley L, Lampkin B, et al. Comparison of allogeneic bone marrow transplantation (BMT) with maintenance chemotherapy in previously untreated childhood acute non-lymphocytic leukemia (ANLL). Proc Am Soc Clin Oncol [Abstract] 1987;6: 163.
81. Reiffers J, Gaspard MH, Maraninchi D, et al. Comparison of allogeneic or autologous bone marrow transplantation and chemotherapy in patients with acute myeloid leukemia in first remission: A prospective controlled trial. Br J Haematol 1989;71:57.
82. Lowenberg B, Verdonck JL, Dekker AW, et al. Autologous bone marrow transplantation in acute myeloid leukemia in first remission: Results of a Dutch prospective study. J Clin Oncol 1990;8:287.
83. Lenarsky C, Weinberg K, Peterson J, et al. Autologous bone marrow transplantation with 4-hydroperoxycyclophosphamide purged marrows for children with acute-nonlymphoblastic leukemia in second remission. Bone Marrow Transplant 1990;6: 425.
84. Ball ED, Mills LE, Cornwell GG III, et al. Autologous bone marrow transplantation for acute myeloid leukemia using monoclonal antibody-purged bone marrow. Blood 1990;75:1199.
85. Huang ME, Ye UC, et al. Use of all-*trans* retinoic acid in the treatment of acute promyelocytic leukemia. Blood 1988;72:567.
86. Castaigne S, Chomienne C, et al. All-*trans* retinoic acid as a differentiation therapy for acute promyelocytic leukemia. I. Clinical results. Blood 1990;76:1704.
87. Smith MA, Adamson PC, Balis FM, et al. Phase I and pharmacokinetic evaluation of all-*trans* retinoic acid in pediatric patients. J Clin Oncol 1992;10(11):1666–1673.
88. Magrath I, Malignant non-Hodgkin's lymphomas in children. In: Pizzo PA, Poplack DG, eds. Principles and practice of pediatric oncology. Philadelphia: JB Lippincott, 1992.
89. Seibel N, Cossman J, Magrath I. Lymphoproliferative disorders. In: Pizzo PA, Poplack DG, eds. Principles and practice of pediatric oncology. Philadelphia: JB Lippincott, 1992.
89a. Rabbitts, TH. Translocations, master genes, and differences between the origins of acute and chronic luekemias. Cell 1991;67:641–646.
90. Magrath IT. The Pathogenesis of Burkitt's Lymphoma. Adv Cancer Res 1990;55: 133–270.
90a. Dahl GV, Rivera, G, Pui CH, et al. A novel treatment of childhood lymphoblastic non-Hodgkin's lymphoma: Early and intermittent use of teniposide plus cytarabine. Blood 1985;66:1110.
91. Link MP, Donaldson SS, Berard CW, et al. Results of treatment of childhood localized non-Hodgkin's lymphoma with combination chemotherapy with or without radiotherapy. N Engl J Med 1990;322, 1169–1174.
91a. Mott MG, Chessells JM, Willoughby ML, et al. Adjuvant low dose radiation in childhood T cell leukaemia/lymphoma (report from the United Kingdom children's cancer study group—UKCCSG). Br J Cancer 1984;50:457.
92. Mauch PM, Weinstein H, Botnick L, et al. An evaluation of long-term survival and treatment complications in children with Hodgkin's disease. Cancer 1983;51:925–932.
93. Donaldson SS, Kaplan HS. A survey of pediatric Hodgkin's disease at Stanford University: Results of therapy and quality of survival. In: Rosenberg SA, Kaplan HS, eds. Malignant lymphomas: Etiology, immunology, pathology, treatment. New York: Academic Press, 1982.
94. Russell KJ, Donaldson SS, Cox RS, Kaplan HS. Childhood Hodgkin's disease: Patterns of relapse. J Clin Oncol 1984;2:80–87.
95. Jenkin D, Doyle J. Paediatric Hodgkin's disease—late results and toxicity. Int J Radiat Oncol Biol Phys 1987;13:92.
96. Lange B, Littman P. Management of Hodgkin's disease in children and adolescents. Cancer 1983;51:1371–1377.
97. Jenkin D, Doyle J, Berry M, et al. Hodgkin's disease in children: Treatment with MOPP and low dose, extended field irradiation without laparotomy. Late results and toxicity. Med Pediatr Oncol 1990;18:265–272.
98. Donaldson SS, Kaplan HS. Complications of treatment of Hodgkin's disease in children. Cancer Treat Rep 1981;66:977–989.
99. Donaldson SS, Whitaker SJ, Plowman PN, et al. Stage I–II pediatric Hodgkin's disease: Long-term follow-up demonstrates equivalent survival rates following different management schemes. J Clin Oncol 1990;8:1128–1137.
100. Longo DK, Glatstein E, Diffey PL, et al. Radiation therapy versus combination chemotherapy in the treatment of early-stage Hodgkin's disease: Seven-year results of a prospective randomized trial. J Clin Oncol 1991;9:906–917.
101. Ekert H, Waters KL, Smith P, et al. Treatment with MOPP or ChlVPP chemotherapy only for all stages of childhood Hodgkin's disease. J Clin Oncol 1988;6:1845–1850.

Cancer: Principles & Practice of Oncology, Fourth Edition,
edited by Vincent T. DeVita, Jr., Samuel Hellman, Steven A. Rosenberg.
J.B. Lippincott Co., Philadelphia © 1993.

Vincent T. DeVita, Jr
Samuel Hellman
Elaine S. Jaffe

CHAPTER 51

Hodgkin's Disease

HISTORY

Thomas Hodgkin's historic paper, "On Some Morbid Appearances of the Absorbent Glands and Spleen," was read before the Medical and Chirurgical Society on January 10 and 24, 1832.[1,2] Hodgkin described six cases of his own and a case described by Thomas Carswell in 1828. A watercolor of the morbid anatomy of this case was on display during Hodgkin's presentations. Like many later discoverers of new diseases, Hodgkin was certain that others must have noticed the disorder; he commented to fellow anatomists that such cases "can scarcely have failed to have fallen under their observation in the course of cadaveric inspection," and such observations had been made.

Hodgkin recognized that he was dealing with a primary disease of the lymphatic glands and not a secondary response to inflammation. His certainty about this was remarkable in its day, especially because he was aware that two of his patients had other illnesses (*i.e.*, tuberculosis, syphilis) that might have accounted for the pathology. Also remarkable is the fact that Hodgkin described the entity based on the natural history of the disease without the aid of a microscope. Subsequent analysis of material from Hodgkin's patients (preserved in the Gordon Museum at Guy's Hospital Medical School, London) confirmed that 4 of 7 patients had Hodgkin's disease; Carswell's case could not be confirmed without tissue, and in the remaining two cases, syphilis and lymphosarcoma were thought to be the causes of the adenopathy.[1]

Hodgkin's contribution would have fallen into oblivion if not for the unselfish behavior of Sir Samuel Wilks. In the course of his description of primary and secondary amyloidosis, also a first, he reported a variant associated with "a peculiar enlargement of lymphatic glands frequently associated with diseases of the spleen." He first thought his observation was original, but by the time he completed writing his paper, he became aware of Hodgkin's work through mention of it in another paper by Bright and diligently tracked it down, noting, "It is only to be lamented that Dr. Hodgkin did not affix a distinct name to this disease, for by so doing, I should not have experienced so long an ignorance (which I believe I share with many others) of a remarkable class of cases."[3] Wilks' paper in 1865 was entitled, "Enlargement of the Lymphatic Glands and Spleen (or, Hodgkin's Disease)," thereby immortalizing Thomas Hodgkin.[4] Nuland questions whether Sir Samuel's seemingly unselfish act was as generous as it appears. He suggests that Sir Richard Bright called to his attention Dr. Hodgkin's priority and pressured his acknowledgment.[5]

Hodgkin's description was the first of a distinct malignancy of the lymphatic system, preceding the description of leukemia by Craigie,[6] Bennett,[7] and Virchow[8] by 61 years and reticulum cell sarcoma by Roulet[9] by 98 years. These important descriptions were largely microscopic delineations of causes of adenopathy other than Hodgkin's disease. Another feat similar to that of Dr. Thomas Hodgkin was not to follow for 126 years, until Burkitt described the lymphoma that bears his name, based on its unique clinical presentation in patients in central Africa.[10]

The history of the discovery of the pathognomonic giant cells of Hodgkin's disease was reviewed by Kaplan.[1] Wilks had the benefit of a microscope and had histologically examined some cases, but observed only that "the microscope showed masses of cells and fibres as of new tissue."[4] Greenfield contributed the first low-power drawings of the appearance of those cells in 1878.[11] Goldmann, using Ehrlich's staining procedures, recognized the acidophilic nature of the nucleolus of the cells in 1892.[12] Sternberg also described the cells in 1898.[13] However, it was Reed who most clearly illustrated the appearance of the multinuclear giant cells with excellent drawings from her 8 patients cases in 1902, and the cells have since been known as Reed-Sternberg cells.[14] The malignant nature of the disease was generally agreed on after the clonal origin of the malignant cell was confirmed by cytogenetic analysis of cell lines by Seif and Spriggs in 1967.[15]

ETIOLOGY AND EPIDEMIOLOGY

In the United States, Hodgkin's disease is diagnosed in 7 of every 100,000 people annually. There is a bimodal incidence pattern for Hodgkin's disease in economically advantaged countries.[16,17] In economically underdeveloped countries, the overall incidence of Hodgkin's disease is lower than in developed countries, but incidence before the age of 15 is higher, with only a modest increase throughout adolescence and young adulthood. Associated with this disparity is a difference in the distribution of histologic subgroups, with nodular sclerosing Hodgkin's disease underrepresented in less developed countries. In Japan, the first peak of Hodgkin's disease usually seen in developed countries is absent. The pattern of Hodgkin's disease varies as the level of development changes within a specific region. Examination of longitudinal data from the Connecticut cancer registry revealed the evolution from an "intermediate" to a typical "developed" pattern between the years 1935 and 1980.[18] There is an increased risk of Hodgkin's disease with increasing educational level of the patient. The relative risk varied from 0.7 to 1.8, depending on the educational level.[18]

The potential infectious nature of Hodgkin's disease has been a topic of discussion since its earliest description. *Mycobacterium tuberculosis* was first suspected to be the etiologic organism because of the high incidence of tuberculosis in patients with this disease.[19–22] Since that time, considerable epidemiologic evidence in support of an infectious cause, particularly a virus, has been found. In several studies that addressed the possibility of an increased risk of Hodgkin's disease associated with infectious mononucleosis, a disease caused by the Epstein-Barr virus (EBV), there was a modest threefold excess in the incidence of Hodgkin's disease among patients with a prior history of mononucleosis over that in controls.[23–27] Serologic and molecular biologic data also provide support for an etiologic role of EBV in Hodgkin's disease. There have been several reports of Hodgkin's disease developing in association with serologically documented primary EBV infection. In serologic studies, the proportion of Hodgkin's patients who have IgG antibody to EBV viral capsid antigens (indicative of prior infection) is similar to controls, but data from the Boston-Worcester case control study show that in young adults with a history of infectious mononucleosis there is a significantly higher geometric mean titer of antibodies against the capsid antigen than controls.[18] The results could reflect reactivation of the virus after development of Hodgkin's disease, but a follow-up study suggested otherwise. Using the resources of five serum banks with 240,000 specimens, 43 patients were identified from whom blood had been drawn and stored an average of 50 months before diagnoses, with results similar to the previous findings. These results imply that, at least for a subset of patients with Hodgkin's disease, endogenous immune stimulation plays a role.

For a short period, there was concern that Hodgkin's disease might be contagious because of reports of clustering of the disease, but that concern has been effectively dispelled.[18] The clustering was first reported by Vianna and associates among high school students exposed to the disease.[28,29] Population-based studies, using cancer registries in Connecticut and California, convincingly made the argument that the reported clusters occurred by chance alone, and a study that repeated the methodology of Vianna and coworkers in a different location also failed to confirm their findings.[31,32] An alternative hypothesis suggested an association between the incidence of Hodgkin's disease and childhood factors that decrease exposure to infectious agents at an early age. Studies showed that the risk of Hodgkin's disease was higher under certain circumstances. Risk-reducing factors that decreased or delayed early exposure to infections included fewer siblings, single-family houses, early birth order, and fewer playmates. The incidence of clinical mononucleosis is also associated with these factors, because the disease becomes clinically relevant only after early childhood. It appears that the infection has different consequences depending on the patient's age at infection and that infection by EBV may parallel that of another agent, with EBV as a cofactor.[33]

Other, unexplained factors are associated with an increased risk of acquiring Hodgkin's disease, including increased risk among woodworkers, elevated rates after tonsillectomy and appendectomy, the familial association of Hodgkin's disease, and its linkage with certain HLA antigens.[34–41]

PATHOLOGY CLASSIFICATION

Hodgkin's disease is unique among cancers because the tumor palpated by the physician largely contains normal lymphocytes, plasma cells, and fibrous stroma of the lymph node, with only a scattering of the characteristic malignant cells of Hodgkin's disease, the Reed-Sternberg cells and their mononuclear variants. The diagnosis of Hodgkin's disease should rarely be made in the absence of Reed-Sternberg cells, although the presence of such a cell by itself is not pathognomonic of the disease. Cells simulating Reed-Sternberg cells have been found in reactive lymphoid hyperplasias, such as infectious mononucleosis, non-Hodgkin's lymphomas, and nonlymphoid malignancies, including carcinomas and sarcomas.[42–45] The historic evolution of the diagnosis and classification of Hodgkin's disease is shown in Table 51–1.

Since the detailed descriptions by Sternberg and Reed, Hodgkin's disease has been recognized as a form of lymphoreticular malignancy with distinctive clinical and pathologic features.[13,14] Histologically, there is a polymorphous admixture of cytologically abnormal cells (*i.e.*, Reed-Sternberg cells and their mononuclear variants) and a variety of apparently normal reactive elements. The Reed-Sternberg cell is large, with two or more mirror-image nuclei, each containing a single, prominent nucleolus (Fig. 51–1).

In the first clinically useful subclassification of Hodgkin's disease developed by Jackson and Parker, cases were divided into three groups: paragranuloma, granuloma, and sarcoma.[50] This classification identified the 10% of patients with the most favorable and least favorable prognoses (*i.e.*, paragranuloma and sarcoma, respectively), but approximately 80% remained

TABLE 51–1. Landmarks in the Description of Hodgkin's Disease

Investigations	*Year*	*Observation*
Hodgkin[2]	1832	"On some morbid appearances of the absorbent glands and spleen"
Wilks[4]	1865	"Cases of the enlargement of the lymph glands and spleen (or Hodgkin's disease)"
Langhans[46] Greenfield[11]	1872 1878	First description of histologic features of Hodgkin's disease, including a description of giant cells and intense fibrous bands
Pell[47]	1887	Described cyclic fever in Hodgkin's disease
Sternberg, Reed[13,14]	1898, 1902	First definitive description of Hodgkin's disease and clear illustrations of the cells bearing their names
Parker, Jackson, Fitzhugh[48]	1932	Described the absence of response to tuberculin in the presence of tuberculosis in Hodgkin's disease
Jackson, Parker[44]	1937	First histopathologic classification of Hodgkin's disease
Lukes[49]	1963	Described the current histopathologic classification of Hodgkin's disease

in the category of granuloma. A major advance occurred in 1966, when Lukes, Hicks, and Butler proposed a new histologic classification that appeared to correlate well with clinical stage and aggressiveness of disease.[45] This scheme was later simplified into the Rye classification, which is now widely employed by pathologists and clinicians. These two classifications are compared in Table 51–2. In the Rye classification, Hodgkin's disease is divided into four categories: lymphocyte predominant, mixed cellularity, lymphocyte depleted, and nodular sclerosis. Although the initial basis of this classification

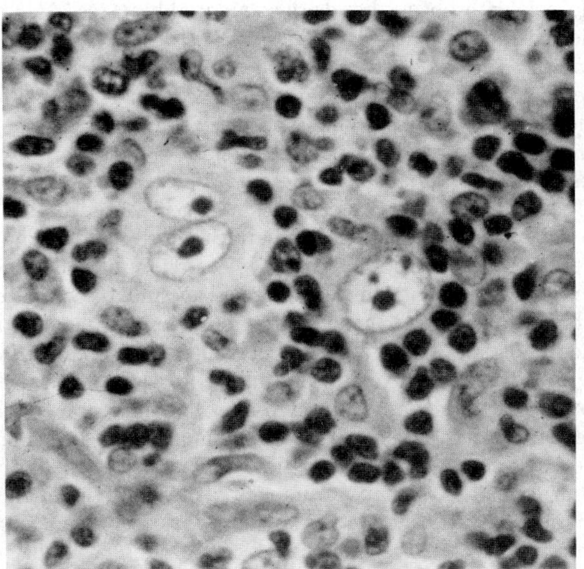

FIGURE 51–1. Characteristic Reed-Sternberg cell and mononuclear variant of Hodgkin's disease (hematoxylin & eosin stain; original magnification × 400).

TABLE 51–2. Histologic Classifications of Hodgkin's Disease

Jackson, Parker[44] *(1944)*	*Lukes, Butler, Hicks*[45] *(1966)*
Paragranuloma (10%)*	Lymphocytic predominant (15%)
	Nodular sclerosis (70%)
Granuloma (80%)	Mixed cellularity (10%)
	Lymphocyte depleted (5%)
	Diffuse fibrosis type
	Reticular type
Sarcoma (10%)	

* The figures in parentheses indicate the percentage of patients in various subcategories in the National Cancer Institute population.

was to divide cases according to the relative proportion of neoplastic mononuclear cells and Reed-Sternberg cells according to reactive elements, especially lymphocytes, in recent years, certain of the forms, such as lymphocyte-predominant Hodgkin's disease, have been shown to have distinctive morphologic, phenotypic, and clinical features. Nodular sclerosing Hodgkin's disease has long been regarded as unique. Its clinical and morphologic features were first hinted at by Greenfield in 1878 but not clearly described until 85 years later by Lukes and colleagues in 1963.[11,49]

The original Lukes and Butler scheme subdivided lymphocyte-predominant Hodgkin's disease (LPHD) into nodular and diffuse subtypes. This distinction was obliterated by the Rye modification but appears to be important in the light of new information that consistently links the nodular subtype to the B-cell arm of the immune system. In LPHD, the lymph node architecture is usually effaced, although a remnant of normal lymph node may remain. The cellular proliferation is composed of benign-appearing lymphocytes with or without benign histiocytes. The growth pattern may be diffuse but is more frequently nodular, and the nodules are considerably larger than those of follicular lymphomas. It is often necessary to examine multiple sections to identify diagnostic Reed-Sternberg cells, and some authorities question whether such cells are necessary for diagnosis in this form.[50] However, L and H variant cells are frequent and are the most characteristic cellular element in the nodular form of LPHD. These cells often have multilobated nuclei and have been called "popcorn" cells because of their resemblance to a popped kernel of corn. Fibrosis is usually not seen. This subtype is more common in male than in female patients and often occurs in the younger age groups (<35 years of age). Most patients have clinically localized disease and are asymptomatic, and the prognosis is usually favorable.

Progressive transformation of germinal centers is linked and often associated with LPHD of the nodular subtype. The nodal architecture is altered by large nodules that contain dispersed follicular center cells in clusters and ill-defined islands; Reed-Sternberg cells and L and H variants are absent. Progressive transformation of germinal centers can be seen with LPHD, precede it, or follow it in other sites.[51–53] The association of this lesion with nodular LPHD has supported the concept that the latter may be closely linked with the B-cell system. The diagnosis of progressive transformation of germinal centers should alert the clinician to the possible development of LPHD. The L and H cells express a B-cell phenotype. In paraffin sections, they are CD20 (Leu-26) positive and CD15 (Leu-M1) negative.[53–56] This phenotype is encountered in most cases of diffuse LPHD, indicating that most cases of the diffuse type represent progression from the nodular variant.[57]

Diffuse large cell lymphomas of B-cell type have been associated with the nodular variant of LPHD.[58] Both processes may occur in the same anatomic site, so-called composite lymphoma, or the large cell lymphomas may occur after the diagnosis of Hodgkin's disease.[59,60] Many of these patients seem to have a better prognosis than those with de novo large cell lymphoma, suggesting it may be a unique variant.[58] The B-cell phenotype lends further support to the B-cell origin of nodular LPHD. Although these lymphomas have been shown to be clonal, clonality has not been proven for the L and H cells of nodular LPHD, phenotypically or genotypically.

In lymphocyte-depleted Hodgkin's disease (LDHD), Reed-Sternberg cells and "pleomorphic" variant cells are plentiful in proportion to normal lymphocytes. The original Lukes and Butler scheme included two subtypes of LDHD: diffuse fibrosis and reticular. The reticular subtype contained sheets of pleomorphic neoplastic cells, making differentiation from a high-grade non-Hodgkin's lymphoma difficult.[61] The currently lower incidence of LDHD than previously reported suggests that some cases previously diagnosed as LDHD may have represented large cell immunoblastic lymphomas.[62] LDHD had been considered as a distinct clinicopathologic entity occurring in older patients with minimal peripheral adenopathy and widespread abdominal disease.[63] However, this syndrome is now in question because misclassification of high-grade diffuse lymphomas such as Hodgkin's disease was common in older series. This same difficulty may be responsible for the association of a significantly worse prognosis with the lymphocyte-depleted type found in these same studies.[62] Using stringent criteria, LDHD accounts for only 5% of all patients in current series.

Most cases of LDHD are the diffuse fibrosis subtype. In this subtype, diffuse fibroblastic proliferation may be prominent, and the process may even have a sarcomatous appearance. Normal lymphocytes are sparse, but neutrophils may be conspicuous, and foci of necrosis are common. Reed-Sternberg cells and variants are present but may be difficult to detect due to the marked fibroblastic reaction. LDHD is the most common category associated with the acquired immunodeficiency syndrome (AIDS). These patients usually have widespread disease with involvement of liver and bone marrow.[64–66] The absence of an effective lymphocytic response may contribute to aggressive clinical and pathologic behavior.

The nodular sclerosis category is distinctive morphologically and clinically. There are two histologic features that differentiate this form of Hodgkin's disease from all others. The first is a variant of the Reed-Sternberg cell, the so-called lacunar cell.[67,68] In formalin-fixed tissue, the abundant pale cytoplasm often retracts and gives the appearance of a cell in space. The second feature, seen in most cases, is a thickened capsule with a proliferation of orderly collagenous bands that divide the lymphoid tissue into circumscribed nodules (Fig. 51–2). In some cases, the sclerosis is absent or minimal, but

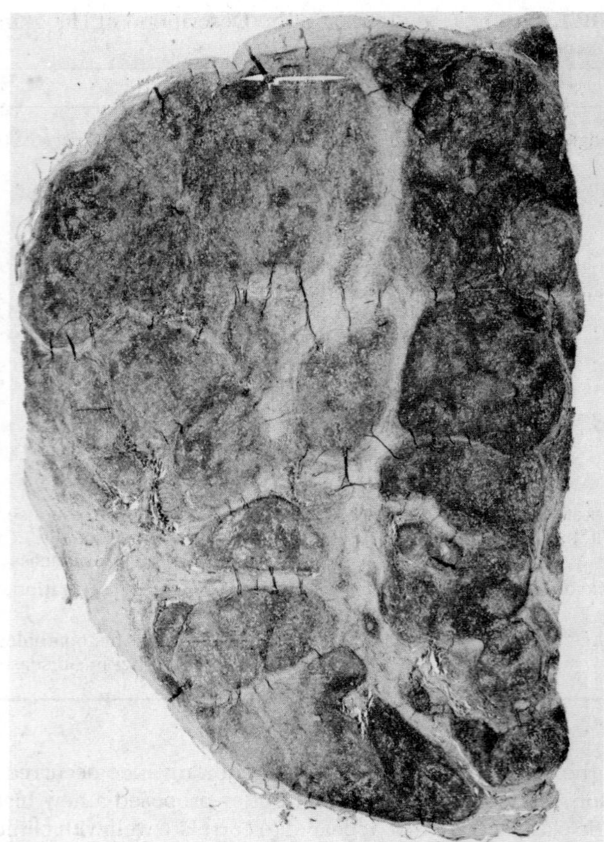

FIGURE 51–2. Lymph node involved by nodular sclerosing Hodgkin's disease. Cellular nodules are surrounded by dense fibrous bands (hematoxylin & eosin stain; original magnification × 8).

the presence of numerous lacunar cells, often in focal nodular aggregates, led some investigators to refer to this as the "cellular phase of nodular sclerosis." Strum and Rappaport observed progression from the cellular phase to classic nodular sclerosis with fibrous bands in sequential biopsies.[69] Nodular sclerosis is the only form of Hodgkin's disease that is more common in female than male patients. It most frequently occurs in adolescents and young adults and is unusual in patients older than 50 years of age. The process has a striking propensity to involve lower cervical, supraclavicular, and mediastinal lymph nodes.

This category can be subclassified according to the frequency of the malignant cells relative to normal lymphocytes. In the lymphocyte-depleted subtype, malignant cells are extremely numerous. Marked necrosis accompanied by acute inflammatory cells is seen in the center of cellular nodules. The neoplastic "histiocytes" palisading this necrosis may, to the unwary, mimic necrotizing granulomas. Fibrous bands may be inconspicuous, although capsular fibrosis is evident. Because of the frequent sheets of malignant cells, this subtype also has been referred to as the syncytial variant. The lymphocyte-depleted subtype, although not clearly an independent prognostic indicator, correlates with advanced stage at presentation and the presence of B symptoms.[62,70,71] Bulky mediastinal disease often is associated with this subtype.[72] MacLennan and coworkers proposed a subclassification scheme for nodular sclerosing Hodgkin's disease, which they believe has clinical and prognostic significance.[73] The type II of Bennett overlaps with the lymphocyte-depleted forms and the syncytial variant.

Mixed-cellularity Hodgkin's disease is characterized by an inflammatory background rich in lymphocytes, plasma cells, eosinophils, and histiocytes.[74,75] The Reed-Sternberg cells and their mononuclear counterparts are of the classic variety with prominent inclusion-like nucleoli, representing 5 to 15 cells per high-power field. Because of the inflammatory background, the differential diagnosis often includes peripheral T-cell lymphoma, and immune markers may be necessary to resolve this point. A relatively high percentage of patients have stage III or IV disease. To some extent. mixed-cellularity Hodgkin's disease has been used to include all cases of Hodgkin's disease that do not readily fall into another category.[45] This wastebasket approach should be avoided, and such cases should be considered "unclassifiable" or "not further subclassified."

Needle-core biopsies of the liver and bone marrow are frequently obtained for staging Hodgkin's disease. To diagnose involvement, the examiner should see atypical mononuclear cells or Reed-Sternberg cells in the appropriate inflammatory environment. In a patient with an established primary diagnosis, Reed-Sternberg cells are not required. However, a polymorphous cellular infiltrate in the absence of atypical cells with prominent nucleoli is a nonspecific finding and should not be considered evidence of disease. In the bone marrow, the atypical cells are frequently distributed in a markedly fibrotic background. The marrow may be replaced by diffuse fibrosis, and atypical cells may be difficult to observe.[76] Bone marrow aspirates are usually not useful in the diagnosis of Hodgkin's disease in the bone marrow. Bone marrow involvement in LPHD is rare and is usually not associated with fibrosis.

Most subtypes of Hodgkin's disease preferentially involve the T-cell-dependent zones of the lymphoid system.[71] In partially involved lymph nodes, the paracortex and the periarteriolar lymphoid sheath and marginal zone of the splenic white pulp are preferentially involved. The thymus gland is frequently involved by nodular sclerosing Hodgkin's disease and may undergo cystic degeneration secondary to involvement.[77] A thymic cyst should be carefully examined microscopically for evidence of occult Hodgkin's disease. Hodgkin's disease tends to involve axial or central lymph node groups. Mesenteric lymph nodes, Waldeyer's ring, and epitrochlear lymph nodes are rarely involved.

A nonnecrotizing epithelioid granulomatous reaction frequently accompanies Hodgkin's disease.[68–78] It may be found in involved lymph nodes and may be extensive enough to obscure the presence of Hodgkin's disease. Sarcoid-like granulomas can be seen throughout the lymphoreticular system in the spleen, liver, and bone marrow. This granulomatous response by itself does not indicate evidence of occult involvement. Patients with granulomas have, stage for stage, better prognoses than patients without this reaction.[75] The granulomas may represent a positive response to the disease.

CELLULAR ORIGIN OF HODGKIN'S DISEASE

The precise cellular origin of Hodgkin's disease is not firmly established, but theories have included derivation from a B lymphocyte or a macrophage-reticulum cell line.[79–82] Origin from a cell of the immune system is strengthened by the observation that Hodgkin's disease is characterized by a functional deficit in T-cell-mediated immune responses early in the course of the disease and before therapy, which persists in cured patients.[83–85] The lymphocytes within Hodgkin's lesions are usually identifiable as predominantly CD4-positive T cells.[86] In the past, a B-cell origin had been proposed based on the presence of surface or cytoplasmic immunoglobulins.[87] However, evidence of monoclonality and synthesis of immunoglobulin associated with Reed-Sternberg cells is lacking. The immunoglobulin is probably passively absorbed by means of IgG Fc receptors on the neoplastic cells and later internalized into the cytoplasm. Internalization of cytophilic antibody occurs in vitro, and similar binding in vivo may produce immunoglobulin on the surface of and within the neoplastic cells.[81]

A hypothesis that received some support was that the Reed-Sternberg cells might be related to the "histiocytic" system, in particular to an antigen-presenting cell rather than a phagocytic cell.[88] Although Reed-Sternberg cells have Ia antigens and Fc receptors, they have never been observed to be phagocytic, and they lack the lysosomal enzymes characteristic of phagocytic cells. The cytochemical profile of Reed-Sternberg cells does resemble that of interdigitating reticulum cells, which is also involved in antigen presentation to T cells. Interdigitating reticulum cells are usually identified in the lymph node paracortex, where Hodgkin's disease is observed to begin in pathologic sections. An interesting feature is the tendency of Reed-Sternberg cells to be rosetted by normal lymphocytes, particularly T cells.[89] This simulates a phenomenon normally demonstrated by T cells and histiocytes.

A useful diagnostic feature, which does not necessarily shed light on the cell of origin of Hodgkin's disease, is the presence of the CD15 antigen in Reed-Sternberg cells and their mononuclear counterparts. Anti-CD15 antibodies, such as Leu-M1, also react with normal granulocytes.[90] Leu-M1 detects a sugar sequence containing lacto-*N*-fucopentose. This reagent works in paraffin-embedded sections and has considerable clinical utility. It is positive in most cases, with the exception of the lymphocyte-predominant variant, which is usually negative.

Established Hodgkin's disease-derived cell lines share many of the phenotypic characteristics of freshly isolated Reed-Sternberg cells.[91] A monoclonal antibody, Ki-1 (CD30), prepared against the cell lines also reacts with Hodgkin's cells in frozen sections of involved nodes.[92] It was hoped that this antibody might shed light on the origin of Reed-Sternberg cells, but subsequent studies showed that it detects an activation antigen without lineage specificity.[93] The CD30 antigen is also expressed on some activated T cells, B cells, EBV-transformed cell lines, and the cells of large cell anaplastic lymphomas, sometimes referred to as Ki-1-positive lymphomas.[94–96]

Although Reed-Sternberg cells do not express lineage-specific markers, they do express antigens characteristic of activated T or B lymphocytes. The cells express interleukin-2 (IL-2) receptors, transferrin receptors, HLA-DR antigens, and Ki-1, all features of activated lymphocytes.[97] The application of molecular probes added support for a lymphoid origin. Clonal rearrangements of antigen receptor genes, most commonly the immunoglobulin genes, have been shown in several instances, especially in cases containing numerous malignant cells or enriched for malignant cells.[98–101] One patient with lymphoid papulosis, a benign cutaneous eruption that can progress to lymphoma, had a t(8:9) translocation in the lymphocytes in the skin lesion and in the cells of a T-cell lymphoma that developed later.[102] This was associated with tumor-specific rearrangement of the α-chain of the T-cell receptor. This patient developed Hodgkin's disease, and the same T-cell receptor rearrangement and translocation were identified in the Reed-Sternberg cells, suggesting a clonal origin from a T-cell line for all these disorders.

One study identified the *BCL2* oncogene in about a third of tested specimens of Hodgkin's tissue using the polymerase chain reaction technique, which suggested a B-cell origin.[103] Another more definitive study showed that although cytogenetic abnormalities are common in Reed-Sternberg cells, the t(14:18) translocation, so common to B-cell lymphomas, is unusual, and *BCL* expression is likely related to bystander normal lymphocytes that carry the 14:18 translocation, which can also be detected in reactive lymphoid tissue.[103a] Another study using antibodies specific for the protein of the *p53* suppressor oncogene found expression common in all types of Hodgkin's disease and neoplastic CD30-positive lymphomas, but not in LPHD, again providing confusing information about the cellular lineage of the Reed-Sternberg cell.[104]

A hypothesis that may explain these diverse bits of evidence of a multilineage origin of the Reed-Sternberg cell is that the malignant cell represents an in vivo hybridoma that occurs in response to the stimulus of an unidentified viral infection that promotes fusion of the interdigitating reticular cell and B, T, or both lymphocytes.[105,106] This hypothesis proposes that the multiple and varied expression of the genome of the Reed-Sternberg cell and its mononuclear variant could represent components of lymphoid cells incorporated into the malignant cell, including the EBV genome, and the described translocations. Using molecular hybridization techniques, the EBV genome was identified in as many as a third of the tissue samples of Hodgkin's and was localized by in situ hybridization to the malignant cells.[107–110] Evidence was provided for clonality of the viral genome in these cases, suggesting that it was incorporated before or at a early stage in the neoplastic transformation. However, these observations are not inconsistent with the incorporation of the EBV genome and that of an infected lymphocyte into an in vivo hybridoma.

In contrast to the other subtypes of Hodgkin's disease, there is a general consensus that the nodular subtype of LPHD is derived from the B-cell system rather than the T-cell system. Affected lymph nodes contain large numbers of polyclonal B lymphocytes, and this subtype of Hodgkin's disease often coexists or is preceded by progressive transformation of germinal centers.[53] The atypical Reed-Sternberg variant cells in this subtype express CD20 and contain the J chain, further supporting a B-cell derivation.[54,111–113] It appears that the cell of origin of Hodgkin's disease may vary in different histologic subtypes, with B and T lymphocytes and interdigitating reticular cells becoming malignant or fusing under different circumstances, suggesting that Hodgkin's disease may represent a generic lymph node reaction to an insult to the immune system.

IMMUNOLOGIC ABNORMALITIES

Hodgkin's disease is associated with a complex deficiency in cellular immunity.[79,81,85,114–116] The panoply of alterations includes impairment of delayed cutaneous hypersensitivity, enhanced immunoglobulin production, high levels of circulating immune complexes, production of antilymphocyte and anti-Ia antibodies, decreased natural killer cell cytotoxicity, enhanced sensitivity to suppressor monocytes and suppressor T cells, and a variety of other disorders of serum factors, including high levels of circulating IL-2 receptors.[85,117,118] In vitro, peripheral blood lymphocytes show spontaneous DNA and IgG synthesis and depressed proliferative response to T-cell mitogen stimulation with impairment of lymphokine production. The data suggest immunosuppression secondary to chronic overstimulation by cytokines, a hypothesis that fits the inflammatory histologic picture, but it is difficult to explain the persistence of these abnormalities in cured patients.

Increasing numbers of long-term survivors provided the opportunity to restudy anergy and in vitro lymphocyte responsiveness in patients who have been successfully treated. Studies at the National Cancer Institute (NCI) in a population of uniformly staged and treated patients showed that anergy did not influence prognosis within a given stage; after successful treatment, anergy to recall antigens was reversible, although response to neonantigens remained suppressed.[83,84,119–121] Fisher and coworkers have shown that, although the total number of circulating lymphocytes in patients who have been in remission for anywhere from 1.3 to 12.8 years (mean, 6.5 years) was not different from normals, the percentage of E-rosetting cells and the response to concanavalin-A and phytohemagglutinin were significantly depressed compared with normal controls.[123] Patients with normal numbers of T cells had depressed in vitro responses to antigens and were abnormally sensitive to the suppressor effects of concanavalin-A-activated lymphocytes and suppressor monocytes compared with normal controls. This defect persisted for long disease-free periods.[122,123] That this defect seems to be related to the disease itself is reinforced by the fact that patients with other types of lymphomas treated with a similar chemotherapy regimen did not have evidence of this defect.[122,124]

Lymphopenia is common in advanced stages of Hodgkin's disease and is also induced by treatment, particularly by radiation therapy. Its most profound effect is in depressing the CD4:CD8 ratio. Radiation therapy-induced lymphopenia returns to normal within 12 to 111 months after cessation of treatment.[124] Because the CD8-positive population appears relatively unaffected by radiation therapy and the CD4-positive lymphocyte population regenerates slowly after treatment is discontinued, the profound deficiency in helper T cells induced by radiation therapy may explain some clinical consequences of immunodeficiency, with an excess of herpes zoster infections during the first and second years after cessation of radiation therapy.[124–127]

Unlike the defects in delayed hypersensitivity, most studies of humoral response have shown that the antibody response of B cells and that B-cell numbers are normal in all but patients with the most advanced Hodgkin's disease. B-cell function is affected by treatment. Although splenectomy alone does not alter B-cell function, the combination of splenectomy and chemotherapy or combined splenectomy, chemotherapy, and radiation therapy does diminish B-cell function, as measured by antibody response to several bacterial antigens.[128,129]

In a study of 51 patients who were vaccinated with the 14-valent pneumococcus vaccine, combined with *Hemophilus influenzae* type B and meningococcus type C, responses were compared with normal control samples and with control patients rendered asplenic for reasons other than the staging of Hodgkin's disease.[130,131] The geometric mean of natural antibodies to these bacterial polysaccharides was not significantly different among the three groups. Persistence of antibody levels in Hodgkin's disease patients was also similar to that of healthy controls, asplenic controls, and patients treated with radiation therapy only. Patients who received chemotherapy or chemotherapy plus radiation therapy had more significant and rapid declines in antibody levels, to 10% to 20% of peak levels, and declines in the levels of natural antibodies. Timing of splenectomy was not important to the development of antibody response, but the timing of initiation of treatment was significant. Patients receiving chemotherapy or combined-modality therapy less than 10 days after vaccination had significantly lower antibody responses. The investigators concluded that the antibody response in patients with untreated Hodgkin's disease was normal and unaffected by the stage or the procedures used for staging the disease. Vaccination of all patients 10 to 14 days before the initiation of chemotherapy is therefore appropriate.[130,131] Because there is no response to booster vaccinations within the first year, boosters are not recommended, although no data are available to evaluate the effect of booster vaccination later. Neither immunization nor antibiotic prophylaxis can be guaranteed to prevent the development of sepsis due to encapsulated microorganisms in patients with Hodgkin's disease whose staging included splenectomy and who have been heavily treated with chemotherapy or radiation therapy. Vaccinated patients and antibiotic-treated patients should remain alert to the risk.

The data indicate that the functional defect in the immune system in Hodgkin's disease appears simultaneously with the appearance of the disease itself. The defect is aggravated by treatment, particularly radiation therapy, and persists in a variable, time-dependent manner, with some recovery occurring after treatment is discontinued. With the exception of rare cases of autoimmune hemolytic anemia and autoimmune thrombocytopenia, a mildly increased incidence of herpes zoster, and the rare occurrence of overwhelming sepsis related to splenectomy and therapy, the immune system of patients with Hodgkin's disease appears to function quite well, given the large number of immune defects that have been described. Opportunistic infections are relatively rare, and second malignancies appear to be more a function of the use of a combined chemotherapy and radiation therapy regimen than the underlying immune defect itself. Placed in the context of the defect found in patients with AIDS, these immunologic abnormalities are more important in the development of the disease itself than as a complicating factor.

CLINICAL IMMUNOLOGIC DISORDERS IN HODGKIN'S DISEASE

Compared with lymphocytic lymphomas, monoclonal protein spikes are less common in Hodgkin's disease.[132] In a study of 71 patients with Hodgkin's disease, unexplained positive Coombs' test results were observed for 7 male patients; all had extensive disease (stages III and IV), and 6 had constitutional symptoms.[133] The Coombs' test results were positive at initial diagnosis for 3 patients and at the time of relapse for 4. Only 3 patients in this group had overt hemolysis. The antibody was characterized in 3 patients, all of whom fulfilled the criteria for IgG with anti-I^t specificity. This antibody may be unique for Coombs-positive hemolytic anemia associated with Hodgkin's disease.[134]

Idiopathic thrombocytopenic purpura (ITP) is uncommonly associated with Hodgkin's disease.[135–137] ITP occurs usually at the time of the diagnosis or later. ITP associated with Hodgkin's disease appears to be more severe and resistant to treatment than ITP alone or associated with other illnesses. Only 6 of 23 patients, for example, responded to steroids, although 6 of 10 patients who underwent splenectomy specifically for ITP appeared to have a good and durable response.[128,129] ITP occurred after splenectomy had been performed for staging purposes in 11 patients. This finding indicates that the antibody responsible for thrombocytopenia can be produced in sites other than the spleen. Most patients develop ITP while in remission after successful radiation therapy or chemotherapy, and the occurrence of ITP does not necessarily indicate relapse. Because most reported cases occurred after splenectomy, the combination of corticosteroids and immunosuppressive drugs is required for treatment, and most patients respond well to this treatment.

Autoimmune neutropenia is rarely associated with Hodgkin's disease. The three reported cases occurred in the absence of active disease after splenectomy, suggesting that the spleen plays no role in this disorder and that splenectomy should not be considered as a form of treatment.[138]

NATURAL HISTORY AND DISEASE EVOLUTION

Hodgkin's disease was first reported to spread by contiguity by the Swiss radiotherapist Gilbert.[139–141] His work was expanded by Peters, Kaplan, and others, who tested the value of prophylactic radiation therapy to lymph nodes adjacent to those involved with disease.[142–145] With the advent of bipedal lymphography in the early 1960s and routine use of staging laparotomy, a better understanding of the evolution of this disease has been reached.[144–150] Although Hodgkin's disease is still thought to be unifocal in origin with spread to contiguous lymph nodes, at some point in the natural history of the disease, the malignant cells become more aggressive, may invade blood vessels, and spread to other organs in a manner similar to visceral malignancies.[145] The champion of this hypothesis was the late Henry Kaplan who was strongly influenced by data of Peters that showed Hodgkin's could be cured by regional radiation therapy, including radiation therapy to contiguous uninvolved nodes. This hypothesis fails, however, to account for some obvious exceptions to the notion of contiguous spread, such as the tendency of the disease to skip the mediastinum but involve the left supraclavicular and periaortic nodes in the abdomen; the involvement of the spleen early in the disease, without other organ involvement, despite the fact that the spleen has no afferent lymphatics; and the involvement of two disconnected sites, such as both axillae.

Sir David Smithers offered another plausible hypothesis.[151] He proposed that Hodgkin's disease, although unifocal in origin, spread quite early through vascular and lymphatic channels like other malignancies, but that its unique pattern of distribution could be explained by the malignant cells involving preferential sites, such as lymph nodes and spleen and only later involving other organs as the disease became more aggressive. Smithers' hypothesis provides an explanation for all of the exceptions to the theory of relentless contiguous spread. To account for the curability of early Hodgkin's disease by regional radiation therapy, Smithers' suggests that radiation therapy works by killing the malignant cell and disrupting its preferential sites of involvement.

Patients with nodular sclerosing Hodgkin's disease tend to have upper thoracic disease that remains localized for longer periods in lymph nodes and adjacent structures. LPHD often presents as solitary peripheral lymph node involvement; extensive workup on such patients may not reveal other sites of disease. However, patients who present with apparently localized LDHD usually do have other, often subdiaphragmatic sites of involvement.

Subdividing lymphocyte-predominant disease into nodular and diffuse forms has resulted in the recognition of quite different clinical behaviors. The diffuse form acts like other Hodgkin's disease types, with relapse infrequent; when it occurs, it occurs early in the posttreatment period. The nodular form is commonly associated with relapses, independent of initial stage, and relapse occurs even after long relapse-free periods.[152]

Histologic evolution of Hodgkin's disease appears to occur concomitantly with progression of disease. For example, as the disease advances there is progressive loss of lymphocytes and an increase in the number of malignant cells and fibrosis. One type of the disease probably begins as LPHD and evolves into mixed cellularity and eventually to LDHD. The reticular form of this LDHD appears to be diminishing due to its correct classification as a diffuse lymphocytic or immunoblastic lymphoma. The nodular sclerosing form of the disease probably begins as a cellular phase that proceeds to the classic picture, showing subdivision of the nodes by fibrous bonds, and then to diffuse fibrosis and necrosis. Histologic characteristics and stage are often correlated. Lymphocyte-predominant and nodular sclerosing disease are more commonly diagnosed in stages I and II, but mixed-cellularity and lymphocyte-depleted disease are more commonly seen in the advanced stages.

DIAGNOSIS AND STAGING

Hodgkin's disease usually arises in lymph nodes. The initial diagnosis of Hodgkin's disease can only be made with a biopsy. Occasionally, multiple biopsies are necessary for proper diagnosis, because reactive hyperplasia of lymph nodes adjacent to those involved by tumor may lead to enlargement and encourage biopsy of a node that is easily accessible but uninvolved.[153] Needle aspiration of lymph nodes is inadequate for initial diagnosis, because it is not usually possible to subclassify the disease among the lymphomas with the limited amounts of biopsy material provided.

Staging is used to differentiate patients who can benefit from extended-field radiation therapy from those who require systemic treatment. Staging systems are anatomic descriptions that describe sites of tumor involvement in relation to the diaphragm. The first useful staging for Hodgkin's disease was developed by Peters and colleagues.[141,154] In 1965, a new staging system was developed at a meeting in Rye, New York, a system that added the designation stage IV to the Peters classification for patients with disseminated disease outside the lymph node system.[155] This was modified at the Ann Arbor Staging Conference in 1970.[156] The Ann Arbor version modified the previous classification in two major ways. First, based on data indicating that localized extensions did not alter prognosis if adequately irradiated, patients whose disease spread contiguously from lymph nodes to adjacent organs were not considered to have diffuse dissemination but were classified only by the extent of lymph node involvement (stages I–III) followed by the subscript *E*, which denoted direct extension.[157] Second, involvement of the spleen is indicated by the subscript *S*. In all systems, patients are classified further as *A* or *B* on the basis of the absence or presence of constitutional symptoms, such as fever higher than 38°C for 3 consecutive days, night sweats, or unexplained loss of more than 10% of body weight in the prior 6 months. At the Ann Arbor meeting, it was decided that pruritus, previously considered an important systemic symptom, did not by itself have prognostic impact and was not sufficient to include a patient in the B category.

In 1989, a new classification was proposed, known as the Cotswald system (Table 51–3).[158] It was developed because of the increasing use of new diagnostic techniques such, as computed tomography (CT) scanning and magnetic resonance

TABLE 51–3. The Cotswald Staging Classification for Hodgkin's Disease

Stage I	Involvement of a single lymph node region or a lymphoid structure (*e.g.*, spleen, thymus, Waldeyer's ring)
Stage II	Involvement of two or more lymph node regions on the same side of the diaphragm (*i.e.*, the mediastinum is a single site, hilar lymph nodes are lateralized). The number of anatomic sites should be indicated by a subscript (*e.g.*, II_2)
Stage III	Involvement of lymph node regions or structures on both sides of the diaphragm: III_1: With or without splenic hilar, celiac, or portal nodes III_2: With paraaortic, iliac, mesenteric nodes
Stage IV	Involvement of extranodal site(s) beyond that designated E:
	A: No symptoms
	B: Fever, drenching sweats, weight loss
	X: Bulky disease: >⅓ the width of the mediastinum >10 cm maximal dimension of nodal mass
	E: Involvement of a single extranodal site, contiguous or proximal to a known nodal site
	CS: Clinical stage
	PS: Pathologic stage

(Lister TA, Crowther D, Sutcliffe SB, et al. Report of a committee convened to discuss the evaluation and staging of patients with Hodgkin's disease: Cotswald meeting. J Clin Oncol 1989;7:1630–1636; J Clin Oncol [Erratum] 1990;8:1602)

imaging (MRI), and because of the greater appreciation of the influence of tumor bulk as a separate prognostic indicator within any given stage. It recognizes mediastinal adenopathy of greater than one third of the widest internal diameter of the chest or any tumor mass greater than 10 cm in diameter by the designation *X*. With the new schema, patients with residual abnormalities after treatment, which cannot be confirmed as benign or malignant, are designated as CRu (u for unconfirmed).

Table 51–4 outlines the recommended staging procedures.[159] Staging starts with a detailed history and physical examination. The history must be careful to determine the presence or absence of systemic symptoms. Physical examination should determine the extent of lymph node involvement. Basic laboratory tests include evaluation of renal and hepatic function, complete blood count, erythrocyte sedimentation rate, and serum lactate dehydrogenase and alkaline phosphatase levels. Roentgenographic studies include the chest radiograph and thoracic CT scan to evaluate mediastinal lymphadenopathy and any extension of such adenopathy into the surrounding viscera. If the chest x-ray film is normal, a CT scan is usually unnecessary. Abdominal involvement is evaluated using the lower-extremity lymphogram and abdominal CT.

With the advent of CT, the routine use of the bipedal lymphogram has been questioned, but it is still the superior staging tool because its sensitivity and specificity are superior to CT scans and because it can determine abnormal architecture of nodes and enlargement.[160–163] Although more labor intensive, the lymphogram has other important features. It can be used as a guide to ensure the removal of involved nodes during laparotomy and confirm their removal afterward, and it can identify abnormal nodes when they are not enlarged. It also is an inexpensive way of monitoring response to treatment. The CT scan is easier to administer and more valuable in the assessment of hepatic portal, mesenteric, and celiac lymph nodes.

Bone marrow biopsy, not aspiration, is required, because Hodgkin's of the marrow is often spotty and associated with fibrosis. Bone marrow biopsy is particularly important in symptomatic patients and in those with bone lesions, bone pain, hypercalcemia, or an elevated level of serum alkaline phosphatase.[164–168]

TABLE 51–4. Required Evaluation Procedures in Staging Hodgkin's Disease

1. Adequate surgical biopsy, reviewed by an experienced hematologist
2. A detailed history recording duration and the presence or absence of fever, unexplained sweating and its severity, unexplained pruritus, and unexplained weight loss
3. A careful and detailed physical examination; special attention to all node-bearing areas, including Waldeyer's ring and determination of size of liver and spleen
4. Necessary laboratory procedures
   a. Complete blood count, including an erythrocytic sedimentation rate
   b. Serum alkaline phosphatase level
   c. Evaluation of renal function
   d. Evaluation of liver function
5. Radiologic studies
   a. Chest radiograph (posteroanterior and lateral)
   b. Chest and abdominal computed tomography scan
   c. Bilateral lower-extremity lymphogram
   d. Views of skeletal system to include thoracic and lumbar vertebrae, the pelvis, proximal extremities, and any areas of bone tenderness

Isotopic scanning of the liver, spleen, and bone may be helpful in defining sites of additional disease. Gallium scanning may be useful, especially the higher-dose (7–10 mCi) imaging on a triple-peak Anger camera. Single-photon emission CT (SPECT) has resulted in the occasional finding of unexpected disease but is more useful in determining suspected recurrence in previously treated patients.[169] Data suggest that lymphomatous involvement of lymph nodes may have a different MRI pattern than fibrosis. This finding, like gallium scanning, may be important in evaluating patients for residual disease or recurrence after treatment.

STAGING LAPAROTOMY

Staging laparotomy is less important than it was 10 years ago.[159,170] It was originally developed by the Stanford group to provide information about the patterns of involvement in subdiaphragmatic Hodgkin's disease.[149] Its justification is that if it alters stage, which it often does, it will alter therapy. The latter should not often be the case, however, because the major determinant of the decision to proceed to laparotomy is whether radiation therapy alone will be used for treatment. Because more stages of Hodgkin's disease are being treated with chemotherapy alone or in combination with radiation therapy, laparotomy need not be done in these patients.[171]

If laparotomy is done, it must be carried out by physicians skilled in the technique, who perform it in a consistent fashion and in conjunction with the treating physician.[172,173] It should include a detailed inspection of the abdomen. The removed spleen should be sectioned in 0.3-cm slices. If disease is identified in the spleen, the total number of nodules should be enumerated. The weight of the spleen should be determined. Examination of the liver should include a wedge biopsy of the right lobe, three needle biopsies of the right and left lobes, and a biopsy of any grossly abnormal hepatic lesions. After inspection and palpation of the nodal groups, a biopsy should be taken of the right and left paraaortic and iliac nodes, regardless of their character on palpation and even if they appear normal on lymphography. Suspicious nodes identified on lymphography should be removed. Lymph nodes should be removed from the splenic hilar, porta, hepatic, mesenteric, and iliac regions. At one time, oophoropexy, the placement of the ovaries out of their normal position to shield them from pelvic irradiation, was recommended routinely for young female patients. This no longer is an indication for laparotomy or necessary for treatment, because the use of pelvic irradiation has been almost eliminated. Iliac bone marrow biopsy should be performed at the time of operation. The early studies employing routine staging laparotomy observed that alterations in clinical stage were made as frequently as 35% of the time as a result of the findings obtained at surgical staging.[174–177] After physical examination and chest x-ray films, approximately 90% of patients are categorized as having early-stage disease (stage I or II). After lymphography, one third of these patients are shown to have more advanced disease. Another one third of patients with clinically diagnosed early-stage disease are placed in higher stages after laparotomy. In the average institution, after all staging procedures are completed, 60% of patients are considered to have stages III or IV disease, and 40% have stages I or II.[159]

Staging laparotomy is a major surgical procedure with established morbidity and mortality.[179–181] Institutions with the most extensive experience report mortality statistics as low as 0.1%, but much higher rates have been reported.[181,182] Morbidity may include wound infection, subphrenic abscess, pulmonary embolus, stress ulcer, gastrointestinal bleeding, pulmonary infection, and wound dehiscence. Staging laparotomy and splenectomy in children require special consideration. Although the complication rate is similar to that observed in adults, there is an increased incidence of severe, sudden, overwhelming infection in children after staging laparotomy and splenectomy.[178–180,183–186] The risk of this complication increases as age decreases below 10 years. It seems prudent to be selective in the use of such procedures in young patients.[187,188]

No evidence suggests that splenectomy improves the ability to administer chemotherapy or radiation therapy, increases the response rate, or alters the survival rate.[189–192] Several studies reported a disconcerting increase in secondary leukemias in patients who have undergone splenectomy compared with similarly treated patients who have not had surgical staging.[193,194] There is no good explanation for this finding, but the consistency of the data between studies suggests it is a real risk. Laparotomy does, however, treat the involved spleen. The reduction of the irradiated field required may permit the physician to avoid irradiating a significant portion of the stomach, intestine, left kidney, and left lower lobe of the lung. Posttreatment laparotomy as a guide to further management has had mixed results and should not be considered a routine procedure.[195,196]

PATTERNS OF CLINICAL PRESENTATION

The clinical presentation of Hodgkin's disease varies in different geographic locations and clinical settings. Reviews of patients seen at the Harvard Joint Center for Radiotherapy in Boston (JCRT) may serve as an example (Table 51–5).[197,198] In this group, 57% of patients were male, 24% had systemic symptoms, 85% were younger than 40 years of age, and 60% had lymphocyte-predominant histology. The predominant sites of lymph node involvement were the mediastinum (59%), left neck (58%), and right neck (55%). One of these sites of involvement existed in 92% of the patients seen. Some sites were positively correlated with each other while others were not (Figs. 51–3 and 51–4), suggesting possible clinical evolution of the disease.[198] Epitrochlear, popliteal, and mesenteric nodes are uncommonly involved. The spleen is involved in approximately 25% of patients.

Liver involvement without splenic involvement is rare in Hodgkin's disease. The risk of liver involvement increases as the size of the involved spleen increases. Liver involvement is also unusual in patients who have normal-sized spleens, ev... spleens are involved in Hodgkin's disease.[141] Bone ...lvement with Hodgkin's disease is associated with ...mor and usually with systemic symptoms.[199,200] ...anemia, or thrombocytopenia are rarely seen, ...vated alkaline phosphatase level may give some hint of bone marrow involvement. The bones themselves may be involved, especially in patients with advanced disease. Rarely, there is invasion of the bone from adjacent lymphadenopathy. The bone lesions are usually osteolytic but may be osteoblastic. Radioisotopic bone scans may reveal focal areas of increased uptake although conventional radiographs

TABLE 51–5. Upstaging of Stage I and II Patients by Clinical Parameters

Subgroup	*No. of Patients*	*PS III-IV (%)*	*p Value (Logistic Regression)*
Sex			
M	296	85 (29%)	0.003
F	256	46 (18%)	
Symptomatic stage			
A	444	94 (21%)	0.027
B	108	37 (34%)	
Sites			
1	171	28 (17%)	0.003
≥2	381	103 (27%)	
Age			
≤39	481	110 (23%)	0.081
≤40	71	21 (30%)	
Histology			
LP/NS	403	91 (23%)	Not significant
MC/LD	149	40 (27%)	

PS, pathologic stage; LP, lymphocyte predominant; NS, nodular sclerosing; MC, mixed cellularity; LD, lymphocyte depleted.
(Mauch P, Larson D, Osteen R, et al. Prognostic factors for positive surgical staging in patients with Hodgkin's disease. J Clin Oncol 1990;8:257–265)

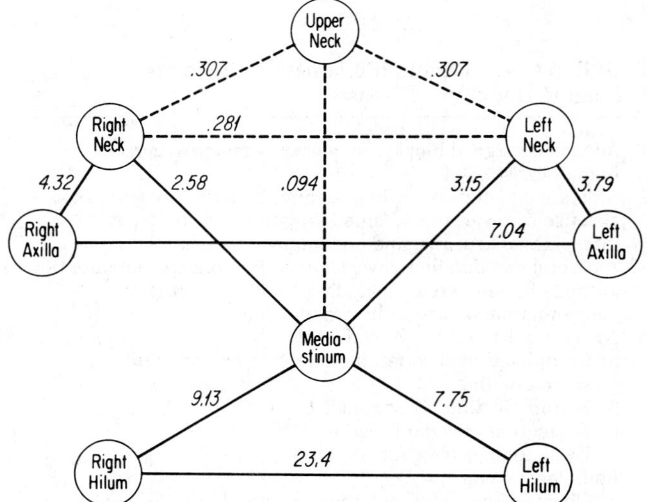

FIGURE 51–3. Patterns of presentation of Hodgkin's disease. Solid lines indicate positive associations, and dotted lines indicate negative associations. Odds ratios are written next to the lines for statistically significant associations ($p \leq 0.01$). (Mauch P, Kalish LA, Kadin M, et al. Patterns of presentation of Hodgkin's disease: Implications for etiology and pathogenesis. Cancer 1992 [in press])

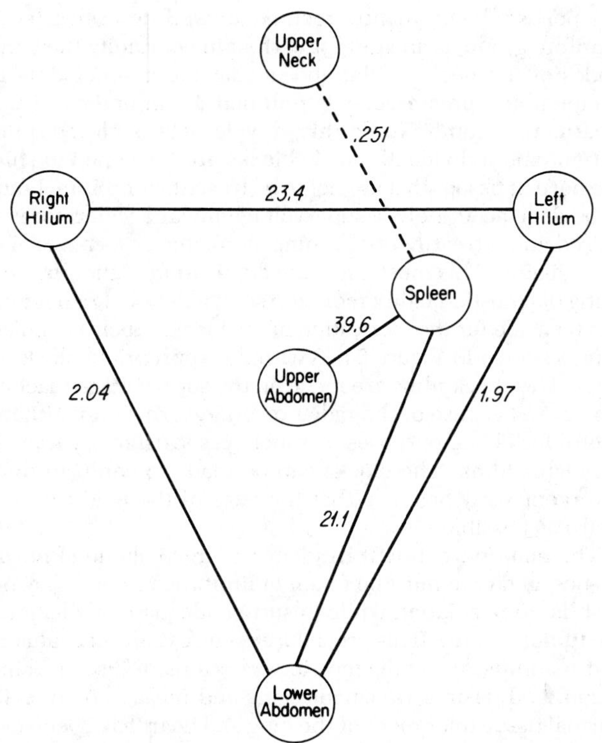

FIGURE 51–4. Patterns of presentation of Hodgkin's disease. Solid lines indicate positive associations, and dotted lines indicate negative associations. Odds ratios are written next to the lines for statistically significant associations ($p \leq 0.01$). (Mauch P, Kalish LA, Kadin M, et al. Patterns of presentation of Hodgkin's disease: Implications for etiology and pathogenesis. Cancer 1992 [in press])

are normal.[201] Such findings are not always evidence of involvement and should be confirmed histologically if possible. Involvement of the bone should not be equated with involvement of the marrow unless there is other evidence of widely disseminated disease. Musshoff and Boutis demonstrated long-term disease-free survival in patients with isolated bone lesions if treated appropriately with radiation therapy.[202]

Involvement of the skin, subcutaneous tissue, and breast can occur with Hodgkin's disease.[203] The disease rarely involves the central nervous system, although invasion of the epidural space can occur by extension through the intervertebral foramina from paraaortic lymph nodes, with neurologic symptoms and pain as the predominant clinical features.[204–206] Unlike other malignant lymphomas, Hodgkin's disease rarely arises in the gastrointestinal tract. Compression of the ureters from lymphadenopathy may occur. Unusual urologic complications of Hodgkin's disease are lipoid nephrosis and amyloid nephrosis, which may occur although no other clinical manifestations of persistence or recurrence are detected.[207,208] They have been reported to regress after effective antitumor treatment. Pleural effusions with low specific gravity and low protein content are usually simple transudates. Neither these nor exudative pleural effusions are indicative of pleural invasion of Hodgkin's disease. Such a diagnosis requires histologic confirmation by pleural biopsy or open thoracotomy. These effusions are often the consequence of hilar or pulmonary involvement. Pericardial involvement may occur as a result of direct invasion from mediastinal lymphadenopathy.

TREATMENT

RADIATION THERAPY

The extreme radiation responsiveness of the lymphomas was noticed shortly after the discovery of x-rays. In 1902, Pusey reported a series of patients with Hodgkin's disease treated with irradiation. In the early part of the century, therapy was limited by the equipment available.[209] The machines had poor depth-dose characteristics and caused extensive skin reactions, limiting their usefulness. Despite this drawback, there was abundant interest in irradiating this tumor. Teschendorf,[210] Voorhoeve,[211] and Kruchen[212] described therapy for these patients. It was Gilbert who laid the foundation for the principles of modern radiation therapy, despite the availability of only orthovoltage radiation therapy.[139,140] Gilbert recognized the importance of treating all involved disease with the maximal dose possible if cure was the goal. He suggested treating adjacent sites, to the extent possible, because of the frequency of adjacent recurrences. These are the principles of radiation therapy today. Gilbert's technique was followed in Toronto and reported by Peters in 1950.[141] She reported patients who were alive as long as 20 years after treatment, indicating that patients could be cured with irradiation, because there were no recurrences in patients who were disease-free 10 years after treatment.[142] The concept of irradiation of adjacent nodal groups with lower doses of radiation was used by Peters.

In 1963, Easson and Russell published an article entitled, "The Cure of Hodgkin's Disease."[213] This work reported the long-term results of local treatment of Hodgkin's disease and localized non-Hodgkin's lymphomas. The paper emphasized that Hodgkin's disease could be cured. Other investigators in the early 1950s and 1960s reported the results of localized irradiation, but it was Kaplan and his group at Stanford who systematically studied the role of radiation therapy in the treatment of Hodgkin's disease and devised new techniques using supervoltage techniques to treat the disease.[214–219] These pioneering studies form the basis of much of what we know today about the curability of Hodgkin's disease.

The information in Figure 51–5 comes from a compilation of studies demonstrating a dose-response association.[220] Although low doses of radiation cause tumors to disappear, high doses are required to ablate them permanently. Hodgkin's disease, like other tumors, has a dose-response curve. This was an important concept, because the prevailing attitude at the time was that, because the disease was responsive to radiation but still incurable, low doses should be given to make local nodal masses regress while "saving" the radiation tolerance for the required subsequent therapies after the disease reappeared. This philosophy of treatment confirmed the self-fulfilling prophecy of the incurability of Hodgkin's disease. However, as seen in the figure, after high doses were given, local recurrence was uncommon.

The Stanford group provided evidence, suspected by Gilbert and Peters, of the orderliness and continuity of the initial presentation of Hodgkin's disease and of its subsequent extension.[217,219] The adaptation of modern supervoltage tech-

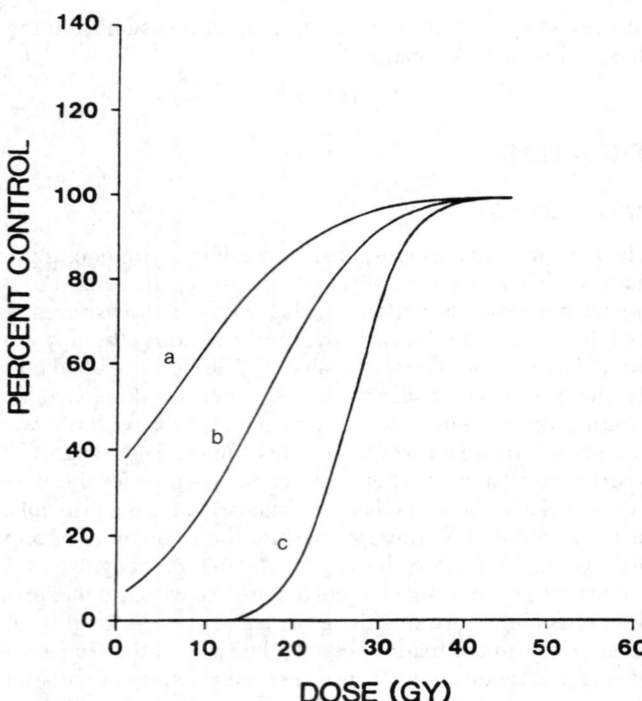

FIGURE 51–5. Dose-response curves (kV and MV data) for subclinical (curve a), <6-cm (curve b) and 6-cm (curve c) nodes. Higher doses are required for equal probabilities of control as disease burden increases. (Vijayakumar S, Myrianthopoulos LC. An updated dose-response analysis in Hodgkin's disease. Radiother Oncol 1992;24:1–13)

niques for the treatment of Hodgkin's disease for the first time allowed high doses of radiation to be given in extensive volumes, and careful beam direction and shielding allowed the treatment to be tolerated by normal tissues.

It is recommended that local tumor masses receive "boost therapy" to a minimal dose of 4000 to 4400 cGy, but apparently uninvolved areas treated for subclinical disease appear to be controlled adequately with doses of 3000 to 3500 cGy. Other data suggest that 3000 cGy may be sufficient.[221] The dose-time relation for Hodgkin's disease is less well known. Because of normal tissue tolerance, patient acceptance, and tumor control, tumor doses of between 150 and 220 cGy per day given five times each week appear to be appropriate. If a significant interruption in treatment occurs, it appears that larger doses should be given.[222] Supervoltage methods must be used to deliver the wide-field radiation required. This method has the advantages of spared skin, increased depth dose, and sharp beam edges with reduced lateral scatter.

A basic tool for the treatment of patients with Hodgkin's disease is the modern linear accelerator, which provides x-ray beams in the 4- to 8-MeV range. Although cobalt units can be used, conventionally available cobalt units have significant limitations. When used at distances of less than 80 cm, they tend to have poor depth-dose characteristics. They often have far less well defined beam edges, because of the large source and short treatment distances. This latter factor causes significantly greater irradiation of adjacent and apparently shielded tissues.

Hodgkin's disease treatment may be divided into three volumes to be irradiated: the mantle, the paraaortic area, and the pelvis.[223] The mantle technique, well described by the Stanford group, is an attempt to treat in continuity the lymph nodes of the neck, axilla, and mediastinum—including the occipital and preauricular lymph nodes—in one contiguous treatment volume. To do this, a wide field is placed on the patient and individually made blocks are fashioned to shield the normal tissues that are not to be treated. For this technique to be done accurately, a supervoltage linear accelerator is required and a treatment-planning simulator or localizer must be available. This must allow the duplication of therapy fields using diagnostic-quality radiation so that detailed radiographs can be made for the fabrication of the blocks. Such a simulator film is shown in Figure 51–6 with the appropriate block outlines. The check films are made on the supervoltage machine. However, because of the radiation energy, this film, although useful for check purposes, is much less satisfactory than the simulator films. The blocks can be made to conform to the divergent x-ray beam so that the edge of the field can be as sharp as possible.

The mantle treatment irradiates a large volume of normal tissues, and care must be taken to limit the unnecessary normal tissue irradiation while ensuring adequate irradiation of the tumor volume. This procedure requires careful evaluation and planning, using diagnostic x-ray films, CT scans, simulation, and dosimetric calculations and measurements. The normal tissue tolerances of the lung and heart have been evaluated in the course of treatment of Hodgkin's disease.[224–226] Whole-lung irradiation, to a maximal dose of 1650 cGy in 150-cGy fractions, is used frequently if the ipsilateral hilum is involved with tumor. The whole heart should not be treated unless evidence of pericardial involvement exists. Under normal circumstances, a significant portion of the cardiac silhouette can be shielded. It is important that the match-line between the mantle and the paraaortic area does not allow overlap of a portion of the spinal cord. If this overlap occurs, the dose that is received can cause significant neurologic

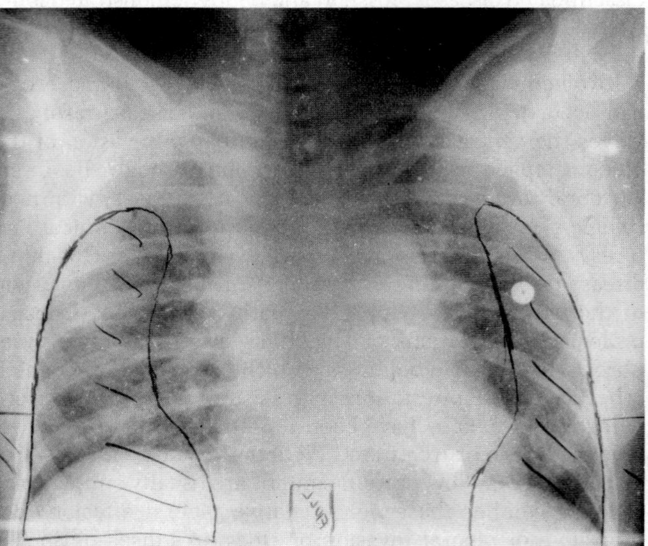

FIGURE 51–6. Simulated film for radiation treatment fields in a patient with mediastinal Hodgkin's disease. Dark lines indicate shielding blocks.

damage. The geometry involved in proper field arrangement for the match-line can be more complicated than is immediately apparent. Techniques to match these fields properly have been described.[227] Farah reported excellent results using a combined mantle and paraaortic field, avoiding any question of overlap at the match-line.[228] The dose per fraction is reduced to 160 cGy, resulting in a shorter treatment course. Treatments of the paraaortic nodes and pelvis are frequently done together as described by the Stanford group.[229,230] It is the experience of others that this treatment is better tolerated if divided into a paraaortic field and a separate pelvic field. In either circumstance, the paraaortic field must be wide enough to include the paraaortic lymph nodes as demonstrated on the lymphogram.

Most modern radiotherapeutic techniques have been influenced by the results of laparotomy. Laparotomy is only of value if the results may alter therapy. It allows removal of the spleen and the placement of radiopaque clips on the splenic pedicle, so that the radiation therapy field may be tailored accurately to this volume. The normal right side of the paraaortic field, as shown in Figure 51–7, does not treat the porta hepatitis; if it is to be treated, the field must be extended laterally. The same considerations for field overlap apply between the paraaortic and pelvic fields; however, these fields are less critical, because this overlap area is below the level of the spinal cord. Considerations for the pelvic field include the treatment of the lymph nodes with as little radiation as possible to important sacral and pelvic bone marrow. The need for pelvic treatment has been markedly reduced, because stages I and II supradiaphragmatic Hodgkin's disease can be treated without pelvic irradiation, and for stage III disease, total nodal irradiation has a limited role. If the pelvic field is to be treated, the amount of marrow irradiated may be greatly reduced by careful blocking and by the use of linear accelerators rather than cobalt units. Adequate covering of the inguinal and femoral lymph nodes must be ensured, and the testes should be shielded. For women, a central block can be placed and the ovaries moved to the midline by tacking them in front or in back of the uterus, a technique first described by Trueblood and colleagues.[231]

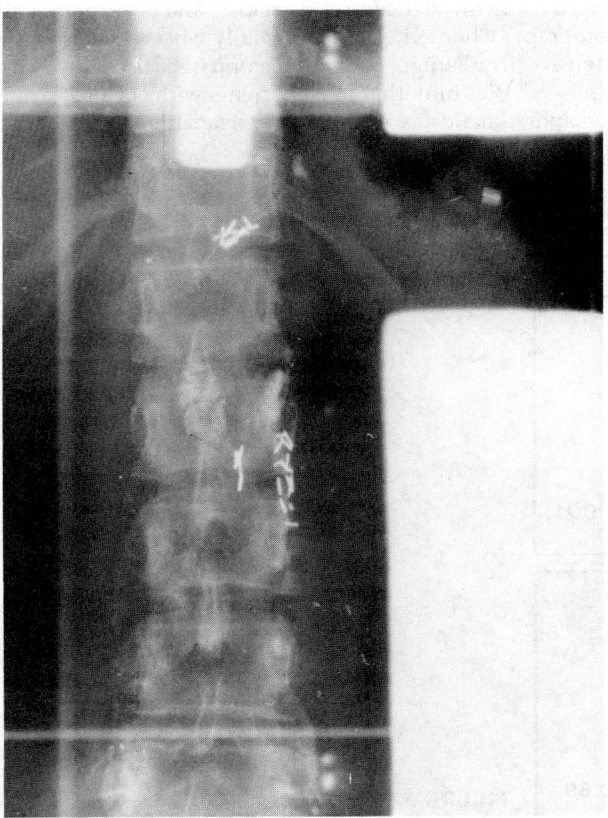

FIGURE 51–7. Normal paraaortic field used in treating a patient with Hodgkin's disease below the diaphragm. The porta hepatic nodes were not involved.

Although individual preference in technique may have a role, most important are the general principles of careful beam definition, detailed patient positioning, use of simulators, individually constructed shielding techniques, and verification of dose, usually using thermoluminescent dosimetry. Small technical considerations, such as the position of the arm, can greatly influence the amount of normal tissue treated and must be considered carefully. Maximal cure with minimal complications can occur only if all the technical aspects of radiation therapy are considered carefully. This fact has been substantiated in a review of the pattern of radiation treatment that related recurrence to technical inadequacies. The facility at which treatment was given significantly affected recurrence rate. Even among university medical centers, technical differences had a significant effect on relapse-free survival. The rates of in-field or marginal recurrence varied from 0% to 11% at different centers among patients with identical-stage disease, and the relapse rate varied from 10% to 39%. These differences did not relate to variations in staging procedures. The portal films of a random sample of patients treated for curative intent were reviewed, and in more than one third of the cases, the treatment portal films did not adequately cover the disease, and more than half of these patients had relapses. For patients with adequate portals, relapse rate was only 14% over a 4-year period.[226,232]

Results of Radiation Therapy

With the results of radiation therapy reported by Peters and associates[142,143] and Easson and Russell,[213] the question of whether uninvolved areas should be irradiated became an important one. In 1966, Peters carefully analyzed her data in an attempt to answer this question.[144] Review of these data makes it difficult to prove that irradiation of the uninvolved lymph nodes in stage I or IIA disease affects the outcome. The Stanford group conducted a randomized, prospective clinical trial (L1) that compared local irradiation with extended-field irradiation for treating stages I and II disease.[141] This study showed no significant difference between involved-field and extended-field irradiation with respect to survival or freedom from relapse. A similar national collaborative study also failed to show significant differences.[233] These studies preceded the use of staging laparotomy and also failed to consider the paraaortic area as a contiguous site for supraclavicular node disease.

A new trial was introduced at Stanford (H1) in which the alternatives for stages I and IIA disease were involved-field irradiation and total nodal irradiation (TNI).[235] This study was

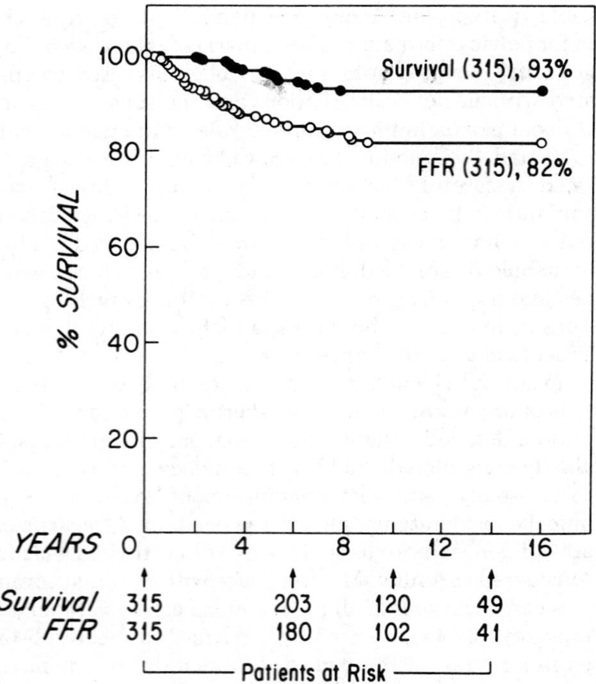

FIGURE 51–8. Survival and freedom from first relapse (FFR) rates for pathologic stage IA and IIA patients treated with mantle and para-aortic–splenic pedicle irradiation. Median follow-up time was 9 years. (Mauch P, Tarbell N, Weinstein, et al. Stage IA and IIA supradiaphragmatic Hodgkin's disease: Prognostic factors in surgically staged patients treated with mantle and para-aortic irradiation. J Clin Oncol 1988;6:1576–1583)

started 1 year before the introduction of laparotomy at Stanford; therefore, most of the patients in this study had staging laparotomies. Results of this study showed a highly significant difference in relapse-free survival in favor of TNI, although overall survival was not affected.[141]

TNI is far more extensive than the intended irradiation of subclinical contiguous disease in stages I and IIA patients. For supradiaphragmatic disease, pelvic irradiation can probably be eliminated. This deletion would greatly reduce the amount of bone marrow irradiated and limit the dose to the gonads. Such a technique for supradiaphragmatic stages I and IIA patients has been recommended at the JCRT.[164,197] The results of such treatment are shown in Figure 51–8. Relapse-free and overall survival rates for stages IA and IIA patients are 82% and 93%, respectively. Review of the 315 patients treated in this manner with a median follow-up of 9 years reveals a 3% rate of pelvic nodal recurrences. This result indicates that the pelvis can be spared irradiation, and the patient still derives the value of extended-field irradiation. This method permits adequate chemotherapy dosage and a decreased likelihood for tumor induction or fatal infection.[234] These studies were done in laparotomy-staged patients in whom the spleen had been removed.

As long-term follow-up increases, it appears that freedom from relapse depends on initial therapy but that survival of patients with early-stage Hodgkin's disease does not, because salvage chemotherapy is so good that overall survival is unaffected. Figure 51–9 describes the results of patients treated at Stanford with involved fields compared with those treated by extended-field irradiation. Chemotherapy with a regimen of nitrogen mustard, vincristine, procarbazine, and prednisone (MOPP) for these radiation therapy failures is quite successful (Table 51–6).[236–238]

The goal of treatment is to cure the most patients with the least therapy to avoid complications. Only 32% of patients treated by involved fields avoid relapse, and 68% require chemotherapy. Chemotherapy, especially when combined with extensive irradiation, may be accompanied by late complications.[239] We think that most patients with stages I or II supradiaphragmatic disease treated by irradiation should receive extended-field irradiation.

Data from the M.D. Anderson Cancer Center,[240] the European Organization for the Research and Treatment of Cancer (EORTC),[241] St. Bartholomew's Hospital,[242] and Memorial

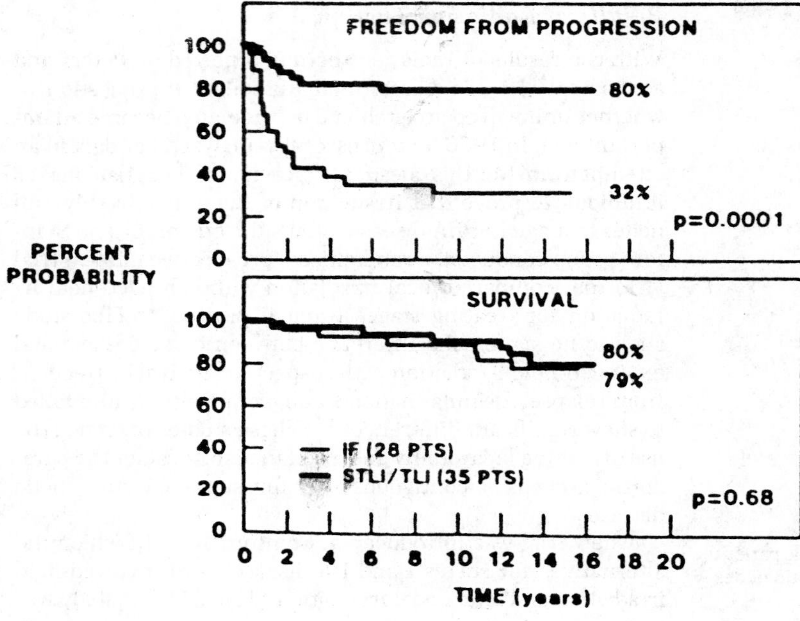

FIGURE 51–9. Involved-field (IF) versus extended-field irradiation. (Rosenberg SA, Kaplan HS. The evolution and summary results of the Stanford randomized clinical trials of the management of Hodgkin's disease: 1962–1984. Int J Radiat Oncol Biol Phys 1985;11:5–22)

TABLE 51–6. MOPP for Hodgkin's Disease Relapse After Initial Radiation Therapy

Investigations	*Initial Stage*	*No. of Patients*	*5-Year Relapse-Free Survival (%)*	*5-Year Survival (%)*
Timothy et al[236]	IA–IIIA	33	85	92
Portlock[237]	IA–IIIA	46	50	58
Mauch et al[238]	IA–IIIA	28	70	70

Hospital pediatric studies[243] have indicated that relapse-free survival was similar in laparotomy-staged patients treated with a mantle field only, compared with those treated more extensively. In these studies, the patients were usually selected for having no or only minimal mediastinal involvement. The EORTC included only patients younger than 40 years of age with nodular sclerosis or lymphocyte-predominant histology, an erythrocyte sedimentation rate of less than 70, and only one or two sites of involvement. These data must be used with caution for patients with more extensive disease.

Although treatment of the paraaortic field is not associated with significant long-term toxic effects, it does cause acute symptoms. It increases the amount of bone marrow irradiated, and in the pediatric patient, it significantly damages growth in the axial spine. It is desirable to avoid the use of the paraaortic field, which may be possible for clinically staged IA patients with lymphocyte-predominant histology and high neck involvement.[244] Its use in patients with more extensive disease results in a greater number of relapses. Although overall survival may be the same, more patients are exposed to chemotherapy. The appropriate treatment of Hodgkin's disease by stage is discussed later in this chapter.

A separate subgroup of patients with stage I or II disease has a higher likelihood for relapse. These patients have large mediastinal masses.[245] Review of such patients at the JCRT revealed that, of 315 stage IA and IIA patients treated with mantle or paraaortic fields, 35 had mediastinal masses greater than one third of the total chest diameter (Table 51–7). Patients relapsed within the initial treatment volume and in adjacent, untreated lymph nodes, and extranodal relapse occurred primarily in the lung. These patients are more likely to experience recurrence, even at involved sites separate from the mediastinum.

TABLE 51–7. Influence of Mediastinal Hodgkin's Disease Treated With Mantle and Paraaortic Irradiation After Relapse

Extent of Disease	*No. of Patients*	*14-Year Relapse Free Survival (%)*
No mediastinal disease	142	87
Mediastinal disease		
≤1/3	138	85
>1/3	35	53

(Mauch P, Gorshein D, Cunningham J, et al. Influence of mediastinal adenopathy on site and frequency of relapse in patients with Hodgkin's disease. Cancer Treat Rep 1982;66:809–817)

Investigators disagree about the best treatment for patients with large mediastinal masses. Significant numbers of patients with large mediastinal masses who fail to respond to irradiation only may be salvaged with chemotherapy, and their ultimate results are similar to patients treated by combined modalities initially. However, treatment with initial irradiation often requires extensive irradiation of the heart and lung to include the large mediastinal mass, which can be the source of significant morbidity. Despite this drawback, with the careful use of thoracic CT scanning, patients may be selected for radiation therapy only.[246] It appears that the treatment of patients with large mediastinal masses needs to be individualized to maximize cure while avoiding unnecessary complications of irradiation or combined-modality treatment.

The prognostic importance of large mediastinal masses has been reported repeatedly.[247–250] Most patients with stage I or IIA disease have no or little mediastinal involvement. For this group, the relapse-free survival rate is 86%, and the overall survival rate is 93%, using a technique that spares the pelvis from irradiation.[251] There appears to be a subgroup of patients with disease limited only to the mediastinum. These patients rarely (2 of 22) have large masses and enjoy excellent prognoses, with an 85% relapse-free rate and 100% overall actuarial survival rate at 8 years.[250–253]

Extensive mediastinal involvement causes several additional problems for patients. They appear to be anesthesia risks, with difficulty occurring during extubation, and the risk-benefit ratio of laparotomy increases.[254] Although this risk can be greatly reduced by irradiating the mass before exploratory laparotomy, the treatment involves a significant amount of heart and lung. This provides another reason for treating these patients with primary chemotherapy, restricting radiation to a limited role as a boost technique at the end of the chemotherapy. Review of three sequential staging and treatment programs—pathologic staging and radiation therapy, pathologic staging and combined-modality treatment, and clinical staging and combined-modality treatment—showed the group receiving only radiation therapy to have the poorest freedom from relapse. They are successfully salvaged with chemotherapy, resulting in similar overall survival rates (Fig. 51–10).[253]

Although the data for subdiaphragmatic-presentation stages I and IIA disease are far more limited, the results of extended-field treatment appear equally satisfactory.[255] In the JCRT experience, there were 15 such patients, with two recurrences. The question of the importance of histology is not certain. It is thought that mixed-cellularity and lymphocyte-depleted disease are more likely present with higher-stage disease when carefully evaluated.

The first curative attempt at treatment of stage III disease

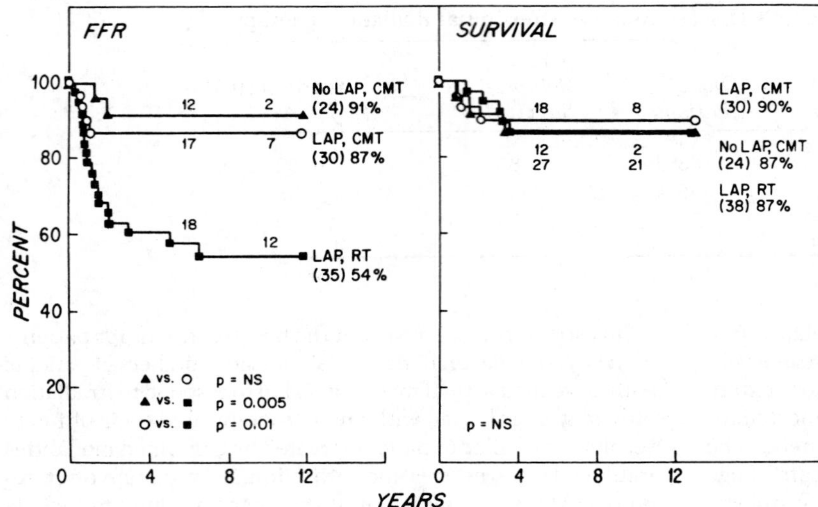

FIGURE 51–10. Actuarial freedom from first relapse (FFR) and survival rates of clinical stage IA and IIB Hodgkin's disease patients undergoing staging laparotomy and radiation therapy, staging laparotomy and combined radiation therapy and chemotherapy (CMT), or CMT without staging laparotomy. (Leopold KA, Canellos GP, Rosenthal D, et al. Stage IA–IIIB Hodgkin's disease: Staging and treatment with large mediastinal adenopathy. J Clin Oncol 1989;7:1059–1065)

was presented in the Stanford (L2) protocol. This protocol compared the conventional low-dose irradiation (*i.e.*, palliative therapy for a disease that was considered to be incurable) with radical irradiation to all lymph node-bearing areas (TNI), including the spleen. Relapses occurred earlier and more frequently in the palliatively treated groups, but their ultimate survival was not statistically significantly lower, presumably because of the success of salvage drug therapy. The success of TNI was the first demonstration that some stage III patients could be cured with irradiation only.[214] Figure 51–11 reveals the actuarial survival and relapse-free survival rates for laparotomy-staged IIIA patients from the JCRT. Despite the increased accuracy of staging, more than 50% of the patients so treated experience relapse.[256] Although many of these patients can be salvaged by subsequent combination chemotherapy, initial treatment with combined-modality therapy is associated with an overall improvement in survival.

Attempts to subdivide these patients into stages IIIA1 and IIIA2 demonstrate the important prognostic significance of this substaging. But even stage IIIA1 patients have a significant likelihood of failure if treated with irradiation only (Fig. 51–12). Perhaps the only group associated with an excellent relapse-free survival rate are the stage IIIA2 patients with fewer than five splenic nodules, because in the JCRT experience, patients treated with radiation only had a 70% rate of freedom from first relapse and an overall survival rate of 100%. Total lymphoid irradiation in the hands of the Stanford group has been associated with a better relapse-free survival rate for stage III patients. These data are better than those from Yale or the JCRT.[257] Possible reasons for this difference include a

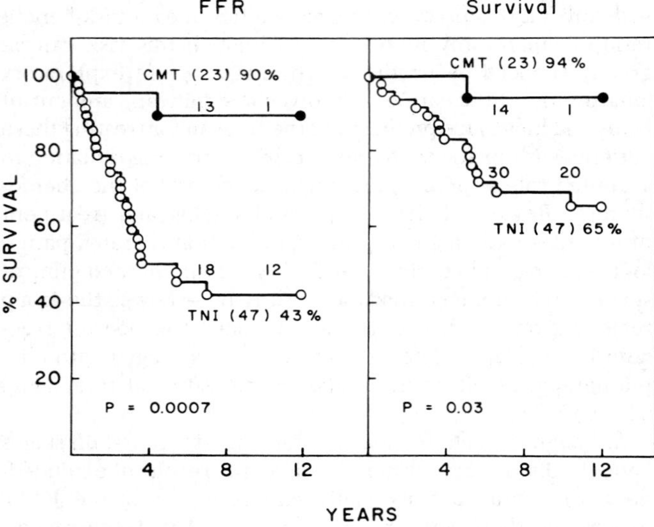

FIGURE 51–11. Actuarial relapse-free survival and survival rates for laparotomy-determined stage IIIA patients treated with combined-modality therapy (CMT) or total nodal irradiation (TNI). (Mauch P, Gorshein D, Cunningham J, et al. Influence of mediastinal adenopathy on site and frequency of relapse in patients with Hodgkin's disease. Cancer Treat Rep 1982;66:809–817)

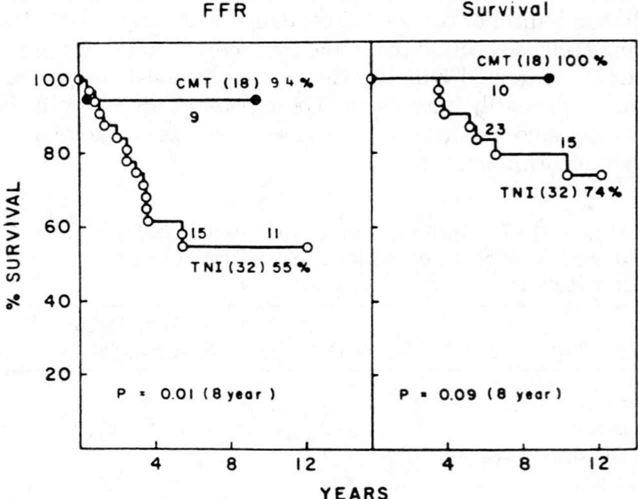

FIGURE 51–12. Freedom from relapse (FFR) and actuarial survival rates after total nodal irradiation (TNI) or combined-modality therapy (CMT) for pathologic stage IIIA1 Hodgkin's disease. (Mauch P, Gorshein D, Cunningham J, et al. Influence of mediastinal adenopathy on site and frequency of relapse in patients with Hodgkin's disease. Cancer Treat Rep 1982;66:809–817)

larger proportion of nodular sclerosis patients seen at Stanford and the routine irradiation of the liver employed there for treating patients with splenic involvement.

Treatment of stages IIB and IIIB Hodgkin's disease with irradiation alone can result in some cases of long-term, relapse-free survival (*i.e.*, approximately 30% in the Stanford L1 and L2 protocols using TNI). Although there is general agreement that radiation therapy alone is unsatisfactory treatment for stage IIIB disease, some data suggest that, in surgical stage IIB disease, irradiation alone may have the same results as combined-modality treatment.[141,256,258] A recent report combines the Stanford and JCRT results for these patients. In this series, 103 patients were treated with radiation therapy only; at 7 years, the rate of freedom from relapse was 74%, and the overall survival rate was 87%. Although the rate of freedom from relapse with combined-modality treatment was better (84%), the overall survival was the same.[259]

Complications of Radiation Treatment

Complications of treatment are related to the technique used, dose administered, and irradiated volume. Most of the complications associated with irradiation are seen in the mantle field.[260] Although no immediate changes are usually apparent on the chest radiograph or in clinical function, a paramediastinal pulmonary density that outlines the irradiated field may be seen on the x-ray film with time. These signs are usually without symptoms, although the patients occasionally may develop dry cough or dyspnea on exertion.

A more important potential complication is acute radiation pneumonitis. This side effect depends on the volume of the lung irradiated and the total dose given. Some changes in pulmonary function after irradiation can be seen if looked for carefully, but symptomatic radiation pneumonitis is much less common if the pulmonary volume irradiated is restricted. If whole-lung irradiation is required, the dose should be restricted to less than 1650 cGy. For example, of 315 patients with stage IA or IIA disease treated with mantle (and paraaortic) irradiation at the JCRT, only 16 (5.1%) developed symptomatic radiation pneumonitis.[251] Symptoms associated with this condition include shortness of breath, cough, and occasional fever. If a large volume of lung has been irradiated to high doses, these changes may become progressive and sometimes fatal.

Several techniques have been used to reduce pulmonary complications. Radiation therapy has been given to large pulmonary masses and interrupted at approximately 1500 cGy to allow time for the mass to shrink; the radiation was continued using smaller fields after a 2- or 3-week hiatus. Similarly, whole-lung irradiation has been given to patients with hilar lymph node involvement, using transmission blocks that allow only a portion of the dose to reach the lungs or fields that include the whole lungs but only to tolerable doses.[141] These techniques have allowed pulmonary irradiation without complications, although long-term follow-up reveals some persistent effects.[261]

Cardiac complications of radiation therapy in Hodgkin's disease were first reported by the Stanford group.[225] When the whole heart is irradiated to doses of greater than 3000 cGy, as many as 50% of the patients develop pericardial complications.[224] By limiting the volume of pericardium irradiated, keeping the radiation fraction less than 250 cGy, and limiting the total dose, such complications have become uncommon, with only 9 cases of pericarditis in 315 patients treated in the JCRT series.[251] It is important to avoid treating the whole pericardium, but if whole-pericardium irradiation is required, the dose must be limited. Technique is also important. If patients are treated primarily through anterior portals, a much larger dose is received by the anterior-placed heart. These techniques have resulted in significant cardiac complications and should be avoided.[262] New methods of cardiac evaluation have revealed abnormal ventricular ejection fractions in some patients long after mediastinal irradiation.[263,264] The symptom complex seen is largely that of pericarditis and, in some patients, continued pericardial fluid causing tamponade or eventual pericardial fibrosis. These conditions can be treated surgically.

Evidence suggests that early coronary artery disease may be a consequence of mediastinal irradiation.[265] One large epidemiologic study shows no significant increase in cardiac-related deaths in Hodgkin's disease patients.[266] However, long-term follow-up data from Stanford revealed disturbing results.[267] Review of the records of 2232 patients treated between 1961 and 1990 revealed 88 deaths, 54 from acute myocardial infarction and 34 from other cardiac complications. The relative risk of death from heart disease is 3.1 compared with age and sex matched controls. The risk was reduced, but still significant, in those who had received less than 3000 cGy to the mediastinum. The relative risk increased with periods of observation, with risk of acute myocardial infarction highest with irradiation of patients younger than 20 years of age ($p<0.01$). A significant decrease in long-term survival occurred as a result of cardiac toxicity.

The most common neurologic complication seen with irradiation is Lhermitte's sign. This transient complication of radiation therapy consists of numbness, tingling, or "electric" sensations, which are produced or exacerbated by head flexion. Carmel and Kaplan reported an incidence of 15% among their patients treated with mantle fields.[224] These symptoms are transitory and are not associated with permanent sequelae. The pathogenesis is unknown. Spinal cord transection can occur when a portion of the spinal cord is included in the mantle and paraaortic fields. If overlap is avoided, this complication does not occur at the doses of 3600 to 4000 cGy used. Radiation fibrosis in the brachial plexus rarely occurs. This complication usually arises if high doses of radiation are given to large neck and axillary tumor masses. Progressive motor and sensory loss have been recorded in patients who have received large doses. Rare malignant tumors of nerve sheaths have been reported long after radiation therapy.[268] These tumors usually are associated with irradiation and chemotherapy.

The thyroid gland is irradiated with the mantle, resulting in about 30% of patients developing an elevated thyroid-stimulating hormone level without T_3 or T_4 reduction.[269] With prompt supplemental thyroid treatment, clinical hypothyroidism has occurred in less than 5% of these patients.[251] Rarely, hyperthyroidism and exophthalmos are seen. Thyroid neoplasms rarely are seen with therapeutic doses of radiation.[270]

Complications related to paraaortic fields are uncommon, and if the doses and fields are as described, gastrointestinal complications are rare. In 315 patients receiving paraaortic field irradiation, there were 8 with complications (*i.e.*, small bowel obstructions) at the JCRT.[251] This 2.5% incidence is similar to that seen with laparotomy without radiation therapy. Pelvic treatment alone may cause persistent thrombocytopenia or leukopenia. This complication is rare with current techniques that use well-collimated linear accelerators and judicious blocks. Infectious complications of treatment occur if TNI and splenectomy are used.

CHEMOTHERAPY

Hodgkin's disease is curable by combination chemotherapy. Single-drug therapy plays a small role in the treatment of newly diagnosed patients, because experienced oncologists usually can select a combination drug program from the options displayed in the tables in this chapter that fit the condition of the patient; the use of drugs in combination is required to effect substantial remission rates and to ensure durable remissions.[271–315] Although remissions are attainable with single agents, they rarely last.

Nitrogen mustard was first used as treatment for lymphomas in 1943 by Goodman and associates.[316] The results, published after World War II, were exciting; they showed marked dissolution of lymph nodes in patients with Hodgkin's disease, but recurrence proved to be the rule. The period between 1942 and 1963 saw the introduction of several new drugs—other alkylating agents, corticosteroids, the antifols, the vinca alkaloids, and a drug almost entirely specific for Hodgkin's disease, procarbazine.[316–323] All were used in the first attempts to cure advanced Hodgkin's disease by combination chemotherapy.

The early studies with single agents did not provide any evidence of the capacity of chemotherapy to cure Hodgkin's disease. Figure 51–13 compares the only available series of untreated patients (all stages included) with the results using alkylating agents alone and with a modern series using all the drugs applied in combination programs given in sequence.[324–326] The shapes of the curves are similar. Median survival was approximately 1 year, and fewer than 5% of patients were alive at 5 years.

The first intensive, four-drug combination program for Hodgkin's disease used vincristine, methotrexate, cyclophosphamide, and prednisone (MOMP) given for 2.5 months.[327] The goal of this pilot protocol was to test the safety of such an approach. Only 14 patients were studied. The data showed the approach was safe and associated with a high complete remission rate (80%). The administration of a two-drug combination, vinblastine and chlorambucil, produced a complete remission rate of approximately 40%. However, this was not a significant improvement over the response achieved with vinblastine alone, and no information on the durability of these remissions—the hallmark of the capacity to cure—was given.[327,328]

In 1964, as experience with procarbazine accrued, the MOMP program was modified in several ways. The duration of treatment was lengthened to 6 months, and procarbazine was substituted for methotrexate.[327] This program was named MOPP.[70,327–333] Each of the agents in the MOPP regimen was selected based on its antitumor activity as a single agent, and the drugs were given in full doses and according to their optimal schedule, with the exception that rest intervals were spaced between cycles and timed, according to available cell kinetics data, to allow marrow recovery between cycles of treatment.[334] Drugs were selected to minimize overlapping toxicity to any single organ. Vincristine was selected over its analog vinblastine, even though vinblastine was the favored drug, because vincristine has less marrow toxicity (although vincristine produced more neurotoxicity). The four drugs were given over a 2-week period. A complete cycle of MOPP took 29 days and consisted of a 2-week treatment period and a 2-week recovery period. A minimum of six cycles was given until the patients achieved a complete remission or tumor grew despite treatment.

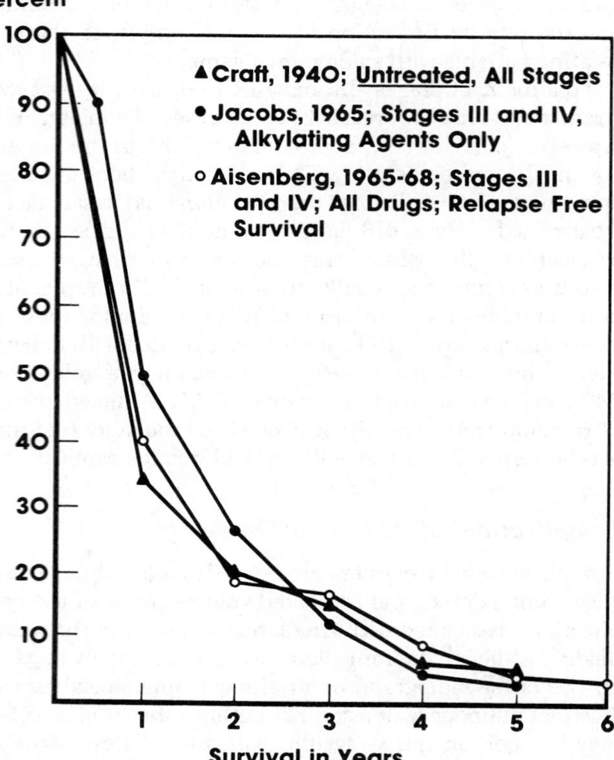

FIGURE 51–13. Two survival curves of patients with advanced Hodgkin's disease treated with single-agent chemotherapy compared with a group left untreated. (DeVita VT. Consequences of the chemotherapy of Hodgkin's disease. Cancer 1981;47:1–13)

Three features of MOPP were unique at the time. The goal of the program was to cure rather than to palliate, as had been the practice in the preceding 2 decades; the cyclic use of combination chemotherapy for 6 months exceeded the duration of any prior treatment of adult tumors; and it was the first regimen to make use of the sliding scale to adjust drug doses for marrow suppression. The sliding scale was designed to permit the administration of each cycle on time, with maximal allowable doses of each agent, and to preserve the dose rate and the integrity of the drug combination.[328] Provisions for delaying subsequent cycles were made only if toxicity was severe enough to require omission of drugs from that cycle. The sliding scale had an interesting effect on dosing in the MOPP regimen and later in other studies of combination chemotherapy. Usually, after two cycles at full or near-full doses,

TABLE 51–8. Twenty-Year MOPP Follow-Up Study by the National Cancer Institute

Number of evaluable patients	188
Number of complete responders	157 (84%)
Number of induction failures	31 (16%)
Number of relapses	56 (34%)
Number continuously free of disease	101 (54%)
Number dead	98 (52%)
Of Hodgkin's disease	68
Free of disease	30
Number alive	90 (48%)
With Hodgkin's disease	2
Free of disease	88

patients had significant myelosuppression, and doses in the third cycle had to be reduced according to the sliding scale to administer the third cycle on schedule and preserve the integrity of the combination (*i.e.*, give some of all four drugs). The impact of reducing doses in the third cycle was to allow the use of full or near-full doses in the fourth or later cycles. The net effect was preservation of dose rate by maintaining tight intervals between cycles.

At NCI, then and now, the dose of vincristine was given on the basis of body surface area and only modified for severe neurotoxicity. The lamentable current practice of capping the dose at a total of 2 mg has no scientific or medical justification and results in a top dose suitable only for persons smaller than 1.43m^2. These types of dose reduction have a deleterious impact on outcome. The standard practice was to administer a minimum of six cycles of treatment or enough cycles to attain a complete remission plus two additional cycles. The average duration of administration for six cycles in the NCI program was 5.8 months, and the omission of any drugs from the program was rare.

The MOPP regimen was considered high-dose, long-duration chemotherapy in 1964. However, subsequent calculations of its dose intensity, using the methods of Hryniuk and Bush[335] and DeVita and colleagues[336] show that it had a dose intensity of 70% of a hypothetical version of MOPP that would use the same four drugs in their full doses continuously, without rest intervals, over 6 months.[336] This type of inadvertent reduction in dose intensity is true of all cyclically administered drug combinations. The early results of the use of MOPP have been confirmed by others, and the durable remissions have been maintained in the NCI study over the past 20 years.[337] Table 51–8 shows the results of the original series after more than 20 years of follow-up. Eighty-four percent of patients attained complete remissions. Of those patients, 64% remain continuously disease-free (Fig. 51–14), and of all treated patients, 54% remain free of disease after a 20-year follow-up. Forty-eight percent of the total population is alive. The relapse-free survival curve illustrates that most negative events took place in the first 4 years of follow-up, after which the curve flattened and relapses were uncommon. The latest relapse in the MOPP study occurred 11 years after treatment was discontinued.

Only 5 (2.5%) patients died of treatment-related toxic effects. Despite the neurotoxicity associated with full doses of vincristine (*i.e.*, 1.4 mg/m^2 with no dose capping), no patients were permanently paralyzed using a sliding-scale adjustment based on the actual appearance of neurotoxic side effects.

The major factors negatively affecting complete response rate in the original study were B symptoms, male sex, advanced-stage disease, and lower than projected rate of vincristine administration for the first six cycles. The most important variables affecting complete remission duration were B symptoms, age, rapidity with which complete response was achieved (patients requiring five cycles or less had significantly longer remissions), number of external sites of disease, and liver or pleural involvement. The impact of being symptom free is dramatic in the NCI study. All asymptomatic patients with stages IIIA (10 patients) and IVA (13 patients)

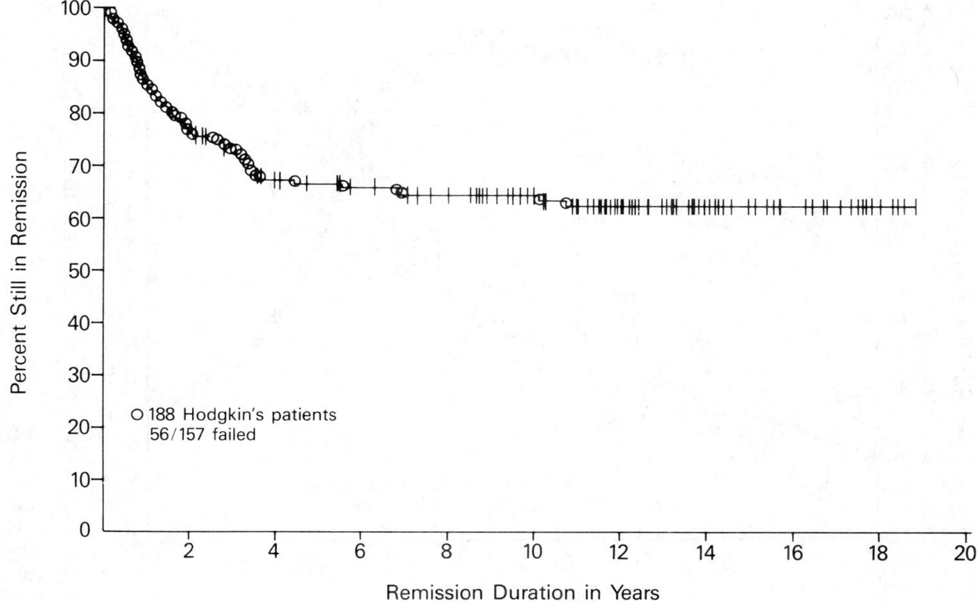

FIGURE 51–14. Remission durations of 188 patients with Hodgkin's disease.

attained complete remissions, and only 2 experienced relapses in more than 20 years of follow-up.

In the 1960s, it was fashionable to give additional continuous "maintenance" chemotherapy after a maximal response was attained to maintain this response, especially because there was little expectation of cure. An NCI study in which patients who achieved complete remission were randomized to additional treatment with MOPP, no further treatment, or treatment with the nitrosourea (BCNU) showed maintenance treatment to be ineffective. Since then, nine studies of maintenance treatment in patients who attained a remission with MOPP showed that it adds nothing to long-term relapse-free survival and survival, and maintenance chemotherapy is not recommended if patients have achieved a complete remission, received a minimum of six cycles of treatment, or two additional cycles of treatment have been given after complete remission was documented.[321–340] As a consequence of the development of a standard treatment for advanced Hodgkin's disease, national mortality decreased approximately 63% during the succeeding decade, and survival rates have increased dramatically. The introduction of MOPP chemotherapy into practice and its effect on national survival and mortality data are illustrated in Figure 51–15.[338]

In the 25 years since the inception and confirmation of the efficacy of the MOPP program, clinical trials of treating advanced Hodgkin's disease have taken three major directions: the development of modifications of MOPP, aimed at retaining efficacy while reducing toxicity; the development of new combinations constructed of drugs with different mechanisms of action and presumed to be noncross-resistant to the drugs in the MOPP program; and the use of these noncross-resistant drug combinations in alternating cycles with MOPP or MOPP modifications to avoid early treatment failures and circumvent the development of drug resistance.[337,341]

The first series of studies that followed the NCI report showed MOPP to be superior to a single agent (*i.e.*, nitrogen mustard) used continuously for 6 months in a controlled trial and superior to a new five-drug combination and to the same five drugs used in a strict sequence, even though the complete remission rates with the latter two regimens was similar to that with MOPP.[271,273] This provided important early evidence that complete remission rates alone did not necessarily reflect the true quality of a remission; duration of remission, after all therapy is discontinued, is the most important indicator of the quality of the induction program. Investigators from Stanford University replicated the results of MOPP, using it as reported from the NCI.[339] However, they thought the toxicity of vincristine at doses used at NCI was too severe, and they recommended the now widely adopted practice of limiting the dose of vincristine to no more than 2 mg/dose regardless of body weight or surface area. Omitting prednisone from MOPP reduced the effectiveness, as was shown in one controlled trial comparing MOPP with MOP.[274] Although one uncontrolled study from Stanford did not confirm this observation, the population of patients at Stanford was composed largely of patients who had relapsed after radiation therapy and is not comparable to most other studies.[340]

In a decade of studies designed to reduce the side effects of MOPP by substituting or adding additional drugs, three four-drug combinations emerged: MVPP, ChlVPP, and BCVPP (Table 51–9) with effects equivalent to MOPP but with different and sometimes fewer side effects, making them useful as alternative treatments.[286,287,292–296] ChlVPP (chlorambucil, vinblastine, procarbazine, prednisone) is an attractive variant of the MOPP program. It substitutes chlorambucil for nitrogen mustard and vinblastine for vincristine. It produces somewhat less nausea and vomiting and much less neurotoxicity, although the degree of myelosuppression is similar. The complete remission rate and fraction of patients who survive continuously free of disease appear equivalent to MOPP. The LOPP variant substitutes chlorambucil for nitrogen mustard. In a controlled trial comparing LOPP with MOPP, the programs were found to be equivalent, but the results with both arms were inferior to those reported elsewhere, a difference

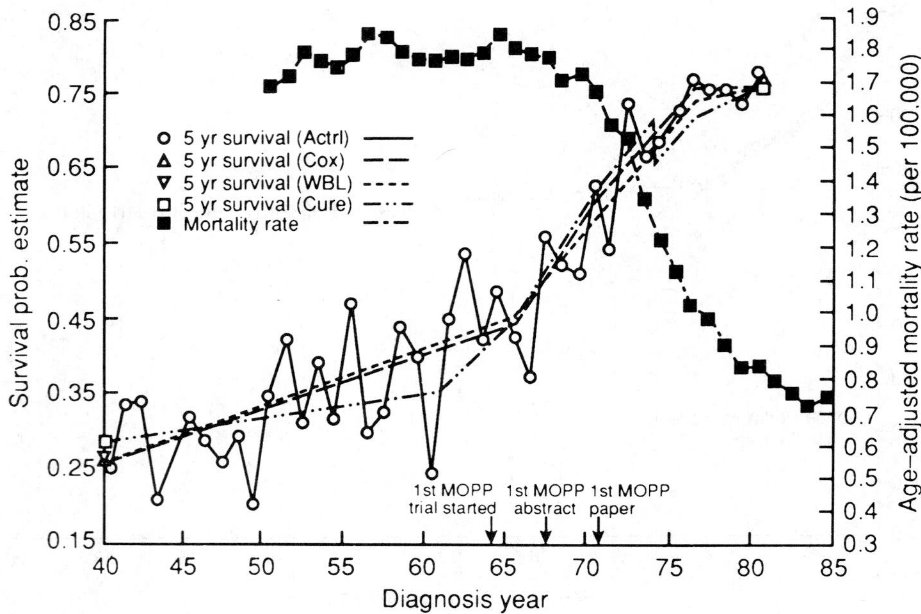

FIGURE 51–15. Hodgkin's disease. The 5-year modeled and actuarial survival rates by the diagnosis year and the U.S. mortality rate by the diagnosis year. (Fuer EJ, Kessler LG, Baker SG, et al. The impact of breakthrough clinical trials on survival in population based tumor registries. J Clin Epidemiol 1991;44:141–153)

TABLE 51–9. Combination Chemotherapy Programs Effective in the Treatment of Advanced-Stage Hodgkin's Disease

Drugs	*Recommended Dose (mg/m^2)*	*Route*	*Days**
MOPP regimen			
Nitrogen mustard	6	I.V.	1, 8
Vincristine	1.4	I.V.	1, 8
Procarbazine	100	PO	1–14
Prednisone†	40	PO	1–14
MVPP regimen			
Nitrogen mustard	6	I.V.	1, 8
Vinblastine	6	I.V.	1, 8
Procarbazine	100	PO	1–14
Prednisone	40	PO	1–14
LOPP regimen			
Chlorambucil	6	PO	1–14
Vincristine	1.4	I.V.	1, 8
Procarbazine	100	PO	1–14
Prednisone	40	PO	1–14
ChlVPP regimen			
Chlorambucil	6	PO	1–14
Vinblastine	6	I.V.	1, 8
Procarbazine	100	PO	1–14
Prednisone	40	PO	1–14
ABVD regimen			
Doxorubicin	25	I.V.	1, 15
Bleomycin	10	I.V.	1, 15
Vinblastine	6	I.V.	1, 15
Dacarbazine	375	I.V.	1, 15
MOPP/ABVD regimen			
Alternating months of MOPP and ABVD			
MOPP/ABV hybrid regimen			
Nitrogen mustard	6	I.V.	1
Vincristine	1.4	I.V.	1
Procarbazine	100	PO	1–7
Prednisone	40	PO	1–14
Doxorubicin	35	I.V.	8
Bleomycin	10	I.V.	8
Vinblastine	6	I.V.	8

* Each cycle lasts 28 days.
† In the original report, prednisone was given only on cycles 1 and 4; it is now given with every cycle.
(Longo D. The use of chemotherapy in the treatment of Hodgkin's disease. Semin Oncol 1990;17: 716–735)

apparently related to inadequate dosing.[282] The results with MVPP, which substitutes vinblastine for vincristine, appear equivalent to those with MOPP but with less neurotoxicity and more myelotoxicity. Interpretation of long-term results of MVPP are complicated by the use of two- and four-drug maintenance treatment in all responders. ChlVPP and MVPP are reasonable alternatives to MOPP, especially for older patients who are less able to tolerate the neurologic side effects of vincristine or for patients with intractable nausea and vomiting related to nitrogen mustard.

The BCVPP regimen substitutes vinblastine and cyclophosphamide for vincristine and nitrogen mustard and adds the nitrosourea BCNU. The Eastern Cooperative Oncology Group (ECOG) conducted a randomized comparison of BCVPP and MOPP in a population of patients with advanced disease, of whom 35% were asymptomatic.[277] Unfortunately, MOPP was used in reduced doses and at wider intervals, with a capping of the vincristine dose at 2 mg. The complete response rates for the two regimens were identical, but the duration of complete remission with BCVPP was significantly longer than with the reduced-dose version of MOPP in previously untreated patients. Life-threatening hematologic toxicity was slightly more severe with BCVPP, probably because of the addition of BCNU, but BCVPP treatment produced less gastrointestinal and neurologic toxicity. Follow-up of this population indicates a higher incidence of acute leukemia in the BCVPP arm than the MOPP arm, which is probably due to the addition of the nitrosourea. The addition of BCNU with greater acute toxicity and long-term side effects makes this combination too toxic for routine use.

In other commonly tested MOPP variants, known by the acronym CVPP, various doses of parenteral cyclophosphamide and vinblastine were combined with various doses of oral procarbazine and prednisone in a variety of schedules. The overall complete remission rate in collected studies is approximately 70% (range, 62–74%), and the actuarial 4-year relapse-free survival rates range from 50% to 60%.[302,341,342] These results do not represent an improvement over MOPP, MVPP, or ChlVPP, because toxicities are similar to that of MOPP, with the exception of peripheral neuropathy and extravasation sequelae. The Cancer and Leukemia Group B (CALGB) studied four-drug regimens in which CCNU was substituted for nitrogen mustard in the CVPP regimen. These studies produced a 68% (average) complete response rate and four-year relapse-free survival rates of 50% to 70%.[341,343,344]

The Southwest Oncology Group (SWOG) conducted a study comparing MOPP with MOPP plus bleomycin.[345,351] In the first SWOG study, the complete response rate with MOPP was 70% and 87% for MOPP plus bleomycin. MOPP plus bleomycin was therefore thought to be the superior treatment, and this program was selected as the control for the next study, which compared it with a new version of MOPP referred to as MOPP-BAP, in which half of the dose of nitrogen mustard was replaced with half of the dose of doxorubicin (Adriamycin).[276] The complete response rate with MOPP plus bleomycin in the second study was not comparable to that of the first SWOG study, decreasing to 67%; it also was inferior to the complete response rate for MOPP-BAP (77%). Based on these results, MOPP-BAP was said to be superior; however, superiority once again came at the expense of a sharp decline in each study in the complete response rate for the control arm (the "best therapy" of the prior study). The complete response rate of MOPP-BAP was not significantly better than that of the MOPP-alone arm in the original SWOG study. Although these trends could be accounted for if the later studies began to include more patients with poorer prognostic factors, the data indicate the opposite. Alterations in doses and schedules seem the more likely explanation, with physicians reducing drug doses as they learn to anticipate the toxicity. The addition of drugs to MOPP, ChlVPP, or MVPP has not made them more useful than the original programs used in adequate doses. Adding drugs adds significant risks and precludes the use of these drugs later if initial treatment fails.

The first new regimen of importance was the ABVD regimen (doxorubicin, bleomycin, vinblastine, dacarbazine) developed by Bonadonna and others.[346–348] In the first comparison of ABVD with MOPP as initial therapy for advanced disease, a 71.5% complete remission rate was obtained with the former, which was not significantly different from the 63% remission rate obtained with the latter. No significant differences in the disease-free or overall survival rates were seen, but ABVD was found to be effective in MOPP failures. ABVD and ABVD variants were subsequently used with MOPP in alternating cycles to improve outcome. Table 51–10 enumerates studies comparing alternating cycles of the two noncross-resistant combinations with MOPP and ABVD.[290,306,307,312–315]

These trials were developed to test the utility of the Goldie-Coldman hypothesis (see Chapter 16). Hodgkin's disease served as a useful model because it is one of the few cancers for which more than one effective drug treatment was available for testing. Interpretations of the data in Table 51–10 should be approached at two levels, the first to evaluate the biologic significance of the Goldie-Coldman hypothesis. Failure to validate the hypothesis should have important implications in the design of future clinical trials in Hodgkin's disease. The second level is a more practical one and relates to the selection of appropriate treatment for patients with advanced Hodgkin's disease to maximize the chances for cure at the time of initial treatment. The data show only a marginal advantage, at best, for eight-drug over four-drug programs, and the studies suffer from design problems.

Bonadonna and associates randomized 88 stage IV patients to alternating monthly cycles of MOPP and ABVD or to MOPP alone.[278–281] The patients received 12 monthly cycles of MOPP—twice the usual duration of treatment—or six cycles of MOPP alternating monthly with six cycles of ABVD. Complete remissions were obtained in 74.4% of the patients with MOPP alone and 88.9% of the patients treated with MOPP and ABVD; the difference was not significant. Greater differences in complete response rate in favor of MOPP and ABVD were noted in patients over age 40 who had no prior radiation therapy, those with lymphocyte-depleted histology or B symptoms, more than three nodal sites involved, or those with bulky tumor. None of these differences were significant. Disease-free and overall survival significantly favored MOPP plus ABVD. The 8-year freedom from progression rates were 35.9% and 64.6% for the MOPP and MOPP plus ABVD groups, respectively. Of the total of 72 complete responders, 45.1% in the MOPP group and 72.6% in the MOPP plus ABVD group were continuously disease free at 8 years. The total survival of the complete responders was significantly different, in favor of MOPP plus ABVD only if death from Hodgkin's disease was considered. If all deaths were considered, the differences were not significant (*i.e.*, 61.9% for MOPP; 76.2% for MOPP plus ABVD) after 8 years of observation.

The toxicity of MOPP plus ABVD was less acceptable to patients than that of MOPP alone. Only 7% of MOPP patients refused to complete treatment, compared with 22% of MOPP plus ABVD patients. The doses in the MOPP arm were, however, markedly reduced, and the results with MOPP in this study were inferior to those at NCI and in prior MOPP studies from the Milan group. The major problem appears to have been the duration of the MOPP program. Patients were unable to tolerate continuous exposure to the MOPP drugs, particularly vincristine, for 12 months, and as a consequence, the dose intensity of MOPP was markedly reduced.

A similar study testing the utility of alternating cycles of two noncross-resistant drug combinations was conducted at the NCI.[315] MOPP was compared, in a randomized trial, with MOPP and CABS (CCNU, doxorubicin, bleomycin, streptozotocin), a program shown to be noncross-resistant to MOPP. In this study, cycles of CABS were alternated with MOPP, but in both arms of the study, the projected number of cycles for remission induction was 6 instead of 12, as in the Milan trial. At total of 127 patients were randomized, 64 to MOPP and 63 to MOPP and CABS, of whom 59 and 56, respectively, were evaluable. The complete response rate was equivalent

TABLE 51–10. Controlled Trials of Alternating, Cyclic Combination Treatment of Advanced Hodgkin's Disease

Investigations	*Regimen*	*Complete Response (%)*	*Relapse-Free Survival (%)*	*Failure-Free Survival (%)*	*Overall Survival (%)*
NCI, Milan[281]	MOPP	74	50	45	64
	vs				
	MOPP/ABVD	89	73*	65*	84
NCI, Bethesda[315]	MOPP	91	65	68	80
	vs				
	MOPP/CABS	92	72	54	72
ECOG[290]	BCVPP	73	56	47	68
	vs				
	BCVPP + RRx	67	61	49	63
	vs				
	MOPP/ABVD	80	61	61	75
CALGB[352]	MOPP	62	48	47	66
	vs				
	ABVD	82	64	57	74
	vs				
	MOPP/ABVD	83*	64	66	76
Intergroup[353]	MOPP → ABVD	73	72	65	82
	vs				
	MOPP/ABV	82*	79*	77*	89*
Canadian[307]	MOPP/ABV	85	75		84
	vs				
	MOPP/ABVD	82	70		84

* $p < 0.05$.

and excellent for both programs, 92% for MOPP and 88% for MOPP and CABS. After more than 5 years of follow-up, the relapse free and overall survival results of both programs were equal and equivalent to or slightly better than the original MOPP study. Dose intensity of the MOPP program in this study exceeded that of the original NCI MOPP study because dose escalation was allowed.

The CALGB recently reported the early results of a comparison of MOPP with ABVD and with MOPP plus ABVD in a group of patients with previously untreated advanced Hodgkin's disease (stages IIIA–IVB).[306] MOPP plus ABVD patients received 6 cycles of each regimen for a total of 12 cycles but, unlike the Milan trial, both four-drug programs were given over 8 rather than 12 months. An extraordinary rate of dose reduction in the MOPP arm was allowed. In addition to capping the vincristine dose, doses of vincristine were reduced by 30% by the third cycle, and the doses of nitrogen mustard and procarbazine were reduced by 56% and 61%, respectively, by the third cycle. Calculations of dose intensity have not been reported, and the impact of prolonging the intervals between cycles was not assessed. The results are mixed and do not support the use of eight drugs over adequate doses of a four-drug program. For example, the complete response rate for MOPP plus ABVD was 82%, compared with 69% for the reduced version of MOPP. However, the complete response rate for ABVD (81%) was identical to that with MOPP plus ABVD. Failure-free survival of 36 months was significantly better with MOPP plus ABVD (64%) than with MOPP (48%), but it was identical to that obtained with ABVD alone (64%). No significant difference in disease-free or overall survival among the regimens has emerged after a follow-up of only 5 years. The data suggest an early failure-free survival advantage for MOPP plus ABVD compared with the reduced version of MOPP but no advantage of MOPP plus ABVD over ABVD given at standard doses.

The ECOG compared MOPP plus ABVD, as used by the Milan group, with their BCVPP regimen, alone or with low-dose radiation therapy added to initially involved sites in patients with advanced Hodgkin's disease.[290] In an interim evaluation of 294 patients, complete response rates among the therapeutic options were found to be similar (68–76%), and no differences in disease-free survival of complete responders (66%) was observed. Because there was no advantage to adding radiation therapy to sites involved by tumor, the two BCVPP arms were combined, and significant advantages were then observed for MOPP plus ABVD in the rates of complete responses, progression free survival, and overall survival. These data do not support the idea that alternating cycles of noncross-resistant combinations provided better results than with adequately used four-drug combination. The data also strongly support the view that investigator bias in regard to anticipated toxicity can radically alter dosing practices and outcome. They suggest that future clinical trials should explore dose modification in initial treatment programs to improve cure rate.

The other two trials shown in Table 51–10 compare different versions of alternating regimens with one another without a four-drug control. The most interesting program studied is that of Connors and Klimo, which featured a MOPP plus ABVD variant in which dacarbazine is omitted, the dose of doxorubicin increased, and all drugs other than prednisone are given within 8 days (MOPP plus ABV hybrid).[307,311,312,314] Partial responders received radiation therapy to nodal areas with residual disease. Complete responses were attained in the original study in 96% of 74 evaluable patients, and the actuarial relapse-free survival rate for complete responders, after more than 5 years off treatment, was 90%. However, the complete response rate includes the 15% of the patients who had radiation therapy to residual disease, and almost 40% of the patients in this study population were in the favorable, asymptomatic group. Longer-term results are more in line with those reported with other drug combination programs. Compared with MOPP plus ABVD in a randomized trial in Canada, the two programs have proven to be equivalent although MOPP plus ABV is somewhat less difficult for patients to tolerate. The Milan group is also testing alternating half cycles of MOPP plus ABVD compared with their original MOPP plus ABVD program; early results show identical response rates and equal durability of responses. The last study in Table 51–10 compares MOPP plus ABVD to the same two programs in sequence with six to eight cycles of MOPP followed by three cycles of ABVD.[307] MOPP plus ABVD was superior to the sequence. This result is not surprising, because the ultimate outcome depends on the initial complete remission rate, which is lower with reduced-dose versions of MOPP. Salvage data from the CALGB trial comparing MOPP plus ABVD with MOPP or with ABVD have some bearing on the interpretation of this study. In the CALGB study, patients who failed ABVD were induced into durable complete remissions twice as often with MOPP as those who failed MOPP and were subsequently treated with ABVD. This suggests that in the Intergroup study the reverse sequence, ABVD followed by MOPP, might be superior to MOPP followed by ABVD.

Two uncontrolled studies routinely added radiation therapy after chemotherapy to sites known to be involved with tumor. Wagener and associates studied 50 advanced-stage patients in a nonrandomized trial in which MOPP was alternated with CAVmP (cyclophosphamide, doxorubicin, VM-26, prednisone).[310] Three cycles of each regimen were given on an alternating schedule, after which consolidation radiation therapy was given to initially involved sites. The complete response after chemotherapy was only 68%; 87% were in complete remission after radiation therapy. The actuarial 3-year survival rate of the total group of complete responders was 94%, and the rate of relapse-free survival was 73%. The investigators concluded that the treatment was no more effective than MOPP in achieving complete remission but that it may be superior in terms of survival. No direct comparison has been made with MOPP. Prosnitz and colleagues periodically update results from a study of a regimen for advanced Hodgkin's disease using combination chemotherapy followed by low-dose irradiation to the initial sites of disease.[308] However, the results of the only controlled trial comparing this approach with radiation therapy alone (see Table 51–10) do not support the use of radiation therapy in adequately dosed patients.[272]

Impact of Dose Intensity on Outcome

Dosing practices in clinical studies have been inconsistent and ignored, despite the fact that retrospective studies of dose intensity consistently show an impact on outcome. Although drugs are added and substituted at will and schedules manipulated frequently, the total dose and dose rate themselves are virtually never examined prospectively as independent variables, nor is actual data on dose intensity given at the time of publication.[337] A retrospective report by Carde and colleagues from Stanford University found that lower doses in the MOPP program correlated with poorer outcome.[349] The dose and dose rate of nitrogen mustard, vincristine, and procarbazine in MOPP, as used at Stanford, were important variables in the ability to attain complete remission and in survival. A regression analysis showed that the mean of the total dose and the dose rate of three cytotoxic agents combined had a significant impact on complete remission rate, particularly in patients with B symptoms, strongly supporting the contention that dose and preservation of the integrity of the combination are important. Patients who received less than 65% of the projected total dose of nitrogen mustard had significantly poorer survival than those who received more than 65% of the projected dose. Another report from Stanford indicated that MOPP failures often achieved good palliation with the use of a single alkylating agent as salvage treatment, which also suggested that significant underdosing with alkylating agents was occurring during their initial treatment with MOPP.[355] These data are bolstered by other reports showing a positive correlation between dose intensity of nitrogen mustard, complete remission rates, and survival free of disease.[356–359]

To compare results across studies in Hodgkin's disease, the NCI group followed the practice of Hryniuk and Bush, converting doses to mg/m^2/week, to obtain an average dose intensity over the 6-month standard MOPP treatment duration.[335] Calculating dose intensity has several advantages over the prevalent practice of comparing percentages of projected dose delivered. Although the percent of projected dose delivered may be high and similar across studies, the projected dose within each study may vary, rendering the comparison useless. A good example is vincristine, for which the percent projected dose delivered is high in most trials, but dose intensity is low because of the routine capping at 2 mg/dose.

Examples of the impact of ad hoc alterations in the MOPP program on dose intensity are shown in Table 51–11.[291] Ver-

TABLE 51–11. Alterations in Relative Dose Intensity of the MOPP Regimen

MOPP Versions	Cycle Intervals (wk) 4	5	6	8
I MOPP, standard	1	0.80	0.67	0.50
II VCR total, 2 mg PCZ scaled up; 14 days	0.92	0.74	0.61	0.46
III VCR total, 2 mg PCZ scaled up; 10 days	0.82	0.66	0.55	0.41

VCR, vincristine; PCZ, procarbazine.

TABLE 51–12. MOPP Regimens for Hodgkin's Disease: Dose Intensity and Outcome

Investigations	*Relative Dose Intensity vs NCI MOPP*	*Actual Relative Dose Intensity*	*Complete Remission (%)*	*% Patients Free of Disease (%)*
NCI/DeVita	1.0	0.85	84	55 (15)
Stanford/Carde	0.95	0.64*	72	30 (5)†
BNLI/Goldman	0.82		52	30 (5)
SEG/Huguley	0.82	0.64	46	16 (2)
CALGB/Nissen	0.81		74	37 (5)
ECOG/Bakemeier	0.77	0.60	73	37 (5)
Milan/Bonadonna	0.76	0.53–0.66	74	36 (8)
SWOG/Frei	0.70		78	31 (5)

* Actual relative dose intensity from a prior study.
† Estimate made from patients with marrow stage IV.

sion I is used at NCI. It has the highest intended dose intensity of any reported program and is used here as the reference standard. Giving version I with an extra week between cycles results in a 20% reduction in the average dose intensity per cycle. Version II, used in most clinical studies, limits the dose of vincristine to a total of 2 mg; procarbazine is scaled up in dose slowly, a practice used in the clinic to reduce nausea and vomiting. If given with the usual 1-week delay between cycles, version II results in a 25% decrease in average dose intensity. MOPP, in practice and in most clinical trials cited, is more often given at 5-week intervals, with a resulting decrease in dose intensity of up to 34%, a reduction in the range that causes a loss of over half of the cure rate in most animal studies. In some human studies, additional significant changes are made, such as omission of a drug entirely, usually vincristine or procarbazine, from the combination, as was done in the Milan study.

Table 51–12 shows data on intended and actual dose intensity of MOPP. It was possible to estimate actual dose intensity in only five of the eight studies shown. There is no consistent effect of intended or actual dose intensity on the complete response rate, a phenomenon seen in animal studies of drug-curable tumors as well.[291] This is an important source of error, because physicians often judge the effectiveness of a new therapy in curable human tumors by its response rate; however, the relation between dose intensity and the fraction of patients who remain free of disease, which is the best indicator of the quality of remission, is more revealing. Reductions in the actual dose intensity of 29% and 38% in the ECOG and Milan studies, respectively, may result in 33% and 35% decreases in overall disease-free survival. Regression analysis yields a correlation coefficient of 0.88 ($p<0.02$) (Fig. 51–16). The difference in outcome between MOPP and the next three programs shown in Figure 51–16 is significant at the $p<0.001$ level.

In the Milan trial comparing MOPP with MOPP plus ABVD, the complete remission and overall survival rates are not significantly different between the two programs, but the relapse-free survival was superior for MOPP plus ABVD.[281] The results with MOPP were poor. Fifty percent of patients in the MOPP arm of the Milan study experienced relapses in the first 24 months, compared with only 34% of patients at NCI over a 14-year follow-up period. In the Milan study, 35% of patients experienced a 50% reduction of the dose of vincristine, and for 9% of patients, the integrity of the combination was entirely disrupted because vincristine was permanently discontinued. The CALGB trial, comparing MOPP with ABVD and with MOPP plus ABVD, suffers from similar dose reductions in the MOPP but not the ABVD arm.

A major reason for treatment failure in Hodgkin's disease may be *underdosing* rather than resistance in the more traditional sense. To test this hypothesis in a clinical trial, all variables but dose must be controlled. The NCI has developed a protocol to test a dose intensified version of MOPP known as Dose Intense MOPP (DIMOPP) in newly diagnosed patients with stage III or IVB disease.[350] The dose intensity of the alkylating agent is increased by two thirds and that of vincristine and procarbazine by one third. The program is given with the support of colony-stimulating factors. This study and others reporting the use of colony-stimulating factors to support standard or increased dosing present opportunities for physicians to finally address the issue of dosing.[351,354]

Chemotherapy for Advanced Hodgkin's Disease

If adjusted for dosing differences, there appear to be no significant differences in long-term outcome when a program from among the following is well administered: MOPP, MVPP, ChlVPP, BCVPP, ABVD, MOPP plus ABVD, and MOPP plus ABV (see Table 51–9). One of these programs should be used as the initial treatment for previously untreated patients with advanced Hodgkin's disease, without the addition of radiation therapy, except in patients with massive mediastinal involvement. The failure to detect a major difference favoring the eight-drug program makes it essential to develop clinical trials examining other variables to improve primary treatment. The choice of a four- or eight-drug program also affects which drugs are available for salvage. If equivalent cure rates can be attained with full doses of a four-drug program, patients who fail can be treated with the alternative program drugs to reduce the body burden of tumor to prepare them for high-dose chemotherapy with marrow or stem cell support.

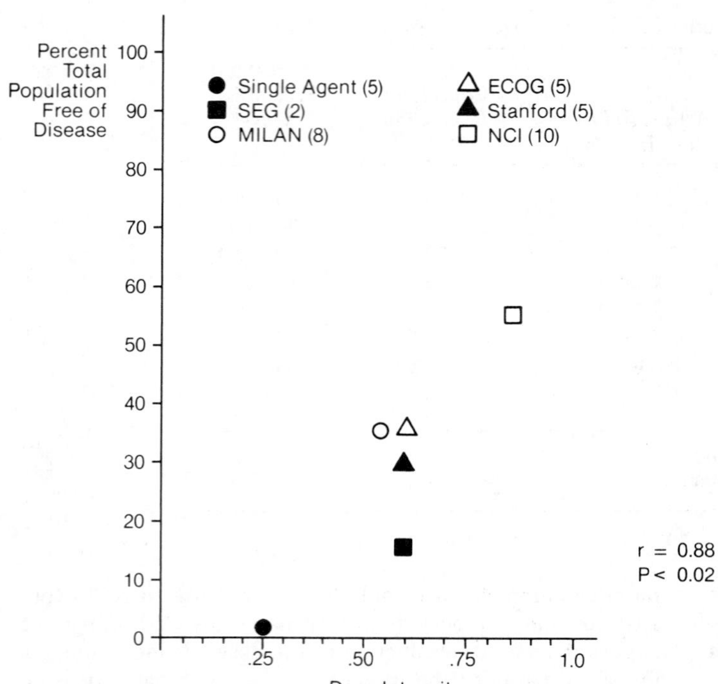

FIGURE 51–16. Relative dose intensity compared with disease-free survival rates of patients with Hodgkin's disease in MOPP programs.

The choice of program should be based largely on toxicity. The acute toxicities of MOPP and ABVD are roughly equivalent but different. The unwarranted fear most physicians have of vincristine-induced neuropathy and the slightly greater nausea and vomiting associated with MOPP often lead to greater dose reductions than with ABVD, with loss of therapeutic effect. A physician is advised to select a program that he or she can faithfully administer in full doses. The most useful MOPP substitute is the ChlVPP regimen, which, if given on the basis of body surface area, appears to preserve dose intensity because it produces fewer acute side effects and to produce equivalent long-term results to MOPP.

The worldwide experience with ChlVPP is minimal. The long-term leukemogenic effect of substituting chlorambucil for nitrogen mustard, while retaining procarbazine, is not yet clear but not likely to be less than with MOPP. MOPP and ChlVPP are reported to be more leukemogenic than ABVD. The limiting and irreversible cardiopulmonary toxicity associated with the use of doxorubicin and bleomycin in ABVD is significant, especially in a young population, and may be an especially serious concern if ABVD is coupled with radiation therapy to the mediastinum. Of the alternating programs, MOPP and ABV is the least emetogenic, because dacarbazine has been omitted, and it is given over a shorter period than MOPP plus ABVD (8 versus 12 months). Because it appears equivalent to MOPP plus ABVD, it may be the program of choice if alternating cyclic chemotherapy is chosen.[307]

Salvage Chemotherapy for Advanced Hodgkin's Disease

One of the most difficult problems faced by oncologists is the proper approach to managing patients with Hodgkin's disease who experience relapse after their primary treatment. It was first observed in 1979 that the length of the prior remission had a marked effect on the ability of patients to respond to subsequent treatment and sustain the response.[360] Patients whose initial remission was longer than 1 year had a greater chance of achieving a second complete remission than newly diagnosed patients of the same stage (95% versus 80%), and their remissions appeared durable. Only about 20% of those who relapsed in less than 1 year attained a second complete remission, and they had a higher risk of relapse. These were important observations for several reasons. They defined subsets of patients with different prognoses who required different approaches to salvage therapy, and they provided information useful in the evaluation of new salvage programs. They also indicated for the first time that drug resistance was probably not the cause of recurrence in patients who had long initial remissions, because they often responded to a second round of the same treatment. The data suggest that undertreatment, particularly underdosing during remission induction, may have led to recurrence, and they provide further support for the notion that dose intensity plays an important role in the outcome of drug-treated patients.[361]

This idea has been significantly bolstered by the results of autologous bone marrow (ABMT) support programs.[362–366] We updated our experience with the long-term follow-up of patients who relapsed from one of several MOPP-based chemotherapy programs at the NCI and were retreated with MOPP.[367] Patients with long initial remissions had a relapse-free survival rate of 45% beyond 10 years, but the development of second cancers and other treatment-related complications reduced the overall survival by almost one half. The disease-free survival rate beyond 11 years from relapse of patients with long initial remissions was only 24%; for those with short initial remissions, it was 11% (Fig. 51–17). The difference was statistically significant. Although long-term survival compatible with cure is possible in patients who relapse after at least 1 year in remission, only about one quarter of the group

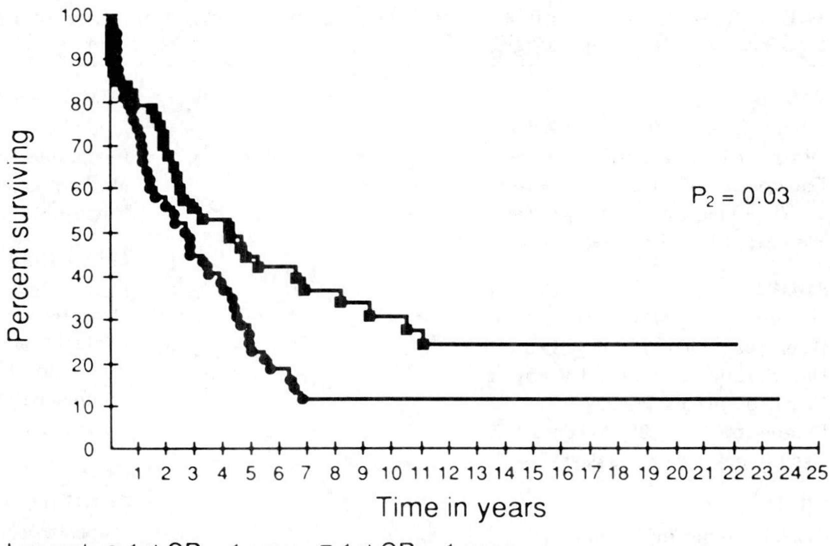

FIGURE 51-17. Kaplan-Meier plot of overall survival from the date of first relapse of patients whose initial remission was shorter than 1 year (●) compared with those whose initial remission was longer than 1 year (■). Survival for patients with short initial remissions is projected to be 11% at 22 years, which is significantly poorer ($p_2 = 0.027$) than the 24% observed for patients with longer initial remissions. (Longo DL, Duffey PL, Young RC, et al. Conventional-dose salvage combination chemotherapy in patients relapsing with Hodgkin's disease after combination chemotherapy: The low probability for cure. J Clin Oncol 1992;10:210–218)

achieve it. The recently published follow-up results from Milan on long-term outcome after ABVD salvage conform to these data.[369] The addition of ABMT or peripheral blood stem cells to support intensification of chemotherapy as salvage treatment has changed the options available for relapsed patients.[362–366] Despite the fact that the patients in ABMT studies were generally resistant to multiple standard drug combinations, the complete remission rates in the various published programs approximates 50%, and a quarter to a half of successfully treated patients remain free of disease, although the follow-up period is still short, with a median of about 3 years.

For the most part, these patients are treated with preparative regimens that contain classes of drugs to which they already have been exposed. The only major new variable is dose intensity—the drugs are given at three to ten times their conventional doses. A major variable that affects outcome is the ability of conventional dose programs to sufficiently reduce tumor volume before transplantation; "responsive failures" make up most of the long-term survivors in transplant programs. Patients who fail a second treatment with a standard program or fail high-dose chemotherapy in the setting of bone marrow support or support with autologous peripheral blood stem cells are candidates for "third-line" programs. Treatment under these circumstances is rarely curative and should be given in the setting of a formal clinical trial, because it provides a way to identify new drug activity that can be used to improve the treatment of newly diagnosed patients.

Patients who fail treatment and are candidates for salvage chemotherapy can be divided into four groups, and their treatment selected accordingly: those initially treated with radiation therapy who recur with systemic disease, patients with advanced disease who fail to attain a complete remission, those who attain a complete remission but whose remission lasts less than 1 year, and patients who relapse after a remission of more than 1 year. Patients who fail radiation therapy should be treated with standard combination chemotherapy as previously outlined. Their response to treatment with chemotherapy is as good as, and in some cases better than, equivalently staged, newly diagnosed patients.[61] Patients who fail to attain a complete remission after treatment with one of the standard programs have the poorest prognosis. Although they sometimes respond to a noncross-resistant standard program (Table 51-13), the remissions are usually brief. This reduction in tumor volume should be exploited, if possible, to prepare them for a program that employs intensive chemotherapy with autologous stem cell or bone marrow support. For patients whose complete remission lasted longer than 1 year, retreatment with the same or a noncross-resistant standard drug combination represents an option that results in satisfactory long-term results compatible with cure in about a quarter of cases.

Because dosing is the most important issue in administering the second set of induction chemotherapy, the choice of which regimen to use should be guided more by the physician's knowledge of the capacity of the particular patient to tolerate the primary treatment. If the patient was treated with MOPP, for example, and marrow suppression was so severe that full doses were not possible, a second six cycles of MOPP is not likely to be any easier to administer, and the selection of ABVD would be a better choice, although marrow sensitivity to drugs is often a generic problem and it would be prudent to augment the treatment with the use of colony stimulating factors. If a patient experienced severe neurotoxicity from the initial treatment with MOPP, MVPP or ChlVPP could be used for retreatment instead of MOPP or ABVD, because vinblastine is substituted for vincristine in these regimens and the general results are roughly equivalent. If nausea and vomiting were the obstacles to administering full doses, as they are occasionally, ChlVPP could be the superior choice for retreatment.

Because the use of high-dose chemotherapy with marrow or stem cell support may reduce the cumulative exposure of the removed bone marrow to drugs and consequently decrease long-term side effects, it is not unreasonable to consider these intensive treatment programs as salvage therapy even for patients who relapse after long remissions, although there are no data on such an approach. It seems wiser to offer patients

TABLE 51–13. Conventional Dose Salvage Combination Chemotherapy Programs for Relapsed, Resistant Hodgkin's Disease

VABCD
Vinblastine 6 mg/m^2 I.V. every 3 weeks
Doxorubicin 40 mg/m^2 I.V. every 3 weeks
Dacarbazine 800 mg/m^2 I.V. every 3 weeks
CCNU 80 mg/m^2 PO every 6 weeks
Bleomycin 15 U I.V. every 1 week

ABDIC
Doxorubicin 45 mg/m^2 I.V. day 1
Bleomycin 5U/m^2 I.V. days 1–5
Dacarbazine 200 mg/m^2 I.V. days 1–5
CCNU 50 mg/m^2 PO day 1
Prednisone 40 mg/m^2 PO days 1–5
Cycle repeats every 28 days

CBVD
CCNU 120 mg/m^2 PO day 1
Bleomycin 15 U I.V. days 1–22
Vinblastine 6 mg/m^2 I.V. days 1–22
Dexamethasone 3 mg/m^2 PO days 1–21
Cycle repeats every 6 weeks

PCVP
Vinblastine 3 mg/m^2 I.V. every 2 weeks
Procarbazine 70 mg/m^2 PO every other day
Cyclophosphamide 70 mg/m^2 PO every other day
Prednisone 8 mg/m^2 PO every other day
Therapy lasts 1 year

CEP
CCNU 80 mg/m^2 PO day 1
Etoposide 100 mg/m^2 PO days 1–5
Prednimustine 60 mg/m^2 PO days 1–5

EVA
Etoposide 200 mg/m^2 PO days 1–5
Vincristine 2 mg I.V. day 1
Doxorubicin 50 mg/m^2 I.V. day 1

MOPLACE
Cyclophosphamide 750 mg/m^2 I.V. day 1
Etoposide 80 mg/m^2 I.V. days 1–3
Prednisone 60 mg/m^2 PO days 1–14
Methotrexate 120 mg/m^2 I.V. days 15, 22 with rescue
Cytarabine 300 mg/m^2 I.V. days 15, 22
Vincristine 2 mg I.V. days 15, 22 every 4 weeks

MIME
Methyl GAG 500 mg/m^2 I.V. days 1–14
Ifosfamide 1 mg/m^2 I.V. days 1–5
Methotrexate 30 mg/m^2 I.V. day 3
Etoposide 100 mg/m^2 I.V. days 1–3, every 3 weeks

MTX-CHOP
Methotrexate 30 mg/m^2 I.V. every 6 hours for 4 days, days 1, 8 with rescue
Cyclophosphamide 750 mg/m^2 I.V. day 15
Vincristine 1 mg/m^2 I.V. days 15, 22
Prednisone 100 mg/m^2 PO days 22–26
Doxorubicin 50 mg/m^2 I.V. day 15 every 4 weeks

CEM
CCNU 100 mg/m^2 PO day 1
Etoposide 100 mg/m^2 PO days 1–3, 21–23
Methotrexate 30 mg/m^2 PO days 1–8, 21, 28 every 6 weeks

CEVD
CCNU 80 mg/m^2 PO day 1
Etoposide 120 mg/m^2 PO days 1–5, 22–26
Vindesine 3 mg/m^2 I.V. days 1, 22
Dexamethasone 3 mg/m^2 PO days 1–8, then 1.5 mg/m^2 PO days 9–26 every 6 weeks

CAVP
CCNU 90 mg/m^2 PO day 1
Melphalan 7.5 mg/m^2 PO days 1–5
Etoposide 100 mg/m^2 PO days 6–10
Prednisone 40 mg/m^2 PO days 1–10 every 6 weeks

EVAP
Etoposide 120 mg/m^2 I.V. days 1, 8, 15
Vinblastine 4 mg/m^2 I.V. days 1, 8, 15
Cytarabine 30 mg/m^2 I.V. days 1, 8, 15
Cisplatin 40 mg/m^2 I.V. days 1, 8, 15 every 4 weeks

(Longo D. The use of chemotherapy in the treatment of Hodgkin's disease. Semin Oncol 1990;17: 716–735)

whose prior remission was shorter than 1 year the opportunity to use their temporary responsiveness to chemotherapy as a way of reducing tumor volume before intensive therapy and marrow or stem cell support.

These data and others indicate the importance of adequate dosing in the successful treatment of advanced Hodgkin's disease. With the advent of colony-stimulating factors to maintain or increase doses of drugs, it may be possible to reduce the primary failure rate in newly diagnosed patients, which also should have the added benefit of reducing the risk of long-term complications.[370–373] Some new studies have incorporated this approach in their design.[361]

For third-line therapy, the selection of a particular salvage treatment program for a patient no longer responsive to standard regimens is complicated by the heterogeneity of the available data. The literature is summarized in Table 51–

13.[347,348,368,374,376,377,382–388] The problem of small patient numbers in all studies is compounded by the extensive mixture of important disease variables and prior response duration. However, the same general theme runs through these data. The best results are attained in patients who experience relapse asymptomatically, who have recurrent nodal disease, and who had attained a prior complete remission of long duration.

The CEP (lomustine, etoposide, prednimustine) salvage program, developed by the Milan group, is the most interesting among those in Table 51–13. It works as well or better than any other regimen, and all the drugs are administered by the oral route.[379–381] CEP has been used effectively with MOPP or ABVD in alternating cycles in patients who fail to respond to ABVD or MOPP, respectively. ABDIC and VABCD contain doxorubicin, bleomycin, dacarbazine, CCNU, and prednisone and resemble ABVD except for the inclusion of a nitrosourea.[375,386] They are most useful in patients not responding to MOPP but may not be superior to ABVD alone; no data are available for comparison. The patient population in the VABCD study was more uniform and the results easier to interpret. Fifteen patients, for example, had stage IV disease, 11 with systemic symptoms. Eight complete remissions occurred in this group and 5 patients remained disease free at the time of the report.

B-CAVE has three of the ABVD drugs plus the nitrosourea, CCNU, but not dacarbazine.[378] Forty-four percent of patients who did not respond to the MOPP regimen had complete remissions, and a quarter of these patients had not progressed at 4 years, although not all were disease free.

No other program has emerged as a major improvement over these regimens. For those who fail to respond to MOPP, the choices are ABVD, ABVD-like combinations, or CEP. For patients who do not respond to ABVD, CEP appears to be the treatment of choice, although the PCVP program (procarbazine, cyclophosphamide, vinblastine, prednisone), which resembles the MOPP program, may be a useful alternative crossover regimen after ABVD failure.[382] Physicians are urged to use these programs in their recommended doses and schedules.

TREATMENT OF STAGE IIIA DISEASE

Several studies support the use of combination chemotherapy alone for treatment of stage IIIA patients who do not have bulky mediastinal disease. A 94% 10-year disease-free survival rate was reported for patients with asymptomatic disease in the original NCI study. Lister[298] and Crowther[299] reported essentially identical results for patients with stage IIIA disease (96% and 91%, respectively) using MVPP. Results in the Lister study were significantly better than the 60% 10-year disease-free survival rate obtained with TNI alone, and the results of the chemotherapy-alone arm were identical to that obtained with combined-modality therapy in the Crowther study. It appears that combination chemotherapy alone is optimal for patients with stage IIIA disease. However, for asymptomatic patients with bulky mediastinal masses or other sites massively involved by tumor, combined-modality treatment is superior to either modality alone.

In the Cotswald system, stage IIIA is divided into IIIA1 and IIIA2 by the extent of disease. IIIA1 is a laparotomy designation of cases, many which would have been clinical stage IIA. In this subgroup, results with radiation therapy alone appear equivalent to chemotherapy.

CHEMOTHERAPY ALONE AND COMBINED-MODALITY TREATMENT IN EARLY-STAGE DISEASE

One principle that has emerged from preclinical animal studies is that curability is inversely related to tumor burden. After there was sufficient evidence that drugs could cure advanced disease, it was logical to explore the use of chemotherapy in early-stage Hodgkin's disease. Adding chemotherapy to radiation therapy in early-stage Hodgkin's disease patients improves disease control, but overall survival is not significantly higher than with radiation therapy alone in patients treated with combined modality therapy, because of the ability to salvage radiation failures with drugs.[389–392] Usually, disease-free survival is about 10% better for patients receiving combined-modality therapy, but about 10% to 20% of these patients die of secondary acute leukemia and solid tumors related to the combined use of chemotherapy with radiation therapy.[393–395]

A prospective randomized study from Stanford suggests that combination chemotherapy may permit the reduction in radiation fields. Horming and colleagues found that patients receiving involved-field radiation therapy plus six cycles of VBM (vinblastine, bleomycin, methotrexate) chemotherapy had a somewhat better freedom from progression and comparable survival than those treated with total or subtotal nodal irradiation.[396] Most of the 67 patients in this small study had stage IA or IIA disease. It is not clear whether VBM, which has not been tested in advanced-stage disease or without radiation therapy, would be effective adjuvant therapy in the subgroup of stage IIB patients felt by the Stanford group to require combined-modality treatment. The virtue of the VBM regimen is its limited toxicity. It spares fertility and is thought to be less carcinogenic than other available standard options.

The first reported experience with combination chemotherapy in early-stage Hodgkin's disease was from the NCI project in Uganda, East Africa, where there were limited diagnostic and radiation therapy facilities.[397] Forty-eight Ugandan children with early clinical stages of Hodgkin's disease were treated with MOPP combination chemotherapy; 42 (88%) achieved a complete response, and 75% of the children were alive and free of disease at 8 years.

Henry Ekert and his colleagues in Australia and New Zealand demonstrated the efficacy of an approach based on the use of combination chemotherapy in clinically staged children.[398] They treated 38 children with stage I or II Hodgkin's disease with MOPP or ChlVPP. Thirty-seven (97%) of these children obtained a complete response to therapy; 1 patient relapsed and was induced into a durable second remission by salvage therapy. The overall survival rate was 94%, and the disease-free survival rate was 97%.

Two prospective randomized studies examined whether combination chemotherapy alone is superior to combined modality therapy in patients with early-stage Hodgkin's disease. Investigators at the University of Maryland Cancer Center randomized 36 patients with stage IB to IIIA disease to receive extended-field radiation therapy followed by MOPP combination chemotherapy or to receive MOPP alone.[399] With a median follow-up of over 6 years, no significant differences occurred between the combined-modality group (75% of patients alive and free of disease) and the group treated with MOPP alone (80% of patients alive and free of disease). However, overall toxicity of the two regimens was different. Viral and fungal infections occurred more frequently in the combined-modality group. Four of the 17 patients treated with combined-modality therapy had toxicities related to the use of radiation therapy; constrictive pericarditis produced limited exercise capacity in 2 patients, and 2 patients developed hypothyroidism. There were three second neoplasms: two squamous cell lung cancers (one on each arm of the study) and one acute leukemia in a patient who had received irradiation and chemotherapy. The study was too small to lead to any conclusions; it provides no evidence that combined-modality therapy is more efficacious than combination chemotherapy alone, and it appears to be associated with more late toxicities.

Pavlovsky and his colleagues performed a prospective, randomized study of clinical stage I and II patients with Hodgkin's disease, comparing CVPP (cyclophosphamide, vincristine, procarbazine, prednisone) chemotherapy alone to CVPP chemotherapy with involved-field radiation therapy administered between the third and fourth cycles of chemotherapy.[400] Although patients were said to be clinically staged, this examination did not include lymphography in one third of the patients. About one third of the patients probably had more advanced stage disease. Another caveat in interpreting this study is related to the fact that the cyclophosphamide and vinblastine were arbitrarily given only once per cycle (intravenously on day 1) in this highly treatable group of patients. This is half as frequent as the usual administration of these agents. Chemotherapy was administered in markedly attenuated doses. Nevertheless, in the patients without poor prognostic factors, those randomized to receive CVPP alone had an 88% complete response rate, 77% 7-year disease-free survival rate, and 92% overall survival rate at 7 years. No significant differences existed between dose-attenuated CVPP alone and dose-attenuated CVPP plus involved-field radiation therapy. The treatment outcome in patients with bulky mediastinal disease favored the use of combined-modality therapy.

These studies provide no evidence that combined-modality therapy is superior to combination chemotherapy alone in the treatment of early-stage Hodgkin's disease.

Two prospective randomized studies compared the efficacy of radiation therapy alone with combination chemotherapy alone in early-stage Hodgkin's disease. Cimino and colleagues randomized 89 patients with pathologic staged IA or IIA disease to receive subtotal nodal radiation therapy or six cycles of MOPP chemotherapy.[401] Complete responses were obtained in all patients treated with radiation therapy and in 40 (91%) of 44 patients treated with MOPP. The disease-free survival and overall survival rates of patients treated with radiation therapy were 74% and 94%, respectively. For patients treated with MOPP, disease-free and overall survival rates were 73% and 87%, respectively. There were no significant differences between the two arms. Relapse on both arms was more common in patients with massive mediastinal disease.

In a follow-up report, it was observed that patients relapsing from chemotherapy-induced complete remission were less responsive to salvage therapy and that their survival from the time of relapse was 15%, compared with 85% for the group relapsing from radiation therapy. This difference was statistically significant, but because the number of patients relapsing is small, the overall results of the study are not altered. As would be expected, infertility was a problem for more patients treated with MOPP chemotherapy. All the men were azoospermic, and half the women developed amenorrhea after MOPP therapy, compared with 0% and 10%, respectively, after irradiation.

The NCI began a prospective, randomized trial comparing subtotal nodal radiation with MOPP in early-stage Hodgkin's disease in 1978.[402,403] The study population included 136 patients with stage IA, IB, IIA, IIB, or IIIA1 Hodgkin's disease. Patients had exploratory laparotomy to complete their staging in most cases (92%). Patients with peripheral stage IA disease (usually defined as stage I disease located above the clavicles) were not randomized and were treated with radiation therapy, because their survival with this approach is 95% or better in most series, and one of these patients failed treatment. Patients with stage IA (central), IB, IIA, IIB, or IIIA1 disease were randomized to receive subtotal nodal radiation therapy (*i.e.*, mantle and paraaortic fields) or MOPP combination chemotherapy precisely as it was administered to patients with advanced-stage disease, with no dose reduction.

In the randomized portion of the NCI study, 49 (96%) of the 51 patients who received radiation therapy achieved complete remissions, but 17 (35%) of the complete responders relapsed, 7 within the treatment portals, 5 outside a treatment portal, and 5 within and outside a treatment portal. Ten (20%) patients randomized to receive radiation therapy died, 7 of Hodgkin's disease and 3 free of Hodgkin's disease. Fifty-two (96%) of the 54 evaluable patients who were randomized to receive MOPP chemotherapy achieved a complete response. A significantly smaller fraction (7 patients, 13%) relapsed, all in previously involved sites of disease. Four (7%) patients died, 3 of Hodgkin's disease and 1 free of disease. Figure 51–18 shows the disease-free survival of the complete responders on the randomized portion of the study. The 10-year disease-free survival rate for MOPP-treated patients was 86%; for radiation therapy-treated patients, it was 60%. The difference between these curves is statistically significant in favor of MOPP treatment (p_2=0.009). Figure 51–19 shows the overall survival for all randomized patients. The 10-year overall survival rate for MOPP-treated patients is 92%; for radiation therapy-treated patients, it is 76%. The difference between the curves is on the borderline for statistical significance in favor of MOPP treatment (p_2=0.051).

In our study, 8 (47%) of 17 patients relapsing after radiation therapy are alive and free of disease after salvage therapy. Three (43%) of the 7 patients relapsing from a MOPP-induced complete response are alive and free of disease after salvage therapy. Although the number of patients relapsing in our study, as in the Cimino study, is small, we do not see evidence that relapsed patients are more refractory to salvage therapy if their primary treatment was combination chemotherapy. Analysis of prognostic factors in the NCI study demonstrated that the advantage of MOPP over radiation therapy was highly significant in two groups of patients: those with massive mediastinal involvement and those with stage IIIA disease. All 11 such patients treated with MOPP are alive and free of disease in their first remission. On the other hand, 6 of 8 patients with massive mediastinal or stage IIIA disease who

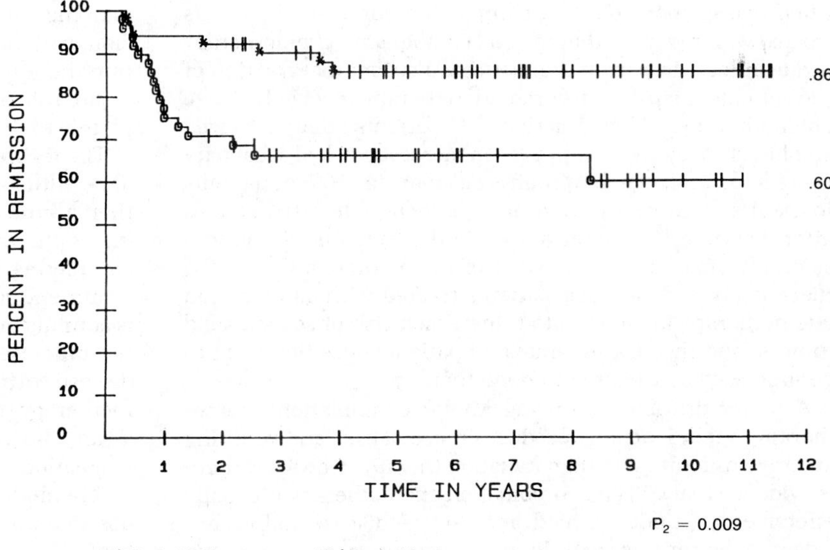

FIGURE 51–18. Kaplan-Meier plot of disease-free survival of patients randomized to receive MOPP (*) or radiation therapy (○) who achieved complete response on the NCI early stage Hodgkin's disease study. The disease-free survival rate was significantly higher among patients treated with MOPP chemotherapy. (Longo DL, DeVita VT. The use of combination chemotherapy in the treatment of early stage Hodgkin's disease. In: DeVita VT, Hellman S, Rosenberg SA, ed. Important advances in oncology. Philadelphia: JB Lippincott, 1992:155–166)

were randomized to receive radiation therapy relapsed, and 5 died (p_2=0.0004 for disease-free survival; p_2=0.0015 for overall survival—both in favor of MOPP). When these two subsets of patients are excluded from both arms of the randomized study, the differences between MOPP and irradiation in disease-free and overall survival rates are no longer significant. In the subsets of patients treated with radiation therapy today, MOPP combination chemotherapy and radiation therapy are equally effective.

These data are sufficiently good to allow the use of combination chemotherapy for patients with early-stage disease, but this population is highly curable by radiation therapy, the delivery of which is better standardized in the United States than chemotherapy. Reducing drug doses arbitrarily in this population reduces the cure rate, and if there is any risk of this occurring, radiation therapy is the better choice for the patient. Theoretically, these data substantiate the inverse rule, because the complete response rate increased from ±80%, achievable in advanced-stage patients, to 96% in early-stage patients with reduced body burden of tumor. There is a commensurate decrease in the relapse rate, from between 35% and 45% to 13%.

The major reason to fear radiation therapy is the development of second solid tumors, although the recently reported risk of premature death from coronary artery disease adds another dimension of concern.[267] By 15 years after treatment, 13% of patients have developed a second solid tumor, and it appears that the risk continues to increase with time.[194] Irradiated patients appear to be at significantly increased risk for lung cancer, melanoma, breast cancer, thyroid cancer, sarcomas, and gastric cancer. Although patients treated with radiation therapy alone have a low risk of developing secondary acute leukemia, about one third of radiation-treated patients relapse and require combination chemotherapy for op-

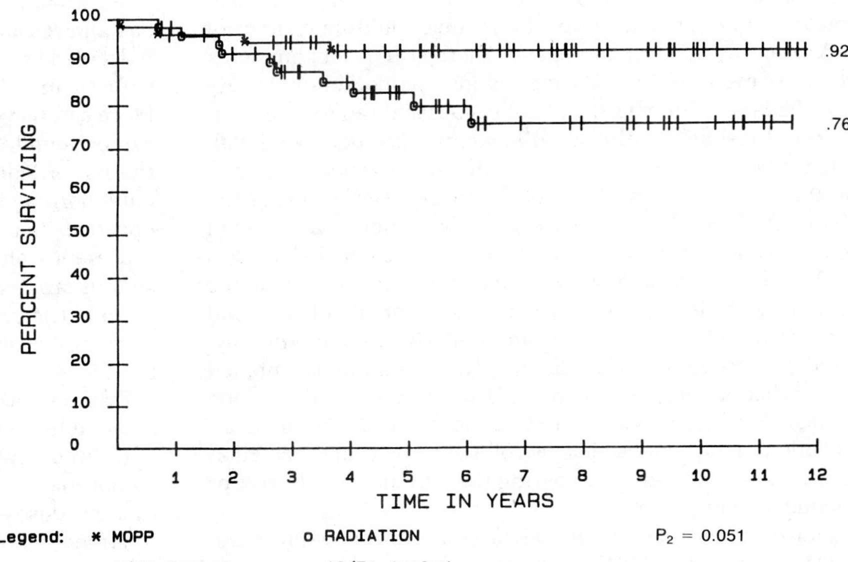

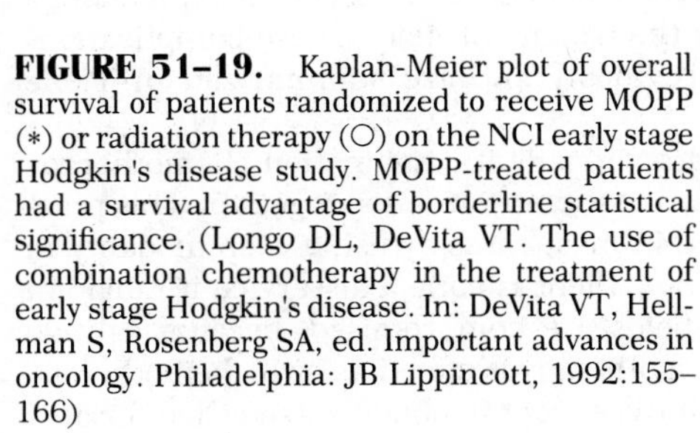

FIGURE 51–19. Kaplan-Meier plot of overall survival of patients randomized to receive MOPP (*) or radiation therapy (○) on the NCI early stage Hodgkin's disease study. MOPP-treated patients had a survival advantage of borderline statistical significance. (Longo DL, DeVita VT. The use of combination chemotherapy in the treatment of early stage Hodgkin's disease. In: DeVita VT, Hellman S, Rosenberg SA, ed. Important advances in oncology. Philadelphia: JB Lippincott, 1992:155–166)

timal disease control. The comparable survival of patients treated with radiation therapy and combination chemotherapy is due at least in part to the fact that a substantial fraction of the patients relapsing after radiation therapy received salvage chemotherapy. This fraction of patients that received combined-modality therapy is at an increased risk of secondary acute leukemia, which may affect as many as 10% of patients in the first decade after treatment, although the risk declines after that time.[394] The magnitude of the leukemic risk is considerably smaller than the risk of other tumors. Currently, there is no evidence that patients treated with combination chemotherapy alone are at an increased risk of second solid tumors, and the risk in irradiated patients does not seem to be increased by the use of chemotherapy.

A major drawback to using MOPP combination chemotherapy is that it acutely produces more nausea and vomiting and myelosuppression than radiation therapy. However, there is evidence that ChlVPP combination chemotherapy is equally effective in patients with advanced-stage disease and is considerably better tolerated. By inference and according to the experience reported by Ekert in children with clinical early-stage disease, ChlVPP should be effective in adults with clinical early-stage disease who have an extraordinary fear of nausea and vomiting.

The major chronic toxic effect of concern with MOPP chemotherapy is infertility, which affects 80% of men and most women older than 26 years of age. Interviews with patients who entered the NCI randomized study suggested that this toxicity may be relevant only for a fraction of patients. Among the 21 men evaluated who were treated with MOPP chemotherapy, only 4 wanted children. Among 30 women treated with MOPP, 10 desired to have children, and 6 were successful. Nevertheless, for patients in whom fertility status is an overriding concern, ABVD chemotherapy appears considerably less toxic to the male and female gonads and should be as effective as MOPP chemotherapy in early-stage disease. Primary fertility-sparing chemotherapy is a valid option for this patient subset.

The concern about secondary acute leukemia in patients treated with MOPP alone is overstated. The major risk of acute leukemia is in patients who are treated with combined-modality therapy and those who receive multiple courses of induction therapy or maintenance therapy. The leukemic risk from six cycles of MOPP combination chemotherapy is very low. Pedersen-Bjergaard and colleagues showed that there is a dose threshold for the small leukemic risk associated with chemotherapy alone and that the threshold generally begins at about eight cycles of MOPP.[402] In 28 years of using the regimen at the NCI, we have seen only a single case of acute leukemia occurring in a patient who received only six cycles of MOPP chemotherapy. However, if a particular patient's fear of acute leukemia is greater than fear of second solid tumors, the physician can recommend ABVD chemotherapy, which is considerably less leukemogenic, even when combined with radiation therapy. The risk of leukemia from ABVD alone is near zero and may be as low as the risk of leukemia from radiation therapy alone. The use of ABVD, instead of radiation therapy, has the virtue of sparing the patient the late risk of secondary solid tumors.

Our current study design, developed as a follow-up to the prior studies, uses ABVD alone for induction therapy for all patients with early-stage disease, and after complete remission, patients are randomized to receive involved-field radiation therapy or to receive no further treatment to assess the future role of radiation therapy in patients who respond completely to drugs.[350]

The techniques of combining irradiation and chemotherapy vary. Although some studies administer all the radiation and then all the chemotherapy, others divide the chemotherapy, giving the radiation after two or three drug cycles, and then completing the chemotherapy. An important principle of treatment is to be sure that at least one treatment modality is administered with appropriate time-dose considerations and the other serves as an adjuvant. For patients with stage II disease with a large mediastinal mass, the full course of chemotherapy should be administered and the irradiation reserved as an adjuvant to the initial site of bulky disease. Extensive irradiation given before chemotherapy may limit the amount of chemotherapy given. This pitfall should be avoided if possible.

HODGKIN'S DISEASE IN HIV-POSITIVE PATIENTS

Although some controversy exists concerning whether Hodgkin's disease is part of the spectrum of AIDS, most epidemiologic studies indicate no evidence to suggest the incidence is higher than might be expected in this young population.[405–410] However, HIV-positive patients with Hodgkin's disease usually present with advanced stage, advanced histology, B symptoms, and unusual patterns of tumor involvement. In contrast to HIV-negative patients, Hodgkin's disease tissues from HIV-positive patients are depleted of helper T lymphocytes and infiltrated with suppressor T cells. Response to chemotherapy has been poor because of poor tolerance to the marrow suppressive effect of drugs and the mucosal toxicity of radiation therapy.[411–413] Outcome is most influenced by whether the HIV-positive patient has clinical manifestations of AIDS at the time of diagnosis.

COMPLICATIONS OF THERAPY

The availability of large populations of long-term survivors has allowed investigators to describe numerous side effects. A detailed list of reported complications in long-term survivors is found in Table 51–14 and reviewed in detail elsewhere.[396] More extensive discussions of the complications of treatment can be found in Chapter 63. Despite the extensive nature of the list of side effects, the lives of long-term survivors are quite normal, because many side effects represent minor annoyances that are easily corrected, occur in few patients, or represent only the potential for future problems. The most serious problem is the risk of developing secondary leukemia or solid tumors in the treatment field. These complications were reviewed previously and are summarized in Table 51–15.

Risk increases dramatically if combination chemotherapy and extensive radiation therapy are used together. This practice can be avoided in most cases by using each modality in its optimal way. The patient is done a disservice if radiation therapy doses or fields are compromised, because salvage treatment with chemotherapy is effective, or if chemotherapy is given concomitantly, except in children (see Chapter 50).

TABLE 51–14. Long-Term Complications in Patients Cured of Hodgkin's Disease

Complication	*Etiology and Risk Factors*	*Management and Prevention*
Immunologic dysfunction	Underlying disease, therapy	Appropriate vaccinations
Herpes zoster-varicella	Underlying disease, therapy	Systemic antiviral therapy, zoster immune globulin
Pneumococcal sepsis	Splenectomy, functional asplenia after radiation therapy (RT)	Pretherapy pneumonococcal vaccine, selected antibiotic prophylaxis, avoid unneccessary staging splenectomy
Nonlymphocytic leukemia	Therapy, older than 40 y	Avoid combined-modality therapy for HD. Supportive care, low-dose chemotherapy, aggressive therapy ± bone marrow transplant
Myelodysplastic syndromes	Therapy, older than 40 y	Same as above
Non-Hodgkin's lymphoma	Therapy	Aggressive combination chemotherapy
Solid tumors	Direct or indirect RT exposure	Conventional management
Thymic hyperplasia	Underlying disease, therapy	Resection
Hypothyroidism	Direct or indirect RT exposure	Hormone replacement, thyroid suppression during therapy (?)
Thyroid cancer	Direct or indirect RT exposure, chronic thyroid stimulation	Thyroid suppression
Male infertility	Therapy, underlying disease	Attempt sperm storage, testicular shielding during RT, suppression of spermatogenesis during CT (?), alternative chemotherapy regimens
Male impotence	Therapy, underlying disease	Counseling, trial of testosterone
Female infertility	Therapy	Oophoropexy, ovarian suppression during therapy (?), cyclic estrogen replacement
Female dyspareunia	Therapy, underlying disease	Counseling, cyclic estrogen replacement
Pericarditis, acute	Mediastinal RT, recall with chemotherapy (CT) after RT	Appropriate RT shielding and technique, avoid doxorubicin after RT, antiinflammatory medication, pericardiocentesis
Pericarditis, chronic	Mediastinal RT	Appropriate RT shielding and technique, pericardiectomy
Cardiomyopathy	Mediastinal RT, doxorubicin, recall with CT after RT	Appropriate RT shielding and technique, avoid doxorubicin after RT, monitor for early signs of toxicity, limit cumulative doxorubicin dose, supportive medical management
Pneumonitis, acute	Direct or indirect RT, bleomycin, nitrosoureas, recall with CT after RT	Appropriate RT shielding and technique, monitor for early signs of toxicity, avoid known toxic drugs, avoid excessive pO_2
Pneumonitis, chronic	Same as above	Supportive management
Avascular necrosis	Steroid therapy, underlying disease (?)	Antiinflammatory medications, joint surgery
Growth retardation	Pediatric RT	Minimize RT, use symmetric RT fields
Dental caries	Salivary change after RT	Maintain good oral hygiene, daily fluoride treatments

Using chemotherapy in full doses minimizes the number of drugs and programs that patients need to be exposed to as well. The problem of fertility and treatment is discussed in Chapter 63.

NEW DRUGS AND BIOLOGICS

The testing of new agents for Hodgkin's disease presents a challenging problem.[414] Because treatment of newly diagnosed patients has been so successful and some patients are curable with second-line therapy or with high doses of chemotherapy with ABMT support, the patient who fails to respond to all available treatment is a poor subject for new agent testing. Bone marrow reserve is usually minimal, and the advanced nature of the disease makes long-term observation difficult. This is a problem faced by oncologists for all tumors that respond well to chemotherapy, such as childhood leukemia and testicular cancer. Patients with advanced Hodgkin's disease should be referred to institutes conducting trials on new drug or biologic therapies.[415–423]

Treatment with biologics should be considered as an alternative to chemotherapy because the side effects of the two modalities are often different. The experience with biologics in Hodgkin's disease is not extensive. Some useful responses and one complete remission have been reported with the use of isotopic immunoglobulins directed against ferritin.[424] Improvement in labeling with isotopes other than iodine 131 may improve the effectiveness of this approach. The use of IL-2 plus lymphokine-activated killer cells in Hodgkin's disease is in its early stages. Some investigators have begun to combine less toxic analogs of active drugs with standard agents in standard combinations to test retention of efficacy with reduced overall toxicity as a way of introducing new agents. Given the heterogeneity of previously treated patients, few useful data have emerged from this approach.

RECOMMENDATIONS FOR TREATMENT OF HODGKIN'S DISEASE BY STAGE

Although the use of laparotomy should be considered as part of the treatment plan, it is unnecessary for patients who receive chemotherapy, regardless of the results of abdominal

TABLE 51–15. Risk Factors for Secondary Acute Myelocytic Leukemia After Therapy for Hodgkin's Disease

Therapy Category	*Relative Risk*	*% Cumulative Risk at 10 Years*
Radiation therapy (RT) alone	Very low	0
Induction chemotherapy alone		
MOPP	Low	2–3
BCNU regimens	Intermediate	3–6
ABVD	Low	?
Combined-modality therapy		
Limited field RT plus MOPP	Low	2–3
Extensive RT plus MOPP	High	4–8
Salvage therapy	High	5–15
Age greater than 40 y	Very high	25–40
Maintenance therapy		
All therapy	High	5–10
Prolonged alkylating agents	Very high	10–30

exploration. It appears that certain early-stage presentations have such a low incidence of abdominal disease that laparotomy is not needed, and these patients may receive radiation therapy alone without surgical staging. Clinical stage I male patients with lymphocyte-predominant or nodular sclerosing histology or with high neck disease and all supradiaphragmatic female stage I patients may receive radiation therapy to the mantle only, without laparotomy, unless there is bulky mediastinal disease. For most of the remainder of the stage I and II patients, laparotomy is required if irradiation alone is contemplated.

Patients with pathologic stage I or IIA Hodgkin's disease with supradiaphragmatic disease and without large mediastinal masses should be treated with mantle irradiation. For most patients, paraaortic fields should be included. Exceptions to this rule may be patients without evidence of any mediastinal disease and nodular sclerosis or lymphocyte-predominant histology. Continued use of the paraaortic field in these patients is uncertain and must be left to individual judgment.

Clinical stage I or IIA patients with massive mediastinal masses should be spared laparotomy and splenectomy and treated with combination chemotherapy initially and then with irradiation to the mediastinum. Laparotomy is not indicated because it does not significantly alter therapy and does have an added anesthesia risk. Full-dose chemotherapy should be given with the radiation volume restricted. The total dose of radiation under these circumstances may be reduced to 3500 to 4000 cGy.

Presentations as subdiaphragmatic disease is almost invariably diagnosed by laparotomy. This disease should be treated with paraaortic and pelvic irradiation for pelvic or inguinal presentation. Patients who present with disease in the periaortic nodes produce a complicated problem, because appropriate treatment would be TNI. Because of complications associated with this technique, especially if chemotherapy must be given for failure, the physician should consider seriously whether they should be treated with primary chemotherapy.

Patients with stage IIB disease should be treated with subtotal nodal radiation. Combined-modality therapy probably should not be used in unless they patients have bulky mediastinal disease or their B symptoms do not abate with the mantle radiation therapy field. Patients with clinical stage IIB disease who have not been evaluated by laparotomy should be treated primarily with chemotherapy.

Radiation therapy alone is not indicated in most stage III patients. The possible exception is stage IIIA patients having only upper abdominal and minimal (<5 tumor nodules) splenic involvement (stage IIIA1); irradiation is administered after laparotomy and splenectomy. For the remainder of stage IIIA patients, chemotherapy alone is the treatment of choice. Irradiation should not be added in these groups: it should be used only in patients with massive mediastinal involvement.

Radiation therapy should be limited in children. The data indicate that the paraaortic fields can be omitted in pathologic stage I or IIA pediatric Hodgkin's disease patients.[244] A treatment volume reduction, even further than the mantle, is desirable, because the radiation produces significant retardation of bone growth. This drawback must be balanced against the risks of recurrence, especially in the very young. The irradiated volume must be limited, and care should be taken to attempt symmetric irradiation to limit the deformities produced by unilateral asymmetric bone growth. For young children, we recommend chemotherapy, with avoidance of irradiation as much as possible. For the young adolescent with supradiaphragmatic presentation after pathologic staging, mantle fields offer the best treatment success with the fewest complications.

Although the data on the successful treatment of early-stage disease with chemotherapy allows substitution of combination chemotherapy for radiation therapy, chemotherapy for stage I and II patients should be used selectively, usually in patients who have limited access to sophisticated radiation therapy equipment and techniques and in some growing children.

REFERENCES

1. Kaplan HS. Hodgkin's disease. 2nd ed. Cambridge: Harvard University Press, 1980.
2. Hodgkin T. On some morbid appearances of the absorbent glands and spleen. Med Chir Trans 1832;17:68–114.
3. Bright R. Observations on abdominal tumours and intumescence. Guy's Hosp Rep 1838;3:401–460.
4. Wilks S. Cases of enlargement of lymphatic glands and spleen (or Hodgkin's disease), with remarks. Guy's Hosp Rep 1865;11:56–67.
5. Nuland SB. The lymphatic contiguity of Hodgkin's disease: A historical study. Bull N Y Acad Med 1981;57:776–789.
6. Craigie D. Case of disease of the spleen, in which death took place in consequence in the presence of purulent matter in the blood. Edinburgh Med Surg J 1845;64:400–413.
7. Bennett JH. Case of hypertrophy of the spleen and liver in which death took place from suppuration of the blood. Edinburgh Med Surg J 1845;64:413–423.
8. Virchow R. Weisses Blut, neue Notizen aus den Geb der Naturund Heikunde. (Froriep's neue Notizen) 1845;36:151–156.
9. Roulet F. Dasprinare Retothelsarkom der Lymphkonten. Virchows Arch [A] 1930;277:15–47.
10. Burkitt D. A sarcoma involving the jaws in African children. Br J Surg 1958;46:218–223.
11. Greenfield WS. Specimens illustrative of the pathology of lymphadenoma and leucocythemia. Trans Pathol Soc London 1878;29:272–304.
12. Goldmann EE. Beitrug zu der Lehre von dem malignen Lymphom. Zentralbl Allg Pathol 1892;3:665–690.
13. Sternberg C. Uber eine Eigenartige unter dem Bilde der Pseudoleukamie verlaufende Tuberculose des lymphatichon Apparates. Z Heilk 1898;19:21–90.
14. Reed DM. On the pathological changes in Hodgkin's disease, with especial reference to its relation to tuberculosis. Johns Hopkins Hosp Rev 1902;10:133–196.
15. Seif GSF, Spriggs AI. Chromosome changes in Hodgkin's disease. JNCI 1967;39:557–470.

16. MacMahon B. Epidemiological evidence of the nature of Hodgkin's disease. Cancer 1957;10:1045–1054.
17. Correa P, O'Conor GT, Berard CW, et al. International comparability and reproducibility in histologic subclassification of Hodgkin's disease. JNCI 1973;50:1429–1435.
18. Mueller NE. Hodgkin's disease. In: Schnottenfeld D, Fraumeni J, eds. Cancer epidemiology and prevention. 2nd ed. New York: Oxford University Press, 1992.
19. Steiner PE. Hodgkin's disease: Search for infective agent and attempts at experimental reproduction. Arch Pathol 1934;17:749–763.
20. L'Esperance ES. Experimental inoculation of chickens with Hodgkin's nodes. J Immunol 1929;16:37–60,.
21. Van Rooyan CE. Etiology of Hodgkin's disease with special reference to *B. tuberculosis avis*. Br Med J 1933;1:50–51.
22. Van Rooyan CE. Recent experimental work on the etiology of Hodgkin's disease. Br Med J 1934;2:519–524.
23. Miller RW, Beebe GW. Infectious mononucleosis and the empirical risk of cancer. JNCI 1973;50:315–321.
24. Connolly RR, Chistene BW. A cohort study of cancer following infectious mononucleosis. Cancer Res 1974;34:1172–1178.
25. Rosdahl N, Larsen SO, Clemmensen J. Hodgkin's disease in patients with previous mononucleosis, 30 years' experience. Br Med J 1974;2:253–256.
26. Munoz N, Davidson RJ, Witthoff B, et al. Infectious mononucleosis and Hodgkin's disease. Int J Cancer 1978;22:10–13.
27. Nonoyama M, Kawai Y, Huang CH, et al. Epstein-Barr virus DNA in Hodgkin's disease, American Burkitt's lymphoma and other human tumors. Cancer Res 1974;34:1228–1231.
28. Vianna NJ, Greenwald P, Davies JNP. Extended epidemic of Hodgkin's disease in high school students. Lancet 1971;1:1209–1210.
29. Vianna JH, Polan AK. Epidemiological evidence for transmission of Hodgkin's disease. N Engl J Med 1973;289:499–502.
30. Smith PG, Pike MC, Kinlam LJ, et al. Contacts between young patients with Hodgkin's disease: A case control study. Lancet 1977;2:59–62.
31. Zack MM, Heath CW Jr, Andrews MD, et al. High school contact among persons with leukemia and lymphoma. JNCI 1977;59:1343–1349.
32. Gutterman S, Cole P, Levitan TR. Evidence against transmission of Hodgkin's disease in high schools. N Engl J Med 1979;300:1000–1011.
33. Gutensohn N, Cole P. Childhood social environment and Hodgkin's disease. N Engl J Med 1981;304:135–140.
34. Milham S Jr, Hesser J. Hodgkin's disease in woodworkers. Lancet 1967;2:136–137.
35. Vianna NJ, Greenwald P, Davies JNP. Tonsillectomy and Hodgkin's disease: The lymphoid tissue barrier. Lancet 1971;1:431–432.
36. Bierman HR. Human appendix and neoplasia. Cancer 1968;21:109–118.
37. Hyams L, Wynder EL. Appendectomy and cancer risk: An epidemiological evaluation. J Chronic Dis 1968;21:319–415.
38. Graff KS, Simon RM, Yankee RA, et al. HLA antigens in Hodgkin's disease: Histopathologic and clinical correlations. JNCI 1974;52:1087–1090.
39. Chakaavarti A, Hallaran SL, Bale SJ et al. Etiological heterogeneity in Hodgkin's disease: HLA linked and unlinked determinants of susceptibility independent of histological concordance. Genet Epidemiol 1986;3:407–415.
40. Gutterman S, Barton JW III, Eby NL. Increased sex concordance of sibling pairs with Becket's disease, Hodgkin's disease, multiple sclerosis, and sarcadosis. Am J Epidemiol 1987;126:365–369.
41. Robertson SJ, Lowman JT, Gutterman S et al. Familial Hodgkin's disease: A clinical and laboratory investigation. Cancer 1987;59:1314–1319.
42. Lukes RJ, Tindle BH, Parker JW. Reed-Sternberg-like cells in infectious mononucleosis. Lancet 1969;2:1000–1004.
43. Strum SB, Dark JK, Rappaport H. Observations of cells resembling Sternberg-Reed cells in conditions other than Hodgkin's disease. Cancer 1970;26:176–190.
44. Jackson H Jr, Parker F Jr: Hodgkin's disease. II. Pathology. N Engl J Med 1944;231: 35–44.
45. Lukes RJ, Butler JJ, Hicks ED. Natural history of Hodgkin's disease as related to its pathologic picture. Cancer 1966;19:317–344.
46. Langhans T. Das Maligne Lymphosarkom (Pseuddukamie). Virchows Arch [A] 1872;54: 509–537.
47. Pell PK. Zur Symptomatologie der sogenannten Pseudoleukamie II. Pseudoleukamie oder chronisches Ruckfallsfieber? Klin Wochenschr 1887;24:644–646.
48. Parker F Jr, Jackson H Jr, Fitzhugh G, et al. Studies of diseases of the lymphoid and myeloid tissues: IV. Skin reactions to human and avian tuberculin. J Immunol 1932;22: 277–282.
49. Lukes RJ. Relationship of histologic features to clinical stages in Hodgkin's disease. AJR 1963;90:944–955.
50. Wright MD. Lymphocyte predominance Hodgkin's disease. N Engl J Med 1988;319: 246 [Letter to the Editor re Regula DP Jr, Hoppe RT, Weiss LM. Nodular and diffuse types of lymphocyte predominance Hodgkin's disease. N Engl J Med 1988;318:214–219].
51. Poppema S, Kaiserling E, Lennert K. Hodgkin's disease with lymphocyte predominance, nodular type (nodular paragranuloma) and progressively transformed germinal centers—a cytohistological study. Histopathology 1979;3:295.
52. Poppema S, Kaiserling E, Lennert K. Nodular paragranuloma and progressively transformed germinal centers. Ultrastructural and immunohistologic findings. Virchows Arch [B] 1979;31:211–225.
53. Burns BF, Colby TV, Dorfman RF. Differential diagnostic features of nodular L&H Hodgkin's disease, including progressive transformation of germinal centers. Am J Surg Pathol 1984;8:253–261.
54. Pinkus GS, Said JW. Hodgkin's disease, lymphocyte predominance type, nodular—a distinct entity? Unique staining profile for L&H variants of Reed-Sternberg cells defined by monoclonal antibodies to leukocyte common antigen, granulocyte-specific antigen, and B-cell-specific antigen. Am J Pathol 1985;118:1–6.
55. Coles FB, Cartun RW, Pastuszak WT. Hodgkin's disease, lymphocyte-predominant type: Immunoreactivity with B-cell antibodies. Mod Pathol 1988;1:274–278.
56. Pinkus GS, Said JW. Hodgkin's disease, lymphocyte predominance type, nodular—further evidence for a B cell derivation. Am J Pathol 1988;133:211–217.
57. Hansmann M-L, Stein H, Dallenbach F, Fellbaum C. Diffuse lymphocyte-predominant Hodgkin's disease (diffuse paragranuloma). A variant of the B-cell-derived nodular type. Am J Pathol 1991;138:29–36.
58. Sundeen JT, Cossman J, Klein M. Lymphocyte predominant Hodgkin's disease nodular subtype with coexistent "large cell lymphoma": Histological progression or composite malignancy? Am J Surg Pathol 1988;12:599–606.
59. Miettinen M, Franssila KO, Saxén E. Hodgkin's disease, lymphocytic predominance nodular. Increased risk for subsequent non-Hodgkin's lymphomas. Cancer 1983;51: 2293–2300.
60. Chittal SM, Alard C, Rossi J-F, et al. Further phenotypic evidence that nodular, lymphocyte-predominant Hodgkin's disease is a large B-cell lymphoma in evolution. Am J Surg Pathol 1990;14:1024–1035.
61. Miller TP, Byrne GE, Jones SE. Mistaken clinical and pathologic diagnoses of Hodgkin's disease: A Southwest Oncology Group study. Cancer Treat Rep 1982;66:645–651.
62. Kant JA, Hubbard SM, Longo DL, et al. The pathologic and clinical heterogeneity of lymphocyte depleted Hodgkin's disease. J Clin Oncol 1986;4:284–294.
63. Neiman RS, Rosen PJ, Lukes RJ. Lymphocyte-depletion Hodgkin's disease. A clinicopathological entity. N Engl J Med 1973;288:751–755.
64. Schoeppel SL, Hoppe RT, Dorfman RF, et al. Hodgkin's disease in homosexual men with generalized lymphadenopathy. Ann Intern Med 1985;102:68–70.
65. Ioachim HL, Cooper MC, Hellman GC. Lymphomas in men at high risk for acquired immune deficiency syndrome (AIDS). Cancer 1985;56:2831–2842.
66. Jaffe ES, Clark J, Steis R, et al. Lymph node pathology of HTLV and HTLV-associated neoplasms. Cancer Res 1985;45:4662S–4664S.
67. Anagnostou D, Parker JW, Taylor CR, et al. Lacunar cells of nodular sclerosing Hodgkin's disease. An ultrastructural and immunohistologic study. Cancer 1977;39:1032–1043.
68. Kadin ME, Glatstein E, Dorfman RF. Clinicopathologic study of 117 untreated patients subject to laparotomy for the staging of Hodgkin's disease. Cancer 1971;27:1277–1294.
69. Strum SB, Rappaport H. Interrelations of the histologic types of Hodgkin's disease. Arch Pathol 1971;91:127–134.
70. DeVita VT Jr, Simon RM, Hubbard SM, et al. Curability of advanced Hodgkin's disease with chemotherapy: Long-term follow-up of MOPP treated patients at NCI. Ann Intern Med 1980;92:587–595.
71. Mann RB, Jaffe, ES, Berard CW. Malignant lymphomas—a conceptual understanding of morphologic diversity. A review. Am J Pathol 1979;94:105–191.
72. Mauch P, Gorshein D, Cunningham J, et al. Influence of mediastinal adenopathy on site and frequency of relapse in patients with Hodgkin's disease. Cancer Treat Rep 1982;66:809–817.
73. MacLennan KA, Bennett MH, Tu A, et al. Relationship of histopathologic features to survival and relapse in nodular sclerosing Hodgkin's disease. A study of 1659 patients. Cancer 1989;64:1686–1693.
74. Lukes RJ. Criteria for involvement of lymph node, bone marrow, spleen, and liver in Hodgkin's disease. Cancer Res 1971;31:1755–1764.
75. Colby TV, Hoppe RT, Warnke RA. Hodgkin's disease: A clinicopathologic study of 659 cases. Cancer 1981;49:1848–1858.
76. Grogan TM. Hodgkin's disease. In: Jaffe ES, ed. Surgical pathology of lymph nodes and related organs. Philadelphia: WB Saunders, 1985:86–134.
77. Rosai J, Levine GD. Tumors of the thymus. In: Atlas of tumor pathology. 2nd series, fasc. 13. Washington, DC: Armed Forces Institute of Pathology, 1975.
78. Kadin ME, Donaldson SS, Dorfman RF. Isolated granulomas in Hodgkin's disease. N Engl J Med 1970;283:859–861.
79. Order SE, Hellman S. Pathogenesis of Hodgkin's disease. Lancet 1972;1:571–573.
80. DeVita VT. Lymphocyte reactivity in Hodgkin's disease: A lymphocyte civil war. N Engl J Med 1973;289:801–802.
81. Kadin ME, Stites DP, Levy R, et al. Exogenous immunoglobulin and the macrophage origin of Reed-Sternberg cells in Hodgkin's disease. N Engl J Med 1978;299:1208–1214.
82. Kaplan HS, Gartner S. "Sternberg-Reed" giant cells of Hodgkin's disease: Cultivation in vitro, heterotransplantation, and characterization as neoplastic macrophages. Int J Cancer 1977;19:511–525.
83. Corder MP, Young RC, DeVita VT. Delayed hypersensitivity in patients with cancer. N Engl J Med 1971;285:522–524.
84. Corder MP, Young RC, Brown RS, et al. Phytohemagglutinin induced lymphocyte transformation: The relationship to prognosis of Hodgkin's disease. Blood 1972;39: 595–602.
85. Slivarck DJ, Ellis TM, Nawrocki, et al. The impact of Hodgkin's disease on the immune system. Semin Oncol 1990;17:673–682.
86. Poppema S, Bhan AK, Reinherz EL, et al. In situ immunologic characterization of cellular constituents in lymph nodes and spleens involved by Hodgkin's disease. Blood 1982;59:226–232.
87. Garvin AJ, Spicer SS, Parmley RT, et al. Immunohistochemical demonstration of IgG in Reed-Sternberg and other cells in Hodgkin's disease. J Exp Med 1974;139:1077–1083.
88. Kadin ME. Possible origin of the Reed-Sternberg cell from an interdigitating reticulum cell. Cancer Treat Rep 1982;66:601–608.

89. Braylan RC, Jaffe ES, Berard CW. Surface characteristics of Hodgkin's lymphoma cells. Lancet 1974;2:1328–1329.
90. Hsu S, Jaffe ES. Leu M1 and peanut agglutinin stain the neoplastic cells of Hodgkin's disease. Am J Clin Pathol 1984;82:29–32.
91. Diehl V, Kirschner HH, Burrighter H, et al. Characteristics of Hodgkin's disease-derived cell lines. Cancer Treat Rep 1982;66:615–632.
92. Stein H, Gerdes J, Schwab U, et al. Identification of Hodgkin's and Sternberg-Reed cells as a unique cell type derived from a newly detected small-cell population. Int J Cancer 1982;30:445–459.
93. Andreesen R, Osterholz J, Lohr GW, et al. A Hodgkin cell-specific antigen is expressed on a subset of auto- and alloactivated T (helper) lymphoblasts. Blood 1984;63:1299–1302.
94. Hecht TT, Longo DL, Cossman J, et al. Production and characterization of a monoclonal antibody that finds Reed-Sternberg cells. J Immunol 1984;134:4231.
95. Stein H, Mason DY, Gerdes J, et al. The expression of the Hodgkin's disease associated antigen Ki-1 in reactive and neoplastic lymphoid tissue: Evidence that Reed-Sternberg cells and histiocytic malignancies are derived from activated lymphoid cells. Blood 1985;66:848–858.
96. Dichl Von Kalle C, Fonatsch, et al. The cell of origin in Hodgkin's disease. Semin Oncol 1990;17:660–672.
97. Hsu S, Yang K, Jaffe ES. Phenotypic expression of Hodgkin's and Reed-Sternberg cells in Hodgkin's disease. Am J Pathol 1985;118:209–217.
98. Weiss L, Strickler JG, Hu E, et al. Immunoglobulin gene rearrangements in Hodgkin's disease. Hum Pathol 1986;17:1009–1014.
99. Sundeen JT, Lipford E, Uppencamp M, et al. Rearranged antigen receptor genes in Hodgkin's disease. Blood 1987;70:96–103.
100. Greisser H, Feller A, Lennert K. Rearrangement of the B chain of the T-cell receptor and immunoglobulin genes in lymphoproliferative disorders. J Clin Invest 1986;78: 1179–1184.
101. Brinker MG, Poppema S, Buys C, et al. Clonal immunoglobulin gene rearrangements in tissues involved by Hodgkin's disease. Blood 1987;70:186–189.
102. Davis TH, Morton CC, Miller-Cassman R, et al. Hodgkin's disease, lymphomatoid papulosis, and cutaneous T-cell lymphoma derived from a common T-cell clone. N Engl J Med 1992;326:1115–1122.
103. Stetler-Stevenson M, Crush-Stanton S, Cossman J. Involvement of the *bcl*-2 gene in Hodgkin's disease. JNCI 1990;82:855–858.
103a. Poppema S, Kaleta J, Hepperle B. Chromosomal abnormalities in patients with Hodgkin's disease: Evidence for frequent involvement of the 14q chromosomal region but infrequent bcl-2 gene rearrangement in Reed-Sternberg cells. JNCI 1992;84:1789–1793.
104. Doglioni C, Pelosio P, Mombello A, et al. Immunohistochemical evidence of abnormal expression of the antioncogene-encoded p53 phosphoprotein in Hodgkin's disease and $CD30^+$ anaplastic lymphomas. Hematol Pathol 1991;5:67–73.
105. Sinkovics JG. Hodgkin's disease revisited: Reed-Sternberg cells as natural hybridomas. Crit Rev Immunol 1991;11:33–63.
106. Drexler HG, Gignac SM, Hoffbrand AV, Minowada J. Formation of multinucleated cells in a Hodgkin's disease-derived cell line. Int J Cancer 1989;43:1083–1090.
107. Mueller N, Evans A, Harris NL, et al. Hodgkin's disease and Epstein-Barr virus. Altered antibody pattern before diagnosis. N Engl J Med 1989;320:689–695.
108. Anagnostopoulos I, Herbst H, Niedobitek G, et al. Demonstration of monoclonal EBV genomes in Hodgkin's disease and KI-1-positive anaplastic large cell lymphoma by combined Southern blot and in situ hybridization. Blood 1989;74:810–816.
109. Weiss LM, Movahed LA, Warnke RA, et al. Detection of Epstein-Barr viral genomes in Reed-Sternberg cells of Hodgkin's disease. N Engl J Med 1989;320:502–506.
110. Pallesen G, Hamilton-Dutoit SJ, Rowe M, et al. Expression of Epstein-Barr virus latent gene products in tumour cells of Hodgkin's disease. Lancet 1991;337(8737): 320–322.
111. Wu T-C, Mann RB, Charache P, et al. Detection of EBV gene expression in Reed-Sternberg cells of Hodgkin's disease. Int J Cancer 1990;46:801–804.
112. Stein H, Hansmann L, Lennert K, et al. Reed-Sternberg and Hodgkin cells in lymphocyte-predominant Hodgkin's disease of nodular subtype contain J chain. Am J Clin Pathol 1986;86:292–297.
113. Timens W, Visser L, Poppema S. Nodular lymphocyte predominance type of Hodgkin's disease is a germinal center lymphoma. Lab Invest 1986;54:457–461.
114. Levy RA, Kaplan HS. Impaired lymphocyte function in untreated Hodgkin's disease. N Engl J Med 1974;290:181–186.
115. Kaplan HS, Smithers DW. Auto-immunity and homologous disease in mice in relation to the malignant lymphomas. Lancet 1959;2:1–4.
116. Schwartz RS, Beldotti L. Malignant lymphomas following allogenic disease: Transition from an immunological to a neoplastic disorder. Science 1965;149:1511–1514.
117. Romagraaic S, Ferrini PW, Ricci M. The immune defect in Hodgkin's disease. Semin Hematol 1985;22:41–45.
118. Pizzolo G, Chilosi M, Vinoutz F, et al. Soluble interleukin-2 receptors in the serum of patients with Hodgkin's disease. Br J Cancer 1987;55:427–428.
119. Bjorkholm M, Holm H, Mellstedt H. Immunologic profile in patients with cured Hodgkin's disease. Scand J Haematol 1977;18:361–368.
120. Young RC, Corder MP, Haynes HA, et al. Delayed hypersensitivity in Hodgkin's disease. A study of 103 patients. Am J Med 1972;52:63–71.
121. King GW, Yanes B, Hurtubise PE, et al. Immune function of successfully treated lymphoma patients. J Clin Invest 1976;57:1451–1460.
122. Van Haelen CP, Fisher RR. Increased sensitivity of T-cells to regulation by normal suppressor cells persist in long-term survivors with Hodgkin's disease. Am J Med 1982;72:385–390.
123. Fisher RI, DeVita VT, Bostick F, et al. Persistent immunologic abnormalities in long-term survivors of advanced Hodgkin's disease. Ann Intern Med 1980;92:595–599.
124. Fisher RI. Implications of persistent T-cell abnormalities for the etiology of Hodgkin's disease. Cancer Treat Rep 1982;66:681–687.
125. Fuks Z, Strober S, Bobrove AM, et al. Long-term effects of radiation on T and B lymphocytes in peripheral blood of patients with Hodgkin's disease. J Clin Invest 1976;58:803–814.
126. Van Rijswijk RE, Sybesma JP, Kater L. A prospective study of the changes in the immune status following radiotherapy for Hodgkin's disease. Cancer 1984;53:62–69.
127. Van Rijswijk RE, Sybesma JP, Kater L. A prospective study of the changes in the immune status before, during and after multiple agent chemotherapy for Hodgkin's disease. Cancer 1983;53:637–644.
128. Weitzman SA, Aisenberg AC, Siber GR, Smith DH. Impaired humoral immunity in treated Hodgkin's disease. N Engl J Med 1977;297:245–248.
129. Minor DR, Schiffman G, McIntosh LS. Response of patients with Hodgkin's disease to pneumococcal vaccine. Ann Intern Med 1979;90:887–892.
130. Hays DM, Ternberg JL, Chen TT, et al. Complications related to 234 staging laparotomies performed in the intergroup Hodgkin's disease in childhood study. Surgery 1984;96:471–478.
131. Donaldson SS, Vosti KL, Berberich FR, et al. Response to pneumococcal vaccine among children with Hodgkin's disease. Rev Infect Dis 1981;3:S133–S143.
132. Ko HS, Pruzanski W. M components associated with lymphoma: A review of 62 cases. Am J Med Sci 1976;272:175–183.
133. Levine AM, Thorton P, Forman SJ, et al. Positive Coombs' test in Hodgkin's disease. Significance and implications. Blood 1980;55:607–611.
134. Booth PB, Jenkins WJ, Marsh WL. Anti-It: A new antibody of the I blood group system occuring in certain Melanesian sera. Br J Haematol 1966;12:341–344.
135. Waddell CC, Cimo PL. Idiopathic thrombocytopenia purpura occurring in Hodgkin's disease after splenectomy. A report of two cases and review of the literature. Am J Haematol 1979;7:381–387.
136. Jones SE. Autoimmune disorders and malignant lymphoma. Cancer 1973;31:1092–1098.
137. Berkman AW, Woog JJ, Kickler TS, et al. Serial determinations of anti-platelet antibodies in a patient with Hodgkin's disease and autoimmune thrombocytopenia. Cancer 1983;51:2057–2060.
138. Heyman MR, Walsh TJ. Autoimmune neutropenia in Hodgkin's disease. Cancer 1987;59:1903–1905.
139. Gilbert R. La roentgentherapie de la granulomatose maligne. J Radiol Electrol 1925;9: 509–513.
140. Gilbert R. Radiotherapy in Hodgkin's disease (malignant granulomatosis): Anatomic and clinical foundations: Governing principles: Results. AJR 1939;41:198–241.
141. Kaplan HS. Hodgkin's disease. 2nd ed. Cambridge: Harvard University Press, 1980.
142. Peters MV. A study of survival in Hodgkin's disease treated radiologically. AJR 1950;63: 299–311.
143. Peters MV, Middlemiss KCH. A study of Hodgkin's disease treated by irradiation. AJR 1958;79:114–121.
144. Peters MV. Prophylactic treatment of adjacent areas in Hodgkin's disease. Cancer Res 1966;26:1232–1243.
145. Kaplan HS. The radical radiotherapy of regionally localized Hodgkin's disease. Radiology 1962;78:553–561.
146. Kinmouth JB, Taylor GW, Harper RK. Lymphography: A technique for its clinical use in the lower limbs. Br Med J 1955;1.930–942.
147. Lee BJ, Nelson JH, Schwarz G. Evaluation of lymphangiography, inferior venacavography and intravenous pyelography in the clinical staging and management of Hodgkin's disease and lymphosarcoma. N Engl J Med 1964;271:327–337.
148. Glatstein E, Guernsey JM, Rosenberg SA, et al. The value of laparotomy and splenectomy in the staging of Hodgkin's disease. Cancer 1969;24:709–718.
149. Glatstein E, Trueblood HW, Enright LP, et al. Surgical staging of abdominal involvement in unselected patients with Hodgkin's disease. Radiology 1970;97:425.
150. Kaplan HS. On the natural history, treatment and prognosis of Hodgkin's disease. Harvey Lectures, 1968–1969. New York: Academic Press, 1970:215–259.
151. Smithers D. Hodgkin's disease. Edinburgh: Churchill-Livingstone, 1973.
152. Regula DP, Hoppe RT, Weiss LM. Nodular and diffuse types of lymphocyte predominant Hodgkin's disease. N Engl J Med 1988;318:214–219.
153. Slaughter DP, Economou SG, Southwick HW. The surgical management of Hodgkin's disease. Ann Surg 1958;148:705–710.
154. Peters MV, Hasselbach R, Brown TC. The natural history of the lymphomas related to the clinical classification. In: Zarafonetis CJD, ed. Proceedings of the International Conference on Leukemia-Lymphoma. Philadelphia: Lea & Febiger, 1968:357–370.
155. Lukes RJ, Craver LF, Hall TC, et al. Report of the nomenclature committee. Cancer Res 1966;26:311.
156. Carbone PP, Kaplan HS, Musshoff K, et al. Report of the committee on Hodgkin's disease staging. Cancer Res 1971;31:1860–1861.
157. Musshoff K, Ronemann H, Bourlis L, et al. Die extranodulare Lymphogranulomatose. Diagnose, Therapie und Prognose bei zwei unterschiedlichen Formen de Organ Befalls. Ein Beitrag zur Stadienein teilung des morbus Hodgkin. Fortschr Geb Roentgenstr Nuklearmed Erganzungsband 1968;109:776–786.
158. Lister TA, Crowther D, Sutcliffe SB, et al. Report of a committee convened to discuss the evaluation and staging of patients with Hodgkin's disease: Cotswald meeting. J Clin Oncol 1989;7:1630–1636; J Clin Oncol [Erratum] 1990;8:1602.
159. Urba W, Longo DL. Hodgkin's disease: Medical progress. N Engl J Med 1992;326: 678–687.
160. Mansfield CM, Fabian G, Jener S, et al. Comparison of lymphography and computer

tomography scanning in evaluating abdominal disease in stages III and IV Hodgkin's disease. Cancer 1990;66:2295–2299.

161. Castellino R, Hoppe RT, Black N. Computed tomography, lymphography and staging laparotomy; correlations in initial staging of Hodgkin's disease. AJR 1984;143:37–41.
162. Hoppe RD, Diehl LF, Lysar M, et al. Hodgkin's disease: Clinical utility of CT in initial staging and treatment. Radiology 1988;169:17–22.
163. Castellino RA. Imaging techniques for staging abdominal Hodgkin's disease. Cancer Treat Rep 1982;66:697–700.
164. Redman HC, Glatstein E, Castellino RA, et al. Computed tomography as an adjunct in the staging of Hodgkin's disease and non-Hodgkin's lymphomas. Radiology 1977;124: 381–385.
165. Breeman RS, Castellino RA, Harell GS, et al. CT-pathologic correlations in Hodgkin's disease and non-Hodgkin's lymphoma. Radiology 1978;126:159–166.
166. Jones SE, Tobias DA, Waldman RS. Complete tomographic scanning in patients with lymphoma. Cancer 1978;41:480–486.
167. Aisenberg AC. The staging of Hodgkin's disease. J Exp Clin Cancer Res 1983;2:209–212.
168. Mellor JA, Simmons AV, Barnard DL, et al. A retrospective evaluation of mediastinal tomograms, isotope liver scans and isotope bone scans in the staging and management of patients with lymphoma. Cancer 1983;52:2227–2229.
169. Tumeh SS, Rosenthal DS, Kaplan WD, et al. Lymphoma: Evaluation with Ga-67 SPECT. Radiology 1987;164:111–114.
170. Delaney TF, Glatstein E. The role of the staging laparotomy in the management of Hodgkin's disease. In: DeVita VT Jr, Hellman S, Rosenberg SA, eds. Cancer: Principles and practice of oncology, vol. 1. Philadelphia: JB Lippincott, 1987:1–44.
171. John RE. Is staging laparotomy routinely indicated in Hodgkin's disease? Ann Intern Med 1971;75:459.
172. Kinsella TJ, Glatstein E. Staging laparotomy and splenectomy for Hodgkin's disease: Current status. Cancer Invest 1983;1:87–91.
173. Lacher MJ. Routine staging laparotomy for patients with Hodgkin's disease is no longer necessary. Cancer Invest 1983;1:93–99.
174. Piro AJ, Hellman S. Laparotomy alters treatment in Hodgkin's disease. NCI Monogr 1973;36:307–311.
175. Kaplan HS, Dorfman RF, Nelson TS, et al. Staging laparotomy and splenectomy in Hodgkin's disease: Analysis of indications and patterns of involvement in 285 consecutive, unselected patients. NCI Monogr 1973;36:291–301.
176. Desser RK, Golomb HM, Ultmann JE, et al. Prognostic classification of Hodgkin's disease in pathologic stage III, based on anatomic considerations. Blood 1977;49: 883–893.
177. Stein RS, Golomb HM, Diggs CH, et al. Anatomic substages of stage III-A Hodgkin's disease. Ann Intern Med 1980;92:159–165.
178. Rosner F, Zarrabi MH. Late infections following splenectomy in Hodgkin's disease. Cancer Invest 1983;1:57–65.
179. Coker DD, Morris DM, Coleman JJ, et al. Infection among 210 patients with surgically staged Hodgkin's disease. Am J Med 1983;75:97–109.
180. Notter DT, Grossman PL, Rosenberg SA, et al. Infections in patients with Hodgkin's disease: A clinical study of 300 consecutive adult patients. Rev Infect Dis 1980;2: 761–800.
181. Desser RL, Ultmann JE. Risk of severe infection in patients with Hodgkin's disease or lymphoma after diagnostic laparotomy and splenectomy. Ann Intern Med 1972;77: 143–147.
182. Meeker WR, Richardson JD, West W, et al. Critical evaluation of laparotomy and splenectomy in Hodgkin's disease. Arch Surg 1972;105:222.
183. Jenkin RRT, Berry MP. Hodgkin's disease in children. Semin Oncol 1980;7:202–211.
184. Chilcote RR, Baehner RH, Hammond D. Septicemia and meningitis in children splenectomized for Hodgkin's disease. N Engl J Med 1976;295:798–800.
185. Slaven R, Nelson TS. Complications of staging laparotomy for Hodgkin's disease. NCI Monogr 1973;36:457.
186. Donaldson SS, Kaplan HS. Complications of treatment of Hodgkin's disease in children. Cancer Treat Rep 1982;66:977–989.
187. Mauch PM, Weinstein H, Botnick L, et al. An evaluation of long-term survival and treatment complications in children in Hodgkin's disease. Cancer 1983;51:925–932.
188. Lange B, Littman P. Management of Hodgkin's disease in children and adolescents. Cancer 1983;51:1371–1377.
189. Salzman JR, Kaplan HS. Effect of splenectomy on hematologic tolerance during total lymphoid radiotherapy of patients with Hodgkin's disease. Cancer 1971;27:471–478.
190. Panattiere RJ, Coltman CA. Splenectomy effects on chemotherapy in Hodgkin's disease. Arch Intern Med 1973;131:363–366.
191. Panattiere RJ, Coltman CA, Delaney FC. Splenectomy, chemotherapy and survival in Hodgkin's disease. Arch Intern Med 1977;137:341–343.
192. Ihde DC, DeVita VT, Canellos GP, et al. Effect of splenectomy on tolerance to combination chemotherapy in patients with lymphoma. Blood 1976;47:211–222.
193. Kaldor JM, Day NE, Clarke A, et al. Leukemia following Hodgkin's disease. N Engl J Med 1990;322:7–13.
194. Tucker MA, Coleman CN, Cox RS, et al. Risk of second cancers after treatment for Hodgkin's disease. N Engl J Med 1988;318:76–81.
195. Sutcliffe SB, Wrigley PFM, Timothy AR, et al. Posttreatment laparotomy as a guide to management in patients with Hodgkin's disease. Cancer Treat Rep 1982;6:759–765.
196. Kostraba NC, Peterson BA, Kennedy BJ, et al. Laparotomy in the reevaluation of patients with advanced Hodgkin's disease. Cancer Treat Rep 1981;65:685–687.
197. Mauch P, Tarbell N, Weinstein, et al. Stage IA and IIA supradiaphragmatic Hodgkin's disease: Prognostic factors in surgically staged patients treated with mantle and paraaortic irradiation. J Clin Oncol 1988;6:1576–1583.
198. Mauch P, Kalish LA, Kadin M, et al. Patterns of presentation of Hodgkin's disease: Implications for etiology and pathogenesis. Cancer (in press).
199. Myers CE, Chabner BA, DeVita VT, et al. Bone marrow involvement in Hodgkin's disease: Pathology and response to MOPP chemotherapy. Blood 1974;44:197–204.
200. Rosenberg SA. Hodgkin's disease of the bone marrow. Cancer Res 1971;31:1733–1736.
201. Ferrant A, Rodhain J, Michaux L, et al. Detection of skeletal involvement in Hodgkin's disease: A comparison of radiography bone scanning and bone marrow biopsy in 38 patients. Cancer 1975;35:1346–1353.
202. Musshoff K, Boutis L. Therapy results in Hodgkin's disease. Cancer 1968;21:1100–1113.
203. Rubins J. Cutaneous Hodgkin's disease: Indolent causes and control with chemotherapy. Cancer 1978;42:1219–1221.
204. Sapozink MD, Kaplan HS. Intracranial Hodgkin's disease. Report of 12 cases and review of the literature. Cancer 1982;52:1301–1307.
205. Valtysson G, Fisher-Beckfield P, Carbone PP. Cerebellar degeneration with Hodgkin's disease. Cancer 1979;29:246–249.
206. Young RC, Howser DM, Anderson T, et al. Central nervous system complications of non-Hodgkin's lymphoma. The potential role for prophylactic therapy. Am J Med 1979;66:246–249.
207. Moorthy AV, Zimmerman SW, Burkholder PM. Nephrotic syndrome in Hodgkin's disease. Evidence for pathogenesis alternative to immune complex deposition. Am J Med 1976;61:471–477.
208. Yum MN, Edwards JL, Kleit S. Glomerular lesions in Hodgkin's disease. Arch Pathol 1975;99:645–649.
209. Pusey WA. Cases of sarcoma and of Hodgkin's disease treated by exposures to x-rays: A preliminary report. JAMA 1902;38:166–170.
210. Teschendorf W. Veber Bestrahlung der ganzen menschluchen Korpers bel Blutkrankheiten. Strahlenther Onkol 1927;26:720–729.
211. Voorhoeve N. La lymphogranulomatose maligne. Acta Radiol 1925;4:567–589.
212. Kruchen C. Beltrag zur Rontgentheraple der Lymphogranulomatose mit besonder Berucksichtigung der neuren klinischen Ergelnisse. Strahlenther Onkol 1929;31: 623–670.
213. Easson EC, Russell MH. The cure of Hodgkin's disease. Br Med J 1963;1:1704.
214. Kaplan HS. Long-term results of palliative and radical radiotherapy of Hodgkin's disease. Cancer Res 1966;26:1250–1252.
215. Kaplan HS. Role of intensive radiotherapy in the management of Hodgkin's disease. Cancer 1966;19:356–367.
216. Kaplan HS. Clinical evaluation and radiotherapeutic management of Hodgkin's disease and the malignant lymphomas. N Engl J Med 1968;278:892–899.
217. Kaplan HS. On the natural history, treatment and prognosis of Hodgkin's disease. Harvey Lectures 1968–1969. New York: Academic Press, 1970:215–259.
218. Kaplan HS. Evidence for a tumoricidal dose level in the radiotherapy of Hodgkin's disease. Cancer Res 1966;26:1221–1224.
219. Rosenberg SA, Kaplan HS. Evidence for an orderly progression in the spread of Hodgkin's disease. Cancer Res 1966;26:1225–1231.
220. Vijayakumar S, Myrianthopoulos LC. An updated dose-response analysis in Hodgkin's disease. Radiother Oncol 1992;24:1–13.
221. Hanks GE, Kinzie JJ, Herring DR, et al. Patterns of care outcome studies in Hodgkin's disease: Results of the national practice and implications for management. Cancer Treat Rep 1982;66:805–808.
222. Landberg T, Liden K, Forslo H. Split-course radiation therapy of mediastinal Hodgkin's disease. TSD and CRE concepts. Acta Radiol 1973;12:33–39.
223. Page V, Gardner A, Karsmark CJ. Physical and dosimetric aspects of the radiotherapy of the malignant lymphomas. I. The mantle technique. Radiology 1970;96:609–618.
224. Carmel RJ, Kaplan HS. Mantle irradiation in Hodgkin's disease. An analysis of technique, tumor irradiation and complications. Cancer 1976;37:2812–2825.
225. Kaplan HS, Stewart HR. Complications of intensive megavoltage radiotherapy for Hodgkin's disease. NCI Monogr 1973;36:439–444.
226. Stewart HR, Cohn KE, Fajardo LF, et al. Radiation-induced heart disease: A study of twenty-five patients. Radiology 1967;89:302–310.
227. Lutz WP, Larsen RD. Technique for match mantle and para-aortic fields. Int J Radiat Oncol Biol Phys 1983;9:1753–1756.
228. Farah R, Ultmann J, Griem M, et al. Extended mantle radiation therapy for pathologic stage I and II Hodgkin's disease. J Clin Oncol 1988;6:1047–1052.
229. Page V, Gardner A, Karsmark CJ. Physical and dosimetric aspects of the radiotherapy of malignant lymphoma. II. The inverted Y technique. Radiology 1970;96:619–626.
230. Lutz WR, Larsen RD. Technique to match mantle and para-aortic fields. Int J Radiat Oncol Biol Phys 1979;5(suppl 2):159.
231. Trueblood HW, Enright LP, Roy GR, et al. Preservation of ovarian function in pelvic irradiation for Hodgkin's disease. Arch Surg 1970;100:236–237.
232. Kinzle JJ, Hanks GE, Maclean CJ, et al. Patterns of care study: Hodgkin's disease relapse rates and adequacy of portals. Cancer 1983;52:2223–2226.
233. Collaborative Group Study. Survival and complications of radiotherapy following involved and extended field therapy of Hodgkin's disease. Stage I and II-A collaborative study. Cancer 1976;38:288–305.
234. Mauch PM, Canellos GP, Rosenthal DS, et al. Reduction of fatal complications from combined modality therapy in Hodgkin's disease. J Clin Oncol 1985;3:501–505.
235. Rosenberg SA, Kaplan HS. The evolution and summary results of the Stanford randomized clinical trials of the management of Hodgkin's disease: 1962–1984. Int J Radiat Oncol Biol Phys 1985;11:5–22.

236. Timothy AR, et al. Hodgkin's disease: Combination chemotherapy for relapse following radical radiotherapy. Int J Radiat Oncol Biol Phys 1979;5:165–169.
237. Portlock CS. Impact of salvage treatment on initial relapses in patients with Hodgkin's disease stages I–III. Blood 1978;51:825–833.
238. Mauch P, Ryback M, Rosenthal D, et al. The influence of initial pathologic stage on the survival of patients who relapse from Hodgkin's disease. Blood 1980;56:892–897.
239. Mauch PM, Canellos GP, Rosenthal DS, et al. Reduction of fatal complications from combined modality therapy in Hodgkin's disease. J Clin Oncol 1985;3:501–505.
240. Hagemeister FB, Fuller LM, Sullivan JA, et al. Treatment of patients with stages I and II non-mediastinal Hodgkin's disease. Cancer 1982;50:2307–2313.
241. Carde P, Burgers JM, Henry-Amar M, et al. Clinical stages I and II Hodgkin's disease: A specifically tailored therapy according to prognostic factors. J Clin Oncol 1988;6: 239–252.
242. Ganesan TS, Wrigley PFM, Murray PA, et al. Radiotherapy for stage I Hodgkin's disease: 20 years' experience at St. Bartholomew's Hospital. Br J Cancer 1990;62: 314–318.
243. Mandell LR, Tan C, Groshen S, et al. Can para-aortic radiation be omitted in pathologically staged IA and IIA pediatric Hodgkin's disease? (in press).
244. Mauch P, Larson D, Osteen R, et al. Prognostic factors for positive surgical staging in patients with Hodgkin's disease. J Clin Oncol 1990;8:257–265.
245. Mauch P, Goodman R, Hellman S. The significance of mediastinal involvement in early stage Hodgkin's disease. Cancer 1978;42:1039–1045.
246. Hoppe RT. The management of stage II Hodgkin's disease with a large mediastinal mass: A prospective program emphasizing irradiation. Int J Radiat Oncol Biol Phys 1985;11:349–355.
247. Thar TL, Million RR, Hausner RJ, et al. Hodgkin's disease stage I and II. Relationship of recurrence to size of disease, radiation dose and number of sites involved. Cancer 1979;43:1101–1105.
248. Hoppe RT, Coleman CN, Kaplan HS, et al. Hodgkin's disease, pathologic stage I and II, the prognostic importance of initial sites of disease and extent of mediastinal involvement. Proc Am Soc Clin Oncol 1980;21:471.
249. Velentjas E, Barrett A, McElwain TJ, et al. Mediastinal involvement in early-stage Hodgkin's disease. Eur J Cancer 1980;16:1065–1068.
250. Mauch P, Gorshein D, Cunningham J, et al. Influence of mediastinal adenopathy on site and frequency of relapse in patients with Hodgkin's disease. Cancer Treat Rep 1982;66:809–817.
251. Leslie NT, Mauch P, Hellman S. Stage IA to IIB supradiaphragmatic Hodgkin's disease: Long-term survival and relapse frequency. Cancer 1985;55:2072–2078.
252. Mauch PM, et al. Stage IA–IIA supradiaphragmatic Hodgkin's disease: Prognostic factors in surgically staged patients treated with mantle and para-aortic irradiation. (in press).
253. Leopold KA, Canellos GP, Rosenthal D, et al. Stage IA–IIIB Hodgkin's disease: Staging and treatment with large mediastinal adenopathy. J Clin Oncol 1989;7:1059–1065.
254. Piro AJ, Weiss DR, Hellman S. Mediastinal Hodgkin's disease: A possible danger for intubation anesthesia. Int J Radiat Oncol Biol Phys 1976;1:415–419.
255. Krikorian JG, Portlock CS, Mauch PM. Hodgkin's disease presenting below the diaphragm: A review. J Clin Oncol 1986;4:1551–1562.
256. Mauch P, Goffman T, Rosenthal DS, et al. Stage III Hodgkin's disease: Improved survival with combined modality therapy as compared with radiation therapy alone. J Clin Oncol 1985;3:1166–1173.
257. Rosenberg SA, Kaplan HS, Gladstein EJ, et al. Combined modality therapy of Hodgkin's disease. A report of the Stanford trials. Cancer 1978;42:991–1000.
258. Goodman R, Mauch P, Piro A, et al. Stages IIB and IIB Hodgkin's disease: Results of combined modality treatment. Cancer 1977;40:8489.
259. Crnkovich MJ, Leopold K, Hoppe RT, et al. Stage I to IIB Hodgkin's disease: The combined experience at Stanford University and the Joint Center for Radiation Therapy. J Clin Oncol 1987;5:1041–1049.
260. Hellman S, Mauch P, Goodman RL, et al. The place of radiation therapy in the treatment of Hodgkin's disease. Cancer 1978;42:971–978.
261. Zucali R, Pagnoni AN, Zanini M, et al. Radiological and spirometric evaluation of mediastinal and pulmonary late effects after radiotherapy and chemotherapy for Hodgkin's disease. J Eur Radiother 1981;2:169.
262. Appelfield MM, Slawson RG, Spicer KM, et al. Long-term cardiovascular evaluation of patients with Hodgkin's disease treated by thoracic mantle radiation therapy. Cancer Treat Rep 1982;66:1003–1013.
263. Mauch P, Hellman S, Belli JA. Cardiac effects of mediastinal irradiation. N Engl J Med 1983;309:378.
264. Burns RJ, Bar-Schlomo BZ, Druck MN, et al. Detection of radionuclide cardiomyopathy by gated radionuclide angiography. Am J Med 1983;74:297–303.
265. Annest LS, Anderson RP, Li W, et al. Coronary artery disease following mediastinal radiation therapy. J Thorac Cardiovasc Surg 1983;85:257–263.
266. Bowin JF, Hutchinson GB. Coronary heart disease after irradiation for Hodgkin's disease. Cancer 1982;49:2470–2475.
267. Hancock SL, Hoppe RT. Heart disease mortality after treatment of Hodgkin's disease. Proc Am Soc Clin Oncol 1952;1155:337.
268. Foley KM, Woodruff J, Ellis F, et al. Radiation induced malignant and typical schwannomas. Ann Neurol 1979;7:311–318.
269. Kinsella TJ, Fraass BE, Glatstein E. Late effects of radiation therapy in the treatment of Hodgkin's disease. Cancer Treat Rep 1982;66:991–1001.
270. McDougall IR, Coleman CN, Burke JS, et al. Thyroid carcinoma after high-dose external radiotherapy for Hodgkin's disease. Cancer 1980;45:2056–2060.
271. Stutzman L, Glidewell O. Multiple chemotherapeutic agents for Hodgkin's disease. JAMA 1973;225:1202–1211.
272. Luce JK, Frei E, Gehan EA, et al. Chemotherapy of Hodgkin's disease. Arch Intern Med 1973;131:391–395.
273. Huguley CM, Durant JR, Moores RR, et al. A comparison of nitrogen mustard, vincristine, procarbazine and prednisone (MOPP) vs nitrogen mustard in advanced Hodgkin's disease. Cancer 1975;36:1227–1240.
274. British National Lymphoma Investigation: Value of prednisone in combination chemotherapy of stage IV Hodgkin's disease. Br Med J 1975;3:413–414.
275. Goldman JM. Combination chemotherapy for stage IV Hodgkin's disease (report #14). Clin Radiol 1981;32:531–535.
276. Jones SE, Haut A, Weick JK, et al. Comparison of Adriamycin-containing chemotherapy (MOP-BAP) with MOPP-bleomycin in the management of advanced Hodgkin's disease. Cancer 1983;51:339–347.
277. Bakemeier RF, Anderson JR, Costello W, et al. BCVPP chemotherapy for advanced Hodgkin's disease: Evidence for greater duration of complete remission, greater survival and less toxicity than with a MOPP regimen. Ann Intern Med 1984;101:447–456.
278. Straus DJ, Myers J, Lee BJ, et al. Treatment of advanced Hodgkin's disease with chemotherapy and irradiation. Am J Med 1984;76:270–278.
279. Haybittle JL, Eastering MJ, Hudson BV, et al. Review of British National Lymphoma Investigation studies of Hodgkin's disease: Development of a prognostic index. Lancet 1985;1:967–972.
280. Santoro A, Bonadonna G, Bonfante V, et al. Alternating drug combinations in the treatment of advanced Hodgkin's disease. N Engl J Med 1982;306:770–775.
281. Bonadonna G, Valagussa P, Santoro A. Alternating non-cross-resistant combination chemotherapy with ABVD or MOPP in stage IV Hodgkin's disease: A report of eight year results. Ann Intern Med 1986;104:739–746.
282. Hancock BW, Hudson GV, Hudson BV, et al. British National Lymphoma investigation randomized study of MOPP against LOPP in advanced Hodgkin's disease—long-term results. Br J Cancer 1991;63:578–582.
283. Somers R, Henry-Amar M, Carde P, et al. MOPP vs alternating MOPP/ABVD in advanced Hodgkin's disease (HD). Proc Am Soc Clin Oncol 1988;7:236.
284. Canellos GP, Propert K, Cooper R, et al. MOPP vs ABVD vs MOPP alternating with ABVD in advanced Hodgkin's disease: A prospective CALGB trial. Proc Am Soc Clin Oncol 1988;7:230.
285. Brusamolino E, Lazzarino M, Canevari A, et al. Alternating non-cross-resistant chemotherapy (MOPP-ABVD) in advanced Hodgkin's disease. Proc Am Soc Clin Oncol 1988;7:239.
286. Nicholson WM, Beard MEJ, Crowther D, et al. Combination chemotherapy in generalized Hodgkin's disease. Br Med J 1970;3:7–10.
287. Sutcliffe SB, Wrigley PFM, Peto J, et al. MVPP chemotherapy regimen for advanced Hodgkin's disease. Br Med J 1978;1:679–683.
288. Wagstaff J, Steward W, Jones M, et al. Factors affecting remission and survival in patients with advanced Hodgkin's disease treated with MVPP. Hematol Oncol 1986;4: 135–147.
289. Morgenfeld M, Somoza N, Magnasco J, et al. Combined chemotherapy cyclophosphamide, vinblastine, procarbazine and prednisone (CVPP) versus CVPP plus CCNU (CCVPP) in Hodgkin's disease. Cancer 1979;43:1579–1586.
290. Glick J, Tsiatis A, Chen M, et al. Improved survival with MOPP-ABVD compared to BCVPP ± radiotherapy for advanced Hodgkin's disease: 6-year ECOG results. Blood 1990;76(Suppl 1):351a.
291. DeVita VT, Hubbard SM, Longo DL. Treatment of Hodgkin's disease. JNCI Monogr 1990;10:19–28.
292. Durant JR, Gams RA, Velez-Garcia E, et al. BCNU, velban, cyclophosphamide, procarbazine, and prednisone (BVCPP) in advanced Hodgkin's disease. Cancer 1978;42: 2101–2110.
293. Gams RA, Durant JR, Bartolucci AA. Chemotherapy for advanced Hodgkin's disease: Conclusions from the Southeastern Cancer Study Group. Cancer Treat Rep 1982;66: 899–905.
294. McElwain TJ, Toy J, Smith E, et al. A combination of chlorambucil, vinblastine, procarbazine and prednisolone for treatment of Hodgkin's disease. Br J Cancer 1977;36: 276–280.
295. Selby P, Patel P, Milan S, et al. ChlVPP combination chemotherapy for Hodgkin's disease: Long-term results. Br J Cancer 1990;62:279–285.
296. Vose J, Armitage J, Weisenburger D, et al. ChlVPP—an effective and well-tolerated alternative to MOPP therapy for Hodgkin's disease. Am J Clin Oncol 1988;11:423–426.
297. Longo D. The use of chemotherapy in the treatment of Hodgkin's disease. Semin Oncol 1990;17:716–735.
298. Lister TA, Dorreen MS, Faux M, et al. The treatment of stage IIIA Hodgkin's disease. J Clin Oncol 1983;1:745–749.
299. Crowther D, Wagstaff J, Deakin D, et al. A randomized study comparing chemotherapy alone with chemotherapy followed by radiotherapy in patients with pathologically staged IIIA Hodgkin's disease. J Clin Oncol 1984;2:892–897.
300. Gams RA, Omura GA, Velez-Garcia E, et al. Alternating sequential combination chemotherapy in the management of advanced Hodgkin's disease. A Southeastern Cancer Study Group trial. Cancer 1986;58:1963–1968.
301. Cooper MR, Pajak TF, Nissen N, et al. A new effective four-drug combination of CCNU (1-3-cyclohexyl-1-nitrosourea) (NSC-79038), vinblastine, prednisone, and procarbazine for the treatment of advanced Hodgkin's disease. Cancer 1980;46:654–662.
302. Cooper MR, Pajak TF, Gottlieb AJ, et al. The effects of prior radiation therapy and age on the frequency and duration of complete remission among various four-drug treatment for advanced Hodgkin's disease. J Clin Oncol 1984;2:748–755.
303. Propert KJ, Cooper MR, Spurr C, et al. Combination chemotherapy with vinca alkaloids and alkylating agents for stage III and IV Hodgkin's disease (HD): Ten years of follow-up (CALGB 7251). Proc Am Soc Clin Oncol 1986;5:192.

304. Vinciguerra V, Propert KJ, Coleman M, et al. Alternating cycles of combination chemotherapy for patients with recurrent Hodgkin's disease following radiotherapy a prospectively randomized study by the Cancer and Leukemia Group B. J Clin Oncol 1986;4:838–846.
305. Druker BJ, Canellos GP. Chlorambucil, vinblastine, procarbazine and prednisone (ChlVPP): An effective but less toxic regimen than MOPP for advanced stage Hodgkin's disease (HD). Proc Am Assoc Cancer Res 1986;27:198.
306. Canellos GP, Anderson JR, Propert KJ, et al. Chemotherapy of advanced Hodgkin's disease with MOPP, ABVD, or MOPP alternating with ABVD. N Engl J Med 1992;327: 1478–1484.
307. Connors JM, Klimo P, Adams G, et al. MOPP/ABV hybrid versus alternating MOPP/ ABVD for advanced Hodgkin's disease. Proc Am Soc Clin Oncol 1992;11:317.
308. Prosnitz LR, Farber LR, Scott J, et al. Combined modality therapy for advanced Hodgkin's disease: 15-year follow-up data. J Clin Oncol 1988;6:603–612.
309. Wagener DJT, Marion J, Burgers V, et al. Sequential non-cross-resistant chemotherapy regimens (MOPP and CAVmP in Hodgkin's disease stage IIIB and IV. Cancer. 1983;52: 1558–1562.
310. Klimo P, Connors JM. MOPP/ABV hybrid program: Combination chemotherapy based on early introduction of seven effective drugs for advanced Hodgkin's disease. J Clin Oncol 1985;3:1174–1182.
311. Connors JM, Klimo P. MOPP/ABV hybrid chemotherapy for advanced Hodgkin's disease. Semin Hematol 1987;24:35–40.
312. Viviani S, Bonadonna G, Santoro A, et al. Alternating versus hybrid MOPP-ABVD in Hodgkin's disease. The Milan experience. Ann Oncol 1991;2:55–62.
313. Longo DL, Russo A, Duffey PL, et al. Treatment of advanced-stage massive mediastinal Hodgkin's disease: The case for combined modality treatment. J Clin Oncol 1991;9: 227–235.
314. O'Reilly SE, Hoskins P, Klimo P, Connors JM. MACOP-B and VACOP-B in diffuse large cell lymphomas and MOPP/ABV in Hodgkin's disease. Ann Oncol 1991;2(suppl 1):17–23.
315. Longo DL, Duffey PL, DeVita VT, et al. Treatment of advanced-stage Hodgkin's disease: Alternating noncrossresistant MOPP/CABS is not superior to MOPP. J Clin Oncol 1991;9:1409–1420.
316. Goodman LS, Wintrobe MM, Dameshek W, et al. Nitrogen mustard therapy. Use of methyl bis (B-chloroethyl) amine hydrochloride and tris (B-chloroethyl) amine hydrochloride for Hodgkin's disease lymphosarcoma, leukemia, and certain allied and miscellaneous disorders. JAMA 1946;132:126–132.
317. Alpert LP, Petersen SK. The use of nitrogen mustard in the treatment of lymphomata. Bull U S Army Med Dept 1947;7:187–194.
318. Damesheck W, Weisfuse L, Stein T. Nitrogen mustard therapy in Hodgkin's disease. Analysis of 50 consecutive cases. Blood 1949;4:338–379.
319. Bollag W, Grunberg E. Tumor inhibitory effects of a new class of cytotoxic agents: Methyl hydrazine derivatives. Experientia 1963;19:751.
320. Mathe G, Schweisguth O, Schneider M, et al. Methylhydrazine in the treatment of Hodgkin's disease. Lancet 1963;2:1077.
321. Martz G, D'Alessandri A, Keel HJ, et al. Preliminary clinical results with a new antitumor agents RO 4-6467 (NSC 77213). Cancer Chemother Rep 1963;33:5–14.
322. Falkson G, de Villieb PC, Falkson HC. *N*-Isopropyl-(2-methyl-hydrazine)-*p*-toluamide (MIH). Proc Soc Exp Biol Med 1965;120:561–565.
323. DeVita VT, Serpick A, Carbone PP. Preliminary clinical studies with ibenzmethyzin. Clin Pharmacol Ther 1966;7:542–546.
324. Craft CB. Results with roentgen ray therapy in Hodgkin's disease. Bull Staff Meet Univ Miami Hosp 1940;11:391–409.
325. Jacobs EM, Peters FC, Luce JK, et al. Mechlorethamine HCL and cyclophosphamide in the treatment of Hodgkin's disease. Cancer Chemother Rep 1963;27:27–32.
326. Aisenberg AC, Qazi R. Improved survival in Hodgkin's disease. Cancer 1976;37:2323–2329.
327. DeVita VT, Serpick A. Combination chemotherapy in the treatment of advanced Hodgkin's disease. Proc Am Assoc Cancer Res 1967;8:13.
328. DeVita VT, Serpick AA, Carbone PP. Combination chemotherapy in the treatment of advanced Hodgkin's disease. Ann Intern Med 1970;73:891–895.
329. Lowenbraun S, DeVita VT, Serpick AA. Combination chemotherapy with nitrogen mustard, vincristine, procarbazine, and prednisone in previously treated patients with Hodgkin's disease. Blood 1970;36:704–717.
330. DeVita VT. Consequences of the chemotherapy of Hodgkin's disease. Cancer 1981;47: 1–13.
331. Frei E III, Luce JK, Gamble JF, et al. Combination chemotherapy in advanced Hodgkin's disease: Induction and maintenance of remission. Ann Intern Med 1973;79:376–382.
332. Canellos GP, Young RC, DeVita VT, et al. Combination chemotherapy of advanced Hodgkin's disease in relapse following extensive radiotherapy. Clin Pharmcol Ther 1972;13:750–754.
333. Cadman E, Bloom AF, Prosnitz A, et al. The effective use of combined modality therapy for the treatment of patients with Hodgkin's disease who relapsed following radiotherapy. Am J Clin Oncol 1983;6:313–318.
334. DeVita VT. Cell kinetics and the chemotherapy of cancer. Cancer Chemother Rep 1971;3:23–33.
335. Hryniuk W, Bush H. The importance of dose intensity in chemotherapy of metastatic breast cancer. J Clin Oncol 1984;2:1281–1288.
336. DeVita VT, Hubbard SM, Longo DL. The chemotherapy of lymphomas: Looking back, moving forward—the Richard and Hinda Rosenthal Foundation Award Lecture. Cancer Res 1987;47:5810–5824.
337. Longo DL, Young RC, Wesley M, et al. Twenty years of MOPP chemotherapy for Hodgkin's disease. J Clin Oncol 1986;4:1295–1306.
338. Fuer EJ, Kessler LG, Baker SG, et al. The impact of breakthrough clinical trials on survival in population based tumor registries. J Clin Epidemiol 1991;44:141–153.
339. Moore ME, Jones SE, Bull JM, et al. MOPP chemotherapy for advanced Hodgkin's disease: Prognostic factors in 81 patients. Cancer 1973;32:52–60.
340. Jacobs C, Portlock CS, Rosenberg SA. Prednisone in MOPP chemotherapy for Hodgkin's disease. Br Med J 1976;2:1469.
341. Morgenfeld M, Somoza N, Magnasco J, et al. Combined chemotherapy cyclophosphamide, vinblastine, procarbazine and prednisone (CVPP) vs CVPP plus CCNU (CCVPP) in Hodgkin's disease. Cancer 1979;43:1579.
342. Diggs Ch, Wiernik PH, Levi JA, et al. Cyclophosphamide, vinblastine, procarbazine and prednisone with CCNU and vinblastine maintenance for advanced Hodgkin's disease. Cancer 1977;39:1949.
343. Gibbs GE, Peterson BA, Kennedy BJ, et al. Long-term survival of patients with Hodgkin's disease. Arch Intern Med 1981;141:897.
344. Nissen IN, Pajak FT, Glidewell O, et al. A comparative study of a BCNU containing 4-drug program versus MOPP versus 3-drug combinations in advanced Hodgkin's disease. Cancer 1979;43:31–40.
345. Coltman CA Jr, Jones SE, Grozea PN, et al. Bleomycin in combination with MOPP in the management of advanced Hodgkin's disease: A Southwest Oncology Group experience. In: Sikic BI, Rosenscweig M, Carter SK, eds. Bleomycin chemotherapy. Orlando, FL: Academic Press, 1985:137–153.
346. Santoro A, Bonadonna G. Prolonged disease-free survival in MOPP-resistant Hodgkin's disease after treatment with Adriamycin, bleomycin, vinblastine and dacarbazine (ABVD). Cancer Chemother Pharmacol 1979;2:101–105.
347. Santoro A, Bonfante V, Bonadonna G. Salvage chemotherapy with ABVD in MOPP-resistant Hodgkin's disease. Ann Intern Med 1982;96:139–143.
348. Papa G, Mandelli F, Anselmo AP, et al. Treatment of MOPP-resistant Hodgkin's disease with Adriamycin, bleomycin, vinblastine and dacarbazine (ABVD). Eur J Cancer 1982;9:803–806.
349. Carde P, MacKintosh R, Rosenberg SA. A dose and time response analysis of the treatment of Hodgkin's disease with MOPP therapy. J Clin Oncol 1983;1:146–153.
350. DeVita VT. The influence of information on drug resistance on protocol design. Ann Oncol 1991;2:53–106.
351. Devereau S, Linch DC, Gribben JG, et al. GM-CSF accelerates neutrophil recovery after autologous bone marrow transplantation for Hodgkin's disease. Bone Marrow Transplant 1989;4:49–54.
352. Anderson J, Canellos GP. MOPP vs. ABVD vs. MOPP alternating with ABVD in advanced Hodgkin's disease. [Abstract] Presented at the International Conference on Malignant Lymphoma, Lugano, 1990.
353. Glick J, Tsiatis A, Schilsky R, et al. A randomized phase III trial of MOPP/ABVD hybrid vs. sequential MOPP-ABVD in advanced Hodgkin's disease: Preliminary results of the Intergroup Trial. Proc Ann Meet Am Soc Clin Oncol [Abstract] 1991;10:A941.
354. Gulati S, Bennett CL. Granulocyte macrophage colony-stimulating factors as adjunct therapy in relapsed Hodgkin's disease. Ann Intern Med 1992;116:177–82.
355. Mead GM, Harker WG, Kushlan P, et al. Single-agent palliative chemotherapy for end-stage Hodgkin's disease. Cancer 1982;50:829–835.
356. Ruud ENVR, Clemens H, Dekker AW, et al. Dose intensity of MOPP chemotherapy and survival in Hodgkin's disease. J Clin Oncol 7:1776–1782, 989.
357. Gobbi PG, Cavalli C, Rossi A, et al. The role of dose and rate of administration of MOPP drugs in 97 retrospective Hodgkin's patients. Haematologica 1987;72:523–528.
358. Rosso R, Venturini M, Mariani GL. The importance of dose intensity in cancer chemotherapy. Forum. Trends Exp Clin Med 1991;1:264–275.
359. Lagarde P, Bonichon H, Eghbali I, et al. Influence of dose intensity and density on therapeutic and toxic effects in Hodgkin's disease. Br J Cancer 1989;59:645–649.
360. Fisher RI, DeVita VT, Hubbard SM, et al. Prolonged disease-free survival in Hodgkin's disease with MOPP reinduction after first relapse. Ann Intern Med 1979;90:761–763.
361. DeVita VT, Hubbard SM, Longo DL. The chemotherapy of lymphomas: Looking back and moving forward. The Richard and Hinda Rosenthal Foundation Award Lecture. Cancer Res 1987;47:5810–5824.
362. Kessinger A, Bierman PJ, Vose JM, Armitage JO. High-dose cyclophosphamide, carmustine, and etoposide, followed by autologous peripheral stem cell transplantation for patients with relapsed Hodgkin's disease. Blood 1991;77:2322–2325.
363. Vose JM, Bierman PJ, Armitage JO. Hodgkin's disease: The role of bone marrow transplantation. Semin Oncol 1990;17:749–757.
364. Phillips GL, Reece DE, Barnett MJ, et al. Allogeneic marrow transplantation for refractory Hodgkin's disease. J Clin Oncol 1989;7:1039–1045.
365. Desch CE, Lasala MR, Smith TJ, Hillner BE. The optimal timing of autologous bone marrow transplantation in Hodgkin's disease patients after a chemotherapy relapse. J Clin Oncol 1992;10:200–209.
366. Armitage JO, Bierman PJ, Vose JM, et al. Autologous bone marrow transplantation for patients with relapsed Hodgkin's disease. Am J Med 1991;91:605–611.
367. Longo DL, Duffey PL, Young RC, et al. Conventional-dose salvage combination chemotherapy in patients relapsing with Hodgkin's disease after combination chemotherapy: The low probability for cure. J Clin Oncol 1992;10:210–218.
368. Vinciguerra V, Coleman M, Jarowski CI, et al. A new combination chemotherapy for resistant Hodgkin's disease. JAMA 1977;237:33–35.
369. Viviani S, Santoro A, Negretti E, et al. Salvage chemotherapy in Hodgkin's disease. Results in patients relapsing more than twelve months after first complete remission. Ann Oncol 1990;1:123–127.
370. Goldman JM, Dawson AA. Combination chemotherapy for advanced resistant Hodgkin's disease. Lancet 1975;2:1224–1227.
371. Longo DL, Duffey PL, Young RC, et al. Conventional-dose salvage combination che-

motherapy in patients relapsing with Hodgkin's disease after combination chemotherapy: The low probability for cure. J Clin Oncol 1992;10:210–218.
372. Devereau S, Linch DC, Gribben JG, et al. GM-CSF accelerates neutrophil recovery after autologous bone marrow transplantation for Hodgkin's disease. Bone Marrow Transplant 1989;4:49–54.
373. Taylor KM, Jagannath S, Spitzer G, et al. Recombinant human granulocyte colony-stimulating factor hasten granulocyte recovery after high-dose chemotherapy and autologous bone marrow transplantation in Hodgkin's disease. J Clin Oncol 1989;7:1791–1799.
374. Weiss J, von Roemling H, Peters HJ, et al. Chemotherapie bei Vorbehandeltem morbus Hodgkin mit Lomustin, Bleomycin, Vinblastin und Dexamethason. Dtsch Med Wochenschr 1983;108:1428–1432.
375. Tannir N, Hagemeister F, Valasquez W, et al. Long-term follow-up with ABDIC salvage chemotherapy of MOPP-resistant Hodgkin's disease. J Clin Oncol 1983;1:432–439.
376. Einhorn LH, Williams SD, Stevens EE, et al. Treatment of MOPP-refractory Hodgkin's disease with vinblastine, doxorubicin, bleomycin, CCNU, and dacarbazine. Cancer 1983;51:1348–1352.
377. Piga A, Ambrosetti A, Todeschini, et al. Doxorubicin, bleomycin, vinblastine and dacarbazine (ABVD) salvage of mechlorethamine, vincristine, prednisone, and procarbazine (MOPP)-resistant advanced Hodgkin's disease. Cancer Treat Rep 1984;58:947–951.
378. Harker GW, Kushlan P, Rosenberg SA. Combination chemotherapy for advanced Hodgkin's disease after failure of MOPP, ABVD and B-CAV-e. Ann Intern Med 1984;10:440–446.
379. Bonadonna G, Viviani S, Valagussa P, et al. Third-line salvage chemotherapy in Hodgkin's disease. Semin Oncol 1985;12:23–25.
380. Santoro A, Viviani SS, Valagussa P, et al. CCNU, etoposide and prednimustine (CEP) in refractory Hodgkin's disease. Semin Oncol 1986;13:23–26.
381. Cervantes F, Reverter JC, Montserrat E, et al. Treatment of advanced resistant Hodgkin's disease with lomustine, etoposide, and prednimustine. Cancer Treat Rep 1986;70:665–667.
382. Mandelli F, Cimino G, Mauro FR, et al. Prognosis and management of patients affected by multi-pre-treated Hodgkin's disease. Haematology 1986;71:205–208.
383. Richards MA, Waxman JH, Ganesan TS, et al. EVA treatment for recurrent or unresponsive Hodgkin's disease. Cancer Chemother Pharmacol 1986;18:51–53.
384. Garbes ID, Gomez GA, Tan T, et al. Salvage chemotherapy for advanced Hodgkin's disease. Med Pediatr Oncol 1987;15:45–48.
385. Hagemeister FBN, Tannir N, McLaughlin P, et al. MIME chemotherapy (Methyl-GAG, ifosfamide, methotrexate, etoposide) as treatment for recurrent Hodgkin's disease. J Clin Oncol 1987;5:556–561.
386. Tseng A, Jacobs C, Coleman CN, et al. Third-line chemotherapy for resistant Hodgkin's disease with lomustine, etoposide, and methotrexate. Cancer Treat Rep 1987;71:475–478.
387. Schulman P, Propert K, Cooper MR, et al. Phase II study of MOPLACE in previously treated Hodgkin's disease. Proc Soc Clin Oncol 1987;6:A742.
388. Levi JA, Wiernik PH, Diggs CH. Combination chemotherapy of advanced previously treated Hodgkin's disease with streptozoticin, CCNU, Adriamycin and bleomycin. Med Pediatr Oncol 1977;3:33–40.
389. Hoppe RT, Coleman CN, Cox RS et al. The management of stage I–II Hodgkin's disease with irradiation alone or combined modality therapy: The Standford experience. Blood 1982;59:455–465.
390. Hagemeister FB, Fuller LM, Velasques WS, et al. Stage I and II Hodgkin's disease: Involved-field radiotherapy versus extended-field radiotherapy versus involved-field radiotherapy followed by six cycles of MOPP. Cancer Treat Rep 1982;66:789–798.
391. Nissen NI, Nordentoft AM. Radiotherapy versus combined modality treatment of stage I and II Hodgkin's disease. Cancer Treat Rep 1982;66:799–803.
392. Anderson H, Deakin DP, Wagstaff J, et al. A randomized study of adjuvant chemotherapy after mantle radiotherapy in supradiaphragmatic Hodgkin's disease PS IIA-IIB: A report from the Manchester Lymphoma Group. Br J Cancer 1985;49:695–702.
393. Coleman DN, Williams CJ, Flint A, et al. Hematologic neoplasia in patients treated for Hodgkin's disease. N Engl J Med 1977;297:1249–1252.
394. Blayney DW, Longo DL, Young RC, et al. Decreasing risk of leukemia with prolonged follow-up after chemotherapy and radiotherapy for Hodgkin's disease. N Engl J Med 1987;316:710–714.
395. Tucker MA, Coleman CN, Cox RS, et al. Risk of second cancers after treatment for Hodgkin's disease. N Engl J Med 1988;318:75–81.
396. Horning SJ, Hoppe RT, Hancock SL, Rosenberg SA. Vinblastine, bleomycin, and methotrexate: An effective adjuvant in favorable Hodgkin's disease. J Clin Oncol 1988;6:1822–1831.
397. Olweny CLM, Katongole-Mbidde E, Kiive C, et al. Childhood Hodgkin's disease in Uganda: A 10-year experience. Cancer 1978;42:787–792.
398. Ekert H, Waters KD, Smith PJ, et al. Treatment with MOPP or ChlVPP chemotherapy only for all stages of childhood Hodgkin's disease. J Clin Oncol 1988;6:1845–1850.
399. O'Dwyer PJ, Wiernik PH, Steward MB, Slawson RG. Treatment of early stage Hodgkin's disease: A randomized trial of radiotherapy plus chemotherapy versus chemotherapy alone. In: Cavalli F, Bonadonna G, Rozencweig M, eds. Malignant lymphomas and Hodgkin's disease: Experimental and therapeutic advances. Boston: Martinus Nijhoff, 1985:329–336.
400. Pavlovsky S, Maschio M, Santarelli MT, et al. Randomized trial of chemotherapy versus chemotherapy plus radiotherapy for stage I–II Hodgkin's disease. JNCI 1988;80:1466–1473.
401. Cimino G, Biti GP, Anselmo AP, et al. MOPP chemotherapy versus extended field radiotherapy in the management of pathological stages I–IIA Hodgkin's disease. J Clin Oncol 1989;7:732–737.
402. Longo DL, Glatstein E, Duffey PL, et al. Radiation therapy versus combination chemotherapy in the treatment of early stage Hodgkin's disease: Seven-year results of a prospective randomized trial. J Clin Oncol 1991;9:897–901.
403. Pedersen-Bjergaard J, Specht I, Larsen SO, et al. Risk of therapy-related leukaemia and preleukaemia after Hodgkin's disease. Relation to age, cumulative dose of alkylating agents, and time from chemotherapy. Lancet 1987;2:83–88.
404. Longo DL, DeVita VT. The use of combination chemotherapy in the treatment of early stage Hodgkin's disease. In: DeVita VT, Hellman S, Rosenberg SA, ed. Important advances in oncology. Philadelphia: JB Lippincott, 1992:155–166.
405. Biggar RJ. Cancer in acquired immunodeficiency syndrome: An epidemiologic assessment. Semin Oncol 1990;17:251–260.
406. Freter CD. Acquired immunodeficiency syndrome-associated lymphoma. NCI Monogr 1990;10:45–54.
407. Zielgler H, Beckstead JA, Volberding PA, et al. Non-Hodgkin's lymphoma in 90 homosexual men: Relation to generalized lymphadenopathy and acquired immunodeficiency syndrome. N Engl J Med 1984;311:565–570.
408. Remick SC, Diamond C, Migliozzi JA, et al. Primary central nervous system lymphoma in patients with and without the acquired immune deficiency syndrome: A retrospective analysis and review of literature. Medicine (Baltimore) 1990;69:345–360.
409. Serrano M, Bellas C, Campo E, et al. Hodgkin's disease in patients with antibodies to human immunodeficiency virus. Cancer 1990;65:2248–2254.
410. Prior E, Goldberg AF, Conjalka MS, et al. Hodgkin's disease in homosexual men. An AIDS-related phenomenon? Am J Med 1986;81:1085.
411. Gill PS, Levine AM, Kiarlo M, et al. AIDS-related malignant lymphomas: Results of prospective drug trials. J Clin Oncol 1987;5:1322.
412. Unger PD, Strauchen JA. Hodgkin's disease in AIDS complex patients. Cancer 1986;58:821.
413. Bookman MA, Longo DL. Complications in patients treated for Hodgkin's disease. Cancer Treat Rev 1986;13:77–111.
414. Louie AC, Cavalli F, Rozensweig M. New agents for Hodgkin's and non-Hodgkin's lymphoma in malignant lymphomas and Hodgkin's disease: Experimental and therapeutic advances. In: Cavalli F, Bonadonna G, Rozensweig M, eds. Malignant lymphomas in Hodgkin's disease: Experimental and therapeutic advances. Boston: Martinus Nijhoff, 1985:493–511.
415. Warrell RP, Coonley CJ, Straus DJ, et al. Treatment of patients with advanced malignant lymphoma using gallium nitrate administered as a seven-day continuous infusion. Cancer 1983;51:1982–1987.
416. Knight WAT, Fabian C, Costanzi J, et al. Methylglyoxal-bis-guanylhydrazone (methyl GAG, MGBG) in lymphoma and Hodgkin's disease. Invest New Drugs 1983;1:235–237.
417. Espana P, Kaplan R, Robichaud K, et al. Phase II study of spiroglimanium (spiro G) in lymphoma patients. Proc Am Soc Clin Oncol 1982;1:166.
418. Weick JK, Jones SE, Ryan DH. Phase II study of amacrine (m-AMSA) in advanced lymphomas: A Southwest Oncology Group study. Cancer Treat Rep 1983;67:489–492.
419. Case ED, Hayes DM. Phase II study of arizidinybenzoquinone in refractory lymphoma. Cancer Treat Rep 1983;67:993–996.
420. Coltman CA, McDaniel TM, Balcerzak SP, et al. Mitoxantone hydrochloride (NSC-310739) in lymphoma. A Southwest Oncology Group study. Invest New Drug 1983;1:65–70.
421. Warrell RP, Kempen SJ. Clinical evaluation of a new anthracyline antibiotic aclacinomycin-A in patients with advanced malignant lymphoma. Am J Clin Oncol 1983;6:81–84.
422. Coonley CJ, Warrell RP, Straus DJ, et al. Clinical evaluation of 4-demethoxydaunorubicin in patients with advanced malignant lymphoma. Cancer Treat Rep 1983;67:949–950.
423. Rosenweig M, Crespeigne N, Kenis Y. Phase I trial with 4-deoxydoxorubin (esonibicen). Invest New Drug 1983;1:309–313.
424. Vriesendorp HM, Herpst JM, Germack MA, et al. Phase I–II studies of yttrium-labeled antiferritin treatment for end-stage Hodgkin's disease, including Radiation Therapy Oncology Group 87-01. J Clin Oncol 1991;9:918–928.

Cancer: Principles & Practice of Oncology, Fourth Edition,
edited by Vincent T. DeVita, Jr., Samuel Hellman, Steven A. Rosenberg.
J.B. Lippincott Co., Philadelphia © 1993.

Dan L. Longo
Vincent T. DeVita, Jr
Elaine S. Jaffe
Peter Mauch
Walter J. Urba

CHAPTER **52**

Lymphocytic Lymphomas

EPIDEMIOLOGY

Malignant lymphomas are the seventh most common causes of death from cancer in the United States.[1] In 1992, approximately 41,000 new cases were diagnosed, and there were approximately 19,400 deaths from the disease. Because of the young average age (42 years) of the lymphoma population, the total in person-years of life lost each year ranks the lymphomas fourth in terms of economic impact among cancers in the United States. There are two major subgroups of lymphoma: Hodgkin's disease and the non-Hodgkin's lymphomas. The term non-Hodgkin's lymphomas does not adequately describe the larger of these two subsets, and because approximately 98% of these lymphomas are of lymphocyte origin, we call them lymphocytic lymphomas. This designation is also not perfect; it is inaccurate in a small fraction of cases and redundant in the rest. As we use the term, lymphocytic lymphomas are those lymphomas that are not Hodgkin's disease.

The incidence of lymphocytic lymphomas is increasing each year; the 50% increase in incidence between 1973 and 1988 reported by the American Cancer Society was one of the largest increases reported for any cancer.[2,3] A large portion of this increase has been attributed to the lymphocytic lymphomas developing in association with the acquired immunodeficiency syndrome (AIDS). The Centers for Disease Control indicate that 3% of all adult patients with AIDS develop lymphoma.[4] In support of this hypothesis is the reported increase in lymphocytic lymphomas among men between the ages of 20 and 54 in San Francisco, which parallels an increase in Kaposi's sarcoma. None of the other geographic areas included in the Surveillance, Epidemiology and End Results (SEER) Program had such large increases in incidence of lymphocytic lymphoma for men in this age group. The rates for 20- to 54-year-old men in San Francisco County are five times higher than those in SEER areas excluding this region. The inescapable conclusion is that the incidence of AIDS-related lymphomas is increasing. However, the large increase in younger men does not account for the 57% increase in the overall incidence of lymphocytic lymphomas. Increases have been seen for other age groups; the group older than 65 years of age has had a 55% increase in incidence. Although the age-adjusted incidence of lymphomas has increased most for high-grade lymphomas (0.4 to 1.7 per 100,000), as would be expected for AIDS-related lymphomas, the incidence of low- and intermediate-grade lymphomas has also increased.

In the United States, there is a steady increase in the incidence of lymphocytic lymphomas from childhood through 80 years of age. They are more common in males than females (16.6 versus 11.2 per 100,000).[3,5–7] The incidence is higher in whites than blacks (13.7 versus 8.6 per 100,000). Unlike Hodgkin's disease, for which new treatment regimens have been rapidly implemented in the oncologic community and rapid decreases in mortality (50% reduction since 1973) have been observed, there has been a slight increase in mortality rates for the lymphocytic lymphomas. This increase, which occurred despite marked improvements in therapy, remains unexplained.

The lymphocytic lymphomas are found worldwide. Their overall incidence, and the incidence of the various histologic subtypes varies in different parts of the world. Burkitt's lymphoma occurs more frequently in tropical Africa; immunoproliferative small intestine disease in the Middle East; and adult T-cell leukemia-lymphoma in southwest Japan and the Caribbean basin.[8]

ETIOLOGY

A hereditary influence on the incidence of lymphomas is suggested by their higher incidence in patients with inherited immunologic deficiency diseases and by a small increase in the incidence in families of patients with immunologic disorders.[9] One study found a significant increase in the incidence of lymphomas in patients with collagen vascular diseases compared with the general population and adjusted for age.[10] This increased incidence approached 10% in patients with long-standing Sjögren's syndrome who tend to develop diffuse aggressive lymphomas or immunoblastic lymphomas.[11–13] An association between the class I major histocompatibility complex (MHC) antigen HLA-B12 and lymphoma has been reported.[14,15] Klinefelter's syndrome and the Chediak-Higashi syndrome have been associated with an increased risk of lymphoreticular malignancy.[16,17] Several other diseases predispose to the development of lymphomas (Table 52–1). Lymphoma-like syndromes have been found in patients who take phenytoin; in most cases, the disease regresses after the patient stops taking phenytoin, but a small fraction develop malignant lymphomas of several different varieties, including Hodgkin's disease.[18]

Environmental exposures, viruses, chromosomal aberrations, and congenital or acquired immunosuppression have been associated with the development of lymphocytic lymphomas. Despite these associations, the actual cause of most lymphocytic lymphomas remains unknown.

ENVIRONMENTAL EXPOSURE

The increased incidence of lymphoma among Midwestern farmers born after 1900 and dying before age 65 has raised the possibility that relatively recent changes in agricultural techniques and practices, such as the increased use of pesticides and fertilizers after World War II, may play a role in the cause of lymphoid neoplasia.[19] This is supported by case-control studies indicating that occupational exposure to phenoxyherbicides is associated with a twofold to fivefold increase in the risk of developing a lymphocytic lymphoma.[20,21] A dose-response association between lymphoma risk and acres sprayed with herbicides has been reported.[22] The carcinogens are presumed to be 2,3-dichlorophenoxyacetic acid (2,4-D) or 2,4,5-trichlorophenoxyacetic acid (2,4,5-T) and their congeners.[23] A case-control study showed that the risk for non-Hodgkin's lymphoma was increased by 50% among Vietnam veterans.[24] Although Agent Orange, a 1:1 mixture of 2,4-D and 2,4,5-T, was originally implicated, the fact that the greatest risk of lymphoma was found among Navy veterans, most of whom were stationed on ocean-going vessels with little opportunity for exposure to Agent Orange, rather than land-based troops in areas exposed to the defoliant, argues against Agent Orange being the causative agent. A 4.2-fold increased risk for developing lymphoma was reported for employees in the U.S. flour industry.[25] The risk was particularly high among persons working in maintenance and elevator departments of mills. Although environmental exposures are associated with lymphoma, the nature of the risky exposure is poorly defined.

TABLE 52–1. Disease Associated With Lymphoma Predisposition

Klinefelter's syndrome
Chediak-Higashi syndrome
Ataxia-telangiectasia syndrome
Wiscott-Aldrich syndrome
Swiss-type agammaglobulinemia
Common variable immunodeficiency disease
Acquired hypogammaglobulinemia
Iatrogenic immunosuppression (*e.g.*, treatment with anti-CD3 or cyclosporine)
Sjögren's syndrome
Rheumatoid arthritis and systemic lupus erythematosus
Acquired immunodeficiency syndrome
Phenytoin therapy
X-linked lymphoproliferative syndrome

It appears that ionizing radiation can cause malignant lymphoma in humans, but the mechanism of neoplastic transformation and the conditions under which it occurs have not been clearly delineated. An increased prevalence of lymphocytic lymphoma was demonstrated in survivors of the atomic bomb in Hiroshima who were exposed to 100 cGy or more.[26,27] An increased incidence of lymphoma has been demonstrated in patients irradiated for ankylosing spondylitis.[28] In both groups, the ratio of observed to expected cases of lymphoma was 2:1. Patients with Hodgkin's disease treated with radiation therapy and chemotherapy have an increased risk of developing secondary large cell lymphomas, often involving the gastrointestinal tract.

IMMUNOSUPPRESSION

Except for the higher incidence of Hodgkin's disease in siblings and the influence of phenytoin on the development of lymphomas, it is difficult to separate the influence of inheritance from immunosuppression, which is probably of etiologic importance even without an inherited background. For example, lymphomas occur with an increased frequency in many congenital and acquired immunodeficiency diseases.

Patients who are chronically immunosuppressed by drugs, particularly those who have received organ transplants, have a higher incidence of cancer, particularly aggressive lymphoproliferative disorders.[29,30] These lesions may range from benign polyclonal B-cell hyperplasias related to Epstein-Barr virus (EBV) infection to frankly malignant monoclonal B-cell lymphomas. Non-B-cell tumors do occur, but comprise 15% or fewer of all tumors. Posttransplantation lymphomas differ from those developing in the general population; extranodal involvement is found in 69% rather than 24% to 48%, respectively, and central nervous system (CNS) involvement is also more common (28% versus 1%). The immunosuppressive regimen influences the incidence of secondary lymphomas; 11% of second cancers are lymphomas after azathioprine- or cyclophosphamide-based therapy, compared with 26% since cyclosporine-based regimens came into use.[31] The secondary lymphomas occur earlier using cyclosporine-based regimens, with a median of 15 months compared with 48 months for the other regimens. The use of anti-CD3 (OKT3) monoclonal antibodies led to an increase in the incidence of lymphomas to 64% of all secondary tumors and to a decrease in the time to disease occurrence (mean, 7 months).[31,32] The higher the dose of OKT3, the higher was the risk of lymphoma.

It is unlikely that the development of lymphoma is agent specific; the risk for developing a lymphoma probably relates more to the extent of immunosuppression. The clinical outcome for these patients varies, but most fare poorly. Anecdotal instances of complete remissions after removal of immunosuppression or treatment with acyclovir have been reported. Most patients require aggressive therapy for eradication of their disease.[33,34] There may be responses to biologic agents when the tumors are in the polyclonal or oligoclonal phase of their natural history. The antibodies, anti-CD21 and anti-CD24, successfully controlled the B-cell lymphoproliferative syndrome in all 16 patients with oligoclonal proliferation after marrow or organ transplantation, and 11 remained free of disease for a median of 3 years after treatment.[35] Interferon-α (IFN-α) plus intravenous immunoglobulin was active in 5 of these patients.[36]

The increased incidence of lymphoma in patients with graft-versus-host disease, in recipients of mismatched T-cell-depleted bone marrow, in patients with iatrogenic immunosuppression, and in patients with AIDS and autoimmune diseases argues strongly for immune dysregulation in the genesis of lymphoma. Chronic antigenic stimulation has been implicated in the development of lymphomas in certain animals, but there are no convincing data in humans. Some patients with nontropical sprue develop primary T-cell lymphomas in the gastrointestinal tract, perhaps related to the gluten stimulation. The immunoglobulin gene rearrangements in about 25% of patients with chronic lymphocytic leukemia (and by inference, diffuse small lymphocytic lymphomas) result in the production of immunoglobulins that share κ chain idiotypes, the structures unique to the antigen recognition site.[37] These tumors rearrange variable region κ genes nonstochastically. This may represent evidence that tumors in different people result from the transformation of a B cell that recognizes a common or similar antigen.

VIRAL CAUSES

There is convincing evidence that viruses cause certain types of lymphomas in rodents, birds, cats, and cows.[38–41] Marek's disease, a lymphoma of chickens, is caused by a herpes-like DNA virus and can now be prevented by a vaccine.[42] A horizontally transmitted C-type retrovirus is a highly infectious cause of bovine lymphosarcoma.[43] Inbreeding appears to play an important role in the viral initiation of these animal cancers.

In humans, there is a strong association between EBV and Burkitt's lymphoma; molecular biologic techniques have established that 98% of endemic cases of Burkitt's lymphoma contain the EBV genome, but only 15% to 20% of nonendemic Burkitt's lymphomas contain the virus.[44] The lymphomas occurring in patients after organ transplantation or with congenital immune deficiencies are usually associated with EBV.[45] Most patients infected with EBV harbor the virus in latent form in B lymphocytes, which are infected by their cell surface receptor for the C3d component of complement (*i.e.*, CD21). The polyclonal B-cell infection is normally controlled by T lymphocytes that eliminate the infected B cells.[46] The viral nuclear proteins (*e.g.*, EBNA-2, EBNA-3s) and membrane proteins (*e.g.*, LMP-1) that induce proliferation of B cells also display epitopes on the cell surface that can be recognized by T cells. When T-cell deficiency exists, EBV-infected B cells can proliferate, and usually one clone escapes regulation and becomes autonomously proliferating. Males with X-linked lymphoproliferative syndrome fail to recognize EBV, which results in fatal infectious mononucleosis, acquired hypogammaglobulinemia or agammaglobulinemia, virus-associated hemophagocytic syndrome, or malignant lymphocytic lymphoma.[47] EBV has been found in patients with Hodgkin's disease and lymphomatoid granulomatosis, but its etiologic role in these diseases is speculative.

Approximately 50% of the lymphomas occurring in human immunodeficiency virus (HIV)-infected persons harbor the EBV genome.[48] The EBV sequences in a benign lymph node from an HIV-infected patient without AIDS is associated with an increased incidence of concurrent lymphoma at another site and is a marker for the increased risk of developing lymphoma.[49]

Lymphomagenesis seems to require immunodeficiency and cellular proliferation followed by cytogenetic and molecular events. Infection with EBV is postulated to occur early and leads to polyclonal expansion; after a second event, a single clone emerges from the nonmalignant cells.[50] Studies performed during the development of lymphoproliferative disorders support the notion that originally there is a polyclonal population of cells. The immunoglobulin (Ig) genes are present in germline configuration, and there is variability of fragment size in the EBV genome. After a second event, there is evolution into a monoclonal population with a single rearranged Ig gene and a single-size EBV episome.[51] During the polyclonal phase of proliferation, EBV DNA is present in an episomal and linear configuration; the latter form indicates active viral replication. It is at this polyclonal stage that acyclovir treatment and anti-B-cell antibodies have induced remission in lymphoproliferative disorders; these treatments are ineffective after monoclonal proliferations occur and the EBV genome is present only as an episome. The second event required to establish malignancy is thought to be related to protooncogene activation through cytogenetic events, often involving c-*MYC*. These observations support a role for EBV in the development of certain lymphomas in humans, but studies have not proven causality.

The most convincing evidence for a viral cause of human malignant lymphoma is in adult T-cell leukemia-lymphoma (ATL). In 1987, Poiesz and colleagues identified a unique C-type RNA tumor virus in certain patients with mature T-cell malignancies.[52] This retrovirus was called human T-cell leukemia-lymphoma virus (HTLV-I). HTLV-I is a unique, exogenously acquired retrovirus that is not closely related to any known animal retroviruses in terms of antigenicity, amino acid sequence, or nucleic acid sequence homology. Although HTLV-I was first isolated from the neoplastic cells of patients thought to have an aggressive variant of mycosis fungoides, it subsequently was recognized that the disease in these patients was identical to ATL as described in Japan.[53]

Other members of this family of human retroviruses have been described. HTLV-II was identified in a patient with atypical T-cell hairy cell leukemia, but it has been isolated from only a few patients, and it is not clearly associated with a distinct clinicopathologic disease entity.[54] HTLV-III (renamed HIV-1) is a member of a distinct family of viruses and has been shown to be the causative agent of AIDS.[55,56] HTLV-V is the putative etiologic virus for certain cutaneous T-cell lymphomas (CTCL).[57] Data on its epidemiology are not available.

The precise mechanism by which HTLV-I infection leads to malignant transformation in vivo is unknown. HTLV-I does not contain an oncogene, nor do the malignancies arising in various patients have common integration sites. HTLV-I, however, can immortalize lymphoid cells in culture and induce malignancy in an infected human host. A proposed model for HTLV-I-mediated transformation starts with infection of the cell through an unidentified cell surface receptor, followed by viral replication. Viral replication is associated with production of *trans*-activating factors (tax) that lead to expression of a variety of cytokines and receptors including interleukin-1 (IL-1), IL-2, and IL-2 receptor. Data suggest that tax induces *REL* expression, a transcription factor that participates in cell activation. Autocrine stimulation would lead to the polyclonal expansion of infected cells and increase the likelihood of an unidentified secondary event that leads to malignant transformation, monoclonal expansion, and the clinical syndrome of ATL.

Because many patients in endemic areas are infected with HTLV-I, but few develop ATL, there appear to be host factors that affect transformation of lymphocytes by HTLV-I, and strong evidence supporting such host-related genetic factors is emerging. HTLV-I has been isolated from the neurons of patients suffering from tropical spastic paraparesis, a disease epidemiologically similar to ATL.[58] A preliminary study in Japan of patients infected with HTLV-I appears to demonstrate that patients developing ATL have a high prevalence of certain HLA antigens (A26, DQw3), and those developing myelopathy express a distinct HLA haplotype (*e.g.*, A11 or A26, Bw52 or Bw54, Cw1, DQw3).[59] Such strong linkage disequilibrium suggests that the MHC is involved in the pathogenesis of HTLV-I-related disease.

CYTOGENETICS AND MOLECULAR BIOLOGY

Cytogenetic analysis of metaphase chromosomes from lymphocytic lymphomas indicates that more than 90% have chromosomal abnormalities.[60,61] For many, the chromosomal abnormality correlates with histologic subtype, immunophenotype, and with the clinical features of the lymphocytic lymphomas (Table 52–2). The most common abnormalities are sets of reciprocal translocations.[62] Two reciprocal translocations are each involved in more than 10% of all lymphocytic lymphomas; t(8;14)(q24;q32) or one of its variants, t(8;22)(q24;q11) and t(2;8)(p11;q24), are observed in more than 90% of Burkitt's lymphomas, and the t(14;18)(q32;q21) translocation has been detected in 80% to 85% of the follicular lymphomas. These reciprocal translocations result in DNA segments moving from a distant chromosome into the DNA sequences comprising the immunoglobulin genes. This translocation deregulates the expression of the translocated non-immunoglobulin gene. This nonimmunoglobulin gene is often an oncogene, and overproduction of its protein product leads to disordered cellular growth.

A variety of cytogenetic abnormalities that involve the T-cell receptor β or γ genes on chromosome 7 or the T-cell receptor α or δ genes on chromosome 14 have been reported.[63] The t(11;14)(q13;q32) and t(3;22)(q27;q11) translocations occur in 2% to 10% of lymphocytic lymphomas. The t(11;14) translocation and its molecular counterpart, *BCL1* rearrangement, has been found in 50% of diffuse intermediately differentiated lymphomas, and the t(3;22) translocation is usually found in patients with diffuse large cell lymphomas. Several other reciprocal translocations have been described in fewer than 2% of lymphocytic lymphomas (see Table 52–2). Perhaps the most well known is the t(2;5)(p23;q35), identified in the CD30 or Ki-1 positive anaplastic large cell lymphoma.[64]

There are several other cytogenetic abnormalities that have been called "recurring other aberrations" or ROA by Offit that are also listed in Table 52–2.[65] These include abnormalities of chromosomes 6q, 1p, 1q, and 17 and trisomies of 7, 3 and 12. None of these abnormalities appears to be specific for one histologic subtype.

Efforts have been made to relate cytogenetic defects to natural history.[65] Because patients usually received heterogenous treatments and were not balanced for other known prognostic factors, it is difficult to ascertain a distinct contribution of cytogenetics to outcome. However, it appears that chromosome 1 defects or the presence of more than four chromosomal abnormalities is associated with shorter survival among patients with diffuse large cell lymphoma. The appearance of additional genetic aberrations during the natural history of a low-grade lymphoma signifies a worsening prognosis. The acquisition of increasing numbers of clones bearing trisomy 7, trisomy 3, and del(13q32) or trisomy 18 in t(14,18)-bearing lymphomas is associated with evolution to a more aggressive histology.[66] Further refinement of cytogenetic techniques and more detailed study will provide more clinically useful information, but currently, the status of the chromosomes within a patient's tumor has little influence on our treatment selection.

ONCOGENES

The major impact of cytogenetics has been in increasing our understanding of the molecular events associated with lymphomagenesis. For example, the t(8;14), t(11;14), and t(14;18) translocations bring certain DNA segments into proximity with the immunoglobulin genes. These DNA segments appear to contain protooncogenes or growth-regulating genes that under certain conditions can lead to the disordered growth of the affected cell. In most cases, the translocated gene comes under the influence of the immunoglobulin enhancer element, resulting in amplified expression of the translocated gene's product. Almost all patients with endemic or nonendemic Burkitt's lymphoma have a reciprocal translocation between chromosome 8 and chromosome 14, 2, or 22. The t(8;14) translocation moves the *MYC* oncogene into the immunoglobulin heavy chain locus, and the t(8;22) or t(2;8) brings *MYC* into juxtaposition with one of the light chain loci, λ or κ, respectively.[67] This results in the constitutive expression of *MYC,* which codes for a DNA-binding protein that is thought to be important in the regulation of cell proliferation.

TABLE 52–2. Cytogenetic-immunophenotypic Correlations in Lymphocytic Lymphoma

Phenotype	*Rearrangement*	*Involved Genes or Sequences**		*Phenotype*	*Rearrangement*
B(sIg +)	t(8;14)(q24;q32)	*MYC*	IgH	Ki-1+ anaplastic large cell lymphoma	t(2;5)(p23;q32)
	t(2;8)(p11–12;q24)	Ig κ	*MYC*		
	t(8;22)(q24;q11)	*MYC*	Ig λ		
	t(14;18)(q32;q21)	*BCL2*	IgH		
	t(11;14)(q13;q32)	*BCL1*	IgH		
	t(1;14)(q21–25;q32)			Variable or unspecified	del(1)(p32–36)
	t(3;14)(p21;q32)				del(1)(p13)
	t(8;14)(q22;q32)				dup(1q)
	t(1;14)(q42;q32)				i(1q)
	t(3;22)(q27–28;q11)				t(1;17)(pllorq11;pllorq11)
	t(10;14)(p11;q32)				del(1)(q21), del(1)(q32), del(1)(q42)
	t(11;14)(q21;q32)				t(2;18)(p11;q21)
	t(11;14)(q23;q32)				del(2)(q32)
					del(3)(p21)
	t(11;14)(p13;q11)†	*TCL2*	*TCRδ*		del(4)(p13–14)
	t(11;14)(p15;q11)†	*TAL1*	*TCRδ*		del(5)(p13)
	t(8;14)(q24;q11)	*MYC*	*TCRα*		i(6p)
	inv(14)(q11q32)	*TCRα*	IgH		del(6)(q14–27)
	inv(14)(q11q32)	*TCRα*	*TCL1*		del(7)(p13–14)
	t(10;14)(q24;q11)	*TCL3*	*TCRδ*		i(7q)
	t(1;14)(p32;q11)	*TCL5*	*TCRδ*		del(7)(q32)
	t(7;19)(p34–36;p13)†	*TCRβ*	*LYL1*		del(9)(p13)
	t(7;9)(q34–36;q34)†	*TCRβ*			del(10)(q23–24)
	t(7;9)(q34–36;q32)†	*TCRβ*	*TCL4*		dup(11)(q13 $\rightarrow$ q23), dup(11)(q13 $\rightarrow$ q25)
	t(7;7)(p15;q11)	*TCRγ*			del(11)(q23)
	t(14;14)(q11;q32)				del(12)(p11–12)
	t(7;14)(q34–36;q11)				del(12)(q22)
	t(7;14)(p15;q11)				dup(12)(q13 $\rightarrow$ q22)
	t(7;11)(q34–36;p13)†				del(13)(q22)
	del(6)(p21p23)				del(14)(q22q24)
					i(17q)
					i(18q)
					del(22)(q11–12)

* *MYC*, cellular protooncogene, homolog of the transforming sequence of the avian myelocytomatosis virus DNA-binding protein; IgH, immunoglobulin heavy chain gene; Ig κ, immunoglobulin kappa light chain gene; Ig λ, immunoglobulin lambda light gene; *BCL2*, B-cell leukemia-lymphoma gene-2 24-kD protein thought to prevent cell death; *BCL1*, DNA sequences isolated from the translocation breakpoint protein related to the cyclin family of cell cycle control genes; *TCL2*, DNA sequences isolated from the translocation breakpoint (T-cell leukemia-lymphoma gene-2); *TCRδ*, T-cell receptor delta chain gene; *TCRα*, T-cell receptor alpha chain gene; *TCL6*, T-cell leukemia-lymphoma gene-6; *TAL1*, DNA sequences isolated from the translocation breakpoint; *TCL1*, DNA sequences isolated from the translocation breakpoint (T-cell leukemia-lymphoma gene-1); *TCL3*, DNA sequences isolated from the translocation breakpoint (T-cell leukemia-lymphoma gene-3); *TCL5*, DNA sequences isolated from the translocation breakpoint (T-cell leukemia-lymphoma gene-5); *LYL1*, lymphoid leukemia gene-1; TCRβ, T-cell receptor beta chain gene; *TCL4*, DNA sequences isolated from the translocation breakpoint (T-cell leukemia-lymphoma gene-4); *TCRγ*, T-cell receptor gamma chain gene.

† These rearrangements have been identified only in T-cell acute lymphoblastic leukemia.

(Modified from LeBeau MM. Seminars in Oncology 1990;17:20–29)

The t(14;18) translocation brings the B-cell leukemia-lymphoma-2 gene (*BCL2*) from chromosome 18 into the immunoglobulin heavy chain joining region on chromosome 14.[68] When this segment of DNA is transcribed, both gene sequences are found on the same mRNA, a so-called hybrid transcript. The coding regions of the *BCL2* gene are left intact so that the *BCL2/IG* hybrid heavy chain transcript produced continues to encode a normal BCL2 protein. Expression of this hybrid mRNA can be increased by as much as a log over that of normal B cells.[69] Only the *BCL2*-encoded portion of the hybrid mRNA is translated, and this leads to production of excessive levels of BCL2 protein. *BCL2*-encoded mRNA levels are normally high during pre-B-cell development, but with maturation, there is down regulation of expression.[70] The

BCL2 protein is an integral inner mitochondrial membrane protein that can block apoptosis, or programmed cell death, of certain B-cell lymphoma cell lines.[71]

When the *BCL2/IG* fusion gene is introduced into the germline of mice (*i.e.*, transgenic mice), there is a polyclonal expansion of resting but responsive IgM-positive, IgD-positive B cells that display prolonged cell survival but no increase in cell cycling.[72] An indolent lymphoid follicular hyperplasia is seen in these mice, which may progress to a malignant diffuse large cell lymphoma.[73] There is a long latency in progression from polyclonal to monoclonal disease and histologic conversion, which suggests secondary genetic changes in addition to the inserted transgene.

Half the high-grade lymphomas contained rearranged *MYC* genes. It was also demonstrated that retroviral insertion of *BCL2*-encoded complementary DNA into human B-cell lines that constitutively overexpress *MYC* and promotes proliferation and tumorigenicity.[74] Taken together, these findings suggest that BCL2 protein provides a survival advantage to B cells and may contribute to neoplasia by permitting a clone to persist until other oncogenes, such as *MYC*, are activated, resulting in cell transformation.

The t(14;18) translocation is found in 85% of follicular lymphomas and in as many as 35% of diffuse large cell lymphomas.[68] Serial examination of tumor specimens during histologic progression from a follicular low-grade lymphoma to an intermediate-grade diffuse lymphoma shows an identical breakpoint in the *BCL2* translocation, indicating that most of the *BCL2*-positive large cell lymphomas probably arose from a *BCL2*-positive follicular small cleaved cell lymphoma.[75] Although the presence of a *BCL2* translocation does not affect the prognosis of a low-grade tumor, its presence in a more aggressive lymphoma may have negative prognostic significance.[76,77] However, the presence of t(14;18) in patients with aggressive lymphoma in relapse has been associated with more prolonged survival, and some of these patients follow a clinical course more similar to indolent lymphomas, with response to therapy followed by relapse occurring over multiple courses of salvage therapy. Techniques that detect the presence of the t(14;18) translocation have found some utility as sensitive indicators of minimal residual disease in the bone marrow or peripheral blood and as a measure of the efficacy of in vitro purging of bone marrow before autologous transplant.[78,79] The use of the t(14;18) translocation or BCL2 protein as a marker of residual disease depends on the assumption that the DNA rearrangement is not found in normal tissue. Early studies failed to detect BCL2 protein in nodes that contained only normal tissue or reactive follicular hyperplasia, but studies using polymerase chain reaction have shown *BCL2* rearrangements in 54% of lymph nodes and tonsils with follicular hyperplasia.[80,81] No *BCL2* rearrangements were detected in reactive lymph nodes without follicular hyperplasia or in bone marrow cells. The implications of these findings are discussed further in the section on treatment of advanced-stage indolent lymphomas.

The t(11;14) translocation involves *BCL1* on chromosome 11 and the immunoglobulin heavy chain gene on 14.[77] Rearrangement deregulates a nearby oncogene called *PRAD1* (parathyroid adenomatosis).[82] *PRAD1,* which is found on 11q13, was identified as a chromosomal breakpoint region rearranged with the parathyroid hormone gene in a subset of parathyroid adenomas. *PRAD1* codes for a cyclin protein. Cyclin genes are involved in regulation of cell cycle progression. *BCL1* and *PRAD1* are no more than 130 kb apart. *PRAD1*-encoded mRNA was abundantly expressed in 7 of 7 cases of diffuse intermediately differentiated or centrocytic lymphomas. The linkage of a cell cycle-regulated gene to the expression of immunoglobulin in a B cell may lead to uncontrolled growth.

MICROSCOPIC AND FUNCTIONAL ANATOMY OF NORMAL LYMPHOID TISSUES

The principal cellular component of lymphoid tissue is the lymphocyte.[83] Lymphoid cells are widely distributed throughout the body, singly and in centers of aggregation.[84] The primary lymphoid organs in which these cells are generated include the bone marrow and thymus. The secondary lymphoid organs populated by differentiated lymphoid cells include lymph nodes, spleen, Waldeyer's ring (the oropharyngeal lymphoid tissues), and lymphoid aggregates in the lamina propria and submucosa of the respiratory and gastrointestinal tracts. In the gastrointestinal tract, they are referred to as Peyer's patches. Lymphoid elements associated with epithelium in the respiratory and gastrointestinal tracts are sometimes referred to as the mucosa-associated lymphoid tissues (MALT) and gut-associated lymphoid tissues.[85] Lymphoid cells also populate bone marrow, as cohabitants of the numerous hematopoietic elements. In addition to these major sites, lymphoid cells are distributed as normally inconspicuous interstitial elements in essentially all tissues except the CNS.

Other cells of the lymphoreticular system include reticular supporting cells, dendritic and interdigitating reticulum cells, and cells of the monocyte-macrophage series. The reticular cells provide the basic three-dimensional matrix of lymph nodes by virtue of their long cytoplasmic processes joined by tight junctions or desmosomes. Within this matrix, the functional cells of the lymphoid and monocyte-macrophage series migrate, proliferate, and serve as the primary arm of the host immunologic defense apparatus. The lymphoreticular system is the anatomic basis of cellular and humoral immunity.

Normally, the lymphoid and monocytic cells of the lymphoreticular system originate in the bone marrow and from there migrate by way of the blood and lymphatic vessels to populate other lymphoreticular tissues.[83] T cells are processed through the thymus gland, and B cells are processed through the mammalian equivalent of the avian bursa of Fabricius, probably the fetal liver. Although T cells and B cells comprise the two major components of the lymphocyte series, there are minor populations of other lymphocytes, such as natural killer (NK) cells, that may develop independently. Evidence suggests that thymocytes and NK cells share a common progenitor. Monocytes also originate in the bone marrow and, like lymphocytes, circulate and eventually populate extramedullary tissues as cells of the monocyte-histiocytic series.[86] These three populations of lymphoreticular cells (*i.e.*, T cells, B cells, monocyte-macrophages) serve different functions and are to some degree compartmentalized anatomically (Fig. 52–1). The malignant lymphomas frequently mirror these normal anatomic distributions in their spread throughout the lym-

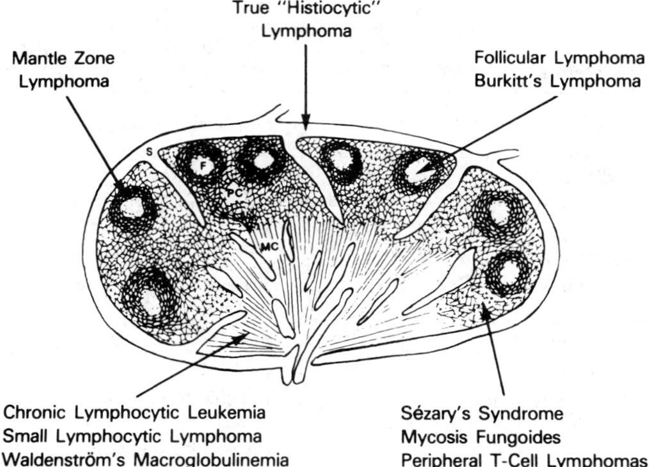

FIGURE 52–1. Schematic diagram of a normal lymph node, illustrating anatomic and functional compartments of the immune system. Malignant lymphomas can be related to these compartments. S, sinuses; F, follicles; PC, paracortex; MC, medullary cords. (Modified from Mann RB, Jaffe ES, Berard CW, et al. Malignant lymphomas: A conceptual understanding of morphologic diversity. Am J Pathol 1979;94:1–3)

phoreticular system.[87] The pattern of spread by the lymphomas is not random, but mimics patterns of normal lymphocyte circulation and distribution.

Functionally, T cells are the basis of the cell-mediated immune system.[88] Cytotoxic T cells directly lyse specific target cells, such as tumor cells or virally infected cells. Other subpopulations of T cells have regulatory functions and act as helpers or suppressors for B cells, macrophages, and other T cells. T lymphocytes recognize antigen when it is associated with the membrane-bound products of the MHC. Some T cells (CD4-positive cells) predominantly recognize antigen in association with class II MHC antigens, and other T cells (CD8-positive cells) recognize antigen in association with class I MHC antigens.

B cells form the basis of the humoral immune system.[89] They express membrane-bound immunoglobulin and, as differentiated B cells or plasma cells, secrete immunoglobulin. The ability to phagocytize particulate material is the hallmark of macrophages and monocytes.[90] These cells play a major role in the processing of antigens and their presentation to lymphocytes. Dendritic reticulum cells and interdigitating reticulum cells are thought to be related to monocyte-macrophages. Although these cells are involved in antigen presentation, they do not serve a phagocytic function.[91,92] The dendritic reticulum cells are localized in lymphoid follicles, and interdigitating reticulum cells are the antigen-presenting cells of the T-cell system and are found in the paracortex. Langerhans cells, most conspicuous in the skin but also found in other sites such as lymph nodes, are closely related to interdigitating reticulum cells and present antigen to T lymphocytes.[93]

IDENTIFICATION OF LYMPHOID CELLS

Normal and neoplastic cells of the immune system can be differentiated by characteristic surface markers. The neoplastic cells frequently retain the phenotypic markers of their normal counterparts. These features can be used to aid in the characterization and subclassification of lymphoid malignancies (Table 52–3). Surface markers are antigens that may be present initially or can be acquired during differentiation. Many of these markers have been functionally characterized and are now recognized as specific membrane receptors or other structures of functional significance, but other antigens are without recognized specific functions.

In 1975, Kohler and Milstein developed a technique for producing an unlimited supply of an antibody of predefined specificity.[94] The resulting monoclonal antibody is one of extraordinary specificity directed against a single antigenic determinant. This technology has produced an ever-increasing battery of reagents that can identify the antigenic determinants of lymphoreticular cells.

These monoclonal antibodies have replaced a complex variety of assays that were previously used to detect lymphocyte surface markers or receptors.[95] A somewhat bewildering aspect of this technology is the enormous number of monoclonal antibodies published and available through commercial and private sources. In many cases, monoclonal antibodies bear different names but immunoprecipitate identical antigens and are of identical specificity. For example, OKT3 and anti-Leu-4 recognize the same antigen, CD3. An international nomenclature has been developed that follows the pattern used for the naming of HLA-related antigens, and the use of such commonly agreed-on terminology is invaluable in comparing reagents and results. Monoclonal antibodies of comparable specificity belong to the same group or "cluster of differentiation" and bear the same "CD" name (Table 52–4).

Monoclonal antibodies can be used in immunofluorescence or immunohistochemical assays to identify normal and neoplastic lymphoid cells. As currently performed, the cell preparation is incubated with an antibody to the molecule of interest, the unbound antibody is washed off, and the bound antibody is detected by fluorescence or a linked enzymatic reaction that gives a colored product. The advantage of immunohistochemical or immunocytochemical techniques (*i.e.*, those on which tissue sections or cytologic preparations from cell suspensions, respectively, are used) is that the in situ organization, cell morphology, and immunologic phenotype can be seen. This is useful because neoplasms rarely are pure populations of neoplastic cells; a variety of normal cell types are usually present. In trying to decide whether a lymphoma is of B- or T-cell origin, a positive result with an antibody to CD3 suggests T-cell origin only if the tumor cells are positive; many B-cell lymphomas contain large numbers of infiltrating T cells. Although not a substitute for hematoxylin-eosin stain morphologic examination, the use of immunohistochemistry is a valuable adjunct to accurate diagnosis.[96]

Complementary information can be gained using flow cytometry to quantitate the expression of surface antigens on cells.[97] Labeling of cells is conceptually the same as in immunohistochemistry, except that the second antibody is conjugated to a fluorescent molecule, such as fluorescein, phycoerythrin, or rhodamine, instead of an enzyme. Cells in suspension are passed single file through a glass chamber through which laser light of an appropriate wavelength is passed. The amount of fluorescence on a given cell, which is sensed quantitatively, is directly proportional to the number

TABLE 52–3. Cellular Origin of Malignant Lymphomas

Neoplasms of B-Cell Origin	*Neoplasms of T-Cell Origin*	*Neoplasms of Histiocytic Reticulum Cell Origin*
Chronic lymphocytic leukemia (98%)	Chronic lymphocytic leukemia (2%)	Monocytic leukemia
	Large granular lymphocyte leukemia‡ (T gamma lymphoproliferative disease)	
Small lymphocytic (well-differentiated) lymphoma	Mycosis fungoides/Sézary syndrome	Malignant histiocytosis
Lymphocytic lymphoma, intermediate or small cleaved cell types (mantle zone lymphoma)	Diffuse aggressive lymphomas of adults (15%)	
	Peripheral T-cell lymphomas	True histiocytic lymphomas
	Mixed cell type	
	Large cell, immunoblastic	
Follicular lymphomas	Adult T-cell leukemia/lymphoma	
Diffuse aggressive lymphomas of adults (85%)	Angiocentric lymphomas (lymphomatoid granulomatosis polymorphic reticulosis)	Dendritic reticulum cell sarcomas
Mixed cell type		Interdigitating reticulum cell sarcomas
Large cell type*		
Large cell immunoblastic		
Small noncleaved cell*		
Burkitt's (small noncleaved cell) lymphoma		
Acute lymphocytic leukemias (75%)†	Acute lymphocytic leukemias (25%)†	
Lymphoblastic lymphomas (10%)†	Lymphoblastic lymphomas (85%)†	

* Majority of cases, 95%.
† These malignancies are of stem cell origin; they have an immature phenotype, but are committed to B- or T-cell differentiation, respectively.
‡ Bears certain T-cell markers, but is probably of NK cell origin.

of antibody molecules bound and therefore proportional to the amount of surface antigen expressed. Measurement of cell size is made at the same time. Current flow cytometers allow the quantitation of two (or three) antigens on a single cell through the concurrent use of two antibodies tagged with molecules that fluoresce at different wavelengths. The flow cytometer provides enumerations of cell size, number, and fluorescent intensity that can be plotted together in various ways. A flow cytometer is used to look at a statistically significant, reproducible sample of tens of thousands of cells in seconds. This allows characterization of a given preparation with numerous antibodies. The optical system is unbiased and sensitive (*i.e.*, it can detect a few thousand molecules on the cell surface with a high-affinity antibody), and the output can be stored in computers as raw data, allowing sophisticated manipulation and analysis.

Most antibodies currently available work only in suspension or in frozen preparations, because the processing for paraffin sections can alter the antigenic determinants significantly. However, some antigens are preserved in paraffin, and the major cell types (*i.e.*, T cells, B cells, mononuclear phagocytes) can be recognized in paraffin sections.[98,99]

T cells have been especially well characterized with monoclonal antibodies; they can be used to identify the cell's stage of differentiation and its functional capabilities (Fig. 52–2).[100] T cells can be divided into two major subsets, the helper/inducer and suppressor/cytotoxic cells.[101,102] Helper T cells are required for the terminal differentiation of a B cell into a plasma cell and provide help for immunoglobulin secretion. Suppressor cells can inhibit antibody production. Helper cells also promote the differentiation of cytotoxic T cells. In normal peripheral blood, the CD4:CD8 ratio is approximately 2:1, and in normal lymph nodes, it is approximately 3.5 or 4:1. Most malignancies of T-cell origin preferentially express a CD4- or a CD8-positive phenotype. However, these antigens are not clonal markers and should not be interpreted as such. For unknown reasons, most mature T-cell malignancies have a CD4-positive phenotype.[103,104]

Monoclonal antibodies can also be used to delineate developmental stages of T-cell differentiation.[105,106] Early T cells lack CD4 and CD8 antigens and later coexpress them. Immature T cells express transferrin receptors identified by CD71.[107] This marker has no lineage specificity, because most proliferating cells have such receptors. Two of the earliest markers with some lineage specificity include the E-rosette receptor (CD2) and CD7. Both of these markers can be expressed before rearrangement of the T-cell antigen receptor.[108] This feature raises a question about marker specificity, and some researchers have reported expression of CD2 and CD7 in acute myelogenous leukemia blasts.[109] The CD1 (T6) antigen is found on cortical thymocytes, but is absent on mature T cells.[105] This antigen is expressed on Langerhans cells of the skin.[93] The CD5 antigen found on all normal T cells is also expressed on a subpopulation of normal B cells.[110] It is useful in the characterization of B-cell malignancies, because it is expressed in some tumors (*e.g.*, B-cell CLL) but not others.[111]

The hallmark of a B lymphocyte is the expression of surface immunoglobulin, which consists of one or more heavy chains and only one type of light chain per lymphocyte. Reactive B-cell proliferations are polyclonal, with a ratio of kappa:lambda expression of approximately 2:1. B-cell lymphomas are monoclonal and express only a single light chain type. When all the cells express a given light chain, the correlation with

TABLE 52–4. Selected CD Markers Expressed on Lymphoid and Hematopoietic Cells

CD Designation	*Common Names*	*Molecular Weight*	*Primary Reactivity*
CD1	Leu-6, T6	43–49	Cortical thymocytes, Langerhans cells
CD2	Leu-5, T11	50	SRBC receptor on T cells; cytoadhesion molecule binding to LFA-3
CD3	Leu-4, T3	20–25	T cells; constant element of T-cell receptor complex
CD4	Leu-3a, T4	59	Helper subset of T cells; cytoadhesion structure binding to MHC class II molecules
CD5	Leu-1, T1, T101	67	T cells and minor subset of B cells (B-CLL)
CD7	Leu-9, 3A1	40	T cells; expressed on prethymic T-cell precursor in bone marrow
CD8	Leu-2a, T8	33	Suppressor subset of T cells; cytoadhesion structure binding to MHC class I molecules
CD10	CALLA, J5	100	Membrane-associated neutral endopeptidase; the common acute lymphoblastic leukemia antigen
CD11a	LFA-1	180/95	Leukocytes, cell adhesion molecule
CD11b	Mo1	155/95	Monocytes, granulocytes, NK cells; C3bi receptor
CD11c	Leu-M5, S-HCL3, KiM1	150/95	α chain of the α/β glycoprotein complex; leukocyte cytoadhesion molecule expressed on monocytes, hairy cell leukemia
CD14	MY4	55	Macrophages
CD15	Leu-M1, My1		X-hapten; expressed in mature granulocytes, Reed-Sternberg cells
CD16	FcRIII	50–65	NK, granulocytes, macrophages Fc receptor for immunoglobulin G
CD18			β-chain to CD11a, b, c
CD19	B4, Leu-12	95	B cells, expressed at time of Ig heavy chain gene rearrangement; member of Ig supergene family
CD20	B1, Leu-16, L26	35–37	B cells, expressed at time of Ig light chain gene rearrangement; L-26 epitope is preserved in paraffin sections
CD21	B2	140	B cells; C3d receptor (CR2); serves as Epstein-Barr virus receptor
CD22	Leu-14, SHCL-1	135	Mature B cells; member of Ig supergene family
CD23	FcϵRII	45–50	Fc receptor for immunoglobulin E
CD25	Tac, IL-2R	55	α-chain of IL-2 receptor complex; low affinity IL-2 receptor; activated T cells
CD30	Ki-1, BerH2 Hefi-1	105	Activated T cells, B cells; found in Reed-Sternberg cells and cells of large cell anaplastic lymphoma; related to the TRK oncogene and nerve growth factor receptor
CD38	T10, Leu-17	45	Plasma cells, activated T cells
CD45	LCA, T29/33	180–220	Common leukocyte antigen; various isoforms are preferentially expressed on different subsets (*e.g.*, CD45R0 [UCHL-1] expressed on memory T cells); functions as a tyrosine phosphatase
CD52	CAMPATH-1	21–28	Lymphocytes and other white cells
CD54	ICAM-1		Cell adhesion molecule
CD56	Leu-19	220/135	NK cells; N-CAM, neural cell adhesion molecule
CD68	KP1, KiM7	110	Macrophages; antigens preserved in paraffin sections
CD71	T9	95	Transferrin receptor; highly expressed on rapidly growing cells
CD74		41/35/33	Invariant chain associated with Ia molecules

malignancy is excellent. However, when using sensitive techniques, such as immunoglobulin gene rearrangement studies, the clinician must be cautious in equating monoclonality with malignancy. Under some conditions, particularly with immunodeficiency, a monoclonal population may be detected and may undergo spontaneous regression.[112]

Fewer monoclonal antibodies have been developed against B cells and B-cell subsets (Fig. 52–3).[113] Monoclonal antibodies with broad reactivity against normal B cells include CD20 (B1), CD19 (B4), and CD22 (Leu-14). These antigens are usually absent at the plasma cell stage. However, they are expressed in immature B cells before the acquisition of immunoglobulin on the cell membrane.[114,115] The so-called common acute lymphoblastic leukemia antigen (CALLA, CD10) was initially described on tumor cells from approximately 70% of patients with acute lymphoblastic leukemias.[116] Immunoglobulin gene rearrangement studies demonstrated that these cells were committed to B-cell differentiation, despite their lack of surface of cytoplasmic immunoglobulin.[117] CD10 is also expressed on Burkitt's lymphoma cells and most follicular lymphomas.[111,118] Although normal peripheral blood B cells do not stain with J5 (antibody to CD10), follicular center cells are positive when sensitive techniques are used.[119] CD10 is neither tumor specific nor lineage specific. It is present on neoplastic cells from 10% to 20% of cases of T-cell lymphoblastic lymphoma and leukemia.[106,118] It also occurs at a low-density on normal peripheral blood polymorphonuclear leukocytes.[120]

Most monoclonal antibodies react with monocytes, and macrophages also react with cells of the granulocytic series.

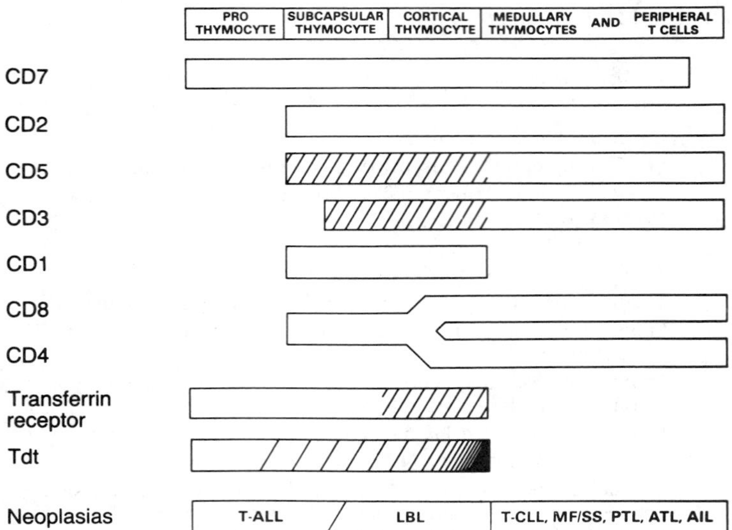

FIGURE 52–2. Monoclonal antibodies can be used to identify different developmental and functional T-cell subpopulations. Monoclonal antibodies are identified according to CD groups established by international nomenclature panel. Neoplasias of T-cell origin can be related to sequential stages of T-cell differentiation. (Modified from Cossman J, Chused T, Fisher R, et al. Diversity of immunologic phenotypes of lymphoblastic lymphoma. Cancer Res 1983;43:4486)

Included in this category are the monoclonal antibodies to CD11 and CD15.[121–123] Antibodies with greater specificity for the monocyte-macrophage fraction include the CD14 group, but these stain many B cells as well.[124] Antibodies to CD68 (KP1) react with macrophages in paraffin and frozen sections.[125]

Several monoclonal antibodies can detect the so-called common leukocyte antigen (CD45).[126,127] This antigen is expressed on all normal lymphoreticular cells. Although these antibodies are not useful in classifying lymphoreticular malignancies, they are useful in differentiating malignant lymphomas from nonlymphoid neoplasms such as carcinomas and sarcomas. All of these antibodies react with an antigen of approximately 200,000 daltons. However, they vary in their ability to stain paraffin-embedded or cryostat sections.

Terminal deoxynucleotidyl transferase (TdT) is a DNA polymerase that catalyses the addition of deoxyribonucleotide triphosphate to the 3′-hydroxy end of single-stranded poly- or oligodeoxyribonucleotide primers.[128] This enzyme is present in immature lymphoid cells of T-cell and B-cell origin. The enzyme is found in low levels in normal bone marrow. Mature peripheral blood B and T lymphocytes and phytohemagglutinin-stimulated lymphocytes do not contain detectable TdT. This enzyme has been identified in the cells of almost all patients with ALL and lymphoblastic lymphoma and in the cells of some patients with chronic myelogenous leukemia in lymphoid blast crisis.[129] TdT determinations may be performed on fresh or frozen tissues in cell suspension and can be identified biochemically or with antisera reactive with TdT antigenically.[130]

The demonstration of various hydrolytic enzymes by cytochemical and histochemical techniques has been useful in

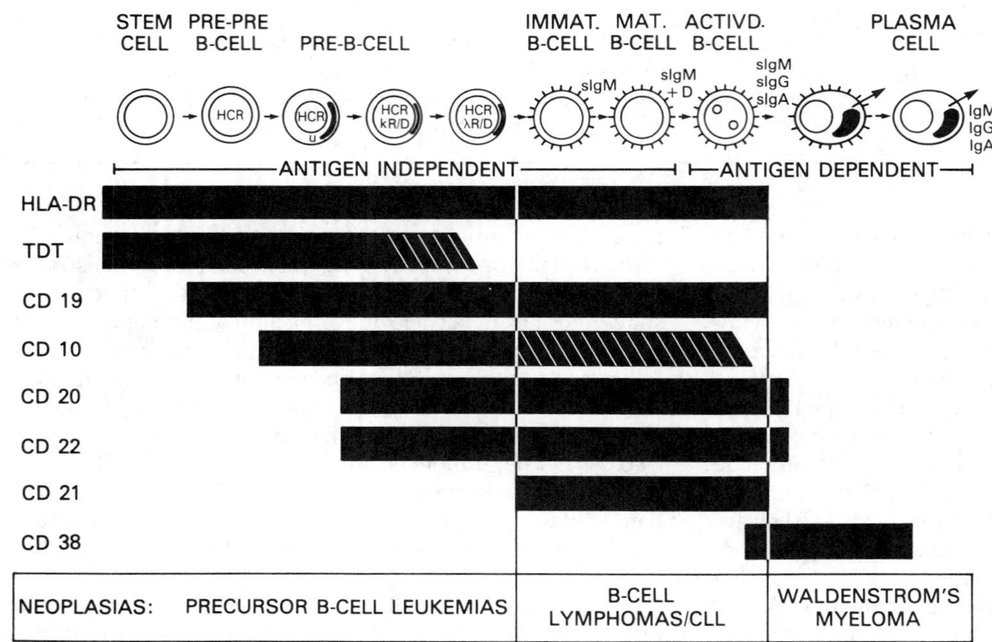

FIGURE 52–3. Diagram demonstrating the molecular genetic and immunophenotypic correlates of normal B-cell differentiation. Monoclonal antibodies are identified according to CD groups established by international nomenclature panel. Steps of heavy and light chain immunoglobulin gene rearrangement are shown. B-cell malignancies are associated with the sequential stages of B-cell differentiation. HCR, heavy chain rearrangement; kappa R/D, kappa light chain rearrangement or deletion; lambda R/D, lambda light chain rearrangement or deletion; μ, mu heavy chain synthesis.

identifying certain cells of the lymphoreticular system.[131] The most helpful assays are those for nonspecific esterase (NSE), acid phosphatase (AP), and tartrate-resistant phosphatase (TRAP). Diffuse activity for NSE and AP is characteristic of monocytes-macrophages; antigen-presenting cells have a more punctate and localized reaction pattern. Normal T lymphocytes display punctate reactivity for NSE (at an acid pH) and AP. However, some reactivity may be seen in normal and neoplastic B lymphocytes. These cytochemical markers are not reliable for the determination of immunologic phenotype of lymphoid cells. TRAP is a characteristic feature of the cells of hairy cell leukemia.[132]

GENE REARRANGEMENT

The technology of molecular biology has provided new methods for detecting lineage, clonality, and minimal residual disease in malignant lymphomas. B cells undergo specific rearrangements of their immunoglobulin genes and T cells their T-cell receptor genes as they are committed to a particular lineage.[133–136] The genes of cells that have not initiated this process are in a germline configuration. As a consequence, the detection of a rearrangement can be used as a tool to determine lineage.[137,138] For example, the cellular origin of hairy cell leukemia was long a subject of speculation, because it had features suggestive of monocytes and B cells. The demonstration of immunoglobulin light chain gene rearrangements resolved the issue.[138] Lymphomas generally can be assigned to T- or B-cell groups by Southern analysis with probes for the T-cell receptor and immunoglobulin subunits. However, certain pitfalls have emerged. Although the finding of rearranged light chain genes appears to be diagnostic of B lineage, heavy chain genes are occasionally rearranged in T or myeloid neoplasms.[139,140] Similarly, the presence of rearranged T-cell receptor genes is not entirely specific for T-cell lineage. Rearranged β chain genes have been seen in otherwise clear cut B-cell lymphomas, and the T-γ gene is problematic as a clonal marker, because its limited number of variable regions gives rise to distinct bands on Southern analysis even in polyclonal populations.[141,142] Nevertheless, only hematopoietic cells rearrange these genes, and therefore, this kind of analysis can be helpful in differentiating between poorly differentiated carcinoma and lymphoma.

The DNA sequences involved in these rearrangements are detected by the Southern blot technique. Intact cellular DNA is isolated and cut into many small fragments by restriction enzymes that are highly specific for certain nucleotide sequences. The restriction fragments can be size separated with agarose gel electrophoresis, and a fragment containing a particular sequence can be detected by using a radioactively labeled, cloned DNA probe that is complementary to the sequence of interest. Because of the innumerable possible rearrangements in a population of normal polyclonal lymphocytes, no single rearrangement pattern would predominate, and a probe would label a smear of fragments of all sizes. However, the nature of the Southern method is such that if more than 1% to 5% of the cells are of monoclonal origin, a single restriction fragment is labeled above the background. In this way, a change in a restriction fragment size from the germline can be used as a marker for a clone of cells derived from a particular lymphocyte.[112] Because each clone has a unique rearrangement pattern, Southern blot analysis is particularly useful in examining sequential specimens. After establishing the rearrangement pattern of the primary lesion, it is possible to determine whether subsequent biopsies contain a clonal population of lymphoid cells and whether the clone is identical to the original one.

Another important potential clinical use is in staging and in the detection of even small numbers of lymphoma cells. For example, clonal populations of T lymphocytes can be detected in lymph nodes from patients with mycosis fungoides that had been called negative for involvement by standard surgical pathology techniques.[143] However, demonstration of a clonal population of lymphocytes is not always proof of malignancy. Lymphomatoid papulosis is a chronic, often self-remitting illness that is limited to the skin, usually without clinical progression to malignancy, despite containing clonally rearranged T cells.[144]

Clonal populations must be viewed with caution, particularly in the setting of immunodeficiency. Patients with the Wiskott-Aldrich syndrome may develop transient serum monoclonal spikes, and in one study, a clonal proliferation of B cells was identified by gene rearrangement in a lymph node from 1 patient.[112] However, this patient never developed a malignant lymphoproliferative disorder. EBV can immortalize B cells in vitro and in vivo, and in the setting of immunodeficiency, these clones may be expanded and identifiable by Southern blot analysis.[145] However, if immunocompetence can be restored, the clones may regress, as has been demonstrated in renal transplant recipients.[33] A second mutational event is probably required for the true malignant transformation of such expanded B-cell clones.

The physician must be careful to use the information these techniques provide only with the benefit of relevant clinical information. The finding of a faint T-β gene rearrangement in a pleural effusion from a patient with a known T-cell lymphoma, in which the rearranging band matches the size of that in the previous biopsy, can be interpreted as diagnostic of lymphoma in the pleural fluid. The same finding in a patient with AIDS is of unknown significance. As these techniques become more widely available, clinical correlation studies will need to be done. For example, it is unknown whether the demonstration of occult disease in lymph nodes of mycosis fungoides patients has any effect on prognosis or whether it is simply a reflection of the ability of the neoplastic cells to circulate throughout the lymphoid system.

Molecular biology techniques have been made dramatically more sensitive for detecting few residual tumor cells, particularly those expressing chromosomal translocations for which there are probes available (*e.g.*, t[14;18] in follicular lymphoma). The polymerase chain reaction (PCR) technique uses in vitro enzymatic synthesis to amplify specific DNA sequences.[146] The reaction is based on the annealing and extension of two oligonucleotide primers that flank the target region in double-stranded DNA. The technique provides extraordinary sensitivity because 20 cycles of the reaction amplify a specific sequence up to 1 million times, enabling the detection of 1 in 10^5 cells bearing that sequence.[147] Cells from 85% or more of cases of follicular lymphoma contain specific sequences as a consequence of the t(14;18)(q32;q21) that transposes the *BCL2* gene from its normal position on chromosome 18 to join it to the gene for the immunoglobulin heavy chain of the joining region (*IGHJ*) on chromosome 14.[148,149] Using primers that recognize sequences specific to the breakpoint, DNA from cells bearing that translocation are amplified but not DNA from unrearranged *BCL2* or *IGHJ* genes in normal cells.

This technique is currently employed to monitor the completeness of purging of tumor cells from bone marrow in extracorporeal depletion experiments, and if applied carefully to bone marrow and lymph node aspirates, it could alter the criterion for determining complete remission in lymphoma.

NORMAL AND MALIGNANT T-CELL AND B-CELL DEVELOPMENT

With a combination of cell surface phenotyping, enzyme histochemistry, and Southern and Northern molecular biology techniques, it is possible to roughly map the stages of differentiation of lymphoid cells and relate the stages to the phenotypes of particular lymphocytic lymphomas (see Figs. 52–2 and 52–3).[150]

T cells arise from a pluripotent stem cell by way of a lymphoid stem cell and undergo maturation in the thymus. The earliest committed T cells express surface receptors for transferrin receptor (CD71) and CD38 and contain terminal transferase. These cells are located in the thymic cortex and comprise about 5% of all thymocytes. With further maturation, these cells lose CD71, acquire CD1, and concurrently express CD38, CD4, and CD8 antigens. The cells contain no terminal transferase, but the message for rearranged β chains of the T-cell antigen receptor and CD3, the nonpolymorphic 7-chain receptor-associated molecule, is detectable in the cytoplasm, but protein is not yet expressed on the cell surface. A fraction of these cells express low-affinity IL-2 receptors. The CD4- and CD8-positive cells (also called double-positive thymocytes) comprise 80% to 85% of thymocytes in the cortex. In the medulla, which makes up about 10% of the thymocyte population, the phenotype of the thymocytes is indistinguishable from peripheral mature T cells. These cells lose CD1, express CD3 and antigen receptors (mainly α chain–β chain heterodimers), and lose CD8 to become class II MHC-restricted helper T cells or CD4 to become class I MHC-restricted suppressor T cells. Throughout their maturation in the thymus, T cells express CD2 and CD7.

Malignancies arising in early or subcapsular cortical thymocytes are usually T-cell ALL. Lymphoblastic lymphomas may have the phenotype of early or common cortical thymocytes. All the other T-cell lymphomas arise from cells with mature or postthymic phenotype. Most tumors arising from mature cells bear CD4 and include ATL, mycosis fungoides, Sézary's syndrome, angiocentric immunoproliferative lesions, most so-called peripheral T-cell lymphomas (*i.e.*, diffuse large cell, immunoblastic and mixed lymphomas by Working Formulation terminology), and about half of the cases of T-cell CLL. A few peripheral T-cell lymphomas, about half of the cases of T-cell CLL, and some cases of T-γ lymphoproliferative disease (*i.e.*, large granular lymphocytic leukemia, T-cell CLL) express CD8. T-γ lymphoproliferative disease is heterogenous, including some CD3-positive and some CD3-negative cases. Its rarity interferes with completely thorough subclassification. However, even those that express CD3 have more similarity to a subset of NK cells than T cells in that they may also express OKM1, CD15, CD38, Fc receptors, asialo-GM1, CD57, and CD56. Those expressing CD3 are usually associated with neutropenia, rheumatoid arthritis, and autoantibody formation, and the CD3-negative tumors are less frequently associated with neutropenia and autoimmune phenomena.[151]

Somewhat less is known about B-cell development and the role of the host in shaping it. Fewer B-cell-specific antibodies are available, and most of what is known about B-cell maturation relates to the steps of immunoglobulin gene rearrangement and expression of surface immunoglobulin. The earliest B cell expresses class II MHC (HLA-DR), CD10, and CD19 on the surface, terminal transferase intracellularly, and has rearranged its heavy chain genes. Subsequently, the cell expresses CD20 and nonsequentially produces cytoplasmic μ heavy chains, rearranges κ light chain genes, rearranges λ light chain genes, and loses terminal transferase. This represents the pre-B-cell stage of development. The cell becomes recognizable as an immature B cell after it loses CD10 expression and expresses surface IgM. The cell then expresses surface CD21 (C3d receptor) and has surface IgD and IgM on the membrane. All subsequent steps in B-cell development are driven by exposure to antigen. After contacting antigen, the immunoglobulin genes undergo a class switch and express the isotype they ultimately secrete. Then they lose CD21, CD20, and surface immunoglobulin, and acquire PC-1 and PCA-1, which are plasma cell markers, and they secrete immunoglobulin. This is the life history of follicular center B cells, the cells most commonly giving rise to lymphocytic lymphomas (see Fig. 52–3).

There is another subpopulation of B cells whose relation to follicular center B cells is unclear. Many of the events in the maturation of follicular center B cells after exposure to antigen are assisted by factors produced by helper T cells. Immunoglobulin class switch is T-cell mediated. However, mantle zone B cells appear to be more independent of the influence of T cells; they express CD5, a pan T-cell marker and do not appear capable of switching to immunoglobulin isotypes other than IgM after exposure to antigen.

Most cases of ALL originate from pre-B cells. Burkitt's lymphoma and leukemia arise from the surface IgM-positive immature B cell. Most follicular and diffuse B-cell lymphomas arise from mature or activated B cells. Waldenström's macroglobulinemia and multiple myeloma originate from cells near terminal differentiation. CLL cells express CD5, as do cells of diffuse intermediately differentiated lymphocytic lymphoma, which are also CD10 positive. This may mean that these tumors derive from mantle zone rather than follicular center B cells.

Although it is possible to phenotype malignancies of lymphocytes, the correlation of the phenotype with histology is not complete. Diffuse large cell lymphomas seem to be the most heterogenous, including tumors of B-cell, T-cell, and histiocyte origin. The clinical course of disease is not accurately predicted by the stage of developmental arrest of a particular tumor. For example, ATL is a tumor of mature, postthymic T cells, but it is every bit as aggressive clinically as a lymphoblastic lymphoma, which is derived from a more immature cell. Although phenotyping can be useful in certain ways, it does not provide information that is more valuable to the clinician than the interpretation of hematoxylin and eosin stained tissue examined under a light microscope by an experienced hematopathologist.

PATHOLOGY OF LYMPHOCYTIC LYMPHOMAS

The classification of neoplastic lymphoid disorders has undergone significant evolution over the past 150 years (Table 52–5).[152–164] The Rappaport classification (Table 52–6) has been the most popular classification for clinicians in the United States.[162,165] Rappaport first divided lymphomas by pattern, whether nodular or diffuse, and then by cytologic subtypes. Tumors were termed poorly or well-differentiated lymphocytic based on the degree to which the neoplastic cells resembled normal lymphocytes. Lymphomas composed of large cells with abundant cytoplasm were termed "histiocytic" and were thought to be derived from histiocytes or phagocytic cells. The term "undifferentiated" was used for lymphomas of intermediate cell size that failed to demonstrate evidence of "lymphoid" or "histiocytic" origin.

Although the Rappaport classification was quite popular among clinicians, it became the subject of considerable controversy, for it was proposed at a time when relatively little was known about the normal immune system. As scientists discovered the functional and ontogenetic heterogeneity of the normal immune system, researchers questioned the scientific validity of the Rappaport approach. The concepts of well differentiated and poorly differentiated were inaccurate as applied in the Rappaport scheme, as was the use of the term "histiocytic" for a tumor of transformed lymphoid cells.

TABLE 52–5. Landmarks in the Description of the Lymphocytic Lymphomas

Investigations	*Observation*
Craigie, 1845[152]	Described the first cases of leukemia
Bennett, 1845[153]	
Virchow, 1845[154]	Differentiated lymphosarcoma from leukemia and included cases described by Hodgkin in the lymphosarcoma group
Billroth, 1871[155]	Coined phrase "malignant lymphomas"
Dreschfeld, 1892[156]	Developed histologic criteria for diagnosing lymphosarcoma
Kundradt, 1893[157]	
Brill et al, 1925[158]	Described giant follicular lymphoma and considered it a benign disease ("Brill-Symmers disease")
Symmers, 1927[159]	
Roulet, 1930[160]	Developed histologic criteria for diagnosing reticulum cell sarcoma and considered it a malignancy of the supporting cells of the lymph node
Gall, Mallory, 1942[161]	Developed criteria for differentiating benign hyperplasia from malignant follicular lymphoma
Rappaport et al, 1956[162]	Described different cell types within follicular lymphomas and named them "nodular lymphomas"
Burkitt, 1958[163]	Described lymphoma of the jaw in Africa, which bears his name
Uchiyama et al, 1977[164]	Described adult T-cell leukemia-lymphoma
Poiesz et al, 1980[52]	Identified HTLV-I as first human retrovirus and the causative agent of adult T-cell leukemia-lymphoma

New classifications attempted to address the scientific inaccuracies of the Rappaport scheme and to relate these tumors more closely to the normal immune system (see Table 52–6).[165–171] For example, the classification of Lukes and Collins proposed that immunologic subtypes could be recognized by morphologic features alone.[168] Although certain features, such as follicle formation by the neoplastic cells, were found to be reliable indicators of follicular B-lymphocyte origin, cytologic features were shown to be unreliable for predicting T- or B-cell phenotype in the diffuse lymphomas.[172,173]

The use of six different pathologic classifications for lymphocytic lymphomas throughout the world makes the international analysis and comparison of clinical trials extremely difficult. A new scheme, called the Working Formulation, is based on an international study comparing the six major systems (Tables 52–6 and 52–7).[174] The basic approach is similar to that of the Rappaport scheme in that lymphomas are classified on the basis of follicular or diffuse pattern and cytologic composition. Although immunologic terminology is not used, correlations with established immunologic phenotypes can be drawn. It has been proposed that this formulation not be viewed as an alternative classification, but rather as a common language that can be used by all clinical investigators to translate from one classification scheme to another. This system is employed throughout this chapter, and we attempt to relate these tumors to the normal immune system if this information is available. The popularity of the Rappaport classification was due to its reproducibility, the fact that it is easily learned, and to the information provided to clinicians, allowing them to relate histology to some reasonable assessment of the likely clinical course. The Working Formulation provides the same clinical information by grouping lymphomas into low-, intermediate-, or high-grade neoplasms based on their untreated or minimally treated natural history (see Table 52–6). Although this has proven to be a useful scheme, we feel that minor modifications are needed to include disease entities that were left out of the original formulation and to improve grouping of the histologic subtypes according to their natural history and the strategies used for their treatment (Table 52–8).

A diagnosis of lymphocytic lymphoma in the Working Formulation is based on morphologic features only, but it has predictive value for survival.[175,176] Low-grade lymphomas are usually characterized by an indolent clinical course and relatively long survival with or without aggressive therapy. Malignant cells are usually found at sites where the normal counterparts of these lymphocytic lymphoma cells are located.[177] For example, follicular lymphomas are derived from follicular B lymphocytes, demonstrate a striking capacity to home to B-cell-dependent portions of the lymphoid system, and have a nondestructive growth pattern.[87] The cells readily circulate or disseminate, and patients with this type of lymphocytic lymphoma usually have stage III or IV disease. However, privileged sites such as testis or CNS are rarely involved by these tumors. Cytologic atypia or anaplasia is not typical of low-grade lymphocytic lymphoma. Follicular lymphomas may respond to normal immunoregulation, unlike the high-grade

TABLE 52–6. Comparison of Commonly Used Classifications for the Lymphocytic Lymphomas

Modified Rappaport Classification (1966)[166,167]	
Nodular	
Lymphocytic, well differentiated	A*
Lymphocytic, poorly differentiated	B
Mixed, lymphocytic and histiocytic	C
Histiocytic	D
Diffuse	
Lymphocytic, well differentiated with plasmacytoid features	A
Lymphocytic, well differentiated with plasmacytoid features	A
Lymphocytic, poorly differentiated	E
Lymphoblastic, convoluted	I
Lymphoblastic, nonconvoluted	I
Mixed, lymphocytic and histiocytic	F
Histiocytic without sclerosis	G
Histiocytic with sclerosis	G
Burkitt's tumor	J
Undifferentiated	J
Malignant lymphoma, unclassified	
Composite lymphoma	

Lukes and Collins Classification (1974)[168]	
Undefined cell type	
T-cell type, small lymphocytic	A
T-cell type, Sézary-mycosis fungoides (cerebriform)	
T-cell type, convoluted lymphocytic	I
T-cell type, immunoblastic sarcoma (T cell)	H
B-cell type, small lymphocytic	A
B-cell type, plasmacytoid lymphocytic	A
Follicular center cell, small cleaved	B–E
Follicular center cell, large cleaved	D–G
Follicular center cell, small noncleaved	J
Follicular center cell, large noncleaved	D–G
Immunoblastic sarcoma (B cell)	
Subtypes of follicular center cell lymphomas	H
1. Follicular	
2. Follicular and diffuse	
3. Diffuse	
4. Sclerotic with follicles	
5. Sclerotic without follicles	
Histiocytic	
Malignant lymphoma, unclassified	

Kiel Classification (1974)[169,170]	
Low-grade malignancy	
Lymphocytic, chronic lymphocytic-leukemia	A
Lymphocytic, other	A
Lymphoplasmacytoid	A
Centrocytic	E
Centroblastic-centrocytic, follicular without sclerosis	B, C, D
Centroblastic-centrocytic, follicular with sclerosis	
Centroblastic-centrocytic, follicular and diffuse, without sclerosis	
Centroblastic-centrocytic, follicular and diffuse, with sclerosis	
Centroblastic-centrocytic, diffuse	F
Low-grade malignant lymphoma, unclassified	
High-grade malignancy	
Centroblastic	G
Lymphoblastic, Burkitt's type	J
Lymphoblastic, convoluted cell type	I
Lymphoblastic, other (unclassified) immunoblastic	H
High-grade malignant lymphoma, unclassified	
Malignant lymphoma, unclassified (unable to specify "high grade" or "low grade")	
Composite lymphoma	

* Letters indicate equivalent or related category in the Working Formulation as shown in Table 52–7.

lymphomas, which are consistently autonomous. Patients with follicular lymphoma may have a history of lymph nodes that wax and wane in size, often for many years before diagnosis.[178] Host immunity has been invoked to explain this phenomenon, and in some cases, the clinical regression has been preceded by bacterial or viral infection. In contrast, the intermediate- and high-grade lymphomas usually have an aggressive and unrelenting natural history unless treated vigorously.[179] Extranodal sites and privileged sites are more frequently involved, and B symptoms are more common.

A further complication in the classification of lymphocytic lymphoma is that a significant fraction of patients with lymphocytic lymphoma have divergent histologies in the same or different biopsy sites, as many as 33% in some series.[180,181] Commonly, there is a follicular pattern in one site and diffuse pattern in another; in such cases, survival is intermediate between the two.[181] Histologic progression from a low-grade lymphoma to one of higher grade during the clinical course is also common in B-cell lymphomas. At the National Cancer Institute (NCI), 37% of patients with a follicular pattern of lymphocytic lymphoma had progression to a diffuse pattern when rebiopsied (>3 months) after initial staging.[182] With modern therapy, eradication of the diffuse aggressive component with only the residual low-grade follicular component remaining is now seen. The term "composite lymphoma" has been used to describe various cases with more than one histologic type; a strict definition of composite lymphoma is a lymphoma consisting of the two distinctly different and well-delineated varieties of lymphoma occurring in a single anatomic site or mass.[183] Most composite lymphomas do not represent two distinct tumors but are different manifestations of the same clonal proliferation. True composite lymphomas, such as the coexistence of Hodgkin's disease and lymphocytic lymphoma in a single site, are identified rarely.

LOW-GRADE LYMPHOMAS

Malignant Small Cell Lymphocytic Lymphoma

Diffuse small lymphocytic lymphoma (*i.e.*, diffuse well-differentiated lymphoma) composed of well-differentiated small lymphocytes is the solid tumor counterpart of CLL.[184] If patients with the usual peripheral blood manifestations of CLL are excluded, these neoplasms constitute approximately 5% of all lymphocytic lymphomas. The patients, even when

TABLE 52–7. Working Formulation of Lymphocytic Lymphoma for Clinical Use: Recommendations of an Expert International Panel and Comparisons to the Rappaport Scheme

Working Formulation	*Rappaport Terminology*
Low Grade	
A. Malignant lymphoma, small lymphocytic	Diffuse well-differentiated lymphocyte
Consistent with chronic lymphocytic leukemia	
B. Malignant lymphoma, follicular, predominantly small cleaved cell	Nodular poorly differentiated lymphocytic
Diffuse areas	
Sclerosis	
C. Malignant lymphoma, follicular mixed, small cleaved and large cell	Nodular mixed lymphocytic histiocytic
Diffuse areas	
Sclerosis	
Intermediate Grade	
D. Malignant lymphoma, follicular	Nodular histiocytic
Predominantly large cell	
Diffuse areas	
Sclerosis	
E. Malignant lymphoma, diffuse small cleaved cell	Diffuse poorly differentiated lymphocytic
F. Malignant lymphoma, diffuse mixed, small and large cell sclerosis	Diffuse mixed lymphocytic-histiocytic
Epitheliod cell component	
G. Malignant lymphoma, diffuse	Diffuse histiocytic
Large cell	
Cleaved cell	
Noncleaved cell	
Sclerosis	
High Grade	
H. Malignant lymphoma large cell, immunoblastic	Diffuse histiocytic
Plasmacytoid	
Clear cell	
Polymorphous	
Epithelioid cell component	
I. Malignant lymphoma lymphoblastic	Diffuse lymphoblastic
Convoluted cell	
Nonconvoluted cell	
J. Malignant lymphoma small noncleaved cell	Diffuse undifferentiated
Burkitt's	
Follicular areas	

aleukemic or subleukemic, often have focal involvement of the bone marrow, liver, and other visceral sites at presentation and usually generalized asymptomatic lymphadenopathy.[185] With time, the natural history of this disease seems to be progression to CLL. In most patients, the malignant cells are monoclonal B lymphocytes and, as in CLL, the neoplastic cells express the p65 membrane protein CD5.[111,186] In one study of small lymphocytic lymphoma and CLL, the lymphoma cells usually expressed LFA-1 (CD11a), a cell adhesion molecule that could affect the propensity of recirculating tumor cells to take up residence in a lymph node.[187] CLL cells usually failed to express these homotypic adhesion molecules. The neoplastic cells of small lymphocytic lymphoma and CLL, like normal medullary cord B lymphocytes, may exhibit some functional differentiation toward plasma cells and can be readily induced to secrete monoclonal immunoglobulin after exposure to the phorbol ester 12-O-tetradecanoylphorbol-13-acetate.[188] The monoclonal protein synthesized and expressed on the cell surface is usually IgM, and the κ light chain is found more often than λ.

The disorder known as Waldenström's macroglobulinemia can be most readily viewed as a form of small lymphocytic

TABLE 52–8. National Cancer Institute Clinical Schema for Lymphocytic Lymphomas Based on Natural History of Untreated or Palliatively Treated Patients

Low Grade or Indolent (median survival measured in years)
Small lymphocytic
Follicular, small cleaved cell
Follicular, mixed
Diffuse, small cleaved cells*
Diffuse, intermediately differentiated (or mantle zone)†
Cutaneous T cell†

Intermediate Grade or Aggressive (median survival measured in months)
Follicular, large cell
Diffuse mixed
Diffuse large cell
Diffuse immunoblastic‡

High Grade (median survival measured in weeks)
Diffuse small noncleaved cell (Burkitt's)
Diffuse small noncleaved cell (non-Burkitt's)
Lymphoblastic
Adult T-cell leukemia-lymphoma†

* Working Formulation intermediate-grade tumor with an indolent natural history.
† Omitted from the Working Formulation.
‡ Working Formulation high-grade tumor with an aggressive natural history.

neoplasia with immunoglobulin secretion as its sine qua non (see Chap. 54). The cells spontaneously secrete immunoglobulin, resulting in a monoclonal IgM serum spike. These cases represent approximately 15% of all small lymphocytic lymphomas. Morphologically, the cells usually demonstrate plasmacytoid features, often exhibiting a spectrum even within a single patient. Unlike CLL and small lymphocytic lymphomas without plasmacytoid differentiation, the cells are CD5 negative. Clinically, the disease presents a spectrum from CLL-like features to a form characterized predominantly by lymphadenopathy and hepatosplenomegaly. Heavy-chain diseases corresponding to the three most plentiful classes of immunoglobulins are also discussed in the chapter on plasma cell neoplasms.

Small lymphocytic lymphomas may contain moderate numbers of larger cells or prolymphocytes, which may accumulate in growth centers, sometimes imparting a pseudofollicular appearance at low power.[189] If the mitotic rate is less than 30 mitoses per 20 high-powered fields, the prognosis is not adversely affected.[189] However, emergence of a monomorphic proliferation of the larger lymphoid cells indicates progression to a diffuse large cell lymphoma, the so-called Richter's syndrome.[190] This transformation occurs in approximately 1% of patients, but a larger proportion of patients undergo a gradual acceleration in the clinical course of their disease over time. Immunologic studies have shown that these large cells bear the same surface determinants as the small lymphoid cells of the original disease.[191]

Mucosal-Associated Lymphoid Tissue Lymphomas

It has been proposed that extranodal small lymphocytic malignancies represent a distinct clinicopathologic entity related to MALT.[192,193] MALT lymphomas are distinctive morphologically, phenotypically, and clinically. Formerly, they were often diagnosed as pseudolymphomas because they contain normal germinal centers and have a somewhat polymorphous cytologic composition.[194] However, phenotypic analysis has shown that the small lymphocytic component is monoclonal. Unlike most small lymphocytic lymphomas, the MALT lymphomas are consistently CD5 negative.[195]

Recognition of the MALT lymphoma concept may be important because a distinctive clinical behavior has been associated with these tumors. Unlike other small lymphocytic malignancies, they seem to have a low risk of dissemination to lymph nodes, bone marrow, or peripheral blood, but they have a high risk of relapse in diverse extranodal sites. The most common sites of involvement include lung, stomach, salivary glands, and lacrimal glands, but almost every extranodal site is at risk.[195] The clinical course is usually indolent, characterized by multiple recurrences over years, but with limited mortality.

Monocytoid B-cell lymphomas appear closely related to MALT lymphomas. Although this process was first described in lymph nodes, it carries a high risk of extranodal disease.[196] These low-grade lymphomas are similar phenotypically, morphologically, and clinically. A close association with Sjögren's syndrome has been demonstrated.[196]

Follicular Lymphomas

Follicular (*i.e.*, nodular) lymphomas are those in which the neoplastic cells form circumscribed aggregates that morphologically resemble germinal centers (Fig. 52–4).[197] The nodular pattern may exist throughout the tumor, or it may be manifested only in a portion of the lymphoma that elsewhere is composed of diffuse cellular proliferation.[180,198] Follicular lymphoma can be differentiated from reactive follicular hyperplasia by the total effacement of lymph node architecture by nodular proliferation. The nodules vary little in size and shape and are crowded together with little intervening normal lymphoid parenchyma. They also lack well-defined lymphoid cuffs. In areas of the nodules, the neoplastic cells may be confined to the nodules with normal-appearing cells in the internodular tissue or present between the nodules. In the former situation, the neoplasms may be mistaken for benign follicular hyperplasia unless careful scrutiny is given to the cells composing the nodules. Although normal germinal centers are composed of cytologically heterogenous populations representing the entire spectrum of proliferating B cells, neoplastic nodules appear more homogenous and "clonal." Other useful differential features include polarization and the presence of a "starry sky" pattern in reactive germinal centers but not in follicular lymphomas. Nodular lymphomas are neoplasms of follicular B cells.[172,199]

The cells of follicular lymphomas can be predominantly small cleaved cells (poorly differentiated lymphocytic), large noncleaved, or large cleaved cells (histiocytic), or a mixture of cell types, such as mixed small cleaved and large cell (mixed

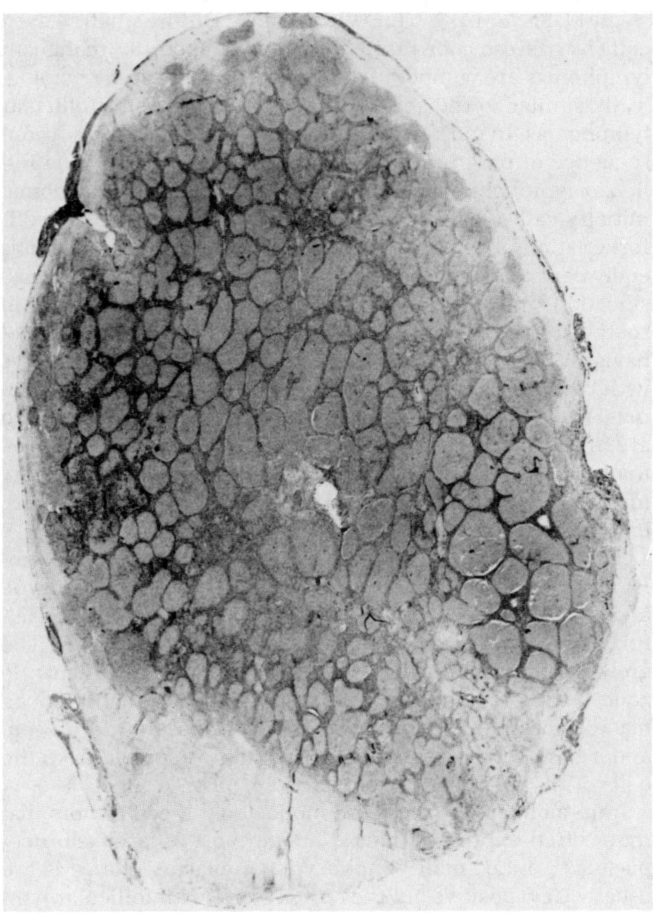

FIGURE 52–4. Effacement of architecture by monotonous nodularity in follicular lymphoma (hematoxylin & eosin stain; original magnification × 10). Compare this with the predominately cortical location of follicles in a normal lymph node shown in Figure 52–1.

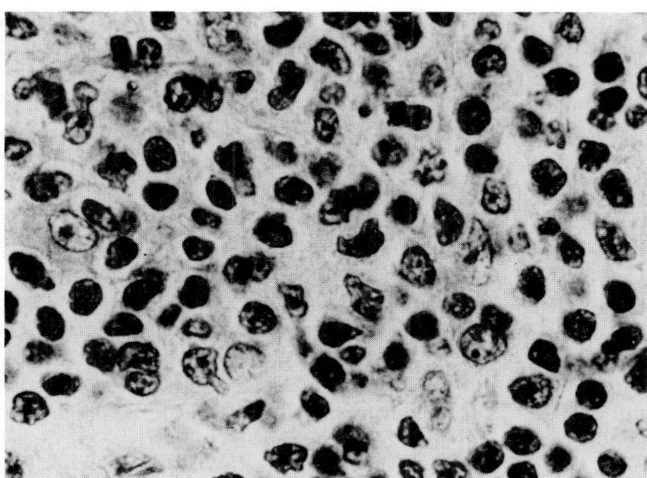

FIGURE 52–5. Follicular lymphoma: predominantly small cleaved cell type. Atypical lymphocytes are indented and angular (hematoxylin & eosin stain; original magnification × 1000).

lymphocytic-histiocytic). The larger cells appear to be the replicative component of the process, and the smaller lymphoid cells are more indolent and perhaps more motile.

FOLLICULAR, PREDOMINANTLY SMALL CLEAVED CELL LYMPHOMA. Follicular, predominantly small cleaved cell lymphoma (*i.e.*, nodular poorly differentiated lymphocytic lymphoma) is the most common type of follicular lymphoma, accounting for approximately 60% of cases. The neoplastic cells usually are small, cleaved, indented lymphocytes with few large cells (Fig. 52–5). Mitotic figures are rare. Monoclonal populations of lymphocytes identical to those found in involved lymph nodes are present in the peripheral blood of many patients with follicular lymphomas who do not otherwise have morphologic evidence of leukemia.[200] When leukemia does appear, the lymphoid cells in the peripheral blood exhibit notches in the nucleus ("buttock cells"). The process has been referred to as lymphosarcoma cell leukemia.[201] However, this term should be avoided because it has been used with biologically and clinically diverse malignant lymphomas that happen to have a leukemic phase.

FOLLICULAR, MIXED SMALL CLEAVED AND LARGE CELL LYMPHOMA. In follicular, mixed small cleaved and large cell (nodular mixed) malignant lymphoma, representing approximately 30% of cases, the large nucleolated cells are more abundant, numbering more than five per high-powered field and, in some cases, appearing to be admixed in almost equal numbers with smaller lymphoid cells.[202] As with most follicular lymphomas, patients usually have easily detectable disseminated disease at presentation, but it is not uncommon to find only the smaller cleaved lymphoid cells in sites distant from the nodes of origin, such as liver or bone marrow. In bone marrow, the characteristic paratrabecular location of the lymphoid infiltrates is useful in differentiating involvement by follicular lymphoma from normal lymphoid nodules that are usually within the marrow space and perivascular in location. This observation underscores the belief that the smaller cells are the migratory component of the normal and malignant lymphoid system and that the large cells are the replicative forms.

FOLLICULAR, PREDOMINANTLY LARGE CELL LYMPHOMA. Follicular, predominantly large cell (nodular histiocytic) malignant lymphoma is the least common form of follicular lymphoma and accounts for only 10% of cases.[203] The motile small lymphoid cells, seen in appreciable numbers in the other nodular lymphomas, are few in these tumors, and the patients often appear to have localized tumors. Despite their earlier clinical stage at diagnosis, they had the least favorable prognosis of all follicular lymphomas, because the localized appearance was deceptive and frequent recurrences and progression to diffuse large cell tumors occurred.

VARIATIONS IN PATTERN AND CYTOLOGY OF FOLLICULAR LYMPHOMAS. In many cases of follicular lymphoma, the nodular growth pattern is seen in only part of the lesion. In such cases, the clinical consequences of the diffuse component vary depending on the cytologic composition of the tumor.[204] In lymphomas composed predominantly of small cleaved cells, the presence of even a major diffuse component does not adversely affect prognosis.[198] However, in follicular lymphomas of the mixed small cleaved and large cell type, if the diffuse phase exceeds 50% of the lesion, the tumor appears to behave in a more aggressive manner. In follicular lymphomas composed predominantly of large cells, even if the diffuse component is only focal, the prognosis approximates that of the diffuse aggressive lymphomas.[203]

Variations in histologic composition can be seen in a single lymph node and in different anatomic sites at the same time. As many as one third of patients with lymphocytic lymphoma who undergo staging laparotomy exhibit some histologic discordance in different sites.[205,206] Usually these differences are minor, such as follicular small cleaved and follicular mixed small cleaved and large cell, and they do not change the prognosis. However, in some cases major histologic discrepancies can be seen, such as follicular mixed small cleaved and large cell and diffuse large cell. In such cases, treatment should be based on the most aggressive histologic subtype encountered.

The natural history of follicular lymphomas results in progression in time from a follicular to a diffuse growth pattern, and a cytologic shift from small, relatively slowly proliferating cells to large, more rapidly proliferating cells. The clinical implications of these histologic transformations are discussed in the following sections.

BIOLOGY OF FOLLICULAR LYMPHOMAS. Follicular lymphomas are monoclonal B-cell lymphomas that express only a single light chain, usually κ, with one or more heavy-chain determinants, most commonly IgM, usually without IgD.[199,207] IgG is the predominant heavy-chain class in fewer than half the cases. The cells are intimately associated with dendritic reticulum cells, the presence of which correlates with a follicular growth pattern.[208] The cells express the B-cell antigens CD19, CD20, and CD22. They also usually express CALLA or CD10. In contrast with the small lymphocytic malignancies, they are consistently CD5 negative.[111]

Suspensions prepared from follicular lymphomas may contain 50% or more T lymphocytes, and these cells are within and between the neoplastic nodules.[209] The T cells are phenotypically normal with a normal lymph node CD4:CD8 ratio, and there is no evidence that they are part of the neoplastic proliferation. However, they are not functionally inert and retain a capacity to modulate immunoglobulin synthesis by the neoplastic B lymphocytes.[210] The presence of numerous T cells in these lesions correlates with the likelihood of responding to antiidiotypic antibody therapy.[211]

Immunologic studies have revealed that most patients with follicular lymphomas exhibit "clonal excess" and excess of cells in the peripheral expressing one light chain in the blood derived from the neoplastic clone.[200] This observation may provide a useful parameter to determine response to treatment or for early detection of recurrence. It also implies that, because of the propensity of the malignant cells to circulate, truly localized disease in follicular lymphomas is extremely rare. PCR analysis of peripheral blood showed that circulating cells with the t(14;18) translocation of follicular lymphoma are present in patients who have been in continuous remission for more than 10 years.[78]

DIFFUSE, SMALL CLEAVED CELL. Diffuse small cleaved cell (*i.e.*, diffuse poorly differentiated lymphocytic) malignant lymphomas are composed of lymphoid cells that are cytologically similar to the small cleaved lymphocytes of follicular lymphomas. In most cases, this neoplasm is not simply a consequence of progression to a diffuse growth pattern in a follicular lymphoma. Most cases represent a B-cell lymphoma, initially called lymphocytic lymphoma of intermediate differentiation or mantle zone lymphoma.[212–214] This tumor is equivalent to diffuse centrocytic lymphoma in the Kiel classification.[215] This lesion seems somewhat more common in southern Europe than in the United States. The clinical behavior is heterogenous, and clinical aggressiveness correlates with the mitotic rate.[213,216] Like the other low-grade lymphomas, patients usually present with disseminated disease and are in the middle-aged or older-aged groups. A male predominance is usually seen. Although there is some heterogeneity in the clinical behavior, sustained complete remissions are uncommon.[216,217]

The term "intermediate" indicates that the tumors cytologically appear intermediate between the small lymphocytic and small cleaved lymphomas. In some cases, there is an admixture of small round and small cleaved lymphocytes. The growth pattern is diffuse or vaguely nodular. The term "mantle zone lymphoma" stems from the observation that residual, naked, normal-appearing germinal centers are often seen, and it has been postulated that the tumor is derived from the cells of the follicular lymphoid cuff or mantle zone.[218]

Immunologically, these are monoclonal B-cell tumors that more often express λ than κ, unlike most other B-cell neoplasms.[216] Like small lymphocytic neoplasms, the cells are usually CD5 positive but they often share with follicular lymphoma the expression of CD10.[111] Correlating with the vaguely nodular growth pattern, a residual meshwork of dendritic reticulum cells may be seen.[208] Because not all mantle zone lymphomas have a mantle zone pattern of growth, the term "mantle cell lymphomas" was recently proposed as an alternative.[219] Cytogenetic and molecular studies finding a high frequency of t(11;14) have lent support to the concept that mantle cell lymphomas are a distinct clinicopathologic entity.

Mycosis Fungoides and Sézary Syndrome

Mycosis Fungoides and Sézary syndrome are referred to collectively as the CTCL. This spectrum of rare T-cell disorders is discussed more fully in Chapter 53.

INTERMEDIATE-GRADE LYMPHOMAS

For clinical purposes, these lymphomas can be thought of as a single group because they share a common clinical presentation and natural history and require similar treatment strategies. They include diffuse mixed cell, diffuse large cell, and immunoblastic lymphomas. They are most common in adults but occur in all age groups and present in nodal (65%) and extranodal (35%) sites. These tumors tend to disseminate rapidly and, unlike the low-grade lymphomas, involve privileged sites such as the CNS and testis. They also have a destructive growth pattern, and regardless of the immunologic phenotype, they uncommonly involve T-cell-dependent or B-cell-dependent zones.[171] Their prognosis is distinctly unfavorable unless modern intensive chemotherapeutic regimens can induce a sustained complete remission. If a complete remission is attained and maintained beyond 2 years, the likelihood of being cured is high.

Immunologically, these lymphomas are heterogenous and are composed of morphologically transformed B (85%) and T (15%) lymphocytes. In fewer than 5% of the patients true histiocytic markers can be demonstrated. Originally, using only limited studies, a large proportion of these tumors appeared to be "null," lacking markers of T or B lymphocytes. However, using a large battery of techniques, including Southern hybridization for immunoglobulin gene rearrangement and T-cell receptor gene rearrangement, the cellular origin can be identified in more than 95% of cases.[220]

Morphologic and immunologic studies have attempted to develop clinically useful subclassifications of these intermediate-grade lymphomas. Most morphologic studies have shown that diffuse lymphomas composed of follicular center cells (*i.e.*, mixed small cleaved and large cell, large cleaved, and large noncleaved) have a somewhat better prognosis than other diffuse aggressive lymphoma.[174] However, these differences have not always achieved statistical significance and should not be interpreted to imply that less than intensive chemotherapy is required for these aggressive lymphomas.[221] Reproducibility of these fine morphologic distinctions among different observers or by the same observer is another problem in developing useful subclassification schemes. Immunologic studies have been useful in illustrating the heterogeneity of this group of tumors. One of the problems of antibody phenotyping is the detection of heterogeneity that simply does not appear to have clinical correlation. T-cell intermediate-grade lymphomas may have a poorer prognosis than their B-cell counterparts, but other evidence suggests that immunologic phenotype has not yet proved useful in delineating clinical and prognostic subtypes.[222,223]

Diffuse, Mixed Small and Large Cell Lymphomas

In approximately 75% of patients, the neoplastic cells of diffuse mixed ("histiocytic") malignant lymphomas are cytologically identical to those of follicular mixed lymphomas, and it is likely that the tumors are diffuse outgrowths of formerly follicular proliferations. B-cell markers, similar to those found on the cells of follicular lymphomas, may be demonstrable on the cells of these diffuse tumors, and the term "histiocytic" is a misnomer for the large nucleolated transformed B cell. Adequate biopsy sampling may even reveal focal residual nodularity. Many of these tumors are composed of large monoclonal B cells and admixed phenotypically normal T cells.[224] The term T-cell-rich B-cell lymphoma has been popularized for this lesion.[225] These lesions frequently contain the *BCL2* translocation.[226] The T-cell component is believed to represent a host response comparable to that seen in many follicular lymphomas. In extranodal sites, particularly in the retroperitoneum and mesentery, these follicular center cell lymphomas may be associated with extensive sclerosis. These patients have an age distribution similar to those with nodular lymphomas, and the disease is often of advanced clinical stage at the time of diagnosis, with occult disease in the liver, bone marrow, and extranodal sites. The natural history of these diffuse lymphomas is more aggressive than their follicular counterparts, but potential for cure exists with appropriate therapy.

In some diffuse lymphomas of mixed cell type (approximately 25%), the cells do not resemble those of nodular lymphomas but appear instead to be a pleomorphic mixture of large and small atypical lymphoid cells. The small cells are atypical but distinctively lymphoid, and the larger cells have prominent central nuclei and abundant cytoplasm. An inflammatory background composed of epithelioid histiocytes, plasma cells, and eosinophils may be present. Binucleated forms of large atypical cells may simulate Reed-Sternberg cells, and these cases may be misdiagnosed as Hodgkin's disease, if the fact that the small lymphoid cells also have a neoplastic appearance, in contrast to Hodgkin's disease, is not recognized. In most cases, the malignant cells bear markers of mature or "peripheral" T lymphocytes.[227,228] Cases in which the epithelioid component is conspicuous have been called "lymphoepithelioid cell lymphomas" or "Lennert's lymphoma" because Lennert first described these tumors and postulated that they might be related to Hodgkin's disease.[229–231] With time, the epithelioid cell component, which is nonneoplastic, is lost, and the tumor may progress to one predominantly composed of the large nucleolated cells, so-called large cell immunoblastic lymphoma. Unlike Hodgkin's disease, these peripheral T-cell lymphomas occur in middle-aged or elderly patients and often present with disseminated disease.[101,232] Clinically, they should be approached as other diffuse aggressive lymphocytic lymphomas.

Diffuse, Large Cell Lymphoma

Diffuse, large cell (*i.e.*, diffuse histiocytic) malignant lymphoma represents one of the two subtypes in the Working Formulation derived from diffuse "histiocytic" lymphoma of Rappaport. These lymphomas are composed of large lymphoid cells with nuclear diameters greater than those of admixed "starry sky" histiocytes. The cells may have cytologic features of large noncleaved or large cleaved follicular center cells. In the noncleaved variant (Fig. 52–6), the nuclei are vesicular with reticulated chromatin and two to three distinct nucleoli, often apposed to the nuclear membrane. The cytoplasm is abundant and slightly amphophilic. The cells of the large cleaved variant have finely dispersed nuclear chromatin, inconspicuous and basophilic nucleoli, and sparse eosinophilic cytoplasm. Sclerosis is frequent in the large cleaved cell variant. Mitoses are usually readily identified in both subtypes. As expected from the follicular center cell characteristics, most cases are of B-cell origin.[220] In some cases, a lymphoma with a follicular pattern can be identified in another anatomic site, and biopsies obtained for staging may indicate other evidence of an underlying follicular lymphoma, such as paratrabecular small cleaved or mixed lymphoid infiltrates in the bone marrow. Cases with this morphology may carry the t(14;18) translocation, further supporting a relation to follicular lymphoma.[233]

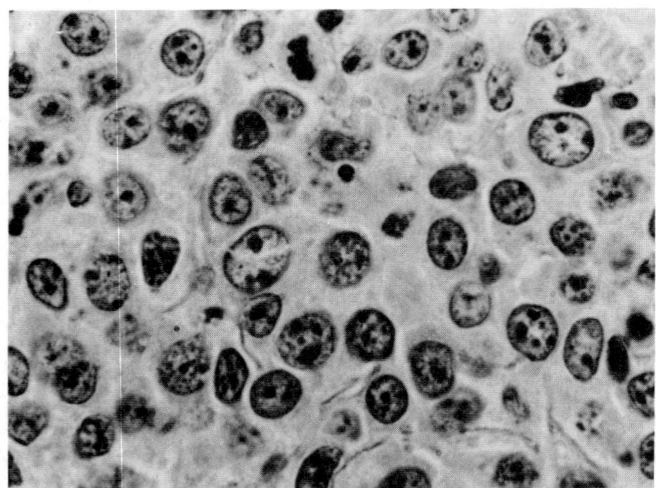

FIGURE 52–6. Malignant lymphoma: diffuse, large cell type. Cells resemble large noncleaved follicular center cells and have multiple, prominent, often membrane-bound nucleoli (hematoxylin and eosin; original magnification × 1000).

Diffuse, Large Cell, Immunoblastic Lymphoma

The category of diffuse, large cell, immunoblastic (diffuse histiocytic) lymphoma is composed of all diffuse histiocytic lymphomas in the Rappaport scheme that do not have the cytologic features of large follicular center cells. Various subtypes are described in the Working Formulation.[174] These are all high-grade (intermediate-grade according to their behavior in most combination chemotherapy clinical trials) neoplasms and commonly exhibit a high mitotic rate.

The *plasmacytoid* subtype is composed of large pleomorphic cells with abundant, deeply amphophilic and pyroninophilic cytoplasm, eccentric nuclei, and prominent central nucleoli. The *clear cell* subtype is composed of cells with abundant, optically clear cytoplasm and distinct nuclear membranes. The *polymorphous* category was proposed to include lymphomas composed of a pleomorphic population of large lymphoid cells, reflecting the morphologic diversity of T-cell lymphomas described in Japan and elsewhere. The term "epithelioid" is used to refer to those large cell lymphomas with a high content of epithelioid histiocytes and represents part of the spectrum of Lennert's lymphomas or lymphoepithelioid cell lymphomas. Similar tumors with a more mixed lymphoid composition are also included in the diffuse, mixed-cell category.

The correlation between morphologic appearance and immunologic subtype is less predictable in these neoplasms. Although plasmacytoid features could indicate a B-cell phenotype, T-cell lymphomas with plasmacytoid features have been described.[173,234] Similarly, the features of the clear cell, polymorphous, and epithelioid subtypes of immunoblastic lymphomas have been most often associated with lymphomas of T-cell origin but can also be encountered in B-cell neoplasms. Moreover, no clinical significance could be demonstrated for these subtypes of large cell immunoblastic lymphoma. The use of these additional descriptive terms is optional.

A variant of immunoblastic lymphoma, large cell anaplastic lymphoma, is characterized by the propensity of the malignant cells to invade lymphoid sinuses.[235] Because of the sinusoidal location of the tumor cells, misdiagnosis as malignant histiocytosis or metastatic carcinoma is common. In most cases studied, the malignant cells express some T-cell antigens, although the cells have a markedly aberrant phenotype. T-cell gene rearrangement has also been shown in some instances. A consistent feature is the expression of the Hodgkin's disease-associated antigen CD30 detected by Ki-1 and Hefi-1 (see Chap. 51).[235,236] This antigen, although present on the malignant cells of Hodgkin's disease, is also found in activated T and B lymphocytes. CD30 bears homology to the nerve growth factor receptor and the related protooncogene *TRK*.[237] This tumor can present in all age groups; but appears relatively common in children and young adults.[235] A high incidence of cutaneous disease has been reported. It is associated with the t(2;5)(p23;q35) translocation.[238] It may follow a more indolent course than other immunoblastic lymphoma types, especially if the disease involves only the skin.

HIGH-GRADE LYMPHOMAS

Diffuse Lymphoblastic Lymphoma

Diffuse lymphoblastic lymphoma is a form of lymphocytic lymphoma common in adolescents and young adults, and it demonstrates a marked male preponderance.[239–241] The neoplastic cells appear blastic with finely distributed nuclear chromatin, small nucleoli, scant cytoplasm, and numerous mitotic figures. The nuclei in some cases are round to oval, but a variable percentage have nuclei with marked lobulations and convolutions. Many of these patients have mediastinal masses, and a relation to the thymus gland was suggested on clinical grounds long before the discovery of T- and B-cell systems.[242] Progression to ALL is a frequent phenomenon in these patients. The enzyme TdT is a ubiquitous feature of all lymphoblastic malignancies and has been demonstrable in virtually all cases studied.[130] The cells from 85% of cases have T-cell surface markers and share many characteristics with the cells from the 20% to 30% of ALL cases of the T-cell type.[106] However, most lymphoblastic lymphoma patients have a slightly more differentiated phenotype than seen in T-cell ALL (see Fig. 52–2). Even in patients who present with soft tissue involvement, a careful workup often reveals occult marrow involvement. There is also a high risk of infiltration of the leptomeninges, with neoplastic cells demonstrable in the cerebrospinal fluid, particularly as a first site of relapse. And as in T-cell ALL, the CNS should be treated prophylactically. Although the disease may appear circumscribed at the time of diagnosis, progression to systemic disease is such a common feature that these patients are now treated with regimens similar to those used for T-cell ALL. This approach has significantly improved the prognosis for this high-grade tumor.

In as many as 10% of patients, the neoplastic cells demonstrate a phenotype similar to that of common ALL or pre-B-cell ALL and are immature lymphoid cells committed to the B-cell lineage.[106] Morphologically, these are indistinguishable from the more frequent T-cell lymphoblastic lymphomas. Clinical differences, however, have been observed in that patients with B-cell tumors usually do not present with mediastinal disease, and isolated lytic bone lesions and skin lesions have been reported.[106,242]

Diffuse Small Noncleaved Cell Lymphoma

Small noncleaved cell (*i.e.,* diffuse, undifferentiated) lymphomas are high-grade malignancies with a high growth fraction and include Burkitt's and non-Burkitt's subtypes. Cytologically, these tumors are composed of cells that resemble small noncleaved follicular center cells. Burkitt's lymphoma is composed of uniform cells of moderate size (15–25 μm) with round to oval nuclei, coarsely reticulated chromatin, and two to five prominent basophilic nucleoli.[243] Each cell possesses a distinct rim of amphophilic and intensely pyroninophilic cytoplasm with the methyl green pyronin stain. Mitoses are numerous, and a starry sky pattern is characteristic but not pathognomonic, because it can be encountered in any rapidly proliferating lymphoma. The growth pattern is usually diffuse, but selective involvement of germinal centers can be seen, further supporting a relation to the B-cell system.[244]

All cases of Burkitt's lymphoma exhibit B-cell markers. The cells usually express a μ heavy chain with a single light-chain type and CD10.[116] The presence of C3d receptors (CD21) varies and correlates with the presence or absence of the EBV genome.[245] Endemic Burkitt's lymphomas, which are usually EBV positive, express C3d receptors, and 85% of nonendemic cases are EBV and C3d receptor negative. The chromosomal abnormalities of Burkitt's lymphoma were previously discussed. The morphologic features of endemic and nonendemic Burkitt's lymphoma are identical. The endemic cases present at a lower median age (7 years) than nonendemic cases (11 years) and more often present in the face and jaw bones. An intraabdominal mass involving the ileocecal region or ovaries is the most common clinical presentation for nonendemic cases. Other extranodal sites frequently involved include kidney, testis, thyroid, and distal long bones. The staging scheme used for Burkitt's lymphoma differs from that used for the other lymphocytic lymphomas. It relates general prognosis to overall tumor burden and bone marrow involvement. As a high-grade lymphoma with a high growth fraction, Burkitt's lymphoma is potentially curable with appropriate combination chemotherapy.[246]

Small noncleaved cell lymphomas of the non-Burkitt's type show a greater degree of nuclear pleomorphism than that considered acceptable to diagnose Burkitt's lymphoma, but they are also high-grade lymphoid neoplasms.[247,248] The mean nuclear diameter is similar to that of Burkitt's lymphoma, 15 to 35 μm, but with greater variation within the tumor cell population; occasional giant cell forms and bizarre cells may be present. The cytologic characteristics are similar to those of Burkitt's, but with greater variation in nuclear shape, chromatin condensation, and nucleolar prominence and number. There is usually a single distinct eosinophilic nucleolus. Small noncleaved cell non-Burkitt's lymphomas present most often in adults (median age, 34 years), and the site of presentation is usually nodal with peripheral lymphadenopathy not uncommon. However, small noncleaved cell lymphomas with nuclear pleomorphism also occur in children, and in this age group, they are virtually indistinguishable clinically and biologically from classic Burkitt's lymphoma.

Neoplastic cells from approximately 95% of cases express B-cell surface markers. Translocations involving the *MYC* oncogene are rare, unlike Burkitt's lymphoma.[249] Both variants of small noncleaved cell lymphomas are the most frequent form of lymphoma seen in association with HIV infection. It has been postulated that the pathogenesis of high-grade B-cell lymphomas in the setting of HIV infection is similar to that of classic Burkitt's lymphoma in Africa.[250] In both settings, polyclonal B-cell proliferation occurs in the absence of effective T-cell regulation, possibly leading to the emergence of a malignant clone.

A mature T-cell phenotype is identified in rare cases of small noncleaved non-Burkitt's lymphoma. This immunologic heterogeneity in concert with some clinicopathologic diversity suggests that, in contrast to Burkitt's lymphoma, this morphologic subtype is not a homogenous clinicopathologic entity.

Adult T-Cell Leukemia-Lymphoma

ATL is a characteristic clinicopathologic entity associated with HTLV-I.[53] The pathologic spectrum of the associated lymphomas is broad and includes several diffuse subtypes in the Rappaport classification and the Working Formulation.[251] The most characteristic morphologic feature is the presence of highly pleomorphic and polylobated cells in the peripheral blood. Polylobated and multinucleated cells can also be seen in the lymph nodes, and by this criterion, many cases have been classified as large cell immunoblastic in the Working Formulation. Approximately 65% of patients present with peripheral blood involvement, and a leukemic phase develops in almost 100% at some time during the clinical course. Other common clinical features include generalized lymphadenopathy, hepatosplenomegaly, cutaneous involvement, hypercalcemia, and lytic bone lesions. Biopsies of lytic lesions do not necessarily show involvement by tumor, and marked osteoclastic activity is seen in lytic lesions and in routine bone marrow biopsies. These observations support the concept that a lymphokine secreted by neoplastic cells, osteoclast activity factor or an osteoclast activating factor-like substance, is responsible for these manifestations. This factor is probably IL-1. The skin lesions are papulonodular with or without ulceration. In two thirds of patients with cutaneous involvement, epidermal infiltration resembling Pautrier's microabscesses is observed. However, most cases can readily be differentiated from mycosis fungoides or Sézary's syndrome on clinical and epidemiologic grounds.

ATL is a postthymic T-cell neoplasm that usually expresses a helper cell surface phenotype. However, in vitro the cells actually function as suppressor cells and suppress immunoglobulin synthesis by B cells.[252] They are strongly positive for acid phosphatase, and the activity is not always entirely inhibited by tartrate.[251] TRAP activity is not pathognomonic of hairy cell leukemia.

MISCELLANEOUS RARE LYMPHOPROLIFERATIVE DISEASES

Angioimmunoblastic Lymphadenopathy

In 1975, a new clinicopathologic entity called angioimmunoblastic lymphadenopathy (AILD) was described.[253,254] It was initially construed as a hyperimmune disorder, but questions have been raised about its potentially neoplastic nature. The mean age of patients is approximately 68 years. The disease has an acute onset with generalized lymphadenopathy. Hepatosplenomegaly and constitutional symptoms occur in most cases. Rashes, a positive Coombs' test, and polyclonal hypergammaglobulinemia are commonly found.

Essential pathologic features include complete architectural effacement; proliferation of arborizing small blood vessels; polymorphous cellular proliferation of lymphocytes, immunoblasts, plasma cells, with or without histiocytes and eosinophils; and absence of germinal centers or a few residual "burned out" or hyalinized germinal centers. Other frequent, but not essential, histologic features are an overall hypocellular appearance with amorphous acidophilic interstitial material. Usually all lymph nodes are involved, and it is important to make the diagnosis only in the appropriate clinical context. Although the disease is progressive and often fatal (median survival, 15 months), the cells are not morphologically malignant. However, as many as 50% of patients are found to have overt lymphomas during the clinical course or at autopsy.[255] The lymphomas are classified as large cell immunoblastic in the Working Formulation.

Cytotoxic treatment has not proved effective in controlling the disease or in preventing progression to lymphoma. Infectious complications often supervene, leading to a high morbidity and mortality after therapy. Corticosteroid therapy, with or without cyclophosphamide, does provide temporary control in some cases.

The polyclonal hypergammaglobulinemia and plasmacytosis found in AILD suggested that it might be a hyperimmune disorder of the B-cell system. However, the immunoblastic cells in AILD and the malignant lymphomas that supervene are Ig negative, and Japanese investigators have described a variant of peripheral T-cell lymphoma that bears a marked resemblance to this lesion.[256] It has been suggested that AILD is a peripheral T-cell lymphoma derived from helper T cells. Cytogenetic investigations that have shown clonal abnormalities in several patients supported a malignant nature for this disease, even early in its course.[257] Clonal rearrangements of the T-cell receptor β chain gene have provided additional evidence for T-cell origin in some cases and further suggest a neoplastic nature.[258,259] However, immunoglobulin gene rearrangements have been found, and sequential analysis has shown spontaneous regression of T-cell and B-cell clones. Others have argued that AILD may be an immunoregulatory disorder.[259] The B-cell clones may be secondary to the expansion of EBV-immortalized B cells as a consequence of the associated immunodeficiency in this disease.[260]

Angiocentric Immunoproliferative Lesions

Although lymphomatoid granulomatosis (LYG), polymorphic reticulosis (PMR), and midline malignant reticulosis (MMR) were initially described as discrete entities in different anatomic sites, they represent the same histologic process. MMR and PMR are associated with the clinical entity lethal midline granuloma and involve the nose, paranasal sinuses, nasopharynx, and palate.[261,262] LYG was first described in the lung, but it also involves the nasopharyngeal sites listed in many patients.[263] Other frequent sites of involvement include skin, kidneys, central and peripheral nervous systems, and gastrointestinal tract. The lesion common to all is an angiocentric and angiodestructive atypical lymphoreticular infiltrate. The vascular involvement often leads to necrosis, which may be extensive. Atypical lymphoid cells are admixed with plasma cells, eosinophils, and histiocytes. Because of these common histologic features, it has been proposed that these lesions represent the same nosologic entity, and the term "angiocentric immunoproliferative lesions" (AIL) has been proposed.[103,264]

LYG was initially described as a benign disorder with a limited risk of progressing to a malignant lymphoma. Similarly, MMR and PMR were believed to be locally invasive and destructive lesions with a low risk of peripheral dissemination. In some series, as many as 50% of patients progress to lymphomas of the large cell immunoblastic type.[265] Moreover, the median survival of LYG patients in one series was only 14 months, and survival was found to be inversely proportional to the number of large, atypical lymphoreticular cells.[266] These observations have prompted the suggestion that these disorders, at least in some cases, may be neoplastic at onset. In the cases studied, the lymphoid cells have had a mature T-cell phenotype, and these processes may represent variants of peripheral T-cell lymphoma.[103,264,267]

Most cases present in adult life (median age, 50 years) and the male to female ratio is 2:1. Presenting complaints are usually related to the involved organs: cough, shortness of breath, and nasal discharge. Systemic symptoms, including fever, weight loss, and malaise, are also common. Approximately 75% of patients with localized upper airway disease respond to radiation therapy without local recurrence or peripheral dissemination. Cyclophosphamide and prednisone have been used in LYG, with as many as 50% sustained complete remissions.[265] Patients who have recurrences or undergo histologic progression require more aggressive multiagent systemic chemotherapy, but survival rates for these patients, who have usually received prior therapy, have been low.

A grading scheme was proposed for AIL.[264] Grade I lesions have a polymorphic cellular composition and no cellular atypia. Grade II lesions demonstrate some cytologic atypia. Grade III lesions represent clear-cut angiocentric lymphoma. Most patients with grade I disease achieved control of their disease with cyclophosphamide and prednisone, unlike patients with grade II disease, most of whom progressed to overt lymphoma within 2 years and died from refractory disease. Patients with grade III disease treated aggressively at onset had a high complete remission rate and prolonged disease-free survival.[264]

EBV is strongly associated with this disease.[268–271] Moreover, by Southern blot analysis the EBV appears to be clonal. Surprisingly, studies to evaluate the clonality of the T-cell antigen receptor genes have not shown clonal arrangements.[270,271] This observation may suggest that the process is not truly of T-cell origin or that the T-cell component is reactive and not neoplastic. In some cases, the cells have exhibited NK cell markers.[272]

True Histiocytic Lymphoma and Malignant Histiocytosis

Malignancies of mononuclear phagocytes include acute monocytic leukemia, malignant histiocytosis, and true histiocytic sarcoma. These three malignancies represent a spectrum in terms of their degree of dissemination and can be conceptually related to different stages of maturation and differentiation in the mononuclear phagocytic series.[273] Acute monocytic leukemia is related to a bone marrow-derived monoblast. This malignancy arises in the bone marrow compartment with secondary involvement of the peripheral blood and usually results in a markedly elevated white blood cell count. Unlike acute myeloid leukemia, there is a somewhat higher incidence of involvement of nonhematopoietic sites, with frequent involvement of skin and gingiva. Hepatosplenomegaly (25%) and lymphadenopathy (50%) are relatively common.[274]

Malignant histiocytosis represents a malignancy of mononuclear phagocytes that are intermediate in differentiation between monocytes and monoblasts and fixed tissue histiocytes. In many instances, the syndromes of acute monocytic leukemia and malignant histiocytosis may merge, and the distinction may be arbitrary and somewhat semantic. Malignant histiocytosis is a systemic malignancy that involves the entire reticuloendothelial system. Within the lymphoreticular system there is preferential involvement of sites normally populated by histiocytes, such as lymph node sinuses, splenic red pulp, and hepatic sinusoids. Bone marrow involvement is common, and although abnormal cells can be seen in the peripheral blood, if peripheral blood involvement is extensive, a diagnosis of acute monocytic leukemia should be considered. Other frequent sites of involvement include skin and bone.

The end point of the spectrum is histiocytic sarcoma or true histiocytic lymphoma, which represents a malignancy of the mononuclear phagocytic series at the stage of the fixed tissue histiocyte. The lesions in histiocytic sarcoma represent localized, relatively discrete tumefactions.[275] In addition to the reticuloendothelial system, common sites of involvement include skin and bone.[276]

Histiocytic sarcomas initially confined to the skin may pursue an indolent clinical course, with spontaneous regression of lesions in some cases.[276] The entity initially described as regressing atypical histiocytosis may represent histiocytic sarcoma with this characteristic presentation.[277] Alternatively, the clinical and pathologic features of these cutaneous lesions are remarkably similar to lymphomatoid papulosis, a chronic self-remitting T-cell lesion of the skin. Poppema had suggested a histiocytic derivation for lymphomatoid papulosis, and because of the high content of lysosomal enzymes in activated T cells, it is not surprising that the distinction between a histiocytic and T-cell origin has been a difficult one.[278] The current molecular and phenotypic evidence supporting a T-cell derivation for lymphomatoid papulosis is strong, and the natures of "regressing atypical histiocytosis" and isolated histiocytic sarcomas of the skin need to be reassessed in light of this new information.[144]

In the absence of special studies, morphologic evidence of phagocytosis by the neoplastic cells, most commonly erythrophagocytosis, has been proposed as a criterion for determining derivation from mononuclear phagocytes. However, phagocytosis is not reliably seen in most mononuclear phagocytic malignancies. Moreover, it is not a specific finding and has been described in lymphoid, plasmacytic, and even epithelial tumors.[267] Even if phagocytosis is observed, it is virtually always clinically insignificant. The clinical syndrome of histiocytic medullary reticulosis, characterized by hepatosplenomegaly, pancytopenia, and jaundice, has been proposed as a manifestation of malignant histiocytosis.[165,279] However, most observers now believe that it is usually a manifestation of a hemophagocytic syndrome, usually seen in association with immunodeficiency or another hematopoietic malignancy.[280,281] This syndrome appears pathogenetically related to excessive production of lymphokines capable of stimulating mononuclear phagocytes.[282]

Because of the misinterpretation of hemophagocytic syndromes in the past as "malignant histiocytosis," many reports of malignant histiocytosis actually represent hemophagocytic syndromes. This appears to be true for many cases of malignant histiocytosis reported in association with ALL. AIL, including LYG, PMR, and MMR, is often associated with a hemophagocytic syndrome as a terminal event that has been misdiagnosed as malignant histiocytosis.[281] These lesions are now recognized as a variant of peripheral T-cell lymphoma. Because of the underlying T-cell malignancy, there may be an associated immunodeficiency and subsequent development of a hemophagocytic syndrome. Alternatively, the hemophagocytic syndrome could be due to lymphokine production by neoplastic cells. Familial erythrophagocytic lymphohistiocytosis is another disorder in which the terminal phase of the disease appears to be a hemophagocytic syndrome. The underlying condition appears to be a poorly characterized immunodeficiency.

True histiocytic lymphomas preferentially involve lymph nodes sinuses. However, this feature is not specific and can be seen in certain T-cell immunoblastic lymphomas. Many instances of so-called malignant histiocytosis appear to represent this variant of Ki-1-positive or large cell anaplastic lymphoma.[236]

Enzyme cytochemistry and histochemistry remain a reliable adjunct to morphology in the diagnosis of malignancies of the mononuclear phagocytic system. The cells have diffuse activity for nonspecific esterase, which is usually at least partially fluoride sensitive. Preferable methods for detection of esterase activity include the α-naphthyl butyrate esterase reaction because activity is not observed in myeloid cells. Myeloid cells also react minimally or not at all with α-naphthyl acetate esterase. The use of the naphthyl ASD acetate requires the use of fluoride to differentiate myeloid and mononuclear phagocytic cells. Activity for acid phosphatase and β-glucuronidase is usually present as well. In all cases, the activity should be relatively diffuse throughout the cytoplasm and not punctate. Punctate reactivity localized to the Golgi region is more characteristic of lymphoid rather than mononuclear phagocytic cells. Caution should be exercised in the use of enzyme cytochemistry because these enzymes are not specific for mononuclear phagocytes and can be seen in certain carcinomas and sarcomas.

Proliferative lesions of antigen-presenting cells are relatively rare. The principal proliferative lesion of the dendritic cell system is histiocytosis X. Most authorities do not consider histiocytosis X to be a malignancy, but rather consider it to be a proliferative lesion, possibly secondary to immunodeficiency.[283,285] The cells of histiocytosis X have the characteristics of Langerhans cells, including CD1 expression and Birbeck granules. Unlike normal Langerhans cells, the cells also express antigens associated with phagocytic histiocytes such as MY4 (CD14) and Leu-M5 (CD11c).

Although the cells of histiocytosis X may sometimes appear cytologically atypical, even with abnormal mitotic figures, histologic features are said not to be an important prognostic indicator in this disease. Prognosis is best correlated with age at presentation and extent of organ system involvement.[284,285] Patients under 2 years of age tend to have a poor prognosis, but those older than 6 years have an excellent prognosis. Clinical staging schemes useful in prognosis correlate with the extent of organ system involvement. The greater the number of organ systems involved, the poorer the prognosis.

Some rare tumors have a proposed derivation from dendritic reticulum cells or interdigitating reticulum cells.[286–288] These lesions are based in lymph nodes and are often associated with an inflammatory background, necrosis, or both. They tend to present as local disease, and although they may be characterized by local recurrence, systemic spread has not been a feature. Because of the rarity of these lesions, it is difficult to make definitive statements about their clinical course.

Castleman's Disease

The eponym of Castleman's disease has been applied to three histologically and clinically distinct lesions. Although these disorders share some morphologic similarities, it is likely that they differ in their pathogenesis and require different therapeutic approaches.[289]

Castleman's disease was initially described as a localized mass lesion to be differentiated from malignant lymphoma or thymoma.[290] The localized form consists of two histologic subtypes: the hyaline vascular variant and the plasma cell type.[291] The hyaline vascular form is by far the most common, representing approximately 90% of cases. Patients are usually asymptomatic, and the process is often detected as an incidental finding or from symptoms secondary to compression by the mass. It occurs primarily in adults with an equal incidence in men and women. Surgical excision is the treatment of choice, and radiotherapy has not been effective. The most common sites of presentation include the mediastinum (52%), abdomen (26%), neck, axilla, or other nodal locations.[289]

The hyaline vascular form of Castleman's disease is composed of altered germinal centers that contain prominent vascular tufts composed of hyperplastic arterioles and sometimes of capillaries. The follicles lack the normal cellular components of the germinal center and are atrophic or regressed in appearance. The follicles are surrounded by a cuff of small lymphocytes that demonstrate an onion skin configuration. The interfollicular region is expanded as well, with numerous postcapillary venules. Plasma cells are relatively sparse.

The plasma cell variant is much less common. Histologically, it resembles a florid follicular hyperplasia with sheets of plasma cells in the interfollicular region. The prominent vascular changes of the hyaline-vascular form are not observed. There are clinical differences as well. Patients are much more likely to be symptomatic from their disease. The clinical presentation includes fever, fatigue, weight loss, with a hemolytic anemia in 90%. Laboratory abnormalities include increased erythrocyte sedimentation rate and polyclonal hypergammaglobulinemia in approximately 80%. These clinical and laboratory abnormalities appear to be mediated in large part by IL-6, which is produced in the germinal centers of the hyperplastic lymph nodes in large quantities.[292] Surgical excision is still the treatment of choice.

Multicentric or generalized Castleman's disease differs from both of the localized forms.[289] Histologically, it often shows some of the vascular lesions characteristic of the hyaline vascular form, but it also contains a marked plasmacytosis, as in the plasma cell variant. In a few cases, a monoclonal population of plasma cells may be identified by immunohistochemical studies.[289] An association with the POEMS syndrome (*i.e.*, *p*olyneuropathy, *o*rganomegaly, *e*ndocrinopathy, *M* protein, *s*kin changes) has been postulated. Additional evidence differentiating the generalized disease from the localized forms is provided by gene rearrangement studies, which have a high incidence of clonal rearrangements (predominantly of the *IG* genes) in the generalized disease, but not in the localized forms.[293] Clinically, the disease occurs in older age groups. Patients present with severe systemic symptoms, generalized lymphadenopathy, and often hepatosplenomegaly.[294,295] There is a 50% mortality, with a median survival of 27 months. Causes of death include sepsis, malignant lymphoma, and other malignancies. Kaposi's sarcoma has also been reported, and it is likely that some cases of the generalized form of Castleman's disease represent the persistent generalized lymphadenopathy syndrome associated with HIV infection. The generalized form of Castleman's disease is not a histologic entity, and the diagnosis should only be made in the appropriate clinical context. Other causes of the lymphadenopathy should be excluded.

DIFFERENTIAL DIAGNOSIS

SUPERFICIAL LYMPH NODE PRESENTATIONS

Eighty percent or more of adult patients with lymphomas present to their physicians with superficial adenopathy. It may have been detected by the patient or found as a result of a physical examination for another reason. Most patients are asymptomatic, although 20% of patients with the lymphocytic lymphomas and as many as 40% of patients with Hodgkin's disease may have some combination of fever higher than 101.5°F, night sweats, or unexplained weight loss of more than 10% of total body weight in the last 6 months, the so-called B symptoms.[296,297] Patients with low-grade lymphomas often give a history of waxing and waning adenopathy over periods extending from months to years before diagnosis, with an average duration of 5 months.

Lymph node enlargement is usually painless, rubbery, discrete, and located in the neck region. Isolated axillary or inguinal lymph node presentations occur but are less common. It is not possible to make accurate distinctions between the various lymphomas by the size, shape, or feel of the lymph nodes. The diagnosis depends on excision of the entire enlarged node and histologic examination by an experienced pathologist. Node aspiration or needle biopsy are inappropriate diagnostic tests. The distribution of peripheral adenopathy can yield diagnostic information (Table 52–9). Involvement of Waldeyer's ring occurs in fewer than 1% of patients with Hodgkin's disease but is identified in 15% to 33% of patients with the lymphocytic lymphomas and often is associated with lymphomas of the gastrointestinal tract.[296–298] Epitrochlear node involvement is unusual in Hodgkin's disease but relatively common in patients with follicular lymphomas. The duration of signs and B symptoms, if present, and a family

TABLE 52–9. Comparison of Lymphocytic Lymphomas and Hodgkin's Disease

Characteristics	*Lymphocytic Lymphoma*	*Hodgkin's Disease*
Presentation	Often extranodal	Usually nodal
Pattern of spread	Hematogenous; noncontiguous nodal spread	Contiguous nodal spread
Extent of disease	Rarely localized nodal disease	Commonly localized nodes
Marrow involvement	Common	Uncommon
Liver involvement	Common	Uncommon
Spleen involvement	Uncommon	Common
Mediastinum	Uncommon (except in lymphoblastic)	Common
Mesenteric disease	Common	Uncommon
Waldeyer's ring	Occasionally	Almost never
Epitrochlear nodes	Occasionally	Almost never
Gastrointestinal involvement	Common	Almost never
Central nervous system involvement	Occasionally	Almost never
Abdominal masses	Common	Uncommon
Skin involvement	Occasionally	Almost never

history of similar or related illnesses such as mononucleosis and immunologic disorders should be documented. During the physical examination, the status of lymph nodes in all peripheral sites, including the spleen, should be determined and recorded for each site separately.

The differential diagnosis of adenopathy depends on the age of the patient; the size, shape, and feel of the lymph nodes; and the location of the adenopathy (Fig. 52–7). Palpable lymph nodes can be a normal finding on careful examination, particularly in the neck region. Soft, flat, elliptical nodes of 0.5 to 1.0 cm are commonly palpable in the submandibular and submental regions and are found by careful examination in as many as 50% of normal people in the superficial jugular or posterior cervical chain.[299] In young patients, superficial adenopathy in the head and neck region is most often related to acute infectious illnesses of the mouth or pharynx. Mononucleosis is a common cause of cervical adenopathy, and although it is often associated with pharyngitis, adenopathy can occur without pharyngeal symptoms. Toxoplasmosis can mimic mononucleosis as well; these disorders can be easily diagnosed by standard methods if suspected. Adenopathy resulting from infection usually causes firm, sometimes tender spherical enlargement of nodes that can be easily confused with lymphomas if they are nontender. A spherical lymph node larger than 1 cm in diameter, thought to be due to an infectious process, and that does not diminish in size over a 4-week period of observation after resolution of the acute pro-

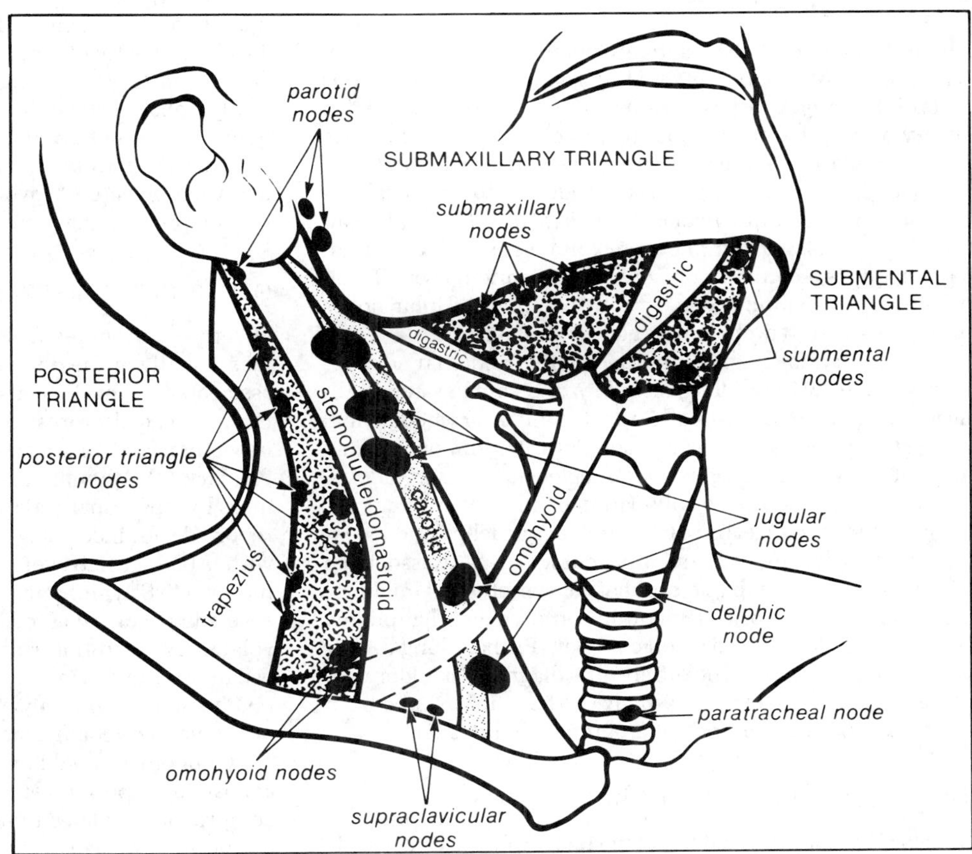

FIGURE 52–7. Anatomic subdivisions of the neck, depicting lymph node areas. (Adapted from Sade HH. Palpable cervical lymph nodes. JAMA 1958;168:496)

cess should be biopsied. Discrete, hard lymph nodes, particularly if fixed or matted, are more worrisome and should be biopsied promptly for diagnosis, particularly in older people. Hard lymph nodes in the submandibular or submental region in older people are more likely related to tumors of the floor of the mouth or larynx. Nasopharyngeal cancers often drain to, and present as, enlarged posterior cervical lymph nodes. Thyroid carcinoma can mimic lymphoma, although the lymph nodes involved with thyroid cancer generally are firmer and are often found in the submental and superficial jugular region, an area less commonly involved in isolation by lymphomas.

Because supraclavicular lymph nodes drain regions of the lung and retroperitoneal space, they can enlarge secondary to lymphomas or other tumors or infectious processes originating in these areas. Isolated axillary lymph node enlargement can be related to local phenomena in the hands or arms, such as infections, trauma (*e.g.*, cat scratch), or insect bites. The clinical presentation affects the likelihood of a specific diagnosis. For example, a young man with an enlarged axillary lymph node is most likely to have a lymphoma or a malignant melanoma, but in a woman, the same two tumors or breast cancer are the most likely diagnoses. Isolated inguinal adenopathy is often difficult to separate from the normal 0.5- to 1.0-cm elliptical lymph nodes found in the region of the inguinal ligament, which are influenced by disorders that occur on the legs and feet. Concomitant enlargement of nodes in the femoral triangle or adenopathy along the external iliac chain should make inguinal adenopathy more suspicious and decrease the threshold for biopsy.

THORACIC PRESENTATIONS

Thoracic adenopathy is relatively common in patients with lymphomas. It may be detected by routine roentgenograms taken for another purpose, such as the workup after the discovery of peripheral adenopathy, or because the patient has had a chronic, dry, nonproductive cough with or without fever. The overall frequency of mediastinal adenopathy in Hodgkin's disease is 50%, but the mediastinum is involved in fewer than 20% of patients with lymphocytic lymphomas.[300] Mediastinal adenopathy is a common presentation in patients with T-cell lymphoblastic lymphomas.[301,302] Involvement of hilar nodes in patients with lymphomas is usually unilateral.

The differential diagnosis of mediastinal and hilar adenopathy includes primary lung disorders and some systemic illnesses that characteristically involve hilar or mediastinal nodes. In the young, mediastinal adenopathy commonly occurs in patients with infectious mononucleosis and sarcoidosis, which in both cases is usually panhilar. In endemic regions, histoplasmosis can cause unilateral paratracheal node enlargement that mimics lymphoma, but it is usually associated with node calcification and esophageal symptoms. Unilateral tuberculous adenopathy is not often confused with lymphoma because of the associated Ghon complex. Primary lung cancer is an important part of the differential diagnosis in older people, especially smokers, and usually can be differentiated from lymphoma by the presence of a parenchymal lesion.

ABDOMINAL PRESENTATIONS

Hodgkin's disease and the lymphocytic lymphomas frequently involve retroperitoneal lymph nodes or the primary lymphatic tissue of the gut and its mesenteric drainage sites. Patients who present with abdominal lymphoma usually have a painless mass discovered on physical examination or pain associated with a palpable mass. Some patients present only with splenomegaly and most often have one of the lymphomas, commonly hairy cell leukemia.[303] Rarely, previously untreated patients may present with perforation of a viscus or hemorrhage from the upper or lower gastrointestinal tract. Previously unsuspected abdominal lymphomas are found more often after the staging workup is completed in patients who have superficial lymph node presentations. Patients whose abdominal disease alone prompts their visit to their physicians most often have one of the lymphomas. It is distinctly unusual to be able to palpate significant abdominal adenopathy in patients with Hodgkin's disease because mesenteric lymph node involvement is uncommon. This is not the case for lymphocytic lymphomas. The so-called Mediterranean lymphoma often presents with disease in the abdomen. Pathologically, these tumors resemble diffuse plasma cell tumors and often are associated with aberrant production of immunoglobulin heavy chains and malabsorption.[304] Abdominal presentations of lymphocytic lymphoma may mimic any type of intraabdominal disease. About two thirds of the lymphocytic lymphomas that involve the gastrointestinal tract originate in the stomach, 25% from the small intestine, and the remainder from the colon and rectum.[305]

CUTANEOUS PRESENTATIONS

Lymphocytic lymphomas may involve the skin primarily or secondarily. Although lymphomas of B-cell or T-cell origin may involve the skin, it is more common for them to be of T-cell origin. Involvement of skin by lymphomas other than CTCL (*e.g.*, mycosis fungoides or Sézary's syndrome) makes the lymphoma stage IV, but the prognosis of the underlying lymphoma is not dramatically affected by cutaneous spread. Skin disease may be indolent regardless of histologic grade if it is the only site of involvement or may be a component of rapidly progressing systemic disease.

OTHER CLINICAL PRESENTATIONS

Seven percent of testicular masses in older men are lymphomas, usually of the diffuse aggressive variety. They often are associated with CNS and Waldeyer's ring involvement.[306] Lymphomas also present as solitary thyroid nodules, usually in women and in association with Hashimoto's thyroiditis. Primary CNS lymphomas presenting as single or multiple mass lesions, usually of intermediate or high grade, are being reported with increasing frequency, particularly in association with AIDS or iatrogenic immunosuppression. More commonly, CNS lymphoma is composed of leptomeningeal disease and occurs in association with bone or bone marrow involvement with intermediate- or high-grade lymphomas, usually in the setting of rapidly progressive disease.[307] CNS involvement commonly presents with symptoms of headache or cranial nerve abnormalities.

Lymphomas should also be included in the differential diagnosis of superior vena cava syndrome, acute spinal cord compression, isolated tumor nodules of the skin, bone tumors, orbital tumors, salivary gland enlargement, sinus problems, and unexplained cytopenias. Some of these manifestations occur with considerable frequency in patients with widespread advancing tumor but are uncommon as initial presentations of the disease.

NATURAL HISTORY AND STAGING OF THE LYMPHOCYTIC LYMPHOMAS

NATURAL HISTORY

With the advent of modern treatment, patients with lymphoma are rarely left untreated, and the natural history is interrupted, often successfully, by treatment. However, there are studies in which patients were followed without treatment or after palliative treatment.[308] What is immediately apparent from these studies is that the natural history of the lymphocytic lymphomas is quite different from that of Hodgkin's disease, but there is a problem in comparing Hodgkin's disease with the lymphocytic lymphomas. Although the behavior of Hodgkin's disease is less affected by the histologic subtype, the lymphocytic lymphomas are a collection of several different diseases with various presentations and natural histories, categorized as low-, intermediate-, and high-grade neoplasms in the Working Formulation. However, certain generalizations are probably appropriate. In contrast to patients with Hodgkin's disease, those with lymphocytic lymphomas most frequently present with advanced disease, commonly with liver or bone marrow involvement. Unlike Hodgkin's disease, in which 50% to 60% of patients have localized disease, only 10% to 15% of lymphocytic lymphoma patients appear to have stage I or II disease.[309–311] Other differences from Hodgkin's disease are also seen. Fewer patients have systemic symptoms, and localized extralymphatic involvement is more common and often occurs as an isolated site of involvement (stage IE) or with adjacent nodes (stage IIE). There is no difference in prognosis for patients with stage I or II localized nodal lymphocytic lymphomas compared with those with extranodal involvement.[312,313]

The clinical features of both diseases are compared in Table 52–9. Lymphocytic lymphomas are probably unifocal in origin, but they remain localized so briefly that widespread disease is the rule at the time of diagnosis rather than the exception. This is particularly true of the low-grade lymphomas. Now that it is accepted that most of the common types of the adult lymphomas originate from a monoclonal population of B cells and the anatomic compartmentalization of these cells in lymph nodes is understood more clearly, certain generalizations can be made about the histologic type of disease to the clinical course of patients with lymphomas.

The most common histologic subgroups are the follicular lymphomas. Patients in this group make up almost half of all cases in most series. The propensity for follicular lymphomas to be associated with widespread disease coincides with the normal tendency of the small untransformed follicular center B cell to migrate in the circulation. These cells have a very small growth fraction, and despite wide dissemination, the follicular small cleaved cell variety of lymphoma is usually clinically indolent. An undetermined fraction of the patients can be left untreated, and approximately 25% evidence waxing and waning adenopathy for months to years before unsightly or painful lymph node enlargement or compression of a vital organ requires treatment.[314] In a few low-grade lymphomas, spontaneous regression can occur and last for many years.[178] Involvement of the bone marrow and liver does not impart the same adverse prognosis as involvement of these organs by Hodgkin's disease or higher-grade lymphocytic lymphomas.

Although intermediate-grade or aggressive lymphomas are most often of B-cell origin, they have a vastly different natural history than nodular lymphomas.[315] In keeping with the lack of motility of transformed follicular B cells, the diffuse large cell lymphomas more often appear to be clinically localized, although the recurrence rate after local treatment indicates otherwise. Unlike patients with follicular small cleaved cell lymphoma, after tumor is identified in organs such as the bone marrow, liver, and bone, patients with diffuse large cell lymphomas have aggressive, rapidly fatal illnesses unless treated successfully.

There is evidence for a link between follicular small cleaved cell lymphomas and the diffuse large cell lymphomas of B-cell origin. The NCI analyzed a series of 515 patients with lymphocytic lymphomas for their frequency of histologic evolution.[182,315] Among patients with follicular lymphoma who had a repeat biopsy more than 3 months after the initial diagnostic biopsy, histologic progression was found in 41%. At Stanford, the actuarial risk of histologic conversion is about 50% at 8 years.[316] An autopsy study of patients at the NCI who initially were diagnosed as having follicular lymphomas revealed that fewer than 10% had evidence of exclusively follicular disease at autopsy. Survival after conversion is short unless complete remission is achieved with chemotherapy. These data indicate that a substantial number of patients have follicular lymphomas that evolve to a diffuse variety as part of the natural history of their disease.

A likely evolution of the lymphoma can be constructed as follows. The follicle-associated cells of B-cell lymphomas (see Fig. 52–1), which initially retain the characteristic of forming follicles, are close to normal tissue in their growth characteristics and migrate easily while minimally differentiated. This accounts for the ease of detectability of these cells in other organs and in the peripheral blood and for the indolent natural history. Their growth rate and invasive potential, for unknown reasons, remain low, and in time, those that are not clonogenic probably die. In time, the malignant clonogenic B cells take on the morphologic characteristics of transformed lymphocytes and presumably acquire additional genetic alterations related to the more rapid proliferation. This transformation may occur slowly over several years or so rapidly that the evolution antedates diagnosis. These transformed cells are less motile, which accounts for the difficulty in detecting them outside the site of origin with normal staging procedures, but they are more invasive, have a higher growth fraction, and are rapidly fatal if growth is unchecked. It also seems likely that the follicular small cleaved cell lymphoma subtype evolves to follicular mixed and follicular large cell lymphomas as the percentage of large cells increases until effacement of the lymph node occurs, and a pathologic picture of diffuse large cell lymphoma is observed. As with the evolution of the histologic effacement of a lymph node in Hodgkin's disease, the reasons for the varying rate of transformation from nodule-forming indolent lymphocytes to large transformed cells are unknown. However, increased cytogenetic abnormalities have been observed with histologic progression.[66,317] Lymphomas of diffuse small lymphocytic cells disseminate widely at an early stage but have an indolent course, in keeping with their benign histologic appearance. They evolve to large cell B neoplasms with much less frequency and usually kill patients by causing bone marrow failure, with hypogammaglobulinemia leading to fatal infections.

STAGING

Classification Systems

The standard staging system for the lymphocytic lymphomas is the same as that proposed for Hodgkin's disease at the Ann Arbor Conference in 1971 (Table 52–10).[318] This system reflects the number of sites of involvement and their relation to the diaphragm, the existence of B symptoms, and the presence of extranodal disease. Patients can be assigned a clinical stage and a pathologic stage. The clinical stage is based on initial tissue biopsy studies, physical examination, bone marrow biopsy, and radiographic evaluation. The pathologic stage includes information obtained by means of invasive procedures such as additional extranodal tissue biopsies, laparoscopy-directed biopsies or, rarely, staging laparotomy, and splenectomy. Some of these factors are relevant to the low-grade lymphomas, but their major relevance is in the intermediate-grade lymphomas. These clinical prognostic factors are much more important in determining treatment outcome than Ann Arbor stage.

Although the Ann Arbor staging scheme is extremely useful in defining patient composition for clinical trials, it is not as prognostically important for the lymphocytic lymphomas as it is for Hodgkin's disease. For the low-grade lymphomas, it is important to identify patients with stage I or II disease, because radiation therapy may be curative. Careful staging is required to identify the 10% to 15% of patients with limited-stage disease. Formerly, it was thought to be unimportant to differentiate stage III from stage IV disease in the remaining 85%, but recent treatment advances may make this a relevant distinction.

The Ann Arbor staging classification is inadequate for the diffuse intermediate- and high-grade lymphomas. Localized disease is rare (<20% of all patients) for these lymphomas. To say that a patient has a stage II diffuse large cell lymphoma conveys little useful prognostic information. The patient may have small cervical and axillary lymph nodes and an excellent probability of successful treatment outcome or may have a bulky abdominal disease refractory to treatment. The actual stage of a patient without localized disease (*i.e.,* stage II intermediate or high grade; stage III or IV of any histologic subtype) is probably less important than the presence or absence of several other clinical prognostic factors.[319–327] These factors include performance status, systemic symptoms, tumor burden (*i.e.,* an abdominal mass more than 10 cm in diameter or three or more extranodal sites of disease), bone marrow involvement, and serum LDH and β_2-microglobulin levels. Some series have suggested that age over 55 years is a poor prognostic factor, and others include the speed of response to therapy as a prognostic factor, but these are not universally used in patients with aggressive histology lymphoma.[321,328]

A modification of the Ann Arbor Classification was proposed at the Cotswolds Meeting.[329] One reason for modifying the original scheme was to recognize the prognostic significance of tumor burden. The changes do not make the classification any more relevant to the lymphocytic lymphomas, but the goal of incorporating well-described prognostic factors in the staging classification also makes sense for the lymphocytic lymphomas. For intermediate-grade lymphomas, a three-stage system seems most appropriate. Stage I is the same as Ann Arbor stage I; stage II is the involvement of two of more lymph node regions or localized extralymphatic organ or site (IIE) with none of the poor prognostic factors (*e.g.,* poor performance status, B symptoms, mass more than 10 cm, three or more extranodal sites, marrow involvement, LDH >500); and stage III is stage II with one or more of the poor prognostic factors (Table 52–11).

The lymphocytic lymphomas are a diverse group of lymphoid neoplasms with varied natural histories and patterns of clinical presentation, and it is not possible to recommend a uniform approach to disease staging that can be applied to all patients. Staging issues depend on the individual patient, the histologic subtype of lymphoma, and its likely distribution (Table 52–12). Recommendations for staging procedures modified from those made at the Ann Arbor symposium are shown in Tables 52–13 and 52–14.[330,331]

Clinical Staging

The date the lymph node enlargement was first observed and the rate of subsequent tumor growth should be documented. This information may influence the choice of therapy and, in patients with low-grade lymphomas, influence the decision to institute treatment at all. The history should determine the

TABLE 52–10. Ann Arbor Staging Classification for Hodgkin's Disease

Stage	*Characteristics*
I	Involvement of a single lymph node region (I) or a single extralymphatic organ or site (IE)
II	Involvement of two or more lymph node regions on the same side of the diaphragm (II) or localized involvement of an extralymphatic organ or site (IIE)
III	Involvement of lymph node regions on both sides of the diaphragm (III) or localized involvement of an extralymphatic organ or site (IIIE) or spleen (IIIS) or both (IIISE)
IV	Diffuse or disseminated involvement of one or more extralymphatic organs with or without associated lymph node involvement. The organ(s) involved should be identified by a symbol: A, asymptomatic; B, fever, sweats, weight loss > 10% of body weight.

TABLE 52–11. National Cancer Institute Modified Staging for Intermediate- and High-Grade Lymphomas

Stage	*Characteristics*
I	Localized nodal or extranodal disease (Ann Arbor stage I or IE)
II	Two or more nodal sites of disease or a localized extranodal site plus draining nodes with none of the following: performance status ≤ 70, B symptoms, any mass > 10 cm in diameter (particularly gastrointestinal), serum lactate dehydrogenase > 500, three or more extranodal sites of disease
III	Stage II plus any poor prognostic features

TABLE 52–12. Histologic and Pathologic Stages of Lymphocytic Lymphomas

Grade	*Stage I (%)*	*Stage II (%)*	*Stage III and IV (%)*	*Common Extranodal Sites**
High grade				
Small noncleaved cell	13	21	66	Gastrointesinal tract, lung/pleura, marrow (14%)
Lymphoblastic	7	20	75	Liver, spleen, lung/pleura, skin, marrow (50%)
Large cell, immunoblastic	23	29	48	Liver, spleen, Waldeyer's ring or GI tract, marrow (12%)
Intermediate grade				
Large cell, diffuse	16	30	54	Liver, spleen, Waldeyer's ring or GI tract, lung/pleura, marrow (10%)
Mixed cell, diffuse	19	26	55	Liver, spleen, Waldeyer's ring or GI tract, bone marrow (14%)
Small cleaved cell, diffuse	9	19	72	Liver, spleen, Waldeyer's ring or GI tract, skin, marrow (32%)
Large cell, follicular	15	12	73	Liver, spleen, Waldeyer's ring or GI tract, marrow (34%)
Low grade				
Mixed cell, follicular	15	12	74	Liver, spleen, marrow (30%)
Small cleaved cell, follicular	8	10	82	Liver, spleen, marrow (51%)
Small lymphocytic	3	8	89	Liver, spleen, marrow (71%)

*Percentages indicate incidence of each stage at presentation.

presence or absence of systemic B symptoms and the presence of symptoms that suggest extralymphatic involvement (*e.g.*, bone pain, gastrointestinal complaints). Particular attention should be given to recording the site and size of all abnormal lymph nodes, including the epitrochlear, femoral, and popliteal sites that are not usually involved in Hodgkin's disease. The presence or absence of hepatosplenomegaly needs to be determined, because unlike Hodgkin's disease, enlargement of these organs in patients with lymphocytic lymphoma correlates with tumor involvement. Preauricular nodal enlargement is often associated with disease in the Waldeyer's ring area, making indirect laryngoscopy an absolute requirement of the staging workup in these patients. Waldeyer's ring involvement is often associated with involvement of the intestine, and gastrointestinal contrast studies are indicated if the patient appears to have localized disease. Primary lesions in extranodal sites such as bone or skin are frequently associated with involvement of regional nodes. Many patients with skin lesions that occur as primary or secondary lesions have multiple cutaneous lesions that may be remote from one another. A careful inspection of the skin and a biopsy of suspicious lesions are necessary, especially in patients with diffuse lymphomas.

The correlation between peripheral blood counts and bone

TABLE 52–13. Required Evaluation Procedures for Staging Lymphocytic Lymphomas

1. Adequate surgical biopsy, reviewed by an experienced hematopathologist
2. Detailed history recording duration and the presence or absence of fever, unexplained sweating and its severity, unexplained pruritus, and unexplained weight loss
3. Detailed physical examination; special attention to all node-bearing areas, including Waldeyer's ring (indirect laryngoscopy is the procedure of choice) and determination of size of liver and spleen
4. Necessary laboratory procedures
   a. Complete blood count, including an erythrocytic sedimentation rate
   b. Serum alkaline phosphatase
   c. Evaluation of renal function
   d. Evaluation of liver function
   e. Serum lactate dehydrogenase and β_2-microglobulin levels
5. Radiologic studies include
   a. Chest roentgenogram (posteroanterior and lateral)
   b. Bilateral lower extremity lymphogram
   c. Abdominal-pelvic computed tomography scan
6. Bilateral bone marrow needle biopsies (not just aspirates; biopsy should be performed before aspirate, if both are done together)

TABLE 52–14. Procedures Required Under Certain Circumstances for Staging Lymphocytic Lymphomas

1. Computed tomography (CT) scans of the thorax if any abnormality is found or suspected on the routine chest roentgenogram
2. Abdominal ultrasonogram, inferior cavography, intravenous pyelogram or upper and lower gastrointestinal contrast studies to supplement lymphographic findings or investigate sites of unexplained symptoms
3. Plain bone radiographs of symptomatic or tender areas
4. Head or spinal CT for neurologic signs or symptoms
5. Exploratory laparotomy and splenectomy, if management decision depends on identification of abdominal involvement (decision to proceed with laparotomy requires knowledge of treatment plan used at the institution of record)
6. Magnetic resonance imaging to detect bone marrow involvement
7. Gallium whole-body scans
8. Skeletal scintigrams
9. Useful ancillary procedures not required for staging
   a. Hepatic and spleen scintigrams
   b. Serum chemistries including serum calcium and uric acid for overall management of patient
   c. Assessment of the patient's delayed hypersensitivity response to recall antigens

marrow involvement with lymphoma is poor. Abnormal blood counts are found in only 37% of patients with bone marrow infiltration by lymphoma and approximately one half of patients with abnormal blood counts have uninvolved bone marrows. Examination of the peripheral smear in patients with lymphoma may yield evidence of malignant cells in approximately 10% of patients; these patients usually have low-grade, small lymphocytic or follicular center cell lymphomas. However, small numbers of occult circulating monoclonal B cells can be identified by immunologic analysis of the ratio of expression of κ or λ light chains on peripheral blood lymphocytes by flow cytometry; significant deviations from the normal 2:1 κ:λ ratio suggest the presence of an abnormal cell (*i.e.*, clonal excess).[332] Southern hybridization looking for rearranged immunoglobulin genes or PCR analysis may also detect lymphoma cells.[333] Southern analysis has been reported to detect as few as 1 in 100 malignant cells, an improvement of approximately 10-fold over methods using clonal excess.[333] Despite this theoretical advantage, no diagnostic gain was identified when comparing the two methods for detection of occult lymphoma in the peripheral blood.[334]

Lymphoma cells can be detected in the peripheral blood of many patients in whom morphologic analysis of a peripheral blood smear is negative. The incidence of peripheral blood involvement at diagnosis is influenced by histologic subtype and stage. Horning and coworkers documented gene rearrangements in 34% of patients with low-grade lymphomas (80% in the small lymphocytic subtype) and 8% in patients with intermediate-grade lymphoma at diagnosis.[333] Occult lymphoma was identified in 12% of patients with stage I or II disease and in 35% of patients with stage IV disease (45% if the bone marrow was involved). The incidence of occult lymphoma reached almost 50% in patients with recurrent disease. PCR analysis is even more sensitive, capable of detecting 1 in 10^5 to 10^6 cells.[148]

Although more sensitive techniques can detect occult disease more frequently, there are insufficient data to enable us to base therapeutic decisions on the presence of malignant cells in the peripheral blood. Although 10% to 15% of patients with stage I or II disease have circulating lymphoma cells, it is not clear that local radiotherapy should be withheld solely on that basis. Nor does the presence of these cells necessarily portend clinical relapse. Among 63 patients with low-grade lymphoma in clinical remission, only 6 had rearrangements in one study. Nineteen patients relapsed, but only 1 relapsed patient had a gene rearrangement in the peripheral blood before relapse. The other patients with circulating abnormalities had been followed a median of 2 years without relapsing.

Serum chemistries are important because the creatinine may indicate renal insufficiency, suggesting obstruction from retroperitoneal tumor; the uric acid and lactate dehydrogenase (LDH) can be indirect indicators of tumor burden and can be of prognostic value and enable the physician to assess the need for hydration before treatment. Tumor lysis syndrome is an avoidable complication of treatment that is most commonly observed in the treatment of high-grade lymphomas or aggressive lymphomas that are growing rapidly. Liver enzymes, bilirubin, and alkaline phosphatase elevations can occasionally be a sign of liver or bone involvement. Serum β_2-microglobulin may be a good predictor of complete response and time to treatment failure in patients with low-grade lymphomas.[325]

Chest roentgenograms yield positive information in about one fourth of patients. The most frequent abnormality is hilar or mediastinal adenopathy (18% of patients), followed by pleural effusions (8%) and parenchymal involvement (4%). Parenchymal lesions and pleural effusions usually require pathologic verification. A chylous or transudative effusion that lacks malignant cells does not change the pathologic stage of the patient. As in Hodgkin's disease, pulmonary parenchymal lesions are usually associated with concurrent hilar or bulky mediastinal lymph node involvement. If only one hemithorax is involved, the parenchymal lesions can be considered an extension from the lymph nodes and do not necessarily change the patient's stage, except for the E designation.

The use of chest computed tomography (CT) scans is not well defined. In patients with stage III and IV disease, routine CT scans are not performed because systemic treatment is already indicated. If the chest x-ray film is definitely abnormal, CT can confirm this and often identify additional sites of involvement. These sites are usually in the chest and rarely change the stage of disease. If radiation therapy is contemplated, CT of the chest is indicated for optimal design of the treatment portals. CT is also useful for monitoring the response to treatment of mediastinal, pericardial, and hilar disease, which may be difficult to follow on routine chest x-ray films. In a patient with a normal radiograph, a CT scan is not required for routine staging purposes.[335]

As in Hodgkin's disease, an accurate noninvasive evaluation of the abdomen remains a problem. Bipedal lymphangiography had been the standard procedure for this task. In experienced hands, lymphangiography has an overall accuracy of 90% for the evaluation of the paraaortic and iliac lymph node regions.[336,337] However, because of the differing natural histories, it is not as reliable in patients with lymphocytic lymphomas as it is in patients with Hodgkin's disease. A negative lymphangiogram in 147 patients with Hodgkin's disease was associated with only one false-negative study for paraaortic or iliac lymph nodes. Bone marrow and liver involvement were found in only 1% and 3% respectively, and no cases of mesenteric adenopathy were found. There was involvement of the spleen or splenic hilar nodes in 24% and 19% of patients, respectively. In lymphocytic lymphomas, there is a much higher incidence of involvement of upper abdominal nodes (particularly mesenteric nodes), even if the lymphangiogram is negative. In the follicular subtypes, approximately 50% of patients have disease in the upper abdomen even in the presence of a negative lymphangiogram. For diffuse intermediate-grade lymphomas, a negative lymphangiogram is a more reliable indicator of the absence of subdiaphragmatic disease, because 10% or fewer of these patients have abdominal disease.

Even though it provides a better architectural assessment of the paraaortic and pelvic nodes than the CT scan, the lymphangiogram is complemented by the CT scan's ability to visualize other abdominal structures.[337,338] Because it provides such an accurate assessment of lymphomatous involvement of the abdominal and pelvic lymph nodes and is so useful in routine follow-up, the lymphangiogram remains a valuable study. The lymphangiogram is an accurate predictor of the likelihood of finding intraabdominal lymphoma in extranodal sites or in splenic, portal, or mesenteric sites. As many as 80% of patients with positive lymphangiograms have disease in the liver or lymph nodes outside the paraaortic region at laparotomy, and 18% to 50% of patients with negative lymphangiograms have similar findings.

The standard test for diagnosing mesenteric, porta hepatic, and splenic hilar nodal involvement is the abdominopelvic CT scan.[339] This test is particularly useful for patients with follicular lymphomas in whom mesenteric nodal involvement is common. The abdominopelvic CT scan can also identify retrocrural nodal involvement, and it is more accurate than the lymphangiogram in determining the size of nodal disease. Involvement of the kidney, bone, and bulky splenic and liver disease, frequently present in patients with aggressive large cell lymphomas, can also be seen on CT scanning but not on bipedal lymphangiography.[338,340,341] CT scanning appears to document disease below the diaphragm in approximately 10% of patients with a negative lymphangiogram.[331] Lymphangiography has a similar incidence of abnormal findings in patients with negative abdominopelvic CT scans.[341] The two studies appear to be complementary in defining the extent of abdominal disease. A reasonable course of action is to perform the CT scan initially and perform a lymphangiogram if this study is entirely negative. However, a lymphangiogram should be performed on most patients. The dye is retained for many months and is useful in following response to therapy with just a flat plate of the abdomen.

The role of magnetic resonance imaging (MRI) in the identification of lymphomatous involvement of abdominal nodes, kidney, liver, and spleen still must be determined. It does appear to be valuable for the detection of bone marrow involvement in patients with lymphoma. When marrow involvement is suspected, even when random marrow biopsies have been negative, the MRI can be used to identify focal areas of involvement which can then be confirmed by biopsy.[342,343]

Gallium 67 (^{67}Ga) scanning is not performed routinely in all patients at most centers. It is of limited use for diagnostic purposes because of its low sensitivity, 18% in one study.[344] In this study, only 1 of 122 patients had their disease upstaged. Although the reliability of ^{67}Ga imaging has been improved by increasing the dose to between 8 and 11 mCi, using spot imaging, double or triple peak angle cameras, single photon emission computed tomography (SPECT), and delayed view of the abdomen, its utility for the diagnosis or staging of lymphocytic lymphomas has not been extensively assessed.[345] ^{67}Ga is more frequently taken up by tumors of intermediate or high grade.[345–347] The sensitivity of ^{67}Ga imaging is affected by tumor location. Lesions within or near the spleen and liver frequently are missed because of the normal uptake by the liver. The normal uptake exhibited by the cecum and sigmoid colon can mask involved sites particularly the iliac region. ^{67}Ga scanning is well suited for the evaluation of the mediastinum and most useful in the evaluation of patients with residual radiographic abnormalities, particularly in the mediastinum or abdomen.[345,347] Because ^{67}Ga is taken up in cells by the transferrin receptor, a potential surrogate measure of cellular proliferation, the conversion of a group of nodes from low to high ^{67}Ga intensity may herald progression to more aggressive histology. ^{67}Ga scanning may be a useful radiographic marker to measure response to chemotherapy and to identify early relapse.[347–349] We do not recommend ^{67}Ga scanning routinely in the initial staging workup or during treatment. Baseline ^{67}Ga scanning should be considered in the initial workup of patients with intermediate-grade lymphomas and bulky disease, for whom evaluation of response might be anticipated to be complicated by a residual mass after chemotherapy. Patients whose tumor mass remains ^{67}Ga positive after combination chemotherapy have an extremely poor prognosis with additional conventional treatment, and they should be considered for high-dose chemotherapy and rescue with autologous bone marrow transplantation (ABMT).[348]

Bone lesions are found in 5% to 15% of all patients at presentation and are more common in patients with diffuse large cell lymphomas. Bone scans have a sensitivity and specificity greater than 95% and have replaced routine roentgenographic studies in detecting occult bone lesions.[350] Routine bone scanning for all patients is not recommended, because it is rare that a change in stage or treatment is required based on its results alone. However, if there is bone pain, a bone scan is recommended. A positive bone scan should be confirmed by plain films and the area biopsied if needed for determination of treatment.

Approximately 50% of patients with lymphocytic lymphoma have bone marrow or hepatic involvement on presentation.[351] The incidence of bone marrow metastasis is highest in patients with the small cell lymphocytic lymphomas, follicular or diffuse (40–100%, depending on the type) and lowest in those with diffuse large cell lymphoma (5–15%). Each subtype of disease tends to have an identifiable pattern of bone marrow involvement.[351] The follicular lymphomas are characterized by a paratrabecular location of involvement, but T-cell lymphomas infiltrate the marrow space. Bone marrow involvement in patients with diffuse, aggressive lymphomas is usually widespread and may be associated with focal or diffuse myelofibrosis. Although bone marrow involvement is less frequent in diffuse large cell lymphoma, its detection is important because of its strong correlation with subsequent spread of disease to the CNS. As many as 35% of patients with large cell lymphomas and positive bone marrow biopsies develop CNS spread.[352] Some of these patients have solitary relapses in the CNS, but most have widespread advanced disease. Cytologic examination of the spinal fluid should be performed in all patients with diffuse types of lymphoma with bone marrow involvement, because therapy of the CNS is indicated if positive.[353]

As with Hodgkin's disease, aspiration of the bone marrow is inadequate for staging purposes. Marrow aspirates are insensitive and detect disease in less than 30% of all biopsy-positive marrows. In view of the clinical importance of bone marrow evaluation and the focal nature of metastases, more than one biopsy should be obtained for evaluation. For patients having two biopsies, as many as 30% have positive findings in a single biopsy.[309] Assuming an even chance of obtaining the positive biopsy on the first attempt, a second biopsy should increase the number of positives by up to 15%. Overall, bilateral bone marrow biopsies can be expected to advance the stage in approximately 25% of patients to stage IV, because some of those with marrow disease were previously classified as stage IV on the basis of other extranodal sites. The shift to stage IV predominantly occurs in patients with stage III disease and in those with follicular and small cell lymphocytic lymphomas.

Lymphomatous involvement of the bone marrow can be detected by morphologic assessment alone if there is 5% or greater infiltration by malignant cells. Newer techniques, such as flow cytometric analysis, clonal excess, and Southern blot analysis, have improved the detection level to 1%.[334] The PCR technique for the t(14;18) translocation is capable of reproducibly detecting one tumor cell with a *BCL2* rearrangement in 10^5 to 10^6 normal cells.[148] Studies of limited numbers of patients have shown that morphologically normal peripheral blood and bone marrow may show infiltration with lymphoma when assessed by PCR.[148,149,354]

The utility of PCR for staging the bone marrow has been examined in 152 patients with advanced-stage lymphocytic lymphomas referred to a tertiary care center for bone marrow transplantation.[79] In this skewed population, PCR appeared to add little to morphologic analysis when both tests were performed before therapy. Among 88 patients with low-grade lymphoma, nine marrows that were positive by morphologic assessment were negative by PCR. All nine marrows and lymph node samples obtained from the same patients lacked PCR-amplifiable breakpoints. Therefore, PCR cannot be used alone because 15% of low-grade lymphomas lack the t(14;18) translocation and understaging would result. However, PCR did detect disease in some patients whose marrows were read as negative for lymphoma. Therefore, PCR would upstage 10% of patients from stage III to stage IV disease.

Unless upstaging affects therapy, there is little reason to go to the added expense of PCR analysis. What effect PCR will have on the staging of patients with stage I and II disease is unknown. Between 10% and 15% of these patients contain cells in their peripheral blood with immunoglobulin gene rearrangements detected by Southern analysis, and it is likely that a higher incidence would be found if PCR was used to test the peripheral blood or bone marrow of these patients.[333] Whether detection of the malignant cells in the peripheral blood or bone marrow by PCR should change our approach to these patients requires further study.

One study indicated that PCR analysis can detect *BCL2* rearrangements in hyperplastic lymph tissues from nontumor-bearing persons.[81] The meaning of this is unclear, but if "nonmalignant" cells undergo rearrangement of *BCL2,* the PCR amplification of *BCL2* sequences would have little value as a diagnostic or staging tool. However, it does not appear that *BCL2* rearrangements in "nonmalignant" cells explain the findings discussed previously. Normal bone marrow and bone marrow from more than 200 specimens from patients with non-*BCL2*-containing tumors, were always negative for *BCL2,* and in each case for which bone marrow and lymph node samples were available, PCR detected the same breakpoint in both.

These data suggest that PCR may be a valuable tool in detecting minimal residual disease after chemotherapy. When multiple marrow aspirates and biopsies obtained at the bone marrow harvest are examined for minimal residual disease by morphology and PCR, patients with overt or minimal histologic involvement were all positive by PCR. Patients with no involvement morphologically were also all positive by PCR. However, involvement of the bone marrow by lymphoma can be patchy. Although all bone marrows were positive by PCR, unless overt involvement was present, not all marrow samples obtained from the same patient at different sites were positive. Only 50% to 60% of the individual samples were positive. Bone marrow biopsies and aspirates were equally effective in permitting PCR analysis. This sampling problem must be addressed before this technique can be used widely. A positive finding from a good lab may well be an important finding, but there is a real question about how many negative findings are needed to be confident of the absence of disease.

Hepatic involvement with lymphocytic lymphoma has been identified in 11% to 42% of patients.[302,355–359] The frequency of identification of liver involvement increases as the size (*i.e.,* from percutaneous biopsies to peritoneoscopy-directed biopsies to staging laparotomies) and number of biopsy specimens increases. Regardless of the biopsy technique, patients with diffuse large cell lymphoma have a much lower incidence of liver metastases than patients with lymphoma in the other major histologic categories of disease. The need for liver biopsy should be determined by the likelihood that the findings will affect treatment. Most patients upstaged after peritoneoscopy-directed liver biopsies were from stage III to stage IV. Because liver involvement is rarely seen in a patient with a negative lymphangiogram, it does not seem sensible to biopsy the liver under these circumstances. Because of the use of effective combination chemotherapy for most stages of aggressive large cell lymphomas and because of the lack of consistent evidence that other subtypes of intermediate- and low-grade lymphomas are adversely affected by minimal initial treatment, the use of percutaneous liver biopsies should be limited to special circumstances.

Staging laparotomy and splenectomy were routinely performed in patients with lymphocytic lymphoma in several centers in the late 1960s and early 1970s. They provided considerable information on the patterns and distribution of disease and uniform staging for early clinical trials. However, staging laparotomy is no longer performed routinely in patients with lymphocytic lymphomas. The current treatment strategies have reduced the number of clinical situations in which a staging laparotomy is required.[302,309,355–359]

For intermediate-grade lymphomas, which often involve the gastrointestinal tract, laparotomies may be performed for diagnostic purposes, and if feasible, complete resection with appropriate staging can be performed. Primary gastric lymphomas are not resected if the extent of tumor requires a total gastrectomy because the morbidity of the procedure is high. However, masses involving other gastrointestinal sites may have improved outcome after resection. Laparotomy upstages a small but significant percentage of patients with low-grade lymphomas. Most upgrades are from stage III to stage IV disease because of occult disease in the liver. Because an advance from stage III to stage IV has minimal impact on therapy, invasive procedures to document hepatic disease are not routinely warranted for patients with stage III disease. Even in patients with stage I or II disease, laparotomy is not performed. Patients with lymphocytic lymphomas tend to be older than those with Hodgkin's disease, and they experience more operative complications. Patients with early-stage low-grade disease are treated with radiation therapy with the full understanding that one third or more have occult disease in the abdomen. Although surgical mortality is approximately 0.5%, significant morbidity, primarily pneumonia, pulmonary embolism, pancreatitis, subdiaphragmatic abscesses, or gastrointestinal bleeding, has been reported in 11% to 40% of patients in three larger series.[302]

The primary factor that accounts for the limited need for laparotomy in lymphocytic lymphoma is the high yield of less morbid procedures and the recognition that precise definition of involvement probably has limited importance in treatment planning for most patients. Laparotomy has been used as a diagnostic tool in patients with residual abdominal masses after treatment. One study showed that CT scans, lymphograms, and gallium scans overpredict for residual disease, and more patients are actually in complete remission than appears to be the case after routine restaging.[360] An NCI study of reexploration of residual abdominal masses that had been stable for at least two cycles of chemotherapy demonstrated that the procedure was not necessary because the abdomens of 21 of the 22 patients did not contain residual lymphoma.[361]

IMMUNOLOGIC ABNORMALITIES IN PATIENTS WITH LYMPHOMA

Clinically apparent immunologic abnormalities, especially of T cells, may precede the development of malignant lymphomas, but for most lymphoma patients the usual measures of immunity are normal. Because the early studies of delayed hypersensitivity in lymphoma patients did not reveal distinct abnormalities in patients with lymphocytic lymphomas, there have been fewer studies in these patients and data are surprisingly scarce. Interpretation of results of available studies needs to be qualified as well because investigators have not allowed for differences among the various histologic subtypes and stages of lymphocytic lymphoma.

The most common immunologic abnormality found in patients with lymphoma is a monoclonal immunoglobulin peak in the serum. A clinically significant monoclonal gammopathy occurs in 6% to 8% of patients with diffuse lymphomas but in 1% or fewer of the patients with follicular lymphomas.[362] These incidence figures reflect the origin of the diffuse lymphomas from the immunoglobulin-producing cells of the medullary cords (see Fig. 52–1). This region is thought to be the site of origin of the cells of Waldenström's macroglobulinemia, chronic lymphocytic leukemia, and the diffuse small lymphocytic lymphomas. With increasingly sophisticated detection methods, it appears that most patients with B-cell lymphoma have microgram or milligram quantities of monoclonal immunoglobulin (M-component) in the serum that is identical in isotype and idiotype to that borne by the malignant cells.[363] However, most patients with an M-component in their serum do not have a lymphoma. Among 1246 patients identified in a screening process to have serum M-components, only 67 (0.05%) had lymphomas.[364] Thirty-three had an elevated level of IgM, 20 had elevated IgG levels, 5 had elevated IgA levels, and 1 had a Bence Jones protein spike. Most patients had diffuse lymphomas. Nine patients had Hodgkin's disease. An associated decrease in the normal serum globulin levels was found in one third of the patients. Seven patients had cryoglobulinemia, and 6 patients had cold agglutinins. The malignant B cells of lymphoma patients do not serve any normal or abnormal immunologic functions, and the paraprotein is not present in sufficient quantity to affect antibody responses to neoantigens. Rare lymphomas may produce factors with biologic activity. For example, there have been reports of patients with lymphoma and leukopenia whose tumor cells produced an inhibitor of myelopoiesis.[365]

Other immune disorders found in patients with lymphoma include Coombs'-positive autoimmune hemolytic anemia (AIHA) in 1% to 2% of patients and idiopathic thrombocytopenia purpura in fewer than 1.0%.[366] AIHA was associated with splenomegaly, systemic symptoms, and 8 of 9 patients with diffuse lymphomas had widely disseminated disease. No patient in this series died of the autoimmune disorder, which could usually be controlled with the drugs used to treat the underlying lymphoma.

Although patients with systemic symptoms or malnutrition may have generalized immunosuppression, there is no consensus that a particular abnormality can be related to the lymphoma.[367] Jones and colleagues demonstrated pretreatment abnormalities in 38 patients with diffuse large cell lymphoma.[368] These abnormalities, which included low IgA levels, poor skin test reactivity, and low lymphocyte counts, were more common in patients who had advanced-stage disease or B symptoms. Patients with follicular lymphoma had only skin test abnormalities, and the defects were more selective (*e.g.*, only 2 of 6 antigens failed to elicit a response). Similar findings were reported by Advani and associates.[369] Because skin tests are an in vivo measure of CD4-positive helper T-cell function, it appears that lymphoma is associated with some compromise of helper T cells. Other investigators have demonstrated mildly defective in vitro function of helper T cells from patients with lymphoma, but increases of in vitro function of peripheral blood T cells from lymphoma patients have also been reported.[370–372] All of this work is highly phenomenologic. Variations in outcome between assay systems do not allow definitive conclusions, but for most patients with lymphoma, immune defects do not seem to be an important cause of the disease. Nevertheless, rare patients do manifest significant immune abnormalities that appear to be a consequence of the disease rather than a cause of it. Certain T-cell malignancies, most notably some patients with CTCL, continue to provide immune functions such as helper activity or suppressor activity.[373,374] Patients with HTLV-I-related ATL have functional helper T-cell deficits that are comparable to those seen in HIV infection and are associated with a significant risk of opportunistic infections from a variety of pathogens, including *Pneumocystis carinii*.[375]

TREATMENT OF LYMPHOCYTIC LYMPHOMAS

The treatment approach to a particular patient with a lymphocytic lymphoma is determined by the tumor histology, the stage of disease, and the physiologic status of the patient.

The influence of tumor histology on the natural history of the lymphocytic lymphomas was described earlier. Years of clinical trials have established that the histologic diagnosis is perhaps the best single predictor of the outcome of the disease. The Working Formulation divides the lymphocytic lymphomas into histologic grades: low, intermediate, and high. The classification employed at the NCI also divides the lymphocytic lymphomas into three groups, but it has additions and minor alterations to the Working Formulation (see Table 52–8). The changes in the Working Formulation include addition of diffuse intermediately differentiated (or mantle zone) lymphoma, diffuse small cleaved cell lymphomas, and CTCL to the low-grade group; adult T-cell leukemia lymphoma to the high-grade group, and switching the immunoblastic lymphomas from the high-grade to the intermediate-grade group. We think that when treatment selection is considered, this classification is the most useful. The intermediate-grade lymphomas (including immunoblastic subtypes) tend to do well with standard combination chemotherapy, but the high-grade aggressive lymphomas require specialized leukemia-like therapy, including CNS prophylaxis, to achieve the best results. The primary determinant of the treatment approach to an individual patient is the natural history of the particular histologic subtype of lymphocytic lymphoma.

The second major determinant is the extent of disease. The staging issues vary with the natural history (*i.e.*, histologic subtype) of the lymphoma. For the indolent lymphomas, it is important to identify the 10% to 15% of patients with stage I or II disease, because radiation therapy may be curative. It is currently controversial as to whether it is also important to differentiate between stage III and stage IV disease in the remaining 85%; some studies suggest that this is an important distinction.[376–379]

Localized disease (stage I) is diagnosed in fewer than 20% of presenting patients with intermediate-grade lymphomas, but it is important to document because it affects therapy. The actual stage of a patient without localized disease (*i.e.*, II, III, IV) is probably less important than several other prognostic factors that are discussed later. For the high-grade lymphomas, most patients have disseminated disease at diagnosis, and there is no evidence that clinical staging makes an impact on the treatment approach, which in all cases, includes high-dose combination chemotherapy.

The final determinant of the treatment approach to an individual patient is their physiologic status. There is no question that the treatments for lymphoma are toxic, but the toxicities are usually dose-related and predictable. The age range for patients with lymphoma is quite large, and many patients are older than 65 years at the time of diagnosis. Lymphomas that occur in older patients are disproportionately those that may be curable with aggressive combination chemotherapy programs. Advanced age is not a contraindication to using an effective combination chemotherapy program. Clinical experience suggests that older patients may experience somewhat more myelotoxicity than younger patients when drug doses are administered on the basis of body surface area. Older patients are more sensitive to the marrow-suppressive effects of radiation therapy. However, myelotoxicity from chemotherapeutic agents is related to dose, and there is usually a particular dose of drugs that can be safely administered to a patient whose marrow is extremely sensitive. It has been our practice to administer the first cycle of drugs to older patients in full doses or rarely at 80% to 90% of the full dose and to modify subsequent cycles based on the nadir counts, similar to what is done in younger patients.

There is some evidence that the speed of response is an important factor in long-term disease-free survival, and the poorer treatment outcome that has been seen in some series of older patients may be related more to the delivery of inadequate doses of drugs in the first few cycles of treatment than to any feature of the tumor in an older patient.[328] Patients with aggressive lymphomas who do not achieve complete remissions have a short and unpleasant life because of the lymphoma. Patients with potentially curable disease should not be treated gently out of fear of toxic effects, which in most patients are completely reversible. The alternative to effective therapy—gentle palliation—has a uniformly fatal outcome and offers the patient treatment- and disease-related toxicity with no prospect for prolonged survival. Treatment priorities must be adjusted to the seriousness of the disease. With the most recent treatment programs, treatment-related death is far less common than treatment-induced long-term complete remission. A different philosophy would be appropriate in the same patient if the diagnosis was a low-grade lymphoma.

The existence of serious underlying medical problems may complicate the choice of therapy for patients with lymphoma. Patients with severe chronic obstructive pulmonary disease, renal failure, cardiomyopathy, or severe hepatic dysfunction should probably not receive bleomycin, high-dose methotrexate, or doxorubicin, respectively.

Another increasingly common clinical dilemma is the treatment of an intermediate- or high-grade lymphoma in the setting of an underlying immunodeficiency. Lymphomas are the most common malignancy seen in immunodeficient patients. Intensive treatment may be associated with complete responses, but the probability of long-term survival often depends more on the natural history of the underlying immune defect than on the lymphoma.

If an underlying medical problem alters the choice of therapy, it is probably best to choose an alternate regimen that does not contain the threatening drug rather than to modify a program on an ad hoc basis by omitting the dangerous drug. No one knows the contribution to the overall success of a program that is related to the effects of an individual agent in that program or whether the modified regimen would have the potential to induce long-term disease-free survival. Without such information, it would seem prudent to use an alternative regimen with a known (although perhaps lower) success rate than to create a new program with no record of success.

TREATMENT OF LOW-GRADE LYMPHOCYTIC LYMPHOMAS

The tumors that comprise the low-grade lymphomas are listed in Table 52–8. Experience in treating patients with diffuse small lymphocytic lymphoma, diffuse small cleaved cell lymphoma, and diffuse intermediately differentiated lymphoma is not extensive, and most of the information about these entities is hidden in larger studies including the more common subtypes such as follicular small cleaved cell and follicular mixed lymphomas. However, there is no evidence that the rarer forms of low-grade lymphomas (except CTCL) require an approach distinct from that used to treat the more common varieties.

There is no area of lymphoma treatment that is more controversial than the treatment of patients with low-grade lymphomas. The central question is whether any treatment can induce long-term disease-free survival and alter the natural history of this indolent neoplasm in patients with advanced-stage disease. However, there is no significant controversy about treating patients with early-stage disease; radiation therapy is potentially curative in this setting. The major decision in early-stage patients relates to the extent of irradiation required and whether the addition of combination chemotherapy improves survival. Although some authors maintain that there are no curative treatments for patients with advanced-stage lymphoma, there are studies indicating that intensive treatment may be curative for certain subsets (particularly stage III) of patients with advanced-stage disease.[376–380] If a lymph node biopsy reveals a low-grade lymphoma, the initial response should not be one of therapeutic nihilism resulting in no or conservative treatment, but it should be considered a call to perform complete staging because the patient is potentially curable if stage I or II disease is found.

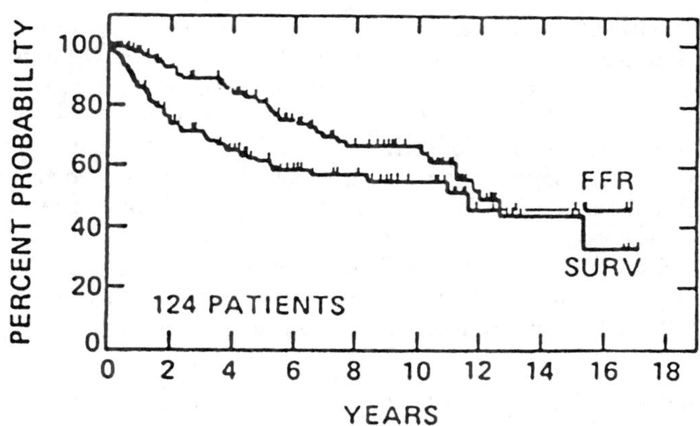

FIGURE 52–8. Survival and freedom from progression curves for extensively staged patients with stage I or II follicular lymphoma managed with radiation therapy at Stanford University.

Early-Stage Low-Grade Indolent Lymphoma

Clinical trials with early-stage low-grade lymphomas (Ann Arbor stages I, II) are composed mainly of patients with follicular small cleaved cell and follicular mixed lymphomas, because the other low-grade histologic varieties are rare and are rarely localized at presentation. Several studies have demonstrated the efficacy of radiation therapy in the treatment of clinically staged patients with localized disease.[381–385] In an extensively staged group of patients from Stanford (41% had staging laparotomies), actuarial survival of patients with clinical stage I or II follicular lymphoma at 5, 10, and 15 years was 84%, 68%, and 42%, respectively (Fig. 52–8).[381] Freedom from relapse at 5 and 10 years was 62% and 54%, respectively. Eighty percent of patients who were 40 years old or younger appeared to be cured with involved-field, extended-field, or total nodal radiation (TNI) therapy. There were no recurrences in this subgroup of patients after 4 years. There was no plateau on the freedom from relapse curve for patients older than 40 years, and the survival for this subgroup of patients was significantly less than for the younger patients.

In the Princess Margaret experience with more than 200 stage I and II follicular lymphomas, the overall survival rate at 10 years was 60% with a relapse-free survival rate of approximately 55% for patients receiving adequate radiotherapy.[383] Prognostic factors in this study included age, stage, histology, tumor bulk, and presence of B symptoms. In the NCI series, overall survival and disease-free survival rates at 10 years were 69% and 48%, respectively.[384] Patients with stage I disease appeared to have a plateau on the disease-free survival curve, with no relapses after 7 years, but there appeared to be a continua of relapses past 18 years for stage II patients. Similar to the Stanford University study, the disease-free and overall survival rates of patients younger than 45 years appeared significantly greater than for patients older than 45. Despite the apparent incurability of most patients who present with advanced disease, these studies indicate that a significant proportion of patients with early-stage disease may be cured, particularly if they are young (≤45 years) and have small-volume stage I disease.

There is some controversy regarding the appropriate radiotherapy field size for the treatment of the early-stage low-grade lymphomas. Because patients with these lymphomas who are treated with less than TNI often relapse in nodal sites distant from the field edge, some physicians have suggested the use of TNI or total-lymphoid irradiation (TLI) for these patients.[386,387] Support for this approach can be found in the Stanford study, which found that freedom from relapse was higher in patients treated with TLI than for those treated with involved-field or extended-field irradiation. However, if only patients who underwent laparotomy are considered, there is no difference in survival or freedom from relapse for patients receiving involved-field irradiation or TLI.[381] The more extensive the staging evaluation, the less extensive the radiation therapy needs to be. It is not recommended that patients undergo staging laparotomy simply to receive less radiation therapy. The data supporting more extensive irradiation are based on small numbers of patients, and current practice is to employ extended-field radiotherapy in these patients. This should provide adequate therapy while minimizing the potential adverse consequences of extensive irradiation on subsequent treatment that is eventually required for many patients who relapse.

A role for combination chemotherapy alone or in combination with radiotherapy in patients with early-stage low-grade lymphoma has not been established. Three randomized studies failed to demonstrate that the use of chemotherapy plus radiation therapy is superior to radiation therapy alone.[387–389] However, it is difficult to draw conclusions from these studies because each trial only included 4 to 26 patients with low-grade histologies, and the power to detect any significant difference between treatment groups was low. Investigators at M.D. Anderson Cancer Center have investigated a combined-modality approach in sequential nonrandomized trials.[390,391] Patients with clinically staged stage I or II low-grade lymphoma received sequential chemotherapy with cyclophosphamide, vincristine, prednisone, and bleomycin (COP-Bleo regimen), or if adverse prognostic features (*e.g.,* high LDH, extranodal sites, bulky nodes) were present, they received the same regimen plus doxorubicin (CHOP-Bleo). Among 44 patients, the 5-year overall survival and failure-free survival rates were 89% and 74%, respectively.[391] These results are superior to those of historic controls receiving involved-field radiotherapy alone.[390] The results from a nonrandomized series of stage I and II patients treated at St. Bartholomew's Hospital with radiotherapy alone or in combination with CVP indicate identical overall survivals but a markedly superior freedom from relapse among the group that received adjuvant chemotherapy.[385]

Without a randomized study, it is impossible to recommend combined treatment for all patients. The best therapy for an individual patient requires a careful assessment of prognostic factors in addition to stage. Most patients with Ann Arbor clinical stage I or II follicular small cleaved cell and follicular mixed lymphomas should have a good prognosis after locoregional radiation therapy (>3000 cGy) alone. For patients whose prognoses are less certain, such as patients with stage II disease with multiple sites of involvement or bulky nodes or patients with follicular large cell histology, chemotherapy followed by involved-field irradiation may improve results.

Advanced-Stage Low-Grade Lymphoma

The optimal treatment strategy for patients with advanced-stage low-grade lymphoma (Ann Arbor stages III, IV) is controversial.[380,392] Treatment generally follows one of two divergent approaches—an aggressive approach that may include extensive radiation therapy, combination chemotherapy, or both, and a conservative approach that consists of no initial treatment followed by palliative single-agent chemotherapy or involved-field radiotherapy when treatment is needed. This dichotomy exists because more than 20 years of painstaking clinical investigation have failed to prove that immediate aggressive therapy improves patient survival compared with conservative therapy.[380] This is despite repeated demonstrations that the advanced-stage low-grade lymphomas are responsive to single and multiple-agent chemotherapy, radiation therapy, and combined-modality treatment approaches.[380] Unfortunately, the responses last only a median of 2 years; in many studies, 10% or fewer patients with low-grade lymphomas remain in remission for 5 years.[393] This is an unusual advanced malignancy, because even without durable complete remissions, median survival is more than 9 years in many series.[394–396] However, the paradox of the low-grade lymphomas is that all patients ultimately die of their disease and usually do so earlier than patients with aggressive lymphomas.[392]

Figure 52–9 illustrates the survival of 147 previously untreated patients enrolled at St. Bartholomew's Hospital in

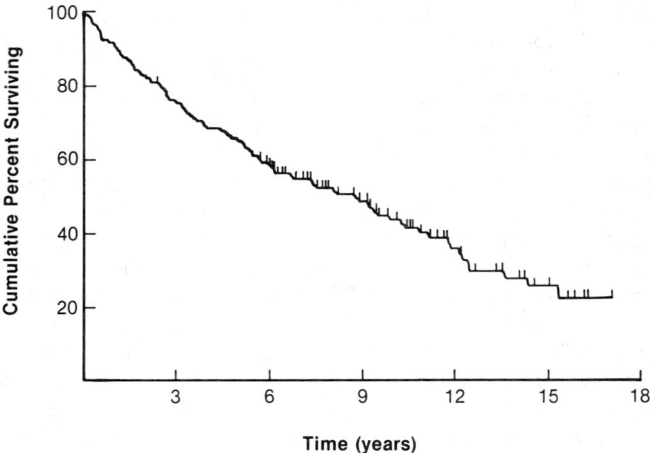

FIGURE 52–9. Overall survival rates for 147 previously untreated patients with stage III or IV indolent lymphoma managed with various treatments at St. Bartholomew's Hospital.

various protocols, ranging from no initial therapy to conservative treatment with single alkylating agents.[396] Only 53 of 147 patients remain alive; 94 patients have died, and only 18 patients died of causes unrelated to lymphoma. This pattern has been seen so often that it is the expected outcome for patients with advanced-stage low-grade lymphomas. One can immediately see positive aspects for the elderly patient (>65 years), but for the younger patient, this curve implies almost certain death from lymphoma. A variety of strategies have been used in an attempt to alter this inexorable natural history.

DIVERSE APPROACHES. The experience with single-agent or combination chemotherapy or TLI or whole-body irradiation (TBI) alone at several selected institutions is summarized in Table 52–15. Complete responses have been observed with all treatment modalities, but continual relapse at a rate of approximately 10% to 15% per year is found regardless of therapy. Combination chemotherapy induces complete remissions more rapidly than single-agent chemotherapy, but if single-agent chemotherapy is given for adequate periods (≥1 year), there is no difference in complete response rate, disease-free survival, or overall survival compared with combination regimens such as CVP. The use of newer combination regimens appears to increase the complete response rate, but they have not been compared directly with single-agent therapy. Neither TLI nor TBI resulted in durable complete remissions when used alone. For the most part, relapses after chemotherapy occur in previously involved sites and relapses after radiation therapy are in previously unirradiated areas.[412] It is logical to combine both modalities. Randomized trials comparing chlorambucil or CVP to CVP plus TLI and combination chemotherapy (CVP) with the same regimen with TBI failed to show significant improvements in relapse-free or overall survival after the addition of radiotherapy (see Table 52–15).[398,408,413,414] When the Stanford group examined actuarial survival and disease-free survival of 114 patients with stage IV low-grade lymphoma randomized to four treatment protocols (*i.e.*, single alkylating agent, TBI plus boost, combination chemotherapy, and combined-modality [TLI and CVP]), there were no significant differences in complete remission rates or actuarial freedom from progression (Fig. 52–10).[380] The disease-free survival was only 25% at 8 years, but 76% of patients survived 8 years, and 55% survived 10 years. The median survival of all patients was between 10 and 11 years (Fig. 52–11).

The failure to detect treatment-related improvements in disease-free and overall survival and the observations that many patients not eligible for these trials or relapsing after a remission obtained from a previous therapy exhibited stable disease or even underwent spontaneous regression led Rosenberg and his colleagues to follow selected asymptomatic patients with advanced-stage disease without treatment.[314,394] Eighty-three patients were carefully selected based on features felt to be consistent with a good prognosis or because they were felt to be too old or had medical problems precluding more aggressive therapy.[394] Patients were excluded if they had bulky peripheral adenopathy, massive retroperitoneal adenopathy with ureteral deviation or obstruction, B symptoms, or splenomegaly causing symptoms or cytopenia. On comparison of these eligibility criteria with patients on their treatment protocols, 56% of the patients referred to Stanford were

TABLE 52–15. Treatment of Advanced-Stage Low-Grade Lymphomas

Treatment	*No. of Patients*	*Complete Response (%)*	*Remission Duration (median, months)*	*Actuarial Survival (median, months)*	*References*
Single alkylating agent	13	46	25+	30	397
	20	65	50	60+	398, 399
	31	13	12	48+	400
	33	33	40	60+	401
Combination chemotherapy					
CVP	49	67	16	83	402
CVP	23	83	50	60+	398
COPP	27	56	84	90	403
BVCP	53	53	26	90	403
CHOP	92	68	?	?	404
CHOP-Bleo	96	77	30	96	405
BACOP	9	89	?	?	406
M-BACOD	10	60	?	?	407
Total-body irradiation (TBI)	33	85	26	26+	408
	31	84	24	48+	409
	28	85	30	48+	410
	17	71	12	48+	399
Combined modality					
CVP vs	23	78	36	—	
CVP + TLI	20	65	48	96+	398
CVP vs	16	67	15+	24+	
CVP + TBI	16	64	15+	24+	408
ProMACE-MOPP + TLI	51	71	45+	60+	411

candidates for no initial therapy. Treatment was withheld until the rate of growth or total bulk of disease was deemed excessive or the patient developed systemic symptoms, anemia, thrombocytopenia, or involvement of new extranodal sites.

Fifty-one of 83 patients eventually required treatment, with a median time to therapy of 33 months. The most common reason for initiating therapy was slowly progressive lymphadenopathy, and treatment usually consisted of single alkylating agents. The length of time a patient could be followed without treatment depended on the histologic subtype; patients with follicular mixed lymphoma required treatment significantly earlier (16.5 months) than patients with follicular small cleaved (48 months) or small lymphocytic subtypes (72 months). The five-year survival rate for patients with follicular mixed disease (66%) was shorter than patients with follicular small cleaved (92%) and small lymphocytic subtypes (92%). Overall survival for patients was 82% at 5 years and 73% at 10 years. The median survival of 11 years compares favorably to the results achieved with a variety of different treatments (see Table 52–15). A comparison of similar patients on treatment protocols performed concurrently at Stanford failed to detect an effect of treatment on survival.

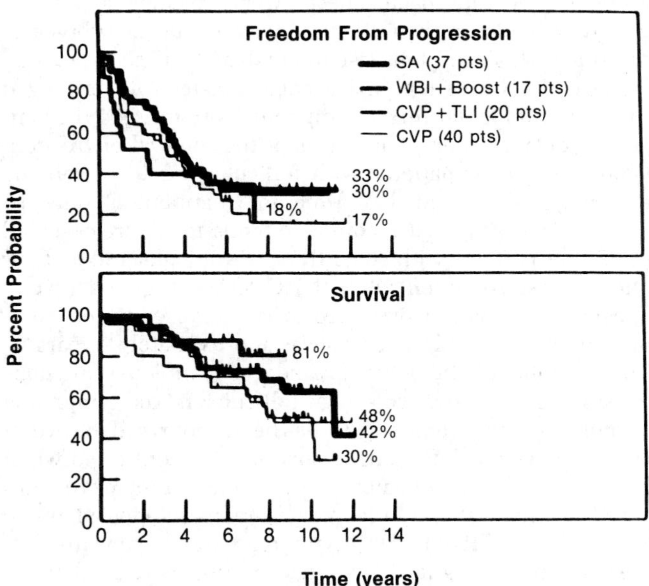

FIGURE 52–10. Freedom from progression (*top panel*) and survival (*bottom panel*) curves of patients with advanced-stage indolent lymphoma treated with different strategies at Stanford University.

An interesting feature of the low-grade lymphocytic lymphomas is their propensity over time to progress to a more aggressive lymphoma. Although some cases may represent outgrowth of a higher-grade tumor that was initially present but undetected at diagnosis (*i.e.*, divergent histologies), most cases represent true transformation from a low-grade subtype. The histology usually changes to a diffuse pattern or a large cell type.[182,316] The transformation rate varies from study to study, but histologic transformation is found in approximately 30% of patients who are rebiopsied and in as many as 90% of patients with lymphoma at postmortem who were initially diagnosed with a low-grade lymphoma.[415] Treatment had been implicated as the cause of histologic progression, but the Stanford study clearly documents that histologic transformation occurs in untreated patients at the same frequency as

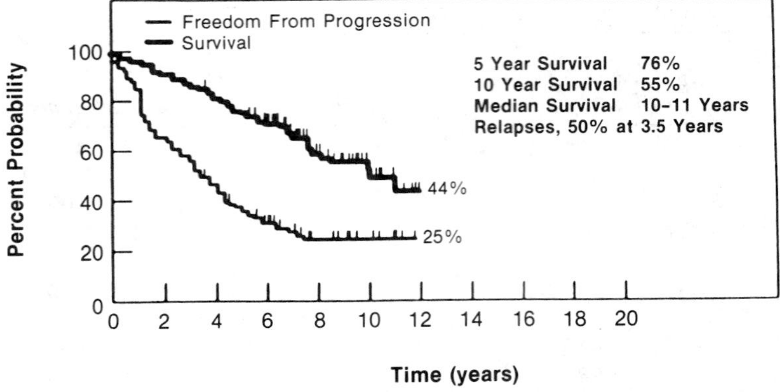

FIGURE 52–11. Data for the patients from Figure 52–10 who received different treatments were merged to obtain freedom from progression and survival curves for all the treatment groups.

in treated patients. The median time to transformation is approximately 57 months. No features have been identified that allow the clinician to predict which patient will undergo transformation. After transformation has occurred, treatment with regimens active against intermediate-grade lymphomas is needed. Complete responses can be achieved, but they appear to be less durable than complete remissions obtained after treatment of de novo large cell lymphomas. Patients who have received previous chemotherapy for their low-grade lymphoma fare particularly poorly.[182,416]

Another interesting feature of the low-grade lymphomas is the occurrence of spontaneous regressions.[178,394] Spontaneous regressions, even complete regressions, were observed in 30% of patients with follicular small cleaved lymphoma followed without initial therapy.[394] The median duration of the spontaneous remissions was more than 13 months, and some patients maintained their remissions for more than 6 years. Regressions in peripheral nodes and intraabdominal sites were observed. Other investigators, including those at the NCI, have seen occasional spontaneous regression of low-grade lymphomas, but not with the frequency reported in this study.

There appear to be several advantages to no initial therapy or the "watch and wait" approach. Foremost is that asymptomatic patients avoid the side effects of therapy, including myelosuppression and the possibility of second tumors. A few patients experience spontaneous regressions and do not require therapy, and a significant number of patients transform to a higher-grade lymphoma, some of whom may be curable with combination chemotherapy.

Several findings color the catholicity of the Stanford experience. In many centers, patients with low-grade lymphomas do not fare as well without therapy as the selected group of Stanford patients. For example, patients with advanced-stage disease at the Memorial Sloan-Kettering Cancer Center[417] had a median survival of only 4 years with conservative treatment, and O'Brien and colleagues[418] reported a median survival of 5 years in initially untreated patients. Although their median time to treatment of 33 months was similar to the Stanford trial, only 11% of patients in the study have not required therapy at 5 years. No spontaneous regressions were observed in this trial. Despite the shorter median survival, there was no survival disadvantage for untreated patients compared with their counterparts receiving treatment with single-agent or combination chemotherapy or with irradiation.

There are certain disadvantages associated with the conservative approach.[392,419] Many patients are adversely affected by the constant and visible enlargement of lymph nodes, which serves as an ever-present reminder of their illness and the uncertainties associated with no therapy. When therapy is finally given, it is often in the form of chronic administration of daily oral alkylating agents with or without radiation therapy, treatment that seriously depletes the nonrenewable marrow stem cell pool and can lead to subsequent intolerance to combination chemotherapy or to secondary acute leukemia or myelodysplastic syndromes.[420–425] This conservative therapy may be associated with even greater iatrogenic problems than aggressive cyclic combination chemotherapy. A subset of patients with low-grade lymphomas can be successfully watched, but even in the Stanford study, this represented only 50% to 60% of the patient population. Therefore, 40% to 50% of patients require immediate therapy because of symptoms or bulky disease.

Data suggest that at least two groups of patients with low-grade lymphoma that would otherwise appear eligible for no initial therapy actually may experience long-term disease-free survival after appropriate therapy, and on that basis, they should be considered for immediate therapy rather than a watch and wait approach. These two groups include patients with lymphomas of the follicular mixed histologic subtype or patients with stage III disease of any histologic subtype.

The conservative approach is not associated with prolonged survival of follicular mixed lymphoma patients, and the benefits of delayed therapy in terms of the interval of freedom from therapy for patients with follicular mixed lymphoma are marginal; the median time to treatment is only 16 months.[380,394] At the NCI, complete remissions were observed in 72% of patients with stage III or IV follicular mixed lymphoma after treatment with the C-MOPP regimen (cyclophosphamide, vincristine, procarbazine, prednisone): the median duration of remissions was approximately 7 years.[426] The durability of chemotherapy-induced complete remissions in patients with advanced-stage follicular mixed lymphoma initially reported from the NCI has been confirmed in several other studies.[405,426] Prolonged survival was confirmed when patients treated with combination chemotherapy were compared with patients receiving oral cyclophosphamide alone.[400,427–429] High LDH, B symptoms, and marrow involvement are poor prognostic factors. Because there are late relapses (6–8 years) in these patients, it is difficult to predict confidently the potential for cure. However, even if cure is not achieved in most of these patients, the long initial complete remissions deserve attention because they minimize the number of treatments that patients need and potentially decrease the risk for development of a second hematologic malignancy.

The application of the more sophisticated measures of complete remission (*i.e.,* measurement of clonal excess in peripheral blood cells) confirms that remissions in follicular mixed lymphoma are durable and complete.[430,431] The circulating abnormal clone that is readily detectable in almost 70% of patients with advanced-stage follicular lymphoma disappears with the achievement of clinical complete remission in patients with follicular mixed lymphoma. In follicular small cleaved cell lymphoma, clinical complete remission is often not accompanied by clearing the malignant clone, and it now appears that this may be the harbinger of relapse.[431] The same data are not available using PCR amplification of the *BCL2* translocation.

There has been little experience with the more recently developed lymphoma treatment programs in advanced-stage follicular mixed lymphoma, but extrapolating from the effects of C-MOPP in diffuse large cell lymphoma and the general correlation between the presence of a large cell component and curability with combination chemotherapy, it seems likely that the second- and third-generation combination chemotherapy programs would be excellent therapy for patients with advanced-stage follicular mixed lymphoma. We currently recommend that patients with advanced-stage follicular mixed lymphoma receive initial therapy at diagnosis with a regimen found to be effective for intermediate-grade lymphoma.

The cell cycle kinetics of the individual histologic subtypes is rather distinct.[432] Follicular small cleaved cell lymphomas have the lowest growth fraction and the lowest percentage of cells expressing the transferrin receptor, a rough immunologic correlate of growth fraction. Follicular mixed lymphomas may have a higher growth fraction and more transferrin receptor-positive cells than follicular small cleaved cell lymphomas, and the follicular and diffuse large cell lymphomas have the highest growth fraction of tumors of follicular center cell origin. As the fraction of large cells in the follicular lymphoma rises, the growth fraction of the tumor increases, the clinical pace of disease becomes more rapid, and the tumor becomes more susceptible to eradication by combination chemotherapy.

The behavior of the follicular lymphomas is analogous to bone marrow, another stem cell compartment with two stem cells. In this analogy, the tumor has two stem cell populations, the small cleaved lymphocytic stem cell that is not in cycle, but is renewable and sensitive to inhibition but not eradication by combination chemotherapy, and a second stem cell that becomes more prominent as the fraction of large cells increases and is nonrenewable, in cell cycle, and sensitive to combination chemotherapy.[420] The explanation for the more indolent growth and the more remote curability of the follicular small cleaved cell lymphomas relates to cell kinetics and the resistance of the stem cell. The analogy to bone marrow seems appropriate. Although most chemotherapeutic agents at conventionally tolerable doses can produce transient cytopenias, the marrow stem cell population usually fully recovers and repopulates the marrow to the normal level. Similarly, the stem cell for follicular small cleaved cell lymphoma usually responds to chemotherapy but continues to regrow and repopulate. A large fraction of follicular mixed lymphoma patients are curable with combination chemotherapy, which correlates with the larger fraction of large cells and the kinetic advantage to treating a nonrenewable stem cell population. This model is speculative but has the advantage of accurately describing the clinical spectrum and response to treatment of the follicular lymphomas. If the stem cell compartment of follicular small cleaved cell lymphomas is analogous to that of the bone marrow, it is possible that treatment capable of ablating bone marrow may also ablate follicular lymphoma. This model provides conceptual support for treating follicular small cleaved cell lymphoma with a high-dose therapy, perhaps with TBI and ABMT.

Patients with stage III disease may also experience long-term disease-free survival. The Stanford experience with TLI (TBI in some) in patients with stage III disease (approximately 50% had staging laparotomies) is instructive.[376,377] The 10-year relapse-free survival rate for stage III patients treated with radiation therapy at Stanford was 40%, with an apparent plateau on the disease-free and overall survival curves (Fig. 52–12). For those with limited stage III disease (*i.e.,* no B symptoms, less than five sites of involvement, maximum size of disease <10 cm), the 15-year freedom from relapse rate was 88%.[377] Most patients relapsed in previously unirradiated lymph node groups, suggesting that the addition of epitrochlear, mesenteric, and Waldeyer's ring fields might have further improved the outcome. Similar excellent results were reported by Cox and colleagues for a study in which the dis-

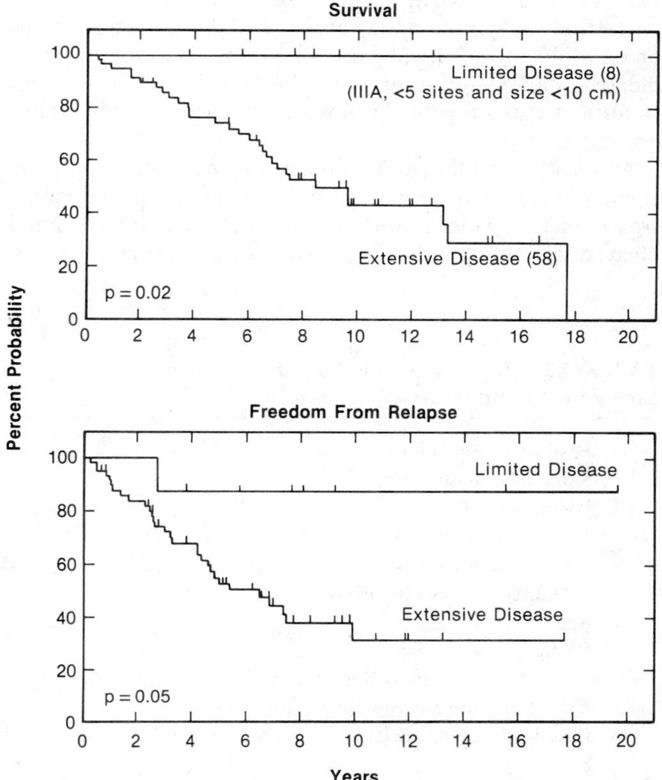

FIGURE 52–12. Disease-free and overall survival curves for patients with stage III indolent lymphoma treated with radiation therapy at Stanford University.

ease-free survival rate was 61% and the actuarial survival rate was 78% at 5 years.[378]

Investigators at M.D. Anderson Cancer Center reported durable remissions in patients with stage III follicular lymphoma using a sequential chemotherapy-radiotherapy sandwich program with CHOP-Bleo and involved-field radiotherapy of 3000 cGy to the abdomen and pelvis and 4000 cGy to peripheral nodes and mediastinum if it is involved.[379,433] This approach resulted in an 81% complete remission rate, a 5-year survival rate of 75%, and 5-year disease-free survival rate of 52% for all patients. Stage III patients without large cell histology, in whom there was no bulky abdominal disease and who had normal LDH levels, did particularly well.

These data strongly suggest that patients with asymptomatic stage III disease, with nonbulky disease involving limited sites should be considered for immediate therapy and are not appropriate candidates for "watch and wait," which merely allows them to progress from a potentially curable to an incurable tumor burden. Extensive radiotherapy with or without chemotherapy is a reasonable option.

Several attempts have been made to discover other useful prognostic factors for patients with low-grade lymphomas.[325–327,403,434–436] The factors that have been most often identified as predictors of complete remission rate or overall survival are listed in Table 52–16. The data are difficult to interpret because the different studies include patients with a variety of stages of disease that are staged according to the institution's own standards (*i.e.*, no liver biopsies or bone marrow examinations in some), and that are untreated, minimally treated, or aggressively treated. These differences may explain the disparity in results observed among these trials. Nevertheless, symptomatic patients with large tumor masses or multiple sites of involvement are clearly a group of candidates suitable for immediate therapy. However, current treatment cures few of these patients, and new approaches are required.

Application of the more recent advances in lymphoma treatment (*e.g.*, active regimens in diffuse large cell lymphoma treatment) to patients with advanced-stage follicular small cleaved cell lymphoma has been slow. However, CHOP, CHOP-Bleo, BACOP (bleomycin, doxorubicin, cyclophosphamide, vincristine, prednisone), and M-BACOD (methotrexate, bleomycin, doxorubicin, cyclophosphamide, vincristine, dexamethasone) have been used in patients with advanced-stage follicular small cleaved cell lymphoma (see Table 52–15). Few patients have been treated, and long-term follow-up is often incomplete. Complete response rates appear higher, and they are attained more quickly than if single agent or more conservative regimens were used. There may be a modest improvement in disease-free survival, but there is still a pattern of continual relapse with no evidence of a plateau.

One exception is the Eastern Cooperative Oncology Group trial that demonstrated that COPP (cyclophosphamide, vincristine, procarbazine, prednisone) induced complete remissions in 56% of patients with advanced follicular small cleaved cell lymphoma, and 57% of the complete remissions lasted more than 5 years.[403] The results of treatment in advanced-stage follicular small cleaved cell lymphoma may be improved by using more active combination chemotherapy programs. None of these putative improvements in complete remission rates or duration have translated into survival advantages for treated patients. Because the median survival of even palliated patients is more than 8 years, such a stringent criterion for efficacy takes many years to meet. Nevertheless, survival without disease off all treatment is also an important goal, and the availability of a treatment approach that can achieve durable complete remissions in most patients would probably change the clinical approach to these patients even before the demonstration of a survival advantage.

In an effort to examine the alternative approaches to low-grade lymphoma treatment prospectively, the NCI initiated a prospective randomized study comparing conservative treatment (no initial therapy) with aggressive combined-modality therapy with ProMACE/MOPP flexitherapy followed by low-dose (2400 cGy) TLI.[411] The patients randomized to receive initial treatment test the hypothesis that the reason for the inability of drug combination programs to produce a significant fraction of long-term disease-free survivors is due to the failure in dose escalation. The group receiving no initial therapy is closely followed to determine the overall survival; the fraction of patients with low-grade follicular lymphomas that can be followed without drug treatment; the number of patients that evolve to follicular mixed, follicular, or diffuse large cell lymphoma over time; and the success of delayed aggressive treatment in achieving long-term disease-free survival. Clinically aggressive tumor masses are biopsied at intervals to determine the histology. If therapy is required and the histology remains low-grade, small-field palliative radiation therapy is used as long as possible. If chemotherapy is required for control of systemic symptoms or for histologic evolution, patients are crossed over to the same treatment as those initially randomized to ProMACE/MOPP flexitherapy.

More than 100 patients have been entered on this study since 1978.[411] Eighty-four percent of all patients presenting with low-grade histologic subtypes were eligible for randomization to aggressive or conservative therapy. The other 16% had serious enough symptoms at presentation that local treatment was not thought to be appropriate. Among the patients randomized to aggressive combination chemotherapy, 74% achieved complete remissions, and 67% of those achieving complete remission remain in their initial remission with a

TABLE 52–16. Prognostic Factors for Advanced-Stage Low-Grade Lymphoma

Histology (follicular mixed)
Stage III disease
B symptoms
Bulk of disease
Large tumor mass
Number of sites involved
Age
Performance Status
Levels of lactate dehydrogenase and B_2-microglobulin
Extent of bone marrow involvement
Histologic transformation
Sex
Aggressive chemotherapy
Anemia

median follow-up of more than 6 years. This is in contrast to a median remission duration in previous treatment programs of about 2 years (see Table 52–15). With median follow-up more than twice as long as the average remission duration from previous treatments, only 33% of the complete responders have relapsed.

Fifty-three percent of the patients randomized to conservative treatment were crossed over to aggressive therapy a median of 23 months after randomization. Among the 47% of patients who have not required systemic treatment, 39% required local irradiation to control symptomatic local disease. The 53% of patients who have crossed over to receive aggressive therapy did so a median of 23 months after randomization. About 40% of those crossing over did so because of progressive systemic symptoms, 33% because of histologic conversion to diffuse large cell or other aggressive lymphoma, and 27% because they had exhausted the limits of local irradiation for symptom control. The complete remission rate after crossover was only 40%, significantly less than the complete remission rate seen in patients who received therapy at diagnosis. Only 4 of the complete responders have relapsed, but there is not enough information to predict whether the responses will be as durable with delayed treatment as with immediate treatment. There is no significant difference in overall survival between the two groups, but there is considerable difference between the two approaches in terms of patients alive and free of disease. Nevertheless, it appears that improvements in therapy can result in prolonged disease-free survival in some patients with follicular and low-grade lymphomas.

The conclusion that emerges from this study is that aggressive therapy at diagnosis may be curative. It appears that delaying therapy until symptoms demand systemic intervention substantially reduces the chances for a successful treatment outcome. More data on the negative impact of delaying treatment were generated by a retrospective analysis of patients treated at the University of Chicago.[437] Initial aggressive therapy achieved a complete remission rate of 71%, but aggressive therapy delivered after initial conservative management achieved a complete remission rate of only 25%. It appears that delaying aggressive therapy results in some patients becoming less responsive to therapy. It may be that the decision about a palliative or curative approach must be made at diagnosis. Failing to decide between these options initially is to decide, because palliation is all that can be done if the decision is delayed.

Although PCR analysis has not been performed on patients after ProMACE/MOPP flexitherapy, there is a strong possibility that malignant cells persist at completion of therapy, even in complete responders. After CHOP chemotherapy, all patients harbor *BCL2*-positive cells in their marrow even when by morphologic assessment they appear to be in complete remission.[79] These residual lymphoma cells may be resistant to standard-dose chemotherapy and responsible for the constant relapse rates seen in patients with advanced low-grade lymphoma. This has led some researchers to employ high-dose chemotherapy with ABMT, an approach that is effective salvage therapy for many patients with intermediate-or high-grade lymphomas.[438]

There have been two major obstacles to ABMT for patients with low-grade lymphomas. First is the observation that a very long natural history can be expected even without therapy, making the excessive treatment-related toxicities associated with transplantation unacceptable. However, the long survival may be reassuring to many older patients with low-grade lymphoma, but to our younger patients, little solace can be derived from the survival curve in Figure 52–9. Moreover, improvements in transplant techniques and supportive therapy have made ABMT a safe procedure.[439] The foreshortened life expectancy with conservative management and the low (4%) mortality from high-dose therapy programs has been used to justify high-dose experimental therapy for younger patients. The second obstacle has been the high incidence of bone marrow involvement with indolent lymphoma. It is possible to exclude patients with involved marrows, as some studies did, but this limits the approach to a rather small fraction of patients with advanced-stage lymphocytic lymphoma.

Trials have used bone marrow that has been "purged" of malignant cells by multiple cycles of ex vivo treatment with specific antibody and complement.[440–442] High-dose chemotherapy with ABMT has been tested by several groups in patients with low-grade lymphomas.[442,443] Schouten and colleagues treated 10 patients after histologic transformation of their low-grade lymphoma.[443] These patients were heavily pretreated and tolerated the ABMT rather poorly; only 1 of the 10 patients remains alive and in a complete remission. Much better results were observed in 8 patients whose tumors had retained their original low-grade histology after relapse from their initial response. All 8 patients achieved complete remissions; 6 patients remained in their initial complete remissions from 1 to 5 years, and all 8 were alive at the time of the report. All bone marrows were free of tumor at the time of harvest and no in vitro purging was attempted.

Investigators at the Dana-Farber Cancer Institute treated 69 patients with low-grade lymphomas in sensitive relapse or incomplete first remission with cyclophosphamide 60 mg/kg on two successive days followed by 1200 cGy of TBI and reinfusion of bone marrow that had been purged of malignant cells with the anti-CD20 (B1) monoclonal antibody alone or as part of a cocktail with anti-B5 and anti-CD10 (CALLA), all with complement.[441] Patients were in complete remission or had achieved a minimal disease state (all involved lymph nodes $\leq$2 cm and bone marrow involvement <20%) before marrow harvest. There were 51 patients with low-grade lymphomas at the time of ABMT and 18 patients whose tumors had undergone histologic transformation. More than 85% of the patients were 50 years of age or younger. After a short follow-up, there was no significant difference in 2-year disease-free survival between patients with low-grade or transformed lymphomas, with 53% and 88% of patients disease-free, respectively. There were 23 relapses, most in previously involved sites, suggesting that resistant lymphoma, not reinfusion of malignant cells with the marrow, was responsible for the relapse. The only significant prognostic factor for disease-free survival was the state of disease at the time of transplant; patients in complete remission did significantly better than partial responders. Rohatiner and colleagues used identical induction and purging regimens in 38 patients who were in their second or subsequent remissions.[442] There were two treatment-related deaths. Median follow-up is only 22 months, but 26 patients remain in remission. Despite bone marrow involvement in almost one half of all patients, ABMT with purged marrow can be performed safely and most patients remain disease free for at least 2 years.

Interesting results regarding purging were reported by Gribben and his colleagues.[79] Among more than 200 patients who had undergone ABMT with in vitro purged marrow, there were 114 whose tumors contained the t(14;18) translocation and who had marrow samples from before and after purging available for PCR analysis. All marrow samples were PCR positive for tumor before purging. No lymphoma cells could be detected after purging in 57 patients. The disease-free survival in these 57 PCR-negative patients was significantly superior to the 57 patients whose marrows could not be cleared of lymphoma cells by purging (Fig. 52–13). The risk of relapse in patients with residual detectable lymphoma cells was 10 times higher than that for patients receiving lymphoma-free marrows. Patients with the least bone marrow involvement and patients who were in complete remission at the time of transplant did well, but the most important prognostic factor was the ability to purge the marrow completely of malignant cells. Follow up is still relatively short, but relapse rates of 7% for recipients of PCR-negative compared with 46% for PCR-positive marrows are impressive.

These data imply that successful purging is an important aspect of therapy. The fact that most patients, even after ABMT, relapse in previously involved sites would seem to argue against the transferred marrow as the source of relapse, but it is possible that it is the microenvironment that is important to relapse and that the most conducive microenvironment is in previously involved sites. These data suggest that a reasonable endpoint for experimental therapy designed to cure this disease is attainment of a completely PCR-negative state in the bone marrow. Others may argue with this approach, because it is clear that the presence of PCR-positive cells in the peripheral blood does not preclude a healthy, long-term survival.[78] PCR-positive cells have been found in the peripheral blood of patients who have been in continuous

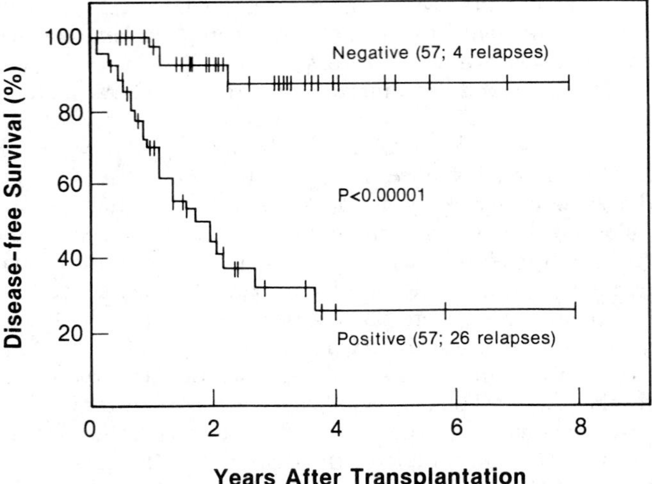

FIGURE 52–13. Disease-free survival rates for patients with indolent lymphoma whose marrow could be purged of polymerase chain reaction-amplified t(14;18)-bearing cells compared with those of patients with indolent lymphoma whose marrow could not be completely purged. This study was conducted at the Dana-Farber Cancer Institute.

complete remissions for more than 10 years. Appearance of PCR-positive cells did not predict for progression of disease. The value of their presence as a predictor of relapse has to be verified in prospective trials, but until further information is obtained, we think a reasonable goal of curative therapy in young patients with low-grade lymphoma is the induction of a PCR-negative state.

BIOLOGIC THERAPY. Biologic therapy has been extensively tested in patients with low-grade lymphomas.[444,445] Nonspecific immune stimulants such as bacillus Calmette-Guérin and levamisole have failed to have reproducible effects on complete remission rates or remission duration.[444] The interferons have activity against the lymphocytic lymphomas.[446,447] Interferon has little antitumor activity in intermediate- or high-grade lymphomas, but response rates of approximately 46% (11% complete remissions) are seen in patients with low-grade lymphomas.[446,447] The median time to achieve remission is approximately 3 months; most remissions are partial and last for a median of 8 months. Three preparations of IFN-α (*i.e.*, natural or lymphoblastoid; recombinant IFN-α2a and IFN-α2b) have been used at doses ranging from 1 million units daily to 50×10^6 U/m^2 3 times weekly. The highest response rates have been reported at the highest doses, but the higher the IFN dose, the more severe is the toxicity, and few patients can tolerate 50×10^6 U/m^2 for any significant period.

Combined treatment with IFN-α and chemotherapy has not improved complete remission rates.[448–450] Hawkins and colleagues administered COPA (cyclophosphamide, vincristine, prednisone, doxorubicin) with IFN-α and described excessive myelosuppression at IFN doses of 12×10^6 U/m^2 or larger.[448] Chlorambucil and IFN-α can be given safely for prolonged periods, but randomized trails have shown that overall response rates with the combination are not superior to chlorambucil alone.[450,451] When patients achieving complete remissions after chlorambucil alone or with IFNα are randomized to maintenance therapy with IFNα or no additional therapy, lower relapse rates were observed in IFN-treated patients.[450,451] It is too early to determine whether there is an effect on overall survival, but the early data are promising.

Several phase II studies of IL-2 with or without lymphokine-activated killer (LAK) cells have been performed in heavily pretreated patients with refractory lymphoma, and responses have been seen in about 27% of treated patients with low-grade lymphoma.[452–455] IL-2 exhibits little activity in patients with intermediate- or high-grade lymphomas or Hodgkin's disease. Responses have been observed in patients receiving IL-2 at high and low doses, by bolus and continuous intravenous infusion, and with or without LAK cells. The responses are usually partial and have a median duration less than 1 year, although long-lasting remissions have been observed. As is the case with IFN-α, the single agent response rate of IL-2 is lower than that expected with chemotherapy in the same patients, but the probability that these biologic agents work by mechanisms entirely different from chemotherapeutic agents makes them attractive for potential combination with other forms of therapy and as therapeutic options to be used much earlier in the course of disease when the host's immune system is minimally compromised.

Monoclonal antibodies have been used with some success

in patients with lymphocytic lymphomas. There are four major classes of mechanisms by which monoclonal antibodies may kill tumor cells: by activating host immune system tumor cell lysis mechanisms (*e.g.*, complement, antibody-dependent cellular cytotoxicity); by triggering or interfering with the function of a physiologically important receptor; by targeting biologically active moieties to tumor cells (*e.g.*, toxins, isotopes, drugs, cytokines); and by eliciting an antitumor response indirectly by inducing autoantibodies or by activating cellular responses to the tumor antigen (*i.e.*, antibody functioning as a biologic response modifier).

Since 1980, patients with B-cell lymphoma have been treated with murine or rat monoclonal antibodies directed against the idiotype of the surface immunoglobulin, CD20 (1F5), a panlymphoid cell antigen (CAMPATH-1), and the Epstein-Barr virus receptor (OKB-7).[456–460] With the exception of a single patient (the *first* patient) treated with antiidiotypic antibody, whose response was complete and lasted 50 months with no further therapy, few patients treated with antibody alone experience tumor regressions that meet criteria for partial responses, and such responses are generally short-lived. There are many reasons for this lack of efficacy. There have been essentially no studies of antibodies in lymphoma patients that have taken a particular antibody and developed it in a fashion analogous to the development of other directly acting antitumor agents. In most cases, maximal tolerated doses have not been determined, and optimal pharmacokinetic parameters are unknown. In some cases (particularly in solid tumors), expression of the target antigen is heterogenous in the tumor cell population. Antibodies cannot activate killing mechanisms or exert direct effects on cells to which they cannot bind. Often the target antigen is shed, down-modulated, or altered during the course of antibody therapy. Circulating antigen makes it extremely difficult for the antibody to find the tumor-bound target. Any change in the tumor that makes it more difficult for the antibody to bind to it compromises the efficacy of the therapy. Murine and rat antibodies commonly elicit a host antibody response, usually within 2 weeks of the first exposure to the therapeutic antibody. This represents yet another distracting influence to systemically administered antibody. Murine and rat antibodies activate human effector mechanisms variably, but often poorly.

Antiidiotype therapy is an elegant approach to tumor-specific therapy. Most other tumor-associated target antigens are not tumor specific. However, there have been technical and logistic problems in the implementation of this clever idea. First, each patient's tumor is derived from a single clone. This implies that each tumor requires the generation of a special reagent specific for a particular patient. The labor involved in generating a unique hybridoma for each patient is onerous. Second, the capacity to change the structure of their immunoglobulin molecule appears to be an essential adaptive feature of human B cells. Alteration in the idiotype of a particular tumor occurs even in the absence of therapy, and it appears that most tumors that have lost responsiveness to antiidiotype therapy have developed an idiotype-negative tumor that nevertheless expresses a clonally related immunoglobulin molecule, which has somatically mutated its antigen combining site.[461,462] This genetic flexibility allows us to make antibodies to antigens that have not been invented yet, which is wonderful for our defense system. However, it means that a single-pronged attack on an idiotypic determinant is unlikely to have a lasting impact on the growth of a B-cell tumor. Strategies to circumvent these two problems include the development of panels of antiidiotypic antibodies that are common to many tumors so that treatment does not have to be individualized, and treatment with multiple antiidiotypic antibodies together or in series minimize the problem of idiotype negative variants.[463]

The problem of antigenic heterogeneity could be overcome by the use of "cocktails" composed of several antibodies. This approach has not yet been tried in humans. Another strategy to overcome heterogeneity is the use of radiolabeled antibody. ^{131}I-labeled antibodies are capable of eradicating a subpopulation of tumor cells lacking the target antigen when they are interspersed with tumor cells bearing the target antigen in mice with lymphoma.[464] Data suggest that the dose rate of radiation delivered to tissue by antibodies may result in antitumor effects better than with the delivery of a maximal tolerated dose of external-beam irradiation.[465]

There have been several studies using radiolabeled antibodies to treat lymphoma in humans. Press and colleagues administered ^{131}I-labeled anti-CD37 (MB-1) antibody to several patients with relapsed lymphoma.[466] With initial tracer doses of antibody, they found that in 5 patients with splenomegaly and high tumor burdens the antibody did not distribute to tumor in a way that would result in the tumor receiving more radioactivity than normal organs. However, 4 other patients showed good tumor localization of the tracer. These 4 patients received 232 to 608 mCi of labeled antibody that was thought to deliver 850 to 4260 cGy of radiation to sites of tumor. Because of the difficulties with dosimetry, these values must be considered estimates. All 4 patients achieved complete remissions, and 2 patients remain in remission at 8+ and 11+ months. However, myelosuppression occurred 3 to 5 weeks after treatment in all cases and required ABMT in two cases. Two patients became hypothyroid. The improved antitumor effects of radiolabeled antibodies have come at the cost of toxicity, but the toxic effects may be anticipated and effectively managed in most cases. There is no evidence to suggest that a maximal tolerated dose of radiation delivered by antibody is superior to a maximal tolerated dose of radiation delivered by external-beam in patients with lymphoma.

De Nardo and colleagues treated 20 B-cell lymphoma patients with ^{131}I-labeled Lym-1 antibody.[467,468] They reported that 65% of the patients obtained responses; three were complete. The response rate was dose related. Patients were more likely to respond after receiving 100 mCi or greater doses of ^{131}I. Rosen and colleagues treated 5 patients with CTCL with ^{131}I-labeled T101.[469] Patients had subjective improvement in pruritus and objective responses lasting 3 weeks to 3 months. At the highest doses (144–150 mCi), myelosuppression was dose limiting. It appears that the cytoreductive power of antibodies has been augmented by conjugating them to radioisotopes.

One of the most potent ways of augmenting the efficacy of monoclonal antibody therapy is to conjugate the antibody to a toxin or chemotherapeutic agent. The preclinical data on the use of immunotoxins are enormous, but there are many fewer relevant clinical studies. Stone and colleagues treated 23 B-cell lymphoma patients with an anti-CD22 antibody conjugated to ricin A chain. The maximal tolerated dose for bolus therapy was 75 mg/m^2.[470] Only 1 patient had an antitoxin response, and no patient had a response to the antibody. Perhaps all the B cells that make such antibodies express CD22 and are eliminated by the immunotoxin, an idea that needs more extensive study. About half the patients achieved short-term partial responses. Nadler and colleagues used an anti-CD19 antibody (anti-B4) conjugated to an intact ricin molecule whose B chain binding site is blocked in 19 lymphoma patients.[471] One of the problems with the A chain ricin toxin has been its relatively inefficient internalization, which is facilitated greatly by the B chain. They administered the immunotoxin by 7-day continuous infusion and have not reached the maximal tolerated dose at 70 μg/kg/day. There have been one complete and four partial responses at the suboptimal doses used. About half the patients developed an antibody response to the immunotoxin.

NEW ACTIVE AGENTS IN INDOLENT LYMPHOMA. New active agents include the purine analogs 2-deoxycoformycin, fludarabine, and 2′-chlorodeoxyadenosine, and there are new methods of administering older drugs, such as oral etoposide and idarubicin (Table 52–17). The three purine analogs are structurally similar compounds that share important features but have distinct mechanisms of action.[472] They are inactive against most common solid tumors and are effective against the same indolent lymphoproliferative disorders, hairy cell leukemia, chronic lymphocytic leukemia, and low-grade lymphocytic lymphomas. Deoxycoformycin is a potent irreversible inhibitor of adenosine deaminase, and when administered at low doses (4–5 mg/m^2 given every other week), it has almost a 50% response rate in patients with low-grade lymphomas.[472,473] One third of the responses were complete. Fludarabine is an analog of the antiviral agent vidarabine, which is resistant to deamination. It appears to function analogously to ara-C. Phase II studies of fludarabine at 18 to 25 mg/m^2 for 5 days have shown overall response rates of 50% in previously treated patients; complete remissions are seen in approximately 20% of patients.[474,475] 2′-Chlorodeoxyadenosine is a synthetic purine analog that is resistant to degradation by adenosine deaminase. It can kill dividing and nondividing cells, a property that makes it particularly suited for neoplasms with a low growth fraction, such as the indolent lymphomas. Kay and colleagues administered 2′-chlorodeoxyadenosine by continuous infusion at a dose of 0.1 mg/kg/day for 7 days.[476] This dose and schedule induced a 95% complete remission rate in patients with hairy cell leukemia. An overall response rate of 43% was achieved in 40 patients with low-grade lymphomas refractory to or relapsed from previous chemotherapy. Complete responses were seen in 20% of patients.

TABLE 52–17. Newer Treatments for Lymphoma

New Single Aspects	*Complete Response (%)*	*Partial Response (%)*	*References*
Deoxycoformycin	20	40	472, 473
Fludarabine	22, 20	26, 32	474, 475
2′-Chlorodeoxyadenosine	20	22	476
Oral etoposide	0	67	477
Oral idarubicin	0, 22	26, 36	478, 479

All three analogs appear to have similar activity in patients with low-grade lymphomas. Although complete responses are observed and some of them have been long-lasting, they are usually temporary, and none of these agents appears to be curative for previously treated patients. Treatment earlier in the natural history of the disease is under investigation, as are combinations with alkylators, anthracyclines, and biologicals. All three drugs are potentially valuable as palliative therapy for relapsing patients.

Etoposide is an effective drug against lymphocytic lymphomas and is a component of many current front-line regimens for the treatment of large cell lymphoma. Hainsworth and his colleagues showed that oral etoposide given at 50 mg/m^2 daily for 21 days results in a 67% partial remission rate, with a median time to progression of 8 months, in patients with low-grade tumors.[477] Responses were seen in patients with disease resistant to regimens containing etoposide given by intravenous infusion. Similar results were described using oral 4-demethoxydaunorubicin (idarubicin).[478,479] These newer drugs and methods are potentially useful for the palliation of patients who have become resistant to other treatments, and they are currently being evaluated as components of front-line therapy.

MANAGEMENT STRATEGY. No initial therapy is an acceptable management approach to patients with advanced-stage follicular small cleaved cell lymphoma, but there is mounting evidence that aggressive treatment at diagnosis may permit a large fraction of patients to enjoy prolonged disease-free survival. Patients younger than 50 years for whom a median survival of 10 years or less represents a significant foreshortening of life expectancy; patients without intercurrent illness; patients with B symptoms, abnormal liver function tests, effusions, or other suggestions of more aggressive disease; and patients initially treated conservatively who undergo histologic conversion to a more aggressive lymphoma should probably receive treatment with one of the newer combination chemotherapy programs with or without TNI for those who achieve complete remission (unnecessary in patients with converted histology).

The decision about whether to treat aggressively should not be indefinitely delayed after diagnosis. Postponing the decision until symptoms demand treatment appears to substantially reduce the efficacy of the treatment program. Those who believe that they must manage patients conservatively should consider the use of cyclical combination chemotherapy such as CVP to control the disease, because the use of chronic oral alkylating agents such as chlorambucil, although it is well tolerated, is associated with irreversible damage to the marrow stem cells, the possible development of a myelodysplasia or secondary leukemia, and a reduction in the capacity to deliver curative therapy if histologic progression should occur. CVP is not associated with chronic marrow damage.

Patients with follicular mixed lymphoma fare worse with a conservative approach and appear to be curable with the chemotherapy programs that have been used in patients with aggressive lymphoma.

Patients with diffuse indolent histologic subtypes may be best managed symptomatically because there are not yet convincing data that therapy leads to cure. The efficacy of fludarabine in CLL makes it an attractive agent for testing in small lymphocytic and mantle zone lymphoma.

TREATMENT OF AGGRESSIVE LYMPHOMAS

The aggressive lymphomas include diffuse large cell (all varieties, including immunoblastic), diffuse mixed, and follicular large cell lymphomas. They constitute about 60% of all lymphocytic lymphomas. Most are of B-cell origin, but about 20%, including some diffuse mixed, diffuse large cell, and immunoblastic lymphomas, are of T-cell origin and are sometimes called peripheral T-cell lymphomas. The designation "peripheral" refers to the cell-surface phenotype mimicking mature postthymic or peripheral T cells (*i.e.*, CD4 or CD8 positive but not both) and differentiates the cells from cortical thymocytes or thymic T cells, which are positive for both CD4 and CD8. However, the term peripheral T-cell lymphoma is of little use in that it does not describe a discrete clinicopathologic entity.[480,481]

The Ann Arbor staging classification is used to stage patients with lymphocytic lymphoma. However, unlike Hodgkin's disease, which has a pattern of spread well suited to an anatomic site lymph node-based staging schema, lymphocytic lymphomas have a propensity to originate in extranodal sites or to spread hematogenously early in their course. Although the Ann Arbor staging classification defines prognosis quite poorly in patients with aggressive lymphoma, there has been no unanimity on what features should be used to identify prognostic groups. There are data suggesting that features of the tumor itself, clinical factors, and treatment-related variables contribute significantly to patient survival.

Several features of the tumor itself may influence treatment outcome, including cell-surface phenotype, growth fraction, and cytogenetic abnormalities. In several series, patients with T-cell tumors fare more poorly than patients with B-cell tumors.[482,483] In one series, the poorer prognosis for patients with T-cell tumors was found only in patients with stage IV disease, but there were only 8 patients with T-cell tumors of stage IV extent, too few cases from which to extrapolate broadly.[222] Other groups have not found significant differences between patients with B-cell or T-cell aggressive lymphomas.[220,223] As suggested by Stein and colleagues, it may be that apparent differences based on T-cell or B-cell phenotype are related to differences in the treatment regimen.[484] At the NCI, we have not found significant differences in outcome based on T- or B-cell phenotype in patients treated with the ProMACE-based regimens. Miller and colleagues suggested that large cell lymphomas that do not express HLA-DR antigens have a poorer prognosis than those that do.[485] However, the Eastern Cooperative Oncology Group has not found such a correlation.[486] There is no consensus that immunologic phenotype should be used to determine prognosis of aggressive lymphoma patients.

The assessment of proliferation index by staining of tissue with Ki-67, by counting mitoses, or by flow cytometric assessment of S-phase fraction seems to be able to separate good-prognosis (*i.e.*, low proliferation index) from poor-prognosis (*i.e.*, high proliferation index) patients.[487–490] There is evidence that the study of cell adhesion molecules on the surface of the tumor may reveal its propensity to spread.[490–492] Tumors expressing high amounts of CD44, the lymphocyte homing receptor, appear to be more likely to spread than those expressing low or no CD44. Such data have not been generated on homogenously staged and treated patients. However, there are sufficient data on the role of Ki-67 staining that it would seem necessary to include this feature of the tumor in any new staging system that is developed.

Another feature of the tumor that appears to have prognostic importance is cytogenetic abnormalities.[493] One convincing study demonstrated that patients with follicular lymphoma that progressed to a diffuse aggressive histology developed an extra chromosome 7, an additional chromosome 17, or an isochromosome 17.[66] These patients appear to have a poorer prognosis than patients without these genetic abnormalities. Cabanillas and colleagues observed a similar poor prognosis for patients with diffuse large cell lymphoma presenting with chromosome 7 or 17 abnormalities, at least some of whom may have had a clinically silent period of follicular lymphoma.[494] Schouten and colleagues at the University of Nebraska confirmed and extended those observations.[495,496] Patients with chromosome 6 abnormalities had a higher incidence of immunoblastic histology and were more likely to have B symptoms. Shorter survival was seen among patients whose tumors had abnormalities in chromosome 17 and 5 or had extra chromosomes 6 and 18. In multivariate analysis, these cytogenetic correlations were stronger than the usual clinical prognostic factors. It appears that any new staging system may also need to consider cytogenetic features of the tumor cells, if such data can be generated in a clinically appropriate time frame.

Clinical prognostic factors for aggressive histology lymphoma have been surrogate measures of the physiologic reserve of the patient (*e.g.*, performance status, age) or tumor bulk (*e.g.*, large masses, multiple extranodal sites, high LDH, B symptoms). In patients with good physiologic reserve and low tumor burden, the response to therapy is excellent. If physiologic reserve is poor and tumor burden is large, response and survival are lower. Several research groups analyzed their treatment results and derived prognostic factor models that separate patients into distinct groups.[320,322–324,497–500] Although the criteria defining poor prognosis differ somewhat in their specifics across the models generated by separate groups, they tend to produce similar groupings when the various models are applied to a single large population of patients distinct from those from whom the criteria were initially derived.[322,500]

A major difficulty has been to obtain a reliable measure of tumor burden. Swan and colleagues from M.D. Anderson Cancer Center suggested that serum β_2-microglobulin might be a reliable serum marker for tumor burden.[501] In their 86 patients in whom LDH and β_2-microglobulin were measured, these factors seemed to be independent prognostic factors. All 27 patients with LDH levels of 250 U/L or less and β_2-microglobulin levels of 3 mg/L or less were alive in first remission; 75% of the group with both markers elevated were dead. Other candidate soluble markers associated with tumor burden have been suggested, such as serum soluble IL-2 receptors, urinary neopterin levels, serum CA 125, but the data in support of β_2-microglobulin are currently stronger.[502–504] A major international collaborative project is underway to pool data on patients with aggressive lymphoma and devise a new clinical staging system.[505]

A third category of prognostic factors includes treatment-related variables, such as the delivered dose intensity of therapy. Treatment-related variables are more difficult to assess because their independence from pretreatment characteristics is not entirely clear.

Treatment of Localized Aggressive Lymphomas

The treatment of choice for localized aggressive histology lymphoma is primary combination chemotherapy with or without involved-field radiation therapy. CHOP or modified ProMACE-MOPP regimens have obtained the best results.[506–509] Cabanillas and colleagues reported that stage I patients treated with CHOP had a 100% 5-year disease-free survival rate, and stage II patients had an 80% 5-year survival rate.[506] Connors and colleagues used three cycles of CHOP followed by involved-field radiation therapy in 78 patients with stage I or stage II (without poor prognostic factors) disease.[508] The complete response rate was 99%, and the long-term survival rate was 85%.

The role of adjuvant radiation therapy is unclear. Jones and colleagues reported an amalgamation of the Arizona and Vancouver experiences.[510] All the Vancouver patients received radiation therapy to the involved field after completing CHOP chemotherapy (usually three cycles). At Arizona, radiation therapy was used in certain patients whose tumor masses were not responding promptly to chemotherapy or who required significant dose modifications of their chemotherapy. Patients who were not treated with radiation therapy usually received eight cycles of CHOP. When patients who received radiation therapy were compared with those who did not, there were no significant differences in relapse rate or survival. The relapse rate among those who received radiation therapy was 14% (15 of 107); for those who did not receive radiation therapy, 24% (8 of 33) relapsed. The 10% difference in relapse rate is worrisome, although not statistically significant.

At the NCI, we administered four cycles of chemotherapy with ProMACE-MOPP with the myelotoxic drugs reduced about 25% from the standard ProMACE-MOPP regimen used in patients with advanced-stage disease; after completing the chemotherapy, patients then received 4000 cGy to the involved field in 20 fractions over 4 weeks.[509] Forty-seven of 49 patients with stage I or IE aggressive histology lymphoma achieved complete remissions, and all 47 complete responders have remained in complete remission, with a median follow-up of about 4 years. The only deaths are the 2 patients who failed to achieve an initial complete response and a 68-year-old woman who died free of disease during her second operation for coronary artery disease after having been in complete remission over 3 years. With a long-term survival rate of 94% with minimal toxicity, we concluded that the combined-modality regimen was effective and well tolerated and have little enthusiasm about asking whether the results would be as good without radiation therapy.

Results using radiation therapy alone are clearly inferior to chemotherapy or combined-modality results in localized aggressive lymphoma when patients are clinically staged. In the classic series of Stanford, the 5-year survival rate for patients with stage I or IE disease was 65%, and for patients with stage II or IIE disease, the rate was 25%.[511] Those results were not due to technical deficiencies that have been improved over the last 20 years. Reddy and colleagues reported a 10-year relapse-free survival rate of 66% for stage I diffuse aggressive lymphoma patients treated with radiation therapy alone.[512] Hagberg and colleagues reported a 60% 10-year disease-free survival rate for clinically staged patients.[513] However, when patients are staged pathologically by performing an exploratory laparotomy, radiation therapy results are improved. Vokes and colleagues[514] from the University of Chicago reported a 70% 10-year survival rate for laparotomy-staged stage I patients, and Hallahan and colleagues[515] reported a 91% 10-year disease-free survival rate among stage I patients pathologically staged. The Stanford group found that the use of larger radiation fields resulted in some improvement in outcome in clinically staged patients.[516] However, even better results were obtained by combined-modality therapy.[517] The five-year survival rate of stage I patients was 81%, but with a subset of 21 patients who received chemotherapy sandwiching radiation therapy, there were no relapses and no deaths.

The morbidity associated with an exploratory laparotomy does not seem to be justified in patients with clinical early-stage disease. The results with radiation therapy alone in pathologically staged patients are not superior to the results of combination chemotherapy in clinically staged patients. When patients relapse from a radiotherapy-induced complete response, they do so in sites not previously involved with lymphoma or in extranodal sites, suggesting that more extensive radiation therapy would not have been of value. There is evidence that patients who relapse after radiation therapy-induced complete response are refractory to salvage combination chemotherapy; relapse is usually fatal.[515,518] The problem with the use of radiation therapy alone is that aggressive-histology lymphoma appears to disseminate hematogenously early in the natural history of the disease. Aggressive lymphoma is best viewed as a systemic disease requiring systemic therapy. Primary combination chemotherapy is of proven efficacy. The role of adjuvant involved-field radiation therapy is not universally agreed on, but its use appears to permit the delivery of fewer cycles of chemotherapy to obtain excellent results. It appears that primary chemotherapy followed by radiation therapy is generally associated with a better outcome than the opposite sequence.

Each year, there are dozens of reports of one or more cases of localized aggressive histology lymphoma involving a particular organ or extranodal site. We think that all patients can be approached with a standard staging evaluation, and if they are found to have localized disease, they can be managed with primary chemotherapy and involved-field radiation therapy. It is helpful to know certain disease predilections; for example, Waldeyer's ring involvement may be accompanied by gastrointestinal tract involvement, and sinus involvement can lead to CNS disease. A systematic approach to staging should reveal any occult sites of disseminated disease that would necessitate more aggressive therapy. The job of the oncologist is to protect the patient with an unusual site of lymphoma from being managed idiosyncratically by a well-meaning subspecialist whose expertise is not lymphoma management.

A particularly common site of localized aggressive lymphoma is the gastrointestinal tract. For patients with palpable abdominal masses, there are at least 15 studies in the literature demonstrating superior survival when patients have surgical resection of the primary lesion followed by systemic chemotherapy (see examples in the reference list[519–522]). However, this conclusion may be based on an unintentional bias related to the clinical decision to operate, which was not standardized. None of the studies involving surgical debulking have been prospective randomized trials. Nevertheless, the data supporting surgical debulking in aggressive lymphoma appears to be at least as good as data supporting surgical debulking in Burkitt's lymphoma. Use of radiation therapy alone after surgery, use of surgery alone, or failure to remove as much of the disease as possible appears to be associated with suboptimal cure rates.[523–526]

Fifteen percent to 20% of primary gastrointestinal lymphomas involve the colon; about 60% involve the stomach; and about 15% involve the small bowel. Small intestinal involvement with lymphoma can be due to distinct clinical entities. In Western countries, segmental involvement of the small bowel can be surgically debulked and treated similar to the more common gastric and colonic lesions. However, in the Middle East, there are two forms of small intestinal lymphoma, immunoproliferative small intestinal disease (IPSID) with or without secretion of immunoglobulin α heavy chains. Both entities commonly involve the mesenteric nodes. The nonsecreting IPSID has a predilection for extension into the gastric mucosa. In α-heavy-chain disease, the lymphoma commonly involves the entire length of the small bowel making surgical resection impractical.[527] Both forms of IPSID respond well to state-of-the-art chemotherapy.[528] The surgical debulking of gastric lymphomas is controversial. Although removal of the tumor may improve response to therapy, the morbidity and mortality associated with total gastrectomy are too great, and results with effective chemotherapy programs suggest that gastric sparing is associated with an excellent prognosis.[529] However, if the disease can be totally removed with a subtotal gastrectomy, such a procedure may be indicated.

Ann Arbor stage II patients are heterogenous. Some with bulky disease or other poor prognostic factors behave more like advanced-stage patients, and others with less tumor bulk respond to treatments that are successful in localized disease. We recommend that patients with localized aggressive lymphoma not undergo laparotomy to stage the extent of disease. Although the best treatment program has not been defined conclusively by prospective randomized trial, we suggest that clinically staged patients with fewer than three sites of disease and no bulky masses receive CHOP or modified ProMACE-MOPP combination chemotherapy for four to six cycles followed by involved-field radiation therapy. Patients with three or more sites of disease, any bulky mass (>10 cm), or other poor-prognostic factors should be managed similarly to patients with advanced-stage disease.

Treatment of Advanced-Stage Aggressive Lymphomas

We define advanced-stage aggressive lymphoma as all Ann Arbor stage III or IV patients plus patients with stage II disease with one or more of the poor prognostic factors, such as three or more sites of disease, bulky disease, B symptoms, poor performance status, or high serum LDH levels. The treatment of choice for advanced-stage aggressive lymphoma is combination chemotherapy. Treatment has improved since the mid-1970s. Before the introduction of combination chemotherapy, 5-year survival was essentially zero. The first significant improvement in treatment outcome came with the use of MOPP and C-MOPP, which induced complete responses in about 45% of patients, and most patients who achieved complete remission remained disease free for as long as 24 years.[179] After a median follow-up of 15 years, 37% of patients remain free of disease. The durability of the complete remissions stood in contrast to the brief remissions seen in patients with indolent lymphoma. It is the experience among physicians who treat lymphoma patients that those with aggressive lymphoma are frequently cured of disease. A patient diagnosed with an aggressive lymphoma has a greater likelihood of living 10 years than a patient diagnosed with an indolent lymphoma. Research on the development of curative programs for indolent lymphoma has proceeded much more slowly, partially because of the widespread use of a palliative approach to its treatment.

On the other hand, treatment programs for aggressive lymphoma have progressed to the point that more than 60% of patients with advanced-stage disease are being cured (Tables 52–18 and 52–19). Treatment programs have become more aggressive but only a little more toxic and have produced substantial increases in the fraction of patients achieving complete response. Unlike indolent lymphoma patients who may live several years with active disease, survival with aggressive lymphoma is short. The only chance for prolonged survival in patients with aggressive lymphoma is to obtain a durable complete response.

During the 17 years since the initial success of C-MOPP was reported, the development of new chemotherapy programs has burgeoned. The treatment outcome with these regimens has generally fallen into three groups. The first group of regimens includes C-MOPP, BACOP (in two different dose schedules), COMLA, and CHOP.[179,406,530–534] They produce complete response rates of 45% to 55% and long-term survival rates of 30% to 35%. The second group of regimens includes M-BACOD, m-BACOD, COP-BLAM, CAP-BOP, ACOMLA, ProMACE/MOPP flexitherapy, and ProMACE-MOPP.[534–541] They produce complete response rates of 70% to 75% and long-term survival rates of 45% to 50%. The third group of regimens includes COP-BLAM III, Mega-COMLA, MACOP-B, ProMACE-CytaBOM, F-MACHOP, VACOP-B, and LNH-84.[538,541–547] They produce complete response rates over 80% and long-term survival rates of 60% to 65%.

A fourth group may have begun. Gulati and his colleagues at Memorial Sloan-Kettering Cancer Center have conducted a pilot study with poor-prognosis patients using high-dose therapy with cyclophosphamide plus TBI followed by ABMT.[548] All the patients achieved complete responses, and 79% are long-term disease-free survivors. A common thread through the development of improved treatment approaches is the augmentation of the dose intensity of the treatment program (Table 52–20).

Despite the accumulated experience suggesting that the likelihood of a favorable treatment outcome has improved over the last 17 years, there has been some resistance to this idea. Critics have pointed out the absence (until recently) of controlled trials showing that one regimen is superior to another. Others observed that some of the regimens have been reported by referral centers whose patient population may not reflect the same proportion of poor-prognosis patients seen

TABLE 52–18. The Most Active Chemotherapy Programs for Intermediate-Grade Lymphoma

COP-BLAM	*Day 1*	*Day 10*	*Day 14*	*Days 15–21*
Cyclophosphamide 400 mg/m² I.V.	×			No therapy
Doxorubicin 40 mg/m² I.V.	×			
Vincristine 1 mg/m² I.V.	×			
Procarbazine 100 mg/m² PO	×-------	-------×		
Prednisone 40 mg/m²	×-------	-------×		
Bleomycin 15 mg I.V.			×	

COP-BLAM III	*Day 1*	*Day 2*	*Day 3*	*Day 4*	*Day 5*
Cycle A					
Vincristine 1 mg/m²/day I.V. infusion	×-------	-------×			
Bleomycin 7.5 mg/m² I.V. bolus, then 7.5 mg/m²/day I.V. infusion	×-------	-------	-------	-------	-------×
Cyclophosphamide 350 mg/m² I.V.	×				
Doxorubicin 35 mg/m² I.V.	×				
Prednisone 40 mg/m² PO	×	×	×	×	×
Procarbazine 100 mg/m² PO	×	×	×	×	×

Cycle B

Like Cycle A without bleomycin and without day 2 of vincristine infusion

Week	1	3	7	10	13	16	19	22	25	28	31	34
Cycle	A	B	A	B	A	B	A	B	A	B	A	B

CAP-BOP	*Day 1*	*Day 7*	*Day 15*	*Day 21*
Cyclophosphamide 650 mg/m² I.V.	×			
Doxorubicin 50 mg/m² I.V.	×			
Procarbazine 100 mg/m² PO	×-------	-------×		
Vincristine 1.4 mg/m²			×	
Bleomycin 10 U/m² SC			×	
Prednisone 100 mg PO			×-------	-------×
Cycles repeated every 3–4 weeks				

ProMACE-CytaBOM	*Day 1*	*Day 8*	*Day 14*	*Day 15–21*
Cyclophosphamide 650 mg/m² I.V.	×			No therapy
Doxorubicin 25 mg/m² I.V.	×			
Etoposide 120 mg/m² I.V.	×			
Cytarabine 300 mg/m² I.V.		×		
Bleomycin 5 mg/m² I.V.		×		
Vincristine 1.4 mg/m² I.V.		×		
Methotrexate 120 mg/m² I.V.		× with leucovorin rescue		
Prednisone 60 mg/m² PO	×-------	-------	-------×	
Cotrimoxazole 2 PO bid throughout 6 cycles of therapy				

MACOP-B *Week*	*1*	*2*	*3*	*4*	*5*	*6*	*7*	*8*	*9*	*10*	*11*	*12*
Cyclophosphamide 350	×		×		×		×		×		×	
Doxorubicin 50 mg/m² I.V.	×		×		×		×		×		×	
Vincristine 1.4 mg/m² I.V.		×		×		×		×		×		×
Methotrexate 400 mg/m² I.V.*		×				×				×		
Bleomycin 10 mg/m² I.V.				×				×				×
Prednisone 75 mg/m² PO od	×-------	-------	-------	-------	-------	-------	-------	-------	-------	-------	-------	-------taper
Cotrimoxazole 2 PO bid	×-------	-------	-------	-------	-------	-------	-------	-------	-------	-------	-------	-------×

(continued)

TABLE 52–18. *(Continued)*

VACOP-B Week	1	2	3	4	5	6	7	8	9	10	11	12
Etoposide 50 mg/m² I.V. day 1			×				×				×	
100 mg/m² PO days 2, 3			×				×				×	
Doxorubicin 50 mg/m² I.V.	×		×		×		×		×		×	
Cyclophosphamide 350 mg/m² I.V.	×				×				×			
Vincristine 1.2 mg/m² I.V.*		×		×		×		×		×		×
Bleomycin 10 U/m² I.V.		×		×		×		×		×		×
Prednisone 45 mg/m² PO daily × 1 wk, then qod × 11 wk												
Cotrimoxazole double strength PO bid × 14 wk												
Ketoconazole 200 mg PO daily × 1 wk, then qod × 11 wk												
Cimetidine 600 mg PO bid × 1 wk, then qod × 11 wk												

LNH-84	*Day 1*	*Day 2*	*Day 3*	*Day 4*	*Day 5*
Induction					
Adriamycin 75 mg/m²	×				
Cyclophosphamide 1200 mg/m²	×				
Vindesine 2 mg/m²	×				×
Bleomycin 10 mg	×				×
Prednisone 60 mg/m²	×	×	×	×	×
Methotrexate 12 mg IT			×		

Week	8	9	10	11	12	13	14	15	16	17	18	19	20	21
Consolidation														
Methotrexate 3 g/m²	×		×											
Ifosfamide 1.5 g/m²					×		×							
Etoposide 300 mg/m²					×		×							
L-asparaginase 50,000 U/m²									×	×				
Cytarabine 100 mg/m² × 4 d												×		×

F-MACHOP *Hours*	0	12	36	42	48	60	66
Vincristine 0.5 mg/m²	×	×					
Cyclophosphamide 800 mg/m²			×				
5-Fluorouracil 15 mg/kg			×	×			
Cytosine arabinoside 1000 mg/m²				×	×		
Adriamycin 60 mg/m²					×		
Methotrexate 500 mg/m²						×	×
Prednisone 60 mg/m²	from day 1 to day 14						
Folinic acid 20 mg/m² I.V. q 12 h × 4 starting on hour 84							

* With leucovorin rescue.

in a population of patients not referred to secondary and tertiary care centers. It has been disconcerting that the originally reported results may not be replicated by others. For example, the MACOP-B regimen in the hands of its originators induced a complete response rate of 84% and an 8-year overall actuarial survival rate of 62%.[545] In other series, results varied widely with MACOP-B. Schneider and colleagues obtained a complete response in only 20 (53%) of 38 HIV-negative patients with diffuse large cell lymphoma, and the survival rate at short follow-up was 50%.[549] Similarly, SWOG investigators using MACOP-B reported complete responses in 54 (50%) of 109 patients with aggressive lymphoma, and a 51% survival rate at 3 years.[550] Vitolo and colleagues reported a 71% complete response rate (127 of 180) in patients with diffuse large cell lymphoma, and the overall survival rate was 60% at 3 years.[551]

Although lower response rates are often expected in group studies, one of the poorest results with MACOP-B was reported from a single-institution study, and an excellent result confirming the original report came from a multicenter study.

TABLE 52–19. Prospect for Long-term Survival With Recent Treatment Programs for Diffuse Aggressive Lymphoma

*Regimen**	*Complete Responses (CR)*	*Relapse Rate (RR)*	*Potential for Long-Term Survival (CR) × (1-RR)*
ProMACE/MOPP flexitherapy	60/75 (80%)	21/60 (35%)	52%
m-BACOD	59/86 (70%)	15/59 (25%)	52%
COP-BLAM	24/33 (73%)	4/24 (17%)	61%
CAP-BOP	37/51 (73%)	11/37 (30%)	51%
COP-BLAM III	43/51 (84%)	4/43 (9%)	76%
MACOP-B	104/125 (84%)	23/104 (21%)	66%
ProMACE/CytaBOM	80/95 (84%)	20/80 (25%)	63%
F-MACHOP	88/113 (78%)	17/88 (19%)	63%
LNH-84	553/737 (75%)	139/553 (25%)	56%

* These studies were conducted and reported at different times. The relapse rates cannot be considered to have reached the maximal level, because the denominators probably still include some patients who remain at risk of relapse. The calculated potential for long-term disease-free survival for these treatment programs probably overestimates the actual potential for cure in some studies, particularly those with the shortest patient follow-up. The dose and schedule of drugs in the regimens is given in Table 52–18.

One of the most active regimens, LNH-84, was originally described by results obtained in a multicenter study. The observed variability in outcome in different series using the same treatment regimen defies simple answers.

One important issue in the interpretation of clinical results is the degree to which the technology of delivering the regimen has been mastered. This issue has been effectively addressed in the radiation therapy community, in which the lack of standardization of technical issues was found to have a dramatic effect on the treatment outcome. The issue has not been addressed in a meaningful way for the delivery of chemotherapeutic agents, but systematic and periodic adjustments to published regimens are frequently made. Sometimes body surface area is rounded down (*i.e.*, calculated at 1.84, rounded to 1.8). A calculated dose of 11.5 mg of a drug may be delivered at 10 mg if the drug is packaged in 10-mg vials. Delays in

TABLE 52–20. Nine-Drug Relative Dose Intensities of 15 Primary Programs for Diffuse Aggressive Lymphomas

*Regimen**	*Duration of Treatment (mo)*	*Percentage of Long-Term Survival*	*9 Drugs*	*Drug Exposure During First 2 Weeks*
MACOP-B	3	62	0.51	5/6
ProMACE-CytaBOM	4.5	69	0.48	8/8
ProMACE-MOPP	6	54	0.44	6/7
ProMACE/MOPP flexitherapy	8	48	0.43	5/7
M-BACOD	7	48	0.42	5/6
COP BLAM III	9	65	0.40	6/6
BACOP	6	35	0.39	3/5
COP BLAM I	6	55	0.39	6/6
MOPP	6	35	0.36	4/4
COMLA	9	<33	0.28	2/4
CHOP	6	<30	0.26	4/4
LNH-84	4	67	0.70	5/5
F-MACHOP	5	68	0.64	7/7
VACOP-B	3	60	0.43	5/6
High-dose chemotherapy plus total-body irradiation	—	79	ablation	—

*The dose and schedule of drugs in the regimens is given in Table 52–18.

treatment not mandated by resolving toxicities are frequently made. All of these seemingly minor adjustments can accumulate to produce a serious compromise in dose intensity.

A major problem in the reporting of clinical trial results is that the actual dose intensity with which a regimen is delivered is not routinely given. A paper attempting to confirm a result may claim that the regimen was given as originally reported, but no objective data are presented to confirm the assertion. SWOG reported their results in a series of 78 patients treated with ProMACE-CytaBOM.[552] Ninety-seven patients were initially entered on the study from 43 institutions, but 19 patients (20%) were found in retrospect to be ineligible. The complete response rate in the eligible patients was 65%, 21% lower than that obtained at the NCI, a difference that was found to be statistically significant.[553] The SWOG researchers stated that 84% of the ProMACE-CytaBOM cycles were given "precisely as described and consistent with explicit rules for dose modification." However, SWOG capped vincristine at 2 mg rather than delivering the protocol dose of 1.4 mg/m^2. In contrast to the claim, none of the cycles were given as originally reported. It is not clear whether there were other significant modifications. In an effort to make objective comparisons, the SWOG investigators reported actual dose intensity of the therapy but used a method that did not account for delays in treatment and has been said to overestimate the delivered dose intensity.[554] This makes comparisons between the SWOG and NCI cohorts difficult. The use of the SWOG method for both cohorts found that SWOG patients received at least 12% less dose intense therapy. It is not known whether this magnitude of difference is biologically significant. Analysis of response rates by prognostic subset should control for the often claimed differences in prognostic factor composition between referral and cooperative group patient populations. Statistically significant differences between the complete response rates in the two cohorts were still seen after taking distinct prognostic factors into account. Perhaps there are quantifiable differences in drug delivery that may account for the differences in outcome. In the SWOG group, the average number of patients treated at any center was fewer than 3. There may be important aspects of delivering a regimen that are gained with experience. These factors should be examined before a failure to confirm high response rates is used to justify the use of an older treatment regimen for patients with a curable tumor.

Those who believe that the therapy for advanced-stage aggressive histology lymphoma has not improved obtained support for their view from the results of SWOG's randomized comparison of CHOP, m-BACOD, MACOP-B, and ProMACE-CytaBOM reported at the 1992 meeting of the American Society of Clinical Oncology.[555] The study shows no difference among the regimens. This conclusion is based on CHOP results at least 15% better than any previously published (overall survival of 45% rather than 30%), and results with the other regimens 15% to 20% poorer than previously reported. The expected 30% difference was not seen. Those who wish to place their faith in the results of this study must do so in preference to an increasing body of data showing that dose intensity is an important determinant of treatment outcome in this disease. In every tumor type in which chemotherapy is curative, there is evidence for a dose-response association with the outcome.

Meyer and colleagues reviewed the evidence from previously published randomized studies to assess the role of dose intensity in treatment outcome.[556] None of the studies directly addressed the role of dose intensity, but a metaanalysis of 14 trials involving over 2300 patients revealed that patients receiving the regimen with a higher projected dose intensity in a comparative trial were about one third more likely to achieve complete remission than those on the lower dose intensity regimen.

We previously analyzed the influence of projected dose intensity on the likelihood of survival among published regimens.[557] It is difficult to compare the dose intensity of regimens composed of different agents. However, for a hypothetical nine-drug regimen with optimal doses of all the agents, each regimen can be assigned a relative dose intensity in proportion the hypothetical standard. As shown in Figure 52–14, there is a significant linear relation between projected relative dose intensity and long-term survival. This method of examining results is interesting but limited. Some studies have begun reporting actual dose intensity data, which may provide a better idea of the role of dose intensity in outcome.

Kwak and colleagues reviewed the outcome of 115 patients treated at Stanford with CHOP, M-BACOD, or MACOP-B and found that an actual relative dose intensity of doxorubicin delivered in the first 12 weeks of therapy greater than 75% of the projected dose was the single most important predictor of survival.[558] Other clinical prognostic factors included performance status, high LDH levels, and extranodal sites of disease. However, this is the first study to demonstrate the prognostic significance of delivered dose intensity in aggressive lymphoma. It is tempting to suggest that administration of a higher dose intensity of doxorubicin would improve the outcome of patients who received lower-dose-intensity doxorubicin, but the data do not permit that extrapolation. It is presumed that doxorubicin was dose modified on the basis of encountered toxicity. There may be other biologic features of the lymphoma or the patient that affected the ability to deliver full doses of therapy. Higher doses of doxorubicin may not have improved the response. Nevertheless, the results certainly support the notion that dose intensity is an important determinant of treatment outcome, even though this treatment-related variable is not a prognostic factor in the usual sense of the term. Classic prognostic factors are features of the patient or the tumor determined before therapy.

Epelbaum and colleagues reviewed the contribution of dose intensity to the treatment outcome of 95 patients treated with CHOP.[559] They found that age over 60 years, advanced stage, male sex, and receiving less than the median dose intensity of any of the four drugs were significantly associated with a poorer survival. Using multivariate analysis, the average relative dose intensity below the median was the strongest prognostic factor predicting poor survival, followed by age over 60 years. Dose intensity appears to contribute to CHOP treatment outcome.

Banavali and colleagues attempted to improve on CHOP by altering the schedule of administration.[560] They administered cyclophosphamide (600 mg/m^2 given intravenously weekly for eight doses), doxorubicin (50 mg/m^2 given intravenously, weeks 1 and 5), vincristine (1.4 mg/m^2 given intravenously weekly for eight doses), and prednisone (40 mg/m^2 given orally daily for 4 weeks, then tapered). This was followed by

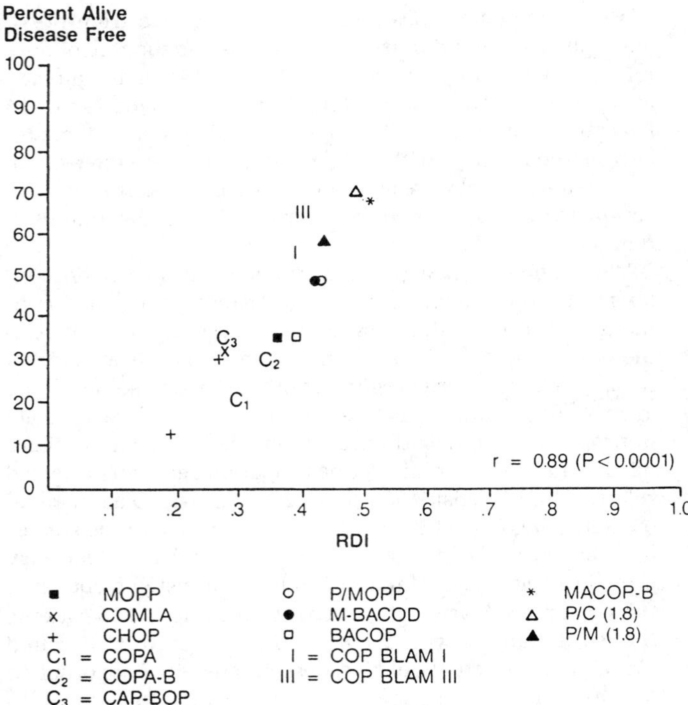

FIGURE 52–14. Relation between normalized nine-drug relative dose intensity (RDI) and disease-free survival of patients with diffuse large cell lymphomas. The 14 most extensively studied treatment programs for diffuse large cell lymphomas use nine drugs in some combination. Each regimen was evaluated for its relative dose intensity based on delivery of full doses of all nine drugs, although none of the programs achieved this ideal; they used four to eight drugs. The regimen that had the highest relative dose intensity was MACOP-B. Its dose intensity was arbitrarily rated as 1, and the other regimens were normalized to MACOP-B, giving a normalized nine-drug relative dose intensity. The long-term survival of each regimen was plotted against the normalized nine-drug relative dose intensity. A statistically significant correlation was found between dose intensity and disease-free survival.

CHOP therapy for 4 weeks every 2 months for 12 to 18 months. The dose intensity of cyclophosphamide, vincristine, and prednisone in the first 8 weeks were significantly augmented over standard CHOP. The complete response rate in 108 patients was 78%, with a 5-year survival rate of 53%. These results compare favorably to the 50% complete response rate and 30% long-term survival rate previously reported for CHOP. Similar increments in response rates and survival were found with Mega-COMLA compared with COMLA.[543] The dose intensity of the cyclophosphamide was doubled by shortening the cycle to 6 weeks from 12. In a small number of patients, the complete response rate was 80%, and 25% of the complete responders relapsed within a median follow-up of 26 months. Conclusions are difficult because of the sporadic use of radiation therapy and CHOP consolidation therapy. However, the results appeared to be an improvement over conventional COMLA.

Improving the dose intensity of CHOP-bleo did not appear to improve the treatment outcome in a series of patients treated at the M.D. Anderson Cancer Center.[561] Nonconcurrent series of patients were treated with conventional doses or maximal tolerated doses (with laminar flow room support) of CHOP-bleo. The conventional-dose regimen was given at about 80% of the dose intensity of the high-dose regimen. Yet the complete response rates (75% for conventional dose; 81% for high dose) and overall survival (53% for conventional dose; 48% for high dose) were not significantly different. There were more good-prognosis patients on the conventional-dose regimen, but it appears that the 20% difference in dose intensity did not translate into an improved outcome. It seems clear that lowering the dose intensity of a regimen can adversely alter its efficacy. The administration of half-dose CHOP to patients, as was routinely done for patients over age 65, resulted in long-term survival in only 12% of patients, compared with 41% in those given full-dose CHOP. Of course, it is also possible that this poorer result was related to differences in the older patient population.

No prospective randomized study with dose intensity as the only variable has been conducted. However, two prospective randomized trials comparing two regimens with substantial overlap in active agents show significant advantages to the regimen with the higher dose intensity. At the NCI, we compared ProMACE-MOPP to ProMACE-CytaBOM in 193 patients with advanced-stage aggressive lymphoma.[541] The complete response rate was significantly higher for ProMACE-CytaBOM (86%) than ProMACE-MOPP (74%), and the projected 8-year survival rate was significantly higher for ProMACE-CytaBOM (69%) than ProMACE-MOPP (53%) (Fig. 52–15). The two regimens share six drugs; five of the six are delivered with greater dose intensity in ProMACE-CytaBOM, and the sixth, methotrexate, has been demonstrated by the Dana-Farber group to make no significant impact on outcome when its dose intensity is reduced (M-BACOD and m-BACOD are similar in efficacy but differ in methotrexate dose intensity).[563] It is possible that the cytarabine and bleomycin in ProMACE-CytaBOM are more active than the mechlorethamine and procarbazine in ProMACE-MOPP, but it seems more likely that the advantage to ProMACE-CytaBOM is related to dose intensity. This is the first randomized study in aggressive lymphoma to demonstrate the superiority of one doxorubicin-containing regimen over another.

Comparison of ProMACE-MOPP to the early NCI study of ProMACE/MOPP flexitherapy allows some evaluation of the Goldie-Coldman hypothesis.[540,562] The Goldie-Coldman hypothesis predicted that earlier exposure of the tumor to non-cross-resistant agents would result in a lower probability of

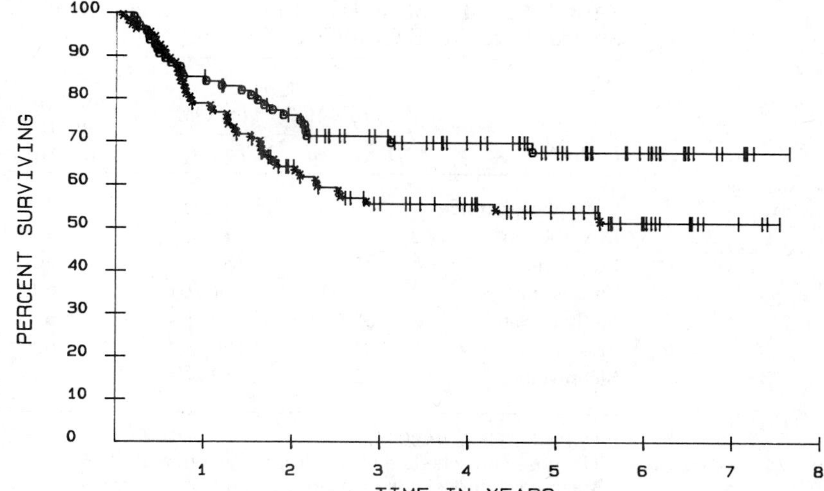

FIGURE 52–15. Survival for patients with advanced-stage lymphoma treated with ProMACE-MOPP (*), for which 44 of 99 failed, or ProMACE-CytaBOM (○), for which 28 of 94 failed, is plotted from the first treatment date to the death date. Four patients died of intercurrent conditions unrelated to lymphoma or its treatment and are censored. All deaths related to lymphoma or lymphoma treatment are plotted. Mantel-Haenszel test for a difference between treatments showed that $p_2 = 0.046$.

developing drug resistance. If this were true, ProMACE-MOPP, which brings the MOPP drugs into the first cycle, should be more effective than ProMACE/MOPP flexitherapy, in which exposure to the MOPP drugs is delayed for 2 or 3 months. However, the results of the two regimens were almost identical: complete response rates were 75% and 74%, and long-term survival rates were 50% and 53% for ProMACE/MOPP flexitherapy and ProMACE-MOPP, respectively. These results represent an excellent internal standard for the consistency of the NCI treatment effects, but they appear to cast some doubt on the ability to improve treatment on the basis of the Goldie-Coldman predictions.

The European Organization for Research and Treatment of Cancer conducted a prospective randomized trial comparing their CHOP-related regimen, CHVmP (in which teniposide replaces vincristine) to the same regimen with vincristine and bleomycin added (CHVmP+VB).[563] CHVmP+VB was significantly better than CHVmP in complete response rate and survival. The complete response rate to CHVmP+VB was 80%, and the 5-year survival rate was 53%. These values were significantly better than the 50% complete response rate and 29% survival rate seen on the CHVmP arm. The improved outcome is clearly related to adding two active agents without compromising the doses of the other four drugs and with no significant additional toxicity. The durability of the complete remissions was comparable with the two regimens, suggesting that the major benefit was obtained because more patients achieved a complete response.

Pilot studies of newer regimens suggest that survival of patients with aggressive lymphoma is improving, and a feature of all the newer regimens is increased dose intensity. COP-BLAM III achieves high-dose intensity partially through the use of infusional drug delivery. MACOP-B involves the weekly delivery of agents. ProMACE-CytaBOM delivers eight active drugs 2 weeks out of 3. F-MACHOP consists of seven drugs administered sequentially within the first 3 days of a treatment cycle. All of these regimens achieve complete responses in 80% or more of patients, and long-term survival rates of 60% or more.

Another treatment experience that favors a role for dose intensity is that of Gulati and colleagues who used myeloablative doses of therapy to treat a group of poor-prognosis patients at Memorial Sloan-Kettering Cancer Center.[548] CHOP therapy and other less aggressive conventional-dose regimens had obtained a 20% survival rate for patients with high LDH levels, large abdominal masses, and B symptoms. However, when treated with high-dose cyclophosphamide plus TBI and ABMT, survival was 79%. This study and those plotted in Figure 52–14 support the conclusion that there is a linear relation between dose intensity and treatment outcome. The data imply that further augmentation of dose intensity may lead to improvements in treatment outcome. However, it may also be true that the dose intensity–survival curve is about to change slopes or plateau and that additional increases in dose intensity would not improve survival.

Although these data seem to support the importance of dose intensity in the treatment of aggressive lymphoma, proof requires a prospective randomized trial in which the only variable is the delivered dose intensity. The availability of colony-stimulating factors may permit dose escalation of the myelotoxic agents, but most of the agents active in lymphoma produce thrombocytopenia and neutropenia. The approved colony-stimulating factors are not effective at preventing or promoting the recovery from thrombocytopenia.

There are other ways of augmenting dose intensity than increasing the doses of the myelotoxic agents. The major variables in dose intensity are amount of drug delivered and time between drug administrations. It is possible to increase dose intensity by increasing individual doses or by administering the drugs closer together. Weekly therapy or continuous infusion therapy are two approaches to augmenting dose intensity that do not require intensive marrow support with factors or transplantation. At the NCI, we have shortened the ProMACE-CytaBOM treatment cycle to 2 weeks by lowering the dose of the myelotoxic agents but have increased their dose intensity by moving their delivery closer together. Table 52–21 compares the delivered dose intensity of the short-cycle ProMACE-CytaBOM with standard ProMACE-CytaBOM. Each agent was delivered with significantly higher dose intensity in the 2-week cycle regimen. Of the first 45 patients, 41 (92%) achieved a complete response, and 7 (17%) of the complete responders relapsed, with a median follow-

TABLE 52–21. Mean Dose Intensity of Short Course Versus Standard ProMACE-CytaBOM

Drugs*	Short ProMACE-CytaBOM Delivered	Short ProMACE-CytaBOM (Projected)	Increased Actual Dose Intensity† Compared With Standard P-C	ProMACE-CytaBOM Delivered	ProMACE-CytaBOM (Projected)
Cyclophosphamide	220.4	(237.5)	27%	173.7	(217)
Doxorubicin	9.5	(10)	44%	6.6	(8.3)
Etoposide	47.6	(50)	46%	32.7	(40)
Vincristine	.64	(.70)	60%	0.40	(.46)
Methotrexate	53.1	(60)	52%	34.9	(40)
Ara-C	136	(150)	65%	82.6	(100)
Bleomycin	2.3	(2.5)	64%	1.4	(1.7)

P-C, ProMACE-CytaBOM.
* The dose and schedule of the drugs is given in Table 52–18.
† Mean dose intensity is measured in units of mg/m^2/week.

up of 18 months. Although it is still early in the course of this pilot study, it is clear that dose intensity has been increased, myelotoxicity is actually somewhat reduced, and high response rates have been maintained. A randomized study comparing the two methods of delivering ProMACE-CytaBOM would probably represent a true test of the dose intensity question.

Toxicities of Therapy for Aggressive Lymphomas

All of the effective treatment programs for the aggressive lymphomas produce myelosuppression. In general, the degree of myelosuppression is a function of the manner in which the drugs are given. The recommended doses are normalized to body surface area, but these starting guidelines may be adjusted up or down based on the response of the individual patient. We recommend 10% upward adjustment of doses if the patient does not develop a leukocyte nadir below 2000/mm^3 or a platelet nadir below 100,000/mm^3. More commonly, it is necessary to reduce the doses of myelotoxic agents because of granulocyte nadirs below 500/mm^3 or platelet count nadirs below 20,000/mm^3 or prolonged duration of nadir. The regimens are published with a sliding scale for modification of each agent based on nadir depth or duration. Patients with cytopenias based on bone marrow involvement should not undergo dose reduction but should receive full dose therapy with appropriate hospitalization and expectant management of febrile neutropenia and thrombocytopenia.

If a patient does not experience myelosuppression during treatment for aggressive lymphoma, the patient is not receiving enough therapy. Infectious complications from myelosuppression occurring in the MACOP-B, VACOP-B, and ProMACE-CytaBOM regimens appear to be significantly reduced by including cotrimoxazole prophylaxis. The treatment-related mortality rate from MACOP-B and VACOP-B was 3%. The treatment-related mortality rate for ProMACE-CytaBOM was 6% because of deaths early in the study from *Pneumocystis carinii* pneumonia.[564] After institution of cotrimoxazole prophylaxis, there were no toxic deaths in the last 59 patients. Another useful effect of the antibiotic treatment was a significant reduction in episodes of febrile neutropenia.[541] Many patients with a history of sulfa allergy are able to tolerate the cotrimoxazole, perhaps because of the concomitant administration of prednisone. However, for patients who cannot take sulfa, monthly aerosolized pentamidine has been used anecdotally with success in preventing interstitial pneumonitis, but it does not reduce episodes of febrile neutropenia. No patient should receive ProMACE-CytaBOM without some form of *Pneumocystis* prophylaxis.

Other toxic effects depend on the regimen. MACOP-B and m-BACOD induce mucositis in 40% or more of patients. This side effect can be reduced in frequency and severity with the use of prophylactic ketoconazole, careful oral hygiene, removal of dentures, particularly if they are ill fitting, and the use of acyclovir in patients with perioral herpes simplex infection. VACOP-B, F-MACHOP, and ProMACE-CytaBOM are associated with much lower rates of mucositis. Skin rashes may occur in 2% to 10% of patients, usually related to bleomycin or procarbazine. Bleomycin, particularly when used with methotrexate, may contribute to mucositis, but the most serious toxic effect is the induction of pulmonary infiltrates in as many as 20% of patients on the m-BACOD program; other regimens are associated with a frequency of 5% or less. Vincristine may be associated with paresthesias or gait disturbances, all of which are reversible. The most serious toxic effect of vincristine other than skin infiltration with local necrosis is obstipation. Stool softeners and laxatives may prevent or ameliorate vincristine-induced bowel problems.

Doxorubicin is contraindicated in patients with congestive heart failure, but the dose and schedule employed in most of the regimens is rarely associated with the induction of heart failure in the absence of a preexisting cardiomyopathy. Mitoxantrone can effectively replace doxorubicin in some lymphoma treatment programs without loss of efficacy, and mitoxantrone is much less cardiotoxic (conversion factor: 1 mg mitoxantrone = 5 mg doxorubicin).[565]

Prednisone administered intermittently may uncover latent diabetes or make glucose control in known diabetics somewhat more difficult. Continuous prednisone for more than a month, as used in MACOP-B and VACOP-B, can be associated with peptic ulcer disease. Prophylaxis with H_2-blockers may be prudent. The doses of cyclophosphamide used in most lymphoma regimens only rarely induce hemorrhagic cystitis. Substitution of an alternative alkylating agent such as chlorambucil may be done in this setting.

Treatment of the Older Patient With Aggressive Lymphoma

The age range for patients with aggressive lymphoma is quite large, and many patients are older than 65 at diagnosis. Advanced age is not a contraindication to using an effective combination chemotherapy program. Age is generally a surrogate measure for physiologic reserve. A 50-year-old patient with diabetes, hypertension, and a myocardial infarction within the last year may do considerably more poorly than an 80-year-old patient who mowed his own grass until last month. Prognostic factor analysis may demonstrate that age makes a significant impact on outcome, but this piece of data may have diverse contributions. For example, some studies have given older patients 50% of the projected dose of a regimen to avoid toxicity. In other studies, deaths from intercurrent illness have not been identified specifically and may look like treatment-related deaths or treatment failures. Vose and colleagues analyzed 112 patients older than 60 years at diagnosis and found that their complete response, disease-free survival, and overall survival rates were not different from those of younger patients if deaths unrelated to lymphoma or its treatment were excluded.[566] SWOG data demonstrate that anticipatory dose reductions compromise treatment efficacy.[567] Although there are no prospective studies on this topic, clinical experience suggests that older patients may experience somewhat more myelotoxicity than younger patients when drug doses are administered on the basis of body surface area. Although the myelotoxicity from the drugs is dose related, it should be possible to find a dose of the drugs that can be safely administered.

Some investigators have attempted to develop special treatment programs for older patients.[568,569] Most of these therapies are lower in drug dose intensity than standard regimens, and they are associated with poorer results. We recommend that older patients receive standard chemotherapy regimens. If there are legitimate concerns about toxicity because of an existing comorbid condition, a 10% to 20% dose reduction may be used initially. However, further treatment should be based on toxicities actually experienced by the patient rather than making anticipatory dose reductions. Many older patients are willing to cope with acute toxicity for the prospect of prolonged disease-free survival.

TREATMENT OF HIGHLY AGGRESSIVE LYMPHOMAS

The highly aggressive lymphomas are the diffuse small noncleaved cell lymphomas, which include Burkitt's and non-Burkitt's subsets, lymphoblastic lymphoma, and HTLV-I-related adult T-cell lymphoma. These are rare tumors in adults. The diffuse small noncleaved cell lymphomas and lymphoblastic lymphomas are more common in children than in adults, and the most successful approaches to their treatment in adults are those that have been proven effective in children. HTLV-I-related ATL is moderately common in regions where the virus is endemic. It has been estimated that the cumulative lifetime risk of developing ATL among HTLV-I-infected persons in Saga, Japan, is about 4.5% for men and 2.6% for women.[570] Because the highly aggressive lymphomas are frequently disseminated at diagnosis, the application of a rigid staging schema is not useful.

The diffuse small noncleaved cell lymphomas (non-Burkitt's) have often been lumped together with diffuse large cell lymphomas in series reporting treatment results. These lymphomas account for fewer than 10% of the cases of diffuse lymphomas. In the older literature, they were called diffuse undifferentiated lymphomas. The small number of homogenously treated patients prohibits making definitive conclusions about their response to treatment. In the last 14 years, the NCI has obtained a complete response rate of 84% for patients with this histology treated with ProMACE-based chemotherapy regimens; 14% of the complete responders have relapsed, and the long-term survival rate is 67%.

Much depends on the reproducibility of the histologic diagnosis. Burkitt's and non-Burkitt's varieties are often difficult to differentiate. The major difference involves the degree of homogeneity of the nuclear size; Burkitt's tumors are highly homogenous, and non-Burkitt's are more heterogenous. Both tumor types have a high growth fraction and may show rapid clinical progression. A review of the molecular genetics of these two entities lent credence to the notion that they can be reliably separated. Seventeen of 18 Burkitt's tumors were found to have *MYC* rearrangements; none of 11 non-Burkitt's tumors had *MYC* rearrangements.[571] These genetic results and the excellent clinical results obtained with second- and third-generation aggressive lymphoma treatment regimens may mean that the subtle histologic differences in these entities are biologically and clinically significant.

McMaster and colleagues devised a high-intensity, brief-duration combination chemotherapy program for diffuse small noncleaved cell lymphomas that includes cyclophosphamide, doxorubicin, etoposide, vincristine, bleomycin, methotrexate, and prednisone.[572] In 20 adult patients (16 were stage IV), the complete response rate was 85%, and with a median follow-up of 29 months, 65% of patients remain disease free. On the basis of current information, this program or one of the more recent regimens used in aggressive histology lymphoma appear to be excellent choices for the therapy of this rare lymphoma subtype.

Several treatment programs have been effective for patients with Burkitt's lymphoma. Straus and colleagues treated 28 adult patients with an intensive chemotherapy program also used in patients with lymphoblastic leukemia.[573] Fifty-nine percent of the HIV-negative patients with Burkitt's lymphoma were long-term disease-free survivors. The CHOMP regimen of Magrath has a similar level of efficacy; almost 60% of patients can be cured.[574] Patients in whom bulky disease could be surgically removed have an even better outcome (81% 3-year survival).

Schwenn and colleagues performed a pilot study with high-intensity short-duration therapy for children with advanced-stage Burkitt's lymphoma.[575] The regimen included cyclophosphamide, high-dose methotrexate, high-dose cytarabine, and vincristine; the complete response rate for the first 20 patients was 95%, and the survival rate at a median follow-up of 3 years is 75%. This regimen is promising because of the high response rate and because of the short duration of the therapy. Most of the other effective regimens in Burkitt's lymphoma have treated patients for 1 to 2 years.

Lymphoblastic lymphoma is overwhelmingly a tumor of thymocyte origin. It is difficult to differentiate from acute lymphoblastic leukemia on morphologic grounds. Many workers use the degree of bone marrow involvement as the criterion to separate lymphoblastic lymphoma from lymphoblastic leukemia; leukemia is present if neoplastic cells account for 25% or more of the marrow cells. Lymphoblastic lymphoma has a high propensity to involve the mediastinum (presumably related to thymus origin or tropism), the bone marrow, and the CNS and has a high male preponderance.[576] Lymphoma treatment regimens may induce responses, but the responses are generally short.[577]

Many of the regimens that are active in Burkitt's lymphoma are also active in lymphoblastic lymphoma, including CHOMP. The APO regimen and the LSA_2-L_2 regimen are the most widely used and result in long-term survival of as many as 75% of patients.[578,579] Application of these regimens to adults has been slow, and the results have not been uniform. Complete response rates are high, but it appears that adults require early CNS prophylaxis to minimize the risk of CNS relapse.[580] However, when the dose of systemic therapy is modified to accommodate early CNS prophylaxis, systemic relapse is more common. The high relapse rate seen in adults with lymphoblastic lymphoma has prompted some workers to perform high-dose therapy with autologous or allogeneic bone marrow transplantation in patients in first remission. Among 36 adult patients treated with an LSA_2-L_2-type protocol, 18 patients in first remission underwent high-dose cyclophosphamide therapy plus TBI and autologous marrow reinfusion.[581] Fourteen of the 18 patients are alive and continue in remission a median of 46 months off therapy. These promising results suggest that the optimal treatment approach in the adult would be to use CHOMP, APO, or LSA_2-L_2 to obtain a complete response and then administer high-dose cyclophosphamide plus TBI followed by ABMT.

HTLV-I-related ATL is a rare disease that is highly responsive to chemotherapy. However, aggressive therapy is poorly tolerated because of the underlying immunodeficiency in ATL patients. Aggressive treatment generally leads to a treatment-related death from opportunistic infection. The clinical events in HTLV-I-related ATL are not very different from those seen in patients with HIV-associated lymphoma. Long-term disease-free survival has not been reported for ATL patients. The clinical syndrome has different prognostic factors based on whether a leukemia picture or a lymphoma picture predominate: leukocyte count and percentage of neoplastic cells in the circulation are prognostic factors for leukemic patients; serum calcium level is prognostic for lymphoma patients.[582] Waldmann pioneered the clinical use of antibodies directed against the IL-2 receptor with some transient responses.[583] Yttrium 90-labeled antibodies have shown more significant antitumor effects in a few patients. There is evidence that IL-1 may be an autocrine stimulating factor for ATL.[584] If this is true, there may be clinical efficacy with the use of the naturally occurring IL-1 antagonists. It seems unlikely that a chemotherapy-based approach can be successful unless it becomes possible to reverse the underlying immunodeficiency. Biologic approaches to treatment may hold more promise for success.

CENTRAL NERVOUS SYSTEM LYMPHOMA

Lymphomas may involve the CNS in two ways: primary CNS lymphoma, which causes mass lesions and usually is not associated with systemic lymphoma, and secondary lymphoma, which most often involves the meninges without mass lesions and usually occurs in the setting of relapsed or growing systemic lymphoma, usually involving bone or bone marrow, testes, or sinuses. Primary CNS lymphoma is increasing in frequency. It complicates the course of immunodeficiency diseases, including AIDS, which are increasing in frequency, but also there is an increase in the incidence of primary CNS lymphoma in immunocompetent persons.[585] Secondary CNS lymphoma is decreasing in frequency, largely due to the incorporation of high-dose methotrexate in the treatment programs and the use of CNS prophylaxis in patients with known risk factors for secondary CNS involvement.

Primary CNS lymphoma accounts for about 2% of brain tumors and 2% of all lymphomas. Most CNS lymphomas are of B-cell origin and are diffuse aggressive lymphomas histologically. In immunosuppressed patients, EBV is frequently detected and implicated in the cause. It appears on CT scan as a lesion of increased density in at least two thirds of patients and uniformly enhances with contrast, usually homogenously.[586] The lymphoma often occurs in the frontal lobes or involves deep central brain structures and may produce multiple lesions, leading to confusion with metastatic carcinoma.

The most common symptoms of CNS lymphoma are headache, visual disturbances (*e.g.,* blurred or double vision), mental changes (*e.g.,* memory loss, dementia, personality changes), nausea, vomiting, and seizures. The major neurologic findings are hemiparesis, papilledema, visual field defects, and cranial nerve palsies. The cerebrospinal fluid usually has a high protein level but no malignant cells.

CNS lymphoma is responsive to radiation therapy, but intracranial relapses are common, and the median survival is 12 to 18 months, not much greater than the survival of other primary brain neoplasms.[587] After surgical removal of as much tumor as possible, patients are usually treated with whole-brain irradiation to about 4000 cGy, with a boost to the primary lesion of about 1500 cGy. Some have advocated irradiating the spinal axis, but with a clinical failure rate in the spinal cord of only 4%, this practice seems unwarranted. About 90% of primary CNS lymphoma relapses are in the CNS; fewer than 10% of patients have relapses outside the CNS. Improved survival has been reported with the use of chemotherapy in addition to radiation therapy, including VEPA (cyclophosphamide, doxorubicin, vincristine, prednisone), high-dose methotrexate, and DHAP (dexamethasone, high-dose cytarabine, cisplatin).[588–590] Efforts to osmotically open the blood-brain barrier have been claimed to improve outcome.[591] Chamberlain and Levin administered irradiation with hydroxyurea as a radiation sensitizer and then gave adjuvant chemotherapy with procarbazine, CCNU, and vincristine.[592] The median survival of their 10 patients was 30 months, which seems significantly longer than that seen with radiation therapy alone. However, most of the reported treatment experiences are elaborate anecdotes without appropriate controls, and although there is appropriate optimism about the use of drugs, it is not yet clear whether systemic chemotherapy with or without radiation therapy is superior to radiation therapy alone. Nevertheless, efforts to improve the results with radiation therapy are needed.

Secondary CNS lymphoma usually occurs in patients with diffuse lymphoma. If a patient with indolent lymphoma develops CNS signs and symptoms, it usually represents histologic progression to aggressive lymphoma. The usual treatment approach is to administer methotrexate, cytarabine, or thiotepa alone or in combination into the spinal canal by repeated spinal taps (which requires concurrent cranial irradiation to treat the meninges over the convexities) or by way of an indwelling Ommaya reservoir.[593] The CNS disease is usually treated at the same time that therapy is administered for peripheral disease. Meningeal lymphoma can usually be eradicated, but survival is limited due to uncontrolled systemic disease. CNS symptoms can be produced by expanding nodal or extranodal masses that cause cord compression. This complication occurs in about 2% of lymphoma cases and is best managed by local radiation treatment together with systemic treatment, if the symptoms have an acute onset, but combination chemotherapy alone may be used if the symptoms developed gradually and have not progressed to complete cord block. The decision about whether to use radiation therapy is usually aided by obtaining a MR scan to better define the anatomy of the spinal cord involvement.

Orbital lymphomas are rare and can be a site of spread to or from the CNS. Local control may be achieved with radiation therapy, but CNS relapse is common. Orbital lymphomas should be treated with combined-modality therapy.

HIV-ASSOCIATED LYMPHOCYTIC LYMPHOMAS

Within 5 years of the original description of AIDS, it was found that HIV infection was associated with an increased incidence of malignant lymphoma.[594] Lymphocytic lymphomas occur approximately 60 times more frequently in AIDS patients than in the general population.[595] Approximately 3% of all cases of AIDS reported to the Centers for Disease Control had an associated lymphocytic lymphoma. Nineteen percent were primary lymphomas of the brain. Lymphomas occurred in all risk groups, but most occurred in homosexuals. This is probably due to the high prevalence of homosexuals in the U.S. AIDS population, but the incidence of lymphoma is also highest in hemophiliacs and homosexuals and lowest in intravenous drug abusers and persons who acquired HIV by heterosexual contact.[595] The incidence of lymphoma in AIDS patients appears to be increasing. Pluda and coworkers estimate that the probability of AIDS patients on antiretroviral therapy developing a lymphoma by 36 months is 29%.[596,597] The rising incidence is probably related to the prolonged immunosuppression that accompanies the increased survival, which is a consequence of the improvements in treating HIV-associated infectious complications and HIV itself. However, the possibility of a direct etiologic role for antiretroviral therapy in lymphomagenesis cannot be excluded. These data predict that almost 4000 excess cases of lymphocytic lymphoma occurred in 1992 because of HIV infection. This represents almost 10% of all cases of lymphocytic lymphomas.

Lymphomas occur in patients across the entire spectrum of HIV infection.[594,598–604] They are seen in patients with AIDS, AIDS-related complex, progressive generalized lymphadenopathy and in asymptomatic HIV-positive patients. In the early descriptions of lymphoma in AIDS patients, most had already experienced an AIDS-defining illness, such as an opportunistic infection or Kaposi's sarcoma at the time the lymphoma was identified, but some reports described a greater occurrence in HIV-positive asymptomatic patients.[594,600,605,606] Currently, the initial AIDS-defining illness is lymphoma in 3% of all HIV-infected patients.

The spectrum of lymphomas observed in HIV-infected patients is different from that seen in the nonimmunosuppressed population but similar to what is observed in patients with congenital immunodeficiencies or those receiving immunosuppressive therapy after organ transplantation. The most common histologic subtypes are diffuse small noncleaved cell, immunoblastic, and large cell lymphomas.[598–604] Most tumors are high grade according to the Working Formulation and are of B-cell origin; only rare T-cell tumors have been identified. Low-grade lymphomas have been described, but they do not necessarily occur at a higher frequency than in the normal population. The lymphomas occurring in the less symptomatic population (*i.e.*, higher CD4 cell count) are most often of the diffuse small noncleaved cell type, and those occurring in patients with AIDS (*i.e.*, lowest CD4 cell count) tend to be extranodal presentations of immunoblastic and large cell histologic subtypes.[604–607]

Although the exact pathogenesis of AIDS-related lymphomas is unknown, many interrelated factors appear to be involved. As in other lymphomas, EBV and the *MYC* oncogene have been implicated.[608] However, EBV is found in fewer than 50% of HIV-related lymphomas, and *MYC* gene rearrangements are found in a minority of tumors.[48] Shiramizu and colleagues performed a molecular analysis of 40 HIV-positive lymphomas to determine clonality, EBV infection, and the status of the *MYC* oncogene.[608] All were B-cell tumors whose cells were not infected with HIV. Six different tumor types were identified. They observed polyclonal lymphomas that were EBV positive or EBV negative; they observed monoclonal EBV-positive and EBV-negative tumors that had unrearranged, germline *MYC;* and they identified monoclonal EBV-positive and EBV-negative tumors that had undergone characteristic rearrangements of the *MYC* oncogene. There appear to be multiple mechanisms of lymphomagenesis in AIDS patients.

The clinical characteristics of patients with HIV-associated lymphoma differ markedly from those seen in the healthy population.[598–605] The median age at diagnosis is 38 years, compared with 56 years for HIV-negative patients. Patients present with advanced symptomatic disease with frequent involvement of extranodal sites. Between 64% and 83% of patients have stage III or IV disease, and 65% to 91% have involvement of extranodal sites. The most frequently involved extranodal sites include the CNS in 26% (*i.e.*, parenchymal, leptomeningeal), bone marrow in 22%, gastrointestinal tract in 17%, and liver in 12%.[603,606] Involvement with lymphoma has been identified in some unusual sites: lung, oral cavity, Waldeyer's ring, rectum, salivary glands, heart, bone, kidney, adrenal, and orbit.[7,15]

As many as 30% of patients present with stage IE disease, and most of these patients have primary lymphoma of the brain. These patients tend to be the sickest; they have the lowest CD4 cell counts; they have usually already had one or more opportunistic infections; and a significant number of them are not diagnosed with lymphoma until postmortem examination. The delay in diagnosis is probably related to the combination of an insufficient suspicion of the possibility and the difficult differential diagnosis. Most patients with primary CNS lymphoma have symptoms.[603] Focal findings such as hemiparesis or aphasia occur in 35%, seizures in 15%, and cranial nerves palsies in 10%. However, more subtle symptoms, such as confusion, lethargy, or memory loss, may be the only abnormality. It is important to remain alert to the possibility of primary CNS lymphoma in HIV-infected patients.

Radiologic studies are not diagnostic, and lymphoma can easily be confused with toxoplasmosis, a common opportunistic pathogen in AIDS patients. Both can present as space-occupying, contrast-enhancing lesions that may be associated with edema. Lymphomas are more often solitary and usually bigger than the lesions of toxoplasmosis, but this is not absolute. The diagnosis of lymphoma may be strongly suspected by scans, but a definitive diagnosis can only be obtained by brain biopsy. Current practice is to empirically treat equivocal lesions as if they were toxoplasmosis for 1 week, after which a repeat CT scan is performed and followed by a brain biopsy if improvement is not observed.[603]

The treatment of primary CNS lymphoma in an immunocompetent person is unsatisfactory. The use of radiotherapy can be associated with complete remissions, but long-term survival of these patients is rare. AIDS patients with CNS lymphoma are usually extremely ill at diagnosis with poor performance status, and 50% or more die of opportunistic infections.

AIDS patients with disseminated lymphoma have been treated with standard combination chemotherapy regimens that have proven to be effective in nonimmunosuppressed patients with intermediate-grade lymphomas.[598–604,609,610] This approach has been unsuccessful with few long-term disease-free survivors. Many regimens have been used, and complete remission rates of approximately 50% and median survival of 5 to 7 months have been produced. Treatment is poorly tolerated in most of these patients, many of whom have bone marrow involvement and most of whom have poor bone marrow reserve. Multiple dose reductions were given, and limited numbers of cycles could be given. Opportunistic infections occurred in more than half the patients during treatment without *Pneumocystis carinii* pneumonia (PCP) prophylaxis, and although the incidence of PCP can be reduced by as much as 50% if prophylaxis is employed, it cannot be eliminated. Relapse from complete remission is common (33–50%), and in the early studies, relapse in the CNS was not uncommon. Attempts to use more aggressive chemotherapy appear to have actually reduced overall survival in at least two trials. Granulocyte-macrophage colony-stimulating factor (GM-CSF) administered after chemotherapy reduces the granulocyte nadir, reduces the number of days that granulocytes are below 500/mm^3, and reduces the frequency of hospitalization for fever and granulocytopenia.[609]

A study employed low-dose M-BACOD with CNS prophylaxis followed by antiretroviral therapy for 42 patients.[610] A complete remission rate of 46% was observed, with a median overall survival of only 5.6 months. There were 4 relapses in the 16 complete remissions but none in the CNS. Opportunistic infections occurred in 21% of patients despite PCP prophylaxis, and deaths on study were split equally between lymphoma and infection.

Treatment of HIV-related lymphoma is difficult, because the patient has two fatal conditions. Current standard regimens are probably as effective against AIDS-related lymphomas as they would be against the same lymphomas in nonimmunosuppressed patients if they could be given with the same intensity, but they cannot. By decreasing the intensity, the regimen is made more tolerable, but it becomes less effective (*e.g.*, complete remission rates ≤50%). Colony-stimulating factors may improve this somewhat. Alternatively, infusional regimens that may have lower toxicity because of lower peak plasma concentrations of drugs may maintain antitumor efficacy at acceptable toxicity. CNS prophylaxis is an essential component of treatment. Prophylaxis against opportunistic infection, if possible, should improve the outcome. The optimal use of antiretrovirals is unknown and principally untested. What they can add, beyond more toxicity, during lymphoma-directed chemotherapy is unknown.

If patients are optimally treated and they survive without a fatal infection, a few patients survive for more than 1 year without lymphoma. Patients with CD4 numbers higher than 200/mm^3, good performance status, and with lymphoma as their initial AIDS-defining condition have the greatest likelihood of surviving tumor free. However, these patients eventually die of some other complication of AIDS. Biologic approaches that may exert antitumor effects without worsening the immunosuppression have not been extensively tested. In light of the antitumor effects that accompany reversal of immunosuppression in some transplant patients, the best approach to managing AIDS-associated lymphoma may be to focus efforts on immune restoration so that existing active chemotherapy regimens may be administered more safely.

SALVAGE TREATMENT OF LYMPHOMAS

Patients with indolent lymphoma who relapse from complete remission with an indolent lymphoma histology usually receive symptomatic treatment. If indolent lymphoma patients relapse with an aggressive lymphoma, an attempt at curative therapy with an aggressive lymphoma treatment program appears warranted. However, some of these patients may have acquired genetic abnormalities that adversely affect the probability of cure.

The advent of high-dose therapy with or without radiation therapy followed by ABMT, peripheral blood stem cell, or allogeneic bone marrow transplantation has changed the prognosis of patients with relapsed aggressive histology lymphoma from uniformly fatal to potentially curable.[611] Clinical experience with high-dose therapy is rapidly growing. However, it remains somewhat difficult to estimate the fraction of all patients who may benefit from this approach because of variability in patient selection criteria. Nevertheless, several consistent findings have been made. First, patients have a higher likelihood of cure if they enter the high-dose phase of therapy with no or minimal residual disease. Second, high-dose cyclophosphamide plus TBI is a well-tolerated and effective marrow ablative regimen in lymphoma, and it appears that certain other agents, such as etoposide, carboplatin, and cytarabine, may be added to it without significant increase in toxicity. It is not yet clear that such manipulations of the preparative regimen have a favorable impact on treatment outcome. Third, allogeneic transplantation may have a higher rate of treatment-related fatality; but a graft-versus-lymphoma effect may make second remission more durable. Fourth, patients with disease progression in the days before high-dose therapy are unlikely to benefit from the therapy and are significantly more likely to have fatal complications.

Only a subset of relapsed patients are selected for such rigorous, life-threatening treatment. Age over 55 years disqualifies about half of all relapsed patients. It appears that the probability of success is related mainly to two features: response to initial therapy and response to conventional-dose salvage therapy before the transplantation. Gribben and colleagues found that 60% of responding patients had complete responses to high-dose therapy, and none experienced treatment-related death.[612] Resistant relapsers had an approximately 10% complete response rate, and 31% of them died of treatment-related complications. Approximately 30% to 60% of complete responders relapse. Because of the selection process for choosing suitable candidates, about 20% of relapsed patients with aggressive lymphoma can be salvaged with high-dose therapy. Such data strongly support augmentation of dose intensity to yield better results in the primary treatment of aggressive lymphoma.

Several approaches are being taken to improve the results. Efforts are being made to induce a complete response with conventional-dose regimens before taking the patient to high-dose therapy. DHAP produced responses in 58% of patients, and complete responses in 15%.[613] CEPP(B) (cyclophosphamide, etoposide, procarbazine, and prednisone or bleomycin) produced complete responses in 31%.[614] MIME (methyl GAG, ifosfamide, methotrexate, etoposide) produced complete responses in 33%, and a variety of other regimens have been tested with roughly comparable response rates.[615] It remains unclear whether the combination of conventional-dose and high-dose therapy is superior to high-dose therapy alone. In light of the patient selection that takes place before entry onto high-dose protocols, it is not clear whether high-dose therapy is as much of a treatment advance as it may appear.

To address this important question, the PARMA cooperative group has undertaken a prospective randomized trial in which patients with aggressive lymphoma who relapsed after a prior complete response are enrolled at the time of their first or second relapse. Patients older than 60 years and those with CNS or bone marrow relapses are excluded. All patients receive two cycles of DHAP. Responding patients are then randomly allocated to receive four additional cycles of DHAP or high-dose BEAC (carmustine, etoposide, cytarabine, cyclophosphamide) and ABMT.[616] Preliminary data on the first 128 patients have shown no significant differences in the 1-year survival or toxic death rates. This important study should shed light on the contribution of high-dose therapy to the salvage treatment of aggressive lymphoma.

A second modification in salvage therapy that is being evaluated is in the myeloablative regimen. The PARMA group are using BEAC; Moormeier et al[617] tested three alkylating agents together (cyclophosphamide, thiotepa, carmustine) without irradiation; and Glenn and associates[618] are studying BECH (carmustine, etoposide, cyclophosphamide, hydroxyurea). It is too early to say whether these and the other reported preparative regimens have improved efficacy; no controlled trials have been performed.

A third strategy for improvement involves evaluation of bone marrow purging techniques using chemotherapeutic agents or antibody cocktails plus complement, toxins, isotopes, or attached magnetic beads. Patients who relapse after ABMT usually do so in previously involved sites of disease. There is not much evidence that any tumor cells contaminating the donor bone marrow influence sites of relapse. There is no evidence that bone marrow purging techniques make an impact on survival in relapsed patients with aggressive histology lymphoma. Evidence supporting a role for purging in patients with indolent lymphoma was previously discussed.

Although high-dose therapy may be life threatening, Freedman and colleagues reported a toxic death rate of only 4% among 100 patients with relapsed lymphoma sensitive to conventional-dose salvage therapy who were subsequently treated with high-dose cyclophosphamide plus TBI.[439] This toxic death rate for patients with sensitive relapse is comparable to that seen with conventional-dose combination chemotherapy used in primary treatment.

Perhaps the most serious risk from high-dose therapy is the problem of marrow graft failure. Marrow purged with drugs in vitro may be slow to engraft. The number of salvage chemotherapy cycles delivered before marrow harvest may contribute to slow engraftment.[619] Different approaches to promoting engraftment are being explored. For example, the use of peripheral blood stem cells with or without a source of marrow may reduce the number of days of granulocytopenia and thrombocytopenia.[620] Pretreatment with GM-CSF increases the number of circulating stem cells, making stem cell harvest by cytapheresis more efficient.[621] These procedures make bone marrow purging techniques of less relevance because peripheral blood stem cells are not as commonly contaminated by tumor cells. Administration of GM-CSF after transplantation also modestly accelerates engraftment and can permit the use of high doses of single-agent and combination chemotherapy without hematopoietic support. The capacity of IL-1 to promote platelet recovery after high doses of carboplatin therapy may lead to cocktails of colony-stimulating factors that affect all lineages.[622–625]

Another strategy under evaluation for the treatment of relapsed patients with aggressive lymphoma is the reversal of drug resistance mediated by the p170 glycoprotein. Salmon and associates found expression of the p170 glycoprotein efflux pump in three of six samples from relapsed lymphoma patients.[626] They administered high-dose verapamil to 18 patients with refractory lymphoma in addition to CVAD combination chemotherapy (cyclophosphamide bolus on day 1, infusional doxorubicin and vincristine for 4 days, and oral dexamethasone).[627] There were five complete and eight partial responses; median response duration was about 6 months. Unfortunately, the investigators never established that the patients were resistant to CVAD, and it is therefore unclear whether verapamil added anything to this combination.

At the NCI, an infusional combination chemotherapy program called EPOCH (infusional etoposide, doxorubicin, and vincristine, bolus cyclophosphamide, oral prednisone) is being evaluated in relapsed patients.[628] When patients stop responding to the regimen, another cycle of the therapy is given together with r-verapamil, a stereoisomer that reverses drug resistance but has little effect on the heart. This study should assist in evaluating the degree to which p170 is involved in drug resistance in lymphoma.

TREATMENT OF RARE PROLIFERATIVE DISORDERS OF THE LYMPHATIC SYSTEM

Angioimmunoblastic lymphadenopathy is a rare disease with histologic features that resemble Hodgkin's disease without the Reed-Sternberg cells. In some series, life expectancy is less than 1 year.[629] The disease is idiopathic, and it is associated with diffuse adenopathy, polyclonal serum immunoglobulin elevations, and often a history of allergic or autoimmune disease.[630] Transient responses have been obtained after plasmapheresis, but more typically the disease evolves into an aggressive lymphoma. The cells can express elevated levels of *NRAS*-encoded mRNA, the significance of which is unknown.[631] The disease may respond to prednisone or to combination chemotherapy. It bears features suggestive of excess cytokine production or responsiveness (*e.g.*, polyclonal gammopathy). Inhibiting cytokine action with cyclosporin A may be therapeutic, but there is insufficient clinical experience to recommend its routine use.

Castleman's disease (*i.e.*, angiofollicular lymph node hyperplasia) is most often an asymptomatic condition diagnosed incidentally in young men on chest x-ray film as enlarged mediastinal nodes. Sometimes the adenopathy is accompanied by systemic symptoms of fever and weight loss. There is a systemic form of the illness associated with malaise, fever, adenopathy, hepatosplenomegaly, rashes, hypergammaglobulinemia, and occasionally CNS symptoms.[294] Many of the manifestations of the disease may be related to the overproduction of IL-6. The median survival was only 30 months. A case report of a successfully treated case suggests that aggressive therapy may be lifesaving.[632]

Angiocentric immunoproliferative lesions (AIL) are a collection of entities classified as peripheral T-cell disorders and include lymphomatoid granulomatosis, midline granuloma, lymphomatoid papulosis, and polymorphic reticulosis.[633] The disease is characterized by extranodal sites of involvement such as the skin, lungs, kidneys, sinuses, and other organs. The lesions are composed of T cells, and they are divided into three histologic grades ranging from benign to frankly malignant. Treatment of grade 1 lesions with cyclophosphamide and prednisone resulted in a 45% long-term survival; the survival rate for patients with grade 2 lesions was 33%. Most of the deaths in grade 1 and 2 patients were from treatment-refractory lymphoma. Grade 3 lesions, which were considered frank lymphoma and treated like aggressive histology lymphomas, had an 87% long-term survival. It appears that even the low-grade AIL could benefit from aggressive therapy with a lymphoma regimen, because they evolve to lymphoma with a high frequency, and their previous treatment appears to result in the emergence of drug-resistant neoplasms. Such a clinical trial is under way.

Acknowledgments

This research was partially sponsored by the National Cancer Institute, Department of Health and Human Services, under contract N01-C0-74102 with Program Resources, Inc./DynCorp. The contents of this publication do not necessarily reflect the views or policies of the Department of Health and Human Services, nor does mention of trade names, commercial products, or organizations imply endorsement by the U.S. Government.

REFERENCES

1. Cancer facts and figures 1992. New York: American Cancer Society, 1992:4.
2. Devesa SS, Silverman DT, Young JL Jr, et al. Cancer incidence and mortality trends among whites in the United States, 1947–84. JNCI 1987;79:701–770.
3. Ries LAG, Hankey BF, Miller BA, et al. Cancer statistics review, 1973–1988. NIH Pub. No. 91-2789. Bethesda: National Cancer Institute, 1991.
4. Opportunistic non-Hodgkin's lymphomas among severely immunocompromised HIV-infected patients surviving for prolonged periods on antiretroviral therapy—United States. MMWR 1991;40:591–600.
5. Cantor KP, Fraumeni JF. Distribution of non-Hodgkin's lymphoma in the United States between 1950 and 1975. Cancer Res 1980;40:2645–2652.
6. Third National Cancer Survey, 1969 Incidence. Preliminary report. Bethesda: Department of Health, Education and Welfare, 1971:71.
7. Higginson J, Muir CS. Epidemiology. In: Holland JF, Frei E, eds. Cancer medicine. Philadelphia: Lea & Febiger, 1973:241.
8. Shih L-Y, Liang D-C. Non-Hodgkin's lymphomas in Asia. Hematol Oncol Clin North Am 1991;5:983–1001.
9. Vianna NJ, Davies JNP, Polan AK, et al. Familial Hodgkin's disease: An environmental and genetic disorder. Lancet 1974;ii:854–857.
10. Miller DG. The association of immune disease and malignant lymphoma. Ann Intern Med 1967;66:507–521.
11. Zulman J, Jaffe R, Talal N. Evidence that the malignant lymphoma of Sjogren's syndrome is a monoclonal B-cell neoplasm. N Engl J Med 1978;299:1215–1220.
12. Talal N, Sokoloff L, Barth W. Extra salivary lymphoid abnormalities in Sjögren's syndrome (reticulum cell sarcoma, "pseudolymphoma," macroglobulinemia). Am J Med 1967;43:50–65.
13. Kassan SS, Thomas TL, Moutsopoulos HM, et al. Increased risk of lymphoma in Sicca syndrome. Ann Intern Med 1978;89:888–892.
14. Kissmeyer-Nielsen F, Bjorn-Jensen K, Femara RB, et al. HLA phenotypes in Hodgkin's disease: Preliminary report. Transplant Proc 1971;3:1287.
15. Dick FR, Fortuny I, Theologides A, et al. HL-A and lymphoid tumors. Cancer Res 1972;32:2608–2611.
16. MacSween RNM. Reticulum cell sarcoma and rheumatoid arthritis in a patient with XY/XXY/XXX/Y Klinefelter's syndrome and normal intelligence. Lancet 1965;1:460–461.
17. Tan C, Etcubanas E, Lieberman P, et al. Chediak-Higashi syndrome in a child with Hodgkin's disease. Am J Dis Child 1971;121:135–139.
18. Hyman GA, Sommers SC. The development of Hodgkins's disease and other lymphomas during anticonvulsant therapy. Blood J Haematol 1966;28:416–437.
19. Weisenburger DD. Lymphoid malignancies in Nebraska: A hypothesis. Nebr Med J 1985;70:300–305.
20. Hardell L, Eriksonn M, Lenner P, Lundgren E. Malignant lymphoma and exposure to chemicals, especially organic solvents, chlorophenols, and phenoxyacids: A case-control study. Br J Cancer 1981;43:169–176.
21. Hoar SD, Blair A, Holmes FF, et al. Agricultural herbicide use and risk of lymphoma and soft tissue sarcoma. JAMA 1986;256:1141–1147.
22. Wigle DT, Semercin RM, Wilkins K, et al. Mortality study of Canadian male farm operators: Non-Hodgkin's lymphoma and agricultural practices in Saskatchewan. 1990;JNCI 82:575–582.
23. Veneus P, Faggiario F, Tedeschi M, Ciccone G. Incidence rates of lymphomas and soft-tissue sarcomas and environmental measurements of phenoxyherbicides. JNCI 1991;83:362–363.
24. The Selected Cancers Cooperative Study Group. The association of selected cancers with service in the U.S. Military in Vietnam. I. Non-Hodgkin's lymphoma. Arch Intern Med 1990;150:2473–2483.
25. Alavanja MD, Blair A, Masters MN. Cancer mortality in the U.S. flour industry. JNCI 1990;82:840–848.
26. Anderson RE, Nishiyama H, Yohei I, et al. Pathogenesis of radiation related leukemia and lymphoma. Speculations based primarily on experience of Hiroshima and Nagasaki. Lancet 1972;1:1060–1062.
27. Miller RW. Delayed radiation effects in atomic bomb survivors. Science 1969;166: 569–574.
28. Court-Brown WM, Doll R. Leukemia and aplastic anemia in patients irradiated for ankylosing spondylitis. Medical Research Council Special Report Series, No. 295. London: Her Majesty's Stationery Office, 1957.
29. Penn I. The incidence of malignancies in transplant recipients. Transplant Proc 1975;7: 323–326.
30. Matas AJ, Hertel BF, Rosai J, et al. Post-transplant malignant lymphoma. Distinctive morphologic features related to its pathogenesis. Am J Med 1976;61:716–720.
31. Penn I. Cancers complicating organ transplantation. New Engl J Med 1990;323:1767–1769.
32. Swinnen LJ, Costanzo-Nordin MR, Fisher SG, et al. Increased incidence of lymphoproliferative disorder after immunosuppression with the monoclonal antibody OKT3 in cardiac-transplant receipts. New Engl J Med 1990;323:1723–1728.

33. Starzl TE, Nalesnik MA, Porter KA, et al. Reversibility of lymphomas and lymphoproliferative lesions developing under cyclosporine-steroid therapy. Lancet 1984;1: 583–587.
34. Hanto DW, Frizzera G, Gajl-Peczalska KJ, et al. Epstein-Barr virus-induced B-cell lymphoma after renal transplantation: Acyclovir therapy and transition from polyclonal to monoclonal B-cell proliferation. N Engl J Med 1982;306:913–918.
35. Fischer A, Blanche S, LeBidois J, et al. Anti-B-cell monoclonal antibodies in the treatment of severe B-cell lymphoproliferative syndrome following bone marrow and organ transplantation. N Engl J Med 1991;324:1451–1456.
36. Shapiro RS, Chauvenet A, McGuire W, et al. Treatment of B-cell lymphoproliferative disorders with interferon alpha and intravenous gamma globulin. N Engl J Med 1988;318:1334.
37. Kipps TJ, Fong S, Tomhave E, et al. High-frequency expression of a conserved kappa light-chain variable-region gene in chronic lymphocytic leukemia. Proc Natl Acad Sci USA 1987;84:2916–2920.
38. Kaplan HS. Etiology of lymphomas and leukemia: Role of C-type RNA viruses. Leukemia Res 1978;2:253–271.
39. Dmochowski L. Viral studies in human leukemia and lymphoma. In: Zarafonetis CJD, ed. Proceedings of the international conference on leukemia-lymphoma. Philadelphia: Lea & Febiger, 1968:97.
40. Kawakami TG, Theilan GH, Dungworth DL, et al. "C" type viral particles in plasma of cats with feline leukemia. Science 1967;158:1049–1050.
41. Kawakami TG, Hull SD, Buckley DM, et al. C-type virus associated with Gibbon lymphosarcoma. Nature New Biol 1972;235:170–171.
42. Rapp F. Viruses an etiologic factor in cancer. Semin Oncol 1976;3:49–63.
43. Van der Maaten MJ, Miller JM, Booth AD. Replicating type-C virus particles in monolayer cell cultures from cattle with lymphosarcoma. JNCI 1974;52:491–497.
44. Purtilo DT, Stevenson M. Lymphotropic viruses as etiologic agents of lymphoma. Hematol Oncol Clin North Am 1991;5:901–923.
45. List AF, Greco FA, Vogler LB. Lymphoproliferative diseases in immunocompromised hosts: The role of Epstein-Barr virus. J Clin Oncol 1987;5:1673–1689.
46. Tosato G, Blaese RM. Epstein-Barr virus infection and immunoregulation in man. Adv Immunol 1985;37:99–149.
47. Harrington DS, Weisenburger DD, Purtilo DT. Malignant lymphoma in the X-linked lymphoproliferative syndrome. Cancer 1987;59:1419–1429.
48. Boyle MJ, Sewell WA, Scully TB, et al. Subtypes of Epstein-Barr virus in human immunodeficiency virus-associated non-Hodgkin lymphoma. Blood 1991;78:3004–3011.
49. Shibata D, Weiss LM, Nathwani BN, et al. Epstein-Barr virus in benign lymph node biopsies from individuals infected with the human immunodeficiency virus is associated with concurrent or subsequent development of non-Hodgkin's lymphoma. Blood 1991;77:1527–1533.
50. Klein G. Lymphoma development in mice and humans: Diversity of initiation is followed by convergent cytogenetic evolution. Proc Natl Acad Sci USA 1979;76:2442–2446.
51. Patton DF, Wilkowski CW, Hanson CA, et al. Epstein-Barr virus-determined clonality in post transplant lymphoproliferative disease. Transplantation 1990;49:1080–1084.
52. Poiesz BJ, Ruscetti FW, Gazdar AF, et al. Detection and isolation of type C retrovirus particles from fresh and cultured lymphocytes of a patient with cutaneous T-cell lymphoma. Proc Natl Acad Sci USA 1980;77:7415–7419.
53. Blayney DW, Jaffe ES, Blattner WA, et al. The human T-cell leukemia/lymphoma virus associated with American adult T-cell leukemia/lymphoma. Blood 1983;62:401–405.
54. Kalyanaraman VS, Sarngadharan MG, Robert-Guroff M, et al. A new subtype of human T-cell leukemia virus (HTLV-II) associated with a T-cell variant of hairy cell leukemia. Science 1982;218:571–573.
55. Kanki PJ, Barin F, M'Boup S, et al. New human T-lymphotropic retroviruses related to simian T-lymphotropic virus type III (STLV-III-HGM). Science 1986;232:238–243.
56. Clavel F, Guetard D, Brun-Vezinet F, et al. Isolation of a new human retrovirus from West African patients with AIDS. Science 1986;233:343–346.
57. Manzari V, Gismondi A, Barillari G, et al. HTLV-V. A new human retrovirus in Tac-negative T-cell lymphoma/leukemia. Science 1987;238:1581–1583.
58. Jacobson S, Raine CS, Mingioli ES, et al. Isolation of an HTLV-I-like retrovirus from patients with tropical spastic paraparesis. Nature 1988;331:540–543.
59. Sonoda S. Relationship of HTLV-I-related adult T-cell leukemia and HTLV-I associated myelopathy to distinct HLA haplotypes. Jikken Igaku 1987;5:769–771.
60. Fifth International Workshop on Chromosomes in Leukemia-lymphoma. Correlation of chromosome abnormalities with histologic and immunologic characteristics in non-Hodgkin's lymphoma and adult T cell leukemia-lymphoma. Blood 1987;70:1554–1564.
61. LeBeau MM. Chromosomal abnormalities in Non-Hodgkin's lymphomas. Semin Oncol 1990;17:20–29.
62. Offit K, Chaganti RSK. Chromosomal abberrations in non-Hodgkin's lymphoma. Biologic and clinical correlations. Hematol Oncol Clin North Am 1991;5:853–869.
63. Schouten HC, Sanger WG, Weisenburger DD, et al. For the Nebraska Lymphoma Study Group: Chromosomal abnormalities in patients with non-cutaneous T-cell non-Hodgkin's lymphoma. Eur J Cancer 1990;26:618–622.
64. Rimokh R, Magaud J-P, Berger F, et al. A translocation involving a specific breakpoint (q35) on chromosome 5 is characteristic of anaplastic large cell lymphoma (Ki-lymphoma). Br J Haematol 1989;71:31–36.
65. Offit K, Wong G, Filippa DA, et al. Cytogenetic analysis of 434 consecutively ascertained specimens of non-Hodgkin's lymphoma: Clinical correlations. Blood 1991;77:1508–1515.
66. Armitage JO, Sanger WG, Weisenberger DD, et al. Correlation of secondary cytogenetic abnormalities with histologic appearance in non-Hodgkin's lymphomas bearing t(14;18)(q32;121). JNCI 1988;80:576–580.
67. Taub R, Kirsch I, Morton C, et al. Translocation of the c-*myc* gene into the immunoglobulin heavy chain locus in human Burkitt's lymphoma and murine plasmacytoma cells. Proc Natl Acad Sci USA 1982;79:7837–7841.
68. Tsujimoto Y, Yunis JJ, Onaroto-Showe L, et al. Molecular cloning of the chromosomal breakpoints of B-cell leukemias with the t(11;14) chromosomal translocation. Science 1984;224:1403–1406.
69. Cleary ML, Smith SD, Sklar J. Cloning and structural analysis of cDNAs for *bcl-2* and a hybrid *bcl-2*/immunoglobulin transcript resulting from the t(14;18) translocation. Cell 1986;47:19–28.
70. Graniger WB, Seto M, Boutain B, et al. Expression of *bcl-2* and *bcl-2*-Ig fusion transcripts in normal and neoplastic cells. J Clin Invest 1987;80:1512–1515.
71. Hockenberry D, Nunez G, Milliman C, et al. *Bcl-2* is an inner mitochondrial membrane protein that blocks programmed cell death. Nature 1990;348:334–336.
72. McDonnell TJ, Deane N, Platt EM, et al. *Bcl-2*-immunoglobulin transgenic mice demonstrate extended B cell survival and follicular lymphoproliferation. Cell 1989;57:79–88.
73. McDonnell TJ, Korsmeyer SJ. Progression from lymphoid hyperplasia to high grade malignant lymphoma in mice transgenic for the t(14;18). Nature 1991;349:254–256.
74. Nunez G, Seto M, Seremetis S, et al. Growth- and tumor-promoting effects of deregulated *bcl-2* in human B-lymphoblastoid cells. Proc Natl Acad Sci USA 1989;86:4589–4593.
75. Zelenetz AD, Chen TT, Levy R. Histologic transformation of follicular lymphoma to diffuse lymphoma represents tumor progression by a single malignant B cell. J Exp Med 1991;173:197–207.
76. Hardy R, Horning SJ. Molecular biologic studies in the clinical evaluation of non-Hodgkin's lymphoma. Hematol Oncol Clin North Am 1991;5:891–900.
77. Yunis JJ, Mayer MG, Arnescu MA, et al. *Bcl-2* and other genomic alterations in the prognosis of large-cell lymphoma. N Engl J Med 1989;320:1047–1054.
78. Price CGA, Meerabux J, Murtaugh S, et al. The significance of circulating cells carrying t(14;18) in long remission from follicular lymphoma. J Clin Oncol 1991;9:1527–1532.
79. Gribben JG, Freedman AS, Neuberg D, et al. Immunologic purging of marrow assessed by PCR before autologous bone marrow transplantation for B-cell lymphoma. N Engl J Med 1991;325:1525–1533.
80. Ngan B-Y, Chen-Levy Z, Weiss LM, et al. Expression in non-Hodgkin's lymphoma of the *bcl-2* protein associated with t(14;18) chromosomal translocation. N Engl J Med 1988;318:1638–1644.
81. Limpens J, de Jong D, van Krieken JHJM, et al. *bcl-2*/J_H rearrangements in benign lymphoid tissues with follicular hyperplasia. Oncogene 1991;6:2271–2276.
82. Rosenberg CL, Wong E, Petty EM, et al. *PRAD1*, a candidate *bcl-1* oncogene: Mapping and expression in centrogenic lymphoma. Proc Natl Acad Sci USA 1991;88:9638–9642.
83. Greaves MF, Owen JJT, Raff MC. T and B lymphocytes: Origins, properties, and roles in immune responses. New York: American Elsevier, 1974.
84. Weiss L. The cells and tissues of the immune system. Structure, functions, interactions. Englewood Cliffs, NJ: Prentice-Hall, 1972.
85. Bienenstock J, Befus D. Gut- and bronchus-associated lymphoid tissue. Am J Anat 1984;170:437–445.
86. Golde D, Cline MJ. A review and reevaluation of the histiocytic disorders. Am J Med 1973;55:49–60.
87. Mann RB, Jaffe ES, Berard CW. Malignant lymphomas a conceptual understanding of morphologic diversity. A review. Am J Pathol 1979;94:105–191.
88. Royer HD, Reinherz EL. T lymphocytes: Ontogeny, function, and relevance to clinical disorders. N Engl J Med 1987;317:1136–1142.
89. Cooper MD. Current Concepts. B lymphocytes: Normal development and function. N Engl J Med 1987;317:1452——1456.
90. Van Furth R, Raeburn JA, van Zwet TL. Characteristics of human mononuclear phagocytes. Blood 1979;54:485–500.
91. Steinman RM, Nussenzweig MC. Dendritic cells: Features and functions. Immunol Rev 1980;53:127–147.
92. Tew JG, Thorbecke GJ, Steinman RM. Dendritic cells in the immune response: Characteristics and recommended nomenclature. J Reticuloendothel Soc 1982;31:371–380.
93. Wood GS, Turner RR, Shiruba RA, et al. Human dendritic cells and macrophages: In situ immunophenotypic definition of subsets that exhibit specific morphologic and microenvironmental characteristics. Am J Pathol 1985;119:73–82.
94. Kohler G, Milstein C. Continuous cultures of fused cells secreting antibody of predefined specificity. Nature 1975;256:495–497.
95. Ajuti F, Cerottini JC, Coombs RRA, et al. Identification, enumeration and isolation of bone marrow derived and thymus derived T lymphocytes from human peripheral blood. Special technical report. Scand J Immunol 1974;3:521–532.
96. Jaffe ES, Cossman J. Immunodiagnosis of lymphoid and mononuclear phagocytic neoplasms. In: Rose NR, Friedman H, Fahey JL, eds. Manual of clinical laboratory immunology. 3rd ed. Washington, DC: American Society of Microbiology, 1986:779.
97. Lovett EJ, Schnitzer B, Keren DF, et al. Application of flow cytometry to diagnostic pathology. Lab Invest 1984;540:115–140.
98. Norton AJ, Isaacson PG. Lymphoma phenotyping in formalin-fixed paraffin wax-embedded tissues. Range of antibodies and staining patterns. Histopathology 1989;14: 437–446.
99. Norton AJ, Isaacson PG. Lymphoma phenotyping in formalin-fixed paraffin wax-embedded tissues. Profiles of reactivity in the various tumor types. Histopathology 1989;14:557–579.
100. Reinherz EL, Haynes BF, Nadler LM, et al. Leukocyte typing II. Human T lymphocytes, vol 1. New York: Springer-Verlag, 1987.
101. Broder S, Waldmann TA. The Sezary syndrome. A malignant proliferation of helper T cells. J Clin Invest 1976;58:1297–1306.

102. Broder S, Waldmann TA. The suppressor cell network in cancer. N Engl J Med 1978;299:1281–1284.
103. Jaffe ES. Pathologic and clinical spectrum of post-thymic T-cell malignancies. Cancer Invest 1984;2:413–426.
104. Weiss LM, Crabtree GS, Rouse RV, et al. Morphologic and immunologic characterization of 50 peripheral T cell lymphomas. Am J Pathol 1985;118:316–324.
105. Reinherz EL, Kung PC, Goldstein G, et al. Discrete stages of human intrathymic differentiation: Analysis of normal thymocytes and leukemic lymphoblasts of T-cell lineage. Proc Natl Acad Sci USA 1980;77:1588–1592.
106. Cossman J, Chused T, Fisher R, et al. Diversity of immunologic phenotypes of lymphoblastic lymphoma. Cancer Res 1983;43:4486–4490.
107. Goding JW, Burns GF. Monoclonal antibody OKT-9 recognizes the receptor for transferin on human acute lymphocytic leukemic cells. J Immunol 1982;127:1256–1258.
108. Pittaluga S, Uppenkamp M, Cossman J. Development of T3/T cell receptor gene expression in human pre-T neoplasms. Blood 1987;69:1062–1067.
109. Greaves MF, Chan LC, Furley AJW, et al. Lineage promiscuity in hematopoietic differentiation and leukemia. Blood 1986;67:1–11.
110. Caligaris-Cappio F, Gobbi M, Bofill M, et al. Infrequent normal B lymphocytes express features of B-chronic lymphocytic leukemia. J Exp Med 1982;155:623–628.
111. Cossman J, Neckers LM, Hsu SM, et al. Low grade lymphomas: Expression of developmentally regulated B-cell antigens. Am J Pathol 1984;114:117–124.
112. Arnold A, Cossman J, Bakhski A, et al. Immunoglobulin gene rearrangements as unique clonal markers in human lymphoid neoplasms. N Engl J Med 1983;309:1593–1599.
113. Reinherz EL, Haynes BF, Nadler LM, et al. Leukocyte typing II. Human B lymphocytes, vol 2. New York: Springer-Verlag, 1987.
114. Nadler LM, Korsmeyer SJ, Anderson KC, et al. B cell origin of non-T cell acute lymphoblastic leukemia. J Clin Invest 1984;74:332–340.
115. Loken MR, Shah VO, Dattilio KL, et al. Flow cytometric analysis of human bone marrow: II. Normal B lymphocyte development. Blood 1987;70:1316–1324.
116. Greaves MF, Brown G, Rapson NT, et al. Antisera to acute lymphoblastic leukemia cells. Clin Immunol Immunopathol 1975;4:67–84.
117. Korsmeyer SJ, Arnold A, Beach A, et al. Immunoglobulin gene rearrangement and cell surface antigen expression in acute lymphocytic leukemias of T-cell and B-cell precursor origins. J Clin Invest 1983;71:301–313.
118. Ritz J, Nadler LM, Bhan AK, et al. Expression of common acute lymphoblastic leukemia antigen (CALLA) by lymphomas of B cell and T cell lineage. Blood 1981;58:648–652.
119. Hsu SM, Jaffe ES. Phenotypic expression of B lymphocytes. Identification with monoclonal antibodies in normal lymphoid tissues. Am J Pathol 1984;114:387–395.
120. Cossman J, Neckers LM, Leonard WJ, et al. Polymorphonuclear neutrophils express the common acute lymphoblastic leukemia antigen. J Exp Med 1983;157:1064–1069.
121. Breard J, Reinherz EL, Kung PC, et al. A monoclonal antibody reactive with peripheral blood monocytes. J Immunol 1980;124:1943–1948.
122. Todd RF, Nadler LM, Schlossman SF. Antigens on human monocytes by monoclonal antibodies. J Immunol 1981;126:1435–1442.
123. Hanjan SN, Kearney JF, Cooper MD. A monoclonal (MMA) that identifies a differentiation antigen on human myelomonocytic cells. Clin Immunol Immunopathol 1982;23:172–188.
124. Reinherz EL, Haynes BF, Nadler LM, et al. Leukocyte typing II. Human myeloid and hematopoietic cells, vol 3. New York: Springer-Verlag, 1988.
125. Pulford KA, Rigney EM, Micklen KJ, et al. KP1: A new monoclonal antibody that detects a monocyte/macrophage associated antigen in routinely processed tissue sections. J Clin Pathol 1989;42:414–421.
126. Battifora H, Trowbridge IS. A monoclonal antibody useful for the differential diagnosis between malignant lymphoma and nonhematopoietic neoplasms. Cancer 1983;51:816–821.
127. Warnke RA, Gatter KC, Phil D, et al. Diagnosis of human lymphoma with monoclonal antileukocyte antibodies. N Engl J Med 1983;309:1275–1281.
128. Bollum FJ. Terminal deoxynucleotidyl transferase as a hematopoietic cell marker. A review. Blood 1979;54:1203–1215.
129. Kung PC, Long JC, McCaffrey RP, et al. Terminal deoxynucleotidyl transferase in the diagnosis of leukemia and malignant lymphoma. Am J Med 1978;64:788–794.
130. Braziel RM, Keneklis T, Donlon JA, et al. Terminal deoxynucleotidyl transferase in non-Hodgkin's lymphoma. Am J Clin Pathol 1983;80:655–659.
131. Braziel RM, Hsu SM, Jaffe ES. Lymph nodes, spleen, and thymus. In: Spicer SS, ed. Histochemistry in pathologic diagnosis. New York: Dekker, 1986:203.
132. Yam LT, Li CY, Lam KW. Tartrate-resistant acid phosphatase isoenzyme in the reticulum cells of leukemic reticuloendotheliosis. N Engl J Med 1971;284:357–360.
133. Tonegawa S. Somatic generation of antibody diversity. Nature 1983;301:575–581.
134. Yanagi Y, Yoshihai Y, Leggett K, et al. A human T cell-specific cDNA clone encodes a protein having extensive homology to immunoglobulin chains. Nature 1984;308:145–149.
135. Hedrick SM, Cohen DI, Nielsen EA, et al. Isolation of cDNA clones encoding T-cell specific membrane-associated proteins. Nature 1984;308:149–153.
136. Hood L, Kronenberg M, Hunkapiller T. T cell antigen receptors and the immunoglobulin supergene family. Cell 1985;40:225–229.
137. Flug F, Pier-Giuseppe P, Bonetti F, et al. T-cell receptor gene rearrangements as markers of lineage and clonality in T-cell neoplasms. Proc Natl Acad Sci USA 1985;82:3460–3464.
138. Korsmeyer SJ, Greene WC, Cossman J, et al. Rearrangement and expression of immunoglobulin genes and expression of Tac antigen in hairy cell leukemia. Proc Natl Acad Sci USA 1983;80:4522–4526.
139. Cheng GY, Minden M, Toyonaga B, et al. T cell receptor and immunoglobulin gene rearrangements in acute myeloblastic leukemia. J Exp Med 1986;163:414–424.
140. Ha K, Minden M, Hozumi N, et al. Immunoglobulin chain gene rearrangement in a patient with T cell acute lymphoblastic leukemia. J Clin Invest 1984;73:1232–1236.
141. Pelicci PG, Knowles DM, Dalla-Favera R. Lymphoid tumors displaying rearrangements of both immunoglobulin and T cell receptor genes. J Exp Med 1985;162:1015–1024.
142. Uppenkamp M, Pittaluga S, Lipford EH, et al. Limited diversity and selection of rearranged gamma genes in polyclonal T cells. J Immunol 1987;138:1618–1620.
143. Weiss LM, Hu E, Wood GS, et al. Clonal rearrangements of T cell receptor genes in mycosis fungoides and dermatopathic lymphadenopathy. N Engl J Med 1985;313:539–544.
144. Weiss LM, Wood GS, Trela M, et al. Clonal T cell populations in lymphomatoid papulosis: Evidence of a lymphoproliferative origin for a clinically benign disease. N Engl J Med 1986;315:475–479.
145. Shearer WT, Ritz J, Finegold MK, et al. Epstein-Barr virus associated B cell proliferations of diverse clonal origins after bone marrow transplantation in a 12-year-old boy with severe combined immunodeficiency. N Engl J Med 1985;312:1151–1159.
146. Templeton NS. The polymerase chain reaction: History, methods and applications. Diagn Mol Pathol 1992;1:58–72.
147. Stetler-Stevenson MA, Crush-Stanton S, Cossman J. Involvement of *bc1–2* gene in Hodgkin's disease. JNCI 1990;82:855–858.
148. Stetler-Stevenson MA, Raffeld M, Cohen P, et al. Detection of occult follicular lymphoma by specific DNA amplification. Blood 1988;72:1822–1825.
149. Lee M-S, Chang K-S, Cabanillas F, et al. Detection of minimal residual cells carrying t(14;18) by DNA sequence amplification. Science 1987;237:175–178.
150. Urba WJ, Longo DL. Cytologic, immunologic, and clinical diversity in non-Hodgkin's lymphoma: Therapeutic implications. Semin Oncol 1985;12:250–267.
151. Chan WC, Link S, Mawle A, et al. Heterogeneity of large granular lymphocyte proliferations: Delineation of two major subtypes. Blood 1986;68:1142–1153.
152. Craigie D. Case of disease of the spleen, in which death took place in consequence in the presence of purulent matter in the blood. Edinb Med Surg J 1845;64:400–412.
153. Bennett JH. Case of hypertrophy of the spleen and liver in which death took place from suppuration of the blood. Edinb Med Surg J 1845;64:413–423.
154. Virchow R. Weisses Blut, neue Notizen aus den Geb der naturund Heikunde. Froriep's Neue Notizen 1845;36:151.
155. Billroth T. Multiple lymphome. Erfolgreiche Behandlung mit Arsenik. Wien Med Wochenschr 1871;21:1066–1068.
156. Dreschfeld J. Clinical lecture on acute Hodgkin's Disease. Br Med J 1892;1:893–896.
157. Kundrat H. Uber. Lympho-sarcomatosis. Wien Klin Wochenschr 1893;6:211–213.
158. Brill NE, Baehr G, Rosenthal N, et al. Generalized giant lymphfollicle hyperplasia of lymph nodes and spleen, a hitherto undescribed type. JAMA 1925;84:668–671.
159. Symmers D. Follicular lymphadenopathy with splenomegaly. A newly recognized disease of lymphatic system. Arch Pathol Lab Med 1927;3:816–820.
160. Roulet F. Das primäre Retothelsarkom der Lymphkonten. Virchows Arch [A] 1930;277:15–47.
161. Gall EA, Mallory TB. Malignant lymphoma. A clinical pathologic survey of 618 cases. Am J Pathol 1942;18:381–429.
162. Rappaport H, Winter WJ, Hicks EB. Follicular lymphoma. A re-evaluation of its position in the scheme of malignant lymphomas, based on a survey of 253 cases. Cancer 1956;9:792–821.
163. Burkitt D. A sarcoma involving the jaws in African children. Br J Surg 1958;46:218–223.
164. Uchiyama T, Yodoi J, Sagawa K, et al. Adult T-cell leukemia: Clinical and hematologic features of 16 cases. Blood 1977;50:481–492.
165. Rappaport H. Tumors of the hematopoietic system. In: Atlas of tumor pathology, sect III, fasc 8. Washington, DC: Armed Forces Institute of Pathology, 1966.
166. Dorfman RF. Classification of non-Hodgkin's lymphomas. Lancet 1974;1:1295–1296.
167. Bennett MH, Farrer-Brown G, Henry K, et al. Classification of non-Hodgkin's lymphomas. Lancet 1974;2:405–406.
168. Lukes RJ, Collins RD. Immunologic characterization of human malignant lymphomas. Cancer 1974;34:1488–1503.
169. Lennert K, Mohri N, Stein H, et al. Malignant lymphomas other than Hodgkin's disease. Berlin: Springer-Verlag, 1978.
170. Lennert K, Mohri N, Stein H, et al. The histopathology of malignant lymphoma. Br J Haematol 1975;31(suppl 1):193–203.
171. Mathe G, Rappaport H, O'Conor GT, et al. Histological and cytological typing of neoplastic diseases of hematopoietic and lymphoid tissues. In: WHO international histological classification of tumors, no. 14. Geneva: World Health Organization, 1976.
172. Jaffe ES, Shevach EM, Frank MM, et al. Nodular lymphoma: Evidence for origin from follicular B lymphocytes. N Engl J Med 1974;290:813–819.
173. Jaffe ES, Strauchen JA, Berard CW. Predictability of immunologic phenotype by morphologic criteria in diffuse aggressive non-Hodgkin's lymphomas. Am J Clin Pathol 1982;77:46–49.
174. National Cancer Institute sponsored study of classifications of non-Hodgkin's Lymphomas. Summary and description of a working formulation for clinical usage. Cancer 1982;49:2112–2135.
175. Rosenberg SA. Current concepts in cancer. Non-Hodgkin's lymphoma: Selection of treatment on the base of histologic type. N Engl J Med 1979;301:924–928.
176. Jaffe ES. Relationship of classification to biologic behavior of non-Hodgkin's lymphoma. Semin Oncol 1986;13:3–9.
177. Jaffe ES. Follicular lymphomas: Possibility that they are benign tumors of the lymphoid system. JNCI 1983;70:401–403.
178. Krikorian JG, Portlock CS, Cooney DP, et al. Spontaneous regression of non-Hodgkin's lymphomas. A report of nine cases. Cancer Res 1980;46:2093–2099.
179. DeVita VT Jr, Canellos GP, Chabner BA, et al. Advanced diffuse histiocytic lymphoma, a potentially curable disease. Lancet 1975;1:248–250.

180. Warnke RA, Kim H, Fuks Z, et al. The coexistence of nodular and diffuse patterns in nodular non-hodgkin's lymphomas: Significance and clinicopathologic correlation. Cancer 1977;40:1229–1233.
181. Fisher RI, Jones RB, DeVita VT Jr, et al. Natural history of malignant lymphomas with divergent histologies at staging evaluation. Cancer 1981;47:2022–2025.
182. Hubbard SM, Chabner BA, DeVita VT Jr, et al. Histologic progression in non-Hodgkin's lymphoma. Blood 1982;59:258–264.
183. Kim H, Hendrickson MR, Dorfman RF. Composite lymphoma. Cancer 1977;40:959–976.
184. Dick FR, Maca RD. The lymph node in chronic lymphocytic leukemia. Cancer 1978;41: 283–292.
185. Pangalis GA, Nathwani BN, Rappaport H. Malignant lymphoma, well differentiated lymphocytic. Its relationship with chronic lymphocytic leukemia and macroglobulinemia of Waldenström. Cancer 1977;39:999–1010.
186. Royston I, Majda JA, Baird SM, et al. Human T-cell antigens defined by monoclonal antibodies: The 65,000-dalton antigen of T-cells (T65) is also found on chronic lymphocytic leukemia cells bearing surface immunoglobulin. J Immunol 1980;125:725–731.
187. Inghirami G, Wieczorek R, Zhee B-Y, et al. Differential expression of LFA-1 molecules in non-Hodgkin's lymphoma and lymphoid leukemia. Blood 1988;72:1431–1434.
188. Cossman J, Necker LM, Braziel RM, et al. In vitro enhancement of immunoglobulin gene expression in chronic lymphocytic leukemia. J Clin Invest 1984;73:587–592.
189. Evans HL, Butler JJ, Youness EL. Malignant lymphoma, small lymphocytic type. A clinicopathologic study of 84 cases with suggested criteria for intermediate lymphocytic lymphoma. Cancer 1978;41:1440–1455.
190. Richter MN. Generalized reticular cell sarcoma of lymph nodes associated with lymphatic leukemia. Am J Pathol 1928;4:285–292.
191. Trump DL, Mann RB, Phelps R, et al. Richter's syndrome: Diffuse histiocytic lymphoma in patients with chronic lymphocytic lymphoma. A report of 5 cases and review of the literature. Am J Med 1980;68:539–548.
192. Isaacson PG, Spencer J. Malignant lymphoma of mucosa-associated lymphoid tissue. Histopathology 1987;11:445–462.
193. Isaacson PG, Spencer J. Malignant lymphoma of mucosa associated lymphoid tissue (MALT). In: Jones DB, Wright DH, eds. Lymphoproliferative diseases. Immunology in medicine series. Norwell: Kluwer-Academic, 1990;15:123–143.
194. Harris NL. Extranodal lymphoid infiltrates and mucosa-associated lymphoid tissue (MALT). Am J Surg Pathol 1991;15:879–884.
195. Sundeen JT, Longo DL, Jaffe ES. CD5 expression in B-cell small lymphocytic malignancies: Correlations with clinical presentation and sites of disease. Am J Surg Pathol 1992;16:130–137.
196. Sheibani K, Burke JS, Swartz WG, et al. Monocytoid B-cell lymphoma. Clinicopathologic study of 21 cases of a unique type of low-grade lymphoma. Cancer 1988;62:1531–1538.
197. Nathwani BN, Winberg CD, Diamond LW, et al. Morphologic criteria for the differentiation of follicular lymphoma from florid reactive follicular hyperplasia. A study of 80 cases. Cancer 1981;48:1794–1806.
198. Garvin AJ, Simon R, Young RC, et al. The Rappaport classification on non-Hodgkin's lymphomas: A closer look using other proposed classifications. Semin Oncol 1980;7: 234–243.
199. Leech JH, Glick AD, Waldron JA, et al. Malignant lymphomas of follicular center cell origin in man. I. Immunologic studies. JNCI 1975;54:11–21.
200. Ault KA. Detection of small numbers of monoclonal B lymphocytes in the blood of patients with lymphoma. N Engl J Med 1979;300:1401–1405.
201. Come SE, Jaffe ES, Anderson JC, et al. Leukemic progression of non-Hodgkin's lymphoma: Clinicopathologic features and therapeutic implications. Am J Med 1980;69: 667–674.
202. Nathwani BN, Metter GE, Miller TP, et al. What should be the morphologic criteria for the subdivision of follicular lymphomas? Blood 1986;68:837–845.
203. Osborne CK, Norton L, Young RC, et al. Nodular histiocytic lymphoma: An aggressive nodular lymphoma with potential for prolonged disease-free survival. Blood 1980;56: 198–203.
204. Hoppe RT. Histologic variation in non-Hodgkin's lymphomas: Commentary. Cancer Treat Rep 1981;65:935–939.
205. Kim H, Dorfman RF. Morphological studies of 84 untreated patients subject to laparotomy for the staging of non-Hodgkin's lymphomas. Cancer 1974;33:657–674.
206. Lotz MJ, Chabner B, DeVita VT, et al. Pathological staging of 100 consecutive untreated patients with non-Hodgkin's lymphomas. Extramedullary sites of disease. Cancer 1976;37:266–270.
207. Levy R, Warnke R, Dorfman RF, et al. The monoclonality of human B-cell lymphomas. J Exp Med 1977;145:1014–1028.
208. Harris NL, Nadler LM, Bhan AK. Immunohistologic characterization of two malignant lymphomas of germinal center type (centroblastic/centrocytic and centrocytic) with monoclonal antibodies: Follicular and diffuse lymphomas of small-cleaved-cell type are related but distinct entities. Am J Pathol 1984;117:262–272.
209. Jaffe ES, Braylan RC, Nanba K, et al. Functional markers: A new perspective on malignant lymphomas. Cancer Treat Rep 1977;61:953–962.
210. Braziel RM, Sussman E, Neckers LM, et al. Induction of immunoglobulin secretion in follicular non-Hodgkin's lymphomas: Role of immunoregulatory T cells. Blood 1985;66: 128–134.
211. Lowder JN, Meeker TC, Campbell M, et al. Studies on B lymphoid tumors treated with monoclonal anti-idiotype antibodies: Correlations with clinical responses. Blood 1987;69:199–210.
212. Berard CW, Dorfman RF. Histopathology of malignant lymphomas. In: Roschberg SA, ed. Clinics in hematology, vol 3. Philadelphia: WB Saunders, 1974:39.
213. Weisenburger DD, Nathwani BN, Diamond LW, et al. Malignant lymphoma, intermediate lymphocytic type: A clinical-pathologic study of 42 cases. Cancer 1981;48: 1415–1425.
214. Weisenburger DD, Kim H, Rappaport H. Mantle-zone lymphoma: A follicular variant of intermediate lymphocytic lymphoma. Cancer 1982;49:1429–1438.
215. Swerdlow SH, Habeshaw JA, Murray LJ, et al. Centrocytic lymphoma: A distinct clinicopathologic and immunologic entity. Am J Pathol 1983;113:181–197.
216. Bookman MA, Lardelli P, Jaffe ES, Duffey PL, et al. Lymphocytic lymphoma of intermediate differentiation: Morphologic, immunophenotypic, and prognostic factors. JNCI 1990;82:742–748.
217. Jaffe ES, Bookman MA, Longo DL. Lymphocytic lymphoma of intermediate differentiation-mantle zone lymphoma: A distinct subtype of B-cell lymphoma. Hum Pathol 1987;18:877–880.
218. Nanba K, Jaffe ES, Braylan RC, et al. Alkaline phosphatase-positive malignant lymphomas. Am J Clin Pathol 1977;68:535–542.
219. Raffeld M, Jaffe ES. *Bcl-1*, t (11;14) and mantle cell derived lymphomas. Blood 1991;78: 259–263.
220. Cossman J, Jaffe ES, Fisher RI. Immunologic phenotypes of diffuse, aggressive, non-Hodgkin's lymphomas. Correlation with clinical features. Cancer 1984;54:1310–1317.
221. Fisher RI, Hubbard SM, DeVita VT Jr, et al. Factors determining our ability to cure aggressive forms of diffuse lymphomas. Blood 1981;58:45–51.
222. Armitage JO, Vose JM, Linder J, et al. Clinical significance of immunophenotype in diffuse aggressive non-Hodgkin's lymphoma. J Clin Oncol 1989;7:1783–1790.
223. Kwak LK, Wilson M, Weiss LM, et al. Similar outcome of treatment of B-cell and T-cell diffuse large-cell lymphomas: The Stanford experience. J Clin Oncol 1991;9: 1426–1431.
224. Jaffe ES, Longo DL, Cossman J, et al. Diffuse B cell lymphomas with T cell predominance in patients with follicular lymphoma or "pseudo T cell lymphoma." Lab Invest 1984;50: 27A–28A.
225. Ramsay AD, Smith WJ, Isaacson PG. T-cell rich B-cell lymphoma. Am J Surg Pathol 1988;12:433–443.
226. Medeiros LJ, Lardelli P, Stetler-Stevenson M, et al. Genotypic analysis of diffuse, mixed cell lymphomas: Comparison with morphologic and immunophenotypic findings. Am J Clin Pathol 1991;95:547–555.
227. Jaffe ES, Shevach EM, Sussman EH, et al. Membrane receptor sites for the identification of lymphoreticular cells in benign and malignant conditions. Br J Cancer 1975;31: 107–120.
228. Waldron JA, Leech JH, Glick AD, et al. Malignant lymphoma of peripheral T lymphocyte origin. Cancer 1977;40:1604–1617.
229. Lennert K, Mestdagh J. Lymphogranulomatoses mit constant hohem Epitheloidzellgehalt. Virchows Arch [A] 1968;344:1.
230. Burke JS, Butler JJ. Malignant lymphoma with a high content of epithelioid histiocytes (Lennert's lymphoma). Am J Clin Pathol 1976;66:1–9.
231. Kim H, Jacobs C, Warnke RA, et al. Malignant lymphoma with a high content of epithelioid histiocytes. A distinct clinicopathologic entity and a form of so-called "Lennert's lymphoma." Cancer 1978;41:620–635.
232. Levine AM, Taylor CR, Schneider DR, et al. Immunoblastic sarcoma of T-cell versus B-cell origin: I. Clinical features. Blood 1981;58:52–61.
233. Lipford E, Wright JJ, Urba W, et al. Refinement of lymphoma cytogenetics by the chromosome 18q21 major breakpoint region. Blood 1987;70:1816–1823.
234. Muller-Hermelink HK, Steinmann G, Stein H, et al. Malignant lymphoma of plasmacytoid T-cells. Morphologic and immunologic studies characterizing a special type of T-cell. Am J Surg Pathol 1983;7:849–862.
235. Kadin ME, Sako D, Berliner N, et al. Childhood Ki-1 lymphoma presenting with skin lesions and peripheral lymphadenopathy. Blood 1986;68:1042–1049.
236. Stein H, Mason DY, Gerdes J, et al. The expression of Hodgkin's disease associated antigen Ki-1 in reactive and neoplastic lymphoid tissue: Evidence that the Reed-Sternberg cells and histiocytic malignancies are derived from activated lymphoid cells. Blood 1985;66:848–858.
237. Durkop H, Latza U, Hummel M, et al. Molecular cloning and expression of a new member of the nerve growth factor receptor family that is characteristic for Hodgkin's disease. Cell 1992;68:421–428.
238. Mitchell AB, Wilbur AF, Richard AL, et al. Morphology in Ki-1 (CD30)-positive non-Hodgkin's lymphoma is correlated with clinical features and the presence of a unique chromosomal abnormality, t(2;5) (p23;q35). Am J Surg Pathol 1990;14:305–316.
239. Barcos MP, Lukes RJ. Malignant lymphoma of convoluted lymphocytes: A new entity of possible T cell type. In: Sinks LF, Godden JO (eds): Conflicts in childhood cancer: An evaluation of current management: Proceedings. New York: Alan R Liss, 1975: 147.
240. Nathwani BN, Kim H, Rappaport H. Malignant lymphoma, lymphoblastic. Cancer 1976;38:964–983.
241. Smith JL, Barker CR, Clein GP, et al. Characterization of malignant mediastinal lymphoid neoplasm (Sternberg sarcoma) as thymic in origin. Lancet 1973;1:74–77.
242. Sander CA, Medeiros LJ, Abruzzo LV, et al. Lymphoblastic lymphoma presenting in cutaneous sites: A clinicopathologic analysis of six cases. J Am Acad Dermatol 1991;25: 1023.
243. Banks PM, Arseneau JC, Gralnick HR, et al. American Burkitt's lymphoma: A clinicopathologic study of 30 cases: II. Pathologic correlations. Am J Med 1975;58:322–329.
244. Mann RB, Jaffe ES, Braylan RC, et al. Nonendemic Burkitt's lymphoma: A B-cell tumor related to germinal centers. N Engl J Med 1976;295:685–691.
245. Magrath IT, Freeman CB, Pizzo P, et al. Characterization of lymphoma-derived cell lines: Comparison of cell lines positive and negative for Epstein-Barr virus nuclear antigen: II. Surface markers. JNCI 1980;64:477–483.

246. Ziegler JL. Treatment results of 54 American patients with Burkitt's lymphomas are similar to the African experience. N Engl J Med 1977;297:75–80.
247. Grogan TM, Warnke RA, Kaplan HS. A comparative study of Burkitt's and non-Burkitt's "undifferentiated" malignant lymphomas: Immunologic, cytochemical, ultrastructural, cytologic, histopathologic, clinical and cell culture features. Cancer 1982;49:1817–1828.
248. Miliauskas JR, Berard CW, Young RC, et al. Undifferentiated non-Hodgkin's lymphomas (Burkitt's and non-Burkitt's types). The relevance of making this histologic distinction. Cancer 1982;50:2115–2121.
249. Yano T, Van Krieken JHJM, Magrath IT, et al. Histogenetic correlations between subcategories of small non-cleaved cell lymphomas. Blood 1992;79:1282–1290.
250. Croce CM, Tsujimoto Y, Erikson I, et al. Biology of disease: Chromosome translocations and B cell neoplasia. Lab Invest 1984;51:258–267.
251. Jaffe ES, Blattner WA, Blayney DW, et al. The pathologic spectrum of HTLV-associated leukemia/lymphoma in the United States. Am J Surg Pathol 1984;8:263–275.
252. Broder S, Bunn PA Jr, Jaffe ES, et al. T-cell lymphoproliferative syndrome associated with human T-cell leukemia/lymphoma virus. Ann Intern Med 1984;100:543–557.
253. Lukes RJ, Tindle BH. Immunoblastic lymphadenopathy. A hyper-immune entity resembling Hodgkin's disease. N Engl J Med 1975;292:1–8.
254. Frizzera G, Moran EM, Rappaport H. Angioblastic lymphadenopathy: Diagnosis and clinical course. Am J Med 1975;59:803–818.
255. Nathwani BN, Rappaport H, Moran EM, et al. Malignant lymphomas arising in angioimmunoblastic lymphadenopathy. Cancer 1978;41:578–606.
256. Watanabe S, Shimosato Y, Shimoyama M. Adult T-cell lymphoma with hypergammaglobulinemia. Cancer 1980;41:2472–2483.
257. Kaneko Y, Larson RA, Variakojis D, et al. Nonrandom chromosome abnormalities in angioimmunoblastic lymphadenopathy. Blood 1982;60:877–887.
258. Weiss LM, Strickler JG, Dorfman RF, et al. Clonal T cell populations in angioimmunoblastic lymphadenopathy and angioimmunoblastic lymphadenopathy-like lymphoma. Am J Pathol 1986;122:392–397.
259. Lipford EH, Smith HR, Pittaluga S, et al. Clonality of angioimmunoblastic lymphadenopathy and implications for its evolution to malignant lymphoma. J Clin Invest 1987;79:637–642.
260. Weiss LM, Jaffe ES, Liu XF, et al. Detection and localization of Epstein-Barr viral genomes in angioimmunoblastic lymphadenopathy and angioimmunoblastic lymphadenopathy-like lymphoma. Blood 1992;79:1789–1795.
261. Kassel SH, Echevarria RA, Guzzo FP. Midline malignant reticulosis (so-called lethal midline granuloma). Cancer 1969;23:920–935.
262. De Remee RA, Weiland LH, McDonald TJ. Polymorphic reticulosis, lymphomatoid granulomatosis: Two diseases or one? Mayo Clin Proc 1978;53:634–640.
263. Liebow AA, Carrington CB, Friedman RJ. Lymphomatoid granulomatosis. Hum Pathol 1972;3:457–558.
264. Jaffe ES, Lipford EH Jr, Margolick JB, et al. Lymphomatoid granulomatosis and angiocentric lymphoma. A spectrum of post-thymic T cell proliferations. Semin Respir Med 1989;10:167–172.
265. Fauci AS, Haynes BF, Costa J, et al. Lymphomatoid granulomatosis, prospective clinical and therapeutic experience over ten years. N Engl J Med 1982;306:68–74.
266. Katzenstein A, Carrington CB, Liebow AA. Lymphomatoid granulomatosis: A clinicalpathologic study of 152 cases. Cancer 1979;43:360–373.
267. Nichols PW, Koss M, Levine AM, et al. Lymphomatoid granulomatosis: A T-cell disorder. Am J Med 1982;72:467–471.
268. Harabuchi Y, Yamanaka N, Kataura A, et al. Epstein-Barr virus in nasal T-cell lymphomas in patients with lethal midline granuloma. Lancet 1990;335:128–130.
269. Katzenstein AL, Peiper SC. Detection of Epstein-Barr virus genomes in lymphomatoid granulomatosis: Analysis of 29 cases by the polymerase chain reaction technique. Mod Pathol 1990;3:435–441.
270. Ho FCS, Srivastava G, Loke SL, et al. Presence of Epstein-Barr virus DNA in nasal lymphomas of B and T cell type. Hematol Oncol 1990;8:271–281.
271. Medeiros LJ, Peiper SC, Elwood L, et al. Angiocentric immunoproliferative lesions: A molecular analysis of eight cases. Hum Pathol 1991;22:1150–1157.
272. Chan JKC, Ng CS, Path MRC, et al. Most nasal/nasopharyngeal lymphomas are peripheral T-cell neoplasms. Am J Surg Pathol 1987;11:418–429.
273. Jaffe ES. Malignant histiocytosis and true histiocytic lymphomas. In: Jaffe ES, ed. Surgical pathology of lymph nodes and related organs. Philadelphia: WB Saunders, 1985:381.
274. Sultan C, Imbert M, Richard MF, et al. Pure acute monocytic leukemia. A study of 12 cases. Am J Clin Pathol 1977;68:752–757.
275. Van der Valk P, Meijer CJLM, Willemze R, et al. Histiocytic sarcoma (true histiocytic lymphoma): A clinicopathology study of 20 cases. Histopathology 1984;8:105–123.
276. Willemze R, Rinter DJ, Wilem A, et al. Reticulum cell sarcomas (large cell lymphomas) presenting in the skin. High frequency of true histiocytic lymphoma. Cancer 1982;50:1367–1379.
277. Flynn KJ, Dehner LP, Gajl-Peczalska KJ, et al. Regressing atypical histiocytosis: A cutaneous proliferation of atypical neoplastic histiocytes with unexpectedly indolent biologic behavior. Cancer 1982;49:959–970.
278. Poppema S, Van Voorst Vader PC, Rozenboom-Uiterwijk T, et al. Lymphomatoid papulosis. Case report providing evidence for a monocyte-macrophage origin of the atypical cells. Cancer 1983;52:1178–1182.
279. Scott RB, Robb-Smith AHT. Histiocytic medullary reticulosis. Lancet 1939;2:194–198.
280. Risdall RJ, McKenna RW, Nesbit ME, et al. Virus-associated hemophagocytic syndrome—A benign histiocytic proliferation distinct from malignant histiocytosis. Cancer 1979;44:993–1002.
281. Jaffe ES, Costa J, Fauci AS, et al. Malignant lymphoma and erythrophagocytosis simulating malignant histiocytosis. Am J Med 1983;75:741–749.
282. Simrell CR, Margolick JB, Crabtree GR, et al. Lymphokine-induced phagocytosis in angiocentric immunoproliferative lesions (AIL) and malignant lymphoma arising in AIL. Blood 1985;65:1469–1476.
283. Favara BE, McCarthy RC, Mierau GW. Histiocytosis X. In: Finefold M, ed. Pathology of neoplasia in children and adolescents. Philadelphia: WB Saunders, 1986:126.
284. Nezelof C, Frileux-Herbert F, Cronies-Sachet J. Disseminated histiocytosis X, analysis of prognostic factors based on a retrospective study of 50 cases. Cancer 1979;44:1824–1838.
285. Lahey ME. Prognostic factors in histiocytosis X. Am J Pediatr Hematol Oncol 1981;3:57–60.
286. Monda L, Warnke R, Rosai J. A primary lymph node malignancy with features suggestive of dendritic reticulum cell differentiation. A report of 4 cases. Am J Pathol 1986;122:562–572.
287. Feltkamp CA, van Heerde P, Feltkamp-Vroom TM, et al. A malignant tumor arising from interdigitating cells; light microscopical, ultrastructural, immuno- and enzyme histochemical characteristics. Virchows Arch [A] 1981;393:183.
288. Chan W, Zaatari G. Lymph node interdigitating reticulum cell sarcoma. Am J Clin Pathol 1986;85:739–744.
289. Frizzera G. Castleman's disease and related disorders. Semin Diagn Pathol 1988;5:346–364.
290. Castleman B, Iverson L, Menendez V. Localized mediastinal lymph node hyperplasia resembling thymoma. Cancer 1956;9:822–830.
291. Keller AR, Hochholzer L, Castleman B. Hyaline-vascular and plasma-cell types of giant lymph node hyperplasia of the mediastinum and other locations. Cancer 1972;29:670–683.
292. Yashizaki K, Matsuda T, Nishimoto N, et al. Pathogenic significance of interleukin-6 (IL-6/BSF-2) in Castleman's disease. Blood 1989;74:1360–1367.
293. Hanson CA, Frizzera G, Patton DF, et al. Clonal rearrangement for immunoglobulin and T-cell receptor genes in systemic Castleman's disease. Association with Epstein-Barr Virus. Am J Pathol 1988;131:84–91.
294. Frizzera G, Peterson BA, Bayrd ED, et al. A systemic lymphoproliferative disorder with morphologic features of Castleman's disease: Clinical findings and clinicopathologic correlations in 15 patients. J Clin Oncol 1985;3:1202–1216.
295. Weisenburger DD, Nathwani BN, Winberg CD, et al. Multicentric angiofollicular lymph node hyperplasia: A clinicopathologic study of 16 cases. Hum Pathol 1985;16:162–172.
296. Kaplan HS. Hodgkin's disease. 2nd ed. Cambridge, MA: Harvard University Press, 1980:689.
297. Rosenberg SA, Diamond HD, Jaslowitz B, et al. Lymphosarcoma: A review of 1269 cases. Medicine (Baltimore) 1961;40:31–84.
298. Banfi A, Bonadonna G, Riece SB, et al. Malignant lymphomas of Waldeyer's ring: Natural history and survival after radiotherapy. Br Med J 1972;2:140.
299. Sage HH. Palpable cervical lymph nodes. JAMA 1958;168:496–498.
300. Filly R, Blank N, Castellino RA. Radiographic distribution of intrathoracic disease in previously untreated patients with Hodgkin's disease and non-Hodgkin's lymphoma. Radiology 1976;120:277–281.
301. Simone JV, Verzosa MS, Rudy JA. Initial features and prognosis in 363 children with acute lymphoblastic leukemia. Cancer 1975;36:2099–2108.
302. Bitran JD, Golomb HM, Ultmann JE, et al. Non-Hodgkin's lymphoma, poorly differentiated lymphocytic and mixed cell types: Results of sequential staging procedures, response to therapy, and survival of 100 patients. Cancer 1978;42:88–95.
303. Golomb H. "Hairy" cell leukemia: An unusual lymphoproliferative disease. Cancer 1978;42:946–956.
304. Rappaport H, Ramot B, Hulu N, et al. The pathology of so-called Mediterranean abdominal lymphoma with malabsorption. Cancer 1972;29:1502–1511.
305. Dragosics B, Bauer P, Radaszkiweicz T. Primary gastrointestinal lymphomas. A retrospective clinicopathologic study of 150 cases. Cancer 1985;55:1060–1073.
306. Buskirk SJ, Evans RG, Banks PM, et al. Primary lymphoma of the testis. Int J Radiat Oncol Biol Phys 1982;8:1699–1703.
307. Young RC, Howser DM, Anderson T, et al. Central nervous system complications of non-Hodgkin's lymphoma. The potential role for prophylactic therapy. Am J Med 1979;66:435–443.
308. Jones SE, Fuks Z, Bull M, et al. Non-Hodgkin's lymphomas: IV. Clinicopathologic correlation in 405 cases. Cancer 1973;31:806–823.
309. Chabner BA, Johnson RE, Young RC, et al. Sequential non-surgical and surgical staging of non-Hodgkin's lymphoma. Ann Intern Med 1976;85:149–154.
310. Anderson T, Chabner BA, Young RC, et al. Malignant lymphoma: I. The histology and staging of 473 patients at the National Cancer Institute. Cancer 1982;50:2699–2709.
311. DeVita VT, Canellos GP. Treatment of the lymphomas. Semin Hematol 1972;9:193–209.
312. Reddy S, Saxena VS, Pellettiere EV, et al. Early nodal and extra nodal non-Hodgkin's lymphomas. Cancer 1977;40:98–104.
313. Paryani S, Hoppe RT, Burke JS, et al. Extralymphatic involvement in diffuse non-Hodgkin's lymphomas. J Clin Oncol 1983;1:682–688.
314. Portlock CS, Rosenberg SA. No initial therapy for stage III and IV non-Hodgkin's lymphomas of favorable histologic types. Ann Intern Med 1979;90:10–13.
315. DeVita VT. Human models of human disease: Breast cancer and the lymphomas. Int J Radiat Oncol Biol Phys 1979;5:1855–1867.
316. Acker B, Hoppe RT, Colby TV, et al. Histologic conversion in the non-Hodgkin's lymphomas. J Clin Oncol 1983;1:11–16.
317. Rowley JD. Consistent chromosome abnormalities in human leukemia and lymphoma. Cancer Invest 1983;3:267–280.

318. Carbone PP, Kaplan HS, Musshoff K, et al. Report of the committee on Hodgkin's disease staging. Cancer Res 1971;31:1860–1861.
319. Ciampi A, Bush RS, Gospodarowicz M. An approach to classifying prognostic factors related to survival experience for non-Hodgkin's lymphoma patients: Based on a series of 982 patients: 1967–1975. Cancer 1981;47:621–627.
320. Jagannath S, Velasquez WS, Tucker SL, et al. Tumor burden assessment and its implication for a prognostic model in advanced diffuse large-cell lymphoma. J Clin Oncol 1986;2:859–865.
321. Vose JM, Armitage JO, Weisenberger DD, et al. The importance of age in survival of patients treated with chemotherapy for aggressive non-Hodgkin's lymphomas. J Clin Oncol 1988;6:1838–1844.
322. Coiffier B, Gisselbrecht C, Vose JM, et al. Prognostic factors in aggressive malignant lymphomas: Description and validation of a prognostic index that could identify patients requiring a more intensive therapy. J Clin Oncol 1991;9:211–219.
323. Hoskins PJ, Ng V, Spinelli JJ, et al. Prognostic variables in patients with diffuse large-cell lymphoma treated with MACOP-B. J Clin Oncol 1991;9:220–226.
324. Shipp MA, Harrington DP, Klatt MM, et al. Identification of major prognostic subgroups of patients with large cell lymphoma treated with m-BACOD or M-BACOD. Ann Intern Med 1986;104:757–765.
325. Litan P, Swan F, Cabanillas F, et al. Prognostic value of serum β_2-microglobulin in low-grade lymphoma. Ann Intern Med 1991;114:855–860.
326. Gallagher CJ, Gregory WM, Jones AE, et al. Follicular lymphoma: Prognostic factors for response and survival. J Clin Oncol 1986;4:1470–1480.
327. Soubeyran P, Eghbali H, Bonichon F, et al. Low-grade follicular lymphoma: Analysis of prognosis in a series of 281 patients. Eur J Cancer 1991;27:1606–1613.
328. Armitage JO, Weisenburger DD, Hutchins M, et al. Chemotherapy for diffuse large cell lymphoma: Rapidly responding patients have more durable remissions. J Clin Oncol 1986;4:160–164.
329. Lister TA, Crowther D, Sutcliffe SB, et al. Report of a committee convened to discuss the evaluation and staging of patients with Hodgkin's disease: Cotswold meeting. J Clin Oncol 1989;7:1630–1636.
330. Young RC, Anderson T, DeVita VT. The treatment of Hodgkin's disease: Emphasizing programs at the Clinical Center, National Institutes of Health. Curr Probl Cancer 1977;1:1–29.
331. Moormeier JA, Williams SF, Golomb HM. The staging of non-Hodgkin's lymphomas. Semin Oncol 1990;17:43–50.
332. Smith BR, Weinberg DS, Robert NJ, et al. Circulating monoclonal B lymphocytes in non-Hodgkin's lymphoma. N Engl J Med 1984;311:1476–1481.
333. Horning SJ, Galili N, Cleary M, et al. Detection of non-Hodgkin's lymphoma in the peripheral blood by analysis of antigen receptor gene rearrangements: Results of a prospective study. Blood 1990;75:1139–1145.
334. Berliner N, Ault K, Martin P, et al. Detection of clonal excess in lymphoproliferative disease by kappa/lambda analysis: Correlation with immunoglobulin gene DNA rearrangements. Blood 1986;67:80–85.
335. Khoury MB, Godwin JD, Halvorsen R, et al. Role of chest CT in non-Hodgkin's lymphoma. Radiology 1986;158:659.
336. Marglin S, Castellino RA. Lymphographic accuracy in 632 consecutive, previously untreated cases of Hodgkin's disease and non-Hodgkin's lymphoma. Radiology 1981;140:351–353.
337. Castellino RA, Dunnick NR, Goffinet DR, et al. Predictive value of lymphography for sites of supradiaphragmatic disease encountered at staging laporotomy in newly diagnosed Hodgkin's disease and non-Hodgkin's lymphoma. J Clin Oncol 1983;1:532–536.
338. Castellino RA, Marglin SI. Imaging of abdominal and pelvic lymph nodes: Lymphography or computed tomography. Invest Radiol 1982;17:433–443.
339. Lee JK, Stanley RJ, Sagel SS, et al. Accuracy of computed tomography in detecting intraabdominal and pelvic adenopathy in lymphoma. AJR 1978;131:311–315.
340. Neumann CH, Finberg H, Rosenthal DS. The role of computerized body tomography of the abdomen in the management of lymphoma patients. Postgrad Radiol 1982;2/3:225–239.
341. Benson WJ, Ding JC, Cooper IA. Abdominal CT and lymphography in the initial staging of non-Hodgkin's lymphomas. Aust N Z J Med 1987;17:253–254.
342. Shields AF, Porter BA, Churchley S, et al. The detection of bone marrow involvement by lymphoma using magnetic resonance imaging. J Clin Oncol 1987;5:225–230.
343. Hoane BR, Shields AF, Porter BA, et al. Detection of lymphomatous bone marrow involvement with magnetic resonance imaging. Blood 1991;78:728–738.
344. Longo DL, Schilsky RL, Blei L, et al. Gallium-67 scanning has limited usefulness in staging patients with non-Hodgkin's lymphoma. Am J Med 1980;68:695–700.
345. Anderson KC, Leonard RC, Canellos GP, et al. High dose gallium imaging in lymphoma. Am J Med 1981;75:327–331.
346. Moran EJ, Ultmann JE, Ferguson DJ. Staging laparotomy on non-Hodgkin's lymphoma. Br J Cancer 1975;31:228–236.
347. Israel O, Front DM, Lam M, et al. Gallium 67 imaging in monitoring response to treatment. Cancer 1988;61:2439–2443.
348. Kaplan WD, Jochelson MS, Herman TS, et al. Gallium-67 imaging: A predictor of residual tumor viability and clinical outcome in patients with diffuse large-cell lymphoma. J Clin Oncol 1990;8:1966–1970.
349. Weeks JC, Yeop BY, Canellos GP, Shipp MA. Value of follow-up procedures in patients with large-cell lymphoma who achieve a complete remission. J Clin Oncol 1991;9:1196–1203.
350. Anderson KC, Kaplan WD, Leonard RCF, et al. Role of ^{99m}Tc methylene diphosphonate bone imaging in the management of lymphoma. Cancer Treat Rep 1985;69:1347–1351.
351. Chabner BA, Fisher RI, Young RC, et al. Staging of non-Hodgkin's lymphoma. Semin Oncol 1980;7:285–291.
352. Levitt LJ, Dawson DM, Rosenthal DS, et al. CNS involvement in the non-Hodgkin's lymphomas. Cancer 1980;45:545–552.
353. Bunn PA Jr, Schein PS, Banks PM, et al. Central nervous system complications in patients with diffuse histiocytic and undifferentiated lymphoma: Leukemia revisited. Blood 1976;47:3–10.
354. Crescenzi M, Seto M, Herzig GP, et al. Thermostable DNA polymerase chain amplification of t(14;18) chromosome breakpoints and detection of minimal residual disease. Proc Natl Acad Sci USA 1988;85:4869–4873.
355. Veronesi U, Musumeci R, Pizzetti F, et al. The value of staging laparotomy in non-Hodgkin's lymphomas (with emphasis on the histiocytic type). Cancer 1974;33:446–459.
356. Castellani R, Bonadonna G, Spinelli P, et al. Sequential pathologic staging of untreated non-Hodgkin's lymphomas by laparoscopy and laparotomy combined with marrow biopsy. Cancer 1977;40:2322–2328.
357. Goffinet DR, Warnke R, Dunnick NR, et al. Clinical and surgical (laparotomy) evaluation of patients with non-Hodgkin's lymphomas. Cancer Treat Rep 1977;61:981–992.
358. Chabner BA, Johnson RE, DeVita VT, et al. Sequential staging in non-Hodgkin's lymphoma. Cancer Treat Rep 1977;61:993–997.
359. Heifetz LJ, Fuller LM, Rogers RW, et al. Laparotomy findings in lymphangiogram staged I and II non-Hodgkin's lymphomas. Cancer 1980;45:2778–2786.
360. Fuks JA, Aisner J, Wiernik PH. Restaging laparotomy in the management of non-Hodgkin's lymphomas. Med Pediatr Oncol 1982;10:429–438.
361. Surbone A, Longo DL, DeVita VT Jr, et al. Residual abdominal masses in aggressive non-Hodgkin's lymphoma after combination chemotherapy: Significance and management. J Clin Oncol 1988;6:1832–1837.
362. Moore DF, Migliore PH, Shullenberg CC, et al. Monoclonal macroglobulinemia in malignant lymphoma. Ann Intern Med 1970;72:43–47.
363. Levy RL, Miller RA. Biological and clinical implications of lymphocyte hybridomas: Tumor therapy with monoclonal antibodies. Ann Rev Med 1983;34:107–116.
364. Ko HS, Pruzanski W. M components associated with lymphoma: A review of 62 cases. Am J Med Sci 1976;272:175–183.
365. Balentine L, Skikne BS, Park CH, et al. Malignant lymphocytic lymphoma: Demonstration of a serum inhibitor of myelopoiesis and response to combination chemotherapy. Cancer 1983;52:35–38.
366. Jones SE. Autoimmune disorders and malignant lymphoma. Cancer 1973;31:1092–1098.
367. Anderson TC, Jones SE, Soehnlen BJ, et al. Immunocompetence and malignant lymphoma: Immunologic status before therapy. Cancer 1981;48:2702–2709.
368. Jones SE, Griffith K, Dombrowski P, et al. Immunodeficiency in patients with non-Hodgkin's lymphomas. Blood 1977;49:335–344.
369. Advani SH, Dinshaw KA, Nair CN, et al. Immune dysfunction in non-Hodgkin's lymphomas. Cancer 1980;45:2843–2848.
370. Silver BA, Bostick-Bruton FW, Neckers L, et al. Deficient helper cell function as a cause of diminished pokeweed mitogen blastogenic responses in patients with non-Hodgkin's lymphomas. Cancer 1984;54:2936–2942.
371. Gajl-Peczalska KJ, Chartrand SL, Bloomfield CD. Abnormal immunoregulation in patients with non-Hodgkin's malignant lymphomas. Clin Immunol Immunopathol 1982;23:366–378.
372. Whisler RL, Balerzak SP, Murray JL. Heterogeneous mechanisms of impaired lymphocyte responses in non-Hodgkin's lymphomas. Blood 1981;57:1081–1087.
373. Broder S, Edelson RL, Lutzner MA, et al. Sezary syndrome: A malignant proliferation of helper T cells. J Clin Invest 1976;58:1297–1306.
374. Broder S, Uchiyama T, Muul L, et al. Activation of leukemic prosuppressor cells to become suppressor effector cells. Influence of cooperating normal T cells. N Engl J Med 1981;302:1382–1387.
375. Longo DL, Broder S. Human T-cell leukemia/lymphoma virus (HTLV) associated adult T-cell leukemia. Med Grand Rounds 1984;3:239.
376. Glatstein E, Fuks Z, Goffinet DR, et al. Non-Hodgkin's lymphoma of stage III extent. Is total lymphoid irradiation appropriate treatment? Cancer 1976;37:2806–2812.
377. Paryani SB, Hoppe RT, Cox RS, et al. The role of radiation therapy in the management of stage III follicular lymphomas. J Clin Oncol 1984;2:841–848.
378. Cox JD, Komaki R, Kun LE, et al. Stage III nodular lymphoreticular tumors (non-Hodgkin's lymphomas): Results of central lymphatic irradiation. Cancer 1981;47:2247–2252.
379. Flippen T, McLaughlin P, Conrad FG, et al. Stage III nodular lymphomas. Preliminary results of a combined chemotherapy/radiotherapy program. Cancer 1983;51:987–993.
380. Rosenberg SA. The low-grade non-Hodgkin's lymphomas: Challenges and opportunities. J Clin Oncol 1985;3:299–310.
381. Paryani SB, Hoppe RT, Cox RS, et al. Analysis of non-Hodgkin's lymphomas with nodular and favorable histologies, stages I and II. Cancer 1983;52:2300–2307.
382. Gomez GA, Barcos M, Krishnamsetty RM, et al. Treatment of early-stages I and II-nodular, poorly differentiated lymphocytic lymphoma. Am J Clin Oncol 1986;9:40–44.
383. Gospodarowicz MK, Bush RS, Brown TC. Prognostic factors in nodular lymphomas: A multivariate analysis based on the Princess Margaret Experience. Int J Radiat Oncol Biol Phys 1984;10:489–497.
384. Lawrence TS, Urba WJ, Steinberg SM, et al. Restrospective analysis of stage I and II indolent lymphomas at the National Cancer Institute. Int J Radiat Oncol Biol Phys 1988;14:417–424.
385. Richards MA, Gregory WM, Hall PA, et al. Management of localized non-Hodgkin's lymphoma: The experience at St. Bartholomew's Hospital 1972–1985. Hematol Oncol 1989;7:1–18.

386. Fuks Z, Glatstein E, Kaplan HS. Patterns of presentation and relapse in the non-Hodgkin's lymphomata. Br J Cancer 1975;31:286–297.
387. Monfardini S, Banfi A, Bonadonna G, et al. Improved five-year survival after combined radiotherapy-chemotherapy for stage I–II non-Hodgkin's lymphoma. Int J Radiat Oncol Biol Phys 1980;6:125–134.
388. Landberg TG, Hakansson LG, Moller TR, et al. CVP remission maintenance in stage I or II non-Hodgkin's lymphomas: Preliminary results of a randomized study. Cancer 1979;44:831–838.
389. Toonkel LM, Fuller LM, Gamble JF, et al. Laparotomy staged I and II non-Hodgkin's lymphomas: Preliminary results of radiotherapy and adjunctive chemotherapy. Cancer 1980;45:249–260.
390. McLaughlin P, Fuller LM, Velasquez WS, et al. Stage I–II follicular lymphoma. Treatment results for 76 patients. Cancer 1986;58:1596–1602.
391. McLaughlin P, Fuller L, Redman J, et al. Stage I–II low-grade lymphomas: A prospective trial of combination chemotherapy and radiotherapy. Ann Oncol 1991;2(suppl 2): 137–140.
392. Longo DL, Young RC, DeVita VT Jr. What is so good about the good prognosis lymphomas? In: Williams CJ, Whitehouse JMA, eds. Recent advances in medical oncology. Edinburgh: Churchill Livingstone, 1982:223.
393. Matis LA, Young RC, Longo DL. Nodular lymphomas: Current concepts. Crit Rev Oncol Hematol 1986;5:171–197.
394. Horning SJ, Rosenberg SA. The natural history of initially untreated low-grade non-Hodgkin's lymphomas. N Engl J Med 1984;311:1471–1475.
395. Anderson T, DeVita VT Jr, Simon RM, et al. Malignant lymphoma II. Prognostic factors and response to treatment of 473 patients at the National Cancer Institute. Cancer 1982;50:2708–2721.
396. Lister TA. The management of follicular lymphoma. Ann Oncol 1991;2(suppl 2):131–136.
397. Kennedy BJ, Bloomfield CD, Kiang DT, et al. Combinations versus successive single agent chemotherapy in lymphocytic lymphoma. Cancer 1978;41:23–28.
398. Portlock CS, Rosenberg SA, Glatstein E, et al. Treatment of advanced non-Hodgkin's lymphomas with favorable histologies. Preliminary results of a prospective trial. Blood 1976;47:747–756.
399. Hoppe RT, Kushlan P, Kaplan HS, et al. The treatment of advanced stage favorable non-Hodgkin's lymphoma: A preliminary report of a randomized trial comparing single agent chemotherapy, combination chemotherapy, and whole body radiation. Blood 1981;58:592–598.
400. Lister TA, Cullen MH, Beard MEJ, et al. Comparison of combined and single-agent chemotherapy in non-Hodgkin's lymphoma of favorable histological type. Br Med J 1978;6112:533–537.
401. Portlock CS, Fischer DS, Cadman E, et al. High-dose pulse chlorambucil in advanced, low-grade non-hodgkin's lymphoma. Cancer Treat Rep 1987;71:1029–1031.
402. Anderson T, Bender RA, Fisher RI, et al. Combination chemotherapy in non-Hodgkin's lymphomas: Results of long-term follow-up. Cancer Treat Rep 1977;61:1057–1066.
403. Ezdinli EZ, Anderson JR, Melvin F, et al. Moderate versus aggressive chemotherapy of nodular lymphocytic poorly differentiated lymphoma. J Clin Oncol 1985;3:769–775.
404. Jones SE, Grozea PN, Metz EN, et al. Superiority of adriamycin-containing combination chemotherapy in the treatment of diffuse lymphoma. A Southwest Oncology Group study. Cancer 1979;43:417–425.
405. Romaguera JE, McLaughlin P, North L, et al. Multivariate analysis of prognostic factors in stage IV follicular low-grade lymphoma: A risk model. J Clin Oncol 1991;9:762–769.
406. Skarin AT, Rosenthal DS, Malloney WC, et al. Combination chemotherapy of advanced non-Hodgkin's lymphoma with bleomycin, Adriamycin, cyclophosphamide, vincristine and prednisone (BACOP). Blood 1977;49:759–770.
407. Licht JD, Bosserman LD, Anderson JW, et al. Treatment of low-grade and intermediate-grade lymphoma with intensive combination chemotherapy results in long-term disease-free survival. Cancer 1990;66:632–639.
408. Young RC, Johnson RE, Canellos GP, et al. Advanced lymphocytic lymphoma. Randomized comparisons of chemotherapy and radiotherapy alone or in combination. Cancer Treat Rep 1977;61:1153–1159.
409. Choi NC, Timothy AR, Kaufman SA, et al. Low dose fractionated whole body irradiation in the treatment of advanced non-Hodgkin's lymphoma. Cancer 1979;43:1636–1642.
410. Thar TL, Million RR, Noyes WD. Total body irradiation in non-Hodgkin's lymphoma. Int J Radiat Biol 1979;5:171–176.
411. Young RC, Longo DL, Glatstein E, et al. The treatment of indolent lymphomas: Watchful waiting v. aggressive combined modality treatment. Semin Hematol 1988;25(suppl 2):11–16.
412. Schein PS, Chabner BA, Canellos GP, et al. Non-Hodgkin's lymphoma: Patterns of relapse from complete remission after combination chemotherapy. Cancer 1975;35: 354–357.
413. Portlock CS. Management of the indolent non-Hodgkin's lymphomas. Semin Oncol 1980;7:292–301.
414. Brereton HD, Young RC, Longo DL, et al. A comparison between combination chemotherapy and total body radiation plus combination chemotherapy in non-Hodgkin's lymphoma. Cancer 1979;43:2227–2231.
415. Garvin AJ, Simon RM, Osborne CK, et al. An autopsy study of histologic progression in non-Hodgkin's lymphoma: 192 cases from the National Cancer Institute. Cancer 1983;52:393–398.
416. Armitage JO, Dick FR, Corder MP. Diffuse histiocytic lymphoma after histologic conversion: A poor prognostic variant. Cancer Treat Rep 1981;65:413–418.
417. Straus DJ, Gaynor JJ, Lieberman PH, et al. Non-Hodgkin's lymphomas: Characteristics of long-term survivors following conservative treatment. Am J Med 1987;82:247–256.
418. O'Brien MER, Easterbrook P, Powell J, et al. The natural history of low grade non-Hodgkin's lymphoma and the impact of a no initial treatment policy on survival. Q J Med 1991;292:651–660.
419. Chabner BA. Nodular non-Hodgkin's lymphoma: The case for watchful waiting. Ann Intern Med 1979;90:115–117.
420. Botnick LE, Hannon EC, Hellman S. Limited proliferation of stem cells surviving alkylating agents. Nature 1976;262:68–70.
421. Hellman S, Reincke V, Botnick LE, et al. Functional organization of the hematopoietic stem cell compartment: Implications for cancer and its therapy. J Clin Oncol 1983;1: 227–284.
422. Dumont J, Thiery JP, Mazabrand A, et al. Acute myeloid leukemia following non-Hodgkin's lymphoma: Danger of prolonged use of chlorambucil as maintenance therapy. Nouv Rev Fr Hematol 1980;22:391–404.
423. Cameron S. Chlorambucil and leukemia. N Engl J Med 1977;296:1065.
424. Casciata DA, Scott DA. Acute leukemia following prolonged cytotoxic agent therapy. Medicine (Baltimore) 1979;58:32–47.
425. Lerner HJ. Acute myelogenous leukemia in patients receiving chlorambucil as long term adjuvant chemotherapy for stage II breast cancer. Cancer Treat Rep 1978;62: 1136–1138.
426. Longo DL, Young RC, Hubbard SM, et al. Prolonged initial remission in patients with nodular mixed lymphoma. Ann Intern Med 1984;100:651–656.
427. Ezdinli EZ, Costello WG, Icli F, et al. Nodular mixed lymphocytic-histiocytic lymphoma (NM): Response and survival: Eastern Cooperative Oncology Group. Cancer 1980;45: 261–267.
428. Merchant N, McLaughlin P, Fuller L, et al. Follicular (nodular) mixed lymphoma: A review of 65 cases. Proc Am Soc Clin Oncol 1984;3:249.
429. Peterson BA, Anderson JR, Frizzera G, et al. Combination chemotherapy prolongs survival in follicular mixed lymphoma (FML). Proc Am Soc Clin Oncol 1990;9:259.
430. Sobel RE, Dillman RO, Collins H, et al. Applications and limitations of peripheral blood lymphocyte immunoglobulin light chain analysis in the evaluation of non-Hodgkin's lymphoma. Cancer 1985;56:2005–2010.
431. Lindemalm C, Mellstedt H, Biberfeld P, et al. Clonal blood B-cell excess in relation to prognosis in untreated non-leukemic patients with non-Hodgkin's lymphoma. In: Cavalli F, Bonadonna G, Rozencweig M, eds. Malignant lymphomas and Hodgkin's disease: Experimental and therapeutic advances. Boston: Martinus-Nijhoff, 1985:225.
432. Hansen H, Koziner B, Clarkson B. Marker and kinetic studies in the non-Hodgkin's lymphomas. Am J Med 1981;71:107–123.
433. McLaughlin P, Fuller LM, Velasquez WS, et al. Stage III follicular lymphoma: Durable remissions with a combined chemotherapy-radiotherapy regimen. J Clin Oncol 1987;5: 867–874.
434. Leonard RCF, Hayward RL, Prescott RJ, et al. The identification of discrete prognostic groups in low grade non-Hodgkin's lymphoma. Ann Oncol 1991;2:655–662.
435. Bastion Y, Berger F, Bryon P-A, et al. Follicular lymphomas: Assessment of prognostic factors in 127 patients followed for 10 years. Ann Oncol 1991;2(suppl 2):123–129.
436. Cabanillas F, Smith T, Bodey GP, et al. Nodular malignant lymphomas. Factors affecting complete response rate and survival. Cancer 1979;44:1983–1989.
437. Samuels B, Ultmann J, Pearson M, et al. Favorable non-Hodgkin's lymphoma: A fifteen year experience. Proc Am Soc Clin Oncol 1987;6:206.
438. Philip T, Armitage JO, Spitzer G, et al. High dose therapy and autologous bone marrow transplantation after failure of conventional chemotherapy in adults with intermediate grade or high grade non-Hodgkin's lymphoma. N Engl J Med 1987;316:1493–1498.
439. Freedman AS, Takvorian T, Anderson KC, et al. Autologous bone marrow transplantation in B-cell non-Hodgkin's lymphoma: Very low treatment-related mortality in 100 patients in sensitive relapse. J Clin Oncol 1990;8:784–791.
440. Freedman AS, Ritz J, Neuberg D, et al. Autologous bone marrow transplantation in 69 patients with a history of low-grade B-cell non-Hodgkin's lymphoma. Blood 1991;77: 2524–2529.
441. Gribben JG, Freedman AS, Sunhee D, et al. All advanced stage non-Hodgkin's lymphomas with a polymerase chain reaction amplifiable breakpoint of *bcl-2* have residual cells containing the *bcl-2* rearrangement at evaluation and after treatment. Blood 1991;78:3275–3280.
442. Rohatiner AZS, Price CGA, Arnott S, et al. Myeloablative therapy with autologous bone marrow transplantation as consolidation of remission in patients with follicular lymphoma. Ann Oncol 1991;2(suppl 2):147–150.
443. Schouten LC, Bierman PJ, Vaughan WP, et al. Autologous bone marrow transplantation in follicular non-Hodgkin's lymphoma before and after histologic transformation. Blood 1989;74:2579–2584.
444. Longo DL. Biologic agents and approaches in the management of patients with lymphoma. A critical appraisal. Hematol Oncol Clin North Am 1991;5:1067–1087.
445. Gilewski TA, Richards JM. Biologic Response modifiers in non-Hodgkin's lymphomas. Semin Oncol 1990;17:74–87.
446. Gaynor ER, Fisher RI. Clinical trials of α-interferon in the treatment of non-Hodgkin's lymphoma. Semin Oncol 1991;18(suppl 7):12–17.
447. Urba WJ, Longo DL. Alpha-interferon in the treatment of nodular lymphomas. Semin Oncol 1986;13:40–47.
448. Hawkins MJ, O'Connell MJ, Schiller JH, et al. Phase I evaluation of recombinant A interferon alpha in combination with COPA chemotherapy. Proc Am Soc Clin Oncol 1985;4:229.
449. Rohatiner AZS, Richards MA, Barnett MJ, et al. Chlorambucil and interferon for low grade non-Hodgkin's lymphoma. Br J Cancer 1987;55:225–226.
450. Non-Hodgkin's Lymphoma Cooperative Study Group. Randomized study of chlorambucil (CB) compared to interferon (alfa-2b) combined with CB in low-grade non-Hodgkin's lymphoma: An interim report of a randomized study. Eur J Cancer 1991;27(suppl 4): 31–33.

451. Price CGA, Rohatiner AZS, Steward W, et al. Interferon-α2b in the treatment of follicular lymphoma: Preliminary results of a trial in progress. Ann Oncol 1991;2(suppl 2):141–145.
452. Tourani J-M, Levy V, Briere J, et al. Interleukin-2 therapy for refractory and relapsing lymphomas. Eur J Cancer 1991;27:1676–1680.
453. Weber JS, Yang JC, Topalian SL, et al. The use of interleukin-2 and lymphokine-activated killer cells for the treatment of patients with non-Hodgkin's lymphoma. J Clin Oncol 1992;10:33–40.
454. Bernstein ZP, Vaickus L, Friedman N, et al. Interleukin-2 lymphokine-activated killer cell therapy of non-Hodgkin's lymphoma and Hodgkin's disease. J Immunotherapy 1991;10:141–146.
455. Margolin KA, Aronson FR, Sznol M, et al. Phase II trial of high-dose interleukin-2 and lymphokine activated killer cells in Hodgkin's disease and non-Hodgkin's lymphoma. J Immunotherapy 1991;10:214–220.
456. Meeker T, Lowder J, Maloney DG, et al. A clinical trial of anti-idiotype therapy for B cell malignancy. Blood 1985;65:1349–1363.
457. Rankin EM, Hekman A, Somers R, et al. Treatment of two patients with B cell lymphoma with monoclonal anti-idiotype antibodies. Blood 1985;65:1373–1381.
458. Press OW, Appelbaum F, Ledbetter JA, et al. Monoclonal antibody 1F5 (anti-CD20) serotherapy of human B cell lymphomas. Blood 1987;69:584–591.
459. Dyer MJS, Hale G, Hayhoe FGJ, et al. Effects of CAMPATH-1 antibodies in vivo in patients with lymphoid malignancies: Influence of antibody isotype. Blood 1989;73:1431–1439.
460. Scheinberg SA, Straus DJ, Yeh SD, et al. A phase I toxicity, pharmacology, and dosimetry trial of monoclonal antibody OKB7 in patients with non-Hodgkin's lymphoma: Effects of tumor burden and antigen expression. J Clin Oncol 1990;8:792–803.
461. Meeker T, Lowder J, Cleary ML, et al. Emergence of idiotype variants during treatment of B-cell lymphoma with anti-idiotype antibodies. N Engl J Med 1985;312:1658–1665.
462. Raffeld M, Neckers L, Longo DL, et al. Spontaneous alteration of idiotype in a monoclonal B-cell lymphoma: Escape from detection by anti-idiotype. N Engl J Med 1985;312:1653–1658.
463. Zelenetz AD, Campbell MJ, Bahler DW, et al. Follicular lymphoma: A model of lymphoid progression in man. Ann Oncol 1991;2(suppl 2):115–122.
464. Nourigat C, Badger CC, Bernstein ID. Treatment of lymphoma with radiolabeled antibody: Elimination of tumor cells lacking target antigen. JNCI 1990;82:47–50.
465. Knox SJ, Levy R, Miller RA, et al. Determinants of the antitumor effect of radiolabeled monoclonal antibodies. Cancer Res 1990;50:4935–4940.
466. Press OW, Eary JF, Badger CC, et al. Treatment of refractory non-Hodgkin's lymphoma with radiolabeled MB-1 (anti-CD37) antibody. J Clin Oncol 1989;7:1027–1038.
467. DeNardo GL, DeNardo SJ, O'Grady LF, et al. Fractionated radioimmunotherapy of B-cell malignancies with ^{131}I-Lym-1. Cancer Res 1990;50:1014S–1016S.
468. O'Grady L, DeNardo S, Lewis J, et al. Radioimmunotherapy of lymphoma. Blood [Abstract 1452] 1990;76(suppl 1):365a.
469. Rosen ST, Zimmer AM, Goldman-Leikin R, et al. Radioimmunodetection and radioimmunotherapy of cutaneous T cell lymphomas using an ^{131}I-labeled monoclonal antibody: An Illinois Cancer Council study. J Clin Oncol 1987;5:562–573.
470. Stone M, Amlot P, Fay J, et al. Immunotoxin therapy of B cell lymphoma. Blood [Abstract 1488] 1990;76:374a.
471. Nadler L, Beitmeyer J, Grossbard M, et al. Anti-B4 blocked ricin immunotherapy for patients with B-cell malignancies: Phase I trial of 7 day continuous infusion. Blood [Abstract 1448] 1990;76:364a.
472. Cheson BD. The purine analogs—A therapeutic beauty contest. J Clin Oncol 1992;10:352–355.
473. Grever MR, Leiby JM, Kraut EH, et al. Low-dose deoxycoformycin in lymphoid malignancy. J Clin Oncol 1985;3:1196–1201.
474. Hochster HS, Kim K, Green MD, et al. Activity of fludarabine in previously treated non-Hodgkin's low-grade lymphoma: Results of an Eastern Cooperative Oncology Group study. J Clin Oncol 1992;10:28–32.
475. Whelan JS, Davis CL, Rule S, et al. Fludarabine phosphate for the treatment of low grade lymphoid malignancy. Br J Cancer 1991;64:120–123.
476. Kay AC, Saven A, Carrera CJ, et al. 2-Chlorodeoxyadenosine treatment of low-grade lymphomas. J Clin Oncol 1992;10:371–377.
477. Hainsworth JD, Johnson DH, Frazier SR, et al. Chronic daily administration of oral etoposide in refractory lymphoma. Eur J Cancer 1990;26:818–821.
478. Steward WP, Smith DB, Crowther D. Weekly oral 4-demethoxydaunorubicin in patients with relapsed low grade non-Hodgkin's lymphoma. Ann Oncol 1991;2:605–606.
479. Case DC Jr, Hayes DM, Gerber M, et al. Phase II study of oral idarubicin in favorable histology non-Hodgkin's lymphoma. Cancer Res 1990;50:6833–6835.
480. Greer JP, York JC, Cousar JB, et al. Peripheral T-cell lymphoma: A clinicopathologic study of 42 cases. J Clin Oncol 1984;2:788–798.
481. Pinkus GS, O'Hara CJ, Said JW. Peripheral/post-thymic T-cell lymphomas: A spectrum of disease. Clinical, pathologic, and immunologic features of 78 cases. Cancer 1990;65:971–998.
482. Lippman SM, Miller TP, Spier CM, et al. The prognostic significance of the immunotype in diffuse large-cell lymphoma: A comparative study of the T-cell and B-cell phenotype. Blood 1988;72:436–441.
483. Coiffier B, Brousse N, Peuchmaur M, et al. Peripheral T-cell lymphomas have a worse prognosis than B-cell lymphomas: A prospective study of 361 immunophenotyped patients treated with the LNH-84 regimen. Ann Oncol 1990;1:45–50.
484. Stein RS, Greer JP, Flexner JM, et al. Large cell lymphomas: Clinical and prognostic features. J Clin Oncol 1990;8:1370–1379.
485. Miller TP, Lippman SM, Spier CM, et al. HLA-DR (Ia) immune phenotype predicts outcome for patients with diffuse large cell lymphoma. J Clin Invest 1988;82:370–372.
486. O'Keane JC, Mack C, Lynch E, et al. Prognostic correlation of HLA-DR expression in large cell lymphoma as determined by LN3 antibody staining. An Eastern Cooperative Oncology Group (ECOG) study. Cancer 1990;66:1147–1153.
487. Hall PA, Richards MA, Gregory WM, et al. The prognostic value of Ki67 immunostaining in non-Hodgkin's lymphoma. J Pathol 1988;154:223–235.
488. Slymen DJ, Miller TP, Lippman SM, et al. Immunobiologic factors predictive of clinical outcome in diffuse large-cell lymphoma. J Clin Oncol 1990;8:986–993.
489. Brandt L, Johnson A, Olsson H, et al. Mitotic activity and survival in advanced non-Hodgkin's lymphoma of unfavourable histology. Eur J Cancer 1990;26:227–230.
490. Jalkanen S, Joensuu H, Klemi P. Prognostic value of lymphocyte homing receptor and S phase fraction in non-Hodgkin's lymphoma. Blood 1990;75:1549–1556.
491. Jalkanen S, Joensuu H, Soderstrom K-O, et al. Lymphocyte homing and clinical behavior of non-Hodgkin's lymphoma. J Clin Invest 1991;87:1835–1840.
492. Horst E, Meijer CJLM, Radaszkiewica T, et al. Adhesion molecules in the prognosis of diffuse large-cell lymphoma: Expression of a lymphocyte homing receptor (CD44), LFA-1 (CD11a/18), and ICAM-1 (CD54). Leukemia 1990;4:595–599.
493. Levine EG, Arthur DC, Frizzera G, et al. Cytogenetic abnormalities predict clinical outcome in non-Hodgkin's lymphoma. Ann Intern Med 1988;108:14–20.
494. Cabanillas F, Pathak S, Grant G, et al. Refractoriness to chemotherapy and poor survival related to abnormalities of chromosomes 17 and 7 in lymphoma. Am J Med 1989;87:167–172.
495. Schouten HC, Sanger WG, Weisenburger DD, et al. Chromosomal abnormalities in untreated patients with non-Hodgkin's lymphoma: Associations with histology, clinical characteristics, and treatment outcome. Blood 1990;75:1841–1847.
496. Schouten HC, Sanger WG, Weisenburger DD, et al. Abnormalities involving chromosome 6 in newly diagnosed patients with non-Hodgkin's lymphoma. Nebraska Lymphoma Study Group. Cancer Genet Cytogenet 1990;47:73–82.
497. Fisher RI, Hubbard SM, DeVita VT Jr, et al. Factors predicting long-term survival in diffuse mixed, histiocytic or undifferentiated lymphoma. Blood 1981;58:45–51.
498. Danieu L, Wong G, Koziner B, et al. Predictive model for prognosis in advanced diffuse histiocytic lymphoma. Cancer Res 1986;46:5372–5379.
499. Velasquez WS, Jagannath S, Tucker SL, et al. Risk classification as the basis for clinical staging of diffuse large-cell lymphoma derived from 10-year survival data. Blood 1989;74:551–557.
500. Coiffier B, Lepage E. Prognosis of aggressive lymphomas: A study of five prognostic models with patients included in the LNH-84 regimen. Blood 1989;74:558–564.
501. Swan F Jr, Velasquez WS, Tucker S, et al. A new serologic staging system for large cell lymphomas based on initial beta$_2$-microglobulin and lactate dehydrogenase levels. J Clin Oncol 1989;7:1518–1527.
502. Harrington DS, Patil K, Lai PK, et al. Soluble interleukin 2 receptors in patients with malignant lymphoma. Arch Pathol Lab Med 1988;112:597–601.
503. Abate G, Coimella P, Marfella A, et al. Prognostic relevance of urinary neopterin in non-Hodgkin's lymphomas. Cancer 1989;63:484–489.
504. Sebban C, Lasne Y, Bernguer V, et al. CA 125 and malignant lymphomas. J Clin Oncol 1990;8:359–360.
505. Coiffier B, Shipp MA, Cabanillas F, et al. Report of the first workshop on prognostic factors in large-cell lymphoma. Ann Oncol 1991;2(suppl 2):213–217.
506. Cabanillas F, Bodey GP, Freireich EJ. Management with chemotherapy only of stage I and II malignant lymphoma of aggressive histologic types. Cancer 1980;46:2356–2361.
507. Miller TP, Jones SE. Initial chemotherapy for clinically localized lymphomas of unfavorable histology. Blood 1984;62:413–417.
508. Connors JM, Klimo P, Fairey RN, et al. Brief chemotherapy and involved field radiation therapy for limited-stage histologically aggressive lymphoma. Ann Intern Med 1987;107:25–29.
509. Longo DL, Glatstein E, Duffey PL, et al. Treatment of localized aggressive lymphomas with combination chemotherapy followed by involved-field radiation therapy. J Clin Oncol 1989;7:1295–1302.
510. Jones SE, Miller TP, Connors JM. Long-term follow-up and analysis for prognostic factors for patients with limited-stage diffuse large-cell lymphoma treated with initial chemotherapy with or without adjuvant radiotherapy. J Clin Oncol 1989;7:1186–1191.
511. Jones SE, Fuks Z, Kaplan HS, et al. Non-Hodgkin's lymphomas. V. Results of radiotherapy. Cancer 1973;32:682–691.
512. Reddy S, Saxena VS, Pelletiere EV, et al. Stage I and II non-Hodgkin's lymphomas: Long-term results of radiation therapy. Int J Radiat Oncol Biol Phys 1989;16:687–692.
513. Hagberg H, Pettersson U, Glimelius B, et al. Prognostic factors in non-Hodgkin lymphoma stage I treated with radiotherapy. Acta Oncol 1989;28:45–50.
514. Vokes EE, Ultmann JE, Golomb HM, et al. Long-term survival of patients with localized diffuse histiocytic lymphoma. J Clin Oncol 1985;3:1309–1317.
515. Hallahan DE, Farah R, Vokes EE, et al. The patterns of failure in patients with pathological stage I and II diffuse histiocytic lymphoma treated with radiation therapy alone. Int J Radiat Oncol Biol Phys 1989;17:767–771.
516. Kaminski MS, Coleman CN, Colby TV, et al. Factors predicting survival in adults with stage I and II large-cell lymphoma-treated with primary radiation therapy. Ann Intern Med 1986;104:747–756.
517. Prestidge BR, Horning SJ, Hoppe RT. Combined modality therapy for stage I–II large cell lymphoma. Int J Radiat Biol Oncol Phys 1988;15:633–639.
518. Armitage JO, Wen BC. Chemotherapy in patients who fail radiotherapy for diffuse aggressive non-Hodgkin's lymphoma. Int J Radiat Oncol Biol Phys 1987;13:1351–1354.
519. Shepherd FA, Evans WK, Kutas G, et al. Chemotherapy following surgery for stages IE and IIE non-Hodgkin's lymphoma of the gastrointestinal tract. J Clin Oncol 1988;6:253–260.

520. Azab MB, Henry-Amar M, Rougier P, et al. Prognostic factors in primary gastrointestinal non-Hodgkin's lymphoma. A multivariate analysis, report of 106 cases, and review of the literature. Cancer 1989;64:1208–1217.
521. Bellesi G, Alterini R, Messori A, et al. Combined surgery and chemotherapy for the treatment of primary gastrointestinal intermediate-or high-grade non-Hodgkin's lymphomas. Br J Cancer 1989;60:244–248.
522. Romaguera JE, Velasquez WS, Silvermintz KB, et al. Surgical debulking is associated with improved survival in stage I–II diffuse large cell lymphoma. Cancer 1990;66: 267–272.
523. Burgers JMV, Taal BG, vanHeerde P, et al. Treatment results of primary stage I and II non-Hodgkin's lymphoma of the stomach. Radiother Oncol 1988;11:319–326.
524. Jones RE, Willis S, Innes DJ, et al. Primary gastric lymphoma. Problems in staging and management. Am J Surg 1988;155:118–122.
525. Mentzer SJ, Osteen RT, Pappas TN, et al. Surgical therapy of localized abdominal non-Hodgkin's lymphoma. Surgery 1988;103:609–614.
526. Kajanti M, Karkinen-Jaaskelainen M, Rissanen P. Primary gastrointestinal non-Hodgkin's lymphoma. A review of 36 cases. Acta Oncol 1988;27:51–55.
527. Tabbane F, Mourali N, Cammoun M, et al. Results of laparotomy in immunoproliferative small intestinal disease. Cancer 1988;61:1699–1706.
528. Rogers P, Hill I, Sinclair-Smith C, et al. Clinical and pathological evolution of alpha chain disease to immunoblastic lymphoma and response to COMP chemotherapy. Med Pediatr Oncol 1988;16:128–131.
529. Maor MH, Velasquez WS, Fuller LM, et al. Stomach conservation in stages IE and IIE gastric non-Hodgkin's lymphoma. J Clin Oncol 1990;8:266–271.
530. Schein PS, DeVita VT Jr, Hubbard SM, et al. Bleomycin, Adriamycin, cyclophosphamide, vincristine, and prednisone (BACOP) combination chemotherapy in the treatment of advanced diffuse histiocytic lymphoma. Ann Intern Med 1976;85:417–422.
531. Berd D, Cornog J, De Conti RC, et al. Long-term remission in diffuse histiocytic lymphoma treated with combination sequential chemotherapy. Cancer 1975;35:1050–1054.
532. Gaynor ER, Ultmann JE, Golomb HM, et al. Treatment of diffuse histiocytic lymphoma (DHL) with COMLA (cyclophosphamide, oncovin, methotrexate, leucovorin, cytosine arabinoside): A 10-year experience in a single institution. J Clin Oncol 1985;3:1596–1604.
533. McKelvey EM, Gottlieb JA, Wilson HE, et al. Hydroxydaunomycin (Adriamycin) combination chemotherapy in malignant lymphoma. Cancer 1976;38:1484–1493.
534. Coltman CA Jr, Dahlberg S, Jones SE, et al. CHOP is curative in 30 percent of patients with large cell lymphoma: A 12-year Southwest Oncology Group follow-up. In: Skarin AT, ed. Advances in cancer chemotherapy: Update on treatment for diffuse large cell lymphoma. New York: Park Row, 1986:71–77.
535. Skarin AT, Canellos GP, Rosenthal DS, et al. Improved prognosis of diffuse histiocytic and undifferentiated lymphoma by use of high-dose methotrexate alternating with standard agents (M-BACOD). J Clin Oncol 1983;1:91–98.
536. Shipp MA, Yeap BY, Harrington DP, et al. The m-BACOD combination chemotherapy regimen in large-cell lymphoma: Analysis of the completed trial and comparison with the M-BACOD regimen. J Clin Oncol 1990;8:84–93.
537. Laurence J, Coleman M, Allen SL, et al. Combination chemotherapy of advanced diffuse histiocytic lymphoma with the six-drug COP-BLAM regimen. Ann Intern Med 1982;97:190–195.
538. Coleman M, Gerstein G, Topilow A, et al. Advances in chemotherapy for large cell lymphoma. Semin Hematol 1987;24:8–20.
539. Todd M, Cadman E, Spiro P, et al. A follow-up of a randomized study comparing two chemotherapy treatments for advanced diffuse histiocytic lymphoma. J Clin Oncol 1984;2:986–993.
540. Fisher RI, DeVita VT Jr, Hubbard SM, et al. Diffuse aggressive lymphomas: Increased survival after alternating flexible sequences of ProMACE and MOPP chemotherapy. Ann Intern Med 1983;98:304–309.
541. Longo DL, DeVita VT Jr, Duffey PL, et al. Superiority of ProMACE-CytaBOM over ProMACE-MOPP in the treatment of advanced diffuse aggressive lymphoma: Results of a prospective randomized trial. J Clin Oncol 1991;9:25–28.
542. Boyd DB, Coleman M, Papish SW, et al. COPBLAM III: Infusional combination chemotherapy for diffuse large-cell lymphoma. J Clin Oncol 1988;6:425–433.
543. Baer MR, Stein RS, Greer JP, et al. Modified cyclophosphamide, vincristine, methotrexate, leucovorin, and cytarabine (COMLA) in intermediate-and high-grade lymphoma: An effective short course regimen. Cancer Treat Rep 1986;70:785–787.
544. Klimo P, Connors JM. MACOP-B chemotherapy for the treatment of diffuse large-cell lymphoma. Ann Intern Med 1985;102:596–602.
545. O'Reilly SE, Hoskins P, Klimo P, et al. MACOP-B and VACOP-B in diffuse large cell lymphomas and MOPP/ABV in Hodgkin's disease. Ann Oncol 1991;2(suppl 1):17–23.
546. Guglielmi C, Amadori S, Martelli M, et al. The F-MACHOP sequential combination chemotherapy regimen in advanced diffuse aggressive lymphomas: Long-term results. Ann Oncol 1991;2:365–371.
547. Coiffier B, Gisselbrecht C, Herbrecht R, et al. LNH-84 regimen: A multicenter study of intensive chemotherapy in 737 patients with aggressive malignant lymphoma. J Clin Oncol 1989;7:1018–1026.
548. Gulati SC, Shank B, Black P, et al. Autologous bone marrow transplantation for patients with poor-prognosis lymphoma. J Clin Oncol 1988;6:1303–1313.
549. Schneider AM, Straus DJ, Schluger AE, et al. Treatment results with an aggressive chemotherapeutic regimen (MACOP-B) for intermediate- and some high-grade non-Hodgkin's lymphomas. J Clin Oncol 1990;8:94–102.
550. Weick JK, Dahlberg S, Fisher RI, et al. Combination chemotherapy of intermediate-grade and high-grade non-Hodgkin's lymphoma with MACOP-B: A Southwest Oncology Group study. J Clin Oncol 1991;9:748–753.
551. Vitolo U, Bertini M, Brusamolino E, et al. MACOP-B treatment in diffuse large-cell lymphoma: Identification of prognostic groups in an Italian multicenter study. J Clin Oncol 1992;10:219–227.
552. Miller TP, Dahlberg S, Weick JK, et al. Unfavorable histologies of non-Hodgkin's lymphoma treated with ProMACE-CytaBOM: A group-wide Southwest Oncology Group study. J Clin Oncol 1990;8:1951–1958.
553. Longo DL, Duffey PL, DeVita VT Jr, et al. The calculation of actual or received dose intensity: A comparison of published methods. J Clin Oncol 1991;9:2042–2051.
554. Hryniuk WM, Goodyear M. The calculation of received dose intensity. J Clin Oncol 1990;8:1935–1937.
555. Fisher RI, Gaynor E, Dahlberg S, et al. A phase III comparison of CHOP vs. m-BACOD vs. ProMACE-CytaBOM vs. MACOP-B in patients with intermediate or high-grade non-Hodgkin's lymphoma: Preliminary results of SWOG-8516 (Intergroup 0067), the national high priority lymphoma study. Proc Am Soc Clin Oncol [Abstract 1067] 1992;11: 315.
556. Meyer RM, Hryniuk WM, Goodyear MDE. The role of dose intensity in determining outcome in intermediate-grade non-Hodgkin's lymphoma. J Clin Oncol 1991;9:339–347.
557. DeVita VT Jr, Hubbard SM, Longo DL. The chemotherapy of lymphomas: Looking back, moving forward—The Richard and Linda Rosenthal Foundation Award lecture. Cancer Res 1987;47:5810–5824.
558. Kwak LW, Halpern J, Olshen RA, et al. Prognostic significance of actual dose intensity in diffuse large-cell lymphoma: Results of a tree-structured survival analysis. J Clin Oncol 1990;8:963–977.
559. Epelbaum R, Faraggi D, Ben-Arie Y, et al. Survival of diffuse large cell lymphoma. A multivariate analysis including dose intensity variables. Cancer 1990;66:1124–1129.
560. Banavali SD, Advani SH, Gopal R, et al. Continuous cyclophosphamide, doxorubicin, vincristine, and prednisolone. A new, innovative protocol for diffuse aggressive lymphomas. Cancer 1990;65:1704–1710.
561. Lee R, Cabanillas F, Bodey GP, et al. A 10-year update of CHOP-bleo in the treatment of diffuse large-cell lymphoma. J Clin Oncol 1986;4:1455–1461.
562. Goldie JH, Coldman AJ. The genetic origin of drug resistance in neoplasms: Implications for systemic therapy. Cancer Res 1984;44:3643–3653.
563. Carde P, Meerwaldt JH, van Glabbeke M, et al. Superiority of second over first generation chemotherapy in a randomized trial for stage II-IV intermediate and high-grade non-Hodgkin's lymphoma: The 1980–1985 EORTC trial. Ann Oncol 1991;2:431–435.
564. Browne MJ, Hubbard SM, Longo DL, et al. Excess prevalence of *Pneumocystis carinii* pneumonia in patients treated for lymphoma with combination chemotherapy. Ann Intern Med 1986;104:338–344.
565. Gherlinzoni F, Guglielmi C, Mazza P, et al. Phase III comparative trial (M-BACOD v M-BNCOD) in the treatment of stage II to IV non-Hodgkin's lymphomas with intermediate- or high-grade histology. Semin Oncol 1990;17(suppl 10):3–8.
566. Vose JM, Armitage JO, Weisenburger DD, et al. The importance of age in survival of patients treated with chemotherapy for aggressive non-Hodgkin's lymphoma. J Clin Oncol 1988;6:1838–1844.
567. Dixon DO, Neilan B, Jones SE, et al. Effect of age on therapeutic outcome in advanced diffuse histiocytic lymphoma: The Southwest Oncology Group experience. J Clin Oncol 1986;4:295–305.
568. O'Reilly SE, Klimo P, Connors JM. Low-dose ACOP-B and VABE weekly chemotherapy for elderly patients with advanced-stage diffuse large-cell lymphoma. J Clin Oncol 1991;9:741–747.
569. Sonneveld P, Michiels JJ. Full dose chemotherapy in elderly patients with non-Hodgkin's lymphoma: A feasibility study using a mitoxantrone containing regimen. Br J Cancer 1990;62:105–108.
570. Tokudome S, Tokunaga O, Shimamoto Y, et al. Incidence of adult T-cell leukemia/lymphoma among human T-lymphotropic virus type I carriers in Saga, Japan. Cancer Res 1989;49:226–228.
571. Yano T, van Krieken JHJM, Magrath IT, et al. Histogenetic correlations between subcategories of small noncleaved cell lymphomas. Blood 1992;79:1282–1290.
572. McMaster ML, Greer JP, Greco FA, et al. Effective treatment of small-noncleaved-cell lymphoma with high-intensity, brief duration chemotherapy. J Clin Oncol 1991;9: 941–946.
573. Straus DJ, Wong GY, Liu J, et al. Small non-cleaved-cell lymphoma (undifferentiated lymphoma, Burkitt's type) in American adults: Results with treatment designed for acute lymphoblastic leukemia. Am J Med 1991;90:328–337.
574. Magrath IT, Janus C, Edwards BK, et al. An effective therapy for both undifferentiated (including Burkitt's) lymphomas and lymphoblastic lymphomas in children and young adults. Blood 1984;63:1102–1108.
575. Schwenn MR, Blattner SR, Lynch E, et al. HiC-COM: A 2-month intensive chemotherapy regimen for children with stage III and IV Burkitt's lymphoma and B-cell acute lymphoblastic leukemia. J Clin Oncol 1991;9:133–138.
576. Nathwani BN, Diamond LW, Winberg CD, et al. Lymphoblastic lymphoma: A clinicopathologic study of 95 patients. Cancer 1981;48:2347–2356.
577. Voakes JB, Jones SE, McKelvey EM. The chemotherapy of lymphoblastic lymphoma. Blood 1981;57:186–191.
578. Weinstein HJ, Cassady JR, Levey R. Long-term results of the APO protocol (vincristine, doxorubicin [Adriamycin], and prednisone) for the treatment of mediastinal lymphoblastic lymphoma. J Clin Oncol 1983;1:537–544.
579. Wollner N, Wachtel AE, Exelby PR, et al. Improved prognosis in children with intra-abdominal non-Hodgkin's lymphoma following LSA_2-L_2 protocol chemotherapy. Cancer 1980;45:3034–3039.
580. Coleman CN, Picozzi VJ Jr, Cox RS, et al. Treatment of lymphoblastic lymphoma in adults. J Clin Oncol 1986;4:1628–1636.
581. Santini G, Coser P, Chisesi T, et al. Autologous bone marrow transplantation for advanced

stage adult lymphoblastic lymphoma in first complete remission. Report of the Non-Hodgkin's Lymphoma Cooperative Study Group. Ann Oncol 1991;2(suppl 2):181–185.

582. Shimamoto Y, Ono K, Sano M, et al. Difference in prognostic factors between leukemia and lymphoma type of adult T-cell leukemia. Cancer 1989;63:289–294.
583. Waldmann TA. Multichain interleukin-2 receptor: A target for immunotherapy in lymphoma. JNCI 1989;81:914–923.
584. Sirakawa F, Tanaka Y, Oda S, et al. Autocrine stimulation of interleukin-1α in the growth of adult human T-cell leukemia cells. Cancer Res 1989;49:1143–1147.
585. Eby NL, Grufferman S, Flannelly CM, et al. Increasing incidence of primary brain lymphoma in the US. Cancer 1988;62:2461–2465.
586. Jack CR Jr, Reese DF, Scheithauer BW. Radiographic findings in 32 cases of primary CNS lymphoma. AJR 1986;146:271–279.
587. Pollack IF, Lunsford LD, Flickinger JC, et al. Prognostic factors in the diagnosis and treatment of primary central nervous system lymphoma. Cancer 1989;63:939–947.
588. Shibamoto Y, Tsutsui K, Dodo Y, et al. Improved survival rate in primary intracranial lymphoma treated by high-dose radiation and systemic vincristine-doxorubicin-cyclophosphamide-prednisolone chemotherapy. Cancer 1990;65:1907–1912.
589. Gabbai AA, Hochberg FH, Linggood RM, et al. High-dose methotrexate for non-AIDS primary central nervous system lymphoma. Report of 13 cases. J Neurosurg 1989;70:190–194.
590. McLaughlin P, Velasquez WS, Redman JR, et al. Chemotherapy with dexamethasone, high-dose cytarabine, and cisplatin for parenchymal brain lymphoma. JNCI 1988;80:1408–1412.
591. Neuwelt EA, Dahlberg SA, Goldman D, et al. Significant prolongation of survival of primary CNS lymphoma patients by combination chemotherapy given in association with osmotic blood-brain barrier disruption. Proc Am Assoc Cancer Res [Abstract 1050] 1989;30:264.
592. Chamberlain MC, Levin VA. Adjuvant chemotherapy for primary lymphoma of the central nervous system. Arch Neurol 1990;47:1113–1116.
593. Giannone K, Greco FA, Hainsworth JD. Combination intraventricular chemotherapy for meningeal neoplasia. J Clin Oncol 1986;4:68–74.
594. Ziegler JL, Beckstead JA, Volberding PA, et al. Non-hodgkin's lymphoma in 90 homosexual men. Relation to generalized lymphadenopathy and the acquired immunodeficiency syndrome. N Engl J Med 1984;311:565–570.
595. Beral V, Peterman T, Berkelman R, et al. AIDS-associated non-Hodgkin lymphoma. Lancet 1991;337:805–809.
596. Pluda JM, Yarchoan R, Broder S. The occurrence of opportunistic non-Hodgkin's lymphomas in the setting of infection with the human immunodeficiency virus. Ann Oncol 1991;2(suppl 2):191–200.
597. Pluda JM, Yarchoan R, Jaffe ES, et al. Development of non-Hodgkin lymphoma in a cohort of patients with severe human immunodeficiency virus (HIV) infection on long-term antiretroviral therapy. Ann Intern Med 1990;113:276–282.
598. Gill PS, Levine AM, Krailo M, et al. AIDS-related malignant lymphoma: Results of prospective treatment trials. J Clin Oncol 1987;5:1322–1328.
599. Knowles, DM, Chamulak GA, Subar M, et al. Lymphoid neoplasia associated with the acquired immunodeficiency syndrome (AIDS). Ann Intern Med 1988;108:744–753.
600. Lowenthal DA, Straus DJ, Campbell SW, et al. AIDS-related lymphoid neoplasia. Cancer 1988;61:2325–2337.
601. Kaplan LD, Abrams DI, Feigal E, et al. AIDS-associated non-Hodgkin's lymphoma in San Francisco. JAMA 1989;261:719–724.
602. Bermudez MA, Grant KM, Rodvien R, et al. Non-Hodgkin's lymphoma in a population with or at risk for acquired immunodeficiency syndrome: Indications for intensive chemotherapy. Am J Med 1989;86:71–76.
603. Levine AM. Lymphoma in acquired immunodeficiency syndrome. Semin Oncol 1990;17:104–112.
604. Roithmann S, Toledano M, Tourani JM, et al. HIV-associated non-Hodgkin's lymphomas: Clinical characteristics and outcome. The experience of the French registry of HIV-associated tumors. Ann Oncol 1991;2:289–295.
605. Gill PS, Levine AM. HIV-related malignant lymphoma: Clinical aspects, treatment and pathogenesis. Cancer Invest 1988;6:413–416.
606. Freter CE. Acquired immunodeficiency syndrome-associated lymphomas. JNCI Monogr 1990;10:45–54.
607. Boyle MJ, Swanson CE, Turner JJ, et al. Definition of two distinct types of AIDS-associated non-Hodgkin lymphoma. Br J Haemtol 1990;76:506–512.
608. Shiramizu B, Herndier B, Meeker T, et al. Molecular and immunophenotypic characterization of AIDS-associated, Epstein-Barr virus-negative, polyclonal lymphoma. J Clin Oncol 1992;10:383–389.
609. Kaplan LD, Kahn JO, Crowe S, et al. Clinical and virologic effects of recombinant human granulocyte-macrophage colony-stimulating factor in patients receiving chemotherapy for human immunodeficiency virus-associated non-Hodgkin's lymphoma: Results of a randomized trial. J Clin Oncol 1991;9:929–940.
610. Levine AM, Wernz JC, Kaplan L, et al. Low-dose chemotherapy with central nervous system prophylaxis and zidovudine maintenance in AIDS-related lymphoma. A prospective multi-institutional trial. JAMA 1991;266:84–88.
611. Armitage JO. Bone marrow transplantation in the treatment of patients with lymphoma. Blood 1989;73:1749–1758.
612. Gribben JG, Goldstone AH, Linch DH, et al. Effectiveness of high-dose combination chemotherapy and autologous bone marrow transplantation for patients with non-Hodgkin's lymphomas who are still responsive to conventional-dose therapy. J Clin Oncol 1989;7:1621–1629.
613. Philip T, Chauvin F, Armitage I, et al. PARMA international protocol: Pilot study of DHAP followed by involved-field radiotherapy and BEAC with autologous bone marrow transplantation. Blood 1991;77:1587–1592.
614. Chao NJ, Rosenberg SA, Horning SJ. CEPP(B): An effective and well-tolerated regimen in poor-risk, aggressive non-Hodgkin's lymphoma. Blood 1990;76:1293–1298.
615. Longo DL, DeVita VT Jr. Lymphomas. Cancer Chemother Biol Response Modif 1992;13:349–403.
616. Philip T, Chauvin F, Bron D, et al. PARMA international protocol: Pilot study on 50 patients and preliminary analysis of the ongoing randomized study (62 patients). Ann Oncol 1991;2(suppl 1):57–64.
617. Moormeier JA, Williams SF, Kaminer LS, et al. High-dose tri-alkylator chemotherapy with autologous stem cell rescue in patients with refractory malignancies. JNCI 1990;82:29–34.
618. Glenn LD, Armitage JO, Bierman PH, et al. High-dose BCNU, etoposide, cytoxan and hydroxyurea (BECH) with autologous hematopoietic stem cell support for poor prognosis non-Hodgkin's lymphoma. Proc Am Assoc Cancer Res [Abstract 929] 1989;30:234.
619. Brandwein JM, Callum J, Sutcliffe SB, et al. Analysis of factors affecting hematopoietic recovery after autologous bone marrow transplantation for lymphoma. Bone Marrow Transplant 1990;6:292–294.
620. Kessinger A, Armitage JO, Smith DM, et al. High-dose therapy and autologous peripheral blood stem cell transplantation for patients with lymphoma. Blood 1989;74:1260–1265.
621. Gianni AM, Siena S, Bregni M, et al. Granulocyte-macrophage colony-stimulating factor to harvest circulating heamopoietic cells for autotransplantation. Lancet 1989;2:580–585.
622. Nemunaitis J, Rabinowe SN, Singer JW, et al. Recombinant granulocyte-macrophage colony-stimulating factor after autologous bone marrow transplantation for lymphoid cancer. N Engl J Med 1991;324:1773–1777.
623. Gianni AM, Bregni M, Siena S, et al. Recombinant human granulocyte-macrophage colony-stimulating factor reduces hematologic toxicity and widens clinical applicability of high-dose cyclophosphamide treatment in breast cancer and non-Hodgkin's lymphoma. J Clin Oncol 1990;8:768–778.
624. Ho AD, Del Valle F, Engelhard M, et al. Mitoxantrone/high-dose ara-C and recombinant human GM-CSF in the treatment of refractory non-Hodgkin's lymphoma. A pilot study. Cancer 1990;66:423–430.
625. Smith JW II, Longo DL, Alvord W, et al. Thrombopoietic effects of IL-1α in combination with high-dose carboplatin. Proc Am Soc Clin Oncol [Abstract 820] 1992;11:252.
626. Salmon SE, Grogan TM, Miller T, et al. Prediction of doxorubicin resistance in vitro in myeloma, lymphoma, and breast cancer by P-glycoprotein staining. JNCI 1989;81:696–701.
627. Miller TP, Grogan TM, Dalton WS, et al. P-glycoprotein expression in malignant lymphoma and reversal of clinical drug resistance with chemotherapy plus high-dose verapamil. J Clin Oncol 1991;9:17–24.
628. Wilson WH, Bryant G, Bates S, et al. Infusional etoposide (E), vincristine (O) and Adriamycin (H) with cyclophosphamide (C), predinsone (P) (EPOCH) and R-verapamil (RV) in relapsed lymphoma. Proc Am Soc Clin Oncol [Abstract 956] 1991;10:275.
629. Schauer PK, Straus DJ, Bagley DM Jr, et al. Angioimmunoblastic lymphadenopathy: Clinical spectrum of disease. Cancer 1981;48:2493–2498.
630. Steinberg AD, Seldin MF, Jaffe ES, et al. Angioimmunoblastic lymphoadenopathy with dysproteinemia. Ann Intern Med 1988;108:575–578.
631. Klinman DM, Steinberg AD, Mushinski JF. Effect of cyclophosphamide therapy on oncogene expression in angioimmunoblastic lymphadenopathy. Lancet 1986;2:1055–1057.
632. Repetto L, Jaiprakash MP, Selby PJ, et al. Aggressive angiofollicular lymph node hyperplasia (Castleman's disease) treated with high dose melphalan and autologous bone marrow transplantation. Hematol Oncol 1986;4:213–217.
633. Lipford EH Jr, Margolick JB, Longo DL, et al. Angiocentric immunoproliferative lesions: A clinicopathologic spectrum of post-thymic T-cell proliferations. Blood 1988;72:1674–1681.

Cancer: Principles & Practice of Oncology, Fourth Edition,
edited by Vincent T. DeVita, Jr., Samuel Hellman, Steven A. Rosenberg.
J.B. Lippincott Co., Philadelphia © 1993.

Paul A. Bunn, Jr
Richard T. Hoppe

CHAPTER **53**

Cutaneous Lymphomas

Investigating the functional, phenotypic, and genotypic properties of normal T lymphocytes and their malignant counterparts produced a better understanding of the biology and classification of T-cell lymphomas.[1–6] Advances in molecular biology and virology led to the discovery of a new T-cell lymphoma called acute T-cell leukemia-lymphoma (ATLL) caused by a type C retrovirus, human T-cell lymphotrophic virus-I (HTLV-I).[7,8] It is possible that other T-cell malignancies, including mycosis fungoides and the Sézary syndrome, are caused by related viruses. HTLV-V, a putative etiologic virus for the cutaneous T-cell lymphomas (CTCL), has been described.[9]

T-cell lymphomas in the United States are much less common than B-cell lymphomas. Peripheral T-cell lymphomas, T-cell chronic lymphocytic leukemia (CLL), and T-γ lymphoproliferative disorders are discussed in other chapters. The age-adjusted incidence of CTCL in the United States is about 4 cases per million persons annually, which is about double the rate from the early 1970s. There are approximately 800 to 1000 total new cases each year.[10–12] The peak incidence is in the sixth decade of life, and onset before age 30 is rare. The disease is slightly more common in men, and there is no racial predilection. Adult T-cell leukemia-lymphoma is rare in the United States. Less than 100 cases are reported in the literature. It is uncertain whether the incidence is rising due to an increased prevalence of HTLV-I infection or other environmental reasons.

Stem cells destined to become T lymphocytes originate in the bone marrow and migrate to the thymus, where they undergo differentiation under the influence of several thymic hormones.[13] During this differentiation, they undergo rearrangement of the T-cell receptor gene loci.[14,15] The exquisite specificity of T cells is a result of this cell surface receptor. The diversity with the ability to recognize millions of antigens is a result of the rearrangement of the gene. The human T-cell receptor (Ti) has two major subunits, Ti-α and Ti-β, which are held together by disulfide bonds. The subunits are closely associated with the T3 molecule that consists of a 25-kd γ-chain and two 20-kd δ- and ϵ-chains (Fig. 53–1). The Ti subunits form a binding site for antigen and major histocompatibility complex molecules through interaction of their variable domains, and the T3 subunits serve a signal transduction function. The Ti subunit proteins are translated from genes that contain variable, diversity, joining, and constant regions (see Fig. 53–1). Southern analysis of DNA from patients' T cells can be used to determine whether malignant cells are T cells and whether there is monoclonal rearrangement of the T-cell receptor gene loci.[6]

Early T cells may express the 3A1 and T11 (CD2) antigens and intracellular terminal deoxyribonucleotide transferase (TdT) before rearrangement of the T-cell receptor gene.[14] The T11 antigen is the sheep erythrocyte receptor. This 50-kd surface glycoprotein facilitates interactions between T lymphocytes and target cells and activates resting T cells.[16] The ability of the T11 antigen to trigger T-cell activation independent of antigen and MHC molecules is important for amplification of the immune response. The T11 antigen is present on T cells throughout their differentiation. The function of the 3A1 antigen is unknown, and it is lost as the cells mature. The transcription of Ti-β precedes Ti-α; T3 transcription first occurs at about the same stage, but surface T3-Ti complex appears in the late thymocyte stage.[14]

The T4 (CD4) and T8 (CD8) surface glycoproteins appear during middle or late thymocyte development, and eventually cells retain or lose one of these antigens.[13] The $CD4^+$ cells, called inducer or helper T cells, comprise approximately 67% of peripheral blood T cells and bind to invariant regions of class II MHC antigens. These cells facilitate the differentiation of B cells into antibody-producing plasma cells and facilitate the function of $T8^+$ cytotoxic or suppressor T cells. The T4

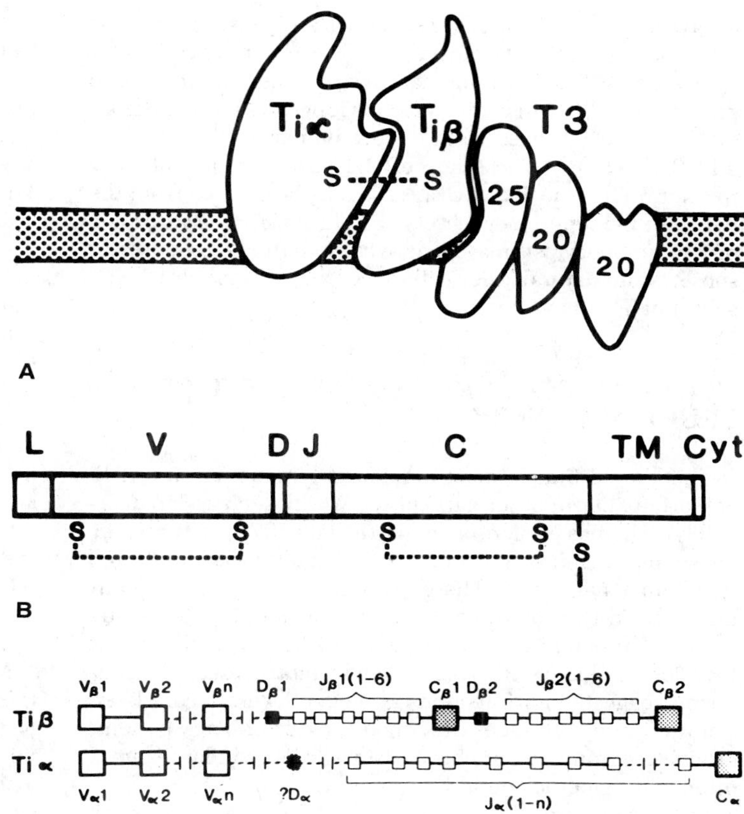

FIGURE 53–1. Structure of the human T-cell receptor and its subunits. **(A)** Subunit composition of the human T-cell receptor. The Ti α and Ti β subunits are held together by S-S bonds and are most closely associated with the 25-kd γ chain of the T3 molecule. The α and β subunits are anchored in the cell membrane with their transmembrane segments. The T3 complex consists of two additional subunits (δ and ϵ) with molecular weights of 20,000. Although not shown, a recently described 16-kd homodimer (32-kd nonreduced), called zeta, is also noncovalently associated with the T3-Ti complex. **(B)** Structure of the Ti subunits. The predicted primary structure of the β-chain subunit after translation from the cDNA sequence is depicted, as are the variable region leader (*L*), V, D, and J segments, a hydrophobic transmembrane segment (*TM*), and cytoplasmic part (*Cyt*) in the C region, potential intrachain sulfhydryl bonds (*S-S*), and the single SH group (*S*) that can form a sulfhydryl bond with the α subunit. **(C)** Scheme of the genomic organization of the human β- and α-chain genes. In the β locus, V indicates the V gene pool located at the 5′ end, at an unknown distance from the $D_{\beta 1}$ element, the $J_{\beta 1}$ cluster, and the $C_{\beta 1}$ constant-region gene. Further downstream, a second $D_{\beta 2}$ element. $J_{\beta 2}$ cluster, and $C_{\beta 2}$ constant-region gene are indicated. A similar nomenclature is used for the Ti α locus in which only a single constant region is found. ?D indicates the uncertainty about the existence of a putative Ti α diversity element. (Reproduced with permission from Royer HD, Reinherz EL. T lymphocytes: Ontogeny. Function, and relevance to clinical disorders. N Engl J Med 1987;317:1136–1142)

molecule is also the receptor for the human immunodeficiency virus (HIV).[17] T8⁺ cytotoxic T cells comprise approximately 33% of peripheral blood T cells and have specificity of antigen and class I MHC antigens. They are responsible for MHC-directed cytotoxicity of virus-infected and malignant cells, for graft rejection, for delayed hypersensitivity reactions and for inhibiting the differentiation of B cells into plasma cells.

T-cell proliferation results from events involving the T3-Ti complex and from binding of interleukin-2 (IL-2), a T-cell growth factor, to IL-2 receptors (IL-2R).[14,18,19] Resting T cells have no IL-2R. After antigen or MHC exposure, the number of surface antigen (Ti) receptors decreases, and the number of IL-2R increases. In contrast to resting lymphocytes and the low-grade T-cell lymphomas, the HTLV-I–infected malignant cells in ATLL constitutively express IL-2R. This may account for the rapid proliferation of these cells.

A small fraction of peripheral blood T cells lack T4 and T8 antigens and express the T3-Ti γ-δ receptor.[20] These cells have broad natural killer activity. Reports of target granular lymphocytic malignancies derived from this population of cells are now appearing.[21]

CLASSIFICATION OF T-CELL MALIGNANCIES

The Rappaport and Working Formulations were not developed for classifying T-cell malignancies.[22,23] Some T-cell malignancies appear in these classifications, and others are omitted. The T-cell malignancies can be separated into low, intermediate, and high grades, as in the Working Formulation, and can be differentiated by their phenotypic properties.

The most immature T-cell malignancies are the lymphoblastic lymphomas and T-cell acute lymphoblastic leukemias.[24–26] The malignant cells in these disorders have prethymic or thymic markers and can be considered to be the leukemic or tissue phases of the same disease process, analogous to chronic lymphocytic leukemia and diffuse well-differentiated lymphocytic lymphoma. The malignant cells in these disorders usually have intracellular TdT and express the 3A1 antigen. Clinically, these disorders are often associated with mediastinal masses and a predilection for central nervous system (CNS) involvement. More detailed descriptions may be found elsewhere in this text. T-cell prolymphocytic leukemia is a rare leukemia derived from intermediate or mature thymocytes and may be T4⁺T8⁺ or T4⁺T8⁻.[27]

Malignancies of mature T cells may be low, intermediate, or high grade. ATLL is a high-grade T-cell leukemia-lymphoma with some distinct clinical features caused by the HTLV-I retrovirus.[1,7,8,28] The cells in ATLL have the helper phenotype and constitutively express IL-2R. All other T-cell lymphomas do not express IL-2R or have low-level expression. The peripheral T-cell lymphomas (including T-cell immunoblastic lymphoma, diffuse large noncleaved, and diffuse large noncleaved types) are intermediate or high grade. These lymphomas do not express immature T-cell markers, almost always express T1, T3, T11, and T4 antigens, and always have monoclonally rearranged T-cell receptor genes.[29]

Low-grade T-cell lymphomas always have a mature T-cell phenotype. CTCL, including mycosis fungoides and the Sézary syndrome, are derived from mature helper T cells (T1, T3, T11, $T4^+$, $T8^-$).[3-5] These cells often lose one or more of these markers. The true T-cell CLL cells may be derived from the helper or the suppressor subsets.[30,31] The cells in the syndrome of T-γ lymphocytosis may be derived from the $T8^+$ suppressor subset, from natural killer cells, or perhaps from the T3-Ti γ subset of T cells.[32-34]

CLINICAL FEATURES OF ADULT T-CELL LEUKEMIA-LYMPHOMA

In the United States, most malignant lymphomas are of B-cell origin, but in other parts of the world, such as Japan, T-cell lymphomas predominate.[1] In the late 1970s, several Japanese investigators recognized a distinct group of T-cell lymphoma patients.[35] These patients were geographically clustered in the southwestern provinces and had acute fulminant lymphomas characterized by leukemic cells, tissue invasion (including skin), and a rapidly fatal course. The clustering suggested an infectious etiology. Several years later, Catovsky and colleagues described a series of black patients originating from the Caribbean basin who had similar features, often with hypercalcemia.[36]

At the same time, a malignant cell line, Hut102, was initiated from a patient with an atypical CTLL at the National Cancer Institute (NCI).[37] This cell line, which grew without exogenous growth factors, produced IL-2, expressed high levels IL-2R, and was infected with HTLV-I.[1,7] Shortly thereafter, antibodies to this virus were detected in 100% of the patients with ATLL in Japan, the Caribbean, and the United States.[1,38] An identical virus was detected in Japanese patients and cell lines.

The HTLV-I retrovirus from Hut102 and other cell lines has been isolated and sequenced completely.[1] It contains 1096 nucleotides. There are long terminal repeats (LTR) positioned at the 5′ and 3′ ends that regulate transcription by providing sites for RNA polymerase attachment. The proviral RNA next contains *GAG*, *POL*, and *ENV* genes that encode for the structural proteins, the reverse transcriptase and the envelope proteins respectively. The most 3′ region termed pX contains a long open reading (LOR) frame that encodes for a protein that acts as a transcriptional activator of the LTR regions and perhaps as an activation for other genes.

There is overwhelming evidence that HTLV-I is the causative agent of ATLL.[1] ATLL occurs in areas endemic for HTLV-I, and ATLL patients have anti-HTLV-I antibodies in their serum. HTLV-I proviral genome is monoclonally integrated in malignant ATLL cells, and infection of normal T4 cells with HTLV-I causes alternations in morphology and independent growth properties characteristic of ATLL cells. Proviral integration into these cells and their descendants is monoclonal. However, the actual site of integration varies among patients and cell lines.

The clinical features of ATLL in the United States and the Caribbean have been described.[8,39] Most patients are from the southeastern United States or Hawaii or have emigrated from other endemic regions, such as Japan or the Caribbean basin. The disease has not been reported in children, and the median age at diagnosis is 35 to 55 years, with a slight male predominance. The disease tends to have a sudden onset, usually with hypercalcemia or rapidly developing skin lesions. The median interval between the onset of symptoms and a diagnosis of lymphoma is short (median, 2 months). Systemic "B" symptoms are common, and all patients are stage IV with involvement of at least one organ, usually the skin, gastrointestinal tract, pulmonary system, or CNS. Lymphadenopathy is invariably present; massive mediastinal node enlargement is uncommon. Opportunistic infections are extremely common because the patients are immunosuppressed.

Hypercalcemia or evidence of bone resorption are common in ATLL. The presence of hypercalcemia imparts a poor prognosis, and the hypercalcemia is difficult to manage without an excellent antitumor response. Osteolytic bone lesions, abnormal bone scans, and elevated alkaline phosphatase levels are other manifestations of the bone-resorbing features of ATLL. It appears that the malignant cells secrete an osteoclast-activating, bone-resorbing protein that is not yet characterized. Vitamin D and parathormone levels are normal.

Many patients with ATLL have T-cell leukemia in which the malignant circulating cells have a characteristic cloverleaf appearance.[28] The peripheral leukocyte count varies from normal to extremely high ($>200,000/\mu l$) in these patients. These cells allow a morphologic diagnosis to be more easily established. The histologic picture of different tissue sites varies. The lymphoma may be described as one of several in the Rappaport classification (*e.g.*, diffuse poorly differentiated lymphocytic, diffuse mixed, diffuse histiocytic), and the cell morphology may be quite pleomorphic.[28]

Few patients infected with HTLV-I develop ATLL. Many HTLV-I-infected patients never develop any disease. Some develop neurologic diseases, such as spastic paraparesis. Some HTLV-I-infected patients develop a chronic low-grade illness with abnormal, circulating cells, sometimes with adenopathy. This disease has been called chronic adult T-cell leukemia. It may persist many years without any sequelae, but it uncommonly may convert to classic ATLL.

CLINICAL FEATURES OF LOW-GRADE T-CELL LYMPHOMAS

CLINICAL FEATURES OF MYCOSIS FUNGOIDES AND THE SÉZARY SYNDROME

The diagnosis of mycosis fungoides (MF) is often preceded by a long (5–10 years) prediagnostic (premycotic) phase marked by the appearance of nonspecific patches, which may be pruritic. Biopsies during this phase are nonspecific. In its earliest diagnostic phase, scaling, erythematous patches or plaques with well-marginated borders but variable size and shape, are seen. They are often in a bathing trunk distribution, although any body surfaces may be affected. Occasionally, there may be a prominent component of poikiloderma, skin atrophy, associated alopecia, or follicular mucinosis.

Skin biopsies demonstrate an infiltrate of mononuclear cells in the epidermis and upper dermis. These mononuclear cells may form intraepidermal clusters, so-called Pautrier microabscesses. The nuclei of these cells are hyperconvoluted (or cerebriform).[55] Cell surface marker studies demonstrate them to be $CD4^+$ (*i.e.*, helper T cells), although further evaluation often demonstrates that they have lost some mature T-cell antigens, such as Leu-8 and Leu-9 (CD7).[40] Eventually, patches may evolve into more numerous, infiltrated plaques, and patients with a long history of plaque disease may develop ulcerated or exophytic tumors. Some patients may present de novo with tumors (d'emblee).

Another variant of skin involvement is generalized erythroderma (l'homme rouge or the red-man syndrome), accompanied by atrophic or lichenified skin. Plaques and tumors may also occur. These patients are intensely symptomatic from pruritus and scaling. If there is peripheral blood involvement, they are considered to have the Sézary syndrome.

Most patients with MF never have any clinical evidence of disease other than skin involvement. However, 10% to 20% of patients eventually develop clinical manifestations of extracutaneous disease.[41] This often manifests initially as regional lymphadenopathy in areas draining extensive skin involvement. Later, visceral involvement may develop. Organs most frequently affected include the lungs, spleen, liver, and gastrointestinal tract. Autopsy studies indicate that involvement of any organ may occur in the final stages of disease.[11]

The Sézary syndrome is a variant of MF in which patients present with erythroderma and abnormal cells (>10%) circulating in the peripheral blood.[42] These cells are identical to the $CD4^+$ helper T cells seen in the cutaneous infiltrates of MF. Lymphadenopathy and splenomegaly are often present.

In large cohorts of patients with long-term follow-up, the median survival after a diagnosis of MF is almost 10 years.[41] Among patients who present with patch or limited plaque disease, most die of unrelated causes, including cardiopulmonary disease or other cancers. However, for patients who present with tumorous involvement or the Sézary syndrome or who develop extracutaneous spread, the prognosis is more dismal. Most patients die of MF or complications related to the disease, such as infection and sepsis, with a median survival of less than 3 years.[11,43–45] Cytologic or histologic transformation into a high-grade lymphoma occurs in some patients and is associated with a poor prognosis.[53] Patients may develop other malignancies, including skin cancers, Hodgkin's disease, and myeloid leukemias.[1,3]

OTHER CUTANEOUS LYMPHOMAS AND LYMPHOMA-LIKE LESIONS

B-cell lymphomas may involve the skin as a primary site of disease or as a manifestation of systemic involvement. Histologically, these can usually be differentiated readily from MF, because the neoplastic infiltrate is usually limited to the dermis, sparing the epidermis and dermal-epidermal junction (Grenz zone) until rather late in the course of disease, when secondary ulceration may occur. Immunophenotyping can confirm the B-cell origin of these lymphomas. These lymphomas may be classified according to the criteria of the Working Formulation, and prognosis is related to histology and stage of disease.[46]

Pagetoid reticulosis (*i.e.*, Woringer-Kolopp disease) is a hyperkeratotic, verrucous form of MF, which presents with limited involvement of a single site, usually an extremity.[47] It has an indolent course, but it may become locally invasive and destructive. It is a monoclonal T-cell lymphoproliferative disease, documented by clonal rearrangements of the T-cell receptor in biopsied tissue.[48]

Lymphomatoid papulosis is a T-cell disease characterized clinically by waxing and waning nodular lesions. Histologic examination reveals atypical cells that resemble Reed-Sternberg cells or hyperconvoluted MF cells. Studies of T-cell receptor gene rearrangements indicate that lymphomatoid papulosis is often a monoclonal T-cell proliferation.[49] There is an increased risk for the development of lymphomatoid papulosis among patients with MF, and patients with lymphomatoid papulosis may later develop frank MF. The relation between these diseases is not clearly understood. Treatment should be symptomatic until a confirmed diagnosis of MF or other lymphoma is clearly established.

STAGING

A staging classification system for MF was proposed at the NCI Workshop on Cutaneous T-Cell Lymphomas in 1978.[50] Table 53–1 summarizes this TNMB system. In large series, approximately 21% of patients present with limited plaque (<10% of the skin surface involved; T1), 36% with generalized plaque (>10% of the skin surface involved; T2), 24% with tumorous involvement (T3), and 19% with erythroderma (T4). The extent of skin involvement has major prognostic importance. The 5- and 10-year survivals for patients with MF, based on the extent of skin involvement, are shown in Table 53–2.

Stage groupings are based on the TNMB criteria. Clinical groupings based on this staging system clearly define patients with a good prognosis (*i.e.*, limited or generalized plaque disease only, with no evidence of extracutaneous spread), who have a median survival greater than 12 years; an intermediate prognosis (*i.e.*, cutaneous tumors, erythroderma, or lymph node involvement), with a median survival of about 5 years; or a poor prognosis (*i.e.*, extracutaneous disease involving viscera), with a median survival less than 3 years.[45] Circulating abnormal cells in the peripheral blood may have little independent effect on prognosis, but this condition is strongly correlated with T stage (usually T4) and extracutaneous disease.

The staging procedures should always include a careful examination of the skin, including the scalp, palms, soles, and perineum. A complete blood count, Sézary cell preparation, screening chemistries, and baseline chest radiograph are reasonable screening studies. Lymph node biopsies should be obtained if there is lymphadenopathy, because lymph node involvement and the lymph node histology affect the stage and prognosis. Visceral biopsies should be considered if there are unexplained clinical findings, such as abnormal liver function studies or an infiltrate on the chest radiograph. Histologically, lymph node biopsies may only reveal nonspecific changes of dermatopathic lymphadenitis. However, even these lymph nodes may show evidence of minimal involvement by MF if DNA content analysis, electron microscopy, or T-cell receptor rearrangements are used.[51,52] The microscopic se-

TABLE 53–1. National Cutaneous T-Cell Lymphoma Workshop Staging Classification

T	*Skin*	*N*	*Lymph Nodes*	*M*	*Visceral Organs**
T1	Limited plaques (<10% BSA)†	N0	No adenopathy; histology negative	M0	No involvement
T2	Generalized plaques	N1	Adenopathy; histology negative	M1	Visceral involvement
T3	Cutaneous tumors	N2	No adenopathy; histology positive		
T4	Generalized erythroderma	N3	Adenopathy; histology positive		

Stage

I	Limited (IA) or generalized plaques (IB) without adenopathy or histologic involvement of lymph nodes or viscera (T1N0M0 or T2N0M0)
II	Limited or generalized plaques with adenopathy (IIA) or cutaneous tumors with or without adenopathy (IIB); without histologic involvement of lymph nodes or viscera (T1–2N1M0, T2N0–1M0)
III	Generalized erythroderma with or without adenopathy; without histologic involvement of lymph nodes or viscera (T4N0–1M0)
IV	Histologic involvement of lymph nodes (IVA) or viscera (IVB) with any skin lesion and with or without adenopathy (T1–4N2–3M0 for IVA; T1–4N0–3M1 for IVB)

* Blood involvement should be recorded as absent (B0) or present (B1) but is not currently used to determine final stage.
† BSA, body surface area.

verity of lymph node involvement may be defined using a "lymph node staging system" that correlates with prognosis.[53] Patients with lymph node biopsies showing dermatopathic changes or small numbers of malignant cells (*i.e.*, LN1 or LN2) had a 5-year survival rate of 80%, those with dermatopathic changes and large clusters of paracortical malignant cells (LN3) had a 5-year survival rate of 30%, and those with effaced nodes had a 5-year survival rate of only 15%.

TREATMENT

THERAPY FOR ADULT T-CELL LEUKEMIA

Therapy for adult T-cell leukemia is unsatisfactory, and patients have a poor prognosis. Complete remissions have been observed in about 50% of patients given intensive combination chemotherapy regimens such as PROMACE/CYTOBOM or M-BACOD.[8] These regimens generally alleviate symptoms such as hypercalcemia and skin lesions, but long-term remissions are not observed. Opportunistic infections, spread to the CNS, and relapse are major problems. Numerous biologic agents have been evaluated. Unlabeled monoclonal antibodies (*e.g.*, T101, anti-Tac), deoxycoformycin, and interferons have not been useful. Antibody conjugates are being evaluated as are antiviral agents.[54] For the rare patients with an indolent asymptomatic course, observation is reasonable.

THERAPY FOR MYCOSIS FUNGOIDES

The essential ingredient for successful management of MF is effective treatment of the skin. Nonspecific topical treatments such as emollients, antipruritics, and antiinflammatories, including hydrocortisone, may provide some relief of symptoms, especially in patients with minimal disease. More effective management demands the use of intensive topical photochemotherapy, nitrogen mustard, or irradiation. With all of these topical therapies, patients may experience an apparent exacerbation of disease at the outset, which is probably related to stimulation of an inflammatory reaction in areas of minimal disease. With continuation of therapy, the skin disease usually responds.

Topical Photochemotherapy

Topical photochemotherapy (*i.e.*, PUVA) includes the oral administration of 8-methoxypsoralen (0.4–0.6 mg/kg) followed 2 hours later by exposure to light in the UVA spectrum.

TABLE 53–2. Survival of 459 Patients With Mycosis Fungoides at Stanford University

T Stage	*Characteristic*	*No. of Patients*	*5-Year Survival (%)*	*10-Year Survival (%)*
T1	Limited plaque	95	91	82
T2	Generalized plaque	167	72	52
T3	Tumorous	112	35	19
T4	Erythroderma	85	46	28

(Hoppe RT, Wood GS, Abel EA. Mycosis fungoides and the Sézary syndrome: Pathology, staging, and treatment. Curr Probl Cancer 1990;14:295–361)

The psoralens intercalate with DNA, and on exposure to ultraviolet light in the 360-nm range, they form monofunctional and bifunctional adducts, which interfere with DNA replication.[55] The UVA does not penetrate beyond the epidermis and upper dermis. Patients receive timed exposure to the UVA (1.5–15 J/cm^2) in a phototherapy unit (PUVA box). Only the eyes are shielded. All other body surfaces may be treated, but certain areas such as the perineum, axillae, and other skin-fold areas may not receive adequate exposure. In the initial clearing phase of treatment, patients are treated two to three times each week. After the skin has cleared, a maintenance program of gradually decreasing frequency is employed. The average time to clearance is 2 to 6 months, with the likelihood of clearance related to the extent of skin involvement. Patients with minimal patch disease achieve complete response rates as high as 90%. Patients with more infiltrated plaques achieve complete response rates of 60% to 80%.[56–60] Maintenance therapy is continued 1 to 4 times per month after the skin has cleared, and if discontinued, most patients relapse. However, resumption of treatment is often associated with a secondary response.

Acute complications of PUVA treatment include mild erythema, pruritus, skin dryness, and nausea. Potential long-term complications include increased risk of cataracts, necessitating the use of UVA-opaque goggles during therapy. Some patients who undergo long-term continuous treatment with PUVA risk developing secondary cutaneous squamoproliferative lesions, including basal cell and squamous carcinomas.[61] Among patients treated for MF, this risk appears to be greatest if multiple topical therapies are used sequentially.[62]

Topical Chemotherapy

The most commonly used topical chemotherapy for MF is nitrogen mustard (HN_2). HN_2 may be prepared in an aqueous solution or in an ointment base, such as aquaphor. The mechanism of action after being applied topically is uncertain.[63] It is not likely that the alkylating agent activity that HN_2 demonstrates when administered systemically is the important factor, because the delay between preparation of the solution and application to the skin far exceeds the half-life of the active ethyleneimonium ion that forms after the HN_2 is put into solution. It is possible that one of the degradation products serves as the active agent or that one or more of these products stimulates an immune response, affecting the disease directly or by some interaction with the epidermal cell–Langerhans' cell–T-cell axis.

Nitrogen mustard is initially applied daily. When the aqueous preparation is used, patients prepare the solution themselves in a 10 to 20 mg per 100 ml solution and apply it to the skin with a cloth or brush. Nitrogen mustard in aquaphor is prepared by the pharmacist in a concentration of 10 to 20 mg per 100 g of aquaphor. The skin may be treated in its entirety, with the exception of the eyelids, lips, and vaginal and anal orifices. Skin-fold areas may be treated intermittently to avoid irritation. The aqueous and aquaphor preparations have similar efficacy, although a randomized trial has not been performed.[64] The choice often depends on convenience or patient preference. Complete response rates from 30% to 60% overall, with the likelihood of response depending on initial extent of skin involvement: about 50% for limited plaque and 25% for generalized plaque disease.[64–66] The median time to skin clearance is about 8 months. Maintenance treatment is continued for 1 to 2 years after skin clearance; the schedule varies. After treatment is discontinued, more than half of patients experience skin relapses, but most respond to resumption of therapy. The overall proportion of patients treated with topical HN_2 who have durable complete responses is about 20%.

The primary complication of topical HN_2 therapy is an acute or delayed hypersensitivity reaction. This may occur in as many as 30% of people treated with the aqueous preparation, but in less than 5% of patients treated with the ointment preparation.[64] Desensitization may be achieved with a variety of topical or systemic desensitization programs. Some patients treated with topical HN_2 have developed secondary squamoproliferative lesions of the skin.[66] This was a problem primarily among patients who were treated with multiple sequential topical therapies for the control of active disease and was observed only occasionally among patients treated with topical HN_2 alone. There is no systemic absorption of topically applied nitrogen mustard, and systemic complications such as hematologic depression or sterility are not potential toxicities.

Another chemotherapeutic agent that has been used topically is carmustine (BCNU).[67] The efficacy of BCNU is similar to topical HN_2, but because of the systemic absorption of BCNU, the potential hematologic complications are greater, and the duration of treatment is limited.

Irradiation

Irradiation has been used in the management of MF for almost a century. Mycosis fungoides is an exquisitely radiosensitive neoplasm, and rather modest doses are capable of achieving long-term control.[68] The responsiveness of MF is related to the intrinsic radiosensitivity of the infiltrating neoplastic lymphocytes. The D_0 of human lymphocytes is less than 100 cGy.

Spot treatment with orthovoltage x-rays (150–250 kV) or low-energy electron-beam therapy (6–9 MeV) may be used in the management of individual plaques or tumors. Fractionated doses of 1500 to 2500 cGy are often adequate for local control. The more important challenge is the effective treatment of large surfaces of skin, as are often involved in patients with the generalized plaque or tumorous phase of skin involvement. Several techniques of total-skin electron-beam therapy (EBT) have been developed. Commonly, patients are treated in the standing position at a distance of 3 to 4 m from a linear accelerator, which is set in the electron mode. This distance enables treatment of large surfaces. Patients stand on a rotating platform or assume several different positions during treatment to treat their entire circumference.[69] The dosimetry of this technique reveals a superficial depth of penetration, which depends on the energy of the incident electrons.[70] For example, using 6-MeV electrons, the 80% depth dose is at 0.3 cm, and the 50% depth dose is at 0.6 cm. For 9-MeV electrons, the corresponding values are 0.7 cm and 1.25 cm.[41] This provides adequate treatment to the depth of most MF patches and plaques, but exophytic or more deeply infiltrating tumors require supplemental boost treatment to achieve local control. The soles of the feet, perineum, and areas under skin folds are treated in a supplementary fashion with orthovoltage x-rays or electrons.

Using total-skin EBT, the usual dose is 2400 to 3600 cGy given in 6 to 12 weeks. In large series, the complete response rate for patients with patch or plaque disease ranges from 71% to 98%.[41,71] The complete response rate for patients who present with tumorous involvement is 60% to 70%. As many as 50% of patients with limited plaque disease and 25% of patients with generalized plaque disease who achieve a complete response enjoy long-term freedom from relapse after the completion of therapy. Relapses usually occur in the skin. Treatment with topical HN_2 at that time can achieve a similar response rate as the de novo use of HN_2. A comparison of response and survival for patients treated with topical HN_2 or EBT is shown in Table 53–3.

The acute complications of EBT include erythema, temporary epilation, temporary loss of fingernails and toenails, and impaired ability to sweat.[41] Chronic complications include dry skin and the development of telangiectasia, which is usually minimal if the techniques of treatment have been appropriate. Cutaneous carcinogenesis is another potential hazard, which is amplified in these patients by the use of multiple sequential therapies.[62]

Radiation may also provide an important palliative benefit for patients with localized extracutaneous disease. Megavoltage photons (≥4 MeV) can be used to treat symptomatic adenopathy or visceral sites of disease, with techniques similar to those used for other lymphomas. The dose should be titrated to the response, but typically it is limited to 2400 to 3600 cGy.

PUVA therapy is highly effective in clearing skin lesions, and approximately 60% of treated patients in all T stages achieve responses.[67–70] However, maintenance therapy is required in all completely responding patients, because its discontinuation results in a prompt relapse. With maintenance therapy, durable remissions are observed with a mean duration after skin clearing of 6 to 16 months.

TABLE 53–3. Results of Topical Therapy for Myocosis Fungoides With Nitrogen Mustard or Electron Beam at Stanford University

T Stage	*Treatment*	*CR (%)*	*PR (%)*	*10-Year FFR (%) (n = 123)*	*10-Year Survival (%) (n = 226)*
T1	HN_2	51	37	30	83
	EBT	98	2	50	80
T2	HN_2	26	43	0	42
	EBT	71	29	25	45
T3	HN_2		33		
	EBT	36	64		25
T4	HN_2	22	44		
	EBT	64	36		

HN_2, topical nitrogen mustard; EBT, total-skin electron-beam therapy; CR, complete response; PR: partial response; FFR, freedom from relapse.

(Hoppe RT, Abel EA, Deneau DG, Price NM. Mycosis fungoides: Management with topical nitrogen mustard. J Clin Oncol 1987;5: 1796–1803 and Hoppe RT, Wood GS, Abel EA. Mycosis fungoides and the Sézary syndrome: Pathology, staging, and treatment. Curr Probl Cancer 1990;14:295–361)

SYSTEMIC THERAPY FOR CUTANEOUS T-CELL LYMPHOMAS

Chemotherapeutic principles in treating CTCL are similar to those employed for the low-grade B-cell lymphomas.[1,3] Objective responses producing palliation of symptoms produced by refractory cutaneous lesions or extracutaneous disease are frequent (70% response rates), but chemotherapy is not curative. The most active agents include methotrexate, alkylating agents (*e.g.*, cyclophosphamide, chlorambucil) etoposide (VP-16), and cisplatin.[1,3,72] Combination chemotherapy produces higher complete response rates but is not curative. Regimens commonly used are similar to those employed for B-cell lymphomas, including chlorambucil plus prednisone, cyclophosphamide plus vincristine plus prednisone (CVP), or similar regimens.[2,3,73,74] No randomized studies have proven the superiority of combinations over single agents. Chemotherapy is often combined with one of the topical therapies previously discussed because of the bulk disease within the skin.[74]

Recombinant interferons are active agents against CTCL, with response rates of about 50% for patients with advanced disease refractory to other treatments and 90% for early-stage untreated patients.[75,76] Whether interferons should be combined with other effective therapies and whether they should be used initially can only be determined by future trials. Initial studies used extremely high doses,but similar response rates were found with lower, more tolerable doses such as 3 to 10 million units every other day or three times weekly.

COMBINED-MODALITY THERAPY

Combined-modality therapy may be considered in the context of combined topical therapies or as combined topical and systemic treatment. Because of the reliably high complete response rate to total-skin EBT and the high risk for relapse after completion of that treatment, combined treatment with EBT and a topical cutaneous adjuvant therapy is a common approach for aggressive initial treatment of the skin. Adjuvant therapies have included topical HN_2 and PUVA.[77,78] Either of these adjuvants may prolong the duration of the disease-free interval, but it is not clear that the long-term rate of relapse is altered.

Topical and systemic therapies have been combined to achieve a better outcome. Phase II reports of successful treatment with combined EBT and systemic chemotherapy led to a randomized trial at the NCI.[79] Patients with all stages of disease were randomized to conservative therapy (*i.e.*, sequential treatment with topical HN_2, PUVA, total-skin EBT, oral methotrexate, and systemic combination chemotherapy) or combined therapy (*i.e.*, total-skin EBT combined with cyclophosphamide, doxorubicin, etoposide, and vincristine) at the outset. The overall response rate was significantly higher in the combined-therapy group (90% versus 65%; $p=0.003$).

However, actuarial plots of disease-free and overall survival rates were similar for either approach. The median survival after combined therapy was 91 months, compared with more than 76 months (median not yet reached) after conservative therapy. Combined chemotherapy and EBT is not recommended as initial therapy unless there is advanced systemic disease or cytologic transformation.

More effective systemic management is needed to improve the efficacy of combined-modality therapy. An innovative approach with excellent preliminary results is the combination of PUVA with interferon.[80] The complete response rate with this combination was higher than reported for PUVA alone, interferon alone, and combined chemotherapy and EBT, and the response duration was longer than with other therapies.[81] Randomized trials comparing this combination with PUVA alone are indicated. Other combinations recently evaluated in small numbers of patients are described under investigational therapies.

BIOLOGIC AND EXPERIMENTAL THERAPIES

Antithymocyte globulin (ATG) and monoclonal antibodies that react with T-cell antigens produced responses, but the therapy was limited by toxicity (especially with ATG) and the brief duration of the responses.[82–85] A chimeric antibody produced less immunotoxicity, but the response rate and duration were still suboptimal.[86] Radiolabeled antibodies in high doses can produce substantial remissions compared with unlabeled antibody.[85] This approach is still highly experimental because of the myelosuppression caused by free radioisotope. Toxin-conjugated antibodies are being evaluated, but their use remains experimental.[87]

Fludarabine is a newly approved chemotherapeutic agent for the treatment of CLL that is also active in CTCL. In a phase II trial using advanced refractory patients, a response rate of 20% was reported.[88] This agent requires additional study for use in CTCL. Deoxycoformycin is a potent inhibitor of adenosine deaminase and has been evaluated in several chronic lymphoid neoplasms. It is active against hairy cell leukemia and CTCL.[89,90] In one series, a 50% response rate and long duration was reported for refractory patients.[90] It is being evaluated in combination with interferon for treatment of both of these disorders, but its use remains investigational. Retinoic acid derivatives such as 13-*cis*-retinoic acid (Accutane), etretinate, and arotinoid-ethylester produce responses in about 50% of patients with advanced disease.[91–93] Like deoxycoformycin, they are being evaluated in combination with interferon. In a trial combining a retinoid with bleomycin, cyclophosphamide, and prednisone, a complete response rate of 80% lasting 8 months was reported.[94] Retinoids have also been combined with PUVA.[95] High response rates were reported, but it is not clear whether the response rates or duration are superior to PUVA alone.

There have been anecdotal reports of responses to acyclovir and cyclosporine.[96–99] The responses observed after acyclovir have been used to support a viral cause for CTCL. These agents remain investigational until larger controlled trials document their value.

Patients with the Sézary syndrome often have many circulating cells that migrate between the skin, peripheral blood, and lymph nodes.[100] Leukophoresis with removal of large numbers of circulating cells causes transient remissions in some cases.[101] After the development of PUVA therapy, Edelson and coworkers evaluated extracorporeal photophoresis by administering oral methoxsalen 2 hours before leukophoresis.[102] The peripheral blood cells were exposed to UVA light during the leukophoresis. Objective responses were observed in 64% of 37 evaluable patients. As with the agents listed earlier, the exact mechanism of action is unknown and further trials are necessary to define the ultimate role of this modality.

The combined use of total-skin electron irradiation combined with wide-field "systemic" irradiation was evaluated in several investigational studies. The Philadelphia group used total-nodal irradiation with skin electron irradiation.[103] Complete responses were observed in most cases. Remission duration was longest in patients with disease confined to the skin. A group in France employed 125 cGy of total-body irradiation (12.5 cGy twice daily three times weekly) before and after 2400 cGy of total-skin electron irradiation.[104] There was considerable myelosuppression, but 8 of 18 patients survived a median of 30+ months without evidence of disease.

REFERENCES

1. Broder S, Bunn PA Jr. Neoplasms of T-cell origin: Immunological aspects and therapy. Semin Oncol 1980;7:310–331.
2. Broder S, Bunn PA Jr, Jaffe ES, et al. T-cell lymphoproliferative syndrome associated with human T-cell leukemia-lymphoma virus. Ann Intern Med 1984;100:543–557.
3. Sausville EA, Bunn PA Jr. Biologic and clinical spectrum of T-cell neoplasms. In: Harrison's principles of internal medicine, update VII, oncology. 1986:159–189.
4. Broder S, Edelson RL, Lutzner M, et al. The Sézary syndrome. A malignant proliferation of helper T cells. J Clin Invest 1976;58:1297–1306.
5. Haynes BR, Metzger RS, Minna JD, Bunn PA Jr. Phenotypic characterization of cutaneous T-cell lymphoma. N Engl J Med 1981;304:1319–1323.
6. Bertness V, Kirsch I, Hollis G, Johnson B, Bunn PA Jr. T-cell receptor gene rearrangements as clinical markers of human T-cell lymphomas. N Engl J Med 1985;313:534–538.
7. Poixsz BJ, Ruscetti FM, Gazdar AF, et al. Detection and isolation of type-c retrovirus particles from fresh and cultured lymphocytes of a patients with cutaneous T-cell lymphoma. Proc Natl Acad Sci USA 1980;77:7415–7419.
8. Bunn PA Jr, Schechter GP, Blayney D, et al. Clinical course of retrovirus-associated adult T-cell lymphoma in the United States. N Engl J Med 1983;309:257–264.
9. Manzari V, Gismondi A, Barillari G, et al. HTLV-V: A new human retrovirus in Tac-negative T cell lymphoma/leukemia. Science 1987;238:1581–1583.
10. Greene MH, Dalager NA, Lamberg SI, et al. Mycosis fungoides. Epidemiologic observations. Cancer Treat Rep 1979;63:596–606.
11. Epstein EH, Levine DL, Croft JD, et al. Mycosis fungoides. Survival prognostic features, response to therapy, and autopsy findings. Medicine (Baltimore) 1972;51:61–72.
12. Weinstock MA, Holm JW. Mycosis fungoides in the United States: Increasing incidence and descriptive epidemiology. JAMA 1988;260:42–46.
13. Reinherz EL, Schlossman SF. Regulation of the immune response: Inducer and suppressor T lymphocyte subsets in human beings. N Engl J Med 1980;303:370–373.
14. Royer HD, Reinherz EL. T lymphocytes: Ontogeny, function, and relevance to clinical disorders. N Engl J Med 1987;317:1136–1142.
15. Davis MM, Chin Y-H, Gascoigne NRJ, Hedrick SM. A murine T cell receptor gene complex: Isolation, structure, and rearrangement. Immunol Rev 1984;81:235–258.
16. Yang SY, Chowaif S, Dont B. A common pathway for T lymphocyte activation involving both CD3-Ti complex and CD2 sheep erythrocyte receptor determinants. J Immunol 1986;137:1097–1100.
17. McDougal JS, Kennedy MS, Sligh JM, et al. Binding of HTL VIII/LAV to T4 and T cells by a complex of the 11K viral protein and the T4 molecule. Science 1986;231:382–385.
18. Smith KA, Baker PE, Gillis S, Ruscetti FW. Functional and molecular characteristics of T cell growth factor. Mol Immunol 1980;17:579–589.
19. Waldmann TA. The structure, function, and expression of interleukin-2 receptors on normal and malignant lymphocytes. Science 1986;232:727–732.
20. Moingeon P, Ythier A, Goubin G, et al. A unique T cell receptor complex expressed on human fetal lymphocytes displaying natural-killer-like activity. Nature 1986;323:638–640.
21. Oshimi K, Hoshino S, Takahashi M, et al. Ti(WT31)-negative, CD3-positive, large granular lymphocyte leukemia with nonspecific cytotoxicity. Blood 1988;71:923–931.
22. Rappaport H. Tumors of the hematopoietic system. In: Atlas of tumor pathology, Sec. III, fasc. 8. Washington, DC: Armed Forces Institute of Pathology, 1966.

23. Rosenberg S, Non-Hodgkin's Lymphoma Pathologic Classification Project. National Cancer Institute sponsored study of non-Hodgkin's lymphoma. Cancer 1982;49:2112–2135.
24. Nathwani BN, Kim H, Rappaport H. Malignant lymphoma, lymphoblastic. Cancer 1976;38:964–983.
25. Catovsky D, Goldman JM, Okos A, et al. T-lymphoblastic leukemia, a distinct variant of acute leukemia. Br Med J 1974;2:643–646.
26. Weiss LM, Bindl J, Picozzi VJ, et al. Lymphoblastic lymphoma, an immunophenotypic study of 26 cases with comparison to T cell acute lymphoblastic leukemia. Blood 1986;67:474–478.
27. Catovsky D, Okos A, Willt-Shaw E, et al. Prolymphocytic leukemia of B and T cell type. Lancet 1973;2:232–235.
28. Jaffe ES, Blattner WA, Blayney DW, Bunn PA, Robert-Guroff M, Gallo RC. The pathologic spectrum of HTLV associated leukemia/lymphoma in the United States. Am J Surg Pathol 1984;8:263–275.
29. Greer JP, York JC, Cousar JB, et al. Peripheral T-cell lymphoma. A clinicopathologic study of 42 cases. J Clin Oncol 1984;2:788.
30. Pandolfi F, De Roossi G, Semenzato G, et al. Immunologic evaluation of T chronic lymphocyte leukemia cells. Correlations among phenotype, functional activities, and morphology. Blood 1982;59:688–695.
31. Reinherz EL, Nadler LM, Rosenthal DS, et al. T-cell subset characterization of human T-CLL Blood 1979;53:1066–1074.
32. Aisenberg AC, Wilkes BM, Harris N, et al. Chronic T-cell lymphocytosis with neutropenia. Report of a case studied with monoclonal antibody. Blood 1981;58:818–822.
33. Kruskall, MS, Weitzman SA, Stossel TP, et al. Lymphoma with autoimmune neutropenia and hepatic sinusoidal infiltration: A syndrome. Ann Intern Med 1982;97:202–206.
34. Rumke HC, Miedema F, Ten Berge IJM, et al. Functional properties of T cells in patients with chronic TG lymphocytosis and chronic T-cell neoplasia. J Immunol 1982;129:419–426.
35. Uchiyama T, Yodoi J, Sagawa K, Takatsuki K, Uchimo H. Adult T cell leukemia: Clinical and hematological features of 16 cases. Blood 1977;50:481–492.
36. Catovsky D, Rose M, Goolden AWG, et al. Adult T cell lymphoma-leukemia in blacks from the West Indies. Lancet 1982;1:639–643.
37. Gazdar AF, Carney DN, Bunn PA, et al. Mitogen requirements for the in vitro propagation of cutaneous T cell lymphomas. Blood 1980;55:409–417.
38. Gallo RC, Kalyanaraman VS, Sarngadharan MG, et al. Association of the human type C retrovirus with a subset of adult T-cell cancers. Cancer Res 1983;43:3892–3899.
39. Gibbs WN, Lofters WS, Campbell M, et al. Non-Hodgkin lymphoma in Jamaica and its relation to adult T cell leukemia-lymphoma. Ann Intern Med 1987;106:361–368.
40. Wood GS, Abel EA, Hoppe RT, Warnke RA. Leu-8 and Leu-9 antigen phenotypes. Immunologic criteria for the distinction of mycosis fungoides from cutaneous inflammations. J Am Acad Dermatol 1986;14:1006–1013.
41. Hoppe RT, Wood GS, Abel EA. Mycosis fungoides and the Sézary syndrome: Pathology, staging, and treatment. Curr Probl Cancer 1990;14:295–361.
42. Wieselthier JS, Koh HK. Sézary syndrome: Diagnosis, prognosis, and critical review of treatment options. J Am Acad Dermatol 1990;22:381–401.
43. Posner LE, Fossieck BE, Eddy JL, et al. Septicemic complications of the cutaneous T-cell lymphomas. Am J Med 1981;71:210–216.
44. Merlo CJ, Hoppe RT, Abel E, et al. Extracutaneous mycosis fungoides. Cancer 1987;60:397–402.
45. Sausville EA, Eddy JL, Makuch RW, et al. Histopathologic staging at initial diagnosis of mycosis fungoides and the Sézary syndrome: Definition of three distinctive prognostic groups. Ann Intern Med 1988;109:372–382.
46. Burke JS, Hoppe RT, Cibull ML, Dorfman RF. Cutaneous malignant lymphoma: A pathologic study of 50 cases with clinical analysis of 37. Cancer 1981;47:300–310.
47. Deneau DG, Wood GS, Beckstead J, Hoppe RT, Price NM. Woringer-Kolopp disease (pagetoid reticulosis). Four cases with histopathologic, ultra-structural, and immunohistologic observations. Arch Dermatol 1984;120:1045–1051.
48. Wood GS, Weiss LM, Hu C-H, et al. T-cell antigen deficiencies and clonal T-cell receptor gene rearrangements in pagetoid reticulosis (Woringer-Kolopp disease). N Engl J Med 1988;318:164–167.
49. Weiss LM, Wood GS, Trela M, et al. Clonal T-cell populations in lymphomatoid papulosis. Evidence for a lymphoproliferative etiology in a clinically benign disease. N Engl J Med 1986;315:475–479.
50. Bunn PA, Lamberg SI. Report of the committee on staging and classification of cutaneous T-cell lymphomas. Cancer Treat Rep 1979;63:725–728.
51. Bunn PA, Huberman MS, Whang-Peng J, et al. Prospective staging evaluation of patients with cutaneous T-cell lymphomas. Demonstration of a high frequency of extracutaneous dissemination. Ann Intern Med 1980;93:223–230.
52. Weiss LM, Hu E, Wood GS, Moulds C, et al. Clonal rearrangements of the T-cell receptor gene in mycosis fungoides and dermatopathic lymphadenopathy. N Engl J Med 1985;313:539–544.
53. Sausville EA, Worsham GF, Matthews MJ, et al. Histologic assessment of lymph nodes in mycosis fungoides/Sézary syndrome (cutaneous T-cell lymphoma): Clinical correlation and prognostic import of a new classification system. Hum Pathol 1985;16:841–849.
54. Kronke M, Pepper JM, Leonard WJ, Vitetta ES, Waldmann T, Greene WC. Adult T cell leukemia: A potential target for ricin A chain immunotoxins. Blood 1985;65:1416–1421.
55. Gilchrest BA. Methoxsalen photochemotherapy for mycosis fungoides. Cancer Treat Rep 1979;63:663–667.
56. Vella Briffa D, Warin AP, Harrington CI, et al. Photochemotherapy in mycosis fungoides. A study of 73 patients. Lancet 1980;2:49–53.
57. Molin L, Thomsen K, Volden G, et al. Photochemotherapy (PUVA) in the pretumour stage of mycosis fungoides: A report from the Scandinavian mycosis fungoides study group. Acta Dermatol Venereal 1980;61:47–51.
58. Honigsmann H, Brenner W, Rauschmeier W, et al. Photochemotherapy for cutaneous T-cell lymphoma. J Am Acad Dermatol 1984;10:238–245.
59. Rosenbaum MM, Roenigk HH, Carol WA, et al. Photochemotherapy in cutaneous T-cell lymphoma and parapsoriasis en plaques. Long-term follow-up in forty-three patients. J Am Acad Dermatol 1985;13:613–622.
60. Abel EA, Sendagorta E, Hoppe RT, Huch M. PUVA treatment of erythrodermic and plaque type mycosis fungoides. Ten-year follow-up. Arch Dermatol 1987;123:897–901.
61. Stern RS, Laird N, Melski J, et al. Cutaneous squamous cell carcinoma in patients treated with PUVA. N Engl J Med 1984;310:1156–1161.
62. Abel EA, Sendagorta E, Hoppe RT. Cutaneous malignancies and metastatic squamous cell carcinoma following therapies for mycosis fungoides. J Am Acad Dermatol 1986;14:1029–1038.
63. Vonderheid EC. Topical mechlorethamine chemotherapy: Considerations on its use in mycosis fungoides. Int J Dermatol 1984;23:180–186.
64. Hoppe RT, Abel EA, Deneau DG, Price NM. Mycosis fungoides: Management with topical nitrogen mustard. J Clin Oncol 1987;5:1796–1803.
65. Ramsay DL, Halperin PS, Zeleniuch-Jacquotte A. Topical mechlorethamine therapy for early stage mycosis fungoides. J Am Acad Dermatol 1988;19:684–691.
66. Vonderheid EC, Tan ET, Kantor AF, et al. Long-term efficacy, curative potential and carcinogenicity of topical mechlorethamine chemotherapy in cutaneous T-cell lymphoma. Am Acad Dermatol 1989;20:416–428.
67. Zackheim HS, Epstein EH, JR, Crain WR. Tropical carmustine (BCNU) for cutaneous T-cell lymphoma. A 15-year experience in 143 patients. J Am Acad Dermatol 1990;22:802–810.
68. Kim JH, Nisce LZ, D'Anglo GJ. Dose-time fractionation study in patients with mycosis fungoides and lymphoma cutis. Radiology 1976;119:439–442.
69. Hoppe RT, Fuks Z, Bagshaw MA. Radiation therapy in the management of cutaneous T-cell lymphomas. Cancer Treat Rep 1979;63:625–632.
70. Cox RS, Heck RJ, Fessenden P, et al. Development of total-skin electron therapy at two energies. Int J Radiat Oncol Biol Phys 1990;18:659–669.
71. Tadros AAM, Tepperman BS, Hryniuk WM, et al. Total skin electron irradiation for mycosis fungoides. Failure analysis and prognostic factors. Int J Radiat Oncol Biol Phys 1983;9:1279–1287.
72. McDonald CJ, Bertino JR. Treatment of mycosis fungoides lymphoma: Effectiveness of infusions of methotrexate followed by oral citrovorum factor. Cancer Treat Rep 1978;62:1009–1011.
73. Grozea PN, Jones SE, McKelvey EM, et al. Combination chemotherapy for mycosis fungoides: A Southwest Oncology Group study. Cancer Treat Rep 1979;63:647–652.
74. Zakem MH, Davis BR, Adelstein DJ, Hines JD. Treatment of advanced stage mycosis fungoides with bleomycin, doxorubicin and methotrexate with topical nitrogen mustard (BAM-M). Cancer 1987;58:2611–2619.
75. Bunn PA Jr, Foon KA, Ihde DC, et al. Recombinant leukocyte A interferon: An active agent in advanced refractory cutaneous T-cell lymphomas (mycosis fungoides and Sézary syndrome). Ann Intern Med 1984;101:484–488.
76. Covielli A, Cavalieri R, Coppola G, et al. Recombinant leukocyte A interferon as initial therapy in mycosis fungoides and Sézary syndrome. Proc Am Soc Clin Oncol 1987;6:189.
77. Price NM, Hoppe RT, Constantine FS, et al. The treatment of mycosis fungoides: Adjuvant topical mechlorethamine after electron-beam therapy. Cancer 1977;40:2851–2853.
78. Spittle MF. Electron-beam therapy in England. Cancer Treat Rep 1979;63:639–641.
79. Kaye FJ, Bunn PA Jr, Steinberg SM, et al. A randomized trial comparing combination electron-beam radiation and chemotherapy with topical therapy in the initial treatment of mycosis fungoides. N Engl J Med 1989;321:1784–1790.
80. Kuzel TM, Gilyon K, Springer E, et al. Interferon alfa-2a combined with phototherapy in the treatment of cutaneous T-cell lymphoma. JNCI 1990;82:203–207.
81. Kuzel TM, Roenigk H Jr, Samuelson E, et al. Therapy of mycosis fungoides with interferon alfa-2a combined with phototherapy: Phase I and II trial long-term follow-up. Proc Am Soc Clin Oncol 1991;10:271.
82. Foon KA, Schroff RW, Bunn PA Jr. Monoclonal antibody therapy for patients with leukemia and lymphoma. In: Foon KA, Morgan AC Jr, eds. Monoclonal antibody therapy for human cancer. Hingham, MA: Martinus Nijhoff, 1985:85–101.
83. Dillman RO, Shawler DL, Dillman JB, et al. Therapy of chronic lymphocytic leukemia and cutaneous T-cell lymphoma with T101 monoclonal antibody. J Clin Oncol 1984;2:881.
84. Carrasquillo JA, Bunn PA Jr, Keenan AM, et al. Radioimmunodetection of cutaneous T-cell lymphoma with ^{111}In-T101 monoclonal antibody. N Engl J Med 1986;315:673.
85. Rosen ST, Zimmer M, Goldman-Leiken R, et al. Radioimmunodetection and radioimmunotherapy of cutaneous T-cell lymphomas using an ^{131}I-labeled monoclonal antibody: An Illinois Cancer Council study. J Clin Oncol 1987;5:562.
86. Knox SJ, Levy R, Hodgkinson S, et al. Observations on the effect of chimeric anti-CD4 monoclonal antibody in patients with mycosis fungoides. Blood 1991;77:20–30.
87. Le Maistre CF, Rosen S, Frankel A, et al. Phase I trial of H-65-RTA immunoconjugates in patients with cutaneous T-cell lymphoma. Blood 1991;78:1173–1182.
88. Von Hoff DD, Cahlberg S, Hartstock RJ, et al. Activity of fludarabine monophosphate in patients with advanced mycosis fungoides: A Southwest Oncology Group study. JNCI 1990;82:1353–1355.
89. Grever MR, Leiby JM, Kraut EH, et al. Low-dose deoxycoformycin in lymphoid malignancy. J Clin Oncol 1985;3:1196–1201.

90. Cummings FJ, Kyungmann K, Nieman RS, et al. Phase II trial of pentostatin in refractory lymphomas and cutaneous T-cell disease. J Clin Oncol 1991;9:565–571.
91. Kessler JF, Meyskens FL, Levine N, et al. Treatment of cutaneous T-cell lymphoma (mycosis fungoides) with 13-*cis*-retinoic acid. Lancet 1983;1:1345–1347.
92. Molin L, Thomsen K, Volden G, et al. Oral retinoids in mycosis fungoides and Sézary syndrome. A comparison of isoretinoin and etretinate. Acta Dermatol Venereol (Stockh) 1987;67:232–236.
93. Hoting E, Meissner K. Arotinoid-ethylester: Effectiveness in refractory cutaneous T-cell lymphoma. Cancer 1988;62:1044–1048.
94. Zachariae H, Thestrup-Pedersen K. Combination chemotherapy with bleomycin, cyclophosphamide, prednisone and etretinate (BCPE) in advanced mycosis fungoides. A six-year experience. Acta Dermatol Venereol (Stockh) 1987;67:433–437.
95. Thomsen K, Hammar H, Molin L, et al. Retinoids plus PUVA (RePUVA) and PUVA in mycosis fungoides, plaque stage: A report from the Scandinavian Mycosis Fungoides Group. Acta Dermatol Venereol (Stockh) 1989;69:536–538.
96. Scheman AJ, Steinberg I, Taddeini, L. Abatement of Sézary syndrome lesions following treatment with acyclovir. Am J Med 1986;80:1199–1202.
97. Resnick L, Schleider-Kushner N, Horwitz SN, Prost P. Remission of tumor stage mycosis fungoides following intravenously administered acyclovir. JAMA 1984;251:1571–1573.
98. Jensen JR, Thestrup-Pedersen K, Zachariae H, Sogaard H. Cyclosporin A therapy for mycosis fungoides. Arch Dermatol 1987;123:160–167.
99. Puttick L, Pollock A, Fairburn E. Treatment of Sézary syndrome with cyclosporin. J R Soc Med 1983;76:1063–1069.
100. Bunn PA Jr, Edelson RL, Ford SS, Shackney SE. Patterns of cell proliferation and migration in patients with Sézary syndrome. Blood 1981;57:452–463.
101. Edelson RL, Facktor M, Andrews A, et al. Successful management of the Sézary syndrome. Mobilization and removal of extravascular neoplastic T-cell by leukapheresis. N Engl J Med 1974;291:293–297.
102. Edelson R, Berger C, Gasparro F, et al. Treatment of cutaneous T-cell lymphoma by extracorporeal photochemotherapy. N Engl J Med 1987;316:297–300.
103. Micaily B, Vonderheid EC, Brady L, et al. Total electron beam and total nodal irradiation for treatment of patients with cutaneous T-cell lymphoma. Int J Radiat Oncol Biol Phys 1985;11:1111–1119.
104. Hariot JC. Personal communication.

Cancer: Principles & Practice of Oncology, Fourth Edition,
edited by Vincent T. DeVita, Jr., Samuel Hellman, Steven A. Rosenberg.
J.B. Lippincott Co., Philadelphia © 1993.

Michael J. Keating
Elihu Estey
Hagop Kantarjian

CHAPTER **54**

Acute Leukemia

Acute leukemia is an uncommon form of malignancy affecting approximately 5 persons per 100,000 in the United States annually.[1] The disproportionate interest in acute leukemia compared with other malignancies over the years is a consequence of the devastating nature of untreated disease, with a 90% mortality rate within 1 year of diagnosis, and the valuable biologic and therapeutic lessons learned from the study of this disease.[2] Many new drugs with proven activity in malignant disease have been discovered initially in treatment of patients with acute leukemia, and the principles of combination chemotherapy were developed in the management of childhood acute lymphocytic leukemia (ALL).

Acute myelogenous leukemia (AML), also called acute nonlymphocytic leukemia, is five times more common than ALL, although the ratio of patients referred to tertiary centers may vary (Table 54–1).[1] AML is proportionately more common in patients older than 50 years of age, as demonstrated by patients referred to the M.D. Anderson Cancer Center (MDACC). Many of the older patients present with a preceding myelodysplastic phase.

Although the prognosis for adults with leukemia improved dramatically during the 1970s, progress was less impressive in the 1980s. However, there were major insights into the biology of acute leukemia. Although formerly the classification of acute leukemia relied entirely on morphology and histochemical stains, there has been a recent explosion of information on the cytogenetic patterns of acute leukemia and correlations with immunophenotype, oncogene expression, and gene mutations. The transformation of acute leukemia from a universally fatal disease to one that is curable in certain subsets of patients is one of the major accomplishments of cancer chemotherapy.

ETIOLOGY

The causes of most acute leukemias, especially adult ALL, are unknown. Epidemiologic studies have concentrated on the usually small variability in the incidence in different countries and within countries.[3,4] The incidence of AML and ALL is consistently higher in men than women, and this sex difference is more striking in older patients, causing speculation about the role of increased exposure to leukemogenic agents in male patients with AML (see Table 54–1). Although the incidence of leukemia overall has been stable for the last 30 years, the increasing age of our population will presumably result in a greater number of cases being reported.[3,5] There are minor ethnic differences. Acute leukemia is less common in blacks than whites, and the incidence for Jews is higher than for non-Jews.[6,7] Acute leukemia is more common in higher socioeconomic settings.

The contribution of heredity to leukemia has been focused on in the last few years as a result of increasing awareness of the importance of genetic rearrangements in acute leukemia. Several families with a clustering of leukemia have been reported, but siblings of patients with leukemia are only twice as likely as others to develop the disease.[8,9] The exception to this is in childhood leukemia, with concordance in identical twins of approximately one in four.[10,11] Parental consanguinity is a common feature in families with genetically related leukemias.[12]

The strongest association of heredity with leukemia is in Down's syndrome (*i.e.*, constitutional trisomy of chromosome 21), for which there is a 20-fold risk of leukemia.[13] Hereditary disorders with a tendency to chromosome breakage, such as Fanconi's anemia and Bloom's syndrome, are associated with

TABLE 54-1. Distribution of Patients

	AML		*ALL*	
*Age (y)**	*Total*	*% Male*	*Total*	*% Male*
<20	19	58	45	60
20–29	88	56	70	60
30–39	94	56	44	75
40–49	83	41	35	66
50–59	95	63	34	53
60–69	104	54	31	61
≥70	60	48	11	64
Total	543	54	270	63

AML, acute myelogenous leukemia; ALL, acute lymphocytic leukemia.
* Patients with leukemia seen at M.D. Anderson Cancer Center, 1980–1990.

an increased risk of AML.[14] Patients with Bruton type X-linked agammaglobulinemia and hereditary ataxia-telangiectasia have an increased risk of lymphoid neoplasms, including leukemia.[4] This increased risk is also associated with congenital agammaglobulinemia, severe combined immune deficiency, and Wiscott-Aldrich syndrome.[15,16]

The dominant piece of evidence for the causal association of radiation with AML and ALL is the markedly increased incidence of these diseases in survivors of the atomic bomb explosions in Japan. The overall incidence increased 10-fold to 15-fold and was greater for ALL than AML. The increased risk was first manifested 1 to 2 years after the explosions, peaked 5 to 6 years later, and then declined to baseline levels over the next 15 years.[17,18] There was no shift in age distribution. No increase in incidence could be demonstrated in patients estimated to be exposed to less than 100 cGy.[19] A possible association of increased risk of leukemia in military personnel present at nuclear bomb tests in Nevada has been reported.[20]

The strongest association of therapeutic irradiation with leukemia is in patients with ankylosing spondylitis who received x-ray therapy between 1935 and 1954, after which there was an overall fivefold increase in cases.[3,21] The time course was similar to that for the atomic bomb explosions. The use of therapeutic irradiation for menorrhagia and thymic enlargement, thorium dioxide (Thorotrast) in radiologic examinations, and ^{32}P for polycythemia vera are associated with an increased risk of AML.[22–25] Workers exposed to radium and U.S. radiologists working in the early part of this century had an increased risk of leukemia.[26,27] The risk of leukemia in children may be increased by parental preconceptual irradiation exposure and by exposure to extremely low-frequency nonionizing radiation.[28,29] Diagnostic radiologic procedures and the use of ^{131}I treatment of thyrotoxicosis and localized radiation for cancer of the cervix have not been associated with an increase incidence of leukemia.[30,31] The role of radiation treatment for other malignancies as a leukemogenic factor is discussed later.

There is substantial evidence for the leukemogenicity of benzene.[32–35] Benzene causes aplastic anemia. Many patients develop leukemia after a protracted period of cytopenia. Most patients developed leukemia within 5 years, but the increased likelihood may persist for 20 years.[35] Most cases have been a variant of AML. Erythroleukemia (M6) appears to be more frequent than expected. The level of exposure of most of these patients had been high for prolonged periods.[33,35] There have been reports of a geographic association of radon levels in homes with the incidence of AML, and investigators from Great Britain suggest that as many as 25% of cases of AML may be caused by radon exposure.[53] A recent report of an excess of radiation exposure in fathers of children with leukemia has not been validated.[54,55]

Little evidence supports the association of leukemia in adults with exposure to phenylbutazone or chloramphenicol, which can cause aplastic anemia, although an increased risk of childhood ALL in China was associated with chloramphenicol use.[30] There have been reports of an increased risk of AML with cigarette smoking, perhaps with a predisposition to certain cytogenetic subgroups.[36,37] Studies seeking an association with the use of pesticides by farmers have not provided strong evidence for increased risk.[38]

The viral cause of leukemia has been strengthened by data demonstrating integration of human T-cell leukemia virus-I (HTLV-I) into the genome of the leukemic cells in patients with adult T-cell leukemia-lymphoma and is supported by several seroepidemiologic studies.[39–42] HTLV-I is a retrovirus with reverse-transcriptase activity that enables the integration of DNA synthesized from the viral RNA template into the human genome. Missense or silent point mutations of the p53 gene were found in 5 of 10 patients with adult T-cell leukemia.[43] Adult T-cell leukemia-lymphoma is associated with mature-looking CD4-positive T cells that commonly invade the skin and is not a typical acute leukemia.[44] Retroviruses can cause acute leukemia in animals, such as the feline leukemia virus.[45] This common cause of leukemia (usually lymphoid) in cats has caused concern that pet owners and veterinarians may have an increased incidence of leukemia, but this has not been supported.[46,47] Leukemia did not increase in incidence after inoculation with polio myelitis and yellow fever vaccines, which contained SV40 viruses and avian leukosis virus, respectively.[48,49] No association of leukemia with the Epstein-Barr virus, which causes infectious mononucleosis, has been found.[50] Although one study associated ALL in Iowa farmers with cattle density and distribution of bovine lymphocytoma in herds, this may be related to other factors, such as the use of agricultural chemicals.[51,52]

SECONDARY LEUKEMIAS

Leukemia occurring after treatment of another malignancy is called secondary acute leukemia (SAL) or treatment-related leukemia. Most cases are AML or myelodysplastic syndrome (MDS).[56–59] Hodgkin's disease, lymphomas, myeloma, ovarian, and breast carcinomas are associated with an increased risk of secondary AML.[57–59] The peak time of development is 4 to 5 years after diagnosis of the initial malignancy.[58] Several factors, such as the causative agent(s) for the original neoplasm, radiation therapy, chemotherapy, immune status, and age of the patient, may affect the risk. Many chemotherapeutic agents, such as alkylating agents and procarbazine, are leukemogenic in animals and cause chromosome damage.[60,61]

The most intensively studied malignancy associated with a secondary AML is Hodgkin's disease.[62–64] Untreated Hodgkin's disease was not associated with secondary AML.[62] Most patients develop AML with their Hodgkin's disease still in remission after treatment.[65] The more intensive the treatment for the Hodgkin's disease, the shorter is the latent period to the second malignancy.[63] The incidence of AML after irradiation alone appears to be low.[65,66] Chemotherapy is more strongly associated with secondary AML in combined-modality therapy with chemotherapy preceding irradiation.[63] Most patients received MOPP chemotherapy (*i.e.*, nitrogen mustard, vincristine, procarbazine, prednisone), with a lower incidence seen with regimens such as ABVD (*i.e.*, doxorubicin, bleomycin, vinblastine, dacarbazine).[67] Older patients with Hodgkin's disease are more likely to develop secondary AML.[57,68] Most cases of secondary AML after myeloma have received melphalan and a disproportionate number have M4 or M5 morphology.[58,70] Most patients with lymphoma and myeloma reported with secondary AML have received chemotherapy and radiation therapy.[58,69,70] A report from the polycythemia vera study group showed that 1% of patients treated with phlebotomy alone developed acute leukemia, compared with 6% for the patients in the ^{32}P group and 11% in the chlorambucil group, within 6 years of initiation of treatment.[71] Morphologically, most patients with secondary AML have myeloblastic subtypes (*i.e.*, M1, M2) with a lower frequency of monocytic forms of leukemia (*i.e.*, M4, M5). Acute promyelocytic leukemia (APL, M3) is rarely seen as a secondary leukemia.[58] AML after chronic lymphocytic leukemia is an uncommon event.[72] Although an acute myeloid transformation is common in chronic myelogenous leukemia, it is considered as an evolutionary step in the disease process rather than a secondary AML.

A 21-fold elevated risk of developing secondary AML after treatment for ovarian cancer has been reported.[73] Alkylating agents are considered far more potent causative factors than irradiation. The only solid tumor associated with secondary AML is breast cancer.[74,75] Several of these patients have been diagnosed simultaneously as having leukemia and breast cancer, an event that is less common in the other associated malignancies. Most of the reported chemotherapeutic agents associated with the development second leukemias are immunosuppressive and cause DNA damage.

The karyotype of the abnormal cells in secondary AML is strikingly different from de novo AML.[58,76] More than 90% of patients with secondary AML have clonal cytogenetic abnormalities. Three quarters of the patients have lost all or part of chromosome 5 or 7. The modal chromosome number is often hypodiploid (<46). Deletion in the leukemic cells in chromosome 7 is from band 3;4 at the end of the long arm of the chromosome. Loss or deletion of chromosomes involving 5q31 appear to be the critical factor in secondary leukemias involving chromosome 5, suggesting that there may be loss of a tumor suppressor gene from this area. Administration of epidophyllotoxins (*i.e.*, etoposide, teniposide) is associated with a secondary AML and chromosome abnormalities involving 11q23.[77,78] For patients referred to the MDACC, classic cytogenetic abnormalities, such as translocation between or within chromosomes, especially t(8;21), t(15;17), and inv(16), are uncommon in secondary AML or in patients who present with prior MDS (Table 54–2).[58,76] The prognosis for response to treatment and survival of secondary AML and secondary MDS is determined by the cytogenetic pattern, patient age, and percentage of blast cells in the bone marrow.[76] The survival of the few patients with secondary AML with a favorable karyotype is good, survival of those with diploid patterns is intermediate, and those with -5/-7 abnormalities have the shortest survival (Fig. 54–1).

DIAGNOSIS AND CLASSIFICATION

CLINICAL FEATURES

Most patients with AML present with nonspecific symptoms of fatigue and malaise.[79,80] The degree of anemia is not closely correlated with the symptoms of fatigue. Only one fourth of the patients have had symptoms for more than 3 months before diagnosis. The relative distribution of clinical characteristics, symptoms, and laboratory findings in patients with AML, ALL, and acute undifferentiated leukemia (AUL) presenting at the MDACC between 1980 and 1990 are illustrated in Table 54–3.

TABLE 54–2. Cytogenetic Abnormalities in AML and MDS

	De Novo AML (%)			*Secondary AML (%)*	*AML After MDS (%)*	*MDS (%)*
Cytogenetics	*(<60 y, 322)**	*(≥60 y, 127)*	*(Total, 449)*	*(101)*	*(219)*	*(536)*
t(8;21)	8	2	7	5	4	1
t(15;17)	13	2	10	2	1	0
Inv(16)	8	1	6	3	3	<1
Diploid	38	50	41	21	37	34
+8	4	7	5	9	12	7
−5, −7	8	15	10	26	19	31
Miscellaneous	14	14	14	25	12	12
Insufficient	6	8	7	8	10	10

AML, acute myelogenous leukemia; MDS, myelodysplastic syndrome.
* Patients seen at M.D. Anderson Cancer Center.

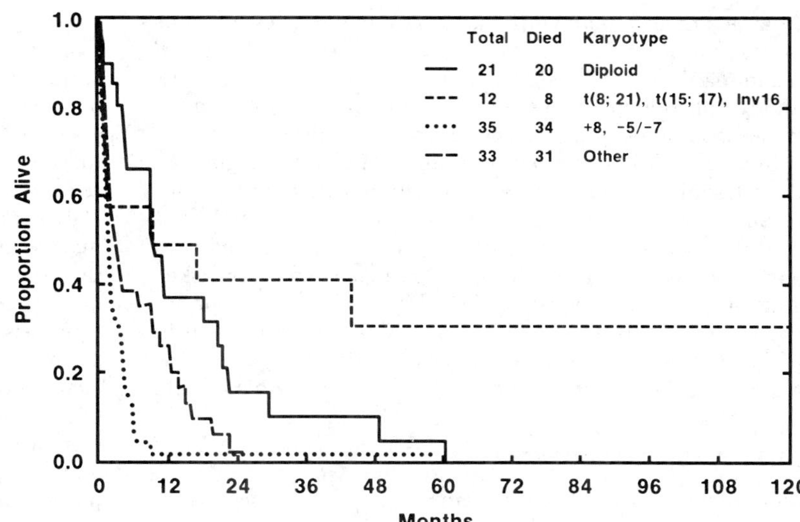

FIGURE 54–1. Survival by cytogenetic pattern of secondary acute myelogenous leukemia patients treated at the M.D. Anderson Cancer Center from 1980 to 1990.

TABLE 54–3. Clinical and Laboratory Features of Adults With AML, ALL, or AUL

	*Percentage With Features**		
Characteristics	*AML*	*ALL*	*AUL*
Male	54	63	65
Age			
<30 y	20	43	14
≥50 y	48	48	51
Presenting symptoms			
Hemorrhage	28	23	16
Bone pain	7	13	6
Infection	30	18	26
Weight loss > 4.5 kg	8	14	14
Presenting signs			
Hepatomegaly	17	26	17
Splenomegaly	11	34	22
Lymphadenopathy	17	37	13
Mediastinal nodes	3	9	0
Gum infiltration	5	2	2
Blood findings			
WBC > 25,000/mm^3	42	36	28
Platelets < 50,000/mm^3	46	49	45
Special stains			
Peroxidase (>3%)	95	0	0
Nonspecific esterase	37	9	11
TdT	15	86	8
Chloroacetate esterase	74	1	9
Acid phosphatase	5	41	17
Auer rods	41	0	0

AML, acute myelogenous leukemia; ALL, acute lymphocytic leukemia; AUL, acute undifferentiated leukemia.
* Patients seen at M.D. Anderson Cancer Center, 1980–1990.

Symptoms of dyspnea, infection, and bleeding are relatively common. The most common infections were relatively minor upper respiratory tract infections or vague flu-like illnesses. Pneumonia was relatively common (~5%) but septicemia was uncommon (<1%) at the time of diagnosis. Many patients who are febrile at the time of presentation have no documented cause of fever. Symptoms of petechiae and ecchymoses are more common in patients with AML. Bleeding symptoms are far more common in patients with APL. Ecchymoses are common only in patients with APL and are associated with the coagulation disturbance rather than the platelet count. The incidence of petechiae correlates well with platelet count but is more common at platelet counts higher than 20,000μl than in other causes of thrombocytopenia, presumably due to impaired platelet function. Anorexia and significant weight loss are relatively uncommon. Bone pain is more common in patients with ALL. Bleeding manifestations and palpable lymph nodes are the only strong features suggesting a diagnosis of leukemia. Many other illnesses can be associated with the nonspecific presenting symptoms observed in most patients.

PHYSICAL FINDINGS

The most common physical finding in leukemia is pallor, and the associated tachycardia is proportionate to the degree of anemia.[79,80] Ecchymoses commonly occur on limbs and are spontaneous or often associated with minor trauma. Petechiae are more common in the lower limbs, presumably because of the hypostatic pressure of dependency. Clinical features of infection are often not striking, because the low neutrophil count and impaired neutrophil function do not allow development of abscesses in many circumstances or consolidation of the lung in patients with pneumonia.[81,82] Throat and gingival infections are relatively common and are often associated with hemorrhagic features. Perianal infections and other soft tissue infections are seldom associated with abscess formation. Hepatomegaly and splenomegaly, uncommon in AML, are more common in ALL (see Table 54–3). Palpable lymph node enlargement is also more prominent in patients with ALL.

Enlarged mediastinal lymph nodes are seen in a few patients on x-ray films and are more common in patients with T-cell leukemia. Within the AML population, hepatosplenomegaly and lymphadenopathy were more common (15–20%) in patients with monocytic differentiation (M4, M5).

Skin infiltration can occur in all AML morphologies, although some series suggest an association with monocytic differentiation. Sternal tenderness occurs in approximately half of the patients. Skeletal pain is not usually associated with abnormalities on x-ray films but can be associated with marked abnormalities on bone scans. Initial clinical presentation involving the central nervous system (CNS) is rare, even in ALL.[83] Initial CNS involvement suggests that the patient has a B-cell ALL, in which the incidence of CNS leukemia is high.

DIFFERENTIAL DIAGNOSIS

Most patients with acute leukemia appear to be acutely or chronically ill, with pallor and often with fever. A complete blood count, differential leukocyte and platelet counts, and blood smear can disclose marked abnormalities in most parameters (Table 54–4). Anemia, thrombocytopenia, elevated leukocyte count with a substantial number of blast cells is almost pathognomonic of acute leukemia. More difficulty is experienced in patients who have pancytopenia without circulating blast cells. Even ALL patients with low leukocyte counts often have a small proportion of circulating blast cells in the peripheral blood. Auer rods in the circulating leukemic cells is almost pathognomonic of AML (see Table 54–3). Auer rods can also be present in some mature cells.

Abnormalities in hematologic counts and the presence of atypical cells should prompt a bone marrow examination. Bone marrow aspiration and biopsy should be performed. In some patients, packing of the marrow with a high proportion of blast cells or development of a reticulin reaction to the presence of the abnormal cells can prevent an adequate bone marrow aspirate.[84] Some patients have hypoplastic bone marrows in association with an increased proportion of blast cells (*i.e.*, hypoplastic acute leukemia) and have inadequate bone marrow aspirates, necessitating a biopsy. In AML and ALL, the bone marrows are usually hypercellular. The proportion of blast cells is usually high (>50%). The major differential diagnosis is between other infiltrative diseases such as lymphoma or other solid tumors such as breast cancer. However, a large proportion of blast cells strongly suggests the diagnosis of acute leukemia.

If there is an increase in the proportion of blast cells to between 5% and 30%, a diagnosis of MDS is suggested.[85] If more than 30% blast cells are present, a diagnosis of acute leukemia is made, with the differential diagnosis among AML, ALL, AUL, or mixed-lineage leukemia. If more than 3% of the blast cells are positive on myeloperoxidase staining, a diagnosis of AML is made.[85,86] If fewer than 3% of the blast cells are peroxidase positive, a terminal deoxynucleotidyl transferase (TdT) stain is performed. If the cells are peroxidase negative and TdT positive, a diagnosis of ALL is likely. Some patients have negative peroxidase and TdT stains, and they are classified as having AUL.

Patients with fever, cytopenia, and a small proportion of circulating blast cells or a minor increase in blast cells in the bone marrow can be difficult to differentiate. Such reactions occasionally occur in tuberculosis, systemic lupus erythe-

TABLE 54–4. Hematologic Values at the Time of Initial Presentation With AML

*Characteristics**	*Value*	*AML (%)*	*ALL (%)*	*AUL (%)*
Hemoglobin (g/dl)	<8	21	15	35
	8–12	71	71	58
	>12	7	14	6
Leukocytes ($\times 10^3/\mu l$)	<10,000	44	48	59
	10–24.9	15	16	14
	25–99.9	29	24	26
	≥100	13	12	2
Platelet count ($\times 10^3/\mu l$)	<25	23	19	24
	25–49	26	23	22
	50–100	27	25	20
	>100	25	29	35
Blasts + promyelocytes (% blood)	0	9	14	20
	1–24	23	25	28
	25–49	15	9	16
	≥50	53	52	37
Neutrophil count ($\times 10^3/\mu l$)	<0.25	33	23	28
	0.25–0.99	21	22	28
	1.0–5.0	27	40	31
	>5.0	19	15	14

AML, acute myelogenous leukemia; ALL, acute lymphocytic leukemia; AUL, acute undifferentiated leukemia.
* Patients (305) seen at M.D. Anderson Cancer Center, 1980–1990.

matosus, paroxysmal nocturnal hemoglobinuria, megaloblastic anemia due to folic acid or vitamin B_{12} deficiency, and aplastic anemia. Patients recovering from the effects of drug-induced marrow suppression often have a transient increase in blast cells during the recovery phase, and differentiation from AML in such patients requires only a repeat bone marrow evaluation after recovery is complete.

Most patients with cytopenias and modest increases in blast cells (5–30%) have features of dysplasia of the erythrocyte, leukocyte, or megakaryocytic series and are classified as MDS patients. These patients often have anemia, neutropenia, monocytopenia, or thrombocytopenia as single or multiple abnormalities. Although the cellularity of the bone marrow is usually increased, it is occasionally decreased. Megaloblastic changes are often prominent in the erythroid series, and care should be taken to separate these patients from folate and vitamin B_{12} deficiency syndromes. Cytogenetic analysis is the single most definitive test to separate MDS from other differential diagnoses. A cytogenetic abnormality occurs in three quarters of MDS patients (see Table 54–2). The finding of the abnormal cytogenetic population supports a strong presumptive diagnosis of a malignant process. The finding of a normal karyotype or insufficient metaphases does not negate the diagnosis of MDS.

The major differential diagnosis for ALL is lymphomas. Most transient viral infections (*e.g.*, infectious mononucleosis) can be sorted out using surface antigen studies, bone marrow aspiration and biopsy, and serologic studies. The differential diagnosis between ALL and lymphoma depends on the clinical pattern of presentation, whether the bone marrow and peripheral blood are involved, and the surface antigen expression. Lymphoblastic lymphoma and ALL appear to be part of the same spectrum of disease, and in adults, they are treated with similar regimens and have similar prognoses. The differential diagnosis between these two categories is less important. If more than one third of the bone marrow is involved, most investigators classify the patients as having ALL.

Difficult morphologic cases can be clarified by the use of electron microscopy. Patients whose cells are undifferentiated on light microscopy can have peroxidase granules detected using electron microscopy. In difficult cases, particularly if a megakaryocytic lineage is involved, electron microscopy studies to identify platelet peroxidase-positive cells is useful to confirm the diagnosis of megakaryocytic leukemia (M7).[87] Other useful stains are the Sudan black stain, the activity of which closely parallels the activity of the myeloperoxidase stain.[86] Cells with acute monocytic leukemia (M5) can be differentiated from AML using a nonspecific esterase stain, such as naphthyl acetate.[88] The esterase activity is inhibited by sodium fluoride in acute monocytic leukemia but not in ALL or other AML subcategories. The periodic acid-Shiff (PAS) reaction is now less commonly used in the diagnosis of acute leukemia. PAS staining is positive in the blast cells of many patients with ALL, in whom blocks of positive staining material are found. The PAS stain is often positive in AML, but the staining pattern is usually more granular than in blocks.[89] TdT staining is not specific for ALL, because the TdT stain is positive (in 5% to 20% of patients with AML; see Table 54–3).

IMMUNOPHENOTYPING

A large literature documents monoclonal antibodies that react with surface antigens expressed on leukemia cell membranes. International workshops have evaluated leukocyte surface antigens and grouped them into 78 cluster designations.[90] The antibodies are useful for confirming the morphologic diagnosis and separating difficult cases. They have limited usefulness in allocating treatment or assessing prognosis. The most commonly used antigens for diagnosing AML are CD11, CD13, CD33, CD14, HLA-DR, CD41, and CD42. CD33 is positive in approximately three quarters of cases, CD13 in two thirds of cases, and CD14 in one third overall and in more than one half of M4 and M5 FAB subtypes. CD11 is positive in half of the cases of monocytic differentiation (Table 54–5). Approximately 20% of cases of AML express lymphoid markers of T-cell lineage.

In T-cell ALL, the most sensitive marker is CD7. CD1, CD2, CD3, and CD5 are other useful confirmatory markers. CD4 and CD8, which identify the helper and suppressor immunophenotypes, are positive in subsets of patients with T-cell ALL. The non-T-cell ALLs react in almost all cases with CD19 and commonly with CD20 and CD22. Most cases are HLA-DR positive. The most mature B cells (L3, Burkitt-type ALL) express surface membrane immunoglobulin of the kappa or lambda phenotype. CD10 (*i.e.*, common acute lymphocytic leukemia antigen or CALLA) is present on most cases of pre-B-cell ALL. The differential diagnosis of the different morphologies can be completed with a relatively defined range of surface antigens. A representative panel of surface markers that can be used to diagnose subtypes of acute leukemia is shown in Table 54–5. In addition, CD41 and CD42 are useful for diagnosing megakaryocytic leukemia and glycophorin, which is specific to red cells, is useful for diagnosing erythroleukemia.

Surface antigens characteristic of T cells exist in approxi-

TABLE 54–5. Surface Markers Useful in the Differential Diagnosis of Acute Leukemias

Leukemia	*HLA-DR*	*CD33*	*CD11*	*CD13*	*CD14*	*CD3*	*CD5*	*CD7*	*TdT*	*CD15*	*CD22*	*CIg*	*SIg*
AML	+*	+	+	+	+†	–	–	+	±	–	–	–	–
T-cell ALL	–	–	–	–	–	+	+	+	++	–	–	–	–
Non-T-cell ALL	+	–	–	–	–	–	–	–	+	+	+	+	+‡

* Except M3.
† M4 or M5.
‡ Mature B cell.

mately 20% of patients with AML, and myeloid antigens occur in 20% of patients with T-cell ALL.[91–93] A combination of morphologic evaluation, special stains, electron microscopy, and surface marker studies can establish the diagnosis of AML or ALL in more than 90% of patients. Other subsets express myeloid and lymphoid characteristics and are often called mixed-lineage leukemias.[94,95] Associations among surface antigen expression, cytogenetic pattern, clinical features, and response are emerging.[95] One study correlated surface antigen expression and response with therapy in AML.[97] Some truly undifferentiated leukemias exist.[96] Many of the undifferentiated leukemias are found to be acute megakaryocytic leukemias if electron microscopy is performed or if studies to detect platelet-specific surface antigens are performed.

Immunoglobulin (Ig) gene rearrangement and T-cell receptor rearrangement studies have been undertaken to separate different types of leukemia. However, 10% to 15% of patients with AML have Ig heavy chain (IgH) gene rearrangements and fewer than 5% have Ig kappa light chain rearrangements. Rearrangement of T-cell receptor genes (*i.e.*, *TCR-β*, *TCR-γ*, and *TCR-δ* genes) are found in 5% to 10% of patients with AML.[98] Ten percent to 15% of patients with T-cell ALL have rearrangements of IgH genes, but *TCR-β*, *TCR-γ*, and *TCR-δ* gene rearrangements or deletions have been found in 33%, 55%, and 80%, respectively, of precursor B-cell ALL.[99–101] The proliferation of methods to delineate lineage has not clarified the area, and few clinical decisions are made on the basis of these sophisticated tests.

LABORATORY FINDINGS

Anemia is found in most patients at the time of initial diagnosis. The erythrocyte morphology is usually normochromic and normocytic in AML and ALL. In AML, moderate macrocytosis can occur. Iron deficiency at the time of diagnosis is rare. Two percent to 5% of patients with AML have nucleated red cells in the peripheral blood smears. Marked anemia is more common in patients with erythroleukemia.

The proportion of patients with high leukocyte counts is similar in AML and ALL (see Table 54–4). Although absence of circulating blast cells are found on routine examination of peripheral blood counts in approximately 10% of patients, close scrutiny often can demonstrate some abnormal blast cells. Within the category of AML, low leukocyte counts are common in APL (M3) and higher counts are observed in monocytic forms (M4, M5) of AML (Table 54–6). Life-threatening thrombocytopenia (<25,000/μl) exists in one fourth of the patients at presentation and is more common in the M3 and M6 varieties of AML. Granulocyte and monocyte morphology is abnormal only in AML cases. Giant platelets or circulating micromegakaryocytes can occasionally be seen in AML. A variety of abnormalities in neutrophil and platelet functions have been described in AML but not in ALL.

BONE MARROW FINDINGS

The cellularity of the bone marrow is best evaluated using the bone marrow biopsy. A bone marrow aspirate with smears evaluates the morphologic type of leukemia better than biopsies. If inadequate aspirates are obtained for smears, a touch preparation of the biopsy material is often useful to allow good morphologic analysis. The causes of difficulty in aspirating marrow are extreme hypercellularity or hypocellularity, increased reticulin or collagen fibrosis, or marrow necrosis. Marrow necrosis is rare in AML and is more common in patients with ALL. Cellularity of the bone marrow is usually higher than 90% in two thirds of patients with AML and 75% of patients with ALL. Hypocellular (<30%) bone marrows are rare (<5%). More than 50% of the nucleated cells are blast cells in 80% to 90% of patients with AML and ALL. Megakaryocytes are usually decreased in number and may have an abnormal morphology in AML.

CLASSIFICATION

In 1976, the French-American British Cooperative Group established classification systems for acute leukemias and MDS.[102] They classified ALL into three morphologic subtypes:

TABLE 54–6. Percentage of Leukemic Patients With Clinical or Laboratory Characteristics According to Morphology

*Characteristics**	*M1 or M2 (n = 53)*	*M3 (n = 62)*	*M4 (n = 107)*	*M5 (n = 40)*	*M6 (n = 5)*	*L1 (n = 47)*	*L2 (n = 153)*	*L3 (n = 18)*
>50 y	53	27	47	48	60	15	28	44
Male	59	55	48	35	60	72	61	78
AHD*	38	10	30	21	45	4	8	6
WBC > 25,000/mm^3	38	11	66	57		34	39	22
Hepatomegaly	16	8	16	20	20	34	22	39
Splenomegaly	9	5	10	20	20	47	37	44
Lymphadenopathy	13	8	30	25	0	40	36	29
Gum infiltration	4	5	8	14	0	4	1	0
Fibrinogen < 150 mg/dl	2	40	3	11	0	4	3	6
Platelets < 25,000/mm^3	22	45	20	7	40	21	18	11
Hyperuricemia	14	10	25	39	40	26	33	83
Creatinine ≥ 1.4 mg/dl	11	8	21	30	12	6	10	28

* Patients seen at the M.D. Anderson Cancer Center, 1980–1990.
† Antecedent Hematologic Disorder for ≥1 month.

L1, L2, and L3. AML was categorized as M1 through M6.[85] Subsequent modifications of the classification has broadened the AML categorization to include M0 (undifferentiated) and M7 (megakaryocytic) and subclassified M5 into M5a and M5b.[89,96,103] Acute myelomonocytic leukemia (AMML, M4) has been subclassified into M4e (*i.e.*, a subset of patients with dysplastic eosinophils).[85,89]

In ALL, the blast cells are usually round with amphophilic cytoplasm.[104] Granules are rarely present in the cytoplasm. The nucleus is usually round and has an open homogenous chromatin network. There are usually one or two small nucleoli. The AML cells are usually larger than in those of ALL, with more variation in the size and shape and with more cytoplasm. Granulation is usually seen. Auer rods are in the cytoplasm of the blasts and sometimes in more differentiated cells (40–45% of patients). Nuclear chromatin is usually reticulated with multiple nucleoli within the nucleus. Sole reliance on morphology and the appearance on Wright-Giemsa stain is inadequate, and ancillary aids such as special stains, immunophenotyping, and cytogenetics are used to establish the cell lineage.

In ALL, the reproducibility of the FAB system has been improved by the addition of a scoring system.[104] Approximately one third of adult patients are L1 type, and most of the others are L2 type. L3 morphology occurs in fewer than 5% of all adults with ALL. The scoring system for separating FAB L1 and L2 relies on the nuclear-cytoplasmic ratio, which tends to be high in L1 (with 0 or 1 nucleoli and small size in L1), the regularity of the nuclear membrane, and the size of the cells.

In AML, the FAB classification runs from M0 to M7. M0 shows minimal evidence of maturation. These cells are peroxidase negative by light microscopy but are often peroxidase positive by transmission electron microscopy, and they have myeloid surface antigens. In FAB M1, the cells tend to have some fine azurophil granules and may have a few Auer rods. There is minimal evidence of differentiation along the rest of the granulocytic or monocytic lineages. In FAB M2, the proportion of blast cells is greater than 30%, and the proportion of monocytic precursors is less than 20%. The cells have abundant cytoplasm and moderate to marked granularity. In FAB M3, otherwise known as APL, the predominant cell is heavily granulated with azurophil granulation. At least some and usually many cells have bundles of Auer rods. The nucleus is often bilobed or kidney shaped. Some cases have less extensive granulation (*i.e.*, microgranular variant). In FAB M4 (formerly AMML), the myeloid precursors (*i.e.*, myeloblast, promyelocytes, myelocytes) and other granulocytic precursors are between 20% to 80% of the nonerythroid nucleated cells. The monocytic cells comprise 20% or more of the nonerythroid nucleated cells. A proportion of these patients have dysplastic eosinophils, and these have been called M4e. In M5 (acute monocytic leukemia), the proportion of granulocyte precursors is less than 20%. In M5a, the blast cells are large with abundant cytoplasm and vacuolated basophilic cytoplasm. In M5b, the cells are more differentiated, and 20% or more of the abnormal cells are recognizable promonocytes or more mature with twisted, folded nuclei. In M6 (acute erythroleukemia), less than 30% of the cells are of myeloid or monocytic lineage, and more than 50% are megaloblastic erythroid precursors. M7 (acute megakaryocytic leukemia) is often associated with extensive marrow fibrosis, with an increase in reticulin or collagen. The bone marrow biopsy often shows clusters of micromegakaryoblasts and other abnormal megakaryoblasts.

In the FAB classification subtypes, M1 and M2 usually stain strongly with peroxidase and chloroacetate esterase. M4 stains with PAS stain and α-naphthyl esterase. M5 stains strongly with PAS, α-naphthyl esterase, and acid phosphatase.

The reproducibility of the FAB myeloclassification is still not high (67%).[105,106] Some subtypes, especially M3, are easily recognized by most cytopathologists. Separation of the other subtypes remains difficult. The approximate distribution of the FAB subgroups in AML are M0<5%, M1=20%, M2=30%, M3=10%, M4=15% to 20%, M4e=5% to 10%, M5a=5%, M5b=5%, M6<5%, and M7<5%. There is little correlation between the FAB subclassification system and the response to treatment or survival.

DIFFICULTIES IN CLASSIFICATION OF ACUTE LEUKEMIA

Acute leukemia is a clonal disease involving stem cells. Supporting evidence for this is obtained from morphologic, cytogenetic, and in vitro growth data and surface antigen expression. The first decisions for the hemopoietic stem cell is whether to differentiate along lymphoid or myeloid lines. Subsequently, the myeloid lineage diverts along erythroid, megakaryocytic, or granulocyte lineages, including monocytic, neutrophilic, eosinophilic, or basophilic lines. Biphenotypic leukemia, in which some cells appear myeloid and others appear lymphoid, presumably arise from pluripotent stem cells. Later steps in the decision-making hierarchy are presumably decided at a nuclear level or under the influence of humoral factors (possibly autoregulatory) that direct the cells to grow along a particular lineage. The cell population can be predominantly eosinophilic, basophilic, monocytic, erythroid, megakaryocytic, neutrophilic, or a combination of these in myeloblastic leukemia. Single cells can demonstrate lineage infidelity, with surface antigens indicating commitments to multiple lines, such as erythroid, granulocytic, megakaryocytic, or even lymphoid lineage.[107–109] The presence of rearranged immunoglobulin genes and T-cell receptor genes in many cases of myelogenous leukemia and expression of myeloid surface antigens in 15% to 20% of cases of ALL emphasize the difficulties in categorizing many of these cases.[98–101]

Acute megakaryocytic leukemia is an uncommon form of leukemia strongly associated with myelofibrosis.[103,110] Detection of platelet peroxidase using transmission electron microscopy, immunohistochemical stains, and monoclonal antibodies against platelet antigens such as CD41 and CD42 have demonstrated that perhaps 5% of patients with AML have megakaryocytic involvement. Megakaryocytic leukemia is characteristically associated with secondary AML and has a high incidence of unfavorable cytogenetic abnormalities. The prognosis is poor.[110] Megakaryocytic hyperplasia often causes myelofibrosis as a reactive process not directly involved in the malignancy, and a normal karyotype has been found in the fibroblasts of these patients.[111]

Eosinophilic leukemia is rare.[112] The eosinophilia may be manifest in the peripheral blood or the bone marrow. There is often infiltration of cardiac, pulmonary, and central nervous systems, as observed in the benign hypereosinophilia syndrome. Most patients with AML with eosinophils in the blood or marrow have M4e associated with inversion of chromosome 16. Eosinophilia can be associated with a diploid karyotype or t(8q;21q) and other chromosomal abnormalities.[113] Reactive eosinophilia can occur in patients with ALL or lymphoma sometimes associated with a hypereosinophilic syndrome, presumably as a result of cytokine production by the lymphoid lineage.[114]

Chronic myelogenous leukemia (CML) presenting de novo in myeloid or lymphoid blast crisis can have substantial eosinophilia. Cytogenetic analysis is important in the evaluation of such patients. Acute basophilic or mast cell leukemia is rare, and most patients have variants of CML in blast crisis. Markedly abnormal basophilic staining can occur in patients with M3 and M4e in association with t(15;17) and inv(16).

MYELODYSPLASTIC SYNDROME

Patients who have cytopenias and persistently abnormal marrows with dysplasia of one or multiple lineages are classified as having MDS.[115] In refractory anemia (RA), there is predominant dysplasia in the erythroid series with less than 5% blast cells in the bone marrow, and less than 1% blast cells in the peripheral blood. In some of these patients, more than 15% of the nucleated erythroid cells are ring-sideroblasts (RASA). Patients with refractory anemia with excess blasts (RAEB) have marked dysplasia of the granulocytes and erythrocytes. The marrow blast cells comprise 5% to 20%. Refractory anemia with excess blasts in transformation (RAEBT) is diagnosed if patients have 20%% to 30% blasts cells in the marrow and sometimes more than 5% blasts in the peripheral blood. Auer rods in MDS patients places them in the RAEBT group. Some patients with MDS have an absolute monocytosis in the peripheral blood of at least 1,000/μl, a condition called chronic myelomonocytic leukemia (CMML). Otherwise, these patients resemble the other MDS groups, and the monocyte count has no prognostic significance.

BIOCHEMICAL AND GENETIC IRREGULARITIES

BIOCHEMICAL ABNORMALITIES

Many patients with leukemia present with abnormalities in a variety of biochemical parameters. The serum uric acid is elevated in 20% of patients with AML, especially M4 and M5 types, and 30% with ALL. It is markedly elevated (>10 mg/dl) in 5% to 10% of patients. Uric acid urinary excretion is almost always increased.[116] Renal impairment due to urate nephropathy is uncommon until treatment is initiated. At that point, rapid lysis of tumor cells can cause a sudden uric acid load for excretion.[117] Tumor lysis syndrome is more common in ALL than AML. A high serum uric acid level is more common in patients with high leukocyte counts, large tumor burden, and monocytic morphology in AML patients. Elevation of the blood urea nitrogen (BUN or serum creatinine) occurs in 10% to 15% of patients at diagnosis. Renal impairment is more common in patients who are elderly or who present with fever or documented infection. Serum muramidase levels are elevated in AML but not ALL and are more strikingly elevated in M4 or M5 patients.[118]

The serum lactate dehydrogenase (LDH) level is elevated in most patients.[118] The most striking elevations appear to occur in patients with ALL, especially B-cell ALL. The serum LDH is an important prognostic factor for remission duration and CNS leukemia in adult ALL.[83,119] The elevated LDH correlates with large tumor burden and a high labeling index in the blast cells.[120]

Mild hepatic dysfunction occurs in a small proportion of patients with acute leukemia. Hypoalbuminemia is common (30–40%) and is an adverse prognostic factor for survival in AML and ALL. The serum calcium level correlates with the serum albumin level and is therefore modestly decreased in a substantial number of patients.

Hypercalcemia rarely occurs in acute leukemia, and if present, suggests ALL, possibly acute T-cell leukemia. The vitamin B_{12}-binding proteins and folic acid-binding proteins are commonly elevated in AML and correlate with the height of the leukocyte count.[121,122] Hypokalemia is commonly found in AML and less commonly in ALL.[123] It is more common in cases with monocytic differentiation. Hypofibrinogenia (<150 mg/dl) occurs in 40% of patients with M3 morphology, 10% of those with M5, and 2% to 5% of other cases of AML and ALL who present to the MDACC (see Table 54–6).

CYTOGENETIC ABNORMALITIES

Most patients with acute leukemia studied with Giemsa or quinacrine banding techniques have an abnormal karyotype in their leukemic cells.[124] High-resolution banding techniques suggest that almost all patients have cytogenetic abnormalities.[125] The changes in chromosome number and structure are not random. Several well-defined clinical syndromes have been described in AML and ALL. The commonest translocations that have been described in AML (5–10% of cases in each) are translocations between chromosomes 8 and 21, t(8q;21q), and between chromosomes 15 and 17, t(15q;17q). Pericentric inversions or translocations of chromosome number 16 also occur in 5% to 10% of patients with AML (see Table 54–2). These three specific translocations occur only in AML and more common in young patients, and overall, they occur in 25% of all patients with de novo AML (see Table 54–2).[124,126] There is a strong association of t(8q;21q) with M2 morphology, presence of Auer rods, and loss of an X or Y chromosome in one half of cases, t(15q;17q) with M3 morphology, and inv(16) in M4e patients.[124]

The breakpoint on chromosome 15 in APL occurs at the PML transcription unit and the retinoic acid receptor-alpha gene is involved in chromosome number 17.[127–130] This generates a chimeric PML-RARA gene product. This chromosome abnormality is associated with a dramatic response of M3 patients to treatment with all-*trans*-retinoic acid.

Trisomy of chromosome 8 or deletions or losses of chromosomes 5 or 7, alone or with additional changes, are common in patients with MDS or secondary AML, are more common in older patients, and are rarely Auer rod positive (see Table 54–2).[126] A small group of male patients with AML demonstrate loss of the Y chromosome in their leukemic cells. These patients tend to behave as if they had no chromosome abnormality.[131]

Two thirds of adults with AML have cytogenetic abnormalities. Abnormalities in chromosome 11 with a breakpoint at 11q23 occur in several cases of monocytic differentiation and biphenotypic cases.[95] The other chromosomes involved in the translocations with chromosome 11 vary but include chromosomes 8, 4, and 9. Inversion in chromosome 3 occurs in a small proportion of patients, and translocation between chromosomes 6 and 9 also occurs in a few patients.[132] Abnormalities in chromosome 20q- are somewhat common in AML and are more common in MDS.[133] The Philadelphia chromosome has been described in a variety of patients with AML.[134] It is described less commonly now in AML than previously for unknown reasons. Several studies confirm the consistent clinical usefulness of the cytogenetic pattern as a prognostic factor in AML.[135–138]

Approximately 10% to 15% of adults with ALL have insufficient metaphases for cytogenetic analysis. Great attention to technique in childhood ALL has been associated with improved ability to document clonal abnormalities, now observed in more than 90% of patients with ALL.[139] The specific cytogenetic abnormalities commonly observed in adult ALL are t(4;11), t(9;22) or t(8;14), t(2;8), and t(8;22).[140,141] Other abnormalities include 14q+ and 6q−. The marked hyperdiploidy (>50 chromosomes) that is common in good-prognosis childhood ALL is rare in adults (<5%).[141] Twenty-five percent of adults have the Philadelphia chromosome present. The abnormality, t(9;22)(q34;q11), has a chromosome break at the breakpoint cluster region (*BCR*) gene in chromosome 22, and the *ABL* protooncogene from chromosome 9 is translocated to the breakpoint in the *BCR* gene. This creates a chimeric *BCR-ABL* gene. In one half of the patients, the chimeric gene ultimately gives rise to the formation of a 210-kd protein (p210) and the other half to a 190-kd protein (p190) in adults. It does not appear that there is a difference in response or survival for the p210 or p190 protein patients.[142]

The t(8;14), t(2;8), and t(8;22) are important although uncommon abnormalities.[141, 143–145] They occur in L3 morphology ALL or Burkitt-type leukemia. In this disease, the *MYC* oncogene on chromosome 8 is brought into apposition with the heavy or light chain regions of the immunoglobulin genes. The t(4;11) is often associated with a biphenotypic leukemia, with features of ALL and monocytic differentiation.[146] All of these cytogenetic abnormalities are associated with a poor prognosis in adult ALL. The t(1;19) that is common in childhood pre-B ALL is uncommon in adults.[147]

GENE REARRANGEMENTS IN LEUKEMIA-ASSOCIATED CHROMOSOMAL TRANSLOCATIONS

Molecular biology has enabled the delineation of specific abnormalities in identified genes. Many of these have been observed in ALL. The *MYC* involvement in t(8;14), t(2;8), and t(8;22) has been well described, as has been the situation with t(15;17) with *PML* and *RARA*. The t(1;19) translocation involves genes *PBX1* on chromosome 1 and *E2A* on chromosome 19. The Philadelphia chromosome abnormality of *ABL* and *BCR* is also well known. Common involvement of chromosome 14q11 in T-cell ALL involves the T-cell receptor genes *TCR-α* and *TCR-δ*. Several other protooncogenes are involved in human malignancies (*e.g.*, *ETS1* oncogene in t(4;11) ALL, *ETS2* in t(8;21) AML (M2), *TCL2* and *TCL3* in T-cell ALL, *PRL* in pre-B t(1;19) ALL, and *CAN* in t(6;9). These specific changes in association with clinical syndromes suggest that they are crucial components in the pathophysiology of some cases of AML and ALL.[148] The specific breakpoints suggest that therapeutic interventions targeted to these abnormalities can be useful.[149]

Structural alterations in protooncogenes and tumor suppressor genes are an area of active exploration. A mutation of the *RAS* genes occurred in 15% to 25% of cases in acute leukemia, more commonly in AML M4 or M5 (33%), and is most common in CMML.[150–152] Fifteen percent to 20% of patients with myelodysplasia and AML have mutations in the *FMS* protooncogene.[153,154] Mutations of the p53 gene have been described in AML and ALL, as have abnormalities in the retinoblastoma (*RB1*) tumor suppressor gene.[155–158] The exact roles of these abnormalities in leukemogenesis require further exploration.

There are additional roles for oncogenes. Qualitative alterations in oncogene expressions, such as mutations, deletions, or rearrangements, and quantitative alterations, such as gene amplification, occur in human leukemia. Because the expression of several of these oncogene products depends on the cell cycle, normal or exaggerated levels of the protein do not necessarily indicate involvement in the disease process. Further work in this area is certain to lead to major advances in our understanding of acute leukemia.

BIOLOGIC FEATURES OF ACUTE LEUKEMIA

AML is characterized not by rapid cell proliferation but a gradual accumulation in the bone marrow or in other organs of undifferentiated cells. The proportion of blast cells in S phase (*i.e.*, undergoing DNA synthesis) or in mitosis in leukemia is lower than in normal bone marrow blasts.[159–162] Considerable heterogeneity exists in the proportion of cells in each cell cycle. Small blast cells tend to have low labeling indices (*i.e.*, percent of cells in S phase), but larger cells are more commonly in S phase.[163] Some cells are considered to be dormant (G_0) but can be recruited into the cycle. Blast cells can recirculate from the peripheral blood to the bone marrow.[164] The proportion of cells in the cell cycle is higher at the time of relapse than at initial presentation.[159,165]

Most antineoplastic agents are more effective on cells participating in the cell cycle. Several agents, such as vincristine, corticosteroids, alkylating agents, and L-asparaginase, appear to cause direct cell lysis of leukemic cells.[166–169] Several drugs, such as cytosine arabinoside (ara-C), amsacrine, 5-azacytidine, and purine analogs, inhibit DNA synthesis, and the anthracyclines arrest cells at the G_2-M interface.[170–175] Vincristine, VP-16, and VM-26 affect cells in mitosis.[176]

Initial attempts at recruiting leukemic cells into the cycle to make them more susceptible to chemotherapy used agents such as ara-C and hydroxyurea.[170,177–180] Growth factors such as (granulocyte-macrophage colony-stimulating factor (GM-CSF) and interleukin-3 (IL-3) stimulate growth and differentiation of leukemic cells.[181–185] Clinical trials have attempted to synchronize the cells into S phase using GM-CSF.[186–190] The results of these trials are equivocal, with some reporting promising results, but others demonstrated a negative impact.[189,190] The clinical concern is that the stimulation of growth of leukemic cells may have a deleterious effect on the patient's outcome.[190]

The prognostic impact of measurements of the cell cycle, such as the percentage of cells in S phase, using flow cytometry or tritiated thymidine labeling indexes has not been reproducible. Some studies correlated a high S-phase percentage with a high complete remission rate, but others have not found this result.[178,179,191,192] A high S-phase percentage has been associated with shorter remission duration.[192] One study demonstrated a discordance of the prognostic impact of S phase on response according to age, with high S-phase percentage associated with a good response in younger patients but a poor response in older patients.[193] The proportion of cells in S phase is higher in bone marrow biopsy specimens than aspirates, because aspirates are diluted with peripheral blood in which a smaller proportion of the blast cells are in the cycle.[194,195] AML appears to be a disease in which cells with limited ability to differentiate accumulate in the bone marrow. Ten percent to 25% of these cells appear to be in G_0 and less susceptible to the effect of chemotherapeutic agents.

Fewer cell cycle studies have been conducted using adults with ALL. Using flow cytometry, the ALL cells show considerable heterogeneity. A high proportion of cells in S phase occurs in B-cell ALL (L3). The mean percentage of cells in S phase is the same as in AML, but there are more cells with high proportions of cells in S phase. The RNA index is lower in ALL than in AML. The results of cell cycle kinetics and the RNA index did not affect outcome for ALL or AML patients in one study.[196]

GROWTH IN CULTURE

Several investigators have attempted to grow leukemic cells in a variety of media. Most studies have used semisolid culture media, such as agar. Normal bone marrow reproducibly grows in agar with colonies of cells (>40 cells) and clusters that are smaller groups of cells.[197] There is no widely used reproducible method of growing ALL cells.[198] A variety of growth stimuli have been applied, such as phytohemaglutinin or placenta conditioned media. GM-CSF has been added alone or with other growth factors to enhance the growth of leukemic cells.[185,199] Similar actions are observed with IL-3.[183] Growth is enhanced with combinations of growth factors compared with the use of single growth factors.[200] The cells that grow from patients with AML can be replated and in some circumstances continue to form colonies and clusters. This is called secondary plating efficiency or the self-renewal capacity and is reported to be a prognostic factor in obtaining a complete remission with chemotherapy. The pattern of growth in agar is reported to indicate a poor prognosis for remission for patients whose cells grow large clusters.[201]

DIFFERENTIATION

Several factors can cause differentiation of AML cells. These include dimethyl sulfoxide, hexamethyl bis-acetamide, and vitamin A and vitamin D analogs.[202–204] G-CSF and GM-CSF caused differentiation of AML cells, and drugs such as ara-C, 5-azacytidine, and aclacinomycin in low doses induced differentiation in some cell lines.[205–209] The most potent evidence for differentiation appears to be with the application of *trans*-retinoic acid to HL60 cells, other cell lines, and patient samples, which translated into therapy to induce complete remissions in APL.[210–213] Few data are available on differentiation of ALL cells in adults.

TREATMENT

Treatment of AML and ALL involves remission induction and postremission therapy. Complications occurring during induction that may be fatal are infection, hemorrhage, and organ failure. Remission is usually obtained by causing severe marrow hypoplasia with high doses of chemotherapy and allowing the normal residual stem cells the opportunity to regrow faster than the leukemic cells, restoring normal neutrophil and platelet counts and the hemoglobin level.

Meticulous surveillance for infection and institution of early vigorous antimicrobial treatment is paramount. The prevention of bleeding from severe thrombocytopenia and coagulation disturbances is crucial. The evaluation of the patient initially should include an estimate of the hemoglobin level, neutrophil count and platelet count, fibrinogen level, and renal and hepatic function. If the patient is febrile and neutropenic, immediate initiation of broad-spectrum antibiotic therapy is mandatory. The risk of dying within 24 hours of untreated gram-negative septicemia is about 20% to 30%.[214] Leukemia alone is seldom a cause of fever at initial diagnosis, and the fever is almost always associated with occult or overt infection. Common sites of infection are the oropharynx, lungs, bloodstream, perirectal areas, and the urinary tract. Chest x-ray films and cultures of the throat, urine, blood, and any obvious lesions must be performed immediately.[214]

If the platelet count is less than 20,000/μl, the patient should receive prophylactic platelet transfusions, and these should be continued as needed (even 1–2 times a day) until the patient achieves complete remission.[215] Most patients need to be transfused with platelets two or three times each week during the remission-induction phase. Approximately 15% to 20% of patients are relatively or absolutely refractory to platelet transfusions at the time of diagnosis. HLA-matched platelets or transfusions from parents, siblings, or children may overcome this resistance.[216]

Disseminated intravascular coagulation (DIC) occurs at the time of presentation, predominantly in patients with APL or those with monocytic morphologies (see Table 54–6). Vigorous treatment with fresh frozen plasma or cryoprecipitate to maintain a fibrinogen level of more than 100 μg/dl and a platelet count above 50,000/μl in patients with evidence of DIC is essential. The role of heparin therapy in DIC in AML is uncertain and has been recently addressed.[217]

Leukostasis occurs in a significant number of patients with high circulating leukemic cell counts (>100,000/μl) and is more common in AML.[218,219] It occurs in 10% to 20% of patients at diagnosis.[220] The most effective way to decrease clinical leukostasis that involves the brain and the lungs is to commence chemotherapy immediately to decrease the cell count and to prevent proliferation of cells that have invaded vessel walls and then grown to form colonies of leukemic cells. Approximately 10% of patients with a leukocyte count of more than 100,000/μl die within the first 10 days of therapy of cerebral or pulmonary hemorrhage.[220] Leukapheresis is also useful in decreasing the circulating blast counts but does not prevent the growth of leukemic cells that have already left the vessel wall and invaded tissues.

Other features requiring effective medical treatment include hepatic and renal insufficiency, which can occur as a result of infiltrating leukemic cells but are more often associated with the presence of infection, hyperuricemia, and dehydration. Organ dysfunction due to proliferation of leukemic cells is an indication for immediate chemotherapy. Hypokalemia occurs frequently and hypocalcemia and hypomagnesemia less frequently, and they should be corrected to prevent arrhythmias, especially if amsacrine is being used.[221] Hyperuricemia should be managed with allopurinol and alkalinization of the urine, particularly in patients with ALL, because tumor lysis is more common in this disease.

CHEMOTHERAPY FOR ACUTE LEUKEMIA

The early treatment of AML and ALL in adults used corticosteroids, methotrexate, 6-mercaptopurine, and vincristine, initially as single agents and subsequently in combinations.[222–224] The emergence of ara-C as the major single agent in the management of AML in the late 1960s converted this incurable disease to a potentially curable condition.[225–227] The subsequent development of the anthracyclines, such as daunorubicin, doxorubicin (Adriamycin), rubidazone, and idarubicin, allowed new combinations with these agents to be developed.[228–232] Representative results of chemotherapy regimens such as the 3/7 regimen, ara-C plus thioguanine, TAD or DAT (daunorubicin, ara-C, thioguanine), and idarubicin plus ara-C regimens are shown in Table 54–7.[233–240]

A study of daunorubicin plus ara-C compared with doxorubicin plus ara-C demonstrated no significant difference in response rate with these regimens.[241] Several studies have substituted mitoxantrone and amsacrine for the anthracycline combination with ara-C.[242,243] Higher doses of ara-C have been studied to overcome pharmacokinetic resistance. The vinca alkaloids, alone or in combination with corticosteroids, and the epidophyllotoxins, methotrexate, 6-mercaptopurine, cyclophosphamide, and L-asparaginase have only minor activity in adult AML, despite marked activity in ALL.

Most regimens in adult ALL incorporate vincristine, corticosteroids, prednisone or dexamethasone, anthracyclines, or L-asparaginase in the initial remission induction phase (see Table 54–7).[248–252] Most remission maintenance therapies rely heavily on 6-mercaptopurine and methotrexate, which are

TABLE 54–7. Commonly Used Remission Induction Regimens for Acute Myelogenous and Lymphocytic Leukemia

Regimen	*Drugs*	*Dose Plus Schedule*	*No. of Patients*	*References*	*Complete Response (%)*	*Comments*
AML						
3/7	Ara-C	100 mg/m²/d × 7 CIVI				
D 3/7	+ Daunorubicin	45 mg/m²/d × 3	646	238, 239, 242, 244, 245	358 (55)	Various studies
I 3/7	+ Idarubicin	12–13 mg/m²/d × 3	161	238, 239	116 (72)	Two randomized studies vs D 3/7
M 3/7	+ (Mitoxantrone)	12 mg/m²/d × 3	98	242	62 (63)	Randomized study vs D 3/7
TAD	Thioiguanine		216	244	123 (57)	Randomized vs 3/7
	ARA-C		576	246	374 (65)	TAD 9
	Daunorubicin		1127	247	757 (67)	D 1/5
ALL						
VAD	Vincristine	0.4 mg/d × 4 CIVI	105	248	(84)	38% CCR at 14 y
	Doxorubicin	12 mg/m²/d × 4 CIVI				
	Dexamethasone	40 mg/d, days 1–4, 9–12, 17–20				
Gimena	Prednisone	40 mg/m²/d × 6 wk	358	249	284 (79)	25% CCR at 4 y, consolidation not helpful
	Vincristine	1.5 mg/m² q w × 6				
	L-Asparaginase	10,000 I.V./m² q wk × 3 (wk 1,2,3)				
	Daunorubicin	40 mg/m² q wk × 3 (wk 3,4,5)				
German	Prednisone	60 mg/m²/d × 28 d	368	250	272 (74)	40% CCR at 4 y
	Vincristine	1.5 mg/m² q wk × 4				
	Daunorubicin	25 mg/m² q wk × 4				
	L-Asparaginase	5000 I.V./m²/d × 14 d				
Linker	Prednisone	60 mg/m²/d × 28 d	109	251	96 (88)	~45% CCR at 4 y for all <50 y of age, 4% induction mortality
	Vincristine	2 mg q wk × 4				
	Daunorubicin	50 mg/m²/d × 3				
	L-Asparaginase	6000 I.V./m²/d × 12 (d 17–28)				

active in adult ALL. Mitoxantrone, amsacrine, and alkylating agents have some activity in salvage therapy of ALL and have been incorporated into combination regimens. VM-26 has been used in children in combination with ara-C as salvage therapy.[253] The clinical pharmacology of these chemotherapeutic agents was discussed in an earlier chapter. Because the regimens used in the management of AML and ALL are different, they are discussed separately.

MANAGEMENT OF ACUTE MYELOGENOUS LEUKEMIA

Most remission induction regimens for AML incorporate a combination of ara-C and an anthracycline. Ara-C is usually given by a 7-day continuous infusion at a dose of 100 to 200 mg/m^2 per day. No advantage was found for the higher dose.[245] Traditionally, daunorubicin at a dose of 45 mg/m^2 per day for 3 days has been added to ara-C to form the traditional 3/7 regimen (see Table 54–7). Attempts to enhance the complete remission rate by extending the duration of infusion to 10 days or adding thioguanine to the regimen has not enhanced the response rate in comparative clinical trials.[244] Subsequently, the 3/7 regimen has become the "gold standard" against which other regimens are compared.

Idarubicin plus ara-C was compared with daunorubicin plus ara-C, with ara-C being maintained at the same schedule and dose.[238–240] One study demonstrated a significantly higher complete remission rate in the idarubicin plus ara-C arm compared with the daunorubicin plus ara-C arm.[238] Two other comparative trials suggested that idarubicin plus ara-C was equivalent or slightly superior to daunorubicin plus ara-C.[239,240] Idarubicin differs from daunorubicin in that its major metabolite (*i.e.*, idarubicinol) has antileukemic activity, but daunorubicinol has no significant antileukemic activity and is still toxic.[238] Idarubicin may be less susceptible to the effect of a multidrug resistance (*MDR1*) gene in terms of accumulation and retention of the drug in cell lines.[238] There is no evidence that doxorubicin or rubidazone have superior activity to daunorubicin. Bishop and colleagues reported that the addition of etoposide to the standard daunorubicin plus ara-C 3/7 regimen is associated with a significantly better remission duration in younger patients.[254]

Mitoxantrone was compared with daunorubicin. There is no significant difference in the complete remission rate in the studies of this agent combined with ara-C.[242]

Ara-C is given by continuous infusion, because there is good evidence for schedule dependency in animal and human clinical studies.[225–227] Ara-C requires uptake by the leukemic cells and activation by an enzyme called deoxycytidine kinase to the triphosphate form.[255] Cytidine deaminase deaminates ara-CMP to ara-UMP and ara-C to ara-U.[255] The triphosphate form of ara-C inhibits DNA synthesis by competitive inhibition of DNA polymerases and by incorporation into DNA.[256–258] It is thought that cells can become resistant to ara-C by lack of an effective level of deoxycytidine kinase, having increased d-CTP to compete for inhibition of DNA polymerase, and rapid egress from the cell of ara-CTP.[259–261] High-dose ara-C regimens are expected to overcome partially the second and third postulated components of resistance. The proposed mechanisms of actions of the various drugs used in the management of AML are discussed in the chapter on pharmacology. The activities of these drugs as single agents are described largely in relapsed patients.

The standard remission induction regimen for treatment of AML can include an anthracycline plus conventional-dose ara-C given by continuous infusion. A complete remission rate of 70% to 80% can be obtained in typical protocol patients. These patients are usually younger than 60 to 65 years of age, with no preceding MDS, no prior malignancy, normal or near-normal hepatic and renal function, and good performance status. Unfortunately, these patients are a minority of patients who present to physicians. Substantially lower response rates are obtained at MDACC in older patients with poor performance status, impaired renal function, MDS, or treatment-associated or secondary AML (Table 54–8 and Fig. 54–2).

The major cause of failure to achieve remission induction is death from infection and hemorrhage (Table 54–9). Ten percent to 20% of patients fail to achieve remission because they are refractory to the chemotherapy administered. Causes of failure to achieve complete remission in patients presenting with de novo acute leukemia, those with secondary AML or a history of MDS, and those with impaired hepatic or renal functional or poor performance status are illustrated in Table 54–9. Nonprotocol patients (groups 2–4) are more likely to fail to achieve remission because of infection (especially fungal), hemorrhage, or organ failure, which occurs during the induction course. Resistance also appears to be more common in these subsets of patients. Questions still remain about the wisdom of treating some nonprotocol-eligible elderly patients with vigorous chemotherapy regimens. There is little evidence

TABLE 54–8. Outcome of Remission Induction Treatment According to Age and Protocol Eligibility Status

Age (y)	*Protocol Eligibility**	*No. of Patients†*	*Complete Response (%)*	*Resistant (%)*	*Death (%)*
<60	Yes	315	81	9	10
<60	No	173	47	19	34
≥60	Yes	101	55	16	29
≥60	Yes	193	36	19	44

* Eligibility criteria: performance status, 0–2 (Zubrod); serum creatinine < 2 mg/dl; bilirubin < 2 mg/dl; no prior myelodysplastic syndrome or secondary acute myelogenous leukemia.
† Patients seen at the M.D. Anderson Cancer Center, 1980–1990.

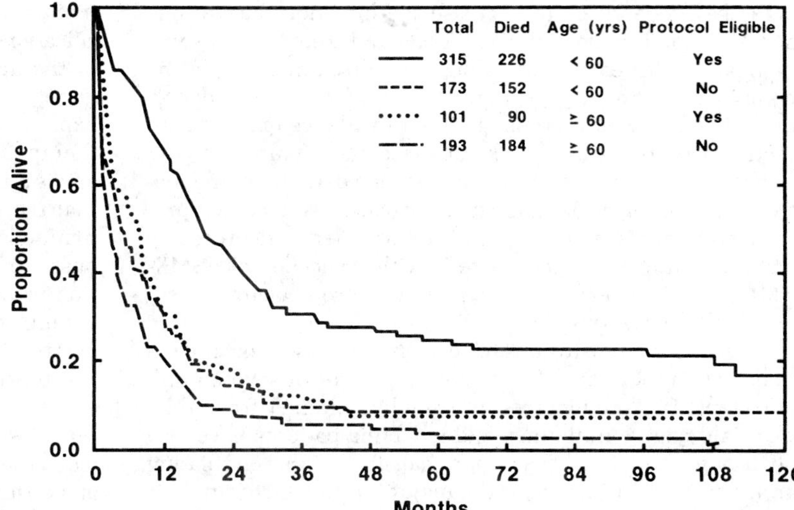

FIGURE 54–2. Survival by age and protocol eligibility groups of patients with acute myelogenous leukemia (AML) patients treated at the M.D. Anderson Cancer Center from 1980 to 1990.

that there is a substantial cure fraction in this group of patients (see Fig. 54–2). However, some patients with advanced age and no prior MDS (group 3) have a smooth remission induction course and a satisfying remission duration. The proportion of patients older than 70 who are cured with chemotherapy is small.[262]

Preisler defined the causes of failure as type 1 or drug resistance with persistence of leukemia after treatment; type 2 or drug resistance with regrowth of leukemia after aplasia; type 3 or regeneration failure with death after prolonged aplasia (>40 days); type 4 or aplastic death with death from hypoplasia (<40 days); and type 5 or early death within 7 days after a course of chemotherapy.[263] Partial remission is defined as type 2 resistance.

The morbidity of induction therapy is predominantly associated with the intensity of the myelosuppression that occurs. Most patients have a period of 3 to 4 weeks of severe neutropenia and thrombocytopenia. Virtually no patient goes through remission induction therapy without having an episode of fever. Organ failure is usually associated with severe infection. Most patients require vigorous support with erythrocyte and platelet transfusions. Hair loss is usually significant because of the doses of anthracyclines that are used.

With the advent of more effective antibacterial agents, the number of patients dying during remission induction from gram-negative bacterial infections is decreasing. However, gram-positive organisms such as methicillin-resistant *Staphylococcus aureus* and *Enterococcus fecalis* are emerging as more frequent contributors to morbidity and mortality.[264–266] The major emerging problem is the development of fungus infections.[267] *Aspergillus* infections are increasing, and many fungal infections that were formerly caused by *Candida albicans* are now associated with a variety of other *Candida* species.[268] The most common site of fatal infections remains the lungs. Most pulmonary infections in which no pathogenic source can be identified are eventually identified at autopsy as fungal infections. Opportunistic infections such as *Pneumocystis carinii*, cytomegalovirus, and herpes simplex are uncommon causes of fatal pneumonias.

Infection Prevention

Early attempts at prevention of death by decreasing infection focused on management in protected environments (PE). Two of three randomized studies demonstrated a higher complete remission rate for patients who were treated in a protected environment.[269–271] The optimal antibiotic regimen to decrease the probability of infection used in conjunction with PEs has not been demonstrated. A variety of regimens incorporating nonabsorbable antibiotics and systemic antibiotics have been used. Oral sulfamethoxazole plus trimethoprim (SMX-TMP) and the quinolones (*e.g.*, ciprofloxacin, norflox-

TABLE 54–9. Factors Contributing to Death During Remission Induction for Acute Myelogenous Leukemia

*No. of Patients**	*Infections (%)*			*Hemorrhage (%)*	*Organ Failure (%)*†
	Bacterial	*Fungal*	*Unknown*		
315	3.2	1.6	1.9	6.0	5.7
173	4.4	14.5	7.5	15.6	25.4
101	6.9	14.9	5.9	14.9	22.8
193	12.4	17.1	12.4	12.4	33.7

* Patients seen at the M.D. Anderson Cancer Center, 1980–1990.

acin) have been used to decrease the infection rate. In one study, a combination of SMX-TMP and ketoconazole was compared with each agent alone or no treatment.[272] In the combination arm, the infection rate was substantially reduced, but in the SMX-TMP group, a higher incidence of fungus infection occurred, and in the ketaconazole-alone arm, a higher incidence of bacterial infection occurred than in the no-treatment group. Quinolones have been studied as prophylactic agents and demonstrated a superior decrease in bacterial infections compared with placebo or SMX-TMP.[273,274] In one randomized study, ciprofloxacin was superior to norfloxacin.[275]

Granulocyte transfusions have been used to support the patients when they are infected during periods of severe granulocytopenia. Granulocytes are usually obtained from relatives, although chronic myeloid leukemia patients have also been used as donors. The short half-life of the circulating granulocytes (<12 hours) is the major limiting factor in their use. It is difficult to harvest enough granulocytes to be useful in sustaining a circulating neutrophil count over a 24-hour period. The prospects of using agents such as G-CSF and GM-CSF to increase the circulating granulocyte count in normal donors is attractive. Randomized trials confirm the beneficial effect of granulocyte transfusions in severe infections in neutropenic patients.[276–278]

The cornerstone of management of infectious complications is to initiate empiric broad-spectrum antibacterial therapy that covers *Pseudomonas* spp., *Klebsiella* spp., and *E. coli.* Although gram-positive infections are becoming more common, they are seldom fatal within the first 48 hours. Fungus infections seldom cause precipitous demise of the patient. Therefore, broad-spectrum gram-negative coverage using a third- or fourth-generation cephalosporin alone or combined with a semisynthetic penicillin or aminoglycoside is satisfactory.[279–282] Regimens incorporating vancomycin to cover gram-positive organisms have been successfully used.[283] If the fever persists for 2 to 4 days and there is evidence of pneumonia, the addition of antifungal therapy with fluconazole, fluorocytosine, or amphotericin-B is recommended.[284] Positive blood cultures for methicillin-resistant *Staphylococcus aureus* or α- or γ-hemolytic streptococci with no response to initial therapy suggests that vancomycin should be added to the regimen.[283]

Fungal infections are more common in older and poor-prognosis patients.[267] *Aspergillus* should be considered in any patient developing a nodular or cavitating pneumonia or a pneumonia associated with a pleural friction rub or sinusitis.[285] Unfortunately, the response to amphotericin-B in fungal infections in the presence of severe neutropenia is poor. Fluconazole has good clinical activity against *Candida* spp. but not against *Aspergillus.*[286]

Postremission Therapy

Many terms have been used to described postremission therapy. These include consolidation, intensification, and maintenance therapy. Consolidation or intensification therapy regimens use doses of chemotherapy that cause severe and often prolonged neutropenia and thrombocytopenia, as occur during remission induction, but maintenance regimens produce low neutrophil counts of the order of 250 to 500/μl and platelet counts of approximately 50,000 to 100,000/μl. Initially, maintenance therapy was continued indefinitely. Late intensification procedures were introduced to decrease the duration of therapy and to eliminate any residual leukemic cells by giving agents to which the patient had not been previously exposed and they demonstrated the ability to discontinue therapy.[287,288] The question of duration of maintenance therapy is still unresolved. Most studies of no maintenance show that the remission duration is usually slightly longer in the maintenance group of patients.[246,289,290] Studies have demonstrated a slight improvement in complete remission duration when maintenance has been given after early consolidation or intensification.[246,291] No significant advantage of postremission therapy for more than 1 year compared with shorter times has been demonstrated.[292,293]

CONSOLIDATION THERAPY. Several studies have evaluated the use of one or two courses of high-dose ara-C, usually at a dose of 3 g/m^2 over 1 to 2 hours every 12 hours for 8 to 12 doses, usually combined with daunorubicin or amsacrine. These are single-arm studies with no comparison with conventional therapy. These strategies have been applied predominantly to patients with AML who were younger than 50 years of age. The probability of being alive and in remission at 3 to 8 years (*i.e.,* potentially cured) varies from 32% to 49%.[294–299] The intensification regimens are associated with considerable morbidity and mortality. One study failed to find an advantage for adding high-dose ara-C to postremission therapy.[295] This was the only comparative study, and there were no differences observed in patients receiving conventional high-dose ara-C regimens. The most popular approach to postremission therapy is to give one or two courses of an intensive postremission regimen incorporating high-dose ara-C. No comparative trials or historically controlled trials have demonstrated convincingly the optimal approach to postremission therapy.

ALLOGENEIC BONE MARROW TRANSPLANTATION AND INTENSIFICATION THERAPY. Several studies of allogeneic transplantation during first remission have been conducted. In one large study from Seattle, the long-term survival rates were 45% to 50%.[300] Similar results were obtained by the International Bone Marrow Transplant Registry (IBMTR).[301] Other studies compared transplantation with intensive chemotherapy. A UCLA study found a significant difference in the probability of remaining in remission at 5 years but no significant difference in survival.[301] A Seattle study compared allogeneic transplant with two consolidation courses of TAD.[302] Some patients in that study elected not to undergo transplantation; 43 patients received chemotherapy because they did not have a donor, and 33 patients received a transplant. There was a higher likelihood of the transplant patients being alive and in remission at 5 years than in the chemotherapy group. There was a slight increase in the 5-year survival rate of 40% in the transplant plus the "assigned to transplant" group compared with 30% in the chemotherapy group, but this was not statistically significant. A subsequent study from UCLA compared 28 adult patients who had a histocompatible transplantation for AML during first remission, with 54 consecutive age-matched adult patients treated with one or more cycles of high-dose ara-C-based consolidation therapy.[297] The relapse rate was significantly lower in the transplant group, but the treatment-related mortality was much higher in the group treated with bone marrow transplantation. There was no significant difference in survival at 5 years for the two groups.

In all reports, it appears that the relapse rate in the transplant population is less, the mortality associated with the transplant is greater, and there is a 5% to 10% higher 5-year survival in the allogeneic transplant group than in the intensive chemotherapy group. The use of partially mismatched related donors and matched unrelated donors is being actively explored.[303]

AUTOLOGOUS BONE MARROW TRANSPLANTATION. Because of the lack of HLA-compatible siblings for allogeneic transplant, there has been considerable interest in the use of autologous bone marrow transplantations in patients during first remission of AML. Several single-arm noncomparative trials show disease-free survival rate of 25% to 60%.[304–308] The largest experience reported suggests that chemopurging is beneficial.[308] The time from complete remission to bone marrow transplantation was usually 3 to 6 months. For this reason, patients at risk of early relapse were excluded from these studies. Not all studies, particularly two from Holland, have demonstrated an improved disease-free survival; in the Holland studies, the proportion of disease-free patients is approximately one in three.[304,307] Comparative trials are underway to document the usefulness of autologous bone marrow transplantation during first remission compared with intensive chemotherapy. The usefulness of bone marrow purging with chemotherapy or monoclonal antibodies and the optimal methodology for purging remain questionable.

MANAGEMENT OF ADULT ALL

As with AML, the phases of treatment of ALL include remission induction and postremission phases. The principles of supportive care apply equally to management of ALL and AML. One difference is that the likelihood of tumor lysis syndrome is higher in patients with ALL, and greater attention should be paid to adequate hydration and monitoring of serum uric acid, phosphate, and potassium levels in the first 3 to 5 days after commencing chemotherapy. Allopurinol should be given prophylactically and the urine alkalinized before chemotherapy. Allopurinol can be given safely except for regimens including 6-mercaptopurine. (Allopurinol markedly increases the serum levels of 6-mercaptopurine.) The tumor lysis syndrome is most frequently observed in patients with B-cell ALL and T-cell ALL and can occasionally occur in non-T, non-B cases with a large tumor burden.

Regimens that incorporate L-asparaginase should have the fibrinogen level monitored, because it can decrease after L-asparaginase therapy. Fibrinogen replacement should be considered if the level falls below 100 mg/dl.

Most regimens are based on the use of vincristine and prednisone or dexamethasone, and most include daunorubicin or doxorubicin (see Table 54–7). Many regimens include L-asparaginase. The usefulness of the addition of L-asparaginase to regimens that use vincristine, prednisone, and an anthracyclines is uncertain. The complete remission rate after chemotherapy is 60% to 85%. The most recent MDACC studies including the VAD regimen report remission rates between 70% and 85% (see Table 54–7).[248–251]

The largest experiences are from the cooperative groups coordinated by Mandelli in Italy and Hoelzer in Germany. In three of these studies, the complete remission rates were 79%, 74%, and 75%. The median remission durations in various studies range from 19 to 27 months, with 22% to 41% of patients predicted to be in complete remission at 5 years. Clarkson and colleagues reported the L10/L10M and L17/L17M protocols in 1985 and obtained complete remission rates of 82% to 85%, with long remission durations and 45% of patients predicted to be in complete remission at 5 years.[309] The remission duration curve and the survival curve of the MDACC VAD regimen patients by age are shown in Figures 54–3 and 54–4.

Of the 20% to 30% of adult ALL patients who do not achieve remission, approximately 10% die during the first 8 weeks of treatment.[250] Most of these patients die of infection, especially fungal infection. The remainder are resistant to chemotherapy, and although some can achieve a remission on salvage therapy, the prospect of cure for this group of patients with chemotherapy is extremely small.

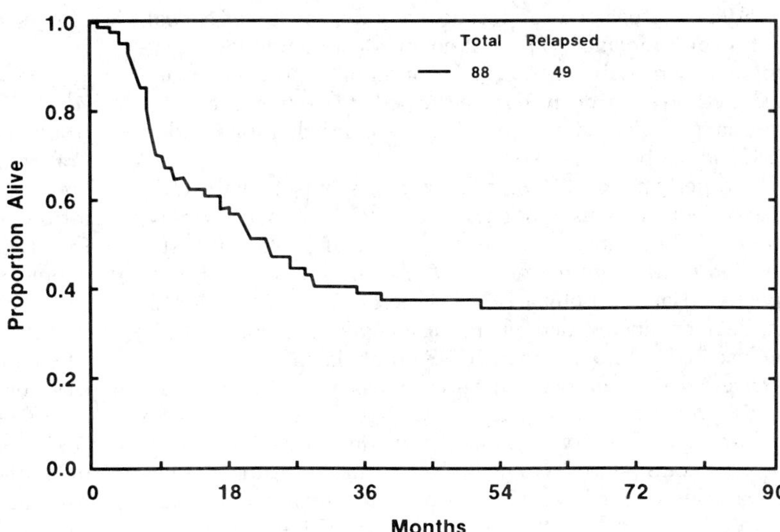

FIGURE 54–3. Remission duration curve for adults with acute lymphocytic leukemia treated with vincristine, doxorubicin, and dexamethasone (VAD) at the M.D. Anderson Cancer Center.

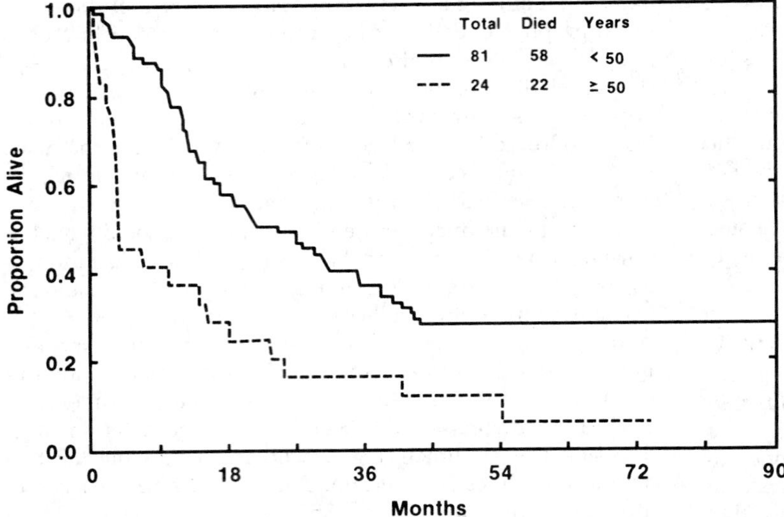

FIGURE 54–4. Survival duration curves for adults with acute lymphocytic leukemia treated with vincristine, doxorubicin, and dexamethasone (VAD) at the M.D. Anderson Cancer Center.

High-dose chemotherapy studies adding methotrexate or rubidazone for treating adult ALL did not improve the complete remission rate in a variety of studies.[310,311] High-dose ara-C has been administered to several patients as the initial therapy.[311–315] The response rate overall is approximately 75%. The median remission duration and proportion of patients in continued complete remissions is not superior to conventional regimens.

Postremission Therapy

Postremission treatment of ALL uses the same terminology as in AML (*i.e.*, intensification, consolidation, maintenance). The regimens are complicated and described in several publications.[248–251,309,312] Intensification strategies using L-asparaginase or ara-C plus cyclophosphamide or ara-C plus daunorubicin have prolonged complete remission durations but have usually not improved overall survival. Two studies of intensification demonstrated prolongation of the median remission duration, and one showed a superior survival for patients receiving consolidation therapy.[311,312] The best combination of drugs and the frequency and intensity of consolidation or intensification is unknown. Most maintenance regimens rely heavily on the combination of 6-mercaptopurine and methotrexate derived from the pediatric experience. The optimal doses and duration of maintenance therapy in adult ALL has not been resolved.

Five percent to 10% of adult patients present with CNS disease, which is usually subclinical.[309,319] Without prophylactic CNS therapy, approximately 40% of adults with ALL develop CNS leukemia.[83,316–318] Only one randomized, prospective trial of prophylactic CNS therapy in adults with ALL has been conducted, demonstrating a higher incidence of CNS relapse in those not receiving CNS prophylaxis, but there was no overall effect on bone marrow remission duration or survival.[318] A variety of approaches to CNS prophylaxis have been undertaken, including cranial irradiation with intrathecal methotrexate (alone by repeated spinal taps or using an Ommaya reservoir) or combinations of methotrexate, ara-C, and hydrocortisone.[309,316–318] The role of cranial irradiation in preventing adult CNS disease has not been prospectively addressed. Different risk features have been identified for the probability of developing CNS disease. A high serum LDH level, high leukocyte count, high percent of cells in S phase in the bone marrow, and B-cell morphology are associated with a high probability of CNS disease.[83,248,250]

If CNS leukemia occurs, treatment is usually undertaken with intrathecal therapy with methotrexate alone or combined with ara-C or hydrocortisone.[249] Many investigators use cranial irradiation, and this is certainly indicated in patients who have cranial nerve or peripheral nerve palsies, because it is likely that there is infiltration of the nerve roots deeper within the nerve than can be reached by topical application of chemotherapeutic agents.[83] CNS therapy is not without side effects.[319,322] Cranial irradiation is associated with somnolence and can aggravate myelosuppression associated with systemic therapy. Repeated spinal taps are associated with the development of arachnoiditis in a small percentage of patients, causing pain in the lumbosacral area, fever, and occasionally meningism. This is less likely if preservative-free saline, Ringers' solution, or Elliot's B solution are used. Demyelinating syndromes have been reported.

Bone Marrow Transplantation

Allogeneic bone marrow transplantation is being used in several patients with ALL.[323] A major Seattle study of allogeneic bone marrow transplantation in ALL found only a 21% long-term disease-free survival.[324] The IBMTR data on 251 patients found a disease-free survival rate of 44%.[325] Comparison of chemotherapy and the IBMTR data suggests that overall disease-free survival was comparable for the two treatments and that the same prognostic factors for failure applied to both. Chao and colleagues reported a disease-free survival rate of 61% for 53 high-risk patients with ALL in first remission, and others reported 40% to 50% disease-free survival rates.[326,327]

Most investigators recommend that bone marrow transplantation be offered during first remission for high-risk adult patients, such as those with high initial leukocyte counts, high serum LDH levels, B-cell ALL, Philadelphia chromosome-positive ALL, and those who take a long time to achieve complete remission.[326,327] The better-risk group of patients have an excellent survival on conventional chemotherapy, and it is recommended that allogeneic transplant be conducted in patients in second remission if necessary.

Autologous bone marrow transplantation is being investigated in adult ALL. Data for second or later remissions have not been promising, with long-term survival rates of less than 20%.[323] There are several difficulties preventing ALL and AML patients from eventually receiving autologous transplants, and these are illustrated by Berman and colleagues.[328]

SALVAGE THERAPY

The prognosis of patients who failed to achieve remissions with their initial therapy (primary refractory) or who relapse after achieving remission (relapsed) remains poor. Overall, only 1 of 3 patients can achieve a second remission, and for most patients, the second remission is shorter than the first. The main prognostic factor associated with the probability of achieving complete remission on the first salvage therapy is response to initial therapy. Patients who have failed initial therapy or relapsed in less than 1 year have a response rate for initial salvage therapy of 25% to 35%.[329,330] Patients whose first complete remission lasted 18 months or longer appear to have a similar prognosis to de novo AML patients. Younger patients with normal organ function, no prior malignancy or MDS, and good performance status have a superior prognosis, as in the initial therapy of AML (Fig. 54–5).[329]

The median survival after initiating salvage therapy is only 14 weeks because of the high mortality during remission induction, and only 15% survived for 1 year. Patients with favorable cytogenetic parameters, such as t(8;21), t(15;17), and inv(16), have the highest probability of obtaining second complete remissions. The second remissions in this subset of patients with long first remissions (particularly >18 months) or favorable karyotypes is associated with a long-term continuous complete remission fraction of 15% to 20%.[330] There is a strong correlation between the duration of first remission and karyotype. Patients with favorable karyotypes of t(8;21), t(15;17), and inv(16) tend to have the longest remissions.

Several regimens have been tried to improve the complete remission rate.[329,330] High-dose cytosine arabinoside, alone or combined with amsacrine or mitoxantrone, has been used.[331–336] New drugs that have activity in AML include idarubicin, mitoxantrone, amsacrine, and diaziquone.[337–341] 5-Azacytidine has modest activity as salvage therapy. Mitoxantrone and VP-16 are commonly used together as a salvage regimen.[343–344] The complete remission rate for amsacrine as a single agent is 20% to 30%. Patients who have Auer rods in their leukemic cells have a markedly high complete remission rate with amsacrine therapy.[345] Mitoxantrone as a single agent has complete remission rates of 10% to 33%.[338–339]

The initial reports on high-dose ara-C (2–3 g/m^2 over 1 to 3 hours for 9 to 12 doses every 12 hours) claimed to have complete remission rates of 50% to 60%.[332–334] More experience with the regimen applied to a nonselected patient population suggests that the first salvage complete remission rate in unselected patients is closer to 33%.[331] Several schedules using lower doses of ara-C with or without asparaginase have produced complete remission rates equivalent to the more toxic high-dose schedules.[333,346] Intermediate doses of ara-C are less toxic and as effective as higher doses when combined with mitoxantrone in relapsed patients with AML.[347] In one of the few randomized studies of salvage therapy for AML, high-dose ara-C and amsacrine were equally disappointing.[348]

Allogeneic transplantation for patients who have disease that is primary refractory or who relapse is an attractive approach, because it is associated with a complete remission rate of approximately 50% to 60% and with 10% to 20% of patients who are long-term survivors.[349] Autologous bone marrow transplantation using bone marrow that has been cryopreserved during first remission has resulted in complete remissions in approximately 50% of patients. Most of these patients relapsed.[350,351] The use of autologous bone marrow transplantation as an intensification strategy for second remissions has been associated with long-term survival for a few patients.[352]

Relatively few salvage regimens have been developed for adult ALL. A variety of programs incorporating high-dose ara-C, alone or with L-asparaginase, amsacrine, mitoxantrone, or idarubicin, have been studied.[353] Great variability in complete

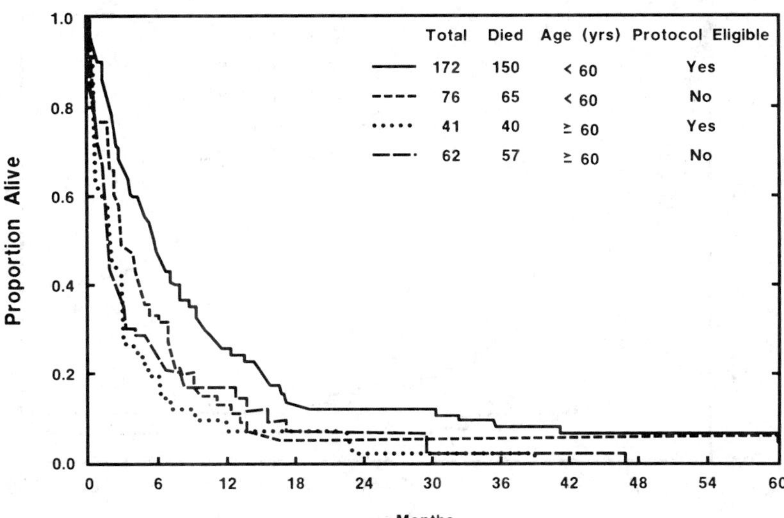

FIGURE 54–5. Survival by age and protocol eligibility status of patients with acute myelogenous leukemia after the first salvage therapy.

remission rates (21–86%) has been reported using these regimens, suggesting a high degree of patient selection. The best results have been reported with a combination of high-dose ara-C with mitoxantrone, idarubicin, or amsacrine.[355–358] Using high-dose ara-C alone, approximately one third of patients achieve remission, but in published series, a combination of high-dose ara-C with mitoxantrone or amsacrine produces a complete remission rate of 50% or greater. The use of GM-CSF after treatment with mitoxantrone and high dose ara-C has decreased the mortality rate but has not increased the complete remission rate.[359]

MANAGEMENT OF ACUTE LEUKEMIA IN THE ELDERLY

Most clinical protocols, particularly those from cooperative groups, address the treatment of AML patients younger than 60. Early trials of chemotherapy failed to achieve remissions in most older patients. The major cause of an adverse outcome was death during remission induction. The complete remission rate with agents such as ara-C and daunorubicin with or without corticosteroids was only 10% to 22%.[360–362] Combinations of ara-C and anthracyclines yielded complete remission rates of approximately 30% in such patients.[363] The 3/7 regimen improved the complete remission rate to 46%, and a combination of rubidizone, ara-C, vincristine, and prednisone achieved a complete remission rate of 48% in patients older than 50 years of age.[241,364,365] The major cause of failure is death during induction due to infection or hemorrhage. Patients older than 60 have a higher likelihood of having a previous MDS, previous malignancy, adverse cytogenetic pattern, reduced performance status, and impaired renal function. All these factors correlate with probability of failure to achieve complete remission in this elderly population.

MANAGEMENT OF MYELODYSPLASTIC SYNDROME

Management of this frustrating group of disorders is limited by the fact that these patients are predominantly elderly and have unfavorable karyotypes (see Table 54–2). Early attempts at chemotherapy resulted in low response rates, primarily because of high mortality during remission induction therapy. This led to attempts at treatment with low-dose cytosine arabinoside, differentiating factors such as *cis*-retinoic acid, and therapeutic strategies using growth factors such as G-CSF, GM-CSF, and erythropoietin.[366–368] The response rate from ara-C has been reported between 20% to 60% but is generally considered to be 20%.[366] The degree of patient selection in these clinical trials presumably explains the variability in complete remission rates.

Although ara-C was thought to function in low doses as a differentiating agent, most of the patients who achieved complete remission developed hypoplastic bone marrows before obtaining complete remissions. None of the differentiation strategies has proven effective in achieving complete remissions in clinical trials with substantial numbers of patients.[368]

G-CSF and GM-CSF can reproducibly improve the neutrophil count in 80% to 90% of patients.[369–372] However, trilineage response involving improvement in hemoglobulin and platelet count are uncommon (<20%). Approximately 20% of patients, usually those with RAEB and RAEBT, have documented leukemia progression when receiving GM-CSF. This has not been observed in patients to whom G-CSF have been administered. G-CSF is usually better tolerated than GM-CSF, which can be associated with fever, lethargy, bone pain, and fluid retention. Trials of IL-3 in MDS results in increase of bone marrow cellularity and increases in neutrophil, eosinophil, basophil, lymphocyte, and monocyte counts. Leukemia progression was not observed. Platelet counts improved in several patients, but erythrocyte production was not increased.[373,374] There is no clinical trial demonstrating a survival advantage for patients treated with growth factors.

One study demonstrated that the survival of patients with MDS when stratified according to karyotype is similar to that of AML.[375] The overall survival of MDS patients at the MDACC according to FAB group is shown in Figure 54–6. Studies were initiated to treat patients with MDS with chemotherapy. Patients with favorable karyotypes have been treated with anthracycline and ara-C combinations.[376–378] More than half of the patients treated on these regimens achieved complete re-

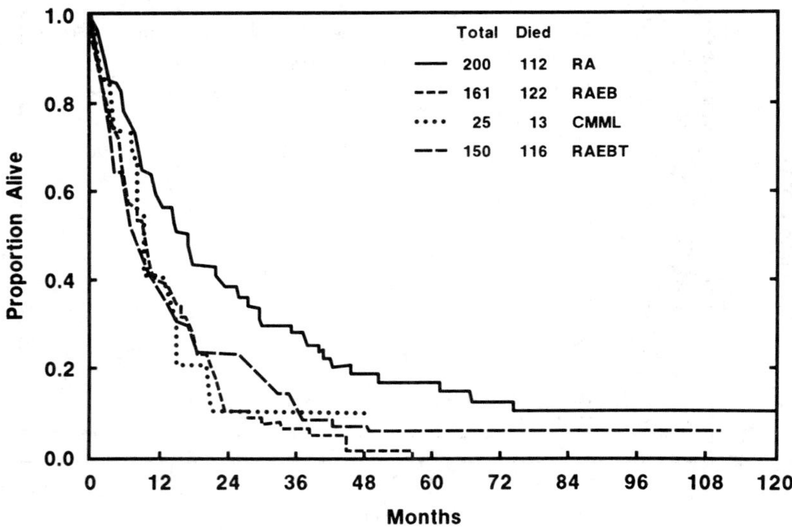

FIGURE 54–6. Survival by FAB group of patients with myelodysplastic syndrome treated at the M.D. Anderson Cancer Center between 1980 and 1990.

missions, suggesting that chemotherapy is an effective strategy in some patients with improved supportive care. Responses after chemotherapy are typical trilineage improvements, with normalization of hemoglobin and of the neutrophil, platelet, and bone marrow differential counts.

USE OF GROWTH FACTORS AS SUPPORTIVE THERAPY

Because of the severe myelosuppression that occurs after intensive chemotherapy in acute leukemia, efforts have been undertaken to increase the speed of recovery of the neutrophil count. High-risk patients have received GM-CSF to enhance recovery of neutrophils.[379] No differences in response rate, duration of neutropenia, or complications were found compared with historic controls. One study administered GM-CSF to poor-prognosis or relapsed AML patients who had hypoplasia after intensive chemotherapy.[380] The 50% complete remission rate compared favorably with a 32% remission rate in historic controls. Two patients had evidence of leukemia regrowth that appeared related to the GM-CSF. A randomized study of G-CSF was conducted by Ohno and colleagues.[381] Patients with refractory or relapsed acute leukemia received chemotherapy and were randomly assigned to receive G-CSF or placebo. The G-CSF-treated group had fewer infectious complications and tolerated higher dose of antileukemic therapy. Recovery of granulocytes was more rapid in the G-CSF group. The complete remission rate was somewhat higher in the G-CSF group (50% versus 36%). No influence on leukemia cell growth was observed.

PROGNOSTIC FACTORS

A variety of prognostic factor analyses have been undertaken for AML and ALL. The patterns have some similarities in the two diseases and distinct differences. Advancing age is an adverse prognostic factor, with patients older than 50 years with either disease faring worse than younger patients.[249,250,382–384]

For each disease, the importance of genetic determination is illustrated by the powerful impact of the cytogenetic profile on probability of outcome.[385] In AML, patients with t(8;21) or inv(16) have an excellent response to therapy (>90% complete remission rate) and a probability of long-term survival of 30% to 40%. Patients with t(15;17) have a complete remission rate of approximately 75%, and if they achieve complete remission have a 30% to 40% probability of long-term survival. Patients who are diploid (*i.e.*, no abnormality detected on cytogenetic analysis) or whose only abnormality is the loss of the Y chromosome have a complete remission rate of 65% to 70%, and approximately 20% of patients remain in complete remission. Patients who have lost part or all of chromosome 5 or 7 or have an additional chromosome 8 as a single chromosome abnormality or combined with other features have response rates of less than 50%, and few of these patients (<5%) remain in complete remission for 3 to 5 years.

A history of MDS is an adverse prognostic factor, as are features of poor performance status or impaired organ function. A low serum albumin level appears to be an adverse prognostic factor in all leukemias.[384,385] Several predictive models have been developed to determine the probability of response based on these variables.

In adult ALL, the major factors predicting response are age, with younger patients having a superior probability of responding, and cytogenetic pattern.[249–251,386] Patients who have the Philadelphia chromosome or have B-cell ALL have a lower complete remission rate. Diploid patients with ALL and those with insufficient metaphases have superior outcomes to those with other abnormalities. There has been no favorable karyotype identified in patients with adult ALL. The favorable karyotype of hyperdiploidy (>50 chromosomes) determined in children is uncommon in adults (<5%). A low serum albumin level and myeloid markers on the blast cells are unfavorable factors for complete remission. L3 morphology (B-cell ALL) is a known adverse factor. Patients with L1 morphology have a higher complete remission rate than patients with L2 morphology. It appears that patients with T-cell ALL may have the best prognosis, with patients with B-cell having the worst prognosis for survival. Prognostic factors for probability of relapse in ALL are dominated by the leukocyte count, serum LDH level, and time to achieving complete remission. All patients with the Philadelphia chromosome eventually relapse.[381,383]

DIFFERENTIATION THERAPY FOR ACUTE PROMYELOCYTIC LEUKEMIA

The use of all-*trans*-retinoic acid in treating promyelocytic leukemia provides a paradigm of differentiation therapy. APL occurs in 5% to 10% of newly diagnosed patients with AML. Huang and colleagues documented the ability to achieve complete remissions in patients with APL, a finding that was subsequently confirmed.[387–389]

Administration of all-*trans*-retinoic acid (ATRA) rapidly corrects coagulation disorders in APL. The leukocyte count increases for the first 3 weeks, and over a period of 2 to 3 months, the bone marrow and blood shows evidence of progressive differentiation into complete remission. No episode of marrow hypoplasia occurs. The response appears to be optimal in previously treated patients with APL.[389] Nineteen of 20 complete remissions were reported in one study.

Use of ATRA as second or third salvage is not as beneficial as for initial salvage therapy. The major complication occurring with this agent is an increase in the circulating leukocyte count, which is more common in patients who commence with elevated leukocyte counts.[390] Some patients develop complications of pulmonary insufficiency, and if the leukocyte count rises above 20,000/μl, treatment with chemotherapy or leukapheresis is recommended. Patients who achieve a complete remission on ATRA relapse if the drug is used alone as maintenance. It is thought that this is, in part, a result of a lowering of plasma ATRA levels with continued therapy. Eventually, the ATRA level becomes too low to have an effect on differentiation.[391]

It is now known that on chromosome 15 is a breakpoint in the *PML* gene (formerly called *MYL*), and the breakpoint on chromosome 17 involves the *RARA* gene, causing a chimeric gene product of PML-RARA.[127–130] The interaction of TRA with the the α, β, and γ receptors for retinoic acid and nuclear retinol binding factors are areas of intense research.

Approximately 75% of patients with newly diagnosed APL

achieve complete remission. Because some patients have been dying of complications of the leukostasis syndrome, combination chemotherapy approaches should be explored. This sequence of investigations demonstrates the need to coordinate clinical observations based on differentiation of cell lines in the laboratory with the molecular genetic findings of specific receptor disturbance. It is hoped that similar observations can be made for other translocations, such as t(8;21), inv(16), t(1;19), and t(9;22).

TRENDS IN THE MANAGEMENT OF LEUKEMIA

The predominant treatments for acute leukemia have been in place for 5 to 15 years. No major new class of drugs for the management of acute leukemia has been discovered. The allogeneic and autologous marrow transplant programs with monoclonal purging and chemotherapy purging have been applied with no major difference in response or survival rates. Development of new drugs that are selected for particular subsets of leukemia patients is of the highest priority.

The availability of hemopoietic tissue growth factors, such as G-CSF, GM-CSF, IL-3, IL-4, IL-6, and stem cell factor, suggests that leukemia cells may be able to be induced into proliferation or differentiation. Explorations of these combinations may lead to new conceptual and therapeutic advances. The ability of the investigators to deliver chemotherapy at maximal doses is enhanced by the availability of the growth factors to accelerate recovery of normal elements. This should enable peripheral blood cells to be collected before intensive chemotherapy for autologous peripheral blood support for chemotherapy.

The discovery that all-*trans*-retinoic acid can achieve complete remissions in APL and the discovery that the *RARA* gene is involved in the specific translocation associated with APL suggests that increased knowledge of the genetic abnormalities observed in leukemia should enhance our ability to delivery specific therapies tailored to the genetic derangement. Further conceptual advances require the dissection of the dysregulation of growth involving growth stimulatory and inhibitory factors. Delineation of risk groups would enable those who are already being cured with conventional treatment to be identified, so that they could be spared aggressive high-dose therapies.

Applications of techniques such as polymerase chain reaction to identify genetic abnormalities should enable selection of patients with minimal residual disease. If subclinical leukemia cell burden under the influence of treatment can be detected before relapse occurs, new treatments can be initiated before the patient has evidence of clinical relapse. Gene therapy or introduction of specific antisense nucleotides into leukemic cells require more refined analysis of the genetic aberrations involved in leukemogenesis.

REFERENCES

1. National Cancer Institute. 1987 Annual cancer statistics review. NIH publication no. 88-2789. Washington, DC: U.S. Department of Health and Human Services, 1988.
2. Tivey H. The natural history of untreated acute leukemia. Ann NY Acad Sci 1954;60:322.
3. Alderson M. The epidemiology of leukemia. Adv Cancer Res 1980;31:1.
4. Heath CW Jr. The leukemias. In: Schottenfeld D, Fraumeni JF Jr, eds. Cancer epidemiology and prevention.
5. Lund E, Lie SO. Incidence of acute leukemia in Norway 1957–1981. Report from the Norwegian Cancer Registry and Pediatric Research Institute, National Hospital of Norway, Oslo, Norway. Scand J Haematol 1983;31:488.
6. McPhedran P, Heath CW Jr, Garcia JS. Racial variations in leukemia incidence among the elderly. JNCI 1970;45:25.
7. Graham S, Gibson R, Lilienfeld A, et al. Religion and ethnicity in leukemia. Am J Public Health 1970;60:266.
8. Gunz FW, Gunz JP, Veale AMO, et al. Familial leukemia: A study of 909 families. Scand J Hematol 1975;15:117.
9. Gunz FW, Gunz JP, Vincent PC, et al. Thirteen cases of leukemia in a family. JNCI 1978;60:1243.
10. Jackson EW, Norris FD, Klauber MR. Childhood leukemia in California-born twins. Cancer 1969;23:913.
11. MacMahon B, Levy MA. Prenatal origin of childhood leukemia. Evidence from twins. N Engl J Med 1964;270:1082.
12. Steinberg A. The genetics of acute leukemia in children. Cancer 1960;13:985.
13. Fraumeni JF Jr, Miller RW. Epidemiology of human leukemia: Recent observations. JNCI 1967;38:593.
14. Miller RW. Radiation, chromosomes and viruses in the etiology of leukemia. N Engl J Med 1964;271:30.
15. Kirkpatrick CH. Cancer in immunodeficiency disease. Birth Defects 1976;12:61.
16. Spector BD, Perry GS, III, Kersey JH. Genetically determined immunodeficiency disease and malignancy. Report from the Immunodeficiency Cancer Registry. Clin Immunol Immunopathol 1978;11:12.
17. Beebe GW, Kato H, Land CE. Studies of the mortality of A-bomb survivors. 6. Mortality and radiation dose, 1950–1974. Radiat Res 1978;75:138.
18. Stewart AM. Delayed effects of A-bomb radiation: A review of recent mortality rates and risk estimates for five-year survivors. J Epidemiol Community Health 1982;36:80.
19. Land CE. Estimating cancer risks from low doses of ionizing radiation. Science 1980;209:1197.
20. Caldwell GG, Kelley D, Zack M, et al. Mortality and cancer frequency among military nuclear test (Smoky) participants, 1957 through 1979. JAMA 1983;250:620.
21. Smith PG, Doll R. Mortality among patients with ankylosing spondylitis after a single treatment course with x-rays. Br Med J 1982;284:449.
22. Smith PG. Leukemia and other cancers following radiation treatment of pelvic disease. Cancer 1977;39:1901.
23. Murray R, Heckel P, Hempelmann LH. Leukemia in children exposed to ionizing radiation. N Engl J Med 1959;261:585.
24. Da Silva Horta J, da Motta LC, Tavares MH. Thorium dioxide effects in man. Environ Res 1974;8:131.
25. Modan B, Lilienfeld AM. Polycythemia vera and leukemia—the role of radiation treatment. Medicine (Baltimore) 1965;44:305.
26. Polednak AP, Stehney AF, Rowland RE. Mortality among women first employed before 1930 in the U.S. radium dialpainting industry. Am J Epidemiol 1978;107:179.
27. March HC. Leukemia in radiologists. Radiology 1944;43:275.
28. Fulton JP, Cobb S, Preble L, et al. Electrical wiring configurations and childhood leukemia in Rhode Island. Am J Epidemiol 1980;111:292.
29. Savitz DA, Wachtel H, Barnes FA, et al. Case-control study of childhood cancer and exposure to 60-Hz magnetic fields. Am J Epidemiol 1988;128:21.
30. Pochin EE. Leukemia following radioiodine treatment of thyrotoxicosis. Br Med J 1960;2:1545.
31. Boice JD, Hutchison GB. Leukemia in women following radiotherapy for cervical cancer: Ten-year follow-up of an international study. JNCI 1980;65:115.
32. Austin H, Delzell E, Cole P. Benzene and leukemia. Am J Epidemiol 1988;127:419.
33. Aksoy M, Dincol K, Erdem S, Dincol G. Acute leukemia due to chronic exposure to benzene. Am J Med 1972;52:160.
34. Vigliani EC, Forni A. Benzene and leukemia. Environ Res 1976;11:122.
35. Rinsky RA, Smith AB, Hornung R, et al. Benzene and leukemia. N Engl J Med 1987;316:1044.
36. Shu XO, Gao YT, Linet MS, et al. Chloramphenicol use and childhood leukemia in Shanghai. Lancet 1987;2:934.
37. Crane MM, Keating MJ, Trujillo JM, et al. Environmental exposures in cytogenetically defined subsets of acute nonlymphocytic leukemia. JAMA 1989;262:634.
38. Severson RK. Cigarette smoking and leukemia. Cancer 1987;60:141.
39. Yoshida M, Seiki M, Hattori S, et al. Monoclonal integration of human T-cell leukemia provirus in all primary tumors of adult T-cell leukemia suggests causative role of HTLV in disease. Proc Natl Acad Sci USA 1984;81:2534.
40. Robert-Guroff M, Nakao Y, Notake K, et al. Natural antibodies to human retrovirus HTLV in a cluster of Japanese patients with adult T-cell leukemia. Science 1982;215:975.
41. Hinuma H, Komoda H, Chosa T, et al. Antibodies to adult T-cell leukemia virus-associated antigen in sera from patients with ATL and controls in Japan: A nationwide seroepidemiologic study. Int J Cancer 1982;29:631.
42. Blattner WA, Blayney DW, Robert-Guroff M, et al. Epidemiology of human T-cell leukemia/lymphoma virus. J Infect Dis 1983;147:406.
43. Sakashita A, Hattori T, Miller CW, et al. Mutations of the p53 gene in adult T-cell leukemia. Blood 1992;79:477.
44. Yamada Y. Phenotypic and functional analysis of leukemic cells from 16 patients with adult T-cell leukemia/lymphoma. Blood 1983;61:192.
45. Essex M. Feline leukemia and sarcoma viruses. In: Klein G, ed. Viral oncology. 1980:205.
46. Blair A, Hayes HM, JR. Cancer and other causes of death among U.S. veterinarians, 1966–1977. Int J Cancer 1980;25:181.

47. Heath CW Jr. The epidemiology of leukemia. In: Schottenfeld D, ed. Cancer and epidemiology and prevention. 1975:316.
48. Fraumeni JF, Ederer F, Miller RW. An elevation of the carcinogenicity of simian virus 40 in man. JAMA 1963;185:713.
49. Waters TD, Anderson PS Jr, Beebe GW, et al. Yellow fever vaccination, avian leukosis virus, and cancer risk in man. Science 1972;177:76.
50. Miller G, Shope T, Heston L, et al. Prospective study of Epstein-Barr virus infections in acute lymphoblastic leukemia of children. J Pediatr 1972;80:932.
51. Blair A, Thomas TL. Leukemia among Nebraska farmers: A death certificate study. Am J Epidemiol 1979;110:264.
52. Blair A, White DW. Death certificate study of leukemia among farmers from Wisconsin. JNCI 1981;66:1027.
53. Henshaw DL, Eatough JP, Richardson RB. Radon as a causative factor in induction of myeloid leukaemia and other cancers. Lancet 1990:1008.
54. Gardner MJ, Snee MP, Hall AJ, et al. Results of case-control study of leukaemia and lymphoma among young people near Sellafield nuclear plant in West Cumbria. Br Med J 1990;300:423.
55. Neel JV. Update on the genetic effects of ionizing radiation. JAMA 1991;266:698.
56. Albain K, LeBeau M, Rowley J, et al. Secondary acute nonlymphocytic leukemia (ANNL) and dysmyelopoietic syndrome (DMPS) in 46 patients: Clinical and cytogenetic correlations. Cancer Genet Cytogenet 1983;8:107.
57. Coltman C Jr. Treatment related leukemias. In: Bloomfield CD, ed. Adult leukemias, vol. 1. 1982:62.
58. Ross HJ, Rowley JD, Koeffler HP. Therapy-related acute nonlymphocytic leukemia. In: Wiernik PH, Canellos GP, Kyle RA, Schiffer CA, eds. Neoplastic diseases of the blood. 1991:303.
59. Kantarjian HM, Estey EH, Keating MJ. Treatment of therapy-related leukemia and myelodysplastic syndrome. Hematol Oncol Clin North Am (in press).
60. Sieber SM, Adamson RH. Toxicity of antineoplastic agents in man: Chromosomal aberrations, antifertility effects, congenital malformations and carcinogenic potential. Adv Cancer Res 1975;22:57.
61. Wantzin GL, Jensen MK. The induction of chromosome abnormalities by melphalan in rat bone marrow cells. Scand J Haematol 1973;11:135.
62. Cadman EC, Capizzi RL, Bertino JR. Acute non-lymphocytic leukemia—a delayed complication of Hodgkin's disease therapy: Analysis of 109 cases. Cancer 1977;40:1280.
63. Valagussa P, Santoro A, Kenda RE, et al. Second malignancies in Hodgkin's disease: A complication of certain forms of treatment. Br Med J 1980;1:216.
64. Kaldor JM, Day NE, Clarke A, et al. Leukemia following Hodgkin's disease. N Engl J Med 1990;322:7.
65. Toland DM, Coltman CA Jr, Moon TE. Second malignancies complicating Hodgkin's disease: The Southwest Oncology Group experience. Cancer Clin Trials 1978;1:21.
66. Coleman CN, Williams CJ, Flint A, et al. Hematologic neoplasia in patients treated for Hodgkin's disease. N Engl J Med 1977;297:1249.
67. Valagussa P, Santoro A, Bellani F, et al. Absence of treatment-induced second neoplasms after ABVD in Hodgkin's disease. Blood 1982;59:488.
68. Pedersen-Bjergaard J, Philip P, Mortensen B, et al. Acute nonlymphocytic leukemia, preleukemia and acute myeloproliferative syndrome secondary to treatment of other malignant disease. Clinical and cytogenetic characteristics and results of in vitro culture of bone marrow and HLA typing. Blood 1981;57:712.
69. Travis LB, Curtis RE, Boice JD Jr, et al. Second cancers following non-Hodgkin's lymphoma. Cancer 1991;67:2002.
70. Bergsagel D, Bailey A, Langley G. The chemotherapy of plasma-cell myeloma and the incidence of acute leukemia. N Engl J Med 1979;300:743.
71. Berk P, Goldberg J, Silverstein M. Increased incidence of acute leukemia in polycythemia vera associated with chlorambucil therapy. N Engl J Med 1981;304:441.
72. McPhedran P, Heath CW. Acute leukemia occurring during chronic lymphocytic leukemia. Blood 1970;35:7.
73. Reimer RR, Hoover R, Fraumeni JF Jr, et al. Secondary primary neoplasms following ovarian cancer. JNCI 1978;61:1195.
74. Rosner F, Carey RW, Zarrabi NH. Breast cancer and acute leukemia: Report of 24 cases and review of the literature. Am J Hematol 1978;4:151.
75. Curtis RE, Boice JD, Moloney WC, et al. Leukemia following chemotherapy for breast cancer. Cancer Res 1990;50:2741.
76. Kantarjian HM, Keating MJ, Walters RS, et al. Therapy-related leukemia and myelodysplastic syndrome: Clinical, cytogenetic, and prognostic features. J Clin Oncol 1986;4:1748.
77. Whitlock JA, Greer JP, Lukens JN. Epipodophyllotoxin-related leukemia. Cancer 1991;68:600.
78. Pin C, Behn F, Raimondi S, et al. Secondary acute myeloid leukemia in children treated for acute lymphoid leukemia. N Engl J Med 1989;321:136.
79. Boggs DR, Sofferman SA, Wintrobe MM, et al. The acute leukemias. Medicine (Baltimore) 1962;41:163.
80. Roath S, Israels MCG, Wilkinson JF. The acute leukemias: A study of 580 patients. Q J Med 1964;33:257.
81. Bodey GP, Buckley M, Sathe YS, et al. Quantitative relationships between circulating leukocytes and infection in patients with acute leukemia. Ann Intern Med 1966;64:328.
82. Suda T, Onai T, Mekawa T. Studies on abnormal polymorphonuclear neutrophils in acute myelogenous leukemia: Clinical significance and changes after chemotherapy. Am J Hematol 1983;15:45.
83. Stewart DJ, Keating MJ, McCredie KB, et al. Natural history of central nervous system acute leukemia in adults. Cancer 1981;47:184.
84. Manoharan A, Horsley R, Ptiney WR. The reticulin content of bone marrow in acute leukaemia in adults. Br J Haematol 1979;43:185.
85. Bennett JM, Catovsky D, Daniel MT, et al. Proposed revised criteria for the classification of acute myeloid leukemia. Ann Intern Med 1985;103:626.
86. Bennett JM, Reed CE. Acute leukemia cytochemical profile: Diagnosis and clinical implications. Blood Cells 1975;1:101.
87. El-Mohandes E, Hayhoe FGJ. 5'-nucleotidase activity of megakaryoblasts in a case of acute megakaryoblastic leukemia. Br J Haematol 1983;53:523.
88. Daniel MT, Flandrin G, Le Jeune F, et al. Les esterases, specifiques moncytaire. Utilization des leucemies, aigues. Nouv Rev Fr Hematol 1971;11:233.
89. Bennett JM. Classification of the acute leukemias: Cytochemical and morphologic considerations. In: Wiernik PH, ed. Neoplastic diseases of the blood. 1991:172.
90. Knapp W, Rieber P, Dorken B, et al. Towards a better definition of human leukocyte surface molecules. Immunol Today 1989;10:253.
91. Rovigatti U, Mirro J, Kitchingman G, et al. Heavy chain immunoglobulin gene rearrangement in acute nonlymphocytic leukemia. Blood 1984;63:1023.
92. Fontenay M, Flandrin G, Baurman H, et al. T cell receptor delta gene rearrangement occurs predominantly in immature myeloid leukemia exhibiting lineage promiscuity. Leukemia 1990;4:100.
93. Sobol RE, Mick R, Royston I, et al. Clinical importance of myeloid antigen expression in adult acute lymphoblastic leukemia. N Engl J Med 1987;316:1111.
94. Mirro J, Zipf TF, Pui C-H, et al. Acute mixed lineage leukemia: Clinicopathologic correlations and prognostic significance. Blood 1985;66:1115.
95. Cuneo A, Michaux J-L, Ferrant A, et al. Correlation of cytogenetic patterns and clinicobiological features in adult acute myeloid leukemia expressing lymphoid markers. Blood 1992;79:720.
96. Lee EJ, Pollak A, Leavitt RD, et al. Minimally differentiated acute nonlymphocytic leukemia: A distinct entity. Blood 1987;70:1400.
97. Griffin JD, Davis R, Nelson DA, et al. Use of surface marker analysis to predict outcome of acute myelogenous leukemia. Blood 1986;68:1232.
98. Adriaansen HJ, Soeting PWC, Wolvers-Tettero ILM, et al. Immunoglobulin and T-cell receptor gene rearrangements in acute non-lymphocytic leukemias. Analysis of 54 cases and a review of the literature. Leukemia 1991;5:744.
99. Kitchingman GR, Rovigatti U, Mauer AM, et al. Rearrangement of immunoglobulin heavy chain genes in T cell acute lymphoblastic leukemia. Blood 1985;65:725.
100. Felix CA, Wright JJ, Poplack DG, et al. T cell receptor α-, β-, and γ-genes in T cell and pre-B cell acute lymphoblastic leukemia. J Clin Invest 1987;80:545.
101. Hara J, Benedict SH, Champagne E, et al. Relationship between rearrangement and transcription of the T-cell receptor α, β, and γ genes in B-precursor acute lymphoblastic leukemia. Blood 1989;73:500.
102. Bennett JM, Catovsky D, Daniel MT, et al. Proposals for the classification of the acute leukaemias. Br J Haematol 1976;33:451.
103. Bennett JM, Catovsky D, Daniel M-T, et al. Criteria for the diagnosis of acute leukemia of megakaryocytic lineage (M7). A report of the French-American-British Cooperative Group. Ann Intern Med 1985;103:460.
104. Bennett JM, Catovsky D, Daniel MT, et al. The morphologic classification of acute lymphoblastic leukaemia: Concordance among observers and clinical correlations. Br J Haematol 1981;47:553.
105. Bennett JM, Begg CB. ECOG study of cytochemistry of acute myeloid leukemia by correlation or subtypes with response and survival. Cancer Res 1981;41:4833.
106. Head DR, Savage RA, Cerezo L, et al. Reproducibility of the French-American-British classification of acute leukemia: The Southwest Oncology Group experience. Am J Hematol 1985;18:47.
107. Cross AH, Goorha RM, Nuss R, et al. Acute myeloid leukemia with T-lymphoid features: A distinct biologic and clinical entity. Blood 1988;72:579.
108. Smith LJ, Curtis JE, Messner HA, et al. Lineage infidelity in acute leukemia. Blood 1983;61:1138.
109. Pui C-H, Dahl GV, Melvin S, et al. Acute leukaemia with mixed lymphoid and myeloid phenotype. Br J Haematol 1984;56:121.
110. Cuneo A, Mecucci C, Kerim S, et al. Multipotent stem cell involvement in megakaryoblastic leukemia: Cytologic and cytogenetic evidence in 15 patients. Blood 1989;74:1781.
111. Van Slyck EJ, Weiss L, Dully M. Chromosomal evidence for the secondary role of fibroblastic proliferation in acute myelofibrosis. Blood 1970;36:729.
112. Benvenisti DS, Ultmann JE. Eosinophilic leukemia. Ann Intern Med 1969;71:731.
113. Holmes R, Keating MJ, Cork A, et al. A unique pattern of central nervous system in acute myelomonocytic leukemia associated with inv(16)(p13a22). Blood 1985;65:1017.
114. Wimmer RS, Raney RB Jr, Naiman JL. Hypereosinophilia with acute lymphocytic and acute myelocytic leukemia in childhood. J Pediatr 1978;92:244.
115. Bennett JM, Catovsky D, Daniel MT, et al. Proposals for the classification of the myelodysplastic syndromes. Br J Haematol 1982;51:189.
116. Hickling RA. Leukaemia and related conditions and the blood-uric-acid. Lancet 1958;1:175.
117. Krakoff IH. Use of allopurinol in preventing hyperuricemia in leukemia and lymphoma. Cancer 1966;19:1489.
118. Levi JA, Speden JB, Vincent PC, et al. Studies on muramidase in hematologic disorders. I. Serum muramidase and serum lactic dehydrogenase in leukemia. Cancer 1973;31:939.
119. Kantarjian HM, Walters RS, Keating MJ, et al. Results of the vincristine, doxorubicin and dexamethasone regimen in adults with standard- and high-risk acute lymphocytic leukemia. J Clin Oncol 1990;8:994.
120. Keating MJ, Smith TL, Gehan EA, et al. A prognostic factor analysis for use in development of predictive models for response in adult acute leukemia. Cancer 1982;50:457.

121. Rachmilewitz D, Rachmilewitz EA, Polliack A, et al. Acute promyelocytic leukemia: A report of five cases on the diagnostic significance of serum vitamin B_{12} determination. Br J Haematol 1972;22:87.
122. Gorst DW, Courtis M, Delamore IW. Folic acid binding protein in acute myeloid leukemia. J Clin Pathol 1976;29:60.
123. Mir MA, Brabin B, Tang OT, et al. Hypokalaemia in acute myeloid leukaemia. Ann Intern Med 1975;82:54.
124. The Fourth International Workshop on Chromosomes in Leukemia, Chicago, IL, September 2–7, 1982. A prospective study of acute nonlymphocytic leukemia. Cancer Genet Cytogenet 1984;11:251.
125. Yunis JJ, Brunning RD, Howe RB, et al. High-resolution chromosome as an independent prognostic indicator in adult acute nonlymphocytic leukemia. N Engl J Med 1984;311: 812.
126. Keating MJ, Cork A, Broach Y, et al. Toward a clinically relevant cytogenetic classification of acute myelogenous leukemia. Leuk Res 1987;11:119.
127. Borrow J, Goddard AD, Sheer D, et al. Molecular analysis of acute promyelocytic leukemia breakpoint cluster region on chromosome 17. Science 1990;249:1577.
128. de The H, Chomienne C, Lanotte M, et al. The t(15;17) translocation of acute promyelocytic leukemia fuses the retinoic acid receptor a gene to a novel transcribed locus. Nature 1990;347:558.
129. Alcalay M, Zangrilli D, Paolo P, et al. Translocation breakpoint of acute promyelocytic leukemia lies within the retinoic acid receptor α locus. Proc Natl Acad Sci USA 1991;88: 1977.
130. Chang K-S, Trjillo JM, Ogura T, et al. Rearrangement of the retinoic acid receptor gene in acute promyelocytic leukemia. Leukemia 1991;5:200.
131. Holmes RI, Keating MJ, Cork A, et al. Loss of the Y chromosome in acute myelogenous leukemia: A report of 13 patients. Cancer Genet Cytogenet 1985;694:10.
132. Vermaelen K, Michaux JL, Louwagie A, et al. Reciprocal translocation t(6;9)(p21;q3): A new characteristic chromosome anomaly in myeloid leukemias. Cancer Genet Cytogenet 1983;10:125.
133. Davis MP, Dewald GW, Pierre RV, et al. Hematologic manifestations associated with deletions of the long arm of chromosome 20. Cancer Genet Cytogenet 1984;12:63.
134. Maddox A-M, Keating MJ, Trujillo J, et al. Philadelphia chromosome-positive adult acute leukemia with monosomy of chromosome number seven: A subgroup with poor response to therapy. Leuk Res 1983;7:509.
135. Bloomfield CD, Secker-Walker LM, Goldman AI, et al. Six-year follow-up of the clinical significance of karyotype in acute lymphoblastic leukemia. Cancer Genet Cytogenet 1989;40:171.
136. Machnicki JL, Bloomfield CD. Clinical significance of the cytogenetics of acute leukemias. Oncology 1990;4:23.
137. Arthur DC, Berger R, Golomb HM, et al. The clinical significance of karyotype in acute myelogenous leukemia. Cancer Genet Cytogenet 1989;40:203.
138. Schiffer CA, Lee EJ, Tomiyasu T, et al. Prognostic impact of cytogenetic abnormalities in patients with de novo acute nonlymphocytic leukemia. Blood 1989;73:263.
139. Williams DL, Raimondi SC, Rivera G, et al. Presence of clonal chromosome abnormalities in virtually all cases of acute lymphoblastic leukemia. N Engl J Med 1985;313: 640.
140. Machnicki JL, Bloomfield CD. Clinical significance of the cytogenetics of acute leukemias. Oncology 1990;4:23.
141. Third International Workshop on Chromosomes in Leukemia. Chromosomal abnormalities and their clinical significance in acute lymphoblastic leukemia. Cancer Res 1983;43:868.
142. Kantarjian HM, Talpaz M, Dhingra K, et al. Significance of the p210 versus p190 molecular abnormalities in adults with Philadelphia chromosome-positive acute leukemia. Blood 1991;78:2411.
143. Kaiser-McCaw B, Epstein AL, Kaplan HS, et al. Chromosome 14 translocation in African and North American Burkitt's lymphoma. Int J Cancer 1977;19:482.
144. Miyoshi I, Hiraki S, Kimura I, et al. 2/8 Translocation in a Japanese Burkitt's lymphoma. Experientia 1979;35:742.
145. Berger R, Bernheim A, Weh HJ, et al. A new translocation in Burkitt's tumor cells. Hum Genet 1979;53:111.
146. Mirro J, Kitchingman G, Williams D, et al. Clinical and laboratory characteristics of acute leukemia with the 4;11 translocation. Blood 1986;67:689.
147. Michael PM, Levin MD, Garson OM. Translocation 1;19—a new cytogenetic abnormality in acute lymphocytic leukemia. Cancer Genet Cytogenet 1984;12:133.
148. Cline MJ, Ahuja H. Oncogenes and anti-oncogenes in the evolution of human leukemia/ lymphoma. Leukemia Lymphoma 1991;4:153.
149. Clarkson B. New pharmacologic approaches to treatment of leukemia. Semin Hematol 1991;28:99.
150. Radich JP, Kopecky KY, William CL, et al. N-ras mutations in adult de novo acute myelogenous leukemia: Prevalence and clinical significance. Blood 1990;76:801.
151. Needleman SW. Ras protooncogene activation in acute myeloid leukemia and related disorders. Leukemia Lymphoma 1991;5:85.
152. Hirsch-Ginsberg C, Le Maistre AC, Kantarjian H, et al. RAS mutations are rare even in Philadelphia chromosome-negative/bcr gene rearrangement-negative chronic myelogenous leukemia, but are prevalent in chronic myelomonocytic leukemia. Blood 1990;76:1214.
153. Ridge SA, Worwood M, Oscier D, et al. FMS mutations in myelodysplastic, leukemic, and normal subjects. Proc Natl Acad Sci USA 1990;87:1377.
154. Tobal K, Pagliuca A, Bhatt B, et al. Mutation of the human FMS gene (M-CSF receptor) in myelodysplastic syndromes and acute myeloid leukemia. Leukemia 1990;4:486.
155. Slingerland JM, Minden MD, Benchimol S. Mutation of the p53 gene in human acute myelogenous leukemia. Blood 1991;77:1500.
156. Fenaux P, Jonveaux P, Quiquandon I, et al. P53 gene mutations in acute myeloid leukemia with 17p monosomy. Blood 1991;78:1652.
157. Gaidano G, Ballerini P, Gong JZ, et al. P53 mutations in human lymphoid malignancies: Association with Burkitt lymphoma and chronic lymphocytic leukemia. Proc Natl Acad Sci USA 1991;88:5413.
158. Ahuja HG, Jat PS, Foti A, et al. Abnormalities of the retinoblastoma gene in the pathogenesis of acute leukemia. Blood 1991;78:3259.
159. Clarkson BD. Review of recent studies of cellular proliferation in acute leukemia. NCI Monogr 1969;30:81.
160. Cronkite EP. Kinetics of leukemic cell proliferation. In: Dameshek W, Dutcher RM, eds. Perspectives in leukemia. New York: Grune & Stratton, 1968.
161. Greenberg ML, Chanana AD, Cronkite EP, et al. The generation time of human leukemic myeloblasts. Lab Invest 1972;26:245.
162. Sjogren U. Mitotic activity in myeloid leukaemias. A study of 277 cases. Scand J Haematol 1977;19:309.
163. Killmann S-A. Acute leukemia: Development, remission/relapse pattern, relationship between normal and leukemic hemopoiesis, and the "sleeper-to-feeder" stem cell hypothesis. Semin Hematol 1968;1:103.
164. Killmann S-A, Karle H, Ernst P, et al. Return of human leukemic myeloblasts from blood to bone marrow. Acta Med Scand 1971;189:137.
165. Dosik G, Barlogie B, Smith TL, et al. Pretreatment flow cytometry of DNA content in adult acute leukemia. Blood 1980;55:474.
166. Hill BT, Baserga R. The cell cycle and its significance for cancer treatment. Cancer Treat Rev 1975;2:159.
167. Stryckmans PA, Lurie PM, Manaster J, et al. Mode of action of chemotherapy in vivo on human acute leukemia. II. Vincristine. Eur J Cancer 1973;9:613.
168. Ernst P, Killman S-A. Perturbation of generation cycle of human leukemic blast cells by cytostatic therapy in vivo: Effect of corticosteroids. Blood 1970;36:689.
169. Ernst P. Perturbation of generation cycle of human leukaemic lymphoblasts in vivo by L-asparaginase. Br J Haematol 1973;25:33.
170. Ernst P, Faille A, Killman S-A. Perturbation of cell cycle of human leukaemic myeloblasts in vivo by cytosine arabinoside. Scand J Haematol 1973;10:209.
171. Furlong NB, Sato J, Brown T, et al. Induction of limited DNA damage by the antitumor agent Cain's acridine. Cancer Res 1978;38:1329.
172. Stryckmans PA, Manaster J, Lachapelle F, et al. Mode of action of chemotherapy in vivo on human acute leukemia. I. Daunomycin, J Clin Invest 1973;52:126.
173. Li LH, Olin EJ, Fraser TJ, et al. Phase specificity of 5-azacytidine against mammalian cells in tissue culture. Cancer Res 1970;30:2770.
174. Le Page GA. Basic biochemical effects and mechanism of action of 6-thioguanine. Cancer Res 1963;23:1202.
175. Ernst P. Perturbation of generation cycle of human leukaemic blast cells in vivo by daunomycin. Scand J Haematol 1973;11:13.
176. Krishan A, Paika K, Frei E. Cytofluorometric studies on the action of podophyllotoxin and epipodophyllotoxins (VM-26, VP-16-213) on the cell cycle traverse of human lymphoblasts. J Cell Biol 1975;66:521.
177. Buchanan JG, Matthews JRD, Postlewaight BF, et al. The proliferative activity of leukaemic myeloblasts following the intravenous infusion of cytarabine. Pathology 1979;11: 349.
178. Vogler WR, Kremer WB, Knospe WH, et al. Synchronization with phase-specific agents in leukemia and correlation with clinical response to chemotherapy. Cancer Treat Rep 1976;60:1845.
179. Vincent PC, Gunz FW, Levi JA, et al. Prognostic value of cytokinetic studies in adult acute leukemia. In: Fliedner TM, Perry S, eds. Workshops in prognostic factors in human acute leukemia. Advances in the Biosciences, vol 14. 1975:345.
180. Smets LA, Taminiau J, Hahlen K, et al. Cell kinetic responses in childhood acute nonlymphocytic leukemia during high-dose therapy with cytosine arabinoside. Blood 1983;61:79.
181. Cannistra SA, Groshek P, Griffin JD. Granulocyte-macrophage colony-stimulating factor enhances the cytotoxic effects of cytosine arabinoside in acute myeloblastic leukemia and in the myeloid blast crisis of chronic myeloid leukemia. Leukemia 1989;3:328.
182. Tafuri A, Andreeff M. Kinetic rationale for cytokine-induced recruitment of myeloblastic leukemia followed by cycle-specific chemotherapy in vitro. Leukemia 1990;4:826.
183. Brach MA, Henschler R, Mertelsmann R, et al. To overcome pharmacologic and cytokinetic resistance to cytarabine in the treatment of acute myelogenous leukemia by using recombinant interleukin-3? Semin Hematol 1991;28:39.
184. Lista P, Brizzi MF, Rossi M, et al. Different sensitivity of normal and leukaemic progenitor cells to ara-C and IL-3 combined treatment. Br J Haematol 1990;76:21.
185. Hoang T, Nara N, Wong G, et al. Effects of recombinant GM-CSF on the blast cells of acute myeloblastic leukemia. Blood 1986;68:313.
186. Cannistra SA, DiCarlo J, Groshek P, et al. Simultaneous administration of granulocyte-macrophage colony-stimulating factor and cytosine arabinoside for the treatment of relapsed acute myeloid leukemia. Leukemia 1991;5:230.
187. Bettelheim P, Valent P, Andreeff M, et al. Recombinant human granulocyte-macrophage colony-stimulating factor in combination with standard induction chemotherapy in de novo acute myeloid leukemia. Blood 1991;77:700.
188. Estey EH, Dixon D, Kantarjian HM, et al. Treatment of poor-prognosis, newly diagnosed acute myeloid leukemia with ara-C and recombinant human granulocyte-macrophage colony-stimulating factor. Blood 1990;75:1766.
189. Maschmeyer G, Ludwig W-D, Sauerland M-C, et al. Recombinant human granulocyte-macrophage colony-stimulating factor after chemotherapy in patients with acute myeloid leukemia at higher age or after relapse. Blood 1991;78:1190.
190. Estey E, Thal PF, Kantarjian H, et al. Treatment of newly diagnosed acute myelogenous leukemia with GM-CSF prior to and during continuous-infusion high-dose ara-C

(CHDAC) + daunorubicin: Comparison to patients treated without GM-CSF. Blood (in press).

191. Hart JS, George SL, Frei E III, et al. Prognostic significance of pretreatment proliferative activity in adult acute leukemia. Cancer 1977;39:1603.
192. Crowther D, Beard MEJ, Bateman CJT, et al. Factors influencing prognosis in adults with acute myelogenous leukaemia. Br J Cancer 1975;32:456.
193. Kantarjian HM, Barlogie B, Keating MJ, et al. Pretreatment cytokinetics in acute myelogenous leukemia: Age-related prognostic implications. J Clin Invest 1985;76:319.
194. Dosik G, Barlogie B, Gohde W, et al. Flow cytometry of DNA content in human bone marrow—a critical reappraisal. Blood 1980;55:734.
195. Hiddemann W, Buchner T, Andreeff M, et al. Cell kinetics in acute leukemia—a critical reevaluation based on new data. Cancer 1982;50:250.
196. Walters RS, Johnston DA, Dixon DO, et al. Nucleic acid flow cytometry—an aid to diagnosis and prognosis in acute leukemia in adults. In: Stass, ed. The acute leukemias—Biologic, diagnostic, and therapeutic determinants. , 1987:203.
197. Moore MAS, Spitzer G, William N, et al. Agar culture studies in 127 cases of untreated acute leukemia: The prognostic value of reclassification of leukemia according to in vitro growth characteristics. Blood 1974;44:1.
198. Estrov Z, Freedman MH. Growth requirements for human acute lymphoblastic leukemia cells: Refinement of a clonogenic assay. Cancer Res 1988;48:5901.
199. Griffin JD, Young D, Herrmann F, et al. Effects of recombinant human GM-CSF on proliferation of clonogenic cells in acute myeloblastic leukemia. Blood 1986;67:1448.
200. Herrmann F, Vellenga E. The role of colony stimulating factors in acute leukemia. J Cancer Clin Oncol 1990;116:275.
201. McCulloch EA, Curtis JE, Messner HA, et al. The contribution of blast cell properties to outcome variation in acute myeloblastic leukemia (AML). Blood 1982;59:601.
202. Sachs L. The differentiation of myeloid leukemia cells: New possibility for therapy. Br J Haematol 1978;40:509.
203. Pegoraro L. Abraham J, Cooper RA, et al. Differentiation of human leukemias in response to 12-O-tetradecanoyl-phorbol-13-acetate in vitro. Blood 1980;55:859.
204. Moore MAS, Gabrilove J, Sheridan AP. Myeloid leukemic cell differentiation induced by human postendotoxin serum and vitamin analogues. In: Neth R, Gallo RC, Greaves MF, Moore MAS, Winkler K, eds. Modern trends in human leukemia. 1983:327.
205. Tomonaga M, Golde DW, Gasson JC. Biosynthetic (recombinant) human granulocyte-macrophage colony-stimulating factor: Effects on normal bone marrow and leukemia cell lines. Blood 1986;67:31.
206. Kelleher C, Miyauchi J, Wong G, et al. Synergism between recombinant growth factors, GM-CSF and G-CSF, acting on the blast cells of acute myeloblastic leukemia. Blood 1987;69:1498.
207. Pinto A, Attadia V, Fusco A, et al. 5-aza-2′-deoxycytidine induces terminal differentiation of leukemic blasts from patients with acute myeloid leukemias. Blood 1984;64:922.
208. Castaigne S, Daniel MT, Tilly H, et al. Does treatment with ara-C in low dosage cause differentiation of leukemic cells? Blood 1983;62:85.
209. Sakurai M, Sampi K, Hozumi M. Possible differentiation of human acute myeloblastic leukemia cells by daily intermittent administration of aclacinomycin A. Leuk Res 1983;7:139.
210. Koeffler HP. Induction of differentiation of human acute myelogenous leukemia cells: Therapeutic implications. Blood 1983;62:709.
211. Breitman TR, Collins SJ, Keen BR. Terminal differentiation of human promyelocytic leukemia cells in primary culture in response to retinoic acid. Blood 1981;57:1000.
212. Chen ZX, Wang W, Wu WL. Heterogenous response of primarily cultured bone marrow cells of patients with variety of leukemias to differentiation inducers. Clin Med J 1989;102:174.
213. Chen ZX, Xue YQ, Zhang R, et al. A clinical and experimental study on all-*trans* retinoic acid-treated acute promyelocytic leukemia patients. Blood 1991;78:1413.
214. Bodey GP, Bolivar R, Fainstein V. Infectious complications in leukemia patients. Semin Hematol 1982;19:193.
215. Gaydos LA, Freireich EJ, Mantel N. The quantitative relation between platelet count and hemorrhage in patients with acute leukemia. N Engl J Med 1962;266:905.
216. Hester JP, Ventura GJ. Characteristics of refractoriness (R) to platelet concentrate transfusions (PC-TX) in newly diagnosed acute myeloid leukemia patients (AML) (PT). Blood 1988;72:278.
217. Tallman MS, Kwaan HC. Reassessing the hemostatic disorder associated with acute promyelocytic leukemia. Blood 1992;79:543.
218. McKee Jr LC, Collins RD. Intravascular leukocyte thrombi and aggregates as a cause of morbidity and mortality in leukemia. Medicine (Baltimore) 1974;53:463.
219. Freireich EJ, Thomas LB, Frei E III, et al. A distinctive type of intracerebral hemorrhage associated with "blastic crisis" in patients with leukemia. Cancer 1960;13:146.
220. Hug V, Keating MJ, McCredie KB, et al. Clinical course and response to treatment of patients with acute myelogenous leukemia presenting with a high white cell count. Cancer 1983;52:773.
221. Legha SS, Latreille J, McCredie KB, et al. Neurologic and cardiac rhythm abnormalities associated with 4′-(9-acridinylamino) methanesulfon-*m*-anisidide (AMSA) therapy. Cancer Treat Rep 1979;63:11.
222. Freireich EJ, Gehan EA, Sulman D, et al. The effect of chemotherapy on acute leukemia in the human. J Chron Dis 1961;14:593.
223. Freireich EJ, Karon M, Frei E III. Quadruple combination therapy (VAMP) for acute lymphocytic leukemia in childhood. Proc Am Assoc Clin Res [Abstract] 1964;5:20.
224. Freireich EJ, Henderson ES, Karon MR, et al. The treatment of acute leukemia considered with respect to cell population kinetics. 21st Annual Symposium on Fundamental Cancer Research: The proliferation and spread of neoplastic cells. 1967:441.
225. Ellison RR, Holland JF, Weil M, et al. Arabinosyl cytosine: A useful agent in the treatment of acute leukemia in adults. Blood 1968;32:507.
226. Bodey GP, Freireich EJ, Monto RW, et al. Cytosine arabinoside (NSC 63878) therapy for acute leukemia in adults. Cancer Chemother Rep 1969;53:59.
227. Bodey GP, Coltman CA, Hewlett JS, et al. Progress in the treatment of adults with acute leukemia: Review of regimens containing cytarabine studied by the Southwest Oncology Group. Arch Intern Med 1976;136:1383.
228. Jacquillat CL, Boiron M, Weil M, et al. Rubidomycin, a new agent active in the treatment of acute leukemia. Lancet 1966;2:27.
229. Weil M, Glidewell OJ, Jacquillat C, et al. Daunorubicin in the therapy of acute granulocytic leukemia. Cancer Res 1973;33:921.
230. Wilson HE, Bodey GP, Moon TE. Adriamycin therapy in previously treated adult acute leukemia. Cancer Treat Rep 1977;61:905.
231. Jacquillat CL, Weil M, Gemon-Auclerc MF, et al. Clinical study of rubidazone (22 040 R.P.), a new daunorubicin-derived compound, in 170 patients with acute leukemias and other malignancies. Cancer 1976;37:653.
232. Daghestani A, Arlin ZA, Leyland-Jones, et al. Phase I and II clinical and pharmaceutical study of 4-demethoxydaunorubicin (idarubicin) in adult patients with acute leukemia. Cancer Res 1985;45:1408.
233. Yates JW, Wallace HJ Jr, Ellison RR, et al. Cytosine arabinoside and daunorubicin therapy in acute nonlymphocytic leukemia. Cancer Chemother Rep 1983;57:485.
234. Clarkson BD, Dowling MD, Gee TS, et al. Treatment of acute leukemia in adults. Cancer 1975;36:775.
235. Rees JKH, Sandler RM, Challener J, et al. Treatment of acute myeloid leukemia with a triple cytotoxic regimen: DAT. Br J Cancer 1977;36:770.
236. Wiernik PH, Glidewell OJ, Hoagland HC, et al. A comparative trial of daunorubicin, cytosine arabinoside, and thioguanine and a combination of the three agents for the treatment of acute myelocytic leukemia. Med Pediatr Oncol 1979;6:261.
237. Finnish Leukemia Group. The effect of thioguanine in a combination of daunorubicine (sic), cytarabine and prednisone in the treatment of acute leukemia in adults. Scand J Haematol 1979;23:124.
238. Berman E, Heller G, Santorsa J, et al. Results of randomized trial comparing idarubicin and cytosine arabinoside with daunorubicin and cytosine arabinoside in adult patients with newly diagnosed acute myelogenous leukemia. Blood 1991;77:1666.
239. Wiernik PH, Banks PLC, Case DC Jr, et al. Cytarabine plus idarubicin or daunorubicin as induction and consolidation therapy for previously untreated adult patients with acute myeloid leukemia. Blood 1992;79:313.
240. Vogler WR, Velez-Garcia E, Omura G, et al. A phase III tiral comparing daunorubicin or idarubicin combined with cytosine arabinoside in acute myelogenous leukemia. Semin Oncol 1989;16:21.
241. Yates J, Glidewell OJ, Wiernik PH, et al. Cytosine arabinoside with daunorubicin or Adriamycin for therapy of acute myelocytic leukemia: A CALGB study. Blood 1982;60:454.
242. Arlin Z, Case DC Jr, Moore J, et al. Randomized multicenter trial of cytosine arabinoside with mitoxantrone or daunorubicin in previously untreated adult patients with acute nonlymphocytic leukemia (ANLL). Leukemia 1990;4:177.
243. Keating M, Gehan E, Smith T, et al. A strategy for evaluation of new treatments in untreated patients: Application to a clinical trial of AMSA for acute leukemia. J Clin Oncol 1987;5:710.
244. Preisler H, Davis RB, Kirshner J, et al. Comparison of three remission induction regimens and two postinduction strategies for the treatment of acute nonlymphocytic leukemia: A cancer and leukemia group B study. Blood 1987;69:1441.
245. Dillman RO, Davis RB, Green MR, et al. A comparative study of two different doses of cytarabine for acute myeloid leukemia: A phase II trial of cancer and leukemia group B. Blood 1991;78:2520.
246. Buchner T, Urbanitz D, Hiddemann W, et al. Intensified induction and consolidation with or without maintenance chemotherapy for acute myeloid leukemia (AML): Two multicenter studies of the German AML Cooperative Group. J Clin Oncol 1985;3:1583.
247. Rees JKH, Swirsky D, Gray RG, et al. Principal results of the Medical Research Council's 8th acute myeloid leukaemia trial. Lancet 1986;2:1236.
248. Kantarjian HM, Walters RS, Keating MJ, et al. Results of the vincristine, doxorubicin, and dexamethasone regimen in adults with standard- and high-risk acute lymphocytic leukemia. J Clin Oncol 1990;8:994.
249. GIMENA Cooperative Group. GIMENA ALL 0183: A multicentric study on adult acute lymphoblastic leukaemia in Italy. Br J Haematol 1989;71:377.
250. Hoelzer D, Thiel E, Loffler H, et al. Prognostic factors in a multicenter study for treatment of acute lymphoblastic leukemia in adults. Blood 1988;71:123.
251. Linker CA, Levitt LJ, O'Donnell M, et al. Treatment of adult acute lymphoblastic leukemia with intensive cyclical chemotherapy: A follow-up report. Blood 1991;78:2814.
252. Schauer P, Arlin ZA, Mertelsmann R, et al. Treatment of acute lymphoblastic leukemia in adults—Results of the L-10 and L-10M protocols. J Clin Oncol 1983;1:462.
253. Rivera GK, Dahl GV, Bowman WP, et al. VM-26 and cytosine arabinoside combination chemotherapy for the initial induction failures in childhood lymphocytic leukemia. Cancer 1980;46:1727.
254. Bishop JF, Lowenthal RM, Joshua D, et al. Etoposide in acute nonlymphocytic leukemia. Blood 1990;75:27.
255. Monparler RL. A model for the chemotherapy of acute leukemia with 1-β-D-arabinofuranosylcytosine. Cancer Res 1974;34:1775.
256. Iwagaki A, Nakamura T, Wakisaka G. Studies on the mechanism of action of 1-β-D-arabinofuranosylcytosine as an inhibitor of DNA synthesis in human leukemic leukocytes. Cancer Res 1969;29:2169.
257. Chu MY, Fisher GA. A proposed mechanism of action of 1-β-D-arabinofuranosylcytosine as an inhibitor of the growth of leukemic cells. Biochem Pharmacol 1962;11:423.

258. Major PP, Egan EW, Beardsley GP, et al. Lethality of human myeloblasts correlated with the incorporation of arabinosylcytosine into DNA. Proc Natl Acad Sci USA 1981;78: 3235.
259. Chu MY, Fisher GA. Comparative studies of leukemic cells sensitive and resistant to cytosine arabinoside. Biochem Pharmacol 1965;14:333.
260. Harris AW, Reynolds EC, Finch LR. Effect of thymidine on the sensitivity of cultured mouse tumor cells to 1-β-D-arabinofuranosylcytosine. Cancer Res 1979;39:538.
261. Rustum YM, Preisler H. Metabolism and intracellular retention of ^{3}H-arabinosylcytosine as predictors of response of animal tumors. Cancer Res 1978;38:543.
262. Walters RS, Kantarjian HM, Keating MJ, et al. Intensive treatment of acute leukemia in adults 70 years of age and older. Cancer 1987;60:149.
263. Preisler HD. Failure of remission induction in acute myelocytic leukemia. Med Pediatr Oncol 1978;4:275.
264. Pizzo PA, Ladisch S, Simon RM, et al. Increasing incidence of gram-positive sepsis in cancer patients. Med Pediatr Oncol 1978;5:241.
265. Wade JC, Schimpff SC, Newman KA, et al. *Staphylococcus epidermidis:* An increasing cause of infection in patients with granulocytopenia. Ann Intern Med 1982;97:503.
266. Pizzo PA, Ladisch S, Witebsky FG. Alpha-hemolytic streptococci: Clinical significance in the cancer patient. Med Pediatr Oncol 1978;4:367.
267. Estey EH, Keating MJ, McCredie KB, et al. Causes of initial remission induction failure in acute myelogenous leukemia. Blood 1982;60:309.
268. Gerson SL, Talbot GH, Hurwitz S, et al. Prolonged granulocytopenia: The major risk factor for invasive pulmonary aspergillosis in patients with acute leukemia. Ann Intern Med 1984;100:345.
269. Schimpff SC, Green WH, Young VM, et al. Infection prevention in acute nonlymphocytic leukemia. Laminar air flow room reverse isolation with oral, nonabsorbable antibiotic prophylaxis. Ann Intern Med 1975;82:351.
270. Bodey GP, Keating MJ, McCredie KB, et al. Prospective randomized trial of antibiotic prophylaxis in acute leukemia. Am J Med 1985;78:407.
271. Rodriguez V, Bodey GP, Freireich EJ, et al. Randomized trial of protected environment-prophylactic antibiotics in 145 adults with acute leukemia. Medicine (Baltimore) 1978;57:253.
272. Estey EH, Maksymiuk A, Smith TL, et al. Infection prophylaxis in acute leukemia: Comparative effectiveness of sulfamethoxazole and trimethoprim, ketoconazole, and a combination of the two. Arch Intern Med 1984;144:1562.
273. Karp JE, Merz WG, Hendricksen C, et al. Oral norfloxacin for prevention of gram-negative bacterial infections in patients with acute leukemia and granulocytopenia. A randomized, double-blind, placebo-controlled trial. Ann Intern Med 1987;106:1.
274. Bow EJ, Rayner E, Louie TJ. Comparison of norfloxacin with cotrimoxazole for infection prophylaxis in acute leukemia. The tradeoff for reduced gram-negative sepsis. Am J Med 1988;84:847.
275. The GIMEMA Infection Program. Prevention of bacterial infection in neutropenic patients with hematologic malignancies—A randomized, multicenter trial comparing norfloxacin with ciprofloxacin. Ann Intern Med 1991;115:7.
276. Vallejos C, McCredie KB, Bodey GP, et al. White blood cell transfusions for control of infections in neutropenic patients. Transfusion 1975;15:28.
277. Vogler WR, Winton EF. A controlled study of the efficacy of granulocyte transfusions in patients with neutropenia. Am J Med 1977;63:548.
278. Alavi JB, Root RK, Djerassi I, et al. A randomized clinical trial of granulocyte transfusions for infection in acute leukemia. N Engl J Med 1977;296:706.
279. Winston DJ, Ho WG, Bruckner DA, et al. Beta-lactam antibiotic therapy in febrile granulocytopenic patients—A randomized trial comparing cefoperazone plus piperacillin, ceftazidime plus piperacillin, and imipenem alone. Ann Intern Med 1991;115: 849.
280. Bodey GP, Elting L, Jones P, et al. Imipenem/cilastatin therapy of infections in cancer patients. Cancer 1987;60:255.
281. Love LJ, Schimpff SC, Hahn DM, et al. Randomized trial of empiric antibiotic therapy with ticarcillin in combination with gentamicin, amikacin or netilmicin in febrile patients with granulocytopenia and cancer. Am J Med 1979;66:603.
282. Bodey GP, Ketchel SJ, Rodriquez V. A randomized study of carbenicillin plus cefamandole or tobramycin in the treatment of febrile episodes in cancer patients. Am J Med 1979;67: 608.
283. Karp JE, Dick JD, Angelopulos C, et al. Empiric use of vancomycin during prolonged treatment-induced granulocytopenia. Am J Med 1986;81:237.
284. Hiddemann W, Essink ME, Fegeler W, et al. Antifungal treatment by amphotericin B and 5-fluorocytosine delays the recovery of normal hematopoietic cells after intensive cytostatic therapy for acute myeloid leukemia. Cancer 1991;68:9.
285. Fisher BD, Armstrong D, Yu B, et al. Invasive asperigillosis: Progress in early diagnosis and treatment. Am J Med 1981;71:571.
286. Grant SM, Clissold SP. Fluconazole—A review of its pharmacodynamic and pharmacokinetic properties, and therapeutic potential in superficial and system mycoses. Drugs 1990;39:877.
287. Bodey GP, Freireich EJ, Gehan EA, et al. Late intensification therapy for acute leukemia in remission. JAMA 1976;235:1021.
288. Bodey GP, Freireich EJ, McCredie KB, et al. Prolonged remissions in adults with acute leukemia following late intensification chemotherapy and immunotherapy. Cancer 1981;47:1937.
289. Embury SH, Elias L, Heller PH, et al. Remission maintenance therapy in acute myelogenous leukemia. West J Med 1977;126:267.
290. Vogler WR, Winton EF, Gordon DS, et al. A randomized comparison of postremission therapy in acute myelogenous leukemia: A southeastern cancer study group trial. Blood 1984;63:1039.
291. Cassileth PA, Begg CB, Bennett JM, et al. A randomized study of the efficacy of consolidation therapy in adult acute nonlymphocytic leukemia. Blood 1984;63:843.
292. Preisler H, Davis R, Kirshner J, et al. Comparison of three remission induction regimens and two postinduction strategies for the treatment of acute nonlymphocytic leukemia: A Cancer and Leukemia Group B study. Blood 1987;69:1441.
293. Kantarjian HM, Keating MJ, Walters RS, et al. Early intensification and short-term maintenance chemotherapy does not prolong survival in acute myelogenous leukemia. Cancer 1986;58:1603.
294. Wolff SN, Herzig RH, Fay JW, et al. High-dose cytarabine and daunorubicin as consolidation therapy for acute myeloid leukemia in first remission: Long-term follow-up and results. J Clin Oncol 1989;7:1260.
295. Preisler HD, Raza A, Early A, et al. Intensive remission consolidation therapy in the treatment of acute nonlymphocytic leukemia. J Clin Oncol 1987;5:722.
296. Phillips GL, Reece DE, Shepherd JD, et al. High-dose cytarabine and daunorubicin induction and postremission chemotherapy for the treatment of acute myelogenous leukemia in adults. Blood 1991;77:1429.
297. Schiller GJ, Nimer SD, Territo MC, et al. Bone marrow transplantation versus high-dose cytarabine-based consolidation chemotherapy for acute myelogenous leukemia in first remission. J Clin Oncol 1992;10:41.
298. Buchner T, Hiddemann W, Loffler G, et al. Improved cure rate by very early intensification combined with prolonged maintenance chemotherapy in patients with acute myeloid leukemia: Data from the AML cooperative group. Semin Hematol 1991;28: 76.
299. Harousseau JL, Milpied N, Briere J, et al. Double intensive consolidation chemotherapy in adult acute myeloid leukemia. J Clin Oncol 1991;9:1432.
300. Clift R, Buckner C, Thomas E, et al. The treatment of acute non-lymphoblastic leukemia by allogeneic marrow transplantation. Bone Marrow Transplant 1987;2:243.
301. Champlin R, Advisory Committee of the International Bone Marrow Transplant Registry. Bone marrow transplantation for acute leukemia: A preliminary report from the International Bone Marrow Transplant Registry. Transplant Proc 1987;19:2626.
302. Champlin R, Ho W, Gale R, et al. Treatment of acute myelogenous leukemia: A prospective controlled trial of bone marrow transplantation versus consolidation chemotherapy. Ann Intern Med 1985;102:285.
303. Beatty PG, Hansen JA, Longton GM, et al. Marrow transplantation from HLA-matched unrelated donors for treatment of hematologic malignancies. Transplantation 1991;51: 443.
304. Lowenberg B, Verdonck LJ, Dekker AW, et al. Autologous bone marrow transplantation and acute myeloid leukemia in first remission: Results of a Dutch prospective study. J Clin Oncol 1990;8:287.
305. Korbling M, Hunstein W, Fliedner TM, et al. Disease-free survival after autologous transplantation in patients with acute myelogenous leukemia. Blood 1989;74:1898.
306. McMillan AK, Goldstone AH, Linch DC, et al. High dose chemotherapy and autologous bone marrow transplantation in acute myeloid leukemia. Blood 1990;76:480.
307. Ferrant A, Doyen C, Delannoy A, et al. Allogeneic or autologous bone marrow transplantation for acute nonlymphocytic leukemia in first remission. Bone Marrow Transplant 1991;7:303.
308. Gorin NC, Labopin M, Meloni G, et al. Autologous bone marrow transplantation for acute myeloblastic leukemia in Europe: Further evidence of the role of marrow purging by mafosfamide. Leukemia 1991;5:896.
309. Clarkson B, Ellis S, Little C, et al. Acute lymphoblastic leukemia in adults. Semin Oncol 1985;12:160.
310. Esterhay RJ, Wiernik PH, Grove WR, et al. Moderate dose methotrexate, vincristine, asparaginase, and dexamethasone for treatment of adult acute lymphocytic leukemia. Blood 1982;59:334.
311. Fiere D, Extra JM, David B, et al. Treatment of 218 adult acute lymphoblastic leukemias. Semin Oncol 1987;14(suppl 1):64.
312. Stryckmans P, de Witte T, Bitar N, et al. Cytosine arabinoside for induction, salvage, and consolidation therapy of adult acute lymphoblastic leukemia. Semin Oncol 1987;14(suppl 1):67.
313. Lister TA, Barnett MJ, Rohatiner AZS, et al. Intensive chemotherapy including high dose cytosine arabinoside for acute lymphoblastic leukemia (ALL). [Abstract] Presented at the 4th International Symposium on Therapy of Acute Leukemias, Rome, 1987: 150.
314. Cassileth P, Anderson J, Hoagland H, et al. Efficacy of high-dose cytarabine in initial therapy of adult acute lymphocytic leukemia (ALL). Proc Am Soc Clin Oncol 1987;6: 158.
315. Boogaerts MA, Emonds MP, Kennes C, et al. Intensive consolidation and maintenance therapy for acute lymphoblastic leukemia in adults. [Abstract] Presented at the 4th International Symposium on Therapy of Acute Leukemias, Rome, 1987:442.
316. Woodruff RK. The management of adult acute lymphoblastic leukemia. Cancer Treat Rev 1978;5:95.
317. Willemze R, Drenthe-Schonk AM, van Rossum J, et al. Treatment of acute lymphoblastic leukaemia in adolescents and adults. Comparison of two schedules for CNS leukaemia prophylaxis. Scand J Haematol 1980;24:421.
318. Omura GA, Moffitt S, Vogler WR, et al. Combination chemotherapy of adult acute lymphoblastic leukemia with randomised central nervous system prophylaxis. Blood 1980;55:199.
319. Kantarjian HM, Walters RS, Smith TL, et al. Identification of risk groups for development of central nervous system leukemia in adults with acute lymphoblastic leukemia. Blood 1988;72:1784.
320. Pochedly C. Neurotoxicity due to CNS therapy for leukemia. Med Pediatr Oncol 1977;3: 101.

321. Radford JE, Burns CP, Jones MP, et al. Adult acute lymphoblastic leukemia: Results of the Iowa HOP-L protocol. J Clin Oncol 1989;7:58.
322. Stewart DJ, Smith TL, Keating MJ, et al. Remission from central nervous system involvement in adults with acute leukemia—Effect of intensive therapy and prognostic factors. Cancer 1985;56:632.
323. Ramsay NKC, Kersey JH. Indications for marrow transplantation in acute lymphoblastic leukemia. Blood 1990;75:815.
324. Doney K, Fisher LD, Appelbaum FR, et al. Treatment of adult acute lymphoblastic leukemia with allogeneic bone marrow transplantation: Multivariate analysis of factors affecting acute graft vs. host disease relapse and relapse-free survival. Bone Marrow Transplant 1991;7:453.
325. Horowitz MM, Messerer D, Hoelzer D, et al. Chemotherapy compared with bone marrow transplantation for adults with acute lymphoblastic leukemia in first remission. Ann Intern Med 1991;115:13.
326. Chao NJ, Forman SJ, Schmidt GM, et al. Allogeneic bone marrow transplantation for high-risk acute lymphoblastic leukemia during first complete remission. Blood 1991;78: 1923.
327. Wingard JR, Piantadosi S, Santos GW, et al. Allogeneic bone marrow transplantation for patients with high risk acute lymphoblastic leukemia. J Clin Oncol 1990;8:820.
328. Berman E, Little C, Gee T, et al. Reasons that patients with acute myelogenous leukemia do not undergo allogeneic bone marrow transplantation. N Engl J Med 1992;326:156.
329. Keating MJ, Kantarjian H, Smith TL, et al. Response to salvage therapy and survival after relapse in acute myelogenous leukemia. J Clin Oncol 1989;7:1071.
330. Kantarjian HM, Keating MJ, Walters RS, et al. The characteristics and outcome of patients with late relapse acute myelogenous leukemia. J Clin Oncol 1988;6:232.
331. Keating MJ, Estey EH, Plunkett W, et al. Evolution of clinical studies with high-dose cytosine arabinoside (ara-C) at the M.D. Anderson Hospital. Semin Oncol 1985;12(suppl 3):98.
332. Herzig RH, Wolff SN, Lazarus HM, et al. High-dose cytosine arabinoside therapy for refractory leukemia. Blood 1983;62:361.
333. Capizzi RL, Poole M, Cooper MR, et al. Treatment of poor-risk acute leukemia with sequential high-dose ara-C and asparaginase. Blood 1984;63:694.
334. Preisler HD, Epstein J, Barcos M, et al. Prediction of response of acute nonlymphocytic leukaemia to therapy with "high-dose" cytosine arabinoside. Br J Haematol 1984;58: 19.
335. Hines JD, Oken MM, Mazza JJ, et al. High-dose cytosine arabinoside and m-AMSA is effective therapy in relapsed acute nonlymphocytic leukemia. J Clin Oncol 1984;2: 545.
336. Hiddemann W, Kreutzmann H, Straif K, et al. High-dose cytosine arabinoside and mitoxantrone: A highly effective regimen in refractory acute myeloid leukemia. Blood 1987;69:744.
337. Carella AM, Santini G, Martinengo M, et al. 4-Demethoxydaunorubicin (idarubicin) in refractory or relapsed acute leukemias—A pilot study. Cancer 1985;55:1452.
338. Larson RA, Daly KM, Choi KE, et al. A clinical and pharmacokinetic study of mitoxantrone in acute nonlymphocytic leukemia. J Clin Oncol 1987;5:391.
339. Koeller J, Eble M. Mitoxantrone: A novel anthracycline derivative. Clin Pharm 1988;7: 574.
340. Legha SS, Keating MJ, Zander AR, et al. 4'-(9-acridinylamino) methanesulfon-*m*-anisidide (AMSA): A new drug effective in the treatment of adult acute leukemia. Ann Intern Med 1980;93:17.
341. Lee EJ, Van Echo DA, Egorin MJ, et al. Diaziquone given as a continuous infusion is an active agent for relapsed adult acute nonlymphocytic leukemia. Blood 1986;67: 182.
342. Schiffer CA, Lee EJ. Approaches to the therapy of relapsed acute myeloid leukemia. Oncology 1989;3:23.
343. Archimbaud E, Leblond V, Michallet M, et al. Intensive sequential chemotherapy with mitoxantrone and continuous infusion etoposide and cytarabine for previously treated acute myelogenous leukemia. Blood 1991;77:1894.
344. Ho AD, Lipp T, Ehninger G, et al. Combination of mitoxantrone and etoposide in refractory acute myelogenous leukemia—An active and well-tolerated regimen. J Clin Oncol 1988;6:213.
345. Estey EH, Keating MJ, Smith TL, et al. Prediction of complete remission in patients with refractory acute leukemia treated with AMSA. J Clin Oncol 1984;2:102.
346. Plunkett W, Iacoboni S, Estey EH, et al. Pharmacologically directed ara-C therapy for refractory leukemia. Semin Oncol 1985;12:20.
347. Hiddemann W, Schleyer E, Uhrmeister C, et al. High-dose versus intermediate-dose cytosine arabinoside in combination with mitoxantrone for the treatment of relapsed and refractory acute myeloid leukemia—Preliminary clinical and pharmacological data of a randomized comparison. Cancer Treat Rev 1990;17:279.
348. Vogler WR, Preisler HD, Winton EF, et al. Randomized trial of high-dose cytarabine versus amsacrine in acute myelogenous leukemia in relapse: A leukemia intergroup study. Cancer Treat Rep 1986;70:455.
349. Thomas ED, Buckner CD, Rudolph RH, et al. Allogeneic marrow grafting for hematologic malignancy using HLA-matched donor recipient sibling pairs. Blood 1971;38:267.
350. Zander AR, Culbert S, Jagannath S, et al. High dose cyclophosphamide, BCNU, and VP-16 (CBV) as a conditioning regimen for allogeneic bone marrow transplantation for patients with acute leukemia. Cancer 1987;59:1083.
351. Maraninchi D, Abecasis M, Gastaut JA, et al. High-dose melphalan and autologous bone marrow transplant for relapsed acute leukaemia. Cancer Chemother Pharmacol 1983;10:109.
352. Yeager AM, Kaizer H, Santos GW, et al. Autologous bone marrow transplantation in patients with acute nonlymphocytic leukemia using ex vivo marrow treatment with 4-hydroperoxycyclophosphamide. N Engl J Med 1986;315:141.
353. Hoelzer D. High-dose chemotherapy in adult acute lymphoblastic leukemia. Semin Hematol 1991;28:84.
354. Capizzi RL, Pool M, Cooper MR, et al. Treatment of poor risk acute leukemia with sequential high-dose ara-C and asparaginase. Blood 1984;63:694.
355. Arlin ZA, Feldman E, Kempin S, et al. Amsacrine with high-dose cytarabine is highly effective therapy for refractory and relapsed acute lymphoblastic leukemia in adults. Blood 1988;72:433.
356. Keating MJ, Kantarjian H, O'Brien S, et al. The M.D. Anderson Cancer Center Experience with mitoxantrone in acute leukemia. Ann Hematol 1991;62:A3.
357. Milpied N, Gisselbrecht C, Harousseau JL, et al. Successful treatment of adult, acute lymphoblastic leukemia after relapse with prednisone, intermediate-dose cytarabine, mitoxantrone, and etoposide (PAME) chemotherapy. Cancer 1990;66:627.
358. Arcese W, Amadori S, Meloni G, et al. Allogeneic or autologous bone marrow transplantation for intensification of salvage therapy in patients with high-risk advanced acute lymphoblastic leukemia. Semin Hematol 1991;28:116.
359. Kantarjian HM, Estey EH, O'Brien S, et al. Intensive chemotherapy with mitoxantrone and high-dose cytosine arabinoside followed by granulocyte-macrophage colony-stimulating factor in the treatment of patients with acute lymphocytic leukemia. Blood 1992;79:876.
360. Bodey GP, Coltman CA, Freireich EJ, et al. Chemotherapy of acute leukemia. Comparison of cytarabine alone and in combination with vincristine, prednisone, and cyclophosphamide. Arch Intern Med 1974;133:260.
361. Wiernik PH, Schimpff SC, Schiffer CA, et al. Randomized clinical comparison of daunorubicin (NSC-82151) alone with a combination of daunorubicin, cytosine arabinoside (NSC-63878), 6-thioguanine (NSC-752), and pyrimethamine (NSC-3061) for the treatment of acute nonlymphocytic leukemia. Cancer Treat Rep 1976;60:41.
362. Peterson BA, Bloomfield CD, Theologides A, et al. Daunorubicin-prednisone in the treatment of acute nonlymphocytic leukemia. Cancer Treat Rep 1981;65:29.
363. Beguin Y, Bury J, Fillet G, et al. Treatment of acute nonlymphocytic leukemia in young and elderly patients. Cancer 1985;56:2587.
364. Rai KR, Holland JF, Glidewell OJ, et al. Treatment of acute myelocytic leukemia: A study by Cancer and Leukemia Group B. Blood 1981;58:1203.
365. Keating MJ, McCredie KB, Benjamin RS, et al. Treatment of patients over 50 years of age with acute leukemia with a combination of rubidazone and cytosine arabinoside, vincristine, and prednisone (ROAP). Blood 1981;58:584.
366. Cheson BD, Simon R. Low-dose ara-C in acute nonlymphocytic leukemia and myelodysplastic syndromes: A review of 20 years' experience. Semin Oncol 1987;14(suppl 1):126.
367. Kizaki M, Koeffler HP. Differentiation-inducing agents in the treatment of myelodysplastic syndromes. Semin Oncol 1992;19:95.
368. Greenberg PL. Treatment of myelodysplastic syndromes with hemopoietic growth factors. Semin Oncol 1992;19:106.
369. Vadhan-Raj S, Keating M, LeMaistre A, et al. Effects of recombinant human granulocyte-macrophage colony stimulating factor in patients with myelodysplastic syndromes. N Engl J Med 1987;317:1545.
370. Ganser A, Volkers B, Greher J, et al. Recombinant human granulocyte-macrophage colony-stimulating factor in patients with myelodysplastic syndromes—A phase I/II trial. Blood 1989;73:31.
371. Thompson JA, Lee DJ, Kidd P, et al. Subcutaneous granulocyte-macrophage colony-stimulating factor in patients with myelodysplastic syndrome: Toxicity, pharmacokinetics, and hematological effects. J Clin Oncol 1989;7:629.
372. Negrin RS, Haeuber DH, Nagler A, et al. Treatment of myelodysplastic syndromes with recombinant human granulocyte colony stimulating factor. Ann Intern Med 1989;110:976.
373. Ganser A, Seipelt G, Lindemann A, et al. Effects of recombinant human interleukin-3 in patients with myelodysplastic syndromes. Blood 1990;76:455.
374. Kurzrock R, Talpaz M, Estrov Z, et al. Phase I study of recombinant human interleukin-3 in patients with bone marrow failure. J Clin Oncol 1991;9:1241.
375. Estey EH, Keating MJ, Dixon DO, et al. Karyotype is prognostically more important than the FAB system's distinction between myelodysplastic syndrome and acute myelogenous leukemia. Hemato Path 1987;1:203.
376. Tricot G, Boogaerts MA. The role of aggressive chemotherapy in the treatment of the myelodysplastic syndromes. Br J Haematol 1986;63:477.
377. Fenaux P, Lai JL, Jouet JP, et al. Aggressive chemotherapy in adult primary myelodysplastic syndromes. Blut 1988;57:297.
378. Aul C, Schneider W. The role of low-dose cytosine arabinoside and aggressive chemotherapy in advanced myelodysplastic syndromes. Cancer 1989;64:1812.
379. Estey EH, Dixon D, Kantarjian HM, et al. Treatment of poor-prognosis, newly diagnosed acute myeloid leukemia with ara-C and recombinant human granulocyte-macrophage colony stimulating factor. Blood 1990;75:1766.
380. Buchner T, Hiddemann W, Koenigsmann M, et al. Recombinant human granulocyte-macrophage colony-stimulating factor after chemotherapy in patients with acute myeloid leukemia at higher age or after relapse. Blood 1991;78:1190.
381. Ohno R, Tomonaga M, Kobayashi T, et al. Effect of granulocyte colony-stimulating factor after intensive induction therapy in relapsed or refractory acute leukemia. N Engl J Med 1990;323:871.
382. Keating MJ, Smith TL, Gehan EA, et al. A prognostic factor analysis for use in development of predictive models for response in adult acute leukemia. Cancer 1982;50: 457.
383. Smith TL, Gehan EA, Keating MJ, et al. Prediction of remission in adult acute leukemia: Development and testing of predictive models. Cancer 1982;50:466.
384. Gaynor J, Chapman D, Little C, et al. A cause-specific hazard rate analysis of prognostic

factors among 199 adults with acute lymphoblastic leukemia: The Memorial Hospital experience since 1969. J Clin Oncol 1988;6:1014.

385. Keating MJ, Smith TL, Kantarjian H, et al. Cytogenetic pattern in acute myelogenous leukemia: A major reproducible determinant of outcome. Leukemia 1988;2:403.

386. Bloomfield CD, Goldman AI, Alimena G, et al. Chromosomal abnormalities identify high-risk and low-risk patients with acute lymphoblastic leukemia. Blood 1986;67: 415.

387. Huang ME, Ye YC, Chai JR, et al. Use of all *trans* retinoic acid in the treatment of acute promyelocytic leukemia. Blood 1988;72:567.

388. Castaigne S, Chomienne C, Daniel MT, et al. All *trans* retinoic acid as a differentiation therapy for acute promyelocytic leukemia: I. Clinical results. Blood 1990;76:1704.

389. Degos L, Chomienne C, Daniel MT, et al. Treatment of first relapse in acute promyelocytic leukemia with all *trans* retinoic acid. Lancet 1990;:1440.

390. Warrel RM, Frankel SR, Miller WH, et al. Differentiation therapy of acute promyelocytic leukemia with tretinoin (all *trans* retinoic acid). N Engl J Med 1991;324:1385.

391. Muindi J, Frankel SR, Miller WH Jr, et al. Continuous treatment with all *trans* retinoic acid causes a progressive reduction in plasma drug concentrations: Implication for relapse and retinoid "resistance" in patients with acute promyelocytic leukemia. Blood 1992;79:299.

Cancer: Principles & Practice of Oncology, Fourth Edition,
edited by Vincent T. DeVita, Jr., Samuel Hellman, Steven A. Rosenberg.
J.B. Lippincott Co., Philadelphia © 1993.

Albert B. Deisseroth
Michael Andreeff
Richard Champlin
Michael J. Keating
Hagop Kantarjian
Issa F. Khouri
Moshe Talpaz

CHAPTER **55**

Chronic Leukemias

During the past 50 years, a major problem facing those responsible for the design and implementation of therapy of the chronic leukemias has been the dose limitations that the nonhematopoietic toxicities of chemotherapy have imposed on therapy. This situation arose in part from the narrow margin of selectivity that conventional chemotherapeutic agents exhibit with respect to chronic leukemia cells, which are often less rapidly proliferating and therefore less sensitive to phase-specific and cycle-dependent chemotherapy than acute leukemia cells. During the 1970s, dose intensification with exogenous hematopoietic reconstitution was used as a means of increasing the safety and effectiveness of therapy. The use of autologous and allogeneic bone marrow transplantation permitted the safe delivery of effective doses of therapy for these diseases. The utility of this approach was limited in part by the medical factors that limit eligibility for this type of therapy in chronic leukemia patients due to their advanced chronologic and physiologic age. During the 1980s, recombinant growth factors were produced in quantities sufficient for therapy. Although these agents were useful adjuncts in limiting the hematopoietic toxicity of conventional-dose therapy, there was no detectable incremental impact of this support modality on survival.

New drugs and molecular approaches to diagnosis are contributing to more selective therapy. It is now possible to define the molecular defects that create leukemic hematopoietic cells, and a new level of selectivity is possible because therapy can be directed to the basic biologic changes that lead to the disease. The ultimate extension of this trend is genetic therapy, which involves the replacement of missing sequences within abnormal cells to correct their defects. In this chapter we review the developments that are permitting the integration of molecular and genetic approaches to therapy with more conventional modalities of chemotherapy, biologic therapy, and molecular and genetic therapy with bone marrow transplantation in the chronic leukemias.

CHRONIC LYMPHOCYTIC LEUKEMIA

Chronic lymphocytic leukemia (CLL) is a monoclonal hematopoietic disorder with expansion of small lymphocytes of B-cell (95%) or T cell lineage (5%). (Other sources provide a more extensive review of this process than can be offered in this chapter.[1,2]) CLL cells accumulate in blood, bone marrow, lymph nodes, and spleen, resulting in enlargement of these organs and decreased bone marrow function.

In 1924, Minot and Isaacs reported the natural history of CLL and described the effects of radiation therapy.[3] In 1975, Rai and colleagues described a clinical staging system and documented the adverse effects of anemia and thrombocytopenia on survival.[4] Another staging system was suggested by Binet.[5]

The monoclonal nature of CLL has been confirmed by surface marker analysis: restriction of light-chain type on the surface of B cells, expression of a single isoenzyme in the lymphocytes of female patients who are heterozygous for glucose-6-phosphate dehydrogenase, immunoglobulin (Ig) gene rearrangements showing single V_L and V_H regions, and by cytogenetic analysis.[6–8]

ETIOLOGY AND INCIDENCE

CLL is the most common leukemia, with an annual incidence of 1.8 to 3.0 per 100,000 population in the United States.[9] Incidence is age related, with 5.2 per 100,000 persons between 35 and 59 years of age and 30.4 per 100,000 persons between 80 and 84 years of age. It affects twice as many men as women.

CLL is less common in Japanese and other Asian populations. Clusters of CLL in families have been reported, and first-degree relatives of patients with CLL have a threefold increased risk for CLL and other lymphoid neoplasms compared with the general population.[10–12] There is no increased incidence after exposure to radiation, and there is no evidence for retroviral initiation of the disease.

CYTOGENETIC ABNORMALITIES

The paucity of metaphases in fresh preparations of CLL cells, which are characterized by a very low mitotic index, makes cytogenetic analysis difficult. B-cell mitogens such as lipopolysaccharide from *E. coli*, 12-0-tetradecanoylphorbol-13-acetate, cytochalasin B, pokeweed mitogen, phytohemagglutinin, and Epstein-Barr virus allow the preparation of metaphases in 90% of cases.[13–16] Using conventional banding techniques, 30% to 50% of patients with CLL have detectable chromosomal abnormalities.[17–21] Patients with clonal chromosomal abnormalities have a poorer prognosis than patients with diploid karyotypes.[16] The most frequent abnormalities involve chromosomes 12 or 14.[22–25] Other changes include −8, iso(2p), 6q−, iso(7p), t(13;21), 14q−, trisomy 18, and −X. At M.D. Anderson Cancer Center, 475 CLL samples were studied with conventional cytogenetic techniques (G-banding) after short-term culture, and abnormal karyotypes were identified in 31% of cases. Of those, 22.8% had trisomy 12 alone or in combination with other abnormalities, and 1.9% had structural abnormalities of chromosome 12. Other abnormalities were 11q− (16.7% of abnormal karyotypes), 14q+ (7.9%), 13q− (7%), t(11;14) (6.1%), 6q− (4.4%), −17 (4.3%), ±19 (4.3%), ±18 (3.5%), ±21 (2.6%), −16 (2.6%), and iso(17q) (1.8%).

The technique of interphase cytogenetics with fluorescence in situ hybridization (FISH) using repetitive DNA sequences as specific probes for the centromeric regions of individual chromosomes is independent of cell division and the presence of metaphases (Fig. 55–1).[26] FISH identified trisomy 12 in 30 (28.6%) of 104 patients.[27] In this study with a short follow-up, there was a significant correlation between the percentage of CD19+ or CD20+ cells and the percentage of cells showing trisomy 12 (R = 0.46, $p < 0.05$). Trisomy 12 was not found in FACS-sorted T cells in B-cell CLL. There was no difference in overall survival between trisomy 12 and diploid patients, but the time to progression of the disease after fludarabine therapy was significantly shorter in patients who had trisomy 12.[27] Trisomy 12 is thought to be associated with early-stage disease, and other abnormalities are acquired in advanced stages.[24,28]

Abnormalities of chromosome 14 include translocations (t[11;14]), deletions (14q−), and inversions (inv[14q]).[29] The presence of 14q+ is associated with a high leukocyte count and poor response to therapy. The genes for the Ig heavy chain (14q32) and for the α-chain of the human T-cell receptor (14q11.2) are localized on chromosome 14.[30] The chromosome 11 segment translocated to the J segment of the heavy chain locus at 14q32 contains the *BCL1* oncogene and results in the production of a novel protein.

Survival of patients with abnormal cytogenetics is significantly shorter than in patients with normal karyotypes. In a study from Roswell Park, there was no correlation of chromosomal abnormalities with age, sex, treatment status, or disease duration, but the 10-year survival rate was 86% for patients with normal karyotypes and 57% for those with abnormal karyotypes.[13] In a study by Juliusson and coworkers of 433 patients with B-cell CLL, 391 patients could be evaluated, and 218 had clonal chromosomal changes.[16] Trisomy of chromosome 12 was found in 30.7% of those with abnormal karyotypes, structural abnormalities of chromosome 13 in 23.4%, and abnormalities of chromosome 14 in 18.8%. Translocations or interstitial deletions involving 13q14, the retinoblastoma gene locus, existed in 35 of 51 patients with abnormalities of chromosome 13. The presence of any clonal abnormalities carried a poor prognosis: survival of these patients was 7.7 years, compared with longer than 15 years for patients with normal karyotypes. Patients with abnormalities of 14q had a poorer survival than those with 13q abnormalities (Fig. 55–2). A high percentage of cells in metaphase with chromosomal abnormalities, perhaps indicating high proliferative activity of leukemic cells, was associated with poor survival ($p < 0.0058$) in multivariate analysis.

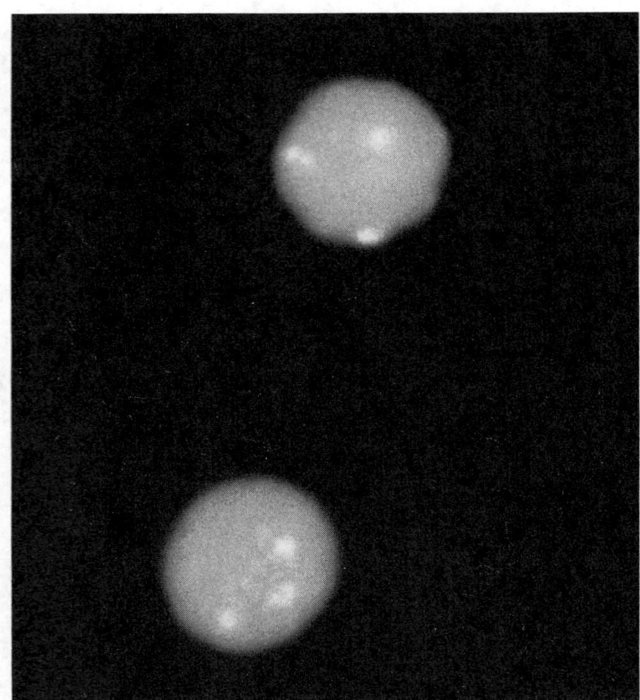

FIGURE 55–1. Detection of trisomy of chromosome 12 in chronic lymphocytic leukemia.

IMMUNOLOGIC PHENOTYPING

B-cell CLL is characterized by clonal B cells carrying only a single Ig light-chain type and single antibody specificity (*i.e.*, idiotype).[31] Cells of most patients have a low number of surface membrane IgM molecules, but serum IgM is found in only a small fraction of samples tested with standard protein electrophoresis techniques. CLL cells have C′3 and Fc receptors and express CD19, CD20, CD21, CD5, and HLA-DR.[32–33] In many patients, CD5, an antigen found on normal adult and fetal B cells but not on mature B lymphocytes, is coexpressed.

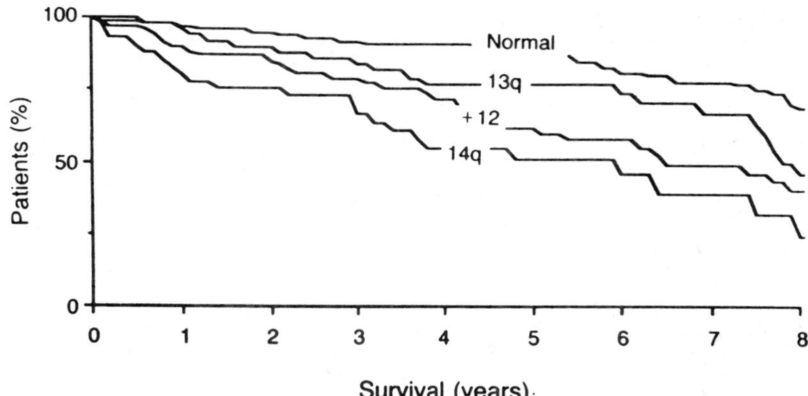

FIGURE 55–2. Survival by karyotype. (Juliusson G, Oscher DG, Fitchett M, et al. Prognostic subgroups in B-cell chronic lymphocytic leukemia defined by specific chromosomal abnormalities. N Engl J Med 1990;323:720)

The monoclonality observed by immunologic phenotyping was confirmed by studies of glucose 6-phosphate dehydrogenase. Although myeloid and T cells are not clonally involved, functional and numeric T-cell abnormalities have been reported in patients with CLL.[34–36] The number of T cells may be increased in absolute numbers, the T4:T8 ratio is decreased, possibly because of an absolute increase in T8 cells. Suppressor T cells may infiltrate the marrow and therefore directly suppress erythropoiesis.[37] The response of circulating T cells to IL-2 is diminished, reflecting functional abnormalities.[38] Lymphokine-activated killer (LAK) cell generation is defective, as is the susceptibility to allogeneic and autologous LAK cells.[39] Clonogenic cells in CLL appear to depend on yet undefined factors provided by activated T cells and conditioned media.[40–41] The complex role of the T-cell compartment in B-cell CLL is not yet fully understood.

Approximately 10% of cases with B-cell CLL show a clonal rearrangement of T-cell receptor consistent with the occurrence of immature B cells.

In half of the patients with CLL, hypogammaglobulinemia is significant and contributes to an increased risk of infection.[42] Decreases in IgM precede deficiencies in IgG and IgA.

The coexpression of CD19, CD20, CD21, or CD24 with CD5 is a useful marker for the detection of minimal disease in B-cell CLL.[43] Patients with no detectable disease by flow cytometry who responded to fludarabine and prednisone therapy with complete remissions had a 2-year disease-free survival rate of 83%, compared with 28% for patients with detectable residual disease ($p < 0.001$).

The cell kinetics of CLL are characterized by a low, almost undetectable number of cells in S phase in peripheral blood and bone marrow (0.2%).[44–45] In one report, however, the labeling index was as high as 60% in CLL lymph nodes.[46] In studies of continuous infusion of ^{3}H-labeled thymidine over 7 days, about 95% of small peripheral blood lymphocytes were long lived, with turnover times of more than 1 year, and CLL can therefore be considered to have an accumulative type of growth. The malignant transformation may protect CLL cells from programmed cell death (*i.e.*, apoptosis), as found for the *BCL2* gene in lymphomas. The notion that most CLL cells are in G_0 may not be correct. Flow cytometric measurements of chromatin structure in intact cells using the acridine orange technique revealed T-α values varying over a large range from "G_0" to G_1. The high expression of the cell cycle-related protooncogene *p53* and high expression of the proliferating cell nuclear antigen (PCNA) suggests that CLL cells are not entirely quiescent.[47–49] Clinically, the determination of lymphocyte-doubling times may provide a measure of net increase in cell mass and may inform the decision about when to initiate treatment.[50]

Expression of the *MDR1* and *MDR3* multidrug-resistance genes have been reported often. Herweijer and colleagues reported *MDR1* positivity in 17 of 17 B-cell CLL patients but in none of 7 B-cell prolymphocytic leukemia (PLL) patients.[51] *MDR3* expression was detected in B-cell CLL (17 of 17), B-cell PLL (7 of 7), and hairy cell leukemia (2 of 2). In these cases, steady-state accumulation of daunorubicin was significantly increased by cyclosporine, an inhibitor of the P-glycoprotein efflux pump, an observation that may be useful for the development of novel therapeutic modalities.

CLINICAL FEATURES AND STAGING

The approach to management of CLL differs from the approach taken in most malignant diseases. The treatment has been palliative, because of the assumption that older patients (most are >60 years) cannot tolerate aggressive chemotherapy. An additional cause for concern was the immunosuppression and myelosuppression associated with CLL, as well as the development of associated hypogammaglobulinemia, T-cell immunodeficiency, neutropenia, and thrombocytopenia. Available treatment (predominantly with alkylating agents such as chlorambucil or cyclophosphamide with or without corticosteroids) seldom achieved complete remissions, and there was no evidence of a cure fraction in CLL.

A major reason for selecting conservative therapy was the observation that many patients with CLL live for long periods without requiring therapeutic intervention. The ability to identify these patients has improved in recent years. The Rai and Binet classifications (Table 55–1) have proven useful in identifying different risk categories.[52,53] Both classifications are based on the presence of marrow compromise (*e.g.*, anemia, thrombocytopenia) in advanced stages and increasing tumor burden in the earlier stages. When applied prospectively, both staging systems yield good prognostic information. Patients who have Rai stage 0 disease at diagnosis have approximately two chances in three of surviving for 20 years or more. In early-stage disease (Rai 0—II, Binet stage A), a group of patients with "smoldering" chronic lymphocytic leukemia have been determined whose hemoglobin is more than 13 g/

TABLE 55–1. Rai and Binet Staging Systems for Chronic Lymphocytic Leukemia

Stage	*Lymphocytosis*	*Lymphadenopathy*	*Hepatomegaly or Splenomegaly*	*Hemoglobin (g/dl)*	*Platelets* $\times 10^3/\mu l$
Rai System					
0	+	−	−	≥11	≥100
I	+	+	−	≥11	≥100
II	+	±	+	≥11	≥100
III	+	±	±	<11	≥100
IV	+	±	±	Any	<100
Binet System					
A	+	± (<3 lymphatic groups* positive)	±	≥10	≥100
B	+	± (≥3 lymphatic groups* positive)	±	≥10	≥100
C	+	±	±	<10	<100

* Cervical, axillary, inguinal nodes; liver; and spleen are each considered one group whether unilateral or bilateral.

dl, platelet count is greater than 150,000, and lymphocyte count is less than 30,000/μl, with a doubling time of peripheral lymphocytes of longer than 1 year and with a nondiffuse bone marrow histology.[54] These patients have a survival equivalent to an age- and sex-matched healthy population.

Overall, the survival of patients seen at the M.D. Anderson Cancer Center before the initiation of any treatment was a median of approximately 6 years. The survival strongly correlates with Rai and Binet stages. Attempts have been made to combine the Rai and Binet stages into a hybrid staging system.[55] Most clinical trials in the United States use the Rai staging system, and those in Europe use the Binet staging system. Important prognostic variables for survival in CLL in addition to stage include the age of the patient, doubling time of the peripheral blood lymphocyte count, and the pattern of bone marrow involvement. The influence of karyotype on survival is uncertain. It appears that patients who have residual normal metaphases or those that are diploid have a better survival than patients who have 100% abnormal metaphases. Different subsets of abnormal cytogenetic patterns are associated with various prognoses.[16]

TREATMENT

Indications

Clinical trials in CLL have been marked by wide diversity of entry criteria and response criteria. Most clinicians treat patients with Rai stage III or IV or Binet stage C at diagnosis, because anemia and thrombocytopenia are adverse prognostic factors (median survival, 18 months to 4 years). Clinicians usually do not treat Rai stage 0 patients. The approach to treatment for patients with adenopathy or hepatosplenomegaly has varied. An National Cancer Institute (NCI) Working Group has come up with indications for treatment in NCI-sponsored clinical trials.[56] In addition to advanced stage, massive adenopathy or massive hepatomegaly or splenomegaly, evidence of progressive enlargement of lymph nodes, liver, or spleen and a doubling time of peripheral blood lymphocytes of less than 6 months are indications for treatment. Development of anemia or thrombocytopenia, which are thought not to be immune mediated, are indications for initiation of treatment. Development of antibody-induced anemia and thrombocytopenia usually triggers treatment with corticosteroids. Most patients responded well to this modality of treatment, but most do not remain stable for long periods, and treatment of the leukemia after correction of the anemia or thrombocytopenia is recommended. Hypogammaglobulinemia or monoclonal gammopathy without symptoms related to these conditions are not considered adequate indications for initiation of treatment.

In addition, the NCI Working Group and the International Working Group for CLL have developed criteria for response to therapy.[57] Many early clinical trials evaluated only clinical examination and peripheral blood findings to evaluate response. In the last decade, increasing emphasis has been placed on the bone marrow as a criterion for remission. The NCI Working Group and International Working Group on CLL require restoration of relatively normal hemoglobin levels and neutrophil and platelet counts, with a decrease in the lymphocyte count to less than 4,000/μl and bone marrow infiltration to lower than 30% lymphocytes for the patient to be considered in complete remission. Both schemes allow persistent lymphoid nodules or aggregates in the bone marrow, because it is uncertain whether these are normal residual lymphoid aggregates or pathologic aggregates. Widespread adoption of these criteria for response should make comparison of clinical trials more reliable.

Conventional Treatment

The workhorse of treatment of CLL has been chlorambucil. Chlorambucil, used in the management of malignant lymphoproliferative disease since the mid-1950s, is available in tablet form and is rapidly and almost completely absorbed from the gastrointestinal tract, with a peak plasma concentration occurring within 1 hour.[58,59] The liver is a predominant metabolic site, and the principal metabolite (*i.e.*, phenylacetic acid mustard) is active against CLL.[60] Fifty percent to 65% of a single oral dose is excreted in the urine within 24 hours. Early studies by Galton and Ezdinli demonstrated that approximately three quarters of patients achieved some response, with two thirds of patients responding to second and subsequent courses.[59,60] The interval between courses of treatment became shorter with a lesser response as the disease progressed. Knospe introduced the concept of intermittent therapy with a single dose of 0.4 mg/kg chlorambucil every 2 weeks.[61] He concluded that biweekly oral administration was effective for CLL, producing less myelosuppression than daily treatment. Before this approach, most patients were treated with a continuous oral dose of 0.1 to 0.4 mg/kg per day for 4 to 8 weeks until response or myelosuppression was observed.

Cyclophosphamide has had minimal evaluation as a single agent but is often combined with vincristine and prednisone in the CVP regimen if chlorambucil fails.[62,63] In single-arm studies of the CVP regimen, the response rates varied from 44% to 77%, with a higher response rate found for patients who had never received previous treatment than for the previously treated group of patients.[62,63]

Corticosteroids have been evaluated over the last 30 years as single agents in doses of 20 to 80 mg per day. Complete responses are rare.[64,65] Decrease in node, liver, and spleen enlargement commonly occur, and improvements in anemia and thrombocytopenia can result. Studies evaluating corticosteroids as single agents focused attention on the incidence of infection with prolonged administration of corticosteroids.[59,64,65]

Since the early 1970s, most investigators have used a combination of chlorambucil and prednisone. This is based on a single small study by Han with 15 patients receiving the combination of chlorambucil and prednisone compared with 11 patients treated with chlorambucil alone.[66] A higher response rate was observed in the combination arm than in the single-agent arm. No significant survival advantage was detected. Prednisone was compared with chlorambucil plus prednisone by the Cancer and Leukemia Group B (CALGB), with chlorambucil given to one group of patients intermittently and to the other group by continuous daily administration.[64] The combination protocols were superior to the prednisone-alone arm, but no difference in the response rate was found for the two schedules of chlorambucil. No survival advantage was found in any arm of the study. Subsequently, most investigators have compared chlorambucil plus prednisone to other regimens. Chlorambucil plus prednisone produced response rates of 64% to 74% in several studies.[67–70] Higher response rates were observed for patients with indolent disease than for patients with active disease defined as those having marrow compromise, constitutional symptoms, bulky disease, or progressive and painful enlargement of lymph nodes or spleen. The median survival in most of these studies is approximately 5 years, with most studies demonstrating better survival for responders than for nonresponders.

Comparative Trials

Several trials have been conducted in which chlorambucil and prednisone were compared with several other regimens. Monserrat compared chlorambucil and prednisone with CVP (see Table 55–1).[68] A higher response rate was observed for chlorambucil and prednisone than for CVP treatment. The same group compared chlorambucil and prednisone with a combination regimen including cyclophosphamide, melphalan, and prednisone (CMP).[69] No superiority was found for the CMP study. The Eastern Cooperative Group in 1991 published comparison of chlorambucil and prednisone with CVP.[70] No significant difference in survival was observed; median values were 4.8 years for chlorambucil and prednisone and 3.9 years for the CVP patients. Complete response rates were 25% and 23% in the two arms of the study. Median survival reported in this study for Rai stage III and IV patients was 4.1 years, which is better than the 18 to 24 months reported in older studies.[52]

The combination of chlorambucil and prednisone has emerged as the gold standard of treatment of CLL. There is no evidence that vincristine has any activity in this disease. The question of dose intensity has been raised by a comparative trial conducted by Jaksic and colleagues.[71] Chlorambucil and prednisone were compared with single-agent continuous chlorambucil at a dose of 15 mg per day. This latter regimen was administered until complete remission or myelosuppression dictated discontinuation of therapy. There was a significant difference in survival between the two groups; the chlorambucil-alone arm produced a median survival of 6 years, and the combination of chlorambucil plus prednisone produced a median survival of 3 years. The intensity of the chlorambucil dose in the single-agent arm was five to six times that used in the combination arm. This study raises the question of a dose-response relation in the treatment of CLL, which has not previously been addressed.

French Cooperative Group Studies

Dr. Binet and his colleagues in the French Cooperative Group for CLL conducted several comparative trials using the Binet staging system.[72–74] For Binet stage A patients, a study of immediate versus delayed continuous oral chlorambucil was conducted.[72] Six hundred twelve patients were randomized. Survival was slightly superior in the 309 patients randomized to delayed treatment. A significantly higher number of epithelial cancers was observed in the group receiving immediate treatment with chlorambucil. Other groups have conducted studies of early and delayed treatment for stage A patients and showed no advantage for earlier treatment.[75] Time to development of progressive disease (stages B and C) is delayed in the immediate-treatment arm, but survival after progression is less, and overall survival was not been influenced. Other trials have not found the increase in incidence of epithelial cancers.[75] For Binet stage B, patients receiving continuous oral chlorambucil were compared with those on the CVP regimen. The study enrolled 191 patients. No difference in survival between the two arms was found before and after adjusting for differences in prognostic factors. The median survival was approximately 5 years.[75]

A surprising outcome was observed in the comparative study conducted using Binet stage C patients.[74] The COP regimen was compared with the CHOP regimen; the COP regimen was fixed and doxorubicin added at a dose of 25 mg/m^2 on day 1 in the CHOP arm. Seventy stage C patients were randomized between the treatments. The overall survival was significantly better for the CHOP group. The median survival was 62 months for the CHOP group and 22 months for the COP group. This well-conducted clinical trial has been criticized because the COP arm had inferior results to those reported in more recent studies of Binet stage C patients.[70] In addition, anthracyclines as single agents do not have marked activity in CLL, and the addition of such a modest dose to COP surprised investigators with the significance of the outcome. Ongoing studies compare CHOP in various dosage regimens to chlorambucil and prednisone in Binet stages B and C.[76,77] Higher remission rates were observed in the CHOP arms, but there were no survival advantages.

Other clinical trials have been conducted with anthracyclines. Two studies from the M.D. Anderson Cancer Center of CAP (cyclophosphamide, doxorubicin [Adriamycin], and prednisone) resulted in 43% of patients achieving complete responses and 23% achieving partial responses, for a total response rate of 66%.[78] The response criteria included bone marrow biopsy. The POACH study, which used the same three drugs with vincristine and cytosine arabinoside, was conducted using 34 previously untreated patients.[79] Fifty-six percent of the patients responded, with 21% obtaining complete remissions. This regimen was also administered to 31 previously treated patients using the same criteria, and 26% of these patients responded, and only 2 patients achieved complete remissions. Median survival of the previously treated patients was 15 months. Chemotherapy regimens including the anthracyclines were well tolerated in both studies.

Multiple Alkylating Agents

Multiple alkylating agents have been combined in the M2 protocol from the Memorial Sloan-Kettering Cancer Center. The regimen uses vincristine, cyclophosphamide, BCNU, melphalan, and prednisone.[80] Of 63 patients studied, 17% obtained complete remissions, and 44% achieved partial responses. The complete response rate was significantly higher for untreated patients than previously treated (11 of 37 versus 0 of 26).

New Agents

Nucleoside analogs are being increasingly studied for the treatment of CLL. Fludarabine and 2-chlorodeoxyadenosine, which are analogs of ara-adenine and pentostatin (an adenosine deaminase inhibitor) have been studied. The most widely studied is fludarabine, which was first evaluated in CLL by Grever and colleagues in 22 patients.[81] In this phase II trial, all patients had received extensive prior treatment. One patient achieved a complete response, 3 patients had excellent partial responses, and 15 had some evidence of response. Larger studies of this agent were conducted at the M.D. Anderson Cancer Center.[82,83] Fludarabine was used as a single agent to treat 68 patients with previously treated CLL. Ten patients (14%) achieved complete responses, and 44% achieved partial responses. Response was higher in the Rai stage O–II patients than for Rai stages III and IV. Using the NCI criteria for complete remission, which allows persistence of residual nodules in the bone marrow, the complete response rate was 29%, and 28% of patients fulfilled the NCI criteria for partial response. The major toxic effects associated with fludarabine were fever and infection. These were much more common in patients with advanced Rai stage and hypoalbuminemia. Myelosuppression was the most common toxic effect. Fifty-six percent of chemotherapy courses were associated with neutropenia and 25% with significant thrombocytopenia. Neurotoxicity, a marked feature of high doses used in the management of acute leukemia, was not observed in these and subsequent studies.

Fludarabine was used to treat 33 previously untreated patients with CLL.[83] The complete remission rate was 75%. Half of these complete responders had residual lymphoid nodules in the bone marrow as the only evidence of disease. Fludarabine is the most effective single agent that has been evaluated in the management of CLL. It is not possible to assess the impact of response on survival at this time. Fludarabine was combined with prednisone in the treatment of 101 previously treated patients.[84] Thirty-six percent of patients achieved complete responses, and 19% achieved partial responses, for a total response rate of 55%. The addition of prednisone did not increase the response rate nor improve survival when compared retrospectively with the fludarabine single-agent study. In the corticosteroid-treated group, *Pneumocystis carinii* and *Listeria* infections occurred, but they did not develop in the single-agent study. Another study using a lower total dose of fludarabine with a continuous infusion reported a response rate above 50%, with no complete remissions reported.[85]

Pentostatin has been studied by several groups, using doses of 4 mg/m^2 every 2 weeks in most studies.[86,87] The response rate with this agent is between 20% and 25%, with few patients achieving complete remissions. A higher response rate was observed in previously untreated patients in a small study conducted by CALGB.[87] Infections were the most common adverse effect in the pentostatin-treated group of patients.

2-Chlorodeoxyadenosine, which is structurally similar to fludarabine, was used to treat 90 patients with refractory CLL.[88] The usual dose was 0.1 mg/kg per day by continuous infusion for 7 days. The median number of cycles was two. All patients had failed prior therapy. It is uncertain whether they were resistant or not. Eighty-seven of the 90 patients had stage C disease. Four patients obtained complete remissions, and 36 patients had partial responses. The median duration of response was 4 months. Thrombocytopenia was dose limiting, and 10 of the 90 patients developed pulmonary infiltrates. Other modalities, total-body irradiation, and splenic irradiation are being studied in the treatment of CLL, with no evidence of a substantial response rate or improvement in survival.

Changing Criteria of Response to Therapy

There are now defined criteria for response to therapy, and increasing emphasis is being given to the documentation of residual disease. Two-parameter flow cytometry is being used to detect residual abnormal cells that coexpress CD5 and CD19 or 20 or 21 surface antigens. Normalization of κ:λ ratio is being studied, as is the prognostic impact of persistent lymphoid aggregates. Lymphoid aggregates may be nodular, interstitial, or mixed nodular and interstitial patterns. Return to a germline pattern for immunoglobulin gene rearrangement is also being studied in several patients.[89] Using the strict criteria, several patients with CLL are achieving true complete remissions.

The ability of a large number of CLL patients to achieve complete responses raises the prospect of conducting autologous bone marrow transplantation, with bone marrows being purged by a variety of monoclonal antibodies against B-cell antigens. These studies are ongoing. Allogeneic bone marrow transplantation has been conducted in a series of patients with CLL.[90] Seventeen patients received an allogeneic transplant. Approximately 45% of the patients are alive and free of disease for as long as 4 years. Fifteen of the 17 patients engrafted. Two patients had early deaths, 4 of the 15 with complete responses died, and 2 relapsed; 9 of 17 patients are alive and in complete remission.

Treatment Prospects

The addition of the nucleoside analogs to the therapeutic armamentarium raises the prospect of achieving complete remissions in most previously untreated patients with CLL. Comparative trials are being conducted under the auspices of the NCI of chlorambucil versus fludarabine versus fludarabine plus chlorambucil to evaluate the role of fludarabine in this disease. The duration of chemotherapy is an unresolved issue. It appears that most patients who achieve complete remission still have significant immunosuppression. Research on immunorestoration in this group is needed.

PROLYMPHOCYTIC LEUKEMIA

PLL is characterized by massive splenomegaly and extremely high circulating lymphocyte counts with B- or T-cell phenotypes.[91] Lymphadenopathy is unusual, and median survival is less than 3 years.[92] The B cells in PLL have abundant surface immunoglobulin. A serum monoclonal protein is seen in 30% of cases, and reactivity with the monoclonal antibody FMC-7 is considered evidence for the relative maturity of PLL cells compared with those of B-cell CLL. PLL B cells do not express CD5 and frequently have a cytogenetic abnormality involving chromosome 14. Other abnormalities involve chromosomes 1, 12, and a specific translocation, t(6;12)(q15;p13).[93] In 20% of PLL patients, T-cell markers are expressed, and the cells also have positivity for α-naphthyl acetate esterase. Splenectomy and chemotherapy with CHOP are effective, but responses are short. Encouraging results have been reported for fludarabine (30 mg/m^2 over 30 minutes daily $\times$ 5 days every 4 weeks with or without prednisone); 35% of patients had complete or partial remissions.[94] These results require longer follow-up.

HAIRY CELL LEUKEMIA

The clinical features of hairy cell leukemia include pancytopenia, splenomegaly, and only infrequent lymphadenopathy.[95] Immunoglobulin genes are rearranged.[96,97] The "hairy" morphology of hairy cell leukemia cell is best appreciated by scanning electron microscopy and positivity for tartrate-resistant acid phosphatase. Hairy cell features can be induced in CLL cells exposed to phorbol esters in vitro.[98]

Historically, splenectomy was the standard approach to therapy. This measure was designed to correct the neutropenia associated with this disease. Interferon-α (INF-α) and 2-deoxycoformycin (pentostatin) supplemented splenectomy because these two therapies reduced the total leukemia cell burden.[99,100] Two groups initiated the use of 2-chlorodeoxyadenosine in the treatment of hairy cell leukemia, one from San Diego and one from Houston, with a complete remission frequency of 11 of 12 (San Diego) and 36 of 46 patients (Houston).[101,102] A dose of 0.1 mg/kg was administered by continuous intravenous infusion for 7 days. Remissions are long lasting, but fever, sepsis, and a reduced CD4:CD8 ratio may be consequences of this therapy. Although it is not possible at this time to ascertain which of the four therapeutic options is most effective for this disease, it is clear that splenectomy has now been supplemented by one type of biologic therapy (INF-α) and two excellent chemotherapeutic options (2-chlorodeoxyadenosine and 2-deoxycoformycin).

T-CELL CHRONIC LYMPHOCYTIC LEUKEMIA

Two percent of cases of CLL have lymphocytes that form rosettes with sheep red blood cells and are classified T-cell CLL.[103–107] Rearrangement of the T-cell receptor β-chain genes reflects clonality, and the phenotypes include CD4 and CD8 forms. CD4 positive CLL patients are characterized by young age, adenopathy, frequent skin involvement, hyperlymphocytosis, and diffuse marrow infiltration. Survival is less than 2 years.

The large granular lymphocytosis syndrome (CD8-positive CLL) is characterized by lymphoid cells with abundant cytoplasms containing azurophilic granules.[107] The neoplastic cells originate from natural killer cells, and patients frequently have neutropenia and less frequently have pure red cell aplasia. Most cases have a rather benign course.[108–111]

The CLL can transform into PLL, acute lymphoblastic leukemia, or diffuse large cell lymphoma (Richter syndrome).[112–116] These transformations are associated with poor survival. The pronounced neutropenia found in T-cell CLL can be treated with corticosteroids and splenectomy, with limited success. The role of cytokines (*e.g.,* rhGM-CSF, rhG-CSF) to stimulate granulopoiesis has not yet been established. The combination chemotherapy used in B-cell CLL is not effective, but new compounds like 2-chlorodeoxyadenosine are promising. Infections require antibiotic therapy, and patients with recurrent infections can be considered. The CD4-positive T-cell CLL patients respond poorly to cytotoxic agents but are amenable to leukapheresis when leukocytosis develops.

CHRONIC MYELOGENOUS LEUKEMIA

Chronic myelogenous leukemia (CML) starts with the acquisition of the Philadelphia chromosome translocation, which generates a chimeric tyrosine-specific protein kinase gene. This gene arises from a chromosomal translocation breakpoint between the second exon of the *BCR* gene on chromosome 22 and the second exon of the *ABL* gene on chromosome 9 or between the third exon of the *BCR* gene and the second exon of the *ABL* gene. The protein product of this chimeric gene, the P210 protein, makes the cell independent of extracellular growth factor stimulation, perhaps due to transcriptional activation of genes that rescue the cell from programmed cell death (*i.e.,* apoptosis), such as *BCL2.*

The *BCR-ABL* rearrangement may be detected by fluorescent in situ hybridization, Southern blot, and by the polymerase chain reaction (PCR)-induced amplification of the reverse transcript generated from the RNA of the CML cells. Although most patients contain a Philadelphia chromosome in all of their CML cells, patients whose disease features suggest CML but in whose cells no Philadelphia chromosome is detectable should be studied by Southern blot analysis for a rearranged *BCR* gene or by the PCR for *BCR-ABL*-encoded mRNA. The latter assay is also useful in following the course of the response to allogeneic bone marrow transplantation. At least 30% of patients have a positive PCR result for several months after an allograft, but most of these eventually convert to a negative assay. Reconversion from the Philadelphia-negative to Philadelphia-positive status is a grave prognostic sign, if it is not due to a contamination of the assay. Rarely, patients with a cytogenetically detectable Philadelphia chromosome but without *BCR-ABL*-encoded mRNA have been detected.

The disease is characterized by a progressive replacement of the normal diploid elements of the marrow with mature myeloid cells that are insensitive to the mechanisms that govern proliferation of normal myeloid cells. This results, in the beginning of the disease, in an ever-increasing ratio of leukemic to normal cells. Because the normal cells are still sensitive to the suppressive effect of an increased level of a circulating myeloid cell mass, without treatment, the disease evolves to greater and greater levels of abnormal cells.

The acquisition of somatic mutations and additional chromosomal abnormalities, such as an extra Philadelphia chromosome, trisomy 8, 17p-, or 22-, decreases the capability of maturation, which terminates in blastic crisis (*i.e.,* blast count in the marrow greater than 30%, severe anemia, and severe thrombocytopenia), often accompanied by basophilia. At this stage, all of the organs of the body are invaded by these blasts, the circulating count can reach several hundred thousand blasts per cubic millimeter, and the patient dies of bleeding, infection, or CNS hemorrhage or thrombosis in organs such as the brain. This process usually evolves in a median of 4 years, and the probability for a given patient for evolving into blastic phase is increased if the following are found at diagnosis: basophilia, additional chromosomal abnormalities, and a blast count that is above 5% in the peripheral blood. There is a 25% probability for blastic conversion for each year of the chronic phase. The phenotype of the blastic conversion is usually myeloid (60%), lymphoid (20%), and smaller percentages of erythroid and megakaryocyte phenotypes.

TREATMENT

Therapy for Chronic-Phase Chronic Myelogenous Leukemia

The criteria for assignment of response are summarized in Table 55–2. Radiation therapy of the spleen and radioactive phosphorous treatment for CML were instituted at the beginning of the century.[117–119] These treatments induced symptomatic relief and improved the quality of life in the chronic phase. Chemotherapeutic agents for the management of CML were introduced in 1952 with busulfan (Myleran or 1,4-dimethanesulfonyloxybutane), a sulfonic acid alkylating agent, and hydroxyurea, a ribonucleotidase inhibitor of DNA synthesis that was evaluated a decade later.[120,121] Both maintained the chronic phase by lowering leukocyte counts, reducing symptoms, and reversing splenomegaly. Although busulfan acts on early progenitor cells, and therefore its effect is prolonged, hydroxyurea induces rapid disease control but shorter remission duration.[122–127] Busulfan is occasionally associated with serious side effects, such as severe myelosuppression in 5% to 10% of patients, pulmonary, endocardial and marrow fibrosis, and an Addison-like wasting syndrome.[128] Survival of CML patients was not affected by either type of therapy, even at higher doses, and only rare cytogenetic remissions were reported after prolonged busulfan, ara-C, or hydroxyurea therapy.[129–141]

Intensive combination chemotherapy did not result in durable suppression of Philadelphia-positive cells.[142–145] Although different programs produced a significant Philadelphia chromosome suppression to less than 35% Philadelphia-positive metaphases in 30% to 50% of patients, these were predominantly transient, lasting for a median of 3 to 9 months.[142,144,146]

TABLE 55–2. Response Criteria for Interferon Therapy for Chronic Myelogenous Leukemia

Cytogenetic or Hematologic Remission	*Leukocyte Count*	*Splenomegaly*	*Bone Marrow With Philadelphia Chromosome (%)*
Complete	$<9 \times 10^3/\mu l$ Normal morphology	None	0
Partial	$<20 \times 10^3/\mu l$	Persistence	≤35
Minor			35–95
Failure or none	$>20 \times 10^3/\mu l$	Persistence	100

(Talpaz M, McCredie KB, Mavligit GM, Gutterman JU. Leukocyte interferon-induced myeloid cytoreduction in chronic myelogenous leukemia. Blood 1983;62:689–692)

Other treatment modalities such as leukapheresis and splenectomy have been used to achieve disease control. Leukapheresis did not alter the course of the disease, and it is used today as an initial measure to prevent leukostasis-related complications and in pregnant patients to avoid fetal teratogenic effects of chemotherapy.[147–150] Splenectomy was added after several studies had demonstrated disease progression in the spleen preceding other disease sites.[151–156] However, controlled studies failed to substantiate an advantageous effect of splenectomy on the onset of blastic phase or on survival.[158,159] Prior splenectomy did not alter the prognosis of blastic crisis patients.[160] Though reported to result in faster recovery after bone marrow transplantation, splenectomy had no effect on posttransplant survival.[161,162] Splenectomy or intraarterial cytarabine perfusion in nonsurgical candidates are now reserved for symptomatic relief in unresponsive patients.[163]

Interferons

Since the discovery of interferon in 1957, it has been learned that interferons are a complex group of naturally occurring proteins produced by eukaryotic cells in response to various stimuli.[164,165] These proteins have pleiotropic biologic activities, among which are antiproliferative, immunomodulatory, antiviral, and differentiation-inducing effects.[166] The interferons consist of three distinct groups of peptides: IFN-α, IFN-β, and IFN-γ. IFN-α and IFN-β are acid stable, bind to the same receptor, and are produced primarily by leukocytes and fibroblasts respectively. IFN-γ is an acid-labile, structurally distinct molecule that binds to a different receptor and is produced mainly by T lymphocytes.[167]

The clinical activity of interferons in CML was first demonstrated with partially pure IFN-α (Finnish Red Cross, Hensinki), given at doses of 3 to 9 $\times$ 10^6 U/day to early-chronic-phase patients. A larger study revealed that laboratory indices of disease activity, such as elevated lactate dehydrogenase and B_{12} levels and increased bone marrow cellularity, normalized among responding patients (70%). Subsequently, cytogenetic responses with various degrees of Philadelphia chromosome suppression were found in 41% of the patients.[168,169]

Studies with the recombinant molecule rIFN-α-2a (Roferon; Hoffman-LaRoche, Nutley, NJ) at a dose of 5 $\times$ 10^6 U/m^2 administered intramuscularly daily demonstrated a 75% response rate (33 of 45 patients) with early Philadelphia-positive CML.[170,171] Eleven patients (23%) achieved complete cytogenetic responses on at least one test. Partial cytogenetic responses were seen in 3 additional patients.[171,172]

Studies with rIFN-α-2b (Intron; Schering, Kenilworth, NJ) demonstrated similar activities to those of rIFN-α2a.[169–172] Niederle and colleagues reported responses for 40 of 59 Philadelphia-positive CML patients treated with rIFN-α-2b with a dose of 4 $\times$ 10^6 U/m^2/day. Thirty-three percent of these patients had cytogenetic responses.[173] Alimena and associates reported a 68% hematologic remission rate and 56% rate of cytogenetic improvements among 63 Philadelphia-positive CML patients administered doses of 2 to 5 $\times$ 10^6 U/m^2 of rIFN-α-2b intramuscularly daily.[174] Similar results were seen by a large cooperative study conducted by the CALGB. Of 47 evaluable patients treated with 5 $\times$ 10^6 U/m^2/day of rIFN-α-2b, 27 (57%) achieved complete hematologic remissions; 40% of the patients had cytogenetic improvements.[175,176]

The relation between response and dose intensity was addressed in the Italian study. Patients were treated with 2 $\times$ 10^6 U/m^2 daily or 5 $\times$ 10^6 U/m^2 daily of rIFN-α-2b, and the results indicated a higher response rate with the higher dose and frequent responses among patients initially assigned to the lower dose and subsequently switched to the higher one.[174] However, there is no evidence that further escalation beyond 5 $\times$ 10^6 U/m^2 can increase response rate. The feasibility of further dose escalation is also questionable because of dose-limiting toxicity. Certain prognostic factors influenced the degree of response. When patients were evaluated according to the multivariate regression model, hematologic and cytogenetic responses were more common in low-risk patients.[169] Time from diagnosis influenced therapy outcome as well; patients who were treated within less than 1 year from diagnosis demonstrated approximately 70% hematologic response rate, in sharp contrast to patients with long-standing disease who exhibited a dramatic decline in the hematologic response rate and for whom complete and partial cytogenetic responses were absent (Table 55–3).[171]

Randomized studies of the course and survival of previously untreated patients assigned to conventional chemotherapy or to interferon therapy are ongoing in different centers.[177,178] Preliminary results of 220 patients randomized to 3 to 9 $\times$ 10^6 U/day of IFN-α-2a versus 102 randomized to conventional chemotherapy demonstrated that after 8, 14, and 24 months, a cytogenetic response occurred in 45%, 47% and 50% of the IFN arm and in 20%, 19% and 0%, respectively, of the conventional chemotherapy arm.[177] Another randomized study that accrued 600 patients failed to show any advantage for interferon over busulfan or hydroxyurea.[183] However, interferon was introduced late in the study. Interferon doses were lower than those in single-arm studies, which may clearly affect incidence and duration of responses.[178,183]

Only one study provides sufficient follow-up to assess re-

TABLE 55–3. Hematologic and Cytogenetic Responses Among Philadelphia-Positive CML Patients Treated With rINF-α2a

	Disease Duration			
Characteristics	*≤1 Year*		*>1 Year*	
Number of patients studied	45		16	
Complete hematologic remission	34	(75%)*	4	(25%)
Philadelphia-chromosome status:				
No cytogenetic response	11	(44%)	1	(25%)
>35% to 95%	9		3	
>5% to <35%	3			
0%		(31%)		(0%)
Partial hematologic remission	11			
Resistant disease	2	(4%)	1	(6%)
	9	(21%)	11	(69%)

* Rate of response is given in parentheses.
(Talpaz M, Kantarjian HM, McCredie KB, Keating MJ, Trujillo J, Gutterman J. Clinical investigation of human alpha interferon in chronic myelogenous leukemia. Blood 1987;69:1280–1288)

mission duration and survival.[172] The overall duration of complete hematologic remission was 41 months. However, the remissions lasted significantly longer in patients who had achieved complete or partial cytogenetic remission compared with patients who achieved minor or no cytogenetic response ($p = 0.02$ by the log rank test; Fig. 55–3).

Lasting complete cytogenetic remission was demonstrated in a group of patients with early Philadelphia-positive CML. Eighteen of 96 patients treated with partially pure IFN-α obtained a complete cytogenetic response. Of these, 11 patients had durable ongoing complete cytogenetic responses from 6 to more than 45 months, as shown in Table 55–3.[172]

Southern blot analysis of DNA extracted from CML patients in complete cytogenetic remission did not reveal any improved sensitivity in detecting residual disease over that of standard cytogenetic analysis.[179] However, a PCR assay provides a means of detecting one Philadelphia-positive cell in 10^5 to 10^6 cells.[180] Eighteen patients in complete cytogenetic remission after therapy with IFN-α were subjected to PCR analysis, revealing that 17 of the patients had evidence of residual disease and 1 patient had no residual disease.[181] However, another laboratory has reported that all patients in cytogenetic remission are PCR positive. The significance of this finding for assessing the risk of relapse in these patients and changes in the residual disease over time is not clear, and the results must be matched to clinical outcome.

The overall survival outlook for IFN-treated CML patients was examined in one study by Talpaz and colleagues.[172] This group found a median survival of 63 months, which is significantly longer than for its matched historic controls. However, factors such as earlier diagnosis and change in the natural history of the disease may have influenced this outcome. The projected survival is excellent for complete and partial cytogenetic responders, and the median survival for this group of patients has not been reached (Fig. 55–4). It is already significantly longer than that of the other responders and the nonresponders.

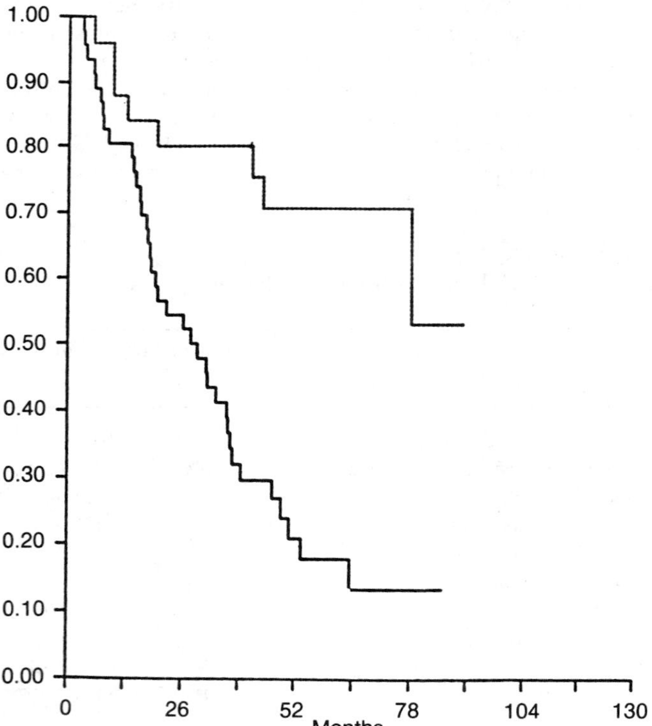

FIGURE 55–3. Kaplan-Meier estimate of the probability of relapse-free survival in patients achieving complete and partial cytogenetic remissions (*dotted line*) compared with that of patients with hematologic remission associated with minor or no cytogenetic response (*solid line*) ($p < 0.001$).

Toxicities to IFN-α can be divided into those observed early in the course of therapy and those developing during the maintenance of the remission.[172] Initially, patients develop fever, chills, malaise, myalgias, fatigue, and headaches, described as an influenza-like syndrome. Acetaminophen or indomethacin can relieve many of these symptoms. Tachyphylaxis usually develops after 1 or 2 weeks of continuous IFN-α administration. Musculoskeletal effects, such as myalgias and arthralgias, are common and transient. However, approximately 10% of the patients develop severe bone pain requiring bed rest. This toxicity was aborted completely with the addition of hydroxyurea, which lowers the initial cell counts (M. Talpaz, unpublished results).

Gastrointestinal toxic effects include elevation of liver transaminase levels to two to three times above baseline values and occasional nausea and diarrhea. Renal toxicity occurs in about 15% of patients and usually manifests as proteinuria. Reversible hair thinning is seen occasionally. Immunomediated hemolysis or thrombocytopenia have been rarely observed.

Perhaps the most significant side effects are neurologic, including impairment of concentration, short-term memory, and other cognitive functions. More serious neurotoxicity with frontal lobe and Parkinsonian syndromes, depression, and psychotic reactions have been observed and mandate discontinuation of therapy.

Late autoimmune side effects such as hypothyroidism and generalized autoimmune phenomena were documented (M. Talpaz, unpublished data). The development of systemic lupus erythematosus in a patient with CML after 45 months of therapy with IFN was reported.[183]

INTERFERON COMBINED WITH OTHER TREATMENT MODALITIES. Combination therapies were initiated to improve the response rate. Maintenance therapy with IFN-α-2b with a dose 2×10^6 U/m^2 three times weekly after remission induction with busulfan was evaluated by Bergsagel and coworkers.[184] With low-dose therapy, these investigators were able to maintain remission in 6 of 8 patients studied for 3+ to 24+ months. Another approach included intensive chemotherapy induction followed by IFN-α.[185] Intensive chemotherapy consisted of three cycles of daunorubicin (120 mg/m^2 on day 1), cytarabine (80 mg/m^2 daily for 10 days), vincristine (2 mg on day 1), and prednisone (100 mg daily for 5 days). Maintenance therapy with IFN-α at doses of 3×10^6 to 5×10^6 U/m^2 daily was adjusted according to cell counts and toxicity. Of the 32 patients studied in the benign phase of the disease, 28 (86%) had Philadelphia chromosome suppression with intensive chemotherapy; 21 (66%) of them had major or complete Philadelphia chromosome suppression. The effect was transient in most the patients, but cytogenetic remission was maintained in 8 patients (31%) for 12+ months, for a range of 22+ to 42+ months.

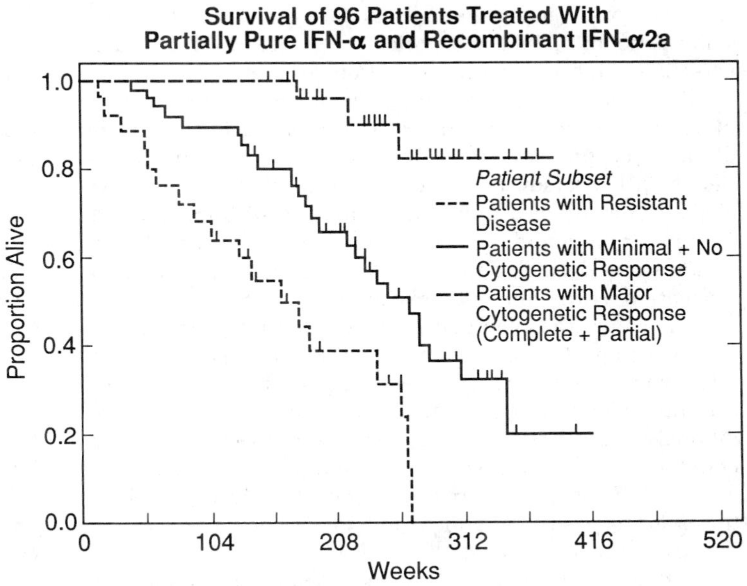

Survival of 96 Patients Treated With Partially Pure IFN-α and Recombinant IFN-α2a

FIGURE 55–4. Survival of complete and partial cytogenetic responders, minor or no cytogenetic responders, and CML patients resistant to interferon therapy.

Concomitant administration of IFN-α with various drugs was studied by several investigators. The combination of IFN-α and low-dose cytarabine or hydroxyurea compares favorably with the results of IFN-α alone. However, the combination-therapy studies have not accrued a sufficient number of patients nor have they been followed long enough to draw conclusions about improvement in the survival rate or the incidence of durable cytogenetic response.[186–188]

IFN-γ suppresses in vitro hematopoietic progenitors in a fashion similar to IFN-α and induces differentiation of leukemia cells.[189–192] A study of IFN-γ (Genentech, South San Francisco, CA) at doses of 0.25 to 0.5 mg/m^2 given intramuscularly daily was conducted in CML Philadelphia-positive patients.[193] Six of 26 patients have achieved a complete hematologic remission; 4 had partial hematologic remissions. Five patients had minor cytogenetic improvements, with emergence of 5% to 45% diploid cells in the bone marrow. Control of thrombocytosis was achieved in all 4 patients with a baseline platelet count of more than $1 \times 10^6/\mu l$. Fever and flu-like symptoms were the most common side effects. The study of combined INF-α and INF-γ in the treatment of CML was prompted by the in vitro synergistic effect of the two molecules.[194,195] Recombinant IFN-α and rIFN-γ were administered on alternating weeks, each at doses ranging from 2 to 10×10^6 U/m^2 given intramuscularly daily. Eleven (41%) of 27 patients achieved complete hematologic remissions, and 3 (11%) achieved partial hematologic remissions. Cytogenetic responses were seen in 6 patients. Niederle and associates found similar results; hematologic responses could be induced in 12 (23%) of 23 patients, with durations of 8+ to 20+ months, and partial hematologic remissions were achieved by another 8 patients.[196] Two patients achieved complete cytogenetic remissions. We and others failed to demonstrate improved response rates with the combination of INF-α and INF-γ, although the schedule used may not have been optimal.

MECHANISMS OF INTERFERON ACTION. The cause of IFN resistance among CML patients is poorly understood. IFN binds to a specific receptor on the cell surface. However, no discernible defects were detected in receptor binding affinity and receptor down regulation after therapy with IFN.[197]

IFN induces multiple genes, commonly known as IFN-stimulated genes (ISG), some with defined function (*e.g.*, 2′,5′-oligoadenylate synthetase [2′,5′A], interferon-associated protein kinase P67; major histocompatibility complex class I; metallothionein II), others with still unknown functions (*e.g.*, ISG-15, ISG-54; genes denoted 6-16, 6-26, and 9-27).[198–202] Studies of cell lines sensitive and resistant to IFN-α have demonstrated a spectrum of defects in induction of 2′,5′A, ISG-15, ISG-54, or 6-16 mRNA in IFN-resistant CML patients.[203–206]

A different approach evaluated the interaction between CML progenitor cells and bone marrow stroma layers.[207] It was suggested that the clinical efficacy of IFN in CML may be due in part to its ability to counteract the defect in attachment of CML progenitor cells to stroma, bringing them under more normal regulatory control. However, no report is available on the changes in IFN-resistant disease. IFN was also shown to interfere with the effect of various growth factors by modulating the receptor to these cytokines or by altering the growth factor-induced cellular signal transduction.[208–210] These studies suggested that resistance may be due to the autonomous production of cytokines by the malignant clone during the progression of CML.[211,212]

Bone Marrow Transplantation

ALLOGENEIC BONE MARROW TRANSPLANTATION. CML is a hematologic malignancy characterized by excessive proliferation of a single clone myeloid cells and their progenitors. The disease can be divided into two phases, an initial chronic phase in which cell maturation is normal, followed by transformation to the acute phase (*i.e.*, blast crisis), characterized by maturation arrest at the level of the myeloblast or lymphoblast.[213] Some patients develop a transient accelerated phase before development of overt blast crisis. Median survival from diagnosis is approximately 4 years. Although some patients may have a prolonged course, CML is a universally fatal disease with conventional therapy.

Allogeneic or syngeneic bone marrow transplantation is an effective treatment for CML, capable of producing long-term disease-free survival.[214,215] The objective is cure of the patient's CML by eradication of the leukemic clone with marrow ablative chemoradiotherapy and restoration of hematopoiesis by transplantation of normal donor-derived stem cells. Most patients receive high-dose cyclophosphamide and total-body irradiation as the antileukemia preparative regimen before bone marrow transplantation. The combination of busulfan and cyclophosphamide without radiotherapy appears equally effective.[216,217] It has not been possible to substantially improve the antileukemia efficacy of the preparation regimen with additional systemic chemotherapy or irradiation without a concomitant increase in toxicity.[218] In addition to the cytotoxic effects of the preparative regimen, considerable data indicate that a graft-versus-leukemia immunologic effect is also important to prevent relapse.[219]

Approximately 20% of syngeneic transplant recipients transplanted in blast crisis have survived free of disease longer than 5 years, demonstrating that the intensive marrow ablative therapy can eradicate even far advanced disease in some patients.[200] Better results have been reported for patients receiving syngeneic bone marrow transplantation while in chronic phase; the actuarial continuous remission rate and survival rate are each approximately 65% at longer than 5 years.

Over 2000 patients with CML have received allogeneic marrow transplantation from an HLA-identical donor.[221–225] For patients transplanted in acute phase, 10% to 20% survive over 5 years in continuous remission; the major cause of treatment failure is leukemia relapse; the actuarial relapse rate is approximately 60%. Patients transplanted while in an accelerated phase or a second chronic phase after blast crisis have had somewhat better results; the actuarial relapse rate is approximately 40%, and the 5-year survival rate is 30%. The best results have been reported with allogeneic bone marrow transplantation for patients in the chronic phase; the actuarial disease-free survival rate is approximately 50% to 60% at 5 years, and fewer than 20% of patients have relapsed. The best results are reported for young patients and those transplanted within 1 year of diagnosis.[226]

Several conclusions can be drawn from these data. Patients with CML in blast crisis or the accelerated phase have a poor prognosis with conventional treatment; median survival is less than 3 months, and few patients survive 1 year. Allogeneic and syngeneic bone marrow transplantations are generally unsuccessful in these patients, but a small proportion may achieve long-term disease-free survival. Results have been better in patients transplanted in chronic phase. The optimal timing of transplantation in chronic-phase patients is controversial. The risks and potential benefits of early bone marrow transplantation must be balanced against the risk of delaying the treatment (*i.e.*, transformation of the leukemia). For patients who are clinically stable, there is a relatively constant risk of transformation to the acute phase; approximately 25% of patients surviving at any point develop acute-phase disease during the ensuing year and die of their disease. Several investigators have reported prognostic factors that may identify good-, average-, and poor-risk groups when treated with conventional treatment.[227,228] Early bone marrow transplantation appears justified in patients with an average or poor prognosis, but a conservative approach may advisable for patients with good prognostic features. This recommendation may need to be reexamined because of the encouraging preliminary data for using INF-α in some patients with early chronic-phase CML.[229]

Most patients who are otherwise appropriate candidates for allogeneic bone marrow transplantation lack an HLA-identical sibling donor. An alternative approach for transplantation involves the use of HLA-nonidentical relatives or unrelated HLA-matched donors. There is a greater risk of acute graft-versus-host disease and graft failure with mismatched or unrelated donor transplants and a higher risk of early mortality. The risk of chronic graft-versus-host disease is also increased with HLA nongenotypically matched transplants.[230–235]

Related donor-recipient pairs that are mismatched for only one A, B, or D HLA locus or HLA phenotypically identical parent-child pairs have survival indistinguishable from transplantation between HLA-identical siblings.[230] Patients mismatched for 2 or more loci have poorer results with a high risk of graft rejection, graft-versus-host disease, and other complications. The development of large registries of potential unrelated donors has allowed evaluation of allogeneic bone marrow transplantation from unrelated HLA phenotypically identical or closely matched donors.[232–235] Approximately 45% of patients transplanted in CML in chronic phase or acute leukemia in remission and 30% with more advanced disease have achieved disease-free survivals of longer than 2 years.[236–237] The higher risks associated with transplants from unrelated or HLA-nonidentical donors have led many centers to reserve this approach for patients who fail to respond to interferon or other more conservative initial therapy.

GRAFT-VERSUS-LEUKEMIA. Allogeneic bone marrow transplantation was originally proposed as a means to escalate the doses of myelotoxic chemoradiotherapy to supralethal levels, using marrow transplantation to restore hematopoiesis. Considerable evidence indicates that the preparative regimen does not usually eradicate the malignancy and an additional immunomediated graft-versus-leukemia effect is important to prevent relapse.

Graft-versus-leukemia is closely associated with the presence of graft-versus-host disease.[238,239] This antileukemic effect correlates best with chronic graft-versus-host disease. The impact of acute graft-versus-host disease is uncertain, but the lowest rate of relapse occurs in patients with acute and chronic graft-versus-host disease. These data suggest that the graft-versus-leukemia effect occurs over many months to years.

Patients receiving transplants from identical twin donors do not develop graft-versus-host disease; these patients have at least twice the risk of relapse of CML as transplant recipients from HLA-identical siblings.[219,224] Conversely, patients transplanted from unrelated donors have a significantly higher rate of graft-versus-host disease; these patients appear to have a lower risk of leukemia relapse than those with transplants from HLA-identical siblings.[235] T-cell depletion of donor bone marrow is the most effective means of preventing acute and chronic graft-versus-host disease, but this benefit has been offset by the substantial increase in the risk of leukemia relapse.[215,234,240–242] The net effect is no change or worsening of disease-free survival.[243] The increase in leukemia relapse is most striking for patients with CML than other forms of leukemia.[243] In a study of the International Bone Marrow Transplant Registry, 12% of patients with CML in chronic phase receiving unmodified HLA-identified bone marrow transplants relapsed, compared with a relapse rate of more than 50% with T-cell-depleted transplants.[244] This marked increase in the rate of relapse is seen in comparing T-cell-depleted recipients who develop graft-versus-host disease with unmodified allograft recipients without graft-versus-host disease. This strongly suggests an effect of T lymphocytes independent of graft-versus-host disease. The high relapse rate for T-cell-depleted transplants indicates that viable leukemia cells survive the preparative regimen and are capable of reestablishing the disease in most patients. Consistent with these data is the observation that after transplantation of unmodified bone marrow, Philadelphia-positive metaphases can be detected intermittently in many patients, even though most never experience a hematologic relapse; growth of these leukemic cells is presumably controlled by the graft-versus-leukemia effect that must be operative over an extended period.[244] It may still be possible to successfully employ T-cell depletion to prevent graft-versus-host disease; several centers are evaluating the use of higher doses of total-body irradiation or the addition of thiotepa or other drugs to the preparative regimen to enhance engraftment and improve the cytotoxicity against leukemia cells.

The recognition and effector mechanisms that mediate graft-versus-leukemia and the cell populations involved are incompletely understood. CD4- and CD8-positive T-cell clones reactive with leukemia cells have been described, and cytotoxic T lymphocytes are likely to be the primary effector cells. LAK and natural killer cells may also be important in this process, and IL-2 may enhance the antileukemic activity.[245–247]

It is uncertain whether the graft-versus-leukemia reaction can be differentiated from graft-versus-host disease in humans or whether the same or different cell populations mediate each process. After allogeneic marrow transplants, stable chimerism with donor-derived hematopoiesis is the rule, although mixed chimerism occurs in some cases. The graft-versus-leukemia effect may result from reactivity directed against host hematopoietic tissue in general. Such an effect would prevent competitive repopulation by normal and leukemic host-derived hematopoietic cells, and this potential mechanism would not require recognition of leukemia-specific antigens.

It is conceivable that different cellular subsets are responsible for graft-versus-host disease and the graft-versus-leukemia effect. CD4-positive T cells recognize antigens presented with class II MHC antigens. CD8-positive lymphocytes recognize antigens presented in the context of class I loci. CD4-positive cells mediate acute graft-versus-host disease in MHC class II disparate recipients, and CD8-positive cells are primarily responsible with class I disparate transplants in mice.[246] Depletion of the CD8-positive suppressor T cells is sufficient to reduce or prevent graft-versus-host disease in most donor-recipient murine strain combinations that are MHC compatible but mismatched for minor histocompatibility loci. We reported that selective depletion of CD8-positive cells in combination with posttransplant cyclosporine resulted in a significantly reduced rate of acute graft-versus-host disease and an increase in the risk of leukemia relapse.[247] Improved methods to selectively enhance the graft-versus-leukemia effect may be possible.

AUTOLOGOUS BONE MARROW TRANSPLANTATION. For the past 2.5 years, patients at the M.D. Anderson Cancer Center who are ineligible for interferon or allograft therapy have been allocated to intensive therapy followed by autologous bone marrow transplantation without purging in an attempt to decrease the evolution of the disease from the early indolent phase to the more aggressive fulminant acute leukemic transformation, which results in death from bleeding and infection. Kantarjian first exposed patients to conventional-dose chemotherapy (*i.e.*, daunomycin, high-dose ara-C), which is designed to reduce the total leukemia cell burden and to permit the regrowth of normal cells in the marrow. In 50% of patients, some degree of cytogenetic remission was achieved. After recovery from this conventional-dose chemotherapy, peripheral blood cells were collected during the stages of early recovery (total leukocyte count between 300/mm^3 and 800/mm^3), because it had been shown by Carella and his colleagues that the probability of collecting circulating diploid early progenitor cells in the peripheral blood was high at this time of early hematopoietic recovery.

The patients then were exposed to total-body irradiation, cyclophosphamide, and VP-16 in doses that would totally ablate endogenous hematopoietic activity. Marrow function was regenerated through infusion of an engrafting dose of the autologous marrow. After recovery of hematopoietic function, interferon maintenance therapy was used. This last stage was designed to provide biologic maintenance therapy that would serve the function associated with the graft-versus-leukemia effect in allograft patients. These patients were treated at a median of 2.5 years from diagnosis. The median follow-up was 800 days for this group of patients. The patients who were given the autologous transplants in first chronic phase with this regimen had a survival rate that was equivalent to patients treated with allografts with the same preparative regimen.

In contrast to the favorable survival (70%) of the first chronic-phase patients, the survival rate of the second chronic-phase accelerated or blast crisis patients given autografts was in the 35% range. There are at least two possible explanations for the adverse lower survival of the second group. First, an overall increase in resistance in advanced disease patients results in persisting systemic disease after delivery of the preparative regimen. Second, the small number of neoplastic cells that are infused in the autologous marrow may have more significant impact on the natural history of the disease in advanced chronic patients.

There are two possible responses to this data: deliver more intensive systemic preparative therapy or increase the stringency of purging. Unfortunately, an increase in treatment-related mortality may accompany the use of more stringent preparative regimens due to an increase in nonextramedullary toxicity. Increasing the stringency of the marrow-cleansing procedures may remove too many reconstituting progenitor cells, delaying recovery and increasing the mortality from infections during neutropenia. It is important to have an assay that can differentiate between a relapse that arose from residual systemic disease or insufficient stringency of bone marrow purging.

RETROVIRAL MARKING TO IDENTIFY ORIGIN OF RELAPSE AFTER MARROW TRANSPLANTATION. As shown in Figure 55–5, retroviral marking is a procedure that can differentiate the origin of relapse in autologous bone marrow transplantation. In this procedure, autologous cells are collected after recovery from conventional-dose therapy that is designed to promote repopulation of the marrow by normal autologous stem cells. The cells are then concentrated and fractionated with monoclonal antibodies that recognize antigens specific for normal or leukemia cells, and the resulting marrow is exposed to a safety-modified retrovirus to mark the leukemia and normal cells in the autologous marrow. The marrow is reinfused, and the patient followed.

If relapse occurs, the cells are assayed for the presence of leukemia cells that contain the viral marker using a PCR assay. The leukemia cells that are marked can be identified by a PCR assay for *BCR-ABL*-encoded mRNA. If the leukemia cells contain the viral marker, we conclude that the relapse arose from residual cells left in the autologous marrow after the purging of the autologous marrow. In that case, we would focus on increasing the stringency of the marrow purging procedure. Our algorithm for this program is summarized in Table 55–4.

GENETIC THERAPY

A natural extension of the marking program in autologous transplantation is the use of autologous transplants for genetic therapy. Genetic therapy involves the replacement of the missing or nonfunctional molecular elements in the DNA of living cells or the introduction of additional genetic elements into these cells. This therapy is designed to correct alterations within living cells that lead to disease in man.

Several steps are required to implement such therapy. The oncologist must have the capability for isolating the progenitor cells, which when modified can contribute to the repopulation of marrow after intensive therapy and which dominate that tissue and the population of cells that arise within it for prolonged periods. The genetic information and introducing the genetic information must not result in undesirable changes within these populations of living cells. The genetic changes introduced must confer a selective advantage for the cell or at least are subject to selective techniques that have limited potential for generating toxicity and at the same time can suppress the unmodified population of cells. The genetic change must involve a single genetic defect that is dominant

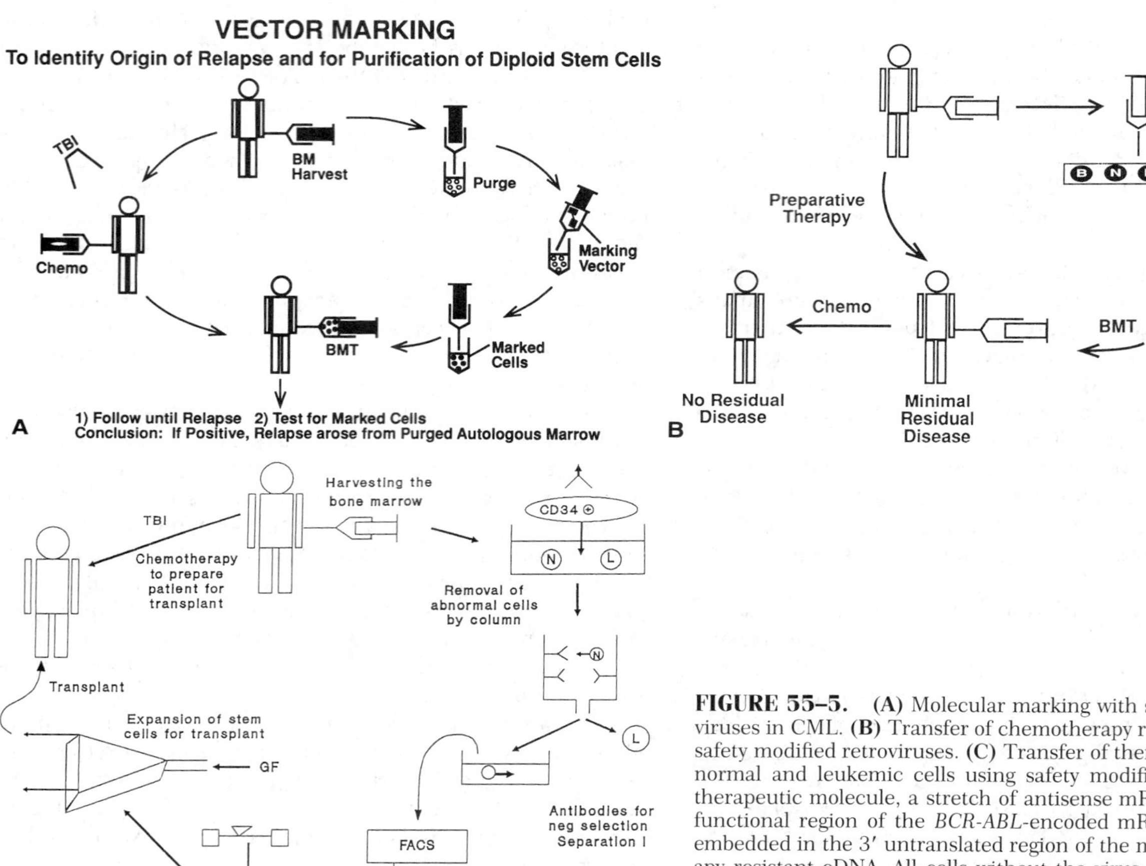

FIGURE 55–5. **(A)** Molecular marking with safety-modified retroviruses in CML. **(B)** Transfer of chemotherapy resistance genes using safety modified retroviruses. **(C)** Transfer of therapeutic molecules to normal and leukemic cells using safety modified retroviruses. The therapeutic molecule, a stretch of antisense mRNA homologous to a functional region of the *BCR-ABL*-encoded mRNA of CML cells, is embedded in the 3′ untranslated region of the multidrug chemotherapy resistant cDNA. All cells without the virus are killed by chemotherapy. The normal cells transduced by the virus are protected from chemotherapy. Although the transduced leukemia cells can acquire drug resistance, they will be suppressed by the antisense ribozyme sequence.

TABLE 55–4. Molecular Marking Program

I. Daunomycin-high dose cytosine arabinoside to induce second chronic phase or cytogenetic remission
II. Harvesting of autologous marrow
III. CD34-positive selection of early progenitor cells
IV. Negative selection
V. Marking with safety-modified retrovirus
VI. Preparative therapy with total-body irradiation, VP-16, and cyclophosphamide
VII. Infusion with marked marrow
VIII. Interferon maintenance therapy after hematopoietic recovery

in the population of hematopoietic cells under consideration for therapy.

CML, because it arises from a single chromosomal translocation that produces a known genetic change within the hematopoietic population of progenitor cells, has been studied as a possible model for this molecular targeting approach. The fact that a single genetic change has occurred within the population of abnormal cells permits the use of molecular assays that are totally specific and unusually sensitive to measure the impact of the genetic therapy on the phenotype of the cell, to optimize the conditions that result in genetic modification, and to evaluate immediately the impact of therapy.

This marking program could be the first stage of a three-step program to use bone marrow transplantation and retroviral marking to develop populations of hematopoietic cells that are enriched in the early pluripotent hematopoietic stem cell and to then genetically modify these cells before autologous transplantation as corrective therapy for the disease:

1. Use of safety-modified retroviruses to mark the autologous cells used for transplant after purging (see Figure 55–5A). This helps identify the origin of relapse, differentiating between residual systemic disease and the neoplastic cells left in the autologous cells after purging and the degree to which the fractionation procedures are enriching the early progenitor cells by the percentage of cells that contain the retroviral transgenome.
2. Use of safety-modified retroviruses to introduce into normal early progenitor cells chemotherapy-resistance genes (see Figure 55–5B). This helps to decrease hematopoietic toxicity after chemotherapy and to establish methods for in vivo selection of genetically modified hematopoietic cells. This would be done in solid tumor patients whose marrow is not involved with cancer.
3. Use of safety-modified retroviruses that contain chemotherapy-resistance genes and therapeutic molecules (see Figure 55–5C) that can be used to control a disease.

The use of fractionation of hematopoietic cells with monoclonal antibodies for purging of leukemia cells and the use of retroviruses in the transplantation setting provide opportunities to develop populations of autologous marrow that are enriched in normal early progenitor cells.

It is possible that investigators will be able to use the percentage of diploid cells that are positive for the retroviral transgenome and the lineage distribution of such cells to monitor the efficiency of fractionation in enriching the hematopoietic stem cell. After fractions of autologous marrow that are sufficiently enriched in early normal progenitor cells are developed by this method, genetic correction models that have shown promise in preclinical or in vitro models will be tested.

CONCLUSION

Major advances are occurring in the therapy for the chronic leukemias. It is likely that these diseases will be a major proving ground for the development of genetic and molecular approaches to therapy, as they have for the established modalities of radiation therapy, chemotherapy, biologic therapy, and bone marrow transplantation during the past 40 years.

REFERENCES

1. Polliack A, Catovsky D, eds. Chronic lymphocytic leukemia. Jerusalem, Israel: Harwood Academic Publishers, 1988.
2. Silber R, Stahl R. Chronic lymphocytic leukemia and related diseases. In: Williams W, Beutler E, Erslev AJ, Lichtman MA, eds. Hematology. New York: McGraw-Hill, 1990:1005.
3. Minot GR, Isaacs R. Lymphatic leukemia: Age incidence, duration and benefit derived from irradiation. Boston Med Surg 1924;191:1.
4. Rai KR, Sawitsky A, Cronkite EP, et al. Clinical staging of chronic lymphocytic leukemia. Blood 1975;46:219.
5. Binet JL, LePorrier M, Dighiero G, et al. A clinical staging system for chronic lymphocytic leukemia. Cancer 1977;40:855.
6. Preud'homme JL, Seligmann M. Surface-bound immunoglobulins as a cell marker in human lymphoproliferative diseases. Blood 1972;40:777.
7. Korsmeyer SJ. Hierarchy of immunoglobulin gene rearrangements in B-cell leukemias. In: Waldman TA, ed. Molecular genetic analyses of human lymphoid neoplasms: Immunoglobulin genes and the c-*myc* oncogene. Ann Intern Med 1985;102:497.
8. Gahrton G, Robert K-H, Friberg K, et al. Nonrandom chromosomal aberrations in chronic lymphocytic leukemia revealed by polyclonal B-cell-mitogen stimulation. Blood 1980;56:640.
9. Surveillance Epidemiology End Results Incidence and Mortality Data: 1973–1977. NCI monograph 57. Bethesda, MD: National Cancer Institute, 1981:10.
10. Gunz FW, Dameshek W. Chronic lymphocytic leukemia in a family including twin brothers and a son. JAMA 1957;164:1323.
11. Reilly EB, Rappaport SI, Karr NW, et al. Familial chronic lymphatic leukemia. Arch Intern Med 1952;90:87.
12. Conley CL, Misiti J, Laster AJ. Genetic factors predisposing to chronic lymphocytic leukemia and to autoimmune disease. Medicine (Baltimore) 1980;5:323.
13. Han T, Ozer H, Sadamori N, et al. Prognostic importance of cytogenetic abnormalities in patients with chronic lymphocytic leukemia. N Engl J Med 1984;310:288.
14. Gahrton G, Robert K-H, Friberg K, Zech L, Bird AG. Nonrandom chromosomal aberrations in chronic lymphocytic leukemia revealed by polyclonal B-cell-mitogen stimulation. Blood 1980;56:640.
15. Hurley JN, Fu SM, Kunkel HG, Chaganti RSK, German J. Chromosome abnormalities of leukaemic B lymphocytes in chronic lymphocytic leukaemia. Nature 1980;283:76.
16. Juliusson G, Oscher DG, Fitchett M, et al. Prognostic subgroups in B-cell chronic lymphocytic leukemia defined by specific chromosomal abnormalities. N Engl J Med 1990;323:720.
17. Han T, Ozer H, Sadamori N, et al. Prognostic importance of cytogenetic abnormalities in patients with CLL. N Engl J Med 1984;310:288.
18. Vahdati M, Graafland H, Emberger JM. Isochromosome 17q in cell lines of two cases of B cell chronic lymphocytic leukemia. Cancer Genet Cytogenet 1983;9:227.
19. Han T, Henderson ES, Emrich LJ, et al. Prognostic significance of karyotypic abnormalities in B-cell chronic lymphocytic leukemia: An update. Semin Hematol 1987;24:257.
20. Callen DF, Ford JH. Chromosome abnormalities in chronic lymphocytic leukemia revealed by TPA as a mitogen. Cancer Genet Cytogenet 1983;10:87.
21. Morita M, Minowada J, Sandberg AA. Chromosomes and causation of human cancer and leukemia. XLV: Chromosome patterns in stimulated lymphocytes of chronic lymphocytic leukemia. Cancer Genet Cytogenet 1981;3:293.
22. O'Donnell PV, Nowinski RC, Stockert E. Amplified expression of murine leukemia virus (MuLV)-coded antigens on thymocytes and leukemia cells of AKR mice after infection by dualtropic (MCF) MuLV. Virology 1982;119:450.
23. Gahrton G, Robert KH, Friberg K, et al. Extra chromosome 12 in chronic lymphocytic leukemia. Lancet 1980;1:146.
24. Knuutila S, Elonen E, Teerenhovi L, et al. Trisomy 12 in B-cells of patients with B-cell chronic lymphocytic leukemia. N Engl J Med 1986;314:865.
25. Erikson J, Finan J, Tsujimoto Y, et al. The chromosome 14 breakpoint in neoplastic B cells with the t(11;14) translocation involves the immunoglobulin heavy chain locus. Proc Natl Acad Sci USA 1984;81:4144.
26. Jones GT, Abramson N. Gastrointestinal necrosis in acute leukemia: A complication of induction therapy. Cancer Invest 1983;1:315.

27. Escudier SM, Pereira-Leahy JM, Goodacre AM, et al. Fluorescence in situ hybridization (FISH) and cytogenetic studies of trisomy 12 in chronic lymphocytic leukemia (CLL). Blood 1991;78(suppl 1):329A.
28. Han T, Emrich LJ, Ozer H, Sandberg AA. Prognostic implications of trisomy 12 and non-trisomy 12 karyotypes in B-cell chronic lymphocytic leukemia. Blood 1985;65: 470.
29. Zech L. Inversion of chromosome 14 marks human T-cell chronic lymphocytic leukaemia. Nature 1984;308:858.
30. Croce CM, Isobe M, Palumbo A, et al. Gene for alpha-chain of human T-cell receptor location on chromosome 14 region involved in T-cell neoplasms. Science 1985;227: 1044.
31. Freedman AS, Boyd AW, Bierber FR. Normal cellular counterparts of B cell chronic lymphocytic leukemia. Blood 1987;70:418.
32. Martin PJ, Hansen JA, Stadak AW, Nowinski RC. Monoclonal antibody recognizing normal human T lymphocytes and malignant human B lymphocytes: A comparative study. J Immunol 1981;127:1920.
33. Perri RT, Royston I, LeBien T, Kay NE. Chronic lymphocytic leukemia progenitor cells carry the antigens T65, BA-1 and Ia. Blood 1983;61:871.
34. Kay NE, Oken MM, Perri RT. The influential T cell in B-cell neoplasms. J Clin Oncol 1983;1:810.
35. Kay NE, Kaplan ME. Defective T cell responsiveness in chronic lymphocytic leukemia: Analysis of activation events. Blood 1986;67:578.
36. Davis S. The variable pattern of circulating lymphocyte subpopulations in chronic lymphocytic leukemia. N Engl J Med 1976;294:1150.
37. Mangan KF, D'Alessandro L. Hypoplastic anemia in B cell chronic lymphocytic leukemia: Evolution of T cell-mediated suppression of erythropoiesis in early-stage and late-stage disease. Blood 1986;66:533.
38. Ayanlar-Bateman O, Ebert E, Hauptman SP. Defective IL-2 production and responsiveness by T cells in patients with chronic lymphocytic leukemia of B cell variety. Blood 1986;67:279.
39. Foa R, Fierro MT, Raspadori D, et al. Lymphokine-activated killer (LAK) cell activity in B and T chronic lymphoid leukemia: Defective LAK generation and reduced susceptibility of the leukemic cells to allogeneic and autologous LAK effectors. Blood 1990;76:1349.
40. Perri RT. Impaired expression of cell surface receptors for B-cell growth factor by chronic lymphocytic leukemia cells. Blood 1986;67:943.
41. Dadmarz R, Rabinowe SN, Cannistra SA, Anderson JW, Freedman AS, Nadler LM. Association between clonogenic cell growth and clinical risk group in B-cell chronic lymphocytic leukemia. Blood 1990;76:142.
42. Rai KR, Sawitsky A. Studies in clinical staging, lymphocyte function, and markers as an approach to the treatment of CLL. In: Silber R, Gordon AS, Lobue J, Muggia FM, eds. Contemporary hematology/oncology. New York: Plenum, 1981:227.
43. Robertson LE, Huh Y, Hirsch-Ginsberg C, et al. Clinical, immunophenotypic and molecular analysis of the completeness of response in chronic lymphocytic leukemia after fludarabine. Blood [Abstract] 1990;76(suppl 1):314A.
44. Andreeff M. Cell kinetics of leukemia. Semin Hematol 1986;23:300.
45. Andreeff M. Flow cytometry of leukemia. In: Melamed MR, Mendelsohn ML, eds. Flow cytometry and cell sorting. New York: Alan R. Liss, 1990:697.
46. Theml H, Trepel G, Schick P, et al. Kinetics of lymphocytes in chronic lymphocytic leukemia: Studies using continuous ^{3}H-thymidine infusion in two patients. Blood 1973;42:623.
47. Squires J, Redner A, Andreeff M. *P53* expression in human leukemia: Restriction to lymphoid cell lineage and potential prognostic importance in acute lymphoblastic leukemia. Proc Am Assoc Cancer Res [Abstract] 1988;29:454.
48. del Giglio A, Zhang W, O'Brien S, et al. Relationship of elevated intranuclear p53 levels in chronic lymphocytic leukemia to marrow architecture and PCNA antigen expression. Proc Am Assoc Cancer Res 1991;32:290.
49. del Giglio A, O'Brien S, Ford R, et al. The prognostic value of proliferating cell nuclear antigen expression in chronic lymphoid leukemia. Blood (in press).
50. Montserrat E, Sanchez-Bisono J, Vinolas N, Rozman C. Lymphocyte doubling time in chronic lymphocytic leukaemia: Analysis of its prognostic significance. Br J Haematol 1986;62:567.
51. Herweijer H, Sonneveld P, Baas F, Nooter K. Expression of *mdr1* and *mdr3* multidrug resistance genes in human acute and chronic leukemias and association with stimulation of drug accumulation by cyclosporine. JNCI 1990;82:1133.
52. Rai KR, Sawitsky A, Cronkit EP, Chanana AD, Levy RN, Pasternack BS. Clinical staging of chronic lymphocytic leukemia. Blood 1975;46:219.
53. Binet J, Auquier A, Dighiero G, et al. A new prognostic classification of chronic lymphocytic leukemia derived from a multivariate survival analysis. Cancer 1981;48:198.
54. Montserrat E, Vinolas N, Reverter JC, Rozman C. Natural history of chronic lymphocytic leukemia: On the progression and prognosis of early clinical stages. Nouv Rev Fr Hematol 1988;30:359.
55. Binet JL, Catovsky D, Chandra P, et al. Chronic lymphocytic leukaemia: Proposals for a revised prognostic staging system, Report from the International Workshop on CLL. Br J Haematol 1981;48:365.
56. Cheson BD, Bennett JM, Rai KR, et al. Guidelines for clinical protocols for chronic lymphocytic leukemia: Recommendations of the National Cancer Institute-sponsored Working Group. Am J Hematol 1988;29:152.
57. International Workshop on Chronic Lymphocytic Leukemia. Chronic lymphocytic leukemia: Recommendations for diagnosis, staging and response criteria. Ann Intern Med 1989;110:236.
58. Galton DAG, Wiltshaw E, Szur L, Dacie JV. The use of chlorambucil and steroids in the treatment of chronic lymphocytic leukemia. Br J Haematol 1961;7:73.
59. Ezdinli EZ, Stutzman L. Chlorambucil therapy for lymphomas and chronic lymphocytic leukemia. JAMA 1965;191:444.
60. Alberts DS, Chang SY, Chen HSG, Larcom BJ, Jones SE. Pharmacokinetics and metabolism of chlorambucil in man: A preliminary report. Cancer Treat Rev 1979;6:9.
61. Knospe WH, Loeb V Jr, Huguley CM Jr. Bi-weekly chlorambucil treatment of chronic lymphocytic leukemia. Cancer 1974;33:555.
62. Liepman M, Votaw ML. The treatment of chronic lymphocytic leukemia with COP chemotherapy. Cancer 1978;41:1664.
63. Oken MM, Kaplan ME. Combination chemotherapy with cyclophosphamide, vincristine, and prednisone in the treatment of refractory chronic lymphocytic leukemia. Cancer Treat Rep 1979;63:441.
64. Sawitsky A, Rai KR, Glidewell O, Silver RT, and participating members of the Cancer and Leukemia Group B. Comparison of daily versus intermittent chlorambucil and prednisone therapy in the treatment of patients with chronic lymphocytic leukemia. Blood 1977;50:1049.
65. Ezdinli EZ, Stutzman L, Aungst CW, Firat D. Corticosteroid therapy for lymphomas and chronic lymphocytic leukemia. Cancer 1969;23:900.
66. Han T, Ezdinli EZ, Shimaoka K, Desai DV. Chlorambucil vs. combined chlorambucil-corticosteroid therapy in chronic lymphocytic leukemia. Cancer 1973;31:502.
67. Keller JW, WH Knospe, Raney M, et al. Treatment of chronic lymphocytic leukemia using chlorambucil and prednisone with or without cycle-active consolidation chemotherapy. Cancer 1986;58:1185.
68. Montserrat E, Alcala A, Parody R, and participating members of Pethema, Spanish Cooperative Group for Hematological Malignancies Treatment, Spanish Society of Hematology. Treatment of chronic lymphocytic leukemia in advanced stages. Cancer 1985;56:2369.
69. Montserrat E, Alcala A, Alonso C, and participating members of Pethema, Spanish Society of Hematology. A randomized trial comparing chlorambucil plus prednisone vs cyclophosphamide, melphalan, and prednisone in the treatment of chronic lymphocytic leukemia stages B and C. Nouv Rev Fr Hematol 1988;30:429.
70. Raphael B, Andersen JW, Silber R, et al. Comparison of chlorambucil and prednisone versus cyclophosphamide, vincristine, and prednisone as initial treatment for chronic lymphocytic leukemia: Long-term follow-up of an Eastern Cooperative Oncology Group randomized clinical trial. J Clin Oncol 1991;9:770.
71. Jaksic B, Brugiatelli M. High dose chlorambucil for the treatment of B-chronic lymphocytic leukemia (CLL). Update of I.G.C.I. CLL trials, Proceedings of the 5th International Workshop on CLL—Sitges, Barcelona, 1991:62.
72. The French Cooperative Group on Chronic Lymphocytic Leukemia. Effects of chlorambucil and therapeutic decision in initial forms of chronic lymphocytic leukemia (stage A): Results of a randomized clinical trial on 612 patients. Blood 1990;75:1414.
73. The French Cooperative Group on Chronic Lymphocytic Leukaemia. A randomized clinical trial of chlorambucil versus COP in stage B chronic lymphocytic leukemia. Blood 1990;75:1422.
74. The French Cooperative Group on Chronic Lymphocytic Leukaemia. Effectiveness of "CHOP" regimen in advanced untreated chronic lymphocytic leukaemia. Lancet 1986: 1346.
75. Catovsky D, Richards S, Fooks J, Hamblin TJ. CLL trials in the United Kingdom—The medical research council CLL trials 1, 2 and 3. Leuk Lymphoma 1991;5:105.
76. Hansen MM, Andersen E, Birgens H, et al. CHOP versus chlorambucil + prednisolone in chronic lymphocytic leukemia. Leuk Lymphoma 1991;5:97.
77. Kimby E, Mellstedt H. Chlorambucil/prednisone versus CHOP in symptomatic chronic lymphocytic leukemias of B-cell type. A randomized trial. Leuk Lymphoma 1991;5: 93.
78. Keating MJ, Hester JP, McCredie KB, Burgess MA, Murphy WK, Freireich EJ. Long-term results of CAP therapy in chronic lymphocytic leukemia. Leuk Lymphoma 1990;2: 391.
79. Keating MJ, Scouros M, Murphy S, et al. Multiple agent chemotherapy (POACH) in previously treated and untreated patients with chronic lymphocytic leukemia. Leukemia 1988;2:157.
80. Kempin S, Lee BH III, Thaler HT, et al. Combination chemotherapy of advanced chronic lymphocytic leukemia: The M-2 protocol (vincristine, BCNU, cyclophosphamide, melphalan and prednisone). Blood 1982;60:1110.
81. Grever MR, Kopecky KJ, Coltman CA, et al. Fludarabine monophosphate: A potentially useful agent in chronic lymphocytic leukemia. Nouv Rev Fr Hematol 1988;30:457.
82. Keating MJ, Kantarjian H, Talpaz M, et al. Fludarabine: A new agent with major activity against chronic lymphocytic leukemia. Blood 1989;74:19.
83. Keating MJ, Kantarjian H, O'Brien S, et al. Fludarabine: A new agent with marked cytoreductive activity in untreated chronic lymphocytic leukemia. J Clin Oncol 1991;9: 44.
84. Keating MJ, Kantarjian H, O'Brien S, Redman J, Childs C, McCredie K. Fludarabine (FLU)–prednisone (PRED): A safe, effective combination in refractory chronic lymphocytic leukemia. Proceedings of the American Society of Clinical Oncology, San Francisco, 1989:210.
85. Puccio CA, Mittelman A, Lichtman SM, et al. A loading dose/continuous infusion schedule of fludarabine phosphate in chronic lymphocytic leukemia. J Clin Oncol 1991;9:1562.
86. Grever MR, Leiby JM, Kraut EH, Wilson HE, Neidhart JA, Wall RL, Balcerzak SP. Low-dose deoxycoformycin in lymphoid malignancy. J Clin Oncol 1985;3:1196.
87. Dillman RO, Mick R, McIntyre OR. Pentostatin in chronic lymphocytic leukemia: A phase II trial of cancer and leukemia group B. J Clin Oncol 1989;7:433.
88. Saven A, Carrera CJ, Carson DA, Beutler E, Piro LD. 2-Chlorodeoxyadenosine treatment of refractory chronic lymphocytic leukemia. Leuk Lymphoma 1991;5:133.
89. Robertson LE, Huh Y, Hirsch-Ginsberg C, et al. Clinical, immunophenotypic, and

molecular analysis of the completeness of response in chronic lymphocytic leukemia after fludarabine. Blood 1990;76:314A.

90. Michallet M, Corront B, Molina L, et al. Allogeneic bone marrow transplantation in chronic lymphocytic leukemia: 17 cases. Report of the EBMT. Leuk Lymphoma 1991;5:127.
91. Jansen J, Schutt HRE, Zwet TL van, Meifer CJLM, Hijmans W. Hairy-cell leukaemia: A B-lymphocytic disorder. Br J Haematol 1979;42:21.
92. Galton DAG, Goldman JM, Wiltshaw E, et al. Prolymphocytic leukemia. Br J Haematol 1974;27:7.
93. Sadamori N, Han T, Minowada J, et al. Possible specific chromosome change in prolymphocytic leukemia. Blood 1983;62:729.
94. Kantarjian H, Childs C, O'Brien S, et al. Efficacy of fludarabine, a new adenine nucleoside analogue in patients with prolymphocytic leukemia and the prolymphocytoid variant of chronic lymphocytic leukemia. Am J Med 1991;90:223.
95. Golomb HM, Catovsky D, Golde DW. Hairy cell leukemia: A clinical review based on 71 cases. Ann Intern Med 1978;89:677.
96. Cleary ML, Good GS, Warnke R, et al. Immunoglobulin gene rearrangements in hairy cell leukemia. Blood 1984;64:99.
97. Golomb HM, Vardiman JW. Response to splenectomy in 65 patients with hairy cell leukemia: An evaluation of spleen weight and bone marrow involvement. Blood 1983;61:349.
98. Caligaris-Cappio F, Pizzolo G, Chilosi M, et al. Phorbol ester induces abnormal chronic lymphocytic leukemia cells to express features of hairy cell leukemia. Blood 1985;66:1035.
99. Quesada JR, Hersh EM, Manning J, et al. Treatment of hairy cell leukemia with recombinant alpha interferon. Blood 1985;68:493.
100. Spiers ASD, Moore D, Cassileth P, et al. Remission in hairy cell leukemia with pentostatin. N Engl J Med 1987;316:825.
101. Piro LD, Carrera CJ, Carson DA, Beutler E. Lasting remissions in hairy cell leukemia induced by a single infusion of 2-chlorodeoxyadenosine. N Engl J Med 1990;322:117.
102. Estey E, Kurzrock R, Kantarjian H, et al. Treatment of hairy cell leukemia with 2-chlorodeoxyadenosine (2-CdA). Blood 1992;79:882.
103. Hoffman R, Kopel S, Hsu SD, Dainiak N, Zanjani ED. T cell chronic lymphocytic leukemia: Presence in bone marrow and peripheral blood of cells that suppress erythropoiesis in vitro. Blood 1978;52:255.
104. Aisenberg AC, Krontiris TG, Mak TW, et al. Rearrangement of the gene for the beta chain of the T-cell receptor in T-cell chronic lymphocytic leukemia and related disorders. N Engl J Med 1985;313:529.
105. Brouet JC, Flandrin G, Sasportes M, et al. CLL of T-cell origin: Immunologic and clinical evaluation in 11 patients. Lancet 1973;2:890.
106. Foa R, Pelicci P-G, Mignone N, et al. Analysis of T-cell receptor beta chain (T-beta) gene rearrangements demonstrates the monoclonal nature of T-cell chronic lymphoproliferative disorders. Blood 1986;67:247.
107. Chan WC, Link S, Mawle A, et al. Heterogeneity of large granular lymphocyte proliferations-delineation of two major subtypes with distinct origins, immunophenotypes, functional and clinical characteristics. Blood 1986;68:1142.
108. Palutke M, Eisenberg L, Kaplan J, et al. Natural killer and suppressor T-cell chronic lymphocytic leukemia. Blood 1983;62:627.
109. Melo JV, Catovsky D, Galton DAG. The relationship between chronic lymphocytic leukaemia and prolymphocytic leukaemia. II. Patterns of evolution of prolymphocytoid transformation. Br J Haematol 1986;64:77.
110. Melo JV, Catovsky D, Galton DAG. The relationship between chronic lymphocytic leukaemia and prolymphocytic leukaemia. IV: Analysis of survival and prognostic features. Br J Haematol 1987;65:23.
111. Zarrabi MH, Grunwald HW, Rosner F. Chronic lymphocytic leukemia terminating in acute leukemia. Arch Intern Med 1977;137:1059.
112. Brouet JC, Preud'homme JL, Seligmann M, et al. Blast cells with monoclonal surface immunoglobulin in two cases of acute blast crisis supervening on chronic lymphocytic leukaemia. Br Med J 1973;4:23.
113. McPhedran P, Heath CW. Acute leukemia occurring during chronic lymphocytic leukemia. Blood 1970;35:7.
114. Januszewicz E, Cooper IA, Pilkington G, et al. Blastic transformation of chronic lymphocytic leukemia. Am J Hematol 1983;15:399.
115. Richter MN. Genealized reticular cell sarcoma of lymph nodes associated with lymphocytic leukemia. Am J Pathol 1928;4:285.
116. Foucar K, Rydell RE. Richter's syndrome in chronic lymphocytic leukemia. Cancer 1980;46:118.
117. Minot GR, Buckman TE, Isaacs R. Chronic myelogenous leukemia: Age, incidence, duration and benefit derived from irradiation. JAMA 1924;82:1489–1494.
118. Reinhard EH, Neely L, Samples DM. Radioactive phosphorus in the treatment of chronic leukemias: Long-term results over a period of 15 years. Ann Intern Med 1959;50:942.
119. Barrett AJ, Longhurst P, Humble JG, Newton KA. Effect of splenic irradiation on circulating colony-forming cells in chronic granulocytic leukaemia. Br Med J 1977;14:1259.
120. Galton DAG. Myleran in chronic myeloid leukemia. Lancet 1953;1:208.
121. Fishbein WN, Carbone PP, Freireich EJ. Clinical trials of hydroxyurea in patients with cancer and leukemia. Clin Pharmacol Ther 1964;5:574.
122. Haut A, Abbott WS, Wintrobe MM, Cartwright GE. Busulfan in the treatment of chronic myelocytic leukemia: The effect of long-term intermittent therapy. Blood 1961;17:1.
123. Sokal JE. Evaluation of survival data from chronic myelocytic leukemia. Am J Hematol 1979;1:493–500.
124. Kennedy BJ, Yarbro JW. Metabolic and therapeutic effects of hydroxyurea in chronic myeloid leukemia. JAMA 1966;195:1038–1043.
125. Kennedy BJ. Hydroxyurea therapy in chronic myelogenous leukemia. Cancer 1972;29:1052–1056.
126. Tanzer J, Briere J, Aucleic A, et al. Long term results for 47 patients with Ph[1]+ chronic myelocytic leukemia given hydroxyurea as major treatment. Blood 1979;54:212A.
127. Schwartz JH, Canellos GP. Hydroxyurea in the management of hematologic complications of chronic granulocytic leukemia. Blood 1975;46:11–16.
128. Feingold ML, Koss LG. Effects of long-term administration of busulfan. Arch Intern Med 1969;124:66–71.
129. Bolin RW, Robinson WA, Sutherland J, Hamman R. Busulfan vs hydroxyurea in long-term therapy of chronic myelogenous leukemia. Cancer 1982;50:1683–1686.
130. Rushing D, Goldman A, Gibbs G, Howe R, Kennedy BJ. Hydroxyurea versus busulfan in the treatment of chronic granulocytic leukemia. Am J Clin Oncol 1982;5:307–313.
131. Sullivan JR, Hurley, Bolton JH. Treatment of chronic myeloid leukemia with repeated single doses of busulfan. Cancer Treat Rev 1977;61:43–45.
132. Vicariot M, Goldman JM, Catovsky D, Galton DAG. Treatment of chronic granulocytic leukaemia with repeated single doses of busulfan. Eur J Cancer 1979;15:559–563.
133. Schwarzenberg L, Mathe G, Pouillart P, et al. Hydroxyurea, leucopheresis, and splenectomy in chronic myeloid leukemia at the problastic phase. Br Med J 1973;1:700–703.
134. Djaldetti M, Padeh B, Pinkhas J, Deries A. Prolonged remission in chronic myeloid leukemia after one course of busulfan. Blood 1966;27:103–109.
135. Finney R, McDonald GA, Baikie AG, Douglas AS. Chronic granulocytic leukaemia with Ph[1] negative cells in hypoplasia. Br J Haematol 1972;23:283–288.
136. Golde DW, Bersch NL, Sparkes RS. Chromosomal mosaicism associated with prolonged remission in chronic myelogenous leukemia. Cancer 1976;37:1849–1852.
137. Brandt L, Mitelman F, Panani A, Lenner HC. Extremely long duration of chronic myeloid leukaemia with Ph[1] negative and Ph[1] positive bone marrow cells. Scand J Haematol 1976;16:321–325.
138. Singer CRJ, McDonald GA, Douglas AS. Twenty-five year survival of chronic granulocytic leukaemia with spontaneous karyotype conversion. Br J Haematol 1984;57:309–313.
139. Zago MA, Costa FF, Bottura C. Cytogenetic remission in a Ph[1]-positive case of chronic myelogenous leukaemia. Scand J Haematol 1977;22:91–95.
140. Sokal JE, Leong SS, Gomez GA. Preferential inhibition by cytarabine of CFU-GM from patients with chronic granulocytic leukemia. Cancer 1987;59:197–202.
141. Spiers ASD, Lorch CA, Harrison BA. Chronic granulocytic leukemia (CGL) in chronic phase with two Ph+ cell lines and suppression of one line by hydroxyurea. Blood Suppl 1986;1:233a.
142. Cunningham I, Gee T, Dowling M, et al. Results of treatment of Ph[1]+ chronic myelogenous leukemia with an intensive treatment regimen (L-5 protocol). Blood 1979;53:375–396.
143. Hester JP, Waddell CC, Coltman CA Jr, et al. Response of chronic myelogeneous leukemia patients to COAP-splenectomy. Cancer 1984;54:1977–1982.
144. Kantarjian HM, Vellekoop L, McCredie KB, et al. Intensive combination chemotherapy (ROAP) and splenectomy in the management of chronic myelogenous leukemia. J Clin Oncol 1985;3:192–300.
145. Brodsky L, Fuscaldo KE, Kahn SB, Conroy JF, Lamping CG. Chronic myelogenous leukemia: A clinical and experimental evaluation of splenectomy and intensive chemotherapy. Semin Hematol 1975;8:143.
146. Got T, Nishikori M, Arlin Z. Growth characteristics of leukemia and normal hematopoietic cells in Ph[1]+ chronic myelogenous leukemia and effects of intensive treatment. Blood 1982;59:793–803.
147. Fitzgerald D, Rowe JM, Heal J. Leukapheresis for control of chronic myelogenous leukemia during pregnancy. Am J Hematol 1986;22:213–218.
148. Lowenthal RM, Buskard NA, Goldman JM, et al. Intensive leukapheresis as initial therapy for chronic granulocytic leukemia. Blood 1975;46:835–844.
149. Vallejos CS, McCredie KB, Brittin GM, Freireich EJ. Biological effects of repeated leukapheresis of patients with chronic myelogenous leukemia. Blood 1973;42:925–933.
150. Goldman JM, Lowenthal RM, Buskard NA, Spiers ASD, Th'ng KH, Park DS. Chronic granulocytic leukemia-selective removal of immature granulocytic cells by leukapheresis. Semin Hematol 1975;8:28–40.
151. Neiman F, Brandt L, Nilsson PG. Cytogenetic evidence for splenic origin of blast transformation in chronic myelogenous leukemia. Scand J Haematol 1974;13:87–90.
152. Baccarani M, Zaccaria A, Santucci AM, et al. A simultaneous study of bone marrow, spleen, and liver in chronic myeloid leukemia: Evidence for differences in cell composition and karyotypes. Semin Hematol 1975;8:81–112.
153. Mitelman F. Comparative cytogenetic studies of bone marrow and extramedullary tissues in chronic myeloid leukaemia. Semin Hematol 1975;8:113–117.
154. Sharp JC, Joyner MV, Wayne AW, et al. Karyotypic conversion in Ph[1]-positive chronic myeloid leukaemia with combination chemotherapy. Lancet 1979;1:1370–1372.
155. Smalley RV, Vogel J, Huguley CM, et al. Chronic granulocytic leukemia: Cytogenetic conversion of the bone marrow with cycle-specific chemotherapy. Blood 1977;50:107–113.
156. Ihde DC, Canellos GP, Schwartz JH, DeVita VT. Splenectomy in the chronic phase of chronic granulocytic leukemia. Effects in 32 patients. Ann Intern Med 1976;84:17–21.
157. Spiers ASD, Ermidou-Szeidis C, Richards HGH. Chronic granulocytic leukaemia: Clinical course, blood and bone marrow changes after chemotherapy and splenectomy. Haematologica 1979;64:616–634.
158. Medical Research Council's Working Party for Therapeutic Trials in Leukemia. Ran-

domized trial of splenectomy in Ph[1] positive chronic granulocytic leukaemia, including an analysis of prognostic factor. Br J Haematol 1983;54:415–430.
159. The Italian Cooperative Study Group on Chronic Myeloid Leukemia. Results of a prospective randomized trial of early splenectomy in chronic myeloid leukemia. Cancer 1984;54:333–338.
160. Kantarjian HM, Keating MJ, Talpaz M, et al. Chronic myelogenous leukemia in blast crisis: An analysis of 242 patients. Am J Med 1987;83:445–454.
161. Goldman JM, Johnson SA, Islam A, Catovsky D, Galton DAG. Haematological reconstitution after autografting for chronic granulocytic leukaemia in transformation: The influence of previous splenectomy. Br J Haematol 1980;45:223–231.
162. Gratwohl A, Goldman J, Gluckman E, Zwann F. Effect of splenectomy before bone-marrow transplantation on survival in chronic granulocytic leukaemia. Lancet 1985;2: 1290–1291.
163. Canellos GP, Sutliffe SB, DeVita VT, Lister TA. Treatment of refractory splenomegaly in myeloproliferative disease by splenic artery infusion. Blood 1979;53:1014–1017.
164. Isaacs A, Lindemann J. Virus interference. 1. The interferons. Proc R Soc Lond (Biol) 1957;147:258–267.
165. Stewart WEI, ed. The interferon system. New York: Springer-Verlag, 1979.
166. Borden EC, Fall LA. Interferons: Biochemical, cell growth, inhibitory, and immunological effects. Prog Hematol 1981;12:299–339.
167. Vilcek J, Gray PW, Rinderknecht E, et al. Interferon-gamma: A lymphokine for all seasons. In: Rick E, ed. Lymphokines, vol 12. Orlando: Academic Press, 1985:1.
168. Talpaz M, McCredie KB, Mavligit GM, Gutterman JU. Leukocyte interferon-induced myeloid cytoreduction in chronic myelogenous leukemia. Blood 1983;62:689–692.
169. Talpaz M, Kantarjian HM, McCredie KB, Keating MJ, Trujillo J, Gutterman J. Clinical investigation of human alpha interferon in chronic myelogenous leukemia. Blood 1987;69:1280–1288.
170. Talpaz M, Kantarjian HM, McCredie KB, Trujillo JM, Keating MJ, Gutterman JU. Hematologic remission and cytogenetic involvement induced by recombinant human interferon alpha in chronic myelogenous leukemia. N Engl J Med 1986;314:1065–1069.
171. Talpaz M, Kurzrock R, Kantarjian H, Gutterman JU. Recent advances in the therapy of chronic myelogenous leukemia. In: DeVita V, ed. Important advances in oncology. Philadelphia: JB Lippincott, 1988:297.
172. Talpaz M, Kantarjian H, Kurzrock R, Trujillo JM, Gutterman JU. Interferon-alpha produces sustained cytogenetic responses in chronic myelogenous leukemia. Philadelphia chromosome-positive patients. Ann Intern Med 1991;114:532–538.
173. Niederle N, Doberauer C, Kloke O, Osieka R, Schweers C, Schmidt CG. Treatment of chronic myelogenous leukemia with recombinant interferon alpha (IFN-α2b). Proc Am Soc Clin Oncol 1986;5:236.
174. Alimena G, Morra E, Lazzarino M, et al. Interferon alpha-2b as therapy for Ph1-positive chronic myelogenous leukemia: A study of 82 patients treated with intermittent or daily administration. Blood 1988;72:642–647.
175. Ozer H, Mick R, Testa J, et al. Subcutaneous α-interferon (α-IFN) shows substantial activity in untreated chronic phase Philadelphia chromosome positive (Ph[1]) chronic myelogenous leukemia (CML). Proc Am Soc Clin Oncol 1988;7:A684.
176. Ozer H. Biotherapy of chronic myelogenous leukemia with interferon. Semin Oncol 1988;15:14–20.
177. Tura S, Russo D, Zuffa E, Fiacchini M. A prospective comparison of human recombinant interferon α-2A (Roferon-A) and conventual chemotherapy in chronic myeloid leukemia (CML). Interim report of the Italian Study. Blood 1990;76(suppl 1):329A.
178. Hehlmann R, Manneheim, Heimpel H, et al. Prospective controlled comparison of busulfan vs hydroxyurea vs interferon alpha in chronic myelogenous leukemia (CML). Blood 1990;76(suppl 1):279A.
179. Yoffe G, Blick M, Kantarjian H, Spitzer G, Gutterman J, Talpaz M. Molecular analysis of interferon-induced suppression of Philadelphia chromosome in patients with chronic myeloid leukemia. Blood 1987;69:961–963.
180. Lee MS, Chang KS, Freireich EJ, et al. Detection of minimal residual bcr/abl transcripts by a modified polymerase chain reaction. Blood 1988;72:893–897.
181. Dhingra K, Kurzrock R, Kantarjian H, et al. Polymerase chain reaction (PCR) for minimal residual disease in 20 CML patients in complete cytogenetic response induced by interferon therapy. Blood 1989;74:235A.
182. Kurzrock R, Gutterman JU, Kantarjian H, Talpaz M. Therapy of chronic myelogenous leukemia with interferon. Cancer Invest 1989;7:83–91.
183. Schilling PJ, Kurzrock R, Kantarjian H, Gutterman JU, Talpaz M. Development of systemic lupus erythematosus after interferon therapy for chronic myelogenous leukemia. Cancer 1991;68:1536–1537.
184. Bergsagel DE, Haas RH, Messner HA. Interferon alpha 2 in treatment of chronic granulocytic leukemia. Semin Oncol 1986;13:29–34.
185. Kantarjian HM, Talpaz M, Keating MJ, et al. Intensive chemotherapy induction followed by interferon-alpha maintenance in patients with Philadelphia chromosome-positive chronic myelogenous leukemia. Cancer 1991;68:1201–1207.
186. Ma DDF, Arthur CK. Treatment of chronic myeloid leukemia (CML) using alpha-interferon (IFN), and low dose cytosine arabinoside (ara-C). Blood 1989;74:363A.
187. Guilhot F, Tanzer J, Brizard A, Huret JL, Dreyfus B. Combination of alpha-2a interferon and chemotherapy in Ph+ chronic myelogenous leukemia (CML) updated results. Proc Am Soc Clin Oncol 1989;8:A788.
188. Kantarjian H, Keating M, McCredie K, et al. Treatment of advanced stages of Philadelphia-chromosome (Ph)-positive chronic myelogenous leukemia (CML) with alpha interferon (IFN-A) and low-dose cytosine arabinoside (ara-C). Blood 1989;7:235A.
189. Klimpel GR, Fleischmann WF Jr, Klimpel KD. Gamma interferon (IFN-gamma) and IFN-alpha/beta suppress murine myeloid colony formation (CFUOC): Magnitude of suppression is dependent upon level of colony-stimulating factor (CSF). J Immunol 1982;129:76–80.
190. Raefsky EL, Platanias LC, Zoumbos NC, Young NS. Studies of interferon as a regulator of hematopoietic cell proliferation. J Immunol 1982;135:2507–2512.
191. Broxmeyer HE, Williams DE, Lu L, et al. The suppressive influences of human tumor necrosis factor on bone marrow hematopoietic progenitor cells from normal donors and patients with leukemia: Synergism of tumor necrosis factor and interferon-gamma. J Immunol 1986;136:4487–4495.
192. Ball ED, Guyre PM, Shen L, et al. Gamma-interferon induces monocytoid differentiation in the HL-60 cell line. J Clin Invest 1984;73:1072–1077.
193. Kurzrock R, Talpaz M, Kantarjian H, et al. Therapy of chronic myelogenous leukemia with recombinant interferon-γ. Blood 1987;70:943–947.
194. Talpaz M, Kurzrock R, Kantarjian H, et al. A phase II study of alternating alpha-2a-interferon and gamma-interferon therapy in patients with chronic myelogenous leukemia. Cancer 1991;68:2125–2130.
195. Czarniecki CW, Fennie CW, Powers DB, Estell DA. Synergistic antiviral and antiproliferative activities of *E. coli* derived human alpha, beta, and gamma interferons. J Virol 1984;49:490–496.
196. Niederle N, Wandl U, Kloke O, et al. Efficacy of interferon alpha (IFN alpha-2b) and IFN gamma in chronic myelogenous leukemia (CML). Proc Am Soc Clin Oncol 1989;8: 185.
197. Maxwell B, Talpaz M, Gutterman JU. Down-regulation of peripheral blood cell interferon receptors in chronic myelogenous leukemia patients undergoing human interferon (HuIFN) therapy. Int J Cancer 1985;36:23–28.
198. Levy D, Larner A, Chaudhuri A, Babiss LE, Darnell JE Jr. Interferon-stimulated transcription: Isolation of an inducible gene and identification of its regulatory region. Proc Natl Acad Sci USA 1986;83:8929–8933.
199. Larner AC, Chaudhuri A, Darnell JE Jr. Transcriptional induction by interferon. New protein(s) determine the extent and length of the induction. J Biol Chem 1986;261: 453–459.
200. Kelly JM, Porter ACG, Chernajovsky Y, Gilbert CS, Stark GR, Kerr IM. Characterization of a human gene inducible by α- and γ-interferons and its expression in mouse cells. EMBO J 1986;5:1601–1606.
201. Rutherford MN, Hannigan GE, Williams BRG. Interferon-induced binding of nuclear factors to promoter elements of the 2-5A synthetase gene. EMBO J 1988;7:751–759.
202. Rice AP, Kerr SM, Roberts WK, Brown RE, Kerr IM. Novel 2',5'-oligoadenylates synthesized in interferon-treated, vaccinia virus-infected cells. J Virol 1985;56:1041–1044.
203. Dron M, Tovey MG, Eid P. Isolation of Daudi cells with reduced sensitivity to interferon. III. Interferon-induced proteins in relation to the phenotype of interferon resistance. J Genet Virol 1985;66:787–795.
204. Reid TR, Race ER, Wolff BH, Friedman RM, Merigan TC, Basham TY. Enhanced in vivo therapeutic response to interferon in mice with an in vitro interferon-resistant B-cell lymphoma. Cancer Res 1989;49:4163–4169.
205. Affabris E, Romeo G, Belardelli F, et al. 2-5A synthetase activity does not increase in interferon-resistant Friend leukemia cell variants treated with α/β interferon despite the presence of high-affinity interferon receptor sites. Virology 1983;125:508–512.
206. Talpaz M, Chernajovsky Y, Troutman-Worden K, et al. Interferon stimulated genes in interferon-sensitive and resistant chronic myelogenous leukemia (CML) patients. Cancer Res (in press).
207. Dowding C, Guo A-P, Osterholz J, Siczkowski M, Goldman J, Gordon M. Interferon-α overrides the deficient adhesion of chronic myeloid leukemia primitive progenitor cells to bone marrow stromal cells. Blood 1991;78:499–505.
208. Pfeffer LM, Donner DB, Tamm I. Interferon-alpha down-regulates insulin receptors in lymphoblastoid (Daudi) cells. Relationship to inhibition of cell proliferation. J Biol Chem 1987;262:3665–3670.
209. Fish EN, Banerjee K. Growth control: Characterizations of the antagonism between growth factors and interferon. J Interferon Res 1989;9:2–7.
210. Pfeffer LM, Tamm I. Interferon-beta inhibition of concanavalin A-stimulated calcium uptake and exchange in HeLa cells. J Interferon Res 1986;6:551–556.
211. Estrov Z, Kurzrock R, Wetzler M, et al. Suppression of chronic myelogenous leukemia colony growth by IL-1 receptor antagonist and soluble IL-1 receptors: A novel application for inhibitors of IL-1 activity. Blood 1991;78:1476–1484.
212. Wetzler M, Kurzrock R, Lowe DG, Kantarjian H, Gutterman JU, Talpaz M. Alteration in bone marrow stromal growth factor expression: A novel mechanism of disease progression in chronic myelogenous leukemia. Blood 1991;78:2400–2406.
213. Champlin RE, Golde DW. Chronic myelogenous leukemia: Recent advances. Blood 1985;65:1039–1047.
214. Thomas ED, Storb R, Clift RA, et al. Bone marrow transplantation. N Engl J Med 1975;292:832–843, 895–902.
215. Champlin RE, Goldman JM, Gale RP. Bone marrow transplantation in chronic myelogenous leukemia. Semin Hematol 1988;25:74–80.
216. Santos GW, Tutschka PJ, Brookmeyer R, et al. Marrow transplantation for acute non-lymphocytic leukemia after treatment with busulfan and cyclophosphamide. N Engl J Med 1983;309:1347.
217. Copelan EA, Grever MR, Kapoor N, Tutschka PJ. Marrow transplantation following busulfan and cyclophosphamide for chronic myelogenous leukaemia in accelerated or blastic phase. Br J Haematol 1989;71:487–491.
218. Clift RA, Buckner CD, Appelbaum FR, et al. Allogeneic marrow transplantation in patients with chronic myeloid leukemia in the chronic phase: A randomized trial of two irradiation regimens. Blood 1991;77:1660–1665.
219. Gale RP, Champlin RE. How does bone marrow transplantation cure leukemia? Lancet 1984;2:28.

220. Fefer A, Cheever MA, Greenberg PD, et al. Treatment of chronic granulocytic leukemia with chemoradiotherapy and transplantation of marrow from identical twins. N Engl J Med 1982;306:63–68.
221. Champlin R, Ho W, Arenson E, Gale RP. Allogeneic bone marrow transplantation in chronic myelogenous leukemia in chronic or accelerated phase. Blood 1982;60:1038–1041.
222. McGlave PB, Arthur DC, Weisdorf D, et al. Allogeneic bone marrow transplantation as treatment for accelerating chronic myelogenous leukemia. Blood 1984;63:219–222.
223. Thomas ED, Clift RA, Fefer A, et al. Marrow transplantation for the treatment of chronic myelogenous leukemia. Ann Intern Med 1986;104:155–163.
224. Goldman JM, Gale RP, Bortin MM, et al. Bone marrow transplantation for chronic myelogenous leukemia in chronic phase: Increased risk of relapse associate with T-cell depletion. Ann Intern Med 1988;108:806–814.
225. Speck B, Bortin MM, Champlin R, et al. Allogeneic bone marrow transplantation for chronic myelogenous leukemia. Lancet 1984;1:665–668.
226. Thomas ED, Clift RA. Indications for marrow transplantation in chronic myelogenous leukemia. Blood 1989;73:861–864.
227. Sokal JE. Evaluation of survival data for chronic myelocytic leukemia. Am J Hematol 1976;1:493–500.
228. Tura S, Baccarni M, Corbelli G, et al. Staging of chronic myeloid leukemia. Br J Haematol 1981;47:105–109.
229. Talpaz M, Kantarjian H, Kurzrock R, Trujillo JM, Gutterman JU. Interferon-alpha produces sustained cytogenetic responses in chronic myelogenous leukemia. Philadelphia chromosome-positive patients. Ann Intern Med 1991;114:532–538.
230. Beatty PG, Clift RA, Mickelson EM, et al. Marrow transplantation from related donors other than HLA-identical siblings. N Engl J Med 1985;313:765.
231. Anasetti C, Amos D, Beatty PG, et al. Effect of HLA compatibility on engraftment of bone marrow transplants in patients with leukemia or lymphoma. N Engl J Med 1989;320:197–204.
232. Beatty PG, Hansen JA, Longton GM, et al. Marrow transplantation from HLA-matched unrelated donors for treatment of hematologic malignancies. Transplantation 1991;51:443–447.
233. Gajewski JL, Ho WG, Feig SA, Hunt L, Kaufman N, Champlin RE. Bone marrow transplantation using unrelated donors for patients with advanced leukemia or bone marrow failure. Transplantation 1990;50:244–249.
234. McGlave PB, Beatty P, Ash R, Hows JM. Therapy for chronic myelogenous leukemia with unrelated donor bone marrow transplantation: Results in 102 cases. Blood 1990;75:1728–1732.
235. Ash RC, Casper JT, Chitambar CR, et al. Successful allogeneic transplantation of T-cell-depleted bone marrow from closely HLA-matched unrelated donors. N Engl J Med 1990;322:485–494.
236. Weiden PL, Sullivan KM, Flournoy N, Storb R, Thomas ED. Antileukemic effect of chronic graft-versus-host disease: Contribution to improved survival after allogeneic marrow transplantation. N Engl J Med 1981;304:1529–1532.
237. Sullivan KM, Weiden PL, Storb R, et al. Influence of acute and chronic graft-versus-host disease on relapse and survival after bone marrow transplantation from HLA-identical siblings as treatment of acute and chronic leukemia. Blood 1989;73:1720–1728.
238. Sullivan KM, Storb R, Buckner CD, et al. Graft-versus-host disease as adoptive immunotherapy in patients with advanced hematologic neoplasms. N Engl J Med 1989;320:828–834.
239. Horowitz MM, Gale RP, Sondel PM, et al. Graft-versus-leukemia reactions after bone marrow transplantation. Blood 1990;75:555–562.
240. Champlin R. T-cell depletion to prevent graft-versus-host disease after bone marrow transplantation. Hematol Oncol Clin North Am 1990;4:687–698.
241. Marmont AM, Horowitz MM, Gale RP, et al. T-cell depletion of HLA-identical transplants in leukemia. Blood 1991;78:2120–2130.
242. Arthur CK, Apperley JF, Guo AP, et al. Cytogenetic events after bone marrow transplantation for chronic myeloid leukemia in chronic phase. Blood 1988;71:1179–1186.
243. Sosman JA, Oettel KR, Smith SD, Hank JA, Fisch P, Sondel PM. Specific recognition of human leukemic cells by allogeneic T-cells: II. Evidence for HLA-D restricted determinants on leukemic cells that are crossreactive with determinants present on unrelated nonleukemic cells. Blood 1990;75:2005–2016.
244. Delmon L, Ythier A, Moingeon P, et al. Characterization of antileukemia cells' cytotoxic effector function. Implications for monitoring natural killer responses following allogeneic bone marrow transplantation. Transplantation 1986;42:252.
245. Hauch M, Gazzola MV, Small T, et al. Anti-leukemia potential of interleukin-2 activated natural killer cells after bone marrow transplantation for chronic myelogenous leukemia. Blood 1990;75:2250–2262.
246. Korngold R, Sprent J. T cell subsets and graft-versus-host disease. Transplantation 1987;44:335–339.
247. Champlin R, Ho W, Gajewski J, et al. Selective depletion of $CD8^+$ T-lymphocytes for prevention of graft-versus-host disease after allogeneic bone marrow transplantation. Blood 1990;76:418–423.

Cancer: Principles & Practice of Oncology, Fourth Edition,
edited by Vincent T. DeVita, Jr., Samuel Hellman, Steven A. Rosenberg.
J.B. Lippincott Co., Philadelphia © 1993.

Sydney E. Salmon
J. Robert Cassady

CHAPTER **56**

Plasma Cell Neoplasms

Plasma cell neoplasms are a group of related disorders, each of which is associated with proliferation and accumulation of immunoglobulin-secreting cells that are derived from the B-cell series of immunocytes. Tumor cells in these neoplasms retain the cytoplasmic differentiation of normal plasma cells and are adapted to high rates of synthesis and secretion of immunoglobulin (Ig). In the normal immune response, individual plasma cells can synthesize and secrete antibody immunoglobulin at rates up to 100,000 molecules each minute.

On the basis of synthesis and secretion of an electrophoretically homogenous immunoglobulin (*i.e.*, M-component or M-protein), plasma cell neoplasms appear to be monoclonal, derived from a single transformed B lymphocyte or plasma cell. Current laboratory data support the concept of the monoclonal origin of B-cell neoplasms. Several synonyms have been applied to plasma cell neoplasms: dysproteinemias, gammopathies, immunoglobulinopathies, monoclonal gammopathies, paraproteinemias, and plasma cell dyscrasias. In terms of incidence and severity, the most important malignant plasma cell neoplasm is multiple myeloma.

The plasma cell neoplasms can be characterized by their monoclonal immunoglobulin products. M-components are seen in the malignant plasma cell disorders (*e.g.*, multiple myeloma, Waldenström's macroglobulinemia) and in clinically ambiguous or idiopathic circumstances, and these products may be associated with benign, premalignant, or early malignant disorders. Idiopathic M-proteins are best described clinically as monoclonal gammopathies of unknown significance (MGUS).[1] Transient M-components have been observed in patients recovering from pneumonia, hepatitis, and other infections; after drug reactions; after other illnesses; or after bone marrow transplantation. The monoclonal immunoglobulins secreted in malignant plasma cell disorders are the equivalent of homogenous normal antibody molecules. The few identified antibody arrangements of M-components appear to be random designs not focused on any specific or tumor-associated antigenic stimulus. An M-component can be detected and differentiated from normal immunoglobulins by serum electrophoresis if the concentration is approximately 0.5 g/dl or higher. Detection of a serum M-component is of major diagnostic value in plasma cell disorders. Quantities of Ig in the range of 0.5 g/dl are the product of approximately 10^9 to 10^{10} monoclonal immunoglobulin-secreting cells in the body.[2] A classification of diseases associated with M-component secretion appears in Table 56–1.

There are five major classes of immunoglobulins synthesized by B lymphocytes and plasma cells: IgG, IgA, IgM, IgD, and IgE. Antibody protein molecules in each of these classes have common monomeric structures. Any one antibody molecule has a monomeric structure composed of two identical heavy (H) chains and two identical light (L) chains, each of which has constant (c) and variable (v) regions of amino acid sequence. The constant regions of the heavy chains for the various classes are γ, α, μ, δ, or ϵ, respectively. There are two types of L chains, κ or λ, and both types are associated with all five immunoglobulin classes.

The constant regions of the molecule define its class specificity and several other biologic characteristics (*e.g.*, the ability to fix complement). Separate genes code for the constant regions of the H and L chains for each H chain class and L chain type. The *variable regions* of H and L chains are considered to be structurally related to the region of the specific antigen-binding site of the molecule and are unique to each specific antibody. A large set of *v* genes code for the variable portions of the Ig molecule, which create the wide variety of antibody specificities in the normal immune response. The variable region of an M-component can be identified immunologically as having a specific *idiotype*, or unique structural region, that

TABLE 56–1. Classification of Disorders Associated With Monoclonal Immunoglobulin (M-Component) Secretion

Disorder	*M-Component*	
Plasma Cell Neoplasms		
Multiple myeloma	IgG > IgA > IgD > IgE; ±free L chain or L chain alone (κ > λ); rarely biclonal or without detectable Ig abnormality	
"Solitary" myeloma of bone		
Extramedullary plasmacytoma		
Macroglobulinemia	IgM ± free L chain (κ > λ)	
Heavy-chain disease	γ, α, or μ chain or fragment; δ, or ε	
Primary amyloidosis	Free L chain (λ > κ) or L chain fragment alone or plus IgG, IgA, IgM, or IgD	
Monoclonal gammopathy of unknown significance	IgG, IgM, IgA, or IgD usually without urinary L chain secretion	
Other B-Cell Neoplasms		
Chronic lymphocytic leukemia	M-component (occasionally secreted) IgM > IgG	
B-cell non-Hodgkin's lymphomas (any morphologic pattern or lymphoid cell types)		
Nonlymphoid Neoplasms		
Chronic myelogenous leukemia	No consistent patterns	
Carcinoma of colon, breast, prostate, or other sites		
"Autoimmune" or Autoreactive Disorders		
Cold agglutinin disease (some characteristics of Waldenström's)	M-component	Antibody activity of M-component
	IgMκ most common	Anti-I antigen of RBC membrane
	IgM	Anti-IgG
Mixed cryoglobulinemia	IgG	Anti-IgG
Hypergammaglobulinemia	IgM	?
Sjögren's syndrome		
Miscellaneous Inflammatory Storage, or Infectious Disorders		
Lichen myxedematosus	IgGλ	
Gaucher's disease	IgG	
Cirrhosis, sarcoid, parasitic diseases, renal acidosis	No consistent pattern	

(Modified from Salmon SE. Plasma cell disorders. In: Wingaarden JB, Smith LH Jr, eds. Cecil textbook of medicine. 18th ed. 1988:1026–1036)

differentiates it from virtually all other immunoglobulin antibody molecules. Table 56–2 summarizes structural and functional properties of normal immunoglobulins. These properties are generally shared by M-proteins.

Although not clinically practical, radioimmunoassay for the idiotype on a serum M-component could detect as few as 10^3 to 10^4 neoplastic cells in the body.[2] For all Ig classes other than IgM, the monomeric form of the Ig is secreted and has a molecular mass (M_r) of approximately 150,000 to 190,000. Immunoglobulin is secreted as a pentameric unit with a M_r of 900,000. As with several other proteins, immunoglobulins are secreted with various amounts of attached carbohydrate; this also applies to M-components. Although myeloma can be diagnosed in patients with any of the Ig types previously summarized, IgM M-components are usually associated with other malignant or benign plasma cell disorders. The synthesis of H and L chains is usually well balanced in normal antibody-producing clones. However, in neoplastic clones, biosynthesis of intracellular H and L chains is sometimes "unbalanced," with an excess synthesis of free L chains that are secreted by the cell as dimers of M_r 60,000. Because of their relatively low molecular mass, L chain dimers are normally filtered by the renal glomerulus, partially reabsorbed and catabolized in the renal tubules, and partially excreted in the urine. Detection of substantial quantities of free light chains in the urine serves as a useful diagnostic test in myeloma and related disorders.

Serum M-components are usually observed as a sharp peak or "spike" in the β- or γ-globulin regions on electrophoresis. Urinary M-components are usually detected in concentrates of 24-hour urine collections, and they migrate similarly on electrophoresis. Definition of an M-component as monoclonal requires H and L chain typing. This is done with immuno-

TABLE 56–2. Properties of Normal Immunoglobulins

Characteristics	*IgG*	*IgA*	*IgM*	*IgD*	*IgE*
Molecular mass	150,000	160,000	900,000	180,000	200,000
Subclasses	4	2	1	2(?)	1
Serum concentration (mg/dl; mean)	1140	180	100	3	0.03
Fixes complement	+	+	+	−	+
Carbohydrate (%)	2.6	5–10	10	10–12	11
$T_{1/2}$ (days)	23.6*	5.8	5.1	2.8	2.3

* Half-life varies proportionally to total serum IgG concentration.

electrophoresis or immunofixation techniques. Examples of serum and urine protein electrophoresis and H and L chain typing by immunofixation in a myeloma case are depicted in Figure 56–1.

HISTORY

Although skeletal evidence for the existence of myeloma in earlier millennia has been obtained from Egyptian mummies and other anthropologic remains, the first published descriptions of major clinical features of a patient with multiple myeloma were made in about 1850 in England. A well-respected tradesman, Thomas Alexander McBean, was seen by Dr. William Macintyre of London in 1845. The patient's symptoms included episodes of fatigue, diffuse bone pain, and urinary frequency. Macintyre treated McBean during the course of that year, and from urinalysis tests, Macintyre detected a urinary protein with the heat properties often observed for urinary L chains. He diagnosed "mollities and fragilitas ossium" based on the patient's bony symptoms and consulted with Dr. Thomas Watson concerning therapy for his patient.[4] Later that year, Dr. Henry Bence Jones also tested urine specimens provided by Macintyre and Watson and corroborated the heat properties of urinary L chains (*i.e.*, now called Bence Jones proteins). Bence Jones thought that the protein was the "hydrated deuteroxide of albumin" and published his findings several years before Macintyre published his case report.[5] Bence Jones also emphasized the potential importance of looking for this urinary protein in other cases with mollities ossium. After the patient died in 1846, a surgeon, Dr. John Dalrymple, examined several bones and made gross and microscopic observations. His drawings are consistent with the morphology of myeloma cells.[6]

In 1873, Rustizky independently described a similar patient and employed the term *multiple myeloma* for the first time to focus on the multiple bone tumors that were present.[7] In 1889, Kahler published a major view on multiple myeloma, and the disease became known, particularly in Europe, as Kahler's disease.[8] Ellinger, in 1899, identified the increased serum proteins and sedimentation rate in myeloma.[9] In 1900, Wright published a case report in which he indicated that myeloma did not arise from the red marrow but was a neoplasm comprising specifically plasma cells.[10] Wright's case was probably the first in which x-ray films were used to show diagnostic abnormalities in the patient's ribs.

Other developments that enhanced the diagnosis or understanding of myeloma included the development of bone marrow aspiration in 1929 and of electrophoresis to separate serum proteins in 1937.[11,12] Within several years after the development of electrophoresis, the tall narrow-based spike in the γ-globulin zone was identified in myeloma.[13] In 1938, Magnus-Levy[14] described amyloidosis as a complication of multiple myeloma, and in 1953, Grabar and Williams[15] developed immunoelectrophoresis, which enabled the precise immunologic identification of the H and L chains in a monoclonal immunoglobulin, enhancing the diagnosis of monoclonality of an Ig. In the 1970s, structural evidence for the relation of amyloid in myeloma to the variable component of L chains was subsequently achieved by Glenner and his colleagues by studying the amino acid sequence of solubilized amyloid fibrils.[16] Other developments included quantitation

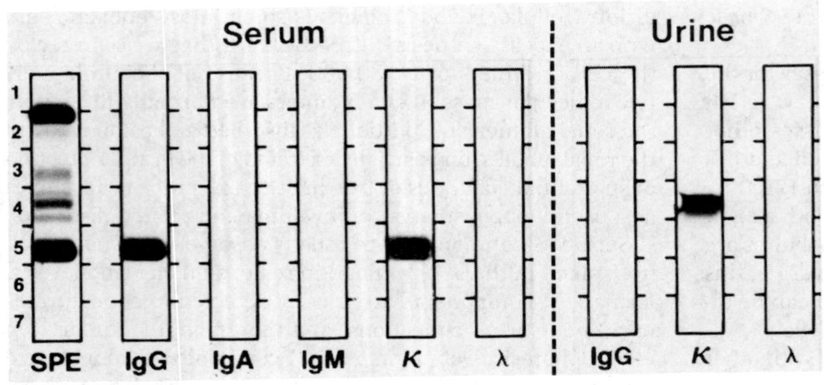

FIGURE 56–1. Identification of serum and urine M-components by the immunofixation technique. The labels indicate the specificity of the antiserum used in developing the immunofixation pattern. In this case, the patient has an IgGκ serum M-component and κ Bence Jones proteinuria.

of the total body burden of tumor cells in myeloma and development of a useful staging system.[17] Several cytokines or interleukins (IL), such as IL-1 and IL-6, have been implicated in myeloma pathophysiology.

Systemic treatment was essentially without effect until 1947, when initial results with urethan in a few patients provided evidence that chemotherapeutic approaches might be of value.[18] A subsequent randomized trial indicated that the survival of patients receiving urethan was inferior to that observed with a placebo.[19] Several other drugs, including nitrogen mustard, 6-mercaptopurine, and 5-fluorouracil, were tried and appeared to be of no value.[20] In 1958, the use of a racemic mixture of D- and L-phenylalanine mustards (Sarcolysine) was reported to be of use in myeloma by Blokhin and colleagues.[21] Subsequently, the D- and L-isomers of phenylalanine mustard were tested separately, and the antimyeloma activity was found to reside in the L-isomer, melphalan. In 1962, Bergsagel and colleagues of the Southwest Oncology Group (SWOG) reported that melphalan could induce remissions in about one third of myeloma patients.[19] Several years later, similar activity was observed with cyclophosphamide.[22] Administration of high doses of the glucocorticoid, prednisone, alone on alternate days, was first reported to induce remissions in relapsing or refractory myeloma in 1967.[23] The use of melphalan in combination with prednisone was then studied extensively.[24,25] A few other single agents with definite activity in myeloma have subsequently been reported, including carmustine (BCNU), doxorubicin (Adriamycin), and interferon-α (INF-α).[26–28]

INCIDENCE AND MORTALITY

Incidence data in the United States as reported by the Surveillance, Epidemiology, and End Result (SEER) program of the National Cancer Institute (NCI) for the period 1973 to 1977 indicate that multiple myeloma accounts for 1.1% of all malignancies in whites and 2.1% in blacks.[29] The average age-adjusted annual incidence for myeloma in whites is 4.3 of 100,000 males and 3.0 of 100,000 females.[29] In blacks, the incidence is higher: 9.6 of 100,000 males and 6.7 of 100,000 females.[29] Myeloma is the most common lymphoid malignancy in blacks and the second most common in whites, for whom non-Hodgkin's lymphoma ranks first. Incidence and mortality rates for myeloma in whites analyzed by SEER rose considerably for both sexes from the late 1940s to the late 1970s, with net increases of 145% or more.[30] In 1983 and 1984, the incidence for whites with myeloma in the United States was 2.8 of 100,000 males and 2.1 of every 100,000 females. Rates for multiple myeloma in Western European countries are similar to those for the American white population, and the incidence is estimated at 2.6 of 100,000 in England and 3.3 of 100,000 in Sweden.[31,32]

The incidence of myeloma in whites and blacks increases with increasing age. Fewer than 2% of the patients are younger than 40 years of age at diagnosis, but the disease has occurred in young adults and children.[33] In the United States, the median age of onset is 68 for men and 70 for women.[28] The mortality patterns closely parallel the incidence curves; the median age at death is 70 years for men and 71 for women.[34] In 1983 and 1984, the mortality rate for the United States white population with multiple myeloma was 8.7 of 100,000 men and 5.1 of 100,000 women.[30] Incidence and mortality appear to be rising, but the data supporting this trend suggest that the apparent increases in myeloma may reflect prior underdiagnosis, rather than a true increase in incidence.[30,35]

A similar age distribution is also observed in the related plasma cell disorders of MGUS and Waldenström's macroglobulinemia.[36] MGUS occurs much more frequently than multiple myeloma, but it can be detected only with specific screening examinations for monoclonal immunoglobulins. Axelsson and colleagues screened for serum M-components in 6995 asymptomatic adults older than 25 who composed most of the adult population in four parishes in Sweden.[37] Sera from 1% of these persons contained M-components. The prevalence of MGUS in this population increased with age, from 2% of those in the eighth decade to almost 6% of those in the ninth decade. Use of more sensitive screening tests for M-components appears to increase the frequency with which MGUS is detected.[38] Because MGUS has a long natural history and cases tend to accumulate over time, the annual age-related incidence is unknown.

PATHOGENESIS

Myeloma occurs in humans and in mice, rats, hamsters, cats, and dogs.[39–45] In rodents, increased susceptibility to plasma cell tumors has been selected fortuitously in some strains as a result of nonrandom breeding patterns used to create genetic uniformity. An additional factor in various domesticated species, which is probably important, is the prevalence of endogenous retroviruses. Retroviruses are associated with the development of B-lymphoid neoplasms through mutagenicity resulting from insertion of viral genomes into cellular DNA and as a result of the transforming ability of certain recombinant retroviruses.[46]

MURINE MODELS OF DISORDERS ASSOCIATED WITH M-COMPONENTS

Study of inbred mouse strains has yielded substantial information on the occurrence of asymptomatic monoclonal gammopathies without obvious tumor formation (perhaps the equivalent of MGUS) and on mechanisms of induction of plasma cell neoplasms.[47] Monoclonal gammopathies (usually IgG) without tumor formation occur spontaneously in approximately 60% of mice of the inbred C57BL/Ka strain within 24 months, but BALB/c and CBA/Rij mice have a low spontaneous incidence of monoclonal gammopathies.[48] Spontaneous plasmacytomas are infrequent findings in old mice, and they are usually encountered as an incidental finding.[48] Unlike the low spontaneous susceptibility of BALB/c mice to monoclonal gammopathy or spontaneous plasma cell tumors, peritoneal plasmacytomas can be readily induced in inbred strains.[49–51] However, the C57BL/Ka strain, which expresses spontaneous monoclonal gammopathies, is relatively resistant to plasmacytoma induction.[52] Plasmacytomas can be induced in BALB/c mice with the intraperitoneal injection of mineral oils or by implantation of solid plastic materials such as Lucite.[53–55] The plasmacytomas develop within oil or foreign-body granulomas in the peritoneum or mesentery, and each plasmacytoma produces a unique M-component. Chemically defined mineral oil alkane components, such as pristane, also induce plasmacytomas, and this process can be facilitated by subsequent infection of the mice with the Abelson virus.[56]

The murine plasmacytomas lead to the production of a growth factor in the peritoneal fluid that sustains the growth of the neoplasm.[57,58] Plasmacytoma growth factors that support the growth of human myeloma cells in culture have been isolated from the splenic macrophages of oil-treated BALB/c mice and from several other sources.[59–62] A human B-cell growth factor, IL-6, has been isolated from Epstein-Barr virus (EBV)-infected B cells or monocytes.[63] IL-6 has been produced by recombinant DNA methods and has been identified as a plasmacytoma growth factor. IL-6 is a 184-amino acid glycoprotein that stimulates the growth of EBV-infected human B cells and mouse and rat plasmacytomas. Another factor that is probably also produced by BALB/c splenic macrophages in plasmacytoma-bearing mice and that inhibits the normal humoral antibody response has been identified.[64]

Antigenic stimulation by normal bacterial flora has a direct or an indirect effect on plasmacytoma formation; there is a marked reduction in the incidence of myeloma in pristane-treated BALB/c mice that have been raised in a germ-free environment, although other lymphoid neoplasms may arise. Germ-free mice have a less-stimulated or less-developed immune apparatus and may lack the B-cell populations most susceptible to myeloma induction.[65] BALB/c mice are known to harbor oncogenic retroviruses, which may play a role in myeloma induction. Mouse plasmacytomas contain large numbers of intracisternal A particles that are not seen in normal plasma cells.[66] These particles are thought to represent a distinct group of retroviruses.[67]

Nonrandom chromosomal translocations and the expression or alteration of specific oncogenes have been observed in murine plasmacytomas. The distal part of chromosome 15 is translocated to chromosome 12 (where the heavy chain genes reside) in several long-term transplanted plasmacytomas.[68,69] A similar phenomenon has been reported in human Burkitt's lymphoma, in which translocations between the long arm of chromosome 8 (band 24) and the bands on chromosomes 14, 2, and 22 that contain the genetic loci for heavy chain, κ light chain, and λ light chain, respectively.[70]

The finding that the translocated component of chromosome 15 in the mouse and of chromosome 8 in man transfers the *MYC* oncogene to the locus of an immunoglobulin gene suggests that the control of *MYC* expression is enhanced by this translocation and leads to increased cell proliferation and tumor formation. Abnormal expression and alterations in *MYC* have been reported in human myeloma.[71,72] However, this gene was detected in about one fourth of the patients studied.[71] These data suggest that the *MYC* oncogene may have some pathologic role in the evolution of myeloma in humans.[71]

ETIOLOGIC CONSIDERATIONS IN HUMANS

Although the cause of multiple myeloma and related plasma cell disorders remains unknown, several factors have been implicated in the pathogenesis. Several lines of evidence suggest that genetic factors may play a role in predisposing persons to developing myeloma or related disorders. One factor that may implicate genetics is race, because of the increased prevalence of the disease in U.S. blacks, but this could also indicate environmental differences.[73,74]

Genetic marker studies have yielded only minimal information on the gammopathies. The frequency of HLA antigens of the 4C group appears to be slightly increased in myeloma.[75–78] The incidence of myeloma appears to be increased in first-degree relatives, and familial myeloma has been the subject of several case reports. At the Mayo Clinic, during one 6-year period, myeloma was diagnosed in 8 siblings of 440 patients with myeloma, an incidence that far exceeds that generally reported.[79] In another study, the median age and sex ratio of 75 reported familial cases resembled those of nonfamilial cases.[80] Because related cases usually have been observed in siblings and only rarely in spouses, it appears that transmission is vertical rather than horizontal.[81,82] Within a given family, the heavy chain types of M-components differ; however, there is concordance in light chain types in 80% of the patients.[80]

Idiopathic monoclonal peaks (*i.e.*, MGUS) have been reported sporadically in relatives of patients with myeloma.[79,83–85] Genetic factors in MGUS are suggested by its relation to selected HLA types, the predominance of the IgG1 subclass, and by reports of the familial occurrence of myeloma and macroglobulinemia.[86–92] At the Mayo Clinic, where 241 patients with MGUS were followed for at least 10 years, MGUS was evaluated as a precursor to myeloma.[1] During this period, 38% of patients had no change in the concentration of the M-component and remained asymptomatic. An additional 35% of the patients died without developing myeloma or any other B-cell neoplasm. In 9%, the M-component increased significantly, but myeloma or a related disorder was not diagnosed. Most importantly, 17% of the 44 patients had a diagnosis of myeloma, macroglobulinemia, amyloidosis, or lymphoma. Multiple myeloma was the diagnosis in 30 (68%) of these patients. This report and anecdotal observations in the literature implicate MGUS as a premalignant condition. In one fascinating case, a patient received passive serotherapy with horse antiserum to tetanus in the 1930s and subsequently developed a serum M-component that persisted for more than 3 decades before overt myeloma developed. After the diagnosis was made, it was determined that the serum IgG M-component exhibited antibody activity with specificity directed toward horse α_2-macroglobulin.[93]

These findings and others have given rise to a "two-hit hypothesis," in which antigenic stimulation in a susceptible host is the first hit, giving rise to a benign monoclone. The second hit is postulated to be a mutagenic or transforming event that gives rise to myeloma from the expanded monoclonal B-cell population.[94]

Environmental or occupational factors in myeloma have been examined in large occupational studies, but these data must be interpreted cautiously because some associations may have occurred by chance alone. A large British case-control study involved 399 myeloma patients and an equal number of matched controls evaluated for a variety of occupational and environmental exposures and for immunization, infection, and immune defects.[95] A strong risk of myeloma (relative risk of 1.8) was associated with agriculture, food processing, and exposure to chemicals. Another case-control study involved 100 white myeloma patients and 100 matched controls in the Baltimore area.[96] Positive associations were documented for a history of occupational exposure to petroleum products, with an observed rate of myeloma that was 3.7 times the expected rate (range, 1.3–10.3), and to asbestos, with an observed rate of 3.5 (range, 1.0–12.0). Among a large number of medications assessed, the use of laxatives appeared to elevate risk of myeloma to 3.5 times the expected rate.

The finding of increased risk with exposure to petroleum products in this study confirms earlier reports of an excessive number of cases of myeloma in workers exposed to petroleum.[1,97] The increased risk of myeloma in petroleum workers correlates well with the mineral oil-induced model for plasma cell neoplasms in BALB/c mice. One patient developed a plasmacytoma in the cutaneous pocket in which a Silastic-covered cardiac pacemaker was installed.[98]

Prior reports of 61 patients with asbestosis have documented the occurrence of four cases of myeloma, one of macroglobulinemia, and one of chronic lymphocytic leukemia (CLL), suggesting that this known carcinogen may be involved in the induction B-cell neoplasms.[99] Although chronic antigenic stimulation in disorders such as cholecystitis, osteomyelitis, and reactions to allergen hyposensitization injections has been suggested as a predisposing factor for human plasma cell neoplasms, data from various studies are inconclusive.[100–117]

As in other hematologic malignancies, a significant association has been observed between radiation exposure and the subsequent development of myeloma. This has been documented in the studies of survivors of the atomic bombs in Hiroshima and Nagasaki.[118,119] Among 109,000 survivors, 29 myeloma deaths were identified between 1950 and 1976. For persons exposed to 100 cGy, the observed rate of myeloma was approximately 4.7 times greater than controls, with the excess risk in this high-dose exposure group becoming apparent after a latent period of about 20 years. Associations between myeloma and low-dose irradiation exposure are more controversial than the atomic bomb casualty reports.[118] However, studies of radiologists have shown excessive mortality resulting from myeloma, as for workers in nuclear plants.[120–123] In an epidemiologic study, there was evidence of an increase in myeloma risk (but not leukemia or lymphoma) with increasing numbers of diagnostic radiographs, but the overall myeloma risk was not high.[124] These findings support the view that even low-level radiation may be a risk factor for myeloma.

PATHOLOGY

The morphologic appearance of plasma cells in malignant and benign disorders are often similar. Plasma cells are at least two to three times the size of peripheral lymphocytes and are round or egg shaped, with one or more eccentrically placed nuclei containing diffuse or clumped chromatin (Fig. 56–2). The light microscopic appearance was first drawn by Dalrymple and published from a woodcut in 1846.[6] Plasma cells contain a highly differentiated cytoplasm that is rich in rough-surfaced endoplasmic reticulum specialized for Ig synthesis. The cytoplasm normally stains blue or blue-purple with Romanovsky-type stains, but some myeloma cells stain red-orange and have been called thesaurocytes or flame cells.[125,126] Once thought to be diagnostic of IgA myeloma, flame cells are now recognized in any plasma cell proliferation in which the M-component has a high carbohydrate content.[126,127] A perinuclear clear zone is usually present in plasma cells and is the site of the Golgi apparatus, wherein Ig is packaged and glycosylated for secretion.[128] Other cytoplasmic findings can include numerous vacuoles (*e.g.*, Mott cells, cells with Russell bodies, grape cells, morula cells).[129] Electron microscopy reveals protein-filled secretion vacuoles or dilated cisternae in the endoplasmic reticulum. Although the cytoplasm is well differentiated, the nucleus in malignant plasma cell disorders can be relatively less differentiated, often has diffuse chromatin, and may have several nucleoli and intranuclear inclusions. None of these features absolutely differentiates benign from malignant plasma cell proliferations.

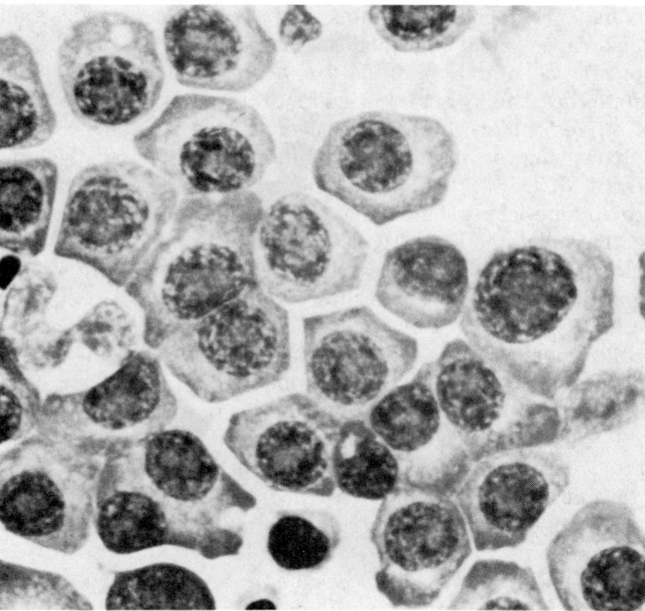

FIGURE 56–2. Bone marrow plasma cell in a patient with IgG myeloma. With the exception of a single cell in the neutrophilic series, the remaining cells are neoplastic plasma cells at various stages of differentiation.

Myeloma patients with large numbers of plasmablasts in their marrow may have a poorer prognosis than those with predominantly mature plasma cells. In macroglobulinemia, cells may have a "lymphoplasmacytic" appearance, with morphologic variations in size and characteristics of those of small lymphocytes to large plasma cells. This pattern is occasionally observed in myeloma. When lymphoplasmacytic cells are examined with immunofluorescence, most contain large amounts of cytoplasmic M-component. Cell surface Ig usually cannot be demonstrated on plasma cells.

In addition to the conventional morphologic assessments of plasma cells, use of monoclonal antibody reagents, histochemical analyses, and other morphologic approaches have been useful in analyzing plasma cells. Several plasma cell-associated antigens have been identified with specific monoclonal antibodies. Some patients' cells react strongly with antibodies to the common acute lymphocytic leukemia antigen (CALLA); these patients may have a poorer prognosis.[130] Immunologic and cytogenetic markers have been used to identify a series of characteristics associated with myeloma stem cells.[131] Histochemical stains, including β-glucuronidase and plasma cell acid phosphatase, have assisted in identifying plasma cells and obtaining prognostic information.[132] Such stains are usually not required for differentiating plasma cells from red cell progenitors; however, the plasma cell acid phosphatase may be of some use in differentiating active myeloma from MGUS.[133,134] Morphologic assessment of the tritiated thymidine-labeling index has been valuable in differentiating active myeloma from MGUS and other entities.[135,136] Monoclonal antibody reagents capable of evaluating cells undergoing DNA synthesis and flow cytometry have been applied to the evaluation of plasma cell disorders.[137,138] The plasma cell β-glucuronidase has been correlated with the extent of disease. With some exceptions, increasing tumor burden is associated with higher plasma cell glucuronidase levels.[139]

Core bone marrow biopsies demonstrate that myeloma cells are present in cords in a reticular network. Involvement of the marrow can be diffuse or nodular, although diffuse involvement with sheets of plasma cells is somewhat more common.

Amyloid deposits can occasionally be found in the bone marrow in the vicinity of myeloma cells or in biopsies of soft-tissue plasmacytomas. Other biopsy sites, such as the abdominal fat and rectal mucosa, have a higher likelihood of demonstrating the presence of amyloid.[140]

The symptoms and signs of multiple myeloma and its effects on the patient result from the secreted products from the myeloma cells, which have a variety of hormonal, immunologic, and physicochemical effects and from the growth kinetics and total-body tumor burden of malignant plasma cells. Several cytokines may play roles in the pathophysiology of myeloma. IL-6 is a major growth factor for myeloma, particularly in the terminal phase of the disease.[141] IL-6 may support myeloma growth through a paracrine mechanism, with its production provided by adherent cells in the monocyte-macrophage series rather than the myeloma cells themselves.[142] In a study using IL-6 antisense oligonucleotides, growth inhibition was observed in human myeloma cells lines, suggesting that IL-6 autocrine mechanisms may also be involved.[141]

HYPERCALCEMIA

In the clinical phase of myeloma, hematogenous dissemination to various skeletal sites is usually extensive and leads to bone pain and hypercalcemia. Radiographic findings of skeletal destruction are depicted in Figure 56–3. In areas of bone resorption, it appears that the cells adjacent to the bony matrix in the resorption lacunae are osteoclasts, which are separated from the myeloma cells by a membrane. This morphologic finding and those of functional studies using myeloma cell secretion products provided the basis for the concept that myeloma cells liberated an osteoclast-activating factor responsible for bone destruction.[143,144] The production of osteoclast-activating factor by a patient's myeloma cells correlates with the extent of skeletal involvement.[145] Several bone-resorbing cytokines have been identified, including lymphotoxin, tumor necrosis factor (TNF) produced by myeloma cells, and IL-1.[146] Antibodies to IL-6 but not to TNF or lymphotoxin partially blocked myeloma osteoclast-activating factor activity, suggesting that IL-1 may play a role in the development of bone lesions.[147]

ANEMIA

Marrow involvement results in the development of a normochromic, normocytic anemia, heralding the symptoms of fatigue and weakness. Reduced erythrocyte production and increased destruction have been observed. High concentrations of serum M-component in the blood lead to rouleaux formation and may lead to blood sludging, which further increases hemolysis.

RENAL FAILURE

Renal failure is a common complication of myeloma that can be significant at the time of clinical presentation. It is an adverse prognostic factor that has a negative impact on overall survival. The renal failure appears to be multifactorial and is most frequently correlated with Bence Jones proteinuria, hypercalcemia, or both. The presence of λ light chains in the urine is more strongly correlated with renal failure than is the excretion of κ chains, suggesting that they often are more nephrotoxic. Light chains normally pass the glomerulus and are reabsorbed and catabolized in the proximal tubules.[148–150] An assay system has been developed to assess the intrinsic nephrotoxic potential of Bence Jones proteins.[151] The excretion of dense (often laminated) tubular casts is a characteristic finding in patients with myeloma kidney.[151] The casts contain albumin, intact Ig molecules, or Bence Jones proteins.[151–161] The proteinuria comprises monoclonal light chains and some albumin. Infection, hyperuricemia, and amyloidosis also contributing to renal failure. Amyloid deposition in the kidney usually appears in the blood vessels, basement membranes of the tubules, interstitium, and occasionally in glomeruli. Proteinuria in patients with renal amyloid is often generalized, and this can provide a clue for differentiating the syndrome from myeloma kidney.

IMMUNODEFICIENCY

Increased susceptibility to bacterial infections, particularly before treatment, is principally due to an acquired hyporesponsiveness to antigenic stimulation. Reduced serum levels of normal serum antibody immunoglobulins are observed in almost all patients with multiple myeloma and in many MGUS patients.[162] The normal pre-B-cell and B-cell compartments are reduced in myeloma.[163] Studies using mice indicate that myeloma cells produce a humoral PC-factor that stimulates monocytes and macrophages to produce a second factor, PIMS, which inhibits normal antigen-stimulated B-cell proliferation after antibody production.[164] Mixing experiments using peripheral blood mononuclear cells from patients with myeloma and those from normal persons indicates that monocytic cells in the myeloma patient's blood can inhibit normal B-cell Ig synthesis induced with pokeweed mitogen.[165] The precise molecular nature of these immunosuppressive cytokines is not established.

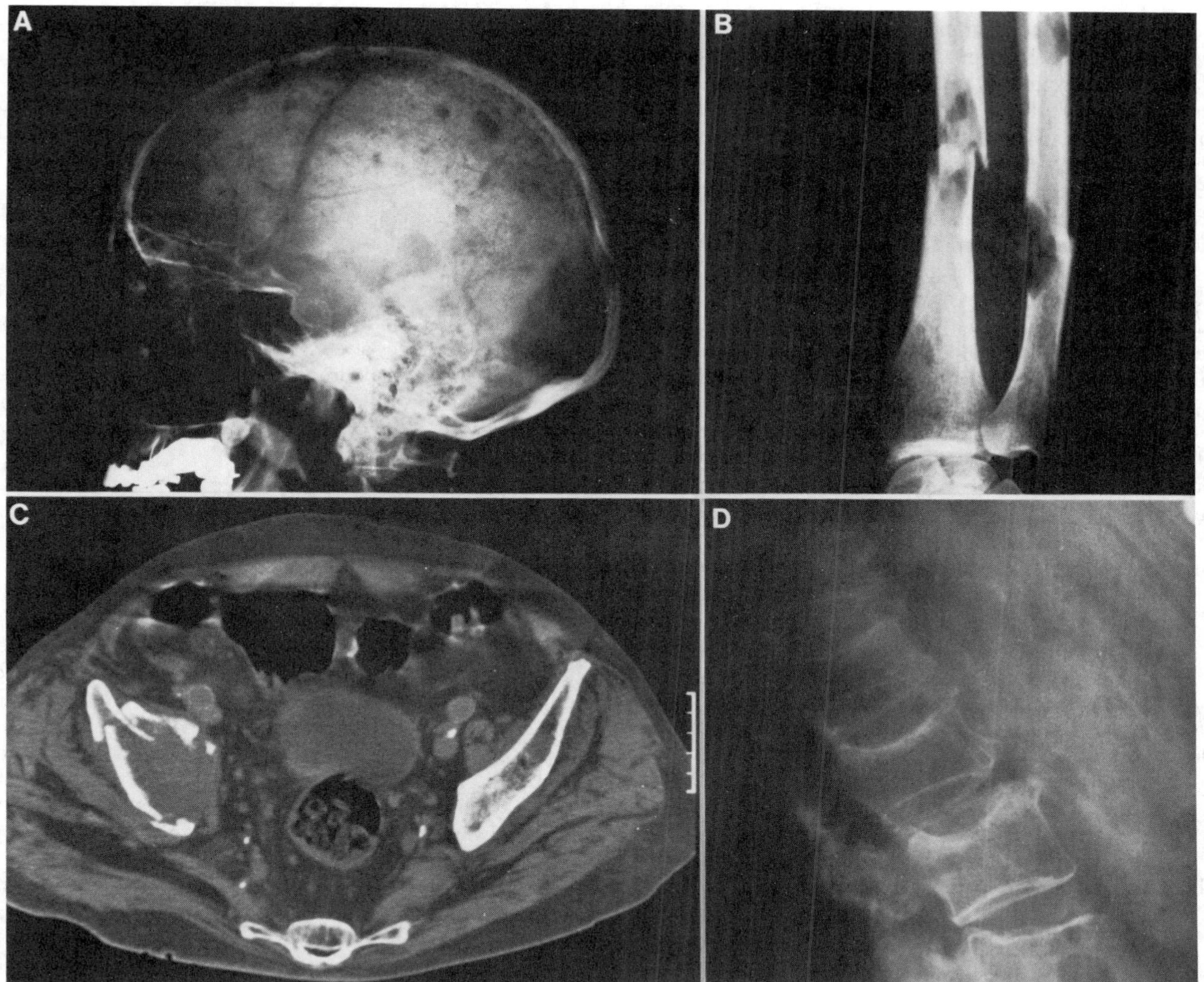

FIGURE 56–3. Typical radiographic evidence of bone involvement in myeloma. **(A)** Punched-out lesions in the skull. **(B)** Intramedullary expansile lesions in a forearm with fracture. **(C)** Pelvic plasmacytoma with a fracture and associated soft tissue mass seen on a computed tomography scan. **(D)** Vertebral compression fractures in the spine.

PHYSICOCHEMICAL OR IMMUNOLOGIC EFFECTS OF M-COMPONENTS

M-components in myeloma and related disorders can cause clinically significant abnormalities in blood flow and function.[166] The most common of these phenomena is the hyperviscosity syndrome. Although more common in macroglobulinemia than in myeloma, it results from a sufficient concentration of an M-protein with a high molecular mass or with a tendency to self-aggregation and a resultant increase in intrinsic viscosity. The hyperviscosity syndrome is rarely seen until the serum viscosity exceeds 4.0 cp units, relative to normal saline, and it is usually manifested by the occurrence of neurologic findings and by spontaneous bleeding phenomena in the absence of thrombocytopenia. In other instances, an M-component exhibits antibody activity, leading to clinical syndromes such as acquired deficiency of factor VIII, with bleeding phenomena and hyperlipidemia.[167–169]

GROWTH KINETICS AND TUMOR BURDEN

Myeloma is a low-growth-fraction tumor, with only a small percentage of tumor cells in the cell cycle at any given time. It is thought to arise from a single transformed cell (10^0 cell). Tritiated thymidine-labeling indices for myeloma cells in patients with active disease usually are in the range of 1% to 3%.[136] Studies of the generation time indicate that the cell cycle time of actively proliferating cells is approximately 1 to 3 days.[170,171] In IgG myeloma, tumor burden ranges from 0.5×10^{12} cells in early asymptomatic cases to 5×10^{12} cells or more in patients with widespread bone destruction.[17]

Studies of growth kinetics have been carried out by measuring the doubling time of serum M-components of patients not actively receiving treatment and by use of mathematical modeling for measurements of progressive tumor growth in patients who have had their total-body tumor burden determined.[170] Using serum M-component doubling times of 4 to

6 months in untreated patients and assuming exponential growth, it was initially proposed that the natural history of myeloma might require 20 to 30 years to evolve from a single malignant plasma cell to clinically evident disease.[172] In some instances, this model would predict that myeloma was initiated before conception! However, subsequent studies using measurements of M-component metabolism and more precise mathematical modeling techniques determined that the growth of myeloma followed Gompertzian kinetics and that the subclinical phase of malignant tumor cell proliferation was about 1 to 3 years before clinical diagnosis.[171] A typical myeloma growth curve is depicted in Figure 56–4.

The phase of myeloma after diagnosis can be viewed as a chronic phase, not dissimilar to that in chronic myeloid leukemia. This chronic phase in myeloma may last from 1 to 10 or more years, during which time treatment is usually beneficial. Late in the course of myeloma, the doubling time (as determined from serum M-component levels) may progressively shorten; this may be analogous to the blast crisis phase of chronic myeloid leukemia.[173] Integration of tritiated thymidine-labeling index and tumor-burden studies defined these patients as having high-growth-fraction, high-tumor-burden myeloma.[136] This patient group has a poor prognosis, with rapid myeloma growth and early death.[136,174] Patients whose myelomas have more rapid growth kinetics have a propensity for extramedullary tumor growth, including soft-tissue plasmacytomas and central nervous system (CNS) involvement. In some instances, the neoplasm takes on a less-differentiated morphologic appearance, similar to that of a large cell lymphoma, with a cell surface Ig that usually corresponds with the prior serum Ig.[94,175,176]

In earlier phases of disease, the quantity of M-component synthesis as determined from serum or urine measurements corresponds with the amount of tumor in the body. However, in the terminal phase, the M-component synthesis rate per tumor may decline or qualitatively change as the tumor progresses, suggesting the development of a mutant clone. Some patients who previously had only a serum M-component switch to primarily urinary light chains, reflecting additional biochemical abnormalities in Ig synthesis and assembly.[177]

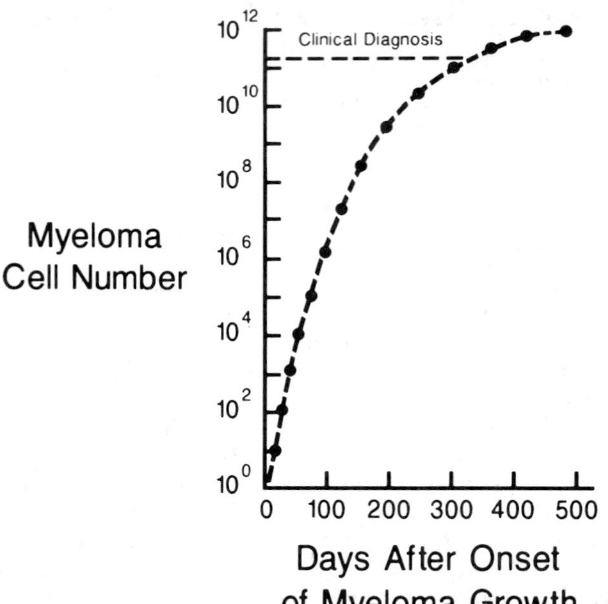

FIGURE 56–4. Gompertzian growth curve in multiple myeloma. In this untreated patient with IgG myeloma, serial measurements of M-component production were used to extrapolate the preclinical phase of myeloma cell proliferation of approximately 1 year.

Unlike the aggressive forms of the disease, another subset of patients have indolent or smoldering myeloma in which, despite evidence of bone lesions, the disease progresses slowly even without treatment. These patients previously could be identified only from their clinical course; however, the use of tritiated thymidine-labeling studies usually identifies these patients as having hypoproliferative myeloma cells, with fewer than 0.5% of the tumor cells labeling and in a range similar to that of MGUS.[135,136]

DIAGNOSIS AND CLINICAL STAGING OF MYELOMA

Presenting symptoms and signs of myeloma usually include bone pain, which may be associated with compression fractures of the spine or pathologic fractures of long bones; weakness and anemia; and infection, usually due to pneumococcal or other gram-positive bacteria. Hypercalcemia, renal failure, spinal cord compression, or a mixture of these findings may be present. Punched-out osteolytic bone lesions are commonly seen on skeletal x-ray films (see Fig. 56–3). A complete skeletal x-ray series, including the axial and appendicular skeleton, should always be obtained at the time of diagnosis. Only in this way can the number and location of lesions be identified to determine if any potentially unstable osteolytic lesions are present.

Studies using magnetic resonance imaging (MRI) scanning suggest that this approach can provide greater detail on myelomatous abnormalities in the vertebral column than conventional radiographs (Fig. 56–5). However, because this procedure is expensive and takes several hours to acquire the imaging information on the entire spine of a single patient, this technique must be used selectively. Bone scans are of no value in the assessment of skeletal involvement in myeloma, because the bone disease is almost purely osteolytic and the nuclear medicine isotopes are taken up only in areas of osteoblastic activity.

An increase in the number of plasma cells is usually demonstrable in the bone marrow or in a biopsy of a plasmacytoma. A serum or urinary M-component can be demonstrated in 99% of the patients. However, in some instances, not all criteria are present, and a mixture of criteria is needed to establish a diagnosis of multiple myeloma and to differentiate it from other plasma cell disorders. Useful diagnostic criteria are summarized in Table 56–3.

A clinical staging system for multiple myeloma was developed at the Arizona Cancer Center by Durie and Salmon by analyzing the presenting features of a series of patients with multiple myeloma who had their tumor burden directly measured using the metabolic techniques.[177] On the basis of these clinical correlations, multiple myeloma was divided into three tumor burden groups: stage I (low), II (intermediate), and III (high). Tumor mass stage alone was predictive of survival.

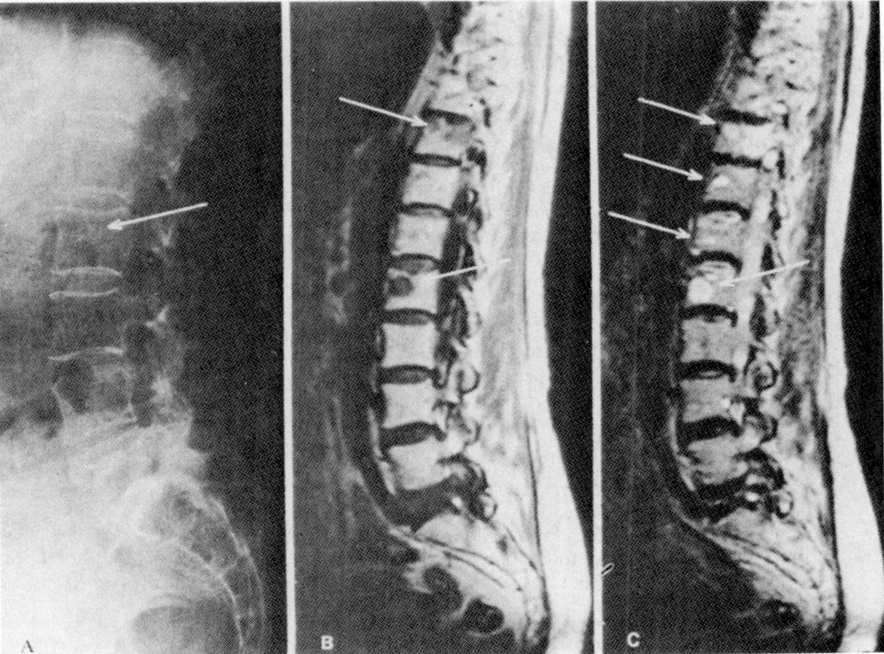

FIGURE 56–5. **(A)** Radiograph of lower spine compared with **(B, C)** magnetic resonance images. The osteolytic lesions in the vertebral bodies of T10–12 and L1 that were poorly visualized on plain films were much more visible on the **(B)** T1-weighted and **(C)** T2-weighted MR images. (Ludwig M, Tscholakoff D, Neuhold A, et al. Magnetic resonance imaging of the spine in multiple melanoma. Lancet 1987;2:364–366)

An additional prognostic factor, renal function, independently impinged on survival and was included in the staging system, with normal renal function (*i.e.*, serum creatinine <2.0 or blood urea nitrogen <30) as substage A and higher values as substage B (Table 56–4).

Several other investigations applied the Durie-Salmon myeloma staging system to evaluate survival by stage in myeloma (Table 56–5). In studies of response to treatment and survival, the clinical features that correlated with a given stage in terms of tumor burden predicted survival in the original patient set and in subsequent reports by other investigative groups.[183,189,190] Figure 56–6 depicts the influence of clinical stage and renal function on the survival of patients with multiple myeloma. In the original study used in developing the Durie-Salmon myeloma staging system, the percentage of bone marrow plasma cells was an important factor, but it was not included in the staging system because it could be replaced by other clinical features and was potentially susceptible to sampling errors. Bone marrow involvement was deleted from the staging criteria after consideration of the potential difficulties that might be encountered in accurately and reproducibly counting plasma cells in the bone marrow differential at different centers. Patients with Bence Jones-only myeloma have been assessed for measured tumor cell burden, and they appear to represent a higher-risk subgroup with a higher tumor cell mass and shorter survival.[192]

DIFFERENTIAL DIAGNOSIS

The criteria shown in Table 56–3 provide the basis for differentiating myeloma from other major plasma cell disorders with M-component secretions other than IgM. The IgM M-components are usually attributable to Waldenström's macroglobulinemia and occasionally to MGUS or other entities. Multiple myeloma with IgM secretion has rarely been reported, and it should be diagnosed only if the patient has multiple osteolytic bone lesions that contain monoclonal plasma cells.[94] Marrow plasmacytosis is observed in several chronic infectious or inflammatory diseases and in hypersensitivity reactions, autoimmune disease, unrelated neoplasms, and occasionally in other conditions; it is not associated with secretion of an M-component, but it is associated with polyclonal hyperglobulinemia.

The major differential diagnosis is usually between myeloma and MGUS. There is an overlap between the findings for patients with MGUS and those with stage I myeloma (or macroglobulinemia) that can often be recognized only by serial follow-up of the patient for at least 1 year without any form of treatment. In MGUS, the M-component level remains constant over many years, but in the malignant plasma cell disorders, the M-component gradually rises, and other symptoms and signs of the disease develop. A policy of watch and wait is completely justifiable, because there is no evidence that treatment improves the outcome in stage I myeloma or MGUS, and the use of chemotherapy has potential hazards that should be avoided if the patient does not have an invasive, progressive plasma cell malignancy. If, after a year's follow-up of the patient's M-component and symptoms and signs at 1- to 2-month intervals, there is no evidence of progression, the most likely diagnosis is MGUS, and follow-up examinations should be done at least annually because approximately 2% of these patients progress to a diagnosis of B-cell neoplasm each year.[1]

Patients presenting with only Bence Jones proteinuria usually have myeloma alone or with amyloidosis.[193,194] It has been stated that its excretion has "sinister significance."[195] However, Bence Jones MGUS has been reported and followed without specific therapy for several years in a few patients.[160,196] It is nonetheless reasonable to have a higher index of suspicion when patients present with idiopathic Bence Jones proteinuria, because it usually progresses within 6 months to 1 year to clearly diagnosed myeloma, which should be treated

TABLE 56–3. Diagnostic Criteria for Multiple Myeloma, Myeloma Variants, and Monoclonal Gammopathy of Unknown Significance (MGUS)

A. Multiple myeloma
   Major criteria
   I. Plasmacytoma on tissue biopsy
   II. Bone marrow plasmacytosis with >30% plasma cells
   III. Monoclonal globulin spike on serum electrophoresis exceeding 3.5 g/dl for G peaks or 2.0 g/dl for A peaks, ≥1.0 g/24 h of κ- or λ-light chain excretion on urine electrophoresis in the presence of amyloidosis
   Minor criteria
   a. Bone marrow plasmacytosis 10% to 30% plasma cells
   b. Monoclonal globulin spike present but less than the level defined above
   c. Lytic bone lesions
   d. Residual normal IgM < 50 mg/dl, IgA < 100 mg/dl, or IgG < 600 mg/dl*
   Diagnosis will be confirmed when any of the following features are documented in symptomatic patients with clearly progressive disease. The diagnosis of myeloma requires a minimum of one major + one minor criterion or three minor criteria that must include a + b, *i.e.*:
   1. I + b, I + c, I + d (I + a not sufficient)
   2. II + b, II + c, II + d
   3. III + a, III + c, III + d
   4. a + b + c, a + b + d
B. Indolent myeloma (same as myeloma except)
   I. No bone lesions or only limited bone lesions (≤3 lytic lesions): no compression fractures
   II. M-component levels: (a) IgG < 7 g/dl; (b) IgA < 5/dl
   III. No symptoms or associated disease features, *i.e.*:
   a. Performance status > 70%
   b. Hemoglobin > 10 g/dl
   c. Serum calcium normal
   d. Serum creatinine < 2.0 mg/dl
   e. No infections
C. Smoldering myeloma (same as indolent myeloma except)
   I. No bone lesions
   II. Bone marrow plasma cells ≤ 30%
D. MGUS
   I. Monoclonal gammopathy
   II. M-component level
      IgG ≤ 3.5 g/dl
      IgA ≤ 2.0 g/dl
      BJ protein ≤ 1.0 g/24 h
   III. Bone marrow plasma cells < 10%
   IV. No bone lesions
   V. No symptoms

* IgA, immunoglobulin A; IgG, immunoglobulin G; IgM, immunoglobulin M; BJ, Bence Jones light chain.
(From references 135, 160, 179, 180)

appropriately. Patients with unrelated metastatic neoplasms occasionally have MGUS, and a series of diagnostic studies and biopsies are required to establish that the patient does not have myeloma. Myeloma and an unrelated metastatic neoplasm may be diagnosed.

β_2-MICROGLOBULIN

β_2-microglobulin is an important prognostic factor in multiple myeloma.[197] It is a low-molecular-mass protein, which is the light chain of the HLA antigen and is synthesized by all nucleated cells.[198] It falls in the class of tubular proteins that pass the glomerulus and are excreted in the urine, but renal functional impairment elevates the serum level of β_2-microglobulin. β_2-Microglobulin can be measured by radioimmunoassay. If corrected for renal function, serum β_2-microglobulin levels correlate strongly with tumor burden in multiple myeloma.[197,199–203] Because the serum levels are a function of myeloma cell mass and renal function, measurement of β_2-microglobulin may provide an alternative to clinical staging for predicting survival.[204] The relation of β_2-microglobulin to survival in myeloma is depicted in Figure 56–7. β_2-Microglobulin can serve as a pretreatment prognostic factor in clinical trials because it permits a more direct comparison of risk factors among the various cooperative groups and institutions interested in myeloma therapy.[205,206] Although it has been proposed that β_2-microglobulin can be used to differentiate between MGUS and myeloma, significant overlap prevents this.[197,200,207] Serial β_2-microglobulin levels have not proven to be as useful as M-component measurements after response to treatment of myeloma. INF-α is reported to raise β_2-microglobulin levels in myeloma.[208] In our own experience, β_2-microglobulin has not proved useful in patients lacking an M-component (nonsecretory myeloma).

TREATMENT

PRINCIPLES

The diagnosis of a monoclonal gammopathy does not represent an immediate mandate for treatment, and patients with MGUS, stage I myeloma, and indolent or smoldering myeloma are often best followed without treatment until it is warranted by the development of clear-cut progression of the disease.

Because multiple myeloma is a disseminated plasma cell neoplasm, the primary approach to treatment is systemic antineoplastic therapy. Symptoms and signs that warrant immediate institution of therapy include the development of bone pain, hypercalcemia, renal failure, severe suppression of bone marrow functions, or spinal cord compression. If the patient has spinal cord compression, completion of local therapy (usually with radiation therapy) should normally precede the initiation of systemic chemotherapy unless other serious complications mandate simultaneous systemic treatment and radiation therapy. Patients presenting with long-bone fractures should have them internally fixed orthopedically before the initiation of chemotherapy. Presentation with constellations of findings, such as marked anemia plus the presence of lytic bone lesions, bacterial sepsis, or Bence Jones proteinuria, provide reasons for initiation of therapy. If there is significant infection, initiation of treatment should usually be delayed until the infection has been controlled. If the clinical findings are ambiguous, a period of observation that includes serial M-component measurements is usually warranted.

Doubling in the M-component in less than 1 year with other clinical findings of myeloma can also be used as a basis for treatment. For example, patients with rising M-component levels or progressive bone lesions are candidates for treatment even if they are asymptomatic. Useful adjuncts to systemic treatment include management of local problems with radiation therapy and a variety of supportive care measures.

Beneficial effects of systemic therapy can be obtained in most patients with newly diagnosed progressive myeloma in

TABLE 56–4. Myeloma Staging System

Criteria	*Measured Myeloma Cell Mass (Cells × $10^{12}/m^2$)*
Stage I	
All of the following:	
Hemoglobin value > 10 g/dl	
Serum calcium value normal (<12 mg/dl)	
On roentgenogram, normal bone structure (scale 0) or solitary bone plasmacytoma only	
Low M-component production rates	<0.6 (low)
IgG value < 5 g/dl*	
IgA value < 3 g/dl	
Urine light chain M-component on electrophoresis < 4 g/24 h	
Stage II	
Overall data not as minimally abnormal as shown for stage I and no single value as abnormal as defined for stage II.	0.6–1.20 (intermediate)
Stage III	
One or more of the following	
Hemoglobin value < 8.5 d/gl	
Serum calcium value > 12 mg/dl	
Advanced lytic bone lesions (scale 3)	
High M-component production rates	>1.20 (high)
IgG value > 7 d/gl	
IgA value > 5 g/dl	
Urine light chain M-component on electrophoresis > 12 g/24 h	
Subclassification	
A = relatively normal renal function (serum creatinine value > 2.0 mg/dl)	
B = abnormal renal function (serum creatinine value ≥ 2.0 gm/dl)	
Examples	
Stage IA = low cell mass with normal renal function	
Stage IIIB = high cell mass with abnormal renal function	

* IgA, immunoglobulin A; IgG, immunoglobulin G.
(Alexanian R, Balcerzak S, Bonnet JD, et al. Prognostic factors in multiple myeloma. Cancer 1975;36: 1192–1201)

TABLE 56–5. Median Survival in Relation to Stage at Diagnosis

		Median Survival (mo)				
		Stage				
Investigations	*No. of Patients*	*I*	*II*	*III*	*A*	*B*
Durie and Salmon[181]	71	>60	50	26		
Alexanian et al[182]	343	39	27	17		
Woodruff et al[183]	237	64	32	6	21	2
Merlini et al[184]	123	76	41	12		
Belpomme et al[185]	118	>60	28	7	>60	12
Gobbi et al[186]	91	>79	51	33		
Santoro et al[187]	81	48	41	23	35	7
Bergsagel et al[188]	364	46	32	23	32	11
Summary	1428	>60	41	23		

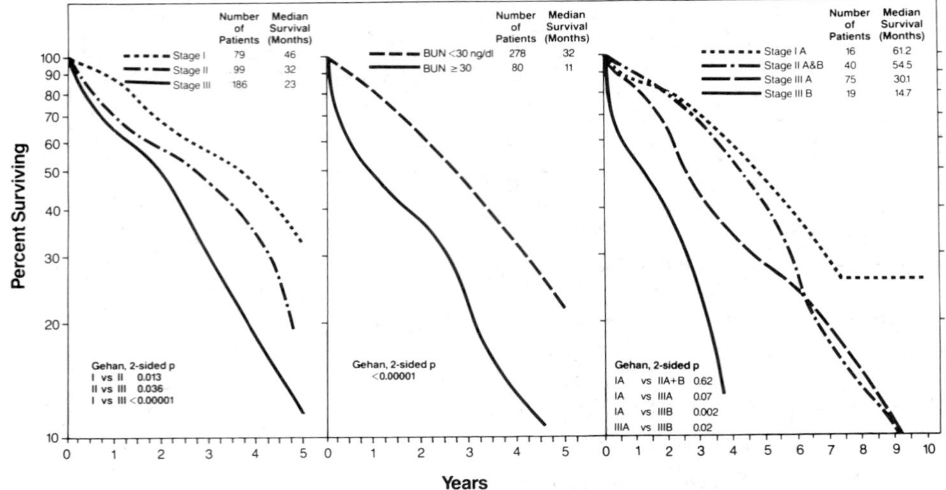

FIGURE 56–6. Influence of clinical stage and renal function on survival of patients with plasma cell myeloma as redrawn from published illustrations. The left two panels are from a Canadian NCI study[189] and show the separate effects of clinical stage and renal function, respectively. The right panel depicts an Arizona Cancer Center study,[191] and the survival curves are shown with clinical stage and renal function integrated with the use of the clinical staging system shown in Table 56-4. Statistical comparisons of survival outcome for the various stages and risk groups in the studies appear in each panel.

clinical stages II or III. The best improvement in survival of patients with myeloma has been obtained for those with stage III disease. The clinical phases of myeloma under treatment include an initial drug sensitive phase, which is observed in most patients; a plateau phase, during which tumor burden is reduced and appears to be stable during maintained or unmaintained remission; and an eventual drug-resistant phase, during which the neoplasm may exhibit altered growth kinetics and resistance to conventional cytotoxic drugs.[2,209] About 15% to 20% of patients manifest resistance even to aggressive parenteral chemotherapy at the time of initial presentation with progressive myeloma.

Systemic therapy usually relieves bone pain relatively promptly, but many other aspects of the disease improve gradually and may require other supportive measures initially. Even with prompt institution of systemic treatment, the drug-sensitive phase of disease usually lasts only 2 to 3 years for most patients before drug resistance manifests. Although the median survival before the era of effective systemic therapy was less than 1 year, it is now in the range of 3 to 4 years. In a few patients, sensitivity to systemic therapy may persist for 5 to 10 years or longer.

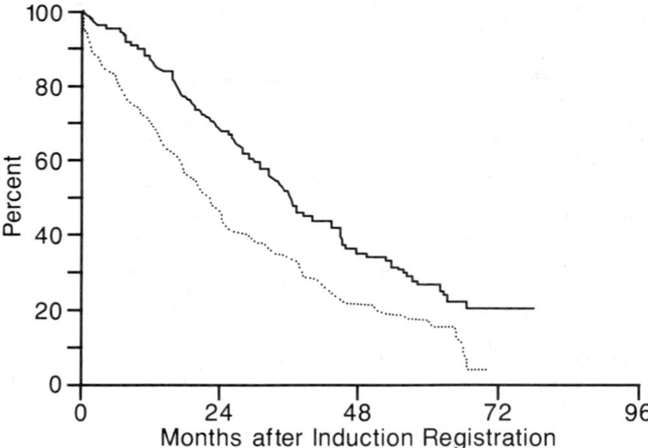

FIGURE 56–7. Life table survival curves in multiple myeloma in relation to serum β_2-microglobulin (β_2M) concentration. The upper curve (*solid line*) is for 324 patients with a serum concentration of less than 6 g/ml (median survival, 36 months). The lower curve (*dotted line*) is for 224 patients with higher serum levels (median survival, 22 months; $p < 0.0001$). (Salmon SE, Tesh D, Crowley J, et al. Chemotherapy is superior to sequential hemibody irradiation for remission consolidation in multiple myeloma: A Southwest Oncology study. J Clin Oncol 1990;8:1575–1584)

Care must include maximal efforts to relieve pain, hypercalcemia, severe anemia, and various local complications promptly to keep the patient from being bedridden, minimizing bone demineralization and superinfections. Patients should be encouraged to drink several liters of fluid daily to avoid dehydration and enhance urinary excretion of light chains and calcium.

EVALUATION OF RESPONSE TO TREATMENT

Because myeloma has a variety of clinical manifestations, a series of initial and follow-up studies are needed to assess the response to systemic treatment. These include a thorough history, physical examination, and following laboratory studies, which include the complete blood count with differential and platelet counts; M-component levels in the serum, 24-hour urine, or both; serum calcium, creatinine, or blood urea nitrogen levels; and skeletal radiographs. Although serum electrophoresis is extremely useful in the initial diagnostic workup, baseline and follow-up quantitation of the serum M-components is most reliably measured using laser nephelometry of the involved immunoglobulin. Serum electrophoresis is sometimes a useful alternative, particularly as the M-component level approaches the normal range for the involved Ig. The radial immunodiffusion test should not be used to measure myeloma immunoglobulins, because it has not proved reliable. Quantitation of urinary Bence Jones protein is best determined by protein electrophoresis using a 24-hour concentrate. The relative value of β_2-microglobulin useful for following the course of myeloma has not been established, but β_2-microglobulin is not as specific as M-component measurements, because its serum concentration is affected by tumor burden and renal function.

In the absence of specific symptoms, follow-up radiographs should be obtained every 6 to 12 months. The initial skeletal x-ray evaluation before therapy should include a complete metastatic survey, because myelomatous involvement can be located in any area of the axial or appendicular skeleton. Isotopic bone scans are of little or no value for myeloma and are not recommended. Bone marrow involvement should be assessed initially with an aspirate and a core bone marrow biopsy. Caution is needed to avoid excessive pressure on the needle when the needle is inserted, because in some myeloma patients, the bone matrix is extremely fragile. Follow-up bone marrow specimens are obtained to confirm remission status after therapy and to explain an unexpected pancytopenia. Marrow involvement with myeloma is usually diffuse, but occasionally it is spotty and may be subject to sampling error for needle aspiration but usually not for core biopsy. "Dry taps" on aspirates can be due to needle placement within a plasmacytoma. Table 56–6 summarizes a useful schedule for obtaining initial and follow-up studies in myeloma patients.

M-component production usually correlates with tumor burden in myeloma patients, and its serial assessment usually provides an excellent guide to the response to treatment or disease progression. Objective response criteria should identify patients who have achieved significant tumor regression and separate them from patients who have only stabilized or who have had symptomatic improvement without having achieved remission status. In 1973, the Leukemia-Myeloma Task Force of the NCI published the criteria for response in myeloma, which required a 50% reduction in the serum or urinary levels of an M-component to define remission.[210] Although the task force criteria were created to identify groups of patients responsive to treatment, they were developed before the acquisition of detailed knowledge of Ig metabolism. Analysis of Ig metabolism led to the recognition that for the major classes of IgG (IgG1, IgG2, and IgG4, which comprise 90% of serum IgG), metabolism is not linear with the serum concentration.[211] With a relatively high serum IgG M-component value, the half-life of IgG may be as short as 8 to 10 days, but with a low value, the half-life may be 40 days or longer. This concentration-dependent phenomenon applies to IgG M-component levels in 90% of patients with IgG myeloma or approximately 50% of all myeloma cases. Comparisons of serum levels in these patients underestimate the degree of change, depending on the initial and follow-up serum M-protein values.[2] Correction can be made for changes in the metabolic rate for IgG through the calculation of a synthetic index from the serum values.[212] A useful nomogram for this purpose has been derived from the metabolic equations.[2] A nomogram with an extended scale for IgG values appears in Figure 56–8.

Assessment of urinary light chain excretion is affected significantly by the degree of catabolism that takes place in the kidney, which is a function of the absolute levels of light chains passing the glomerulus and the degree of renal functional impairment.[192] To avoid difficulties in assessment, criteria for improvement in Bence Jones proteinuria must be quite stringent. The response criteria adopted by SWOG are summarized in Table 56–7. Response in accord with the SWOG criteria is strongly correlated with improvement in survival. When these criteria are applied, reduction in the synthetic index of serum M-proteins to less than 10% of control levels is associated with a better survival than if reduction is 10% to 24%, which is better than a reduction to 24% to 50% of control values. Lesser degrees of reduction in tumor burden are not associated with improvement in survival. Patients whose hemoglobin, renal function, and albumin levels improve have a better outcome than if the clinical variables remain unchanged or worsen. Responsive patients have improvement in general well-being and in ambulation, and they have marked relief of symptoms of bone pain. However, recalcification of osteolytic bone lesions is observed in fewer than 5% of patients who respond to chemotherapy.

A retrospective analysis of 69 stage II and 80 stage III myeloma patients treated at a single institution was evaluated with Myeloma Task Force and SWOG response criteria.[213] In

TABLE 56–6. Checklist of Laboratory Studies for Patients With Multiple Myeloma

Routine Pretreatment Evaluation

- Complete blood count, differential, and platelets
- Serum protein electrophoresis
- Serum immunoglobulins (nephelometry)
- Serum β_2-microglobulin
- 24-h urine for total protein and electrophoresis
- Antigenic typing of serum and urine monoclonal Igs by immunofixation or immunoelectrophoresis
- Bone marrow aspiration and biopsy
- Serum creatinine
- Serum calcium
- Serum electrolytes
- Serum uric acid
- Liver functions
- Chest radiograph
- Skeletal x-ray survey (entire skeleton)
- Electrocardiogram

Specialized Studies for Selected Patients

- Abdominal fat pad or rectal biopsy for amyloid (also tap joint effusions for amyloid)
- Solitary lytic lesion, soft tissue or lymph node biopsy
- Serum viscosity if IgM component present or if any serum M-component > 7.0 g/dl
- Plasma volume if serum relative viscosity > 4.0
- Myelogram (or in some instances MRI) if paraspinal mass or symptoms and signs of spinal cord or nerve root compression. (Spinal fluid should be sent for cell count, cytospin differential, glucose, and protein.)

Routine Follow-Up Studies

- Before every course of treatment
  - CBC, differential, platelets (should be repeated to check nadirs on first few courses)
- At least every 3 months (and on completion of induction or change to alternative therapy for refractory patients)
  - Serum monoclonal Ig by nephelometry or electrophoresis
  - 24-h urine protein electrophoresis (if Bence Jones protein present)
  - Serum chemistry panel
- At least annually
  - Skeletal x-ray survey (entire skeleton), chest film, serum β_2-microglobulin
  - Bone marrow aspiration if any significant abnormality in blood counts, Igs, or new symptoms
  - Serum Igs (nephelometry)

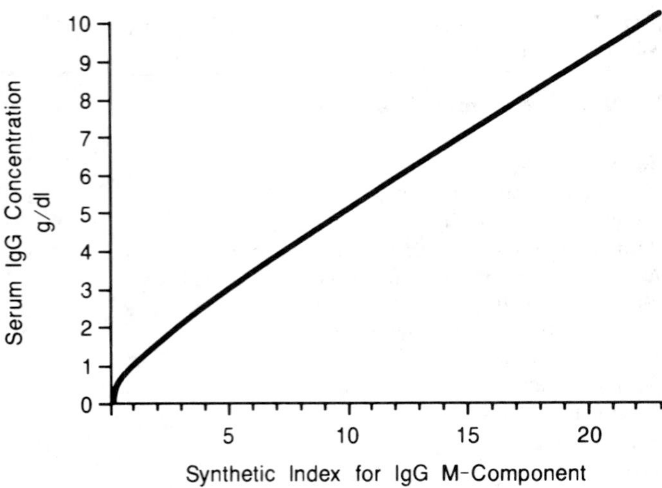

FIGURE 56–8. Nomogram for determining the synthetic index for IgG M-components of subclasses IgG1, IgG2, and IgG4, which comprise 90% of IgG myelomas. Using the patient's initial serum IgG concentration (g/dl) on the vertical axis, read down from the line to the horizontal axis to determine the synthetic index for that IgG value (Syn1). The same procedure is followed for the follow-up value (Syn2). Syn2/Syn1 × 100 = % of baseline synthetic index and tumor burden. This nomogram corrects for concentration-dependent changes in M-component synthesis and myeloma cell mass and gives a more accurate assessment of changes in tumor burden in IgG myeloma than can be calculated directly from the serum levels. The nomogram is not required for IgG3, IgA, IgD, or IgM serum M components, and changes in serum values for these Igs can be used directly to determine the percent change in tumor burden. The equation used to develop this nomogram has been incorporated into a program for a pocket calculator to calculate tumor cell mass. (Salmon SE, Wampler SE. Multiple myeloma: Quantitative staging and assessment of response with a programmable pocket calculator. Blood 1977;49:379–389)

TABLE 56–7. SWOG Myeloma Response Criteria

A. Responsive patients who satisfy all of the following criteria are considered to have achieved definite objective improvement.
   - A sustained decrease in the synthesis index of serum M protein to 25%, or less, of the pretreatment value on at least two measurements separated by 4 wk. For IgA and IgG3 M-proteins, the synthetic index is the same as the serum concentration. For IgG M-proteins of subclasses 1, 2, and 4, the synthetic index must be estimated using the nomogram shown in Figure 47-6.
   - A sustained decrease in 24-h urine globulin to 10%, or less, of the pretreatment value, and to less than 0.2 g/24 h on at least two occasions separated by 4 wk.
   - In all responsive patients the size and number of lytic skull lesions must not increase, and the serum calcium must remain normal. Correction of anemia (hematocrit > 27 vol. %) and hypoalbuminemia (>3.0 g/dl) is required if they are considered to be secondary to myeloma.
   - With equivocal data (*e.g.*, nonsecretors, L chain producers for whom the pretreatment urine collection was lost), the following support the conclusion that an objective response has occurred:
     - Recalcification of lytic skull lesions.
     - Significant increments in depressed normal immunoglobulins (*e.g.*, increments >200 mg/dl IgM, >400 mg/dl IgA, and >4000 mg/dl IgG).

B. Improved patients show a decline in the serum M-protein synthesis rate to less than 50%, but not less than 25% of the pretreatment value.

C. Unresponsive patients fail to satisfy the criteria for responsive or improved patients.

(Alexanian R, Bonnet J, Gehan E, et al. Combination chemotherapy for multiple myeloma. Cancer 1972;30:382–389)

carrying out this analysis, 2 stage II patients and 9 stage III patients who failed to live 3 months were censored to minimize the "guarantee time" inherent in including early deaths as nonresponders by usual statistical methods. The researchers concluded from this analysis of a relatively small series of patients that the Myeloma Task Force criteria of response may have similar predictive value to that of the SWOG for stage II patients. They found that the SWOG criteria had greater predictive value for stage III patients but believed that the latter difference was of questionable significance. Further analysis of significantly larger patient populations is warranted to authenticate the association of M-component reduction and tumor regression in multiple myeloma.

RADIATION THERAPY

Palliation for Bone Pain and Soft Tissue Masses

Radiation therapy has been recognized for many years as a rapid and highly effective palliative agent in the treatment of multiple myeloma.[225–229] Despite advances in the systemic treatment of this disease, radiation therapy continues to be important. It has been estimated that almost 70% of all patients eventually require and potentially benefit from treatment with irradiation.[230]

Treatment of painful, disabling bony sites is usually rapidly successful because of the radioresponsive nature of myeloma. In addition to rapid relief of pain, with accompanying decrease in narcotic requirements, pain relief allows patients to maintain much more normal activity, reducing the structural weakness in bone caused by calcium loss from bedrest. Because treatment is often rapidly effective at relatively modest doses, irradiation can arrest local tumor progression in bone and prevent pathologic fractures, minimizing the morbidity of more invasive therapeutic interventions for these patients. These positive features of irradiation enable a much more normal functional existence for patients.[225–228]

Myeloma is usually quite responsive to radiation therapy, and tumor doses of approximately 2000 to 2400 cGy in five to seven fractions over 1 to 1.5 weeks are usually sufficient.[226,228] Relief of pain is obtained in more than 90% of treated patients.[230,231] From 30% to 65% of responses are complete.[230] An analysis of 100 patients treated at the University of Arizona demonstrated no increase in response probability with doses greater than 1500 cGy. Limited numbers of sites were treated with lower doses. Neither the probability of recurrent symptoms nor the time to relapse at the treated site was influenced by the radiation dose. Except for solitary disease, higher doses have not been advantageous, and because of the generalized nature of the disease and its relatively long natural history, higher doses may preclude a necessary second course of treatment to a site caused by tumor reseeding, extension, or regrowth.

Careful treatment planning is necessary to ensure inclusion

of the entire lesion(s) responsible to the localized problem, and imaging studies such as computed tomography (CT) scans may be helpful in delineating the extent of tumor.

Judgment and experience are necessary in determining when radiation therapy is appropriate (versus systemic treatment), especially early in the course of this often chronic condition. Although irradiation relieves the most disabling symptom(s), a similar result often can be achieved by chemotherapy, especially early in the course of myeloma, with no resultant compromise in future delivery of chemotherapy because of myelosuppression. This is particularly true in the treatment of sites containing considerable bone marrow, such as the pelvis. A Cancer and Leukemia Group B (CALGB) study that attempted "total bone marrow" treatment by sequential irradiation in combination with chemotherapy was not beneficial.[232] Recirculation of myeloma into previously treated sites may partially explain the negative study.[233] Ideal management requires close coordination with the physician administering the patient's systemic chemotherapy.

Structural changes brought about by tumor involvement may, by nerve compression or orthopedic instability, be responsible for a substantial portion of a patient's pain. It is usually a mistake to treat a patient with multiple myeloma to progressively higher doses than those previously used if some level of pain persists, assuming that careful prior imaging studies and treatment planning have been accomplished.

Special Indications for Radiation Therapy

Several other localized manifestations of myeloma may be indications for palliative irradiation, especially in the patient who has proved resistant to most conventional systemic agents. Included are patients who present with proptosis caused by sphenoid or orbital bone involvement, those who present with dental or facial abnormalities caused by maxillary or mandibular involvement, or those who present with CNS symptoms caused by extensive calvarial or base of the skull involvement. A treatment philosophy and approach similar to that for palliation of bone pain is appropriate.

CHEMOTHERAPY

Systemic Chemotherapy

The initial approach to treatment for most patients with symptoms and signs of progressive disease is with systemic chemotherapy. Cycle-nonspecific cytotoxic drugs, particularly alkylating agents, represent the current mainstay of standard therapy.

Bifunctional alkylating agents, particularly melphalan and cyclophosphamide; nitrosoureas, including carmustine and lomustine (CCNU); doxorubicin; and glucocorticoids represent the major active agents used in systemic therapy for multiple myeloma.[23,26,27,214,215] Vincristine has been used in several treatment programs; although there is evidence it can reduce tumor burden somewhat, there is no indication that its addition to other drugs increases survival.[216–218] INF-α has antitumor activity in myeloma and is currently under investigation to determine whether it can play a role with other systemic agents in the drug-sensitive phase of disease.[219–224] All of these agents have been subjected to clinical trials as single agents in myeloma and have been incorporated into various drug combinations for evaluation in previously untreated patients.

Remission-Induction Chemotherapy

ALKYLATING AGENTS WITH OR WITHOUT PREDNISONE. A variety of simple alkylating agent—prednisone combinations and more complex regimens have been used for remission induction for patients with multiple myeloma. Overall objective response rates in various series using single alkylating agents alone or in combination with prednisone usually are 20% to 70%, and the rates are influenced by the response criteria used and the aggressiveness with which the regimens can be administered because of their myelosuppressive effects. Prednisone and other glucocorticoids have been combined with alkylating agents because of their single-agent activity, lack of overlapping toxicity, and the suggestion that they may potentiate the action of other agents. In most instances, patients in these trials received maintenance chemotherapy after remission induction.

Many studies used a variety of schedules of oral administration of melphalan or cyclophosphamide alone or in combination with prednisone, with generally similar therapeutic results. Useful dosage schedules for the commonly used alkylating agents appear in Table 56–8. Dosage adjustments for myelosuppression are commonly employed, but dose escalation in the absence of myelosuppression is not usually followed satisfactorily. Inadequate dose escalation (particularly with melphalan) can produce significant underdosing. Melphalan has variable absorption by the oral route, and the drug is best absorbed when ingested on an empty stomach.[234] Although oral absorption is not usually a problem with oral cyclophosphamide or CCNU, regular monitoring of the leukocyte count and differential count can detect patients with compliance problems with the self-administration of oral agents. Nadir absolute granulocyte counts below 2000/μl should be achieved between intermittent courses of therapy, but with continuous courses, the dosage should be adjusted to

TABLE 56–8. Selected Schedules Using Intermittent or Continuous Schedules of Alkylating Agents for Treatment of Myeloma Alone or in Combination With Prednisone

Intermittent Schedules	
Cyclophosphamide	
I.V.	1000 mg/m^2 (27 mg/kg) q 3 weeks
	(Significantly higher doses now being evaluated)
Oral	250 mg/m^2 per d × 4d q 3 wk
Melphalan	
I.V.	16 mg/m^2 q 2 wk × 4 then q 4 wk
	Reduce initial dosing by 50% if serum creatinine > 2.0 mg/dl (BUN > 30 mg/dl)
Oral	8 mg/m^2 q 3 wk or 9 mg/m^2 q 4 wk
	(Because of varying bioavailability of oral melphalan, the dose must be increased to induce hematologic toxicity or significant underdosing may occur.)
Carmustine (BCNU)	
I.V.	100–150 mg/m^2 q 4–6 wk
Lomustine (CCNU)	
Oral	130 mg/m^2 q 4–6 wk

maintain the leukocyte count between 2000 and 3500/μl. Although intravenous schedules provide more predictable dose delivery, the largest experience has been with oral regimens.

Regardless of the dosage schedules or objective response rates in major clinical trials, the median survival time of patients receiving oral melphalan or cyclophosphamide alone or in combination with prednisone have ranged from 18 to 35 months, with an overall median of about 24 months (Table 56–9). Some "response rates" have varied because different criteria were used to determine objective response in the reported studies. Similar results have been observed with the nitrosoureas, although these agents have not been studied extensively.[26]

The survival outcome in myeloma patients is now clearly superior to that observed before the introduction of alkylating agents, when median survival times from diagnosis were in the range of 3.5 to 11.5 months.[235–237] The improvement in survival that occurred in myeloma after the introduction of the alkylating agents is due to these drugs, rather than to changes in earlier diagnosis or changes in supportive care. Equivalent therapeutic effects have been reported with intermittent and continuous schedules. An initial loading dose followed by a subsequent continuous dose, as used by the CALGB, produced similar results.[25] Intermittent schedules may have advantages in terms of assuring regular monitoring of the patient's progress and avoiding cumulative toxicity.

MULTIAGENT COMBINATION CHEMOTHERAPY. An area of continuing controversy for myeloma therapy is the comparative effectiveness of the simple oral melphalan plus prednisone (MP) or cyclophosphamide plus prednisone (CP) combinations with more complex regimens. Several institutions and cooperative groups have explored a variety of multiagent combinations, with a subset of these studies reporting significantly better survival results than have been observed with the simple combinations; however, this is far from uniform. Multiagent combinations incorporate agents with different mechanisms of action, little or no cross-resistance, and reduced overlapping toxicities, enabling greater cytoreduction of the myeloma cell burden. Some experimental evidence suggests that combinations of alkylating agents may be potentiating because there are different mechanisms of membrane uptake and other potential differences in their mode of action and cellular cytotoxicity.[245]

Some of the most widely used multiagent combinations include the M2 protocol developed at Memorial Sloan-Kettering Cancer Center[246] and the alternating combination chemotherapy regimens developed by SWOG.[190] In the initial SWOG report of alternating combinations, vincristine, melphalan, carmustine, and prednisone (VMCP) was alternated with vincristine, carmustine, doxorubicin, and prednisone (VBAP) or vincristine, cyclophosphamide, doxorubicin, and prednisone (VCAP).[190] In subsequent trials, the alternation has been limited to VMCP and VBAP, because VBAP can reinduce remission in myeloma patients who have previously responded and relapsed from therapy with melphalan or cyclophosphamide combinations.[247] The dosage schedules for these Memorial Sloan-Kettering and SWOG combination programs are summarized in Table 56–10. The fifth Medical Research Council's (MRC5) trial of alternating combination chemotherapy used

TABLE 56–9. Effects of Some Major Trials of Single Alkylating Agents Alone or in Combination With Prednisone on Survival in Multiple Myeloma

Investigations	*Treatment* (Alkylating Agent Scheduled)*	*No. of Patients*	*Response Rate†*	*Median Survival From Start of Therapy (mo)*
Alexanian et al[238]	Melphalan (i)	82	49–59	23
Alexanian et al[239]	Melphalan (d)	35	17–19	18
	Melphalan, prednisone (i)	79	~65	24
Bergsagel et al[21]	Melphalan (d)	165	14	25
Bergsagel et al[189]	Melphalan, prednisone (i)	100	72	28
Costa et al[25]	Melphalan (d)	60	~25	26
	Melphalan, prednisone (d)	71	~48	35
	Melphalan, prednisone + testosterone (d)	58	~54	24
Hoogstraten et al[240]	Melphalan (d)	64	45	23
Hoogstraten et al[241]	Melphalan (i)	48	45	26
Korst et al[22]	Cyclophosphamide (d)	165	~48	24.5
McArthur et al[237]	Melphalan (d)	39	41	28
MRC 1st study[242]	Melphalan (d)	133	NR	18
	Cyclophosphamide (d)	141	NR	18
MRC 2nd study[243]	Melphalan, prednisone (d)	128	NR	20
	Cyclophosphamide (d)	124	NR	20
MRC 3rd study[244]	Melphalan (i)	179	NR	20
	Cyclophosphamide (i) (intravenous)	174	NR	26

* d, daily; i, intermittent; NR, not reported.
† Response rates shown with Myeloma Task Force Criteria or approximated from published data.

TABLE 56–10. Dosage Schedules for the M2, VMCP–VBAP, and ABCM Regimens

Drug Regimen	*Vincristine*	*Melphalan*	*Cyclophosphamide*	*BCNU*	*Doxorubicin*	*Prednisone*
M2 regimen[246]	0.03 mg/kg day 1	0.25 mg/kg days 1–7	10 mg/kg day 1	0.5 mg/kg day 1		1 mg/kg days 1–7
VMCP[190]	1.0 mg day 1	6 mg/m^2/d days 1–4	125 mg/m^2/d days 1–4			60 mg/m^2/d days 1–4
VBAP[190]	1.0 mg day 1			30 mg/m^2 day 1	30 mg/m^2 day 1	
ABCM[248]		6 mg/m^2/d days 1–4	100 mg/m^2/d days 1–4	30 mg/m^2 day 1	30 mg/m^2 day 1	days 1–4

As currently used, the M2 protocol is usually repeated at 4- to 5-wk intervals. The VMCP–VBAP program repeats courses of chemotherapy in 21-day cycles using either a direct alternation of the two regimens or a syncopated alternation wherein VMCP is used for three cycles followed by VBAP for three cycles with similar therapeutic results by either of these schedules. Currently an every-3-week alternation is used. The MRC has used an almost identical schedule to VMCP–VBAP in their alternating program, except that vincristine and prednisone have been deleted. Alternations are also at 3-wk intervals in the MRC's ABCM program.

drug dosages that were essentially identical with that of SWOG, with the deletion of vincristine and prednisone (see Table 56–10).[248]

Slight changes in dosages of the M2 regimen have been used in various series.[206] With the M2 regimen, improved survival has been reported in a nonrandomized study, in which survival was calculated from the date of diagnosis rather than from the onset of therapy.[246] Subsequent randomized studies carried out by the Eastern Cooperative Group (ECOG) in the United States and by a multihospital group from Denmark compared the M2 regimen to melphalan and prednisone.[249,250] Both studies failed to show a survival advantage with the M2 regimen, although good-risk subsets in the ECOG study had improved survival.[249] An update on the ECOG study reported improved survival for stage III patients.[247]

Two successive studies carried out by SWOG compared the alternating combination regimens to a simpler regimen of MP or vincristine, cyclophosphamide, plus prednisone (VCP). In both studies (evaluated by different study coordinators), quite similar advantages in terms of improved response rate and improved median survival were observed with the alternating combination compared with the simpler regimen.[190,251] Results of the first of these studies were reanalyzed in 1985, again demonstrating a survival advantage of alternating combination chemotherapy over MP.[190,251] The second of SWOG's evaluations of alternating combinations demonstrated remarkably similar survival plots for the VMCP plus VBAP compared with the simpler VCP regimen. Analysis of pretreatment prognostic factors showed that the treatment groups were quite comparable. A significantly larger proportion of patients responded to the alternating combinations, suggesting that the additional responsive patients may have required combination therapy to reach remission status and could be anticipated to have had a poorer prognosis and below average remission duration. Analysis of the data on high-risk stage III patients in some studies supports this interpretation and is consistent with the overall remission duration in the VMCP-VBAP group being diluted with the addition of poor-risk patients "recruited into" the responsive category with the aggressive combinations who would not have achieved remission with the simple regimens.[246]

A similar interpretation may apply to studies from ECOG and the CALGB, who found improved response rates, survival time, or both in specific subsets of patients with multiagent combinations compared with the MP regimen.[249,252] In these two studies, overall survival for all patients was not improved, suggesting that the increased toxicity of the aggressive regimens may have a detrimental effect on survival of subsets of patients. The MRC study made a similar observation to that by SWOG. In the MRC study, 627 patients were randomized to receive almost identical schedules of the cytotoxic agents used in the SWOG VMCP-VBAP studies, except that vincristine and prednisone were omitted. The MRC study compared alternating MC and BA to M in a study begun in 1982 and closed in 1986. In the MRC's study, the survival advantage for the 314 patients receiving the alternating combinations was significantly superior (p=0.0003) to that obtained with M alone.[248] Curves for the MRC5 study are similar to the SWOG results despite the omission of vincristine and prednisone. The MRC's comparison of ABCM to M is significantly larger than the SWOG study or other studies comparing multiagent chemotherapy to M or MP.[248] A summary of results from these studies appear in Table 56–11.

Other multicenter randomized trials using VMCP-VBAP or variants of the M2 protocol (VBMCP) failed to show better results than simpler regimens (Table 56–12).[253] Comparison of the different trials is difficult because of different prognostic factors, differences in the treatments used, and differences in dose modifications and other factors. Several studies compared sequential administration of various alkylating agents with simultaneous combinations or MP (data not shown). These studies showed inferiority or no advantage for the sequential regimens.[188,252] Although there are discrepancies between multiagent and simpler regimens in various trails, none of these regimens are curative or control the disease for 4 years or longer. Therefore newer therapeutic approaches are needed.

Although INF-α is known to have some activity in mye-

TABLE 56–11. Results of Recent Alternating Combination Chemotherapy Regimens Used for Remission Induction in Multiple Myeloma in Multicenter Randomized Trials

*Investigations**	*Treatment*	*No. of Patients*	*% Responding† (mo)*	*Median Survival*
SWOG Alternating Combinations vs MP or VCP				
Study 7704[190,251]	VMCP + VBAP or VCAP	160	54	42
	MP	77	32	23
Study 7927[251]	VMCP + VBAP	93	54	48
	VCP	107	28	29
MRC Alternating Combination vs M				
Myelomatosis V[248]	ABCM	314	61	32
	M	316	59	24

* In these studies, patients had a statistically significant improvement in survival with alternating combination chemotherapy as compared with melphalan or MP therapy.
† Response criteria varied between SWOG and the MRC groups but were consistent within each group's trial.

loma patients in relapse, the recombinant forms of IFN-α have had only limited study in previously untreated patients.[219–222,259–261] In an initial report, 7 of 14 patients with previously untreated myeloma with stages I or II myeloma responded to treatment.[223] The response was associated with an increase in residual polyclonal immunoglobulins. However, two randomized trials comparing initial therapy with IFN-α to chemotherapy have shown IFN-α monotherapy to be less active than standard chemotherapy.[262,263] Recombinant IFN-α has also been integrated into combination chemotherapy with alkylating agent and prednisone combinations.[224] On the basis of the initial experience with this approach, the CALGB

TABLE 56–12. Results With Combination Chemotherapy Regimens Used for Remission Induction in Multiple Myeloma in Multicenter Randomized Trials That Failed to Show a Survival Advantage With Multiagent Chemotherapy Compared With Simple Alkylating Agent Regimens

Investigations	*Treatment*	*No. of Patients*	*% Response (mo)*	*Median Survival*
Argentine[255]	MeCCMVP	105	46	41
	MP	129	38	39
CALGB[254]	MCBP (I.V.)	156	56	29
	MCBPA (I.V.)	157	44	26
	MP (I.V.)	146	47	33
Canadian[189]	MCBP	116	47*	31
	MP	125	31*	28
Danish[250]	M2	31	45	21
	VMP	32	73	30
	MP	33	58	21
ECOG[256]	M2	134	74	~31
	MP	131	53	~30
Finnish[257]	MOCCA	64	75	41
	MP	66	54	45
Norwegian[258]	M2	33	74	33
	MP	34	67	33
SECSG[256]	BCP	186	49	36
	MP	187	52	36
Italian[253]	VMCP-VBAP	158	77	32
	MP	146	64	37

MeC, methyl-CCNU; B, BCNU; C, cyclophosphamide; V, vincristine; P, prednisone; A, doxorubicin (Adriamycin); MOCCA, melphalan, vincristine, CCNU, cyclophosphamide, doxorubicin.
* SWOG response criteria (all others reported by Myeloma Task Force Criteria).

initiated a randomized trial comparing the effectiveness of MP to MP plus recombinant IFN-α2.[261] There appears to be no advantage to using aggressive regimens in treatment of stage I patients. The major issue is whether any therapy should be employed until clear evidence of symptomatic disease progression occurs. Application of additional prognostic factors, such as the pretreatment β_2-microglobulin level or evaluation of the proliferative index of myeloma cells, may assist in better identifying the patient groups most likely to benefit from aggressive systemic therapy.

TUMOR CELL REDUCTION WITH INDUCTION CHEMOTHERAPY. The magnitude of tumor cell reduction with chemotherapy can be assessed using the quantitative methods to determine response in terms of the degree of cytoreduction achieved. For myeloma, this was first achieved using a computer-based method in which serial measurements of the amount of M-component produced per cell in vitro, intravascular mass of M-components, and catabolic rate were integrated.[2,170] For the current standard treatment programs and magnitude of cell death determined from M-component-derived measurements, the maximal degree of cytoreduction observed in patients treated with conventional chemotherapy rarely exceeds 90% to 99%. Despite continued treatment, the tumor burden appears to plateau in most cases.[170] Kinetic analysis of the plateau-phase population suggests that the residual tumor cells behave differently from those present before treatment, and they are comparatively hypoproliferative and perhaps less responsive to cytotoxic chemotherapy.[209]

With a total tumor burden in most patients in the range of 10^{12} myeloma cells or more, it is not surprising that there is not a strong correlation between the exact magnitude of cytoreduction (*e.g.*, 75%, 90%, 99%) and overall survival. However, remission durations after induction chemotherapy can vary substantially in comparably staged patients with similar degrees of apparent cytoreduction and the presence of a clearly measurable residual M-component peak in the serum. Although the median duration of unmaintained remission is 11 months, unmaintained remissions after induction chemotherapy in some patients with stage III myeloma may last for 5 years or longer.[264,265] This suggests that there is an alteration in the residual myeloma cell population or in the tumor-host relation. Such observations provide the basis for seriously questioning whether the residual cell mass determined from M-component levels in remission reflects the initial population of malignant plasma cells or a less malignant population more akin to that in patients with MGUS. However, patients regularly relapse with overt myeloma from unmaintained remissions, indicating that an underlying highly malignant monoclone persists but may be submerged under a population of less highly proliferative M-component-secreting cells.

Analysis of the myeloma regrowth rate based on M-component doubling times has been carried out for patients studied sequentially after a series of unmaintained remissions.[169] Even in the presence of continued chemosensitivity (as reflected by cytoreduction after reinstitution of chemotherapy), some patients studied developed a progressive shortening of the M-component doubling time during subsequent unmaintained remissions. Such observations suggest progressive loss of growth control with the emergence of a kinetically more aggressive tumor cell population.

Remission Maintenance Versus Unmaintained Remission

Therapeutic approaches in myeloma have usually been developed in an analogous fashion to those for other advanced neoplasms and have included remission-induction phase and remission-maintenance phase treatments. Myeloma patients who exhibit drug sensitivity and achieve remission usually have been maintained on a similar form of chemotherapy until the time of relapse.

The usefulness of maintenance therapy with cytotoxic drugs has been examined in several studies with similar results.[264,266–268] Patients achieving remission with chemotherapy were randomized to maintenance chemotherapy with MP or to no maintenance therapy. Patients randomized to no maintenance received alkylating agent chemotherapy again at the earliest evidence of relapse as manifested by a rise in M-component levels or recurrent symptoms and signs of active myeloma. There was no overall survival advantage for patients receiving maintenance chemotherapy. Continuation of conventional alkylating agent therapy for patients achieving remission appears to offer no obvious advantage over unmaintained remission, as long as patients are followed closely and have treatment reinstituted when there is laboratory or clinical evidence of reactivation of myeloma. In general, patients followed in unmaintained remission should be followed monthly, with regular monitoring of serum and urine M-components to detect the first signs of relapse. Patients presenting initially with stage III myeloma with heavy Bence Jones proteinuria or amyloidosis must be followed closely, because fulminant relapse from unmaintained remission can lead to irreversible complications unless treatment is reinstituted promptly at the first sign of disease reactivation.

An approach to remission maintenance that used recombinant IFN-α was reported by the Italian Multiple Myeloma Study Group.[269,270] In this study, 70 patients with remissions induced with MP or VMCP-VBAP (on a randomized induction) were re-randomized to maintenance therapy with recombinant IFN-α2 or to no treatment. The IFN-α2 was administered at a dosage of 3×10^6 IU/m^2 subcutaneously three times weekly. After 27 months of follow-up, 8 (24%) of 33 of evaluable patients receiving IFN-α2 and 22 (59%) of 37 patients with no maintenance had relapsed, with a significant difference ($p<0.01$) in the actuarial curves of remission duration in the two groups.[270] A larger study of IFN maintenance conducted by the SWOG with over 200 patients randomized to interferon maintenance or observation using 3×10^6 of IFNα2 given intravenously with the same schedule showed no advantage of IFNα2 over unmaintained remission for remission duration or survival.[271] Further follow-up of these two studies and several other interferon maintenance studies are required before the role for IFN maintenance can be established.

SOLITARY PLASMACYTOMA OF BONE AND EXTRAMEDULLARY PLASMACYTOMA

About 7% of all patients with plasma cell malignancies present with solitary lesions in bone or soft tissues, with bone marrow examinations demonstrating fewer than 5% plasmacytes. Several factors differentiate patients with solitary lesions from those with multiple myeloma. Age at presentation tends to be younger, and a higher percentage are male (70% versus 55%). A smaller fraction (30% versus 97%) present with serum or urinary M-components.

The demonstration that an elevation in M-component may persist after high-dose local irradiation, but may return to normal with subsequent long-term disease-free survival after nonradical surgical excision of Waldeyer's ring material, suggests two alternative possibilities for the response of certain malignant plasma cells to irradiation. One alternative is that a substantial population of cells in certain patients is highly resistant to irradiation. However, several factors mitigate against this explanation, especially the long disease-free survival after a nonradical surgical approach. Because of the monoclonal nature of the disease in these patients and their generally excellent response to irradiation, it seems more likely that these persistent cells represent clonogenically nonviable foci that fail to manifest radiation damage because they divide slowly or not at all. Such behavior is somewhat analogous to functioning pituitary adenomas in which elevated hormone levels may be observed for months or years after radiation therapy without evidence of ultimate progression.

Several studies have shown a relatively favorable course for both these groups of patients, but many long-term studies have demonstrated the distinct difference in ultimate prognosis between patients with solitary lesions in bone and those with extramedullary lesions.[272–275,277] Although they experience significantly longer survivals than patients with classic multiple myeloma, virtually all patients with solitary bone lesions develop systemic disease if followed for sufficient periods.[272–275] In one study, although almost 35% of patients were progression-free at 10 years, by 13 years, more than 90% of patients experienced widespread evidence of disease.[274] The report by Chak and coworkers is slightly more optimistic.[276] More than 80% of patients treated for extramedullary lesions are progression free at periods exceeding 10 years after treatment.[272–274,277]

Despite this difference in ultimate prognosis, long-term survival is observed in substantial numbers in both groups and suggests the desirability for long-term local control. Radiation doses of 3500 to 5000 cGy have been proposed, with doses at the lower end of this spectrum usually applied with shortened treatment times and increased daily radiation fractions. We favor a total dose of 4500 to 5000 cGy in 4.5 to 5 weeks, using megavoltage fields that adequately encompass necessary soft tissue and bony structures. In primary bony lesions, the entire medullary cavity of the bone must be encompassed, as in patients with Ewing's tumor because of the possibility of medullary cavity spread.

Few data are available on the probability of regional lymph node spread, and treatment of nodal sites, in addition to adequately encompassing of the primary lesion, usually is not recommended. The report of Knowling and associates suggests that treatment may be of value in selected patients.[273] Typical survival curves after radiation treatment for these two groups of patients appear in Figure 56–9.[272–274,276,277]

IN VITRO TESTING OF CLONOGENIC MYELOMA CELLS

In vitro methods have been developed to support the growth of colony-forming neoplastic plasma cells from the bone marrows of some patients with multiple myeloma and to assess the response of the clonogenic myeloma cells to a variety of anticancer drugs.[59,278–281] Clonogenic growth of myeloma cells has been applied to in vitro drug testing by several laboratories.[278,279,281,282] At the Arizona Cancer Center, true-positive correlations between in vitro sensitivity and clinical response were obtained in 22 (79%) of 28 instances in which in vitro sensitivity was observed, and true-negative correlations with in vitro drug resistance were observed in 35 (99%) of 37 instances.[281] Although such findings suggest that this assay may have potentially broad application, it is still applicable to only a few of the patients tested, because of inadequate colony growth in many instances. Due to technical limitations, it is currently impractical to routinely test patients' myeloma cells for drug sensitivity. However, in the research setting, we continue to find this approach an aid in the discovery of new drugs with activity against myeloma cells and in identifying potentially active drugs for a selected subset of patients whose cells can be cultivated in vitro. New information on cytokines that support the growth of plasmacytoma cells and the use of more sensitive assays may increase the applicability of this approach to myeloma in the future.[61,63,283–285]

TREATMENT OF REFRACTORY MYELOMA

Patients who relapse after unmaintained remission can often be reinduced into remission with a regimen similar to that used initially and are not considered to be refractory to therapy

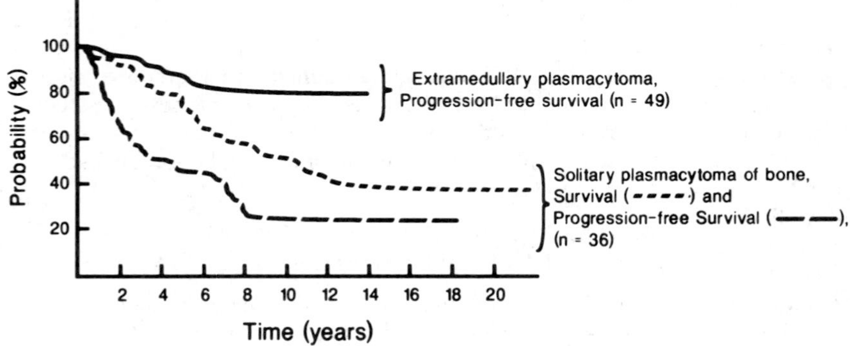

FIGURE 56–9. Survival and disease-free survival for patients with solitary plasmacytoma of bone and disease-free survival of those with solitary soft-tissue disease. Notice the significant advantage for those with soft tissue disease and low disease-free survival (in time) for those with bone disease.

unless they fail to achieve remission on reinduction.[264,286] However, at least one third of patients with multiple myeloma fail to respond to induction chemotherapy, and those who initially achieve remission eventually relapse and require additional treatment. Standard and new agents and approaches have been evaluated in refractory patients.[287,288] Therapeutic agents used for treatment of refractory patients usually include the same drugs used in initial remission-induction therapy (*e.g.,* anthracyclines, glucocorticoids, vinca alkaloids, alkylating agents, nitrosoureas), often given in alternative dosages, schedules, and combinations to those used initially. INF-α has activity as a phase II agent, but remissions are usually short, and IFN-α has yet to be integrated effectively into combination therapy for second-line therapy.[221,222,289–291]

It is important to differentiate between the two subsets of patients who are usually classified as refractory, because their prognoses differ substantially. For simplicity, refractory myeloma patients are usually divided into drug-resistant and relapsing groups. Patients who fail to respond to induction chemotherapy and are drug-resistant have the poorest overall prognosis, and only a few respond to alternate treatments. The second major category comprises relapsing patients who respond to induction chemotherapy but then relapse while still receiving chemotherapy or within a few months thereafter. They have a higher probability of responding to second-line therapy than do the drug-resistant patients.

High-Dose Glucocorticoids

The antitumor activity of single-agent prednisone for a high-dose, alternate-day schedule for resistant and relapsing patients was first reported over 20 years ago.[23] This single-agent activity of high doses of glucocorticoids has been confirmed and extended using prednisone and dexamethasone in alternate-day or pulse schedules.[214,287,292,293] High-dose dexamethasone recently has been studied in previously untreated patients with myeloma and has been found to be active when used as monotherapy.[293a] A P-glycoprotein-expressing multidrug-resistant myeloma cell line was reported to develop collateral sensitivity to glucocorticoids, suggesting that there may be some specificity of steroids for drug-resistant cells.[294] Overall, approximately 40% of resistant and relapsing myeloma patients achieve second remissions with glucocorticoids. Because glucocorticoids are nonmyelosuppressive, they are particularly useful in refractory patients with poor bone marrow reserves. In our experience, some pancytopenic patients have remissions of myeloma for several years with alternate-day prednisone alone. Efforts have been made to quantitate glucocorticoid receptors in myeloma, and these measurements may aid in identifying patients potentially sensitive to glucocorticoids.[295]

Combination Chemotherapy Regimens

Although there were a few initial favorable reports on combination regimens that included primarily alkylating agents, most reports have been less promising, with response rates in the range of 8% for resistant and 22% for refractory patients.[246,297–302] These regimens are far more active for reinducing remissions in patients who have disease reactivation from unmaintained remission.[264,286,303–305]

More favorable results have been obtained with doxorubicin-based combinations. Although doxorubicin alone exhibits activity in only 10% of patients, when combined with BCNU or with BCNU, vincristine, and prednisone (VBAP) or cyclophosphamide instead of vincristine, somewhat better results are obtained.[27,306–310] Approximately 30% of relapsing patients respond to these regimens, but only 10% of resistant patients respond. Although not all studies report the remission durations of responders or overall survival, the remission duration is usually less than 1 year. Significantly better results have been obtained by using the vincristine, doxorubicin, and dexamethasone (VAD) regimen developed at the M.D. Anderson Cancer Center.[311] Vincristine and doxorubicin are administered by continuous infusion over 4 days through an indwelling venous catheter, and dexamethasone is given orally (Table 56–13).

In an initial report, 14 (70%) of 20 patients with refractory myeloma responded to VAD, with a projected survival in excess of 1 year for responders.[311] Although granulocytopenia was only moderate, infection represented the most frequent complication, perhaps because of the large doses of dexamethasone used. In a follow-up report, VAD or dexamethasone were administered on a nonrandom basis to 85 refractory patients.[214] Among relapsing patients, 65% responded to VAD, but only 21% responded to dexamethasone alone. Among resistant patients, only 32% responded to VAD, a result quite similar to the 27% response rate observed with dexamethasone alone. This suggests that response to the VAD regimen in initially unresponsive patients is primarily due to the glucocorticoid in the regimen.[214] Similar therapeutic results have been confirmed with the VAD regimen by other investigators.[312–314] Toxicity has been the major limitation of the VAD regimen, with serious infection attributed primarily to the steroid program. Serious gastrointestinal toxicity, including gastric perforations, and steroid psychoses have been observed. Overall, approximately one third of patients receiving VAD develop moderate to severe toxic effects. Nonetheless, it appears to be the most effective treatment for myeloma relapses.

For patients with primary drug resistance, steroid alone is preferable to VAD. The multidrug resistance mechanism associated with P-glycoprotein expression appears to be frequently expressed by myeloma cells from patients with drug-resistant disease.[329–331] A novel means for reversing resistance to VAD has been reported for relapsing patients who previously

TABLE 56–13. Dosage Schedule for VAD Regimen

Vincristine	0.4 mg/d I.V. for 4 d
Doxorubicin	9 mg/m^2/d I.V. for 4 d
Dexamethasone	40 mg/d orally for 4 d beginning on days 1, 9, and 17 of the first 28-d cycle and on alternate cycles thereafter. On the other cycles dexamethasone is given only on days 1–4.

All patients also received cimetidine for antacid prophylaxis and trimethoprim—sulfamethoxazole as antiinfective prophylaxis.

(Barlogie B, Smith L, Alexanian R. Effective treatment of advanced multiple myeloma refractory to alkylating agents. N Engl J Med 1984;310:1353–1356)

responded to the VAD regimen and subsequently developed multidrug resistance associated with expression of the P-glycoprotein.[315] The P-glycoprotein was detected using a murine monoclonal antibody and by mRNA dot blot analysis. Five refractory myeloma patients were first treated with the VAD regimen, and at the time of relapse or failure to respond to VAD, the calcium channel blocker verapamil was administered at high dosage by continuous infusion along with VAD. Resistance was at least partially reversed in 2 patients, with improvement in M-component and hematologic values. In one patient whose myeloma cells were tested in vitro, verapamil exposure significantly increased intracellular accumulation of doxorubicin, suggesting a possible mechanism by which the verapamil effect was mediated. In a subsequent expansion of this trial, 5 (23%) of 22 VAD-refractory patients achieved remission again after high-dose intravenous verapamil was added to the VAD regimen.[316] However, verapamil is not a good agent to use as a chemosensitizer in myeloma patients, because it induces hypotension that can further compromise renal function in patients with Bence Jones proteinuria and impaired renal function. These studies provide proof that multidrug resistance can be circumvented, but better chemosensitizers are needed. Recently, cyclosporin also has been reported to reverse multidrug resistance when combined with the VAD regimen for use in VAD-resistant myeloma patients.[331a]

SYSTEMIC RADIATION THERAPY

Rider, Bergsagel, and colleagues were instrumental in pioneering wide-field or hemibody irradiation for systemic illness.[317,318] A variety of treatment schemes have been used, but in most, a radiation dose of 750 to 850 cGy in 150-cGy fractions (dose rate of ≥50 cGy/minute) is given to the hemibody (umbilicus used as midpoint) after pretreatment preparation with corticosteroids and antiemetics. Total-body approaches have also been used.[233] Patients have usually been a a poor-prognosis group with stage III disease, who have usually relapsed after first-line chemotherapy.[206] In most patients, the lower hemibody was treated initially. Approximately 50% to 75% of patients complete treatment to hemibody segments in most series.[317,318,320–325]

Because of the incidence of radiation pneumonitis in patients treated initially, cumulative lung doses have been reduced to 600 to 650 cGy (usually not corrected for air transmission) in more recently treated patients.[326] Although laboratory evidence of hematologic toxicity exists for most patients who have received treatment to the whole body, with some patients requiring platelet or erythrocyte transfusions, major clinical morbidity from hematologic toxicity has been moderate. In some instances, it can be prolonged. By using this irradiation approach, approximately half of all treated patients have experienced significant subjective relief.

Median survivals in irradiated patients have averaged 6 months, with mean survival times averaging 12 months. Some patients from this group have survived more than 18 months, and two reports documented more than 24 months of survival in several patients.[327,328]

In an attempt to use this treatment modality for better-prognosis patients, the SWOG carried out a phase III prospectively randomized trial (SWOG 8229/8230) in which previously untreated patients who achieved remission (≥75% tumor mass regression) randomized to maintenance chemotherapy or to sequential hemibody irradiation (750 cGy per five fields for 1 week) with 4 to 6 weeks or more elapsing between the two irradiation courses, depending on the severity and duration of hematologic toxicity.[206]

In the SWOG study, the survival outcome for patients receiving hemibody irradiation was significantly inferior to that of patients receiving maintenance chemotherapy. The difference in survival could be attributed to a shorter relapse-free survival with irradiation. Survival time from relapse to death was identical in both groups.[206,319] Myelosuppression was significantly more severe in patients receiving hemibody radiation therapy than those receiving maintenance chemotherapy. The primary toxicity was prolonged thrombocytopenia. These findings indicate that chemotherapy maintenance is more effective than hemibody irradiation for remission consolidation in myeloma patients who respond to induction chemotherapy.

HIGH-DOSE THERAPY ALONE OR WITH BONE MARROW TRANSPLANTATION

More aggressive approaches to the therapy of multiple myeloma use high-dose chemotherapy alone or high-dose chemotherapy with total-body irradiation and autologous or allogeneic bone marrow transplantation to overcome drug resistance to conventional-dose therapy.[332–346] The drug most commonly used in high doses has been melphalan, administered intravenously in doses ranging from 80 to 140 mg/m^2, without or with bone marrow or peripheral blood stem cell support. With high-dose melphalan alone, a high response rate is observed, including complete remissions associated with complete disappearance of the M-component and normalization of the bone marrow.[338] Unfortunately, the responses to high-dose melphalan alone among relapse patients have usually lasted only 3 months to 1 year. Toxicity has included profound myelosuppression, mucositis, diarrhea, nausea, and vomiting. Treatment-related deaths are not uncommon and are associated with host failure and severe hematologic toxicity. However, because the use of high-dose melphalan is still relatively new, further experience may provide a means to enhance efficacy and reduce toxicity (*e.g.*, with the use of myeloid colony-stimulating factors or by limitation of high-dose melphalan administration to patients with good performance status).

Prognostic factors associated with better outcome with autologous bone marrow transplantation in myeloma include the presence of drug-sensitive disease.[347] The addition of autologous bone marrow transplantation with or without purging has reduced the severity of myelosuppression. When total-body irradiation (usually 200 cGy twice daily for 3 days; total dose, 1200 cGy) delivered at a reduced dose rate (5–50 cGy/minute)) was combined with high-dose melphalan and autologous bone marrow transplantation, significantly longer remissions were observed.[339] In many instances, evidence of a residual M-component was still detected with immunofixation. Efforts to develop purging techniques to remove residual myeloma from the marrow are being attempted to enhance the potential of autologous transplantation. As an alternative to purging, autologous blood stem cells have been used for hematopoietic reconstitution.[348–353] The main limitation appears to be the difficulty of eradicating myeloma with the available preparative regimens for transplantation.

A promising study of 90 patients was published by the European Cooperative Group for Bone Marrow Transplantation.[354] This study showed good outcome for a significant fraction of patients receiving HLA-matched sibling donor marrow. The complete remission rate after marrow transplantation was 43% for all patients and 58% for patients with engraftment. The actuarial survival rate at 76 months was 76% (Fig. 56–10). Of 90 patients undergoing allogeneic bone marrow transplantation, 43% of all patients and 58% of patients who engrafted achieved complete remission. The median duration of relapse-free survival for complete remission patients was 48 months, and overall survival at 76 months was 40% (see Fig. 56–10). Allogeneic transplantation should be considered for selected patients younger than 55 who have an HLA-matched sibling donor.

ACTIVITY OF AGENTS IN PHASE II TRIALS

A few other antitumor agents have induced remissions in 10% or more of myeloma patients in relapse in phase II trials. These include pentostatin,[356] epirubicin, poly (I,C)-LC (an interferon inducer), peptichemio, and teniposide.[355,357–360] Except for the interferon inducer, these agents warrant additional investigation in refractory cases to better define their activity.

Other chemotherapeutic agents that have been subjected to phase II clinical trials in myeloma and found to have minimal activity (with less than a 10% response rate in refractory patients) include aclarubicin, acronine, amsacrine, bleomycin, cisplatin, chlorozotocin, cytarabine, diaziquone, etoposide, hexamethylmelamine, mitoxantrone, prednimustine, procarbazine, pyrazofurin, urethane, vindesine, fludarabine, or amonafide.[19,361–380] Although hexamethylmelamine appeared to exhibit greater than 10% activity, this was probably attributable to the concomitant use of glucocorticoids in the protocol.[381]

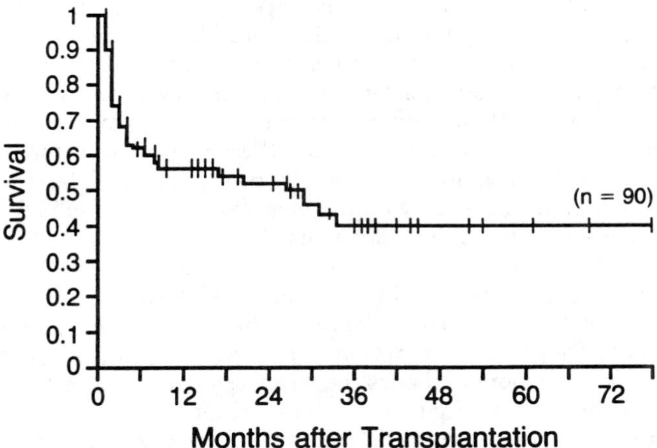

FIGURE 56–10. Actuarial survival after bone marrow transplantation for all 90 patients reported from the European Group for Bone Marrow Transplantation Registry as having allogeneic transplants performed for multiple myeloma. The actuarial survival at 76 months was 40%. The median duration of relapse-free survival among patients who were in complete remission after their transplants was 48 months. (Gahrton G, Sante T, Per L, et al. Allogeneic bone marrow transplantation in multiple myeloma. N Engl J Med 1992;325:1267–1273)

COMPLICATIONS AND SPECIAL PROBLEMS

RENAL FAILURE

In most studies, approximately 20% of patients with multiple myeloma present with renal failure, which adversely affects survival.[382] In one report, patients with stage IIIB myeloma had a median survival of only 4 months.[383] For patients who have normal or minimally impaired renal function, it is important to take actions that minimize the likelihood of subsequent development of renal failure. Myeloma patients should have a high fluid intake (*e.g.,* at least 2 L/day) to facilitate the excretion of calcium, Bence Jones proteins, uric acid, and other nephrotoxic excretory products. Patients with Bence Jones proteinuria and evidence of advanced or progressive myeloma should promptly be started on a chemotherapy regimen.

Adequate chemotherapy and hydration are important in managing myeloma patients with renal failure.[382] Administration of allopurinol with chemotherapy is a worthwhile precaution in stage III patients, at least for the first few courses of therapy. Patients with known myeloma should not be dehydrated for intravenous pyelography, and hypercalcemia and urinary tract infections should be treated promptly. The use of antibiotics with known nephrotoxicity (*e.g.,* the aminoglycosides) should be avoided if possible. Agents causing sustained hypotension and reduced renal blood flow should also be avoided. When melphalan is administered intravenously to patients in renal failure, increased myelosuppression has been observed.[384] Pharmacokinetic studies of intravenous melphalan in dogs and of oral administration in myeloma patients established that melphalan elimination is reduced by renal insufficiency.[385,386] Dose reductions are often needed for melphalan when it is administered intravenously, but because of the varying bioavailability of oral melphalan, dose reductions for renal failure may further compromise its therapeutic activity.

In the fourth MRC myeloma chemotherapy trial, management of renal failure was studied prospectively.[387] Of the 522 patients admitted to the trial, 80 had evidence of renal failure that persisted after an initial 24-hours of rehydration. Seventy-three of the 80 patients who had renal failure were maintained with a fluid intake of at least 3 L/day in addition to receiving chemotherapy. These patients were randomized to receive sodium bicarbonate or no supplement to render the urine pH neutral. The remaining 7 patients had congestive heart failure or required continued dialysis for oliguric renal failure and were not eligible for evaluation of oral fluid supplementation. Of 49 patients who survived more than 100 days, 39 achieved reversal of renal failure (18 complete, 21 partial). Death of 14 of the patients was directly attributable to renal failure rather than other complications or manifestations of myeloma. Patients who received bicarbonate did marginally better than those who did not. The survival outcome of patients with renal failure in the MRC's third myeloma trial appeared to be inferior to that obtained in the fourth trial, in which high fluid intake was mandated. This study showed that, in many cases, renal failure in myeloma can be reversed completely or partially by simple fluid administration, but in oliguric renal failure of myeloma, the glomeruli may open up after a period of dialysis.

Several of the patients who had improvement in renal function with these measures were subsequently able to lead more active lives. However, prolonged survival is not likely unless renal failure can be reversed rapidly.[388] For patients who have myeloma and signs of acute renal failure, dialysis is indicated.[389] Peritoneal and hemodialysis have been used successfully, but continued dialysis is not indicated for patients who have evidence of progressive myeloma while receiving chemotherapy.[390–392] Plasmapheresis can be of temporary benefit to myeloma patients who develop acute renal failure because of an inability to adequately excrete light chains. Plasmapheresis is tenfold more effective than peritoneal dialysis for this acute complication.[393–396] Renal transplantation has been carried out successfully for a patient responsive to chemotherapy.[397] Before considering renal transplantation, the patient's presenting stage, age, response to treatment, and prognosis must be considered in view of the eventual fatal outcome of the disease and the added morbidity and complexities of management associated with transplantation.

HYPERCALCEMIA

About one forth of multiple myeloma patients have hypercalcemia with a serum calcium concentration in excess of 11.5 mg/dl (after correction for the serum albumin), and a significant fraction of patients develop hypercalcemia in the refractory phase of myeloma.[398] The serum calcium concentration should be measured routinely as part of staging evaluation in the initial workup of all patients with myeloma. The physicians should suspect hypercalcemia if the patient complains of polyuria, constipation, nausea or vomiting, lethargy, or mental confusion or has signs of dehydration or coma. The symptoms and signs of hypercalcemia correlate well with the level of ionized calcium rather than with the total calcium level, although the ionized level usually cannot be conveniently measured. Patients with bone pain or fractures who are bedridden or immobilized are also prone to hypercalcemia, and every effort should be made to mobilize them as quickly as possible.

As in other settings of malignant disease in which hypercalcemia occurs, vigorous hydration and diuresis should be used as soon as hypercalcemia is recognized, and the patient should be started promptly on corticosteroid therapy (*e.g.*, 50–100 mg of prednisone per day), because steroids have a direct affect on myeloma cells and in blocking osteoclastic activity and reducing negative calcium balance. Hypercalcemia in newly diagnosed patients and those relapsing from unmaintained remission usually comes promptly under control with institution of systemic chemotherapy for myeloma. Additional useful agents to control severe hypercalcemia (*i.e.*, serum calcium >13.5 mg/dl) or to use for patients in whom fluids, diuretics, and steroids prove inadequate over several days include parenteral mithramycin, gallium nitrate, Pamidronate or other diphosphonates, and calcitonin. For severe hypercalcemia, Pamidronate is administered in a dose of 90 mg as a 24-hour infusion and is more effective than multiple daily doses of etidronate.[399] A dose of 60 mg of Pamidronate is usually sufficient for moderate hypercalcemia, but it must be given by 24-hour infusion. Treatments can be repeated at 7-day intervals if needed. For chronic hypercalcemia, oral phosphates are usually administered in a dosage of 1 to 3 g/day. Phosphate enemas can be used as an alternative to oral phosphate for patients with nausea and vomiting. Phosphates should not be used in patients in renal failure with an elevated serum phosphorus level. When needed, these supplementary agents represent additions to hydration and steroid therapy. When treatment is effective at normalizing the serum calcium, patients usually experience reduction in bone pain and in hypercalciuria and hydroxyproline excretion.

Although calcium binding is primarily attributable to serum albumin, in some myeloma patients, the M-component firmly binds calcium, leading to an asymptomatic elevation in the serum calcium concentration without an increase in the ionized calcium level.[400–402] Myeloma patients who are asymptomatic but have a chronically elevated serum calcium concentration should have the serum level of ionized calcium determined by a reference laboratory.

BONE PAIN

Bone pain is the most common symptom of myeloma and usually results from pathologic fractures. Bone disease in myeloma is the result of increased bone resorption associated with myeloma cell infiltration and osteoclast activation.[403] Skeletal damage in myeloma manifests as generalized osteoporosis or as focal punched-out osteolytic lesions without the rim of new bone formation often observed with metastatic carcinomas. One common bone manifestation of myeloma consists of compression fractures in the thoracic or lumbar spine. Bone density is reduced, resulting in gradual or sudden compression of the vertebral plates, which often results in a "fish-mouth" deformity. Pain is often radicular and lancinating to one or both sides, is aggravated by movement, and probably is related to instability of the weak bone substance. Symptoms usually subside within days to weeks after initiation of systemic chemotherapy. Opiates are often useful for pain control. Nonsteroidal antiinflammatory agents may also relieve pain but are associated with a higher prevalence of renal failure in myeloma patients.[404] For persistent pain despite chemotherapy, localized radiation therapy may be required. Orthopedic back braces are usually poorly tolerated, but the newer lightweight braces with Velcro fasteners are useful for some severely debilitated patients.

The osteolytic lesions commonly observed in the skull, although pathognomonic for myeloma, are usually asymptomatic and normally do not require treatment. Typical examples of bone destruction in myeloma appear in Figure 56–4. Lytic lesions in major long bones should be irradiated if the lesion's diameter is one third to one half of the bone's diameter or if it involves a significant component of the cortex and the risk of pathologic fracture is high. Systemic chemotherapy infrequently leads to significant recalcification of large lesions, and they remain susceptible to pathologic fracture, even after achieving remission with systemic therapy.

Skeletal strength is enhanced by ambulation, which should be encouraged as soon as it is feasible. Internal fixation of a pathologic fracture of the femur should be carried out promptly, because the myeloma patient's general condition usually deteriorates rapidly if they are maintained at bedrest in skeletal traction. Intramedullary fixation of fractures of long bones should be followed with local radiation therapy. Administration of sodium fluoride (50 mg twice daily) with calcium carbonate (1.0 g four times daily) can enhance bone density as determined by quantitative studies on bone biopsies.[405] The addition of 50,000 units of vitamin D twice weekly and of androgens may be beneficial.[406,407] However, in a large randomized chemotherapy trial, fluoride, calcium, and vitamin D did not significantly improve outcome after a trial of chemotherapy alone but were thought to contribute to morbidity.[258] The effects of the oral diphosphonate etidronate were evaluated in a double blind study in newly diagnosed myeloma patients in conjunction with chemotherapy. Unfortunately, etidronate failed to have significant impact on bone disease in myeloma.[408] Several of the newer diphosphonate derivatives that are much more potent than etidronate may enhance bone density, but they are still undergoing clinical trials.

SPINAL CORD COMPRESSION AND OTHER NEUROLOGIC SYNDROMES

Spinal cord compression is a serious complication of multiple myeloma that occurs in 10% to 15% of patients and is usually observed early in the patient's course or in the late relapse phase of the disease. As with other neoplastic causes of spinal cord compression, back pain is usually the initial symptom. The presence of a paraspinal mass suggests that this complication may be imminent. Compression of the spinal cord usually results from ingrowth of the tumor through an intervertebral foramina or by direct extension from a heavily involved vertebra. If initial skeletal x-ray studies obtained for staging indicate a paraspinal mass, follow-up evaluation with an MRI scan or CT scan is warranted to exclude invasion of the spinal canal. The earliest symptom of spinal cord compression often is radicular pain, which is accentuated by coughing or sneezing; motor or sensory loss or abnormality in bowel or bladder function are signs of more extensive compression. Paraplegia is a late and usually irreversible finding.

Any of the symptoms or signs demand imaging of the spinal cord by MRI or CT scanning or myelography. We continue to be impressed with the value and accuracy of myelography, even though lumbar and cisternal introduction of contrast are frequently necessary. Currently available data suggest that noninvasive MRI scanning may provide information that is equally useful, but in some instances, MRI fails to provide the needed information. Controlled studies comparing myelography, CT, and MRI are currently underway. If permanent cord damage has not yet occurred, initiation of emergency radiation therapy and high-dose steroid therapy usually results in marked improvement or complete resolution of the patient's symptoms. If paralysis has occurred, emergency treatment usually only prevents further worsening of the patient's disability. If myelography is performed and demonstrates a partial or complete block, the contrast medium should be left in place to assist in treatment planning and for following the response to treatment.

Steroid dosage for myeloma patients with spinal cord compression should initially be in the range of 16 mg of dexamethasone per day in divided doses, with tapering starting after the completion of radiation therapy. For radiation therapy, wide margins are necessary to encompass the disease, but treatment of the entire vertebral column is rarely indicated because of the palliative treatment philosophy and the need to resume myelosuppressive chemotherapy. Decompression laminectomy is usually not required in the diagnosis or treatment of spinal cord compression syndromes in myeloma, because plasma cell tumors are usually quite radiation sensitive. The acute debilitation resulting from this form of surgery presents a special problem for myeloma patients because of the protracted period of complete bedrest after surgery, which further increases the likelihood of developing infection or hypercalcemia. Nerve root compression syndromes and the few instances of cerebral compression by a cranial or dural plasmacytoma can usually be treated successfully with radiation therapy.[409–416] Because plasmacytomas in the skull are normally chemosensitive and rarely cause substantial cerebral compression, specialized imaging studies and radiation therapy are indicated only if the patient develops localized CNS symptoms and signs of involvement during the course of systemic treatment.

Other neurologic syndromes encountered in myeloma patients include an acute encephalopathy associated with hypercalcemia, hyperviscosity, uremia, or meningitis. A variety of peripheral neuropathies are also encountered, most commonly caused by amyloidosis.[417] In fewer than 1% of patients, a mixed sensory-motor neuropathy develops, usually involving the extremities. It does not appear to be the result of amyloid or direct tumor infiltrate and usually improves after the initiation of chemotherapy.[418–423] The neuropathy can be painful and debilitating. In some instances, the neuropathy may be the result of a direct binding between the M-component and peripheral nerve constituents. It has commonly been reported in patients with macroglobulinemia, but it has also been observed in patients with multiple myeloma, including in some with osteosclerotic myeloma.[419,424–428] The antigen binding in sural nerve biopsies has been seen with myelin-associated glycoprotein and associated with demyelination and, in other cases, with binding to endoneurial constituents.[429] Nerve binding of IgM in patients has been passively transferred to mice with purified IgM fractions, with evidence of specificity.[430]

Another rare neuropathy sometimes associated with myeloma is the POEMS syndrome composed of polyneuropathy organomegaly, endocrinopathy, monoclonal gammopathy, and skin changes.[431] The pathophysiology of this disorder is not understood.

HEMATOLOGIC COMPLICATIONS

Anemia

Anemia is the most common hematologic complication of myeloma, with a hemoglobin level of less than 12 g/dl in 62% of patients at the time of presentation.[432] Severe anemia with a hemoglobin level of less than 8.5 g/dl and a marked reduction in erythrocytes are observed in approximately 25% of patients. The degree of anemia correlates with total-body tumor burden.[181] In patients with the hyperviscosity syndrome, expansion of the plasma volume and its resulting hemodilution can exaggerate the reduction in hemoglobin out of proportion to the reduction in erythrocyte mass.

The anemia of myeloma usually improves significantly with response to chemotherapy unless the patient has persistent renal failure. Severe symptomatic anemia requires transfusion of packed erythrocytes, because the recovery of adequate hemoglobin values usually does not occur until the patient has been receiving chemotherapy for at least 3 months. Recovery of an adequate level of circulating erythrocytes is not enhanced by administration of folic acid, vitamin B_{12}, or iron unless a factor deficiency can be documented. In some instances, folate deficiency may be due to excessive folate use by the myeloma cells.[433]

Some patients whose hemoglobin level does not improve sufficiently with chemotherapy improve after receiving a potent androgen (*e.g.*, testosterone enanthate, 600 mg intramuscularly every 4–6 weeks; fluoxymesterone, 15–30 mg orally daily). Androgen therapy often needs to be continued for 3 to 6 months to see benefit. Recombinant erythropoietin has substantial effect on increasing the erythrocyte mass in noncancer patients with the anemia of renal failure.[434,435] Several reports indicate that it can be useful in correcting anemia in some myeloma patients, even in the absence of renal failure.[436,437]

Granulocytopenia and Thrombocytopenia

Although mild granulocytopenia (<3000 granulocytes/μl) is common in myeloma, moderate to severe granulocytopenia or thrombocytopenia is uncommon, but if present, it is usually attributable to extensive bone marrow involvement with myeloma. If detected at diagnosis, marked granulocytopenia or thrombocytopenia should not lead to reduction in the dosage of induction chemotherapy. Patients should be treated aggressively with myeloma chemotherapy, blood components, and supportive care in a fashion analogous to the management of acute leukemia. Recombinant granulocyte colony-stimulating factor or granulocyte-macrophage colony-stimulating factor can help to normalize the absolute granulocyte count in neutropenic myeloma patients.

Acute Leukemia and Myelodysplastic Syndromes

An association between multiple myeloma and acute leukemia was first reported in 1965, and it has been confirmed extensively since then.[438,439] In the first myeloma trial conducted by the Clinical Trials Group of the NCI of Canada, 15 cases of acute leukemia were observed among 365 myeloma patients treated with combinations of alkylating agents and prednisone.[189,438] The incidence of leukemia in that study was 230 times higher than expected in the normal population.[438] On an actuarial basis, the risk of acute leukemia was projected to be 19.6% at 50 months after the start of treatment. Although it appears that acute leukemia was a more frequent complication in this study than in other reported myeloma trials, it nonetheless underscores the importance of this potential complication. The actual number of cases is significantly less than the actuarial incidence predicted.

There has been much speculation about the cause of acute leukemia in myeloma patients, and the predominant view is that it is a complication of the alkylating agents or radiation therapy.[439,440] However, there also are reports of acute leukemia in patients with myeloma before the general use of alkylating agents for treatment, and myelodysplastic changes have occasionally been observed in the marrow of myeloma patients before treatment.[441,442] Acute leukemia has also been observed in untreated patients with macroglobulinemia or MGUS. Although the actual incidence of acute nonlymphocytic leukemia in untreated myeloma patients is unknown, some researchers have speculated that there may be an intrinsic increased susceptibility to acute leukemia in patients with plasma cell neoplasia.[438]

Analyses of incidence of acute leukemia in cancer trials for myeloma or ovarian cancer in which patients received melphalan or cyclophosphamide therapy strongly incriminate melphalan as a leukemogenic agent. In the MRC's first two trials for myeloma, 12 of 648 patients developed a myelodysplastic syndrome (considered to be preleukemic) or acute leukemia.[443] This corresponds to a 5-year actuarial prevalence of 3% and an 8-year prevalence of 10%. In these two MRC studies, patients were randomized to receive melphalan or cyclophosphamide. A significant association was found with the length of melphalan treatment (p=0.0001) but none for cyclophosphamide. In this analysis, the risk of a secondary hematopoietic neoplasm in myeloma patients after 10 years of follow-up was approximately 3% for each year of melphalan treatment, with much of the risk occurring within 3 years of the last melphalan treatment.[443] It was the the researchers' view that if there was an intrinsic element of increased risk for secondary hematologic neoplasms in myeloma, it would be difficult to explain the association they found with melphalan exposure.

A similar conclusion about the leukemogenicity of melphalan was reached in an analysis of 1794 1-year survivors of ovarian cancer treated with chemotherapy.[444] In the ovarian cancer study, there was a 93-fold increase in the incidence of acute nonlymphocytic leukemia overall, with the greatest risk in the first 5 years after chemotherapy. The 10-year accumulated risk of acquiring leukemia was 11.2% after receiving melphalan and 5.4% after cyclophosphamide. Moreover, there was a definite dose-response relation for melphalan therapy, and women receiving melphalan were two to three times more likely to develop leukemia than those receiving cyclophosphamide.[444]

The results of these studies indicate that the choice of alkylating agent and dose administered may significantly influence the risk for late complications of chemotherapy in myeloma. The effect of melphalan dosage in these studies also suggests that the current trials using high-dose intravenous melphalan in myeloma may be associated with a significant incidence of leukemia as a therapy-related complication.

The acute nonlymphocytic leukemias that evolve in myeloma patients often evolve after a period of bone marrow injury with an associated pancytopenia or morphologic evidence of myelodysplasia. As for other secondary acute leukemias (*e.g.*, in Hodgkin's disease), treatment of the leukemia is difficult because of the preexisting impaired bone marrow reserve resulting from the disease or treatment. In myeloma, advanced age, immunodeficiency, and impaired renal function may further compromise the treatment of acute leukemia. Nonetheless, worthwhile hematologic remissions of secondary leukemia are sometimes achieved in myeloma patients using standard induction chemotherapy regimens incorporating an anthracycline and cytarabine (cytosine arabinoside).

Coagulopathy

Coagulation disorders in the absence of thrombocytopenia occur commonly in patients with macroglobulinemia or cryoglobulinemia and somewhat less often in patients with myeloma. Purpura, epistaxis, and ecchymosis, and retinal hemorrhages or mucosal bleeding caused by coagulopathies may be observed in patients with monoclonal gammopathy. In the syndromes discussed later, the functional abnormality of the bleeding disorder appears related to the presence of the M-component. There are many mechanisms of coagulopathy in patients with M-components. In several case reports, inhibitors of individual coagulation factors have been observed, including inhibitors of factors V, VII, VIII, and X and of the prothrombin complex.[445] In some instances, patients have reductions in multiple coagulation factors, including factors II, V, VII, and VIII and fibrinogen.

The mechanism of multifactor depression is obscure, but it has been suggested that the M-component binds to or coprecipitates with coagulation complexes.[446] In macroglobulinemia, specific M-components appear to interact with or bind to fibrin during the clotting process and inhibit the polymerization of the fibrin monomer. This can be detected as a prolongation in the thrombin time.[447] However, this abnormality usually does not cause clinical bleeding, unless platelet function is also impaired. In some instances, the hemostatic defect is associated with impaired platelet function. Prolonged bleeding time, impaired clot retraction, prolongation of the thromboplastin generation time with the patient's platelets, and defective platelet aggregation are indicators of impaired platelet function.[448,449] In some instances, the M-component appears to coat the platelets, leading to the release of platelet factor III and impaired aggregation.[450–452] A patient with plasma cell leukemia had a circulating heparin sulfate proteoglycan anticoagulant.[453] Fibrinolysis with severe bleeding was reported in a patient with myeloma and amyloidosis who had an associated deficiency of α_2-plasmin inhibitor. Treatment with ϵ-aminocaproic acid reduced bleeding and was associated with recovery of the plasmin inhibitor level.[454]

SYNDROMES RESULTING FROM PHYSICOCHEMICAL PROPERTIES OF M-COMPONENTS

Hyperviscosity

The hyperviscosity syndrome occurs in approximately 50% of patients with macroglobulinemia but in fewer than 5% of patients with multiple myeloma.[455–461] Hyperviscosity results from the protein-protein interactions of large, long molecules with high intrinsic viscosity (*e.g.*, IgM M-components) or from high concentrations of specific IgG or IgA M-components, which have a tendency to form multimolecular aggregates.[455–460] It rarely or never occurs in patients with light-chain-only myeloma because of the small molecular size of Bence Jones proteins. Although plasma viscosity rises with increasing concentration of an M-component, beyond a critical point, viscosity rises much more steeply, even with relatively small additional increments in serum M-component concentration. Variations among patients in the relation of M-component concentration to viscosity make prediction of plasma viscosity difficult without direct measurement.[462]

As a result of poorly understood homeostatic mechanisms, increases in plasma viscosity lead to expansion of the plasma volume.[463] The hemodilution resulting from plasma volume expansion can dilute the circulating erythrocytes, giving the appearance of an anemia. To clarify this situation, use of nuclear medicine techniques to directly measure the plasma volume (with radioiodinated albumin) and the erythrocyte mass (with radiochromate-labeled erythrocytes) are of value. The intrinsic viscosity of serum or plasma can be measured by noting the time necessary for a given volume of serum to pass a constriction in a glass tube (Ostwald viscometer or a leukocyte pipette) and relating the time to that of a normal saline control.

Symptoms and signs of the hyperviscosity syndrome are usually not seen unless the serum relative viscosity is greater than 4.0 cp, and the full-blown classic syndrome is usually not seen unless the viscosity is greater than 5.0 cp (normal human serum relative viscosity is in the range of 1.4–1.8 cp). Clinical symptoms and signs of the hyperviscosity syndrome include bleeding disorders, retinopathy, neurologic findings, and evidence of hypervolemia. Hemorrhagic complications include bruising, purpura, and mucosal bleeding that is often manifest as severe or recurrent bleeding from the nose or uterus. Characteristic ocular findings include marked dilatation and segmentation of the retinal veins (giving the appearance of a line of boxcars or sausage links), retinal hemorrhages, or papilledema. Neurologic abnormalities range from fatigue, weakness, headache, vertigo, nystagmus, and confusion, to transient paralysis and frank coma. Findings of hypervolemia include distension of peripheral blood vessels and symptoms and signs of heart failure.

Therapeutically, the initial approach to patients with the hyperviscosity syndrome is to perform plasmapheresis. Plasmapheresis is performed most effectively with a continuous or a discontinuous flow blood cell separator. Another high-efficiency method uses plasma cascade filtration through a cellulose diacetate membrane that selectively removes the high-molecular-mass M-components while permitting return of the patient's albumin with reasonable efficiency.[463–465] However, if the needed equipment for high-efficiency plasmapheresis or filtration is not available, conventional double-double plasma separation packs can be used with centrifugation.[466] Patients who have acute hyperviscosity usually need treatment of at least 2 to 3 L daily for 4 to 5 days or as long as needed until the viscosity falls below 4.0 cp. Although plasmapheresis relieves the hyperviscosity syndrome on a temporary basis, for long-term control, systemic chemotherapy, as used for multiple myeloma or macroglobulinemia, should be initiated to reduce M-component production and tumor burden. In some drug-resistant cases of macroglobulinemia, satisfactory long-term control of hyperviscosity can be maintained with intermittent plasmapheresis alone at 2- to 3-week intervals.

Cryoglobulinemia

Cryoglobulinemia should be suspected in patients with acrocyanosis or Raynaud's phenomenon alone or with purpura, particularly after cold exposure. Cryoglobulins in macroglobulinemia or myeloma are M-components with low thermal amplitude, which can be readily demonstrated by drawing blood in a warm syringe and allowing it to clot and retract in a 37°C water bath. The serum is then transferred to a clean tube and placed in a refrigerator for 1 to 2 days, after which time the cryoglobulin has formed a flocculent white precipitate or a gel in the bottom of the tube. Cryoglobulins can usually be quantitated by carrying out the cold exposure in hematocrit tubes and centrifuging them to determine a "cryocrit." Cryoglobulins in B-cell neoplasms are usually IgM or IgG M-components; however, IgA M-components and mixed cryoglobulins have also been reported.[467–471]

Treatment with alkylating agents and steroids usually relieves most symptoms of cryoglobulinemia, although some patients continue to need gloves and earmuffs or a move to a warmer climate in the winter. Patients with cryoglobulinemia who present with purpura and other bleeding manifestations or evidence of renal failure should be treated initially with plasmapheresis before the start of chemotherapy.

Anomalous Serum Chemistries

Several abnormalities in serum chemistries are commonly observed in myeloma patients who have high concentrations of serum M-components. These can be confused with abnormalities of clinical significance, but they are usually of little or no clinical importance. These include apparent hyponatremia, hypoglycemia, and the "anion gap."[472–474] The apparent reductions in serum sodium and glucose are attributed to the displacement of the water-based solutes and electrolytes in serum by the large physical mass of the M-component solute, which does not contain sodium or glucose and displaces water in the serum. The reduced serum sodium has been described as "isotonic hyponatremia."[475] An apparent low anion gap has been attributed to the fact that M-components are cationic (*i.e.*, net positive charge). To balance such unmeasured protein cations, chloride and bicarbonate are retained to neutralize the protein's charge. A low anion gap has also been observed in MGUS.[476] The finding of a low anion gap in a patient not known to have an M-component should lead the physician to order appropriate diagnostic studies to look for a monoclonal protein. For patients with known monoclonal gammopathies, saline infusions should not be given for hyponatremia unless there is additional documentation that the patient is sodium and volume depleted. Hyponatremia associated with inappropriate secretion of antidiuretic hormone has been reported in patients with macroglobulinemia.[475]

BACTERIAL SEPSIS

Humoral immunodeficiency is the principal underlying cause for bacterial sepsis in patients with myeloma.[477–482] *Streptococcus pneumoniae* and *Hemophilus influenzae* are the most common pathogens in previously untreated myeloma patients and those nonneutropenic patients responding to chemotherapy. However, in neutropenic patients and in those with refractory disease, *Staphylococcus aureus* and gram-negative bacteria are the preponderant organisms.[483] Patients with fever, productive cough, or other symptoms of bacterial infection should have bacterial culture and appropriate x-ray studies performed as quickly as possible, and bactericidal antibiotic therapy should be started.

If patients present with signs of sinopulmonary infection and are in suitable condition to be treated on an outpatient basis, the combination of amoxicillin and clavulanate usually suffices because its spectrum is broad enough to cover most common organisms. For neutropenic patients or for those whose overall condition requires hospitalization, the use of vancomycin plus a third-generation cephalosporin (*e.g.*, ceftazidime) or an aminoglycoside plus an antipseudomonal penicillin (*e.g.*, ticarcillin) is usually indicated. If an aminoglycoside regimen is used, special attention must be paid to renal function, and the frequency of follow-up doses of the aminoglycoside should be judged based on serum assays and renal function. Patients who have repeated episodes of sinopulmonary infections often benefit from being provided with a supply of a suitable oral cephalosporin (*e.g.*, cefaclor) or the amoxicillin-clavulanate combination or ciprofloxacin so that they can start therapy at the time of initial symptoms. For patients who have difficulties with compliance, prophylactic treatment with benzathine penicillin G should be considered if there has been a history of prior pneumococcal or meningococcal infection.

In a controlled study, intramuscular injection of 20 ml of γ-globulin every 2 weeks did not reduce the frequency of bacterial infections, and it is not indicated for infection prophylaxis in myeloma.[484] Although far larger doses of γ-globulin can be given intravenously, patients with IgG myeloma still catabolize this formulation rapidly. This form of supportive therapy is expensive and has yet to be proven useful in controlled clinical trials in myeloma. Use of pneumococcal vaccination may be worth trying.[485] However, most myeloma patients respond poorly to bacterial antigenic stimulation. Vaccines containing live organisms (*e.g.*, varicella) are contraindicated in patients with myeloma because their immunodeficiencies permit infection to disseminate.

AMYLOIDOSIS

Systemic amyloidosis is a complication that occurs in approximately 15% of patients with multiple myeloma. The fibrillar amyloid protein deposited in myeloma has a pattern of tissue distribution characteristically observed in "primary amyloidosis," a condition with bone marrow plasmacytosis, Bence Jones proteinuria, or a serum M-component but no osteolytic bone lesions. Differentiation of the amyloid associated with myeloma from that of primary amyloidosis is artificial because the amyloid is of similar genesis and tissue distribution, and the conditions are more appropriately considered to be parts of the spectrum of the same basic disease process.[490]

There is a clear structural relation between amyloid fibril deposits and Bence Jones proteins. Amyloid fibrils from primary amyloidosis and amyloidosis associated with myeloma are homogenous and homologous to the variable region fragment of κ or λ light chains, as defined by amino acid sequence analysis of purified amyloid proteins.[486,487] Primary amyloidosis and the amyloidosis associated with myeloma, other monoclonal gammopathies, and agammaglobulinemia have immunoglobulin amyloid fibrils or amyloid L-chain proteins. Most monoclonal L chains do not appear to be amyloidogenic, suggesting that specific structural properties must be present to undergo fibrillar deposition. Although κ-type L chains are more frequent than the λ-type L chains on M-components or as Bence Jones proteins, amyloidogenic L chains of the λ type are significantly more frequent than those of the κ type.[488] Amyloid fibrils are at best sparingly soluble in physiologic saline or plasma, but they can be solubilized in distilled water or low ionic strength media; therefore, it is not surprising that they tend to deposit in tissues. Serum amyloid P component (SAP) has been radioiodinated and its clearance studied in normal persons and patients with systemic amyloid. In these studies, SAP was cleared more rapidly in amyloid patients and accumulated and persisted in their amyloid deposits.[489]

The presenting symptoms of amyloidosis (with or without myeloma) include weakness, weight loss, ankle edema dyspnea, paresthesias, light-headedness, or syncope.[490] Aching in the hands (particularly at night) can be symptomatic of median nerve compression associated with the carpal tunnel syndrome caused by amyloid infiltration of the transverse carpal ligament. Physical findings include enlargement of the tongue and liver, purpura, and ankle edema. Ankle edema is usually due to congestive heart failure or a nephrotic syndrome. A peripheral neuropathy may also be present.[417] Macroglossia occurs in approximately 20% of patients. The tongue frequently shows indentations from the teeth and may prevent closure of the mouth. Splenomegaly (usually slight) affects fewer than 10% of patients. The tissues most subject to amyloid deposition in myeloma include the tongue, gastrointestinal tract, heart, skin, and skeletal muscle. Although macroglossia or periorbital purpura in a myeloma patient should suggest the diagnosis, a knowledgeable and alert physician is needed in most instances. Purpura of the eyelids is characteristic of amyloid, and unilateral or bilateral periorbital purpura ("raccoon eyes") may appear suddenly after placing the head in a dependent position, as during proctoscopy; it has been called postproctoscopic purpura or PPP.[489,491] Other skin manifestations include plaques, papules, or nodules. Joint involvement with amyloid can result in an appearance similar to rheumatoid arthritis.[490,492] Involvement of the glenohumeral joints can give a "shoulder pad" appearance. Low voltage on the electrocardiogram can be suggestive of cardiac involvement. More specific is two-dimensional echocardiographic evidence of amyloidosis involving the heart, with thickening of ventricular walls, septum, papillary muscles, and pericardial effusion, and a characteristic "granular sparkling" appearance of the thickened cardiac walls.[493]

A rectal biopsy has been the classic method of establishing the diagnosis of amyloidosis, and it is positive in more than 60% of patients.[490] Another study showed that abdominal fat aspiration, using a 19-gauge needle, can yield positive results in more than 70% of patients. This procedure can be done at the bedside and is probably the simplest way to diagnose amyloidosis.[140] Resected carpal ligaments should be examined for the presence of amyloid, and the specimens can be evaluated retrospectively from tissue blocks from previously resected ligaments. Amyloid can be demonstrated in needle biopsies of the liver or kidney, but these procedures are more hazardous because of the increased risk of bleeding from vascular wall involvement or from deficiency of factor X. Cracking or rupture of the liver after biopsy has been observed when there is heavy infiltration with amyloid. Amyloid stains pink with hematoxylin and eosin and has metachromatic staining properties with methyl or crystal violet. Congo red stain produces an apple-green birefringence under polarized light and is the most specific stain for amyloid under the light microscope. Electron microscopy may be somewhat more sensitive and has shown the presence of amyloid fibrils even when Congo red staining has not revealed amyloid.[490] Serum β_2-microglobulin levels appear to predict survival in patients with systemic amyloidosis without associated myeloma.[494]

Treatment for amyloidosis with myeloma is essentially the same as the treatment for multiple myeloma, but it usually does not have as great an impact on resolving amyloid deposits as it does in causing tumor regression. However, treatment may stop or slow further amyloid deposition, and this can be important for patients with early cardiac involvement.[495] The authors of a retrospective analysis concluded that a trial of chemotherapy was warranted in patients with myeloma and amyloidosis and that patients with objective response of the myeloma had a better survival than those that did not. Although there were no absolute predictors of response, patients who achieved remission were much less likely to have cardiac amyloid but were more likely to have high β_2-microglobulin or κ L-chain M-component levels.[496] In a double-blind study of primary amyloidosis (without overt myeloma), patients given melphalan and prednisone were able to continue treatment longer than those given placebo, and improvement in nephrotic syndrome or proteinuria was observed, but survival did not differ significantly between the two groups.[497] Detection of a high plasma cell labeling index was reported to be useful for identifying patients with amyloidosis who were responsive to chemotherapy, but their overall survival was still poor (14 months).[498] Colchicine, dimethylsulfoxide, and penicillamine have been tried in treating L-chain amyloid without success. Congestive heart failure caused by amyloid represents a poor prognostic feature of the disease and usually does not respond to cardiac glycosides.[499] Diuretics are useful for relief of edema.

OTHER PLASMA CELL NEOPLASMS

MACROGLOBULINEMIA

In 1944, Waldenström raised the question of whether a new syndrome that differed from multiple myeloma could be identified in the setting of a high-molecular-mass M-component and a bleeding syndrome of the type associated with hyperviscosity.[500] Development of immunodiagnostic techniques, such as immunoelectrophoresis, led to the recognition that a serum IgM M-component was a common feature in patients with the syndrome described by Waldenström.[501] Although the disease was initially thought to occur predominantly in men, later reports suggested an approximately equal sex prevalence.[461,502–505]

Macroglobulinemia is far less common than multiple myeloma.[107,506–508] Pathogenetic mechanisms similar to those in myeloma may be involved, but there is considerable literature indicating an element of familial susceptibility that is more significant than that for myeloma, including families with multiple cases of macroglobulinemia or IgM MGUS in first-degree relatives.[89,509–511] Macroglobulinemia in a pair of monozygotic twins was reported.[512] The case for environmental factors was made for a canary breeder who developed pulmonary symptoms and was found to have a pulmonary infiltrate with IgM-containing cells, Waldenström's macroglobulinemia, and an M-component that exhibited antibody activity against an antigen in canary droppings.[513]

Patients with macroglobulinemia are usually first seen with findings analogous to those of advanced non-Hodgkin's lymphomas: hepatosplenomegaly and lymphadenopathy. The patients often develop the hyperviscosity syndrome, with attendant bleeding manifestations (Table 56–14). The fundi of patients with macroglobulinemia should be examined routinely with an ophthalmoscope for evidence of hyperviscosity. The fundic changes can revert rapidly in response to plasmapheresis.

The presence of a serum IgM M-component is not tantamount to a diagnosis of macroglobulinemia because there are other B-cell neoplasms in which serum IgM M-components exist, but with the exception of macroglobulinemia and myeloma, the levels are usually lower than 1.0 g/dl and almost always lower than 2.0 g/dl. Only 25% of patients with IgM M-components have Waldenström's macroglobulinemia; other entities with IgM secretion include subsets of patients with CLL, non-Hodgkin's lymphomas, the cold hemagglutinin syndrome, and MGUS. Patients with osteolytic bone lesions in addition to an IgM serum M-component are rare, but they are usually classified as having IgM multiple myeloma, rather than macroglobulinemia.[514] Lacking definitive causal agents or other markers to differentiate these entities, this spectrum of neoplasms should be considered as representing various expressions of B-cell lymphoplasmacytic tumors, with their morphology "frozen" at different stages of differentiation and with clinical manifestations that vary as a function of M-component production, tumor cell proliferation, and invasiveness.[94] Supporting that concept is the report on the cytogenetics in a case of Waldenström's macroglobulinemia with an 8:14 translocation with breakpoints (q24;p32) similar to those found in Burkitt's lymphoma.[515]

Hematologic manifestations of macroglobulinemia include anemia in at least 70% of patients (often partially dilutional because of the expanded plasma volume) and some degree of thrombocytopenia in approximately 30% of patients. Bone marrow involvement is common in macroglobulinemia, and the morphologic appearance of the plasma cells is pleomorphic, with a range of light microscopic appearances from small lymphoid cells to mature plasma cells. Immunofluorescent studies have shown that most of the lymphoid cells have cell-surface IgM but lack cytoplasmic Ig, and the plasma cells contain cytoplasmic IgM. In a flow cytometry study, patients with macroglobulinemia usually had circulating lymphoid cells that contained intracytoplasmic μ chains and cell-surface expression of the B-cell-specific antigens B1, B2, and B4 and the plasma cell antigen PCA-1.[516]

As with myeloma, quantitation of the IgM M-component should be performed by laser nephelometry or electrophoresis and not with immunodiffusion methods. Serum viscosity determinations should be performed in all patients at the time of diagnosis and serially in patients who have a serum relative viscosity higher than 3.0 cp. Residual normal immunoglobulins are often depressed, but less severely than in myeloma.[517] In contrast to the high percentage of myeloma patients with urinary light chain excretion, only about 10% of macroglobulinemic patients have Bence Jones proteins detectable in the urine by standard techniques, and tubular casts are absent.[518] Renal disease is seen only infrequently in macroglobulinemia and is markedly different from that seen in myeloma, taking on the appearance of an immunologically mediated glomerulonephritis or nephrotic syndrome.[518–521]

Neurologic syndromes observed in patients with macroglobulinemia include the neurologic entities discussed as myeloma complications, and they are usually due to the hyperviscosity syndrome or occur as peripheral neuropathies. Peripheral neuropathies are seen in approximately 20% of patients with macroglobulinemia.

The treatment of macroglobulinemia is similar to that of other indolent B-cell neoplasms. Oral alkylating agents (*e.g.*, chlorambucil, melphalan, cyclophosphamide) are the mainstays of therapy and are usually used alone or in combination with prednisone, administered with the same dosage schedules as those used in multiple myeloma or CLL.[502,504,505,522–527] Plasmapheresis is often needed initially to treat hyperviscosity. Systemic treatment is normally continued until the serum IgM level plateaus. At that point, treatment can be discontinued until there is evidence of a rising serum viscosity or other evidence of relapse. Although complete remission is rarely achieved, responsive patients have been reported to have median survivals in the range of 50 months, and nonresponsive patients have survivals about half that long.[461,505] Some patients have indolent macroglobulinemia (analogous to indolent myeloma) survive for more than 2 decades.

A case has been made for continuing the use of plasmapheresis and the cytotoxic agents, so that the dose required of the cytotoxic agent or the frequency of plasma exchange can be reduced.[528] Sequential hemibody irradiation has been used with some benefit, but it did not eliminate the patient's requirement for intermittent plasmapheresis.[529] Because of the relative rarity of the disease, comparative evaluations of treatment programs for macroglobulinemia have not been reported, and it is best to use one of the standard regimens for CLL or myeloma. Patients who become refractory to alkylating agents can be maintained effectively on long-term plasmapheresis if the IgM production rate is not too high. One macroglobulinemic patient with alkylating agent resistance has been maintained on plasmapheresis every 2 weeks for the

TABLE 56–14. Clinical Manifestations in 260 Patients With Macroglobulinema

Mean age (y)	
At onset of symptoms	63
At diagnosis	65 (range, 18–92)
Symptoms, % of patients with	
Severe fatigue	85
Bleeding	60
Neurologic	17
Bone pain	10
Signs, % of patients with	
Lymphadenopathy	40
Hepatomegaly	30
Splenomegaly	30
Hepatosplenomegaly	25

(Modified from MacKenzie MR. Macroglobulinemia. In: Wiernik PH, Canelloa GP, Kyle RA, Schiffer CA, eds. Neoplastic diseases of the blood, vol. 2. New York: Churchill-Livingstone, 1985:575–592)

past 12 years. On the basis of our experience and unpublished and published reports by others, patients with refractory macroglobulinemia may achieve drug-induced remissions with fludarabine, doxorubicin, the M2 protocol, VBAP, INF-α, or pentostatin.[530–533] Patients with macroglobulinemia treated with alkylating agents have developed acute leukemia in a fashion analogous to that seen after treatment with melphalan or chlorambucil in myeloma or polycythemia vera.[523,533–537]

LICHEN MYXEDEMATOSUS

Lichen myxedematosus (*i.e.*, papular mucinosis or scleromyxedema) is a rare skin disorder that is usually associated with the presence of a serum IgGλ M-component that is basic and has a marked cathodal electrophoretic mobility.[538] Some cases have been reported with IgA or IgM M-components, usually also with λ L chains. However, osteolytic bone lesions, marrow plasmacytosis, or Bence Jones proteinuria are found only rarely.[539] This dermatologic condition is manifested as raised papules or plaques containing a mucinous material mainly composed of hyaluronic acid. Skin fibroblasts from a patient with typical skin lesions and an IgGμ M-component grew to a lower cell density in culture but produced more glycosaminoglycans (with a higher ratio of hyaluronic acid to sulfated glycosaminoglycans) and less collagen than did normal fibroblasts.[540] Compared with the effect of normal serum, serum from a patient with lichen myxedematosus was found to stimulate hyaluronic acid and prostaglandin E production by normal foreskin or synovial fibroblasts.[541] These data suggest that the serum M-component is acting directly on the skin fibroblasts, altering their metabolism and inducing the skin lesions. Striking cutaneous and systemic improvements have been observed when patients have been treated with melphalan or cyclophosphamide.[542–544] The presence of the monoclonal M-component and the response to alkylating agent therapy suggest that lichen myxedematosus is an unusual plasma cell neoplasm. Isotretinoin therapy was tried in several patients.[545]

HEAVY-CHAIN DISEASES

The heavy-chain diseases are rare lymphoplasmacytic neoplasms in which a fragment of an Ig heavy chain is secreted by the tumor cells and is detected in the serum or in the urine. The heavy-chain fragments have an intact Fc portion but a deletion in the Fd region. The first report on a heavy-chain disease was on γ-heavy-chain disease in 1964 by Franklin and associates, who predicted that α- and μ-chain diseases would also be discovered.[546] This prediction was validated with the subsequent identification of unique syndromes associated with α- and μ-chain fragment secretion. Analysis of the structure of fragments secreted in the heavy-chain diseases has shed some light on normal Ig structure and immunogenetics.[547–550]

γ-*Heavy-Chain Disease*

Since the initial description of γ-heavy-chain disease (γ-HCD), more than 90 additional cases have been reported, mostly as individual case reports.[551] The world literature on this entity was reviewed.[552] In most cases, the clinical description is similar to that of non-Hodgkin's lymphoma, with nodal or external involvement, and in 4 patients, a picture somewhat more like that of multiple myeloma, with osteolytic bone lesions, was reported.[553] γ-HCD is not a specific pathologic process; it is a mutant molecular expression in the spectrum of B-cell neoplasia.[552] In 4 patients, chromosome abnormalities have been reported, but a unique abnormality has yet to be identified.[554] The median age at diagnosis of γ-HCD is 60, but it appears in some patients before the age of 20, and the disease is slightly more common in men than women.[555]

Most patients present with fever, anemia, weakness, and lymphadenopathy, often accompanied with hepatosplenomegaly. Involvement of Waldeyer's ring is relatively common. Leukopenia, eosinophilia, and thrombocytopenia are often present, and atypical lymphocytes and plasma cells may be found in the blood smears. The bone marrow aspirate and biopsy specimens usually show an increase in the lymphoplasmacytic series and occasionally some degree of eosinophilia. Immunofluorescent studies have shown that the cells throughout the lymphoplasmacytic spectrum contain γ chains.[556] However, in some instances, the bone marrow findings are normal.

The γ chain in γ-HCD is incomplete, and because of the major deletions, the molecular mass of the protein is between one half and three quarters that of a normal γ chain.[557] The pattern on serum protein electrophoresis varies, with broad-based increases in γ-globulin, a discrete M-component spike, or a normal or hypogammaglobulinemic pattern. Immunoelectrophoresis has been used to identify most γ-HCD cases, and it is likely that the frequency of this disorder may be underreported because the test is not routinely used in the workup of patients with diffuse lymphomas. Proteinuria may be undetectable or may range up to 20 g/day. Electrophoresis usually shows the presence of an M-component or γ-globulin band that is negative on the heat test for Bence Jones proteins and can be demonstrated antigenically to have γ-type H-chain characteristics but is totally devoid of L-chain antigens. Most patients have less than 1 g/day of urinary protein excretion, and renal failure is uncommon.[546,555,558]

The clinical course of γ-HCD is highly variable, with some patients succumbing to a rapidly progressing neoplasm within weeks to others who survive 5 years or more.[559–561] The median survival for 49 patients for whom data was available was 12 months (range, 1–264 months).[555] Because of the diffuse nature of the disease, most patients are treated with programs similar to those used for patients with non-Hodgkin's lymphomas (*e.g.*, CVP, CHOP). Local radiation therapy may be useful for symptomatic relief of palatal edema and respiratory distress in patients with Waldeyer's ring involvement.

α-*Heavy-Chain Disease*

α-Heavy-chain disease (α-HCD) was first described by Seligmann and associates in an Arab woman with a severe malabsorption syndrome resulting from a lymphoplasmacytic infiltrate in the small bowel and monoclonal α chains in the serum.[562] This disease is the most common of the heavy-chain diseases, and there were more than 150 cases in the literature, including several detailed reviews of this syndrome.[563–568] α-HCD is also known as Mediterranean lymphoma and immunoproliferative small intestinal disease, with several articles appearing in the gastroenterologic and the oncologic literature. Most reports on α-HCD have been of Arab or Jewish patients from the Mediterranean area, including North Africa and the Middle East. However, the disease is not limited to Semitic peoples or to a given geographic area; one case was reported from Taiwan.[569]

In some instances, α-HCD appears to be premalignant, with a complete reversal of the syndrome after antibiotic therapy.[570–573] Often the disease relapses despite antibiotics and takes on a more malignant form.[574] The prevalence is slightly higher in males than in females, and the peak age of incidence is distinctly lower than that for myeloma or macroglobulinemia, with most patients in their twenties or thirties, but with a few children as young as 10 years of age.[575] Most patients with α-HCD are from undernourished populations with poor hygiene and infestation with intestinal parasites. Compared with normal persons and patients with other malabsorption syndromes, patients with α-HCD have a greater association of HLA-AW19 and HLA-B12 antigens, suggesting a genetic element in the disease.[576]

Characteristic symptoms of α-HCD include diarrhea, steatorrhea, weight loss, and abdominal pain. Abdominal masses may be palpable, although hepatosplenomegaly and peripheral lymphadenopathy are uncommon.[577] Clubbing of the fingers and growth retardation (including secondary sex characteristics) may occur.[578] Hypocalcemia and other electrolyte disturbances occur as a result of the diarrhea in this syndrome. X-ray studies and intestinal biopsy specimens demonstrate extensive infiltration and thickening of the mucosa with tumor. On biopsy, the infiltrate is lymphoplasmacytic, and the neoplastic cells usually contain α chains. The lamina propria is infiltrated with plasma cells, and the infiltrate may involve the submucosa and the mesenteric lymph nodes. Chromosomal analysis of mesenteric lymph nodes was reported for 4 patients with α-HCD, and abnormalities were found in 3 of them.[579] In 2 of these patients, there were rearrangements of chromosome 14 (band q32) resulting from translocations that differ from those observed in most other non-Hodgkin's lymphomas. In one prior case, a closely related abnormality in chromosome 14 (14q+) was reported in a patient with α-HCD.[580]

Unlike other monoclonal gammopathies, an M-component spike is normally not seen on electrophoresis in α-HCD. For about one half of the patients, a diffusely increased band is seen in the α_2- or β-globulin zones, but for the remaining patients, there was no overt abnormality on serum electrophoresis. Presumptive diagnosis of α-HCD based on serum protein analysis requires that the α-H chain be identified with anti-α-chain antisera on immunoelectrophoresis or immunofixation without a reaction to anti-L-chain antisera. However, because not all L-chain antisera detect L chains on IgA globulins, definitive diagnosis requires isolation and purification of the protein, followed by reduction and alkylation and demonstration that the reduced monoclonal protein constituents do not contain light chains.[581]

All reported cases of α-HCD have been of the α_1 subtype rather than the α_2 subtype. The molecular mass of the α-HCD proteins is about one half to three quarters that of the intact α chain and appears to result from an internal deletion of most of the variable region in the H chain and the C1α domains.[555] The α chains have a tendency to polymerize to variously sized molecules with different net charges; this property probably accounts for the presence of a diffuse band rather than a characteristic monoclonal spike on electrophoresis. The abnormal α chains have also been found in modest quantities in the patients' urine in the absence of Bence Jones proteinuria.

Treatment of some patients with antibiotics alone (*e.g.*, tetracycline) has resulted in resolution of the syndrome, and α-HCD has therefore been considered a potential example of "immune escalation" from benign monoclonal immunoproliferation to frank neoplastic transformation.[94] In most patients, aggressive therapy with melphalan or cyclophosphamide plus prednisone or multiagent combinations has been required.[582] In some patients, complete remissions have been obtained, primarily for those with stage A disease (*i.e.*, mature plasmacytic or lymphoplasmacytic infiltration limited to the lamina propria).[581,583] Usually the tumor is at a more advanced stage, with involvement of the submucosa or muscularis (stage B), or has undergone conversion to an immunoblastic sarcoma with involvement of the mesenteric nodes and bowel (stage C), for which remissions are only transient, and the disease progresses to a fatal outcome associated with cachexia or sepsis.

μ-Heavy-Chain Disease

The first patient with μ-heavy-chain disease (μ-HCD) was reported by several groups in 1970 and had a clinical picture of CLL.[584,585] In 1975, Franklin reported a series of 7 patients, all but one of whom had CLL.[586] Since that time, most additional reports of cases of μ-HCD have been of CLL. Almost all of the patients with μ-HCD have a clinical picture of CLL, but there is one clearly documented case with a clinical syndrome of myeloma with amyloid and osteolytic bone lesions with a μ-H chain in the serum, and one patient with an apparent μ-chain MGUS has also been identified.[555,587] Although μ-HCD patients usually have a CLL-like picture, the converse is not true. In a detailed immunologic analysis of 120 patients with CLL, none proved to have μ-HCD.[588] A common finding in the bone marrow of patients with μ-HCD is the presence of vacuolated plasma cells, and this finding should lead to a search for this entity. The diagnosis is established by demonstrating the presence of a μ-H chain in the serum by immunoelectrophoresis or immunofixation. Approximately two thirds of patients with μ-HCD have free L chains in the urine (Bence Jones proteins), usually of the κ-type.[588]

Molecular studies of the purified μ chains from these patients have been difficult because of the small amounts usually present and difficulty in isolation, but as with γ-HCD and α-HCD, μ chains in μ-HCD commonly have large deletions in the variable region.[589] In one patient with a leukemic picture, μ-HCD, and free L-chain production, the tumor cells produced a shortened μ chain that lacked the entire variable region.[549] The deletion was further localized to a defect at the level of the Ig gene structure and assembly that deletes coding information and results in aberrant RNA processing, which yields a truncated μ-chain protein that lacks a variable region and cannot assemble with light chains.[550]

The clinical course of patients with μ-HCD is varied but usually follows the course of CLL. When treatment is indicated, patients are usually treated with alkylating agents and prednisone in a fashion similar to that used in the treatment of CLL and with some benefit.

δ-Heavy-Chain Disease

In a single patient who presented with osteolytic bone lesions and renal failure, the serum M-component comprised closed tetramers of δ chains.[590] Monoclonal L chains were not detected with standard immunologic techniques. At autopsy, the patient also had subendothelial deposits on the basement membranes of the renal glomeruli, and the patient was reported as having δ-HCD.[590] The patient's clinical syndrome was consistent with multiple myeloma.

PERSPECTIVE

There has been a substantial advancement in our understanding of multiple myeloma and related plasma cell neoplasms since 1970. This has been the result of increased research efforts in the basic and clinical areas and the major impact of advances in immunobiology. At the clinical level, the development of a useful staging system, the identification of serum β_2-microglobulin as a major pretreatment prognostic factor, and the incorporation of anthracyclines into combination treatment regimens for remission induction in advanced stage and refractory patients offer evidence of progress. Current combination chemotherapy regimens for patients with active disease have achieved better results than the simpler regimens brought into use in the 1960s. However, intrinsic drug sensitivity in plasma cell neoplasms is not as marked as in some of the less-well-differentiated B-cell neoplasms, and kinetic and drug-resistance phenomena appear responsible for the inability to achieve true complete remissions. Higher-dosage alkylating agent regimens with myeloid growth factor support or with bone marrow transplantation may change this picture for good-risk patients. Recent results with allogeneic bone marrow transplants from HLA-matched siblings are encouraging, but this approach is only applicable to younger patients ($\leq$55), and the median age at the time of diagnosis is 62 in most series. The procedure is therefore relevant to 10% or fewer myeloma patients.

The potential role of INF-α for remission maintenance after cytoreduction requires thorough investigation. Because there is now substantial clinical and preclinical evidence that melphalan is more leukemogenic than cyclophosphamide, selection of chemotherapeutic drugs should be guided by the goal of reducing the frequency of late side effects of treatment.

The use of monoclonal antibodies for identification of plasma cell and B-cell-associated cell-surface antigens provides a new approach to classification of patients with plasma cell neoplasms and the basis for developing new therapeutic agents capable of purging marrow of myeloma cells for autologous transplantation and for targeted cytotoxic destruction of residual myeloma-associated antigen-bearing cells in remission patients.

The role of drug-resistance mechanisms in blunting the effectiveness of chemotherapy is only now beginning to be understood at a cellular and molecular level in myeloma. With a better understanding of these mechanisms, development of pharmacologic means to abrogate drug resistance appears to be a realistic possibility that may have a major impact on future management of multiple myeloma. The clinical introduction of recombinant growth factors that stimulate the proliferation of normal progenitor populations in the bone marrow offers the promise that the anemia of myeloma and the granulocytopenia associated with its treatment may prove amenable to therapy for patients entering the next generation of clinical trials. Identification of IL-6 as a major plasmacytoma growth factor opens new avenues of therapy through the development of agents that inhibit the production of IL-6 or block its receptor-mediated effects on myeloma progenitor cells.[141]

REFERENCES

1. Kyle RA. Monoclonal gammopathy of undetermined significance (MGUS): A review. In: Hoffbrand AV, Lasch HG, Nathan DG, Salmon SE, eds. Clinics in Hematology. Eastbourne: WB Saunders, 1982:123–150.
2. Salmon SE. Immunoglobulin synthesis and tumor kinetics of multiple myeloma. Semin Hematol 1973;10:136–147.
3. Salmon SE. Plasma cell disorders. In: Wingaarden JB, Smith LH Jr, eds. Cecil textbook of medicine. 18th ed. 1988:1026–1036.
4. Macintyre W. Case of mollities and fragilitas ossium, accompanied with urine strongly charged with animal matter. Med Chir Trans Lond 1859;33:211.
5. Bence Jones H. On a new substance occurring in the urine of a patient with mollities and fragilitas ossium. Phil Trans R Soc Lond 1848;55:673.
6. Dalrymple J. On the microscopical character of mollities ossium. Dublin Q J Med Sci 1846;2:85.
7. Rustizky J. Multiple myeloma. Deutsch Z Chir 1972;3:162–172.
8. Kahler O. Zur Symptomatologie des multiplen Myeloma: Beobachtung von Albumosurie. Prog Med Wochnschr 1889;14:33–45.
9. Ellinger A. Das Vorkommen des Bence Jones' schen Korpers in Harn bei Tumoren des Knochenmarks und seine diagnostische Bedeutung. Deutsch Arch Klin Med 1899;62:266–278.
10. Wright JH. A case of multiple myeloma. Bull Johns Hopkins Hosp 1933;52:156.
11. Arinkin MI. Die intravitale Untersuchungs—Methodik des Knochenmarks. Folia Haematol (Leipz) 1929;38:233.
12. Tiselius A. Electrophoresis of serum globulin. II. Electrophoretic analysis of normal and immune sera. Biochem J 1937;31:1464.
13. Longsworth LG. Shedlovsky T, MacInnes DA. Electrophoretic patterns of normal and pathological human blood serum and plasma. J Exp Med 1939:70:399.
14. Magnus-Levy A. Multiple myeloma. Acta Med Scand 1938;95:217–280.
15. Grabar P. Williams CA. Methode permettant l'etude conjugee des proprietes electrophoretiques et immunochimiques d'un melange de proteines. Application au serum sanguin. Biochim Biophys Acta 1953;10:193.
16. Glenner GG, Terry W, Harada M, et al. Amyloid fibril proteins: Proof of homology with immunoglobulin light chains by sequence analysis. Science 1971;172:1150–1151.
17. Salmon SE, Smith BA. Immunoglobulin synthesis and total body tumor cell number in IgG multiple myeloma. J Clin Invest 1970;49:1114.
18. Alwall N. Urethane and stilbamidine in multiple myeloma: Report on 2 cases. Lancet 1947;2:388–389.
19. Holland JF, Hosley H, Scharlau C, et al. A controlled trial of urethane treatment in myeloma. Blood 1966;27:328–342.
20. Bergsagel DE, Griffith KM, Haut A, et al. The treatment of plasma cell myeloma. Adv Cancer Res 1967;10:311–359.
21. Bergsagel DE, Sprague CC, Austin C, et al. Evaluation of new chemotherapeutic agents in the treatment of multiple myeloma. IV. L-phenylalanine mustard (NSC-8806). Cancer Chemother Rep 1962;21:87–99.
22. Korst DR, Clifford GO, Fowler WM, et al. Multiple myeloma. II. Analysis of cyclophosphamide in 165 patients. JAMA 1964;189:758–762.
23. Salmon SE, Shadduck RK, Schilling A. Intermittent high-dose prednisone therapy for multiple myeloma. Cancer Chemother Rep 1967;51:179.
24. Alexanian R, Bonnet J, Gehan E, et al. Combination chemotherapy for multiple myeloma. Cancer 1972;30:382–389.
25. Costa G, Engle RL Jr, Schilling A, et al. Melphalan and prednisone: An effective combination for the treatment of multiple myeloma. Am J Med 1973;54:589–599.
26. Salmon SE. Nitrosoureas in multiple myeloma. Cancer Treat Rep 1976;60:789–794.
27. Alberts DS, Salmon SE. Adriamycin (NSC-123127) in the treatment of alkylator-resistant multiple myeloma: A pilot study. Cancer Chemother Rep 1975;59:345–350.
28. Mellstedt A, Aahre A, Bjorkholm M, et al. Interferon therapy in myelomatosis. Lancet 1979;1:245–247.
29. Young JL, Percy CL, Asire AJ. Surveillance, epidemiology, and end results: Incidence and mortality data, 1973–1977. NCI Monograph 57. Bethesda: Department of Health and Human Services, NIH, 1981;81–2330.

30. Devesa SS, Silverman DT, Young JL Jr, et al. Cancer incidence and mortality trends among whites in the United States, 1947–84. JNCI 1987;79:701–770.
31. Martin NH. The incidence of myelomatosis. Lancet 1961;1:237–239.
32. Malignant neoplasms of lymphatic and haematopoietic tissues: Multiple myeloma. WHO Epidemiol Vital Stat Rep 1965;18:414–415.
33. Hewell GM, Alexanian R. Myeloma in young persons. Ann Intern Med 1976;84:441–443.
34. Blattner WA, Blair A, Mason TJ. Multiple myeloma in the United States, 1950–75. Cancer 1981;48:2547.
35. Linos A, Kyle RA, O'Fallon MW, et al. Incidence and secular trend of multiple myeloma in Olmstead County, Minnesota: 1965–77. JNCI 1981;66:17.
36. Blattner WA. Multiple myeloma and macroglobulinemia. In: Schottenfeld D, Fraumeni JF Jr, eds. Cancer epidemiology and prevention. Philadelphia: WB Saunders, 1982: 722.
37. Axelsson U, Bachmann R, Hallen J. Frequency of pathological proteins (M-components) in 6995 sera from an adult population. Acta Med Scand 1966;179:235–247.
38. Englisova M, Englis M, Kyral V, et al. Changes of immunoglobulin synthesis in old people. Exp Gerontol 1968;3:125–127.
39. Bazin H, Deckers C, Beckers A, et al. Transplantable immunoglobulin-secreting tumors in rats. I. General features of Lou/Wsl strain rat immunocytomas and their monoclonal proteins. Int J Cancer 1972;10:568–580.
40. Bazin H, Beckers A, Deckers C, et al. Transplantable immunoglobulin-secreting tumors in rats. V. Monoclonal immunoglobulins secreted by 250 ileocecal immunocytomas in Lou/Wsl rats. JNCI 1973;51:1359–1361.
41. Cotran RS, Fortner JG. Serum-protein abnormality in a transplantable plasmacytoma of the Syrian golden hamster. JNCI 1962;28:1193–1205.
42. Farrow BRH, Penny R. Multiple myeloma in a cat. J Am Vet Assoc 1971;158:606–611.
43. Kehoe JM, Hurvitz Al, Capra JD. Characterization of three feline paraproteins. J Immunol 1972;109:511–516.
44. Osborne CA, Perman V, Sautter JH, et al. Multiple myeloma in the dog. J Am Vet Assoc 1968;153:1300–1319.
45. Hurvitz AI. Animal model for human disease: Canine monoclonal gammopathies/immunoglobulins. Comp Pathol Bull 1971;3:4.
46. Payne GS, Bishop JM, Varmus HE. Multiple arrangements of viral DNA and an activated host oncogene in bursal lymphomas. Nature 1982;295:209.
47. Potter M. Concepts of pathogenesis and experimental models of immunoglobulin-secreting tumors in animals. In: Weirnick PH, Canellos GP, Kyle RA, Schiffer CA, eds. Neoplastic diseases of the blood, vol. 1. New York: Churchill-Livingstone, 1985: 393–412.
48. Radl J. Hollander CF, Van Den Berg P, et al. Idiopathic paraproteinemia. I. Studies in an animal model—the aging C57BL/KaLWRij mouse. Clin Exp Immunol 1978;33: 395.
49. Dunn TB. Plasma cell neoplasms beginning in the ileocecal area in strain 3CH mice. JNCI 1957;19:371.
50. Potter M, Wax JS. Genetics of susceptibility to pristane induced plasmacytomas in BALB/cAN. Reduced susceptibility in BALB/cJ with a brief description of pristane-induced arthritis. J Immunol 1981;127:1591.
51. Potter M, Wax JS. Peritoneal plasmacytomas—genesis in mice. A comparison of three pristane dose regimens. JNCI 1983;71:391.
52. Potter M, Pumphrey JG, Bailey DW. Genetics of susceptibility of plasmacytoma induction. I. BALB/cAnN(C), C57BL/6N(B6), C57BL/Ka(BK), $(C \times B6)F_1$ $(C \times BK)F_1$ and $C \times B$ recombinant inbred strains. JNCI 1975;54:1413.
53. Potter M. Pathogenesis of plasmacytomas in mice. In: Becker FF, ed. Cancer: A comprehensive treatise. New York: Plenum Press, 1982.
54. Potter M, Boyce C. Induction of plasma cell neoplasms in strain BALB/c mice with mineral oil and mineral oil adjuvants. Nature 1962;193:1086.
55. Merwin RM, Redman LW. Induction of plasma cell tumors and sarcomas in mice by diffusion chambers placed in the peritoneal cavity. JNCI 1963;31:998–1007.
56. Anderson PN. Plasma cell tumor induction in BALB/c mice. Proc Am Assoc Cancer Res [Abstract] 1970;11:3.
57. Potter M, Pumphrey JG, Walters JL. Brief communication: Growth of primary plasmacytomas in the mineral oil-conditioned environment. JNCI 1972;49:305–308.
58. Potter M, Walters JL. Effect of intraperitoneal pristane on established immunity to the Adj-PC-5 plasmacytoma. JNCI 1973;51:875–881.
59. Hamburger AW, Salmon SE. Primary bioassay of human myeloma stem cell. J Clin Invest 1977;60:846–854.
60. Namb Y, Hanaoka M. Immunocytology of cultured IgM-forming cells of mouse. I. Requirement of phagocytic cell factor for the growth of IgM-forming tumor cells in tissue culture. J Immunol 1972;109:1193–1200.
61. Nordan RP, Potter M. A macrophage-derived factor required by plasmacytomas for survival and proliferation in vitro. Science 1986;233:566–568.
62. Metcalf D. The serum factor stimulating colony formation in vitro by murine plasmacytoma cells: Response to antigens and mineral oil. J Immunol 1974;113:235–243.
63. Tosato G. Seamon KB, Goldman ND, et al. Monocyte-derived human B-cell growth factor identified as interferon-β_2 (BSF-2, IL-6). Science 1988;239:502–504.
64. Hamburger AW. Inhibition of B lymphocyte clonal proliferation by spleen cells from plasmacytoma-bearing mice. JNCI 1980;65:1337–1343.
65. McIntire KR, Princler GL. Prolonged adjuvant stimulation in germfree BALB/c mice: Development of plasma cell neoplasia. Immunology 1969;17:481–487.
66. Dalton AJ, Potter M, Merwin RM. Some ultrastructural characteristics of a series of primary and transplanted plasma cell tumors of the mouse. JNCI 1961;26:1221–1267.
67. Kuff EL, Smith LA, Lueders KK. Intracisternal A particle genes in *Mus musculus*. A conserved family of retrovirus-like elements. Mol Cell Biol 1981;1:216.
68. Shepard JS, Pettengill OS, Wurster-Hill DH, et al. A specific chromosome breakpoint associated with mouse plasmacytomas. JNCI 1978;61:225.
69. Yosida MC, Moriwaki K, Migita S. Specificity of the deletion of chromosome no. 15 in mouse plasmacytoma. JNCI 1978;60:235–238.
70. Dickman SH, Goldstein M, Kahn T, et al. Amyloidosis: An unusual complication of Gaucher's disease. Arch Pathol Lab Med 1978;102:460–462.
71. Selvaney P, Block M, Narni R, et al. Alteration and abnormal expression of the c-*myc* oncogene in human multiple myeloma. Blood 1988;71:30–35.
72. Palumbo AP, Boccadero M, Battaglo S, et al. Human homologue of Moloney leukemia virus integration-4 locus (MLVI-4) located 20 kilobases 3′ of the *myc* gene, is rearranged in multiple myelomas. Cancer Res 1990;50:6478–6482.
73. MacMahon B, Clark DW. The incidence of multiple myeloma. J Chron Dis 1956;4: 508–515.
74. McPhedran P. Heath CW Jr, Garcia J. Multiple myeloma incidence in metropolitan Atlanta, Georgia: Racial and seasonal variations. Blood 1972;39:866.
75. Bertrams J, Kuwert E, Bohme U, et al. HL-A antigens in Hodgkin's disease and multiple myeloma—increased frequency of W18 in both diseases. Tissue Antigens 1972;2: 41.
76. Jeannet M, Magnin C. HL-A antigens in haematological malignant diseases. Eur J Clin Invest 1971;2:39.
77. Mason DY, Cullen P. HL-A antigen frequencies in myeloma. Tissue Antigens 1975;5: 238.
78. McDevitt HO, Bodner WF. Histocompatibility antigens, immune responsiveness and susceptibility to disease. Am J Med 1972;52:1.
79. Maldonado JE, Kyle RA. Familial myeloma. Report of eight families and a study of serum proteins in their relatives. Am J Med 1974;57:875–884.
80. Blattner WA. Epidemiology of multiple myeloma and related plasma cell disorders: An analytic review. In: Potter M, ed. Progress in myeloma: Biology of myeloma. New York: Elsevier North-Holland, 1980:1.
81. Kyle RA, Heath CW Jr, Carbone P. Multiple myeloma in spouses. Arch Intern Med 1971;127:944–946.
82. Pietruszka M, Rabin BS, Srodes G. Multiple myeloma in husband and wife. Lancet 1976;1:314.
83. Kyle RA. Monoclonal gammopathy of undetermined significance: Natural history in 241 cases. Am J Med 1978;64:814.
84. Meijers KAE, Leeuw B, Voormolen-Kalova M. The multiple occurrence of myeloma and asymptomatic paraproteinaemia within one family. Clin Exp Immunol 1972;12: 185.
85. Youinou P. Genetic propensity to benignity in monoclonal gammopathy. Acta Haematol (Basel) 1979;62:173.
86. Axelsson U, Hallen J. Familial occurrence of pathological serum proteins of different gammaglobulin groups. Lancet 1965;2:369.
87. Williams RC, Erickson JL, Polesky HF, et al. Studies of monoclonal immunoglobulins (M-components) in various kindreds. Ann Intern Med 1967;67:309.
88. Blattner WA, Garber J, Mann DL, et al. Waldenström's macroglobulinemia and autoimmune disease in a family. Ann Intern Med 1980;93:830.
89. Björnsson OG, Arnason A, Gudmundsson S, et al. Macroglobulinema in an Icelandic family. Acta Med Scand 1978;203:283.
90. Fine JM, Lambin P, Valentin L, et al. IgG monoclonal gammopathy in the sister of a patient with Waldenström's macroglobulinemia. Biomedicine 1973;19:117.
91. Fraumeni JF Jr, Wertelecki W, Blattner WA, et al. Varied manifestations of a familial lymphoproliferative disorder. Am J Med 1975;59:145.
92. Kalff MW, Hijmans W. Immunoglobulin analysis in families of macroglobulinemia patients. Clin Exp Immunol 1969;5:479.
93. Seligmann M, Sassy C, Chevalier A. A human IgG myeloma protein with anti-alpha$_2$-macroglobulin antibody activity. J Immunol 1973;110:85.
94. Salmon SE, Seligmann M. B-cell neoplasia in man. Lancet 1974;2:1230.
95. Cuzick J, De Stavola B. Multiple myeloma. A case control study. Br J Cancer 1988;57: 516–520.
96. Linet MS, Sioban DH, McLaughlin JK. A case-control study of multiple myeloma in whites: Chronic antigenic stimulation, occupation and drug use. Cancer Res 1987;47: 2978–2981.
97. Hamaker WR, Lindell ME, Gomez AC. Plasmacytoma arising in a pacemaker pocket. Ann Thorac Surg 1976;21:354.
98. Gerber MA. Asbestosis and neoplastic disorders of the hematopoietic system. Am J Clin Pathol 1970;53:204–208.
99. Kagan E, Jacobson RJ, Yeung K-Y, et al. Asbestosis-associated neoplasms of B cell lineage. Am J Med 1979;67:325–330.
100. Osserman EF, Takatsuki L. Considerations regarding the pathogenesis of the plasmacytic dyscrasias. Semin Hematol 1965;4:28–49.
101. Pratt PW, Estren S, Kochwa S. Immunoglobulin abnormalities in Gaucher's disease: Report of 16 cases. Blood 1968;31:633–640.
102. Wolf P. Monoclonal gammopathy in Gaucher's disease. Lab Med 1973;4:28–29.
103. MacDonald M, McCathie M, Faed MJW, et al. Gaucher's disease with bronchial gammopathy. J Clin Pathol 1975;28:757.
104. Turesson I, Rausing A. Gaucher's disease and benign monoclonal gammopathy. Acta Med Scand 1975;197:507–512.
105. Penny R, Hughes S. Repeated stimulation of the reticuloendothelial system and the development of plasma cell dyscrasias. Lancet 1970;1:77–78.
106. Rosenblatt J, Hall CA. Plasma-cell dyscrasia following prolonged stimulation of reticuloendothelial system. Lancet 1970;1:301–302.

107. Isobe T, Osserman EF. Pathologic conditions associated with plasma cell dyscrasias: A study of 806 cases. Ann N Y Acad Sci 1971;90:507–518.
108. Goldenberg GJ, Paraskevas F, Israels LG. The association of rheumatoid arthritis with plasma cell and lymphocytic neoplasms. Arthritis Rheum 1969;12:569–579.
109. Wegelius O, Skrifvars B. Rheumatoid arthritis terminating in plasmacytoma. Acta Med Scand 1970;187:133–138.
110. Wohlenberg H. Osteomyelitis and plasmacytoma. N Engl J Med 1970;283:822–823.
111. Isomaki HA, Hakulmen T, Joutsenlahti U. Excess risk of lymphomas, leukemias and myelomas in patients with rheumatoid arthritis. J Chron Dis 1978;31:691–699.
112. Imahori S, Moore GE. Multiple myeloma and prolonged stimulation of reticuloendothelial system. N Y State J Med 1972;72:1625.
113. Jancelewicz Z, Takatsuki K, Sugai S, et al. IgD multiple myeloma. Review of 133 cases. Arch Intern Med 1975;135:87.
114. Schafer AI, Miller JB. Association of IgA multiple myeloma with preexisting disease. Br J Haematol 1979;41:19–24.
115. Schafer AI, Miller JB, Lester EP, et al. Monoclonal gammopathy in hereditary spherocytosis: A possible pathogenetic relation. Ann Intern Med 1978;88:45–46.
116. Waldbaum B, Gelfand M. Myelomatosis in the Rhodesian African. Trop Geogr Med 1974;26:26.
117. Krause RM. Factors controlling the occurrence of antibodies with uniform properties. Fed Proc 1970;29:59.
118. Ichimaru M, Ishimaru T, Mikami M, et al. Multiple myeloma among atomic bomb survivors, Hiroshima and Nagasaki, 1950–1976. Radiation effects research foundation technical report no. 9–79. Hiroshima: Radiation Effects Research Foundation, 1979.
119. Cuzik J. Radiation-induced myelomatosis. N Engl J Med 1981;304:204–210.
120. Lewis EB. Leukemia, multiple myeloma, and aplastic anemia in American radiologists. Science 1963;142:1492.
121. Matanoski GM. Risk of cancer associated with occupational exposure in radiologists and other radiation workers. In: Burchenal JH, Oettgen HF, eds. Cancer, achievements, challenges, and prospects for the 1980s. New York: Grune & Stratton, 1982:241.
122. Matanoski GM, Seltzer R, Santwell RE, et al. The current mortality rates of radiologists and other physician specialists: Specific causes of death. Am J Epidemiol 1975;101: 199.
123. Mancuso TE, Stewart A, Kneale G. Radiation exposures of Hanford workers dying from cancer and other causes. Health Phys 1977;33:369.
124. Boice JD Jr, Morin MM, Glass AG, et al. Diagnostic x-ray procedures and risk of leukemia, lymphoma and multiple myeloma. JAMA 1991;265:1290–1294.
125. Hayhoe FGJ, Neuman Z. Cytology of myeloma cells. J Clin Pathol 1976;29:916.
126. Paraskevas F, Heremans J, Waldenström J. Cytology and electrophoretic pattern in γ_1A (B_2A) myeloma. Acta Med Scand 1961;170:575–589.
127. Maldonado JE, Bayrd ED, Brown AL. The flaming cell in multiple myeloma: A light and electron microscopy study. Am J Clin Pathol 1965;44:605.
128. Farquhar MG, Palade GE. The Golgi apparatus (1954–1981) from artifact to center stage. J Cell Biol 1981;91:77–103.
129. Blom J, Mansa B, Wiik A. A study of Russell bodies in human monoclonal plasma cell by means of immunofluorescence and electron microscopy. Acta Pathol Microbiol Scand [A] 1976;84:335.
130. Durie B, Grogan T. CALLA positive myeloma an aggressive subtype with poor survival. Blood 1985;66:229–232.
131. Grogan TM, Durie BGM, Lomen C, et al. Delineation of a novel pre-B cell component in plasma cell myeloma: Immunochemical, immunophenotypic, genotypic, cytologic, cell culture, and kinetic features. Blood 1987;70:932–942.
132. Bataille R, Durie BGM, Sany J, Salmon SE. Myeloma bone marrow acid phosphatase staining: A correlative study of 38 patients. Blood 1980;55:802.
133. Cassuto JP, Hammou JC, Pastorelli E, et al. Plasma acid cell phosphatase, a discriminative test for benign and malignant monoclonal gammopathies. Biomedicine 1977;27: 197.
134. Tortarolo M, Cantore N, Grande M, et al. Plasma cell acid phosphatase an adjunct in the differential diagnosis of monoclonal immunoglobulinemias. Acta Haematol 1981;65:103.
135. Kyle KA, Greipp PR. Smoldering multiple myleoma. N Engl J Med 1980;302:1347–1349.
136. Durie BGM, Salmon SE, Moon TE. Pretreatment tumor mass, cell kinetics, and prognosis in multiple myeloma. Blood 1980;55:364–372.
137. Greipp PR, Witzig TE, Gonchoroff NJ, et al. Immunofluorescence labeling indices in myeloma and related monoclonal gammopathies. Mayo Clin Proc 1987;62:969–977.
138. Barlogie B, Latreille J, Alexanian R, et al. Quantitative cytology in myeloma research. In: Hoffbrand AV, Lasch HG, Nathan DG, Salmon SE, eds. Clinics in Hematology. Eastbourne: WB Saunders, 1982:19–46.
139. Seigneurin D, David J, Sotto JJ, et al. β-Glucuronidases plasmocytaires dans les dysglobulinemias. Interet diagnostique de leur mise en evidence. Pathol Biol 1979;27: 467.
140. Duston MA, Skinner M, Shirahama T, et al. Diagnosis of amyloidosis by abdominal fat aspiration. Am J Med 1987;82:412–414.
141. Levy Y, Tsapis A, Brovet JC. Interleukin-6 antisense oligonucleotides inhibit the growth of human myeloma cell lines. J Clin Invest 1991;88:696–699.
142. Klein B, Zhang XG, Jourdan M, et al. Paracrine rather than autocrine regulation of myeloma-cell growth and differentiation by Interleukin-6. Blood 1989;73:517–526.
143. Mundy GR, Raisz LG, Cooper RA, et al. Evidence for the secretion of an osteoclast stimulating factor in myeloma. N Engl J Med 1974;291:1041–1046.
144. Valentin-Opran A. Charhon SA. Meunier PJ, et al. Quantitative histology of myeloma-induced bone changes. Br J Haematol 1982;52:602–610.
145. Durie BGM, Salmon SE, Mundy GR. Relation of osteoclast activating factor production to the extent of bone disease in multiple myeloma. Br J Haematol 1981;47:21–30.
146. Garret IR, Durie BGM, Nedwin GE, et al. Production of lymphotoxin, a bone-resorbing cytokine by cultured human myeloma cells. N Engl J Med 1987;317:526–532.
147. Cozzolino F, Torcia M, Aldinucci D, et al. Production of interleukin-1 by bone marrow myeloma cells. Blood 1989;74:380–387.
148. Solomon A, Waldmann TA, Fahey JL, et al. Metabolism of Bence Jones proteins. J Clin Invest 1964;43:103–117.
149. Waldmann TA, Strober W, Mogielnicki RP. The renal handling of low-molecular-weight proteins. II. Disorders of serum protein catabolism in patients with tubular proteinuria, the nephrotic syndrome, or uremia. J Clin Invest 1964;51:2162–2174.
150. Wochner RD, Strober W, Waldmann TA. The role of catabolism of Bence Jones proteins and immunoglobulin fragments. J Exp Med 1967;126:207–221.
151. Solomon A, Weiss DT, Kattine AA. Nephro-toxic potential of Bence Jones proteins. N Engl J Med 1991;324:1845–1851.
152. Levi DF, Williams RC Jr, Lindstrom FD. Immunofluorescent studies of the myeloma kidney with special reference to light chain disease. Am J Med 1968;33:92–933.
153. Costanza DJ, Smoller M. Multiple myeloma with the Fanconi syndrome. Study of a case, with electron microscopy of the kidney. Am J Med 1963;34:125–133.
154. Engle RL Jr, Wallis LA. Multiple myeloma and the adult Fanconi syndrome. I. Report of a case with crystal-like deposits in the tumor cells and in the epithelial cells of the kidney. Am J Med 1957;22:5–12.
155. Finkel PN, Kronenberg K, Pesce AJ, et al. Adult Fanconi syndrome, amyloidosis, and marked kappa light chain proteinuria. Nephron 1973;10:1–24.
156. Sirtoa JH, Hamerman D. Renal function studies in an adult subject with the Fanconi syndrome. Am J Med 1954;16:138–152.
157. Preuss HG, Hammack WJ, Murdaugh HV. The effect of Bence Jones protein on the in vitro function of rabbit renal cortex. Nephron 1967;5:210–216.
158. Preuss HG, Weiss FR, Iammarino RM, et al. Effect on rat kidney slice function in vitro of proteins from the urines of patients with myelomatosis and nephrosis. Clin Sci Mol Med 1974;46:283–294.
159. Maldonado JE, Velosa JA, Kyle RA, et al. Fanconi syndrome in adults. A manifestation of a latent form of myeloma. Am J Med 1975;58:354–364.
160. Kyle RA, Greipp PR. "Idiopathic" Bence Jones proteinuria. Long-term follow-up in seven patients. N Engl J Med 1982;306:564–567.
161. Pruzanski W, Ogryzlo MA. Abnormal proteinuria in malignant diseases. Adv Clin Chem 1970;13:335–382.
162. Pruzanski W, Gidon MS, Roy A. Suppression of polyclonal immunoglobulins in multiple myeloma: Relationship to the staging and other manifestations at diagnosis. Clin Immunol Immunopathol 1980;17:280.
163. Duperray C, Bataille R, Boiron JM, et al. No expansion of the pre-B and B cell compartments of the bone marrow in patients with multiple myeloma. Cancer Res 1991;51: 3224–3228.
164. Ullrich S, Zolla-Pazner S. Immunoregulatory circuits in myeloma. In: Hoffbrand AV, Lasch HG, Nathan DG, Salmon SE, eds. Clinics in Hematology. Eastbourne: WB Saunders, 1982:87–111.
165. Broder S, Humphrey R, Durm M, et al. Impaired synthesis of polyclonal (non-paraprotein) immunoglobulin by circulating lymphocytes from patients with multiple myeloma: Role of suppressor cells. N Engl J Med 1975;293:887–892.
166. Salmon SE. Paraneoplastic syndromes associated with monoclonal lymphocyte and plasma cell proliferation. Ann N Y Acad Sci 1974;230:228–239.
167. Bovill EG, Ershler WB, Golden EA, et al. A human myeloma-produced monoclonal protein directed against the active subpopulation von Willebrand factor. Am J Clin Pathol 1986;85:115–123.
168. Merlini G, Farhangi M, Osserman EF. Monoclonal immunoglobulins with antibody activity in myeloma, macroglobulinemia and related plasma cell dyscrasias. Semin Oncol 1986;13:350–365.
169. Kilgore LL, Patterson BW, Parenti DM, et al. Immune complex hyperlipidemia induced by an apolipoprotein-reactive immunoglobulin A paraprotein from a patient with multiple myeloma. J Clin Invest 1985;76:225–232.
170. Sullivan PW, Salmon SE. Kinetics of tumor growth and regression in IgG myeloma. J Clin Invest 1972;51:1597.
171. Drewinko B, Alexanian R, Boyer H, et al. The growth fraction of human myeloma cells. Blood 1981;57:333.
172. Hobbs JR. Growth rates and response to treatment in human myelomatosis. Br J Haematol 1969;16:607.
173. Bergsagel DE. Assessment of the response of mouse and human myeloma to chemotherapy and radiotherapy. In: Drewinko B, Humphreya RM, eds. Growth kinetics and biochemical regulation of normal and malignant cells. University of Texas Cancer Center, M.D. Anderson Hospital and Tumor Institute, 29th Annual Symposium on Fundamental Cancer Research. Baltimore: Williams & Wilkins, 1977:705–717.
174. Bergsagel DE, Pruzanski W. Treatment of plasma cell myeloma with cytotoxic agents. Arch Intern Med 1975;135:172–176.
175. Suchman AL, Coleman M, Mouradian JA, et al. Aggressive plasma cell myeloma: A terminal phase. Arch Intern Med 1981;141:1315–1320.
176. Falini B, DeSolas I, Levine AM, et al. Emergence of B-immunoblastic sarcoma in patients with multiple myeloma: A clinicopathologic study of 10 cases. Blood 1982;59: 923–933.
177. Hobbs JR. Immunocytoma o' mice an' men. Br Med J 1971;2:67.
178. Ludwig H, Tscholakoff D, Neuhold, et al. Magnetic resonance imaging of the spine in multiple myeloma. Lancet 1987;2:364–366.
179. Alexanian R. Localized and indolent myeloma. Blood 1980;56:521.
180. Durie BGM, Salmon SE. Multiple myeloma, macroglobulinaemia and monoclonal

gammopathies. In: Hoffbrand AV, Brain MC, Hirsh J, eds. Recent advances in haematology. Edinburgh: Churchill-Livingstone, 1977:243.

181. Durie BGM, Salmon SE. A clinical staging system for multiple myeloma. Correlation of measured myeloma cell mass with presenting clinical features, response to treatment and survival. Cancer 1975;36:842–852.
182. Alexanian R, Balcerzak S, Bonnet JD, et al. Prognostic factors in multiple myeloma. Cancer 1975;36:1192–1201.
183. Woodruff RK, Wadworth J, Malpas JS, et al. Clinical staging in multiple myeloma. Br J Haematol 1979;42:199–205.
184. Merlini G, Waldenström JC, Jayakar SD. A new improved clinical staging system for multiple myeloma based on analysis of 123 treated patients. Blood 1980;55:1011–1019.
185. Belpomme D, Simon F, Pouillart P, et al. Prognostic factors and treatment of multiple myeloma: Interest of a cyclic sequential chemohormonotherapy combining cyclophosphamide, melphalan and prednisone. Recent Results Cancer Res 1978;65:28–40.
186. Gobbi M, Cavo M, Savelli G, et al. Prognostic factors and survival in multiple myeloma. Analysis of 91 cases treated by melphalan and prednisone. Haematology 1980;65:437–445.
187. Santoro A. Schieppati G, Franchi F, et al. Clinical staging and therapeutic results in multiple myeloma. Eur J Cancer Clin Oncol 1983;19:1353–1359.
188. Bergsagel DE, Phil D, Bailey AJ, et al. The chemotherapy of plasma cell myeloma and the incidence of acute leukemia. N Engl J Med 1979;301:743.
189. Bergsagel DE, Bailey AJ, Langley GR, et al. The chemotherapy of plasma cell myeloma and the incidence of acute leukemia. N Engl J Med 1979;301:743.
190. Salmon SE, Haut A, Bonnet J, et al. Alternating combination chemotherapy improves survival in multiple myeloma. A Southwest Oncology Group study. J Clin Oncol 1983;1:453.
191. Durie BGM. Staging and kinetics of multiple myeloma. In: Hoffbrand AV, Lasch HG, Nathan DG, Salmon SE, eds. Clinics in Hematology. Eastbourne: WB Saunders, 1982:3–18.
192. Durie BGM, Cole PW, Chen HSG, et al. Synthesis and metabolism of Bence Jones protein and calculation of tumour burden in patients with Bence Jones myeloma. Br J Haematol 1981;47:7.
193. Waldenström J. Diagnosis and treatment of multiple myeloma. New York: Grune & Stratton, 1970.
194. Seligmann M, Basch A. The clinical significance of pathological immunoglobulins. In: XII International Congress of Hematology (plenary session papers). New York: International Society of Hematology, 1968:21–31.
195. Hobbs JR. Paraproteins, benign or malignant? Br Med J 1967;3:699–704.
196. Kyle RA, Maldonado JE, Bayrd ED. Idiopathic Bence Jones proteinuria—a distinct entity? Am J Med 1973;55:222–226.
197. Norfolk D, Child JA, Cooper EH, et al. Serum β_2-microglobulin in myelomatosis: Potential value in stratification and monitoring. Br J Cancer 1980;42:510–515.
198. Karlsson FA, Groth T, Sege K, et al. Turnover in humans of β_2-microglobulin: The constant chain of HLA-antigens. Eur J Clin Invest 1980;10:293–300.
199. Cassuto JP, Krebs BJ, Viot G, et al. β_2-microglobulin, a tumour marker of lymphoproliferative disorders. Lancet 1978;2:108.
200. Bataille R, Magullo M, Greinier J, et al. Serum beta-2-microglobulin in multiple myeloma: Relation to presenting factors and clinical status. Eur J Cancer Clin Oncol 1982;18:59–66.
201. Scarffe JH, Anderson H, Palmer MK, et al. Prognostic significant of pretreatment serum β-2-microglobulin levels in multiple myeloma. Eur J Cancer Clin Oncol 1983;19:1361–1364.
202. Bataille R, Magulo M, Greinier J, et al. Serum beta-2-microglobulin in multiple myeloma: A simple, reliable marker for staging. Br J Haematol 1983;55:439.
203. Bataille R, Grenier J. Serum beta-2 microglobulin in multiple myeloma—A critical review. Eur J Cancer 1987;23:1829–1832.
204. Bataille R, Durie BGM, Grenier J, et al. Prognostic factors and staging in multiple myeloma: A reappraisal. J Clin Oncol 1986;4:80–87.
205. Durie BGM, Stock-Novack D, Salmon SE, et al. Prognostic value of pretreatment serum β_2-microglobulin in myeloma: A Southwest Oncology Group study. Blood 1990;75:823–830.
206. Salmon SE, Tesh D, Crowley J, et al. Chemotherapy is superior to sequential hemibody irradiation for remission consolidation in multiple myeloma: A Southwest Oncology study. J Clin Oncol 1990;8:1575–1584.
207. Karlsson FA, Wibell L, Evrin PE. β_2-microglobulin in clinical medicine. Scand J Clin Lab Invest 1980;40(suppl 154):27.
208. Tienharra A, Remes K, Pelliniemi TT. Alpha interferon raises serum beta-2-microglobulin in patients with multiple myeloma. Br J Haematol 1991;77:335–338.
209. Durie BGM, Russell DH, Salmon SE. Reappraisal of plateau phase in myeloma. Lancet 1980;2:65–68.
210. Chronic Leukemia-Myeloma Task Force, National Cancer Institute. Proposed guidelines for protocol studies. II. Plasma cell myeloma. Cancer Chemother Rep 1973;4:145–158.
211. Waldmann TA, Strober W. Metabolism of immunoglobulins. Prog Allergy 1969;13:1.
212. Salmon SE, Wampler SE. Multiple myeloma: Quantitative staging and assessment of response with a programmable pocket calculator. Blood 1977;49:379–389.
213. Palmer M, Belch A, Brox L, et al. Are the current criteria for response useful in the management of multiple myeloma? J Clin Oncol 1987;5:1373–1377.
214. Alexanian R, Barlogie B, Dixon D. High-dose glucocorticoid treatment of resistant myeloma. Ann Intern Med 1983;105:8–11.
215. Sporn JR, McIntyre OR. Chemotherapy of previously untreated multiple myeloma patients: An analysis of recent treatment results. Semin Oncol 1986;13:318–325.
216. Salmon SE. Expansion of the growth fraction in multiple myeloma with alkylating agents. Blood 1975;45:119–129.
217. Jackson DV, Case LD, Pope EK, et al. Single agent vincristine by infusion in refractory multiple myeloma. J Clin Oncol 1985;3:1508–1512.
218. MacLennan IC, Cusick J. Objective evaluation of the role of vincristine in induction and maintenance therapy for myelomatosis. Medical Research Council Working Party on Leukaemia in Adults. Br J Cancer 1985;52:153–158.
219. Mellstedt H, Bjorkholm M, Johansson B. Interferon therapy in myelomatosis. Lancet 1979;1:245–248.
220. Gutterman JU, Blumenschein GR, Alexanian R. Leucocyte interferon-induced tumor regression in human metastatic breast cancer, multiple myeloma, and malignant lymphoma. Ann Intern Med 1980;93:399–406.
221. Costanzi JJ, Cooper MR, Scarffe JH, et al. Phase II study of recombinant alpha-2 interferon in resistant multiple myeloma. J Clin Oncol 1985;3:654–659.
222. Oken MM, Kyle RA, Kay NE, et al. A phase II trial of interferon alpha$_2$ (rIFN$_2$) in the treatment of resistant multiple myeloma. Proc Am Soc Clin Oncol [Abstract 837] 1985;4:215.
223. Quesada JR, Alexanian R, Hawkins M, et al. Treatment of multiple myeloma with recombinant β-interferon. Blood 1986;67:275–278.
224. Cooper MR, Fefer A, Thompson J, et al. Alpha-2-interferon/melphalan/prednisone in previously untreated patients with multiple myeloma: A phase I-II trial. Cancer Treat Rep 1986;70:473–476.
225. Benson WJ, Scarffe JH, Todd IDH, et al. Spinal cord compression in myeloma. Br Med J 1979;1:1541–1544.
226. Mill WB, Griffith R. The role of radiation therapy in the management of plasma cell tumors. Cancer 1980;45:647–652.
227. Mill WB. Radiation therapy in multiple myeloma. Radiology 1975;115:175–178.
228. Garrett MJ. Spinal myeloma and cord compression—diagnosis and management. Clin Radiol 1970;21:42–46.
229. Garland LH, Kennedy BR. Roentgen treatment of multiple myeloma. Radiology 1948;50:297–316.
230. Bosch A, Frias Z. Radiotherapy in the treatment of multiple myeloma. Int J Radiat Oncol Biol Phys 1988;15:1363–1369.
231. Rostom AY. A review of the place of radiotherapy in myeloma with emphasis in whole body irradiation. Hematol Oncol 1988;6:193–198.
232. McIntyre OR, Tefft M, Propert R, et al. Melphalan and prednisone plus total bone marrow irradiation as initial treatment for multiple myeloma. Int J Radiat Oncol Biol Phys 1988;15:1007–1012.
233. Ellwanger FR. Controlling multiple myeloma. Int J Radiat Oncol Biol Phys 1989;16:909.
234. Alberts DS, Chang FY, Chen HSG, et al. Oral melphalan kinetics. Clin Pharmacol Ther 1979;6:737–745.
235. Feinleib M, MacMahon B. Duration of survival in multiple myeloma. JNCI 1960;24:1259–1269.
236. Osgood EE. The survival time of patients with plasmocytic myeloma. Cancer Chemother Rep 1960;9:1–10.
237. McArthur JR, Athens JW, Wintrobe MM, et al. Melphalan and myeloma. Experience with a low-dose continuous regimen. Ann Intern Med 1970;72:665–670.
238. Alexanian R, Bergsagel DE, Migliore PJ, et al. Melphalan therapy for plasma cell myeloma. Blood 1968;31:1–10.
239. Alexanian R, Haut A, Khan AU, et al. Treatment for multiple myeloma. JAMA 1969;208:1680–1685.
240. Hoogstraten B, Sheehe PR, Cuttner J, et al. Melphalan in multiple myeloma. Blood 1967;30:74–83.
241. Hoogstraten B, Costa J. Intermittent melphalan therapy in multiple myeloma. JAMA 1969;209:251–253.
242. Medical Research Council. Myelomatosis: Comparison of melphalan and cyclophosphamide therapy. Br Med J 1971;1:640–641.
243. Medical Research Council. Report on the second myelomatosis trial after five years of follow-up. Br J Cancer 1980;42:813–822.
244. Medical Research Council. Treatment comparisons in the third MRC myelomatosis trial. Br J Cancer 1980;42:823–830.
245. Ogawa M, Bergsagel D, McCulloch E. Chemotherapy of mouse myeloma: Quantitative cell cultures predictive of response in vivo. Blood 1973;41:7–15.
246. Case DC, Lee BJ III, Clarkson BD. Improved survival times in multiple myeloma treated with melphalan, prednisone, cyclophosphamide, vincristine and BCNU: M2 protocol. Am J Med 1977;63:897–903.
247. Bonnet J, Alexanian R, Salmon S, et al. Vincristine-BCNU-Adriamycin-prednisone (VBAP) combination in the treatment of relapsing or resistant multiple myeloma. A Southwest Oncology Group study. Cancer Treat Rep 1982;66:1267–1271.
248. MacLennan IC, Chapman C, Dunn J, Kelly K. Combined chemotherapy with ABCM versus melphalan for treatment of myelomatosis. Lancet 1992;340:433–438.
249. Oken MM, Tsiatis A, Abramson N, et al. Comparison of MP with intensive VBMCP therapy for the treatment of multiple myeloma (MM). Proc Am Soc Clin Oncol [Abstract] 1984;3:270.
250. Hansen OP, Clausen NT, Drivsholm A, et al. Phase II study of intermittent 5-drug regimen (VBCMP) versus intermittent 3-drug regimen (VMP), versus intermittent melphalan and prednisone (MP) in myelomatosis. Scand J Haematol 1985;35:518–524.
251. Durie BGM, Dixon B, Carter S, et al. Improved survival duration with combination chemotherapy induction for multiple myeloma: A Southwest Oncology Group study. J Clin Oncol 1986;4:1127–1237.

252. Harley JB, Pajak TF, McIntyre OR, et al. Improved survival of increased-risk myeloma patients on combined triple alkylating agent therapy: A study of the CALGB. Blood 1979;54:13–22.
253. Boccadero M, Marmont F, Tribalto M, et al. Multiple myeloma: VMCP/VBAP alternating melphalan and prednisone even in high risk patients. J Clin Oncol 1991;9: 444–448.
254. Cooper MR, McIntyre OR, Propert KJ, et al. Single, sequential, and multiple alkylating agent therapy for multiple myeloma: A CALGB study. J Clin Oncol 1986;4:1331–1339.
255. Pavlovsky S, Saslavsky J, Tezanos Pinto M, et al. A randomized trial of melphalan and prednisone versus melphalan, prednisone, cyclophosphamide, MeCCNU, and vincristine in untreated multiple myeloma. J Clin Oncol 1984;2:836–840.
256. Palva IP, Ahrenberg A, Almquist K, et al. Aggressive combination chemotherapy in multiple myeloma. A multicentre trial. Scand J Haematol 1985;35:205–209.
257. Kildahl-Anderson P, Bjark P, Bondevik A, et al. Multiple myeloma in central Norway 1981–1982: A randomized clinical trial of 5-drug combination therapy versus standard therapy. Scand J Haematol 1986;37:243–248.
258. Cohen HJ, Silberman HR, Tornyos K, et al. Comparison of two long-term chemotherapy regimens, with or without agents to modify skeletal repair, in multiple myeloma. Blood 1984;63:639–648.
259. Mettstedt H, Aahre A, Bjorkholm M. Interferon therapy of patients with myeloma. In: Terry WD, Rosenberg SA, eds. Immunotherapy of human cancer. New York: Elsevier, 1982:387–391.
260. Case DC, Sonneborn HL, Paul SD, et al. Phase II study of rDNA alpha-2 interferon (intron A) in patients with multiple myeloma utilizing an escalating induction phase. Cancer Treat Rep 1986;70:1251–1254.
261. Cooper MR, Welander CE. Interferons in the treatment of multiple myeloma. Semin Oncol 1986;13:334–340.
262. Ludwig H, Cortelezzi A, Van Camp BGK, et al. Treatment with recombinant-alpha-2C. Multiple myeloma and thrombocythaemia in myeloproliferative diseases. Oncology 1985;42(suppl 1):19–25.
263. Ahre A, Bjorkholm M, Mellstedt H, et al. Human leukocyte interferon and intermittent high-dose melphalan-prednisone administration in the treatment of multiple myeloma: A randomized clinical trial from the Myeloma Group of Central Sweden. Cancer Treat Rep 1984;68:1331–1338.
264. Alexanian R, Gehan E, Haut A, et al. Unmaintained remissions in multiple myeloma. Blood 1978;51:1005–1011.
265. Alexanian R. Long unmaintained remission in multiple myeloma. Am J Clin Oncol 1986;9:458–460.
266. Southwest Oncology Group study. Remission maintenance therapy for multiple myeloma. Arch Intern Med 1975;135:147.
267. Belch A. White D, Bergsagel D, et al. The role of maintenance chemotherapy for multiple myeloma. Proc Am Soc Clin Oncol [Abstract c1050] 1984;3:268 1984.
268. Cohen JH, Bartolucci AA, Forman WB, et al. Consolidation and maintenance therapy in multiple myeloma: Randomized comparison of a new approach to therapy after initial response to treatment. J Clin Oncol 1986;5:888–899.
269. Tribalto M, Mandelli F, Cantonetti M, et al. In: Bernasconi C, ed. New trends in the therapy of leukemia and lymphoma. Pavia, Italy: Edizione Medic Scientifiche, 1987: 61–68.
270. Mandell F, Tribalto M, Cantonetti M, et al. Recombinant alpha 2β interferon as maintenance therapy in responding multiple myeloma patients. Blood 1987;70(suppl 1):247a.
271. Salmon SE, Crowley J. Impact of glucocorticoids and interferon on outcome in multiple myeloma. Proc Am Soc Clin Oncol [Abstract] 1992;11:316.
272. Crowin J, Lindberg RD. Solitary plasmacytoma of bone vs extramedullary plasmacytoma and their relationship to multiple myeloma. Cancer 1979;43:1007–1013.
273. Knowling M, Harwood A, Bergsagel DE. A comparison of extramedullary plasmacytoma with multiple and solitary plasma cell tumors of bone. J Clin Oncol 1983;1:255–262.
274. Wiltshaw E. The natural history of extramedullary plasmacytoma and its relation to solitary myeloma of bone and myelomatosis. Medicine (Baltimore) 1976;55:217–238.
275. Woodruff RK, Malpas JS, White FE. Solitary plasmacytoma. II. Solitary plasmacytoma of bone. Cancer 1979;43:2344–2347.
276. Chak LY, Cox S, Bostwick DG, et al. Solitary plasmacytoma of bone: Treatment, progression, and survival. J Clin Oncol 1987;5:1811–1815.
277. Woodruff RK, Whittle JM, Malpas JS. Solitary plasmacytoma. I. Extramedullary soft tissue plasmacytoma. Cancer 1979;43:2340–2343.
278. Hamburger AW, Salmon SE. Primary bioassay of human tumor stem cells. Science 1977;197:461–463.
279. Otsuka T, Okamura S, Niho Y. Colony assay in patients with multiple myeloma—relationship between colony growth and clinical stage. Acta Haematol Jpn 1986;49: 1792–1799.
280. Salmon SE, Hamburger AW, Soehnlen BJ, et al. Quantitation of differential sensitivity of human tumor stem cells to anticancer drugs. N Engl J Med 1978;298:1321–1327.
281. Salmon SE. In vitro cloning and chemosensitivity of human myeloma stem cells. In: Hoffbrand AV, Lasch HG, Nathan DG, Salmon SE, eds. Clinics in Hematology. Eastbourne: WB Saunders, 1982:47–64.
282. Ludwig H, Fritz E. Individualized chemotherapy in multiple myeloma by cytostatic drug sensitivity testing of colony-forming stem cells. Anticancer Res 1981;1:329–334.
283. Nordan RP, Pumphrey JG, Rudikoff S. Purification and NH_2-terminal sequence of a plasmacytoma growth factor derived from the murine macrophage cell line P388D1. J Immunol 1987;139:813–817.
284. Van Snick J, Cayphas S, Vink A, et al. Purification and NH_2-terminal amino acid sequence of a T-cell derived lymphokine with growth factor activity for B-cell hybridomas. Proc Natl Acad Sci USA 1986;83:9679–9683.
285. Tanigawa N, Kern DH, Hikasa Y, et al. Rapid assay for evaluating the chemosensitivity of human tumors in soft agar culture. Cancer Res 1982;42:2159–2164.
286. Alexanian R, Salmon S, Gutterman J, et al. Chemoimmunotherapy of multiple myeloma. Cancer 1981;47:1923–1929.
287. Buzaid AC, Durie BGM. Management of refractory myeloma: A review. J Clin Oncol 1988;6:889–905.
288. Kyle RA, Greipp PR, Gertz MA. Treatment of refractory multiple myeloma and considerations for future therapy. Semin Oncol 1986;13:326–333.
289. Medenica R, Slack N. Clinical results of leucocyte interferon-induced tumor regression in resistant human metastatic cancer resistant to chemotherapy and/or radio-therapy-pulse therapy schedule. Cancer Drug Deliv 1985;2:53–76.
290. Wagstaff A, Loynds R, Scarffe JH. Phase II study of rDNA human alpha-2 interferon in multiple myeloma. Cancer Treat Rep 1985;69:495–498.
291. Ohno R, Kimura K, Amaki I, et al. Treatment of multiple myeloma with recombinant human leucocyte α interferon. Cancer Treat Rep 1985;69:1433–1435.
292. Alexanian R, Yap BS, Bodey GP. Prednisone pulse therapy for refractory myeloma. Blood 1983;62:572–577.
293. Alexanian R, Dimopoulos M, Barlogie B. Intermittent dexamethasone as initial chemotherapy for multiple myeloma. Blood 1991;78:174a.
293a. Alexanian R, Dimopoulos MA, Barlogie B. Primary dexamethasone treatment of multiple myeloma. Blood 1992;80:887–890.
294. Dalton WS, Durie BGM, Alberts DS, et al. Characterization of a new drug resistant human myeloma cell line which expresses P-glycoprotein. Cancer Res 1986;45:5125–5130.
295. Murakami T, Togawa A, Satch H, et al. Glucocorticoid receptor in myeloma. Eur J Haematol 1987;39:54–59.
296. Bergsagel DE, Cowan DH, Hasselbach R. Plasma cell myeloma: Response of melphalan-resistant patients to high-dose intermittent cyclophosphamide. Can Med Assoc J 1972;107:851–855.
297. Kyle RA, Sligman BR, Wallace J, et al. Multiple myeloma resistant to melphalan (NSC-8806) treated with cyclophosphamide (NSC-26271), prednisone (NSC-10023), and chloroquine (NSC-187208). Cancer Chemother Rep 1975;59:557–562.
298. Tornyos K, Silberman H, Soloman A. Phase II study of oral methyl-CCNU and prednisone in previously treated alkylating agent-resistant multiple myeloma. Cancer Treat Rep 1977;61:785–787.
299. Buonanno G, Tortarolo M, Valente A, et al. Drug-resistant multiple myeloma. A trial with the M_2 cyclic alkylating agent polychemotherapy. Haematologica (Pavia) 1978;63: 45–55.
300. Kyle RA, Gailani S, Seligman BR, et al. Multiple myeloma resistant to melphalan: Treatment with cyclophosphamide, prednisone, and BCNU. Cancer Treat Rep 1979;63: 1265–1269.
301. Blade J, Feliu E. Rozman C, et al. Cross-resistance to alkylating agents in multiple myeloma. Cancer 1983;52:786–789.
302. Steinke B, Busch FW, Becherer C, et al. Cancer Chemother Pharmacol 1985;14: 279–281.
303. Paccagnella A, Salvagno L, Bolzonella S, et al. Second and third response to M_2 (BCNU, VCR, CTX, PRED) in multiple myeloma. Am Soc Clin Oncol [Abstract] 1985;4:217.
304. Paccagnella A, Cartel G, Fosser V, et al. Treatment of multiple myeloma with M_2 protocol and without maintenance therapy. Eur J Cancer Clin Oncol 1982;19:1345–1351.
305. Belch A, Shelley W, Bergsagel D, et al. A randomized trial of maintenance versus no maintenance melphalan and prednisone in responding multiple myeloma patients. Br J Cancer 1988;57:94–99.
306. Alberts DS, Durie BGM, Salmon SE. Doxorubicin/BCNU chemotherapy for multiple myeloma in relapse. Lancet 1976;1:926–928.
307. Bonnet JD, Alexanian R, Salmon SE, et al. Addition of cisplatin and bleomycin to vincristine-doxorubicin-prednisone (VBAP) combination in the treatment of relapsing or resistant multiple myeloma: A Southwest Oncology Group study. Cancer Treat Rep 1984;68:481–485.
308. Blade J, Rozman C, Montserrat E, et al. Treatment of alkylating resistant multiple myeloma with vincristine, BCNU, doxorubicin and prednisone (VBAP). Eur J Cancer Clin Oncol 1986;22:1193–1197.
309. Present CA, Klahr C. Adriamycin, 1,3-bis-(2-chloroethyl)-1-nitrosourea (BCNU, NSC #409962), cyclophosphamide plus prednisone (ABC-P) in melphalan-resistant multiple myeloma. Cancer 1978;42:1222–1227.
310. Kyle RA, Pajak TF, Henderson ES, et al. Multiple myeloma resistant to melphalan: Treatment with doxorubicin, cyclophosphamide, carmustine (BCNU), and prednisone. Cancer Treat Rep 1982;66:451–456.
311. Barlogie B, Smith L, Alexanian R. Effective treatment of advanced multiple myeloma refractory to alkylating agents. N Engl J Med 1984;310:1353–1356.
312. Sheehan T, Judge M, Parker AC. The efficacy and toxicity of VAD in the treatment of myeloma and related disorders. Scand J Hematol 1986;37:425–428.
313. Monconduit M, Le Loet X, Bernard JF, et al. Combination chemotherapy with vincristine, doxorubicin, dexamethasone for refractory or relapsing multiple myeloma. Br J Haematol 1986;63:599–601.
314. Monconduit M, Bauters F, Najman A. Evaluation of the association vincristine-Adriamycin plus high-dose dexamethasone (VAD) in severe previously treated myeloma. Blood 1986;68(suppl 1):240a.
315. Dalton WS, Grogan TM, Meltzer PS, et al. Resistance in multiple myeloma and non-Hodgkin's lymphoma: Detection of P-glycoprotein and potential circumvention by addition of verapamil to chemotherapy. J Clin Oncol 1989;7:415–424.

316. Salmon SE, Dalton WS, Grogan TM, et al. Multidrug-resistant myeloma: Laboratory and clinical effects of verapamil as a chemosensitizer. Blood 1991;78:44–50.
317. Fitzpatrick PJ, Rider WD. Half-body radiotherapy. Int J Radiat Oncol Biol Phys 1976;1:197–207.
318. Rider WB. Half-body radiotherapy, an update. Int J Radiat Oncol Biol Phys 1978;4(suppl 2):69–70.
319. Salmon SE, Crowley J, Tesh D. Chemotherapy is sequential to hemibody irradiation for remission consolidation in multiple myeloma. J Clin Oncol [Letter to the editor] 1991;9:2234–2235.
320. Jaffe JP, Bosch A, Raich PC. Sequential hemi-body radiotherapy in advanced multiple myeloma. Cancer 1979;43:124–128.
321. Qasim MM. Techniques and results of half-body irradiation (HBI) in metastatic carcinoma and myeloma. Clin Oncol 1979;5:65–68.
322. Rowland CG, Garrett MJ, Crowley, et al. Half-body radiation in plasma cell myeloma. Clin Radiol 1983;34:507–510.
323. Coleman M, Soletan S, Wolf D, et al. Whole bone marrow irradiation for the treatment of multiple myeloma. Cancer 1982;49:1328–1333.
324. Richards JDM, Coates PB, Closs SP, et al. Case of macroglobulinemia treated with hemibody irradiation. Lancet [Letter] 1983;2:844.
325. Tobias JS, Richards JDM, Blackman GM, et al. Hemibody irradiation in multiple myeloma. Radiother Oncol 1985;3:11–16.
326. Prato FS, Kurdyak R, Saibil EA, et al. The incidence of radiation pneumonitis as a result of single fraction, upper half-body irradiation. Cancer 1976;39:71–78.
327. Jacobs P, LeRoux I, King HS. Sequential half-body irradiation as salvage therapy in chemotherapy-resistant multiple myeloma. Am J Clin Oncol 1988;11:104–109.
328. Singer CRJ, Tobias JS, Giles F, et al. Hemibody irradiation: An effective second line therapy in drug resistant multiple myeloma. Cancer 1989;63:2446–2451.
329. Kartner N, Everndaleporelle D, Bradley G, et al. Detection of P-glycoprotein in multidrug-resistant cell lines by monoclonal antibodies. Nature 1985;316:820–823.
330. Dalton WS, Grogan TM, Rybski JA, et al. Immunohistochemical detection and quantitation of P-glycoprotein in multiple drug resistant human myeloma cells: Association with level of drug resistance and drug accumulation. Blood 1989;73:747–752.
331. Salmon SE, Grogan TM, Miller TP, et al. Prediction of doxorubicin resistance in vitro in myeloma, lymphoma and breast cancer by P-glycoprotein staining. JNCI 1989;81:696–701.
331a. Sonneveld P, Durie BG, Lokhorst HM, et al. Modulation of multidrug-resistant multiple myeloma by cyclosporin. Lancet 1992;340(8814):255–259.
332. Perren TJ, Selby PJ, Mbidde EK, et al. High dose chemotherapy of multiple myeloma (MM) with melphalan (HDM) and with methylprednisolone (HDMP). Am Soc Clin Oncol [Abstract] 1986;5:158.
333. McElwain TJ, Powles RL. High-dose intravenous melphalan for plasma-cell leukaemia and myeloma. Lancet 1983;2:822–824.
334. Lenhard RE, Oken MM, Barnes JM, et al. High-dose cyclophosphamide. An effective treatment for advanced refractory multiple myeloma. Cancer 1984;53:1456–1460.
335. Lenhard RE, Tsiatis AA, Oken MM, et al. Time sequential high-dose cyclophosphamide (CY) and vincristine (VCR) treatment of multiple myeloma (MM). Proc Am Soc Clin Oncol [Abstract] 1985;4:217.
336. Barlogie B, Hall R, Zander A, et al. High-dose melphalan with autologous bone marrow transplantation for multiple myeloma. Blood 1986;67:1298–1301.
337. Barlogie B, Alexanian R, Dicke KA, et al. High-dose melphalan (HDM) + total body irradiation (TBI) and bone marrow transplantation (BMT) for refractory myeloma. Blood 1986;68(suppl 1):240a.
338. Selby PJ, McElwain TJ, Nandi AC, et al. Multiple myeloma treated with high dose intravenous melphalan. Br J Haematol 1987;66:55–62.
339. Barlogie B, Alexanian R, Dicke K, et al. High-dose chemoradiotherapy and autologous bone marrow transplantation for resistant myeloma. Blood 1987;70:869–872.
340. Osserman EF, DiRe Lb, DiRe J, et al. Identical twin marrow transplantation in multiple myeloma. Acta Haematol (Basel) 1982;68:215–223.
341. Ozer H, Han T, Nussbaum-Blumenson A, et al. Allogenic bone marrow transplantation and idiotype (ID) monitoring in multiple myeloma. Clin Invest [Abstract] 1984;25:161.
342. Gahrton G, Tura S, Flesch M, et al. Bone marrow transplantation in multiple myeloma: Report from the European Cooperative Group for Bone Marrow Transplantation. Blood 1987;69:1262–1264.
343. Gallamini A, Buffa F, Bacigalupo A, et al. Allogeneic bone marrow transplantation in multiple myeloma. Acta Haematol 1987;77:111–114.
344. Feffer A. Personal communication, 1987.
345. Tura S. Bone marrow transplantation in multiple myeloma: Current status and future perspectives. Bone Marrow Transplant 1986;1:17–20.
346. Gahrton G, Ringden O, Lonnqvist B. Bone marrow transplantation in multiple myeloma. Acta Med Scand 1986;219:523–527.
347. Jagannoth S, Barlogie B, Dicke K, et al. Autologous bone marrow transplantation in multiple myeloma: Identification of prognostic factors. Blood 1990;76:1860–1866.
348. Tong AM, Lee JC, Fay JW, et al. Elimination of clonogenic stem-cells from human multiple myeloma cell lines by a plasma cell-reactive monoclonal antibody and complement. Blood 1987;70:1482–1489.
349. Rhodes EG, Baker P, Rhodes JM, et al. Peanut agglutinin in combination with CD19 monoclonal antibody has potential as a purging agent in myeloma. Exp Hematol 1991;19:833–837.
350. Anderson KC, Barut BA, Ritz J, et al. Monoclonal antibody-purged autologous bone marrow transplantation therapy for multiple myeloma. Blood 1991;77:712–720.
351. Dinota A, Barbieri L, Gobbi M, et al. An immunotoxin containing momordin suitable for bone marrow purging in multiple myeloma patients. Br J Cancer 1989;60:315–319.
352. Shimazaki C, Wisniewski D, Scheinberg DA, et al. Elimination of myeloma cells from bone marrow by using monoclonal antibodies and magnetic immunobeads. Blood 1988;72:1248–1254.
353. Fermand JP, Levy Y, Gerota J, et al. Treatment of aggressive multiple myeloma by high-dose chemotherapy and total body irradiation followed by blood stem cells autologous graft. Blood 1989;73:20–23.
354. Gahrtner G, Tura S, Ljungman P, et al. Allogeneic bone marrow transplantation in multiple myeloma. N Engl J Med 1991;325:1267–1272.
355. Belch AR, Henderson JF, Brox LW. Treatment of multiple myeloma with deoxycoformycin. Cancer Chemother Pharmacol 1985;14:49–52.
356. Grever MR, McGee RA, Kraut ER, et al. Deoxycoformycin in refractory myeloma. Blood 1987;70(suppl 1):246a.
357. Case DC Jr, Oldham F, Ervin T, et al. Phase I–II study of epirubicin in multiple myeloma. Am Soc Clin Oncol [Abstract] 1987;6:146.
358. Durie BGM, Levy HB, Voakes J, et al. Poly (I,C)-LC as an interferon inducer in refractory multiple myeloma. J Biol Response Mod 1985;4:518–524.
359. Paccagnella A, Salvagno L, Chiarion-Sileni V, et al. Peptichemio in pretreated patient with plasma cell neoplasms. Eur J Cancer Clin Oncol 1986;22:1053–1058.
360. Tirelli U, Carbone A, Zagonei V, et al. Phase II study of teniposide (VM-26) in multiple myeloma. Am J Clin Oncol 1985;8:329–331.
361. Gockerman JP, Silberman H, Bartolucci AA. Phase II evaluation of aclarubicin in refractory multiple myeloma: A Southeastern Cancer Study Group trial. Cancer Treat Rep 1987;71:773–774.
362. Scarffe JH, Beaumont AR, Crowther D. Phase I–II evaluation of acronine in patients with multiple myeloma. Cancer Treat Rep 1983;67:93–94.
363. Ahmann FR, Meyskens FL, Jones SE, et al. Phase II evaluation of amsacrine (*m*-AMSA) in solid tumors, myeloma, and lymphoma: A University of Arizona and Southwest Oncology Group study. Cancer Treat Rep 1983;67:697–700.
364. Blum RH, Carter SK, Agre K. A clinical review of bleomycin, a new anti-neoplastic agent. Cancer 1973;31:903–913.
365. Bennett JM, Silber R, Ezdinli E, et al. Phase II study of Adriamycin and bleomycin in patients with multiple myeloma. Cancer Treat Rep 1978;62:1367–1369.
366. Corder MP, Elliot TE, Bell SJ. Dose limiting myelotoxicity and absence of significant nephrotoxicity with the weekly outpatient schedule of *cis*-platinum (II) diamminedichloride. J Clin Hematol Oncol 1977;7:645–651.
367. Cornell CJ Jr, Pajak TF, McIntyre OR. Chlorozotocin: Phase II evaluation in patients with myeloma. Cancer Treat Rep 1984;68:685–686.
368. Forman WB, Cohen HJ, Bartolucci AA, et al. Phase II evaluation of chlorozotocin in refractory multiple myeloma. Cancer Treat Rep 1984;68:1409–1410.
369. Kantarjian H, Dreicer R, Barlogie B, et al. High-dose cytosine arabinoside in multiple myeloma. Eur J Cancer Clin Oncol 1984;20:227–231.
370. Vinciguerra V, Anderson K, McIntyre OR. Diaziquone for resistant multiple myeloma. Cancer Treat Rep 1985;69:331–332.
371. Stuckey WJ, Crowley J, Baker LH, et al. Phase II trial of diaziquone in patients with refractory and relapsing multiple myeloma: A Southwest Oncology Group study. Cancer Treat Rep 1987;71:1095–1096.
372. Gockerman JP, Bartolucci AA, Nelson MO, et al. Phase II evaluation of etoposide in refractory multiple myeloma: A Southeastern Cancer Study Group trial. Cancer Treat Rep 1986;70:801–802.
373. Cohen HJ, Bartolucci AA. Hexamethylmelamine and prednisone in the treatment of refractory multiple myeloma. Am J Clin Oncol 1982;5:21–27.
374. Alberts DS, Balcerzak SP, Bonnet JP, et al. Phase II trials of mitoxantrone in multiple myeloma: A Southwest Oncology Group study. Cancer Treat Rep 1985;69:1321–1323.
375. Tirelli U, Sorio R, Magri MD, et al. Prednimustine in elderly patients with multiple myeloma: A phase II study. Cancer Treat Rep 1986;70:537–538.
376. Moon JH, Edmonson JH. Procarbazine (NSC-77213) and multiple myeloma. Cancer Chemother Rep 1970;54:245–248.
377. Lake-Lewin D, Myers J, Lee BL, et al. Phase II trial of pyrazofurin in patients with multiple myeloma refractory to standard cytotoxic therapy. Cancer Treat Rep 1979;63:1403–1404.
378. Houwen B, Ockhuizen T, Marrink J, et al. Vindesine therapy in melphalan-resistant myeloma. Eur J Cancer 1981;17:227–232.
379. Kraut EH, Crowley JJ, Gever MR, et al. Phase II study of fludarabine phosphate in multiple myeloma. A Southwest Oncology Group study. Invest New Drugs 1990;8:199–200.
380. Hanson KH, Crowley J, Salmon SE, et al. Evaluation of amonafide in refractory and relapsing multiple-myeloma—A Southwest Oncology Group study. Anticancer Drug Des 1991;2:247–250.
381. Oken MM, Lenhard RE, Tslatis AA, et al. Contribution of prednisone to the effectiveness of hexamethylmelamine in multiple myeloma. Cancer Treat Rep 1987;71:807–811.
382. Alexanian R, Barlogie B, Dixon D. Renal failure in multiple myeloma. Ann Intern Med 1990;150:1693–1695.
383. Cavo M, Baccarani M, Galieni P, et al. Renal failure in multiple myeloma. A study of the presenting findings, response to treatment and prognosis in 26 patients. Nouv Rev Fr Hematol 1986;28:147–152.
384. Cornwell CG, Pajak TF, McIntyre OR, et al. Influence of renal failure on the myelosuppressive effects of melphalan: Cancer and Leukemia Group B experience. Cancer Treat Rep 1982;66:475–481.
385. Alberts DS, Chen H-SY, Berg D, et al. Effects of renal dysfunction in dogs on the disposition and marrow toxicity of melphalan. Br J Cancer 1981;43:330–334.
386. Adair CG, Bridges JM, Desai ZR. Renal function in the elimination of oral mephalan in patients with multiple myeloma. Cancer Chemother Pharmacol 1986;17:185–188.

387. MRC Working Party on Leukemia in Adults. Analysis and management of renal failure in fourth MRC myelomatosis trial. Br Med J 1984;288:1411–1416.
388. Bernstein SP, Humes DH. Reversible renal insufficiency in multiple myeloma. Arch Intern Med 1982;142:2083–2086.
389. Coward RA, Mallick NP, Delamore IW. Should patients with acute renal failure associated with myeloma be dialysed? Br Med J 1983;287:1575–1578.
390. Iggo N, Palmer AB, Severn A, et al. Chronic dialysis in patients with multiple myeloma and renal failure: A worthwhile treatment. Q J Med 1989;270:903–910.
391. Johnson WJ, Kyle RA, Pineda AA, et al. Treatment of renal failure associated with multiple myeloma. Plasmapheresis, hemodialysis and chemotherapy. Arch Intern Med 1990;150:863–869.
392. Korzets A, Tam F, Russell G, et al. The role of continuous ambulatory peritoneal dialysis in end-stage renal failure due to multiple myeloma. Am J Kidney Dis 1990;16: 216–223.
393. Russell JA, Fitzharris BM, Corringham R, et al. Plasma exchange vs peritoneal dialysis for removing Bence Jones protein. Br J Med 1978;2:1397.
394. Feest TG, Burge PS, Cohen SL. Successful treatment of myeloma kidney by diuresis and plasmapheresis. Br J Med 1976;1:503–505.
395. Misiani R, Remuzzi G, Bertani T, et al. Plasmapheresis is the treatment of acute renal failure in multiple myeloma. Am J Med 1979;66:684–688.
396. Pasquali S, Cagnoli L, Rovinetti C, et al. Plasma exchange therapy in rapidly progressive renal failure due to multiple myeloma. Int J Artif Organs 1984;8:27–30.
397. Humphrey RL, Wright JR, Zachary JB, et al. Renal transplantation in multiple myeloma. A case report. Ann Intern Med 1975;83:651–653.
398. Payne R, Little A, Williams R, et al. Interpretation of serum calcium in patients with abnormal serum proteins. Br Med J 1973;4:643.
399. Ralston SH, Gallacher SJ, Patel U, et al. Comparison of three intravenous biophosphonates in cancer-associated hypercelcemia. Lancet 1989;2:1180–1182.
400. Lingarde F, Zettervall O. Hypercalcemia and normal ionized serum calcium in a case of myelomatosis. Ann Intern Med 1973;78:396–399.
401. Soria J, Soria C, Dao C. Immunoglobulin bound calcium and ultrafilterable serum calcium in myeloma. Br J Haematol 1976;34:343–344.
402. Jaffe JP, Mosher DF. Calcium binding in a myeloma protein. Am J Med 1979;67: 343–346.
403. Bataille R, Chappard D, Marcelli C, et al. Mechanisms of bone destruction in multiple myeloma. J Clin Oncol 1989;7:1909–1914.
404. Rota S, Mougenot B, Baudouin B, et al. Multiple myeloma and severe renal failure: A clinicopathologic study of outcome and prognosis in 34 patients. Medicine (Baltimore) 1987;66:126–137.
405. Kyle RA, Jowsey J, Kelly PJ, et al. Multiple myeloma bone disease. The comparative effect of sodium fluoride and calcium carbonate or placebo. N Engl J Med 1975;293: 1334–1338.
406. Kyle RA, Jowsey J. Effect of sodium fluoride, calcium carbonate, and vitamin D on the skeleton in multiple myeloma. Cancer 1980;45:1669–1674.
407. Gardner FH. Fluorides for multiple myeloma. N Engl J Med 1972;287:1252–1253.
408. Belch AR, Bergsagel DE, Wilson K, et al. Effect of daily etidronate on the oesteolysis of myeloma. J Clin Oncol 1991;9:1397–1402.
409. Jakubowski J, Kendall BE, Symon L. Primary plasmacytoma of the cranial vault. Acta Neurochir 1980;55:117–134.
410. Stark RJ, Henson RA. Cerebral compression by myeloma. J Neurol Neurosurg Psychiatry 1981;44:833–836.
411. Kohli CM, Kawazu T. Solitary intracranial plasmacytoma. Surg Neurol 1982;17:307–312.
412. Atweh GF, Jabbour M. Intracranial solitary extraskeletal plasmacytoma resembling meningioma. Arch Neurol 1982;39:57–59.
413. Soffer D, Siegal T. Solitary dural plasmacytoma with conspicuous cytoplasmic inclusions. Cancer 1982;49:2500–2504.
414. Mancardi GL, Mandybur TI. Solitary intracranial plasmacytoma. Cancer 1983;51: 2226–2233.
415. Coppeto JR, Monteiro MLR, Collias J, et al. Foster-Kennedy syndrome caused by solitary intracranial plasmacytoma. Surg Neurol 1983;19:267–272.
416. Pritchard PB III, Martinez RA, Hungerford GD, et al. Dural plasmacytoma. Neurosurgery 1983;12:576–579.
417. Benson MD, Brandt KD, Cohen AS, et al. Neuropathy, M components and amyloid. Lancet 1975;1:10–12.
418. Davis LE, Drachman DB. Myeloma neuropathy. Successful treatment of two patients and review of cases. Arch Neurol 1972;27:507–511.
419. Driedger H, Pruzanski W. Plasma cell neoplasia with peripheral neuropathy. A study of five cases and a review of the literature. Medicine (Baltimore) 1980;59:301–310.
420. Reitan JB, Pape E, Fossa SD, et al. Osteosclerotic myeloma with polyneuropathy. Acta Med Scand 1980;208:137–144.
421. Delauche MC, Clauvel JP, Seligmann M. Peripheral neuropathy and plasma cell neoplasias: A report of 10 cases. Br J Haematol 1981;48:384–392.
422. Osby E, Noring L, Hast R, et al. Benign monoclonal gammopathy and peripheral neuropathy. Br J Haematol 1982;51:531–539.
423. Kelly JJ Jr, Kyle RA, Miles JM, et al. Osteosclerotic myeloma and peripheral neuropathy. Neurology 1983;33:202–210.
424. Besinger UA, Toyka KV, Anzil AP, et al. Myeloma neuropathy: Passive transfer from man to mouse. Science 1981;213:1027–1039.
425. Lator N, Sherman WH, Nemni R, et al. Plasma cell dyscrasia and peripheral nerve myelin. N Engl J Med 1980;303:618–621.
426. Lamarca J, Casquero P, Pou A. Mononeuritis multiplex in Waldenström's macroglobulinemia. Ann Neurol 1987;22:268–272.
427. Vital C, Deminiere C, Bourgouin B, et al. Waldenström's macroglobulinemia and peripheral neuropathy: Deposition of M-component and kappa light chain in the endoneurium. Neurology 1985;35:603–606.
428. Ohi T, Kyle RA, Dyck PJ. Axonal attenuation and secondary segmental demyelination in myeloma neuropathies. Ann Neurol 1985;17:255–261.
429. Nobile-Orazio E, Marmiroli P, Baldini L, et al. Peripheral neuropathy in macroglobulinemia: Incidence and antigen-specificity of M-proteins. Neurology 1987;37:1506–1514.
430. Hoppe U, Drager HS, Patzold U, et al. Polyneuropathy in Waldenström's macroglobulinaemia. Passive transfer from man to mouse. Acta Neurol Scand 1987;75:112–116.
431. Schulz W, Domenico P, Nand S. The POEMS syndrome associated with polycythemia vera. Cancer 1989;63:1175–1178.
432. Kyle RA. Multiple myeloma. Review of 869 cases. Mayo Clin Proc 1975;50:29–40.
433. Hoffbrand AV, Hobbs JR, Kremenchuzky S, et al. Incidence and pathogenesis of megaloblastic erythropoiesis in multiple myeloma. J Clin Pathol 1967;20:699–705.
434. Winearls CG, Pippard MJ, Downing MR, et al. Effect of human erythropoietin derived from recombinant DNA on the anaemia of patients maintained by chronic haemodialysis. Lancet 1986;2:1175–1177.
435. Eschbach JW, Egrie JC, Downing MR, et al. Correction of the anemia of end-stage renal disease with recombinant human erythropoietin. Results of a combined phase I and II clinical trial. N Engl J Med 1987;316:73–78.
436. Ludwig H, Fritz E, Kotzmann H, et al. Erythropoietin treatment of anemia associated with multiple myeloma. N Engl J Med 1990;322:1693–1699.
437. Oster W, Herrmann F, Gamm H, et al. Erythropoietin for the treatment of anemia of malignancy associated with neoplastic bone marrow infiltration. J Clin Oncol 1990;8: 956–962.
438. Bergsagel DE. Plasma cell neoplasms and acute leukaemia. In: Hoffbrand AV, Lasch HG, Nathan DG, Salmon SE, eds. Clinics in Hematology. Eastbourne: WB Saunders, 1982:221–234.
439. Holland D, Muller JM, Leger J, et al. Association myeloma, leucose myeloide et lymphosarcome. Reflexions nosologiques. Lyon Med 1965;213:967–974.
440. Kyle RA, Robert MD, Pierre RV, et al. Multiple myeloma and acute myelomonocytic leukemia. N Engl J Med 1970;283:1121–1125.
441. Nordenson NG. Myelomatosis: A clinical review of 30 cases. Acta Med Scand (Suppl) 1966;445:178–186.
442. Mufti GJ, Hamblin TJ, Clein GP, et al. Coexistent myelodysplasia and plasma cell neoplasia. Br J Haematol 1983;54:91–96.
443. Cuzick J, Erskine S, Edelman D, et al. A comparison of the incidence of the myelodysplastic syndrome and acute myeloid leukaemia following melphalan and cyclophosphamide treatment for myelomatosis. Br J Cancer 1987;55:523–529.
444. Green MH, Harris EL, Gershensen DM, et al. Melphalan may be a more potent leukemogen than cyclophosphamide. Ann Intern Med 1986;105:360–367.
445. Lackner H. Hemostatic abnormalities associated with dysproteinemias. Semin Hematol 1973;10:125–133.
446. Henstell HH, Kligerman M. A new theory of interference with the clotting mechanism: The complexing of euglobulin with factor V, factor VII, and prothrombin. Ann Intern Med 1958;49:371–387.
447. Lackner H. Hemostatic abnormalities associated with dysproteinemias. Semin Hematol 1973;10:125–133.
448. Godal HC, Borchgrevink CF. The effect of plasmapheresis on the hemostatic function in patients with macroglobulinemia Waldenström and multiple myeloma. Scand J Clin Lab Invest 1965;17(suppl 84):133–137.
449. Doumenc J, Prost RJ, Samama M, et al. Anomalie de l'agregation plaquettaire au cours de la maladie de Waldenstrom (a propos de 3 cas). Nouv Rev Fr Hematol 1966;6:734–738.
450. Penny R, Castaldi PA, Whitsed HM. Inflammation and hemostasis in paraproteinemias. Br J Haematol 1971;20:35–44.
451. Pachter MR, Johnson SA, Neblett TR, et al. Bleeding, platelets, and macroglobulinemia. Am J Clin Pathol 1959;31:467–482.
452. Pachter MR. Johnson SA. Basinski DH. The effect of macroglobulins and their dissociation units on release of platelet factor 3. Thromb Diath Haemorrh 1959;3:501–509.
453. Khoory MS, Nesheim ME, Bowie EJW, et al. Circulating heparin sulfate proteoglycan anticoagulant from a patient with a plasma cell disorder. J Clin Invest 1980;65:666–674.
454. Meyer K, Williams EC. Fibrinolysis and acquired alpha-2 plasmin inhibitor deficiency in amyloidosis. Am J Med 1985;79:394–396.
455. Somer T. Hyperviscosity syndrome in plasma cell dyscrasias. Adv Microcirc 1975;6: 1–55.
456. Fahey JL. Serum protein disorders causing clinical symptoms in malignant neoplastic disease. J Chron Dis 1963;16:703–712.
457. Fahey JL, Barth WF, Soloman A. Serum hyperviscosity syndrome. JAMA 1965;192: 464–467.
458. Bloch KJ, Maki DG. Hyperviscosity syndromes associated with immunoglobulin abnormalities. Semin Hematol 1973;10:113–124.
459. McGrath MA, Penny R. Paraproteinemia: Blood hyperviscosity and clinical manifestations. J Clin Invest 1976;58:1158–1162.
460. MacKenzie MR, Lee TK. Blood viscosity in Waldenström macroglobulinemia. Blood 1977;49:507–510.
461. MacKenzie MR, Fudenberg HH. Macroglobulinemia: An analysis for forty patients. Blood 1972;39:874.
462. Crawford J, Cox EB, Cohen HJ. Evaluation of hyperviscosity in monoclonal gammopathies. Am J Med 1985;79:13–22.
463. MacKenzie MR, Brown E, Fudenberg HH, et al. Waldenström's macroglobulinemia

correlation between expanded plasma volume and increased serum viscosity. Blood 1970;35:934.
464. Valbonesi M, Tarantino M, Montani F, et al. Biochemical and clinical evaluation of a new cellulose diacetate secondary filter for cascade filtration. Int J Artif Organs 1985;8:105–108.
465. Valbonesi M, Monani F, Guzzini F, et al. Efficacy of discontinuous flow centrifugation compared with cascade filtration in Waldenström's macroglobulinemia: A pilot study. Int J Artif Organs 1985;8:165–168.
466. Avnstorp C, Nielson H, Drachman O, et al. Plasmapheresis in hyperviscosity syndrome. Acta Med Scand 1985;217:133–137.
467. Whittaker JA, Tuddenham EGD, Bradley J. Hyperviscosity syndrome in IgA multiple myeloma. Lancet 1973;2:572.
468. Pruzanski W, Jancelewicz Z, Underdown B. Immunological and physiochemical studies of IgA (λ) cryogelglobulinemia. Clin Exp Immunol 1973;15:181–191.
469. Meltzer M, Franklin EC. Cryoglobulinemia: A study of twenty-nine patients. I. IgG and IgM cryoglobulins and factors affecting cryoprecipitability. Am J Med 1966;40: 828–836.
470. MacKay IR, Erikson N, Motulsky AG, et al. Cryo- and macroglobulinemia: Electrophoretic, ultracentrifugal, and clinical studies. Am J Med 1956;20:564–587.
471. Liss M, Fudenberg HH, Kritzman J. A Bence Jones cryoglobulin: Clinical, physical, and immunological properties. Clin Exp Immunol 1967;2:467–475.
472. Bloth B. Christensson T, Mellstedt H. Extreme hyponatremia in patients with myelomatosis. An effect of cationic paraproteins. Acta Med Scand 1978;203:273–275.
473. Emmett ME, Narins RG. Clinical use of the anion gap. Medicine (Baltimore) 1977;56: 38–54.
474. Murray T, Long W, Narins RG. Multiple myeloma and the anion gap. N Engl J Med 1976;292:574–575.
475. Braden GL, Mikolich DJ, White CF, et al. Syndrome of inappropriate antidiuresis in Waldenström's macroglobulinemia. Am J Med 1986;80:1242–1244.
476. Schnur MJ, Appel GB, Karp G, et al. The anion gap in asymptomatic plasma cell dyscrasia. Ann Intern Med 1977;86:304–305.
477. Jacobson DR, Zolla-Pazner S. Immunosuppression and infection in multiple myeloma. Semin Oncol 1986;13:282–290.
478. Zinneman HH, Wall WH. Recurrent pneumonia in multiple myeloma and some observations on immunologic response. Ann Intern Med 1954;41:1152–1163.
479. Fahey JR, Scoggins R, Utz JP, et al. Infections, antibody response and γ globulin components in multiple myeloma and macroglobulinemia. Am J Med 1963;35:698–707.
480. Meyers BR, Hirschman SZ, Axelrod JA. Current patterns of infection in multiple myeloma. Am J Med 1972;52:87–92.
481. Twomey JJ. Infections complicating multiple myeloma and chronic lymphocytic leukemia. Arch Intern Med 1973;132:562–565.
482. Norden CW. Infections in patients with multiple myeloma. Arch Intern Med [Editorial] 1980;140:1150–1151.
483. Savage DG, Lindenbaum J, Garret TJ. Biphasic pattern of bacterial infection in multiple myeloma. Ann Intern Med 1982;96:47–50.
484. Salmon SE, Samai BA, Hayes DM, et al. Role of gamma globulin for immunoprophylaxis in multiple myeloma. N Engl J Med 1967;227:1336–1340.
485. Nolan CM, Baxley PJ, Frasch CE. Antibody response to infection in multiple myeloma. Implications for vaccination. Am J Med 1979;67:331–334.
486. Glenner GG, Ein D, Eanes ED, et al. The creation of "amyloid" fibrils from Bence Jones protein in vitro. Science 1971;174:712–714.
487. Glenner GG. Amyloid deposits and amyloidosis: The β-fibrilloses. N Engl J Med 1980;302:1283–1292.
488. Cathcart ES, Ritchie RF, Cohen AS, et al. Immunoglobulins and amyloidosis. An immunologic study of sixty-two patients with biopsy-proven disease. Am J Med 1972;52: 93–101.
489. Hawkins PN, Wootton R, Pepys MB. Metabolic studies of radioiodinated serum amyloid P component in normal subjects and patients with systemic amyloidosis. J Clin Invest 1990;86:1862–1869.
490. Kyle RA. Amyloidosis. In: Hoffbrand AV, Lasch HG, Nathan DG, Salmon SE, eds. Clinics in Hematology. Eastbourne: WB Saunders, 1982:151–180.
491. Kyle RA, Bayrd ED. Amyloidosis: Review of 236 cases. Medicine (Baltimore) 1975;54: 271–299.
492. Gordon DA, Pruzanski W, Ogryzlo MA, et al. Amyloid arthritis simulating rheumatoid disease in five patients with multiple myeloma. Am J Med 1973;55:142–154.
493. Siqueria-Filho AG, Cunha CLP, Tajik AJ, et al. M-mode and two dimensional echocardiographic features in cardiac amyloidosis. Circulation 1981;63:188–196.
494. Gertz MA, Kyle RA, Greipp PR. Beta-2-microglobulin predicts survival in primary systemic amyloidosis. Am J Med 1990;89:609–614.
495. Buxbaum JN, Hurley ME, Chuba J, Spira T. Amyloidosis of the AL type: Clinical, morphologic, and biochemical aspects of the response to therapy with alkylating agents and prednisone. Am J Med 1979;67:867–878.
496. Fielder K, Durie BG. Primary amyoloidosis associated with multiple myeloma. Predictors of successful therapy. Am J Med 1986;80:413–419.
497. Kyle RA, Greipp PR. Primary systemic amyloidosis: Comparison of melphalan and prednisone versus placebo. Blood 1978;52:818–827.
498. Gertz MA, Kyle RA, Greipp PR. The plasma cell labeling index: A valuable tool in primary amyloidosis. Blood 1989;74:1108–1111.
499. Kyle RA, Greipp PR, O'Fallon WM. Primary systemic amyloidosis: Multivariate analysis for prognostic factors in 168 cases. Blood 1986;68:220–224.
500. Waldenström J. Incipient myelomatosis or "essential" hyperglobulinemia with fibrogenopenia—A new syndrome? Acta Med Scand 1944;117:216–222.
501. Waldenström J. Macroglobulinemia. Adv Metab Dis 1965;2:115.
502. Carter P, Koval JJ, Hobbs JR. The relation of clinical and laboratory findings to the survival of patients with macroglobulinanemia. Clin Exp Immunol 1977;28:241–249.
503. Stein RS, Ellman L, Bloch KJ. The clinical correlates of IgM M-components: An analysis of thirty-four patients. Am J Med Sci 1975;269:209–216.
504. McCallister BD, Bayrd ED, Harrison EG Jr, et al. Primary macroglobulinemia. Review with a report on thirty-one cases and notes on the value of continuous chlorambucil therapy. Am J Med 1967;43:394–434.
505. Krajny M, Pruzanski W. Waldenström's macroglobulinemia: Review of 45 cases. Can Med Assoc J 1976;114:899–905.
506. Ameis A, Ko HS, Pruzanski W. M components: A review of 1242 cases. Can Med Assoc J 1976;114:889.
507. Benbassat J, Fluman N, Zlotnick A. Monoclonal immunoglobulin disorders: A report of 154 cases. Am J Med Sci 1976;271:325.
508. Peltonen S, Wasastjerna C, Wager O. Clinical features of patients with a serum M component. Acta Med Scand 1978;203:257.
509. Massari R, Find JM, Metais R. Waldenström's macroglobulinaemia observed in two brothers. Nature 1962;196:176.
510. Seligmann M. A genetic predisposition to Waldenström's macroglobulinaemia. Acta Med Scand 1966;445:140.
511. Fine JM, Lambin P, Massari M, et al. Malignant evolution of asymptomatic monoclonal IgM after seven and fifteen years in two siblings of a patients with Waldenström's macroglobulinaemia. Acta Med Scand 1982;211:237.
512. Fine JM, Muller JY, Rochu D, et al. Waldenström's macroglobulinemia in monozygotic twins. Acta Med Scand 1986;220:368–373.
513. James JM, Brouet JC, Orvoenfrija E, et al. Waldenström's macroglobulinemia in a bird breeder: A case history with pulmonary involvement and antibody activity of the monoclonal IgM to canary's droppings. Clin Exp Immunol 1987;68:397–401.
514. Takahashi K, Yamamura F, Motoyama H. IgM multiple myeloma—its distinction from Waldenström's macroglobulinemia. Acta Pathol Jpn 1986;36:1553–1563.
515. San Roman C, Ferro T, Guzman M, et al. Clonal abnormalities in patients with Waldenström's macroglobulinemia with special reference to a Burkitt-type t(8;14). Cancer Genet Gytogenet 1985;18:155–158.
516. Kucharska-Pulczynska M, Ellegaard J, Hokland P. Analysis of leukocyte differentiation antigens in blood and bone marrow from patients with Waldenström's macroglobulinemia. Br J Haematol 1987;65:395–399.
517. MacKenzie MR. Macroglobulinemia. In: Wiernik PH, Canelloa GP, Kyle RA, Schiffer CA, eds. Neoplastic diseases of the blood, vol. 2. New York: Churchill-Livingstone, 1985:575–592.
518. Morel-Maroger L, Basch A, Danon F, et al. Pathology of the kidney in Waldenström's macroglobulinemia: Study of 16 cases. N Engl J Med 1970;283:123–129.
519. Martelo OJ, Schultz DR, Pardo V, et al. Immunologically mediated renal disease in Waldenström's macroglobulinemia. Am J Med 1975;58:567–575.
520. Lindstrome FD, Hed J, Enestrom S. Renal pathology of Waldenström's macroglobulinemia with monoclonal antiglomerular antibodies and the nephrotic syndrome. Clin Exp Immunol 1980;41:196–204.
521. Hory B, Saunier F, Wolff R, et al. Waldenström's macroglobulinemia and nephrotic syndrome with minimal change lesion. Nephron 1987;45:68–70.
522. Bayrd ED. Continuous chlorambucil therapy in primary macroglobulinemia of Waldenström: Report of 4 cases. Proc Mayo Clin 1963;36:40.
523. Bierling P, Rochant H, Brum B, et al. Macroglobulinemie de Waldenström a forme pancytopenique. Remission complete apres polychimiotherapie avec recul de 26 mois. Ann Med Interne (Paris) 1979;130:443.
524. Cass RM, Anderson BR, Vaughan JH. Waldenström's macroglobulinemia with increased serum IgG levels treated with low doses of cyclophosphamide. Ann Intern Med 1969;71: 971.
525. Cohen RJ, Bohannon RA, Wallerstein RO. Waldenström's macroglobulinemia: A study of ten cases. Am J Med 1966;41:274.
526. Heading RC, Girdwood RH, Eastwood MA. Macroglobulinemia treated with prednisone, azathioprine, and folic acid. Br Med J 1970;3:750.
527. Sokalova A, Gazova A, Hrubisko M, et al. Clinical utilization of plasmapheresis and cyclophosphamide in the treatment of malignant lymphoproliferative processes. Neoplasma 1973;20:335.
528. Busnach G, Dal Col A, Brando B, et al. Efficacy of a combined treatment with plasma exchange and cytostatics in macroglobulinemia. Int J Artif Organs 1986;9:267–270.
529. Jacobs P, Wood L, Le Roux I, et al. Waldenström's macroglobulinemia treated with sequential hemibody irradiation. J Clin Apheresis 1987;3:181–184.
530. Kantarjian HM, Alexanian R, Koller CA, et al. Fludarabine therapy in microglobulinemic lymphoma. Blood 1990;75:1928–1931.
531. Clamon GH, Corder MP, Burns CP. Successful doxorubicin therapy of primary macroglobulinemia resistant to alkylating agents. Am J Hematol 1980;9:21.
532. Case DC Jr. Combination chemotherapy (M-2 protocol) (BCNU, cyclophosphamide, vincristine, melphalan and prednisone) for Waldenström's macroglobulinemia. Blood 1982;59:934.
533. Riddell S, Johnston JB, Rayner HL, et al. Response of Waldenström's macroglobulinemia to pentostatin (2′-deoxycoformycin) Cancer Treat Rep 1986;70:546–548.
534. Allen EL, Metz EN, Balcerzak SP. Acute myelomonocytic leukemia with macroglobulinemia, Bence Jones proteinuria, and hypercalcemia. Cancer 1973;32:121.
535. Martelli MF, Falini B, Firenze A, et al. Acute leukemia complicating Waldenström's macroglobulinemia. Haematologica 1981;66:303.
536. Rosner F, Grunwald HW. Multiple myeloma and Waldenström's macroglobulinemia terminating in acute leukemia. N Y State J Med 1980;80:558.
537. Sondergaard Peterson H. Erythroleukaemia in a melphalan-treated patients with primary macroglobulinaemia. Scand J Haematol 1973;10:5.

538. James K, Fudenberg H, Epstein WL, et al. Studies on a unique diagnostic serum globulin in papular mucinosis (lichen myxedematosus). Clin Exp Immunol 1967;2: 153.
539. Cream JJ. Pyoderma gangrenosum with a monoclonal IgM red cell agglomerating factor. Br J Dermatol 1971;84:223–226.
540. Turakainen H, Valimaki M, Penttinen R. Synthesis of glycosaminoglycans and collagen in skin fibroblasts cultured from a patient with lichen myxedematosus. Arch Dermatol Res 1985;277:55–59.
541. Yaron M, Yaron I, Yust I, et al. Lichen myxedematosus (scleromyxedema) serum stimulates hyaluronic acid and prostaglandin E production by human fibroblasts. J Rheumatol 1985;12:171–175.
542. Feldman P, Shapiro L, Pick Al, et al. Scleromyxedema. A dramatic response to melphalan. Arch Dermatol 1969;99:51–56.
543. Degos R, Civatte J, Clauvel JP, et al. Anomalies globuliniques dans les mucinoses cutanees. Bull Soc Fr Dermatol Syphiligr 1970;77:579–591.
544. Truhan AP, Roenigk HH Jr. Lichen myxedematosus. An unusual case with rapid progression and possible internal involvement. Int J Dermatol 1987;26:91–95.
545. Milam CP, Cohen LE, Fenske NA, Ling NS. Schleromxedema: Therapeutic response to isotretinoin in three patients. J Am Acad Dermatol 1988;19:469–477.
546. Franklin EC, Lowenstein J, Bigelow B, et al. Heavy chain disease: A new disorder of serum γ-globulins. Report of the first case. Am J Med 1964;37:332–350.
547. Frangione B, Franklin EC. Heavy-chain diseases: Clinical features and molecular significance of the disordered immunoglobulin structure. Semin Hematol 1973;10: 53–64.
548. Franklin EC, Kyle R, Seligmann M. Correlation of protein structure and immunoglobulin gene organization in the light of two new deleted heavy chain disease proteins. Mol Immunol 1979;16:919.
549. Bakhshi A, Guglielmi P, Coligan JE. A pre-translational defect in a case of human mu heavy chain disease. Mol Immunol 1986;23:725–732.
550. Bakhshi A, Guglielmi P, Siebenlist U, et al. A DNA insertion/deletion necessitates an aberrant RNA splice accounting for a mu heavy chain disease protein. Proc Natl Acad Sci USA 1986;83:2689–2693.
551. Kyle RA, Greipp PR, Banks PM. The diverse picture of gamma heavy-chain disease: Report of seven cases and review of literature. Mayo Clin Proc 1981;56:439.
552. Fermand JP, Brovet JC, Danon F, Seligmann M. Gamma heavy chain "disease": heterogeneity of the clinico-pathologic features. Report of 16 cases and review of the literature. Medicine (Baltimore) 1989;68:321–335.
553. Kanoh T, Nakasato H. Osteolytic gamma chain disease. Eur J Haematol 1987;39: 60–65.
554. O'Connor GT Jr, Wrandt HE, Innes DJ, et al. Gamma heavy chain disease: Report of a case associated with a trisomy of chromosome 7. Cancer Genet Cytogenet 1985;15: 1–5.
555. Kyle RA. The heavy-chain diseases. In: Wiernik PH, Canelloa GP, Kyle RA, Schiffer CA, eds. Neoplastic diseases of the blood, vol. 2. New York: Churchill-Livingstone, 1985:593–605.
556. Buxbaum JN, Preud'homme JL. Alpha and gamma heavy chain diseases in man: Intracellular origin of the aberrant polypeptides. J Immunol 1972;109:1131.
557. Seligmann M, Mihaesco E, Preud'homme JL, et al. Heavy chain diseases: Current findings and concepts. Immunol Rev 1979;48:145–167.
558. Zamadzki ZA, Benedek TG, Ein D, et al. Rheumatoid arthritis terminating in heavy-chain disease. Ann Intern Med 1969;70:335.
559. Block KJ, Lee L, Mills JA, et al. Gamma heavy chain disease—an expanding clinical and laboratory spectrum. Am J Med 1973;55:61.
560. Shirakura T, Kobayshi Y, Murai Y, et al. A case of gamma heavy chain disease associated with autoimmune haemolytic anaemia: Clinical haematological, immunological and pathological details. Scand J Haematol 1976;16:387.
561. Westin J, Eyrich R, Falsen, et al. Gamma heavy chain disease: Reports of three patients. Acta Med Scand 1972;192:281.
562. Seligmann M, Danon F, Hurez D, et al. Alpha-chain disease: A new immunoglobulin abnormality. Science 1968;162:1396.
563. Rambaud JC, Galian A, Matuchansky C, et al. Natural history of alpha-chain disease and the so-called Mediterranean lymphoma. Recent Results Cancer Res 1978;64: 271.
564. Roth S, Riecken EO. Alpha-chain disease: Mediterranean lymphoma and primary intestinal lymphoma in Western countries; a review of the cases in the literature. Ergeb Inn Med Kinderheilkd 1977;39:79.
565. Seligmann M. Immunobiology and pathogenesis of alpha chain disease. Ciba Found Symp 1977;46:263.
566. Selzer G, Sherman G, Callihan TR, et al. Primary small intestinal lymphomas and α-heavy-chain disease: A study of 43 cases from a pathology department of Israel. Isr J Med Sci 1979;15:111.
567. Haghighi P, Wolf PL. Alpha-heavy chain disease. Clin Lab Med 1986;6:477–489.
568. Isaacson PG. Middle Eastern intestinal lymphoma. Semin Diagn Pathol 1985;2:210–223.
569. Shi LY, Liaw SJ, Hsueh S, et al. Alpha-chain disease. Report of a case from Taiwan. Cancer 1987;59:545–548.
570. Monges H, Aubert L, Chamlian A, et al. Maladie des chaines alpha a forme intestinale: Preventation d'un cas traite par antibiotherapie avec remission clinique, histologique et immunologique. Arch Fr Mal Appar Dign 1975;64:223.
571. Roge J, Druet P, Marche C. Lymphome Mediterranean avec maladie des chaines alpha: Triple remission clinique, anatomique et immunologique. Pathol Biol (Paris) 1970;18:851.
572. Roge J, Druet P, Marche C, et al. Alpha-chain disease cured with antibiotics. [Letter] Br Med J 1975;4:225.
573. O'Keefe SJ, Winter TA, Newton KA, et al. Severe malnutrition associated with alpha heavy chain disease: Response to tetracycline and intensive nutritional support. Am J Gastroenterol 1988;83:995–1001.
574. Mir-Madjlessi SH, Mir-Ahmadian M. Alpha-chain disease—A report of eleven patients from Iran. J Trop Med Hyg 1979;82:229.
575. Savilahi E, Brandtzaeg P, Kuitunen P. Atypical intestinal alpha-chain disease evolving into selective immunoglobulin: A deficiency in a Finnish boy. Gastroenterology 1980;79:1303.
576. Nikbin B, Banisadre M, Ala F, et al. HLA AW19, B12 in immunoproliferative small intestinal disease. Gut 1976;20:226.
577. Al-Bahrani Z, Al-Saleem T, Al-Mondiry M, et al. Alpha heavy chain disease (report of 18 cases from Iraq). Gut 1978;19:627.
578. Tabbane S, Tabbane F, Cammoun M, et al. Mediterranean lymphomas with alpha heavy chain monoclonal gammopathy. Cancer 1989;1976;38:1989.
579. Berger R, Bernheim A, Tsapis A, et al. Cytogenetic studies in four cases of alpha chain disease. Cancer Genet Cytogenet 1986;22:219–223.
580. Gafter U, Kessler E, Shabtay F, et al. Abnormal chromosomal marker (D14q+) in a patient with alpha heavy chain disease. J Clin Pathol 1980;33:136.
581. Seligmann M. Immunochemical, clinical, and pathological features of α-heavy chain disease. Arch Intern Med 1975;135:78–82.
582. Doe WF. Alpha chain disease: Clinicopathological features and relationship to so-called Mediterranean lymphoma. Br J Cancer 1975;31(suppl 2):350.
583. Galian A, Lecestre M-J, Scotto J, et al. Pathological study of alpha-chain disease with special emphasis on evolution. Cancer 1977;39:2081.
584. Ballard HS, Hamilton LM, Marcus AJ, et al. A new variant of heavy-chain disease (μ-chain disease). N Engl J Med 1970;282:1060.
585. Forte FA, Prelli F, Yount WJ, et al. Heavy chain disease of the μ (γM) type: Report of the first case. Blood 1970;36:137.
586. Franklin EC. μ-Chain disease. Arch Intern Med 1975;135:71.
587. Pruzanski W, Hasselback R, Ratz A, et al. Multiple myeloma (light chain disease) with rheumatoid-like amyloid arthropathy and μ-heavy chain fragment in the serum. Am J Med 1978;65:334.
588. Brouet J-C, Seligmann M, Danon F, et al. μ-Chain disease: Report of two new cases. Arch Intern Med 1979;139:672.
589. Levo Y, Recht B, Michaelsen T, et al. The interaction of immunoglobulin heavy and light chains in the absence of the V_H domain. J Immunol 1977;119:635.
590. Vilpo JA, Irjala K, Viljanen MK, et al. δ-Heavy chain disease: A study of a case. Clin Immunol Immunopathol 1980;17:584.

Cancer: Principles & Practice of Oncology, Fourth Edition,
edited by Vincent T. DeVita, Jr., Samuel Hellman, Steven A. Rosenberg.
J.B. Lippincott Co., Philadelphia © 1993.

Paul A. Bunn, Jr
E. Chester Ridgway

CHAPTER **57**

Paraneoplastic Syndromes

Tumors produce signs and symptoms in the patient by invasion, obstruction, and bulk mass at the primary tumor site and in regional and distant deposits. Tumors can produce signs and symptoms at a distance from the tumor or its metastases. These are collectively referred to as "paraneoplastic syndromes" or "remote effects" of malignancy.[1–4] By definition, these syndromes are not produced directly by the tumor or its metastases. The best characterized paraneoplastic syndromes are those produced by tumors secreting a polypeptide hormone (*e.g.*, adrenocorticotropin [ACTH] or parathormone [PTH]) that is distributed by the circulation and acts on target organ(s) at a distance from the tumor. In these instances, the course of the paraneoplastic syndrome runs parallel to the course of the underlying malignancy, and removal or destruction of the tumor halts production of the hormone. A thorough review of the response of paraneoplastic syndromes to various therapies was published.[5]

Various nonendocrine paraneoplastic syndromes were thought to be produced by unidentified tumor-secreted proteins. During the past decade, many of these new tumor-secreted proteins were described. Previously described paraneoplastic syndromes can be attributed to these proteins, and new syndromes are being recognized. Newly described tumor-derived proteins responsible for paraneoplastic syndromes include growth factors and cytokines. Many of the hematologic paraneoplastic syndromes are caused by tumor secretion of colony-stimulating factors.[6,7] Tumor secretion of transforming growth factor-α (and possibly epidermal growth factor) by malignant melanoma cells was shown to produce acanthosis nigricans, the sign of Leser-Trelat, and multiple acrochordons.[8]

Paraneoplastic syndromes may also be caused by proteins produced by normal cells in response to the tumor. Molecular studies demonstrated that the monokines, tumor necrosis factor, and cachectin, are identical proteins.[9–11] Cachectin may be responsible for the cachexia syndrome in some patients with malignancy. Antibodies produced in response to malignancy are responsible for many of the neurologic paraneoplastic syndromes, including cerebellar degeneration, the Eaton-Lambert syndrome, paraneoplastic retinopathy, and sensory neuronopathy.[12–15] There are many paraneoplastic syndromes of unknown cause that may be produced by tumor-secreted proteins. Some of these syndromes may be caused by nonparaneoplastic factors.

Progressive multifocal leukoencephalopathy (PML) was initially described as a neurologic paraneoplastic syndrome.[16] PML is caused by a virus, and although patients with malignancy may be prone to develop this viral syndrome, PML is not truly paraneoplastic.[17]

Endocrine tumors can be functional, and their hormonal products (*e.g.*, polypeptide, catecholamines, iodothyronine, steroids) give symptoms at a distance from the primary tumor, but for practical purposes, this chapter deals only with syndromes produced by tumors arising in sites other than the pituitary, adrenals, endocrine pancreas, endocrine cells of the gastrointestinal tract, and endocrine cells of the ovaries and testes and all forms of the carcinoid syndrome. These are discussed in other chapters.

Paraneoplastic syndromes develop in a minority of cancer patients. Their exact frequency is difficult to determine for a variety of reasons, including various definitions, unknown causes, and lack of systematic case-control studies. For example, in an uncontrolled study, Croft and Wilkinson reported that 7% of cancer patients have neurologic paraneoplastic syndromes, but in a case-control study, Brody found no difference in the frequency of neurologic syndromes in patients with lung cancer and controls with benign chronic lung disease.[18,19] The frequency figures given in this chapter are usually from uncontrolled studies.

The importance of the paraneoplastic syndromes (including

hormones detected by immunoassay) and the elucidation of their mechanisms are important for many reasons. Their appearance may be the first sign of a malignancy, which allows its early detection in a curable state. They may simulate metastatic disease and prevent patients from having curative therapy. Conversely, treatable complications of malignancy (*e.g.*, metastatic disease, infection) may be ascribed to a paraneoplastic syndrome, leading to the withholding of appropriate therapy. They can be used as tumor markers in previously treated patients to detect early recurrence or in patients undergoing adjuvant therapy to guide further therapy. In patients with metastatic disease, their syndromes can be disabling, and appropriate treatment of the paraneoplasia may be the best means of palliating patients. The hormones released by tumors may be required for tumor growth (*i.e.*, the tumor may produce its own growth factors and "autostimulate"), and appropriate identification of such hormones may allow a new rational therapeutic approach to treatment of the neoplasms.[20]

Because of their importance, numerous articles and reviews describing paraneoplastic syndromes have been published in the past 20 years.[1–4,21,22]

ETIOLOGY AND PATHOGENESIS OF PARANEOPLASTIC SYNDROMES

Paraneoplastic syndromes can arise in several ways:

1. Tumor-produced biologically active proteins or polypeptides, including peptide hormones, their precursors, growth factors, interleukins, cytokines, prostaglandins, fetal proteins such as carcinoembryonic antigen (CEA) or α-fetoprotein (AFP), other proteins such as immunoglobulins, and enzymes produced and released by tumors
2. Autoimmunity or immune complex production and immune suppression
3. Ectopic receptor production or a competitive blockade of normal hormone action by tumor-produced biologically inactive hormones
4. "Forbidden contact" in which there is release of enzymes (*e.g.*, placental alkaline phosphatase) or other products that normally are not circulated but that takes place because of abnormal tumor vasculature or disrupted basement membranes, allowing antigenic reactions, inappropriate initiation of normal physiologic functions, and other toxic manifestations to occur
5. Unknown causes.

DIFFERENTIAL DIAGNOSIS

The importance and frequency of paraneoplastic syndromes make it imperative to establish the appropriate diagnosis. If the cause of the paraneoplastic syndrome is unknown, this may mean excluding all other known causes of the syndrome. Each section of this chapter includes a listing of the differential diagnoses. In general, paraneoplastic syndromes must be differentiated from

1. Direct invasion by the primary tumor or its metastases
2. Obstruction caused by tumor or tumor products
3. Vascular abnormalities
4. Infections
5. Fluid and electrolyte abnormalities
6. Toxicity of cancer therapy, including cytotoxic chemotherapy, radiation therapy, immunotherapy, or antibiotic therapy.

ENDOCRINOLOGIC MANIFESTATIONS OF MALIGNANCY

Paraneoplastic syndromes caused by the production of polypeptide hormones are the most frequent and best understood paraneoplastic syndromes. To establish a paraneoplastic cause for alterations in hormone production, conclusive evidence that the hormone is produced by the tumor must be established. The differential diagnosis of endocrinologic abnormalities in the cancer patient is shown in Table 57–1.

The laboratory evaluation begins after a complete history and physical examination. Abnormal levels of the hormone in question should be documented, usually by radioimmunoassay. Paraneoplastic hormone production usually is independent of the normal regulatory mechanisms. There is other direct evidence that a tumor produces a hormone causing the paraneoplastic syndrome:

1. Fall in hormone levels after removal or treatment of the tumor
2. Maintenance of elevated hormone levels after extirpation of the "normal" gland of origin of the hormone
3. Demonstration of an arteriovenous gradient of hormone levels across the tumor
4. Demonstration of synthesis and secretion of the hormone by tumor tissue in vitro
5. Demonstration of hormone synthesis and secretion by in vitro clonal tissue culture isolates of the tumor cells.

Secretion of polypeptide hormones by tumors has been known for most of this century to cause recognized paraneoplastic syndromes. In the past 10 years, many previously unknown polypeptide hormones have been discovered. Most of these peptides have been identified within the central nervous system (CNS) or the gastrointestinal tract.[24,25] Table 57–2 lists the categories of mammalian polypeptide hormones; some cause known paraneoplastic syndromes, and some are produced by human tumor cells. The function of many of the hormones, such as neurophysin, bombesin, and physalaemin, is unknown. However, they are produced by human tumors,

TABLE 57–1. Endocrinologic Manifestations of Malignancy: Differential Diagnosis

1. Hormone production by benign cells (*e.g.*, parathyroid adenoma)
2. Hormone production by a malignancy of an endocrine organ (*e.g.*, MEN)
3. Alterations in hormone production as a direct result of infiltration of an endocrine gland by a primary tumor or its metastases
4. Alterations in hormone production by therapy
5. Alterations in hormone production by infection
6. Paraneoplastic

TABLE 57–2. Categories of Mammalian Brain Peptides Producing Proven or Potential Paraneoplastic Syndromes

Hypothalamic-Releasing Hormones	**Gastrointestinal Peptides**
Thyrotropin-releasing hormone	Vasoactive intestinal peptide*†
Gonadotropin-releasing hormone	Cholecystokinin
Somatostatin	Gastrin
Corticotropin-releasing hormone	Substance P
Growth hormone-releasing hormone	Neurotensin†
	Met-enkephalin
Neurohypophyseal Hormones	Leu-enkephalin
Vasopressin*†	Insulin
Oxytocin	Glucagon†
Neurophysin(s)†	Bombesin†
	Gastrin-releasing peptide†
Pituitary Peptides	Secretin
Adrenocorticotropic hormone*†	Somatostatin†
β-Endorphin†	Thyrotropin-releasing hormone
Melanocyte-stimulating hormone*†	Motilin
Prolactin	
Luteinizing hormone	**Others**
Growth hormone†	Angiotensin II
Thyrotropin	Bradykinin
	Carosine
Invertebrate Peptides	Sleep peptide(s)
FM RT amide	Calcitonin†
Hydra head activator	CGRP
	Neuropeptide Y
Nonbrain Hormones	Physalaemin†
Parathormone*†	Neuron-specific enolase†
β-hCG*†	
T_3	

* Produces a proven paraneoplastic syndrome.
† Produced by small cell lung cancer or carcinoid tumors.
(Kreiger DT, Martin JB. Brain peptides. N Engl J Med 1981;304:876–885; Kreiger DT. Brain peptides: What, where, and why? Science 1983;222:975–985)

such as small cell lung cancer.[26–28] Some of the paraneoplastic syndromes for which the cause is unknown and perhaps some unrecognized paraneoplastic syndromes will probably be ascribed to these hormones after more is learned of their function.

The endocrine paraneoplastic syndromes, the responsible hormone, the most frequently associated tumor types, and incidence are shown in Table 57–3.[23,29] With the development of radioimmunoassays and screening of cancer patients, it was found that hormone production in cancer patients (presumably from their tumors) was much more frequent than previously realized.[3,23] Table 57–4 lists screening studies of lung cancer patients or tumor extracts for the presence of various hormones using radioimmunoassays.[30–35] These frequencies are much higher than those of the clinically recognized paraneoplastic syndromes related to these hormones because the large-molecular-weight hormone precursors, fragments, or subunits secreted by tumors are often biologically inactive. Other factors that obscure the true frequency of hormone secretion by tumors include inadequate clinical follow-up (*e.g.*, spot-checks of patients rather than observation throughout the clinical course); production of a hormone that does not have easily recognizable clinical effect (*e.g.*, acromegalic effects of growth hormone, which may take years to manifest); operation of normal physiologic feedback mechanisms, which suppress normal hormone production; secretion of multiple hormones (*e.g.*, secretion of ACTH obscuring the clinical effect of simultaneous arginine vasopressin [AVP] secretion); and investigator and laboratory facility bias.

ACTH AND CUSHING'S SYNDROME

Evidence from analysis of cultured tumor cells, pituitary extracts, and recombinant DNA work demonstrates that the prohormone (*i.e.*, stem hormone) molecule of ACTH contains the following in sequence from the NH_2-terminal to the COOH-terminal end (Fig. 57–1).[24,25,36–38]

1. A putative signal peptide (amino acid position −141 to −110)
2. A NH_2-terminal region with unknown function (position −110 to −53)
3. γ-MSH (position −53 to −48)
4. A region with unknown function (position −48 to −1)
5. ACTH (position 1 to 39) or "classic" ACTH, which contains within it α-MSH (position 1 to 13) and corticotropin-like intermediate lobe peptide (position 18 to 39)
6. β-Lipotropin hormone (β-LPH; position 42 to 134), which contains within it γ-LPH (position 42 to 101) and β-MSH (position 84 to 101)

TABLE 57–3. Endocrine Paraneoplastic Syndromes

Syndrome	*Hormone*	*Tumor*	*Incidence (%)*
Cushing's syndrome	ACTH	Lung cancer—all types	0–2.0
		Small cell lung cancer	6
Inappropriate antidiuresis	AVP	Lung cancer—all types	0.9–2.0
	ANP	Small cell lung cancer	9
Nonmetastatic hypercalcemia	PTH	Lung cancer—all types	1.0–7.5
		Squamous cell lung cancer	15
		Other tumors	14
Gynecomastia		Lung cancer—all types	0.5–0.9
		Small cell lung cancer	2.0
Hyperthyroidism		Lung cancer	0–1.4
Calcitonin		Medullary carcinoma of the thyroid	
		Small cell lung cancer	
		Other lung cancer types	
		Breast cancer	
Acromegaly	GHRH	Carcinoids, pheochomocytoma—rare	
		Pancreatic cancer	

(Lees LH. The biosynthesis of hormones by nonendocrine tumours—A review. J Endocrinol 1975;67: 143–175; Richardson RL, Greco FA, Oldhan RK, Liddle GW. Tumor products and potential markers in small cell lung cancer. Semin Oncol 1978;5:253–262)

7. Met-enkephalin (position 104 to 108)
8. β-Endorphin (position 104 to 134)

The prohormone molecule has been called "big ACTH" or proopiocortin and contains four repetitive sequences based on the ACTH-MSH core, with these sequences separated by paired basic residues. The importance of the promolecule is that it can be split into many biologically active fragments. These activities include adrenal gland stimulation to make corticosteroids and androgens (*e.g.*, by ACTH); melanocyte stimulation-hyperpigmentation activity (*e.g.*, by MSH-containing peptides); and opiate-like activity (*e.g.*, β-LPH, β-endorphin, met-enkephalin). There has been an explosion of knowledge concerning the biologic activity of fragments of this molecule, particularly the opioid peptides (*e.g.*, β-LPH, β-endorphin, met-enkephalin), which mimic morphine in their action.[39–41] The paired basic residues flank the biologically active sequences. Proteolytic processing takes place at these sites that determines the biologic activities and the paraneoplastic syndromes seen in humans. The regulation of cleavage of the promolecule in neoplastic states is important. The cleavage patterns change during development and may

TABLE 57–4. Frequency of Peptide Hormone Elevation in the Blood of Lung Cancer Patients

	*Patients With Significantly Elevated Levels (%)**			
Hormone	*Small Cell*	*Epidermoid*	*Adenocarcinoma*	*Large Cell*
ACTH	30–69	0–80	17–75	26
LPH	54	33	20	Not done
Calcitonin	48–64	9	0	11
ADH	32			
PTH	27	32	0	17
β-hCG	1–32	19	17	26
GH	0	3	0	0
GRP	74	17	20	7
SLI	27	11	Not done	Not done
NSE	69	Not done	Not done	Not done
Neurophysins	65	14	29	20

* Not all studies were done in all patients.
(Data from references 30–35)

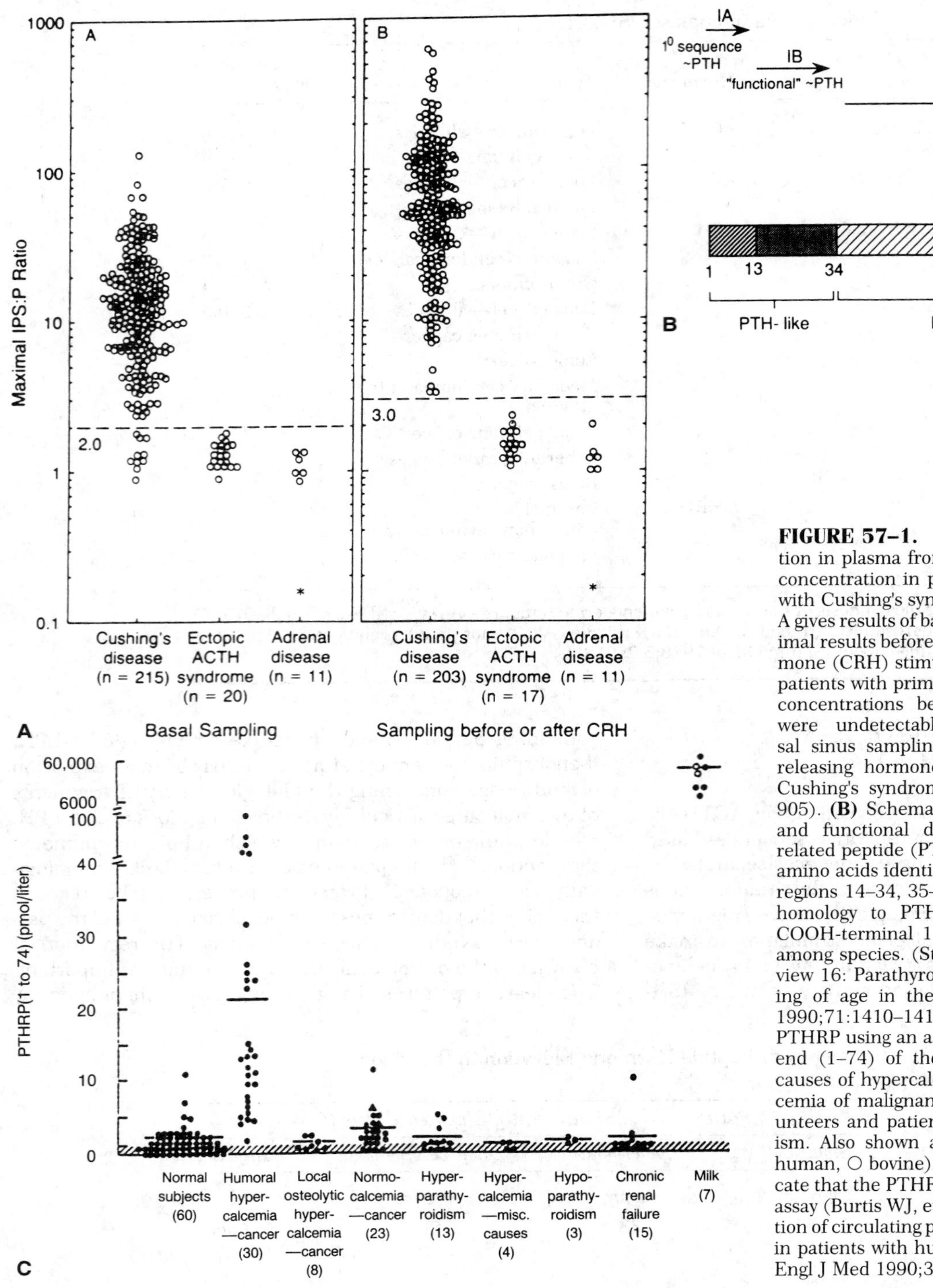

FIGURE 57–1. **(A)** The ratio of ACTH concentration in plasma from one inferior petrosal sinus to the concentration in peripheral blood (IPS:P) in patients with Cushing's syndrome due to various causes. Panel A gives results of basal samples, and Panel B gives maximal results before or after corticotropin-releasing hormone (CRH) stimulation. The asterisks represent five patients with primary adrenal disease in whom ACTH concentrations were undetectable. (Oldfield EH, et al. Petrosal sinus sampling with and without corticotropin-releasing hormone for the differential diagnosis of Cushing's syndrome. N Engl J Med 1991;325:897–905). **(B)** Schematic representation of the structural and functional domains of parathyroid hormone-related peptide (PTHRP). The 1–13 region contains 8 amino acids identical with the PTH sequence, but the regions 14–34, 35–111, and 112–141 bear little or no homology to PTH or other known peptides. The COOH-terminal 112–141 region is poorly conserved among species. (Stewart AF, Broadus AE. Clinical review 16: Parathyroid hormone related proteins: Coming of age in the 1990s. J Clin Endocrinol Metab 1990;71:1410–1414). **(C)** Plasma concentrations of PTHRP using an assay directed to the amino-terminal end (1–74) of the molecule. Patients with various causes of hypercalcemia including humeral hypercalcemia of malignancy are compared with healthy volunteers and patients with primary hyperparathyroidism. Also shown are the PTHRP levels in milk (● human, ○ bovine). Symbols in the hatched area indicate that the PTHRP level could not be detected in the assay (Burtis WJ, et al. Immunochemical characterization of circulating parathyroid hormone-related protein in patients with humoral hypercalcemia of Cancer. N Engl J Med 1990;322:1106–1112)

be different in tumors than in adult pituitary tissue.[41] Proopiocortin is a glycosylated peptide, and glycosylation may play an important role in proteolysis, packaging, and storage. Classically, ectopic ACTH production is thought to be unregulated, but some tumor tissues studied in vitro continue to show some control over ACTH secretion by means of a cyclic AMP-dependent mechanism.[42]

Clinical Features of Ectopic Proopiocortin Excess

The clinical features of the ectopic ACTH syndrome include hypokalemia, hyperglycemia, edema, muscle weakness or atrophy, hypertension, and weight loss. Other features seen in pituitary Cushing's disease or exogenous corticosteroid excess (*e.g.,* centripetal obesity, cutaneous striae, moon facies, buffalo hump, pigmentation) are uncommonly seen in highly malignant tumors (*e.g.*, oat cell lung cancer) but are more frequent in the indolent carcinoids, thymomas, and pheochromocytomas. Although the cases first reported involved men, the increased prevalence of lung cancer in women may be associated with more features seen in women, including hirsutism, which was seen in Brown's original patient.[43]

FREQUENCY OF ECTOPIC PROOPIOCORTIN PRODUCTION BY TUMORS. The major clinical association of ectopic ACTH production is with lung cancer, particularly of the small cell histologic type.[3,23,38] Clinically apparent Cushing's syndrome is found in 0.4% to 2% of patients with lung cancer of all histologic types (see Table 57–3).[23,29,44,45] In small cell lung cancer, 5.5% of 473 patients in several large series had clinical manifestations of Cushing's syndrome.[46–48] Lung cancer represents more than 50% of the clinically obvious cases, carcinoids and neural crest tumors (*e.g.*, pheochromocytomas, neuroblastomas, medullary carcinomas of the thyroid) amount to 15% each, and bronchial carcinoid and thymomas represent 10% each. The frequency of significantly elevated levels of ACTH by radioimmunoassay (RIA) in the blood and tumor extracts of lung cancer patients (Table 57–5) is much higher than the frequency of the ectopic Cushing's syndrome.[49–57] Similarly, the frequency of increased fasting morning cortisol levels with dexamethasone suppression (49–71%) or without dexamethasone suppression (38%) is higher than the frequency of the ectopic syndrome.[23,31,57–59] Although these differences could be due to the presence of inactive proACTH or stress, Bondy and Gilby suggest that the tumors secrete only small amounts of excess hormone.[57]

The ectopic ACTH is not secreted under feedback control, enters the plasma without normal diurnal variations, and is not suppressed normally by exogenous dexamethasone, but it is not sufficient to cause clinical abnormalities. The clinical syndrome occurs only in the uncommon tumors that secrete large excesses of active hormone. Most extracts of small cell lung cancer tumors have increased levels of ACTH and LPH detected by RIA. The other histologic types vary in positivity between 6% and 40%. Although non-small cell lung cancer types have increased cortisol levels, the mechanism of this is unknown.[22,23,49] The frequency of ectopic ACTH-associated clinical syndromes and adrenal function is not well described for other tumor types.[38]

HISTOLOGY OF ACTH-PRODUCING TUMORS. Azzopardi and Williams reviewed the world's literature on the ectopic syndrome and found that 112 of 130 cases arose in the lung, pancreas, or thymus.[60] The most frequent histologic finding was a small cell cancer or a carcinoid structure. Other tumors included pheochromocytomas, related tumors, and certain ovarian tumors. Ten years later, Skrabanek and Powell continued the literature review of cases with ectopic ACTH and Cushing's syndrome and found that all such tumors with clinically apparent ACTH excess could be grouped into a carcinoid-oat cell (small cell) group and a pheochromocytoma-neuroblastoma class based on histologic appearance.[61] They thought that tumors found in organs other than the lung (*e.g.*, thymus, all thymic carcinoids rather than epithelial thymoma), thyroid (*e.g.*, medullary carcinoma), esophagus, stomach, pancreas, small intestine, appendix, salivary gland, ovary, testis, uterine cervix, and prostate had a carcinoid or a small cell lung cancer-type tissue structure.[62,63] They and others postulated that these tumors arose only where normal Kulchitsky-type cells occur and could potentially have a common origin.

If a histologic type other than these described is suggested (*e.g.*, adenocarcinoma), the finding should be viewed with skepticism and carefully documented. The histologic material should be reviewed and more obtained, if necessary. The extrapulmonary cancers with small cell structure should be treated as if they were small cell carcinoma of the lung, and

TABLE 57–5. Frequency of ACTH Elevation in Blood and Tumor Extracts Detected by RIA in Lung Cancer Patients Without Clinically Evident Ectopic ACTH Syndrome

Source of Material Tumor Type	*Patients (n)*	*Positive (%)*	*References*
Patient's Blood			
All histologic types	290	19, 41, 42, 88	49, 50, 51, 52
Epidermoid	88	0–50	49, 51
Adenocarcinoma	25	17–26	49, 51
Large cell carcinoma	28	26–49	49, 51
Small cell carcinoma	49, 51	11, 29–30	49, 51
Chronic obstructive pulmonary disease	101	25*	49, 50, 52
Tumor Extracts (Surgical Specimens)			
All histologic types	127	31, 58, 93, 100	49, 50, 53, 54
Epidermoid	49	49	49
Adenocarcinoma	17	6	49
Large cell carcinoma	8	25	49
Small cell carcinoma and carcinoid	12	100	55, 56

* Seventeen percent of patients with elevated ACTH levels developed lung cancer within 2 years.
(Data from references 49–57)

those with a carcinoid tissue structure should be dealt with as carcinoids.[64,65] It is important to obtain more studies on the efficacy of chemotherapy on tumors producing ACTH that do not have typical small cell or carcinoid tissues.

DIAGNOSIS OF ECTOPIC CUSHING'S SYNDROME. About 40% of patients presenting with overt Cushing's syndrome have pituitary Cushing's with an obvious tumor, 28% have pituitary Cushing's syndrome without tumors (both of these usually occur in women of childbearing age), 17% have adrenal Cushing's (usually in children), and 15% have the ectopic Cushing's syndrome (usually in adult men). Although the production of proopiocorticoid molecule may have unrecognized clinical effects, the diagnosis of clinically significant ectopic ACTH excess begins with thinking about the possibility in the appropriate clinical setting, such as an older man with small cell lung cancer or a patient with unexplained hypokalemic alkalosis, particularly if it is accompanied by edema, hypertension, profound muscular weakness or atrophy, mental changes, or glucose intolerance. Patients with ectopic ACTH from thymic tumors and bronchial carcinoids are usually younger and present with more classic features of Cushing's syndrome, primarily because of the more indolent course of the neoplasms. When clinical features are present, a plasma ACTH value of over 200 pg/ml suggests ectopic ACTH production.

The biochemical diagnosis of Cushing's syndrome that results from ectopic ACTH production involves the demonstration of excessive cortisol production by measuring a 24-hour urinary free cortisol. Abnormal values are higher than 100 μg/day, and values as high as 1000 μg/day may be seen. A simultaneous plasma ACTH value of over 200 pg/ml suggests ectopic ACTH production. However, many cases of ectopic ACTH production due to a bronchial or thymic carcinoid may have ACTH values between 20 and 200 pg/ml. Abnormal suppression of elevated cortisol production is documented by showing that plasma cortisol levels do not suppress after administering dexamethasone, 2 mg every 6 hours for 48 hours, or after giving a single 8-mg dose of dexamethasone at midnight before obtaining a sample to test the plasma cortisol level at 8:00 A.M. the next morning. Elevations in the 24-hour urinary free cortisol, elevations in the plasma ACTH concentration, and abnormal dexamethasone suppressibility are highly suggestive of the ectopic ACTH syndrome. Unfortunately, these diagnostic criteria are not perfect in making the diagnosis of ectopic ACTH production. For example, a high-dose dexamethasone suppression test suppresses cortisol production in almost half the patients with ectopic ACTH tumors caused by bronchial carcinoids.[66,67] A high-dose dexamethasone suppression test fails to suppress cortisol production in about 20% of patients with Cushing's disease due to a pituitary tumor.[67a]

To improve the precision in diagnosing ectopic ACTH production and differentiating it from pituitary-dependent Cushing's disease, the simultaneous sampling of ACTH from the inferior petrosal sinuses has provided a major advance.[68,69,69a] If the source of ACTH is from a pituitary tumor, plasma ACTH levels in the petrosal venous sinuses should be much higher than peripheral levels. If the ACTH source is from a tumor distant from the pituitary, ACTH levels in petrosal venous sinuses and peripheral venous blood should be similar. This procedure has been validated in a large group of patients at the National Institute of Health for whom ACTH levels measured in the inferior petrosal sinuses (IPS) are related to ACTH levels in peripheral blood plasma (P) and expressed as an IPS:P ratio.[69a] An IPS:P ratio of 2 or more in basal samples correctly identified the source of ACTH in patients with Cushing's disease with a sensitivity of 95% and no false-positive results. Results were improved if the sampling was performed after the administration of corticotropin-releasing hormone (CRH) in which a peak IPS:P ratio of 3 or more identified the source of ACTH in 100% of Cushing's disease with no false-positive results. Patients with ectopic ACTH syndrome uniformly had IPS:P ratios less than 2 in basal samples and less than 3 in CRH-stimulated samples (see Fig. 57–1A). In patients with benign or malignant adrenal tumors, the ACTH levels in plasma are low or undetectable, and the cortisol levels are not suppressed with dexamethasone. The IPS:P ratio in these cases is always below 2 or 3 in basal or CRH-stimulated samples.

Other sources of difficulty in the correct diagnosis of ectopic Cushing's syndrome can occur with the simultaneous production of two hormones (*e.g.*, ACTH and AVP) or of a peptide hormone or amine product.[23,70] Multiple hormone secretion indicates a nonpituitary tumor. Other cases of dexamethasone suppression of ectopic ACTH production have been linked to secretion of CRH itself by the tumor.[71,72] Well-defined cases of Cushing's syndrome resulting from tumor production of CRH have been documented.[73–75] The CRH is postulated to act on the pituitary to stimulate pituitary ACTH release or at the tumor level to stimulate tumor cell ACTH production.

Treatment of Ectopic ACTH and Related Syndromes

The treatment of ectopic proopiocorticoid syndromes should be directed primarily at the tumor. In carcinoids, this can involve surgery, and with thymomas, surgery or radiotherapy. With appropriate therapy, the syndrome is usually cured, and the high levels of ACTH are reduced in most patients.[76] Although previous reviews have stated that a prognosis of less than 4 months is expected for the ectopic ACTH syndrome with small cell lung cancer, these predated the substantial gains in treatment and potential cure of some patients with small cell carcinoma. (The principles of the treatment of small cell lung carcinomas with combination chemotherapy is discussed in detail in Chap. 23). If the histologic appearance of any mediastinal or extrathoracic tumor is compatible with a small cell tumor, we favor treating the patient as though he had small cell lung cancer. The data on response to therapy of Cushing's syndrome in small cell cancer patients are anecdotal, but reports of a fall in ACTH levels after combination chemotherapy, with or without radiotherapy, have appeared.[30,48] If treatment of the tumor fails, drugs that inhibit adrenal corticoid production may be used, such as aminoglutethimide, metyrapone, or mitotane.[68,77–79] (The reader should review appropriate endocrinology sources for directions in using these adrenal suppressants.) After drug treatment, patients should be treated with supplemental steroids to avoid hypoadrenalism. Because of the increasing use of aminoglutethimide in breast cancer patients, this drug is probably the first choice. Another possibility is combining aminoglutethimide and metyrapone to lower the dose-related toxicity of both agents with dexamethasone and fludrocortisone.[80] In rare cases, with chronic ectopic ACTH excess and indolent tumors, bilateral adrenalectomy can be considered.

Use of proACTH and β-Lipotropin Hormone for Early Cancer Detection

Odell and associates found significant blood elevations of proACTH in 92% of pancreatic cancers, 72% of lung cancers, 54% of gastric or esophagus cancers, 41% of breast cancers, and 27% of colon cancers, and the corresponding values for elevated LPH were 25%, 36%, 14%, 0%, and 10%, respectively, for these tumor types.[32] In general, the quantitative levels of proACTH-ACTH and LPH were correlated. Some 20% of patients with chronic obstructive pulmonary disease had blood elevations of proACTH, whereas 13% had elevations of LPH. Other studies found proACTH elevations in chronic lung disease, suggesting that the lung may produce or bind proACTH or LPH in response to injury.[50–52] Five of 20 of the patients with elevated proACTH in chronic obstructive pulmonary disease eventually developed lung cancer, but only 2 of 81 of the patients with normal plasma levels of ACTH developed lung cancer.[45]

When ACTH, calcitonin, and hCG were measured simultaneously, significant elevated levels were found in 65% of 109 lung cancer patients and 78% of small cell cancer patients, suggesting the usefulness of several markers in concert to detect lung cancer.[31] More studies are needed to know if the proACTH-LPH or other peptide hormone assays are predictors of the development of lung cancer and if they can be useful in following the course of the disease. Extracts of tumors other than lung cancer showed significant elevations (>1 ng/g tissue) of proACTH or LPH: 6 of 16 colon cancers, 3 of 4 breast cancers, and 22 of 31 miscellaneous tumors and metastatic lesions. Although elevated levels of immunoreactive material were found, there is no direct evidence that the tumors produced the peptides. Many tumors may make preopiocorticoid, but only some have the ability to cleave it appropriately into biologically active forms. The expression of the syndromes may depend more on the promolecule processing than the presence of the ectopic prohormone itself.[2]

With the development and use of RIAs for measuring lipotropin and β-endorphin and receptor assays for measuring endogenous opiate peptides in human cerebrospinal fluid and plasma, it may become possible to correlate unusual neurologic syndromes and mental behavior directly with fragments derived from the proopiocorticoid molecule.[32,39,81] It is reasonable to start applying these assays to patients with such symptoms and appropriate tumor settings (*e.g.*, lung cancer). Circulating immune complexes of ACTH and human immunoglobulins have been reported.[82] ACTH also may be involved in an immune complex paraneoplastic syndrome. A portion of the ACTH promolecule with opioid activity undergoes a striking increase in the pituitary of newborn monkeys. This increase in endogenous opioid may help the fetus withstand the stress of parturition.[41] Likewise, tumor production of an analgesic-like material such as β-endorphin may allow the cancer patient a measure of relief from tumor-related symptoms. Additional work quantitating the amount and nature of such endogenous analgesics is necessary.

SYNDROME OF INAPPROPRIATE SECRETION OF ANTIDIURETIC HORMONE

Hyponatremia was first associated with lung cancer in 1938; the syndrome of "inappropriate secretion" of antidiuretic hormone (SIADH; ADH = arginine vasopressin [AVP]) was postulated by Schwartz and coworkers in 1957 to be caused by stimulation of the posterior pituitary to secrete AVP by a thoracic tumor.[83,84] In 1963, Amatruda and coworkers showed it to be related to tumor production of AVP.[85] AVP, oxytocin, and neurophysins have been found by RIA in tumors, and the AVP is bioactive and immunoreactive.[23,86] The neurophysins normally are synthesized, stored, and secreted in parallel with AVP and oxytocin.[87] These polypeptides function as binding proteins for AVP and oxytocin; there are different neurophysins for AVP and oxytocin.[88] Whether AVP and oxytocin actually form a promolecule with their respective neurophysins is under investigation.[23] Currently, there are no recognized syndromes related to tumor production of neurophysins or oxytocin, but tumor production of AVP results in hyponatremia.

Clinical Findings and Pathophysiology

Continuous tumor production, exogenous administration, and posterior pituitary production of AVP all result in a syndrome of hyponatremia, urine inappropriately higher in osmolality than the plasma, and high urinary sodium concentrations in the face of serum hyponatremia.[2,3,23] This is thought to result from the action of AVP on the renal tubule with resultant water retention. The hyponatremia comes from renal sodium loss and dilution by water retention. The mechanism of the natriuresis is not defined but could include an increased filtered sodium load, a decreased aldosterone secretion, or a decreased tubular reabsorption of sodium. The major clinical symptoms are caused by water intoxication (*i.e.*, hypoosmality and hyponatremia) and manifested by altered mental status, confusion, lethargy, psychotic behavior, seizures, coma, or occasionally death.[2,3,23,89] Focal neurologic findings can be associated with water intoxication from SIADH alone without brain metastases.[89] Because of the predominant occurrence of SIADH with small cell lung cancer and the frequent presence of brain metastases in this cancer, all patients with neurologic syndromes in small cell lung cancer should have serum sodium levels checked for hyponatremia, and all small cell cancer patients with hyponatremia and neurologic syndromes should be evaluated for brain metastases.

Diagnosis of Ectopic Arginine Vasopressin Production

Hyponatremia is the usual mode of presentation of SIADH because of the routine use of serum electrolytes in patient evaluation (Table 57–6). Some patients present with neurologic symptoms. The first major problem is to differentiate SIADH from the multiple other causes of hyponatremia, such as diuretic use; cardiac, hepatic, and renal failure; dilutional causes; diminished function of adrenals, anterior pituitary, or thyroid. Various drugs can impair free water excretion by acting on the renal tubule or by inducing pituitary AVP, including chlorpropamide, thiazide diuretics, cyclophosphamide, vincristine, and morphine.[90–92] To separate these causes of hy-

TABLE 57–6. Differential Diagnosis for the Syndrome of Inappropriate Antidiuretic Hormone

Tumors
- Small cell lung cancer
- Other types

Pulmonary, chest conditions
- Infection (tuberculosis, abscess, pneumonia—viral or bacterial), mitral stenosis (status after surgical correction)

Central nervous system
- Trauma (skull fracture, subdural, concussion, subarachnoid hemorrhage, thrombosis)
- Intracranial space-occupying lesions (primary and metastatic tumor)
- Infections (meningitis, encephalitis, lues)
- Vasculitis (lupus)
- Guillian-Barré
- Acute intermittent porphyria
- Pain and emotional stress

Drugs
- Chlorpropamide
- Morphine
- Nicotine
- Ethanol
- Cyclophosphamide
- Vincristine
- Idiopathic

ponatremia from SIADH, it is mandatory to demonstrate the following:

1. Hypoosmolality (usually <280 mOsm/kg)
2. Urinary osmolality greater than the plasma (≥500 mOsm/kg)
3. Continued urinary excretion of sodium (>20 mEq/L) although taking no diuretics
4. Absence of signs of volume depletion
5. Normal renal function
6. Normal adrenal and thyroid function.

Fichman and Bethune studied 86 patients with SIADH and found serum sodium levels of 88 to 126 mEq/L, urine sodium levels of 35 to 175 mEq/24 hours, serum osmolalities of 190 to 273 mOsm/kg, and urine osmolalities of 332 to 780 mOsm/kg.[92] The most common mistake in diagnosis of SIADH is failing to notice the previous administration of a diuretic or of occult volume depletion with resulting dilutional hyponatremia. Repeat clinical examinations can exclude these causes. Although AVP can be measured by RIA, this is not routinely available, and many conditions can be associated with the "appropriate" and the "inappropriate" secretion of AVP.

The most common disorders associated with SIADH besides small cell lung cancer include CNS diseases (*e.g.*, CNS infection, head trauma, intracranial space-occupying lesions, subarachnoid hemorrhage, acute intermittent porphyria, pain, emotional stress) and pulmonary infections (see Table 57–6). If any of these affect patients with SIADH and malignant disease (including small cell cancer), they should be treated in an effort to control the SIADH. Water loading can elicit clinically occult SIADH but can be dangerous in patients with hyponatremia and probably should not be done if the serum sodium concentration is 125 mEq/L or less.[90]

In studies of lung cancer patients with SIADH and high levels of AVP by RIA, fluid restriction further increased the already elevated AVP level, probably from stimulation of the pituitary to release AVP.[93] The other causes of SIADH (particularly drugs) account for some of the SIADH seen in tumor patients without small cell lung cancer or carcinoid histologic findings and stress the need for biosynthetic studies of AVP by cultured tumor cells to prove the source of the AVP. Other complications (*e.g.*, pneumonia) usually occur because of the cancer, and the development of SIADH represents a "secondary" paraneoplastic syndrome. For example, cyclophosphamide and vincristine are used to treat small cell lung cancer. When cyclophosphamide is given in high doses and the patient is hydrated to prevent cystitis, the combined effect of cyclophosphamide to decrease free water clearance and the water load can lead to SIADH.[92,94,95] Whether this represents release of pituitary AVP or a direct effect of cyclophosphamide metabolites on the renal tubules is unknown.[94]

If the histology of the tumor-associated SIADH is small cell cancer, the cancer is treated and correlation is made between the tumor response and the SIADH. If the tumor's histologic structure is other than small cell or carcinoid, the physician should be skeptical about tumor production of AVP until all causes of the SIADH are sought. If no other causes of SIADH are apparent, the physician should consider obtaining more tumor tissue, because a component of small cell carcinoma may be present. This dictates a more aggressive chemoradiotherapy approach than that for an "unresponsive" non-small cell tumor type.

If a patient presents with idiopathic SIADH, a careful search and follow-up for small cell tumor must be maintained; although cases like this are uncommon, the workup probably should include a full staging evaluation for small cell cancer, including fiberoptic bronchoscopy and computed tomography (CT) scans of the chest and abdomen to locate small tumor masses. The tumor should declare itself within a few months. In comparing tumor-related SIADH and SIADH resulting from other causes, serum and urinary sodium levels, osmolality, blood urea nitrogen, plasma AVP, and renin levels all failed to differentiate neoplastic from nonneoplastic causes.[94] The speed of rise in serum sodium concentration with water restriction supposedly is faster (3 days versus 7–10 days) for nonneoplastic causes than for neoplastic causes of SIADH.[96] However, this distinction may not be clear enough to be useful clinically.

Frequency and Tumor Types

Almost all of the tumors that produce AVP are small cell carcinomas of the lung.[2,3,23,29] However, SIADH has been seen with other tumor types, including carcinomas of the prostate, adrenal cortex, esophagus, pancreas, duodenum, colon, bronchial carcinoids, thymomas, head and neck, Hodgkin's disease, and non-Hodgkin's lymphomas.[2,3,23] At least some of these may have had a nonpulmonary small cell or carcinoid histologic structure. Small cell lung cancer lines grown in tissue culture make immunologically detectable AVP.[97,98] There have been no clear biosynthetic studies of cultured tumor cells of other histologic types.

Collected series show that 9% of 523 small cell lung cancer patients have clinically evident SIADH with hyponatremia.[23,46,59,99,100] Like ACTH, measurement of blood AVP by RIA has shown significant elevations in an even larger fraction of cases (32–44%).[31,100] Evidence of SIADH by water loading of patients showed that 53% to 68% had subclinical but evocable SIADH.[31,100] Odell and associates found 41% of lung cancer patients of all histologic types and 43% of colon cancer patients to have significantly elevated blood AVP levels without clinically evident SIADH.[2] North's group studied neurophysins in 72 small cell cancer patients and found significantly elevated levels of one or both (AVP or oxytocin) neurophysins in 65%.[88]

Treatment

The fundamental principle of the treatment of tumor-associated SIADH involves successful treatment of the underlying cancer (see Chap. 23).[99] If chemotherapy is not effective, radiotherapy of bulk tumor mass or, in selected cases of non-small cell lung cancer limited to the chest, surgical removal of the tumor may be considered. There are several major decisions that are influenced by antitumor treatment:

1. The problem of water restriction and high-dose chemotherapy
2. Management of severely symptomatic hyponatremia
3. The problem of differentiating SIADH that develops during treatment from other causes and true tumor relapse
4. Treatment of recurrent SIADH with tumor progression on primary therapy.

For symptomatic hyponatremia and serum sodium levels of less than 130 mEq/L, fluid restriction to less than 500 ml/24 hours allows patients to increase their plasma osmolality slowly over 7 to 10 days. If chemotherapy requires hydration and the chemotherapy could induce more hyponatremia (*e.g.*, cyclophosphamide in high doses), this usually can be handled by careful monitoring of body weight, input and output, daily or more frequent serum sodium determinations, and urine sodium and potassium measurements while giving normal saline with furosemide diuretics and electrolyte replacement.[95,101,102] If the patient is severely hyponatremic or symptomatic (*e.g.*, serum sodium <125 mEq/L), correction of this over several days may be required before instituting chemotherapy. An excellent correlation of antitumor response to chemoradiotherapy and disappearance of SIADH was reported by the National Cancer Institute group for 7 of 7 patients and by the Vanderbilt group for 16 of 17 newly diagnosed small cell cancer patients.[102] North and coworkers studied 18 patients with elevated neurophysins (some of which represent elevated AVP) by RIA and found complete agreement between tumor and neurophysin levels and response to chemotherapy (reduction of neurophysin levels in 12 patients with complete or partial remissions and rise in 6 patients with progressive tumor).[103] Because these latter markers occur in 65% of small cell cancer patients initially, the neurophysins may prove to be excellent tumor markers.

When a patient presents severely symptomatic from SIADH (*e.g.*, comatose), more acute measures are needed. The procedure of Hantman and associates involves using 3% hypertonic saline and intravenous furosemide to increase the net free water clearance.[104] Furosemide (1 mg/kg body weight) is given intravenously and subsequent doses are given as needed to obtain the desired negative fluid balance. Besides routine vital signs, urinary losses of sodium and potassium are measured hourly and replaced by an infusion of appropriate amounts of hypertonic sodium chloride solution, to which appropriate amounts of potassium chloride are added. Using an estimated total-body water content of 60% of female body weight and 70% of male body weight, the negative fluid balance necessary to raise the plasma osmolality to 270 mOsm/kg water is calculated for an individual patient by the following formula:

$$\begin{aligned}&\text{Desired negative water balance in liters}\\&\quad = \text{total body water (TBW)}\\&\quad = \text{weight in kg}\\&\quad \times 0.6 \text{ or } 0.7 - \frac{\text{TBW} \times \text{plasma osmolality}^{104}}{270}\end{aligned}$$

This approach resulted in the serum sodium concentrations rising from 120 to 133 mEq/L in 6 to 8 hours.[104] Although none of these patients had small cell carcinoma, the Johns Hopkins group has used this regimen successfully in small cell cancer.[89] This procedure also could be used to prepare patients for chemotherapy.

In patients who have relapsed and who have recurrent SIADH with no or only minimally effective chemotherapy available, therapy with demeclocycline or urea can be tried. Demeclocycline is more effective in treating SIADH than lithium carbonate.[105–107] Demeclocycline blocks AVP action at the level of the renal tubule by inhibiting AVP-induced cAMP formation and blocking the effect of any cAMP generated with more reproducibility than lithium carbonate. A positive correlation between serum sodium and blood urea was found in patients with SIADH, suggesting the use of urea therapy to correct SIADH. Urea given in dosages of 30 g/day corrected the salt-losing tendency of SIADH in 2 patients with small cell cancer and in normal persons given exogenous AVP.[108] Because it induces an osmotic diuresis, urea therapy allows a normal daily intake of water despite continued SIADH. Thirty grams of urea (99% pure crystalline material) is dissolved in 100 ml of water with 15 g of magnesium and aluminum hydroxide (Maalox) and is taken at noon; this has been maintained for as long as 11 weeks without water restriction.[108] The urea is taken orally because of good gastrointestinal absorption and because cells are freely permeable to urea. There is no risk of cardiac failure from rapid shifts of water, as is possible in a mannitol-induced diuresis.

Although hyponatremia and SIADH are the classic presenting features of tumor secretion of AVP, other paraneoplastic syndromes may occur, because at much higher concentrations, AVP acts on the cardiovascular system and other smooth muscles throughout the body.[91]

Hyponatremia Secondary to Ectopic Atrial Natriuretic Peptide Secretion

Atrial natriuretic peptide (ANP), produced by human atrial tissue has potent natriuretic activity. Several series demonstrated that it may be a circulating hormone producing hyponatremia and SIADH.[109] Kamoi and coworkers described a patient with small cell lung cancer and hyponatremia who had sustained high plasma levels of ANP, but normal levels of AVP, suggesting the ANP produced the hyponatremia.[110] In this case, evaluation of tumor tissue showed no ANP, indicating an increased secretion by atrial tissue. The overall frequency of ANP-induced hyponatremia in cancer patients is unknown.

HYPERCALCEMIA

Hypercalcemia is common in cancer patients; about 10% of patients with cancer have hypercalcemia, and 10% to 15% of these do not have associated bone metastases.[111,112] The most common tumor types associated with hypercalcemia are breast cancer (15%, usually associated with bone metastases), lung cancer (10%), and multiple myeloma (>50%, usually associated with bone involvement). Although most breast cancer patients with hypercalcemia have bone metastases, a prospective series showed that 24% had no bone metastases and a purely hormonal mechanism was postulated.[113] Patients with squamous cell carcinomas, especially of lung, head, neck, and esophagus have a high frequency of paraneoplastic hypercalcemia.[114,115] This is rare in small cell lung cancer. Hypercalcemia with or without bone metastases is seen in most patients with adult T-cell leukemia, and it occurs in lower frequency in other lymphomas.[116]

There are several documented mechanisms of hypercalcemia in cancer patients, including bone metastases, the simultaneous occurrence of primary hyperparathyroidism, ectopic tumor-produced parathormone-like substances, tumor-produced prostaglandins (*e.g.*, PGE_1,PGE_2), tumor-produced osteoclast-activating factor, tumor growth factor-α, 1,25-dihydroxyvitamin D, and other osteolytic factors.[23,111,115,117–119] In normal persons, calcium is maintained by a series of control mechanisms that govern bone resorption and osteolysis, which are stimulated by PGE, PTH, osteoclast-activating factor, thyroxine (T_4), and a monocyte-derived osteolytic factor and are inhibited by calcitonin and estrogen. Absorption of calcium from the gastrointestinal and renal tubular tracts is stimulated by PTH, growth hormone, and vitamin D.[111] Production by tumors of any of these materials could cause hypercalcemia. Although paraneoplastic syndromes usually are considered to be those humorally mediated at a distance from the primary tumor or its metastases, in hypercalcemia the mediators released by the tumor cells may act locally, as with PGE and osteoclast-activating factor.

The most frequent cause of paraneoplastic hypercalcemia is tumor secretion of a parathyroid hormone-related peptide (PTHRP).[120–122] This fascinating protein is derived from a gene that has been identified in multiple species. The gene for PTHRP is different from that of PTH. They reside on different chromosomes, and the two genes may have developed by an evolutionary duplication. The human gene expresses three mRNAs that encode three distinct peptides, all different at the COOH-terminal region of the molecule consisting of amino acids of 139, 141, and 173 residues. However, 8 of the first 13 amino acids are the same as PTH (see Fig. 55–1B). The PTHRP gene is expressed in many normal tissues, including the keratinocyte, the pancreas islet cells, normal parathyroid cells, cells of pituitary, adrenal, ovarian, testicular, and brain origin, and the placenta and lactating breast. In normal persons, the PTHRP protein is low or not detected in the circulation, suggesting that expression of the gene gives rise to a protein that serves an autocrine or paracrine role in local calcium homeostasis. For example, the highest levels of PTHRP protein reported in normal humans is in breast milk, and its concentration there is presumably a reflection of important calcium-modulating roles related to breast milk. High circulating levels of PTHRP in humans are found in the syndrome of humeral hypercalcemia of malignancy. In these circumstances, the circulating levels of PTHRP are similar to those of PTH. This is reported most often in squamous cell carcinoma of the head, neck, and lung and for a variety of adenocarcinomas, including breast cancer (see Fig. 57–1C). Approximately 50% to 80% of cases of humeral hypercalcemia of malignancy have abnormal levels of PTHRP in the serum, depending on the specific assay. These patients have increased levels of cAMP, increased serum levels of calcium, and low serum levels of phosphorous. The level of intact PTH measured by new immunoradiometric assays is low or undetectable in these cases, unlike patients having primary hyperparathyroidism, in which high levels of intact PTH are found. The development of new assays for PTHRP and PTH have facilitated the diagnosis of primary hyperparathyroidism and humeral hypercalcemia of malignancy.

The hypercalcemia in multiple myeloma and lymphomas is usually ascribed to osteoclast-activating factors.[116,123–127] These cases have normal or low levels of PTH, cAMP, 1,25-dihydroxyvitamin D, and evidence of osteoclast activation on bone biopsy. The osteoclast-activating factor appears to be a locally secreted lymphokine. It is not clear whether the lymphokine is the same or is different in various lymphomas and myelomas. Interleukin-1β (IL-1β) may also be a bone-resorbing lymphokine secreted by some of the lymphoproliferative malignancies.

Tumor secretion of PGE is rare and is associated with normal or low PTH, cAMP, and vitamin D levels. Such secretion has been reported in hypernephomas and rarely in other tumor types.[117,118,128–133] It is important to recognize because prostaglandin inhibitors, such as indomethacin (Indocin), may be successful therapeutically.

Active metabolites of vitamin D have also been produced by some malignancies including lymphoma, small cell lung cancer, and melanoma. In general, these cases show hypercalcemia, elevated 1,25-dihydroxyvitamin D levels, low PTH, and low urinary and AMP excretion.[134–136] Treatment of the tumors surgically or by chemotherapy usually reverses the chemical abnormalities. In some instances, vitamin D metabolites have been purified from tumor cells or shown to be synthesized in vitro by the tumor cells.

Transforming growth factors α and β have also been associated with hypercalcemia of malignancy.[120] Transforming growth factor α has been isolated from squamous cell carcinomas of the lung, head and neck, kidney, and breast. It is a 5000 Da protein with 50 amino acids. It mediates its effect predominantly through the EGF receptor and antibodies; the EGF receptors can block the bone-resorbing activity.

All of the mechanisms of hypercalcemia should be considered in cancer patients, and determining the cause of the hypercalcemia is important because of the therapeutic implications. The pathophysiology, clinical manifestations, and treatment are discussed in Chapter 60.

HYPOCALCEMIA

In patients with bone metastases, hypocalcemia occurs in 16% and hypercalcemia only in 9%.[137–140] Hypocalcemia commonly occurs with osteoblastic metastases of the breast, prostate, and lung.[138,141] Only rarely is tetanic hypocalcemia seen with these osteoblastic metastases.[142] However, with more refined studies of nerve, muscle, or other physiologic function testing, hypocalcemia may be found to impair a patient's neuromuscular function. Hypocalcemia may be mediated by way of tumor-secreted calcitonin, although there is no direct evidence for this. No specific therapy is indicated, except in the rare case of tetany, for which calcium can be given.

HYPOPHOSPHATEMIC OSTEOMALACIA ASSOCIATED WITH BENIGN MESENCHYMAL TUMORS

An acquired, adult-onset, vitamin D-resistant rickets with bone pain, severe phosphaturia, renal glycosuria, hypophosphatemia, normocalcemia (normal PTH levels), low 1,25-dihydroxyvitamin D levels, and increased alkaline phosphatase levels is associated with benign mesenchymal tumors that occur in soft tissues or bone (*i.e.*, tumoral osteomalacia, oncogenic osteomalacia).[143–146] They are also called ossifying mesenchymal tumors, giant cell tumors of bone, sclerosing hemangioma, cavernous hemangioma, or reparative giant cell granuloma.[147] The syndrome often precedes the discovery of the tumor by several years.[25] The basis of treatment is resection of the mesenchymal tumor, which results in resolution of the syndrome.[143,144,148] Otherwise, treatment requires large doses of vitamin D and phosphate. The proposed mechanisms include inhibition of the conversion of 25-hydroxyvitamin D to 1,25-dihydroxyvitamin D and a tumor-secreted "phosphaturic substance." It is possible that a single protein produces both of these effects. Active osteoclastic bone resorption has been reported. Rarely, this syndrome has been reported with lung and prostate cancers.[149,150] The importance of recognizing this syndrome is its cure with surgical resection. Sometimes multiple osteolytic lesions or osteoblastic-like lesions are seen in sclerosing hemangiomas of bone. These require treatment with oral phosphate and vitamin D, which give relief of bone pain and weakness.[145] These bone lesions can resemble diffuse metastases on a roentgenogram, and careful pathologic examination is required.

CALCITONIN PRODUCTION BY TUMORS

The polypeptide hormone calcitonin normally is produced by the C cells of the thyroid. It prevents calcium release from bone and causes an increase in renal excretion of calcium, sodium, and phosphate.[151] However, no described clinical syndromes are associated with tumor production of calcitonin, although one small cell cancer patient with high calcitonin levels had hypocalcemia.[30] The major clinical use of calcitonin assay is in monitoring patients with medullary carcinoma of the thyroid. This tumor produces large amounts of calcitonin without clinical signs or symptoms.[151] Calcitonin is an extremely sensitive indicator of residual tumor after surgery.[89] It is useful in identifying patients with type II multiple endocrine neoplasia, a familial disorder involving an association of medullary carcinoma of the thyroid, pheochromocytoma, and parathyroid adenomas. These are described in detail in Chapter 41. Because of the excellent clinical correlation of calcitonin with medullary thyroid cancer, the hormone has been studied in other tumor types.

Elevated plasma calcitonin levels are consistently found in 48% to 64% of patients with small cell lung cancer and at other rates with the other lung cancer cell types (see Table 57–4).[22,30,31,152] Urinary calcitonin is elevated in 75% of lung cancer patients: 53% of epidermoid, 45% of adenocarcinomas, 20% of large cell cancers, but surprisingly only 17% of small cell cancers.[153] When antiserum detecting the COOH-terminal end and midportion of the calcitonin molecule was used on serum and urine samples, more than 90% of lung cancer patients had abnormal values.[153] Calcitonin levels mirrored clinical tumor status 67% of the time in lung cancer patients, but selective venous sampling showed tumoral and thyroidal production of the elevated calcitonin levels.[152] Its usefulness as a marker of lung cancer is not yet established. Other tumor types associated with increased plasma calcitonin levels include carcinoids, breast cancer (in some studies, up to 100%), colon cancer (24%), and gastric cancer (38%). High calcitonin levels do not correlate with bone metastases.[152] However, a variety of nonneoplastic conditions are associated with elevated calcitonin levels, including hypercalcemia, chronic renal failure, pregnancy, pernicious anemia, Zollinger-Ellison syndrome, and pancreatitis.[22,152] Its use as a screen for the early detection of cancer is problematic.

Because of the several possible sources of calcitonin, biosynthetic studies would be useful. Immunoreactive calcitonin has been found in many tumor extracts, including small cell cancer, pheochromocytomas, malignant carcinoids, other types of lung cancer, breast, melanoma, colon, gastric, esophagus, and pancreatic cancer.[97,154,155] These studies failed to show that calcitonin and ACTH were on a common precursor molecule, as predicted by some, but they did show a high-molecular-mass form of calcitonin.[156,157] The nature of the calcitonin precursor molecule is unknown. Calcitonin is a polypeptide hormone, apparently produced by many cancers, waiting for definition of a clinically evident paraneoplastic syndrome and prospective documentation as a marker of response to therapy.

CHROMOGRANIN A PRODUCED BY TUMORS

Chromogranin A is a 48,000-d acidic glycoprotein, which may account for as much as 10% of the weight of cells of the neuroendocrine system.[158] It is secreted by several neuroendocrine tumors, especially small cell lung cancer.[158–160] It is stored in vesicles of chromaffin cells and released with catecholamines after splanchnic stimulation. It may act in neuroendocrine secretion by binding intravesicular calcium. Its sequence is almost identical to pancreastatin, which inhibits insulin and somatostatin secretion from the pancreas.[161,162] Pancreastatin may be generated from chromogranin A or from a chromogranin A-like precursor. Like calcitonin, it is unknown whether there is an associated paraneoplastic syndrome.

HUMAN PLACENTAL AND PITUITARY GLYCOPROTEIN HORMONES PRODUCED BY TUMORS

Gonadotropins

Precocious puberty in children, gynecomastia in men, and oligomenorrhea in premenopausal women may result from excessive gonadotropin production by tumors.[2,3,23,163] Very high levels of gonadotropin secretion may result in thyroid stimulation and hyperthyroidism.[164,165] Gonadotropin secretion may occur in pituitary tumors, gestational trophoblastic tumors (*e.g.*, choriocarcinoma, hydatidiform mole), germ cell tumors of testis and ovary, germ cell tumors arising or presenting in extragonadal primary sites, or hepatoblastomas in children and large cell and adenocarcinoma of the lung in adults.[2,3,23,163,166,167]

The tumors arising in gestational tissue, testis, ovary, and endocrine organs are discussed in other chapters, in which the great value of gonadotropin measurement as a marker in the treatment of gestational trophoblastic tumors and testicular cancer is discussed.[168,169] Their usefulness as a marker in these tumors stimulated intense study of gonadotropin expression in other tumors to see if they could be used as markers for early diagnosis or monitoring of subsequent treatment.[170]

The human hormones with gonadotrophic properties are follicle stimulating hormone (FSH), luteinizing hormone (LH), and human chorionic gonadotropin (hCG).[163] These three hormones are composed of two polypeptide chains, α- and a β-subunits. The α-subunit is common to all the hormones, and the β-subunit confers immunologic and biologic specificity. Both subunits are required for bioactivity.[163] Radioimmunoassay can differentiate between the various types of β-subunits.[163] In normal persons, FSH and LH are produced by the pituitary and are normally present in serum, but biologically active hCG is produced by the placenta and usually is found only in pregnant women. Because levels of FSH and LH vary widely under normal physiologic conditions, the assay for β-hCG is theoretically the best hormone to use for following patients with suspected paraneoplastic production of gonadotropin excess. An hCG-like material has been found in extracts of all normal tissue by RIA and radioreceptor assay, calling into question the use of hCG in cancer patients. However, this hCG is carbohydrate-free, and that produced by the placenta and many tumors contains carbohydrate. Carbohydrate-free hCG is cleared rapidly from the circulation and has marked loss of bioactivity.[163,171]

Many studies have looked at "elevations" of hCG, β-hCG, and α-hCG (Table 57–7). Many of the common tumors (*e.g.*, lung, colorectum, breast) had frequent elevations of these markers. However, 5% to 10% of patients with nonmalignant chronic disease also had hormone elevations, calling the specificity of the findings in tumor patients into doubt. In pursuing this, Blackman and coworkers conducted a detailed study of human placental and pituitary glycopeptide hormones and their subunits in the sera of patients with lung cancer, gastrointestinal cancer, malignant carcinoid, and malignant islet cell tumors and compared their results with 579 appropriately matched controls (Table 57–8).[170,173,174] Values for the α- and β-subunit of hCG were significantly higher in the cancer patients, and elevations of FSH-β, TSH-β, and LH-β were not observed. The sensitivity of detection of cancer patients increased by combining the results from the two tests. They and others found differences in the ratio of α-hCG/β-hCG positivity between sexes and among cancer groups, a finding that is unexplained.

TABLE 57–7. Elevations of Human Chorionic Gonadotropin or its β-Subunit and the α-Subunit of Placental and Pituitary Glycoprotein Hormones in Various Tumors

	% Elevated	
Tumor Type	*hCG or β-hCG*	*α-Subunit*
Lung*	0–12	3–30
Colorectal	0–20	20–26
Breast	7–50	30
Pancreatic adenocarcinoma	11–50	
Gastric carcinoma	0–24	
Prostate cancer	1	0
Islet cell carcinoma	22–50	52
Carcinoid of gut and lung		16
Small intestine	13	
Hepatoma	17–20	
Nonmalignant lung disease	7	
Nonmalignant GI disease	9	
Nonmalignant breast disease	4	

* Within lung, there were 32% epidermoid cancers; 27% small cell lung cancers; 13% large cell lung cancers; 11% adenocarcinoma; and 17% miscellaneous and undetermined histologic malignant diseases. Within GI cancer, there were 13% pancreatic adenocarcinomas; 8% gastric cancers; 4% hepatomas; 10% other types of upper GI cancer; and 65% lower GI cancers. Carcinoid lesions included 80% of GI origin; malignant islet cell neoplasms included 28% insulinomas and 40% gastrinomas. Normal controls included 299 healthy subjects, 123 patients with chronic lung disease, 110 with benign GI disease, and 47 with benign endocrine diseases.

(Winkler WA, Crankshaw OF. Chloride depletion in conditions other than Addison's disease. J Clin Invest 1938;17:1–6; Thomas TH, Morgan DB, Swaminathan R, et al. Severe hyponatremia. Lancet 1978;1:621–624)

Because of the frequency of elevation in common tumors, such as lung and gastrointestinal cancers, and because of the correlation with response in trophoblastic disease and testicular tumors, it is important to test prospectively the roles of α-hCG and β-hCG in monitoring the therapy of common tumors. In some nontrophoblastic tumors, these markers have been valuable in monitoring therapy.[172,176] However, these reports are still anecdotal. For example, Broder and associates reported a patient with prostatic cancer and elevated hCG whose serum hCG levels mirrored the clinical course more reliably than the concomitant acid phosphatase levels.[175] Muggia and coworkers reported 4 patients with metastatic cancer, and in seven of nine episodes, clinical remission was associated with marker decrease or exacerbation associated with marker increase.[172] Metz and coworkers reported a patient with an hCG-secreting large cell carcinoma of the lung with painful gynecomastia and testicular atrophy.[176] Investigation revealed elevated levels of β-hCG subunits and elevated

TABLE 57–8. Elevations of the β-Subunits of Chorionic Gonadotropin or the α-Subunit of Glycoprotein Hormones in Patients With Lung and Gastrointestinal Cancer

	% of Tumor Patients With Hormone Elevations Over 95th Percentile of Normal Controls			
*Tumor Type**	*Patients (n)*	*α-Subunit*	*β-hCG*	*α-Subunit or BhCG*
Lung cancer				
Men	269	11	41	45
Women	31	16	16	29
Gastrointestinal cancer				
Men	92	32	28	48
Women	71	18	34	41
Carcinoid				
Men	25	50	0	50
Women		13	50	50
Malignant islet cell				
Men	40	61	6	61
Women		38	19	43

* Within lung cancer 32% were epidermoid.
(Blackman MR, Weintraub BD, Rosen SW, et al. Human placental and pituitary glycoprotein hormones and their subunits as tumor markers: A quantitative assessment. JNCI 1980;65:81–93)

α-subunits, normal estradiol levels, low-normal testosterone levels, and abnormal (delayed) pituitary response to LHRH. These abnormal findings reverted to normal after surgical resection of the tumor (shown to contain high levels of hCG), recurred with tumor regrowth, and regressed again with the addition of combination chemotherapy, which produced a complete clinical remission of the tumor and the biochemical parameters.[176] The β-hCG level was more sensitive than gynecomastia in predicting recurrence. This was an important case because it demonstrated the usefulness of the β-hCG marker in a common solid tumor to monitor therapy and achieve potential cure with the use of chemotherapy in a semiadjuvant setting.

Studies of tumor lines in vitro agree with these studies of serum samples. The β- and α-subunits of hCG are produced by human tumor cell lines in vitro.[170,177,178] Unbalanced synthesis of α- and β-subunits is seen, but no evidence of production of FSH-β or TSH-β existed,and only rarely and at low levels was LH-β found.

Although tumor-produced α- and β-hCG are found frequently, there are no definitive reports of tumor-produced FSH, TSH, or LH.[3,23] Patients with suspected tumor production of these hormones should be carefully documented and reported. Some elevations of LH and FSH may occur in cancer patients, probably as the result of gonadal failure related to age, stress, chronic illness, or treatment.[170] Blackman and associates showed that 50% to 59% of men with malignant lung disease, 28% to 32% of men with benign lung disease, but only 10% of normal persons had evidence of hypogonadism when assessed with serum testosterone, LH, and FSH.[179] Obviously other causes of elevated hormones, such as those seen in physiologic causes of hypergonadotropinemia, hyperthyrotropinemia, pituitary adenomas, pregnancy, and uremia, must be excluded.[170]

DIFFERENTIAL DIAGNOSIS. The exact frequency of symptoms associated with tumor-produced gonadotropin is unknown, although an intact hormone (both subunits) and an appropriate host (*i.e.*, child for precocious puberty, man for gynecomastia, premenopausal women for oligomenorrhea) are required simultaneously for clinical expression. A detailed discussion of the differential diagnosis of these conditions is beyond the scope of this chapter. However, the most common problem is a male patient presenting with unexplained gynecomastia. In this situation, a β-hCG determination should be performed and a careful examination of the testes and radiographic examination of the chest and mediastinum should be done. It is important to use an RIA, because routine urinary pregnancy tests are not sensitive enough to detect many hCG secretory neoplasms.[176] Germ cell tumors of the testis or extragonadal sites and lung cancers are the most frequent cause of the combination of gynecomastia and hCG elevation, and these men should be persistently and thoroughly evaluated, because this syndrome can present before a clinically evident cancer is found.[179a]

Other tumors associated with biologically active hCG are rare. Skrabanek and associates found only 44 extragonadal cases in the world's literature, and these involved the lung, adrenal gland, liver, gastrointestinal tract, and nongonadal portions of the genitourinary tract.[180] Analysis of the histologic specimens revealed that all contained syncytial giant cells or frankly choriocarcinomatous elements similar to classic trophoblastic germ cell tumors. Greco and associates found that 40% of patients with extragonadal germ cell tumors, "masquerading" as poorly differentiated carcinomas, had immunochemical tumor staining for β-hCG and AFP without serum elevations of the markers.[181] Many patients responded to combination chemotherapy. These results suggest that immunohistochemistry and a chemotherapy approach similar to that for histologically classic germ cell tumors are warranted for the potentially curable poorly differentiated midline carcinomas in young adults.

Precocious puberty has been found in children with hepatoma or hepatoblastomas. In these children, secondary sexual characteristics developed prematurely, with advanced skeletal maturation and hyperplasia of prostatic and testicular interstitial cells.[23,182–184] Abnormal endocrine manifestations consisting of precocious puberty, irregular bleeding, amenorrhea, and hirsutism occurred in 9 (60%) of 15 patients with tumors of the ovary, and biopsy specimens stained immunohistochemically for hCG in syncytiotrophoblast-like cells and for AFP in embryonal carcinoma cells.[185]

TUMOR-PRODUCED HUMAN PLACENTAL LACTOGEN, GROWTH HORMONE, GROWTH HORMONE-RELEASING HORMONE, PROLACTIN, AND THYROTROPIC SUBSTANCE

Human placental lactogen (hPL) was detected in the sera of 5% to 8% of patients with nontrophoblastic nongonadal tumors.[186,187] Many of these patients with elevated hPL also had elevated levels of estrogens and had gynecomastia. Some of these patients also have elevated hCG levels. When hPL is found in nonpregnant women, it is a specific indication of malignancy.[187]

Elevated growth hormone levels have been reported in patients with lung cancer and gastric cancer, but that may be uncommon. Although patients with these neoplasms may not live long enough to develop acromegaly, it has been speculated that growth hormone may cause hypertrophic pulmonary osteoarthropathy, and the syndrome has been reversed by resection of lung tumors.[187a] However, a study of patients with and without osteoarthropathy failed to reveal any relation between the syndrome and elevated plasma growth hormone levels, and none were acromegalic.[188]

Acromegaly has been produced by tumor secretion of growth hormone-releasing hormone (GHRH).[189–193] The GHRH is a 44-amino acid peptide that has been isolated from two GHRH-secreting pancreatic tumors. A GHRH-induced acromegaly was reported with bronchial carcinoids. The clinical symptoms of acromegaly decreased after surgical resection. The secretion of GHRH can also be controlled by administration of long-acting somatostatin analogs.

Three patients with elevated prolactin levels (*i.e.*, undifferentiated lung cancer, small cell lung cancer, and hypernephroma) were reported, only one of whom had associated galactorrhea.[3,23] Resection or irradiation decreased the levels of prolactin in all patients. Cases of nonpituitary prolactin-secreting tumors are rare, and any suspected cases should be differentiated carefully from pituitary lesions and reported.

Cancer patients frequently have a "hypermetabolic state" that may resemble hyperthyroidism, and 1.4% of lung cancer patients reportedly are hyperthyroid, but documentation of tumor-caused syndromes is uncommon.[194] Four substances that could stimulate the thyroid gland are pituitary-like TSH, chorionic thyrotropin, hCG, and long-activating thyroid-stimulating substances (LATS). Documented examples of hyperthyroidism produced by TSH, LATS, and chorionic thyrotropin probably do not exist. Isolated reports of tumor-associated TSH without thyrotoxicosis have been made.[195] However, a definite association is found between hyperthyroidism and gestational trophoblastic disease (*e.g.*, choriocarcinoma, hydatidiform mole), in which 8% of cases can have biochemical evidence of hyperthyroidism. This is also seen in testicular tumors.[23,196] In all cases, the relation seems to be between trophoblastic tumors and very high levels of hCG, in which the thyroid-stimulating substance occasionally was hCG.[164,165,197]

HYPOGLYCEMIA

Hypoglycemia frequently is caused by insulinomas. Hypoglycemia associated with non-islet cell tumors is an uncommon and poorly characterized paraneoplastic syndrome. Other types of neoplasms associated with hypoglycemia are mesenchymal (64%), including mesothelioma, fibrosarcoma, neurofibrosarcoma, and hemangiopericytoma; hepatomas (21%); adrenal carcinomas (6%); gastrointestinal tumors (5%); and miscellaneous (5%), including anaplastic carcinomas of unknown primary, pseudomyxoma, hypernephromas, lymphomas, pheochromocytomas.[2,3,78,198]

The tumors usually are quite large (1–10 kg; average, 2.4 kg), often invade the liver, and often have protracted courses over many years.[2,3] Hypoglycemia may be the presenting symptom of a tumor.[2] Mesotheliomas are the most common cause of hypoglycemia, and about 50% of these occur in the abdomen, and the remainder occur in the chest. The signs and symptoms are those of hypoglycemia with neurologic findings (*e.g.*, stupor, coma, focal findings, agitated behavior) predominating until the hypoglycemia is discovered.[89]

Tumors can cause hypoglycemia by ectopic insulin production, production of nonsuppressible insulin-like activity (NSILA) or insulin-like growth factors I and II, overuse of glucose, production of a material stimulating ectopic insulin release, massive infiltration of the liver or production of an inhibitor of hepatic glucose output, insulin binding by an M-protein in myeloma, or insulin receptor proliferation.[199,200]

Tumor use of glucose to a degree that causes hypoglycemia has not been substantiated, and only rarely is liver infiltration by tumor massive enough to cause hypoglycemia.[2,3,201] There are rare reports of insulin production by non-islet cell tumors but no definitive biosynthetic studies to prove this.[202] A massive thoracic mesothelioma associated with hypoglycemia and very low glucagon levels was postulated as the source of a factor that suppresses glucagon secretion.[203] Artifactual hypoglycemia may occur in acute leukemia if the high number of circulating leukemia cells metabolizes the plasma glucose while standing in the collection tube.[204]

The most likely mechanism is tumor production of somatomedins, also called NSILA, and insulin-like growth factors.[2,3,89,205–207] Somatomedins are a family of peptide hormones normally produced by the liver under growth hormone regulation.[208] By current definitions, substances with identical bioassay properties of insulin in the rat diaphragm or epididymal fat pad and that also react in insulin radioreceptor assays (RRA) but do not react in insulin RIA, are somatomedins. Approximately half of the 200 μU of biologically active insulin and insulin-like activity in normal human serum is related to NSILA-somatomedin activity.[209] Hypoglycemia associated with cancer generally occurs after fasting and physical exertion, but reactive postprandial hypoglycemia usually is not part of the paraneoplastic syndrome.[89] Some cancer patients with hypoglycemia have elevated tumor extract levels of biologically active insulin-like activity that is not suppressed or reactive with antiinsulin antibodies but is reactive in the RRA.[209,210] These patients appear to have tumors producing NSILA, and it is important to study tissue culture lines of tumors from them to see if they produce this substance. The evaluation of these patients is experimental after the common causes of severe hypoglycemia (*e.g.*, exogenous insulin or sulfonylureas, insulinoma, islet cell tumor, adrenal or pituitary insufficiency, ethanol abuse, poor nutrition) have been excluded.

Initially, the treatment of paraneoplastic hypoglycemia involves glucose infusion to control the acute symptoms. Reduction of tumor bulk, usually by surgical resection, should then be carried out. However, there are no good data on the long-term effectiveness of any surgical, radiotherapy, or chemotherapy approach. If tumor treatment is not possible or is inadequate, other possibilities include the use of intermittent subcutaneous or long-acting intramuscular glucagon or high-dose corticosteroids.[89] However, there are few data on the long-term effectiveness of these agents in controlling hypoglycemia.

NEUROGASTROINTESTINAL PEPTIDES UNASSOCIATED WITH KNOWN PARANEOPLASTIC SYNDROMES

Neurogastrointestinal peptides have important roles in the perception of pain; in memory, learning, and behavior, in psychiatric diseases; and in temperature and blood pressure regulation.[24,25] Changes in levels of somatostatin, cholecystokinin, substance P, VIP, and enkephalin have been reported in two major idiopathic neurologic diseases: Alzheimer's disease and Huntington's disease.[211-215] In a patient with subacute necrotizing encephalopathy, naloxone administration reversed the symptoms of apnea, unconsciousness, hypothermia, and restlessness.[216] Analysis of spinal fluid showed an increased level of an uncharacterized opioid-like activity, and autopsy examination revealed increased concentrations of met- and leu-enkephalin in the cortex. Ectopic tumor production of these hormones may produce previously described neurologic paraneoplastic syndromes of unknown cause such as limbic encephalitis or other previously undescribed syndromes.

NEUROLOGIC MANIFESTATIONS OF MALIGNANCY

Neurologic problems occur frequently in patients with cancer. In the experiences of Posner and coworkers at Memorial Hospital, 17% of all patients at admission have neurologic symptoms and signs requiring neurologic consultation.[217] In patients with established cancer, true paraneoplastic syndromes account for a minority of neurologic problems, and the diagnosis of paraneoplastic syndrome can be established only after other diagnoses are excluded. The differential diagnosis of the cancer patient with neurologic signs and symptoms is provided in Table 57–9. Most frequently, neurologic complications are caused directly by the tumor or its metastases. For example, 40% to 65% of lung cancers metastasize to the brain, and overall Posner and Chernick reported that intracranial metastases were found in 24% of autopsies at Memorial Sloan-Kettering Cancer Center.[219-220]

Neurologic syndromes caused by endocrine, fluid, and electrolyte abnormalities are the second most common cause of neurologic symptoms and signs in cancer patients. Hepatic encephalopathy and hypercalcemia are the most frequent of these. Cerebral and spinal vascular disease are common in cancer patients and are found in 13% of autopsied cancer patients.[217] The causes of the vascular problems in these autopsied patients are shown in Table 57–10. Clearly the causes of stroke in these patients are strikingly dissimilar from those in the general population. Marantic and septic emboli, disseminated intravascular coagulation, tumor-related hemorrhage, superior sagittal sinus occlusion, and many of the cases of subarachnoid hemorrhage were directly tumor related and account for more than 50% of strokes.[220-224] Risk factors for the general population, including hypertension, atherosclerotic heart disease, and diabetes, are less important in the cancer patient.

TABLE 57–9. Differential Diagnosis of Neurologic Syndromes

Syndromes due to effects of primary or metastatic tumor
Syndromes due to endocrine or metabolic tumor products (*e.g.*, ADH, calcium, glucose, electrolytes)
Syndromes due to cerebral and spinal vascular disease
Syndromes due to toxicity of primary treatment (chemotherapy, radiotherapy)
Syndromes due to CNS infections
Paraneoplastic syndromes associated with malignancy with unknown mechanisms

TABLE 57–10. Causes of Stroke in Cancer Patients

Cause	*Frequency (%)*
Embolic infarction	27
Septic	13
Marantic	12
Tumor	2
Thrombotic infarction	19
Atherosclerotic	10
Disseminated intravascular coagulation	9
Miscellaneous infarction	6
Intraparenchymal hemorrhage	32.5
Spontaneous	13
Tumor related	13
Hypertension	5
Unknown	1.5
Subdural hemorrhage	8.5
Subarachnoid hemorrhage	3
Superior sagittal sinus occlusion	4
Total	100

(From studies by Allen,[217] Rosen,[221] Collins,[222] and Sigsbee[223])

Several associations of cancer and neurologic vascular disease are noteworthy. Marantic endocarditis with emboli (*i.e.*, nonbacterial thrombotic endocarditis) occurs predominantly in patients with adenocarcinoma, especially of the lung, and may present neurologically as multifocal abnormalities, focal abnormalities or progressive encephalopathy without any focal deficits.[221,224] Hemorrhage is seen most often in the leukemias, especially acute nonlymphocytic leukemia.[222] Fungi are the most frequent cause of septic emboli. Paraneoplastic thrombosis of cerebral venous structures, a part of the hypercoagulable state associated with malignancy, produces headaches, followed by the abrupt onset of CNS dysfunction.[225] This may include motor abnormalities, sensory complaints, vision and speech abnormalities, rapid mental deterioration, and seizures. The diagnosis is made by angiography. Angioendotheliosis may be another neurologic paraneoplastic syndrome associated with vascular disease produced by endothelial cell proliferation and causing silent strokes and dementia.[226-229]

Paraneoplastic syndromes or remote effects of tumors on the CNS are uncommon, although the incidence varies considerably in different reports. Croft and Wilkinson found neuromyopathies in 7% of 1476 cancer patients; lung cancers were the most frequent.[18] Brody, however, found no difference in the frequency of neurologic syndromes between patients with lung cancer and controls with chronic lung disease.[19] Some specific neurologic syndromes occur exclusively or with much higher frequency in cancer patients. The patient with no known cancer who develops one of these syndromes should alert the physician to suspect an occult cancer, and a full evaluation for cancer is warranted. These syndromes include subacute cerebellar degeneration, subacute motor neuropathy, dermatomyositis in older men, Eaton-Lambert syndrome, and dorsal root ganglionitis. If a patient not known to have cancer develops a neurologic syndrome less often associated with malignancy, a careful history and physical examination should be performed, but exhaustive laboratory and radiologic searches for tumor are not indicated (Table 57–11). In these instances and for a highly suspect syndrome with negative evaluation result, careful patient follow-up is required.

Most paraneoplastic syndromes run a course parallel to the underlying tumor. This is less often the case in neurologic paraneoplastic syndrome, in which the course of the neurologic abnormalities is frequently independent of the underlying tumor. In many instances, this can be attributed to the inability of the nervous tissue to divide and repair damage. In some instances, such as the myasthenic syndrome and polymyositis, cases of a parallel course of tumor and syndrome have been documented.

Many neurologic paraneoplastic syndromes are produced by "autoimmune" immunologic reactions, in which the tumor shares antigens with normal nervous tissue.[230–232] The host immune response to the tumor then produces immunologic damage of the nervous system. Evidence suggests that subacute cerebellar degeneration, optic neuritis, sensory carcinomatous neuropathy, and the Eaton-Lambert syndrome may be caused by immunologic cross-reactions.[12–15,233,238,245,272] The antineuronal antibodies may have diagnostic and therapeutic implications. In a large series, Moll and colleagues reported finding antineuronal antibodies in 38% of patients with paraneoplastic syndromes with a high specificity (98.6%).[233a] The sensitivity may increase as other antibody-antigen reagents are used. Plasmapheresis has been used to remove the antibodies from the serum or cerebrospinal fluid.[233b] Only limited success was reported, and treatment of the tumor remains the primary approach.

Numerous neurologic syndromes have been described. For convenience they are listed in Table 57–11, which is divided by area within the nervous system.

REMOTE EFFECTS ON THE CEREBRUM AND CRANIAL NERVES

Remote paraneoplastic syndromes involving the brain and cranial nerves are less common than those involving other areas of the neuraxis. In one large series involving 1476 cancer patients, only 162 had neurologic abnormalities, and of these, only 15 had lesions of the brain.[18] These 15 had subacute cerebellar degeneration, which is one of the syndromes with a strong association with malignancy.

Subacute cerebellar degeneration is commonly associated with lung cancer, but many other tumor types have been described. It is characterized by a subacute and progressive, bilateral, symmetric cerebellar failure with ataxia, dysarthria, hypotonia, and pendular reflexes.[234–238e] Dementia may occur. Frequently present are a cerebrospinal fluid lymphocytosis and elevated protein levels. Pathologically, there is atrophy with loss of Purkinje cells.

Paraneoplastic cerebellar degeneration is one of the neurologic syndromes caused by antineuronal antibodies.[12,238a–d] These antibodies were reported to be specific for Purkinje cells, but they may react with other neurons. The anti-Yo antibody described in patients with gynecologic cancers reacts with antigens of 62-kd and 34-kd. The gene encoding the 34-kd antigen was cloned and shown to be a leucine-zipper DNA-binding protein, which may play a role in gene expression. Another antibody was shown to react with a 51-kd antigen whose gene was cloned and was unique and separate from the anti-Yo 34-kd protein. Another group isolated an antibody that reacts with the repeat hexapepticle Phe-Leu-Glu-Asp-Val-Asp. This hexapepticle is almost identical to the sequence in α_2-macroglobulin and α_1-trypsin inhibitor. This led to speculation that the presence of these antibodies may confer a better outcome. Improvement in paraneoplastic cerebellar degeneration was observed after removal of the primary tumor, corticosteroid administration, plasmapheresis, and effective therapy of Hodgkin's disease.

Dementia is probably the most frequent cerebral abnormality in cancer patients. Because it is also frequent in the general population, its association with malignancy is attenuated. Dementia is often associated with abnormalities in other areas of the nervous system. The electroencephalograph shows generalized slowing, and a cerebrospinal fluid pleocytosis may exist. In some instances, rapid-onset dementia may be caused by angioendotheliomatosis. This syndrome is a proliferative disorder of endothelial cells of blood vessels and may produce a clinical picture of multiple infarct dementia with edema.[226–228] It has been described as a primary endothelial disorder, perhaps even malignant. More likely, it is produced by tumor secretion of an angiogenic peptide.[228,229] Angiogenic peptides include fibroblast growth factors (acidic and basic), tumor necrosis factor, transforming growth factors-α and -β, and IL-1β. Acidic fibroblast growth factor and IL-1β are quite homologous. The syndrome has responded to high-dose steroids, chemotherapeutic agents, and radiation.

Limbic encephalitis is characterized by a progressive dementia associated with degenerative changes in the hippocampus and amygdaloid nuclei. Pathologically, there are inflammatory and degenerative changes. The cerebrospinal fluid may be normal or show a pleocytosis. In one case, magnetic resonance (MR) imaging showed signal abnormalities in the medial portions of both temporal lobes, the amygdaloid nuclei, and the hypothalamus. An MR-guided biopsy confirmed the presence of encephalitis.[243a] The syndrome does not appear to improve with removal of the primary tumor and did not improve after resection of primary lung tumors; it has been reported to improve after successful chemotherapy for small cell lung cancer, Hodgkin's disease, and testicular cancer.[241–243] Viral and immunologic causes have been postulated.

Optic neuritis is characterized by scotomas, decreased vision, and papilledema, which may be unilateral or bilateral. Pathologically, demyelination is found. This syndrome is related to the visual paraneoplastic syndrome characterized by binocular loss of vision in patients with small cell lung cancer.[13,245,246] The triad of photosensitivity, ring scotomatous

TABLE 57–11. Paraneoplastic Syndromes of the Nervous System

Site	*Syndrome*	*Investigations*	*Clinical Features*	*Associated Neoplasms*	*Comments*
Brain	Subacute cerebellar degeneration*	Brain[234] Paone[235] Victor[236] Steven[237] Greenlee[12] Dropcho[238] Furneaux[238a] Shaykh[238b] Duncan[238c] Sakai[238d]	Subacute, progressive, bilateral, symmetric, cerebellar failure often with dementia, dysarthria, CSF lymphocytosis, and elevated protein	Lung Prostate Colorectal Ovary Cervix Hodgkin's Other	Some reports of improvements with removal of primary tumor; no other known treatment; caused by specific anti-Purkinje cell antibodies
	Dementia	Shapiro[239] Dorfman[240]	Variable presentation, acute to slowly progressive; often associated with abnormalities in other areas of the neuraxis; EEG shows slowing; CSF pleocytosis sometimes seen	Lung	Relatively common (30–40%)
	Limbic encephalitis	Corsellis[241] Dorfman[240] Brennan[242] Carr[293] Lacomis[243a] Burton[243b]	Dementia with degenerative changes in the hippocampus and amygdaloid nuclei; often associated with inflammatory and degenerative lesions in other areas of the neuraxis	Lung Hodgkin's Testicular Other	May or may not improve with removal of primary tumor (Ophelia syndrome); MRI may be useful for diagnosis
	Optic neuritis/visual retinopathy	Sawyer[244] Grunwald[13,245] Pillay[246] Thirkill[246a] Jacobson[246b]	Decrease in vision, photosensitivity, ring scotomatous field loss, attenuated retinal arteriole caliber, papilledema; unilateral or bilateral	Small-cell lung cancer	Rare; produced by antiretinal antibodies; improves after immunosuppressive therapy
	Opsoclonus/ataxia	Lugue[246c]	Eye movement disorder (opsoclonus) and ataxia	Breast Gynecologic	Produced by anti-Ri antibody
	Progressive multifocal leukoencephalopathy	Padgett[247] Richardson[16] Weiner[17]	Dementia, paralysis, aphasia, ataxia, dysarthria, visual field defects, blindness, coma, seizures; demyelination of white matter; CSF often normal; death usually rapid	Leukemias, lymphomas, sarcomas, other	Caused by papova viruses of 2 types: JC virus or SV-40-like virus
	Angioendotheliosis	Petito[227] Person[226] Gallego[228] Folkman[229]	Rapid onset of multiple infarct dementia; CT/MRI findings consistent with multiple strokes	Lymphomas, other	Not proved; may be caused by angiogenic peptides
Spinal cord	Amyotropic lateral sclerosis (ALS)	Norris and Engel[248]	Upper and lower motoneuron disease with spasticity, extensor plantar responses, wasting, and fasciculations		Syndrome similar to that in patients without cancer but sometimes progresses more slowly; cancer found in 10% of ALS patients in one report, but others find cancer less frequently
	Subacute necrotic myelopathy	Mancall[249] Handforth[250] Dansey[250a]	Rapid ascending motor and sensory paralysis to thoracic level; elevated CSF protein	Lung Kidney Hodgkin's	Severe tissue destruction of grey and white matter

(continued)

TABLE 57-11. *(Continued)*

Site	*Syndrome*	*Investigations*	*Clinical Features*	*Associated Neoplasms*	*Comments*
	Subacute motor neuropathy*	Walton[251]	Slowly developing lower motoneuron weakness without sensory changes; most often in irradiated patients with lymphoma	Lymphoma	No known treatment; occasional spontaneous recovery; ? viral origin
Peripheral nerves	Sensory neuropathy*	Horwich[252] Henson[253] Graus[14]	Subacute onset of sensory loss including deep tendon reflexes, with normal strength and normal motor conduction velocity; elevated CSF protein	Lung Other	Uncommon, also called dorsal root ganglionitis may be caused by antineuronal antibody
	Sensorimotor peripheral neuropathy	Croft[254] Dayan[255] Newman[256] Victor[257] Forman[257a]	Distal weakness and wasting, areflexia, distal sensory loss; elevated CSF protein; single-fiber electromyography may help in diagnosis	Lung GI Breast Other	Quite common; recovery rare even with removal of primary tumor
	Ascending acute polyneuropathy (Guillian–Barré)	Lisak[258]	Bilateral, usually symmetric weakness (flaccid), usually beginning in lower extremities and ascending; sensory symptoms and signs usually develop as well; elevated CSF protein	Lymphoma	Association not definite
	Autonomic and gastrointestinal neuropathy	Schuffer[259] Siemsen[260] Park[261] Ahmed[262] Ogilvie[263]	Orthostatic hypotension; neurogenic bladder; intestinal pseudo-obstruction	Lung (small cell)	Many cases of Ogilvie's syndrome (colonic pseudo-obstruction) may be paraneoplastic
Muscle and neuromuscular junction	Dermatomyositis and polymyositis*	DeVere[264] Barnes[265] Williams[266] Sigurgeirsson[266a]	Progressive muscle weakness developing gradually over weeks to months (proximal > distal); usually not disabling; elevated muscle enzymes and sedimentation rate	Lung Stomach Ovary Other	Stringent association in older males; less frequent in colorectal tumors
	Myasthenic syndrome* (Eaton-Lambert syndrome)	Lambert[267,268] Simpson[269] Cherrington[270] Jenkyn[271] Fukunaga[15] Login[272] McEvoy[272a]	Weakness and fatigability of proximal muscles, especially pelvic girdle and thigh; dryness of mouth; dyspagia, dysarthria, and peripheral paresthesias common; EMGs show a facilitated response in active muscles	Lung (small cell) Stomach Ovary Other	Poor response to Tensilon; should respond to therapy of primary tumor; guanidine and 3,4-diaminopyridine may also be useful
	Myasthenia gravis	Tyler[273]	Weakness with predilection for ocular and cranial muscles, tendency for fluctuation and partial reversibility by cholinergic drugs	Thymoma Lymphomas Breast Other	Except for thymoma, association not proved

* These syndromes are so strongly associated with malignancy that a thorough investigation for malignancy is indicated when they develop in patients not known to have cancer.

visual field loss, and attenuated arteriole caliber were reported.[246a] There is specific loss of retinal ganglion cells and their processes due to immune deposits of antibodies that react with antigens shared by normal retinal and small cell lung cancer cells.[246d]

A syndrome of opsoclonus (eye movement disorder) and ataxia in patients with breast cancer and gynecologic cancers was reported.[246c] Opsoclonus can be diagnosed at the bedside by the presence of spontaneous, large amplitude conjugate saccades occurring in all directions of gaze without a saccadic interval. An antibody called anti-Ri was found in these patients.

Progressive multifocal leukoencephalopathy is included in this section, although multiple areas of the neuraxis are involved and it is not a true paraneoplastic syndrome because a viral cause has been established. The syndrome is characterized by dementia, paralysis, aphasia, ataxia, dysarthria, visual field defects, blindness, and sometimes coma or seizures. It usually is rapidly progressive, with death occurring within 6 months. The cerebrospinal fluid is usually normal. This syndrome occurs most often in malignancies associated with impaired immunity (*e.g.*, leukemias, lymphomas) but also occurs in many benign conditions with altered immunity (*e.g.*, sarcoidosis, steroid therapy). Pathologically, demyelination of white matter is found throughout the nervous system. Evidence suggests the illness is caused by one or two types of papovavirus.[17,247]

REMOTE EFFECTS INVOLVING THE SPINAL CORD

In the large series of Croft and Wilkinson, paraneoplastic syndromes primarily involving the spinal cord accounted for only 9% of all nervous system syndromes.[18] From a different perspective, Norris and Engel reported that 10% of 130 patients with amyotrophic lateral sclerosis (ALS) had underlying malignancies.[248]

ALS is characterized by widespread lower motor neuron muscle weakness, atrophy, spasticity, hyperreflexia, extensor plantar responses, and fasciculations. If associated with cancer, the sex distribution is predominantly male, and the age is older. The course of ALS may progress more slowly in cancer patients. Despite the report of Norris and Engel, many observers feel that far fewer than 10% of ALS patients have underlying cancers.[248]

Subacute necrotic myelopathy is characterized by a rapidly ascending motor and sensory paralysis, which is most severe in the thoracic region. It usually terminates in death in a matter of days or weeks. There are often degenerative lesions in other areas of gray and white matter. The cerebrospinal fluid protein level usually is elevated. In one case of Hodgkin's disease, an elevated cerebrospinal fluid level of B_2-microglobulin was reported. The syndrome improved, and the cerebrospinal fluid B_2-microglobulin level decreased after treatment with intrathecal corticosteroids.[250a] The syndrome is most often associated with lung cancer, but other tumors have been reported.

Subacute motor neuropathy is strongly associated with malignancy, particularly the lymphomas. It is characterized by slowly developing but progressive lower motor weakness without sensory changes. It occurs most often in irradiated patients. Although the course often progresses slowly, it may wax and wane, and there may be spontaneous recovery. A viral cause has been speculated.

REMOTE EFFECTS ON THE PERIPHERAL NERVOUS SYSTEM

Paraneoplastic syndromes involving the peripheral nerves are the most frequent site in the nervous system. The association was first reported in the late 1800s, and several reports appeared in the late 1940s and early 1950s. A large series was reported by Croft and Wilkinson in 1965, who divided these neuropathies into two groups: a symmetric sensory peripheral neuropathy that usually developed late in the course of the neoplasm and an acute or subacute severe sensory motor neuropathy that often progresses to paralysis before other signs of malignancy.[18] The cerebrospinal fluid protein often is elevated in these syndromes. Single-fiber electromyography may be useful for diagnosis.[257a] The neurologic abnormalities may wax and wane, and steroids are occasionally associated with clinical improvement. In one small cell lung cancer patient for whom combined therapy with chemoradiotherapy and plasma exchange was used, neurologic recovery occurred.[257b] However, surgical removal of the tumor rarely leads to improvement. The syndrome has been reported with a wide variety of neoplasms, most commonly lung cancer.[273]

Pure sensory neuropathy associated with degeneration of dorsal root ganglia (*i.e.*, dorsal root ganglionitis) is strongly associated with malignancy. In most instances, the tumor is located in the chest (*e.g.*, lung cancer, thymoma, lymphomas involving the mediastinum, laryngeal or esophageal carcinomas). The syndrome is characterized by the subacute development of distal sensory loss, especially proprioception, and loss of deep tendon reflexes with normal muscle strength. Motor nerve conduction velocities are normal. The cerebrospinal fluid protein often is elevated. The illness usually precedes the development of cancer, leaves the patient severely disabled, and rarely improves. An immunologic mechanism has been postulated for these sensory neuropathies because organ-specific antibrain antibodies have been reported in sera and cerebrospinal fluid.[14] In 1 patient with a plasma cell dyscrasia and peripheral neuropathy, pathologic and immunologic studies indicated that an IgM κ-antibody directed against peripheral nerve myelin produced the neuropathy.[274]

Ascending acute polyneuropathy (*i.e.*, Guillain-Barré syndrome) has been reported in some patients with malignancy, particularly Hodgkin's disease and malignant lymphomas.[233] The syndrome has been clinically similar to that found in patients without malignancy. Because both are relatively common and parallel clinical courses have not been demonstrated, the association may be coincidental. Autonomic neuropathy has been associated most commonly with lung cancer, usually small cell lung cancer.[259,263] The most frequently reported syndrome has been orthostatic hypotension. Neurogenic bladder, disordered peristalsis of the esophagus, stomach, and intestine, and intestinal pseudo-obstruction (*i.e.*, Olgivie's syndrome) have been reported. The neuropathologic findings in these cases have resembled those in other neurologic paraneoplastic syndromes with neuronal and axonal degeneration associated with infiltration by lymphocytes, plasma cells, and histiocytes.[259]

Peripheral nerve abnormalities may be found as a result of other phenomena associated with the cancer. For example, patients with multiple myeloma may have neuropathies secondary to amyloid deposition. Johnson and coworkers reported 3 patients who developed peripheral neuropathy (*i.e.*, mononeuritis multiplex) as a result of tumor-related vasculitis limited to the peripheral nervous system.[275] Neuropathies secondary to hemorrhage into the nerves have been reported in leukemic patients.

REMOTE EFFECTS ON MUSCLE AND NEUROMUSCULAR FUNCTION

Dermatomyositis and Polymyositis

In large series, 7% to 34% of patients with dermatomyositis or polymyositis also have cancer. The patients with these disorders have five to seven times the incidence of malignancy as the general population.[264,266] In a Swedish population-based study, the relative risk of cancer was 1.75 in patients with polymyositis and 2.9 in patients with dermatomyositis compared with the normal population.[266a] Both were statistically significant increases. It appears from these retrospective series that the association is most striking in men older than 50, of whom more than 70% have developed cancer.

The syndrome is characterized by gradually progressive muscle weakness occurring over weeks to months. The weakness eventually stabilizes and usually is not disabling. The weakness involves the proximal musculature. Reflexes usually are present but diminished. Muscle enzymes and sedimentation rate usually are elevated. The electromyogram tracing is abnormal, and muscle biopsies show muscle fiber necrosis with minimal inflammatory changes.

In most instances, the myopathy and cancer appear within 1 year of each other. In one long-term follow-up study, patients with dermatomyositis continued at risk for developing cancer for longer than 5 years.[266a] Most reported cases do not relate the temporal cause of the tumor and the dermatomyositis. Barnes was able to find 29 reports of improvement in tumor and dermatomyositis and seven reports of worsening of both in a review of 258 cases.[265] Steroids have been useful, although this is controversial, and there are no well-controlled therapeutic studies.

Myasthenic Syndrome

The myasthenic syndrome (*i.e.*, Eaton-Lambert syndrome) is uncommon but strongly associated with small cell undifferentiated bronchogenic carcinoma. The syndrome is characterized by muscle weakness and fatigue, which are most pronounced in the pelvic girdle and thigh, making it difficult to climb stairs or get out of a chair. Other features include dryness of mouth, dysarthria, dysphagia, blurred vision or diplopia, ptosis, paresthesias, and muscle pain. In contrast to true myasthenia gravis, muscle strength improves with exercise, and there is poor response to edrophonium (Tensilon). The electromyogram confirms the increase in muscle action potential with repeated nerve stimulation at rates faster than 10 per second. Most patients have lung cancer, particularly small cell lung cancer. Lambert and associates reported that fewer than 1% of all lung cancer patients, but 6% of all small cell lung cancer patients, have this syndrome.[267,268] In the authors' experience, these syndromes are infrequent in lung cancer patients. There are a few reports of the relation between response to antitumor therapy and improvement in the syndrome.[271] Recovery from the syndrome has been observed in patients with small cell lung cancer treated with combination chemotherapy. Because more than 90% of patients with small cell lung cancer respond to combination chemotherapy, this should be tried as a first measure. For patients failing chemotherapy or having no improvement in muscle strength with response to chemotherapy, guanidine and 3,4-diaminopyridine have been reported to be useful.[270] There are accumulating data that the Eaton-Lambert syndrome is an autoimmune condition. This is supported by the ability to transfer the syndrome to mice by the administration of immunoglobulin or purified IgG from patients' serum.[15] Studies suggest that IgG autoantibody inhibits acetylcholine release through a functional blockade of calcium channels.[272] Alternatively, the autoantibodies may induce excess production of acetylcholinesterase.[269]

Myasthenia Gravis

The association of myasthenia gravis and thymoma is well established. Several tumors including lymphomas, pancreas, breast, prostate, ovary, thyroid, cervix, kidney, rectum, and palate have been associated with myasthenia gravis, but many researchers conclude that the incidence is no greater than that expected in the normal population.[273]

HEMATOLOGIC MANIFESTATIONS OF MALIGNANCY

Abnormalities in all the hematopoietic cell lines and in the clotting proteins have been reported in cancer patients. As with the other paraneoplastic syndromes, these abnormalities are most often produced as a direct result of marrow infiltration by the tumor or its metastases. Infection and the toxic effects of cancer therapies are more common than true paraneoplastic effects. As our understanding of hormones and protein factors regulating hematopoiesis has increased in recent years with newer in vitro cell culture techniques, the mechanisms for hematologic paraneoplastic syndromes, particularly increases in cell numbers, appear to be caused by aberrant production of hematopoietic colony-stimulating factors.[6,7,270,276]

ERYTHROCYTOSIS

Common Forms

Tumor-associated erythrocytosis is well documented in the literature. In a review of 340 cases of tumor-associated erythrocytosis, 35% were hypernephromas, 14% were benign renal problems (*e.g.*, cystic kidneys, hydronephrosis), 3% were other tumors involving the kidney (*e.g.*, Wilms' tumor, hemangioma, adenomas, sarcomas), 19% were hepatomas, 15% were cerebellar hemangioblastomas, 7% were uterine fibroids (often aldosterone-secreting adenomas), 3% were adrenal (often aldosterone-secreting adenomas) tumors and pheochromocytomas, and 3% were miscellaneous tumors (*e.g.*, ovary, lung, thymus).[277] Overall, 53% of cases had some renal involvement. About 1% to 5% of patients with renal tumors and 9% to 20% of patients with cerebellar hemangioblastomas have erythrocytosis.[278] The erythrocytosis usually regresses with removal of the primary tumor and recurs with tumor progression.[277]

Increased erythropoietin levels were found in 64% of the tumor extracts of cystic fluids tested, but no erythropoietin was detected in normal tissues. Elevated serum erythropoietin levels were found in 53% of patients. Although Wilms' tumor usually is not associated with erythrocytosis, elevated plasma erythropoietin levels have been found in patients without erythrocytosis, but the exact frequency of this is unknown.[277] All of this suggests that about half of certain tumors associated with erythrocytosis make erythropoietin.[277]

Erythropoietin normally is produced by the kidney but may be produced by the liver in anephric persons.[23] It is not surprising that certain renal and liver tumors may produce erythropoietin. Direct production of erythropoietin activity by human renal cell carcinomas in vitro has been demonstrated.[279] There are various mechanisms by which tumors could cause elevated erythropoietin levels: tumor production of erythropoietin; induction of local kidney or systemic hypoxia by tumor mass effect, vascular obstruction, or hypoxia; secretion by the tumor of a factor that stimulates the release of ectopic erythropoietin; and change in the metabolism of erythropoietin by the tumor.[277]

With renal cysts, local renal hypoxia is a likely cause, but most cases are probably a result of tumor production of erythropoietin.[277]

Other Mechanisms Generating Erythrocytosis in Cancer Patients

Because not all cancer patients with erythrocytosis have elevated tumor levels of erythropoietin, other mechanisms that cause erythrocytosis must exist. Adrenal cortical tumors and virilizing ovarian tumors can produce androgenic hormones with erythropoietic effects.[23] This may be the mechanism of erythrocytosis associated with Cushing's syndrome. Although pheochromocytomas and aldosterone-producing adrenal adenomas may cause erythrocytosis by this mechanism, the exact hormonal basis has not been defined.[277]

Another possible mechanism is tumor-produced prostaglandins, because prostaglandins enhance the effects of erythropoietin on erythroid differentiation.[23] This is likely because elevated prostaglandin levels associated with hypercalcemia usually were found in patients with renal tumors.[129,130] It would be interesting to consider a trial of indomethacin for cancer-associated erythrocytosis in patients without elevated erythropoietin levels.

By convention, erythrocytosis is diagnosed if there is increased red cell mass, usually associated with hematocrit values over 55% for a man and over 50% for a woman.[280] Elevated but lower hematocrits in the setting of appropriate tumors (*e.g.*, hypernephromas, hepatomas, CNS tumors) should alert suspicion of a paraneoplastic syndrome. The differential diagnosis of erythrocytosis includes the panmyelosis (all blood elements) and splenomegaly of polycythemia vera, stress polycythemia, arterial desaturation from many causes, a hemoglobinopathy with aberrant oxygen-binding features, and dehydration with hemoconcentration.[280] A physical examination, arterial Po_2 determination, a hemoglobin electrophoresis, and family history can resolve most of these. Demonstration of elevated erythropoietin in the blood would confirm the diagnosis, but this test is usually not performed because of the difficulty bioassay. If a tumor is evident, it is probably wise to rule out other causes of erythrocytosis; an intravenous pyelogram (looking for cysts or other benign abnormalities), careful pelvic examination (looking for fibroids), and neurologic examination for cerebellar signs should always be performed.

The erythrocytosis usually does not need treatment, and phlebotomy is rarely used.[277] Tumor resection is successful in controlling the erythrocytosis in more than 97% of resectable cases; this should be the primary approach.[277] There are no good data on the response of erythrocytosis to chemotherapy (*e.g.*, of a hepatoma). Because only half of the patients with resectable tumors had increased serum or tumor extract erythropoietin levels before surgery and because the erythrocytosis corrected with resection, nonerythropoietin-mediated tumor erythrocytosis should be treated primarily with resection, if possible.

ANEMIA ASSOCIATED WITH CANCER

Anemia occurs frequently in cancer patients. Various mechanisms may explain the anemias, including the anemia of chronic disease; bone marrow invasion; blood loss; marrow suppression by chemoradiotherapy; hypersplenism; immune hemolysis of warm and cold antibody types; megaloblastic anemia; vitamin and iron deficiency; microangiopathic hemolytic anemia; and pure red cell aplasia.[281–303] The reader is referred to other general hematologic sources for the general evaluation of anemia in cancer patients, but the mechanisms of anemia associated with cancer usually have not been elucidated.[281,282]

Anemia found in leukemias probably is not explained by "crowding out" of normal marrow.[281] For many patients, a good explanation of anemia cannot be found, and the diagnosis of anemia of chronic disease is given. Although this is easy to treat with transfusions, the cause is unknown and probably represents a remote effect of the tumor on bone marrow function, red cell metabolism, or cell kinetics. The anemia of chronic malignancy has no associated cancer types and is usually normocytic and normochromic or hypochromic states, with normal iron stores (but low serum iron levels and low total iron-binding capacity), normal reticulocyte count, normal red cell maturation, moderately increased erythropoiesis, and slightly shorter red cell survival.[281,283,284] New approaches to finding the mechanisms include study of red cell production in nude mice bearing human tumors associated with malignancy or cocultivation of in vitro erythropoiesis systems with human tumor cells.

Pure red aplasia with a severe anemia is associated with a variety of tumors, with about one half having thymomas.[285–287] A selective absence of marrow erythropoiesis occurs, and hypogammaglobulinemia may occur.[285,286] Reports of pure red cell aplasia associated with carcinomas have included gastric and breast adenocarcinomas, adenocarcinomas of unknown primary site, lung and skin squamous cell carcinomas, anaplastic lung cancers, and T-γ lymphoproliferative diseases.[288] In the latter cases, T-cell-mediated suppression of erythropoiesis was demonstrated, and the anemia improved after cyclophosphamide therapy. Many patients with and without thymomas have responded to cyclophosphamide therapy, and the mechanism of the aplasia may be through some T-lymphocyte-mediated system.

Megaloblastic anemia without folate or vitamin B_{12} deficiency is seen in the bone marrow of cancer patients before chemotherapy; this is unexplained. A macrocytic anemia of unknown origin occasionally is associated with multiple myeloma. The marrow is megaloblastic and the serum vitamin B_{12} levels low, but the patients fail to respond to B_{12}.[289]

Hypersplenic anemia with shortened erythrocyte survival probably is not a paraneoplastic syndrome because it usually occurs with myelofibrosis or, rarely, with a chronic granulocytic leukemia.[280] However, the cause of the fibrosis in the marrow and the spleen may be a humoral factor.

Autoimmune hemolytic anemias (AHA) associated with tumors usually are found with B-cell lymphoproliferative neoplasms.[290,292] The mechanisms by which the B-cell neoplasms upset the normal immunoregulatory circuits are unidentified. However, the monoclonal immunoglobulins produced by the B-cell neoplasms on their surface membranes probably are not themselves responsible for the hemolysis.

Rarely, AHA are associated with solid tumors. In a review of a large series of patients with AHA, only 2% had associated solid tumors.[296–298] In these cases, the mean age is 10 years older than in patients presenting with idiopathic AHA.[295] When AHA presents in the elderly, it is important to consider the possibility of an underlying carcinoma. A wide variety of tumor types are reported to be associated with AHA, including lung cancer of all histologic types, hypernephromas, ovarian, breast, stomach, uterine cervix, colon, and cecal cancer, seminoma, dermoid cysts of the ovary, and microcysts in adenomas of the pancreas.

In tumor-associated AHA, anemia is often the presenting symptom, with mean hemoglobin levels of 7.4 g/dl and frequent reticulocytosis. Splenomegaly is common. Response to corticosteroids is infrequent, in contrast to the high response seen in idiopathic AHA. However, successful treatment of the primary tumor with resection, radiation therapy, or chemotherapy usually leads to improvement or cure of the AHA.[295,300] In some cases, recurrent tumor was associated with recurrent AHA. Definitive tumor treatment should be the first approach, rather than corticosteroids or splenectomy. If this fails, splenectomy can be tried and does work in some patients. The two most likely causes are immune response to antigens shared by the tumor with erythrocytes (but exposed on the erythrocyte in a nonstimulating form) or attachment of immune complexes to erythrocytes. Evans' syndrome is characterized by the simultaneous occurrence of AHA and immune thrombocytopenia (ITP).[298,299] It occurs less often than AHA or ITP alone and has been observed with various carcinomas and lymphomas. The syndrome could be caused by cross-reacting antibodies, tumor production of autoantibodies, or tumor production of a substance altering erythrocytes and platelets, rendering them immunogenic to the host immune system.

Microangiopathic hemolytic anemia (MAHA) has been associated with 55 cancer patients in a comprehensive review.[301] By definition, the peripheral blood smear in MAHA contains fragmented erythrocyte forms.[302] Severe MAHA is rare in cancer patients, in one series occurring in only 8 of 3200 patients.[303] However, Antman and associates postulate that a careful search of the peripheral blood film for signs of microangiopathy (*e.g.*, schistocytosis) may uncover many more cases of a milder nature.[301] In the reported MAHA patients, the hemolysis was abrupt and severe, requiring several units of transfused blood daily to maintain a 20% hematocrit. The mean hemoglobin level was 7 g/dl, the mean percentage of nucleated erythrocytes was 30%, elevated bilirubin levels were found in 93%, and a leukoerythroblastic blood film was found in 35% of patients. The mean number of days from diagnosis of MAHA to death was 21 (range, 2–90 days). The Coombs' test result was always negative. Associated laboratory findings of disseminated intravascular coagulation (DIC) were found in 50% to 60%, and some of the patients had migratory thrombophlebitis. However, some of the patients with MAHA did not have signs of DIC.

Most of the tumors were mucin-producing adenocarcinomas; 55% were gastric cancer, 10% were of unknown primary (possibly gastric), and breast and lung accounted for 13% and 7%, respectively. The remainder were divided among prostate, ovary, pancreas, colon, hepatoma, cholangiocarcinoma, and seminal vesicle tumors.[301] Several of the gastric primaries were occult and found only at autopsy.

MAHA is easily diagnosed by the presence of a severe hemolytic anemia, with fragmented erythrocyte forms on the peripheral blood smear and a negative Coombs' test result. The causes of the MAHA syndrome represent various diseases associated with lesions of small blood vessels, including thrombotic thrombocytopenic purpura (TTP); congenital vascular abnormalities, such as the Kasabach-Merritt syndrome; hemolytic-uremic syndrome; DIC; malfunction at an aortic valve prosthesis; and neoplastic disease. The differentiating MAHA caused by neoplastic diseases from TTP or DIC may be impossible because TTP and DIC have been reported in association with malignancy.[304,305] The renal function of patients with MAHA associated with malignancy was not indicated but supposedly was not unusual.

Although heparin has been used to treat other causes of MAHA, particularly the hemolytic uremic syndrome, it appears ineffective when given alone in MAHA of neoplastic disease. In contrast, in 7 of 9 patients, the MAHA syndrome responded to hormonal anticancer therapy (for breast and prostate cancer) or chemotherapy.[301] However, if DIC is associated with MAHA, it would appear reasonable to treat with heparin to control the immediate DIC problem while instituting appropriate anticancer therapy, as is done in acute promyelocytic leukemia.[305]

The pathophysiology of MAHA associated with cancer may represent various causes of erythrocyte shearing, including fibrin strands from DIC; pulmonary intraluminal tumor emboli (31% of MAHA patients); and narrowing of pulmonary arterioles by intimal proliferation or a side effect of chemotherapy.[301] The presence of tumor emboli diffusely involving pulmonary arterioles occurs in about 1% of cancer patients.[301] Association of MAHA with gastric cancer may be explained by its tendency for widespread vascular metastasis and mucin production. Mucin can act as a procoagulant and potentially cause DIC. The occurrence of intimal proliferation is thought to cause pulmonary hypertension and increase the shearing force on the erythrocyte.[301]

GRANULOCYTOSIS ASSOCIATED WITH NONHEMATOLOGIC MALIGNANCIES

Elevation in the peripheral granulocyte count to more than 20,000/μl without overt infection or leukemia occurs in association with several neoplasms.[6,280,306–309] Monocyte elevation may be seen.[310] Neoplasms associated with a granulocytosis syndrome are gastric, lung, pancreas, melanoma, and brain tumors; Hodgkin's disease; and diffuse histiocytic lymphoma (*i.e.*, reticulum cell sarcoma).[280,311] The exact frequency in each histologic type is unknown, but many cases have been reported during the past 50 years.[280] The granulocytosis usually is asymptomatic and consists of mature neutrophils.[282]

Although there are many potential causes of neutrophilia in cancer patients (*e.g.*, infection, inflammatory disorders, drugs, metabolic disorders, physical and emotional stimuli), the major diagnostic problem for a persistently high neutrophil count is to differentiate it from coexistent chronic myelogenous leukemia (CML).[280] The major features differentiating a paraneoplastic "leukemoid reaction" in the cancer patient from CML are a leukocyte count less than 100,000/μl; no left shift to blast or progranulocytic forms; normal platelet and basophil levels; absent splenomegaly; elevated leukocyte alkaline phosphatase levels; normal serum B_{12} levels; and no Philadelphia chromosome.[282] After other disorders and coexistent CML are ruled out in cancer patients, a paraneoplastic granulocytosis is likely.

The mechanism behind tumor-associated granulocytosis is most often tumor production of a colony-stimulating factor (CSF).[282a] The colony-stimulating factors include granulocyte CSF (G-CSF), granulocyte-macrophage CSF (GM-CSF), macrophage CSF (M-CSF; CSF-1), interleukin-3 (IL-3), and interleukin-1 (IL-1).[276] The genes for these proteins have been cloned, and probes for DNA and RNA expression are available, as are antibodies to the factors. Future studies will establish exactly which protein is responsible for these syndromes. Prior studies were concluded before these tools were available. For example, Robinson tested the serum and urine of 12 patients with cancer and unexplained sustained granulocytosis for CSF activity using in vitro bone marrow culture assays.[306] In his series, there were five lung cancers (type unspecified), two melanomas, two adrenal cancers, an unknown primary, hepatoma, and multiple myeloma. He found elevated CSF levels in all of these patients, and the levels correlated with the degree of elevation of the peripheral neutrophil count. The two adrenal tumors did not make CSF in culture; the other tumors were not tested. Several laboratories have reported establishing cultures of human tumor cell lines of lung cancer (squamous), oral cavity (squamous), and fibrous histiocytoma, which produce large amounts of a CSF-like factor.[312–314] The activity can be demonstrated in marrow cultures in vitro, and after the human tumors are heterotransplanted, they cause neutrophilia in athymic nude mice.[312,313] Neutrophilia is frequent in Sweet's syndrome, characterized by pyrexia, neutrophilia, and painful cutaneous plaques.[315] It is likely that this syndrome is also caused by tumor production of a CSF, perhaps IL-1. There is no specific therapy for the granulocytosis other than to treat the underlying malignancy.[282] Paraneoplastic syndromes with hypercalcemia and granulocytosis were attributed to tumor production of IL-1, G-CSF, and parathyroid hormone-related protein.[315a]

GRANULOCYTOPENIA AS A PARANEOPLASTIC SYNDROME

Granulocytopenia associated with cancer usually is the result of chemotherapy, radiotherapy, other drugs, or severe infection.[311] Granulocytopenia rarely has been reported with thymomas and may have the same immunologic basis as pure red cell aplasia.[311] Neutropenia alone may develop with marrow involvement by carcinoma, lymphoma, myeloma, or leukemia, but a pancytopenia is more common.[371] With the exception of leukemia, the neutropenia usually is not life threatening. Despite the frequent involvement of the bone marrow with cancer, significant granulocytopenia unrelated to therapy must be uncommon in cancer patients. However, experimental evidence suggests that a paraneoplastic syndrome involving granulopoiesis may exist. When 10^5 normal bone marrow cells are plated in semisolid medium with CSF, 20 to 100 hematopoietic colonies (containing 40 or more cells) and five to ten times that number of "cluster" (aggregates of 3–40 cells) are found.[316] In contrast, when marrow from patients with acute leukemia, preleukemic states, and CML in blast transformation are plated, mainly clusters and only rare colonies are found, suggesting that the leukemic process may inhibit the activity of the exogenously added CSF in some unknown way. Similar findings occur with solid tumors.

McCarthy and coworkers studied 9 small cell lung cancer patients for bone marrow colony formation with CSF.[316] The marrows of 2 of these patients (1 with and 1 without small cell cancer marrow involvement) were not able to form colonies in agar but had large numbers of clusters with or without CSF. The patient with marrow involvement had neutrophilia, and the one without marrow involvement had neutropenia.[316] It is likely that some tumors may suppress granulopoiesis by interfering with the action of CSF on marrow progenitor cells. Neutropenia is associated with T-γ lymphoproliferative diseases.[317] It is thought that the abnormal T cells interfere directly with granulocyte production. Corticosteroids and alkylating agents have led to improvement in some patients.

EOSINOPHILIA AND BASOPHILIA ASSOCIATED WITH NEOPLASMS

Eosinophilia is associated with nonleukemic neoplasms, particularly Hodgkin's disease (in as many as 20% of cases) and mycosis fungoides, but it has been found with other lymphomas, melanoma, brain tumors, and other cancers. The exact frequency in these tumors is not documented.[280,311,318]

It is possible that the eosinophilia itself may be symptomatic if the cell count is sufficiently high and an allergic or Loeffler's-like syndrome (*i.e.*, fleeting nodular pulmonary infiltrates with eosinophilia [PIE syndrome], with mild cough, lassitude, and low-grade fever) is produced in cancer patients. A small peptide that acts as an eosinophilopoietin has been described, and the tumor cells may be producing or stimulating the secretion of this factor.[319] Slungaard and associates found that serum and tumor extracts from a patient with large cell bronchogenic carcinoma and eosinophilia markedly stimulated the growth of eosinophil colonies from human bone marrow.[320] The tumor-associated eosinophilopoietic factor was found to be a glycoprotein of M_r 45 kd.

Therapy should be directed against the tumor, particularly in cases of the malignant lymphomas that are potentially curable. If this does not work or if pulmonary symptoms are troublesome, a trial of corticosteroids could be given because this sometimes gives dramatic results in other forms of the PIE syndrome, but data for cancer patients are lacking.[318]

Eosinopenia as a tertiary result of tumor secretion of ACTH or other hormones is possible but should give no clinical symptoms. Basophilia commonly is associated with CML, myelofibrosis, and polycythemia vera, but it has not been reported with other malignancies, and there now is no recognized basophilic paraneoplastic syndrome.[280]

THROMBOCYTOSIS ASSOCIATED WITH CANCER

Thrombocytosis (platelet count $>400{,}000/\mu l$) is said to occur in as many as 30% to 40% of cancer patients.[321–323] The differential diagnosis of thrombocytosis in the cancer patient includes myeloproliferative disorders (which may represent a paraneoplastic syndrome); acute and chronic inflammatory disorders; acute hemorrhage, iron deficiency; hemolytic anemias; postsplenectomy and other surgical procedures; and responses to vincristine or epinephrine.[321] Thrombocytosis has been seen with carcinomas, leukemias, Hodgkin's disease, and non-Hodgkin's lymphomas; a fall in the platelet count is associated with a response to therapy.[282] Although not characterized, there is a "thrombopoietin" that regulates normal megakaryocyte production and maturation.[324] Patients with neoplasms and thrombocytosis should have serum and tumor levels of thrombopoietin assayed. Although platelet counts above 1×10^6 cells/μl may lead to thrombosis or hemorrhage, these are rarely seen associated with malignancy, and such symptoms do not appear to occur with any regularity with the thrombocytosis of malignancy. No specific treatment of the thrombocytosis is indicated, except to treat the underlying malignancy.

UNEXPLAINED THROMBOCYTOPENIA IN CANCER PATIENTS

Thrombocytopenia commonly is seen in cancer patients and usually is related to chemotherapy, radiotherapy, acute leukemia, or DIC. A syndrome resembling ITP occasionally is seen associated with malignancy.[325–330] This association is uncommon, and in one study of ITP, it represented 4% of 381 patients with otherwise unexplained thrombocytopenia; all of these patients had lymphomas.[326] In another evaluation of patients with ITP, 9 of 52 had cancer.[325]

The diagnosis of an ITP-like syndrome is made by finding thrombocytopenia without anemia and with normal or increased numbers of normal erythrocytes on a peripheral smear; no evidence of DIC; and no evidence of a drug-induced thrombocytopenia.[325] The types of neoplasms associated with this syndrome are Hodgkin's disease; chronic lymphocytic leukemia; non-Hodgkin's lymphoma; acute lymphoblastic leukemia; immunoblastic sarcomas; and carcinomas of the lung, breast, rectum, gallbladder, and testis.[283,284] The association with chronic lymphocytic leukemia and Hodgkin's disease is widely known, and the syndrome occurs in approximately 30% of patients with immunoblastic lymphadenopathy.[328–330] However, the association with other tumors is less widely recognized. The mean age of patients is older (54 years) than the mean age of patients with ITP alone. About 80% of patients are symptomatic, with bleeding, petechiae, or purpura. Most have platelet counts under $30{,}000/\mu l$.[325] Response of platelet counts to high-dose (60 mg/day) prednisone is common but transient. However, 6 of 10 patients had a complete and apparently permanent response to splenectomy.[325]

The syndrome is called ITP-like because the course is much like classic ITP, but an immune mechanism has not been demonstrated. In the future, studies of antiplatelet antibodies will have to be done with tests of antibody cross-reactivity with tumor cells. Most patients have been treated with splenectomy in addition to various antineoplastic therapies; the effect of tumor treatment alone on the thrombocytopenia is unknown.[325] Other causes of thrombocytopenia need to be excluded, particularly the use of thiazide diuretics and quinidine or the presence of DIC or severe infection. In thrombocytopenic patients receiving antineoplastic therapy, ITP-like syndromes should be considered. The clues are thrombocytopenia disproportionate to granulocytopenia, normal or increased numbers of marrow megakaryocytes, and a rapid fall in transfused platelets. This diagnosis should be remembered particularly in lymphoproliferative disorders. Therapy consists of platelet transfusions, initial corticosteroids, and then splenectomy. Because of the poor response to steroids and inconsistent response to treatment of the underlying malignancy, a reasonable approach is to take the patient directly to splenectomy after other causes of thrombocytopenia have been excluded.

Abnormalities of platelet function sometimes are associated with plasma cell dyscrasias and are thought to result from the interference of the monoclonal protein with platelet function.[292]

MIGRATORY THROMBOPHLEBITIS, DISSEMINATED INTRAVASCULAR COAGULATION, AND NONBACTERIAL THROMBOTIC ENDOCARDITIS

Hemorrhage, thrombotic, and embolic complications occur frequently in cancer patients.[304,305,331] These may arise from a variety of specific mechanisms, including treatment-related thrombocytopenia, local tissue disruption from tumor or therapy, infection, vitamin deficiency, liver disease, circulating anticoagulants, and DIC. Usually, there is no specific cause, and successful therapy of the underlying malignancy alleviates the problem. The clinical association between cancer and thrombophlebitis was first observed by Trousseau.[332] In 1949, Marder and colleagues reported afibrinogenemia in metastatic prostate cancer.[333] Other abnormalities in clotting characteristics, frank DIC, and nonbacterial thrombotic endocarditis (NBTE) were later recognized to occur with greater than expected frequency in patients with cancer.[334–352] Sack and coworkers recognized that thrombophlebitis, DIC, coagulation abnormalities, and NBTE often occurred in the same patient and that each was part of a spectrum of the hypercoagulable state in cancer.[304] Many theories on mechanisms of activation of the coagulation system have been postulated and are reviewed by Rickles and Edwards.[349]

Thrombophlebitis

The incidence of clinical episodes of thrombophlebitis in cancer patients varies from 1% to 11%, and the incidence has been even higher in autopsy studies.[334] Many years ago, Trousseau recognized that cancer patients frequently have multiple episodes of thrombophlebitis and that these often occurred in veins in which deep venous thromboses were uncommon.[332] This syndrome of migratory thrombophlebitis is referred to as Trousseau's syndrome, a syndrome that he developed after its description. Migratory thrombophlebitis may occur before or after malignancy is documented. Like many paraneoplastic syndromes, its presence should lead to an investigation for occult cancer. For patients presenting with a deep venous thrombosis, one series showed that patients subsequently shown to have cancer were older, had lower hemoglobin levels, and had higher eosinophil counts than patients who did not develop cancer.[352] These factors can be used to select patients for a workup for occult cancer.

Mucin-secreting adenocarcinomas of the gastrointestinal tract most frequently are associated with migratory thrombophlebitis, but lung, breast, ovarian, prostate, and other tumors also are associated.[349] Although the greatest risk may be associated with pancreatic cancer (a prevalence of up to 57% or 50 times higher than control subjects with chronic pancreatitis), lung cancer is the most common association because of its greater prevalence. The treatment of migratory thrombophlebitis usually is difficult; acute episodes require heparin therapy. Long-term therapy with warfarin generally is unsuccessful, and extended subcutaneous heparin therapy has met with only limited success.[304,353] Treatment of the underlying malignancy is the mainstay of treatment.

Coagulation Abnormalities and Disseminated Intravascular Coagulation

DIC may present as a chronic coagulation disorder, usually of a thrombotic nature as an acute hemorrhage diathesis, or as a coagulation abnormality detected by laboratory tests alone (Table 57–12).[304,305,331–342,354] Abnormalities of routine blood coagulation tests have been reported in as many as 92% of cancer patients.[349] The most common abnormalities are elevated levels of fibrin or fibrinogen degradation products, thrombocytosis, and hyperfibrinogenemia.[349] These abnormalities are consistent with overcompensated intravascular coagulation with fibrinolysis. The low-grade coagulation with accelerated factor use may be accompanied by increased synthesis rates for fibrinogen, clotting factors, and platelets, resulting in actual increases in their circulating levels. Overt DIC with consumption of platelets and clotting factors and resultant bleeding is rare. The most commonly associated neoplasms are acute promyelocytic leukemia and adenocarcinomas.[349] The DIC may be exacerbated in patients with acute promyelocytic leukemia after treatment with cytotoxic agents.

For cancer patients suspected of having DIC or other

TABLE 57–12. Frequency of Different Cancer Types Associated With Disseminated Intravascular Coagulopathy

		*% of Tumors Making Up Various DIC Series**	
Tumor Type	*Chronic DIC (n = 213)*[304]	*Bleeding Disorder (n = 134)*[305]	*Coagulation Abnormality (n = 86)*[354]
Pancreas	24	2	0
Lung	20	1.5	12
Prostate	13	18	8
Stomach	12	4	0
Acute leukemia	9	64	19
Colon	5	0.7	6
Unknown primary	5	0	0
Ovary	4	0.7	1
Gallbladder (cholangiocarcinoma)	4	0.7	2
Lymphomas	1	1.5	16
Breast	0.5	0	10
Melanomas	0.5	0	3
Miscellaneous others	3	3	10

* Some of the cases in refs. 304 and 305 may overlap. The data in ref. 304 were obtained from a literature review from 1960–1970 looking for the association of malignancy and thrombophlebitis, hemorrhagic diathesis, DIC, arterial embolism, or nonbacterial thrombotic endocarditis. The data in ref. 305 are based on a literature review to find cases to permit a tentative diagnosis of DIC. The data in ref. 354 come from review of the coagulation laboratory and medical records from 1971–1974 at the Memorial Sloan-Kettering Cancer Center looking for laboratory evidence of DIC.

thrombotic or hemorrhagic phenomena, Sack and coworkers stressed the need for sequential monitoring of coagulation tests and the striking decreases that occurred in fibrinogen and platelet levels associated with the acute vascular events.[304] They postulated that this was due to a shift from a "compensated" to a "decompensated" coagulation status engendered by the tumor.[304] Although the thrombotic events of chronic DIC are clearly related to the coagulation disorder, the relation is not so clear for the multiple organ system dysfunction seen in acute (often hemorrhagic) DIC.[305] The situations that appear most related to DIC are the adult respiratory distress syndrome; oliguric renal insufficiency with gram-negative sepsis, and the hemolytic-uremic syndrome; neurologic syndromes related to intracranial bleeding and thrombosis; pulmonary hemorrhage syndrome; and the infarcted skin of purpura fulminans.[305] Autopsy studies show DIC usually contributes strongly to patient morbidity and mortality, particularly with thrombosis or bleeding in the lung, CNS, or gastrointestinal tract.[305]

MANAGEMENT OF DISSEMINATED INTRAVASCULAR COAGULATION IN MALIGNANCY. There is universal agreement that identification and treatment of all precipitating factors is the keystone to DIC management.[260,293] This should include not only treatment of cancer, but evaluation of patients with DIC for other precipitating factors (*e.g.*, sepsis, volume deficit, hypotension, hypoxemia, acidosis, fungus infection, transfusion reactions, vessel manipulation). Other hemostatic deficits should be identified and corrected. A response of the malignancy to tumor treatment often is associated with response of the DIC, and the long-term goal is appropriate antineoplastic therapy.[304,347]

A major controversy is whether heparin should be used.[305,335] There is a tendency to use heparin more in DIC with thrombotic, thromboembolic, or necrotizing complications, as is often seen in the chronic DIC of malignancy.[305,306] However, randomized trials of heparin therapy in the DIC of malignancy have not been conducted. After the association between DIC and acute promyelocytic leukemia (APL) was established, Gralnick and associates showed that heparin could improve the coagulation abnormalities.[336] Subsequently, nonrandomized trials suggested that heparin should be used prophylactically in all APL patients.[341,342] Later studies suggest heparin need not be given to all patients.[343] The liberal use of fresh-frozen plasma and platelets was suggested by the researchers. Until randomized trials are conducted, coagulation values should be monitored closely in APL patients. Heparin should be considered if there is overt bleeding or a change in laboratory evaluations.

Sack and associates, in their review of the literature on chronic DIC in malignancy, found positive responses to anticoagulant therapy (defined as cessation of signs or symptoms of thrombophlebitis, hemorrhage, or arterial emboli) in 65% of 55 patients treated with heparin initially and 33% of 26 patients treated with heparin after failing warfarin therapy.[304] Only 19% of 32 patients treated with warfarin alone responded. In addition, 53% of 36 patients had recurrence of symptoms of the thrombotic-hemorrhage disorder after the heparin was stopped, suggesting a therapeutic role of heparin in control of the DIC. Table 57–13 summarizes the results of anticoagulant and antineoplastic therapy in the treatment of the chronic DIC of malignancy. All combinations of antineoplastic and anticoagulant therapy were associated with response of the DIC symptoms in more than half of the cases, but only 10% to 20% of patients had long-term control, presumably reflecting the lack of control of the underlying tumor. Although in many patients the temporal correlation of heparin therapy with cessation of DIC is persuasive, spontaneous remission of DIC occurring with persistent cancer has been reported.[348]

After DIC associated with malignancy is diagnosed and other factors corrected, it is wise to establish the tempo of the DIC. If the DIC is acute with life-threatening symptoms (*e.g.*, uncontrolled bleeding) or if it is chronic and the symptoms debilitating (*e.g.*, recurrent thromboembolic lesions), a trial of heparin therapy should be given. The doses used in the literature range from 300 to 600 U/kg per 4 hours. Bell and associates showed that heparin prevented thrombotic events in several patients and that sudden catastrophic events occurred when it was discontinued.[353] They recommended continuous intravenous heparin (administered by an external pump connected to an indwelling catheter) if the heparin requirements (to maintain the PTT at 1.5 to 2 times normal) exceed 40,000 U/day. Otherwise, intermittent subcutaneous or intravenous (every 6–8 hours) heparin was satisfactory. After heparin therapy has begun, the repletion of coagulation factors with platelets, cryoprecipitates, and whole blood can be used, particularly in highly symptomatic, hemorrhagic,

TABLE 57–13. Treatment of Chronic Disseminated Intravascular Coagulopathy in Malignancy

Treatment Given		*No. of Patients*	*% Response**	
Antineoplastic	*Anticoagulant†*		*Short-Term*	*Long-Term*
+	+	27	52	15
+	−	22	55	18
−	+	48	60	10
+	+	12‡	75	?

* Data from ref. 304. Response is defined as cessation of signs or symptoms of thrombophlebitis, hemorrhage, or arterial emboli. Long-term indicates for over 250 days or until death.
† In most cases, the anticoagulant therapy was heparin; 81 of 87 patients reported for anticoagulant response received heparin.
‡ Patients with recurrent DIC after stopping heparin therapy were again given heparin.

acute DIC.[305] Although heparin treatment may be maintained for weeks, it is only a temporary measure, and control of the underlying malignancy affords the only long-term control of chronic DIC.

NONBACTERIAL THROMBOTIC ENDOCARDITIS

NBTE, another cause of thrombotic or hemorrhagic complications, may occur with or without DIC and is characterized by the presence of sterile verrucous, bland, fibrin-platelet lesions in the left-side heart valves.[221,304,344–346] Patients often present with emboli to the brain and to other organs. The brain emboli may have an abrupt or a gradual onset of neurologic symptoms with development of focal neurologic deficits or diffuse abnormalities such as confusion, disorientation, generalized seizure, or disturbances in consciousness. Neurologic signs are often the only evidence of thromboembolism.[224] For these patients cerebral angiography showing multiple arterial occlusions is the definitive diagnostic test.[224] Only one third or fewer of the patients have heart murmurs, usually systolic. Patients are usually afebrile, but all patients should have blood cultures if emboli are suspected. Echocardiography may be of diagnostic use for vegetations larger than 2 mm, but most lesions are smaller and are not detected by echocardiography. Arterial emboli can go to the CNS, heart, spleen, kidneys, and peripheral sites. Occlusion of large and small vessels is detected pathologically in the brain. Myocardial infarction can result from emboli to coronary arteries.[344,345] Paraneoplastic endocarditis can present with early malignancy or in later stages and does not mean incurability.[346]

In Rosen's series, the autopsy incidence of NBTE in patients with adenocarcinoma of the lung (7.5%) was twice that of adenocarcinomas of the prostate or pancreas (3–4%) and more than seven times that of other solid tumors, lymphomas, or leukemias.[350] In Goodnight's review of NBTE, bleeding frequently was found in the skin (77–100%), CNS (22–49%), genitourinary tract (38–42%), eye, ear, nose, and mouth (31–47%), and gastrointestinal (24–56%) and respiratory (20–31%) tracts in leukemias and solid tumor patients, respectively.[334] Of the leukemias and solid tumor patients, 37% had autopsy evidence of fibrin thrombi, but only 1% had evidence of NBTE.

The principles of treating NBTE are similar to those in treating other aspects of the hypercoagulable state. Treatment of the underlying malignancy is the primary therapy. In anecdotal cases, warfarin has been unsuccessful; heparin has been used with limited success. There are no studies reporting the use of antiplatelet drugs or fibrinolytic agents.

RENAL MANIFESTATIONS OF MALIGNANCY

Numerous problems involving the kidneys develop in patients with malignancies. The causes of these complications are listed in Table 57–14. In most instances, the renal abnormalities are not paraneoplastic in origin. Only the glomerular lesions and obstruction by tumor products can be considered to be true paraneoplastic syndromes.

Massive proteinuria with the nephrotic syndrome is the major consequence of these paraneoplastic glomerular lesions, although renal failure may develop later. In patients with malignancy, the nephrotic syndrome may develop as a result of neoplastic infiltration of the kidneys, renal vein thrombosis, or amyloid infiltration. Besides these established causes of the nephrotic syndrome, there does seem to be a true paraneoplastic syndrome. Until 1966, there were only a few scattered case reports of an association between idiopathic nephrotic syndrome and malignancy. In 1966, Lee and associates reported that among 101 patients with the nephrotic syndrome of unknown cause, 11 were found to have cancer.[355] The neoplastic syndrome preceded discovery of the cancer in 7 of these 11 patients, who were all over the age of 40. Since that time, the nephrotic syndrome has been associated with several cancers, although recent studies suggest the incidence is lower than that reported by Lee and associates.[356]

TABLE 57–14. Differential Diagnosis of Renal Abnormalities in Patients With Malignancy

Direct infiltration of the kidney by tumor
Obstruction of the urinary tract by tumor
Electrolyte imbalances, many of which are caused by the tumor or its treatment (*e.g.*, calcium, uric acid, potassium)
Fluid imbalances induced by the tumor or its treatment (prerenal)
Infection
Toxicity of therapy (chemotherapy, radiotherapy, immunotherapy, antibiotics)
Glomerular lesions of uncertain cause (usually associated with nephrotic syndrome), paraneoplastic
Obstruction by tumor products

Clinical and immunologic evidence supports the true paraneoplastic nature of this syndrome.[355–362] The nephrotic syndrome may precede the development of neoplastic disease.[358] Surgical removal of tumor or response to radiotherapy or chemotherapy usually is associated with dramatic diminution in proteinuria, but recurrence of the neoplasm is followed by increased proteinuria.[357,359,360] Tumor-specific antigens and antibodies and carcinoembryonic antigen have been found in the glomeruli of some patients.[361–363]

The most frequently reported associated neoplasm is Hodgkin's disease.[357,358,360,364–366] In patients with Hodgkin's disease, the most common (80%) renal lesion is lipoid nephrosis (minimal glomerular changes).[364–367] In most of these instances, the renal findings have been similar to those seen in idiopathic lipoid nephrosis, including an absence of electron-dense deposits on electron microscopy and an absence of immunoglobulin deposits.[364] In the remaining 20% of cases, lesions typical of membranous glomerulopathy, focal sclerosis, or a membranoproliferative glomerulonephritis have been observed.[357,360,365]

In the non-Hodgkin's lymphomas (*i.e.*, Burkitt's lymphomas, lymphocytic and histiocytic lymphomas), the frequency of the nephrotic syndrome appears to be lower than that in Hodgkin's disease and some other carcinomas, although there are numerous case reports.[369,374] In 35 patients in the literature, 5 had minimal-change lesions, 7 had membranous, and 7 had membranoproliferative lesions.[369] In several of the patients with non-Hodgkin's lymphomas, immunoglobulin deposits have been identified, suggesting an immune complex as the cause of the syndrome.[373,374]

There is a striking difference in the type of renal lesions described in patients with carcinomas when compared with Hodgkin's disease. The most frequently observed glomerular lesion in patients with carcinomas is membranous glomerulonephritis.[368,370–372,375,376] Membranous glomerulonephritis is characterized by subepithelial electron-dense deposits and granular peripheral capillary deposits of IgG with or without C3.[357] It occurs in 80% to 90% of patients with carcinoma and nephrotic syndrome. The remaining patients have lipoid nephrosis or proliferative glomerulonephritis.[357,368,372] Patients with neoplasia account for 5% to 10% of all patients with membranous glomerulonephritis.[377,378]

There is a similarity between the immunopathologic features of the membranous glomerulonephritis associated with carcinomas and experimentally induced immune complex nephritis in animals. It has been suggested that there is a common pathophysiologic mechanism with glomerular deposition of circulating antigen-antibody complexes.[357,370] Tumor-specific antibodies have been eluted from the kidneys of 2 patients with lung cancer and the nephrotic syndrome, and a tumor-specific antigen was demonstrated in the glomeruli of a patient with colonic carcinoma.[357,362,370] In another patient with colon cancer, carcinoembryonic antigen-antibody complexes were found in the glomeruli, and a patient with prostate cancer had positive immunoperoxidase staining for prostate-specific acid phosphate, prostate-specific antigen, and immune deposits detected by electron microscopy in the glomerulus.[363,363a]

The pathogenesis of lipoid nephrosis in patients with Hodgkin's disease seems to have a different mechanism. There is some evidence that lipoid nephrosis may be a result of deficient T-cell function, and abnormalities of T-cell function are common in Hodgkin's disease.[379]

Other renal abnormalities caused directly or indirectly by tumor products include renal dysfunction in patients with multiple myeloma amyloidosis; renal potassium wasting and hypocalcemia related to lysozyme in acute monocytic or myelomonocytic leukemia; intrarenal obstruction by mucoprotein in pancreatic carcinoma; and nephrogenic diabetes insipidus with leiomyosarcoma.[380–399]

The renal problems of myeloma are discussed in Chapter 60.

PARANEOPLASTIC LESIONS INVOLVING THE SKIN

A long list of fascinating cutaneous syndromes have been reported with malignancies.[399] The salient features of these syndromes are outlined in Tables 57–15 through 57–20. There is great variation in the associations among the cutaneous lesions and the malignancies. In some instances (*e.g.,* acanthosis nigricans, tripe palms, erythema gyratum repens) the cutaneous syndrome is uncommon but usually associated with cancer. In other instances the cutaneous lesions may be common (*e.g.,* bullous lesions, exfoliative dermatitis, erythema multiforme) and be associated with benign disorders or cancers. In some instances (*e.g.,* bullous lesions), the association of the skin lesions and cancer may not be proved. The cutaneous syndrome may always be associated with a particular tumor (*e.g.,* esophageal cancer, tylosis), or the cutaneous lesions may be associated with various neoplasms (*e.g.,* dermatomyositis). The cause of the cutaneous lesion is well known in some instances (*e.g.,* hirsutism in adrenal or ovarian tumors or flushing in carcinoid tumors), but in most, the mechanism is unknown.

Because many cutaneous paraneoplastic syndromes are proliferative, a causal role for tumor-secreted growth factors has been suggested. Ellis and coworkers demonstrated that malignant melanoma cells secreted transforming growth factor-α (TGF-α). This growth factor bound to normal epidermal growth factor receptor-bearing epidermal cells, producing acanthosis nigricans, the sign of Leser-Trelat, and multiple acrochordons.[8] As with some neurologic paraneoplastic syndromes, there may be an immunologic mechanism, as described with paraneoplastic pemphigus.

PATIENT EVALUATION

The evaluation of cutaneous lesions suspected of being paraneoplastic begins with the clinical history, with particular emphasis on drug and other exposures, associated medical conditions, and family history. An evaluation for an underlying cancer should be undertaken only if there is no evidence of drug exposure. Many of the cutaneous syndromes are hereditary. The onset of symptoms in the paraneoplastic cutaneous lesions often is more rapid than in other benign conditions (*e.g.,* dermatomyositis, malignant down, or erythema gyratum repens). The physical examination is of critical importance. For example, while café au lait spots are not always associated with von Recklinghausen's disease, the finding of six or more café au lait spots greater than 1.5 cm in diameter or the presence of axillary freckling are diagnostic aids for the earlier recognition of neurofibromatosis.[402]

Laboratory evaluations are helpful for cutaneous lesions suspected of being metabolic (*e.g.,* hyperpigmentation in Cushing's and Addison's disease). Skin biopsy is the most important procedure for establishing the correct diagnosis and should be performed in most instances; it may provide important information. For example, exfoliative dermatitis in patients with mycosis fungoides may be associated with infiltration of the skin, as in the Sézary syndrome, but may occur in patients with uninvolved skin areas. It may occur in these patients as a result of treatment with chemotherapy or electron-beam radiotherapy.

The differential diagnosis for cutaneous lesions of possible paraneoplastic origin includes benign, nonrelated skin conditions, cutaneous lesions resulting from a primary tumor or its metastases, cutaneous infections, and toxicity from anticancer therapy (particularly cytotoxic chemotherapy or radiotherapy). Numerous cytotoxic chemotherapeutic agents have mucocutaneous toxicities. Although a detailed discussion is beyond the scope of this chapter, an excellent review is available.[403]

Pigmented Lesions

Of special interest is acanthosis nigricans.[8,404–406] This skin lesion is characterized by the presence of symmetric brown areas of hyperpigmentation with hyperkeratosis, exaggerated skin markings, and warty lesions, particularly in the intertriginous and flexural areas such as the axilla, neck, anogenital

TABLE 57–15. Pigmented Lesions and Keratoses

Disorder	*Investigations*	*Description*	*Predominant Malignancy*	*Cause*	*Comments*
Acanthosis nigricans*	Brown[404] Curth[405] Ellis[8] Matsuoka[406]	Hyperkeratosis and pigmentation, especially of axillae, neck, flexures, and anogenital region	Gastric 60%; abdominal 90%; other	Unknown	Important to differentiate benign forms present from birth and benign forms associated with various syndromes
Tripe palms	Cohen[406a]	Exaggerated ridges and tumors on palms	Lung; gastric	Unknown	Often associated with acanthosis nigricans. Strongly associated with comar (94%).
Leser-Trelat*	Dantzig[408] Ronchese[409] Snedden[407] Holdiness[410] Curry[411]	Sudden showing of large numbers of seborrheic (wart-like) keratoses	NHL; miscellaneous GI adenocarcinomas	Unknown	Must be differentiated from multiple seborrheic keratoses, which are common and may not be associated with malignancy; occasionally associated with acanthosis nigricans
Bowen's disease	Graham[412] Anderson[413]	A persistent, progressive, nonelevated red, scaly, or crusted plaque caused by an intraepidermal neoplasm	Lung; GI; GU; skin	Generally unknown; arsenic exposure in some cases	25% developed systemic cancers an average of 5 years after initial skin lesions, but significance of association has been questioned
Chronic arsenism	Minkowsky[414]	A corn-like, punctate keratosis more profuse on the extremities and characteristically affecting the palms and feet	Lung; miscellaneous	Chronic exposure to arsenic	Not a true paraneoplastic lesion
Generalized melanosis	Fitzpatrick[415] Helm[400]	A diffuse darkening of the skin with a ruddy gray color secondary to chronic liver disease; generalized blue-gray appearance	Lymphoma; hepatoma; metastatic liver tumors, melanoma	Melanin deposits in dermis	Also seen in a variety of benign conditions; may be rapid at onset
Paget's disease	Ashikari[416]	Erythematous keratotic patch over areola, nipple, or accessory breast tissue	Breast	Paget cells are either migrants from the carcinoma or Langerhans' cells	Occurs in fewer than 3% of breast cancers
Bazex's disease*	Braverman[401] Witkowski[417] Wishart[418] Bolognia[418a]	Erythema hyperkeratosis with scales and pruritus predominantly on palms and soles.	Head and neck, esophagus, lung, especially squamous histology, GI	Unknown, may be immunologic	Males only; responds to removal of primary tumor and may respond to etretinate (Tegason)
Sweet's syndrome*	Cohen[315]	Fever, neutrophilia, multiple painful cutaneous plaques and neutrophilic dermal infiltrate	Hematologic malignancies, various carcinomas	Section of a lymphokine such as IL-1 (?)	Rapid response to steroids; 10–15% associated with cancer

* True paraneoplastic syndromes.[315]

TABLE 57–16. Erythemas

Disorder	*Investigations*	*Description*	*Predominant Malignancy*	*Cause*	*Comments*
Erythema gyratum repens*	Purdy[420] Gammell[419] Summerly[421] Appell[421a]	Rapidly changing and advancing gyri with scaling and pruritus; wood grain appearance	Breast, lung, other	Unknown	Almost always associated with malignancy
Erythema annulare centrifugum	Lazar[422]	Slowly migrating annular and configurate erythematous lesions	Prostate, myeloma, other	Unknown	Occurs also with infections and other disorders
Necrolytic migratory erythema (glucagonoma)*	Wilkinson[423] Church[424]	Circinate and gyrate areas of blistering and erosive erythema on limbs; stomatitis	Islet cell on pancreas	Glucagonoma or other metabolic product	See chapter on islet cell tumors
Flushing*	Sjoerdsma[425] Mason[426]	Episodic flushing of face and neck	Carcinoids, medullary carcinoma of thyroid	Serotonin or other vasoactive peptides	See chapter on carcinoids
Exfoliative dermatitis†	Abrahams[427] Nicolis[428] Helm[400]	Progressive erythema followed by scaling	Cutaneous T-cell lymphomas, NHL, Hodgkin's disease, non-Hodgkin's lymphoma	Unknown	Account for 10–20% of all exfoliative dermatitis
Erythema multiforme	Elias[429]	Distinctive target lesions in symmetric distribution, sometimes with plaques or bullae			

* True paraneoplastic syndromes.
† True neoplastic syndrome only in some instances.

TABLE 57–17. Endocrine and Metabolic Lesions

Disorder	*Investigations*	*Description*	*Predominant Malignancy*	*Cause*	*Comments*
Systemic nodular panniculitis* (nodular relapsing fat necrosis; Weber-Christian disease*)	Fitzpatrick[430]	Recurrent crops of tender erythematous subcutaneous nodules; may be accompanied by abdominal pain, fat necrosis in bone marrow, lungs, and other organs	Adenocarcinoma of pancreas	Effect of pancreatic enzymes released into circulation on fatty tissues	Usually associated with pancreatic disease but may be benign pancreatic disease
Porphyria cutanea tarda*	Weddington[431] Thompson[432]	Photosensitive skin lesions, often painful or pruritic	Liver	Increased porphyrins in skin tissues	Rare
Cushing's syndrome		Broad purple striae, atrophy, hyperpigmentation (uncommon), plethora, telangiectasia, mild hirsutism	Ectopic lung (small cell), thyroid, testes, ovary, adrenal tumors; pancreatic islet cell, pituitary, other	Increased ACTH	
Addison's syndrome		Generalized hyperpigmentation, especially scars, pressure points, points of friction; increased amounts of hair	Adrenal gland invasion, lymphomas or carcinomas	Decreased glucocorticoids	Rarely caused by tumors invading the adrenal
Hirsutism			Adrenal tumors, ovarian tumors	Increased glucocorticoid, increased testosterone	Associated with virilism

* True paraneoplastic syndrome.

TABLE 57–18. Bullous and Urticarial Lesions

Disorders	*Investigations*	*Description*	*Predominant Malignancy*	*Cause*	*Comments*
Pemphigoid	Stone[433] Anhalt[433a]	Large tense bullae with histologically absent acantholysis	Lymphomas, miscellaneous	Autoantibodies that react with an antigen complex composed of desmoplakin I, the bullous pemphigoid antigens and two unidentified antigens	Although the clinical association of bullous pemphigoid and malignancy was once accepted, recent age-matched studies have failed to support the association
Dermatitis herpetiformis	Tobias[434] Helm[400]	Pleomorphic symmetric subepidermal bullae particularly with scarring	Lymphomas, miscellaneous	Related to autoantibodies	

region, umbilicus, and areola. The salient features are shown in Table 57–15. The lesions of Leser-Trelat with multiple seborrheic keratoses have been described in patients with acanthosis nigricans (see Table 57–15), and both may be produced by tumor secretion of TGF-α.[8,407] There is a strong association between acanthosis nigricans and malignancy, with more than half of all reported cases having cancer. However, the acanthosis nigricans may precede, occur simultaneously with, or occur after the diagnosis of malignancy has been made. There are several documented cases of regression after surgical tumor removal. The most frequent association is with adenocarcinomas of the gastrointestinal tract (92%), particularly of the stomach (50–60%). However, the lesions have been reported in a variety of other tumors, including breast cancer, lymphomas, and squamous carcinomas.[404,405]

The most important part of the differential diagnosis is to differentiate between true acanthosis nigricans associated with malignancy, benign acanthosis, and pseudoacanthosis. Benign acanthosis is a nevoid condition present at birth or beginning in childhood and associated with several benign syndromes. Pseudoacanthosis occurs in obese persons, especially those with dark complexions. It may occur in patients with gigantism, acromegaly, Stein-Leventhal syndrome, or diabetes mellitus. It may develop after prolonged administration of corticosteroids, diethylstilbestrol, or nicotinic acid. Insulin resistance is common in these patients. However, insulin resistance caused by the development of antibodies against the insulin receptor has been reported in acanthosis nigricans associated with malignancy (*e.g.*, pheochromocytoma).[406] Because of the strong association of acanthosis and cancer, patients developing true acanthosis nigricans after the age of 40 should be evaluated for malignancy, including a thorough evaluation of the gastrointestinal tract, lymph nodes, and breasts. Tripe palms is the appearance of exaggerated dermatoglyphics on the palmar surfaces of the palms and fingers.[406a] The palms may have a thickened velvety appearance, exaggeration of ridges and furrows and brown hyperpigmentation. In a review of the world's literature, 94% of cases occurred in patients with cancer.[406a] Tripe palms occurred with acanthosis nigricans in 77% of patients and alone in 23%. The common malignancies were lung and gastric cancers in about half the cases. Trip palms were the presenting feature of a previously undiagnosed cancer in 40% of cases.[406a]

Although more rare than acanthosis nigricans, the sudden development and rapid increase in size of seborrheic keratoses (sign of Leser-Trelat) are strongly associated with malignancy, particularly of the gastrointestinal tract.[407,408] As with many cutaneous paraneoplastic syndromes, the most important feature is the rapid change, because multiple seborrheic keratoses may be common, especially in older age groups.

Salient features of other pigmented or proliferative lesions are summarized in Table 57–15.

Erythemas

The major features of erythemas associated with malignancy are summarized in Table 57–16. Erythema gyratum repens is usually associated with malignancy, and necrolytic migratory erythema is pathognomonic of glucagonoma. Exfoliative dermatitis can be caused by a variety of malignancies, drug reactions, or unknown causes.[400,427,428] Various studies report that 10% to 20% of cases may be associated with malignancy, particularly lymphomas. In some instances, the skin lesions are not paraneoplastic, because cutaneous infiltration of the skin can be documented by skin biopsy. In some instances, there is no demonstrable cutaneous tumor, and the condition may improve after therapy, and the skin condition appears to be a true paraneoplastic syndrome. Although the mechanism is unknown, some have speculated that there is an immunologic response to some antigenic material derived from the tumor.[400]

Endocrine and Metabolic Lesions and Bullous and Urticarial Lesions

Important skin lesions associated with endocrine and metabolic tumors (Table 57–17) are systemic nodular panniculitis, with adenocarcinoma of the pancreas, and porphyria cutanea tarda, with hepatomas. The associations of malignancy with bullous and urticarial lesions are not completely proven (Table 57–18). However, Anhalt and colleagues described 5 patients with cancer who had a novel acantholytic skin disease char-

TABLE 57–19. Miscellaneous Lesions

Disorder	*Investigations*	*Description*	*Predominant Malignancy*	*Cause*	*Comments*
Dermatomyositis*	Williams[465] Arundell[435] DeVere[264] Barnes[265]	Purplish pink erythema, especially of eyelids, neck, and hands	Miscellaneous	Unknown	Malignant disease reported in 7–50%; precedes carcinoma by days to years with an average of 6 mo
Hypertrichosis languginosa* (malignant down)	Lyell[436] Hegedus[437]	Rapid development of fine, long, silky hair, especially on ears and forehead and may involve the entire body	Lung, colon, bladder, uterus, gall bladder	Unknown	High association with cancer
Acquired ichthyosis*	VanDijk[438] Flint[439]	Generalized dry, crackling skin, hyperkeratotic palms and soles, rhomboidal scales	Hodgkin's disease, other lymphomas, multiple myeloma, other	Unknown	Should be differentiated from hereditary form, which occurs before age 20
Pachydermoperi-ostosis*	Vogl[440]	Thickening of skin and creation of new folds; thickened lips, ears, and lids; macroglossia; thick forehead and scalp; clubbing; excessive sweating	Lung (uterus)	Unknown	Occurs also in lung abscess and benign tumors
Pruritus*	Rajka[441] Cormia[442]	Failure to determine an overt or covert cutaneous cause of generalized pruritus necessitates evaluation for a possible underlying systemic disease	Lymphomas, leukemias, multiple myelomas, CNS tumors, abdominal tumors	Unknown	Also associated with many benign diseases
Amyloid deposits		Macroglossia, pinch purpura, superficial waxy yellow and pink elevated nodules	Multiple myeloma, Waldenström's macroglobulinemia	Amyloid deposition in blood vessels and dermis	Also associated with primary systemic amyloid and other benign conditions
Herpes zoster	Schimpff[443] Dolin[444] Huberman[445]	Vesicular eruption in a dermatomal distribution	Hodgkin's disease, non-Hodgkin's lymphomas, chronic lymphocytic leukemia, small cell lung cancer	Immunosuppression	Increased incidence in cancers associated with immunosuppression and after severely immunosuppressive therapy
Caput medusa					
Thrombophlebitis					
Gynecomastia					

* True paraneoplastic syndrome.

acterized by autoantibodies that were pathogenic after passive transfer to mice.[433a] The autoantibodies reacted with an antigen complex composed of desmoplakin I, a 230-kd antigen of bullous pamphizoid, and two unidentified epithelial antigens (Table 57–18).

Miscellaneous Lesions

The cutaneous lesions in dermatomyositis are characterized by purple-pink heliotrope erythema of the face with edema of the eyelids, with spread to the neck and arms (Table 57–19). Erythematous purplish papules and plaques over the knuckles and interphalangeal joints (*i.e.*, Grotton's sign) may be characteristic but usually occur late. All types of malignancies have been reported.[264–266,435] Overall, cancers are reported in 7% to 52% of patients with dermatomyositis. There are reports of dramatic improvement in dermatomyositis after antitumor therapy, supporting its identification as a true paraneoplastic syndrome.[266,435]

An important feature of paraneoplastic acquired ichthyosis

TABLE 57–20. Hereditary Disorders

Disorders	*Investigations*	*Description*	*Predominant Malignancy*	*Heredity*	*Comments*
Gardner's syndrome	Gardner[446] Bussey[447] Jones[448]	Epidermal cysts, sebaceous cysts, dermoid tumors, lipomas, fibromas	Adenocarcinoma of large or small bowel	Autosomal dominant	Associated with polyposis of colon and bony exostoses
Peutz-Jeghers syndrome	Jeghers[449] Riley[450]	Pigmentation of lips, face, oral mucosa, and digits	GI adenocarcinomas	Autosomal dominant	Low (2–3%) incidence
Tylosis (palmaris and plantaris)	Howel-Evans[451]	Hyperkeratosis of palms and soles after age 10	Esophageal carcinoma	Autosomal dominant	95% incidence of carcinoma by age 65
Multiple mucosal neuromas	Williams[452]	Neuromas of eyelids, lips, tongue, and oral mucosa	Pheochromocytoma, medullary carcinoma of thyroid (MEN II)	Autosomal dominant	Parathyroid adenomas, hypertension common
Cowden's disease—multiple harmartoma syndrome	Lloyd[435]	Fibromas of oral mucosa, acral verucous papulas, trichilemmomas of the face	Thyroid, breast carcinomas	Autosomal dominant	Associated with multiple hamartomas, lipomas, neuromas, hemangiomas, thyroid adenomas
Multiple basal cell neuromas syndrome	Solomon[454]	Multiple basal cell carcinomas, pits on soles and palms	Medulloblastoma, fibrosarcoma (jaw)	Autosomal dominant	Infrequent association with internal malignancy
Neurofibromatosis (von Recklinghausen)	Crowe[402]	Neurofibromas, café au lait spots	Pheochromocytoma	Autosomal dominant	Malignancies develop in a minority of patients
Tuberous sclerosis (Bourneville)	Butterworth[455]	Lipopigmented macules, adenomas, fibromas	Neurologic malignancies	Autosomal dominant	Malignancies develop in a minority of patients
Cerebelloretinal hemangioblastoma (von Hippel-Lindau)	Christoferson[456]	Retinal malformation, papilledema	Neurologic malignancies	Autosomal dominant	Malignancies develop in a minority of patients
Encephalotrigeminal syndrome (Sturge-Weber)	Doll[457]	Capillary or cavernous hemangiomas within the cutaneous distribution of the trigeminal nerve	Neurologic malignancies	Autosomal dominant	Malignancies develop in a minority of patients
Ataxia-telangiectasia	Doll[457] Frizzera[458]	Telangiectasias	Lymphomas, leukemias	Autosomal recessive	IgA ± IgE deficiency; sinopulmonary infections, tumors in <10%
Bloom's syndrome	Helm[402]	Photosensitivity, telangiectasias, erythema of face	Leukemia	Autosomal recessive	Stunted growth, high incidence
Fanconi's anemia	Helm[400]	Patchy hyperpigmentation	Leukemias	Autosomal recessive	High incidence
Chédiak-Higashi syndrome	Doll[456]	Recurrent pyoderma, giant melanosomes, dilution of skin and hair color	Lymphomas	Autosomal recessive	High incidence
Werner's syndrome (adult progeria)	Epstein[459]	Scleroderma-like changes, premature aging, leg ulcers, short stature	Sarcomas, meningiomas, others	Autosomal recessive	Cancers in about 10%
Wiskott-Aldrich syndrome	Doll[457] Frizzeria[458]	Eczematous dermatitis, pyroderma	Lymphomas	Sex linked (males)	>10% incidence
Bruton's sex-linked agammaglobulinemia	Helm[400]	Recurrent infections	Lymphoma, leukemias	Sex linked	>5% incidence

is the rapid development of the lesions. The lesions are characterized by generalized dry cracking skin with hyperkeratotic palms and soles. The acquired forms are associated most often with Hodgkin's disease and other malignant lymphomas, although associations with solid tumors have been reported.[438,439] The acquired forms can be differentiated from genetic forms by the fact that the latter arise usually before the age of 20. A parallel course of the malignant lymphoma and acquired ichthyosis has been reported for many patients.[439]

Hereditary Disorders

Many hereditary disorders associated with malignant disease and skin lesions of presumed paraneoplastic nature are summarized in Table 57–20.

GASTROINTESTINAL PARANEOPLASTIC SYNDROMES

The Zollinger-Ellison, carcinoid, and other syndromes resulting from hormone-producing endocrine tumors are discussed in Chapter 41. One of the most frequent of all the paraneoplastic syndromes is the malignancy associated anorexia and cachexia. It may be caused by a tumor-secreted cytokine, TNF-α.[8–11]

PROTEIN-LOSING ENTEROPATHIES ASSOCIATED WITH MALIGNANCY

More than 90% of cancer patients have low serum albumin levels.[412] Metabolic studies show that this can be due to decreased albumin synthesis, abnormal distribution of albumin in effusions, or increased loss of protein into the gastrointestinal tract (*e.g.*, protein-losing enteropathy).[460] The most common mechanism is decreased albumin synthesis, but why this is so is unknown.[460] Although patients usually present with other signs of malignancy, unexplained edema and hypoproteinemia were the initial manifestations of malignancy in a few patients.

The mechanisms of protein-losing enteropathy include inflammation and ulceration of the gastrointestinal mucosa and exudative loss of proteins; disorders of the intestinal lymphatic channels from neoplastic obstruction (*e.g.*, with lymphomas); congestive failure (*e.g.*, in patients with carcinoid or pericardial construction) with resultant loss of protein and lymphocytes rich in lymph into the gastrointestinal lumen; and a group of undefined mechanisms. The resulting hypoalbuminemia leads to edema, and the lymphopenia decreases cellular immunity with impaired skin test reactivity.[460] Although these syndromes may not fulfill all of the criteria for paraneoplasia (*i.e.*, acting at a distance from the tumor), anecdotal case reports indicate that protein-losing enteropathy can be reversed by appropriate treatment of the underlying tumor. Profuse watery diarrhea, hypokalemia, and hypochlorhydria usually are associated with pancreatic non-β-islet cell tumors or villous adenomas of the rectum. This syndrome can be found in patients with lung cancer, but the mechanism is unknown.[461]

MALABSORPTION

Malabsorption syndromes for several or specific substances may occur by a variety of mechanisms in cancer patients, including side effects of surgery, irradiation, and chemotherapy. Malabsorption often is associated with lymphoma involving the small bowel or with gastric, hepatic, or biliary tract tumors, particularly if biliary obstruction exists. These examples are not remote effects of the tumor. However, some malabsorption syndromes may be paraneoplastic, as suggested by finding histologic abnormalities of the small bowel in as many as 62% of various cancers in some studies.[462–464] Although the exact frequency of the histologic types is unknown, the abnormalities include "flat" mucosa with simple or partial villous atrophy. Subtotal villous atrophy is less common. However, the severity of associated malabsorption does not correlate with the severity of the small bowel histologic changes.[462] The tumors associated with small bowel abnormalities are colon, lung, prostate, and pancreatic cancers and lymphomas. The mechanisms behind the loss of villous height are unknown. Treatment should be directed at the underlying tumor plus administration of exogenous nutrients and vitamins to bypass the malabsorption.

HEPATOPATHY AS A PARANEOPLASTIC SYNDROME

An elevated hepatic alkaline phosphatase level has occurred with a malignant schwannoma and disappeared with surgical resection.[465] This also occurs in hypernephroma, in which there can be reversible abnormalities of liver function not associated with liver metastases.[465–468] Decreased albumin synthesis rises to normal after resection of the renal tumor. Biochemical abnormalities, such as elevated alkaline phosphatase levels or hyperglobulinemia, hypocholesterolemia, and prolonged prothrombin time, and hepatosplenomegaly, have disappeared after primary tumor removal in 4 of 6 patients.[466,468] The mechanisms for the hepatopathy associated with hypernephroma are unknown, but they may include hepatic amyloid or be related to the generalized hepatic hypervascularity seen on angiography or the nonspecific focal periportal inflammation seen on biopsy.[466,467,469] It is important to recognize the hepatopathy syndrome so that these signs are not confused with metastases to the liver. Biopsy confirmation of liver metastases from renal carcinoma is highly desirable if this metastatic site alone would preclude resection of the primary renal tumor for cure.

ANOREXIA, CACHEXIA, AND TASTE ABNORMALITIES AS PARANEOPLASTIC MANIFESTATIONS

Problems with anorexia, taste, weight loss, and cachexia are common in cancer patients.[470,476] One third or more of cancer patients are in negative nitrogen balance; they can even be in positive nitrogen balance and still maintain a caloric deficit.[472] The syndrome comprises anorexia, cachexia, asthenia, loss of body tissue, and inability to conserve normal regulatory functions of metabolism and bears no correlation to the amount, type, or site of neoplastic tissue.[473] It can occur as an early symptom of disease or appear in the presence of bulk neoplasms. The best evidence of the paraneoplastic nature of the anorexia-cachexia syndrome comes when it appears before the malignancy is discovered and disappears with the resection or control of the tumor.[472] Obviously, cancer patients can have these symptoms as a result of therapy toxicity, gross invasion, or obstruction of structures by tumor. Cachexia may result from decreased caloric intake, malabsorption, loss of material from the body (*e.g.*, from effusions, hemorrhage, ulcers), or a change in the body metabolism. Anorexia and taste changes may result in decreased caloric intake. However, a variety of experimental evidence suggests that malnutrition alone cannot explain the cachexia of malignancy.[472] In malignancy and cachexia, the caloric expenditure remains high, and the basal metabolic rate is increased despite the reduced dietary intake, indicating a profound systemic derangement of host metabolism.[472] These findings are in contrast to the lower metabolic rates and adaptation that normal subjects make after starvation.[473] With starvation in normal persons, the caloric expenditure is lowered, amino acids cease being used for gluconeogenesis, and exogenous glucose is readily oxidized, but it is not in malignancy. Protein synthesis is maintained in malignancy rather than reduced as in starvation.

Studies demonstrated that circulatory factors could produce cancer anorexia-cachexia.[474] Other studies demonstrated that the cytokines, TNF-α and IL-1β, could produce a similar syndrome in animals.[475] TNF-α was shown to be identical with cachectin.[8–11] This cytokine inhibits lipoprotein lipase activity in peripheral tissues and may orchestrate the metabolic changes leading to tumor cachexia-anorexia.[457a] Other hypolytic factors produced by tumor cells may be responsible for cancer cachexia in some patients.[475b]

Aversion to meats and other protein-containing food frequently occurs in cancer patients. DeWys found that 16 of 50 cancer patients of various types had an aversion to meat; this was correlated with a lowered threshold for bitter taste (*i.e.*, urea).[471] These patients had elevated thresholds for sweet (*i.e.*, sucrose) substances. The taste abnormalities were correlated with a patient's body burden of tumor and then normalized after response to treatment.[471]

The regulation of hunger and satiety is complex and involves a CNS "satiety" center in the ventromedial nuclei of the hypothalamus and a "feeding" center in the lateral hypothalamic nuclei.[472] Alimentary tract regulation; glucostatic, lipostatic, thermostatic, and osmotic regulation; hormone regulation by insulin; regulation of growth hormone, glucagon, enterogastrone, adrenal corticosteroids, amino acid levels, and of an as yet unidentified anorexigenic pituitary polypeptides take place.[479] It appears likely that mechanisms underlying the paraneoplastic anorexia-cachexia syndrome involve molecules produced by the tumor that impinge on one or more of the regulatory mechanisms of hunger, satiety, metabolism, or taste and cause the organism to falsely disrupt these patterns and enter into a metabolically chaotic state.[472] The treatment of the underlying tumor appears to be the best general approach to reversing the state of cancer cachexia. The progestin megace may be used in symptomatic patients.

MISCELLANEOUS PARANEOPLASTIC SYNDROMES

FEVER AS A PARANEOPLASTIC SYNDROME

Fever occurs frequently in cancer patients and usually is caused by infection. Although other noninfectious causes (*e.g.*, drug toxicity, adrenal insufficiency) exist, certain tumors are associated with fever.[477] Of 351 cancer patients, Petersdorf found that 30% developed fever and 5% had fever that could be related only to their cancer.[494] The major associations are with Hodgkin's disease, myxomas, hypernephromas, osteogenic sarcomas, and a variety of other tumors.[478,479] Tumor-associated fever usually is defined as unexplained fever that coincides with tumor growth, disappears promptly on tumor removal or control, and reappears with tumor regrowth. Alternatively, when the fever persists with uncontrolled tumor without any other reasonable cause, the tumor is a likely cause of the fever.[477] In Hodgkin's disease, fever as a systemic symptom suggests a worse prognosis stage-by-stage, and its disappearance is required to document remission of tumor and subsequent cure. There are no data about the influence on prognosis of fever associated with other tumors.

The cause of the tumor-associated fever may be release of pyrogen from tumor cells, normal leukocytes, or a variety of other normal cells that have endogenous pyrogen. For example, the Kupffer cells of the liver contain endogenous pyrogen that could cause fever with hepatoma or with metastases to the liver from other tumors.[480] The pyrogen acts on the hypothalamus to cause some reset of temperature regulation. Tumor cells can produce pyrogen. Bodel showed that five of six hypernephromas placed in vitro released pyrogen into the supernatant medium (detected by injection into a rabbit).[477] Similarly, spleen and lymph node tissue from Hodgkin's disease patients produce pyrogen when cultured into the medium in vitro. However, pyrogen production, although correlated with lymph node involvement, did not correlate with histologic involvement of the spleen or with fever in the patient.[477] It is still unknown whether tumor cells themselves or other normal cells mixed in the incubated specimens produce the pyrogen. IL-6 has been implicated as the pyrogen in some cases and was shown to be released by tumor cells.[477a] Treatment should be directed at the underlying tumor, and the most dramatic remissions of paraneoplastic fever come in successfully treated patients with Hodgkin's disease or hypernephroma.

LACTIC ACIDOSIS

Lactic acidosis usually is associated with acute lymphatic or myelogenous leukemia, Hodgkin's disease, and other lymphomas and responds in parallel with tumor regression to therapy.[481–483] Bicarbonate therapy is often needed.

HYPERLIPIDEMIA

Hyperlipidemia frequently is seen in lymphoma-bearing hamsters and normalizes after tumor treatment.[480] Hyperlipidemias have been seen in multiple myeloma, hepatoma, and colon cancer.[484–486] Total lipid levels of 2 g/dl, cholesterol levels above 500 mg/dl, and triglyceride levels of 580 mg/dl have been found. However, no associated vascular abnormalities have been reported. With myeloma, monoclonal proteins sometimes have reacted with α- or β-lipoproteins or with lipolytic enzymes. The mechanism in the other tumor types is obscure but may involve invasion by tumor.

HYPERTENSION AND HYPOTENSION

Malignant hypertension and hypokalemia associated with apparent tumor production of renin have been reported with lung cancer, hypernephroma, and Wilms' tumor.[487–490] Hypertension recedes with control of the tumor. Endothelin-1 is a potent vasoconstrictor peptide produced by endothelial cells. It has been implicated in the hypertension produced by some cases of hemangioendothelioma, a malignant vascular neoplasm.[490a]

An antihypertension syndrome has been seen with a PGA-secreting renal cell tumor, and abnormally low baroreceptor pressure responses have been seen with intrathoracic carcinomas.[491,492] The latter syndrome appears related to interference of transmission of impulses from intrathoracic stretch receptors, resulting in orthostatic hypotension and abnormalities of sodium excretion.

AMYLASE ELEVATION

Synthesis and secretion of amylase by tumors are uncommon; the tumors have all been lung cancer, usually adenocarcinoma.[493] These tumors make the salivary type of amylase, which allows differentiation from a pancreatic source of the amylase evaluation. The tumor-produced amylase itself apparently does not cause symptoms, but its appearance can lead to great concern and medical evaluation for the presence of pancreatitis or various types of pancreatic fistulas.[493]

HYPERTROPHIC PULMONARY OSTEOARTHROPATHY

Hypertrophic pulmonary osteoarthropathy (HPO) is a paraneoplastic syndrome comprising clubbing of the fingers and toes, periostitis of the long bones, and sometimes a polyarthritis resembling rheumatoid arthritis.[494–497] Periostitis-arthritis produces pain in the knees, wrists, and ankles with tenderness and swelling of the affected bones. Involved bones usually include the distal ends of the tibia, fibula, humerus, radius, or ulna. Hyperemia of the affected joints or hands and feet is seen.[494] The syndrome may precede the discovery of the neoplasm by several months and usually has a fairly defined onset. Patients often do not present with clubbing but appear with joint pain or polyarthritis, and in adult patients presenting with unexplained polyarthritis or joint pain, the HPO syndrome should be kept in mind.[494] Pathologic examination of the joints may show pannus formation; however, most joints show only hyperemia.[494] If polyarthritis is present, joint effusions, particularly of the knees, with noninflammatory synovial fluid and good mucin clot are present. Ossifying periostitis is seen on roentgenogram at the distal end of the shafts of long bones as a thin opaque line of new bone formation, separated from the underlying denser cortex by a narrow radiolucent band. Radionuclide bone scans often are positive over the bones involved with periostitis before the other radiologic changes appear.[498] In advanced cases, other bones (*e.g.*, the ribs, clavicle, iliac crests, vertebral column) may be involved.

Hypertrophic pulmonary osteoarthropathy is encountered most frequently in lung cancer, occurring in 12% of patients with adenocarcinoma and less frequently in other cell types; HPO is almost nonexistent in small cell lung cancer.[499,500] Of interest, the HPO syndrome occurs often with benign mesothelioma and the rare neurolemmomas of the diaphragm, but malignant mesotheliomas are thought never to produce HPO.[494] Other tumors metastatic to the chest can cause HPO, including metastases from renal cancer, thymoma, leiomyoma of the esophagus, intrathoracic Hodgkin's disease, osteogenic sarcoma, fibrosarcoma, and the undifferentiated nasopharyngeal tumors of young people after the tumors metastasize to mediastinal lymph nodes.[501–507]

The diagnosis is made by physical findings, radionuclide bone scan, and radiographic appearance of the bones. Although benign causes should be considered, the bone changes of hyperparathyroidism can simulate HPO and should be ruled out, although it is possible for HPO and ectopic PTH to coexist. The cause is unknown, although estrogens, circulatory factors, neurogenic factors, and growth hormone have been postulated to play a role.[452,457,508–510] Other arthropathies associated with cancer include secondary gout and carcinoma polyarthritis.[507a]

AMYLOIDOSIS

Amyloid deposition (*i.e.*, paraneoplastic β-fibrils) is a pathologic process whose manifestations depend on the formation of a specific, unique protein conformation—the twisted β-pleated sheet fibril.[511] Histochemically, these fibrils have green polarization color after Congo red staining. This structure normally is not found in mammalian tissues and can occur with a variety of proteins produced by several different pathogenic mechanisms. Immunoglobulin fragments produced by plasma cell dyscrasias are the most common neoplastic mechanism. Because of the β-pleated structure, the fibrils are resistant to normal proteolytic digestion under physiologic conditions and accumulate as inert fibrils in tissues. This causes pressure atrophy, morbidity, and death from interference of normal physiologic processes of the affected vital organs (*e.g.*, heart, kidneys, nerves, joints).

Although amyloidosis may have several nonmalignant causes, 15% of cases occur with malignant disease, including multiple myeloma, lymphomas, and carcinomas.[511,513] Amyloid occurs in 6% to 15% of multiple myeloma and Waldenström's macroglobulinemia, in 4% of Hodgkin's disease, and 1% of other lymphomas, and probably all B-cell lymphomas can give rise to amyloidosis. Carcinomas associated with amyloidosis are hypernephromas, bladder and renal pelvic cancer, uterine cervix cancer, and biliary tract cancer.[512] Hypernephroma is reported to represent more than 25% of all tumors associated with amyloidosis, but the nature of the protein in the amyloid deposit of hypernephromas is unknown.[511,512]

The "amyloidogenic" protein can be monoclonal light chains (designated AL) or other proteins (designated AA).[511] Amyloid fibrils from medullary carcinoma of the thyroid contain part of the calcitonin molecule; peptides produced by several tumors, if they contain sequences that can form β-pleated sheets, may cause amyloid.[511] In amyloidosis with multiple myeloma, Bence Jones proteinuria is usually present, and the occurrence is higher in free light-chain myeloma.[511]

The signs and symptoms of amyloidosis of malignancy, particularly with myeloma, are a peripheral neuropathy (*e.g.*, painful stocking-glove condition), autonomic nervous symptoms of sexual impotence, gastrointestinal motility disturbances, orthostatic hypotension, and dyshidrosis.[511] Motor function is impaired from median nerve entrapment, and weight loss is frequent. A restrictive cardiomyopathy, with signs and symptoms of right heart failure with only minimal radiographic evidence of cardiomegaly, occurs. Low-voltage electrocardiographic changes, arrhythmias, conduction disturbances, and electrocardiographic pattern-simulating myocardial infarction may occur. The patients are extremely sensitive to digitalis, and several toxic deaths from this have been reported. Pinch purpura, periorbital purpura after procedures, macroglossia, waxy cutaneous papules, subcutaneous nodules, alopecia, and scleroderma-like skin infiltration may occur. Joint infiltration often produces painless limitation of the range of motion. The large joints are affected in amyloid arthropathy, and the "shoulder pad" sign develops, with massive infiltration of the glenohumeral articulation. Carpal and tarsal tunnel syndromes occur with infiltration of these regions.

The diagnosis of amyloid is made by the demonstration of the characteristic emerald-green birefringence of tissue specimens stained by Congo red and examined by polarization microscopy.[511] Biopsies of infiltrated lesions, gingiva, skin, bone marrow, or rectum can be used. The prognosis of clinically evident amyloidosis with malignancy is poor, and in myeloma, median survival from diagnosis is 14 months or less.[511] There is not good evidence that treatment of myeloma or other neoplastic disorders can reverse the amyloid already deposited, but it probably halts amyloid progression. Supportive care problems abound because the congestive heart failure from amyloid does not respond to digitalis. (Amyloid patients started on digitalis therapy should be hospitalized because of potential toxicity.) Diuretics can cause dehydration and cardiovascular collapse because of concurrent renal damage, postural hypotension, adrenal insufficiency, autonomic neuropathy, and low cardiac output. Mineralocorticoids, elastic stockings, broad-spectrum antibiotics for bacterial overgrowth in bowel with disturbed motility, gastrostomy and tracheostomy for macroglossia, hemodialysis, and surgical decompression of carpal tunnel syndrome have been used.[511]

PALMAR FASCIITIS AND ARTHRITIS

The shoulder-hand syndrome, a variant of reflex sympathetic dystrophy has been reported with malignancy.[514–516] Brain and lung cancers were reported most often, although cancers of the bladder, uterus, breast, and esophagus were described. Palmar fasciitis and arthritis associated with ovarian carcinoma have more dramatic and progressive findings with complete loss of upper-extremity function and contracture. The severe syndrome has been reported in patients with small cell lung cancer, adenocarcinoma of the pancreas, CML, and Hodgkin's disease. The cause is unknown, but immunoglobulin deposits were found in the fascial tissue of a patient, suggesting an immunologic cause. The syndrome often preceded the diagnosis of malignancy and improved after successful antitumor therapy.

ARTHRITIS, POLYMYALGIA RHEUMATICA, SYSTEMIC LUPUS ERYTHEMATOSUS, VASCULITIS

Rheumatoid arthritis or asymmetric polyarthritis may occur with malignancy or may be related by chance.[4,517–519] Joint manifestations regress on removal or control of the underlying malignancy in 48% of patients. About 80% of female patients with asymmetric polyarthritis and malignancy had breast cancer. Some 83% of patients with polymyalgia rheumatica are said to develop a malignancy within 3 months, and some of these cases may represent arterial emboli to muscle from nonbacterial thrombotic endocarditis. Lymphomas may be associated with systemic rheumatic disease.[519,520] In Sjögren's syndrome, a spectrum of benign to malignant lymphoproliferations can be seen, but whether this is "at a distance from the tumor" remains to be determined.[521] Metastases to joints can simulate rheumatoid arthritis, and cytologic studies should be done on joint effusions in cancer patients.[522,523]

Systemic lupus erythematosus (SLE) is associated with lymphomas, lymphoblastic leukemia, thymomas, testicular and ovarian tumors, and lung cancer, and remission of the SLE often occurs with tumor treatment.[521,524] The syndrome may be caused by an antinuclear antibody recognizing a novel antigen.[575]

In a study of 222 patients with vasculitis, 11 were found to have an associated malignancy.[526] Hematologic malignancies were most common in this and other similar series. The cause of the vasculitis is uncertain but may have an immunologic basis.

REFERENCES

1. Hall TC, ed. Paraneoplastic syndromes. Ann N Y Acad Sci 1974;230:1–577.
2. Odell WD, Wolfsen AR. Humoral syndromes associated with cancer. Ann Rev Med 1978;29:379–406.
3. Blackman MR, Rosen SW, Weintraub BD. Ectopic hormones. Adv Intern Med 1978;23: 85–113.
4. Shneider BS, Manalo A. Paraneoplastic syndromes. Unusual manifestations of malignant disease. Dis Month 1979;Feb:1–60.
5. Markman M. Response of paraneoplastic syndromes to antineoplastic therapy. West J Med 1986;144:580–585.
6. Ascensao JL, Oken MM, Ewing SL, et al. Leukocytosis and large cell lung cancer. A frequent association. Cancer 1987;60:903–905.
7. Hocking W, Goodman J, Golde D. Granulocytosis associated with tumor cell production of colony stimulating activity. Blood 1983;61:600–603.
8. Ellis DL, Kafka SP, Chow JC, et al. Melanoma, growth factors, acanthosis nigricans, the sign of Leser-Trelat, and multiple acrochordons. A possible role of alpha-transforming growth factor in cutaneous paraneoplastic syndromes. N Engl J Med 1987;317: 1582–1587.
9. Beutler B, Greenwald D, Hulmes JD, et al. Identity of tumor necrosis factor and the macrophage-secreted factor cachectin. Nature 1985;316:552–554.
10. Torti FM, Dieckmann B, Beutler B, et al. A macrophage factor inhibits adipocyte gene expression: An in vitro model of cachexia. Science 1985;229:867–870.
11. Theologides A. Anorexins, asthenins, and cachectins in cancer. Am J Med 1986;81: 696–698.
12. Greenlee JE, Lipton HL. Anticerebellar antibodies in serum and cerebrospinal fluid of a patient with oat cell carcinoma of the lung and paraneoplastic cerebellar degeneration. Ann Neurol 1986;19:82–85.
13. Grunwald GB, Kornguth SE, Towfighi J, et al. Autoimmune basis for visual paraneoplastic syndrome in patients with small cell lung carcinoma. Cancer 1987;60:780–786.
14. Graus F, Elkon KB, Cordon-Cardo C, Posner J. Sensory neuronopathy and small cell lung cancer. Antineuronal antibody that also reacts with the tumor. Am J Med 1986;80: 45–52.
15. Fukunaga H, Engel AG, Lang B, et al. Passive transfer of Eaton-Lambert myasthenic syndrome with IgG from man to mouse depletes the presynaptic membrane active zones. Proc Natl Acad Sci USA 1983;80:7636–7640.
16. Richardson EP. Progressive multifocal leukoencephalopathy. In: Vinken PJ, Bruryn GW, eds. Handbook of clinical neurology. Amsterdam: Elsevier North-Holland, 1970: 485–499.
17. Wiener LP, Henden RM, Narayan O, et al. Virus related to SV40 in patients with progressive multifocal leukoencephalopathy. N Engl J Med 1972;286:385–390.
18. Croft P, Wilkinson M. The incidence of carcinomatous neuromyopathy in patients with various types of carcinoma. Brain 1965;88:427–434.
19. Wilner EC, Brody JA. An evaluation of the remote effects of cancer on the nervous system. Neurology 1967;18:1120–1124.
20. De Larco JE, Todaro GJ. Growth factors from murine sarcoma virus-transformed cells. Proc Natl Acad Sci USA 1978;75:4001–4005.
21. Waldenström JG. Paraneoplasia, biological signals in diagnosis of cancer. New York: John Wiley & Sons, 1978.
22. Odell WD, Wolfsen AR. Hormones from tumors: Are they ubiquitous? Am J Med 1980;68:317–318.
23. Lees LH. The biosynthesis of hormones by nonendocrine tumours—A review. J Endocrinol 1975;67:143–175.
24. Kreiger DT, Martin JB. Brain peptides. N Engl J Med 1981;304:876–885.

25. Kreiger DT. Brain peptides: What, where, and why? Science 1983;222:975–985.
26. Moody TW, Pert CS, Gazdar AF, et al. High levels of intracellular bombesin characterize human small-cell lung carcinoma. Science 1981;214:1246–1248.
27. Maurer LH, O'Donnell JF, Kennedy S, et al. Human neurophysins in carcinoma of the lung. Relation to histology, disease stage, response rate, survival and syndrome of inappropriate antidiuretic hormone secretion. Cancer Treat Rep 1983;67:971–976.
28. Lazarus LH, Di Augustine RP, Jahnke CD, Hernandez O. Physalaemin: An amphibian tachykinin in human lung small cell carcinoma. Science 1983;219:79–81.
29. Richardson RL, Greco FA, Oldhan RK, Liddle GW. Tumor products and potential markers in small cell lung cancer. Semin Oncol 1978;5:253–262.
30. Gropp C, Havemann K, Scheuer A. Ectopic hormones in lung cancer patients at diagnosis and during therapy. Cancer 1980;46:347–354.
31. Hansen M, Hansen HH, Hirsch FR, et al. Hormonal polypeptides and amine metabolites in small cell carcinoma of the lung, with special reference to stage and subtypes. Cancer 1980;45:1432–1437.
32. Odell WD, Wolfsen AR, Bachelot I, Hirose FM. Ectopic production of lipotropin by cancer. Am J Med 1979;66:631–638.
33. Roos BA, Lindall AW, Ells J, et al. Increased plasma and tumor somatostatin-like immunoreactivity in medullary thyroid carcinoma and small cell lung cancer. J Clin Endocrinol Metab 1981;52:187–194.
34. Yamaguchi K, Abe K, Kameya T, et al. Production and molecular size heterogeneity of immunoreactive gastrin-releasing peptide in fetal and adult lungs and primary lung tumors. Cancer Res 1983;43:3932–3939.
35. Carney DN, Ihde DC, Cohen MH, et al. Serum neuron-specific enolase: A marker for disease extent and response to therapy of small cell lung cancer. Lancet 1982;1:583–585.
36. Nakanishi S, Inoue A, Kita T, et al. Nucleotide sequence of cloned cDNA for bovine corticotropin-β-lipotropin precursor. Nature 1979;278:423–427.
37. Bertagna XY, Nicholson WE, Pettengill OS, et al. Corticotropin, lipotropin, and β-endophin production by a human nonpituitary tumor in culture: Evidence for a common precursor. Proc Natl Acad Sci USA 1978;75:5160–5164.
38. Jeffcoate WJ, Rees LH. Adrenocorticotropin and related peptides in nonendocrine tumors. Curr Top Exp Endocrinol 1978;3:57–74.
39. Guillemin R. Endorphins, brain peptides that act like opiates, N Engl J Med 1977;296:226–228.
40. Huges J. Opioid peptides and their relatives. Nature 1979;278:394–395.
41. Silman RE, Holland D, Chard T, et al. The ACTH "family tree" of the rheusus monkey changes with development. Nature 1978;276:526–528.
42. Hirata Y, Yamamoto H, Matsukura S, Imura H. In vitro release and biosynthesis of tumor ACTH in ectopic ACTH producing tumors. J Clin Endocrinol Metab 1975;41:106–114.
43. Brown WH. A case of pluriglandular syndrome: Diabetes of bearded women. Lancet 1928;2:1022–1023.
44. Rassam JW, Anderson G. Incidence of paramalignant disorders in bronchogenic carcinoma. Thorax 1975;30:86–90.
45. Ross EJ. Endocrine syndromes of non-endocrine origin: Cancer and the adrenal cortex. Proc R Soc Med 1966;59:335–338.
46. Lokich JJ. The frequency and clinical biology of the ectopic hormone syndromes of small cell carcinoma. Cancer 1982;50:2111–2114.
47. Singer W, Kovacs K, Ryan N, Horvath E. Ectopic ACTH syndrome. Clinicopathological correlation. J Clin Pathol 1978;31:591–598.
48. Abeloff MD, Trump DL, Baylin SB. Ectopic adrenocorticotrophic (ACTH) syndrome and small cell carcinoma of the lung: Assessment of clinical implications in patients on combination chemotherapy. Cancer 1981;48:1082–1087.
49. Yallow RS, Eastridge CE, Higgins G Jr, Wolf J. Plasma and tumor ACTH in carcinoma of the lung. Cancer 1979;44:1789–1792.
50. Wolfsen AR, Odell WD. ProACTH. Use for early detection of lung cancer. Am J Med 1979;66:765–772.
51. Liddle GW, Island D, Meador CK. Normal and abnormal regulation of corticotropin secretion in man. Recent Prog Horm Res 1962;18:125–166.
52. Ayvazian LF, Schneider B, Gewirtz G, Yalow RS. Ectopic production of big ACTH in carcinoma of the lung. Its clinical usefulness as a biologic marker. Am Rev Respir Dis 1975;3:279–287.
53. Ratcliff JG, Knight RA, Besser GM. Tumour and plasma ACTH concentrations in patients with and without the ectopic ACTH syndrome. Clin Endocrinol 1972;1:27–44.
54. Gewirtz G, Yalow RS. Ectopic ACTH production in carcinoma of the lung. J Clin Invest 1974;53:1022–1032.
55. Abe K, Adachi I, Miyakawa S, et al. Production of calcitonin, adrenocorticotropic hormone, and β-melanocyte stimulating hormone in tumors derived from amine precursors uptake and decarboxylation cells. Cancer Res 1977;37:4100–4194.
56. Bloomfield GA, Holdaway IM, Corrin B, et al. Lung tumours and ACTH production. Clin Endocrinol 1977;6:95–104.
57. Gilby ED, Rees LH, Bondy PK. Ectopic hormones as markers of response to therapy in cancer. In: Proceedings of the Sixth International Symposium of Biological Characterizations of Human Tumors. New York: American Elsevier, 1976:132–138.
58. Amatruda TT, Upton GV. Hyperadrenocorticism and ACTH-releasing factor. Ann N Y Acad Sci 1974;230:168–180.
59. Eagan RT, Maurer LH, Forcier RJ, Tulloh M. Small cell carcinoma of the lung: Staging, paraneoplastic syndromes, treatment and survival. Cancer 1974;33:527–532.
60. Azzopardi JG, Williams ED. Pathology of "nonendocrine" tumors associated with Cushing's syndrome. Cancer 1968;22:273–286.
61. Skrabanek P, Powell D. Unifying concept of non-pituitary ACTH secreting tumors: Evidence of common origin of neural-crest tumors, carcinoids, and oat-cell carcinomas. Cancer 1978;42:1263–1269.
62. Lojek MA, Fer MF, Kasselberg AG, et al. Cushing's syndrome with small cell carcinoma of the uterine cervix. Am J Med 1980;69:140–144.
63. Matsuyama M, Inoue T, Ariyoshi Y, et al. Argyrophil cell carcinoma of the uterine cervix with ectopic production of ACTH, β-MSH, serotonin, histamine, and amylase. Cancer 1979;44:1813–1823.
64. Levenson RM, Ihde DC, Matthews MJ, et al. Small cell carcinoma presenting as an extrapulmonary neoplasm: Sites of origin and response to chemotherapy. J Natl Cancer Inst 1981;67:607–612.
65. Remick SC, Ruckdiscel JC. Extrapulmonary and pulmonary small cell carcinoma: Tumor biology, therapy and outcome. Med Pediatr Oncol 1992;20:89–99.
66. Rees LH, Ratcliffe JG. Ectopic hormone production by nonendocrine tumors. Clin Endocrinol 1974;3:263–299.
67. Bailey RE. Periodic "hormonogenesis"—a new phenomenon. Periodicity in function of a hormone-producing tumor in man. Clin Endocrinol 1971;32:317–327.
67a. Nieman LK, Chrousos GP, Oldfield EH, et al. The ovine corticotropin-releasing hormone stimulation test and the dexamethasone suppression test in the differential diagnosis of Cushing's syndrome. Ann Intern Med 1986;105:862–867.
68. Gold EM. The Cushing syndromes: Changing views of diagnosis and treatment. Ann Intern Med 1979;90:829–844.
69. Howlett TA, Perry L, Rees LH, et al. Diagnosis and management of ACTH dependent Cushing's syndrome: Comparison of the features in ectopic and pituitary ACTH production. Clin Endocrinol 1986;24:699–713.
69a. Oldfield EH, Deppman JL, Nieman LK, et al. Petrosal sinus sampling with and without corticotropin-releasing hormone for the differential diagnosis of Cushing's syndrome. N Engl J Med 1991;325:897–905.
70. Hattori M, Imura H, Matsukura S, et al. Multiple hormone-producing lung carcinoma. Cancer 1979;43:2429–2437.
71. Mason AMS, Ratcliffe JA, Buckly RM, Mason AS. ACTH secretion by bronchial carcinoid tumors. Clin Endocrinol 1972;1:3–25.
72. Imura H, Matsukura S, Yamamoto H, et al. Studies on ectopic ACTH-producing tumors. II. Clinical and biochemical features of 30 cases. Cancer 1975;35:1430–1437.
73. Corey RM, Varma SK, Drake CR, et al. Ectopic secretion of corticotropin-releasing factor as a cause of Cushing's syndrome. A clinical, morphologic and biochemical study. N Engl J Med 1984;311:13.
74. Belsky JL, Cuello B, Swanson LW, et al. Cushing's syndrome due to ectopic production of corticotropin-releasing factor. J Clin Endocrinol Metab 1985;60:496.
75. Schleingart DE, Lloyd RV, Akil H, et al. Cushing's syndrome secondary to ectopic corticotropin-releasing hormone—adrenocorticotropin secretion. J Clin Endocrinol Metab 1986;63:770.
76. Orth DN, Liddle GW. Results of treatment of 108 patients with Cushing's syndrome. N Engl J Med 1971;285:243–247.
77. Gordon P, Becker CE, Levey GS, Roth J. Efficacy of aminoglutethimide in the ectopic ACTH syndrome. J Clin Endocrinol Metab 1968;28:921–923.
78. Carey RM, Orth DN, Hartmann WH. Malignant melanoma with ectopic production of adrenocorticotrophic hormone: Palliative treatment with inhibitors of adrenal steroid biosynthesis. J Clin Endocrinol Metab 1973;36:482–487.
79. Vaughn CB, Pearson S, Chapman J, et al. The treatment of ACTH paraneoplastic syndrome with aminoglutethimide. J Natl Med Assoc 1979;71:21–23.
80. Child DF, Burke CW, Burley DM, et al. Drug control of Cushing's syndrome. Combined aminoglutethiamide and metapyrone therapy. Acta Endocrinol 1976;82:330–341.
81. Naber D, Pickar D, Dionne RA, et al. Assay of endogenous opiate receptor ligands in human CSF and plasma. Subst Alcohol Actions Misuse 1980;1:83–91.
82. Gropp C, Havemann K, Scharfe T, Ax W. Incidence of circulating immune complexes in patients with lung cancer and their effect on antibody dependent cytotoxicity. Oncology 1980;37:71–76.
83. Winkler WA, Crankshaw OF. Chloride depletion in conditions other than Addison's disease. J Clin Invest 1938;17:1–6.
84. Schwartz WDF, Bennett W, Curelop S, Bartter F. A syndrome of renal sodium loss and hyponatremia probably resulting from inappropriate secretion of antidiuretic hormone. Am J Med 1957;23:529–542.
85. Amatruda TT, Mulrow PJ, Gallagher JC, Sawyer WH. Carcinoma of the lung with inappropriate antidiuresis. N Engl J Med 1963;269:544–549.
86. Hamilton BPM, Upton GV, Amatruda TT. Evidence for the presence of neurophysins in tumors producing the syndrome of inappropriate antidiuresis. J Clin Endocrinol Metab 1972;35:764–767.
87. Cheng KW, Friesen HG. Physiological factors regulating secretion of neurophysin. Metabolism 1970;19:876–890.
88. Maurer LH, O'Donnell JF, Kennedy S, et al. Human neurophysins in carcinoma of the lung: Relation to histology, disease stage, response rate, survival and syndrome of inappropriate anti-diuretic hormone secretion. Cancer Treat Rep 1983;67:970–976.
89. Trump DL, Baylin SB. Ectopic hormone syndromes. In: Abeloff MD, ed. Complications of cancer: Diagnosis and management. Baltimore: Johns Hopkins University Press, 1979:211–241.
90. Moses AM, Miller M, Streeten DHP. Pathophysiologic and pharmacologic alterations in the release and action of ADH. Metabolism 1976;25:697–721.
91. Goodman LS, Gilman A, Gilman AG, Koelle GB. The Pharmacological basis of therapeutics. 5th ed. New York: MacMillan, 1975.
92. Fichman M, Bethune J. Effects of neoplasms on renal electrolyte function. Ann N Y Acad Sci 1974;230:448–472.

93. Padfield PL, Morton JJ, Brown JJ, et al. Plasma arginine vasopressin in the syndrome of antidiuretic hormone excess associated with bronchogenic carcinoma. Am J Med 1976;61:825–831.
94. Harlow PJ, DeClerck YA, Shore NA, et al. A fatal case of inappropriate ADH secretion induced by cyclophosphamide therapy. Cancer 1979;44:896–898.
95. DeFronzo RA, Braine H, Colvin OM, Davis PJ. Water intoxication in man after cyclophosphamide therapy: Time course and relation to drug activation. Ann Intern Med 1973;78:861–869.
96. Thomas TH, Morgan DB, Swaminathan R, et al. Severe hyponatremia. Lancet 1978;1: 621–624.
97. Radice PA, Dermody WC. Clonal heterogeneity of hormone produced by continuous cultures of small cell carcinoma of the lung. Proceedings of the American Association for Cancer Research and American Society of Clinical Oncology 1980;21:41.
98. Pettengill OS, Caulkner CS, Wurster-Hill DH, et al. Isolation and characterization of a hormone-producing cell line from human small cell anaplastic carcinoma of the lung. JNCI 1977;58:511–518.
99. Hainsworth JD, Workman R, Greco FA. Management of the syndrome of inappropriate antidiuretic hormone secretion in small cell lung cancer. Cancer 1983;51:161–165.
100. Comis RL, Miller M, Ginsberg SJ. Abnormalities in water homeostasis in small cell anaplastic lung cancer. Cancer 1980;45:2414–2421.
101. Munro AHG, Crompton GK. Inappropriate antidiuretic hormone secretion in oat cell carcinoma of bronchus: Aggravation of hyponatremia by intravenous cyclophosphamide. Thorax 1972;27:640–642.
102. Cohen MH, Bunn PA Jr, Ihde DC, et al. Chemotherapy rather than demeclocycline for inappropriate secretion of antidiuretic hormone. N Engl J Med 1978;298:1423.
103. North WG, Maurer H, O'Donnell JF. Human neurophysins and small cell carcinoma. Clin Res 1979;27:390A.
104. Hantman D, Rossier B, Zohlman R, Schrier R. Rapid correction of hyponatremia in the syndrome of inappropriate secretion of antidiuretic hormone. An alternative treatment to hypertonic saline. Ann Intern Med 1973;78:870–875.
105. Forrest JN Jr, Cox M, Hong C, et al. Superiority of demeclocycline over lithium in the treatment of chronic syndrome of inappropriate secretion of antidiuretic hormone. N Engl J Med 1978;298:173–177.
106. DeTroyer A. Demeclocycline treatment for syndrome of inappropriate antidiuretic hormone secretion. JAMA 1977;237:2823–2826.
107. White MG, Fetner DC. Treatment of the syndrome of inappropriate secretion of antidiuretic hormone with lithium carbonate. N Engl J Med 1975;292:390–392.
108. Decaux G, Brimioulle S, Genette F, Mockel J. Treatment of the syndrome of inappropriate secretion of antidiuretic hormone by urea. Am J Med 1980;69:99–106.
109. Cogan E, Debieve M-F, Philipart I, et al. High plasma levels of atrial natriuretic factor in SIADH. Lancet 1986;2:1258–1259.
110. Kamoi K, Ebe T, Hasegawa A, et al. Hyponatremia in small cell lung cancer. Mechanisms not involving inappropriate ADH secretion. Cancer 1987;60:1089–1093.
111. Trump DL. Abnormalities of bone and mineral metabolism. In: Abeloff MD, ed. Complications of cancer. Diagnosis and management. Baltimore: Johns Hopkins University Press, 1979:263–281.
112. Myers WPL. Differential diagnosis of hypercalcemia and cancer. CA 1977;27:258–272.
113. Isales C, Carcangiu ML, Stewart AF. Hypercalcemia in breast cancer. Reassessment of the mechanism. Am J Med 1987;82:1143–1147.
114. Holtz G, Johnson TR Jr, Schrock ME. Paraneoplastic hypercalcemia in ovarian tumors. Obstet Gynecol 1979;54:483–487.
115. Cryer PE, Kissane JM. Clinicopathologic conference. Malignant hypercalcemia. Am J Med 1979;65:486–494.
116. Bunn PA, Schechter GP, Blayney DP, et al. Clinical course of retrovirus-associated adult T-cell lymphoma in the United States. N Engl J Med 1983;309:257–262.
117. Moseley JM, Kubota M, Diefenbach-Jagger H, et al. Parathyroid hormone related protein purified from a human lung cancer cell line. Proc Natl Acad Sci USA 1987;84: 5048–5052.
118. Tashjian AH, Voelkel EF, Levine L. Evidence that the bone resorption-stimulating factor produced by mouse fibrosarcoma cells is prostaglandin E_2: A new model for the hypercalcemia of cancer. J Exp Med 1972;135:1329–1343.
119. Voelkel EF, Tashjian AH Jr, Franklin R, et al. Hypercalcemia and tumor-prostaglandins: The VX2 carcinoma model in the rabbit. Metabolism 1975;24:973–986.
120. Budayr WJ, Nissenson RA, Klein RF, et al. Increased serum levels of a parathyroid hormone-like protein in malignancy-associated hypercalcemia. Ann Intern Med 1989;111:807–812.
121. Stewart AF, Broadus AE. Clinical review 16: Parathyroid related proteins: Coming of age in the 1990s. J Clin Endocrinol Metab 1990;71:1410–1414.
122. Burtis WJ, Brady TG, Orloff JJ, et al. Immunochemical characterization of circulating parathyroid hormone-related protein in patients with humoral hypercalcemia of malignancy. N Engl J Med 1990;322:1106–1112.
123. Horton JE, Raisz LG, Simmons HA, et al. Bone resorbing activity in supernatant fluid from cultured human peripheral blood leukocytes. Science 1972;177:793–795.
124. Luben RA, Mundy GR, Trummel CL, Raisz LG. Partial purification of osteoclast-activating factor from phytohemagglutinin-stimulated human leukocytes. J Clin Invest 1974;53:1473–1480.
125. Mundy GR, Raisz LG, Cooper RA, et al. Evidence for the secretion of an osteoclast stimulating factor in myeloma. N Engl J Med 1974;291:1041–1046.
126. Elion G, Mundy GR. Direct resorption of bone by human breast cancer cells in vitro. Nature 1978;276:726–728.
127. Koeffler HP, Mundy GR, Golde DW, Cline MJ. Production of bone-resorbing activity in poorly differentiated monocytic malignancy. Cancer 1978;41:2438–2443.
128. Seyberth HW. Prostaglandin-mediated hypercalcemia: A paraneoplastic syndrome. Klin Wochenschr 1978;56:373–387.
129. Brereton HD, Halushka PV, Alexander RW, et al. Indomethacin-responsive hypercalcemia in a patient with renal-cell adenocarcinoma. N Engl J Med 1975;29:83–85.
130. Robertson RP, Baylink DJ, Marini JJ, Adkison HW. Elevated prostaglandins and suppressed parathyroid hormone associated with hypercalcemia and renal cell carcinoma. J Clin Endocrinol Metab 1975;41:164–167.
131. Ito H, Sanada T, Katayama T, Shimazaki J. Indomethacin-responsive hypercalcemia. N Engl J Med 1975;293:558–559.
132. Seyberth HW, Segre GV, Morgan JL, et al. Prostaglandins as mediators of hypercalcemia associated with certain types of cancer. N Engl J Med 1975;293:1278–1283.
133. Tashjian AH Jr. Prostaglandins, hypercalcemia and cancer. N Engl J Med 1975;293: 1317–1318.
134. Shigeno C, Yamamoto I, Dokoh S, et al. Identification of 1,24-dihydroxyvitamin D_3-like bone-resorbing lipid in a patient with cancer-associated hypercalcemia. J Clin Endocrinol Metab 1985;61:761–768.
135. Rosenthal N, Insogua KL, Godsall JW, et al. Elevations in circulating 1,25-dihydroxyvitamin D in three patients with lymphoma-associated hypercalcemia. J Clin Endocrinol Metab 1985;60:29–33.
136. Frankel TL, Mason RS, Hersey P, et al. The synthesis of vitamin D metabolites by human melanoma cells. J Clin Endocrinol Metab 1983;57:627–630.
137. Raskin P, McClain CJ, Medsger TA. Hypocalcemia associated with metastatic bone disease. Arch Intern Med 1973;132:539–543.
138. Sackner MA, Spivak AP, Balian LJ. Hypocalcemia in the presence of osteoblastic metastases. N Engl J Med 1960;262:173–176.
139. Hall TC, Griffiths CT, Petranek JR. Hypocalcemia: An unusual metabolic complication of breast cancer. N Engl J Med 1966;275:1474–1477.
140. Jackson HJ, Taylor FHL. Calcium, potassium, and inorganic phosphate content of the serum in cancer patients. Effect of roentgen ray radiation on the level of these substances in the blood of cancer patients. Am J Cancer 1933;19:379–388.
141. Ehrlich M, Goldsten M, Heinemann HO. Hypocalcemia, hypoparathyroidism and osteoblastic metastases. Metabolism 1963;12:516–526.
142. Gordon GS. Hyper-and hypocalcemia: Pathogenesis and treatments. Ann N Y Acad Sci 1974;230:181–186.
143. Salassa RM, Jowsey J, Arnaud C. Hypophosphatemia osteomalacia associated with "nonendocrine" tumors. N Engl J Med 1970;283:65–69.
144. Stanbury W. Tumor-associated hypophosphatemia, osteomalacia and rickets. Clin Endocrinol Metabol 1972;1:256–259.
145. Daniels RA, Weisenfeld I. Tumorous phosphaturic osteomalacia. Report of a case associated with multiple hemangiomas of bone. Am J Med 1979;67:155–159.
146. Siris ES, Clemens TL, Dempster DW, et al. Tumor-induced osteomalacia. Kinetics of calcium, phosphorus, and vitamin D metabolism and characteristics of bone histomorphometry. Am J Med 1987;82:307–312.
147. Olefsky J, Compson R, Jones H, Reaven G. "Tertiary" hyperparathyroidism, and apparent "cure" of vitamin D resistant rickets after removal of an ossifying mesenchymal tumor of the pharynx. N Engl J Med 1972;286:740–746.
148. Evans DJ, Azzopardi JG. Distinctive tumours of bone and soft tissue causing acquired vitamin-D-resistant osteomalacia. Lancet 1972;1:353–354.
149. Taylor HC, Velasco ME, Fallan MD. Oncogenic osteomalacia and inappropriate antidiuretic hormone secretion due to oat cell carcinoma. Ann Intern Med 1984;101: 786–788.
150. Ryan EA, Reiss E. Oncogenous osteomalacia. Review of the world literature of 42 cases and report of two new cases. Am J Med 1984;77:501–512.
151. Tashjian AH, Wolfe HJ, Voelkel EF. Human calcitonin: Immunologic assay, cytologic localization and studies of medullary thyroid carcinoma. Am J Med 1974;56:840–849.
152. Silva OL, Broder LE, Doppman JL, et al. Calcitonin as a marker for bronchogenic cancer: A prospective study. Cancer 1979;44:680–684.
153. Becker KL, Nash DR, Silva OL, et al. Urine calcitonin levels in patients with bronchogenic carcinoma. JAMA 1980;243:670–672.
154. Ellison M, Woodhouse D, Hillyard C, et al. Immunoreactive calcitonin production by human lung carcinoma cells in culture. Br J Cancer 1975;32:373–379.
155. Bertagna XY, Nicholson WE, Pettengill OS, et al. Ectopic production of high molecular weight calcitonin and corticotropin by human small cell carcinoma cells in tissue culture: Evidence for separate precursors. J Clin Endocrinol Metab 1978;47:1390–1393.
156. Lips CJ, Vander Sluys V, Van Der Donk JA, Van Dam RH. Common precursor molecule as origin for the ectopic-hormone-producing tumor syndrome. Lancet 1978;1:16–18.
157. Hillyard V, Coombes RC, Greenberg PB, et al. Calcitonin in breast and lung cancer. Clin Endocrinol 1976;5:1–8.
158. Iacangelo A, Affolter HV, Eiden LE, et al. Bovine chromogranin A sequence and distribution of its messenger RNA in endocrine tissues. Nature 1986;323:82–86.
159. Sobol RE, O'Connor DT, Addison J, et al. Elevated serum chromogranin A concentrations in small cell lung cancer. Ann Intern Med 1986;105:698–700.
160. O'Connor DT, Deftos LI. Secretion of chromogranin A by peptide producing endocrine neoplasms. N Engl J Med 1986;314:1145–1151.
161. Huttner WB, Benedum UM. Chromogranin A and pancreastatin. Nature 1987;325: 305.
162. Eiden LE. Is chromagranin a prohormone? Nature 1987;325:301.
163. Vaitukaitis JL, Ross GT, Braunstein GD, Rayford PL. Gonadotropins and their subunits: Basic and clinical studies. Recent Prog Horm Res 1976;32:289–321.
164. Kenimer JG, Hershman JM, Higgins HP. The thyrotropin in hydatidiform moles is human chorionic gonadotropin. J Clin Endocrinol Metab 1975;40:481–491.

165. Nisula BC, Ketelslegers JM. Thyroid-stimulating activity and chorionic gonadotropin. J Clin Invest 1974;54:494–499.
166. Faiman C, Colwell JA, Ryan RJ, et al. Gonadotropin secretion from a bronchogenic carcinoma. N Engl J Med 1967;277:1395–1399.
167. Fusco FD, Rosen SW. Gonadotropin-producing anaplastic large-cell carcinomas of the lung. N Engl J Med 1966;275:507–515.
168. Anderson T, Waldmann TA, Javadpour N, Glatstein E. Testicular germ-cell neoplasms: Recent advances in diagnosis and therapy. Ann Intern Med 1979;90:373–385.
169. Lewis JL. Chemotherapy of gestational choriocarcinoma. Cancer 1972;30:1517–1521.
170. Blackman MR, Weintraub BD, Rosen SW, et al. Human placental and pituitary glycoprotein hormones and their subunits as tumor markers: A quantitative assessment. JNCI 1980;65:81–93.
171. Tsuruhara T, Dufau ML, Hickman J, Catt KJ. Biological properties of hCG after removal of terminal sialic acid and galactose residues. Endocrinology 1972;91:296–301.
172. Muggia FM, Rosen SW, Weintraub BD, Hansen HH. Ectopic placental proteins in nontrophoblastic tumors: Serial measurements following chemotherapy. Cancer 1975;36:1327–1337.
173. Kahn CR, Rosen SW, Weintraub BD, et al. Ectopic production of chorionic gonadotropin and its subunits by islet cell tumors: A specific marker for malignancy. N Engl J Med 1977;197:565–569.
174. Bender RA, Weintraub BD, Rosen SW. Prospective evaluation of two tumor-associated proteins in pancreatic adenocarcinoma. Cancer 1979;45:591–595.
175. Broder LE, Weintraub BD, Rosen SW, et al. Placental proteins and their subunits as tumor markers in prostatic carcinoma. Cancer 1977;40:211–216.
176. Metz SA, Weintraub B, Rosen SW, et al. Ectopic secretion of chorionic gonadotropin by a lung carcinoma. Pituitary gonadotropin and subunit secretion and prolonged chemotherapeutic remission. Am J Med 1978;65:325–333.
177. Tashjian AH Jr, Weintraub BD, Barowksy NJ, et al. Subunits of human chorionic gonadotropin: Unbalanced synthesis and secretion by clonal cell strains derived from a bronchogenic carcinoma. Proc Natl Acad Sci USA 1973;70:1419–1422.
178. Rosen SW, Weintraub BD, Aaronson SA. Nonrandom ectopic protein production by malignant cells: Direct evidence in vitro. J Clin Endocrinol Metab 1980;50:834–841.
179. Blackman MR, Weintraub BD, Rosen SW, Harmen SM. Comparison of the effects of lung cancer, benign lung disease, and normal aging on pituitary—gonadal function in men. J Clin Endocrinol Metab 1988;66:88–95.
179a. Rudnick P, Odell WD. In search of a cancer. N Engl J Med 1971;284:405–408.
180. Skrabanek P, Kirrane J, Powell D. A unifying concept of chorionic gonadotropin production in malignancy. Invest Cell Pathol 1979;2:75–85.
181. Greco FA, Fer MF, Oldham RD, et al. Intracytoplasmic localization of ectopic β-human chorionic gonadotropin and α-fetoprotein in suspected extragonadal germ cell cancers by immunohistochemical methods. Clin Res 1980;28:415A.
182. Novarro C, Sancho A, Morales L, et al. Paraneoplastic precocious puberty. Report of a new case with hepatoblastoma and review of the literature. Cancer 1985;56:1725–1729.
183. Root AW, Bongiovanni AM, Eberlein WR. A testicular-interstitial-cell stimulating gonadotropin in a child with hepatoblastoma and sexual precocity. J Clin Endocrinol Metab 1968;28:1317–1322.
184. McArthur J, Toll GD, Russfield AB, et al. Sexual precocity attributable to ectopic gonadtropin secretion by hepatoblastoma. Am J Med 1973;54:390–403.
185. Kurman RJ, Norris HJ. Embryonal carcinoma of the ovary: A clinicopathologic entity distinct from endodermal sinus tumor resembling embryonal carcinoma of the adult testes. Cancer 1976;38:2420–2433.
186. Weintraub BD, Rosen SW. Ectopic production of human chorionic somatomammotrophin by nontrophoblastic cancers. J Clin Endocrinol Metab 1971;32:94–101.
187. Rosen SW, Weintraub BD, Vaitukaitis JL, et al. Placental proteins and their subunits as tumor markers. Ann Intern Med 1975;82:71–83.
187a. Steiner H, Dahlback O, Waldenstrom J. Ecotpic growth-hormone production and osteoarthropathy in carcinoma of the bronchus. Lancet 1968;1:783–785.
188. Ennis CG, Cameron DP, Burger HG. On the etiology of hypertrophic pulmonary osteoarthropathy in bronchogenic carcinoma: Lack of relationship to elevated growth hormone levels. Aust N Z J Med 1973;3:157–161.
189. Sonksen PH, Ayres AB, Braimbridge M, et al. Acromegaly caused by pulmonary carcinoid tumors. Clin Endocrinol 1976;5:505–513.
190. Scheithauer BW, Bloch B, Carpenter PC, Brazeau P. Ectopic secretion of a growth hormone-releasing factor. Report of a case of acromegaly with bronchical carcinoid tumor. Am J Med 1984;76:605–616.
191. Thorner MO, Vance ML, Kovacs K. Ectopic growth hormone-releasing hormone (GHRH) syndrome and significance. Proc Int Chemother Cong [Abstract] 1986:5051.
192. Boizel R, Labat F, Bachelot I, et al. Acromegaly due to a growth hormone releasing hormone secreting bronchial carcinoid tumor. Further information on the abnormal responsiveness of the somatotroph cells and their recovery after successful treatment. J Clin Endocrinol Metab 1987;64:304–308.
193. Roth KA, Eberwine J, Kovacs K, et al. Acromegaly and pheochromocytoma: A multiple endocrine syndrome caused by a plurihormonal adrenal medullary tumor. J Clin Endocrinol Metab 1986;63:1421–1426.
194. Anderson G. The incidence of paramalignant syndromes. In: Anderson G, ed. Paramalignant syndromes in lung cancer. London: William Heinemann, 1973:4.
195. Hennen G. Characterization of a thyroid-stimulating factor in human cancer tissue. J Clin Endocrinol Metab 1967;27:610–614.
196. Odell WD, Bates RW, Rivlin RS, et al. Increased thyroid function without clinical hyperthyroidism in patients with choriocarcinoma. J Clin Endocrinol Metab 1963;23:658–668.
197. Cave WT Jr, Dunn JT. Choriocarcinoma with hyperthyroidism: Probable identity of the thyrotropin with human chorionic gonadtropin. Ann Intern Med 1976;85:60–63.
198. Bommer G, Altenahr E, Kuhnau J Jr, Kloppel G. Ultrastructure of hemangiopericytoma associated with paraneoplastic hypoglycemia. Z Krebsforsh 1976;85:231–241.
199. Sluiter WJ, Marrink J, Houwen B. Monoclonal gammopathy with an insulin binding IgG(κ) M-component associated with severe hypoglycemia. Br J Haematol 1986;62:679–687.
200. Stuart CA, Prince MJ, Peters EJ, et al. Insulin receptor proliferation: A mechanism for tumor-associated hypoglycemia. J Clin Endocrinol Metab 1986;63:879–885.
201. Younus S, Soterakis J, Sossi AJ, et al. Hypoglycemia secondary to metastases to the liver. A case report and review of the literature. Gastroenterology 1977;72:334–337.
202. Kiang DT, Bauer GE, Kennedy BJ. Immunoassayable insulin in carcinoma of the cervix associated with hypoglycemia. Cancer 1973;31:801–805.
203. Silvert CK, Rossini AA, Ghazvinian S, et al. Tumor hypoglycemia: Deficient splanchnic glucose output and deficient glucagon secretion. Diabetes 1976;25:202–206.
204. Solomon J. Case report: Spurious hypoglycemia and hypperkalemia in myelomonocytic leukemia. Am J Med Sci 1974;267:359–363.
205. Zapf J, Walter H, Froesch ER. Radioimmunological determination of insulin-like growth factors I and II in normal subjects and in patients with growth disorders and extrapancreatic tumor hypoglycemia. J Clin Invest 1981;68:1321–1330.
206. Gorden P, Hendricks CM, Kahn CR, et al. Hypoglycemia associated with non-islet cell tumor and insulin like growth factors. N Engl J Med 1981;305:1452–1455.
207. Li TCM, Reed C, Stubenbard WT, et al. Surgical cure of hypoglycemia associated with cystosarcoma phylloides and elevated NSILP. Am J Med 1983;74:1080–1084.
208. Van Wyk JJ, Underwood LE, Hintz RL, et al. The somatomedins: A family of insulin-like hormones under growth hormone control. Recent Prog Horm Res 1974;30:259–318.
209. Chandalia HB, Boshell BR. Hypoglycemia in association with extrapancreatic tumors. Arch Intern Med 1972;129:447–456.
210. Megyesi K, Kahn CR, Roth J, Gordon P. Hypoglycemia in association with extrapancreatic tumors: Demonstration of elevated plasma NSILA-S by a new radioreceptor assay. J Clin Endocrinol Metab 1974;38:931–934.
211. Farsang C, Ramirez-Gonzalez MD, Mucci L, Kunos G. Possible role of an endogenous opiate in the cardiovascular effects of central α-adrenoceptor stimulation in spontaneously hypertensive rats. J Pharmacol Exp Ther 1980;214:203–208.
212. Davies P, Joseph J, Thompson A. Anterior to posterior variations in the concentration of somatostatin-like immunoreactivity in human basal ganglia. Brain Res Bull 1981;7:365–368.
213. Perry RH, Dockray GJ, Dimaline R, et al. Neuropeptides in Alzheimer's disease, depression and schizophrenia. J Neurol Sci 1981;51:465–472.
214. Emson PC, Arregui A, Clement-Jones V, et al. Regional distribution of methionine-enkephalin and substance P-like immunoreactivity in normal brain and in Huntington's disease. Brain Res 1980;199:147–160.
215. Aronin N, Cooper PE, Lorenz LJ, et al. Somastostatin is increased in the basal ganglia in Huntington disease. Ann Neurol 1983;13:519–526.
216. Brandt NJ, Teremius L, Jacobsen BB, et al. Hyper-endorphin syndrome in a child with necrotizing encephalomyelopathy. N Engl J Med 1980;303:914–916.
217. Allen JC, Deck MDF, Foley KM, et al. Neuro-oncology, vol 2. New York: Memorial Sloan-Kettering Cancer Center, 1979.
218. Newman SJ, Hansen HH. Frequency, diagnosis, and treatment of brain metastases in 247 consecutive patients with bronchogenic carcinoma. Cancer 1974;33:492–496.
219. Nugent JL, Bunn PA Jr, Matthews MJ, et al. CNS metastases in small cell bronchogenic carcinoma. Increasing frequency and changing pattern with lengthening survival. Cancer 1979;44:1855–1893.
220. Posner JB, Chernik NL. Intracranial metastasis from systemic cancer. Adv Neurol 1978;19:575–587.
221. Rosen P, Armstrong D. Nonbacterial thrombotic endocarditis in patients with malignant neoplastic disease. Am J Med 1973;54:23–29.
222. Collins RC, Al-Mondhiry H, Chernik NL, Posner JB. Neurologic manifestations of intravascular coagulation in patients with cancer: A clinical-pathological analysis of 12 cases. Neurology 1975;25:795–806.
223. Sigsbee B, Deck MDF, Posner JB. Non-metastatic superior saggital sinus thrombosis complicating systemic cancer. Neurology 1979;29:139–146.
224. Rogers LR, Cho ES, Kempin S, Posner JB. Cerebral infarction from nonbacterial thrombotic endocarditis. Clinical and pathologic study including effects of anticoagulation. Am J Med 1987;83:746–756.
225. Hickey WF, Garnick MB, Henderson IC, Dawson DM. Primary cerebral venous thrombosis in patients with cancer—A rarely diagnosed paraneoplastic syndrome. Am J Med 1982;73:740–750.
226. Persen JR. Systemic angioendotheliosis: A possible disorder of a circulating angiogenic factor. Br J Dermatol 1977;96:329–331.
227. Petito CK, Gottlieb GJ, Dougherty JH, Petito FH. Neoplastic angioendotheliosis: Ultrastructural study and review of the literature. Ann Neurol 1978;3:393–399.
228. Gimenez-Gallego G, Rodkey J, Bennett C, et al. Brain derived acidic fibroblast growth factor: Complete amino acid sequence and homologies. Science 1985;230:1385–1833.
229. Folkman J. A family of angiogenic peptides. Nature 1987;329:671–672.
230. Bell CE Jr, Seetharam S. Expression of endodermally derived and neural crest-derived differentiation antigens by human lung and colon tumors. Cancer 1979;44:12–18.
231. Bunn PA, Gazdar AF, Carney DN, Minna JD. Small cell lung carcinoma and natural killer cells share an antigen determinant, Leu-7. Clin Res 1984;32:413A.
232. Schuller-Petrovic S, Gebhart W, Lassmann H, Rumpold H, Kraft D. A shared antigenic determinant between natural killer cells and nervous tissue. Nature 1983;306:179–181.

233. Wilkinson PC, Zeroniski J. Immunofluorescent detection of antibodies against neurones in sensory carcinomatoms neuropathy. Brain 1965;88:529–538.
233a. Moll JWB, Henzen-Logmans SC, Splinter TAW, van der Burg MEL, Vecht CJ. Diagnostic value of anti-neuronal antibodies for paraneoplastic disorders of the nervous system. J Neurol Neurosurg Psychiatry 1990;53:940–943.
233b. Grause F, Abos J, Roquer J, Mazzara R, Pereira A. Effect of plasmapheresis on serum and CSF auto-antibody levels in CNS paraneoplastic syndromes. Neurology 1990;40: 1621–1623.
234. Brain WR, Wilkinson M. Subacute cerebellar degeneration associated with neoplasms. Brain 1965;88:465.
235. Paone JF, Jeyasingham K. Remission of cerebellar dysfunction after pneumonectomy for bronchogenic carcinoma. N Engl J Med 1980;302:156–157.
236. Victor M, Adams RD, Mancall EL. A restricted form of cerebellar cortical degeneration occurring in alcoholic patients. Arch Neurol 1959;1:579–688.
237. Steven MM, Carnegie PR, Mackay IR, et al. Cerebellar cortical degeneration with ovarian carcinoma. Postgrad Med J 1982;58:47–51.
238. Dropcho EJ, Chen Y-T, Posner JB, Old LB. Cloning of a brain protein identified by autoantibodies from a patient with paraneoplastic cerebellar degeneration. Proc Natl Acad Sci USA 1987;84:4552–4556.
238a. Furneaux HM, Rosenblum MK, Dalmau J, et al. Selective expression of purkinje-cell antigens in tumor tissue from patients with paraneoplastic cerebellar degeneration. N Engl J Med 1990;322:1844–1851.
238b. Fathallah-Shaykh H, Wolfs, Wang E, Posner JB, Furneaux HM. Cloning of a leucine-zipper protein recognized by the sera of patients with antibody-associated paraneoplastic cerebellar degeneration. Proc Natl Acad Sci USA 1991;88:3451–3454.
238c. Duncan MB, Cobos E, Maccario M. Paraneoplastic cerebellar degeneration due to Hodgkin's Disease. West J Med 1989;150:463–465.
238d. Sakai K, Mitchell DJ, Tsudamoto T, Steinman L. Isolation of a complementary DNA clone encoding an autoantigen recognized by an anti-neuronal cell antibody from a patient with paraneoplastic cerebellar degeneration. Ann Neurol 1990;28:692–698.
238e. Komguth SE. Neuronal proteins and paraneoplastic syndromes. N Engl J Med 1989;321:1607–1608.
239. Shapiro WR. Remote effects of neoplasm on the central nervous system: Encephalopathy. Adv Neurol 1976;15:101–117.
240. Dorfman LH, Forno LS. Paraneoplastic encephalomyelitis. Acta Neurol Scand 1972;48: 556–574.
241. Corsellis JAN, Goldberg GJ, Norton AR. "Limbic encephalitis" and its association with carcinoma. Brain 1968;91:481–497.
242. Brennan LV, Craddock PR. Limbic encephalopathy as a nonmetastatic complication of oat cell lung cancer. Am J Med 1983;75:518–520.
243. Carr I. The Ophelia syndrome: Memory loss in Hodgkin's disease. Lancet 1982;1: 844–845.
243a. Lacomis D, Khoshbin S, Schick RM. MR imaging of paraneoplastic limbic encephalitis. J Comput Assist Tomogr 1990;14:115–117.
243b. Burton GV, Bullard DE, Walther PJ, Burger PC. Paraneoplastic limbic encephalopathy with testicular carcinoma. A reversible neurologic syndrome. Cancer 1988;62:2248–2251.
244. Sawyer RA. Blindness caused by photoreceptor degeneration as a remote effect of cancer. Am J Ophthalmol 1976;81:606–613.
245. Grunwald GB, Simmonds MA, Klein R, Kornguth SE. Autoimmune basis for visual paraneoplastic syndrome in patients with small cell lung carcinoma. Lancet 1985;1: 658–661.
246. Pillary N, Ebers GC, Gilbert JJ, Brown JD. Internuclear opthalmoplegia and "optic neuritis": Paraneoplastic effects of bronchial carcinoma. Neurology 1984;34:788–791.
246a. Thirkill CE, FitzGerald P, Sergott RC, et al. Cancer-associated retinopathy (CAR syndrome) with antibodies reacting with retinal, optic nerve, and cancer cells. N Engl J Med 1989;321:1589–1594.
246b. Jacobson DM, Thirkill CE, Tipping SJ. A chemical triad to diagnose paraneoplastic retinopathy. Ann Neurol 1990;28:162–167.
246c. Luque FA, Furneaux HM, Ferziger R, et al. Anti-Ri: An antibody associated with paraneoplastic opsoclenus and breast cancer. Ann Neurol 1991;29:241–251.
247. Padgett BL. JC papovavirus in progressive multifocal leukoencephalopathy. J Infect Dis 1976;133:686–690.
248. Norris FH Jr, Engel WK. Carcinomatous amyotrophic lateral sclerosis. In: Brain WR, Norris FH Jr, eds. The remote effects of cancer on the nervous system. New York: Grune & Stratton, 1965.
249. Mancall EL, Rosales RK. Necrotizing myelopathy associated with visceral carcinoma. Brain 1964;87:636–639.
250. Handforth A, Nag S, Sharp D, Robertson DM. Paraneoplastic subacute necrotic myelopathy. Can J Neurol Sci 1983;10:204–207.
250a. Dansey RD, Hammond-Tooke GD, Lai K, Bergwoda WR. Subacute myelopathy: An unusual paraneoplastic complication of Hodgkin's disease. Med Pediatr Oncol 1988;16: 284–286.
251. Walton JN, Tomlinson BE, Pearce GW. Subacute "poliomyelitis" and Hodgkin's disease. J Neurol Sci 1968;6:435–445.
252. Horwich MS, Cho L, Porro RS, Posner JB. Subacute sensory neuropathy: A remote effect of carcinoma. Ann Neurol 1977;1:7–19.
253. Henson RA, Hoffman HL, Urich H. Encephalomyelitis with carcinoma. Brain 1965;88: 449–464.
254. Croft PB, Urich H, Wilkinson M. Peripheral neuropathy of sensorimotor type associated with malignant disease. Brain 1967;90:31–66.
255. Dayan AD, Croft PB, Wilkinson M. Association of carcinomatous neuromyopathy with different histological types of carcinoma of the lung. Brain 1965;88:435–448.
256. Newman MK, Gugino RJ. Neuropathies and myopathies associated with occult malignancies. JAMA 1964;190:575–577.
257. Victor M, Banker BQ, Adams RD. The neuropathy of multiple myeloma. J Neurol Neurosurg Psychiatry 1958;21:73–88.
257a. Founan A. Peripheral neuropathy in cancer patients: Incidence, features, and pathophysiology. Oncology 1990;4:57–62, 85–89.
257b. Weissman DE, Gottshall JL. Complete remission of paraneoplastic sensorimotor neuropathy: A case associated with small cell lung cancer responsive to chemotherapy, plasma exchange and radiotherapy. J Clin Apheresis 1989;5:3–5.
258. Lisak RP. Gullain-Barre syndrome and Hodgkin's disease: Three cases with immunological studies. Ann Neurol 1977;1:72–78.
259. Schuffer MD, Baird HW, Fleming CR, et al. Intestinal pseudo-obstruction as the presenting manifestation of small cell carcinoma of the lung. Ann Intern Med 1983;98: 129–134.
260. Siemsen JK, Meister L. Bronchogenic carcinoma associated with severe orthostatic hypotension. Ann Intern Med 1963;58:669–676.
261. Park DM, Johnson RH, Crean GP, Robinson JF. Orthostatic hypotension in bronchial carcinoma. Br Med J 1972;3:510–511.
262. Ahmed MN, Carpenter S. Autonomic neuropathy and carcinoma of the lung. Can Med Assoc J 1975;113:410–412.
263. Ogilvie H. Large intestine colic due to sympathetic deprivation. Br Med J 1948;2: 671–673.
264. DeVere R, Bradley WG. Polymyositis: Its presentation, morbidity and mortality. Brain 1976;98:637–666.
265. Barnes BE. Dermatomyositis and malignancy. A review of the literature. Ann Intern Med 1976;84:68–76.
266. Williams RC Jr. Dermatomyositis and malignancy: A review of the literature. Ann Intern Med 1959;50:1174–1181.
266a. Sigurgeirsson B, Lindelof B, Edhag O, Allander E. Risk of cancer in patients with dermatomyositis or plymyositis. A population-based study. N Engl J Med 1992;326: 363–367.
267. Lambert EH, Eaton LM, Rooke ED. Defect of neuromuscular conduction associated with malignant neoplasms. Am J Physiol 1956;187:612.
268. Lambert EH, Rooke ED. Myasthenic state and lung cancer. In: Brain WR, Norris FH Jr, eds. The remote effects of cancer on the nervous system. New York: Grune & Stratton, 1965:67–80.
269. Simpson JA. The myasthenic (Eaton-Lambert) syndrome associated with carcinoma: Enzyme induction as a possible mechanism of paraneoplastic syndromes. Scott Med J 1982;27:220–228.
270. Cherington M. Guanidine and germline in Eaton-Lambert syndrome. Neurology 1976;26:944–946.
271. Jenkyn LR, Brooks PL, Forcier RJ, et al. Remission of the Lambert-Eaton syndrome and small cell anaplastic carcinoma of the lung induced by chemotherapy and radiotherapy. Cancer 1980;46:1123–1127.
272. Login IS, Kim YI, Judd AM, et al. Immunoglobulins of Lambert-Eaton myasthenic syndrome inhibit rat pituitary hormone release. Ann Neurol 1987;22:610–614.
272a. McEvoy KM, Windebank AS, Draube JR, Low PSA. 3,4-Diaminopyricline in the treatment of Lambert-Eaton myasthenic syndrome. N Engl J Med 1989;321:1567–1571.
273. Tyler HR. Paraneoplastic syndromes of nerve, muscle, and neuromuscular junction. Ann N Y Acad Sci 1974;230:348–357.
274. Latov N, Sherman WH, Nemni R, et al. Plasma cell dyscrasia and peripheral neuropathy with a monoclonal antibody to peripheral-nerve myelin. N Engl J Med 1980;303: 618–621.
275. Johnson PC, Rolak LA, Hamilton RH, Laguna JF. Paraneoplastic vasculitis of nerve: A remote effect of cancer. Ann Neurol 1979;5:437–444.
276. Clark SC, Kamen R. The human hematopoietic colony stimulating factors. Science 1987;236:1229–1237.
277. Hammond D, Winnick S. Paraneoplastic erythrocytosis and ectopic erythropoietins. Ann N Y Acad Sci 1974;230:219–227.
278. Valentine WN, Hennessy TG, Lang E, et al. Polycythemia: Erythrocytosis and erythremia. Ann Intern Med 1968;69:587–606.
279. Sytkowski AJ, Richie JP, Bicknell KA. New human renal carcinoma cell line established from a patient with erythrocytosis. Cancer Res 1983;43:1415–1419.
279a. Da Silva JL, Lacombe C, Bruneval P, et al. Tumor cells are the site of erythropoietin synthesis in human renal cancers associated with polycythemia. Blood 1990;75:577–582.
280. Williams WJ, Beutler E, Erslev AJ, Rundles RW. Hematology. 2nd ed. New York: McGraw-Hill, 1977.
281. Berlin NI. Anemia of cancer. Ann N Y Acad Sci 1974;230:209–211.
282. Waterbury L. Hematologic problems. In: Abeloff MD, ed. Complications of cancer: Diagnosis and management. Baltimore: Johns Hopkins Press, 1979:121–145.
282a. Hocking W, Goodman J, Golde D. Gramulocytosis associated with tumor production of colony stimulating factor. Blood 1983;61:600–609.
283. Cartwright GE, Lee GR. The anemia of chronic disorders. Br J Haematol 1971;21: 147–152.
284. Crowthers D, Bateman CJT. Hematological aspects of systemic disease-malignant disease. Clin Haematol 1972;1:447–455.
285. Jacobs EM, Hutter RVP, Pool JL, Ley AB. Benign thymoma and selective erythroid aplasia of the bone marrow. Cancer 1959;12:47–57.
286. Vasavada PJ, Bournigal LJ, Reynolds RW. Thymoma associated with pure red cell aplasia and hypogammaglobulinemias. Postgrad Med 1973;54:93–98.

287. Guthrie TH, Thornton RM. Pure red cell aplasia obscured by a diagnosis of carcinoma. South Med J 1983;76:632–634.
288. Akard LP, Brandt J, Lee L, et al. Chronic T cell lymphoproliferative disorder and pure red cell aplasia. Am J Med 1987;83:1069–1074.
289. Hoffbrand AV, Hobbs JR, Kremenchuzky S, Mallin DL. Incidence and pathogenesis of megaloblastic erythropoiesis in multiple myeloma. J Clin Pathol 1967;20:699–705.
290. Pirofsky B. Clinical aspects of autoimmune hemolytic anemia. Semin Hematol 1976;13:251–265.
291. Ludwin D, Sacks P, Lynch S, et al. Autoimmune hematological complications occurring during the treatment of malignant lymphoproliferative diseases. S Afr Med J 1974;48:2143–2145.
292. Lackner H. Hemostatic abnormalities associated with dysproteinemias. Semin Hematol 1973;10:125–133.
293. Burkert L, Becker G, Pisciotta AV. Ovarian malignancy and hemolytic anemia. Ann Intern Med 1970;73:91–93.
294. Dawson MA, Tolbert W, Yarbro JW. Hemolytic anemia associated with an ovarian tumor. Ann J Med 1971;50:552–556.
295. Spira MA, Lynch EC. Autoimmune hemolytic anemia and carcinoma: An unusual association. Am J Med 1979;67:753–758.
296. Dacie JV. The hemolytic anemias: Congenital and acquired. Part III: Secondary and symptomatic hemolytic anemias. New York: Grune & Stratton, 1967.
297. Pirofsky B. Autoimmunization and the autoimmune hemolytic anemias. Baltimore: Williams & Wilkins, 1968.
298. Evans RS, Takahasi K, Duane RT, et al. Primary thrombocytopenic purpura and acquired hemolytic anemia. Evidence for a common etiology. Arch Intern Med 1957;87:48–65.
299. Doll DC, List AF, Yarbro JW. Evans' syndrome associated with microcystic adenoma of the pancreas. Cancer 1987;59:1366–1368.
300. Barry KG, Crosby WH. Autoimmune hemolytic anemia arrested by removal of an ovarian teratoma: Review of the literature and report of a case. Ann Intern Med 1957;47:1002–1007.
301. Antman KH, Skarin AT, Mayer RJ, et al. Microangiopathic hemolytic anemia and cancer: A review. Medicine (Baltimore) 1979;58:377–384.
302. Brain MC, Dacie JV, Hourihane OB. Microangiopathic hemolytic anemia: The possible role of vascular lesions in pathogenesis. Br J Haematol 1962;8:358–374.
303. Lohrmann HP, Adam W, Heymer B, Kubanek B. Microangiopathic hemolytic anemia in metastatic carcinoma: Report of eight cases. Ann Intern Med 1973;79:368–375.
304. Sack GH, Levin J, Bell WR. Trousseau's syndrome and other manifestations of chronic disseminate coagulopathy in patients with neoplasms. Medicine (Baltimore) 1977;56:1–37.
305. Colman RW, Robboy SJ, Minna JD. Disseminated intravascular coagulation: A reappraisal. Ann Rev Med 1979;30:359–374.
306. Robinson WA. Granulocytosis in neoplasia. Ann N Y Acad Sci 1974;230:212–218.
307. Meyer LM, Rotter SD. Leukemoid reaction (hyperleukocytosis) in malignancy. Am J Clin Pathol 1942;12:218–222.
308. Fahey RJ. Unusual leukocyte response in primary carcinoma of the lung. Cancer 19521;4:930–935.
309. Hughes WF, Highley CS. Marked leuckocytosis resulting from carcinomatosis. Ann Intern Med 1952;37:1095–1098.
310. Barrett O Jr. Monocytosis in malignant disease. Ann Intern Med 1970;73:991–992.
311. Finch SC. Granulocytopenia and granulocytosis. In: Williams WJ, Beutler E, Erslev AJ, Rundles RW, eds. Hematology. 2nd ed. New York: McGraw-Hill, 1977.
312. Asano S, Urabe A, Okabe T, et al. Demonstration of granulopoietic factor(s) in the plasma of nude mice transplanted with a human lung cancer and in the tumor tissue. Blood 1977;49:845–852.
313. Okabe T, Sato N, Kondo Y, Asano S, Ohsawa N, Kosaka K, Ueyama Y. Establishment and characterization of a human cancer cell line that produces human colony-stimulating factor. Cancer Res 1978;38:3910–3917.
314. Di Persio JF, Brennan JK, Lichtman MA, Speiser BL. Human cell lines that elaborate colony-stimulating activity for the marrow cells of man and other species. Blood 1978;51:507–519.
315. Cohen PR, Kurzrock R. Sweet's syndrome and malignancy. Am J Med 1987;82:1220–1226.
315a. Sato K, Fujii Y, Kakiuchi T, et al. Paraneoplastic syndrome of hypercalcemia and leukocytosis caused by squamous carcinoma cells (T3M-1) producing parathyroid hormone-related protein, interleukin 2, and granulocyte colony stimulating factor. Cancer Res 1989;49:4740–4746.
316. McCarthy JH, Sullivan JR, Ungar B, Metcalf D. Two cases of carcinoma of the lung characterized by a bone marrow agar culture pattern resembling acute myeloid leukemia. Blood 1979;54:530–533.
317. Aisenberg AC, Wilkes BM, Harris N, et al. Chronic T-cell lymphocytosis with neutropenia: Report of a case studied with monoclonal antibody. Blood 1981;58:818–823.
318. Knowles JH. Miscellaneous disorders of the lung. In: Harrison TR, Adams RD, Bennett IL, et al, eds. Harrison's principles of internal medicine. 5th ed. New York: McGraw-Hill, 1966:955–957.
319. Liddle GW, Nicholson WE, Island DP, et al. Clinical and laboratory studies of ecotopic humoral syndromes. Recent Prog Horm Res 1969;25:283–314.
320. Slungaard A, Ascensao J, Zanjani E, Jacob HS. Pulmonary carcinoma with eosinophilia: Demonstration of a tumor-derived eosinophilopoietic factor. N Engl J Med 1983;309:778–781.
321. Williams WJ. Thrombocytosis. In: Williams WJ, Beutler E, Erslev AJ, Rundles RW, eds. Hematology. 2nd ed. New York: McGraw-Hill, 1977.
322. Levin J, Conley CL. Thrombocytosis associated with malignant disease. Arch Intern Med 1964;114:497–500.
323. Davis RB, Theologides A, Kennedy BJ. Comparative studies of blood coagulation and platelet aggregation in patients with cancer and nonmalignant disease. Ann Intern Med 1967;71:67–80.
324. Aster RH. Control of platelet production. In: Williams WJ, Beutler E, Erslev AJ, Rundles RW, eds. Hematology. 2nd ed. New York: McGraw-Hill, 1977.
325. Kim HD, Boggs DR. A syndrome resembling idiopathic thrombocytopenic purpura in 10 patients with diverse forms of cancer. Am J Med 1979;67:371–377.
326. Doan C, Bouroncle BA, Wiseman BK. Idiopathic and secondary thrombocytopenic purpura. Clinical study and evaluation of 381 cases over a period of 28 years. Ann Intern Med 1960;53:861–876.
327. Bellone JD, Kunicki TS, Aster RH. Immune thrombocytopenia associated with carcinoma. Ann Intern Med 1983;99:470–472.
328. Kaden BR, Rosse WF, Hauch TW. Immune thrombocytopenia in lympho proliferative diseases. Blood 1979;53:545–551.
329. Khilanani P, Al-Sarraf M. The association of autoimmune thrombocytopenia and Hodgkin's disease. Oncology 1973;28:238–245.
330. Jones SE. Autoimmune disorders and malignant lymphoma. Cancer 1973;31:1092–1098.
331. Bowie EJW, Owen CA Jr. Hemostatic failure in clinical medicine. Semin Hematol 1977;14:341–364.
332. Trousseau A. Phlegmasia alba dolens. Clinique medicale de l'Hotel-Dieu de Paris. London. N Sydenham Soc 3:94, 1865.
333. Marder M, Weiner M, Shulman P, Shapiro S. Afibrinogenemia occurring in a case of malignancy of the prostate with bone metastases. N Y State J Med 1949;49:1197–1198.
334. Goodnight SH Jr. Bleeding and intravascular clotting in malignancy: A review. Ann N Y Acad Sci 1974;230:271–288.
335. Sharp AA. Diagnosis and management of disseminated intravascular coagulation. Br Med Bull 1977;33:265–272.
336. Gralnick HR, Abrell E. Studies of the procoagulant and fibrinolytic activity of promyelocytes in acute promyelocytic leukemia. Br J Hematol 1973;24:59–99.
337. Colman RW, Robby SJ, Minna JD. Disseminated intravascular coagulation (DIC): An approach. Am J Med 1972;52:679–689.
338. Siegal T, Seligsohn U, Aghai E, Modan M. Clinical and laboratory aspects of dessem-inated intravascular coagulation (DIC): A study of 118 cases. Thromb Haemost 1978;39:122–134.
339. Merskey C, Johnson AJ, Kleiner GJ, Wohl H. The defibrination syndrome: Clinical features and laboratory diagnosis. Br J Haematol 1967;13:528–549.
340. Owen CA Jr, Bowie EJ. Chronic intravascular coagulation syndromes: A summary. Mayo Clin Proc 1974;49:673–679.
341. Drapkin RL, Gee TS, Dowling MD, et al. Prophylactic heparin therapy in acute promyelocytic leukemia. Cancer 1978;41:2484–2490.
342. Gralnick HR, Sultan C. Acute prolmyelocytic leukemia: Haemorrhagic manifestation and morphologic criteria. Br J Haematol 1975;29:333–336.
343. Goldberg MA, Ginsberg D, Mayer RJ, et al. Is heparin administration necessary during induction chemotherapy for patients with acute promyelocytic leukemia? Blood 1987;69:187–191.
344. Fayemi AO, Deppisch LM. Nonbacterial thrombotic endocarditis and myocardial infarction. Am Heart J 1979;97:405–406.
345. MacDonald RA, Robbins SL. The significance of nonbacterial thrombotic endocarditis: Autopsy and clinical study of 78 patients. Ann Intern Med 1957;46:255–273.
346. Studdy P, Wiloughby JMT. Non-bacterial thrombotic endocarditis in early cancer. Br J Med 1976;1:752.
347. Susens GP, Hendrickson C, Barto DA, Sams BJ. Disseminated intravascular coagulation syndrome with metastatic melanoma: Remission after treatment with 5-(3,3-dimethyl-l-traizeno)-imidazole-4-carboxamide (DTIC). Ann Intern Med 1976;84:175.
348. Alving BM, Abeloff MD, Bell W. Spontaneous remission of recurring disseminated intravascular coagulation associated with prostatic carcinoma. Cancer 1976;37:928–930.
349. Rickles FR, Edwards RL. Activation of blood coagulation in cancer: Trousseau's syndrome revisited. Blood 1983;63:14–31.
350. Rosen P, Armstrong D. Nonbacterial thrombotic endocarditis in patients with malignant neoplastic disease. Am J Med 1973;54:23–29.
351. Sun NC, McAfee WM, Hum GJ, Weiner JM. Hemostatic abnormalities in malignancy: A prospective study in one hundred eight patients: I. Coagulation studies. Am J Clin Pathol 1979;71:10–16.
352. Aderka D, Brown A, Zelikovski A, Pinkhas J. Idiopathic deep vein thrombosis in an apparently healthy patient as a premonitory sign of occult cancer. Cancer 1986;57:1846–1849.
353. Bell WR, Starksen NF, Tang S, Porterfield JK. Trousseau's syndrome. Devastating coagulopathy in the absence of heparin. Am J Med 1985;79:423–430.
354. Al-Mondhiry H. Disseminated intravascular coagulation: Experience in a major cancer center. Thromb Diathes Haemorrh 1975;34:181–193.
355. Lee JC, Yamuchi H, Hopper J Jr. The association of cancer and the nephrotic syndrome. Ann Intern Med 1966;64:51.
356. Alpers CE, Cotran RS. Neoplasia and glomerular injury. Kidney Int 1986;30:465–473.
357. Glassock RJ, Friedler RM, Massry SG. Kidney and electrolyte disturbances in neoplastic diseases. Contrib Nephrol 1977;7:2–41.
358. Ghosh L, Meuhrhe RC. The nephrotic syndrome: A prodrome to lymphoma. Ann Intern Med 1970;72:379–382.

359. Cantrell EG. Nephrotic syndrome cured by removal of gastric carcinoma. Br Med J 1969;2:739.
360. Plager J, Stutzman L. Acute nephrotic syndrome as a manifestation of active Hodgkin's disease. Am J Med 1971;50:56–66.
361. Lewis MG, Loughridge LW, Phillips TM. Immunological studies in nephrotic syndrome associated with extrarenal malignant disease. Lancet 1971;2:134–185.
362. Couser WG, Wagonfeld JB, Spargo BH, Lewis EJ. Glomerular deposition of tumor antigen in membranous nephropathy associated with colonic carcinoma. Am J Med 1974;57:962–970.
363. Costanza ME, Perin V, Schwartz RS, Nathansen L. Carcinoembryonic antigen-antibody complexes in a patient with colonic carcinoma and nephrotic syndrome. N Engl J Med 1973;289:520–522.
363a. Haskell LP, Fusco MJ, Wadler S, Sablay LB, Mennemeyer RP. Crescentic glomerulonephritis associated with prostatic carcinoma: Evidence of immune-mediated glomerular injury. Am J Med 1990;88:189–192.
364. Sherman RL, Susin M, Weksler ME, Becker EL. Lipoid nephrosis in Hodgkin's disease. Am J Med 1972;52:699–706.
365. Lokich JJ, Galvanek EG, Moloney WC. Nephrosis of Hodgkin's disease. Arch Intern Med 1973;132:597–600.
366. Moorthy AV, Zimmerman SW, Burkholder PM. Nephrotic syndrome in Hodgkin's disease. Am J Med 1976;61:471–477.
367. Carpenter CB. Case records of the Massachusetts General Hospital. N Engl J Med 1973;289:1241–1247.
368. Richard-Mendes da Costa C, Dupont E, Hamers R, et al. Nephrotic syndrome in bronchogenic carcinoma: Report of two cases with immunochemical studies. Clin Nephrol 1974;2:245–251.
369. Dobbs DJ, Striker LM, Mignon F, Striker G. Glomerular lesions in lymphomas and leukemias. Am J Med 1986;80:63–70.
370. Gagliano RG, Costanzi JJ, Beathard GA, et al. The nephrotic syndrome associated with neoplasia: An unusual paraneoplastic syndrome: Report of a case and review of the literature. Am J Med 1976;60:1026–1031.
371. Moorthy AV. Minimal change glomerular disease: A paraneoplastic syndrome in 2 patients with bronchogenic carcinoma. Am J Kidney Dis 1983;3:58–62.
372. Jermanovich NB, Glammarco R, Ginsberg SJ, et al. Small cell anaplastic carcinoma of the lung with mesangial proliferative glomerulonephritis. Arch Intern Med 1982;142: 397–399.
373. Cameron JS. Nephrotic syndrome in chronic lymphatic leukemia. Br Med J 1974;4: 164–167.
374. Hyman LR, Burkholder PM, Joo PA, Segar WE. Malignant lymphoma and the nephrotic syndrome: A clinicopathologic analysis with light immunofluorescence and electron microscopy of the renal lesions. J Pediatr 1973;82:207–217.
375. Higgins MR, Randall RE, Still WJS. Nephrotic syndrome with oat-cell carcinoma. Br Med J 1974;3:450.
376. Karpen HO, Bhat JG, Feiner HD, Baldwin DS. Membranous nephropathy associated with renal cell carcinoma: Evidence against a role of renal tubular or tumor antibodies in pathogenesis. Am J Med 1978;64:864–867.
377. Hopper JH Jr. Tumor related renal lesions. Ann Intern Med 1974;81:550–551.
378. Row PG, Cameron JS, Turner DR, et al. Membranous nephropathy: Long-term follow-up and association with neoplasia. Q J Med 1975;44:207–239.
379. Shalhoub RJ. Pathogenesis of lipoid nephrosis: A disorder of T-cell function. Lancet 1974;2:556–558.
380. Osserman EF, Lawlor DP. Serum and urinary lysozyme (muramidase) in monocyte and monomyelocytic leukemia. J Exp Med 1966;124:921–951.
381. Pruzanki W, Platts MF. Serum and urinary proteins, lysozyme (muramidase) and renal dysfunction in mono- and myelomonocytic leukemia. J Clin Invest 1970;49: 1694–1707.
382. Hobbs JR, Evans DJ, Wrong OM. Renal tubular obstruction by mucoprotein from adenocarcinoma of pancreas. Br Med J 1974;2:87–89.
383. Freibusch J, Barbosa-Saldivar JL, Bernstein RS, Robertson GL. Tumor-associated nephrogenic diabetes insipidus. Ann Intern Med 1980;92:797–798.
384. Kyle RA. Multiple myeloma: Review of 869 cases. Mayo Clin Proc 1975;50:29–40.
385. DeFronzo RA, Cooke CR, Wright JR, Humphrey RL. Renal function in patients with multiple myeloma. Medicine (Baltimore) 1978;57:151–161.
386. Zlotnick A, Rosenmann E. Renal pathologic findings associated with monoclonal gammopathies. Arch Intern Med 1975;135:40–45.
387. Schubert GE, Viegel J, Lennert K. Structure and function of the kidney in multiple myeloma. Virchows Arch [A] 1972;355:135–137.
388. Brown WW, Herbert LA, Piering WF, et al. Reversal of chronic and stage renal failure due to myeloma kidney. Ann Intern Med 1979;90:793–794.
389. Leech SH, Polesky HF, Shapiro FL. Chronic hemodialysis in myelomatosis. Ann Intern Med 1972;77:239–242.
390. Richmond J, Sherman RS, Diamond HD, Craver LF. Renal lesions associated with malignant lymphomas. Am J Med 1962;32:184–207.
391. Martinez-Maldonado M, Ramirez de Arellano GA. Renal involvement in malignant lymphomas: A survey of 49 cases. J Urol 1966;95:485–488.
392. Matthews MJ. Problems in morphology and behavior of monchopulmonary malignant disease. In: Israel L, Chanimian P, eds. Lung cancer, facts, problems and perspectives. New York: Academic Press, 1976:23–62.
393. Brin EN, Schiff M Jr, Weiss RM. Palliative urinary diversion for malignancy. J Urol 1975;113:619–622.
394. Fichman M, Bethune J. Effects of neoplasms on renal electrolyte function in paraneoplastic syndromes. Ann N Y Acad Sci 1974;230:448–472.
395. Garnic MB, Mayer RJ. Acute renal failure associated with neoplastic disease and its treatment. Semin Oncol 1976;5:155–165.
396. Keane WF, Crosson JT, Staley NA, et al. Radiation-induced renal disease: A clinicopathologic study. Am J Med 1967;60:127–137.
397. Dosik GM, Gutterman JE, Hersh EM, et al. Nephrotoxicity from cancer immunotherapy. Ann Intern Med 1978;89:41–46.
398. Bennett WM, Muther RS, Parker RA, et al. Drug therapy in renal failure: Dosing guidelines for adults. Ann Intern Med 1980;93:286–325.
399. Kierland RR. Cutaneous signs of internal malignancy. South Med J 1972;65:563–568.
400. Helm F, Helm J. Cutaneous markers of internal malignancies. In: Helm F, ed. Cancer dermatology. Philadelphia: Lea & Febiger, 1979:247–283.
401. Braverman IM. Skin signs of systemic disease. Philadelphia: WB Saunders, 1970.
402. Crowe FW. Axillary freckling as a diagnostic aid in neurofibromatosis. Ann Intern Med 1964;61:1142–1143.
403. Levine N, Greenwald ES. Mucocutaneous side effects of cancer chemotherapy. Cancer Treat Rev 1978;5:67–84.
404. Brown J, Winkelmann RK. Acanthosis nigricans: A study of 90 cases. Medicine (Baltimore) 1968;47:33–51.
405. Curth HO. Classification of acanthosis nigricans. Int J Dermatol 1976;15:592.
406. Matsuoka MY, Goldman J, Wortsman J, et al. Antibodies against the insulin receptor in paraneoplastic acanthosis nigricans. Am J Med 1987;82:1253–1256.
406a. Cohen PR, Grossman ME, Almeida L, Kurzrock R. Tripe palms and malignancy. J Clin Oncol 1989;7:669–678.
407. Sneddon IB, Roberts JBM. An incomplete form of acanthosis nigricans. Gut 1962;3: 269–272.
408. Dantzig PI. Sign of Leser-Trelat. Arch Dermatol 1973;108:700–701.
409. Ronchese F. Keratoses, cancer and "the sign of Leser-Trelat." Cancer 1965;18:1003–1006.
410. Holdiness MR. The sign of Leser-Trelat. Int J Dematol 1986;25:564–572.
411. Curry SS, King LE. The sign of Leser-Trelat. Arch Dermatol 1980;116:1059–1060.
412. Graham JH, Helwig EB. Bowen's disease and its relationship to systemic cancer. Arch Dermatol 1961;83:738–758.
413. Anderson SL, Nielsen A, Reymann F. Relationship between Bowen's disease and internal malignancy. Arch Dermatol 1973;108:367–370.
414. Minkowsky S. Multiple carcinomata following the ingestion of medicinal arsenic. Ann Intern Med 1964;61:296–299.
415. Fitzpatrick TB, Montgomery H, Lerner AB. Pathogenesis of generalized dermal pigmentation secondary to malignant melanoma and melanuria. J Invest Dermatol 1954;22:163–172.
416. Ashikari R, Park K, Huvos AG, Urban JA. Paget's disease of the breast. Cancer 1970;26: 680–685.
417. Witkowski JA, Parish LC. Bazex's syndrome: Paraneoplastic acrokeratosis. JAMA 1983;248:2883–2884.
418. Wishart JM. Bazex paraneoplastic acrokeratosis: A case report and response to Tagason. Br J Dermatol 1986;115:595–599.
418a. Bolognia JL, Brewer YP, Cooper DL. Bazex syndrome (acroheratosis paraneoplastica): An analytical review. Medicine (Baltimore) 1991;70:269–280.
419. Gammel JA. Erythema gyratum repens: Skin manifestations of patients with carcinoma of breast. Arch Dermatol 1952;66:494–505.
420. Purdy MJ. Erythema gyratum repens: Report of a case. Arch Dermatol 1959;80:590–591.
421. Summerly R. The figurate erythemas and neoplasia. Br J Dermatol 1964;80:370–373.
421a Appell ML, Ward W, Tyring SK. Erythema gyratum repens. A cutaneous marker of malignancy. Cancer 1988;62:548–550.
422. Lazar P. Cancer, erythema annulare centrifugum and autoimmunity. Arch Dermatol 1963;87:246–253.
423. Wilkinson DS. Necrolytic migrating erythema with pancreatic carcinoma. Proc R Soc Med 1971;64:1197–1198.
424. Church RE, Crane WAJ. A cutaneous syndrome associated with islet cell carcinoma of the pancreas. Br J Dermatol 1967;79:284–286.
425. Sjoerdsma A, Weissbach H, Udenfriend S. A clinical, physiologic, and biochemical study of patients with malignant carcinoid (argentaffinoma). Am J Med 1956;21: 520–532.
426. Mason DT, Melmon KL. New understanding of the mechanism of the carcinoid flush. Ann Intern Med 1966;65:1334–1339.
427. Abrahams F, McCarthy JT, Sanders SL. 101 Cases of exfoliative dermatitis. Arch Dermatol 1963;87:96–103.
428. Nicolis GD, Helwig EB. Exfoliative dermatitis: A clinicopathologic study of 135 cases. Arch Dermatol 1973;108:788–979.
429. Elias PM, Fritsch PO. Erythema multiforme. In: Fitzpatrick TB, Eisen AZ, Wolf K, et al, eds. Dermatology in general medicine. 2nd ed. New York: McGraw-Hill, 1979: 295–303.
430. Fitzpatrick TB, Clark WH Jr. Recurrent attacks of abdominal pain and cutaneous lesions. N Engl J Med 1964;270:1248–1251.
431. Waddington RT. A case of primary liver tumor associated with porphyria. Br J Surg 1972;59:653–654.
432. Thompson RPH, Nicholson DC, Farman T, et al. Cutaneous porphyria due to a malignant primary hepatoma. Gastroenterology 1970;59:779–783.
433. Stone SP, Schroeder AL. Bullous pemphigoid and associated malignant neoplasms. Arch Dermatol 1975;111:991–994.
433a. Anhalt GJ, Kim SC, Stanley JR, et al. Paraneoplastic pemphigus. An autoimmune microcutaneous disease associated with neoplasia. N Engl J Med 1990;323:1729–1735.

434. Tobias N. Dermatitis herpetiformis associated with visceral malignancy. Urol Cutan Rev 1951;55:352.
435. Arundell FD, Wilkinson RD, Haserick Jr. Dermatomyositis and malignant neoplasm in adults. Arch Dermatol 1960;82:772–775.
436. Lyell A, Whittle CH. Hypertrichosis languginosa acquired type. Br J Dermatol 1951;63: 411–413.
437. Hegedus SI, Schorr WF. Acquired hypertrichosis lanquinosa and malignancy. Arch Dermatol 1972;106:84–88.
438. Van Dijk E. Ichthyosiform atrophy of the skin with internal malignant diseases. Dermatologica 1963;127:413–428.
439. Flint GL, Flam M, Soter NA. Acquired ichthyosis. Arch Dermatol 1975;111:1446–1447.
440. Vogl A, Goldfischer S. Pachydermoperiostosis. Primary or idiopathic hypertrophic osteoarthopathy. Am J Med 1962;33:166–187.
441. Rajka G. Investigation of patients suffering from generalized pruritus, with special references to systemic diseases. Acta Dermato-Venereol 1966;46:190–194.
442. Cormia FE. Pruritus, an uncommon but important symptom of systemic cancer. Arch Dermatol 1965;92:36–39.
443. Schimpff S, Serpick A, Stoler B, et al. Varicella-zoster infection in patients with cancer. Ann Intern Med 1972;76:241–254.
444. Dolin R, Reichman RC, Mazur MH, Whitley RJ. Herpes zoster-varicella infections in immunosuppressed patients. Ann Intern Med 1978;89:375–388.
445. Huberman M, Fossieck BE Jr, Bunn PA Jr, et al. Herpes zoster and small cell bronchogenic carcinoma. Am J Med 1980;68:214–218.
446. Gardner EJ. Follow-up study of a family group exhibiting dominant inheritance for a syndrome including intestinal polyps, osteomas, fibromas, and epidermal cysts. Am J Hum Genet 1962;16:376–390.
447. Bussey HJR. Gastrointestinal polyposis. Gut 1970;11:970–978.
448. Jones EL, Cornell WP. Garnder's syndrome: Review of the literature and report on a family. Arch Surg 1966;92:287–300.
449. Jeghers H, McKusick VA, Katz KH. Generalized intestinal polyposis and melanin spots of the oral mucosa, lips and digits: A syndrome of diagnostic significance. N Engl J Med 1949;241:933–1005, 1031–1036.
450. Riley E, Swift M. A family with Peutz-Jeghers syndrome and bilateral breast cancer. Cancer 1980;46:815–817.
451. Howel-Evans W, McConnell RR, Clarke CA, Sheppard PM. Carcinoma of the esophagus with keratosis palmaris et plantaris (tylosis). Q J Med 1958;27:413–429.
452. Williams ED, Pollock DJ. Multiple mucosal neuromata with endocrine tumors: A syndrome allied to Von Recklinghausen's disease. J Pathol Bacteriol 1966;91:71–80.
453. Lloyd KM, Dennis M. Cowden's disease, a possible new symptom complex with multiple system involvement. Ann Intern Med 1963;58:136–142.
454. Solomon LM, Fretzin DF, Dewald RL. The epidermal nevus syndrome. Arch Dermatol 1968;97:273–285.
455. Butterworth T, Wilson M Jr. Dermatologic aspects of tuberous sclerosis. Arch Dermatol Syph 1941;43:1–41.
456. Christoferson LA, Gustafson MB, Petersen AG. Von Hippel-Lindau's disease. JAMA 1961;178:280–282.
457. Doll R, Kinlen L. Immunosurveillance and cancer: Epidemiologic evidence. Br Med J 1970;4:420–422.
458. Frizzera G, Rosai J, Dehner LP, et al. Lymphoreticular disorders in primary immunodeficiencies: New findings based on an up-to-date histologic classification of 35 cases. Cancer 1980;46:692–699.
459. Epstein CJ, Martin GM, Schultz AL, Motulsky AG. Werner's syndrome: A review of the symptomatology, natural history, pathologic features, genetics, and relationship to the natural aging process. Medicine (Baltimore) 1966;45:177–221.
460. Waldman TA, Broder S, Strober W. Protein-losing enteropathies in malignancy. Ann N Y Acad Sci 1974;230:306–317.
461. Lucy K, Scobie BA. Watery diarrhoea (WDHA) syndrome associated with carcinoma of the lung. Aust N Z J Med 1976;6:490–491.
462. Troncale FJ. Distant manifestations of colonic carcinoma. Ann N Y Acad Sci 1974;230: 332–347.
463. Klipstein FA, Smorth G. Intestinal structure and function in neoplastic disease. Am J Dig Dis 1969;14:887–889.
464. Gilat T, Fischel B, Danon J, Lowewnthal M. Morphology of small bowel mucosa and malignancy. Digestion 1972;12:147–155.
465. Henderson AR, Grace DM. Liver-originating isoenzymes of alkaline phosphatase in the serum: A paraneoplastic manifestation of a malignant schwannoma of the sciatic nerve. J Clin Pathol 1976;29:237–240.
466. Walsh PN, Kissane JM. Nonmetastatic hypernephroma with reversible hepatic dysfunction. Arch Intern Med 1968;122:214–222.
467. Utz DC, Warren MM, Gregg JA, et al. Reversible hepatic dysfunction associated with hypernephroma. Mayo Clin Proc 1970;45:161–169.
468. Cronin RE, Kaehny WD, Miller PD, et al. Renal cell carcinoma: Unusual systemic manifestations. Medicine (Baltimore) 1976;55:291–311.
469. Mena E, Bull FE, Bookstein JJ, et al. Angiography of the nephrogenic hepatic dysfunction syndrome. Radiology 1974;111:65–68.
470. DeWys WD. Working conference on anorexia and cachexia of neoplastic disease. Cancer Res 1970;30:2816–2818.
471. De Wys WD. Abnormalities of taste as a remote effect of a neoplasm. Ann N Y Acad Sci 1974;230:427–434.
472. Theologides A. The anorexia-cachexia syndrome: A new hypothesis. Ann N Y Acad Sci 1974;230:14–22.
473. Waterhouse C. How tumors affect host metabolism. Ann N Y Acad Sci 1974;230:86–93.
474. Beck SA, Tisdale MJ. Production of lipolytic and proteolytic factors by a murine tumor producing cachexia in the host. Cancer Res 1987;47:5919–5923.
475. Ternell M, Moldawer LC, Lonnroth C, et al. Plasma protein synthesis in experimental cancer compared to paraneoplastic conditions, including monokine administration. Cancer Res 1987;47:5825–5830.
475a. Yoneda T, Alsina MA, Chavez JB, et al. Evidence that tumor necrosis factor plays a role in the paraneoplastic syndromes of cachexia, hypercalcemia, and leukocytosis in a human tumor in nude mice. J Clin Invest 1991;87:977–985.
475b. Beck SA, Mulligan HD, Tisdale MJ. Lipolytic factors associated with murine and human cancer cachexia. JNCI 1990;82:1922–1926.
476. Gold J. Cancer cachexia and gluconeogenesis. Ann N Y Acad Sci 1974;230:103–110.
477. Bodel P. Tumors and fever. Ann N Y Acad Sci 1974;230:6–13.
477a. Fukumoto s, Matsumoto T, Harada S, et al. Pheochromocytoma with pyrexia and marked inflammatory signs: A paraneoplastic syndrome with possible relation to interleukin-6 production. J Clin Endocrinol Metab 1991;73:877–881.
478. Petersdorf RG. Fever and cancer. Hosp Med 1965;1:2–10.
479. Lobell M, Boggs DR, Wintrobe MM. The clinical significance of fever in Hodgkin's disease. Arch Intern Med 1966;117:335–342.
480. Gluckman JB, Turner MD. Systemic manifestations of tumors of the small gut and liver. Ann N Y Acad Sci 1974;230:318–331.
481. Block JB. Lactic acidosis in malignancy and observations on its possible pathogenesis. Ann N Y Acad Sci 1974;230:94–102.
482. Nadiminti Y, Wang JC, Chou S, et al. Lactic acidosis associated with Hodgkin's disease: Response of chemotherapy. N Engl J Med 1980;303:15–17.
483. Spechler SJ, Esposito AL, Koff RS, Hong WK. Lactic acidosis in oat cell carcinoma with extensive hepatic metastases. Arch Intern Med 1978;138:1663–1664.
484. Eridani S, Burdick L, Periti M, Arosio A, Libretti A. Primary carcinoma of the colon and hyperlipemia: A paraneoplastic syndrome. Biomedicine 1976;25:324–326.
485. Glueck HL, MacKenzie M, Glueck CJ. Crystalline IgG protein in multiple myeloma: Identification of effects on coagulation and on lipoprotein metabolism. J Lab Clin Med 1972;79:731–744.
486. Santer MA, Waldmann TA, Fallon HJ. Erythrocytosis and hyperlipemia as manifestations of hepatic carcinoma. Arch Intern Med 1967;120:735–739.
487. Gangulu A, Gribble J, Tune B, et al. Renin-secreting Wilms' tumor with severe hypertension: Report of a case and brief review of renin-secreting tumors. Ann Intern Med 1973;79:835–837.
488. Genest J, Rojo-Ortega JM, Kuchel O, et al. Malignant hypertension with hypokalemia in a patient with renin-producing pulmonary carcinoma. Trans Assoc Am Physicians 1975;88:192–201.
489. Aurell M, Rudin A, Tisell LE, et al. Captopril effort on hypertension in patient with renin-producing tumor. Lancet 1979;2:149–150.
490. Hollifield JW, Page DL, Smith C, et al. Renin-secreting clear cell carcinoma of the kidney. Arch Intern Med 1975;135:859–864.
490a. Yokokawa K, Tahara H, Kohno M, et al. Hypertension associated with endothelin-secreting malignant hemangioendothelioma. Ann Int Med 1991;114:213–215.
491. Zusman RM, Snider JJ, Cline A, et al. Antihypertensive function of renal-cell carcinoma: Evidence for a prostaglandin A secreting tumor. N Engl J Med 1974;290: 843–845.
492. Boasberg PD, Henry JP, Rosenbloom AA, et al. Case reports and studies of paraneoplastic hypotension: Abnormal low pressure baroreceptor responses. Med Pediatr Oncol 1977;3:59–66.
493. Braganza JM, Butler EB, Fox H, et al. Ectopic production of salivary type amylase by a pseudomesotheliomatous carcinoma of the lung. Cancer 1978;41:1522–1525.
494. Mills JA. A spectrum of organ systems that respond to cancer: The joints and connective tissue. Ann N Y Acad Sci 1974;230:443–447.
495. Greenfield GB, Schorsch HA, Shkolnik A. The various roentgen appearance of pulmonary hypertrophic osteoarthropathy. Am J Roentgenol Radium Ther Nucl Med 1967;101:927–931.
496. LeRoux BT. Bronchial carcinoma with hypertrophic pulmonary osteoarthropathy. S Afr Med J 1968;42:1074–1075.
497. Jao JY, Barlow JJ, Krant MKJ. Pulmonary hypertrophic osteoarthropathy, spider angiomata and estrogen hypersecretion in neoplasms. Ann Intern Med 1969;70:580–584.
498. Donnelly B, Johnson PM. Detection of hypertrophic pulmonary osteoarthropathy by skeletal imaging with ^{99m}Tc-labeled diphosphonate. Radiology 1975;114:389–391.
499. Green N, Kurohara SS, George FW III, Crews QE Jr. The biologic behavior of lung cancer according to histologic type. Radiol Clin Biol 1972;41:160–170.
500. Yesner R. Spectrum of lung cancer and ectopic hormones. In: Sommers SC, Rosen PP, eds. Pathology annual, vol 12. New York: Appleton-Century-Crofts, 1978:217–240.
501. Goldstraw P, Walbraun PR. Hypertrophic pulmonary osteoarthropathy and its occurrence with pulmonary metastases from renal carcinoma. Thorax 1976;31:205–211.
502. Miller ER. Carcinoma of the thymus with marked pulmonary osteoarthropathy. Radiology 1939;32:651–660.
503. Ullal SR. Hypertrophic osteoarthropathy and leiomyoma of the oesophagus. Am J Surg 1972;123:356–358.
504. Shapiro RF, Zvaifler NJ. Concurrent intrathoracic Hodgkin's disease and hypertrophic osteoarthropathy. Chest 1973;63:912–916.
505. Howard CP, Telander RL, Hoffman AD, Burgert EO Jr. Hypertrophic osteoarthropathy in association with pulmonary metastasis from osteogenic sarcoma. Mayo Clin Proc 1978;53:538–541.
506. Papavasiliou C, Pavlatou M, Pappas J. Nasopharyngeal cancer in patients under the age of thirty years. Cancer 1977;40:2312–2316.
507. Ellouz R, Cammoun M, Attia RB, Bahi J. Clinical aspects: Nasopharyngeal carcinoma

in children and adolescents in Tunisia: Clinical aspects and the paraneoplastic syndrome. IARC Sci Pub 1978;20:115–129.

507a. Thomas CR Jr, Rest EB, Brown CR Jr. Rheumatologic manifestations of malignancy. Med Pediatr Oncol 1988;18:146–158.

508. Cudkowicz L, Armstrong JB. Finger clubbing and changes in the bronchial circulation: Arterio-venous shunts in hypertrophic pulmonary osteoarthropathy. Br J Tuberc 1953;47:227–232.

509. Carroll KB, Doyle L. A common factor in hypertrophic osteoarthropathy. Thorax 1974;29:262–264.

510. Riyami AM, Anderson EG. Hypertrophic pulmonary osteoarthropathy: A clinical and biochemical study. Br J Dis Chest 1974;68:193–196.

511. Glenner GC. Amyloid deposits and amyloidosis: The β-fibriloses. N Engl J Med 1980;303:1283–1292, 1333–1347.

512. Azzopardi JG, Lehner T. Systemic amyloidosis and malignant disease. J Clin Pathol 1966;19:539–548.

513. Kyle RA, Bayrd ED. Amyloidosis: Review of 236 cases. Medicine (Baltimore) 1975;54: 271–547.

514. Shiel WC, Prete PE, Jason M, Andrews BS. Palmar fasciitis and arthritis with ovarian and non-ovarian carcinomas. Am J Med 1985;79:640–644.

515. Pfinsgraff J, Buckingham RB, Killian PJ, et al. Palmar fasciitis and arthritis with malignant neoplasms: A paraneoplastic syndrome. Semin Arthritis Rheum 1986;16: 118–125.

516. Michaels RM, Sorber JA. Reflex sympathetic dystrophy as a probable paraneoplastic syndrome: Case report and literature review. Arthritis Rheum 1984;27:1183–1185.

517. Mills JA. Connective tissue disease associated with malignant neoplastic disease. J Chron Disi 1963;16:797–811.

518. Calabro J. Cancer and arthritis. Arthritis Rheum 1967;10:553–567.

519. Cammarata R, Rodnan GP, Jensen WM. Systemic rheumatic disease and malignant lymphoma. Arch Intern Med 1963;111:112–119.

520. Miller D. The association of immune disease and malignant lymphoma. Ann Intern Med 1967;66:507–521.

521. Anderson LG, Talal N. The spectrum of benign to malignant lymphoproliferation in Sjögrens syndrome. Clin Exp Immunol 1971;9:199–221.

522. Murray GC, Persellin RH. Metastatic carcinoma presenting as nonarticular arthritis: A case report and review of the literature. Arthritis Rheum 1980;23:95–100.

523. Karten I, Bartfield H. Bronchogenic carcinoma simulating early rheumatoid arthritis. JAMA 1962;179:160–161.

524. Tumulty PA. Systemic lupus erythematosus. In: Wintrobe MM, Thorn GW, Adams RD, Brauwald E, Isselbacher KJ, Petersdorf RG, eds. Harrison's principles of internal medicine. 6th ed. New York: McGraw-Hill, 1971:1962–1967.

525. Freundlich B, Makover D, Maul GG. A novel antinuclear antibody associated with a lupuslike paraneoplastic syndrome. Ann Intern Med 1988;109:295–297.

526. Sanchez-Guerro J, Gutierrez-Vrena S, Vidaller A, et al. Vasculitis as a paraneoplastic syndrome. Report of 11 cases and review of the literature. J Rheumatol 1990;17: 1458–1462.

Cancer: Principles & Practice of Oncology, Fourth Edition,
edited by Vincent T. DeVita, Jr., Samuel Hellman, Steven A. Rosenberg.
J.B. Lippincott Co., Philadelphia © 1993.

F. Anthony Greco
John D. Hainsworth

CHAPTER **58**

Cancer of Unknown Primary Site

Patients with cancer of unknown primary site are common, representing 5% to 10% of all cancer patients. Within this heterogenous patient group there are several clinical presentations and histologic tumor types. The largest group of patients have metastatic carcinoma of unknown primary site. Others have equivocal histologic diagnoses and tumors that are difficult to classify using the time-honored method of light microscopic examination. Specialized pathologic studies are essential in delineating the type of neoplasm present in many of these patients, and at times may suggest the site of origin. Extreme heterogeneity in clinical presentations, histologic appearances, and natural histories has made systematic evaluation of these patients difficult, and an established base of knowledge has developed slowly. Only a few investigators have been interested in detailed studies of these patients. Therefore, past information suffers from many generalizations and is not representative of the entire patient population. These data are derived from grouping all patients and deal primarily with results of various chemotherapeutic regimens.

Over the past few decades several important issues have changed in oncology. Combination chemotherapy, often used with surgery or radiation therapy, has proved to be potentially curative for several metastatic tumors of known primary site. In addition, palliation and prolongation of survival has been demonstrated with systemic therapy for many other tumor types. These therapeutic improvements have relevance for patients with cancers of unknown primary site, because some have these responsive neoplasms (*i.e.,* with occult primaries or atypical histologies).

Diagnostic pathology has improved remarkably. The more routine use of electron microscopy and the emerging fields of immunohistochemistry and molecular genetics are contributing to the more precise diagnosis of neoplasms. It is possible to define more reliably the histology and, at least in selected patients, the origin and biology of their neoplasms. In concert with the evolving diagnostic techniques, several clinical syndromes and features are being recognized and are helping physicians to better understand and manage these patients. Oncologists are rethinking the issues with respect to patients with cancers of unknown primary site.

Appropriate patient management requires an understanding of several clinicopathologic features that help to identify patients with responsive tumors. A patient with cancer of unknown primary site typically develops symptoms or signs at a metastatic site, and the diagnosis is made by biopsy of a metastatic lesion. History, physical examination, chest radiograph, and laboratory studies fail to identify the primary site. The initial biopsy should be generous because many studies may be required. Routine light microscopic histology establishes the neoplastic process and provides a practical classification system on which the patient can be subsequently evaluated and managed. In the broad category of cancers of unknown primary site, there are four major light microscopic diagnoses:

1. Poorly differentiated neoplasms
2. Well-differentiated and moderately well-differentiated adenocarcinoma
3. Squamous cell carcinoma
4. Poorly differentiated carcinoma and poorly differentiated adenocarcinoma

These diagnoses vary with respect to clinical characteristics, recommended diagnostic evaluation, treatment, and prognosis.

POORLY DIFFERENTIATED NEOPLASMS OF UNKNOWN PRIMARY SITE

If the pathologist is confident of a cancer but cannot differentiate a general category of neoplasm (*e.g.*, carcinoma, lymphoma, melanoma, sarcoma), it is designated a poorly differentiated neoplasm of unknown primary site. A more precise diagnosis is essential in this group of patients because many have responsive tumors. About 5% of all patients with cancers of unknown primary site present with this diagnosis. The number will decrease as specialized pathology is more widely used. The most frequent tumor for which specific effective therapy is available is non-Hodgkin's lymphoma. In reported series, 35% to 65% of poorly differentiated neoplasms were found to be lymphomas after further pathologic study.[1–4] Most of the remaining tumors in this group are carcinomas. Melanoma and sarcoma together account for less than 15% of all patients.

The evaluation of poorly differentiated tumors requires specialized pathologic studies. Immunoperoxidase tumor staining, electron microscopy, and genetic analysis can be helpful in the differential diagnosis. The most common cause of a nonspecific light microscopic diagnosis is an inadequate biopsy specimen. Fine-needle aspiration biopsy should not be performed in these patients as an *initial* diagnostic procedure, because the histology is poorly preserved and the ability to perform special studies is limited. Frequently, a definitive diagnosis can be made by obtaining a larger biopsy. Communication with the pathologist is important if repeat biopsy is performed, because some pathologic studies require special tissue processing. Some neoplasms remain unclassifiable by light microscopy, even with an adequate biopsy specimen. Additional pathologic study is always indicated in these tumors.

TABLE 58–1. Immunoperoxidase Tumor Staining Patterns Useful in the Differential Diagnosis of Poorly Differentiated Neoplasms

Tumor Type	*Immunoperoxidase Staining*
Carcinoma	Epithelial stains (*e.g.*, cytokeratin, EMA; +)
	CLA, S-100, vimentin (−)
Lymphoma	CLA (+)
	EMA occasionally (+)
	All other stains (−)
Sarcoma	
Mesenchymal	Vimentin (+)
	Epithelial stains usually (−)
Rhabdomyosarcoma	Desmin (+)
Angiosarcoma	Factor VIII antigen (+)
Melanoma	S-100, vimentin (+)
	NSE often (+)
	Epithelial stains (−)
	HMB-45 (+)
Neuroendocrine tumor	NSE, chromogranin (+)
	Epithelial stains (+)
Germ cell tumor	HCG, AFP (+)
	Epithelial stains (+)
Prostate cancer	PSA (+)
	Epithelial stains (+)
Breast cancer	ER, PR (+)
	Epithelial stains (+)

+, positive result; −, negative result; AFP, α-fetoprotein; CLA, common leukocyte antigen; EMA, epithelial membrane antigen; ER, estrogen receptor; HCG, human chorionic gonadotropin; NSE, neuron-specific enolase; PR, progesterone receptor; PSA, prostate-specific antigen.

IMMUNOPEROXIDASE TUMOR STAINING

Immunoperoxidase staining is the most widely available specialized technique for the classification of neoplasms. Immunoperoxidase staining often can be done on formalin-fixed, paraffinized tissue, which broadens its applicability, making repeat biopsy unnecessary in some patients. Immunoperoxidase antibodies are either monoclonal or polyclonal and are directed at cell components or products, which can include enzymes (*e.g.*, prostatic acid phosphatase, neuron-specific enolase [NSE]), normal tissue components (*e.g.*, keratin, desmin, vimentin, neurofilaments, common leukocyte antigen [CLA]), hormones and hormone receptors (*e.g.*, estrogen receptor), oncofetal antigens (*e.g.*, α-fetoprotein [AFP], carcinoembryonic antigen [CEA]), and other substances (*e.g.*, S-100 protein, chromogranin). Many new antibodies are being developed and appear almost monthly, making this area of diagnostic pathology a dynamic and evolving field. Specific diagnoses usually cannot be made on the basis of immunoperoxidase staining alone, because none of these reagents is directed at tumor-specific antigens. Therefore, results must be interpreted in conjunction with the light microscopic appearance and the clinical picture. Immunoperoxidase staining patterns that are useful in the differential diagnosis of poorly differentiated neoplasms are outlined in Table 58–1.

Several important questions can usually be answered by immunoperoxidase staining (see Table 58–1). The CLA stain usually can be used to make the important distinction between lymphoma and carcinoma.[5–6] Staining for NSE and chromogranin can suggest a neuroendocrine carcinoma (*e.g.*, small cell lung cancer, carcinoid, islet cell tumor).[7–8] Staining for prostate-specific antigen (PSA) strongly suggests prostate carcinoma in a male with metastatic adenocarcinoma.[9] Certain staining characteristics can suggest amelanotic melanoma (*e.g.*, positive staining for S-100 protein, vimentin, HMB-45) or sarcoma (*e.g.*, positive staining for desmin, vimentin, factor VIII antigen).[10–13] Staining for human chorionic gonadotropin (HCG) or AFP can suggest the diagnosis of a germ cell tumor in an appropriate clinical situation.[14,15]

Several problems are associated with immunoperoxidase stains. Technical expertise is required to perform these tests accurately and reproducibly, and proper interpretation requires an experienced pathologist. Appropriate control slides are stained and examined concurrently because nonspecific staining occasionally is a problem. Care must be taken to avoid overinterpretation, because no staining pattern is entirely specific. Certain stains, particularly CLA and PSA are specific; however, false-positive and false-negative results can occur with any of these stains. For example, some carcinomas stain with vimentin, some sarcomas stain with keratin, and a wide variety of carcinomas (other than neuroendocrine and germ cell tumors) stain with NSE and HCG, respectively.

In some circumstances, diagnoses based on immunoperoxidase staining in patients with poorly differentiated neoplasms of unknown primary site can be used to plan therapy and predict outcome. Undifferentiated neoplasms identified as lymphoma on the basis of positive CLA staining respond well to the combination chemotherapy used for non-Hodgkin's lymphoma.[1] In 35 patients with equivocal routine light microscopic histology and positive CLA staining, treatment with a variety of standard lymphoma regimens resulted in an actuarial disease-free survival of 45% at 30 months. Their outcome was similar to a group of concurrently treated patients who had non-Hodgkin's lymphomas with typical light microscopic histology. In patients diagnosed on the basis of immunoperoxidase staining with tumors other than lymphoma, only limited data exist concerning treatment outcome. These data are discussed later concerning patients with poorly differentiated carcinoma.

ELECTRON MICROSCOPY

A diagnosis can be made by electron microscopy in some poorly differentiated neoplasms. Electron microscopy is not widely available, requires special tissue fixation, is relatively expensive, and should be reserved for the study of neoplasms whose lineage is unclear after routine light microscopy and immunoperoxidase staining. Like immunoperoxidase staining, electron microscopy is reliable in differentiating lymphoma from carcinoma. It may be superior to immunoperoxidase staining for the identification of poorly differentiated sarcoma. Other specific structures such as neurosecretory granules (neuroendocrine tumors) or premelanosomes (melanoma) can suggest a particular tumor. Undifferentiated tumors often have nonspecific ultrastructural features; therefore, the absence of a particular ultrastructural finding cannot be used to rule out a specific diagnosis. Some neoplasms defy further classification despite specialized pathologic study.

In some instances, electron microscopy provides evidence for adenocarcinoma or squamous cell carcinoma. Features of adenocarcinoma include intercellular and intracellular lumina and surface microvilli. Squamous carcinomas are characterized by frequent and prominent desmosomes and by prominent bundles of prekeratin filaments in the adjacent cytoplasm. It usually is not possible to determine the origin of poorly differentiated adenocarcinoma or squamous carcinoma by electron microscopic features. Treatment implications for adenocarcinoma and squamous carcinoma recognized only by ultrastructural features are unclear (see the section on poorly differentiated carcinoma).

GENETIC ANALYSIS

The identification of chromosomal abnormalities and genetic changes associated with neoplasms is becoming increasingly important in predicting prognosis. The use of tumor-specific chromosomal abnormalities in diagnosis is still limited, but it is likely that future research will identify many additional specific genetic abnormalities.

Chromosomal abnormalities have been best studied in hematopoietic neoplasms. Most B cell non-Hodgkin's lymphomas are associated with tumor-specific immunoglobulin gene rearrangements, and typical chromosomal changes have been identified in some B cell and T cell lymphomas and in Hodgkin's disease.[16–17] In the rare instance when the diagnosis of lymphoma cannot be definitively established with either immunoperoxidase staining or electron microscopy, detection of chromosomal translocations t(14:18); t(8:14) or the presence of an immunoglobulin gene rearrangement provides definitive diagnostic information.

Two specific chromosomal rearrangements associated with nonlymphoid tumors have been identified. A specific chromosomal translocation, t(11:22), has been found in peripheral neuroepitheliomas and frequently in Ewing's tumor.[18,19] An isochromosome of the short arm of chromosome 12 (i12p) and other chromosome 12 abnormalities are found in a large percentage of testicular and extragonadal germ cell tumors in men.[20–22] Because these tumor types are poorly differentiated and are often metastatic at the time of diagnosis, identification of these chromosomal abnormalities may provide a specific diagnosis. Genetic analysis has been applied successfully to a subset of patients with carcinoma of unknown primary site (see the section on poorly differentiated carcinoma).

ADENOCARCINOMA OF UNKNOWN PRIMARY SITE

CLINICAL CHARACTERISTICS

Well-differentiated or moderately well-differentiated adenocarcinoma is the most frequent light microscopic diagnosis in patients with carcinoma of unknown primary site, accounting for about 60% of patients. Typically, patients with this diagnosis are elderly and have metastatic tumors at multiple sites. The sites of tumor involvement frequently determine the clinical presentation; common metastatic sites include liver, lung, and bone.

The clinical course is often dominated by symptoms and signs related to the metastases. The primary site becomes obvious in only 15% to 20% of patients during life.[23] At autopsy, however, 70% to 80% of patients have a primary site detected. The most common primaries identified at autopsy are the lung and pancreas, accounting for about 40%.[24] Other gastrointestinal sites (*e.g.*, stomach, colon, liver) are frequent, although adenocarcinomas from a wide variety of other primary sites are encountered occasionally. Adenocarcinomas of the breast, prostate, and ovary are rare in this group of patients.[24]

As a group, patients with metastatic adenocarcinoma of unknown primary site have a poor prognosis, with inexorable progression and a median survival of only 3 to 4 months. Many patients in this group have widespread metastases and poor performance status at the time of diagnosis. However, it is an error to stereotype *all* patients with carcinoma of unknown primary site, because within this large group are subsets of patients with more favorable prognoses. These patients often can be identified, as is discussed later in this chapter.

PATHOLOGY

The diagnosis of well-differentiated or moderately well-differentiated adenocarcinoma is based on light microscopic features, particularly the formation of glandular structures by neoplastic cells. We have considered patients with well-differentiated or moderately well-differentiated adenocarcinoma as one group. These histologic features are shared by all adenocarcinomas, and the site of the primary tumor usually cannot be determined by histologic examination. Certain histologic features typically are associated with a particular tumor type (*e.g.*, papillary features with ovarian cancer, and signet ring cells with gastric cancer). However, these characteristics are not specific enough to be used as definitive evidence of the primary site. Immunoperoxidase stains and electron microscopy are of limited use in identifying the site of origin of most well-differentiated or moderately well-differentiated adenocarcinomas. The stain for PSA is an exception because it is specific for prostate cancer, and it should be used in men with suggestive clinical findings. Positive immunoperoxidase staining for estrogen receptor suggests metastatic breast cancer in women with metastatic adenocarcinoma. Rarely, neuroendocrine stains (*e.g.*, NSE, chromogranin) can identify an unsuspected neuroendocrine neoplasm.

The diagnosis of poorly differentiated adenocarcinoma should be viewed differently, because some of these patients may be distinctive in tumor biology and responsiveness to systemic therapy (see the section on poorly differentiated carcinoma). This diagnosis is usually made when only minimal glandular formation is seen on histologic examination or, on occasion, when tumors exhibit positive staining for mucin but have no glandular features. Well-differentiated adenocarcinoma, poorly differentiated adenocarcinoma, and poorly differentiated carcinoma are diagnoses that probably represent parts of a spectrum of tumor differentiation rather than specific, sharply demarcated entities. These histologies represent a heterogenous group of tumors with various biologic properties. Different pathologists may use slightly different criteria for making each of these three diagnoses. It is therefore appropriate to perform additional study with immunoperoxidase staining or electron microscopy in all poorly differentiated adenocarcinomas. Guidelines for the evaluation and treatment of patients with poorly differentiated adenocarcinoma are provided later in this chapter.

DIAGNOSTIC EVALUATION

An exhaustive search for the primary site is not indicated because it rarely can be found. Therefore, the clinical evaluation should be performed to evaluate any suspicious clinical symptoms or signs and to determine the extent of metastatic disease. Routine initial evaluation should include a thorough history and physical examination, standard laboratory screening tests (*i.e.*, complete blood count, liver function tests, serum creatinine, urinalysis), and chest radiography. All men should have a serum PSA or acid phosphatase determination, and all women should undergo mammography. Computed tomographic (CT) scans of the abdomen can identify a primary site in 10% to 35% of patients and frequently are useful in identifying additional sites of metastatic disease.[25,26] Additional symptoms, signs, or abnormal physical and laboratory findings should be evaluated with appropriate diagnostic studies. Extensive radiologic evaluation of asymptomatic areas is rarely useful in identifying a primary site, is expensive, and often results in confusing or false-positive results.

TREATMENT

The group of patients with adenocarcinoma of unknown primary site contains several clinically defined subgroups for which useful therapy can be given. Effective therapy does not exist for most patients who do not fall into one of these subgroups, although some patients benefit from empiric hormonal therapy or chemotherapy.

Peritoneal Carcinomatosis in Women

Adenocarcinoma causing diffuse peritoneal involvement is typical of ovarian carcinoma, although carcinomas from the gastrointestinal tract or breast can occasionally produce this clinical picture. Several women have been described with diffuse peritoneal carcinomatosis who had no primary site found in the ovaries or elsewhere in the abdomen at the time of laparotomy.[27–33] These patients frequently had histologic features typical of ovarian carcinoma, such as papillary configuration or psammoma bodies. This syndrome has been termed "multifocal extraovarian serous carcinoma" or "peritoneal papillary serous carcinoma." In the early 1980s, several anecdotal case reports documented excellent responses to cisplatin-based chemotherapy in women with this syndrome.[27–30]

Recently, larger series of patients have been described (Table 58-2).[31–33] Eighteen women with abdominal carcinomatosis and no primary site documented at laparotomy were reported from Vanderbilt University.[32] The clinical features in these patients were similar to those seen in patients with advanced ovarian carcinoma. Metastases outside the peritoneal cavity were unusual. The histologic features were similar to ovarian carcinoma; however, only 7 of 18 patients had serous adenocarcinoma. Patients were managed as if they had advanced ovarian cancer, using initial surgical cytoreduction followed by cisplatin-based combination chemotherapy. The median survival for the entire group was 23 months. Seven of 18 patients had complete clinical response to chemotherapy, and 3 have remained continuously disease free for more than 4 years after completing treatment.

A second group of 31 patients with extraovarian peritoneal serous papillary carcinoma was reported recently.[31] All these patients underwent initial surgical cytoreduction followed by chemotherapy. Most patients in this group received single-agent chemotherapy with chlorambucil or cisplatin or both. Ten of 31 patients responded to treatment; 3 had complete response and 2 are long-term disease-free survivors.

A third series by Ransom and colleagues described 33 patients with papillary adenocarcinoma of the peritoneum.[33] All but 2 patients had debulking surgical procedures. All received cisplatin-based combination chemotherapy. Several patients responded, and 2 had a negative second look laparotomy. Three patients remain alive 7 years after therapy, and the median survival of the entire group was 17 months.

TABLE 58–2. Therapy for Women With Peritoneal Adenocarcinomatosis of Unknown Primary Site

Investigations	*No. of Patients*	*Therapy*	*Complete Response Rate (%)*	*Long-Term Survival (%)*	*Median Survival (mo)*
Strand et al, 1989[32] (Vanderbilt)	18	Surgical cytoreduction and cisplatin-based chemotherapy	39	17	23
Dalrymple et al, 1989[31] (King George Hospital)	31	Surgical cytoreduction and chemotherapy*	10	6	11
Ransom et al, 1990[33] (Mayo Clinic)	33	Surgical cytoreduction and cisplatin-based chemotherapy	13†	9	17

* Single-agent chlorambucil or cisplatin-based chemotherapy.
† Sixteen of 33 patients had laparotomy to evaluate response; 2 of these patients had complete response.

Women with metastatic adenocarcinoma involving the peritoneal surface and no obvious primary site have tumors that are distinct in biology and are often responsive to chemotherapy. Many of these patients have elevations of serum CA 125 levels. The site of origin of these carcinomas is unknown, but some may arise from the peritoneal surface. Because ovarian epithelium is in part an extension of the mesothelial surface, some carcinomas arising from the peritoneal (mesothelial) surface may share a similar lineage (müllerian derivation) and biology with ovarian carcinoma. There is some question whether men can develop this tumor. Certainly, this possibility should be considered and would not be surprising (*e.g.*, papillary mesothelioma). Optimal management of these patients includes aggressive surgical cytoreduction followed by postoperative chemotherapy. The intensive cisplatin-based regimens considered optimal for the treatment of advanced ovarian cancer would seem a reasonable choice for initial chemotherapy. Some patients in this group have complete responses to therapy, and a small percentage have prolonged disease-free survival.

Women With Axillary Lymph Node Metastases

Breast cancer should be suspected in women who have axillary lymph node involvement with adenocarcinoma. Men with occult breast cancer could present in this fashion but would be rare. The initial lymph node biopsy should include measurement of estrogen and progesterone receptors. Elevated levels provide strong evidence for the diagnosis of breast cancer.[34] If no other metastases are identified, these patients may have stage II breast cancer with an occult primary, which is potentially curable with appropriate therapy. Modified radical mastectomy has been recommended in such patients, even when physical examination and mammography are normal. An occult breast primary has been identified after mastectomy in 44% to 68% of patients.[35,36] Primary tumors are usually less than 2 cm in diameter; in occasional patients, only noninvasive tumor is identified in the breast.[37] Prognosis after primary therapy is similar to that of other patients with stage II breast cancer.[35–37] Radiation therapy to the breast after axillary lymph node dissection may be an effective alternative primary therapy. Adjuvant systemic chemotherapy after primary therapy appears indicated in this setting.

Women with metastatic sites in addition to the axillary lymph nodes may have metastatic breast cancer with an occult primary. These women should be managed as if they have metastatic breast cancer. Elevated serum levels of CA 15-3 suggest the possibility of breast cancer. Estrogen and progesterone receptor status is of particular importance in these patients, because those with positive hormone receptors may derive major palliative benefit from hormonal therapy or chemotherapy or both.

Men With Skeletal Metastases

Metastatic prostate carcinoma should be suspected with adenocarcinoma involving predominantly bone, particularly if the metastases are blastic. In this setting, elevated levels of serum acid phosphatase of PSA or tumor staining with PSA provides confirmatory evidence of prostate cancer. Hormonal therapy may provide effective palliation.

Chemotherapy for Metastatic Adenocarcinoma of Unknown Primary Site

Most patients with well-differentiated or moderately differentiated adenocarcinoma of unknown primary site are not in one of the three clinical subgroups outlined above. Chemotherapy has been ineffective in most of these patients, producing low response rates and few complete responses. The results of chemotherapy in reported series of 10 or more patients are summarized in Table 58–3. Some patients with poorly differentiated carcinomas of unknown primary site were included in some of these series. Most of these patients did not receive cisplatin-based chemotherapy. The only drug that has been studied adequately as a single agent is 5-fluorouracil (5-FU); response rates ranged from 0% to 16%.[23,38,39] The FAM regimen (5-FU, doxorubicin, mitomycin C) and various modifications have been used frequently, based on the demonstrated activity of these regimens against some gastrointestinal cancers.[40–46] Response rates varied from 7% to 39%, median survival remained in the 4 to 11 month range,

TABLE 58–3. Empiric Chemotherapy Results in Series of Patients With Adenocarcinoma of Unknown Primary Site

Investigations	*Chemotherapy Regimen*	*No. of Patients*	*Response Rate (%)*	*Median Survival (mo)*
Single-Agent Trials				
Schildt et al, 1983[23]	F	20	0	3.5
Johnson et al, 1964[38]	F	65	6	—
Moertel et al, 1972[39]	F	88	16	4
Combination Chemotherapy				
Woods et al, 1980[42]	AM	25	36	4.2
Eagan et al, 1987[43]	AM	28	7	5.5
Milliken et al, 1987[40]	AM	51	39	4.5
McKeen et al, 1980[41]	FAM	28	21	8+
Goldberg et al, 1986[44]	FAM	43	30	11
Fiore et al, 1985[46]	A + vindesine	38	13	8+
Kambhus et al, 1986[45]	AM + vindesine	55	26	6
Woods et al, 1980[42]	CMeF	22	5	3
Schildt et al, 1983[23]	CAF	16	0	3
Anderson et al, 1983[63]	CAV	20	50	8
Eagan et al, 1987[42]	AMP	27	19	5
Pasterz et al, 1986[64]	CAFP	47	28	7
Milliken et al, 1987[40]	PVeB	50	39	5

A, doxorubicin (Adriamycin); B, bleomycin; C, cyclophosphamide; F, 5-fluorouracil; M, mitomycin C; Me, methotrexate; P, cisplatin, V, vincristine; Ve, vinblastine; —, no data.

and long-term disease-free survivors were not reported. Cisplatin does not appear to have a major role in the treatment of well-differentiated adenocarcinoma of unknown primary site. In two randomized studies comparing a cisplatin-containing regimen to doxorubicin plus mitomycin C, no difference in median survival was observed, and increased toxicity occurred in the cisplatin-containing arm.[40,43] The combination of cisplatin and etoposide has not been evaluated adequately in patients with adenocarcinoma of unknown primary site, nor has the combination of 5-FU and leucovorin.

Patients with good performance status should be considered for a trial of chemotherapy. Regimens containing doxorubicin and mitomycin C have usually produced partial responses in 20% to 40% of patients. Complete responses are rare. No compelling evidence exists to include cisplatin in these regimens unless the histology is poorly differentiated (see the section on poorly differentiated carcinoma). Cisplatin-containing regimens have been studied in too few patients to make firm conclusions. In patients with widespread metastases and poor performance status, systemic chemotherapy is unlikely to be of benefit. In these patients it has been our policy to administer tamoxifen (for women) and megestrol acetate (for women and men) as a therapeutic trial.

SQUAMOUS CARCINOMA OF UNKNOWN PRIMARY SITE

Squamous carcinoma at a metastatic site represents about 5% of all patients with unknown primary carcinomas. Effective treatment is available for patients with certain clinical syndromes, and appropriate evaluation of these patients is important.

SQUAMOUS CARCINOMA INVOLVING CERVICAL AND SUPRACLAVICULAR LYMPH NODES

The cervical lymph nodes are the most common metastatic site. Patients are usually middle-aged or elderly, and frequently they have abused tobacco or alcohol. When the upper or middle cervical lymph nodes are involved, a primary tumor in the head and neck region should be suspected. Clinical evaluation should include an examination of the oropharynx, hypopharynx, nasopharynx, larynx, and upper esophagus by direct endoscopy, with biopsy of any suspicious areas. When the lower cervical or supraclavicular lymph nodes are involved, a primary lung cancer should be suspected. Fiberoptic bronchoscopy should be performed if the chest radiograph and head and neck examination are normal. Of patients presenting with squamous carcinoma in cervical lymph nodes, 20% to 40% will subsequently have a primary site documented during the clinical course. In these patients, most primary sites become manifest in the head and neck region.

When no primary site is identified, local treatment should be given to the involved neck. The reported results involve retrospective, single-institution experiences, often using a variety of treatment modalities (Table 58–4). In most reports, a substantial percentage of patients achieved long-term disease-free survival after local treatment modalities. The results obtained using radical neck dissection, high-dose radiation

TABLE 58–4. Squamous Carcinoma of Unknown Primary Site Involving Cervical Lymph Nodes: Summary of Results, 1970–1990

Investigations	*No. of Patients*	*Treatment*	*5-Year Survival (%)*
Barrie et al, 1970[47]	104	Surger ± RT	31
Jessie et al, 1973[48]	184*	Surgery, RT, surgery + RT	43
Coker et al, 1977[49]	39	Surgery + RT	54
Jose et al, 1979[50]	54*	RT ± surgery	29
Nordstrom et al, 1979[51]	51*	Surgery, RT, surgery + RT	29
Fermont et al, 1980[52]	139*	RT	5
Leipzig et al, 1981[53]	32	Surgery, RT, surgery + RT	32 (3-y)
Pacini et al, 1981[54]	42	RT	23
Spiro et al, 1983[55]	79	Surgery, RT, surgery + RT	29
Mobit-Tabatabasi et al, 1986[56]	46	Surgery, RT, surgery + RT	18
Yang et al, 1983[57]	80	RT	37
Yang et al, 1983[57]	33	Chemotherapy	5
Carlson et al, 1986[58]	93†	RT ± surgery	70
McCunniff et al, 1986[59]	25	RT ± surgery	48
Bataini et al, 1987[60]	138	RT ± surgery	35
De Braud et al, 1989[61]	25	Surgery, RT, surgery + RT	44
De Braud et al, 1989[61]	16	Chemotherapy + RT + surgery	69 (3-y)

RT, radiation therapy.
* Includes patients with poorly differentiated carcinoma and adenocarcinoma.
† Excludes patients with massive neck involvement (*i.e.*, "incurable" patients).

therapy, or a combination of these modalities have been similar. The volume of tumor in the involved neck influences outcome, with N1 or N2 disease having a significantly higher cure rate than N3 or massive neck involvement. When resection alone is used as the primary treatment modality, a primary tumor in the head and neck subsequently becomes obvious in 20% to 40% of patients. Primary tumors surface less commonly when radiation therapy is used, presumably due to the eradication of occult head and neck primary sites within the radiation field. Radiation therapy dosages and techniques should be similar to those used in patients with primary head and neck cancer,[58] and the nasopharynx, oropharynx, and hypopharynx should be included in the irradiated field.

Patients with low cervical and supraclavicular nodes do not do as well because lung cancer is a frequent site of occult primary tumors. Patients with no detectable disease below the clavicle should be treated with aggressive local therapy because 10% to 15% of these patients will have long-term disease-free survival.

The role of chemotherapy for metastatic squamous carcinoma in cervical lymph nodes is undefined. One small nonrandomized comparison of patients treated with local modalities alone or with local modalities combined with chemotherapy (cisplatin and 5-FU) showed a higher complete response rate (81% versus 60%) and longer median survival time (>37 months versus 24 months) in patients also receiving chemotherapy.[61] Larger, randomized studies are necessary to verify the role of chemotherapy. The role of neoadjuvant chemotherapy in locally advanced head and neck carcinoma remains unproved; the role in this more unusual patient group is unlikely to be clarified soon.

SQUAMOUS CARCINOMA INVOLVING INGUINAL LYMPH NODES

Most patients with a tumor in inguinal lymph nodes have a detectable primary site in the genital or anorectal areas. Careful examination of vulva, vagina, cervix, penis, and scrotum is important, with biopsy of any suspicious areas. Digital examination and anoscopy should be performed to exclude lesions in the anorectal area. Identification of a primary site in these patients is important, because curative therapy is available for carcinomas of the vulva, vagina, cervix, and anus, even after spread to regional lymph nodes. For the patient in whom no primary site is identified, surgical resection with or without radiation therapy to the inguinal area sometimes results in long-term survival.[62]

SQUAMOUS CARCINOMA METASTATIC TO OTHER SITES

Metastatic tumor in areas other than the cervical or inguinal lymph nodes usually represents metastasis from an occult primary lung cancer. CT scans of the chest and fiberoptic bronchoscopy should be considered. Chemotherapy with regimens employed in the treatment of non-small cell lung cancer may be considered in patients with good performance status.

Patients with the diagnosis of poorly differentiated squamous carcinoma should be evaluated carefully, particularly if other clinical features are atypical for lung cancer (*i.e.*, young patient, nonsmoker, unusual metastatic sites). Occasionally, adenocarcinomas, particularly in the breast, undergo squamous differentiation at metastatic sites. As with the diagnosis of poorly differentiated adenocarcinoma, this histologic diagnosis is sometimes based on minimal histologic findings. Additional pathologic evaluation with immunoperoxidase stains or electron microscopy should be considered. When the diagnosis remains unclear, such patients should be considered for a trial of therapy for poorly differentiated carcinoma as discussed later in this chapter.

POORLY DIFFERENTIATED CARCINOMA AND ADENOCARCINOMA OF UNKNOWN PRIMARY SITE

Patients with poorly differentiated carcinoma or adenocarcinoma of unknown primary site appear to represent distinctive subgroups with specific therapeutic implications. They account for about 30% of all patients with carcinoma of unknown primary site; about 20% have poorly differentiated carcinoma, and 10% have poorly differentiated adenocarcinoma. Chemotherapy trials in the past often included these patients along with the more common patients with well-differentiated adenocarcinoma of unknown primary. All these patients were assumed to be similar, and they experienced a poor response to 5-FU-based chemotherapy and a short survival (see Table 58–3).[23,38–46,63,64] These chemotherapy trials included drugs likely to be useful in a palliative sense for patients with gastrointestinal and breast carcinomas. Some patients with poorly differentiated carcinomas have responsive neoplasms, and some are curable with cisplatin-based combination chemotherapy.[65–72] Clinical and pathologic evaluation is therefore crucial in patients with poorly differentiated carcinoma.

CLINICAL CHARACTERISTICS

The clinical characteristics in this diverse group of patients appears to differ substantially from the characteristics of patients with well-differentiated adenocarcinoma. The median age of this patient group is younger, although both groups have a wide age range. Patients with poorly differentiated carcinoma often give a history of rapid progression of symptoms (often <30 days) and have objective evidence of rapid tumor growth.[24,65,73] Most importantly, the location of metastases differs, and the predominant sites of involvement are frequently lymph nodes, mediastinum, and retroperitoneum, occurring much more commonly than in well-differentiated adenocarcinoma.

PATHOLOGIC EVALUATION

Light microscopic features that can differentiate chemotherapy-responsive tumors from nonresponsive tumors have not been identified.[66] Even with careful retrospective review of these tumors, responsive tumors of well-defined types (*e.g.*, germ cell tumor, lymphoma) are only rarely identified.

These tumors should undergo additional pathologic study with immunoperoxidase staining, electron microscopy, and genetic analysis. The use of routine light microscopy alone is not adequate to assess these tumors. The information provided by these additional pathologic studies has been summarized previously (see the section on poorly differentiated neoplasms). The frequency of more specific diagnoses, particularly lymphoma, is much lower in the carcinoma group than in the group initially diagnosed by routine light microscopy as poorly differentiated neoplasm. This is not surprising because carcinoma is a more specific diagnosis. Other diagnoses may still be suggested.

To assess the clinical utility of immunoperoxidase tumor-cell staining in patients with poorly differentiated carcinoma of unknown primary site, we retrospectively performed a battery of stains on archival tumors in 1989 from 87 patients treated between 1978 and 1983.[67] Poorly differentiated carcinoma or poorly differentiated adenocarcinoma was diagnosed on the basis of routine light microscopic examination, and all patients were treated before the technology of immunoperoxidase staining was routinely used. Therefore, results of immunoperoxidase staining could be correlated with clinical outcome in this group of similarly treated patients with a long median follow-up. Immunoperoxidase staining confirmed the diagnoses of poorly differentiated carcinoma in 49 patients (56%) and yielded other diagnoses in 14 patients (16%): melanoma (in 8 patients), lymphoma (4), prostatic carcinoma (1), and yolk sac carcinoma (1). In 24 patients (28%), the immunoperoxidase staining pattern was inconclusive; electron microscopy was occasionally helpful in clarifying the diagnosis in these patients. Seventy-five patients (86%) received combination chemotherapy with a cisplatin-based regimen, and 24 patients (28%) had a complete response. Nine of these patients were later given specific diagnoses by immunoperoxidase staining; lymphoma was diagnosed in 4 patients, melanoma in 4 patients, and yolk sac tumor in 1 patient. All patients with an immunoperoxidase diagnosis of lymphoma had clinical features compatible with lymphoma and are long-term survivors. Patients with immunoperoxidase features suggesting melanoma were surprisingly responsive to chemotherapy, with 3 of 7 complete responses and 2 long-term survivors. Patients with melanoma diagnosed by immunoperoxidase staining alone should not be excluded from a trial of cisplatin-based therapy. Immunoperoxidase staining is useful in the routine evaluation of metastatic poorly differentiated carcinoma of unknown primary site, as it can occasionally suggest the lineage of the tumor and have specific therapeutic implications.

Immunoperoxidase staining should be used in the evaluation of poorly differentiated carcinomas to do the following:

1. Confirm the diagnosis of carcinoma
2. Identify a primary site of a recognized carcinoma (*e.g.*, prostate)
3. Identify patients who may have other neoplasms, such as lymphoma or melanoma (although therapeutic recommendations for neoplasms other than lymphoma identified in this manner remain to be established)
4. Identify a group of patients in whom electron microscopy may provide important additional information

Electron microscopy can be useful for a small minority of these carcinomas. In general, electron microscopy should be reserved for those tumors not diagnosed by immunoperoxidase stains. Lymphoma can be diagnosed reliably in most instances in those tumors mistakenly believed to be carcinoma. In addition, sarcoma, melanoma, mesothelioma, and neuroendocrine tumors occasionally are defined by subcellular features. Neuroendocrine differentiation is particularly important and is discussed later in this chapter.

Chromosomal analysis is becoming an increasingly important method of diagnosis. Specific abnormalities have been identified in some leukemias, lymphomas, germ cell tumors, peripheral neuroepithelioma, and Ewing's sarcoma.[16–22,74] Evaluation for these specific abnormalities may be useful in patients with poorly differentiated carcinoma of unknown primary site. In reference to germ cell tumors, Motzer and colleagues performed genetic analysis (cytogenetic study and Southern blot analyses) on tumors in 8 patients with midline carcinomas of uncertain histology.[22] In 4 of the 8 patients with poorly differentiated carcinoma, abnormalities of chromosome 12 (*e.g.*, i[12p]; del [12 q]; multiple copies of 12 p) were diagnostic of germ cell tumor. Three of the 4 patients diagnosed on basis of genetic analysis achieved a complete response to cisplatin-based chemotherapy. This confirms the previously formulated hypothesis that some of these patients have histologically atypical germ cell tumors.[69] These genetic findings can be diagnostic in these patients. Additional specific chromosomal abnormalities in other solid tumors probably will be identified in the future, further improving the ability to establish tumor lineage.

Autopsy data looking specifically at patients with poorly differentiated carcinoma of unknown primary site are limited. Unfortunately, the number of postmortem examinations in medicine in general is declining. Based on the limited necropsy data we have accumulated, it appears that primary sites are found only occasionally in these patients (<35%). These findings are contrary to those for well-differentiated adenocarcinoma of unknown primary site, in which the primary site is found in most patients (>75%) at autopsy.[24]

DIAGNOSTIC EVALUATION

The clinical evaluation of these patients is similar to that described for patients with well-differentiated adenocarcinoma of unknown primary site. A history, physical examination, routine laboratory testing, and chest radiograph should be obtained in each patient. Any clues are followed with appropriate diagnostic testing. CT scans of the chest and abdomen should be performed in all patients in this group, due to the frequency of mediastinal and retroperitoneal involvement. Serum levels of HCG and AFP should be measured because substantial elevations of these markers suggest the diagnosis of germ cell tumor. The correlation of other serum tumor markers, such as CEA, CA 125, CA 19-9, and CA 15-3 with response to chemotherapy has not been established.

TREATMENT

When additional pathologic studies identify a specific neoplasm (*e.g.*, lymphoma, sarcoma), appropriate therapy can be administered. Patients with elevated serum levels of HCG or AFP and clinical features suggestive of extragonadal germ cell tumor (*e.g.*, mediastinal or retroperitoneal mass) should be treated with chemotherapy effective for germ cell tumors, even when pathologic examination is not diagnostic.

Most patients have multiple metastases and only the nonspecific diagnoses of poorly differentiated carcinoma or poorly differentiated adenocarcinoma despite additional pathologic study. The first reports showing that some of these patients (a small subset) have highly responsive tumors appeared about a decade ago.[68–71] Most of these patients were young men with mediastinal tumors; serum levels of HCG or AFP were frequently elevated. These patients initially were thought to have histologically atypical extragonadal germ cell tumors.

Further evidence for the responsiveness of other tumors in patients with poorly differentiated carcinoma of unknown primary site has accumulated during the last decade. The large prospectively collected group of patients from Vanderbilt University Medical Center will be discussed in detail because this group of patients is by far the largest group evaluated and treated in a similar fashion. Many recommendations for management are derived from this experience. Several other smaller patient groups have been reported recently and will be discussed briefly.

Prospective Series of Patients Compiled at Vanderbilt University Medical Center

Between 1978 and 1989, a series of 220 patients with poorly differentiated carcinoma of unknown primary site was prospectively compiled. Of these patients, 170 were initially seen and evaluated at Vanderbilt Medical Center. One hundred forty-two patients received their entire course of chemotherapy at Vanderbilt, and 28 patients were treated elsewhere according to our initial recommendations. After consultation, these patients were treated according to our recommendations, and detailed treatment records were obtained. Because of our ongoing interest in these patients, we frequently receive telephone consultations from oncologists practicing elsewhere. We have included 50 such patients from various regions of the United States in this series. These patients represent all telephone consultation patients during the years of this study who met entrance criteria and were treated (at our recommendation) with cisplatin-based chemotherapy. Therefore, the group of 220 patients includes all patients with poorly differentiated carcinoma or poorly differentiated adenocarcinoma of unknown primary site seen at Vanderbilt and all similar patients made known to us by telephone consultation during this 12-year period. Sixty-four of these 220 patients were evaluated and treated between 1978 and 1982 and were reported thereafter.[65]

Patients were included in this series if they had metastatic tumor at one or more sites and had one of the following light microscopic diagnoses: poorly differentiated carcinoma, poorly differentiated adenocarcinoma, poorly differentiated squamous carcinoma, or poorly differentiated small cell (questionable neuroendocrine) carcinoma. A few patients with the initial light microscopic diagnosis of poorly differentiated malignant neoplasm were included; in each of these tumors, specialized pathologic testing had confirmed the diagnosis of carcinoma. Between 1978 and 1982, at least one of the following clinical features was also required for inclusion: patient younger than 50 years, tumor involving primarily midline structures, elevated serum levels of HCG or AFP, clinical evidence of rapid tumor growth, or tumor responsive to previously administered radiation therapy or chemotherapy. After 1982, patients were included on the basis of histologic diagnosis alone, and no additional clinical feature was required.

PRETREATMENT EVALUATION. Because of the great variability in clinical presentation, diagnostic and staging procedures in these patients varied. All patients had a thorough history and physical examination, routine laboratory studies (complete blood counts, electrolytes, urinalysis, SMA12), and chest roentgenograms. Most patients also had CT scans of the chest and abdomen, and most had pretreatment determinations of serum HCG and AFP. Specific abnormalities identified by history, physical examination, or routine laboratory tests were investigated with further diagnostic studies in an attempt to identify a primary site. Fiberoptic bronchoscopy was performed in patients with radiographic evidence suggesting a lung cancer; patients with endobronchial lesions compatible with lung cancer were excluded from this series. In general, patients did not undergo an exhaustive radiologic search for a primary site in the absence of specific signs and symptoms, because this approach has not been found useful.

Biopsy specimens from all patients were examined at Vanderbilt University Medical Center. The initial diagnosis was always made on the basis of either an excisional biopsy or a core needle biopsy. Cytologic analysis alone (*e.g.*, fine-needle aspiration) was not used for diagnosis in any patient. Histochemical staining from mucin (or mucicarmine) was performed in 187 patients (85%). Most biopsies were evaluated further with immunoperoxidase staining or electron microscopy or both. A few tumors were studied by genetic analysis. During the first several years of this study, immunoperoxidase staining was not a standard part of the evaluation of poorly differentiated tumors because the antibodies were not available. Immunoperoxidase stains were subsequently performed on paraffin-fixed tumor specimens from many patients in this series, as part of a separate retrospective study.[67] Most of the patients in whom neither electron microscopy nor immunoperoxidase staining was performed had poorly differentiated adenocarcinoma by light microscopy; in these patients, the pathologist believed that further study was unlikely to result in additional useful information. Subsequently, several of these tumors were better defined by specialized pathology (see the summary of pathology studies below).

The light microscopic diagnosis of poorly differentiated carcinoma was based on the finding of a pleomorphic population of large cohesive malignant cells growing with no definable histologic pattern. Poorly differentiated adenocarcinoma was diagnosed if any adenomatous differentiation occurred, such as rudimentary gland formation or polarity of cells. In addition, some tumors with histologic features of poorly differentiated carcinoma were called poorly differentiated adenocarcinoma if the histochemical staining for mucin was strongly positive. All tumors with features of well-differentiated or moderately well-differentiated adenocarcinoma (*i.e.*, well-formed glandular structures, ducts with lumina, and mucin evident from hematoxylin-eosin staining) were excluded from this series. Poorly differentiated small cell carcinomas (questionable neuroendocrine) had a cohesive, homogenous population of small cells, with a high nucleus-to-cytoplasm ratio and dispersed chromatin in the nucleus.

CLINICAL CHARACTERISTICS. The clinical characteristics of the 220 patients are summarized in Table 58–5. The median age was 39 years, and 76% of the patients were younger than 50 years. Males outnumbered females by about 3 to 1. There were only 9 blacks (4%), which may reflect patterns of patient referral or rarity in blacks. One hundred seventeen patients (53%) had a history of tobacco use (more than 10 pack-years). Most patients were ambulatory and had only mild to moderate symptoms at the time of diagnosis.

Serum levels of HCG, AFP, and lactic dehydrogenase (LDH) were measured in most patients. HCG and AFP levels were infrequently elevated. Serum LDH levels were elevated in 48% of patients; however, 32 of 96 patients (33%) with elevated levels also had liver metastases as a possible source for LDH. Serum CEA levels were measured in 127 patients and were elevated in 47 (37%). Other more recently available markers (*e.g.*, CA 125, CA 15-3, CA 19-9) were measured in only a few patients.

Staging evaluation revealed metastases in two or more sites in 74% of patients. Many of the patients with metastases in only one site also had extensive tumor; for example, patients with multiple liver metastases or multiple bone metastases as the only site of tumor involvement were included in this group. In none of these patients was the single site of tumor believed to be a primary site, and in only 4 of the 57 patients in this group could a complete resection be accomplished. These 4 patients had tumor involving a single peripheral lymph node area.

Patients were categorized according to their predominant site of tumor involvement (see Table 58–5). Because most patients had two or more sites of metastases, assignment of a dominant site was sometimes arbitrary but was based on the site containing the greatest bulk of tumor. For example, a patient with a large retroperitoneal mass and several small liver defects on CT scan was classified as having predominant disease in the retroperitoneum. One hundred five patients (48%) had predominant tumor involvement in the mediastinum, retroperitoneum, or other peripheral lymph node groups. Patients with predominant lung involvement usually had multiple lung masses, and most had normal fiberoptic bronchoscopy. Fifty patients had tumor involving multiple metastatic sites, without an identifiable dominant site of involvement.

SUMMARY OF PATHOLOGY STUDIES. Based on initial routine light microscopic evaluation, 193 patients (88%) were given the diagnoses of poorly differentiated carcinoma (142 patients) or poorly differentiated adenocarcinoma (51 patients). Histochemical staining for mucin or mucicarmine was performed in 187 patients as a part of the initial evaluation. This test was positive in 47 patients (25%); most tumors with positive staining were called poorly differentiated adenocarcinomas. The remaining 27 patients were given the following diagnoses by light microscopy: poorly differentiated small cell carcinoma or poorly differentiated carcinoma with neuroendocrine features (12 patients), poorly differentiated malignant

TABLE 58–5. Clinical Characteristics of 220 Patients With Poorly Differentiated Carcinoma of Unknown Primary Site Treated at Vanderbilt University Medical Center

Characteristics	*No. of Patients (%)*
Sex	
Female/male	54/166
Race	
White	209
Black	9
Asian	2
Performance Status	
ECOG 0, 1	188
ECOG 2, 3	32
Dominant Metastatic Site	
Mediastinum	43 (20)
Retroperitoneum	42 (19)
Lung	29 (13)
Lymph nodes (cervical, axillary, inguinal)	20 (9)
Liver	11 (5)
Pleura/peritoneum	6
Bone	5
Pelvic mass	4
Pancreas	3
Soft tissue	2
Brain	2
Other (1 each)	3
Multiple sites (no dominant site)	50 (23)
Serum Tumor Markers	
HCG (N = 206)	
• Normal	174
• Elevated	32 (16)
AFP (N = 201)	
• Normal	190
• Elevated	11 (5)
LDH (N = 199)*	
• Normal	103
• Elevated	96 (48)
CEA (N = 127)	
• Normal	80
• Elevated	47 (37)
No. of Metastatic Sites	
1	57 (26)
2	67 (31)
3	60 (27)
>3	36 (16)

AFP, α-fetoprotein; CEA, carcinoembryonic antigen; ECOG, Eastern Cooperative Oncology Group; HCG, human chorionic gonadotropin; LDH, lactic dehydrogenase.
* Thirty-two of 96 patients had liver metastases as possible source for elevated LDH.

neoplasm (11 patients), and poorly differentiated squamous carcinoma (4 patients).

In most patients, other specialized pathologic studies were performed in addition to light microscopy. Immunoperoxidase studies were performed on 147 tumors and electron microscopy on 96 tumors. In only 46 cases was the final diagnosis based on light microscopic appearance alone. Immunoperoxidase studies in 32 patients were performed later (retrospectively) when the technology become available,[67] long after these patients had been treated. Patients in whom specialized pathologic evaluation before therapy resulted in a tumor diagnosis with specific therapeutic implications (*e.g.*, lymphoma) were not included in the series and received appropriate tumor-specific therapy.

In only 30 patients (13%) was the primary site or tumor type eventually identified (Table 58–6). In 17 of these 30 patients, the definitive diagnosis was made at repeat biopsy later during the course of the disease or at autopsy. In the remainder, retrospective specialized pathology studies provided the basis for diagnosis. All six lymphomas were identified retrospectively: 4 by immunoperoxidase staining, 1 by repeat biopsy at the time of tumor relapse, and 1 by genetic analysis (detection of an immunoglobulin gene rearrangement). Unfortunately, only 26 autopsies were done, and in only 9 (34%) was a primary site identified. In the remainder, metastatic poorly differentiated carcinoma or poorly differentiated adenocarcinoma with no primary site was found. In addition, 9 patients were thought to have melanoma on the basis of pathologic review or special pathologic studies; however, none of these patients had a known primary site, and none had typical light microscopic findings of melanoma.

THERAPY. At the time of identification, 198 patients had received no previous treatment for their cancer, whereas 22 patients had received radiation therapy (10 patients), chemotherapy (10 patients), or both (2 patients). In addition, 2 patients had a distant history of a previous neoplasm for which they had received radiation therapy (1 patient) or chemotherapy (1 patient).

All patients were treated with cisplatin-based combination chemotherapy (Table 58–7). One hundred sixteen patients treated between 1978 and 1984 received the cisplatin, vinblastine, bleomycin regimen (PVB) or a doxorubicin-containing modification of the PVB regimen. In 1985, etoposide was substituted for vinblastine in the treatment regimen, due to the synergy of etoposide with cisplatin and the demonstration of reduced toxicity and at least equivalent results.[75] Since 1985, 104 patients have received regimens including cisplatin and etoposide. In most patients, cisplatin and etoposide were administered for 5 days (cisplatin 20 mg/m^2 intravenously daily for 5 days, and etoposide 100 mg/m^2 intravenously daily for 5 days). In 55 patients, bleomycin (30 units weekly) was added to cisplatin and etoposide. Nine patients received regimens that included other agents in addition to cisplatin and etoposide.

Patients received two courses of therapy at 3-week intervals and were then evaluated for response. All patients showing any evidence of response after two courses received a total of four courses of therapy. Patients who failed to show any initial response were treated with alternative therapy.

TABLE 58–6. Specific Pathologic Diagnoses Confirmed

			Method of Diagnosis				
Diagnosis	*Autopsy*	*Rebiopsy (After Initial Therapy)*	*Review of Light Microscopy*	*Electron Microscopy*	*Immunoperoxidase Staining*	*Genetic Analysis*	*Total*
Lymphoma		1			4	1	6
Sarcoma (no primary site)		1		5			6
Lung							
Adenocarcinoma	5						5
Mixed adenocarcinoma and small cell carcinoma		1					1
Germ cell tumor							
Extragonadal		2	1				3
Testis		1					1
Carcinoid tumor*	2	1					3
Peripheral neuroepithelioma						1	1
Kidney carcinoma	1						1
Pancreatic carcinoma	1						1
Prostatic carcinoma					1		1
Breast carcinoma		1					1
Total	9	8	1	5	5	2	30

* Primary sites identified in 2 of 3 patients (rectum 1, lung 1).

Complete reevaluation was performed after completion of four courses of chemotherapy. All previously abnormal radiographic studies were repeated, and some patients had exploratory surgery for resection or biopsy of residual masses to better define tumor response. Patients were considered complete responders if no residual evidence of malignancy was found at reevaluation (*i.e.*, normalization of all previously abnormal physical or radiographic findings and normalization of biochemical findings). Partial response was defined as an objective decrease of 50% or greater in tumor size (product of perpendicular diameters), without interval appearance of any new lesions. All remaining patients were considered nonresponders. Duration of survival was calculated from the first day of treatment.

TABLE 58–7. Combination Chemotherapy in 220 Patients With Poorly Differentiated Carcinoma/ Adenocarcinoma

Chemotherapy	*No. of Patients*
Cisplatin, vinblastine, bleomycin (PVB regimen)	107
PVB + doxorubicin	9
Cisplatin, etoposide, bleomycin	55
Cisplatin, etoposide	40
Cisplatin, etoposide, vinblastine	3
Cisplatin, etoposide, bleomycin, vinblastine	2
Cisplatin, etoposide, ifosfamide	2
Cisplatin, etoposide, cyclophosphamide, vincristine, methotrexate	2

TREATMENT RESULTS. Two hundred nine patients received at least two courses of treatment and were evaluable for response to therapy. Eleven patients were inevaluable for response, for the following reasons: 6 died of treatment-related complications before the second course, 3 died of unrelated intercurrent illnesses during chemotherapy, and 2 refused treatment after only one course. These patients are all considered treatment failures in calculating the actuarial survival curve.

Fifty-eight patients (26%) had complete response to cisplatin-based therapy, whereas 80 patients (36%) had a partial response. An additional 4 patients were treated after surgical excision of their metastatic lesion, at a time when they had no evaluable tumor. Three of these 4 patients had tumor at the margins of the resection and therefore were known to have residual local disease. These patients were not assessed for response to chemotherapy but are included in the overall survival curve. Thirty-six patients (16% of the entire group) were free of disease at a median of 61 months following therapy (range 11 to 142 months). Thirty-two of these patients have been continuously disease free since completion of chemotherapy. Three patients relapsed after an initial complete response and are in a second complete response after salvage chemotherapy. One patient had a partial response to initial cisplatin-based chemotherapy but achieved complete response with subsequent resection of residual tumor followed by local radiation therapy. In addition to the 36 patients known to be disease free, 2 patients were lost to follow-up while in complete remission 28 and 42 months after completion of therapy. Twenty-four of 27 patients (89%) who relapsed after achieving complete remission did so during the first 12 months after treatment; only 1 patient has relapsed more than 24 months after completing therapy.

The actuarial survival curves for the entire group of patients and for the subset of patients who achieved complete remission are shown in Figures 58–1 and 58–2. Median survival for the entire group is 12 months, with an actuarial 16% 12-year survival. The actuarial survival at 12 years for patients achieving complete response is 62%. Treatment results do not differ significantly after deletion of the 30 patients in whom specific diagnoses were eventually made. In the remaining 190 patients, 49 (26%) had complete response, 70 (37%) had partial response, and 30 (16%) are long-term disease-free survivors.

Results in the 170 patients seen or treated at Vanderbilt were compared with the 50 patients seen and treated elsewhere. The complete response rate was significantly higher in patients treated elsewhere (21 of 50 [42%] versus 41 of 170 [24%], $p<0.05$). The percentage of long-term survivors was higher in the group treated elsewhere but did not attain statistical significance at the $p<0.05$ level (13 of 50 [26%] versus 24 of 170 [14%]. These results further clarify that these patients are being seen and managed appropriately in the community.

Treatment Results From Other Recent Series

Other investigators have demonstrated the responsiveness of these tumors.[73, 76–78] Van der Gaast and colleagues from Holland treated 40 patients with either poorly differentiated carcinoma or poorly differentiated adenocarcinoma; combination chemotherapy included bleomycin, etoposide, and cisplatin.[73] Eighteen of 34 patients (53%) responded, with 4 (12%) complete responses and 2 long-term disease-free survivors.

In the report of Raber and colleagues at the M.D. Anderson Cancer Center, 36 evaluable patients (21 patients with adenocarcinoma, 14 with undifferentiated carcinoma, and 1 with squamous cell carcinoma) received cisplatin, 5-FU, and etoposide.[76] Eight patients (22%) responded, but 4 (11%) had complete responses with durations of 19, 19, 24+ and 37+ months. Briassoulis and colleagues from Greece treated 42 patients (31 patients with poorly differentiated carcinoma and 11 with adenocarcinoma) with either cisplatin-based or carboplatin-based combination regimens. Nine of 42 (21%) responded with 3 (7%) complete responders.[77] Zarba and colleagues from France reported 22 evaluable patients (all adenocarcinoma) treated with 5-FU, mitomycin C, epirubicin, and cisplatin.[78] Nine patients (40%) responded with 2 (10%) complete responders. In each of these series, with the exception of the series by van der Gaast and colleagues, some patients had well-differentiated or moderately well-differentiated adenocarcinoma.

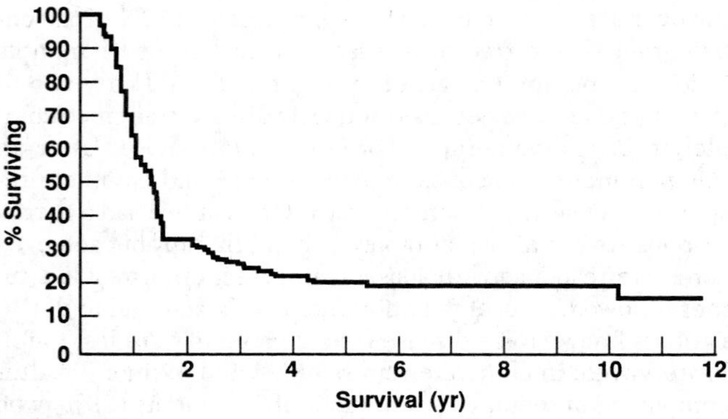

FIGURE 58–1. Twelve-year actuarial survival curve for all 220 patients with poorly differentiated carcinoma of unknown primary site (16% at 12 years).

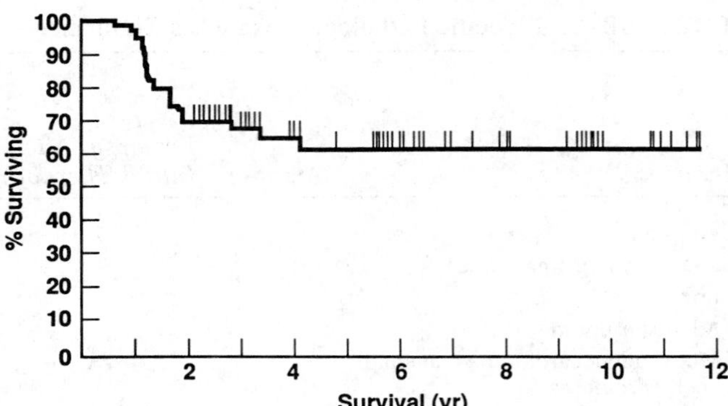

FIGURE 58–2. Actuarial survival curve of complete responders (62%). Tick marks indicate patients free of tumor.

The achievement of complete remissions in a minority of these patients is reproducible, as is a small cohort (5% to 15%) of long-term disease-free survivors. Combination chemotherapy should include cisplatin and etoposide with or without bleomycin. Results for this combination are at least as good as previous results using cisplatin, vinblastine, and bleomycin and are achieved with less toxicity. A therapeutic trial of two courses should be given. Responders should complete a total of four treatment courses. No evidence exists that more prolonged treatment will improve results, and nearly all long-term survivors have received only four treatment courses. In patients with residual palpable or radiographic abnormalities, surgical resection should be contemplated.

Although these results represent marked improvement when compared with the dismal historical results, this group of patients is heterogenous, and there are many patients with unresponsive tumors. Many of these patients should be considered for investigational trials of newer approaches. Several responsive subsets can be identified using clinical and pathologic features.

CLINICAL AND PATHOLOGIC CHARACTERISTICS PREDICTIVE OF RESPONSIVE TUMORS

A detailed analysis of the series of 220 patients compiled at Vanderbilt has revealed several important features. Table 58–8 shows the relation of response and long-term survival to the site of dominant tumor involvement. Most groups of patients had high overall response rates. Tumor responses usually correlate with good palliation and prolongation of survival. Complete responses and long-term survival were more frequent when tumor involved predominantly the retroperitoneum or peripheral lymph node areas (*e.g.,* cervical, axillary, or inguinal). Patients with multiple visceral sites of involvement had only a small chance of long-term disease-free survival.

TABLE 58–8. Chemotherapy Response, Survival, and Predominant Site of Tumor

Dominant Tumor Site	*No. of Patients*	*Overall Response Rate (CR + PR) (%)*	*No. of Complete Responders (%)*	*No. of Disease-Free Survivors (%)*
Retroperitoneum	42	35 (83)	21 (50)	13 (31)
Peripheral lymph nodes (cervical, axillary, inguinal)	20	14 (70)	11 (55)	9 (45)
Mediastinum	43	29 (67)	13 (30)	7 (16)
Bone	5	3 (60)	1 (20)	1 (20)
Pelvic mass	4	4 (100)	1 (25)	1 (25)
Lung	29	21 (72)	6 (21)	2 (7)
Liver	11	5 (45)	1 (9)	1 (9)
Pleura/peritoneum	6	2 (33)	1 (17)	0
Multiple sites (no dominant site)	50	25 (50)	5 (10)	2 (4)
Other sites*	10	4 (40)	2 (20)	1 (10)
Total	220	142 (65)	62 (28)	37 (17)

* Sites include pancreas (3 patients), brain (2), subcutaneous tissue (2), stomach (1), parotid (1), and nasopharynx (1).

The chance for complete response and long-term survival depends on several clinical and pathologic characteristics (Table 58–9). The following clinical features are highly predictive of an excellent therapeutic outcome, as determined by univariate analysis:

1. Predominant tumor location in the retroperitoneum or peripheral lymph nodes
2. Tumor limited to one or two metastatic sites
3. Normal serum CEA level
4. Normal serum LDH level
5. No history of cigarette use

Other characteristics, including age, sex, light microscopic histology, and cisplatin-based regimen had no significant influence on treatment outcome.

A Cox multivariate regression analysis was performed using the following prognostic factors: age, sex, smoking history, light microscopic histology (poorly differentiated carcinoma versus poorly differentiated adenocarcinoma), predominant tumor location (retroperitoneum or peripheral lymph nodes versus all other sites), number of metastatic sites (1 or 2 versus >2), LDH level, CEA level, and tumor marker (HCG, AFP) levels. The following factors were shown to have favorable prognostic significance: predominant tumor location in the retroperitoneum or peripheral lymph nodes ($p<0.001$), limited (1 or 2) metastatic sites ($p<0.001$), negative smoking history ($p=0.003$), and younger age ($p=0.028$).

Finally, a group of patients with clinical features highly suggestive of extragonadal germ cell tumors was analyzed for response to therapy and long-term survival. This group included 34 men younger than 45 years who had predominant disease in the mediastinum or retroperitoneum. Six of these men had elevated serum levels of AFP, HCG, or both. The histologic features of all tumors in this group were re-reviewed, and only one had typical features of a germ cell tumor (yolk sac tumor).[66] In this group, 29 of 34 patients (85%) responded to therapy, with 17 patients (50%) having complete response. Ten patients in this group (29%) remain disease free. Therefore, selection of patients with *clinical features* suggestive of extragonadal germ cell tumor, despite the nondiagnostic histology, defines a subgroup with a higher complete response rate and long-term survival than the group as a whole (see the section on special issues in cancer of unknown primary site).

Neuroendocrine Carcinomas of Unknown Primary Site

Electron microscopic examination of poorly differentiated carcinomas identifies neurosecretory granules in about 10% of tumors. These tumors are called "poorly differentiated neuroendocrine tumors" or "primitive neuroectodermal tumors" on this basis. Neuroendocrine features are suggested occasionally by light microscopic examination in some of these tumors. In most tumors, however, the light microscopic diagnosis is poorly differentiated carcinoma. A group of 29 patients with poorly differentiated neuroendocrine tumors was reported from Vanderbilt University (Table 58–10).[72] Most patients had clinical evidence of a high-grade tumor, and most had metastases in multiple sites. The retroperitoneum, lymph nodes, and mediastinum were frequently involved. Eighteen of 23 evaluable patients responded to chemotherapy with either a cisplatin-based combination or a combination regimen useful for patients with small cell lung cancer. Six patients had complete responses, and 3 patients remain continuously disease free more than 2 years after completion of therapy. Four other patients with limited involvement at only one site were treated with local modalities only (surgical excision in 3 patients and radiation therapy in 1 patient). All 4 patients have had long-term disease-free survival.

The nature and lineage of these tumors in most patients remains unclear. In 4 patients, specific diagnoses were made later in their clinical course or at autopsy. Two patients were found to have carcinoid tumors with undifferentiated growth pattern (both presented with abdominal carcinomatosis), 1

TABLE 58–9. Clinical and Pathologic Characteristics Predictive of Chemotherapy Responsiveness

Clinical/Pathologic Characteristics	*No. of Patients*	*No. of Complete Responders (%)*	*p Value*	*No. of Disease-Free Survivors (%)*	*p Value*
Age					
≤35 y	81	28 (35)	NS	18 (22)	
>35 y	139	34 (24)		19 (14)	NS
Sex					
Male	166	48 (29)	NS	29 (17)	NS
Female	54	14 (26)		8 (15)	
Dominant Tumor Location					
Retroperitoneum/peripheral nodes	62	32 (52)	<0.001	22 (35)	<0.001
All others	158	30 (19)		15 (9)	
Smoking History					
>10 pack-years	117	24 (21)	0.007	14 (12)	0.038
≤10 pack-years	103	38 (37)		23 (22)	
Light Microscopic Histology					
PDC	142	43 (30)	NS	28 (20)	NS
PDA	51	9 (18)		5 (10)	
No. of Metastatic Sites					
1 or 2	124	46 (37)	<0.001	32 (26)	<0.001
>2	96	16 (17)		5 (5)	
Chemotherapy					
PVB ± A	116	29 (25)		15 (13)	NS
Cisplatin/etoposide	104	33 (32)	NS	22 (21)	
Serum Markers					
LDH: Normal	103	36 (35)	0.01	25 (24)	0.018
Elevated	96	18 (18)		11 (11)	
CEA: Normal	80	26 (33)	<0.001	17 (21)	0.003
Elevated	47	2 (4)		1 (6)	

A, doxorubicin (Adriamycin); CEA, carcinoembryonic antigen; LDH, lactic dehydrogenase; NS, not significant; PDA, poorly differentiated adenocarcinoma; PDC, poorly differentiated carcinoma; PVB, cisplatin, vinblastine, and bleomycin.

patient had small cell lung cancer, and 1 patient had an extragonadal germ cell tumor with predominant neuroendocrine differentiation. A few similar patients, some with long-term survival after chemotherapy, have been reported and classified as "extrapulmonary small cell carcinoma."[79,80] The histology of these tumors was always small cell carcinoma and most of these patients had a recognized primary site (*e.g.,* head and neck, salivary gland, esophagus, bladder). Because most of our patients did not have small cell carcinoma histology and primary sites were not identified, it is unlikely their tumors represent this entity. Similarly, it is possible that some patients had unrecognized small cell lung cancer with an occult primary. The histology was usually not typical, and almost half of the patients had no smoking history. This finding, coupled with the lack of pulmonary involvement, makes this possibility unlikely. The clinical and biologic behavior of these poorly differentiated tumors is not typical of most of the other known types of neuroendocrine tumors in adults (*e.g.,* carcinoid tumors, islet cell tumors, medullary carcinoma of the thyroid, paraganglioma), which are well-defined clinical entities with typical histologic appearance and often indolent biology.

Perhaps some of these tumors represent an undifferentiated form of a well-recognized type of neuroendocrine tumor (*e.g.,* carcinoid, peripheral neuroepithelioma), albeit without a recognizable primary site. In the undifferentiated form, the clinical and pathologic characteristics no longer resemble the characteristics of the more differentiated counterpart. Some of these neoplasms may represent a newly defined (previously unrecognized) type of neuroendocrine tumor. It is likely, but not confirmed, that most of these tumors may be recognized by immunoperoxidase staining with chromogranin and NSE.

Although the nature of these tumors remains undefined,

TABLE 58–10. Poorly Differentiated Neuroendocrine Tumors of Unknown Primary Site in 29 Patients

	No. of Patients
Clinical Characteristics	
Male/female	21/8
Smoking (>10 pack-years)	17
Dominant Tumor Site	
Retroperitoneum	8
Lymph nodes	7
Mediastinum	3
Bone	2
Liver	2
Other	4
Multiple sites without dominant site	3
Treatment	
Cisplatin-based combinations	19
Cyclophosphamide, doxorubicin, vincristine ± etoposide	6
Surgical excision	3
Radiation therapy	1
Response to Chemotherapy	
Complete response	6
Partial response	12
No response or inevaluable	7
Continuously disease-free	3

(Data from Hainsworth JD, Johnson DH, Greco FA. Poorly differentiated neuroendocrine carcinoma of unknown primary site: A newly recognized clinicopathologic entity. Ann Intern Med 1988;109:364–371)

the presence of neuroendocrine differentiation (as determined by electron microscopy or immune staining) identifies a highly treatable subgroup. Chromosome studies of these tumors may be helpful if an 11:22 translocation is found, because this would support a diagnosis of peripheral neuroepithelioma or soft tissue Ewing's sarcoma. All of these patients should be considered for a trial of cisplatin-based chemotherapy. Some patients with limited single-site involvement may be curable with local treatment modalities alone.

SUMMARY OF DATA ON POORLY DIFFERENTIATED CARCINOMA

These treatment results provide evidence that patients with poorly differentiated carcinoma or poorly differentiated adenocarcinoma of unknown primary site are distinct from other patients with carcinoma of unknown primary site. In these data collected prospectively over 12 years from the group of 220 patients at Vanderbilt, an overall response rate of 62% with intensive cisplatin-based chemotherapy was achieved. More importantly, 26% of patients had complete response to therapy, and the 12-year actuarial survival is 16%. Many of the complete responders have been continuously disease free for more than 5 years and are undoubtedly cured. Long-term survivors were included in the groups treated at Vanderbilt and elsewhere, and somewhat better results were achieved in patients in the outside group, who were treated by oncologists from various regions of the United States. Similar results have been reported in small groups of patients identified prospectively using similar criteria and treated with cisplatin-based regimens.[73,76–78] Results in all these groups of patients contrast sharply with those previously reported for adenocarcinoma of unknown primary site, where the overall response rate was less than 30%, with rare complete responses and no long-term survivors.

The initial light microscopic diagnosis can reliably define this patient subgroup. About 60% of patients with carcinoma of unknown primary site have carcinomas with easily identified glandular features; these well-differentiated adenocarcinomas were excluded from our series, but some of these patients were included in other recent reports of cisplatin-based therapy.[76–78] Patients with only minimal histologic features of adenocarcinoma, or those with positive mucin stains as the only evidence of adenocarcinoma (poorly differentiated adenocarcinoma) have been included. Patients with the initial diagnosis of poorly differentiated neoplasm were excluded, unless additional pathologic studies provided evidence of carcinoma. Therefore, the identification of patients has relied primarily on well-defined, traditional histologic criteria, and consequently should be generally applicable and reproducible.

Despite detailed and specialized pathologic study, few tumors previously known to be potentially curable with chemotherapy can be defined. Only 4 patients with germ cell tumors and 1 patient with peripheral neuroepithelioma were eventually identified. Five patients with lymphoma are free of disease; however, the other 31 disease-free patients in this series had no well-defined tumor type.

The clinical characteristics of patients with poorly differentiated carcinoma differ from those previously described in the literature for patients with carcinoma of unknown primary site. This may be explained by the fact that the groups previously analyzed were comprised largely of patients with well-differentiated adenocarcinoma. The median age of patients in the Vanderbilt series was 39 years, substantially younger than reported for patients with adenocarcinoma of unknown primary site. The dominant site of metastatic tumor was frequently the mediastinum, retroperitoneum, or peripheral lymph nodes (50% of patients). These are uncommon sites of tumor involvement in patients with well-differentiated adenocarcinoma of unknown primary site, who usually have metastases involving liver, lungs, or bone. Considerable overlap exists between these two patient groups, and about 25% of the poorly differentiated carcinomas had metastases at multiple visceral sites.

Because most of the highly responsive tumors cannot be identified despite extensive pathologic evaluation, a variety of clinical features have been found to be useful as prognostic indicators (see Tables 58–8 and 58–9). Although evaluation of these clinical features enables the identification of patients with a higher chance of complete response, none of these indicators is specific enough to be able to exclude a patient from a therapeutic trial reliably.

Twelve years ago, we hypothesized that the highly responsive carcinomas probably were unrecognized or histologically atypical extragonadal germ cell tumors. We still believe that some of the highly responsive tumors are germ cell tumors that are marker negative and are not identifiable using all available pathologic methods. Strong support for this hypothesis has been provided by Motzer and colleagues, who demonstrated chromosome 12 abnormalities diagnostic of germ cell tumors in several young men with poorly differentiated midline carcinomas.[22] The excellent response to treatment and survival (50% complete responders, 29% disease-free survival) for patients with clinical features highly suggestive of extragonadal germ cell tumor suggests that these are germ cell tumors, albeit histologically atypical. These treatment results do not differ greatly from those in patients with known extragonadal germ cell tumors treated with standard cisplatin-based therapy.[81,82] If feasible, chromosomal analysis on tumor tissue should be done as a diagnostic test for selected patients with carcinoma of unknown primary site.

The responsive tumors in this patient group are heterogenous in their origin, and probably only a small subset of patients have histologically atypical germ cell tumors. A few of the patients have non-Hodgkin's lymphoma. Certain lymphomas are recognized to be confused with anaplastic carcinomas; some lymphomas, notably the Ki-1 lymphomas, also can stain positively with epithelial membrane antigen, further complicating their differentiation from carcinomas.[83] Hopefully, this confusion will be minimized or eliminated with the routine use of immunoperoxidase staining for CLA. A second group of highly responsive patients have poorly differentiated neuroendocrine tumors. The origin of such tumors remains speculative but may be an anaplastic variant of occult primary carcinoid. Metastatic poorly differentiated neuroendocrine carcinomas with known gastrointestinal or pancreatic primary sites have demonstrated marked sensitivity to chemotherapy with cisplatin and etoposide.[84]

The nature of the other responsive tumors in this heterogenous group of patients remains even more speculative. Malignant thymoma is a tumor recently recognized to be responsive to cisplatin-based therapy, with some patients experiencing long-term complete remissions.[85] Some patients with poorly differentiated carcinoma located predominantly in the mediastinum may have thymoma. A few patients in the Vanderbilt series who were long-term survivors were identified as having melanoma on the basis of immunoperoxidase stains. This diagnosis seems unusual because melanoma is a tumor that is usually unresponsive to chemotherapy. It is possible that melanomas identifiable only by immunoperoxidase staining or electron microscopy represent a uniquely chemotherapy-sensitive subset. Finally, it is possible that some responsive tumors represent a heretofore undefined tumor type. Alternatively, some may represent highly undifferentiated, and therefore perhaps chemotherapy-sensitive, epithelial tumors from occult primary sites, which are usually much less responsive to systemic therapy. It is likely that future knowledge and refinements in genetic diagnosis will establish the identity of many of these tumors.

The large series of patients compiled at Vanderbilt and smaller recent series provide firm evidence that patients with poorly differentiated carcinoma or poorly differentiated adenocarcinoma of unknown primary site require specific evaluation and treatment. Most of these patients have a major tumor response to cisplatin-based therapy, and a few are cured with such treatment. The fact that 220 patients with poorly differentiated carcinoma were collected in a 12-year period at a single institution indicates these tumors are not rare. Many such patients continue to be treated with supportive care only, with local radiation therapy, or with 5-FU-based regimens, as a result of previous pessimism and data concerning patients with adenocarcinoma of unknown primary site. Patients evaluated and treated by several oncologists from around the United States (compiled at Vanderbilt) did as well as those patients treated at a single institution. This confirms that these patients can be identified appropriately and treated successfully outside an academic setting. Multivariate analysis of a large group of patients has identified important prognostic factors. The lack of importance of other factors (*i.e.*, sex, light microscopic histology, serum HCG and AFP levels) has been documented. Poorly differentiated carcinomas evaluated with state-of-the-art pathologic techniques have shown that *most* responsive tumors in this group are *not* misdiagnosed or poorly diagnosed but are truly of unknown origin and biology.

It is imperative to consider the large group of patients with well-differentiated or moderately well-differentiated adenocarcinoma as clinically distinct from those with poorly differentiated carcinomas. All patients with poorly differentiated carcinoma should be considered for a therapeutic trial with cisplatin-based chemotherapy. Those with favorable prognostic features are likely to respond well. Although treatment results appear similar with the cisplatin-based regimens, the combination of cisplatin, etoposide, and bleomycin has been shown to have less toxicity than the cisplatin, vinblastine, and bleomycin regimen and is therefore preferred. The usefulness of cisplatin-based therapy for patients with no favorable prognostic features is less certain. Responses are frequent, and a few long-term survivors have been seen even in poor prognostic groups (see Tables 58–8 and 58–9). Responses usually occur rapidly, and a brief therapeutic trial should be considered. If no response is observed after one or two courses, therapy should be discontinued and alternate approaches considered. Poorly differentiated carcinoma of unknown primary site should be viewed as a highly responsive tumor to appropriate combination chemotherapy. Many patients can enjoy substantial clinical benefit, prolongation of survival, and, at times, cure.

SPECIAL ISSUES IN CARCINOMA OF UNKNOWN PRIMARY ORIGIN

EXTRAGONADAL GERM CELL CANCER SYNDROME

Selected patients with poorly differentiated carcinoma almost certainly have germ cell tumors, although the histologic features are atypical, even when generous pathologic specimens are available for study. Chromosomal analysis may provide a definitive diagnosis in some of these patients, particularly if their tumor cells contain specific chromosome 12 abnormalities. Even if not found or in the absence of tumor karyotypic study, young people who have mediastinal or retroperitoneal masses with or without elevated serum levels of HCG or AFP should be suspected of harboring a germ cell tumor. Lymphoma should be ruled out by immunoperoxidase stains, electron microscopy, or, if necessary, cytogenetic studies (*e.g.*, chromosome analysis and immunoglobulin gene rearrangement evaluation). The clinical extragonadal germ cell cancer syndrome was described in 1979.[68,69] The full syndrome has the following features:

1. The syndrome usually occurs in young men (<50 years).
2. Tumors are predominantly located in the midline (mediastinum, retroperitoneum) or multiple pulmonary nodules.
3. The symptom interval is short (<3 months), and there is a history of rapid tumor growth.
4. Serum levels of HCG, AFP, or both are elevated.
5. There is a good response to previously administered radiation therapy or chemotherapy.

Few patients have all elements of this syndrome. These clinical features are those of extranodal germ cell tumors, but without definitive histology the diagnosis is not unequivocal. In rare cases, women can have these tumors, and the other features are not absolute. Any one feature suggests the possibility of a germ cell tumor. It is prudent to treat patients having these atypical germ cell tumors with cisplatin-based therapy.

A SINGLE SITE OF NEOPLASM

In the unusual situation where only one site of neoplasm is identified (*e.g.*, one node group or one large mass), the possibility of an unusual primary tumor mimicking metastatic disease should be considered. Several unusual tumors could present in this fashion, including Merkel's cell tumors, skin adnexal tumors (*e.g.*, apocrine, eccrine, and sebaceous carcinomas), and even sarcomas or melanomas that are mistakenly interpreted as metastatic carcinoma (pathologically and clinically). Patients with one site of involvement usually have metastatic carcinoma, and many other sites are present but are not detectable. In the absence of any other documented metastatic disease, these patients should be treated with aggressive local therapy (*i.e.*, resection, radiation therapy, or both) because a minority will enjoy long-term disease-free survival. If a definitive diagnosis cannot be established, and the neoplasm is poorly differentiated, we believe these patients should receive adjuvant cisplatin-based chemotherapy, but it is difficult to know if this treatment is superior to local therapy alone.

On occasion, patients will present with apparent solitary metastasis of adenocarcinoma or poorly differentiated carcinoma in the brain, liver, subcutaneous tissue, lymph nodes, or other areas. In most instances, other metastases will become clinically apparent with time. There are certainly examples of resection or radiation of these single areas and of patients doing well with no evidence of recurrence. At times, the resection may be planned as palliative, particularly with a brain metastases. The method of choice in managing these patients is to resect the single lesion. After resection and depending on the other clinical circumstances, patients may be candidates for chemotherapy, particularly if their histology is poorly differentiated carcinoma. In those patients with single metastases (*i.e.*, brain), it would be prudent to consider radiation therapy after surgical resection. Isolated axillary adenocarcinoma in women often arises from an occult breast cancer (see the section on adenocarcinoma).

PROSTATE CANCER WITH ATYPICAL METASTASES

There have been patients with clinical presentations atypical for prostate cancer in whom the diagnosis was suggested only by tumor staining for PSA.[86,87] These patients usually presented with adenocarcinoma metastases to the lung, mediastinal lymph nodes, or upper abdominal lymph nodes, with no obvious involvement of bone or pelvic lymph nodes. Some of these patients respond to therapy for metastatic prostate cancer.

UNSUSPECTED GESTATIONAL CHORIOCARCINOMA

In young women with poorly differentiated carcinoma or anaplastic neoplasms, particularly with lung nodules, be aware of the possibility of metastatic gestational choriocarcinoma. The history of recent pregnancy, spontaneous abortion, or missed menstrual periods should suggest the possibility. In this group of patients, serum HCG levels are invariably elevated. On occasion, biopsy specimens do not show the classic appearance of choriocarcinoma but simply that of metastatic carcinoma, usually poorly differentiated. Ultrasound or CT scan of the abdomen may show an enlarged uterus, and a dilation and curettage may be indicated in these patients. Most of these patients are curable with single-agent methotrexate.

ISOLATED PLEURAL EFFUSION

An isolated pleural effusion containing carcinoma in women will occasionally represent metastatic disease from occult ovarian carcinoma or be accompanied by peritoneal carcinomatosis. Even when the patient has no symptoms or signs and an abdominopelvic CT scan is normal, the primary may reside in the abdomen or pelvis. These occult abdominal neoplasms may arise from the ovary or the peritoneal surface and most characteristically cause a right pleural effusion. Should there be no clue of neoplasm in the abdomen, an elevated plasma CA 125 level suggests the possibility of this phenomena. In the absence of clinical findings in the abdomen, laparoscopy or exploratory laparotomy might be diagnostic, but these procedures are not therapeutic in this setting. Some of these tumors are particularly responsive to cisplatin-based treatment.

An isolated pleural effusion can be a manifestation of a peripheral lung carcinoma (usually adenocarcinoma) or a mesothelioma. Diagnosis may be difficult; at times the primary is not apparent even after chest tube drainage. Cytology usually shows adenocarcinoma. Electron microscopy may reveal ultrastructural features diagnostic of mesothelioma. The therapy of these patients is difficult. In those with poor performance status or advanced age, a trial of tamoxifen or megestrol acetate is reasonable. In fit patients, a trial of cisplatin-based chemotherapy should be considered.

TABLE 58–11. Carcinoma of Unknown Primary Site: Summary of Evaluation and Therapy of Responsive Subsets

	*Clinical Evaluation**	*Special Pathologic Studies*	*Subsets*	*Therapy*	*Prognosis*
Adenocarcinoma (well-differentiated or moderately differentiated)	Abdominal CT scan Men: Serum PSA Women: Mammogram Serum CA 15-3 Serum CA 125 Additional studies to evaluate symptoms, signs	Men: PSA stain Women: ER, PR	1. Women, axillary node involvement	Treat as primary breast cancer	Poor for entire group (median survival: 4 mo); better for subgroups
			2. Women, peritoneal carcinomatosis	Surgical cytoreduction + chemotherapy effective in ovarian cancer	
			3. Men, blastic bone metastases, high serum PSA, or PSA tumor staining	Hormonal therapy for prostate cancer	
			4. Single peripheral nodal site of involvement	Lymph node dissection ± radiotherapy	
Squamous carcinoma	Cervical node presentation Panedoscopy	None	Cervical adenopathy	Radiation therapy ± neck dissection	25–50% 5-y survival
	Supraclavicular presentation Bronchoscopy		Supraclavicular	Radiation therapy	5–15% 5-y survival
	Inguinal presentation Pelvic, rectal exams, anoscopy		Inguinal adenopathy	Inguinal node dissection ± radiation therapy	Potential long-term survival
Poorly differentiated carcinoma, poorly differentiated adenocarcinoma	Chest, abdominal CT scans; serum HCG, AFP; additional studies to evaluate symptoms, signs	Immunoperoxidase staining Electron microscopy Genetic analysis	1. Atypical germ cell tumors (identified by chromosomal abnormalities only)	Treatment for germ cell tumor	40–50% cure rate
			2. Neuroendocrine tumors	Cisplatin-based therapy	High response rate
			3. Predominant tumor location in retroperitoneum, peripheral nodes	Cisplatin/etoposide/bleomycin	50% prolongation of survival; 10–20% cured

AFP, α-fetoprotein; ER, estrogen receptor; HCG, human chorionic gonadotropin; PR, progesterone receptor; PSA, prostate-specific antigen.
* In addition to history, physical examination, routine laboratory tests, and chest x-ray films.

GERM CELL TUMORS WITH METASTASES OF OTHER HISTOLOGIES

On occasion, patients with germ cell tumors, particularly extragonadal primaries, may have a metastatic lesion that consists of only somatic tumor cells. This is particularly true for neuroendocrine or sarcomatous differentiation. Patients therefore may be diagnosed as having a neuroendocrine tumor or sarcoma. In these rare instances, a primary germ cell tumor (usually extragonadal) is present elsewhere and subsequently will be clinically apparent. It is difficult to make the diagnosis initially. An elevated plasma AFP or HCG level is suggestive. The presence of a mediastinal, retroperitoneal, or testicular mass support this possibility. Chromosomal analysis of tumor tissue may be diagnostic if a specific chromosome 12 abnormality is found. If the patient has metastatic germ cell tumor with metastases of other histologies, the treatment of choice is cisplatin-based chemotherapy. These patients appear to have a worse prognosis than those with typical germ cell tumors because the somatic cell tumors are less sensitive to chemotherapy.

CARCINOID TUMORS OF UNKNOWN PRIMARY SITE

In rare instances, patients have metastatic typical carcinoid tumors but with an unknown primary site. This is more likely to manifest as multiple liver metastasis with an occult primary in the intestinal tract, usually in the ileum or rectum. These patients should be managed no differently than those with known primaries. In the event of a solitary lesion in a node, bone, liver, lung, or elsewhere, aggressive local therapy (*i.e.*, resection and radiation therapy) is indicated because there is a possibility of long-term control. If the histology is poorly differentiated, cisplatin-based chemotherapy is likely to be beneficial. Most of these patients with typical carcinoids (well-differentiated pattern) have indolent tumors, and recurrence over years is likely. The primary never becomes apparent in some patients, but the bronchus and gastrointestinal tract eventually reveal the primary in most cases.

SMALL CELL CARCINOMAS OF UNKNOWN PRIMARY SITE

Tumors with typical histologic features of small cell carcinomas of unknown primary site are not rare. These patients usually have an occult primary in the lung (bronchus), and CT chest scan or bronchoscopy may find the primary. Postmortem examination has disclosed clinically undetectable primaries in some patients. In rare instances, the occult primary arises from extrapulmonary sites (*e.g.*, salivary gland, esophagus, bladder). Poorly differentiated or atypical carcinoid tumors can mimic these tumors, as can other anaplastic neuroendocrine lesions. A poorly differentiated neuroendocrine carcinoma subset has been defined by electron microscopy and immunoperoxidase stains (see the section on poorly differentiated carcinoma). These patients usually do *not* have the classic or typical histologic features of small cell carcinomas. Patients with small cell carcinoma of unknown primary site should receive aggressive local therapy with resection or radiation therapy or both, followed by chemotherapy known to be useful in small cell lung cancer.

SUMMARY

The recognition of subsets of responsive tumors in patients within the large heterogenous population of cancers of unknown primary site represents an improvement in the management of these patients. These patients with responsive tumors can often be defined with appropriate clinical and pathologic evaluation. A summary of several subsets and an outline of the evaluation necessary for their identification is given in Table 58–11. A therapeutic trial is the only absolute method to determine if a patient has a responsive tumor, and some patients who do not conform to a defined subset do respond to chemotherapy. Even for responsive carcinomas, the tumor biology and lineage continue to be an enigma. Unfortunately, a large group of patients with insensitive tumors remains. Improved therapy for these patients will probably follow advances in the treatment of non-small cell lung cancer, pancreatic cancer, and the other gastrointestinal cancers, because most insensitive adenocarcinomas probably arise from these occult primary sites.

A registry has been established at Vanderbilt, and an attempt is being made to collect and catalog patients from other physicians around the country. Pathologic material, clinical summaries, and follow-up data on all such patients are being requested. A bank of unstained slides currently exists, and special stains developed in the future may be evaluated rapidly. These data eventually may provide a better assessment of the frequency and spectrum of these neoplasms and allow for more specific diagnoses and therapy.

REFERENCES

1. Horning SJ, Carrier EK, Rouse RV, et al. Lymphomas presenting as histologically unclassified neoplasms: Characteristics and response to treatment. J Clin Oncol 1989;7:1281–1287.
2. Hales SA, Gatter KC, Heryet A, Mason DY. The value of immunocytochemistry in differentiating high-grade lymphoma from other anaplastic tumours: A study of anaplastic tumours from 1940 to 1960. Leuk Lymphoma 1989;1:59–63.
3. Gatter KC, Alcock C, Heryet A, Mason DY. Clinical importance of analysing malignant tumours of uncertain origin with immunohistochemical techniques. Lancet 1985;2:1302–1305.
4. Azar HA, Espinoza CG, Richman AV et al. "Undifferentiated" large cell malignancies: An ultrastructural and immunocytochemical study. Hum Pathol 1982;13:323–333.
5. Warnke RA, Gatter KC, Falini B, et al. Diagnosis of human lymphoma with monoclonal antileukocyte antibodies. N Engl J Med 1983;209:1275–1281.
6. Battifora H, Trowbridge IS. A monoclonal antibody useful for the differential diagnosis between malignant lymphoma and nonhematopoietic neoplasms. Cancer 1983;51:816–821.
7. Tapra FJ, Polak JM, Barbosa AJA, et al. Neuron-specific enolase is produced by neuroendocrine tumors. Lancet 1981;1:808–811.
8. O'Connor DT, Burton D, Deftos LJ. Immunoreactive human chromogranin A in diverse polypeptide hormone producing human tumors and normal endocrine tissues. J Clin Endocrinol Metab 1983;57:1084–1086.
9. Allhof EP, Proppe KH, Chapman CM. Evaluation of prostate-specific acid phosphatase and prostate-specific antigen. J Urol 1983;129:316–319.
10. Denk H, Knepler R, Artlieb U, et al. Proteins of intermediate filaments: An immunohistochemical and biochemical approach to the classification of soft tissue tumors. Am J Pathol 1983;110:193–208.
11. Osborn M, Weber K. Biology of disease: Tumor diagnosis by intermediate filament type—a novel tool for surgical pathology. Lab Invest 1983;48:372–394.
12. Kahn HJ, Marks A, Thom H, et al. Role of antibody to S-100 protein in diagnostic pathology. Am J Clin Pathol 1983;79:341–347.
13. Gown AM, Vogel AM, Hoak D, et al. Monoclonal antibodies specific for melanocytic tumors distinguish subpopulations of melanocytes. Am J Pathol 1986;123:195–203.
14. Bosman FT, Giard RWM, Nieuwenhuijen-Kruseman AC, et al. Human chorionic gonadotrophin and alpha fetoprotein in testicular germ cell tumors: A retrospective immunohistochemical study. Histopathology 1980;4:673–684.
15. Kurman KJ, Scardino PT, McIntire KR, et al. Cellular localization of alpha fetoprotein and human chorionic gonadotropin in germ cell tumors of the testis using an indirect immunoperoxidase technique: A new approach to classification utilizing tumor markers. Cancer 1977;40:2136–2151.

16. Arnold A, Cossman J, Bakhshi A, et al. Immunoglobulin-gene rearrangements as unique clonal markers in human lymphoid neoplasms. N Engl J Med 1983;309:1593–1599.
17. Rowley JD. Recurring chromosome abnormalities in leukemic and lymphoma. Semin Hematol 1990;27:122–130.
18. Turc-Carel C, Philip I, Berger MP, et al. Chromosomal translocation in Ewing's sarcoma. N Engl J Med 1983;309:497–498.
19. Whang-Peng J, Triche TJ, Knutsen T, et al. Chromosome translocation in peripheral neuroepithelioma. N Engl J Med 1984;311:584–585.
20. Bosl GJ, Dmitrovsky E, Reuter V, et al. i(12p): A specific karyotypic abnormality in germ cell tumors. Proc Am Soc Clin Oncol [Abstract] 1989;8:131.
21. Atkin NB, Baker MC. Specific chromosome change, i(12p), in testicular tumors. Lancet 1982;2:1349–1356.
22. Motzer RJ, Rodriguez E, Reuter VE, et al. Genetic analysis as an aid in diagnosis for patients with midline carcinomas of uncertain histologies. JNCI 1991:83:341–346.
23. Schildt RA, Kennedy PS, Chen TT, et al. Management of patients with metastatic adenocarcinoma of unknown origin: A Southwest Oncology Group study. Cancer Treat Rep 1983;67:77–79.
24. Nystrom JS, Weiner JM, et al. Metastatic and histologic presentations in unknown primary cancer. Semin Oncol 1977;4:53–58.
25. McMillan JH, Levine E, Stephens RH. Computed tomography in the evaluation of metastatic adenocarcinoma from an unknown primary site. Radiology 1982;143:143–146.
26. Karsell PR, Sheedy PF, O'Connell MJ. Computerized tomography in search of cancer of unknown origin. JAMA 1982;248:340–343.
27. Hochster H, Wernz JC, Muggia FM. Intra-abdominal carcinomatosis with histologically normal ovaries. Cancer Treat Rep [Letter] 1984;68:931–932.
28. Gooneratne S, Sassone M, Blaustein A, Talerman A. Serous surface papillary carcinoma of the ovary: A clinicopathologic study of 26 cases. Int J Gynecol Pathol 1982;1:258–269.
29. Chen KT, Flam MS. Peritoneal papillary serous carcinoma with long-term survival. Cancer 1986;58:1371–1373.
30. August CZ, Murad TM, Newton M. Multiple focal extraovarian serous carcinoma. Int J Gynecol Pathol 1985;4:11–23.
31. Dalrymple JC, Bannatyne P, Russell P, et al. Extraovarian peritoneal serous papillary carcinoma: A clinicopathologic study of 31 cases. Cancer 1989;64:110–115.
32. Strnad CM, Grosh WW, Baxter J, et al. Peritoneal carcinomatosis of unknown primary site in women. Ann Intern Med 1989;111:213–217.
33. Ransom DT, Patel SR, Keeney GL, et al. Papillary serous carcinoma of the peritoneum: A review of 33 cases treated with cisplatin-based chemotherapy. Cancer 1990;66:1091–1094.
34. Bhatia SK, Saclarides TJ, Witt TR, et al. Hormone receptor studies in axillary metastases from occult breast cancers. Cancer 1987;59:1170–1172.
35. Ashikari R, Rosen PP, Urban JA, Senoo T. Breast cancer presenting as an axillary mass. Ann Surg 1976;183:415–417.
36. Patel J, Nemoto T, Rosner D, et al. Axillary lymph node metastases from an occult breast cancer. Cancer 1981;47:2923–2927.
37. Rosen PP. Axillary lymph node metastases in patients with occult noninvasive breast carcinoma. Cancer 1980;46:1298–1306.
38. Johnson RO, Castro R, Ansfield FJ. Response of primary unknown cancers to treatment with 5-fluorouracil. Cancer Chemother Rep 1964;38:63–64.
39. Moertel CG, Reitemeier RJ, Schutt AJ, Hahn RG. Treatment of the patient with adenocarcinoma of unknown origin. Cancer 1972;30:1469–1472.
40. Milliken ST, Tattersall MHN, Woods RL, et al. Metastatic adenocarcinoma of unknown primary site: A randomized study of two combination chemotherapy regimens. Eur J Cancer Clin Oncol 1987;23:1645–1648.
41. McKeen E, Smith F, Haidak D, et al. Fluorouracil, adriamycin and mitomycin-C for adenocarcinoma of unknown origin. Proc Am Assoc Cancer Res [Abstract] 1980;21:358.
42. Woods RL, Fox RM, Tattersall MHN, et al. Metastatic adenocarcinomas of unknown primary: A randomized study of two combination-chemotherapy regimens. N Engl J Med 1980;303:87–89.
43. Eagan RT, Thernean TM, Rubin J, et al. Lack of value for cisplatin added to mitomycin-doxorubicin combination chemotherapy for carcinoma of unknown primary site. Am J Clin Oncol 1987;10:82–85.
44. Goldberg RM, Smith FP, Ueno W, et al. Fluorouracil, adriamycin and mitomycin in the treatment of adenocarcinoma of unknown primary. J Clin Oncol 1986;4:395–399.
45. Kambhus, Kelsen D, Niedzwiecki D, et al. Phase II trial of mitomycin C, vindesine, and adriamycin and predictive variables in the treatment of patients with adenocarcinoma of unknown primary site. Proc Am Assoc Cancer Res [Abstract] 1986;27:734.
46. Fiore JJ, Kelsen DP, Gralla RJ, et al. Adenocarcinoma of unknown primary origin: Treatment with vindesine and doxorubicin. Cancer Treat Rep 1985;69:591–594.
47. Barrie JR, Knapper WH, Strong EW. Cervical nodal metastases of unknown origin. Am J Surg 1970;120:466–470.
48. Jesse RH, Perez CA, Fletcher GH. Cervical lymph node metastasis: Unknown primary cancer. Cancer 1973;31:854–859.
49. Coker DD, Casterline PF, Chambers RG, Jacques DA. Metastases to lymph nodes of the head and neck from an unknown primary site. Am J Surg 1977;134:517–522.
50. Jose B. Bosch A, Caldwell WL, Frias Z. Metastasis to neck from unknown primary tumor. Acta Radiol Oncol 1979;18:161–170.
51. Nordstrom DG, Tewfik HH, Latourette HB. Cervical lymph node metastases from an unknown primary. Int J Radiat Oncol Biol Phys 1979;5:73–76.
52. Fermont AC. Malignant cervical lymphadenopathy due to an unknown primary. Clin Radiol 1980;31:355–358.
53. Leipzig B, Winter ML, Hokanson JA. Cervical nodal metastases of unknown origin. Laryngoscope 1981;91:593–598.
54. Pacini P, Olmi P, Cellai E, Chiavacci A. Cervical lymph node metastases from an unknown primary tumour. Acta Radiol Oncol 1981;20:311–314.
55. Spiro RH, DeRose G, Strong EW. Cervical node metastasis of occult origin. Am J Surg 1983:146:441–446.
56. Mobit-Tabatabasi MA, Dasmaphapatra KS, Rush BF Jr, Ohanian M. Management of squamous cell carcinoma of unknown origin in cervical lymph nodes. Am Surg 1986;52:152–154.
57. Yang ZY, Hu YH, Yan JH, et al. Lymph node metastases in the neck from an unknown primary: Report on 113 patients. Acta Radiol Oncol 1983;22:17–22.
58. Carlson LS, Fletcher GH, Oswald MJ. Guidelines for the radiotherapeutic techniques for cervical metastases from an unknown primary. Int J Radiat Oncol Biol Phys 1986;12:2101–2110.
59. McCunniff AJ, Raber M. Metastatic carcinoma of the neck from an unknown primary. Int J Radiat Oncol Biol Phys 1986;12:1849–1852.
60. Bataini JP, Rodriguez J, Jaulerry C, et al. Treatment of metastatic neck nodes secondary to an occult epidermoid carcinoma of the head and neck. Laryngoscope 1987;97:1080–1084.
61. De Braud F, Heilbrun LK, Ahmed K, et al. Metastatic squamous cell carcinoma of an unknown primary localized to the neck: Advantages of an aggressive treatment. Cancer 1989;64:510–515.
62. Guarischi A, Keane TJ, Elhakim T. Metastatic inguinal nodes from an unknown primary neoplasm: A review of 56 cases. Cancer 1987;59:572–577.
63. Anderson H, Thatcher N, Rankin E, et al. VAC (vincristine, Adriamycin and cyclophosphamide) chemotherapy for metastatic carcinoma from an unknown primary site. Eur J Cancer Clin Oncol 1983;19:49–52.
64. Pasterz R, Savoraj N, Burgess M. Prognostic factors in metastatic carcinoma of unknown primary. J Clin Oncol 1986;4:1652–1657.
65. Greco FA, Vaughn WK, Hainsworth JD. Advanced poorly differentiated carcinoma of unknown primary site: Recognition of a treatable syndrome. Ann Intern Med 1986;104:547–556.
66. Hainsworth JD, Wright EP, Gray GF Jr, Greco FA. Poorly differentiated carcinoma of unknown primary site: Correlation of light microscopic findings with response to cisplatin-based combination chemotherapy. J Clin Oncol 1987;5:1275–1280.
67. Hainsworth JD, Wright E, Davis B, Johnson D, Greco FA. Immunoperoxidase staining in the evaluation of poorly differentiated carcinoma of unknown primary site. Proc Am Soc Clin Oncol [Abstract] 1989;8:11.
68. Richardson RL, Greco FA, Wolff S, et al. Extragonadal germ cell malignancy: Value of tumor markers in metastatic carcinoma in young males. Proc Am Assoc Cancer Res [Abstract] 1979;20:204.
69. Richardson RL, Schoumacher RA, Fer MF, et al. The unrecognized extragonadal germ cell cancer syndrome. Ann Intern Med 1981;94:181–186.
70. Hainsworth JD, Greco FA. Poorly differentiated carcinoma of unknown primary site. In: Fer MF, Greco FA, Oldham R, eds. Poorly differentiated neoplasms and tumors of unknown origin. Orlando: Grune & Stratton, 1986:189–202.
71. Fox RM, Woods RL, Tattersall MHN. Undifferentiated carcinoma in young men: The atypical teratoma syndrome. Lancet 1979;1:1316–1318.
72. Hainsworth JD, Johnson DH, Greco FA. Poorly differentiated neuroendocrine carcinoma of unknown primary site: A newly recognized clinicopathologic entity. Ann Intern Med 1988;109:364–371.
73. Van der Gaast A, Verweij J, Henzen-Logmans SC, et al. Carcinoma of unknown primary: Identification of a treatable subset. Ann Oncol 1990;1:119–123.
74. Kurzrock R, Gutterman JU, Talpazm P. The molecular genetics of Philadelphia chromosome-positive leukemias. N Engl J Med 1988;319:990–998.
75. Williams SD, Birch R, Einhorn LH, et al. Treatment of disseminated germ-cell tumors with cisplatin, bleomycin, and either vinblastine or etoposide. N Engl J Med 1987;316:1435–1440.
76. Raber MN, Faintuch J, Abbruzzese J, et al. Continuous infusion 5-fluorouracil, etoposide and cis-diamminedichloroplatinum in patients with metastatic carcinoma of unknown primary site. Ann Oncol 1991;2:519–520.
77. Briassoulis E, Foutzilas G, Theoharis D, et al. The role of platinum-containing chemotherapy in carcinoma of unknown primary: A Hellenic Cooperative Oncology Group study. Eur J Cancer [Abstract] 1991;27(Suppl 2):1347.
78. Zarba J, Izzo J, Hahjoubi R, et al. Treatment of unknown primary adenocarcinoma with fluorouracil, mitomycin, epirubicin and platinum. Eur J Cancer [Abstract] 1991;27(Suppl 2):1350.
79. Van der Gaast A, Verwey J, Prins E, Splinter TAW. Chemotherapy as treatment of choice in extrapulmonary undifferentiated small cell carcinomas. Cancer 1990;65:422–424.
80. Kasimis BS, Wuerker RB, Malefatto JP, Moran EM. Prolonged survival of patients with extrapulmonary small cell carcinoma arising in the neck. Med Pediatr Oncol 1983;11:27–32.
81. Hainsworth JD, Einhorn LH, Williams SD, et al. Advanced extragonadal germ-cell tumors: Successful treatment with combination chemotherapy. Ann Intern Med 1982;97:7–11.
82. Israel A, Bosl GJ, Golbey RB, et al. The results of chemotherapy for extragonadal germ-cell tumors in the cisplatin era: The Memorial Sloan Kettering Cancer Center experience (1975–1982). J Clin Oncol 1985;3:1073–1078.
83. Agnarsson BA, Kadin ME: Ki-1 positive large cell lymphoma: A morphologic and immunologic study of 19 cases. Am J Surg Pathol 1988;12:264–274.
84. Moertel CG, Kovals LK, O'Connell MJ, et al. Treatment of neuroendocrine carcinomas with combined etoposide and cisplatin: Evidence of major therapeutic activity in the anaplastic variants of these neoplasms. Cancer 1991;68:227–233.
85. Loehrer PJ, Perez CA, Roth LM, et al. Chemotherapy for advanced thymoma: Preliminary results of an intergroup study. Ann Intern Med 1990;113:520–524.
86. Tell DT, Khoury JM, Taylor HG, et al. Atypical metastasis from prostate cancer: Clinical utility of the immunoperoxidase technique for prostate-specific antigen. JAMA 1985;253:3574–3575.
87. Gentile PS, Carloss HW, Huang T-Y, et al. Disseminated prostatic carcinoma simulating primary lung cancer. Cancer 1988;62:711–715.

Cancer: Principles & Practice of Oncology, Fourth Edition,
edited by Vincent T. DeVita, Jr., Samuel Hellman, Steven A. Rosenberg.
J.B. Lippincott Co., Philadelphia © 1993.

Judith E. Karp
Jerome E. Groopman
Samuel Broder

CHAPTER **59**

Cancer in AIDS

The relation between immunodeficiency and cancer has been well documented for several decades. The predisposition to develop neoplasia was perhaps first clearly detected in patients with genetically determined disorders of cellular and humoral immunity, in particular ataxia-telangiectasia and Wiskott-Aldrich syndrome, and then, not surprisingly, in patients receiving immunosuppressive therapies for autoimmune disorders or transplantation. The malignancies arising in the context of insufficient immune function are frequently of lymphoid origin, most commonly B-cell, but epithelial and endothelial-related cancers (in particular, Kaposi's sarcoma [KS]) occur as well. The common themes underlying the emergence and perpetuation of the diverse cancers in these heterogenous immunocompromised states include three major factors: the absence of protective immune surveillance to recognize and eradicate abnormal clones; disruption of the normal balance between cell proliferation and differentiation that, in part, may be augmented by abnormal growth-factor expression; and chronic antigenic stimulation, sometimes accompanied by infection with "oncogenic" viruses, that leads to expansion of one or more cell cohorts. The uncovering of the molecular lesions that cause immune dysfunction, whether inherited or acquired, and the elucidation of mechanisms that permit malignant transformation in this setting will lead to the development of targeted molecular strategies that may be applicable to the therapy and prevention of cancers in general.

This association is being detected in patients with acquired immunodeficiency syndrome (AIDS), caused by infection with the pathogenic retrovirus known as human immunodeficiency virus (HIV). The multiple factors that operate to promote or permit the emergence of cancers in other immunodeficiency disorders also operate in AIDS. Further, the types of malignancies and their incidence rates are increasing in AIDS as the development of effective antiretroviral therapies and prophylaxis against opportunistic infections leads to prolonged survival in what would otherwise be a lethal immunocompromised state.

Although there is not yet a cure for HIV infection, there are now a number of therapies, the dideoxynucleoside zidovudine (azidothymidine; AZT) being the first and dideoxyinosine (ddI) being the second of several antiretroviral agents capable of suppressing viral replication and consequently prolonging survival for AIDS patients. Before 1986 (before the wide availability of AZT), the median survival of AIDS patients was less than 1 year.[1–3] With the use of AZT in conjunction with prophylaxis against *Pneumocystis carinii* and herpesvirus suppressive therapy, the duration of survival has more than doubled[2–7] and is likely to lengthen dramatically in the near future. Moreover, Rosenberg and colleagues[8] found that starting between 1987 and 1988 (the first year after AZT was approved by the Food and Drug Administration), there has been a sharp decrease in the quarterly incidence of new AIDS cases (but not in HIV seropositivity) in white gay men, for whom the incidence has fallen by nearly 30%. This decrease likely reflects the ability of AZT and other medical interventions to delay progression of HIV infection to AIDS. In early disease, AZT also delays the loss of CD4-positive cells.

It is, however, the net prolongation of survival in the face of impaired immunity that may drive the increasing incidence of malignancies in the AIDS population. For example, the risk for development of non-Hodgkin's lymphoma (NHL) is not uniform over time but, rather, appears to increase at around 2 years after AZT institution for full-blown AIDS.[7,9,10] This is worth noting because studies that do not provide follow-up data for more than 2 years will not detect this association accurately. Recent projections estimate that about 4700 new cases of AIDS lymphomas (range, 2900–9800) will occur annually in the near future, and some projections suggest that

10% to 20% of all new NHL cases may eventually be related to AIDS in the United States.[3]

We will discuss the major opportunistic malignancies associated with HIV infection in the approximate order in which each has been recognized as a significant and related complication: KS, human papillomavirus (HPV)-associated anogenital carcinoma, and AIDS-related NHL (AIDS-NHL).

AIDS-RELATED KAPOSI'S SARCOMA

Kaposi's sarcoma was initially described in 1872 by Moricz Kaposi[11] (a pseudonym) as "idiopathic, multiple pigmented sarcomas of the skin." The classic KS is a rare tumor with an indolent clinical course that occurs in elderly men (usually of Mediterranean or Ashkenazi Jewish descent) and is characterized by lower-extremity skin nodules caused by blood vessel proliferation. An endemic KS variant is prevalent in Central Africa (mainly Kenya, Tanzania, and Zaire) and accounts for 10% of all neoplasms in that region, with striking male predominance. In contrast to classic KS, the endemic form occurs mainly in younger black male adults and has a clinical spectrum that ranges from a benign, localized, nodular disease to an aggressive, locally invasive malignancy. The lymphadenopathic variant of endemic KS occurs in black African children of both sexes as a highly aggressive, widely disseminated tumor with extensive lymph node and deep visceral involvement that has a rapidly progressive and ultimately fatal course.[12] The epidemiologic and clinical features of these and other KS variants are summarized in Table 59–1.

The etiologic linkage between KS and immunodeficiency was first recognized in settings of iatrogenic immunosuppression, including organ transplantation, where the incidence of KS is about 200 to 400 times higher than expected in the general population. In addition, KS can arise in the presence of other malignancies that compromise the integrity of immunologic function, for example, B-cell malignancies such as NHL and multiple myeloma or adult T-cell leukemia caused by the human T-cell leukemia type 1 retrovirus.[13,14] In the milieu of immunocompromise, the clinical presentation can resemble the indolent classic KS or the highly malignant lymphadenopathic KS variant. With the AIDS epidemic, KS has risen from an interesting but unusual neoplasm to a prominent challenge, occurring in about 20% of all AIDS patients. Until recently, KS was the first manifestation of AIDS in 30% to 40% of patients; now, KS is the AIDS-defining illness in only about 10%.[12,15] The decrease in KS as the presenting feature of AIDS may relate to several factors, including a change in sexual practices that have been associated with KS development, changing demographics, increasing numbers of HIV-positive women, the increasing ability to detect HIV infection before immune impairment, and the advent of effective antiretroviral therapies, which can delay HIV disease progression. However, although the incidence of KS as the initial, AIDS-defining opportunistic event is declining, KS remains a prevalent and life-threatening complication of AIDS.

ETIOLOGY AND PATHOGENESIS

A number of genetic factors and environmental cofactors have been examined for their relative contributions to KS development in HIV-infected patients, which occurs almost exclusively (at least 95%) in homosexual males.[15,16] There appear a few predisposing genetic factors, including race (black) and ethnicity (Haitian).[17] The original suggestion, however, that HLA-DR5 conferred heightened susceptibility and an increased severity of classic KS[18] and epidemic AIDS-related KS (AIDS-KS) has not been substantiated as the number of affected people has increased over time. Behavioral cofactors associated with the development of AIDS-KS include homosexuality (as opposed to intravenous drug use) and specific sexual practices (including anal-receptive intercourse and the use of various inhaled nitrate aphrodisiacs).[15,19]

The role of cytomegalovirus (CMV) as a critical cofactor in the emergence and perpetuation of KS in HIV-infected men is controversial. All KS variants are associated with a high incidence of CMV seropositivity.[20,21] It is also likely that CMV, like other DNA viruses of the herpesvirus family, encodes transcriptional activators capable of enhancing HIV gene expression and increasing HIV-related immunosuppression.[20,22] On the other hand, the presence or absence of anti-CMV antibodies in HIV-positive homosexual men does not usefully discriminate among those who will or will not develop AIDS-KS. Furthermore, molecular studies have not detected the presence of CMV DNA sequences in AIDS-KS or endemic (African) KS tumor tissue.[23] Although it is intriguing to postulate that CMV infection enhances HIV disease progression and facilitates the development of KS through that route, the direct role of CMV in the pathogenesis of KS remains undetermined.

AIDS-RELATED KAPOSI'S SYNDROME AS A PARADIGM OF NEOPLASIA DRIVEN BY GROWTH FACTORS

One of the most intriguing aspects of AIDS-KS pathogenesis is the sensitivity of this malignancy to numerous growth factors. The origin of the AIDS-KS cell, specifically the transformed spindle cell, is as yet undetermined, but likely candidates are endothelial cells (vascular or lymphatic) and pluripotent mesenchymal cells (Schwann cells). A major pathophysiologic component of AIDS-KS is angiogenesis and the production of multiple growth factors that promote new blood vessel formation. The transformed spindle cell, whatever its origin, is a potent source for such factors.

The initial polyclonal expansion of multiple interactive cell types—namely, T cells, monocytes, and vascular endothelial cells—is likely driven by the diverse cytokines produced by host cells (neoplastic and virus-infected) and by HIV. In addition to the potpourri of cytokines produced by HIV-infected T cells and monocytes (in particular, interleukin-6 [IL-6]),[24,25] AIDS-KS cells, when exposed to soluble factors liberated from activated CD4-positive T cells, produce at least eight growth factors that induce autocrine and paracrine growth stimulation. These growth factors include the basic and a unique KS-derived fibroblast growth factor (FGF), platelet-derived growth factor (PDGF), endothelial growth factor (which is identical to acidic-FGF), transforming growth factor-β, IL-1, IL-6, and granulocyte-macrophage colony-stimulating factor (GM-CSF).[26–29] Many of these are angiogenesis factors, which stimulate vascular endothelial cell proliferation and new blood vessel formation, and lymphohematopoietic stimulators.

TABLE 59–1. Distinctive Clinical Features of Classic, Endemic, Iatrogenic, and Epidemic Variants of Kaposi's Sarcoma

	Epidemiology			*Clinical Manifestations*			*Clinical Course*	
Type	*Major Population Affected*	*Age (y)*	*Male/ Female Ratio*	*Mucocutaneous*	*Lymph Node*	*Visceral*	*Behavior*	*Survival (y)*
Classic	Mediterranean Ashkenazi Jewish	50–80	10–15:1	Patches, plaques and nodules, localized to lower extremities	Rare (late-onset)	Occasional (late-onset)	Indolent	10–15—up to one third develop lymphoma
Endemic	Black men in Central Africa	25–40	13–17:1	Nodules localized to lower extremities	Rare	Rare	Indolent	8–10
				Aggressive exophytic lesions with underlying bone invasion	Rare	Occasional	Progressive	5–8
				Florid, widely disseminated nodular lesions	Occasional	Common	Rapidly progressive	3–5
	Children (lymphadenopathic variant)	2–13	3:1	Minimal	Generalized	Common	Virulent and rapidly progressive	1–3
Iatrogenic	Patients receiving immunosuppressive therapy (*e.g.*, renal transplantation, autoimmune disorders)	20–60	2.3:1	Patches, plaques and nodules, usually localized but can disseminate	Rare	Common	Indolent or rapidly progressive; may reverse with reduction or discontinuation of immunosuppression	30% fatal within 2–3
Epidemic AIDS	Homosexual men	18–65	>100:1	Irregular fusiform plaques and nodules; multifocal	Common	Common (gastrointestinal, lung)	Fulminant	<2

AIDS-KS cells respond to corticosteroids by expressing cytokines that induce proliferation and vascular permeability and also express angiogenic activity in chicken chorioallantoic membrane, nude mouse, and guinea pig in vivo assay systems.[30] Corticosteroids may predispose to the development of AIDS-KS by two distinct mechanisms: growth perturbation (by growth-factor induction) and immunosuppression (*e.g.*, by direct lymphocytolysis).

Of particular interest is the KS-specific FGF (K-FGF), a member of the heparin-binding FGF cytokine family that shares partial homology with basic and acidic FGF and has related angiogenic activities. K-FGF is encoded by the KS oncogene, which is identical to the *HST* oncogene (found in human stomach cancers) located on chromosome 11q12-13 and to the mouse *INT*2 oncogene (the site of mouse mammary tumor virus integration).[26] The KS oncogene is constitutively expressed in AIDS-KS, and its K-FGF product may contribute to an autocrine mechanism of tumor proliferation.[27] K-FGF is also secreted extracellularly, where it may stimulate capillary endothelial cell proliferation in paracrine fashion. When the K-FGF gene is transfected into cultured human adrenocortical carcinoma cells, and the gene-transfected cells are then transplanted into athymic nude mice, the transplanted cells secrete large amounts of K-FGF and undergo KS-like cell growth, with development of rapidly growing, highly vascularized tumors (rather than growth typical of the parent tumor cell line).[31] These findings lend credence to the hypothesis that the KS oncogene and its K-FGF gene product might play important roles in the growth dysregulation, malignant transformation, and pathogenesis of AIDS-KS.

Like K-FGF, the gene encoding basic FGF (b-FGF) is expressed at high levels in AIDS-KS cells, resulting in synthesis of large quantities of b-FGF, which is then secreted extracellularly and can induce autocrine effects on tumor cells and paracrine effects on endothelial cells.[28] It has been shown that b-FGF can stimulate the gene expression and secretion of macrophage CSF (M-CSF or CSF-1) from bone marrow stromal cells, which, in turn, may serve as a positive feedback mediator for the production of several "inflammatory" cytokines.[32] M-CSF also enhances replication of a monocytotropic strain of HIV-1 in infected bone marrow stem cells that are undergoing macrophage differentiation.[33] This may be a key mechanism of action for many of the heparin-binding growth factors, and as such, it may contribute to autocrine and paracrine aspects of proliferation in AIDS-KS and to the progression of HIV disease activity.

Similarly, IL-1 (mainly the IL-1β form) is expressed in high amounts in AIDS-KS cells[28] and may also induce a cascade of cytokines in multiple cell types involved in the pathogenesis and progression of AIDS-KS. IL-1 stimulates the synthesis and release of many growth-modulating cytokines (*e.g.*, PDGF, GM-CSF, M-CSF, and IL-6) in a variety of cell types, including vascular endothelial cells, mesenchymal cells, and fibroblasts from several sources (notably bone marrow and skin). IL-1 also increases the expression of adhesion molecules by endothelial cells.[34] Studies demonstrate the expression of functional IL-1 receptors of the type expressed on T cells and fibroblasts on human vascular endothelial and smooth muscle cells.[35] It is logical to surmise that these receptors mediate the autocrine and paracrine growth-promoting effects of IL-1 on vascular cells. The discovery and recombinant production of an IL-1 receptor antagonist (IL-1ra) that competitively inhibits IL-1 binding to its receptors (especially the receptors found on T cells and fibroblasts)[34] offers a potential therapeutic tool for diseases such as AIDS-KS in which IL-1 may play a pathogenic role, and is worthy of further exploration. Some patients with HIV-associated KS have extensive edema and tissue swelling, and it is thought that such sequelae are mediated by IL-1.

Of the many other cytokines produced by AIDS-KS, HIV-infected, fibroblastic, and endothelial cells, IL-6 is secreted by all such cell types (in some instances, induced by IL-1) and is autostimulatory for AIDS-KS cells, monocytes, and HIV replication.[24,29] Of particular relevance is the mechanism for the positive feedback loop in AIDS-KS, namely the IL-6-induced upregulation of the IL-6 receptor.[29] This mechanism is perhaps similar to the one detected for multiple myeloma, in which IL-6 is constitutively expressed by the dysregulated plasma cells, acts as an autocrine growth factor, and likely facilitates eventual transformation or expansion of neoplastic clones.[36–38]

AIDS-KS cells may also proliferate in response to HIV regulatory proteins. Specifically, AIDS-KS cells respond to the HIV TAT protein.[39] The HIV transactivating gene, *TAT*, and its protein product (TAT) are essential for viral gene expression and replication and may contribute to immunodeficiency by modulating host cell gene expression and T-cell antigenic response. In addition, and perhaps more important for the growth of AIDS-KS, HIV-infected CD4 cells and monocytes may release biologically active TAT. This extracellular TAT can then be taken up by cells in close proximity. After uptake, extracellular TAT localizes in the nucleus and transactivates HIV-1 long-terminal-repeat-directed gene expression, can stimulate growth of AIDS-KS and mesenchymal cell types, and mediates cell attachment to culture plates through binding to cell surface integrins expressed by mesenchymal cells and other cell types.[39] This latter activity may be especially important to the proliferation of AIDS-KS cells. Therefore, the HIV-1 TAT protein may have a pivotal role in the pathogenesis and clonal expansion of AIDS-KS, particularly as an extracellular product. By stimulating proliferation of AIDS-KS cells and normal mesenchymal cells and by inducing HIV-1 viral replication, extracellular TAT may act as a promoting or progression factor in KS development and in the immunodeficiency occurring in HIV-1 infected patients. These are interesting possibilities, but they cannot be taken as clinical facts because further research is needed.

HISTOPATHOLOGY

The microscopic appearances of the cutaneous lesions from the classic, endemic, and epidemic forms of KS are remarkably similar. The clinical spectrum of cutaneous and mucosal lesions is paralleled histologically in terms of features connoting aggressiveness. Histopathology of early macular patches, with involvement limited to the upper portion of the reticular dermis, demonstrates irregular and dilated vascular spaces as a result of blood vessel proliferation but not much evidence for angiogenesis, inflammation, or cellular dysplasia. Progression to papules and plaques that extend into the subcutis is accompanied by increasing numbers and aggregates of spindle cells (the presumptive AIDS-KS cell), erythrocyte extravasation, and intense inflammatory cell infiltration. Ultimately, these lesions develop into deeply invasive nodules that, on histologic examination, evince significant nuclear atypia, dense infiltration and active proliferation of spindle cells, intense inflammation and erythrophagocytosis, exuberant neoangiogenesis, and obliteration of vascular spaces.

CLINICAL MANIFESTATIONS AND STAGING

As noted previously, AIDS-KS commonly presents as an aggressive and widely disseminated neoplasm, arising in multiple foci from vascular endothelium or lymphatic tissue in skin, mucosal surfaces, lymph nodes, and visceral organs, including liver, spleen, gastrointestinal (GI) tract, and lung. In some patients, KS is confined to the skin and may not require therapy per se. In many cases, however, the tumor parallels the clinical course seen in the lymphadenopathic variant of endemic KS and aggressive variants of KS emerging from the background of immunosuppression. Lesions at all sites (skin and viscera) commonly progress from macules to plaques and nodules, often coalesce, and ultimately develop into fungating or ulcerated masses (Fig. 59–1).

Multiorgan involvement occurs in most AIDS-KS patients at initial clinical presentation. Although virtually any organ can be involved by KS, the most common (and most life-threatening) are the GI tract and the lung. GI tract lesions, submucosal or nodal, have been detected in 50% to 70% of KS patients and are frequently associated with enteropathic and hemorrhagic symptoms;[40] however, they can also be clinically silent. Pulmonary involvement, a particularly ominous development, has been reported in 20% to 50% of patients and often mimics (and can occur concomitantly with) opportunistic infections on clinical grounds.[41] The definitive diagnosis of pulmonary KS is further complicated by recurrent episodes of hemorrhage that can acutely exacerbate pulmonary compromise. The discrimination of pulmonary KS from infectious complications has been facilitated by lung computed tomography (Fig. 59–2) and may obviate the need to pursue invasive diagnostic techniques in some patients.[42] Pulmonary KS is exceedingly difficult to treat with any modality.

Because AIDS-KS appears to arise from multiple foci, classic oncologic staging criteria have not adequately characterized the extent of the disease process in an entirely satisfactory way.[43] Furthermore, any staging classification of AIDS-KS, if it is going to be relevant to overall prognosis and therapeutic outcome, should incorporate measurements of immunologic function and other parameters of virus activity and extent of tumor involvement.[44] Krown and colleagues[43] developed a system for uniform staging and evaluation of clinical trials outcomes for AIDS-KS patients based on the three broad stratification criteria: extent of tumor involvement, immunologic status, and systemic illness (including other opportunistic infections or HIV-related malignancies; Table 59–2). Such standardization will facilitate the interpretation of clinical results, the evaluation of innovative anti-KS therapies, and the appropriate application of specific therapies, such as interferon (detailed later), on the basis of clearly defined prognostic criteria.

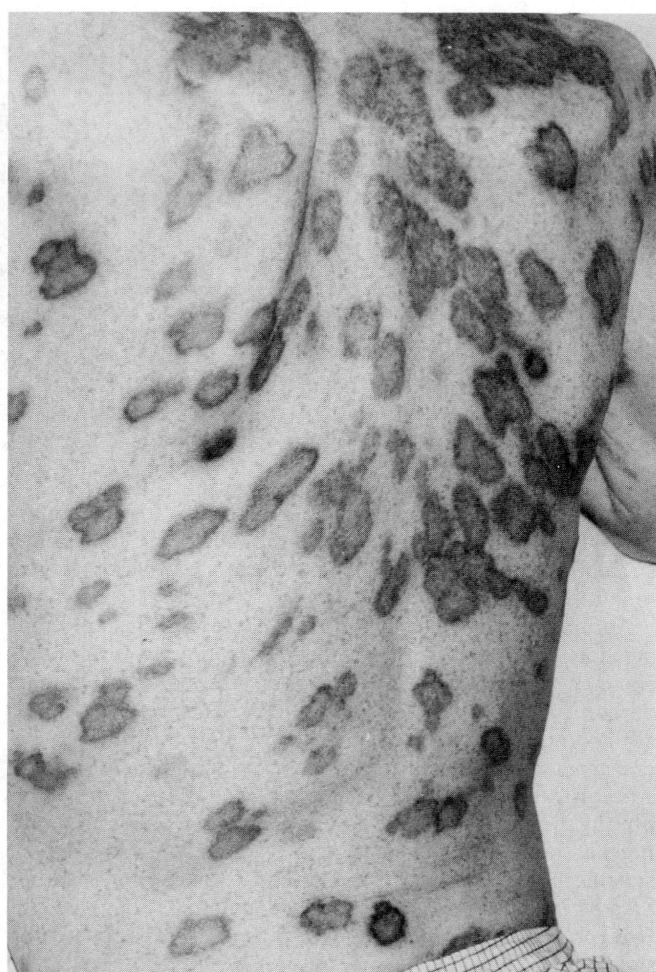

FIGURE 59–1. Extensive cutaneous plaques on the trunk of a patient with HIV-associated Kaposi's sarcoma. Several plaques have coalesced and are irregular and fusiform in shape. Notice the bilateral symmetry and the prominence at sites of skin cleavage. (Courtesy of James M. Pluda, MD)

LOCAL AND SYSTEMIC THERAPEUTIC APPROACHES

Like other malignancies arising in the immunocompromised host, the therapy of AIDS-KS is a multifaceted challenge. The complexity of this challenge is conferred by the multiple levels of dysregulation exerted by the interactions between HIV and the host. The net result in many patients is aggressive tumor behavior and increased host cell toxicity in response to chemotherapy- or radiation therapy-induced cell damage. Some of the local and systemic therapeutic approaches to AIDS-KS are delineated in Table 59–3.

Local therapies have been useful for palliation of localized cutaneous or mucosal lesions or for mass lesions producing obstructive findings such as lymphedema.[44,45] Radiation therapy (1500–2200 cGy) for all such lesions and carbon dioxide and neodymium:yttrium-aluminum-garnet laser therapy for more isolated lesions (*e.g.*, oral or urethral meatus) bring about significant but often incomplete and temporary resolution. Local recurrence is common. Whole-lung irradiation also

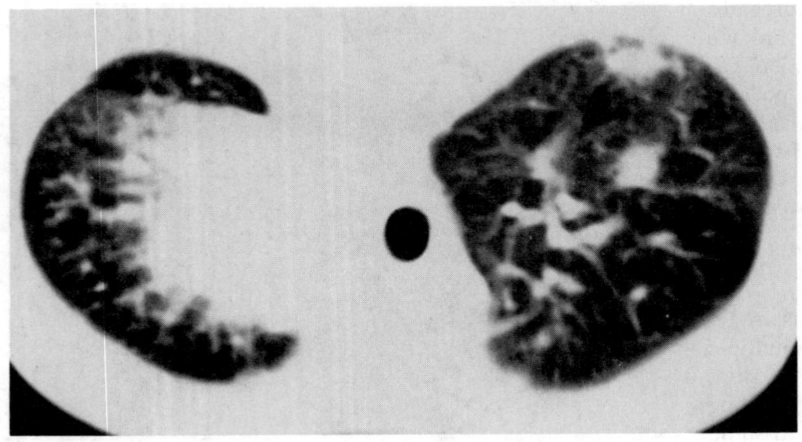

FIGURE 59–2. Chest CT scan of a patient with HIV-associated pulmonary Kaposi's sarcoma, demonstrating massive hilar involvement with extension into the pulmonary parenchyma and multiple pulmonary nodules. (Courtesy of James M. Pluda, MD)

provides palliation but not long-term control for pulmonary KS lesions. Radiation therapy is complicated by a heightened susceptibility of uninvolved host tissue to radiation-related toxicities.

A number of novel radiation-related approaches are being developed for AIDS-KS. Photodynamic therapy has shown significant antitumor activity in diverse cancers such as bladder, ovary, esophagus, and lung cancers. This modality, aimed at maximizing toxicity to tumor foci while concomitantly decreasing toxicity to nontumorous tissues, employs the systemic administration of a photosensitizing agent (*e.g.*, hematoporphyrin) that is selectively retained by tumor cells and not by normal host cells. The compound is activated on exposure to specific light wavelengths delivered to a well-circumscribed area by laser and, when activated, is cytotoxic. Early results from preliminary trials demonstrate tumor regression in multiple KS nodules.

An important form of local therapy for cutaneous and mucosal KS involves intralesional drug administration.[44,45] Local injection of cytotoxic agents (*e.g.*, vinblastine or bleomycin) or biomodulatory agents, such as interferon or tumor necrosis factor (TNF), have met with tumor regression and minimal systemic toxicity. Other agents that might be experimental candidates for this innovative approach to mucocutaneous tumor suppression could be targeted to the autocrine and paracrine growth factors operating in AIDS-KS. Examples include IL-1 receptor antagonists[34]; various derivatives of retinoic acid, which, as discussed in more detail later, may interdict IL-6-mediated autostimulation[46]; immunotoxin molecules, for instance, b-FGF conjugated to a *Pseudomonas* exotoxin (b-FGF-PE-40); or monoclonal antibodies directed against stimulatory factors, such as anti-IL-6.[47] Such compounds have potential to effect significant local tumor control, perhaps with additional salutary effects on involved accessory cell types near

TABLE 59–2. Staging Classification for AIDS-Related Kaposi's Sarcoma

	Good Risk (0) (all *the parameters listed)*	*Poor Risk (1)* (any *of the parameters listed)*
Tumor (T)	Small tumor burden with limited involvement of one or more: Skin Lymph nodes Oral*	Large tumor burden: Oral Gastrointestinal Pulmonary Other visceral involvement Tumor-associated edema or ulceration
Immune system (I)	CD4+ cells ≥ 200/mm^3	CD4+ cells < 200/mm^3
Systemic illness (S)	No opportunistic infection (including thrush) or B symptoms†	History of opportunistic infection or thrush B symptoms Other HIV-related illness (*e.g.*, NHL or other malignancy, neurologic disease, wasting syndrome)

* Limited oral disease is confined to the palate and is not nodular.
† B symptoms are unexplained fever, night sweats, weight loss of more than 10% body weight, or diarrhea persisting for longer than 2 weeks.
(Modified from Krown SE, Metroka C, Wernz JC. Kaposi's sarcoma in the acquired immunodeficiency syndrome: A proposal for uniform evaluation, response, and staging criteria. J Clin Oncol 1989;7: 1201)

TABLE 59–3. Promising Therapeutic Strategies for AIDS-Related Kaposi's Sarcoma

Therapeutic Strategy	*Specific Modality*
Current Approaches	
Local interventions	Radiation therapies
	Fractionated radiation
	Whole-body electron beam
	Laser (including photodynamic therapy)
	Intralesional therapies
	Cytotoxic drugs (vinblastine, bleomycin)
	Biomodulators (IFN-α, tumor necrosis factor)
	Topical
	Liquid nitrogen
Systemic chemotherapies	
Cytotoxic chemotherapies	Single-agent
	Vinca alkaloids, VP-16, anthracyclines, cisplatin, bleomycin; response rate 40–50% (complete responses up to 25%)
	Combination
	Doxorubicin + bleomycin + vincas or VP-16 ± methotrexate; response rate 60–85% (complete responses up to 40%)
Antiviral therapies	Single-agent
	IFN-$\alpha \geq 20 \times 10^6$ U/m²/d; response rate 25–40% (complete responses up to 25%)
	Combination
	IFN-α 9–18 $\times 10^6$ U/m²/d + AZT 600 mg/d; response rate 45–55% (complete responses up to 40%)
Biomodulation	
Marrow protection during systemic therapies	Granulocyte-macrophage or granulocyte colony-stimulating factors
Antiangiogenesis and growth-factor inhibition	IFN-α, heparin analogs (suramin, pentosan)
Future Approaches	
Local interventions	Growth-factor inhibition
	IL-1 receptor antagonists
	Anti-IL-6 (monoclonal antibodies, retinoids)
	Immunotoxins (*e.g.*, b-FGF-PE-40, IL-6-PE-40)
Systemic interventions	
New antiretrovirals	Dideoxynucleosides (AZT, ddI, ddC) in combination with IFN-α or other antivirals
	TAT gene or TAT protein inhibitors
Antiangiogenesis and growth-factor inhibition	Angioinhibins (fumagillin analogs)
	Tissue inhibitor of metalloproteinase-2
	IL-1 receptor antagonists
	Anti-IL-6 (retinoids, pentoxifylline)
	Immunotoxins

IFN-α, interferon-α; PE, *pseudomonas* exotoxin.

tumor mass (endothelial or stromal cells, as examples) and are worthy of further clinical investigation.

AIDS-KS, like KS arising in other settings of immunodeficiency and in contrast to the classic KS of elderly Mediterranean or Ashkenazi Jewish men, is characterized by extensive mucocutaneous involvement and is frequently associated with deep tissue involvement, in particular the lung and the GI tract. Although local modalities can confer local disease control for a limited tumor burden, AIDS-KS patients usually require systemic therapy for widespread superficial or tissue-invasive tumor at some point in the clinical course. Systemic treatment of disseminated KS has evolved from initial trials of single cytotoxic or antiviral agents to the development of non-cross-resistant drug combinations and antiviral combinations (*i.e.*, anti-HIV and interferon).

Several individual antitumor agents (especially vinca alkaloids, epipodophyllins such as VP-16, anthracyclines, cisplatin, and bleomycin) have demonstrated anti-KS activity, each inducing tumor responses in 40% to 50% of patients. Combinations of these active agents—most commonly, doxorubicin, bleomycin, a vinca alkaloid (vincristine or vinblastine), and VP-16, with or without methotrexate—have led to responses in 60% to 85% of patients with widespread KS. Gill and coinvestigators[48] demonstrated remarkable efficacy of low-dose combination chemotherapy with doxorubicin (Adriamycin), bleomycin, and VP-16 (ABV). This regimen yields complete responses in almost 40% of patients (including patients with pulmonary involvement) and has an overall response rate of more than 80%. Further, in their randomized, prospectively stratified clinical trial comparing ABV with doxorubicin alone, disease-free survival in the ABV-treated patients was significantly prolonged (median 9 months versus 3.5 months, $p = 0.004$). To date, however, ABV has not had a major impact on overall survival in these heterogenous AIDS patients with extensive KS. As with all other regimens, the overriding determinants of clinical response and survival are the manifestations of deep immunocompromise and HIV activity, namely the extent of CD4 cell destruction and the prior history of opportunistic infections.

With respect to antiviral therapy, the use of interferon-α (IFN-α) as a single agent has produced clinically significant responses in about 30% of AIDS-KS patients (range, 20–50%), especially in those patients treated with at least 20×10^6 U/m^2/d and in those with less extensive immunosuppression.[49] Other IFN species (IFN-β and IFN-γ preparations) have not yielded clinically meaningful antitumor responses, although IFN-β has shown some suppression of HIV activity (decreases in HIV p24 antigenemia) in patients with relatively early HIV disease.[50] In a trial conducted by Lane and colleagues,[51] high-dose IFN-α (35×10^6 U/d) induced complete remissions in 24% and partial remissions in another 14% of patients, for an overall response rate of 38%. All patients with CD4 counts higher than 400/mm^3, but none with CD4 counts lower than 150/mm^3, had a meaningful response. In addition, there was evidence of HIV suppression in clinical responders, as manifested by at least a 75% decrease in HIV p24 antigenemia.

The relation between CD4 count and probability of response to IFN is noteworthy. In all trials using adequate dosage, it was clear that IFN-α possesses antitumor and anti-HIV activity, particularly in those patients whose immune function is relatively well preserved (*i.e.*, CD4 count higher than 400/mm^3).[49,52] Tumor responses may not occur before 1 to 2 months of therapy, and maximal responses require 6 or more months. In general, the parameters associated with clinical refractoriness to IFN therapy parallel those that determine a poor response to cytotoxic therapies, namely, visceral tumor, deep HIV-related immunosuppression, and features of progressive HIV activity (constitutional symptoms and high levels of serologic markers such as β_2-microglobulin, neopterin, and endogenous IFN levels). Side effects of IFN therapy include constitutional influenza-like symptoms (malaise, fever, chills, myalgia, arthralgia) and transient hypotension, which frequently occur when IFN is initiated, are partly dose-related, and subside with continued IFN administration.[44,49] The development of tachyphylaxis allows patients to tolerate gradual increases in IFN dosage. Myelosuppression (mainly neutrophils and platelets) and hepatic enzyme elevations (transaminases in particular) are commonly transient and reversible with attenuation of IFN dose.[49,52,53]

IFN antiretroviral activity differs from that of AZT or other dideoxynucleosides such as ddI and dideoxycytidine (ddC). IFN appears to act late in the HIV life cycle, specifically on viral packaging and budding of infectious particles from the host cell membrane. By contrast, the dideoxynucleosides act early in the process of HIV replication by inhibiting the HIV reverse-transcriptase enzyme.[2,4] In contrast to IFN-α, the antiretroviral drug AZT has not shown any antitumor effect against AIDS-KS when used as a single agent, despite suppression of HIV activity. When AZT is combined with IFN-α, however, there is evidence of synergy with respect to anti-KS and anti-HIV effects. Krown and colleagues[52] and Fischl[53] documented significant tumor regression in 45% to 55% of patients, which occurred within 3 to 4 months of combination therapy (3 to 6 months earlier than with IFN-α alone), a notably sustained (longer than 40 weeks) increase in CD4 cell counts with a concomitant heightened skin test reactivity, sustained suppression of HIV p24 antigenemia in a high proportion of patients, and prevention of emergence of AZT resistance. Major dose-limiting toxicities, namely, AZT-related neutropenia and IFN-related hepatotoxicity, were effectively abrogated by using attenuated doses of both agents without compromising antitumor, immunologic, or virologic effects. The regimen based on these trials to provide an optimal therapeutic ratio is AZT 600 mg/d plus IFN-α 9 to 18×10^6 U/d.

Scadden and colleagues[54] added the hematopoietic stimulator GM-CSF to AZT 1200 mg/d plus IFN-α 9×10^6 U/d. GM-CSF permitted the administration of full-dose AZT. With this approach, tumor responses occurred in half of patients receiving GM-CSF (80% of whom were poor-risk), without an obvious negative impact on immunologic or virologic modulation. As in all other clinical therapy trials in AIDS-KS, the most salutary results are achieved in patients with less HIV-related immune impairment (*i.e.*, CD4 counts higher than 200/mm^3). Overall, these results are encouraging and support the need for early therapeutic intervention at a time when tumor burden is low and some immune function persists. Future trials of other hematopoietic stimulators or reverse-transcriptase inhibitors associated with less myelosuppression, specifically ddI and ddC, may be used in combination or alternating with AZT.[2,4] Such approaches are unproved and should be undertaken only in an approved protocol. The use of multiple antiretroviral agents may permit the administration of higher doses of IFN-α, perhaps with cycles of cytotoxic combinations such as ABV. The potential improved tolerance for therapy and non-cross-resistant HIV suppression might facilitate the implementation of multimodal regimens aimed at curing AIDS-KS.

BIOMODULATION AND ANTIANGIOGENESIS APPROACHES

Theoretically, the multiple diverse pathogenic factors that may contribute to the emergence and perpetuation of KS in AIDS patients can serve as targets for therapy. Some of these factors are being addressed through combined antiviral therapies aimed at the control of HIV replication and the replication of potential viral cofactors, such as Epstein-Barr virus (EBV) or CMV. Other targets, such as the enhancement of immune function, inhibition of angiogenic factors such as FGF, inhibition of stimulatory cytokines such as IL-1 and IL-6, inhibition of viral proteins such as TAT, and hormonal manipulations, are or will become the focus of innovative anti-KS therapy and prevention measures.

The striking production of autostimulatory and angiogenic growth factors by KS cells suggests that these factors should be an important target for therapy. To this end, pentosan (a heparin analog related to the growth-factor inhibitor suramin) inhibits angiogenesis and the proliferative effects of KS-specific FGF on the autocrine growth of AIDS-KS cells and has anti-HIV activity that is synergistic with AZT in vitro.[55] Although early clinical trials have not demonstrated an antitumor activity, second- and third-generation compounds are worth exploring. Fumagillin, a unique angiogenesis inhibitor derived from the fungus *Aspergillus fumigatus*, and its synthetic analogs ("angioinhibins") block endothelial cell proliferation, tumor-induced neovascularization, and in vivo growth of diverse tumors in mice.[56,57] The human protein known as tissue inhibitor of metalloproteinase-2 (TIMP-2) blocks tumor cell invasion by complexing with and blocking the action of collagenase enzymes.[58] TIMP-2 also inhibits angiogenesis in an in vitro assay and in animal models, apparently by a direct action on human endothelial cells. Each of these novel biomodulators provides important approaches for future development.

One cytokine that likely has a pivotal role in autocrine stimulation of host cell proliferation and viral expression is IL-6. IL-6 may be a critical factor in the genesis and clonal expansion of AIDS-KS and B-cell malignancies, in particular NHL. The role of IL-6 in lymphomagenesis and the possible clinical application of IL-6 inhibitors to antilymphoma therapy are addressed later in this chapter. IL-6 inhibitors may have potential therapeutic value in AIDS-KS as well. For example, studies by Sidell and colleagues[46] of multiple myeloma cells demonstrate that retinoic acid can down-regulate IL-6 receptors and inhibit IL-6-mediated autocrine growth stimulation. This mechanism of inhibition may also apply to AIDS-KS, which, like multiple myeloma, appears to be driven by IL-6 in an autostimulatory fashion through upregulation of tumor cell IL-6 receptors. Along similar lines, the methylxanthine pentoxifylline (Trental) inhibits intracellular HIV replication by inhibiting TNF-α synthesis.[59] Since IL-6 expression is linked to TNF production through an autocrine loop, it is intriguing to speculate that pentoxifylline might provide antiretroviral and anti-IL-6 effects in AIDS-KS (and perhaps in AIDS-lymphomas).

AIDS-RELATED ANOGENITAL CANCERS

Anogenital tumors, in particular those associated with HPV, have a notably aggressive course in patients infected with HIV.[60–62]. At least two mechanisms may operate, in theory, to predispose HIV-infected patients to HPV-induced malignant transformation. The HPV oncoproteins E6 and E7, especially those from the transforming HPV types 16 and 18, bind to or degrade the tumor suppressor proteins p53 and RB.[63,64] The potential importance of the loss of normal tumor suppressor mechanisms to the pathogenesis of AIDS lymphomas is discussed later. Further, HPV and HIV act synergistically through their respective transactivating factors (*i.e.*, products of the *E2* and *TAT* genes) to increase cellular transcription and to augment each other's gene expressions.[20] The enhanced expression of viral proteins that increase viral replication, abrogate host tumor suppressor functions, and further exacerbate cellular immunodeficiency contribute to the high incidence of advanced-stage disease that is rapidly progressive and refractory to therapy.

Kiviat and colleagues[60] and Palefsky and colleagues[62] detected the presence of anal HPV, in particular the oncogenic strains 16 and 18, in more than half of HIV-seropositive gay men. Moreover, abnormal anal cytology occurs in about 40% and anal intraepithelial neoplasia in 15% of these men, particularly in those with CD4 counts lower than 200/mm^3 and with severe HIV infection.[60] The presence of DNA from a single HPV strain confers about a fivefold increased risk for developing preneoplastic cytopathology; however, infection with multiple strains, a common finding in this patient cohort, confers a dramatically increased (up to 40-fold) risk of detecting cytologic abnormalities, which, in turn, are directly associated with the development of an intraanal neoplastic lesion. The presence and magnitude of the constellation of findings related to HPV-induced anal squamous cell cancer is linked to the presence and severity of HIV infection.

Similarly, advanced cervical cancer is emerging as a major complication as HIV affects increasing numbers of women.[61] In this regard, cervical cancer is an opportunistic cancer, much like KS, NHL, and the related HPV-associated anal squamous cell cancers in HIV-infected men. HPV coinfection is common in women with HIV; in fact, 60% of HIV-infected women have cervical dysplasia noted on Papanicolaou tests (similar to anal epithelial dysplasia in men). Studies to define the true incidence and natural history of concomitant HPV and HIV infections, cervical intraepithelial neoplasia (an early or premalignant lesion), and cervical cancer will lay the groundwork for effective strategies aimed at early detection and prevention.

AIDS-RELATED NON-HODGKIN'S LYMPHOMAS

Even before AIDS, NHL was an increasing problem. The National Cancer Institute Surveillance, Epidemiology, and End Results (SEER) data base is informative.[65] The incidence of NHL in the United States and other Western countries has risen steadily over the past decade and is still largely unexplained. This increase in NHL has not been accompanied by an increased incidence of Hodgkin's disease (Fig. 59–3). Hodgkin's disease can occur in the setting of HIV infection, however, specifically in intravenous drug users. Predominant histologic subtypes are mixed cellularity and lymphocyte depletion, and more than 80% of Hodgkin's disease patients present with advanced-stage disease.[66] The apparent propensity of HIV-infected patients who use drugs to develop Hodgkin's disease, in contrast to gay men who acquire AIDS by sexual transmission (and who seem to preferentially develop NHL) is unexplained and is a topic for future investigation.

EPIDEMIOLOGY AND CLINICAL MANIFESTATIONS

In the United States, there has been about a 50% increase in incidence and a 22% increase in the death rate of NHL since

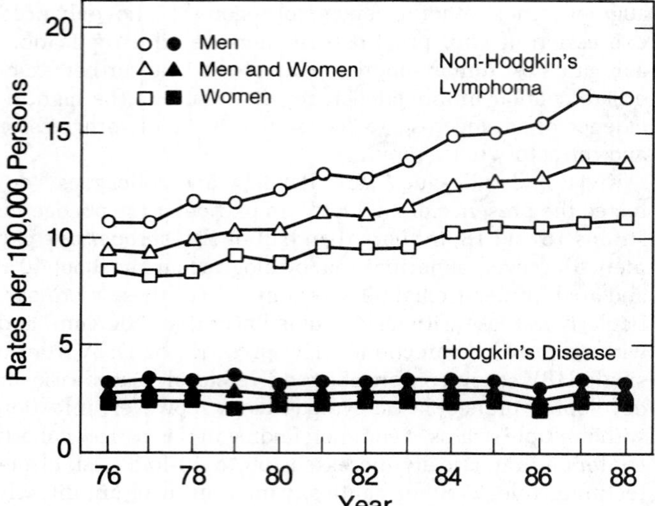

FIGURE 59–3. Incidence rates for non-Hodgkin's lymphoma (NHL) and Hodgkin's disease (HD) in men and women of all ages from 1976 to 1988. The incidence of NHL increased by about 50% during this period, substantially due to an increased incidence in men, and is still not explained. This increase antedated the AIDS pandemic, but AIDS has aggravated these statistics (see Fig. 59–5). In contrast, no such increase was detected in the incidence of HD for either men or women during this time frame. (Courtesy of Edward J. Sondik, PhD)

the early 1970s.[65] About 38,000 cases of NHL are reported per year in the United States alone, and this disease entity can no longer be considered minor or rare. In more recent years, a significant new component of this increase reflects the emergence of lymphomas associated with AIDS.[9,10,67,68] The SEER program has been able to track the unexpected increase in incidence of specific types of NHL.[65] The connection between AIDS and NHL was first reported in 1982. Beginning in 1983, a sharp rise in the incidence of NHL has been detected exclusively for men aged 20 to 54 years (Fig. 59–4). In an analysis of almost 100,000 unselected AIDS patients from 1981 to 1989, about 3% had NHL, a 60-fold increase over that expected for the general population.[69] Further, in an autopsy series of 101 AIDS patients from 1981 to 1987, lymphomas were detected in 20 patients: five tumors were located in the brain, and eight (including four of the brain tumors) were detected only at autopsy.[70]

The increase in AIDS-NHL has occurred predominantly in high-grade B-cell types, with large cell immunoblastic and small noncleaved lymphomas comprising about 70% of AIDS-NHL and with the intermediate-grade diffuse large cell lymphomas making up the remaining 30%.[9,67] Frequently, AIDS-related lymphomas have the histology and cytogenic pattern characteristic of Burkitt's lymphoma.[67,69]

AIDS lymphomas resemble NHL occurring in other severely immunocompromised settings by their frequent involvement of extranodal sites (particularly GI tract and brain) and by the high incidence of stage IV disease, especially in Burkitt's lymphoma (in which bone marrow infiltration is common).[9,67,68] In particular, primary central nervous system (CNS) lymphoma may occur with striking frequency in large cell immunoblastic or small noncleaved cell types, usually as mass lesions (Fig. 59–5) but on occasion as a more diffuse leptomeningeal process.[71] Pluda and colleagues[9] described 5 of 8 AIDS patients with NHL at the National Cancer Institute who had primary CNS involvement, and Moore and colleagues[72] described 10 of 24 AIDS patients with NHL from a multicenter study who had primary CNS involvement. Like NHL that arises from a background of chronic immunosuppression and unlike NHL that occurs outside a known immunosuppressed state, AIDS lymphomas demonstrate a high frequency of multiclonality. A 2-year (1987–1989) prospective multicenter study of over 1000 patients with advanced HIV who received AZT detected an overall 2.3% prevalence of NHL, rising to 3.2% after 2 years of antiretroviral therapy.[72] The median CD4 cell count at the start of AZT therapy was 104/mm^3, and, as in other series of AIDS patients undergoing AZT treatment, the probability of survival at 2 years was 50%.[2,4,9] In this group, risk factors for NHL development can be explained by immunosuppression and infection with other viruses, namely the presence of prior KS, CMV infection, and oral hairy leukoplakia (an EBV-related lesion). The modest overall proportion of NHL cases in this patient cohort may relate to two factors: (1) the median observation period of 600 days with a maximum of 2 years, which is when NHL occurrence in AZT-treated patients began to escalate in the studies by Pluda and colleagues[9]; and (2) the relative preservation of CD4 count (higher than 100/mm^3) at study entry. Analyses by Yarchoan and colleagues[7] and the Centers for Disease Control[10] suggest that the greatest risk for NHL development and death from any cause occurs when there is a substantial impairment of cellular immunity, represented by CD4 counts less than 50/mm^3.

NHL is likely to be a particular problem for patients with CD4-positive lymphocyte counts less than 50/mm^3.[7,10] In the analysis by Pluda and colleagues[9], 8 of 55 (14.5%) AIDS patients undergoing antiretroviral therapy at the National Cancer

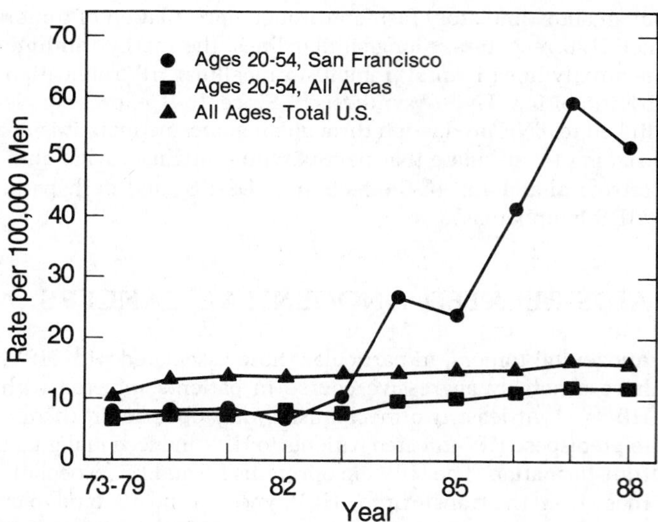

FIGURE 59–4. The increasing incidence of non-Hodgkin's lymphoma in men 20 to 54 years old since 1983. The incidence is particularly striking for men of this age group in San Francisco and is clearly associated with the AIDS pandemic. (Courtesy of Edward J. Sondik, PhD)

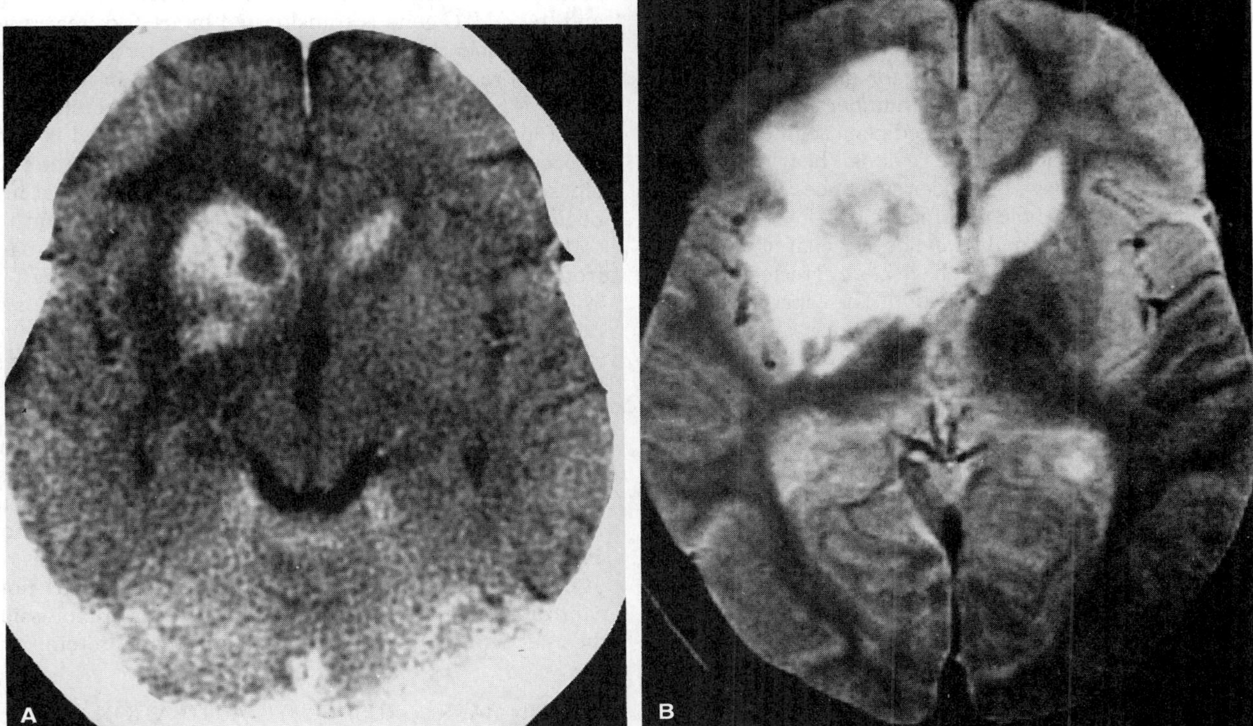

FIGURE 59–5. **(A)** CT scan of the brain (with intravenous contrast dye injection) of an AIDS patient with primary central nervous system lymphoma, small noncleaved cell morphology. **(B)** T2-weighted spin echo magnetic resonance image of the same patient. (Courtesy of Irwin Feuerstein, MD)

Institute developed aggressive B-cell NHL (extranodal involvement, especially CNS) an average of 2 years after beginning AZT therapy, with the estimated actuarial probability of developing NHL rising to about 30% after 3 years of antiretroviral therapy. The median CD4 count at the onset of AZT therapy was 74/mm^3, and at the time of NHL development it was 6/mm^3. All eight patients had serologic evidence of EBV infection, and two patients developed primary CNS lymphoma in the setting of prior toxoplasmosis; it is reasonable to speculate that these infections led to polyclonal B-cell activation, a prelude to malignant transformation (discussed later). In this closely followed cohort of patients, where consistent and frequent observations were made over an extended period, virtually all who developed NHL did so with CD4 counts higher than 50/mm^3 for 12 months or more (median 18 months) before NHL emerged. The depth of immunocompromise—as specifically reflected by a CD4 cell count higher than 50/mm^3—appears to be a critical factor in the emergence of opportunistic NHL in the setting of AIDS.[7,9,10] Lymphomas can and do occur with CD4 counts higher than 50/mm^3; however, the risk is significantly elevated once this threshold is crossed. Ultimately, prevention of NHL development may hinge on an ability to restore immune function or at least maintain it at a critical protective level.

A primate model in cynomolgus monkeys infected with simian immunodeficiency virus (SIV) may provide a close parallel to human AIDS.[73] In this model, high-grade B-cell NHL develops 5 to 15 months after SIV inoculation, in conjunction with severe immunodeficiency. Median CD4 counts at the time of NHL onset are 80/mm^3, similar to the AZT-treated patient cohort from the National Cancer Institute series.[9] As with humans, there is a disproportionate incidence of Burkitt's lymphomas with wide dissemination, and some tumors demonstrate integration of the EBV genome in tumor cell DNA. The primate model validates the association of retrovirus-induced profound immunosuppression and a propensity for NHL development and is important for future studies of pathogenesis, treatment, and prevention that may extrapolate to HIV-infected humans.

GENE REARRANGEMENTS IN NORMAL AND MALIGNANT B-CELL DEVELOPMENT

Normal B- and T-lymphocyte differentiation is accomplished through rearrangements of gene sequences that encode antigen receptors, namely immunoglobulin and T-cell-receptor genes, respectively. The process of gene rearrangements in these antigen receptor genes, accomplished through DNA breakage and rejoining and mediated by recombinase enzymes, confers diversity in the repertoire of specialized immune responses to a variety of antigens. Focusing specifically on B-lineage development, molecular rearrangement of the three gene segments encoding the variable regions of the immunoglobulin heavy chain—variable (V), diversity (D), and joining (J)—takes place in early precursors, namely pre-B and immature B cells.[74,75] The three gene segments, located on discontinuous portions of the long arm of chromosome 14 (14q32), are joined in a specific pattern (V_H-D-J_H). The sequence of recombination events is orderly, but juxtaposition of specific molecular sequences within each region is random, providing the first element of diversity in the generation of an antibody response. The capacity for diversity is further increased by variation in nucleotide number and type within the joining regions of the recombined gene segments. In addition, all immunoglobulin gene regions (heavy and light chains, both κ and λ) have enhancer sequences that activate transcription over the whole chromosome.

Lymphohematopoietic malignancies are characterized by the clonal expansion of cells that have been arrested at a specific developmental stage of maturation. The capacity for self-renewal is preserved, but the capacity for terminal differentiation is blocked. In this regard, the finding by Berberian and colleagues[76] of a clonal deficit in rearrangements of a specific subfamily of the genes encoding the variable region of the immunoglobulin heavy chain, specifically the VH3L subfamily, in B cells of HIV-infected patients is provocative. The clonal defect reflects B-cell maturation arrest within lymph node germinal centers and results in a deficit in memory B cells.[77] This impaired B-cell differentiation is accompanied by an increase in circulating levels of IL-6,[78] which may provide a chronic proliferative stimulus for the arrested B-cell clone and thereby drive expansion of certain B-cell clones.

One pathogenic mechanism underlying the malignant transformation of lymphoid precursors in general and of B cells specifically is the translocation of a normal growth-promoting gene (or *protooncogene*) to the lineage-specific antigen receptor genes (in the case of B cells, the immunoglobulin genes). The juxtaposition of the protooncogene segment with the immunoglobulin gene, in particular its transcriptionally active enhancer sequences, results in deregulation of the translocated growth-promoting gene, which (by virtue of overexpression) now functions as a true oncogene. This process does not require literal proximity. In addition, aberrant recombinase function may contribute to the pathogenesis of lymphoid malignancies by catalyzing chromosomal breaks and translocations that involve 14q32 (the locus of the heavy-chain gene), especially those occurring at the 5′ region of the J_H segment of the gene.[75,79]

A classic example of oncogene activation resulting from this type of chromosomal rearrangement occurs in Burkitt's lymphoma, in which the c-*MYC* gene, located on the long arm of chromosome 8 (8q24),[80] participates in a translocation to the immunoglobulin gene heavy-chain locus on 14q32. There are a number of mechanisms by which *MYC* activation can ensue, all of which may operate to some degree in t(8;14).[81–83] Transcriptional activation of c-*MYC* can occur from juxtaposition to immunoglobulin gene enhancer sequences or from the action of long-range enhancers on chromosome 14. Inactivation of the 5′ regulatory sequences of the c-*MYC* gene locus can occur through point mutations or truncation of the 5′ region or by separation of the regulatory region from the rest of the gene. The translocated portion of c-*MYC* can be rearranged, for example, by inverting itself on insertion into the breakpoint on 14q32. All these mechanisms permit *MYC* overexpression.

The translocation and recombination of 8q24 and 14q32 typify Burkitt's lymphoma in its endemic (African) and sporadic (American) forms; however, the c-*MYC* gene may behave differently in the two variants.[79,82,83] In the endemic form, the breakpoint on chromosome 8q24 is outside the *MYC* region, and the c-*MYC* gene is translocated intact (not rearranged), albeit frequently with point mutations, to a break in the V_H-D-J_H recombination, most commonly in the J_H segment.[75,82] This translocation occurs in a nonsecretory pre-B-cell (an early stage of B-cell differentiation) and is thought to occur in conjunction with aberrant function of the recombinase enzyme in the process of completing normal immunoglobulin gene rearrangement.[79,84] In the sporadic form, the c-*MYC* gene is disrupted within its 5′ portion and separated from its regulatory (or *repressor*) region. The first *MYC* exon is translocated in some instances to a break in the switch region of the heavy-chain gene (S_μ) and is inverted (rearranged) on translocation.[81–85] The breakpoint on 14q32 results from an error in the action of isotype-switching enzymes in a more mature B cell that is capable of immunoglobulin secretion. The net result of c-*MYC* translocation to the immunoglobulin gene locus for the endemic or sporadic type is the abrogation of the effects of negative regulatory elements on c-*MYC* transcription. More than transcriptional activation or amplification of *MYC* per se, these gene rearrangements result in constitutive *MYC* expression and a failure of the normal control mechanisms, which leads to a net overexpression of the c-*MYC* mRNA-and DNA-binding phosphoprotein.[75,80]

EPSTEIN-BARR VIRUS, C-*MYC* ACTIVATION, AND B-CELL LYMPHOMAGENESIS

The role of EBV in B-cell lymphomagenesis has been established for endemic (African) Burkitt's lymphoma and postulated for many of the B-cell malignancies that arise in the setting of chronic immunosuppression. In the case of EBV-associated endemic Burkitt's lymphoma, c-*MYC* breakpoints occur outside the 5′ regulatory region, and the c-*MYC* gene is altered mainly through mutations within its first exon (most commonly at Pvu site II) rather than through truncation or rearrangement on translocation.[83] In the absence of EBV DNA, in the sporadic form, c-*MYC* breakpoints occur within the 5′ region of the gene and commonly result in truncation of the gene when it is translocated. Translocation to the nonswitch region of 14q32 results in transcription activation by immunoglobulin gene enhancer sequences; alternatively, translocation of the disrupted c-*MYC* gene to the switch region of 14q32 is accompanied by c-*MYC* gene inversion or true rearrangement, which results in direct oncogene overexpression. Nonetheless, for EBV-related Burkitt's lymphomas, c-*MYC* deregulation must involve other mechanisms. In this regard, EBV latent genes encode viral nuclear antigens (EBNAs) that act as transcriptional activators to enhance the survival and self-renewal capacities of EBV-infected host cells and viral genome.[86] EBNAs may also interact with the c-*MYC* regulatory region to effect gene overexpression and may further augment the effects of any point mutations occurring within the 5′ regulatory region.

Yet another mechanism of EBV-induced B-cell stimulation may operate through BCRF-1, an EBV-encoded protein that shares remarkable structural and functional homology with IL-10.[87,88] BCRF-1 causes a decrease in T-cell (and possibly natural killer-cell) synthesis of IFN-γ and perhaps IL-2, the net result of which is functional suppression of T-cell antiviral activity. Consequently, viral survival is enhanced as the byproduct of BCRF-1-related immunomodulation. B-cell activation and polyclonal B-cell expansion are promoted as a result of ongoing EBV propagation.

EBV has also been implicated in the cause of non-Burkitt's B-cell lymphomas, most commonly those that occur in the setting of chronic, profound immunosuppression. In contrast to Burkitt's lymphomas, these lymphoproliferative malignancies are often characterized by the presence of multiple neoplastic clones and by an immunoblastic large cell morphology with plasmacytoid features.[89–91] In this situation, EBV may provoke polyclonal B-cell activation, which, in the absence of normal T-cell controls, permits unopposed B-cell expansion with increased numbers of cells susceptible to destabilizing genetic events such as chromosomal breaks and recombinations. The etiologic effects of EBV have been demonstrated by inducing lymphomas in mice with severe combined immunodeficiency disease (SCID) that have been reconstituted with EBV-negative human peripheral or nodal lymphocytes (SCID/hu chimeric mice) and subsequently infected with EBV[92] or with peripheral blood lymphocytes from EBV-seropositive donors.[93] Of note is the absence of c-*MYC* and *BCL2* translocations or rearrangements. This animal model parallels the large cell immunoblastic B lymphomas that occur in humans with severe immunodeficiency (*e.g.*, after organ transplantation)[89,91,94] and in primary CNS lymphomas (now recognized as an AIDS-associated lesion).[20,71,90] In the human tumors, as in the SCID/hu mouse model, EBV genome is present in tumor cells, and the tumors (often with multiclonal origin) develop from a background polyclonal activation that is likely a consequence of EBV infection.

The mechanisms by which EBV may induce B-cell malignant transformation in the setting of AIDS are reminiscent of the mechanisms that operate in other states of chronic immunosuppression. Despite these similarities, however, the direct etiologic role of EBV in AIDS-related lymphomas remains a focus of investigation. It is likely that EBV is but one of many possible inducers of malignant transformation. Other DNA viruses of the herpesvirus family—most notably, CMV and human herpesvirus type 6 (HHV-6)—may also enhance B-cell activation and promote B-cell clonal expansion. These potential cofactors interact with HIV in ways that may enhance transcriptional activation and HIV replication.[20,22,95] Herpesviruses, like HIV, upregulate the expression of several cytokines by virus-infected lymphocytes and monocytes. These cytokines can induce host cell proliferation and viral replication through a positive feedback mechanism and, in this way, may provide a chronic stimulus for B-cell proliferation and activation.

Cells from about half (up to as many as 80%, in some series) of AIDS-NHL contain EBV DNA sequences.[20,96] Studies examining EBV genomic termini as clonal markers of infection have demonstrated the presence of the monoclonal episomes of EBV DNA, usually in the form of closed circles.[97] Of eight peripheral (nonprimary CNS) AIDS-associated lymphomas at the National Cancer Institute, seven were shown to contain EBV genomic sequences in the configuration of monoclonal episomes.[97a] Nevertheless, at least in selected human Burkitt's lymphoma and other B-lymphoblastoid cell lines, the EBV genome has been found to be integrated into host DNA, preferentially being inserted into segments of numerous chromosomes (in particular, 1, 5, and 13).[98] Whatever the structural particulars, all these findings are consistent with the hypothesis that EBV precedes and probably causes clonal expansions in AIDS-NHL and in endemic and some cases of sporadic Burkitt's lymphomas.[97] In addition, when EBV DNA and EBNAs are detected in nodes from HIV-positive patients with generalized lymphadenopathy, their presence signifies the likely emergence of NHL (with persistence of the EBV genome in the malignant clones); in contrast, cells from patients with EBV-negative lymphadenopathy do not appear to undergo malignant transformation,[99] supporting the notion that EBV has a direct etiologic role in NHL development in at least some AIDS patients.

In most cases in which NHL cells from AIDS patients contain the EBV genome or its protein products, there is concomitant alteration and deregulation of the c-*MYC* gene. However, there is not an inextricable linkage between EBV and c-*MYC* perturbations in AIDS-NHL.[100–102] In a few cases of phenotypically unusual B-lineage AIDS-NHL, EBV DNA sequences, gene products, and virus-induced surface antigens (*e.g.*, Ki-24) are detectable without associated c-*MYC* alterations.[101] More commonly, when there is dissociation of EBV and c-*MYC*, c-*MYC* mutations or rearrangements (present in about 70% of all large cell AIDS-NHL) occur in the absence of detectable EBV DNA or EBNAs.[100,102] Most cases of non-EBV, non-Burkitt's NHL have c-*MYC* rearrangements and 14q32 switch region breaks that mimic the sporadic Burkitt-type; but endemic-type breakpoints in c-*MYC* and 14q32 occur in about one fourth of cases of non-EBV AIDS-NHL and are accompanied by similar point mutations in the first *MYC* exon.[81] In terms of c-*MYC* breakpoints and the sites of c-*MYC* translocation to the heavy-chain gene (J_H versus S_u), AIDS lymphomas show both patterns. Overall, the prevalence of abnormalities in c-*MYC* structure and function is consistent with the notion that c-*MYC* has a central role in the malignant transformation and clonal expansion of B-cell lymphomas in AIDS.

POTENTIAL ROLE OF ABERRANT TUMOR SUPPRESSION IN THE PATHOGENESIS OF AIDS LYMPHOMAS

The loss of normal tumor suppressor gene and gene product function is thought to be a critical step in the pathogenesis and progression of diverse epithelial and lymphohematopoietic cancers.[103] Investigations have uncovered losses or mutations in specific tumor suppressor genes, particularly the retinoblastoma (*RB*) gene on chromosome 13q14 and the *p53* gene on chromosome 17p13, in myeloid and lymphoid leukemias and lymphomas.[103–105] The presence of *RB* and *p53* abnormalities is associated with clonal evolution and increasing aggressiveness of these malignancies, and there is a suggestion that the altered tumor suppressor genes may act in concert with activated oncogenes to effect the full transformation process.

The interaction between viral proteins and tumor suppressor proteins has been documented for several oncogenic DNA viruses and for RB and p53, the nuclear phosphoprotein products of the *RB* and *p53* genes.[106,107] In fact, the roles that tumor suppressors play in cell cycle regulation—in particular, their inhibition of movement from G1 into S phase—have been defined by the binding of viral proteins, such as SV40 large T antigen (for RB and p53) and adenovirus E1A (for RB) or E1B (for p53) to suppressor proteins and inactivation of their antiproliferative effects.[106,108] The blocking effects of HPV oncoproteins on RB and p53 activity may be important to the induction of anogenital cancers by HPV.[63,64] Studies of herpes simplex virus type 1 suggest that the virus may induce relocation of RB and p53 from their usual nuclear compartments to the sites of viral DNA replication, thereby facilitating host cell and virus replication.[107] Abrogation of tumor suppression may be a common mechanism by which any or all herpesviruses (including EBV) could operate in the pathogenesis of AIDS lymphomas and other AIDS-related cancers.

The sequential acquisition of aberrant oncogene and tumor suppressor gene and gene product function may be especially relevant to the process of viral tumorigenesis. In such cases, viruses might enhance the process of transformation and growth dysregulation through any one of several mechanisms: chromosomal breakage and translocation, leading to c-*MYC* or other oncogene activation; or production of viral proteins that bind to and alter the function of tumor suppressors that normally control transition through the cell cycle. These interactions may contribute to the pathogenesis of AIDS lymphomas through a direct effect of HIV or through other viruses, such as EBV, CMV, or HHV-6. Along these lines, the finding that exogenous HIV infection of EBV-seropositive, HIV-seronegative human peripheral blood B lymphocytes enhance EBV and endogenous c-*MYC* gene expression, in association with in vitro transformation of a subpopulation of those B cells to a malignant phenotype capable of B-lymphoma formation in SCID mice,[109] is provocative but requires confirmation. Theoretically, under some conditions that could have clinical relevance, HIV might act synergistically with EBV to exert a direct transforming effect, perhaps through transcriptional activation.

INTERLEUKINS AND THE DEVELOPMENT OF AIDS LYMPHOMAS

The proliferation and differentiation of lymphohematopoietic elements from pluripotent stem cells into mature end-stage cells is directed by a "family" of interactive glycoproteins, the *hematopoietic growth factors,* or *cytokines.* More than 20 cytokines—interleukins, colony-stimulating factors, interferons, and other growth factors—have been identified and characterized with respect to molecular and mechanistic features. Heightened cytokine production in response to HIV infection (and perhaps to other viruses) may contribute to the development of lymphomas in AIDS. The major cellular sources of production are T cells, monocytes, and bone marrow stromal cells of mesenchymal origin (namely fibroblasts), which can be infected by HIV and respond to HIV or other virus infection by increasing cytokine production.[24,25] Of the many lymphohematopoietic growth factors liberated under normal and virus-perturbed conditions, IL-6 may be especially relevant to pre-malignant polyclonal B-cell expansion and to eventual malignant transformation in AIDS-NHL. IL-6 promotes the growth and differentiation of B cells, particularly the induction of immunoglobulin gene expression and the final differentiation from immature B-cell precursors to plasma cells.[36,110] IL-6 also plays a role in the recruitment of resting T cells to the proliferative state and their differentiation along the cytotoxic T-lymphocyte pathway. IL-6 has major effects on the proliferation, differentiation, and net expression of multiple arms of the immune response. The increase in serum IL-6 levels that accompanies the HIV-associated clonal VH3L defect in B-cell maturation[76,78] may represent an attempt (albeit abortive) to drive the differentiation of the arrested B-cell clone. The B-cell maturation arrest occurs early in HIV infection, even before subclinical evidence for cellular immune impairment,[76] suggesting that the compensatory increase in circulating IL-6 levels also occurs early in HIV infection and can drive B-cell proliferation chronically over a long period of time. Further, IL-6 may augment HIV replication (and hence disease progression) in an autocrine loop through its enhancement of T-cell and monocyte growth.[24] Similar autocrine growth may exist in other tissues, such as brain. The production of IL-6 by brain tissue, particularly virus-infected tissue, is intriguing in light of the proclivity of AIDS-NHL to involve the CNS. Additionally, the production of IL-6 from HIV-infected monocytes promotes the proliferation of activated B cells (*e.g.*, by EBV), thereby driving immunoglobulin synthesis and causing the nonspecific hyperimmunoglobulinemia commonly seen in early HIV infection.[24,111]

In addition to mechanisms that directly stimulate B-cell expansion, suppression of helper T-cell antiviral or cytotoxic surveillance activities can permit the establishment of malignant clones. The recently described IL-10, called *cytokine synthesis inhibitory factor,* is such a suppressor of T-cell function.[87,88] IL-10 shares significant homology with the EBV protein BCRF-1 and likewise impairs T-cell synthesis of IFN-γ and IL-2. Besides their antiviral activities, IFN-γ and IL-2 upregulate major histocompatibility complex II surface antigen expression (which provokes the generation of cytotoxic T lymphocytes, a major effector of antitumor immune surveillance) and support the clonal expansion of immune-activated T cells in autocrine fashion. Excess IL-10 may permit viral replication (particularly EBV and possibly HIV) to go unchecked, which promotes the cascade of events that culminates in the establishment of clonal B-cell malignancy.

OPPORTUNITIES FOR THERAPEUTIC INNOVATION

Like other lymphomas arising in immunodeficient hosts, AIDS-NHL is a resilient, clinically aggressive therapeutic challenge. AIDS lymphomas are histologically high-grade tumors that usually present with multiorgan involvement and a substantial tumor burden. CNS tumor is especially common and, partly because it is protected as a sanctuary site, a frequent site of relapse. HIV-related bone marrow suppression (likely a consequence of direct progenitor cell infection or stromal cell infection with attendant suppression of hematopoietic growth factors)[25] and the presence of multiple chronic opportunistic infections act in concert to limit the host's ability to tolerate full cytotoxic therapy. Moreover, the absence of any antitumor immunity permits the expansion of tumor cells remaining after therapy to proceed unchecked.

As a result, multidrug regimens effective in de novo NHL—for example, ProMACE-MOPP (prednisone, methotrexate, doxorubicin [Adriamycin], cyclophosphamide [Cytoxan], etoposide–mechlorethamine, vincristine, procarbazine, prednisone) or variants containing bleomycin (MACOP-B, M-BACOD) and cytosine arabinoside (ProMACE-CytaBOM)

TABLE 59–4. Hematopoietic Growth Factors in the Therapy of AIDS and AIDS-Related Malignancies

	Erythropoietin	*Granulocyte-CSF*	*GM-CSF*	*Macrophage-CSF*	*IL-3*
Hematopoietic target cell	Erythrocyte	Granulocyte	Granulocyte, eosinophil, monocyte	Monocyte	Granulocyte, eosinophil, monocyte, platelets?
Amelioration of AZT-induced myelosuppression (in vivo)	+	+	+	?	?
Enhanced viral replication in monocyte/macrophage target cells	−	−	+	+	+
Enhanced AZT antiretroviral activity		+	−	+	
Marrow-protective effects demonstrated during antitumor chemotherapy		+ (KS)	+ (KS, NHL)		

—have met with variable results in AIDS lymphomas. Such combinations of alternating non-cross-resistant agents that reproducibly achieve complete remission rates of 70% to 90%, median disease-free survivals longer than 3 to 5 years, and median overall survivals exceeding 5 to 7 years in patients with advanced-stage aggressive NHL[112] have yielded remission rates of 20% to 50%, with overall survivals far less than 1 year for AIDS-associated lymphomas.[113] A potentially significant factor in the poor responses for AIDS-NHL is the attenuation or complete omission of therapy cycles on the basis of functionally impaired marrow reserve or uncontrollable opportunistic infection. The roles of marrow-protective hematopoietic growth factors in antiretroviral therapies for HIV infection and in antitumor therapies for AIDS-related malignancies are being defined through integrated laboratory and clinical investigations[33,54,114-118] (Table 59–4). Multiagent chemotherapy regimens combined with CNS therapy, antiretroviral therapy, anti-*Pneumocystis* prophylaxis, and marrow-protective colony-stimulating factors[114,116] are being tested in clinical trials (Table 59–5). A clinical trial by McMaster and colleagues[119] employing two cycles of intensive, multiagent non-cross-resistant cytoreductive therapy (including CNS therapy) to patients with high-grade, extensive small noncleaved cell lymphomas yielded promising results. Each of three HIV-infected patients in this trial achieved complete remission, and two were alive and well 2 to 3 years after therapy; however, none of these patients had full-blown preexisting AIDS.

A multimodality approach combines intensive cytotoxic antilymphoma therapy, antiretroviral therapy, and allogeneic or syngeneic bone marrow transplantation aimed at hematopoietic and immune reconstitution.[120] The net effects of allogeneic transplantation on immunocompetence are complex, but the ability to reinitiate some capacity for immune responsiveness seems crucial to the achievement of long-lasting antitumor effects. In this respect, transplantation of pluripotent stem cells offers the potential for long-term control of HIV infection and AIDS-NHL. Such approaches would likely require antiretroviral coverage.

For AIDS-NHL, it is likely that IL-6, alone or in concert with other B-stimulatory and T-suppressing lymphokines, chronically drives B-cell clonal expansion.[4,24] As discussed for AIDS-KS, it is logical to search for therapeutic agents that might inhibit net IL-6 activity, such as retinoic acid, pentoxifylline, anti-IL-6 antibodies, or for other molecular modifications that might block IL-6 binding and signaling. The ability to target and modify the activity of specific overexpressed genes with antisense oligodeoxynucleotides offers a novel approach to anti-HIV[121,122] and anticancer therapies.[123–125] At least in theory, this form of gene-directed therapy suppresses

TABLE 59–5. National Cancer Institute Protocol Therapy for AIDS-Related Non-Hodgkin's Lymphoma

I. Cyclic Chemotherapy (Cycles Repeated Every 21 Days)

Day One

Cyclophosphamide, 500 mg/m^2

VP-16, 100 mg/m^2

Doxorubicin, 15 mg/m^2

Day Eight

Vincristine, 1.4 mg/m^2

Methotrexate, 120 mg/m^2

Leucovorin, 25 mg/m^2 q6h × four doses (beginning 24 h after methotrexate)

All drugs are given intravenously.

II. Prophylaxis and Therapy for CNS Lymphoma

Intrathecal methotrexate, 12.5 mg, and cytosine arabinoside, 70 mg, are given weekly × 6.

For lymphomatous meningitis, intrathecal therapy is given twice weekly until clear, then weekly × 6. In addition, whole-brain irradiation, 3600 cGy, is administered daily in 180 cGy fractions.

III. Marrow-Protective Therapy

Granulocyte-macrophage colony-stimulating factor (GM-CSF), 10 μg/kg/d, is administered subcutaneously on days 2 through 7 and 9 through 14 of each cycle.

IV. Antiretroviral Therapy

AZT 500 mg PO, is administered daily

V. Anti-*Pneumocystic Carinii* Pneumonia Prophylaxis

Aerosolized pentamidine inhalation therapy is given monthly.

TABLE 59–6. Potential Factors Involved in the Pathogenesis of AIDS-Related Lymphomas

Pathogenic Factor	*Specific Host or Virus Effector*	*Mechanism for Malignant Transformation*	*Mechanism for (Poly) Clonal Expansion*
Oncogene activation	c-*MYC*	Chromosomal translocation	Deregulated (constitutive?) gene expression Blockade of apoptosis
Tumor suppressor inactivation	*RB, p53*	Gene loss or mutation Binding inactivation by viral oncoproteins	Loss of cell cycle regulation at G_1 and S boundary
HIV	*VH3L* gene	Maturation arrest in germinal center B cells	(Compensatory) increase in IL-6 production
	Transcriptional activation?	c-*MYC*	*EBV* gene expression
Oncogenic viral cofactors	DNA viruses (*e.g.*, EBV, CMV, HHV-6)	c-*MYC* breakage, mutation, translocation, and deregulation	Transcriptional activation Blockage of T-cell antiviral lymphokines Synergy with HIV Growth-factor induction Chronic antigenic stimulation
Lymphokines	IL-6	Enhanced gene expression Genetic instability?	Autocrine growth stimulation
	IL-10	Enhanced viral replication or expression	Inhibition of T-cell synthesis of IFN-γ and IL-2
DNA damage or repair	Aberrant recombinase activity	Maturational arrest?	?
	HIV	Replication of damaged or abnormally rearranged DNA	?

the malignant clone while sparing normal host tissues. Antisense oligomers can be made complementary to a specific aberrant mRNA transcribed from aberrant gene segments, for example, the fusion *BCR-ABL* gene that typifies chronic myelogenous leukemia[125] or the first intron of a translocated c-*MYC* gene present in a Burkitt's lymphoma cell line.[123] In both instances, the antisense constructs selectively inhibit the net expression of the targeted tumor cell gene, tumor cell proliferation, and survival without affecting normal cell counterparts. The development of diffusible phosphodiester and phosphorothioate oligodeoxynucleotides complementary to specific sequences in the *BCL2* protooncogene and the demonstration that incubation of these antisense compounds with leukemic lymphoblasts results in growth inhibition and eventual cytotoxicity is a template for future gene-targeted therapies.[124] *BCL2*, however, is discussed only as a model since it is not known to be abnormally expressed in AIDS-related lymphomas.

FUTURE DIRECTIONS: PREVENTION

As with all malignancies, the most effective strategies are those targeted to prevention. The ability, early in the course of active HIV infection, to interfere with mechanisms that promulgate B-cell hyperproliferation and clonal expansion—especially growth factors (IL-6, in particular) and concomitant viral infections (mainly EBV, but also CMV and HHV-6)—might decrease the occurrence or prolong the time to development of AIDS-related malignancies. Ultimately, however, the key strategies will be those directed toward maintaining the CD4 cell count at a level that prevents the establishment and perpetuation of transformed clones. From the studies of Yarchoan and colleagues,[7] the critical level for NHL development appears to be a CD4 count of about 50/mm^3. The identification of factors that portend a significant risk of cancer development for an HIV-infected patient (Table 59–6) and the development of antiretroviral strategies that confer long-term suppression of HIV activity and relative preservation of immune function (perhaps in combination with specific antigrowth-factor or other antiviral therapies) are essential to the ultimate prevention of all malignancies that arise as a consequence of HIV-induced immunosuppression. Although much remains to be done, we have a strong foundation to build new approaches for preventing and treating these important neoplastic complications of AIDS.

REFERENCES

1. Siegal B, Levinton-Kriss S, Schiffer A, et al. Kaposi's sarcoma in immunosuppression. Cancer 1990;65:492.
2. Broder S, Mitsuya H, Yarchoan R, et al. Antiretroviral therapy in AIDS. Ann Intern Med 1990;113:604
3. Gail MH, Pluda JM, Rabkin CS, et al. Projections of the incidence of non-Hodgkin's lymphoma related to acquired immunodeficiency syndrome. J Natl Cancer Inst 1991;83:695
4. Yarchoan R, Pluda JM, Perno C-F, et al. Antiretroviral therapy of HIV infection: Current strategies and challenges for the future. Blood 1991;78:859.
5. McKinney RE, Maha MA, Connor EM, et al. A multicenter trial of oral zidovudine in children with advanced human immunodeficiency virus disease. N Engl J Med 1991;324:1018.
6. Moore RD, Hidalgo J, Sugland BW, et al. Zidovudine and the natural history of the acquired immunodeficiency syndrome. N Engl J Med 1991;324:1412.
7. Yarchoan R, Venzon DJ, Pluda JM, et al. CD4 count as a mortality risk indicator in human immunodeficiency virus (HIV)-infected patients receiving antiretroviral therapy: Experience in a research hospital. Ann Intern Med 1991;115:184.

8. Rosenberg PS, Gail MH, Schrager LK, et al. National AIDS incidence trends and the extent of zidovudine therapy in selected demographic and transmission groups. J AIDS 1991;4:392.
9. Pluda JM, Yarchoan R, Jaffe ES, et al. Development of non-Hodgkin's lymphoma in a cohort of patients with severe immunodeficiency virus (HIV) infection on long-term antiretroviral therapy. Ann Intern Med 1990;113:276.
10. Centers for Disease Control. Current trends: Opportunistic non-Hodgkin's lymphomas among severely immunocompromised HIV-infected patients surviving for prolonged periods on antiretroviral therapy—United States. MMWR 1991;40:591.
11. Kaposi M. Idiopathisches multiples pigmentsarkom der haut. Arch Dermatol Syph 1872;4:265.
12. Friedman-Kien AE, Saltzman BR. Clinical manifestations of classical, endemic African, and epidemic AIDS-associated Kaposi's sarcoma. J Am Acad Dermatol 1990;22:1237.
13. Greenberg SJ, Jaffe ES, Ehrlich GD. Kaposi's sarcoma in human T-cell leukemia virus type I-associated adult T-cell leukemia. Blood 1990;76:971.
14. Lind SE, Gross PL, Andiman WA, et al. Malignant lymphoma presenting as Kaposi's sarcoma in a homosexual man with the acquired immunodeficiency syndrome. Ann Intern Med 1985;102:338.
15. Haverkos HW, Friedman-Kien AE, Drotman P. The changing incidence of Kaposi's sarcoma among patients with AIDS. J Am Acad Dermatol 1990;22:1250.
16. Krigel RL, Friedman-Kien AE. Epidemic Kaposi's sarcoma. Semin Oncol 1990;17: 350.
17. Pitchenik AE, Fischl MA, Dickinson GM, et al. Opportunistic infections and Kaposi's sarcoma among Haitians: Evidence of a new acquired immunodeficiency state. Ann Intern Med 1983;98:277.
18. Marmor M, Friedman-Kien AE, Zolla-Pazner S, et al. Kaposi's sarcoma in homosexual men. Ann Intern Med 1984;100:809–819.
19. Jaffe HW, Choi K, Thomas PA, et al. National case-control study of Kaposi's sarcoma and *Pneumocystis carinii* pneumonia in homosexual men: Part 1, epidemiologic results. Ann Intern Med 1983;99:145.
20. Cremer KJ, Spring SB, Gruber J. Role of human immunodeficiency virus type I and other viruses in malignancies associated with acquired immunodeficiency disease syndrome. J Natl Cancer Inst 1990;82:1016.
21. Rogers MF, Morens DM, Steward JA, et al. National case-control study of Kaposi's sarcoma and *Pneumocystis carinii* pneumonia in homosexual men: Part 2, laboratory results. Ann Intern Med 1983;99:151.
22. Laurence J. Molecular interactions among herpesviruses and human immunodeficiency virus. J Infect Dis 1990;162:338.
23. Ambinder RF, Newman C, Hayward GS, et al. Lack of association of cytomegalovirus with endemic African Kaposi's sarcoma. J Infect Dis 1987;156:193.
24. Birx DL, Redfield RR, Tencer K, et al. Induction of interleukin-6 during human immunodeficiency virus infection. Blood 1990;76:2303.
25. Scadden DT, Zeira M, Woon A, et al. Human immunodeficiency virus infection of human bone marrow stromal fibroblasts. Blood 1990;76:317.
26. Delli Bovi P, Curatola AM, Kern FG, et al. An oncogene isolated by transfection of Kaposi's sarcoma DNA encodes a growth factor that is a member of the FGF family. Cell 1987;50:729.
27. Delli-Bovi P, Curatola AM, Newman KM, et al. Processing, secretion, and biologic properties of a novel growth factor of the fibroblast growth factor family with oncogenic potential. Mol Cell Biol 1988;8:2933.
28. Ensoli B, Nakamura S, Salahuddin SZ, et al. AIDS-Kaposi's sarcoma-derived cells express cytokines with autocrine and paracrine growth effects. Science 1989;243: 223.
29. Miles SA, Rezai AR, Salazar-Gonzalez JF, et al. AIDS Kaposi sarcoma-derived cells produce and respond to interleukin 6. Proc Natl Acad Sci USA 1990;87:4068.
30. Salahuddin SZ, Nakamura S, Biberfeld P, et al. Angiogenic properties of Kaposi's sarcoma-derived cells after long-term culture in vitro. Science 1988;242:430.
31. Wellstein A, Lupu R, Zugmaier G, et al. Autocrine growth stimulation by secreted Kaposi fibroblast growth factor but not by endogenous basic fibroblast growth factor. Cell Growth Differ 1990;1:63.
32. Abboud SL, Pinzani M. Peptide growth factors stimulate macrophage colony-stimulating factor in murine stromal cells. Blood 1991;78:103.
33. Kitano K, Abboud CN, Ryan DH, et al. Macrophage-active colony-stimulating factors enhance human immunodeficiency virus type I infection in bone marrow stem cells. Blood 1991;77:1699.
34. Dinarello CA. Interleukin-1 and interleukin-1 antagonism. Blood 1991;77:1627.
35. Boraschi D, Rambaldi A, Sica A, et al. Endothelial cells express the interleukin-1 receptor type I. Blood 1991;78:1262.
36. Hirano T. Interleukin 6 (IL-6) and its receptor: Their role in plasma cell neoplasias. Int J Cell Cloning 1991;9:166.
37. Schwab G, Siegall CB, Aarden LA, et al. Characterization of an interleukin-6-mediated autocrine growth loop in the human multiple myeloma cell line U266. Blood 1991;72: 587.
38. Zhang XG, Klein B, Bataille R. Interleukin-6 is a potent myeloma-cell growth factor in patients with aggressive multiple myeloma. Blood 1989;73:11.
39. Ensoli B, Barillari G, Salahuddin SZ, et al. Tat protein of HIV-1 stimulates growth of cells derived from Kaposi's sarcoma lesions of AIDS patients. Nature 1990;345:84.
40. Friedman SL. Kaposi's sarcoma and lymphoma of the gut in AIDS. Bailliere's Clin Gastroenterol 1990;4:455.
41. Ognibene FP, Steis RG, Macher AM, et al. Kaposi's sarcoma causing pulmonary infiltrates and respiratory failure in the acquired immunodeficiency syndrome. Ann Intern Med 1985;102:471.
42. Heitzman ER. Pulmonary neoplastic and lymphoproliferative disease in AIDS: A review. Radiology 1990;177:347.
43. Krown SE, Metroka C, Wernz JC. Kaposi's sarcoma in the acquired immune deficiency syndrome: A proposal for uniform evaluation, response, and staging criteria. J Clin Oncol 1989;7:1201.
44. Pluda JM, Brawley OW, Yarchoan R, et al. Neoplasms associated with AIDS. In: Calabresi P, Schein PS, eds. Medical oncology: Basic principles and clinical management of cancer. Elmsford, UK: Pergamon Press, 1992 (in press).
45. Northfelt DW, Kahn JO, Volberding PA. Treatment of AIDS-related Kaposi's sarcoma. Hematol Oncol Clin North Am 1991;5:297.
46. Sidell N, Taga T, Hirano T, et al. Retinoic acid-induced growth inhibition of a human myeloma cell line via down-regulation of IL-6 receptors. J Immunol 1991;146:3809.
47. Waldmann TA. Monoclonal antibodies in diagnosis and therapy. Science 1991;252: 1657.
48. Gill PS, Rarick M, McCutchan JA, et al. Systemic treatment of AIDS-related Kaposi's sarcoma: Results of a randomized trial. Am J Med 1991;90:427.
49. Krown SE. Interferon and other biologic agents for the treatment of Kaposi's sarcoma. Hematol Oncol Clin North Am 1991;5:311.
50. Miles SA, Wang H, Cortes E, et al. Beta-interferon therapy in patients with poor-prognosis Kaposi sarcoma related to the acquired immunodeficiency syndrome (AIDS): A phase II trial with preliminary evidence of antiviral activity and low incidence of opportunistic infections. Ann Intern Med 1990;112:582.
51. Lane HC, Kovacs JA, Feinberg J, et al. Antiretroviral effects of interferon-alpha in AIDS-associated Kaposi's sarcoma. Lancet 1988;ii:1218.
52. Krown SE, Gold JWM, Niedzwiecki D, et al. Interferon-a with zidovudine: Safety, tolerance, and clinical and virologic effects in patients with Kaposi sarcoma associated with the acquired immunodeficiency syndrome (AIDS). Ann Intern Med 1990;112: 812.
53. Fischl MA. Antiretroviral therapy in combination with interferon for AIDS-related Kaposi's sarcoma. Am J Med 1991;90:2S.
54. Scadden DT, Bering HA, Levine JD, et al. Granulocyte-macrophage colony-stimulating factor mitigates the neutropenia of combined interferon alfa and zidovudine treatment of acquired immune deficiency syndrome-associated Kaposi's sarcoma. J Clin Oncol 1991;9:802.
55. Wellstein A, Zugmaier G, Califano JA III, et al. Tumor growth dependent on Kaposi's sarcoma-derived fibroblast growth factor inhibitied by pentosan polysulfate. J Natl Cancer Inst 1991;83:716.
56. Folkman J, Weisz PB, Joullie MM, et al. Control of angiogenesis with synthetic heparin substitutes. Science 1989;243:1490.
57. Ingber D, Fujita T, Kishimoto S, et al. Synthetic analogues of fumagillin that inhibit angiogenesis and suppress tumor growth. Nature 1990;348:555.
58. Albini A, Melchiori A, Santi L, et al. Tumor cell invasion inhibited by TIMP-2. J Natl Cancer Inst 1991;83:775.
59. Fazely F, Dezube BJ, Allen-Ryan J, et al. Pentoxifylline (Trental) decreases the replication of the human immunodeficiency virus type I in human peripheral blood mononuclear cells and in cultured T cells. Blood 1991;77:1653.
60. Kiviat N, Rompalo A, Bowden R, et al. Anal human papilloma-virus infection among human immunodeficiency virus-seropositive and -seronegative men. J Infect Dis 1990;162:358.
61. Maiman M, Fruchter RG, Serur E, et al. Human immunodeficiency virus infection and cervical neoplasia. Gynecol Oncol 1990;38:377.
62. Palefsky JM, Gonzales J, Greenblatt RM, et al. Anal intraepithelial neoplasia and anal papillomavirus infection among homosexual males with group IV HIV disease. JAMA 1990;263:2911.
63. Dyson N, Howley PM, Munger K, et al. The human papilloma virus-16 E7 oncoprotein is able to bind to the retinoblastoma gene product. Science 1989;248:934.
64. Werness BA, Levine AJ, Howley PM. Association of human papillomavirus types 16 and 18 E6 proteins with p53. Science 1990;248:76.
65. Cancer Statistics Review 1973-1988. National Cancer Institute, Division of Cancer Prevention and Control. NIH publication No. 91-2789, 1991.
66. Monfardini S, Tirelli U, Vaccher E, et al. Hodgkin's disease in 63 intravenous drug users with human immunodeficiency virus. Ann Oncol (Supplement) 1991;2:201.
67. Knowles DM, Chamulak GA, Subar M, et al. Lymphoid neoplasia associated with the acquired immunodeficiency syndrome (AIDS). Ann Intern Med 1988;108:744.
68. Ziegler JL, Beckstead JA, Volberding PA, et al. Non-Hodgkin's lymphoma in 90 homosexual men: Relation to generalized lymphadenopathy and the acquired immunodeficiency syndrome. N Engl J Med 1984;211:565.
69. Beral V, Peterman T, Berkelman R, et al. AIDS-associated non-Hodgkin lymphoma. Lancet 1991;337:805.
70. Wilkes MS, Fortin AH, Felix JC, et al. Value of necropsy in acquired immunodeficiency syndrome. Lancet 1988;ii:85.
71. Gill PS, Levine AM, Meyer PR, et al. Primary central nervous system lymphoma in homosexual men: Clinical, immunologic and pathologic features. Am J Med 1985;78: 742.
72. Moore RD, Kessler H, Richman DD, et al. Non-Hodgkin's lymphoma in patients with advanced HIV infection treated with zidovudine. JAMA 1991;265:2208.
73. Feichtinger H, Putkonen P, Parravicini C, et al. Malignant lymphomas in cynomolgus monkeys infected with simian immunodeficiency virus. Am J Pathol 1990;137:1311.
74. Waldmann TA, Korsmeyer SJ, Bakhshi A, et al. Molecular genetic analysis of human lymphoid neoplasms: Immunoglobulin genes and the *c-myc* oncogene. Ann Intern Med 1985;102:497.
75. Croce CM, Nowell PC. Molecular basis of human B cell neoplasia. Blood 1985;65:1.
76. Berberian L, Valles-Ayoub Y, Sun N, et al. A VH clonal deficit in human immunodeficiency virus-positive individuals reflects a B-cell maturational arrest. Blood 1991;78: 175.

77. Braun J, Galbraith L, Valles-Ayoub Y, Saxon A. Human immunodeficiency resulting from maturational arrest of germinal center B cells. Immunol Lett 1991;27:205.
78. Breen EC, Rezai AR, Nakajima K, et al. Infection with HIV is associated with elevated IL-6 levels and production. J Immunol 1990;144:480.
79. Haluska FG, Tsujimoto Y, Croce CM. Mechanisms of chromosome translocation in B- and T-cell neoplasia. Trends Genet 1987;3:11.
80. Dalla-Favera R, Bregni M, Erikson J, et al. Human *c-myc* oncogene is located on the region of chromosome 8 that is translocated in Burkitt lymphoma cells. Proc Natl Acad Sci USA 1982;79:7824.
81. Ladanyi M, Offitt K, Jhanwar SC, et al. MYC rearrangement and translocations involving band 8q24 in diffuse large cell lymphomas. Blood 1991;77:1057.
82. Pellici PG, Knowles DM, Magrath I, et al. Chromosomal breakpoints and structural alterations of the *c-myc* locus differ in endemic and sporadic forms of Burkitt lymphoma. Proc Natl Acad Sci USA 1986;83:2984.
83. Shiramizu B, Barriga F, Neequaye J, et al. Patterns of chromosomal breakpoint locations in Burkitt's lymphoma: Relevance to geography and Epstein-Barr virus association. Blood 1991;77:1516.
84. Klein G. Multiple phenotypic consequences of the Ig/Myc translocation in B-cell-derived tumors. Genes Chromosomes Cancer 1989;1:3.
85. Gauwerky CE, Croce CM. Molecular biology of leukemias and lymphomas. In: Broder S, ed. Molecular foundations of oncology. Baltimore, MD: Williams and Wilkins, 1991:295–310.
86. Gregory CD, Dive C, Henderson S, et al. Activation of Epstein-Barr virus latent genes protects human B cells from death by apoptosis. Nature 1991;349:612.
87. Hsu D-H, Malefyt RD, Fiorentino DF, et al. Expression of interleukin-10 activity by Epstein-Barr virus protein BCRF1. Science 1990;250:830.
88. Moore KW, Vieira P, Fiorentino DF, et al. Homology of cytokine synthesis inhibitory factor (IL-10) to the Epstein-Barr virus gene BCRF1. Science 1990;248:1230.
89. Hanto DW, Frizzera G, Gajl-Peczalska KJ, et al. Epstein-Barr virus-induced B-cell lymphoma after renal transplantation: Acyclovir therapy and transition from polyclonal to monoclonal B-cell proliferation. N Engl J Med 1982;306:913.
90. Hochberg FH, Miller G, Schooley RT, et al. Central-nervous-system lymphoma related to Epstein-Barr virus. N Engl J Med 1983;309:745.
91. Shearer WT, Ritz J, Finegold MJ, et al. Epstein-Barr virus associated B-cell proliferations of diverse clonal origins after bone marrow transplantation in a 12-year-old patient with severe combined immunodeficiency. N Engl J Med 1985;312:1151.
92. Cannon MJ, Pisa P, Fox RI, et al. Epstein-Barr virus induces aggressive lymphoproliferative disorders of human B cell origin in SCID/hu chimeric mice. J Clin Invest 1990;85:1333.
93. Rowe M, Young LS, Crocker J, et al. Epstein-Barr Virus (EBV)-associated lymphoproliferative disease in the SCID mouse model: Implications for the pathogenesis of EBV-positive lymphomas in man. J Exp Med 1991;173:147.
94. Penn I. Tumors arising in organ transplant recipients. Adv Cancer Res 1978;28:31.
95. Lusso P, De Maria A, Malnati M, et al. Induction of CD4 and susceptibility to HIV-1 infection in human CD8+ T lymphocytes by human herpesvirus 6. Nature 1991;349:533.
96. Hamilton-Dutoit SJ, Pallesen G, Karkov J, et al. Identification of EBV-DNA in tumour cells of AIDS-related lymphomas by in-situ hybridisation. Lancet 1989;i:554.
97. Neri A, Barriga F, Inghirami G, et al. Epstein-Barr virus infection precedes clonal expansion in Burkitt's and acquired immunodeficiency syndrome-associated lymphomas. Blood 1991;77:1092.
97a. Raffeld M. Personal communication. National Cancer Institute, January 1992.
98. Trescol-Biemont MC, Biemont C, Daillie J. Localization polymorphism of EBV DNA genomes in the chromosomes of Burkitt lymphoma cell lines. Chromosoma 1987;95:144.
99. Shibata D, Weiss LM, Nathwani BN, et al. Epstein-Barr virus in benign lymph node biopsies from individuals infected with the human immunodeficiency virus is associated with concurrent or subsequent development of non-Hodgkin's lymphoma. Blood 1991;77:1527.
100. Groopman JE, Sullivan JL, Mulder C, et al. Pathogenesis of B cell lymphoma in a patient with AIDS. Blood 1986;67:612.
101. Knowles DM, Inghirami G, Ubriaco A, et al. Molecular genetic analysis of three AIDS-associated neoplasms of uncertain lineage demonstrates their B-cell derivation and the possible pathogenetic role of the Epstein-Barr virus. Blood 1989;73:792.
102. Subar M, Neri A, Inghirami G, et al. Frequent c-myc oncogene activation and infrequent presence of Epstein-Barr virus genome in AIDS-associated lymphoma. Blood 1988;72:667.
103. Stanbridge EJ, Nowell PC. Origins of human cancer revisited. Cell 1990;63:867.
104. Ginsberg AM, Raffeld M, Cossman J. Inactivation of the retinoblastoma gene in human lymphoid neoplasms. Blood 1991;77:833.
105. Hollstein M, Sidransky D, Vogelstein B, Harris CC. p53 Mutations in human cancers. Science 1991;253:49.
106. Hollingsworth RE, Lee WH. Tumor suppressor genes: New prospects for cancer research. J Natl Cancer Inst 1991;83:91.
107. Wilcock D, Lane DP. Localization of p53, retinoblastoma and host replication proteins at sites of viral replication in herpes-infected cells. Nature 1991;349:429.
108. DeCaprio JA, Ludlow JW, Lynch D, et al. The product of the retinoblastoma susceptibility gene has properties of a cell cycle regulatory element. Cell 1989;58:1085.
109. Laurence J, Astrin SM. Human immunodeficiency virus induction of malignant transformation in human B lymphocytes. Proc Natl Acad Sci 1991;88:7635.
110. Kishimoto T. The biology of interleukin-6. Blood 1989;74:1.
111. Yarchoan R, Redfield RR, Broder S. Mechanisms of B cell activation in patients with acquired immunodeficiency syndrome and related disorders. J Clin Invest 1986;78:439.
112. Longo DL, DeVita VT, Duffey PL, et al. Superiority of ProMACE-CytaBOM over ProMACE-MOPP in the treatment of advanced diffuse aggressive lymphoma: Results of a prospective randomized trial. J Clin Oncol 1991;9:25.
113. Raphael BG, Knowles DM. Acquired immunodeficiency syndrome-associated non-Hodgkin's lymphoma. Semin Oncol 1990;17:361.
114. Kaplan LD, Kahn JO, Crowe S, et al. Clinical and virologic effects of recombinant granulocyte-macrophage colony stimulating factor in patients receiving chemotherapy for human immunodeficiency virus-associated non-Hodgkin's lymphoma: Results of a randomized trial. J Clin Oncol 1991;9:929.
115. Koyanagi Y, O'Brien WA, Zhao JQ, et al. Cytokines alter production of HIV-1 from primary mononuclear phagocytes. Science 1988;241:1673.
116. Perno CF, Cooney DA, Currens MJ, et al. Ability of anti-HIV agents to inhibit HIV replication in monocyte/macrophages or U937 monocytoid cells under conditions of enhancement by GM-CSF or anti-HIV antibody. AIDS Res Hum Retroviruses 1990;6:1051.
117. Pluda JM, Yarchoan R, Smith PD, et al. Subcutaneous recombinant granulocyte-macrophage colony-stimulating factor used as a single agent and in an alternating regimen with azidothymidine in leukopenic patients with severe human immunodeficiency virus infection. Blood 1990;76:463.
118. Schuitemaker H, Kootstra NA, van Oers MHJ, et al. Induction of monocyte proliferation and HIV expression by IL-3 does not interfere with anti-viral activity of zidovudine. Blood 1990;76:1490.
119. McMaster ML, Greer JP, Greco A, et al. Effective treatment of small-non-cleaved-cell lymphoma with high-intensity, brief-duration chemotherapy. J Clin Oncol 1991;9:941.
120. Holland HK, Saral R, Rossi JJ, et al. Allogeneic bone marrow transplantation, zidovudine, and human immunodeficiency virus type 1 (HIV-1) infection: Studies in a patient with non-Hodgkin's lymphoma. Ann Intern Med 1989;111:973.
121. Stein CA, Ranajit P, DeVico AL, et al. Mode of action of 5'-linked cholesteryl phosphorothioate oligodeoxy-nucleotides in inhibiting syncytia formation and infection by HIV-1 and HIV-2 in vitro. Biochemistry 1991;30:2439–2444.
122. Sullenger BA, Gallardo HF, Ungers GE, et al. Overexpression of TAR sequences renders cells resistant to human immunodeficiency virus replication. Cell 1990;63:601.
123. McManaway ME, Neckers LM, Loke SL, et al. Tumour-specific inhibition of lymphoma growth by an antisense oligodeoxynucleotide. Lancet 1990;335:808.
124. Reed JC, Stein C, Subasinghe C, et al. Antisense-mediated inhibition of *BCL-2* protooncogene expression and leukemic cell growth and survival: Comparisons of phosphodiester and phosphorothioate oligodeoxynucleotides. Cancer Res 1990;50:6565.
125. Szczylik C, Skorski T, Nicolaides NC, et al. Selective inhibition of leukemic cell proliferation by BCR-ABL antisense oligodeoxynucleotides. Science 1991;253:562.

Cancer: Principles & Practice of Oncology, Fourth Edition,
edited by Vincent T. DeVita, Jr., Samuel Hellman, Steven A. Rosenberg.
J.B. Lippincott Co., Philadelphia © 1993.

CHAPTER 60

Oncologic Emergencies

SECTION 1

JOACHIM YAHALOM

Superior Vena Cava Syndrome

Superior vena cava syndrome (SVCS) is the clinical expression of obstruction of blood flow through the superior vena cava (SVC). Characteristic symptoms and signs may develop quickly or gradually when this thin-walled vessel is compressed, invaded, or thrombosed by processes in the superior mediastinum. The first pathologic description of SVC obstruction in a patient with syphilitic aortic aneurysm appeared in 1757.[1] In 1954, Schechter reviewed 274 well-documented cases of SVCS reported in the literature; 40% of them were due to syphilitic aneurysms or tuberculosis mediastinitis.[2] These entities have since virtually disappeared, and cancer of the lung is now the underlying process in approximately 70% of the patients with SVCS.

ANATOMY AND PATHOPHYSIOLOGY

The SVC is the major vessel for drainage of venous blood from the head, neck, upper extremities, and upper thorax. It is located in the middle mediastinum and is surrounded by relatively rigid structures such as the sternum, trachea, right bronchus, aorta, pulmonary artery, and the perihilar and paratracheal lymph nodes. The SVC extends from the junction of the right and left innominate veins to the right atrium for a distance of 6 to 8 cm. The distal 2 cm of the SVC is within the pericardial sac, with a point of relative fixation of the vena cava at the pericardial reflection. The azygos vein, the main auxiliary vessel, enters the SVC posteriorly, just above the pericardial reflection. The SVC maintains blood at a low pressure. It is large but thin-walled, compliant, and easily compressible, and it is vulnerable to any space-occupying process in its vicinity. The SVC is completely encircled by chains of lymph nodes that drain all the structures of the right thoracic cavity and the lower part of the left thorax. The auxiliary azygos vein is also threatened by enlargement of paratracheal nodes. Other critical structures in the mediastinum, such as the main bronchi, esophagus, and the spinal cord, may be involved by the same process that led to obstruction of the SVC.[3–5]

When the SVC is fully or partially obstructed, an extensive venous collateral circulation may develop. The azygos venous system is the most important alternative pathway. Carlson found that dogs could not survive sudden ligation of the SVC below the level of the azygos vein, but they tolerated well ligation of the SVC above it.[6] He could, however, successfully obstruct the SVC and the azygos vein in operations performed in two stages, presumably by allowing time for collaterals to form. Other collateral systems are the internal mammary veins, lateral thoracic veins, paraspinous veins, and the esophageal venous network. The subcutaneous veins are important pathways, and their engorgement in the neck and thorax is a typical physical finding in SVCS. Despite these collateral pathways, venous pressure is almost always elevated in the upper compartment if there is obstruction of the SVC. Venous pressures have been recorded as high as 200 to 500 cm H_2O in severe SVCS.[7]

ETIOLOGY AND NATURAL HISTORY

The syndrome usually has an insidious onset and progresses to typical symptoms and signs. Review of the data from three

TABLE 60–1. Common Symptoms and Physical Findings of Superior Vena Cava Syndrome

Symptoms	*Patients Affected* (%)*	*Physical Findings*	*Patients Affected (%)*
Dyspnea	63	Venous distention of neck	66
Facial swelling or head fullness	50	Venous distention of chest wall	54
Cough	24	Facial edema	46
Arm swelling	18	Cyanosis	20
Chest pain	15	Plethora of face	19
Dysphagia	9	Edema of arms	14

* Analysis based on data from 370 patients.[8–10]

recent series (Table 60–1) shows dyspnea to be the most common symptom.[8–10] Dyspnea occurred in 63% of the patients with SVCS. A sensation of fullness in the head and facial swelling was reported by 50% of the patients. Other complaints were cough (24%), arm swelling (18%), chest pain (15%), and dysphagia (9%). The characteristic physical findings were venous distention of the neck (66%) and chest wall (54%), facial edema (46%), plethora (19%), and cyanosis (19%). These symptoms and signs may be aggravated by bending forward, stooping, or by lying down.

Malignant disease is the most common cause of SVCS. The percentage of patients in different series with a confirmed diagnosis of malignancy varies from 78% to 86% (Table 60–2).[3,9–11] Lung cancer was diagnosed in 65% of 415 patients analyzed in these series.[3,9–11] Armstrong and Perez did a retrospective review of 4100 cases treated for bronchogenic carcinoma between 1965 and 1984, and identified 99 patients (2.4%) with SVCS.[8] Salsali observed SVCS in 4.2% of 4960 patients with lung cancer; 80% of the tumors inducing SVCS were of the right lung.[12] Small cell lung cancer is the most common histologic subtype (Table 60–3), and it was found in 38% of the patients who had lung cancer and SVCS. Among 225 consecutive patients with small cell cancer, 26 (11.5%) had SVCS when the malignancy was diagnosed.[13] The second most common histologic subtype is squamous cell carcinoma, found in 26% of lung cancer patients with SVCS.

Lymphoma involving the mediastinum was the cause of SVCS in 8% of the patients reported in the series (see Table 60–2). Armstrong and Perez found SVCS in 1.9% of 952 lymphoma patients.[8] Perez-Soler identified 36 cases (4%) of SVCS among 915 patients with non-Hodgkin's lymphoma (NHL) treated at the M.D. Anderson Cancer Center.[14] Twenty-three patients (64%) had diffuse large cell lymphoma, 12 (33%) had lymphoblastic lymphoma, and 1 patient had follicular large cell lymphoma. Of their patients with diffuse large cell lymphoma and lymphoblastic lymphoma, 7% and 21% had SVCS, respectively. Hodgkin's lymphoma commonly involves the mediastinum, but it rarely causes SVCS. Other primary mediastinal malignancies that cause SVCS are thymoma and germ cell tumors. Breast cancer is the most common metastatic disease that causes SVCS.[3,9,11]

Nonmalignant conditions causing SVCS are not as rare as previously reported.[8,15] When the data were collected from general hospitals, as many as 22% of the patients had noncancerous causes of SVCS.[3,9,11] Parish[9] reported 19 patients with benign causes of SVCS, and Schraufnagel[3] included 16 such patients in his series. Fifty percent of the patients in both reports had a diagnosis of mediastinal fibrosis, which was probably due to histoplasmosis. Parish reported 6 patients with thrombosis of SVC, and in 5, thrombosis developed in the presence of central vein catheters or pacemakers.[9] Sculier reviewed 24 cases of central venous catheter-induced SVC.[16] Of these, 18 were caused by pacemaker catheters. LeVeen shunts, Swan-Ganz catheters, and hyperalimentation catheters were also involved. The increasing use of these devices for the delivery of chemotherapy agents or for hyperalimentation contributes to the development of SVCS in the cancer patient.[17]

Obstruction of SVC in the pediatric age group is rare and has a different etiologic spectrum. The causative factors are mainly iatrogenic, secondary to cardiovascular surgery for congenital heart disease, ventriculoatrial shunt for hydro-

TABLE 60–2. Primary Pathologic Diagnoses for Superior Vena Cava Syndrome

Histologic Diagnosis	*Bell[10] 159 Patients (%)*	*Schraufnagel[3] 107 Patients (%)*	*Parish[9] 86 Patients (%)*	*Yellin[11] 63 Patients (%)*	*Total 415 Patients (%)*
Lung cancer	129 (81)	67 (63)	45 (52)	30 (48)	271 (65)
Lymphoma	3 (2)	10 (9)	8 (9)	13 (21)	34 (8)
Other malignancies (primary or metastatic)	4 (3)	14 (13)	14 (16)	8 (13)	40 (10)
Nonneoplastic	2 (1)	16 (15)	19 (22)	11 (18)	50 (12)
Undiagnosed	21 (13)				21 (5)

TABLE 60–3. Lung Cancer Subtypes Associated With Superior Vena Cava Syndrome

Histology	*No. of Patients (%)*
Small cell	142 (38)
Squamous cell	97 (26)
Adenocarcinoma	52 (14)
Large cell	43 (12)
Unclassified	34 (9)
Total	370 (100)

cephalus, and SVC catheterization for parenteral nutrition.[18] In a report of 175 children with SVCS, 70% were iatrogenic. Of the remaining 53 cases, 37 (70%) were caused by mediastinal tumors, 8 (15%) were caused by benign granuloma, and 4 (7.5%) by congenital anomalies of the cardiovascular system. Two thirds of the tumors causing SVCS in childhood are lymphomas.[18,19] Of 16 children reported from St. Jude Children's Research Hospital with SVCS at presentation, 8 were diagnosed with NHL, 4 had acute lymphoblastic leukemia, 2 had Hodgkin's disease, 1 had neuroblastoma, and 1 had a yolk sac tumor.[20] Most children who developed SVCS late in the course of their malignancy had recurrent solid tumors.[20] Issa reported that mediastinal fibrosis secondary to histoplasmosis caused SVCS in 7 (5%) of the 150 patients reviewed.[18]

DIAGNOSTIC PROCEDURES

The SVCS has long been considered to be a potentially life-threatening medical emergency.[4,15,21] It was common practice to immediately apply radiation therapy with initial high-dose fractions, sometimes even before the histologic diagnosis of the primary lesion was established.[15,21,22] Diagnostic procedures, such as bronchoscopy, mediastinoscopy, thoracotomy, or supraclavicular lymph node biopsy, were often avoided because they were considered to be hazardous in the presence of SVCS.[4,15] The traditional therapeutic philosophy was recently challenged.[3,23,24] The reported clinical experience was reassessed, and the safety and importance of diagnostic procedures were reevaluated. Multidrug chemotherapy, sometimes combined with radiation therapy, is potentially curative for small cell carcinoma of the lung and non-Hodgkin's lymphoma even when presented as SVCS. The current practice of using different modalities for different primary causes of SVCS makes the accurate histologic diagnosis of SVCS invaluable. Mediastinal irradiation before biopsy precludes proper interpretation of the specimen in almost half of the patients.[25]

The clinical identification of SVCS is simple, because the symptoms and signs are typical and unmistakable. The chest film shows a mass in most patients. Only 16% of the patients studied by Parish had normal chest films.[9] The most common radiographic abnormalities are superior mediastinal widening and pleural effusion (Table 60–4). A computed tomography (CT) scan provides more detailed information about the SVCS, its tributaries, and other critical structures, such as the bronchi

TABLE 60–4. Chest Radiographic Findings for 86 Patients With Superior Vena Cava Syndrome

Finding	*No. of Patients (%)*
Superior mediastinal widening	55 (64)
Pleural effusion	22 (26)
Right hilar mass	10 (12)
Bilateral diffuse infiltrates	6 (7)
Cardiomegaly	5 (6)
Calcified paratracheal nodes	4 (5)
Mediastinal (anterior) mass	3 (3)
Normal	14 (16)

(Parish JM, et al. Etiologic considerations in SVCS. Mayo Clin Proc 1981;56:407–413)

and the cord.[26] The additional information is necessary because involvement of these structures requires prompt action for relief of pressure. Moncada outlined the advantages of combining a CT scan with CT digital phlebography in SVCS[27]:

1. Detailed resolution of the intrathoracic structures and musculoskeletal anatomy
2. Accurate identification of the site and extent of obstructing thrombus in the SVC and of external compression or invasion by a mediastinal mass
3. Contrast opacification of the venous trunks and collateral circulation sufficient to make confident surgical decisions and to determine late graft patency
4. Accurate guidance for percutaneous biopsy techniques
5. Guidance for radiation therapy to ensure that radiation ports fully encompass the disease
6. Monitoring the effect of therapy.

The role of magnetic resonance imaging (MRI) has been insufficiently investigated but appears promising, especially because this modality is totally noninvasive.[28]

Contrast venography is controversial.[5,29] It provides important information for determining if the vena cava is completely obstructed or remains patient and extrinsically compressed.[29] Dyet and Moghissi demonstrated by venography that 41% of patients with SVCS have patent SVCs that are displaced or involved but not obstructed by tumor.[30] Another 19% have SVC obstruction below the azygos vein, for which collateral venous compression should be adequate. Venography is valuable if surgical bypass is considered for the obstructed vena cava.[31] Lokich stated that venograms are relatively contraindicated because interruption of the integrity of the vessel wall, in the presence of increased intraluminal pressures, may result in excessive bleeding from the puncture site.[15] However, there is no evidence of this complication. Although venography can confirm the clinical diagnosis and outline the anatomy, priority should still be given to procedures that help establish the histolytic diagnosis. Radionuclide technetium 99m venography is an alternate, minimally invasive method of imaging the venous system.[32,33] Although images that are obtained by this method are not as well defined as those that are achieved with contrast venography, they demonstrate patency and flow patterns. Collateral circulation can be evaluated in a general manner and quantified to some degree by radionuclide venography.

In 58% of 107 patients reported by Schraufnagel, SVCS developed before the primary diagnosis was established.[3] The diagnostic procedures that were employed in different studies are summarized in Table 60–5. Sputum cytology established the diagnosis for almost half of the patients. Cytologic diagnosis is as accurate as tissue diagnosis in small cell carcinoma.[35] Bronchoscopy supplies the malignant cells for cytologic evaluation in most cases of small cell disease.[36] In the presence of pleural effusion, thoracocentesis established the diagnosis of malignancy in 71% of the patients. Biopsy of a supraclavicular node, especially if there was a suspicious palpatory finding, was rewarding in two thirds of the reported attempts. Small cell carcinoma of the lung and non-Hodgkin's lymphoma often involve the bone marrow. A biopsy of the bone marrow may provide the diagnosis and stage for these patients.

Mediastinoscopy has a high success rate in providing a diagnosis, but Painter reported complications in five of nine procedures attempted.[34] In 2 patients, the procedure had to be terminated before completion. In 3 patients, complications occurred after the mediastinoscopy, but these complications were managed successfully, and the procedure was diagnostic in each case. Lewis and associates reported their experience in performing cervical mediastinoscopies in 15 patients with SVCS.[37] All mediastinoscopies were diagnostic, and no complications were observed.

Percutaneous transthoracic (CT-guided fine-needle biopsy) is emerging as an effective and safe alternative to an open biopsy or mediastinoscopy.[38] Successful diagnostic transluminal atherectomy has also been reported.[39] A thoracotomy is diagnostic if all other procedures have failed.

Ahmann examined the traditional opinion that diagnostic procedures carry with them significant hazard, primarily excessive bleeding.[15,21,23] He reviewed 843 invasive and semiinvasive diagnostic procedures and found only 10 reported complications, none of them fatal. Ahmann and others found minimal evidence to suggest that diagnostic procedures such as venographies, thoracotomies, bronchoscopies, mediastinoscopies, and lymph node biopsies carry an excessive risk in patients with SVCS.[11,24]

TABLE 60–5. Positive Yield of Diagnostic Procedures for Patients With Superior Vena Cava Syndrome

Procedure	*No. of Procedures*	*No. Positive*	*Percent Positive*
Sputum cytology	59	29	49
Thoracocentesis	14	10	71
Bone marrow biopsy	13	3	23
Lymph node biopsy	95	64	67
Bronchoscopy	124	65	52
Mediastinoscopy	54	44	81
Thoracotomy	49	48	98

TREATMENT

The goals of treatment of SVCS are to relieve the symptoms and to attempt the cure of the primary malignant process. Small cell carcinoma of the lung, non-Hodgkin's lymphoma, and germ cell tumors constitute almost half of the malignant causes of SVCS. These disorders are potentially curable, even in the presence of SVCS. The treatment of SVCS should be selected according to the histologic disorder and stage of the primary process. The prognosis of patients with SVCS strongly correlates with the prognosis of the underlying disease.

SMALL CELL LUNG CANCER

Combination chemotherapy alone or in conjunction with radiation therapy is considered to be the standard treatment for small cell lung cancer. Dombernowsky reported the results of the treatment of 26 patients with small cell carcinoma of the lung presenting with SVCS.[13] Of these 26 patients, 22 were initially treated with combination chemotherapy alone and, in all these patients, the resolution of the SVCS was prompt (median, 7 days). Maddox reported on 56 patients with small cell lung cancer who presented with SVCS.[40] Correction of SVCS was obtained in 64% (9 of 16) of patients treated with radiation alone, in 100% (23 of 23) of those given chemotherapy, and in 83% (5 of 6) of patients receiving combined therapy. The type of treatment did not substantially influence survival.

Among 643 patients with small cell lung cancer, Sculier identified 55 patients (8.5%) with SVCS.[41] One half of the patients developed the manifestations of SVCS before the histologic diagnosis was established. In the rest of the patients, the syndrome developed after the pathologic diagnosis of small cell lung cancer was made but before specific treatment was started. Symptomatic relief of SVCS was obtained in 35 (73%) of 48 patients initially treated with chemotherapy and in 3 (43%) of 7 patients who were initially treated with radiation. Relief of SVCS occurred within 7 to 10 days after initiation of therapy. Fourteen patients had recurrent SVCS after initial treatment. Improvement of recurrent SVCS was obtain in 8 of 12 patients treated with radiation, one of two patients treated with chemotherapy, and three of four patients treated with combined modality.

Spiro analyzed 37 patients with SVCS who, after initial chemotherapy for small cell lung cancer, were randomized to receive chemotherapy alone or radiation therapy followed by more chemotherapy.[42] The addition of a radiation dose of 4000 cGy to the mediastinum did not increase the protection from local recurrence or improve the survival. In several reports, SVCS was not found to be an adverse prognostic for patients with small cell lung cancer.[13,41–43]

Three randomized trials have shown that there is an advantage for combining radiation therapy with chemotherapy over chemotherapy alone in the treatment of limited-disease small cell cancer of the lung.[44–46] The optimal sequence of the two modalities and the dose and fractionation of radiotherapy have not been established. However, the use of combination chemotherapy as the initial modality, with subsequent rapid shrinkage of the tumor, may eliminate the necessity of irradiating a large volume of lung tissue. When chemotherapy is administered, the arm veins should be avoided. Veins of the lower extremities provide an alternative simple venous access.

NON-HODGKIN'S LYMPHOMA

The most extensive experience of treating SVCS secondary to non-Hodgkin's lymphoma is reported from the M. D. Anderson Cancer Center.[14] Twenty-two patients with diffuse large cell lymphoma, and 8 patients with lymphoblastic lymphoma were evaluated for the results of treatment. The patients were treated with chemotherapy alone, chemotherapy combined with irradiation, or with radiotherapy alone. All patients achieved complete relief of SVCS symptoms within 2 weeks of the onset of any type of treatment. No treatment modality appeared to be superior in achieving clinical improvement. The presence of dysphagia, hoarseness, or stridor was a major adverse prognostic factor for patients with lymphoma presenting with SVCS. Eighteen (81%) of 22 patients with large cell lymphoma achieved complete response. Relapse occurred in all 6 patients treated with irradiation alone, in 4 of 7 patients treated with chemotherapy alone, and in 5 of 9 patients treated with chemotherapy and radiotherapy. The median survival was 21 months. All 8 patients with lymphoblastic lymphoma achieved complete response. Six relapses occurred in this group, and all were in sites not initially involved. Median survival was 19 months.

From these results, the researchers concluded that SVCS secondary to lymphoma is rarely an emergency that requires treatment before a histologic diagnosis is made. They recommended that the choice of treatment should be based on the histologic diagnosis and that the patients should undergo, if possible, a complete staging workup before therapy. However, lymphangiography should be avoided to prevent embolization of contrast material that could result in respiratory failure. They advocated chemotherapy as the treatment of choice, because it provides both local and systemic therapeutic activity. They suggested that local consolidation with radiation therapy may be beneficial in patients with large cell lymphoma with mediastinal masses larger than 10 cm.

NONMALIGNANT CAUSES

Patients with nonmalignant causes of SVCS differ significantly from patients with malignant disease. If the cause is not malignant, the patients often have symptoms long before they seek medical advice, it takes more time to establish the diagnosis, and their survival is markedly longer.[3] Schraufnagel reported that the average survival was 9 years if the primary process was benign, compared with an average survival of 5 months for patients with lung cancer.[3] Mahajan reviewed the literature of benign SVCS and reported 16 new cases.[47] Twelve (75%) of these 16 patients had a mediastinal granuloma that was attributed to histoplasmosis. Most patients had an insidious onset of SVCS and were relatively young. Ten patients who were available for a follow-up of 1 to 11 years were all doing well at the time of the report. It was suggested that the good prognosis of patients with benign SVCS caused by fibrosing mediastinitis does not provide a role for SVC bypass surgery.[47,48] However, Nieto and Doty advocate surgery for SVCS caused by benign disorders if the syndrome develops suddenly, progresses, or persists after 6 to 12 months of observation for possible collateral vessel development.[29] In patients whose histoplasmosis complement fixation titers suggest active disease, ketoconazole treatment may prevent recurrent SVCS.[49]

CATHETER-INDUCED OBSTRUCTION

In catheter-induced SVCS, the mechanism of obstruction is usually thrombosis. Streptokinase, urokinase, or recombinant tissue-type plasminogen activator may cause lysis of the thrombus early in its formation.[16,50–53] Heparin and oral anticoagulants may reduce the extent of the thrombus and prevent its progression. Removal of the catheter, if possible, is another option and should be combined with anticoagulation to avoid embolization. In patients for whom electrodes of a pacemaker must be changed, the broken wire should be removed to prevent the risk of developing SVCS.[16,50,54] Percutaneous transluminal angioplasty with or without thrombolytic therapy has been successfully used to open catheter-induced SVC obstructions.[50,55,56]

RADIATION THERAPY

In patients with SVCS as a result of non-small cell carcinoma of the lung, radiotherapy is the primary treatment. The likelihood of relieving the symptoms and signs of SVCS is high, but the overall prognosis for these patients is poor.[3,4,8,23] In Armstrong's series, the 1-year survival for these patients was 17%, and the survival at 2 years declined to 2%.[8]

Radiotherapy has been advocated as standard treatment for most patients with SVCS.[15,21,22] It is employed as the initial treatment if a histologic diagnosis cannot be established and the clinical status of the patient is deteriorating. However, recent reviews suggest that SVC obstruction alone rarely represents an absolute emergency that requires treatment without a specific diagnosis.[11,23,24] The syndrome may be the earliest manifestation of invasive involvement of additional critical structures in the thorax (Table 60–6), such as the bronchi. Under such circumstances, prompt treatment with irradiation may be required without any delay.

TABLE 60–6. Complications of Malignant Invasion

Complication	*No. of Patients* (%)*
Esophagus	
Symptoms of dysphagia or esophageal dysfunction	26 (24)
Anatomic evidence of esophageal invasion	6 (6)
Trachea	
Displaced on examination or roentgenogram	7 (7)
Compressed or invaded by lesion	14 (13)
Vocal cord paralysis	
Unilateral	6 (6)
Bilateral	3 (3)
Pericardium	
Tamponade	3 (3)
Neoplastic invasion at necropsy	6 (6)

* Some patients may have had more than one complication.
(Schraufnagel DE, et al. Superior vena caval obstruction. Am J Med 1981;70:1169–1174)

The fractionation schedule of radiation usually includes two to four large initial fractions of 300 to 400 cGy, followed by conventional fractionation to a total dose of 3000 to 5000 cGy.[4,15,21] Patients treated with initial high-dose fractions showed a slightly faster symptomatic improvement than patients receiving conventional-dose radiation.[8] Improvement within 2 weeks or less was observed in 70% of those treated with initial high-dose fractions and in 56% of patients receiving conventional-dose therapy. This difference was not statistically significant. Serial venograms and autopsies suggest that the symptomatic improvement achieved by radiotherapy is not always due to improvement of flow through the SVC, but it is probably also a result of the development of collaterals after the pressure in the mediastinum is eased.[23]

The field of radiation for SVCS induced by lung cancer should encompass the gross tumors with appropriate margins and the mediastinal, hilar, and supraclavicular lymph nodes. In Armstrong's series, supraclavicular failures occurred in 8 (9%) of 91 patients receiving radiation therapy to the supraclavicular fossae, and 2 (33%) of 6 patients not receiving therapy to these lymph nodes failed at this site.[8]

TRANSLUMINAL ANGIOPLASTY

Percutaneous transluminal angioplasty using balloon technique or insertion of expandable wire stents has been successfully used to open and maintain the patency of the SVC even after maximal-tolerance radiation therapy.[55–60] In two cases, percutaneous atherectomy was used for establishing the histologic diagnosis of SVCS and treatment of the obstruction.[39] In catheter-induced SVCS, administering a thrombolytic agent through the angioplasty device may be therapeutically beneficial.[56]

SURGERY

The experience with successful direct bypass graft for SVC obstruction is limited. It was recommended that autologous grafts of almost the same size as the SVC should be used.[61] Doty used a composite spiral graft, which was constructed from the patient's saphenous vein.[62] He reported 15 years of experience with this procedure in 9 patients with benign obstruction of SVC. Seven maintained patent SVCs, and all patients were relieved of symptoms of SVCS. Avashti reported four successful bypasses of obstructed SVCs using Dacron prostheses.[63]

The preferred bypass route is between an innominate or jugular vein on the left side and the right atrial appendage, using an end-to-end anastomosis.[29] Piccione used the autologous pericardium to reconstruct the SVC after resection for malignant obstruction.[64] In a patient with malignancy-induced SVCS, surgical intervention should be considered only after other therapeutic maneuvers with irradiation and chemotherapy have been exhausted. Most patients with SVCS of benign origin have long survivals without surgical intervention.[47,48] However, if the process progresses rapidly or if there is a retrosternal goiter or aortic aneurysm, surgical intervention may relieve the obstruction.

THROMBOLYTIC THERAPY

Successful experience with thrombolytic agents is limited to the treatment of catheter-induced SVCS.[16,53,65] A review of the response of SVCS to thrombolytic therapy from the Cleveland Clinic showed that the thrombus was effectively lysed in 8 (73%) of 11 patients with a central venous catheter, compared with only 1 of 5 patients who responded to thrombolytic therapy in the absence of a central catheter.[53,66] The higher yield of thrombolytic therapy in patients with catheters is probably related to the mechanism of obstruction, the ability to deliver the agent directly to the thrombus, and to earlier recognition of SVCS in patients with malfunctioning catheters. In the Cleveland Clinic experience, urokinase was more effective than streptokinase, and a delay administering therapy beyond 5 days of symptoms onset was associated with a treatment failure.[53] Favorable experience with recombinant tissue-type plasminogen activator as a thrombolytic agent for catheter-induced SVCS has been reported.[51,52]

GENERAL MEASURES

Medical measures other than specific chemotherapy may be beneficial in temporarily relieving the symptoms of SVCS. Bed rest with the head elevated and oxygen administration can reduce the cardiac output and venous pressure. Diuretic therapy and a reduced-salt diet to reduce edema may have an immediate palliative effect, but the risk of thrombosis enhanced by dehydration should not be ignored. Steroids are commonly used, but their effectiveness has never been properly evaluated. They may improve obstruction by decreasing a possible inflammatory reaction associated with tumor or with irradiation. However, Green and Rubin demonstrated the lack of inflammatory reaction and edema after radiotherapy for experimental SVCS, but documentation in a controlled fashion is lacking.[67] Thrombolytic therapy with urokinase, streptokinase, and recombinant tissue-type plasminogen activator was effective in catheter-induced SVCS.[51–53,65,66]

MANAGEMENT RECOMMENDATIONS

In patients without a clear cause of SVCS, an efficient diagnostic effort should be attempted before any specific treatment. Three deep-cough sputum specimens should be obtained for cytologic analysis. A positive cytologic evaluation provides reliable pathologic information, particularly in the diagnosis of small cell lung carcinoma.[35] If there is pleural effusion, thoracocentesis should be performed and the centrifuge-prepared specimen examined for the presence of malignant cells. If a suspicious lymph node is palpable, particularly in the supraclavicular area, a needle or an open biopsy should be the next diagnostic step. In the absence of positive sputum results, pleural effusion, or accessible suspicious lymph node analysis, a bronchoscopy should be performed, and brushing, washing, and biopsy samples should be obtained for cytologic and histologic analysis. If these efforts do not provide the histologic diagnosis of the primary process, percutaneous transthoracic fine-needle biopsy under CT or fluoroscopic guidance is safe and highly effective.[38,39] In the rare patient for whom less-invasive procedures have failed to establish the diagnosis, the location of the suspicious lesion in the chest and the experience of the surgical team should determine whether mediastinoscopy or thoracotomy be performed.

During the diagnostic process, the patient can benefit from bed rest with the head elevated and with oxygen administration. Some clinicians advocate the use of diuretics and steroids (*e.g.*, 6–10 mg of dexamethasone given orally or intravenously every 6 hours) as a temporary palliative measure if the patient is uncomfortably symptomatic. Anticoagulation is of no proven benefit and may interfere with diagnostic procedures. After the cause of SVCS has been established, treatment of the primary process should promptly follow. Combination chemotherapy with an appropriate regimen is the treatment of choice for small cell lung cancer or non-Hodgkin's lymphoma. Radiation therapy of the lesion and adjacent nodal areas may enhance control after initial response to chemotherapy. Non-small cell lung cancer causing SVCS is best treated with radiation therapy. The incorporation of CT scan information into a carefully designed treatment plan may enable the administration of a total radiation dose above 5000 cGy, which may provide long-term local control for some patients.

Most patients with nonmalignant causes for SVCS have an indolent course and a good prognosis. Percutaneous transluminal angioplasty should be considered an effective alternative to surgery. Surgery is indicated only when the process is rapidly progressing or caused by a retrosternal goiter or an aortic aneurysm. If SVCS is induced by a catheter, the catheter should be removed if possible. Heparin should be administered during the removal of the catheter to prevent embolization. In catheter-induced SVCS, urokinase, streptokinase, or recombinant tissue-type plasminogen activator are of value if used early in the thrombotic process.[51–53,65]

The clinical course of SVCS rarely represents an absolute emergency. In these situations, the bronchus is likely to be obstructed by the same basic process, and irradiation may have to be started immediately, even before the histologic diagnosis is established.

REFERENCES

1. Hunter W. The history of an aneurysm of the aorta, with some remarks on aneurysms in general. Med Observ Inq 1757;1:323–357.
2. Schechter MM. The superior vena cava syndrome. Am J Med Sci 1954;227:46–56.
3. Schraufnagel DE, Hill R, Leech JA, Pare JAP. Superior vena caval obstruction. Is it an emergency? Am J Med 1981;70:1169–1174.
4. Davenport D, Ferree C, Blake D, Raben M. Radiation therapy in the treatment of superior vena caval obstruction. Cancer 1978;42:2600–2603.
5. Rubin P, Hicks GL. Biassociation of superior vena caval obstruction and spinal-cord compression. N Y State J Med 1973;73:2176–2182.
6. Carlson HA. Obstruction of the superior vena cava: An experimental study. Arch Surg 1934;29:669–677.
7. Roswit B, Kaplan G, Jacobson HG. The superior vena cava syndrome in bronchogenic carcinoma. Radiology 1953;61:722–737.
8. Armstrong BA, Perez CA, Simpson JR, Hederman MA. Role of irradiation in the management of superior vena cava syndrome. Int J Radiat Oncol Biol Phys 1987;13:531–539.
9. Parish JM, Marschke RF, Dines DE, Lee RE. Etiologic considerations in superior vena cava syndrome. Mayo Clin Proc 1981;56:407–413.
10. Bell DR, Woods RL, Levi JA. Superior vena caval obstruction: A 10-year experience. Med J Aust 1986;145:566–568.
11. Yellin A, Rosen A, Reichert N, Lieberman Y. Superior vena cava syndrome. The myth—the facts. Am Rev Respir Dis 1990;141:1114–1118.
12. Salsali M, Cliffton EE. Superior vena caval obstruction in carcinoma of lung. N Y State J Med 1969;69:2875–2880.
13. Dombernowsky P, Hansen HH. Combination chemotherapy in the management of superior vena caval obstruction in small-cell anaplastic of the lung. Acta Med Scand 1978;204:513–516.
14. Perez-Soler R, McLaughlin P, Velasquez WS, et al. Clinical features and results of management of superior vena cava syndrome secondary to lymphoma. J Clin Oncol 1984;2: 260–266.
15. Lokich JJ, Goodman R. Superior vena cava syndrome: Clinical management. JAMA 1975;231:58–61.
16. Sculier JP, Feld R. Superior vena cava obstruction system: Recommendation for management. Cancer Treat Rev 1985;12:209–218.
17. Bertrand M, Presant CA, Klein L, Scott E. Iatrogenic superior vena cava syndrome. A new entity. Cancer 1984;54:376–378.
18. Janin Y, Becker J, Wise L, et al. Superior vena cava syndrome in childhood and adolescence: A review of the literature and report of three cases. J Pediatr Surg 1982;17: 290–295.
19. Issa PY, Brihi ER, Janin Y, Slim MS. Superior vena cava syndrome in childhood: Report of ten cases and review of the literature. Pediatrics 1983;71:337–341.
20. Ingram L, Rivera GK, Shapiro DN. Superior vena cava syndrome associated with childhood malignancy: Analysis of 24 cases. Med Pediatr Oncol 1990;18:476–481.
21. Perez CA, Presant CA, Van Amburg AL III. Management of superior vena cava syndrome. Semin Oncol 1978;5:123–134.
22. Scarantino, C, Salazar OM, Rubin R, et al. The optimum radiation schedule in the treatment of superior vena caval obstruction: Importance of ^{99m}Tc scintinangiograms. Int J Radiat Oncol Biol Phys 1979;5:1987–1995.
23. Ahmann FR. A reassessment of the clinical implications of the superior vena cava syndrome. J Clin Oncol 1984;2:961–969.
24. Shimm DS, Lugue GL, Tigsby LC. Evaluating the superior vena cava syndrome. JAMA 1981;245:951–953.
25. Loeffler JS, Leopold KA, Recht A, et al. Emergency prebiopsy radiation for mediastinal masses: Impact on subsequent pathologic diagnosis and outcome. J Clin Oncol 1986;4: 716–721.
26. Yedlicka JW, Schultz K, Moncada R, Flisak M. CT findings in superior vena cava obstruction. Semin Roentgenol 1989;24:84–90.
27. Moncada R, Cardella R, Demos TC, et al. Evaluation of superior vena cava syndrome by axial CT and CT phlebography. AJR 1984;143:731–736.
28. Hansen ME, Spritzer CE, Sostman HD. Assessing the patency of mediastinal and thoracic inlet veins: Value of MR imaging. AJR 1990;155:1177–1182.
29. Nieto AF, Doty DB. Superior vena cava obstruction: Clinical syndrome, etiology and treatment. Curr Probl Cancer 1986;10:442–484.
30. Dyet JF, Moghissi K. Role of venography in assessing patients with superior vena cava obstruction caused by bronchial carcinoma for bypass operations. Thorax 1980;35:628–630.
31. Stanford W, Jolles H, Ell S, Chiu LC. Superior vena cava obstruction: A venographic classification. AJR 1987;148:259–262.
32. Son YH, Wetzel RA, Wilson WA. ^{99m}Tc pertechnetate scintiphotography as diagnostic and follow-up aids in major vascular obstruction due to malignant neoplasm. Radiology 1968;91:349–375.
33. Van Houtte P, Fruhling J. Radionuclide venography in the evaluation of superior vena cava syndrome. Clin Nucl Med 1981;6:177–183.
34. Painter TD, Karpf M. Superior vena cava syndrome: Diagnostic procedures. Am J Med Sci 1983;285;2–6.
35. Yesner R, Gersti B, Auerbach O. Application of the World Health Organization classification of lung carcinoma to biopsy material. Ann Thorac Surg 1965;1:33–49.
36. Ihde DC, Cohen MH, Bernath AM, et al. Serial fiberoptic bronchoscopy during chemotherapy of small cell carcinoma of the lung. Chest 1978;74:531–536.
37. Lewis RJ, Sisler GE, Mackenzie JW. Mediastinoscopy in advanced superior cava obstruction. Ann Thorac Surg 1981;32:458–462.
38. Cosmos L, Haponik EF, Dariak JJ, Summer WR. Neoplastic superior vena caval obstruction: Diagnosis with percutaneous needle aspiration. Am J Med Sci 1987;293:99–102.
39. Dake MD, Zemel G, Dolmatch BL, Katzen BT. The cause of superior vena cava syndrome diagnosis with percutaneous atherectomy. Radiology 1990;174:957–959.
40. Maddox AM, Valdivieso M, Lukeman J, et al. Superior vena cava obstruction in small cell bronchogenic carcinoma. Cancer 1983;52:2165–2172.
41. Sculier JP, Evans WK, Feld R, et al. Superior vena caval obstruction in small cell lung cancer. Cancer 1986;57:847–851.
42. Spiro SG, Shah S., Harper PG, et al. Treatment of obstruction of the superior vena cava by combination chemotherapy with and without irradiation in small-cell carcinoma of the bronchus. Thorax 1983;38:501–505.
43. Van Houtte P, De Jager R, Lustman-Marechal J, Kenis Y. Prognostic value of the superior vena cava syndrome as the presenting sign of small-cell anaplastic carcinoma of the lung. Eur J Cancer 1980;16:1447–1450.
44. Perez CA, Einhorn LH, Oldham RK, et al. Randomized trial of radiotherapy to the thorax in limited small cell carcinoma of the lung treated with multiagent chemotherapy and elective brain irradiation: A preliminary report. J Clin Oncol 1984;2:1200–1208.
45. Perry MC, Eaton WL, Chahinian P, et al. Chemotherapy with or without radiation therapy in limited small cell cancer of the lung. Proc Am Soc Clin Oncol 1986;5:173.
46. Bunn P, Cohen M, Lichter A, et al. Randomized trial of chemotherapy versus chemotherapy plus radiotherapy in limited stage small cell lung cancer. Proc Am Soc Clin Oncol 1983;2:200.
47. Mahajan V, Strimlan V, Van Ordstrand HS, Loop FD. Benign superior cava syndrome. Chest 1975;68:32–35.

48. Effler DB, Groves LK. Superior vena caval obstruction. J Thorac Cardiovasc Surg 1962;43: 574–584.
49. Urshel HC Jr, Razzuk MA, Netto GJ, Disiere J, Chung SY. Sclerosing mediastinitis: Improved management with histoplasmosis titer and ketoconazole. Ann Thorac Surg 1990;50:215–221.
50. Goudevonos JA, Reid PG, Adams PC, Holden MP, Williams DO. Pacemaker-induced superior vena cava syndrome: Report of four cases and review of the literature. PACE 1989;12:1890–1895.
51. Fine DG, Shepherd RF, Welch TJ. Thrombolytic therapy for superior vena cava syndrome. Lancet [Letter] 1989;1:1200–1201.
52. Greenberg S, Kosinski R, Daniels J. Treatment of superior vena cava thrombosis with recombinant tissue type plasminogen activator. Chest 1991;99:1298–1301.
53. Gray BH, Olin JW, Grador RA, Young JR, Bartholomew JR, Ruschhaupt WF. Safety and efficacy of thrombolytic therapy for superior vena cava syndrome. Chest 1991;99: 54–59.
54. Blackburn T, Dunn M. Pacemaker-induced superior vena cava syndrome: Consideration of management. Am Heart J 1988;116:893–896.
55. Grace AA, Sutters M, Schofield PM. Balloon dilation of pacemaker-induced stenosis of the superior vena cava. Br Heart J 1991;65:225–226.
56. Montgomery JH, D'Souza VJ, Dyer RB, et al. Non-surgical treatment of the superior vena cava syndrome. Am J Cardiol 1985;56:829–830.
57. Ali MK, Ewer MS, Balakrishnan PV, et al. Balloon angioplasty for superior vena cava obstruction. Ann Intern Med 1987;107:856–857.
58. Walpole HT Jr, Lovett KE, Chuang VP, West R, Clements SD Jr. Superior vena cava syndrome treated by percutaneous transluminal balloon angioplasty. Am Heart J 1988;115:1303–1304.
59. Capek P, Cope C. Percutaneous treatment of superior vena cava syndrome. AJR 1989;152: 183–184.
60. Putnam JS, Uchida BT, Antonovic R, Rosch J. Superior vena cava syndrome associated with massive thrombosis: Treatment with expandable wire stents. Radiology 1988;167: 727–728.
61. Scherck JP, Kerstein MD, Stansel HC. The current status of vena caval replacement. Surgery 1974;76:209–233.
62. Doty DB, Doty JR, Jones KW. Bypass of superior vena cava. Fifteen years' experience with spiral vein graft for obstruction of superior vena cava caused by benign disease. J Thorac Cardiovasc Surg 1990;99:889–896.
63. Avashti RB, Moghissi K. Malignant obstruction of the superior vena cava and its palliation. J Thorac Cardiovasc Surg 1977;74:244–248.
64. Piccione W Jr, Faber LP, Warren WH. Superior vena caval reconstruction using autologous pericardium. Ann Thorac Surg 1990;50:417–419.
65. Meister FL, McLaughlin TF, Tenney RD, Sholkoff SD. Urokinase. A cost-effective alternative treatment of superior vena cava thrombosis and obstruction. Arch Intern Med 1989;149:1209–1210.
66. Comerota AJ. Safety and efficacy of thrombolytic therapy for superior vena caval syndrome. Chest [Editorial comment] 1991;99:3–4.
67. Green J, Rubin P, Holzwasser G. The experimental production of superior vena cava obstruction. Radiology 1963;81:406–414.

SECTION **2**

THOMAS F. DELANEY
EDWARD H. OLDFIELD

Spinal Cord Compression

Spinal cord or cauda equina compression frequently complicates uncontrolled cancer. It is the second most common neurologic complication of cancer after brain metastasis. At autopsy, its occurrence is documented in approximately 5% of patients with malignancies.[1] Black estimated an annual incidence of 18,000 new cases in the United States.[2] The incidence of spinal cord compression will increase as palliative, noncurative therapies evolve and the population continues to age. Patients rarely die of spinal cord compression, but it is a medical emergency, because delay in treatment often results in irreversible paralysis and loss of sphincter control.

The neurologic status at initiation of treatment is the most significant factor influencing neurologic outcome. This is true despite the tumor type, level of spinal axis involved, degree of systemic tumor involvement, or treatment by radiotherapy or by surgery and radiotherapy. Because successful treatment is much more likely in ambulatory patients who retain intact bowel and bladder control at the start of treatment, early recognition of the problem and initiation of therapy is essential.[3–5] Fortunately, most patients with spinal metastasis have pain and characteristic physical and diagnostic findings that prompt early diagnosis by the astute clinician before significant and irreversible loss of neurologic function occurs. Patients who receive treatment while they are still ambulatory remain ambulatory. Despite this understanding, as many as 80% of patients treated in the last half of the 1980s could not walk at presentation.[6] Patients with a diagnosis of cancer must be advised that the development of back pain is a potentially ominous symptom that should be brought to the attention of their doctors without delay.

PATHOPHYSIOLOGY

Although compression of the spinal cord or the cauda equina can arise from intradural metastases, the spinal involvement is usually extradural.[7,8] Compression usually results from tumor involvement of the vertebral column, affecting a vertebral body or a neural arch.[85] Most often, tumor in the vertebral body presses on the anterior aspect of the dural sac (Fig. 60–1). Progressive tumor expansion posteriorly compresses the spinal cord (or the cauda equina in lesions below the L1–L2 vertebral level) and produces neurologic impairment. Tumor occasionally metastasizes to the epidural space without bone involvement.[9] Paraspinal tumors, such as malignant lymphoma or neuroblastoma, may invade through the intervertebral foramen and compress the cord without bony involvement. No difference in treatment or functional outcome has been reported for lesions involving the cauda equina, and they are discussed with spinal cord compression.[9]

Several models have been used to study the pathophysiology of neurologic dysfunction from compression of the spinal cord by tumor. Tarlov related neurologic recovery after release of mechanically induced cord compression in dogs to the rate of induction and the duration of compression.[10–12] After gradual induction, decompression could be delayed and neurologic function still return. Rapid compression required rapid decompression if paralysis was to be reversed. The recovery of neurologic function was greatly enhanced with incomplete cord compression. Ushio and colleagues induced spinal cord compression by transplanting Walker 256 carcinoma cells into the paravertebral area of rats.[13] They found vasogenic edema in the compressed cord and histologic evidence of neuronal injury. Spinal cord edema and neurologic signs were transiently improved by treating symptomatic animals with dexamethasone.

Siegal and associates demonstrated in rats with neoplastic spinal cord compression that edema in compressed spinal cord segments was associated with a consistent increase in prostaglandin estradiol (PGE_2) production.[14–16] Increased PGE_2 production also occurred in rats with early neurologic dysfunction before development of cord edema.[14] PGE_2 is a

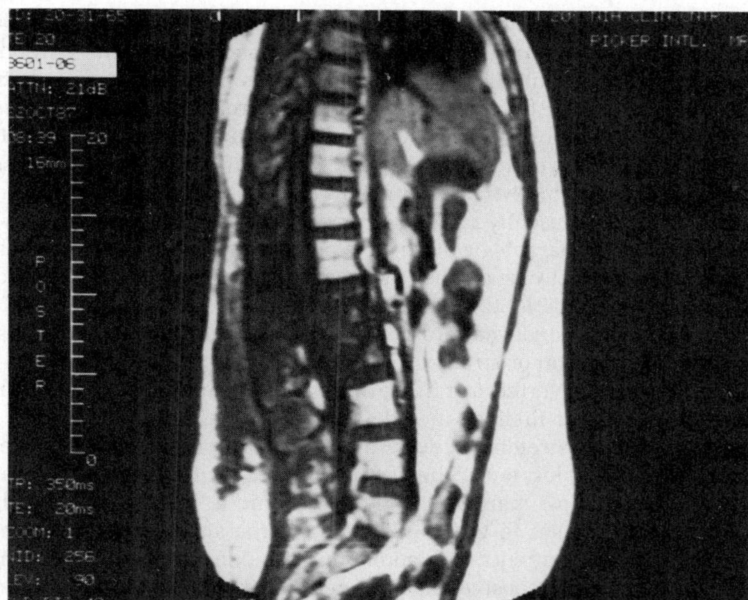

FIGURE 60–1. T1-weighted, sagittal magnetic resonance image of a 21-year-old woman with a Ewing's sarcoma involving the first and second lumbar vertebrae, which appear darker than the uninvolved spine. Tumor has produced structural deformities in the involved vertebral bodies and is compressing the dural sac.

mediator of inflammation and edema.[17] The researchers found that spinal cord specific gravity was higher in untreated rats than in normal controls and that it appeared to be the sum expression of multiple tissue changes.[16] They reported that dexamethasone and indomethacin corrected specific gravity abnormalities and delayed onset of paraplegia.[16] Methylprednisolone, which decreases edema but does not normalize tissue specific gravity, failed to delay the onset of paraplegia.[18]

CLINICAL PRESENTATION

The most common tumors causing spinal cord compression are listed in Table 60–7.[19] Depending on the institution, 8% to 47% of patients present with spinal cord compression as the initial clinical manifestation of malignancy.[1,3,7] More commonly, spinal cord compression occurs in patients with previously diagnosed cancer. The interval from primary diagnosis to epidural cord compression from metastatic disease varies widely with different tumors. Patients with lung cancer usually develop epidural cord compression within a few months after the diagnosis of the primary lesion (average, 6 months).[7] Patients with breast cancer manifest spinal cord compression as long as 20 years (average, 4 years) after presentation of the primary tumor.[3]

The segment of spine involved—approximately 10% cervical, 70% thoracic, and 20% lumbosacral—reflects the number and volume of vertebral bodies in each anatomic segment.[1,3,19–21] Epidural cord compression at one site frequently accompanies spinal involvement elsewhere, which may also threaten the cord. This is particularly true with widely disseminated breast and prostate cancer and with myeloma. Many patients with spinal epidural metastases subsequently develop a second site of epidural metastases. Reported frequencies of second epidural metastases range from 8% to 37%.[22–24] More than 90% of patients present with pain, which is often localized to the spine.[9,80]

Pain, which is usually from involved bone, may be exacerbated by movement, recumbency, cough, sneeze, or strain. The distribution of pain may be radicular.[3,78] Radicular pain localizes the lesion to within one or two vertebral segments. Most patients have pain for weeks to months before the onset of neurologic symptoms.[83] The development of neck or back pain in a patient with cancer should be considered an ominous symptom that requires prompt investigation. Without treatment, the next symptom is usually weakness. This is often accompanied or occasionally preceded by sensory loss.

TABLE 60–7. Relation Between Tumor Type and Spinal Cord Compression

Patients With Cord Compression	*Lung*	*Breast*	*Unknown Primary*	*Lymphoma*	*Myeloma*	*Sarcoma*	*Prostate*	*Kidney*	*Gastro-intestinal*	*Thyroid*	*Other Tumors*
Number	129	94	91	86	68	65	52	44	34	24	116
Percent	16	12	11	11	9	8	7	6	4	3	15

(Adapted from Bruckman JE, Bloomer WD. Management of spinal cord compression. Semin Oncol 1978;5:135–140)

Numbness usually begins in the toes and gradually ascends to the level of cord compression. Weakness combined with sensory loss, particularly loss of proprioception, may produce ataxia. Autonomic dysfunction with urinary retention and constipation usually appears late. Although pain usually precedes the other symptoms by days or weeks, after sensory, motor, or autonomic symptoms or signs develop, progression of myelopathy is usually rapid. Without treatment, complete and irreversible paraplegia often develops over hours to days. Examination usually establishes the level of cord compression and, in a cancer patient, the likely diagnosis.

Signs include tenderness to percussion over the involved spine. Neck flexion or straight leg raising may produce pain over the involved vertebra or in the distribution of an involved nerve root. Motor findings include weakness, spasticity, abnormal muscle stretch reflexes, and extensor plantar responses. Sensory loss occurs below the involved cord segment and is usually most marked distally. If present, a "level" of decreased sensation in the trunk indicates the site of cord compression. In patients with autonomic dysfunction, a palpable bladder, large postvoid urinary residual, or diminished anal tone may be present.

DIAGNOSTIC EVALUATION

The patient's neurologic status influences the nature and tempo of the diagnostic evaluation. Patients with signs or symptoms of spinal cord compression, such as motor impairment, urinary urgency or retention, or ascending numbness, require emergent evaluation and treatment. Patients should be seen by the oncologist, neurologist, radiation oncologist, and neurosurgeon. Dexamethasone should be administered immediately if the history and neurologic examination suggest cord compression.[25] High-dose intravenous dexamethasone (10 mg intravenously followed by 4 mg every 6 hours) may rapidly relieve pain and improve function.[3,21] Animal studies demonstrate reduction in cord edema and a diminished rate of loss of neurologic function with high-dose steroids.[26] The optimal steroid dose in patients has not been established.[86] A small, randomized study found no difference in pain relief and neurologic improvement between a single high-dose intravenous dexamethasone bolus of 10 or 100 mg if followed by 4 mg every 6 hours after the initial bolus.[27] The steroid dosage is tapered after radiation therapy or surgery, as soon as clinical circumstances permit. The serious complications of high-dose steroids (*e.g.*, infection, myopathy, ulcer) can be avoided if the duration of use is not prolonged.[28]

More than two thirds of patients with cord compression have bony abnormalities seen on plain radiographs of the spine.[20,29–31] Spine radiographs are accurate in detecting spinal epidural metastases in as many as 83% of patients with back pain.[22] Findings diagnostic of spinal tumor include erosion and loss of pedicles, partial or complete collapse of vertebral bodies, and paraspinous soft tissue masses. Normal spine films, however, do not exclude epidural metastases. In patients with lymphoma, more than 60% of patients with epidural tumor may have normal spine radiographs.[22]

Although the myelogram has been the standard for diagnosis and localization of epidural cord compression, magnetic resonance imaging (MRI) is increasingly used as the primary study to diagnose and localize spinal metastases.[22,25,32–37] Although several early studies suggested that myelography is slightly more sensitive than MRI (especially if small epidural masses or root compressions are responsible for symptoms), MRI has several advantages over myelography that have led most investigators to recommend MRI as the initial study, to be followed by myelography and computed tomography (CT) only if the MRI is nondiagnostic.[35–39,77]

There are other advantages for MRI.[35,37] Lumbar puncture, which is required for myelogram, is associated with a 16% to 24% rate of rapid neurologic deterioration requiring surgery in patients with complete subarachnoid block.[40] Patients with coagulopathies may experience local bleeding complications with myelography. MRI is noninvasive, less uncomfortable, and safer. MR examinations require 60 to 90 minutes, compared with 90 to 120 minutes for myelography or CT plus myelography.

Identification of paravertebral tumor extension by MRI can be used in designing the fields for radiation therapy and in planning surgery. Because MR images the entire spine and is sensitive in demonstrating bone metastases, it provides important information for designing radiation therapy fields. MRI allows visualization of areas of spinal cord compression that occur between sites of myelographic blocks. In patients with a complete myelographic block, routine myelography after lumbar injection fails to demonstrate the upper extent of the lesion that blocks the flow of contrast and additional rostral lesions that compromise the subarachnoid space, which are present in about 15% of patients. Because such information is important for treatment planning, myelographic demonstration of such lesions requires that contrast be introduced from above through a C1–C2 puncture to demarcate the upper border of the myelographic block and define any other lesions. An alternative approach is CT after metrizamide myelography to define the extent of epidural compressions in patients with complete blocks.[33] Although this approach is less uncomfortable than performing a C1–C2 puncture, it is often less satisfactory in the patient with another spinal lesion above the block.[41]

MRI can differentiate extradural from extramedullary and intramedullary intradural lesions. MRI for suspected epidural cord compression can generally be performed without gadolinium (Gd-DTPA) contrast, although gadolinium enhancement helps differentiate disk herniation, indicates regions of more active tumor for biopsy, and delineates response to therapy.[42] Gadolinium is an essential component of the imaging process for intramedullary and extramedullary intradural lesions. If the MRI is diagnostic, no further imaging is required. If it is negative or equivocal in the face of neurologic signs or symptoms, myelography, with or without CT scanning, is recommended.

Although MRI and CT have eliminated the need for myelography in most patients, myelography is occasionally employed according to the previously outlined guidelines. A spinal needle with a small diameter, 22 gauge or smaller, is used for myelography. Just before instillation of the contrast agent, a small cerebrospinal fluid sample (<2 ml) should be drawn for cytologic, protein, and glucose evaluations. Because of its low viscosity and water solubility, Metrizamide (Amipaque), a nonirritant water-soluble agent, mixes readily with cerebrospinal fluid, travels freely in the subarachnoid space, and provides homogenous diffusion in the cerebrospinal fluid that can be used for CT imaging of the spine after conventional myelography.

For patients with back pain but no neurologic signs the diagnostic evaluation can be performed on an outpatient basis in an expedient manner. Patients with abnormalities on plain films should undergo MRI, because as many as 81% of these patients have epidural tumors.[22] If bone films are normal, bone scintigraphy is indicated, because it is more sensitive than plain films in detecting bony involvement by tumor. Although epidural metastases are uncommon with an abnormal bone scan and normal plain radiographs, the information that the bone scan provides about other bony areas involved by the tumor are helpful in planning and assessing the results of treatment.[22]

TREATMENT

The goals of therapy for patients with epidural spinal neoplasms are recovery or preservation of normal neural function, local tumor control, spinal stability, and pain relief. Because cure is currently not possible for most patients with advanced cancer, palliation is a reasonable objective in the management of spinal metastases.

Several important points about the anticipated response to treatment merit emphasis. Approximately 40% to 60% of all patients treated for epidural cord compression by radiotherapy alone or combined laminectomy and irradiation are ambulatory after treatment.[3,28,21,29–31,43,44,87] The outcome after treatment closely correlates with the degree of neurologic impairment before therapy (Table 60–8). Most ambulatory patients treated with irradiation alone or surgery followed by postoperative irradiation remain ambulatory after treatment.[4–6,28] Paraplegia is a grave prognostic feature; fewer than 10% of adult patients with no voluntary movement in their lower extremities become ambulatory after treatment.[28,30,31] Early diagnosis and initiation of treatment is essential.

For many years, treatment for spinal metastases implied decompressive laminectomy. Laminectomy entails removal of the spinous processes and laminae overlying and one level above and below the site of cord compression (Fig. 60–2). If the tumor involves the posterior bony elements or the tumor is visible in the spinal canal, it is removed. The theoretical basis of the universal application of this procedure, regardless of whether the patient had tumor anterior or posterior to the spinal cord, was that it permitted the cord to move dorsally away from compression by anterior lesions or allowed removal of the offending tumor mass for lesions located posteriorly. However, the results of laminectomy were disappointing. Approximately 30% of patients improved (*i.e.*, ambulatory after treatment), and operative mortality averaged 9%, 11% had nonfatal complications, and 12% were worse after surgery (Table 60–9).[2]

By the early 1980s, several retrospective reviews that compared laminectomy with radiation therapy had demonstrated that irradiation alone produces similar or superior results and less morbidity and mortality than treatments that included laminectomy.[2,3,43,45,46] If all patients are considered, radiotherapy was shown by Gilbert and colleagues[3] and by Black[2] (in a review of reports before 1979) to provide benefit comparable to surgery plus radiation therapy, and irradiation alone and surgery followed by irradiation were superior to surgery alone (see Table 60–9). This finding also applied when patients were analyzed according to the degree of neurologic deficit before treatment. The better the neurologic status of the patient before treatment, the better was the outcome, despite the choice of treatment (see Table 60–8).

As a result of these studies, radiation therapy combined with steroids became the treatment used for most patients. Surgery was recommended only for patients with no previous tissue diagnosis, progressive neurologic dysfunction during irradiation, or recurrent cord compression after previous radiation therapy. However, that surgical management should be limited to decompressive laminectomy to relieve cord compression, regardless of the site of pressure at the circumference of the cord, has been questioned.[47–50] Surgery selected on the basis of the site of tumor involvement in the spinal column (see Fig. 60–2), such as anterior or anterolateral resection of the tumor and involved vertebral body for tumor anterior to the cord and laminectomy only for tumor posterior to the cord, yields results greatly superior to those obtained previously with laminectomy alone.[47–56] For these reasons, the role of surgery in patients with epidural cord compression and metastatic tumor is being reconsidered.

Because there is no definitive prospective study that compares current treatments under similar conditions, absolute recommendations for management of patients with spinal metastases cannot be made. Clinical experience and published reports indicate that radiotherapy and surgery are effective treatments to be used alone or in combination as required by the circumstances of the patients. Chemotherapy is effective treatment for selected patients. The choice of treatment depends on the clinical presentation, the availability of a his-

TABLE 60–8. Effect of Pretreatment Motor Function on Treatment Outcome

	Laminectomy and Irradiation		*Irradiation Only*	
Pretreatment Condition	*No. Ambulatory/ No. Treated*	*Percent Ambulatory*	*No. Ambulatory/ No. Treated*	*Percent Ambulatory*
Ambulatory	14/22	64	46/58	79
Paraparetic	15/33	45	37/83	45
Paraplegic	1/10	10	1/29	3

(Adapted from Gilbert RW, Kim JH, Posner JB. Epidural spinal cord compression from metastatic tumor: Diagnosis and treatment. Ann Neurol 1978;3:40)

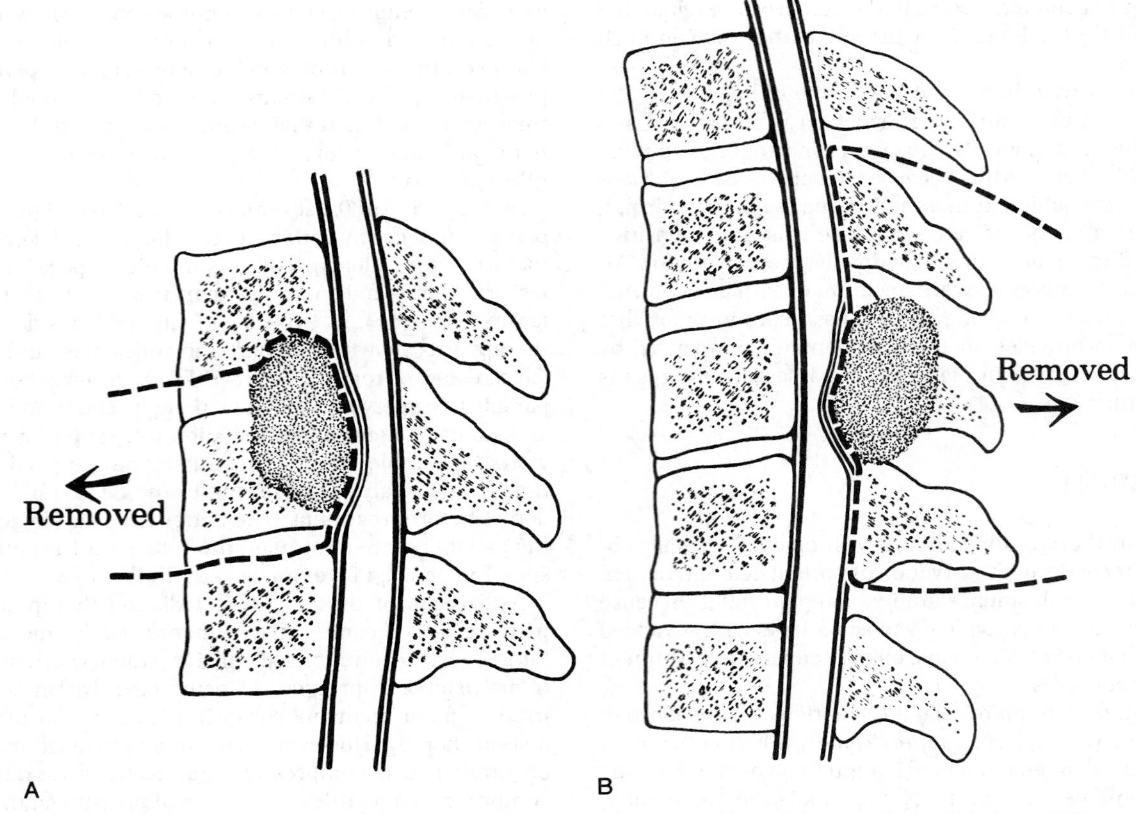

FIGURE 60–2. **(A)** Most spinal metastases occur in the vertebral column anterior to the spinal canal. If surgery is indicated for tumors anterior to the spinal canal, surgical excision of the tumor and involved vertebral body with immediate stabilization of the spinal column effectively reverses compression of the spinal cord. **(B)** Spinal cord compression by tumors posterior to the spinal canal can be successfully relieved by laminectomy (*i.e.*, removal of the laminae and spinous processes one level above and one level below the site of tumor) and tumor excision.

tologic diagnosis, the rapidity of the clinical course, the tumor type, the site of spinal involvement, the stability of the spine, and the nature of any previous treatment. However, it is reasonably clear when irradiation or surgery should be used, and definite recommendations can be made for the management of most patients.

SURGERY

Although epidural tumors located lateral or posterior to the spinal canal in the laminae or pedicles can be readily removed by laminectomy, tumor involvement of the vertebral body limits the potential for improvement after laminectomy. This was observed by Wright as early as 1963.[30] In 81 patients with metastatic spinal tumor treated with laminectomy, 38% of the patients with lateral or posterior compartment tumor had a satisfactory outcome, but only 19% with vertebral involvement were improved. Correlation of tumor location with outcome after laminectomy was studied by Hall and McKay, who found that 35% to 39% of patients with tumors in the posterior elements of the spinal canal (*i.e.*, removable by laminectomy) improved compared with only 9% with tumors anterior to the spinal canal.[57]

Laminectomy frequently fails to relieve neurologic deficits or myelographic block in patients with ventral compression of the spinal cord due to tumor in a vertebral body or due to pathologic collapse of a vertebra with posterior migration of the bony elements into the anterior aspect of the spinal canal. Many patients with radiosensitive tumors with associated structural changes in the spine and cord compression cannot be relieved, even if the local tumor is effectively treated by irradiation. Removal of the neural arches at laminectomy can produce spinal instability and increase neurologic deficits.[58] In patients with structural instability of the spinal column as a result of metastatic tumor, restoration and maintenance of spinal stability represents an important goal of therapy and one that can only be successfully accomplished with surgery.[79] The overall unsatisfactory results with laminectomy may not reflect the potential results of surgery, but those produced by an unselective surgical strategy.

Several reports indicate the importance of selecting the surgical approach on the basis of location of the tumor mass or bone encroachment on the spinal canal.[47–56,59,82] Because 85% of epidural tumors arise in a vertebral body and remain largely anterior to the spinal cord, the focus of the surgical procedure for most patients should be the involved vertebral body. A posterolateral approach is used for thoracic lesions and for many lumbar lesions. For cervical and certain lumbar lesions, a more direct anterior approach is used. The intervertebral disks and the vertebral body are removed. All tumor

TABLE 60–9. Results of Therapies for Spinal Cord Compression

Treatment	*No. of Patients*	*Ambulatory Patients After Treatment*	
		No.	*Mean %*
Laminectomy*	275	85	31
Radiotherapy*	387	176	45
Laminectomy plus radiotherapy*	216	111	51
Vertebral body resection†‡	101	78	78
Selective surgery†§	140	117	84
Vertebral body resection for anterior tumor	108	101	94
Laminectomy for posterior tumor	32	16	50

* Cumulative data from several published series. Each series consisted of a heterogenous group of metastatic tumors. (Adapted from Black P. Spinal metastasis: Current status and recommended guidelines for management. Neurosurgery 1979;5:726)
† Radiotherapy in addition to surgery in most patients.
‡ Includes only patients with vertebral body involvement with tumor. (Data from Sundaresan N, Galicich JH, Lane JM, et al. Treatment of neoplastic epidural cord compression by vertebral body resection and stabilization. J Neurosurg 1985;63:676)
§ Treatment selected on basis of site of spinal involvement—whether the vertebral body or the neural arch was involved by tumor. (Data combined from Siegal T, Siegal T. Surgical decompression of anterior and posterior malignant epidural tumors compressing the spinal cord: A prospective study. Neurosurgery 1985;17:424 and Sundaresan N, Digiacinto GV, Hughes JEO, et al. Treatment of neoplastic spinal cord compression: Results of a prospective study. Neurosurgery 1991;29:645)

and devitalized bone are removed down to the dura. Various techniques for spinal stabilization permit tumor excision and structural stabilization of the spine during the same operation and with one operative approach.[47–56,59,60]

Sundaresan and associates treated 101 consecutive patients with epidural cord compression by vertebral body resection, tumor excision, and immediate stabilization.[50] Patients received surgery who had a pathologic compression fracture as the presenting feature of malignancy, a solitary site of tumor relapse, destruction of the spine by a paraspinous tumor, a known radioresistant tumor (*e.g.*, melanoma, sarcoma, kidney tumor), a structural abnormality of the spine producing compression of the spinal cord, or segmental instability of the spine after previous local treatment with irradiation. Of the 101 patients, 78 (78%) left the hospital walking (including 51 patients who had local tumor relapse after a full course of radiation therapy). Thirty-two (70%) of 46 patients who were nonambulatory before treatment were ambulatory, with or without support, at hospital discharge. Pain relief was achieved in 85% of the patients with significant back or radicular pain. The incidence of complications—8 patients died within 30 days and 10% had nonfatal complications—was considered acceptable. The median survival of all patients was 8 months, and 37% lived longer than 1 year after treatment. Similar results were reported by Harrington.[47]

Siegal and Siegal treated 167 episodes of cord compression prospectively by a standard protocol in which the selection of the surgical approach, when surgery was indicated, depended on the tumor location.[70] This was the first study in which selection of the appropriate surgical approach (*i.e.*, anterior versus posterior based on the site of neoplastic cord compression) was carried out according to strict criteria. Because most tumors arise anteriorly, most patients received vertebral body resection. Irradiation was the primary therapy for patients who had poor general medical status, had multiple myelographic blocks, were paraplegic for longer than 72 hours, or had previously diagnosed radiosensitive tumors without previous radiation treatment. Of the 18 patients with radiosensitive tumors who were treated only with irradiation, 13 (72%) were ambulatory after treatment. Surgical treatment was assigned primarily to 86 patients who had no previous histologic diagnosis of their tumor, who received previous treatment with irradiation at the involved site, who had a known radioresistant tumor (*e.g.*, osteogenic sarcoma, melanoma, giant cell tumor of bone), or who developed neurologic deterioration during radiation treatment. Twenty-five patients had posterior or posterolateral tumor and received laminectomy for tumor removal, decompression of the spinal cord, and if indicated, spinal fixation with spinal rods and bone cement for instability. Although 25% of this group deteriorated as a direct result of surgery, 40% were ambulatory after surgery (92% of this group were nonambulatory before surgery), and normal sphincter control was achieved in 57% (76% were incontinent preoperatively).

Sixty-one patients had anterior tumors and received vertebral body resections; 55 (91%) had spinal instability and received immediate internal spinal fixation using acrylic replacement of the involved vertebral body. The 30-day mortality rate for this group was 7%, 80% were ambulatory within 30 days (72% of this group were nonambulatory preoperatively), 93% had normal sphincter control (41% were incontinent preoperatively), and although 97% had persistent pain before treatment, complete pain relief was obtained in 56% after surgery. The median survival of these patients was 16 months. The high ambulation rate, which was superior to that generally reported for irradiation alone, occurred although more than half of the patients treated by vertebral body resection had relapsed after receiving previous irradiation.

In a study of 54 patients who prospectively received surgery with a approach based on the tumor site, all patients were ambulatory after surgery, including the 24 patients who could not walk before surgery (completely paraplegic patients were excluded from the study prospectively).[51] Twenty-three of the 25 patients who survived at 2 years continued to be ambulatory.

These studies indicate that proper patient selection and the choice of surgical approach based on the tumor location are prerequisites for successful surgery. Laminectomy, which is the generally accepted surgical approach to the treatment of metastatic epidural mass lesions, is ineffective and can be harmful when the pathologic process is anterior to the spinal cord. The outcome of a selective surgical approach (*i.e.*, 80% ambulation and 93% sphincter control) is superior to results obtained by irradiation alone or irradiation combined with laminectomy (see Tables 60–8 and 60–9). It remains to be determined if similar results can be achieved in the unselected population of cancer patients seen at most general hospitals, where most patients are treated.

If surgical decompression is to be used, excision of the tumor, adequate decompression of the spinal cord, and correction of any significant spinal deformity must be accomplished. To ensure optimal exposure for tumor removal and decompression at the site of direct pressure on the spinal cord, posterior lesions are approached posteriorly by a wide laminectomy, and anterior and anterolateral lesions receive anterior or anterolateral resection of the tumor and the involved vertebral body. Complete tumor removal should be attempted, because early relapse of myelopathy after radiotherapy usually occurs in the same region from regrowth of residual tumor.[23] For instability of the spine, fusion should be performed during the same procedure by instrumentation with or without methylmethacrylate reconstruction, which produce immediate stability. Neurologic improvement is due to correctly directed and efficient decompression of the spinal cord and to immediate stabilization of the spinal column. Local pain in patients with spinal metastases often results from segmental spinal instability. This is suggested by demonstration of a collapsed vertebra and by pain that is relieved by immobilization, bed rest, or traction. Immediate spinal stability enhances rehabilitation by permitting immediate ambulation, if neurologic recovery allows, and eliminates pain from segmental instability.

Children with metastatic sarcoma (*e.g.*, Ewing's sarcoma, soft tissue sarcoma, osteogenic sarcoma, rhabdomyosarcoma) seem to be an exception to the previously described recommendations. Pediatric tumors frequently enter the spinal canal by the intervertebral foramen and compress the cord circumferentially, which permits laminectomy to accomplish decompression. In one large series, 66% of children (all tumor types) with no motor or sensory function below the level of compression became ambulatory after laminectomy combined with irradiation or medical therapy.[61]

RADIATION THERAPY

Response to treatment with irradiation alone is well established. An early report by Mones and colleagues described a favorable response, defined as the ability to ambulate, in 14 (34%) of 41 patients with epidural cord compression treated only with radiation therapy.[45] Response to treatment was excellent in their patients with radioresponsive tumors, such as lymphoma, Ewing's sarcoma, and neuroblastoma, less satisfactory in patients with metastatic breast cancer and poor in patients with lung cancer.[45] Complete or partial reversal of neurologic deficits occurred in 41% of 82 additional patients treated similarly at the same hospital.[62] Paraplegic patients had limited responses, with only 16% improved compared with 58% of patients with some initial motor function.

Gilbert and associates at Memorial Hospital retrospectively reviewed the clinical findings and results of treatment in 130 consecutive patients who were treated for epidural spinal cord compression by irradiation alone or laminectomy followed by irradiation.[3] No significant differences in treatment outcomes were seen. After treatment, 49% of patients who received irradiation alone walked, compared with 46% of those who received surgery and postoperative irradiation. The duration of improvement in the two treatment groups was similar, with approximately 75% of patients ambulatory after treatment remaining so for 6 months or longer. Patients with radioresponsive tumors generally received irradiation, as did most who were paraplegic at presentation and felt to have little chance to recover after laminectomy. Patients without prior histologic diagnosis, those who had previously received spinal irradiation, and patients with rapidly progressing myelopathy usually received surgery. Regardless of the treatment chosen, 73% of ambulatory patients remained so, 36% of the paraparetic patients (*i.e.*, nonambulatory but able to lift the legs) regained ambulation, but only 1 of 39 paraplegic patients improved. Tumors considered radioresponsive (*e.g.*, seminoma, lymphoma myeloma, Ewing's sarcoma, neuroblastoma) responded better to either therapy than less radioresponsive tumors (*e.g.*, carcinomas, melanoma, soft tissue sarcomas). Patients with rapid progression of spinal cord dysfunction, formerly considered an indication for surgery, improved more often with irradiation alone than with decompressive laminectomy followed by irradiation. Of the 9 patients with weakness that developed over less than 48 hours who underwent surgical decompression, none improved, but 7 of 13 patients irradiated without surgery improved. Autonomic dysfunction predisposed to a worse outcome after treatment. Of 65 patients with urinary incontinence or retention before treatment, 43 (66%) were or became nonambulatory, but inability to walk occurred in fewer than 50% of patients without autonomic dysfunction.

Recovery of motor function and ambulation in patients presenting with complete paralysis may be delayed for some time after irradiation. Helweg-Larsen reported recovery of ambulation in 5 patients and recovery of motor function in a sixth among 15 patients who presented with total leg paralysis and underwent irradiation.[63] Recovery in these patients occurred 3 to 18 months after treatment. The duration of paralysis before treatment ranged from 1 to 10 days. The median time from initial motor symptoms to total paralysis was longer (45 days) in the 6 patients who recovered than the 9 who remained paralyzed (9 days). This observation is consistent with the experimental observations of Tarlov for mechanically induced cord compressions in dogs.[10–12]

Greenberg and colleagues administered high-dose dexamethasone (100 mg) at diagnosis and began radiation therapy within several hours.[21] After daily doses of 500 cGy for the first 3 days of treatment, 300 cGy/day were given to a total dose of 3000 cGy. Dexamethasone was continued at 96 mg daily in divided doses for 3 days and then tapered during the course of radiation therapy if symptoms permitted. They compared their results with those from the same institution by Gilbert and associates and reported no differences in outcome with the new treatment program.[3] They did, however, find a substantial reduction in pain in 64% of patients in the first day of treatment, which they attributed to dexamethasone, because improvement occurred even before the initiation of irradiation in 6 patients. The optimal steroid regimen is not established.

Cobb and colleagues reported the retrospective analysis of 44 patients with epidural cord compression from metastatic breast cancer, 26 of whom received initial laminectomy and 18 of whom received initial radiotherapy.[43] No significant difference in treatment outcome occurred, with 75% of ambulatory patients remaining so. Deterioration of neurologic function developed in 6 patients undergoing initial radiation therapy. Two of these patients underwent decompressive laminectomy, with a favorable outcome for 1 patient. The researchers highlight the need for close neurologic examination during radiotherapy and recommend surgery in patients who show evidence of neurologic deterioration during irradiation.

Although the number of patients is small, one randomized, prospective study compared the outcome in 16 patients who underwent decompressive laminectomy plus radiotherapy with 13 patients who received irradiation only.[46] There were no significant differences in outcome between the two groups.

The effect of the type of tumor on outcome of treatment with irradiation is difficult to assess, because of the relatively small numbers of patients with each specific histologic diagnosis in any single series. Pooled data may not account for difference in ambulatory status, treatment techniques, and dose. Nevertheless, the results reported suggest excellent outcomes after irradiation with lymphomas and myelomas, good results in patients with prostate, breast, and renal cancers and generally disappointing results in patients with lung carcinomas.[3,19,21,28,43,45,46,64,65] Herbert and associates reported that a treatment program of radiation therapy with or without laminectomy was effective in palliating the symptoms of epidural cord compression caused by metastatic melanoma.[66] Improvement was seen in 86% of treated sites and was complete in 30%. A radiation dose of more than 3000 cGy was significantly associated with the probability of a complete response.

Radiation therapy portals are designed using information from the history and physical examination, spine radiographs, MRI or myelography, bone scan if available, and CT scans if indicated. MRI scans or myelograms are mandatory for radiation therapy treatment planning for patients with neurologic symptoms or signs. Calkins and colleagues showed that myelography influenced field size in 69% of patients.[32] Even in patients with discrete bony lesions, results of myelography affected treatment 45% of the time.

After the diagnosis of spinal cord compression is established, high-dose steroid therapy should be started. Patients who are to undergo irradiation should start treatment immediately after diagnosis. The radiation portal includes the site of the epidural disease and in addition should extend two vertebral bodies above and below.[3,23] Because in one series all second subsequent sites of epidural metastasis occurring within 7 months of initial treatment appeared within two vertebral bodies of the original site of disease, these guidelines appear prudent.[23] Modification may be necessary, depending on previous radiation portals and other sites of tumor seen on bone radiographs or scans. Paravertebral tumor should be included if possible in the treatment field. For cervical spine lesions, parallel-opposed lateral portals are usually employed. Most thoracic lesions can be treated with a single posterior field, generally prescribing to a depth of 6 cm.[84] Because the anterior edge of the lumbar spine is near the midline, lesions of the lumbar spine generally require parallel-opposed anteroposterior fields. This technique avoids overdosage to the spinal cord from a single posterior field.

The optimal radiation dose and fractionation scheme have not been established, but several guidelines are available. Spinal cord tolerance to irradiation cannot be exceeded. The radiation therapy should be delivered such that the rapidity of tumor regression and the probability of disease control in the irradiated volume is maximized. Friedman and associates demonstrated a good response in 71% of patients who received more than than 2500 cGy for epidural cord compression from malignant lymphoma, compared with 34% in the group that received 2500 cGy or less.[67] No clear dose-response relation has been demonstrated for other histologies except melanoma, although higher doses (time-dose fraction >60.5) appear to reduce the rate of recurrence within the original treatment field.[24] Commonly employed doses are 3000 to 4000 cGy over 2 to 4 weeks.

Experimental data for rats with epidural cord compression secondary to lymphoma or carcinoma demonstrate more rapid neurologic recovery after large daily fractions of radiation (500 cGy) than after smaller daily doses (100–200 cGy).[26,68] Fractionated doses provide more prolonged functional improvement than large single-dose treatment in rats.[26] Large initial fractions (300–400) cGy are advocated for the first 3 days of therapy, which are followed by smaller daily doses (150–300 cGy).[21,69] Despite concerns about irradiation-induced edema from large fractions, experimental evidence fails to confirm its development.[68,71,81]

CHEMOTHERAPY

Several reports describe successful chemotherapy for epidural cord compression for tumors known to be responsive to chemotherapy (*e.g.*, lymphomas, germ cell neoplasms, neuroblastoma, Ewing's sarcoma).[70,72–74] Experiments with the Walker 256 carcinoma cell line in the rat show that cyclophosphamide is more effective for relieving the neurologic signs of cord compression than laminectomy or 1500 cGy of irradiation delivered in three fractions.[26] Hayes and colleagues reported 9 children with neuroblastoma and 5 children with Ewing's sarcoma who had epidural cord compression by tumor.[70] Five children received laminectomy before referral, but only 1 had neurologic recovery. The other 9 patients did not undergo surgery. All 14 patients received chemotherapy with rapid regression of tumor and neurologic deficits.

Chemotherapy is a feasible alternative to laminectomy and irradiation in the management of certain types of epidural tumors. In infants and children, in whom growth inhibition from irradiation may be significant, it seems reasonable to consider chemotherapy for sensitive tumors, as long as the patients are closely monitored by the oncologist, radiation oncologist, and neurosurgeon so that other interventions may be quickly undertaken if needed. Children with severe canal encroachment by tumor (near complete or complete) demonstrated by myelography or filling more than 50% of the spinal canal on MR scans should be considered for laminectomy. Twenty-five of 26 such patients undergoing laminectomy improved or stabilized, compared with 4 of 7 patients who were treated without surgery in one report.[75]

Friedman and associates reported 2 adult patients with testicular cancers who had neurologic recovery after successful decompression of an epidural cord compression by chemotherapy with cyclophosphamide, bleomycin, vinblastine, and cisplatin.[73] In the adult patient with epidural cord compression from metastatic tumor that is responsive to chemotherapy, the physician should consider adding chemotherapy to surgery or irradiation or using chemotherapy if surgery or irradiation are not tenable.

CONCLUSION

Epidural spinal cord compression is an oncologic emergency that requires prompt evaluation and treatment. Because the best results of treatment of spinal metastases are obtained if there is minimal loss of neurologic function, early diagnosis and treatment are the most important elements of successful treatment. Evaluation should include a careful physical examination, complete spine radiographs, spinal MRI or complete myelography (including cervical myelography in cases of complete block), and if indicated, bone scintigraphy or CT. Patients should be assessed at presentation by the medical or pediatric oncologist, neurologist, radiation oncologist, and neurosurgeon. Corticosteroids should be started after the diagnosis is established.

Although there is no definitive prospective study that compares current treatments under similar conditions, it is reasonably clear when irradiation or surgery should be used, and recommendations can be made for the management of most patients as outlined in Table 60–10. Radiation therapy is recommended as initial treatment for patients with cord compression who have radiation-sensitive tumors that are not associated with spinal instability. Patients who have spinal involvement by tumor that is neither causing neurologic symptoms nor spinal instability should be treated initially with radiation therapy. Patients whose neurologic status deteriorates during radiation therapy and patients who relapse at the site of previous irradiation should undergo surgery. Surgery should be the initial treatment for patients with a pathologic fracture resulting in spinal instability or compression of the spinal cord by bone and in patients with radiation-resistant tumors. Surgery has traditionally been the initial treatment in patients without a previous tissue diagnosis. The use of percutaneous needle biopsy to determine the histology has been proposed as a reliable and logical approach to deciding on the treatment modality.[76] If surgery is indicated, the surgical procedure should be based on the site of tumor involvement by using the appropriate anterior or posterior approach. Because of the difficulty of completely resecting tumor adjacent to the spinal cord, surgery should be followed by postoperative radiation therapy as long as the spinal cord tolerance is not exceeded.

Chemotherapy may be used as an adjuvant in adult patients with tumors responsive to chemotherapy or as primary therapy if irradiation or surgery are not tenable. In selected pediatric patients with chemosensitive tumors, chemotherapy may be considered for initial treatment if the patients are closely monitored for any signs of progressive neurologic dysfunction during chemotherapy. We emphasize that the most appropriate treatment in each case is also the most effective if instituted before major neurologic dysfunction develops.

TABLE 60–10. Recommendations for Management of Patients With Spinal Metastases*

Radiation Therapy Only

Known radiation-sensitive tumor and no spinal instability (regardless of rate of progression or neurologic condition)

Spinal involvement without spinal instability or neurologic deficit

Surgery† Followed by Radiation

Pathologic fracture with spinal instability or compression of the spinal cord by bone

Radiation-resistant tumor with neurologic deficit

Unknown tissue diagnosis (if a radiosensitive tumor is suspected, needle biopsy can provide the diagnosis)

Surgery† Only

Relapse at the site of previous irradiation

Failure to respond to radiation therapy

Chemotherapy

Pediatric patients with responsive tumors

Adjuvant treatment in adult patients with responsive tumors

Relapse of a responsive tumor at site of previous irradiation and surgery

* Steroid therapy should be used in the early phases of therapy with radiation, surgery, or chemotherapy.

† Surgery should be based on the site of tumor (anterior versus posterior).

REFERENCES

1. Barrons KD, Hirano A, Araki S, Terry RD. Experiences with metastatic neoplasms involving the spinal cord. Neurology (Minn) 1959;9:91.
2. Black P. Spinal metastasis: Current status and recommended guidelines for management. Neurosurgery 1979;5:726.
3. Gilbert RW, Kim JH, Posner JB. Epidural spinal cord compression from metastatic tumor: Diagnosis and treatment. Ann Neurol 1978;3:40.
4. Sorensen PS, Borgensen SE, Rohde K, et al. Metastatic epidural spinal cord compression: Results of treatment and survival. Cancer 1990;65:1502.
5. Maranzano E, Latini P, Checcaglini F, et al. Radiation therapy in metastatic cord compression. A prospective analysis of 105 consecutive patients. Cancer 1991;67:1311.
6. Kim RY, Spencer SA, Meredith RF, et al. Extradural spinal cord compression: Analysis of factors determining functional prognosis. Radiology 1990;176:279.
7. Stark RJ, Henson RA, Evans SJW. Spinal metastases. A retrospective survey from a general hospital. Brain 1982;105:189.
8. Meyer PC, Reah TG. Secondary neoplasms of the central nervous system and meninges. Br J Cancer 1953;7:438.
9. Posner JB. Spinal cord compression: A neurologic emergency. Clin Bull 1971;1:65.
10. Tarlov IM, Klinger H, Vitale S. Spinal cord compression studies. I. Experimental techniques to produce acute and gradual compression. Arch Neurol Psychiatry 1957;70:813.
11. Tarlov IM, Klinger H. Spinal cord compression studies. II. Time limits for recovery after acute compression in dogs. Arch Neurol Psychiatry 1954;71:271.
12. Tarlov IM. Spinal cord compression studies. III. Time limits for recovery after gradual compression in dogs. Arch Neurol Psychiatry 1954;71:588.
13. Ushio Y, Posner R, Posner JB, Shapiro WR. Experimental spinal cord compression by epidural neoplasms. Neurology 1977;27:422.
14. Siegal T, Shohami E, Siegal TZ. Indomethacin and dexamethasone treatment in experimental spinal cord compression. Part II. Effect on edema and prostaglandin synthesis. Neurosurgery 1988;22:334–339.
15. Siegal T, Siegal TZ, Shapira Y, et al. Experimental neoplastic spinal cord compression. Evoked potentials, edema, prostaglandins, and light and electron microscopy. Spine 1987;12:440.
16. Siegal T, Siegal TZ, Sandbank U, et al. Indomethacin and dexamethasone treatment in experimental spinal cord compression. Part I. Effect on water content and specific gravity. Neurosurgery 1988;22:328.
17. Johnson M, Corey F, McMillan RM. Alternative pathways of arachidonate metabolism: Prostaglandins, thromboxane, and leukotrienes. Essays Biochem 1983;19:41.
18. Siegal T, Siegal TZ. Current considerations in the management of neoplastic spinal cord compression. Spine 1989;14:223.
19. Bruckman JE, Bloomer WD. Management of spinal cord compression. Semin Oncol 1978;5:135.
20. Torma T. Malignant tumors of the spine and the spinal epidural space. A study based on 250 histologically verified cases. Acta Chir Scand 1957;225:1.
21. Greenberg HS, Kim JH, Posner JB. Epidural spinal cord compression from metastatic tumor: Results with a new treatment protocol. Ann Neurol 1980;8:361.
22. Rodichok LD, Harper GR, Ruckdeschel JC, et al. Early diagnosis of spinal epidural metastases. Am J Med 1981;70:1181.
23. Kaminski HJ, Diwan VG, Ruff RC. Second occurrence of spinal epidural metastases. Neurology 1991;41:744.
24. Loeffler JS, Glicksman AS, Tefft M, Gelch M. Treatment of spinal cord compression: A retrospective analysis. Med Pediatr Oncol 1983;11:347.

25. Portenoy RK. Lipton RB, Foley KM. Back pain in the cancer patient: An algorithm for evaluation and management. Neurology 1987;37:134.
26. Ushio Y, Posner R, Kim J, et al. Treatment of experimental spinal cord compression caused by extradural neoplasms. J Neurosurg 1977;47:380.
27. Vecht CJ, Haaxma-Reiche H, Van Putten WLJ, et al. Initial bolus of conventional versus high-dose dexamethasone in metastatic spinal cord compression. Neurology 1989;39: 1255.
28. Martenson JA Jr, Evans RG, Lie MR, et al. Treatment outcome and complications in patients treated for malignant epidural spinal cord compression (SCC). J Neurol Oncol 1985;3:77.
29. Wild WO, Porter RW. Metastatic epidural tumor of the spine. A study of 45 cases. Arch Surg 1963;87:137.
30. Wright RL. Malignant tumors in the spinal extradural space: Results of surgical treatment. Ann Surg 1963;157:227.
31. White WA, Patterson RH, Bergland RM. Role of surgery in the treatment of spinal cord compression by metastatic neoplasm. Cancer 1971;27:55B.
32. Calkins AR, Olson MA, Ellis JH. Impact of myelography on the radiotherapeutic management of malignant spinal cord compression. Neurosurgery 1986;19:614.
33. Fink IJ, Garra BS, Zabell A, Doppman JL. Computed tomography with metrizamide myelography to define the extent of spinal canal block due to tumor. J Comput Assist Tomogr 1984;8:1072.
34. Aichner F, Poewe W, Rogalsky W, et al. Magnetic resonance imaging in the diagnosis of spinal cord diseases. J Neurol Neurosurg Psychiatry 1985;48:1220.
35. Harnsberger HR, Dillon WP. The radiologic role in diagnosis, staging and follow-up of neoplasia of the brain, spine, and head and neck. Semin Ultrasound CT MR 1989;10: 431.
36. Smoker WRK, Godersky JC, Knutzon RK, et al. The role of MR imaging in evaluating metastatic spinal disease. AJNR 1987;8:901.
37. Sarpel S, Sarpel G, Yu E, et al. Early diagnosis of spinal-epidural metastasis by magnetic resonance imaging. Cancer 1987;59:1112.
38. Hagenau C, Grosh W, Currie M, et al. Comparison of spinal magnetic resonance imaging and myelography in cancer patients. J Clin Oncol 1987;5:1663.
39. McAfee PC, Bohlman HH, Han JS, Salvagno RT. Comparison of nuclear magnetic resonance imaging and computed tomography in the diagnosis of upper cervical spinal cord compression. Spine 1986;11:295.
40. Hollis PH, Malis LI, Zappullo RA. Neurological deterioration after lumber puncture below complete spinal subarachnoid block. J Neurosurg 1986;64:253.
41. Johansen JG, Orrison WW, Amundsen P. Lateral C1–2 puncture for cervical myelography. Part 1: Report of a complication. Radiology 1983;146:391.
42. Sze G, Krol G, Zimmerman RD, et al. Malignant extradural spinal tumors: MR imaging with Gd-DTPA. Radiology 1988;167:217.
43. Cobb CA III, Leavens ME, Eckles N. Indications for nonoperative treatment of spinal cord compression due to breast cancer. J Neurosurg 1977;47:653.
44. Raichle ME, Posner JB. The treatment of extradural spinal cord compression. Neurology 1970;20:391.
45. Mones RJ, Dozier D, Berrett A. Analysis of medical treatment of malignant extradural spinal cord tumors. Cancer 1966;19:1842.
46. Young RF, Post EM, King GA. Treatment of spinal epidural metastases: Randomized prospective comparison of laminectomy and radiotherapy. J Neurosurg 1980;53:741.
47. Harrington KD. Anterior cord decompression and spinal stabilization for patients with metastatic lesions of the spine. J Neurosurg 1984;61:107.
48. Sundaresan N, Galicich JH. Treatment of spinal metastases by vertebral body resection. Cancer Invest 1984;2:383.
49. Siegal T, Siegal T. Surgical decompression of anterior and posterior malignant epidural tumors compressing the spinal cord: A prospective study. Neurosurgery 1985;17: 424.
50. Sundaresan N, Galicich JH, Lane JM, et al. Treatment of neoplastic epidural cord compression by vertebral body resection and stabilization. J Neurosurg 1985;63:676.
51. Sundaresan N, Digiacinto GV, Hughes JEO, Cafferty M, Vallejo A. Treatment of neoplastic spinal cord compression: Results of a prospective study. Neurosurgery 1991;29:645.
52. Shaw B, Mansfield FL, Borges L. One-stage posterolateral decompression and stabilization for primary and metastatic vertebral tumors in the thoracic and lumbar spine. J Neurosurg 1989;70:405.
53. Cybulski GR, Stone JL, Opesanmi O. Spinal decompression via a modified costotransversectomy approach combined with posterior instrumentation for management of metastatic neoplasms of the thoracic spine. Surg Neurol 1991;35:280.
54. Johnston FG, Uttley D, Marsh HT. Synchronous vertebral decompression and posterior stabilization in the treatment of spinal malignancy. Neurosurgery 1989;25:872.
55. Moore AJ, Uttley D. Anterior decompression and stabilization of the spine in malignant disease. Neurosurgery 1989;24:713.
56. Manabe S, Tateishi A, Abe M, Ohno T. Surgical treatment of metastatic tumors of the spine. Spine 1989;14:41.
57. Hall AJ, MacKay NNS. The results of laminectomy for compression of the cord and cauda equina by extradural malignant tumor. J Bone Joint Surg [Br] 1973;55:497.
58. Findlay GF. Adverse effects of the management of malignant spinal cord compression. J Neurol Neurosurg Psychiatry 1984;47:761.
59. Hall DJ, Webb JK. Anterior plate fixation in spine tumor surgery: Indications, technique, and results. Spine 1991;16:S80.
60. Haid RW Jr, Carter RL, MacMillan M. Cotrel-Dubousset instrumentation for spinal neoplasms. J Neurosurg 1990;72:350A.
61. Klein SL, Sanford RA, Muhlbauer MS. Pediatric spinal epidural metastases. J Neurosurg 1991;74:70.
62. Zevallos M, Chan PYM, Munoz L, et al. Epidural spinal cord compression from metastatic tumor. Int J Radiat Oncol Biol Phys 1981;13:875.
63. Helweg-Larsen S, Rasmusson B, Sorensen PS. Recovery of gait after radiotherapy in paralytic patients with metastatic epidural spinal cord compression. Neurology 1990;40: 1234.
64. Haddad P, Thael JF, Kiely JM, et al. Lymphoma of the spinal extradural space. Cancer 1976;38:1862.
65. Khan FR, Glicksman AS, Chu FCH, Nickson JJ. Treatment by radiotherapy of spinal cord compression due to extradural metastases. Radiology 1967;89:495.
66. Herbert SH, Solin LJ, Rate WR, et al. The effect of palliative radiation therapy on epidural compression due to metastatic malignant melanoma. Cancer 1991;678:2472.
67. Friedman M, Kim TM, Panahon AM. Spinal cord compression in malignant lymphoma. Cancer 1976;37:1485.
68. Rubin P. Extradural spinal cord compression by tumor. Part I. Experimental production and treatment trials. Radiology 1969;93:1243.
69. Rubin P, Mayer E, Poutter C. Exrtradural spinal cord compression by tumor. Part II. High daily dose experience without laminectomy. Radiology 1969;93:1243.
70. Hayes FA, Thompson EL, Avizdala E, et al. Chemotherapy as an alternative to laminectomy and radiation in the management of epidural tumor. J Pediatr 1984;104:221.
71. Redmond H. Effects of whole-brain irradiation. Presented at the Work in Progress Session of the 52nd Scientific Assembly and Meeting of the Radiological Society of North America, Chicago, 1966.
72. Silverberg IJ, Jacobs EM. Treatment of spinal cord compression in Hodgkin's disease. Cancer 1971;27:308.
73. Friedman HM, Sheetz S, Levine HC, et al, eds. Combination chemotherapy and radiation therapy. The medical management of epidural spinal cord compression from testicular cancer. Arch Intern Med 1986;146:509.
74. Gale GB, O'Connor DM, Chu J-Y, et al. Successful chemotherapeutic decompression of epidural malignant germ cell tumor. Med Pediatr Oncol 1986;14:97.
75. Raffel C, Neave VCD, Lavine S, McComb JG. Treatment of spinal cord compression by epidural malignancy in childhood. Neurosurgery 1991;28:349.
76. Findlay GFG, Sandeman DR, Buxton P. The role of needle biopsy in the management of malignant spinal compression. Br J Neurosurg 1988;2: 479.
77. Bosley TM, Cohen DA, Schatz NJ, et al. Comparison of metrizamide computed tomography and magnetic resonance imaging in the evaluation of lesions at the cervicomedullary junction. Neurology 1985;35:485.
78. Brady LW, Asbell SO, Antoniades J, et al. The treatment of metastatic disease of the nervous system by radiation therapy. In: Seydel HG, ed. Tumors of the nervous system. New York; John Wiley & Sons, 1975:177–188.
79. Cybulski GR. Methods of surgical stabilization for metastatic disease of the spine. Neurosurgery 1989;25:240.
80. Elsberg CA. Surgical diseases of the spinal cord membranes and nerve roots: Symptoms, diagnosis, and treatment. New York: Hueber, 1941:501.
81. Gregersen MI, Pallavicini C, Chien S. Studies on the chemical composition of the central nervous system in relation to the effects of x-irradiation and of disturbances in water and salt balance. Radiat Res 1962;17:209.
82. Kostiuk JP. Anterior spinal cord decompression for lesions of the thoracic and lumber spine, techniques, new methods of internal fixation, results. Spine 1983;8:512.
83. Livingston KE, Perrin RG. The neurosurgical management of spinal metastases causing cord and cauda equina compression. J Neurosurg 1978;49:839.
84. Millburn L, Hibbs GG, Hendrickson FR. Treatment of spinal cord compression from metastatic carcinoma. Cancer 1969;21:447.
85. Mullan J, Evans JP. Neoplastic disease of the spinal extradural space. Arch Surg 1957;74: 900.
86. Renaudin J, Fewer D, Wilson CB, et al. Dose dependence of Decadron in patients with partially excised brain tumors. J Neurosurg 1973;39:302.
87. Smith R. An evaluation of surgical treatment of spinal cord compression due to metastatic carcinoma. J Neurol Neurosurg Psychiatry 1965;28:152.

SECTION **3**

RAYMOND P. WARRELL, JR

Metabolic Emergencies

Patients with cancer present a microcosm of the metabolic and endocrinologic problems encountered in internal medicine, albeit frequently to an extreme degree. Grouped among the paraneoplastic syndromes are metabolic disorders associated with cancer or its treatment that require urgent medical therapy for treatment or prevention.

HYPERCALCEMIA

EPIDEMIOLOGY

Hypercalcemia is the most common life-threatening metabolic disorder associated with cancer. The most reasonable estimates of the prevalence of this disorder in the United States and Western Europe range from 15 to 20 cases per 100,000 persons.[1,2] The incidence of hypercalcemia varies with the underlying cancer diagnosis; it is highest in myeloma and breast cancer (40–50%), intermediate in non-small cell lung cancer, and rare in small cell carcinoma of the lung and colon cancer.[3–6]

DIFFERENTIAL DIAGNOSIS

Hypercalcemia is associated with a wide variety of pathologic states (Table 60–11). Several excellent reviews discuss the diagnostic evaluation and differential diagnosis of patients with hypercalcemia.[7–10] Primary hyperparathyroidism and cancer are the two most common causes of hypercalcemia, and both diseases are prevalent.[11,12] The differential diagnosis of hypercalcemia in cancer and hyperparathyroidism has been linked to changes in serum chloride, phosphorus, "nephrogenous" cyclic adenosine monophosphate (cAMP), immunoreactive parathyroid hormone (PTH), and the results of steroid suppression tests.[13–15] A patient who presents with a recent onset of symptomatic hypercalcemia and weight loss is more likely to have a malignant disorder. In hypercalcemic patients who require hospitalization, cancer has been previously diagnosed or becomes apparent after minimal diagnostic evaluation in most cases.[1] Asymptomatic hypercalcemia and chronic symptoms are the most common presentations of primary hyperparathyroidism.[2] With current assays, a low or normal serum immunoreactive PTH level, especially when combined with elevated serum PTH-related protein, can reliably exclude the diagnosis of primary hyperparathyroidism.[16,17]

Serum calcium is highly bound to albumin, and measurements of total serum calcium fluctuate with changes in serum protein concentrations. Some patients with myeloma present with striking elevations of total serum calcium due solely to an increase in serum proteins that bind calcium.[18–20] Measurements of ionized calcium by ion-specific electrode are essential in such cases. However, for most patients, an approximate estimate of the severity of hypercalcemia can be made by using one of several formulas that adjust serum calcium levels for serum albumin concentration, as follows:

$$\text{Corrected [calcium] (mg/dl)} = \text{measured [calcium] (mg/dl)} - \text{[albumin] (g/dl)} + 4.0 \quad (20)$$

In this equation, concentrations in mg/dl can be converted to SI units by multiplication with 0.2495, yielding concentrations expressed in mmol/L.

TABLE 60–11. Diseases Associated With Hypercalcemia

- Endocrine or metabolic diseases:
  - Primary hyperparathyroidism
  - Hyperthyroidism
  - Pheochromocytoma
  - Osteopetrosis
  - Infantile hyperphosphatasia
  - Familial hypercalcemia with hypercalciuria
- Cancer
- Infectious diseases:
  - Tuberculosis
  - Coccidioidomycosis
  - HIV infection
- Renal insufficiency
- Granulomatous diseases:
  - Sarcoidosis
  - Berylliosis
- Dietary or drug-related:
  - Vitamin D intoxication
  - Vitamin A intoxication
  - Calcium supplements
  - Lithium
  - Milk-alkali syndrome

CLINICAL MANIFESTATIONS

Patients with hypercalcemia can present with a wide variety of symptoms affecting multiple organs (Table 60–12). The severity of the presentation is not exclusively related to the degree of elevation of serum calcium. Patients with slight or moderate elevations (12–13 mg/dl) may become obtunded if the increase occurs acutely. Conversely, patients with long-standing hypercalcemia (*e.g.*, those with parathyroid carcinoma) may tolerate a serum calcium level of more than 14 mg/dl with few symptoms. Other factors, especially age, performance status, sites of metastases, and hepatic or renal dysfunction, contribute to the severity of symptoms.

TABLE 60–12. Clinical Manifestations of Cancer-Related Hypercalcemia

General: dehydration, weight loss, anorexia, pruritus, polydipsia
Neuromuscular: fatigue, lethargy, muscle weakness, hyporeflexia, confusion, psychosis, seizure, obtundation, coma
Gastrointestinal: nausea, vomiting, constipation, obstipation, ileus
Genitorenal: polyuria, renal insufficiency
Cardiac: bradycardia, prolonged P-R interval, shortened Q-T interval, wide T-wave, atrial or ventricular arrhythmias

In patients with evolving hypercalcemia, fatigue, lethargy, constipation, nausea, and polyuria are the most common initial complaints. It is important to evaluate the serum calcium of patients who have these relatively nonspecific complaints, because the combination of polyuria and nausea can lead to rapid dehydration and substantial worsening of the hypercalcemic state. Patients in late stages may present in stupor or coma, and the condition is easily mistaken for diabetic ketoacidosis or drug overdose.

PATHOPHYSIOLOGY

In the past, cancer-related hypercalcemia was conveniently categorized according to the presence or absence of bone involvement. Hypercalcemia in the former group was believed to be associated with direct bone destruction by cancer cells, and the second group was characterized by various humorally mediated mechanisms. It is now evident that hypercalcemia—even in patients with extensive osteolysis—is probably mediated by factors released from or induced by malignant cells that ultimately act to resorb calcium from bone.

Parathyroid Hormone and the PTH-Related Protein

Some patients with cancer-related hypercalcemia have biochemical characteristics suggesting PTH stimulation, including increased tubular reabsorption of calcium, hypophosphatemia with phosphaturia, and elevated levels of nephrogenous cAMP.[21–23] However, most studies of ectopic hyperparathyroidism have been based on bioassays or measurements of immunoreactive material that do not satisfy current criteria of proof for ectopic hormone production.[24] Studies examining PTH-specific mRNA in tumors have confirmed that ectopic PTH production is not a common cause of hypercalcemia.[25] Convincing evidence for tumor secretion of authentic PTH has been presented in only two case reports.[26,27] True ectopic hyperparathyroidism is an exceptionally rare event.

In the mid-1980s, a PTH-related protein was isolated, and this factor has been fully characterized.[28–34] PTH-related protein and authentic human PTH are homologous for only 8 of the first 13 amino acids in the amino-terminal portion. Like the recently cloned receptor for PTH, screening studies have shown that PTH-related protein is widely distributed in normal tissues, such as brain, kidney, parathyroid, skin, uterus, and breast.[35–40] The specific function of the this factor in normal physiology remains uncertain, but it appears likely that the protein is involved only in local signaling and that it probably is not released into the general circulation under normal conditions.

PTH-related protein appears to be the most common mediator of cancer-related hypercalcemia.[41–45] In a study using immunoassay detection of PTH-related protein (Fig. 60–3), the factor was strikingly elevated in patients with solid tumors, particularly patients with squamous (epidermoid) carcinomas.[43] The factor is not associated with most hematologic cancers, such as myeloma or lymphoma, although high levels have been reported in HTLV-I associated T-cell lymphoma and non-Hodgkin's lymphomas associated with human immunodeficiency virus infection. Elevated serum PTH-related protein levels have been found in 30% to 50% of hypercalcemic patients with breast cancer.[41–43,46] The factor is elaborated at sites of bone metastases.[47,48] These data have clearly indicated that previous classifications of hypercalcemic syndromes based on the presence or absence of bone metastases were erroneous.

Prostaglandins

Prostaglandins have long been implicated as circulating mediators of cancer-related hypercalcemia, and certain prostaglandins, especially the E series, have potent bone-resorptive activity in vitro.[49–52] Although occasional hormonally induced flares of hypercalcemia in breast cancer have been linked to prostaglandin release, hypercalcemia rarely responds to cyclooxygenase inhibition, and circulating levels of prostaglandin E in hypercalcemic patients are far too low to account for the observed degree of accelerated bone resorption.[53–56] Prostaglandins may have an important role in cancer-related osteolysis but one that is distinctly time-dependent and highly focal.[57,58]

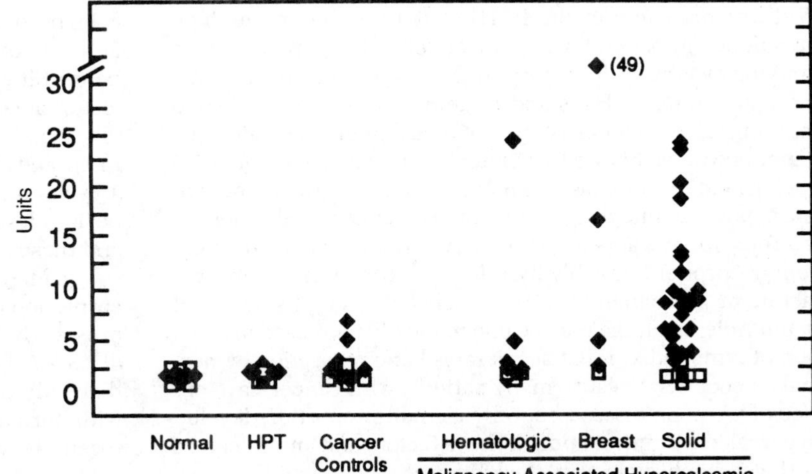

FIGURE 60–3. Serum levels of parathyroid hormone-related protein in normal controls, patients with primary hyperparathyroidism, and patients with diseases associated with cancer-related hypercalcemia. (Budayr AA, Nissenson RA, Klein RF, et al. Increased serum levels of a parathyroid hormone-like protein in malignancy-associated hypercalcemia. Ann Intern Med 1989;111: 807–812)

Cytokines

Factors with osteoclast-activating activity were originally isolated from lymphoid cells.[59,60] This activity is now understood to be associated with a wide variety of cytokines. The transforming growth factors (TGFs) are released in an autocrine manner by a variety of cancer cells and appear to be important regulatory factors for normal bone resorption and formation.[61] TGF-α shares partial similarity of amino acid sequence with epidermal growth factor (EGF), binds to the EGF receptor, and is a potent inducer of bone resorption in vitro.[62–64] Conversely, TGF-β is secreted by osteoblasts and may regulate osteoblast growth and differentiation.[65,66] Dysregulated TGF secretion may lead to uncoupling of bone resorption and formation and could partially account for the mixed lytic and blastic appearance of skeletal metastases in diseases such as carcinoma of the breast and prostate. Other cytokines, including interleukin-1, platelet-derived growth factor, tumor-derived hematopoietic colony-stimulating factors, tumor necrosis factor (TNF), particularly TNF-β (lymphotoxin), are potent inducers of bone resorption in vitro.[67–74] Although the local interaction of these factors in vivo is complex, there is little evidence that circulating cytokines are important mediators of cancer-related hypercalcemia.

Vitamin D

Elevated serum 1,25-dihydroxy vitamin D_3 levels have been reported in patients with Hodgkin's disease, non-Hodgkin's lymphoma, myeloma, and some patients with solid tumors.[75–80] These effects may result from increased enzymatic conversion of 25-OH-vitamin D by 1-α-vitamin D-hydroxylase, similar to patients with granulomatous disease. However, these observation do not prove an etiologic association; the observed elevations in serum vitamin D have generally been well below levels that are known to cause hypercalcemia in patients with vitamin D intoxication. Whether vitamin D plays an important physiologic role or acts merely as a marker of tumor burden is unknown. Normalization of serum vitamin D levels and resolution of hypercalcemia occurs with control of the underlying disease.

Mechanism of Cancer-Related Hypercalcemia

With the discovery of the PTH-related protein and its high prevalence in patients with cancer-related hypercalcemia, a unifying hypothesis for the cause of this syndrome has become more apparent. PTH-related protein, not normally released into general circulation, is a potent mediator of hypercalcemia. Patients who elaborate this factor, particularly patients with epidermoid carcinomas, are more resistant to treatment with antihypercalcemic drugs. Most breast cancers and other osteotropic tumors appear to require proximity to bone to effect bone resorption, possibly by release of transforming growth factors or prostaglandins. The extensive osteolysis observed in multiple myeloma may be due to focally increased production of lymphotoxin that accelerates bone resorption by normal osteoclasts. Because many patients with cancer have obvious lytic bone disease but only a small proportion develop hypercalcemia, interaction of these factors and amplification of the pathophysiology by the kidney also undoubtedly occur.

TREATMENT

General Measures

Although the best treatment for cancer-related hypercalcemia is therapy directed at the underlying disease, hypercalcemia most commonly occurs in patients with advanced disease who have failed prior therapy. The usual therapies for hypercalcemia are directed at decreasing serum calcium by increasing urinary calcium excretion or decreasing bone resorption by inhibition of osteoclast function. For practical purposes, increased intestinal absorption of calcium does not make an important contribution to hypercalcemia in patients with cancer; thus, low-calcium diets are ineffective.

Immobilization should be minimized because inactivity tends to aggravate hypercalcemia. Drugs that inhibit urinary calcium excretion (especially thiazides) should be discontinued.[81] Nonsteroidal antiinflammatory drugs and H_2-receptor antagonists (*e.g.*, cimetidine, ranitidine) decrease renal blood flow and should be avoided if possible. The patient should be carefully interviewed with respect to dietary aberrations. Medications containing calcium, vitamin D, vitamin A, and retinoids should be stopped.[82–84]

Specific Measures

The literature on the treatment of cancer-related hypercalcemia contains few controlled studies. Interpretation of clinical trial results has been confounded by tremendous variability in patient selection, underlying diagnoses, severity of hypercalcemia, and unique methods of reporting results.[85] Table 60–13 summarizes current therapies and provides an estimate of the relative potency of particular therapies.

INTRAVENOUS FLUIDS AND DIURETICS. Hypercalcemic patients frequently present with loss of intravascular volume because of vomiting and obligate water losses associated with calciuresis. Intravenous rehydration, preferably with isotonic saline, is the mainstay of acute therapy for hypercalcemia. Volume expansion and natriuresis increase renal blood flow and enhance calcium excretion due to ionic exchange of calcium for sodium in the distal tubule.[86–88] The rate of fluid administration depends on a clinical estimate of the extent of dehydration, cardiovascular function, and renal excretory capacity. Assuming renal function has previously been normal and cardiac reserves are adequate, saline infusion at a rate of 300 to 400 ml/hour is recommended for 3 to 4 hours. Slower hydration is indicated for less severe metabolic disturbances or in the settings of congestive heart failure or oliguria. After several hours, serum levels of calcium, creatinine, and electrolytes should be reassessed, and urinary output and cardiac status should be reevaluated. Potassium and magnesium losses frequently occur with hydration and diuretics, and these should be replaced as needed.

The effectiveness of hydration with or without diuretics for correction of clinically significant hypercalcemia is low. In a prospective study of patients with serum calcium of 13.0 mg/dl (3.25 mmol/L) or more, Hosking and colleagues found that only 5 of 16 patients (31%) achieved normocalcemia with normal saline (4000 ml/day for 2 days).[89] Although furosemide-induced natriuresis theoretically enhances urinary calcium excretion, no controlled studies have been conducted

TABLE 60–13. Therapy for the Treatment of Cancer-Related Hypercalcemia

Treatment Characteristics	*Normal Saline*	*Oral Phosphorus*	*Corticosteroids*	*Calcitonin*	*Etidronate*	*Plicamycin*	*Gallium Nitrate*	*Pamidronate*
Dose	200–400(+) ml/h	1–3 g/d orally, divided doses	40–100 mg/d prednisone or equivalent	2–8 U/kg SC or IM every 6–12 h	7.5 mg/kg I.V. over 4 h daily for 3–5 d	10–50 (usually 25) micrograms/kg I.V. by brief infusion	100–200 mg/m^2/ day by continuous I.V. infusion up to 5 d	60–90 mg I.V. over 24 h
Indications	Hypovolemia, dehydration	Mild or moderate hypercalcemia, hypophosphatemia	Hypercalcemia from myeloma, lymphoma, hormonal flare	Mild or moderate hypercalcemia; acute control	Mild or moderate hypercalcemia	Moderate or severe hypercalcemia	Moderate or severe hypercalcemia	Moderate or severe hypercalcemia
Onset of action	12–24 h	24–48 h	3–5 d	1–4 h	48 h	24–48 h	24–48 h	24–48 h
Relative potency*	20%	30%	0–40%, depending on disease	30%	30–40%	80%	80%	70–80%
Advantages	Corrects dehydration	Orally available; minimal toxicity	Orally available	Minimal toxicity	Usually well tolerated; decreases bone resorption	Highly effective	Highly effective, decreases bone resorption	Highly effective, decreases bone resorption
Disadvantages/ toxicity	Pulmonary edema, hypernatremia, fluid overload	Nausea, diarrhea, extraosseous calcification	Hyperglycemia, gastritis, osteopenia	Nausea, hypersensitivity	Occasional nephrotoxicity	Nausea, nephrotoxicity, hepatotoxicity, thrombocytopenia, coagulopathy	Prolonged infusion, nephrotoxicity, hypophosphatemia	Fever, venous irritation

* Potency is defined as the expected proportion of patients with a serum calcium ≥12.0 mg/dl who will achieve normocalcemia.

to indicate that hypercalcemic patients benefit from routine furosemide treatment. The drug also increases the risk for developing hypovolemia; the resultant decrease in glomerular filtration may actually stimulate renal calcium reabsorption.[90]

The heroic degrees of saline hydration and forced diuresis that comprised past therapy for cancer-related hypercalcemia are no longer indicated.[91] Such treatment frequently results in problems with fluid overload, including life-threatening pulmonary edema and massive weight gain, that are exceptionally difficult to resolve. Except in uncomplicated patients with mild hypercalcemia, fluid administration with or without diuretics should not be solely relied on unless early intervention with systemic anticancer treatment is also contemplated. Treatment with antiresorptive drugs should be initiated promptly after rehydration for control of hypercalcemia in most hospitalized patients.

PHOSPHATES. An increase in serum phosphorus concentration decreases osteoclastic activity, inhibits calcium resorption from bone, and causes a significant reduction in urinary calcium excretion.[92–94] However, administration of exogenous phosphate to hypercalcemic patients also shifts calcium from blood to other tissues, which can result in severe toxicity. Oral phosphate (0.5–3 g/day) may be highly effective, particularly in mild forms of hypercalcemia.[95–98] Principal side effects are diarrhea and nausea, which may lead to noncompliance. For patients with nausea or impaired mental status, phosphate can be administered rectally by retention enema at a dose of 1.5 g twice per day. Serum phosphorus concentrations should be monitored in all patients who receive oral phosphorus, especially patients with decreased renal function or preexisting hyperphosphatemia.[99] Serum creatinine should be regularly monitored to avoid renal insufficiency. When the calcium × phosphorus product (expressed in mg/dl) exceeds 60, phosphates are usually discontinued.

Intravenous phosphate is highly effective, and the onset of hypocalcemic action occurs more rapidly than with any other hypocalcemic therapy.[100,101] However, renal failure, hypotension, extraskeletal calcification, and severe hypocalcemia are common sequelae of parenteral phosphate therapy, and the use of intravenous phosphate has largely been abandoned.[102–106] Although uncommon, these effects have occasionally been seen with oral phosphates.

PROSTAGLANDIN INHIBITORS. Inhibitors of prostaglandin synthesis may reduce serum calcium in some patients, but fewer than 5% of unselected patients with cancer-related hypercalcemia respond to such drugs, and it is not possible to predict which patients will respond based on clinical findings.[107–109] Because most nonsteroidal antiinflammatory drugs decrease renal blood flow, the use of these drugs for treatment of hospitalized patients or those with compromised renal function is not recommended.[110,111]

SULFATE, CITRATE, AND EDTA. Sodium sulfate and sodium citrate have been used to increase natriuresis and to complex with calcium in urine.[112] However, these therapies are associated with substantial toxicity, including hypervolemia, pulmonary edema, and renal failure.[113,114] EDTA (ethanediamine tetraacetate), a calcium chelating agent, has been associated with a particularly high incidence of renal failure when used in patients with hypercalcemia.[115] These agents are of historical interest only, and their use is no longer recommended.

CORTICOSTEROIDS. Steroids acutely inhibit osteoclast-mediated bone resorption in vitro and decrease gastrointestinal calcium resorption.[116–118] Corticosteroids are most useful in patients whose underlying tumor is responsive to the cytostatic action of these drugs. This group includes patients with myeloma, lymphoma, leukemia, and some patients with carcinoma of the breast, particularly those who have a hypercalcemic flare due to treatment with hormones.[119,120] Steroids do not have consistent hypocalcemic activity in other diseases, and the use of steroids is associated with a variety of undesirable consequences, such as hyperglycemia, hyperosmolar states, gastrointestinal hemorrhage, and osteopenia.[121–123] Prednisone (40–100 mg/day or equivalent) is usually effective in controlling hypercalcemia due to hematologic cancers. Lower doses (15–30 mg/day) may suffice for patients with hypercalcemic flares due to breast cancer.

CALCITONIN. Pharmacologic doses of calcitonin reduce serum calcium by increasing renal calcium excretion and inhibiting bone resorption.[124,125] Calcitonin is especially advantageous due to its rapid onset of action (2–4 hours) and its lack of serious toxicity other than rare hypersensitivity reactions.[126–129] The hypocalcemic effect of calcitonin is relatively weak; the acute response peaks at 48 hours and diminishes thereafter despite continued treatment (*i.e.*, "escape").[130,131] Fewer than 30% of hypercalcemic patients treated with calcitonin as a single agent achieve a normal serum calcium value. Maximally recommended doses of calcitonin (8 IU/kg every 6 hours) should be employed for acute treatment of hypercalcemia. If there is no thrombocytopenia, the drug should be administered intramuscularly rather than subcutaneously to ensure complete absorption. For chronic use, lower doses (4 IU/kg) can be injected subcutaneously once or twice per day on an ambulatory basis. Corticosteroids do not appear to enhance the hypocalcemic effects of calcitonin in patients whose underlying disease is not steroid responsive.[130] Due to its rapid action, calcitonin has been increasingly used in combination with more potent antiresorptive drugs such as gallium nitrate and the bisphosphonates. These combinations may represent optimal treatment of patients with acute severe hypercalcemia.

BISPHOSPHONATES. Bisphosphonates (formerly diphosphonates) are chemical analogs of pyrophosphate. These compounds are not susceptible to hydrolysis by pyrophosphatase and are stable for long periods in vivo. Bisphosphonates adsorb to the surface of crystalline hydroxyapatite and directly inhibit calcium release from bone.[132,133] The main compounds in clinical use are etidronate, clodronate, pamidronate, and alendronate.[134,135]

Oral etidronate has been used for the treatment of Paget's disease of bone and postmenopausal osteoporosis; the drug has also been approved for intravenous therapy of cancer-related hypercalcemia.[136] Reports of the effectiveness of etidronate have varied.[137,138] In a randomized study against saline placebo, normocalcemia was achieved in 27% of patients treated with intravenous etidronate—a degree of potency comparable to calcitonin.[130,139] Etidronate has been compared with gallium nitrate and pamidronate in randomized, double-blind studies; the response to high doses of etidronate in both studies was similar: 43% and 42%, respectively (Fig. 60–4).[140,141] Etidronate is administered intravenously at a maximal dose of 7.5 mg/kg/day for 3 to 5 days. The drug should be given as a slow infusion over 4 hours to avoid renal insufficiency.[142] Similar to all antiresorptive drugs except calcitonin, the drug should not be given until hydration has been initiated and adequate urinary output has been established. Despite the activity of oral etidronate in Paget's disease and osteoporosis, controlled studies do not suggest the oral formulation is useful for prolonging the duration of normocalcemia.[143]

Pamidronate and alendronate are the most potent bisphosphonates currently available. Like etidronate, both of these agents are generally well tolerated. Acute side effects are limited to infusion-site irritation and fever that occurs after the first infusion in approximately 20% of patients. Multiple doses and schedules of pamidronate were employed during its clinical development.[144–147] The recommended dose schedule for pamidronate is 60 mg infused over 24 hours for patients with mild or moderate hypercalcemia. A dose of 90 mg has been recommended for patients with more severe hypercalcemia (total calcium >13.0 mg/dl).[147] The recommended dose of alendronate is 10 or 15 mg, depending on the initial level of serum calcium.[148] Both agents have been used in clinical studies that employed shorter infusion times (2–6 hours) without excessive toxicity.

GALLIUM NITRATE. Gallium nitrate is another potent inhibitor of bone resorption.[149–153] Elemental gallium is incorporated into bone and renders hydroxyapatite less soluble and more resistant to cell-mediated resorption.[154,155] The agent impairs osteoclast acidification of bone matrix by decreasing proton transport across the cell membrane; it may also enhance bone formation by stimulation of bone collagen synthesis and by increasing calcium accretion into bone.[155–157] Two randomized, double-blind studies have demonstrated superiority of gallium nitrate compared with calcitonin and etidronate (see Fig. 60–4B) for acute treatment of resistant hypercalcemia.[130,140] After administration as a continuous intravenous infusion (100–200 mg/m^2/day over 24 hours for up to 5 days), gallium nitrate induces normocalcemia in approximately 80% to 90% of patients.[130,140,158] The maximal hypocalcemic effect may occur several days after the drug has been discontinued. In studies using high doses of gallium nitrate for cancer treatment, nephrotoxicity was dose limiting, but the incidence of renal toxicity in studies of hypercalcemia was similar to etidronate and calcitonin and was not appreciably different from the background incidence of renal insufficiency in this disorder.[130,140] Like the bisphosphonates, gallium nitrate should be administered after the patient has been rehydrated. A daily urinary output of 2000 ml should be maintained during the infusion, and highly nephrotoxic drugs such as aminoglycosides and cisplatin should not be administered concurrently.

PLICAMYCIN. Plicamycin (mithramycin) is an antitumor antibiotic with substantial activity in testicular cancer.[159] Hypocalcemia was observed as an unexpected side effect and current use of this agent is limited to treatment of resistant Paget's disease and hypercalcemia.[160–165] Plicamycin acts directly by killing osteoclasts, thereby decreasing cell-mediated bone resorption.[166–168] Plicamycin is administered at doses ranging from 10 to 50 μg per kilogram of body weight. The usual dose is 25 μg/kg or a total dose of 1.5 to 2.0 mg given

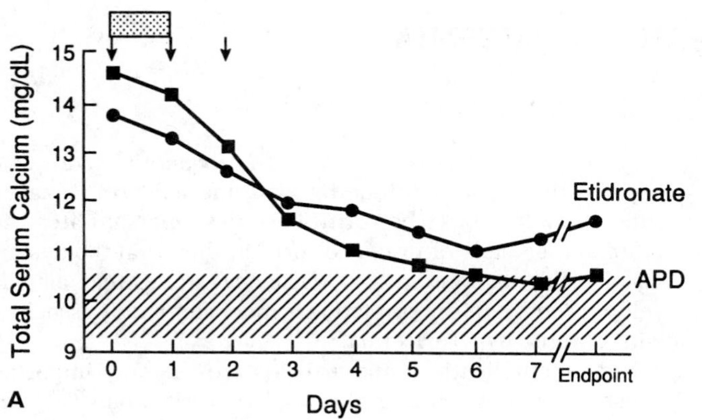

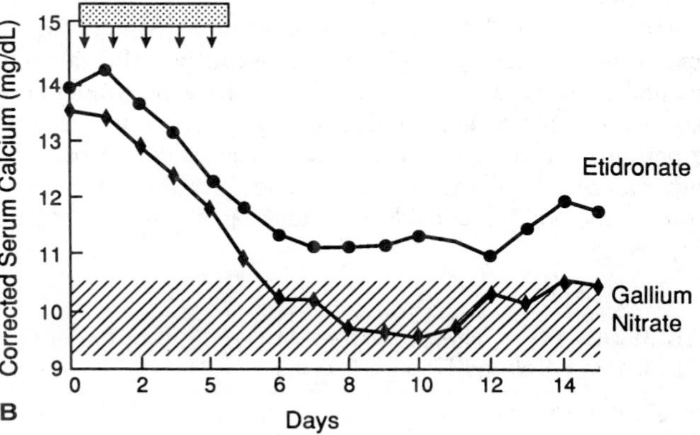

FIGURE 60–4. **(A)** The top graph shows the relative hypocalcemic effects of pamidronate (APD) compared with etidronate in a randomized, double-blind study. Solid squares represent mean daily concentrations of serum calcium for patients receiving APD; solid circles represent data for patients receiving etidronate. Duration or frequency of infusion times are indicated at the top left; APD was administered as a single 24-hour infusion, and etidronate was administered as a 4-hour infusion daily for 3 days. The normal range for total serum calcium is indicated by the shaded area. (Gucalp R, Ritch P, Wiernik PH, et al. Comparative study of pamidronate disodium and etidronate disodium in the treatment of cancer-related hypercalcemia. J Clin Oncol 1992;10:134–142). **(B)** The bottom graph shows the relative hypocalcemic effects of gallium nitrate compared with etidronate in a randomized, double-blind study. (Warrell RP Jr, Heller G, Murphy WP, Schulman P, O'Dwyer P. A randomized double-blind study of gallium nitrate compared to etidronate for acute control of cancer-related hypercalcemia. J Clin Oncol 1991;9:1467–1475)

as a brief infusion. Because the onset of action occurs after 24 to 48 hours, doses should not be repeated more frequently than every 2 days. Except for nausea, single injections are generally well tolerated; the incidence of adverse effects (*e.g.*, renal insufficiency, hepatotoxicity, thrombocytopenia, hemorrhagic diathesis) increase with multiple injections.[169]

Management Approach

Patients with hypercalcemia can be grouped according to those who require urgent in-hospital therapy and those for whom out-patient therapy can be considered. Table 60–14 presents a list of considerations that influence this decision. Hospitalization should be considered for any patient with a serum calcium level greater than 12.0 mg/dl or for any patient who is symptomatic. Hospitalization is especially indicated for patients who are dehydrated or who have a significant degree of nausea that precludes increased oral hydration. Hypercalcemia that has evolved slowly may rapidly progress after a patient begins vomiting or if mentation is impaired.

EMERGENCY TREATMENT OF HOSPITALIZED PATIENTS. Intravenous hydration is the initial treatment of choice for all patients who require hospitalization. Furosemide should be given only if diuresis is inadequate or to treat problems related to fluid retention. Most patients with significant hypercalcemia (total calcium ≥12.0 mg/dl) do not respond satisfactorily if acute treatment is limited to intravenous fluids and diuretics, no matter how aggressive. Given the toxicity of aggressive hydration, the use of other newly available antiresorptive drugs should be considered after hydration has been started and satisfactory urinary output established. Calcitonin (4–8 U/kg as an intramuscular injection every 6–8 hours) can be given immediately to provide an immediate but short-lived and incomplete hypocalcemic effect. However, optimal treatment probably combines hydration, calcitonin, with a potent bisphosphonate (pamidronate or alendronate) or gallium nitrate.[170,171] Corticosteroids are distinctly beneficial if the primary disease is steroid responsive. Mithramycin should be reserved for patients without thrombocytopenia or significant renal or hepatic dysfunction who do not respond to pamidronate or gallium nitrate. Hypercalcemic patients with marked renal insufficiency, especially those with myeloma, should be considered candidates for immediate dialysis.[172]

TABLE 60–14. Criteria for the Management of Patients With Cancer-Related Hypercalcemia

Out-Patient Criteria	*In-Patient Criteria*
Serum calcium <12.0 mg/dl	Serum calcium ≥12.0 mg/dl
No significant nausea	Nausea or vomiting
Able to ingest fluids	Dehydration
Fatigue	Altered mental status
Normal renal function	Renal insufficiency
Stable cardiac rhythm	Cardiac arrhythmia
Mild constipation	Obstipation, ileus
Companion for supervision	Lives alone
Access to emergency care	Limited access to medical care

AMBULATORY MANAGEMENT OF HYPERCALCEMIC PATIENTS. Treatment of ambulatory patients is preferably undertaken in conjunction with specific cytotoxic therapy, such as irradiation or chemotherapy. Certain anticancer drugs (*e.g.*, dactinomycin, doxorubicin, cisplatin) have hypocalcemic actions independent of demonstrable effects on the primary tumor.[173] The hypocalcemic mechanism is the same as with mithramycin: lethal toxicity to bone cells.[174]

Ambulatory patients must receive clear instructions regarding increased oral fluid intake. The amount of fluid should be stated in terms that the patient and family can understand. It is imperative that a family member or companion attend the patient to ensure that nausea due to worsening hypercalcemia does not lead to further dehydration. Diuretics such as furosemide should not be added because the risk of dehydration outweighs theoretical benefits in ambulatory patients who are not edematous. Oral phosphate can be an extremely useful adjunct. One to 3 g/day of oral phosphorus in divided doses are usually well tolerated. Patients who receive phosphorus must not have preexisting hyperphosphatemia nor any significant degree of renal impairment (*e.g.*, creatinine clearance <30 ml/minute). Corticosteroids are helpful if the underlying disease is responsive. Subcutaneous injections of calcitonin (100–200 U/day) may be useful for mild forms of hypercalcemia. Although oral etidronate is probably not effective, intermittent infusions (once per week) of pamidronate or alendronate may be useful for out-patient treatment. Low doses of gallium nitrate (20 mg/m^2/day) have been administered with some success after acute normalization with intravenous therapy. Plicamycin can be administered in doses of 10 to 25 μg/kg once or twice weekly. Patients who receive plicamycin therapy as outpatients must be closely monitored for evidence of myelosuppression and for changes in renal or hepatic function.

HYPERURICEMIA

PATHOPHYSIOLOGY

Uric acid is formed as a result of the sequential catalysis of hypoxanthine and xanthine by xanthine oxidase. Renal insufficiency develops when urine becomes supersaturated with urate and crystals of uric acid form in the renal tubules and distal collecting system.[175,176] Uric acid stones may also develop, although this presentation is more commonly associated with chronic hyperuricemia.

Renal complications and arthritis are the only important consequences of acute or chronic hyperuricemia.[177–181] The disorder occurs most commonly in hematologic neoplasms, particularly the leukemias, high-grade lymphomas, and myeloproliferative diseases such as polycythemia vera.[178–181] Acute urate nephropathy has been reported after chemotherapy for solid tumors.[182] Patients at highest risk include those with bulky high-grade lymphomas, patients with high leukocyte counts undergoing remission-induction chemotherapy for acute or chronic leukemia, and persons with preexisting renal impairment, especially those with ureteral obstruction. Hyperuricemia is a side effect of certain agents, notably diuretics (*e.g.*, thiazides, furosemide), antituberculosis drugs (*e.g.*, pyrazinamide, ethambutol, and nicotinic acid), and the cytotoxic agent tiazofurin.[183]

TREATMENT

Recognition of patients at risk is essential for proper therapy. It is essential that prophylactic measures be undertaken *before* cytotoxic therapy is initiated. Drugs that tend to elevate serum urate or that produce an acidic urine (*e.g.*, thiazides, salicylates) should be withdrawn. All patients should receive intravenous hydration to correct preexisting deficits of intravascular volume and to ensure continued urinary output. Increased urinary volume decreases the concentration of urate in urine and minimizes problems with respect to urate solubility.[184] Although furosemide theoretically promotes increased tubular urate reabsorption, this effect is outweighed by its acute diuretic action; the drug can be used to maintain satisfactory urine output if urine volume and electrolytes are monitored and replaced. Alkalinization of the urine should be initiated to maintain a urine pH of 7.0 or higher. Although oral sodium bicarbonate can be used, it is usually simpler to add sodium bicarbonate solution (50–100 mmol/L) to intravenous fluids and adjust the admixture so that an alkaline urine pH is maintained. Acetazolamide, an inhibitor of carbonic anhydrase, may be used to increase the effects of alkalinization. However, it should be recognized that alkalinization is secondary to the overall goal of decreasing urinary uric acid concentration by increasing urinary volume.[230]

The mainstay of current drug therapy is allopurinol.[185,186] Initially developed as a method of cancer treatment, allopurinol was incidentally found to cause hypouricemia, and this indication represents its principal current use.[187,188] Allopurinol inhibits xanthine oxidase and consequently increases plasma and urinary concentrations of xanthine and hypoxanthine. Although xanthine is somewhat more soluble than uric acid, allopurinol has occasionally been associated with renal failure due to xanthine nephropathy.[189,190]

Allopurinol is generally well tolerated. The most common adverse reaction is a blanching, erythematous skin rash that indicates hypersensitivity. The onset of this reaction is usually delayed for several days after initial administration, and the drug can usually be continued throughout periods of greatest risk in patients who have not had prior exposure. In acute situations, the drug is administered orally once or twice daily in total daily doses ranging from 300 to 900 mg. Intravenous allopurinol is available on an investigational basis.[191] The dose of certain drugs (*e.g.*, 6-mercaptopurine) that are metabolized by xanthine oxidase must be substantially reduced during treatment with allopurinol.

Patients in renal failure and allopurinol-sensitive persons represent uncommon but difficult management problems.[192] Azapropazone, merbarone, and benzbromarone are effective hypouricemic drugs that are available on an investigational basis.[193–195] Intravenous administration of uricase has also been useful in certain circumstances.[196] In the face of acute oliguria, ultrasonography or computed tomography (CT) scanning should be used to evaluate possible ureteral obstruction by urate calculi. Administration of intravenous contrast agents for pyelography should be avoided because of an increased risk of acute tubular necrosis.[197] Peritoneal dialysis or hemodialysis are effective in reversing renal failure due to urate deposition.[198]

TUMOR LYSIS SYNDROME

PATHOPHYSIOLOGY

The tumor lysis syndrome occurs as a result of the rapid release of intracellular contents into the bloodstream, which may then increase to life-threatening concentrations. The syndrome is characterized by hyperuricemia, hyperkalemia, hyperphosphatemia, and hypocalcemia. Lethal cardiac arrhythmias are the most serious consequences of hyperkalemia. Hyperphosphatemia may result in acute renal failure.[199–201] Elevated serum phosphorus may decrease renal function, which can further reduce urinary potassium and phosphate excretion. Hypocalcemia—a result of hyperphosphatemia—may cause muscle cramps, cardiac arrhythmias, and tetany.

The tumor lysis syndrome occurs most commonly in diseases with large tumor burdens and high proliferative fractions that are exquisitely sensitive to cytotoxic treatment. These disorders include high-grade lymphomas, leukemias with high leukocyte counts, and much less commonly, solid tumors.[202–209] The syndrome has been observed with agents that have potent myelosuppressive activity and with drugs such as interferon-α, tamoxifen, and intrathecal methotrexate.[210–212] Although technically not related to tumor lysis, severe hypocalcemia has been associated with cisplatin treatment, estrogenic treatment of prostate cancer, and accelerated bone formation in patients with leukemia.[213–215]

TREATMENT

Recognition of risk and prevention are essential to management. Patients at risk should be identified before the initiation of chemotherapy. If possible, intravenous hydration should be started 24 to 48 hours before the administration of chemotherapy. Any acid-base or electrolyte disorders should be corrected, although intravenous administration of sodium bicarbonate may aggravate symptoms of hypocalcemia. Treatment with allopurinol should be undertaken with other measures to minimize hyperuricemia as described previously. Serum electrolytes, uric acid, phosphorus, calcium, and creatinine should be checked repeatedly for 3 to 4 days after initiating cytotoxic treatment. The frequency of monitoring depends on the clinical condition of the patient. If hyperkalemia or hypocalcemia become evident, an electrocardiogram should be obtained, and the cardiac rhythm should be monitored while these abnormalities are corrected. Hypocalcemia can be corrected with intravenous administration of calcium gluconate, but hypocalcemia may persist for several days despite continued therapy. Hyperkalemia (serum $[K^+] \geq 5.0$ mg/dl) should be treated with an oral sodium-potassium exchange resin (*e.g.*, 15 g of Kayexalate given orally every 6 hours) or with combined insulin and glucose therapy.

In the face of acutely worsening renal function after administration of chemotherapy, consideration should be given to *early* initiation of renal dialysis to rapidly control serum concentrations of potassium, calcium, phosphate, and uric acid and other problems related to uremia. The dose of many drugs, especially antineoplastics, requires substantial modification for renal insufficiency.[216]

HYPOGLYCEMIA

Insulin-producing islet cell tumors are the most frequent cause of hypoglycemia in patients with cancer, but more than 250 cases of hypoglycemia associated with non-islet cell tumors have been reported.[217,218] Non-islet cell tumors associated with hypoglycemia tend to be large. Mesenchymal tumors (*e.g.*, fibrosarcomas, leiomyomas, rhabdomyosarcomas, liposarcomas, mesotheliomas) comprise approximately 50% of cases; another 25% are hepatomas.[217] Classic symptoms of hypoglycemia (*e.g.*, weakness, dizziness, diaphoresis, nausea) are nonspecific and may develop slowly. In the initial phases, symptoms tend to be worse in the early morning due to overnight fasting and improve after ingestion of food. However, patients may present with seizures, coma, and focal or diffuse neurologic deficits.

PATHOPHYSIOLOGY

Several etiologic mechanisms for cancer-related hypoglycemia have been proposed: secretion of insulin-like substances; excessive glucose use by the tumor that exceeds hepatic production; and failure of counter-regulatory mechanisms that usually prevent hypoglycemia. Substances with nonsuppressible insulin-like activities (NSILAs) have been detected in serum from patients with hypoglycemia. These factors are composed of two general classes: relatively low-molecular-weight substances that are soluble in acid and ethanol, and high-molecular-weight substances that are acid-ethanol precipitable. The low-molecular-weight compounds consist of four peptides, the insulin-like growth factors (*e.g.*, IGF-I, IGF-II, somatomedin A, somatomedin C).[219–221] IGF-I and II share a high degree of amino acid similarity with proinsulin, but they do not react with antiinsulin antibodies, and they have only 1% to 2% of the specific metabolic activity of insulin.[220] The NSILAs with high molecular weights are less well characterized.[222] Approximately 40% of cancer patients with symptomatic hypoglycemia have elevated plasma levels of low-molecular-weight NSILAs.[218,223] These observations suggested that humoral mechanisms (*i.e.*, tumor production of IGFs) might be responsible for hypoglycemia in a significant proportion of patients.

Accelerated glucose use by large tumors could account for cancer-related hypoglycemia. It has been estimated that a 1 kg tumor may use 50 to 200 g of glucose daily.[224] Because the liver can produce approximately 700 g of glucose daily, hepatic production should theoretically be sufficient to prevent hypoglycemia. However, many patients with hypoglycemia have primary tumors that weigh several kilograms and extensive hepatic metastases; the combination of accelerated glucose use with impaired production may lead to hypoglycemia.

Failure of the usual counter-regulatory mechanisms in patients with large tumors may induce hypoglycemia.[225] Impaired liver function can decrease glycogenolysis and gluconeogenesis. Certain patients with cancer have a depressed hyperglycemic response to the administration of glucagon; depressed secretion of counter-regulatory hormones such as glucagon, ACTH, glucocorticoids, and growth hormone has been reported. Insufficient data currently exist to establish the importance of these mechanisms as independent causes of hypoglycemia.

TREATMENT

The therapy for hypoglycemia should match the severity of the condition. As with most paraneoplastic syndromes, specific antitumor therapy is the preferred treatment. Chemotherapeutic agents that are cytotoxic for islet cells or that block insulin release or activity have had little effect on production, release, or activity of NSILAs. Mild hypoglycemia can usually be managed by increasing the frequency of meals. In patients with more severe or unpredictable symptoms, the administration of corticosteroids and glucagon may afford symptomatic relief. Intravenous infusions of glucose provide temporary support while other specific treatment (*e.g.*, surgery, chemotherapy, irradiation) is administered. Under certain circumstances, continuous infusions of glucagon using portable pumps have been used with some success.[226]

ADRENAL FAILURE

Symptomatic adrenocortical insufficiency due to destruction of cortical tissue by metastatic carcinoma is uncommon. More common are iatrogenic causes, such as surgical adrenalectomy, treatment with mitotane and inhibitors of steroid synthesis like aminoglutethimide, and chronic corticosteroid therapy.[227,228] Nonetheless, technical improvements in CT and magnetic resonance imaging have increased the likelihood of making an antemortem diagnosis of adrenal metastases. In one study, 19% of patients with metastatic cancer and enlargement of the adrenal glands detected by CT scans developed symptoms of adrenal insufficiency.[229] In a separate study in which 15 patients with metastatic cancer and adrenal enlargement on CT scan were evaluated by ACTH stimulation, one third were judged to have adrenal insufficiency. Further clinical study revealed symptoms of nausea, anorexia, and orthostatic hypotension in all of these patients.[230] Adrenal insufficiency may develop insidiously in patients with adrenal metastasis, and CT scans and ACTH testing may be useful diagnostic tools.

CLINICAL MANIFESTATIONS

Classic signs and symptoms of adrenal insufficiency include weakness, weight loss, anorexia, hyperpigmentation, and postural hypotension. At least one of these symptoms is evident in most patients, but the onset of symptoms is frequently insidious. Circulatory collapse and shock are uncommon but may develop with the onset of infection. Biochemical evaluation frequently reveals a mild acidosis without an anion gap, hyponatremia, and hypokalemia.

EVALUATION AND TREATMENT

Because an ACTH-stimulation test is a benign procedure, this test is recommended when symptoms suggestive of adrenal insufficiency are evident. Typically, patients receive Cosyntropin (0.25 mg intravenously), and serum cortisol is monitored at baseline, 30 minutes, and 1 hour. An increase in serum cortisol of 5 to 7 μg/dl over baseline levels (to a minimum of 15 μg/ml) is considered normal. If adrenal insufficiency is strongly suspected on clinical grounds, steroid replacement or stress doses of steroids should be started immediately, and subsequent therapy can be reevaluated after results of the ACTH test become available.

Physiologic glucocorticoid replacement is attained by administration of cortisone acetate (25 mg in the morning and 12.5 mg in the early evening). During periods of stress (*e.g.*, operative procedures, infection), these doses may need to be doubled or tripled. Occasionally, mineralocorticoid replacement (*e.g.*, 0.05–0.1 mg of fludrocortisone) is required in addition to cortisone acetate. In patients with no adrenocortical function whatsoever, maintenance doses of dexamethasone or prednisone do not provide adequate mineralocorticoid coverage, and fludrocortisone must be given. Pharmacologic doses of parenteral glucocorticoids are required in the setting of acute adrenal failure and circulatory collapse. Typically, aqueous-soluble forms of hydrocortisone (*e.g.*, sodium succinate salt) at doses of 100 mg intravenously every 8 hours are required. Thereafter, the patient should be monitored for evidence of hyperglycemia, hypokalemia, or hypernatremia.

LACTIC ACIDOSIS

Lactic acidosis is a rare but potentially severe metabolic complication in patients with cancer. Type A lactic acidosis is due to impaired delivery of oxygen to peripheral tissue and is commonly seen with shock and septicemia. Type B lactic acidosis is associated with a variety of diseases, including diabetes, renal failure, liver disease, infection, and cancer, and with drugs, toxins, and hereditary conditions.[231–234] Lactic acidosis is characterized by decreased arterial pH (<7.37) secondary to accumulation of blood lactate (>2 mEq/L). The disorder is a consequence of increased lactate production and impaired use. Lactate is a metabolite of pyruvate and is produced in a cytosolic reaction catalyzed by lactic dehydrogenase—an enzyme with an absolute requirement for nicotinamide adenine dinucleotide (NAD). Consequently, the concentrations of pyruvate, hydrogen ion, and NAD regulate lactate metabolism. Accelerated glycogenolysis increases pyruvate production and decreases tissue oxygen, which decreases levels of NAD. As NAD is depleted, gluconeogenesis is halted and pyruvate increases. Anaerobic metabolism of pyruvate to lactate is increased, which leads to accumulation of NADH and hydrogen ions.

Sculier and colleagues reviewed 25 cases of lactic acidosis in which the underlying tumor was believed to represent the primary etiologic factor.[235] More than two thirds of these cases were associated with leukemia or lymphoma, and the remainder were associated with various solid tumors. The development of lactic acidosis coincided with the onset of progressive disease, and most patients with solid tumors had extensive liver metastases. Typically, the patient with lactic acidosis presents with hyperventilation and hypotension. Nonspecific clinical symptoms such as tachycardia, weakness, nausea, and stupor may proceed to frank shock as the acidosis worsens. Laboratory studies show decreased blood pH, a widened anion gap, and a low serum bicarbonate level.

The prognosis for patients with a serum lactate concentration greater than 4 mEq/L is exceedingly poor, but the outcome is largely determined by the underlying disease and not the acidosis. Several reports suggested that administration of sodium bicarbonate increases production of lactate and CO_2 and impairs oxygen delivery without improving survival.[236–239] Detrimental effects of severe acidemia on cardiovascular function can probably be ameliorated by bicarbonate administration, and this temporizing measure may be useful while effective anticancer therapy is attempted.[240–244]

REFERENCES

1. Fisken RA, Heath DA, Bold AM. Hypercalcemia—a hospital survey. Q J Med 1980;49:405–418.
2. Mundy GR. Primary hyperparathyroidism: Changes in the pattern of clinical presentation. Lancet 1980;1:1317–1320.
3. Brada M, Rowley M, Grant DJ, Ashley S, Powles TJ. Hypercalcemia in patients with disseminated breast cancer. Acta Oncol 1990;29:577–580.
4. Bender RA, Hanson H. Hypercalcemia in bronchogenic carcinoma: A prospective study of 200 patients. Ann Intern Med 1974;80:205–208.
5. Coggeshall J, Merrill W, Hande K, Des Prez R. Implications of hypercalcemia with respect to diagnosis and treatment of lung cancer. Am J Med 1986;80:325–328.
6. Hayward ML Jr, Howell DA, O'Donnell JF, Maurer LH. Hypercalcemia complicating small cell carcinoma. Cancer 1981;48:1643–1646.
7. Strewler GJ, Nissenson RA. Nonparathyroid hypercalcemia. Adv Intern Med 1987;32:235–258.
8. Insogna KL, Broadus AE. Hypercalcemia of malignancy. Annu Rev Med 1987;38:241–256.
9. Boyd JC, Ladenson JH. Value of laboratory tests in the differential diagnosis of hypercalcemia. Am J Med 1984;77:863–872.
10. Lafferty FW. Differential diagnosis of hypercalcemia. J Bone Miner Res 1991;6(suppl 2):S51–S59.
11. Heath HH III, Hodgson SF, Kenedy MA. Primary hyperparathyroidism: Incidence, morbidity, and potential economic impact on the community. N Engl J Med 1980;302:189–193.
12. Axelrod DM, Bockman RS, Wong GY, Osborne MP, Kinne DW, Brennan MF. Distinguishing features of primary hyperparathyroidism in patients with breast cancer Cancer 1987;60:60:1620–1624.
13. Wills MR. Value of plasma chloride concentration and acid-base status in the differential diagnosis of hyperparathyroidism from other causes of hypercalcaemia. J Clin Pathol 1971;24:219–227.
14. Lufkin EG, Kao PC, Heath H. Parathyroid hormone radioimmunoassays in the differential diagnosis of hypercalcemia due to primary hyperparathyroidism or malignancy. Ann Intern Med 1987;106:559–560.
15. Watson L, Moxham J, Fraser P. Hydrocortisone suppression test and discriminant analysis in differential diagnosis of hypercalcemia. Lancet 1980;1:1320–1325.
16. Ratcliffe WA, Hutcheson ACJ, Bundred NJ, Ratcliffe JG. Role of assays for parathyroid hormone-related protein in investigation of hypercalcaemia. Lancet 1992;339:164–167.
17. Nussbaum SR, Potts JT Jr. Immunoassays for parathyroid hormone 1-84 in the diagnosis of hyperparathyroidism. J Bone Miner Res 1991;6(suppl 2):S43–S50.
18. Hazani A, Silvian I, Tatarsky I, Spira G. Non-symptomatic hypercalcemia in a myeloma patient. Am J Med Sci 1982;283:169–273.
19. Annesley TM, Burritt MF, Kyle RA. Artifactual hypercalcemia in multiple myeloma. Mayo Clin Proc 1982;57:572–575.
20. Payne RB, Carver ME, Morgan DB. Interpretation of serum total calcium: Effects of adjustment for albumin concentration on frequency of abnormal values and on detection of change in the individual. J Clin Pathol 1979;32:56–60.
21. Rizzoli R, Caverzasia J, Fleisch H, Bonjour JP. Parathyroid hormone-like changes in renal calcium and phosphate reabsorption induced by Leydig cell tumor in thyroparathyroidectomized rats. Endocrinology 1986;119:1004–1009.
22. Stewart AF, Horst R, Deftos LJ, Cadman EC, Lang R, Broadus AE. Biochemical evaluation of patients with cancer-associated hypercalcemia: Evidence for humoral and nonhumoral groups. N Engl J Med 1980;303:1377–1383.
23. Kukreja SC, Shemerdiak WP, Lad TE, et al. Elevated nephrogenous cyclic AMP with normal serum parathyroid hormone levels in patients with lung cancer. J Clin Endocrinol Metab 1980;52:765–771.
24. Skrabanek P, McPartlin J, Powell D. Tumor hypercalcemia and "ectopic hyperparathyroidism." Medicine (Baltimore) 1980;59:262–282.
25. Simpson EL, Mundy GR, D'Souza SM, Ibbotson KJ, Bockman RS, Jacobs JW. Absence of parathyroid messenger RNA in nonparathyroid tumors associated with hypercalcemia. N Engl J Med 1983;309:325–330.
26. Nussbaum SR, Gaz RD, Arnold A. Hypercalcemia and ectopic secretion of parathyroid hormone by an ovarian carcinoma with rearrangement of the gene for parathyroid hormone. N Engl J Med 1990;323:1324–1328.
27. Strewler GJ, Budayr AA, Bruce RJ, Clark OH, Nissenson RA. Secretion of authentic parathyroid hormone by a malignant tumor. Clin Res 1990;38:462A.
28. Broadus AC, Goltzman D, Webb AC, Kronenberg HM. Messenger ribonucleic acid from tumors associated with humoral hypercalcemia of malignancy directs the synthesis of a secretory parathyroid hormone-like peptide. Endocrinology 1985;117:1661–1666.
29. Strewler GJ, Williams RJ, Nissenson RA. Human renal carcinoma cells produce hypercalcemia in the nude mouse and a novel protein recognized by parathyroid hormone receptors. J Clin Invest 1983;71:769–774.
30. Burtis WJ, Wu T, Bunch C, et al. Identification of a novel 17,000-dalton parathyroid

hormone-like adenylate cyclase-stimulating protein from a tumor associated with humoral hypercalcemia of malignancy. J Biol Chem 1987;262:7151–7156.
31. Moseley JM, Kubota M, Dieffenbach-Jagger H, et al. Parathyroid hormone-related protein purified from a human lung cancer cell line. Proc Natl Acad Sci USA 1987;84:5048–5052.
32. Suva LJ, Winslow GA, Wettenhall REH, et al. A parathyroid hormone-related protein implicated in malignant hypercalcemia: Cloning and expression. Science 1987;237:894–897.
33. Mangin M, Webb AC, Dreyer BE, et al. Identification of a cDNA encoding a parathyroid hormone-like peptide from a human tumor associated with humoral hypercalcemia of malignancy. Proc Natl Acad Sci USA 1988;85:597–601.
34. Mangin M, Ikeda K, Dreyer BE, Broadus AE. Isolation and characterization of the human parathyroid hormone-like peptide gene. Proc Natl Acad Sci USA 1989;86:2408–2412.
35. Abou-Samra AB, Jueppner H, Freeman MW, et al. Expression and cloning of the parathyroid hormone (PTH) bone receptor cDNA. Clin Res 1991;39:342A.
36. Merendino JJ Jr, Insogna KL, Milstone LM, Broadus AC, Stewart AF. A parathyroid hormone-like protein from cultured human keratinocytes. Science 1986;231:288–290.
37. Weir EC, Brines ML, Ikeda K, Burtis WJ, Broadus AE, Robbins RJ. Parathyroid hormone-related peptide gene is expressed in the mammalian central nervous system. Proc Natl Acad Sci USA 1990;87:108–112.
38. Broadus AE, Mangin M, Ikeda K, et al. Humoralhypercalcemia of cancer. Identification of a novel parathyroid hormone-like peptide. N Engl J Med 1988;319:556–562.
39. Thiede MA, Rodan GA. Expression of a calcium-mobilizing parathyroid hormone-like peptide in lactating mammary tissue. Science 1988;242:278–280.
40. Thiede MA, Daifotis AG, Weir EC, et al. Intrauterine occupancy controls expression of the parathyroid hormone-related peptide gene in preterm rat myometrium. Proc Natl Acad Sci USA 1990;87:6969–6973.
41. Burtis WJ, Brady TG, Orloff JJ, et al. Immunochemical characterization of circulating parathyroid hormone-related protein in patients with humoral hypercalcemia of cancer. N Engl J Med 1990;322:1106–1112.
42. Budayr AA, Nissenson RA, Klein RF, et al. Increased serum levels of a parathyroid hormone-like protein in malignancy-associated hypercalcemia. Ann Intern Med 1989;111:807–812.
43. Henderson JE, Shustic C, Kremer R, Rabbani SA, Hendy GN, Goltzman D. Circulating concentrations of parathyroid hormone-like peptide in malignancy and hyperparathyroidism. J Bone Miner Res 1990;5:105–113.
44. Insogna KL. Humoral hypercalcemia of malginancy. The role of parathyroid hormone-related protein. Endocr Metab Clin North Am 1989;18:779–794.
45. Kao PC, Klee GG, Taylor RL, Heath H. Parathyroid hormone-related peptide in plasma of patients with hypercalcemia and malignant lesions. Mayo Clin Proc 1990;65:1399–1407.
46. Motokura T, Fukumoto S, Matsumoto T, et al. Parathyroid hormone-related protein in adult T-cell leukemia-lymphoma. Ann Intern Med 1989;111:484–488.
47. Southby J, Kissin MW, Danks JA, et al. Immunohistochemical localization of parathyroid hormone-related protein in human breast cancer. Cancer Res 1990;50:7710–7716.
48. Powell GJ, Southby J, Danks JA, et al. Localization of parathyroid hormone-related protein in breast cancer metastases: Increased incidence in bone compared with other sites. Cancer Res 1991;51:3059–3061.
49. Seyberth HW, Segre GV, Morgan JL, Sweetman BJ, Potts JT Jr, Oates JA. Prostaglandins as mediators of hypercalcemia associated with certain types of cancer. N Engl J Med 1975;293:1278–1283.
50. Tashjian AH Jr. Prostaglandins, hypercalcemia and cancer. N Engl J Med 1975;293:1317–1318.
51. Tashjian AH Jr, Tice JE, Sides R. Biological activities of prostaglandin analogues and metabolites on bone resorption in vitro. Nature 1977;266:645–647.
52. Raisz LG, Dietrich JW, Simmons HA, et al. Effects of prostaglandin endoperoxides and metabolites on bone resorption in vitro. Nature 1977;267:532–535.
53. Valentin-Opran A, Eilon G, Saez S, et al. Estrogens and antiestrogens stimulate release of bone-resorbing activity by cultured human breast cancer cells. J Clin Invest 1985;75:726.
54. Brenner BE, Harvey HA, Lipton A, Demers L. A study of prostaglandin E_2, parathormone, and response to indomethacin in patients with hypercalcemia of malignancy. Cancer 1982;49:556–561.
55. Metz SA, McRae JR, Robertson RP. Prostaglandins as mediators of paraneoplastic syndromes: Review and update. Metabolism 1981;30:299–316.
56. Robertson RB, Baylink DJ, Metz SA, Cummings KB. Plasma prostaglandin E in patients with cancer with and without hypercalcemia. J Clin Endocrinol Metab 1976;43:1330–1335.
57. Lau K-HW, Lee MY, Linkhart TA, et al. A mouse tumor-derived osteolytic factor stimulates bone resorption by a mechanism involving local prostaglandins production in bone. Biochim Biophys Acta 1985;840:56–68.
58. Bringhurst FR, Bierer BE, Godeau F, Neyhard N, Varner V, Segre GV. Humoral hypercalcemia of malignancy: Release of a prostaglandin-stimulating bone resorbing factor in vitro by human transitional-cell carcinoma cells. J Clin Invest 1986;77:456–464.
59. Mundy RR, Raisz LG, Cooper RA, Schechter GP, Salmon SE. Evidence for the secretion of an osteoclast stimulating factor in myeloma. N Engl J Med 1974;291:1041–1046.
60. Mundy GR, Luben RA, Raisz LG, Oppenheim JJ, Buell DN. Bone-resorbing activity in supernatants from lymphoid cell lines. N Engl J Med 1974;290:867–871.
61. Sporn MB, Roberts AB. Autocrine growth factors and cancer. Nature 1985;313:745–747.
62. Todaro GJ, Fryling C, De Larco JE. Transforming growth factors produced by certain human tumor cells: Polypeptides that interact with epidermal growth factor receptors. Proc Natl Acad Sci USA 1980;77:5258–5262.
63. Ibbotson KJ, Twardzik DR, D'Souza SM, et al. Stimulation of bone resorption in vitro by synthetic transforming growth factor-alpha. Science 1985;228:1007–1009.
64. Stern PH, Krieger NS, Nissenson RA, et al. Human transforming growth factor-alpha stimulates bone resorption in vitro. J Clin Invest 1985;76:2016–2019.
65. Sporn MB, Roberts AB, Wakefield LM, de Crombrugghe B. Some recent advances in the chemistry and biology of transforming growth factor-beta. J Cell Biol 1987;105:1039–1045.
66. Robey PG, Young MF, Flanders KC, et al. Osteoblasts synthesize and respond to TGF-beta in vitro. J Cell Biol 1987;105:457–463.
67. Gowen G, Wood DD, Ihrie EJ, McGuire MKB, Russell RGG. An interleukin 1-like factor stimulates bone resorption in vitro. Nature 1983;306:378–380.
68. Dewhirst FE, Stashenko PP, Mole JE, et al. Purification and partial sequence of human osteoclast activating factor: Identity with interleukin-1 beta. J Immunol 1985;135:2562–2568.
69. Stashenko P, Dewhirst FE, Peros WJ, Kent RL, Ago JM. Synergistic interactions between interleukin-1, tumor necrosis factor, and lymphotoxin in bone resorption. J Immunol 1987;138:1464–1468.
70. Mundy GR, Ibbotson KJ, D'Souza DM. Tumor products and the hypercalcemia of malignancy. J Clin Invest 1985;76:391–394.
71. Lee MY, Liu CC, Lottsfeldt JL, Judkins SA, Howard GA. Production of granulocyte-stimulating and bone cell-modulating activities from a neutrophilia hypercalcemia-inducing murine mammary cancer cell line. Cancer Res 1987;47:4059–4065.
72. Sato K, Mimura H, Han DC, et al. Production of bone-resorbing activity and colony-stimulating activity in vivo and in vitro by a human squamous cell carcinoma associated with hypercalcemia and leukocytosis. J Clin Invest 1986;78:145–154.
73. Bertolini DR, Nedwin GE, Bringman TS, Smith DD, Mundy GR. Stimulation of bone resorption and inhibition of bone formation in vitro by human tumor necrosis factors. Nature 1986;319:516–518.
74. Garrett IR, Durie BGM, Nedwin GE, et al. Production of lymphotoxin, a bone-resorbing cytokine, by cultured human myeloma cells. N Engl J Med 1987;317:526–532.
75. Davies M, Mawer EB, Hayes ME, Lumb GA. Abnormal vitamin D metabolism in Hodgkin's lymphoma. Lancet 1985;1:1186–1188.
76. Rieke JW, Donaldson SS, Horning SJ. Hypercalcemia and vitamin D metabolism in Hodgkin's disease. Is there an underlying immunoregulatory relationship? Cancer 1989;63:1700–1707.
77. Breslau NA, McGuire JL Zerwekh JE, Frenkel EP, Pak CYC. Hypercalcemia associated with increased serum calcitriol levels in three patients with lymphoma. Ann Intern Med 1984;100:1–7.
78. Adams JS, Fernandez M, Gacad MA, et al. Hypercalcemia and hypercalciuria associated elevated serum 1,25-dihydroxyvitamin D concentrations in patients with AIDS and non-AIDS-related lymphoma. Blood 1989;73:235–239.
79. Helikson MA, Harvey AD, Zerwekh JE, Breslau NA, Gardner DW. Plasma cell granuloma producing calcitriol and hypercalcemia. Ann Intern Med 1986;105:379–381.
80. Shigeno H, Yamamoto I, Dokoh S, et al. Identification of 1,24-(R)-dihydroxyvitamin D_3-like-bone-resorbing lipid in a patient with cancer-associated hypercalcemia. J Clin Endocrinol Metab 1985;61:761–768.
81. Stote RM, Smith LH, Wilson DM, et al. Hydrochlorothiazide effects on serum calcium and immunoreactive parathyroid hormone concentration: Studies in normal subjects. Ann Intern Med 1972;77:587–591.
82. Mawer EB, Hann JT, Berry JL, et al. Vitamin D metabolism in patients intoxicated with ergocalciferol Clin Sci 1985;68:135–141.
83. Katz CM, Tzagournis M. Chronic adult hypervitaminosis A with hypercalcemia. Metabolism 1972;21:1171–1176.
84. Valentic JP, Elias AN, Weinstein GD. Hypercalcemia associated with oral isotretinoin in the treatment of severe acne. JAMA 1983;250:1899–1900.
85. Warrell RP Jr. Questions about clinical trials in hypercalcemia. J Clin Oncol [Editorial] 1988;6:759–761.
86. Blythe WB, Gitelman HJ, Welt LG. Effect of expansion of the extracellular space on the rate of urinary excretion of calcium. Am J Physiol 1968;214:52–57.
87. Massry SG, Coburn JW, Chapman LW, et al. Effect of NaCl infusions on urinary Ca^{++} and Mg^{++} during reduction in their filtered loads. Am J Physiol 1967;213:1218–1224.
88. Massry SG, Friedler RM, Coburn JW Excretion of phosphate and calcium: Physiology of their renal handling and relation to clinical medicine. Arch Intern Med 1973;131:828–836.
89. Hosking DJ, Cowley A, Bucknall CA. Rehydration in the treatment of severe hypercalcemia. Q J Med 1981;200:473–481.
90. Suki WN, Hull HR, Rector FC Jr, et al. Mechanism of the effect of thiazide diuretics on calcium and uric acid. J Clin Invest 1967;46:1121.
91. Suki WN, Yium JJ, Von Minden M, et al. Acute treatment of hypercalcemia with furosemide. N Engl J Med 1970;283:836–840.
92. Yates AJ, Oreffo ROC, Mayor K, Mundy GR. Inhibition of bone resorption by inorganic phosphate is mediated by both reduced osteoclast formation and decreased activity of mature osteoclasts. J Bone Miner Res 1991;6:473–478.
93. Herbert LA, Lemann J, Peterson JR, et al. Studies of the mechanism by which phosphate infusion lowers serum calcium concentration. J Clin Invest 1966;45:1886–1894.
94. Eisenberg E. Effect of intravenous phosphate on serum strontium and calcium. N Engl J Med 1970;282:889–892.
95. Spaulding SW, Walser M. Treatment of experimental hypercalcemia with oral phosphate. J Clin Endocrinol 1970;31:531–538.
96. Mundy GR, Wilkinson R, Heath DA. Comparative study of available medical therapy for hypercalcemia of malignancy. Am J Med 1983;74:421–432.

97. Heath DA. The use of inorganic phosphate in the management of hypercalcemia. Metab Bone Dis Rel Res 1980;2:213–215.
98. Thalassinos N, Joplin GF. Phosphate treatment of hypercalcemia due to carcinoma. Br Med J 1968;4:14–19.
99. Ayala G, Chertow BS, Shah JH, et al. Acute hyperphosphatemia and acute persistent renal insufficiency induced by oral phosphate therapy. Ann Intern Med 1975;83:520–521.
100. Goldsmith RS, Ingbar SH. Inorganic phosphate in the treatment of hypercalcemia of diverse etiologies. N Engl J Med 1966;274:1–7.
101. Massry SG, Mueller E, Silverman AG, et al. Inorganic phosphate treatment of hypercalcemia. Arch Intern Med 1968;121:307–312.
102. Shackney S, Hasson J. Precipitous fall in serum calcium, hypotension, and acute renal failure after intravenous phosphate therapy for hypercalcemia: Report of two cases. Ann Intern Med 1967;66:906–916.
103. Carey RW, Schmott GW, Kopald HH, et al. Massive extraskeletal calcification during phosphate treatment of hypercalcemia. Arch Intern Med 1968;122:150–155.
104. Dudley FJ, Blackburn CRB. Extraskeletal calcification complicating oral neutral phosphate therapy. Lancet 1970;2:628–630.
105. Laflamme GH, Jowsey J. Bone and soft tissue changes with oral phosphate supplements. J Clin Invest 1972;51:2834–2840.
106. Breuer RI, LeBauer J. Caution in the use of phosphates in the treatment of severe hypercalcemia. J Clin Endocrinol Metab 1967;27:695–698.
107. Seyberth HW, Segre GV, Hamet P, Sweetman BJ, Potts JT Jr, Oates JA. Characterization of the group of patients with the hypercalcemia of cancer who respond to treatment with prostaglandin synthesis inhibitors. Trans Assoc Am Physicians 1976;89:92–104.
108. Brenner DE, Harvey HA, Lipton A. A study of prostaglandin E_2, parathormone, and response to indomethacin in patients with hypercalcemia. Cancer 1982;49:556–561.
109. Coombes RC, Neville AM, Bondy PK, et al. Failure of indomethacin to reduce hydroxyproline excretion or hypercalcemia in patients with breast cancer. Prostaglandins 1976;12:1027–1035.
110. Sandler DP, Burr R, Weinberg CR. Nonsteroidal anti-inflammatory drugs and the risk for chronic renal disease. Ann Intern Med 1991;115:165–172.
111. Whelton A, Stout RL, Spilman PS, Klassen DK. Renal effects of ibuprofen, piroxicam, and sulindac in patients with asymptomatic renal failure. A prospective, randomized, crossover comparison. Ann Intern Med 1990;112:568–576.
112. Chakmajian ZH, Bethune JE. Sodium sulfate treatment of hypercalcemia. N Engl J Med 1966;275:862–869.
113. Heckman BA, Walsh JH. Hypernatremia complicating sodium sulfate therapy for hypercalcemic crisis. N Engl J Med 1967;276:1082–1083.
114. Kahill M, Orman B, Gyorkey F, Brown H. Hypercalcemia—experience with phosphate and sulphate therapy. JAMA 1967;201:721–724.
115. Spencer H, Greenberg J, Berger E, Perrone M, Laszlo D. Studies on the effect of ethylenediaminetetraacetic acid in hypercalcemia. J Lab Clin Med 1956;47:29–41.
116. Raisz LG, Trummel CL, Wener JA, et al. Effect of glucocorticoids on bone resorption in tissue culture. Endocrinology 1972;90:961–967.
117. Bentzel CJ, Carbone PP, Rosenberg L. The effect of prednisone on calcium metabolism and ^{47}Ca kinetics in patients with multiple myeloma and hypercalcemia. J Clin Invest 1964;43:2132–2145.
118. Kimberg DB, Baerg RD, Gershon E, et al. Effect of cortisone treatment on the active transport of calcium by the small intestine. J Clin Invest 1971;50:1309–1321.
119. Muggia FM, Heinemann HO. Hypercalcemia associated with malignant disease. Ann Intern Med 1970;73:281–290.
120. Myers WPL. Cortisone in the treatment of hypercalcemia in neoplastic disease. Cancer 1958;11:83–88.
121. Percival RC, Yates AJP, Grey RES, et al. Role of glucocorticoids in the management of malignant hypercalcemia. Br Med J 1984;289:287.
122. Ashkar FS, Miller R, Katins RB. Effect of corticosteroids on the hypercalcemia of malignant disease. Lancet 1971;1:41.
123. Thalassinos NC, Joplin G. Failure of corticosteroid therapy to direct the hypercalcemia of malignant disease. Lancet 1970;2:537–538.
124. Austin LA, Heath H III. Calcitonin: Physiology and pathophysiology. N Engl J Med 1981;304:269–278.
125. Krane SM, Harris ED Jr, Singer FR, et al. Acute effects of calcitonin on bone formation in man. Metabolism 1973;22:51–58.
126. Vaughn CB, Vaitkevicius K. The effects of calcitonin in hypercalcemia in patients with malignancy. Cancer 1974;34:1268–1271.
127. Hosking DJ. Treatment of severe hypercalcemia with calcitonin. Metab Bone Dis Rel Res 1980;2:207–212.
128. Wisneski LA, Groom WP, Silva DL, Becker KL. Salmon calcitonin in hypercalcemia. Clin Pharmacol Ther 1978;23:219–222.
129. Wisneski LA. Salmon calcitonin in the acute management of hypercalcemia. Calcif Tissue Int 1990;46:S26–S30.
130. Warrell RP Jr, Israel R, Frisone M, Snyder T, Gaynor JJ, Bockman RS. A randomized double-blind study of gallium nitrate versus calcitonin for acute treatment of cancer-related hypercalcemia. Ann Intern Med 1988;108:669–674.
131. Wener JA, Gorton SJ, Raisz LG. Escape from inhibition of resorption in cultures of fetal bone treated with calcitonin and parathyroid hormone. Endocrinology 1978;90: 752–759.
132. Reitsma PH, Teitelbaum SL, Bijvoet OLM, Kahn AJ. Differential action of the bisphosphonates (3-amino-1-hydroxypropylidene)-1,1-biphosphonate (APD) and disodium dichloromethylidene biphosphonate (Cl_2MDP) on rat macrophage-mediated bone resorption in vitro. J Clin Invest 1982;70:927–933.
133. Carano A, Teitelbaum SL, Konsek JD, Schlesinger PH, Blair HC. Bisphosphonates directly inhibit the bone resorption activity of isolated avian osteoclasts in vitro. J Clin Invest 1990;85:456–461.
134. Witte RS, Koeller J, Davis TE, et al. Clodronate: A randomized study in the treatment of cancer-related hypercalcemia. Arch Intern Med 1987;147:937–939.
135. Bonjour J-P, Rizzoli R. Clodronate in hypercalcemia of malignancy. Calcif Tissue Int 1990;46:S20–S25.
136. Storm T, Thamsborg G, Steiniche T, Genant HK, Sorensen OH. Effect of intermittent cyclical etidronate therapy on bone mass and fracture rate in women with postmenopausal osteoporosis. N Engl J Med 1990;322:1265–1271.
137. Hasling C, Charles P, Mosekilde L. Etidronate disodium for treating hypercalcaemia of malignancy: A double blind, placebo-controlled study. Eur J Clin Invest 1986;16: 433–437.
138. Ryzen E, Martodam RR, Troxell M, et al. Intravenous etidronate in the management of malignant hypercalcemia. Arch Intern Med 1985;145:449–452.
139. Singer FR, Ritch PS, Lad TE, et al. Treatment of hypercalcemia with intravenous etidronate: A controlled multicenter study. Arch Intern Med 1991;151:471–476.
140. Warrell RP Jr, Heller G, Murphy WP, Schulman P, O'Dwyer P. A randomized double-blind study of gallium nitrate compared to etidronate for acute control of cancer-related hypercalcemia. J Clin Oncol 1991;9:1467–1475.
141. Gucalp R, Ritch P, Wiernik PH, et al. Comparative study of pamidronate disodium and etidronate disodium in the treatment of cancer-related hypercalcemia. J Clin Oncol 1992;10:134–142.
142. Bounameaux HM, Schifferli J, Monatni J-P, Chatelanat F. Renal failure associated with intravenous diphosphonates. Lancet 1983;1:471.
143. Schiller JM, Rasmussen P, Benson AB, et al. Maintenance etidronate in the prevention of malignancy-associated hypercalcemia. Arch. Intern Med 1987;147:963–966.
144. Thiebaud D, Jaeger P, Jacquet AF, et al. Dose response in the treatment of hypercalcemia of malignancy by a single infusion of the bisphosphonate AHPrBP J Clin Oncol 1988;6: 762–768.
145. Body JJ, Magritte A, Seraj F, Sculier JP, Borkowski A. Aminohydroxypropylidene bisphosphonate (APD) treatment for tumor-associated hypercalcemia: A randomized comparison between a 3-day treatment and single 24-hour infusions. J Bone Miner Res 1989;4:923–928.
146. Body JJ, Pot M, Borkowski A, Sculier JP, Klastersky J. Dose-response study of aminohydroxypropylidene bisphosphonate in tumor-associated hypercalcemia. Am J Med 1987;82:957–963.
147. Nussbaum SR, Mallette L, Gagel R, et al. Single dose treatment of hypercalcemia of malignancy with aminohydroxypropylidene bisphosphonate (APD). J Bone Miner Res 1989;4:S313.
148. Adami S, Bolzicco GP, Rizzo A, et al. The use of dichloromethylene bisphosphonate and aminobutane bisphosphonate in hypercalcemia of malignancy. Bone Miner 1987;2: 395–404.
149. Warrell RP Jr, Bockman RS, Coonley CJ, Isaacs M, Staszewski H. Gallium nitrate inhibits calcium resorption from bone and is effective treatment for cancer-related hypercalcemia. J Clin Invest 1984;73:1487–1490.
150. Bockman RS, Boskey A, Alcock N, Bullough P, Warrell R. Gallium nitrate inhibits bone resorption, increases bone calcium content, but is not cytotoxic to bone cells. J Bone Miner Res 1985;1:65.
151. Cournot-Witmer G, Bourdeau A, Lieberherr M, et al. Bone modeling in gallium-nitrate-treated rats. Calcif Tissue Int 1987;40:270–275.
152. Hall TJ, Chambers TJ. Gallium inhibits bone resorption by a direct effect on osteoclasts. Bone Miner 1990;8:211–216.
153. Warrell RP Jr, Alcock NW, Skelos A, Bockman RS. Gallium nitrate inhibits accelerated bone turnover in patients with bone metastases. J Clin Oncol 1987;5:292–298.
154. Bockman RS, Repo MA, Warrell RP, et al. Distribution of trace levels of therapeutic gallium in bone as mapped by synchrotron x-ray microscopy. Proc Natl Acad Sci USA 1990;87:4149–4153.
155. Bockman RS, Bosley A, Blumenthal NC, Alcock NW, Warrell RP. Gallium increases bone calcium and crystallite perfection of hydroxyapatite. Calcif Tissue Int 1986;39: 376–381.
156. Schlesinger PH, Teitelbaum SL, Blair HC. Osteoclast inhibition by Ga^{3+} contrasts with bisphosphonate metabolic suppression: Competitive inhibition of H^+ ATPase by bone-bound gallium. J Bone Miner Res 1991;6(suppl 1):S127.
157. Bockman RS, Israel R, Alcock N, Ferguson R, Warrell RP. Gallium nitrate stimulates bone collagen synthesis. Clin Res 1987;35:620A.
158. Warrell RP Jr, Skelos A, Alcock NW, Bockman RS. Gallium nitrate for acute treatment of cancer-related hypercalcemia: Clinicopharmacologic and dose-response analysis. Cancer Res 1986;46:4208–4212.
159. Brown JH, Kennedy BJ. Mithramycin in the treatment of disseminated testicular neoplasms. N Engl J Med 1965;272:111–118.
160. Kennedy BJ. Metabolic and toxic effects during mithramycin therapy. Am J Med 1970;49: 494–503.
161. Lebbin D, Ryan WG, Schwartz TB. Outpatient treatment of Paget's disease of bone with mithramycin. Ann Intern Med 1974;81:635–637.
162. Perlia CP, Gubisch NJ, Wolter J, et al. Mithramycin treatment of hypercalcemia. Cancer 1970;25:389–394.
163. Elias EG, Evans JT. Hypercalcemic crisis in neoplastic diseases: Management with mithramycin. Surgery 1972;71:631–635.
164. Stapleton FB, Linshaw MA. Treatment of hypercalcemia associated with osseous metastases. J Pediatr 1976;89:1209–1030.
165. Coombes RC, Dady P, Parsons C, et al. Mithramycin therapy: An adjunct to conventional treatment of hypercalcemia and bone metastases in breast cancer. Metab Bone Dis Rel Res 1980;2:199–202.

166. Kiang DT, Loken MK, Kennedy BJ. Mechanism of the hypocalcemic effect of mithramycin. J Clin Endocrinol Metab 1979;48:341–344.
167. Minkin C. Inhibition of parathyroid hormone stimulated bone resorption in vitro by the antibiotic mithramycin. Calcif Tissue Int 1973;13:249–257.
168. Parsons DM, Baum M, Self M. Effect of mithramycin on calcium and hydroxyproline metabolism in patients with malignant disease. Br Med J 1967;1:474–477.
169. Green L, Donehower RC. Hepatic toxicity of low doses of mithramycin in hypercalcemia. Cancer Treat Rep 1984;68:1379–1381.
170. Ralston SH, Gardner MD, Dryburgh FJ, Jenkins AS, Cowan RA, Boyle IT. Comparison of aminohydroxypropylidene diphosphonate, mithramycin, and corticosteroids/calcitonin in treatment of cancer-associated hypercalcemia. Lancet 1985;2:907–910.
171. Thiebaud D, Jacquet AF, Burckhardt P. Fast and effective treatment of malignant hypercalcemia: Combination of suppositories of calcitonin and a single infusion of 3-amino-1-hydroxypropylidene-1-bisphosphonate. Arch Intern Med 1990;150:2125–2128.
172. Miach PJ, Dawborn JK, Martin TJ, et al. Management of the hypercalcemia of malignancy by peritoneal dialysis. Med J Aust 1975;1:782–784.
173. Lad TE, Mishoulam HM, Shevrin DH, Kukla LJ, Abramson EC, Kukreja SC. Treatment of cancer-associated hypercalcemia with cisplatin. Arch Intern Med 1987;147:329–332.
174. Bockman RS, Bohnsack R, Warrell RP. Effect of metal-based compounds on bone resorption. Clin Res 1986;34:390A.
175. Robinson RR, Yarger WE. Acute uric acid nephropathy. Arch Intern Med 1977;137:839–840.
176. Klinenberg JR, Kippen I, Bluestone R. Hyperuricemic nephropathy: Pathophysiologic features and factors influencing urate deposition. Nephron 1975;14:88–98.
177. Crittendon DR, Ackerman GL. Hyperuricemic acute renal failure in disseminated carcinoma. Arch Intern Med 1977;137:97–99.
178. Maidemont CG, Greaves MF, Black AJ. T-cell leukemia presenting with hyperuricaemia, acute renal failure, and gout. Clin Lab Haematol 1983;5:423–426.
179. Cohen LF, Balow JE, Magrath IT, Poplack DG, Ziegler JL. Acute tumor lysis syndrome. A review of 37 patients with Burkitt's lymphoma. Am J Med 1980;68:486–491.
180. Garnick MB, Mayer RB. Acute renal failure associated with neoplastic disease and its treatment. Semin Oncol 1978;5:155–165.
181. Yu T-F. Secondary gout associated with myeloproliferative diseases. Arthitis Rheum 1965;8:765–771.
182. Ultmann J. Hyperuricemia in disseminated neoplastic disease other than lymphomas or leukemias. Cancer 1962;15:122–129.
183. Melink TJ, Von Hoff DD, Kuhn JG, et al. Phase I evaluation and pharmacokinetics of tiazofurin (2-beta-D-ribofuranosylthiazole-4-carboxamide, NSC 286193). Cancer Res 1985;45:2859–2865.
184. Conger JD, Falk SA. Intrarenal dynamics in the pathogenesis and prevention of acute urate nephropathy. J Clin Invest 1977;59:786–793.
185. Muggia FM, Ball TJ Jr, Ultmann JE. Allopurinol in the treatment of neoplastic disease complicated by hyperuricemia. Arch Intern Med 1967;120:12–18.
186. Krakoff IH, Meyer RL. Prevention of hyperuricemia in leukemia and lymphoma. JAMA 1965;193:1–6.
187. Skipper HE, Robins RK, Thomson JR, et al. Structure-activity relationships observed on screening a series of pyrazolopyrimidines against experimental neoplasms. Cancer Res 1957;17:579–596.
188. Rundles RW, Wyngaarden JB, Hithcings GH, Elion GB, Silberman HR. Effects of a xanthine oxidase inhibitor on thiopurine metabolism, hyperuricemia, and gout. Trans Assoc Am Physicians 1963;76:126–140.
189. Band PR, Silbverberg DS, Henderson JF, et al. Xanthine nephropathy in a patient with lymphosarcoma treated with allopurinol. N Engl J Med 1970;283:354–357.
190. Hande KR, Hixson CV, Chabner BA. Postchemotherapy purine excretion in lymphoma patients receiving allopurinol. Cancer Res 1981;41:2273–2279.
191. Ortega JA, Ruccione K, Weinberg K, Sato J, Lammers P. Use of an investigational form of intravenous (IV) allopurinol for the treatment of hyperuricemia in children with malignancy. Proc Am Soc Clin Oncol 1985;4:257.
192. Simmonds HA, Cameron JS, Morris GS, Davies PM. Allopurinol in renal failure and the tumor lysis syndrome. Clin Chim Acta 1986;160:189–195.
193. Templeton JS. Azapropazone or allopurinol in the treatment of chronic gout and/or hyperuricemia. A preliminary report. Br J Clin Pract 1982;36:353–358.
194. Gibson T, Simmonds HA, Armstrong RD, Fairbanks LD, Rodgers AV. Azapropazone—a treatment for hyperuricaemia and gout? Br J Rheumatol 1984;23:44–51.
195. Warrell RP Jr, Muindi J, Stevens Y-W, Isaacs M, Young CW. Induction of profound hypouricemia by a non-sedating C-5 monosubstituted thiobarbiturate. Metabolism 1989;38:550–554.
196. Jankovic M, Zurlo MG, Rossi E, et al. Urate-oxidase as hypouricemic agent in a case of acute tumor lysis syndrome. Am J Pediatr Hematol Oncol 1985;7:202–204.
197. Mandell GA, Swacus JR, Rosenstock J, Buck BE. Danger of urography in hyperuricemic children with Burkitt's lymphoma. J Can Assoc Radiol 1983;34:273–277.
198. Steinberg SM, Galen MA, Lazarus JM. Hemodialysis for acute uric acid nephropathy. Am J Dis Child 1975;129:956–958.
199. Monballyou J, Zachee P, Verherckmoes R, Boogaerts MA. Transient acute renal failure due to tumor lysis-induced severe phosphate load in a patient with Burkitt's lymphoma. Clin Nephrol 1984;22:47–50.
200. Wollner A, Shalit M, Brezis M. Tumor genesis syndrome. Hypophosphatemia accompanying Burkitt's lymphoma cell leukemia. Miner Electrolyte Metab 1986;12:173–175.
201. Boles JM, Dutel JL, Briere J, et al. Acute renal failure caused by extreme hyperphosphatemia after chemotherapy of an acute lymphoblastic leukemia. Cancer 1984;53:2425–2429.
202. Tsokos GC, Balow JE, Speigel RJ, et al. Renal and metabolic complications of undifferentiated and lymphoblastic lymphomas. Medicine (Baltimore) 1981;60:218–229.
203. Cervantes F, Ribera JM, Granena A, et al. Tumor lysis syndrome with hypocalcemia in chronic granulocytic leukemia. Acta Haematol 1982;68:157–159.
204. Boccia RV, Longo DL, Lieher ML, Jaffe ES, Fisher RI. Multiple recurrences of acute tumor lysis syndrome in an indolent non-Hodgkin's lymphoma. Cancer 1985;56:2295–2297.
205. Zusman J, Brown DM, Nesbit ME. Hyperphosphatemia, hyperphosphaturia, and hypocalcemia in acute lymphoblastic leukemia. N Engl J Med 1973;289:1335–1340.
206. Ettinger DS, Harker WG, Gerry HW, Sanders RC, Saral R. Hyperphosphatemia, hypocalcemia, and transient renal failure: Results of cytotoxic treatment of acute lymphoblastic leukemia. JAMA 1978;239:2472–2474.
207. Gomez GA, Han T. Acute tumor lysis syndrome in prolymphocytic leukemia. Arch Intern Med 1987;147:375–376.
208. Vogelzang NJ, Nelimark RA, Nath KA. Tumor lysis syndrome after induction chemotherapy of small cell bronchogenic carcinoma. JAMA 1983;249:513–514.
209. Stark ME, Dyer MC, Coonley CJ. Fatal acute tumor lysis syndrome with metastatic breast carcinoma. Cancer 1987;60:762–764.
210. Fer MF, Bottino GC, Sherwin SA, et al. Atypical tumor lysis syndrome in a patients with T-cell lymphoma treated with recombinant leukocyte interferon. Am J Med 1984;77:953–956.
211. Cech P, Block JB, Cone IA, Stone R. Tumor lysis syndrome after tamoxifen flare. N Engl J Med 1986;315:263–264.
212. Simmons ED, Somberg KA. Acute tumor lysis syndrome after intrathecal methotrexate administration. Cancer 1991;67:2062–2065.
213. Gonzalez C, Villasanta U. Life-threatening hypocalcemia and hypomagnesemia associated with cisplatin chemotherapy. Obstet Gynecol 1982;59:732–734.
214. Harley HA, Mason R, Phillips PJ. Profound hypocalcemia associated with oestrogen treatment of carcinoma of the prostate. Med J Aust 1983;2:41–41.
215. Schenkein DP, O'Neill WC, Shapiro J, Miller KB. Accelerated bone formation causing profound hypocalcemia in acute leukemia. Ann Intern Med 1986;105:375–378.
216. Schilsky RL. Renal and metabolic complications of cancer chemotherapy. Semin Oncol 1982;9:75–83.
217. Papaioannou AN. Tumors other than insulinoma associated with hypoglycemia. Surg Gynecol Obstet 1966;123:1093–1109.
218. Daughaday WH. Hypoglycemia in patients with non-islet cell tumors. Endocrinol Metab Clin North Am 1988;18:91–101.
219. Hall K, Takano K, Fryklund L, Sievertsson H. Somatomedins. Adv Metab Disorders 1975;8:19–46.
220. Rinderknecht E, Humbel RE. The amino acid sequence of human insulin-like growth factor I and its structural homology with proinsulin. J Biol Chem 1978;253:2769–2776.
221. Zapf J, Schmid C, Guler HP, et al. Regulation of binding proteins for insulin-like growth factors (IGF) in humans. Increased expression of IGF binding protein 2 during IGF I treatment of healthy adults and in patients with extrapancreatic tumor hypoglycemia. J Clin Invest 1990;86:952–961.
222. Shapiro ET, Bell GI, Polonsky KS, Rubenstein AH, Kew MC, Tager HS. Tumor hypoglycemia: Relationship to high molecular weight insulin-like growth factor-II J Clin Invest 1990;85:1672–1679.
223. Axelrod L, Ron D. Insulin-like growth factor II and the riddle of tumor-induced hypoglycemia. N Engl J Med 1988;319:1477–1479.
224. Tisdale MJ, Brennan RA. Metabolic substrate utilization by a tumour cell line which induces cachexia in vivo. Br J Cancer 1986;54:601–606.
225. Davis MR, Shamoon H. Deficient counterregulatory hormone responses during hypoglycemia in a patient with insulinoma. J Clin Endocrinol Metab 1991;72:788–792.
226. Samaan NA, Pham FK, Sellin RV, Fernandez JF, Benjamin RS. Successful treatment of hypoglycemia using glucagon in a patient with and extreapancreatic tumor. Ann Intern Med 1990;113:404–406.
227. Hoffken K, Kemf H, Miller AA, et al. Aminoglutethimide without hydrocortisone in the treatment of postmenopausal patients with advanced breast cancer. Cancer Treat Rep 1986;70:1153–1157.
228. Spiegel RJ, Oliff AI, Bruton J, et al. Adrenal suppression after short-term corticosteroid therapy. Lancet 1979;1:630–633.
229. Seidenwurm DJ, Elmer EB, Kaplan LM, Williams EK, Morris DG, Hoffman AR. Metastases to the adrenal glands and the development of Addision's disease. Cancer 1984;54:552–557.
230. Redman DG, Pazdur R, Zingas AP, Loredo R. Prospective evaluation of adrenal insufficiency in patients with adrenal metastasis. Cancer 1987;60:103–107.
231. Frommer JP. Lactic acidosis. Med Clin North Am 1983;67:815–829.
232. Mizock BA. Controversies in lactic acidosis. Implications in critically ill patients. JAMA 1987;258:497–501.
233. Doolittle GC, Wurster MW, Rosenfeld CS, Bodensteiner DC. Malignancy-induced lactic acidosis. South Med J 1988;81:533–536.
234. Madias NE. Lactic acidosis. Kidney Int 1986;29:752–754.
235. Sculier JP, Nicaise C, Klastersky J. Lactic acidosis: A metabolic complications of extensive metastatic cancer. Eur J Clin Oncol 1983;19:597–601.
236. Fraley, DS, Adler, R, Bruns, FJ, Zetts, B. Stimulation of lactate production by administration of bicarbonate in a patient with a solid neoplasm and lactic acidosis. N Engl J Med 1980;303:1100–1102.
237. Cooper DJ, Walley KR, Wiggs BR, Russell JA. Bicarbonate does not improve hemodynamics in critically ill patients who have lactic acidosis. A prospective controlled clinical study. Ann Intern Med 1990;112:492–498.

238. Stacpoole PW. Lactic acidosis: The case against bicarbonate therapy. Ann Intern Med [Editorial] 1986;105:276–279.
239. Ritter JM, Doktor HS, Benjamin N. Paradoxical effect of bicarbonate on cytoplasmic pH. Lancet 1990;335:1243–1246.
240. Androgue HJ, Brensilver J, Cohen JJ, et al. Influence of steady-state alterations in acid-base equilibrium on the fate of administered bicarbonate in the dog. J Clin Invest 1983;71:867–879.
241. Graf L, Leach WJ, Arieff AI. Metabolic effects of sodium bicarbonate in hypoxic lactic acidosis in dogs. Am J Physiol 1985;249:F630–F635.
242. Narins RC, Cohen JJ. Bicarbonate therapy for organic acidosis: The case for its continued use. Ann Intern Med 1987;106:615–618.
243. Narins RG, Jones ER, Dornfield LP. Alkali therapy of the organic acidoses: A critical assessment of the data and the case for judicious use of sodium bicarbonate. In: Narins RG, ed. Controversies in nephrology and hypertension. New York: Churchill-Livingstone, 1984:359.
244. Stacpoole PW, Wright EC, Baumgartner TG, et al. A controlled clinical trial of dichloroacetate for treatment of lactic acidosis in adults. N Engl J Med 1992;327:1564–1569.

SECTION **4**

ALAN R. BAKER

Surgical Emergencies

The patient with cancer is potentially susceptible to a constellation of physical insults. Some arise as a direct consequence of the primary tumor or its metastatic sequelae; some appear in the aftermath of treatment and are toxicity related. Still others arise completely independent of the malignancy. For the surgeon called on to evaluate an emergency in a patient with cancer, a thorough understanding of the natural history of the specific tumor and an appreciation of where he or she intercepts the patient in the course of that neoplastic encounter help to clarify problems that otherwise can be quite perplexing. No effort is made in this chapter to summarize general surgery or physical diagnosis, because good references abound for these topics.[1–3] The natural histories of the many different tumor types are discussed in the chapters on specific diseases in this text. This chapter examines the clinically pressing circumstances that arise in the context of successful or failed treatment of the tumor. Diagnostic manipulations and therapeutic maneuvers that have proven useful adjuncts to difficult judgment making at the bedside are presented. Although there exist few texts covering these topics, three good references should be reviewed.[4–6]

DIAGNOSIS AND CONSULTATION

Pain, tenderness, fever, chills, nausea, vomiting, diarrhea, obstipation, distension, and blood, whether occult or frank, issuing from mouth or anus are the often cited problems that invite surgical consultation. These symptoms and signs must be taken with utmost seriousness and should prompt the surgeon to a thorough understanding of the patient's total problem. A meticulous history must be elicited from the patient and the family, and the patient's records must be queried for specific information. This is the time to read the pertinent prior operative notes and pathology reports and examine the details of recent and remote treatment measures. How much radiation therapy has the patient received and to what portals? Which antineoplastic agents has the patient been given in the past 6 weeks? What other drugs, with particular emphasis on narcotics, steroids, and diuretics, has the patient been taking?

With the chart in hand, the patient's recent laboratory data are reviewed to determine the impact of treatment and the extent of aberration caused by acutely deranged physiology. Bone marrow reserve and response are assessed through determinations of hemoglobin or hematocrit, leukocyte count and differential, and platelet count. Serum electrolytes, particularly potassium and magnesium, amylase, BUN, creatinine, and liver function tests including prothrombin time and, if pertinent, serum tumor marker levels are observed. Recent data from the microbiology laboratory are reviewed with particular reference to positive blood cultures and possibly stool *Clostridium difficile* titers.

A diligent but directed physical examination, usually coupled with rectal and, for women, pelvic assessment should be performed. Extra time spent in eliciting evidence of peritoneal irritation, as manifested by cough or shake tenderness and truly absent bowel sounds, is well spent.

Although the data afforded by the history, physical examination, and laboratory studies frequently does not completely reveal the problem, they can provide direction about which more elaborate, more expensive, and often more invasive additional studies should be obtained. They provide important baseline information, because changes in the patient's clinical condition over time measured in hours often weigh heavily in making the decision about whether to proceed to operation. Alternatively, changes sometimes proceed more slowly than expected, and fully appreciating them requires once or twice daily visits, stretched over a couple of weeks, as host defenses recover and homeostatic integrity is restored.

For most problems, it is usual to obtain initial plain roentgenograms of the chest (posteroanterior [PA] and lateral views) and abdomen (supine and upright views). When these x-ray films are examined, it is always profitable to take the extra time to compare them with prior similar films and review all contrast-enhanced fluoroscopic studies and CT and MR scans.

The complexity of the cancer patient's clinical story creates and contributes to uncertainty and confusion. Determining whether the apparent urgent situation is a consequence of the tumor or the therapy directed at it can be quite difficult. Leukemic or lymphomatous organ infiltration can simulate the pain that results from a myriad of other causes of the acute surgical abdomen.[7–12] Steroids occasionally mask the usual response to peritoneal soilage and make the most sinister of circumstances seemingly serene.[13] The fever, chills, and rigors associated with severe chemotherapy-induced neutropenia can deceptively mimic the sepsis picture of bowel perforation or undrained accumulations of pus.[14] Some paraneoplastic factors and certain antineoplastic agents can produce a profound degree of gut neuropathy that simulates mechanical intestinal obstruction.[15,16] Resolving these kinds of ambiguity can prove a significant clinical challenge but must be done to determine whether the urgent circumstance warrants or demands surgical intervention. Additional diagnostic tests are usually needed.

The past two decades have witnessed a technologic explosion in the number, kind, and complexity of tests available for sorting out difficult problems. The astute clinician must decide which tests to do, when to obtain them, and reckon the cost of the information derived in terms of time, effort, dollars, and potential morbidity. Subtle problems in communication among the subspecialists involved can make this task more difficult. Every test or study ordered should be directed at answering a question. Couched in these terms, the consultant diagnostic or invasive radiologist, nuclear medicine specialist, or endoscopist can better understand the problem and nature of the help sought and be better able to assist in the determination of which of the available options can most expeditiously provide the needed information.

DECIDING TO OPERATE

Many cancer patients, particularly those in therapy, are significantly depleted, immunologically compromised hosts with exceedingly limited reserves. Compound their chronic illness with an acute, catabolic, and occasionally catastrophic insult, and the stage is set for significant morbidity and high mortality rate outcomes.

In a survey by Turnbull and Starnes at Memorial Sloan-Kettering Cancer Center, one third (66 of 200) of the urgent procedures were done to manage the cancer or a complication of chemotherapy.[5] Forty-four percent (88 of 200) were performed to manage a complication of the prior cancer surgery, and 21% (42 of 200) of the laparotomies were necessitated by nonneoplastic or antineoplastic treatment related diagnoses. In fact, 13 of these 42 procedures were done in patients without evidence of cancer. Laparotomy failed to reveal an urgent problem in the remaining 2% (4 of 200).

Salvage after surgery to manage these urgent problems was disappointing, although not unexpectedly so. In 36% (72 of 200) of the cases, the patient died before discharge from the hospital. If postprocedure recovery led to discharge, survival was less than 3 months for roughly 10% (19 of 200) of procedures, between 3 and 6 months for 11% (22 of 200) of procedures, between 6 and 12 months for 11% (22 of 200) of procedures, and exceeded 1 year for the remaining 32% (65 of 200).

That cancer patients receiving chemotherapy are acutely vulnerable to insults that necessitate operation is highlighted by the fact that 45% (64 of 140) of the procedures had to be done in this setting. That their expectation for survival is poor is additionally reflected in the experience reported by Ferrara.[17] Of 21 patients actively in treatment who suffered catastrophic perforative (15) or hemorrhagic (6) complications, 17 died (81%) after operation. An additional 2 patients died within 1 month of hospital discharge: 1 patient survived 5 months, and the last remained alive and disease free 9 months after discharge at the time of the report. Nineteen of these 21 patients suffered a total of 51 postoperative complications that included pneumonia or respiratory failure (15), septicemia (9), hemorrhage (7), hepatic failure (3), bone marrow failure (3), wound infection (5), and nonspecified problems (5). The four second operations were categorized as complications.

Because oncologic patients can ill afford a procedure that creates more problems than it solves, the surgeon before proceeding to operation must clarify or resolve several important questions.[18] What is the exact nature of the problem? What surgically, in specific terms, must be done to provide remedy? Are there any less invasive, equally suitable alternatives to operation available? In this setting, I think the role of the purely exploratory laparotomy is of questionable value.

URGENT CONDITIONS

The urgent problems surgeons most often confront in cancer patients can be grouped as obstruction, perforation, hemorrhage, and infection. Some overlap syndromes are seen, but usually one of these four clinical features becomes dominant and compelling. Table 60–15 summarizes the results reported by Turnbull and Starnes of the urgent reasons for which cancer patients required surgery.[5] Instructive representative clinical examples within each category are examined later in this section.

PERFORATION

A perforated intestinal viscus and the attendant peritonitis it causes almost always produces a clinically dramatic picture. Severe, constant abdominal pain with associated diffuse tenderness, guarding, and often rigidity, profound ileus with consequent distension and quiet to absent bowel sounds, fever and the hemodynamic sequelae of third space fluid accumulation, and bacteremia with resultant tachycardia, hypotension, and oliguria contribute to an appropriate sense of bedside urgency. The upright chest x-ray film or left-side-down lateral decubitus view, which usually demonstrates free intraabdominal air, strongly favors colonic or gastroduodenal perforation and usually demands urgent exploration.[19] I have never regretted making some preoperative effort to determine the site of perforation. Moderate or severely edematous bowel, covered by a fibrinopurulent exudate in the setting of multiple adhesions from the usual prior abdominal procedure, can make finding the site of perforation quite difficult. Being able to proceed directly to the sigmoid colon or to an initial look at the distal stomach and duodenum permits the physician to make the optimal incision, saves operative time, and minimizes the chance for unintended injury to structures encountered during a tedious, otherwise undirected exploration.

TABLE 60–15. Gastrointestinal or Intraabdominal Problems Requiring Operation in 310 Patients With Cancer

Problem	*No. of Patients (%)*
Obstruction	89 (29)
Perforation	66 (21)
Hemorrhage	85 (28)
Infection	47 (15)
Other	23 (7)
Total	310 (100)

(Turnbull ADM. Surgical emergencies in the cancer patient. Chicago: Year Book Medical Publishers, 1987:157;195)

If the clinical history favors gastroduodenal perforation (*e.g.*, steroids, prior ulcer disease, hematemesis or occult blood in the stool), it is wise to proceed with a Gastrografin study by mouth or through the nasogastric tube that had initially been placed. If the findings favor a colonic lesion (*e.g.*, prior diverticular disease, antecedent crampy lower abdominal pain), it is better to start with a Gastrografin enema. With a positive initial study, the surgeon can proceed directly to operation. If the initial study is negative and the patient's clinical condition permits, the alternative examination is done. During the 2 hours required and after blood cultures have been obtained, broad-spectrum antibiotics (*e.g.*, gentamycin, ampicillin, clindamycin) are instituted and energetic intravascular volume resuscitation initiated.

Alternatively, the perforation may not be into the free peritoneal cavity. If it occurs into another hollow viscus, it produces an enteroenteric, enterovessical, enterovaginal, or enteroureteral fistula.[20] If the leak tracks to an external surface, an enterocutaneous fistula results. Perforation into the vascular tree produces an arterioenteric fistula with clinical manifestations of intermittent sepsis and episodes of sentinel or massive hemorrhage.[21] Retroperitoneal tumors can on occasion erode into the gut.[22] The clinical picture in this circumstance is similar to that seen if the leak from an intestinal segment is contained or walled off by surrounding structures, and it heralds itself as an abscess with septic features.

Clinically significant acute pancreatitis can mimic the acute abdomen seen with bowel infarction and impending or frank nonfree gut perforation. Although most often idiopathic, alcohol, or gallstone related, it can be seen after the administration of chemotherapeutic agents, most notably L-asparaginase.[23,24] Because it is usually desirable to avoid operation for patients with acute pancreatitis, it is helpful to obtain a serum amylase and lipase preoperatively. Normal values virtually exclude acute pancreatitis, and significantly elevated values make the diagnosis likely. Because some amylase can be released from infarcting intestine, the minimally elevated value leaves the physician in a diagnostic quandary. If intraperitoneal fluid is present, it can be helpful to tap it by paracentesis or culdocentesis; measure amylase, lipase, glucose, and lactic acid dehydrogenase levels in it; examine the fluid by Gram's stain; and culture for organisms and quantitate the numbers of leukocytes and erythrocytes. The laboratory profile is usually diagnostic.

Most perforations occur through a portion of bowel wall involved by a clinically known or undiagnosed tumor. Mural involvement by lymphoma at the level of the colon, small intestine, or stomach can perforate spontaneously or in the wake of effective antitumor chemotherapy.[25–27] Several nongut primary tumors, including lung, breast, melanoma, and kidney, can metastasize to bowel wall, undergo necrosis, and produce perforative sequelae.[28] Primary gastric and colon cancer can present as gut perforations. The site of the perforation is usually at the tumor, although sometimes a more distally located colon tumor produces sufficient closed-loop obstructive difficulty (in the presence of a competent ileocecal valve) and distension to lead to cecal perforation.

A host of other etiologic factors may play a role, particularly if the site of perforation is through bowel wall uninvolved by tumor. Included among these are acid-peptic, diverticular, and benign gastric ulcer disease associated with or without concomitant steroids.[13,29] Toxic colitis or typhlitis, often seen in the context of drug-related (*e.g.*, cytarabine, vinca alkaloids, taxol) profound neutropenia, can lead to appendiceal or colonic perforation.[30–33] Similarly, cytomegalovirus infection associated with human immunodeficiency virus infection or with tumor- or drug-induced immunocompromise can produce incipient or frank gut perforation as can severe *C. difficile* toxin-associated enterocolitis.[34,35] Immunotherapy with interleukin-2 has produced this complication.[36] On occasion, a suture line leak or disruption at the site of enterotomy closure or formal anastomosis, particularly if the bowel has been subjected to significant prior irradiation, can produce the clinical picture of bowel perforation.[37,38] A summary of the complex constellation of etiologically associated factors is provided in Table 60–16.

Perforative problems and their sequelae can be dire clinical events in cancer patients, with an associated mortality rate in excess of 50%.[13,17,39–42] Because these hosts often exhibit a diminished capacity to provide hemostasis, resist microbial attack, and repair injured tissue, several principles of management must be remembered. These are summarized in Table 60–17. The surgeon must remember that the surgical procedure does not have to solve all the patient's problems at once. It should instead strive to eradicate only the most life-threatening problems identified and restore the patient to a condition that permits continued attention to and therapy for the primary disease. Liberal provision of blood and blood product support, nutritional supplementation, and aggressive antimicrobial drug administration are critical elements in bolstering weakened host defenses.

The following cases and pertinent associated diagnostic studies illustrate several features and issues encountered in relation to the patient with perforative pathology.

Patient No. 1

Six years earlier, a 49-year-old woman had undergone a complete hysterectomy for a high-grade uterine leiomyosarcoma. A large, left-sided malignant pleural effusion and pulmonary metastases were proven at diagnostic thoracotomy 2 months before referral. After receiving a hematoporphyrin photosensitizer on April 23, 1991, she underwent median sternotomy, left pneumonectomy, right middle lobe nodule wedge excision, and photodynamic therapy to the

TABLE 60–16. Etiologic Factors in Gut Perforation

Tumor at Site of Perforation	*Perforation Through Noninvolved Gut Wall*
Primary colon	Cecal perforation with distal obstructing colon cancer
Primary stomach	Acid-peptic, diverticular disease (±steroids)
Lymphoma	Colitis
Leukemia	Neutropenic enterocolitis (drug)
	Viral (CMV)
	Bacterial (*C. difficile*)
	Interleukin-2
Primary small bowel	Gastric ulcer
Metastatic cancer from lung, breast, melanoma, kidney	Failure of anastomosis or enterotomy closure (±irradiation)

TABLE 60–17. Surgical Principles in the Management of Gut Perforations in Cancer Patients

1. Eliminate the source of continued septic insult by resecting the site of perforation. Exteriorization/resection, particularly for colonic perforation, is preferred. Suture plication should be used for benign duodenal ulcer, benign gastric ulcer, and traumatic perforation only.
2. Be conservative in immediately restoring bowel continuity. Stomas (*e.g.*, colostomy, ileostomy, mucous fistula) are recommended. Anastomotic leaks should be avoided.
3. Copiously irrigate the peritoneal cavity with antibiotic solutions to reduce the burden of contamination.
4. Place drains so that enteric leaks can be comfortably converted to controlled fistulas.
5. Achieve adequate hemostatis using electrocautery, sutures, hemoclips, and topical thrombin or Gelfoam as needed.
6. Minimize wound complications by delayed primary closure techniques and the use of retention sutures.
7. Use liberal tube decompression to avoid adverse impact of distension on healing bowel or abdominal incision. These tubes can later be used for enteral feeding.

chest cavity. On her third postoperative day, she developed severe abdominal pain. A chest x-ray film (Fig. 60–5A,B) showed new, free intraperitoneal air, and a Gastrografin swallow (see Fig. 60–5C,D) revealed contrast extravasation through a perforated duodenal ulcer. The problem was managed at laparotomy with plication and an omental patch graft. Her subsequent recovery proved uneventful, and she was discharged home on the 13th postlaparotomy day. She remained well until 8 months later, when recurrent chest, axillary,and neck nodal metastatic disease developed.

Patient No. 2

An 11-year-old boy with an abdominal mass underwent right colectomy for mural and mesenteric nodal involvement by diffuse histiocytic lymphoma. He received 2100 cGy of postoperative abdominal radiotherapy and multidrug chemotherapy consisting of cyclophosphamide, vincristine, methotrexate, and prednisone. One week after the administration of cycle three, he developed severe abdominal pain, nausea, and vomiting. A chest x-ray film and Gastrografin swallow revealed free intraperitoneal air and contrast agent extravasation similar to that seen in patient #1. A gastric perforation through an area of lymphomatous involvement (Fig. 60–6) was found at laparotomy and handled with resection by partial gastrectomy and splenectomy. On recovery from surgery, two additional cycles of chemotherapy were administered, followed by autologous bone marrow transplantation. Despite this approach, his lymphoma progressed, and he died 5 months after the gastric perforative catastrophe.

OBSTRUCTION

The patient with intestinal obstruction suffers symptoms of spectral severity ranging from "can't eat to can't drink to can't handle endogenous secretions, swallowed air, or gut elaborated gases." Partial or complete deprivation of oral intake imposes a significant quality of life debit and leaves the patient anywhere from mildly distressed to deeply miserable. The accompanying, usually crampy abdominal pain, nausea, vomiting, obstipation, absent flatus, distension, and usually hyperactive (with rushes and tinkles) or dystonic (amphoric and resonant) bowel sounds invite surgical consultation and force the need to pose and methodically answer the following questions. Is there a mechanical impediment or problem present? At what and how many sites is it located? To what functional degree is the lumen compromised? Is bowel viability threatened as a consequence of distension? What is or are the causes of the blockage? What is the likelihood of spontaneous resolution?

Plain films of the abdomen (supine and upright) and chest (PA and lateral) should demonstrate the absence of free air and usually show luminal distension which, depending on degree, distribution, and the presence of differential air-fluid levels, permit inferences about whether the obstruction is partial or complete, its site, and its mechanism. Unless early in its evolution, gas seen in the rectum and rectosigmoid colon strongly suggest an incomplete blockage. Extensive colonic and small bowel dilation suggest a distal colonic site, and differential air-fluid levels favor a mechanical rather than a metabolic cause.

Significant hypokalemia, hypomagnesemia, and hypocalcemia and the recent intake of narcotics or administration of vinca alkaloids can severely impair neuromuscular function and produce profound and ubiquitous gut distension. These kinds of drug-associated toxicity represent an often seen constellation in the cancer patient and can contribute significantly to what may prove a multifactor basis for an obstructive picture. A normal serum amylase or lipase reassuringly rules out pancreatitis with its attendant ileus.

Unless there is fever, focal tenderness, and significant leukocytosis, any of which create a sense of urgency by provoking concern about gut ischemia and infarction, the passage of a nasogastric tube usually provides some degree of decompression, buys time, and permits repletion of third space fluid losses and a decision about which additional diagnostic studies or procedures to perform.[43] Serial plain films of the abdomen are quite useful and provide a sense about whether the situation is getting better or worse.

A colonic component in any obstructive picture significantly complicates the workup and management of the problem and must be appreciated before surgery. For the cancer patient, if time and circumstances permit, the colon should be "prepped" before any operation directed at relieving obstruction. Meaningfully obstructed colon is difficult to prepare well for surgery. Cathartics like GoLytely, castor oil, or magnesium citrate are contraindicated. Depending on how proximal the obstruction is and its degree, enemas may be inefficient in evacuating feces upstream of it. Nonabsorbable antibiotics given by mouth may never reach the colon. Dealing with an unprepared colon at surgery is a major hazard. Obstipated feces themselves can compound the mechanical obstructive problem and potentially threaten the integrity of a proximal anastomosis or enterotomy closures and provide significant peritoneal contamination if the colon is inadvertently entered. Colonic pathology in the unprepared colon is usually managed with a colostomy, the surgical alternative that virtually every patient dreads.

Because primary colonic inflammatory pathology, such as diverticulitis, focal ischemic colitis, Crohn's disease, or a walled-off perforative neoplasm, often deceptively mimics pure small bowel obstruction, it is usually wise to rule out a large bowel component to the obstructive picture. Sigmoid-

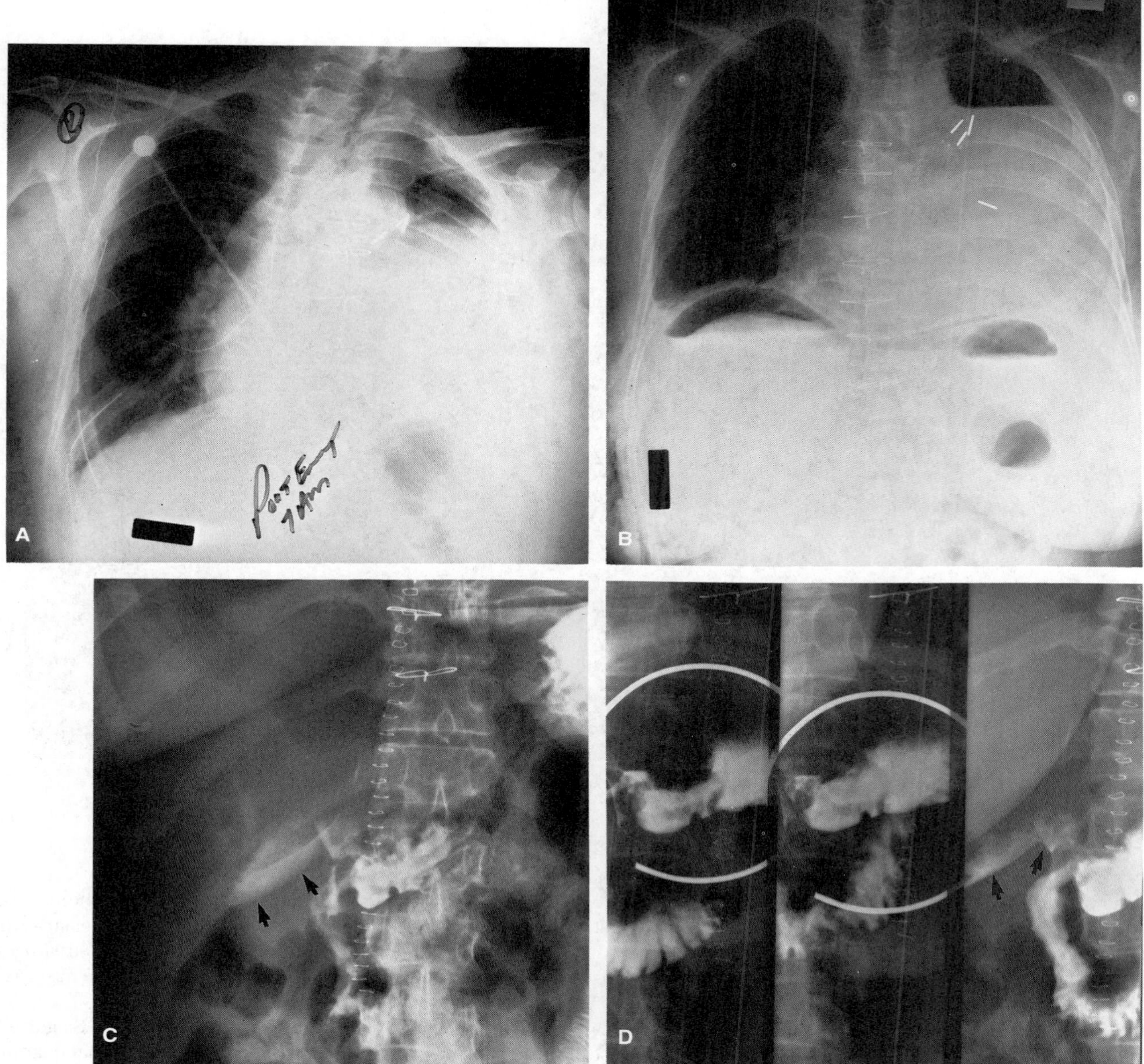

FIGURE 60–5. **(A)** Poststernotomy chest x-ray film that shows no free intraperitoneal air. **(B)** B) Radiograph taken 2 days later, shortly after the abdominal pain developed, shows free intraperitoneal air. **(C, D)** Extravasation of contrast agent (*arrows*) through the perforated duodenal ulcer.

oscopy followed by barium enema suitably accomplishes this objective. If on fluoroscopy a significant obstructive colonic process is seen, the radiologist must terminate the study and try to minimize the quantity of barium sulfate permitted to go proximal to it. Water absorbed by the colon from the barium sulfate suspension proximal to an even partially obstructive colonic problem will make it impossible to adequately prepare the bowel.

If the barium enema acquits the colon of playing any pathogenetic role in the obstructive picture, it becomes safe and often useful to later perform an upper gastrointestinal series with small bowel follow through or a similar prograde study done through a long gastrointestinal tube (*e.g.*, Miller-Abbott, Cantor). The long tube minimizes the amount of information-obscuring barium sulfate required and makes it easier to delineate the areas of obstructive pathology. In this instance, barium sulfate is much preferred to a water-soluble contrast agent like Gastrografin, which tends to become progressively more dilute, with resultant loss of information, as it flows distally into fluid filled loops. Unlike the colon, the small intestine is unable to absorb significant water from the barium sulfate suspension used. Even if it remains upstream of a complete block for a significant period, barium concretions never form, and no iatrogenic compounding of the problem ensues. The upper gastrointestinal series (Fig. 60–7), done in error as the initial study for presumptive small bowel ob-

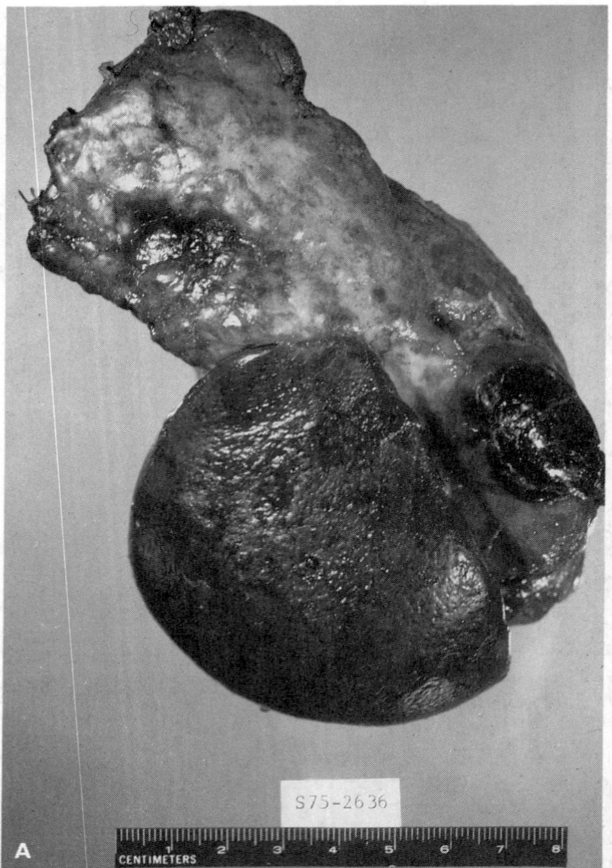

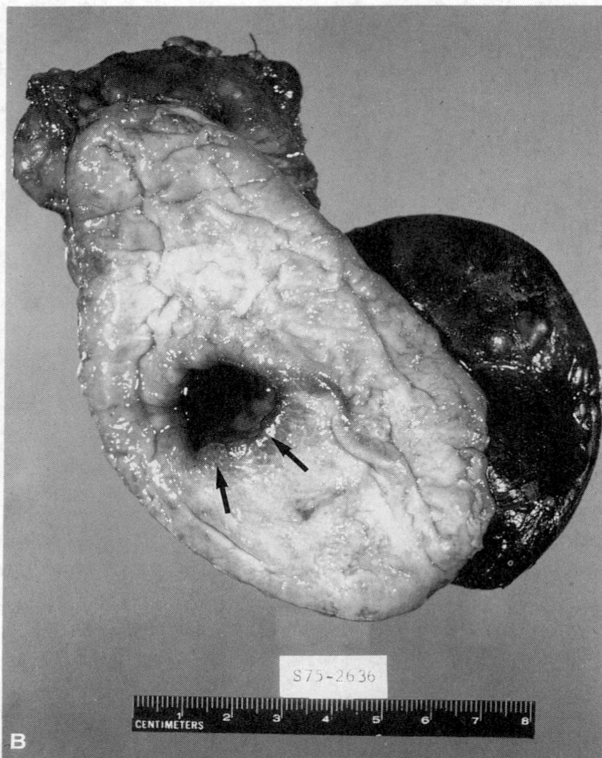

FIGURE 60–6. (A) Photograph of the resected specimen, consisting of a portion of the greater curvature of stomach and spleen. (B) The stomach has been opened, and the lymphomatous ulcer (*arrows*) is readily seen.

struction, illustrates the problem created when barium sulfate irretrievably impacts in a markedly distended cecum just proximal to an obstructing primary colon cancer.

Somewhat perversely, a swallowed barium sulfate meal often passes through and clears the gut of a patient who is intermittently vomiting and unable to adequately aliment. Regrettably, the barium meal, a not quite stringent enough test for the problem, neither pleases the palate nor has any nutritional value. The fluoroscopist may be unable to identify one or more focal points of obstruction. He should however, provide qualitative information about the amount and coherence of peristaltic activity and provide a measure of gut transit time. In this situation, it can be particularly helpful to pass a long gastrointestinal tube. The Miller-Abbott or Cantor tube is an almost too stringent test for mechanical obstruction. Although it may hang up prematurely in a proximal small bowel loop, it often proceeds quite a distance into the jejunum. Every loop the tube does traverse is a functionally unobstructed loop. At later operation, when virtually unrecognizable, matted, and plastered bowel loops can create much confusion and consternation, the palpable presence of the tube helps to identify the location in the gut and permits bypass of the obstructive problem by performing an anastomosis between the most distal tube-containing (*i.e.*, unobstructed) small bowel loop and some anatomically convenient portion of the colon, previously shown to be unobstructed by barium enema. I have no preference for the long tube over the nasogastric tube, aside from its unique utility in the just described situation. Both fairly efficiently decompress the gut, but the nasogastric tube is easier to place and maintain.

The information summarized in Table 60–18, garnered from nine reports spanning the past 2 decades that examined populations of cancer patients who developed intestinal obstruction, helps to put any given patient in clinical perspective.[44–52] Although the number of patients reported in each series is modest, a total of 583 patients were tracked. In most instances, the percentage of patients falling within each subgroup is provided; notice that these percentages do not always sum to 100% due to using denominators in subgroup calculations that differ from the total number of patients in the actual series.

The history of a prior malignancy or the presence of recurrent tumor, even if at sites outside the abdomen, substantially increase the probability that a bout of intestinal obstruction is due to tumor. The proportion with malignant causes for their obstructions is between 59% and 97% (mean, 78%).[44,45,47,48,50–52] This figure contrasts strikingly to the roughly 10% of patients with a malignant cause for the problem reported in nonselective series of patients with gut obstruction, for whom the far more frequent cause is benign

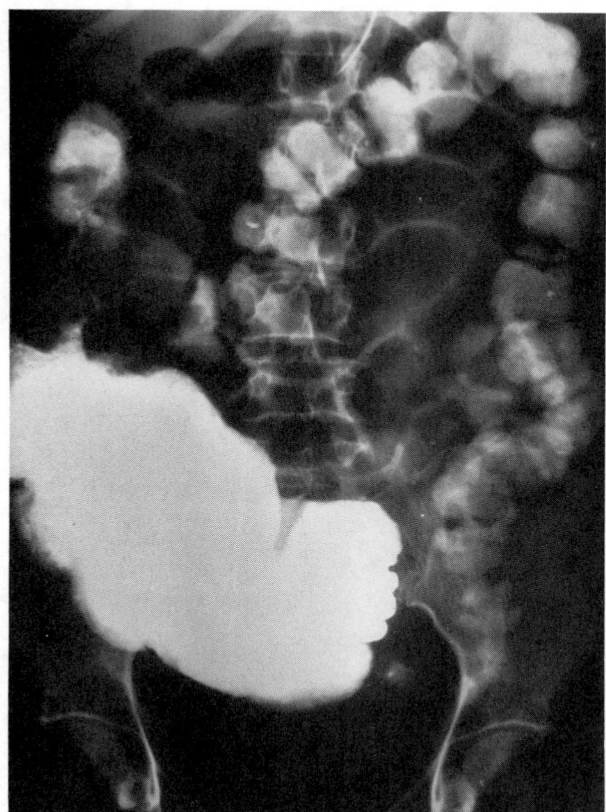

FIGURE 60–7. Irretrievable, orally administered barium sulfate is impacted in the cecum and ascending colon of a patient with an obstructing colonic cancer.

postoperative adhesions.[49,53] Cancer patients can have benign causes for their intestinal obstructions; between 3% and 38% (mean, 23%) were in this group.[44–48,50–52] If radiation therapy had been employed, radiation enteritis was more often implicated as a cause.[44,47]

The primary tumors most commonly predisposing to obstruction were of colorectal, ovarian, gastric pancreatic, uterine, and bladder lesions. Lymphoma was frequently found, as were tumors arising outside the abdominal cavity, such as breast, melanoma, and sarcoma.

Clinically appreciated persistent or recurrent cancer and a short free interval between treatment for the primary lesion and the presentation of the obstructive problem seem to increase the likelihood of a malignant cause for the blockage.[45,50,51]

Reliable differentiation before operation of patients with ischemic or infarcted gut can be exceedingly difficult.[54] Experienced clinical judgment is at best faulty. None of our tests are adequately sensitive or specific. Because the morbidity and mortality of operations complicated by this finding are higher than for those that deal with simple obstruction, the expectant or nonoperative management of the obstructed patient is somewhat anxiety provoking. Fortunately and reassuringly, most series of bowel obstruction in cancer patients report a relatively small proportion of patients, usually between 0% and 5%, with strangulation.[49–52] The highest figure, an anomalous 19%, was reported by Butler.[44]

Between 12% and 28% of cancer patients spontaneously resolve their obstructive difficulties.[44,46,49,50] Even those who seemingly resolve on gut decompression and intravenous fluid support can develop a recurrent bout, often soon after the initial episode that necessitated surgery.[44,46,50]

Probably little is lost with conservative management for 3 to 10 days. During that interval, the patient's anatomic problem can be better defined and initial efforts made at physiologically and psychologically preparing him for what lies ahead.

If surgery becomes necessary, the technical options include lysis of adhesions, gut bypass, bowel resection, or fashioning of a colostomy, ileostomy, or jejunostomy. A combination of these alternatives is often required by the anatomic sites and etiologic circumstances of blockage. Often difficult to detect preoperatively is extensive carcinomatosis, with multiple sites of obstruction, foreshortened mesentery, and presumed neural plexus infiltration. In this context, the meaningful options are exceedingly limited. When nothing can apparently be done to relieve the obstruction, placement of a palliative gastrostomy can be helpful.

For the cancer patient with intestinal obstruction, the realistic prospects for surgical intervention are rather grim. Operative mortality is high, 9% to 35% (average, 19%), as is the corresponding operative morbidity rate of 15% to 49%.[44–52] Between 4% and 45% (average, 15%) of the operations fail to resolve the obstructive problem, or it recurs soon after surgery. Repeated operations, although occasionally done, rapidly approach diminishing returns.[50–52] Unless a benign cause for the obstruction is found, survival for these patients is on the order of several months.[45,46,48,50] A small proportion of patients do survive for prolonged periods, and those fortunate enough to be relieved of their obstructive distress enjoy far better quality of life. Baines and coworkers at St. Christopher's Hospice, London, in an enlightening report, detailed the "aggressive medical measures" that can be done to optimize the quality of a patient's remaining life if surgery fails or is not undertaken.[55] Pharmacologic manipulations with a variety of agents, often administered by patient-controlled, continuous, parenteral infusion, permit comfortable nasogastric tube-free existence for periods ranging between 1 and 12 months.

The previous comments do not apply to intestinal obstruction in the cancer patient in the perioperative context. In this setting, most bouts of apparent bowel obstruction respond to conservative measures and often need to be patiently waited out. Without clinical findings to suggest causes such as bowel suture line leak, volvulus, retention suture bowel loop entrapment, or incarcerated gut with an internal hernia, I have let periods as long as 21 days go by, awaiting spontaneous lysis of these presumed perioperative, filmy adhesions. The judicious use of parenteral, centrally, or peripherally administered hyperalimentation ensures minimal further loss of nutritional ground during this period.

Pseudo-obstruction involving the small or large intestine is a pathogenetically, poorly understood entity that has been reported with increasing frequency in the recent literature.[56–58] Although it occasionally is seen in cancer patients, it more commonly afflicts those with collagen-vascular and metabolic diseases. Affection of the small bowel can often be satisfactorily managed with long tube decompression, and

TABLE 60–18. Experiences With Intestinal Obstruction in Cancer Patients

Characteristics	*Butler, 1991*[44] (*n* = 54)	*Clarke, 1987*[45] (*n* = 49)	*Gallick, 1986*[46] (*n* = 84)	*Walsh, 1984*[47] (*n* = 53)	*Aabo, 1984*[48] (*n* = 41)	*Bizer, 1981*[49] (*n* = 35)	*Osteen, 1980*[50] (*n* = 66)	*Annest, 1979*[51] (*n* = 34)	*Ketcham, 1970*[52] (*n* = 117)
Known or recurrent cancer (%)	48	92					59	100	
Benign cause of obstruction (%)	32	14	26	32	17		38	3	18
Malignant cause of obstruction (%)	68	86		68	83		59	97	82
Gut strangulation (%)	19		Rare			3	2	0	5
Spontaneous resolution (%)	28		12			14	24		Seldom, temporary
Subsequently recurred (%)	45		41				41		
Recurrent or persistent obstruction after surgical treatment (%)	32	27	45	4	33	13	20	38	33
Operative mortality (%)	22	14	35	14	24		9	18	14
Operative morbidity (%)	49	49				20	15 wound	44	
Survival for all patients (mo)		5.7 (7 pts >1 y)	2.5	11 (15 pts >1 y)	4.5			4	(13% >3 y)
Survival with benign cause (mo)	49				36		5.5		(38% >3 y)
Survival with malignant cause (mo)	4.9				3		3 (6 pts >6 mo)		11 (4% >3 y)

similar, viability-threatening colonic involvement can usually be therapeutically decompressed with the colonoscope. Figure 60–8 illustrates an example of what was thought to be a severe case of vincristine-induced gut neuropathy.

A case is presented to illustrate the obstructive picture complex.

Patient No. 3

Eighteen years earlier, this 80-year-old man underwent abdominoperineal resection for adenocarcinoma of the rectum. A diagnosis of Wegener's granulomatosis was made 5 years ago on open lung biopsy; the hospital course was complicated by sepsis and pulmonary insufficiency that required a lengthy intensive care unit stay. Three years ago, the patient developed prostate cancer with extensive bony metastases treated with 7200 cGy to the prostate, 5400 cGy to pelvic lymph nodes, and bilateral orchiectomy. His disease remained stable for the next 3 years until he developed gross hematuria. At cystoscopy, bullous edema was found, and a mass was seen elevating the floor of the bladder. Biopsies revealed adenocarcinoma that stained immunohistochemically positive for carcinoembryonic antigen (CEA). Serum CEA was elevated to 144 ng/ml, and serum prostate specific antigen and acid phosphatase levels were normal. Chest x-ray films showed about 20 new pulmonary nodules. After suffering several weeks of intermittent abdominal distension and crampy pain, the patient developed frank small bowel obstruction confirmed on flat and upright abdominal films (Fig. 60–9A,B). A Gastrografin enema revealed no obstructive colonic component, refluxed the ileocecal valve, and showed a critically stenotic segment of distal ileum (see Fig. 60–9C,D). This finding was corroborated on abdominal CT scan (see Fig. 60–9E). At exploratory laparotomy numerous adhesions were lysed, a 6 × 8 cm pelvic mass identified, and a segment of strictured distal small bowel, presumably secondary to prior radiation therapy, bypassed with an ileoascending colostomy. Meaningful palliation was achieved when gastrointestinal integrity and function resumed uneventfully after operation. The patient died about 4 months later with progressive pulmonary metastatic disease and inanition.

HEMORRHAGE

Spontaneous hemorrhage of massive proportions from neoplastic lesions is a relatively uncommon problem. It can arise from a tumor, usually metastatic in nature and involving the mucosa of some portion of the gastrointestinal tract; from an extraluminal site, usually a hepatoma or hepatic adenoma; or more rarely a hepatic metastasis.[59–64] Occasionally, lymphomatous or leukemic gut infiltrative disease can produce this same problem.[25,65,66]

Far more common are episodes of hemorrhage that occur in an iatrogenically flavored context: postoperative bleeding after surgery for the primary lesion, a metastasis, or a treatment-related complication; spontaneous hemorrhage from an intercurrent benign lesion in the setting of chemotherapy-associated thrombocytopenia or clotting factor coagulopathy; or after percutaneous liver biopsy or central access line placement.[67]

The thought process triggered by most of these situations addresses several critical questions. What is the specific site of the hemorrhage? Point-source hemorrhage is far easier to control than diffuse bleeding. Ligatures are effective only when

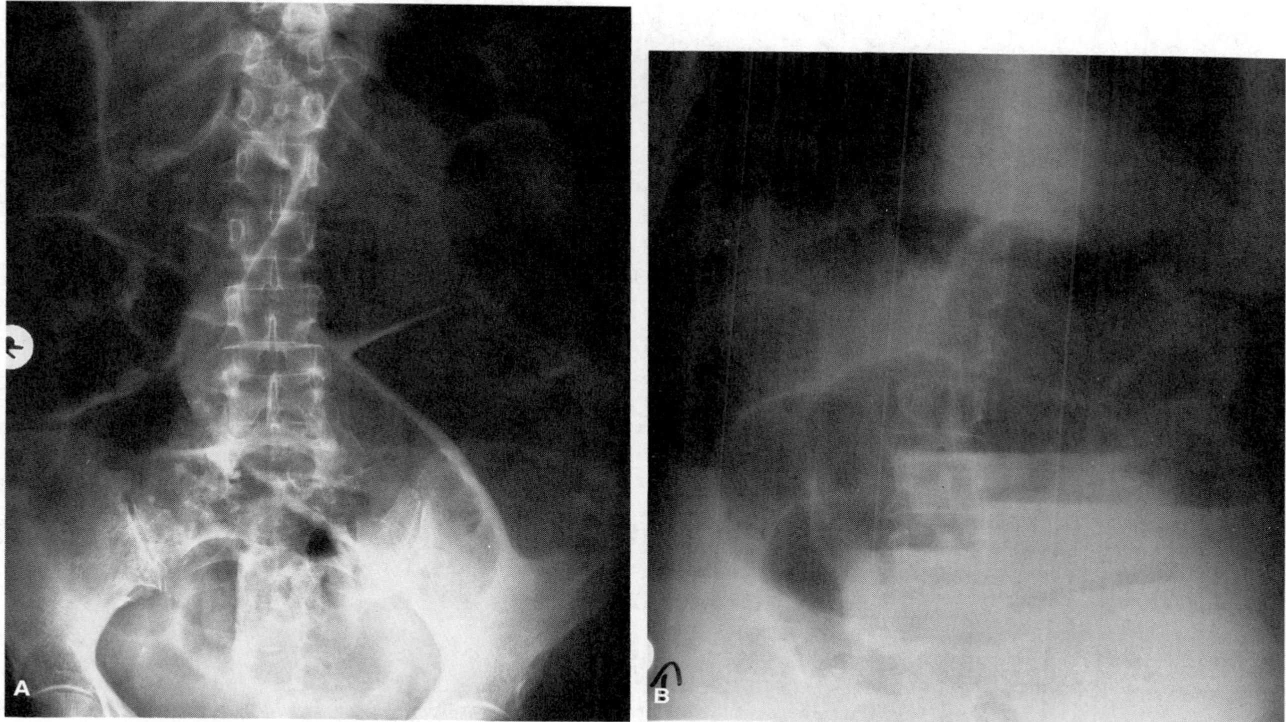

FIGURE 60–8. **(A, B)** Plain abdominal films illustrate a severe vincristine-induced ileus that persisted for several weeks.

thrown about the bleeding vessel rather than in rough proximity to it. Are coagulopathic problems identifiable and will correction of them result in cessation of the hemorrhage? Is the bleeding of sufficient magnitude that specific therapeutic measures should be initiated to control it?

The stigmata of hemorrhage are tempo driven. Hemodynamic instability, ranging from tachycardia, mild weakness, and orthostatic pressure changes to frank shock with profound hypotension, is seen. Intravascular volume and erythrocyte support must be expeditiously provided. A useful approach to the patient suffering a bout of hemorrhage is summarized in Table 60–19. Several points deserve emphasis and elaboration. Although listed serially, the enumerated maneuvers are usually made concomitantly.

In a gratifying proportion of instances, with volume support and coagulopathy correction, the bleeding spontaneously remits. If it does not and its site can be determined, the less invasive alternatives usually undertaken to define the site often control or stop the hemorrhage.

In experienced hands, endoscopically performed injection, electrocoagulation, or photocoagulation of bleeding gastroduodenal lesions provides definitive control of hemorrhage in about 75% of the patients.[68–70] Forceps or brush biopsy of suspicious looking lesions can provide additional information about benign, neoplastic, fungal, or viral causes.

Continuing hemorrhage, at a rate of about 1 ml per minute in the colon or small intestine is best evaluated by angiography. The more actively bleeding the lesion, the easier it is to angiographically demonstrate. Unwisely administered gut contrast agents, until cleared, preclude this option. Patients who are hemodynamically unstable, particularly if oliguric because of the contrast dye load needed, are stressful to study. The overall complexity of the effort required makes multiple studies difficult to accomplish and probably unwise and unreasonable to attempt. Because of these practical limitations, the timing of the study is critical, and this decision should be shared by surgeon and angiographer. Because a complete study may require several hours for runs of the inferior mesenteric artery, superior mesenteric artery, and celiac axis and a substantial administered dye load, it is wise to evaluate first the site most likely to be bleeding. If a diagnostic angiographic blush is identified, judgments can then be made about vasopressin infusion therapy (Athanasoulis) or transcatheter instillation of materials capable of producing vessel occlusion. Autogenous clot, Gelfoam torpedoes, Ivalon sponge, and metallic coils have been used with various degrees of success.[72,73] End-artery occlusion can produce significant organ ischemia and lead to complicating bowel infarction and perforation.

The importance of the invasive radiologist's technical virtuosity and judgmental expertise cannot be overstated. The former permits him to catheterize successfully and selectively the bleed vessel at a most distal or peripheral site, and the latter dictates which vessels can be successfully occluded without organ infarction.

If the less invasive therapeutic alternatives are not successful or not recommended, at least prior identification of the bleeding site lets the surgeon operate with the intent to suture-ligate or resect the affected tissues.

Hemorrhage into the free abdominal cavity, into the liver, or from the retroperitoneum or rectus sheaths is best evaluated by an abdominopelvic CT scan.[74] Spontaneous bleeding into the psoas or rectus muscles usually tamponades itself, can be

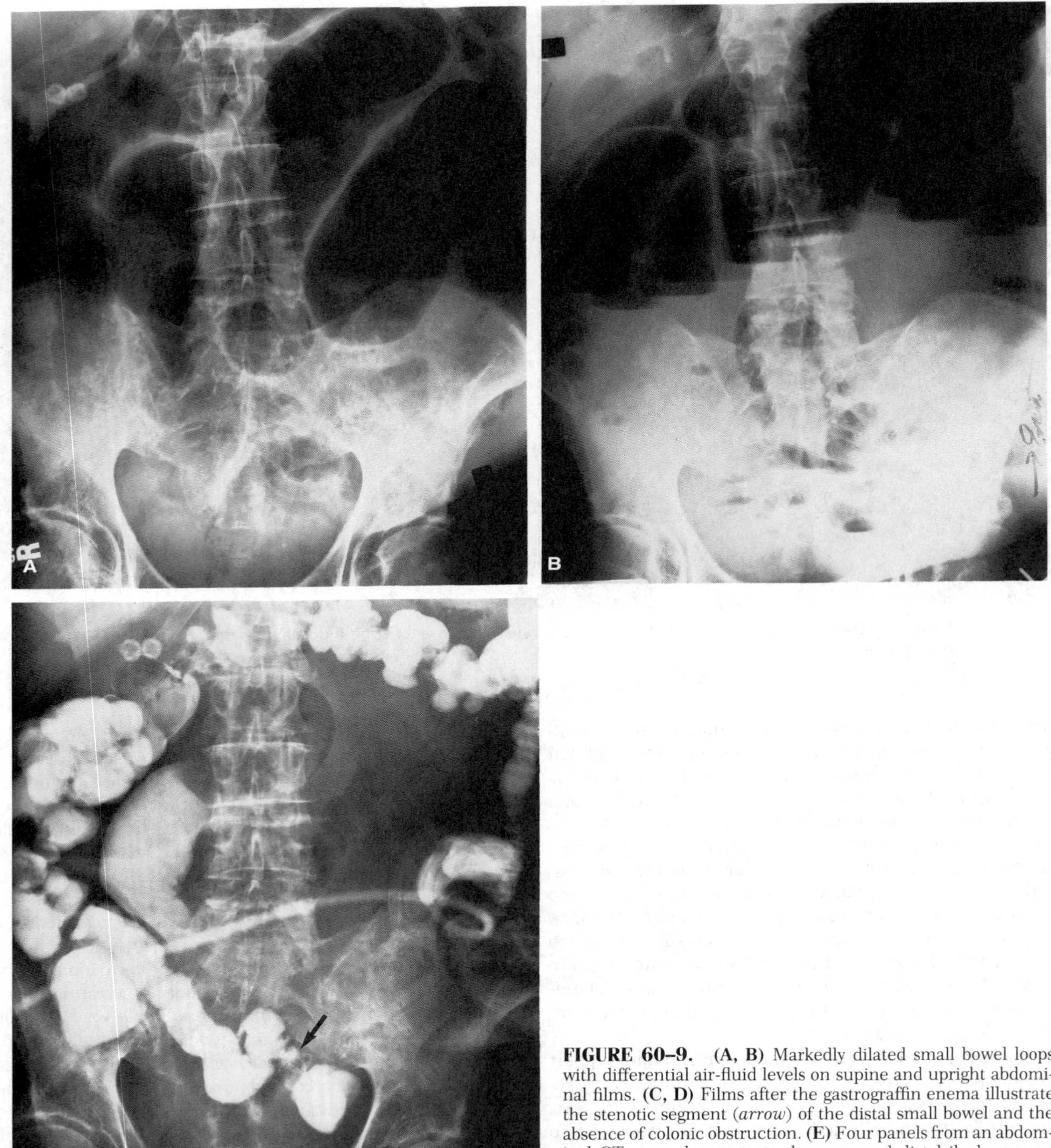

FIGURE 60–9. **(A, B)** Markedly dilated small bowel loops with differential air-fluid levels on supine and upright abdominal films. **(C, D)** Films after the gastrograffin enema illustrate the stenotic segment (*arrow*) of the distal small bowel and the absence of colonic obstruction. **(E)** Four panels from an abdominal CT scan, demonstrate the narrowed distal ileal segment (*arrow*).

managed expectantly, and resorbs in time. After needle biopsy, liver hemorrhage usually remits, but it occasionally becomes a hemodynamic threat. Angiographic approaches, as previously described, can permit the patient to escape surgical intervention. Figure 60–10A illustrates a contrast-enhanced abdominal CT scan obtained hours after percutaneous needle biopsy of the liver and shows a large right lobe hematoma. Figure 60–10B is a cut from an arteriogram done several hours later because of persistent hemorrhage. A dye blush shows the site of continued active bleeding, which was satisfactorily controlled by instillation of multiple Gelfoam torpedoes into the right hepatic artery.

The cancer patient deserves the time-tested surgical approaches to control free intraperitoneal hemorrhage from spleen, liver, aorta, or other sources. Fibrin glue, delivered as an aerosolized spray at surgery, has helped to control diffuse surface hemorrhage from the liver, spleen, and retroperitoneum.[75]

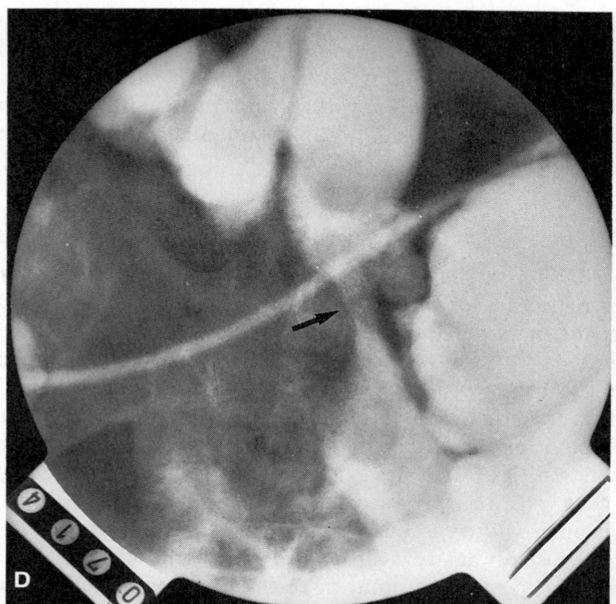

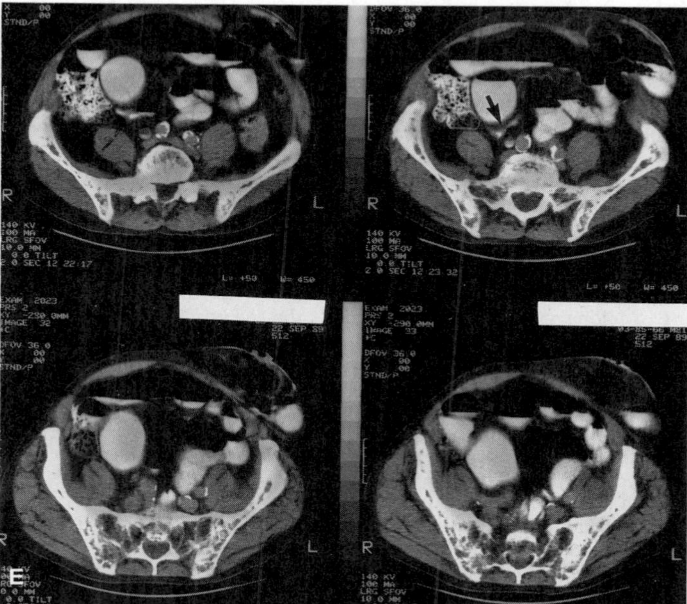

FIGURE 60–9. *(Continued)*

Anemia with subtly presenting symptoms of lassitude, fatigue, weakness, palpitations, and breathlessness is the result of slow chronic gut blood loss secondary to mucosal involvement by primary or metastatic tumor. Melanoma, metastatic to the bowel, often produces this sinister symptomatic picture and, after anatomic localization, can be palliated by segmental resection of the involved site.[76]

The following case presentation and accompanying studies reinforce several important points in regard to the urgent situation heralded by hemorrhage.

Patient No. 4

A 58-year-old man underwent subtotal gastrectomy for adenocarcinoma of the stomach in 1979. He observed bright red blood from the rectum 7 months earlier, and 4 weeks before the National Institutes of Health (NIH) referral, a large rectal cancer, fixed to the left pelvic sidewall was biopsied. Cystoscopy showed no bladder invasion, and the patient was treated with from 3600 cGy of preoperative pelvic irradiation complicated by urinary retention, proctitis, and severe perianal inflammation. In December of 1984, abdominoperineal resection was done in conjunction with placement of afterloading catheters and a silicone-gel-filled pelvic prosthesis, the latter to displace small bowel out of the pelvis and protect it from further radiation injury. Four months later, an upper gastrointestinal series suggested partial small bowel obstruction, and an abdominal CT scan showed a hydronephrotic left kidney (Fig. 60–11A). The patient was admitted to the hospital, where he suffered a massive (18 units of blood) lower gastrointestinal hemorrhage. An arteriogram revealed an arterioenteric fistula from the left internal iliac artery to small bowel (see Fig. 60–11B–D). Exsanguinating hemorrhage was controlled with transient balloon inflation and methylmethacrylate instillation into the internal iliac artery (see Fig. 60–11E). One day later, the patient developed a cold, pulseless, insensate foot and required Fogarty catheter thrombectomy. Spiking temperatures ensued, and three blood cultures positive for *Streptococcus fecalis* were obtained. Three days after methylmethacrylate occlusion, the patient rebled, and an urgent laparotomy was performed. Takedown of the internal iliac artery to small bowel fistula was accomplished by ligating the internal iliac artery and resecting the involved small bowel segment. The silicone gel pelvic prosthesis was removed, a left nephrostomy performed, and the severely damaged, obstructed, distal left ureter ligated. Five weeks later, a recurrent, severe, acute left foot and ischemic leg was managed with a femorofemoral Gortex bypass graft. In November 1985, 5 months later, cystoscopy revealed a fibrotic, small, nonfunctional bladder, and the patient underwent jejunal loop diversion. In April 1986, he developed multiple pulmonary metastases and progressive cachexia. He died several months later.

INFECTION

Sepsis represents a constant threat to the patient with a malignancy. This often older population frequently has a host of chronic problems that can include malnutrition, diabetes, relatively asymptomatic periodontal disease, sinusitis, cholelithiasis, diverticulosis, and anorectal pathology. Although capable of erupting at any time, the patient is at greatest risk for a clinically problematic episode of infection during periods of treatment related vulnerability.

Febrile Neutropenia

Empiric antibiotic therapy has become the standard management approach to the common episodes of febrile granulocytopenia in cancer patients undergoing intensive chemotherapy.[77,78] Antifungal agents are often added to the therapy regimen if the patient fails to initially respond to treatment.[79] These patients can appear systemically quite ill with a paucity of focal findings, and surgical consultation is often sought. Infectious agents are frequently identified and presumably often arise from endogenous sources. Handled in this fashion,

TABLE 60–19. Evaluation and Treatment of Cancer Patients With Hemorrhage

1. Define the site, source, and cause. Consider the less invasive therapeutic alternatives.
   A. Hematemesis is almost always from the stomach, duodenum, or proximal-most jejunum. Pass nasogastric or larger bore orogastric tube to evacuate clot. Perform upper gastrointestinal endoscopy. Consider injection, electrocoagulation, photocoagulation for lesions of acid-peptic disease, gastritis, Mallory-Weiss tear, or sclerotherapy for varices.
   B. Melena or bright red blood around the rectum. Perform sigmoidoscopy to rule out source in distal 25 cm of colon if no blood is found in nasogastric aspirate. Consider angiogram. If actively bleeding lesion is seen in small bowel or colon consider infusional or occlusional therapy. Consider radionuclide-labeled erythrocyte scan as a diagnostic alternative to angiogram. Consider colonoscopy, which is occasionally helpful if the rate of bleeding permits cleansing of the colon for adequate inspection.
   C. Extraluminal hemorrhage. CT scan of abdomen or pelvis to rule out intraperitoneal, retroperitoneal, or rectus sheath bleeds.
2. Determine and correct all coagulopathic problems: platelet count, prothrombin time, partial thromboplastin time, bleeding time, other coagulation factor level assessment. Consider platelet transfusion, vitamin K, fresh frozen plasma, or factor concentrates as appropriate.
3. Eliminate the chemical offenders: aspirin, nonsteroidal antiinflammatory agents, heparin (sometimes only by line flush), Coumadin, alcohol, and caffeine.
4. Initiate the surface protective agents (for gastroduodenal bleeding): H_2-receptor blockers or sucralfate.
5. Surgical intervention for recalcitrant bleeding. Use suture ligation or resection as appropriate for the site or cause.

with bone marrow recovery and the restoration of more normal neutrophil numbers, most episodes remit, and there is no need for surgical intervention.

Persistent fever with or without continued neutropenia, the appearance of jaundice, or the development of focal signs invite further diagnostic study.

Jaundice

In addition to the more common specific causes of biliary obstruction secondary to tumor or stone disease, extensive hepatic metastases, cirrhosis, hepatitis, or hepatotoxic drugs, jaundice occurs as a poorly understood consequence of sepsis. Pancreatitis can produce sufficient gland edema to impede bile drainage and cause mild to modest elevation in the serum bilirubin and must be ruled out. The diagnostic question of cholecystitis of the calculous or more treacherous acalculous variety must be addressed. An ultrasound of the biliary tree, particularly if the serum bilirubin has reached the level of 10 mg/dl, usually answers the question of whether there is ductal dilation, the often unremitting result of mechanical blockage. The study is the best test for the presence of gallstones, the inciter of cholecystitis and, if causing common ductal obstruction, cholangitis. Even without stones, if the gallbladder appears to be thick walled, enlarged, and full of sludge, the possibility of acalculous infection exists and can often be addressed with a radionuclide HIDA (*N*-[2,6-diethylacetanilido]-iminodiacetic acid) scan. Nondilated ducts and a normal HIDA scan reassuringly eliminate the need to contemplate cholecystectomy or a biliary drainage procedure. A CT scan of the liver makes useful complementary comments on the gallbladder and biliary ductal tree.

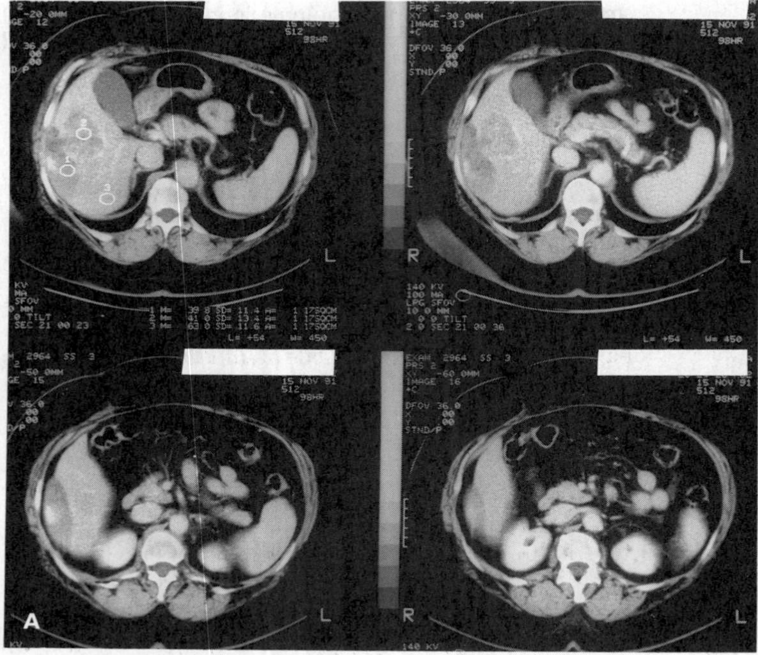

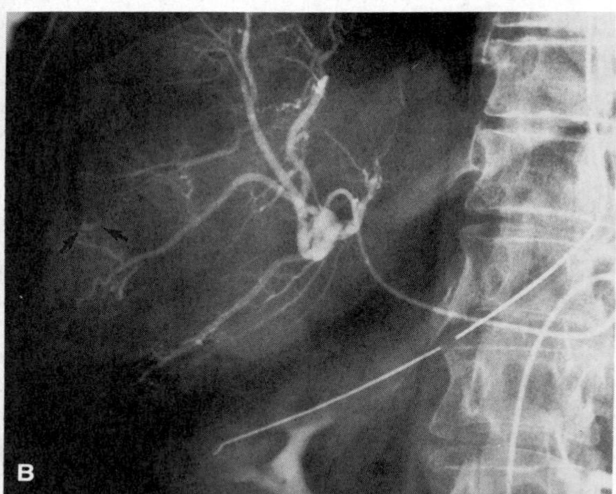

FIGURE 60–10. **(A)** Four panels from a contrast-enhanced abdominal CT scan illustrate the large right lobar hepatic hemorrhage. **(B)** A cut from the hepatic arteriogram demonstrates a dye blush (*arrow*), representing continued bleeding.

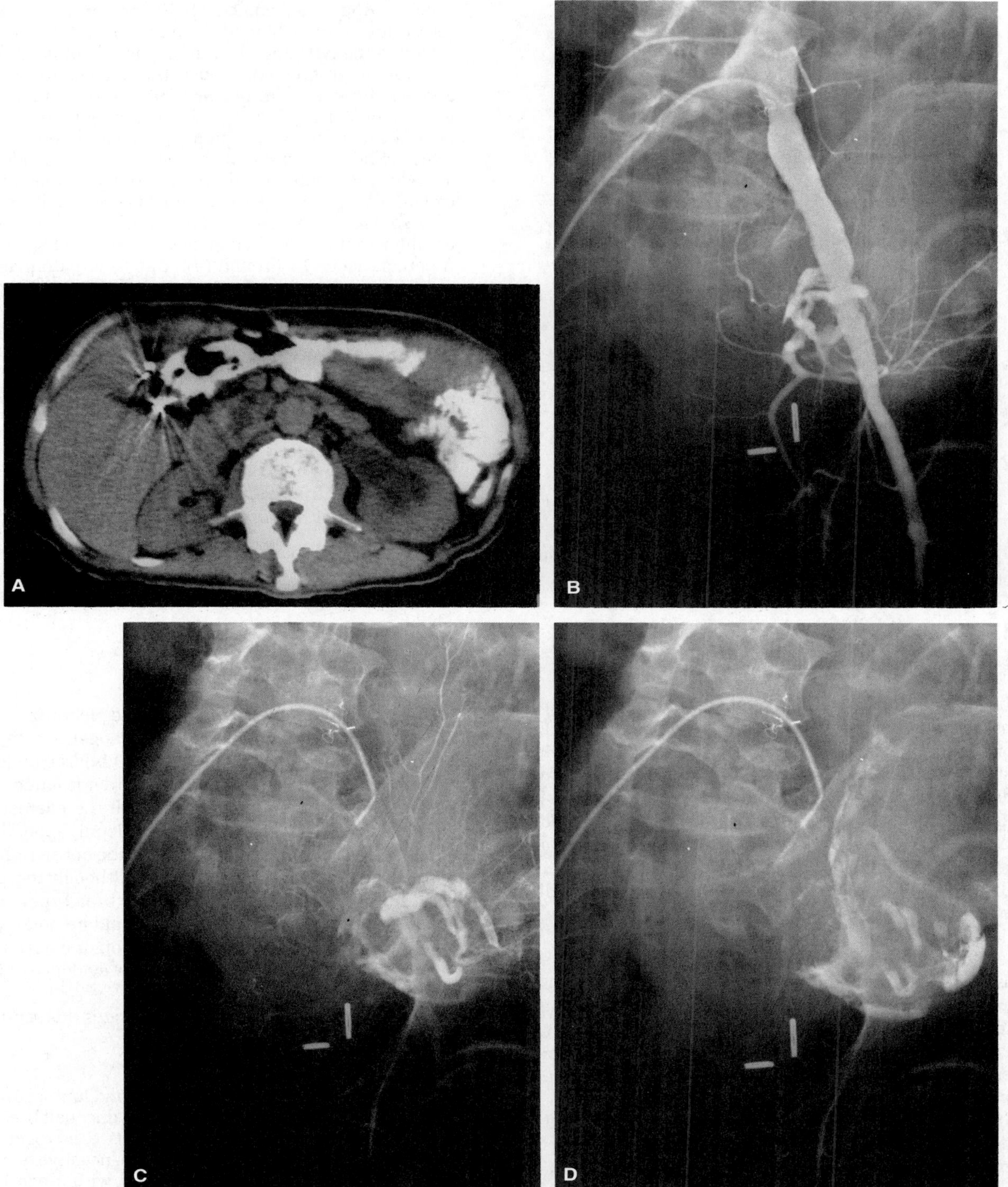

FIGURE 60–11. **(A)** A panel from the abdominal CT scan illustrates the left hydronephrosis. **(B–D)** Arteriographic cuts demonstrate arteriovenous shunting and the arterioenteric fistula. **(E)** The angiogram balloon occludes the left internal iliac artery before methylmethacrylate instillation. *(continued)*

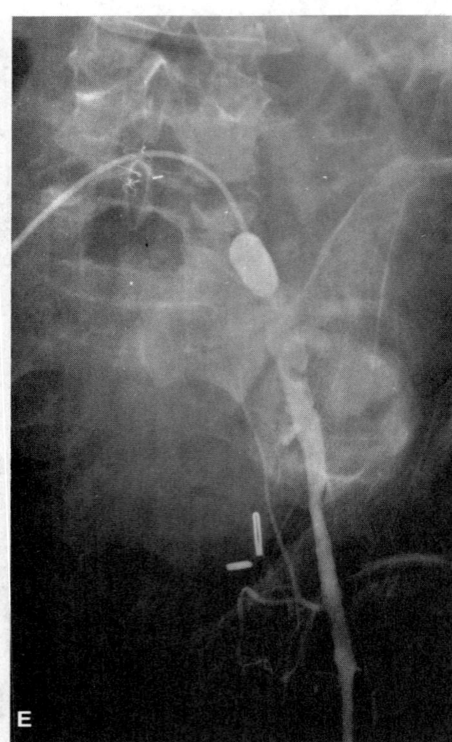

FIGURE 60–11. *(Continued)*

Gallbladder or biliary tree infection, particularly associated with stones, that does not quickly respond to antibiotics and supportive therapy requires drainage. Percutaneous cholecystostomy with or without an endoscopic retrograde common duct drainage procedure can, particularly in the high-risk patient, represent a salutary alternative to laparotomy, cholecystectomy, and possibly common duct exploration and drainage.[80–82] Malignant biliary obstructive problems, even if complicated by infection, can often be satisfactorily handled by the interventional radiologist with a percutaneous transhepatic approach.[83,84]

Like ultrasound, the abdominal CT scan can detect mass lesions, such as abscess or tumor, in the liver. Hepatic abscesses caused by bacterial or fungal infection are being seen with increasing frequency in patients with leukemia or lymphoma and gastrointestinal malignancy.[85] For one to four abscesses, the patient, can often be well managed by percutaneous drainage and escape laparotomy.[86,87]

If the initial assessments of the hepatobiliary tree fail to provide an explanation for the jaundice, a more thorough CT scan of the abdomen and pelvis, particularly in the patient recovering from a laparotomy classified as contaminated, can prove useful. An otherwise occult intraabdominal or pelvic abscess is being sought, and if found, it can often be handled by percutaneous drainage.[88–93]

A case illustrates the diagnostic utility of the CT scan and salutary problem resolution through invasive percutaneous radiologic intervention.

Patient No. 5
A 62-year-old woman with obstructive jaundice underwent laparotomy for unresectable pancreas cancer in August 1985. A Roux-en-Y choledochojejunostomy and gastroenterostomy were fashioned. Two months later, she was referred to the NIH and given monoclonal antibody therapy. Her tumor progressed, eroded the duodenum, ulcerated, and actively bled and, in April 1986, required laparotomy to control the hemorrhage. In September 1986, she appeared for a follow-up clinic visit severely obtunded and febrile. She was profoundly hypoglycemic and acidotic, had a tender right upper quadrant, and required fluid and electrolyte resuscitation. An abdominal CT scan done in pursuit of a source for her septic picture demonstrated a large, complex multiloculated hepatic abscess (see Fig. 60–12A). A percutaneous 14 French (4.6 mm) sump drainage catheter was placed into the abscess (see Fig. 60–12B) and 2.1 L of pus evacuated, which on culture grew *E. coli, Klebsiella pneumoniae, Streptococcus fecalis,* and *Bacteroides melanogenicus*. The patient's postdrainage course was complicated by the development of adult respiratory distress syndrome and coagulopathy. She recovered after a 2-week stay in the intensive care unit and was discharged home for continued supportive care.

Central Access Line Sepsis and Suppurative Thrombophlebitis

The diagnosis and management of central access line sepsis and suppurative thrombophlebitis, an increasingly common surgical emergency, are thoroughly discussed elsewhere in the book.

Enterocolitis

Typhlitis, neutropenic enterocolitis, and necrotizing enteropathy are terms used to describe a pathogenetically poorly understood syndrome seen most often in children undergoing chemotherapy for leukemia, but the disorder is found in some adults with solid malignancies. Although the edematous involvement can be limited to the distal ileum, appendix, and cecum alone, it often extends to involve the entire right colon and sometimes the transverse colon. Although the process often remits on supportive therapy and broad-spectrum antibiotics, the conservative approach should be quickly abandoned in favor of laparotomy and resection or exteriorization and resection of the afflicted tissues if any evidence of further clinical deterioration becomes apparent.[30,32,33,94,95]

The following case presentation illustrates this septic complication of treatment.

Patient No. 6
A 36-year-old women was 2 years beyond lumpectomy and axillary adenectomy for an infiltrating duct cell breast cancer. After operation for her node-negative, estrogen receptor-negative, and progesterone receptor-negative tumor, she received breast irradiation (4500 cGy with a boost to the tumor bed to 5940 cGy) and six cycles of adjuvant therapy with cyclophosphamide, methotrexate, and 5-fluorouracil (CMF). Two months earlier, a chest CT scan showed bilateral pulmonary nodules, one of which proved cytologically positive for breast cancer on fine-needle aspiration. Eight days after starting taxol, doxorubicin, and granulocyte colony-stimulating factor therapy, she developed crampy abdominal pain, distension, diarrhea, and severe febrile neutropenia. Broad-spectrum antibiotics were started, and because of marked lower abdominal tenderness, an abdominal CT scan was obtained (Fig. 60–13A) which suggested

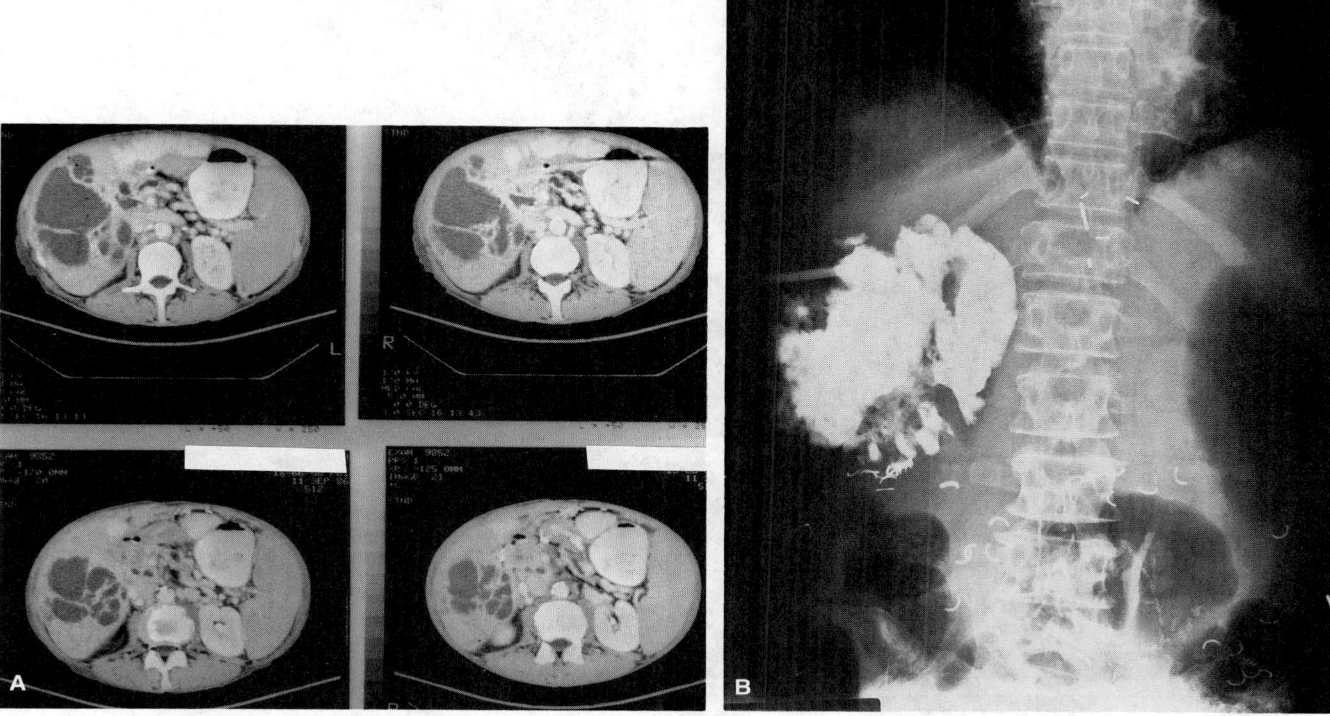

FIGURE 60–12. **(A)** Four panels from an abdominal CT scan demonstrate the large, complex, multiloculated hepatic abscess. **(B)** X-ray film illustrates the drainage catheter in the abscess that was filled with contrast material.

an inflammatory process involving bowel in the right lower quadrant. Because insufficient orally ingested contrast opacified these bowel loops, dilute gastrograffin was administered by enema and fluoroscopy and additional CT images obtained (see Fig. 60–13B–D). A phlegmonous, ulcerated process involving the cecum was clearly delineated that, on continued supportive care, slowly resolved clinically and roentgenographically over the next 3 weeks.

Perirectal Infection

Anorectal symptoms are common among cancer patients; pain, with or without bowel movements is the most frequent complaint. Hemorrhoidal pathology is exceedingly common and often made more problematic by the bouts of diarrhea and constipation that complicate chemotherapy and the use of narcotic pain medication. Anal fissuring, probably secondary to constipation, is slow to heal in the catabolic patient. Although underreported in the literature, anal gland inflammation in the neutropenic patient can rapidly progress to extensive perirectal cellulitis or frank abscess formation.[96]

Perirectal infection, particularly when the patient is febrile and neutropenic, can be quite difficult to sort out. Inspection, facilitated by buttock cheek retraction and a Valsalva maneuver, and gentle external palpation sometimes reveals a thrombosed or ulcerative internal hemorrhoid, a fissure, point tenderness, or an indurated bulge. Often nothing is appreciated on this kind of limited assessment. A pelvic CT scan that permits evaluation of the perirectal spaces and fat pyramids for symmetry, inflammatory streaking, edematous change, or frank abscess formation can be helpful. Ambiguous findings often dictate whether to proceed immediately with a digital rectal examination and anoscopy. These assessments usually cannot be made without giving the patient an anesthetic.

An initial period of conservative local management is usually tried. Warm Sitz baths, Tucks to promote local hygiene, stool softeners, or antidiarrheal agents as indicated and analgesics are helpful. If stability or slight clinical improvement is not seen after 24 to 48 hours, the more invasive diagnostic efforts can be made.

Perianal cellulitis, particularly in the face of neutropenia and thrombocytopenia, is initially best managed with intravenously administered, high-dose, broad-spectrum antibiotics. Abscesses characterized by frank fluctuance require incision and drainage by standard surgical approaches. Infrequently, the infection becomes so locally and systemically aggressive that fecal diversion becomes necessary.

Soft Tissue Infection

In addition to the usual array of soft tissue infections that include acne-like pustules, furuncles, carbuncles, paronychia, felons, foreign-body-related infections, and cellulitis, which are handled in standard surgical fashion, several unusual circumstances merit consideration.

After axillary or groin lymphadenectomy, the extremity becomes particularly susceptible to an aggressive, virulent streptococcal (often mixed streptococcal and staphylococcal)

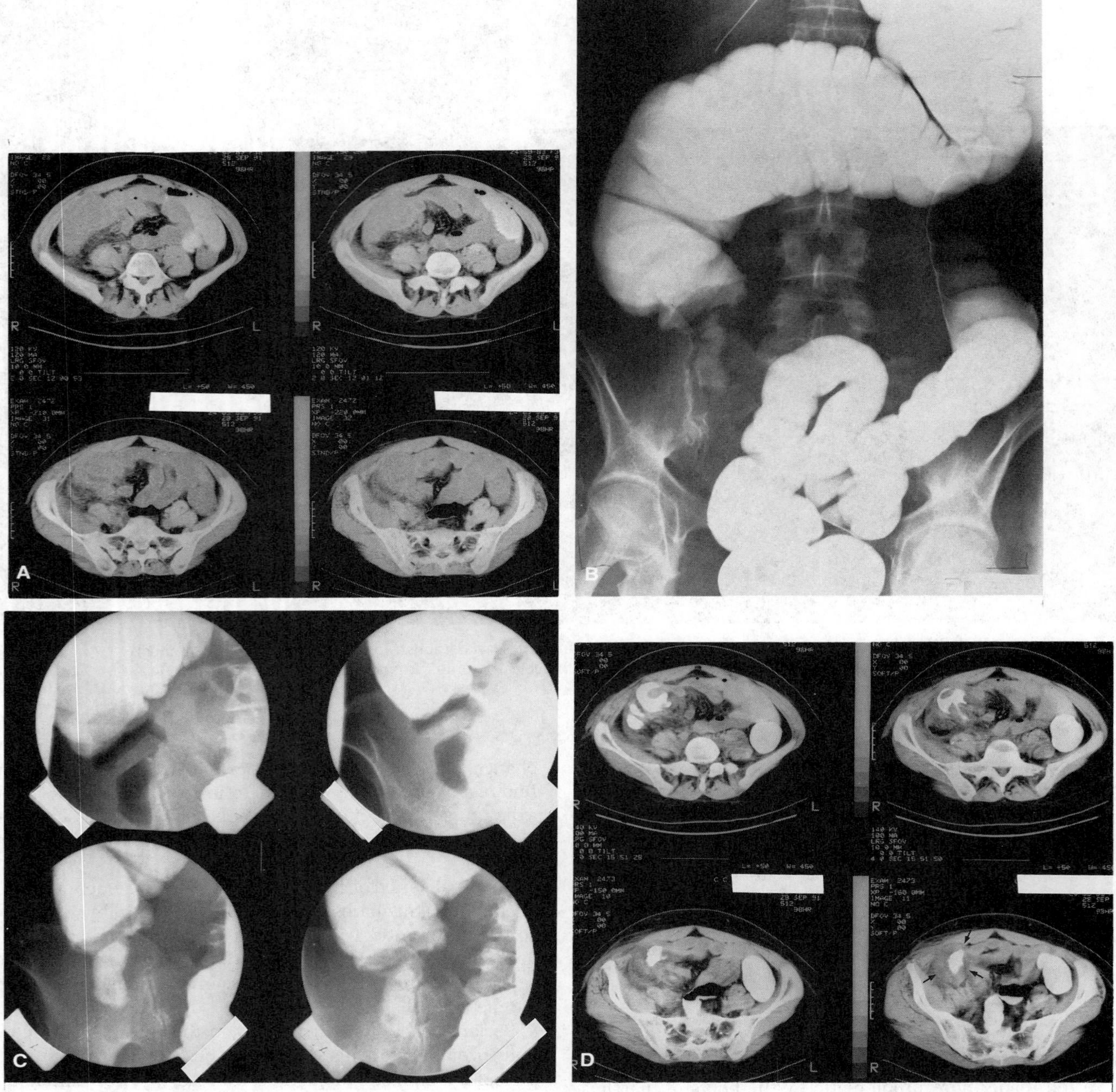

FIGURE 60–13. **(A)** Four panels from the initial abdominal CT scan that demonstrates only dilated, fluid-filled bowel loops and suggest an edematous, inflammatory process involving bowel in the right lower quadrant. **(B, C)** X-ray films obtained after a gastrograffin enema show a large, ulcerated area involving the cecum. **(D)** Abdominal CT scan cuts obtained after a gastrograffin enema corroborate the markedly edematous, thick-walled, ulcerated cecum (*arrows*) seen in typhlitis.

cellulitis called erysipelas. An initial innocuous-appearing patch of cutaneous erythema, sometimes after an otherwise harmless scratch, can progress in several hours with significant swelling to involve the entire extremity and leave the patient markedly febrile, prostrate, and systemically toxic. No portal of entry for the bacteria is identified for many cases, although the cutaneous cracks consequent to preventable foot fungal infection can admit the organisms. Successful treatment rests on early recognition of the infection's virulent potential. Intravenous administration of high-dose antibiotics directed at both potentially offending organisms, extremity elevation, and rest are the therapy cornerstones. Due to the adenectomy-imposed compromise to lymphatic fluid return, I usually omit warm compresses or soaks, which encourage increased blood flow into the tissues and contribute to potentially problematic edema formation.

The chronic and intermittently acute immunocompromised nature of the cancer patient makes him susceptible to an additional group of gangrene-producing, exceedingly virulent soft tissue infections that, depending on the organisms involved and tissues affected, go by the names of necrotizing fasciitis, anaerobic cellulitis, gas gangrene, bacterial synergistic gangrene, or necrotizing cutaneous mucormycosis. These entities are thoroughly considered in a text by Howard and Simmons.[97] The infection commonly follows a contaminated surgical procedure and usually involves the wound. This life-threatening infection characteristically produces extensive tissue necrosis, potentially involving skin, fat, fascia, and muscle. Prompt, aggressive, and wide surgical incision, drainage, and debridement coupled with broad-spectrum antibiotics that include anaerobic coverage is imperative. Hyperbaric oxygen administration can probably help if clostridial myonecrosis is involved.

Because of their heightened susceptibility to the unusual and the usually identified organisms, it is essential to pursue infections in these hosts with energetic efforts to culture and identify the offender. An unsuspected but treatable fungus, like *Aspergillus,* is sometimes found.

DECIDING ON AGGRESSIVE OR CONSERVATIVE MANAGEMENT

Regrettably, cancer patients often succumb to medically recalcitrant progressive disease. This circumstance is understandably trying, tension provoking, and frustrating for the patient, the family, and the physician. If inanition, pulmonary infection, and metabolic derangement are the terminal issues, the surgeon remains uninvolved, but if obstruction, hemorrhage, or the consequences of a progressive mass are the insults provoking a sense of urgency, the surgeon will be asked to intervene. This situation, perhaps more than any other, tests the judgmental acumen of the surgeon and demands from him or her an honest assessment of what a surgical undertaking potentially affords. If the expectations for serious-minded palliation are realistic and not insubstantial, proceeding to operation is reasonable, but if the likelihood of minimally deferring the inevitable while protracting the burden of suffering at ever increasing cost is more likely, than alternative, pain-alleviating measures should be liberally instituted.

NUTRITION AND OTHER SUPPORT

Cancer and the treatments we direct at it invariably represent a catabolic insult. Resultant malnutrition, poor wound healing, and immunocompromise are the almost inescapable consequences. "Food is medicine" is the message that must be tirelessly preached to patient and family alike. The liberal use of high-calorie enteral supplements and a multivitamin preparation should be regularly encouraged.

Constipation, often associated with narcotic usage and poor fluid intake, contributes to the development of symptomatic anorectal difficulty and should be anticipated and prevented through the use of stool softeners and bulk-restoring agents. The conscientious physician must provide the patient with a mild cathartic to facilitate elimination of the barium burden administered with fluoroscopic gastrointestinal studies. Obstipation, impaction, and painful and unpleasant digitally assisted evacuation or stercoral colonic ulceration and perforation are preventable.

Stress-related anxiety and depression are associated with cancer. Anxiety contributes to erosive, acid-peptic gastroduodenal bleeding and can be managed effectively with mucosal surface-protective agents, like sucralfate or the H_2-receptor blockers, and depression adversely affects the patient and the family's quality of life and saps strength that might otherwise be marshaled in the struggle to survive.[98] Group support systems, professional psychiatric help, and mood-impacting medicines can be quite helpful and should not be forgotten.

Treatment-complicating intercurrent problems or issues like symptomatic gallstones, diverticular disease, anorectal pathology, or the threat of an unwanted pregnancy should be anticipated. Often the nonvulnerable period before treatment or the quiescent intervals between treatments can be use to surgically address and prevent problems that may later erupt in far more morbid, unmanageable forms. The advent of less invasive, safer surgical procedures, like laparoscopic cholecystectomy, with rapid postprocedure recovery, will doubtless encourage these preventive considerations.[99]

REFERENCES

1. Botsford TW, Wilson RE. The acute abdomen: An approach to diagnosis and management. 2nd ed. Philadelphia: WB Saunders, 1977.
2. Dunphy RE, Botsford TW. Physical examination of the surgical patient: An introduction to clinical surgery. 4th ed. Philadelphia: WB Saunders, 1975.
3. Schwartz SI, Shires GT, Spencer FC, eds. Principles of surgery. 5th ed. New York: McGraw-Hill, 1989.
4. Shiloni E, Weiss CM, Baker AR. Surgical management of the critically ill immunocompromised patient. In: Parillo JE, Masur H, eds. The critically ill immunocompromised patient: Diagnosis and management. Bethesda, MD: Aspen Publication, 1987:557–584.
5. Turnbull ADM, Starnes HF Jr. Surgical emergencies in the cancer patient. Chicago: Year Book Medical Publishers, 1987.
6. Wilson RE. Surgical problems in immuno-depressed patients. In: Major problems in clinical surgery, vol 30. Philadelphia: WB Saunders, 1984.
7. Sherlock P. The gastrointestinal manifestations and complications of malignant lymphoma. Schweiz Med Wochenschr 1980;110:1031–1037.
8. Herrmann R, Panahon AM, Barcos MP, et al. Gastrointestinal involvement in non-Hodgkin's lymphoma. Cancer 1980;46:215–222.
9. Lewin KJ, Ranchod M, Dorfman RF. Lymphomas of the gastrointestinal tract—a study of 117 cases presenting with gastrintestinal disease. Cancer 1978;42:693–707.
10. Sherman NJ, Wooley MM. The ileocecal syndrome in acute childhood leukemia. Arch Surg 1973;107:39–42.
11. Klener P, Donner L, Bocanova M, et al. Gastronintestinal lesions and complications in hemoblastoses. Folia Haematol (Leipz) 1973;100:57–66.
12. Lee JR, Gray SW, Brown BC, et al. Diffuse histiocytic lymphomas of the gastrointestinal tract in the adult. Surg Gynecol Obstet 1983;157:286–300.
13. Remine SG, McIlrath DC. Bowel perforation in steroid treated patients. Ann Surg 1980;192:581–586.
14. Pizzo PA. Granulocytopenia and cancer therapy—past problems, current solutions, future challenges. Cancer 1984;54:2649–2661.
15. Shuffler MD, Baird HW, Fleming CR, et al. Intestinal pseudoobstruction as the presenting manifestation of small cell carcinoma of the lung. A paraneoplastic neuropathy of the gastrointestinal tract. Ann Intern Med 1983;98:129–134.
16. Rosenthal S, Kaufman S. Vincristine neurotoxicity. Ann Intern Med 1974;80:733–737.
17. Ferrara JJ, Martin EW, Carey LC. Morbidity of emergency operations in patients with metastatic cancer receiving chemotherapy. Surgery 1982;92:605–609.
18. Pauker SG, Kopelman RI. Clinical problem solving—Trapped by an incidental finding. N Engl J Med 1992;326:40–43.
19. Roh JJ, Thompson JS, Harned RK, et al. Value of pneumoperitoneum in the diagnosis of visceral perforation. Am J Surg 1983;146:830–833.
20. Zer M, Wolloch Y, Lombrozo MD, et al. Palliative treatment of duodenoenteric fistulas. World J Surg 1980;4:131–135.
21. Vetto JT, Culp SC, Smythe TB, et al. Iliac aterial-enteric fistulas occurring after pelvic irradiation. Surgery 1987;101:643–647.
22. Kostroff KM, Turnbull AD, Rotstein LE, et al. Duodenojejunostomy and stapled occlusion for distal duodenal perforation from malignant retroperitoneal tumors. J Surg Oncol 1984;26:252–255.
23. Bertolone SJ, Fuenfer MM, Groff DB, et al. Delayed pancreatic pseudocyst formation—Long-term complication of L-asparaginase treatment. Cancer 1982;50:2964–2966.
24. Puckett JB, Butler WM, McFarland JA. Pancreatitis and cancer chemotherapy. Ann Intern Med [Letter] 1982;97:453.

25. Hande KR, Fisher RI, DeVita VT, et al. Diffuse histiocytic lymphoma involving the gastrointestinal tract. Cancer 1978;41:1984–1989.
26. Weingrad DN, DeCosse JJ, Sherlock P, et al. Primary gastrointestinal lymphoma: A 30-year review. Cancer 1982;49:1258–1265.
27. Rajagopalan AE, Pickleman J. Free perforation of the small intestine. Ann Surg 1982;196: 576–579.
28. Leidich RB, Rudolf LE. Small bowel perforation secondary to metastatic lung carcinoma. Ann Surg 1981;193:67–69.
29. Perkins JD, Shield CF III, Chang FC, et al. Acute diverticulitis—Comparison of treatment in immunocompromised and nonimmunocompromised patients. Am J Surg 1984;148: 745–748.
30. Shamberger RC, Weinstein HJ, Delorey RN, et al. The medical and surgical management of typhlitis in children with acute nonlymphocytic (myelogenous) leukemia. Cancer 1986;57:603–609.
31. Sauter ER, Vauthey JN, Bolton, et al. Selective management of patients with neutropenic enterocolitis using peritoneal lavage. J Surg Oncol 1990;45:63–67.
32. Wade DS, Douglas H Jr, Nava HR, et al. Abdominal pain in neutropenic patients. Arch Surg 1990;125:1119–1127.
33. Starnes HF, Moore FD, Mentzer S, et al. Abdominal pain in neutropenic cancer patients. Cancer 1986;57:616–621.
34. Frank D, Raicht RF. Intestinal perforation associated with cytomegalovirus infection in patients with acquired immune deficiency syndrome. Am J Gastroenterol 1984;79: 201–205.
35. Rosenberg JM, Walker M, Welch JP, Mullany L. *Clostridium difficile* colitis in surgical patients. Am J Surg 1984;147:486–491.
36. Schwartzentruber D, Lotze MT, Rosenberg SA. Colon perforation—An unusual complication of therapy with high-dose interleukin-2. Cancer 1988;62:2350–2353.
37. Galland RB, Spencer MS. Surgical management of radiation enteritis. Surgery 1986;99: 133–138.
38. Morganstern L, Hart M, Lugo D, Friedman NB. Changing aspects of radiation enteropathy. Arch Surg 1985;120:1225–1228.
39. Lundy J, Sherlock P, Kurtz R, et al. Spontaneous perforation of the gastrointestinal tract in patients with cancer. Am J Gastroenterol 1975;63:447–450.
40. Isabella V, Marotta E, Bianchi F. Ischemic necrosis of proximal gastric remnant following subtotal gastrectomy with splenectomy. J Surg Oncol 1984;25:124–132.
41. Koretz MJ, Neifeld JP. Emergency surgical treatment for patients with leukemia. Surg Gynecol Obstet 1985;161:149–151.
42. Vaughn EA, Key CR, Sterling WA Jr. Intraabdominal operations in patients with leukemia. Am J Surg 1988;156:51–53.
43. Dunn JT, Halls JM, Berne TV. Roentgenographic contrast studies in acute small bowel obstruction. Arch Surg 1984;119:1305–1308.
44. Butler JA, Brian CL, Morrow M, Kahng K, et al. Small bowel obstruction in patients with a prior history of cancer. Am J Surg 1991;162:624–628.
45. Clarke-Pearson DL, Chin NO, DeLong ER, et al. Surgical management of intestinal obstruction in ovarian cancer. 1. Clinical features, postoperative complications and survival. Gynecol Oncol 1987;26:11–18.
46. Gallick HL, Weaver DW, Sachs RJ, Bouwman DL. Intestinal obstruction in cancer patients: An assessment of risk factors and outcomes. Am Surg 1986;52:434–437.
47. Walsh HPJ, Schofield PF. Is laparotomy for small bowel obstruction justified in patients with previously treated malignancy. Br J Surg 1984;71:933–935.
48. Aabo K, Pedersen H, Bach F, Knudsen J. Surgical management of intestinal obstruction in the late course of malignant disease. Acta Chir Scand 1984;150:173–176.
49. Bizer LS, Liebling RW, Delany HM, Gleidman ML. Small bowel obstruction. Surgery 1981;89:407–413.
50. Osteen RT, Guyton S, Steele G Jr, Wilson RE. Malignant intestinal obstruction. Surgery 1980;87:611–615.
51. Annest LS, Jolly PC. The results of surgical treatment of bowel obstruction caused by peritoneal carcinomatosis. Am Surg 1979;45:718–721.
52. Ketcham AS, Hoye RC, Pilch YH, Morton DL. Delayed intestinal obstruction following treatment for cancer. Cancer 1970;25:406–410.
53. Stewardson RH, Bombeck T, Nyhus LM. Critical operative management of small bowel obstruction. Ann Surg 1978;187:189–193.
54. Sarr MG, Bulkley GB, Zuidema GD. Preoperative recognition of intestinal strangulation obstruction: Prospective evaluation diagnostic capability. Am J Surg 1983;145:176–182.
55. Baines M, Oliver DJ, Carter RL. Medical management of intestinal obstruction in patients with advanced malignant disease. Lancet 1985;2:990–993.
56. Richards WO, Williams LF Jr. Obstruction of the large and small intestine. Surg Clin North Am 1988;68:355–376.
57. Geelhoed GW. Colonic pseudo-obstruction in surgical patients. Am J Surg 1985;149: 258–265.
58. Nivatvongs S, Vermeulen FD, Fang DT. Colonic decompression of acute pseudo-obstruction. Ann Surg 1982;196:598–600.
59. Gordon B, Lossef SV, Jelinger E, et al. Embolotherapy for small bowel hemorrhage from Metastatic renal cell carcinoma: Case report. Cardiovasc Intervent Radiol 1991;14: 311–313.
60. Plukker JT, Koops HS, Sleijfer DT, et al. Intestinal hemorrhages in patients with a nonseminomatous testicular tumor. Cancer 1991;68:2630–2632.
61. Harris MN. Massive gastrointestinal hemorrhage. Arch Surg 1964;88:1049–1051.
62. Okasaki M, Higashihara H, Koganemaru F, Nakamura T. Intraperitoneal hemorrhage from hepatocellular carcinoma: Emergency chemoemboliztion or embolization. Radiology 1991;180:647–651.
63. Foster JH, Berman MM, eds. Solid liver tumors. In: Major problems in clinical surgery, vol XXII. Philadelphia: WB Saunders, 1977:79, 155.
64. Erb RE, Gibler WB. Massive hemoperitoneum following rupture of hepatic metastases from unsuspected choriocarcinoma. Am J Emerg Med 1989;7:196–198.
65. Rosenfelt F, Rosenberg SA. Diffuse histiocytic lymphoma presenting with gastrointestinal tract lesions: The Stanford experience. Cancer 1980;45:2188–2193.
66. Schaller RT, Schaller JF. The acute abdomen in the immunologically compromised child. J Pediatr Surg 1983;18:937–944.
67. McGill DB, Rakela J, Zinmeister AR, Ott BJ. A 21-year experience with major hemorrhage ager percutaneous liver biopsy. Gastroenterology 1990;99:1396–1400.
68. Cook DJ, Guyatt GH, Salena BJ, Laine LA. Endoscopic therapy for acute nonvariceal upper gastrointestinal hemorrhage: A meta-analysis. Gastroenterology 1992;102:139–148.
69. Waring JP, Sanowski RA, Sawyer RL, et al. A randomized comparison of monopolar electrocoagulation and injection sclerosis for the treatment of bleeding peptic ulcer. Gastrointest Endosc 1991;37:295–298.
70. Hui WM, Ng MMT, Lok ASF, Lai CL. A randomized comparative study of laser photocoagulation, heater probe, and bipolar electrocoagulation in the treatment of actively bleeding ulcers. Gastrointest Endosc 1991;37:299–304.
71. Athanasoulis CA, Baum S, Waltman AC, et al. Control of acute gastric mucosal hemorrhage. N Engl J Med 1974;290:597–603.
72. Pisco JM, Martins JM, Correia MG. Internal iliac artery: Emobolization to control hemorrhage from neoplasms. Radiology 1989;172:337–339.
73. Chuang VP, Wallace S, Gianturco C. A new improved coil for tapered-tip catheter for arterial occlusion. Radiology 1980;135:507–509.
74. Jeffrey RB Jr, Cardoza JD, Olcott EW. Detection of active intraabdominal arterial hemorrhage: Value of dynamic contrast-enhanced CT. AJR 1991;156:725–729.
75. Kram HB, Shoemaker WC, Clark SR, Macabee JR. Spraying of aerosolized fibrin glue in the treatment of nonsuturable hemorrhage. Am Surg 1991;57:381–384.
76. Das Gupta TK, Brasfield RD. Metastatic melanoma of the gastrointestinal tract. Arch Surg 1964;88:969–973.
77. Gucalp R. Management of the febrile neutropenic patient with cancer. Oncology 1991;5: 137–147.
78. Pizzo PA, Hathorn JW, Hiemenz J, et al. A randomized trial comparing ceftazidime alone with combination antibiotic therapy in cancer patients with fever and neutropenia. N Engl J Med 1986;315:552–558.
79. Pizzo PA, Robichaud KJ, Wesley R, Commers JR. Fever in the pediatric and young adult patient with cancer. Medicine (Baltimore) 1982;61:153–165.
80. Klimberg S, Hawkins I, Vogel SB. Percutaneous cholecystostomy for acute cholecystitis in high-risk patients. Am J Surg 1987;153:125–129.
81. van Sonnenberg E, Wittich GR, Casola G, et al. Diagnostic and therapeutic gallbladder procedures. Radiology 1986;160:23–26.
82. Frazee RC, Nagorney DM, Mucha P Jr. Acute acalculous cholecystitis. Mayo Clin Proc 1989;64:163–167.
83. Ring EJ. Radiologic approach to malignant biliary obstruction: Review and commentary. Cardiovasc Intervent Radiol 1990;13:217–222.
84. Walta DC, Fausel CS, Brant B. Endoscopic biliary stents and obstructive jaundice. Am J Surg 1987;153:444–447.
85. Thaler M, Pastakia B, Shawker TH, et al. Hepatic candidiasis in cancer patients: The evolving picture of the syndrome. Ann Intern Med 1988;108:88–100.
86. Haaga JR. Imaging intraabdominal abscesses and nonoperative drainage. World J Surg 1990;14:204–209.
87. Pruett TL, Simmons RL. Status of percutaneous catheter drainage of abscesses. Surg Clin North Am 1988;68:89–105.
88. Olak J, Christou NV, Stein LA, et al. Operative vs percutaneous drainage of intra-abdominal abscesses: Comparison of morbidity and mortality. Arch Surg 1986;121:141–146.
89. Johnson WC, Gerzof SG, Robbins AH, Nabseth DC. Treatment of abdominal abscesses: Comparative evaluation of operative versus percutaneous catheter drainage by guided computed tomography or ultrasound. Ann Surg 1981;194:510–552.
90. Lurie K, Plzak L, Deveney CW. Intra-abdominal abscessess in the 1980s. Surg Clin North Am 1987;67:621–632.
91. Flancbaum L, Nosher JL, Brolin RE. Percutaneous catheter drainage of abdominal abscesses associated with perforated viscus. Am Surg 1990;56:52–56.
92. Lent WM, Goldman MJ, Bizer LS. An objective appraisal of the role of computed tomographic (CT) guided drainage of intraabdominal abscesses. Am Surg 1990;56:688–690.
93. Stabile BE, Puccio E, van Sonnenberg E, Neff CC. Preoperative percutaneous drainage of diverticular abscesses. Am J Surg 1990;159:99–105.
94. Alt B, Glass NR, Sollinger H. Neutropenic enterocolitis in adults. Am J Surg 1985;149: 405–408.
95. Villar HV, Warneke JA, Peck MD, et al. Role of surgical treatment in the management of complications of the gastrointestinal tract in patients with leukemia. Surg Gynecol Obstet 1987;165:217–222.
96. Sehdev MK, Dowling MD Jr, Seal SH, Stearns MW Jr. Perianal and anorectal complications in leukemia. Cancer 1973;31:149–152.
97. Howard RJ, Simmons RL, eds: Surgical infectious disease. 2nd ed. Norwalk, CT: Appleton & Lange, 1988:377–442.
98. McCarthy DM. Sucralfate. N Engl J Med 1991;235:1017–1025.
99. Southern Surgeons Club: A prospective analysis of 1518 laparoscopic cholecystectomies. N Engl J Med 1991;324:1074–1078.

SECTION 5

PAUL RUSSO

Urologic Emergencies

Urologic emergencies are common in the cancer patient and are related mainly to complications of bladder hemorrhage, upper or lower urinary tract obstruction, urinary tract infection, and priapism. The causes, clinical presentations, and management of these emergencies are the focus of this chapter.

BLADDER HEMORRHAGE

Urinary tract hemorrhage can occur in a variety of clinical settings in the cancer patient and can rapidly evolve into a life-threatening emergency. Gross hematuria is often the presenting sign of a urologic malignancy (*e.g.*, kidney, urothelial, prostatic) or may be secondary to direct invasion of colonic and gynecologic cancers or pelvic sarcomas into the urinary tract. Occasionally, a benign process, such as a renal angiomyolipoma or arteriovenous malformation, bleeds massively into the urinary tract. Hemorrhagic cystitis after chemotherapy or radiation therapy or secondary to viral infection in an immunocompromised host can also cause life-threatening hemorrhage. Disorders in hemostasis due to the systemic manifestations of cancer (*e.g.*, thrombocytopenia, disseminated intravascular coagulation) can cause occult tumors or damaged urothelium to bleed. More than one etiologic factor may be responsible for the bleeding.

PATHOPHYSIOLOGY AND ETIOLOGY

Drug-Induced Hemorrhagic Cystitis

Hemorrhagic cystitis is defined as an acute or insidious diffuse bladder inflammation with hemorrhage that can be caused by numerous toxic agents. Metabolites of chemotherapeutic agents, bladder injury secondary to radiation therapy, and viral infection account for most cases of hemorrhagic cystitis encountered in cancer patients.[1,2]

In the early experience with cyclophosphamide used as a chemotherapeutic agent or in preparation for bone marrow transplantation, the incidence of hemorrhagic cystitis was as high as 40% to 68%.[3,4] When massive bladder hemorrhage occurred in the bone marrow transplant population, a mortality rate as high as 75% was reported.[5]

There are no clinical predictors to indicate which patient will experience this complication. Acute hemorrhage usually occurs during or shortly after treatment, and delayed hemorrhage is most common in patients on chronic long-term oral cyclophosphamide.[1] With acute hemorrhage, the patient may complain of dysuria and urinary frequency. Microscopic hematuria due to a hyperemic, edematous, and ulcerated bladder mucosa may precede serious bladder hemorrhage.[6] Of 100 patients treated with cyclophosphamide at the Mayo Clinic who developed hemorrhagic cystitis, bleeding sufficient enough to require transfusion occurred in 20%. Hemorrhagic cystitis developed after a mean cumulative oral dose of 90 g and a mean cumulative intravenous dose of 18 g of cyclophosphamide. Three patients developed hemorrhagic cystitis after a single intravenous dose. Although most of the patients recovered, cystectomy with urinary diversion was performed as a lifesaving measure in 9 patients, and death secondary to exsanguinating bladder hemorrhage or complications of hemorrhage occurred in 10 patients.[6]

Liver metabolites of cyclophosphamide and its analog ifosfamide, are phosphoramide mustard and acrolein. Acrolein is the urinary metabolite that has been implicated as the urotoxic substance, but the exact mechanism by which it damages the urothelium is unknown.[7] Overhydration to dilute urinary acrolein is successful in reducing the incidence of major bladder hemorrhage associated with cyclophosphamide.[5] Sodium 2-mercaptoethane sulfonate (mesna) is an effective uroprotectant that does not interfere with the chemotherapeutic efficacy of cyclophosphamide.[8,9] Within minutes of its intravenous administration, mesna is oxidized in the serum to a stable, inactive disulfide that is activated in the kidney and binds to urinary acrolein to form an inert thioether. Mesna slows the degradation of the 4-hydroxy-metabolites of ifosfamide and cyclophosphamide, further inhibiting their breakdown and the release of acrolein. The only side effects associated with its administration are mild nausea and occasional vomiting.[1] The serum half-life of mesna is 90 minutes, and that of cyclophosphamide is 6 hours.[1,10] To be effective, mesna must be present in the bladder at the time the acrolein comes into contact with the urothelium. Mesna must be administered before the first dose of cyclophosphamide and continued after the last dose, using one of several schedules that employ continuous infusion or intravenous bolus methods.[11–13] The use of mesna has dramatically reduced the incidence of hematuria and hemorrhagic cystitis after cyclophosphamide-based chemotherapy to less than 5%, has reduced cyclophosphamide-induced complications of bone marrow transplantation, and has obviated the need for chemotherapy dose reductions.[11–16]

Radiation-Induced Cystitis

Approximately 20% of patients receiving definitive radiation therapy for gynecologic, genitourinary, and rectal cancers experience bladder complications.[17,18] Although symptoms of urinary urgency, frequency, and urinary retention may occur after pelvic irradiation, serious bladder hemorrhage is an unusual acute event.[1] The small vessel injury caused by irradiation leads to interstitial bladder wall fibrosis, reduced bladder capacity, and the formation of friable, telangiectatic blood vessels that course the bladder mucosa and can spontaneously rupture leading to massive hemorrhage.

Although there are no specific measures to prevent radiation-induced cystitis, acute symptoms of urgency, dysuria, and frequency may be relieved by topical analgesics (*e.g.*, phenazopyridine hydrochloride) and antispasmodics (*e.g.*, oxybutynin chloride). A period of bladder catheterization may be necessary to relieve symptoms of bladder irritability or treat acute urinary retention. Currently under clinical investigation for the treatment of radiation-induced hemorrhagic cystitis are sodium pentosulfanpolysulfate, hyperbaric oxygen, and conjugated estrogen—each of which attempts to stabilize the damaged urothelium and promote healing.[19–21]

Virus-Induced Hemorrhagic Cystitis

Efforts to understand the late onset of hemorrhagic cystitis in bone marrow patients focused on a possible viral infection. Although hemorrhagic cystitis secondary to adenovirus type 11 was reported in immunologically competent children, this virus was infrequently detected in the urine of bone marrow transplant patients.[22–24] Rice and colleagues identified the BK type of human polyomavirus in the urine of 5 of 6 bone marrow recipients, 2 of whom had hemorrhagic cystitis.[25] The BK virus in healthy people is ubiquitous, persists in the kidney after primary infection, and is only occasionally associated with a mild respiratory illness.[26] The BK virus is activated during periods of immunosuppression (*e.g.*, organ and marrow transplantation) and is recoverable in the urine.[27] A prospective study of 53 bone marrow recipients demonstrated BK virus in the urine of 47%.[28] Hemorrhagic cystitis lasting longer than 7 days occurred four times as frequently in patients who excreted BK virus than in those who did not. Urinary BK virus was identified in 55% of patients during episodes of hemorrhagic cystitis but in only 11% of patients who were cystitis free. Despite the use of mesna and overhydration during bone marrow transplantation, BK virus activation remains a major factor in the evolution of hemorrhagic cystitis in this group of cancer patients.

TREATMENT

If bladder hemorrhage is massive and intractable, the patients develop clot urinary retention and complain of severe suprapubic and flank pain. The urologist must reestablish urinary outflow quickly by inserting a large diameter, multiple hole urethral catheter into the bladder and initiate a saline lavage and clot evacuation. Often the hemorrhage slows or ceases after removing the clots and decompressing the bladder. When the lavage has a clear or pink-tinged return, continuous bladder irrigation using a three-way Foley catheter can be effective in removing any residual small clots and maintaining free bladder drainage.

Bedside lavage is not always effective in evacuating all clots, especially if they have been present for many hours. Continued irrigation in this setting may increase intravesical pressure and cause bladder rupture (Fig. 60–14A,B). Instead, the patient should be taken to the operating room for an endoscopic clot evacuation under anesthesia. Under direct vision, the urologist can mechanically disrupt the clots, inspect the bladder for a controllable source of bleeding, and fulgurate any bleeding vessels or tumor.

Diffuse bleeding from any cause that persists despite clot evacuation and fulguration is an indication for intravesical instillation of a hemostatic agent such as formalin, which acts

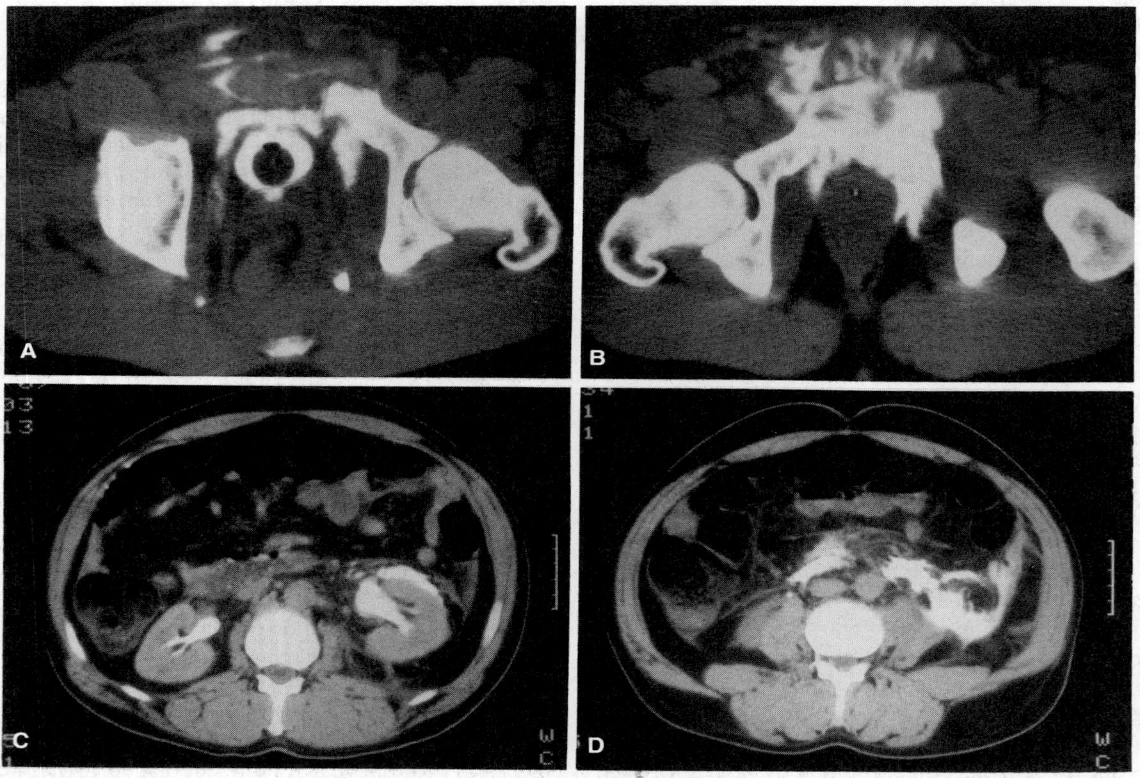

FIGURE 60–14. **(A, B)** Pelvic CT scans demonstrate extraperitoneal bladder rupture with urinary extravasation into the retropubic space and abdominal wall soft tissues after unsuccessful bedside lavage for a patient with clot urinary retention. **(C, D)** Abdominal CT scans demonstrate rupture of the renal calyceal fornix from acute distal ureteral obstruction, leading to extravasation of urine into perinephric fat and retroperitoneal soft tissues. (Courtesy of Dr. Susan Hilton, Department of Radiology, Memorial Sloan-Kettering Cancer Center, New York, NY)

as chemical cautery to control bleeding from submucosal and mucosal vessels.[1,2] In 1969, the use of a 10% formalin instillation was reported effective in controlling intractable bladder hemorrhage in 24 patients treated with radiation therapy for bladder cancer.[29] Complications of renal papillary necrosis, renal failure, ureteral stenosis, bladder contracture, and bladder rupture with fatal intraperitoneal extravasation tempered the initial enthusiasm for the use of 10% formalin.[2,30] In 1974, Fair reported the use of a 1% to 2% formalin solution to treat hemorrhagic cystitis and found it to be effective without the toxicity of 10% formalin.[31] Complications of formalin appear infrequently if concentrations of 4% or less are used. More than 75% of patients with hemorrhagic cystitis have their bleeding controlled by this method.[32] The technique of formalin instillation currently used at our institution is as follows:

1. Spinal or general anesthesia is required because formalin is caustic to sensory nerves within the bladder. Cystoendoscopy is performed to evacuate clots and fulgurate bleeding vessels.
2. A cystogram is performed to identify vesicoureteral reflux or evidence of bladder perforation. If reflux is documented, the involved ureteral orifice(s) must be occluded with a Fogarty balloon-tip catheter before formalin instillation. Any evidence of bladder perforation is an absolute contraindication to formalin instillation.
3. Formalin and formaldehyde are not equivalent compounds. Formalin is a 37% solution of formaldehyde. The stock solution is diluted with sterile water to the desired concentration as follows: 10% formalin is 3.7% formaldehyde and 1% formalin is a 0.37% formaldehyde solution. The order to the pharmacy for the preparation of the desired formalin solution must be explicitly written and the solutions checked by the operating team to avoid serious error.
4. An 18 French (6 mm) Foley catheter is used to catheterize the bladder, and a 1% solution of formalin (500–1000 ml) is instilled under gravity at no higher than 15 cm above the pubis for an overall contact time of approximately 10 to 15 minutes. During the instillation, the catheter should not be clamped, because formalin induced bladder contraction may occur increasing the likelihood of reflux or intravascular absorption. In the female patient, the perineum should be painted with petroleum jelly and the vagina packed with petroleum gauze to prevent skin irritation from formalin.
5. After the formalin instillation, the bladder is thoroughly irrigated with at least 1 L of distilled water, and a Foley catheter is left indwelling for 24 to 48 hours.
6. The instillation of 2.0%, 4%, and rarely 10% formalin using the steps outlined may be necessary to control persistent hemorrhage. Retreatment with formalin should be avoided for at least 48 hours, because its favorable effects may not be apparent for that time. Concentrations of greater than 10% formalin should not be administered.[32]

Other methods of controlling bleeding in hemorrhagic cystitis, including intravesical alum, prostaglandins, phenol, intravesical silver nitrate, hydrostatic distention, iced saline lavage, and parenteral or oral aminocaproic acid have been used with various degrees of success.[1,2] Of these agents, intravesical 1% alum and prostaglandin E_2 and F_2, each of which can be instilled without anesthesia, are the most effective. A 1% alum solution (*i.e.*, the ammonium or potassium salt dissolved in water) delivered by continuous bladder irrigation causes protein precipitation, vasoconstriction, and decreased capillary permeability.[33–35] During instillation, bladder spasms may occur but are usually well controlled by antispasmodic medication. The principal advantage to alum in the treatment of hemorrhagic cystitis is that it can be delivered at the bedside using a three-way indwelling catheter without the need for anesthesia. Some urologists recommend the initial use of alum for massive bladder hemorrhage with formalin as second line treatment. A significant disadvantage of alum irrigation is that it may take as long as 7 days to effectively control the bleeding. Serum aluminum levels should be monitored as rare cases of alum-induced encephalopathy have been reported.[36]

Prostaglandin E_2 and F_2 can also be instilled intravesically without anesthesia and have been reported to be effective in controlling intractable hemorrhagic cystitis, possibly by protecting the microvasculature and epithelium and inhibiting the development of tissue edema.[37,38] Prostaglandin induced severe bladder spasms may limit their overall utility.

Despite all conservative efforts, exsanguinating hemorrhage from the bladder may persist, necessitating open surgical attempts to control the bleeding. Control of the bleeding may require open cystotomy with bladder packing, cutaneous ureterostomy, hypogastric artery embolization, or cystectomy with urinary diversion.[6,39–41] Surgical intervention in these already critically ill patients should be performed only if conservative measures have failed. Surgical control of hemorrhage may still not be possible.

OBSTRUCTIVE UROPATHY

UPPER TRACT OBSTRUCTION

Obstruction of one or both ureters in the cancer patient may be secondary to direct tumor invasion, compression of the ureter by a retroperitoneal tumor, encasement of the ureter by retroperitoneal or pelvic lymph nodes involved with metastatic disease, or rarely by direct metastases to the ureter. Seventy percent of tumors causing ureteral obstruction are genitourinary (*e.g.*, cervical, bladder, prostate) in origin (Fig. 60–15), with breast, gastrointestinal, and lymphoma comprising most of the remainder (Fig. 60–16).[42,43] Ureteral obstruction may be secondary to retroperitoneal fibrosis after combinations of surgery, chemotherapy, or pelvic radiation therapy.[44] Acute ureteral obstruction usually causes flank pain and colic typical of the symptoms of urolithiasis. In contrast, chronic unilateral obstruction is usually a silent event—often detected incidentally as hydronephrosis with renal cortical atrophy on upper abdominal imaging studies (Fig. 60–17).

Acute or chronic bilateral ureteral obstruction is associated with decreased urine output and symptoms of uremia. In one study of 50 patients with acute renal failure secondary to bilateral ureteral obstruction, 76% of the patients had malignant disease as the cause of the obstruction, and half of these patients had uremia as the presenting sign of their cancer.[45] Increased renal pelvic pressure may cause rupture of the renal calyceal fornix, leading to extravasation of urine into the renal

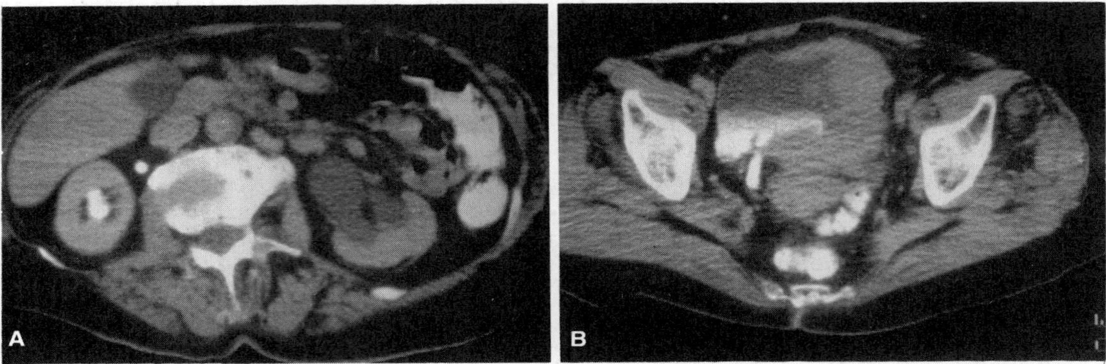

FIGURE 60–15. **(A)** Abdominal CT scan demonstrates the lack of function of the left kidney with hydronephrosis. **(B)** Pelvic CT demonstrates a large, invasive bladder tumor with extravesical extension responsible for distal left ureteral obstruction.

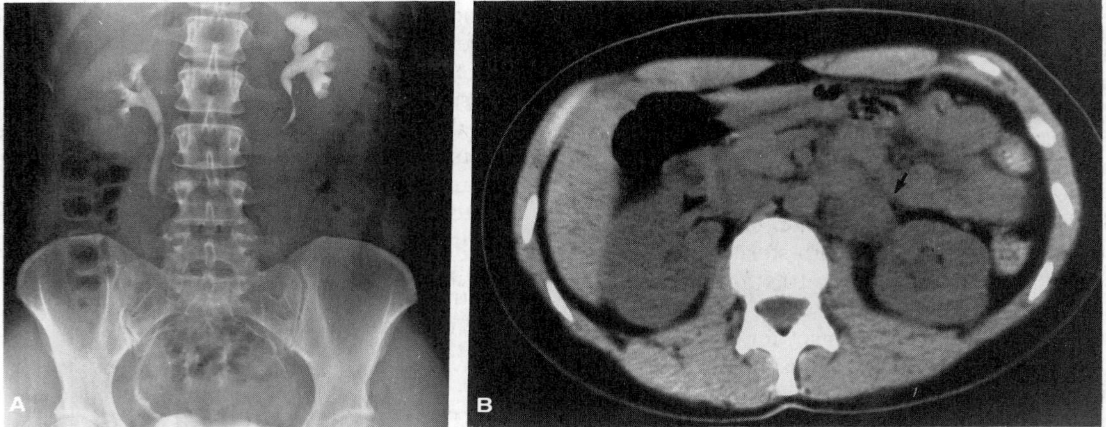

FIGURE 60–16. **(A)** Intravenous urogram of a 30-year-old woman with a history of invasive breast cancer demonstrates left hydronephrosis. **(B)** Abdominal CT scan demonstrates a metastatic deposit (*arrow*) in the area of the left proximal ureter that is responsible for obstruction.

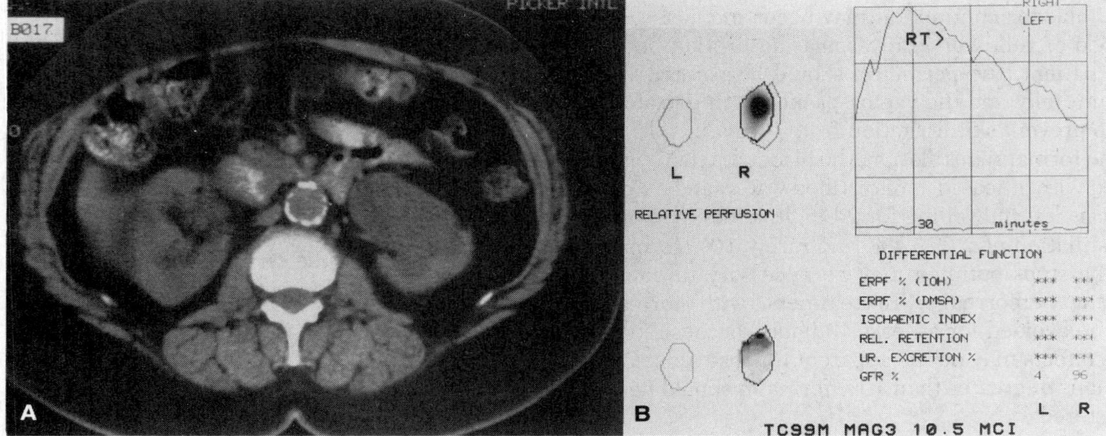

FIGURE 60–17. **(A)** CT scan of the abdomen demonstrates left hydronephrosis with cortical atrophy secondary to a pelvic recurrence of cervical cancer in a 58-year-old woman. **(B)** Radionuclide renogram (DMSA) demonstrates a nonfunctioning left kidney and normal function of the right. Because of the documented lack of function in the left kidney, decompression was not advised.

sinus with the formation of a perinephric urinoma (Figure 60–14C,D).[46] If infected urine exists in the obstructed system, fever, chills, and eventual urosepsis may ensue, requiring emergency urologic decompression. The diagnosis of ureteral obstruction may be made by intravenous urogram, computed tomography (CT) scan, renal ultrasound, retrograde pyelogram, or radionuclide renography.[47] Of these, abdominal CT has the advantage of better defining any extrarenal pathology that may account for the obstruction.

A difficult ethical question arises with the diagnosis of ureteral obstruction in the patient with an incurable malignancy. Is decompression going to facilitate treatment with chemotherapy and palliate symptoms or will it merely address a short-term problem and prolong the patient's suffering? Palliative urinary diversion or decompression with ureteral stents is justified if improvement in renal function facilitates the use of chemotherapy or if symptoms of ureteral obstruction (*e.g.*, pain, urosepsis) can be alleviated.

Malignant ureteral obstruction was previously managed by open surgical placement of a nephrostomy tube, a procedure associated with a major complication rate of up to 45%.[42] Approximately 25% of patients undergoing open nephrostomy died within 30 days of operation, and the average survival after the procedure was approximately 6 months. In the last 10 years, techniques have evolved using percutaneous and endoscopic techniques to decompress the obstructed urinary tract. Using these "endourologic" techniques, decompression of obstructed kidneys, removal of obstructing ureteral stones, and dilation of ureteral strictures can be performed without an open operation. The percutaneous tubes and stents are composed of flexible synthetic materials (*e.g.*, polyurethane) that minimize migration within the urinary tract due to the "double J" configuration of the stents (*i.e.*, one end coiled in the bladder and the second end coiled in the renal pelvis) (Fig. 60–18). Stents of this type cause less encrustation and are easy to change.[48] Flexible guidewires can negotiate narrowed ureteral lumens and sharp bends in the obstructed ureter and aid in the placement of the stents during retrograde cystoscopic or antegrade percutaneous procedures. Recent reports of experience with endourologic decompression of ureteral obstruction in prostate cancer, gynecologic tumors, colorectal cancer, and breast cancer confirm the value of these techniques.[49–52] A mean survival in the range of 10 months can be obtained after diversion or stenting in patients with advanced malignancy and ureteral obstruction. In patients with bilateral ureteral obstruction, significant palliation and return of near-normal renal function is possible after decompression of the obstructed kidney, with more substantial remaining cortex as determined by CT or ultrasound examination.

Endourologists can incise or balloon dilate and stent benign ureteral strictures or ureteral enteric stenoses after urinary diversion (Fig. 60–19).[53,54] After a ureteral stent or percutaneous nephrostomy is placed, subsequent management requires meticulous follow-up, including periodic monitoring of renal function, upper tract imaging (*e.g.*, CT, renal ultrasound), frequent urine cultures, and periodic stent or tube replacement (every 4–6 months). If chemotherapy or radiation therapy directed at the primary tumor successfully eliminates the lesion responsible for the ureteral obstruction, such as retroperitoneal adenopathy from breast cancer or leukemic infiltrates of the ureter (Fig. 60–20), removal of the percutaneous nephrostomy or ureteral stents can be done if imaging studies document the restoration of normal urinary drainage from the involved kidney.[52,55]

Complications of endourologic procedures include gross hematuria with perinephric hematoma, splenic or bowel injury, and hemothorax or pneumothorax.[56] Indwelling ureteral stents can migrate, obstruct with proteinaceous encrustations, become infected, fragment, cause uncomfortable vesicoureteral reflux, and erode through the urinary tract.[48] Patients may complain of bladder spasm from irritation of the trigone, which generally subsides within several weeks of stent placement. Open nephrostomy, cutaneous ureterostomy, or operative urinary diversion should be reserved for unusual cases in which endourologic techniques are not successful, the patients are in satisfactory medical condition, and for patients with life expectancies that do not preclude major surgical procedures.[57] Major operative reconstruction (*e.g.*, revision of ileal ureteral anastomosis, ureteral reimplantation, ileal ureter interposition) may be considered in this setting.

BLADDER OUTLET OBSTRUCTION AND URINARY RETENTION

Acute urinary retention and bladder outlet obstruction (*e.g.*, hesitancy, dribbling, incomplete bladder emptying, overflow

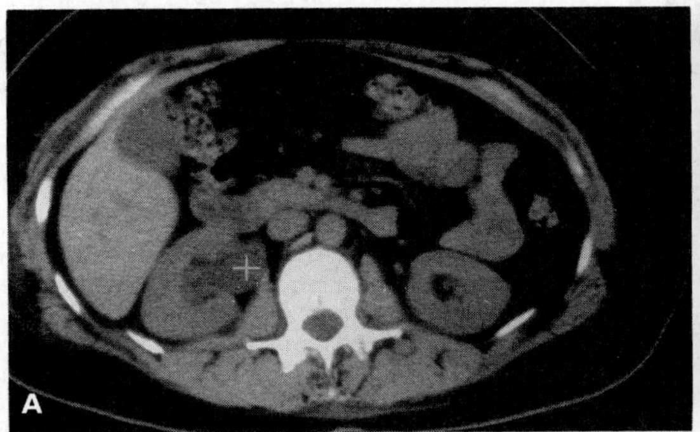

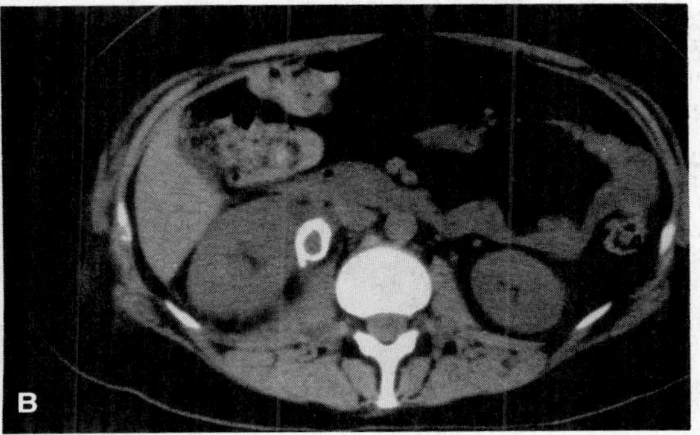

FIGURE 60–18. **(A)** CT scan of the abdomen demonstrates right hydronephrosis in a 48-year-old women with pelvic recurrence of cervical cancer. **(B)** CT scan of the abdomen demonstrates decompression of an obstructed kidney with a cystoscopically placed double J ureteral stent, which is seen coiled in the right renal pelvis.

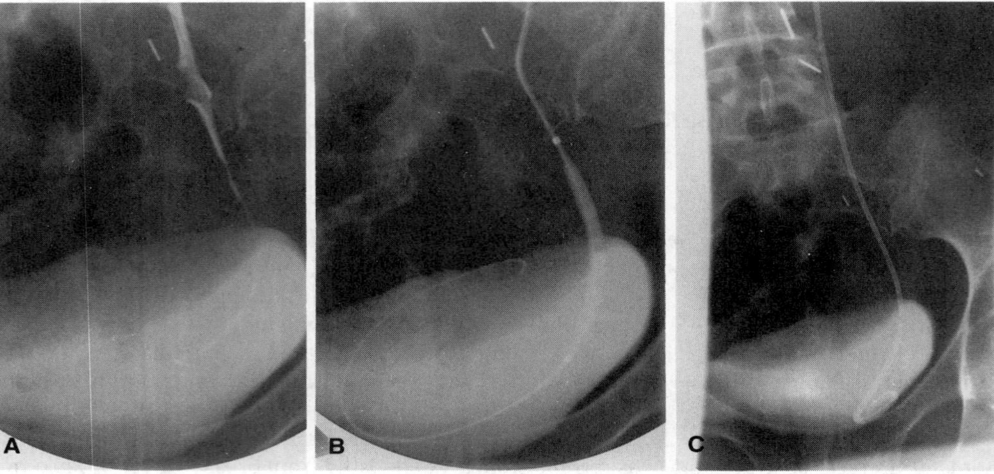

FIGURE 60–19. **(A)** Antegrade ureterogram demonstrates a benign stricture of the distal left ureter in a 54-year-old woman treated with pelvic irradiation for cervical cancer. **(B)** Balloon dilation of a ureteral stricture is performed over a flexible guidewire, which is coiled in the bladder. **(C)** Antegrade placement of double J stent through a previous ureteral stricture.

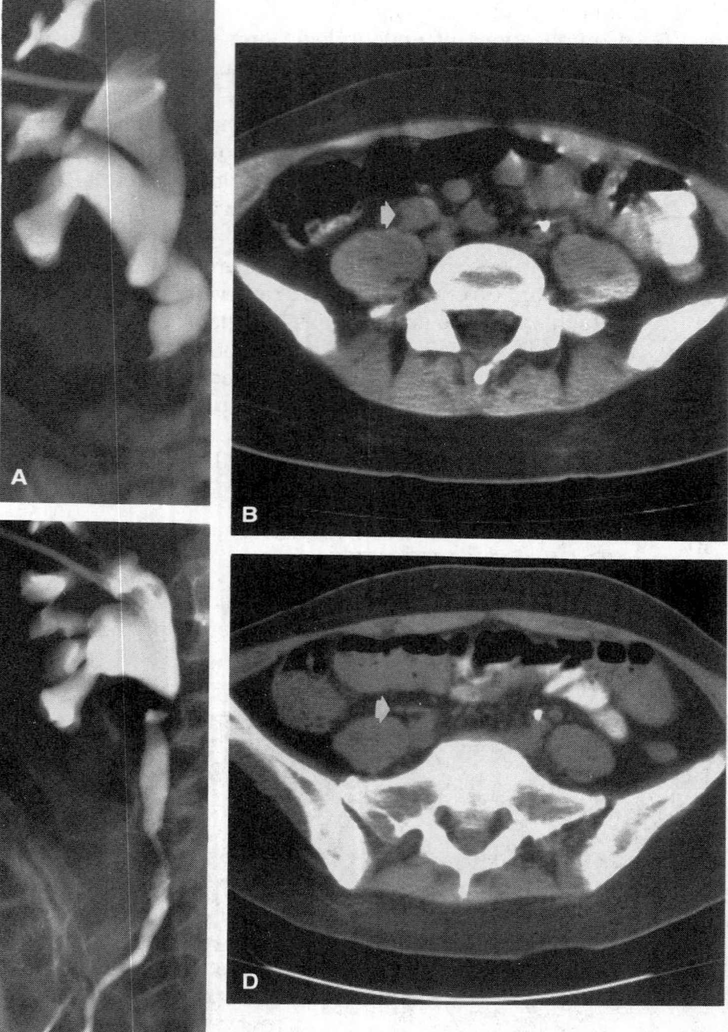

FIGURE 60–20. **(A)** Right hydronephrosis with complete distal ureteral obstruction. The kidney is decompressed with percutaneous nephrostomy. **(B)** Abdominal CT scan demonstrates a leukemic infiltrate (*arrow*) in the area of the proximal ureter that is responsible for the obstruction. **(C)** Antegrade nephrostogram demonstrates the patency of the distal ureter after systemic chemotherapy. **(D)** Complete resolution of the infiltrate responsible for the obstruction after chemotherapy.

incontinence, decrease in the force of the voided stream) can be caused by mechanical or neurophysiologic factors. These factors may be primary manifestations of the malignancy, secondary to treatment, or due to preexisting benign conditions involving the lower urinary tract. A patient with urinary retention complains of severe suprapubic pain and has a palpable suprapubic fullness secondary to a distended bladder. Pelvic and rectal examination may reveal a genitourinary or rectal tumor that is responsible for obstructing the bladder outlet. Complete bladder outlet obstruction can lead rapidly to bilateral hydroureteronephrosis with renal insufficiency and should be treated emergently.

If a malignant cause of bladder outlet obstruction is excluded, a preexisting benign mechanical condition, such as benign prostatic hyperplasia (BPH) or urethral stricture, may be the cause. Less likely causes of retention include constipation and neurologic disorders.[58] It is estimated that 5% to 10% of men at age 40 and 80% of men at age 80 have BPH, although the symptoms vary widely and do not correlate directly with prostate size by digital rectal examination.[59] Many patients have significant obstructive symptoms and may compensate by limiting their fluid intake. During chemotherapy, the combination of antiemetic medication and hydration may precipitate urinary retention in patients with preexisting prostatism.

Improved understanding of the neurophysiology of micturition has allowed us to more precisely diagnose and treat acute nonmechanical causes of bladder outlet obstruction. Urodynamic evaluation, including uroflow, cystometrogram, and perineal sphincter electromyography, are useful in assessing the micturition reflex, which includes sensory nerves in the bladder wall, voluntary cerebral control over the pontine micturition center, sacral parasympathetic nerves (S2–S3), cholinergic nerves to the external sphincter, and sympathetic nerves to the bladder neck.[60–62] Anatomic or neuropharmacologic interference with the micturition reflex occurs frequently in the cancer patient and can lead to acute urinary retention. For example, postoperative urinary retention, often attributed to prostatism, can be caused by the use of certain anticholinergic anesthetic agents that depress detrusor contractility, pain and stress-induced sympathetic activity that increase tone in the bladder neck and proximal urethral muscles, and perioperative pain medications (*e.g.*, opiates) that directly inhibit the pontine micturitional center and depress the urge to void.[63]

Tumors arising in or metastasizing to the brain and or spinal cord can directly interfere with the central voluntary control of micturition and the coordination of bladder emptying and sphincter muscle relaxation. This condition, detrusor external sphincter dyssynergia, can lead to a functional bladder outlet obstruction characterized by bladder wall hypertonicity and hypertrophy with reduced capacity, vesicoureteral reflux, and incomplete bladder emptying. Hypotonic bladder dysfunction may occur in as many as 50% of patients undergoing abdominoperineal resection for rectal carcinoma or radical hysterectomy in which extensive pelvic dissection can disrupt the pelvic parasympathetic nerves necessary for normal detrusor muscle contraction.[64] This effect is usually permanent in only 10% of patients. Viral radiculomyelitis secondary to herpes simplex in an immunocompromised host can cause a flaccid neurogenic bladder, which is usually self-limiting, with the return of normal bladder function expected in approximately 2 weeks.[65]

The first step in the management of urinary retention is the passage of a small (14 French or 4.6 mm) urethral catheter into the bladder. In a male patient, distal urethral obstruction from preexisting stricture disease may be encountered. The urologist may dilate the stricture using filiforms and followers—a procedure that should be rapidly terminated if blood appears at the urethral meatus. A curved urethral catheter (Coudé tip) may be required to pass an enlarged benign or malignant prostate. In the male patient, a Foley catheter should be passed to its hub, with urine return observed before inflating the balloon. This maneuver avoids the inadvertent inflation of the catheter balloon in the prostatic urethra and subsequent brisk bleeding. Forcing a catheter that is not passing easily may cause urethral lacerations and create false passages beneath the prostatic capsule, allowing blood and urine to extravasate into the pelvis and perineum. Should infected urine extravasate, a case of urinary retention can rapidly be converted iatrogenically into urosepsis and soft tissue infection. If transurethral catheterization is not easily accomplished, a percutaneous suprapubic cystotomy tube should be placed, allowing a more orderly approach to the diagnosis and treatment of the underlying obstruction.

In the case of long-standing and complete urinary retention, elevations in ureteral pressure can cause a secondary decrease in renal blood flow, a decrease in glomerular filtration rate, renal tubular dysfunction, and cellular atrophy. The abrupt relief of lower urinary obstruction can initiate a postobstructive diuresis, during which the urine output can be as great as 200 ml/hour for 6 to 12 hours. This initial diuresis is a normal physiologic response to the relief of bladder outlet obstruction, with the kidneys appropriately excreting retained urea, salt, and water. Excessive supplementary intravenous fluids should be avoided, because this tends to prolong the period of diuresis. A pathologic response can occur in patients with more extensive renal tubular damage and nephrogenic diabetes insipidus can develop. In these patients, excessive water loss continues even after the retained water and solutes have been eliminated. The urine remains dilute with low osmolality, and the administration of antidiuretic hormone is ineffective. Normally, the conscious patient retains a normal thirst mechanism and is able to avoid dehydration until renal tubular function normalizes. Rarely, a salt-losing nephropathy occurs, leading to hypotension and hyponatremia. Close monitoring and fluid resuscitation with normal or hypertonic saline must be undertaken until tubular function normalizes.[66]

Treatment of the cancer patient in urinary retention should be conservative. Patients are often debilitated from the effects of the primary tumors and treatment, and they are further frustrated by the new inability to urinate. Many patients, when given another chance to void after a period of catheter decompression, are able to urinate normally and may be spared any invasive procedures.[67]

After bladder decompression is accomplished, the decision about when to give the patient another voiding trial should be based on the patient's clinical status. In the postoperative patient in urinary retention, it is prudent to wait for some recovery from the operation, a decrease in the requirement for pain medication, and the ability to ambulate before another voiding trial is initiated. In the chemotherapy patient in urinary retention, the voiding trial should be delayed until the period of hydration is passed and the need for antiemetic medication is lessened. There is no role for "bladder training" (*i.e.*, clamping and unclamping of the catheter to give the bladder more tone), which was previously advocated by some for patients in retention.

During periods of bladder catheterization, urine cultures should be obtained every 3 days. If colonization of the urine occurs, an appropriate antibiotic to which the organism is sensitive can be administered at the time of the voiding trial. The use of continuous antibiotics in the catheterized patient should be avoided because this will lead to colonization by resistant organisms. If the colonizing organism is urease-producing (*e.g.*, *Proteus mirabilis*), the urine can become alkaline, and magnesium ammonium phosphate (struvite) calculi can form. To prevent this, a short course of an appropriate antibiotic should be administered.[68]

The male patient with a significant antecedent history of prostatism may remain in urinary retention despite voiding trials. Radiologic imaging of the upper urinary tract with intravenous urography, ultrasound, or CT scan can determine if hydronephrosis or renal cortical atrophy exist.[69] Ultrasound has emerged as the most cost effective means of evaluating the urinary tract and has the added appeal of avoiding the use of iodinated contrast materials, which can occasionally cause nephrotoxicity.[70,71] Most patients can have their bladder outlet obstructions relieved by transurethral resection of the prostate (TURP) with acceptable morbidity, although complications of bleeding, clot retention, infection, and persistent failure to void make careful case selection in the cancer patient population important.[72–74] Alternatives to prostatectomy under clinical investigation include luteinizing hormone-releasing hormone analogs, inhibition of 5α-reductase and androgen ablation, α-adrenergic blockers, urethral stents, local microwave hyperthermia, and balloon dilation.[75–80] Although select patients may benefit from these techniques alone or in combination, their overall efficacy appears to be less than standard prostatectomy in the short term, and long-term follow-up data is unavailable.

After a neurologic cause for urinary retention is diagnosed, the mainstay of treatment is clean intermittent self-catheterization, which is performed every 4 to 6 hours.[81] This method of alleviating urinary retention can preserve kidney function, reduce infection rates, reduce stone formation, and improve the quality of patients' lives compared with chronic indwelling Foley catheters. In a report of 75 patients with neurogenic bladders followed for a mean of 7 years, all patients had preservation of upper urinary tract function. Complications occurred in 20% and included urethral injury or stenosis (13), epididymitis (6), bladder calculi (3), and pyelonephritis (1).[82] Antibiotics are not given prophylactically to patients on intermittent self-catheterization, because they have not been shown to lower the incidence of clinical urinary tract infection.[83]

URINARY TRACT INFECTION

Urinary tract infections occur in the cancer patient when normal defense barriers are disrupted during hospitalization.[84] These barriers include normal perineal flora (*e.g.*, lactobacilli, streptococci, coagulase-negative staphylococcus) and an anatomically intact urinary tract with normal micturitional reflexes. Most urinary tract infections are ascending, with the presence of an indwelling bladder catheter the principal portal of entry.[85] The approximately 5% incidence of urinary tract infection in neutropenic and bone marrow transplant patients is directly related to the frequency and duration of bladder catheterization.[84] The bladder catheterization procedure may introduce bacteria into the bladder at rates as high as 20% in the hospitalized patient.[86] Closed catheter drainage systems have reduced bacteriuria, but hospital-acquired bacteria still gain access to the system. After periurethral colonization, pathogenic bacteria can track along the catheter causing urethritis and eventual bladder infection. The risk of bacteriuria increases 5% to 10% for each day of catheterization, a fact that should provide the impetus for early catheter removal or the institution of intermittent catheterization.[87] Cancer patients receiving systemic antibiotics have alterations in periurethral flora favoring colonization with enteric organisms and resistant organisms prevalent in the hospital environment, such as *Pseudomonas aeruginosa* and *Candida albicans*.

The most common pathogens causing urinary tract infection are gram-negative bacteria, with *E. coli* responsible for 50% to 75% of cases of clinical pyelonephritis.[88] Bacteria can adhere to mucosal and catheter surfaces in a biofilm (*e.g.*, glycocalyx), which protects them from the mechanical flow of urine, inflammatory defenses, and antibiotics.[89] Bacterial bladder infection causes an initial inflammatory response that results in acute and chronic cystitis but is usually not associated with fever or an elevated leukocyte count. With longer catheterization, bacteria can ascend into the ureters and invade the renal epithelium causing inflammatory infiltrates in the kidneys. Acute pyelonephritis is marked by fever, flank pain, bacteremia, and an elevated leukocyte count.[90] Upper tract infection can lead to stone formation due to urea-splitting organisms such as *Proteus mirabilis*, xanthogranulomatous pyelonephritis (Fig. 60–21A), renal cortical abscess (Fig. 60–21B), perinephric abscess, renal carbuncle, emphysematous pyelonephritis, and urosepsis.[91]

The diagnostic approach to the patient with renal infection should begin with a plain film radiograph of the abdomen to detect calculi or abnormal gas collections overlying the kidney. Contrast-enhanced CT scans and renal ultrasound can precisely identify cortical or perinephric abscess or acute focal bacterial nephritis and have supplanted ^{67}Ga citrate or ^{111}In-labeled white blood cell scans in the diagnosis of kidney abscess.[92]

The prevention of urinary tract infection in the cancer patient begins with the selective use of indwelling catheters for the treatment of urinary retention, the assessment of hourly urine output when critical, or in the immediate postoperative period. The catheter should be removed as soon as possible to limit the chances of bacterial colonization. Systemic antibiotics should be avoided during periods of indwelling catheterization to prevent the emergence of resistant organisms. At the end of a long period of urinary catheterization, a urine culture should be obtained and a short course (3–5 days) of an appropriate oral antibiotic prescribed to sterilized the urine.

A common complication of long-term bladder catheterization in the presence of systemic antibiotics is candiduria.[90] This form of bladder colonization is usually asymptomatic

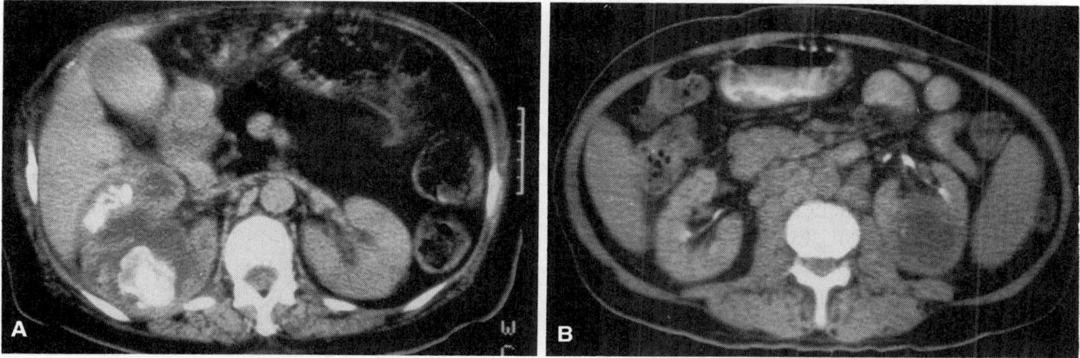

FIGURE 60–21. **(A)** CT scan of the abdomen demonstrates right xanthogranulomatous pyelonephritis with several large struvite calculi in a patient with a long-standing foley catheter. **(B)** CT scan of the abdomen demonstrates a left renal cortical abscess.

and resolves on removal of the catheter. If prolonged catheterization is required and candiduria is persistent, continuous bladder irrigation through a three-way catheter using amphotericin B (50 mg dissolved in 1 L of sterile water) usually eradicates the infection. Persistent candiduria with budding yeast forms should prompt upper tract imaging studies and cystoendoscopy to rule out the presence of fungal balls that would require urgent surgical removal.

If acute pyelonephritis occurs, a 10-day course of parenteral antibiotics should be administered—a treatment duration effective in curing 90% of uncomplicated cases.[93] Before blood and urine culture data are available, a combination of an aminoglycoside to cover enteric gram-negative rods and *Pseudomonas* and ampicillin to cover enterococcus should be started. When the antibiotic sensitivities are known, the choice of antibiotic should be made based on degree of effectiveness, potential nephrotoxicity, allergic history, and cost.[88] Failure to respond to appropriate antibiotics within 48 hours should raise the possibility of septic ureteral obstruction, renal cortical abscess, perinephric abscess, or renal carbuncle. An ultrasound or CT scan of the kidney should be performed to rule out these conditions. If an abscess is diagnosed, prompt open surgical drainage or CT-guided percutaneous drainage is required.[94] If a septic course is prolonged and imaging studies reveal a nonfunctional kidney without abscess formation consistent with a renal carbuncle, emergency nephrectomy may be required to eliminate the infection.

Secondary infections of the prostate and epididymis can occur as urethral or bladder pathogens pass through the vas deferens and prostatic ducts, causing acute epididymitis or acute prostatitis. These infections can cause painful febrile illnesses that can result in abscess formation requiring emergency surgical drainage or orchiectomy (Fig. 60–22A).[95,96] It is often difficult to culture the offending pathogen, and empiric antibiotic treatment for 10 to 14 days and local measures (*e.g.*, scrotal elevation, warm sitz baths, antiinflammatory agents) are often effective in alleviating symptoms. The most common urologic manifestation of acquired immunodeficiency syndrome-related tuberculosis is an epididymo-orchitis with abscess formation and a draining scrotal sinus (Fig. 60–22B). The involved testicle is usually completely destroyed by tuberculous granulomas, and orchiectomy in conjunction with systemic antituberculous therapy is the treatment of choice.[97]

Rarely, extravasation of infected urine from the anterior

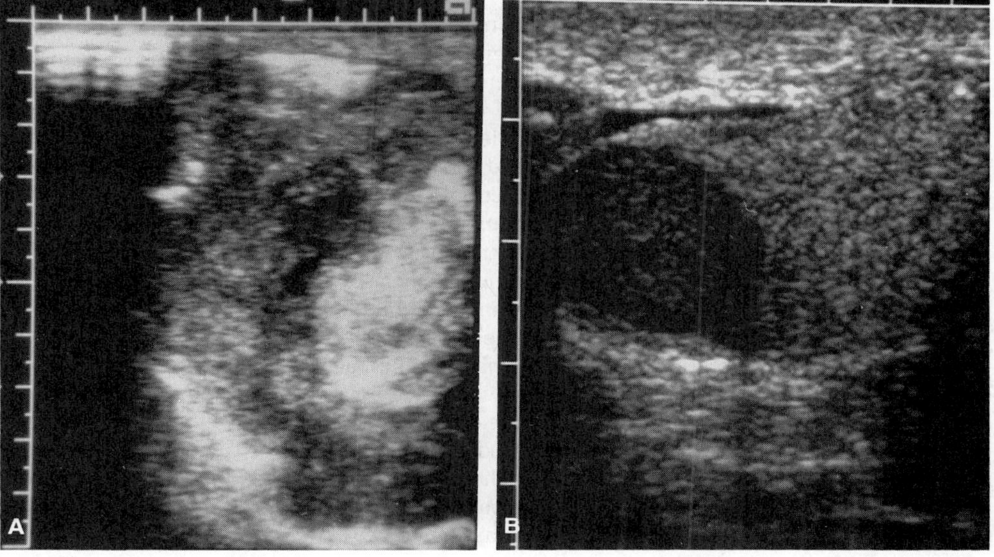

FIGURE 60–22. **(A)** Scrotal ultrasound, transverse section, demonstrates a testicular abscess after an episode of epididymal orchitis. **(B)** Scrotal ultrasound, longitudinal section, demonstrates a tuberculous abscess in the right testicle of a 26-year-old man with AIDS.

urethra into perineal soft tissues (*e.g.*, after traumatic dilation of a urethral stricture or infection of periurethral glands) or the perineal extension of a perirectal abscess can cause a polymicrobial infection involving enteric gram-negative and gram-positive anaerobes. This synergistic infection, marked by early fever, chills, and genital discomfort out of proportion to physical findings, causes an obliterating end-arteritis, which can lead rapidly to subcutaneous ischemia, evolving necrosis of the penile, scrotal, and perineal skin with the anaerobic production of hydrogen and nitrogen gas. The gas is clinically detectable as subcutaneous crepitus and plain x-ray films of the pelvis show air in the soft tissues. Aggressive medical and surgical management must be instituted as soon as the diagnosis of scrotal (Fournier's) gangrene is entertained. Triple antibiotic therapy, including an aminoglycoside, high dose-penicillin, and clindamycin, covers aerobic and anaerobic components of the infection. All nonvital genital tissue must be widely debrided and, depending on the source of the infection, urinary or fecal stream diversion should be performed. Aggressive wound debridement, often requiring repeated operations, can be followed later by skin grafts or myocutaneous flaps for skin coverage. Despite early recognition and aggressive treatment of Fournier's gangrene, mortality rates as high as 33% are reported. In immunocompromised and neutropenic patients, the mortality rate is higher.[98,99]

PRIAPISM

Priapism is defined as a persistent state of painful erection associated with elevated intracavernous pressures not due to sexual stimulation. If left untreated, priapism can cause endothelial damage, thrombosis, and fibrosis leading to impotency. Most cases of priapism have no discernible cause. In the United States, however, sickle cell anemia accounts for approximately 20% of adult cases and 60% of pediatric cases.[100] In the cancer patient, priapism may be due to a primary hematologic malignancy (*e.g.*, leukemia, myeloma), metastatic disease to the corporal bodies of the penis, disruption of venous outflow from the penis secondary to a pelvic tumor, or intracavernous drug therapies used in the treatment of impotence.

Schreibman and colleagues reported priapism in 4 patients with chronic granulocytic leukemia; the priapism resolved after the institution of effective systemic chemotherapy for their underlying disease and normalization of the leukocyte count.[101] Metastatic disease to the corporal bodies of the penis has been reported in cases of clinically advanced genitourinary (*e.g.*, bladder, prostate, kidney) or gastrointestinal (*e.g.*, colorectal) cancer.[102] Although the exact mechanism whereby the metastatic deposits cause priapism is unknown, thrombosis, perhaps in conjunction with a malignancy-associated hypercoagulable state, occurs, and venous drainage from the corporal bodies is blocked. Treatment directed toward the primary tumor (*e.g.*, androgen deprivation in the case of metastatic prostate cancer) may improve or resolve the state of priapism. Occasionally, radiation therapy to the corporal bodies can be effective. In cases of priapism secondary to malignancy, corporal shunting procedures used in idiopathic cases are usually ineffective; treatment should be palliative, with relief of pain and urinary obstruction the primary objectives.

Urologists treating patients who are impotent after radical pelvic surgery with intracavernous injections of papaverine or prostaglandin E_1 face an 8% incidence of pharmacologically induced priapism.[103] When this occurs, corporal aspiration to reduce intracavernous pressures and remove excess vasoactive agent in conjunction with the injection of an α-adrenergic agent (*e.g.*, phenylephrine hydrochloride) is usually effective treatment. Shantha and colleagues reported the use of a 5-mg oral dose of terbutaline, a β_2-agonist, to be effective in rapidly reversing pharmacologically induced priapism.[104]

REFERENCES

1. DeVries CR, Freiha FS. Hemorrhagic cystitis: A review. J Urol 1990;143:1–9.
2. Levine LA, Richie JP. Urologic complications of cyclophosphamide. J Urol 1989;141: 1063–1069.
3. Watson NA, Noteley RG. Urologic complications of cyclophosphamide. Br J Urol 1973;45:606.
4. Texter JH, Koontz WW, McWilliams NB. Hemorrhagic cystitis as a complication of the management of pediatric neoplasm. Urol Surv 1979;29:47.
5. Droller MJ, Saral S, Santos, G. Prevention of cyclophosphamide-induced hemorrhagic cystitis. Urology 1982;20:256.
6. Stillwell TJ, Benson RC. Cyclophosphamide induced hemorrhagic cystitis. A review of 100 patients. Cancer 1988;61:451–457.
7. Cox PJ. Cyclophosphamide-induced cystitis-identification of acrolein as the causative agent. Biochem Pharmacol 1979;28:2045.
8. Freedman A, Ehrlich RM, Ljung BM. Prevention of cyclophosphamide cystitis with 2-mercaptoethane sodium sulfonate: A histologic study. J Urol 1984;132:580.
9. Ehrlich RM, Freedman A, Goldsobel AB, et al. The use of sodium 2 mercaptoethane sulfonate to prevent cyclophosphamide cystitis. J Urol 1984;131:960.
10. Jardine I, Ferselau C, Appler M, et al. Quantification by gas chromatography, chemical ionization, mass spectrometry of cyclophosphamide, phosphoramide mustard and nitrogen mustard in the plasma and urine of patients cyclophosphamide therapy. Cancer Res 1978;38:408–415.
11. Antman KH, Ryan L, Elias A, et al. Response to ifosfamide and mesna: 124 previously treated patients with metastatic or unresectable sarcoma. J Clin Oncol 1989;7:126–131.
12. Pratt CB, Horowitz ME, Meyer WH, et al. Phase 2 trial of ifosfamide in children with malignant solid tumors. Cancer Treat Rep 1987;71:131.
13. Williams SD, Munshi, N, Einhorn LH, et al. Cyclophosphamide and ifosfamide: Role of uroprotective agents. Cancer Invest 1990;8:269.
14. Andriole GL, Sandlund JT, Miser JS, et al. The efficacy of mesna (2-mercaptoethane sodium sulfonate) as a uroprotectant in patients with hemorrhagic cystitis receiving further oxazaphosphorine chemotherapy. J Clin Oncol 1987;5:799–803.
15. Brugieres L, Hartmann JP, Travagli E, et al. Hemorrhagic cystitis following high-dose chemotherapy and bone marrow transplantation in children with malignancies: Incidence, clinical course, and outcome. J Clin Oncol 1989;7:194–199.
16. Shepherd JD, Pringle LE, Barnett MJ, et al. Mesna versus hyperhydration for the prevention of cyclophosphamide-induced hemorrhagic cystitis in bone marrow transplantation. J Clin Oncol 1991;9:2016–2020.
17. Dean RJ, Lytton B. Urologic complications of pelvic irradiation. J Urol 1978;119:64.
18. Schellhammer PF, Jordan GH, El-Mahdi AM. Pelvic complications after interstitial and external beam irradiation of urologic and gynecologic malignancy. World J Surg 1986;10:259–268.
19. Parsons CL. Successful management of radiation cystitis with sodium pentosanpolysulfate. J Urol 1986;136:813.
20. Weiss JP, Boland FP, Mori H, et al. Treatment of radiation induced cystitis with hyperbaric oxygen. J Urol 1986;134:352–354.
21. Liu YK, Harty JI, Steinbock GS, et al. Treatment of radiation or cyclophosphamide induced cystitis using conjugated estrogen. J Urol 1990;144:41–43.
22. Numazaki Y, Shigeta S, Kumaska T, et al. Acute hemorrhagic cystitis in children: Isolation of adenovirus type 11. N Engl J Med 1968;278:700–704.
23. Mufson MA, Belshe RB. A review of adenoviruses in the etiology of acute hemorrhagic cystitis. J Urol 1976;115:191–194.
24. Ambinder RF, Burns W, Forman M, et al. Hemorrhagic cystitis associated with adenovirus infection in bone marrow transplantation. Arch Intern Med 1986;146:1400–1401.
25. Rice SJ, Bishop JA, Apperley J, et al. BK virus as cause of hemorrhagic cystitis after bone marrow transplantation. Lancet 1985;2:844–845.
26. Shah KV, Daniel RW, Warszawski RM. High prevalence of antibodies to BK virus, an SV40-related papovavirus, in residents of Maryland. J Infect Dis 1973;128:784–787.
27. Heritage J, Chesters PM, McCance DJ. The persistence of papovavirus BK DNA sequences in normal human renal tissue. J Med Virol 1981;8:143–150.
28. Arthur RR, Shah KV, Baust SJ, et al. Association of BK viuruia with hemorrhagic cystitis in recipients of bone marrow transplants. N Engl J Med 1986;315:230–234.
29. Brown RB. A method of management of inoperable carcinoma of the bladder. Med J Aust 1969;1:23.
30. Donahue LA, Frank IN. Intravesical formalin of hemorrhagic cystitis: Analysis of therapy. J Urol 1989;141:809.

31. Fair WR. Formalin in the treatment of massive bladder hemorrhage. Techniques, results, and complications. Urology 1974;3:573.
32. Godec CJ, Gleich P. Intractable hematuria and formalin. J Urol 1983;130:688.
33. Ostroff EB, Chenault OW. Alum irrigation for the control of massive bladder hemorrhage. J Urol 1982;128:929–930.
34. Goel AK, Rao MS, Bhagwat AG, et al. Intravesical irrigation with alum for the control of massive bladder hemorrhage. J Urol 1984;133:956–957.
35. Arrizabalga M, Extramiana JL, Parra JL, et al. Treatment of massive hematuria with aluminous salts. Br J Urol 1987;60:223–226.
36. Kavoussi LR, Gelstein LD, Andriole GL. Encephalopathy and an elevated serum aluminum level in a patient receiving intravesical alum irrigation for severe urinary hemorrhage. J Urol 1986;136:665.
37. Mohuiddin J, Prentice HG, Schey S, et al. Treatment of cyclophosphamide-induced cystitis with prostaglandin E_2. Ann Intern Med 1984;101:142.
38. Shurafa M, Shumaker E, Cronin S. Prostaglandin F_2-alpha bladder irrigation for control of intractable cyclophosphamide-induced hemorrhagic cystitis. J Urol 1987;137:1230.
39. Andriole GL, Yuan JJ, Catalona WJ. Cystotomy, temporary urinary diversion and bladder packing in the management of severe cyclophosphamide-induced hemorrhagic cystitis. J Urol 1990;143:1006.
40. Pomer S, Karcher G, Simon W. Cutaneous ureterostomy as last resort treatment of intractable hemorrhagic cystitis following radiation. Br J Urol 1983;55:392.
41. Golin AI, Benson RC. Cyclophosphamide hemorrhagic cystitis requiring urinary diversion. J Urol 1977;118:110.
42. Holden S, McPhee M, Grabstald H. The rationale of urinary diversion in the cancer patient. J Urol 1979;121:19.
43. Zadra JA, Jewett, MA, Keresteci AG, et al. Nonoperative urinary diversion for malignant ureteral obstruction. Cancer 1987;60:1353.
44. Montana GS, Fowler WC. Carcinoma of the cervix: Analysis of bladder and rectal radiation dose and complications. Int J Radiat Oncol Biol Phys 1989;16:95.
45. Norman RW, Mack FG, Awad SA, et al. Acute renal failure secondary to bilateral ureteral obstruction: Review of 50 cases. Can Med Assoc J 1982;127:601.
46. Rose BS, Ragosin R, La Rosa JL, et al. Pyelosinus extravasation and urinoma associated with malignancy. Urology 1988;31:349.
47. Cronan JJ. Contemporary concepts in imaging urinary obstruction. Radiol Clin North Am 1991;29:527.
48. Saltzman B. Ureteral stents: Indications, variations, and complications. Urol Clin North Am 1988;15:481.
49. Chiou RK, Chang WY, Horan J. Ureteral obstruction associated with prostate cancer. The outcome after percutaneous nephrostomy. J Urol 1990;143:957.
50. Soper JT, Blaszczyk TM, Oke E, et al. Percutaneous nephrostomy in gynecologic oncology patients. Am J Obstet Gynecol 1988;158:1126.
51. Lee PH, Khauli RB, Baker S, et al. Prognostic and therapeutic observations of manifestations in the genitourinary tract of adenocarcinoma of the colon and rectum. Surg Gynecol Obstet 1989;169:511.
52. Reloux P, Weiser M, Piccart M, et al. Ureteral obstruction in patients with breast cancer. Cancer 1988;61:1904.
53. Meretyk S, Albala DM, Kavoussi LR. Endosurgery: Noncalculus application in the upper urinary tract. Monogr Urol 1991;12:67.
54. Meretyk S, Clayman RV, Kavoussi LR, et al. Endourologic treatment of ureteroenteric anastomotic strictures: Long-term follow-up. J Urol 1991;145:723.
55. Blumenthal D, Russo P, Orr J. Unilateral ureteral obstruction in a patient with acute leukemia. Urol Radiol 1990;12:61.
56. Brannen GE, Bush WH. Complications of endourology. AUA Update Series 9, Lesson 3. Houston: American Urological Association, 1985.
57. MacGregor PS, Montie JE, Straffon RA. Cutaneous ureterostomy as palliative diversion in adults with malignancy. Urology 1987;30:31.
58. Murray K, Massey A, Feneley RCL. Acute urinary retention—A urodynamic assessment. Br J Urol 1984;56:468.
59. Christensen MM, Bruskewitz RC. Clinical manifestations of benign prostatic hyperplasia and indications for therapeutic intervention. Urol Clin North Am 1990;17:509.
60. Chancellor MB, Blaivis JG, Kaplan SA, et al. Bladder outlet obstruction versus impaired detrusor contractility: The role of uroflow. J Urol 1991;145:810.
61. Blaivas JG. Multichannel urodynamic studies in men with benign prostatic hyperplasia. Urol Clin North Am 1990;17:543.
62. Blaivas JG. The neurophysiology of micturition. A clinical study of 550 patients. J Urol 1982;127:958.
63. Anderson JB, Grant JBF. Postoperative retention of urine: A prospective urodynamic study. Br Med J 1991;302:894.
64. Eickenberg HU, Amin M, Klompus W, et al. Urologic complications following abdominoperineal resection. J Urol 1976;115:180.
65. Steinberg J, Rukstalis DB, Vickers MA. Acute urinary retention secondary to herpes simplex meningitis. J Urol 1991;145:359.
66. Loo MH, Vaughan ED. Obstructive nephropathy and postobstructive diuresis. AUA Update Series 4, Lesson 9. Houston: American Urological Association, 1985.
67. Taube M, Gajraj H. Trial without catheter following acute retention. Br J Urol 1989;63: 180.
68. Russo P, Packer MG, Fair WR. Prophylactic antibiotics in urological surgery. Semin Urol 1983;1:155.
69. McClennan BL. Diagnostic imaging evaluation of benign prostatic hyperplasia. Urol Clin North Am 1990;17:517.
70. Reisman ME, Kennedy TJ, Roehrborn CG, et al. A prospective study of urologist-performed sonographic evaluation of the urinary tract in patients with prostatism. J Urol 1991;145:1186.
71. Bryd L, Sherman RL. Radiocontrast induced acute renal failure. Medicine (Baltimore) 1979;58:270.
72. Mebust WK. Transurethral prostatectomy. Urol Clin North Am 1990;17:575.
73. Mebust WK, Holtgrewe HL, Cockett ATK, et al. Transurethral prostatectomy: Immediate and postoperative complications. A cooperative study of 13 participating institutions evaluating 3885 patients. J Urol 1989;141:243.
74. Meyerhoff HH, Gleason DM, Bottaccini MR. The effects of transurethral resection on the urodynamics of prostatism. J Urol 1989;142:785.
75. Keane PF, Timoney AG, Kiely E, et al. Response of benign hypertrophied prostate to treatment with LHRH analogue. Br J Urol 1988;62:163.
76. McConnell JD. Androgen ablation and blockade in the treatment of benign prostatic hyperplasia. Urol Clin North Am 1990;17:661.
77. Caine M. The present role of alpha adrenergic blockers in treatment of benign prostatic hypertrophy. J Urol 1986;136:1.
78. Nissenkorn I. Experience with a new self-retaining intraurethral catheter in patients with urinary retention: A preliminary report. J Urol 1989;142:942.
79. Strohmaier WL, Bichler KH, Flucter SH, et al. Local microwave hyperthermia of benign prostatic hyperplasia. J Urol 1990;144:913.
80. Dowd JB, Smith JJ. Balloon dilation of the prostate. Urol Clin North Am 1990;17:671.
81. Lapides J, Diokno AC, Silber S, et al. Clean intermittent self-catheterization in the treatment of urinary tract disease. J Urol 1972;107:458.
82. Wyndaele JJ, Maes D. Clean intermittent self-catheterization: A 12-year follow-up. J Urol 1990;143:906.
83. Maynard F, Diokno A. Urinary infection and complications during clean intermittent catheterization following spinal cord injury. J Urol 1984;132:943.
84. Korzeniowski OM. Urinary tract infection in the impaired host. Med Clin North Am 1991;75:391.
85. Warren JW. The catheter and urinary tract infection. Med Clin North Am 1991;75: 481.
86. Garibaldi RA, Burke JP, Dickman ML, et al. Factors predisposing to bacteriuria during indwelling urethral catheterization. N Engl J Med 1974;291:215.
87. Stamm WE. Nosocomial infections: Etiologic changes, therapeutic challenges. Hosp Pract 1981;16:75.
88. Fierer J. Acute pyelonephritis. Urol Clin North Am 1987;14:251.
89. Nickel JC, Ruseska I, Wright JB, et al. Tobramycin resistance of *Pseudomonas aeruginosa* cells growing as a biofilm on urinary catheter material. Antimicrob Agents Chemother 1985;27:619.
90. Warren JW, Muncie HL, Hall-Craggs M. Acute pyelonephritis associated with bacteriuria of long-term catheterization: A prospective clinico-pathological study. J Infect Dis 1988;158:1341.
91. Roberts JA. Pyelonephritis, cortical abscess, perinephric abscess. Urol Clin North Am 1986;13:637.
92. Merenich WM, Popky GL. Radiology of renal infection. Med Clin North Am 1991;75: 425.
93. Sheenan G, Harding G, et al. Advances in the treatment of urinary tract infection. Am J Med 1984;15:141.
94. Kuligowska E, Newman B, White SJ, et al. Interventional ultrasound in detection and treatment of renal inflammatory disease. Radiology 1983;147:521.
95. Berger RE. Acute epididymitis: Etiology and therapy. Semin Urol 1991;9:28.
96. Pfau A. Prostatitis: A continuing enigma. Urol Clin North Am 1986;13:695.
97. Vapnek JM. Urologic disease in HIV infection. Infect Urol 1991;4:104.
98. Cohen MS. Fournier's gangrene. AUA Update Series 5, Lesson 6. Houston: American Urological Association, 1986.
99. Jones RB, Hircschmann JV, Brown GS, et al. Fournier's syndrome: Necrotizing subcutaneous infection of the male genitalia. J Urol 1979;122:279.
100. Nelson JH, Winter CC. Priapism: Evolution of management in 48 patients in a 22-year series. J Urol 1977;117:455.
101. Schreibman SM, Gee TS, Grabstaldt H. Management of priapism in patients with chronic granulocytic leukemia. J Urol 1974;111:786.
102. Powell BL, Craig JB, Muss HB. Secondary malignancies of the penis and epididymis: A case report and review of the literature. J Clin Oncol 1985;3:110.
103. Nolens RE, Ells L, Crammer-Levied D. pharmacologic erection: Diagnosis and treatment applications in 69 patients. J Urol 1987;138:52.
104. Shantha TR, Finnerty DP, Rodriquez AP. Treatment of persistent penile erection and priapism using terbutaline. J Urol 1989;141:1427.

Cancer: Principles & Practice of Oncology, Fourth Edition,
edited by Vincent T. DeVita, Jr., Samuel Hellman, Steven A. Rosenberg.
J.B. Lippincott Co., Philadelphia © 1993.

CHAPTER 61

Treatment of Metastatic Cancer

DONALD C. WRIGHT
THOMAS F. DELANEY
JAN C. BUCKNER

SECTION 1

Treatment of Metastatic Cancer to the Brain

Physicians caring for patients with oncologic disease face a daunting challenge when invasion of the nervous system by generalized cancers becomes evident. The appearance of neurologic symptoms in this setting evokes a feeling of dread in patients and in their families and occasionally prompts a concealed nihilism among the treating physicians. Successful, appropriate management of cerebral metastatic spread requires rapid diagnosis and institution of therapy to minimize neurologic injury and maximize the duration and quality of survival. Selected patients derive tremendous benefit from combined treatment approaches, and careful management limits the neurologic impairment in many others. Extending this success to the majority of patients with brain metastases, however, remains an elusive goal.

Metastases to the central nervous system (CNS), a favored site for metastatic spread among the more common cancers affecting the U.S. population, occur in 25% to 35%[1] of all cancer patients. This chapter focuses on the treatment of *parenchymal* metastases to the nervous system, the more common mode of CNS involvement by cancer. Epidemiologic estimates of CNS involvement by cancer in the 1992 U.S. population (Table 61–1)[2] forecast that more than 152,600 patients, or 13.5% of the total U.S. cancer population, will develop symptomatic metastasis to the brain.[1–6]

CLASSIFICATION AND EPIDEMIOLOGY OF CEREBRAL METASTASES

ANATOMIC DISTRIBUTION

The specific anatomic site(s) or "compartments" involved in a metastatic process, as well as the primary histologic type, temporal profile, and clinical status of the patient at the time of diagnosis, are useful criteria in determining prognosis and the most efficacious therapy. The anatomic cerebral compartments commonly involved by metastasis (Fig. 61–1) are the skull, dura, leptomeninges (arachnoid and pia), and parenchymal substance of the brain (pituitary and extracranial sites are omitted in this chapter). Central nervous system involvement in cancer ranges from 20% to 30%, reflecting the difference between clinical detection during life and careful necropsy examination.[1,5,7] *Intracranial* involvement is estimated as 25%, with *intradural* (parenchymal and leptomeningeal) deposits affecting 20% and *parenchymal* involvement only present in 10% of patients.[5,8]

Clinical series indicate that multiple deposits are present in 53% of patients. Autopsy examination and increasingly sensitive diagnostic studies suggest that the frequency of multiple tumors is higher.[4,5,8,9] Certain tumor types are typically associated with single (renal, ovarian, osteogenic sarcoma, breast) and multiple (lung, melanoma, seminoma) metastases.[5] The detection of multiple metastatic deposits plays a critical role in the choice of therapy, because most authors restrict surgery to single metastases.

HISTOPATHOLOGY: FREQUENCY OF METASTASES BY TUMOR TYPE

Parenchymal patterns of metastases are determined by the general incidence of a specific cancer and the relative ten-

TABLE 61–1. Epidemiologic Estimates of Brain Metastases—1992

Site or Type	*Systemic Cancer 1992: New Cases*	*Frequency of Symptomatic Metastases**	*New Cases: Symptomatic Metastases†*	*1992 Deaths*	*Deaths With Symptomatic Metastases‡*
All sites	1,130,000	0.135	152,600	520,000	70,200
Lung	168,000	0.263	44,200	146,000	38,400
Breast	181,000	0.158	28,600	45,300	7200
Colon and rectum	156,000	0.045	7000	58,300	2600
Urinary organs	78,100	0.128	10,000	20,200	2600
Melanoma	32,000	0.37	11,800	6700	2500
Prostate	132,000	0.053	7000	34,000	1800
Pancreas	28,300	0.04	1100	25,000	1000
Leukemia	28,200	0.06	1700	19,200	1200
Lymphoma§	44,400	0.038	1800	20,900	800
Liver	15,400	0.04	600	12,300	500
Female genital	71,500	0.015	1100	24,000	400

* Symptomatic parenchymal location only (does not include skull, dura, or leptomeninges).
† Estimated by (new 1992 cases) × (metastatic frequency).
‡ Estimated by (1992 cancer deaths) × (metastatic frequency of symptomatic parenchymal metastases).
§ Includes all lymphoma (Hodgkin's and non-Hodgkin's types).
(Boring CC, Squires TS, Tong R. Cancer statistics, 1992. CA 1992;42:19–38; Hildebrand J. Lesions of the nervous system in cancer patients. Monograph series of the European Organization for Research on Treatment of Cancer. Vol 5. New York: Raven Press, 1978; Takakura K, Sano K, Hoho S, et al. Metastatic tumors of the central nervous system. Tokyo: Igaku-Shoin, 1982; Galicich JH, Sundaresan N. Metastatic brain tumors. In: Wilkins RH, Rengachary SS, eds. Neurosurgery. New York: McGraw-Hill, 1985:597–610)

dency for cerebral spread. Table 61–2 indicates the parenchymal metastatic patterns for the most common cancers in a large autopsy series.[5] Lung, gastrointestinal, and urinary tract primary tumors account for 80% of metastases in men, whereas breast, lung, gastrointestinal tract, and melanoma account for 80% of metastases in women.

Lung carcinoma, by virtue of its relative frequency, is the most common metastasis, accounting for 40% to 60% of all parenchymal deposits in the U.S. population.[5,6,10] Melanoma has the highest likelihood of cerebral spread, with 65% of patients developing this complication during the course of the disease. The relative metastatic attack rates for breast (51%) and lung (41%) are lower, but they contribute a greater number of patients by virtue of their greater overall prevalence.

TEMPORAL PATTERNS OF PRESENTATION

Brain metastasis may present in three distinct temporal profiles: *precocious* (occult primary), *synchronous* (simultaneous primary), and *metachronous* (antecedent primary).[7] Lung, melanoma, and renal tumors tend to have brief intervals from the time of initial diagnosis to evolution of a brain metastasis, whereas breast, colon, and sarcomas have long intervals. The majority of patients (81%) present with an antecedent (*metachronous*) primary tumor before development of cerebral spread.

Other clinical classification approaches are useful (see section on Clinical Aspects of Brain Metastases) for prognosis and as an aid in choosing the most efficacious treatment modality for a given patient.

PATHOGENESIS AND PATHOPHYSIOLOGY OF CEREBRAL METASTASES

The general concepts of tumor metastasis are germane to cerebral metastasis[11]; the brain, however, has a unique anatomic, physiologic, and immunologic organization that influences the localization, growth pattern, and spread of metastases.[12,13] Cerebral metastases are generally a "tertiary" phenomenon of metastatic spread more commonly arising after secondary metastatic sites (*e.g.*, lung, liver) have developed.[14] Brain metastases arise either from hematogenous dissemination of circulating tumor cells or, less commonly, by contiguous spread from adjacent sites (skull, basal foraminae, and soft tissues of the head and neck). Hematogenous spread occurs when tumor cells are passively disseminated into the bloodstream.[5,7,15–17] The distribution patterns for parenchymal metastases (Fig. 61–2) generally correlate with the regional brain weight and blood flow, with approximately 80% of metastases occurring in the supratentorial compartment.[3] A preferential distribution by metastases for the superficial distal arterial fields (watershed areas) was noted in an antemortem study[13] that also demonstrated a posterior fossa predilection by metastases from pelvic and gastrointestinal primary tumors. Another explanation for nonrandom or preferential involvement of the brain by certain primary tumors (*e.g.*, melanoma and small cell carcinoma of the lung) is the observation that primary tumors have metastatic cell subpopulations with "site-specific" characteristics that favor the brain as a preferential site for metastatic spread.[18–21]

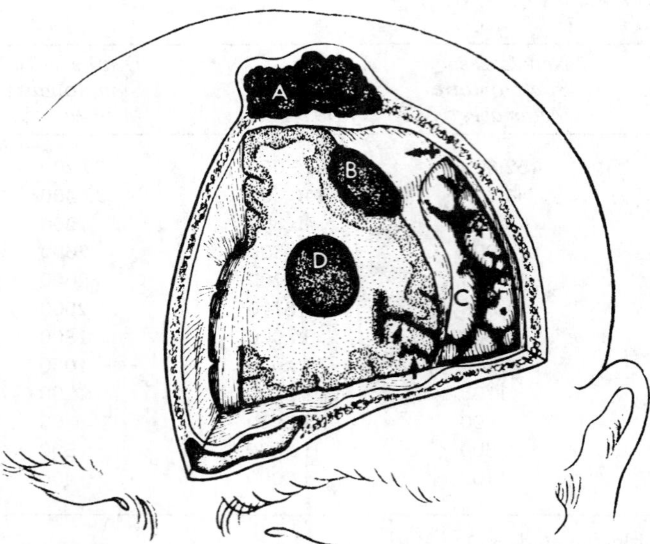

FIGURE 61–1. Anatomic classification of brain metastases. Three-quarter view of left frontal cranium, showing **(A)** a large metastasis to the skull diploë; **(B)** a dural metastasis; **(C)** superficial leptomeningeal invasion; and **(D)** a parenchymal metastasis (revealed by a coronal cut made at the posterior border of the frontal lobe). Open arrows indicate areas of leptomeningeal spread. Crossed arrow indicates the convex surface of the brain with dura intact. Solid arrows indicate leptomeningeal spread into several sulci. (Courtesy of Pat Kenny, Medical Illustration Section, National Institutes of Health, Bethesda, MD) (Wright DC. Surgical treatment of brain metastases. In: Rosenberg SA, ed. Surgical treatment of metastatic cancer. Philadelphia: JB Lippincott, 1987:165–222)

CEREBRAL PATHOPHYSIOLOGY IN METASTASIS

Clinical symptoms from brain metastases arise by impairment of the homeostatic mechanisms necessary for maintenance of normal brain function. Mechanical distortion and displacement (herniations) by a progressively increasing neoplastic mass; increases in intracranial pressure (ICP) and decreases in cerebral blood flow (CBF); propagation of vasogenic cerebral edema; and derangement of metabolic energy processes represent the major pathophysiologic changes that can occur.

Brain swelling occurs as a result of mass lesions (*e.g.*, neoplasm, hematoma), obstruction of cerebrospinal fluid (CSF) pathways (hydrocephalus), alterations in cerebrovascular regulation (*e.g.*, hyperemia, local dysregulation of vascular tone or blood flow), and propagation of cerebral edema.

Rapid changes in the intracranial volume-pressure relation by progressive neoplastic growth result in elevated intracranial pressure if the normal buffering system of the brain cannot compensate by reciprocal reductions in CSF and vascular and extracellular volumes.[22–25] Various stereotypical clinical herniation syndromes[26] arise when severe mechanical distortions occur and frequently result in permanent neurologic injury or death of the patient.

Brain edema is an increase in brain water and ions (primarily sodium)[27] arising either by direct injury to cells (cytotoxic edema) or from injury to the vascular endothelium (vasogenic edema).[27,28] Direct injury to the endothelium by compressing or invading tumor, dysplastic vascular structures present within tumors,[29] and biochemically mediated alterations of capillary permeability[30–33] contribute to the development of vasogenic edema. Water and ions passively diffuse into the brain extracellular space in areas of increased vascular permeability, primarily affecting the cerebral white matter. Edema fluid may travel along longitudinally oriented white

TABLE 61–2. Brain Metastases by Histologic Type*

Site of Primary Neoplasm	*No. of Patients*	*No. of Metastases**	*% Total†*	*Relative Frequency (%)‡*
Lung	774	266	7.9	48
Breast	526	111	3.3	20
Gastrointestinal	773	43	1.3	8
Urinary	199	34	1.0	6
Melanoma	69	34	1.0	6
Prostate	140	10	0.3	2
Liver & pancreas	293	14	0.4	3
Other	585	43	1.3	8
Total	3359	555	16.5	100

* Parenchymal metastases only.

† Expressed as $\frac{\text{number (parenchymal) metastases}}{\text{total number of cancer autopsies}}$

‡ Relative frequency $= \frac{\text{number (parenchymal) metastases by tumor type}}{\text{total number of parenchymal metastases}} \times 100$

(Modified from Takakura K, Sano K, Hoho S, et al. Metastastic tumors of the central nervous system. Tokyo: Igaku-Shoin, 1982)

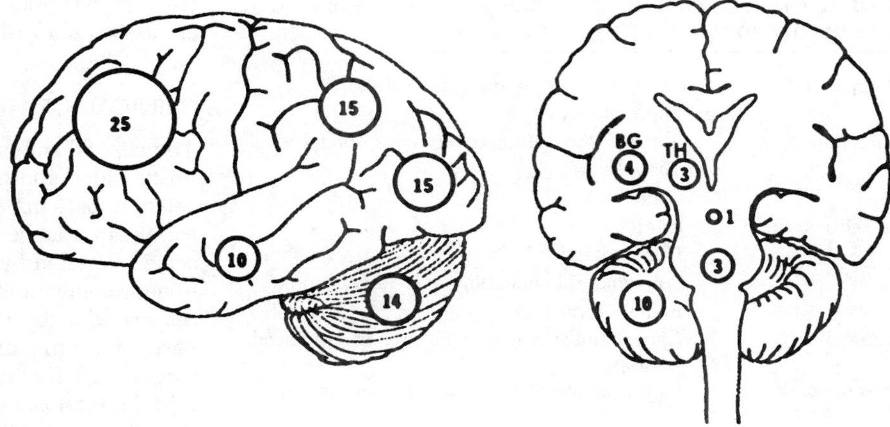

FIGURE 61–2. Parenchymal distribution of brain metastases. The distribution and relative frequency (%) are diagrammed according to metastatic site. The subcortical gray structures (BG, basal ganglia; Th, thalamus) receive 7% of metastases, and cerebellar hemispheres receive 10% of metastases. (Adapted from Takakura K, Sana K, Hoho S, et al. Metastatic tumors of the central nervous system. Tokyo: Igaku-Shoin, 1982. Reproduced from Wright DC. Surgical treatment of brain metastases. In: Rosenberg SA, ed. Surgical treatment of metastatic cancer. Philadelphia, JB Lippincott, 1987:165–222)

matter tracts at great distances (Fig. 61–3) from the focal "source" of increased capillary permeability[34] with ultimate deterioration in neurologic function.

CLINICAL ASPECTS OF BRAIN METASTASES

The definitive diagnosis of brain metastasis cannot be made solely on the basis of the clinical examination,[6] because the presenting symptoms and signs are not distinct from those of other intracranial mass lesions (Table 61–3). Various disease processes mimic brain metastases both clinically and by diagnostic studies. Benign, treatable conditions simulating a metastasis must be identified (even in the patient with an established diagnosis of cancer) to avoid inappropriate or dangerous therapy.[9,35,36] Those patients without a prior diagnosis of cancer require an unequivocal pathologic diagnosis. Complications of disease or iatrogenic injuries (infectious, cerebrovascular, toxic) are common in the cancer patient and frequently account for neurologic symptoms rather than the primary disease process and require specific evaluation and treatment.

PRESENTATION: SYMPTOMS AND SIGNS

The presenting neurologic symptoms and signs (Table 61–4) of brain metastases are headache, weakness, cognitive or affective disturbance, and seizures.[4,10,37–42] The pathogenesis of neural injury previously discussed can be aligned with presenting symptoms in a general way: focal symptoms and signs (unilateral headache, weakness, seizures) generally result from direct parenchymal injury by neoplasm, whereas diffuse symptoms and signs (generalized headache, cognitive or behavioral changes, papilledema) reflect the global effects of cerebral edema, metabolic dysfunction, or CSF obstruction.

Headaches, the most common (≥50%) presenting symptom, arise as a result of either direct injury, such as traction or distortion of pain-sensitive structures (dura, dural venous sinuses, large blood vessels, cranial nerves), or indirect mechanisms (edema, CSF obstruction). The headache is usually remitting, occurring in the morning or early hours and

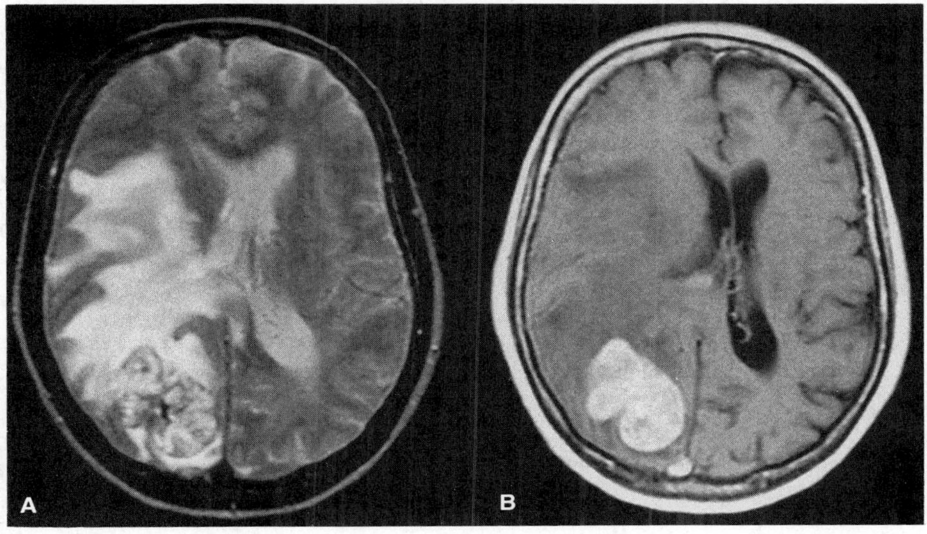

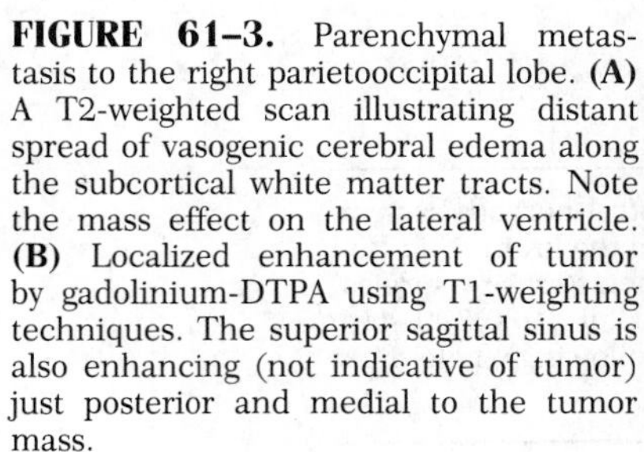

FIGURE 61–3. Parenchymal metastasis to the right parietooccipital lobe. **(A)** A T2-weighted scan illustrating distant spread of vasogenic cerebral edema along the subcortical white matter tracts. Note the mass effect on the lateral ventricle. **(B)** Localized enhancement of tumor by gadolinium-DTPA using T1-weighting techniques. The superior sagittal sinus is also enhancing (not indicative of tumor) just posterior and medial to the tumor mass.

TABLE 61–3. Differential Diagnosis of Neurologic Dysfunction in the Cancer Patient

Neoplastic*	Primary brain tumors (glial series)
	Meningioma
Infectious	Abscess—pyogenic, tuberculous, fungal
	Toxoplasma
	Other
Cerebrovascular	Infarction
	Hemorrhage
	Sub, epidural collection; acute and chronic
Toxic	Radiation necrosis
Metabolic	Encephalopathy (organ failure, drug-induced, sepsis)
Paraneoplastic syndromes	Eaton-Lambert syndrome, polyneuropathy

* Partial listing; not intended to serve as complete differential diagnostic list.
(Modified from Weiss HD. Neoplasms. In: Samuels MA, ed. Manual of neurologic therapeutics. Boston: Little, Brown, 1986)

gradually increasing in duration and frequency until associated with symptoms and signs of increased intracranial pressure (ICP). Paroxysmal headache, when present, is occasionally accompanied by fluctuating neurologic signs (*e.g.*, hemiparesis) and reflects abnormalities of intracranial pressure dynamics (plateau waves).[37] Unilateral headaches, when present, are of localizing value in the majority of patients.[10]

Weakness, the most common focal sign, is symptomatic in 40% of patients and elicitable on examination in 65%.[37] Ataxia may be present in patients with CSF obstruction and is associated with cerebellar deposits. Disturbances in mental functions (changes in behavior, memory, speech, and cognitive skills) appear in a third of patients as presenting symptoms and are demonstrated on psychological testing in 50% to 75% of patients.[37,43]

Seizures account for the most common acute onset of symptoms and, if focal, are of localizing value. Certain tumors (melanoma) and tumor patterns (leptomeningeal deposits) are associated with a high incidence of seizures.[37,44]

CLINICAL GRADING

The clinical status of patients at initial treatment is of prognostic value and has a positive correlation with outcome in selected patients subjected to surgery.[6,38,45,46] Most classification approaches employ the long-standing performance scale instituted by Karnofsky[47] supplemented by a measure of neurologic function.[1,48] The extent of disseminated disease associated with cerebral metastasis also has prognostic value, particularly in patients subjected to the physiologic stress of surgery. Such clinical grading of patients at the time of cerebral metastasis greatly facilitates risk evaluation and guides the clinician in choosing a rational approach to treatment; likewise, the comparison of various treatment modalities in matched patient groups is facilitated by this clinical classification.

SPECIALIZED NEURODIAGNOSTIC EVALUATION

In addition to standard screening diagnostic and laboratory studies routinely performed for patients with cancer, neurodiagnostic studies are increasingly employed in routine evaluation because of the high incidence of cerebral metastases in the more common cancers affecting the U.S. populations. Computed tomographic (CT) scanning, magnetic resonance imaging (MRI), and arteriography constitute the primary studies currently employed in neurodiagnostic evaluation for cerebral metastases. These imaging studies provide diagnostic information and, more important, anatomic localization of the mass lesion(s). This localization is critical to the radiation therapist for treatment planning and to the surgeon for accurate placement of scalp flaps, bone openings, and cortical incisions.[6,25]

Contrast CT scanning has, until recently, been the single most important neurodiagnostic study in patients with suspected brain metastases. Contrast (gadolinium-DTPA) MRI scanning, now widely available, is currently the most sensitive

TABLE 61–4. Symptoms and Signs of Cerebral Metastases

Symptoms	*Frequency (%)*	*Signs*	*Frequency (%)*
Headache	53	Hemiparesis	66
Weakness, focal	40	Impaired cognition	77
Mental disturbance	31	Sensory loss, unilateral	27
Seizures	15	Papilledema	26
Gait disorder	20	Ataxia	24
Visual disturbance	12	Aphasia	19
Language disturbance	10		

(Data from Takakura K, Sano K, Hoho S, et al. Metastatic tumors of the central nervous system. Tokyo: Igaku-Shoin, 1982; Posner JB. Diagnosis and treatment of metastases to the brain. Clin Bull 1974;4:47–57; Gamache FW Jr, Posner JB, Galicich JH. Treatment of brain metastases by surgical extirpation. In: Weiss L, Gilbert H, Posner J, eds. Brain metastases. Boston: GK Hall, 1980:390–414; Order SE, Hellman S, Von Essen CF, et al. Improvement in quality of survival following whole-brain irradiation for whole-brain metastasis. Radiology 1968;91:149–153)

study for detection of metastases,[49] although CT scanning is still preferred by many radiation therapists and surgeons because of the superior diagnostic specificity and depiction of bone (localization) detail. Parenchymal metastases are typically spheroidal, with peritumoral edema formation, and located in the gray matter-white matter junction (see Fig. 61–3).[13] Enhancement (both CT and MRI) occurs because of permeability changes in the "blood-brain" and "blood-tumor" vascular endothelium[50,51] and because of the increased vascular volumes (neovascularity) characteristically found in metastatic tumors, which prolong the transit times for water-soluble conjugates (meglumine–iodine and gadolinium-DTPA) used clinically as contrast agents. The value of CT or MRI scanning extends beyond the initial evaluation; serial scanning is a very effective means to monitor tumor development, progression, response to therapy, and detection of secondary complications.

Arteriography provides neoplastic and normal vascular detail, such as the origin of arterial supply, routes of venous drainage, and degree of neovascularity. Because of the wide availability of CT and MRI scanners, arteriography is generally reserved for the patient in whom tumor vascular characteristics play an important role in surgical planning.

Emphasis should be made regarding caution in the performance of lumbar puncture in the setting of cerebral metastasis. This procedure is hazardous in any patient with increased intracranial pressure, particularly where focal masses produce regional transients of increased tissue pressure, a common situation in brain metastasis. Lumbar puncture has diagnostic value in situations where infectious or neoplastic involvement of the CSF space is suspected. These represent the only entities where a *specific* diagnosis can be inferred from examination of the cerebrospinal fluid. Neurologic consultation and CT scanning should be performed in a patient with known or suspected cancer before performance of a lumbar puncture.

Specialized neurodiagnostic studies have dramatically altered the immediate hazards of therapy by minimizing the morbidity of neoplastic and treatment-related complications. This ability has vastly improved selection of the most appropriate therapy by localizing lesions to the specific anatomic compartment(s) involved, and it has allowed identification of metastatic complications (hemorrhage, hydrocephalus, edema, infection) arising from treatment (surgical complications, radiation necrosis).

PRINCIPLES OF MANAGEMENT

THERAPEUTIC GOALS

Secondary spread of a generalized cancer to the brain places the patient in a precarious situation demanding urgent treatment to prevent or minimize progressive neurologic injury. Neurologic dysfunction arising from cerebral metastases, particularly of cognitive and motor systems, has a disproportionate impact on the functional performance of the patient when compared with the disability arising from systemic metastases elsewhere. The principal therapeutic goals for patients with brain metastasis are to maximize and maintain the highest neurologic function attainable; the quality of survival for most patients is dramatically improved if control of intracranial metastases is achieved.

The principal treatment regimens applied specifically toward cerebral metastasis are radiation therapy alone or surgery combined with adjunctive postoperative radiation therapy. The therapeutic approach varies for a given patient with cerebral metastases depending on the tumor type and clinical setting. All patients should receive general supportive care, steroids, and radiation therapy; selected patients should undergo surgical resection followed by radiation therapy. Surgery may be employed as primary treatment for attempted total resection of a single metastasis or as a secondary procedure for diagnostic biopsy. Adjunctive chemotherapy is indicated in selected patients and specific tumor types. Seizure prophylaxis is indicated for patients who present with seizures[52] and those patients subjected to surgery.

PHARMACOLOGIC THERAPY OF ELEVATED INTRACRANIAL PRESSURE

Effective treatment of the various causes of elevated intracranial pressure (ICP) associated with cerebral metastases contributes to the emergent palliation of neurologic dysfunction and reduces the morbidity associated with definitive treatment (surgery or radiation therapy). Specifically, the means to control vasogenic cerebral edema guided the progressive advances in therapy since the introduction of glucocorticoids and other agents in this role.[53–55] Steroids (dexamethasone, methylprednisolone, prednisone) exert rapid clinical responses (6–24 hours)[56,57] benefiting 60% to 80% of patients in resolving or reducing clinical symptoms.[9,53,58] Steroids are used empirically because their optimal dose is unknown and their mechanism of action only partially understood.[25] Typically, starting doses (Table 61–5) for dexamethasone (or equivalent doses of other steroids) of 16–24 mg/day are used[59] (with or without a bolus loading dose), and higher doses (100 mg/day) are sometimes effective in patients without benefit at lower doses.[58] Steroids are used for both acute and chronic relief of generalized symptoms of increased ICP (headache, papilledema, confusion), but benefit is usually transient if no additional therapy is employed.

Osmotherapy, commonly used in the emergent control of ICP, reduces brain extracellular water and total body water. ICP is lowered by a reduction of brain extracellular volume, which also promotes movement of edema fluid out of the brain.[60] Diuretics (*e.g.*, furosemide, acetazolamide) and hyperosmolar solutions (mannitol, urea) are used acutely to lower ICP by reducing brain extracellular volume in areas with intact blood–brain barrier. Mannitol also has direct rheologic effects that increase local cerebral blood flow. Clinical dosages (see Table 61–5) for mannitol are 1.0 to 1.5 g/kg intravenous bolus, or intermittent intravenous administration to maintain serum osmolality between 295 and 320 mOsm. Furosemide is given in intermittent intravenous doses of 10 to 20 mg (40–80 mg/day) to achieve a brisk diuresis.

NEUROLOGIC EMERGENCIES IN CEREBRAL METASTASES

Patients with cerebral metastases may develop neurologic deficits acutely (seizure, cerebral hemorrhage, CSF outflow ob-

TABLE 61–5. Common Pharmacologic Measures in Cerebral Metastases

Drug	*Use or Indications*	*Mode of Administration*	*Dose**	*Therapeutic Range Comments*
Dexamethasone	Vasogenic cerebral edema	I.V. or PO	16–24 mg	Empiric
Prednisolone	Vasogenic cerebral edema	I.V. or PO	105–160 mg	Empiric
Mannitol	Cerebral edema mass effect	I.V	1.0–1.5 g/kg	Maintain serum osmolality > 295 < 320
Furosemide	Cerebral edema mass effect	I.V. or PO	40–80 mg/d	Empiric; maintain osmolality > 295 < 320
Acetazolamide	Cerebral edema mass effect	I.V. or PO	500–1000 mg/d	Empiric; maintain osmolality > 295 < 320
Phenytoin	Anticonvulsant	I.V. or PO	200–400 mg/d (5 mg/kg/d)	5–20 μg/ml; loading dose is 15 mg/kg
Carbamazepine	Anticonvulsant	PO	600–800 mg/d (7–15 mg/kg/d)	3–12 μg/ml

(Samuels MA, ed. Manual of neurologic therapeutics. Boston: Little, Brown, 1986:1–424)

struction)[61,62] or manifest a deteriorating neurologic syndrome (cerebral edema, rapidly expanding neoplasm, communicating hydrocephalus). The former situation generally arises in patients with unsuspected or occult cerebral lesions, whereas the latter is a common feature of patients with relapsing tumors in whom initial therapeutic measures are ineffective. In either setting, rapid diagnostic evaluation and initiation of therapy is paramount. Examination of the patient (general and neurologic systems), diagnostic imaging (CT or MRI), and other specialized diagnostic studies (*e.g.*, electroencephalogram [EEG]) are required to identify the etiology of the deterioration. Focal neurologic symptoms and signs generally arise from intracranial pressure shifts that result in various herniation syndromes. Global, nonspecific alterations in neurologic function (headache, nausea and vomiting, impaired mental status, cognitive dysfunction, and so forth) usually result from a generalized increase in intracranial pressure or an encephalopathic process (metabolic disturbances of electrolytes, hepatic/renal dysfunction, CNS infection). Treatment is directed toward correction of the underlying cause and may require medical care, surgical intervention, or both.

Immediate, nonspecific measures[61] may be necessary to stabilize neurologic function in a patient before clinical evaluation until a specific diagnosis and appropriate therapy can be formulated. Such maneuvers include hyperventilation (decreases pCO_2), osmotherapy, steroids, and seizure control (see Table 61–5), if indicated. Occasionally, neurologic resuscitation for severely ill or rapidly deteriorating patients requires airway protection (intubation) and ventilatory support. Neurosurgical intervention may be required for neurologic monitoring (ventricular catheter for drainage; placement of ICP monitoring devices) or, more common, to correct underlying treatable causes of increased ICP (tumoral hemorrhage, ventricular obstruction, and so forth). Rational therapy requires a specific diagnosis as well as knowledge of the extent of systemic disease processes. Surgical indications and the results of emergent surgery are discussed in the following sections.

RADIATION THERAPY APPROACHES IN CEREBRAL METASTASES

Radiation is employed in nearly all patients with cerebral metastases, either as primary therapy or as an adjunct to surgical excision of a neoplastic mass. Numerous studies[42,63–68] have established the efficacy of radiation therapy and have identified specific factors influencing the radiation response for a given histologic tumor type and patient profile.[69]

Randomized prospective clinical trials[70] have investigated the optimal time-dose schedules for patients with cerebral metastases stratified according to histology of the primary site and the presence or absence of metastases to sites other than the brain. While no differences were seen in the randomized groups with respect to response or median survival, the shorter time-dose fractionation schemes had equal efficacy and less expense over longer treatment schedules. A program of 30 Gy/2 weeks (1 Gy = 100 rads) to the entire cranial cavity is generally well tolerated and can be followed by a boost of 9 Gy in three additional fractions to areas of gross disease as defined by diagnostic images.

These initial studies suggested significantly longer survivals in both ambulatory and nonambulatory patients when the brain was the only site of metastases or when the primary lesion was controlled, and they prompted an additional trial to investigate higher radiation doses. Patients with brain metastases and no evidence of other sites of disseminated disease were randomized to receive 50 Gy/4 weeks or 30 Gy/2 weeks. This study group was predominated by patients with aggressive cancers (80% had lung cancer) and demonstrated no statistically significant advantage of one treatment over the other for symptom relief, median survival, or prevention of death by brain metastases.[71]

Very rapid fractionation programs (*e.g.*, 10 Gy in one fraction) have also been tested for palliation of brain metastases. Response rates, promptness of neurologic improvement, treatment morbidity, and median survival were comparable to those of patients receiving higher doses in multiple fractions. However, the duration of improvement, time to deterioration of neurologic status, and rate of complete disappearance of neurologic symptoms were generally less for those patients who received 10 or 12 Gy, suggesting that ultra-rapid, high-dose irradiation schedules might not be as effective as conventionally fractionated higher dose schedules in the palliation of brain metastases.[70,72] A high complication rate has been associated with this strategy, especially in moribund patients with evidence of increased intracranial pressure, who should be considered unsuitable for rapid, high-dose schedules.[65,73]

Specialized Radiation Approaches to Brain Metastases

Because 30% to 50% of patients treated with conventional external radiation therapy for brain metastases will develop progressive intracranial disease, there has been considerable interest in combination therapy (surgery plus radiation therapy) and innovative radiation approaches. Normal tissue (brain) irradiation tolerance limits the dose (55–70 Gy) that can be safely delivered with conventional external radiation techniques. *Focal* radiation delivered either by tightly collimated, multiple trajectory ports (stereotactic radiosurgery) or by image-directed brachytherapy (interstitial radiation) increases the tumor dose without exceeding normal tissue tolerance. Brachytherapy allows local application of continuous radiation exposure during the treatment interval (typically between 7 and 60 days), which is analogous to delivering the radiation dose in a large number of very small fractions. Radiation sources are surgically implanted within the tumor borders and configured to deliver doses (80–150 Gy) higher than those possible with conventional external radiation techniques.[74] The physical characteristic of the isotope used determines such factors as the dose rate and distance the emitted radiation travels in tissue, permitting relative control over the dose distribution. This strategy aims to achieve a high-dose "local boost" to the tumor, creating a focal area of radiation necrosis within the borders of the neoplasm while minimizing radiation exposure to normal tissues. Response is determined by such factors as tumor size and geometry, ability to accurately image the tumor-brain interface, and tumor radiosensitivity.

This approach has been used for reirradiation in a small number of patients with recurrent metastases[74–76] or to deliver "boost" treatment in addition to external cranial irradiation in selected patients with brain metastases at presentation.[75] Some patients with recurrent disease have been noted to remain free of progressive intracranial tumor for over a year and up to 4 years after brachytherapy.[75,76] Neurologic function is generally preserved, but there is a risk of focal radiation necrosis when implants are used in this setting.

Recently, stereotactic external irradiation ("stereotactic radiosurgery," Gamma knife, linear accelerator [LINAC], and so forth) has been used to treat patients with brain metastases.[77–79] This technique uses single high doses of irradiation from a specially designed cobalt source or from a modified linear accelerator. Multiple, nonplanar, narrow beams are stereotactically directed to the site of metastatic disease by use of sophisticated radiation dosimetry techniques. Because the whole-brain dose of irradiation increases rapidly with increases in the target volume, the technique is limited to small, circumscribed lesions, generally $\leq$3.5 cm in diameter. A recent analysis indicated that radiosurgery of intracranial tumors is associated with a low risk of complications for lesions $<$10 ml treated with a single isocenter to maximum tumor doses $<$25 Gy with a tumor dose inhomogeneity $<$10 Gy.[80] Clinical experience with this technique, although limited, demonstrated that the majority of patients improved neurologically and could be withdrawn from corticosteroid therapy. Patients with adenocarcinomas demonstrated radiographic regression of treated lesions. The procedure was well tolerated, and no patients developed symptomatic radiation necrosis.

While these reports hold promise, the technical demands of such approaches will probably limit application to selected patients with a single recurrent or unresectable, isolated brain metastasis ($<$3.5 cm in size and not involving the corpus callosum) in the setting of controlled systemic disease.

CHEMOTHERAPY FOR CEREBRAL METASTASES

The role of chemotherapy in the treatment of brain metastases has not been clearly defined. In the past, the assumption that the blood–brain barrier prevents the passage of most chemotherapeutic agents into cerebral tumors discouraged clinical investigation. Recently, clinical studies have demonstrated tumor regressions with intravenous administration of conventional chemotherapeutic agents. The extent to which tumor regression influences overall control of brain metastases remains uncertain.

Microcirculation and Drug Delivery

The microcirculation of cerebral metastases differs substantially from that of the normal blood–brain barrier. Capillaries within brain metastases contain membrane fenestrations, gap junctions, and open endothelial junctions.[81] The clinical correlation of the ultrastructural anatomy is illustrated by the passage of CT and MRI scan contrast media into cerebral metastases and by laboratory studies that have demonstrated the presence of chemotherapeutic agents within resected and autopsy specimens of patients with metastatic and primary brain tumors. Clinical drug uptake studies in patients with primary and metastatic tumors[82] show variable biodistribution of drug (*e.g.*, cisplatin) to tumor and cerebrospinal fluid. Significant regional variation of drug concentration within tumor was also demonstrated, suggesting a variable degree of disruption of the normal cerebral vasculature. Other preliminary studies suggest that various chemotherapeutic agents (etoposide,[83] teniposide,[84] pentamethylmelamine,[85] 3-deazauridine,[86] AZQ,[87] MGBG,[88] vinblastine,[89] PALA,[90] ANCU,[91] and TCNU[92]) can reach sufficient concentrations in tumor tissue to be cytotoxic.

Tumor Response: Inherent and Acquired Chemoresistance

Apart from issues of drug delivery, there are two other factors that may prevent successful treatment of brain metastases with chemotherapy. First, the histologic types of primary malignancies that most frequently metastasize to brain are themselves chemoresistant. Almost half of all cases of brain metastases result from lung primaries, and the non-small cell histologic forms will predominate. Because only 20% to 40% of primary non-small cell lung cancer patients respond to current chemotherapy regimens,[93] the likelihood of response in the brain is also low. Although breast carcinoma, the second most common source of brain metastases, is relatively responsive to chemotherapy, 25% to 50% of patients will not respond.[94] The third, fourth, and fifth most common sources of brain metastases are gastrointestinal carcinomas, urinary (particularly renal) malignancies, and melanoma. Colorectal carcinoma, by far the most common gastrointestinal cancer, responds to current regimens in approximately 20% to 40% of cases.[95] Both renal cell carcinoma and melanoma are notably chemoresistant, usually responding to chemotherapy or immunotherapy in less than 20% of patients.[96–98] Given the limited success of chemotherapy for the primary malignancies that most commonly spread to the brain, one would expect limited success in treating brain metastases with chemotherapy.

Second, most patients (81%) develop brain metastases after diagnosis and treatment of the primary tumor.[46] Metastases that appear despite prior drug therapy are likely to be more resistant to subsequent chemotherapy. Relapse in the brain is most commonly part of widespread drug-resistant systemic relapse rather than an isolated phenomenon. The majority of patients with brain metastases die of systemic manifestations of disease rather than the brain metastases.[63]

SURGICAL MANAGEMENT OF CEREBRAL METASTASES

Perioperative Care

The most important prognostic factor influencing the results for patients subjected to surgery is the preoperative state.[6,38,45,46,48,99] Morbidity, 30-day mortality, and the postoperative neurologic functional level are directly related to the preoperative classification of patients[6]; maximal benefit is achieved for surgically treated patients when preoperative steps to optimize the general condition and neurologic performance are taken. Careful preoperative assessment of cardiopulmonary function and other potential medical problems (coagulopathy, abnormalities of electrolytes and water balance, malnutrition, infectious hazards) and management of vasogenic cerebral edema are necessary preludes to successful surgery. Measures to resist brain swelling in the perioperative period are begun before surgery (24–48 hours) and reduce the morbidity substantially (see Table 61–5). Stabilizing decompensated patients medically has superior results compared with emergent surgical decompression in unstable, postherniated, or moribund patients.[38,100]

Surgical Indications, Goals, Benefits

Surgery, when appropriate, is generally employed to achieve an accurate diagnosis based on pathologic examination of tissue, to remove or reduce a mass lesion, or to relieve CSF obstruction (Table 61–6). The indications for surgery are related to the therapeutic goals and are dependent on the clinical setting. Gross total removal of a metastasis is achieved in 80% or more of selected patients,[5,6,45] with this as a preoperative goal, and has superior benefit over subtotal removal or biopsy.[48,99,101–103]

TABLE 61–6. Selection Criteria for Surgical Therapy of Brain Metastases*

Diagnostic uncertainty
Solitary metastasis
Life-threatening or critically located multiple metastases
Recurrent or persistent symptoms after nonsurgical therapy
Clinically resistant tumors
Treatment of metastatic complications—hemorrhagic, infectious, CSF obstruction
Placement of delivery devices for intrathecal access (Ommaya reservoir)

* Criteria are suggested guidelines rather than absolute indications; see text.

Technical Aspects: Application of Microsurgical Technique

Consistent application of advanced surgical technique and use of available technical aids are not always routinely considered. Most metastases are sizable "macroscopic" lesions (≥3 cm) and have historically been resected without sophisticated techniques. Preservation of the normal brain and microcirculation adjacent to metastasis is routinely possible and should be the technical goal in all surgical patients.[25] Precise preoperative and intraoperative localization (CT, MRI, stereotaxis, ultrasound) allows accurately placed scalp, bone, and cortical incisions, and use of standard microsurgical techniques to preserve local microcirculation (*e.g.,* longitudinal rather than transverse gyral incisions)[6,25,104] minimizes morbidity from the surgical procedure. Gross total removal in selected patients with such techniques has superseded the era when regional surgical procedures with sacrifice of normal tissue (wide tumor margins, lobectomy) were required to control postoperative edema. Surgical biopsy for diagnosis (*e.g.,* precocious presentation) and clinical staging has achieved impressive levels of safety and diagnostic accuracy since the introduction of various image-guided stereotactic systems.[25]

CEREBRAL METASTASES: RESULTS OF THERAPY

Modern-era expectations for patients with cerebral metastatic disease have gradually translated into modest benefit for the majority of patients and guarded optimism for selected patients with favorable prognostic factors. Treatment modalities (surgery, radiation therapy) have changed only marginally, but advances in perioperative care, application of microsurgical technique, and highly accurate diagnostic imaging devices have had a significant impact on management. Relatively few definitive conclusions can be drawn as to the effectiveness of a particular treatment approach for cerebral metastases, despite the existing literature since 1960. With several notable exceptions,[36] these studies lack comparable matched treatment groups and differ in defining such variables as clinical–anatomic classification, response to therapy, quality of survival, relapse rates, morbidity, mortality, and cause of death (neurologic versus systemic disease). Despite these difficulties, several generalizations can be drawn from these clinical reports (Tables 61–7 and 61–8). The natural history of untreated cerebral metastases is one of progressive neurologic deterioration, with a median survival of 1 to 2 months.[5,41,63,105] Steroids sustain neurologic performance and extend median survival to 2.5 months,[106] and the use of radiation therapy further increases median survival to 3 to 6 months. Selected patients treated with surgery, radiation therapy, and steroids[36,38] have a median survival exceeding 6 months.

RADIATION THERAPY

Although the majority of patients (80%) treated with radiation therapy have an initial response, a surprisingly modest gain in survival ensues when they are compared with untreated and steroid groups. Morbidity and mortality (5%) during the course of radiation further reduce benefit, because 10% to 20% of patients fail to complete the prescribed course of therapy.[36,70,107] A strict interpretation of these reports (see Table 61–8) can be misleading, because this group tends to have unselected patients with poor prognostic factors and high mortality from uncontrolled systemic disease. Improvement in functional neurologic performance was noted in 50% to 60% of patients treated with whole-brain irradiation, and, not surprisingly, those patients with mild deficits had the greatest benefit. Sustained neurologic performance was relatively brief in those responders surviving to 6 months after therapy, illustrating a failure to control intracranial disease in a substantial proportion of patients treated.[70]

A favorable subgroup of patients irradiated for brain metastases has been identified by the Radiation Therapy Oncology Group (RTOG).[69] The favorable prognostic factors include: Karnofsky performance status of 70 to 100, an absent/controlled primary tumor, age <60 years, and metastatic spread limited to the brain. Patients with all four favorable factors had a 52% predicted probability of 6-month survival from the start of treatment. Patients with three of the four characteristics had a 33% to 40% probability of 6-month survival, and patients with none of the four had only an 8% chance of surviving 6 months. Fifty-three percent of patients were in a poor prognostic group with a median survival of 3.1 months. Radiation alone in this setting fails to permanently control intracranial disease in a substantial proportion of treated patients.

Two trials of radiation sensitizers have failed to demonstrate either improved local control or improved survival in patients with brain metastases undergoing cranial irradiation. The RTOG studied misonidazole and found no improvement over radiation therapy alone.[108] Lonidamine, an indazole carboxylic acid shown to be synergistic with radiotherapy in tissue culture and animal models, failed to improve response rate or survival.[109]

Because of the high frequency of uncontrolled tumor in the brain (50–70%), the issue of retreatment with irradiation will arise in many patients with brain metastases. The use of stereotactic radiosurgery in this role has been discussed above. Several reports[42,64,110,111] describe neurologic improvement in

TABLE 61–7. Treatment for Selected Combined Therapy* Series of Brain Metastases

Investigations	*Collection Interval*	*Cases*	*Mortality (%)*†	*Survival*	
				Median‡	*1-Year (%)*
Stortebecker, 1954[39]	1922–1951	125	25	3.6	21
Richards and McKissock, 1963[103]	1946–1960	108	32	5.0	17
Lang and Slater, 1964[41]	1933–1963	208	22	4.0	20
Vieth and Odom, 1965[116]	1938–1962	155	15	6.0	13
Raskind et al, 1971[149]	1959–1968	51	12	6.0	30
Haar and Paterson, 1972[102]	1933–1968	167	11	6.0	22
Ransohoff, 1975[120]	1970–1973	100	10	6.0	28
Winston et al, 1980[45]	1967–1977	79	10	6.0	22
Gamache et al, 1980[46]	1968–1977	94	8.5	6.0	25
Galicich, 1981[104]	1977–1980	75	9	9.0	45
Takakura et al, 1982[5]	1960–1981	259	14§	9.1	26
Smalley et al, 1987[140]	1972–1982	85	—	13.5‖	59‖

* The majority of patients in combined therapy series were treated with surgery and postoperative radiation therapy.
† Reported as 30-day mortality, except Stortebeck (20 days), Vieth (14 days), and Raskind (14 days).
‡ Median survival is given in months.
§ All mortality occurred before 1976 (prior use of CT scanning for patient selection).
‖ Overall results: results of surgery plus adjuvant radiation therapy (34 patients) were superior to those of surgery alone (51 patients), 21 months versus 11.5 months median survival.

TABLE 61–8. Treatment for Selected Radiation Therapy Series* of Brain Metastases

Investigations	*Collection Interval*	*Cases*	*Mortality (%)*	*Survival*		
				Median (mo)	*Mean (mo)*	*1-Year (%)*
Order et al, 1968[107]	1958–1966	108	—	3–6.0	6.3	9
Deeley and Edwards, 1968[147]	Not given	88	—	<6.0	—	14
Hindo et al, 1970[65]	Not given	54	—		5.6	9
Nisce et al, 1971[42]	Not given	560	—	6.0	—	16
Montana et al, 1972[121]	1966–1971	47	—	3.0	—	10
Young et al, 1974[73]	1967–1972	162	4.3	3.0	3.4	
Deutsch et al, 1974[66]	1962–1971	88	36†	3–6.0	—	10
Berry et al, 1974[67]	1964–1973	124	—	4	—	9
Hendrickson, 1977[68]	1971–1976	1001	—	5.8	—	15
Cairncross et al, 1980[63]	1977–1978	183	4.0	4.0	—	8
Kurtz et al, 1981[71]	1976–1979	309	4.0	4.5	—	—

* Majority of patients treated by radiation therapy only, except Order (26), Deeley (7), Nisce (376), Young (89), Deutsch (17), and Berry (29), where parentheses indicate total cases subjected to surgery before radiation.
† Includes patients unable to complete therapy.

patients retreated by external-beam irradiation, with an average remission of 4 months. Others are less sanguine about the prospects of retreatment,[72] citing a risk of radiation necrosis and only transient benefit, with a median survival after retreatment of only 8 weeks.[112] Selection of patients probably accounts for the difference in reported results of reirradiation. Cooper and colleagues selected patients for reirradiation who had remained in good general condition for at least 4 months after their initial course of radiation therapy and had then experienced neurologic deterioration from recurrent brain metastases.[113] Forty-two percent of treated patients experienced improvement in neurologic function, and the survival after retreatment averaged 5 months. The benefits of reirradiation appear modest, but it may be appropriate for selected patients who remain in good general condition for some months after initial irradiation and who have limited extracranial disease.

SURGERY

Surgery for cerebral metastases was generally regarded as a futile endeavor in the era before modern-day diagnostic and perioperative management methods.[114,115] As morbidity and mortality declined for neurosurgical procedures, it became evident that meaningful benefit and prolongation of survival were possible for selected patients.[10,39,41,103,116–119]

Over the last 30 years, clinical investigators have established the efficacy of various treatment approaches and clarified the role of surgery for this group of patients. The principal surgical gains during this period have been dramatic reductions in operative morbidity and mortality, largely by improved selection of patients and advances in tumor localization, neuroanesthesia, surgical technique, and perioperative care. The overall 30-day mortality associated with surgery for cerebral metastasis has fallen tenfold during this period from approximately 30%[103] to 3%,[5,6,36,46] with similar progress in associated morbidity.

A small, uncontrolled group of patients subjected to surgery alone for metastases, as well as surgery combined with radiation therapy, gradually led clinical investigators to a general recognition that surgical therapy, when indicated, had a modest advantage over irradiation alone, particularly with respect to long-term survival.[5,9,38,46,100,107,120–122]

CHEMOTHERAPY TRIALS IN CEREBRAL METASTASES: PRELIMINARY RESULTS

Despite obstacles to successful treatment of brain metastases with chemotherapy, there are several reports of favorable results.[123–130] As one might expect, combination regimens effective for diffuse systemic metastases yield the greatest benefit for patients harboring chemosensitive tumors or malignancies with brain metastases present at the time of diagnosis of the primary disease. Small cell carcinomas of the lung are particularly responsive to combination chemotherapy,[123–125] with response rates of 64% to 78% in patients with metastatic disease to the brain and extracerebral sites. These reported response rates in the brain and periphery are quite similar to the expected response rates for first-line and salvage-treatment regimens for small cell lung carcinoma in general.[131] Notable successes have also been achieved in germ cell tumors[126] and gestational choriocarcinoma.[127]

Each of the studies involving very chemosensitive malignancies, such as small cell lung carcinoma, germ cell tumors, and gestational choriocarcinoma, reported favorable outcome when the patients were treated at presentation with agents known to be effective against the primary tumor. Salvage chemotherapy, on the other hand, was much less effective. Studies reporting results of chemotherapy for less chemosensitive tumors follow a similar pattern.

Breast carcinoma is considered to be relatively chemosensitive, with approximately 50% to 75% of patients with metastatic breast carcinoma expected to respond to first-line combination chemotherapy regimens. Rosner and colleagues reported the results of treating 100 breast cancer patients with brain metastases who had received no prior chemotherapy.[128] Although the results have not been confirmed by other investigators, there were 10 complete and 40 partial responders (N = 100), the best responses (52%) occurring in the group treated with cyclophosphamide, fluorouracil, and prednisone (CFP). All but 6 of the 100 patients treated with first-line chemotherapy received prednisone as part of the regimen, and the degree to which corticosteroid use affected interpretation of response is unknown. Recently, Cocconi and colleagues reported an overall response rate of 55% (5 complete and 7 partial responses) in 22 consecutive patients with brain metastases from breast carcinoma treated with etoposide and cisplatin.[129] Responses in the brain paralleled responses of systemic metastases, and all responses occurred while patients remained on stable or decreased corticosteroid doses.

Results of chemotherapy for brain metastases in less chemosensitive tumors are difficult to assess. Most reports include a few cases of various histologic types of malignancies treated with a single type of chemotherapy in previously treated patients.[130,132–139] The majority of patients had non-small cell lung or breast carcinomas, and responses were infrequent in those malignancies known to be chemoresistant. Jacquillat and colleagues, in a large phase II trial of fotemustine (an investigational nitrosourea) for patients with disseminated melanoma and no prior therapy, demonstrated parallel response rates in brain compared with other organs (cerebral metastatic response, 25%; visceral metastatic response, 19.2%).[130]

Based on the limited information currently available in the literature, chemotherapy can effect regression of brain metastases if regimens known to be effective in the treatment of chemosensitive malignancies are used before the development of widespread drug-resistant disease. Significant neurologic deterioration during chemotherapy and before radiotherapy has not been reported under these circumstances. Studies comparing cranial irradiation with chemotherapy alone or chemotherapy followed by radiation therapy have not been performed. It would appear that such studies could be performed safely in chemosensitive tumors. The contribution of chemotherapy toward reducing morbidity and prolonging survival in patients with brain metastases remains to be defined.

COMBINED THERAPY

The decline of morbidity associated with surgery and the relatively high rate of uncontrolled cerebral deposits after radiation therapy alone form the basis for a combined treatment approach in suitable patients. Retrospective studies[45,99,101,140,141] have strongly supported a combined approach, and a recent randomized study[36] lends further support.

As alluded to previously, comparison of nonrandomized studies lacking comparable treatment groups has long been recognized[9,38,63] to be of limited value; fortunately, preliminary results of controlled trials[36,142–144] are becoming available to supplement the existing literature regarding the respective roles of surgery, radiation therapy, and chemotherapy. Careful evaluation of selected clinical studies (see Tables 61–7 and 61–8) and newly available randomized trials provides some reliable conclusions regarding the expected results of therapy for brain metastases.

The Patchell study consisted of patients with a single metastasis randomly assigned to a surgical group (treated by surgical removal and postoperative radiation therapy) and a radiation group (treated with diagnostic biopsy and radiation therapy).[36] The study group included 48 adult patients with Karnofsky performance status ≥70 and excluded patients with tumors that were highly radiosensitive (small cell lung cancer, germ cell tumors, lymphoma, myeloma). All patients on study were biopsied before randomization. Six patients (11% of total) with solitary brain lesions and a prior cancer diagnosis were in fact noted on biopsy *not* to have a metastatic lesion (and were excluded from the study). The six nonmetastatic lesions included two glioblastomas, one low-grade astrocytoma, two abscesses, and one nonspecific inflammatory reaction, emphasizing the importance of biopsy in this setting.

Survival was longer in the surgery group (median, 40 weeks) compared with the radiation group (median, 15 weeks), and recurrence at the site of the original metastasis was less frequent (Fig. 61–4) in the surgery group (20%) compared with the radiation group (52%). Patients treated with surgery remained functionally independent longer (median, 38 weeks) compared with the radiation group (median, 8 weeks). Only surgical treatment and the absence of other systemic metastases were associated with a decreased risk of recurrence of the original brain metastasis. Fifty percent of radiation patients died from neurologic causes, compared with 29% of surgery patients, although this was not significant. Operative mortality was 4% and morbidity 8%, which was similar to the 30-day mortality and morbidity rates of 4% and 17% in the radiation group. Multivariate analysis showed that surgical treatment was associated with longer survival in patients with a long interval between the primary diagnosis and the development of the brain metastasis. The presence of disseminated cancer and older age were associated with declining survival. Nevertheless, survival was still less than 10% in both the surgery and radiation groups by 90 weeks after treatment, underlining the guarded prognosis in these patients, even with aggressive treatment.

Several retrospective studies have examined the role of postoperative radiation after surgical resection of solitary brain metastatic lesions. All but one demonstrate improved control of intracranial disease with the combination of surgery and radiation therapy compared with surgery alone. In the one negative study, Dosoretz and colleagues found no significant difference in survival or local recurrence rate in the brain when comparing patients receiving adjuvant whole-brain irradiation with those patients who were observed (no radiation) after complete resection of tumor.[145] A larger retrospective review (85 patients, 1972–1982) of a similar patient group rendered clinically disease-free by the resection of a solitary cerebral metastasis demonstrated a significant reduction of brain relapse in the 34 patients who received adjuvant whole-brain radiotherapy compared with the surgery-only group (21% versus 85%, respectively).[140] The median survival in the group receiving adjuvant radiotherapy (21 months) exceeded that of the surgery-only group (11.5 months). Those patients who received adjuvant radiation doses ≥39 Gy had an 11% rate of subsequent brain failure, as contrasted with a 31% relapse rate seen in patients receiving <39 Gy, suggesting that higher doses may be appropriate for these prognostically favored patients with solitary brain metastases and no other clinical evidence of systemic disease.

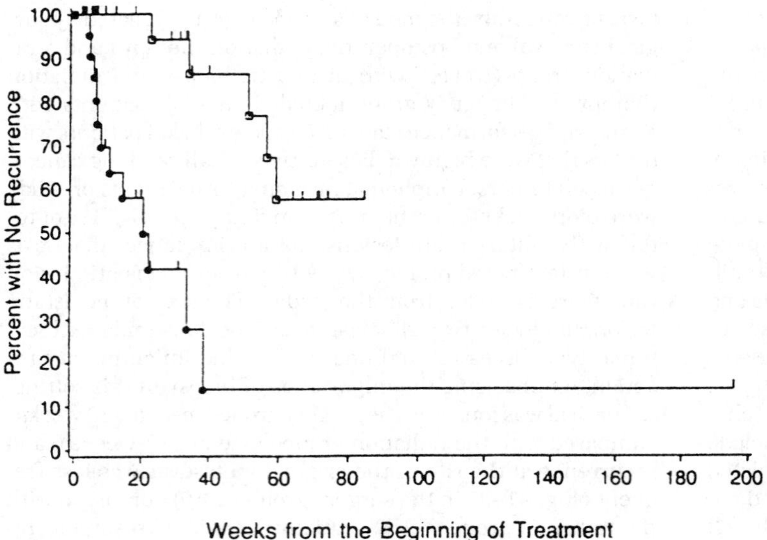

FIGURE 61–4. Length of time to local recurrence by treatment group. Open circles represent patients treated with surgery and postoperative radiation. Solid circles represent patients treated with diagnostic biopsy and radiation alone. Median time to recurrence was longer than 59 weeks (surgery) versus 21 weeks (radiation). Recurrence was defined as the reappearance of a metastasis at the same site as the initial cerebral deposit. (Patchell RA, Tibbs PA, Walsh JW, et al. A randomized trial of surgery in the treatment of single metastases to the brain. N Engl J Med 1990;322:494–500)

DeAngelis and associates found that postoperative whole-brain irradiation after resection of a solitary brain metastasis significantly prolonged the time to neurologic relapse, with a 1-year recurrence rate of 22% in the irradiated group and 46% in the surgery-alone patients.[109] Radiation appeared to decrease the likelihood of recurrence at the site of the resected metastasis but did not seem to affect the relapse rate elsewhere in the brain. The median survival in the irradiated group was 20.6 months compared with 14.4 months in the surgery-alone group, but this was not statistically significant. Eleven percent of the irradiated patients developed severe radiation-induced neurologic toxicity, with dementia, ataxia, and urinary incontinence. This was seen only with large-fraction (4–6 Gy), short-course radiation programs.

Hagen and colleagues reported a reduction in death from neurologic causes and a longer interval to CNS relapse in patients receiving postoperative whole-brain irradiation after resection of a single brain metastasis from melanoma.[146] Eighty-five percent of the surgery-only group died of neurologic causes, whereas 24% of the surgery-plus-radiation therapy patients died of neurologic causes. Neurologic relapse also occurred earlier in the operative group, but overall survival was no different, because patients in the combined group would continue to die from uncontrolled systemic disease.

In spite of the encouraging results with a combined therapeutic approach, the majority (≥60%) of patients are unsuited for surgery and undergo irradiation (with or without steroids) as the primary treatment for intracranial metastatic disease. This direction in patient management is influenced by the clinical profile of the patients with brain metastases. Although approximately 50% of patients harbor solitary brain metastases,[8] nearly one half of this group with solitary deposits will not be candidates for operation because of widespread systemic disease, major neurologic dysfunction, poor performance status, or other factors.[36] In addition, the lack of effective systemic therapy for many malignancies limits an aggressive surgical and radiotherapeutic approach for those patients with the combination of brain metastases and uncontrolled systemic disease.

PROGNOSTIC FACTORS: EXTENDED SURVIVAL IN BRAIN METASTASES

The *preoperative neurologic condition* and *extent of systemic disease* are the two most important prognostic factors influencing the short-term results for combined treatment (surgery, radiation therapy, and steroids) and also correlate with the long-term survival. Figures 61–5 and 61–6 reflect the influence of these two prognostic variables in the results for combined therapy. Patient age and the interval from the detection of a primary tumor to the development of a symptomatic metastasis also have a strong correlation with survival.

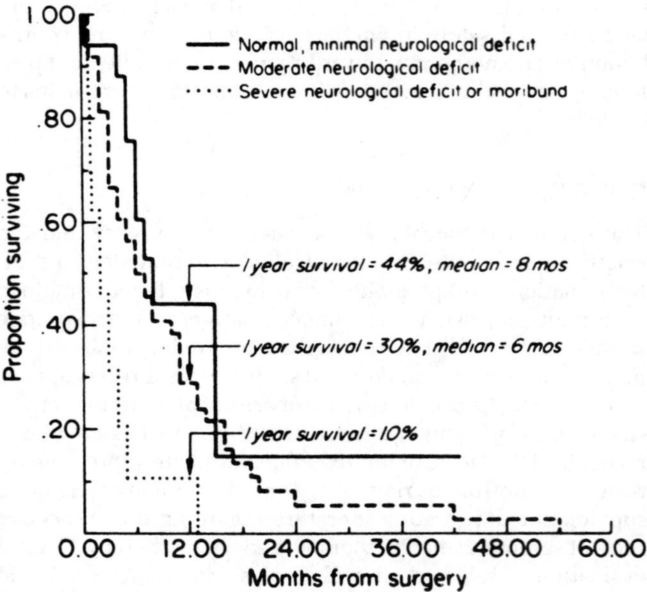

FIGURE 61–5. Survival curve for patients treated with surgery and irradiation according to preoperative patient status. (Galicich JG, Sundaresan N, Arbit E, et al. Surgical treatment of single brain metastasis: Factors associated with survival. Cancer 1980;45:381–386)

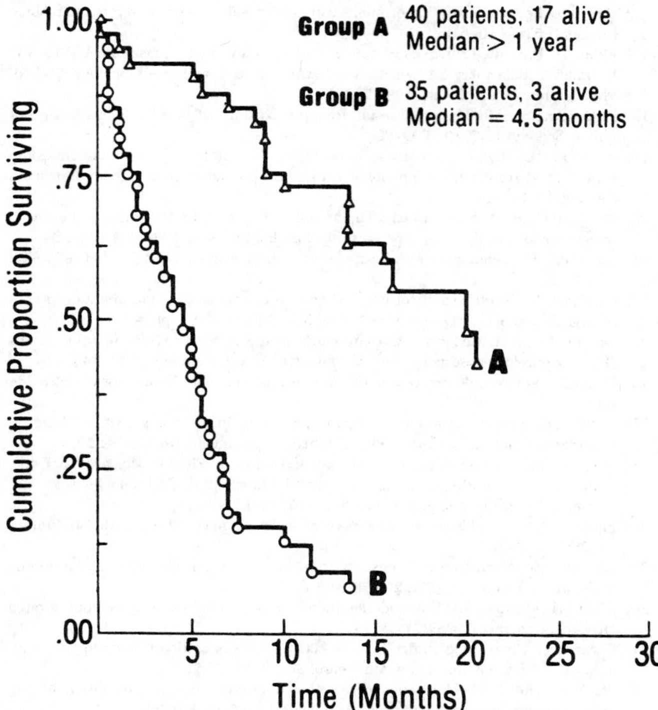

FIGURE 61–6. Survival plot according to extent of disease. Group A represents patients without evidence of extra-CNS disease. Group B had evidence of disseminated disease outside the CNS. All patients were treated with surgery and irradiation. CNS, central nervous system. (Galicich JH, Sundaresan N. Metastatic brain tumors. In: Wilkins RH, Rengachary SS, eds. Neurosurgery New York: McGraw-Hill, 1985:597–610)

Extended survival (greater than 2 years)[5,10,41,45,63,99,102,118,122,140,147,148] is an occasional feature of clinical reports, and the majority of long survivors have been subjected to various forms of combined therapy (surgery, radiation therapy, steroids, chemotherapy), although numerous anecdotal reports document long survival with surgery as the only therapy.[41,45,116,140,145,149] The more indolent tumors constitute the largest group of extended survivors (*e.g.*, breast carcinoma has a 38% 2-year survival rate). Long-term survival (≥5 years), however, is not exclusively restricted to patients with less malignant tumors. A precocious presentation with an occult systemic primary tumor and no evidence of extraneural metastases is associated with long survivals in a fraction of patients.[45,99] Definitive identification of prognostic factors for extended survival beyond 3 to 5 years is not currently possible, but subjecting patients with favorable clinical profiles to aggressive combined therapy may provide further insight to this occasional phenomenon.

RELATIVE INDICATIONS FOR SURGICAL INTERVENTION

Surgical indications (see Table 61–6) have been previously discussed, and these general guidelines serve for most clinical settings, with only occasional exceptions. Emergent situations sometimes arise where rapid neurologic compromise has occurred because of progressive tumor growth in patients in whom maximal medical therapy has failed or metastatic complications (*e.g.*, hemorrhage, abscess formation, CSF obstruction) arise. In such situations, urgent surgical intervention is only occasionally appropriate for patients in poor neurologic condition and multiple medical problems arising from uncontrolled or widespread systemic metastases. Such patients are best managed with aggressive neurologic and medical resuscitation measures when appropriate, and they should be subjected to surgery only when they are stabilized and their preoperative state improves.[6] Metastatic complications should be promptly treated as if metastases were a secondary problem, unless severe risks attend a surgical approach. Dramatic benefit can be realized from correction of CSF obstruction (external/internal shunting) or drainage of hemorrhagic and infectious (abscess) complications.

Patients with multiple metastases who progressively deteriorate (neurologically) despite the best available nonsurgical therapy, or after completion of medical therapy, represent an unsolved problem in the management of metastases. If favorable prognostic factors are present (*e.g.*, good neurologic status, minimal or controlled extra-CNS disease), surgery may represent the only treatment option. Surgery is generally not indicated for multiple metastases or leptomeningeal spread, other than diagnostic biopsy, because mortality is significantly increased. Critically located deposits (*e.g.*, posterior fossa mass obstructing CSF pathways) are occasionally appropriate for resection despite the increased risk if other (supratentorial) deposits are small or clinically silent.

Lastly, surgical resection of dominant hemispheric masses in critically functional brain areas is not necessarily associated with increased morbidity.[6,48] The preoperative neurologic performance largely determines the risk in these patients; if careful microtechnique with precise localization and intraoperative monitoring is used, the discrete nature of most metastases allows gross total removal with minimal morbidity in such locations.

CEREBRAL METASTASES: SUMMARY

The potentially severe consequences of brain involvement by cancer is a common problem confronting the oncologic specialties. Symptomatic parenchymal lesions are projected to afflict 152,600 patients in the United States annually, with lung, breast, gastrointestinal, renal, and melanoma contributing the majority of lesions coming to clinical attention. Timely, effective therapy for brain metastases can restore neurologic function or prevent the neurologic complications of cancer for the duration of survival. Limiting the disability of metastases is difficult, and available therapy is not fully effective.

Since the previous edition of this text, important contributions have been made in regard to the role of surgery in selected patients,[36] advances in radiation techniques,[69,75,79,109] and preliminary results of chemotherapy trials.[144,150] The surgery plus radiation group reported by Patchell and colleagues had advantages over radiation alone in neurologic relapse, length and quality of survival, and deaths by neurologic cause (uncontrolled brain metastases).[36] The optimal radiation time-dose regimen has been further developed, and progress in more effective control (combination chemotherapy) of both systemic and metastatic sites has been noted.

Rational selection of the appropriate therapy for patients with brain metastases requires accurate diagnosis, localization, and determination of prognostic criteria. The major prognostic variables for this group are the pretreatment neurologic state, the metastatic interval, and the extent of systemic disease.

Surgery combined with adjuvant radiation therapy for selected patients achieves the best results in therapy of resistant malignancies of the lung, kidney, thyroid, colon, and skin, as well as many soft tissue sarcomas. The indications for surgery are well established; the most suitable surgical patients have a single lesion with minimal neurologic impairment, limited extra-CNS disease, a prolonged antecedent (metachronous) tumor history before cerebral metastasis, or a precocious presentation with occult systemic disease. The risks of surgery are generally determined by the preoperative state and the extent of systemic disease. Superior results are realized when the dual goals of total gross resection and minimal brain injury are achieved. Surgery for brain metastases is applicable to only 10% to 30% of patients, with the use of conservative selection criteria; the majority have unfavorable neurologic impairment, uncontrolled systemic tumor, and other factors increasing the risk and reducing the potential benefit of a combined approach.

Patients with prohibitive risk factors should have maximal medical management including radiation therapy delivered with one of the shorter treatment programs. Consideration of the novel radiation therapy approaches recently described[75,79] may be warranted, but experience in the use of these approaches is limited. Chemotherapy, particularly for sensitive tumors without prior drug therapy, offers increasing efficacy and safety.

A multidisciplinary approach in this patient population is mandatory, with cooperating specialists fully cognizant of the limitations of their respective therapeutic measures.

REFERENCES

1. Posner JB. Brain metastases: A clinician's view. In: Weiss L, Gilbert HA, Posner JB, eds. Brain metastases. Boston: GK Hall, 1980:2–29
2. Boring CC, Squires TS, Tong T. Cancer statistics, 1992. CA 1992;42:19–38.
3. Walker AE, Robins M, Weinfeld FD. Epidemiology of brain tumors: The national survey of intracranial neoplasms. Neurology 1985;35:219–226.
4. Hildebrand J. Lesions of the nervous system in cancer patients. Monograph series of the European Organization for Research on Treatment of Cancer. Vol 5. New York: Raven Press, 1978.
5. Takakura K, Sano K, Hoho S, et al. Metastatic tumors of the central nervous system. Tokyo: Igaku-Shoin, 1982.
6. Galicich JH, Sundaresan N. Metastatic brain tumors. In: Wilkins RH, Rengachary SS, eds. Neurosurgery. New York: McGraw-Hill, 1985:597–610.
7. Rubin R, Green J. Solitary metastases. Springfield, IL: Charles C Thomas, 1968.
8. Posner JB, Chernik NL. Intracranial metastases from systemic cancer. Adv Neurol 1978;19:575–587.
9. Posner JB. Diagnosis and treatment of metastases to the brain. Clin Bull 1974;4:47–57.
10. Simionescu MD. Metastatic tumors of the brain. A follow-up study of 195 patients with neurosurgical considerations. J Neurosurg 1960;17:361–373.
11. Liotta LA, Kohn E. Cancer invasion and metastases. JAMA 1990;263:1123–1126.
12. Katz DA, Liotta LA. Tumor invasion and metastasis in the central nervous system. In: Zimmerman HM, ed. Progress in neuropathology. Vol 6. New York: Raven Press, 1986:119–131.
13. Delattre JY, Krol G, Thaler HT, Posner JB. Distribution of brain metastases. Arch Neurol 1988;45:741–744.
14. Weiss L. Metastatic brain tumors. Factors that govern the metastatic process. In: Wilkins RH, Rengachary SS, eds. Neurosurgery. New York: McGraw-Hill, 1985:591–596.
15. Warren BA. Arrest and extravasation of cancer cells with special reference to brain metastases and the microinjury hypothesis. In: Weiss L, Gilbert HA, Posner JB, eds. Brain metastases. Boston: GK Hall, 1980:81–99.
16. Coman D, DeLong R. The role of the vertebral venous system in the metastasis of cancer to the spinal cord: Experiments with tumor-cell suspension in rats and rabbits. Cancer 1951;4:610–618.
17. Fidler IJ, Hart IR. Principles of cancer biology: Cancer metastasis. In: DeVita VT, Hellman S, Rosenberg SA, eds. Cancer. Principles & Practice of Oncology. 2nd ed. Philadelphia: JB Lippincott, 1985:113–124.
18. Fidler IJ, Kripke ML. Metastasis results from pre-existing variant cells within a malignant tumor. Science 1977;197:893–895.
19. Nicolson GL. Organ specificity of tumor metastasis: Role of preferential adhesion, invasion and growth of malignant cells at specific secondary sites. Cancer Metastasis Rev 1988;7:143–188.
20. Nicolson GL. Cancer metastasis: Tumor cell and host organ properties important in metastasis to specific secondary sites. Biochim Biophys Acta 1988;948:175–224.
21. Zetter BR. The cellular basis of site-specific tumor metastasis. N Engl J Med 1990;322:605–612.
22. Lundberg N. Continuous recording and control of ventricular fluid pressure in neurosurgical practice. Acta Psychiatr Neurol Scand 1960;36(Suppl 149):1–193.
23. Langfitt TW. Increased intracranial pressure and the cerebral circulation. In: Youmans JR, ed. Neurological surgery. 2nd ed. Philadelphia: WB Saunders, 1982:846–930.
24. Miller JD. Volume and pressure in the craniospinal axis. Clin Neurosurg 1975;22:76–105.
25. Wright DC. Surgical treatment of brain metastases. In: Rosenberg SA, ed. Surgical treatment of metastatic cancer. Philadelphia: JB Lippincott, 1987:165–222.
26. Plum F, Posner JB. The diagnosis of stupor and coma. In: Plum F, McDowell FH, eds. Contemporary neurology series no. 19. 3rd ed. Philadelphia: FA Davis, 1980.
27. Fishman RA. Brain edema. N Engl J Med 1975;293:706–711.
28. Fishman RA. Steroids in the treatment of brain edema. N Engl J Med [Editorial] 1982;306:359–360.
29. Hirano A, Zimmerman HM. Fenestrated blood vessels in a metastatic renal carcinoma in the brain. Lab Invest 1972;26:465–468.
30. Chan PH, Fishman RA. Brain edema: Induction in cortical slices by polyunsaturated fatty acids. Science 1978;201:358–360.
31. Caronna JJ, Chan PH, Fishman RA. Protective effects of corticosteroids on fatty acid-induced cerebral edema. Trans Am Neurol Soc 1980;105:200–202.
32. Black KL, Hoff JT. Leukotrienes increase blood–brain barrier permeability following intraparenchymal injections in rats. Ann Neurol 1985;18:349–351.
33. Senger DR, Galli SJ, Dvorak AM, et al. Tumor cells secrete a vascular permeability factor that promotes accumulation of ascites fluid. Science 1983;219:983–985.
34. Blasberg RG, Gazendam J, Patlak CS, Fenstermacher JD. Quantitative autoradiographic studies of brain edema and a comparison of multi-isotope autoradiographic techniques. Adv Neurol 1980;28:255–270.
35. Raskind R, Weiss SR. Conditions simulating metastatic lesions of the brain. Report of eight cases. Int Surg 1970;43:40–42.
36. Patchell RA, Tibbs RP, Walsh JW, et al. A randomized trial of surgery in the treatment of single metastases to the brain. N Engl J Med 1990;322:494–500.
37. Posner JB. Clinical manifestations of brain metastasis. In: Weiss LGH, Posner JB, eds. Brain metastasis. Boston: GK Hall, 1980:189–207.
38. Gamache FW Jr, Posner JB, Patterson RH. Metastatic brain tumors. In: Youmans JR, ed. Neurological surgery. 2nd ed. Vol 4. Philadelphia: WB Saunders, 1982:2872–2898.
39. Stortebecker TP. Metastatic tumors of the brain from a neurosurgical point of view: A follow-up study of 158 cases. J Neurosurg 1954;11:84–111.
40. Paillas JE, Pellet W. Brain metastases. In: Vinken PJ, Bruyn GW, eds. Handbook of clinical neurology. Vol 18. Amsterdam: North-Holland Publishing Co., 1975:201–232.
41. Lang EF Jr, Slater J. Metastatic brain tumors. Results of surgical and non-surgical treatment. Surg Clin North Am 1964;44:865–872.
42. Nisce IZ, Hilaris BS, Chu FCH. A review of experience with irradiation of brain metastasis. AJR 1971;111:329–333.
43. Strub RL, Black RW. The mental status examination in neurology. Philadelphia: FA Davis, 1977.
44. Hayward RD. Secondary malignant melanoma of the brain. Clin Oncol 1976;2:227–232.
45. Winston KR, Walsh JW, Fischer EG. Results of operative treatment of intracranial metastatic tumors. Cancer 1980;45:2639–2645.
46. Gamache FW Jr, Posner JB, Galicich JH. Treatment of brain metastases by surgical extirpation. In: Weiss L, Gilbert H, Posner JB, eds. Brain metastases. Boston: GK Hall, 1980:390–414.
47. Karnofsky DA, Burchenol JH. The clinical evaluation of chemotherapeutic agents in cancer. In: McLeod CN, ed. Evaluation of chemotherapeutic agents. New York: Columbia University Press, 1949:191–205.
48. Galicich JH, Sundaresan N, Arbit E, Pase A. Surgical treatment of single brain metastasis: Factors associated with survival. Cancer 1980;45:381–386.
49. Sze G, Milano E, Johnson C, Heier L. Detection of brain metastases: Comparison of contrast-enhanced MR with unenhanced MR and enhanced CT. Am J Neuroradiol 1990;11:785–791.
50. Gado MH, Phelps ME, Coleman RE. An extravascular component of contrast enhancement in cranial computed tomography (parts I and II). Radiology 1975;117:589–597.
51. Takeda N, Tanaka R, Nakai O. Dynamics of contrast enhancement in delayed computed tomography of brain tumors: Tissue-blood ratio and differential diagnosis. Radiology 1982;142:663–668.
52. Cohen N, Strauss G, Lew R, Silver D, Recht L. Should prophylactic anticonvulsants be administered to patients with newly-diagnosed cerebral metastases: A retrospective analysis. J Clin Oncol 1988;6:1621–1624.
53. Galicich JH, French LA, Ueki K, Melby JC. Use of dexamethasone in the treatment of cerebral edema associated with brain tumors. Lancet 1961;81:46–53.

54. French LA. The use of steroids in the treatment of cerebral edema. Bull NY Acad Med 1966;42:301–311.
55. Renaudin J, Fewer D, Wilson CB, et al. Dose dependency of Decadron in patients with partially excised brain tumors. J Neurosurg 1973;39:302–305.
56. Gutin PH. Corticosteroid therapy in patients with cerebral tumor: Benefits, mechanisms, problems, practicalities. Semin Oncol 1975;2:49–56.
57. Ransohoff J. The effects of steroids on brain edema in man. In: Reulen HJ, Schurmann K, eds. Steroids and brain edema. Berlin: Springer-Verlag, 1972:211–221.
58. Ehrenkranz JRL, Posner JB. Adrenocorticosteroid hormones. In: Weiss L, Gilbert H, Posner JB, eds. Brain metastasis. Boston: GK Hall, 1980:340–363.
59. Samuels MA, ed. Manual of neurologic therapeutics: With essentials of diagnosis. 3rd ed. Boston: Little, Brown and Co., 1986:1–424.
60. Fenstermacher JD. Volume regulation of the central nervous system. In: Staub NC, Taylor AE, eds. Edema. New York: Raven Press, 1984:383–404.
61. Weiss HD. Neoplasms. In: Samuels MA, ed. Manual of neurologic therapeutics: With essentials of diagnosis. 3rd ed. Boston: Little, Brown and Co., 1986.
62. Quest DO. Increased intracranial pressure, brain herniation, and their control. In: Wilkins RH, Rengachary SS, eds. Neurosurgery. New York: McGraw-Hill, 1985:332–342.
63. Cairncross JG, Kim J-H, Posner JB. Radiation therapy for brain metastases. Ann Neurol 1980;7:529–541.
64. Chu FCH, Hilaris BB. Value of radiation therapy in the management of intracranial metastasis. Cancer 1961;14:577–581.
65. Hindo WA, DeTrana FA, Lee MS, et al. Large dose increment irradiation in treatment of cerebral metastases. Cancer 1970;26:138–141.
66. Deutsch M, Parsons JA, Mercado R Jr. Radiotherapy for intracranial metastases. Cancer 1974;34:1607.
67. Berry HC, Parke RG, Gerdes AJ. Irradiation of brain metastases. Acta Radiol Ther 1974;13:535–544.
68. Hendrickson FR. The optimum schedule for palliative radiotherapy for metastatic brain cancer. Int J Radiat Oncol Biol Phys 1977;2:165–168.
69. Diener-West M, Dobbins TW, Phillips TL, Nelson DF. Identification of an optimal subgroup for treatment evaluation of patients with brain metastases using RTOG study 7916. Int J Radiat Oncol Biol Phys 1991;16:669–673.
70. Borgelt B, Gelber R, Kramer S, et al. The palliation of brain metastases: Final results of the first two studies by the Radiation Therapy Oncology Group. Int J Radiat Oncol Biol Phys 1980;6:1–9.
71. Kurtz JM, Gelber R, Brady LW, et al. The palliation of brain metastases in a favorable patient population: A randomized clinical trial by the Radiation Therapy Oncology Group. Int J Radiat Oncol Biol Phys 1981;7:891–895.
72. Harwood AR, Simpson WF. Radiation therapy of cerebral metastases. A randomized prospective clinical trial. Int J Radiat Oncol Biol Phys 1977;2:1091–1094.
73. Young DF, Posner JB, Chu FCH, et al. Rapid-course radiation therapy of cerebral metastases: Results and complications. Cancer 1974;34:1069–1076.
74. Gutin PH, Phillips TL, Hosobuchi Y, et al. Permanent and removable implants for the brachytherapy of brain tumors. Int J Radiat Oncol Biol Phys 1981;7:1371–1381.
75. Prados M, Leibel S, Barnett CM, Gutin PH. Interstitial brachytherapy for metastatic brain tumors. Cancer 1989;63:657–660.
76. Heros DO, Kasdon DL, Chun M. Brachytherapy in the treatment of recurrent solitary brain metastases. Neurosurgery 1988;23:733–737.
77. Sturm V, Kober B, Hover KH, et al. Stereotactic percutaneous single dose irradiation of brain metastases with a linear accelerator. Int J Radiat Oncol Biol Phys 1987;13: 279–282.
78. Loeffler JS, Kooy HM, Wen PY, et al. The treatment of recurrent brain metastases with stereotactic radiosurgery. J Clin Oncol 1990;8:576–582.
79. Coffey RJ, Flickinger JC, Bissonette DJ, Lunsford LD. Radiosurgery for solitary brain metastases using the cobalt-60 gamma unit: Methods and results in 24 patients. Int J Radiat Oncol Biol Phys 1991;20:1287–1295.
80. Nedzi LA, Kooy H, Alexander E III, et al. Variables associated with the development of complications from radiosurgery of intracranial tumors. Int J Radiat Oncol Biol Phys 1991;21:591–599.
81. Long DM. Capillary ultrastructure in human metastatic brain tumours. J Neurosurg 1979;51:53–58.
82. Stewart DJ, Leavens M, Maor M, et al. Human central nervous system distribution of cis-diamminedichloroplatinum and use as a radiosensitizer in malignant brain tumors. Cancer Res 1982;42:2472–2479.
83. Stewart DJ, Richard MR, Hugenholtz H, et al. Penetration of VP-16 (etoposide) into human intracerebral and extracerebral tumors. J Neurooncol 1984;2:133–139.
84. Stewart DJ, Richard MR, Hugenholtz H, et al. Penetration of teniposide (VM-26) into human intracerebral tumors. J Neurooncol 1984;2:315–324.
85. Stewart DJ, Benvenuto JA, Leavens M, et al. Human central nervous system pharmacology of pentamethylmelamine and its metabolites. J Neurooncol 1983;1:357–364.
86. Stewart DJ, Benvenuto J, Leavens M, et al. Penetration of 3-deazauridine in human brain, intracerebral tumor, and cerebrospinal fluid. Cancer Res 1979;39:4119–4122.
87. Savaraj N, Lu K, Feun LF, et al. Intracerebral penetration and tissue distribution of 2,5-diaziridinyl 3,6-bis (carboethoxyamino) 1,4-benzoquinone, (9AZQ NSC 182986). J Neurooncol 1983;1:15–20.
88. Rosenblum M, Stewart DJ, Yap BS, et al. Penetration of methylglyoxal bis-(guanylhydrazone) into intracerebral tumor in humans. Cancer Res 1981;41:459–462.
89. Stewart DJ, Lu K, Benjamin RS, et al. Concentrations of vinblastine in human intracerebral tumor and other tissues. J Neurooncol 1983;1:139–144.
90. Stewart DJ, Leavens M, Friedman J, et al. Penetration of N-(phosphyonacetyl)-L-aspartate into human central nervous system and intracerebral tumor. Cancer Res 1980;40:3163–3166.
91. Hori T, Muraoka K, Yoshikazu S, et al. Influence of modes of ACNU administration on tissue and blood drug concentration in malignant brain tumors. J Neurosurg 1987;66: 372–378.
92. Whittle IR, MacPherson JS, Miller JD, et al. The disposition of TCNU (tauromustine) in human malignant glioma: Pharmacokinetic studies and clinical implications. J Neurosurg 1990;72:721–725.
93. Mulshine J, Ruckdeschel JC. The role of chemotherapy in the management of disseminated non-small cell lung cancer. In: Roth J, Ruckdeschel J, Weisenburger T, eds. Thoracic oncology. Philadelphia: WB Saunders, 1989:220–228.
94. Henderson IC. Chemotherapy of breast cancer. A general overview. Cancer 1983;51: 2553–2559.
95. Poon MA, O'Connell MJ, Moertel CG, et al. Biochemical modulation of fluorouracil: Evidence of significant improvement of survival and quality of life in patients with advanced colorectal carcinoma. J Clin Oncol 1989;7:1407–1417.
96. Creagan ET. Regional and systemic strategies for metastatic malignant melanoma. Mayo Clin Proc 1989;64:852–860.
97. Harris DT. Hormonal therapy and chemotherapy for renal cell carcinoma. Semin Oncol 1983;10:422–430.
98. Muss HB. The role of biological response modifiers in metastatic renal cell carcinoma. Semin Oncol 1988;15(Suppl 5):30–34.
99. Ransohoff J. Surgical therapy of brain metastases. In: Weiss L, Gilbert HA, Posner JB, eds. Brain metastases. Boston: GK Hall, 1980:380–389.
100. Posner JB. Management of central nervous system metastases. Semin Oncol 1977;4: 81–91.
101. Galicich JH, Sundaresan N, Thaler HT. Surgical treatment of single brain metastasis: Evaluation of results by computerized tomography scanning. J Neurosurg 1980;53: 63–67.
102. Haar F, Paterson R Jr. Surgery for metastatic intracranial neoplasm. Cancer 1972;30: 1241–1245.
103. Richards P, McKissock W. Intracranial metastases. Br Med J 1963;1:15–18.
104. Galicich JH. Surgery of malignant brain tumors. In: Vick NA, ed. Seminars in neurology. Vol 1. New York: Thieme-Stratton, 1981:159–168.
105. Posner JB. Neurological complications of systemic cancer. Med Clin North Am 1971;55: 625–646.
106. Horton J, Baxter DD, Olson DB, et al. The management of metastases to the brain by irradiation and corticosteroids. AJR 1971;111:334–336.
107. Order SE, Hellman S, Von Essen CF, et al. Improvement in quality of survival following whole-brain irradiation for whole brain metastasis. Radiology 1968;91:149–153.
108. Kamarnicky LT, Phillips TL, Martz K, et al. A randomized phase III protocol for the evaluation of misonidazole combined with radiation in the treatment of patients with brain metastases (RTOG-7916). Int J Radiat Oncol Biol Phys 1991;20:53–58.
109. DeAngelis LM, Mandell LR, Thaler HT, et al. The role of postoperative radiotherapy after resection of single brain metastases. Neurosurgery 1989;24:798–805.
110. Shehata WM, Hendrickson FR, Hindo WA. Rapid fractionation technique and retreatment of cerebral metastases by irradiation. Cancer 1974;34:257–261.
111. Kurup P, Reddy S, Hendrickson FR. Results of re-irradiation for cerebral metastases. Cancer 1980;46:2587–2589.
112. Hazuka MB, Kinzie JJ. Brain metastases: Results and effects of re-irradiation. Int J Radiat Oncol Biol Phys 1988;15:433–437.
113. Cooper JS, Steinfeld R, Lerch IA. Cerebral metastases: Value of reirradiation in selected patients. Radiology 1990;174:883–885.
114. Grant FC. Concerning intracranial malignant metastases; their frequency and the value of surgery in their treatment. Ann Surg 1926;84:635–646.
115. Dandy WE. Brain tumors—General diagnosis and treatment. In: Lewis JR, ed. Practice of surgery. Vol 12. New York: Harper & Row, 1932:443–674.
116. Vieth R, Odom G. Intracranial metastases and their neurosurgical treatment. J Neurosurg 1965;23:375–383.
117. Bakay L. Results of surgical treatment of intracranial metastasis from pulmonary cancer. Report of a case with five-year survival. J Neurosurg 1958;15:338–341.
118. Lang EF Jr. Neurosurgical management of intracranial metastatic malignancy. Surg Clin North Am 1967;47:737–742.
119. Olivecrona H. The metastatic tumors. In: Olivecrona HTW, ed. Handbuch der Neurochirurgie. Berlin: Springer-Verlag, 1967:292–298.
120. Ransohoff J. Surgical management of metastatic tumor. Semin Oncol 1975;2:23–27.
121. Montana GS, Meacham WF, Caldwell WL. Brain irradiation for metastatic disease of lung origin. Cancer 1972;29:1477–1480.
122. Modesti LM, Feldman RA. Solitary cerebral metastasis from pulmonary cancer. Prolonged survival after surgery. JAMA 1975;231:1064.
123. Lee JS, Murphy WK, Glisson BS, et al. Primary chemotherapy of brain metastasis in small-cell lung cancer. J Clin Oncol 1989;7:916–922.
124. Twelves CJ, Souhami RL, Harper PG, et al. The response of cerebral metastases in small cell lung cancer to systemic chemotherapy. Br J Cancer 1989;61:147–150.
125. Postmus PE, Haaxma-Reiche H, Sleijfer DT, et al. High dose etoposide for brain metastases of small cell lung cancer. A phase II study. Br J Cancer 1989;59:254–256.
126. Rustin GJS, Newlands ES, Bagshawe KD, et al. Successful management of metastatic and primary germ cell tumors in the brain. Cancer 1986;57:2108–2113.
127. Rustin GJS, Newlands ES, Begent RHJ, et al. Weekly alternating etoposide, methotrexate, and actinomycin/vincristine and cyclophosphamide chemotherapy for the treatment of CNS metastases for choriocarcinoma. J Clin Oncol 1989;7:900–903.

128. Rosner D, Nemoto T, Lane WW. Chemotherapy induces regression of brain metastases in breast carcinoma. Cancer 1986;58:832–839.
129. Cocconi G, Lottici R, Bisagni G, et al. Combination therapy with platinum and etoposide for brain metastases from breast carcinoma. Cancer Invest 1990;8:327–334.
130. Jacquillat C, Khayat D, Banzet P, et al. Chemotherapy by fotemustine in cerebral metastases of disseminated malignant melanoma. Cancer Chemother Pharmacol 1990;25:263–266.
131. Bunn PA. Recent advances in the biology and treatment of small cell lung cancer. Adv Oncol 1986;2:9–15.
132. Cascino TL, Bryn TN, Deck MDF, et al. Intra-arterial BCNU in the treatment of metastatic brain tumors. J Neurooncol 1983;1:211–218.
133. Madajewicz S, West CR, Park HC, et al. Phase II study: Intra-arterial BCNU therapy for metastatic brain tumors. Cancer 1981;47:653–657.
134. Feun LG, Wallace S, Stewart DJ, et al. Intracarotid infusion of cis-diamminedichloroplatinum in the treatment of recurrent malignant brain tumors. Cancer 1984;54: 794–799.
135. Stewart DJ, Grahovac Z, Hugenholtz H, et al. Intraarterial mitomycin-C for recurrent brain metastases. Am J Clin Oncol 1987;10:432–436.
136. Feun LG, Lee Y, Yung WKA, et al. Intracarotid VP-16 in malignant brain tumors. J Neurooncol 1987;4:397–401.
137. Kolaric K, Roth A, Jelicic I, et al. Phase II clinical trial of cis-dichlorodiammine platinum (cis-DDP) in metastatic brain tumours—A preliminary report. In: Davis W, Maltoni C, Tanneberger S, eds. The control of tumour growth and its biological bases. Boston: Martinus Nijhoff Publishers, 1983:287–291.
138. Neuwelt EA, Dahlborg SA. Chemotherapy administered in conjunction with osmotic blood–brain barrier modification in patients with brain metastases. J Neurooncol 1987;4: 195–207.
139. Conte PF, Giaccone G, Musella R, et al. Combination chemotherapy for metastatic brain tumors. Tumori 1981;67:559–562.
140. Smalley SR, Schray MF, Laws ER, O'Fallon JR. Adjuvant radiation therapy after surgical resection of solitary brain metastasis: Association with patterns of failure and survival. Int J Radiat Oncol Biol Phys 1987;13:1611–1616.
141. Sause WT, Crowley JJ, Morantz R, et al. Solitary brain metastasis: Results of an RTOG/ SWOG protocol evaluation: Surgery + RT versus RT alone. Am J Clin Oncol 1990;13: 427–432.
142. Otter R, Hermans J, Brand R, et al. Solitary brain metastasis treatment: A randomized trial. Neurology 1988;38(Suppl 1):393.
143. Posner JB. Surgery for metastases to the brain. N Engl J Med 1990;322:544–545.
144. Ushio Y, Arita N, Hayakawa T, et al. Chemotherapy of brain metastases from lung carcinoma: A controlled randomized study. Neurosurgery 1991;28:201–205.
145. Dosoretz DE, Blitzer PH, Russell AH, et al. Management of solitary metastasis to the brain: The role of elective brain irradiation following complete surgical resection. Int J Radiat Oncol Biol Phys 1980;6:1727–1730.
146. Hagen NA, Cirrincione C, Thaler HT, DeAngelis LM. The role of radiation therapy following resection of single brain metastasis from melanoma. Neurology 1990;40: 158–160.
147. Deeley TJ, Edwards JM. Radiotherapy in the management of cerebral secondaries from bronchial carcinoma. Lancet 1968;1:1209–1213.
148. Dayes LA, Rouhe SA, Barnes RW. Excision of multiple intracranial metastatic hypernephroma: Report of a case with a 7-year survival. J Neurosurg 1977;46:533–535.
149. Raskind R, Weiss RS, Manning JJ, et al. Survival after surgical excision of single metastatic brain tumors. Am J Roentgenol Rad Ther Nucl Med 1971;111:323–328.
150. Siegers HP. Chemotherapy for brain metastases: Recent developments and clinical considerations. Cancer Treat Rev 1990;17:63–76.

SECTION **2**

HARVEY I. PASS

Treatment of Metastatic Cancer to the Lung

There have been numerous reports regarding an aggressive approach for the management of metastases to the lung. The value of complete resection of isolated pulmonary metastases from soft tissue sarcoma and osteogenic sarcoma has been documented with improved survival compared with patients whose disease could not be totally extirpated. The magnitude of the problem of pulmonary metastases can be appreciated when one considers that the lungs are the second most common site of metastases for all histologies[1] and that the lungs serve as the most common site of first recurrence in patients with sarcomas.[2] Moreover, up to 20% of cases with pulmonary metastases at autopsy have no other detectable tumor in other sites.[3]

HISTORY

Weinlechner is credited with the first removal of a pulmonary metastasis in 1882, with the resection accomplished en bloc during a chest wall sarcoma excision.[4] Concomitant excision of a lung nodule at the time of resection of a chest wall sarcoma was reported by Krolein shortly thereafter in 1884. Divis in 1926 removed a right lower lobe metastasis at a separate procedure. In 1939, Barney and Churchill resected a solitary renal adenosarcoma pulmonary metastasis.[5] The long duration of survival (23 years) coupled with the patient's death from unrelated causes (coronary artery disease) gave credibility to the concept of metastasectomy. In 1947, Alexander and Haight reported apparent cures in 3 of 6 patients after resection of metastases.[6]

Although these efforts clearly intimated a survival benefit from pulmonary metastasectomy, it was not until the maturation of techniques in thoracic surgery and anesthesia in the 1950s and 1960s that efforts to treat large numbers of patients began. Thomford and colleagues found comparable postthoracotomy survival rates for patients with excision of a solitary or multiple carcinomas and sarcoma lung metastases, justifying a more aggressive approach to resection.[7] Martini and colleagues[8] and Morton and associates[9] confirmed these observations by reporting comparable survival rates after resection of solitary or bilateral multiple metastases.

PATHOPHYSIOLOGY

ROUTES OF PRODUCTION

The most common pathway for true pulmonary metastatic disease is by way of *hematogenously disseminated malignant emboli* arising from invasion of thin-walled capillaries,[10] with transportation through the pulmonary artery. Most of these cells are destroyed in the bloodstream, and the number of tumor emboli correlate not only with the primary tumor duration and size but also with the probability of producing pulmonary metastases.[11] Other pathways include *endobronchial metastases* by way of a parenchymal or mediastinal nodal mass with secondary bronchial invasion, direct *lymphatic* spread, transbronchial *aspiration*, and *bronchial arterial* spread.[12–14] *Lymphangitic spread,* also by way of hematogenous dissemination, can occur by retrograde lymphatic spread through involved abdominal lymph nodes to hilar and mediastinal nodes.[12,15,16] *Pleural fluid* associated with parietal pleural metastases may be due to increased capillary permeability due to obstructive pneumonitis, decreased absorption, or erosion of vessels.[17]

MORPHOLOGIC CHARACTERISTICS

The number and morphology of nodules are important considerations in the evaluation of the etiology of pulmonary metastases. A solitary nodule in a patient with known extracellular malignancies is usually a second primary tumor if the original cancer was a squamous carcinoma. It is a metastasis or a second primary tumor if the original lesion was adenocarcinoma, but it is virtually always a metastasis if the original was melanoma or sarcoma.[18]

There is no predilection for laterality of pulmonary metastases,[19] and tumor distribution is usually greater at the bases, reflecting the flow characteristics of the pulmonary circulation.[2] The exception to this is choriocarcinoma, which, because of trophoblastic dissemination at the time of curettage, is posteriorly distributed to the upper lobes.[20,21]

The size of the metastasis is related to its detection during its natural history, and virtually 80% to 90% of these metastases are found in the periphery or outer third of the lung in a subpleural position.[22,23] Large peripheral lesions can actually assume a plaque-like shape that conforms to the shape of the chest wall and visceral pleura.

SIGNS AND SYMPTOMS

Because of the peripheral, subpleural, or parenchymal location of metastases, 85% to 95% of patients with metastases are asymptomatic.[24–26] Slow development of *dyspnea* may be due to airway obstruction, pleural effusion, or parenchymal replacement by innumerable lesions. Sudden shortness of breath may be due to hemorrhage into a lesion with space occupation or pleural effusion, or due to the development of a pneumothorax. The nature of the metastatic pneumothorax is unexplainable but may be due to rupture of subpleural blebs by growth of the lesion.[27–29] *Hemoptysis* demands bronchoscopic examination to rule out endobronchial tumor. Patients with increasing dyspnea, with diminished diffusing capacity and arterial desaturation in the absence of radiographic findings, may have lymphangitic spread of tumor.[30,31] The appearance of *chest pain* usually portends an ominous situation with discontinuous parietal pleural metastases.

ROENTGENOGRAPHIC APPEARANCE

Most pulmonary metastases, independent of histology, present as nodules (*i.e.*, increased densities that are roughly spherical in shape, are not associated with linear densities, and are sharply demarcated).[2] Pulmonary lesions with an irregular border usually imply primary lung cancer or infection,[12] but lesion age, hemorrhage, and previous treatment (see below) may influence the appearance of the metastases.

Cavitation may occur in approximately 5% of metastases, chiefly with sarcoma or squamous histologies due to central necrosis with liquefaction from rapid growth or treatment.[12] *Bleb formation* can be associated with testicular metastases.[32] *Calcification* may also be noted in metastases; therefore, calcification in a lesion must not be dismissed as a benign occurrence. Osteogenic sarcoma, chondrosarcoma, and synovial sarcoma are all associated with calcification, and infrequently calcified lung metastases are seen in thyroid, ovarian, and mucinous gastrointestinal malignancies and breast tumors.

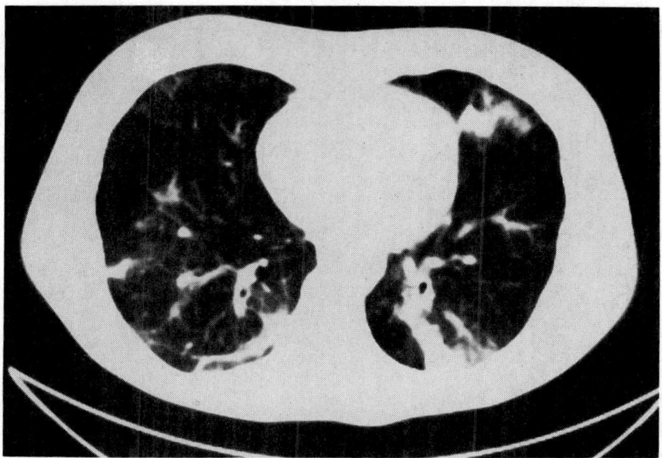

FIGURE 61–7. Computed tomographic scan of a patient with lymphangitic metastases from breast cancer. Notice the patchy, linear densities extending toward the hilum.

Postchemotherapeutic or postradiotherapeutic manipulation causing degeneration of metastases may result in calcification in a variety of pulmonary metastases.[33–38]

Lymphangitic carcinomatosis from lung, gastric, breast, pancreatic, or prostatic cancer may have minimal chest radiographic findings.[11,15] In the late stages there will be linear markings and possibly enlarged hilar nodes. Computed tomographic (CT) findings are much more specific for lymphangitic spread than are the plain radiographic findings (Figs. 61–7 and 61–8).

Lobar or total collapse is usually associated with endobronchial metastases from kidney, breast, colon, rectum, female genital tract, thyroid, or melanoma (Figs. 61–9 and 61–10). The frequency of metastatic involvement of the bronchus is approximately 2% to 28% of cancer patients.[39–41]

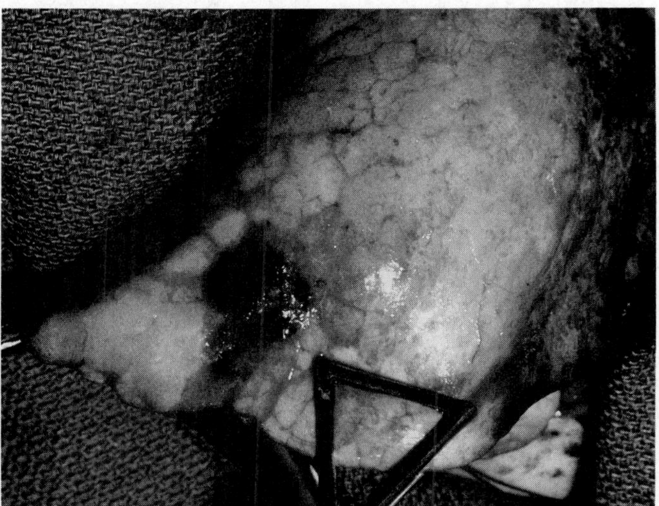

FIGURE 61–8. Operative photograph of patient with chest computed tomographic scan seen in Figure 61–7. The darkened area on the visceral pleura is a confluence of lymphatic channels plugged with tumor.

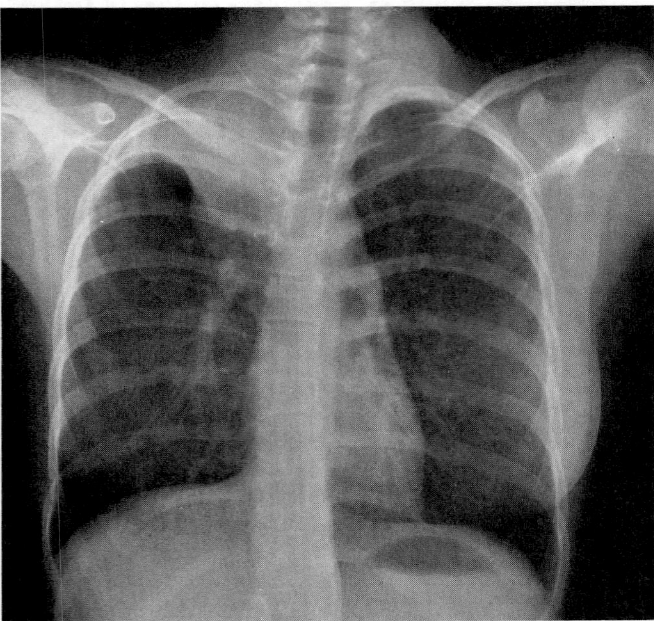

FIGURE 61–9. Right upper lobe collapse in a child with osteogenic sarcoma metastatic to the bronchus. The lesion was visible on bronchoscopy.

ROENTGENOGRAPHIC EXAMINATION

In any patient with extrathoracic malignant disease, either at the time of primary resection or during follow-up in the surveillance for pulmonary metastases, posteroanterior and lateral chest radiography is mandatory. In the initial evaluation of a patient, the chest radiograph serves as a useful baseline and also indicates coexisting benign cardiopulmonary disease. An abnormality on chest radiography in the initial examination demands the diligent examination of previous chest radiographs to define the morphologic characteristics of the abnormality and to document any change in the appearance of the lesion over time. Nevertheless, *computed tomography* (CT) of the chest has become the standard of care for the detection, operative planning, and follow-up of patients at risk for the development of pulmonary metastases. The ideal CT should be able to detect the smallest of abnormalities, be specific enough to pinpoint malignancy either on initial nodule examination or on follow-up, and be cost-effective so it can be repeated at frequent intervals without subjecting the patient to excessive irradiation. Unfortunately, such a standard does not exist at this time; however, more recent developments with the "fast CT" scanners may impart greater nodule differentiation with less distortion because of volume averaging. Certainly, CT has surpassed the use of conventional linear tomograms in the documentation of pulmonary metastases[42] because of the elimination of structural overlap and shadows by the cross-sectional depiction in CT scanning (Figs. 61–11 and 61–12). Subpleural abnormalities are easily detected, and contrast resolution exceeds conventional techniques by at least a factor of 10.[2] More lesions can be detected on CT, and lesions as small as 3 mm can be detected.[2] Partial volume averaging, in which a lesion is not fully in the CT volume and is not shown as an area of increased attenuation because of abutting of aerated lung, usually underestimates the number of lesions. Moreover, small nodules close to vessels are sometimes difficult to identify, but this has been improved with contrast enhancement.[43-48]

The real use of CT is its ability to take small nodules and define their natural history over a short time interval. The temporal pattern of appearance of hematogenous pulmonary metastases is variable. The appearance of the lung at any particular time is a cumulative phenomenon depending on

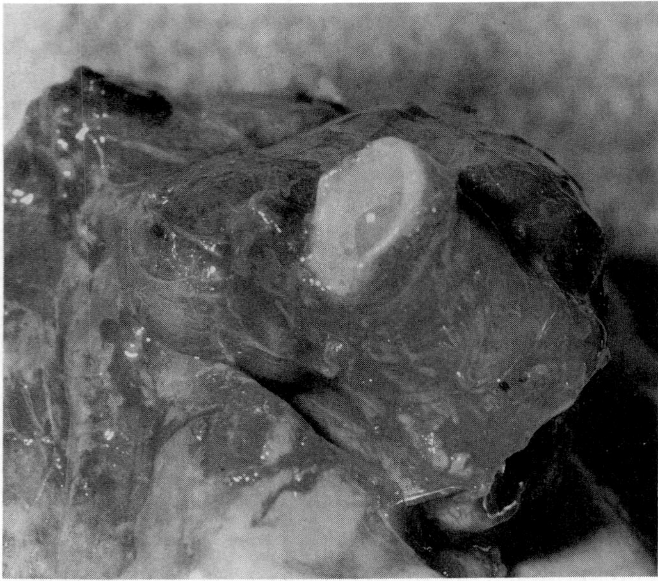

FIGURE 61–10. Operative photograph of the resected bronchus as a sleeve lobectomy (sparing the middle and lower lobe) in the patient with the chest radiograph seen in Figure 61–9. The bulbous lesion is seen just inside the superior cut end of the bronchus.

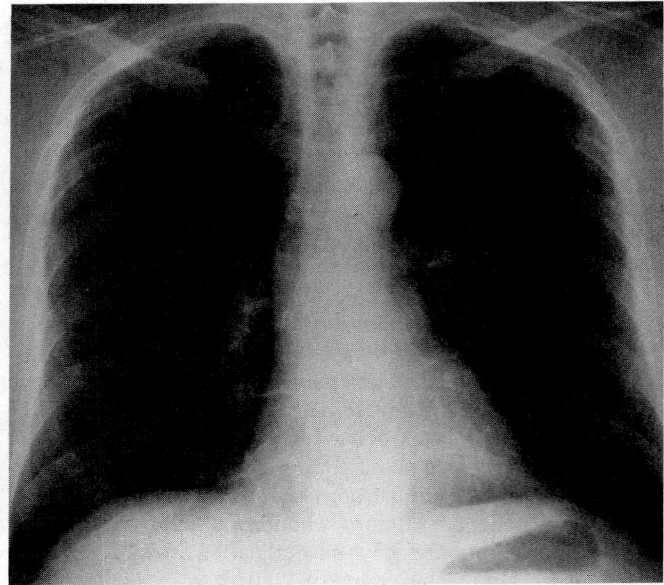

FIGURE 61–11. Routine surveillance chest radiograph in a patient with soft tissue sarcoma. No abnormality was detected.

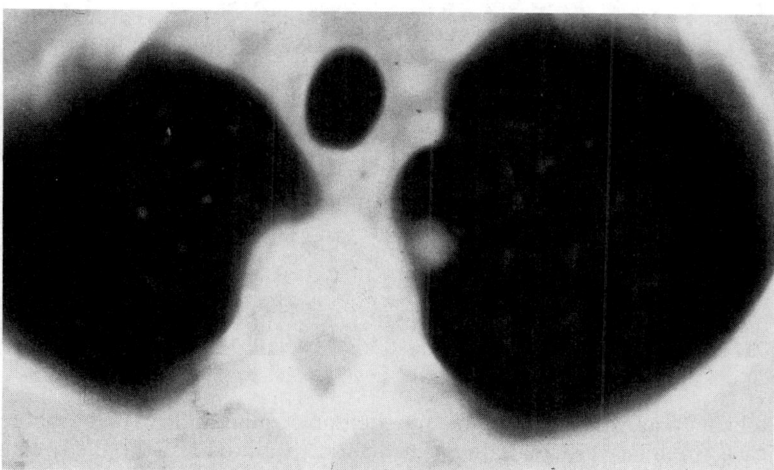

FIGURE 61–12. Computed tomographic scan reveals a lesion in the left upper lobe in the patient with the normal-appearing radiograph in Figure 61–11.

the frequency and intensity of the embolic showers, the capacity of the metastases to colonize, and the duration of the patient's disease. In the surveillance of pulmonary metastases, the problem is essentially to distinguish between benign and malignant processes. Usually the benign nodule is static in growth. Serial CT scanning can determine the dynamic properties of the pulmonary lesions, specifically in a homogenous patient population. Nodules can be classified as *stable, developing, or growing.* The predictive value of CT in defining a nodule as a malignancy is not as high in stable nodules on sequential scans.[2] The development of a new CT abnormality, however, in the sarcoma population or growth of a previous nodule will be histologically documented as malignant with a 90% confidence level. Questionable abnormalities demand repeat CTs at 2- to 3-month intervals to document any biologic change that would justify exploration.

USE OF CT IN MONITORING SPECIFIC HISTOLOGIES

If a nodule appears questionable on conventional studies, CT should be performed not only to verify the finding but also to document other possible lesions. In patients known to have an extrathoracic tumor that is likely to metastasize first to the lung (*i.e.,* testicular carcinoma, soft tissue sarcoma, or choriocarcinoma), chest CT should be performed initially as a baseline. This is especially true if an aggressive approach to the resection of metastases from these histologic types is to be maintained. In patients who present with extrathoracic tumors and multiple nodules on chest radiography, CT is of questionable usefulness except for the documentation of response to therapies. Chest radiography can probably suffice for more frequent examinations in these patients.

If CT of the liver is negative and there is no clinical or laboratory evidence of hepatic metastases in patients with cancers whose first metastases would be to the liver (*i.e.,* cancers of the colon, rectum, pancreas, or stomach), pulmonary metastases are unlikely. In this setting, a negative chest radiograph is probably most likely a true negative finding.[49] Similarly, if a bone scan is negative in patients with a high probability of first metastases to bone (*i.e.,* those with prostate cancer), CT of the thorax should be reserved for evaluation of abnormalities seen on the chest radiograph.

Surveillance intervals for the detection of pulmonary metastases depend on the probability that a given histologic type will metastasize to the lung. For lesions such as soft tissue sarcoma and osteogenic sarcomas, which are most likely to metastasize within the first 2 years of diagnosis, 3-month intervals are usually recommended.

NEWER ROENTGENOGRAPHIC METHODS

Because a considerable amount of radiation is delivered to patients in an attempt to detect pulmonary metastases, a sensitive screening modality free of ionizing radiation would be of value, especially in young persons. *Magnetic resonance imaging* (MRI) has made considerable diagnostic strides for the diagnosis of chest diseases, yet few studies have addressed its use in the detection of pulmonary metastases. A prospective trial was recently completed at the National Cancer Institute (NCI), where MRI, chest radiography, computed tomography, and surgical verification of disease were all obtained in 12 patients.[50] All images were interpreted in a blinded fashion (Fig. 61–13). For individual nodules, MRI was at least as sensitive as CT for nodules greater than 5 mm, and significantly more sensitive than chest radiographs. The sequences of the MRI could be changed for added sensitivity, as was the addition of contrast enhancement with gadopentetate dimeglumine. Future studies with higher generation MRI scanners will be needed, however, to displace CT as the "gold standard" for detection and surveillance of pulmonary metastases.

INVASIVE DIAGNOSTIC MEANS EXCLUSIVE OF THORACOTOMY

The pursuit of a histologic diagnosis of the undiagnosed chest nodule will depend on the equivocality of the radiographic studies, the physiologic reserve of the patient, the location of the lesions, the histology of the primary focus, and whether the surgeon feels the patient could be rendered free of disease. Certainly any pleural effusion associated with nodules in the chest demands cytologic verification of malignancy, and possibly pleural biopsy. Patients with poor performance status who cannot tolerate thoracotomy but need histologic verification of disease for further management may require his-

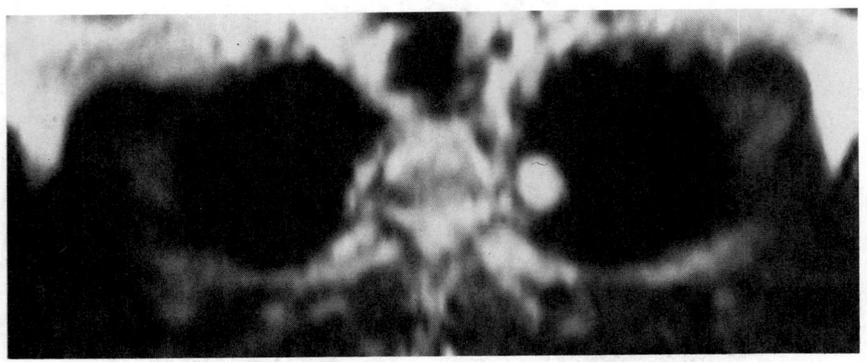

FIGURE 61–13. Magnetic resonance image reveals the lesion seen in the computed tomographic scan of Figure 61–12. The T2-weighted image highlights the lesion. (Photograph courtesy of Dr. Irwin Feuerstein, Department of Diagnostic Radiology Clinical Center, National Institutes of Health, Bethesda, MD)

tologic inquiries. Finally, if documentation of metastatic disease would have a major impact on the magnitude of the primary operation (limb salvage versus amputation for cure in the patient with multiple pulmonary nodules), verification of diagnosis as well as feasibility of complete resection need to be documented.

Diagnostic studies that are useful in other thoracic neoplasms are of limited value in the diagnosis of pulmonary metastases. In one series, *sputum cytologic examination* revealed malignant cells in only 5% of patients, and *bronchoscopy* provided notable findings in only 10% of patients with documented pulmonary metastases.[51] Bronchoscopies *should* be performed, however, to verify endobronchial metastases to define whether operative intervention is possible. In the case of an isolated metastasis seen by bronchoscopy, lobectomy or sleeve lobectomy may be performed with favorable survival. If resection is not possible, endobronchial management with or without laser ablation may be of great palliative interest (see later).

In general, there are few indications for *fine-needle aspiration biopsies (FNAB)* to avoid open thoracotomy for diagnosis, for if the primary lesion is favorable for resection, there is no reason for fine-needle aspiration biopsy. If the patient is unable to undergo thoracotomy, and histologic verification is necessary to guide treatment options, fine-needle aspiration is a reasonable alternative.[52] High sensitivity (88%) of FNAB for melanoma,[53] breast cancer, gastrointestinal cancer, germinal tumors,[53,54] and soft tissue sarcomas[55–57] has been reported in those series in which the aspirate can be compared with the primary tumor. Major complications include a 4% chance of a pneumothorax requiring chest tube treatment,[58] transient hemoptysis (2–4%), and, rarely, air embolism. Needle track implantations are rare.[59]

THORACOSCOPY

The use of thoracoscopy to diagnose pleural effusions and pulmonary metastases has increased and is now combined with video monitoring for documentation and ease of exploration. The multiple trocar technique and newly designed instruments for endoscopic surgery, including instruments to accomplish wedge resection of lung, have made this technique very popular for thoracic diseases. Certainly, for lesions on the surface of the visceral pleura, resection can be performed, although the length of time that these endoscopic resections require seems to be minimized in the literature. The ability of video thoracoscopy to ensure a complete resection of pulmonary metastases, however, remains to be demonstrated, because, as described in the following sections, deeper parenchymal lesions must be palpated in order to be found, and the technology of the endoscopic instruments for resection at this time is applicable for only the most superficial of lesions.[60–63]

SURGICAL RESECTION OF PULMONARY METASTASES

ELIGIBILITY FOR SURGICAL RESECTION

The selection of patients for thoracotomy for pulmonary metastasectomy must fulfill basic criteria, because only a portion of the patients will derive a survival benefit, and fewer will be cured of their disease. These criteria include: (1) local control of the primary tumor or the ability to gain local control if pulmonary exploration is performed first; (2) absence of metastatic lesions in nonpulmonary sites; (3) radiologic findings consistent with metastases; (4) potential for operative resection to preserve adequate functioning lung tissue; (5) ability of the pulmonary metastatic disease to be completely resected; and (6) lack of any other effective antitumor therapy. Occasionally, if a patient presents with synchronous pulmonary lesions and a lesion that could be handled by amputation or marginal limb-sparing option, it is preferable to determine complete resectability in the chest before committing the patient to an amputation in the face of unresectable pulmonary disease. Of the 30% of patients with malignant disease who develop pulmonary metastases, only one third will meet the defined basic treatment criteria of primary disease control and lack of metastases in other sites.[41]

In order to satisfy the above criteria, an extensive functional and staging workup is usually required. Computed tomography, magnetic resonance imaging, or appropriate endoscopic or barium studies must be performed to rule out evidence of disease at the primary site. *Sarcomas* will usually metastasize to the lungs in preference to other sites, so the primary site evaluation and radionuclide bone scans are all that are needed in these patients before the resection. *Carcinomas* and *melanomas* require a more extensive evaluation of peripheral sites, including the liver, adrenal glands, and brain.

A thorough functional evaluation must also be performed to determine whether the patient can safely withstand thoracotomy with low cardiopulmonary risk. Patients with carcinoma will tend to be older than sarcoma patients, necessitating a workup directed toward the cardiovascular/renal/pulmonary axis. Patients who have had cytotoxic chemotherapy must have recovery of their marrow to ensure the absence of bleeding, and it is necessary to search for clinical and subclinical evidence of cardiomyopathy or congestive heart failure in sarcoma patients and other patients who have had doxorubicin (Adriamycin),[64] particularly if the dose exceeds 500 mg/m^2.[65] Such assessment can be accomplished by measurement of ejection fraction at rest and during exercise.[66]

The majority of patients will simply require wedge resections for their lesions, but in the occasional patient who requires lobectomy or multiple wedge resections, a thorough evaluation of respiratory reserve must be performed by pulmonary function testing. In general, a patient must have postoperative FEV_1 of 800 to 1000 ml to avoid prolonged respiratory management after resection. The use of quantitative ventilation perfusion scanning may assist in determining residual FEV_1 after resection.[67] Diligent workup of a patient's pulmonary function should also be routine in patients who are having repeated thoracotomies for metastasis resection, or who have been previously exposed to pulmonary fibrotic inducing agents under high inspired oxygen conditions, such as bleomycin. Preexposure to bleomycin will dictate low inspired oxygen concentrations during and after the resection.

PROGNOSTIC FACTORS FOR THE RESECTION OF PULMONARY METASTASES

In the ideal situation, independent of histology, there would be a number of factors that would define preoperatively or intraoperatively who the best candidates would be for long-term survival after pulmonary metastasectomy. Unfortunately, despite a significant number of publications that have attempted to define such parameters, there is no uniform agreement as to which are the most important factors that predict a successful (*i.e.,* long-term survival) outcome. Many of the factors are based on biologic characteristics of the tumor, including disease-free interval and tumor doubling time, whereas other factors are based on the sensitivity of present radiographic studies, which will detect only 50% of the metastases found at operation. Moreover, different histologies seem to have varying factors that may prognosticate survival, and, unfortunately, uniform agreement does not appear in the literature, even with the same histology. The following discussion of prognostic factors, therefore, must serve only as a *superficial guide* to the practitioner to advise his patient regarding the possible outcome of metastasectomy before operation.

RESECTABILITY

There is almost uniform agreement that the ability to completely resect all nodules that are metastases (as opposed to an incomplete or unresectable situation) will be associated with an improved outcome compared with patients who remain with disease. This has been confirmed for carcinoma,[68] sarcoma,[25,69,70] osteogenic sarcoma[24,70] and other histologies.[71,72] Unfortunately, because of the limited sensitivity of the present radiographic studies, as well as the differing philosophies among different thoracic surgeons regarding how many nodules to remove, such a factor cannot be predicted unless the patient undergoes exploration. One must, therefore, define what *is* resectability in this situation. Any disease outside the confines of the visceral envelope (*i.e.,* pleural metastases, diaphragmatic involvement, discontinuous pericardial involvement, presence of pleural effusion histologically positive for malignancy, and tumor involvement of lymph nodes) must be considered unresectable disease and must be recorded as such. Moreover, if the patient's pulmonary functions are limiting and one cannot remove all disease for fear of irreversible pulmonary compromise, this is also an unresectable situation.

NUMBER OF METASTASES RESECTED

It would seem logical that the presence of a large number of metastases would have a more grave prognosis for patients undergoing metastasectomy than for those with few metastases. Indeed, in the early studies from the National Cancer Institute, longer postthoracotomy survival time was associated with fewer metastases.[25] Patients with resectable disease and 15 or fewer metastases had a longer postthoracotomy survival than did patients with 16 or more. Unfortunately, only 3 patients had 16 or more nodules. In a more recent study of 74 patients over a more modern era (1982–1987), however, no differences in long-term survival were found in completely resected patients who had one to four metastases as opposed to five or more metastases (Fig. 61–14).[69] The absence of correlation with number of metastases removed at operation, at least for the sarcoma patient, has also been pointed out in other more recent studies.[70] In osteogenic sarcoma[24] and Ewing's sarcoma,[71] if four or more nodules are resected there will likely be increased survival with less burden of disease. In colon cancer, a poor prognosis has been noted when there is more than one metastasis.[73] In patients with breast carcinoma, however, there does not seem to be a correlation with survival and number of metastases resected.[74] No correlation between solitary or multiple metastases and survival has been reported in other series with varying histologies (Table 61–9).[75]

The survival of patients after pulmonary metastasectomy *may* be more influenced by the completeness of resection, regardless of the number of nodules, in the face of extrathoracic disease control. Such an aggressive approach, however, still needs to be tempered by the biology of the metastasis kinetics, as seen with disease-free interval.

DISEASE-FREE INTERVAL

With the exception of the report by Pastorini,[70] there is general agreement that the resection of pulmonary metastases from osteogenic and soft tissue sarcoma is influenced by the disease-free interval from the time of the primary tumor resection to the removal of the pulmonary metastases (see Table 61–9). An original series of 93 patients with soft tissue sarcoma metastases from 1974 to 1982[25] and a second series resected from 1982 to 1987 both confirmed that a disease-free interval of less than a year was associated with a poor survival after metastasectomy (Fig. 61–15).[69] Other studies have confirmed this finding.[68,76] The importance of the disease-free interval was not seen in Ewing's sarcoma,[71] or most recently in me-

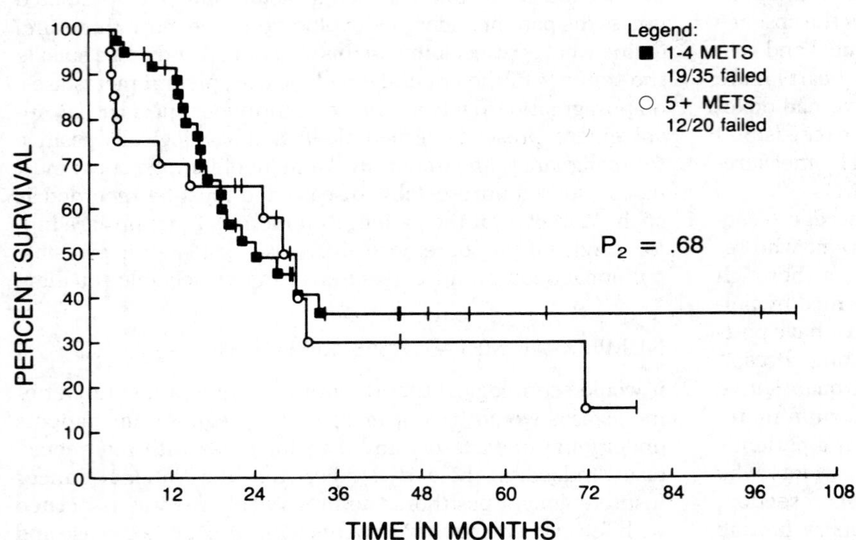

FIGURE 61–14. Survival rates of sarcoma patients. No difference in survival was noted in patients who were completely resected of pulmonary metastases from soft tissue sarcoma at the National Cancer Institute (NCI) from 1982 to 1987. (Reproduced with permission from Jablons D, Steinberg SM, Roth J, Pittaluga S, Rosenberg SA, Pass HI. Metastasectomy for soft tissue sarcoma. J Thorac Cardiovasc Surg 1989;97:695–705)

tastasectomy for colon cancer.[73] Breast cancer metastases that occurred less than 1 year after the primary resection were associated with a decreased survival after metastasectomy.[74]

One of the more intriguing subcategories of biologic factors involves patients with *synchronous lung metastases* at the time of the primary tumor resection. Putnam found that only 46% of such patients with synchronous pulmonary metastases in primary tumors could have their pulmonary metastases resected.[25] However, those patients with synchronous presentation who were completely resected had the same survival as patients with metachronous metastases. Such a finding has been documented in Ewing's sarcoma[71] and carcinoma,[68] as well as in renal cell cancer metastases.[77]

TUMOR DOUBLING TIME

There has been much effort to document that tumor doubling time correlates positively with prognosis after resection (*i.e.*, the shorter the doubling time, the shorter the survival). One must consider whether it is wise to measure tumor doubling

TABLE 61–9. Prognostic Factors for Pulmonary Metastasectomy

Histology	*Investigations*	*No. of Patients*	*Correlation With Survival*
Disease-Free Interval			
Carcinoma–Sarcoma	Vogt-Moykopf[68]	368	Negative ≤3 y vs >3 y
Sarcoma	Liennard[76]	19	Negative ≤1 y vs >1 y
Sarcoma	Jablons[69]	74	Negative ≤1 y vs >1 y
Sarcoma	Pastorini[87]	56	None
Ewing's sarcoma	Lanza[71]	19	None
Melanoma	Pogrebniak[106]	33	None
Colon	McAfee[73]	139	None
Breast	Lanza[74]	44	Negative ≤1 y vs >1 y
Renal cell	Pogrebniak[77]	23	None
Number of Metastases Resected			
Carcinoma–Sarcoma	Vogt-Moykopf[68]	386	None
Carcinoma–Sarcoma	Venn[75]	118	None
Sarcoma	Jablons[69]	74	None
Sarcoma	Pastorini[87]	56	None
Ewing's sarcoma	Lanza[71]	19	Negative >4 y
Melanoma	Pogrebniak[106]	33	None
Colon	McAfee[73]	139	Negative >1 y
Breast	Lanza[74]	44	None
Renal cell	Pogrebniak[77]	23	None

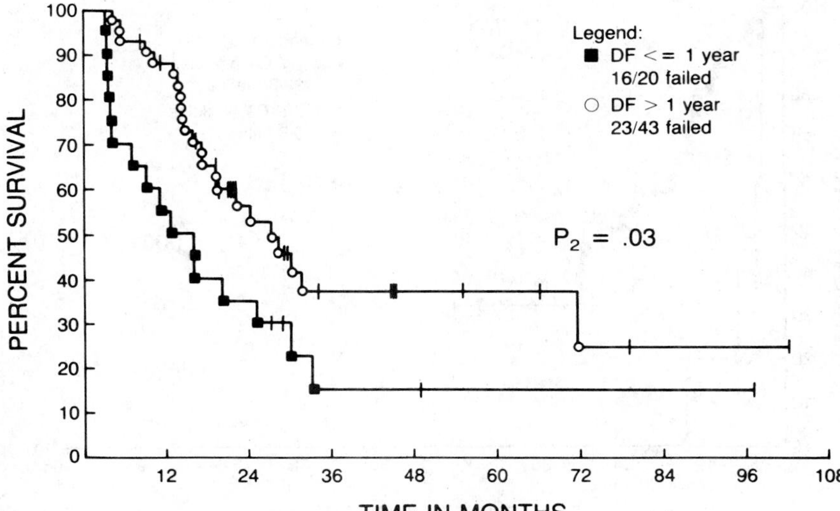

FIGURE 61–15. Survival rates of sarcoma patients. A disease-free interval of less than 1 year correlated with shorter long-term survival in patients resected for metastatic soft tissue sarcoma. (Reproduced with permission from Jablons D, Steinberg SM, Roth J, Pittaluga S, Rosenberg SA, Pass HI. Metastasectomy for soft tissue sarcoma. J Thorac Cardiovasc Surg 1989;97:695–705)

time in these patients, especially if the patient has a resectable number of metastases on preoperative studies, is able to tolerate thoracotomy, and has a substantial disease-free interval. Without denying that there is probably prognostic significance for a rapidly doubling tumor,[25,78,79] it is probably safe to say that serial examination of CT scans in patients with a known or developing abnormality should be reserved only for those rare instances when the nodule is not distinct, or where there is a history (*i.e.*, pneumonitis, septic emboli) that would suggest that the abnormality may resolve within a period of 1 or 2 months. In most patients considered for metastasectomy, the nodule will be of new onset, no other standard therapies will be available, and the procedure will be possible if the patient has the physiologic reserve and his peripheral workup is negative. Therefore, delaying the surgery (especially with a risk of mortality of less than 1%) in order to document a tumor doubling time seems unnecessary. An examination of the recent literature also reveals this "deemphasis" on the tumor doubling time as a useful prognostic factor.[80]

PREOPERATIVE RADIOGRAPHIC STUDIES

It seems pointless to use the preoperative number of nodules as a prognostic factor because the absolute number of metastases resected may not correlate with long-term survival as long as the patient can be rendered completely free of disease. At the time the preoperative studies are performed, however, it is not known with 100% certainty that the patient is, indeed, resectable. Moreover, the number of nodules seen on the preoperative studies will always underestimate the number of nodules resected by as much as a factor of 2.[2] Unfortunately, a systematic analysis of the number of nodules on preoperative studies has been performed only in the osteogenic and soft tissue sarcoma situation. Putnam found, in his analysis on the number of nodules on preoperative conventional lung tomograms, that survival was significantly prolonged in patients with osteogenic and soft tissue sarcoma if there were four or fewer nodules.[25] Jablons noted in a follow-up report that when computed tomography was adopted as standard for roentgenographic surveillance at the National Cancer Institute, patients with six or more CT nodules had a significantly decreased survival (Fig. 61–16).[69] One must remember, however, that these numbers are somewhat artificial because they include patients who were found to be unresectable at the time of thoracotomy.

OTHER PROGNOSTIC VARIABLES EXAMINED

NODAL STATUS

It is rare that the nodal status of patients with resection of pulmonary metastases is noted, because if they are deemed to have mediastinal disease on preoperative studies, they are not offered surgery. Nevertheless, the survival of patients with soft tissue sarcoma found to have hilar or mediastinal involvement is significantly poorer than that of patients not found to have nodal involvement.[25,69,79]

UNILATERAL VERSUS BILATERAL METASTASES

No correlation of unilaterality or bilaterality with survival is noted if the patients are completely resected.[25]

AGE/SEX

Neither age nor sex correlates with survival after metastasectomy.

ADJUVANT CHEMOTHERAPY

There are no randomized studies to compare survival of patients who receive postoperative or preoperative adjunctive chemotherapy along with metastasectomy with survival of those who do not receive this treatment. Nevertheless, in a subset of 32 patients from the National Cancer Institute who did not receive chemotherapy after their primary sarcoma

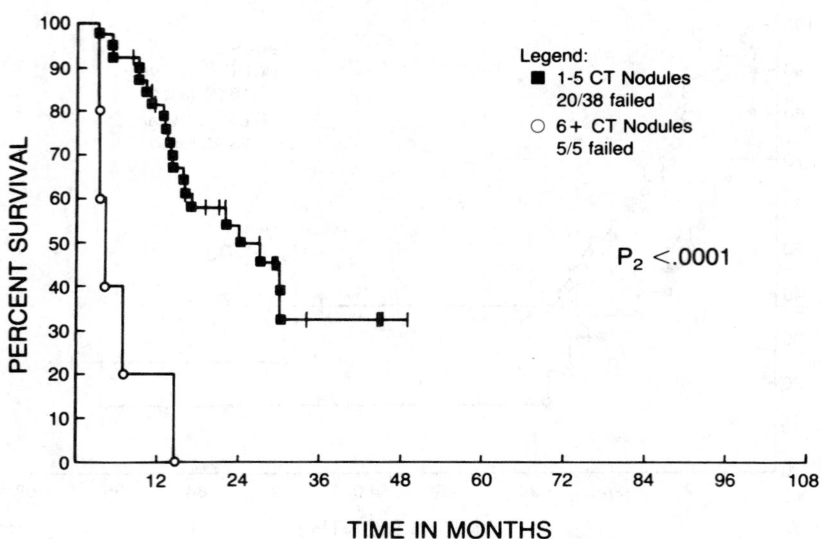

FIGURE 61–16. Survival rates of sarcoma patients. Patients with six or more nodules from metastatic soft tissue sarcoma to the lungs have decreased survival compared with patients with five or fewer nodules noted by computed tomography. (Reproduced with permission from Jablons D, Steinberg SM, Roth J, Pittaluga S, Rosenberg SA, Pass HI. Metastasectomy for soft tissue sarcoma. J Thorac Cardiovasc Surg 1989;97:695–705)

was resected, 15 received chemotherapy after the metastases and 17 did not. No survival differences were noted between the two groups.[69] Similarly, in a study from the M.D. Anderson Cancer Center, the survival after resection of pulmonary metastases from soft tissue sarcoma could not be accurately predicted based on the clinical response to the preoperative chemotherapy.[81]

TECHNIQUE OF PULMONARY METASTASECTOMY

The technique of pulmonary metastasectomy has been standardized and essentially involves the median sternotomy or lateral thoracotomy approach. Double-lumen endotracheal tubes (Fig. 61–17) are used to totally collapse the lung for a thorough exploration. The thoracic cavity, including the mediastinum, the chest wall, and the hilar nodes are thoroughly explored. Palpable abnormalities that do not appear to be obvious granulomas or intrapulmonary lymph nodes are excised with the automatic stapling device (Fig. 61–18). For peripheral lesions, a Duval lung clamp can be positioned on either side of the nodule, and for small nodules, the nodule can be positioned in the cutout portion of the clamp. The 30-, 55-, or 90-mm automatic stapling device is then placed across the base of the lesion depending on its size. Deeper lung lesions may require use of the GIA (gastrointestinal anastomosis) stapler, which simultaneously cuts and staples. Resection of metastases with the lung inflated will prevent removal of excessive lung tissue and still provide an adequate margin. For lesions that cannot be removed by wedge resection without ensuring a negative margin, lobectomy or segmentectomy can be performed if the patient's pulmonary reserve is adequate to support such anatomic resection.

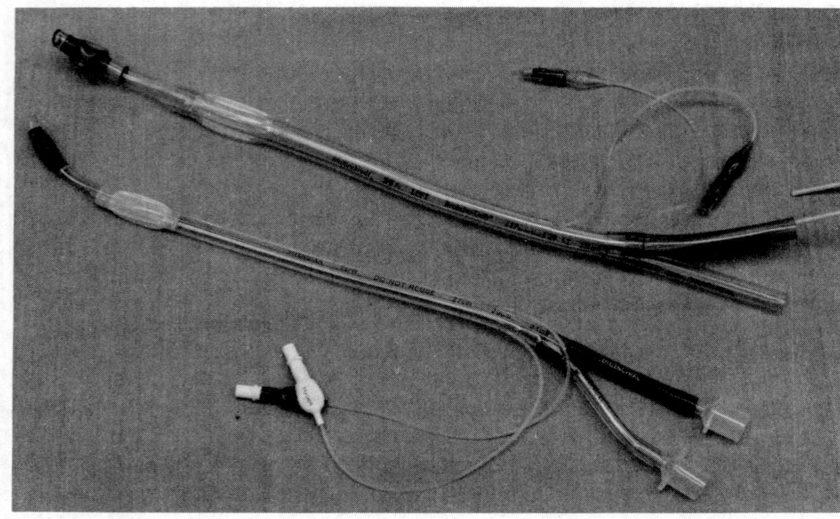

FIGURE 61–17. Double-lumen endotracheal tubes, both adult and child size, are a prerequisite to the proper performance of pulmonary metastasectomy. Other bronchial blockade methods can be used; however, these tubes are the most convenient technique for one-lung anesthesia.

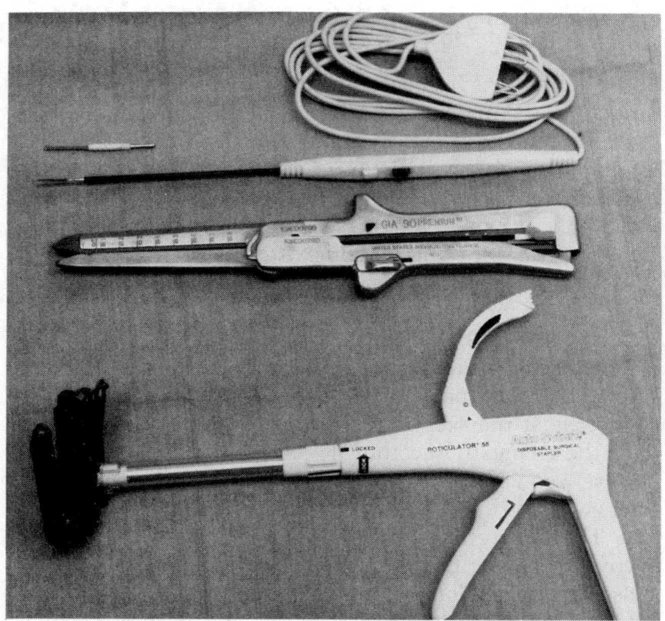

FIGURE 61–18. The long-handled electrocautery, the gastrointestinal anastomosis stapling device, and the standard or roticulated stapling machines are the surgeon's primary tools for accomplishing metastasectomy.

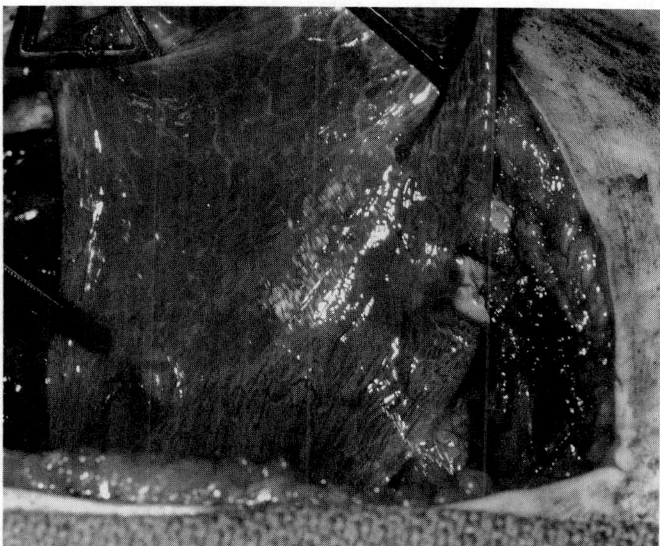

FIGURE 61–20. Typical appearance, by the use of double-lumen anesthesia, of a nodular pulmonary metastasis in a lung that is collapsed.

MEDIAN STERNOTOMY OR THORACOTOMY?

The desired approach, if feasible, for the removal of pulmonary metastases is the use of the median sternotomy.[69,70,72] Both lungs can be palpated simultaneously, and frequently unsuspected metastases not detected by radiographic methods will be found (Fig. 61–19). There are no differences, however, with regard to long-term survival advantage, morbidity, or mortality when comparing median sternotomy with lateral thoracotomy.[19] The avoidance of a second procedure (because of the necessity for staged thoracotomies for patients with bilateral disease), however, is probably advantageous. Moreover, with few exceptions, any procedure related to the eradication of pulmonary metastatic disease can be performed by sternotomy once the surgeon becomes comfortable with the approach. Wide mediastinal exposure, complete lung collapse, placement of posterior packs and elevation of the lung with lung clamps, and release of the inferior pulmonary ligament are all maneuvers to facilitate the operation. The anesthesiologist must be alerted when the surgeon is placing traction on the pulmonary vein so that he can carefully monitor blood pressure and rhythm changes. Early decisions should be made regarding the necessity for a formal resection, and if there are ten or more nodules on one side, or a lesion requires anatomic lobectomy or segmentectomy, the contralateral lung should be explored for location, size, and number of nodules before resecting the first side, to rule out an unresectable situation (Fig. 61–20). Concomitant procedures, such as chest wall resection (Fig. 61–21), can be performed through the

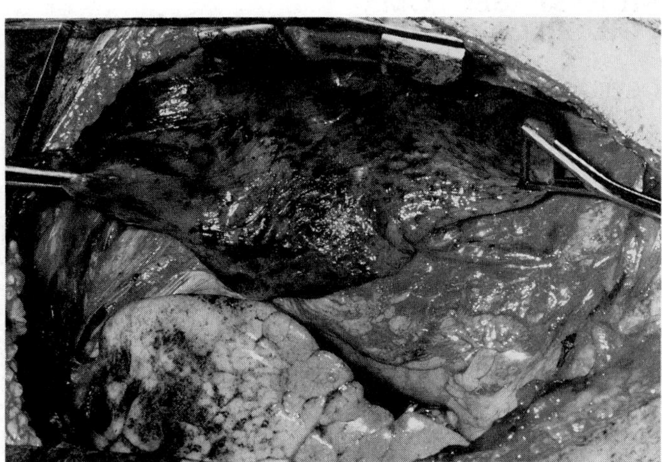

FIGURE 61–19. Wide exposure by way of the median sternotomy. The patient's head is to the left; the left upper lobe is collapsed and grasped with lung clamps. Inferiorly and to the right, the right lung is expanded, as seen through the widely opened pleura.

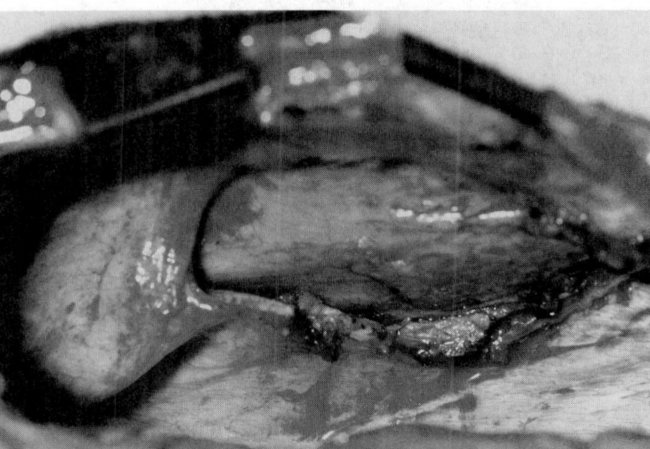

FIGURE 61–21. View from the median sternotomy to the left chest. A chest wall resection has been accomplished completely through the sternotomy, and just above the resected pleura is the posterior fascia of the pectoralis major.

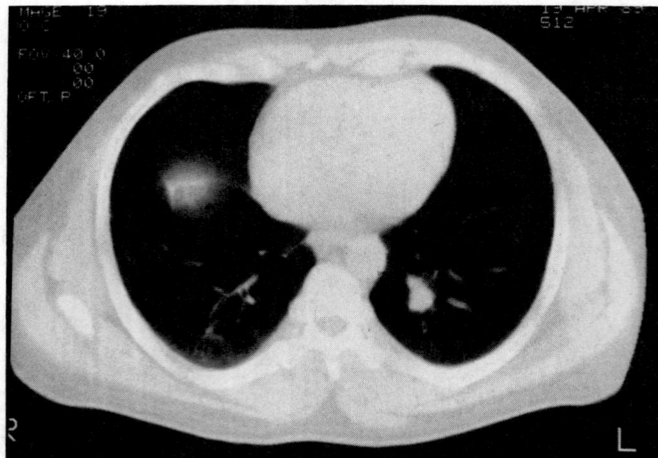

FIGURE 61–22. Computed tomographic scan of a parenchymal renal cell metastasis in the basilar segment of the left lower lobe.

median sternotomy approach. The most difficult resection by this technique, of course, is a left lower lobectomy, but even this can be performed in most patients without difficulty (Figs. 61–22 and 61–23).

There are a few preoperative hints, however, that may make lateral thoracotomy preferable to median sternotomy. Very large posterior or central lesions, specifically in the left lower lobe, may force one to abandon the median sternotomy approach and perform initial or concomitant left lateral thoracotomy. Previous sternal irradiation should probably be an absolute contraindication to the midline approach because of poor wound healing. Central staple line recurrences, posteromedial chest wall disease, and the preoperative assessment of the necessity for a sleeve-type resection also usually dictate a lateral thoracotomy approach. Finally, exposure of the mediastinum becomes difficult in obese individuals with a large heart and a narrow retrosternal space, and these patients should probably be explored through a lateral thoracotomy.

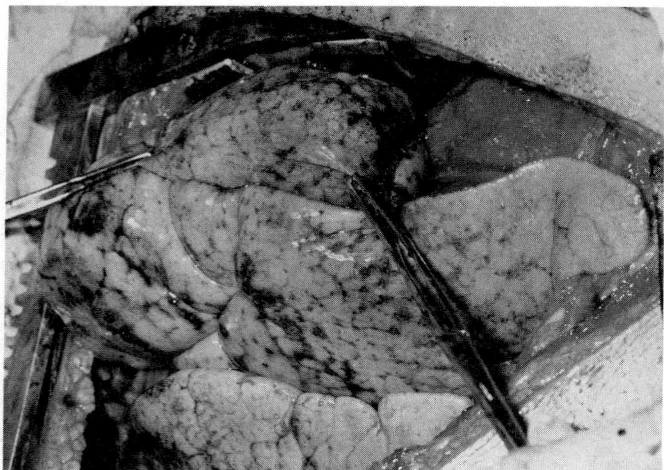

FIGURE 61–23. Operative photograph of the completed resection of the basilar segment of the left lower lobe of the patient whose computed tomographic scan is depicted in Figure 61–22. The lung clamps are holding the superior segment of the left lower lobe, just medial to which is the left upper lobe. The right lung is seen inferiorly.

REOPERATIVE METASTASECTOMY

Some institutions have attempted to define an aggressive approach for the management of patients who present with recurrent pulmonary metastases.[82–84] In most histologies, it is unknown whether reresection of pulmonary metastases is associated with a long-term survival benefit. There are data, however, that support the reresection of pulmonary metastases in metastatic soft tissue sarcoma. At the National Cancer Institute since 1976, 43 patients have had two or more thoracic explorations for the purpose of resecting pulmonary metastases by way of 89 reexplorations through either a median sternotomy or a lateral thoracotomy. There was an operative mortality of 0%, and 31 of the 43 patients were rendered free of disease at the second thoracotomy. The median survival from the second thoracotomy for the patients with resectable disease was 25 months, whereas the median survival of patients who had unresectable disease was 10 months (Fig. 61–24). There were no fixed guidelines with regard to the operative approach; however, after four median sternotomies, subsequent resections were performed by the lateral thoracotomy. The majority of these resections, despite reexploration, were wedge resections. A disease-free interval of more than 18 months between the first and second thoracotomies was associated with prolonged survival after the second thoracotomy. Other than resectability and disease-free interval (Fig. 61–25), no other factors in an unvaried analysis could foretell the long-term survival benefit.[83] A similar series of patients from the M.D. Anderson Cancer Center with adult soft tissue sarcoma have also been analyzed with regard to reoperative pulmonary metastasectomy. In the series of 39 patients undergoing two or more metastasectomies, a significantly longer median survival was found for the 34 patients whose recurrent metastases could be completely resected.[84] In that particular series, the only factor predicting longer postthoracotomy survival was the resection of a solitary metastatic nodule. Patients who had two or more recurrent nodules resected had a median survival of 14 months only.

METASTASECTOMY FOR SPECIFIC HISTOLOGIES

OSTEOGENIC SARCOMA

Before the use of aggressive resection of pulmonary metastases from osteogenic sarcoma, the survival of amputated patients was poor, with 5-year disease-free survival rates of 17% (Table 61–10).[85] The development of pulmonary metastases in 80% of these patients within the first year was associated with a 50% death rate in that first year after the primary resection. When resection was coupled with neoadjuvant or adjuvant programs including methotrexate, vincristine, and doxorubicin, a significant increase in salvage of these patients was documented by Telander at the Mayo Clinic (1946–1974: 5-year survival, 23%; versus 1974–1977: 5-year survival, 57%)86 and Pastorini (1970–1983: 3-year survival, 20%; versus 1984–1988: 3-year survival, 46%).[87] It is impossible, however, to sort out the relative contribution of the intensive chemotherapeutic approach or the aggressive surgical resection to the prolongation of survival in these patients. The gen-

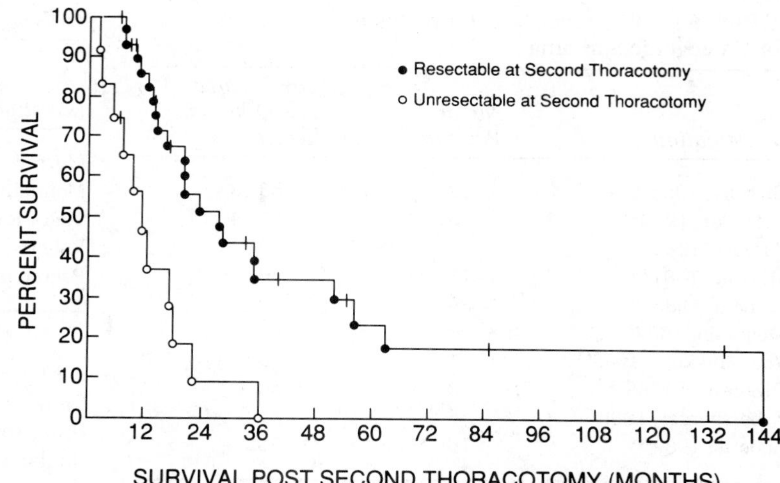

FIGURE 61–24. Reoperative metastasectomy in patients with soft tissue sarcoma can provide long-term survival in completely resected individuals.

erally accepted 5-year salvage rate for osteogenic sarcoma is now 35% to 40%, justifying initial and repeated metastasectomies in this patient population.[24,68,88–95]

SOFT TISSUE SARCOMA

Metastases from soft tissue sarcomas occur within the first 2 years of the primary tumor management and are confined to the lung in the majority of patients. Multiple series have now documented that approximately a 33% salvage rate with aggressive or repeated metastasectomies can be accomplished (Table 61–11).[25,68,69,95–97] At the National Cancer Institute, two time periods with separate groups of patients have confirmed a 32% and 35% 3-year survival rate from the initial thoracotomy in the soft tissue sarcoma population.[25,69] The disease-free interval, the ability to render patients free of disease, and possibly the number of nodules in preoperative studies seem to correlate with survival. No correlation with the number of metastases resected has been seen in the most recent study of patients rendered free of disease with soft tissue sarcoma; therefore, there are no guidelines regarding an unresectable number of nodules as long as the patient has been left with sufficient pulmonary reserve at the completion of the resection.

URINARY TRACT CANCER

Approximately half of all patients with renal cell cancer will present with or develop pulmonary metastases.[77] There have been multiple reports of the efficacy of resection of renal cell pulmonary metastases, with 5-year survival ranging from 13% to 50% and median survival ranging from 23 to 33 months (Table 61–12).[68,77,90,92,93] Unfortunately, however, in addition to analyzing patients having resection of pulmonary metastases, the majority of these studies also include patients who underwent resection of isolated extrapulmonary metastases in the brain, in bone, or in adrenal, subcutaneous, or other sites. Pogrebniak analyzed the results of metastasectomy in 23 patients who underwent resection of pulmonary metastases from renal cell carcinoma between 1985 and 1991.[77] Mean survival from exploration was 43 months, and survival after resection did not correlate with the number of nodules on preoperative tomograms, the number of nodules resected, or the disease-free interval. Patients who underwent complete

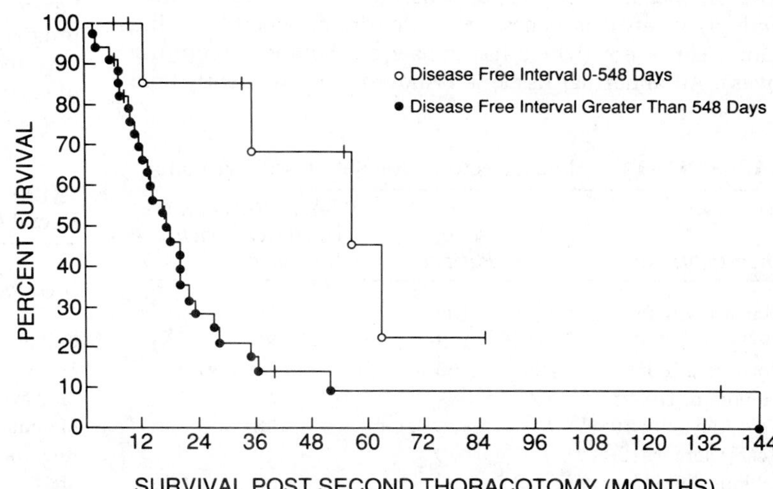

FIGURE 61–25. A disease-free interval of more than 1.5 years between thoracotomies is associated with longer survivals in patients having re-resection of soft tissue sarcoma pulmonary metastases.

TABLE 61–10. Metastasectomy Results for Osteogenic Sarcoma

Investigations	*No. of Patients*	*5-Year Survival (%) Unless Otherwise Indicated*
Giritsky, 1986[88]	12	58 (3 y)
Telander, 1978[86]	28	57 (4 y)
Burgess, 1980[89]	6	60
Morrow, 1981[90]	11	36
Putnam, 1983[24]	39	40
Mountain, 1984[26]	56	51
Vogt-Moykopf, 1988[68]	41	33 (3 y)
DiLorenzo, 1988[94]	10	50
Eckersberger, 1988[95]	6	31
Roberts, 1989[93]	16	23

resection of metastatic disease had a significantly longer survival (mean of 49 months) than did patients who were incompletely resected (median of 16 months). There is no general agreement in other studies regarding the importance of synchronous versus metachronous lesions, number of nodules on preoperative studies, or number of nodules resected. The number of metastases resected in Pogrebniak's study did not correlate with survival as long as the patient could be rendered free of disease at exploration. The majority of the patients in Pogrebniak's studies received biologic modifiers (*i.e.*, interleukin-2 [IL-2]). The contribution of this therapy to long-term survival cannot be sorted out at this time, but future studies, specifically in renal cell cancer patients who receive immunotherapy, may point to synergistic benefits of treatment with immunotherapy and metastatic pulmonary resection.[98]

TESTICULAR CANCER

Nonseminomatous germ cell tumors of the testis are characterized by wide dissemination, including pulmonary metastases and extreme sensitivity to chemotherapy. Indications for thoracotomy in these patients are: (1) when there is no response to chemotherapy, (2) when there is partial response followed by recurrence while on chemotherapy, (3) when there are no chemotherapy options, but markers begin to rise, and (4) when it is necessary to determine whether viable tumor is present (which has impact on therapeutic alternatives). All abnormal tissue is removed, and frequently only

TABLE 61–11. Metastasectomy for Soft Tissue Sarcoma

Investigations	*No. of Patients*	*5-Year Survival (%) Unless Otherwise Indicated*
Martini, 1978[96]	102	26
Creagen, 1979[97]	112	29
Putnam, 1984[25]	63	30 (3 y)
Mountain, 1984[26]	49	33
Vogt-Moykopf, 1988[68]	56	33
Eckersberger, 1988[95]	29	18
Jablons, 1989[69]	68	33

TABLE 61–12. Metastasectomy for Urinary Tract Cancer

Investigations	*No. of Patients*	*5-Year Survival (%) Unless Otherwise Indicated*
Morrow, 1981[90]	30	24
Mountain, 1984[26]	20	54
Vogt-Moykopf, 1988[68]	42	42
Roberts, 1989[93]	33	24
Pogrebniak, 1991[77]	23	43 mo (mean)

benign teratomas (because of successful chemotherapy) are found.[68,75,90,92] In a recent report, 24 patients with both retroperitoneal disease and metastatic pulmonary disease of testicular germ cell cancer who received preoperative chemotherapy had synchronous sternotomy and retroperitoneal lymph node dissection.[99] Overall, chemotherapy altered metastases to mature teratomas in the majority of patients, and among 22 patients with necrotic masses, 19 were long-term survivors. The overall cure rate for patients with this disseminated testicular cancer was approximately 80%, and that of the entire thoracic surgical group was 74%.

HEAD AND NECK

With the exception of the lip, tonsil, and adenoid, the lung is the first site of recurrence for head and neck cancer including the nose, nasopharynx, larynx, mouth, tongue, salivary glands, and oropharynx. In these patients, there is a high prevalence for second primary lung cancers. Resection is indicated to rule out either the possibility of a new primary tumor or metastases, with 5-year salvage rates of close to 44%.[68,92,100]

COLORECTAL CANCER

A minority of patients with colorectal cancer (1%) will present with isolated pulmonary metastases (as opposed to the liver) as the first site of recurrence. Although certain authors have stressed a difference in survival when comparing resection of colon with resection of rectal metastases, most series have not separated their results, and survival rates are 13% to 61% (Table 61–13).[73,90,92,93,100,101] The largest series of patients has recently demonstrated a 5-year survival of 31%.[73] Poor prognostic indicators include more than one metastasis and elevated carcinoembryonic antigen. Aggressive management of extrapulmonary disease, in addition to the pulmonary metastases, also results in equal 5-year survival rates.

TABLE 61–13. Metastasectomy for Colon and Rectal Cancer

Invesigations	*No. of Patients*	*5-Year Survival (%)*
Cahan, 1974[101]	31	31
McCormack, 1979[103]	40	15
Morrow, 1981[90]	16	13
Mountain, 1984[26]	28	28
Roberts, 1989[93]	13	23
McAfee, 1991[73]	139	30

BREAST

Approximately 21% of breast cancer patients will die of isolated metastases to the lung that were potentially resectable during the course of the disease, and despite the large number of cases of breast cancer, there are few reports concerning the efficacy of metastasis resection. Mountain and colleagues originally reported a 5-year survival rate of 27%,[92] while Wright[102] and McCormack[103] had 5-year survival rates of 27% and 30%, respectively. A recent series from the M.D. Anderson Cancer Center reports a 50% 5-year survival in 37 patients after complete resection of their metastatic breast cancer.[74] A disease-free interval of more than 1 year correlated with enhanced survival. Such increases in survival may also relate to improved and more intensive chemotherapy regimens, yet the individual contributions of surgery and chemotherapy cannot be separated.

MELANOMA

As seen in Table 61–14, metastasectomy for malignant melanoma has been generally unrewarding.[90,92,104,105] This has been recently documented at the National Cancer Institute, where 49 patients had resection of presumed pulmonary metastases from melanoma between 1970 and 1986.[106] Median survival for all patients with malignant disease was 13 months, and survival after resection did not correlate with Clark level, lymph node status, disease-free interval, or number of nodules on preoperative tomogram. Two of 10 patients with one nodule resected were long-term survivors. Nevertheless, 16 patients were found to have only benign disease, despite the appearance of a new nodule in 13. Hence, exploration in patients with presumed metastases from melanoma may be justified simply to rule out benign disease, even if a new solitary nodule is detected. In general, however, the multiplicity of nodules, as well as the unfavorable natural history independent of pulmonary disease, rules out melanoma as a favorable histology for metastasectomy.

TABLE 61–14. Metastasectomy for Other Histologies

Investigations	*No. of Patients*	*5-Year Survival (%) Unless Otherwise Indicated*
Testicular Cancer		
Morrow, 1981[90]	6	30
Mountain, 1984[26]	20	54
Venn, 1989[75]	42	84
Vogt-Moykopf, 1988[68]	42	82 (2 y)
Head and Neck Cancers		
McCormack, 1979[103]	25	44
Mountain, 1984[26]	48	41
Vogt-Moykopf, 1988[68]	12	44
Uterine–Cervical Cancer		
Morrow, 1981[90]	22	8
Mountain, 1984[26]	34	24
Breast Cancer		
McCormack, 1979[103]	34	30
Mountain, 1984[26]	30	27
Wright, 1982[102]	18	27
Lanza, 1991[74]	37	50
Melanoma		
Morrow, 1981[90]	12	12
Dahlback, 1980[104]	8	7-mo median
Cahan, 1973[105]	12	33
Mountain, 1984[26]	58	13-mo median
Pogrebniak, 1988[106]	33	13-mo median

REFERENCES

1. Willis RA. Secondary tumors of the lung. In: The spread of tumors in the human body. London: Butterworths, 1973:167–174.
2. Pass HI, Dwyer A, Makuch R, Roth JA. Detection of pulmonary metastases in patients with osteogenic and soft tissue sarcoma: The superiority of CT scan compared with conventional linear tomograms using dynamic analyses. J Clin Oncol 1985;3:1261–1265.
3. Viadana E, Irwin D, Bross J, Pickren JW. Cascade spread of blood-borne metastases in solid and non-solid cancers of humans. In: Weiss L, Gilbert H, eds. Pulmonary metastasis. Boston: GK Hall, 1978:143–167.
4. van Dongen JA, van Slooten EA. The surgical treatment of pulmonary metastases. Cancer Treat Rep 1978;5:29–48.
5. Barney JD, Churchill ED. Adeno-carcinoma of the kidney with metastasis to the lungs treated by pulmonary resection. J Urol 1939;42:269–276.
6. Alexander J, Haight C. Pulmonary resection for solitary metastatic sarcomas and carcinomas. Surg Gynecol Obstet 1947;85:129–135.
7. Thomford NR, Wodner LB, Clagett OT. The surgical treatment of metastatic tumors in the lungs. J Thorac Cardiovasc Surg 1965;49:357–363.
8. Martini N, Huvos AG, Mike V, et al. Multiple pulmonary resections in the treatment of osteogenic sarcoma. Ann Thorac Surg 1971;12:271–280.
9. Morton DL, Joseph WL, Ketcham AS, et al. Surgical resection and adjunctive immunotherapy for selected patients with multiple pulmonary metastases. Ann Surg 1973;178:360–365.
10. Liotta LA, Kleinerman J, Saidel FM. The significance of hematogenous tumor cell clumps in the metastatic process. Cancer Res 1976;36:889.
11. Dwyer AJ, Reichert CM, Woltering EA, et al. Diffuse pulmonary metastasis in melanoma: Radiographic pathologic correlation. AJR 1984;143:983.
12. Libshitz HI, North LB. Pulmonary metastases. Radiol Clin North Am 1982;20:437.
13. Berg HK, Petrelli NJ, Herrera L, et al. Endobronchial metastasis from colorectal carcinoma. Dis Colon Rectum 1984;27:745.
14. Shapshay SM, Strong MS. Tracheobronchial obstruction from metastatic distant malignancies. Ann Otol Rhinol Laryngol 1982;91:648.
15. Janower ML, Blennerhassett HJB. Lymphangitic spread of metastatic cancer to the lung. Radiology 1971;101:267.
16. Heitzman ER, Markarian B, Raasch BN, et al. Pathways of tumor spread through the lung: Radiologic correlations with anatomy and pathology. Radiology 1982;144:3.
17. Naidich DP, Zerhouni EA, Siegelman SS. Pleura and chest wall. In: Naidich DP, Zerhouni EA, Siegelman SS, eds. New York: Raven Press, 1984:261.
18. Cahan WG, Shah JP, Castro ELB. Benign solitary lung lesions in patients with cancer. Ann Surg 1978;187:241.
19. Roth JA, Pass HI, Wesley MN, et al. Comparison of median sternotomy and thoracotomy for resection of pulmonary metastases in patients with adult soft tissue sarcomas. Ann Thorac Surg 1986;42:134.
20. Hendin AS. Gestational trophoblastic tumors metastatic to the lung. Cancer 1984;53:58.
21. Wagner D. Trophoblastic cells in the blood stream in normal and abnormal pregnancy. Acta Cytol 1968;12:137.
22. Crow J, Slavin G, Kreel L. Pulmonary metastasis: A pathologic and radiologic study. Cancer 1981;47:2595.
23. Scholten ET, Kreel L. Distribution of lung metastases in the axial plane. Radiol Clin North Am 1977;46:248.
24. Putnam JB, Roth JA, Wesley MN, et al. Survival following aggressive resection of pulmonary metastases from osteogenic sarcoma: Analysis of prognostic factors. Ann Thorac Surg 1983;36:516.
25. Putnam JB, Roth JA, Wesley MN, et al. Analysis of prognostic factors in patients undergoing resection of pulmonary metastasis from soft tissue sarcomas. J Thorac Cardiovasc Surg 1984;87:260.
26. Mountain C. Surgery for pulmonary metastasis. Ann Thorac Surg 1984;38:323.
27. D'Angio GJ, Iannoccone G. Spontaneous pneumothorax as a complication of pulmonary metastases in malignant tumors of childhood. AJR 1961;86:1092.
28. Lodmell EA, Capps SC. Spontaneous pneumothorax associated with metastatic sarcoma: Report of three cases. Radiology 1949;52:88.
29. Macklin MT, Macklin CC. Malignant interstitial emphysema of the lungs and mediastinum as an important occult complication in many respiratory diseases and other conditions. Medicine 1944;23:281.
30. Lome LG, John T. Pulmonary manifestations of prostatic carcinoma. J Urol 1973;109:680.
31. Schwarz MI, Waddell LC, Dombeck DH, et al. Prolonged survival in lymphangitic carcinomatosis. Ann Intern Med 1969;71:779.

32. Sarno RC, Carter BL. Bullous change by CT heralding metastatic sarcoma. Comput Radiol 1985;9:115.
33. Morse D, Reed JO, Bernstein J. Sclerosing osteogenic sarcoma. AJR 1963;88:491.
34. Fraser RG, Pare JAP. Neoplastic disease of the lung. In: Fraser RG, Pare JAP, eds. Diagnosis of diseases of the chest. Philadelphia: WB Saunders, 1989:1630.
35. Zollikofer C, Castaneda-Zuniga W, Stenlund R, et al. Lung metastases from synovial sarcoma simulating granulomas. AJR 1980;135:161.
36. Rosenfield AT, Sanders RC, Custer LE. Widespread calcified metastases from adenocarcinoma of the jejunum. Am J Dig Dis 1975;20:990.
37. Fraley EE, Lange PH, Kennedy BJ. Germ cell testicular cancer in adults. N Engl J Med 1979;301:1370.
38. Panella J, Mintzer RA. Multiple calcified pulmonary nodules in an elderly man. JAMA 1980;244:2559.
39. King DS, Castleman B. Bronchial involvement in metastatic pulmonary malignancy. J Thorac Surg 1943;12:305.
40. Braman SS, Whitcomb ME. Endobronchial metastases. Arch Intern Med 1975;135: 543.
41. Shepherd MP. Endobronchial metastatic disease. Thorax 1982;37:362.
42. Pass HI, Roth JA. Diagnosis of pulmonary metastases. In: Rosenberg SA, ed. Surgical treatment of metastatic cancer. Philadelphia: JB Lippincott, 1987:37–67.
43. Cohen M, Grosfeld J, Baehner R, et al. Lung CT for detection of metastases: Solid tissue neoplasms in children. AJR 1982;139:895.
44. Piekarski JD, Schlumberger M, Leclere J, et al. Chest computed tomography (CT) in patients with micronodular lung metastases of differentiated thyroid carcinoma. Int J Radiat Oncol Biol Phys 1985;11:1023.
45. Lund G, Heilo A. Computed tomography of pulmonary metastases. Acta Radiol 1982;23: 617.
46. Sones PJ, Torres WE, Colvin RS, et al. Effectiveness of CT in evaluating intrathoracic masses. AJR 1982;139:469.
47. Krudy AG, Doppman JL, Herdt JR. Failure to detect a 1.5 cm lung nodule by chest computed tomography. J Comput Assist Tomogr 1982;6:1178.
48. Kuhns LR, Borlaza G. The "twinkling star" sign. An aid in differentiating pulmonary vessels from pulmonary nodules on computed tomograms. Radiology 1980;135:763.
49. Chiles C, Ravin CE. Intrathoracic metastasis from an extrathoracic malignancy: A radiographic approach to patient evaluation. Radiol Clin North Am 1985;23:427.
50. Feuerstein I, Jicha D, Pass HI, et al. A comparison of computerized tomography and magnetic resonance imaging for diagnosis of pulmonary metastases. Radiology 1992;182:123–129.
51. Vincent RG, Choksi LB, Takita H, et al. Surgical resection of the solitary pulmonary metastases. In: Weiss L, Gilbert HA, eds. Pulmonary metastases. Boston: GK Hall, 1978:224.
52. Johnston WW. Percutaneous fine needle aspiration biopsy of the lung: A study of 1,015 patients. Acta Cytol 1984;28:218.
53. Poellein S, Rothenberg J, Penkava RR. Metastatic malignant melanoma in the lung: Diagnosis by thin-needle aspiration biopsy. Arch Pathol Lab Med 1982;106:119.
54. Pilotti S, Rilke F, Gribaudi G, et al. Transthoracic fine needle aspiration biopsy in pulmonary lesions, updated results. Acta Cytol 1984;28:225.
55. Silverman JF, Weaver MD, Gardner EW, et al. Aspiration biopsy cytology of malignant schwannoma metastatic to the lung. Acta Cytol 1984;29:15.
56. Nieberg RK. Fine needle aspiration cytology of alveolar soft-part sarcoma. Acta Cytol 1984;228:198.
57. Nguyen GK, Jeannot A. Cytopathologic aspects of pulmonary metastasis of malignant fibrous histiocytoma, myxoid variant. Acta Cytol 1982;26:349.
58. Crosby JH, Hager B, Hoeg K. Transthoracic fine-needle aspiration. Cancer 1985;56: 2504.
59. Nordenstrom BEW. Technical aspects of obtaining cellular material from lesions deep in the lung. Acta Cytol 1984;28:233.
60. Page RD, Jeffrey RR, Donnelly RJ. Thoracoscopy: A review of 121 consecutive surgical procedures. Ann Thorac Surg 1989;48:66–68.
61. Bonniot JP, Homasson JF, Roden SL, Angebault ML, Renault PC. Pleural and lung cryobiopsies during thoracoscopy. Chest 1989;95:492–493.
62. Lewis RJ, Caccavale RJ, Sisler GE. Special report: Video-endoscopic thoracic surgery. N J Med 1991;88:473–475.
63. Inderbitzi R, Molnar J. Experiences in the diagnostic and surgical video-endoscopy of the thoracic cavity. Schweiz Med Wochenschr 1990;120:51–52.
64. Dresdale A, Bonow RO, Wesley R, et al. Prospective evaluation of doxorubicin-induced cardiomyopathy resulting from post-surgical adjuvant treatment of patients with soft tissue sarcomas. Cancer 1983;52:51–60.
65. Gottindiener JS, Mathisen DJ, Borer JS, et al. Doxorubicin cardiotoxicity: Assessment of late left ventricular dysfunction by radionuclide cineangiography. Ann Intern Med 1981;94:430–435.
66. Mason JW, Bristow MR, Billingham ME, et al. Invasive and noninvasive methods of assessing Adriamycin cardiotoxic effects in man: Superiority of histopathologic assessment using endomyocardial biopsy. Cancer Treat Rep 1978;62:857–864.
67. Boysen PG, Block AJ, Olsen GN, et al. Prospective evaluation for pneumonectomy using the 99m technetium quantitative perfusion lung scan. Chest 1977;72:422–425.
68. Vogt-Moykopf I, Bulzebruck H, Merkle NM, Probst G. Results of surgical treatment of pulmonary metastases. Eur J Cardiothorac Surg 1988;2:224–232.
69. Jablons D, Steinberg SM, Roth J, Pittaluga S, Rosenberg SA, Pass HI. Metastasectomy for soft tissue sarcoma. J Thorac Cardiovasc Surg 1989;97:695–705.
70. Pastorini U, Valente M, Gasparini M, et al. Median sternotomy and multiple lung resections for metastatic sarcomas. Eur J Cardiothorac Surg 1990;4:477–481.
71. Lanza LA, Miser JS, Pass HI, Roth JA. The role of resection in the treatment of pulmonary metastases from Ewing's sarcoma. J Thorac Cardiovasc Surg 1987;94:181–187.
72. Regal A-M, Reese P, Antkowiak J, Hart T, Takita H. Median sternotomy for metastatic lung lesions in 131 patients. Cancer 1985;55:1334–1339.
73. McAfee MK, Allen MS, Trastek VF, Ilstrup DM, Deschamps C, Pairolero PC. Colorectal lung metastases: Results of surgical excision. Ann Thorac Surg 1992;53:780–786.
74. Lanza LA, Natarajan G, Roth JA, Putnam JB Jr. Long-term survival following resection of pulmonary metastases from carcinoma of the breast. Ann Thorac Surg 1992;54: 244–247.
75. Venn GE, Sarin S, Goldstraw P. Survival following pulmonary metastasectomy. Eur J Cardiothorac Surg 1989;3:105–110.
76. Linard D, Rocmans P, Lejeune FJ. Resection of lung metastases from sarcomas. Eur J Surg Oncol 1989;15:530–534.
77. Pogrebniak HW, Haas G, Linehan WM, Rosenberg SA, Pass HI. Renal cell carcinoma: Resection of solitary and multiple metastases. Ann Thorac Surg 1992;54:33–38.
78. Joseph WL, Morton DL, Adkins PC. Prognostic significance of tumor doubling time in evaluating operability in pulmonary metastatic disease. J Thorac Cardiovasc Surg 1971;61:23–32.
79. Takita H, Edgerton F, Karakousis C, et al. Surgical management of metastases to the lung. Surg Gynecol Obstet 1981;152:191–194.
80. Yellin A, Lieberman Y. Surgery for pulmonary metastases: Review of literature and experience at the Shaba Medical Center. In: Martini N, Vogt-Moykopf I, eds. Thoracic surgery: Frontiers and uncommon neoplasms. St. Louis: CV Mosby, 1989:275–284.
81. Lanza LA, Putnam JB Jr, Benjamin RS, Roth JA. Response to chemotherapy does not predict survival after resection of sarcomatous pulmonary metastases. Ann Thorac Surg 1991;51:219–224.
82. Rizzoni WE, Pass HI, Wesley MN, et al. Reoperative pulmonary metastasectomies in patients with adult soft-tissue sarcomas. Ann Thorac Surg 1986;121:1248–1252.
83. Pogrebniak HW, Roth JA, Steinberg SM, Rosenberg SA, Pass HI. Reoperative pulmonary resection in patients with metastatic soft tissue sarcoma. Ann Thorac Surg 1991;52: 197–203.
84. Casson AG, Putnam JB, Natarajan G, et al. Efficacy of pulmonary metastasectomy for recurrent soft tissue sarcoma. J Surg Oncol 1991;47:1–4.
85. Marcove RC, Mike V, Hajek JV, et al. Osteogenic sarcoma under the age of 21: A review of 145 operative cases. J Bone Joint Surg 1970;52:411–421.
86. Telander RL, Pairolero PC, Pritchard DJ. Resection of pulmonary metastatic osteogenic sarcoma in children. Surgery 1978;84:335–341.
87. Pastorini U, Valente M, Santoro A, et al. Results of salvage surgery for metastatic sarcomas. Annals of Oncology 1990;1:269–273.
88. Gritsky AS, Etcubanas E, Mark JBD. Pulmonary resection in children with metastatic osteogenic sarcoma. J Thorac Surg 1986;75:354–362.
89. Burgers JMV, Breur K, Van Dobbenburgh OA, et al. Role of metastasectomy without chemotherapy in the management of osteosarcoma in children. Cancer 1980;45:1664–1668.
90. Morrow CE, Vassilopoulos P, Grage TB. Surgical resection for metastatic neoplasms of the lung. Cancer 1981;45:2981–2985.
91. Meyer WH, Schell MJ, Kumar AP, et al. Thoracotomy for pulmonary metastatic osteosarcoma: An analysis of prognostic indicators of survival. Cancer 1987;59:374–379.
92. Mountain CF, McMurtrey MJ, Hermes KE. Surgery for pulmonary metastases: A 20-year experience. Ann Thorac Surg 1984;38:323.
93. Roberts DG, Lepore V, Cardillo G, Dernevik L, et al. Long-term follow-up of operative treatment for pulmonary metastases. Eur J Cardiothorac Surg 1989;3:292–296.
94. DiLorenzo M, Collin PP. Pulmonary metastases in children: Results of surgical treatment. J Pediatr Surg 1988;23:762–765.
95. Eckersberger F, Moritz E, Wolner E. Results and prognostic factors after resection of pulmonary metastases. Eur J Cardiothorac Surg 1988;2:433–437.
96. Martini N, McCormack PM, Bains MS, et al. Surgery for solitary and multiple pulmonary metastasis. N Y State J Med 1978;78:1711–1713.
97. Creagan ET, Fleming TR, Edmonson JH, Pairolero PC. Pulmonary resection for metastatic nonosteogenic sarcoma. Cancer 1979;44:1908–1912.
98. Sherry RM, Pass HI, Rosenberg SA, Yang JC. Surgical resection of metastatic renal cell carcinoma and melanoma after response to interleukin-2 based immunotherapy. Cancer 1992;69:1850–1855.
99. Mandelbaum I, Yaw PB, Einhorn LH, Williams SD, et al. The importance of one-stage median sternotomy and retroperitoneal node dissection in disseminated testicular cancer. Ann Thorac Surg 1983;36:524–528.
100. McCormack PM, Attiyeh FF. Resection of pulmonary metastases from colorectal cancer. Dis Colon Rectum 1979;22:553–556.
101. Cahan WG, Castro EB, Hajdu SI. The significance of a solitary lung shadow in patients with colon carcinoma. Cancer 1974;33:414–421.
102. Wright JO, Brandt B, Ehrenhaft JL. Results of pulmonary resection for metastatic lesions. J Thorac Cardiovasc Surg 1982;83:94–99.
103. McCormack PM, Martini N. The changing role of surgery for pulmonary metastases. Ann Thorac Surg 1979;41:833–840.
104. Dahlback O, Hafstrom L, Johnsson PE, et al. Lung resection for metastatic melanoma. Clin Oncol 1980;6:15–20.
105. Cahan WG. Excision of melanoma metastases to lung: Problems in diagnosis and management. Ann Surg 1973;178:703–709.
106. Pogrebniak HW, Stovroff M, Roth JsA, Pass HI. Resection of pulmonary metastases from malignant melanoma: Results of a 16-year experience. Ann Thorac Surg 1988;46: 20–23.

SECTION **3**

JOHN E. NIEDERHUBER
WILLIAM D. ENSMINGER

Treatment of Metastatic Cancer to the Liver

The spread of malignant cells from a primary tumor to the liver and their growth therein carry a grave prognosis for the patient. While these metastatic liver tumors may be the first evidence of the progression of a patient's cancer, and often—especially in colorectal cancer—are the only tumors detected, they almost always signal widespread dissemination of the malignancy. Despite improvements in early detection of liver metastases, new drug development, improved surgical techniques for resection, and innovative targeted therapies, most patients will not survive.

In spite of the gravity of the diagnosis of liver metastases, those responsible for treating such patients know of the occasional success of surgical resection with resultant long-term survival. It is this observation more than any other that has suggested the existence of at least a subset of patients whose metastases reach biologic significance only in their liver. The existence of such a subset of patients has been essentially the exclusive property of colorectal cancer. As such, it has been the rationale behind much of the effort to provide long-term survival and even cure for patients with isolated liver metastases by aggressive resection of their metastases and by innovative regional infusion of active agents.

An extensive literature documents the history of these efforts now spanning several decades. The task here is to provide a meaningful and timely review.

LIVER METASTASES FROM COLORECTAL CANCER

INCIDENCE

In 1992, more than 150,000 Americans will be diagnosed with colorectal cancer, and over 60,000 will die from this tumor. The incidence of colorectal cancer remains quite constant and is exceeded only by cancers of the breast, lung, and prostate.[1] At the time of diagnosis, 15% to 25% will have hepatic metastases, and another 20% to 30% will develop metastatic lesions subsequent to resection of their primary tumors. Ultimately, at least 50% of these 150,000 patients will die secondary to metastatic disease, and for many, progressive involvement of the liver will be a major determinant, or the only determinant, of their survival.[1–4] Although the overall mortality from colorectal cancer has decreased in recent years, patients with metastatic disease continue to face a grim prognosis.

NATURAL HISTORY

Metastatic tumors to the liver develop a rich blood supply and tend to grow rapidly. The natural progression of these lesions depends on a number of factors, including primary histologic type, extent of hepatic involvement, physiologic status of the liver parenchyma, and growth properties of the tumor cells. In addition, the extent of the primary lesion and whether local recurrences can be prevented (especially for rectal cancer) affect the overall survival of the patient.[5–9] Left untreated, metastatic lesions to the liver from colorectal cancers are associated with survival of 3 to 24 months.

Hepatic resection of colorectal metastases may be the only hope for "cure" in a select subgroup of patients. As a result, it has been difficult to subject patients with potentially "curable" hepatic metastases to prospective randomized trials where these lesions are left untreated in order to determine the natural progression of the disease and the ultimate survival benefit of resection. Historically, high operative mortality and morbidity rates associated with hepatic resections discouraged many physicians and surgeons from offering resection as a treatment option. Retrospective reviews, therefore, have provided some insight into the natural history of these lesions by analyzing groups of patients with tumors that would now be deemed "resectable" (Table 61–15).[2,7–19]

Table 61–15 summarizes multiple reports illustrating the poor clinical outcome in patients with intrahepatic metastases from colorectal cancers not surgically resected. It is important to note that these collective data are not categorized by extent of the primary lesions or extent of hepatic involvement. In some reports, patients with extensive metastatic disease (both intrahepatic and extrahepatic) were included. Although there are anecdotal reports of long-term survivors with hepatic lesions left untreated, it is clear from these reports that most patients die within 2 years of diagnosis—median survival for cited reviews is 6 months.[2,7–20] It is of interest to note that the recently published series have patients with longer median length of survival. This most likely reflects earlier detection of metastatic lesions secondary to the use of newer diagnostic modalities, and more aggressive monitoring of patients after resection of their primary tumor.

TABLE 61–15. Survival of Patients With Intrahepatic Colorectal Metastases

Investigations	*No. of Patients*	*Median Survival (mo)*	*5-Year Survivors*
Steele, 1991[7]	47	16.5	NA
Scheele, 1990[10]	983	6.9–14.2	0
Finan, 1985[11]	86	8–15.5	0
Wagner, 1984[12]	252	11–21	<5%
Lahr, 1983[13]	147	4.5–12	1
Goslin, 1982[9]	125	10–24	0
Boey, 1981[14]	73	6–9	0
Bengtsson, 1981[15]	25	3–6	0
Wood, 1976[2]	113	3–17	1
Baden, 1975[16]	105	10	1
Abrams, 1971[17]	58	7	0
Cady, 1970[8]	241	13	2
Bengmark, 1970[18]	38	6 (mean)	0
Sterns, 1954[19]	22	11	1

NA, not available.

DIAGNOSIS

The largest solid organ in the human body is the liver, and it is the most common site for many hematogenously disseminated tumors, with gastrointestinal tumors being the most frequent.[21–27] Modern modalities have aided early detection of colonic lesions, but until recently, secondary hepatic tumors were frequently diagnosed at advanced stages.

Physical findings and clinical symptoms are, perhaps, the least accurate means of diagnosing liver involvement by metastatic tumors. Clinical symptoms such as ascites, jaundice, and pain associated with large or rapidly growing hepatic tumors are a late and ominous sign. Other physical signs of metastatic disease, such as palpable nodularity at the liver edge or an audible bruit, are also late findings, and all carry a dismal prognosis, with most patients dying soon after diagnosis.[2,12,18,21]

Laboratory measurements of various tumor markers and liver enzymes are easily obtainable, and many patients can be screened with little expense and relative ease. Among those most commonly used are γ-glutamyl transpeptidase, aspartate aminotransferase, alkaline phosphatase, and carcinoembryonic antigen (CEA). Even though Wanebo and colleagues reported elevated CEA levels in approximately 90% of patients with metastases from colorectal cancer, most authors have been unable to correlate the extent of CEA elevation with prognosis.[7,28–30] Although there is some controversy as to the prognostic significance of these various laboratory values, CEA levels can be especially helpful when tracking patients after primary tumor resection and may be the first indication of potential recurrence of metastasis.

Preoperative assessment of liver function is often difficult when clinical evidence of cirrhosis is absent. Many authors have studied liver enzyme tests in an attempt to quantitate parenchymal reserve; however, it remains difficult to correlate these laboratory tests with capacity of the liver parenchyma to regenerate after resection. A multivariate regression analysis by Lahr and colleagues showed that abnormal liver function tests are independent factors that may predict median survival of patients with colorectal metastases to the liver.[13] They found that hyperbilirubinemia (1–5 mg/dl) was associated with a median survival of 2.5 months and a 1-year survival rate of 7%. Elevated alkaline phosphatase levels also predicted a poor prognosis, with a median survival of 2.5 months compared with 9.2 months in patients with normal values.[13,29] A commonly used assessment of liver function in selecting patients and assessing operative risk relies on Child's classification, and patients judged as Child's class A or B (Table 61–16) have a better prognosis.[64–66]

TABLE 61–16. Assessment of Liver Function With the Modified Child Classification

	Score		
Parameter	*1*	2	3
Serum bilirubin (mg/100 ml)	1–2	2–3	>3
Albumin (g/L)	>35	28–35	<28
Prothrombin time (seconds prolonged)	1–4	4–6	>6
Encephalopathy (grade)	—	1–2	3–4
Ascites	Absent	Slight	Moderate

Child group equivalents: A, 5–6 points; B, 7–9 points; C, 10–15 points. (Pugh RNH, Murray-Lyon IM, Danson JL, Pietroni MC, Williams R. Transsection of esophagus for bleeding varices. Br J Surg 1973;60: 646)

Improvements in radiographic studies of the liver, such as preoperative and intraoperative ultrasonography, contrast-enhanced computed tomography (CT), magnetic resonance imaging (MRI), and arteriography, have helped define the extent of metastatic disease and have aided the surgeon in planning resection of potentially "curable" lesions.

Ultrasound is the least expensive noninvasive radiologic test available to aid in the diagnosis of intrahepatic disease. Ultrasonic examination is highly dependent on the sophistication of the equipment used and the experience of the clinician interpreting the findings. In addition, results may vary in relation to patient obesity, amount of "bowel gas," and inability to detect lesions in anatomic regions of the liver that may be difficult to image. Nonetheless, preoperative ultrasound is very effective in detecting tumors 1 to 2 cm in size and in distinguishing solid from cystic (possibly benign) lesions.

Ultrasonic guidance is frequently used for directing percutaneous needle biopsies to obtain histologic diagnosis before operation. Intraoperative ultrasound can be extremely helpful in guiding the surgeon through segmental resections and can often identify metastases 2 to 4 mm in size deep within the liver parenchyma that would be missed by palpation. Recent experience with intraoperative ultrasound has supported the importance of this modality as the definitive step in assessing resectability.[22,31,36,70–72]

The early-generation CT scanners and many present scanners can detect intrahepatic lesions approximately 1 to 2 cm in diameter, but it is not uncommon for metastases to be missed on routine scanning. Enhancement of intraabdominal CT scans with intravenous contrast agents improves these results, and smaller liver tumors (0.5 cm) may be reliably detected.[32,67] Caution must be used when employing intravenous dyes because they can be associated with severe allergic reactions. CT scan also allows for assessment of other potential sites of metastases (*i.e.*, celiac, perihepatic, paraaortic lymph nodes, etc.) that may preclude or alter the possibility of a "curative" resection.

Magnetic resonance imaging can be very useful in visualizing hepatic tumors, and, as with CT, these images can be enhanced with specific contrast agents.[33–35] The role of MRI in the screening and staging of metastatic lesions in the liver is an evolving one, and determining surgical resectability of limited hepatic metastases by preoperative radiographic studies is an area of intense research. Several investigators have compared the sensitivity and specificity of CT versus MRI scans.[35,67–69] For example, Sitzmann and colleagues compared MRI, arteriographically enhanced CT, and routine CT screening of 100 patients with suspected hepatic metastases.[34] Enhanced CT (with portal arteriography) detected 94% of lesions, compared with 70% by MRI and 66% by routine CT. In particular, the sensitivity of enhanced CT was significantly greater than the sensitivity of MRI for lesions $\leq$1 cm (82% versus 20%). MRI, however, was significantly more accurate than CT in demonstrating vascular involvement.[67]

Some authors recommend MRI in the initial evaluation of hepatic lesions when trying to distinguish benign cysts or hemangiomas from malignant disease. There are several advantages to MRI in this setting: (1) intravenous contrast agents are not always needed, and (2) MRI can distinguish between benign and malignant tumors with a high degree of specificity (93%) and sensitivity (89%).[67,68] New techniques using superparamagnetic particulate iron oxide contrast agents are being studied to increase the accuracy of MRI scanning in detecting small metastatic hepatic lesions.[35,69]

The role of scintigraphy and angiography in the preoperative evaluation of hepatic tumors has changed dramatically because of the improvements in CT, MRI, and ultrasound. The present and future focus of research with scintigraphy is to develop immunologic markers that can be used to aid in the clinical staging of patients with metastatic disease.[37,38] A recent multicenter study demonstrated that radiolabeled antibody imaging may be helpful as an adjunct in the preoperative assessment of patients with colorectal cancer. Immunoscintigraphy was used in 116 patients and correlated with the pathologic diagnoses in 70% of patients with metastases and 90% of patients who were disease free.[38] Although these new techniques have limited clinical significance at this time, they may soon serve as a useful tool in the preoperative workup of patients with malignant disease.

Knowledge of arterial and venous structures before hepatic resection is most helpful when embarking on segmental or anatomic resections, whereas wedge resection of peripheral lesions does not necessarily require preoperative angiography. Preoperative angiography continues to be the best method of determining arterial anatomy and assessing tumor involvement of hepatic vein(s) or the portal venous system.

Although these radiologic tests are extremely useful in determining the stage and extent of disease, they should be used selectively. In most situations it will not be necessary to use multiple imaging techniques for the accurate evaluation of patients with colonic tumors or with metastases to the liver.

The imaging methods described are critical to the decision of recommending operative exploration, but the most accurate assessment of hepatic metastases occurs at the time of laparotomy when the surgeon can palpate all areas of the liver. An experienced surgeon can palpate most superficial lesions and some deeper lesions (particularly those in the left lobe). Intraoperative ultrasonography can detect lesions 2 to 4 mm in diameter within the liver parenchyma.[71] Intraoperative ultrasonic evaluation of hepatic tumors can delineate the extent of tumor invasion, can illustrate relations to vital vascular and biliary structures, and can be used to direct needle biopsies of intrahepatic lesions.

Use of an appropriate combination of imaging techniques provides the best opportunity for early detection and subsequent resection of small metastatic tumors. Earlier surgical intervention combined with second-line adjuvant therapy could increase overall survival of these patients.

TREATMENT OPTIONS

Treatment options for hepatic metastases include aggressive surgical resection of all gross tumor, administration of regional chemotherapeutic agents, arterial embolization, systemic chemotherapy, radiotherapy, or other palliative and investigational procedures.[53,73–80] To date, the only means shown to prolong survival in patients with limited metastatic disease from colorectal cancer (potential for "cure") is surgical resection.[7] Future combinations of treatment modalities may ultimately define other options as well. Unfortunately, fewer than 10% of patients with metastatic colorectal cancers are candidates for surgical resection.[4] To determine the feasibility and potential benefit from hepatic resection of secondary tumors, a thorough preoperative evaluation is essential. Systemic treatment of liver metastases and other locoregional therapeutic options are addressed in subsequent sections of this chapter.

LIVER METASTASES FROM NONCOLORECTAL TUMORS

A clear understanding of the properties that allow tumor cells to become blood borne and establish a new nest of tumor cells (metastasize) does not exist. There is, however, no doubt that many tumors have a propensity for implantation and growth within the liver. Although primary tumors arising from the gastrointestinal tract are the ones most likely to invade the liver, many other secondary tumors are detected as isolated liver metastases or as part of disseminated tumor. Once diagnosis of these lesions is established, the natural history of these tumors lends an equally grim or worse prognosis than

TABLE 61–17. Histology of Hepatic Metastases Resected in 153 Patients

Type of Lesion	*No. of Patients*
Secondary hepatic malignancy	153
Colorectal cancer	118
Intestinal cancer	6
Carcinoid	4
Spindle cell sarcoma	1
Leiomyosarcoma	1
Kidney cancer	5
Renal cell cancer	3
Wilms' tumor	2
Adrenal cancer	5
Adrenocortical carcinoma	4
Neuroblastoma	1
Breast cancer	4
Adenocarcinoma	2
Comedocarcinoma	1
Angiosarcoma	1
Gastric leiomyosarcoma	2
Ovarian adenocarcinoma	2
Uterus cancer	2
Squamous cell cancer	1
Endometrial sarcoma	1
Melanoma	2
Glucagonoma, pancreas	1
Leiomyosarcoma, rectum	1
Thyroid medullary carcinoma	1
Ewing's sarcoma	1
Mesothelioma	1
Rhabdomyosarcoma, colon	1
Adenocarcinoma, stomach	1

(Iwatsuki S, Sheahan DG, Starzl TE. The changing face of hepatic resection. Curr Probl Surg 1989;26[5]:283–379)

TABLE 61–18. Survival After Liver Resection of Noncolorectal, Nonendocrine Liver Metastases

Cancer Type	*Postoperative Survivors*	*5-Year Survivors*	*Died of Recurrence After 5 Years*
Wilms' tumor[12,13,16,18]	20	6 (14, 17 y)	?
Renal cell cancer[12,13,15–17]	11	3 (5 y, 7 y, and 12 y)	0
Adrenal carcinoma[12,16,19]	4	2 (6 y and 7 y)	0
Leiomyosarcoma[12,13,16–19]	16	2 (12 y)	1
Melanoma[12,18]	13	1	1
Pancreatic cancer[12,16,17]	8	1	1
Stomach cancer[12,15–17]	23	0	—
Other adult sarcomas[12,17,18]	9	0	—
Breast cancer[6,12,15,17]	7	0	—
Ovarian cancer[12,15,18]	5	0	—
Uterine and cervical cancer[12,13,18]	7	0	—
Lung cancer[12,15]	2	0	—
Esophageal cancer[15,16,74]	3	1 (13 y)[74]	—
Rhabdomyosarcoma[16]	1	0	—
Neuroblastoma[12]	1	0	—
Thyroid cancer[12]	1	0	—
Choriocarcinoma[13]	1	0	—
Periampullary cancer[17]	1	0	—

(Sugarbaker PH, Reinig JW, Hughes KS. Diagnosis of hepatic metastases. In: Rosenberg SA, ed. Surgical treatment of metastatic cancer. Philadelphia: JB Lippincott, 1987)

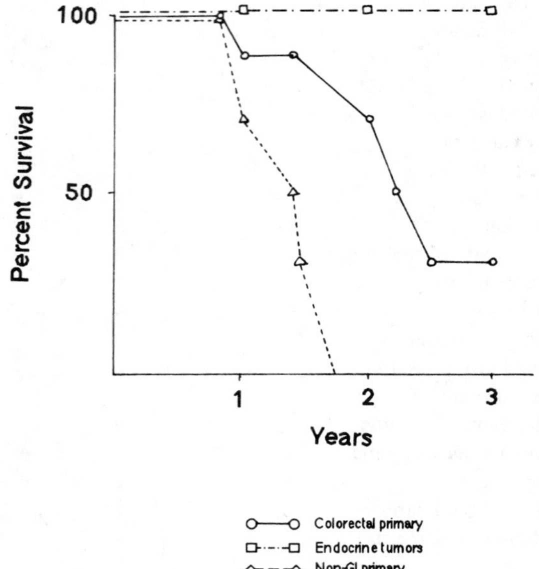

FIGURE 61–26. Percent survival after resection of intrahepatic metastases. (Adapted from Gozetti G, Mazziotti A. Expectations and possibilities of liver resection in the management of secondary liver tumors. In: Lygidakis NJ, Tytgat GNJ, eds. Hepatobiliary and pancreatic malignancies. Diagnosis, medical and surgical management. New York: Georg Thieme Verlag Stuttgart, Thieme Medical Publishers, 1989:183–190)

that of metastatic colorectal cancer. An exception appears to be metastatic neuroendocrine tumors, and a few anecdotal reports exist regarding long-term survivors after resection of liver metastases arising from neuroendocrine primaries.

There are limited reports in the literature regarding survival after resection of non-gastrointestinal-tract metastatic tumors to the liver. Unlike the reports for metastatic colorectal cancer, most reports collecting information regarding other liver metastases do not give a favorable outcome. Table 61–17, summarizing 153 hepatic tumors that were resected, is a representative sampling of the frequency with which secondary tumors from other sites occur.[40] Table 61–18 shows the poor results seen in patients after resection of noncolorectal, nonendocrine metastases, and Figures 61–26 and 61–27 illustrate similar findings.[2,7–20,41,81] In general, patients with neuroendocrine tumors (*i.e.*, carcinoid) that are resected have the best long-term survival rates, even if gross tumor is left unresected. In contrast, although the data are not conclusive, most studies indicate poor prognosis and lack of survival benefit after resection of secondary tumors originating from noncolorectal primaries[6,20,41]

HEPATIC RESECTION OF SECONDARY TUMORS

HISTORICAL PERSPECTIVES

The earliest surgical experiences with hepatic surgery dealt with traumatic injuries. Later, surgeons attempted elective hepatic resections, and Langenbruch is credited with the first

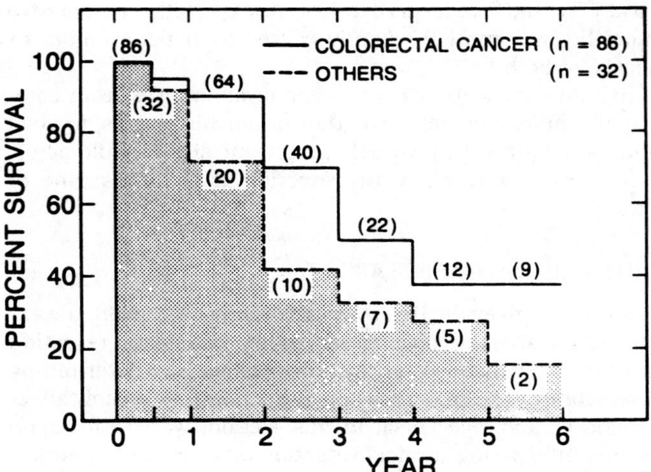

FIGURE 61–27. Actuarial survival after resection of intrahepatic metastases. (Iwatsuki S, Sheahan DG, Starzl TE. The changing face of hepatic resection. Curr Probl Surg 1989;26[5]:283–379. Reproduced with permission)

successful hepatic resection for tumor in 1888.[21,42] Several reports by Keen, Wendell, and others followed in later years, but with little knowledge of the segmental anatomy and physiology of the liver, results were not optimal. Hemorrhage was one of the greatest obstacles facing these surgical pioneers, as is evident by Keen's remark, ". . . the whole question of the operative surgery of the liver practically is one of haemostasis."[21,42,43] A major contribution to hepatic surgery was made by Couinauld with his description of the "segmental" anatomy of the liver (Fig. 61–28). He described anatomically distinct areas, each supplied by a separate arterial branch and biliary radical, each with a venous tributary of the right, middle, or left hepatic vein.[44–46] This allowed for control of these major structures during segmental/anatomic resections, thereby decreasing blood loss and postoperative complications.

In recent years, the number of hepatic resections has markedly increased because of advances in surgical and anesthetic techniques, the use of intraoperative autotransfusion devices, and the extensive preoperative evaluation and careful selection of surgical candidates. In addition, operative techniques and experience with postoperative care used in the management of patients undergoing orthotopic liver transplantation have contributed greatly to improvements in surgical outcome after major liver resections. As a result, the operative morbidity and mortality associated with hepatic surgery has significantly decreased, with most current studies reporting operative mortality rates between 2% and 7%.[3–8,10,20,39–41,60,62] Although operative mortality is low, liver resections are major undertakings for the patients and their families. Surgical intervention for metastatic disease should be offered only when the potential to extend the patient's disease-free survival exists. A thorough evaluation will aid in selecting those patients who will gain maximum benefit from resection of metastatic lesions.

PREOPERATIVE EVALUATION

Before any major abdominal surgery, a careful diagnostic workup, with particular attention to the patient's general health and cardiovascular and pulmonary status, is essential. The patient's age is of consideration in relation to the above; however, advanced age itself has not been shown to increase operative mortality after liver resection.[6,20] An extensive search for extrahepatic metastases is mandatory because this may contraindicate hepatic resection or the option of regional infusion therapy. Preoperative evaluation should include laboratory tests to determine hepatic reserve and renal function, and radiographic studies to determine the extent of intrahepatic and extrahepatic metastases. As mentioned earlier, arteriography, including a venous phase depicted on subtraction films, is helpful in delineating the vascular anatomy of the tumor as well as the native vascular anatomy of the liver, because anatomic variants are common (Table 61–19 and Fig. 61–29).[73,74]

Liver resection in the face of compromised hepatic function can be disastrous. One of the most important factors influencing major hepatic resection is the underlying physiologic

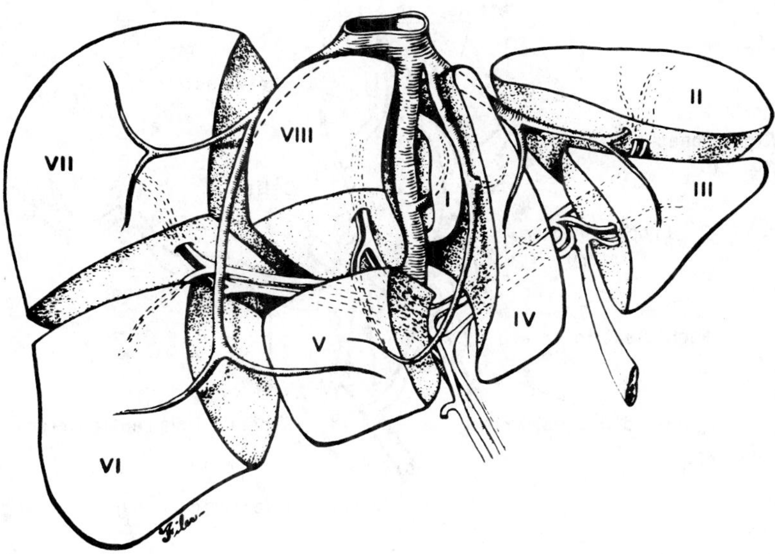

FIGURE 61–28. Segmental anatomy of the liver as described by Couinauld. There are eight segments numbered I through VIII. (Iwatsuki S, Sheahan DG, Starzl TE. The changing face of hepatic resection. Curr Probl Surg 1989;26[5]:283–379. Reproduced with permission)

TABLE 61–19. Hepatic Artery Anatomy in 232 Patients (University of Michigan)

Anatomy	*No. of Patients*
Standard	137 (59%)
Trifurcation	38 (16%)
RRHA*	36 (16%)
LHA replaced to LGA†	15 (6%)
Other‡	6 (3%)

* Right hepatic artery replaced to superior mesenteric artery. This includes one RRHA originating from the aorta.
† Left hepatic artery (LHA) replaced to the left gastric artery (LGA).
‡ A variety of anomalous origins of right and left hepatic arteries.
(Niederhuber JE. Colorectal cancer metastatic to the liver: Hepatic artery chemotherapy. In: Cameron JL, ed. Current surgical therapy. 3rd ed. Toronto, Philadelphia: BC Decker, 1989:222–233)

state of the normal liver parenchyma and its capacity to regenerate and function after surgery. Patients with significant hepatic impairment face increased morbidity secondary to hemorrhage, poor nutritional status, compromised immune and renal function, and poor regenerative capacity of the liver, all of which will affect their intraoperative or postoperative course. It is difficult to quantitate hepatic reserve with the use of liver enzyme studies. Most surgeons are willing to undertake hepatic resection in patients assessed as Child's class A or B. Prolongation of prothrombin time that does not correct with administration of vitamin K suggests poor synthetic capacity of the liver and may be suggestive of cirrhosis. These patients have significantly higher mortality rates, and most authors agree that major hepatic resections should be avoided in the face of poor hepatic function.[21] In contrast, a recent study that examined 123 cirrhotic patients with hepatocellular carcinoma indicates that limited resection of small, peripherally located tumors in this select group of patients may be appropriate. Overall operative mortality rate was 13%, 1-year survival 77%, and 5-year survival 49%. As expected, postoperative mortality was most frequently caused by hepatic failure or sepsis, or both.[47]

In summary, patients with hepatic metastases from colorectal tumors, and selected other tumor histologies, in good general health with favorable prognostic signs should be offered the option of hepatic resection as their first line of therapy.

DETERMINING RESECTABILITY

After thorough evaluation by an experienced surgeon, the extent of intrahepatic disease and timing of hepatic resection must be determined. Many factors considered in determining resectability of secondary hepatic tumors will ultimately affect prognosis, and vice versa. In this section, we will focus on factors influencing surgical resection of secondary tumors.

When hepatic metastases are found at the time of initial resection of a colorectal primary tumor, the lesions should be carefully examined, their size and location should be noted, and intraoperative biopsy should be performed. It should be stressed that all patients diagnosed as having a resectable primary tumor should be completely staged preoperatively. There should rarely be the surprise of finding an unexpected liver metastasis. In such instances, however, intraoperative ultrasonic evaluation should be considered to determine the full extent of hepatic involvement. Although many surgeons will delay resection of hepatic metastases until a later date, a well-prepared experienced surgeon can easily and safely accomplish resection of the primary as well as the secondary liver metastasis. If resection of liver metastases is deferred, it appears that a short period of delay will not affect prognosis.[6,20,41,48,49] Certainly when a single small peripheral tumor, confirmed by frozen section, is noted, it should be resected at the time of initial laparotomy. Experience with patients who present with synchronous metastases in the liver indicates that they have a worse overall prognosis. However, this prognosis does not appear to be related to surgical resection of these lesions but rather to the properties of the underlying disease.[6,20,39,61,82]

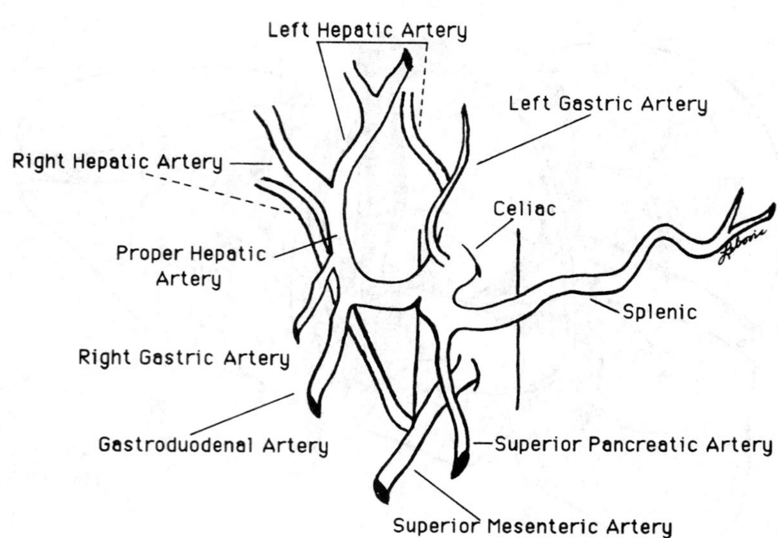

FIGURE 61–29. Schematic drawing of hepatic arterial blood supply and common aberrant origins of the right and left hepatic arteries (indicated by dotted line).

Patients being evaluated for resection of secondary hepatic tumors that become evident months to years after resection of their primary tumors should undergo a comprehensive workup to ensure that the liver is the only site of metastasis. If deemed resectable, surgical strategy for excision of the hepatic lesions is planned, and exploratory laparotomy with careful examination for evidence of extrahepatic metastases is performed. Particular attention is given to the primary site of the colorectal tumor, as well as to regional, mesenteric, celiac, and perihepatic lymph nodes. Any suspicious tissue is examined by frozen section. The presence of extrahepatic disease has been associated with early recurrence and may affect the overall length of survival after resection of hepatic metastases.

It should be emphasized that the presence of extrahepatic disease is not an absolute contraindication to hepatic resection.[6,10,20,39,49,50] Once abdominal exploration is complete, the liver is thoroughly examined, and the results are compared with the preoperative radiographic studies. Intraoperative ultrasound is used to visualize deep parenchymal lesions, to define the relation of the tumor(s) to vascular and biliary structures, and to rule out the presence of other metastases not detected before surgery. Present information, primarily from the prospective evaluation conducted by the Gastrointestinal Tumor Study Group (GITSG), suggests that it is possible to resect up to four lesions, even if they are bilobar.[7] When dealing with a healthy, noncirrhotic liver, as much as 50% to 80% of the liver can be removed with a large tumor mass while maintaining acceptable liver function and parenchymal regeneration. Taking all of this information into account, the surgeon determines the extent of, feasibility of, and technical approach to resection.

TECHNICAL ASPECTS OF RESECTION

There are many excellent surgical atlases, well-written manuscripts, and monographs that can provide the reader with an in-depth description on how to perform hepatic resections. Such a discussion is beyond the scope of this chapter, and the reader is referred to the following sources for additional information: references 20, 21, 23, 24, 40, 42, and 44. Some comments here regarding the segmental anatomy of the liver, and special surgical techniques that allow safe surgical intervention in the treatment of hepatic metastases, may, however, be of value.

The surgical anatomy of the liver has been described by many authors, and there are some discrepancies in the nomenclature as it pertains to surgical resection. For the purposes of this discussion, we will use terminology most frequently used in the United States.

On gross examination, it is tempting to divide the liver into right and left lobes along the falciform ligament; however, the true anatomic division of the right and left lobes is defined along "Cantlie's" line, a sagittal plane passing through the gallbladder bed posteriorly toward the vena cava.[51] To the right of this line lies the entire right lobe of the liver. The portion of tissue between Cantlie's line and the falciform ligament is the medial segment of the left lobe, and all tissue to the left of the falciform ligament constitutes the lateral segment of the left lobe. The right lobe can be further divided into an anterior and posterior segment by a coronal plane, and Couinauld's further division of both lobes into four subsegments creates a total of eight distinct anatomic segments of the liver (see Figs. 61–28 and 61–30).[4]

Identifying and controlling the arterial and venous structures within the liver parenchyma are crucial to minimizing blood loss, and the surgeon must be well versed in normal as well as variant anatomy. Most metastatic tumors derive 90% to 95% of their blood supply from the hepatic artery and only a small fraction from the portal venous system.[52–57] In over 59% of cases, the common hepatic artery arises from the celiac axis, traverses the upper border of the antrum of the stomach in the lesser omentum where it gives rise to the right gastric and gastroduodenal arteries, and then becomes known as the proper hepatic artery.[73,74] The proper hepatic artery lies medial to the common bile duct and anterior to the portal vein within the hepatoduodenal ligament. Later, it branches into the right and left hepatic arteries, each of which gives rise to terminal segmental arteries. A number of anatomic variants exist. In roughly 16% to 20% of cases, the right hepatic artery arises directly from the superior mesenteric artery and courses anteriorly and to the right of the portal vein in the hepatoduodenal ligament.[21,58,73,74] The most common aberrant site of origin of the left hepatic artery is the left gastric artery (see Fig. 61–29). Preoperative angiography can be most useful in defining the vascular anatomy so that the surgeon may plan appropriately for resection. The venous phase of the arteriogram is even more valuable in delineating both the portal and hepatic venous structures.

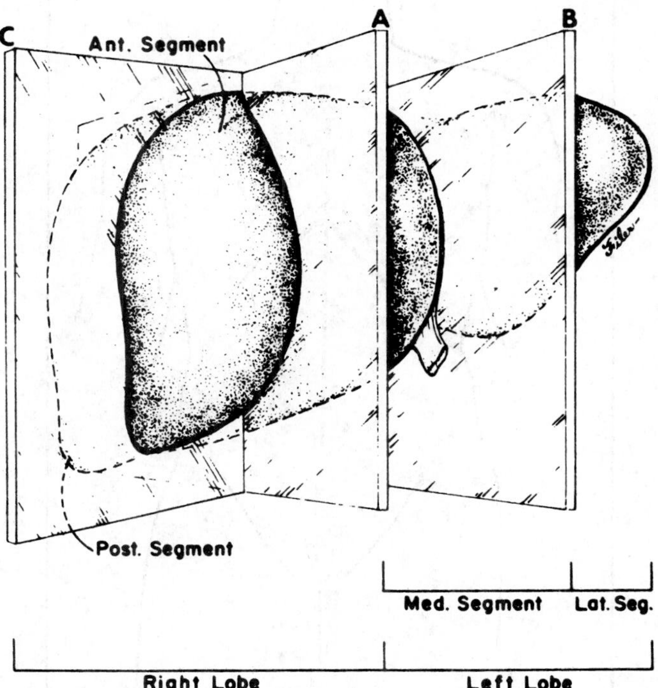

FIGURE 61–30. Anatomic divisions of the liver. **(A)** Cantlie's line divides the right and left lobe. **(B)** Left lobe subdivided into medial and lateral segments. **(C)** Right lobe divided into anterior and posterior segments by a coronal plane. (Iwatsuki S, Sheahan DG, Starzl TE. The changing face of hepatic resection. Curr Probl Surg 1989;26[5]:283–379. Reproduced with permission)

In preparation for hepatic resection, the patient is positioned in the supine position with slight extension of the torso. It is prudent to prep the entire chest and abdomen in the event that greater exposure becomes necessary. Most hepatic resections can be achieved through a generous midline incision, although some surgeons use an extended right subcostal approach. Additional exposure can be obtained by extension of the incision superiorly in the midline, splitting the sternum, or extension into the right thoracic cavity (Fig. 61–31).[21] After abdominal exploration, the liver is mobilized by detachment of its ligamentous reflections to the diaphragm. The anterior and posterior coronary ligaments, present on both the right and left sides, are divided. Attention is then directed toward dissection and identification of all structures within the hepatoduodenal ligament, with complete exposure of the hepatic arteries, the right and left bile ducts, and the right and left portal veins.

A formal lobectomy or trisegmentectomy will require careful bisection of the liver from the inferior vena cava. Each small branch is meticulously ligated in continuity and then divided. A second figure-of-eight 5-0 proline suture is placed in the inferior vena cava to secure these vessels. At this point, the major hepatic veins are exposed and enough of the vena cava is isolated above and below the liver to ensure rapid control if the situation requires. If possible, it is much safer to take the major hepatic veins just within the liver parenchyma.

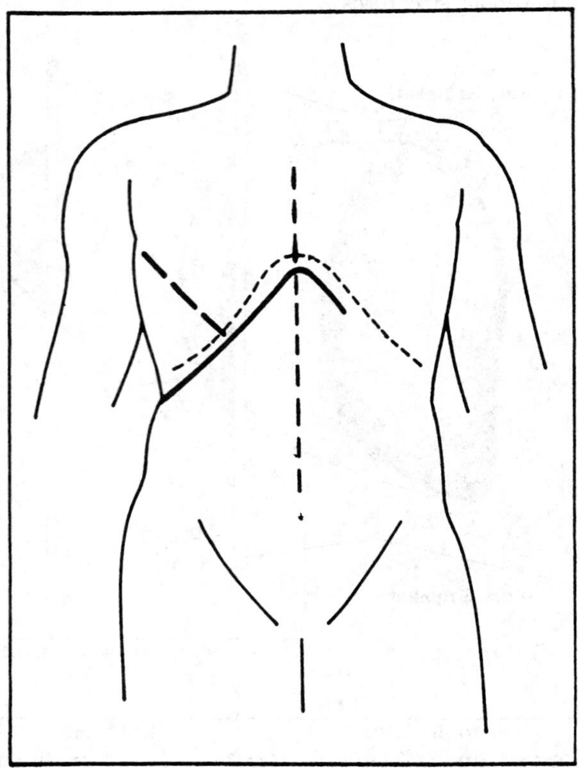

FIGURE 61–31. Extended right subcostal incision. Also shown are incisions into chest, which may be used for additional exposure as needed. (Schwartz SI. Primary and metastatic hepatic malignant tumors, and hepatic resection. In: Seymour I, Schwartz SI, Ellis H, eds. Maingot's abdominal operations. 9th ed. Norwalk, CT: Appleton & Lange, 1989:1253–1290. Reproduced with permission)

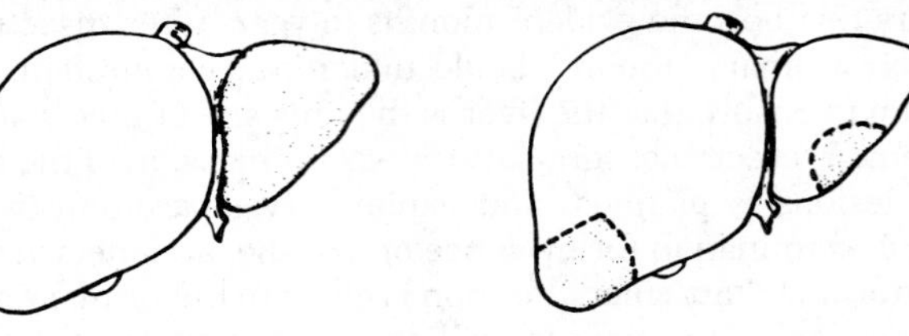

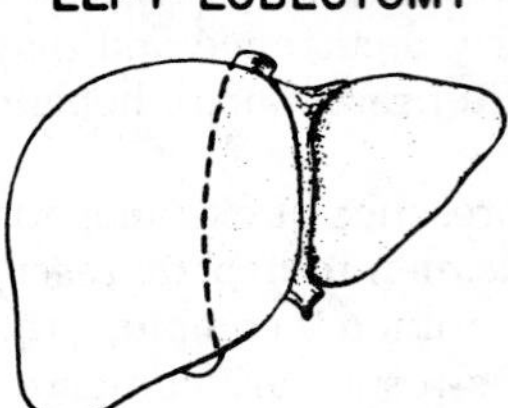

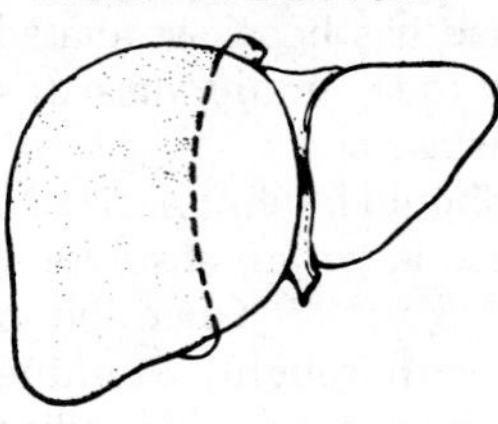

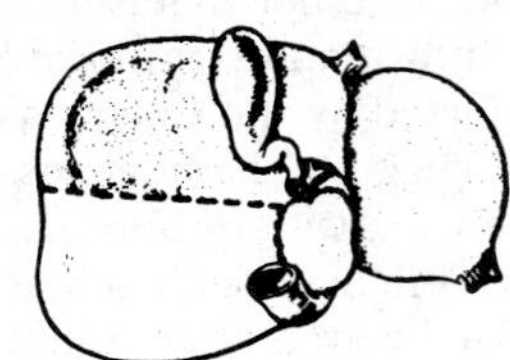

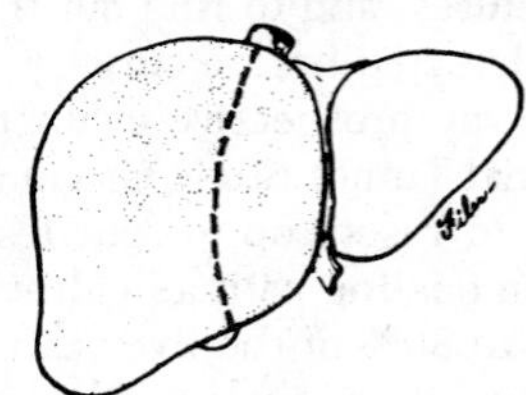

FIGURE 61–32. Anatomic hepatic resections commonly performed (right trisegmentectomy = extended right lobectomy/hepatectomy). (Iwatsuki S, Sheahan DG, Starzl TE. The changing face of hepatic resection. Curr Probl Surg 1989;26[5]:283–379. Reproduced with permission)

More limited resections such as nonanatomic wedge excisions do not require this degree of dissection and isolation of the structures cited above.

Depending on the type of resection to be performed, the surgeon uses a number of special techniques designed to allow for disruption of the liver parenchyma while permitting controlled dissection, ligation, and transection of vascular and biliary radicals. Finger fracture is a useful technique that permits isolated ligation of critical structures after manually disrupting the surrounding liver tissue.[21] More sophisticated devices, such as the Cavitron ultrasonic aspirator (CUSA; Valleylab, Boulder, CO) ultrasonic dissector, use this same principle. The metal tip vibrates at an ultrasonic frequency that shatters the hepatocytes because of the relatively high water content and aspirates the debris, leaving vascular and biliary structures intact to be properly ligated and divided.[59] Electrocautery and the argon-beam laser coagulator are also helpful in controlling bleeding from the raw surfaces of the transected liver tissue.

Figure 61–32 illustrates several anatomic and segmental hepatic resections commonly performed. The choice of resection is dependent on the extent of tumor involvement, as described in earlier sections. Evidence supports the conclusion that modest resection affecting a margin of 1 to 2 cm of normal liver provides results similar to those of more extensive resections.[7]

TABLE 61–20. Survival After Resection of Intrahepatic Colorectal Metastases

Investigations	*No. of Patients*	*5-Year Survival*	*Operative Mortality (%)*
Steel, 1991[7]	87	Median survival 29 mo	2.7
Scheele, 1990[10]	183	40/27% at 5/10 y	5.5
Lise, 1990[3]	39	32%	5
Iwatsuki, 1989[40]	86	38%	0
Hughes, 1989[6]	800	32%	NA
Gozzetti, 1989[41]	45	30% (3 y)	2.2
Butler, 1986[200]	62	34%	10
Gennari, 1986[5]	48	Median survival 30 mo	2
Coppa, 1985[201]	25	25%	4
Adson, 1984[39]	141	25%	4
August, 1985[4]	33	35%	0
Cady, 1970[8]	23	40%	0
Fortner, 1984[60]	65	40%	0–9 (0 since 1980)
Foster, 1981[62]	231	23%	6

NA, not available.

RESULTS

Surgical resection of colorectal metastases to the liver improves overall survival as well as disease-free survival and may provide a significant chance for "cure" in carefully selected patients. Many series have consistently reported these findings with acceptable operative morbidity and mortality rates. Table 61–20 summarizes the results of studies published during the past decade. These data indicate that 5-year actuarial survival rates after hepatic resection for colorectal metastases range from 23% to 40%, with operative mortality between 0% and 10%. This contrasts sharply with the data in Table 61–15, which reflects the dismal outcome of these patients when hepatic metastases are not resected.

Many factors may affect a patient's outcome after resection of hepatic metastases, but perhaps the most important is the clinician's judgment in properly selecting appropriate surgical candidates. Large retrospective studies have provided information regarding metastatic tumors to the liver that can be used to identify appropriate patients for resection. Much of these data were gathered and entered into the multiinstitutional "Registry of Hepatic Metastases." Hughes, Scheele, and Sugarbaker have made a significant contribution by analyzing this large body of information.[6,20,22] In addition, an extensive review of the literature suggests that the following factors may affect the prognosis (5-year survival and disease-free interval) of patients with metastatic lesions to the liver undergoing resection.

Stage of Primary Tumor. Most studies suggest that patients with Dukes' B carcinomas have a significantly improved 5-year survival when compared with patients with Dukes' C primary lesions (Fig. 61–33).[20,39,60,61]

Number of Metastases. Data suggest that patients with one or two metastases have the same 5-year survival. Those with three or four lesions, even if bilobar, have a slightly worse prognosis, but there is no clear cutoff. Most authors agree that resection of up to four metastases is reasonable.[4,6,8,20,25,39,62]

Size of Metastases. Size of metastatic lesions has been considered an important variable, and some studies have shown that patients with large (>5 cm) solitary metastases appear to have a worse prognosis.[5,6,20,25,62] This should not preclude surgical resection if technically feasible, and in some cases, resection of large symptomatic lesions may be considered as a means of palliation.

Extrahepatic Metastases. Though controversial, there appears to be no significant difference in overall survival when limited "nonnodal" extrahepatic metastases are resected at the time of hepatic resection (*i.e.*, a solitary pulmonary nodule). However, the *disease-free* 5-year survival rates of these patients are significantly decreased compared with those of patients free of

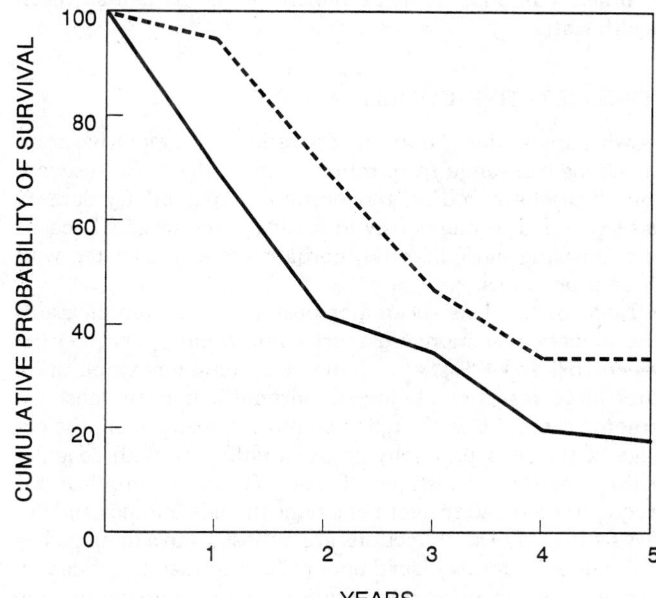

FIGURE 61–33. Survival curves for patients after hepatic resection. *Dashed line,* Dukes' stage B; *solid line,* Dukes' stage C.

extrahepatic disease at the time of hepatic resection.[6,10,20,39,49,50,85]

Surgical Resection. Several authors have noted that clear pathologic margins surrounding resected metastases significantly improve patients' survival. A margin of at least 1 cm of normal liver parenchyma should be excised with the specimen. The specific type of surgical resection (anatomic versus segmental or wedge resection) does not appear to affect survival when treating lesions <4 cm in diameter. Anatomic lobectomy for larger lesions has been associated with improved outcome, which may relate to obtaining adequate surgical margins.[4,6,8,20]

Disease-Free Interval. Studies have shown that patients who present with metastatic disease more than 1 year after resection of the primary tumor have a better prognosis than those who present with synchronous lesions or develop metastases during the 12 months after resection of a primary tumor. This most likely reflects the biologic properties of the tumor, and rapid growth or obvious spread that occurs after resection of a primary colorectal tumor may preclude resection.[6,20,39,61,82]

Nodal Status. Patients with tumor involvement of the celiac or hepatic nodes have a significantly decreased 5-year survival rate, even when all gross tumor is removed at the time of hepatic resection.[6,20]

Cirrhosis. Many studies have shown that patients with poor hepatic function have a higher morbidity and mortality rate after hepatic resection. Useful indicators of acceptable parenchymal function are patients classified as Child's (modified classes A and B) and a minimum rate of urea-nitrogen synthesis of 6 g/day. Patients with normal liver function may present with evidence of portal hypertension and ascites secondary to compression from a large tumor mass, and this does not necessarily contraindicate resection.[47,64–66]

Other Factors. Patients with CEA levels <5 ng/ml may have a better overall prognosis; however, these findings are inconsistent throughout the literature. Chronologic age does not appear to affect prognosis in patients with good general health.

Most series indicate that in carefully selected patients, 5-year survival rates of 20% to 40% are attainable, and the experienced surgeon should aggressively pursue resection of secondary tumors from colorectal cancers unless deemed technically impossible or prohibited by the patient's overall health status.

POSTOPERATIVE COMPLICATIONS

As with any major abdominal operation, postoperative complications can range from minor wound infections to severe complications requiring reoperation. Hepatobiliary surgery has expanded tremendously in recent years, largely because of decreasing mortality and morbidity rates associated with these procedures.

Table 61–21 lists the major postoperative complications after hepatic resection. Most series report morbidity rates between 15% and 43%,[20,84] with the most common complication after large resections being subphrenic hematoma/abscess. In some cases this is related to continued oozing from the cut edge of the liver parenchyma in combination with coagulopathies seen in the postoperative period. Other complications frequently seen after liver resections include bilomas and biliary fistulae. These collections are almost always managed by percutaneous drains placed under CT or ultrasonic guidance. Percutaneous transhepatic biliary catheter drainage may be necessary.

Intraoperative blood loss can be significant with major hepatic resections, and some authors have suggested a direct relation between intraoperative blood loss and postoperative morbidity.[5,64,83,84] The use of new operative techniques and equipment, such as the argon-beam coagulator and CUSA ultrasonic dissector, have helped to decrease intraoperative blood loss substantially, thereby decreasing operative morbidity.

Most patients are monitored in the intensive care unit postoperatively, and coagulopathies are aggressively treated. Hepatic failure due to inadequate functioning of the remaining parenchyma is another cause for postoperative morbidity, and this is often accompanied by renal failure. It is essential to avoid renal failure in these patients, because their mortality rates are very high when this complication occurs.

TABLE 61–21. Postoperative Complications Commonly Seen After Hepatic Resections

Subphrenic abscess
Intraabdominal hemorrhage at operative site
Bile leak (bilomas and biliary fistulae)
Hepatic failure
Coagulopathies
Transfusion reaction
Pulmonary complications/pleural effusion
Renal failure
Cardiac arrhythmias/myocardial infarction
Gastrointestinal bleeding
Small-bowel obstruction
Wound infection
Wound dehiscence
Deep venous thrombosis

(Hughes KS, Sugarbaker PH. Resection of the liver for metastatic solid tumors. In: Rosenberg S, ed. Surgical treatment of metastatic cancer. Philadelphia: JB Lippincott, 1987; Iwatsuki S, Sheahan DG, Starzl TE. The changing face of hepatic resection. Curr Probl Surg 1989; 26[5]:283–379; Vetto JT, Hughes KS, Rosenstein R, Sugarbaker PH. Morbidity and mortality of hepatic resection for metastatic colorectal carcinoma. Dis Colon Rectum 1990;33[5]:409–413)

PATTERNS OF FAILURE

Unfortunately, the natural progression of colorectal cancer will ultimately lead to recurrence of disease, and even after removal of all grossly visible hepatic metastases, most patients will return with metastatic disease again in the liver. There are many reports of resection of these recurrent tumors as well, but the majority of these patients will again return with liver metastases. The length of time before recurrence, the site of recurrence, and the extent of recurrence are intimately linked to the biologic behavior of the primary tumor. Patients with stage I lesions appear to have a better disease-free interval.[50]

Close follow-up of patients with colorectal cancers is essential. Most clinicians recommend colonoscopy every 6 to 12 months, frequent CEA levels, and close monitoring of hepatic function tests. Detection of recurrent disease in these patients is most reliably found by a persistent clinician looking for signs of recurrence long before the patient becomes symptomatic. Rising CEA levels may be the first indication of a recurrence, and follow-up studies, such as CT scans, should be pursued without hesitation.

CONCLUSIONS

Hepatic resection for metastatic colorectal cancer has become a widely accepted procedure with the ability to prolong overall and disease-free survival in patients who would otherwise face a grim prognosis. In properly selected patients, 5-year actuarial survival rates range from 20% to 40%, with very acceptable mortality and morbidity rates. Nonetheless, many of these patients remain daunted by the ultimate return of their tumors and will face death secondary to recurrent disseminated disease. There is little doubt that surgical management of metastatic colorectal cancer affects the natural course of disease significantly; however, surgery alone is not enough. It is important to note an intergroup study currently in progress (ECOG-9288, INT-0103). This study has been designed to prospectively evaluate: (1) resection of limited hepatic metastases from colon cancer alone versus (2) resection in combination with continuous hepatic arterial infusion of FUDR (floxuridine) plus systemic infusion of 5-FU (5-fluorouracil). Continued research will hopefully define a role for innovative adjuvant treatment options and aggressive systemic therapy of disseminated disease that can be combined with surgical management to provide optimal curative treatment of primary and metastatic cancers.

SYSTEMIC CHEMOTHERAPY

For several reasons, systemic chemotherapy represents the modality most frequently used in the treatment of hepatic metastases. Although hepatic metastases are often predominant in the generation of morbidity, the liver is rarely the sole site of metastatic disease. Liver involvement with breast cancer, lung cancer, melanoma, and even pancreatic and gastric cancer either occurs with or heralds the subsequent development of tumor in multiple metastatic sites. Application of systemic chemotherapy has the potential to reach all sites of disease. In addition, for those tumors that are responsive to systemic chemotherapy, intravenous drug treatment represents the most convenient, cost-effective, and efficient approach. The relative ease with which hepatic metastases can be evaluated with modern radiologic techniques makes liver tumor nodules useful as indicator lesions for response evaluation with systemic therapies.

Colorectal cancer frequently metastasizes to the liver. As demonstrated by surgical resection for cure, the liver may truly represent the sole site of metastatic disease in a minority of patients. The majority of patients with hepatic metastases from colorectal cancer either have or will develop extrahepatic tumor and therefore are reasonable candidates for systemic chemotherapy. The standard chemotherapeutic agent for advanced colorectal cancer has been 5-FU, which generates a response rate of about 20% as a single agent when used intensively (Table 61–22). Prolonged continuous infusions of 5-FU have been shown to generate a higher response rate (30%) when compared with an equitoxic bolus regimen (7%).[104]

A variety of combination chemotherapy regimens based on 5-FU have been evaluated in advanced colorectal cancer. Table 61–22 illustrates that hepatic metastases from colorectal cancer respond to systemic therapy with rates similar to those found in general with each specific regimen. Drug treatments using biochemical modulation of 5-FU with leucovorin (LV) have become standard in practice based on multiple phase III studies demonstrating superiority in response rate of 5-FU plus LV over 5-FU alone.[97,105–107] More important, the regimen of 5-FU plus low-dose LV has been shown to produce a significant improvement in median survival (12 months) over that resulting from 5-FU alone (7.7 months).[108]

Pancreatic and gastric adenocarcinomas represent the two other common gastrointestinal malignancies that frequently metastasize to the liver as well as to multiple other sites. Response rates to systemic chemotherapy for hepatic metastases in these diseases are low (~25%) and are associated with a short survival of 3 to 4 months.[109]

Carcinoid tumors and islet cell carcinomas frequently metastasize to the liver. Compared with other neoplasms of the gastrointestinal tract, these neuroendocrine tumors are rare yet notable for their relative indolence and production of hormone-related symptoms. Combination chemotherapy for carcinoid tumors produces response rates of approximately 30% with durations of response of less than 9 months.[110,111] The octapeptide somatostatin analog, octreotide acetate (Sandostatin), has become standard therapy for symptomatic control of the carcinoid syndrome, such as occurs with liver metastases. Islet cell tumors appear to be more responsive to systemic chemotherapy, with responses of up to 60% and response durations of up to several years.[110,111]

Systemically administered chemotherapy used to treat hepatic metastases is limited by and generates the customary systemic toxicities of the agents applied. Usually mucositis, diarrhea, and myelosuppression are dose-limiting, with little or no limitation of therapy due to liver toxicity.

Most patients developing liver metastases from gastrointestinal cancers will ultimately die in a manner causally related to the disease within the liver. In other cancers such as breast cancer, lung cancer, and melanoma, progression in multiple sites generates morbidity and mortality coincidental to hepatic progression.

After initial systemic therapy has failed to control growth of liver metastases, second-line therapeutic options are determined by the type of cancer and the extent of extrahepatic disease. For nongastrointestinal cancers, systemic chemotherapy options should be foremost and should be selected from historical experience or available research regimens. For colorectal cancer, carcinoid, and islet cell hepatic metastases, regional treatment options as discussed below may be of benefit.

REGIONAL CHEMOTHERAPY

RATIONALE AND PHARMACOLOGY

The direct injection of chemotherapeutic agents into the blood supply of the liver has received much attention over the years. The goal of such regional chemotherapy has been to provide higher drug exposures to tumor within the liver with concurrently lower systemic exposures. Based on dose-response effects, improved selectivity of drug exposure should increase the regression of hepatic cancer while decreasing systemic toxicities.[112,113] In the last 15 years, application of regional chemotherapy to the treatment of metastatic disease within the liver has been spurred on by developments in pharmacokinetics, drug delivery, and methods of tumor evaluation.

TABLE 61–22. Response of Liver Metastases From Colorectal Carcinoma to Systemic Chemotherapy

Investigations	*No. of Patients*	*Response (%)*	*No. With Liver Metastases*	*Response (%)*
FU				
Moertel, 1969[87]	144	15	118	24
Baker, 1976[88]	42	10	11	0
Siefert, 1975[89]	36	17	5	20
Grage, 1979[90]	31	23	31	23
FU + MeCCNU ± VCR				
MacDonald, 1976[91]	25	40	14	43
Baker, 1976[88]	152	32	41	31
Buroker, 1978[92]	133	16	93	18
Kemeny, 1979[93]	69	11	41	11
FU + MeCCNU + VCR + strep				
Kemeny, 1983[94]	35	34	29	30
Kemeny, 1980[95]	74	32	58	45
FU + LV				
Machover, 1986[96]	86	39	73	30
Petrelli, 1989[97]	109	30	85	27
Ardalan, 1991[98]	22	45	18	44
FU + MTX				
Kemeny, 1984[99]	43	32	33	31
FU + MTX + LV				
Nordic Group, 1989[100]	119	17	84	18
FU + Mito + DDP + VCR				
Pandya, 1986[101]	23	48	15	30
FU + DDP				
Leohrer, 1985[102]	38	29	22	16
Kemeny, 1987[103]	105	28	77	20

FU, 5-fluorouracil; LV, leucovorin; DDP, cisplatin; Mito, mitomycin C; strep, streptozotocin; MTX, methotrexate; MeCCNU, methylcyclohexylnitrosurea; VCR, vincristine.

Although the liver receives most of its nutrient blood flow by way of the portal vein, there is considerable evidence that macroscopically detectable cancers derive their blood supply directly from the hepatic artery.[56–58,114] Based on such evidence, the administration of continuous hepatic arterial chemotherapy was introduced by Sullivan and associates in the early 1960s.[115] Considering the diseases in question, the response rates achieved exceeded rates with standard intravenous chemotherapy by twofold to threefold. Over the subsequent two decades, many reports demonstrated that, for colorectal cancer in particular, higher response rates could be achieved by hepatic arterial therapy than were found with standard intravenous therapy with 5-FU (Table 61–23).

Interest in hepatic arterial chemotherapy was rekindled and broadened during the late 1970s for a variety of reasons. The disease most frequently metastatic to the liver, colorectal cancer, was found to be extremely refractory, with a lack of success in the development of new agents. Clearly, any ap-

TABLE 61–23. Intraarterial Therapy of Hepatic Metastases With Use of External Pumps in Patients With Colorectal Cancer

Investigations	*Drugs Used*	*No. of Evaluable Patients*	*Response Rate (%)*
Sullivan, 1965[116]	Multiple regimens	39	62
Watkins, 1970[117]	FUDR	82	73
Cady, 1974[118]	FUDR	51	57
Buroker, 1976[119]	FUDR	21	35
Grage, 1979[90]	FU	30	34
Oberfield, 1979[120]	FU/FUDR	48	75
Patt, 1979[121]	Mitomycin/FUDR	12	83
Reed, 1981[122]	FUDR	77	76

FUDR, floxuridine; FU, 5-fluorouracil.

proach having higher activity than was achievable with intravenous therapy was felt to have a role in the treatment of colorectal liver metastases.

Other developments during the late 1970s provided added impetus to hepatic arterial chemotherapy. Pharmacologic studies were carried out with a variety of antineoplastic drugs (Table 61–24). Clinical pharmacologic investigation of 5-fluoro-2′-deoxyuridine (5-FUDR) and 5-FU demonstrated that high hepatic extraction could lead to reduced systemic drug levels, validating the rationale for the use of these agents.[123] 5-FUDR was found to be 97% to 99% extracted by the liver when given by the hepatic artery, whereas hepatic extraction of 5-FU was less efficient at 25% to 30%. These data suggested that 5-FUDR was the more selective of the two agents for regional chemotherapy by the hepatic artery.

Important refinements in pharmacokinetic theory were subsequently defined.[124,125] It was shown that the relative advantage (R_d) of hepatic arterial infusion (in terms of regional drug exposure to tumor fed by the hepatic artery) versus an intravenous infusion of a given drug is determined by the drug's total body clearance (CL_{TB}), the arterial blood flow (Q), and the fraction of drug extracted across the liver (E_H). The relation was shown to be:

$$R_d = 1 + \frac{CL_{TB}}{Q(1 - E_H)}$$

Table 61–24 illustrates the estimated exposure advantage for a number of agents. It should be noted that the high hepatic extraction of 5-FUDR generates negligible systemic exposure, particularly in comparison to the related, but much less effectively extracted drug, 5-FU. In light of these pharmacologic studies, the earlier reports of high response rates with hepatic arterial chemotherapy could be viewed as a logical extension of dose-response effects for the fluorinated pyrimidines. However, when considering the increased exposures possible with hepatic arterial infusion, it must be recognized that there is not likely to be a linear pharmacodynamic relation between target organ effect (or response) and concentration.[124] For example, preclinical studies of 5-bromo-2′-deoxyuridine (5-BUDR), an agent similar to 5-FUDR in some respects, have demonstrated that incorporation of the 5-BUDR into DNA is nonlinear and levels off at higher concentrations.[126] Extension of such investigations into hepatic arterial 5-BUDR infusions with the VX-2 tumor grown in rabbit liver demonstrates a marked decline in regional selectivity with increasing rates of drug infusion.[127]

Developments in nuclear medicine have affected hepatic arterial therapy as well. During the late 1970s, nuclide angiography was developed as a technique to define and mimic drug flow distribution patterns during the slow fluid infusion rates used in hepatic arterial chemotherapy.[128] Radioactively labeled, γ-emitting particles (^{99m}Tc-macroaggregated albumin, TcMAA) were injected at slow flow rates through the hepatic artery. It was found that the pattern of flow distribution, as seen by the entrapment of these microparticulates within the first capillary bed of the liver, correlated with the pattern of regression of tumor. Nuclide flow to a particular region of the liver was correlated with a high probability of response for tumors in that region, whereas a lack of direct drug flow was found to correlate with a lack of response. This raised the possibility that response rates would actually be higher if catheters were always positioned within the hepatic artery such that there was direct drug infusion to the entire tumor-bearing liver. Recognition of the important roles of catheter position and infusion patterns meant that more attention had to be paid to these variables during surgical and radiologic catheter placement (see below). Recent studies have suggested that the intensity of tumor uptake of TcMAA with arterial nuclide flow scans can be predictive of tumor response: 16 of 31 patients with increased TcMAA uptake relative to liver responded to arterial chemotherapy, whereas only 1 of 16 responded to arterial chemotherapy when there was decreased TcMAA uptake.[129]

A recent important nuclear medicine study performed by the Memorial Sloan Kettering group in patients with colorectal liver metastases used radioactive (tritiated) 5-FUDR.[130] Tumor uptake of the agent was determined after hepatic arterial or portal venous administration. Liver and tumor biopsies demonstrated that the mean tumor 5-FUDR level after hepatic arterial infusion was 12.4 mmol/g, whereas the mean level after portal venous infusion of a similar 5-FUDR dose was 0.8 mmol/g. This crucial study validated the choice of the hepatic arterial route for chemotherapy with 5-FUDR for macroscopic liver metastases. It is noteworthy that radiola-

TABLE 61–24. Pharmacokinetically Rational Agents for Hepatic Arterial Infusion

Drug	*Estimated Increased Hepatic Exposure With Hepatic Arterial Infusion*	*Retained Systemic Exposure Relative to Intravenous Use (%)*	*Dose-Limiting Toxicity of Hepatic Arterial Therapy*
Fluorouracil (5-FU)	50–100-fold	60–70	Mucositis/diarrhea
Floxuridine (5-fluoro-2′-deoxyuridine; 5-FUDR)	100–400-fold	<5	Hepatobiliary
Carmustine (bischlorethyl-nitrosourea; BCNU)	7–13-fold	~100	Myelosuppression
Mitomycin	3–5-fold	80–90	Myelosuppression
Cisplatin	2–4-fold	~100	Renal

(Adapted from Ensminger WD, Gyves JW. Regional cancer chemotherapy. Cancer Treat Rep 1984;68: 101–115)

beled TcMAA was administered in the same solution with 5-FUDR in this study and that tumor uptake of 5-FUDR correlated directly and significantly with TcMAA retention by tumor.

CLINICAL THERAPEUTICS

External Drug Delivery Systems

Until the early 1980s, hepatic arterial infusions used externalized catheters and external pumps (see Table 61–23). However, the use of externalized catheters placed either at operation or by the Seldinger radiologic technique resulted in high complication rates, including catheter displacement, sepsis, and gastrointestinal hemorrhage. For example, Oberfield and colleagues reported complications in 80% of cases, with complete or partial hepatic artery thrombosis in 39% and catheter displacement in 33% of patients.[120] Reed and colleagues reported on 109 patients who had hepatic artery catheters either placed with the Seldinger technique or directly inserted at laparotomy.[122] Complications resulting in interruption of therapy occurred in 35% of patients, with catheter or arterial thrombosis and catheter displacement accounting for most of the complications. Although published data suggested that direct hepatic arterial infusion could generate improved tumor response rates, difficulties in achieving and sustaining hepatic arterial infusions with the available options in externalized systems prevented widespread use of such therapy.

Implanted Drug Delivery Systems

In the late 1970s and early 1980s, interest in hepatic arterial infusions was stimulated by the development of an implantable pump that, when attached to a surgically implanted catheter, constituted a totally implanted system.[131] In 1980, Buchwald and associates at the University of Minnesota reported on the application of an implantable pump they had invented for heparin infusion for hepatic arterial therapy of 5 patients with 5-FUDR.[132] In 1981, investigators at the University of Michigan described their results in 13 patients using the commercial variant of the Minnesota pump, denoted the model 400 Infusaid pump.[133] The model 400 INFUSAID pump (INFUSAID, Norwood, MA) had a SIDEPORT that bypassed the pumping mechanism and allowed direct injection into the catheter for nuclide angiography with TcMAA, for bolus drug administration, and for clearing of obstruction in the catheter. The limiting toxicities of continuous-infusion 5-FUDR were defined in this initial study and were found to be gastrointestinal and hepatic. Infusion system problems were minimal compared with prior external systems. The response rate in the 13 patients, with the use of physical examination and nuclide liver scans, was found to be 85% when mitomycin was given by the Sideport on failure of single-agent 5-FUDR.

Interest stirred by the initial, albeit limited, positive results with use of the implanted drug delivery system generated additional phase II studies focused on colorectal cancer (Table 61–25). Subsequent phase II studies used more restrictive and defined criteria of response, leading to lower response rates that were, nonetheless, considerably higher than those described for most studies of systemic chemotherapy (see Table 61–22). Unfortunately, survival impact and the role of patient selection in achieving improved response rates could not be distinguished in these phase II studies.

Prospective, randomized trials were developed to compare hepatic arterial FUDR with systemic chemotherapy in the treatment of liver metastases from colorectal cancer. The results of the four major published studies are noted in Table 61–26. It should be pointed out that mitomycin was not used in any of these randomized studies, whereas most of the earlier phase II studies used hepatic arterial mitomycin in addition to 5-FUDR. The results of these four studies define a significant and greater than twofold improvement in response rate with hepatic arterial 5-FUDR as compared with intravenous infusions of 5-FUDR or 5-FU. The NCI and Mayo Consortium trials examined survival in the two treatment groups and found no significant difference.[143,144] The NCI trial enrolled patients both with and without hepatic lymph nodes positive for tumor. When survival of the subset of patients with negative hepatic lymph nodes was examined, the 2-year actuarial survival for the arterial group (47%) was improved over that for the intravenous group (13%) (p = 0.03). The Mayo consortium trial included 5 patients who did not receive hepatic arterial therapy and 7 patients with documented extrahepatic intraabdominal cancer in the hepatic arterial group (33 patients) for survival analysis comparison. It was noted that the 7 patients with extrahepatic disease had a significantly shorter

TABLE 61–25. Phase II Studies With Use of an Implanted Drug Delivery System for Hepatic Metastases From Colorectal Cancer

Investigations	*No. of Patients*	*Drugs Used*	*Response Rate (%)*
Balch, 1983[134]	81	FUDR/Mito	88
Niederhuber, 1984[135]	93	FUDR/Mito	78
Kemeny, 1984[136]	41	FUDR/Mito	44
Shepard, 1985[137]	40	FUDR/Mito	20
	13	FUDR/DichloroMTX	69
Kemeny, 1985[138]	24	FUDR	73
Patt, 1986[139]	29	FUDR/Mito/Cisplatin	52
Cohen, 1986[140]	36	FUDR/Mito/BCNU	70

FUDR, floxuridine; Mito, mitomycin C; MTX, methotrexate; BCNU, carmustine.

TABLE 61–26. Randomized Studies of Intrahepatic Chemotherapy Versus Systemic Chemotherapy for Hepatic Metastases From Colorectal Cancer

Group	No. of Patients	*Intrahepatic*		*Systemic*	
		Drug	*Response (%)*	*Drug*	*Response (%)*
MSKCC[141]	99	FUDR	50	FUDR	20 $p = 0.001$
NCOG[142]	115	FUDR	42	FUDR	10 $p = 0.001$
NCI[143]	64	FUDR	62	FUDR	17 $p = 0.003$
Mayo consortium[144]	60	FUDR	48	FU	21 $p = 0.02$

MSKCC, Memorial Sloan-Kettering Cancer Center; NCOG, Northern California Oncology Group; NCI, National Cancer Institute; FUDR, floxuridine; FU, 5-fluorouracil.

survival ($p = 0.04$) and shorter time to overall (any site) progression ($p = 0.01$) than did patients without extrahepatic disease. The Mayo investigators noted that the significantly higher response rate of hepatic tumor to hepatic arterial therapy provided a rationale for further studies combining hepatic arterial and systemic chemotherapy to provide control of both hepatic and extrahepatic disease. In this regard, the efficient hepatic extraction of 5-FUDR would be expected to lead to negligible systemic effects on extrahepatic tumor when the agent is given into the hepatic artery (see Table 61–24).

Technical Considerations for Establishing Arterial Access

Hepatic arterial infusions may be accomplished with either percutaneous angiographic placement or surgical placement at laparotomy. Angiographic catheters are of necessity stiffer than the silicone rubber catheters used in operative placement. In general, the stiffness of the angiographic catheter and the motion of the tip of the catheter have made radiologic placement most suitable for short-duration (up to 2 weeks) infusions. Repeated angiographic insertions for repeated courses of therapy generate a progressive probability for arterial thrombosis and intimal damage. In addition, although blood flow distribution can be changed from an unfavorable to a favorable pattern (*i.e.,* one where a single catheter infuses the entire liver and nothing outside of the liver) with angiographic embolic techniques, the skills involved are considerable.[145] As described below, surgical techniques for achieving protracted hepatic arterial access are much more refined at present.

Proper placement of the hepatic arterial catheter is critical to ensure equal distribution of chemotherapeutic agents to the right and left lobes of the liver and to minimize the extent of extrahepatic perfusion. This procedure may seem straightforward; however, the operation can be much more difficult than is generally appreciated. The liver may be increased in size, making exposure difficult; there may be extensive adhesions from previous operations; and the arterial blood supply may be complex and difficult to define.

Preoperative preparation includes a complete workup to determine the extent of metastatic disease, hepatic angiography, a complete bowel prep, and administration of intravenous antibiotics. This brief section will describe the basic principles for catheter placement in the patient with "standard" hepatic arterial anatomy. Several anatomic variants are illustrated in Figures 61–34 through 61–37, and for further details the reader is referred to previous reports.[146,147]

Abdominal exploration is performed through a standard midline incision. Careful exposure of the portal triad with definition of the hepatic arterial anatomy is essential, because placement of the perfusion catheter will vary depending on the patient's particular anatomy. Elective cholecystectomy is routinely done at the beginning of the operation. This facilitates exposure of the hepatic arteries and will eliminate the problem of chemical cholecystitis in the postoperative period. After cholecystectomy, attention is directed toward proper placement of the silicon catheter. In general, the gastroduodenal artery is the vessel used for catheter placement, and it is ligated distal to the point of insertion (see Fig. 61–34). To

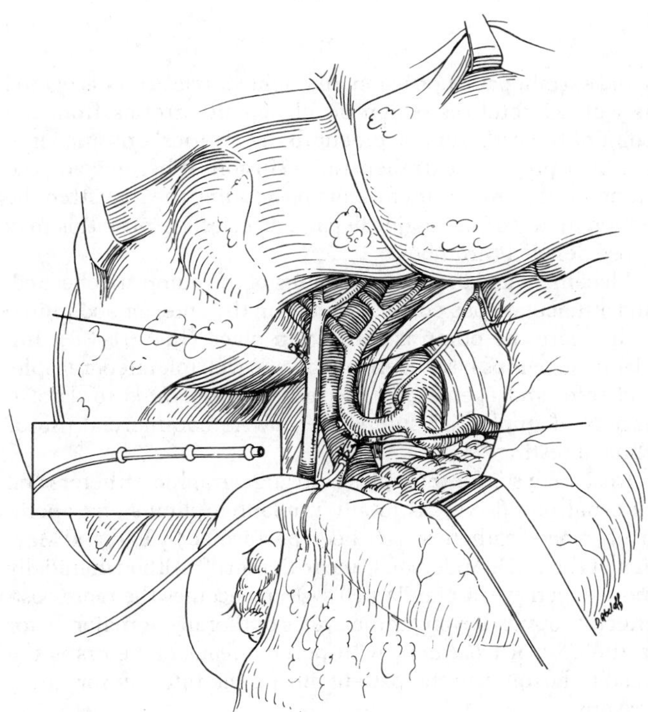

FIGURE 61–34. The patient has "standard" hepatic arterial anatomy permitting the catheter to be placed in the gastroduodenal artery. Note that the tip of the catheter is positioned just at the junction of the gastroduodenal artery with the hepatic artery. A close-up view of the beaded catheter is shown in the inset. The silicone rubber catheter has an outer diameter of 2.3 mm and an inner diameter of 0.63 mm.

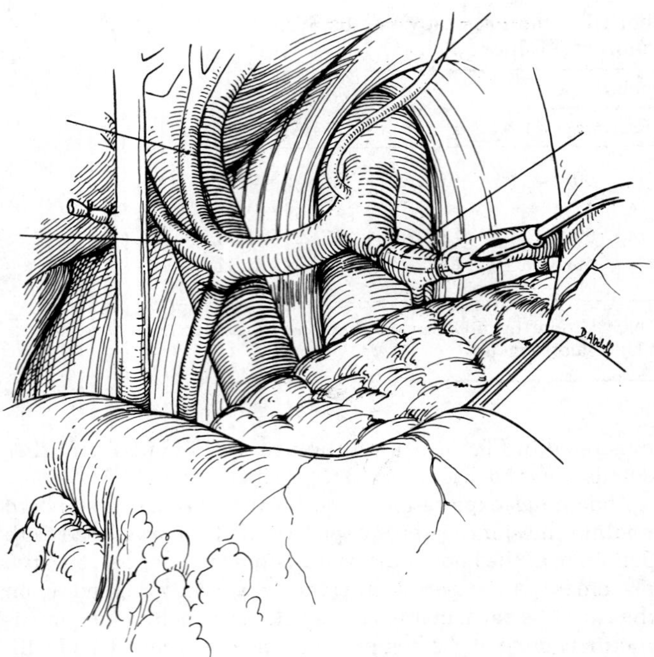

FIGURE 61–35. In this patient, the right and left hepatic arteries originate too close to the gastroduodenal artery to allow its use for the catheter placement. A catheter placed in the gastroduodenal artery would not permit adequate mixing of the drug in the arterial blood to provide equal distribution to right and left lobes of the liver. Thus, the splenic artery has been isolated and ligated for catheter placement. The gastroduodenal artery and all other branches have been carefully identified and ligated to prevent extrahepatic distribution of drug.

avoid extrahepatic perfusion, the right gastric artery is ligated as well. Careful dissection of all hepatic arteries from the point of the catheter placement to the arteries' entrance into the liver prevents extrahepatic perfusion. When placing the catheter, it is important to avoid positioning the tip within the lumen of any of the major hepatic arteries, because this may cause delayed thrombosis.

Placement and proper functioning of the pump are checked, and a subcutaneous pocket is made on the anterior abdominal wall where the pump is secured in place (Fig. 61–38). Implantable pumps have been found to be well tolerated, reliable, and safe, and over 25,000 have been implanted to date. A variety of implanted pumps are now in commercial use or clinical testing.[148]

Cost analyses for therapies with angiographic catheters and external pumps versus totally implanted pumps and operatively placed catheters have been performed by Patt and Mavligit at the M.D. Anderson Cancer Center.[149] Although initially more expensive, an implanted system becomes the more cost-effective option beyond three cycles of therapy. A major factor in the cost of treatment with percutaneous catheters is the need to hospitalize the patient during the infusion for safety reasons.

Toxicities

Hepatic arterial therapy has a number of toxicities or complications not seen with conventional intravenous therapy.[148] These include thrombosis of the hepatic artery or other visceral arteries with resultant pain and inability to use further arterial therapy. Placement (radiologically) and maintenance of a transbrachial or transfemoral percutaneous catheter are associated with the risk of thrombosis of the vessels through which the catheter passes and of embolic damage to the extremity with the insertion site. Embolic injury from fibrin sheaths or clots forming on the catheter can involve varied internal organs and the brain, causing temporary ischemia or infarction. Thrombosis related to entrance into the brachial or femoral artery may cause ischemia of the extremity and may necessitate thrombectomy. Infection initiated at the entrance site can also occur, usually with *Staphylococcus aureus.* For implanted systems, additional complications include permanent occlusions of the implanted catheter, catheter rupture when attempting to clear such occlusions, and pump pocket seromas, hematomas, and infections. The risk and severity of complications bear some relation to the experience, skill, and dedication of the radiologists, surgeons, and medical oncologists involved in such treatment.

The lowered risks associated with totally implanted systems for hepatic arterial 5-FUDR infusion made it possible for a large number of centers to administer chronic, protracted therapy, which had not been possible with externalized systems. In contrast to the toxicity of systemically administered chemotherapy, which is frequently myelosuppression, the toxicity of chronic hepatic arterial chemotherapy was found

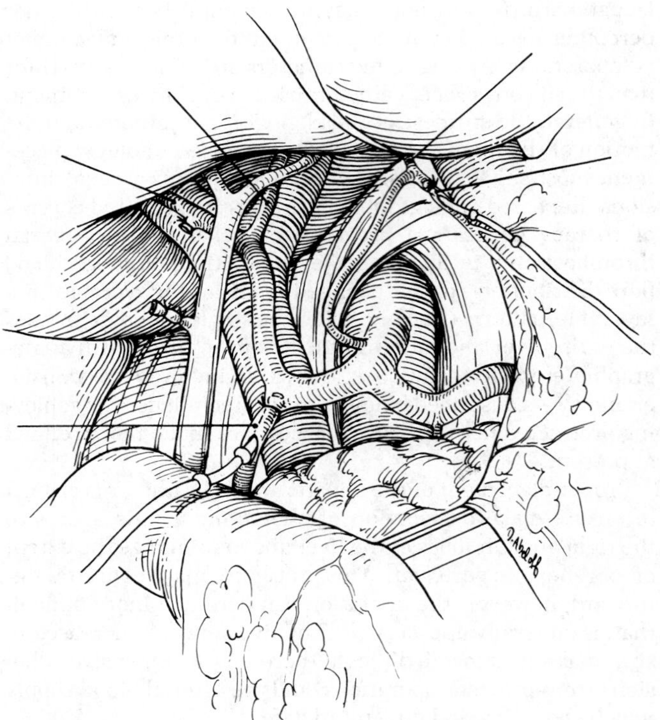

FIGURE 61–36. The left hepatic artery in this patient arises from the left gastric artery. The middle and right hepatic arteries have their normal origins from the proper hepatic artery. This situation requires a dual-catheter pump. One catheter is positioned in the left gastric artery and inserted so the tip is just at the left hepatic artery, with care being taken not to obstruct flow. The right lobe is perfused by way of a second catheter positioned in the gastroduodenal artery.

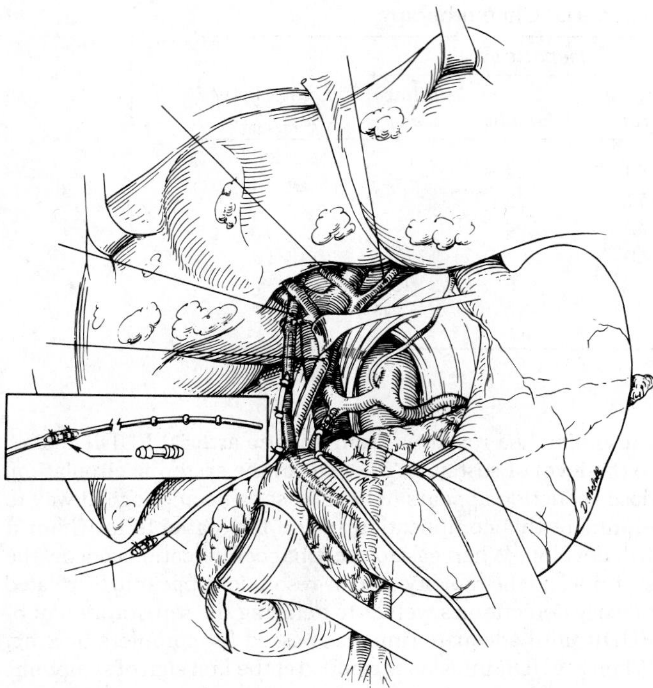

FIGURE 61–37. Two catheters are also required in patients with a right hepatic artery replaced to the superior mesenteric artery. There are no significant accessible branches of the RRHA, making it necessary to introduce a special thin-walled catheter directly into the lumen. The introduction of the catheter is accomplished by inserting an 18-gauge needle into the lateral wall of the exposed vessel. A guide wire is passed through the needle. The needle is removed and a beaded catheter is passed over the wire and threaded for a short distance into the lumen of the artery until the first catheter bead rests against the adventitia. A silk stitch is placed through the adventitia of the artery just behind the first catheter bead and is used to secure the catheter alongside the RRHA. This special thin-walled catheter is connected to one of the two pump catheters.

to relate primarily to the regionally high (and protracted) exposure to 5-FUDR or 5-FU. In early studies, the incidence of symptomatic gastric injury and of hepatobiliary damage, the major regional toxicities associated with hepatic arterial infusion of 5-FUDR, was approximately 50% for each (Table 61–27).

The primary mechanism for gastric toxicity with hepatic arterial infusion appears to be direct blood flow to the stomach through vessels distal to the site of drug entrance into the hepatic artery (*i.e.*, distal to the catheter tip). Gastric toxicity was described earlier for hepatic arterial infusion that used percutaneous angiographically placed hepatic arterial catheters. One study described the development of gastric ulcers in 8 of 251 patients who received intrahepatic infusion of 5-FU by way of a catheter inserted percutaneously and positioned in the hepatic artery.[151] None of these patients had a history of ulcers. Four of the patients developed bleeding, and there was gastric perforation in 1 patient. In every patient with ulceration, the catheter tip had become dislodged and was found to be either directly infusing the left gastric artery or proximal to the right gastric artery or to the gastroduodenal artery, allowing direct flow of 5-FU to the stomach. Each of the patients was symptomatic for several days before the documentation of the diagnosis of gastric ulcer. A subsequent study documented the development of severe dyspepsia in 18 of 124 patients receiving hepatic arterial chemotherapy through percutaneous, angiographically positioned catheters.[152] Ten of the 18 patients had documented gastrointestinal pathology: 6 had gastric ulcers and gastritis, 2 had duodenal ulcers, 1 had pyloroduodenitis, and 1 had pancreatitis. Investigators in the study noted that endoscopically defined ulceration and gastritis caused by hepatic arterial infusion chemotherapy were confined to the distribution of the infused arteries. Nine of the 10 patients with toxicity had received 5-FUDR as well as mitomycin C through the hepatic artery catheter.

Initial results with the totally implanted drug delivery system showed significant gastrointestinal (GI) toxicity (see Table 61–27). Fortunately, however, the report by Hohn and associates, describing their experience with 35 patients who received hepatic arterial FUDR administered with the implanted infusion pump, demonstrated that gastric ulceration could be prevented.[153] These investigators found that none of the 35 patients in their study developed signs or symptoms of gastritis or ulcer attributable to chemotherapy because particular care was taken at surgery to identify and divide those vessels arising from the hepatic artery (distal to the point of cannulation) that supplied the superior border of the distal stomach and proximal duodenum. They found that, despite the standard approach of meticulous devascularization of the upper border of the distal stomach and proximal duodenum, infusion of fluorescein intraoperatively into the pump Sideport demonstrated residual gastroduodenal perfusion requiring further dissection and ligation of previously unrecognized

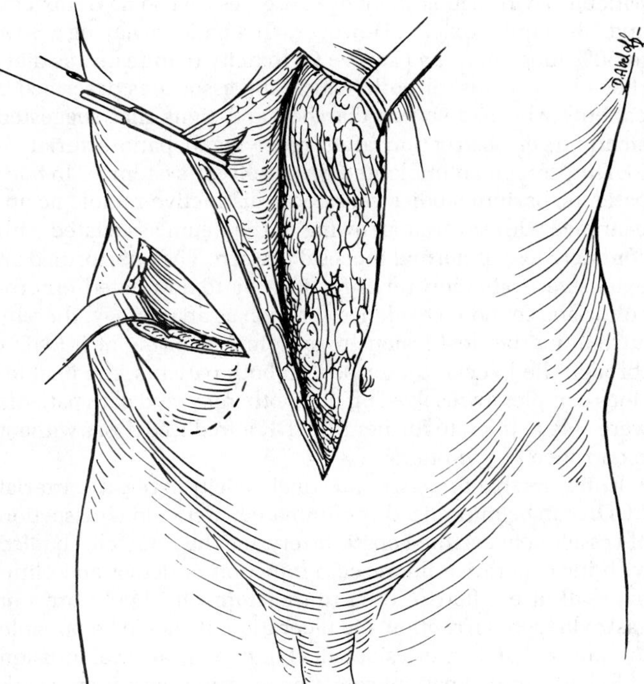

FIGURE 61–38. A midline incision with a subcutaneous pocket for the implanted pump positioned in the right lower quadrant of the abdomen.

TABLE 61–27. Toxicities of Chronic Hepatic Arterial Chemotherapy

	Gastric (%)		Hepatic (%)			
Investigations	*Symptoms*	*Ulcers*	*Enzyme Elevation*	*Jaundice*	*Biliary Stenosis*	*Cholecystitis (%)*
Niederhuber, 1984[135]	56		54	24		
Kemeny, 1984[136]	46	29	71	22		
Shepard, 1985[137]		18	49	24		
Kemeny, 1985[138]	15	4	59		17	13
Hohn, 1986[150]	0	0	56	5	29	
Kemeny, 1987[141]		17	42	19	8	

blood vessels in 7 patients. Residual vessels were most commonly identified adjacent to the common bile duct and portal vein. As will be described below, it is noteworthy that these same investigators describe a relatively high incidence of biliary sclerosis, perhaps related, in part, to a more efficient devascularization of proximal parts of the biliary tree.

It is probable that the maintenance of a low level of 5-FUDR in the systemic circulation can, by itself, inflict a different form of gastrointestinal toxicity, namely, diarrhea. Studies in which 5-FUDR has been administered intravenously for 14 days have described a high incidence of significant diarrhea.[141,142] Although the efficiency of hepatic extraction of 5-FUDR exceeds 95%, this holds true only when there is a low percentage of arteriovenous (AV) shunting. Using hepatic arterial angiography with TcMAA, Kaplan and associates found a correlation between lung shunting (*i.e.*, the percentage of a dose of hepatic arterial TcMAA that goes through AV shunts in the liver and is trapped in the lung) and diarrhea.[154] In 10 patients having a lung shunt of 15% or less, 8 had no GI toxicity and 2 had mild toxicity. However, all 4 patients having a 30% to 50% lung shunt had severe GI toxicity manifested as diarrhea or mucositis, or both. Gluck and associates described 2 patients who had severe diarrhea and signs that suggested small-bowel obstruction after receiving hepatic arterial 5-FUDR through an implanted drug delivery system.[155] In both patients, barium studies revealed a distinctive radiologic appearance with severe narrowing of the ileum associated with complete loss of normal mucosal pattern. They performed an extensive evaluation for infectious or toxin-related enterocolitis and found no evidence for such as an etiology, thereby attributing the ileal lesions to systemic shunting of 5-FUDR through the liver or tumor bed. In both patients, the ileal lesions completely resolved off chemotherapy, and both patients were able to tolerate further 5-FUDR at reduced doses without recurrence of symptoms.

It appears that the gastrointestinal toxicity of hepatic arterial FUDR can be minimized or eliminated. Meticulous dissection of vessels between the hepatic artery and the stomach, coupled with intraoperative fluorescein injection to detect and eliminate all direct flow of drug to the stomach, should prevent gastroduodenal irritation and ulceration. It should be possible to remove diarrhea as a side effect of hepatic arterial infusion of FUDR through patient selection, eliminating patients with AV shunts through the liver that are of such magnitude that 20% or more of TcMAA injected into the hepatic artery flows directly through the liver into the pulmonary circulation. Because diarrhea resulting from hepatic arterial FUDR relates to the level of sustained 5-FUDR in the systemic circulation, dose reduction appears to be a reasonable and logical way to eliminate this complication in the few patients in whom it will develop. When gastrointestinal complications occur, the severity and the rapidity of their resolution appear to be related to early detection as well as to delaying the reinstitution of 5-FUDR until adequate time has passed for complete healing. When 5-FUDR infusion is stopped at the first sign of symptoms that may be related to gastrointestinal irritation, such symptoms tend to rapidly resolve. Further administration of drug in the face of the development of such symptoms tends to make the symptoms much more intense and their resolution much more protracted. Avoiding the reinstitution of 5-FUDR for at least a month after resolution of symptoms and then reinstituting infusion at a lower dose or for a shorter duration appears to be prudent. Any severe symptoms or protracted symptoms mandate the use of endoscopy to document gastrointestinal pathology.

The major and most severe toxicity of chronic hepatic arterial FUDR is hepatobiliary damage. There are three elements to hepatobiliary damage: cholecystitis, biliary stricture/sclerosis, and hepatitis.[147,156] The incidence of hepatobiliary toxicity appears relatively uniform from study to study and seems to affect approximately 50% of patients (see Table 61–27). Cholecystitis, previously noted to occur with hepatic arterial chemotherapy with 5-FUDR and mitomycin C administered through percutaneous angiographic catheters,[154] may develop in as many as 33% of patients receiving chronic FUDR treatment with the implanted drug delivery system.[138] The symptoms generated by a chemically induced cholecystitis can become quite confusing in the care of patients who have metastatic cancer within the liver. The relatively high incidence of cholecystitis and associated morbidity have led to the recommendation for a prophylactic cholecystectomy at the time of hepatic arterial catheter implantation.

The gallbladder and the biliary tree are thought to receive their total blood supply directly from the hepatic artery, whereas hepatocytes receive a mixed blood supply, with about 33% from the hepatic artery and 66% from the portal vein.[157] Hence, with hepatic arterial chemotherapy, the gallbladder and biliary tree will be exposed to protracted drug levels that are some threefold higher than those of the hepatocytes. Removal of the gallbladder is a reasonable solution to the problem of chemical cholecystitis. On the other hand, toxicity of 5-FUDR to the biliary tree is a much more serious problem.

During initial studies with the implanted drug delivery system for hepatic arterial chemotherapy, it was noted that approximately 25% of patients would become jaundiced during treatment and that generally jaundice would resolve when there was a protracted drug-free period.[133] In some patients, however, jaundice did not resolve. Kemeny and associates reported that 8 of 46 (17.4%) patients treated with continuous hepatic arterial infusion of FUDR developed biliary strictures.[158] They noted that the lesions were clinically, radiographically, and pathologically identical to the idiopathic sclerosing cholangitis frequently seen in association with inflammatory bowel disease. Two of their 8 patients died of the complication. All 35 patients receiving intraarterial 5-FUDR in the study of Hohn and associates developed significant increases in alkaline phosphatase, and 7 of the patients who were studied cholangiographically had sclerosis of the intrahepatic or extrahepatic bile ducts, or both.[159] Liver biopsies done on these patients showed cholestasis and pericholangitis with minimal hepatocyte damage.

Although Hohn and colleagues suggest that "biliary sclerosis" rather than "chemical hepatitis" is the predominant toxicity associated with hepatic arterial infusions of 5-FUDR,[159] Doria and associates describe additional liver histopathology and clinical features of 8 patients who developed hepatitis while receiving hepatic arterial chemotherapy.[160] All 8 patients who developed hepatitis had responded to the treatment. Clinical findings included nausea, vomiting, abdominal pain, and jaundice. Serum transaminases, alkaline phosphatase, and bilirubin levels were increased. Pathologic examination of biopsies revealed hepatocyte necrosis, steatosis, cholestasis, central vein sclerosis, and alterations in the portal triad (primarily fibrosis). In addition, central vein lesions like those accompanying venoocclusive disease and micronodular sclerosis as induced by alcohol were encountered. These latter investigators noted that the degree of damage appeared to be related to the dose and duration of hepatic arterial infusion.

Biliary sclerosis is a serious toxicity that may greatly compromise the life of patients who otherwise may have benefited from significant tumor reduction. The development of biliary sclerosis is uniformly preceded by an elevation in liver function tests, particularly alkaline phosphatase. Careful monitoring of the liver function tests over cycles of therapy can sort out those patients who are most susceptible to this toxicity. The manipulation that is available to the physician to deal with hepatobiliary toxicity is an alteration of dose-schedule. For example, 1 week of 5-FUDR instead of 2 weeks of 5-FUDR with longer drug-free intervals between the infusions may be more tolerable in susceptible patients. Reductions in the dose rate of 5-FUDR to levels of 0.1 or 0.05 mg/kg/day may lower the incidence of hepatobiliary toxicity.

In an effort to study the effect of altering dose schedule on biliary toxicity and in an attempt to increase cumulative drug tolerated, a phase I and II clinical trial was initiated at Johns Hopkins Oncology Center under the direction of Louise Grochow.[53] This trial has studied weekly 48-hour infusions of FUDR using an implanted drug delivery system. This initial infusion dose was 0.2 mg/kg/day for 48 hours each week. Doses were escalated in cohorts of 3 new patients. At 0.5 mg/kg/day, 2 of 2 patients had grade IV hepatic toxicity. At 0.4 mg/kg/day, no patient had dose-limiting hepatic toxicity. Two of 35 patients experienced complete response and 51% had partial response. The median duration of response was greater than 20 months. As experience has accumulated, it has become clear that patients treated less aggressively and monitored more closely tend to do better in the long run. Although the overall incidence of hepatobiliary toxicity may not be decreasing, the severity of the toxicity appears to be declining to a more tolerable level with accumulating experience.[141,142] Studies in a dog model may ultimately define the mechanism of this toxicity and how to control it more effectively.[161] A recent clinical study suggests that dexamethasone may play a role in decreasing such toxicity as well.[162]

Patterns of Failure

Colorectal cancer represents the only type of metastatic liver disease consistently treated in a defined manner, with hepatic arterial therapy making it possible to evaluate for sites of disease control and failure. Aggressive hepatic arterial therapy can generate hepatic tumor control such that extrahepatic tumor progression is the cause of death in ~75% of patients.[135] The lung is the most frequent site of extrahepatic disease at death in patients initially presenting with metastatic colorectal cancer confined to the liver. Patients with evidence for extrahepatic disease at the time of pump implantation have a high incidence of progressive disease in the lung and in extrahepatic abdominal sites at time of death. In the Memorial Sloan Kettering study of hepatic arterial versus intravenous 5-FUDR, failure within the liver occurred in only 37% of patients on arterial treatment as compared with 82% of patients on intravenous treatment.[140] Extrahepatic failure was found to occur in 56% of patients on arterial therapy and 37% of patients on the intravenous arm. In this regard, it is relevant that the high hepatic extraction of over 95% of 5-FUDR means that little drug goes into the systemic circulation with hepatic arterial infusion.

It is interesting to compare hepatic arterial therapy for colorectal cancer with surgical resection in terms of sites of failure. In the largest multiinstitutional study of resection, 55% of patients had extrahepatic failure either alone or with failure in the liver.[163] Of total failures, 78% were extrahepatic. It is reasonable to assume that patients undergoing hepatic resection of colorectal metastases have disease of decreased metastatic potential. It is likely that such patients should have less propensity to develop extrahepatic disease as compared with patients receiving hepatic arterial therapy alone. In summary, the data on sites of failure with regional treatments indicate that the achievement of survival benefit in the majority of patients with colorectal liver metastases will require the application of more effective systemic therapies to control extrahepatic disease.

Hepatic Arterial Therapy Plus Systemic Chemotherapy

Extrahepatic tumor growth occurring frequently in the setting where intrahepatic tumor is controlled by hepatic arterial FUDR has led to several clinical trials in which additional systemic therapy was added. In one study, dual-catheter implanted pumps were used to simultaneously deliver hepatic arterial and intravenous 5-FUDR.[164] Although extrahepatic spread of tumor during therapy occurred less frequently with combined treatment (33%) than with hepatic arterial treatment (61%) in this randomized study, survival was the same for both treatment groups. In a small phase I trial, the addition of a 5-day infusion of systemic 5-FU immediately after a standard 14-day infusion of hepatic arterial 5-FUDR was shown to be feasible, although systemic toxicities (mucositis, diarrhea) appeared to be moderately increased.[165] A shortened duration (7 days) of hepatic arterial 5-FUDR combined with bolus injections of hepatic arterial 5-FU by way of the Sideport of the Infusaid pump (days 15, 22, and 29 of a 35-day cycle) was found to produce less hepatobiliary toxicity while retaining a high response rate (50%) and a prolonged survival (26.6 months).[166] In this latter study, the first evidence of disease progression occurred in the liver in 50% of patients, in an extrahepatic site in 35% of patients, and in the liver plus an extrahepatic site in 15% of patients. The less efficient hepatic extraction of 5-FU means that more systemic effect will occur with this agent than with the highly extracted agent 5-FUDR. Unfortunately, the solubility and potency of 5-FU necessitate use of an external pump for high-volume infusions of 5-FU through either surgically placed port-catheter systems or radiologically placed catheters.[148,167] One such study using 5-FU with leucovorin and mitomycin C reported a 58% response rate.[168] Yet, despite the potential of this regimen to produce systemic effects, extrahepatic tumor, primarily in the lung and peritoneum, developed during treatment in 58% of patients.

SUMMARY OF CURRENT HEPATIC ARTERIAL THERAPY FOR COLORECTAL HEPATIC METASTASES

There is recognition, supported by the phase II and III studies described above, that the response rate for regression of colorectal cancer within the liver is greater for hepatic arterial 5-FUDR than for systemically administered 5-FU or 5-FUDR. A survival benefit for hepatic arterial 5-FUDR has not been demonstrated because of limitations imposed on hepatic arterial therapy by hepatobiliary toxicity and because of a lack of control of systemic disease with such regionally focal treatment. The technology for hepatic arterial therapy has been refined with improved drug delivery systems and mechanisms for ensuring and defining infusion such that all hepatic tumor sees the higher drug exposures generated thereby. It is anticipated that progress will be made in terms of understanding and controlling hepatobiliary toxicity and in combining systemic with regional treatment to control all sites of disease. Further additions to the therapeutic armamentarium are likely to be created out of attempts to develop innovative second-line treatments as described below.

CURRENT HEPATIC ARTERIAL THERAPY FOR NONCOLORECTAL LIVER METASTASES

There are no randomized, controlled studies of hepatic arterial therapy in diseases other than colorectal cancer. The number of patients with liver metastases as the sole site of disease with other tumor types is extremely small. In actual practice, such patients are often considered together with colorectal patients in phase II studies and treated in the same manner. Nonetheless, for centers skilled in the delivery of hepatic arterial therapy, other agents such as doxorubicin (Adriamycin) and cisplatin have been used in addition to 5-FUDR, 5-FU, and mitomycin C.[139,169] Although of low incidence, hepatic involvement with carcinoid and nonfunctional islet cell neuroendocrine tumors represents a situation where hepatic arterial therapy is applicable. Infusional hepatic arterial chemotherapy with agents such as 5-FU and streptozocin can produce responses.[110,111,170,171] The relative hypervascularity of neuroendocrine tumors within the liver appears to make them especially susceptible to vascular occlusion with use of hepatic arterial embolization with Gelfoam or polyvinyl alcohol particles.[172–175] The majority of patients treated with embolization are reported to have symptomatic improvement as well as evidence of reduction in bulk hepatic tumor.

SECOND-LINE THERAPEUTIC OPTIONS

Radiation Therapy Combined With Hepatic Arterial Therapy

Although it has long been recognized that 5-FU has radiosensitizing properties, only recently has it been demonstrated that 5-FUDR is also capable of producing radiosensitization at clinically achievable concentrations.[176] A variety of studies have been conducted using primarily hepatic arterial 5-FU or 5-FUDR with external beam radiotherapy (Table 61–28). Generally, these treatment schemes have used total radiation doses of less than 3000 cGy to limit the potential for radiation hepatitis such as occurs with larger doses.[184,185] Recently, the development of computer-assisted three-dimensional (3D) radiotherapy planning has made it possible to exceed the 3000 cGy dose by giving focal radiotherapy to tumor-bearing partial liver volumes.[183,186] With the sparing of volumes of normal liver, as is made possible by dose-volume histogram analyses, Lawrence and associates found no hepatic toxicity with the delivery of up to 6000 cGy to localized hepatic tumors despite concurrent hepatic arterial 5-FUDR (Fig. 61–39).[186–188] The delivery of such high doses of radiotherapy to focal hepatic tumor nodules is a step in developing a radiotherapy equivalent to surgical metastasectomy. It is highly likely that the more effective radiosensitizers, 5-iodo-2′-deoxyuridine (5-IUDR) and 5-bromo-2′-deoxyuridine (5-BUDR), can be administered in hepatic arterial therapy combined with high-dose, three-dimensionally planned focal radiotherapy for improved therapeutic potential.[189–191]

Hepatic Arterial Microsphere Therapy

Several less conventional forms of hepatic arterial therapy have used microspheres to deliver either radiotherapy or chemotherapy to hepatic tumors. Most neuroendocrine hepatic metastases and some colorectal metastases can be relatively hypervascular when evaluated through use of tracer microparticles such as TcMAA.[52,129]

Yttrium 90 (^{90}Y) incorporated into microspheres has been used as a radiotherapeutic agent for hepatic arterial therapy of metastatic tumors.[192,193] It is not yet understood why liver tolerance to ^{90}Y microsphere therapy is such that doses of 10,000 cGy and higher produce little or no hepatic damage. Y-90 microsphere therapy has received approval for use as a conventional therapy in Canada.

TABLE 61–28. Hepatic Irradiation and Infusional Chemotherapy

Investigations	*Drug*	*Total Radiation Dose*	*No. of Patients*	*Response (%)*	*Hepatic Toxicity (%)*
Barone, 1982[177]	FUDR or FU	3000 cGy	18	56	20
Herbsman, 1978[178]	FUDR	2500–3000 cGy	13	46	30
Webber, 1978[179]	FUDR	2500 cGy	25	33	1
Lokich, 1982[180]	FU	2500–3000 cGy	15	75	
Raju, 1987[181]	FUDR or FU	2100 cGy	12	83	
Friedman, 1979[182]	FU, Ad	1350–2100 cGy	22	55	0
Lawrence, 1991[183]	FUDR	3300 cGy	20	39	
		4500–6000 cGy (by DVH)	13	64	

FU, fluorouracil; FUDR, floxuridine; Ad, doxorubicin (Adriamycin); DVH, dose determined by dose-volume histogram.

Biodegradable starch microspheres were investigated as a means to deliver more chemotherapy to hepatic tumor in the early 1980s in the United States, and investigations still continue outside of the United States.[194–196] Pharmacologic studies demonstrated the ability of hepatic arterial injection of starch microspheres within a chemotherapeutic drug solution (a form of chemoembolization) to reduce systemic drug exposure and to increase drug delivery to hepatic tumor.[196]

The use of hepatic arterial microsphere therapy as described above carries with it an even greater need for precise delivery of agent than that seen with fluoropyrimidine infusions. The therapeutic agent is administered in a very short time period (several minutes) in a highly potent suspension. Maldistribution in the delivery pattern could lead to high concentrations of the cytotoxic agent directly reaching the stomach or duodenum and inflicting severe damage. Alternatively, if the flow distribution is such that all of the hepatic tumor is not directly infused, essentially no therapeutic effect can be expected.

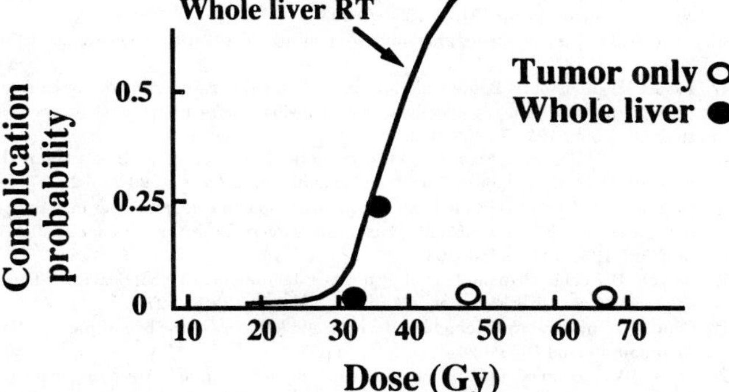

FIGURE 61–39. Ability to deliver high doses of radiation to intrahepatic tumors using three-dimensionally planned radiation therapy based on dose volume histogram analysis. Solid symbols represent observed complication probability for patients who received whole-liver irradiation; open symbols show data from patients receiving focal irradiation to tumor with sparing of 33% (48 Gy) and 66% (66 Gy) of normal liver.[185] Solid line represents compilation of complication probabilities derived from the literature.[186]

Focal Treatments for Hepatic Tumors

Treatments that are applicable when there are small numbers of hepatic metastases include surgical resection and focal external beam radiotherapy as described previously. The delivery of tissue-destroying agents to intrahepatic tumors localized by direct observation, ultrasound, or CT by way of needles inserted into such lesions extends the concept of metastasectomy to nodules not amenable to resection and to patients unable to tolerate major surgery. Radioactive seeds can be positioned for interstitial, focal radiotherapy.[197] Alternatively, direct instillation of absolute alcohol or liquid nitrogen into tumor nodules can be used to achieve focal destruction through fixation and freeze-thawing, respectively.[198,199] Although abscess formation is a possible concern, a major limitation of such approaches is that such debulking treatment does not address the subclinical presence of other metastatic tumor. With focal treatments, it is especially important that adjunctive chemotherapy regimens be considered to deal with occult metastatic tumor likely to be present elsewhere in the liver and in extrahepatic sites.

CONCLUSIONS

The importance of hepatic metastases transcends even the high frequency of morbidity and mortality associated with the disease. The fact that, under defined circumstances, the resection of metastatic nodules leads to a cure in an appreciable proportion of patients (30% in colorectal cancer) has provided hope for patients, an impetus for aggressive surgical resection, and some insight into relevant tumor biology. The unique ability to deliver therapeutic agents in high concentrations directly to the metastatic tumor using the hepatic artery has validated concepts in regional pharmacokinetics and dose-response effects. In addition, hepatic arterial chemotherapy has been pivotal in the technologic development of implantable drug delivery pumps and ports for vascular access. Distinguishing aspects of tumor blood supply have proved useful in tumor detection and in various forms of embolic therapies. The circumscribed and often isolated nature of hepatic tumor nodules, which makes them sometimes resectable, also makes them amenable to attack with direct implantation of therapeutic agents as well as with high-dose, focal external beam radiotherapy. It is likely that future integration of these regional technologies will increase the potential for cure (in some patients) or, at least, for significant palliation (in most patients).

Unfortunately, the subsequent development of extrahepatic tumor continues to frustrate cure in most instances. Nonetheless, recent advances in the adjuvant therapy of colorectal cancer suggest that the debulking induced by hepatic tumor removal or sterilization might be reasonably combined with adjunctive systemic therapy. In such efforts, progress will require the cooperation of surgical, medical, and radiation therapists working together, driven by a dissatisfaction with current outcomes that is coupled with optimism from successes to date.

REFERENCES

1. NIH Consensus Conference. Adjuvant therapy for patients with colon and rectal cancer. JAMA 1990;264(11):1444–1450.
2. Wood CB, Gillis CR, Blumgart LH. A retrospective study of patients with liver metastases from colorectal cancer. Clin Oncol 1976;2:285–288.
3. Lise M, Dabian PP, Nitti D, et al. Colorectal metastases to the liver: Present status of management. Dis Colon Rectum 1990;35(8):688–694.
4. August DA, Sugarbaker PH, Ottow RT. Hepatic resection of colorectal metastases. Ann Surg 1985;201:210–218.
5. Gennari L, Doi R, Bignami P, Bozzetti F. Surgical treatment of hepatic metastases from colorectal cancer. Ann Surg 1986;203(1):49–54.
6. Hughes K, Scheele J, Sugarbaker PH. Surgery for colorectal cancer metastatic to the liver. Surg Clin North Am 1989;69(2):339–359.
7. Steele G Jr, Bleday R, Mayer RJ, et al. A prospective evaluation of hepatic resection for colorectal carcinoma metastases to the liver: Gastrointestinal Tumor Study Group Protocol, 6584. J Clin Oncol 1991;9(7):1105–1112.
8. Cady B, Monson DO, Swinton NW. Survival of patients after colonic resection for carcinoma with simultaneous liver metastases. Surg Gynecol Obstet 1970;131:697–700.
9. Goslin R, Steele G Jr, Zamcheck N, et al. Factors influencing survival in patients with hepatic metastases from adenocarcinoma of the colon and rectum. Dis Colon Rectum 1982;25:749–754.
10. Scheele J, Stangl R, Altendorf-Hofmann A. Hepatic metastases from colorectal carcinoma: Impact of surgical resection on the natural history. Br J Surg 1990;77(11):1241–1246.
11. Finan PJ, Marshall RJ, Cooper EH, et al. Factors affecting survival in patients with synchronous hepatic metastases from colorectal cancer: A clinical and computer analysis. Br J Surg 1985;72:373–377.
12. Wagner JS, Adson MA, vanHeerden JA, et al. The natural history of hepatic metastases from colorectal cancer. Ann Surg 1984;199:502.
13. Lahr CJ, Scong SJ, Cloud G, et al. A multifactorial analysis of prognostic factors in patients with liver metastases from colorectal carcinoma. J Clin Oncol 1983;1:720–726.
14. Boey J, Choi TK, Wong J, et al. Carcinoma of the colon and rectum with liver involvement. Surg Gynecol Obstet 1981;153:864–868.
15. Bengtsson G, Carlson G, Hofstrom L, et al. Natural history of patients with untreated liver metastases from colorectal cancer. Am J Surg 1981;141:586–589.
16. Baden H, Anderson B. Survival of patients with untreated liver metastases from colorectal cancer. Scand J Gastroenterol 1975;10:221–223.
17. Abrams MS, Lerner HJ. Survival of patients at Pennsylvania Hospital with hepatic metastases from carcinoma of the colon and rectum. Dis Colon Rectum 1971;14:431–434.
18. Bengmark S, Hofstrom L. The natural history of primary and secondary malignant tumors of the liver: I. The prognosis for patients with hepatic metastases from colonic and rectal carcinoma by laparotomy. Cancer 1970;23:198–202.
19. Sterns MW, Binkley GE. Palliative surgery for cancer of the rectum and colon. Cancer 1954;7:1016–1019.
20. Hughes KS, Sugarbaker PH. Resection of the liver for metastatic solid tumors. In: Rosenberg SA, ed. Surgical treatment of metastatic cancer. Philadelphia: JB Lippincott, 1987.
21. Schwartz SI. Primary and metastatic hepatic malignant tumors, and hepatic resection. In: Schwartz SI, Ellis H, eds. Maingot's abdominal operations. 9th ed. Norwalk, CT: Appleton & Lange, 1989:1253–1290.
22. Sugarbaker PH, Reinig JW, Hughes KS. Diagnosis of hepatic metastases. In: Rosenberg SA, ed. Surgical treatment of metastatic cancer. Philadelphia: JB Lippincott, 1987.
23. Foster JH, Ensminger WF. Treatment of metastatic cancer to the liver. In: DeVita VT Jr, Hellman S, Rosenberg S, eds. Cancer principles and practice of oncology. 2nd ed. Philadelphia: JB Lippincott, 1985.
24. Kemeny N, Sugarbaker PH. Treatment of metastatic cancer to the liver. In: DeVita VT Jr, Hellman S, Rosenberg S, eds. Cancer principles and practice of oncology. 3rd ed. Philadelphia: JB Lippincott, 1989.
25. Foster JH. Surgical treatment of metastatic liver tumors. Hepatogastroenterology 1990;37:182–187.
26. Weiss L, Grundman E, Torkorst J, et al. Hematogenous metastatic patterns in colonic carcinoma: An analysis of 1541 necropsies. J Pathol 1986;150:195–203.
27. Welch JP, Donaldson GA. The clinical correlation of an autopsy study of recurrent colorectal cancer. Ann Surg 1979;189:496.
28. Wanebo JH, Rao B, Pinsky CM, et al. Preoperative carcinoembryonic antigen level as a prognostic indicator in colorectal cancer. N Engl J Med 1978;299:448–451.
29. Roh MS. Hepatic resection for colorectal liver metastases. Hematol Oncol Clin North Am 1989;3(1):171–181.
30. Klose G, Schmiegel W. Laboratory investigations in hepatobiliary and pancreatic malignancies: The role of tumor markers. In: Lygidakis NJ, Tytgat GNJ, eds. Hepatobiliary and pancreatic malignancies. Diagnosis, medical and surgical management. New York: Georg Thieme Verlag Stuttgart, Thieme Medical Publishers, 1989:157–161.
31. Rosenbusch G, Smits NJ, Reeders JWAJ. Ultrasonography in hepatobiliary and pancreatic malignancies. In: Lygidakis NJ, Tytgat GNJ, eds. Hepatobiliary and pancreatic malignancies. Diagnosis, medical and surgical management. New York: Georg Thieme Verlag Stuttgart, Thieme Medical Publishers, 1989:51–65.
32. Strake LTE, Reeders JWAJ. Computed tomography in hepatobiliary and pancreatic malignancies. In: Lygidakis NJ, Tytgat GNJ, eds. Hepatobiliary and pancreatic malignancies. Diagnosis, medical and surgical management. New York: Georg Thieme Verlag Stuttgart, Thieme Medical Publishers, 1989:79–89.
33. Engelholem L, Mathieu D, Segebarth C, et al. Magnetic resonance imaging (MRI) in hepatobiliary and pancreatic malignancies. In: Lygidakis NJ, Tytgat GNJ, eds. Hepatobiliary and pancreatic malignancies. Diagnosis, medical and surgical management. New York: Georg Thieme Verlag Stuttgart, Thieme Medical Publishers, 1989:90–99.
34. Sitzmann JV, Coleman JA, Pitt HA, et al. Preoperative assessment of malignant hepatic tumors. Am J Surg 1990;159:137–142.
35. Laufer I, Braffman B, Gefter W. Diagnosis and imaging of gastrointestinal tract cancers. Curr Opin Oncol 1991;3(4):730–736.
36. Castaing D, Edmond J, Kunstlinger F, Bismuth H. Utility of operative ultrasound in the surgical management of liver tumors. Ann Surg 1986;204:600–605.
37. Takahashi H, Carlson R, Ozturk M, Sun S, et al. Radioimmunolocation of hepatic and pulmonary metastasis of human colon adenocarcinoma. Gastroenterology 1989;96:1317–1329.
38. Doerr RJ, Abdel-Nabi H, Kray D, Mitchell E. Radiolabelled antibody imaging in the management of colorectal cancer. Ann Surg 1991;214(2):118–124.
39. Adson MA, vanHeerden JA, Adson MH, Wagner JS, Ilstrup DM. Resection of hepatic metastases from colorectal cancer. Arch Surg 1984;119:647.
40. Iwatsuki S, Sheahan DG, Starzl TE. The changing face of hepatic resection. Curr Probl Surg 1989;26(5):283–379.
41. Gozzetti G, Mazziotti A. Expectations and possibilities of liver resection in the management of secondary liver tumors. In: Lygidakis NJ, Tytgat GNJ, eds. Hepatobiliary and pancreatic malignancies. Diagnosis, medical and surgical management. New York: Georg Thieme Verlag Stuttgart, Thieme Medical Publishers, 1989:183–190.
42. Meyers WC. Neoplasms of the liver. In: Sabiston D Jr, ed. Textbook of surgery. The biological basis of modern surgical practice. 13th ed. Philadelphia: WB Saunders, 1986:1079–1092.
43. Ravitch MM. Chapter 22. In: Ravitch MM, ed. A century of surgery. Philadelphia: JB Lippincott, 1982:318–319.
44. Kremer B, Henne-Burns D. Surgical techniques. In: Lygidakis NJ, Tytgat GNJ, eds. Hepatobiliary and pancreatic malignancies. Diagnosis, medical and surgical management. New York: Georg Thieme Verlag Stuttgart, Thieme Medical Publishers, 1989:195–218.
45. Couinauld C. Bases anatomiques des hepatectomies gauche et droit reglees: Techniques qui en decoulent. J Chir (Paris) 1954:70:933.
46. Couinauld C. Le foie: Etudes anatomiques et chirugicales. Paris: Masson & Cis, 1957:3–9.
47. Paquet KJ, Koussouris P, Mercado MA, et al. Limited hepatic resection for selected cirrhotic patients with hepatocellular or cholangiocellular carcinoma: A prospective study. Br J Surg 1991;78:459–462.
48. Sitzmann JV. Colorectal cancer metastatic to the liver: Resection. In: Cameron JL, ed. Current surgical therapy. 3rd ed. Philadelphia: BC Decker, 1989:220–225.
49. Nordlinger B, Parc R, Delva E, et al. Hepatic resection for colorectal liver metastases. Influence on survival of preoperative factors and surgery for recurrences in 80 patients. Ann Surg 1986;305(3):256–263.
50. Bozzetti F, Doci R, Bignami P, et al. Patterns of failure following surgical resection of colorectal cancer liver metastases. Ann Surg 1986;305(3):264–270.
51. Cantlie J. On a new arrangement of the right and left lobes of the liver. Proc Anat Soc Gr Britain Ireland 1898:32:4–9.
52. Gyves JW, Ziessman HA, Ensminger WD, et al. Definition of hepatic tumor microcirculation by single photon emission computerized tomography (SPECT). J Nucl Med 1984;25:972.
53. Niederhuber JE, Grochow LB. Status of infusion chemotherapy for the treatment of liver metastases. Principles and Practices of Oncology (Updates) 1989;3(3):1–9.
54. Breedes C, Young G. The blood supply of neoplasms in the liver. Am J Pathol 1954;30:227.
55. Hesly JE. Vascular patterns in human metastatic liver tumors. Surg Gynecol Obstet 1965;120:1187.
56. Lin B, Lunderquist A, Hogersteand L, et al. Postmortem examination of the blood supply and vascular pattern of small liver metastases in man. Surgery 1984;96:517.

57. Ridge JA, Bading JR, Gelbard AS, et al. Perfusion of colorectal hepatic metastases: Relative distribution of flow from the hepatic artery and portal vein. Cancer 1987;59: 1547.
58. Schuur KH, Reeders JWAJ. Angiography in the preoperative staging of hepatobiliary and pancreatic malignancies. In: Lygidakis NJ, Tytgat GNJ, eds. Hepatobiliary and pancreatic malignancies. Diagnosis, medical and surgical management. New York: Georg Thieme Verlag Stuttgart, Thieme Medical Publishers, 1989:136–146.
59. Putnam CW. Techniques of ultrasonic dissection in resection of the liver. Surg Gynecol Obstet 1982;157:475.
60. Fortner JG, Silva JS, Golbey RB, et al. Multi-variate analysis of a personal series of 247 consecutive patients with liver metastases from colorectal cancer. Ann Surg 1984;199:306.
61. Attiyeh FF, Wanebo HJ, Stearns MW. Hepatic resection for metastasis from colorectal cancer. Dis Colon Rectum 1978;21:160.
62. Foster JH, Lundy J. Pathology of liver metastasis. Curr Probl Surg 1981;18:157.
63. Tomas-de la Vega JE, Donahue EJ, Doolas A, et al. A ten year experience with hepatic resection. Surg Gynecol Obstet 1984;159:223–228.
64. Bismuth H, Houssin D, Ornowski J, Meriggi F. Liver resections in cirrhotic patients: A Western experience. World J Surg 1986;10:311–317.
65. Kanematsu T, Takenake K, Matsumata T, et al. Limited hepatic resection effective for selected cirrhotic patients with primary liver cancer. Ann Surg 1984;199:51–56.
66. Yomanaka N, Okamoto E, Kuwata K, Tanaka N. A multiple regression equation for prediction of posthepatectomy liver failure. Ann Surg 1984;200:658–663.
67. Sitzmann JV, Coleman JA, Pitt HA, et al. Preoperative assessment of malignant hepatic tumors. Am J Surg 1990:159:137–142.
68. Egglin TK, Rummeny E, Stark DD, et al. Hepatic tumors: Quantitative tissue characterization with MR imaging. Radiology 1990;176:107–110.
69. Hahn PF, Stark DD, Weissleder R, et al. Clinical application of superparamagnetic iron oxide in MR imaging of tissue perfusion in vascular liver tumors. Radiology 1990;174:361–366.
70. Charnley RM, Morris DL, Dennison AR, et al. Detection of colorectal liver metastases using intraoperative ultrasonography. Br J Surg 1991;78(1):45–48.
71. Steele G Jr, Ravikumar TS. Resection of hepatic metastases from colorectal cancer. Ann Surg 1989;210(2):127–138.
72. Brower ST, Dumistrescu O, Rubinoff S, et al. Operative ultrasound establishes resectability of metastases by major hepatic resection. World J Surg 1989;13(5):649–657.
73. Niederhuber JE. Surgical aspects of intrahepatic artery therapy. In: Bottino JC, Opfell RW, Muggia FM, eds. Liver cancer. Boston: Martinus Nijhoff Publishing, 1985:179–194.
74. Niederhuber JE. Colorectal cancer metastatic to the liver: Hepatic artery chemotherapy. In: Cameron JL, ed. Current surgical therapy. 3rd ed. Philadelphia: BC Decker, 1989: 222–233.
75. Szakacs JG, Szakacs JE, Karl RC. Surgical resection versus perfusion in the treatment of metastatic and primary liver tumors. Ann Clin Lab Sci 1990;20(4):245–257.
76. Kuroda C, Sakurai M, Monden M, et al. Transcatheter arterial embolization for metastatic liver tumors: A study in resected cases. Cardiovasc Intervent Radiol 1989;12:72–75.
77. Akuta K, Ahe M, Kondo M, et al. Combined effects of hepatic arterial embolization using degradable starch microspheres in hyperthermia for liver cancer. Int J Hyperthermia 1991;7(2):231–242.
78. Vetter D, Wenger JJ, Bergier JM, et al. Transcatheter oily chemoembolization in the management of advanced hepatocellular carcinoma in cirrhosis: Results of a Western comparative study in 60 patients. Hepatology 1991;13(3):427–433.
79. Livraghi T, Vettori C, Lazzaroni S. Liver metastases: Results of percutaneous ethanol injection in 14 patients. Radiology 1991;179:709–712.
80. Onik G, Rubinsky B, Zemel R, et al. Ultrasound-guided hepatic cryosurgery in the treatment of metastatic colon carcinoma. Cancer 1991;67(4):901–907.
81. Iwatsuki S, Starzl TE. Hepatic resection for metastatic tumor. In: Lygidakis NJ, Tytgat GNJ, eds. Hepatobiliary and pancreatic malignancies. Diagnosis, medical and surgical management. New York: Georg Thieme Verlag Stuttgart, Thieme Medical Publishers, 1989:191–194.
82. Schlag P, Hohenberger P, Herfath C. Resection of liver metastases in colorectal cancer—Competitive analysis of treatment results in synchronous versus metachronous metastases. Eur J Surg Oncol 1990;16:360–365.
83. Brown DA, Pomnier RF, Woltering EA, et al. Nonanatomic hepatic resection for secondary hepatic tumors with special reference to hemostatic technique. Arch Surg 1988;123:1063.
84. Vetto JT, Hughes KS, Rosenstein R, Sugarbaker PH. Morbidity and mortality of hepatic resection for metastatic colorectal carcinoma. Dis Colon Rectum 1990;33(5):409–413.
85. Murray KD. Excision of pulmonary metastasis of colorectal cancer. Semin Surg Oncol 1991;7:157–161.
86. Pugh RNH, Murray-Lyon IM, Danson JL, Pietroni MC, Williams R. Transsection of esophagus for bleeding varices. Br J Surg 1973;60:646.
87. Moertel CG, Reitemeier RJ. Advanced gastrointestinal cancer—Clinical management and chemotherapy. New York: Harper & Row, 1969.
88. Baker LH, Talley RW, Maiter R, et al. Phase III comparison of the treatment of advanced gastrointestinal cancer with bolus weekly 5-FU vs methyl-CCNU plus bolus weekly 5-FU. Cancer 1976;38:1–7.
89. Siefert P, Baker LH, Reed MD, et al. Comparison of continuously infused 5-fluorouracil with bolus injection in treatment of patients with colorectal adenocarcinoma. Cancer 1975;36:123–128.
90. Grage TG, Vassilopoulos P, Shingleton WW, et al. Results of a prospective randomized study of hepatic artery infusion with 5-fluorouracil vs intravenous 5-fluorouracil in patients with hepatic metastases from colorectal cancer. A Central Oncology Group study. Surgery 1979;86:550–555.
91. MacDonald JS, Kisner DF, Smythe T, et al. 5-Fluorouracil (5-FU), methyl-CCNU and vincristine in the treatment of advanced colorectal cancer. Phase II study utilizing weekly 5-FU. Cancer Treat Rep 1976;60:1597–1600.
92. Buroker J, Kim PN, Groppe C, et al. 5-FU infusion with methyl-CCNU in the treatment of advanced colon cancer. Cancer 1978;42:1228–1233.
93. Kemeny N, Yagoda A, Golbey RB. A randomized study of two different schedules of methyl-CCNU, 5-FU and vincristine for metastatic colorectal carcinoma. Cancer 1979;43:78–82.
94. Kemeny N, Yagoda A, Braun D. Metastatic colorectal carcinoma: A prospective randomized trial of methyl-CCNU, 5-fluorouracil (5-FU) and vincristine (MOF) versus MOF plus streptozotocin (MOF-strep). Cancer 1983;51:20–25.
95. Kemeny N, Yagoda A, Braun D. Therapy for metastatic colorectal carcinoma with a combination of methyl-CCNU, 5-fluorouracil, vincristine, and streptozotocin (MOF-strep). Cancer 1980;45:876–881.
96. Machover D, Goldschmidt E, Chollet P, et al. Treatment of advanced colorectal and gastric adenocarcinoma with 5-fluorouracil and high-dose folinic acid. J Clin Oncol 1986;4:685–696.
97. Petrelli N, Douglass HO Jr, Herrera L, et al. The modulation of fluorouracil with leucovorin in metastatic colorectal carcinoma: A prospective randomized phase III trial. J Clin Oncol 1989;7:1419–1426.
98. Ardalan B, Chua L, Tian EM, et al. A phase II study of weekly 24-hour infusion with high-dose fluorouracil with leucovorin in colorectal carcinoma. J Clin Oncol 1991;9: 625–630.
99. Kemeny N, Ahmed T, Michaelson R, et al. Activity of low dose methotrexate and fluorouracil in advanced colorectal carcinoma: Attempted correlation with tissue and blood levels of phosphoriboxylpyrophosphate. J Clin Oncol 1984;2:311–315.
100. Nordic Gastrointestinal Tumor Adjuvant Therapy Group. Superiority of sequential methotrexate, fluorouracil, and leucovorin to fluorouracil alone in advanced symptomatic colorectal carcinoma: A randomized trial. J Clin Oncol 1989;7:1437–1446.
101. Pandya KJ, Chan AYU, Qazi R, et al. Combination chemotherapy for advanced colorectal cancer. A pilot study. Am J Clin Oncol 1986;9:31–34.
102. Loehrer PJ Sr, Einhorn LH, Williams SD, et al. Cisplatin plus 5-FU for the treatment of adenocarcinoma of the colon. Cancer Treat Rep 1985;69:1359–1363.
103. Kemeny N, Reichman B, Botet J, et al. Continuous infusion 5-fluorouracil (FU) and bolus cisplatin (DDP) for metastatic colorectal cancer. Proc Am Soc Clin Oncol 1987;6: 86.
104. Lokich JJ, Ahlgren JD, Gullo JJ, et al. A prospective randomized comparison of continuous infusion fluorouracil with a conventional bolus schedule in metastatic colorectal carcinoma: A Mid-Atlantic Oncology Program study. J Clin Oncol 1989;7:425–432.
105. Erlichman C, Fine S, Wong A, Elhakim T. A randomized trial of fluorouracil and folinic acid in patients with metastatic colorectal carcinoma J Clin Oncol 1988;6:469–475.
106. Doroshow JH, Multhauf P, Leong L, et al. Prospective randomized comparison of fluorouracil versus fluorouracil and high-dose continuous infusion leucovorin calcium for the treatment of advanced measurable colorectal cancer in patients previously unexposed to chemotherapy. J Clin Oncol 1990;8:491–501.
107. Bruckner HW, Motwani BT. Chemotherapy of advanced cancer of the colon and rectum. Semin Oncol 1991;18:443–461.
108. Poon MA, O'Connell MJ, Moertel CG, et al. Biochemical modulation of fluorouracil: Evidence of significant improvement of survival and quality of life in patients with advanced colorectal carcinoma. J Clin Oncol 1989;7:1407–1417.
109. Kemeny N. The systemic chemotherapy of hepatic metastases. Semin Oncol 1983;10: 148–159.
110. Kvols LK, Buck M. Chemotherapy of endocrine malignancies: A review. Semin Oncol 1987;14:343–353.
111. Ajani JA, Carrasco CH, Samaan NA, Wallace S. Therapeutic options for patients with advanced islet cell and carcinoid tumors. Reg Cancer Treat 1991;3:235–242.
112. Ensminger WD, Gyves JW. Regional cancer chemotherapy. Cancer Treat Rep 1984;68: 101–115.
113. Frei E III, Canellos GP. Dose: A critical factor in cancer chemotherapy. Am J Med 1980;69:585–594.
114. Bierman HR, Byron RL, Kelly KH, Grady A. Studies on the blood supply of tumors in man III. Vascular patterns of the liver by hepatic arteriography in vivo. JNCI 1951;12: 107–117.
115. Sullivan RD, Norcross JW, Watkins E. Chemotherapy of metastatic liver cancer by prolonged hepatic-artery infusion. N Engl J Med 1964;270:321–327.
116. Sullivan RD, Zurek WZ. Chemotherapy for liver cancer by protracted ambulatory infusion. JAMA 1965;194:481–486.
117. Watkins E, Khazei AM, Nahra KS. Surgical basis for arterial infusion chemotherapy of disseminated carcinoma of the liver. Surg Gynecol Obstet 1970;130:581–605.
118. Cady B, Overfield RA. Regional infusion chemotherapy of hepatic metastases from carcinoma of the colon. Am J Surg 1974;127:220–227.
119. Buroker T, Samson M, Correa J, et al. Hepatic artery infusion of 5-FUDR after prior systemic 5-fluorouracil. Cancer Treat Rep 1976;60:1277–1279.
120. Oberfield RA, McCaffrey JA, Polio J, et al. Prolonged and continuous percutaneous intra-arterial hepatic infusion chemotherapy in advanced metastatic liver adenocarcinoma from colorectal primary. Cancer 1979;44:414–423.
121. Patt YZ, Mavligit GM, Chuang VP, et al. Percutaneous hepatic arterial infusion (HAI) of mitomycin C and floxuridine (FUDR): An effective treatment for metastatic colorectal carcinoma in the liver. Cancer 1979;46:261–265.
122. Reed ML, Vaitkevicius VK, Al-Sarraf M, et al. The practicality of chronic hepatic artery

infusion therapy of primary and metastatic hepatic malignancies; ten-year results of 124 patients in a prospective protocol. Cancer 1981;47:402–409.

123. Ensminger WD, Rosowsky A, Raso V, et al. A clinical-pharmacological evaluation of hepatic arterial infusions of 5-fluoro-2′-deoxyuridine and 5-fluorouracil. Cancer Res 1978;38:3784–3792.
124. Collins JM. Pharmacologic rationale for regional drug delivery. J Clin Oncol 1984;2: 498–504.
125. Collins JM. Pharmacokinetics and clinical monitoring. In: Chabner BA, Collins JM, eds. Cancer chemotherapy principles & practice. Philadelphia: JB Lippincott, 1990.
126. Stetson PL, Maybaum J, Wagner JW, et al. Tissue-specific pharmacodynamics of 5-bromo-2′-deoxyuridine incorporation into DNA in VX 2 tumor-bearing rabbits. Cancer Res 1988;48:6900–6905.
127. Knol JA, Stetson PL, Wagner JG, et al. 5-Bromo-2′-deoxyuridine incorporation into DNA in hepatic VX2 tumor-bearing rabbits. J Surg Res 1989;47:112–116.
128. Kaplan WD, Ensminger WD, Come SE, et al. Radionuclide angiography to predict patient response to hepatic artery chemotherapy. Cancer Treat Rep 1980;64:1217–1222.
129. Daly JM, Butler J, Kemeny N, et al. Predicting tumor response in patients with colorectal hepatic metastases. Ann Surg 1985;202:384–393.
130. Sigurdson ER, Ridge JA, Kemeny N, Daly JM. Tumor and liver drug uptake following hepatic artery and portal vein infusion. J Clin Oncol 1987;5:1836–1840.
131. Blackshear PJ, Dorman FD, Blackshear PL Jr, et al. The design and initial testing of an implantable infusion pump. Surg Gynecol Obstet 1972;134:51–56.
132. Buchwald H, Grage TB, Vassilopoulos PP, et al. Intra-arterial infusion chemotherapy for hepatic carcinoma using a totally implantable infusion pump. Cancer 1980;45: 866–869.
133. Ensminger WD, Niederhuber J, Dakhil S, et al. Totally implanted drug delivery system for hepatic arterial chemotherapy. Cancer Treat Rep 1981;65:393–400.
134. Balch CM, Urist MM, Soong SJ, McGregor M. A prospective phase II clinical trial of continuous FUDR regional chemotherapy for colorectal metastases to the liver using a totally implantable drug infusion pump. Ann Surg 1983;198:567–573.
135. Niederhuber JE, Ensminger WD, Gyves J, et al. Regional chemotherapy of colorectal cancer metastatic to the liver. Cancer 1984;53:1336–1343.
136. Kemeny N, Daly J, Oderman P, et al. Hepatic artery pump infusion: Toxicity and results in patients with metastatic colorectal carcinoma. J Clin Oncol 1984;2:595–600.
137. Shepard KV, Levin B, Karl RC, et al. Therapy for metastatic colorectal cancer with hepatic artery infusion chemotherapy using a subcutaneous implanted pump. J Clin Oncol 1985;3:161–169.
138. Kemeny MM, Goldberg DA, Browning S, et al. Experience with continuous regional chemotherapy and hepatic resection as treatment of hepatic metastases from colorectal primaries. Cancer 1985;55:1265–1270.
139. Patt YZ, Boddie AW Jr, Charnsangavej C, et al. Hepatic arterial infusion with floxuridine and cisplatin: Overriding importance of antitumor effect versus degree of tumor burden as determinants of survival among patients with colorectal cancer. J Clin Oncol 1986;4: 1356–1364.
140. Cohen AM, Schaeffer N, Higgins J. Treatment of metastatic colorectal cancer with hepatic artery combination chemotherapy. Cancer 1986;57:1115–1117.
141. Kemeny N, Daly J, Reichman B, et al. Intrahepatic or systemic infusion of fluorodeoxyuridine in patients with liver metastases from colorectal carcinoma. Ann Intern Med 1987;107:459–465.
142. Hohn DC, Stagg RJ, Friedman MA, et al. A randomized trial of continuous intravenous versus hepatic intraarterial floxuridine in patients with colorectal cancer metastatic to the liver: The Northern California Oncology Group trial. J Clin Oncol 1989;7:1646–1654.
143. Chang AE, Schneider PD, Sugarbaker PH, et al. A prospective randomized trial of regional versus systemic continuous 5-fluorodeoxyuridine chemotherapy in the treatment of colorectal liver metastases. Ann Surg 1987;206:685–693.
144. Martin JK, O'Connell MJ, Wieand HS, et al. Intra-arterial floxuridine vs systemic fluorouracil for hepatic metastases from colorectal cancer. Arch Surg 1990;125:1022–1027.
145. Chuang VP, Wallace S. Hepatic arterial redistribution for intraarterial infusion of hepatic neoplasms. Radiology 1980;135:295–299.
146. Daly JM, Kemeny N. Therapy of colorectal hepatic metastases. In: DeVita VT Jr, Hellman S, Rosenberg SA, eds. Important advances in oncology. Philadelphia: JB Lippincott, 1986.
147. Niederhuber JE, Ensminger WD. Surgical considerations in the management of hepatic neoplasia. Semin Oncol 1983;10:135–147.
148. Ensminger WD. Intraarterial therapy. In: Perry MC, ed. The chemotherapy sourcebook. Baltimore: Williams & Wilkins, 1992.
149. Patt YZ, Mavligit GM. Arterial chemotherapy in the management of colorectal cancer: An overview. Semin Oncol 1991;18:478–490.
150. Hohn DC, Rayner AA, Economou JS, et al. Toxicities and complications of implanted pump hepatic arterial and intravenous floxuridine infusion. Cancer 1986;57:465–470.
151. Narsete T, Ansfield F, Wirtanen G, et al. Gastric ulceration in patients receiving intrahepatic infusion of 5-fluorouracil. Ann Surg 1977;186:734–736.
152. Chuang VP, Wallace S, Stroehlein J, et al. Hepatic artery infusion chemotherapy: Gastroduodenal complications. Am J Radiol 1981;137:347.
153. Hohn DC, Stagg RJ, Price DC, et al. Avoidance of gastroduodenal toxicity in patients receiving hepatic arterial 5-fluoro-2′-deoxyuridine. J Clin Oncol 1985;3:1257–1260.
154. Kaplan WD, Come SE, Takvorian RW, et al. Pulmonary uptake of technetium 99m macroaggregated albumin: A predictor of gastrointestinal toxicity during hepatic artery perfusion. J Clin Oncol 1984;2:1266–1269.
155. Gluck WL, Akwari OE, Kelvin FM, et al. A reversible enteropathy complicating continuous hepatic artery infusion chemotherapy with 5-fluoro-2′-deoxyuridine. Cancer 1985;56:2424–2427.
156. Carrasco CH, Freeny PC, Chuang VP, et al. Chemical cholecystitis associated with hepatic artery infusion chemotherapy. AJR 1983;141:703–706.
157. Northover JMA, Terblanche J. A new look at the arterial supply of the bile duct in man and its surgical implications. Br J Surg 1979;66:379–384.
158. Kemeny MM, Battifora H, Blayney DW, et al. Sclerosing cholangitis after continuous hepatic artery infusion of FUDR. Ann Surg 1985;202:176–181.
159. Hohn D, Melnick J, Stagg R, et al. Biliary sclerosis in patients receiving hepatic arterial infusions of floxuridine. J Clin Oncol 1985;3:98–102.
160. Doria MI Jr, Shepard KV, Levin B, et al. Liver pathology following hepatic arterial infusion chemotherapy. Cancer 1986;58:855–861.
161. Andrews JC, Knol J, Wollner I, et al. Floxuridine-associated sclerosing cholangitis. A dog model. Invest Radiol 1989;24:47–51.
162. Kemeny N, Seiter K, Niedzwiecki D, et al. A randomized trial of intrahepatic infusion of fluorodeoxyuridine with dexamethasone versus fluorodeoxyuridine alone in the treatment of metastatic colorectal cancer. Cancer 1992;69:327–334.
163. Hughes KS, Simon R, Songhorabodi S, et al. Resection of the liver for colorectal carcinoma metastases: A multi-institutional study of patterns of recurrence. Surgery 1986;100:278–284.
164. Safi F, Bittner R, Roscher R, et al. Regional chemotherapy for hepatic metastases of colorectal carcinoma (continuous intraarterial versus continuous intraarterial/intravenous therapy). Cancer 1989;64:379–387.
165. Seiter K, Kemeny N, Sigurdson E, et al. A phase I trial of hepatic artery fluorodeoxyuridine combined with systemic 5-fluorouracil for the treatment of metastases from colorectal cancer. Reg Cancer Treat 1991;3:293–297.
166. Stagg RJ, Venook AP, Chase JL, et al. Alternating hepatic intra-arterial floxuridine and fluorouracil: A less toxic regimen for treatment of liver metastases from colorectal cancer. JNCI 1991;83:423–428.
167. Sheen MC, Wang YW. Complications of port-catheter systems in intra-arterial infusion chemotherapy. Reg Cancer Treat 1991;4:92–97.
168. Walther H, Kahle M, Filler RD. Hepatic artery infusion via an implantable catheter system using the 5-fluorouracil, leucovorin, mitomycin C regimen. Reg Cancer Treat 1991;4:136–139.
169. Khayat D, Le Cesne A, Weil M, et al. Intra-arterial treatment of hepatic metastases using the 5-fluorouracil, Adriamycin, mitomycin C (FAM) chemotherapeutic regimen. Reg Cancer Treat 1988;1:62–64.
170. Gyves JW, Stetson P, Ensminger WD, et al. Hepatic arterial streptozocin: A clinical pharmacologic study in patients with liver tumors. Cancer Drug Delivery 1983;1:63–68.
171. Reed ML, Kuipers FM, Vaitkevicius VK, et al. Treatment of disseminated carcinoid tumors including hepatic-artery catheterization. Treat Carcinoid Tumors 1963;269: 1005–1010.
172. Ajani JA, Carrasco CH, Charnsangavej C, et al. Islet cell tumor metastatic to the liver: Effective palliation by sequential hepatic artery embolization. Ann Intern Med 1988;108: 340–344.
173. Mitty HA, Warner RRP, Newman LH, et al. Control of carcinoid syndrome with hepatic artery embolization. Radiology 1985;155:623–626.
174. Allison DJ, Modlin IM, Jenkins WJ. Treatment of carcinoid liver metastases by hepatic artery embolisation. Lancet 1977;2:1323–1325.
175. Carrasco CH, Chuang VP, Wallace S. Apudomas metastatic to the liver: Treatment by hepatic artery embolization. Radiology 1983;149:79–83.
176. Bruso CE, Shewach DS, Lawrence TS. Fluorodeoxyuridine-induced radiosensitization and inhibition of DNA double strand break repair in human colon cancer cells. Int J Radiat Oncol Biol Phys 1990;19:1411–1417.
177. Barone RM, Byfield JE, Goldfarb PB, et al. Intra-arterial chemotherapy using an implantable infusion pump and liver irradiation for the treatment of hepatic metastases. Cancer 1982;50:850–862.
178. Herbsman H, Gardner B, Harshaw D, et al. Treatment of hepatic metastases with a combination of hepatic artery infusion chemotherapy and external radiotherapy. Surg Gynecol Obstet 1978;147:13–17.
179. Webber BM, Soderberg CH, Leone LA, et al. A combined treatment approach to management of hepatic metastases. Cancer 1978;42:1087–1095.
180. Lokich JJ, Kinsella T, Perri J, et al. Concomitant hepatic radiation and intra-arterial fluorinated pyrimidine therapy: Correlation of liver scan, liver function tests, and plasma CEA with tumor response. Cancer 1982;48:2569–2574.
181. Raju PI, Maruyama Y, DeSimone P, MacDonald J. Treatment of liver metastases with a combination of chemotherapy and hyperfractionated external radiation therapy. Am J Clin Oncol 1987;10:41–43.
182. Friedman M, Cassidy M, Levine M, et al. Combined modality therapy of hepatic metastasis. Cancer 1979;44:906–913.
183. Lawrence TS, Dworzian LM, Walker-Andrews S, et al. Treatment of cancers involving the liver and porta hepatis with external beam irradiation and intraarterial hepatic fluorodeoxyuridine. Int J Radiat Oncol Biol Phys 1991;20:555–561.
184. Ingold JA, Reed GB, Kaplan HS, Bagshaw MA. Radiation hepatitis. Am J Roentgenol 1965;93:200–208.
185. Wharton JT, Declos L, Gallager W, Smith JP. Radiation hepatitis induced by abdominal irradiation with cobalt 60 moving strip technique. AJR 1973;117:73–80.
186. Lawrence TS, Kessler ML, Lavigne ML, et al. The use of 3-D dose volume analysis to predict radiation hepatitis. Proceedings of the American Society for Therapeutic Radiology and Oncology 1991;21:187.

187. Lawrence TS, TenHaken RK, Kessler ML, et al. The use of 3-D volume analysis to predict radiation hepatitis. Int J Radiat Oncol Biol Phys 1992;23(4):781–788.
188. Emani B, Lyman J, Brown A, et al. Tolerance of normal tissue to therapeutic irradiation. Int J Radiat Oncol Biol Phys 1991;21:109–122.
189. Chang AE, Collins JM, Speth PAJ, et al. A phase I study of intraarterial iododeoxyuridine in patients with colorectal liver metastases. J Clin Oncol 1989;7:662–668.
190. Speth PAJ, Kinsella TJ, Chang AE, et al. Selective incorporation of iododeoxyuridine into DNA of hepatic metastases versus normal human liver. Clin Pharmacol Ther 1988;44:369–375.
191. Ensminger WD, Andrews JC, Walker-Andrews S, et al. Clinical pharmacology of hepatic arterial 5-bromo-2′-deoxyuridine (BUDR). In: Ensminger WD, Selam JL, eds. Update in drug delivery systems. New York: Futura, 1989.
192. Herba MJ, Illescas FF, Thirlwell MP, et al. Hepatic malignancies: Improved treatment with intraarterial Y-90. Radiology 1988;169:311–314.
193. Andrews JC, Shapiro B, Walker-Andrews SC, Ensminger WD. Hepatic radioembolization with Y-90 microspheres: Initial results. Radiology 1990;177:257–258.
194. Gyves JW, Ensminger WD, VanHarken D, et al. Improved regional selectivity of hepatic arterial BCNU with degradable microspheres. Clin Pharmacol Ther 1983;34:259–265.
195. Lorenz M, Herrmann G, Kirkowa-Reimann M, et al. Temporary chemoembolization of colorectal liver metastases with degradable starch microspheres. Eur J Surg Oncol 1989;15:453–462.
196. Civalleri D, Esposito M, Fulco RA, et al. Liver and tumor uptake and plasma pharmacokinetics of arterial cisplatin administered with and without starch microspheres in patients with liver metastases. Cancer 1991;68:988–994.
197. Dritschilo A, Grant EG, Harter KW, et al. Interstitial radiation therapy for hepatic metastases: Sonographic guidance for applicator placement. AJR 1986;147:275–278.
198. Livraghi T, Festi D, Monti F, et al. US-guided percutaneous alcohol injection of small hepatic and abdominal tumors. Radiology 1986;161:309–312.
199. Ravikumar TS, Kane R, Cady B, et al. Hepatic cryosurgery with intraoperative ultrasound monitoring for metastatic colon carcinoma. Arch Surg 1987;122:403–409.
200. Butler J, Attiyeh FF, Daly JM. Hepatic resection for metastases of the colon and rectum. Surg Gynecol Obstet 1986;162:109–113.
201. Coppa GF, Eng K, Ranson JHC, et al. Hepatic resection for metastatic colon and rectal cancer: An evaluation of preoperative and postoperative factors. Ann Surg 1985;202:203–208.

SECTION **4**

MARTIN M. MALAWER
THOMAS F. DELANEY

Treatment of Metastatic Cancer to Bone

Metastatic cancer is the most common neoplasm involving the skeletal system. Of approximately 965,000 new cancer patients per year in the United States, about 30% to 70% will develop involvement.[1–3] Like primary bone tumors, metastatic skeletal cancer is best treated with a multimodality approach that involves the combined expertise of the medical, surgical, and radiation oncologist. Major advances have been made in the early detection, diagnosis, and surgical/radiotherapeutic treatment of metastatic bone disease. The use of bone scintigraphy, computed tomography (CT), and magnetic resonance imaging (MRI) permits extremely early detection and localization of bony lesions and aids in treatment and preoperative planning.[4–9] During the early 1970s, paralleling the development of joint replacements and the use of a bone cement, polymethylmethacrylate (PMMA), orthopedic surgeons for the first time had a relatively simple and reliable method of treating patients with pathologic fractures.[10,11] The use of PMMA and prosthetic replacements allowed reconstruction of large tumor defects without having to depend on bone healing. This permitted immediate and reliable stabilization of tumor defects and increased early function and ambulation. As these techniques have developed, so has an interest in identifying patients at high risk for pathologic fracture, and thereby the concept of prophylactic fixation has developed. Similarly, improved techniques of spinal surgery have been applied to the treatment of metastatic cancer of the spine, resulting in marked improvement in the ability to decompress and stabilize the spine involved by tumor, with resultant improvement of neurologic status.[12,13]

Most patients do not require surgery; radiation therapy and medical management generally suffice. Megavoltage irradiation, along with radioisotopes for specific tumor types, is permitting a significant number of patients to be treated successfully.[14–20]

This chapter concentrates on the metastatic carcinoma. Sarcomas, melanomas, and the hematogenous malignancies are described briefly. Radiographic imaging techniques, mechanisms of bony metastases and biomechanical effects, biopsy/histologic techniques, and surgical/radiotherapeutic management are described. Specific emphasis is placed on the unique considerations of the different carcinomas and the different anatomic sites.

INCIDENCE AND ANATOMIC SITES OF SKELETAL METASTASES

Bony metastases occur primarily to the axial skeletal and lower extremities. Abrams and colleagues analyzed 1000 consecutive autopsies of patients who died of neoplasms of epithelial origin and reported bone metastasis in 272 cases.[2] The sites of the primary tumors associated with bony metastasis were breast (73.1%), lung (32.5%), kidney (24%), rectum (13%), pancreas (13%), stomach (10.9%), colon (9.3%), and ovary (9%). Clain analyzed 2000 patients who died of cancer with bone metastasis and reported involvement of the following sites: vertebra (69%), pelvis (41%), femur (especially the hip) (25%), and skull (14%).[20] The upper extremity is much less commonly involved; approximately 10% to 15% of bony metastasis occur at this site.[2] The pattern of involvement is similar for most carcinomas, although some tumors show a predilection for specific skeletal sites (*e.g.*, prostate tumors for the pelvic bones).

Pathologic fractures requiring surgical intervention occur in approximately 9% of patients with metastatic bone disease.[21] Higinbotham and Marcove reported that 165 of 1800 patients with solitary or multiple metastatic cancer to bone treated at the Bone Tumor Service at Memorial Sloan-Kettering Hospital between 1931 and 1965 required surgery for fracture; 150 had metastatic carcinoma, and 15 had metastatic sarcoma or myeloma.[21] Most of these fractures were of the femur, humerus, or both. Four types of tumors accounted for nearly 80% of the fractures: breast (53%), kidney (11%), lung (8%), and thyroid (5%). Many studies have shown a similar distribution.[2,10,11,22,23]

GENERAL CONSIDERATIONS

CLINICAL CHARACTERISTICS

The hallmark of skeletal metastases, irrespective of histogenesis, is localized pain. The pain pattern is similar to that of primary bone tumors (*i.e.*, initially intermittent, unrelated to activity, and eventually becoming continuous and unrelenting). Many metastatic lesions, however, are not painful and are detected only by radiographic or bone scintigraphy.[9,24] Additional characteristics are related to the specific sites involved. Shoulder girdle metastases often present as a "frozen" shoulder, whereas thoracic and vertebral body involvement may cause referred pain to the chest wall and the lower extremities, respectively. Lumbar vertebral disease often presents as "low back pain," sciatica, or both. The most serious complication of vertebral metastases is secondary epidural compression of the spinal cord or cauda equina. Early cord compression is heralded by increasing back pain, and the patient must be immediately evaluated for this complication. Any cancer patient who develops skeletal pain should undergo plain radiography of the affected area and bone scintigraphy.

LABORATORY EVALUATION

Laboratory evaluation for the detection of skeletal disease includes serum calcium/phosphorus, alkaline and acid phosphatase, and carcinoembryonic antigen (CEA) assays. None of these tests is specific for bony metastases. Hypercalcemia is not directly related to the extent of bony disease, although patients with bony metastases often have high serum calcium levels.[3,25,26]

DIAGNOSIS

The clinical presentation, plain radiography, and bone scintigraphy findings are usually typical of metastatic disease. A confirmatory pathologic evaluation is performed by simple needle or aspiration biopsy in most anatomic sites.[7,27] In the adult, entities that may be confused with metastatic cancer are the hematologic malignancies (myeloma, leukemia, lymphoma) and Paget's disease of bone. A primary sarcoma of bone may occasionally be mistaken for a metastatic cancer; therefore, solitary metastases must be appropriately staged and biopsied. Radiation-induced sarcomas should also be considered if a bony lesion arises in a previous radiation therapy field after an appropriate latency period.

GOALS AND TYPES OF TREATMENT

Most skeletal metastases do not require surgery. Radiation therapy, chemotherapy, and hormonal manipulation provide good symptomatic relief. A pending or actual pathologic fracture requires operative fixation, because fractures through a tumor-bearing bone rarely heal without such intervention.

The goals of fixation are to relieve pain, to improve function and ambulation, to facilitate medical and nursing care, and to improve psychologic well-being.[28] This requires a surgical approach different from that used for nonneoplastic lesions. Immediate fixation must be provided. A variety of techniques are in use, including replacement by a prosthesis (especially about the hip) or a combination of internal fixation and PMMA.[10,22,23,28] Both provide immediate stability. In general, radiation therapy is used after wound healing to arrest local tumor growth, permit bony repair, and prevent regrowth of tumor around the fixation device.

MECHANISM AND PATHOGENESIS OF SKELETAL METASTASIS

The way in which tumor cells travel to the skeletal system and establish metastases, their relation to the primary tumor, and the way in which they destroy normal bone are poorly understood. Attempts to explain the phenomenon have focused on the unique nature of the venous system, the bony microvascular structure, and, recently, the relation of tumor cell to bone, termed the microenvironment.[29–31]

VASCULAR AND MICROVASCULAR CONSIDERATIONS

Normal bone does not contain lymphatic channels. Skeletal metastases occur hematogenously.[29,32] The peculiarities of the venous system[33–40] are considered the main pathway of mechanical transport of cancer cells to the skeletal system.

Batson initially emphasized the significant role of a complex network of vertebral, epidural, and perivertebral veins, a system heretofore not appreciated or named, in the transport of cancer cells to the skeleton (Fig. 61–40).[31,33,41,42] This system parallels, joins, and also *bypasses* the other three venous systems. External pressure, not valves, determines the flow within this system. Blood within this system flows in different directions, depending on the pressure exerted by physiologic activity. This network partially explains the frequency and distribution of metastases along the vertebral column, in the

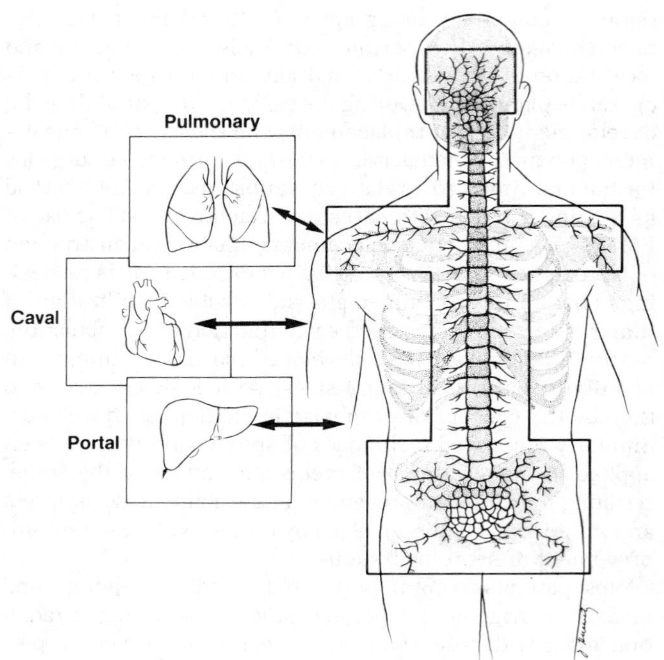

FIGURE 61–40. Batson's plexus. (Modified from Batson OV. The function of the vertebral veins and their role in the spread of metastases. Ann Surg 1940;112:138–149)

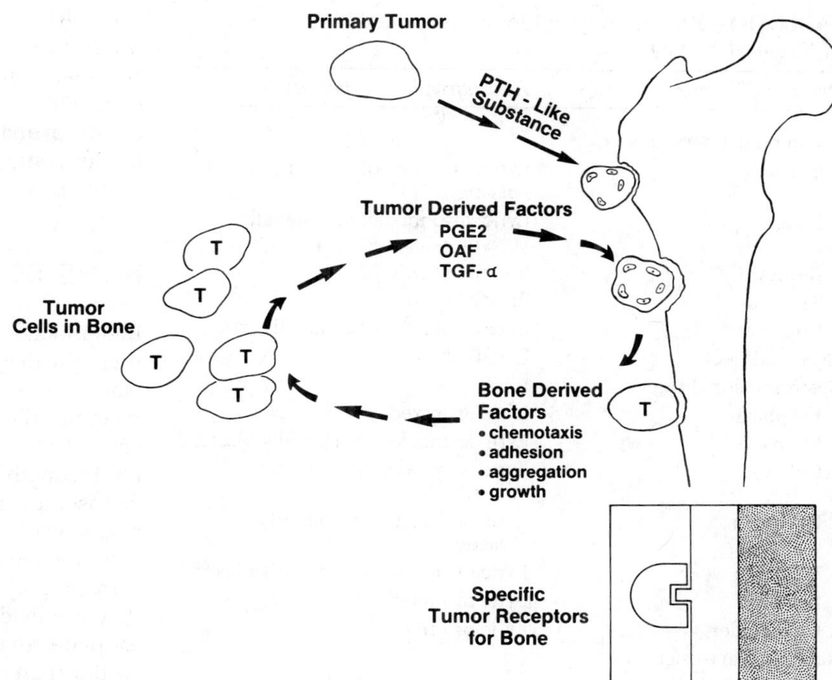

FIGURE 61–41. Mechanisms of tumor cell growth and bone destruction. (Modified from Manishen WJ, Sivananthan K, Orr WF. Resorbing bone stimulates tumor cell growth. A role for the host microenvironment in bone metastasis. Am J Pathol 1986;123:39–45)

pelvic and shoulder girdle, and in apparent "aberrant" sites. In addition, the increased susceptibility of red marrow is related to the special hemodynamic and microanatomic aspects of its vasculature.[4,29] Its unique cellular structure contributes to the propensity of tumor cell extravasation and to the formation of foci of tumor cells within the red marrow.[43]

TUMOR CELL-HOST BONE RELATION

Tumor cells may destroy bone directly, produce mediators that stimulate resorption by osteoclasts, or produce other newly described mediators such as transforming growth factor (TGF) and prostaglandins (PGE_1 and PGE_2) (Fig. 61–41).[3,30,44] Much of this information comes from studies of patients with malignant hypercalcemia. Prostaglandins in bone act similarly to parathormone (*i.e.,* they stimulate cAMP, activate collagenase synthesis, and increase osteoclast number and activity).[32] Galasko demonstrated that osteoclastic proliferation and subsequent bony resorption occurred quite soon after tumor invasion.[3] An osteoclast-activating factor (OAF) has been identified (from lymphoma and myeloma cells) that might be dependent on prostaglandins.[45] It has been suggested that tumor cells may have specific receptors for bone marrow.[46] Another possibility is that resorbing bone itself can release chemoattractants that will cause tumor cell adherence and migration.[47]

RADIOGRAPHIC DIAGNOSIS AND EVALUATION OF METASTASES

The diagnosis of metastatic cancer to the skeletal system is based on one of several radiographic imaging studies, followed by a definitive biopsy. The skeletal system can be easily and accurately imaged by several imaging modalities. The choice, indications, and advantages of each are summarized.

RADIOGRAPHY

Plain radiographs are highly accurate in differentiating metastatic carcinoma from other benign or malignant lesions of bone. In many cases, no other tests may be required. Wilner described the general characteristics of these lesions.[48]

Location

The most common sites of metastasis are the spine, hip, and femur. When long bones are involved, the metaphyseal area and, less commonly, the middiaphyseal area are affected. Tumor generally reaches the medullary area before invading the cortex; primary cortical metastases are rare.

Size, Shape, and Number

Multiple bony lesions are the hallmark of metastatic disease. Solitary metastases occur occasionally and are difficult to differentiate from a primary bone tumor. In general, metastatic carcinomas are small (1–3 cm) and well defined. Lesions of the hip and pelvis may be larger. Appreciation of tumor size and shape, in conjunction with multiplicity, usually enables one to diagnose metastatic cancer with confidence. Extraosseous extension (*i.e.,* a soft tissue component) rarely occurs with metastatic cancer; it is largely a characteristic of primary sarcomas of bone. Among the primary multiple tumors of bone that might be confused with metastatic carcinoma are histiocytosis, enchondromatosis, and fibrous dysplasia. Each of these tends to occur in the younger patient.

Radiographic Pattern

Bone that is invaded by metastatic cancer typically exhibits three patterns: osteolytic, osteoblastic, and, less commonly, mixed (Table 61–29). A given patient may demonstrate a

TABLE 61–29. Radiographic Appearance of Skeletal Metastases

Primary Tumor	*Radiographic Appearance*
Common primary cancer	
Breast	Lytic; also mixed; frequently blastic
Lung	Lytic; also mixed; occasionally blastic
Kidney	Invariably lytic
Thyroid	Invariably lytic
Prostate	Usually blastic; occasionally lytic
Head and neck	Usually lytic
Gastrointestinal tract	
Esophagus	Lytic or mixed
Stomach	Lytic or mixed; occasionally blastic
Colon	Lytic or mixed; infrequently blastic
Rectum	Lytic or mixed; infrequently blastic
Pancreas	Lytic or mixed; occasionally blastic
Liver	Lytic or mixed
Gallbladder	Lytic or mixed
Genitourinary tract	
Urinary bladder	Lytic; infrequently blastic
Adrenal	Lytic
Reproductive system	
Uterine cervix	Lytic or mixed; occasionally blastic
Uterine corpus	Lytic
Skin	
Squamous and basal cell carcinoma	Lytic
Malignant melanoma	Lytic
Carcinoid tumors	
Bronchial and abdominal	Blastic; frequently mixed

(Modified from Wilner D. Cancer metastasis to bone. In: Wilner D, ed. Radiology of bone tumors and allied disorders. Philadelphia: WB Saunders, 1982:3646)

combination of patterns, often even within one bone. There are three types of osteolytic patterns: (1) moth-eaten (multiple, small-to-medium-sized lesions that may coalesce to form large defects such as those often seen with breast cancer); (2) diffuse infiltrative (often seen with round cell tumors such as lymphoma, neuroblastoma, and Ewing's sarcoma); and (3) large, expansile lesions (thyroid, hypernephroma) (Fig. 61–42).

Osteoblastic metastases, which are less common, are frequently seen in conjunction with cancers of the prostate and breast. They tend to be smaller than osteolytic lesions. There are three types of osteoblastic patterns: (1) rounded, discrete (well-circumscribed, uniform density); (2) mottled (irregular areas with varying sclerosis); and (3) diffuse (large lesions). The osteoblastic component is *not* neoplastic osteoid tissue but rather represents the reaction of normal bone to the metastatic cancer. The amount and pattern of sclerosis indicate the growth rate of tumor: the denser the pattern, the slower the growth. If growth is fast, a mixed dense and lytic pattern is seen. Increasing sclerosis is a sign of repair.

Involvement of the cortex adjacent to metastatic cancer *rarely* causes periosteal elevation; when it does, one should consider cancer of the prostate or lung. In general, periosteal elevation is associated with primary bony neoplasms. In addition, primary tumors such as Paget's sarcoma, malignant fibrous histiocytoma (MFH) of bone, or primary fibrosarcoma should be considered if periosteal elevation is present.

BONE SCINTIGRAPHY

Radionuclide imaging of the skeletal system is extremely useful in the diagnosis and management of the patient with skeletal metastasis.[2,8,9,24,49–51] With the development of whole-body imaging, the Gamma camera, and a reliable bone imaging agent (^{99m}Tc-diphosphonate), bone scanning has become a routine method of evaluating the skeletal system for metastatic disease. It is used for detection and staging, for following the response of a bone lesion to treatment, and as a guide in performing needle biopsies for difficult lesions.[2,7–9,50,51]

In general, bone scans will detect metastatic lesions before they are evident on plain radiographs (Fig. 61–43). Wilner estimates that bone scans will detect lesions about 3 months earlier than plain radiographs.[48] Galasko reported a range of 2 months to 18 months, with 75% of breast cancer patients developing corresponding changes within 6 months.[32] Bone scans are most reliable for tumors of the breast, prostate, lung, and kidney. They are least accurate for the diagnosis of round cell tumors, myeloma, lymphoma, and the leukemias.[32] Areas of *decreased* uptake ("photopenic" areas) are often observed with myeloma and, occasionally, with breast and lung cancers.

THE SOLITARY LESION

A unique problem with bone scintigraphy in following patients with a known cancer is the appearance of a solitary lesion. This occurs in 6% to 8% of all patients.[9] McNeil reviewed 273 reports of such cases and reported that 55% represented metastatic disease.[9] Trauma (25%), infection (10%), and miscellaneous factors (10%) accounted for the nonmalignant causes. McNeil emphasized that anatomic site is important in this differentiation; 80% of the vertebral lesions, compared with 18% of the rib lesions, proved to be metastatic in patients with a known primary tumor. If scintigraphy reveals a solitary lesion, additional evaluation, including high-resolution plain radiographs, CT, and possibly biopsy, is recommended.

BONE SCAN-GUIDED NEEDLE BIOPSY

Within the past few years, several reports[3,4] have described the use of bone scintigraphy as an aid to biopsy.[7,8] The scan may be used to mark an area of abnormality before biopsy or may confirm that the correct area has been biopsied intraoperatively. These techniques have enhanced the accuracy of the biopsy in cases in which other modalities have not demonstrated a lesion. Zegel and colleagues described a technique of localizing "hot" rib lesions with nuclear medicine guidance by the use of a lead ring.[7] Percutaneous biopsies reported in conjunction with positive scans revealed that 13 of 14 patients had metastatic tumor. Little and associates described a tech-

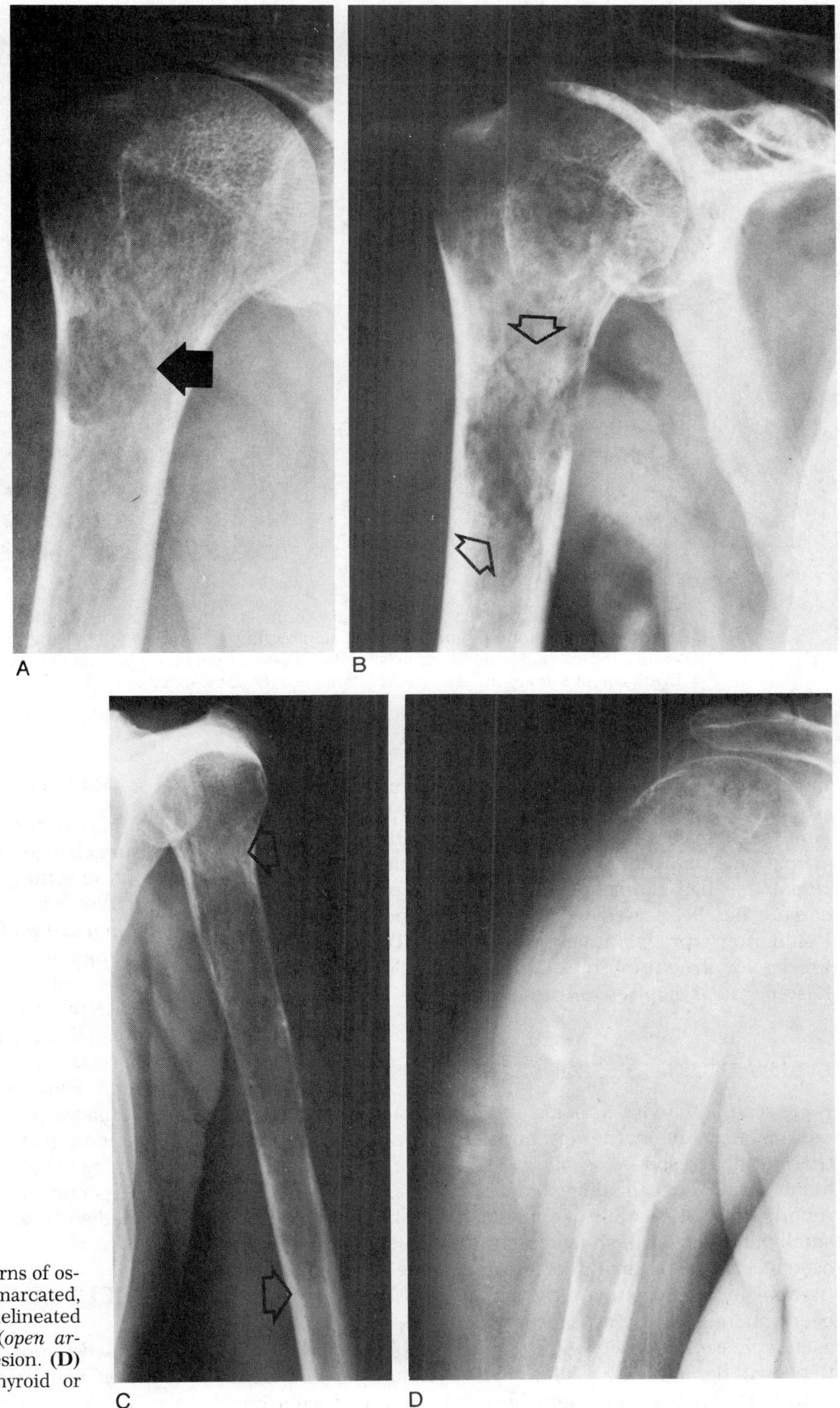

FIGURE 61–42. Different radiographic patterns of osteolytic metastatic cancer. **(A)** Sharply demarcated, punched-out defect (*solid arrow*) with well-delineated borders. **(B)** Diffuse but well-localized lesion (*open arrows*). **(C)** Large, diffuse, extensive osteolytic lesion. **(D)** Large, expansile lesion, usually seen with thyroid or hypernephroma.

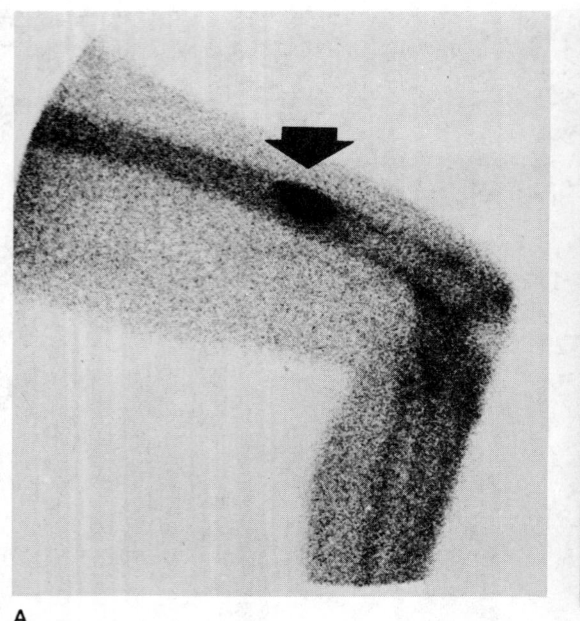
A

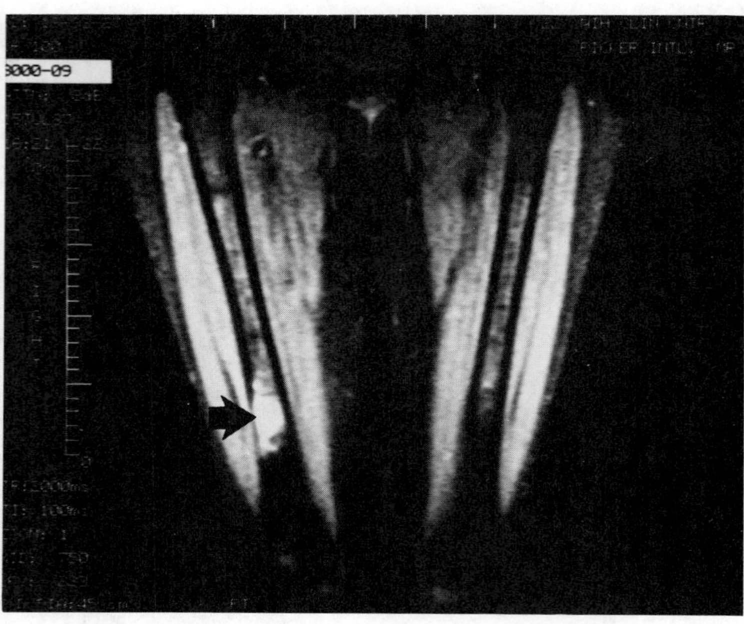
B

FIGURE 61–43. Radiographic imaging for metastatic cancer. Plain radiograph of the femur failed to demonstrate a metastatic lesion. **(A)** Bone scintigraphy (lateral view) showing increased uptake in the anterior cortex of the distal femoral diaphysis. **(B)** A T2-weighted image that demonstrates an area of medullary tumor involvement seen as an area (*solid arrow*) of increased signal (*white*).

nique of marking the suspected rib under scintigraphic control with methylene blue and surgically excising the marked area.[8] None of their 15 patients had a grossly identifiable lesion, yet 10 patients had metastatic disease. Abnormal scans in the remainder had nonneoplastic causes. A portable Gamma camera has been used in the operating room to localize a lesion after a preoperative injection of ^{99m}Tc-diphosphonate for deeper structures (hip, femur, acetabulum). It prevents false-negative biopsies for these lesions.

EVALUATION OF RESPONSE TO TREATMENT

Bone scan activity of a metastatic bony lesion generally decreases after chemotherapy/hormone therapy or radiation therapy if a response is obtained.[9] Plain radiographs may demonstrate bone healing and reossification within a few months. The limitation of plain radiographs is that only a small percentage will show reossification, and changes in the osteoblastic lesions are difficult to determine. With bone scintigraphy, one can compare the activity. Most experience has been obtained with breast cancer patients. Healing is indicated as a decrease in activity. Approximately 10% to 15% of patients will demonstrate a "flare" phenomenon (*i.e.*, a period of increased uptake is presumably due to new, nonneoplastic reparative bone attempting to heal the tumor defect). Occasionally, this response is associated with pain. After this period, a repeat bone scan will show decreased uptake with no new lesions. In rare cases, previously unappreciated lesions will ossify, suggesting a new lesion; in retrospect, these can usually be identified as old lesions.

QUANTITATIVE BONE SCANNING

Quantitative bone scanning (QBS) is a technique used to measure changes in bone scans to avoid the variations obtained in routine scintigraphy. The proportion of increased uptake in the diseased region is compared with the average uptake in the normal regions.[6] It gives an objective measurement of the change of activity in any region relative to normal for a given patient. This technique has been used for comparing response to treatment in patients with metastatic and other diseases. Drelichman and colleagues described 10 patients with prostate carcinoma in whom sequential QBS was performed.[6] Those patients with more than a 50% average decrease had a partial remission, as defined by their criteria. All patients had an increase within the first month (corresponding to the "flare" phenomenon), and no significant decrease occurred until 3 months. Similar results have been obtained with patients with breast carcinoma.[9]

COMPUTED TOMOGRAPHY

Computed tomography has not been used in the evaluation of metastatic skeletal cancer as commonly as it has in other organ systems, although the literature on the usefulness of CT for malignant and benign primary bone neoplasms is extensive. Recently, CT has proved useful in evaluating "hot" spots to confirm the presence of metastatic or other disease.[5] During and associates evaluated 44 breast cancer patients with positive bone scans and negative radiographs; 25 of these patients presented with solitary hot spots on bone scans, and 19 became positive after definitive treatment of their primary disease. Seventy-six percent (19/25) of those presenting with a positive bone scan and a normal radiograph had a benign cause identified by CT. Similar to surgical staging for primary bone tumors, CT is used in the preoperative evaluation of metastatic spinal disease and tumors of the pelvis.[52]

MAGNETIC RESONANCE IMAGING

Magnetic resonance imaging (MRI) accurately images the medullary (marrow) component of bone and is therefore ideal for the early detection of metastatic cancer, especially primary infiltrative neoplasms such as leukemia, lymphoma, and multiple myeloma (see Fig. 61–43).[4,5] Its ability to detect such lesions is due to the high signal intensity (brightness) of normal marrow, which is mostly fat. Because of increased cellularity and therefore a higher water content, infiltrating neoplasms will appear as a darker area on T1-weighted images. Lesions within the skeletal system that are most difficult to image by other modalities (*e.g.*, round cell tumors) are accurately detected by MRI. Daffner and colleagues reported a prospective study of 80 patients with known malignancies; 50 had suspected metastases and 30 had multiple myeloma.[5] All patients who were evaluated with plain radiographs and bone scintigraphy (80%) were shown to have disease.[40] Ten (20%) had no evidence of metastasis, and the abnormalities on bone scintigraphy were shown to be due to other causes. Of the 30 patients with multiple myeloma, 6 (20%) had positive scans, 20 (67%) had abnormal radiographs, and 11 (37%) had abnormal CT scans. MRI demonstrated abnormalities in all 30 patients; these were confirmed by needle aspiration. These authors emphasize the importance of correlating MRI with other studies, because infection, infarction, and other entities can also yield a decreased signal. In general, they recommend that MRI studies of the coronal sections of the pelvis and hips and sagittal sections of the spine (*i.e.*, the hematopoietic-active sites) be performed when evaluating for metastatic cancer.

ANGIOGRAPHY

Angiography is rarely used for diagnosis of metastases to bone. Its main use is for preoperative assessment of large lesions and for embolization of vascular tumor (see Preoperative Evaluation).[53–56]

BIOMECHANICAL AND HEALING CONSIDERATIONS OF TUMOR DEFECTS AND PATHOLOGIC FRACTURES

BIOMECHANICAL CONSIDERATIONS

The strength of normal bone depends on the continuity of the cortex and the underlying medullary/metaphyseal trabecular structure.[57,58] The torsional (rotational), compressive, and bending forces are transmitted and absorbed by both components. A typical metastatic lesion of a long bone destroys a segment of the medullary structure and the corresponding cortical bone (Fig. 61–44). Cortical defects greatly weaken a bone to torsional forces. A defect whose length is less than the diameter of the bone (termed a "stress riser") decreases torsional strength by 70%, whereas a defect larger than the diameter of the bone (termed an "open section," and the most common defect encountered clinically) effects a 90% reduction in strength.[57,58] The aim of an orthopedic procedure is to convert an open section to a closed section so as to allow significant axial and torsional loads to be carried.

HEALING CONSIDERATIONS

The determinants of bony union after a pathologic fracture are quite different from those associated with nonneoplastic fracture. Bony union almost never occurs without surgical or radiotherapeutic treatment. Although pathologic fractures are quite common, few investigators have evaluated the rate and determinants of union. Gainor and Buchert reviewed 129 fractures of long bones in 123 patients treated between 1955

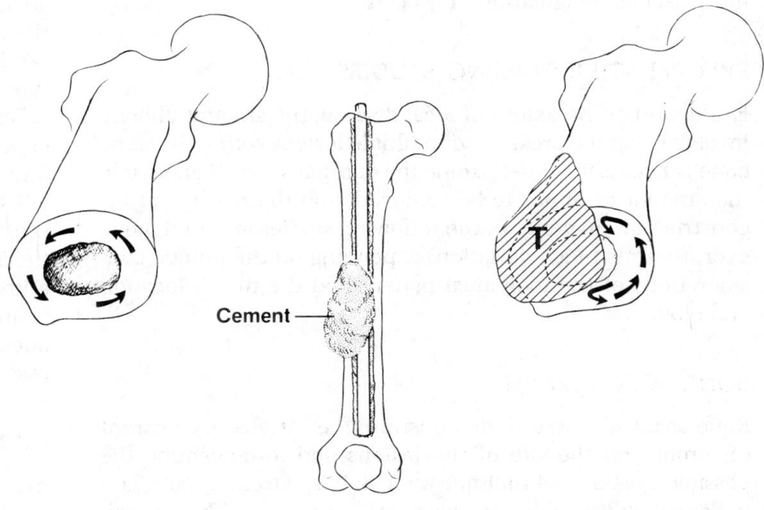

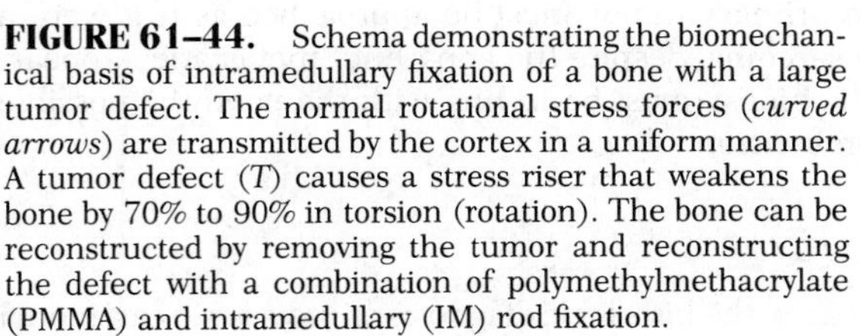

FIGURE 61–44. Schema demonstrating the biomechanical basis of intramedullary fixation of a bone with a large tumor defect. The normal rotational stress forces (*curved arrows*) are transmitted by the cortex in a uniform manner. A tumor defect (*T*) causes a stress riser that weakens the bone by 70% to 90% in torsion (rotation). The bone can be reconstructed by removing the tumor and reconstructing the defect with a combination of polymethylmethacrylate (PMMA) and intramedullary (IM) rod fixation.

and 1979.[59] The overall healing rate was 36% (45 of 129 fractures). Individual healing rates were: multiple myeloma (67%), hypernephroma (44%), and breast cancer (37%). None of the patients with lung cancer healed. The length of patient survival was the main determinant of fracture healing. Fracture healing was found to be multifactorial. Determinants of bony union of pathologic fractures are summarized[59]:

1. *Type of Tumor:* Lung and colorectal tumors and melanomas tend not to heal. Multiple myelomas, tumors of the breast, and hypernephromas have the highest rate of healing.
2. *Type of Fixation:* Internal fixation combined with PMMA significantly increases the chance of osseous union.
3. *Duration of Survival:* Longer survival (greater than 6 months) increases the rate of union.
4. *Amount of Postoperative Radiation Therapy:* High-dose postoperative radiation therapy (greater than 3000–3500 rads) is associated with poorer healing.
5. *Effects of Chemotherapy:* There is little evidence regarding the impact of chemotherapy on bony repair.

PREOPERATIVE EVALUATION, LOCAL STAGING, AND BIOPSY CONSIDERATIONS

PREOPERATIVE CONSIDERATIONS

Special preoperative considerations are needed in cases of metastasis to bone because these patients often have extensive underlying metabolic, hematologic, and nutritional deficits. The risk of infection is increased because of multiple sources of possible sepsis (*e.g.*, colostomy, urinary tract infection), neutropenia from chemotherapy or other adjuvant modalities, and poor local skin condition from prior radiation therapy or other procedures. Perioperative antibiotics are recommended for all patients. All patients should have hematologic and clotting evaluation. Adequate blood replacement should be available, because curettage of many carcinomas, especially myeloma, thyroid tumor, and renal cell carcinoma, often leads to significant blood loss. Thrombocytopenia occasionally occurs intraoperatively and should be monitored. Disseminated intravascular coagulation may occur.[60]

PREOPERATIVE STAGING STUDIES

Evaluation of the extent of local disease, the amount of bone involved, and the presence of multiple lesions within the same bone is necessary to determine the optimal surgical approach, the amount of tumor to be removed, and the method of reconstruction. In general, the following studies are used; however, there is much variation, depending on the unique considerations of the individual patient and the tumor location and type.

BONE SCINTIGRAPHY

Bone scans are used to demonstrate the intraosseous extent of tumor and the site of the lesions and to determine the possible existence of multiple tumors. It is extremely common to detect additional lesions within the same bone. In general, all lesions within the same bone require simultaneous treatment; usually this requires placement of an intramedullary (IM) rod.

CT/MRI

Computed tomography is usually required for lesions of the pelvis and spine; it is rarely required for extremity lesions. Tumors of the bony pelvis often have large soft tissue components that may bleed excessively or lead to mechanical failure of reconstruction if they are not recognized preoperatively. Vertebral body lesions are best evaluated by CT, MRI, or both. The amount of destruction and extent of epidural disease are best estimated with these studies.[13,52,61] Soft tissue components rarely occur with carcinomas of the extremities; however, they are common with metastatic sarcoma (*e.g.*, primary sarcomas), some hypernephromas, and melanomas.

ANGIOGRAPHY

Angiography is not routinely performed; specific indications are pelvic tumors with large extraosseous components and lesions in which preoperative embolization is considered. Patients with metastatic hypernephroma should undergo angiography with embolization.[53–55,62,63]

BIOPSY: TECHNIQUE AND CONSIDERATIONS

There are three situations in which a biopsy is warranted: (1) to confirm metastatic disease in a patient with a known primary tumor; (2) to evaluate a "suspicious" radiographic lesion; and (3) to obtain tissue for hormonal/immunohistochemical evaluation. The technique of biopsy varies, depending on the tumor location and the specific answers sought.

In general, needle aspiration and cytologic evaluation can reliably confirm the diagnosis of cancer.[8,60,64–64B] If the radiograph demonstrates a lesion, biopsy should be performed under fluoroscopic guidance. Permanent x-ray films should be obtained to document that the correct area has been sampled. Several aspirations or cores should be obtained. The material should routinely be sent for culture, because indolent infections occasionally can present as metastatic lesions. Frozen sections or touch preps should be obtained to determine the types of cells present. If the primary tumor is unknown, sufficient tissue should be obtained for special stains (see later), especially immunohistochemical studies. This may require a large sample. If there is excessive bleeding, an absorbable gelatin sponge (Gelfoam) or PMMA should be packed into the defect. One must not assume that all "solitary" lesions in the adult are metastatic. A solitary lesion in the adult without a known primary tumor must be approached as if it were a primary sarcoma, despite the apparent "metastatic" appearance. The biopsy must be in line with the potential possible resection incision.

HISTOLOGY

In most cases, the histologic diagnosis of metastatic carcinoma to bone is easily established. This depends on the recognition of squamous patterns of glandular structures, the features of which are highly typical of the carcinomas that most frequently metastasize to bone. This diagnosis is further facilitated when representative microscopic slides from the primary neoplasm are available for comparison.

Metastatic poorly differentiated carcinomas, and some melanomas (particularly those containing abundant spindled and pleomorphic cells), can closely mimic primary bone sarcomas such as fibrosarcoma or MFH. This pitfall is most often encountered with renal cell carcinoma. The application of selected histochemical studies to demonstrate cellular products has been helpful to confirm the presumption of metastatic carcinoma and to aid in determining the source of an unknown primary lesion. Alcian blue and mucicarmine stains will reveal the presence of epithelial mucins in some adenocarcinomas of the breast, lung, and gastrointestinal tract. Abundant cytoplasmic glycogen typically occurs in renal cell carcinoma and in some clear cell neoplasms from other organs. The demonstration of cytoplasmic melanin granules with the Fontana stain supports the diagnosis of melanoma.

The recent development of immunohistochemical techniques that can be applied to paraffin-embedded tissues has created a powerful diagnostic tool.[65,66] With this procedure, peroxidase-conjugated antibodies, directed against a variety of known antigenic markers, are detected at antibody-antigen reaction sites by the addition of peroxidase-sensitive chromogens. For example, an epithelial tumor (carcinoma) can contain a variety of cytokeratins, epithelial membrane antigen, or carcinoembryonic antigen. The application of an appropriately selected panel of antibodies will produce a recognizable pattern of positive staining of tumor cells that confirms the presence of carcinoma.[67] Similarly, there are antibodies available to identify specific markers of neuroendocrine tumors and melanoma (anti-S-100 protein and anti-melanoma-specific antigens).[68] Metastatic carcinoma and adenocarcinoma of the prostate and metastatic follicular carcinoma of the thyroid can appear quite similar. Immunohistochemical studies to detect prostatic-specific acid phosphatase or thyroglobulin will usually resolve this problem in differential diagnosis.[69] It must be noted, however, that immunohistochemical techniques require meticulous methodology and are fraught with numerous artifacts and interpretive pitfalls.[70]

PRINCIPLES OF SURGICAL TREATMENT FOR SKELETAL METASTASIS

Within the past 20 years, the surgical treatment of metastatic cancer involving the skeletal system has undergone dramatic change as a result of the development of techniques to replace and stabilize large segments of abnormal bone.[11,19,21,22,28,33,61,71a] These techniques have been paralleled by developments in total joint replacements and by procedures developed by the orthopedic oncologist in the treatment of primary bone tumors. Prosthetic replacements now permit the removal and immediate reconstruction of destroyed bone.[23] PMMA, when combined with various metallic rods or prostheses, or both, permits immediate filling and reconstruction of large defects and immediate stabilization.

The common local surgical procedures for metastatic tumors of the extremities are:

1. *Composite Osteosynthesis:* curettage of tumor combined with internal fixation, either bone plates and screws (composite osteosynthesis) or intramedullary fixation with IM rods. This technique is most often used for the shaft (diaphysis) of long bones, most commonly the humerus and femur.[22,28,71a]
2. *Hemijoint Replacement:* resection of a joint with reconstruction by an endoprosthesis combined with PMMA. This technique is most often used for tumors of the hip (Fig. 61–45).[23]
3. *Segmental Resection:* resection of a large segment of bone combined with custom segmental prosthetic replacement and PMMA. This technique is less common and involves substantially more surgical morbidity. It is most often used when no significant bone remains that can be reconstructed by the techniques mentioned above.
4. *Cryosurgery:* Cryosurgery may be combined with any of the above procedures in order to increase local tumor control and control hemorrhage.[71b,72]
5. *Amputations:* Amputations are occasionally necessary to control serious complications of extremity lesions, usually after inadequate tumor control.[73]

The general principles of management of pathologic or pending fractures are:

1. Preoperative embolization for suspected vascular lesions
2. Perioperative antibiotics
3. Adequate hematologic evaluation and blood and component replacement
4. Modification of standard incisions, if necessary, to avoid prior radiation fields and to provide adequate soft tissue coverage and adequate closure to ensure healing
5. Curettage and removal of all gross disease, if possible
6. Composite reconstruction with internal fixation or prosthetic replacement and PMMA. Assurance that PMMA fills the defect and extends proximal and distal to the abnormal area
7. Postoperative radiation therapy for local control

AMPUTATIONS

Amputations are rarely required today for metastatic cancer. Occasionally, radical amputation is indicated when advanced cancer of an extremity results in uncontrollable, intractable pain, a necrotic or functionless extremity, fungation and sepsis, or erosion and hemorrhage of a major vessel at the tumor site. These complications occur after inadequate tumor con114trol. Elimination of pain and sepsis with restoration of function may be achieved by amputation.[73]

CRYOSURGERY

Cryosurgery is the use of liquid nitrogen as a surgical adjunct to tumor curettage to freeze (cryonecrosis) any residual tumor cells. The aim is to enhance local control.[71,72,74] Necrosis is obtained by a double or triple freeze-thaw cycle requiring temperatures between −20° and −40°C. Marcove at Memorial Sloan-Kettering Hospital has treated several hundred patients with this technique since 1964.[71,72] It is useful for tumors that have recurred despite radiation therapy and those in difficult anatomic locations, and in the treatment of hypernephromas.

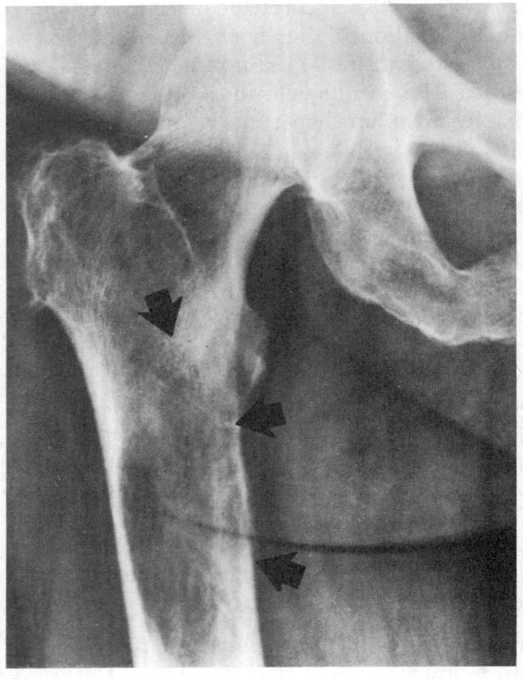

A

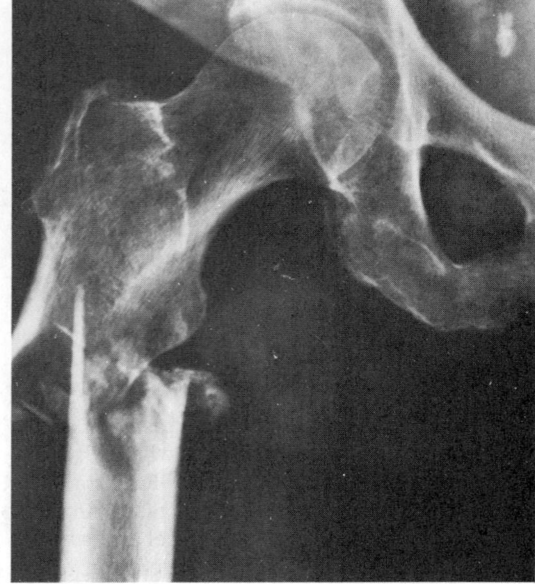

B

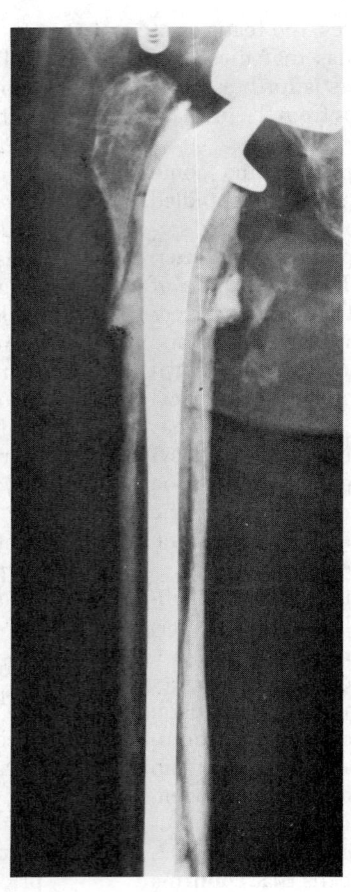

C

FIGURE 61–45. Typical pathologic hip fracture. **(A)** Large subtrochanteric lesion (*solid arrows*) with medial cortical destruction from a metastatic breast cancer. **(B)** A subtrochanteric fracture occurred during administration of radiation therapy. **(C)** The tumor was curetted and a long-stem endoprosthesis was used with PMMA for fixation. The patient was allowed to ambulate several days after surgery. Postoperative radiation therapy to the entire femur is routinely recommended. A long-stem prosthesis with PMMA is recommended for all pathologic fractures of the hip.

GENERAL PRINCIPLES OF RADIATION THERAPY FOR SKELETAL METASTASIS

Radiation is an effective treatment for cancer that has metastasized to bone. Aims of treatment include pain relief, elimination or reduction of the need for narcotics, improvement in ambulation, and arrest of local tumor growth that might otherwise lead to intractable pain, cord compression, or pathologic fracture. With thoughtful treatment planning and appropriate high-energy equipment, localized treatment can usually be delivered to symptomatic sites with minimal morbidity. The efforts of the radiation oncologist should be closely coordinated with those of other physicians and health care personnel. Careful consideration of the nature of the patient's disease is important in determining the most appropriate radiation therapy strategy and technique.

Eighty to ninety percent of patients with a limited number of sites of disease can be effectively treated with external-beam irradiation.[75–82] If there is a single site of bony metastatic disease, high-dose radiation therapy may render the patient disease free for an extended period of time. For patients with symptoms of disease at multiple sites, systemic therapy with chemotherapy or endocrine therapy should be instituted. If symptoms persist, several approaches should be considered. These include localized external radiation therapy to the most symptomatic areas or, for patients with widely disseminated disease, hemibody irradiation or internally administered radionuclide treatment.

TREATMENT PLANNING

The radiation fields should be planned with the use of data from the history and physical examination, the bone scan, plain skeletal films, and, where indicated, myelograms, CT scans, and MRI (see Preoperative Staging Studies, earlier). Soft tissue masses, most often associated with bony metastases to the vertebral bodies or pelvis, must be included in the radiation therapy fields. The distribution of bone marrow is an important consideration, because irradiation for bony metastases will suppress hematopoiesis in the treatment field (Table 61–30). Bone marrow suppression secondary to irradiation is more significant in patients who have received or are receiving myelosuppressive chemotherapy. Blood counts should be monitored closely during treatment. All previous radiation treatment portals must be reviewed. Damage to normal tissue can result from improperly matched or overlapping fields.

Lesions not responding to treatment should prompt another review of the diagnostic studies, particularly in a patient with multiple metastases in whom a lesion not in the treatment field might in fact be causing persistent symptoms. Another possibility is that a soft tissue mass adjacent to the bony lesion being radiated is not completely encompassed by the treatment field.

TABLE 61–30. Marrow Distribution in the Adult

Anatomic Site	*% of Total Red Marrow*
Head	13.1
Cranium	12.0
Mandible	1.1
Upper limbs	8.3
2 humeri	2.0
2 scapulae	4.8
2 clavicles	1.5
Sternum	2.3
Ribs	7.9
Vertebrae	42.3
Cervical	3.4
Thoracic	14.1
Lumbar	10.9
Sacrum	13.9
Lower limb girdle	26.1
2 os coxae	22
Femoral head and neck	4

(Extracted from Ellis RE. The distribution of active bone marrow in the adult. Phys Med Biol 1961;5:255)

PAIN RELIEF

Approximately 80% to 90% of patients undergoing radiation therapy for pain from osseous metastases will have partial pain relief.[75–82] Most patients will begin to experience some pain relief 10 to 14 days after the start of therapy. In one study, 70% of patients had pain relief by 2 weeks after the completion of treatment; 90% had relief within 1 to 3 months.[81] A sudden increase in pain during treatment should raise concern about a pathologic fracture, and appropriate films and orthopedic evaluation should be done. In a recent study, 70% of patients experiencing pain relief did not develop recurrent pain in the treatment field.[75] Another study noted sustained relief of pain in 55% to 65% of patients during the first year after treatment.[83]

In spite of the clinical impression that painful osseous metastases from the thyroid, lung, and kidney are more difficult to palliate with radiation, several small studies have failed to document any clear differences in overall response rates among different histologies.[81,83,84] It has been observed, however, that the time to achieve pain relief after treatment was longer with slowly proliferating tumors such as prostate cancer.[84] The final report from the large, randomized study by the Radiation Therapy Oncology Group (RTOG) indicated that a significantly higher percentage of patients with metastases from breast and prostate primary tumors achieved complete pain relief when compared with patients with lung and other primary tumors.[75] The sites of metastases have not been shown to correlate with the degree of pain relief.[18,75] Severe and frequent pain has been shown to be a poor prognostic feature.[75]

BONE HEALING

Radiation affects both tumor and adjacent bone. The presence of tumor, however, is a significant threat to the structural integrity of bone, and this is worse than the adverse effects of radiation on bone healing. Bone reossification will often occur after tumor eradication. Seventy-eight percent of osteolytic lesions treated in one study recalcified, and another 15% showed no further progression after radiation therapy.[80,85,86] In a study of bone reformation at the base of the skull after irradiation for carcinoma of the nasopharynx, 11 patients showed apparent bone reformation within 4 to 6 months of treatment.[87] These patients received treatment with doses of 5000 to 7000 cGy, which are higher than those used in patients treated for metastatic lesions to the bone.

DOSE, FRACTIONATION, AND TYPES OF RADIATION

There is considerable debate among radiation oncologists about the optimal dose and fractionation scheme for delivering radiation therapy to metastatic lesions in bone. Total dose, fraction size, and duration of treatment are the major issues. In patients with metastatic cancer in whom life expectancy is limited, one would like to deliver effective treatment with minimal morbidity over as short a time span as possible. The RTOG studied pain relief in 759 patients randomized to a variety of dose-fractionation schedules: 270 cGy × 15 fractions, 300 × 10, 300 × 5, 400 × 5, and 500 × 5. No significant difference in response was seen, although an independent reanalysis of the data suggested that the protracted fractionation schemes (270 × 15 or 300 × 10) were more likely to provide complete pain relief with cessation of the use of narcotics.[88]

Several other reported randomized trials do not indicate a clear advantage for the longer, multiple-fraction regimens when compared with shorter or single-course regimens.[89–91] In a study at the Royal Marsden Hospital, 288 patients with painful bony metastases were randomized to receive either 800 cGy in one fraction or 3000 cGy in ten fractions.[79,92] There was no difference in the percentage of patients responding to treatment (80%), the rapidity of response, or the duration of pain relief between the two regimens. A larger number of patients who received the single treatment were subsequently retreated with irradiation to the same site. This was also noted in the RTOG trial, where substantially more patients in the short-course regimens were reirradiated. This, however, may only reflect the reluctance of radiation oncologists to reirradiate areas that received prior high-dose, multifractionated regimens. No late normal tissue complications were seen in the single-fraction group. Other trials have shown equivalent pain relief when comparing 400 cGy × 6 fractions with 1000 cGy × 2, 400 cGy × 6 with 800 cGy × 1, and 200 cGy × 15 with 450 cGy × 5.[121–123] Four retrospective studies of single (400–1500 cGy) versus multiple (2000–4000 cGy) treatment regimens have not shown any striking differences between the two.[16,17,80,93]

While it has been supposed that tumor shrinkage is responsible for pain relief in this setting, the very rapid pain relief associated with orchiectomy or hemibody irradiation for prostate cancer and hypophysectomy for breast cancer does raise the possibility that pain relief might in fact be due to a cytotoxic effect on host cells secreting chemical mediators of the pain response.[89] Even lower doses of single-fraction irradiation for palliation of pain relief are also currently being studied. Single fractions of 400 cGy were recently reported to produce partial pain relief in 9 of 21 (43%) evaluable patients and complete relief in 1 of 21 (5%), with responses occurring within 3 weeks.[94] Seven of the ten responders, however, subsequently developed recurrent pain at the irradiated site.

It might be expedient to give single-fraction irradiation to a debilitated patient for whom repeated, daily trips for treatment would be burdensome. Single large fractions, however, to the abdomen and brain may not be well tolerated acutely. Therefore, each radiation oncologist must consider the site of disease, the patient's performance status and social situation, and any normal tissue in the treatment field when deciding on a treatment regimen. Patients with one or few sites of metastases who have a good performance status and a primary disease that responds well to systemic therapy may live for many years after irradiation for bony pain. Therefore, large fractions that are known to produce more late effects in normal tissue must be used with considerable caution, especially when radiation fields include the brain, spinal cord, kidneys, or significant portions of the liver or bowel. Such patients may also survive long enough to have problems with recurrent tumor in bones that have not been irradiated to high doses. Patients with bony metastases producing spinal cord compression are not suitable for single-fraction treatment because of the obvious neurologic risks of recurrent tumor at this site.

It has been difficult to demonstrate a clear dose-response relation in the treatment of bone metastases, often because the groups studied have been heterogenous, with different histologies and survival times after treatment. Arcangeli reported a higher frequency of complete pain relief when doses of ≥4000 cGy were employed.[95] In patients with good performance status, limited metastatic disease, and long expected survival after palliative irradiation, doses of ≥4000 cGy with conventional fractionation are recommended. For patients whose expected survival is short, a high dose is probably less important because they will not live long enough to manifest recurrent tumor.

HEMIBODY IRRADIATION

Sequential hemibody irradiation has been used as an alternative to localized radiation therapy directed at specific sites of metastatic disease for patients with widely disseminated bony metastases.[15,18] It is designed to avoid repeated trips to the hospital for multiple courses of irradiation in such patients. One study reported complete relief of pain in 21% and partial relief in 77% of patients, most of whom had breast, prostate, or lung cancer.[15] Pain control was achieved rapidly, with improvement noted within 2 days among half of the patients experiencing pain relief. Patients received 600 to 800 cGy of irradiation to either the upper, middle, or lower portions of the body. Patients treated for metastases of the upper body were hospitalized for a day, hydrated, and premedicated with antiemetics and corticosteroids: those undergoing midbody and lower body therapy were premedicated as outpatients to minimize nausea and vomiting. Treatment to the lower body and midbody was tolerated relatively well, with severe or life-threatening nausea and vomiting, diarrhea, and hematologic toxicity occurring in 2%, 6%, and 8% of patients, respectively. Upper body treatment induced severe or life-threatening nausea and vomiting, fever, and hematologic toxicity in 15%, 4%, and 32% of the patients, respectively. Hematologic complications were worse in patients who had received prior intensive courses of chemotherapy and had started treatment with low peripheral blood counts. There were no fatalities related to treatment, yet side effects as described above were prominent, especially with the upper body treatment. Kuban reported good palliation with hemibody irradiation in patients with disseminated prostate cancer.[96] Palliative effects were maintained until death in 82% of the patients treated in the upper half of the body and 67% of the patients treated in the lower half of the body. Doses of 600 to 800 cGy to the upper and 800 cGy to the lower hemibody were well tolerated. Fractionated hemibody irradiation has been reported to yield more durable pain relief by a group from Memorial Sloan-Kettering Cancer Center without any increase in complications.[97]

SYSTEMIC RADIONUCLIDES

Systemically administered isotopes have been used to palliate pain caused by widespread osseous metastases. Iodine 131 (^{131}I) can provide pain relief in patients with well-differentiated thyroid carcinoma, and radioactive phosphorus (^{32}P) and subsequently strontium 89 (^{89}Sr) and ^{131}I-diphosphonates have been used to treat patients with other histologies. ^{32}P-orthophosphate has been the most commonly administered form of ^{32}P. Localization studies show that it is primarily taken up in bone spicules adjacent to the site of metastatic cancer cells.[98] Pain relief responses of varying durations in the range of 60% to 90% have been reported, which is similar to that noted for sequential hemibody irradiation.[99] ^{32}P tends to cause worse bone marrow suppression but does not have the concomitant risk of nausea, vomiting, pneumonitis, and alopecia seen with hemibody irradiation.[93,99] Some have advocated the use of priming with testosterone to increase uptake in prostate tumor, or parathyroid hormone to increase uptake in bone.[19,102–105] Response rates with endocrine priming do not appear substantially different from those with ^{32}P alone. Moreover, testosterone priming followed by ^{32}P therapy has been reported to cause transient exacerbation of pain, irreversible morbidity such as spinal cord compression, or even death.[103,105] Most investigators currently do not advocate endocrine priming.[99]

Recently, several groups have employed ^{89}Sr, a bone-seeking radionuclide with a lower energy beta emission than ^{32}P. Two groups reported favorable response rates ranging from 72% to 91%, while a third institution noted improvement in 51% of patients so treated.[106–108] Less bone marrow toxicity has been reported in these patients. Therefore, this isotope may prove to be a useful therapy for patients with widespread bony metastases. A recent phase I study of ^{131}I-diphosphonates, which also have a high affinity for bone, showed complete pain relief in 44% of patients, substantial pain relief in 6%, minimal improvement in 22%, and no change in 28%. Systemic toxicity and marrow toxicity were minimal.[19A] Other new isotopes under investigation include rhenium 185 (tin) and hydroxyethylidene diphosphonate (^{153}Sm-EDTMP).[109,110] Both are bone seekers, emit gammas that permit imaging, have favorable beta emissions for therapy, and have favorable half-lives for radiation safety purposes. Early studies show responses in the 65% to 80% range. Controlled trials will be needed to determine the optimal role for these newer radionuclides in the treatment of patients with symptomatic, advanced bony metastatic disease.

SPECIFIC TUMORS: UNIQUE CLINICAL AND MANAGEMENT CONSIDERATIONS

In general, the medical management of bony metastases is similar to that of disseminated disease for each individual tumor type.[108] The unique clinical characteristics and surgical and radiotherapeutic aspects of management of bony metastases are summarized for the most common tumors.

BREAST CANCER

Between 50% and 85% of all breast cancer patients will develop bony metastases.[2,9,32,50,51,111] In general, bony lesions respond well to radiation therapy, hormonal therapy, or chemotherapy, or all three.[75,108]

Radiation therapy is recommended for lesions not responding to endocrine therapy or chemotherapy, for sites of pathologic fracture after fixation, and for areas such as the femoral neck and vertebral bodies, which are prone to complication in the event of tumor progression. The intent of radiation therapy should be to provide long-term control of symptomatic sites and to prevent late complications in normal tissue. This generally means fractionated, high-dose treatment to appropriately planned fields with megavoltage machines. To avoid any injury to normal tissue, one should be aware of any overlap with previous radiation fields involving the breast or draining nodal areas. Early (prophylactic) surgery is recommended for large lesions of the hip or femur, or both, to avoid fracture (see Indications for Prophylactic Fixation, later), especially for those who remain symptomatic despite radiation therapy. Pathologic fractures of the long bones are treated by a combination of intramedullary rod fixation and PMMA. A subgroup of breast cancer patients (with skeletal metastases only) has been been recently described.[14,112,113] Because of their prolonged survival, it is recommended that these patients undergo aggressive management of skeletal metastases.[14]

RENAL CELL CARCINOMA (HYPERNEPHROMA)

Approximately 25% of patients with hypernephroma develop bony metastases.[115–117] One significant surgical consideration of metastatic hypernephromas is that they are extremely vascular; life-threatening hemorrhage can easily occur from a small incision. A second consideration is that, unlike other metastatic carcinomas, hypernephromas are often associated with a large extraosseous component. Therefore, before any surgical intervention, CT and angiography are recommended. Biopsy of a suspected hypernephroma should be undertaken only after careful planning; a needle biopsy is recommended. If an open biopsy is required, preoperative embolization should be performed. The need for surgery is indicated by large lesions, progressive bony destruction, instability, or pending fracture. Preoperative embolization and proximal vascular control are mandatory to avoid extensive hemorrhage.[46,63] Cryosurgery has been used as a surgical adjuvant in decreasing bleeding and in increasing local tumor control.[118,119] Palliative embolization alone (without surgery) for large tumors, especially those of the pelvis, has been reported to effect good pain relief.[63] Transient increases in pain and fever may occur as a postinfarction syndrome.

Many radiation oncologists believe that pain from renal call carcinoma metastatic to bone is difficult to palliate. Arcangeli reported a lower rate of complete pain relief in patients with this histology.[95] Improved results were seen with doses of 4000 cGy or more.[120] Other authors do not describe a significant impact of histology on response rate.[92,114]

COLORECTAL CARCINOMA

Skeletal metastases (4%) occur infrequently from colorectal cancer; when they do, it is usually late in the course of the disease.[121] The most common sites of metastases are the lumbar spine and sacrum. Radiation therapy is the most effective mode of palliation in these anatomic sites.[121,122] Long-bone fractures are rare.

LUNG CARCINOMA

Metastatic bony disease occurs in 20% to 40% of lung cancer patients.[115,123] Palliative radiation therapy is usually successful in 60% to 80% of patients.[92,95] A dose of 3000 rads in ten fractions is frequently employed. Fractures are less common in these patients than in others with osteolytic lesions, probably because the bony lesions do not have time to grow. When fractures do occur, treatment is similar to that of the other carcinomas.[22]

THYROID CANCER

McCormack reported bone metastases in 33 of 259 patients (12.7%) with thyroid cancer.[124] Most metastatic bony lesions can be treated with radioisotopes or external irradiation, or both.

Well-differentiated thyroid tumors, follicular carcinomas, and some papillary tumors often retain their affinity for iodine. It is therefore possible to deliver localized radioactive ^{131}I to these lesions when they have metastasized to bone after appropriate surgical ablation of normal thyroid.[19,20] Effective treatment with ^{131}I usually requires several doses given at 3-month intervals. Therefore, sites of severe bone pain should be managed with local external-beam irradiation to achieve early pain relief.[33] For thyroid lesions that do not take up iodine, external-beam irradiation usually provides relief. Pathologic fracture is rare. If surgery is required, bleeding may be excessive. Preoperative angiography and embolization may be useful. For the rare situation of a solitary bone metastasis, Niederle and colleagues have recommended surgical removal in lieu of radioiodine, especially for follicular or papillary carcinoma.[125]

MELANOMA

Stewart and associates reported an overall incidence of bony involvement in melanoma of 6.9%.[126,127] The authors emphasized that these patients may not go through the sequential stage devised for the characterization of melanomas; approximately half of the patients they studied were clinically stage I before the detection of a bony lesion. Bone involvement is a grave prognosis; mean survival was only 3.6 months.[127] They strongly recommended nonoperative management unless the fracture was unstable, because radiation therapy provided good symptomatic relief and expected survival was short.

PROSTATE CANCER

Metastatic prostate cancer most often involves the axial skeleton and pelvis. Typically, bony metastases are osteoblastic (dense), multiple, and small. Occasionally, difficulty arises in distinguishing Paget's disease from metastatic lesions, and solitary metastases from a primary sarcoma. Acid phosphatase is almost always elevated in the presence of bony metastases and is helpful in these differentiations. Pathologic fractures tend not to occur because of the osteoblastic reaction. Despite the frequency of prostate cancer, only 4% of patients in most large series of pathologic fractures have prostate cancer.[9,10,22,23] Prophylactic surgery is rarely required.[19,102,104,105] Localized external irradiation will palliate most sites of bony metastatic disease.[95] Hemibody irradiation or radioisotopes should be considered for patients with multiple sites of symptomatic bony metastases.[97]

LEUKEMIA, LYMPHOMA, AND MYELOMA

The leukemias and lymphomas, while exquisitely sensitive to irradiation, are usually managed with systemic chemotherapy when metastases are present. Pathologic fractures are uncommon, except with multiple myeloma. If surgery is required, the major problem is excessive bleeding due to thrombocytopenia, unexpected coagulopathy, and, rarely, disseminated intravascular coagulopathy. Multiple myeloma tends to be notoriously vascular.

Should a metastasis involve a vertebral body with potential compromise of the spinal cord or nerve roots, localized radiation is recommended. Sites refractory to drug therapy can also be irradiated. For the indolent lymphomas and the leukemias, 2000 to 2500 cGy should provide excellent palliation. For the aggressive lymphomas, doses in the range of 3000 to 4000 cGy should be used. Radiation treatment can provide excellent palliation for patients with symptomatic bony diseases from multiple myeloma.[75–77]

SARCOMAS

Pathologic fracture through a primary sarcoma of bone is rare. In general, a pathologic fracture through a spindle cell sarcoma requires an amputation (see Bone Sarcomas). Radiation therapy generally offers good palliation for metastatic sarcomas to bone.[100] If surgery is required, a primary prosthetic replacement is preferred to internal fixation to avoid progressive local disease.

SPECIFIC ANATOMIC SITES: CLINICAL, SURGICAL, AND RADIOTHERAPEUTIC CONSIDERATIONS

The surgical and radiotherapeutic considerations for metastatic tumors of the most common anatomic sites are discussed.

PROXIMAL FEMUR (HIP)

The hip is the most common site of pathologic fracture (see Fig. 61–4).[10,22,23,32] The aim of treatment is to reduce pain and to keep the patient ambulatory. In general, all pathologic fractures of the hip require surgical reconstruction followed by postoperative radiation therapy. Even in the weakened, nonambulatory patient, surgery is often warranted to relieve pain, to permit simple nursing care, and to enable the patient to sit in a chair.

Indications for Prophylactic Fixation

Firm indications for pending fracture of the hip have not been established; criteria for operative repair based on the experience at Memorial Sloan-Kettering Hospital are summarized here.[23] These authors noted that whenever one of the following three circumstances was present, significant loss of bone substance and continuity was found at surgery:

1. A painful intramedullary lytic lesion equal to or greater than 50% of the cross-sectional diameter of the bone
2. A painful lytic lesion involving a length of cortex equal to or greater than the cross-sectional diameter of the bone or larger than 2.5 cm in axial length
3. A lesion of bone in which pain was unrelieved after radiation therapy

Several investigators have described similar radiographic criteria for the high-risk fracture.[10,128,129] In the largest study to date, Keene and colleagues attempted to identify the clinical and radiographic risk factors for pathologic fracture of the femur.[129] The authors reviewed the skeletal surveys of 2673 patients with breast cancer. Eleven percent (293) of the patients had proximal femoral metastases; 203 of these patients were evaluable. Overall, only 11% of these patients sustained pathologic fracture. There was no difference in the average age, height, weight, pain pattern, or response to radiation therapy between those sustaining fracture and those who did not. These authors were unable to identify either a specific percent involvement of the bone or a critical diameter for metastasis to fracture. The 12 measurable lesions that fractured had the same degree of involvement as the 208 measurable lesions that did not fracture. There are no accurate criteria to select the patient at risk. Keene and colleagues concluded that radiographic measurements alone cannot identify the high-risk patient. To date, exact criteria for prophylactic fixation have not been determined.

Because of this difficulty in predicting which patients might fracture through a long-bone metastasis, Mirels and associates developed a weighted scoring system to quantify the risk of fracture.[130] This system analyzes and combines four roentgenographic and clinical factors into a single score (range, 3–12). The four clinical factors are: anatomic site, pain pattern, type of lesion, and size (Table 61–31).

Seventy-eight lesions were analyzed. Fifty-one lesions did not fracture in the subsequent 6 months and 27 lesions did fracture. The nonfracture group had a mean score of 7 versus a mean score of 10 for the fracture group. As the score increased above 7, so did the risk of fracture. The authors concluded that the lesions of long bones with scores below 7 could safely be irradiated, whereas those with a score of 8 or higher should be treated by internal fixation before irradiation (see Table 61–31). They noted that a score of 9 had a 33% fracture rate and a score of 10 had an 82% fracture rate. Analysis of their results shows that the rate of fracture was small (5%) when the size of the lesion was less than two thirds of the diameter of the bone but increased to 81% for lesions larger than two thirds. They emphasized the difficulty of using standard roentgenograms and recommended the use of CT in difficult cases. They also noted that pain alone was not a major determinant, but if it were "functional" pain (*i.e.*, made worse by use of the extremity), almost all went on to fracture. Importantly, these lesions measured greater than two thirds of the diameters of the involved bones. The probability of fracture with nonfunctional pain was 10%. This system is the first attempt to score and predict potential fractures.

TABLE 61–31. Scoring System for Pathologic Fractures

	Score		
Variable	*1*	*2*	*3*
Site	Upper limb	Lower limb	Peritrochanter
Pain	Mild	Moderate	Functional
Lesion	Blastic	Mixed	Lytic
Size*	<⅓	⅓–⅔	>⅔

* In relation to the diamter of the bone.
(Mirels H. Metastatic disease in long bones. A proposed scoring system. Clin Orthop 1989;249:256–265)

Radiographs and bone scans of the entire femur and acetabulum must be obtained before surgery. It is not uncommon to detect other lesions farther down the shaft, a situation that indicates the need for simultaneous fixation. In general, a long-stem prosthesis will treat both the femoral neck and the diaphyseal lesion. The acetabulum must be evaluated. If there is substantial disease, surgery should include curettage of that lesion and total replacement of the hip and acetabulum. Harrington emphasizes the need for removal of all gross disease and replacement with PMMA and internal fixation (see next section).[11,61] Significant bleeding may occur, especially in patients with myelomas, thyroid tumors, and hypernephromas. Preoperative angiography and embolization of the profundus femoris artery should be considered.

Surgical Treatment

Metastatic fractures of the hip may be intracapsular, intertrochanteric, or subtrochanteric (see Fig. 61–45). Surgical treatment of intracapsular fractures entails endoprosthetic replacement (usually long stem) or total hip replacement. The treatment of intertrochanteric and subtrochanteric fractures varies; plate and screw fixation (with PMMA) and Zickel rods (Howmedica, Rutherford, NJ), respectively, have been described with good success. Recently, Lane has recommended long-stem prostheses with PMMA for any of these three areas.[23] Endoprosthetic replacement has many advantages. It is reliable and simple, avoids late failure or fixation seen with other devices, simultaneously treats lesions more distal in the shaft, and permits early mobilization. Lane reported no instances of loosening or dislocation and only two infections in 167 patients (1.2%). A bicentric device is now preferred in lieu of a fixed-head endoprosthesis.[23]

Similarly, Rinkes and colleagues evaluated the treatment of manifest and pending fractures of the femoral neck in 34 patients.[131] They emphasized the use of cemented hemiarthroplasty for immediate fixation and early mobilization (average, 9 days). All patients experienced pain relief. Mean survival was 17.6 months (12 months for manifest and 40 months for impending fracture). They emphasized the necessity for complete tumor curettage and filling of the defect with PMMA. It is important to note that segmental resections were not required. PMMA was used to fill large tumor defects. We agree with the authors that proximal femoral lesions should be treated aggressively to improve function, ambulation, nursing management, and pain relief.

Technique

A standard posterolateral approach is used. The trochanter should not be osteotomized. The head and neck are removed and the canal is reamed with *flexible* reamers; solid reamers may perforate abnormally thin bone. The length of the stem of the prosthesis should be at least to the isthmus or distal to any shaft lesions, or both. The incision may be extended to curette all gross tumor. Any absent bone can be reconstructed with PMMA. It is extremely important to obtain a good cement mantle around the stem of the prosthesis and distal to the tip. The PMMA should be cooled before injection to increase the time of polymerization. The patient is mobilized within 2 to 3 days. If there is extensive loss of proximal bone, a segmental prosthesis is used. This technique is associated with significant operative morbidity and is not routinely performed. When required, however, it can successfully reconstruct large proximal defects.

Radiation Therapy

Radiation portals should encompass the involved area of the proximal femur and extend distally to any sites of involvement of the femoral shaft. If surgery has been performed, radiation therapy should be started after the surgical wound has healed. Intramedullary or other fixation devices are generally included in the radiation field to encompass any microscopic tumor that might be dislodged by the surgery. Radiation fields should spare the knee joint unless there is frank tumor involvement of the adjacent distal femur. As is customary in other extremity sites, a strip of soft tissue should be left unirradiated to preserve lymphatic drainage.

FEMORAL SHAFT

Fractures of the femoral shaft should be treated by IM fixation and PMMA (Fig. 61–46). Combined osteosynthesis (*i.e.*, plate and screw fixation and PMMA) may be successful; however, it is not preferred because of the risk of fracture proximal and distal to the plate, increased operative time, and the need for a more extensive surgical exposure. In general, IM rod fixation is performed by the "open" method: the tumor/fracture site is exposed, the tumor is curetted, PMMA is injected proximal and distal, and the IM rod is inserted. The proximal and distal fragments should be carefully reamed of all gross disease to permit easy insertion of the PMMA and rod. A uniform cement mantle should be obtained around the rod. Immediate ambulation with full weight bearing is permitted a few days after surgery.

Prophylactic Femoral Shaft Fixation

Small lesions of the femoral shaft may be treated before fracture by the "closed" method (*i.e.*, fluoroscopically inserting an IM rod from a small incision at the tip of the greater trochanter and passing through the lesion to obtain good distal fixation). When using this procedure, it is difficult to insert PMMA. This method is indicated only for small lesions of the femoral shaft with normal bone proximal. Interlocking the rod is useful. Careful preoperative evaluation of the hip is required, because progression and subsequent treatment of an undetected hip lesion would be extremely difficult with an IM rod in place.

Supracondylar Femoral Fixation

Healy and Lane evaluated the Zickel supracondylar device for patients with difficult metastatic lesions of the distal femoral diaphysis (Fig. 61–47).[132] They reported good functional and symptomatic relief in 11 of 14 patients. They emphasized that both medial and lateral incisions were necessary. They also stressed that no matter what the size of the defect, PMMA was used to obtain immediate fixation and stability in all cases. This device is not indicated for distal femoral metaphyseal lesions. This situation is best treated by a custom distal femoral replacement.

PELVIS AND ACETABULUM

Metastatic tumors of the pelvis usually present with progressive pain; fractures are rare. The pelvis can be successfully treated nonoperatively with radiation therapy. Fortunately, marked bony destruction is uncommon; when it occurs, surgery can provide pain relief and enable the patient to walk again. Harrington classified and described the surgical management of 58 patients with severe acetabular insufficiency (classes I, II, III).[11,61] This classification is based on the amount and location of bony destruction and the surgical procedure required for stabilization.

Extensive preoperative evaluation of the bony pelvis, ex-

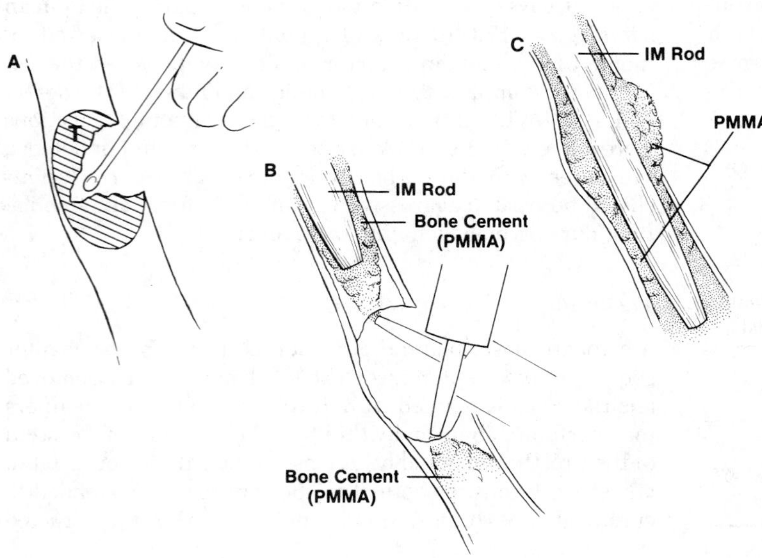

FIGURE 61–46. Diaphyseal reconstruction for metastatic cancer. Long bones (femur and humerus) with metastatic tumors of the shafts (diaphysis) are reconstructed by intramedullary (IM) rod fixation combined with polymethylmethacrylate (PMMA). **(A)** Curettage of the tumor. **(B)** It is important to get the PMMA proximal and distal to the site of the tumor or fracture site, or both, in addition to filling the tumor defect. **(C)** Stable fixation depends on this combined fixation. Small diaphyseal tumors may be treated prophylactically without opening the fracture site by using fluoroscopic control.

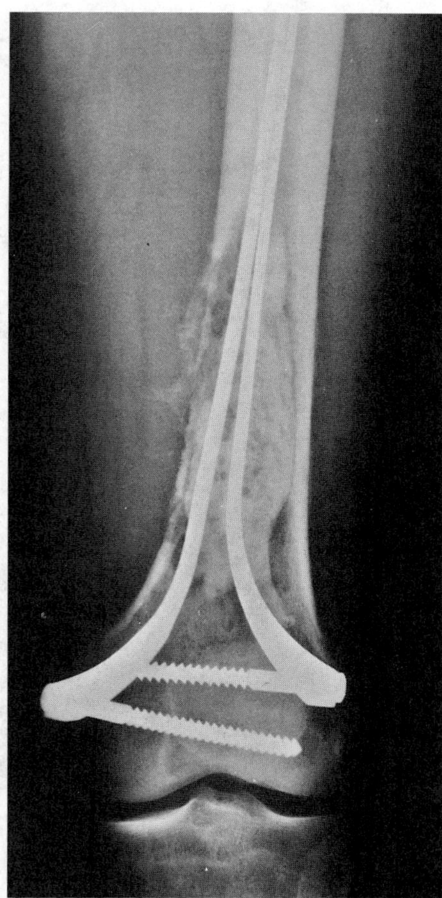

FIGURE 61–47. Zickel (Howmedica, Rutherford, NJ) supracondylar rod fixation of a distal femoral metastatic lesion.

traosseous tumor extension, and tumor vascularity is required. CT/MRI is more reliable than bone scintigraphy for evaluating pelvic tumor extent and is recommended for all patients. Angiography should be performed on all patients before surgery, with embolization of the vascular tumors. Significant blood loss must be anticipated; Harrington reported a mean blood loss of 1800 ml each for classes I and II and a loss of 2790 ml for class III (range, 1125–8550 ml).[61] He emphasized that these procedures are indicated only in a *highly* select group of patients with a predictive long-term survival. For this select group, results are quite good. Sixty-seven percent of the patients reported excellent or good pain relief at 6 months, and 43% at 2 years. Eighty percent were ambulatory at 6 months.

Surgical Treatment

The surgical solution for overcoming the insufficiency of the roof or bony rim is to transmit the forces away from the local periacetabular bone into the superior part of the ilium and sacrum, which is still structurally intact. A standard anterior approach is used. It is unnecessary to enter the retroperitoneal space unless there is a large extraosseous component. All gross disease must be curetted. Hemostasis can be obtained by rapid tumor curettage and PMMA. Reconstruction is accomplished with a combination of Steinmann pins (Howmedica, Rutherford, NJ), protrusio cups, and wire mesh. The trochanter should not be osteotomized. Close intraoperative monitoring of blood loss and hematologic parameters is required.

Malawer and colleagues recently reported a new technique for the treatment of large acetabular lesions that require surgery. This technique curettes out gross tumor and reconstructs the defect with a Saddle prosthesis (Waldermar-Link, Hamburg, Germany), which articulates with the remaining ilium. No other reconstruction is required (Fig. 61–48).[133] This technique avoids the difficult reconstructions using PMMA, screws, and special acetabular components. Reported operative time and surgical blood loss for the Saddle prosthesis have been less than those reported by Harrington for acetabular reconstruction.[61,133]

Pelvic Radiation Therapy

Radiation therapy is recommended for all symptomatic pelvic and acetabular lesions after surgical procedures. Radiation therapy fields must encompass the area of bone involved by tumor and yet spare bone not grossly infiltrated by tumor to minimize irradiation of the marrow. Consideration of the effect of irradiation on bone marrow will be particularly important in patients receiving chemotherapy. If only a portion of the pelvis is treated, field edges should be designed to facilitate matching, in case treatment elsewhere in the pelvis is required at a later date. Pelvis fields will necessarily include some small bowel; the dose and fractionation must be within the limits of small bowel tolerance.

SPINE

The vertebral bodies are most often affected by metastatic cancer (Fig. 61–49). Pain may be secondary to intraosseous disease, instability, collapse or pathologic fracture, or epidural compression, with or without nerve root involvement. Most vertebral pain can be treated with nonoperative modalities such as chemotherapy, radiation therapy, and an external orthosis. The "radiosensitive" solid tumors, lymphomas, and myelomas will respond with decreased pain and reossification. Indications for surgery include progressive neurologic symptoms, intractable pain, and progressive deformity. The traditional aim of such treatment has been decompression of the spinal canal by a posterior laminectomy and, occasionally, posterior stabilization with Harrington rods and PMMA. Recently, significant disagreement has arisen regarding the efficacy of posterior decompression.[12,13,134,135] It is based on the fact that the site of metastatic disease to the spine is anterior, primarily involving the vertebral body. Several reports have described an anterior approach to the affected vertebrae, with removal of all gross disease, that permits decompression of the spinal cord and nerve roots and immediate stabilization by use of PMMA for vertebral body reconstruction.[12,13,134]

Computed tomography, MRI, and myelography are required before surgery. The CT scan demonstrates the amount of bony destruction, while the MRI and myelogram localize the level and extent of epidural disease. The indications for anterior decompression are progressive neurologic deficit after surgery or radiation therapy, and kyphosis with significant deformity (especially of the cervical spine).[12,13] All authors emphasize that this procedure is technically demanding, with significant

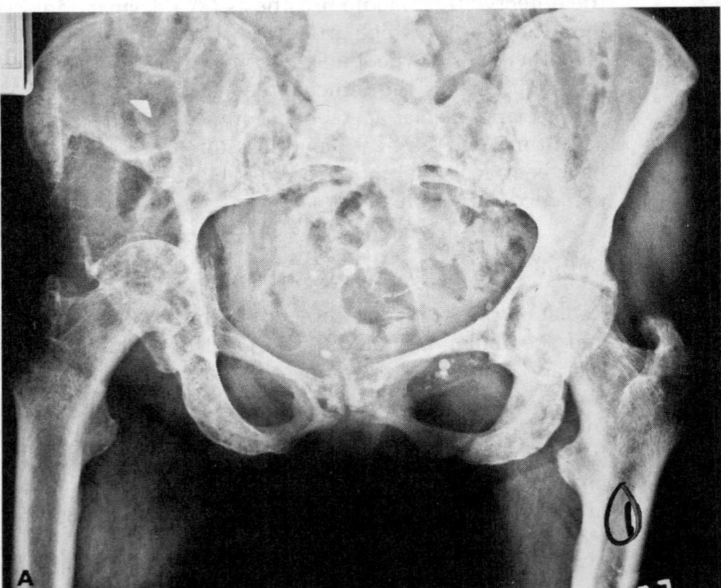

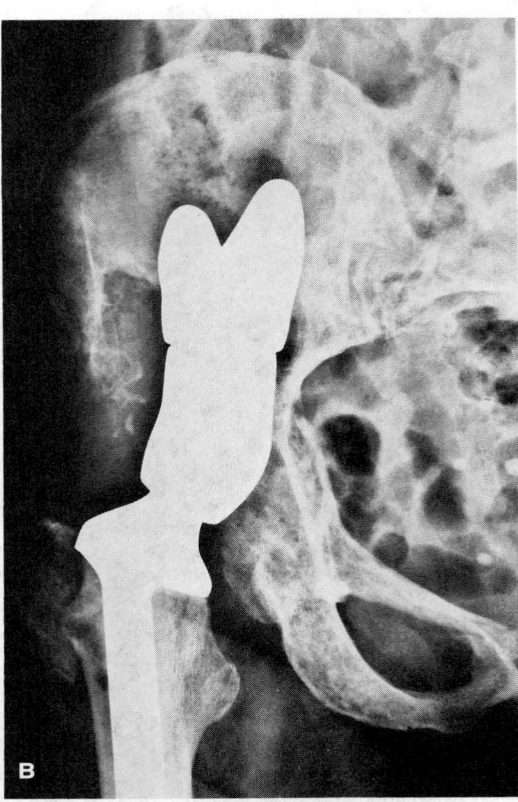

FIGURE 61–48. **(A)** Multiple myeloma of the pelvis with marked destruction of the right acetabulum. This represents a difficult reconstructive problem. **(B)** A saddle prosthesis is used to reconstruct the hip after curettage of the tumor.

morbidity and blood loss. It should be used only in highly selected patients by skilled surgeons. Harrington initially reported 14 patients treated by vertebral body resection and PMMA replacement; 9 of 12 patients with major preoperative neurologic impairment recovered completely, 2 recovered partially, and 1 had no change.[12] Thirteen of the 14 patients had excellent pain relief. Average blood replacements for the cervical/thoracic and lumbar procedures were 200 and 1200 ml, respectively. Sundaresan and associates have performed 100 vertebral body resections and stabilizations for spinal metastases.[13] Eighty percent of these patients had significant pain relief immediately. Complications were related to previous treatment with intensive chemotherapy or radiation therapy. Minimal morbidity occurred in the de novo case.

Recently, Rosenthal and associates (1991) reviewed their experience with anterior corpectomy for metastatic cancer at Memorial Sloan-Kettering Cancer Center.[136] They evaluated 53 patients and concluded that, in addition to anterior decompression, posterior stabilization is required in all patients undergoing decompression, except patients with thoracic lesions. They noted a loss in neurologic and functional status due to tumor progression or collapse of the anterior reconstruction between 7.1 and 8.2 months, whereas the average patient survival was 16 months (range, 1–47 months). They emphasized that these procedures were difficult, with an overall mortality of 5% to 10%.

Surgical Technique

A thoracic or thoracolumbar approach is used. The lumbar vertebrae are approached from the left side, and the aorta is mobilized and retracted. Care must be taken not to injure the segmental vessels, which must be carefully ligated. All gross disease is removed from the affected vertebral body, and the adjacent disks are removed (Fig. 61–50). Gelfoam and continuous irrigation are used to protect the dura from the heat of polymerization before placing the PMMA. Steinmann pins or short distraction rods are placed as vertical supports between the vertebral bodies and then embedded within the PMMA.[12,134] The adjacent bodies are undercut to permit snug PMMA fixation. Care must be taken not to put pressure on the cord.

Newer techniques and concepts of metastatic disease of the spine continue to evolve. Techniques based on advances in spinal surgery, instrumentation, and prosthetic design have permitted various radical methods of vertebral body resection to be performed for selected patients with vertebral body metastases. It must be emphasized that these procedures are performed in highly selected spinal treatment and cancer centers.[137] The overall goals of surgical treatment are:

1. To decompress the spinal cord
2. To leave the patient with a stable spine
3. To leave the patient with a painless spine

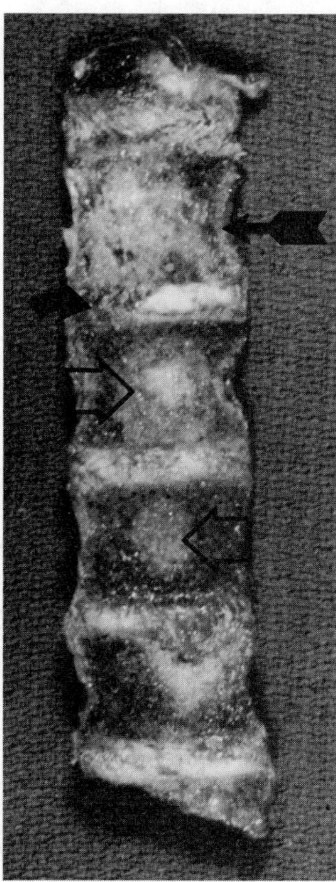

FIGURE 61–49. Metastatic spinal disease. The spine is the most common site of metastatic disease. Metastatic cancer characteristically involves the anterior portion (vertebral body) of the spine. Shown is a gross specimen of the lumbar vertebra with characteristic metastatic tumor deposits within the vertebral bodies (*arrows*). The top vertebra (*straight solid arrow*) is almost completely replaced by tumor, and the adjacent disk space is being destroyed (*short curved arrow*). The lower two vertebrae show small, rounded central deposits of metastatic cancer (*open arrows*).

Cochran and colleagues described a single posterior approach for total vertebrectomy with vertebral body replacement.[137] They reported the largest series to date with 13 patients. This technique permits complete spinal cord decompression with immediate stability. Significant pain relief and preservation of neurologic function were reported.

Radiation Therapy

Radiation therapy is recommended for symptomatic lesions and after surgical decompression. Radiation portals should include sites of symptomatic vertebral disease and other involved vertebrae that can be conveniently included without undue morbidity. Spinal cord tolerance must not be exceeded. Treatment of a portion of a vertebral body is not recommended because of the inherent danger of matching later treatment fields over the spinal cord should disease recur in the untreated portion of the vertebra. Paravertebral soft tissue masses should be included in the treatment field.

HUMERUS

Small lesions can be treated nonoperatively with radiation therapy and sling immobilization. Large lesions or those with a pathologic fracture are best treated by curettage, intramedullary fixation, and PMMA.[28] Proximal humeral lesions are approached through the standard deltopectoral interval. Tumors of the shaft require two incisions: one should be proximal, over the greater tuberosity, and the second should be over the tumor. Lesions of the supracondylar area are best treated by two rods inserted through the epicondyles. If the patient also has lower extremity lesions, early surgery for the humerus is recommended to permit crutch use and protect the lower extremities.

LESIONS DISTAL TO THE KNEE AND ELBOW

Leeson reported that 7% (57/827) of patients with metastatic cancer had distal extremity involvement.[138] The most common primary cancers associated with distal metastases are lung, breast, kidney, and gastrointestinal tract. Tumors of the forearm or tibia are best treated by intramedullary fixation with PMMA. A recent poll of 163 hand surgeons showed that amputation of the digit was recommended in lieu of complicated surgical procedures and difficult radiation. Tumors of the hand may require amputation for local control and palliation, although substantial experience with extremity preservation has been accumulated with combined modality therapy for primary sarcomas of the hand and foot.[139] Patients with metastatic disease to the hand or foot should undergo irradiation for attempted palliation. Amputation can be used for patients not palliated with irradiation.

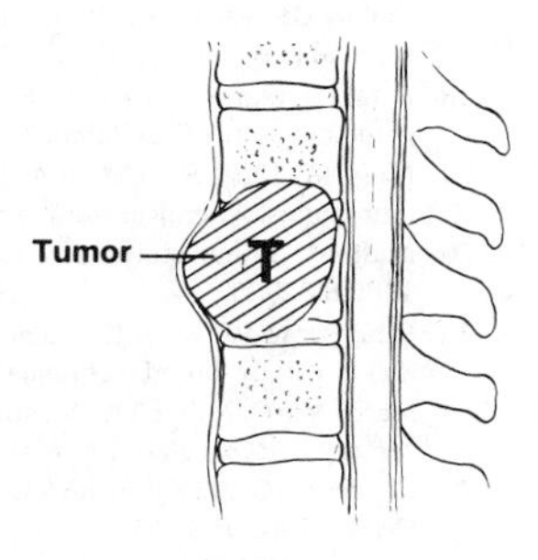

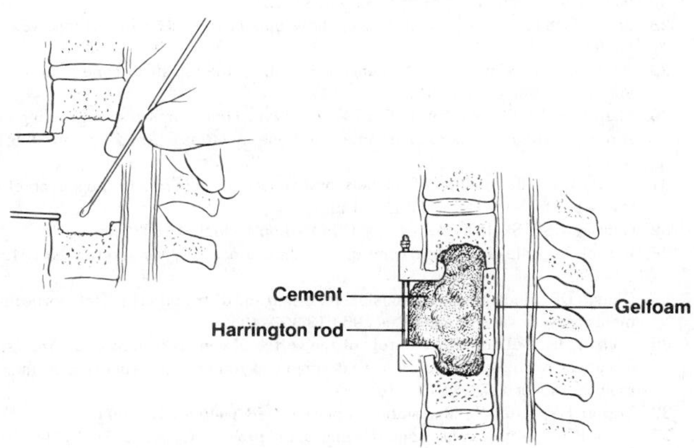

FIGURE 61–50. Technique of vertebral body reconstruction. The anterior aspect of the spine (vertebral bodies) can be approached successfully with reliable tumor removal, decompression of the spinal cord, and reconstruction in carefully selected patients. Significant morbidity and bleeding must be anticipated.

REFERENCES

1. Silverberg E, Lubera J. Cancer statistics, 1987. CA 1987;37:2–20.
2. Abrams HL, Spiro R, Goldstein N. Metastases in carcinoma. Analysis of 1000 autopsied cases. Cancer 1950;23:74–85.
3. Galasko CSB. Mechanisms of lytic and blastic metastatic disease of bone. Clin Orthop 1982;169:20–27.
4. Porter BA, Sheilds AF, Olson DO. Magnetic resonance imaging of bone marrow disorders. Radiol Clin North Am 1986;24:269–288.
5. Daffner RH, Lupetin AR, Dash N, Sefczek RJ, Schapiro RL. MRI in the detection of malignant infiltration of bone marrow. Am J Radiol 1986;146:353–358.
6. Drelichman A, Decker DA, Al-Sarraf M, et al. Computerized bone scan. A potential useful technique to measure response in prostatic carcinoma. Cancer 1984;53:1061–1065.
7. Zegel HG, Turner M, VelchiK MG, et al. Percutaneous osseous needle aspiration biopsy with nuclear medicine guidance. Clin Nucl Med 1984;9:89–91.
8. Little AG, DeMeester TR, Kirchner PT, et al. Guided biopsies of abnormalities on nuclear bone scans. Technique and indications. J Thorac Cardiovasc Surg 1983;85: 396–403.
9. McNeil BJ. Value of bone scanning in neoplastic disease. Semin Nucl Med 1984;14: 277–286.
10. Harrington KD, Johnston JJ, Turner RH, Green DL. The use of methylmethacrylate as an adjunct in the internal fixation of malignant neoplastic fractures. J Bone Joint Surg [Am] 1972;54:1665–1676.
11. Harrington KD. New trends in the management of lower extremity metastasis. Clin Orthop 1982;169:53–61.
12. Harrington KD. The use of methylmethacrylate for vertebral-body replacement and anterior stabilization of pathological fracture-dislocations of the spine due to metastatic malignant disease. J Bone Joint Surg [Am] 1981;63:36–46.
13. Sundaresan N, Galicich JH, Lane JM, et al. Treatment of neoplastic epidural cord compression by vertebral body resection and stabilization. J Neurosurg 1985;63:676–684.
14. Sherry MM, Greco FA, Johnson DH, Hainsworth JD. Metastatic breast cancer confined to the skeletal system, an indolent disease. Am J Med 1986;81(3):381–386.
15. Salazar OM, Rubin P, Hendrickson FR, et al. Single-dose half-body irradiation for palliation of multiple bone metastases from solid tumors: Final Radiation Therapy Oncology Group report. Cancer 1986;58:29.
16. Vargha ZO, Glicksman AS, Boland J. Single-dose radiation therapy in the palliation of metastatic disease. Radiology 1969;93:1180.
17. Penn CRH. Single dose and fractionated palliative irradiation for osseous metastases. Clin Radiol 1976;27:405.
18. Fitzpatrick PJ, Rider WD. Half-body radiotherapy. Int J Radiat Oncol Biol Phys 1976;1: 197.
19. Lawrence JH, Tobias CA. Radioactive isotopes and nuclear radiations in the treatment of cancer. Cancer Res 1956;16:185.

19a. Eisenhut M, Berberich R, Kimming B, Oberhausen E. Iodine-131-labelled diphosphonates for palliative treatment of bone metastases: II. Preliminary clinical results with iodine-131 BDP3. J Nucl Med 1986;27:1255.

20. Clain A. Secondary malignant disease of bone. Br J Cancer 1965;19:15.
21. Higinbotham NL, Marcove RC. The management of pathological fractures. J Trauma 1965;5:792–798.
22. Haberman ET, Sachs R, Stern RE, et al. The pathology and treatment of metastatic disease of the femur. Clin Orthop 1982;169:70–82.
23. Lane JM, Sculco TP, Zolan S. Treatment of pathological fractures of the hip by endoprosthetic replacement. J Bone Joint Surg [Am] 1980;62:954–959.
24. Goris ML, Bretille J. Skeletal scintigraphy for the diagnosis of malignant metastatic diseases of bone. Radiother Oncol 1985;4:319–329.
25. Mundy GR, Ibbotson KJ, D'Souza SM. Tumor products and hypercalcemia of malignancy. J Clin Invest 1985;76:391–394.
26. Beard DB, Haskell CM. Carcinoembryonic antigen in breast cancer. Clinical review. Am J Med 1986;80:241–245.
27. El-Khoury GY, Terepka RH, Mickelson MR, et al. Fine-needle aspiration biopsy of bone. J Bone Joint Surg [Am] 1983;65:522–525.
28. Sim F, Pritchard D. Metastatic disease of the upper extremity. Clin Orthop 1982;169: 83–94.
29. Berrettoni BA, Carter JR. Mechanisms of cancer metastasis to bone. J Bone Joint Surg [Am] 1986;68:308–311.
30. Manishen WJ, Sivananthan K, Orr FW. Resorbing bone stimulates tumor cell growth. A role for the host microenvironment in bone metastasis. Am J Pathol 1986;123: 39–45.
31. Batson OV. The function of the vertebral veins and their role in the spread of metastases. Ann Surg 1940;112:138–149.
32. Galasko CSB. Skeletal metastases. Clin Orthop 1986;210:18–30.
33. Batson OV. Role of vertebral veins in metastatic processes. Ann Intern Med 1942;16: 38–45.
34. Coman DR. Mechanisms responsible for origin and distribution of blood-borne tumor metastases. Review. Cancer Res 1953;13:397–404.
35. Coman DR, DeLong RP. The role of the vertebral venous system in the metastasis of cancer to the spinal column. Experiment of tumor-cell suspension in rats and rabbits. Cancer 1951;4:610–618.
36. Turner JW, Jaffe HL. Metastatic neoplasms. AJR 1940;43:479–494.
37. Clark RL. Systemic cancer and the metastatic process. Cancer 1979;43:790.
38. Hollinshead WH, McFarlane JA. A collateral venous drainage system from kidney following occlusion of renal vein in dog. Surg Gynecol Obstet 1953;97:213–219.
39. Brookes M. Blood vessels in bone marrow. In: The blood supply of bone. An approach to bone biology. London: Butterworths, 1971:67–91.
40. Enneking WF. Metastatic carcinoma. In: Enneking WF, ed. Musculoskeletal tumor surgery. vol 2. New York: Churchill Livingstone, 1983:1541.
41. Dodds PR, Cardie VJ, Lytton B. The role of the vertebral veins in the dissemination of prostatic carcinoma. J Urol 1981;126:753–755.
42. del Regato JA. Pathways of metastatic spread of malignant tumors. Semin Oncol 1977;4:33–38.
43. Brookes M. Blood vessels in bone marrow. In: The blood supply of bone. An approach to bone biology. London: Butterworths, 1971:67–91.
44. Gephardt M, et al. Prostaglandins. Clin Oreth and Rel Res
45. Mundy GR, Raisz LG, Cooper RA, et al. Evidence for the secretion of an osteoclast-stimulating factor in myeloma. N Engl J Med 1974;291:1041–1046.
46. Kamenov B, Kiernan MW, Barrington-Leight, et al. Homing receptors as functional markers for classification, prognosis and therapy of leukemias and lymphomas. Proc Soc Exp Biol Med 1984;177:211–219.
47. Lam WC, Delikatny JE, Orr FW, et al. The chemotactic response of tumor cells. A model of cancer metastasis. Am J Pathol 1981;104:69–76.
48. Wilner D. Cancer metastasis to bone. In: Wilner D, ed. Radiology of bone tumors and allied disorders. Philadelphia: WB Saunders, 1982:3641–3908.
49. Pollne JJ, Witztum KF, Ashburn WL. The flare phenomenon of radionuclide bone scan in metastatic prostate cancer. Am J Radiol 1984;142:773–776.
50. Hortobagyi GN, Lipshitz HI, Seabod JE. Osseous metastases of breast cancer. Clinical, biochemical, radiographic, and scintigraphic evaluation of response to therapy. Cancer 1984;53:577–582.
51. Hayward RB, Frazier TG. A re-evaluation of bone scans in breast cancer. J Surg Oncol 1985;28:111-113.
52. Weissman DE, Gilbert M, Wang H, Grossman SA. The use of computed tomography of the spine to identify patients at high risk for epidural metastases. J Clin Oncol 1985;3:1541–1544.
53. Wallace S, Granmayeh M, DeSantos LA, et al. Arterial occlusion of pelvic bone tumors. Cancer 1979;43:322–328.
54. Wallace S, Charnsangavej C, Carrasco H, Bechtel W. Infusion-embolization. Cancer 1984;54:2751–2765.
55. Jonsson K, Johnell O. Preoperative angiography in patients with bone metastases. Acta Radiol Diagn 1982;23:485–489.
56. Bowers TA, Murray JA, Charnsangavej C, Soo C, et al. Bone metastases from renal carcinoma, the preoperative use of transcatheter arterial occlusion. J Bone Joint Surg [Am] 1982;64:749–754.
57. Pugh J, Sherry H, Futterman B, et al. Biomechanics of pathologic fractures. Clin Orthop 1982;169:109–114.
58. Ryan JR, Begeman PC. The effects of filling experimental large cortical defects with methylmethacrylate. Clin Orthop 1984;185:306–310.
59. Gainor BJ, Buchert P. Fracture healing in metastatic bone disease. Clin Orthop 1983;178:297–302.
60. Unger AS, Boothe RE. Disseminated intravascular coagulopathy in a patient undergoing total hip arthroplasty. A case report. Clin Orthop 1984;183:76–78.
61. Harrington KD. The management of acetabular insufficiency secondary to metastatic malignant disease. J Bone Joint Surg [Am] 1981;63:653–663.
62. Schobinger R. The arteriographic picture of metastatic bone disease. Cancer 1958;11: 1265–1268.
63. Varm J, Huben RP, Wajsman Z, Pontes JE. Therapeutic embolization of pelvic metastases of renal cell carcinoma. J Urol 1984;131:647–649.
64. Mink J. Percutaneous bone biopsy in the patient with known or suspected osseous metastases. Radiology 1986;161:191–194.

64a. Michele AA, Krueger FJ. Surgical approach to the vertebral body. J Bone Joint Surg [Am] 1949;31:873–878.

64b. Schajowicz F, Derequic JC. Puncture biopsy in lesions of the locomotor system. Review of results in 4050 cases, including 941 vertebral punctures. Cancer 1968;21:531–548.

65. Taylor CR, Kledzik G. Immunohistologic techniques in surgical pathology—A spectrum of "new" special stains. Hum Pathol 1981;12:590–596.
66. Pinkus GS. Diagnostic immunocytochemistry of paraffin-embedded tissues. Hum Pathol 1982;13:411–415.
67. Pinkus GS, Kurtin PJ. Epithelial membrane antigen—A diagnostic discriminant in surgical pathology. Hum Pathol 1985;16:929–940.
68. Kahn HJ, Marks A, Thom H, Baumal R. Role of antibody to S100 protein in diagnostic pathology. Am J Clin Pathol 1983;79:341–347.
69. Nadji M, Tabei SZ, Castro A, Chu TM, Morales AR. Prostatic origin of tumors. An immunohistochemical study. Am J Clin Pathol 1980;73:735–739.
70. Nadji M. Immunoperoxidase techniques I. Facts and artifacts. Am J Dermatopathol 1986;8:32–36.

71a. Sangeorzan BJ, Ryan JR, Salciccioli GG. Prophylactic femoral stabilization with the Zickel nail by closed technique. J Bone Joint Surg [Am] 1986;68:991–999.

71b. Marcove RC, Miller TR. Treatment of primary and metastatic bone tumors by cryosurgery. JAMA 1969;207:1890.

72. Marcove RC. A 17-year review of cryosurgery in the treatment of bone tumors. Clin Orthop 1982;163:231.
73. Malawer MM, Baker A. Amputations for tumors. In: Evarts CM, ed. Surgery of the musculoskeletal system. 2nd ed. New York: Churchill Livingstone, 1990.
74. Malawer MM, Marks MR, McChecney D, et al. The effect of cryosurgery and polymethylmethacrylate (PMMA) in dogs with experimental bone defects comparable to tumor defects. Clin Orthop 1988;226:229–310.

75. Tong D, Gillick L, Hendrickson FR. The palliation of symptomatic osseous metastases: Final results of the Radiation Therapy Oncology Group. Cancer 1982;50:893.
76. Delclos L. New and old concepts in radiotherapeutic treatment. Int J Radiat Oncol Biol Phys 1976;1:1217.
77. Hendrickson FR, Sheinkop MB. Management of osseous metastases. Semin Oncol 1975;2:399.
78. Weber DA. The quantitative measurement of the response to treatment. Int J Radiat Oncol Biol Phys 1976;1:1221.
79. Yarnold JR. Role of radiotherapy in the management of bone metastases from breast cancer. J R Soc Med 1985;78(Suppl):23.
80. Garmatis CJ, Chu FCH. The effectiveness of radiation therapy in the treatment of bone metastases from breast cancer. Radiology 1978;126:235.
81. Allen KL, Johnson TW, Hibbs GG. Effective bone radiation as related to various treatment regimens. Cancer 1976;37:984.
82. Twycross RG. Analgesics and relief of pain. In: Stoll BA, Parbhoo S, eds. Bone metastasis: Monitoring and treatment. New York: Raven Press, 1983.
83. Gilbert HA, Kagan HR, Nussbaum H, et al. Evaluation of radiation therapy for bone metastases: Pain relief and quality of life. AJR 1977;129:1095–1096.
84. Hendrickson FR, Shehata WM, Kirchner AR. Radiation therapy for osseous metastasis. Int J Radiat Oncol Biol Phys 1976;1(3–4):275–278.
85. Bhadrwaj S, Holland JF. Chemotherapy of metastatic cancer to bone. Clin Orthop 1982;169:28–37.
86. Greenberg EJ, Chu FCH, Dwyer AJ, et al. Effects of radiation therapy on bone lesions as measured by 47-Ca and 85-Sr local kinetics. J Nucl Med 1972;13:747.
87. Unger JD, Chiang LC, Unger GF. Apparent reformation of the base of the skull following radiotherapy for nasopharyngeal carcinoma. Radiology 1978;126:779.
88. Blitzer PH. Reanalysis of the RTOG study of the palliation of symptomatic osseous metastasis. Cancer 1985;55:1468.
89. Madsen EL. Painful bone metastasis: Efficacy of radiotherapy assessed by the patients: A randomized trial comparing 4 Gy × 6 versus 10 Gy × 2. Int J Radiat Oncol Biol Phys 1983;9:1775–1779.
90. Cole DJ. A randomized trial of a single treatment versus conventional fractionation in the palliative radiotherapy of painful bone metastases. Clin Oncol 1989;1:59–62.
91. Okawa T, Kita M, Goto M, et al. Randomized prospective clinical study of small, large and twice-a-day fraction radiotherapy for painful bone metastases. Radiother Oncol 1988;13:99–104.
92. Price P, Hoskin PJ, Easton D, et al. Prospective randomised trial of single and multifraction radiotherapy schedules in the treatment of painful bony metastases. Radiother Oncol 1986;6:247–255.
93. Qasim MM. Single dose palliative irradiation for bony metastases. Strahlentherapie 1977;153:531.
94. Price P, Hoskin PJ, Easton D, et al. Low dose single fraction radiotherapy in the treatment of metastatic bone pain: A pilot study. Radiother Oncol 1988;12:297–300.
95. Arcangeli G, Micheli A, Arcangeli G, et al. The responsiveness of bone metastases to radiotherapy: The effect of site, histology and radiation dose on pain relief. Radiother Oncol 1989;14:95–101.
96. Kuban DA, Delbridge T, El-Mahdi AM, Schellhammer PF. Half-body irradiation for treatment of widely metastatic adenocarcinoma of the prostate. J Urol 1989;141:572–574.
97. Zelefsky MJ, Scher HI, Forman JD, et al. Palliative hemiskeletal irradiation for widespread metastatic prostate cancer: A comparison of single dose and fractionated regimens. Int J Radiat Oncol Biol Phys 1989;17:1281–1285.
98. Kaplan E, Miree J, Hirsh E, et al. Autoradiographic localization of 32P phosphate in metastatic carcinoma of the breast to bone. Int J Appl Radiat Isot 1959;5:94–98.
99. Montebello JF, Hartson-Eaton M. The palliation of osseous metastasis with 32P and 89Sr compared with external beam and hemibody irradiation. Cancer Invest 1989;7(2): 139–160.
100. McKenna WG, Barnes MM, Kinsella TJ, et al. Combined modality treatment of adult soft tissue sarcomas of the head and neck. Int J Radiat Oncol Biol Phys 1987;13:1127.
101. Ellis RE. The distribution of active bone marrow in the adult. Phys Med Biol 1961;5: 255.
102. Maxfield JR, Maxfield JJG, Maxfield WS. The use of radioactive phosphorus and testosterone in metastatic bone lesions from breast and prostate. South Med J 1958;51: 320.
103. Ariel IM, Hassouna H. Carcinoma of the prostate: The treatment of bone metastases by radioactive phosphorus (32P). Int Surg 1985;70:63.
104. Aziz H, Choi K, Sohn C, et al. Comparison of 32P therapy and sequential hemibody irradiation (HBI) for bony metastases as methods of whole body irradiation. Am J Clin Oncol 1986;9:264.
105. Fowler JE Jr, Whitmore WF Jr. Considerations for the use of testosterone with systemic chemotherapy in prostatic cancer. Cancer 1982;49:1373.
106. Firusian N, Mellin P, Schmidt CG. Results of 89 strontium therapy in patients with carcinoma of the prostate and incurable pain from bone metastases: A preliminary report. J Urol 1976;116:764.
107. Reddy EK, Robinson RG, Mansfield CM. Strontium-89 therapy for palliation of bone metastases. J Natl Med Assoc 1986;78:27.
108. Bhadrwaj S, Holland JF. Chemotherapy of metastatic cancer to bone. Clin Orthop 1982;169:28–37.
109. Maxon HR III, Schroeder LE, Thomas SR, et al. Re-186(Sn) HEDP for treatment of painful osseous metastases: Initial clinical experience in 20 patients with hormone-resistant prostate cancer. Radiology 1990;176:155–159.
110. Turner JH, Claringbold PG, Hetherington EL, et al. A phase I study of samarium-153 ethylenediaminetetramethylene phosphonate therapy for disseminated skeletal metastases. J Clin Oncol 1989;7:1926–1931.
111. Miller F, Whitehill R. Carcinoma of the breast metastatic to the skeleton. Clin Orthop 1984;184:121–127.
112. Sherry MM, Greco A, Johnson DH, Hainsworth JD. Breast cancer with skeletal metastases at initial diagnosis. Cancer 1986;58:178–182.
113. Scheid V, Buzdar AU, Smith TL, et al. Clinical course of breast cancer patients with osseous metastasis treated with combination chemotherapy. Cancer 1986;58:2589–2593.
114. Arkless R. Renal carcinoma: How it metastasizes. Cancer 1965;84:496–501.
115. Garfield DH, Kennedy BJ. Regression of metastatic renal cell carcinoma following nephrectomy. Cancer 1972;30:190–196.
116. Dorn W, Gladden MP, Rankin EA. Regression of a renal-cell metastatic osseous lesion following treatment. J Bone Joint Surg [Am] 1975;57:869–870.
117. Chute R, Houghton JD. Solitary distant metastases from unsuspected renal carcinomas. J Urol 1958;80:420–424.
118. Marcove RC, Sadrieh J, Huvos AG, et al. Cryosurgery in the treatment of solitary or multiple bone metastases form renal cell carcinoma. J Urol 1972;108:540.
119. Marcove RC, Searfoss RC, Whitmore WF, et al. Cryosurgery in the treatment of bone metastases from renal cell carcinoma. Clin Orthop 1972;127:220.
120. Delaney TF. Personal experience.
121. Bonnheim DC, Petrelli NJ, Herrera L, Walsh D, Mittelman A. Osseous metastases from colorectal carcinoma. Am J Surg 1986;151:457–459.
122. Seife B. Osseous metastases from carcinoma of the large bowel. Cancer 1973;119: 414–418.
123. Napoli LD, Hansen HH, Muggia FM, et al. The incidence of osseous involvement in lung cancer, with special reference to the development of osteoblastic changes. Radiology 1973;108:17–21.
124. McCormack KR. Bone metastases from thyroid carcinoma. Cancer 1966;19:181–184.
125. Niederle B, Roka R, Schemper M, et al. Surgical treatment of distant metastases in differentiated thyroid cancer: Indications and results. Surgery 1986;100:1088–1097.
126. Wilner D, Breckenridge RL. Bone metastasis in malignant melanoma. 1949;62:388–394.
127. Stewart WR, Gelerman RH, Harrelson JM, et al. Skeletal metastases of melanoma. J Bone Joint Surg [Am] 1978;60:645–649.
128. Beals RK, Lawton GD, Snell WE. Prophylactic internal fixation of the femur in metastatic breast cancer. Cancer 1971;28:1350–1354.
129. Keene JS, Sellinger DS, McBeath AA, Engber WD. Metastatic breast cancer in the femur. A search for the lesion at risk of fracture. Clin Orthop 1986;203:282–288.
130. Mirels H. Metastatic disease in long bones, a proposed scoring system. Clin Orthop 1989;249:256–265.
131. Rinkes IHB, Wiggers T, Bouma WH, Van Geel AN, Boxma H. Treatment of manifest and impending pathological fractures of the femoral neck by cemented hemiarthroplasty. Clin Orthop 1990;260:220–223.
132. Healy JH, Lane JM. Treatment of pathological fractures of the distal femur with the supracondylar nail. Clin Orthop 1990;250:216–220.
133. Aboulafia AJ, Faulks W, Li W, Buch R, Matthews J, Malawer MM. Reconstruction using the Saddle prosthesis following excision of malignant periacetabular tumors. In: Brown KLB, ed. Complications of limb salvage: Prevention, management and outcome. Montreal: International Society of Limb-Sparing Surgery, 1991.
134. Siegal T. Vertebral body resection of epidural compression by malignant tumors. Results of forty-seven consecutive operative procedures. J Bone Joint Surg [Am] 1985;67: 375–382.
135. Harrison KM, Muss HB, Ball MR, et al. Spinal cord compression in breast cancer. Cancer 1985;55:2839–2844.
136. Rosenthal HG, Healy JH, Peterson M, et al. Outcome analysis of corpectomy without posterior instrumentation. In: Brown KLB, ed. Complications of limb salvage: Prevention, management and outcome. Montreal: International Society of Limb-Sparing Surgery, 1991.
137. Cochran JM, Keppler L, Biscup RS, Brantigan JW, Enker P, Steffee AD. Total posterior vertebrectomy with vertebral body replacement. In: Brown KLB, ed. Complications of limb salvage: Prevention, management and outcome. Montreal: International Society of Limb-Sparing Surgery, 1991.
138. Leeson MC, Makley JT, Carter JR. Metastatic disease distal to the elbow and knee. Clin Orthop 1986;206:94–99.
139. Kinsella TJ, Miser JS, Waller B. Extremity preservation by combined modality therapy in sarcomas of the hand and foot: An analysis of local control, disease free survival and functional results. Int J Radiat Oncol Biol Phys 1983;9:1115–1119.

SECTION **5**

HARVEY I. PASS

Treatment of Malignant Pleural and Pericardial Effusions

The occurrence of a new pleural or pericardial effusion in a cancer patient merits complete investigation by the oncologist. The degree of symptoms attending such effusions is variable, and the cause may not be due to malignancy. Appropriate therapy, however, must be dictated by objective documentation of a cause, especially when treatment may involve operative intervention or innovative therapy.

PLEURAL EFFUSIONS

PATHOPHYSIOLOGY

Five to 10 L of fluid move through the pleural space in 24 hours, of which 35% to 75% is turned over each hour, leaving 5 to 20 ml of fluid with a protein content of less than 2 g/dl.[1] Eighty percent to 90% of the fluid is reabsorbed, and abnormal fluid collections result from increased capillary permeability, increased hydrostatic pressure (congestive heart failure), increased negative intrapleural pressure (atelectasis), decreased oncotic pressure (hypoalbuminemia), or increased pleural fluid oncotic pressure (pleural tumor growth).[2] Processes that impair pleural lymphatic drainage also lead to effusion. There is a strong relation between carcinomatous infiltration of mediastinal lymph nodes and pleural effusion; however, the extent of direct pleural involvement by metastases bears no relation to the development of pleural effusion.[3] Therefore, the key elements in *malignant* pleural effusions include increased capillary permeability through inflammation or disruption of the capillary endothelium or impaired lymphatic drainage secondary to obstruction by tumor.[2] Although cancer patients may have transudative effusions on the basis of hypoalbuminemia, heart failure, or liver disease, malignant effusions are classically described as exudative with a protein content of >3 g/dl, specific gravity >1.015, pleural protein/serum protein ratio >0.5, and pleural lactate dehydrogenase (LDH)/serum LDH ratio >0.6. As protein concentration in the pleura increases, pleural osmotic pressure increases, which impedes efflux of pleural fluid. Pleural tumor involvement leads to mesothelial shedding and subsequently pleural thickening. Capillary engorgement and lymphocyte infiltration of the pleura commonly lead to a lymphocyte-abundant, bloody pleural effusion from tumor directly invading the blood vessels, from occlusion of venules, or from capillary dilation by vasoactive substances. A bloody effusion is the single strongest positive predictive element of malignancy.[4,5]

SYMPTOMS AND SIGNS

Twenty-three percent of patients are asymptomatic at the time of presentation, and 50% to 90% of patients with primary or metastatic pleural malignancy will have pleural effusion as their initial presenting manifestation.[6] Most (90%) will have effusions of more than 500 ml, and approximately 33% will have bilateral effusions at the time of presentation.

Dyspnea, cough, and *chest pain* are the common presenting complaints. The degree of symptom severity is related to the rapidity with which the fluid develops rather than the amount of fluid present.[7] Dyspnea is related to pulmonary compression. Pleuritic chest wall pain occurs with parietal pleural inflammation, whereas dull continuous pain is usually associated with parietal pleural metastases.[1] Diaphragmatic pleural irritation may be referred to the ipsilateral shoulder. Cough is usually dry and nonproductive and is due to compression of bronchial walls by fluid.[7]

Objective findings include tachypnea, labored breathing, and restricted chest wall expansion. Dullness to percussion, decreased fremitus, increased intercostal fullness, and undetectable diaphragmatic excursion may be present. Massive effusions may cause contralateral tracheal deviation.

DIAGNOSTIC TECHNIQUES

Radiography

Blunting of the costophrenic angle seen in the upright posteroanterior (PA) x-ray film will be observed with as little as 175 to 525 ml of fluid, and a lateral decubitus film will detect as little as 100 ml.[8–11] Fluid can be loculated within pulmonary fissures (pseudotumors) or between the lung and the diaphragm (Fig. 61–51).

An opacified hemithorax with mediastinal shift usually indicates massive effusion (>1500 ml). Opacification without shift should alert one to the possibility of mainstem bronchial obstruction, mediastinal fixation with malignant lymph nodes, or malignant mesothelioma.[3]

Small pleural effusions can be detected on computed tomography (CT), and CT can sometimes delineate an underlying pleural malignancy. The use of CT attenuation numbers (Hounsfield units) for the differentiation of pleural fluid from pleural tumors is controversial.[12] The usual place for CT in

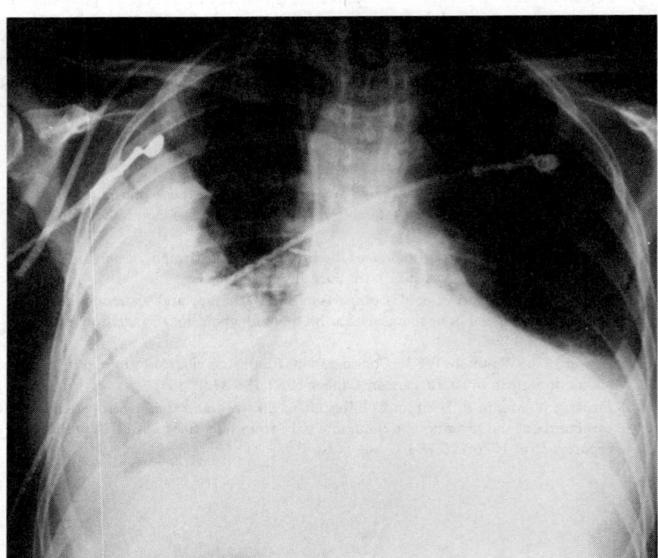

FIGURE 61–51. Patient with right-side pseudotumor, pleural effusion, and large pericardial effusion from breast cancer.

the management of malignant pleural effusions is *after* pleural drainage, which then allows the radiologist to evaluate subtle changes in pleural structure, new parenchymal infiltrates or masses, or enlargement of mediastinal lymph nodes. This is especially useful if previous chest tomograms are available from before the development of the effusion. Ultrasound techniques with the use of both A- and B-mode scans have been widely used to detect and sample pleural effusions.[13] Ultrasonography can identify pleural fluid and can differentiate between pleural thickening and pleural fluid.[5] The use of ultrasonic guidance to determine the proper site for thoracentesis and establish the depth of the fluid decreases the risk of complications, especially in small effusions demonstrated by radiographic techniques.[5,14]

Cytology

Demonstration of malignant cells in pleural fluid is the sine qua non of a malignant pleural effusion. Samples prepared for examination of pleural fluid include wet mounts stained with toluidine blue; smears fixed in 95% alcohol or air dried; membrane-filtered, cytocentrifuge preparations; and cell blocks for paraffin embedding and sectioning. Staining is by the modified Papanicolaou method, cytocentrifuge specimens by Wright-Giemsa, and paraffin sections by hematoxylin-eosin.

The rate of positivity for pleural cytologic specimens varies among large series. Sears,[15] Lopes-Cardozo,[16] and Johnston[17] have reported positive pleural cytologic appearances in 44%, 29% and 9%, respectively, of all pleural specimens submitted. The results of the cytologic examination vary according to the site of the effusion, the type and site of the primary neoplasm, and the method of processing the specimen.[15,16,18–20] Cytologic specimens from patients *known to have neoplasms* have given positive results in 42% to 96% of patients, whereas the false-positive rates have ranged from 0% to 3%.[16,18,19,21,22]

Recognition of cancer cells by cytopathologic techniques has become highly accurate when performed by an experienced clinical morphologist. Difficulties arise when trying to differentiate cancer cells from reactive mesothelial cells or when trying to classify the organ of origin. The use of immunocytochemical techniques as an adjunct to the diagnosis of malignant pleural effusions has, until recently, been limited by the availability, sensitivity, and specificity of the assays using polyclonal sera or monoclonal antibodies. Immunochemical techniques are now routinely performed in the diagnosis of malignancy. Anti-carcinoembryonic antigen (anti-CEA) heteroantisera has demonstrated reactivity with approximately 50% of cancer cells, whereas no reactivity is noted with mesothelial cells or benign effusions.[23] Polyclonal antisera to epithelial membrane antigen has demonstrated reactivity with 54% of carcinomatous effusions and no reactivity with benign effusions.[24–26] B72.3, an IgG1 monoclonal antibody, has recently been shown to recognize 100% of adenocarcinomas in patients with effusions from cancers of breast, ovary, and lung, and when additional metastatic adenocarcinomas from other sites are considered, overall recognition is 95%, including poorly differentiated squamous cell lung cancer.[27,28] Cytochemical staining with acid phosphatase, α-naphthylacetate esterase, and periodic acid-Schiff, as well as sheep erythrocyte rosetting, is useful in recognizing malignant lymphocytes.[29]

Cytogenetic analysis of pleural effusions combining cytologic and chromosome analyses of pleural effusions has correctly diagnosed 83% to 91% of malignant effusions, a result that was better than that with either technique alone[30]; however, the false-positive rate is higher in chromosome analysis than in ordinary cytology.[5] Other studies[31,32] have yielded nearly a 90% positive diagnosis of malignancy, with a 3% false-negative rate. Pleural cytogenetics, however, is limited by expense and time consumption.

Biochemical Analysis

The CEA levels in pleural fluid may be useful in detecting malignancy,[5] with a pleural fluid level of >20 ng/ml having a 91% sensitivity and 92% specificity in effusions caused by adenocarcinoma. In patients with metastatic bronchogenic adenocarcinoma in the pleura, the CEA level is higher than 10 ng/ml in 90% of the patients. Reported sensitivities in malignant effusion range from 25% to 57%, with cutoff values between 10 and 20 ng/ml.[33–35] The CEA level assays are expensive, are time-consuming, and lack sensitivity and specificity for malignancy in general. Hyaluronic acid levels have been noted to be elevated in patients with mesothelioma[15]; however, this assay lacks sensitivity and will not provide a definitive diagnosis.[36]

Thoracentesis

Thoracentesis of suspected malignant pleural effusions can be both diagnostic and therapeutic, although the symptomatic relief of fluid removal is usually short-lived without other adjuvant measures. Bleeding, pneumothorax with peripheral bronchopleural fistula, and "pleural shock," an exaggerated vagal response as the needle passes through the parietal pleura, causing bradycardia, are possible complications. The latter is easily reversed with intravenous fluids, atropine, and Trendelenberg positioning. Oxygen therapy and narcotics may be necessary because of the pain of reexpansion. Thoracentesis of volumes larger than 1500 ml may cause reexpansion pulmonary edema.[37–39]

The fluid withdrawn is sent for cytologic and bacteriologic determinations, and for levels of protein, LDH, glucose, specific gravity, and cell count to determine the transudative or exudative nature of the fluid.

Pleural Biopsy

Closed pleural biopsy is a relatively easy technique that can be coordinated with CT guidance to try to decrease sampling error. The pleural biopsy should be done before fluid aspiration to avoid pulmonary injury. Cytologic examination of pleural fluid alone has a higher sensitivity than needle biopsy,[40,41] and the yield of diagnosis of pleural neoplasm by needle biopsy alone ranges from 40% to 69%.[42–46] When pleural biopsy is combined with cytology, however, the diagnostic yield is increased from 81% to 90%.[47,48]

The morbidity of pleural biopsy is 0.6%,[49] with the most commonly reported complications being pneumothorax, pleural shock, hemothorax, subcutaneous emphysema, and inadequate biopsy. Cancer implantation, associated with the use of larger needles and hematoma formation, occurs in 4.1% of patients.[50]

Thoracoscopy

In undiagnosed suspected malignant pleural effusions with persistently negative cytologic results, thoracoscopy has been useful in establishing the diagnosis in 93% to 96% of the patients (Fig. 61–52).[51–53] Recently, video thoracoscopy, employing television monitoring of the procedure and transthoracic trocars to aid in lung manipulation, has been used to enhance the efficacy of malignant effusion treatment. With the use of lateral decubitus positioning and double-lumen endotracheal intubation with ipsilateral lung collapse, the videoscope, retractors, and instruments are introduced through separate 10-mm incisions. Greater documentation of disease extent, and the ability to perform pleurectomy for increased sclerosis efficacy, may make this rapidly developing technique invaluable in the future. Synchronous sclerosis of malignant pleural effusions at the time of thoracoscopy has been reported with good success.[54,55]

Thoracotomy

The need for open thoracotomy in the management of malignant pleural effusion is reserved for the rare case of nondiagnostic studies and continued suspicion of malignant disease. Even after thoracotomy, a significant number of patients will be found not to have malignant disease.[2,5]

PROGNOSIS AND TREATMENT

The prognosis of patients who develop malignant pleural effusions varies with the histologic type of the primary tumor. When one considers all effusions regardless of the histologic type, 65% of the patients will be dead within 3 months and 80% within 6 months. Patients with breast cancer will have a mean survival of 7 to 15 months posteffusion[15,56] and a 3-year survival of 20%.[57] Mean survival time in patients with lung cancer has been reported to be as low as 2 months from the time of diagnosis of malignant pleural effusion,[56] and 66% of the patients will be dead by 3 months. Thirty-three percent of patients with ovarian cancer will die within a mean time of 10 months after the diagnosis of malignant effusion, and the mean survival time is 3 months.[15]

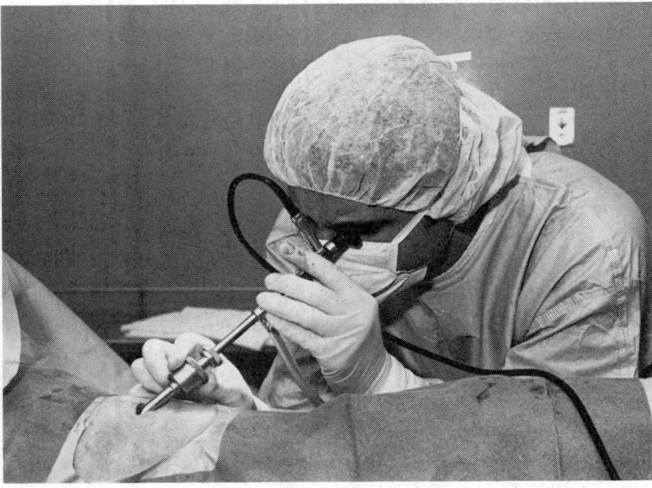

FIGURE 61–52. Thoracoscopy with the rigid thoracoscope permits visualization of pleural abnormalities and direct biopsy.

Treatment should palliate symptoms in the most reliable, least complicated, and, hopefully, most durable manner. In selected instances, local treatment can be combined with systemic regimens (*i.e.*, testicular carcinoma, lymphoma, breast cancer), depending on the efficacy of the systemic agents for a given malignant histologic type. In most cases of solid tumors with malignant effusions, only local therapy is considered, to control reaccumulation of pleural fluid and diminish or eliminate the need for repeated thoracenteses required by repeated bouts of respiratory compromise.

From the literature, it is difficult to objectively evaluate composites of large series for the success of treatment of malignant pleural effusions because of the differing criteria used to denote responsitivity. Moreover, time endpoints for evaluation differ among studies. The most useful criterion has been a failure of the effusion to recur at 4 to 6 weeks, because patients treated by simple thoracentesis and followed for 1 month have a 97% recurrence rate. Some of the newer strategies (*e.g.*, the use of bacillus Calmette-Guérin [BCG] vaccine and *Corynebacterium parvum*), which do not employ tube thoracostomy, define a complete response as no reaccumulation after one thoracentesis employing intrapleural treatment.

METHODS OF TREATMENT

Sclerotherapy

The management of malignant pleural effusions involves the proper technique of sclerotherapy after space obliteration by placement of a large-bore thoracostomy tube. Initial removal of the effusion allows the visceral pleura to come into contact with the chest wall parietal pleura and thereby obliterates, by continuous, underwater-seal suction drainage, the space occupied by the effusion. A sclerosing agent (*i.e.*, antibiotic, antineoplastic, or radioactive) can then be delivered intrapleurally to produce mesothelial fibrosis and obliterate small pleural blood vessels, rather than produce specific antineoplastic activity.[58] Table 61–32 represents a survey of the available literature on the efficacy of intrapleural sclerotherapy. Some groups have attempted to relate the outcome of sclerosis (specifically with talc) to alterations in pleural fluid chemistry.[50] Glucose levels less than 60 mg/dl in the pleural fluid seem to correlate with the extent of pleural disease, and the cytology yield will be positive for malignancy in 87% of such neoplastic pleural effusions. Moreover, patients with a low glucose level or a low pH (*i.e.*, less than 7.3) had significantly worse results with regard to achieving pleural symphysis with successful effusion management, with a 50% failure rate. These findings, although interesting, require verification in larger numbers of patients.

TECHNIQUE OF PLEURAL SCLEROTHERAPY. The intrapleural instillation of agents in patients with neoplastic pleural disease has been fairly standardized. The first order of business is a careful examination of the available roent-

TABLE 61–32. Management of Malignant Pleural Effusions*

Treatment	*Histologic Type*					
	Lung	*Breast*	*Lymphoma*	*Ovary*	*Other*	*Overall (%)*
Chest tube alone	1/6	18/38	—	—	1/10	20/54 (37)
Tetracycline	17/28	24/44	0/1	0/1	20/40	61/114 (54)
Quinacrine	30/37	39/49	7/9	5/8	19/26	100/129 (78)
Bleomycin	7/11	33/38	4/6	5/6	32/55	81/116 (70)
Nitrogen mustard	35/53	109/225	7/19	8/11	24/50	183/358 (51)
5-FU						23/35 (66)
Thiotepa	0/1	11/21		2/2	0/2	14/26 (54)
Talc	54/59	71/75	4/4	8/9	71/90	208/237 (88)
Irradiation	8/10	2/3	9/10	—	11/15	30/38 (79)
Isotopes	102/190	234/413	22/44	32/54	85/177	475/878 (54)
BCG						5/9 (56)
Corynebacterium parvum						57/70 (81)

BCG, bacillus Calmette-Guérin vaccine.
* Number successful/number reported.

genographic studies, including lateral decubitus films, upright PA films, lateral chest films, and chest CT scans (if available). One must first determine whether or not this is a free-flowing pleural effusion without loculations, which may have developed because of initial multiple thoracenteses. The development of loculations in such a situation makes it difficult for a single chest tube placement to obtain adequate evacuation of the fluid. Fortunately, however, most patients have free-flowing pleural effusions without loculations.

Placement of the chest tube should be done by an experienced physician to minimize the patient's discomfort. The chest tube can usually be placed laterally in the sixth or seventh interspace, in a position lying in the anterior axillary line, such that the patient will not be lying on the chest tube when he is supine. Premedication with 75 to 100 mg of meperidine (Demerol) or 6 to 8 mg of morphine, subcutaneously, will relax the patient and decrease discomfort. The appropriate chest is sterilely prepared with an iodine-based cleansing solution, and sterile towels are placed. The skin is infiltrated locally with 1% lidocaine (Xylocaine) at the appropriate site for chest tube placement. Usually 10 to 30 ml of 1% lidocaine, placed intradermally and subdermally and down to the chest wall, will provide a satisfactory local block. Once the skin and chest wall are anesthetized, a quick thoracentesis is performed to document good flow of effusion in this designated area. If free flow of fluid is not obtained, another site that will guarantee good flow of fluid should be chosen for chest tube placement. A short 1- to 3-cm incision is then made in the skin and carried down to the subcutaneous tissues. A curved scissors is then used to create a tunnel through the chest wall musculature, directly down to the interspace of choice. The more care that is taken with the development of this subcutaneous tunnel down to the intercostal muscles over the appropriate rib, the less discomfort the patient will have when the chest tube is placed. Some physicians prefer the use of a trocar chest tube; however, the use of a surgical clamp to open into the pleural space under controlled conditions will allow the finger to be placed into the chest to assure that there are no adhesions that could be violated by chest tube placement. An appropriate-sized chest tube, either 28 or 32 French, is then placed through the subcutaneous tunnel into the pleural cavity and directed cephalad by having a clamp on the introducing end of the chest tube and a clamp at the end of the chest tube, closing it off to prevent open pneumothorax and a rush of fluid out of the chest tube. The chest tube is then connected to an underwater-seal drainage system, using any of a variety of systems. A stitch of heavy silk is used to anchor the chest tube to the skin, and sterile dressings are applied. A chest x-ray film is then obtained and viewed for proper tube placement. We repeat chest radiographs daily after chest tube placement and subsequent sclerosis therapy.

For the first 24 hours, the chest tube should be connected to underwater-seal drainage with negative suction (approximately 15–20 cm H_2O) applied to the device. This will ensure maximum expansion of the compressed, underlying lung and total evacuation of the fluid. Because the use of a chest tube alone is associated with a low success rate (see Table 61–32), we always approach the patient who has a chest tube placed for neoplastic pleural disease as a candidate for intrapleural therapy. If the chest x-ray film, taken 24 hours after the placement of the chest tube, shows total evacuation of fluid with good lung expansion, the sclerotherapy can be started. Sclerotherapy should not be performed if the patient has a large volume of residual fluid left in the chest. Doing this will doom the treatment to failure because of dilution of the sclerosing medium and the insufficient expansion of the underlying lung.

When the decision is made to give sclerotherapy, the patient is medicated 30 minutes before treatment with a narcotic agent. The sclerosing drug is then instilled directly through the chest tube with an irrigating catheter, followed by clamping of the chest tube and connection of the end of the chest tube back to the drainage system. Essentially, the sclerosing agent remains in the chest cavity because the chest tube is clamped, and the patient is instructed to change positions every 15 minutes for 4 hours (*i.e.*, lying flat, right-side-up, left-side-up, head-down, and head-up) to equally distribute this 100 ml throughout the pleural cavity. At the end of this 4 hours, the chest tube clamp is removed and the fluid is allowed to drain, with suction for another 24 hours.

Twenty-four hours after the sclerotherapy, the patient is disconnected from suction and the chest is allowed to drain by gravity. The patient is maintained connected to this underwater-seal system, with daily monitoring of the amount of effluent. When the drainage has decreased substantially (*e.g.*, to 50–100 ml/24 hours) and the lung remains reexpanded (as seen on x-ray films) with the chest tube in, the tube is removed and the site is closed with a stitch of 3-0 silk or with gauze. We prefer suture closure of the chest tube site to ensure the absence of continued drainage onto the skin or a sucking chest wound. Twenty-four hours after chest tube removal, the patient should have a chest radiograph that reveals no further accumulation of fluid and total lung expansion, at which point the patient can be considered for discharge. A follow-up radiographic examination should be performed 1 month later.

Specific Sclerosing Agents

TETRACYCLINE. Intrapleural tetracycline (TCN) has gained popularity because of its overall efficiency, convenience, low cost, and minimal morbidity. Prospective trials comparing TCN with quinacrine,[59] with a comparable pH placebo,[60] or with tube thoracostomy alone[61] show consistently better results with intrapleural TCN, with significantly less fever and pleuritic chest pain. Premedication of the patient with a narcotic, and the addition of lidocaine (150 mg) to the sclerosis medium,[62] may abate the pleurisy. Experimental models reveal that TCN increases pleural capillary permeability, allowing an accumulation of clotting factors in the pleural space and inactivation of the common fibrinolytic mechanism of pleural fluid. The fibrin matrix allows fibroblast attachment.[63] The effusion recurrence rate after TCN sclerosis is related to progression of the underlying malignancy, and the optimum dose of tetracycline for instillation is not clear.[64] In a 10-year retrospective review with only 59% of the patients classified as a treatment success, the authors commented that the dose of tetracycline was an important factor in predicting outcome, with a significantly higher complete response rate noted. No recurrence of effusion at 30 days was noted for the patients who were treated with more than 1 g of tetracycline.[65] Patients may be successfully retreated with TCN sclerosis.

The era of tetracycline sclerosis, however, may be completed, because the availability of intravenous tetracycline will be severely limited in the future. In the absence of randomized trials, it is difficult to recommend a viable alternative; nevertheless, the chief contenders for comparable sclerotherapy efficacy are sterilized (baked) talc, bleomycin, and doxycycline.

TALC. The administration of intrapleural talc, either at the time of thoracoscopy under general anesthesia or by aerosolization through a chest tube, has been a popular means of controlling malignant pleural effusions in Great Britain and Europe, despite the absence of randomized trials.[53,66–70] In selected studies, talc sclerotherapy has proved more effective than tetracycline in patients with pleural effusion from breast cancer.[71] An insufflation catheter is introduced through the thoracoscope. The talc should be free of asbestos and incubated in a dry-heat oven at 125°C for 12 hours and then cultured; it should show no bacterial or fungal contamination over a 7-day period before it is released for operative use. No more than 10.5 g of the talc is routinely used in adult patients. When performed under general anesthesia at the time of thoracotomy or thoracoscopy, talc administration is 85% to 100% effective if there is complete expansion of the underlying lung.[72]

ANTINEOPLASTIC AGENTS. Cytotoxic drugs most likely are effective by inducing inflammatory pleurodesis in the pleural space. Nitrogen mustard, thiotepa, bleomycin, doxorubicin, and 5-fluorouracil have been used for intrapleural management of malignant effusions, with the major side effects being bone marrow depression and leukopenia. Bleomycin seems to be the most successful. It has the fewest side effects at an instillation dose of 60 mg[73] and has minimal myelosuppressive problems and minimal fever and pain. An older randomized study comparing bleomycin with TCN revealed equal response rates.[74] Fortunately, with the limited availability of TCN in the future, a recent trial compared 85 patients with documented malignant pleural effusion who were randomized to treatment with either intrapleural bleomycin (60 U; 44 patients) or intrapleural tetracycline (1 g; 41 patients) after the pleural cavity was drained of accumulated fluid.[75] Sixty-seven percent of the tetracycline patients had recurrent effusion within 30 days, compared with 36% who received bleomycin. Unfortunately, not all patients were restudied in the first 30 days. At 90 days, 19/36 tetracycline patients had recurrent effusion compared with 11/37 bleomycin patients ($p = 0.047$). These data imply, at least, that bleomycin will be a viable alternative to tetracycline for sclerotherapy on a consistent basis in the future, despite the cost considerations that at one time made this agent a less desirable therapy than TCN.

A more aggressive approach with combination intrapleural agents, including cisplatin and cytarabine, has been used by some groups (overall response rate at 3 weeks = 49%).[76]

BIOLOGIC AGENTS. Intrapleural instillation of *C. parvum*, 5 to 10 mg, streptococcal preparation OK432, and BCG cell wall skeleton have demonstrated promising results in the management of malignant effusion. Recently, however, a randomized trial of *C. parvum* versus bleomycin revealed a higher but not statistically significant percentage of responses in the bleomycin group (74% versus 43%).[77] The *C. parvum* effect is not associated with evidence of enhancement of local cell-mediated immunity.[78]

The most recent developments in the use of biologic therapies for pleural effusions involve the use of the interferons or interleukins for intracavitary treatment. Five to 20 million units of interferon-β for a maximum administration of three doses was delivered by way of an intracavitary route in 32 patients with recurrent pleural effusions. Eleven (28%) showed complete remission and three (10%) showed partial remission.[79] Small effusion size (<1000 ml) correlated with treatment efficacy. Intrapleural infusion of interferon-γ twice a week over 2 months in stage I patients with diffuse pleural mesotheliomas yielded four thoracoscopic histopathologic responses and one partial response (56%).[80] Patients with higher-stage disease had minimal responses.

Recent reports from China demonstrate disappearance of effusion in 9 of 15 patients with malignant pleurisy, with significant decreases in the other 6 patients with the use of lymphokine-activated killer cells combined with recombinant interleukin-2 (rIL-2) or rIL-2 alone.[81] No serious side effects were found except for transient fever in 7 patients. In a series of 11 patients with malignant pleurisy due to lung cancer, pleural effusions and cancer cells disappeared after intrapleural instillations of recombinant IL-2.[82] Such studies require verification in larger numbers of patients.

External Radiation

Only lymphomatous pleural effusions seem to respond favorably to external-beam irradiation. Close to 90%[1,83] of malignant lymphoma effusions were controlled in a small series of patients with the use of mediastinal and hemithorax irradiation (1.4–2.3 Gy). Systemic chemotherapy is also used.[84]

Surgical Interventions

PLEURECTOMY. Stripping of the parietal pleura from the rib cage and mediastinum, essentially removing 90% of the pleura, is infrequently used because of the modern-day success of sclerotherapy. Its limited reported applications[85–87] include highly selected patients who have failed all other approaches, usually because of the presence of trapped or nonexpansile lung. A 23% complication rate and a 9% mortality are reported. Control of effusion is reported to be 87% to 100%.

PLEUROPERITONEAL SHUNTING. Internal drainage of malignant pleural effusions to the abdomen was first described in 1984. The valved, pumping chamber of a Denver shunt (Denver Biomaterials, Evergreen, CO) was placed subcutaneously with a proximal limb in the pleural effusion and a distal limb in the abdomen (Fig. 61–53). The pleuroperitoneal shunt can be used in instances for which sclerotherapy has failed, particularly when the failure is due to inability of the lung to expand. The procedure can be performed under local anesthesia, and complications are minimal. Patients must be sufficiently strong to pump the device, or the family must be taught to do this.

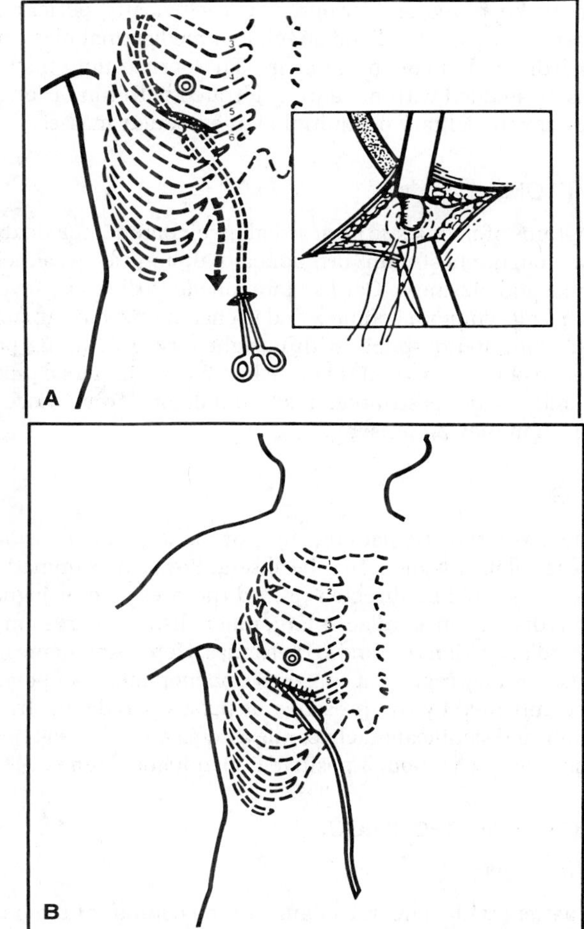

FIGURE 61–53. **(A)** Placement of pleuroperitoneal shunt for drainage of intractable pleural effusions from chest to abdominal cavity. (**Insert**) A small pursestring suture seals the entry site into the peritoneum. **(B)** View of the completed procedure. (Reprinted with permission of Denver Biomaterials, Evergreen, CO)

PERICARDIAL EFFUSIONS

INCIDENCE

Malignant involvement of the heart or pericardium is not uncommon in patients with advanced cancer, and its prevalence has been described in a number of autopsy studies. The prevalence of combined metastasis to the pericardium and heart has ranged from 0.1% to 21%.[88–91] In a series of 3327 autopsies, tumor lesions of the heart were detected in 5.1% of the cases.[92] When such data are available from autopsy series,[89,92–94] the pericardium is solely involved in 45% of the cases, the myocardium alone in 32%, and the myocardium and pericardium in 22%.

The most common malignancies involving the heart or pericardium include lung, breast, leukemia, Hodgkin's and non-Hodgkin's lymphoma, melanoma, gastrointestinal primaries, and sarcomas. Lung and breast predominate all autopsy series as the most likely neoplasms to cause myopericardial metastases, and it is estimated that 35% of patients with lung cancer will be found to have pericardial metastases at autopsy,[95] whereas as many as 25% of patients with breast cancer will have pericardial involvement at autopsy.[96–98]

PATHOPHYSIOLOGY

In the pericardial sac there is usually no more than 50 ml of pericardial fluid, which serves as a lubricant. The increase in pericardial fluid seen in malignant pericardial effusions is due to obstruction of lymphatic and venous drainage of the heart, and this disturbs the level of intrapericardial pressure, depending on the rate of fluid accumulation, pericardial compliance, ventricular mass, and intravascular volume. Mediastinal nodal involvement, frequently seen with lung and breast cancer, disturbs lymphatic drainage through the cardiac nodes from the heart and pericardium.[99] Pathologically, pericardial metastases may extend and attach to a mediastinal mass and pericardium alone or to the heart. The pericardium may be diffusely studded with nodules, infiltrated with tumor, or associated with solitary or multiple large nodular masses.[92]

SYMPTOMS

Symptoms of neoplastic pericardial involvement include dyspnea, cough, chest pain, orthopnea, palpitations, weakness, fatigue, and dizziness. Cardiac tamponade is the most severe presenting symptom complex and is characterized by anxiety, chest pain, and dyspnea, with upright forward-leaning posturing to obtain maximal relief. Ashen faces with facial plethora and vague gastrointestinal complaints from visceral congestion may be present.[94]

SIGNS

In the asymptomatic patient, signs of malignant pericardial/myocardial involvement may be absent. Physical examination, however, should be directed toward the presence of jugular venous distension, cardiac enlargement, distant heart sounds, pericardial friction rub, and arrhythmias. Hepatosplenomegaly and ascites may represent congestive phenomena. Tamponade is accompanied by the presence of pulsus paradoxus, hypotension, and significant tachycardia associated with weak heart sounds with or without a positive hepatojugular reflex.

DIAGNOSTIC TECHNIQUES

Radiography

In a patient with cancer, a change in the contour of the heart shadow on an upright AP x-ray film of the chest, in association with the aforementioned symptoms, should alert the clinician to the possibility of neoplastic pericarditis. A normal chest roentgenogram, however, does not exclude the possibility of effusion.[100] Classically, there is an enlargement of the cardiopericardial silhouette, described as a water-bottle heart, with bulging and loss of the normal contours of the pericardial reflection. The regular use of CT in diagnosing and staging lymphoma demonstrates pericardial involvement earlier and with greater accuracy than conventional radiography.[101] Effusions that are difficult to detect, such as those distorted by pneumonectomy for lung cancer, are more readily detected by CT.[102] Malignant pericardial disease is suspected by CT criteria, including: (1) pericardial effusion with high CT density, (2) localized or diffuse pericardial thickening, (3) masses from or contiguous with the pericardium, and (4) obliteration of normal tissue planes between a paracardiac mass and the heart or pericardium.[103,104]

Echocardiography (ECHO) represents the least invasive, least time-consuming, and most precise method for rapid demonstration and quantitation of malignant pleural effusion. Precise bedside confirmation of placement of pericardial catheters can also be accomplished with ECHO.

ELECTROCARDIOGRAPHIC ABNORMALITIES

The electrocardiogram (ECG) changes seen with neoplastic pericarditis include tachycardia, premature contractions, low QRS voltage, and nonspecific ST-segment and T-wave changes.[1] The alternans pattern will disappear with appropriate therapy for the effusion.[94]

Pericardiocentesis

TECHNIQUE AND USE IN DIAGNOSIS. The use of percutaneous pericardiocentesis guided by two-dimensional echocardiography is associated with a high diagnostic yield, a low frequency of complications, and rapid amelioration of symptoms of tamponade in patients with malignant pericardial effusions.[105] The risk of pericardiocentesis is dependent on the amount and location of the fluid. Patients with loculated effusion in a posterior position usually cannot be drained by the routine approaches. The use of fluoroscopy or ECHO guidance decreases, to a minimum, the previously reported risk of cardiac chamber puncture, ventricular tachycardia, and tension pneumothorax.[106,107]

USE OF PERICARDIOCENTESIS FOR CYTOLOGIC DIAGNOSIS. Hemorrhagic fluid is usually associated with positive pericardial cytologic results, especially in lung cancer, and cytologic examination will demonstrate malignant cells in 80% to 90% of the patients with neoplastic pericarditis. There is, however, a significant percentage of false-negative cytologic results observed, and a negative report does not eliminate cancer from the differential diagnosis.[108,109] There is a definite frequency of late effusive constructive pericarditis that is seen in patients with lymphoma who have received mediastinal irradiation. A frequency of radiation-related pericardial effusion of 31% has been reported after upper-mantle radiation therapy for Hodgkin's disease.[110] These patients will usually present with negative cytologic evaluations yet will require management of the effusion and the possible constrictive symptoms.

TREATMENT

The ultimate outcome for patients with malignant pericardial disease will depend on the performance status of the patients, the presence of metastatic disease, the availability of adjuvant systemic therapy, and the local management of the pericardial effusion for the long-term abolition of tamponade-like symptoms. Despite the prevalence of this manifestation of malignant disease, there are no prospective randomized trials comparing methods of local therapy to evaluate long-term effectiveness or survival.

Catheter Drainage Alone

The use of pericardial drainage alone has met with equivocal success in a small number of patients, as reported in the literature. Of 6 patients having a single pericardiocentesis or 24 to 48 hours of pericardial drainage, 4 had effusion control for 1 month or longer.[111] Of 16 patients with malignant effusions in another study,[106] only 2 required subsequent pericardiectomy for recurrence. Nine of the 16, however, had other nonsurgical therapy. In a more recent study of patients with histologically confirmed neoplastic (breast) pericarditis, all 3 patients treated by pericardiocentesis alone relapsed, at 11, 40, and 1462 days, respectively, after the tap. One of these patients died, in relapse or tamponade, and the other two required surgery.

Instillational Local Therapy

Nitrogen mustard, thiotepa, and quinacrine were all used for intrapericardial instillation in the 1970s, but they were associated with severe pain and bone marrow toxicity. Treatment with TCN instillation usually requires multiple instillations for it to be effective. Of the 28 patients described, each treated with a mean TCN instillation of 500 mg/instillation, a success rate of longer than 1 month was seen in 75%, with a mean of 120 days without recurrence.[111,112] Complications included mild fever, arrhythmias, and pain. Bleomycin (4 patients),[113] cisplatin (1 patient),[114] and vinblastine (1 patient)[115] have also been used for local instillation. These studies further verify that the pericardial catheter can be successfully left in place longer than 72 hours without infection and that catheter occlusion is more prevalent with continuous drainage as opposed to intermittent flushing.[106]

Radiation Therapy

Although formerly used for pericardial effusions related to various histologic types of carcinoma, pericardial radiation is most suited for the management of pericardial effusions from lymphoma.[116] Recommended dosages are 2.0 to 3.0 Gy, fractionated over a 2- to 3-week period.

Surgery

Most of the patients will be able to have emergent placement of a pericardial catheter to relieve tamponade symptoms and be more favorable surgical-anesthetic candidates. It is generally agreed that surgical intervention should be considered in those medically fit patients whose effusive pericarditis is unresponsive to radiation therapy or to intrapericardial therapy, or who have required repeated pericardiocentesis. Finally, patients with constrictive pericarditis caused by radiation or neoplastic pericardial constriction, documented hemodynamically by catheterization, and who would be expected to have a reasonable long-term survival, should have pericardial resection.

The subxiphoid approach has received many enthusiastic commendations in the literature, from a number of institutions, as being the procedure of choice in the management of malignant effusions. The use of local anesthesia; direct exposure of the pericardium; complete drainage of the pericardial space by chest tubes, allowing pericardial and epicardial symphysis; and the avoidance of a thoracotomy have all been expounded as the advantages of this technique. When one examines the reports in the literature and defines the subset of patients with malignant effusions who had subxiphoid drainage (Table 61–33), it is difficult to label this procedure as the "cure all to end all" for neoplastic pericarditis. Ideally, the minimum mortality in cancer patients is 8%, and the ideal described recurrence rate is 7%. This procedure is probably superior to simple window formation by a left thoracotomy, relative to mortality and recurrence. Moreover, the type of pericardiectomy does not seem to have any influence on the postoperative survival in patients with malignant disease. Survival in patients with malignant disease is affected by the tumor cell type, with lung cancer having a mean survival of 3.5 months; breast cancer, after surgical intervention, having a survival of 9.3 to 18.5 months; and lymphoma having a survival of approximately 10 months. The amount of pericardium remaining after surgical drainage, however, does impinge directly on the development of late postoperative complications (*e.g.*, recurrence of effusion). Patients who have a complete pericardiectomy have significantly fewer late failures than those who have a window pericardiectomy. Therefore, in patients who have other salvage therapies, either radiation or chemotherapy, or those expected to have a longer survival (*e.g.*, lymphoma or breast cancer), the widest pericardial resection should be considered to prevent future recurrence. Moreover, radiation-induced effusions should not be managed by a subxiphoid window because of a high late-failure rate.

TABLE 61–33. Subxiphoid Approach for Malignant Pericardial Effusion

Investigations	*No. of Patients*	*Mortality*	*Recurrence*
Ghosh, 1985[117]	20	0	1
Hankins, 1980[118]	13	0	0
Raza, 1980[118]	49	0	3
Williams, 1980[118]	26	0	3
Osuch, 1985[119]	12	1	0
Berman, 1984[120]	3	0	0
Little, 1984[121]	19	6	0
Piehler, 1985[122]	10	1	3
Miller, 1985[122]	3	2	—
Prager, 1982[123]	6	3	—
Total	161	13 (8%)	10 (7%)

REFERENCES

1. McKenna RJ, Ali MK, Ewer MS, et al. Pleural and pericardial effusions in cancer patients. Curr Probl Cancer 1985;9:1.
2. Hausheer FH, Yarbro JW. Diagnosis and treatment of malignant pleural effusion. Semin Oncol 1985;12:54.
3. Sahn SA. Malignant pleural effusions. Clin Chest Med 1985;6:113.
4. Martensson G, Pettersson K, Thiringer G. Differentiation between malignant and non-malignant pleural effusion. Eur J Respir Dis 1985;67:326.
5. Dhillon DP, Spiro SG. Malignant pleural effusions. Br J Hosp Med 1983;29:506.
6. Chernow B, Sahn SA. Carcinomatous involvement of the pleura: An analysis of 96 patients. Am J Med 1977;63:695.
7. Zehner LC, Hoogstraten B. Malignant effusions and their management. Semin Oncol Nurs 1985;1:259.
8. Austin EH, Flye MW. The treatment of recurrent malignant pleural effusion. Ann Thorac Surg 1979;28:190.
9. Kaunitz J. Landmarks in simple pleural effusions. JAMA 1939;113:1312.
10. Peterson JA. Recognition of infrapulmonary pleural effusion. Radiology 1960;74:34.
11. Woodring JH. Recognition of pleural effusion on supine radiographs: How much fluid is required? AJR 1984;142:59.
12. Salonen O, Kivisaari L, Nordenstam G, et al. Computed tomography of pleural lesions with special reference to the mediastinal pleura. Acta Radiol Diagn 1986;27:527.
13. Doust BD, Baum JK, Maklad NF, et al. Ultrasonic evaluation of pleural opacities. Radiology 1975;114:135.
14. Ravin CE. Thoracentesis of loculated pleural effusions using grey scale ultrasonic guidance. Chest 1977;71:666.
15. Sears D, Hajdu SI. The cytologic diagnosis of malignant neoplasm in pleural and peritoneal effusions. Acta Cytol 1987;31:85.
16. Lopes-Cardozo PL. A critical evaluation of 3000 cytologic analyses of pleural fluid, ascitic fluid, and peritoneal fluid. Acta Cytol 1966;10:455.
17. Johnston WW. The malignant pleural effusion: A review of cytopathologic diagnosis of 584 specimens from 472 consecutive patients. Cancer 1985;56:905.
18. Jarvi OH, Kunnas RJ, Laitio MT, et al. The accuracy and significance of cytologic cancer diagnoses in pleural effusions. Acta Cytol 1972;16:152.
19. Johnson WD. The cytologic diagnosis of cancer in serous effusions. Acta Cytol 1966;10:161.
20. Melamed MR. The cytologic preparation of malignant lymphomas and related disease in effusions. Cancer 1963;16:413.

21. Ceelen GH. The cytologic diagnosis of ascitic fluid. Acta Cytol 1964;8:175.
22. Spriggs AL. Br Med J [Letter] 1981;282:1972.
23. Schested M, Ralfkiaer E, Rasmussen J. Immunoperoxidase demonstration of carcinoembryonic antigen in pleural and peritoneal effusions. Acta Cytol 1983;27:124.
24. To A, Coleman V, Dearnaley DP, et al. Use of antisera to epithelial membrane antigen for the cytodiagnosis of malignancy in serous effusions. J Clin Pathol 1981;24:1326.
25. To A, Dearnaley DP, Ormerod G, et al. Epithelial membrane antigen: Its use in the cytodiagnosis of malignancy in serous effusions. Am J Clin Pathol 1982;77:214.
26. Walts AE, Said JW, Banks-Schlegel S. Keratin and carcinoembryonic antigen in exfoliated mesothelial and malignant cells: An immunoperoxidase study. Am J Clin Pathol 1983;80:671.
27. Johnston WW, Szpak CA, Lottich SC, et al. Use of a monoclonal antibody (B72.3) as an immunocytochemical adjunct to diagnosis of adenocarcinoma in human effusions. Cancer Res 1985;45:1894.
28. Martin SE, Moshiri S, Thor A, et al. Identification of adenocarcinoma in cytospin preparations of effusions using monoclonal antibody B72.3. Am J Clin Pathol 1986;86:10.
29. Das DK, Gupta SK, Ayzagari S, et al. Pleural effusions in non-Hodgkin's lymphoma: A cytomorphologic, cytochemical, and immunologic study. Acta Cytol 1987;31:119.
30. Musilova J, Michalova K. Cytogenetic study of cancer cells in effusions. Cancer Genet Cytogenet 1986;19:271.
31. Carlevaro C, Rossi GA, Cerri E, et al. Cytogenetic study of pleural effusions. Tumori 1978;64:335.
32. Fraisse J, Brizard CO, Emonot A, et al. Diagnosis of malignancy by cytogenetic means in effusions. Clin Genet 1978;14:288.
33. McKenna JM, Chandraesekhar AJ, Henkin RE. Diagnostic value of carcinoembryonic antigen in exudative pleural effusion. Chest 1980;78:587.
34. Rutgers RA, Loewenstein MS, Feinerman AE, et al. Carcinoembryonic antigen levels in benign and malignant pleural effusions. Ann Intern Med 1978;88:631.
35. Vladutin AO, Brason FW, Adler RH. Differential diagnosis of pleural effusions: Clinical usefulness of cell marker quantitation. Chest 1981;79:297.
36. Rasmussen KN, Faher V. Hyaluronic acid in 247 pleural fluids. Scand J Respir Dis 1967;48:366.
37. Ratliff JL, Chavez CM, Hamchuk A, et al. Reexpansion pulmonary edema. Chest 1973;64:654.
38. Trapnell DH, Thurston JGB. Unilateral pulmonary edema after pleural aspiration. Lancet 1970;1:1367.
39. Yamazaki S, Ogawa J, Shohyu A, et al. Pulmonary blood flow to rapidly re-expanded lung on spontaneous pneumothorax. Chest 1982;81:118.
40. Prakash UBS. Malignant pleural effusions. Postgrad Med 1986;80:201.
41. Prakash UBS, Reiman HM. Comparison of needle biopsy with cytologic analysis for the evaluation of pleural effusion: Analysis of 414 cases. Mayo Clin Proc 1985;60:158.
42. Hanson G, Philips T. Pleural biopsy in diagnosis of thoracic disease. Br Med J 1962;2:300.
43. Sisson BS, Weiss W. Needle biopsy of the parietal pleura in patients with pleural effusion. Br Med J 1962;2:298.
44. Scerbo J, Keltz H, Stone DJ. A prospective study of closed pleural biopsies. JAMA 1971;218:377.
45. Liss HP. Cope needle biopsy. South Med J 1984;77:837.
46. Bevelaque FA, Aranda C, Leon W. The role of closed pleural biopsy in suspected malignant effusions. N Y State J Med 1984;84:229.
47. Salyer WR, Eggleston JC, Eroyan YS. Efficacy of pleural needle biopsy and pleural fluid cytopathology in the diagnosis of malignant neoplasm involving the pleura. Chest 1975;67:536.
48. Winkelman M, Pfitzer P. Blind pleural biopsy in combination with cytology of pleural effusions. Acta Cytol 1981;25:373.
49. Schools GS. Needle biopsy of parietal pleura: Current status. Tex State J Med 1963;59:1056.
50. Jones FL. Subcutaneous implantation of cancer: A rare complication of pleural biopsy. Chest 1970;57:189.
51. Boutin C, Cargrino P, Viallat JR. Thoracoscopy in the early diagnosis of malignant pleural effusions. Endoscopy 1980;12:155.
52. Weissburg D, Kaufman M, Zurkowski Z. Pleuroscopy in patients with pleural effusions and pleural masses. Ann Thorac Surg 1980;29:205.
53. Weissburg D, Kaufman M. Diagnostic and therapeutic pleuroscopy: Experience with 127 patients. Chest 1980;78:732.
54. Oakes DD, Sherck JP, Brodsky JB, et al. Therapeutic thoracoscopy. J Thorac Cardiovasc Surg 1984;87:269.
55. Weissburg D. Diagnostic and therapeutic pleuroscopy. Chest 1980;5:732–735.
56. Chernow B, Sahn SA. Carcinomatous involvement of the pleura. Am J Med 1977;37:291.
57. Roy RH, Can DT, Payne WS. The problem of chylothorax. Mayo Clin Proc 1967;42:457.
58. Leff A, Honeywell PC, Costello J. Pleural effusion from malignancy. Ann Intern Med 1978;88:532.
59. Bayly TC, Kisner DL, Sybert A, et al. Tetracycline and quinacrine in the control of malignant pleural effusions: A randomized trial. Cancer 1978;41:1188.
60. Zaloanek AJ, Oswald SG, Langin M. Intrapleural tetracycline in malignant pleural effusions: A randomized study. Cancer 1983;51:752.
61. O'Neill W, Spurr C, Muss H, et al. A prospective study of chest tube drainage and tetracycline sclerosis versus chest tube drainage in the treatment of malignant pleural effusion. Proc Am Soc Clin Oncol 1979;21:349.
62. Wallach H. Chest [Letter] 1978;73:246.
63. Sahn SA, Good JT. The effect of common sclerosing agents on the rabbit pleural space. Am Rev Respir Dis 1981;124:65.
64. Dunkel TB. Intrapleural tetracycline in the treatment of malignant pleural effusions. Minn Med 1986;69:717.
65. Gravelyn TR, Michelson MK, Gross BH, Sitrin RG. Tetracycline pleurodesis for malignant pleural effusions. Cancer 1987;59:1973–1977.
66. Sorensen PG, Svendsen TL, Enk B. Treatment of malignant pleural effusion with drainage, with and without instillation of talc. Eur J Respir Dis 1984;65:131.
67. Adler RH, Sayek I. Treatment of malignant pleural effusion: A method using tube thoracostomy and talc. Ann Thorac Surg 1976;22:8.
68. Starkey GW. Recurrent malignant pleural effusions. N Engl J Med 1964;270:436.
69. Jones GR. Treatment of malignant pleural effusion by iodized talc pleurodesis. Thorax 1969;24:69.
70. Shedbalker AR, Head JM, Head LR, et al. Evaluation of talc pleural symphysis in management of malignant pleural effusion. J Thorac Cardiovasc Surg 1971;61:492.
71. Fentiman IS, Rubens RD, Hayward JI. A comparison of intracavitary talcum and tetracycline for the control of pleural effusion secondary to breast cancer. Eur J Cancer Clin Oncol 1986;22:1079.
72. Daniel TM, Tribble CG, Rodgers BM. Thoracoscopy and talc poudrage for pneumothoraces and effusions. Ann Thorac Surg 1990;50:186–189.
73. Ostrowski M. An assessment of the long term results of controlling the reaccumulation of malignant effusions using intracavitary bleomycin. Cancer 1986;57:721.
74. Gupta N, Opfell RW, Padova C, et al. Intrapleural bleomycin vs tetracycline for control of malignant pleural effusions. A randomized study. Am Soc Clin Oncol [Abstract] 1980;C-189:366.
75. Moores DWO. Malignant pleural effusion. Semin Oncol 1991;18:59–61.
76. Rusch VW, Figlin R, Godwin D, Piantadosi S. Intrapleural cisplatin and cytarabine in the management of malignant pleural effusions: A Lung Cancer Study Group trial. J Clin Oncol 1991;9:313–319.
77. Ostrowski MJ, Priestman TJ, Houston RF, Martin WMC. A randomized trial of intracavitary bleomycin and *Corynebacterium parvum* in the control of malignant pleural effusions. Radiother Oncol 1989;14:19–26.
78. Rossi GA, Felletti R, Balbi R, et al. Symptomatic treatment of recurrent malignant pleural effusions with intrapleurally administered *Corynebacterium parvum*. Am Rev Respir Dis 1987;135:885.
79. Rosso R, Rimoldi R, Salvati F, et al. Intrapleural natural beta interferon in the treatment of malignant pleural effusions. Oncology 1988;45:253–256.
80. Boutin C, Viallat JR, Van Zandwijk N, et al. Activity of intrapleural recombinant gamma-interferon in malignant mesothelioma. Cancer 1991;67:2033–2037.
81. Dianjun L, Yaorong W, Ziaodong Y, Jie S, Yunfu C, Denian B. Treatment of patients with malignant pleural effusions due to advanced lung cancer by transfer to autologous LAK cells combined with rIL-2 or rIL-2 alone. Proc Chin Acad Med Sci Peking Union Med Coll 1990;5:51–55.
82. Yasumoto K, Miyazaki K, Nagashima A, et al. Induction of lymphokine-activated killer cells by intrapleural instillations of recombinant interleukin-2 in patients with malignant pleurisy due to lung cancer. Cancer Res 1987;47:2184–2187.
83. Weick JK, Killy JM, Harison EG, et al. Pleural effusion in lymphoma. Cancer 1973;31:848.
84. Xaubet A, Duimenjo MC, Maren A, et al. Characteristics and prognostic value of pleural effusion in non-Hodgkin's lymphoma. Eur J Respir Dis 1985;66:135.
85. Martini N, Bains M, Beattie EJ. Indications for pleurectomy in malignant effusion. Cancer 1975;35:734.
86. Jensik R, Cagle JE, Melloy F, et al. Pleurectomy in the treatment of pleural effusion due to metastatic malignancy. J Thorac Cardiovasc Surg 1963;46:322.
87. Anderson CB, Philpott GW, Ferguson TB. The treatment of malignant pleural effusions. Cancer 1974;33:916.
88. Yates WM. Tumors of the heart and pericardium. Arch Intern Med 1931;48:627.
89. Scott RW, Garvin CF. Tumors of the heart and pericardium. Am Heart J 1939;17:431.
90. Bisel HF, Wroblewski F, LaDue JS. Incidence and clinical manifestations of cardiac metastases. JAMA 1953;153:712.
91. Thurber DL, Edwards JE, Achor RWP. Secondary malignant tumors of the pericardium. Circulation 1962;26:228.
92. Skhvatsabaju LV. Secondary malignant lesions of the heart and pericardium in neoplastic disease. Oncology 1986;43:103.
93. Goudie RB. Secondary tumors of the heart and pericardium. Br Heart J 1955;17:183.
94. Theologides A. Neoplastic cardiac tamponade. Semin Oncol 1978;5:181.
95. Shenkai T, Tomenagu K, Saijo N, et al. The incidence of cardiac metastases in primary lung cancer and the management of malignant pericardial effusion. Jpn J Clin Oncol 1982;12:23.
96. Buck M, Ingle JN, Guilani ER, et al. Pericardial effusion in women with breast cancer. Cancer 1987;60:263.
97. Hagemeister FB, Buydan AU, Luna MA, et al. Causes of death in breast cancer. Cancer 1980;46:162.
98. Nakayama R, Yoneyama T, Takatani O, et al. A study of metastatic tumors to the heart, pericardium and great vessels. Jpn Heart J 1966;7:227.
99. Oruigbo WIB. The spread of lung cancer to the heart, pericardium, and great vessels. Jpn Heart J 1974;15:234.
100. Pories WJ, Gaudiani VA. Cardiac tamponade. Surg Clin North Am 1975;55:573.
101. Jochelson MS, Balikian JP, Mauch P, et al. Peri- and paracardial involvement in lymphoma: A radiographic study of 11 cases. AJR 1983;140:483.
102. Dighton DH, Golding R, de Feytes PJ. Post-pneumonectomy pericardial effusion. Chest 1982;82:389.

103. Golding RD, Zanten TEG. Computed tomography in malignant conditions affecting the pericardium. J Belge Radiol 1984;67:371.
104. Johnson FE, Wolverson MIL, Sundaram M, et al. Unsuspected malignant pericardial effusion causing cardiac tamponade. Chest 1982;82:501.
105. Callahan JA, Seward JB, Nishimura RA, et al. Two-dimensional echocardiographically guided pericardiocentesis: Experience in 117 consecutive patients. Am J Cardiol 1985;55:476.
106. Kopecky SL, Callahan JA, Tajek AJ, et al. Percutaneous pericardial catheter drainage: Report of 42 consecutive cases. Am J Cardiol 1986;58:633.
107. Wong B, Murphy J, Chang CJ, et al. The risk of pericardiocentesis. Am J Cardiol 1979;44:1110.
108. Zepf RE, Johnston WW. The role of cytology in the evaluation of pericardial effusions. Chest 1972;62:593.
109. Reyes CV, Strinden C, Banerji M. The role of cytology in neoplastic tamponade. Acta Cytol 1982;26:299.
110. Applefeld MM, Cole JF, Pollock SH, et al. The late appearance of chronic pericardial disease in patients treated by radiotherapy for Hodgkin's disease. Ann Intern Med 1981;94:338.
111. Pavis S, Sharma SM, Blumberg ED, et al. Intrapericardial tetracycline for the management of cardiac tamponade secondary to malignant pericardial effusion. N Engl J Med 1978;299:1113.
112. Shephard FA, Ginsberg JS, Evans WR, et al. Tetracycline sclerosis in the management of malignant pericardial effusion. J Clin Oncol 1985;3:1678.
113. Maher FR, Buckman R. Intrapericardial instillation of bleomycin in malignant pericardial effusion. Am Heart J 1986;111:613.
114. Markman M, Howell SB. Intrapericardial instillation of cisplatin in a patient with a large malignant effusion. Cancer Drug Deliv 1985;2:49.
115. Primrose WR, Clee MD, Johnston RN. Malignant pericardial effusion managed with vinblastine. Clin Oncol 1983;9:67.
116. Terry LN, Klegerman MM. Pericardial and myocardial involvement by lymphomas and leukemias: The role of radiotherapy. Cancer 1970;25:1003.
117. Ghosh SC, Larrieu A, Ablaza S, et al. Clinical experience with subxyphoid pericardial decompression. Int Surg 1985;70:5.
118. Hankins JR, Sattersfield JR, Aisner J, et al. Pericardial window for malignant pericardial effusion. Ann Thorac Surg 1980;30:465.
119. Osuch JR, Khandehar JN, Fry WA. Emergency subxyphoid pericardial decompression for malignant pericardial effusion. Am Surg 1985;51:298.
120. Berman K, Fielding MB, Richi AA. Diagnosis and treatment of malignant pericardial effusion: The subxyphoid approach. Conn Med 1984;48:701.
121. Little AG, Krimser PC, Wade JL, et al. Operation for diagnosis and treatment of pericardial effusions. Surgery 1984;96:738.
122. Piehler JM, Pluth JR, Schaff HV, et al. Surgical management of effusive pericardial disease. J Thorac Cardiovasc Surg 1985;90:506.
123. Prager PL, Wilson CH, Bender AW. The subxyphoid approach to pericardial disease. Ann Thorac Surg 1982;34:6.

SECTION **6**

ALAN R. BAKER
JEFFREY S. WEBER

Treatment of Malignant Ascites

MALIGNANT ASCITES

The development of a malignant peritoneal effusion or disseminated peritoneal carcinomatosis is a prognostically adverse event in the natural history of a number of tumors, particularly ovarian, colorectal, gastric, and uterine cancer. Anorexia, early satiety, difficulty with ambulation, and respiratory compromise are associated with significant intraperitoneal disease or ascites. Although the median survival is about several months (Table 61–34), mechanical intervention to drain ascitic fluid can provide good palliation, and newer therapeutic approaches with the use of intracavitary chemotherapy and aggressive surgery have resulted in prolonged survival for selected patients in small phase I and II studies. Numerous therapies have historically been tested in patients with malignant ascites and intraperitoneal disease,[1] such as systemic and intraperitoneal chemotherapy, external-beam and intracavitary radiocolloid instillation, intraperitoneal instillation of biologic response modifiers with and without lymphokine-activated killer (LAK) cells, and internal ascitic fluid shunting. However, internal peritoneovenous shunting is still the standard of care for patients with malignant ascites, and promising initial results with local instillation of chemotherapy or immunotherapeutic reagents need to be tested in expanded phase II and III studies.

The pathogenesis of malignant ascites is multifactorial. Tumor cells can be shown to invade the subdiaphragmatic lymphatic channels and plexuses as shown by Feldman[2,3] and others,[4,5] and this can compromise drainage of the peritoneal cavity. Although excess fluid generation is probably a more important factor in the genesis of cirrhotic ascites, Hirabayashi[6] has demonstrated that it occurs in the setting of ovarian cancer, and Garrison and colleagues[7] have suggested that tumors can elaborate humoral factors that cause increased capillary leakage, even across normal peritoneal surfaces and omentum. The hydrodynamic disequilibria caused by hypoalbuminemia, portal venous obstruction, or hepatic venous obstruction, noted when the liver is extensively replaced by metastatic tumor, probably promotes the formation of ascitic fluid as well.

DIAGNOSIS AND WORKUP

Ascites and increasing abdominal girth from bulky intraperitoneal tumor are often presenting signs of advanced ovarian cancer but more often are harbingers of relapse and metastatic disease in patients with ovarian, uterine, colorectal, or gastric carcinoma. Nonneoplastic causes for ascites, such as congestive heart failure, cirrhosis, or nephrosis with protein wasting, and, less frequently, complications of radiation therapy or chemotherapy can occur and should be ruled out.

Abdominal paracentesis should be performed in cancer patients with ascites to assess the chemistry profile of the fluid and its cell count, differential, cytology, Gram's stain, and culture. Removal of as much fluid as possible will temporarily reduce symptoms and give an opportunity to assess the time for reaccumulation. To prevent infrequently seen orthostatic changes from rapid intravascular fluid shifts, or electrolyte aberrations that follow removal of a large volume of ascitic fluid, an intravenous line should be in place, or the patient should be encouraged to take fluids liberally. Patients should also be cautioned about dizziness or lightheadedness, reflecting intravascular depletion after a paracentesis.

The character of the aspirated fluid can offer clues to its etiology. Malignant collections are often bloody or serosanguineous; serous fluid is consistent with a cirrhotic, nephrotic, pancreatic, or cardiac origin; turbid or cloudy fluid can be indicative of infectious peritonitis; and chylous fluid suggests lymphoma, gut lymphatic injury, or thoracic duct injury.

No single feature in the biochemical profile of ascitic fluid is diagnostic for a malignant etiology, although the presence of an elevated ascitic/serum protein ratio (>0.4), increased ascitic/serum lactic dehydrogenase (LDH) ratio (>1.0), in-

TABLE 61–34. Reported Experience With Peritoneovenous Shunt Management of Malignant Ascites

	Underlying Malignancy						*Patient Survival*	
Investigations	*Ovary*	*GI*	*Breast*	*Unknown Adenocarcinoma*	*Other*	*Comments*	*Median (wk)*	*% Alive at 1 y*
Straus, 1979[56]	13	10	3	2	9	27/37 (73%) Good shunt function and palliation	8	
Osterlee, 1980[57]	6	7	2	1	4	13/20 (65%) Good shunt function and palliation	7	5
Raaf, 1980[58]		2	1	1	1	5/5 (100%) Ascites controlled	5	0
Lokich, 1980[59]	3		3	1	1	6/8 (75%) Ascites controlled and meaningful palliation	8	12
Lund, 1982[61]	14	9	5		7	Excellent initial and long-term therapy for ascites	16	11
Qazi, 1982[62]	28	4	8			28/40 (70%) Effective palliation		
Cheung, 1982[63]	2	7	4		9		5	10
Reinhold, 1983[64]	6	3	6		4	6/19 (32%) Excellent symptomatic relief	6	
Souter, 1983[65]	9	4	4	4	5	23/26 (88%) Satisfactory palliation	16	12
Gough, 1984[66]	4	4	2		7	13/17 (76%) Ascites controlled, worthwhile palliation	13	6
Downing, 1984[60]		2	3	1	1	4/7 (57%) Good shunt function and palliation	13	0
Kostroff, 1985[67]	11	8	5		7		8	0
Campioni, 1986[68]	8	14	7	7	6	Safe and effective way to improve quality of life	7	7
Sonnenfeld, 1986[69]		16		5	6	19/27 (70%) Good palliation	8	0
Roussel, 1986[70]	12	10	11		3	Effective palliation for most patients	13	0
Soderlund, 1986[71]	7	15			2	No benefit for patients with GI malignancy	7	4
Shepherd, 1988[72]	2	8	1		3	Majority of patients got little benefit	6	7
Edney, 1989[73]	8	24	8		5	75% experience relief of symptoms	33	13+
Smith, 1989[74]	3	23	9	5	10	36/50 (72%) Adequate palliation	22	4+
Total	136	170	82	27	90		5–33	0–12

GI, gastrointestinal (colon, stomach, pancreas, hepatobiliary).

creased carcinoembryonic antigen (CEA) (>10), OC-125 or other tumor markers favor neoplasia.[7-10] Greater than 10,000 erythrocytes/μL, and more than 1000 leukocytes/μL, in the absence of bacteria or fungus on Gram stain and a sterile fluid culture characterize a malignant effusion. Papanicolaou stain of the ascitic cells from a spun pellet or cell block will show malignant cells on cytology 50% or more of the time, and this will confirm the diagnosis. The information in Table 61–35 summarizes important features in the workup of a patient with suspected malignant peritoneal effusion.

TREATMENT

To date, no well-controlled, randomized trials have been performed in cancer patients comparing the alternative methods of managing malignant ascites. In many studies, the reported median survival for patients with newly diagnosed malignant ascites is approximately 2 months (see Table 61–34), suggesting that for most patients it is an indicator of end-stage disease. Therefore, therapy for malignant ascites, and for patients diagnosed with diffuse intraperitoneal carcinomatosis, has focused on palliation of symptoms as opposed to attempts at achieving a long-term regression of bulky tumor masses and large peritoneal effusions. While it is true that efforts in these patients should be directed at maximizing ambulatory out-of-hospital time and minimizing treatment-induced morbidity, newer, more experimental approaches to malignant ascites and intraperitoneal disease will also be discussed in this section. With these considerations in mind, we will describe the current therapeutic options, proceeding from the less invasive to the more invasive and more morbid alternatives.

DIET AND DIURESIS

Although a useful maneuver in the management of cirrhotic ascites, dietary salt restriction, aldosterone-inhibiting diuretics, and loop diuretics have little impact on malignant ascites. Sodium retention is less important as a pathologic factor than increased fluid elaborated from the tumor-involved peritoneal surface and lymphatic obstruction that inhibits fluid resorption. However, Greenway and colleagues[11] have reported decreased malignant peritoneal effusions in 13 of 15 patients treated with high doses of spironolactone (150–450 mg/day).

TABLE 61–35. Assessment of the Patient With a Peritoneal Effusion

Diagnosis/Workup
- History
  - Increasing abdominal girth—"clothes don't fit"
  - Indigestion and early satiety
  - Ankle swelling
  - Easy fatigability
  - Shortness of breath
- Physical examination
  - Fluid wave
  - Shifting dullness
- Radiographic studies
  - Abdominal flat plate: generalized ground-glass appearance; air-filled small bowel loops occupy central position and are separated by fluid between loops; psoas shadows obscured
- Ultrasound, abdominal CT: both are sensitive tests that definitively diagnose small amounts of ascites
- Paracentesis
  - Gross character on inspection: bloody, serous, milky, turbid
  - Cell count and differential
  - Chemistries: Total protein, LDH, CEA, OC-125, amylase
  - Cytology
  - Microbiology: Gram's stain and culture

CT, computed tomography; LDH, lactic dehydrogenase; CEA, carcinoembryonic antigen.

The only treatment-related toxicity noted was nausea in 2 of 15 patients. Baseline elevated plasma renin levels were measured in 5 of 5 patients, with elevated aldosterone levels noted in 3 of the 5 tested.

REPEATED PARACENTESIS AND EXTERNAL DRAINS

Frequently reported abdominal taps, while a commonly used technique to palliate the discomfort, bloating, and shortness of breath caused by malignant ascites,[12,13] can lead to protein depletion, postural hypotension, and electrolyte abnormalities. In addition, the frequent insertion of a catheter into the sterile intraperitoneal space can lead to visceral injury and bleeding, as well as bacterial inoculation and subsequent peritonitis.

A newer approach to external drainage of ascites is a permanently implanted abdominal drain.[14] In one small series, 17 patients with intractable ascites had a Silastic catheter permanently implanted in the peritoneal space; relief of symptoms was obtained in the 15 patients who had patent catheter function, although bacterial growth was eventually seen in the peritoneal fluid of 8. In addition, there have been isolated case reports of the use of implanted Tenckoff catheters (Davol, Cranston, RI) to drain malignant ascites.[15]

INTRACAVITARY THERAPY

Intraperitoneal therapy to treat malignant ascites or diffuse peritoneal tumor was initially described over 40 years ago by Muller,[16] who used radioactive ^{63}Zn. ^{198}Au later became the instilled isotope of choice,[17] but colloidal suspensions of $^{32}CrPO_4$ have been used mainly in the last decade or two. At least two series of patients have been studied,[18,19] suggesting that half of those treated with radiocolloid ^{32}P derive palliative benefit from this approach while suffering minimal treatment-related toxicity.

Chemotherapeutic agents were initially studied as long ago as 1955, when Weisberger reported the results of intraperitoneal nitrogen mustard treatment of 7 patients with ovarian cancer.[20] Diminution of ascites was seen in all patients, albeit with a significant amount of toxicity—mainly abdominal pain. Further interest in direct intracavitary instillation of chemotherapy drugs was generated at the National Cancer Institute (NCI) by Dedrick and colleagues,[21] who hypothesized that a 2 to 3 log higher local concentration of drug could be achieved by intraperitoneal rather than systemic administration, without causing unacceptable systemic toxicity from high serum levels. This theory was initially tested by Ozols and colleagues at the NCI[22]; they demonstrated that in patients with ovarian cancer who had ascites or diffuse intraperitoneal disease, or both, there was a significant pharmacokinetic advantage over the intravenous route for chemotherapy agents instilled intraperitoneally. There was a significant and large ratio of the "area under the curve" (AUC) or drug concentration versus time for the peritoneal cavity as opposed to plasma. Agents known to be metabolized during first passage through the liver, such as doxorubicin or 5-FU, or drugs that have limited systemic clearance, such as mitoxantrone, can have mean peritoneal to plasma AUC ratios of up to 1400, suggesting a significant advantage to the intraperitoneal route.[23,24] The development of the indwelling Port-A-Cath system (Pharmacia, St. Paul, MN) has led to minimal discomfort and increased compliance by patients receiving intraperitoneal therapy,[25] but there is still potential for bleeding, infection, or chemical peritonitis as a significant source of morbidity.[26]

A large number of phase I and II studies have demonstrated that single agents, particularly cisplatin,[27] as well as others[28,29] and combinations of up to three[30,31] drugs, can be given safely to patients with advanced ovarian and colorectal cancer who have diffuse intraperitoneal disease. With cisplatin, the single most active agent in ovarian cancer, several groups have performed phase II studies and have demonstrated a 30% pathologically confirmed complete response rate in patients with small-volume residual disease (<2 cm) who had failed first-line platinum-containing systemic regimens.[32] It is likely, however, that patients with bulky disease (defined as >2 cm), after a second- or third-look laparotomy, will not respond to intraperitoneal therapy. In one study by Howell and colleagues, a group of 25 patients with microscopic residual (<0.5 cm) disease after first-line chemotherapy were treated with intraperitoneal instillation of cisplatin and achieved a median survival of greater than 49 months, with 74% having a 4-year survival.[33] In the most recent platinum combination intraperitoneal trials, patients who fail first-line chemotherapy but have microscopic residual disease (<0.5 cm) at laparotomy can achieve 45% to 50% pathologic complete response rates. However, these encouraging results should be interpreted with caution, because randomized phase III studies to compare survival in patients treated with systemic or intraperitoneal second-line therapies have not matured. In addition, other phase III studies are currently in progress comparing intraperitoneal chemotherapy in previously untreated patients with advanced ovarian cancer with standard systemic therapy.[34] Other studies to evaluate the use of intraperitoneal chemotherapy as an adjuvant in early- or late-stage disease after definitive surgical or systemic chemotherapeutic management are being performed. Some investigators have recommended that intraperitoneal chemotherapy be a standard treatment option in patients with persistent microscopic residual disease (<0.5 cm) after cisplatin- or carboplatinum-based chemotherapy who have shown a response to the initial systemic therapy.[35] Certainly, no established therapy has shown superior results in this scenario, but a randomized phase III trial is needed to demonstrate that a survival advantage exists for the intraperitoneal option.

A number of biologic response modifiers such as interferon-α (INF-α)[36,37] and interleukin-2 (IL-2) with or without LAK cells have been administered intraperitoneally to patients with ascites or disseminated carcinomatosis, or both, caused by ovarian or colorectal cancer. Interferon-α2b was administered to 13 patients with ovarian carcinoma and ascites, and there was a significant decrease in ascites in 5 of the 13 who had microscopic disease.[36] Berek and colleagues treated 14 patients with residual disease after first-line chemotherapy and second-look laparotomy with escalating doses of intraperitoneal INF-α and achieved a 45% pathologically confirmed response rate (4 complete and 1 partial); all patients had less than 0.5 cm of disease.[37]

Both allogeneic and syngeneic LAK cells have been employed with intraperitoneal IL-2 to treat patients with ovarian and colorectal cancer. Steis and colleagues[38] treated 24 patients who had diffuse peritoneal carcinomatosis, mostly from ovarian, colorectal, or uterine cancer, with IL-2 and LAK cells instilled intraperitoneally by way of a Tenckoff catheter. Seven of 24 patients had pathologically confirmed partial responses, albeit with significant morbidity that limited therapy, including peritoneal fibrosis in 10 patients and significant abdominal pain in 22 patients.[37,38]

Finally, while interferon-γ (INF-γ) has been instilled intraperitoneally in a phase I trial[39] and has been shown to have no significant antitumor activity, it may have clinical utility in immunotherapy for its ability to locally upregulate major histocompatibility complex (MHC) and tumor antigen expression on ascites tumor cells from patients exposed to the drug intraperitoneally. Subsequent therapy with tumor-specific T cells administered into the peritoneum may allow increased recognition and killing of tumor cells.

RADICAL SURGERY

Sugarbaker and colleagues have studied small numbers of patients with disseminated carcinomatosis from colorectal and gastric cancer who received aggressive debulking surgery followed by early postoperative intraperitoneal chemotherapy and, in some cases, abdominal radiation.[40,41] They claim that the majority of patients receiving intraperitoneal chemotherapy and aggressive debulking with use of a ball-type electrocautery device have disease-free survival of greater than 3 years. Although these results may be impressive for patients with uniformly lethal gastrointestinal malignancies, they need to be confirmed in larger follow-up phase III studies. The same group has studied 50 patients with cystadenocarcinoma limited to peritoneal surfaces; 26 had massive ascites. All were treated with radical debulking surgery and early (within 72 hours of surgery) intraperitoneal chemotherapy; 36 are alive 1 to 8 years after therapy.

PERITONEOVENOUS SHUNTING

Although the concept of returning an ascitic fluid collection to the intravascular space is over 75 years old,[42,43] the technology to accomplish this objective in a minimally cumbersome fashion with continuous reinfusion has evolved significantly over the past 25 years.[44–47] The availability of several relatively simple, reasonably effective peritoneovenous (PV) shunt devices (LeVeen, Becton-Dickenson and Leveen, Rutherford, NJ and Denver; Johnson and Johnson, Evergreen, CO) has led to their fairly widespread use. The devices consist of (1) a length of multiply perforated tubing to be implanted in the free peritoneal cavity, (2) a length of tubing to be inserted into the superior vena cava or right atrium, and (3) a unidirectional flow valve connecting the two limbs.

The principal difference between the LeVeen and Denver shunts is that the one-way valve in the Denver shunt can be manually pumped by physician or patient to flush it clear of possibly accumulating debris at periodic intervals. Despite this potentially theoretic advantage, the literature fails to demonstrate functional superiority for one or the other of these devices; either may be chosen on the basis of personal preference. This approach, with substantial pathophysiologic rationale,[48] was initially applied to the management of intractable ascites from cirrhosis.[49–55] Numerous series that address its applicability in the management of malignant ascites have been recently published.[56–74]

In principle, the PV shunt takes advantage of the fact that a 5- to 15-cm H_2O pressure head exists between the ascites-laden peritoneal cavity and the central venous circulation. On inspiration, when intrathoracic pressure becomes more negative, the pressure differential further increases. Whenever the pressure gradient exceeds about 3 to 5 cm H_2O, the unidirectional flow valve opens, and ascitic fluid moves through the tubing from peritoneal cavity to central circulation. Several excellent reports that describe details of shunt placement are available[46,47,50,75–77] and might profitably be perused by the uninitiated in an effort to avoid any one of the numerous technical pitfalls responsible for early shunt malfunction.

Figure 61–54 represents a schematic illustration of the shunt in place. In brief, the operation may be performed under general anesthesia or under local anesthesia supplemented with sedation. Prophylactic antibiotics are used. The peritoneal limb of the shunt is placed first through a roughly 7.6-cm-long, muscle-splitting, subcostal incision. A nonabsorbable pursestring suture, which includes some transversus abdominus muscle, secures this limb in a watertight fashion. If the Denver shunt is used, a subcutaneous pocket overlying the lower rib cage is made for the pump device, and it is secured in position. Free flow of ascitic fluid is demonstrated by holding the open end of the venous limb several inches below heart level. Most surgeons remove about 50% of the patient's ascitic fluid burden at this point, submitting some for culture and perhaps the rest for cytologic analysis. A cervical incision is then made exposing the internal jugular vein, and a fine Prolene pursestring suture (Ethicon, Somerville, NJ) is placed in its anterior wall. A uterine sound can then be used to make

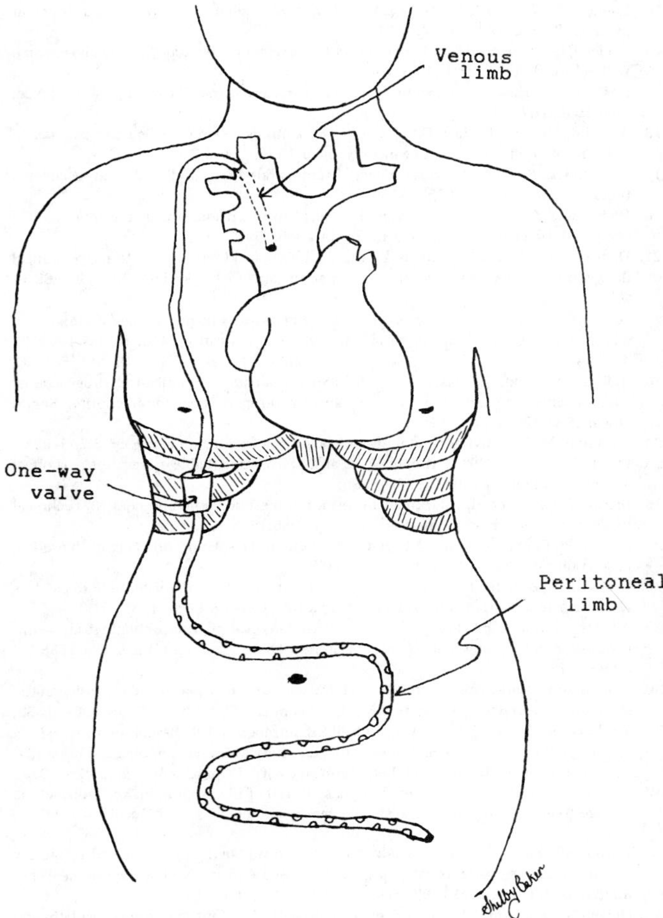

FIGURE 61–54. The peritoneovenous shunt in situ.

a graceful subcutaneous tunnel linking the abdominal and neck incisions such that all tubing will lie in a kink-free manner. The venous limb is then passed through the tunnel, exiting into the cervical incision. After free flow of ascitic fluid is again demonstrated and the venous limb is cut to permit its tip to lie in the superior vena cava or right atrium, the venous limb is placed through a stab wound in the internal jugular vein and advanced centrally. It is useful to confirm the position of the PV shunt at this point, either fluoroscopically or with portable chest and abdominal x-ray films. The wounds are then irrigated with antibiotic solution and inspected, perfect hemostasis is assured, and the wounds are closed.

Although able to afford palliation, PV shunting is no panacea. Before a PV shunt procedure is attempted, the patient's ascites, at the very least, should have proved refractory to first-line treatment for the underlying malignant condition. This is particularly true in the setting of ovarian cancer, for which ascites can be a component of relatively early stage (IC or IIC) disease and can come under control with hysterectomy-salpingo-oophorectomy alone. Furthermore, multidrug regimens have proved quite successful, at least initially, in controlling the manifestations of much more extensive intra-abdominal dissemination and may significantly impinge on the ascitic fluid component of the tumor-imposed burden.

The data in Table 61–34 summarize the results of 19 reported studies of patients managed by placement of a PV shunt to control malignant ascites. Although each includes only a modest number of patients, 505 patients in all are reported, with the majority suffering cancer of the gastrointestinal tract (34%), ovary (27%), and breast (16%). The fact that end-stage illness is an apt characterization of the patient population's clinical condition is attested to by the median survivals of about 2 to 6 months and the 1-year survivals of about 10%. Although, for the most part, the authors emphasize that patients derive significant symptomatic relief and improvement in qualitative existence, this regrettably translates into substantial quantitative postshunt survival only anecdotally.

COMPLICATIONS

Although the litany of potential and reported complications is long, with the exception of shunt malfunction, they tend to occur infrequently and, on occasion, are preventable.

Shunt occlusion with flow cessation can occur at any time after insertion. Ten percent to 42% of shunts placed stop functioning before the patient's death.[56–61,66,67,69,70,77,78] Immediate malfunction often is due to technical factors, such as tube kinking or tip malposition. Later failures may be secondary to fibrin clot formation and debris accumulation at the valve. Heavily blood-tinged ascites, particularly rich in protein with a somewhat viscous character, portend this complication. Valve chamber pumping (Denver) and shunt flushing with thrombolytic agents[61] can, on occasion, restore flow, but revision or replacement, if clinically indicated, is usually required. Late occlusion may also reflect thrombosis of the venous system around that limb of the PV shunt.

Ascitic fluid leakage at the peritoneal insertion site predisposes to infection, and it is perhaps best prevented by using a double-pursestring suture buttressed by transversus abdominus muscle and fascia at this location.[50,69]

Acute postinsertion problems with fluid overload, pulmonary congestion, and respiratory insufficiency occur infrequently.[61,67] To help avoid this problem, most authors recommend removing about 50% of the ascitic fluid accumulation at the time of shunt placement. Careful postoperative monitoring is required and includes central venous pressure assessment, input-output determination, daily weight, and abdominal girth measurement. A Foley catheter facilitates management of the often brisk, post-PV shunt insertion, diuretic-abetted diuresis and can help to more accurately monitor fluid fluxes. Judicious intravenous fluid support and the liberal use of diuretics and potassium replacement are often necessary to prevent intravascular volume overload and hypokalemia. Because shunt flow volume is hydrostatically determined, simply raising or lowering the head of the patient's bed will alter significantly the flow pressure gradient. Need for this maneuver can be monitored by central venous pressure determination, and change can be made accordingly.

Although disseminated intravascular coagulation (DIC) and bleeding diatheses occur often[79–81] after PV shunt management of cirrhotic ascites, they are rarely a clinical problem when shunts are placed in the neoplastic ascites context.[56,62,79] Laboratory evidence for the ongoing process at a subclinical level is readily demonstrable. Mild decreases in platelet count, slight prolongation in prothrombin and partial thromboplastin time, and measurable increases in fibrin degradation products have been reported.[62,81,82] Significant preshunt hepatic dysfunction, particularly as evidenced by a serum bilirubin level higher than 3 mg/dl, may well presage clinical coagulopathy and probably will contraindicate the procedure.[80,83]

Although shunt-induced tumor dissemination is a potentially adverse complication, it appears more of a theoretic consideration than a clinical contraindication. Although several reports, particularly in the setting of ovarian malignancy, suggest that this can occur and can produce serious consequences,[57,59,78,84,85] in most instances this problem has not occurred. Tarin and colleagues prospectively studied a series of 29 PV shunt recipients, 15 of whom came to autopsy.[86,87] All had large numbers of viable malignant cells ($8–600 \times 10^6$/100 ml ascites—95+% viable) in their ascitic fluid. Most formed colonies when grown in soft agar. Postshunt peripheral blood samples often revealed bizarre multinucleated cells, morphologically suggestive of tumor. Eight of the 15 patients had no evidence of hematologic dissemination at postmortem examination. The longest survivor, a patient with an ovarian primary lesion, lived 27 months after initial shunt placement. The 7 patients with evidence of hematogenous spread survived 1 to 9 months after shunt placement; 6 of the 7 had evidence of multiple, uniform-sized, small pulmonary nodules, possibly of iatrogenic origin but clinically not felt to have caused the patient's death. It may well be that the otherwise limited longevity of the PV shunt recipient precludes this theoretic difficulty from becoming a problematic clinical reality. Not unexpectedly, tumor growth along the subcutaneous shunt tunnel[58,88] and at the venotomy site of the venous limb[49,62] has been reported.

Although fever in the immediate postoperative period has been noted by most authors,[66,67] it usually remits spontaneously and is only rarely the harbinger of serious sepsis.[51,63]

REFERENCES

1. Lacy JH, Wieman TJ, Shively EH. Management of malignant ascites. Surg Gynecol Obstet 1984;159:397–412.
2. Feldman GB, Knapp RC, Order SE, Hellman S. The role of lymphatic obstruction in the formation of ascites in a murine ovarian carcinoma. Cancer Res 1972;32:1663–1666.
3. Feldman GB, Knapp RC. Lymphatic drainage of the peritoneal cavity and its significance in ovarian cancer. Am J Obstet Gynecol 1974;119:991–994.
4. Coates G, Bush RS, Aspin N. A study of ascites using lymphoscintigraphy with 99 Tc sulfur colloid. Radiology 1973;107:577–583.
5. Bronskill MJ, Bush RS, Ege GN. A quantitative measurement of peritoneal drainage in malignant ascites. Cancer 1977;40:2375–2380.
6. Hirabayashi K, Graham J. Genesis of ascites in ovarian cancer. Am J Obstet Gynecol 1970;106:492–497.
7. Garrison RN, Kaelin LD, Heusser LS, Galloway RH. Malignant ascites. Ann Surg 1986;203:644–651.
8. Greene LS, Levine R, Gross MJ, Gordon S. Distinguishing between malignant and cirrhotic ascites by computerized step-wise discriminant functional analysis of its biochemistry. Am J Gastroenterol 1978;70:448–454.
9. Nystrom JS, Dyce B, Wada J, et al. Carcinoembryonic antigen titers on effusion fluid. Arch Intern Med 1977;137:875–879.
10. Lowenstein MS, Rittgers RA, Kupchik HZ, et al. Improved detection of malignant ascites and pleural effusions by combined assay of fluid CEA and cytology. Clin Res 1975;23:596A.
11. Greenway B, Johnson PJ, Williams R. Control of malignant ascites with spironolactone. Br J Surg 1982;69:441–442.
12. Appleqvist P, Silvo J, Salmela L, Kostiainen S. J Surg Oncol 1982;20:238–242.
13. Lifshitz S. Ascites, pathophysiology and control measures. Int J Radiat Oncol Biol Phys 1982;8:1423–1426.
14. Belfort MA, Stevens RJ, DeHaek K, Soeters R, et al. A new approach to the management of malignant ascites. A permanently implanted abdominal drain. Eur J Surg Oncol 1990;16:47–53.
15. Lomas DA, Willis PJ, Stockley RA. Palliation of malignant ascites with a Tenckoff catheter. Thorax 1989;44:828–831.
16. Muller JH. Zur medizinisch-therapoeutischen verwendung der kunstlichen radioaktivitat. Bull Schweiz Akad Wiss 1949;5:584.
17. Rose RG. Intracavitary radioactive colloidal gold: Results in 257 cancer patients. J Nucl Med 1962;3:323–331.
18. Ariel IM, Oropeza R, Pack GT. Intracavitary administration of radioactive isotopes in the control of effusions due to cancer. Cancer 1966;19:1096–1102.
19. Jackson GL, Blosser NM. Intracavitary chromic phosphate (32-P) colloidal suspension therapy. Cancer 1981;48:2596–2598.
20. Weisberger AS, Levine B, Storasli JP. Use of nitrogen mustard in the treatment of serous effusions of neoplastic origin. JAMA 1955;159:1704–1707.
21. Dedrick RL, Myers CE, Bungay PM, et al. Pharmacokinetic rationale for peritoneal drug administration in the treatment of ovarian cancer. Cancer Treat Rep 1978;62:1–9.
22. Ozols RF, Young RC, Speyer JL, et al. Phase I and pharmacological studies of Adriamycin administered intraperitoneally to patients with ovarian cancer. Cancer Res 1982;42:4265–4269.
23. Alberts DS, Young L, Mason N, et al. In vitro evaluation of anticancer drugs against ovarian cancer at concentrations achievable by intraperitoneal administration. Semin Oncol 1985;12(Suppl 4):38–42.
24. Markman M. Intracavitary chemotherapy. Crit Rev Oncol Hematol 1985;3:205–233.
25. Pfeifle CE, Howell SB, Markman M, et al. Totally implantable system for peritoneal access. J Clin Oncol 1984;2:1277–1280.
26. Piccart MJ, Speyer JL, Markman M, et al.Intraperitoneal chemotherapy: Technical experience at five institutions. Semin Oncol 1985;12:90–96.
27. Howell SB, Pfeifle CE, Wang WE, et al. Intraperitoneal cisplatin with systemic thiosulfate protection. Ann Intern Med 1982;97:845–851.
28. Ozols RF, Speyer JL, Jenkins J, et al. Phase II trial of 5-FU administered IP to patients with refractory ovarian cancer. Cancer Treat Rep 1984;68:1229–1232.
29. Alberts DS, Surwit EA, Peng Y-M, et al. Phase I clinical pharmacokinetic study of mitoxantrone given to patients by intraperitoneal administration. Cancer Res 1988;48:5874–5877.
30. Reichman B, Markman M, Hake T, et al. Intraperitoneal cisplatin and etoposide in the treatment of refractory recurrent ovarian carcinoma. J Clin Oncol 1989;7:1327–1332.
31. Markman M, Cleary S, Lucas WE, Howell SB. Intraperitoneal chemotherapy with high dose cisplatin and cytosine arabinoside for refractory ovarian carcinoma and other malignancies principally involving the peritoneal cavity. J Clin Oncol 1985;3:925–931.
32. Kirmani S, Lucas WE, Kim S, et al. A phase II trial of IP cis platinum and etoposide as salvage treatment for minimal residual ovarian carcinoma. J Clin Oncol 1991;9:649–657.
33. Howell SB, Zimm S, Markman M, et al. Long term survival of advanced refractory ovarian carcinoma patients with small-volume disease treated with intraperitoneal chemotherapy. J Clin Oncol 1987;5:1607–1612.
34. Howell SB, Kirmani S, Lucas WE, et al. A phase II trial of intraperitoneal cisplatin and etoposide for primary treatment of ovarian epithelial cancer. J Clin Oncol 1990;8:137–145.
35. Markman M. Intraperitoneal chemotherapy. Semin Oncol 1991;18:248–254.
36. Bezwoda WR, Seymour L, Dansey R. Intraperitoneal recombinant interferon-alpha 2b for recurrent malignant ascites due to ovarian cancer. Cancer 1989;64:1029–1033.
37. Berek JS, Hacker HF, Lichtenstein A, et al. Intraperitoneal recombinant alpha-interferon for "salvage" immunotherapy in stage III epithelial ovarian cancer. A Gynecologic Oncology Group study. Cancer Res 1985;45:4447–4453.
38. Steis RG, Urba WJ, Vander Molan LA, et al. Intraperitoneal lymphokine-activated killer cell and interleukin-2 therapy for malignancies limited to the peritoneal cavity. J Clin Oncol 1990;8:1618–1629.
39. D'Acquisto R, Markman M, Hakes T, et al. A phase I trial of intraperitoneal recombinant gamma-interferon in advanced ovarian carcinoma. J Clin Oncol 1988;6:689–695.
40. Sugarbaker PH. Surgical treatment of peritoneal carcinomatosis: 1988 DuPont Lecture. Can J Surg 1989;32:164–170.
41. Sugarbaker PH. Mechanisms of relapse for colorectal cancer: Implications for intraperitoneal therapy. J Surg Oncol 1991;52:36–41.
42. Routte M. De l'abouchement des veines saphenes internes au peritoine abdominal dans certains cas d'ascite a reproduction. Lyon Med 1910;114:911–921.
43. Evler T. Autoserotherepie bei bauchfelltuberkulose durch dauerdrainage des Aszites unter die haut. Med Klin 1910;16:627–628.
44. Hyde GL, Eisman B. Peritoneal atrial shunt for intractable ascites. Arch Surg 1967;95:369–373.
45. Pollock AV. The treatment of resistant malignant ascites by insertion of a peritoneo-atrial Holter valve. Br J Surg 1975;62:104–107.
46. LeVeen HH, Christoudias G, Ip M. Peritoneo-venous shunting for ascites. Ann Surg 1974;180:580–591.
47. Lund RH, Newkirk JB. Peritoneo-venous shunting system for surgical management of ascites. Contemp Surg 1979;14:31–45.
48. Stanley MM. Treatment of intractable ascites in patients with alcoholic cirrhosis by peritoneovenous shunting (LeVeen). Med Clin North Am 1979;63:523–536.
49. LeVeen HH, Wapnick S, Grosberg S, et al. Further experiences with peritoneo-venous shunt for ascites. Ann Surg 1976;184:574–581.
50. Reinhardt GF, Stanley MM. Peritoneovenous shunting for ascites. Surg Gynecol Obstet 1977;145:419–424.
51. Greig PD, Langer B, Blendis LM, et al. Complications after peritoneovenous shunting for ascites. Am J Surg 1980;139:125–131.
52. Greenlee HB, Stanley MM, Reinhardt GF. Intractable ascites treated with peritoneovenous shunts (LeVeen). Arch Surg 1981;116:518–524.

53. Bernhoft RA, Pelligrini CA, Way LW. Peritoneovenous shunts for refractory ascites. Arch Surg 1982;117:631–635.
54. Stanley MM, Shigeru O, Lee KK, Nemchausky BA, et al. Peritoneovenous shunting as compared with medical treatment in patients with alcoholic cirrhosis and massive ascites. N Engl J Med 1989;321:1632–1638.
55. Gines P, Arroyo V, Vargas V, Planas R, et al. Paracentesis with intravenous infusion of albumin as compared with peritoneovenous shunting in cirrhosis with refractory ascites. N Engl J Med 1991;325:829–835.
56. Straus AK, Roseman DL, Shapiro RM. Peritoneovenous shunting in the management of malignant ascites. Arch Surg 1979;114:489–491.
57. Osterlee J. Peritoneovenous shunting for ascites in cancer patients. Br J Surg 1980;67: 633–666.
58. Raaf JH, Stroehlein JR. Palliation of malignant ascites by the LeVeen peritoneo-venous shunt. Cancer 1980;45:1019–1024.
59. Lokich J, Reinhold R, Silverman M, et al. Complications of peritoneovenous shunt for malignant ascites. Cancer Treat Rep 1980;64:305–309.
60. Downing R, Black J, Windsor CW. Palliation of malignant ascites by the Denver peritoneovenous shunt. Ann R Coll Surg Engl 1984;66:340–343.
61. Lund RH, Moritz MW. Complications of Denver peritoneovenous shunting. Arch Surg 1982;117:924–928.
62. Qazi R, Savlov ED. Peritoneovenous shunt for palliation of malignant ascites. Cancer 1982;49:600–602.
63. Cheung DK, Raaf JH. Selection of patients with malignant ascites for a peritoneovenous shunt. Cancer 1982;50:1204–1209.
64. Reinhold RB, Lokich JJ, Tamashefski J, et al. Management of malignant ascites with peritoneovenous shunting. Am J Surg 1983;145:455–457.
65. Souter RG, Tarin D, Kettlewell MGW. Peritoneovenous shunts in the management of malignant ascites. Br J Surg 1983;70:478–481.
66. Gough IR. Control of malignant ascites by peritoneovenous shunting. Cancer 1984;54: 2226–2230.
67. Kostroff KM, Ross DW, Davis JM. Peritoneovenous shunting for cirrhotic versus malignant ascites. Surg Gynecol Obstet 1985;161:204–208.
68. Campioni N, Pasquali, Lasagni RP, Vitucci C, et al. Peritoneovenous shunt and neoplastic ascites: A 5 year experience report. J Surg Oncol 1986;33:31–35.
69. Sonnenfeld T, Tyden G. Peritoneovenous shunts for malignant ascites. Acta Chir Scand 1986;152:117–121.
70. Roussel JGJ, Kroon BBR, Hart GAM. The Denver type for peritoneovenous shunting of malignant ascites. Surg Gynecol Obstet 1986;162:235–240.
71. Soderlund C. Denver peritoneovenous shunting for malignant or cirrhotic ascites. Scand J Gastroenterol 1986;21:1161–1172.
72. Shepherd KE, Miller BJ. Peritoneovenous shunts—Devices of last resort. Can J Surg 1988;31:444–447.
73. Edney JA, Hill A, Armstrong D. Peritoneovenous shunts palliate malignant ascites. Am J Surg 1989;158:598–601.
74. Smith DAP, Weaver DW, Bouman DL. Peritoneovenous shunts (PVS) for malignant ascites: An analysis of outcome. Am Surg 1989;55:445–449.
75. Hyde GL, Dillon M, Bivins BA. Peritoneal venous shunting for ascites: A 15 year perspective. Am Surg 1982;48:123–127.
76. Holman JM, Albo D Jr. Peritoneovenous shunting in patients with malignant ascites. Am J Surg 1981;142:774–776.
77. LeVeen HH, Vujic I, D'Ovidio NG, Hutto RB. Peritoneovenous shunt occlusion—Etiology, diagnosis and therapy. Ann Surg 1984;200:212–223.
78. Souter RG, Wells C, Tarin D, et al. Surgical and pathologic complications associated with peritoneovenous shunting in the management of malignant ascites. Cancer 1985;55: 1973–1978.
79. Ragni MV, Lewis JH, Spero JA. Ascites-induced LeVeen shunt coagulopathy. Ann Surg 1983;198:91–95.
80. Schwartz ML, Swaim WR, Vogel SB. Coagulopathy following peritoneovenous shunting. Surgery 1979;85:671–676.
81. Harmon DC, Demirjian Z, Ellman L, Fischer JE. Disseminated intravascular coagulation with the peritoneovenous shunt. Ann Intern Med 1979;90:774–776.
82. Glysteen JJ, Hussey CV, Heckman MG. The cause of coagulopathy after peritoneovenous shunt for malignant ascites. Arch Surg 1990;125:474–477.
83. Tempero MA, Davis RB, Reed E, et al. Thrombocytopenia and laboratory evidence of disseminated intravascular coagulation after shunts for ascites in malignant disease. Cancer 1985;55:2718–2721.
84. Maat B, Osterlee J, Sapps JAJ, et al. Dissemination of tumor cells via LeVeen shunt. Lancet 1979;1:988.
85. Smith RRL, Sternberg SS, Paglia MA, et al. Fatal pulmonary tumor embolization following peritoneovenous shunting for malignant ascites. J Surg Oncol 1981;16:27–35.
86. Tarin D, Price JE, Kettlewell MGW, et al. Mechanisms of human tumor metastasis studied in patients with peritoneovenous shunts. Cancer Res 1984;44:3584–3592.
87. Tarin D, Vass ACR, Kettlewell MGW, et al. Absence of metastatic sequellae during long term treatment of malignant ascites by peritoneo-venous shunting. Invasion Metastasis 1984;4:1–12.
88. Berger A, Goldberg MI. Subcutaneous cancer growth complicating the peritoneovenous shunting of malignant ascites. Surgery 1983;93:374–376.

Cancer: Principles & Practice of Oncology, Fourth Edition,
edited by Vincent T. DeVita, Jr., Samuel Hellman, Steven A. Rosenberg.
J.B. Lippincott Co., Philadelphia © 1993.

CHAPTER 62

Bone Marrow Dysfunction in the Cancer Patient

SECTION 1 Use of Blood and Blood Products

RALPH O. WALLERSTEIN, JR
ALBERT B. DEISSEROTH

As the intensity of cancer chemotherapy has increased, the need for skilled use of blood and blood products has increased. The improved technologies for leukocyte depletion, testing of blood products for infectious agents and for preventing their transmission, and for the collection and manipulation of bone marrow and peripheral blood stem cells must be understood by the practicing oncologist.

ERYTHROCYTE TRANSFUSION

INDICATIONS

The indications for erythrocyte transfusion depend on the physiologic status of the host, the cause of anemia, and the rate of development of the anemia. Before ordering a transfusion, it is useful to recall that anemia is a laboratory finding (*i.e.*, hemoglobin <2 SD below normal for the population group being studied) for which an explanation should be sought and not a diagnosis. It is not sufficient to attribute the anemia to cancer. A minimal evaluation should include review of the mean corpuscular volume, the reticulocyte count, and the morphology of the peripheral smear and determination of the platelet count, leukocyte count, and differential count.[1] A systematic approach to the laboratory evaluation of anemia ensures appropriate specific therapy and prevents serious morbidity due to delayed diagnosis, such as autoimmune hemolytic anemia complicating lymphoma or chronic lymphocytic leukemia or hemolytic-uremic syndrome after bone marrow transplantation or administration of mitomycin C.

Most patients tolerate a hemoglobin level of 10 g/dl. Because cardiac output begins to increase as the hemoglobin drops below 10 g/dl, patients with cardiopulmonary, renal, hepatic, or cerebral vascular disease should be maintained at or above this level. Younger patients may tolerate a hemoglobin as low as 6 or 7 g/dl, but most cancer patients are transfused when their hemoglobin is 8 g/dl or less.

For most transfusions, the physician should order packed cells. The use of specific blood components rather than whole blood limits the volume of the transfusion and allows the plasma and platelets to be used for other patients. In patients who are expected to have a chronic transfusion requirement over many years, such as those with myelodysplasia of the refractory anemia or refractory anemia with ringed sideroblasts subtypes, prophylactic desferrioxamine therapy should be considered.

ADVERSE REACTIONS

The most common reactions after transfusion of erythrocytes are fever and chills (Table 62–1). Most fevers are caused by febrile nonhemolytic transfusion reactions (FNHTRs) due to antibodies in the recipient directed against granulocyte-specific and HLA antigens on leukocytes in the donor blood.[2]

TABLE 62–1. Differential Diagnosis of Acute Transfusion Reactions

Symptoms	*Possible Diagnosis*
Fever and chills	Major hemolytic transfusion reaction
	Reaction to foreign HLA and granulocyte-specific antigens on transfused leukocytes and platelets
Dyspnea	Fluid overload
	Major hemolytic transfusion reaction
	Contaminated blood
	Air embolism
	Anaphylactic reaction due to transfusion of IgA-containing plasma to IgA-deficient recipient with anti-IgA
Bleeding	Disseminated intravascular coagulation due to major hemolytic transfusion reaction or contaminated blood
	Thrombocytopenia due to massive transfusion of packed erythrocytes
	Washout of coagulation factors due to massive transfusion of packed erythrocytes
Arrhythmia	Circulatory overload
	Hyperkalemia
	Hyperthermia
	Hypocalcemia
	Major hemolytic transfusion reaction
	Contaminated blood
	Air embolism
Hypotension	Major hemolytic transfusion reaction
	Contaminated blood
	Anaphylaxis due to IgA deficiency
Hemoglobinuria	Major hemolytic transfusion reaction
	Excessive infusion pressure through small-bore needle
	Overheating with blood warmer
	Contaminated blood

In most cases, the chills do not start until at least 30 minutes into the transfusion and often not until 1 to 2 hours into the transfusion. These FNHTRs are uncommon in children but may occur in 20% of multiparous females due to prior sensitization and in as many as 79% of multiply transfused patients. Although these reactions can be treated or in some cases prevented by the use of acetaminophen before transfusion, some patients still experience recurrent severe chills and fever with packed erythrocytes. For these patients, the use of leukocyte-poor or leukocyte-depletion methods is indicated.

A unit of packed cells contains about 1 to 3×10^9 leukocytes, depending on the donor's white count. If leukocyte contamination is reduced to less than 5×10^8 per unit, the incidence of chill or fever reactions is markedly reduced.[3] This one-log reduction of leukocytes may be accomplished by several means, including differential centrifugation, freezing with glycerol as a cryoprotectant (which appears to protect only the erythrocytes so that the leukocytes are lysed) followed by washing to remove the leukocyte debris, or use of leukocyte depletion filters. Leukocyte depletion filters may be employed at the time of collection, in the blood bank before issuing, or at the bedside. By preventing granulocyte disintegration, which occurs during the first 2 days of storage, depletion at the time of collection may decrease the amount of soluble granulocyte membrane antigens in the plasma. It is possible that these soluble antigens account for some of the chill and fever reactions that continue to occur despite leukocyte filtration at the time of administration. The current generation of leukocyte depletion filters result in a 99.3% to 99.5% depletion (2 logs) with 87.4% to 92.2% erythrocyte recovery.[4] For patients who still experience severe chill or fever reactions with leukocyte-depleted erythrocytes, a trial of frozen deglycerolized erythrocytes should be considered.

The physician must always consider the possibility of a major hemolytic transfusion reaction in the differential diagnosis of chill and fever reactions, particularly if the chills occur in the first 30 minutes, if the patient is nulliparous and has never been transfused, or if there are other associated systemic symptoms like low back pain, chest pain, restlessness, dyspnea, and pain at the site of transfusion. Signs include tachycardia, hypotension, oliguria, hemoglobinuria, tachypnea, and generalized bleeding (if disseminated intravascular coagulation [DIC] has developed). Most major hemolytic transfusion reactions result from human error, particularly at the time the clot is drawn for type and crossmatch tests if the specimen is mislabelled.

Bacterial contamination is another cause for chill and fever reactions, and the onset may be acute or delayed, depending on the amount of contamination and whether the bacteria have produced a toxin. Contamination of packed erythrocytes is uncommon because of the rigorous antiseptic techniques used in blood collection, the storage of blood at 4°C, and the natural antibacterial properties of blood. Bacterial contamination is more of a problem with platelets, because they are stored at room temperature. Nevertheless, certain cryopathic organisms, mostly gram-negative organisms, can proliferate at 4°C. Several cases of *Yersinia enterocolitica* (which can cause minimal symptoms in the donor even when bacteremic and which can proliferate at 4°C) sepsis transmitted by transfusion have been reported, some of which were fatal.[5–6] Aber recommended excluding donors with gastrointestinal symptoms in the 4 weeks before donation and minimizing the period of storage at 4°C as a means of risk reduction, although others have been concerned that this would exclude many potential donors.[7] It does seem prudent to consider bacterial contamination in the differential diagnosis of severe chill and fever reactions, to obtain blood cultures of the patient and the unit of blood, and to consider empiric antibiotic coverage pending the results of culture.

Allergic reactions, including urticaria and hives, may occur in 3% to 5% of transfused patients. Some of these reactions are due to recipient antibodies against immunoglobulin components or other soluble proteins in the plasma. The best defined of these reactions occurs in patients with congenital deficiency of IgA (1 of 800 people). Some of these patients develop IgG or IgE antibodies against IgA, and when transfused with any blood product containing even small amounts of plasma, they may develop severe allergic or even fatal anaphylactic reactions. These patients should receive extensively washed erythrocytes or preferably blood from IgA-deficient donors. Most urticarial reactions, however, occur in non-IgA-deficient recipients and are rarely life threatening. The transfusion is temporarily stopped, the patient is treated with intravenous diphenhydramine, and the transfusion is resumed in 30 minutes. If the allergic reactions recur or increase, transfusion of that unit should be discontinued and further use of that donor for that patient stopped. Such urticarial reactions generally do not recur. For the few patients who experience recurrent or severe urticarial reactions, the physician should measure the quantitative immunoglobulins to exclude IgA deficiency and order washed erythrocytes from which virtually all of the plasma has been removed (Table 62–2).

TRANSFUSION-INDUCED GRAFT-VERSUS-HOST DISEASE

All blood products given to severely immunocompromised patients should be treated with 1500 cGy of gamma radiation to prevent viable T lymphocytes from causing transfusion-induced graft-versus-host disease (GVHD) in the recipient.[8,9] The clinical manifestations of GVHD when caused by transfusion include the rash, diarrhea, and abnormal liver function seen after allogeneic bone marrow transplant. In addition,

TABLE 62–2. Blood Component Therapy Indications and Complications

Component	*Indications*	*Complications*
Packed erythrocytes	Anemia	Fever, volume overload, hepatitis and other infections
		Urticaria, hemolytic transfusion reaction
Leukocyte-poor packed erythrocytes	Prior febrile reactions to packed erythrocytes	Increased viscosity
	May delay alloimmunization	
Washed or plasma-poor packed erythrocytes	Prior urticarial reactions, IgA deficiency, need to avoid complement transfusion	
Frozen packed erythrocytes	Rare blood types, autologous donations, process also removes leukocytes and plasma	
Whole blood	None	
Random-donor platelets	Bleeding with platelet count $<100,000/mm^3$, bleeding and qualitative platelet dysfunction	Fever
		Urticaria
	Elective surgery and thrombocytopenia	Hepatitis
	Prophylactic for platelets $<10,000–20,000/mm^3$	Bacterial contamination
Single-donor platelets	May delay alloimmunization	
	Lower risk of infection because exposed to one donor	
Leukoctye-poor platelets	Prior febrile reactions to packed erythrocytes or platelets	
HLA-matched single-donor platelets	Poor response to platelet transfusion due to alloimmunization	
Autologous frozen platelets	Refractoriness to HLA-matched platelets	
Granulocytes	Documented bacterial infection not responding to appropriate antibiotics, with severe neutropenia not expected to recover for several days.	Fever
Respiratory distress		
Alloimmunization		
Fresh-frozen plasma	Coagulation factor deficiency, including rapid warfarin reversal with plasmapheresis for TTP	Hepatitis and other infections
Volume overload		Hypernatremia
Cryoprecipitate	Severe von Willebrand's disease	Hypocalcemia
Hepatitis and other infections	Hypofibrinogenemia	
	Uremic bleeding	
Intravenous immunoglobulin	Hypogammaglobulinemia	Systemic reactions
	Idiopathic thrombocytopenic purpura	Local venous reaction
	Bleeding and alloimmunization, even to HLA-matched platelets	Anaphylaxis
	Passive immunization	
	Prevention of GVH	
Heat-treated lyophilized factor VIII	Hemophilia A	
Non-A, non-B hepatitis		
Heat-treated lyophilized prothrombin	Hemophilia B	
Non-A, non-B hepatitis complex	Factor VIII inhibitor	Thrombosis
Albumin	Volume expansion	

pancytopenia occurs because the hematopoietic cells are foreign to the attacking lymphocytes, but in allogeneic transplant the attacking lymphocytes and marrow are both of donor origin. There is no effective treatment, and the mortality is 85% to 90% after a median of 21 days.

Lymphocyte proliferation in response to allogeneic cells is completely abolished after 500 cGy. After 1500 cGy, there was a 90% reduction in mitogen-stimulated ^{14}C-thymidine incorporation in one study and an 85% reduction in mitogen-induced blast transformation in another. A dose of 5000 cGy decreased these to 97% and 98.5%, respectively.

Other cells are less sensitive than lymphocytes to irradiation. Erythrocytes are unaffected by doses up to 20,000 cGy, but platelets may suffer after exposure to 5000 cGy. Granulocyte function may be affected above 2000 to 5000 cGy. Although 500 cGy may be sufficient to inhibit some lymphocyte functions, a dose of 1500 cGy provides a safe and effective dose, and there have been no documented transfusion-related GVHD cases reported from large centers using this dose. Although there have been no adverse reactions reported from the use of irradiated blood products, their use is associated with additional expense, because the cost of the irradiator and the radiation source is $50,000. Irradiated pluripotent stem cells may survive with sublethal damage, which may allow mutated stem cells to survive. Although the likelihood of harm is remote, because of theoretical concerns and real cost concerns, irradiated blood products should only be used for the specific indications mentioned.

Patients at risk of GVHD include those with profound immunosuppression due to cancer and its treatment, such as allogeneic and autologous (especially with total-body irradiation [TBI] in the preparative regimen) transplant recipients, those undergoing combined modality treatment for Hodgkin's and non-Hodgkin's lymphoma, patients with acute lymphocytic leukemia, those with congenital immunodeficiency, and neonatal patients receiving large volume exchange transfusions. GVHD has occurred in patients with Hodgkin's disease receiving chemotherapy alone. Fatal transfusion-induced graft-versus-host disease may occur in nonimmunocompromised patients, if the blood donor is homozygous for one of the HLA haplotypes of the recipient. This situation is most likely to occur with designated donor transfusions from first-degree relatives or in geographic areas with less genetic diversity.

Other possible complications of transfusions are listed in Table 62–3. The signs and symptoms of a major hemolytic transfusion reaction have been discussed. If the reaction is suspected, the physician should stop the blood transfusion immediately and notify the blood bank. Verification of the identification on the blood unit and the patient should be sought. Remaining blood in the bag should be returned to the blood bank, and repeat blood samples should be drawn from the recipient to repeat the type and crossmatch and to determine if there is pink or brown plasma that would indicate hemoglobinemia. A urine sample should be tested for hemoglobinuria. If the plasma is pink or brown, suggesting intravascular hemolysis has occurred, the physician should order tests for DIC, including partial thromboplastin time (PTT), platelet count, fibrinogen, fibrin monomer, and fibrin-split products. If the patient is bleeding and has DIC, replace clotting factors and platelets if a significant deficiency is documented. Blood pressure should be maintained with intravenous fluids and

TABLE 62–3. Complications of Transfusion

Fever or chills
Allergy
Urticaria
Anaphylaxis
Infection
Hepatitis
Human immunodeficiency virus
Cytomegalovirus
Bacterial contamination
Parasites
Volume overload
Major hemolytic transfusion reaction
Delayed hemolytic transfusion reaction
Graft-versus-host disease
Posttransfusion purpura
Hypocalcemia
Hyperkalemia
Hypothermia
Respiratory distress
Iron overload
Air embolism
Alloimmunization

pressors, and a urine output greater than 100 ml/hour should be maintained with intravenous fluids. If needed, mannitol or Lasix should be used to prevent oliguric acute tubular necrosis. The physician should monitor input, output, and serum electrolytes, blood urea nitrogen (BUN), and creatinine. A nephrologist should be consulted if renal failure occurs. Most major hemolytic transfusion reactions are due to a clerical error, which occurs at the time the initial blood type and crossmatch sample is drawn and labeled.

Delayed hemolytic transfusion reactions occasionally occur if the recipient has a titer of alloantibody that is too low to be detected in the antibody screen and crossmatching procedure but develops a strong anamnestic antibody response that causes a fall in hemoglobin and an increase in bilirubin and lactate dehydrogenase (LDH) 5 to 10 days after transfusion. This is particularly common for alloantibodies to antigens of the Kidd blood group system.[10]

Patients who develop profound thrombocytopenia 5 to 8 days after transfusion should be suspected of having posttransfusion purpura. Two percent of people lack the platelet antigen $P1^{A1}$. $P1^{A1}$-negative patients, when transfused with blood containing platelets or soluble platelet antigen, particularly if they have been previously immunized by prior transplacental contamination from a $P1^{A1}$-positive fetus or by prior transfusion, may develop severe thrombocytopenia. The intriguing aspect is that the patient's own $P1^{A1}$-negative platelets are destroyed as well, a process that may continue for several weeks if untreated. Suspected cases of posttransfusion purpura are confirmed by measuring antibody to $P1^{A1}$ in the recipient's serum. Plasmapheresis is the treatment of choice for this problem. The cause of the destruction of the patient's own platelets is unclear. Some investigators suspect that the $P1^{A1}$ antigen is soluble and circulates and binds to the patient's own platelets, causing their destruction. Other investigators feel that the development of the alloantibody to $P1^{A1}$ causes the simultaneous development of an autoantibody.

Although massive transfusions (>10 units in 1–6 hours) have been associated with hypocalcemia, hyperkalemia, hypothermia, and bleeding due to coagulation factor and platelet washout, these reactions are relatively uncommon in patients with cancer. Low levels of ionized calcium are due to the citrate in the anticoagulated packed erythrocytes. Except in severe liver dysfunction, citrate usually is rapidly metabolized. Although stored erythrocytes progressively increase the extracellular potassium concentration, it is unusual to see clinical hyperkalemia, except with renal failure. Coagulation factor washout has occurred in patients with trauma, in whom accelerated consumption due to DIC is probably more of a factor than dilution. Prophylactic transfusion of fresh-frozen plasma is not indicated, but the decision should be guided by the PT and activated PTT. Platelet washout is a potential problem with massive transfusion, but the physician should follow the specific platelet count as a guide to platelet repletion.

TRANSMISSION OF INFECTIOUS AGENTS

Bacterial contamination has already been discussed. Other infections that may be transmitted through blood include human immunodeficiency virus (HIV); hepatitis A, B, or C; cytomegalovirus (CMV); human T-cell lymphotropic virus type I (HTLV-I); and parasites.

The risk of HIV infection in a recipient of blood from an infected donor is substantial. Perkins and colleagues identified patients with newly diagnosed acquired immunodeficiency syndrome (AIDS) reported to the San Francisco Public Health Department who had donated blood before the diagnosis of AIDS.[11] Sixty-two percent of the recipients of blood from these donors showed evidence of infection, including recipients of whole blood, erythrocytes, platelet concentrates, and fresh-frozen plasma. The closer the donation was given before the diagnosis of AIDS in the donor, the higher the risk of infection. Nine of 10 recipients from donations given in the 12 months immediately before AIDS diagnoses became infected. Recipients younger than 11 years of age or older than 79 were more likely to have developed AIDS or AIDS-related complex (ARC) at the time of follow-up.[12] Other investigators reported an 89% incidence of infection after transfusion of HIV-seropositive blood. A recent projection by Medley suggests that the mean incubation period for transfusion associated with AIDS is 1.97 years for children younger than 5 and 8.23 years for persons 5 to 59 years old.[13]

HIV infection from blood transfusion has been significantly reduced because blood banks excluded high-risk groups from donating in March 1983 and began screening donated blood for antibody to HIV in the spring of 1985. The physician must be alert for the development of HIV-related disorders in patients transfused between 1976 and 1985, with the peak risk of transmission occurring in 1982 with an estimated risk of 1.1% per transfused unit.[14] Because some donors acutely infected with HIV may not develop an antibody response for a few weeks or months, the risk of acquiring HIV infection from blood products, although quite small (Table 62–4), is not zero.[15]

A recent report from the Centers for Disease Control found

TABLE 62–4. Risk of Viral Infection From Blood Products

Infection	*Risk (%)*
Human immunodeficiency virus	<0.001
Hepatitis C	0.1

(Herbert A. Perkins, MD, personal communication)

an overall prevalence of HIV positivity among blood donors of only 0.038%.[16] Improvements in methods to exclude persons at risk (*e.g.*, avoiding pressure to donate in blood drives) should reduce the number of persons who are infected but not yet antibody positive.[17] Improvements in the sensitivity of the enzyme immunoassay (EIA) are possible by detection of IgM or IgA to HIV in addition to the IgG that current kits detect.[18] In a report of 127 persons who were positive by EIA, 95 were positive on repeat EIA, and 32 were negative on repeat testing.[19] Of the 95 repeatedly positive, 9 were positive by Western blot, 31 were indeterminate, and 55 were negative. EIA was repeated 3 to 12 months later. All 32 who were negative on the initial repeat by EIA remained negative. All 55 who were HIV positive by EIA but negative by Western blot remained negative. Of the 31 indeterminate, 1 tested positive by polymerase chain reaction (PCR) amplification of conserved sequences of HIV specific nucleic acids (*i.e.*, *POL* gene) and subsequently converted to positive on Western blot when retested 3 to 12 months later. All 9 who were HIV positive by EIA and by Western blot were also positive by PCR amplification. Patients who are HIV positive but indeterminate by Western Blot should be periodically retested. PCR testing, although expensive and labor intensive, remains of interest in the evaluation of patients with equivocal results or those who may be passively antibody positive (*e.g.*, newborns of infected mothers).

The incidence of posttransfusion hepatitis depends on the effort taken to detect hepatitis, the adequacy of follow-up of patients, and the prevalence of the disease in the donor population. Before 1986, it was estimated that the incidence of posttransfusion hepatitis was 5% to 20%. At that time, many blood banks instituted a new policy of testing donated blood for elevations of alanine aminotransferase (ALT) and hepatitis B core antibody as "surrogate markers" for non-A, non-B hepatitis. In 1989, the hepatitis C virus (HCV) was isolated, and an enzyme linked immunoassay for a nonstructural antigen of HCV was approved by the FDA in May 1990. Because seroconversion to antibody positivity may take up to 1 year, the continued use of surrogate testing has been advocated. Recent estimates suggest that 91% of cases of posttransfusion non-A, non-B hepatitis are caused by HCV.[20]

HTLV-I is an RNA tumor virus that appears to cause adult T-cell leukemia-lymphoma and tropical spastic paraparesis.[21] The lifetime risk for HTLV-I-positive persons is estimated to be 2% to 5% for adult T-cell leukemia-lymphoma and 0.25% for the neurologic disorder.[22] In November 1988, a serologic test for HTLV-I was approved by the FDA. This test also detects HTLV-II, which has not been proven to cause any disease, although the ability to differentiate between the two viruses is fairly recent and more data are necessary to determine the effects of HTLV-II. Both viruses can be transmitted through transfusions. Erythrocytes stored for less than 4 days and platelets may be particularly infections due to the death of infected lymphocytes during prolonged refrigerator storage.[23] The ability of leukocyte depletion filters to prevent transmission is currently an area of research.

Because blood banks now routinely screen donors for HTLV-I and notify them of the results and because of the small but documented long-term risk of HTLV-I, three methods have been developed to differentiate HTLV-I from HTLV-II.[22] One method looks at the differential Western blot reactivity to specific viral antigens; reactivity to HTLV-I p19 antigen equal to or greater than to p24 favors HTLV-I, but if p24 is greater than p19, HTLV-II is favored. A second method uses an enzyme-linked immunoassay for HTLV-I gp46^{env} or HTLV-II gp52^{env}. The "gold standard" method uses PCR amplification in the viral regulatory genes with sequence-specific oligonucleotide hybridization to differentiate the two viruses.

The use of leukocyte filtration of blood products appears to decrease the transmissibility of CMV and possibly other viruses.[24–28] Although CMV primary infection and reactivation are of most concern in allogeneic transplantation, CMV interstitial pneumonitis does occur after autologous transplantation. It is likely that CMV contributes significantly to unexplained fevers, hepatitis, gastroenteritis, immunosuppression, and delayed hematopoietic recovery, which complicate intensive therapy. For CMV-negative recipients of allogeneic marrow from CMV-negative donors, the exclusive use of CMV-negative blood almost totally prevents CMV infection and pneumonitis. Even after CMV-negative patients receive allogeneic bone marrow transplants from CMV-positive donors, 25% do not seroconvert.[29]

Theoretically, a rationale for limiting CMV exposure through blood exists for this group. As high-dose therapy with autologous bone marrow transplantation (particularly when TBI is part of the preparative regimen) becomes more widely applied in the treatment of relapsed or refractory Hodgkin's and non-Hodgkin's lymphoma and solid tumors (*e.g.*, breast cancer, ovarian cancer), CMV infection and interstitial pneumonia are growing problems. Because the availability of exclusively CMV-negative blood products is limited, alternative strategies are necessary to support CMV-negative patients who are undergoing intensive therapy or who may undergo intensive therapy in the future. It is our policy to routinely leukocyte filter all blood products for these patients to decrease the likelihood or prevent primary CMV infection. We continue to provide CMV-negative blood products with intravenous IgG for CMV-negative allogeneic patients. Even in these patients, there may be a rationale for leukocyte depletion, depending on the rate of false-negative CMV serologies (reported sensitivities of the serologic tests are 89–93%) in the donor population.

Parasite transmission through blood transfusion is uncommon in the United States. As a result of excluding donors who have been in endemic malarial areas, only about 3 cases per year of transfusion-transmitted malaria occur in the United States.[30] Babesiosis transmission appears to be even less common. Travelers to the Middle East, including service personnel who served in Operation Desert Storm, are being excluded from donation because of the risk of leishmaniasis, which is transmitted by the bite of the sand fly. Transfusion-transmitted Chagas' disease, particularly in immunocompromised patients, is of some concern, even though the documented cases are few, because of the increasing number of Central and South Americans emigrating to this country.[31] In areas with a high prevalence of at-risk donors, a combination of donor screening with questions and serologic evaluation has been implemented.

PLATELET TRANSFUSIONS

INDICATIONS

Platelet transfusions are indicated for prophylaxis or treatment of bleeding due to decreased number or function of platelets. As with anemia, it is important to have a systematic method for the laboratory evaluation of the bleeding patient to direct specific therapy and avoid missing factors contributing to the bleeding.[32]

The bleeding time increases linearly as the platelet count falls from 100,000 to 10,000, below which it tends to be prolonged indefinitely.[33] If the platelet count is greater than 100,000 and the bleeding time is prolonged, the patient has von Willebrand's disease or a qualitative platelet defect.[34,35] If von Willebrand's disease has been excluded by normal factor VIII antigen, factor VIII activity, ristocetin cofactor activity, and multimer analysis, the patient has a qualitative platelet defect. Patients with life-threatening bleeding due to a qualitative platelet defect should be given a platelet transfusion. For patients with qualitative platelet dysfunction due to uremia, transfused platelets will acquire the same qualitative defect, and the treatment of choice is vigorous hemodialysis. For patients already being dialyzed, desmopressin acetate (DDAVP) or cryoprecipitate may be useful. For patients with other than life-threatening bleeding due to qualitative platelet dysfunction, a trial of DDAVP is indicated because it is not associated with the risk of viral infection seen with cryoprecipitate and platelets.[36]

In 1962, Gaydos and coworkers documented a quantitative relation between platelet counts and hemorrhages in patients with acute leukemia (Fig. 62–1).[37] In these patients, the incidence of hemorrhage of any kind, including gross hemorrhage, rose dramatically as platelet counts declined, especially to levels less than 20,000/mm^3. They also observed that bleeding episodes associated with thrombocytopenia frequently follow a decline in platelet count. They reported that of 8 patients with intracranial hemorrhage unassociated with high blast counts and intracerebral leukostasis, 7 patients had platelet counts of less than 5000/mm^3. No intracranial bleeding was observed at a platelet count of 10,000/mm^3 or more.

Retrospective and prospective studies have shown a decreased incidence of bleeding episodes when platelets were transfused prophylactically for patients with platelet counts less than 20,000 to 30,000/mm^3 (Table 62–5).[38] At any given level, patients with thrombocytopenia due to decreased platelet production have a more prolonged bleeding time than patients with thrombocytopenia due to increased destruction, probably because with accelerated destruction there is usually accelerated production and release of young, hemostatically effective platelets. In the case of decreased production, the circulating platelets are several days old and less effective.

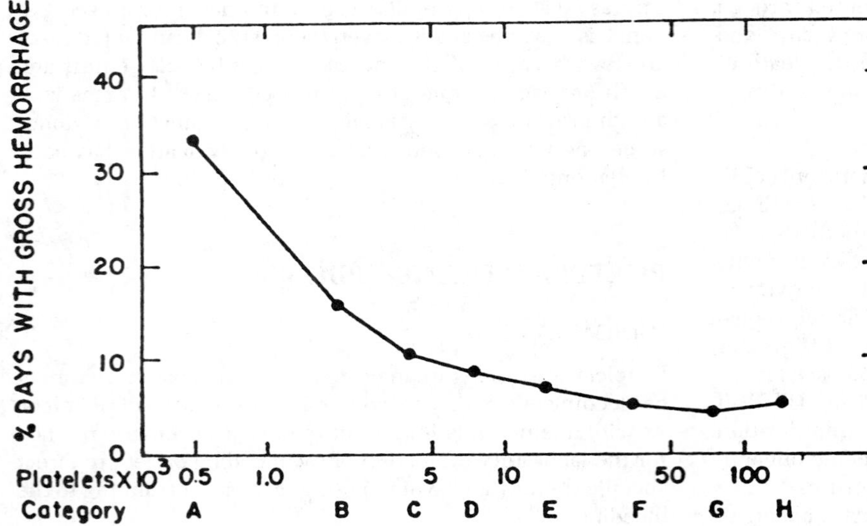

FIGURE 62–1. Relation between platelet counts and the number of days patients had grossly visible hemorrhage. Capital letters along the abscissa refer to the following categories of platelet counts: A, less than 1000/mm^3; B, 1000–3000/mm^3; C, 3000–5000/mm^3; D, 5000–10,000/mm^3; E, 10,000–20,000/mm^3; F, 20,000–50,000/mm^3; G, 50,000–100,000/mm^3; H, >100,000/mm^3.

The benefit of preventing bleeding by prophylactic platelet transfusions must be balanced against the risk of the patient developing alloantibodies to the transfused platelets, and if bleeding occurs in the future, transfused platelets may be less effective. In practice, when thrombocytopenia is expected to be limited (*e.g.*, induction chemotherapy for acute leukemia), prophylactic platelet transfusions are given to keep the platelet count above 10,000 to 20,000/mm^3. For chronic thrombocytopenia (*e.g.*, myelodysplasia) most clinicians reserve platelet transfusions for bleeding episodes.

Platelets are prepared from differential centrifugation of donated whole blood or from platelet pheresis of single donors. Platelet concentrates can be administered through a standard blood bank filter (170 micropore size) during 10 to 20 minutes. Because platelets are stored at room temperature, small amounts of contaminating microorganisms present on day 1 may reach high titers by days 5 to 7.[39–41] At some major centers, platelet concentrates became the major source for transfusion-induced sepsis, and storage of platelets beyond 5 days is no longer permitted.[42]

ALLOIMMUNIZATION

A major limitation to the prevention of bleeding through the use of prophylactic platelet transfusions is the development of platelet alloimmunization. The likelihood of platelet alloimmunization may be decreased for diseases and treatments that decrease the immune response. For example, the incidence in acute lymphocytic leukemia and lymphoma patients undergoing intensive therapy is less than for patients with aplastic anemia or autotransplants for breast cancer.[43] HLA exposure through prior transfusions or pregnancy increases the incidence of alloimmunization. Individual immune response genes appear important, because the occurrence of alloimmunization has been reported to be independent of the number of transfusions and tends to occur within the first few weeks if it is going to occur at all.[44]

Development of alloimmunization requires the presence of class I antigens and class II antigens. Platelets alone do not result in the development of antibodies because they carry only class I HLA antigens and platelet-specific antigens. The class II antigens necessary for the development of alloimmunization are provided by monocytes, lymphocytes, and dendritic cells.[45,46] Although not rigorously proven, it appears that if the number of leukocytes can be reduced to less than 10^6 per bag of platelets and erythrocytes, alloimmunization to platelets can be markedly delayed or prevented.[50–64] Another approach to preventing alloimmunization under investigation is ultraviolet irradiation.[65–70]

For patients who become refractory to random-donor platelets, single-donor platelets are used. For patients refractory to single-donor platelets, partial HLA matching may identify donors who will provide a better increment. In the absence of facilities for HLA typing, if several different single donors are tried and posttransfusion increments measured, a donor may be found empirically whose platelets are less rapidly destroyed. For allogeneic bone marrow transplantation, the marrow donor may be used as the source of HLA-identical platelet transfusions after the preparative regimen has begun. Some centers are developing methods for platelet cross-matching for alloimmunized patients.[71] After every platelet transfusion, a repeat platelet counts should be obtained within 10 to 60 minutes after transfusion and 24 hours later.[72] A poor increment ($<10,000/\mu l/m^2$ of body surface area per unit of platelets) at 1 hour is seen with splenomegaly or alloimmunization. A good 1-hour count that returns to baseline by 24 hours is much less specific and can be seen with bleeding, infection, poor-quality platelets, autoimmune or drug-induced immune thrombocytopenia, DIC, or any cause for accelerated platelet consumption.[47–49]

An alternative approach for patients who have recovered from a cycle of therapy during which they demonstrated platelet refractoriness is to collect and cryopreserve autologous platelets while in remission.[73,74] Over time, patients who have been previously refractory to random-donor or single-donor platelets may lose their alloimmunization, possibly as a result of disease progression, intensive therapy, or natural antibody decline with time, and it is worthwhile to periodically transfuse these patients and measure their 1-hour and 24-hour posttransfusion increments.

TABLE 62–5. Transfusion Guidelines for Commonly Encountered Hematologic Problems

Chronic Anemia

No significant cardiopulmonary compromise; stable patient.

No absolute indication for transfusion if hemoglobin is above 6 to 7 g/100 mg.

Consider transfusion for otherwise unexplained lassitude, malaise, tachycardia, dyspnea in association with hemoglobin less than 9 to 10 g/100 ml.

Cardiopulmonary disease; fever, surgery. Maintain hemoglobin level at 10 g/100 ml.

If management protracted (years), monitor for evidence of iron overload (secondary hemochromatosis).

Thrombocytopenia

Thrombocytopenia due to failure of platelet production.

Platelet count >20,000/mm^3; stable patient without retinal hemorrhages.

Platelet transfusion probably not necessary.

Platelet count <20,000/mm^3; patient not bleeding: Provide prophylactic platelet transfusion unless thrombocytopenia expected to be chronic, in which case transfuse only for bleeding.

Platelet count <50,000/mm^3; patient bleeding or surgery anticipated: Use local measures to control bleeding; look for defects in coagulation pathways; maintain platelet counts at 50,000/mm^3 or above with transfusion every 12 to 24 hours.

Platelet count <20,000/mm^3; patient refractory to random platelet transfusion: Consider transfusion for evidence of bleeding, if retinal hemorrhages noted, or if platelet count is <10,000/mm^3; use HLA-match platelets.

Granulocytopenia

Patient candidate for aggressive supportive care.

Granulocytes <500/mm^3; afebrile, stable patient: No established indication for granulocyte transfusion.

Granulocytes <500/mm^3; patient febrile, but cultures negative and no clinical evidence of infected area or tissue: No established indication for granulocyte transfusion.

Documented bacterial infection not improving after 48 hours of antibiotics to which the organism is sensitive in a patient with <500 neutrophils/mm^3 and who is expected to have marrow aplasia for more than 1 week: Granulocyte transfusion indicated.

Some patients become refractory to HLA-matched platelets. Although this may be caused by antibodies to platelet-specific antigens, the physician should also consider the possibility of a drug-induced immune thrombocytopenia (*e.g.*, heparin or vancomycin) or the development of an autoantibody.[75] Although small randomized studies have not shown general benefit, high-dose intravenous immunoglobulin (400 mg/kg/day for 5 days) occasionally permits better platelet increments in platelet-refractory patients.[76–78] The patients who benefit possibly have a different mechanism of accelerated platelet destruction than the usual alloimmunized patient. Without a way to prospectively identify those who will benefit, given the minimal disadvantages of intravenous immunoglobulin other than cost, and because there are few alternative approaches,[79,80] an empiric trial of IgG seems reasonable for severely thrombocytopenic platelet refractory patients especially if they are bleeding.[112,113] For patients with no response to intravenous IgG, an empiric trial of plasmapheresis may be tried.

The physician must remain alert for DIC, thrombotic thrombocytopenia purpura (TTP), or hemolytic uremic syndrome (HUS) presenting as refractory thrombocytopenia. Particularly in advanced solid tumors (especially adenocarcinomas) DIC may present with thrombocytopenia, a normal or even short PT and PTT, and a normal or elevated fibrinogen, but the fibrin split products or D-dimer are usually elevated. A HUS-TTP-like syndrome may occur after allogeneic transplantation, possibly related to cyclosporine or TBI, and may mimic platelet refractoriness, but there is a concurrent microangiopathic hemolytic anemia with elevated LDH and schizocytes on the peripheral smear.

GRANULOCYTE TRANSFUSION

The frequency and severity of infection is inversely related to the number of circulating neutrophils and the duration of neutropenia. In 1966, Bodie and coworkers showed that, for patients with acute leukemia, the incidence of infection began to increase as the absolute neutrophil count fell below 1000/mm^3.[81] For patients with breast cancer undergoing chemotherapy, the incidence of infection appears to increase below an absolute neutrophil count of 500/mm^3.[82] It is likely that these differences are related to the immunosuppressive effect of the disease and to the concomitant mucositis often seen with induction therapy of acute leukemia, which increases the likelihood that intestinal bacteria will invade the bloodstream.

With the use of prophylactic platelet transfusions to prevent death due to bleeding, infection is the major cause of death for patients with acute leukemia, for whom pancytopenia lasts for several weeks.[83] There are no data that justify the use of prophylactic granulocyte transfusions. Several older prospective, randomized studies of the use of granulocyte transfusions reported an increase in survival rates, but the aggressive use of more potent antibiotics have markedly diminished the need for granulocyte transfusions.[84–87,99,100] However, for the severely neutropenic patient (<200/mm^3), not expected to recover neutrophil counts for 1 week and with a documented bacterial or fungal infection not responding to appropriate antibiotics, granulocyte transfusions are still indicated. Profoundly neutropenic patients with progressive local infections such as cellulitis or perirectal infections may benefit from granulocyte transfusion.[88–96] For alloimmunized recipients, HLA-matched and granulocyte-compatible donors should be found.[97] CMV-seronegative donors should be used for seronegative recipients.[98] The granulocytes should be irradiated for severely immunosuppressed patients.

INTRAVENOUS IMMUNOGLOBULIN

Intravenous immunoglobulin is used to decrease the incidence of infection in cancer patients with hypogammaglobulinemia or impaired humoral immunity, to prevent and treat cytomegalovirus infection in bone marrow transplant patients, to treat several autoimmune disorders that may complicate particularly hematologic malignancies, and in some other selected situations.

The theoretical basis for the use of intravenous IgG in chronic lymphocytic leukemia, multiple myeloma, and low-grade lymphoma is the hypogammaglobulinemia, impaired antibody response to challenge even in the absence of lowered antibody levels, and possibly IgG subclass deficiency seen in these disorders and the high incidence of infection and death due to infection.[101,102] Because the major randomized study of intravenous IgG in chronic lymphocytic leukemia showed fewer moderate infections (*i.e.*, those requiring oral antibiotics) but not major infections (*e.g.*, those requiring intravenous antibiotics or hospitalization), and in view of the expense ($12,000–$16,000/year cost to the pharmacy) and inconvenience of prophylactic intravenous IgG, it would appear that the use of intravenous IgG should continue to be on a selective basis (*e.g.*, patients with recurrent sinopulmonary infections not responding to prophylactic oral antibiotics).

Another group of patients with apparently diminished B-cell reactivity are patients recovering from autologous or allogeneic bone marrow transplantation. After an uncomplicated allogeneic bone marrow transplantation, the total number of B cells return to normal in about 1 month, but the serum concentrations of IgG and IgM do not return to the normal range until 9 months, apparently due to delayed recovery of helper T cells.[103] Antibody production in response to antigenic stimulation is severely impaired in the first 3 months after allogeneic and syngeneic transplantation, indicating that it is not simply due to GVHD prophylaxis. Patients who develop acute or chronic GVHD experience substantial further delays in immune system reconstitution.

In a randomized prospective trial from Seattle, intravenous IgG (500 mg/kg weekly until day 90 and then monthly until day 360) reduced the incidence grade II through IV acute GVHD in patients older than 20 years of age, but no difference was observed in younger patients, possibly because of the low incidence in this group and the lack of adequate numbers to detect a difference; the results confirmed an earlier study of Winston and colleagues.[104,105] No increase in the rate of relapse or graft rejection was seen in the patients older than 20 in whom there was a reduction in GVHD. For those younger than 20 (in whom there had not been a reduction in GVHD), there was a 78% relapse rate compared with 47% for controls, but this difference appeared to be due to a larger number of advanced-stage patients in the immunoglobulin group. Determining whether the reduction in GVHD comes without an increase in graft rejection or relapse, as is the case with other measures that prevent GVHD, will need further confirmation. The incidence of gram-negative septicemia (positive culture with hypotension), but not bacteremia, was reduced. Overall, there was a reduction in the incidence of local infection from 144 (78%) in 185 control patients to 94 (51%) of 184 treated patients. No effect on the incidence of gram-positive or fungal septicemia was observed. In patients older than 20, there was a substantial reduction in the incidence of interstitial pneumonia (primarily due to CMV). Platelet recovery was accelerated (*i.e.*, median day of last platelet transfusion was 52 days in controls and 31 days in treated) and total platelet transfusion requirement reduced (*i.e.*, control patients required an average of 51 more units of platelets). This study is in line with most studies of intravenous IgG in the bone marrow transplantation setting in not finding a reduction of CMV infection but observing a modification of the severity of disease, primarily a reduced incidence of interstitial pneumonia and death.[106–108]

For CMV-seronegative recipients from CMV-seronegative donors, the exclusive use of CMV-negative blood products markedly reduces the incidence of CMV infection. For most transplants in which the donor or recipient is CMV positive, IgG is considered the standard of practice. There is great interest in the use of leukocyte-depleted blood products to decrease additional CMV exposure and the use of prophylactic ganciclovir to further reduce the incidence and severity of CMV infection. For the treatment of CMV pneumonia, intravenous immunoglobulin is generally given every other day concurrently with twice-daily full-dose ganciclovir. Prior studies had not shown a benefit for either agent alone. Although the ganciclovir prevents viral DNA replication, it does not prevent the host T-cell-mediated response to viral induced antigens on the surface of the lung cells. The IgG in this setting possibly coats the viral antigens or otherwise modifies the immunomediated lung parenchymal damage.

Intravenous immunoglobulin may be useful if autoimmune hemolytic anemia or thrombocytopenia complicate chronic lymphocytic leukemia, low-grade lymphoma, or other hematologic malignancies and for pure red cell aplasia due to persistent parvovirus B19.[109,110]

The consensus is that the current immunoglobulin preparations do not transmit HIV or hepatitis B or C.[114] Because of high levels of hepatitis B antibody, seronegative patients may become passively antibody positive for hepatitis B after infusion. A similar situation probably applies for hepatitis C, but this information is not yet available.

Adverse reactions to intravenous IgG are a function of the rate of infusion and the immunocompetence of the recipient. Overall, fewer than 1% of patients experience adverse reactions to IgG infusion, but approximately 10% of hypogammaglobulinemic patients who receive intravenous IgG for the first time or whose last treatment was over 6 to 8 weeks before infusion experience adverse reactions if the initial flow rate exceeds 1 ml per minute. Flushing of the face, chest tightness, chills, fever, nausea, vomiting, diarrhea, dizziness, wheezing, diaphoresis, and hypotension are the most common symptoms. When such symptoms occur, the infusion should be slowed or stopped. Pretreatment with steroids may be useful in the rare patient with recurrent symptoms. The explanation for the first dose effect is unknown, but it is thought that patients with low levels of immunoglobulin may build up an antigen load and that the first infusion of intravenous IgG results in the formation of a large number of antigen-antibody complexes and complement activation. With subsequent infusions, the rate can be increased, and for selected patients using 12% formulations and dissolving with water instead of saline, it may be possible to administer the IgG in 1 hour or less.[115] Because each lot of IgG is obtained from thousands of donors, any erythrocyte alloantibodies in the donors should be highly diluted, but occasionally, patients develop positive Coombs' tests or have frank hemolysis after IgG infusion.

APHERESIS

INDICATIONS

Apheresis, using the current generation of cell separators, has a limited but specific role to play in the management of malignant disease (Table 62–6).[116–128]

TABLE 62–6. Indications for Apheresis

Technique	*Indications*
Plasmaphersis	Hyperviscosity[114] syndrome in myeloma or Waldenstrom's with staph A column,[124–128] TTP/HUS
Leukapheresis	Hyperleukocytosis,[117] DIC in acute promyelocytic leukemia, CML in pregnancy,[121] to harvest lymphocytes for LAK cell production, for granulocyte transfusions
Platelet pheresis	Thrombocytosis with acute symptoms in polycythemia vera or essential thrombocytosis, for platelet transfusion
Photopheresis	Cutaneous T-cell lymphoma,[123] chronic graft-versus-host disease
Peripheral blood stem cell collection	Source of hematopoietic progenitor cells

In experienced hands, apheresis is a relatively safe procedure with minimal morbidity. Because citrate is used as an anticoagulant, hypocalcemia can develop, which usually manifests as paresthesias but can result in tetany or arrhythmias. Vasovagal reactions can result in hypotension, and this usually responds to volume infusion. If fresh-frozen plasma is used (*e.g.*, in the treatment of TTP), patients can have allergic reactions to the plasma and may acquire viral infections. Because of the catheters used for vascular access, complications may include thrombosis, bleeding, and infection. Overall, the incidence of minor morbidity is approximately 10%. Because at least 10 deaths have been reported with cytopheresis and more than 50 with plasmapheresis, this procedure should be reserved for specific, appropriate indications and only performed under the direction of physicians skilled in the use of this technique.[129,130]

PERIPHERAL BLOOD STEM CELLS

One of the newest and most exciting uses for apheresis is for the collection of peripheral blood stem cells (PBSC). Studies in the 1970s in mice, dogs, and humans demonstrated hematopoietic stem cells in the peripheral blood. It was subsequently observed that after moderate to high doses of chemotherapy, there was a rebound increase in the number of these hematopoietic stem cells in the peripheral blood for a few days. With the introduction of granulocyte-macrophage colony-stimulating factor (GM-CSF), granulocyte colony-stimulating factor, and interleukin-3 into clinical trials, it has been learned that these factors increase the number of stem cells in the peripheral blood. The combination of a stem cell-sparing chemotherapeutic agent (*e.g.*, cyclophosphamide) followed by growth factor in previously untreated patients dramatically increased PBSCs.[131]

PBSCs have been used primarily as a substitute for autologous marrow in patients with prior pelvic irradiation or for those with involvement of the marrow by tumor.[132] Many centers have reported engraftment rates similar to those obtained with autologous marrow. A second clinical use of major interest is the use of PBSCs to bone marrow and hematopoietic growth factors to accelerate neutrophil and platelet recovery after high-dose chemotherapy.[133,134]

The advantages of PBSCs over bone marrow include avoiding a general anesthetic, possibly accelerated hematopoietic recovery, the infusion of cryopreserved platelets with the stem cells, and the possible ability to exploit differences between peripheral blood and bone marrow stem cells with regard to cell number or function. Without chemotherapy or growth factor priming, 8 to 10 4-hour sessions are needed to collect an adequate number of cells. If chemotherapy priming is used, it generally must be intense enough to induce profound neutropenia, which may result in infection necessitating intravenous antibiotics and hospitalization. Heavily pretreated patients tend to show markedly diminished responses to growth factor priming. Some concern remains about the ability of PBSCs and particularly primed PBSCs to produce sustained engraftment of all cell lines after truly myeloablative preparative regimens.

BONE MARROW TRANSPLANTATION

AUTOLOGOUS BONE MARROW

The standard approach for autologous bone marrow harvesting is to perform multiple bone marrow aspirations from the posterior iliac crests in the prone position in the operating room under general anesthesia.[135] If one hemipelvis has been irradiated or the yield from the pelvis is poor, the patient can be turned and additional marrow aspirated from the anterior iliac crests and sternum. Generally, 1000 to 1200 ml of marrow are aspirated; 1500 to 2000 ml may be needed if the marrow will be purged because of loss of normal stem cells. The aspirated marrow is mixed with tissue culture medium and anticoagulated. A concentrate of mononuclear cells is often prepared by density-gradient centrifugation or by machine processing on a blood cell separator.[136–138] Next, purging is performed. In most cases, the marrow is then frozen using dimethyl sulfoxide (DMSO) or glycerol as a cryoprotectant and using a freezer that carefully controls the rate of freezing.[139] The marrow is stored in liquid nitrogen or in an electric freezer, but care must be taken with the latter to avoid power failure and accidental thawing. DMSO, in the concentrations used for cryopreservation, is toxic to normal stem cells at room temperature. Thawing should be accomplished rapidly at the patient's bedside and the marrow rapidly reinfused. Patients are routinely premedicated before autologous marrow infusion with hydrocortisone, diphenhydramine, and acetaminophen. Oxygen, intravenous fluids, and advanced cardiac life support medications are closely available.

Most patients experience some adverse reactions, which are thought to be due to the DMSO.[140,141] Most commonly, patients may have chills, fever, nausea, flushing, abdominal cramps, or vomiting. Dyspnea and a decrease in forced vital capacity may occur, which rarely results in respiratory failure. An increase in blood pressure and a decrease in heart rate are fairly common. Rarely, patients develop frank anaphylactic shock and death.[142] In patients who receive a double transplant, who develop urticarial or anaphylactic symptoms during the first transplant, consideration should be given to using glycerol as the cryoprotectant for subsequent harvests. Hematopoietic growth factors are now commonly given after autologous marrow infusion to accelerate neutrophil recovery.

MARROW PURGING

Most investigators think the primary reason for relapse after high-dose chemotherapy is the failure of the preparative regimen to eradicate disease in the patient and not due to reinfusion of a few malignant cells in the marrow. Nevertheless, marrow purging is an area of intense research interest and one that patients frequently focus on.

There are several ways to prevent reinfusion of malignant cells. One of the first methods used was monoclonal antibodies specific for antigens on the tumor cells but not on the pluripotent stem cells. These monoclonal antibodies are incubated with the mononuclear cell fraction in vitro before the addition of DMSO and freezing. In some cases, complement is added to causes cytolysis of the antibody coated cells; in others, the antibody is coupled to toxins (*e.g.*, ricin). The antibodies may be bound to magnetic spheres and the marrow subsequently passed through a strong magnetic field to extract the tumor cells. One of the limitations of negative purging is antigenic heterogeneity of the tumor cells and the possibility that the tumor stem cells may not express the antigens seen on the more differentiated cells, which are the primary cells represented when a tumor is screened.

Another method that uses monoclonal antibodies is called positive stem cell selection. In this approach, the antibodies are specific for antigens on the pluripotent stem cells but not on the tumor cells (*e.g.*, CD34). The antibodies may be attached to a column or bound to a specialized pan and the mononuclear cell fraction then poured in. Problems with this approach include nonspecific binding of tumor cells and the need to release the stem cells without damage. The magnetic bead approach can be adapted for positive stem cell collection. In this case, after separation of the normal stem cells in the magnetic field, a second monoclonal reagent is added that binds to the first near the Fab portion and alters its antigen binding site, releasing the stem cell unharmed.

Another strategy involves the in vitro incubation of the marrow with chemotherapy. The most commonly used agent has been 4-hydroperoxycyclophosphamide, which tends to spare the normal stem cells. In preclinical animal experiments, this approach eradicated leukemic cells in transplanted animals. One of the major problems with chemopurging is to ensure that the collateral damage to the normal stem cells is not so severe as to compromise hematopoietic recovery. The Seattle group reported that, if patients have graft failure after a chemopurged marrow autograft, GM-CSF frequently can not salvage the graft, presumably because there are not enough committed progenitors on which the growth factor can act.[143]

Although experience with autologous bone marrow transplantation after intensive therapy is improving with the advent of purging, relapses still occur. After relapse occurs, it is impossible to determine whether the origin of relapse arises from residual neoplastic cells in the purged bone marrow or from cells that escaped the cytotoxic effect of systemic preparative regimens. To resolve this problem and to provide a mechanism to monitor in vitro marrow manipulations, we and others have initiated the use of neutral safety-modified retroviruses for marking stem cells that are infused from purged autologous marrow. If the relapsed cells contain the genetic marker of the viral transgenome, relapse occurred from cells residual in the marrow after purging, suggesting that the methods used to purge the marrow were inadequate. This marking procedure can be used to follow individual steps in the purging or positive stem cell selection process. Carried to its ultimate, this technique can lead to the purification of the hematopoietic progenitor cell if the infused marked populations are used for the transplantation after chemotherapy. By following the percentage of cells in each lineage and the lineage distribution of the retroviral transgenome, the researcher can identify the relative impact of a fractionation on the frequency representation of the hematopoietic progenitor cell.

ALLOGENEIC BONE MARROW

Another means for restoring marrow function in situations of marrow failure or after high-dose chemotherapy is the use of allogeneic bone marrow. The greatest experience has been using HLA-matched sibling marrow, although HLA-matched unrelated and HLA partially matched related (*e.g.*, from parent, child, or extended family) marrow are increasingly being used as techniques for preventing GVHD improve.

High-dose chemotherapy, with or without TBI, is given to the patient before the transplant to prevent graft rejection, to create space in the marrow, and to eradicate or cytoreduce the hematologic malignancy. The donor marrow is generally harvested as described for autologous transplantation about 1 week after the start of the high-dose chemoradiation preparative regimen, and the marrow is infused the same day as harvest without freezing. In some cases, the marrow is processed to partially deplete T cells or subsets of T cells to decrease the incidence and severity of GVHD. Immunosuppressive treatment, such as cyclosporine, methotrexate, or steroids, is usually given to the patient to prevent GVHD. The allogeneic marrow reconstitutes hematopoiesis, restoring leukocytes, platelets, and erythrocytes (often more quickly than with autologous transplant because the allogeneic marrow has not been exposed to cytotoxic agents), and provides a new immune system. It is this latter feature which differentiates allogeneic from autologous bone marrow transplantation, giving rise to the substantial morbidity and mortality of acute and chronic GVHD and to the graft-versus-leukemia (GVL) effect.

The cure rate with allogeneic bone marrow transplantation for severe aplastic anemia, leukemia, lymphoma, and other hematopoietic neoplasms is at least 50%. New methods of donor-recipient compatibility phenotyping (*e.g.*, polymorphism analysis with oligonucleotide and PCR or isoelective focusing analysis of HLA antigens) should reduce the incidence of GVHD as will new immunosuppressive drugs and tolerance induction regimens. Methods for stem cell fractionation using positive and negative selection procedures should decrease the morbidity and mortality of GVHD while preserving the GVL effect. Improvements in supportive care, such as new growth factors, ex vivo expansion of stem cells, and T-cell depletion, should improve the outcome of allogeneic bone marrow transplantation and expand its applicability.

CONCLUSION

An increasing number of patients will be eligible for intensive therapies in the future. Matched unrelated allogeneic transplantation is making transplant an option for patients without an HLA-matched sibling. Improved methods for the prevention and treatment of GVHD are increasing the upper age limit for this procedure. Autologous transplantation, which has established itself in the treatment of relapsed Hodgkin's and intermediate-grade non-Hodgkin's lymphoma, is increasingly applied in other hematologic malignancies and solid tumors. Conventional-dose chemotherapy is being intensified through the use of hematopoietic growth factors. For centers that deliver intensified therapies, the use of irradiated leukocyte-filtered blood products to prevent transfusion-induced GVHD decrease the incidence of chill and fever reactions, delay or prevent the development of platelet alloimmunization, and prevent the acquisition of CMV infection has become standard. It is essential for the initial treating physicians to be aware of these issues so that patients are not already CMV positive and alloimmunized by the time they are referred for more intensive therapies. Particularly for patients in whom prognostic variables at the time of diagnosis predict a high risk for relapse, consideration should be given early to the optimal timing for collection of bone marrow or peripheral blood stem cells and for employing all of the methods discussed to preserve the best opportunity for treatment with minimal morbidity and mortality.

It is anticipated that the next decade will bring tremendous technologic advances in our ability to collect, manipulate, and use stem cells, which undoubtedly represent the most pluripotent blood product.

REFERENCES

1. Wallerstein R Jr. Laboratory evaluation of the bleeding patient. West J Med 1989;150: 51–58.
2. Brubaker DB. Clinical significance of white cell antibodies in febrile nonhemolytic transfusion reactions. Transfusion 1990;30:733–737.
3. Perkins HA, Payne R, Ferguson J, et al. Nonhemolytic febrile transfusion reactions. Quantitative effects of blood components with emphasis on isoantigenic incompatibility of leukocytes. Vox Sang 1966;11:578–600.
4. Bodensteiner DC. Leukocyte depletion filters: A comparison of efficiency. Am J Hematol 1990;35:184–186.
5. Grossman BJ, Kollins P, Lau PM, et al. Screening blood donors for gastrointestinal illness: A strategy to eliminate carriers of *Yersinia enterocolitica.* Transfusion 1991;31: 500–501.
6. Tipple MA, Bland LA, Murphy JJ, et al. Sepsis associated with transfusion of red cells contaminated with *Yersinia enterocolitica.* Transfusion 1990;30:207–213.
7. Aber RC. Transfusion-associated *Yersinia enterocolitica.* Transfusion 1990;30:193–195.
8. Vogelsang GB. Transfusion-associated graft-versus-host disease in nonimmunocompromised hosts. Transfusion 1990;30:101–103.
9. Anderson KC, Weinstein HJ. Transfusion-associated graft-versus-host disease. N Engl J Med 1990;323:315–321.
10. Mollison PL. Blood transfusion in clinical medicine. Oxford: Blackwell Scientific, 1979: 578–583.
11. Perkins HA, Samson S, Garner J, et al. Risk of AIDS for recipients of blood components from donors who subsequently developed AIDS. Blood 1987;70:1604–1610.
12. Curran JW, Jaffe HW, Hardy AM, et al. Epidemiology of HIV infection and AIDS in the United States. Science 1988;239:610–616.
13. Medley GF, Anderson RM, Cox DR, et al. Incubation period of AIDS in patients infected via blood transfusion. Nature 1987;328:719–721.
14. Busch MP, Young MJ, Samson SM, et al. Risk of human immunodeficiency virus transmission by blood transfusions before the implementation of HIV-1 antibody screening. Transfusion 1991;31:4–11.
15. Busch MP, Eble BE, Khayam-Bashi H, et al. Evaluation of screened blood donations for human immunodeficiency virus type 1 infection by culture and DNA amplification of pooled cells. N Engl J Med 1991;325:1–5.
16. Petersen LR, Doll LS, et al. Human immunodeficiency virus type 1-infected blood donors: Epidemiologic, laboratory, and donation characteristics. Transfusion 1991;31: 698–703.
17. Doll LS, Peterson LR, White CR, et al. Human immunodeficiency virus type 1-infected blood donors: Behavioral characteristics and reasons for donation. Transfusion 1991;31: 704–709.
18. Epstein JS. Sensitivity and consistency of screening tests for antibodies to human immunodeficiency virus type 1. Transfusion 1991;31:388–389.
19. Perrin LH, Yerly S, Adami N, et al. Human immunodeficiency virus DNA amplification and serology in blood donors. Blood 1990;76:641–645.
20. Aach RD, Stevens CE, Hollinger FB, et al. Hepatitis C virus infection in post-transfusion hepatitis. N Engl J Med 1991;325:1325–1329.
21. Manns A, Blattner WA. The epidemiology of the human T-cell lymphotropic virus type I and type II. etiologic role in human disease. Transfusion 1991;31:67–75.
22. Hjelle B, Cyrus S, Swenson S, et al. Serologic distinction between human T-lymphotropic virus (HTLV) type I and HTLV type II. Transfusion 1991;31:731–736.
23. Donegan E, Busch MP, Galleshaw JA, et al. Transfusion of blood components from a donor with human T-lymphotropic virus type II (HTLV-II) infection. Ann Intern Med 1990;113:555–556.
24. Verdonck LF, Graan-Hentzen YC, Dekker AW, et al. Cytomegalovirus seronegative platelets and leukocyte poor red blood cells from random donors can prevent primary cytomegalovirus infection after bone marrow transplantation. Bone Marrow Transplant 1987;2:73–78.
25. Murphy MF, Metcalfe P, Thomas H, et al. Use of leukocyte-poor blood components to prevent primary cytomegalovirus (CMV) infection in patients with acute leukemia. Br J Haematol 1988;70:253–255.
26. De Gran-Hatzen YCE, Gratama JW, Mudde GC, et al. Prevention of primary cytomegalovirus infection in patients with hematologic malignancies by intensive white cell depletion of blood products. Transfusion 1989;29:757–760.
27. Gilbert GL, Hayes K, Hudson I, et al. Prevention of transfusion-acquired cytomegalovirus infection in infants by blood filtration to remove leukocytes. Lancet 1989;:1228–1231.
28. Bowden RA, Slichter SJ, Sayers MH, et al. Use of leukocyte-depleted platelets and cytomegalovirus-seronegative red blood cells for prevention of primary cytomegalovirus infection after marrow transplant. Blood 1991;78:246–250.
29. Hillyer CD, Snydman DR, Berkman EM. The risk of cytomegalovirus infection in solid organ and bone marrow transplant recipients: Transfusion of blood products. Transfusion 1990;30:659–666.
30. Shulman IA. Parasitic infections, an uncommon risk of blood transfusion in the United States. Transfusion 1991;31:479–480.
31. Schmuñis GA. Trypanosoma cruzi, the etiologic agent of Chagas' disease: Status of the blood supply in endemic and nonendemic countries. Transfusion 1991;31:547–557.
32. Wallerstein R Jr. Laboratory evaluation of the bleeding patient. West J Med 1989;150: 51–58.
33. Harker LA, Slichter SJ. The bleeding time as a screening test for evaluation of platelet function. N Engl J Med 1972;287:155–159.
34. Malpass TW, Harker LA. Acquired disorders of platelet function. Semin Hematol 1980;17:242–258.
35. Day HJ, Rao AK. Platelets and megakaryocytes: Semin Hematol 1986;23:89–101.
36. Kobrinsky NL, Gerrard JM, Watson CM, et al. Shortening of bleeding time by 1-deamino-8-D-arginine vasopressin in various bleeding disorders. Lancet 1984;1:1145–1148.
37. Gaydos LS, Freireich EJ, Mantel N. The quantitative relation between platelet count and hemorrhage in patients with acute leukemia. N Engl J Med 1962;266:905–909.
38. Menitove JE, Aster RH. Transfusion of platelets and plasma products. Clin Haematol 1983;12:239–266.
39. Gottschall JL, Rzad L, Aster RH. Studies of the minimum temperature at which human platelets can be stored with full maintenance of viability. Transfusion 1986;26:460–462.
40. Simon TL, Nelson EJ, Murphy S. Extension of platelet concentrate storage to 7 days in second-generation bags. Transfusion 1987;26:6–19.
41. Heal JM, Singal S, Sardisco E, et al. Bacterial proliferation in platelet concentrates. Transfusion 1986;26:388–390.
42. Braine HG, Kickler TS, Charache P, et al. Bacterial sepsis secondary to platelet transfusion: An adverse effect of extended storage at room temperature. Transfusion 1986;268:391–393.
43. Holohan TV, Terasaki P, Deisseroth A. Suppression of transfusion-related alloimmunization in intensively treated cancer patients. Blood 1981;58:122–128.
44. Dutcher JP, Schiffer CA, Aisner J, et al. Alloimmunization following platelet transfusion: The absence of a dose-response relationship. Blood 1981;57:395.
45. Claas FHJ, Smeenk RJT, Schmidt R, et al. Alloimmunization against the MHC antigens after platelet transfusions is due to contaminating leukocytes in the platelet suspension. Exp Hematol 1981;9:84–89.
46. Eernisee JG, Brand A. Prevention of platelet refractoriness due to HLA antibodies by administration of leukocyte-poor blood components. Exp Hematol 1981;9:77–83.
47. Daly PA, Schiffer CA, Aisner J, et al. Platelet transfusion therapy. One-hour post-transfusion increments are valuable in predicting the need for HLA-matched preparations. JAMA 1980;243:435–438.
48. Bishop JF, McGrath K, Wolf MM, et al. Clinical factors influencing the efficacy of pooled platelet transfusion. Blood 1988;71:383–387.
49. Schiffer CA. Prevention of alloimmunization against platelets. Blood [Editorial] 1991;77: 1–4.
50. Andreu G, Dewailly J, Leberre C, et al. Prevention of HLA immunization with leukocyte-poor packed red cells and platelet concentrates obtained by filtration. Blood 1988;72: 964–969.
51. Murphy MF, Metcalfe P, Thomas H, et al. Use of leukocyte-poor blood components and HLA-matched platelet donors to prevent HLA alloimmunization. Br J Haematol 1986;62:529–534.
52. Sniecinski I, O'Donnell MR, Nowicki B, et al. Prevention of refractoriness and HLA alloimmunization using filtered blood products. Blood 1988;71:1402–1407.
53. Saarinen UM, Kekomaki R, Siimes MA, et al. Effective prophylaxis against platelet

refractoriness in multitransfused patients by the use of leukocyte-free blood components. Blood 1990;75:512.

54. Van Marwijk Kooy M, van Prooijen C, Moes M, et al. Use of leukocyte-depleted platelet concentrates for the prevention of refractoriness and primary HLA alloimmunization: A prospective, randomized trial. Blood 1991;77:201–205.
55. Bock M, Wagner M, Knuppel W, et al. Preparation of white cell-depleted blood: Comparison of two bedside filter systems. Transfusion 1990;30:26–29.
56. Bodensteiner DC. Leukocyte depletion filters: A comparison of efficiency. Am J Hematol 1990;35:184–186.
57. Sirchia G, Wenz B, Rebulla P, et al. Removal of white cells from red cells by transfusion through a new filter. Transfusion 1990;30:30–33.
58. Van Marwijk Kooy M, van Prooijen HC, Borghuis L, et al. Filtration: A method of prepare white cell-poor platelet concentrates with optimal preservation of platelet viability. Transfusion 1990;30:34–38.
59. Steneker I, Biewenga J. Histologic and immunohistochemical studies on the preparation of white cell-poor red cell concentrates: The filtration process using three different polyester filters. Transfusion 1991;31:40–46.
60. Brecher ME, Pineda AA, Zylstra-Halling VW, et al. In vivo viability and functional integrity of filtered platelets. Transfusion 1990;30:718–721.
61. Rawal BD, Schwadron R, Busch MP, et al. Evaluation of leukocyte removal filters modelled by use of HIV-infected cells and DNA amplification. Blood 1990;76:2159–2161.
62. Sloand EM, Klein HG. Effect of white cells on platelets during storage. Transfusion 1990;30:333–338.
63. Högman CF, Gong J, Eriksson L, et al. White cells protect donor blood against bacteria contamination. Transfusion 1991;31:620–626.
64. Heal JM, Cohen HJ. Do white cells in stored blood components reduce the likelihood of post-transfusion bacterial sepsis? Transfusion [Editorial] 1991;31:581–583.
65. Capon SM, Sacher RA, Deeg HJ. Effective ultraviolet irradiation of platelet concentrates in Teflon bags. Transfusion 1990;30:678–681.
66. Deeg HJ. Ultraviolet irradiation in transplantation biology. Transplantation 1988;5: 845–851.
67. Andreu G, Boccaccio C, Lecrubier C, et al. Ultraviolet irradiation of platelet concentrates: Feasibility in transfusion practice. Transfusion 1990;30:401.
68. Pamphilon DH, Potter M, Cutts M, et al. Platelet concentrates irradiated with ultraviolet light retain satisfactory in vitro storage characteristics and in vivo survival. Br J Hematol 1990;75:240.
69. Boccaccio C, Garcia I, Klaren J, et al. Ultraviolet irradiation of platelet concentrates: In vitro and in vivo preclinical evaluation. Transfus Sci 1990;11:141–147.
70. Pamphilon DH. Platelet concentrates and ultraviolet light. Transfus Sci 1990;11:149–152.
71. O'Connell BA, Schiffer CA. Donor selection for alloimmunized patients by platelet crossmatching of random-donor platelet concentrates. Transfusion 1990;30-4:314–317.
72. Daly PA, Schiffer CA, Aisner J, et al. Platelet transfusion therapy. One-hour post-transfusion increments are valuable in predicting the need for HLA-matched preparations. JAMA 1980;243:435–438.
73. Schiffer CA, Aisner J, Wiernik PH. Frozen autologous platelet transfusion for patients with leukemia. N Engl J Med 1978;299:7–12.
74. Dullemond AC, Prooijen HC, Riemens MI, et al. Cryo-preservation disturbs stimulus-response coupling in a platelet subpopulation. Br J Haematol 1987;67:325–333.
75. Christie DJ, Buren N, Lennon SS, Putnam JL. Vancomycin-dependent antibodies associated with thrombocytopenia and refractoriness to platelet transfusion in patients with leukemia. Blood 1990;75:518–523.
76. Berkman SA, Lee ML, Gale RP. Clinical uses of intravenous immunoglobulins. Ann Intern Med 1990;112:278–292.
77. Zeigler ZR, Shadduck RK, Rosenfeld CS, et al. High-dose intravenous gamma globulin improves responses to single-donor platelets in patients refractory to platelet transfusion. Blood 1987;70:1433–1436.
78. Lee EJ, Norris D, Schiffer CA. Intravenous immune globulin for patients alloimmunized to random-donor platelet transfusion. Transfusion 1987;27:245–247.
79. Sindet-Pederson S, Ramstrom G, Bernvil S, et al. Hemostatic effect of tranexamic acid mouthwash in anticoagulant-treated patients undergoing oral surgery. N Engl J Med 1989;320:840–843.
80. Mannucci PM. Desmopressin: A non-transfusional form of treatment for congenital and acquired bleeding disorders. Blood 1988;72:1449–1455.
81. Bodey GP, Buckley M, Sathe YS, et al. Quantitative relationships between circulating leukocytes and infection in patients with acute leukemia. Ann Intern Med 1966;64: 328–340.
82. Esparza L, Yap HY, Smith T, et al. Quantitative relationship between degree of myelosuppression and infection in patients with metastatic breast cancer (MBC). Proc Am Soc Clin Oncol [Abstract C-348] 1983;2:39.
83. Bodey GP. Infection in cancer patients: A continuing association. Am J Med 1986;81: 11–26.
84. Clift RA, Buckner CD. Granulocyte transfusions. Am J Med 1984;76:631–636.
85. Wright DG. Leukocyte transfusions: Thinking twice. Am J Med 1984;76:637–644.
86. Young LS. The role of granulocyte transfusions in treating and preventing infection. Cancer Treat Rep 1983;67:109–111.
87. Winston DJ, Ho WG, Gale RP. Therapeutic granulocyte transfusions for documented infections. Ann Intern Med 1982;97:509–515.
88. Strauss RG, Hester JP, Vogler WR, et al. A multicenter trial to document the efficacy and safety of a rapidly excreted analog of hydroxyethyl starch for leukapheresis with a note on steroid stimulation of granulocyte donors. Transfusion 1986;26:258–264.
89. Strauss RG, Goeken JA, Eckermann I, et al. Effects of intensive granulocyte donation on donors and yields. Transfusion 1986;26:441–445.
90. Robinson EAE. Single donor granulocytes and platelets. Clin Haematol 1984;13:186–216.
91. Strauss RG, Goeken JA, Imig KM. Effects on immunity of multiple leukapheresis using a rapidly excreted analog of hydroxyethyl starch. Transfusion 1986;26:265–268.
92. Hersman J, Meyers JD, Thomas E, et al. The effect of granulocyte transfusions on the incidence of cytomegalovirus infection after allogeneic marrow transplantation. Ann Intern Med 1982;96:149–152.
93. Dutcher JP, Schiffer CA, Johnson GS, et al. Alloimmunization prevents the migration of transfused indium-111-labeled granulocytes to sites of infection. Blood 1983;62: 354–360.
94. Wright DG, Robichaum KJ, Pizzo PA, et al. Lethal pulmonary reactions associated with the combined use of amphotericin B and leukocyte transfusions. N Engl J Med 1981;304:1185–1189.
95. Dana BW, Durie GBM, White RF, et al. Concomitant administration of granulocyte transfusions and amphotericin B in neutropenic patients: Absence of significant pulmonary toxicity. Blood 1981;57:90–94.
96. Schiffer CA. Granulocyte transfusion therapy. Cancer Treat Rep 1983;67:113–119.
97. Buckner CD, Clift RA. Prophylaxis and treatment of infection of the immunocompromised host by granulocyte transfusions. Clin Haematol 1984;13:557–572.
98. Bowden RA, Sayers M, Flournoy N, et al. Cytomegalovirus immune globulin and seronegative blood products to prevent primary cytomegalovirus infection after marrow transplantation. N Engl J Med 1986;314:1006–1010.
99. Herzig RH, Herzig GP, Graw RG, et al. Successful granulocyte transfusion therapy from gram-negative septicemia. N Engl J Med 1977;296:701–705.
100. Alavi JB, Root RK, Djerassi I, et al. A randomized clinical trial of granulocyte transfusions for infection in acute leukemia. N Engl J Med 1977;296:706–711.
101. Berkman SA, Lee ML, Gale RP. Clinical uses of intravenous immunoglobulins. Ann Intern Med 1990;112:278–292.
102. Cooperative Group for the Study of Immunoglobulin in Chronic Lymphocytic Leukemia. Intravenous immunoglobulin for the prevention of infection in chronic lymphocytic leukemia. N Engl J Med 1988;319:902–907.
103. Atkinson K. Reconstruction of the haemopoietic and immune systems after marrow transplantation. Bone Marrow Transplant 1990;5:209–226.
104. Sullivan KM, Kopecky KJ, Jocom J, et al. Immunomodulatory and antimicrobial efficacy of intravenous immunoglobulin in bone marrow transplantation. N Engl J Med 1990;323: 705–712.
105. Winston DJ, Ho WG, Lin C-H, et al. Intravenous immune globulin for prevention of cytomegalovirus infection and interstitial pneumonia after bone marrow transplantation. Ann Intern Med 1987;106:12–18.
106. Bowden RA, Sayers M, Flournoy, N, et al. Cytomegalovirus immune globulin and seronegative blood products to prevent primary cytomegalovirus infection after marrow transplantation. N Engl J Med 1986;314:1006–1010.
107. Verdonch LF, Middeldorp JM, Kreeft HAJG, et al. Primary cytomegalovirus infection and its prevention after autologous bone marrow transplantation. Transplantation 1985;39:455–457.
108. Levin MJ, Zaia JA, Spector SA, et al. Current approaches to the prevention and treatment of cytomegalovirus disease after bone marrow transplantation: An overview. Semin Hematol 1990(suppl 1);27:2.
109. Anderson LJ. Human parvoviruses. J Infect Dis 1990;161:603–608.
110. Frickhofen N, Abkowitz JL, Safford M, et al. Persistent B19 parovirus infection in patients infected with human immunodeficiency virus type I (HIV-I): A treatable cause of anemia in AIDS. Ann Intern Med 1990;113:926–933.
111. Berkman SA, Lee ML, Gale RP. Clinical uses of intravenous immunoglobulins. Ann Intern Med 1990;112:278–292.
112. Zeigler ZR, Shadduck RK, Rosenfeld CS, et al. High-dose intravenous gamma globulin improves responses to single-donor platelets in patients refractory to platelet transfusion. Blood 1987;70:1433–1436.
113. Lee EJ, Norris D, Schiffer CA. Intravenous immunoglobulin for patients alloimmunized to random-donor platelet transfusion. Transfusion 1987;27:245–247.
114. Wells MA, Wittek AE, Epstein JS, et al. Inactivation and partition of human T-cell lymphotropic virus, type III, during ethanol fractionation of plasma. Transfusion 1986;26: 210–213.
115. Schiff RI, Sedlak D, Buckley RH. Rapid infusion of Sandoglobulin in patients with primary humoral immunodeficiency. J Allergy Clin Immunol 1991;88:61–67.
116. Linker CL. Plasmapheresis in clinical medicine. West J Med 1983;138:60–69.
117. Bunin NJ, Pui CH. Differing complications of hyperleukocytosis in children with acute lymphoblastic or acute nonlymphoblastic leukemia. J Clin Oncol 1985;3:1590–1595.
118. Gale RP, Foon KA. Chronic lymphocytic Leukemia. Ann Intern Med 1985;103:101–120.
119. Yam LT, Klock JC, Mielke CH. Therapeutic leukapheresis in hairy cell leukemia: Review of literature and personal experience. Semin Oncol 1984;11:493–501.
120. Golomb HM. The treatment of hairy cell leukemia. Blood 1987;69:979–983.
121. Fitzgerald D, Rowe JM, Heal J. Leukapheresis for control of chronic myelogenous leukemia during pregnancy. Am J Hematol 1986;22:213–218.
122. Rosenberg SA, Lotze MT, Muul LM, et al. A progress report on the treatment of 157 patients with advanced cancer using lymphokine-activated killer cells and interleukin-2 or high-dose interleukin-2 alone. N Engl J Med 1987;316:889–897.
123. Edelson R, Berger C, Gasparro F, et al. Treatment of cutaneous T-cell lymphoma by extracorporeal photochemotherapy. N Engl J Med 1987;316:297–303.
124. Ventura GJ, Buzdar AU, Kau S, et al. Clinical trail of plasma perfusion over immobilized staphylococcal protein A in metastatic breast cancer. Cancer Treat Rep 1987;71:411–413.

125. MacKintosh FR, Bennett K, Schiff S, et al. Treatment of advanced malignancy with plasma perfused over staphylococcal protein A. West J Med 1983;139:36–40.
126. Messerschmidt GL, Henry DH, Snyder HW, et al. Protein A immunoadsorption in the treatment of malignant disease. J Clin Oncol 1988;6:203–212.
127. Murgo AJ. Thrombotic microangiopathy in the cancer patient including those induced by chemotherapeutic agents. Semin Hematol 1987;24:161–177.
128. Korec S, Schein PS, Smith FP, et al. Treatment of cancer-associated hemolytic syndrome with staphylococcal protein A immunoperfusion. J Clin Oncol 1986;4:210–215.
129. Hazards of apheresis. Lancet 1982;2:1025–1026.
130. Council on Scientific Affairs. Current status of therapeutic plasmapheresis and related techniques: Report of the AMA panel on therapeutic plasmapheresis. JAMA 1985;253:819–825.
131. Siena S, Bregni M, Brando B, et al. Circulation of CD34+ hematopoietic stem cells in the peripheral blood of high-dose cyclophosphamide-treated patients: Enhancement by intravenous recombinant human granulocyte-macrophage colony-stimulating factor. Blood 1989;74:1905–1914.
132. Kessinger A, Armitage JO. The evolving role of autologous peripheral stem cell transplantation following high-dose therapy for malignancies. Blood 1991;77:211–213.
133. Gianni AM, Bregni M, Siena S, et al. Rapid and complete hemopoietic reconstitution following combined transplantation of autologous blood and bone marrow cells. A changing role for high-dose chemo-radiotherapy? Hematol Oncol 1989;7:139–148.
134. Siena S, Bregni M, Brando B, et al. Flow cytometry for clinical estimation of circulating hematopoietic progenitors for autologous transplantation in cancer patients. Blood 1991;77:400–409.
135. Thomas ED, Storb R. Technique for human marrow grafting. Blood 1970;36:507–515.
136. Beaujean F, Gourdin MF, Farcet JP, et al. Separation of large quantities of mononuclear cells from human blood using a blood processor. Transfusion 1985;25:152–154.
137. English D, Lamberson R, Graves V. Semiautomated processing of bone marrow grafts for transplantation. Transfusion 1989;29:12–16.
138. Areman EM, Cullis H, Spitzer T, et al. Automated processing of human bone marrow can result in a population of mononuclear cells capable of achieving engraftment following transplantation. Transfusion 1991;31:724–730.
139. Gorin NC. Collection, manipulation and freezing of haemopoietic stem cells. Clin Haematol 1986;15:19–48.
140. Davis JM, Rowley SD, Braine HG, et al. Clinical toxicity of cryopreserved bone marrow graft infusion. Blood 1990;75:781–786.
141. Stroncek DF, Fautsch SK, Lasky LC, et al. Adverse reactions in patients transfused with cryopreserved marrow. Transfusion 1991;31:521–526.
142. Rapoport AP, Rowe JM, Packman CH, et al. Case report: Cardiac arrest after autologous marrow infusion. Bone Marrow Transplant 1991;7:401–403.
143. Nemunaitis J, Singer JW, Buckner CD, et al. Use of recombinant human granulocyte-macrophage colony-stimulating factor in graft failure after bone marrow transplantation. Blood 1990;76:245–253.

SECTION 2

JANICE L. GABRILOVE
DAVID W. GOLDE

Hematopoietic Growth Factors

The cellular elements of the blood are essential to life and may be viewed as operating centrally in host defense. The erythrocytes protect against hypoxia and function solely to deliver oxygen to the tissues. Erythrocytes are anucleate and survive for about 120 days in the peripheral blood. Platelets defend against bleeding and play a primary role in the initiation of hemostasis and clotting; they circulate in the blood for approximately 8 days.

Neutrophils are primarily concerned with defense against microorganisms, particularly bacteria and fungi and they have a half-life in the peripheral blood of only about 8 hours. The other granulocytes include the eosinophils and basophils whose role in host defense is not clearly defined although the eosinophils function importantly in extracellular killing of large parasites.

The monocytes are the blood form of the mononuclear phagocyte system and are important in antimicrobial function and the removal of organic and inorganic debris. The tissue component of the mononuclear phagocyte system comprises the resident macrophages in most tissues and organs, including the Kupffer cell of the liver, the alveolar macrophage of the lung, and the Langerhans cell of skin. Tissue macrophage populations can be self-sustaining and are not critically dependent on an influx of precursor cells from the bone marrow.

The circulating T and B lymphocytes respectively comprise the cell-mediated and humoral arms of the immune system. Some T and B cells may live for many years, perhaps for the person's life span.

Surprisingly, this diverse and highly specialized array of blood cells originates from a common stem cell in the bone marrow. A stem cell may be defined as a cell with extensive ability to reproduce itself and to differentiate along several lineages.[1] The totipotent hematopoietic stem cell is normally quiescent but is capable of giving rise to all hematopoietic lineages and repopulating lethally irradiated recipients. This repopulating property of stem cells is critical to the success of bone marrow transplantation. The mouse hematopoietic stem cell has been enriched to high purity, and human stem cells thought to have pluripotent repopulating capability have been isolated.[2] The ability to isolate and cryopreserve human stem cells will have considerable impact on autotransplantation for cancer and for allogeneic procedures. Positive selection of stem cells may be a potent means of purging bone marrow of malignant cells and reducing the incidence of graft-versus-host disease in the allogeneic situation.

As pluripotent stem cells differentiate, they become restricted to one or more hematopoietic lineages. Ultimately, commitment to a single lineage occurs, such as for the erythroid lineage. The process of stem cell differentiation is poorly understood, although the "decision" along which lineage to differentiate is thought to be stochastic (*i.e.*, random). However, the microenvironment can influence this decision, and environmental influences probably play an important role in initiating stem cell replication. The important manifestation of lineage commitment is the expression of receptors for specific hematopoietic hormones. The expression of receptors allows the cell to respond to hormonal signals in the environment and ultimately produce mature cells in appropriate numbers for the specific function required.

HUMORAL REGULATION OF HEMATOPOIESIS

Mature blood cells are produced at a prodigious rate. Approximately 10 billion erythrocytes, neutrophils, and platelets are produced in the average person every hour, and this baseline production can be increased many fold in times of need. Most of the regulation of mature blood cell production occurs in the morphologically identifiable pools in the bone marrow, and under stable conditions, it is thought that few stem cells enter the active cell cycle.

The various hormones that regulate hematopoiesis are known as hematopoietic growth factors or hematopoietins, and considerable information has been obtained about their molecular biology, biochemistry, and therapeutic use. Substantially less is known about the physiology of the hematopoietic growth factors, particularly their function in daily regulation of hematopoiesis. Erythropoietin is clearly identified as the major regulator of erythrocyte production, but relatively little is known about the specific hormones regulating the production of platelets.

PRINCIPLES OF THERAPY WITH HEMATOPOIETIC GROWTH FACTORS

Because the blood cells are concerned with host defense, the primary reason for giving growth factors is to improve or optimize the patient's host defense capabilities. Although most clinicians are comfortable with the concept of replacement therapy, such an approach does not play a major role in hematopoietic growth factor treatment in cancer. For growth factors other than erythropoietin, serum levels may be difficult to measure, or the hormone may not circulate, and measurement may provide little guide to therapy. The clinician must think in terms of regulating blood cell production in the face of complex circumstances, frequently involving the administration of chemotherapy, infection, and bone marrow failure.

Physiologic responses, although normal, are seldom optimal. The erythropoietic response to an important change in altitude occurs over time and not with sufficient rapidity to be optimal. Adaptation to altitude could be optimized by erythropoietin administration, and similarly, host defense against microorganisms and tumors must aim at an optimal response. Such principles may be difficult to put into practice because the ideal blood counts for a patient at a given time can be difficult to ascertain. A normal neutrophil count may be inadequate in some circumstances. Despite incomplete information, the physician must decide the appropriate level of circulating mature cells for a given situation. Using the hematopoietic growth factors, we can regulate the production of erythrocytes, neutrophils, eosinophils, and monocytes, but we still do not have a growth factor to regulate thrombopoietin, although interleukin-3 (IL-3) shows some potential in this regard. Because the hematopoietic growth factors also regulate mature cell function, the therapist must consider the number of effector cells and their level of activation. The identification of functional defects usually requires special testing, but the oncologist should be aware of the specific alterations in mature cell function induced by administration of the hematopoietic growth factors.

Because the host defense system marshals cellular defenses against a biologically hostile environment, recognition becomes the crucial element in directing effector cell function. In autoimmunity, recognition is confused, and the host defense system may be subverted to attack normal tissue. Because several hematopoietic growth factors play a crucial role in inflammation, the possibility of host defense cell damage to normal tissues is an important complicating issue that should be considered. Activated mature host defense cells may cause appropriate inflammation, and hematopoietic growth factors may have effects on nonhematopoietic tissues that could be therapeutically deleterious. To be effective, the hematopoietic hormones must have target cells expressing appropriate receptors, and if they are absent due to bone marrow aplasia, therapeutic intervention is ineffective. The clinician must decide with incomplete information how the use of hematopoietic growth factors can optimize the cancer patient's ability to fight infection, transport oxygen, and prevent bleeding. Ultimately, strategies for using hematopoietic growth factors to treat cancer itself will depend on appropriately directing the immune system and the various effector cells.

ERYTHROPOIETIN

Erythropoietin is the circulating hormone primarily responsible for regulating the rate of red blood cell production in the bone marrow (Fig. 62–2).[3] Erythropoietin is a glycoprotein hormone, approximately 90% of which is produced in the kidneys and 10% in the liver. The hormone was purified in 1977 from human urine, and its molecular mass was about 34 kd.[4] In 1985, the gene for human erythropoietin and its cDNA was molecularly cloned. The gene is single copy and consists of five exons. The cDNA sequence predicts a molecule of 18,398 d, and the most highly purified protein has a specific activity approaching 200,000 units per milligram of protein. Erythropoietin for clinical use is produced in Chinese hamster ovary cells and is glycosylated with a total molecular weight of about 29,900 and a specific activity of 120,000 units per milligram of protein.

Erythropoietin interacts with precursor cells in the bone marrow expressing the erythropoietin receptor. The erythropoietin receptor has been molecularly cloned and is part of the hemopoietin receptor superfamily. It has an extracellular ligand binding domain, a transmembrane region, and an intracellular portion that lacks an intrinsic tyrosine kinase domain. The erythropoietin receptor is expressed by cells committed to erythroid differentiation under control of specific transcription factors. Erythroid precursors respond to erythropoietin by replication and maturation, and erythropoietin is necessary for cellular development to the mature erythrocyte. Under conditions of maximal erythropoietin stimulation, erythropoiesis can be expanded approximately tenfold.

Erythropoietin produced in the kidney is synthesized and elaborated largely in response to the need for oxygen-carrying capacity. The oxygen "sensor" links erythropoietin synthesis to oxygen-carrying demand. If a normal person moves to a higher altitude, relative hypoxemia is sensed, and erythropoietin elaboration is increased, which leads to increased erythrocyte production and homeostasis being achieved at the higher hematocrit necessary for normal oxygen-carrying capacity. After the person returns to sea level, erythropoietin elaboration is decreased in response to excess oxygen-carrying capacity, and the hematocrit drops appropriately. The relation between the hematocrit and plasma erythropoietin concentration is shown in Figure 62–3. Physiologic responses tend to be suboptimal, and in disease states, compensatory mechanisms are often inadequate. In the anemia of chronic inflammation, for example, plasma erythropoietin levels are low relative to the degree of anemia.[5–7]

Anemia in cancer patients is common, and the specific causes should be determined by careful investigation. Blood loss, iron deficiency, vitamin B_{12} or folate deficiency, hemolysis, chemotherapy, drug toxicity, hypersplenism, and tumor involvement of the bone marrow may occur in various combinations. There is an entity known as the anemia of cancer. Although this may not be a specific process, careful study of

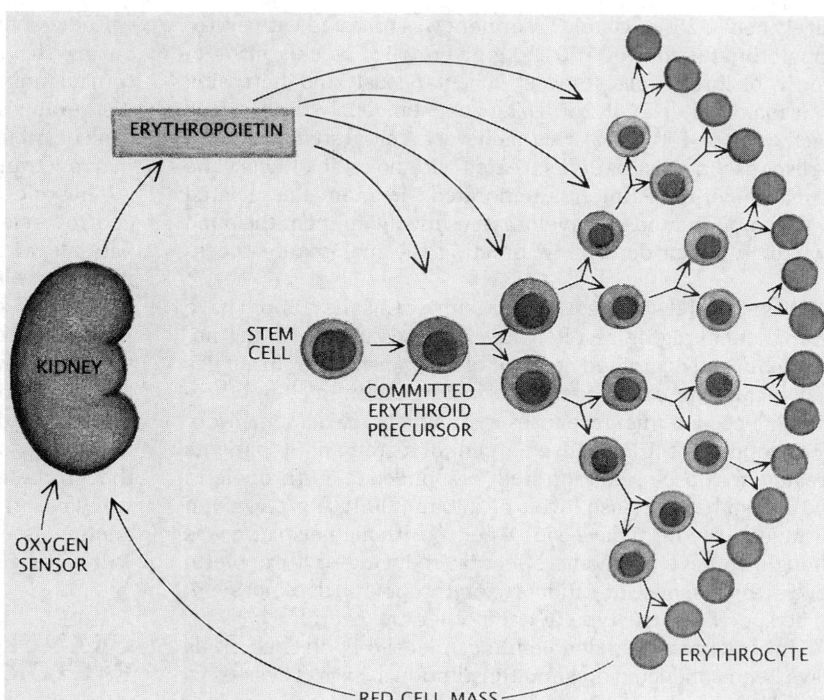

FIGURE 62–2. Regulation of red cell mass by erythropoiesis. (Golde DW. Hormones that stimulate the growth of blood cells. Sci Am 1988;259:62–70)

these patients has shown that they have an inadequate erythropoietin response for a given degree of anemia.[7] Relative erythropoietin deficiency may exist in otherwise hematologically uncomplicated tumors. Malignancies of hematopoietic tissue clearly interfere with normal erythrocyte production, but pharmacologic doses of erythropoietin can be effective. A central element in considering the potential benefit of erythropoietin therapy is the adequacy of the endogenous erythropoietin response, which is best evaluated by a plasma erythropoietin concentration interpreted with regard to the hematocrit.

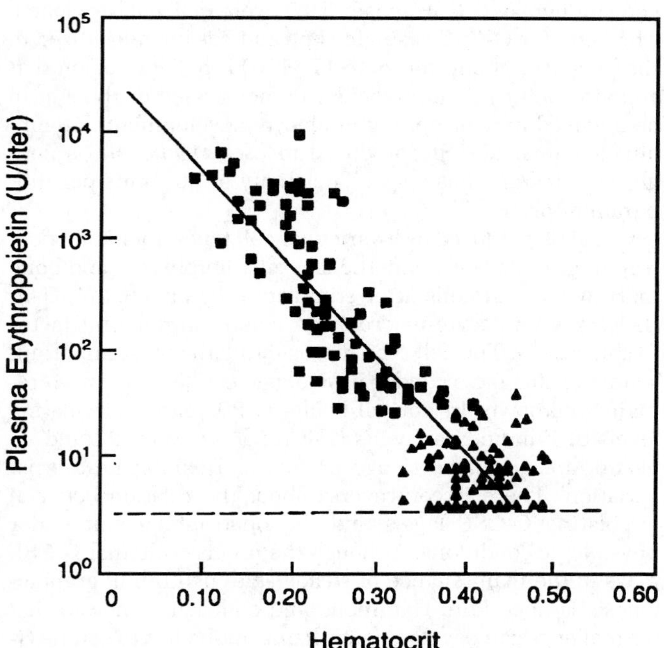

FIGURE 62–3. Relation of plasma erythropoietin concentration to hematocrit in 175 persons. (Erslev AJ. Erythropoietin. N Engl J Med 1991;324:1339–1344)

In addition to impaired erythropoietin response to anemia in cancer patients, there may be a diminished responsiveness of bone marrow erythroid precursors to erythropoietin. The cause of this reduced responsiveness of the bone marrow to erythropoietin is uncertain, but inflammatory cytokines such as interleukin-1 (IL-1) and tumor necrosis factor (TNF) elaborated in association with malignant disease can impair erythropoiesis. Erythropoietic impairment may be due to decreased responsiveness and decreasing elaboration of erythropoietin.[8] The anemia of cancer is pathophysiologically similar to the anemia of chronic inflammation, as occurs in active rheumatoid arthritis. The cancer patient may have reduced hematopoietic progenitors because of cytotoxic chemotherapy, radiation therapy, or disruption of the marrow architecture by invasion of malignant cells.

Recombinant erythropoietin is cleared from the circulation in an exponential fashion with a half-life of 9.3 ± 3.2 hours. After seven treatments with erythropoietin, the half-life tends to decrease by about 30%. In normal persons, the mean half-life is 4 to 6 hours after intravenous injection. Subcutaneous delivery results in peak serum levels of about 5% of those achieved after an equivalent intravenous dose, and the time necessary to reach peak serum levels is 5 to 24 hours. Peak levels after intravenous administration are achieved in 0.5 hour. The disposal of erythropoietin is poorly understood. Less than 10% is excreted by the kidneys, and small amounts are cleared by the liver. No dose modifications are recommended for renal or hepatic failure.

Early trials of erythropoietin in cancer involved patients with anemia associated with marrow infiltration with non-Hodgkin's lymphoma and multiple myeloma.[8–11] These patients had modestly elevated endogenous erythropoietin levels rarely above 200 mU/ml. Treatment was initiated with erythropoietin at a dose of 150 U/kg given twice weekly intravenously or three times per week subcutaneously and increasing to a maximal dose of 250 U/kg subcutaneously three times each week or 450 U/kg twice each week. Initial studies showed a response in most patients treated with no toxic effects. The erythropoietin treatment ameliorated the anemia associated with lymphomatous or myelomatous involvement of the bone marrow without detectably affecting the malignant process itself.

Phase I and II studies using patients with solid tumors have shown encouraging results with increases in circulating hemoglobin and decreased need for blood transfusion.[8] In studies specifically aimed at the use of erythropoietin in chemotherapy-induced anemia, responses in relatively few patients were dose dependent. Eighty-five percent of a group of 30 patients treated in a dose-escalation study responded to erythropoietin in the two highest dose levels of 200 to 300 IU/kg/day given intravenously for 5 days each week.[12] Although cisplatin was thought to have a specific effect on reducing erythropoietin levels, the response of patients to erythropoietin does not seem to be specific to the type of chemotherapy given.[13]

Three large-scale, double-blind, placebo-controlled trials have been conducted on a multiinstitutional basis. These trials enrolled a total of 413 patients, including 124 patients in a no-chemotherapy group, 157 patients in a no-cisplatin group, and 132 patients in a cisplatin-receiving group of patients. In each of these trials, patients randomized to erythropoietin treatment had a significantly greater increase in hematocrit than patients receiving placebo. In analyzing the two chemotherapy trials, there was a significantly lower transfusion requirement in the erythropoietin-treated patients during the second or third month of the trial. Quality of life parameters were improved for patients receiving erythropoietin whose hematocrit increased by 6% or more.[8]

The studies indicate that erythropoietin treatment can ameliorate the anemia associated with cancer and chemotherapy, reduce the need for transfusions, and possibly enhance the quality of life. The reduced need for transfusion is the major objective of erythropoietin therapy, reducing the cost, inconvenience, and potential toxicity of blood transfusions.

The question of dose is problematic because efficacy depends in part on the relative impairment of erythropoietin elaboration with respect to the degree of anemia and in part on the level of impaired responsiveness of the bone marrow.[14] A reasonable starting point is 150 U/kg subcutaneously thee times each week. This amounts to approximately 10,000 U for a 70-kg person. Patients with lower plasma erythropoietin concentrations may respond to lower doses of erythropoietin, and higher doses may be needed in patients with apparent bone marrow resistance to erythropoietin. The timing of erythropoietin administration with respect to chemotherapy or radiation therapy has not been sufficiently studied. Most investigations have involved erythropoietin administration concomitantly with chemotherapy. Given our current understanding of the physiology and pathophysiology of erythropoietin responses, this approach does not appear to be ideal. Subsequent investigations may show high-dose administration of erythropoietin for a limited time after chemotherapy to be more efficacious and cost effective.

Endogenous erythropoietin responses tend to be blunted during the 2 or 3 weeks immediately after bone marrow transplantation preceded by intensive chemotherapy and radiotherapy, suggesting that impaired erythropoietin response can contribute to the delayed erythrocyte recovery after bone marrow transplantation.

The role of erythropoietin therapy in myelodysplasia is controversial, with some studies showing responses only in patients with the lowest pretreatment endogenous erythropoietin levels.[15–18] Intensive, high-dose erythropoietin therapy has shown responses in a higher percentage of patients with myelodysplasia. One study showed responses in 24% of patients receiving erythropoietin at a dose of 1200 to 1600 U/kg intravenously twice weekly.[19]

None of the studies of erythropoietin in cancer have reported any significant toxicity due to the erythropoietin, although the cost is significant. It appears that erythropoietin will have an important role in ameliorating the multifactorial anemia associated with cancer, and ultimately, this efficacy will be judged by the decreased need for transfusion.

GRANULOCYTE COLONY-STIMULATING FACTOR

Granulocyte colony-stimulating factor (G-CSF) is a glycoprotein that regulates the production and function of neutrophil granulocytes. G-CSF was originally identified as a leukemia differentiation factor that could be detected in murine serum or lung-conditioned medium after endotoxin administration.[20] Purification revealed that this leukemia differentiation activity was identical to a colony-stimulating factor that exclusively supported the growth of neutrophil granulocyte precursors. Human G-CSF was first purified to homogeneity from the human bladder carcinoma cell line, 5637; subsequently, the gene for human G-CSF and its cDNA were molecularly cloned. The gene for G-CSF is single copy and has been localized to the long arm of chromosome 17 (17q11–q23), a region that contains other genes previously demonstrated or thought to be involved in neutrophil granulocyte development. Recombinant human G-CSF, produced in *Escherichia coli*, is nonglycosylated and has a specific activity of 10^8 units per milligram of protein.[21]

G-CSF is produced by a variety of cell types, including neutrophil granulocytes, endothelial cells, fibroblasts, and bone marrow stromal cells after stimulation by endotoxin, TNF, IL-1, or granulocyte-macrophage colony-stimulating factor (Table 62–7). The cell type representing the most important source of this factor under physiologic conditions in vivo remains unknown. In normal adults (>20 years), circulating levels of immunoreactive G-CSF range between 20 and 95 pg/ml, are unrelated to age or sex, and exhibit no diurnal variation. There is controversy about the relation between circulating G-CSF levels and the neutrophil count under physiologic conditions. Although the precise role that G-CSF plays in the maintenance of steady-state neutrophil granulopoiesis is uncertain, Hammond and colleagues showed that normal dogs can develop neutralizing antibodies to canine G-CSF after administration of human recombinant G-CSF, and they develop profound neutropenia.[22] This result suggests that G-CSF is critical for the regulation and production of neutro-

TABLE 62–7. Sources of Colony-Stimulating Factors

Cell Type	*Stimulus*	*G-CSF*	*GM-CSF*	*IL-3*	*M-CSF*
T-lymphocytes	Antigen, lectin IL-1		+	+	
			+		
B-lymphocytes	LPS, TPA		+		
Natural killer cells	IL-2/CD16 phorbol diester,		+		+
	calcium ionophore			+	
Macrophages	LPS, IL-3, γIFN, GM-CSF	+*			+
		+			
		+			+
Mast cells	IgE, calcium ionophore		+		
Osteoblasts	PTH, LPS		+		
Mesothelial cells	EGF, TNF		+		
Endothelial cells	IL-1	+	+		
Fibroblasts	TNF	+			
	IL-1		+		
Neutrophils	γIFN, GM-CSF	+			
Bone marrow stroma	IL-1	+	+		+

G-CSF, granulocyte colony-stimulating factor; GM-CSF, granulocyte-macrophage colony-stimulating factor; IL-3, interleukin-3; M-macrophage colony-stimulating factor; LPS, lipopolysaccharide; TPA, 12 tetradecanoylphorbol 13 acetate; IL-1, interleukin-1; IL-2, interleukin-2; γIFN, gamma interferon; PTH, parathyroid hormone; EGF, endothelial growth factor; TNF, tumor necrosis factor.
* +, possesses this biologic activity.

phil granulocytes. In bacteremia, in which the characteristic leukocytosis is neutrophilic, G-CSF levels have exceeded 2000 pg/ml, providing additional evidence that G-CSF is systemic regulator of neutrophil production.[23]

G-CSF promotes the survival and stimulates the growth and expansion of immature neutrophil granulocyte precursor cells, enriched promyelocytes, and myelocytes. G-CSF enhances the effector cell capability of the neutrophil granulocyte (Table 62–8) and functions as a weak chemoattractant for these same terminally differentiated cells. G-CSF induces human vascular endothelial cells to proliferate and migrate.

Low numbers of high-affinity receptors for G-CSF exist on normal and malignant myeloid cells and on endothelial cells, placenta, and certain nonhematopoietic tumor cell lines.[24]

TABLE 62–8. Effects of Colony-Stimulating Factors on Myeloid Cells

		Mature Cells			
Factor	*Progenitors*	*Neutrophil*	*Eosinophil*	*Basophil*	*Monocyte*
GM-CSF	Stimualtes CFU-GEMM, CFU-GM, and BFU-E	ADCC, phagocytosis, degranulation, superoxide production, viability, arachidonic acid release, Mo1 expression, cytokine production, changes in cell surface receptor (FMLP) expression, leukotriene and PAF synthesis chemoattractant migration inhibition	ADCC, phagocytosis, viability, cytotoxicity, leukotriene production	Histamine release	ADCC, cytotoxicity, cytokine production, oxidative metabolism, adherence, chemoattractant
G-CSF	Stimulates CFU-G and pre-CFU	ADCC, enhances migration, changes in cell surface receptors for FMLP, weak chemoattractant			
IL-3	Stimulates CFU-GEMM, CFU-GM, BFU-E, CFU-blast		ADCC, cytotoxicity, phagocytosis	Histamine release	ADCC, cytotoxicity
M-CSF	Stimulates CFU-M				ADCC, cytotoxicity

CFU-GEMM, colony-forming unit granulocyte erythroid, megakaryocyte monocyte macrophage; CFU-GM, colony-forming unit granulocyte macrophage; BFU-E, burst forming unit erythroid; CFU-G, colony-forming unit granulocyte; CFU, colony-forming unit; CFU-M, colony forming unit monocyte macrophage; ADCC, antibody-dependent cellular cytotoxicity; FMLP, F-MET-LEU-PHE; PAF, platelet-activating factor.

The molecular mass of the receptor observed in cross-linking experiments is about 150 kd. The high-affinity receptor for human G-CSF has been cloned and found to have an amino-terminal immunoglobulin domain, three fibronectin type III regions, and four conserved cysteine residues characteristic of the cytokine receptor superfamily. A portion of the extracellular domain of the G-CSF receptor exhibits a striking similarity to the prolactin receptor and some similarity to the NCAM family of adhesion molecules. A G-CSF receptor molecule with a deleted transmembrane domain has been cloned, suggesting that it is secreted and can function as a soluble binding protein.[24]

Preclinical studies demonstrated the ability of G-CSF to augment the number of functionally normal neutrophil granulocytes in normal and tumor-bearing mice, hamsters, and cynomolgus monkeys. This neutrophil granulocytosis results from an augmentation in the number of divisions and a reduction (from 96 to 24 hours) in the time required for maturing neutrophil granulocyte precursors to develop into terminally differentiated cells released into the circulation.[25] G-CSF reduced the period of neutropenia in cynomolgus primates treated with high-dose cyclophosphamide, busulfan, or total-body irradiation with autologous marrow reinfusion and in dogs given DLA-identical littermate transplants. G-CSF is radioprotective and can augment survival in murine and canine models of supralethal irradiation without bone marrow rescue.[26]

Three initial human studies revealed that an intravenous bolus, continuous intravenous infusion, subcutaneous injection, or continuous subcutaneous infusion of G-CSF resulted in a dose-dependent increase in the circulating neutrophil granulocyte count.[27–29] This increase in absolute neutrophil count was due primarily to an increase in mature segmented polymorphonuclear leukocytes and was associated with an expansion of the bone marrow myeloid compartment. Morphologic changes (*e.g.*, Döhle bodies, toxic granulations, decreased nuclear lobulation) observed in neutrophil granulocytes after G-CSF are consistent with the marked reduction in the bone marrow transit time of neutrophil precursors mediated by G-CSF. Neutrophil granulocytes produced in response to G-CSF have been shown to be functionally normal, as measured by phagocytic, in vitro, or in vivo migration assays, or to be activated, as evidenced by an increase in leukocyte alkaline phosphatase. An intravenous dose of G-CSF results in an initial decline in the circulating neutrophil count followed by a subsequent rise, with a peak value achieved 4 to 6 hours after G-CSF treatment. After a subcutaneous injection, no initial decline in the neutrophil count is observed, and the maximal neutrophil count achieved is observed 10 to 12 hours after the administered dose of G-CSF. The time at which a blood count is drawn must be taken into account when evaluating a patient's neutrophil response to G-CSF treatment. On discontinuation of G-CSF, neutrophil counts decrease by one half daily and generally return to baseline within 4 days of discontinuing treatment.

Other hematopoietic cell lineages are unaffected by the administration of G-CSF except at higher doses (>60 μg/kg/day, intravenously), for which an increase in circulating monocytes has been reported.[27]

Intravenous and subcutaneous administration of G-CSF is effective for rapidly elevating G-CSF levels in serum. After a single intravenous injection, the peak serum concentration achieved and area under the concentration-time curve are dose dependent. The elimination half-life is about 3.5 hours.[27] After subcutaneous injection, peak levels are achieved within 4 to 6 hours, and levels of more than 10 ng/ml are maintained for 10 to 16 hours thereafter.[30] The mode of G-CSF clearance is unknown.

Neutropenia in cancer patients is a major cause of morbidity and mortality and results from malignant disease and its treatment. Phase I and II studies using a broad spectrum of commonly employed chemotherapeutic regimens demonstrated the ability of G-CSF to accelerate recovery from chemotherapy-induced neutropenia (Table 62–9). In all of these studies, G-CSF was administered 24 hours after cessation of chemotherapy. Optimization of timing and duration of G-CSF treatment has been investigated in patients receiving high-dose melphalan.[31] This study demonstrated accelerated recovery from neutropenia even when G-CSF treatment was begun 8 days after chemotherapy. The ability to delay the use of G-CSF, but not GM-CSF, and commence treatment closer to the time of expected nadir most likely results from the ability of G-CSF to rapidly mobilize neutrophil granulocytes from the bone marrow mitotic compartment. These data suggest that the rate limiting step for G-CSF-mediated recovery from neutropenia is the availability of G-CSF-responsive progenitors.

Based on the phase I and II trials, a randomized, double-blind, placebo-controlled trial of G-CSF was designed to definitively evaluate the incidence of infection as manifested by fever with neutropenia (absolute neutrophil count <1000 cells/μl at 38.2°C).[32] A total of 211 patients were randomly assigned to receive placebo (110) or G-CSF (101), of which 199 were evaluable for efficacy. At least one episode of fever with neutropenia occurred in 77% of placebo group and 40% of the G-CSF-treated group. Over all cycles of chemotherapy, the median duration of severe neutropenia (<500 cells/μl) was 6 days with placebo and 1 day with G-CSF. During cycles of blinded treatment, the days of intravenous antibiotic use, hospitalization, and the incidence of confirmed infections were reduced by 50% with G-CSF administration compared with placebo.

This pivotal phase III trial and earlier studies led to the approval of G-CSF in the United States, Europe, and Japan to reduce the incidence of infection manifested by febrile neutropenia in adult and pediatric patients with nonmyeloid malignancies receiving myelosuppressive chemotherapy. Although only limited data exist for the use of G-CSF for myelosuppressive chemotherapy in the pediatric population, considerable data show a comparable safety profile of G-CSF for children and adults. The recommended starting dose is 5 μg/kg/day subcutaneously to begin after the cessation of chemotherapy, with careful monitoring of blood counts thereafter to avoid leukocytosis. Treatment should be discontinued when the absolute neutrophil count is more than 10,000 cells/μl, after the expected chemotherapy-induced nadir.

Although G-CSF has been of clinical benefit in the treatment of chemotherapy-induced myelosuppression, the use of G-CSF after myeloablative chemotherapy for acute myelogenous leukemia is more controversial. Ohno and colleagues conducted a prospective randomized trial of G-CSF in patients with de novo acute myelogenous leukemia, leukemic trans-

TABLE 62–9. Clinical Trials of G-CSF in Cancer Treatment

Investigations	*Phase*	*G-CSF Dose + Route*	*Tumor Type*	*Chemotherapy*	*No. of Patients*	*Major Findings*
Chemotherapy						
Bronchud[29]	I–II	1–40 μg/kg I.V. 14 days	Small cell lung cancer	Doxorubicin (50 mg/m²), Ifosfamide (5 g/m²), Mesna (8 g/m²) day 1; Etoposide (120 mg/m²/d) days 1–3; repeat q 21 days	12	Decrease in the days of neutropenia, decrease in febrile neutropenia, decrease antibiotic use
Gabrilove[27]	I–II	1–60 μg/kg/d I.V. 8 days (d 4–11)	Transitional cell urothelial carcinoma	Methotrexate (30 mg/m²) days 0, 14, 21; Vinblastine (3 mg/m²) days 1, 14, 21; Doxorubicin (30 mg/m²) and Cisplatin (70 mg/m²) day 1; repeat q 28 days	40	Decrease in days of neutropenia, decrease in febrile neutropenia, decrease antibiotic use, decrease mucositis, increase in patients qualified to receive full dose chemotherapy on schedule
Morstyn[28]	I–II	0.3, 1 or 3 μg SC or 3–10 μg/kg CSCl	Metastatic malignancies	Melphalan (25 mg/m²) day 1	15	Decreased leukopenia
Morstyn[31]	I–II	0.3–10 μg/kg/d SC 5 schedules 1) d 2–13 2) d 8–13 3) d 2–18 4) d 8–18 5) −9 to −2 + d 2–13	Metastatic malignancies	Melphalan (25 mg/m²) day 1	31	Decreased leukopenia
Crawford[32]	III double-blind, randomized, placebo-controlled trial	5 μg/kg/day	Small cell lung cancer	Cyclophosphamide (1 g/m²); Etoposide (120 mg/m² d 1–3) Doxorubacin (50 mg/m²d 1)	210	Statistically significant decrease in days of neutropenia, statistically significant decrease in febrile neutropenia, statistically significant decrease in documented infections
Dose-Intensified Chemotherapy						
Bronchud[37]	I–II	5 μg/kg/day C1 × 11 d	Ovarian and breast carcinoma	Doxorubacin 75, 100, 125, or 150 mg/m² q 14 days	21	Dose escalation of doxorubacin to 100 mg/m² q 2 weeks
Neidhart[38]	I–II	23–69 μg/kg I.V. d 8–28	Refractory malignancy	Cisplatin (105 mg/m²) Etoposide (1500 mg/m²) Cyclophosphamide (5 g/m²)	18	Dose intensity able to be delivered
Bone Marrow Transplantation						
Sheridan[34]	I–II	20 μg/kg/d SC: scheduled dose reductions: 5 μg/kg/d ANC >1000 × 3 days; 1 μg/kg/d if ANC >1000 × 3 days on 5 μg/kg/d 28 days total treatment	Hodgkin's/non-Hodgkin's lymphoma, germ cell, ALL, ANLL	Busulfan (4 mg/kg/d) days −7 to −4; Cyclophosphamide (60 mg/kg/d) days −3 and −2	15	Reduction in days of neutropenia compared to historic controls

(continued)

TABLE 62–9. *(Continued)*

Investigations	*Phase*	*G-CSF Dose + Route*	*Tumor Type*	*Chemotherapy*	*No. of Patients*	*Major Findings*
Taylor[35]	I–II	60 μg/kg/d scheduled dose reductions: 30 μg/kg/d if ANC >2500 × 3 days, 8 μg/kg/d if ANC increase further on 30 μg/kg/d 28 days (max)	Hodgkin's disease	Cyclophosphamide (1.5 g/m²/d) days −6 to −3; carmustine (300 mg/m²); day −6; etoposide (125 mg/m² q 12 h) days −6 to −4	18	Reduction in days of severe neutropenia (<200 cells/μl and <500 cells/μl)
Peters[36]	I–II	16–64 μg/kg C1 × 14 days	Breast cancer or melanoma	Cyclophosphamide (5625 mg/m²), cisplatin (165 mg/m²), carmustine (600 mg/m²)	15	Reduction in days of neutropenia

formation from myelodysplastic syndrome (MDS), acute lymphocytic leukemia, or blastic phase of chronic myelogenous leukemia after mitoxantrone, etoposide, and bentenoyl-cytosine arabinoside therapy.[33] G-CSF significantly accelerated the recovery of neutrophils, reduced the incidence of documented infection, and did not preferentially promote the regrowth of leukemic cells.

G-CSF has been used in patients with breast carcinoma, Hodgkin's disease, and non-Hodgkin's lymphoma undergoing autologous bone marrow transplantation.[34–36] The G-CSF administered after ablative therapy was effective in augmenting recovery from neutropenia compared with historic controls.

Although treatment with G-CSF has rendered standard cancer treatment more tolerable with respect to neutropenia and its complications, a larger question remains about whether it will permit significant intensified therapy and whether such therapy will contribute to improved survival for cancer patients. Bronchud and colleagues demonstrated that G-CSF allowed administration of dose-intensified doxorubicin (100 mg/m² every 2 weeks) for three cycles to patients with ovarian or breast carcinoma refractory to standard-dose chemotherapy.[37] Treatment resulted in a response rate of 80%. Neidhart and coworkers demonstrated the ability of G-CSF to reduce grade IV neutropenia and antibiotic requirements in patients treated with dose-intensified cisplatin (150 mg/m²), etoposide (150 mg/m²), and cyclophosphamide (5 g/m²).[38] These two studies show that dose-intensified chemotherapy is feasible, but a significant period of neutropenia was observed despite concomitant treatment with G-CSF. The use of earlier-acting hematopoietic growth factors or specific progenitor populations harvested from the peripheral blood will probably be required to provide greater protection from myelosuppression and permit safe study of dose-intensified regimens.

Neutropenia is an important problem in hematopoietic malignancies, pancytopenic states, acquired immunodeficiency syndrome (AIDS), and genetic disorders of granulocyte production. Pilot studies of G-CSF in patients with hairy cell leukemia, myelodysplastic syndrome, and aplastic anemia have demonstrated improvements in circulating neutrophil counts associated in some instances with a decrease in the incidence of or enhanced recovery from active infection.[39–41] No evidence of treatment-induced proliferation of the malignant clone has been observed. G-CSF, administered alone or in combination with erythropoietin, can ameliorate zidovudine-induced myelotoxicity in patients with AIDS without stimulating p24 antigen expression.[42] Initial pilot studies of G-CSF in patients with primary neutropenic disorders (*e.g.*, cyclic neutropenia, congenital neutropenia, idiopathic neutropenia) demonstrated the ability of G-CSF to augment circulating neutrophil counts, reduce the incidence of infection and mucositis, and improve quality of life parameters.[43–45] These preliminary findings have been confirmed by a phase III randomized trial of G-CSF in patients with severe chronic neutropenia, suggesting that this hematopoietic growth factor can play an important role in the management and treatment of these disorders.

Treatment with G-CSF is generally well tolerated, with the most consistent and significant clinical side effect being "medullary" bone pain. This bone discomfort is felt most in the lower back, pelvis, and sternum and is usually experienced within a 24-hour period as the neutrophil count begins to recover. It is observed most commonly after intravenous administration. Chronic G-CSF administration in patients with primary neutropenia has been associated with the detection of clinically inapparent splenomegaly as measured by magnetic resonance imaging or computed tomography scanning in 13% of patients. This effect of G-CSF is more commonly seen in children. Other unusual side effects, reported in single patients, have included a flare in psoriasis, recurrence of Sweet's syndrome (*i.e.*, cutaneous neutrophilic vasculitis) and cutaneous vasculitis.

GRANULOCYTE-MACROPHAGE COLONY-STIMULATING FACTOR

Granulocyte macrophage colony-stimulating factor (GM-CSF) is one of a family of glycoproteins that have potent effects in stimulating the proliferation and function of hematopoietic cells. Human GM-CSF was purified by Gasson and colleagues from a human T-cell leukemia virus (HTLV-II)-infected T-lymphoblastoid cell line.[46] The purified protein was identical to the previously described T-lymphocyte-derived lymphokine referred to as neutrophil-migration inhibition factor. Human GM-CSF is highly and variably *N*- and *O*-glycosylated, accounting for a wide range in reported molecular weights (14–35 kd). The complementary cDNA encoding the human GM-CSF protein was molecularly cloned by Wong and coworkers.[47] The gene for human GM-CSF is single copy and has been mapped by in situ hybridization to the long arm of chromosome 5 (5q23–31). This region contains a number of growth factors and receptors that are involved in the regulation of hematopoiesis and the inflammatory response. Complementary DNA encoding GM-CSF has been expressed in Chinese hamster ovary cells (CHO cells), yeast, and *E. coli*. The three forms of recombinant GM-CSF, which have been produced for clinical use, have specific acclivities of 4.4×10^6 units, 5×10^7 units, and 2×10^8 units per milligram of protein, respectively.

GM-CSF is produced by activated T lymphocytes, B lymphocytes, endothelial cells, mast cells, fibroblasts, macrophages, mesothelial cells, and osteoblasts in response to specific activating agents (see Table 62–7). GM-CSF is also constitutively produced by a number of tumor cell lines and placenta. Unlike G-CSF, GM-CSF is not detectable in serum under physiologic conditions, suggesting that GM-CSF normally acts in a paracrine fashion. Analogous to IL-1, GM-CSF has been detected in synovial fluid from patients with inflammatory arthropathies, suggesting that it might play a role in the tissue damage associated with the inflammatory process.

GM-CSF supports the in vitro growth of uncommitted multilineage precursors (in the presence of erythropoietin) and committed cells (*i.e.*, granulocyte, monocyte) precursor cells (see Table 62–8). In addition to its effects on bone marrow progenitors, GM-CSF enhances the function of mature neutrophil and eosinophil granulocytes and monocytes and macrophages. The effects of GM-CSF on mature effector cells of several lineages, in contrast to G-CSF, may reflect the wide role of this cytokine in host defense and the inflammatory response (see Table 62–8). GM-CSF directly affects neutrophil expression of cellular adhesion molecules, locomotion, responsiveness to chemotactic factors, biosynthetic function, and tumoricidal and phagocytic activity. Priming effects of GM-CSF on neutrophils include stimulation of the respiratory burst, degranulation and enhanced synthesis of mediators of inflammation such as leukotrienes, platelet-activating factor, and elaboration of cytokines such as TNF, M-CSF, IL-1, and G-CSF. In the presence of GM-CSF, mature eosinophils and macrophages demonstrate enhanced tumoricidal and phagocytic activity. In contrast to M-CSF, GM-CSF is a more potent inducer of secondary cytokines secreted by monocytes, such as IL-1 and TNF-α, perhaps accounting for the difference in side effects reported in vivo with these two molecules. GM-CSF has enhanced the replication of human immunodeficiency virus (HIV) in normal monocytes and macrophages and potentiated the anti-HIV activity of zidovudine by facilitating drug entry and subsequent phosphorylation.

Similar to G-CSF, M-CSF, and IL-3, GM-CSF was produced by some blasts obtained from patients with acute myelogenous leukemia. Controversy exists about whether this represents constitutive production or induction secondary to in vitro cell manipulation. GM-CSF has also been shown, as have G-CSF and IL-3 but not M-CSF, to augment the proliferation of myeloid leukemic cells. Progenitors derived from patients with juvenile chronic myelogenous leukemia exhibit an enhanced sensitivity to the stimulatory effects of GM-CSF.[48] Overexpression of GM-CSF in murine bone marrow results in a myeloproliferative syndrome that is fatal but nonneoplastic.[49] A comparable model employing G-CSF results in sustained neutrophilia and organ infiltration by neutrophilic granulocytes without organ damage or premature death.[50] A role for GM-CSF in the pathogenesis of myeloid leukemias is uncertain.

Receptors for GM-CSF exist on normal neutrophils and their precursors, eosinophils, and monocytes and macrophages.[24,51] These cells normally express a low number of high-affinity binding sites with dissociation constants of 30 to 100 pM. High-affinity receptors have been found on cell lines derived from small cell carcinoma, malignant myeloid (HL-60 and KG-1), and monocytoid (U937) leukemias and on nonhematopoietic tissue, such as placenta and endothelial cells.[24] Low-affinity binding sites have been identified on malignant hematopoietic cells and on COS cells, human melanoma, osteogenic sarcoma, and breast carcinoma cell lines and primary melanoma.[24] Controversy exists about whether these low-affinity receptors mediate proliferation in all cells in which it is expressed. The low-affinity human GM-CSF receptor (α subunit) has been cloned and sequenced and localized to the pseudoautosomal region of the sex chromosomes. Hayashida and colleagues isolated a human homolog of the murine IL-3 receptor cDNA, which encodes a 120-kd transmembrane adapter protein (β subunit) that confers high-affinity binding to the low-affinity (α) GM-CSF receptor.[51] Specific α subunits exist for GM-CSF, IL-5, and IL-3 receptors, but they share and may compete for the same B subunit.

In preclinical studies, the administration of human GM-CSF to normal rhesus monkeys resulted in a dramatic leukocytosis consisting initially of only neutrophil granulocytes and monocytes followed by an additional substantial increase in eosinophil granulocytes.[52] Treatment was associated with significant reticulocytosis, but no changes in hemoglobin or hematocrit were observed. A model of pancytopenia induced by simian type D retrovirus in rhesus monkeys provided data supporting the clinical application of GM-CSF in patients with AIDS, bone marrow failure states, and infectious disease.[52] Models investigating the utility of GM-CSF after total-body irradiation and autologous bone marrow reinfusion demonstrated the myelorestorative effect of GM-CSF in the transplant setting and provided the framework for designing clinical trials with humans.

The initial clinical investigation of GM-CSF, which was the first clinical study of a hematopoietic growth factor in humans, was conducted using 16 relatively well patients with AIDS and leukopenia.[53] Continuous intravenous infusion of CHO cell-derived recombinant GM-CSF (0.3–4.5 μg/kg/day for 14 days) resulted in a dramatic augmentation in circulating granulocytes and with a lesser increase in monocytes. Neutrophils produced in 6 of these patients exhibited improved phagocytosis and antibody-dependent cellular cytotoxicity. Additional studies evaluating the safety of *E. coli*-derived GM-CSF and the chronic subcutaneous administration of CHO cell-derived GM-CSF showed improved leukocyte counts and enhanced monocyte function in treated patients with AIDS; however, treatment has been associated with an increase in serum HIV p24 antigen in some cases, suggesting stimulation of HIV replication.[54] In patients randomized to receive GM-CSF after chemotherapy for HIV-associated non-Hodgkin's lymphoma, there was a more than twofold increase in HIV p24 compared with controls.[55] In contrast, the subcutaneous administration of nonglycosylated GM-CSF to HIV patients receiving ganciclovir or yeast-derived GM-CSF to patients with AIDS-associated Kaposi's sarcoma receiving zidovudine and interferon-α has not been associated with any discernible stimulation of HIV replication and has resulted in the abrogation of therapy-associated neutropenia.[56] Similarly, the administration of zidovudine alternating with GM-CSF in patients previously treated with GM-CSF alone is associated with a return to baseline of serum HIV p24 values, permitting patients to receive zidovudine who otherwise could not tolerate conventional doses of antiviral medication. These data suggest that, although GM-CSF holds promise for use in AIDS in combination with antiviral agents, there are a number of complex interactions that still require investigation. The impressive leukocyte responses observed in these studies also underscores the remarkable sensitivity of leukopenic AIDS patients to low doses of GM-CSF. Although these patients are highly responsive to GM-CSF, they also seem to be more sensitive to toxic effects and often do not tolerate chronic administration well.

In hematologically normal and leukopenic cancer patients, a dose-dependent increase in neutrophils is observed after short or continuous intravenous infusion and subcutaneous injection of CHO cell, yeast, and bacterially derived GM-CSF; intravenous bolus of nonglycosylated GM-CSF appears to be less efficacious. Patients who have received extensive prior chemotherapy or radiotherapy exhibit the smallest elevations in circulating leukocytes in response to GM-CSF treatment. The neutrophils produced in response to GM-CSF appear to function normally, as measured by phagocytosis and generation of superoxide; however, impaired migration in vivo has been reported in patients receiving continuous intravenous infusions of CHO cell-derived GM-CSF but not bacterially derived GM-CSF administered as a 4-hour infusion.[57,58]

After the administration of CHO cell or bacterially derived GM-CSF (given as a short or continuous intravenous infusion), there is an immediate transient neutropenia, eosinopenia, and monocytopenia. The time of maximal nadir is 30 minutes, with a rebound in leukocyte count to baseline or above baseline by 2 hours. Radionucleotide labeling studies show that this leukopenia is due primarily to sequestration within the lungs.[59] After subcutaneous administration, the nadir occurs 60 minutes after treatment and can persist for up to 4 hours.

In addition to neutrophilia, treatment with GM-CSF results in an augmentation of circulating monocytes with, in some instances, enhanced tumoricidal activity. The ability to stimulate monocyte-macrophage number and function may be responsible for the reported serum cholesterol lowering activity of GM-CSF. Eosinophils also increase after 7 days of treatment with GM-CSF. No consistent effects on hemoglobin, reticulocyte, or platelet counts have been found after treatment with GM-CSF; however, the occurrence of thrombocytopenia secondary to reactivation of idiopathic thrombocytopenic purpura has been reported.

The augmentation in circulating leukocyte counts after glycosylated and nonglycosylated GM-CSF administration is associated with an 18-fold and eightfold increase in circulating myeloid and erythroid hematopoietic precursor cells, respectively.[60] Additional studies in chemotherapy-naive patients demonstrated impressive mobilization of peripheral blood progenitors (up to 1000-fold) when GM-CSF is administered after myelosuppressive chemotherapy.[61] No comparable changes in bone marrow progenitors have been reported, although marrow cellularity and myeloid-to-erythroid cell ratios are increased; however, an increase in the percentage of bone marrow-derived myeloid and erythroid progenitors, myeloblasts, promyelocytes and myelocytes in S phase has been observed in patients receiving 3 and 6 days of yeast-derived GM-CSF.[62] An increase in the rate of hematopoietic cells entering the cell cycle, a decrease in the actual cell cycle time, and a decrease in the duration of the S-phase portion of the cell cycle has also been reported. After discontinuation of GM-CSF, the proportion of cells in S phase decreases to values below that observed before treatment. These findings suggest a period where hematopoietic cells may exhibit relative refractoriness to cell-cycle-specific antineoplastic agents.

The pharmacokinetics of glycosylated GM-CSF and nonglycosylated GM-CSF have been extensively studied. A two-compartment model has been determined for both with comparable elimination times: $T_{1/2}\alpha$ of 10 ± 3 minutes and a $T_{1/2}\beta$ of 85 ± 35 minutes for yeast-derived GM-CSF; $T_{1/2}\alpha$ of 5 minutes and $T_{1/2}\beta$ of 150 minutes for bacterially derived GM-CSF.[30] In contrast, a rise in detectable GM-CSF levels occurs within 1 hour, peaks in 2 to 4 hours, and declines 2 to 12 hours after subcutaneous administration of nonglycosylated GM-CSF. The time during which nonglycosylated GM-CSF remains detectable is dose dependent. After the injection of 10 μg/kg nonglycosylated GM-CSF, plasma levels of GM-CSF equivalent to the maximal activity required to stimulate progenitor cell development and granulocyte-monocyte function are achieved and are detectable for 12 hours.

Several studies have explored the role of glycosylated and nonglycosylated GM-CSF in ameliorating the myelosuppression associated with autologous bone marrow transplantation for breast carcinoma, melanoma, lymphoid malignancies, and non-Hodgkin's lymphoma (Table 62–10).[63–65] The first trial in this clinical setting demonstrated that CHO cell-derived GM-CSF, administered as a continuous intravenous infusion beginning 3 hours after autologous marrow infusion, resulted in accelerated recovery of circulating leukocyte counts and reduced bacteremia, hepatotoxicity, and nephrotoxicity compared with historic controls.[63] A second historically controlled trial of yeast-derived GM-CSF administered as a daily 2-hour infusion for 14 days, beginning 1 hour after completion of autologous or allogeneic bone marrow transplantation, demonstrated that treatment (at doses >60 μg/m^2) resulted in fewer days of neutropenia (neutrophil count <500 cells/μl), fever, and required platelet transfusions.[64] No enhancement of graft-versus-host disease was found in the few patients receiving allogeneic transplants.

A randomized, double-blind, placebo-controlled trial of yeast-derived GM-CSF after autologous bone marrow transplantation for lymphoid cancer was later completed.[65] Sixty-three patients received daily 2-hour infusions of GM-CSF for 21 days, beginning within 4 hours of marrow infusion, and 63 patients received placebo. The patients treated with GM-CSF had a recovery of neutrophils to 500 cells/μl 7 days earlier than patients who received placebo, 3 fewer days of antibiotics,

(text continues on page 2288)

TABLE 62–10. Clinical Trials of GM-CSF in Cancer Treatment

Investigations	*Phase*	*GM Prep*	*GM Dose + Route*	*Tumor Type*	*Chemotherapy*	*No. of Patients*	*Results*
Chemotherapy							
Antman[63]	I–II	Glycosylated CHO cell	CI	Sarcoma	Isofamide, doxorubicin, dacarbazine	16	Less severe and shorter neutropenia: no difference in febrile neutropenia
Gianni[65]	I–II	Glycosylated (CHO)	CI 5.5 μg/kg/d d 1–14	Breast, non-Hodgkin's lymphoma	Cyclophosphamide (7 g/m^2)	15	Reduction in the duration of neutropenia, decrease in infections complications
De Vries[67]	II	Glycosylated (CHO)	SC 0.25–0.75 μg/m^2	Ovarian carcinoma	Carboplatin, cyclophosphamide	15	Improved hematologic (neutrophil and platelet count) recovery after successive cycles of chemotherapy
Morstyn[64]	I–II	Nonglycosylated	SC 5–15 μg/kg/d d 7–21	Small Cell Lung carcinoma	CBDCA Etoposide	18	Improved neutrophil counts
Hermann[67]	II	Nonglycosylated	SC 6.1 μg/kg/d 10 days	Various	Several regimens	22	Reduction in duration neutropenia earlier neutrophil nadir improved delivery of chemotherapy on schedule reduction in infectious episodes
Barloggie[66]	I–II	Nonglycosylated	SC 0.25–0.75 mg/m^2	Multiple myeloma	Melphalan	23	Reduction in duration of neutropenia in younger patients with adequate hematopoietic reserve
Logethetis[69]	I	Nonglycosylated	SC or Cl d 3–13 120–500 μg/m^2	Bladder carcinoma	Methotrexate, vinblastine	32	Reduction in severity and duration of granulocytopenia
Bone Marrow Transplantation							
Nemunaitis[61]	I	Glycosylated (yeast)	I.V. (2h) 1–250 μg/m^2 × 21 days	Lymphoid cancers	Cyclophosphamide and total-body irradiation	15	In patients receiving ≥60 μg/m^2, the following was observed: enhanced neutrophil count recovery, decrease in episodes of infection, reduction in days of hospitalization, and decrease in the number of days to become platelet transfusion independent
Brandt[60]	I	Glycosylated (CHO)	Continuous I.V.	Breast carcinoma and melanoma	Cyclophosphamide, cisplatin, carmustine	19	Enhanced recovery of neutrophil count, decrease in transplant-associated morbidity with decrease in elevations of creatinine and bilirubin and decrease in bacteremia
Nemunaitis[62]	III (randomized, double blind)	Glycosylated (yeast)	250 μg/m^2 2-h I.V. infusion × 21 days	Lymphoid cancers		126	Decrease in neutropenic (<500 cells/μl) days, decrease in infectious episodes, decrease in antibiotic requirements, decrease in the days of hospitalization

TABLE 62–11. Clinical Trials of Hematopoietic Growth Factors in Myelodysplastic Syndrome

Investigations	*Growth Factor*	*Dose*	*Route and Schedule*	*No. of Patients*	*Prior Therapy*	*MDS Subtype*	*Blasts in Bone Marrow (%)*	*Blasts in Blood (%)*	*Results: Decreased RBC TX*	*Decreased Platelets TX*	*Other Findings*	*POD to AML*
Vadhan-Raj	Glycosylated GM (yeast)	30–500 μg/m²	Continuous infusion (CI) × 14 d every 2 wk	8	2 hormonal/ vitamin 4 Dauna/Ara-C	1 RA 3 RAEB 3 RAEBIT 1 Hypoplasia after Chemo RX	>10% (6)	0/8 with circulating blasts	2/4 (1 who had hypoplasia p RX)	2/8 (1 had hypoplasia p RX)	Increase WBC and ANC	0
Rifkin	Glycosylated GM (yeast)	30–480 μg/m²	Subcutaneous 4 wk	11	NA	RA RAEB + RAEBT	NA	NA		1	Increase in ANC (10/11) Increase in retics (2/11) 2 patients progressed to acute leukemia	
Antin	Glycosylated GM (yeast)	15–480 μg/m²	Short intravenous infusion 7 or 14 d	7	NA	2 RA 4 RAEB	NA	NA	No change	No change	Increase in ANC, monocytes and reticulocytes (6/7) increase in eosinophils (2/7) increase in blasts (2/7)	0
Ganser	Nonglycosylated GM (*E. coli*)	15–50 μg/m²	Intravenous (I.V.) bolus day 1: 8 hour infusion, thereafter ×	11	1 LDAra-C	3 RA 4 RAEB 2 CMMOL	>14% (4)	4/11	No change	No change	Increase WBC and ANC (8/11), increase bone marrow and circulating blasts in 1 patient with no prior circulating blasts: increase circulating blasts in 1 patient with prior circulating blasts	5
Thompson	Nonglycosylated GM (*E. coli*)	0.3–10 μg/kg/d	Subcutaneous (SC) daily × 28 d	16	7 hormonal/ vitamin 1 LDAra-C	7 RA 8 RAEB 1 RAEBIT	≥10% (8)	NA	No change	No change	Increase ANC (12/16): increase monos/eos (10/16), transient increase in retics (2).	1

											Increase in bone marrow blasts (5) decrease bone marrow blasts (4)
Estey	Glycosylated GM	120 $\mu g/m^2$	CI	22	NA	17 RAEBT	NA	NA	NA	2	Increase in ANC in all patients Increase bone marrow blasts (4/22); increase platelets (2/22)
Hermann	Nonglycosylated GM and yeast-derived GM (*E. coli*)	5–750 $\mu g/m^2$ × 5	I.V. q 5 h q 10 d × 11	4	1 HDAra-C 3 LDAra-C 1 Mithramycin	1 RAEB 1 RAEBT 2 CMML	17–29%			No change	Increase in ANC with >500 $\mu g/m^2$ yeast GM or >250 *E. coli* GM Increase × >2-fold in circulating blasts Increase in bone marrow blasts
Kobaychi	G-CSF nonglycosylated (*E. coli*)	50–1600 $\mu g/m^2$	I.V.	5	NA	RAEB	0–67% before treatment	NA	NA	NA	Increase in ANC
Negrin	G–CSF nonglycosylated	0.1–3.0 $\mu g/kg/d$	SC × 6–8 wk	13	Retinoic Acid Danozol	2 RA 8 RAEBT	≥21%	0–13% peripheral blood myeloblasts	2/9 transfusion dependent	0	Increase ANC (11/13) Increase retics (5/13)
Ganser	IL-3 nonglycosylated	250–500 $\mu g/m^2$	SC daily × 15 d	9	GM-CSF (2) Steroids (2) Ara-C (1) Androgens (1)	6 RA 3 RAEB	NA	>10% (1)	1	2	Increase WBC 1.3- to 3.6-fold Increase platelets in 7/9 Decrease platelets transiently 2/9

Dauna/Ara-C, Daunorubicin, cytosine arabinoside; NA, not available; HD, high dose; RX, treatment; RA, refractory anemia; RAEB, refractory anemia with excess blasts; CMMOL, chronic myelomonocytic leukemia; Ara-C, cytosine arabinoside; LD, low dose; RAEBT, refractory anemia with excess blasts in transformation; Chemo RX, chemotherapy; ANC, absolute neutrophil count; WBC, white blood cell count; retics, reticulocyte count; GM, granulocyte macrophage colony-stimulating factor; G-CSF, granulocyte colony-stimulating factor; IL-3, interleukin-3; TX, transfusion; POD, progression of disease.

and 6 fewer days of initial hospitalization; however, no difference in survival was observed at 100 days after transplantation. Based on these data, yeast-derived GM-CSF was approved in the United States to reduce infection in the setting of autologous bone marrow transplantation.

The therapeutic utility of glycosylated and nonglycosylated GM-CSF in ameliorating myelosuppressive toxicity of chemotherapy, in the absence of marrow reinfusion, has been investigated in patients with sarcoma, small cell carcinoma of the lung, non-Hodgkin's lymphoma, myeloma, ovarian carcinoma, other advanced solid tumors, and acute myelogenous leukemia (see Table 62–10).[66–72] The results of these nonrandomized trials suggest that treatment with GM-CSF hastens the recovery of granulocytes but not platelets or erythrocytes.

GM-CSF used after chemotherapy for acute nonlymphocytic leukemia has not been associated with an increased incidence of relapse or induction failure. In these trials, GM-CSF was begun immediately after the administration of chemotherapy. Gianni and coworkers compared the granulocyte recovery observed when CHO cell-derived GM-CSF was administered 1 day or 5 days after high-dose cyclophosphamide (7 g/m^2). In this study, no accelerated leukocyte recovery was observed when GM-CSF treatment was delayed, suggesting that the immediate administration of GM-CSF after completion of chemotherapy is critical if a therapeutic benefit is to be preserved. Three additional studies examined the therapeutic contribution of GM-CSF to the successful implementation of dose-intensified chemotherapeutic regimens, with conflicting results.[73–75] Although the administration of nonglycosylated GM-CSF permitted dose-intensified M-VAC regimen to be safely administered, resulting in significant tumor responses in previously unresponsive patients, the coadministration of this same preparation of GM-CSF did not maintain the initial hematologic improvement observed over multiple 21-day cycles of doxorubicin (75 mg/m^2) plus cyclophosphamide (750 mg/m^2) therapy in patients with advanced breast carcinoma.[73,74] GM-CSF did not permit additional dose escalation of these two agents. Similarly, treatment with GM-CSF (125 μg/m^2 over 6 hours on days 6 through 21) resulted in significantly more erythrocyte and platelet transfusions and infectious episodes in patients treated with high-dose etoposide (800 mg/m^2 continuous infusion × 96 hours), cisplatin (100 mg/m^2 by continuous infusion × 96 hours), Solu-Medrol (500 mg by intravenous bolus on days 1–5), and cytosine arabinoside (1.5 g/m^2 on day 5), compared with the prophylactic antibiotics ketoconazole (200 mg/day) and ciprofloxacin (750 mg orally twice daily on days 6 through 21).

Clinical investigations of GM-CSF in aplastic anemia indicate that treatment results in augmentation of circulating monocytes and granulocytes, in patients with some evidence of residual myelopoiesis but does not affect consistent changes in platelet count, erythrocytes, or transfusion requirements.[76–79] Prior treatment has no effect on therapeutic response, and most patients require continued treatment to maintain the desired hematologic effect. Discontinuation of treatment is associated with a return to baseline peripheral blood counts and bone marrow cellularity.

Nonrandomized clinical trials investigating the role of yeast and bacterially derived GM-CSF in patients with myelodysplastic syndrome reported similar increases in granulocyte counts, without consistent improvements in other hematopoietic lineages (Table 62–11).[80–84] In patients with more advanced disease (*e.g.*, refractory anemia with excess blasts or refractory anemia with excess blasts in transformation) or chronic myelomonocytic leukemia, treatment is associated with an increase in circulating and bone marrow blasts, although in most cases, the blast count returned toward pretreatment values after discontinuation of treatment. Initial results from a phase III randomized trial in patients with refractory anemia and severe neutropenia, receiving 6 months of GM-CSF or no treatment demonstrate that GM-CSF does accelerate transformation to acute leukemia within the time frame studied and augments neutrophil counts. Whether treatment results in a significant reduction in serious infection in this category of patients remains to be determined.

Several side effects have been reported in patients receiving glycosylated and nonglycosylated GM-CSF. Fever and bone pain are the most common side effects observed in patients treated with nonglycosylated GM-CSF. Pericarditis was dose limiting in patients treated with 20 to 30 μg/kg/day, but this side effect was not observed in 16 patients treated with lower doses. In patients receiving nonglycosylated GM-CSF, a peculiar first-dose reaction including flushing, hypotension, transient hypoxia, and tachycardia has been described.[85] Subsequent doses do not elicit this response; however, if treatment is discontinued for 10 or more days and GM-CSF is reintroduced, the first dose again may produce this reaction. Morstyn and colleagues reported that the reaction appears to occur predominantly in patients receiving short infusions and perhaps more commonly in patients with active pulmonary disease.[85]

The major side effects associated with glycosylated GM-CSF appear to be fever, bone pain, myalgia, and constitutional symptoms. The fever observed secondary to CHO cell-derived GM-CSF can be abrogated by the concomitant administration of indomethacin, suggesting that it is mediated by prostaglandins. Short intravenous infusion of yeast-derived GM-CSF has been associated with dose-limiting epigastric distress, nausea, and vomiting. In two studies, higher doses (>32 μg/kg/day) of CHO cell-derived GM-CSF used before chemotherapy or after autologous bone marrow transplantation resulted in generalized edema, thrombophlebitis, hypotension, and acute renal failure. Comparable side effects with yeast-derived GM-CSF have not been reported, but comparable doses have not been explored in equivalent clinical settings. The side effects have been minimal for yeast-derived GM-CSF used in the setting of autologous bone marrow transplantation for lymphoid malignancies. Treatment with glycosylated and nonglycosylated GM-CSF has been associated with a transient decline in platelet count and with reactivation of idiopathic thrombocytopenic purpura.

MACROPHAGE COLONY-STIMULATING FACTOR

Macrophage colony-stimulating factor (M-CSF or CSF-1) is a mononuclear phagocyte-specific growth factor first identified and purified from mouse L cells and human urine.[86] M-CSF is a heavily glycosylated disulfide-linked homodimer biochemically related to the insulin-relaxin family of hormones. Complementary cDNAs have been cloned that encode two different biologically active forms of M-CSF, resulting from differential splicing. The larger M-CSF precursor (mRNA,

4.0 kb) encodes a protein that is proteolytically cleaved within the cell; the resulting 70,000-kd glycoprotein product is secreted from the cell. This M-CSF is the major form excreted in human urine. The smaller precursor (mRNA, 2.0 kb) encodes a membrane-bound protein from which multiple forms of soluble extracellular M-CSF are generated by proteolytic cleavage. Removal of carbohydrate does not affect the biologic function of M-CSF, but treatment with disulfide-reducing agents abolishes activity. Human M-CSF is coded for by a single gene, which was initially localized to the long arm of chromosome 5 (5q33.1), but which recently has been reassigned to the short arm of chromosome 1 (1p13–21). Recombinant human M-CSF for clinical use is produced in *E. coli* and CHO cells and has a specific activity 1×10^7 units and 0.8×10^6 units per milligram of protein, respectively.

M-CSF is constitutively produced by fibroblasts and bone marrow stromal cells. Monocyte-macrophages and endothelial cells also synthesize M-CSF in response to activators involved in the inflammatory response. Uterine glandular epithelial cells express M-CSF in response to ovarian hormones, suggesting that M-CSF may be of importance in placental development or function.[86] M-CSF is normally detected in human serum and appears to be increased in patients with myeloproliferative disorders.

Radiolabeled M-CSF-binding studies demonstrate a single class of high-affinity receptors on the surface of mononuclear phagocytes and trophoblasts.[24] This cell-surface receptor is now known to be the *CSF1R* (formerly *FMS*) protooncogene product, an integral transmembrane glycoprotein with ligand stimulated protein-tyrosine kinase activity. Binding of M-CSF to its receptor activates the kinase resulting in autophosphorylation of the receptor and phosphorylation of other cellular proteins on tyrosine residues. The physiologic substrates for the receptor kinase activity have not been identified.

In vitro, M-CSF stimulates the growth and maturation of monocyte and macrophages. M-CSF also enhances macrophage migration, expression of Fc receptors and adhesion molecules, cytotoxicity and respiratory burst activity, and bacterial and fungal killing in vitro. M-CSF primes but does not directly induce monocytes to secrete cytokines such as TNF and IL-1. M-CSF has been implicated in the growth, maturation, and function of osteoclasts, and alterations in the M-CSF gene are responsible for congenital osteopetrosis in op/op mutant mice.[87]

In vivo, M-CSF increases circulating monocytes that are functionally activated and exhibit enhanced tumoricidal cytotoxicity.[88] There is an associated expansion of bone marrow monocytic elements. M-CSF protects mice from lethal infection after challenge with *Candida albicans*.

The first clinical trials of M-CSF employed highly purified human urinary CSF and demonstrated some myelorestorative activity.[89] The administration of recombinant glycosylated and nonglycosylated M-CSF in cancer patients stimulates a prominent increase in the number of circulating monocytes.[90,91] Monocytes induced by M-CSF display enhanced antibody-dependent cellular cytotoxicity, respiratory burst activity, migration, and degranulation and ingestion of *Candida*. The ability of M-CSF to augment intracellular killing of fungal organisms prompted a trial designed to evaluate the ability of M-CSF to enhance recovery from invasive fungal infection in marrow transplant recipients receiving conventional antifungal therapy. The results suggest that M-CSF may be useful in this setting, but further investigation is needed to establish its therapeutic benefit. In these initial clinical investigations, adverse events included bone pain and thrombocytopenia due presumably to peripheral destruction of platelets. Administration of glycosylated M-CSF has also been associated with a marked reduction in serum cholesterol. Additional studies designed to explore this biologic property should prove informative.

INTERLEUKIN-3

IL-3 (multi-CSF) is a glycoprotein hormone related to GM-CSF that supports the growth of multilineage colonies in vitro. Murine IL-3 was identified and characterized by Ihle and associates, and the human IL-3 cDNA was isolated by expression cloning of mRNA from a Gibbon T-cell line.[92] Human IL-3 exists as a single copy gene mapped to the long arm of chromosome 5 (5q23–31) within 9 kb of the gene for GM-CSF. IL-3 and GM-CSF share conserved regions in their promoter sequences, suggesting a common regulatory mechanism for their expression. Recombinant human IL-3 for clinical use is produced in *E. coli* and yeast and has a specific activity of 4.3×10^6 units and $0.9–6.7 \times 10^8$ units per milligram of protein, respectively.

IL-3 is a lymphokine and is produced primarily by activated T lymphocytes and natural killer cells. IL-3 supports the growth of early hematopoietic progenitors in vitro. IL-3 augments the functional activity of monocytes, macrophages, and eosinophils, and it stimulates the growth of basophils and the production of intracellular histamine.

IL-3 administration to normal primates results in a modest and delayed leukocytosis with increases in neutrophil, eosinophil, and basophil granulocytes and a dose-dependent increase in intracellular and plasma histamine levels.[93] Increases in corrected reticulocyte counts and variable increases in platelets have been observed. The administration of IL-3 to cynomolgus monkeys after treatment with cyclophosphamide or 5-fluorouracil significantly reduced the duration of severe neutropenia (neutrophil count <500 cells/μl). Platelet recovery appears to occur earlier in animals treated with IL-3.

The ability of glycosylated and nonglycosylated IL-3 to abrogate chemotherapy-induced myelosuppression, alone or in combination with more lineage-specific factors, is under investigation in humans. Several trials exploring the therapeutic utility of IL-3 in correcting the pancytopenia associated with aplastic anemia or myelodysplastic syndrome have been conducted (see Table 62–11).[94,95] In these studies, IL-3 administration resulted in an increase in neutrophil and eosinophil granulocyte counts, with increases in basophil granulocytes, erythrocytes, and platelets being more variable. Studies in humans have shown relatively modest toxicities including fever, headaches, and flushing, but the toxicity profile has not been determined at high doses.

HEMATOPOIETIC GROWTH FACTORS IN COMBINATION

It is clear that the regulation of hematopoietic cell development is sensitivity controlled by an intricate network of positive and negative influences. To optimally enhance host defense and to effect more complete hematopoietic reconstitution, we will probably need to employ a combination of regulatory factors that act at different levels along the pathway of blood cell development. Considerable in vitro evidence suggests that synergism is achieved when certain hematopoietic growth factors are employed in combination. IL-3, an early-acting factor, synergizes with GM-CSF and G-CSF to enhance the proliferation and differentiation of myeloid committed progenitors, suggesting that combinations of early-acting and lineage-restricted regulatory molecules may have clinical utility in patients with iatrogenic or disease-related myelosuppression. Because individual CSFs enhance monocyte and neutrophil effector cell function, combinations may better augment host defenses.

Preclinical studies exploring the combination of GM-CSF or G-CSF plus IL-3 have demonstrated that IL-3 potentiates the myeloid responsiveness of the host to subsequent administration of the lineage specific growth factor. Combinations of low concentrations of IL-3 and M-CSF, which by themselves were inactive, increased the percentage and cycle status of macrophage high-proliferative and low-proliferative potential colony-forming cells. The combination of IL-1 and G-CSF enhanced neutrophil recovery in murine and primate nontumor-bearing and tumor-bearing models of chemotherapy-induced myelosuppression compared with the administration of each growth factor alone.[96,97]

Colony-stimulating factors have reduced treatment-related neutropenia and infectious morbidity, but thrombocytopenia remains a significant clinical problem. It is likely that the clinical application of hematopoietic growth factors, which stimulate uncommitted progenitors and promote megakaryocyte formation, such as stem cell factor and IL-1, -4, -6 and -11, will reduce this complication. The use of these newer regulatory molecules in combination with colon-stimulating factors and "primed" progenitors harvested from the peripheral blood should enable more complete hematopoietic reconstitution and permit the successful implementation of dose-intensified regimens designed to cure malignant disease.

REFERENCES

1. Golde DW. The stem cell. Sci Am 1991;265:86–93.
2. Spangrude GJ, Smith L, Uchida N, et al. Mouse hematopoietic stem cells. Blood 1991;78:1395–1402.
3. Krantz SB. Erythropoietin. Blood 1991;77:419–434.
4. Miyake T, Kung CKH, Goldwasser E. Purification of human erythropoietin. J Biol Chem 1977;252:5558.
5. Boyd HK, Lappin TRJ. Erythropoietin deficiency in the anaemia of chronic disorders. Eur J Haematol 1991;46:198–201.
6. Schilling RF. Anemia of chronic disease: A misnomer. Ann Intern Med 1991;115:572–573.
7. Miller CB, Jones RJ, Piantadosi S, et al. Decreased erythropoietin response in patients with the anemia of cancer. N Engl J Med 1990;322:1689–1992.
8. Doweiko JP, Goldberg MA. Erythropoietin therapy in cancer patients. Oncology 1991;5:31–37.
9. Abels RI, Rudnick SA. Erythropoietin: Evolving clinical applications. Exp Hematol 1991;19:842–850.
10. Ludwig H, Fritz E, Kotzmann H, et al. Erythropoietin treatment of anemia associated with multiple myeloma. N Engl J Med 1990;322:1693–1699.
11. Oster W, Herrmann F, Gamm H, et al. Erythropoietin for the treatment of anemia of malignancy associated with neoplastic bone marrow infiltration. J Clin Oncol 1990;8:956–962.
12. Platanias LC, Miller CB, Mick R, et al. Treatment of chemotherapy-induced anemia with recombinant human erythropoietin in cancer patients. J Clin Oncol 1991;9:2021–2026.
13. Smith DH, Goldwasser E, Vokes EE. Serum immunoerythropoietin levels in patients with cancer receiving cisplatin-based chemotherapy. Cancer 1991;68:1101–1105.
14. Abels RI, Larholt KM, Krantz KD, Bryant EC. Recombinant human erythropoietin (r-HuEPO) for the treatment of the anemia of cancer. Data on file: RW Johnson Pharmaceutical Research Institute, Raritan, NJ.
15. Bowen D, Culligan D, Jacobs A. The treatment of anaemia in the myelodysplastic syndromes with recombinant human erythropoietin. Br J Haematol 1991;77:419–423.
16. Hirashima K, Bessho M, Susaki K, et al. Improvement of anemia by intravenous injections of recombinant erythropoietin in patients with myelodysplastic syndromes and aplastic anemia. Exp Hematol 1989;17:657.
17. Van Kamp H, Prinsze-Postema TC, Kluin PM, et al. Effect of subcutaneously administered human recombinant erythropoietin on erythropoiesis in patients with myelodysplasia. Br J Haematol 1991;78:488–493.
18. Hellström E, Birgegård G, Lockner D, et al. Treatment of myelodysplastic syndromes with recombinant human erythropoietin. Eur J Haematol 1991;47:355–360.
19. Stein RS, Abels RI, Krantz SB. Pharmacologic doses of recombinant human erythropoietin in the treatment of myelodysplastic syndromes. Blood 1991;78:1658–1663.
20. Burgess A, Metcalf D. Characterization of a serum factor stimulating the differentiation of myelomonocytic leukemic cells. Int J Cancer 1980;26:647–654.
21. Souza LM, Boone TC, Gabrilove J, et al. Recombinant pluripotent human granulocyte colony stimulating factor: Effects on normal and leukemic myeloid cells. Science 1986;232:61–65.
22. Hammond WP, Boone TC, Donahue RE, Souza LM, et al. A comparison of treatment of canine cyclic hematopoiesis with recombinant human granulocyte-macrophage colony-stimulating factor (GM-CSF), G-CSF, interleukin-3, and canine G-CSF. Blood 1990;76:523–532.
23. Kawakami M, Tsutsumi H, Kumakawa T, et al. Levels of serum granulocyte colony-stimulating factor in patients with infections. Blood 1990;76:1962–1964.
24. Kaczmarski RS, Mufti GJ. The cytokine receptor superfamily. Blood Rev 1991;5:193–203.
25. Lord BI, Molineux G, Pojda Z, et al. Myeloid cell kinetics in mice treated with recombinant interleukin-3, granulocyte colony-stimulating factor (CSF), or granulocyte-macrophage CSF in vivo. Blood 1991;77:2154–2159.
26. Schuening FG, Storb R, Goehle S, et al. Recombinant human granulocyte colony-stimulating factor accelerates hematopoietic recovery after DLA-identical littermate marrow transplants in dogs. Blood 1990;76:636–640.
27. Gabrilove JL, Jakubowski A, Fain K, et al. Phase I study of granulocyte colony-stimulating factor in patients with transitional cell carcinoma of the urothelium. J Clin Invest 1988;82:1454–1461.
28. Morstyn G, Souza LM, Keech J, et al. Effect of granulocyte colony stimulating factor on neutropenia induced by cytotoxic chemotherapy. Lancet 1988;1:667–672.
29. Bronchud MH, Scarffe JH, Thatcher N, et al. Phase I/II study of recombinant human granulocyte colony-stimulating factor in patients receiving intensive chemotherapy for small cell lung cancer. Br J Cancer 1987;56:809–813.
30. Layton JE, Hockman H, Sheridan WP. Evidence for a novel in vivo control mechanism of granulopoiesis: Mature cell-related control of a regulatory growth factor. Blood 1989;74:1303–1307.
31. Morstyn G, Campbell L, Lieschke G, et al. Treatment of chemotherapy-induced neutropenia by subcutaneously administered granulocyte colony-stimulating factor with optimization of dose and duration of therapy. J Clin Oncol 1989;7:1554–1562.
32. Crawford J, Ozer H, Stoller R, et al. Reduction by granulocyte colony-stimulating factor of fever and neutropenia induced by chemotherapy in patients with small-cell lung cancer. N Engl J Med 1991;325:164–170.
33. Ohno R, Tomonaga M, Kobayashi T, et al. Effect of granulocyte colony-stimulating factor after intensive induction therapy in relapsed or refractory acute leukemia. N Engl J Med 1990;323:871–877.
34. Sheridan WP, Wolf M, Lusk J, et al. Granulocyte colony-stimulating factor and neutrophil recovery after high-dose chemotherapy and autologous bone marrow transplantation. Lancet 1989;1:891–894.
35. Taylor KM, Jagannath S, Spitzer G, et al. Recombinant human granulocyte colony-stimulating factor hastens granulocyte recovery after high-dose chemotherapy and autologous bone marrow transplantation in Hodgkin's Disease. J Clin Oncol 1989;7:1791–1799.
36. Petros W, Rabinowitz J, Stuart A, et al. Comparative pharmacokinetics of granulocyte colony-stimulating factor (rHuGM-CSF) in patients receiving high-dose chemotherapy and autologous bone marrow support. Proc Am Assoc Clin Oncol 1991;10:97.
37. Bronchud MH, Howell A, Crowther D, et al. The use of granulocyte colony-stimulating factor to increase the intensity of treatment with doxorubicin in patients with advanced breast and ovarian cancer. Br J Cancer 1989;60:121–125.
38. Neidhart J, Mangalik A, Kohler W, et al. Granulocyte colony-stimulating factor stimulates recovery of granulocytes in patients receiving dose-intensive chemotherapy without bone marrow transplantation. J Clin Oncol 1989;7:1685–1692.
39. Glaspy JA, Baldwin GC, Robertson PA, et al. Therapy for neutropenia in hairy cell leukemia with recombinant human granulocyte colony-stimulating factor. Ann Intern Med 1988;109:789.
40. Greenberg P, Negrin R, Nagler A, et al. Effects of prolonged treatment of myelodysplastic syndromes with recombinant human granulocyte colony-stimulating factor. Int J Cell Cloning 1990;8:293–302.
41. Kojima S, Fukuda M, Miyajima Y, et al. Cyclosporine and recombinant granulocyte colony-stimulating factor in severe aplastic anemia. N Engl J Med 1990;323:920–921.
42. Miles SA, Mitsuyasu RT, Lee K, et al. Recombinant human granulocyte colony-stimulating factor increases circulating burst forming unit-erythron and red blood cell production in patients with severe human immunodeficiency virus infection. Blood 1990;75:2137–2142.
43. Hammond WP, Price TH, Souza LM, et al. Treatment of cyclic neutropenia with granulocyte colony-stimulating factor. N Engl J Med 1989;320:1306–1311.
44. Bonilla MA, Gillio AP, Ruggeiro M, et al. Effects of recombinant human granulocyte

colony-stimulating factor on neutropenia in patients with congenital agranulocytosis. N Engl J Med 1989;320:1574–1580.

45. Jakubowski AA, Souza L, Kelly F, et al. Effects of human granulocyte colony-stimulating factor in a patient with idiopathic neutropenia. N Engl J Med 1989;320:38–42.
46. Gasson JC, Weisbart RH, Kaufman S, et al. Purified human granulocyte macrophage colony stimulating factor: Direct action on neutrophils. Science 1984;226:1339–1349.
47. Wong GG, Witek JS, Temple PA, et al. Human GM-CSF. molecular cloning of complementary DNA and purification of the natural and recombinant proteins. Science 1985;228:810–815.
48. Emanuel PD, Bates LJ, Castleberry RP, et al. Selective hypersensitivity to granulocyte-macrophage colony-stimulating factor by juvenile chronic myeloid leukemia hematopoietic progenitors. Blood 1991;77:925–929.
49. Johnson GR, Gonda TJ, Metcalf D, et al. A lethal myeloproliferative syndrome in mice transplanted with bone marrow cells infected with a retrovirus expressing granulocyte-macrophage colony stimulating factor. EMBO J 1989;8:441.
50. Chang JM, Metcalf D, Gonda TJ, et al. Long-term exposure to retrovirally expressed granulocyte-colony-stimulating factor induces a nonneoplastic granulocytic and progenitor cell hyperplasia without tissue damage in mice. J Clin Invest 1989;84:1488.
51. Hayashida K, Kitamura T, Gorman DM, et al. Molecular cloning of a second subunit of the receptor for human granulocyte-macrophage colony-stimulating factor (GM-CSF): Reconstitution of a high-affinity GM-CSF receptor. Proc Natl Acad Sci USA 1990;87:9655–9659.
52. Donahue RE, Wang EA, Stone DK, et al. Stimulation of haematopoiesis in primates by continuous infusion of recombinant human GM-CSF. Nature 1986;321:872–875.
53. Groopman JE, Mitsuyasu RT, De Leo MJ, et al. Effect of recombinant human granulocyte-macrophage colony-stimulating factor on myelopoiesis in the acquired immunodeficiency syndrome. N Engl J Med 1987;317:593–598.
54. Pluda JM, Yarchoan R, Smith PD, et al. Subcutaneous recombinant granulocyte-macrophage colony-stimulating factor used as a single agent and in an alternating regimen with azidothymidine in leukopenic patients with severe human immunodeficiency virus infection. Blood 1990;76:463–472.
55. Kaplan LD, Kahn JO, Crowe S, et al. Clinical and virologic effects of recombinant human granulocyte-macrophage colony-stimulating factor in patients receiving chemotherapy for human immunodeficiency virus-associated non-Hodgkin's lymphoma: Results of a randomized trial. J Clin Oncol 1991;9:929–940.
56. Scadden DT, Bering HA, Levine JD, et al. Granulocyte-macrophage colony-stimulating factor mitigates the neutropenia of combined interferon alfa and zidovudine treatment of acquired immune deficiency syndrome-associated Kaposi's sarcoma. J Clin Oncol 1991;9:802–808.
57. Peters WP, Stuart A, Affronti ML, et al. Neutrophil migration is defective during recombinant human granulocyte-macrophage colony-stimulating factor infusion after autologous bone marrow transplantation in humans. Blood 1988;72:1310–1315.
58. Toner GC, Gabrilove JL, Gordon M, et al. Phase I/II study of intraperitoneal and intravenous granulocyte-macrophage colony stimulating factor. Proc Am Assoc Cancer Res 1990;31:1042.
59. Devereux S, Linch DC, Campos Costa D, et al. Transient leukopenia induced by granulocyte-macrophage colony-stimulating factor. Lancet 1987;1:1523–1524.
60. Socinski MA, Elias A, Schnipper L, et al. Granulocyte-macrophage colony stimulating factor expands the circulating haemopoietic progenitor cell compartment in man. Lancet 1988;1:1194–1198.
61. Gianni AM, Bregni M, Stern AC, et al. Granulocyte-macrophage colony-stimulating factor to harvest circulating hematopoietic stem cells for autotransplantation. Lancet 1989;1:580–584.
62. Aglietta M, Piacibello W, Sanavio F, et al. Kinetics of human hemopoietic cells after in vivo administration of granulocyte-macrophage colony-stimulating factor. J Clin Invest 1989;83:551–557.
63. Brandt SJ, Peters WP, Atwater SK, et al. Effect of recombinant human granulocyte-macrophage colony-stimulating factor on hematopoietic reconstitution after high-dose chemotherapy and autologous bone marrow transplantation. N Engl J Med 1988;318:869–876.
64. Nemunaitis J, Singer JW, Buckner CD, et al. Use of recombinant human granulocyte-macrophage colony-stimulating factor in autologous marrow transplantation for lymphoid malignancies. Blood 1988;72:834–836.
65. Nemunaitis J, Rabinowe SN, Singer JW, et al. Recombinant granulocyte-macrophage colony-stimulating factor after autologous bone marrow transplantation for lymphoid cancer. N Engl J Med 1991;324:1773–1778.
66. Antman KS, Griffin JD, Elias A, et al. Effect of recombinant human granulocyte-macrophage colony-stimulating factor on chemotherapy-induced myelosuppression. N Engl J Med 1988;319:593–598.
67. Morstyn G, Stuart-Harris R, Bishop J, et al. Optimal scheduling of granulocyte macrophage colony stimulating factor (GM-CSF) for the abrogation of chemotherapy induced neutropenia in small cell lung cancer (SCLC). Proc Am Soc Clin Oncol 1989;8:850.
68. Gianni AM, Bregni M, Siena S, et al. Recombinant human granulocyte-macrophage colony-stimulating factor reduces hematologic toxicity and widens clinical applicability of high-dose cyclophosphamide treatment in breast cancer and non-Hodgkin's lymphoma. J Clin Oncol 1990;8:768–778.
69. Barlogie B, Jagamath S, Dixon DO, et al. High dose melphalan and granulocyte-macrophage colony stimulating factor for refractory multiple myeloma. Blood 1990;76:677.
70. De Vries EGE, Biesma B, Willemse PHB, et al. A double-blind placebo controlled study with granulocyte-macrophage colony stimulating factor during chemotherapy for ovarian carcinoma. Cancer Res 1991;51:116–122.
71. Herrmann F, Schulz G, Wieser M, et al. Effect of granulocyte-macrophage colony-stimulating factor on neutropenia and related morbidity induced by myelotoxic chemotherapy. Am J Med 1990;88:619–624.
72. Buchner T, Hiddemann W, Koenigsmann M, et al. Recombinant human granulocyte-macrophage colony stimulating factor after chemotherapy in patients with acute myeloid leukemia at higher age or after relapse. Blood 1991;78:1190–1197.
73. Logothelis L, Dexeus F, Sella A, et al. Escalated (ESC) M-VAC (MTX 30 $\mu g/m^2$, Adriamycin 60 $\mu g/m^2$, vinblastine 4 $\mu g/m^2$, cisplatin 100 $\mu g/m^2$) with recombinant human granulocyte macrophage stimulating factor (rhGM-CSF) for patients with advanced and chemotherapy refractory urothelium tumors: A phase I study. Proc Am Soc Clin Oncol 1989;8:514.
74. Hoekman K, Wagstaff J, van Groeningen CJ, et al. Effects if recombinant human granulocyte-macrophage colony-stimulating factor on myelosuppression induced by multiple cycles of high-dose chemotherapy in patients with advanced breast cancer. JNCI 1991;83:1546–1533.
75. Rodriquez MA, Swan F, Hagemeister F, et al. High-dose ESHAP with GM-CSF vs. prophylactic antibiotics. Blood 1990;76(suppl 1):10.
76. Champlin RE, Nimer SD, Ireland P, et al. Treatment of refractory aplastic anemia with recombinant human granulocyte-macrophage-colony-stimulating factor. Blood 1989;73:694–699.
77. Antin JH, Smith BR, Holmes W, et al. Phase I/II study of recombinant human granulocyte-macrophage colony-stimulating factor in aplastic anemia and myelodysplastic syndrome. Blood 1988;72:705–713.
78. Vadhan-Raj S, Buescher S, Broxmeyer HE, et al. Stimulation of myelopoiesis in patients with aplastic anemia by recombinant human granulocyte-macrophage colony-stimulating factor. N Engl J Med 1988;319:1628–1634.
79. Guinan EC, Sieff CA, Oette DH, et al. A phase I/II trial of recombinant granulocyte-macrophage colony-stimulating factor for children with aplastic anemia. Blood 1990;76:1077–1082.
80. Vadhan-Raj S, Keating M, LeMaistre A, et al. Effects of recombinant human granulocyte-macrophage colony-stimulating factor in patients with myelodysplastic syndromes. N Engl J Med 1987;317:1545–1551.
81. Ganser A, Völkers B, Greher J, et al. Recombinant human granulocyte-macrophage colony-stimulating factor in patients with myelodysplastic syndromes—A phase I/II trial. Blood 1989;73:31–37.
82. Rifkin RM, Hersh EM, Hultquist KN, et al. Therapy of the myelodysplastic syndrome (MDS) with subcutaenously (SC) administered recombinant human granulocyte-macrophage colony-stimulating factor. Proc Am Soc Clin Oncol 1989;8:178.
83. Thompson JA, Lee DJ, Kidd P, et al. Subcutaneous granulocyte-macrophage colony-stimulating factor in patients with myelodysplastic syndrome: Toxicity, pharmacokinetics, and hematological effects. J Clin Oncol 1989;7:629–637.
84. Herrmann F, Lindemann A, Klein H, et al. Effect of recombinant human granulocyte-macrophage colony-stimulating factor in patients with myelodysplastic syndrome with excess blasts. Leukemia 1989;3:335–338.
85. Lieschke GJ, Maher D, Cebon J, et al. Effects of bacterially synthesized recombinant human granulocyte-macrophage colony-stimulating factor in patients with advanced malignancy. Ann Intern Med 1989;110:357–364.
86. Rettenmier CW, Sherr C. The mononuclear phagocyte colony-stimulating factor (CSF-1, M-CSF). Hematol Oncol Clin North Am 1989;3:479–493.
87. Wiktor-Jedrzejczak W, Bartocci A, Ferrante AW Jr, et al. Total absence of CSF-1 in macrophage deficient osteopetrolic (op/op) mice. Proc Natl Acad Sci USA 1987;87:4828–4832.
88. Munn DH, Garnick MB, Cheung NKV. Effects of parenteral macrophage colony-stimulating factor (M-CSF) on circulating monocyte number, immunophenotype and anti-tumor activity in cynomolgus monkeys. Blood 1988;72:127a.
89. Motoyoshi K, Takaku F, Miura Y. High serum colony-stimulating activity of leukocytopenic patients after intravenous infusions of human urinary colony-stimulating factor. Blood 1983;62:685–688.
90. Bajorin DF, Jakubowski A, Cody B, et al. Phase I trial of recombinant macrophage colony stimulating factor (rhM-CSF) in patients (pts) with melanoma (MEL). Blood 1989;74:1222.
91. Nemunaitis J, Meyers J, Buckner CD, et al. Phase I/II trial of recombinant human macrophage-colony stimulating factor (M-CSF) in patients with invasive fungal infection. Blood 1990;76:2065.
92. Ihle JN, Keller J, Henderson L, et al. Procedures for the purification of interleukin-3 to homogeneity. J Immunol 1982;129:2431.
93. Donahue RE, Seehra J, Metzger M, et al. Human IL-3 and GM-CSF act synergistically in stimulating hematopoiesis in primates. Science 1988;241:1820–1823.
94. Ganser A, Seipelt G, Lindemann A, et al. Effects of recombinant human interleukin-3 in patients with myelodysplastic syndromes. Blood 1990;76:455–462.
95. Ganser A, Lindmann A, Seipelt G, et al. Effects of recombinant human interleukin-3 in aplastic anemia. Blood 1990;76:1297–1292.
96. Warren DJ, Moore MAS. Synergism among interleukin-1, interleukin-3, and interleukin-5 in the production of eosinophils from primitive hemopoietic stem cells. J Immunol 1988;140:94–99.
97. Moore MAS, Stolfi RL, Martin DS. Hematologic effects of interleukin-1β, granulocyte colony-stimulating factor, and granulocyte-macrophage colony-stimulating factor in tumor-bearing mice treated with fluorouracil. Exp Hematol 1990;82:1031–1037.

PHILIP A. PIZZO
JOEL MEYERS
ALISON G. FREIFELD
THOMAS WALSH

SECTION **3**

Infections in the Cancer Patient

The associations among malignancy, immunocompromise, and infectious morbidity and mortality are established.[1–4] More intensive treatment regimens have produced more patients with cancer who are immunocompromised. The life-threatening infectious complications can limit the benefits of antineoplastic therapy. The oncologist must be familiar with the risk factors contributing to infection and knowledgeable about the infectious syndromes and the available therapies.

The patient with cancer may be immunocompromised because of the underlying malignancy or the antineoplastic therapy. Specific malignancies may be associated with immune deficits that predispose to infection with particular pathogens. For example, patients with Hodgkin's or non-Hodgkin's lymphomas tend to have abnormalities of the cellular immune system that heighten their risk for viral and fungal infections. Therapeutic modalities such as corticosteroids, cytotoxic chemotherapy, and localized or widespread irradiation result in additional deficiencies of host defense. The consequence of these interrelated abnormalities of immune function is the immunocompromised cancer patient.

IMPAIRED HOST DEFENSES OF THE CANCER PATIENT

INTEGUMENTARY AND MUCOSAL BARRIERS

The skin and mucosal surfaces constitute the primary host defense against invasion by endogenous and acquired microorganisms. The integrity of this physical barrier can be disrupted by the patient's tumor or by its treatment. Mucosal and epithelial cells contain specific and nonspecific receptors for the attachment or adherence of microorganisms.[5,6] These receptors can be altered by disease and by certain therapies, particularly antibiotics, permitting colonization of the immunosuppressed cancer patient with new pathogens.[6–8] Colonization is influenced by suppression of the host's anaerobic microflora, because these organisms can resist colonization by aerobic pathogens.[9] The anaerobic flora are suppressed by many antibiotics, particularly the β-lactams. The mucosal changes provide a nidus for microbial colonization, a focus for local infection, and a portal for systemic invasion.

PHAGOCYTIC DEFENSES

The neutrophil and the monocyte-macrophage are the major cellular defenses against most bacteria and fungi.[10] Whether disease related or as a consequence of therapy, the degree of severe neutropenia is inversely related to the risk of serious infection (Table 62–12).[11] To meet rapidly changing needs, there is normally a large bone marrow granulocyte reserve that exceeds the circulating pool of neutrophils that is distributed equally between the blood stream and a marginating pool. The half-life of cells in the circulating granulocyte pool is 6 to 7 hours, after which the cells marginate along the vascular endothelial surfaces or move into extravascular spaces. If granulopoiesis is depressed by disease or treatment, the granulocyte reserves are rapidly depleted, with severe granulocytopenia ensuing within 5 to 7 days.

Several glycoprotein hormonal growth factors integral to granulopoiesis have been characterized, their genes cloned, and recombinant proteins purified. It has become apparent that various cells, including T and B lymphocytes, monocytes, fibroblasts, and endothelial cells, produce cytokines that are integral to hematopoiesis. The colony-stimulating factors (CSF) include the granulocyte-macrophage CSF (GM-CSF), granulocyte CSF (G-CSF), macrophage CSF (M-CSF), and multiprotein CSF (*i.e.*, IL-3).[12,13] These hematopoietic growth factors affect many target cells, and some (*e.g.*, IL-3, GM-CSF) stimulate several blood cell lineages. Cloned GM-CSF and G-CSF can shorten the recovery of neutrophils after chemotherapy-induced or radiation-induced myelosuppression. In addition to accelerating neutrophil recovery, these cytokines can enhance phagocyte activity, including superoxide generation, phagocytosis, and antibacterial activity.[15–18]

Several cytokines appear to be interlinked in generating GM-CSF or in initiating cell reactivity. Included among these are tumor necrosis factor (TNF or cachectin), interleukin-1 (IL-1), interleukin-2, and interferon.[19–28] A variety of cytokines play an integral role in host defense and cell regulation. The characterization, purification, cloning, and production of these growth factors offer new prospects for studying the biology of hematopoiesis and for bolstering host defenses that are altered in patients undergoing treatment for cancer.[29]

In addition to quantitative defects, qualitative abnormalities of neutrophil function have been described in patients with hematologic malignancies. These include defects in chemotaxis, phagocytosis, bactericidal capacity, and the absence of the respiratory burst that usually accompanies phagocytosis.[30] Although phagocytic capacity remains normal, decreased spontaneous migratory and chemotactic leukocyte functions have been described in untreated patients with lymphoma and carcinoma, suggesting the presence of a circulating inhibitor in the sera of these patients,[31,32]

Cancer chemotherapy may produce defects of neutrophil function. Corticosteroids, for example, can decrease phagocytosis and neutrophil migration. The combination of prednisone with vincristine and asparaginase or 6-mercaptopurine and methotrexate can produce a significant decrease in the phagocytic and killing capability.[33] Although the mechanism is not understood, bactericidal activity may be transiently impaired within the 3 months after craniospinal irradiation in patients with leukemia, which may contribute to the infectious complications that occur during that period.[34] Analgesic narcotics such as morphine can cause a dose-dependent suppression of granulocytes and can exacerbate infections in experimental animals.[35]

The mature macrophage is more resistant to cytotoxic che-

This chapter is dedicated in memory of Joel Meyers (deceased, October 1991), who contributed so much to the prevention and management of infectious complications in cancer patients, especially those undergoing bone marrow transplantation.

TABLE 62–12. Percentage of Cancer Patients Who Develop Serious Infections With Granulocytopenia and the Cumulative Risk of Infection With Prolonged Granulocytopenia

Granulocyte Level (per mm³)		*Percentage of Serious Infections (duration of granulocytopenia in weeks)*							
Initial	*Change*	*1*	*2*	*3*	*4*	*6*	*10*	*12*	*14*
Any level	Any fall	12							
Any level	Fall to 2000	2							
Any level	Fall to 1500	5							
Any level	Fall to 1000	10	30	45	50	65	70	85	100
Any level	Fall to 500	19							
Any level	Fall to <100	28	50	72	85	100			

(Adapted from Bodey GP, Buckley M, Sathe YS, et al. Quantitative relationships between circulating leukocytes and infection in patients with acute leukemia. Ann Intern Med 1966;61:328–340)

motherapy than the granulocyte and provides some residual phagocytic capacity during periods of severe neutropenia. The activated macrophage is an important defense against mycobacteria, *Listeria, Brucella,* and several fungi, protozoans, and viruses. Macrophages are important in the initiation of the immune responses, because they are triggered into a metabolically active state by antigenic stimuli and subsequently process and present these antigens to T and B lymphocytes. Macrophages produce a variety of low-molecular-weight polypeptide hormones (*i.e.*, monokines) that regulate lymphocyte function and CSFs that are important in granulopoiesis.[12,13] If macrophage function is altered, as with steroids, the primary defense against fungal pathogens is altered, further aggravating the altered host defense of the neutropenic host.[36]

CELLULAR AND HUMORAL IMMUNITY

Patients with lymphoid malignancies, especially Hodgkin's disease, may have abnormalities of cell-mediated immunity, such as anergy and decreased phytohemagglutinin responsiveness, which may persist even after the underlying malignancy has been treated.[37] These defects are aggravated by chemotherapy with glucocorticosteroids and by infections like disseminated histoplasmosis, making patients susceptible to viral (*e.g.*, herpes zoster) or fungal (*e.g.*, *Cryptococcus*) infections.[38]

Cytotoxic chemotherapy adversely affects B-cell and T-cell functions, resulting in diminished opsonizing activity, inadequate agglutination and lysis of bacteria, and deficient neutralization of bacterial toxins.[39] Impaired antibody production has been described in untreated patients with chronic lymphocytic leukemia, multiple myeloma, or Hodgkin's disease.[40] Suppressor lymphocytes may contribute to impaired antibody production in patients with multiple myeloma and Hodgkin's disease and may relate to the fungal infections that occur in some of these patients.[41] In animal studies, the glucocorticoid-induced defects in lymphocyte function and decreased neutralizing-antibody formation contribute to the increased lethality of fungal, protozoan, and viral infections.

The importance of humoral defenses in the cancer patient has become apparent from several lines of evidence.[42–46] First, patients with defective antibody production (*e.g.*, chronic lymphocytic leukemia and multiple myeloma) have an increased frequency of pyogenic infections, even if they are not neutropenic. Patients with acute leukemia have lower levels of antibody to the core glycolipid of the Enterobacteriaceae than noncancer patients, and the antibody level falls in patients receiving cytotoxic therapy.[47] The protective role of this antibody is based on the fact that gram-negative bacteria share in common a core glycolipid composed of 2-keto-3-deoxy-octonate (KDO) and lipid A (endotoxin). A rough mutant of *Escherichia coli* 0111 exposes this core glycolipid and has been used to prepare a vaccine and antisera, known as the J5 antisera, which has protected rabbits challenged with endotoxin and has improved survival in nonneutropenic patients with gram-negative sepsis.[48,49] Monoclonal antibodies to J5 have been developed and evaluated in the clinic.

RETICULOENDOTHELIAL SYSTEM AND SPLENECTOMY

The spleen serves as a mechanical filter and an early source of opsonizing activity. Splenectomized patients manifest diminished antibody production when challenged with particulate antigens, are deficient in tuftsin (phagocytosis-promoting peptide), and have decreased levels of IgM and properdin.[50] Consequently, splenectomized patients are at increased risk for septicemia with encapsulated bacteria, particularly *Streptococcus pneumoniae, Neisseria meningitis,* and *Hemophilus influenzae*, and with *Babesia microti*.[51] Septicemia in these patients is characteristically fulminant, with large numbers of organisms in the blood stream. Although the incidence of postsplenectomy septicemia is especially significant in children and adolescents (1.4–20%) receiving chemotherapy, bacteremia with *S. pneumoniae* or *H. influenzae* can occur even when patients are not granulocytopenic, suggesting that splenectomy is an important independent risk factor for cancer patients.[52–54] Splenectomy does not appear to enhance the risk for most nonbacterial infections.[55]

NUTRITION

Malnutrition is a frequent complication of cancer, and its treatment contributes to the loss in integrity of the integumentary and mucosal barrier, to impaired phagocytic capacity, to decreased macrophage mobilization, and to depressed lymphocyte function.[56] Total parenteral nutrition to attenuate drug-induced bone marrow suppression or decrease mucosal cell damage has produced mixed results in clinical trials.[57]

EXOGENOUS AND ENDOGENOUS MICROBIAL FLORA

Unperturbed, the endogenous microbial flora exists as a carefully balanced, synergistic microenvironment within the host. However, more than 80% of the infections that occur in cancer patients arise from endogenous microbial flora, almost half of which are acquired by the patient during hospitalization. The most frequent isolates are gram-negative and gram-positive bacteria and *C. albicans*.[58–62] Numerous sources contribute to the colonization of the hospitalized patient, including transmissions from staff to patient and from patient to patient; contamination of food, air, water, special equipment such as catheters, respirators, or humidifiers; and medical or surgical procedures (Fig. 62–4).[63,64] These inanimate reservoirs of microorganisms require human vectors for transmission, particularly furnished by poor hand-washing techniques.[65] Fewer than 30% of physicians caring for seriously ill patients wash their hands between patient contacts.[66] This emphasizes the need for continued education and reinforcement of this important infection-control practice.

Current technology has provided new routes for the transmission of microorganisms, particularly the increased use of indwelling catheters, hyperalimentation lines, and hemodynamic monitoring devices.[67,68] Even the disinfectants and antiseptics used to cleanse the skin before an invasive procedure are occasionally contaminated.[69]

Interface of Colonization and Infection

Contact with microorganisms does not necessarily result in colonization or infection; hospital workers or psychiatric patients rarely become colonized with gram-negative organisms.[70] However, more than 80% of seriously ill noncancer patients eventually become colonized in the oropharynx with gram-negative bacteria, presumably due to alterations in the epithelial adherence of these organisms.[5] Attachment is mediated by a specific lock-and-key mechanism, in which ligand molecules (adhesions) on the surface of the microbe interact with complementary molecules (receptors) on the epithelial cell surface. The biochemical structures of adhesions include proteins *(e.g., E. coli, Neisseria gonorrhoeae),* the lipid protein of a glycolipid (*e.g., S. pyogenes*), and carbohydrates (*e.g.,* many cariogenic streptococci). In healthy persons, integumentary and mucosal attachment sites are populated with relatively innocuous normal flora, consisting predominantly of aerobic gram-positive and a variety of anaerobic organisms.[5,6]

In cancer patients, a decrease in the normal aerobic gram-positive flora and colonization of the oropharynx and stool with aerobic gram-negative organisms is observed soon after hospitalization, even before the patient receives antibiotics, although antibiotics enhance colonization.[8] Endogenous properties of the microorganisms are important for colonization and infection. For example, certain biotypes of Enterobacteriaceae are more capable of colonizing the host than others, and certain colonizing organisms are more likely to result in infection, presumably because of their inherent virulence.[59,60] Although *E. coli* is the most frequently isolated organism, few of the patients who become colonized develop infections. In contrast, 40% to 68% of patients who are colonized with or who acquire *Pseudomonas aeruginosa* while in the hospital develop serious infections with this organism during subsequent periods of granulocytopenia.[60,61] Antibiotic regimens can influence colonization and infection, as evidenced by the increase in streptococcal infections in patients receiving quinolone antibiotics (*e.g.*, cyprofloxacin) for prophylaxis.

The relation between colonization and infection also applies to nonbacterial organisms. For example, *Candida albicans* is ubiquitous and can be cultured from the oropharynx and stool of more than 80% patients who have received broad-spectrum antibiotics.[62] Although *C. tropicalis* is less frequently isolated

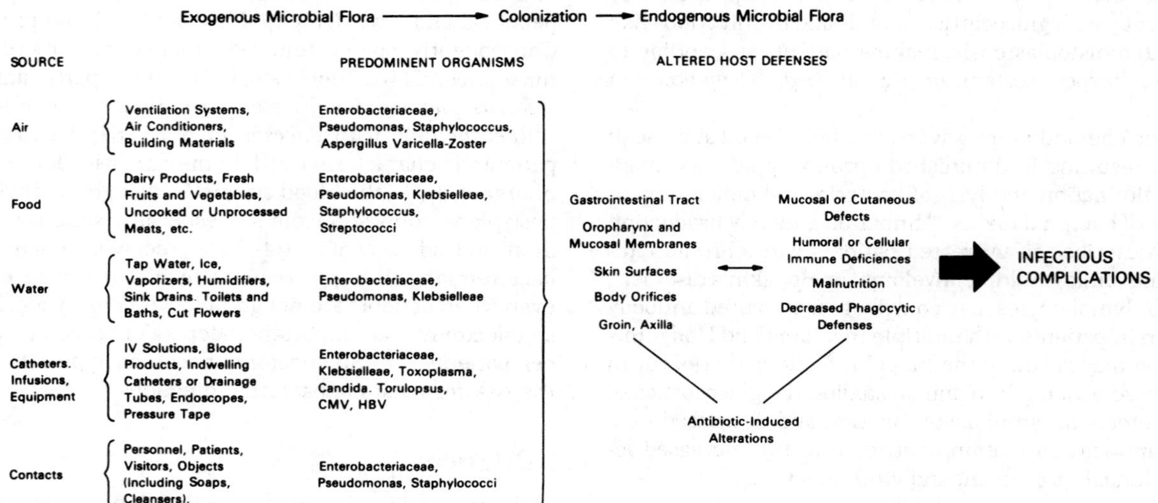

FIGURE 62–4. Sources of nosocomial infection in high-risk patients and interactions between colonization and infection.

and causes fewer overall infections, it appears to be more pathogenic, because 14 of the 25 patients colonized by *C. tropicalis* in the series reported by Wingard and colleagues developed an infection with this organism.[71] The reservoir for organisms may vary among institutions and can be influenced by changes in antimicrobial practice. For example, *Candida krusei* has been observed in cancer patients receiving fluconazole for antifungal prophylaxis.[72]

Interactions among different components of the host's endogenous microflora (*e.g.*, viruses with bacteria or protozoa) may result in alterations of the microenvironment and consequent infectious complications, such as the increase in α-streptococcal infections in cancer patient with oral herpes simplex virus (HSV) who are also receiving cytotoxic therapy with cytosine arabinoside. Viruses can suppress or alter immune functions, which has been appreciated since the advent of the acquired immunodeficiency syndrome (AIDS) and its etiologic agent, the human immunodeficiency virus (HIV). Other human viruses, including parvoviruses and herpesviruses (*e.g.*, HSV, Epstein-Barr virus, cytomegalovirus), can be immunosuppressive. This can result from destruction of a specific lymphocyte or macrophage target or from the release of soluble factors or activated suppressor cells that alter host immunity while responding to the viral infection.[73]

Predominant Pathogens in the Cancer Patient

The spectrum of infecting organisms has changed during the last 3 decades. During the 1950s and early 1960s, *Staphylococcus aureus* was the most frequent bacterial isolate in immunosuppressed patients. When the β-lactamase-resistant antistaphylococcal penicillins were introduced and provided effective therapy for *S. aureus*, gram-negative bacillary organisms became the predominant bacterial pathogens (especially *E. coli*, *Klebsiella* species, and *P. aeruginosa*).[1–4] During the 1980s, infections with *P. aeruginosa* have inexplicably decreased in many institutions, a phenomenon that affects the selection and the probable success of initial empiric antibiotics. Increased infections due to nonaeruginosa pseudomonads (*e.g.*, *P. maltophilia*, *P. cepacia*, *P. stutzeri*) have been observed in cancer patients as nosocomial infections or as a consequence of antibiotic resistance.[74] In some centers, an increase in multiply-resistant gram-negative bacterial isolates (*e.g.*, *Enterobacter* species, *Citrobacter* species, *Acinetobacter* species, *S. marcescens*) are presumably a consequence of antibiotic use and misuse.

In most centers, gram-positive bacteria became the common isolates during the 1980s.[75] *S. aureus* and the coagulase-negative staphylococci were the predominant isolates, especially in patients with indwelling intravenous catheters.[76–78] Although some centers experienced major problems with methicillin-resistant *S. aureus*, most were able to contain the spread of the isolates with careful infection control practices, especially hand washing.[79–81] During the last decade, the coagulase-negative staphylococci became increasingly resistant to all β-lactam antibiotics, making vancomycin the drug of choice. There was a report of a coagulase-negative staphylococcal isolate that was resistant to vancomycin.[82] Although some investigators reported serious infectious complications, including pneumonia, endocarditis, meningitis, with coagulase-negative staphylococci, most found this organism to be less virulent and only rarely associated with serious sequelae.[83–86]

Alpha-hemolytic, viridans streptococci, and corynebacteria, some of which are multiply-antibiotic-resistant diphtheroids (CDC group JK), can result in serious infections, particularly in patients with prolonged granulocytopenia.[87–92]

Although anaerobes play a lesser role than aerobes in primary infections in cancer patients, they are responsible for approximately 5% of bacteremias and are responsible for mixed infections in the mouth and perianal area. *Clostridia perfringens* and *C. septicum* are well-described isolates, but *C. tertium*, previously considered a contaminant, has been associated with serious infection.[93] Only half of the isolates of *C. tertium* are sensitive to standard antianaerobic agents (*e.g.*, clindamycin, metronidazole), but most are sensitive to vancomycin. *Bacillus* species have been associated with infection in cancer patients and are difficult to eradicate in patients who have indwelling Silastic catheters, unless the venous access device is removed.[94]

Mycobacterial infections are uncommon in cancer patients, although *M. avium-intracellulare* has become a highly prevalent pathogen in patients with AIDS.[95,96] Infections with rapid growers (*e.g.*, *M. chelonei*, *M. fortuitum*) have been observed in patients with indwelling catheters.[97]

Fungi are major pathogens, especially in immunosuppressed patients who have prolonged granulocytopenia and who receive protracted courses of antibiotics.[98] The predominant fungal pathogens are *Candida* species, *Aspergillus* species, *Cryptococcus neoformans*, and the *Phycomycetes*. There is considerable institutional variation in the predominant fungal pathogens, although in many centers, *Aspergillus* infections have increased in frequency.[98] Although their incidence is less common, the *Mucoraceae* (*Mucor*, *Absidia*, and *Rhizopus* species) can cause pulmonary disease or invade the sinuses, causing rhinocerebral syndrome. *Cryptococcus* is a noteworthy pathogen for patients with lymphoma, and it is responsible for disseminated infection in AIDS patients.[99] *Trichosporon* species, an arthrospore-forming yeast, can cause local skin lesions and invasive disease.[100] Infections due to *Fusarium* species, *Dreschlera*, *Pseudoallescheria boydii*, and *Malassezia furfur* have been described in cancer patients.[98] Although geographic mycoses such as *Histoplasma*, *Coccidioides*, and *Blastomyces* have not increased in frequency, there is an increase in their severity and invasiveness when infection occurs.

In addition to bacteria and fungi, parasitic and viral infections are important primary or secondary complications. *P. carinii* is an important cause of pneumonia, particularly in patients on corticosteroids or with AIDS. Viral infections represent a considerable source of morbidity in immunosuppressed hosts. The herpesviruses HSV, varicella-zoster virus (VZV), and CMV are particularly important. Rodents infected with CMV have a higher mortality rate when challenged with *P. aeruginosa* or *Candida* species than noninfected controls; the clinical corollary of this is that patients who become infected with CMV have a higher incidence of bacterial superinfections.[101,102]

The immunosuppressed host is at risk for a staggering array of infectious complications. Often, the same patients have multiple infections, further confounding their management.

EVALUATION AND MANAGEMENT OF THE FEBRILE CANCER PATIENT

FEVER AND GRANULOCYTOPENIA

Fever is common in cancer patients and can result from tumor necrosis, inflammation, transfusions, and chemotherapeutic or antimicrobial drugs. Although the patient's underlying malignancy can cause fever, 55% to 70% of the fevers that occur in cancer patients are caused by infections, especially in patients who are granulocytopenic, defined as having fewer than 500 polymorphonuclear leukocytes and bandforms per 1 mm^3.[103] The activated monocyte-macrophage is thought to be the most important source of physiologically relevant IL-1, but other phagocytic cells, including polymorphonuclear leukocytes, fixed tissue cells of the reticuloendothelial system, keratinocytes, gingival and corneal epithelial cells, renal mesangial cells, and astrocytes, are capable of producing IL-1-like molecules.[28] IL-1 and TNF mediate an array of metabolic, endocrinologic, neurologic, and immunologic functions common to the acute-phase inflammatory response, the effect of which is a unified host response against an infectious insult. Directly or indirectly, these include the production of fever, polymorphonuclear leukocytosis, hepatic synthesis of acute-phase reactants, activation of T and B lymphocytes, and the metabolic changes (*e.g.*, mobilization of amino acids, decreased serum iron and zinc, increased serum copper) that inhibit bacterial replication.

The initial evaluation and management of the febrile patient depends on the underlying malignancy and the degree of treatment-induced host compromise. For example, altered cellular immunity places the patient with Hodgkin's disease at increased risk for *H. zoster* infection or cryptococcal meningitis; patients who have undergone allogeneic bone marrow transplantation are at risk for severe interstitial pneumonia, especially with CMV.[104–106]

Although evaluation of the nonimmunosuppressed febrile cancer patient can proceed according to general medical principles, the detection of infection and the management of the febrile granulocytopenic patient is complicated by two important factors. First, granulocytopenia markedly alters the host's inflammatory response, making it difficult to detect the presence of infection. Second, an undetected and untreated infection can be rapidly fatal in the granulocytopenic cancer patient.[107]

Because the classic signs and symptoms of infection often are missing in the granulocytopenic cancer patient (*e.g.*, pyuria may be detectable in only 11% of patients with a urinary tract infection or purulent sputum in only 8% of patients with pneumonia), the physician must take a careful history and perform a scrupulous physical examination, being especially attentive to subtle signs of inflammation.[108] The physical examination may need to be repeated frequently, especially if an initial source of infection is not discernible.

All granulocytopenic cancer patients deserve prompt empiric antibiotic management when they become febrile. Adults with solid tumors are at risk for fever when rendered neutropenic and appear to do well when treated empirically with antibiotics.[109] In a survey of 1001 consecutive episodes of fever in 324 pediatric and young adult cancer patients treated at the National Cancer Institute (NCI), 39.5% had at least one febrile episode while they were granulocytopenic. There was no apparent difference in the incidence, pattern, or severity of infectious complications that occurred, regardless of the patient's underlying malignancy, after they became granulocytopenic. All granulocytopenic patients should be considered to be at risk for infection and, once febrile, should be considered as candidates for early empiric therapy.

Although some investigators recommend starting antibiotics if the granulocyte count falls below 1000/mm^3, the Consensus Conference of the Infectious Diseases Society of America and the Immunocompromised Host Society have agreed that the risk is really increased if the granulocyte count is less than 500/mm^3.[110a,110b] The incidence of bacteremia is particularly increased if the granulocyte count is less than 100/mm^3. Perhaps more important than the absolute nadir is the rate at which the counts are falling.

The level of fever that should prompt therapy has been defined. In general, two or three low-grade elevations above 38°C (taken orally) or a single elevation above 38.5°C in concert with a granulocyte count of less than 500/mm^3 are sufficient criteria to begin empiric therapy. Fever should not be caused by blood products, cancer, or medications, and the physician should ascertain if the patient is receiving drugs that mask a febrile response (*e.g.*, steroids, antipyretic-containing analgesics). Institutional criteria for fever and granulocytopenia should be defined and rigidly adhered to. Such a policy plays an important role in reducing infection-related morbidity and mortality.

PREANTIBIOTIC EVALUATION

In a prospective evaluation of 140 febrile granulocytopenic patients, it was not possible to differentiate patients with bacteremia-induced fever from those with unexplained fever by their age, sex, underlying malignancy, or the types of therapeutic modalities or invasive diagnostic procedures they had received.[110] The absence of physical findings suggesting infection did not exclude a potentially life-threatening bacteremia, because more than half of the bacteremic patients in this study lacked any specific physical findings.

Patients about to receive empiric therapy should have a baseline chest radiograph, urinalysis, at least two sets of preantibiotic blood cultures, and aspirate or biopsy cultures from any accessible sites suggesting infection. If blood cultures are obtained from an indwelling Silastic catheter, it is essential to obtain additional cultures from a peripheral vein. It is important to obtain blood cultures from each port in patients with multilumen catheters.

Even with a comprehensive evaluation, an infectious cause is demonstrated in only 30% to 40% of febrile granulocytopenic patients.[111,112] Moreover, definitive diagnosis may take days, presumably because of the low microbial inoculum. This probably reflects the short period that elapses between the onset of fever and evaluation and initiation of empiric therapy. Even subtle indications of inflammation must be considered as sites of infection in the context of granulocytopenia. For example, minimal perirectal erythema and tenderness may be the harbinger of a perirectal cellulitis. Minimal erythema and serious discharge at the site of a Hickman catheter exit may herald a tunnel or exit site infection. Accordingly, any clinically suspicious and accessible site of infection in the neutropenic patient should be aspirated for culture and tested with Gram's stain. It is generally not possible to differentiate granulocytopenic patients who have a bacteremia from those with unexplained fever (FUO).[110]

Because the patients' colonizing flora frequently can be implicated as the cause of infection, some have advocated surveillance cultures as an aid to diagnosis and antibiotic management. To assess this approach, we evaluated serial surveillance cultures of the nose, throat, urine, and stool from 271 patients at the NCI during 652 episodes of fever and neutropenia.[62] Sixty-two percent of these patients were colonized with the organism ultimately found to be responsible for the infection. However, the clinical usefulness of these surveillance cultures was limited, because there was not any one body site that was consistently predictive, and invariably other potential pathogens were isolated, making it difficult to differentiate prospectively the true pathogen. By the time the results from a routine surveillance culture (stool) were known, the true pathogens had been found in pure growth in blood cultures. The cost of routine surveillance is enormous. Even knowing the colonizing flora is unlikely to have a tremendous impact on initial antibiotic management, because most clinicians routinely employ broad-spectrum antibiotics for empiric treatment of febrile granulocytopenic patients. Routine surveillance cultures should not be part of the patients' evaluations. Exceptions to this may be patients in protected isolation, where stool cultures may be of use, or centers with a high incidence of *Aspergillus* infections, where nasal swabs may be helpful in identifying high-risk patients.[64]

Nuclear scanning with indium 111 has been used to define occult sites of infection.[113,114] Rubin described a method for linking ^{111}In to IgG, increasing its sensitivity in detecting sites of inflammation or infection.[115] The use of this technique for patients with fever and neutropenia must be further explored.

Although rapid diagnostic assays, such as the limulus assay for endotoxin, the enzyme-linked immunosorbent assay, and latex particle agglutination, have been successfully employed in certain common infections, they have had little impact on the rapid diagnosis of the bacterial and fungal infections that occur in cancer patients. This is primarily a consequence of the many antigenically diverse pathogens that can infect the cancer patient. Because of the difficulty in diagnosing fungal infections in cancer patients, several nonculture-dependent, rapid diagnostic techniques have been investigated. The detection of *Candida* enolase, especially if coupled with blood cultures, provides high specificity and sensitivity for detecting invasive candidiasis.[116] Sensitive methods for detecting *Aspergillus* are critically needed.[98]

EMPIRIC ANTIBIOTIC THERAPY

The prompt initiation of empiric antibiotics when the neutropenic cancer patient becomes febrile has been the single most important advance in the management of the immunocompromised host (Fig. 62–5).[108] Before this policy, the mortality of gram-negative infections, especially with *P. aeruginosa, E. coli,* and *K. pneumoniae,* approached 80%.[117,118] Since the widespread use of effective empiric antibiotics, the overall survival rate is between 60% and 90%.[119,120]

What are the criteria for an empiric antibiotic regimen? Between 85% and 90% of pathogens proven or associated with new fevers in the immunosuppressed patients are bacteria.[110,120] However, because gram-positive and gram-negative bacteria can be responsible for these initial infections, the empiric regimen must be broad, achieve high bactericidal levels, and be as nontoxic and as simple to administer as possible. This has usually necessitated the combination of two or more antibiotics. The availability of third-generation cephalosporins and carbapenems offers an alternative to combination regimens, because many of these single-agent antibiotics provide an exceedingly broad range of activity and high bactericidal levels (see Table 62–12).[121–123] Unlike the aminoglycosides, these newer β-lactam antibiotics do not require monitoring of serum levels and have minimal toxicity.

No particular combination has been shown to be clearly superior, and the regimen that is chosen at a given institution should reflect specific epidemiologic considerations (*e.g.,* local resistance patterns) and cost.[124–127]

Despite the proven efficacy of combination therapy, the potential of a single antibiotic for the empiric management of the febrile neutropenic patient is attractive for its ease of administration, cost, and lack of toxicity. To assess the efficacy of a monotherapeutic regimen, a prospective randomized trial was initiated at the NCI that compared monotherapy using ceftazidime with combination therapy using cephalothin, carbenicillin, and gentamicin for the initial empiric management of 550 episodes of fever and neutropenia.[112] The early evaluation at 72 hours was performed to assess the efficacy of the antibiotics during the period when they were used in an empiric manner (*i.e.,* before definitive microbiologic data). The overall evaluation was performed at the resolution of the neutropenic episode. The responses were categorized as "successes" (with or without modification of the initial regimen) if the patients survived the episode of neutropenia and as "failures" if the patients died while neutropenic. The importance of including additions to or modifications of the initial antibiotic regimen in the analysis of studies evaluating empiric antibiotic therapy has been underscored by the Immunocompromised Host Society's Consensus conference.[110b]

In the NCI study, there was no significant difference in terms of success for patients randomized to ceftazidime or the combination regimen among patients classified as FUO or as having a clinically or microbiologically documented infections. A significantly greater number of modifications were required among the patients randomized to ceftazidime: 58 (21%) of 282, compared with 29 (11%) of 268 (p^2=0.002 by chi-square).[115] This increased need for antibiotic modifications at the early evaluation reflected the need for anaerobic coverage in patients randomized to ceftazidime who developed necrotizing gingivitis or perirectal cellulitis and the greater need for vancomycin in patients with documented gram-positive infections, especially those due to *S. epidermidis.*

The result at the overall evaluation demonstrated equivalent success rates for the two regimens for patients with FUO or with documented infections. The percentage of patients treated successfully without modification of the initial antimicrobial therapy was predictably less than that at the early evaluation (Table 62–13). Patients with documented infections required changes in antimicrobial therapy more often than FUO patients, but the need for modifications of the initial therapy for patients randomized to monotherapy (59%) and those randomized to combination therapy (59%). In terms of

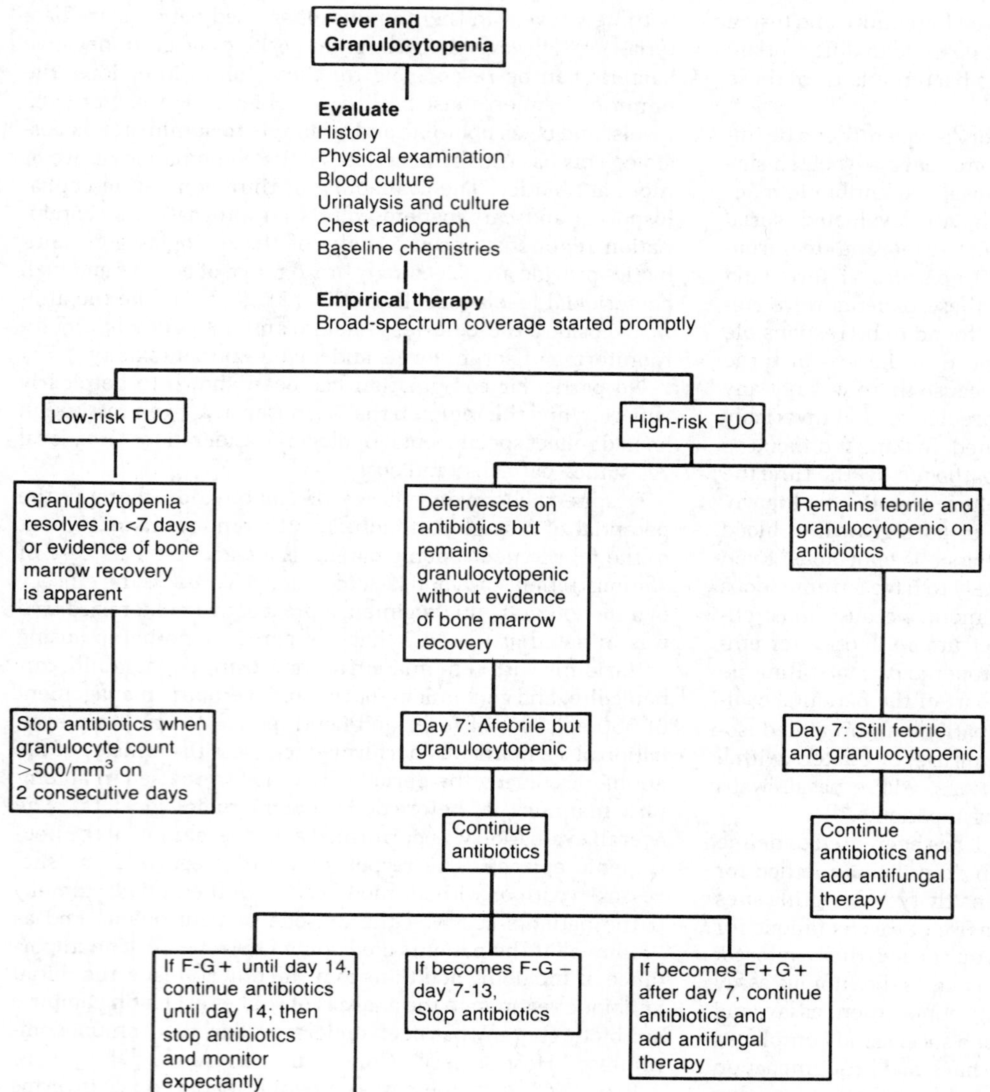
Fever and Granulocytopenia
Evaluate
History
Physical examination
Blood culture
Urinalysis and culture
Chest radiograph
Baseline chemistries
Empirical therapy
Broad-spectrum coverage started promptly
Low-risk FUO
High-risk FUO
Granulocytopenia resolves in <7 days or evidence of bone marrow recovery is apparent
Defervesces on antibiotics but remains granulocytopenic without evidence of bone marrow recovery
Remains febrile and granulocytopenic on antibiotics
Stop antibiotics when granulocyte count >500/mm³ on 2 consecutive days
Day 7: Afebrile but granulocytopenic
Day 7: Still febrile and granulocytopenic
Continue antibiotics
Continue antibiotics and add antifungal therapy
If F-G+ until day 14, continue antibiotics until day 14; then stop antibiotics and monitor expectantly
If becomes F-G – day 7-13, Stop antibiotics
If becomes F+G+ after day 7, continue antibiotics and add antifungal therapy

FIGURE 62–5. Algorithm for the initial management of the patient who has unexplained fever and neutropenia.

the overall outcome and the frequency with which modifications of the initial empiric regimen were necessary, monotherapy with ceftazidime was as effective as combination therapy with cephalothin (Keflin), carbenicillin, and gentamicin for these patients.

Other antibiotics are being evaluated for use as monotherapy in patients with neutropenia. Among the most important is imipenem, a member of the carbapenem class of antibiotics, that provides activity against most gram-positive bacteria (including the enterococci), the Enterobacteriaceae, P. aeruginosa (but not not *Pseudomonas maltophilia*), and anaerobes.[122] Overall, it has the broadest spectrum of activity of any available antibiotic. Early results of a randomized study comparing ceftazidime with imipenem at the NCI demonstrate to corroborate is efficacy in this setting. More than 500 episodes of fever and neutropenia have been enrolled in an NCI study that randomly assigned pediatric and adult patients to receive monotherapy with ceftazidime or imipenem and cilastatin; the data suggest that the overall outcome is comparable. More gram-positive infections have been observed in patients randomly assigned to receive ceftazidime and a significantly higher incidence of *Clostridium difficile* colitis occurred in patients randomly assigned to receive imipenem. Despite its broad spectrum of activity, imipenem has several potential drawbacks, including the emergence of resistant strains of *P. aeruginosa* (caused by alterations of the organism's porin channels), the risk for breakthrough infections with *Pseudomonas* (*Xanthomonas*) *maltophilia* resistant to imipenem, and the potential for imipenem to decrease the seizure threshold in patients with central nervous system abnormalities. We have observed unexpectedly frequent nausea and vomiting in patients receiving imipenem, despite a slow rate of infusion.

Because of the increasing incidence of gram-positive infections in patients with cancer during the 1980s and because of the increased resistance to β-lactam antibiotics, several groups suggested that vancomycin or teicoplanin (a new glycopeptide antibiotic with activity similar to that of vancomycin) be included in initial empiric regimens.[128–130] Conversely, it has been argued that many of these bacteria are relatively low in virulence and that vancomycin may be safely withheld until the gram-positive isolate has been identified microbiologically.

Although two randomized studies have demonstrated a reduction in gram-positive infections in patients receiving a vancomycin regimen, no significant differences in survival were observed in patients who received vancomycin in a pathogen-directed manner. A retrospective analysis from the NCI of 550 patient episodes indicated that no excess morbidity occurred as a result of delaying the institution of vancomycin to wait for a microbiologic or clinical indication for its use (*i.e.*, a positive culture for a resistant gram-positive organism, or a clinical infection developing during other antibiotic therapy).[131] A study by the European Organization for Research and Treatment of Cancer and the National Cancer Institute of Canada evaluated data on 747 febrile patients with granulocytopenia and failed to demonstrate a benefit derived from empiric vancomycin therapy.[132] Comparable results were obtained in children with fever and neutropenia. Moreover, a study of teicoplanin as an alternative to vancomycin failed to demonstrate a significant benefit when teicoplanin was administered empirically.[133]

It seems reasonable not to include vancomycin routinely in all empiric antibiotic regimens. Its use should be guided by institutional experience and sensitivity patterns. Patterns of infecting microorganisms may fluctuate. For example, penicillin-resistant α-hemolytic streptococci are particularly virulent pathogens in some centers, perhaps related to the use of high-dose cytosine arabinoside therapy or to alteration of the oral mucosa by infection with HSV.[134] Centers with a high frequency of infection with methicillin-resistant *S. aureus* should routinely use vancomycin empirically. The emergence of new pathogens or of pathogens with altered sensitivity profiles may force changes in our use of antibiotics.

NEWER ANTIBIOTICS FOR THE COMPROMISED HOST

The monobactams are another novel group of antibiotics, of which aztreonam is the prototype.[135,136] Susceptible organisms include most enteric gram-negative rods, including *P. aeruginosa.* Aztreonam has no significant activity against any of the clinically important gram-positive aerobic organisms or against anaerobes. A particularly useful feature of aztreonam is its apparent lack of cross-reactivity to the other β-lactams in patients who have penicillin or β-lactam allergies. It may be most useful for the treatment of the patient with a significant allergy to β-lactams for whom therapy with an anti-*Pseudomonas* β-lactam antibiotic is still desirable or who requires a bacterial agent

β-Lactams are combined with β-lactamase inhibitors (*e.g.*, clavulanic acid and sulbactam). Three preparations are now available: amoxicillin plus clavulanic acid (oral formulations only), ticarcillin plus clavulanic acid, and ampicillin plus sulbactam. Others, such as piperacillin plus sulbactam, are under development.

The quinolones represent a group of structurally distinct synthetic synthetic antibiotics with a broad spectrum of activity and a unique mechanism of action characterized by the inhibition of DNA gyrase.[137] The spectrum of activity of the fluoroquinolones includes most gram-negative organisms encountered in neutropenic hosts. However, the currently available quinolones have only moderate activity against many species of streptococci, including *Enterococcus* species and *Streptococcus pneumoniae*, and are virtually devoid of activity against the clinically important anaerobic bacteria.[138,139]

The appropriate role for the quinolones in the patient with neutropenia has yet to be defined. Because of their relatively limited activity against certain gram-positive organisms, they should not be used alone for empiric therapy. They may be useful for the completion of therapy in patients who initially responded to intravenously administered antibiotics and who have had a fever of undetermined origin or a susceptible bacterial isolate, an issue that is currently under study at the NCI. However, with expanded use the resistant isolates have emerged. Moreover, the quinolones are not approved for use in the pediatric population because of articular abnormalities observed in the weight-bearing joints in the young of some experimental animals, although phase I and II trials are in progress in children with cancer and cystic fibrosis.

MANAGEMENT APPROACHES

Prolonged Granulocytopenia

The question of the duration of empiric antibiotic therapy in patients with persistent neutropenia is a matter of practical significance. This can be approached by placing patients in one of two categories: those whose initial examination (at the time of presentation with fever and neutropenia) did not reveal a source of infection and those whose initial studies revealed a documented infection to account for the fever (*i.e.*, positive culture, clinically infected site) At most centers, the majority of patients are in the unexplained-fever category, although this proportion varies with the institution, the therapy, and the patient population.

UNEXPLAINED FEVER. For patients whose granulocytopenia is of short duration (<1 week), stopping antibiotic therapy after recovery of the leukocyte count can be practical and effective. Some studies suggest that afebrile patients recovering from their neutropenia (but whose absolute granulocyte count remains below 500/mm^3) can have their antibiotics discontinued with adverse sequelae.[140] However, a problem arises in the population with more prolonged granulocytopenia. In a study from the NCI, patients with unexplained fever and persistent granulocytopenia were randomly selected to discontinue the use of antibiotics on day 7 of therapy or to continue under the resolution of the neutropenia. Almost 40% of afebrile patients who stopped antibiotic therapy had recurrent fever subsequently, and 38% of febrile patients whose antibiotic therapy was discontinued had hypotensive episodes. It was concluded that day 7 was too early to discontinue antibiotic treatment in this group.

A subsequent study conducted at the NCI randomly selected afebrile patients with persistent neutropenia to continue or discontinue antibiotic therapy on day 14. Analysis showed no difference between the two groups; approximately one third of patients became afebrile again regardless of whether they stopped or continued treatment with antibiotics.[142] However, those whose fevers recurred after discontinuation of antibiotic therapy responded to reinstitution of their initial regimens, but those continuing to receive antibiotics required the addition of amphotericin B. On this basis, it seems reasonable to discontinue antibiotic therapy on day 14 in patients who

(text continues on page 2308)

TABLE 62–13. Antimicrobial Agents Commonly Used in Cancer Patients

Antimicrobial Agent	*Trade Name*	*Major Indications*	*Usual Daily Dosage (I.V.)*	*Daily Dosage Schedule*	*Usual Maximal Adult Dose per Day*
Penicillins					
Penicillin G	Benzathin Permapen Bicillin	*S. pneumoniae, S. pyogenes, S. viridens, S. bovis, Neisseria,* most anaerobes (except *B. fragilis*)	25–500,000 units/kg	q 4 h	20 g
Penicillinase resistant					
Methicillin	Straphcillin, celbenin	*S. aureus,* streptococci	1–300 mg/kg	q 4 h	12 g
Nafcillin	Unipen		1–300 mg/kg	q 4 h	12 g
Oxacillin	Prostaphin, bactocill		1–300 mg/kg	q 4 h	12 g
Aminopencillin					
Ampicillin	Omipen Prinipen Polycillin Penbritin	*S. fecalis, L. monocytogenes, Hemophilus, E. coli, Salmonella, Proteus*	2–400 mg/kg	q 4 h	12 g
Ampicillin/ sulbactam	Unasyn	Same as ampicillin but with more reliable gram-negative activity and broader anaerobic activity	100–400 mg/kg	q 6 h	12 g
Carboxy penicillins					
Carbenicillin	Pyopen, Geopen	*P. aeruginosa, Enterobacter, Proteus, Serrata, Acinetobacter, Providentia.*	500 mg/kg	q 4 h	36 g
Ticarcillin	Ticar	Anaerobes including some *Bacteroides* sp., some *Clostridium* sp. *Peptostreptococcus, Fusobacterium*	300 mg/kg	q 4 h	21 g
Extended-spectrum					
Mezlocillin	Mezlin	Same as carboxy penicillin plus *Klebsiella* sp.	300 mg/kg	q 4 h	21 g
Piperacillin	Pipercil	Same as mezlocillin plus increased activity against *P. aeruginosa*	300 mg/kg	q 4 h	21 g
Azlocillin	Azlin	Same as piperacillin	300 mg/kg	q 4 h	21 g
Cephalosporins					
First generation:					
Cephalothin	Keflin	*E. coli, Klebsiella, Proteus, Hemophilus, S. aureus, S. epidermidis,* streptococci	170 mg/kg	q 4 h	12 g
Cefazolin	Kefzol, Ancef	Similar to cephalothin, more active against *Klebsiella, E. coli*	50 mg/kg	q 6 h	2–6 g
Second generation:					
Cephamandole	Mandol	More active against *Hemophilus, Klebsiella, E. coli, Enterobacter* sp., *Proteus;* less active against gram-positive cocci	100–200 mg/kg	q 4 h	6–12 g
Cefoxitin	Mefoxitin	Same as cephalothin plus *Proteus* sp., and anaerobes, including *B. fragilis*	200 mg/kg	q 4 h	6–12 g

Peak Serum Level ($\mu g/ml$)	$T_{1/2}$ (h) Normal	Renal Failure	Modifications for Renal Failure (adults) Moderate C_{CR} 10–50 ml/min	Severe C_{CR} <10 ml/min	Comments
2	0.5	2.5	NC	1,600,000 units q 6 h	
40	0.5	4	NC	2 g q 8 h	Rare nephritis
6	0.5	1.5	NC	NC	Rare SGOT elevation
2.6	0.5	1.0	NC	NC	Rare neutropenia, hepatotoxicity
3.5	1.0	8	NC	0.5–1 g q 8 h	Diarrhea common Synergistic with aminoglycoside for *Enterococcus*
Same as ampicillin	1.0	9	C_{CR} 15–29: 1.5–3.0 g q 12 h	C_{CR} 5–14: 1.5–3.0 q 24 h	
200	1.1	15	3 g q 4 h	2 g q 8 h	Synergistic with gentamicin for *Pseudomonas* Higher sodium load (carbticar)—hypokalemia
140	1.2	15	2 g q 4 h	2 g q 8 h	Rare platelet dysfunction Should never be mixed in same bottle with aminoglycosides
100–110	0.8	1.6	NC	25 mg/kg/dose q 6 h	Similar to carboxy penicillins Bleeding reactions not described
100–110	1.0	3.1	NC	25 mg/kg/dose q 6 h	The extended-spectrum penicillins have a lower sodium content (1.8–2.0 mEq g)
100–110	0.8	4	NC	45 mg/kg/dose q 12 h	They have a lower protein binding and higher biliary excretion than the carboxy penicillins.
80	0.5–0.8	2	1 g q 4–6 h	1 g q 8 h	Most gram-positive activity among cephalosporins
135	1.5	20–40	0.5 g q 6–12 h	0.5 g q 24–48 h	Longer half-life than cephalothin
36	0.9–1.5		1.2 g q 6–8 h	0.5 g q 8–12 h	Cefuroxime (Zinacef) provides comparable coverage with a slightly longer half-life
20–23	0.75	22	15–30 mg/kg/dose q 12–24 h	15 mg/kg/dose q 24 h	Cefoxitin can induce production of β-lactamases which can hydrolyze other β-lactam antibodies used in combination

(continued)

TABLE 62–13. *(Continued)*

Antimicrobial Agent	*Trade Name*	*Major Indications*	*Usual Daily Dosage (I.V.)*	*Daily Dosage Schedule*	*Usual Maximal Adult Dose per Day*
Cefuroxime	Zinacef	Similar to cefamandole, penetrates into CSF	0.75–1.5 g	q 8 h	5–9 g
Third generation:					
Cefotaxime	Claforan	Same as cephalothin plus *Enterobacter* sp., indole positive *Proteus, H. influenzae, Citrobacter* sp., *Serratia* sp., and some *P. aeruginosa* and *Bacteroides* sp.	200 mg/kg	q 4 h	12 g
Ceftriaxone	Rocephin	Similar to cefotaxime	1–2 g	q 12–24 h	2 g
Cefoperazone	Cefaloid	Same as cefotaxime but with better *P. aeruginosa* activity	200 mg/kg	q 8 h	12 g
Ceftizoxime	Cefizox	Same as cefotaxime	200 mg/kg	q 8 h	12 g
Ceftazidime	Fortaz	Same as cefoperazone but with less anaerobic activity. Most active agent against *P. aeruginosa*	100 mg/kg	q 8 h	6 g
Carbapenems					
Imipenem/cilastatin	Primaxin	In addition to the Enterobacteriaceae and *P. aeruginosa,* primaxin has efficacy against *S. aureus,* group D streptococci, many coagulase-negative staphylococci, listeria, and anaerobes. Only *P. maltophilia* and *P. cepacia* are not covered.	50–60	q 6 h	3–4
Monobactams					
Monobactems					
Aztreonam	Azactam	Broad gram-negative but no gram-positive coverage. Is not cross-reactive with other β-lactams so can be used in penicillin or cephalosporin allergic patients	100–150	q 6 h	4–6
Aminoglycosides					
Gentamicin	Garamycin	*P. aeruginosa,* Enterobacteriaceae, Enterococcus (with ampicillin)	3–6 mg/kg	q 6–8 h	

Peak Serum Level (μg/ml)	$T_{1/2}$ (h) Normal	Renal Failure	Modifications for Renal Failure (adults) Moderate C_{CR} 10–50 ml/min	Severe C_{CR} <10 ml/min	Comments
100	1–2	15	0.75–1.5 g q 8–12 h	0.75–1.5 q 24 h	Cefuroxime also is dispensed in an oral formulation
125–175	1.3–1.6	27	NC	30 mg/kg q 12 h	All third-generation cephalosporins have less gram-positive activity than first-generation agents. None are effective against enterococci or *Listeria*. They have variable coverage against pseudomonads and anaerobes
270	8	11.9–15.4	0.5–1 g q 12–24 h	0.5–1 g q 12–24 h	Longest half-life of third-generation cephalosporins, permits once- or twice-daily dosing. Also has activity against *N. gonorrhoeae*
175–225	1.6–2.1	4.2	NC	20 mg/kg dose q 12 h	Highest biliary excretion of the third generation group. It contains the methylthiotetrazole group and may cause serious bleeding
150–200	2.1–2.8	19.3	1 g q 12	0.5 g q 24 h	
150–200	1.6–2.1		C_{CR}31–50: 1 g q 12 h C_{CR}16–30: 1 g q 24 h	C_{CR}6–15: 0.5 mg q 24 h C_{CR}5: 0.5 mg q 48 h	Best activity against *P. aeruginosa*
43–78	1	4	0.5–1 g q 6–12 h	0.5–1 g q 12–24 h	Can cause seizures in patients with preexisting CNS disease or in patients with altered renal functions. Higher doses can cause nausea and vomiting
125	1.7–2	6–8.7	0.5–2 g q 12–24 h	0.5–2 g q 12–24 h	Not cross-rective with β-lactams and can be used in the penicillin or cephalosporin allergic patient.
4–8	2.3	45–55	Monitor serum levels		All aminoglycosides synergistic or additive with penicillins or cephalosporins against *Pseudomonas*, enterococcus, staph., strep., Enterobacteriaceae

(continued)

TABLE 62–13. *(Continued)*

Antimicrobial Agent	*Trade Name*	*Major Indications*	*Usual Daily Dosage (I.V.)*	*Daily Dosage Schedule*	*Usual Maximal Adult Dose per Day*
Tobramycin	Nebicin	Similar to gentamicin (except not as active against enterococcus with ampicillin)	3–6 mg/kg	q 6–8 h	
Amikacin	Amikin	*Serratia, Proteus, Pseudomonas,* Enterobacteriaceae, *Providentia*	15 mg/kg	q 8–12 h	
Miscellaneous					
Chloramphenicol	Chloromycetin	*Hemophilus, B. fragilis, S. pneumoniae, Neisseriae, Salmonella, Klebsiella,* most anaerobes, *Rickettsia*	50–100 mg/kg	q 6 h	3–6 g
Erythromycin	Ilotycin Gluceptate	*Legionella* *Mycoplasma*	30–50 mg/kg	q 6 h	6 g
Clindamycin	Cleocin	*B. fragilis, Clostridia, S. pneumoniae, S. viridens, S. pyogenes, S. aureus*	30 mg/kg	q 6 h	2400 mg
Vancomycin	Vancocin	*C. difficile, S. aureus, S. epidermidis, S. fecalis,* multiply resistant *Corynebacteria, S. bovis*	25–40 mg/kg	q 8–12 h	3 g
Trimethoprim-Sulfamethoxazole (1:5 ratio)	Bactrim Septra	*P. carinii, S. aureus, S. pneumoniae, S. pyogenes, Salmonella, Listeria, E. coli, Proteus, Serratia, Hemophilus, Neisseria*	10–20 mg/kg as trimethoprim	q 8–12 h	960 g
Ciprofloxacin	Cinoxacin	Gram negatives including Enterobacteriaceae, *P. aeruginosa, Hemophilus, Branhamella,* gonococci. Also active against *Chlamydia,* some mycoplasma, *Legionella.* Less active against gram-positive bacteria, especially streptococci	250–500 mg	q 6–12 h	1.5 g
Antiparasitics					
Pentamidine Isethionate	Lomidine	*P. carinii*	4 mg/kg IM	Once/day	
Thiabendazole	Mintezol	*Strongyloides,* visceral larva migrans	50 mg/kg 2 days	q 12 h	3 g
Antifungal Agents					
Amphotericin B	Fungizone	*Candida, Aspergillus, Zygomycetes, Torulopsis, Cryptococcus, Histoplasma*	0.5–1.0 mg/kg	Once/day	

Peak Serum Level (μg/ml)	$T_{1/2}$ (h) Normal	Renal Failure	Modifications for Renal Failure (adults) Moderate C_{CR} 10–50 ml/min	Severe C_{CR} <10 ml/min	Comments
4–8	2.3	45–55	Monitor serum levels		All have renal and ototoxicity
15–25	2.3	50–80	Monitor serum levels		
12	4.1	4.2	NC	NC	Both idiosyncratic and dose-related bone marrow toxicity Dosage must be reduced with hepatotoxicity
0.4–1.8	1.4	5	NC	NC	Burning and phlebitis intravenously
10	2.4	6	NC	NC	Risk for pseudomembranous enterocolitis (Treat with vancomycin or metronidazole)
25–50	6	9 d	1 g q 36 h	1 g q 10–14 d	Drug of choice for antibiotic (*C. difficile*) induced colitis but must be given orally (125 mg PO q 6 h). Also drug of choice for *S. epid.* and methicillin-resistant staph (I.V.)
1.6–3.2 trimethoprim	7½	25	10 mg/kg q 12 h	5 mg/kg q 12 h	May be useful for prophylaxis against *P. carinii* May result in myelosuppression, particularly in AIDS
2.4	3.9	5–10	250 mg q 12–24 h	Not recommended	Both oral and parenteral formulations available. Accumulates in cartilage and not approved for children
0.2	Very short		q 36 h	q 48 h	Very toxic: hypotension, renal damage, sterile abscesses, hypo- and hyperglycemia Available only through CDC
	1				Rare hepatoxicity. May cause nausea, vomiting, headache, dizziness
0.5–2.0	24	NC	NC	0.5 mg/kg/q 36 h	Dose modification necessary for patients with hepatic abnormalities Major toxicities are fever, electrolyte disturbances. May be combined with 5-FC to treat cryptococcal meningitis

(continued)

TABLE 62–13. *(Continued)*

Antimicrobial Agent	*Trade Name*	*Major Indications*	*Usual Daily Dosage (I.V.)*	*Daily Dosage Schedule*	*Usual Maximal Adult Dose per Day*
5-Fluorocytosine	Flucytosine Ancobon	*Cryptococcus, Candida, Torulopsis, Chromomycosis*	50–150 mg/kg	q 6 h	
Clotrimazole	Lotrimin	*Candida* sp., dermatophytes	50 mg (troche)	q 6 h	
Miconazole	Monistat	*Candida* sp., *Aspergillus* sp., *Zygomycetes, Torulopsis, Cryptococcus, Petrielldium, Blastomyces, Coccidioides, Histoplasma, Paracoccidiides, Sporothrix*	1500–3600 mg/d		
Ketoconazole	Nizoral	Similar to miconazole	2–400 mg/d	q d	400 (higher doses are being investigated)
Fluconazole	Diflucan	*Candida, Crytococcus, Histoplasma, Blastomyces, Coccidioides*	100–400 mg/d (oral or I.V.)	q d	Excellent penetration into CSF
Antiviral Agents					
Adenosine arabinoside	Vidarabine	H. simplex varicella-zoster	10–15 mg/kg/d	12-h infusion	
Acycloguanosine	Acyclovir	H. simplex, varicella-zoster	750 mg/m²/d (H. simplex) 1500 mg/m²/d (VZV)	q 8 h	
Ganciclovir	Cytovene	Cytomegalovirus reninitis, pneumonia, colitis	5 mg/kg q 12 h × 14–21 day induction then 5 mg/kg q d or 6 mg/kg 5 d/wk for maintenance.	Induction	
Interferons (α, β, γ)		H. simplex, VZV	1 × 10⁴ 5 × 10⁵ units/kg/d	q d	

NC, no change.

Peak Serum Level (μg/ml)	$T_{1/2}$ (h) Normal	Renal Failure	Modifications for Renal Failure (adults) Moderate C_{CR} 10–50 ml/min	Severe C_{CR} <10 ml/min	Comments
30	3.4	200	12–25 mg/kg once	Not given	Rapid resistance develops when used alone Normal use is in conjunction with amphotericin Parenteral form investigational For topical use only (*e.g.*, oral troche). If systemically absorbed, is inactivated by hepatic enzymes
2–8 μg	0.4, 2.1, 24.2 h (3 compartments)		NC	NC	No proven efficacy in invasive fungal infections in immunocompromised hosts Can cause hyponatremia, anemia, thrombocytosis, nausea, vomiting, cardiac arrhythmias. Less than 1% excreted in urine. 50% excreted in feces
2–13 μg	2–8 h (biphasic)		NC	NC	No proven value in immunocompromised hosts. May cause nausea, vomiting, hepatic enzyme elevation, dizziness, gynecomastia, adrenal insufficiency. Antacids and cimetidine impede absorption
4–8 μg/ml	3–5 h		No established guidelines. Reduce by 25% in severe renal failure and monitor metabolites		No activity against CMV Anorexia, nausea, vomiting, diarrhea. Rare myelosuppression, neurotoxicity. Excessive fluid requirements
30–50 μM	2.2–5 h		5–10 mg/kg q 12 h for C_{CR} 25–50.; 5–10 mg/kg q 24 h for C_{CR} 10–25	2.5–5 mg/kg q 24 h	Twice maintenance fluids necessary with higher doses to avoid renal toxicity Neurotoxicity (at high doses) Thymidine kinase resistant mutants have been described
8–11 μg/ml	3–4 h		28–5 h	Dose adjustments necessary	Poace and bioavailabiilty require maintenance in HIV patients, can cause marrow suppression Local pain, fever, alopecia, fatigue, anorexia, bone marrow suppression

have remained consistently afebrile during empiric therapy, recognizing that when the antibiotics are withdrawn, these patients must be closely monitored for recurrent fever or infection until the resolution of their granulocytopenia. The question of whether the antibiotic therapy could be delivered orally for these patients is being explored by the NCI Pediatric Branch. The results of this study will help to define the safety of ciprofloxacin in children and its utility for simplifying continuation of therapy for patients with prolonged neutropenia.

DOCUMENTED INFECTIONS AT PRESENTATION. For patients with persistent neutropenia who have had clinical and microbiologic resolution of their infection, and who are afebrile at day 14 (for a minimum of 7 days), antibiotic therapy may be discontinued. The ultimate decision of whether to continue or discontinue antibiotic therapy depends on potential antibiotic toxicity, the predicted duration of neutropenia, the seriousness of the initial infection, and the presence or absence of other factors predisposing the patient to subsequent infection. Antibiotics are usually administered for 10 to 14 days unless there is a residual site of infection (*e.g.*, perianal cellulitis) and the neutropenia persists. In such cases, antibiotic therapy should be continued until resolution of the signs of infection or recovery from neutropenia.

The question of whether the spectrum of antibiotics can be narrowed when a specific isolate is determined is of practical relevance.[143] Although a primary infection caused by an identified organism can be treated successfully with a broad-spectrum or a pathogen-specific antibiotic, the risk of second (or breakthrough) infections is increased in patients with prolonged neutropenia (>7 days) who receive a narrow-spectrum antibiotic.

Therapy Modifications During the Granulocytopenic Course

Empiric antibiotic therapy has its greatest impact early in the course of neutropenia. It should not be assumed that a regimen demonstrating initial efficacy will suffice as the sole antimicrobial therapy throughout a protracted course of neutropenia. During a prolonged granulocytopenic episode, the patient is at increased risk for secondary infections or superinfections; this risk increases the longer that the neutropenia persists. Throughout the course of the patient's disease, the persistence of fever and changing clinical findings may dictate that modifications be made to ensure a successful outcome. Few of these new infections represent a failure of the initial therapy. Most should be viewed as part of the "natural history" of patients with prolonged neutropenia, and needed modifications of the initial regimens should be expected and planned, with the goal of maximizing the patient's chance for survival.

Bacterial isolates that are resistant or that become resistant to the initial empiric regimen are invariably encountered in patients with neutropenia. Some of them can be anticipated; others emerge sporadically. For example, at most centers, the majority of coagulase-negative staphylococci are resistant to β-lactams, and breakthrough infections with these organisms should be anticipated if a regimen not containing vancomycin is employed. Fortunately, coagulase-negative staphylococci are relatively low in virulence. For patients with evidence of gram-positive infection during therapy with one or more β-lactam antibiotics or for those with evidence of a catheter-site infection, vancomycin should usually be added to the initial antibiotic regimen.

Breakthrough bacteremia with gram-negative organisms, particularly *Enterobacter, Serratia,* and *Citrobacter*, are of concern, especially if a β-lactam antibiotic is used alone. Many of the organisms likely to break through an antibiotic regimen can often be predicted from an understanding of the defined limitations of the antibiotic.

The appearance of a new site of infection (*e.g.*, cellulitis, pneumonia) and the progression of infection at a previously documented site are additional reasons for modifications of the antimicrobial regimen.

Empiric Antifungal Therapy

Patients who have prolonged periods of profound neutropenia after intensive cytotoxic chemotherapy or ablative irradiation are at increased risk of acquiring invasive fungal infections.[144] The early diagnosis of invasive fungal infections in children with granulocytopenia can be difficult, and fever may be the only manifestation of infection. Moreover, withholding antifungal therapy until infection is proved by culture or histologic examination increases the likelihood of disseminated infection. This has led to the concept of employing empiric antifungal therapy to prevent fungal overgrowth in patients with prolonged granulocytopenia and to provide early treatment of clinically occult infection.[145] Two randomized clinical trials demonstrated that the use of empirically administered amphotericin B in persistently or recurrently febrile patients with granulocytopenia decreases the frequency, morbidity, and mortality rates for invasive fungal infections, especially in patients with profound granulocytopenia who are not receiving antifungal prophylaxis.[146,147] The morbidity and mortality rates for untreated or undertreated invasive fungal infections in patients with granulocytopenia usually supersede the toxic effects of amphotericin B, which are usually reversible.

Treatment with amphotericin B (0.5 mg/kg/day) should be instituted in patients with granulocytopenia who remain persistently or recurrently febrile after 7 days. Nonetheless, because of the side effects associated with amphotericin administration, less toxic alternatives are highly desirable. Orally administered ketoconazole is comparable to amphotericin B in preventing the onset of a fungal disease, but after infection does arise, it invariably progresses unless the patient is given amphotericin B.[148] Fluconazole, a new antifungal triazole with significant activity against *Candida,* is currently being evaluated for empiric antifungal therapy in children.[149,150] However, the absence of activity against *Aspergillus* is likely to limit the value of fluconazole. This limitation underscores the need for newer antifungal agents with broader profiles.

Even empiric amphotericin B therapy does not completely prevent the development of fungal infections; invasive infection with organisms more resistant to amphotericin B (*e.g., Aspergillus, Pseudallescheria, Trichosporon, Fusarium)* has been reported in patients who were receiving the drug at dosages of 0.5 to 0.6 mg/kg per day.[151] Higher dosages of empiric amphotericin (1.0–1.5 mg/kg/day) may be necessary for patients with more prolonged neutropenia or who develop recurrent fever and pulmonary signs and symptoms while receiving standard dosages of amphotericin B.

TREATMENT OF INFECTIOUS COMPLICATIONS

BACTEREMIA

Approximately 10% to 20% of febrile neutropenic cancer patients have bacteremia at the time of presentation. Among immunocompromised patients, the respiratory tract is the most common initial site of sepsis (25%), followed by a perianal and perioral cellulitis, the gastrointestinal tract, and the genitourinary tract (each approximately 10%). Indwelling intravascular devices have become a common source of bacteremias. Unfortunately, there is no clinically reliable method for prospectively identifying febrile neutropenic patients who are bacteremic.[62,110]

Until the late 1970s, gram-negative aerobic organisms were the most frequently isolated pathogens. The pattern of infections has shifted, and gram-positive bacteria now are isolated as often as gram-negative bacteria at most cancer centers. Among the gram-positive pathogens, *S. aureus, S. epidermidis,* and *Streptococcus* species (including the viridans and group D) are the most commonly isolated. Documented septicemia with *S. bovis,* although uncommon, is important because of its close association with carcinoma of the colon and should heighten the clinician's suspicion of an undetected neoplasm.[152] Species of *Corynebacterium* (*e.g.,* CDC group JK, *C. diphtheriae, C. equi*) and *Bacillus* are less frequently isolated and tend to occur in patients with prolonged episodes of granulocytopenia or indwelling vascular access devices, respectively. *E. coli, K. pneumoniae,* and *P. aeruginosa* are the most frequently isolated gram-negative bacilli, although more resistant species (*e.g.,* nonaeruginosa Pseudomonades, *Serratia marcescens, Enterobacter* species, *Citrobacter* species) are also found.

Primary bacteremia due to anaerobic organisms are uncommon, accounting for less than 5% of the septicemia in cancer patients. For reasons that are unclear, the incidence of infections due to *P. aeruginosa* has been decreasing in recent years. The morbidity and mortality rates due to gram-positive bacteria, especially the coagulase-negative staphylococci, are less than those due to gram-negative pathogens.

The most important therapeutic intervention for patients ultimately shown to be bacteremic is the prompt initiation of empiric antibiotics when fever and neutropenia occur. Modifications of the regimen should be based on the microbiologic sensitivity pattern of the bloodstream isolate (Table 62–14). The minimal duration of therapy for bacteremic patients is 10 to 14 days, although patients with persistent neutropenia or a persistent site of infection are likely to require longer treatment.

TABLE 62–14. Modification of Therapy

Clinical Event	*Possible Modifications of Therapy*
Breakthrough bacteremia	If gram-positive isolate (*e.g., S. epidermidis*), add vancomycin If gram-negative isolate (*i.e.,* presumably resistant), switch to regimen containing noncross-resistant antibiotics (*e.g.,* aminoglycoside plus a carbapenem or extended-spectrum penicillin).
Catheter-associated infection	Add vancomycin (and gram-negative coverage if not already being given).
Severe oral mucositis or necrotizing gingivitis	Add specific antianaerobic agent (*e.g.,* clindamycin or metronidazole)
Esophagitis	Trial of oral clotrimazole, ketoconazole, or I.V. amphotericin B.
Pneumonitis	
Diffuse or interstitial	Trial of trimethoprim-sulfamethoxazole and erythromycin (plus broad-spectrum antibiotics if the patient is granulocytopenic).
New infiltrate in a granulocytopenic patient also receiving antibiotics	If granulocyte count is rising, watch and wait. If granulocyte count is not recovering, biopsy to establish diagnosis; if biopsy cannot be done, add amphotericin B empirically.
Perianal tenderness	If patient is already receiving broad-spectrum antibiotics, add a specific antianaerobic agent. If patient is not on antibiotics, begin broad-spectrum therapy with anaerobic coverage.
Persistent fever and neutropenia	Continue antibiotics after 1 week of persistent fever and neutropenia; add systemic antifungal therapy empirically.

Catheter-Associated Bacteremias

Catheter-related bacteremias have become increasingly important during the past several years, largely because of the increased use of indwelling right atrial Hickman-Broviac catheters.[68] Although the benefit of these catheters in providing venous access to patients is enormous, the frequency of catheter-associated bacteremia and other problems is significant. Complication rates have been between 3% and 60%, which may be caused by different techniques of catheter insertion, care, and maintenance. Differences in patient populations, their therapies, degree of catheter use, and definition of catheter-related infection and complications also influence the rates of complications.

The diagnosis of a catheter-related bacteremia is made by documenting positive blood cultures from the catheter lumen(s) and a peripheral venous site. The colony count from the lumen sample is ordinarily greater than that from the peripheral site. Most catheter-associated infections are caused by the coagulase-positive staphylococci, but other gram-positive bacteria (*e.g., S. aureus,* streptococci), gram-negative organisms (*Acinetobacter* species, *P. aeruginosa, Bacillus* species, *Corynebacterium* species), and *Candida* can cause infection. *Malassezia furfur* has been isolated in compromised hosts, particularly where hyperalimentation and intralipids were being delivered. Polymicrobial infections occur in rare cases. An outbreak of catheter-exit site infections due to *Aspergillus flavus* was described in association with air contamination in an operating room.[153] Local skin infections due to mycobacteria, particularly *M. fortuitum* and *M. chelonei,* also were described, although these were geographically distributed.[97]

It is important to obtain blood cultures from all ports and from peripheral sites. Careful inspection of the catheter exit site and the subcutaneous tunnel for Hickman-Broviac catheters or the subcutaneous reservoir for implanted Port-a-Cath and Med-I-Port catheters is imperative in management of infections.

If bacteremia occurs in a patient with a foreign body, the device or catheter usually should be removed to ensure eradication of the infection. However, it has become apparent that more than 80% of catheter-associated bacteremias caused by coagulase-negative staphylococci can be treated without removing the catheter if a 10-day course of vancomycin is infused through the catheter (Fig. 62–6). If the patient has a multilumen catheter, the antibiotic infusion should be rotated to include all ports and lumens. Catheter and peripheral venous samples must be obtained after therapy is started. If the cultures remain positive despite 24 hours of appropriate therapy, the catheter should be removed and vancomycin continued; the possibility of endocarditis should be considered for patients with persistent positive blood cultures, and a cardiac echo should be performed. If there is evidence of tenderness or induration along the subcutaneous track of the catheter from its exit to its insertion into the subclavian or jugular vein ("tunnel infection"), the catheter should be removed because these infections are not otherwise treatable.

Not all organisms are as treatable as the coagulase-negative staphylococci. For example, catheter-associated bacteremia caused by *Bacillus* species or by *Candida* usually necessitates catheter removal, even if the organisms are sensitive to the antibiotics being administered.[94] To determine if the type of catheter influences the incidence of infection or ease of the treatment, we compared the incidence of infectious complications in patients randomized to receive Hickman-Broviac or subcutaneously implanted Port-a-Caths. No differences in the incidence of infectious or noninfectious catheter-related complications were observed.

The presence of an indwelling catheter influences the use of antibiotics for a febrile cancer patient. Data for nonneutropenic patients with catheters are lacking, but because of the morbidity associated with untreated gram-negative infection, we recommend that these patients should have cultures obtained and then receive a 48-hour trial of antibiotics (we use ceftraxone because of its ease of administration until it is determined that the fever was not due to a catheter-associated infection. If the cultures are negative, the antibiotics are discontinued; if positive, a full course of treatment is administered.

If the patient is neutropenic and has a catheter and becomes febrile, the empirical use of vancomycin would seem appropriate. We reviewed our experiences at the NCI and found that, although gram-positive and gram-negative bacteremias are more common in patients with indwelling catheters than without, there was no apparent advantage from the addition of vancomycin to the broad-spectrum regimen. We treat neutropenic patients who become febrile without empiric vancomycin, regardless of whether they have an indwelling catheter.

Antibiotic Considerations for the Septicemia Patient

The optimal management of the neutropenic patient with a defined infection poses a dilemma. Should the patient continue to receive a broad-spectrum antibiotic regimen or can the antibiotics be narrowed to a pathogen-directed therapy? Continuing broad-spectrum therapy maintains antimicrobial activity against a wide range of gram-positive and gram-negative pathogens and may effectively eradicate or suppress second bacterial infections. However, this approach may allow the proliferation of resistant bacteria and fungi and result in secondary bacteremias or disseminated mycoses. The advantage of pathogen-directed therapy is less disturbance of the patient's microbial flora, potentially decreasing the risk of infection with multiply-resistant bacteria or fungi.

A study conducted at the NCI reviewed 78 neutropenic patients with gram-positive (primarily *S. aureus*) bacteremia who received specific therapy with nafcillin or oxacillin or continued broad-spectrum therapy. Patients who remained granulocytopenic for less than 1 week did well regardless of the therapy chosen. Among patients with more prolonged granulocytopenia, 47% of those who received specific therapy developed a second infection due to a gram-negative aerobe.[154]

A prospectively randomized trial revealed no significant difference between patients treated with narrow- or broad-spectrum coverage with respect to second infections, new fevers, or mortality. However, many patients treated with a narrowed antibiotic regimen required subsequent modification of the therapy.[143]

Current recommendations for the management of immunosuppressed and neutropenic patients with documented bacterial infections can be summarized as follows. For patients whose neutropenia is expected to last less than 7 days, a narrowed antimicrobial regimen may be safely employed. For patients with more prolonged neutropenia, there seems to be no advantage to narrowing the initial empiric antibiotic regimen. If the empiric regimen is narrowed (*e.g.,* simplification of fluid administration, cost constraints), the patient's course must be carefully monitored for evidence of recrudescent fever, progression of an infection, or clinical deterioration. Any change should immediately prompt the reexpansion of antimicrobial coverage.

As a supplement to antimicrobial therapy, high doses of corticosteroid have been administered to patients with shock or with the adult respiratory distress syndrome associated with sepsis. Controlled clinical trials, however, have failed to demonstrate the benefit of high-dose steroids in either of these clinical settings.[155,156] Monoclonal antibodies (HA-1A) against the J5 core glycolipid have reduced mortality among patients with documented gram-negative bacteria. Whether these benefits will apply to neutropenic patients is unknown. Monoclonal antibody against TNF will soon be available with other

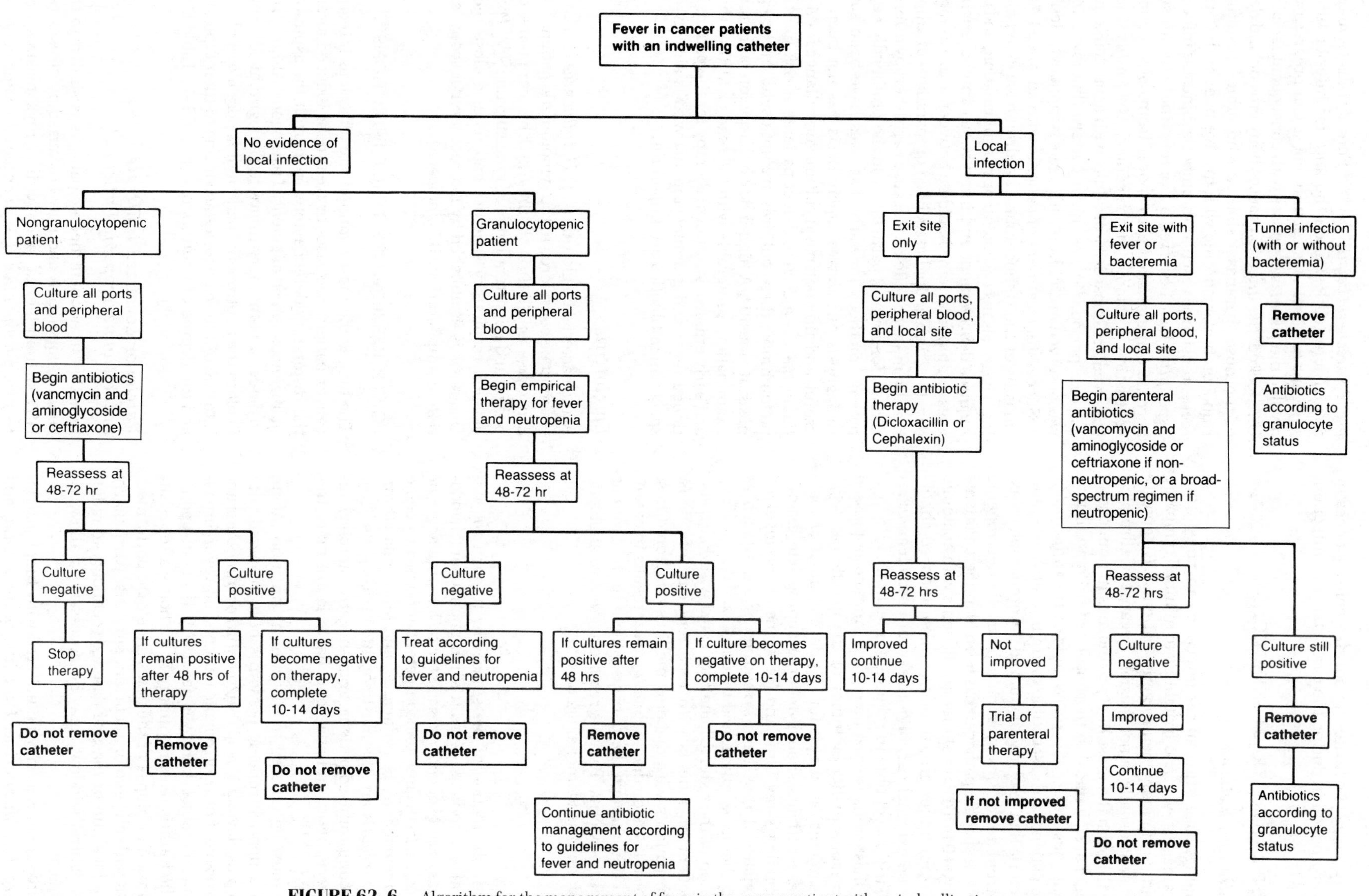

FIGURE 62–6. Algorithm for the management of fever in the cancer patient with an indwelling intravenous catheter.

biologicals that may modulate the adverse consequences of cytokine overproduction during the early stages of infection.

UPPER RESPIRATORY TRACT INFECTIONS

Otitis Media and Externa

Clinical findings suggesting an ear infection can range from ear pain, drainage, fever, and irritability to minimal tympanic erythema in profoundly neutropenic patients. Diagnostic tympanocentesis usually is not feasible because of thrombocytopenia. Although the most likely pathogens in nonneutropenic patients are identical to those isolated from an immunocompetent host (*i.e., S. pneumoniae, H. influenzae*), neutropenic patients are susceptible to gram-positive or gram-negative bacteria that may have colonized the oronasopharynx. Broad-spectrum antibiotics must be used in the neutropenic patient unless a specific pathogen has been identified. Patients should receive 10 to 14 days of therapy. Patients with anatomic alterations from tumor growth or treatment-induced abnormalities of the external ear, middle ear, or eustachian tubes are particularly susceptible to recurrent infections.

Although mastoiditis is uncommon, the immunosuppressed host with an abnormality or tumor of the middle ear (*e.g.,* rhabdomyosarcoma) is at risk for the development of mastoiditis. These patients should undergo appropriate examinations, including x-ray films and CT scans of the involved area, particularly if they have symptoms or signs, such as localized erythema, swelling, and tenderness.

Colonization of the external auditory canal with *P. aeruginosa* is frequent in patients with recurrent ear infections. However, in patients with diabetes mellitus or altered host defenses, local invasion due to *Pseudomonas* results in extension of infection through the petrous bone into the brain as malignant otitis externa. Patients require aggressive antibiotic therapy with antipseudomonal agents.

Sinusitis

Patients with obstruction of the sinuses by tumor (*e.g.,* nasopharyngeal carcinomas, Burkitt's lymphoma, or rhabdomyosarcomas) are especially at risk for developing acute or chronic sinusitis. In the immunocompetent or nonneutropenic patient, *S. pneumoniae, H. influenzae,* and Moraxella (*Branhamella*) *catarrhalis* are the most common pathogens.[182] In an immunocompromised patient, gram-negative aerobes, including *P. aeruginosa,* and anaerobic bacteria are more frequently found.[157–159]

Therapy must be tailored to the clinical situation. Acute sinusitis in a nonneutropenic person is best managed with amoxicillin plus clavulanic acid (Augmentin) or trimethoprim-sulfamethoxazole. For neutropenic patients, however, broad-spectrum antimicrobial therapy is necessary. If a neutropenic patient with sinusitis does not improve 72 hours after treatment, aspiration or biopsy of the sinus should be performed. For patients with chronic or recurrent sinusitis, particularly those with a local tumor mass or damage secondary to radiotherapy, an "antral window" may be necessary to allow adequate drainage.

The paranasal sinuses may be infected with fungi, particularly *Aspergillus, Mucoraceae, Fusarium, Exserohilum,* and *Pseudoalescheria boydii.*[98,160–163] Fungal sinusitis may begin as a small crusted lesion on the anterior inferior turbinate or adjacent cartilaginous septum, but it can progress rapidly to involve the paranasal sinuses with consequent facial swelling. Unchecked, the infection causes bony erosion and destruction of the nose, paranasal sinuses, and orbits, resulting in the rhinocerebral syndrome with involvement of the brain by direct extension or vascular thrombosis. Sinusitis infections with *Aspergillus* have occurred in centers where the air supply has become contaminated with spores from construction dust or ventilation problems. At one center, *Aspergillus* sinusitis was observed in almost 20% of adults with acute leukemia during a 5-year period.[163,164] A similar pattern (but lower incidence) was observed in children with acute lymphocytic leukemia.[165]

Successful treatment of patients with advanced *Aspergillus* sinusitis or the rhinocerebral syndrome has been disappointing. Diagnosis necessitates biopsy confirmation, and treatment requires debridement and intravenous amphotericin B. Dosages of amphotericin should be between 1 to 1.5 mg/kg each day. If available, lipid-associated preparations of amphotericin may be more beneficial. Because early therapy offers the best chance for control, particularly in the profoundly neutropenic patient, methods for early diagnosis have been sought. Serodiagnosis of invasive aspergillosis has not been clinically useful, and although nasal culture surveillance for *Aspergillus flavus* has been used to detect patients at risk for *Aspergillus* pneumonitis, these cultures are not useful in the early diagnosis of sinusitis. A high index of suspicion, a thorough nasal examination, preferably with CT scan or MRI of the sinuses, and early empiric antifungal therapy for the patient with continued fever and granulocytopenia who is already on broad-spectrum antibiotics are important.

Epiglottitis

Acute bacterial epiglottitis (*e.g., H. influenzae*) is rare in adults but must be considered in the symptomatic patient.[166] *Candida* can cause epiglottitis, hallmarked by symptoms of odynophagia and persistent hypopharyngeal pain.[167,168] Patients can develop respiratory stricture and require close monitoring. Diagnosis is established by indirect laryngoscopy, and initiation of amphotericin B is indicated.

LOWER RESPIRATORY TRACT INFECTIONS

The lung is the most common site of serious infection in the cancer patient. Disease- or treatment-induced alterations of the respiratory defense network permit the aspiration or hematogenous spread of potential pathogens. Although the ability to detect a pulmonary infiltrate radiographically may be difficult in the neutropenic patient, it is possible to place patients into one of four categories according to their type of infiltrate and the degree of neutropenia (Fig. 62–7, Table 62–15).

Patchy or Localized Infiltrate in the Nonneutropenic Patient

Infection in nonneutropenic patients is similar to that in the general population and may be caused by viruses (*e.g.,* RSV, HSV, parainfluenza, adenovirus), mycoplasma, or bacteria (*e.g., S. pneumoniae, H. influenzae*). In some centers, *Legion-*

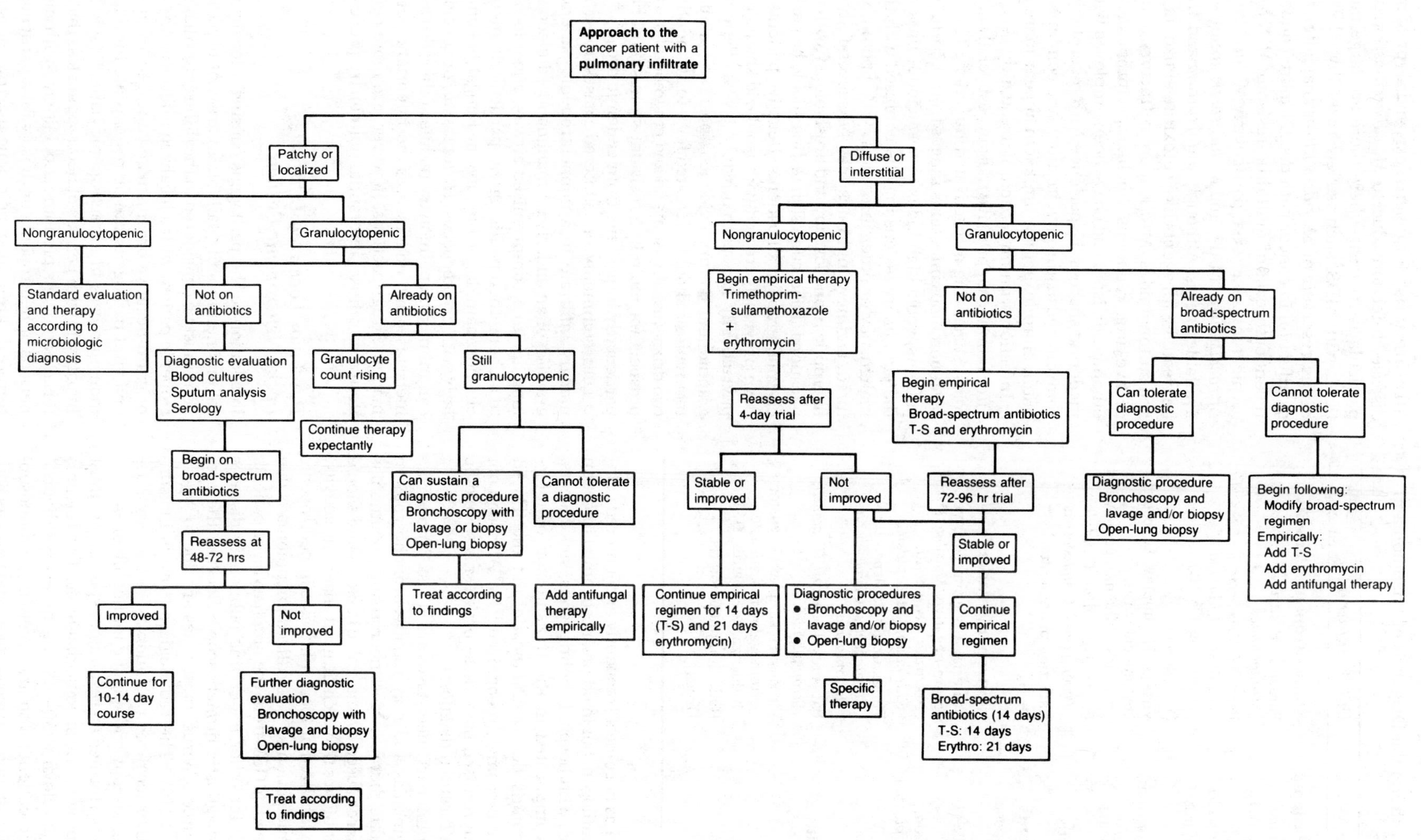

FIGURE 62–7. Algorithm for the management of the cancer patient with a pulmonary infiltrate.

TABLE 62–15. Differential Diagnosis of Pneumonia in Cancer Patients

Localized Infiltrate	*Diffuse Infiltrate*
Nonneutropenic Patients	**Nonneutropenic Patients**
Bacteria: *S. pneumoniae, Hemophilus, Mycobacteria*	Parasites: *P. carinii, T. gondii, Strongyloides*
Fungi: *Cryptococcus, Histoplasma, Coccidioides*	Bacteria: *Mycobacteria, Nocardia, Legionella, Chlamydia* (including TWAR)
Viruses: RSV, adenovirus	*Mycoplasma*
Underlying tumor	Viruses: H. simplex, V. zoster, cytomegalovirus, measles, influenza, adenovirus
Drugs: busulfan, bleomycin, cyclophosphamide, methotrexate, cytosine arabinoside	Fungi: *Aspergillus, Candida, Zygomycetes, Cryptococcus*
Radiation pneumonitis	Radiation pneumonitis
	Drugs
Neutropenic Patients	**Neutropenic Patients**
Bacteria: Any gram-positive or gram-negative, *Mycobacteria, Nocardia*	Bacteria: Any gram-positive or gram-negative, *Mycobacteria, Nocardia, Legionella, Chlamydia, Mycoplasma*
Fungi: *Aspergillus, Zygomycetes, Candida, Cryptococcus, Histoplasma*	Fungi: *Candida, Aspergillus, Zygomycetes, Cryptococcus, Histoplasma*
Viruses: H. simplex, V. zoster	Parasites: *P. carinii, T. gondii, Strongyloides*
Drugs (see above)	Viruses: H. simplex, V. zoster, cytomegalovirus, measles, influenza, adenovirus, RSV
Radiation pneumonitis	Radiation pneumonitis
	Drugs

ella pneumophila has become a frequently encountered community-acquired pathogen, but in others, nosocomial infection has been observed, with hospital cooling tanks, sink faucets, and showerheads implicated in the transmission of infection.[169,170] Pneumonitis due to *Chlamydia* and the TWAR strain, have been increasingly recognized.[171,172] Although not unique to the compromised host, these organisms should be included in the differential diagnosis.

Patients with pulmonary metastases are at risk for obstructive bronchopneumonias and may require bronchoscopy in addition to antibiotic therapy. Most necrotizing pneumonias or lung abscesses are caused by anaerobic bacteria and should be treated with antibiotics that include good anaerobic activity.

HSV may cause localized or focal infiltrates in neutropenic and nonneutropenic patients.[173] Localized pneumonia is due to contiguous spread of HSV from the oropharynx of patients who are intubated for other underlying pulmonary diseases or who undergo diagnostic bronchoscopy. Because the oropharynx is the source of virus, most cases are due to type 1 rather than type 2 HSV. The radiologic picture is indistinguishable from other localized pneumonias, and appropriate studies (*e.g.*, bronchoscopy and specific immunofluorescence and virus cultures performed on respiratory specimens) must be carried out to provide the specific diagnosis. Treatment is with intravenous acyclovir (250–500 mg/m^2 every 8 hours).

Nonneutropenic patients who are receiving immunosuppressive therapy (including corticosteroids) and patients with AIDS are at risk for tuberculosis and atypical mycobacterial disease. Infections due to *M. tuberculosis* have increased, particularly in areas where there are large numbers of patients with AIDS, such as New York City.[174,175] This change in the reservoir of *M. tuberculosis* may alter the incidence of infection in cancer patients. Of more concern have been recent outbreaks of multidrug-resistant *M. tuberculosis*. The atypical mycobacteria, particularly *M. fortuitum, M. avium-intracellulare* (MAI), and *M. kansasii,* are often resistant to available agents. Although *M. fortuitum* and *M. chelonei* can be treated with agents like cefoxitin, amikacin, tetracycline, and sulfonamides, MAI is more refractory to therapy. Four- or five-drug regimens (including ciprofloxacin, amikacin, ethambutol, isoniazid) have been employed with minimal to moderate success. Experience with macrolides like clarithromycin and azithromycin, alone and combined with ethambutol, ciprofloxacin or amikacin appear more promising.

Infection with mycobacteria frequently becomes apparent after immunosuppressive therapy, especially after corticosteroids, suggesting a reactivated infection. The mortality rate for tuberculous infections ranges from 17% to 50% in cancer patients, and a high index of suspicion is important, because the pulmonary lesions may be confused with the underlying malignancy or other infections.[176,177] Sputum should be cultured, and new infiltrates may be successfully diagnosed by fiberoptic bronchoscopy and brush biopsy with minimal complications. Tuberculin skin testing should be performed before chemotherapy in all patients. Reactive patients who have not been previously treated with isoniazid should be treated prophylactically for approximately 1 year. Patients with radiographic and culture evidence (positive sputum) for typical tuberculosis should be treated for 9 to 12 months with at least two drugs (usually isoniazid and ethambutol or rifampin). The prospect for multidrug resistant strains must be entertained, particularly in patients from endemic areas.

Less commonly encountered causes for a localized pulmonary infiltrate in a nonneutropenic patient include progression of an underlying malignancy, atelectatic segment of lung due to a compromised airway, and a localized reaction to a chemotherapeutic agent, particularly methotrexate, cyclophosphamide, or bleomycin. Fungal pneumonia, particularly with cryptococcus, *Histoplasma,* or coccidioidomycosis, can mimic the pulmonary nodules otherwise associated with metastases and underscores the importance of tissue confirmation. Drug reactions, however, are more commonly manifested as diffuse, interstitial pulmonary processes.

Patchy or Localized Infiltrates in the Neutropenic Patient

In addition to the pathogens causing a localized infiltrate in the nonneutropenic patient, an array of opportunistic pathogens must be considered in the differential diagnosis of a neutropenic patient with a localized infiltrate. Any gram-positive or gram-negative organism and a variety of fungal, parasitic, and viral pathogens can be responsible for a localized pneumonic process in a neutropenic patient (see Table 62–15). In patients with periods of neutropenia less than 14 days, bacterial pathogens predominate. Patients with more prolonged periods of neutropenia or those with a particular clinical pattern (*e.g.*, after allogeneic bone marrow transplantation) are more prone to develop a fungal (*Candida* or *Aspergillus*) or viral infection (CMV).

Unless the clinical presentation suggests otherwise, it is appropriate to initiate 48 to 72 hours of broad-spectrum antibiotic therapy before proceeding to an invasive diagnostic procedure (see Fig. 62–7). If the patient has stabilized or improved by 72 hours, continuing treatment for 10 to 14 days is necessary. If the patient has not stabilized or improved after broad-spectrum antibiotics, further evaluation is mandatory to exclude other potentially treatable organisms. Although diagnostic material occasionally can be obtained with transtracheal aspiration, bronchoscopy, or percutaneous needle biopsy, the yield with these procedures rarely approaches 50%.

The bronchoalveolar lavage (BAL) has come into vogue because it has a low morbidity and can be safely performed by experienced hands in neutropenic patients with platelet counts as low as 30,000/mm^3.[178–181] A transbronchial biopsy, however, should not be performed during the BAL in patients whose platelet count is less than 50,000/mm^3.

If the diagnosis cannot be established with BAL, the next procedure to consider is the open lung biopsy. Unlike the minithoracotomy, which can be performed for the patient with a diffuse infiltrate, a more complete thoracotomy is often necessary for the patient with a localized infiltrate.[208] It is important that the biopsy be obtained from the center of the lesion and from its outer borders to decrease the chance for a false-negative biopsy. Biopsy or tissue samples, touch preps, ground material, and sections should be comprehensively analyzed microscopically by Gram's stain, wet mount, toluidine blue, modified methylene blue, acid-fast, methenamine silver, Dieterle or Gimenez, and if necessary, *Legionella*-direct immunofluorescent antibody and electron microscopy. Routine aerobic, anaerobic, acid-fast, fungal, and supplemented charcoal-yeast extract cultures should be made. After a comprehensive analysis, the diagnostic yield from an open lung biopsy is very high, unless the patient is already receiving multiple antimicrobial therapies.

LEGIONELLA. Although not common at most centers, an important pathogen to consider as the cause of localized pneumonia in an immunosuppressed host is *Legionella*.[182] *Legionella* species are ubiquitous and usually found in water, including air conditioning cooling towers and hospital shower heads.[4] Aerosolization of contaminated water is probably the most common mechanism of transmission, and nosocomial infections have been described.

Although legionellosis is a multisystem disease, the lung represents the primary target organ. Incubation ranges from 2 to 10 days (median, 4 days), although immunosuppressed patients tend to have shorter incubation periods and a more abrupt onset of symptoms. The initial symptoms are generally nonspecific and include malaise, anorexia, lethargy, and headache. A nonproductive cough develops in 90% of patients, although it usually follows the initial symptoms by 2 to 3 days. Diarrhea, which occurs in approximately 50% of patients, may proceed or follow the respiratory symptoms.

Fever is usually the initial sign of *Legionella* and is normally unremitting until institution of effective therapy. Two-thirds of patients manifest a pulse deficit (*i.e.*, relative bradycardia) and one third have some degree of neurologic dysfunction, ranging from disorientation, depression, hallucinations, and seizures to lethargy, stupor, and coma. Physical examination may reveal hyperreactive or hyporeactive deep tendon reflexes, nystagmus, peripheral sensory or motor neuropathies, and rarely, signs of meningeal irritation.

The initial radiographic abnormality is a patchy, alveolar infiltrate involving a single lobe. If translobar consolidation occurs, it usually involves contiguous segments. Cavitary lesions or abscess formation is unusual except for *L. micdadei*.

The most rapid and accurate means of diagnosis is a direct fluorescent antibody (DFA) or DNA probe test performed on respiratory tract secretions, pulmonary tissue from biopsy specimens, pleural fluid, or pus or urine antigen test. However, not all serotypes are detectable, and a negative DFA does not eliminate *Legionella* as a diagnostic consideration. Culturing of the organism on a charcoal-yeast extract medium requires 2 to 7 days.

Erythromycin (40–50 mg/kg/day, with a maximum of 4 g in four divided doses for 3 weeks) is the treatment of choice. Therapy should be administered intravenously for the first several days in seriously ill patients; subsequent therapy may be oral. Patients unable to tolerate erythromycin should receive doxycycline (5 mg/kg/day in two divided doses). Rifampin (20 mg/kg/day in two divided doses) may be given in addition to erythromycin or doxycycline for seriously ill patients. Response to therapy is normally prompt, with a resolution of fever and subjective improvement within 24 to 48 hours.

Nocardia asteroides and *N. brasiliensis* may present as localized pulmonary infiltrates, although miliary and microcavitary patterns have been described in cancer patients.[21,183] Approximately 30% of patients with a pulmonary infection due to *N. asteroides* have associated cutaneous and central nervous system (CNS) infection, usually brain abscesses. Diagnosis depends on positive cultures or histopathologic demonstration of tissue invasion by the organisms. Microscopically, the gram-positive organisms are irregularly stained, beaded or branching, and partially acid-fast staining and filamentous. Skin lesions, usually subcutaneous abscesses, are associated with *Nocardia*. Sulfonamides (*e.g.*, sulfadiazine, 4–6 g/day for 4–6 months) provide the most effective therapy for this infection, but mortality is significant (30%) after the infection has become disseminated. Favorable responses have been observed with ampicillin plus erythromycin or with minocycline. Trimethoprim-sulfamethoxazol has in vitro activity and has been used clinically, although late relapses have been reported.

FUNGI. Fungal infections constitute the greatest threat for the neutropenic patient who develops a new or progressive pulmonary infiltrate while receiving broad-spectrum antibiotic therapy, often occurring as part of a disseminated infection (see Table 62–15).[184] Two groups can be identified patients who developed a new infiltrate while the granulocyte count was rising and patients who developed a new infiltrate while they were granulocytopenic.[185] Patients who developed infiltrates in conjunction with bone marrow recovery did well without therapeutic modifications. In contrast, the patients who developed a new and progressive infiltrate while on antibiotics and while still granulocytopenic were likely to have a fungal cause for their new infiltrates. Ideally, an open lung biopsy should be performed in these patients to establish the diagnosis and guide the therapy. If a biopsy cannot be performed, amphotericin B should be instituted empirically, because a significant survival advantage can be observed for patients who received early, empiric antifungal therapy. In such cases, higher doses of amphotericin B (1–1.5 mg/kg/day) should be administered.

The presence of *Candida* in the sputum correlates poorly with overt infection. Although a positive blood culture for *Candida* is highly correlated with invasive or disseminated infection in the immunocompromised patient, negative blood cultures are not infrequent. Measurement of the *Candida* enolase may provide a means for early diagnosis of invasive candidiasis. Isolation of *C. tropicalis* from multiple body sites (*e.g.,* sputum, urine, and stool) has been correlated with invasive disease.[71] Definitive diagnosis usually requires histopathologic confirmation.

Endophthalmitis, characterized by focal, white, fluffy, mound-like retinal lesions that can extend rapidly into the vitreous, has been associated with disseminated candidiasis.[186]

In many treatment centers, the incidence of aspergillosis in cancer patients from *A. fumigatus, A. flavus, A. niger,* and *A. terreus* has increased over the last decade. The upper airway is the most frequent route of entry of these organisms, and clusters of nosocomial aspergillosis have occurred in hospitals in which construction materials have been contaminated with *Aspergillus* spores. The pathologic hallmark of aspergillosis is blood vessel invasion, with consequent thrombosis and infarction. *Aspergillus* pneumonia in the immunocompromised host is a rapidly invasive, necrotizing bronchopneumonia or a hemorrhagic infection with thrombosis of the pulmonary arteries and veins, with a possibility for life-threatening hemoptysis. Approximately half of the patients are also infected with other organisms, especially *Pseudomonas.*

A characteristic radiographic appearance for *Aspergillus* pneumonia has not been described, but the development of a new pulmonary infiltrate in a neutropenic patient who is receiving broad-spectrum antibiotics, especially if accompanied by new or persistent fever despite antibiotics, chest pain, or hemoptysis, should raise suspicion. Patients receiving low-dose empiric amphotericin B (0.5 mg/kg/day) may break through with pulmonary aspergillosis. Blood cultures are rarely positive, even though disseminated infection occurs in 30% of patients. Extrapulmonary sites include the sinuses, CNS, liver, kidney, skin, and heart valves. Diagnosis of aspergillosis by noninvasive measures is suboptimal, although reports suggest that positive sputum or BAL cultures in a patient with prolonged fever, neutropenia, and a progressive infiltrate is highly correlated with a diagnosis of *Aspergillus* pneumonia.[187] Despite initially optimistic reports, antigen and antibody methods of detection have not been as sensitive as had been hoped and are associated with too many false-negative results. Studies with mannitol offer some encouragement, but definitive confirmatory data are still lacking. A definitive diagnosis still requires histologic confirmation or a positive BAL culture obtained in a clinically relevant setting.

Treatment of *Aspergillus* pneumonia requires an early diagnosis and prompt intervention. Optimal therapy is amphotericin B. Although standard dosages of amphotericin B have ranged between 0.5 and 1.0 mg/kg/day, 14 patients treated with high-dose amphotericin (1–1.5 mg/kg/day) had an exceptional survival rate.[188] Controlled clinical trials are needed to test this approach and to test amphotericin B encapsulated into liposomes because of the encouraging results obtained in preclinical models and early clinical trials. Although not proven, the addition of 100 to 150 mg/kg/day of 5-fluorocytosine (5-FC) in three divided doses to amphotericin B may be helpful. If 5-FC is given, blood levels should be measured. Even with appropriate pharmacologic intervention, the most important prognosticator of a successful outcome is the return of adequate levels of granulocytes. Infrequently, *Aspergillus* causes a mycetoma or fungus ball in immunocompromised patients, and resection is usually recommended.

The *Phycomycetes* (especially *Mucor* and *Rhizopus*) are the third most frequent cause of invasive fungal infection in cancer patients.[184] Like *Aspergillus,* the *Phycomycetes* are acquired by way of the respiratory tract and cause a necrotizing bronchopneumonia or infarction after vascular invasion and thrombosis. Dissemination to the kidney, gastrointestinal tract, CNS, liver, pancreas or heart may occur in 50% of patients with *Phycomycetes* infections. Early biopsy of suspicious lesions and aggressive therapy with amphotericin B and surgical debridement are essential.

Histoplasmosis can cause serious pneumonia in the cancer patient, usually manifested as a military infiltrate.[190] Infection is usually disseminated, and the reticuloendothelial system is generally so heavily infected that the resultant adenopathy, hepatosplenomegaly, and bone marrow involvement can sometimes be confused with the underlying malignancy. Consequently, careful histologic examination of biopsies from the nodes, liver, or bone marrow for the intracellular yeast forms, using Giemsa or methenamine-silver staining, is extremely important in evaluating suspected patients or those from endemic areas.

Coccidioides immitis and *Cryptococcus neoformans* can result in serious pneumonia and disseminated infections in cancer patients and can mimic nodules that appear to be tumor metastases. *Torulopsis* (or *Candida*) *glabrata* has been isolated increasingly from cancer patients and associated with serious fungal infections. Infection with *T. glabrata* occurs predominantly in debilitated, neutropenic patients, but it has also been associated with a foreign body (*e.g.,* hyperalimentation catheter, urinary catheter). The most common sites of infection are lung, kidney, and gastrointestinal tract. Fungemia with this organism may occasionally produce an endotoxin-like shock syndrome. Because of its similarity to *Candida,* diagnosis of *T. glabrata* is difficult, and differentiation rests on its smaller size and lack of pseudomycelia. *Trichosporon* species, an arthrospore-forming yeast, can cause local skin lesions and invasive disease in cancer patients.[98] *T. beigelii* is the cause of white piedra in noncompromised hosts but can involve the lungs, kidneys, skin, and eyes in immunocompromised patients. The serum from patients with trichosporosis can react with the cryptococcal latex agglutination test due to shared antigens between *T. beigelii* and *C. neoformans.* Successful therapy depends on the early initiation of amphotericin B and, most importantly, recovery from neutropenia. Although rare, serious pulmonary infection can result from *Fusarium* and *Pseudoallecheria boydii,* both of which can mimic *Aspergillus.*

Treatment options for the patient with serious fungal disease are currently limited to a few drugs, the most reliable of which is still amphotericin B (see Table 62–12). Although amphotericin achieves a concentration in excess of the minimum inhibitory concentration of most major fungal pathogens, it is associated with significant acute and delayed toxicity, and there is a spectrum of sensitivity. For example, some isolates of *Candida* appear tolerant to amphotericin B, and all isolates of *Pseudoallescheria boydii* are resistant to amphotericin B, although sensitive to miconazole.

Most patients receiving amphotericin B experience fever, chills (sometimes with rigors), nausea, and vomiting. Less commonly, hypotension, bronchospasm, or seizures may occur. With continued administration, nephrotoxicity, including azotemia, elevated creatinine, renal tubular acidosis, and cylindruria, and electrolyte disturbances, especially hypokalemia, occur. Particular attention should be paid to hydration and salt loading, because this can decrease the nephrotoxicity. A decreased erythrocyte production and thrombocytopenia may occur after 22 to 35 days of amphotericin B therapy. Because most immunosuppressed patients who become candidates for amphotericin are already receiving nephrotoxic antibiotics, the decision to initiate therapy is often difficult.

When therapy is instituted in the cancer patient, it is important to achieve an effective serum concentration of amphotericin as rapidly as possible. We initially administer a test dose of 1 mg; if tolerated, the remaining dose of 0.5 mg/kg/day is given within 2 to 4 hours. Premedication with acetaminophen and the addition of hydrocortisone sodium succinate (25–50 mg) to the infusion bottle may reduce toxicity. The dose of 0.5 mg/kg (therapeutic range, 0.4–0.6 mg/kg) is administered over 2 to 3 hours daily for routine empiric therapy. Patients with lesions suggesting (or confirmed to be) aspergillosis or mucormycosis should receive 1 to 1.5 mg/kg/day. The infusion should not be interrupted because of fever and chills, because this is a self-limited reaction. Meperidine (Demerol, 0.5–1 mg/kg intravenously) is helpful in controlling the rigors, although the mechanism of action is unknown. Potassium supplementation is important with hydration and NaCl loading, and if toxicity is excessive, an every-other-day amphotericin schedule may help.

The total dose for disseminated infection often averages 1.5 to 2 g (30–40 mg/kg). Recommended doses of amphotericin B are not based on controlled clinical trials and depend on the site and nature of infection. For example, a short course (5–7 days) of low-dose amphotericin B (0.1–0.3 mg/kg) may be adequate for patients with oral or esophageal mucosal candidiasis.[191] For uncomplicated candidemia, a course of 500 mg/kg (10 mg/kg total dose) is successful in treating the fungemia and preventing endophthalmitis. More protracted and higher doses of amphotericin B (*e.g.*, 5–7 g) may be necessary for the treatment of hepatic candidiasis. The combination of amphotericin B with other agents, such as rifampin or 5-FC, is frequently considered, but demonstrable efficacy with amphotericin B plus 5-FC has been shown only for the treatment of patients with cryptococcal meningitis.[192–194] The therapeutic index in experimental candidiasis was improved when amphotericin B was encapsulated into liposomes, and preliminary reports suggest enhanced clinical efficacy, particularly in hepatic candidiasis.[163,164] Unfortunately, difficulties in formulating a standard liposomal preparation have hampered controlled clinical trials, although multicenter studies are underway.

5-FC is an antimetabolite that has demonstrable in vitro efficacy against most fungi.[195] It can be administered orally (100–150 mg/kg/day every 6 hours) and is well absorbed. The data to support its efficacy as a single agent for the treatment of serious fungal infections in humans are meager. In vivo resistance to 5-FC develops rapidly, but 5-FC may be additive or synergistic with amphotericin B.[196] Toxic effects from 5-FC include nausea, vomiting, hepatotoxicity, and bone marrow depression.

Alternative antifungal drugs are the imidazoles and the azoles, a group of synthetic agents with in vitro activity against most fungi.[197] Clotrimazole has efficacy for the treatment of chronic mucocutaneous candidiasis, but it does not appear to be useful for systemic therapy.[198] Clotrimazole may be useful in preventing oral *Candida* infections, and we have found it helps some patients with esophagitis.

Miconazole has in vitro activity against almost all pathogenic fungi except *Mucor* and *Rhizopus.* The most extensive clinical experience with miconazole has been for patients with chronic or disseminated coccidioidomycoses. Miconazole has shown some efficacy against paracoccidioidomycosis, South American blastomycosis, chronic mucocutaneous candidiasis, esophageal candidiasis, and petriellidosis, although frequent relapse remains a problem.

The role of miconazole in cancer patients with invasive fungal infection has been limited. Toxic effects with miconazole has included nausea, phlebitis, anemia, hyponatremia, and pruritus; anaphylaxis and cardiac arrhythmia have also been observed during infusion. Miconazole is poorly absorbed, necessitating parenteral administration for prolonged periods. Coupled with its limited efficacy and high relapse rate, miconazole cannot be considered a first-line antifungal drug for cancer patients.

Ketoconazole has been evaluated in cancer patients. In vitro testing has documented sensitivity for a variety of fungi, including *Candida* species, *Paracoccidioides, Coccidioides, Cryptococcus,* and *Histoplasma.* Human trials have used ketoconazole has a single daily oral dose of 200 to 1200 mg and estimated the half-life range from 4 to 12 hours. However, ketoconazole is not effective against *Aspergillus* and *Mucor,* and its spectrum against *Candida* species is not complete. For example, *C. tropicalis* and *T. glabrata* are not covered by ketoconazole.

Despite the advantages of the oral preparation and although relatively nontoxic, a range of problems includes poor intestinal absorption, nausea and vomiting, dizziness, lethargy, headache, and confused states. Hepatic enzyme elevation is common, and one case of fatal hepatic necrosis has been reported. Prolonged use may result in gynecomastia, azoospermia, depressed adrenal and testosterone synthesis, and decreased libido.

Although ketoconazole appears useful for the treatment of patients with mucosal infections (*e.g.*, oral mucositis, esophagitis), its efficacy for immunosuppressed patients with invasive mycoses is unestablished. Studies suggest that ketoconazole should not be used for invasive mycoses and should be restricted to use in patients with superficial mycoses. Ketoconazole has been evaluated for antifungal prophylaxis, but its efficacy is limited.

Itraconazole is a triazole that inhibits steroid synthesis, is available with an oral formulation, and has a broad spectrum of antifungal activity that includes *Candida* and *Aspergillus.*

Although available in Europe, itraconazole has not yet been approved for use in the United States. Fluconazole has a narrower spectrum of activity that includes *Candida* and *Cryptococcus* but does not include *Aspergillus*. However, it has a long half-life and high bioavailability, and it crosses the blood-brain barrier avidly. Fluconazole has assumed an important role in the maintenance treatment of AIDS patients with cryptococcal meningitis and *Candida* esophagitis and severe oral mucositis. The role of fluconazole for the treatment of invasive candidiasis or hepatic candidiasis remains less well defined. As with other imidazoles, breakthrough infection (*e.g.*, *C. krusei*) has been observed when fluconazole was used for oral prophylaxis.

Interstitial Infiltrates in the Nonneutropenic Patient

Diffuse pulmonary infiltrates can be caused by bacterial, viral, fungal, and protozoal pathogens and are influenced by whether or not the patient is neutropenic (see Table 62–15).

PNEUMOCYSTIS PNEUMONIA. A nonneutropenic patient with diffuse pulmonary infiltrate is unlikely to have a bacterial or fungal process. Perhaps the most commonly encountered infection in this setting is *Pneumocystis carinii* pneumonia.[199] This infection is thought to result from a reactivation of latent cysts, because almost 100% of normal children possess detectable antibody to *P. carinii*.[200] Patient-to-patient transmission has been suggested by reports on nosocomial clusterings of cases.[201] The natural reservoir of *P. carinii* remains undefined.

Certain chemotherapeutic regimens may predispose patients to interstitial infiltrates caused by *P. carinii*.[202] For example, an increased prevalence of *P. carinii* pneumonia was observed at the NCI in a group of non-Hodgkin's lymphoma patients receiving combination chemotherapy. Patients had been randomized to one of two treatment arms, and only in the one containing cytosine arabinoside and bleomycin, in addition to drugs shared in common in both treatment arms, was the prevalence of *P. carinii* pneumonia increased. Whether this chemotherapy regimen enhanced reactivation of latent organisms or made patients more susceptible to reinfection from ambient organisms is unclear. This problem, however, has been abrogated by the prophylactic administration of trimethoprim-sulfamethoxazole to patients receiving this treatment regimen.

The most common clinical manifestations of *Pneumocystis* in cancer patients include fever, cough, and tachypnea, generally with intercostal retractions and the absence of detectable rales. A chest radiograph shows a hazy, bilateral alveolar infiltrate, which often begins at the hilus and spreads to the periphery. Arterial blood gases reflect a low PaO_2, normal $PaCO_2$, and alkaline pH. The clinical presentation can be indolent (1–2 months) but more often is fulminant (4–5 days). The chest roentgenographic findings may occasionally be atypical (*e.g.*, lobar consolidation, effusion, and even nodular) and, in rare cases, the radiograph may appear normal despite the presence of pneumocysts on biopsy. *P. carinii* pneumonia in cancer patients differs from that in AIDS patients by having a more smoldering and indolent course; the median duration of symptoms is 28 days in AIDS patients, but 5 days for non-AIDS patients.[203]

Diagnosis of *P. carinii* pneumonia requires demonstration of cysts or trophozoites in pulmonary material from patients with a clinically compatible course; cysts have been found in asymptomatic, previously healthy persons autopsied after traumatic deaths. In patients with AIDS, positive specimens may be obtained from sputum samples because the "cyst burden" is high.[204] In cancer patients, induced sputum can be positive, but cysts may be best demonstrated by BAL or open lung biopsy. The sensitivity of these examinations is enhanced by the use of special strains and monoclonal antibodies with indirect immunofluorescence. Serologic confirmation is of questionable value.

If the likelihood of *P. carinii* pneumonia is great, the choice is to proceed with diagnostic procedure or to administer an empiric course of therapy with trimethoprim-sulfamethoxazole (see Fig. 62–7). If induced sputum or BAL is readily available, it is the procedure of choice for establishing the diagnosis. However, if induced sputum or BAL is not available or if the patient's clinical or hematologic status does not permit a BAL, an empiric trial of trimethoprim-sulfamethoxazole (20 mg/kg/day of trimethoprim) plus erythromycin (for *Legionella*) is recommended, rather than proceeding directly to open lung biopsy. This is based on the results of a randomized NCI trial demonstrating that in nonneutropenic patients with diffuse infiltrates, empiric therapy is as safe and effective an open lung biopsy.[205] However, a response may not be apparent for 4 to 5 days, although stabilization or slight improvement in alveolar air exchange generally occurs within 72 to 96 hours.[206] Failure to improve (*e.g.*, continued fever, depressed PaO_2, progressive infiltrates) after 4 days of therapy serves as an indication to modify therapy, usually with the addition of pentamidine (4 mg/kg/day as a 1–2-hour infusion). The early use of steroids has been shown to improve the outcome of AIDS patients with moderate to severe *P. carinii* pneumonia (as evidenced by a room air arterial PO_2 of 75 mm Hg or less on presentation).[207,208] Whether early steroid use will benefit cancer patients with *P. carinii* pneumonia is unknown, but many advocate its use for cancer patients.

If a histologic diagnosis is necessary and not achievable by BAL, not all procedures, such as transtracheal aspirate, transbronchial biopsy or aspirate, or open lung biopsy, are of comparable diagnostic accuracy. Burt and colleagues examined each of 17 patients having an open lung biopsy for the diagnosis of a diffuse interstitial infiltrate with a transthoracic needle aspirate and a transbronchial brush and biopsy.[209] The patients in this unique study served as their own controls. A diagnosis was established from only 30% of the aspirates and from 59% of the transbronchial biopsy samples; it suggests that the open lung biopsy is the procedure of choice. Open lung biopsy provides the best guidance for patient management, especially if the patient is neutropenic and requires multiple antimicrobial agents. The role of open lung biopsy for neutropenic patients already receiving antibiotic and antifungal therapy appears less defined because the diagnostic yield is low and therapeutic modifications are minimal.[210]

Because the patients who are candidates for open lung biopsy are often thrombocytopenic, appropriate hematologic preparation for surgery is vital. Elevation of the platelet count to a surgically safe level of $30,000/mm^3$ or greater can usually be accomplished by the infusion of 4 to 8 units of platelet concentrates 1 hour before surgery. Maintenance of the platelet count at this level for 24 hours after surgery with additional platelet concentrates minimizes any postoperative bleeding complications.

Because of the importance the *P. carinii* has assumed in patients with AIDS, the search for new therapeutic agents has intensified. Other agents that have been explored include trimetrexate, primaquine plus clindamycin, and the quinone, 566C80, which has shown promising activity in adults with AIDS.

The appropriate course of treatment in the cancer patient with proved or putative *P. carinii* pneumonia is to begin with trimethoprim-sulfamethoxazole and, if the patients has not stabilized or improved by day 4 of therapy, to add pentamidine. If there is no improvement after 4 days of pentamidine, trimetrexate should be substituted.

VIRAL PNEUMONIAS. CMV has been a cause of severe interstitial pneumonia, especially among patients receiving allogeneic marrow transplants for hematologic malignancies. Renal, cardiac, and liver allograft recipients and patients with lymphoma or leukemia are also at risk, albeit at a lower incidence. Although the pathogenesis of CMV pneumonia is incompletely defined, several risk factors for CMV pneumonia after allogeneic marrow transplant have been identified.[211,212] These include being seropositive for antibody to CMV before transplant, undergoing allogeneic or autologous transplantation, receiving total-body irradiation as part of the conditioning regimen, and developing acute graft-versus-host disease (GVHD) after transplant.

In addition to active CMV infection, disordered immune function undoubtedly underlies the development of CMV pneumonia. For example, the lack of GVHD, which is as immunosuppressive as its treatment, is the putative explanation for the paucity of CMV pneumonia after syngeneic or autologous transplantation. However, whether it is the lack of specific immune responsiveness to CMV or an immunopathologic immune response directed at CMV antigens in pulmonary tissue is undefined. Investigation of pulmonary immune responses may clarify the pathogenesis of this syndrome.

Depending on the various risk factors, as many as 50% of marrow allograft recipients develop interstitial pneumonia, 70% of which is associated with CMV. CMV pneumonia characteristically occurs within the first 3 months after transplantation, with a median onset of 50 to 70 days. Late cases developing after 100 days occur among patients with chronic GVHD. Diffuse infiltrates are most common, but localized and nodular infiltrates have been described. However, patients with apparently localized disease have diffuse involvement when other portions of lung are examined by sensitive virologic techniques. Pleural effusions are rare.

CMV pneumonia is clinically indistinguishable from other causes of diffuse infiltrates in the compromised host, especially *Pneumocystis carinii,* and specific virologic studies must be done to provide the diagnosis. Rising antibody titers to CMV or excretion of virus in throat, urine, or blood are not of sufficient to obviate the need for direct examination of pulmonary specimens.[213] Open lung biopsy was previously considered the necessary diagnostic procedure, but BAL has shown high sensitivity among marrow transplant patients with pulmonary infiltrates.[212] Specificity and negative predictive value are of concerns, and results in marrow transplant patients cannot necessarily be extrapolated to other immunocompromised patients, especially those with AIDS. If BAL is not diagnostic, open lung biopsy should be performed. Specimens obtained by open biopsy or BAL should be examined by rapid virologic techniques because conventional cultures usually do not become positive for CMV for 2 to 3 weeks, and 4 to 5 weeks is sometimes required. Direct examination of specimens by specific immunofluorescence using murine monoclonal antibodies is rapid (2–4 hours), but has a sensitivity of only about 60% depending on the quality of the specimen. Inoculation of viral cultures by centrifugation followed by immunofluorescent staining for immediate or early CMV antigens (centrifugation or "shell vial" cultures) is extremely sensitive (>95%), specific, and rapid, with results available within 24 hours; some specimens may be positive as soon as 4 hours.[214] Other techniques include standard histologic staining for intranuclear inclusions and cytomegalic cells. Nucleic acid hybridization remains investigational and may not be more sensitive than centrifugation cultures.

CMV may involve other organs, including the liver, spleen, kidney, adrenal, gastrointestinal tract, heart, CNS, and the eye. Enteritis and retinitis have been particularly common among patients with AIDS, but they also occur in organ allograft recipients. CMV has been associated with other organisms including *P. carinii,* bacteria, fungi, and other viruses.

Therapy for CMV pneumonia after marrow transplant combines ganciclovir and intravenous CMV immunoglobulin, with survival rates of 50% to 70% reported for a previously virtually untreatable infection.[215,216] Foscarnet has entered the antiviral armamentarium and has demonstrated benefit for patients with CMV retinitis alone or, in a few cases, in combination with ganciclovir. The specific role of these agents for cancer patients with CMV pneumonitis is less well defined, but they appear to add to the therapeutic options.

The sole use of seronegative blood products can eliminate primary CMV infection in seronegative marrow transplant recipients who have seronegative marrow donors.[278] Similar observations have been made after cardiac and renal transplants. Although passive immunoprophylaxis with intravenous immunoglobulins continues to be studied in seronegative patients, results of clinical trials have been conflicting, and this modality should not be used in place of seronegative blood products. Other approaches to prophylaxis, such as use of interferon, have not been successful after marrow transplantation. Effective prophylaxis has been observed with high doses of acyclovir and with ganciclovir.[217,218]

Other viruses may cause severe, diffuse pneumonias. HSV can cause diffuse pulmonary infiltrates. The pathogenesis includes viremia and involvement of other organs, including liver or brain; type 1 and type 2 HSV have been implicated. Because of clinical similarity to other viral pneumonias like CMV, bronchoscopy or open biopsy is needed for diagnosis. VZV can cause severe, diffuse pneumonia, although this is rare in the absence of cutaneous manifestations of disseminated VZV infection. Treatment of HSV and VZV pneumonia is with intravenous acyclovir (500 mg/m^2 every 8 hours).

The measles virus can cause severe pneumonia in immunocompromised patients. The incidence of measles in young children and adolescents has increased sharply in recent years throughout the United States because of the failure to vaccinate young infants or the loss of vaccine protection among teenagers and young adults. The oncologist must be aware that measles may be more likely now than during the past 20 years. It may occur concomitantly with the initial illness with fever, coryza, and rash, or it may develop as long as 6 months after initial infection.[281] Diagnosis may require open lung biopsy for specific immunofluorescence and culture. Immunosuppressed patients who have never received measles vaccine and are seronegative for antibody to measles and who have contact with measles should receive prophylactic γ-globulin (0.5 ml/kg, maximal dose of 15 ml) as soon after exposure as possible. Treatment of measles is supportive. Live virus vaccines should not be used in immunocompromised patients.[282]

Although the incidence of influenza and other common respiratory viruses (*e.g.*, parainfluenza 1 and 3, respiratory syncytial virus, rhinoviruses) does not appear to be increased in the cancer patient, infection due to these viruses may be severe.[219] Both primary viral pneumonias and secondary bacterial infections may occur. With adenoviruses, increased severity and an increased incidence due to reactivation of latent viruses may occur. Disseminated adenovirus infection commonly involves lung, liver, and kidney, although hemorrhagic cystitis with or without nephritis may occur without other manifestations. Specific immunofluorescence performed on respiratory specimens and virus cultures are necessary for diagnosis. Respiratory syncytial virus (RSV) pneumonia in immunocompromised patients occurs in children and adults with severe clinical courses and high mortality rates.

The synthetic nucleoside, ribavirin, given by aerosol, has been used for treatment of RSV, influenza, and parainfluenza infections and should be given to children or adults with cancer who develop symptomatic infection.[220] Amantadine (or rimantadine) has prophylactic efficacy against influenza A and may have some therapeutic efficacy as well. Some centers routinely use the killed influenza vaccine for cancer patients, although the antibody response to this vaccine may be diminished in patients receiving chemotherapy.[288,289]

Interstitial Infiltrate in the Neutropenic Patient

In addition to *P. carinii* and CMV, gram-positive and gram-negative bacteria and several fungi can cause interstitial infiltrates in neutropenic patients. Broad-spectrum antibiotics and trimethoprim-sulfamethoxazole are necessary for empiric therapy in these patients. Failure of the patient to improve necessitates lung biopsy and consideration of antifungal therapy.

CARDIOVASCULAR INFECTIONS

Cardiovascular infections are relatively uncommon among cancer patients, probably because of the early institution of broad-spectrum antimicrobial therapy. However, cancer patients who have predisposing factors for cardiovascular infections (*e.g.*, dental abscesses, intravenous drug abuse, congenital cardiac anomalies) are at risk. Guidelines for dental prophylaxis should be followed, and procedures should be avoided in patients who are neutropenic. If however, dental work is essential in a patient who is neutropenic, broad-spectrum antibiotic prophylaxis should be used.

Endovascular infections are more likely with the increased use of indwelling venous access catheters. Although gram-positive bacteria (*e.g.*, enterococcus, viridans streptococci, β-hemolytic streptococci, and *S. aureus*) most commonly cause endovascular infections, aerobic gram-negative bacilli (*e.g.*, *P. aeruginosa*) and fungal organisms (*Candida, Aspergillus*) may also cause disease. Diagnosis can be difficult and can be enhanced by using esophageal probes for ultrasonography. These pathogens are particularly difficult to eradicate, and morbidity and mortality rates are discouragingly high. Myocardial microabscesses occur more frequently (*Candida*), and myocarditis may be associated with viruses and protozoa (*Toxoplasma*). Endocarditis may suggest an underlying malignancy (*e.g.*, association of *S. bovis* with colon cancer).

The clinical manifestations of endocarditis in the immunosuppressed patient are similar to those in an immunocompetent patient. Nonspecific complaints of fever, chills, malaise, fatigue, night sweats, and weight loss are common. Unfortunately, these complaints are not diagnostically specific. In most instances, the diagnosis of an endovascular infection in an immunocompromised patient must be made based on physical and laboratory evaluation. The numerous physical stigmata of endocarditis should be sought (*e.g.*, heart murmurs, splinter hemorrhages, Roth's spots, splenomegaly), but the diagnosis is confirmed by the isolation of an organism from multiple blood cultures. The complications of endovascular infections are similar to those described for noncancer patients. Valvular insufficiency resulting in congestive heart failure, embolic phenomenon, and renal failure are the most serious complications. Fungal endocarditis is particularly likely to cause large vessel embolization. Patients with *Candida* or *Aspergillus* endocarditis are candidates for valve replacement.

Therapy must be directed at the specific pathogen. The isolation of *S. aureus* or *S. epidermidis* from multiple blood samples, even if the patient has an indwelling catheter, is not sufficient criteria for prolonged antibiotic therapy unless confirmation of a valvular infection can be made. Standard therapy of 10 to 14 days suffices for these patients.[221]

GASTROINTESTINAL TRACT INFECTIONS

The gastrointestinal tract is a major reservoir of microorganisms, is associated with several characteristic infectious complications, and serves as a major portal for systemic infection during periods of host compromise.

Oral Mucositis

Ulceration of the oral mucosa frequently occurs with chemotherapy. Colonization of drug-induced lessons by the indigenous aerobic or anaerobic oral flora may result in local infection and may provide portal for septicemia in the neutropenic patient. Mucositis, gingivitis, and other dental-related problems may occur in as many as 85% of leukemic patients during the course of their disease.

Measures have been sought to lower the risk of oral gingivitis and mucositis. Peterson and coworkers evaluated 38 febrile patients undergoing treatment for acute nonlymphocytic leukemia and found a 32% incidence of local oral infections, more than half of which were thought to cause the patients' fevers.[222] The periodontium was the most common site of infection, cultures of which usually revealed mixed flora, including many of the organisms associated with systemic infection in cancer patients (*e.g., S. aureus, S. epidermidis, C. albicans, P. aeruginosa*). In adults, preexisting periodontitis is common (>90%) and is exacerbated with immunosuppression. The presence of marginal or necrotizing gingivitis, characterized by an erythematous periapical gingiva, is caused by mouth anaerobes and should be treated with specific antianaerobic agents (*e.g.,* clindamycin or metronidazole). The vigorous use of mouth cleansing salts and solutions (*e.g.,* equal parts of a nonirritating mouth wash, hydrogen peroxide, and water swished every 2 hours) may decrease or control the mucositis.

The oral mucosa is a difficult site to decontaminate fully, and several organisms, such as *C. albicans,* are especially problematic. Although oral candidiasis (thrush) is predominantly a superficial infection, it may serve as a portal for systemic invasion in severely neutropenic patients. Oral nystatin is of only minimal benefit. Oral clotrimazole troches (10 mg, 5 troches daily) has been used successfully in patients with mild to moderate infection. Patients with more extensive oral candidiasis, may benefit from fluconazole at dosages of 200 to 400 mg/day or from a short course of amphotericin B (0.1–0.5 mg/kg/day for 7 days).

HSV may cause significant oral disease. Oral HSV infection may not manifest with typical cutaneous or intraoral vesicles and may not be distinguishable from radiation-induced or chemotherapy-induced mucositis. Viral cultures or immunofluorescence or both must be performed for diagnosis. Intravenous acyclovir and vidarabine have demonstrated efficacy in the treatment of immunosuppressed patients with proven mucocutaneous HSV infection.[223,224] Results are better with acyclovir. Treatment with intravenous acyclovir (250 mg/m^2 every 8 hours for 7 days) shortened the period of virus shedding by almost 2 weeks and the period of healing by 1 week.[225] Orally administered acyclovir (400 mg 5 times daily for 7–10 days) appears comparable to intravenous acyclovir among patients who can comply with oral drugs. Topical acyclovir ointment is beneficial, but it is only effective against external lesions and is less effective than oral or intravenous acyclovir.[226] Patients who are seropositive for antibody to HSV have a 70% to 80% incidence of HSV reactivation during leukemic induction therapy or after organ allografting.[227] They may be protected against virus reactivation with intravenous (250 mg/m^2 every 8–12 hours) or oral (400 mg 4–5 times daily or 800 mg every 12 hours) acyclovir given during the period of major risk, usually defined as the period of leukopenia.[228,229] Reduction in streptococcal superinfection and bacteremia has been reported among patients receiving prophylaxis.[230]

Esophagitis

Clinically significant esophagitis may be the result of infectious and noninfectious causes. For example, a syndrome clinically identical to an infectious esophagitis occurs in patients who have received extensive chest wall or mediastinal irradiation. An infectious esophagitis most commonly occurs among patients who have been granulocytopenic and receiving antibiotics for several days. Patients most often present with a subacute onset of retrosternal, burning chest pain and odynophagia. Fungal, viral, and bacterial organisms can all cause an infectious esophagitis in the immunocompromised host.[231,232]

The occurrence of an infectious esophagitis in the nonneutropenic person is rare. In nonneutropenic patients, esophagitis is most commonly due to chemical irritation of the distal esophagus by refluxed gastric contents (*e.g.,* chemotherapy-induced emesis). These patients are best managed with judicious use of antacids or histamine antagonists. If the nonneutropenic patient has persistent esophageal discomfort, esophagoscopy with brushings for culture and a biopsy should be done. In nonneutropenic patients with AIDS, herpetic or candidal esophagitis are common.

For the neutropenic patient who is already receiving broad-spectrum antibiotic therapy, *Candida* is the most likely cause of esophagitis, but severe esophagitis with fatal hematemesis has been reported with *Aspergillus.* HSV, alone or with *Candida,* and bacteria also deserve careful consideration. CMV has emerged as a frequent cause of esophagitis in AIDS patients or marrow allograft recipients. A common dilemma is whether endoscopy and biopsy should be performed to establish the diagnosis. Although barium swallow or simple fiberoptic esophagoscopy can demonstrate cobblestoning or the putative "white curtain" associated with *Candida,* both are nonspecific and are associated with false-positive and false-negative results. The only definitive way to establish the diagnosis is with biopsy, culture, and histologic examination. For example, when patients with acute nonlymphocytic leukemia with symptomatic esophagitis were endoscoped, 3 of 7 cases that appeared to be *Candida* were shown by biopsy to be nonfungal.

It is not always possible or safe to biopsy the patient with esophagitis, particularly if the patient is profoundly thrombocytopenic. An alternative to biopsy is a short course of empiric therapy. Patients with esophageal candidiasis usually respond within 48 hours to oral clotrimazole, ketoconazole, or fluconazole. If patients have persistence or worsening of the esophageal complaints after 48 hours of therapy, they should be given a trial of low-dose amphotericin B (0.1–0.5 mg/kg/day for 5 days). If the patient has persistent symptoms after 48 hours of intravenous amphotericin B, it is unlikely that *Candida* is the cause. Although some physicians advocate esophagoscopy at this point, an alterative is an empiric course of acyclovir (750 mg/m^2/day, at 8-hour intervals), because the second most likely pathogen or copathogen is HSV. If the patient responds, acyclovir should be given for 5 to 7 days.

Intraabdominal Infections

The clinical presentation of even common intraabdominal processes (*e.g.,* appendicitis, infectious diarrheal syndromes) can be altered by granulocytopenia and compounded by complications of cancer or its treatment. For example, obstructive lesions may be due to primary or metastatic cancer (*e.g.,* lymphoma); cholangitis or a conjugated hyperbilirubinemia may be due to extrahepatic biliary obstruction by tumor (*e.g.,* rhabdomyosarcoma); and chronic abdominal pain or diarrheal syndromes may be caused by bowel wall infiltration by malignant disease or infection.

Intraabdominal complaints must be expeditiously evaluated with a thorough abdominal and pulmonary examination, including a judiciously performed rectal examination. Repetitive rectal examinations must not be performed in the neutropenic patient, because bacteremia and local infection may result. Appropriate laboratory studies include routine hematologic and serum chemistry values, tests for amylase and total and direct bilirubin, and flat and upright abdominal radiographs. Additional diagnostic procedures (*e.g.*, abdominal or pelvic ultrasound, CT scans) should be pursued if appropriate. As a general rule, invasive diagnostic or radiographic procedures (*e.g.*, barium enema, endoscopy) should be avoided in the neutropenic patient unless absolutely required.

Foremost among the intraabdominal infections that are unique to the cancer patient is typhlitis (*i.e.*, necrotizing enterocolitis), an inflammatory cellulitis involving the cecum.[233,234] Typhlitis most commonly occurs in association with prolonged episodes of granulocytopenia and broad-spectrum antimicrobial therapy in patients with acute leukemia, although any granulocytopenic patient is at risk. Patients normally present with subacute or acute onset of right lower quadrant abdominal pain, which frequently becomes generalized over several hours with the development of fever, diarrhea, and prostration. The agents responsible for typhlitis include gram-negative bacteria, especially *P. aeruginosa*. Abdominal ultrasonography reveals bowel wall thickening and ascites and can help in the differential diagnoses. Optimal management includes supportive care, including appropriate hydration, nasogastric suction, adjustments of antimicrobial therapy to cover resistant gram-negative and anaerobic species, and if necessary, aggressive surgical intervention to resect a necrotic bowel. Proposed indications for surgery include evidence of persistent gastrointestinal bleeding despite resolution of hematologic abnormalities; evidence of an intraperitoneal perforation; clinical deterioration suggesting uncontrolled sepsis (*e.g.*, need for vasopressors, large fluid volume replacement); or development of symptoms compatible with an acute abdomen that would otherwise indicate a need for surgery. Despite aggressive measures, mortality rates are 30% to 50%.

An infrequently encountered clinical syndrome is peritonitis and bacteremia due to *Clostridia*. Patients with clostridial peritonitis classically have a fulminant clinical course with fever, tachycardia, abdominal wall ecchymoses and crepitance, and significant hemolysis. *C. perfringens* and *C. septicum* are the two most frequently isolated organisms. A less fulminant bacteremic syndrome due to *C. tertium* has been described.[93] Most patients have been granulocytopenic children with acute leukemia maintained on broad-spectrum antimicrobial therapy for prolonged periods (*e.g.*, 17 days). The gastrointestinal tract has most often implicated as the source of infection. Most patients with *C. tertium* have been relatively resistant to the penicillins, cephalosporins, and clindamycin, and they require the use of vancomycin for successful therapy.

Antibiotic-associated colitis (AAC) has long been associated with the administration of clindamycin, ampicillin, and broad-spectrum β-lactam antibiotics. *Clostridium difficile* has been isolated in most cases.[235] The symptomatic disease is related to toxin production by the organism. In cancer patients, antineoplastic agents and antibiotics increase the risk for AAC. Patients with AAC classically present with acute, generalized abdominal pain, fever, leukocytosis, and watery or mucoid, foul-smelling diarrhea. A high index of suspicion is necessary because of similar abdominal symptoms in cancer patients receiving chemotherapy or periabdominal radiation therapy. Cancer patients with diarrhea should be evaluated with stool cultures for *C. difficile* and with toxin assays. Toxin production, not just a positive culture for *C. difficile*, is necessary for diagnosis of ACC, because as many as 42% of hospitalized patients receiving antibiotics will be culture positive, but not toxin positive, for *C. difficile*.

Treatment of documented *C. difficile*-associated colitis requires oral vancomycin (125 mg four times daily for 10–14 days) or metronidazole (250 mg four times daily for 10 days). There is a 10% to 20% rate of relapse, although most patients respond to a second course with the same or alternative therapy. *C. difficile* may be nosocomically transmitted, and patients who are culture and toxin positive for *C. difficile* should be placed on enteric precautions.

Hyperinfection syndrome is an infrequently encountered clinical problem. It is caused by the intestinal nematode, *Strongyloides stercoralis*.[235,236] The clinical syndrome of fever, nausea, vomiting, diarrhea, and abdominal pain is caused by the invasion and ulceration of the gastrointestinal mucosa by the filariform larvae. Chemotherapy promotes the maturation of these filariform larvae from a quiescent rhabditiform stage. Polymicrobial sepsis may accompany the stage of intestinal invasion, presumably as a result of the ulcerated intestinal mucosa. Overwhelming pulmonary and meningeal involvement has been described in immunocompromised patients. Diagnosis requires demonstration of the larvae in feces or duodenal fluid and should be sought in patients who have resided in subtropical climates or endemic regions. Treatment of asymptomatic infestation is accomplished with the administration of thiabendazole (25 mg/kg twice daily for 2 days). Immunocompromised patients with the hyperinfection syndrome should be treated for 2 to 3 weeks, although the mortality rate is high despite long-term treatment.

Hepatitis may be caused by a variety of infectious agents, including those that infect the liver primarily (*e.g.*, hepatitis A, B, C and the delta agent) and secondarily (*e.g.*, HSV, CMV, EBV, coxsackievirus B, adenoviruses, toxoplasmosis). Hepatitis C (HCV), previously referred to as non-A, non-B hepatitis, is a small single-stranded RNA virus that is the most commonly encountered cause of blood-bone hepatitis in cancer patients.[237] Antibody to HCV has been found in 80% to 100% of persons who develop histologically confirmed non-A, non-B hepatitis. Clinically, hepatitis C closely resembles hepatitis B, with an insidious onset and a prolonged, relapsing course. There is substantial evidence for a chronic carrier state, and chronic sequelae may occur in as many as 50% of infected persons. The development of antibody after infection with hepatitis C is usually delayed, with an average interval of 20 or more weeks, making serologic testing late during the clinical course important. Interferon-α has been effective in patients with hepatitis C, with dosages of 3 million units three times per week resulting in normalization of amino transferases and improvement in histologic findings in almost 50% of the treated patients.[238]

Hepatitis B infection (HBV) may result in acute and chronic infections, including chronic active, chronic persistent, and an asymptomatic carrier state. Diagnosis is aided by detection of specific viral antigens in the serum of infected patients, especially hepatitis B surface antigens (HBsAg), DNA polymerase, and the hepatitis Be antigen, all of which are present before and at the onset of clinical symptoms. HBsAg may be detected in the serum as early as 6 days after infection with HBV, although it is usually observed 29 to 43 days after parenteral exposure and 67 to 82 days after oral exposure. In patients with self-limited HBV infection, the DNA polymerase titer falls early, and the HBsAg titer falls later in the clinical disease course, eventually being replaced by antibody to HBsAg and HBeAg.

HBV may result in acute infection, chronic infection, or a symptomatic carrier state, with or without hepatic disease. Although the frequency of HBsAg is approximately 0.1% in the general population of the United States, it has been detected in 10% to 20% of children or adults with cancer.[239,240] This is a consequence of multiple transfusions, although currently available sensitive screening tests have reduced this risk dramatically. Nonparenteral transmission (*e.g.*, saliva, urine, feces, semen, effusions, cerebrospinal fluid) constitutes an important vector. Immunosuppressive therapy may increase the risk of hepatitis, and enhance the development of a chronic carrier state and can reactivate HBV infections in asymptomatic chronic carriers.[241,242]

Because many of the chemotherapeutic agents currently used in cancer treatment are metabolized or excreted by the liver, altered hepatic function caused by HBV hepatitis can seriously compromise the pharmacokinetics of administered chemotherapy. This is most pronounced for patients with chronic hepatitis, in whom even reduced dosages of chemotherapy may permit the maintenance of the viral carrier state and aggravate drug-induced hepatic injury.

The delta agent, an incomplete RNA virus, requires existing or co-infection with the hepatitis B virus for clinical expression. Hepatitis due to the delta agent only occurs in three circumstances: as a superimposed infection in a patient with active hepatitis B; as an acute delta hepatitis in a chronic hepatitis B carrier; and as a chronic delta infection in a chronic hepatitis B carrier. Although hepatitis due to the delta agent has been noticed among multiply-transfused patients, its incidence should decrease as the prevalence of hepatitis B diminishes.

Treatment of the patient with chronic active hepatitis is controversial. The current recommendation is that immunosuppressive therapy be restricted to patients who are symptomatic and who have subacute hepatitis with multilobular necrosis and active cirrhosis. Encouraging therapeutic results have been observed using human leukocyte and fibroblast interferon for patients with chronic hepatitis.[243] A short course (10–14 days) of interferon leads to a decreased serum levels of DNA polymerase, HBsAg, and anti-HBsAg; HBeAg remains unchanged; and all virologic markers again become elevated after the termination of the interferon therapy. However, with 4 to 5 months of continuous interferon therapy, HBsAg may be eliminated in some patients without rebound after discontinuing therapy. Further study of the dose and schedule of interferon may enhance this therapy.

Because of the morbidity of HBV, trials using standard serum immunoglobulin have been compared with serum globulin containing a high titer or an intermediate titer of antibody to HBsAg for patients or medical staff who have been potentially inoculated with HBV. Although earlier studies suggested that the high-titer globulin was effective, subsequent observations suggest that it may merely delay the onset of hepatitis as long as 9 months, with the incidence of hepatitis remaining unchanged at 7%. High-titer globulin (0.07 mg/kg) is, however, currently recommended for patients or staff who have had a significant inoculation or ingestion of HBV and who are also negative for anti-HBsAg. Hepatitis B vaccine produced by recombinant technology (Recombivax) is strongly recommended for seronegative hospital personnel at high risk for hepatitis B.

Several viruses may secondarily affect the liver as part of a more widespread systemic infection. EBV, CMV, HSV, rubella, rubeola, mumps, adenovirus, and coxsackie virus B have been associated with hepatic enzyme elevation. The hepatic dysfunction with these secondary infections is generally self-limited and less severe than that associated with primary viral hepatitis. However, fulminant hepatic necrosis, coma, and death have been described with several of these agents, especially the herpesvirus group, in the immunocompromised host.

All cancer patients with clinical or biochemical evidence of hepatitis should undergo a serologic evaluation to characterize the cause. Serum tests for anti-HAV (IgM), HBsAg, and anti-HBC (IgM) can identify patients with hepatitis A or B. Patients who test negative for hepatitis A or B should be evaluated repeatedly for anti-HCV, because it can take months antibody to develop.[244] Patients who remain negative to all of these viruses may have non-A, non-B, non-C hepatitis and may have a delta virus infection or hepatitis due to some other infectious or noninfectious cause. Hepatitis enzyme elevation or hyperbilirubinemia can occur with bacterial sepsis, fungal infection of the liver (especially *Candida* or *Aspergillus*), or toxoplasmosis.

In addition to the morbidity and mortality directly attributable to the hepatitis, significant alteration in hepatic function can affect the pharmacokinetics of antineoplastic agents, especially those metabolized or excreted by the liver (*e.g.*, methotrexate, doxorubicin).

Therapy for patients with hepatitis is primarily supportive, with bed rest and avoidance of further hepatic insult. Patients with hepatitis due to HSV should receive acyclovir. Chronic B or C hepatitis can be treated with interferon-α.

Hepatic candidiasis is increasingly diagnosed and is characterized by the presence of "bull's eye" lesions in the liver on ultrasound or CT scans (Fig. 62–8).[245,246] These lesions are not apparent in patients who are neutropenic but become recognizable at the time of neutrophil recovery. The MRI scan may be the most sensitive imaging technique, but variations among patients determines which imaging study is best. It is important to recognize that hepatic lesions may be smaller than the degree of resolution of current imaging techniques and in high-risk patients with a negative abdominal ultrasound or CT scans, a biopsy may still be necessary to confirm or rule out hepatic candidiasis. Patients are characterized by the persistence of fever at the time of recovery from an episode of neutropenia, frequently with right upper quadrant discomfort, nausea, and an elevated level of alkaline phosphatase and a leukocytosis. The lesions are granulomas, consisting of an inner core of central necrosis (where the yeast and pseudohyphae can be found), surrounded by a ring of inflammatory cells and an outer ring of fibrosis. To confirm the diagnosis, a liver biopsy is necessary. Because of the focality of the le-

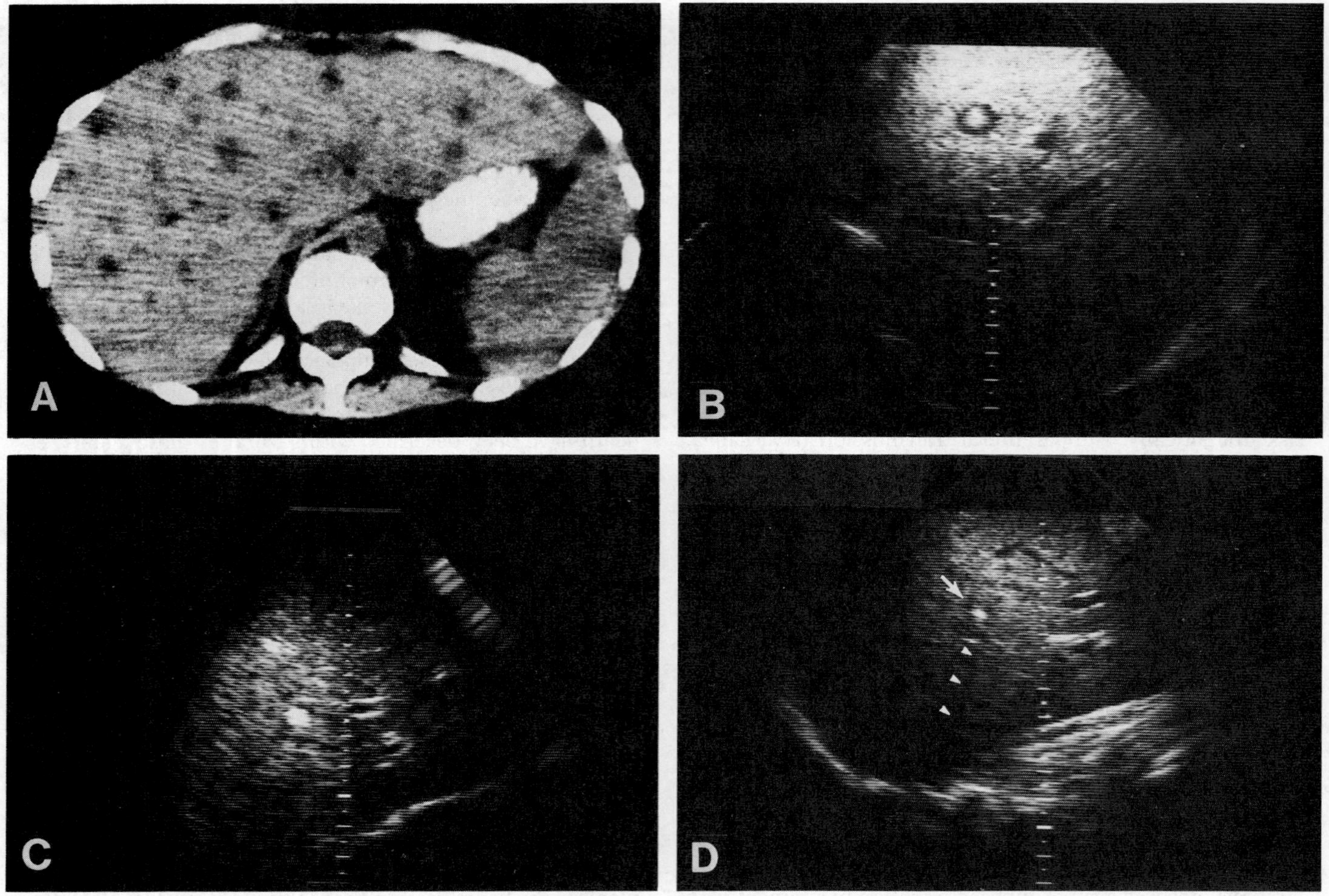

FIGURE 62–8. **(A)** CT scan of the liver shows numerous rounded areas of decreased attenuation compatible with the diagnosis of hepatic candidiasis. This is a nonspecific finding. **(B)** Ultrasound examination in the same patient shows the typical bull's eye lesion of candidiasis, characterized by a central echogenic nidus surrounded by a radiolucent halo. This is seen early in the natural history of the disease. **(C)** The radiolucent halo is now less obvious than in B. This illustrates the variable appearances of *Candida* abscesses on ultrasound studies at different times in the same patient. **(D)** Late in the course of the disease, the microabscesses become denser (*arrow*). The acoustic shadow posterior to the lesion was caused by attenuation of the sound beam (*arrow heads*). (Thaler M, Pastakia B, Shawker TM, et al. Hepatic candidiasis in cancer patients: The evolving picture of the syndrome. Ann Intern Med 1988;108:88–100)

sions, an open biopsy or peritoneoscopy guarded procedure is preferable. Cultures of the lesions are likely to be negative, and diagnosis requires demonstration of yeast forms or pseudohyphae. Serial sections of the biopsy may be necessary to confirm the presence of yeasts. These imaged lesions change over time and with treatment; on resolution, they become calcified, an important endpoint of therapy.

Hepatic candidiasis poses a therapeutic challenge because long courses of treatment are necessary, and the average dose of amphotericin B is 5 g. Experimental data suggest that the combination of amphotericin B with 5-FC is preferable. Serial biopsy may be necessary to confirm the resolution of infection. Although experience is limited, several investigators have suggested that lipid associated complexes or liposomal amphotericin B may be more effective and less toxic than deoxycholate amphotericin. The total dosage of amphotericin can be delivered much more rapidly. Although experience is limited, fluconazole has been given to patients who have failed to respond to amphotericin B and has been used for combination therapy in patients who have received short courses of amphotericin B.[247,248]

Perirectal Cellulitis

The overall incidence of perirectal cellulitis has decreased in recent years, presumably due to the early use of empiric antibiotic therapy when granulocytopenic patients become febrile. Nonetheless, there is still a risk for perianal cellulitis, especially for patients with prolonged (>7 days) and profound degrees (<100/mm^3) of granulocytopenia. Predisposing factors include perirectal mucositis due to chemotherapy or localized radiotherapy, hemorrhoids, anal fissures, and any type of rectal manipulation (*e.g.,* barium enema, anoscopy, sigmoidoscopy). Constipation should be avoided with stool softeners because passage of hard stool promotes the formation of anal fissures and increases the risk for perianal infections.

The most common pathogens in perirectal cellulitis are aerobic gram-negative bacilli (*e.g., P. aeruginosa, K. pneumoniae, E. coli*), the group D streptococci, and bowel anaerobes.[249] Because of the involvement and anaerobic organisms, antibiotic coverage must include a specific antianaerobic agent (*e.g.*, clindamycin or metronidazole) in addition to the broad-spectrum aerobic coverage. Therapy should commence at the time of the first complaints of tenderness, ideally before florid symptoms of cellulitis develop. Additional supportive measures include the use of sitz baths three or four times daily, stool softeners, a low-bulk diet, and avoidance of unnecessary rectal manipulation, especially repetitive digital examinations. Surgical intervention should be restricted to patients who demonstrate persistence of erythema or induration or progressive involvement of ischiorectal fossa despite optimal antimicrobial therapy.[249,250]

GENITOURINARY TRACT INFECTIONS

The genitourinary tract is infrequently the source of infection in the immunocompromised child. However, local obstruction due to tumor, neurologic dysfunction mediated by spinal cord compression or medications (*e.g.*, vincristine, narcotics), and local therapeutic maneuvers (*e.g.*, radiotherapy, surgery, bladder catheterization) can predispose cancer patients to genitourinary infections. Most commonly, gram-negative aerobic bacilli (*e.g., E. coli, Klebsiella* species, *Proteus* species, *P. aeruginosa*) and enterococci are the causative agents.

An important distinction must be made between a pathogen and colonizing organism when interpreting the results of the urine cultures obtained from an immunocompromised patient. In a nonneutropenic patient, a single organism colony count of greater than 10^5/ml is considered diagnostic of a urinary tract infection in a symptomatic person. In neutropenic patients, a colony count greater than 10^3/ml of a single organism may be considered diagnostic of a urinary tract infection if the patient is symptomatic (*e.g.*, dysuria, urgency, frequency, fever), and a colony count greater than 10^5/ml of a single organism should prompt antibiotic intervention whether or not the patient is symptomatic. Leukocytes in the urine must not be relied on as a diagnostic criterion in the neutropenic patient.

The distinction between colonization and tissue invasion is particularly difficult for fungal pathogens. Fungal colonization is especially prevalent among patients with indwelling urinary catheters or in patients receiving broad-spectrum antimicrobial therapy. Unlike the typical situation with bacterial pathogens, in which clinical signs and symptoms are present, fungal invasion of the genitourinary tract may be insidious. The repetitive isolation of a particular fungal species (usually *C. albicans, C. tropicalis,* or *T. glabrata*) in association with fever, deteriorating renal function, or flank pain should prompt the institution of systemic amphotericin B. Heavily colonized or superficial bladder infections, manifested by the persistence of positive urine cultures despite removal of predisposing factors, may be effectively treated with a single dose of amphotericin B and fluconazole or, in refractory cases, with instillation of amphotericin B (50 mg in 1 L D5W daily) into the bladder.

CUTANEOUS INFECTIONS

The integrity of this primary physical defense barrier is frequently disrupted in the cancer patient (*e.g.*, needle punctures, biopsies, surgery, irradiation, chemotherapy). Local cutaneous infections with bacteria or fungi are common and may result in disseminated infection during periods of immunosuppression. Vigilant skin cleansing with iodophor solutions is essential before any procedure that may permit pathogens. Careful attention to the physical examination of the skin in febrile cancer patients may yield a lesion from which a specific diagnosis can be made.[251]

The skin can become infected during bacteremia (*e.g., P. aeruginosa, A. hydrophilia, C. equi, S. marcescens*); fungemia (*e.g., Aspergillus, Candida, Mucor, C. neoformans, H. capsulatum*); or viremia (*e.g.*, HSV, VZV). There are noninfectious processes that mimic infection (*e.g.*, pyoderma gangrenosa, Sweet's syndrome). Skin lesions may permit the early diagnosis of generalized infection, and fresh lesions should be aspirated or biopsied and the material cultured and examined with Gram's stain, potassium hydroxide, methylene blue, and modified acid-fast stain.

If a viral infection is suspected, the base of several fresh vesicles should be scrapped with a Dacron swab, which should then be used to prepare microscope slides and placed into appropriate viral transport media for subsequent virus culture. The microscope slides should be examined by specific immunofluorescence for HSV and VZV. Immunofluorescence performed on appropriately prepared slides remains the most sensitive (approximately 85%) diagnostic test for varicella or herpes zoster. Viral cultures are useful for diagnosis if immunofluorescence is negative or if the slides are not adequate for examination, although cultures may not be positive for 2 to 4 weeks in the case of VZV. Wright-Giemsa staining (Tzanck test) of the microscope slides for detection of multinucleated giant cells may be performed, but the process does not differentiate between HSV and VZV infections. The diagnosis of vesicular lesions in the cancer patient is important for appropriate patient management and permits the physician to decide if isolation is necessary for the protection of other patients and staff members.

Primary varicella (chicken pox) is the most serious vesicular eruption in pediatric cancer patients, with a mortality rate of 7%. The major complication is the visceral dissemination that occurs in 32% of patients. Pneumonia occurs in 79% of patients with visceral varicella, generally developing 3 to 7 days after the onset of skin lesions, usually presenting as bilateral, "fluffy," nodular infiltrates. Other target organs during disseminated VZV infection include the liver, spleen, CNS, gastrointestinal tract, bone marrow, and lymph nodes. Secondary bacterial infections account for the additional severity of varicella dissemination. The risk for visceral dissemination is increased in patients receiving chemotherapy at the time of infection, especially if they are also lymphopenic (<500/mm^3). In children with AIDS, recurrent or chronic cutaneous varicella has been observed, in which lesions can range from verrucous to pyoderma gangrenosa and which can be a source of shedding virus.

Because of the severity of varicella infection in patients with cancer, attention has been directed at immunoprophylaxis. The most effective regimen is varicella-zoster immunoglobulin (VZIG), prepared from the sera of patients who have recently recovered from zoster and provided through the American Red Cross Blood Services. Administered within 72 hours of exposure, VZIG usually modifies the infection to a mild or subclinical form. If VZIG is not available, an alternative is one of the licensed intravenous immunoglobulins or zoster immune plasma (ZIP); the former is preferred.

Management of the seronegative patient exposed to varicella, commonly from a household or playmate contact, should include the discontinuation of all chemotherapy and the administration of VZIG, intravenous immunoglobulin, or ZIP within 72 hours of exposure. Chemotherapy should be withheld in patients with documented exposure until the end of the average incubation period, which is 21 days. In patients who develop overt varicella, immunosuppressive therapy should not be reinstituted until all the skin lesions have dried and scabbed.

Acyclovir, vidarabine, and interferon have been evaluated in the treatment of varicella and herpes zoster infections in immunocompromised patients. All have been effective compared with placebo.[252–255] Acyclovir (1500 mg/m^2/day in three divided doses) administered parenterally is the treatment of choice. Hydration should be maintained above baseline to avoid crystalluria. Therapy should be continued for a minimum of 7 of 10 days and potentially longer if the lesions have not become dry and scabbed. Orally administered acyclovir has been used for treatment of varicella in immunocompromised children, but it is poorly absorbed and produces plasma levels substantially lower than with intravenous acyclovir. Until controlled trials proving efficacy are available, oral acyclovir cannot be recommended for this purpose. Supportive management and early treatment of secondary bacterial infections are crucial for patients with established varicella.

Because varicella is highly contagious, there is a considerable risk for spread to other seronegative immunosuppressed patients. Varicella may be transmitted for 2 days before the appearance of rash. Extreme caution must be exercised in the management of potentially or overtly infected patients. Careful patient, parent, and staff education is essential. Absence from school where chicken pox has occurred may be necessary, usually for the 21-day incubation period. Parents should be alerted not to bring their children to the clinic waiting room area if chicken pox is suspected, and if hospitalization is required, reverse isolation should be undertaken, ideally on a hospital floor where immunosuppressed patients are not located.[342] Staff members should be checked for a history of chicken pox or tested serologically using the fluorescent antibody against membrane antigen or immune adherence hemagglutination technique to further minimize the possibility of nosocomial transmission.

A live attenuated chicken pox vaccine has been tested extensively in Japan, with demonstrable protection in normal and immunosuppressed children.[256] Although most active immunizations in patients receiving chemotherapy have been unsuccessful because of the inability to maintain effective antibody titers, current data suggest that children receiving maintenance chemotherapy can mount an antibody response if they can be vaccinated at a time when chemotherapy is stopped for 2 weeks.[257] Whether a similar response can be obtained in more intensively treated patients has not been established, and the consequences of administering a live vaccine to seriously immunosuppressed patients must be carefully considered.

The incidence of reactivation infection with VZV (*i.e.*, herpes zoster or shingles) among patients with previous varicella infections ranges from 5% to 10% among patients with solid tumors to 35% to 50% among patients treated for Hodgkin's disease or who have received marrow allografts. Most cases occur within the first 2 years after treatment. Herpes zoster is due to reactivation of VZV that had been latent in dorsal root ganglia. The likelihood of reactivation increases with intensity of immunosuppression, with the suppression of cell-mediated immunity more important than humoral immunity. Local irradiation may have a role in reactivation of virus, with disease occurring in the irradiated dermatome. The most important complication of herpes zoster is dissemination outside of the original dermatome, which occurs 4 to 9 days after onset. Some patients with cutaneous dissemination develop manifestations of visceral dissemination, most commonly including pneumonia, hepatitis, and encephalitis. Cutaneous dissemination rates of 5% to 50% have been observed, with higher rates among patients with more severe immunosuppression. Some patients develop cutaneously disseminated disease without an initial dermatome infection (*i.e.*, atypical disseminated zoster), and they have higher mortality rates than patients with initial localization. The overall mortality of herpes zoster is lower than that of primary varicella, although mortality rates as high as 10% have been observed in some series. Death is usually due to VZV pneumonia, although encephalitis due to direct invasion of the CNS may occur.

The local morbidity of herpes zoster may be considerable, due to acute pain, secondary bacterial infection, or neurologic complications, including peripheral neuropathies, aseptic meningitis, or myelitis. Encephalitis may occur by direct involvement of the CNS by VZV or may be postinfectious. Zoster encephalitis usually appears within 2 weeks of the rash, although it may occur from 1 week before rash to 8 weeks after.

Ophthalmic zoster is associated with involvement of the nasociliary nerve and is suggested by lesions on the tip of the nose. A unique syndrome of ophthalmic zoster with contralateral hemiplegia has been described. Herpes zoster of the ophthalmic division of the trigeminal nerve may be especially troublesome because of acute pain and corneal involvement with scarring and subsequent blindness.

Another zoster syndrome is abdominal pain occurring before or without development of a rash. Because of obvious difficulties in diagnosis, these patients may have many diagnostic procedures performed, including laparotomy, before herpes zoster becomes apparent as the cause. The most common problem is postherpetic neuralgia, particularly in older patients; it has been reported in as many as 45% of patients in some treatment trials. Pain may last for months or years in some cases. Treatment of postherpetic neuralgia is often unsatisfactory, although some patients may derive benefit from phenytoin (Dilantin) or carbamazepine (Tegretol).

Diagnosis of varicella or herpes zoster is based on the characteristic appearance of the skin lesions, on the distribution of lesions, and on immunofluorescent staining of material from the base of the vesicles. HSV can cause localized cutaneous disease and dermatomal-appearing rashes, which may be mistaken for herpes zoster. Wright-Giemsa staining of vesicle scrapings or electron microscopy do not differentiate HSV from VZV, and specific immunofluorescence and viral cultures should be performed for diagnosis.

Local skin care and observation for secondary bacterial infections are important. Data about therapy with antiviral agents are similar to those for varicella. Although interferon, vidarabine, and acyclovir are effective when compared with placebo, acyclovir appears to be the agent of choice. A direct comparison of acyclovir (500 mg/m^2 every 8 hours) and vidarabine for treatment of herpes zoster, conducted primarily among marrow transplant recipients, showed acyclovir to be superior, with shorter durations of fever, new lesion formation, and acute pain and more rapid healing and elimination of cutaneous dissemination.[258] Acyclovir appears to be effective among patients in whom cutaneous dissemination has already occurred, although initiation of treatment within 48 to 72 hours of onset is highly desirable. VZV resistance to acyclovir has not been observed in vivo and continuation of new lesion formation and cutaneous dissemination occurring within the first 2 to 3 days after initiation of treatment should not be interpreted as treatment failure. Acyclovir treatment should be continued for 7 days or for 2 days after the last new lesion, whichever is longer. In severely immunosuppressed patients, acyclovir should be administered parenterally. In less immunosuppressed patients, oral acyclovir has been given, although validating clinical trials are lacking. Because of failure to develop adequate specific immune responses, some patients who have received acyclovir treatment for herpes zoster have "relapses" of herpes zoster within the succeeding 2 months; they should receive another treatment course. Attention must be paid to adequate hydration, because renal insufficiency and other side effects such as nausea have been observed more frequently among patients who become dehydrated during treatment.

Patients with lymphomas or leukemia or who have received marrow allografts, who are at highest risk of cutaneous and visceral dissemination, should be treated with intravenous acyclovir if they develop herpes zoster. Because of the potential for spread of VZV to other immunosuppressed patients, all patients with herpes zoster should be kept in single rooms, and glove and gown precautions should be used; strict isolation may be appropriate in some circumstances or institutions. Susceptible patients and hospital staff can acquire primary varicella after exposure to herpes zoster.

MUSCULOSKELETAL INFECTIONS

The musculoskeletal system is an uncommon primary site of infection in cancer patients. However, atypical infections such as deep pyomyositis due to *S. aureus* or gram-negative organisms or psoas muscle abscesses have been described in neutropenic and nonneutropenic leukemic patients. Treatment includes incision and drainage and appropriate antibiotic therapy.

Crepitance and soft tissue tenderness suggests an anaerobic infection with *Clostridia* or with the toxin-producing *Bacillus cereus.* Necrotizing fascitis due to *S. pyogenes* represents a potentially life-threatening infection, rarely caused by nonsteroidal antiinflammatory drugs.[259] Immediate intervention with debridement and antibiotics is essential, and hyperbaric oxygen may be used in some cases. Other gas-forming organisms (*e.g., E. coli*) may cause a similar clinical syndrome.

Septic arthritis or osteomyelitis in the cancer patient may be caused by gram-negative organisms (*e.g., Pseudomonas, Klebsiella, Salmonella, Eikenella*), fungi (*e.g., Candida*), or the more common gram-positive bacterial pathogens. Patients with local skeletal defects or who have undergone extensive surgery, such as amputation or soft tissue dissection, and patients with bacteremia or fungemia are considered to be at high risk. Occasionally, it may be difficult to differentiate osteomyelitis from Ewing's sarcoma or radionecrosis.

CENTRAL NERVOUS SYSTEM INFECTIONS

Infections of the CNS are surprisingly infrequent in patients with cancer, but patients who present with symptoms or signs suggesting CNS dysfunction must be expeditiously evaluated with the appropriate physical, laboratory, and radiographic examinations. Evaluation of cerebrospinal fluid from cancer patients should include aerobic culture and Gram's stain, cryptococcal antigen determination, fungal culture, and cytologic examination in addition to the routine cerebrospinal fluid tests. Potential infections include shunt (*e.g.,* Ommaya reservoir) infections, meningitis or meningoencephalitis, encephalitis, and brain abscesses.

Shunt Infections

Intraventricular shunts and Ommaya reservoirs are associated with an increased incidence of CNS infection. The responsible pathogens are most commonly those colonizing the adjacent skin: coagulase-positive and coagulase-negative staphylococci, *Propionibacterium acnes, Corynebacterium* species, enterococci, and gram-negative bacilli. Patients may be totally asymptomatic, or they may have fever, headache, increased intracranial pressure, and meningism. Most patients with Ommaya reservoir infections can be successfully treated without removing the device.

Meningitis

Meningitis or meningoencephalitis is most frequently encountered in patients with impaired cell-mediated immunity and is typically caused by *Cryptococcus neoformans* or *Listeria monocytogenes. C. neoformans* causes a meningoencephalitis that is typically indolent. The presenting complaints include headaches, altered mental status, low-grade, intermittent fevers, or meningism. Examination of the cerebrospinal fluid demonstrates a mild mononuclear pleocytosis (40–400 leukocytes/mm^3) and minimally decreased glucose. Only 50% of patients have a detectable organism by an India ink preparation, and the most reliable means of diagnosis is documentation of cryptococcal antigen in serum or cerebrospinal fluid. Therapy for *C. neoformans* meningitis or meningoencephalitis includes the combination of amphotericin B (0.3–0.5 mg/kg/day) and oral 5-FC (150 mg/kg/day every 6 hours) for 4 to 6 weeks. Although a multicenter trial in adults with AIDS and cryptococcal meningitis found fluconazole to be comparable amphotericin B, the time to negative of cerebrospinal fluid cultures was longer for patients receiving fluconazole.

Listeria monocytogenes is a motile, gram-positive rod that causes several distinct clinical syndromes, including meningitis. Patients with impaired cell-mediated immunity and especially those with defects of T-cell-mediated immune function are susceptible. Although the organism can be isolated from soil, dust, water, sewage, and contaminated foods (especially cheese and dairy products), the exact mode transmission in most immunocompromised patients is unclear. Community outbreaks have occurred and hospital-associated clustering in immunosuppressed patients has been described. The most common presentation includes a subacute course of low-grade fevers and personality changes. Focal neurologic signs are occasionally present. Laboratory findings include a mild to moderate cerebrospinal fluid pleocytosis (6–12,000 cells/mm^3) and may include a predominance of polymorphonuclear leukocytes or mononuclear cells. Protein levels are generally elevated (100–300 mg/100 ml), and cerebrospinal fluid glucose levels are usually decreased. Diagnosis depends on a high index of suspicion. Ampicillin or penicillin provide the optimal treatment and should be continued for 3 to 6 weeks, because relapses have been reported with shorter therapy. Third-generation cephalosporins are inactive against *Listeria*.

Encephalitis

HSV, VZV, and measles are the most likely causes of sporadic viral encephalitis. HSV encephalitis, which may present as a focal or generalized process, responds to acyclovir treatment; acyclovir is also appropriate treatment for VZV encephalitis.

Patients with encephalitis or encephalomyelitis commonly present with signs of meningeal irritation (*e.g.*, fever, headache, nuchal rigidity) and evidence of altered mentation. Confusion may progress to stupor and to coma. Focal neurologic signs and seizures are relatively common. Cerebrospinal fluid examination may demonstrate a pleocytosis (10–2000 cells/mm^3), with a predominance of mononuclear cells. An increased number of cerebrospinal fluid red cells has been reported with HSV encephalitis. Cerebrospinal fluid protein levels are normally elevated, and the glucose characteristically remains within the normal range, except for a decreased level in mumps infection.

For the cancer patient with focal neurologic deficits or altered mentation, it is important to differentiate between an infectious, metabolic, toxic, or neoplastic causes. Unfortunately, diagnosis of the specific cause of encephalitis in an immunocompromised patient is difficult. Acute and convalescent serum antibody titers should be obtained, and specific cerebrospinal fluid antibody may be detected in cases of mumps, HSV, and varicella zoster. Although definitive diagnosis of HSV encephalitis requires a brain biopsy and because the clinician's therapeutic armamentarium against most causes of encephalitis is limited, empiric administration of acyclovir (500 mg/m^2 given every 8 hours) to the cancer patient with signs and symptoms suggesting of encephalitis seems warranted.

A treatable CNS infection that can present as an encephalitis in an immunosuppressed patient or as a mass lesion in the AIDS patient is due to the obligate intracellular parasite *Toxoplasma gondii*. Toxoplasmosis may represent newly acquired or reactivated infection and is rarely limited to the CNS, usually occurring in concert with fever, lymphadenopathy, hepatitis, pneumonitis, myocarditis, and pericarditis. The cerebrospinal fluid typically manifests a mononuclear pleocytosis, elevated protein levels, and a normal glucose concentration. A battery of serologic tests are available for the diagnosis of toxoplasmosis in the immunocompetent host, but most of these are limited in their applicability to the immunosuppressed patient due to suboptimal antibody responses. The definitive diagnosis requires demonstration of the parasite within tissue sections.

Treatment of active toxoplasmosis should include the combination of pyrimethamine and sulfadiazine or "triple sulfa" therapy—trisulfapyrimidines-sulfamerazine, sulfamethazine, and sulfadiazine. In immunodeficient patients, therapy should be continued for 4 to 6 weeks after the resolution of all clinical symptoms and signs. Clindamycin and pyrimethamine also benefit AIDS patients with central toxoplasmosis. The 566C80 quinone that has demonstrated activity against *P. carinii* also offers some benefit to patients with toxoplasmosis.

The important differential diagnosis in a cancer patient with evidence of a focal lesion (mass) within the CNS is between metastatic or primary malignancy and a brain abscess. Predisposing factors for brain abscesses include contiguous sites of infection (*e.g.*, otitis, sinusitis, dental abscesses), a history of penetrating cranial trauma, congenital cardiac disease, bacterial endocarditis, and pulmonary infections. In addition to the usual aerobic and anaerobic bacteria responsible for abscesses in immunocompetent patients, fungal and nocardial species are particularly prone to cause disease in an immunosuppressed patient. In patients with disseminated candidiasis, almost half may have CNS involvement, although this is usually unrecognized. In AIDS patients, CNS lesions may be caused by lymphoma or *T. gondii*. The association of pulmonary lesions with focal neurologic findings suggests *Nocardia, Aspergillus, Mucor,* or *Candida*.

Early evaluation and specific diagnosis are crucial in the management of brain abscesses, because effective antimicrobial or neurosurgical therapy is available. Diagnosis is commonly made by radiographic demonstration of a localized CNS mass, followed by an open or closed neurosurgical procedure to aspirate or resect the localized lesion.

Dementias

One of the disconcerting sequelae of modern chemotherapy has been the occurrence of leukoencephalopathy. Many of these dementing processes can be linked to intrathecal chemotherapy, especially the combination of irradiation and methotrexate. However, awareness that slow virus infections can produce CNS deterioration in humans has raised concern that some dementing processes may have a viral cause. Adults with lymphoma and symptoms of progressive mental and emotional deterioration, including decreased visual acuity, aphasia, and sensory and cerebellar signs, may have antibody to the human papillomavirus JC and isolation of virus from infected mononuclear cells, suggesting the diagnosis of progressive multifocal leukoencephalopathy.[260]

PREVENTING INFECTION IN CANCER PATIENTS

Despite a multitude of clinical trials investigating the efficacy of various measures to prevent or reduce the occurrence of infection, the most important antiinfective measure identified has been the simplest—careful hand-washing practices.[66] Several approaches have been taken to decrease the acquisition of new organisms or suppress those already colonizing the cancer patient (Table 62–16). Unfortunately, no method is singularly effective, each having promise and problems (Tables 62–17 and 62–18). As new preventive strategies are evaluated, they initially appear promising, but as additional studies are conducted, their beneficial results become less convincing.[261]

PREVENTING ACQUISITION OF NEW ORGANISMS

Because almost 85% of the organisms responsible for infections among patients with cancer are derived from the endogenous flora and almost half of these are acquired from the hospital environment, much attention has been directed toward preventing the acquisition of potential pathogens.

Inanimate objects within the hospital environment (*e.g.*, faucet aerators, shower heads, respirators, plants, floors) are reservoirs of pathogenic organisms. However, most epidemiologic studies suggest that transmission from such inanimate sources usually requires a human vector.[65] The simplest yet most efficacious intervention that can be performed is adherence to strict hand-washing precautions.[66] The easiest way to enforce such a policy is to educate the child and parents to disallow contact with anyone who has neglected to wash his hands.

A second maneuver to decrease the acquisition of new organisms is to maintain a cooked diet during periods of granulocytopenia, with avoidance of fresh fruits and vegetables and nonprocessed dairy products, because these foods are naturally contaminated with gram-negative bacteria, especially *K. pneumoniae, E. coli,* and *P. aeruginosa.* However, the true benefits of such a diet in reducing the acquisition of new organisms and the incidence of infection has not been proven.

Environmental sources can contribute to fungal (*e.g.*, *Aspergillus*) and bacterial (*e.g.*, *Legionella*) colonization and infection. In centers where *Aspergillus* is a significant problem, special air filtration systems (*e.g.*, high-efficiency particulate air filters) or water purification systems may help.

Although the technique of reverse isolation has often been used, it does not significantly reduce the acquisition of new organisms in an environment where hand-washing techniques are strictly followed.[262] There is no compelling reason to enforce this policy.

The total protective environment (TPE) is a comprehensive antiinfective regimen designed to reduce the patient's endogenous microbial burden while preventing the acquisition of new organisms (see Table 62–17). A sterile environment is created in a clean air room with constant positive air flow and is maintained by an aggressive program of surface decontamination, sterilization of all objects that enter the room, and an intensive regimen to disinfect the patient, including oral, nonabsorbable antibiotics, skin antiseptics, antibiotic sprays and ointments, and a low-microbial diet. Several studies have documented that the TPE can reduce infections in profoundly granulocytopenic patients. However, the TPE is expensive, and because of the improvement in treating established infections, it does not offer a survival advantage to patients. TPE is not necessary for the routine care of cancer patients and, with newer and less expensive modalities, is less frequently used in current clinical practice (see Table 62–18).

TABLE 62–16. Methods for Preventing Infection in Cancer Patients

Prevent Acquisition and/or Suppress or Eliminate Microbial Flora	*Improve or Modify Host Defenses*
Isolation	**Immunization**
Simple or reverse isolation	Active
Isolation with HEPA air filtration	*Pseudomonas*
	Pneumococcus
Prophylactic Antibiotics	Passive
Nonabsorbable antibiotics	J-5 Core glycolipid
Trimethoprim-sulfamethoxazole	Pooled immunoglobulins
Selective decontamination	Specific monoclonal
Quinolones	**Cell-Component Replacement**
Prophylactic Antivirals	Leukocyte transfusions
Acycloguanosine (Acyclovir)	Accelerate granulocyte recovery
Gangciclovir	GM-CAF
Amantadine	G-CSF
Prophylactic Antifungals	IL-3
Nystatin	Peripheral stem cells
Imidazoles	
Prophylactic Antiparasitics	
Thiabendazole	
Trimethoprim-sulfamethoxazole	
Combination—Comprehensive	
Total protection isolation	

ANTIMICROBIAL PROPHYLAXIS

Antibacterial Prophylaxis

Many clinical trials have been conducted to investigate the utility of prophylactic antibiotic regimens in immunocompromised patients. Several strategies have been explored, including systemic prophylaxis, gastrointestinal decontamination, and selective gastrointestinal decontamination (*i.e.*, maintenance of "colonization resistance"). Unfortunately, the interpretation of many of these trials is difficult due to poor study design, nonuniform patient groupings, and failure to report or document compliance with the prophylactic regimens.[264]

Because the gastrointestinal tract is the source for many of the pathogens causing microbiologically defined infections, investigators have evaluated the efficacy of reducing the en-

TABLE 62–17. Antimicrobial Activity of Various Prophylactic Regimens Against Exogenous and Endogenous Microorganisms

Sources	*Total Protected Environment*	*Nonabsorbable Antibiotics*	*Trimethoprim-Sulfamethoxazole*	*Selective Decontamination*	*Quinolones*
Exogenous Sources					
Air, food, water contacts	Yes	No	No	No	No
Endogenous Sources					
Nares	Yes	No	No	No	Yes
Oropharynx	Yes	+/−	No	Yes	Yes
Lower respiratory tract	+/−	No	+/−	+/−	Yes
Gastrointestinal tract	Yes	Yes	Yes	Yes	Yes
Perianal area	Yes	+/−	+/−	+/−	+/−
Skin	Yes	No	No	No	No
Central venous catheter	No	No	No	No	No
Peripheral catheters	No	No	No	No	No
Systemic effect	+/−	No	Yes	Yes	Yes

dogenous gastrointestinal flora by the administration of oral, nonabsorbable antibiotics. This technique has not been especially valuable and is fraught with problems. The antimicrobial agents used (*e.g.*, vancomycin, gentamicin, polymyxin B, nystatin, framycetin, colistin) are unpalatable and are generally poorly tolerated, making compliance difficult, especially among patients receiving emetogenic chemotherapy (see Table 62–17). Equally disturbing has been the emergence of resistant bacterial strains when aminoglycoside-containing regimens have been used. Prophylactic regimens aimed solely at reducing the endogenous gastrointestinal flora cannot be recommended (see Table 62–18).

A modified technique is the "selective decontamination" of the gastrointestinal tract, employing antibiotics that preserve the anaerobic flora but reduce the aerobic bacteria. Data show that the preservation of the anaerobic flora of the gas-

TABLE 62–18. Effectiveness and Limitations of Various Strategies in Preventing Infection in Cancer Patients

Qualities Assessed	*Total Protected Environment*	*Nonabsorbable Antibiotics*	*Trimethoprim-Sulfamethoxazole*	*Selective Decontamination*	*Quinolones*
Efficacy					
Reduced infection	Yes	No	+/−	+/−	Yes
Decreased in fever	Yes	No	No	No	Yes
Decrease or shorten need for antibiotics and antifungals	No	No	No	+/−	Yes
Contributed to survival	No	No	No	No	No
Compliance					
Well tolerated?	No	No	+/−	+/−	Yes
Impact on efficacy	Yes	Yes	Yes	+/−	No
Liabilities					
Emergency of resistant organisms	Yes	Yes	Yes	Yes	Yes
Organ side effects:					
Interference with other drugs	Yes	Yes	Yes	No	No
BM suppression	No	No	Yes	Yes	No
Specific organ toxicity	No	No	Yes	Yes	Yes
Cost					
For the drugs or regimens	Yes	Yes	No	Yes	Yes
Surveillance or monitoring	Yes	Yes	Yes	Yes	Yes
Reducing need for hospitalization or need for drugs	No	No	No	+/−	+/−

trointestinal tract provides a colonization resistance against aerobic and fungal organisms.[265,266] Although initial clinical trials provided evidence of a reduction of infections in patients undergoing induction therapy for acute leukemia, clearly defined efficacy has not been established.[267,268] The most commonly investigated agent used for selective decontamination has been trimethoprim-sulfamethoxazole. Early trials investigating this antibiotic in children and adults demonstrated a reduction in all infections and in bacteremic episodes, but many follow-up clinical trials yielded conflicting results.[269–275] The reasons for the contradictory results are unclear, although factors such as variability in study design, nonuniform patient populations, and failure to properly monitor compliance have played a part. The potential for reduction in infectious morbidity and mortality must be balanced against the prolongation of granulocytopenia and emergence of resistant organisms.[276] Successful use of this approach requires close monitoring to properly adjust the antimicrobial regimen for resistant or newly emerging species, and this surveillance is expensive and time consuming.

Prophylactic antibiotic trials employing a derivative of nalidixic acid, the quinolone antibiotic norfloxacin, have shown promising results in a population of bone marrow transplant patients. Although fluoroquinolones such as ciprofloxacin can decrease the incidence of gram-negative bacteria, the use of these agents has not been associated with a reduction in infection-related mortality.

Although some investigators have suggested that the time the initiation of parenteral therapy is lengthened with the use of oral ciprofloxacin, two problems have been observed with prophylactic quinolones.[277,278] One is breakthrough infection with gram-positive organisms, a problem that can potentially be overcome with the addition of penicillin or amoxicillin with clavulanic acid. Of more concern is the increasing incidence of quinolone-resistant organisms.[263] The inappropriate use of these agents for prophylaxis can jeopardize the long-term benefits of this class of antibiotics. The quinolones cannot be used in children younger than 18 years of age because of putative joint toxicity, although studies evaluating their safety in pediatric patients are ongoing.

Antifungal Prophylaxis

Because of the increasing incidence of invasive mycoses in immunocompromised hosts, antifungal prophylaxis has been studied. The most frequently evaluated antifungal agents have included nystatin, amphotericin B, miconazole, clotrimazole, and ketoconazole. Most prophylactic regimens have been aimed at a reduction of invasive infections due to *Candida*, and by virtue of the antifungal activity of the agents employed, they would not be expected to have a significant impact against *Aspergillus* or *Mucormycoses*.

Interpretation of existing data is difficult, because studies suffer from different patient criteria, disparate dosage regimens, nonuniform response criteria, and lack of appropriate controls. An added problem is the inherent difficulty in the definitive diagnosis of a fungal infection in an immunocompromised patient.

Within the context of these limitations, several conclusions about antifungal prophylaxis can be offered. First, after an adequate dose of antifungal agent (*e.g.*, amphotericin B, ketoconazole, clotrimazole) has been administered, there has been a consistent decrease in fungal colonization.[279] However, decreased colonization has not clearly resulted in a decreased incidence of invasive mycotic disease, although a decrease in superficial infection has been found in some studies. Second, several studies employing prophylactic and empiric antifungal regimens have reported a shift in the colonization pattern of fungal organisms, mostly toward more resistant fungi. The prophylactic regimens may successfully eradicate the susceptible fungi (particularly *C. albicans*) but may permit the overgrowth and ultimate invasion by more resistant species, especially *Aspergillus*. This was recently observed with fluconazole, one of the newest antifungal agents to be introduced into clinical practice. Patients undergoing bone marrow transplantation and who received fluconazole prophylaxis had an increased incidence of infection with *Candida krusei*, a more resistant and difficult to treat organism. This trend must be closely monitored.

The potential benefits of prophylactic antifungal therapy must be balanced against the toxicities, epidemiologic considerations, and relative efficacy of the regimen employed. Until clear benefit can be proven, widespread chemoprophylaxis against fungi should not be attempted.

Antiviral Prophylaxis

Intravenous and oral formulations of acyclovir can prevent reactivation of HSV and resultant stomatitis among patients undergoing induction therapy for leukemia or lymphoma or marrow allografting.[280] Twice-daily administration of intravenous acyclovir appears to be almost as effective as use three times daily and is more convenient and less expensive. Prophylactic acyclovir may increase the development of acyclovir resistance. Prevention of CMV infection has been more problematic. Although primary CMV infection among seronegative patients can be prevented by use of screened seronegative blood products, use of CMV immunoglobulins or the licensed intravenous immunoglobulins remains controversial. Interferon-α has a prophylactic benefit in renal allograft patients, although this effect was not reproduced in one study among marrow allograft recipients. Intravenous acyclovir may have some effect against CMV if used prophylactically. Ganciclovir is beneficial if administered prophylactically in reducing the incidence of CMV pneumonitis.

Antiparasitic Prophylaxis

In centers where *P. carinii* occurs with some frequency, the administration of trimethoprim-sulfamethoxazole has convincingly reduced the incidence of infection. However, not all children undergoing cancer treatment require prophylactic treatment. It should be influenced by the patients underlying disease (*e.g.*, leukemia, solid tumors), the intensity or immunosuppression of the therapy being delivered, and the center where treatment is being administered. Current recommendations for children are for trimethoprim-sulfamethoxazole (150 mg/m^2) or trimethoprim in two divided doses on 3 consecutive days. In adults, two double-strength (check) tablets, twice daily on 3 consecutive days, is the recommended treatment. These schedules appear to be less associated with hematologic complications (*e.g.*, neutropenia) than daily therapy. Studies of adults with AIDS have demonstrated that trimethoprim-sulfamethoxazole is superior to aerosolized pentamidine in preventing *P. carinii* pneumonia. However, aerosolized pentamidine can be an alternative for patients unable to tolerate trimethoprim-sulfamethoxazole. Other alternatives include dapsone, and the reports of 566C80 suggest that it may be an important component of the anti-*P. carinii* repertoire.

Active and Passive Immunization and Biologicals

Fatal infections due to measles, polio, and vaccinia have occurred as a consequence of live virus immunizations in patients with impaired immune function. Although an initial antibody response may be elicited, the concurrent administration of cytotoxic chemotherapy is usually associated with a rapid decline of titers. Inactivated polio vaccine should be given to the immunologically deficient host and his or her siblings and other household contacts, because oral poliovirus vaccine strains are transmissible to the immunocompromised person. Live virus vaccines may be administered at least 3 months after all immunosuppressive therapy has ceased. An important exception to this rule appears to be the use of the live attenuated varicella vaccine that, despite a being associated with a relatively high incidence of adverse effects (primarily mild to moderate rash), appears to be effective in protecting children with cancer from severe natural varicella infection.

Inactivated vaccines may not yield protective immunity in immunosuppressed patients. Clinical trials have indicated that the efficacy of immunizations against influenza, pneumococcus, and *H. influenzae* type B given during the course of cancer chemotherapy are often impaired because of inadequate antibody responses.

Passive immunization with VZIG reduces the incidence of pneumonitis and encephalitis and decreases the mortality rate from between 5% and 7% to 0.5% in immunocompromised patients with primary varicella infection. Immunosuppressed persons who are seronegative or possess low-titer antivaricella antibody should receive 1 vial of globulin per 15 kg of body weight within 72 hours after exposure to a potentially infectious source.

Immunotherapy for gram-negative septic shock is a strategy based on the hypothesis that passive immunization with antibody against endotoxin, the lipopolysaccharide component of the gram-negative cell wall, can block the endotoxin-triggered release of factors that mediate shock and tissue damage. Initial studies employed high-titer human polyclonal antiserum directed against endotoxin core determinants of the J5 mutant of *E. coli* 0111:B4. Polyclonal J5 antiserum has decreased mortality in patients with documented gram-negative bacteremia and protected high-risk surgical patients from complications due to gram-negative infections.

A human monoclonal IgM antibody, HA-1A, binds specifically to the toxic moiety of endotoxin. In a large randomized, double-blind, placebo-controlled trial, HA-1A antibody significantly reduced mortality in patients who were ultimately proven to have gram-negative bacteremia.[281] However, the clinical criteria used to enroll patients in this study were only able to identify patients with a 30% to 40% probability of having gram-negative sepsis. Most patients in the study did not have gram-negative sepsis, and in those patients, HA-1A antibody had no impact on mortality. Moreover, no benefit has yet been observed for neutropenic patients. Until better clinical criteria are developed to accurately predict gram-negative bacteremia, the widespread use of HA-1A antibody for all critically ill patients with presumed sepsis cannot be supported.

The therapeutic use of intravenous immunoglobulins is based on the observations that antibody deficiency and increased susceptibility to bacterial infections may occur in patients with hematologic cancers or in those who receive immunosuppressive therapies for cancer or in preparation for bone marrow transplantation. In a large, double-blind trial, intravenous immunoglobulin significantly decreased the number of bacterial infections in patients with chronic lymphocytic leukemia.[282] An extensive cost and benefit analysis of this study, however, revealed that this frequent administration of immunoglobulin over a long period did not improve the quality or length of life in patients with chronic lymphocytic leukemia and that it is an extremely expensive intervention compared with other generally accepted treatments.[283]

In the setting of allogeneic bone marrow transplantation, the prophylactic use intravenous immunoglobulins has significantly reduced the incidence and severity of acute GVHD and associated interstitial pneumonia related to cytomegalovirus and significantly decreased the frequency of sepsis and local infections. A decrease in transplant-related mortality was observed among patients older than 20 years of age who had received immunoglobulin.[284] These encouraging results suggest that the expense of intravenous immunoglobulin therapy in certain bone marrow transplant recipients may be justified. Further study is required to identify to the optimal dose, schedule and population for passive immunotherapy.

Perhaps the most exciting development is the cloning, purification, and clinical application of the hematopoietic growth factors, including the CSFs and several of the interleukins. These glycoproteins endogenously stimulate the proliferation and maturation of bone marrow progenitor cells into fully differentiated circulating blood cells. The two growth factors most intensively studied are G-CSF and GM-CSF. G-CSF specifically promotes the proliferation and maturation of neutrophilic precursors, and the function of mature neutrophils. GM-CSF additionally enhances the number and function of cells of the monocyte-macrophage lineage. The potential utility of the CSFs to attenuate the marrow toxic effects of cancer chemotherapy and radiotherapy has been assessed in several trials. Early, uncontrolled studies indicated that administration of recombinant human (rh)GM-CSF or rhG-CSF administration can decrease the duration and severity of neutropenia in patients after intensive chemotherapy for small cell lung cancer, bladder cancer, metastatic sarcomas, and other neoplasms and in those undergoing autologous bone marrow transplantation.[285–289] One trial showed a reduction in the number of days of neutropenia associated with rhG-CSF use during chemotherapy for relapsed or refractory acute myelogenous leukemia.

Data from several studies suggested that patients treated with CSFs experienced fewer infectious complications than historic controls. Two large, randomized, double-blind, placebo-controlled trials substantiated these results. Nemunaitis and colleagues observed that patients undergoing autologous bone marrow transplantation for lymphoid cancers who received rhGM-CSF had accelerated neutrophil recovery by 1 week, a reduced incidence of culture-proven infections, and a decreased duration of required antibiotic administration and hospitalization.[284] Similar findings were reported with the use of rhG-CSF in patients receiving chemotherapy for small cell lung cancer.[285] In these studies, rhGM- and G-CSF were well-tolerated, although others have reported significant toxicities associated with rhGM-CSF including fevers, rashes, malaise, arthralgias and myalgias, and a capillary leak syndrome, generally at high doses. Very few adverse effects have been seen with rhG-CSF. The encouraging results led to the licensing of G-CSF and GM-CSF as adjuncts to some of the highly marrow-suppressive cancer therapies.

These trials indicate that by minimizing the chemotherapy-induced toxicities of prolonged neutropenia and complicating infections, the CSFs may permit the delivery of chemotherapy in schedules and doses that maximize tumoricidal activity. With the identification and purification of an increasing array of immunomodulatory substances, (*e.g.*, interleukins, interferons, TNF) there is the potential for improving the altered host defenses of the cancer patient and reducing the complications and limitations of chemotherapy.[290]

REFERENCES

1. Bodey G. Infection in cancer patients: A continuing association. Am J Med 1986;81(suppl 1A):11–26.
2. Sculier JP, Weerts D, Klastersky J. Causes of death in febrile granulocytopenic cancer patients receiving empiric antibiotic therapy. Eur J Cancer Clin Oncol 1984;20:55–60.
3. Pizzo PA, Rubin M, Freifeld A, Walsh TJ. The child with cancer and infection. I. Empirical therapy for fever and neutropenia, and preventive strategies. J Pediatr 1991;119:676–694.
4. Pizzo PA, Rubin M, Freifeld A, Walsh TJ. The child with cancer and infection. II. Nonbacterial infections. J Pediatr 1991;119:845–857.
5. Beachey EH. Bacterial adherence: Adhesin-receptor interactions mediating the attachment of bacteria to mucosal surfaces. J Infect Dis 1981;143:325–345.
6. Schoolnik GK, Lark D, O'Hanley P. Bacterial adherence and anticolonization vaccines. In: Remington JS, Schwarz NM, eds. Current clinical topics in infectious diseases, vol 6. New York: McGraw Hill, 1985:85–102.
7. Johanson WG, Pierce AK, Sanford JP. Changing pharyngeal flora of hospitalized patients: Emergence of gram-negative bacilli. N Engl J Med 1969;281:1137–1140.
8. Fainstain V, Rodriguez V, Turk, et al. Patterns of oropharyngeal and fecal flora in patients with leukemia. J Infect Dis 1981;144:10–18.
9. Van der Waaij D. Gut resistance to colonization: Clinical usefulness of selective use of orally administered antimicrobial and antifungal drugs. In: Klastersky J, ed. Infection in cancer patients. New York: Raven Press, 1982:73–86.
10. Spitznagel JK, Shafer WM. Neutrophil killing of bacteria by oxygen-independent mechanism: A historical summary. Rev Infect Dis 1985;7:398–403.
11. Bodey GP, Buckley M, Sathe YS, et al. Quantitative relationships between circulating leukocytes and infection in patients with acute leukemia. Ann Intern Med 1966;64: 328–340.
12. Sieff CA. Hematopoietic growth factors. J Clin Invest 1987;79:1549–1557.
13. Roilides E, Pizzo PA. Modulation of host defenses by cytokines. Evolving adjuncts in prevention and treatment of serious infection in immunocompromised hosts. Clin Infect Dis (in press).
14. Nienhuis AW, Donahue RE, Karisson S, et al. Recombinant human granulocyte-macrophage colony-stimulating factor (GM-CSF) shortens the period of neutropenia after autologous bone marrow transplantation in a primate model. J Clin Invest 1987;80: 573–577.
15. Mayer P, Lam C, Obenaus H, et al. Recombinant human GM-CSF induces leukocytosis and activates peripheral blood polymorphonuclear neutrophils in nonhuman primates. Blood 1987;70:206–213.
16. Lopez AF, Williamson D, Gamble R, et al. Recombinant human granulocyte-macrophage colony-stimulating factor stimulates in vitro mature human neutrophil and eosinophil function, surface receptor expression, and survival. J Clin Invest 1986;78:1220–1228.
17. Weisbart RH, Kwan L, Golde DW, et al. Human GM-CSF primes neutrophils for enhanced oxidative metabolism in response to the major physiological chemoattractants. Blood 1987;69:18–21.
18. Glasson JC, Weisbard RH, Kaufman SE, et al. Purified human granulocyte-macrophage colony-stimulating factor: Direct action on neutrophils. Science 1984;226:1339–1342.
19. Lynch HT, Katz DA, Bogard PJ, Lynch JF. The sarcoma, breast cancer, lung cancer, and adrenocortical carcinoma syndrome revisited: Childhood Cancer. Am J Dis Child 1985;139:134–136.
20. Beutler B, Milsard IW, Cerami A. Passive immunization against cachectin/tumor necrosis factor protects mice from lethal effect of endotoxin. Science 1985;229:869–871.
21. Dinarello CA. Interleukin-1. Rev Infect Dis 1984;6:51–59.
22. Estrov Z, Roifman C, Mills G, et al. The regulatory role of interleukin-2 responsive T lymphocytes on human marrow granulopoiesis. Blood 1987;69:1161–1166.
23. Cannistra SA, Rambaldi A, Spriggs DR, et al. Human granulocyte-macrophage colony-stimulating factor induces expression of the tumor necrosis factor gene by the U937 cell line and by normal human monocytes. J Clin Invest 1987;79:1720–1720.
24. Zucali JR, Dinarello CA, Oblon DJ, et al. Interleukin-1 stimulates fibroblasts to produce granulocyte-macrophage colony-stimulating activity and prostaglandin E_2. J Clin Invest 1986;77:1857–1863.
25. Perfect JR, Granger DL, Durack DT. Effects of antifungal agents and γ-interferon on macrophage cytotoxicity for fungi and tumor cells. J Infect Dis 1987;156:316–323.
26. Wilson CB, Westall J. Activation of neonatal and adult human macrophages by alpha, beta, and gamma interferons. Infect Immunol 1985;49:351–356.
27. Dinarello CA, The proinflammatory cytokones interleukin 1 and tumor necrosis factor and treatment of nil septic shock syndrome. J Infect Dis 1991;163:1177–1184.
28. Dinarello CA, Mier JW. Lymphokines. N Engl J Med 1987;317:940–945.
29. Nathan DG. Hope for hematopoietic hormones. N Engl J Med 1987;317:626–628.
30. Curnette JT, Boxer LA. Clinically significant phagocytic cell defects. In: Remington J, Swartz M, eds. Current clinical topics in infectious diseases, vol 6. New York: McGraw Hill, 1985:103–156.
31. McCormack RT, Nelson RD, Bloomfield CD, et al. Neutrophilic function in lymphoreticular malignancy. Cancer 1979;44:920–926.
32. Snyderman R, Seigler HF, Meadows L. Abnormalities of monocyte chemotaxis in patients with melanoma. Effects of immunotherapy and tumor removal. JNCI 1977;58: 37–41.
33. Pickering LK, Ericsson CD, Kohl S. Effect of chemotherapeutic agents on metabolic and bactericidal activity of polymorphonuclear leukocytes. Cancer 1978;42:1741–1746.
34. Baehner RL, Neiburger RG, Johnson DG, et al. Transient bactericidal defect of peripheral blood phagocytes from children with acute lymphoblastic leukemia receiving craniospinal irradiation. N Engl J Med 1973;289:1209–1213.
35. Tubaro E, Borelli G, Croce C, et al. Effect of morphine on resistance to infection. J Infect Dis 1983;148:656–666.
36. Schaffner A, Douglas H, Braude A. Selective protection against *Candidia* by mononuclear and against mycelia by polymorphonuclear phagocytes in resistance to *Aspergillus*. J Clin Invest 1982;69:617–631.
37. Fisher RI, DeVita VT, Bostick F. Persistent immunologic abnormalities in long term survivors of advanced Hodgkin's disease. Ann Intern Med 1980;92:595–599.
38. Dale DC, Petersdorf RG. Corticosteroids and infectious disease. Med Clin North Am 1973;57:1277–1287.
39. Nossai GJV. Current concepts: Immunology: The basic components of the immune system. N Engl J Med 1987;316:1320–1325.
40. Fahey JL, Scoggins R, Utz JP, et al. Infection, antibody response and gamma globulin components in multiple myeloma and macroglobulinemia. Am J Med 1973;35:698–707.
41. Stobo JD, Paul S, Von Scoy RE, et al. Suppressor thymus-derived lymphocytes in fungal infection. J Clin Invest 1976;57:319–328.
42. Zinner SH, McCabe WR. Effect of IgM and IgG antibody in patients with bacteremia due to gram-negative bacilli. J Infect Dis 1976;133:37–45.
43. Siber GR, Weitzman SA, Aisenberg AC, et al. Impaired antibody response to pneumococcal vaccine after treatment for Hodgkin's disease. N Engl J Med 1978;299: 442–448.
44. Pier G, Thomas DM. Characterization of the human immune response to a polysaccharide vaccine from *Pseudomonas aeruginosa*. J Infect Dis 1983;148:206–213.
45. Schildt RA, Boyd JF, McCracken JF, et al. Antibody response to pneumococcal vaccine in patients with solid tumors and lymphomas. Med Pediatr Oncol 1983;11:305–309.
46. Cooper M. B lymphocytes: Normal development and function. N Engl J Med 1987;317: 1452–1456.
47. Peter G, Pizzo PA, Robichaud KR, et al. Possible protective effect of circulating antibodies to the shared glycolipid of enterobacteriaceae in children with malignancy. Pediatr Res 1979;13:466.
48. Braude AI, Douglas H, Davis CE. Treatment and prevention of intravascular coagulation with antiserum to endotoxin. J Infect Dis 1973;128:S157–S164.
49. Ziegler EJ, McCutchan JA, Fierer S, et al. Successful treatment of gram-negative bacteremia and shock with human antiserum to a UPD-GAL epimerase-deficient mutant *Escherichia coli*. N Engl J Med 1982;307:1225–1230.
50. Rosse WF. The spleen as a filter. N Engl J Med 1987;317:705–706.
51. Sun T, Tenenbaum MJ, Greenspan J, et al. Morphologic and clinical observations in human infection with *Babesia microti*. J Infect Dis 1983;148:239–248.
52. Donaldson SS, Glatstein E, Vosti KL. Bacterial infections in pediatric Hodgkin's disease. Relationship to radiation, chemotherapy and splenectomy. Cancer 1978;41:1949–1958.
53. Chilcote RR, Baehner RL, Hammond D, et al. Septicemia and meningitis in children splenectomized for Hodgkin's disease. N Engl J Med 1976;295:798–800.
54. Weitzman S, Aisenberg AC. Fulminant sepsis after the successful treatment of Hodgkin's disease. Am J Med 1977;62:47–50.

55. Schimpff SC, O'Connell MJ, Greene WH, et al. Infections in 92 splenectomized patients with Hodgkin's disease. A clinical review. Am J Med 1975;59:695–701.
56. Keusch GT. Nutrition and infection. In: Remington JS, Swartz NM, eds. Current clinical topics in infectious disease, vol 5. New York: McGraw-Hill, 1984:106–123.
57. Shamberger RC, Pizzo PA, Goodgame JT, et al. The effect of total parenteral nutrition on chemotherapy induced myelosuppression: A randomized study. Am J Med 1983;74:40–48.
58. Schimpff SC, Young VM, Greene WH, et al. Origin of infection in acute nonlymphocytic leukemia: Significance of hospital acquisition of potential pathogens. Ann Intern Med 1972;77:707–714.
59. Van der Waaij D, Tielemons-Speltie TM, de Houban-Roech AMJ. Infection by and distribution of biotypes of enterobacteriaceae species in leukaemic patients treated under ward conditions and in units for protective isolation in seven hospitals in Europe. Infection 1977;5:3–10.
60. Schimpff SC, Greene WH, Young VM, et al. Significance of *Pseudomonas aeruginosa* in the patient with leukemia or lymphoma. J Infect Dis 1974;130:S24–S31.
61. Kurrle E, Bhaduri S, Krieger D, et al. Risk factors for infections of the oropharynx and the respiratory tract in patients with acute leukemia. J Infect Dis 1981;144:128–136.
62. Kramer BK, Pizzo PA, Robichaud KJ, et al. Role of serial microbiological surveillance and clinical evaluation in the management of cancer patients with fever and granulocytopenia. Am J Med 1982;72:561–568.
63. Pizzo PA, Levine AS. The utility of protected environment regimens for the compromised host: A critical assessment. In: Progress in hematology, vol X. New York: Grune & Stratton, 1977:311–332.
64. Aisner J, Murillo J, Schimpff SC, et al. Invasive *Aspergillus* in acute leukemia: Correlation with nose cultures and antibiotic use. Ann Intern Med 1979;90:4–9.
65. Maki DG, Alvarado CJ, Hessewer CH, et al. Relation of the inanimate hospital environment to endemic nosocomial infection. N Engl J Med 1982;307:1562–1565.
66. Albert RK, Condie F. Handwashing patterns in medical intensive care units. N Engl J Med 1981;304:1465–1466.
67. Maki D. Infections associated with intravascular lines. In: Remington JS, Swartz M, eds. Current clinical topics in infectious disease. New York: McGraw Hill, 1982:309–363.
68. Hiemenz J, Skelton J, Pizzo PA. Perspective on the management of catheter related infections in cancer patients. Pediatr Infect Dis 1986;5:6–11.
69. Craven DE, Moody B, Connolly MG, et al. Pseudobacteremia caused by povidone-iodine solution contaminated with *Pseudomonas cepacia*. N Engl J Med 1981;305:621–623.
70. Johanson WG, Pierce AK, Sanford JP, et al. Nosocomial respiratory infections with gram-negative bacilli. The significance of colonization of the respiratory tract. Ann Intern Med 1972;77:701–706.
71. Wingard JR, Merz WG, Saral R. *Candida tropicalis:* A major pathogen in immunocompromised patients. Ann Intern Med 1979;91:539–543.
72. Wingard JR, Merz WG, Rinaldi MG, et al. Increase in *Candida krusei* infection among patients with bone marrow transplantation and neutropenia treated prophylactically with fluconazole. N Engl J Med 1991;325:1274–1277.
73. Rouse BT, Horohov DW. Immunosuppression in viral infections. Rev Infect Dis 1986;8:850–873.
74. Todeschini G, Rubin M, Gill V, et al. Non-aeruginosa bacteremias in cancer patients. Review of 10 years' experience at the National Cancer Institute. Proceedings of the 27th Interscience Conference on Antimicrobial Agents and Chemotherapy, New York: 1987:265.
75. Pizzo PA, Ladisch SL, Gill F, et al. Increasing incidence of gram-positive sepsis in cancer patients. Med Pediatr Oncol 1978;5:241–244.
76. Wade JC, Schimpff SC, Newman KA, et al. *Staphylococcus epidermidis:* An increasing cause of infection in patients with granulocytopenia. Ann Intern Med 1982;97:507–508.
77. Lowder JN, Lazarus HM, Herzig RH. Bacteremias and fungemias in oncologic patients with central venous catheters. Changing spectrum of infection. Ann Intern Med 1982;142:1456–1459.
78. Winston DJ, Dudnick FV, Chapin M, et al. Coagulase-negative staphylococcal bacteremia in patients receiving immunosuppressive therapy. Arch Intern Med 1983;143:32–36.
79. Myers JP, Linneman CC. Bacteremia due to methicillin-resistant *Staphylococcus aureus.* J Infect Dis 1982;145:532–536.
80. Haley RW, Hightower AW, Khabbaz RF, et al. The emergence of methicillin-resistant *Staphylococcus aureus* infections in United States' hospitals. Ann Intern Med 1982;97:297–308.
81. Walsh TJ, Vlahov D, Hansen SL, et al. Prospective surveillance in control of nosocomial methicillin-resistant *Staphylococcus aureus.* Infect Control 1987;8:7–14.
82. Schwabe RS, Stapleton JT, Gilligon PH. Emergence of vancomycin resistance in coagulase-negative staphylococci. N Engl J Med 1987;316:927–931.
83. Lowry FD, Hammer SM. *Staphylococcus epidermidis* infection. Ann Intern Med 1983;99:834–839.
84. Joshi J, Newman K, Tenny J, et al. *Staphylococcus epidermidis* pneumonia in granulocytopenic patients with acute leukemia. Proc Am Soc Clin Oncol 1983;2:90.
85. Thaler M, Gill V, Pizzo PA. Staphylococcal bacteremias in a cancer research hospital. Proceedings of the 26th Interscience Conference on Antimicrobial Agents and Chemotherapy, New Orleans, 1986.
86. Rubin M, Hathorn JW, Marshall D, et al. Gram-positive infections and the use of vancomycin in 550 episodes of fever and neutropenia. Ann Intern Med 1988;108:30–35.
87. Pizzo PA, Ladish SL, Witebsky F. Alpha-hemolytic streptococci: Clinical significance in cancer patients. Med Pediatr Oncol 1978;4:367–370.
88. Cohen J, Donnelly JP, Worsley AM, et al. Septicemia caused by viridans streptococci in neutropenic patients with leukaemia. Lancet 1983;2:1452–1454.
89. Von Etta LL, Filica GA, Ferguson RM, et al. *Corynebacterium equi:* A review of 12 cases of human infection. Rev Infect Dis 1983;5:1012–1018.
90. Hande KR, Witebsky FG, Brown MS, et al. Sepsis with a new species of *Cornyebacterium.* Ann Intern Med 1976;85:423–426.
91. Berg R, Chmel H, Mayo J, et al. *Corynebacterium equi* infection complicating neoplastic disease. Am J Clin Pathol 1977;68:73–77.
92. Gill VJ, Manning C, Lamson M, et al. Antibiotic-resistant group JK bacteria in hospitals. J Clin Microbiol 1982;13:472–477.
93. Thaler M, Gill V, Pizzo PA. Emergence of *Clostridium tertium* as a pathogen in neutropenic patients. Am J Med 1986;81:596–600.
94. Cotton DJ, Gu V, Hiemenz J, et al. *Bacillus* bacteremias in an immunocompromised patient population: Clinical features, therapeutic interventions, and relationship to chronic intravascular catheters in sixteen cases. J Clin Microbiol 1987;25:672–674.
95. Harsburg CR Jr. Mycobacaterium avium complex infection in the acquired immunodeficiency syndrome. N Engl J Med 1991;324:1332–1338.
96. Macher AM, Kovacs JA, Gill V, et al. Bacteremia due to *Mycobacterium avium-intracellulare* in the acquired immunodeficiency syndrome. Ann Intern Med 1983;99:782–785.
97. Hoy JF, Rolston KVI, Hopfer RL, et al. *Mycobacterium fortuitum* bacteremia in patients with cancer and long-term venous catheters. Am J Med 1987;83:213–217.
98. Walsh T, Pizzo PA. Nosocomial mycoses in immunocompromised patients. Annu Rev Microbiol (in press).
99. Macher AM. Infection in the acquired immunodeficiency syndrome. In: Fauci AJ, moderator. Acquired immunodeficiency syndrome: Epidemiologic, clinical, immunologic, and therapeutic considerations. Ann Intern Med 1984;100:92–106.
100. Walsh TJ, Newman KR, Moody M, et al. Trichosporonosis in patients with neoplastic disease. Medicine (Baltimore) 1986;65:268–279.
101. Hamilton JR, Overall JC, Glasgow LA. Synergistic effect on mortality in mice with murine cytomegalovirus and *Pseudomonas aeruginosa, Staphylococcus aureus* or *Candida albicans* infections. Infect Immunol 1976;14:982–989.
102. Rand KH, Pollard RB, Merigan TC. Increased pulmonary superinfections in cardiac transplant patients undergoing primary cytomegalovirus infection. N Engl J Med 1978;298:951–953.
103. Browder AA, Hoff JA, Petersdorf RG. The significance of fever in neoplastic disease. Ann Intern Med 1961;55:932–942.
104. Goodman R, Jaffe N, Filler R, et al. Herpes zoster in children with stage I–III Hodgkin's disease. Radiology 1976;118:429–431.
105. Kaplan MS, Rosen PP, Armstrong D. Cryptococcosis in a cancer hospital. Clinical and pathological correlates in forty-six patients. Cancer 1977;39:2265–2274.
106. Winston DJ, Gale RP, Meyer DV. Infectious complications of human bone marrow transplantation. Medicine (Baltimore) 1979;58:1–31.
107. Sickles EA, Green WH, Wiernik PH. Clinical presentation of infection in granulocytopenic patients. Arch Intern Med 1975;135:715–719.
108. Schimpff SC, Satterlee W, Young VM, et al. Empiric therapy with carbenicillin and gentamicin for febrile patients with cancer and granulocytopenia. N Engl J Med 1971;284:1061–1065.
109. Markman M, Abeloff M. Management of hematologic and infectious complications of intensive induction therapy for small cell carcinoma of the lung. Am J Med 1983;74:741–746.
110. Pizzo PA, Robichaud KJ, Wesley R, et al. Fever in the pediatric and young adult patient with cancer. A prospective study of 1001 episodes. Medicine (Baltimore) 1982;61:153–165.
110a. Hughes WT, Armstrong D, Bodey GP, et al. Guidelines for the use of antimicrobial agents in neutropenic patients with unexplained fever. A statement by The Infectious Disease Society of America. J Infect Dis 1990;161:381–396.
110b. Pizzo PA, Armstrong D, Bodey GP, et al. The design, analysis and reporting of clinical trials in the empirical antibiotic management of the neutropenic patient. J Infect Dis 1990;161:397–401.
111. The EORTC International Antimicrobial Therapy Project Group. Three antibiotic regimens in the treatment of infection in febrile granulocytopenic patients with cancer. J Infect Dis 1978;137:14–29.
112. Pizzo PA, Hathorn JW, Hiemenz JW, et al. A randomized trial comparing ceftazidime alone with combination antibiotic therapy in cancer patients with fever and neutropenia. N Engl J Med 1986;315:552–558.
113. Anstall HB, Coleman RE. Donor-leukocyte imaging in granulocytopenic patients with suspected abscesses: Concise communication. J Nucl Med 1978;23:319–321.
114. Dutcher JP, Schiffer CA, Johnston GS. Rapid migration of ^{111}In-labelled granulocytes to sites of infection. N Engl J Med 1981;304:586–589.
115. Rubin E, Farber JL. Pathology. Philadelphia: JB Lippincott, 1988.
116. Walsh TJ, Hathorn JW, Sobel JD, et al. Antigenemia due to Candida enolase during invasive candidiasis in patients with neoplastic diseases: A prospective multicenter study. N Engl J Med 1991;324:1026–1031.
117. McCabe WR, Jackson GG. Gram-negative bacteremia. Arch Intern Med 1982;110:847–855.
118. Bryant RE, Hood AF, Hood CE, et al. Factors affecting mortality of gram-negative bacteremia. Arch Intern Med 1971;127:120–128.
119. Love LJ, Schimpff SC, Schiffer CA, et al. Improved prognosis for granulocytopenic patients with gram-negative bacteremia. Am J Med 1980;68:643–648.
120. Schimpff SC. Overview of empiric antiobiotic therapy for the febrile neutropenic patient. Rev Infect Dis 1985;7(suppl 4):5734–5740.

121. Pizzo PA, Thaler M, Hathorn J, et al. New β-lactamase antibiotics in the granulocytopenic patient: New options and new questions. Am J Med 1985;79:75–82.
122. Huijgens PC, Ossenkoppele GJ, Weijers TF, et al. Imipenem-citastatin for empirical therapy in neutropenic patients with fever: An open study in patients with hematologic malignancies. Eur J Haematol 1991;46:42–46.
123. Neu HC. β-lactam antibiotics: Structural relationships affecting in vitro activity and pharmacologic properties. Rev Infect Dis 1986;8(suppl 3):S237–S259.
124. The EORTC International Antimicrobial Therapy Cooperative Group. Ceftazidime combined with a short or long course of amikacin for empirical therapy of gram-negative bacteremia in cancer patients with granulocytopenia. N Engl J Med 1987;317:1692–1698.
125. Pizzo PA. After empiric therapy. What to do until the granulocyte comes back. Rev Infect Dis 1987;9:214–219.
126. DePauw BE, Kauw F, Muytjens H, et al. Randomized study of ceftazidime versus gentamicin plus cefotaxime for infections in severely granulocytopenic patients. J Antimicrob Chemother 1983;12(suppl A):593–599.
127. Young L. Empirical antimicrobial therapy in the neutropenic host. N Engl J Med [Editorial] 1986;315:580–581.
128. Karp JE, Dick JD, Angelopoulos C, et al. Empiric use of vancomycin during prolonged treatment-induced granulocytopenia. Randomized, double-blind, placebo-controlled clinical trial in patients with acute leukemia. Am J Med 1986;81:237–242.
129. Kramer BJ, Ramphal R, Rand K. Randomized comparison between two ceftazidime containing regimens and cephalothin-gentamicin-carbenicillin in febrile granulocytopenic cancer patients. Antimicrob Agents Chemother 1986;30:64–68.
130. Shenep JL, Hughes WT, Roberson PK, et al. Vancomycin, ticarcillin and amikacin compared with ticarcillin-clavulanate and amikacin in the empirical treatment of febrile neutropenic children with cancer. N Engl J Med 1988;317:1053.
131. Rubin M, Hathorn JW, Marshall D, Gress J, Steinberg S, Pizzo PA. Gram-positive infections and the use of vancomycin in 550 episodes of fever and neutropenia. Ann Intern Med 1988;108:88–100.
132. European Organization for Research and Treatment of Cancer (EORTC), International Antimicrobial Therapy Cooperative Group and the National Cancer Institute of Canada-Clinical Trials Group. Vancomycin added to empirical combination therapy for fever in granulocytopenic cancer patients. J Infect Dis 1991;163:951–958.
133. Novakova I, Donnelly JP, DePauw B. Ceftazidime as monotherapy or combined with teicoplanin for initial empiric treatment of presumed bacteremia in febrile granulocytopenic patients. Antimicrob Agents Chemother 1991;35:672–678.
134. Dybedal I, Lomuik J. Respiratory insufficiency in acute leukemia following treatment with cytosine arabinoside and septicemia with *Streptococcus viridans*. Eur J Hematol 1989;42:405–406.
135. Sobel J. Imipenem and aztreonam. Infect Dis Clin North Am 1989;3:613–24.
136. Neu H. Aztreonam activity, pharmacology, and clinical uses. Am J Med 1990;88(suppl 3C):2S–6S.
137. Neu H. The quinolones. Infect Dis Clin North Am 1989;3:625–39.
138. Smith G, Leyland M, Farrell I, Geddes A. A clinical, microbiological and pharmacokinetic study of ciprofloxacin plus vancomycin as initial therapy of febrile episodes in neutropenic patients. J Antimicrob Chemother 1988;21:647–55.
140. Mullen CA, Buchanan GR. Early hospital discharge of children with cancer treated for fever and neutropenia: Identification and management of the low-risk patient. J Clin Oncol 1990, 8:12;1998–2004.
141. Pizzo PA, Robichaud KJ, Gill FA, et al. Duration of empiric antibiotic therapy in granulocytopenic cancer patients. Am J Med 1979;67:194–200.
142. Pizzo PA, Commers J, Cotton D, et al. Approaching the controversies in the antibacterial management of cancer patients. Am J Med 1984;76:436–449.
143. Cotton D, Marshall D, Gress J, et al. Pathogen-specific vs broad-spectrum antibiotics for granulocytopenic patients with proven infection. Proceedings of the 24th Interscience Conference on Antimicrobial Agents and Chemothererapy, Washington, DC, 1984:158.
144. Walsh TJ, Pizzo PA. Fungal infections in granulocytopenic patients: Current approaches to classification, diagnosis, and treatment. In: Holmberg K, Meyer R, eds. Diagnosis and therapy of systemic fungal infections. New York: Raven Press, 1989:47–70.
145. Walsh TJ, Lee J, Lecciones J, et al. Empiric therapy with amphotericin B in febrile granulocytopenic patients. Rev Infect Dis 1991;13:496–503.
146. Pizzo PA, Robichaud RJ, Gill FA, et al. Empiric antiobiotic and antifungal therapy for cancer patients with prolonged fever and granulocytopenia. Am J Med 1982;72:101–111.
147. EORTC International Antimicrobial Therapy Cooperative Group. Empiric Antifungal Therapy in Febrile Granulocytopenic Patients. Am J Med 1989;86:668–672.
148. Walsh TJ, Rubin M, Hathorn J, et al. Amphotericin B vs high-dose ketoconazole for empirical antifungal therapy among febrile, granulocytopenic cancer patients: A prospective, randomized study. Arch Intern Med 1991;151:765–770.
149. Fluconazole. Med Lett 1990;32:50–52.
150. Meunier F, Aoun M, Gerard M. Therapy for oropharyngeal candidiasis in the immunocompromised host: A randomized double-blind study of fluconazole vs. ketoconazole. Rev Infect Dis 1990;12(suppl 13):364–368.
151. Navarro E, Lecciones JA, Lee JW, et al. Invasive pulmonary aspergillosis developing during empirical antifungal therapy in febrile cancer patients (in press).
152. Klein RS, Catalona MT, Edberg SC, et al. *Streptococcus bovis* septicemia and carcinoma of the colon. Ann Intern Med 1979;91:560–562.
153. Mueller B, Skelton J, Callender D, et al. A prospective randomized trial comparing the infectious and non-infectious complications of externalized (Hickman-Broviac) versus subcutaneously implanted (Port-a-Cath) devices in cancer patients. J Clin Oncol 1992;10:1943–1948.
154. Pizzo PA, Ladisch SL, Robichaud K. Treatment of gram-positive septicemia in cancer patients. Cancer 1980;45:206–207.
155. Bone RC, Fisher CJ, Clemmer TP, et al. A controlled clinical trial of high-dose methylprednisolone in the treatment of severe sepsis and septic shock. N Engl Med 1987;317:653–658.
156. Bernard GR, Luce JM, Sprung CL, et al. High-dose corticosteroids in patients with the adult respiratory distress syndrome. N Engl J Med 1987;317:1565–1570.
157. Frederick J, Braude AI. Anaerobic infection of the paranasal sinuses. N Engl J Med 1974;290:135–137.
158. Caplan ES, Hoyt NJ. Nosocomial sinusitis. JAMA 1982;247:639–641.
159. McGill TJ, Simpson G, Healy GB. Fulminant aspergillosis of the nose and paranasal sinuses: A new clinical entity. Laryngoscope 1980;90:748–754.
160. Meyer RD, Rosen P, Armstrong D. Phycomycosis complicating leukemia and lymphoma. Ann Intern Med 1972;77:871–879.
161. Eden OB, Santos J. Effective treatment for rhinopulmonary mucormycosis in a boy with leukemia. Arch Dis Child 1979;54:557–559.
162. Viollier AF, DeJongh C, Newman K, et al. *Aspergillus* sinusitis in cancer patients. Proceedings of the 21st Interscience Conference on Antimicrobial Agents and Chemotherapy, Chicago, Illinois, 1981:801.
163. Mahoney DH, Steuber CP, Starling KA, et al. An outbreak of aspergillosis in children with acute leukemia. J Pediatr 1979;95:70–71.
164. Berkow RL, Weisman SJ, Provisor AJ, et al. Invasive aspergillosis of paranasal tissues in children with malignancies. J Pediatr 1983;103:49–53.
165. Swerdlow B, Doresinski S. Development of *Aspergillus* sinusitis in a patient receiving amphotericin B. Treatment with granulocyte transfusions. Am J Med 1984;76:162–166.
166. Mayosmith MF, Hirsch PJ, Wodzinski SF, et al. Acute epiglottitis in adults. An eight-year experience in the state of Rhode Island. N Engl J Med 1986;314:1133–1139.
167. Cole S, Zawin M, Lundberg B, et al. *Candida* epiglottitis in an adult with acute non-lymphocytic leukemia. Am J Med 1987;82:662–663.
168. Walsh TJ, Gray W. *Candida* epiglottitis in immunocompromised patients. Chest 1987;9:482–485.
169. Arnow PM, Chou T, Weil D, et al. Nosocomial legionnaires: Disease caused by aerosolized tap water from respiratory devices. J Infect Dis 1982;146:460–467.
170. Helms CM, Massanari RM, Zeitter R, et al. Legionnaires' disease associated with a hospital water system: A cluster of 24 nosocomial cases. Ann Intern Med 1983;99:172–178.
171. Grayston TJ, Kuo CC, Wong SP, et al. A new *Chlamydia psittaci* strain, TWAR, isolated in acute respiratory tract infections. N Engl J Med 1986;315:161–168.
172. Marrie TJ, Grayston JT, Wong SP, et al. Pneumonia associated with the TWAR strain of *Chlamydia*. Ann Intern Med 1987;106:507–511.
173. Ramsey PG, Fife KH, Hackman RC, et al. Herpes simplex virus pneumonia: Clinical, virological and pathological features in 20 patients. Ann Intern Med 1982;97:813–820.
174. Barnes PF, Block AB, Davidson PT, Snider DE Jr. Tuberculosis in patients with human immunodeficiency virus infection. N Engl J Med 1991;324:1644–1650.
175. Daley CL, Small PM, Schecter GF, et al. An outbreak of tuberculosis with accelerated progression among persons infected with the human immunodeficiency virus. An analysis using restriction-fragment-length polymorphisms. N Engl J Med 1992;326:231–235.
176. Feld R, Bodey GP, Groschel D. Mycobacteriosis in patients with malignant disease. Arch Intern Med 1976;136:67–70.
177. Ludmerer KM, Kissnae JM. Fulminant pneumonia and death in an immunocompromised woman. Am J Med 1983;75:1043–1052.
178. Stover DE, Zamm MB, Hajdu SI, et al. Bronchoalveolar lavage in the diagnosis of diffuse pulmonary infiltrates in the immunocompromised host. Ann Intern Med 1984;101:1–6.
179. Thorpe JE, Baughman RP, Frame PT, et al. Bronchoalevolar lavage for diagnosing acute bacterial pneumonia. J Infect Dis 1987;155:855–861.
180. Kahn FW, Jones JM. Diagnosing bacterial respiratory infection by bronchoalveolar lavage. J Infect Dis 1987;155:862–869.
181. Levine SJ, Stover DE. Bronchoscopy and related techniques. In: Shelhamer J, Pizzo PA, Parrillo JR, Masur H, eds. Respiratory disease in the immunosuppressed host. Philadelphia: JB Lippincott, 1991:94–104.
182. Meyer RD, Ching WTW. *Legionella* pneumonia. In: Shelhamer J, Pizzo PA, Parrillo JR, Masur H, eds. Respiratory disease in the immunosuppressed host. Philadelphia: JB Lippincott, 1991:286–297.
183. Goldberg MB, Simm HB. Pneumonia due to *Nocardia* and *Actinomyces*. In: Shelhamer J, Pizzo PA, Parrillo JR, Masur H, eds. Respiratory disease in the immunosuppressed host. Philadelphia: JB Lippincott, 1991:330–337.
184. Jones JM. Pneumonia due to *Candida, Aspergillus* and *Mucaroles* species. In: Shelhamer J, Pizzo PA, Parrillo JR, Masur H, eds. Respiratory disease in the immunosuppressed host. Philadelphia: JB LIppincott, 1991:338–354.
185. Commers JC, Robichaud K, Pizzo PA. New pulmonary infiltrates in granulocytopenic patients being treated with antibiotics. Pediatr Infect Dis 1984;3:423–428.
186. Edwards JE. *Candida* endophthalmitis. In: Remington JS, Swartz MN, eds. Current clinical topics in infectious diseases. New York: McGraw Hill, 1982:381–397.
187. Yu VL, Muder RR, Poorsattar A. Significance of isolation of *Aspergillus* from the respiratory tract in diagnosis of invasive pulmonary aspergillosis. Results from a three-year prospective study. Am J Med 1986;81:249–251.
188. Burch PA, Karp JE, Merz WG, et al. Favorable outcome of invasive aspergillosis in patients with acute leukemia. J Clin Oncol 1987;5:1985–1993.
189. Lopez-Berestein G, Bodey GP, Fainstein V, et al. Treatment of systemic fungal infections with liposomal amphotericin B. Arch Intern Med 1989;149:2533–2536.

190. Drutz DJ. Pneumonia due to endemic fungi. In: Shelhamer J, Pizzo PA, Parrillo JR, Masur H, eds. Respiratory disease in the immunosuppressed host. Philadelphia: JB Lippincott, 1991:355–385.
191. Medoff G. Controversial areas in antifungal chemotherapy: Short course and combination therapy with amphotericin B. Rev Infect Dis 1987;9:403–407.
192. Bennett JE, Dismukes WE, Duma RJ, et al. Amphotericin B flucytosine in cryptococcal meningitis. N Engl J Med 1979;301:126–131.
193. Dismukes WE, Cloud G, Gallis HA, et al. Treatment of cryptococcal meningitis with combination amphotericin B and flucytosine for four as compared with six weeks. N Engl J Med 1987;317:334–341.
194. Thaler M, Bacher J, O'Leary T, et al. Evaluation of single-drug and combination antifungal therapy in an experimental model of candidiasis in rabbits with prolonged neutropenia. J Infect Dis 1988;158:80–88.
195. Bennett JF. Flucytosine. Ann Intern Med 1977;86:319–322.
196. Stiller RL, Bennett JE, Scholer HJ, et al. Correlation of in vitro susceptibility test results with in vivo response: Flucytosine therapy in a systemic candidiasis model. J Infect Dis 1983;147:1070–1077.
197. Saag MS, Dismukes WE. Azole antifungal agents: Emphasis on new triazoles. Antimicrob Agents Chemother 1988;32:1–8.
198. Shechtman LB, Funaro L, Robin T, et al. Clotrimazole treatment of oral candidiasis in patients with neoplastic disease. Am J Med 1984;76:91–91.
199. Masur H. *Pneumocystis carinii* pneumonia. In: Shelhamer J, Pizzo PA, Parrillo JR, Masur H, eds. Respiratory disease in the immunosuppressed host. Philadelphia: JB Lippincott, 1991:409–427.
200. Meuwissen JH, Tauber I, Leewenberg AD, et al. Parasitologic and serologic observations of infection with *Pneumocystis* in humans. J Infect Dis 1977;136:4349.
201. Ruebush TK, Weinstein RA, Baehner RL, et al. An outbreak of *Pneumocystis* pneumonia in children with acute lymphocyte leukemia. Am J Dis Child 1978;132:143–148.
202. Browne M, Hubbard SM, Longo DL, et al. Excess prevalence of *Pneumocystis carinii* pneumonia in lymphoma patients with chemotherapy. Ann Intern Med 1986;104:338–344.
203. Kovacs JA, Hiemenz JW, Macher AM, et al. *Pneumocystis carinii* pneumonia: A comparison of clinical features in patients with the acquired immune deficiency syndrome and patients with other immune diseases. Ann Intern Med 1984;100:663–671.
204. Lipschik GY, Kovacs JA. Sputum evaluation and nonbronchoscopic lavage. In: Shelhamer J, Pizzo PA, Parrillo JR, Masur H, eds. Respiratory disease in the immunosuppressed host. Philadelphia: JB Lippincott, 1991:64–72.
205. Browne MJ, Potter D, Gress J, et al. A randomized trial of open lung biopsy versus empiric antimicrobial therapy in cancer patients with diffuse pullmonary infiltrates. J Clin Oncol 1990;8:222–229.
206. Masur H. Prevention and treatment of Pneumocystis pneumonia. N Engl J Med 1992;327:1853–1860.
207. Gagnon S, Boota AM, Fischl MA, et al. Corticosteroids as adjunctive therapy for severe *Pneumocystis carinii* pneumonia in the acquired immunodeficiency syndrome. N Engl J Med 1990;323:1444–1450.
208. Bozzette SA, Sattler FR, Chiu J, et al. A controlled trial of early adjunctive treatment with corticosteroids for *Pneumocystis carinii* pneumonia in the acquired immunodeficiency syndrome. N Engl J Med 1990;323:1451–1457.
209. Burt ME, Flye MW, Webber BL, et al. Prospective evaluation of aspiration needle, cutting needle, transbronchial and open lung biopsy in patients with pulmonary infiltrates. Ann Thorac Surg 1981;32:146–153.
210. McCabe RE, Remington JS. Open lung biopsy. In: Shelhamer J, Pizzo PA, Parrillo JR, Masur H, eds. Respiratory disease in the immunosuppressed host. Philadelphia: JB Lippincott, 1991:105–117.
211. Schooley RT. Pneumonia due to herpesviruses. In: Shelhamer J, Pizzo PA, Parrillo JR, Masur H, eds. Respiratory disease in the immunosuppressed host. Philadelphia: JB Lippincott, 1991:386–397.
212. Crawford JW, Meyers JD. Respiratory disease in bone marrow transplant patients. In: Shelhamer J, Pizzo PA, Parrillo JR, Masur H, eds. Respiratory disease in the immunosuppressed host. Philadelphia: JB Lippincott, 1991:595–623.
213. Meyers JD, Flournoy N, Thomas ED. Risk factors for cytomegalovirus infection after human marrow transplantation. J Infect Dis 1986;153:478–488.
214. Gleaves CA, Meyers JD. Rapid diagnosis of invasive cytomegalovirus infection by examination of tissue specimens in centrifugation culture. Am J Clin Pathol 1987;88:354–358.
215. Emanuel D, Cunningham I, Jules-Elysee K, et al. Cytomegalovirus pneumonia after bone marrow transplantation successfully treated with the combination of ganciclovir and high dose intravenous immune globulin. Ann Intern Med 1988;109:777–782.
216. Reed EC, Bowden RA, Dandliker PS, Lilleby KE, Meyers JD. Treatment of cytomegalovirus pneumonia with ganciclovir and intravenous cytomegalovirus immunoglobulin in patients with bone marrow transplantation. Ann Intern Med 1988;109:783–788.
217. Meyers JD, Reed EC, Shepp DH, et al. Acyclovir for prevention of cytomegalovirus infection and disease after allogeneic marrow tansplantation. N Engl J Med 1988;318:70–75.
218. Schmidt GM, Horak DA, Niland JC, et al. A randomized, controlled trial of prophylactic ganciclovir for cytomegalovirus pulmonary infection in recipients of allogeneic bone marrow transplants N Engl J Med 1991;324:1005–1011.
219. Dolin R. Pneumonia caused by viruses other than herpes viruses. In: Shelhamer J, Pizzo PA, Parillo JR, Masur H, eds. Respiratory disease in the immunosuppressed host. Philadelphia: JB Lippincott, 1991:398–408.
220. Smith DW, Frankel LR, Mathers LH, et al. A controlled trial of aerosolized ribavirin in infants receiving mechanical ventilation for severe respiratory syncytial virus infections. N Engl J Med 1991;325:24–29.
221. Ladisch S, Pizzo PA. *S. aureus* sepsis in children with cancer. Pediatrics 1978;61:231–234.
222. Peterson DE, Minah GE, Overholser CD, et al. Microbiology of acute periodontal infection in myelosuppressed cancer patients. J Clin Oncol 1987;5:1461–1468.
223. Meyers JD, Wade JC, Mitchell CD, et al. Multicenter collaborative trial of intravenous acyclovir for the treatment of mucocutaneous herpes simplex virus infection in the immunocompromised host. Am J Med 1982;73:229–235.
224. Whitley RJ, Spruance S, Hayden FC, et al (NIAID Collaborative Antiviral Study Group). Vidarabine therapy for mucocutaneous herpes simplex virus infection in the immunocompromised host. J Infect Dis 1984;149:1–8.
225. Shepp DH, Newton BA, Dandliker PS, et al. Oral acyclovir therapy for mucocutaneous herpes simplex virus infections in immunocompromised marrow transplant recipients. Ann Intern Med 1985;102:783–785.
226. Whitley RJ, Levin M, Barton N, et al. Infections caused by herpes simplex virus in the immunocompromised host: Natural history and topical acyclovir therapy. J Infect Dis 1984;150:323–329.
227. Meyers JD, Flournoy N, Thomas ED. Infection with herpes simplex virus and cell-mediated immunity after marrow transplant. J Infect Dis 1980;142:338–346.
228. Saral R, Ambinder RF, Burns WH, et al. Acyclovir prophylaxis against herpes simplex virus infection in patients with leukemia. Ann Intern Med 1983;99:773–776.
229. Wade JC, Newton B, Flournoy N, et al. Oral acyclovir for prevention of herpes simplex virus reactivation after marrow transplant. Ann Intern Med 1984;100:823–828.
230. Ringden O, Heimdahl A, Lonnqvist B, et al. Decreased incidence of viridans streptococcal septicaemia in allogeneic bone marrow transplant recipients after the introduction of acyclovir. Lancet [Letter] 1984;1:744.
231. McDonald GB, Sharma P, Hackman RC, et al. Esophageal infections in immunosuppressed patients after marrow transplant. Gastroenterology 1985;88:1111–1117.
232. Walsh TJ, Belitsos N, Hamiltol SR. Bacterial esophagitis in immunocompromised patients. Arch Intern Med 1986;146:1345–1348.
233. Varki AP, Armitage JO, Feagler JR. Typhlitis in acute leukemia: Successful treatment by early surgical intervention. Cancer 1979;43:695–697.
234. Skibber JM, Matler GJ, Lotze MT, et al. Right lower quadrant complications in young patients with leukemia: A surgical perspective. Ann Surg 1987;206:711–716.
235. McFarland LV, Mulligan ME, Kwok RYY, Stamm WE. Nosocomial acquisition of Clostridium difficile infection. N Engl J Med 1989;320:204–210.
236. Armstrong D, Paredes J. Strongyloidiasis. In: Shelhamer J, Pizzo PA, Parrillo JR, Masur H, eds. Respiratory disease in the immunosuppressed host. Philadelphia: JB Lippincott, 1991:428–432.
237. Choo Q-L, Kuo G, Weiner AM, et al. Isolation of a cDNA clone derived from a blood-borne non-A, non-B viral hepatitis genome. Science 1989;244:359–362.
238. Hoofnagle JH, Mullen KD, Jones B, et al. Treatment of chronic non-A, non-B hepatitis with recombinant human alpha interferon. A perliminary report. N Engl J Med 1986;315:1575–1578.
239. Tabor E, Gerety JR, Mott M, et al. Prevalence of hepatitis B in a high-risk setting: A serologic study of patients and staff in a pediatric oncology unit. Pediatrics 1978;61:711–715.
240. Wade JC, Gaffey M, Wiernik PH, et al. Hepatitis in patients with acute nonlymphocytic leukemia. Am J Med 1983;75:413–422.
241. Berk PD, Jones A, Plotz PH, et al. Corticosteroid therapy for chronic active hepatitis. Ann Intern Med 1976;85:523–524.
242. Hoofnagle JH, Dusheiko GM, Schafer DF, et al. Reactivation of chronic hepatitis B virus infection by cancer chemotherapy. Ann Intern Med 1982;96:447–449.
243. Davis GL, Balart LA, Schiff ER, et al. Treatment of chronic hepatitis C with interferon alpha. A multicenter randomized, controlled trial. N Engl Med 1989;321:1501–1506.
244. After HJ, Purcell PH, Shih JW, et al. Detection of antibody to hepatitis C virus in prospectively followed transfusion recipients with acute and chronic non-A, non-B hepatitis. N Engl J Med 1989;321:1494–1500.
245. Haron E, Feld R. Tuffnell P, et al. Hepatic candidiasis: An increasing problem in immunocompromised patients. Am J Med 1987;83:17–26.
246. Thaler M, Pastakia B, Shawker TH, et al. Hepatic candidiasis in cancer patients: The evolving picture of the syndrome. Ann Intern Med 1988;108:88–100.
247. Kauffman CA, Bradley SF, Ross SC, Weber DR. Hepatosplenic candidiasis: Successful treatment with fluconazole. Am J Med 1991;91:137–141.
248. Anaissie E, Bodey GP, Kantarjian H, et al. Fluconazole therapy for chronic disseminated candidiasis in patients with leukemia and prior amphotericin B therapy. Am J Med 1991;91:142–150.
249. Glenn J, Cotton D, Wesley R, et al. Anorectal infections in patients with malignant diseases. Rev Infect Dis 1988;10:42–52.
250. Barnes SG, Sattler FR, Ballard JO. Improved survival after drainage of perirectal infections in patients with acute leukemia. Ann Intern Med 1984;100:515–518.
251. Kingston ME, Mackey D. Skin clues in the diagnosis of life-threatening infections. Rev Infect Dis 1986;8:1–11.
252. Whitley R, Hilty M, Haynes R, et al. Vidarabine therapy for varicella in immunosuppressed patients. J Pediatr 1982;101:125–131.
253. Prober CG, Kirk LE, Keeney RE. Acyclovir therapy of chickenpox in immunosuppressed children—a collaborative study. J Pediatr 1982;101:622–625.
254. Arvin AM, Feldman S, Merigan TC. Human leukocyte interferon in the treatment of varicella in children with cancer in preliminary controlled trial. Antimicrob Agents Chemother 1978;13:605–607.
255. Arvin AM, Kushner JH, Feldman S, et al. Human leukocyte interferon for the treatment of varicella in children with cancer. N Engl J Med 1985;306:761–765.
256. Takahashi M, Otsuka T, Okuno Y, et al. Live vaccine used to prevent the spread of varicella in children in the hospital. Lancet 1974;2:1288–1290.
257. Gershon A. Live attenuated varicella vaccine. J Pediatr 1987;110:154–157.

258. Shepp DH, Dandliker PS, Meyers JD. Treatment of varicella-zoster virus infection in severely immunocompromised patients: A randomized comparison of acyclovir and vidarabine. N Engl J Med 1986;314:208–212.
259. Rimailho A. Fulminant necrotizing fascitis and nonsteroidal anti-inflammatory drugs. J Infect Dis 1987;155:143–146.
260. Houff S, Major EO, Katz DA, et al. Involvement of JC virus-infected mononuclear cells from the bone marrow and spleen in the pathogenesis of progressive multifocal leukoencephalopathy. N Engl J Med 1988;318:301–305.
261. Pizzo PA. Considerations for preventing infectious complications in cancer patients. Rev Infect Dis 1989;11:S1551–S1563.
262. Nauseef WM, Maki DG. A study of the value of simple protective isolation in patients with granulocytopenia. N Engl J Med 1981;304:448–453.
263. Kotilainen P, Nikoskelainen J, Huovinen P. Emergence of ciprofloxacin-resistant coagulase-negative staphylococcal skin flora in immunocompromised patients receiving ciprofloxacin. J Infect Dis 1990; 161:41–44.
264. Pizzo PA. Antibiotic prophylaxis in the immunosuppressed patient with cancer. In: Remington JS, Swartz MN, eds. Current clinical topics in infectious Diseases. 4th ed. New York: McGraw Hill, 1983:153–167.
265. Van der Waaij D, Berghuis de Vries JN, Lekkerkerk van der Wees JEC, et al. Colonization resistance of the digestive tract in conventional and antibiotic treated mice. J Hyg (Lond) 1971;69:405–411.
266. Van der Waaij D, Berghuis de Vries JN. Selective elimination of enterobacteriae species from the digestive tract in mice and monkeys. J Hyg (Lond) 1974;72:205–211.
267. Guiot HFL, van der Brock PJ, van der Meer JWM, et al. Selective antimicrobial modulation of the intestinal flora of patients with acute nonlymphocytic leukemia. A double-blind placebo-controlled study. J Infect Dis 1983;147:615–623.
268. Sleijfer DT, Mulder NK, de Vries-Hospers HG, et al. Infection prevention in granulocytopenic patients by selective decontamination of the digestive tract. Eur J Cancer 1980;16:859–869.
269. Gurwith MJ, Brunton JL, Lank BA. A prospective controlled investigation of prophylactic trimethoprim-sulfamethoxazole in hospitalized granulocytopenic patients. Am J Med 1979;66:248–256.
270. Pizzo PA, Robichaud KJ, Edwards BK, et al. Oral antibiotic prophylaxis in patients with cancer: A double-blind randomized placebo-controlled trial. J Pediatr 1983;102: 125–133.
271. Weiser B, Lange M, Fialkow MA, et al. Prophylactic trimethoprim-sulfamethaxozole during consolidated chemotherapy for acute leukemia: A controlled trial. Ann Intern Med 1981;95:436–438.
272. Dekker A, Rozenberg-Arska M, Sixma JJ, et al. Prevention of infection by trimethoprim-sulfamethoxazole plus amphotericin B in patients with acute nonlymphocytic leukemia. Ann Intern Med 1981;95:555–559.
273. Kauffman CA, Leipman MJ, Bergman AG, et al. Trimethoprim-sulfamethoxazole prophylaxis in neutropenic patients: Reduction of infections and effect on bacterial and fungal flora. Am J Med 1983;74:599–607.
274. Gaultieri RJ, Donowitz GR, Kaiser CE, et al. Double-blind randomized study of prophylactic trimethoprim-sulfamethaxozole in granulocytopenic patients with hematoloic malignancies. Am J Med 1983;74:934–940.
275. Wade JC, DeJongh CA, Newman KA, et al. Selective antimicrobial modulation as prophylaxis against infection during granulocytopenia: Trimethoprim-sulfamethoxazole versus nalidixic acid. J Infect Dis 1983;147:624–634.
276. Wilson JM, Guinery DG. Failure of oral trimethoprim-sulfamethoxazole prophylaxis in acute leukemia: Isolation of resistant plasmids from strains of enterobacteriaceae causing bacteremia. N Engl J Med 1982;306:16–20.
277. Karp JE, Merz WG, Hendricksen C, et al. Oral Norfloxacin for prevention of gram-negative bacterial infections in patients with acute leukemia and granulocytopenia. Ann Intern Med 1987;106:1–7.
278. Dekker AW, Rozenberg-Arska M, Verhoef J. Infection prophylaxis in acute leukemia: A comparison of cifrofloxacin with trimethoprim-sulfamethoxazole and colistin. Ann Intern Med 1987;106:7–12.
279. Meunier F. Prevention of mycoses in immunocompromised patients. Rev Infect Dis 1987;9:408–416.
280. Saral R, Bruns WH, Laskin OL, et al. Acyclovir prophylaxis of herpes simplex virus infections: A randomized, double-blind controlled trial in bone marrow transplant recipients. N Engl J Med 1981;305:63–67.
281. Zeigler EKJ, Fisher CJ, Sprung CL, et al. Treatment of gram-negative bacteremia and septic shock with HA-1A human monocular antibody against endotoxin. N Engl J Med 1991;324:429–436.
282. Cooperative Group for the Study of Immunoglobulin in Chronic Lymphocytic Leukemia. Intravenous immunoglobulin for the prevention of infection in chronic lymphocytic leukemia: A randomized, controlled clinical trial. N Engl J Med 1988;319: 902–907.
283. Weeks JC, Tierney MR, Weinstein MC. Cost effectiveness of prophylactic intravenous immune globulin in chronic lymphocytic leukemia. N Engl J Med 1991;325:81–86.
284. Sullivan KM, Kopecky KJ, Jocom J, et al. Immunomodulatory and antimicrobial efficacy of intravenous immunoglobulin in bone marrow transplantation. N Engl J Med 1990;323:705–712.
285. Crawford J, Ozer H, Stoller R, et al. Reduction by granulocyte colony-stimulating factor of fever and neutropenia induced by chemotherapy in patients with small-cell lung cancer. N Engl J Med 1991;325:164–170.
286. Gabrilove J, Jakubowski A, Scher H, et al. Effect of granulocyte colony-stimulating factor on neutropenia and associated morbidity due to chemotherapy for transitional cell carcinoma of the urothelium. N Engl J Med 1988;318:1414–1422.
287. Brandt S, Peters W, Atwater S, et al. Effect of recombinant human granulocyte-macrophage colony-stimulating factor on hematopoietic reconstitution after high-dose chemotherapy and autologous bone marrow transplantation. N Engl J Med 1988;318:869–876.
288. Ohno R, Tomonaga M, Kobayashi T, et al. Effect of granulocyte colony-stimulating factor after intensive induction therapy in relapsed or refractory acute leukemia. N Engl J Med 1990;323:871–877.
289. Nemunaitis J, Rabinowe SN, Singer JW, et al. Recombinant granulocyte-macrophage colony-stimulating factor after autologous bone marrow transplantation for lymphoid cancer. N Engl J Med 1991;324:1773–1778.
290. Peters WP, Kurtzberg J, Kirkpatrick G, et al. GM-CSF primed peripheral blood progenitor cells coupled with autologous bone marrow transplantation will eliminate absolute leukopenia following high dose chemotherapy. Blood 1989;743(suppl 1): 50a.

Cancer: Principles & Practice of Oncology, Fourth Edition,
edited by Vincent T. DeVita, Jr., Samuel Hellman, Steven A. Rosenberg.
J.B. Lippincott Co., Philadelphia © 1993.

CHAPTER 63

Adverse Effects of Treatment

SECTION 1

RICHARD J. GRALLA

Antiemetic Therapy

Control of chemotherapy-induced emesis is a standard of care; however, this represents a marked change that has occurred over the past 10 to 12 years. This change resulted from oncologists recognizing the increasing need for emetic control and developing a logical clinical research program emphasizing careful methodology. Interest and advances in related basic sciences were then stimulated by the clinical improvements. Increased knowledge in neuropharmacology has further enhanced the control of emesis.

With the potential to achieve complete control of nausea and vomiting in most patients comes the responsibility of the clinician to possess a deeper understanding of the problem. This increases the likelihood of controlling emesis and permits more appropriate and cost-effective approaches.

Progress has included the recognition of different emetic problems, the identification of effective agents, the establishment of appropriate doses and schedules for these agents, the testing of combination regimens of greater efficacy, the synthesis of newer agents with an improved therapeutic index, and the application of a useful study methodology.

PHYSIOLOGY AND PHARMACOLOGY IN CONTROLLING EMESIS

The mechanism by which chemotherapy induces emesis is not completely understood. Older studies of Borison and McCarthy[1] have had an important influence that has provided a framework for further research. Questions that remain include: Why is there a delay from the administration of chemotherapy to the onset of emesis? Is it the chemotherapy drug itself, a metabolite, or a neurotransmitter that stimulates a receptor and causes emesis? Why do different chemotherapy agents with similar intracellular effects have such varying potentials for inducing emesis?

Studies support the hypothesis that emesis is caused by stimulation of receptors in the central nervous system or in the gastrointestinal tract. Receptor areas have been identified in the medulla that are of particular interest. An area called the *vomiting* or *emetic center* is found in the lateral reticular formation. Once receptors in this region are stimulated, the complicated act of vomiting then follows. An important area also located in the medulla is the chemoreceptor trigger zone (CTZ), in the area postrema.[2] The CTZ is sensitive to chemical stimuli from both the blood and the cerebrospinal fluid.

Chemotherapeutic agents, their metabolites, or a neurotransmitter may stimulate receptors (such as dopamine or serotonin receptors) in the CTZ. Impulses generated in the CTZ and transmitted to the vomiting center may then lead to the initiation of emesis. Neuroreceptors in the gastrointestinal tract, which has afferents to the vomiting center, may also play a role in chemotherapy-induced nausea and vomiting.

The theory developed that drugs that bind to neurotransmitter receptors in the CTZ, the vomiting center, or the gastrointestinal tract have the potential to interrupt the process leading to emesis. Interest initially focused on agents that bind to dopamine receptors in that these receptors are found in high concentration in the CTZ. In the 1950s and 1960s, agents such as phenothiazines, butyrophenones, and substituted benzamides, which affect these receptors, became available.

Early trials with phenothiazines indicated some antiemetic

activity. As newer chemotherapy agents with emesis as a prominent side effect were introduced, the marked limitations of the phenothiazines became apparent. Unlike the phenothiazines, the substituted benzamide metoclopramide can be given in high intravenous doses without causing hypotension or other hazardous side effects.[3] This method of administration of metoclopramide demonstrated a high degree of efficacy with this agent known to block dopamine (D2) receptors.

Although the effectiveness of high-dose metoclopramide represented an important improvement in the control of chemotherapy-induced emesis, it was not clear why the elevated doses of the agent proved so effective. Metoclopramide binds avidly to dopamine receptors, and it was thought that even small doses of the drug would saturate the receptors, eliminating the need for very high doses. An important clue came with the investigation of serotonin (5-hydroxytryptamine, or 5-HT) receptors.[4,5] Metoclopramide blocks serotonin receptors (specifically the type 3, or 5-HT3, receptor) but with less affinity than it has for dopamine receptors or than the newer agents have for 5-HT3 receptors.[6] Therefore, very high doses of metoclopramide are required for it to prevent emesis as a 5-HT3 antagonist. It appears that metoclopramide may have served in a transitional role between the older dopamine-blocking agents and the newer, more selective 5-HT3 antiemetics. The antiemetic activity of metoclopramide may be exerted primarily through 5-HT3 receptors, while its side effects are the result of its interaction with dopamine receptors.

Does the importance of the role of serotonin receptors help answer some of the questions remaining in the neuropharmacology of chemotherapy-induced emesis? It has been suggested that this phenomenon may be mediated by serotonin itself; that is, a chemotherapeutic agent may have a direct effect on the small bowel, resulting in the liberation of a large amount of endogenous serotonin. This liberated serotonin then stimulates the 5-HT3 receptors in the central nervous system, resulting in emesis. The effect of the serotonin may be mediated through vagal nerves or through direct stimulation of the receptors by an elevated blood level of serotonin.

Cisplatin causes many rapid physiologic alterations, and one of those is an increased excretion of 5-HIAA, indicating a liberation of endogenous serotonin.[7,8] Certainly, the increased levels of serotonin and the association with cisplatin indicate the possibility that the hypothesis may be correct. Several arguments remain against the hypothesis that serotonin liberation mediates chemotherapy-induced emesis. These objections include the following:

1. Although 5-HIAA excretion is increased after cisplatin, the increase is generally only double that of baseline (often remaining in the normal range) and far less than levels frequently observed in carcinoid syndrome.[9]
2. Emesis is not a prominent finding in carcinoid syndrome.[9]
3. If the lack of emesis in carcinoid is due to a decreased sensitivity after prolonged exposure to serotonin, it is curious that patients with malignant carcinoid treated with cisplatin often are troubled by emesis.
4. The reflex may be mediated by vagal afferents from the gut, yet after the radical vagotomy involved in esophagectomy, emesis still results with cisplatin treatment.[10]
5. If the liberation of serotonin after cisplatin were sufficient to cause emesis, the full carcinoid syndrome would likely occur, especially in patients given 5-HT3-blocking agents, which do not inhibit serotonin release[7,8] and only affect the type 3 serotonin receptor.

Many questions remain concerning the mediation of chemotherapy-induced emesis and the neuropharmacology of the phenomenon.

EMETIC PROBLEMS

In patients receiving chemotherapy, three types of emetic problems have been identified. Careful attention to which problem is to be treated or prevented is significant since causes of and treatments for the various problems may differ. These emetic syndromes include acute chemotherapy-induced emesis, delayed emesis, and anticipatory emesis. An additional problem is that patients may have emesis for reasons other than their chemotherapy.

Patients with cancer have a variety of reasons for emesis that are not associated with chemotherapy. Prominent causes are medications. These particularly involve pain medications, bronchodilators (especially long-acting preparations), and antibiotics. Other common problems causing emesis include intestinal obstruction, brain metastases, ileus, and azotemia. In these instances, adjustment of medications or treatment of the complications of the tumor may be more important than the selection of the proper antiemetic drug.

Most antiemetic studies have investigated acute chemotherapy-induced emesis. This is the major topic of the subsequent discussion, with separate sections concerning delayed and anticipatory emesis.

ACUTE CHEMOTHERAPY-INDUCED EMESIS

The chemotherapeutic agent, its dose, and the route of administration can affect the incidence of nausea and vomiting (Table 63–1). With most agents, emesis begins between 1 and 2 hours after starting chemotherapy, in patients who have not previously received chemotherapy. Important exceptions to this pattern occur with cyclophosphamide and carboplatin, which can cause a late onset of emesis (a problem different than delayed emesis, which is discussed later). When cyclophosphamide is given intravenously in high doses, emesis often does not begin until 9 to 18 hours after chemotherapy.[11] Several studies have indicated that carboplatin also induces a late onset of emesis.[12] Although carboplatin is somewhat less emetic than cisplatin, it still can cause significant nausea and vomiting. A recent report concluded that a similar degree of good antiemetic control could be achieved with either of these platinum-containing drugs if appropriate antiemetic regimens are used.[13]

The late onset of emesis emphasizes two important principles. First, to be effective, an antiemetic regimen must consider the individual pattern and potential for causing emesis of the chemotherapeutic drug. Second, when combination chemotherapy is used, each of the drugs must be individually considered. Therefore, a regimen that is effective against cisplatin may not be well designed for the patient receiving cy-

TABLE 63–1. Emetic Potential of 25 Chemotherapeutic Agents

Most likely to result in emesis	Cisplatin
↑	Dacarbazine
	Dactinomycin
	Nitrogen mustard
	Hexamethylmelamine
	Cyclophosphamide*
	Carboplatin*
	Lomustine
	Carmustine
	Doxorubicin
	Daunorubicin
	Idarubicin
	Ifosfamide
	Cytosine arabinoside
	Vinorelbine
	Mitomycin C
	Etoposide
	Vindesine
	Bleomycin
	Methotrexate
	5-Fluorouracil
	Chlorambucil
↓	Vincristine
Least likely to result in emesis	Vinblastine
	Tamoxifen

* Associated with the late onset of emesis.

clophosphamide. Careful testing of antiemetic regimens for particular chemotherapeutic combinations is necessary before acceptance of a regimen as a standard. Activity of the antiemetic at the receptor is of greater importance than simply the blood level of the drug.

The differences in the likelihood of chemotherapeutic drugs to result in emesis are given in Table 63–1. In general, the agents most often associated with emesis also induce the greatest severity of this side effect. Differences occur among patients and even among treatment courses in the same patient.

Emesis and its control are best studied in patients given cisplatin. This has occurred for several reasons. First, cisplatin causes emesis in all patients if effective antiemetics are not given, and it results in a median of over ten episodes in those receiving this agent in high doses. Second, cisplatin is an important neoplastic agent in several malignancies. Third, antiemetics effective against cisplatin are useful with chemotherapeutic agents of lesser emetic potential. Therefore, cisplatin provides a model for the testing of antiemetics for all chemotherapy treatment regimens.

DELAYED EMESIS

Early into the use of cisplatin, it was clear that all patients experienced nausea and vomiting.[10,14,15] This emesis cleared after several hours in many patients; however, others continued to be troubled for many days. These were not considered to be separate events until after effective antiemetic regimens were introduced and carefully studied. Delayed emesis is now defined as nausea or vomiting beginning 24 hours or more after chemotherapy administration.

This problem is best described in patients treated with high total doses of cisplatin (100 mg/m^2, or more, given as a single dose or over several days). Whether other agents or lower doses of cisplatin cause this problem is unknown; consequently, statements made about this phenomenon that are not based on patients receiving these high doses of cisplatin may not be appropriate to generalize. The time of observation for the onset of emesis (24 hours after chemotherapy) is arbitrary. The phenomenon may begin earlier in some patients, and this may be important in planning for prevention of the phenomenon.

A natural history study observed that delayed emesis is less severe than acute chemotherapy-induced emesis and is not simply a deferral of the acute problem to a later period.[16] Nonetheless, delayed emesis still causes a great deal of discomfort as well as difficulties with hydration and nutrition. Although it occurs less often in those patients who have complete emetic control on the day of chemotherapy, delayed emesis is not necessarily eliminated, even in this most favorable group. Most patients treated with cisplatin at doses greater than 100 mg/m^2 experience some degree of delayed emesis. The onset is most frequent 48 to 72 hours after chemotherapy,[16] and the phenomenon gradually diminishes over the next 1 to 3 days. Although treatment is not ideal, appropriate regimens, as discussed later, can significantly reduce the incidence of delayed emesis.

ANTICIPATORY EMESIS

This problem is defined as nausea or vomiting beginning before the administration of chemotherapy.[17] It typically occurs in patients with poor control of emesis with past chemotherapy. This poor control can be with acute chemotherapy-induced emesis or with delayed emesis. Since this is a conditioned response, the hospital environment or other treatment-related associations may trigger the onset of emesis. The administration of the chemotherapy itself may bring on this response as a chemical stimulus or as a psychologic factor. The various contributing factors illustrate the difficulty with the definition of the problem and with determining the incidence of anticipatory emesis. Patients who have emesis before chemotherapy may have greater difficulty, but those who have conditioned emesis after chemotherapy administration are also troubled. The poorer control observed with subsequent cycles of chemotherapy may, at least in part, be related to conditioning. Anxiety or insomnia 1 or 2 days before a scheduled treatment may be a less dramatic expression of the same phenomenon. The stronger the likelihood of emesis and the poorer the control, the greater is the chance of developing anticipatory emesis.[17,18]

CONTROL OF EMESIS AND PATIENT CHARACTERISTICS

Several aspects of a patient's prior experience or characteristics may influence emetic outcome. Studies to date have indicated that alcohol intake history, prior experience with

TABLE 63–2. Factors Associated With Control of Emesis

Patients
Emesis with past chemotherapy
Chronic alcohol use history
Gender
Age
Chemotherapy
Agent
Dose
Schedule
Route
Antiemetic
Agent
Dose
Schedule

chemotherapy, age, and gender are important factors (Table 63–2).

ALCOHOL INTAKE HISTORY

Studies have indicated that emesis is more easily controlled in patients with chronic heavy alcohol use histories (more than 100 g/day, or about five mixed drinks) than in those without this past experience.[19,20] In a prospective evaluation in 52 patients receiving high-dose cisplatin and an appropriate combination antiemetic regimen, 93% of those with the high alcohol history had no emesis, as opposed to 61% ($p < 0.01$) of the other patients.[19] Subsequent trials examining this variable have confirmed the greater ease of controlling emesis in this population.[21] Patients do not have to continue to use alcohol to be considered as having a high chronic alcohol history and to be easier to treat. Also, patients with this history are at high risk of having emesis if the most effective antiemetic regimens are not used; however, their response to these regimens is enhanced. The alcohol usage history needs to be outlined for each treatment group in comparison trials.

PRIOR CHEMOTHERAPY EXPERIENCE

Poor control of emesis with past courses of chemotherapy predisposes a patient to unsatisfactory antiemetic results with subsequent similar chemotherapy. A report[3] of a trial in which patients received their initial treatment with the same antiemetic noted that major control was three times more likely in those who had not previously had chemotherapy. Whether this is due to the development of conditioned anticipatory emesis or to other possible factors is not clear.

AGE

Older age appears not to be a direct concern with the control of emesis; instead, younger age implies a predilection to experience acute dystonic reactions when receiving antiemetics with dopamine-receptor blocking as a mechanism of action.[22] This category of antiemetics includes such valuable agents as substituted benzamides, butyrophenones, and phenothiazines. In a report[22] summarizing the experience of nearly 500 patients receiving metoclopramide, the incidence of trismus or torticollis was only 2% in those over 30 years of age; a 27% occurrence was reported in younger patients. In addition, when dopamine-blocking antiemetics are given on several consecutive days, dystonic reactions are also more common.[23] This can be especially important for younger patients in that several regimens for malignancies of this age group use chemotherapy on a daily schedule.

Many of the newer antiemetic agents exert their activity by blocking 5-HT3 receptors. Agents that are specific for this mechanism do not cause dystonic reactions. Although only a few pediatric studies with these agents have been conducted, the initial good results and lack of dystonic reactions already indicate that these are the drugs of choice for children receiving chemotherapy likely to result in emesis.

Formal antiemetic trials in older patients are unusual. Those patients over age 70 who have been treated with metoclopramide or ondansetron have generally tolerated the agents well at the same doses given to younger patients, and efficacy has been preserved. With the aging population in many continents and with the increasing incidence of many malignancies with age, formal analysis and testing of antiemetic regimens in the geriatric population is a mandatory objective for the near future.

GENDER

Several studies have suggested that it is more difficult to control emesis in women than in men. This is a complicated issue.[24] Women enlisted in antiemetic studies are more likely to be receiving two or more emetic agents given in combination (especially cisplatin plus cyclophosphamide) and are less likely to have histories of heavy alcohol usage. It is possible that factors other than gender are of greater importance in affecting the control of emesis. Multivariate analyses of large, well-conducted trials are needed to answer this question. One recent study suggests that gender is indeed an independent variable.[21]

NEW ANTIEMETIC AGENTS

Several agents have been synthesized that bind with greater affinity and specificity to 5-HT3 receptors than metoclopramide. As illustrated in Table 63–3, five agents (ondansetron, granisetron, tropisetron, dolasetron, and RG 12915) are at various stages of development. Factors varying among these agents include short (2- to 4-hour) versus moderate (9- to 16-hour) half-lives. Most of these drugs have good bioavailability, and studies only employing oral administration may prove useful.

Three of the agents are commercially available, and the remainder are in phase II or III trials. Research with this new class of antiemetic is directed toward preserving or improving the efficacy of metoclopramide and eliminating dopamine-related side effects.

Ondansetron has become widely available for the prevention of nausea and vomiting associated with emetic chemotherapy. In the United States, the dose and schedule recommended for ondansetron is 0.15 mg/kg intravenously for three doses, with

TABLE 63–3. Frequently Used Antiemetic Agents and Classes With Commonly Administered Doses

Antiemetic	*Class*	*Dose and Schedule*
Ondansetron	Serotonin-receptor antagonist	0.15 mg/kg I.V. × three doses every 2–4 h
		8 mg I.V. × 1
		32 mg I.V. × 1
		Various oral regimens
Granisetron	Serotonin-receptor antagonist	10–40 μg/kg I.V. × 1
		3 mg I.V. × 1
Tropisetron	Serotonin-receptor antagonist	5 or 10 mg I.V. × 1
Dolasetron	Serotonin-receptor antagonist	1.8–3.0 mg/kg I.V. × 1
RG 12915	Serotonin-receptor antagonist	5–25 mg PO × 1
Metoclopramide	Substituted benzamide	1–3 mg/kg I.V. × two to three doses every 2 h
Haloperidol	Butyrophenone	1–3 mg I.V. × two to three doses every 2–4 h
Prochlorperazine	Phenothiazine	10–20 mg PO every 3–6 h
		25 mg PR every 4–6 h
		10 mg I.V. every 4–6 h
Dexamethasone	Corticosteroid	10–20 mg I.V. × 1 given over 5 min
Dronabinol	Cannabinoid	2.5–5 mg PO every 3–6 h

the initial dose administered 30 minutes before chemotherapy and the two subsequent doses repeated every 4 hours thereafter. Somewhat different regimens are recommended in other countries. Of interest, studies have indicated that schedules of every 2 or 4 or 6 or 8 hours all have similar efficacy.[25,26] This flexibility allows patients to receive this agent in a variety of treatment settings where the length of treatment may be an important factor. This lack of schedule dependency supports preliminary studies indicating efficacy with 8 mg and 32 mg single-dose schedules. Because early clinical trials noted important dose-efficacy relations, it is surprising that the above two doses (8 mg and 32 mg) were chosen for further study. In particular, doses above or below the 0.15 mg/kg level (about 10–12 mg) either showed no advantage or were less effective.[27]

Trials comparing ondansetron with metoclopramide in patients receiving high doses of cisplatin have yielded similar results,[28–30] as outlined in Table 63–4. In an illustrative study, ondansetron was given at 0.15 mg/kg intravenously every 4 hours for a total of three doses, and metoclopramide was given at 2 mg/kg intravenously every 2 to 3 hours for a total of six doses.[29] The median number of emetic episodes was less with ondansetron (one versus two, $p = 0.005$). The difference in complete control did not reach significance (40% versus 30%); however, the major control rate difference (fewer than three episodes) of 65% versus 51% with metoclopramide was significant ($p = 0.016$) in the 307 patients. No akathisia or dystonic reactions occurred in those given ondansetron (versus 10% and 8%, respectively, in those receiving metoclopramide). Headache was more common on the ondansetron arm

TABLE 63–4. Random Assignment Trials With Ondansetron and Metoclopramide in Previously Untreated Patients Receiving Cisplatin

Investigations	*No. of Evaluable Patients*	*Cisplatin Dose*	*Antiemetic Regimen*	*Major Control Rate (0–2 Episodes; $p < 0.02$)*
Hainsworth et al, 1991[29]	307	≥100 mg/m²	Ondansetron: 0.15 mg/kg I.V. q 4 h × 3 doses vs Metoclopramide: 2 mg/kg I.V. q 3 h × 6 doses	Ondansetron: 65% Metoclopramide: 51%
Marty et al, 1990[28]	76	80–100 mg/m²	Ondansetron: 8 mg I.V. followed by 1 mg/h × 24 h by continuous infusion vs	Ondansetron: 75% Metoclopramide: 42%
DeMulder et al, 1990[30]	95	50–100 mg/m²	Metoclopramide: 3 mg/kg I.V. followed by a continuous infusion of 5 mg/kg over 8 h	Ondansetron: 72% Metoclopramide: 42%

of the study (24% versus 11%, $p = 0.005$). This trial has been criticized for blinding only the patients and not the evaluating staff, for using an outdated metoclopramide regimen, and for having a somewhat better patient population for antiemetic control on the ondansetron arm (fewer women and more patients with a heavy alcohol history). All comparison studies, however, have yielded the same results favoring ondansetron.

The other agents listed in Table 63–5 are generally given in single-dose schedules. Granisetron has been registered in several countries and, after ondansetron, is the best studied agent. Several agents have been studied as both intravenous and oral agents, with the latter route emphasized in the development of RG 12915.

Antiemetic efficacy reported to date in patients receiving moderate to high doses of cisplatin and other emetic chemotherapy is similar among these agents, with complete control rates of 40% to 60% and major control rates of 60% to 80%.[31–36]

The side-effect profile of the serotonin antagonists provides a distinct advantage over the more conventional antiemetics. Extrapyramidal side effects, including acute dystonic reactions and akathisia, are not observed in patients receiving these serotonin antagonists. The lack of central nervous system effects with these agents is especially important for pediatric patients and young adults—those most prone to experience extrapyramidal side effects. Mild headaches and transient transaminase elevations have been characteristically yet inconsequentially associated with the serotonin antagonists.[25–37] Typically, the headache requires no treatment or the use of a mild analgesic, such as acetaminophen.

With efficacy clearly outlined for chemotherapy regimens containing high-dose cisplatin, patients receiving lesser emetic chemotherapy agents have even more favorable control of nausea and vomiting.[25,31,37]

The rationale for using combination antiemetic regimens as applied to conventional agents is being used with the 5-HT3 antagonists. Further improvement of response rates with serotonin antagonists can be accomplished with antiemetic combinations plus a corticosteroid. One report outlines a significant improvement in the complete control rate when 20 mg of dexamethasone was given intravenously in conjunction with 0.15 mg of ondansetron given intravenously three times over a 4-hour period.[37] Eighty-one percent of patients had complete control of both nausea and vomiting with the combination, as opposed to 56% who received ondansetron as a single agent.[37] Further combination antiemetic trials are confirming the results of safety and efficacy.[38,39] For use in current practice situations, the best results continue to be obtained by those who apply carefully established regimens in a precise manner.

STANDARD ANTIEMETIC AGENTS

Several antiemetic agents have been shown to be safe and effective (see Table 63–5). Among the best studied of the more effective agents are those that exert their activity by blocking dopamine receptors. These include such classes and agents as: (1) substituted benzamides (metoclopramide and alizapride), (2) butyrophenones (haloperidol and droperidol), and (3) phenothiazines (prochlorperazine and chlorpromazine). Additionally, corticosteroids (dexamethasone and methylprednisolone) are effective agents, and benzodiazepines and cannabinoids may also have a role.

TABLE 63–5. Metoclopramide Combination Regimens

Chemotherapy Indication	*Antiemetic Regimen*
Highly Emetogenic Agents	
Cisplatin, ≥70 mg/m² or Cyclophosphamide, 750 mg/m² or Carboplatin or dacarbazine	Metoclopramide, 3 mg/kg I.V. × 2 doses, every 2 h plus Dexamethasone, 20 mg I.V. × 1 plus Lorazepam, 1–2 mg I.V × 1
Moderately Emetogenic Agents	
Cisplatin, ≤60 mg/m² or Cyclophosphamide, ≤600 mg/m² or Doxorubicin or ifosfamide	Metoclopramide, 1–2 mg/kg I.V. × 2–3 doses, every 2 h plus Dexamethasone, 20 mg I.V. × 1 plus Lorazepam 1–2 mg I.V. × 1

SUBSTITUTED BENZAMIDES

The most commonly used and most effective drug of this class is metoclopramide. Although some controversy exists, a pharmacologic study demonstrated that efficacy was correlated with high blood levels (more than 850 ng/ml) of metoclopramide in patients receiving cisplatin.[40] Maintaining an adequate level of metoclopramide at the time of emetic vulnerability through the use of an appropriate dosing schedule may be important. In preventing emesis induced by cisplatin or by cyclophosphamide plus doxorubicin, metoclopramide administration every 2 hours (beginning shortly before chemotherapy) appears to be the most effective schedule. Unlike the selective 5-HT3 antagonists, metoclopramide is schedule-dependent. Doses and schedules of metoclopramide are outlined in Tables 63–5 and 63–6.

Random-assignment studies have shown metoclopramide to be superior to, or at least equivalent to, all other standard antiemetic agents that it has been compared with in cisplatin-

TABLE 63–6. Combination Antiemetic Regimens for High-Dose Cisplatin

Regimen A

Metoclopramide, 3 mg/kg I.V. every 2 h for 2 doses, plus
Dexamethasone, 20 mg I.V. × 1 dose (over 5 min), plus
Lorazepam, 1–2 mg I.V. × 1 dose

Regimen B

Serotonin-receptor antagonist (See Table 63–3 for dose and schedule), plus
Dexamethasone, 20 mg I.V. × 1 (over 5 min)

(Data from references 37, 48, and 64)

induced emesis.[10,14,15,41] Several reports have indicated useful activity against the emesis associated with a number of other chemotherapeutic agents.[44–46]

A recent study[47] explored markedly higher doses of metoclopramide (4 to 6 mg/kg) given only once in patients receiving cisplatin. Although the original antiemetic phase I trials did not exceed 3 mg/kg per dose, the total amount administered was as high as 15 mg/kg given over 10 hours.[3] The rationale behind the single very-high-dose study included several points: (1) a single dose of metoclopramide (in this case in combination with dexamethasone plus lorazepam) given before chemotherapy would be convenient and economical, with fewer administration charges, (2) a high peak level of the agent would be ensured, and a therapeutic level would likely be maintained throughout the period of emetic vulnerability, and (3) such high levels would be likely to saturate 5-HT3 receptors. The results of the trial indicated that these very-high-dose metoclopramide regimens are as safe and effective as lower-dose combinations and that the single prechemotherapy dose of each of the agents was convenient and cost-effective. These findings have been confirmed in a randomized comparison trial.[48] The recommended single-dose regimen is as follows: lorazepam, 1.5 mg/m^2 given intravenously 30 minutes before chemotherapy, plus dexamethasone, 20 mg given intravenously over 5 minutes at 25 minutes before chemotherapy, followed by a 20-minute intravenous infusion of metoclopramide, 4 mg/kg given immediately before chemotherapy.[47]

The side effects commonly associated with metoclopramide include mild sedation, dystonic reactions (age-related), akathisia (restlessness), and diarrhea (which may be an effect of specific chemotherapeutic agents, such as cisplatin).[49] In general, the side effects are easy to control or prevent. Akathisia is prevented or treated with a benzodiazepine; dystonic reactions can be dealt with similarly or with diphenhydramine. As is discussed in the section on combinations of antiemetics, dexamethasone, in addition to metoclopramide, improves efficacy and reduces diarrhea.[50]

BUTYROPHENONES

Haloperidol and droperidol were shown in initial trials to be active antiemetics.[51,52] Since substantial differences have not been demonstrated between these two butyrophenones, most of the subsequent comments refer to studies conducted with haloperidol. A formal study comparing haloperidol with metoclopramide in patients receiving cisplatin reported that both antiemetics are effective, although a trend toward greater activity was seen with metoclopramide.[42] Doses of 1 to 3 mg of haloperidol given intravenously every 2 to 6 hours are used most commonly (see Table 63–5); the higher doses and more frequent schedules more often are associated with better results. Toxicity commonly includes sedation, dystonic reactions, and akathisia, with hypotension occasionally observed.

PHENOTHIAZINES

The unsatisfactory results observed with oral and intramuscular phenothiazines encouraged the need for new studies to examine other classes of agents, different administration schedules, and higher dosage regimens. Structure-activity studies indicated that variations of the side chain at position 10 of the phenothiazine ring affect the antiemetic properties of these drugs.[53] Agents such as prochlorperazine would be predicted to have greater activity than other commonly used phenothiazines, such as chlorpromazine. This predicted difference has not been established in patients receiving chemotherapy.

Prochlorperazine given in typical oral and intramuscular doses in random-assignment trials has been found to be less active than metoclopramide[10] or dexamethasone[54] and equivalent to or less active than tetrahydrocannabinol.[55–57] A study using intravenous prochlorperazine in comparison with metoclopramide has indicated more encouraging results.[58] Two problems with this trial should be considered: (1) an imbalance in the arms of the study (concerning additional cyclophosphamide with the late onset of emesis), and (2) failure to evaluate adequately the incidence of orthostatic blood pressure changes, which is an important side effect of phenothiazines with major implications for outpatient usage. Other side effects are similar to those listed for haloperidol.

CORTICOSTEROIDS

Although several theories exist, the antiemetic mechanism of action of corticosteroids remains unclear. Several open studies and random-assignment trials have confirmed their utility.[54,59–62] Dexamethasone doses generally have been in the range of 4 to 20 mg per dose. In most trials in which a corticosteroid was added to an effective agent of another class, improved antiemetic efficacy for the combination resulted. This improvement has been evident in trials combining corticosteroids with metoclopramide or butyrophenones or ondansetron.

Toxicity has generally been mild with short courses of dexamethasone or methylprednisolone. There has been no indication of a lessening of chemotherapeutic effect through the use of steroids as antiemetics. With the low degree of toxicity, the low cost of generic dexamethasone, and a different mechanism of action than other agents, corticosteroids are ideal candidates for use in combination antiemetic regimens.

BENZODIAZEPINES AND CANNABINOIDS

Benzodiazepines can be useful additions to antiemetic regimens. Trials with lorazepam have shown a high degree of patient acceptance with a marked decrease in akathisia and in anxiety.[63,64] Additionally, lorazepam may add a small degree of objective antiemetic efficacy.[64] In a phase I trial, only modest major antiemetic activity was observed, but the subjective benefits appeared to make it an agent worth considering for use in combination.[65] A major difficulty in evaluating this agent's true activity is that it produces a dose-related memory loss.[63,65]

Most cannabinoid trials have included δ9-tetrahydrocannabinol (THC)[14,55,66,67]; two synthetic cannabinoids, nabilone and levonantradol, have also been tested clinically,[68–70] as has inhalant marijuana.[72] THC has been tried at many doses with differing schedules. Doses in the range of 5 to 10 mg/m^2 given orally every 3 to 4 hours appear to be among the most useful.[14,66,67] In general, THC has been found to be superior to placebo and equivalent to or superior to oral prochlorperazine.[55,57] Similar results have been reported with nabilone.[68,69] Side effects are frequent but generally manageable and include sedation, dry mouth, orthostatic hypotension, ataxia, dizziness, a "high," and euphoria or dysphoria.

The popular press has carried several stories extolling the properties of crude smoked marijuana for a variety of indications in patients with cancer or acquired immunodeficiency syndrome (AIDS). The most prominent of the indications is as an antiemetic. No cannabinoid has had efficacy close to that observed with the more effective agents (including those available for more than a decade) in patients given highly emetic chemotherapy.[14] Reputed benefits include the ability for the patient to titrate the dose independently, although no study has demonstrated this to be achievable.[72] Objections include the fact that marijuana includes dozens of chemicals without antiemetic properties, that microorganisms are found in the leaves and can be inhaled, and that there is no evidence to support efficacy superior to any other cannabinoid.[72]

The question of whether marijuana is superior to THC capsules was addressed in a double-blind, randomized, crossover trial.[72] Patients were given inhalant marijuana plus a placebo THC capsule, or THC plus an inhalant placebo cigarette, with their initial course of cisplatin or cyclophosphamide, and they were given the opposite with the next course. Overall, efficacy was poor on both arms of the trial.[72] There was a trend toward a patient preference for the THC in this blinded study; no superiority in blood levels or efficacy was seen for the patients titrating their own marijuana. The role of the cannabinoids remains unclear. It is apparent that such agents as ondansetron (as one of several effective and safe 5-HT3 antagonists), metoclopramide, and corticosteroids are superior antiemetics and have fewer side effects.[14,37,64]

TABLE 63–7. Regimens for Delayed Emesis in Patients Receiving High Cisplatin Doses

Recommended Regimen

To start 24 hours after cisplatin administration:

- Metoclopramide, 0.5 mg/kg PO, 4 times per day for 2 days, plus
- Dexamethasone, 8 mg PO, 2 times per day for 2 days, then 4 mg PO, 2 times per day for 2 additional days

Regimen for Consideration for Clinical Investigation

To start 16 hours after cisplatin administration:

- Oral 5-HT3 receptor antagonist at full established dose for 2 days plus
- Dexamethasone, 8 mg PO, 2 times per day for 2 days, then 4 mg PO, 2 times per day for 2 additional days

(Data from references 80 to 83)

ANTIEMETIC COMBINATIONS

Trials of single agents have indicated which are the most effective antiemetics and which are most likely to be compatible with other active drugs. Guidelines for effective combination regimens include the following:

1. Regimens should combine agents that have different mechanisms of activity without overlapping toxicities.
2. The drugs should be active as single agents, with the optimal doses, best route of administration, and proper schedules used in the combination.
3. Agents added to the combination may be useful if they lessen the side effects of the regimen or if they reduce other toxicities of the chemotherapy.

Studies have compared the activity of metoclopramide with the combination of metoclopramide plus a corticosteroid. In each of these studies, the combination of the two active antiemetics has been superior to the single agent.[50,73–75] In addition to improved antiemetic efficacy with the steroid plus metoclopramide, the incidence of diarrhea was significantly reduced.[50,73] An open study combining a butyrophenone with a corticosteroid also reported favorable results.[76] Recently, combination studies of ondansetron with dexamethasone have been completed.[37,39] In the larger of these studies, the combination was superior to ondansetron alone, with complete control of both nausea and vomiting achieved in 81% of the cisplatin-treated patients[39] (see the section on new antiemetic agents for dosing details, or Table 63–7).

Regimens for patients receiving high doses of cisplatin (120 mg/m^2) should generally include a corticosteroid plus either a selective 5-HT3 antagonist (such as ondansetron or granisetron) or metoclopramide, as outlined in Table 63–6.

Metoclopramide plus dexamethasone regimens benefit from the addition of a benzodiazepine such as lorazepam. The latter agent adds some subjective benefits, prevents akathisia and dystonic reactions, and appears to add a small amount of efficacy over similar combinations with diphenhydramine.[64] The recommended regimen is listed in Table 63–6. This table also outlines recommended regimens and alternatives for use with a variety of chemotherapeutic drugs. These regimens have all been tested, either in formal comparison studies or in open trials. It is clear from this table that in nearly all instances, unless an agent is contraindicated for a specific patient, combinations are recommended.

Chemotherapy regimens that involve several consecutive days of treatment present a special problem in controlling emesis. The antiemetics that block dopamine receptors appear to result in a greater incidence of dystonic reactions when given on multiple consecutive days.[23] When agents such as cisplatin or dacarbazine are given over several days without effective antiemetics, the emesis gradually lessens. Regimens with ondansetron have been tried in patients receiving chemotherapy in this setting. Paradoxically, efficacy is greatest over the first 1 or 2 days and then diminishes.[77] When ondansetron is given intravenously at 0.15 mg/kg for three doses per day, the agent is well tolerated with no change in its side-effect pattern.[25]

A regimen under investigation in patients over age 30, who are given cisplatin at 25 to 33 mg/m^2/day for 3 to 4 days, gives gradually decreasing doses of antiemetics. Patients are given 20 mg of dexamethasone intravenously 30 minutes before chemotherapy on each day. Metoclopramide also is given at 2 mg/kg at 30 minutes before cisplatin administration. On the first and second treatment days, the same metoclopramide dose is repeated 90 minutes after cisplatin; on the third day, the metoclopramide dose is repeated, but only at 1 mg/kg, and no repeat dose is given on the fourth day. Diphenhydramine is given intravenously at 50 mg with the first metoclopramide dose each day. A recent multicenter study compared the ondansetron plus dexamethasone regimen (as in regimen B in Table 63–6) with a metoclopramide and dexamethasone combination (similar to regimen A in Table 63–6, but using diphenhydramine 50 mg intravenously instead of lorazepam). Overall, both regimens were effective in the previously untreated patients receiving cisplatin, who were the subjects in the trial. However, a significant advantage emerged for those patients assigned to the serotonin antagonist combination.[78]

CONTROLLING EMESIS IN SPECIAL SITUATIONS

Lessons learned in treating acute chemotherapy-induced emesis can be valuable when considering the approach to delayed or anticipatory emesis, as long as the differences are respected.

DELAYED EMESIS

Only a few facts are known about this phenomenon. First, it is associated with high total cisplatin doses (more than 100 mg/m^2); and second, the incidence peaks about 2 days after chemotherapy. The pathophysiology of delayed emesis remains unclear.

Two preliminary open trials indicated that steroids plus either metoclopramide or prochlorperazine can be useful in controlling this problem.[79,80] A random assignment comparison study was done in which all patients received cisplatin, 120 mg/m^2, as their initial chemotherapy and received high-dose intravenous metoclopramide plus dexamethasone for acute emesis on the day of cisplatin administration.[81] Beginning 24 hours after chemotherapy, patients were assigned to receive oral placebo, oral dexamethasone for 4 days, or the combination of the oral dexamethasone regimen plus oral metoclopramide. Significantly greater complete control over the 4-day period was observed for those receiving the oral combination (57%) over placebo (11%). Side effects were generally mild.[81] The recommended regimen for delayed emesis is given in Table 63–7.

Only a limited amount of experience in delayed emesis with selective 5-HT3 antagonists exists. As a single agent, given orally, ondansetron's activity has not been encouraging in this setting.[82,83] Little information can be found for the other 5-HT3 antagonists. There is no reason to expect that a single dose of these agents on the day of chemotherapy will protect against both acute and delayed emesis.

An important finding comes from the phase II studies in acute chemotherapy-induced emesis with the 5-HT3 antagonists. In most trials, the time of onset of emesis, in the 60% who vomit with high-dose cisplatin, is between 16 and 20 hours. This is not, however, the time defined as the beginning of delayed emesis. Rather, the definition of this phenomenon beginning at 24 hours after chemotherapy is solely an arbitrary one of convenience. The implication is that the delayed emesis prevention regimen, as outlined previously, should be started earlier. A trial comparing the start of delayed emesis medications at 24 hours versus 14 hours would be warranted to test this hypothesis and to try to improve on the 50% control rate. An additional study of interest would be to test an oral regimen of dexamethasone plus a 5-HT3 antagonist versus the dexamethasone plus metoclopramide regimen shown in Table 63–6.

ANTICIPATORY EMESIS

Although treatment of this problem is important, prevention is imperative. The difficulties of anticipatory emesis underscore the importance of giving the most effective antiemetics with the initial course of emesis-producing chemotherapy.

Studies have indicated that behavior therapy can be helpful for patients with anticipatory emesis[84]; however, patients with this problem will need effective control of emesis with the next chemotherapy administration if further anticipatory emesis is to be avoided. In addition to behavior therapy, the use of antianxiety agents has been suggested. Benzodiazepines, especially lorazepam, may be helpful in patients with anticipatory emesis; however, formal trials have not carefully studied this question. When should these agents be started? Are they effective for patients who exhibit signs of anxiety a day or two before chemotherapy? Appropriate studies may allow a clearer approach to this problem.

COST OF TREATING EMESIS

Since effective antiemetics became available with high doses of metoclopramide, the question of the cost has been raised. Certainly, there is a great need to control this most disturbing and feared toxicity. It is important to reassure patients that helpful medicines are available. Chemotherapy patients should be reassured of the likelihood of control of nausea and vomiting.

A justification that has been given for high antiemetic costs has been that shortened hospital stays can result when effective agents are used. Additionally, convenient regimens with only single antiemetic doses can be cost-effective in that, for some agents, the cost of drug preparation and administration can exceed the actual cost of the drug.

Charges for drugs differ markedly among institutions, by reimbursement plans, and from country to country. This was illustrated in a recent survey showing a broad range of charges for the same doses of metoclopramide plus dexamethasone plus lorazepam among three different institutions in the United States.[85] The cost of an agent to the pharmacist or practice may vary by the market or nation but may be relatively constant within a market (especially when only a single supplier is available). When high-quality generic agents or competing agents are available, a variety of prices may be found.

Another factor of importance is the treatment regimen. When approval for marketing a drug is granted, the Food and Drug Administration typically approves the schedule and doses for the trials it has reviewed. If subsequent studies indicate that more practical schedules are available, these newer, more economical, and possibly more effective regimens are not necessarily indicated in the package labeling.

As seen in Table 63–8, several factors can influence the cost of antiemetic treatment. If the single low-dose serotonin antagonists plus steroid regimens prove to be as effective as multiple dose schemes, then the simpler regimen may be

TABLE 63–8. Factors Influencing the Cost of Antiemetic Treatment

Factor	*Comment*
Hospitalization	Effective control can decrease or eliminate hospitalization.
Chemotherapy	Appropriate regimens (fewer days of treatment) can enhance antiemetic efficacy, lower costs, and maintain antitumor activity.
Antiemetic schedule	Single-dose schedules reduce nursing and pharmacy charges (which may exceed drug costs).
Cost of antiemetic agents	The lowest, equally effective dose should be used. Of the 5-HT3 antagonists (if of equal efficacy), a single-dose lower-unit cost agent should be the drug of choice. Generic drugs should be used.
Institutional markup	Markup often ranges between 50% and 300% and can exceed the cost of the antiemetic agent.

competitive with metoclopramide combinations. Knowledge of alternative regimens can result in substantial savings for patients, payers, and medical institutions.

CONCLUSION

The last 10 years have seen major improvements in the control of emesis. Effective antiemetic regimens have become part of a standard of care in most major cancer treatment hospitals and clinics. Efforts to control emesis have presented an ideal situation for the collaboration of physicians and nurses who are oncology specialists. More new agents are soon to be introduced and are likely to be helpful, and better application of available techniques can result in major improvements in patient care. The newer 5-HT3 inhibitors are contributing to the successful control of emesis. The goal of optimal control of emesis requires knowledge of the more active drugs, experience with their use in combination, and consideration of the emetic problem of each patient.

New studies, however, must be accurately interpreted. Precision in evaluation techniques is mandatory if accurate results are to be obtained. Additionally, attention to the differing patient characteristics and to specific emetic patterns of individual chemotherapeutic agents must be considered in the design of trials and in the planning of an individual patient's treatment regimen.

The control of emesis is one of many important topics in the supportive care of patients with cancer. The considerable research efforts of the past decade in this area have resulted in improvements; the application of these findings continues to be the responsibility of all of us in clinical oncology.

REFERENCES

1. Borison HL, McCarthy LE. Neuropharmacology of chemotherapy induced emesis. Drugs 1983;25:8–17.
2. Borison HL. Role of the area postrema in vomiting and related functions. Rev Pharmacol Clin Exp 1986;3:7–8.
3. Gralla RJ, Braun TJ, Squillante A, et al. Metoclopramide: Initial clinical studies of high dosage regimens in cisplatin-induced emesis. In: Poster D, ed. The treatment of nausea and vomiting induced by cancer chemotherapy. New York: Masson, 1981:167–176.
4. Fozard JR, Mobarok A. Blockade of neuronal tryptamine receptors by metoclopramide. Eur J Pharmacol 1978;49:109–112.
5. Ireland SJ, Straughan OW, Tyers MB. Influence of 5-HT uptake on the apparent 5-HT antagonist potency of metoclopramide on the rat isolated superior cervical ganglion. Br J Pharmacol 1987;90:151–160.
6. Miner WD, Sanger GJ, Turner DH. Evidence that 5-hydroxytryptamine 3 receptors mediate cytotoxic drug and radiation-evoked emesis. Br J Cancer 1987;56:159–162.
7. Cubbedu LX, Hoffman IS, Fuenmayor NT, et al. Efficacy of ondansetron (GR38032F) and the role of serotonin in cisplatin-induced nausea and vomiting. N Engl J Med 1990;327:810–816.
8. Gralla RJ, Clark RA, Lohman TP. Does serotonin mediate chemotherapy-induced emesis? Proc Am Soc Clin Oncol 1991;10:324.
9. Engelman K. Malignant carcinoid syndrome. In: DeGroot LG, Besser GM, Cahill GF, eds. Endocrinology. Philadelphia: WB Saunders, 1989:2649–2657.
10. Gralla RJ, Itri LM, Pisko SE, et al. Antiemetic efficacy of high-dose metoclopramide: Randomized trials with placebo and prochlorperazine in patients with chemotherapy-induced nausea and vomiting. N Engl J Med 1981;305:905–909.
11. Fetting JH, Grochow LB, Folstein MF, et al. The course of nausea and vomiting after high-dose cyclophosphamide. Cancer Treat Rep 1982;66:1487–1493.
12. Martin M, Diaz Rubio E, Sanchez A, et al. The natural course of emesis after carboplatin treatment. Acta Oncol 1990;29:593–596.
13. Mangioni C, Bolis G, Pecorelli S, et al. Randomized trial in advanced ovarian cancer comparing cisplatin and carboplatin. J Natl Cancer Inst 1989;81:1464–1471.
14. Gralla RJ, Tyson LB, Borden LA, et al. Antiemetic therapy: A review of recent studies and a report of a random assignment trial comparing metoclopramide with delta-9-tetrahydrocannabinol. Cancer Treat Rep 1984;68:163–172.
15. Homesley HD, Gayney JM, Jobsen VN, et al. Double-blind placebo-controlled study of metoclopramide in cisplatin-induced emesis. N Engl J Med 1982;307:250–251.
16. Kris MG, Gralla RJ, Clark RA, et al. Incidence, course, and severity of delayed nausea and vomiting following the administration of high-dose cisplatin. J Clin Oncol 1985;3:1379–1384.
17. Morrow GR. Prevalence and correlates of anticipatory nausea and vomiting in chemotherapy patients. J Natl Cancer Inst 1982;68:585–588.
18. Wilcox PM, Fetting JH, Nettesheim KM, et al. Anticipatory vomiting in women receiving cyclophosphamide, methotrexate and 5-FU (CMF) adjuvant chemotherapy for breast carcinoma. Cancer Treat Rep 1982;66:1601–1604.
19. D'Acquisto RW, Tyson LB, Gralla RJ, et al. The influence of a chronic high alcohol intake on chemotherapy-induced nausea and vomiting. Proc Am Soc Clin Oncol 1986;5:257.
20. Sullivan JR, Leyten MJ, Bell R. Decreased cisplatin induced nausea and vomiting with alcohol ingestion. N Engl J Med 1983;309:13, 796.
21. Roila F, Tonato M, Basurto C, et al. Protection from nausea and vomiting in cisplatin-treated patients: High dose metoclopramide combined with methyl prednisolone versus metoclopramide combined with dexamethasone and diphenylhydramine. A study of the Italian Oncology for Clinical Research. J Clin Oncol 1989;7:1693–1700.
22. Kris MG, Tyson LB, Gralla RJ, et al. Extrapyramidal reactions with high-dose metoclopramide. N Engl J Med 1983;309:433.
23. Allen JC, Gralla RJ, Reilly C, et al. Metoclopramide: Dose-related toxicity and preliminary antiemetic studies in children receiving cancer chemotherapy. J Clin Oncol 1985;3:1136–1141.
24. Gralla RJ, Clark RA, Kris MG, Tyson LB. Methodology in antiemetic trials. Eur J Cancer 1991;27:55–58.
25. Kris MG, Gralla RJ, Clark RA, et al. Phase II trials of the serotonin antagonist GR38032F for the control of vomiting caused by cisplatin. J Natl Cancer Inst 1989;81:42–46.
26. Hesketh PJ, Murphy WK, Lester RP, et al. GR38032F: A novel compound effective in the prevention of acute cisplatin-induced emesis. J Clin Oncol 1989;7:700–705.
27. Kris MG, Gralla RJ, Clark RA, et al. Dose ranging evaluation of the serotonin antagonist GR-C507/75 (GR38032F) when used as an antiemetic in patients receiving cancer chemotherapy. J Clin Oncol 1988;6:659–662.
28. Marty M, Pouillart P, Scholl S, et al. Comparison of the 5-hydroxytryptamine 3 (serotonin) receptor antagonist ondansetron (GR38032F) with high-dose metoclopramide in the control of cisplatin-induced emesis. N Engl J Med 1990;332:816–821.
29. Hainsworth J, Harvey W, Pendergrass K, et al. A single-blind comparison of intravenous ondansetron, a selective serotonin antagonist, with intravenous metoclopramide in the prevention of nausea and vomiting associated with high-dose cisplatin chemotherapy. J Clin Oncol 1991;9:721–728.
30. DeMulder PHM, Deynaere C, Vermorken JB, et al. Ondansetron compared with high-dose metoclopramide in prophylaxis of acute and delayed cisplatin-induced nausea and vomiting. Ann Intern Med 1990;113:834–840.
31. Baltzer L, Tyson LB, Kris MG, et al. Oral antiemetics for lung cancer chemotherapy: Studies with metoclopramide and RG12915. Proc 6th World Conf Lung Cancer 1991;7:148.
32. Clark RA, Gralla RJ, Tyson LB, et al. Controlling emesis with serotonin antagonists: Experience with 5 new agents in 109 patients. Proc 6th World Conf Lung Cancer 1991;7:148.
33. Grunberg SM, Kris MG, Gralla RJ, et al. High dose MDL 73, 147EF for the prevention of cisplatin-induced emesis. Proc 6th World Conf Lung Cancer 1991;7:148.
34. Kaplan HG, Jofthagen C. Use of granisetron to prevent platinol induced nausea and vomiting. Proc Am Soc Clin Oncol 1991;10:339.
35. Tyson LB, Gralla RJ, Kris MG, et al. Phase I antiemetic study of the serotonin antagonist ICS 205–930. Proc Am Soc Clin Oncol 1989:8:331.

36. Clark RA, Kris MG, Gralla RJ, et al. Serotonin antagonists demonstrate antiemetic effectiveness without extrapyramidal symptoms: Analysis of studies with 3 new agents in 155 patients. Proc Am Soc Clin Oncol 1990;9:332.
37. Roila F, Tonato M, Cognetti F, et al. Prevention of cisplatin-induced emesis: A double-blind multicenter randomized crossover study comparing ondansetron and ondansetron plus dexamethasone. J Clin Oncol 1991;9:674–678.
38. Tyson LB, Kris MG, Baltzer L, et al. Combining ondansetron with dexamethasone: A randomized antiemetic trial comparing two ondansetron schedules in patients receiving cisplatin. Proc Am Soc Clin Oncol 1991;10:341.
39. Smith DB, Newland ES, Rustin GJS, et al. Comparison of ondansetron and ondansetron plus dexamethasone as antiemetic prophylaxis during cisplatin-containing chemotherapy. Lancet 1991;338:487–498.
40. Meyer BR, Lewin M, Dreyer DE, et al. Optimizing metoclopramide control of cisplatin-induced emesis. Ann Intern Med 1984;100:393–395.
41. Frustacci S, Tumolo S, Tirell U, et al. High dose metoclopramide versus dexamethasone in the prevention of cisplatin induced vomiting. Proc Am Soc Clin Oncol 1983;2:87.
42. Grunberg Sm, Gala KV, Lampenfeld M, et al. Comparison of the antiemetic effect of high-dose intravenous haloperidol: A randomized double-blind crossover study. J Clin Oncol 1984;2:782–787.
43. Richards PD, Flaum MA, Bateman M, et al. The antiemetic efficacy of secobarbital and chlorpromazine compared to metoclopramide, diphenhydramine, and dexamethasone: A randomized trial. Cancer 1986;58:959–962.
44. Gralla RJ, Tyson LB, Clark RA, et al. An all oral combination antiemetic regimen for patients receiving Cytoxan + Adriamycin + vincristine. Proc Am Soc Clin Oncol 1985;4: 267.
45. Strum SB, McDermed JE, Opfell RW, et al. Intravenous metoclopramide: An effective antiemetic in cancer chemotherapy. J Am Med Assoc 1982;247:2683–2686.
46. Tyson LB, Clark RA, Gralla, RJ. High dose metoclopramide: Control of dacarbazine-induced emesis in a preliminary trial. Cancer Treat Rep 1982;66:2108.
47. Clark RA, Gralla RJ, Kris MG, et al. Exploring very high doses of metoclopramide (4–6 mg/kg): Preservation of efficacy and safety with only a single dose in a combination regimen. Proc Am Soc Clin Oncol 1989;8:1286.
48. Basuto C, Roila F, Bracarda S, et al. Single vs divided dose of metoclopramide in a combined regimen of treatment of cisplatin induced emesis: A double-blind prospective comparative trial. Perugia International Cancer Conference III. In: Supportive therapy: Challenges for the '90s. 1990:109.
49. Von Hoff DD, Schilisky R, Reichert CM, et al. Toxic effects of disdichlorodiammine-platinum (II) in man. Cancer Treat Rep 1979;63:1527–1531.
50. Kris MG, Gralla RJ, Tyson LB, et al. Improved control of cisplatin-induced emesis with high-dose metoclopramide and with combinations of metoclopramide, dexamethasone, and diphenhydramine: Results of consecutive trials in 255 patients. Cancer 1985;55: 527–534.
51. Grossman B, Lessen LS, Cohen P. Droperidol prevents nausea and vomiting from cisplatinum. N Engl J Med 1979;301:47.
52. Neidhart J, Gayen M, Metz E. Haldol and mustard induced vomiting when other agents fail. Proc Am Soc Clin Oncol 1980;21:365.
53. Wampler G. The pharmacology and clinical effectiveness of phenothiazines and related drugs for managing chemotherapy-induced emesis. Drugs 1983;25:31–51.
54. Markman M, Sheidler V, Ettinger DS, et al. Antiemetic efficacy of dexamethasone: Randomized, double-blind, crossover study with prochlorperazine in patients receiving cancer chemotherapy. N Engl J Med 1984;311:549–552.
55. Frytak S, Moertel CG, O'Fallon J, et al. Delta-9-tetrahydrocannabinol as an antiemetic in patients treated with cancer chemotherapy: A double-blind comparison with prochlorperazine and a placebo. Ann Intern Med 1979;91:825–830.
56. Orr LE, McKerman JF, Bloone B. Antiemetic effect of tetrahydrocannabinol. Arch Intern Med 1980;140:1431–1433.
57. Sallan SE, Cronin CM, Zelen M, et al. Antiemetics in patients receiving chemotherapy for cancer: A randomized comparison of delta-9-tetrahydrocannabinol and prochlorperazine. N Engl J Med 1980;302:135–138.
58. Carr BI, Bertrand M, Browning S, et al. A comparison of the antiemetic efficacy of prochlorperazine and metoclopramide for the treatment of cisplatin-induced emesis: A prospective randomized double-blind study. J Clin Oncol 1985;3:1127–1132.
59. Aapro MS, Alberts DS. High dose dexamethasone for prevention of cisplatinum-induced vomiting. Cancer Chemother Pharmacol 1981;7:11–14.
60. Aapro MS, Plezia PM, Alberts DS, et al. Double-blind crossover study of the antiemetic efficacy of high-dose dexamethasone vs high-dose metoclopramide. Proc Am Soc Clin Oncol 1983;2:93.
61. Cassileth PA, Lusk EJ, Torri S, et al. Antiemetic efficacy of dexamethasone therapy in patients receiving cancer chemotherapy. Arch Intern Med 1983;143:1347–1349.
62. Lee BJ. Methylprednisolone as an antiemetic. N Engl J Med 1981;304:486.
63. Kris MG, Gralla RJ, Clark RA, et al. Consecutive dose-finding trials adding lorazepam to the combination of metoclopramide plus dexamethasone: Improved subjective effectiveness over the combination of diphenhydramine plus metoclopramide plus dexamethasone. Cancer Treat Rep 1985;69:1257–1262.
64. Kris MG, Gralla RJ, Clark RA, et al. Antiemetic control and prevention of side effects of anticancer therapy with lorazepam or diphenhydramine when used in conjunction with metoclopramide plus dexamethasone: A double-blind, randomized trial. Cancer 1987;69:1353–1357.
65. Laszlo J, Clark RA, Hanson DC, et al. Lorazepam in cancer patients treated with cisplatin: A drug having antiemetic, amnesic, and anxiolytic effects. J Clin Oncol 1985;3:864–869.
66. Chang AE, Shilling DJ, Stillman RC, et al. Delta-9-tetrahydrocannabinol as an antiemetic in patients receiving high-dose methotrexate: A prospective randomized evaluation. Ann Intern 1979;91:819–824.
67. Vincent BJ, McQuistion DJ, Einhorn LH, et al. Review of cannabinoids and their antiemetic effectiveness. Drugs 1983;25:52–62.
68. Herman TS, Einhorn LH, Jones SE. Superiority of nabilone over prochlorperazine as an antiemetic in patients receiving cancer chemotherapy. N Engl J Med 1979;300: 1295–1297.
69. Steele N, Gralla RJ, Braun DW, et al. Double-blind comparison of the antiemetic effects of nabilone and prochlorperazine on chemotherapy-induced emesis. Cancer Treat Rep 1980;64:219–224.
70. Tyson LB, Gralla RJ, Clark RA, et al. Phase I trial of levonantradol in chemotherapy induced emesis. Am J Clin Oncol 1985;8:528–532.
71. Venner P, Bruera E, Diebrt D, et al. Intensive treatment scheduling of nabilone plus dexamethasone vs metoclopramide plus dexamethasone in cisplatinum-induced emesis. Proc Am Soc Clin Oncol 1986;5:253.
72. Levitt M, Faiman C, Hawks R, et al. Randomized double-blind comparison of delta-9-tetrahydrocannabinol (THC) and marijuana as chemotherapy antiemetics. Proc Am Soc Clin Oncol 1984;3:91.
73. Allan SG, Cornbleet MA, Warrington PS, et al. Dexamethasone and high-dose metoclopramide: Efficacy in controlling cisplatin-induced nausea and vomiting. Br Med J 1984;289:878–879.
74. Rosell R, Abad-Esteve A, Ribas-Mundo M, et al. Evaluation of a combination antiemetic regimen including IV high-dose metoclopramide, dexamethasone, and diphenhydramine in cisplatin-based chemotherapy regimens. Cancer Treat Rep 1985;69:909–910.
75. Grunberg SM, Akerley WL, Baker C, et al. Comparison of metoclopramide and metoclopramide + dexamethasone in complete prevention of cisplatinum induced emesis. Proc Am Soc Clin Oncol 1985;4:262.
76. Mason BA, Dambra J, Grossman B, et al. Effective control of cisplatin-induced nausea using high-dose steroids and droperidol. Cancer Treat Rep 1982;66:243–245.
77. Hainsworth JD, Omura GA, Khojasteba, et al. Ondansetron (GR 38032F): A novel antiemetic effective in patients receiving a multiple-day regimen of cisplatin chemotherapy. Am J Clin Oncol 1991;14:336–348.
78. Roila F, Tonato M, Favalli G, et al. A multi-center double-blind study comparing the antiemetic efficacy and safety of ondansetron (OND) plus dexamethasone (DEX) vs metoclopramide (MTC) plus DEX and diphenhydramine (DIP) in cisplatin (CDDP) treated cancer patients (PTS). Am Soc Clin Oncol 1992;11:394.
79. Clark RA, Kris MG, Tyson LB, et al. Antiemetic trials to control delayed vomiting following high-dose cisplatin. Proc Am Soc Clin Oncol 1986;5:257.
80. Strum S, McDermed J, Abrahano-Umali R, et al. Management of cisplatin-induced delayed-onset nausea and vomiting: Preliminary results with two drug regimens. Proc Soc Am Clin Oncol 1985;4:263.
81. Kris MG, Gralla RJ, Tyson LB, et al. Controlling delayed vomiting: Double-blind randomized trial comparing placebo, dexamethasone alone, and metoclopramide plus dexamethasone in patients receiving cisplatin. J Clin Oncol 1989;7:108–114.
82. Grunberg SM, Groshen S, Stevenson LI, et al. Double-blind randomized study of two doses of oral ondansetron for the prevention of cisplatin-induced delayed nausea and vomiting. Proc Am Soc Clin Oncol 1990;9:327.
83. Kris MG, Tyson LB, Clark RA, et al. Oral ondansetron for the control of delayed emesis after cisplatin: Report of a phase II study and a review of completed trials to manage delayed emesis. Cancer 1992;70:1012–1016.
84. Morrow GR, Morrell C. Behavioral treatment for the anticipatory nausea and vomiting induced by cancer chemotherapy. N Engl J Med 1982;307:1476–1480.
85. Muller RJ, Gralla RJ, Kris MG, et al. Administration of effective antiemetic regimens: Marked differences in patient changes among different institutions. Proc Am Soc Clin Oncol 1990;9:334.

SECTION **2**

RAYMOND B. WEISS
NICHOLAS J. VOGELZANG

Miscellaneous Toxicities

Chemotherapeutic agents can produce a variety of acute and chronic organ toxicities. Besides heart and lung toxicities, which are covered in other sections, damage to the kidneys, nerve tissue, liver, and blood vessels may occur. In addition, acute hypersensitivity reactions may produce immediate life-threatening problems, such as hypotension and respiratory distress. Such hypersensitivity reactions may necessitate cessation of treatment with the precipitating drug, or at least means must be found to minimize or prevent the problem. Acute hepatic, renal, or central nervous system toxicity may also be life-threatening but in a less immediate manner. If the offending drug is discontinued before irreversible damage occurs, the manifestations of toxicity usually wane. As patients live longer after receiving cancer chemotherapy, chronic toxicities such as Raynaud's phenomenon may become evident and sometimes debilitating and irreversible.

Antitumor drugs are often used in combination, and it may be difficult to determine which drug is most responsible for a particular form of tissue injury. Other medical conditions such as infections or the cancer itself may cause tissue injury during chemotherapy, and the antitumor agent may be blameless. Whether the toxicity is acute or chronic, awareness of the potential for toxicity with each agent in use is important, and appropriate monitoring (which may be simple patient questioning about symptoms or laboratory testing) must be accomplished. If not, severe and irreversible tissue injury may occur.

NEPHROTOXICITY

The kidneys are the elimination pathway of many drugs and their metabolites and therefore are vulnerable to injury. The entire anatomic renal pathway from glomerulus to distal tubule is at risk, depending on the drug involved. The symptoms vary from an asymptomatic rise in serum creatinine or mild proteinuria to acute renal failure with anuria requiring dialysis.

PLATINUM COMPOUNDS

The nephrotoxicity of cisplatin has been well known since it was first used in clinical trials in the early 1970s.[1,2] This obstacle to its use has been so profound that hundreds of cisplatin analogs have been synthesized in the hope of finding a less nephrotoxic compound of equal antitumor efficacy. Fortunately, a means was found to avoid nephrotoxicity from cisplatin by forcing diuresis and enhancing drug excretion.[3]

The renal toxicity is dose-related, cumulative, and manifested primarily by a rise in serum creatinine. Single doses under 40 mg/m^2 usually cause little renal injury, but higher doses require aggressive hydration, or abrupt irreversible renal failure may occur.[4] The hydration used most successfully is normal saline because the high chloride concentration possibly inhibits cisplatin hydrolysis in the tubules, providing a measure of nephrotoxicity protection. Mannitol is also used to stimulate diuresis, but there is no evidence that mannitol is necessary. A urine output of at least 100 ml/hour for 2 to 4 hours before and 4 to 6 hours after cisplatin doses of 40 to 75 mg/m^2 reduces, but does not eliminate, nephrotoxicity. More intensive hydration schedules are necessary when higher cisplatin doses are used.

The pathologic lesion of cisplatin renal damage is primarily in the proximal and distal tubules but also may involve the collecting ducts,[5] while glomeruli are unaffected. This extensive area of tissue injury helps explain why electrolyte abnormalities, such as hyponatremia and hypomagnesemia, are so common after cisplatin administration.[6,7] The hypomagnesemia is usually asymptomatic, but it can last months to years.[8] The hyponatremia has been reported to cause persistent orthostatic hypotension.[7]

The precise mechanism of the tubular injury continues to be the subject of research. It is not simply the tubular handling of a heavy metal, because the *trans* isomer of cisplatin is not nephrotoxic.[9] Cisplatin produces DNA intrastrand crosslinks as one of its mechanisms of antitumor effect, and the same damage to DNA in tubular cells probably also occurs.

A variety of substances have been tested to minimize cisplatin nephrotoxicity, besides using the often inconvenient hydration and diuresis. These include probenecid, superoxide dismutase, amifostine (WR 2721), mesna, sodium thiosulfate, diethyldithiocarbamate, and hypertonic saline. None of these substances has achieved acceptance as a substitute for hydration. One simple technique for additional nephrotoxicity protection, besides hydration, is to administer cisplatin in the evening to take advantage of circadian rhythm effects that have been shown to reduce renal injury.[10]

A final measure of protection is to be certain that normal renal function is present initially by performing a pretreatment 24-hour urine creatinine clearance. A result of less than 70 ml/minute, especially in patients over age 60, probably precludes cisplatin administration without an inordinate risk of nephrotoxicity.[11] In addition, other renal tubular toxins, such as aminoglycoside antibiotics, should be avoided whenever possible to obviate additive tubular damage.

Carboplatin was synthesized as a cisplatin alternative with less nephrotoxicity. It is less nephrotoxic,[12] but it is not free of potential for renal injury, especially in patients who previously have received nephrotoxins or when given in high doses.[13,14] Usually, carboplatin-related dysfunction is detectable only by the sensitive means of measuring urine tubular enzyme excretion or glomerular filtration rate.[15] The serum creatinine and creatinine clearance are rarely affected.

MITOMYCIN

The capacity of mitomycin to produce renal toxicity has been known for over 20 years.[16] Renal effects from mitomycin are not as common as from the platinum compounds, but they can be immediately life-threatening in some cases.

The clinical manifestations vary from a chronic progressive rise in serum creatinine[17] without thrombocytopenia to microangiopathic hemolytic anemia (MAHA), which is usually fulminant in onset. MAHA has been reported in a large number of anecdotal cases,[18] but in one study[19] of adjuvant mitomycin, a 10.7% incidence occurred.

The MAHA toxicity is cumulative dose-related, but even one to three doses of mitomycin can initiate it. It also can develop a few months after mitomycin has been discontinued.[18,20] The incidence has been reported to rise to 25% to 30% if the cumulative mitomycin dose is over 70 mg/m^2.[20]

The clinical presentation of MAHA is an abrupt and often severe hemolytic anemia that usually precedes the renal dysfunction by 1 or 2 weeks. The peripheral blood smear shows schistocytes, and thrombocytopenia becomes apparent as renal failure develops. The thrombocytopenia is not part of a generalized coagulopathy because laboratory evidence of disseminated intravascular coagulation is usually not observed. Other accompanying abnormalities are rash, fever, arterial hypertension, central neurologic dysfunction, pericarditis, interstitial pneumonitis, hematuria, and proteinuria.[18,20] A high rate (65%) of patients have noncardiogenic pulmonary edema.[20] A prominent feature of this syndrome is the fact that it is often precipitated or worsened by blood transfusions, suggesting that blood product use should be avoided as much as possible when administering mitomycin. The outcome is often (over 50%) death, despite vigorous treatment.[19,20]

Treatment includes hemodialysis and plasmapheresis.[21] The most successful treatment has been plasma perfusion over filters containing staphylococcal protein A, a method of removing immune complexes from the blood.[20,22]

The pathogenesis of this acute form of nephrotoxicity is not certain. Cattell[23] showed that mitomycin caused glomerular endothelial damage when directly injected into the renal arteries of rats. Such vascular endothelial injury may activate platelets and lead to fibrin thrombi deposition in the microvasculature of the kidney, initiating renal dysfunction and hemolysis.

METHOTREXATE

When methotrexate is administered in conventional oral or intravenous doses, nephrotoxicity is only an occasional problem. If high doses are used, along with folinic acid rescue, acute nephrotoxicity can pose a greater danger.

Methotrexate is excreted rapidly in the urine whether it is administered orally or parenterally. Both parent compound and the main metabolite, 7-hydroxymethotrexate, are filtered by the glomeruli and actively secreted by the tubules. At physiologic pH, the drug is fully ionized, but in acidified form (pH less than 5.7), the parent drug and main metabolite are less ionized and may precipitate.[24] During urinary excretion, drug precipitation occurs as the urine is concentrated and acidified in the tubules. The solubility of 7-hydroxymethotrexate is only one fourth that of methotrexate, providing further potential for drug precipitation within the tubules and resulting in acute renal dysfunction.

Acute methotrexate nephrotoxicity produces abrupt renal insufficiency. The patient may complain of costovertebral angle pain while the serum creatinine and blood urea nitrogen rise rapidly. Dehydration, oliguria, and even anuria may occur.

Since methotrexate nephrotoxicity is largely a physical process of tubular drug precipitation, the incidence can be kept low by means of precipitation prevention. The two main methods are hydration and urine alkalinization.[25] Whenever a methotrexate dose high enough to require folinic acid rescue is being given, the urine should be kept alkaline (pH greater than 8) with sodium bicarbonate administration, and a urine output of over 100 ml/hour should be maintained. Serial serum methotrexate levels should be monitored until the concentration reaches 10^{-8} molar or less, 24 to 48 hours after administration.[25]

If renal clearance of methotrexate is impaired by renal dysfunction already present or by concurrently administered drugs, nephrotoxicity can be initiated or enhanced. Prior treatment with cisplatin may contribute to nephrotoxicity from methotrexate.[26] In addition, concurrent administration of nonsteroidal antiinflammatory drugs can provoke serious, and even fatal, methotrexate nephrotoxicity. Indomethacin,[27] ketoprofen,[28] diclofenac,[28] and naproxen[29] have been reported to increase the risk of such renal problems, whether the methotrexate is being given in a high dose[28] or low dose.[29] The mechanism of this drug interaction is not known, but it is probably mediated by a reduced methotrexate clearance through the kidney.

Treatment of acute nephrotoxicity from high methotrexate doses by hemodialysis and peritoneal dialysis has been minimally successful.[30] Charcoal hemofiltration by methods similar to those used to remove barbiturates from overdosed patients has been more effective.[31]

NITROSOUREAS

Streptozocin has the most potential for nephrotoxicity in this drug class, and this is its dose-limiting form of toxicity. The incidence rises with prolonged drug administration so that most patients eventually display it if therapy continues.

The kidneys are the major excretion pathway for both parent drug and metabolites, which may be the main factor in the pathogenesis of the renal toxicity. The sites of streptozocin injury are both the glomerulus and tubules (primarily the proximal) where histologic changes have been observed.[32] The mechanism of this injury, however, is not known. Hypophosphatemia and proteinuria are early indications of renal effect.[33] Renal tubular acidosis, with its characteristic abnormalities of glycosuria, acetonuria, hyperchloremia, and aminoaciduria, is seen frequently. If the drug is discontinued, these findings usually resolve. A rising serum creatinine is a later, and sometimes irreversible, finding. Hydration and diuresis have occasionally minimized renal dysfunction during therapy.[34]

The other two nitrosoureas in clinical use (carmustine and lomustine) are much less nephrotoxic. Carmustine usually causes problems of interstitial pneumonitis before it causes any renal toxicity. Lomustine has caused only rare instances of nephrotoxicity when large cumulative doses were administered.[35]

IFOSFAMIDE

Cyclophosphamide and ifosfamide are analogs with similar chemical structures. Both produce the metabolite acrolein, which causes hemorrhagic cystitis during urinary excretion. Despite similarities in structure, toxicity, and antitumor efficacy, they differ significantly in their ability to cause nephrotoxicity. Cyclophosphamide produces no kidney toxicity of clinical consequence, while ifosfamide produces a variety of renal abnormalities, some of which have been fatal.[36]

Early studies with ifosfamide showed that single high doses could result in acute tubular necrosis and renal failure within a few days of drug administration.[37] Such outcomes were one reason that a fractionated dose schedule was developed for this drug. Administration over five consecutive days reduced both renal and bladder toxicity. The most effective measure for reducing urinary tract toxicity was the development of mesna as a means of cystitis prevention. Mesna is now a standard accompaniment to ifosfamide use, but it does not obviate nephrotoxicity.[38]

The incidence of nephrotoxicity varies from several percent up to 33%, a level seen in young children.[39] Clinical manifestations include tubular dysfunction, Fanconi's syndrome, and a rising serum creatinine resulting in renal failure. The tubular injury is manifested by glycosuria, renal tubular acidosis, hypokalemia, proteinuria, and hypophosphatemia, which can even result in rickets in children.[40,41]

PLICAMYCIN

The first antitumor agent recognized to have nephrotoxicity potential was plicamycin (mithramycin).[42] Acute renal failure was a common toxicity when this drug was used for treating testicular cancer. Although it now is used only for its therapeutic effect in hypercalcemia, renal toxicity can still occur, even after only a single drug dose.[43] An acute rise in serum creatinine is the usual manifestation of such toxicity.

OTHER AGENTS

Table 63–9 lists antitumor agents that have been reported to cause renal injury. They are categorized by the risk of such toxicity from occasional anecdotal reports to high risk of severe damage.

Not only can individual drugs cause nephrotoxicity, but also combinations of agents can occasionally cause serious reactions, such as microangiopathic hemolytic anemia. The combination of cisplatin, bleomycin, and methotrexate or vincristine has initiated such toxicity in similar fashion to mitomycin.[44,45]

TABLE 63–9. Antitumor Agents That Cause Nephrotoxicity

High Potential for Nephrotoxicity	
Azacitidine	Methotrexate (in high doses)
Cisplatin	Mitomycin
Diaziquone (in high doses)	Pentostatin
Gallium nitrate	Plicamycin
Ifosfamide	Streptozocin
Interleukin-2	
Azotemia Without Nephrotoxicity	
Dacarbazine	
L-Asparaginase	
Occasional Irreversible Nephrotoxicity	
Cisplatin	Mitomycin
Gallium nitrate	Streptozocin
Lomustine	
Low Potential for Nephrotoxicity	
Azathioprine	Lomustine
Carboplatin	6-Mercaptopurine
Interferons	Methotrexate (in low doses)

NEUROTOXICITY

VINCA ALKALOIDS

The first drug class to be recognized as having neurotoxicity was the vinca alkaloids, especially vincristine. Vincristine is unique among the antitumor agents in that neurotoxicity is dose-limiting. The neurologic injury can be to the peripheral, central, or autonomic nervous systems.[46,47]

The most common and initial manifestations of neurotoxicity are depression of the deep tendon reflexes and paresthesia of the distal extremities. The Achilles tendon reflexes and the fingertips are the respective initial sites of abnormalities. Loss of the Achilles tendon reflex is usually asymptomatic. The paresthesia commonly progresses proximally as vincristine therapy is continued and may involve the entire hands or feet. The hyporeflexia spreads to other sites, and areflexia develops next. Surprisingly, despite the presence of peripheral paresthesia, vibration sense, position sense, pinprick sensation, and two-point discrimination are generally unaffected.

Motor dysfunction and gait disorders are initially manifested as lower extremity weakness. Footdrop and a slapping gait may ensue, and if vincristine is continued, weakness to the point of paraparesis may develop. Severe bone pain and pain in the mandible region may occur acutely a few hours after vincristine administration. It usually subsides after a few days.

Cranial nerves may be affected and cause ophthamoplegia and facial palsy. Ataxia is seen rarely. The parasympathetic nervous system can be affected also, so that constipation and difficult micturation may develop. These symptoms can progress to paralytic ileus with obstipation and bladder atony. Autonomic neuropathy can manifest as orthostatic hypotension, which can be symptomatic or clinically silent.[48] Vocal cord paralysis producing hoarseness and dysphagia may occur. The risk of vincristine neurotoxicity is enhanced by certain underlying neuropathies, such as diabetic neuropathy and Charcot-Marie-Tooth disease.[49]

No effective treatment has been developed for the neurotoxicity except to stop vincristine therapy and wait for neurologic recovery. Depending on the severity of the neurologic dysfunction, recovery may take weeks or months to occur. Residual minor abnormalities sometimes persist indefinitely. Empiric vitamin therapy is ineffective. Intestinal dysfunction from autonomic neuropathy may be improved by metoclopramide use.[50]

Vincristine binds to the β-subunit of tubulin, causing disruption of microtubule function in neuronal axons. Electrophysiologic studies indicate distal axonal degeneration, and nerve conduction testing shows that sensory nerves are most affected with a reduced amplitude of nerve action potentials. Histologic changes are generally those of axonal degeneration.

The vincristine analog vinblastine also has potential for causing neurotoxicity, although it is less common, and the dose-limiting toxicity of vinblastine is myelosuppression, not neurotoxicity. The clinical manifestations are similar to those of vincristine. The degree of neurologic injury is related to both individual and cumulative doses.

CISPLATIN

Although nephrotoxicity is a major and cumulative dose-limiting toxicity for cisplatin, neurotoxicity is also a common toxicity and can be dose-limiting for both single and cumulative doses.[51–54] Cisplatin-induced neuropathy can be manifested as peripheral neuropathy, Lhermitte's sign,[55] autonomic neuropathy,[56] grand mal or focal seizures,[57] encephalopathy,[53] transient cortical blindness,[58] retrobulbar neuritis,[53] and retinal injury.[59]

The incidence ranges up to 50% but depends on individual and cumulative dose, duration of treatment, concomitant or prior neurotoxic drugs used, the presence of other medical conditions, and possibly gender (women being more sensitive).[51,52] If very high doses (200 mg/m^2 over 5 days) are used, the incidence rises to nearly 100%.[52] A cumulative cisplatin dose of 300 to 500 mg/m^2 raises the incidence significantly.[51,53]

Peripheral neuropathy similar to that induced by vincristine is the most common form of cisplatin neurotoxicity. Vincristine produces initial paresthesia in the fingers, while cisplatin most often affects the toes and feet.[54] Loss of the Achilles tendon reflexes is also an early sign, and continued treatment leads to loss of deep tendon reflexes at more proximal sites, loss of vibration sense, and sensory ataxia (from loss of sensation in the feet). Although muscle cramps are a common symptom, motor function is usually not affected.

The pathophysiology of the neurotoxicity is not known, but it may be related to the accumulation of inorganic platinum within neurons. Large sensory nerves are affected most and show axonal demyelination. Treatment is discontinuation of cisplatin, but the symptoms, particularly of the peripheral neuropathy, may take months to resolve, and may never resolve.[60] The symptoms and signs may even progress despite discontinuing treatment.[61] Because treatment of the neurotoxicity is of limited benefit, prevention has been explored using protective agents. Two investigational drugs, amifostine (WR 2721) and an adrenocorticotropic hormone analog called Org 2766, have demonstrated promise in delaying or preventing cisplatin neurotoxicity.[62,63]

CYTARABINE

This drug is administered both intravenously and intrathecally, and both routes produce neurotoxicity. The manifestations include cerebellar dysfunction, seizures, generalized encephalopathy, peripheral neuropathy, necrotizing leukoencephalopathy, spinal cord myelopathy, and pseudobulbar palsy.[64]

The highest incidence (15–37%) occurs in patients receiving high-dose therapy (*i.e.*, over 1 g/m^2 in multiple doses).[64,65] Generally, the toxicity is acute and not cumulative, in contrast to vincristine and cisplatin.

Cerebellar effects (dysarthria, ataxia, and dysmetria) are the most common form of neurotoxicity. These symptoms often occur within days of first treatment and are accompanied by somnolence, memory loss, altered mentation, and headache. Seizures have rarely occurred. These neurologic abnormalities can progress to coma and even death.

Peripheral neuropathy is rare. Symptoms range from a purely sensory neuropathy to sensorimotor polyneuropathies in a stocking-glove distribution.[64] Even this form of neurotoxicity can be severe and fatal,[66] by inducing a polyneuropathy causing flaccid paralysis and respiratory arrest.

Risk factors for neurotoxicity are age over 60, drug dose, prior cytarabine treatment, and renal dysfunction.[64,67] Although the risk for neurologic problems increases when high cytarabine doses are given to patients over age 60, it is not prohibitive, and older patients should be treated if indicated.[64]

Recovery from the neurologic effects usually occurs within a few days after discontinuing therapy. Most patients should probably not be retreated with cytarabine after recovery, unless special circumstances exist. There is no known therapy.

The mechanism of such neurologic toxicity is not known. Research suggests that cytarabine inhibits survival of neurons by blocking an essential deoxynucleoside[68] or by inducing production of large amounts of choline acetyltransferase enzyme.[69] Also unknown is why the cerebellum has a particular sensitivity to intravenous cytarabine. Intrathecal administration, which can cause myelopathy, spares the cerebellum in its toxic effect.

IFOSFAMIDE

Ifosfamide and cyclophosphamide have similar chemical structures, but ifosfamide induces neurotoxicity, while cyclophosphamide does not. Acute symptoms are hallucinations, vivid dreams, confusion, anxiety and restlessness, personality changes, seizures, cerebellar and cranial nerve dysfunction, hemiparesis, coma, and occasionally death.[70–72] The onset is a mean of 46 hours (and up to 5 days) after beginning ifosfamide,[70,71] and recovery usually occurs within a few days. Occasionally, memory and affect disorders may persist.[73] No cumulative-dose effects of ifosfamide on neural tissue have been reported.

The incidence has been reported to vary from 5% to 70%, depending on how carefully patients were monitored and results recorded.[70,71,73,74] The intensity of neurologic dysfunction is also variable, but an overall incidence of significant symptoms is 10% to 25%. The neurotoxicity is possibly due to high blood levels of a metabolite of ifosfamide, chloracetaldehyde.[75] It is not the uroprotective agent mesna.[70]

Factors that increase the risk of encephalopathy are low serum albumin, any degree of renal dysfunction, prior administration of cisplatin (resulting in subclinical renal abnormalities), and perhaps age. Giving ifosfamide in a 5-day continuous infusion appears to reduce the frequency of neurotoxicity.[76]

5-FLUOROURACIL

5-Fluorouracil (5-FU) has been known to cause neurotoxicity since the earliest clinical trials conducted with this drug.[77] Cerebellar dysfunction with findings of gait ataxia, nystagmus, dysmetria, and dysarthria is the most common form of neurotoxicity. Confusion and cerebral cognitive defects have also been reported.[78] A rare problem is optic neuropathy and decreased vision.[79]

The incidence is 5% to 10% and occurs with all schedules of administration in common use. This toxicity is acute in onset, and a cumulative-dose effect has not been observed.

The cause is not well understood. A 5-FU metabolite, fluorocitrate, was believed to induce the neurotoxicity,[80] but several patients have been reported who developed severe toxic symptoms due to an enzyme deficiency for metabolizing 5-FU.[81] This toxicity appears to be due to the parent compound and not metabolites. Patients with complete or partial deficiency of the enzyme, dihydropyrimidine dehydrogenase, appear particularly subject to 5-FU neurotoxicity.[81]

This neurotoxicity is usually reversible by discontinuing 5-FU. Since there is no cumulative effect, therapy can be resumed later if desired, usually with either a lower dose or a less frequent dosing schedule to prevent recurrence.

METHOTREXATE

Neurotoxicity from methotrexate drug can manifest as meningeal irritation, transient paraparesis, or encephalopathy.

When methotrexate is administered intrathecally, it can induce headache, nausea and vomiting, lethargy, nuchal rigidity, and other features of meningeal irritation.[82] A subacute set of abnormalities include paraparesis, cranial nerve palsies, and cerebellar symptoms, which can develop days to several weeks after therapy. If methotrexate is given repetitively, especially if it is administered through an intraventricular device, progressive necrotizing leukoencephalopathy may rarely develop. Symptoms include initial memory loss with later progression to severe dementia and seizures. Risk factors are cranial irradiation, presence of neoplastic cells in the spinal fluid, and cumulative dose.

Intravenous methotrexate also can produce encephalopathy, especially if cranial irradiation is used concomitantly or high methotrexate doses are given. The manifestations and risk factors are similar to those of intrathecal methotrexate. The neurologic dysfunction may be acute and transient with full recovery[83] or delayed in onset with personality changes.[84] The incidence varies from 5% to 15%. Neuroradiologic scans often show white matter abnormalities that are probably irreversible.[85]

The neurotoxic effect of methotrexate is probably a direct effect of high drug concentrations in the central nervous system. Neurotransmitter substance synthesis may be impeded by methotrexate.

PACLITAXEL (TAXOL)

This agent causes neurotoxicity similar to that of cisplatin and vincristine in the form of a peripheral neurotoxicity that can be a treatment-limiting effect.[86] The clinical manifestations are glove-stocking or perioral paresthesia, burning pain in the plantar surfaces of the feet, loss of vibration sense, loss of deep tendon reflexes, and orthostatic hypotension.[86,87] The symptoms may be greater than the degree of objective abnormalities found either on physical examination or by neurometric testing. Motor dysfunction is uncommon but has been severe when it occurs.[86] The onset of neurotoxicity can be rapid, with development of symptoms within a few days of receiving the drug.[87]

The neurotoxicity is both individual and cumulative dose-related.[86,88] Individual doses over 170 mg/m^2 and four or more courses are most often associated with neurotoxic manifestations. The incidence varies but has been reported to be as high as 25%.[87] Risk factors include the presence of preexisting alcoholic or diabetic neuropathy and the concomitant administration of cisplatin.[87,88] The mechanism of Taxol neurotoxicity is likely due to drug effect on neuronal and Schwann cell microtubules, causing axonal degeneration and demyelination. Neurometric testing demonstrates decreased nerve conduction velocities and absent sural nerve action potentials.[86,87] Sometimes abnormal test results are demonstrated in the absence of neurologic symptoms.

The only effective treatment, as with other neurotoxic drugs, is discontinuation of therapy. The symptoms usually resolve after a few months. Amitriptyline may help with symptomatic relief.

ALTRETAMINE (HEXAMETHYLMELAMINE)

This drug causes a variety of peripheral and central nervous system toxicities. Peripheral neuropathy is the most common form and manifests as paresthesia, hyperesthesia, hyporeflexia, and diminished proprioception.[89] Central nervous effects are confusion, dysphasia, personality changes, ataxia, somnolence, seizures, respiratory dyskinesia, and parkinsonian tremors.[89]

Neurotoxicity is related to both individual and cumulative doses. Intermittent dosing schedules help reduce this side effect. The incidence varies depending on the dose but can be as high as 40%.[89] Altretamine can be safely administered to patients who have been treated previously with cisplatin,[90] but not if significant cisplatin neuropathy is present.

Administration of pyridoxine has been used as neurotoxicity prophylaxis but has provided modest efficacy, and at least one study[91] suggested that pyridoxine can reduce antitumor effect. The most effective treatment is discontinuation of altretamine therapy. Symptoms, especially the severe ones, usually then resolve.

PROCARBAZINE

Neurotoxicity from this agent has been known since it was first used clinically.[92] Both central and peripheral neurotoxicity symptoms can occur. Cerebral symptoms predominate and consist of lethargy, depression, confusion, hallucinations, agitation, and rarely psychosis. Extremity paresthesia and depressed deep tendon reflexes are the manifestations of peripheral neuropathy.

Since this drug is most commonly used in combination with the vinca alkaloids, it is difficult to determine which agent is causing peripheral neuropathy symptoms. The incidence of neuropathy induced by procarbazine alone is 20% or less. It is much higher when procarbazine and vincristine are administered together.

Treatment is discontinuation of therapy. Cerebral symptoms usually resolve promptly, but peripheral neuropathy may last for weeks to months.

FLUDARABINE

When this agent was tested in phase I and II trials in acute leukemia, central nervous system toxicity was so severe that the studies had to be closed. Altered mental status, photophobia, amaurosis, generalized seizures, spastic or flaccid paralysis, quadriparesis, and coma occurred at doses over 90 mg/m² given for 5 to 7 days.[93,94] Despite discontinuing therapy, some patients had progressive neurologic abnormalities and died. Since such severe toxicity is clearly dose-related, the recommended fludarabine dose is 25 mg/m² daily for 5 days, monthly. Such doses usually cause no more than mild neurologic symptoms.[95] Even doses in this range, however, can occasionally cause severe, and even fatal, central nervous system toxicity.[94,96]

Fludarabine specifically affects the optic nerves and causes optic demyelination. It also can cause demyelination in the cerebral peduncles and pons.

OTHER AGENTS

Table 63–10 lists other drugs that can produce neurotoxicity and categorizes them based on the risk for this side effect. The manifestations are similar to those described for the individual drugs.

HEPATOTOXICITY

A number of antitumor agents cause hepatic injury (Table 63–11). This toxicity takes three main forms: hepatocellular dysfunction and chemical hepatitis, venoocclusive disease (VOD), and chronic fibrosis.

HEPATOCELLULAR DYSFUNCTION

This form of hepatic injury is usually due to a direct effect of either parent drug or a metabolite and is an acute event. Serum hepatic enzymes rise as cellular damage occurs. Fatty infiltration and cholestasis may occur as the toxic effect progresses. Since hepatic metastases, viral hepatitis, and drugs administered for other therapeutic purposes (*e.g.*, antiemetics) can cause similar enzymatic abnormalities, the clinical picture, appropriate laboratory or radiologic studies, and the pattern of abnormal liver function tests must be analyzed to identify the cause of the hepatic changes.

The drugs most likely to cause enzymatic abnormalities are L-asparaginase, carmustine in high doses, cytarabine, dactinomycin, diaziquone, etoposide, azathioprine and 6-mercaptopurine, methotrexate in high doses, plicamycin (mithramycin), streptozocin, and vincristine. All these drugs can cause rises in the serum glutamic-oxaloacetic transaminase, serum glutamic pyruvate transaminase, and serum bilirubin, but the feature of azathioprine and 6-mercaptopurine toxicity is most often cholestatic jaundice.

L-Asparaginase causes the widest spectrum of liver abnormalities and has the highest incidence of toxicity. It produces changes in liver enzymes and in hepatic protein synthesis, resulting in low plasma levels of albumin, lipoproteins, and clotting factors.[97] Prolongation of the thrombin and prothrombin times occurs as a result. Fatty metamorphosis is commonly seen,[97] and these changes may persist for several months after discontinuing treatment.[98]

Cytarabine hepatotoxicity is a common event in the treatment of acute leukemia, especially when high doses are used.[99] Since patients with acute leukemia are subject to transfusion-related hepatitis and receive a variety of potentially hepatotoxic drugs, it is always difficult to establish cytarabine as the sole hepatotoxin. However, hyperbilirubinemia developing in temporal relation to cytarabine administration, accompanied by histologic abnormalities on liver biopsy, has demonstrated the hepatotoxicity potential of this agent.[100]

TABLE 63–10. Antitumor Agents That Cause Neurotoxicity

High Potential for Neurotoxicity	
Altretamine	Interferons (in high doses)
L-Asparaginase	Methotrexate
Carboplatin	Pentostatin
Cisplatin	Procarbazine
Cytarabine	Suramin
Fludarabine	Taxol
5-Fluorouracil	Vincristine and vinblastine
Ifosfamide	
Occasional Irreversible Neurotoxicity	
Cisplatin	Suramin
Cytarabine	Taxol
Ifosfamide	
Low Potential for Neurotoxicity	
Amsacrine	Nitrosoureas
Dacarbazine	Teniposide
Etoposide	Thiotepa (intrathecal)
Interferons (in low doses)	

TABLE 63–11. Antitumor Agents That Cause Hepatotoxicity

High Potential for Hepatotoxicity	
L-Asparaginase	Methotrexate (long-term therapy)
Cytarabine	Plicamycin (mithramycin)
Interferons (in high doses)	Streptozocin
High Potential for Hepatotoxicity With High Doses	
Busulfan	Dactinomycin (in single doses)
Carmustine	Diaziquone
Cyclophosphamide	Methotrexate
Cytarabine	Mitomycin
Occasional Irreversible Hepatotoxicity	
Azathioprine	Dacarbazine
Busulfan (in high doses)	Methotrexate
Carmustine (in high doses)	Mitomycin
Cytarabine	
Low Potential for Hepatotoxicity	
Azathioprine	6-Mercaptopurine
Dacarbazine	Pentostatin
Hydroxyurea	6-Thioguanine
Interferons (in low doses)	Vincristine

VENOOCCLUSIVE DISEASE

Venoocclusive liver disease results from blockage of venous outflow in the small centrilobular and sublobular hepatic vessels. Antitumor drugs known to produce this form of hepatotoxicity are azathioprine and 6-mercaptopurine, cytarabine, dacarbazine, and 6-thioguanine. In addition, busulfan, carmustine, cyclophosphamide, and mitomycin given in high doses can cause VOD.

Dactinomycin in combination with vincristine has been recognized to cause this severe hepatotoxicity, especially when dactinomycin is administered in single doses rather than over 5 days.[101] The clinical features are marked elevations in serum enzymes, ascites, hepatomegaly, and hepatic encephalopathy. The onset is often abrupt and the clinical course fulminant. In some cases, the histologic features are those of hepatic VOD, and in others, there is hepatocellular injury.[101]

Busulfan, carmustine, cyclophosphamide, and mitomycin all can produce hepatic VOD when they are administered in high doses for marrow transplantations. The incidence in transplantation settings is about 20%, and the mortality is high.[102,103] All the drugs reported to induce VOD at high doses have been alkylating agents. This may not be due to any unusual tendency of alkylating agents to cause VOD but rather to the fact that these are the drugs used in very large doses in marrow transplantation.

VOD is initiated by injury to hepatic venous endothelium, which then precipitates thrombosis and hepatocellular necrosis. There is probably also a component of hepatocellular injury directly related to the high-dose drug and not mediated by thrombosis.[103]

Conventional doses of certain antitumor agents (*e.g.*, dacarbazine, 6-mercaptopurine, 6-thioguanine) can also cause hepatic VOD. Dacarbazine has been recognized to have this toxicity most often, although only sporadic cases have been reported. Use of dacarbazine both alone and in combination with other drugs has been associated with hepatic VOD.[104] It is unknown why only some patients develop this life-threatening complication of dacarbazine, but a form of allergic or hypersensitivity reaction has been speculated as the mechanism.[105]

CHRONIC FIBROSIS

Methotrexate dosing schedules used for cancer treatment can produce acute and reversible hepatocellular injury and elevations of serum enzymes. Intermittent dosing seems to obviate chronic hepatic toxicity; however, long-term use of methotrexate for the treatment of nonmalignant disease (*e.g.*, psoriasis and rheumatoid arthritis) poses a greater hazard for development of hepatic fibrosis. Since patients with autoimmune diseases may already have underlying histologic abnormalities, there is controversy regarding how much hepatic damage methotrexate causes and whether periodic liver biopsies are necessary for patient monitoring.[106] It is clear, however, that a few patients suffer severe cirrhosis from this drug and require liver transplantation.[107]

HYPERSENSITIVITY REACTIONS

Most of the available antitumor drugs can produce hypersensitivity reactions, and a substantial minority cause such reactions in as many as 5% of patients treated. There are two agents for which hypersensitivity reactions are frequent enough to be a major treatment-limiting toxicity: L-asparaginase and Taxol. Most other agents produce such reactions only sporadically. The mechanism of these hypersensitivity reactions is often unknown or evaluated only in a single patient, and it is rarely possible to prevent them.

L-Asparaginase produces hypersensitivity reactions in 10% to 20% of patients, and it can be immediate and life-threatening with all the components of anaphylaxis. This high rate is undoubtedly related to the fact that L-asparaginase is a polypeptide of bacterial origin, displaying multiple antigenic sites.

The clinical manifestations are typical of type I reactions with acute onset of wheezing, pruritus, rash, angioedema, extremity pain, agitation, and hypotension.[97,108] A number of factors increase the risk for hypersensitivity reactions, including history of atopy or other drug allergy, prior L-asparaginase therapy (including even several years previously), high drug doses, and intravenous route of administration. Intramuscular administration often reduces the severity of reactions,[109] but they still can occur and may do so several hours after the drug is given. Concomitant treatment with prednisone and vincristine (for the acute leukemia being treated) also appears to reduce the risk of reactions.[108]

No reliable method has been developed to determine who is going to have a reaction with any dose of L-asparaginase. Intradermal skin testing can give both false-negative and false-positive results, and test doses of the drug are valueless.[108] Therefore, one must approach each dose of L-asparaginase as the one that could initiate a hypersensitivity reaction and be prepared to treat it. Antianaphylaxis medication must be close at hand, and the patient should be observed for about 1 hour after the drug is administered.

When a hypersensitivity reaction occurs with the *Escherichia coli* source of L-asparaginase, one can substitute the *Erwinia chrysanthemia* form and continue therapy. This form of drug is immunologically distinct[110] and appears to have a lower degree of immunogenicity. Patients may still sustain a hypersensitivity reaction from the *Erwinia* sp form, but most (75%) do not and can complete the planned therapy.[108] Precautions for treating anaphylaxis are as necessary for the *Erwinia* sp substitute as for the *E. coli* product. A third form of L-asparaginase has been developed that provides another alternative for the patient who is reactive to the other two forms and still needs L-asparaginase therapy. This form, a conjugate with polyethylene glycol (pegaspargase), may be the least immunogenic and has lower degrees of all toxicities.[111]

The mechanism of L-asparaginase reactions appears to be mediated by an immunoglobulin (Ig) E antibody in at least some cases.[112] There is also evidence that complement activation occurs, perhaps induced by specific IgG or IgM antibodies.[110]

Taxol is a newly approved drug that has high promise for being an effective addition to the oncologist's therapeutic arsenal. One of its toxicities has been hypersensitivity reactions, and it is standard procedure to administer drugs as prophylaxis for such reactions.[113]

The clinical manifestations are those of any type I hypersensitivity reaction and include bronchospasm and wheezing, rash, agitation, angioedema, and hypotension. These symptoms most often occur with the first or second drug exposure. The onset is usually within minutes of starting a drug infusion, and even very small drug doses are capable of initiating a hypersensitivity reaction.[113]

To prevent or assuage these reactions, Taxol is usually infused over 6 to 24 hours. In addition, premedication with corticosteroids and antihistamines is standard procedure. Such measures reduce the risk but do not fully prevent reactions.

It is unclear whether Taxol itself or the excipient, Cremophor EL, is the cause of hypersensitivity. Cremophor EL induces histamine release and could be responsible for acute reactions. The mechanism of these reactions has not been well studied, but the fact that they can occur with the first Taxol dose suggests a nonimmunologic one.

A number of other chemotherapeutic agents (Table 63–12) are known to produce hypersensitivity reactions in at least sporadic instances.[114] Most of these reactions have the features of a type I hypersensitivity, whether mediated by IgE or nonimmunologically. Hemolytic anemia (type II reaction) is an uncommon form of toxicity.[18] Some drugs, such as procarbazine and methotrexate, produce acute episodes that are typical of a type III reaction and cause interstitial pneumonitis and vasculitis.[114] In most cases of hypersensitivity reactions from antitumor drugs, only isolated cases are studied adequately to define the cause of the reaction, and it is not possible to rule out the excipients used in drug formulation (*e.g.*, benzyl alcohol and dimethylacetamide) or other drugs used concomitantly (*e.g.*, mesna and mannitol) as the source of the reactivity.[114] When reactions occur from one drug, it is often possible to continue therapy by either substituting another drug in the same class or administering premedication as prophylaxis.

VASCULAR TOXICITY

Three main forms of vascular toxicity are produced by chemotherapeutic agents: VOD, venous or arterial thrombosis, and vascular ischemia (involving cerebral, myocardial, or extremity arterial vessels).

TABLE 63–12. Antitumor Agents That Cause Hypersensitivity Reactions

High Potential for Hypersensitivity Reactions	
L-Asparaginase	Teniposide
Elliptinium	Taxol
Procarbazine	
Low Potential for Hypersensitivity Reactions	
Anthracyclines	Ifosfamide
Azathioprine	Interferons
Bleomycin	Interleukin-2
Carboplatin	Mechlorethamine
Chlorambucil	Melphalan
Cisplatin	6-Mercaptopurine
Cyclophosphamide	Methotrexate
Cytarabine	Mitomycin
Dacarbazine	Mitoxantrone
Etoposide	Pentostatin
5-Fluorouracil	Vinca alkaloids
Hydroxyurea	

VOD of the hepatic vein is discussed under the section on hepatotoxicity. This acute venous toxicity can also involve pulmonary vessels as a rare toxicity of chemotherapy.[115] It may be just one manifestation of pulmonary toxicity from such drugs as bleomycin and mitomycin.

Venous thrombosis in association with metastatic cancer has long been recognized (Trousseau's syndrome). Chemotherapeutic agents can also induce venous thrombosis in the form of extremity thromboses and pulmonary emboli, even in the absence of demonstrable metastatic cancer.[116,117] Although it is less common, thromboses of extremity arteries can also be initiated by chemotherapy, again in the absence of demonstrable cancer.[117,118] No one drug seems to be at fault, and the mechanism of thrombosis induction is unknown.

Arterial ischemia or thrombosis can be induced by chemotherapy in major coronary or cerebral vessels and in the small vessels of the extremities. Cerebrovascular accidents have been reported in association with the use of cisplatin and bleomycin in young men without other risk factors for such events.[119] In similar circumstances, acute myocardial infarction has occurred.[6,120] Myocardial ischemia and infarction occur in about 10% of patients who receive infusional 5-FU, and sudden death has occurred.[121] These events occur in patients who have no known underlying coronary vessel disease, and the pathogenesis seems to be coronary artery spasm. Anginal symptoms are often a precursor, which can be relieved by discontinuing the 5-FU therapy. Raynaud's phenomenon occurs as a chronic toxicity in about 40% of young men treated with cisplatin-based combination chemotherapy for testicular cancer.[6] Cigarette smoking increases the risk for this toxicity. Clinical manifestations are painful digits and paresthesia occurring a mean of 10 months after starting chemotherapy and lasting for 5 or more years. Patients often are unable to work outside in cold weather. The mechanism appears to be a vasospastic phenomenon, without any vascular obstruction, in the terminal arterioles due to impaired smooth muscle function.[122] It is not known which of the drugs used for testicular cancer is most involved in the cause of this toxicity, but bleomycin is the most likely candidate because it can cause Raynaud's phenomenon when used alone.[123]

REFERENCES

1. Rossof AH, Slayton RE, Perlia CP. Preliminary clinical experience with *cis*-diamminedichloroplatinum II (NSC 119875). Cancer 1972;30:1451–1456.
2. Talley RW, O'Bryan RM, Gutterman JU, et al. Clinical evaluation of toxic effects of *cis*-diamminedichloroplatinum (NSC-119875): Phase I clinical study. Cancer Chemother Rep 1973;57:465–471..
3. Hayes DM, Cvitkovic E, Golbey RB, et al. High dose cis-platinum diammine dichloride: Amelioration of renal toxicity by mannitol diuresis. Cancer 1977;39:1372–1381.
4. Hardaker WT, Stone RA, McCoy R. Platinum nephrotoxicity. Cancer 1974;34:1030–1032.
5. Tanaka H, Ishikawa E, Teshima S, et al. Histopathological study of human cisplatin nephropathy. Toxicol Pathol 1986;14:247–257.
6. Vogelzang NJ, Torkelson JL, Kennedy BJ. Hypomagnesemia, renal dysfunction, and Raynaud's phenomenon in patients treated with cisplatin, vinblastine, and bleomycin. Cancer 1985;56:2765–2770.
7. Hutchison FN, Perez EA, Gandara DR, et al. Renal salt wasting in patients treated with cisplatin. Ann Intern Med 1988;108:21–25.
8. Markman M, Rothman R, Reichman B, et al. Persistent hypomagnesemia following cisplatin chemotherapy in patients with ovarian cancer. J Cancer Res Clin Oncol 1991;117:89–90.
9. Leonard BJ, Eccleston E, Jones D, et al. Antileukaemic and nephrotoxic properties of platinum compounds. Nature 1971;234:43–45.

10. Hrushesky WJM. Circadian timing of cancer chemotherapy. Science 1985;228:73–74.
11. Hargis JB, Anderson JR, Propert KJ, et al. Predicting genitourinary toxicity in patients receiving cisplatin-based combination chemotherapy: A Cancer and Leukemia Group B study. Cancer Chemother Pharmacol 1992;30:291–296.
12. Mangioni C, Bolis G, Pecorelli S, et al. Randomized trial in advanced ovarian cancer comparing cisplatin and carboplatin. J Natl Cancer Inst 1989;81:1464–1471.
13. McDonald BR, Kirmani S, Vasquez M, et al. Acute renal failure associated with the use of intraperitoneal carboplatin: A report of two cases and review of the literature. Am J Med 1991;90:386–391.
14. Reed E, Jacob J. Carboplatin and renal dysfunction. Ann Intern Med 1989;110:409.
15. Sleijfer DT, Smit EF, Meijer S, et al. Acute and cumulative effects of carboplatin on renal function. Br J Cancer 1989;60:116–120.
16. Liu K, Mittelman A, Sproul EE, et al. Renal toxicity in man treated with mitomycin C. Cancer 1971;28:1314–1320.
17. Hanna WT, Krauss S, Regester RF, et al. Renal disease after mitomycin C therapy. Cancer 1981;48:2583–2588.
18. Doll DC, Weiss RB. Hemolytic anemia associated with antineoplastic agents. Cancer Treat Rep 1985;69:777–782.
19. Allum WH, Hallissey MT, Kelly KA for the British Stomach Cancer Group. Adjuvant chemotherapy in operable gastric cancer. Lancet 1989;1:571–574.
20. Lesesne JB, Rothschild N, Erickson B, et al. Cancer-associated hemolytic-uremic syndrome: Analysis of 85 cases from a national registry. J Clin Oncol 1989;7:781–789.
21. Chow S, Roscoe J, Cattran DC. Plasmapheresis and antiplatelet agents in the treatment of the hemolytic uremic syndrome secondary to mitomycin. Am J Kidney Dis 1986;7: 407–412.
22. Korec S, Schein PS, Smith FP, et al. Treatment of cancer-associated hemolytic uremic syndrome with staphylococcal protein A immunoperfusion. J Clin Oncol 1986;4:210–215.
23. Cattell V. Mitomycin-induced hemolytic uremic kidney: An experimental model in the rat. Am J Pathol 1985;121:88–95.
24. Stoller RG, Jacobs SA, Drake JC, et al. Pharmacokinetics of high-dose methotrexate (NSC-740). Cancer Chemother Rep 1975;6:19–24, 1975.
25. Ackland SP, Schilsky RL: High-dose methotrexate: A critical reappraisal. J Clin Oncol 1987;5:2017–2031.
26. Goren MP, Wright RK, Horowitz ME, et al. Enhancement of methotrexate nephrotoxicity after cisplatin therapy. Cancer 1986;58:2617–2621.
27. Ellison NM, Servi RJ. Acute renal failure and death following sequential intermediate-dose methotrexate and 5-FU: A possible adverse effect due to concomitant indomethacin administration. Cancer Treat Rep 1985;69:342–343.
28. Thyss A, Kubar J, Milano G, et al. Clinical and pharmacokinetic evidence of a life-threatening interaction between methotrexate and ketoprofen. Lancet 1986;1:256–258.
29. Singh RR, Malaviya AN, Pandey JN, et al. Fatal interaction between methotrexate and naproxen. Lancet 1986;1:1390.
30. Thierry FX, Vernier I, Dueymes JM, et al. Acute renal failure after high-dose methotrexate therapy: Role of hemodialysis and plasma exchange in methotrexate removal. Nephron 1989;5:416–417.
31. Bouffet E, Frappaz D, Laville M, et al. Charcoal haemoperfusion and methotrexate toxicity. Lancet 1986;1:1497.
32. Loftus L, Cuppage FE, Hoogstraten B. Clinical and pathological effects of streptozotocin. J Lab Clin Med 1974;84:407–413.
33. Broder LE, Carter SK. Pancreatic islet cell carcinoma. II. Results of therapy with streptozotocin in 52 patients. Ann Intern Med 1973;79:108–118.
34. Tobin MV, Warenius HM, Morris AI. Forced diuresis to reduce nephrotoxicity of streptozotocin in the treatment of advanced metastatic insulinoma. Br Med J 1987;294: 1128.
35. Ellis ME, Weiss RB, Kuperminc M. Nephrotoxicity of lomustine: A case report and literature review. Cancer Chemother Pharmacol 1985;15:174–175.
36. Focan C, Boossy J, Focan-Henrard D, et al. Phase II trial with high-dose ifosfamide and mesna given in a 24-h infusion for advanced GI tract cancer. Cancer Chemother Pharmacol 1989;23:192–193.
37. van Dyk JJ, Falkson HC, van der Merwe AM, et al. Unexpected toxicity in patients with iphosphamide. Cancer Res 1972;32:921–924.
38. Sangster G, Kaye SB, Calman KC, et al. Failure of 2-mercaptoethane sulphonate sodium (mesna) to protect against ifosfamide nephrotoxicity. Eur J Cancer Clin Oncol 1984;20: 435–436.
39. Shore RW, Geary D, Koren G, et al. Iphosphamide (IP) related nephrotoxicity in children. Proc Am Soc Clin Oncol 1991;10:311.
40. Patterson WP, Khojasteh A. Ifosfamide-induced renal tubular defects. Cancer 1989;63: 649–651.
41. Pratt CB, Meyer WH, Jenkins JJ, et al. Ifosfamide, Fanconi's syndrome, and rickets. J Clin Oncol 1991;9:1495–1499.
42. Parker GW, Wiltsie DS, Jackson CB. The clinical evaluation of PA-144 (mithramycin) in solid tumors of adults. Cancer Chemother Rep 1960;8:23–26.
43. Benedetti RG, Heilman KJ, Gabow PA. Nephrotoxicity following single dose mithramycin therapy. Am J Nephrol 1983;3:277–278.
44. Gradishar WJ, Vokes EE, Ni K. Chemotherapy-related hemolytic-uremic syndrome after the treatment of head and neck cancer: A case report. Cancer 1990;66:1914–1918.
45. Gardner G, Mesler D, Gitelman HJ. Hemolytic uremic syndrome following cisplatin, bleomycin, and vincristine chemotherapy: A report of a case and a review of the literature. Renal Failure 1989;11:133–137.
46. Weiden PL, Wright SE. Vincristine neurotoxicity. N Engl J Med 1972;286:1369–1370.
47. Weiss HD, Walker MD, Wiernik PH. Neurotoxicity of commonly used antineoplastic agents (second of two parts). N Engl J Med 1974;291:127–133.
48. Roca E, Bruera E, Politi PM, et al. Vinca alkaloid-induced cardiovascular autonomic neuropathy. Cancer Treat Rep 1985;69:149–151.
49. Griffiths JD, Stark RJ, Ding JC, et al. Vincristine neurotoxicity in Charcot-Marie-Tooth syndrome. Med J Aust 1985;143:305–306.
50. Garewal HS, Dalton WS. Metoclopramide in vincristine-induced ileus. Cancer Treat Rep 1985;69:1309–1311.
51. Gerritsen van der Hoop R, van der Burg MEL, ten Bokkel Huinink WW, et al. Incidence of neuropathy in 395 patients with ovarian cancer treated with or without cisplatin. Cancer 1990;66:1967–1702.
52. Legha SS, Dimery IW. High dose cisplatin administration without hypertonic saline: Observation of disabling neurotoxicity. J Clin Oncol 1985;3:1373–1378.
53. Cersosimo RJ. Cisplatin neurotoxicity. Cancer Treat Rev 1989;16:195–211.
54. Thompson SW, Davis LE, Kornfeld M, et al. Cisplatin neuropathy: Clinical, electrophysiologic, morphologic, and toxicologic studies. Cancer 1984;54:1269–1275.
55. Eeles R, Tait DM, Peckham MJ. Lhermitte's sign as a complication of cisplatin-containing chemotherapy for testicular cancer. Cancer Treat Rep 1986;70:905–907.
56. Cohen SC, Mollman JE. Cisplatin-induced gastric paresis. J Neurooncol 1987;5:237–240.
57. Mead GH, Arnold AM, Green JA, et al. Epileptic seizures associated with cisplatin administration. Cancer Treat Rep 1982;66:1719–1722.
58. Pippitt CH, Muss HB, Homesley HD, et al. Cisplatin-associated cortical blindness. Gynecol Oncol 1981;12:253–255.
59. Wilding G, Caruso R, Lawrence TS, et al. Retinal toxicity after high-dose cisplatin therapy. J Clin Oncol 1985;3:1683–1689.
60. Greenspan A, Treat J. Peripheral neuropathy and low dose cisplatin. Am J Clin Oncol (CCT) 1988;11:660–662.
61. Siegal T, Haim N. Cisplatin-induced peripheral neuropathy: Frequent off-therapy deterioration, demyelinating syndromes, and muscle cramps. Cancer 1990;66:1117–1123.
62. Mollman JE, Glover DJ, Hogan WM, et al. Cisplatin neuropathy: Risk factors, prognosis, and protection by WR 2721. Cancer 1988;61:2192–2195.
63. Gerritsen van der Hoop R, Vecht CJ, van der Burg MEL, et al. Prevention of cisplatin neurotoxicity with an ACTH (4–9) analogue in patients with ovarian cancer. N Engl J Med 1990;322:89–94.
64. Baker WJ, Royer GL, Weiss RB. Cytarabine and neurologic toxicity. J Clin Oncol 1991;9:679–693.
65. Graves T, Hooks MA. Drug-induced toxicities associated with high-dose cytosine arabinoside infusions. Pharmacotherapy 1989;9:23–28.
66. Nevill TJ, Benstead TJ, McCormick CW, et al. Horner's syndrome and demyelinating peripheral neuropathy caused by high-dose cytosine arabinoside. Am J Hematol 1989;32: 314–315.
67. Damon LE, Mass R, Linker CA. The association between high-dose cytarabine neurotoxicity and renal insufficiency. J Clin Oncol 1989;7:1563–1568.
68. Wallace TL, Johnson EM. Cytosine arabinoside kills postmitotic neurons: Evidence that deoxycytidine may have a role in neuronal survival that is independent of DNA synthesis. J Neurosci 1989;9:115–124.
69. Patel AJ, Hunt A, Seaton P. The mechanism of cytosine arabinoside toxicity on quiescent astrocytes in vitro appears to be analogous to in vivo brain injury. Brain Res 1988;450: 378–381.
70. Weiss RB. Ifosfamide vs cyclophosphamide in cancer therapy. Oncology (Williston Park) 1991;5:67–76.
71. Watkin SW, Husband DJ, Green JA, et al. Ifosfamide encephalopathy: A reappraisal. Eur J Cancer Clin Oncol 1989;25:1303–1310.
72. Merimsky O, Inbar M, Reider-Grosswasser I, et al. Ifosfamide-related acute encephalopathy: Clinical and radiological aspects. Eur J Cancer 1991;27:1188–1189.
73. Heim ME, Fiene R, Schick E, et al. Central nervous side effects following ifosfamide monotherapy of advanced renal carcinoma. J Cancer Res Clin Oncol 1981;10:113–116.
74. Pratt CB, Green AA, Horowitz ME, et al. Central nervous toxicity following treatment of pediatric patients with ifosfamide/mesna. J Clin Oncol 1986;4:1253–1261.
75. Goren MP, Wright RK, Pratt CB, et al. Dechloroethylation of ifosfamide and neurotoxicity. Lancet 1986;2:1219–1220.
76. Cerny T, Castiglione M, Brunner K, et al. Ifosfamide by continuous infusion to prevent encephalopathy. Lancet 1990;1:175.
77. Moertel CG, Reitemeier RJ, Bolton CF, et al. Cerebellar ataxia associated with fluorinated pyrimidine therapy. Cancer Chemother Rep 1964;41:15–18.
78. Lynch HT, Droszcz CP, Albano WA, et al. "Organic brain syndrome" secondary to 5-fluorouracil toxicity. Dis Colon Rectum 1981;24:130–131.
79. Adams JW, Bofenkamp TM, Kobrin J, et al. Recurrent acute toxic optic neuropathy secondary to 5-FU. Cancer Treat Rep 1984;68:565–566.
80. Koenig H, Patel A. Biochemical basis for fluorouracil neurotoxicity: The role of the Krebs cycle inhibition by fluoroacetate. Arch Neurol 1970;23:155–160.
81. Diasio RB, Beavers TL, Carpenter JT. Familial deficiency of dihydropyrimidine dehydrogenase: Biochemical basis for familial pyrimidinemia and severe 5-fluorouracil-induced toxicity. J Clin Invest 1988;81:47–51.
82. Nelson RW, Frank JT. Intrathecal methotrexate-induced neurotoxicities. Am J Hosp Pharm 1981;38:65–68.
83. Walker RW, Allen JC, Rosen G, et al. Transient cerebral dysfunction secondary to high-dose methotrexate. J Clin Oncol 1986;4:1845–1850.
84. Kramer ED, Lewis D, Raney B, et al. Neurologic complications in children with soft tissue and osseus sarcoma. Cancer 1989;64:2600–2603.
85. Lien HH, Blomlie V, Saeter G, et al. Osteogenic sarcoma: MR signal abnormalities of

the brain in asymptomatic patients treated with high-dose methotrexate. Radiology 1991;179:547–550.

86. Rowinsky EK, Cazenave LA, Donehower RC. Taxol: A novel investigational antimicrotubule agent. J Natl Cancer Inst 1990;82:1247–1259.
87. Lipton RB, Apfel SC, Dutcher JP, et al. Taxol produces a predominantly sensory neuropathy. Neurology 1989;39:368–373.
88. Rowinsky EK, Gilbert MR, McGuire WP, et al. Sequences of Taxol and cisplatin: A phase I and pharmacologic study. J Clin Oncol 1991;9:1692–1703.
89. Weiss RB. The role of hexamethylmelamine in advanced ovarian carcinoma treatment. Gynecol Oncol 1981;12:141–149.
90. Manetta A, MacNeill C, Lyter JA, et al. Hexamethylmelamine as a single second-line agent in ovarian cancer. Gynecol Oncol 1990;36:93–96.
91. Wiernik PH, Yeap B, Vogl E, et al. Hexamethylmelamine and low or moderate dose cisplatin with or without pyridoxine for treatment of advanced ovarian carcinoma: A study of the Eastern Cooperative Oncology Group. Cancer Invest 1992;10:1–9.
92. Brunner KW, Young CW. A methylhydrazine derivative in Hodgkin's disease and other malignant neoplasms: Therapeutic and toxic effects studied in 51 patients. Ann Intern Med 1965;63:69–86.
93. Warrell RP, Berman E. Phase I and II study of fludarabine phosphate in leukemia: Therapeutic efficacy with delayed central nervous system toxicity. J Clin Oncol 1986;4:74–79.
94. Chun HG, Leyland-Jones BR, Caryk SM, et al. Central nervous system toxicity of fludarabine phosphate. Cancer Treat Rep 1986;70:1225–1228.
95. Puccio CA, Mittelman A, Lichtman SM, et al. A loading/continuous infusion schedule of fludarabine phosphate in chronic lymphatic leukemia. J Clin Oncol 1991;9:1562–1569.
96. Merkel DE, Griffin NL, Kagen-Hallet K, et al. Central nervous system toxicity with fludarabine. Cancer Treat Rep 1986;70:1449–1450.
97. Oettgen HF, Stephenson PA, Schwartz MK, et al. Toxicity of E. coli L-asparaginase in man. Cancer 1970;25:253–278.
98. Pratt CB, Johnson WW. Duration and severity of fatty metamorphosis of the liver following L-asparaginase therapy. Cancer 1971;28:361–364.
99. Herzig RH, Wolff SN, Lazarus HM, et al. High-dose cytosine arabinoside therapy for refractory leukemia. Blood 1983;62:361–369.
100. Pizzuto J, Avilés A, Ramos E, et al. Cytosine arabinoside induced liver damage: Histopathologic demonstration. Med Pediatr Oncol 1983;11:287–290.
101. Green DM, Norkool P, Breslow NE, et al. Severe hepatic toxicity after treatment with vincristine and dactinomycin using single-dose or divided-dose schedules: A report from the National Wilms' Tumor Study. J Clin Oncol 1990;8:1525–1530.
102. Jones RJ, Lee KSK, Beschorner WE, et al. Venoocclusive disease of the liver following bone marrow transplantation. Transplantation 1987;44:778–783.
103. Rollins BJ. Hepatic veno-occlusive disease. Am J Med 1986;81:297–306.
104. Marsh JC. Hepatic vascular toxicity of dacarbazine (DTIC): Not a rare complication. Hepatology 1989;9:790–792.
105. Erichsen C, Jönsson PE. Veno-occlusive liver disease after dacarbazine therapy (DTIC) for melanoma. J Surg Oncol 1984;27:268–270.
106. Kaplan MM. Methotrexate hepatotoxicity and the premature reporting of Mark Twain's death: Both greatly exaggerated. Hepatology 1990;12:784–786.
107. Gilbert SC, Klintmaln G, Menter A, et al. Methotrexate-induced cirrhosis requiring liver transplantation in three patients with psoriasis. Arch Intern Med 1990;150:889–891.
108. Evans WE, Tsiatis A, Rivera G, et al. Anaphylactoid reactions of *Escherichia coli* and *Erwinia* asparaginase in children with leukemia and lymphoma. Cancer 1982;49:1378–1383.
109. Eden OB, Shaw MP, Lilleyman JS, et al. Non-randomized study comparing toxicity of *Escherichia coli* and *Erwinia* asparaginase in children with leukaemia. Med Pediatr Oncol 1990;18:497–502.
110. Fabry U, Körholz D, Jürgens H, et al. Anaphylaxis to L-asparaginase during treatment for acute lymphoblastic leukemia in children–evidence of a complement-mediated mechanism. Pediatr Res 1985;19:400–408.
111. Kurtzberg J, Friedman H, Asselin B, et al. The use of polyethylene glycol conjugated L-asparaginase (PEG-ASP) in pediatric patients with prior hypersensitivity to native L-asparaginase. Proc Am Soc Clin Oncol 1990;9:219.
112. Khan A, Hill JM. Atopic hypersensitivity to L-asparaginase: Resistance to immunosuppression. Int Arch Allergy 1971;40:463–469.
113. Weiss RB, Donehower RH, Wiernik PH, et al. Hypersensitivity reactions from Taxol. J Clin Oncol 1990;8:1263–1268.
114. Weiss RB. Hypersensitivity reactions. Semin Oncol 1992;19:458–477.
115. Joselson R, Warnock M. Pulmonary veno-occlusive disease after chemotherapy. Hum Pathol 1983;14:88–91.
116. Weiss RB, Tormey DC Holland JF, et al. Venous thrombosis during multimodal therapy of primary breast carcinoma. Cancer Treat Rep 1981;65:677–679.
117. Saphner T, Tormey DC, Gray R. Venous and arterial thrombosis in patients who received adjuvant therapy for breast cancer. J Clin Oncol 1991;9:286–294.
118. Wall JG, Weiss RB, Norton L, et al. Arterial thrombosis associated with adjuvant chemotherapy for breast carcinoma: A Cancer and Leukemia Group B study. Am J Med 1989;87:501–504.
119. Doll DC, List AF, Greco FA, et al. Acute arterial ischemic events following cisplatin-based combination chemotherapy for germ cell tumors of the testis. Ann Intern Med 1986;105:48–51.
120. Samuels BL, Vogelzang NJ, Kennedy BJ. Severe vascular toxicity associated with vinblastine, bleomycin, and cisplatin chemotherapy. Cancer Chemother Pharmacol 1987;19:253–256.
121. Gradishar WJ, Vokes EE. 5-fluorouracil cardiotoxicity: A critical review. Ann Oncol 1990;1:409–414.
122. Hansen SW, Olsen N, Rossing N, et al. Vascular toxicity and the mechanism underlying Raynaud's phenomenon in patients treated with cisplatin, vinblastine and bleomycin. Ann Oncol 1990;1:289–292.
123. Epstein E. Intralesional bleomycin and Raynaud's phenomenon. J Am Acad Dermatol 1991;24:785–786.

SECTION **3**

McCLELLAN M. WALTHER

Cystitis

Cystitis, defined symptomatically as an irritation of the bladder, manifests itself with suprapubic discomfort, frequency, dysuria, and urgency. Severe cases may include urge incontinence and hematuria. The cause may be related to a chemical agent that is toxic to the bladder, radiation, thrombocytopenia with subsequent bleeding, or myelosuppression with associated infection. Patients may present with acute exsanguinating hematuria (discussed in Chapter 50, section 5) but more commonly develop milder symptoms and pathologic disease.

General measures taken in the initial evaluation of patients with cystitis should exclude urinary infection and the presence of malignancy. Symptomatic relief of discomfort on voiding can be obtained with urinary analgesics such as phenazopyridine hydrochloride (Pyridium). Suprapubic discomfort, frequency, urgency, and urge incontinence require antispasmodics to obtain relief. Oxybutynin chloride (Ditropan), propantheline bromide (Pro-banthine), hyoscyamine sulfate (Cysto-spaz, Levsin), and flavoxate hydrochloride (Urispas) are used for this purpose. Combinations of drugs, sometimes including antiseptics, are often helpful. These include methenamine, methylene blue, phenyl salicylate, benzoic acid, atropine sulfate, and hyoscyamine (Urised); phenazopyridine, hyoscyamine, and butabarbital (Pyridium Plus); and sulfisoxazole and phenazopyridine (Azo Gantrisin). Severe symptoms may require belladonna and opium rectal suppositories. Treatment measures unique to each cause are discussed next.

CHEMICAL CYSTITIS

OXAZAPHOSPHORINES

Cyclophosphamide (Cytoxan), the most commonly used oxazaphosphorine, is an alkylating agent first used in the treatment of malignant tumors in Europe in 1957. Cyclophosphamide has a role in the treatment of solid tumors and lymphomas as well as benign inflammatory states, most commonly Wegener's granulomatosis and rheumatoid arthritis. Other oxazaphosphorines—ifosfamide, trofosfamide, and sufosfamide—have been used since the 1970s for the treatment of solid malignancies and lymphomas. Dose-limiting toxicity with these compounds is usually urinary tract toxicity.

After treatment with these compounds, urinary symptoms (frequency, urgency, dysuria, and nocturia) develop in as many as 24% of patients treated with oral cyclophosphamide.[1] Microhematuria occurs in 7% to 53% of patients, and gross hematuria occurs in 0.6% to 15% of patients.[1–3] Gross hematuria can range from lightly stained urine to exsanguinating hemorrhage. Symptoms usually occur soon after cyclophosphamide is given but may occur years later.[2] Prolonged use can lead to chronic fibrosis or hemorrhage. Malignant lesions, usually transitional cell carcinoma, occur in 2% to 5% of patients who receive oral cyclophosphamide for nonmalignant disease.[1,4] The entire urothelium can be effected, but the bladder is the most frequently involved area.

Bladder pathology has been attributed to toxic metabolites of these compounds. Cyclophosphamide is broken down by hepatic microsomal cells to hydroxycyclophosphamide, then by target cells to aldophosphamide, and then to phosphoramide mustard, the active antineoplastic metabolite, and acrolein, which has no significant antitumor activity.[5–7] Similarly, ifosfamide is metabolized to ifosforamide mustard and acrolein.[6] Urinary excretion of acrolein is believed to be the major source of urothelial toxicity.[6] Most normal cells are able to break down the toxic metabolites and diminish their effect. Glutathione is a naturally occurring thiol that can confer such protection in most cells, but it is present in low levels in urine.[5] Oxazaphosphorine toxicity has been demonstrated in several animal models with systemic administration and by instillation of normal metabolic products directly into the bladder.[8,9] Urine from animals given these agents, when placed in other animal bladders, reproduces these findings, while instillation of cyclophosphamide does not.[9,10] Electron microscopy suggests that the initial toxic effect is disruption of the plasma membrane and cytoplasmic matrix.[11]

Bladder damage from these compounds is cumulative and is generally dose-related. Cyclophosphamide-induced cystitis occurs frequently and early after intravenous therapy, especially dose-intensive regimens. Cystitis usually takes weeks to develop after oral treatment but has been seen after as little as one dose.[12] Fibrosis has been found in as many as 25% of children receiving high-dose cyclophosphamide.[13] Severe hematuria and telangiectasia are more common in these patients.[13] Oxazaphosphorine-induced cystitis is potentiated by prior pelvic irradiation.[2,14]

Laboratory values reveal normal coagulation profiles, normal platelet count, and negative urine culture. Because these patients are at risk for developing urothelial malignancies, these episodes of cystitis and hematuria must be evaluated judiciously. Initial evaluation includes urinalysis and urine cytology. Patients receiving cyclophosphamide develop markedly abnormal urinary cytologic analyses demonstrating marked atypia, increased nuclear size, and bizarrely shaped cytoplasm, which frequently resolves with cessation of the drug.[15] These findings can be suggestive of malignancy and need to be interpreted with caution.[16] Patients who have abnormal urinary cytology that has not been investigated previously should undergo a thorough urologic evaluation. Cystoscopy may reveal a tumor or changes compatible with cyclophosphamide-induced cystitis. Acutely diffuse inflammation is seen. Chronic changes include a pale bladder mucosa with telangiectasia. Areas of edema can be present with patchy hemorrhagic areas that stain with methylene blue, an indicator of mucosal injury.[8] Biopsy specimens reveal hyperemia, hemorrhage, edema, mucosal thinning, and ulceration of the urothelium. Necrosis of mucosa, muscle, and small arterioles and telangiectasia can be present.[8,10,11] Atypia can be prominent, and abundant mitoses often occur.[10,11,15] These finding are similar to those seen after radiation therapy.

Hemorrhagic cystitis is managed by stopping or reducing the drug. Replacing the drug, usually with azathioprine, is necessary in as many as one third of patients who develop severe cystitis.[17] Hydration and diuresis are routinely used to dilute the metabolites in the urine and minimize their toxicity.[7] Because high-dose oxazaphosphorines cause accumulation of free water, patients can develop fluid overload with hyponatremia, seizures, or death if furosemide is not used.[18,19] Potassium levels need to be followed in patients on this regimen. The cystitis usually improves within several days after cessation of the drug but occasionally persists for months. Patients receiving high doses of oxazaphosphorines require additional measures to counter the effects.[19] Bladder irrigation is helpful in many of these patients.[20]

Development of drugs that can neutralize the toxic metabolites has been an important addition to treatment of cyclophosphamide-induced cystitis. Sodium 2-mercaptoethane sulfonate (mesna) was designed to function in the urinary tract to detoxify oxazaphosphorine metabolites with urothelial toxicity. Mesna is a sulfhydryl compound that is administered intravenously and rapidly excreted by the urinary tract. After intravenous administration, mesna undergoes oxidation, forming disulfide bonds and making an unreactive dimer (dimesna). One concern regarding such a class of drugs is that they might effect the antineoplastic properties of oxazaphosphorines. Mesna and dimesna are hydrophilic and do not normally penetrate cells, explaining their antineoplastic-sparing effect.[7] The unreactive form, dimesna, is filtered by the kidneys and undergoes tubular reabsorption, where one third of it is reduced to its active form, mesna, by glutathione reductase.[7] In the urinary tract, the sulfhydryl group of mesna complexes with the terminal methyl group of acrolein, joining the compound to the double bond of acrolein and forming a nontoxic thioether.[7] The presence of mesna also inhibits spontaneous breakdown of cyclophosphamide to acrolein in the urine.[21] In addition to decreasing chemical cystitis, the risk of bladder cancer is significantly reduced when mesna is used in the Sprague-Dawley rat model.[22] This is an important argument for its use whenever possible.

Oral mesna is well absorbed but slow to achieve adequate urinary concentrations. It has an unpleasant taste, which makes patient tolerance poor, particularly when there is concomitant administration of a chemotherapy that induces nausea.[5] Mesna is best given intravenously, and the manufacturer recommends three doses. A loading dose equivalent to 20% (wt/wt) of the ifosfamide dose, given 15 minutes before the ifosfamide, is followed by two similar doses 4 and 8 hours after the ifosfamide.[7] Doses as high as 60% to 120% (wt/wt) have been used with cyclophosphamide, given at a similar schedule. The timing of dosages of mesna is important because the half-life of mesna is 35 minutes, while that of cyclophosphamide is 4 hours.[7,23] Mesna toxicity is minimal, and its major side effects are diarrhea, headache, and limb pain.[5]

Another thiol compound, *N*-acetyl cysteine (NAC), has been used less extensively to ameliorate the effects of oxazaphosphorines. Animal data demonstrate that the bladder is protected when given at a dose of 1:1 (wt/wt) with cyclophosphamide in a similar schedule as mesna.[24] Problems with NAC include a wide distribution in the body, with low urinary levels. High intravenous doses or intravesical administration are required to reach effective concentrations.[25] Conflicting data concerning impairment of antitumor activity have not been resolved.

BONE MARROW TRANSPLANTATION

Hemorrhagic cystitis occurs in about 2% of conditioning regimens that do not contain cyclophosphamide and is frequently related to thrombocytopenia.[14] The incidence of hemorrhagic cystitis in regimens with cyclophosphamide is 13% to 56%.[14,26,27] Prior cyclophosphamide, radiation, urethral catheterization, infection (bacterial or previous viral), concurrent medication, or coagulation disorders (thrombocytopenia) can all contribute to the development of hemorrhagic cystitis in these patients. Prior administration of busulfan, an alkyl sulfonate, increases the risk of hemorrhagic cystitis to as high as 36%, compared with 4% in patients receiving the same regimen without prior exposure.[26] Concomitant use of these agents is associated with hemorrhagic cystitis in 0.5% to 50% of patients.[14,27,28]

Several viruses have been implicated in the cause of hemorrhagic cystitis in patients undergoing bone marrow transplantation, either as viral reactivation or a new infection. These include polyma (BK) virus[14,29]; adenovirus, especially adenovirus 11[29,30]; papovavirus; influenza A; and cytomegalovirus.[27,29] Patients in whom viral particles were recovered developed hematuria later after transplantation (55 days)[29] than did patients with so-called idiopathic hemorrhagic cystitis (25–27 days).[14] The viral type also had a longer duration than idiopathic cystitis.[29,30]

It has been recommended patients receiving the combination of cyclophosphamide and busulfan should receive continuous bladder irrigation during treatment.[27] Prophylactic treatment with mesna is efficacious and does not appear to effect engraftment.[31] A dose of 60% (wt/wt) has been adequate in children, but adults appear to require a higher dose (120–160% [wt/wt]).[31]

INTRAVESICAL CHEMOTHERAPY

Intravesical treatment of superficial bladder tumors with chemotherapeutic agents or biologic modifiers may cause chemical cystitis or an inflammatory response with marked symptoms. Several agents are commonly employed. Thiotepa is well tolerated, although 2% to 49% of patients experience cystitis[32,33] and about one third develop hematuria.[32] One third of patients receiving epodyl[33] and 26% to 50% of patients receiving doxorubicin develop cystitis.[33,34] Mitomycin C is best tolerated, with 6% to 33% of patients developing cystitis and one third developing hematuria.[32–34] Most hematuria is microscopic. Significant hemorrhagic cystitis is uncommon with any of these agents. Bladder contractures have rarely been reported in patients receiving thiotepa or mitomycin.

Most patients receiving bacillus Calmette-Guérin develop irritative voiding symptoms, which can be the most severe of all intravesical treatments. Biopsy specimens from these patients reveal acute and chronic inflammatory changes and granuloma formation. Urinary analgesics and antispasmodics are particularly helpful in this group. If symptoms are prolonged, isoniazid and acetaminophen or ibuprofen are given until symptoms resolve. It is uncommon for treatment regimens to be stopped because of toxicity.[35]

OTHER

Other chemotherapeutic regimens that do not include agents with known bladder toxicity appear to be able to induce cystitis and hematuria without associated thrombocytopenia.[36] The mechanism in these patients is not clear, although bleomycin has been suggested to be the culprit.[36,37]

Busulfan, an alkyl sulfonate used in the treatment of chronic granulocytic leukemia, has also been reported as a cause of hemorrhagic cystitis.[26,38] As many as 16% of patients in regimens with intravenous busulfan, and without cyclophosphamide, develop hemorrhagic cystitis.[14] Cystoscopy in these patients reveals generalized inflammation and edema. Biopsy specimens demonstrate metaplastic changes in the urothelium, submucosal inflammation, and telangiectasia.[38] Cystoscopic and histologic findings are similar to those for radiation or oxazaphosphorine cystitis. Bladder malignancies have not been associated with busulfan. Given orally, a cumulative dose of 2 to 5 kg appears necessary to induce these changes.[38,39] Stopping the drug and alleviation of irritative symptoms are the primary treatment.

INTRAVESICAL PHOTOTHERAPY

Treatment of superficial bladder tumors with phototherapy was first performed by Kelly and Snell in 1975. Treatment involves administration of an intravenous photosensitizer (usually a hematoporphyrin derivative), waiting 2 days, and then activation of the compound with light. The time lag allows preferential retention of sensitizer by tumor, with normal tissue levels decreasing, thus increasing the therapeutic index. An optical fiber placed in the bladder through a cystoscope transmits light to activate the sensitizer. Patients whose entire bladder mucosa is illuminated develop marked bladder irritation with suprapubic discomfort, urgency, and urge incontinence. Symptoms can be surprisingly mild the first day after activation but peak on the second or third day. Symptoms improve quickly and usually resolve after 4 to 6 weeks. Cystoscopy initially reveals exuberant local reaction and edema.[40] Biopsy specimens initially reveal coagulative necrosis and hemorrhage.[40] Later, acute and chronic inflammation and atypia are present.[41] The acute response can resolve with little residual effect visually apparent. Bladder fibrosis and reflux are unpredictable side effects of this therapy. Treatment of the acute symptoms includes drainage with a Foley catheter to put the bladder to rest and B&O suppositories to control bladder discomfort.

RADIATION

Patients undergoing primary radiation therapy of malignant pelvic tumors, most commonly uterine, bladder, and prostate neoplasms, can suffer direct or incidental damage to the bladder. The risk is increased when urinary infection is present or radiation therapy is repeated, when high-dose radiation therapy is given, or when surgery has been performed in the area. Cyclophosphamide, given systemically in combination with pelvic irradiation, greatly increases the risk for radiation cystitis.[42]

In the first 4 to 6 weeks after treatment, an acute inflammatory response with resultant irritative symptoms or hematuria develops. Mild symptoms occur in as many as 50% to 82% of patients and generally do not require medication.[43,44] Hemorrhagic cystitis can occur later, even years after successful treatment,[44] and frequently is associated with tumor recurrence.[45] The time between treatment and development of delayed symptoms (frequency, dysuria, and hematuria), is proportional to the dose received.[44] Patients with late cystitis develop bladder ulcers, bladder fibrosis, and ureteral strictures. These patients require thorough evaluation because they are at increased risk for developing transitional cell carcinoma of the bladder. Bladder biopsies should be done sparingly because the bladder mucosa heals poorly.

Some 3.7% of patients receiving intravaginal intracavitary irradiation alone (3200 cGy) for stage I endometrial carcinoma, after transabdominal hysterectomy and bilateral salpingo-oopherectomy, develop cystitis.[46] When external-beam irradiation (4000–5400 cGy) is added, 4% to 6.5% of patients develop cystitis.[46,47] Patients undergoing definitive radiation treatment of cervical carcinoma have a risk of cystitis that is dose-related.[45,48] At doses less than 6000 cGy, the development of cystitis has been strongly linked to recurrent tumor.[45] The incidence of cystitis in this group is 2.8% to 8%.[44,49,50] From 1.2% to 18% of patients receiving external-beam irradiation (3000–8500 cGy) for bladder cancer developed cystitis,[45,51,52] 8% hematuria,[45] and 5% a contracted bladder.[52] Chronic cystitis develops in 15% of patients. Radiation therapy to the prostate (5000–7200 cGy) and draining of the lymph nodes (5000 cGy) for cure of prostate cancer elicits dysuria and mild to moderate hematuria in 18% to 40% of patients.[53,54] Of these patients, 0.8% to 8.3% develop severe dysuria or hematuria, and 3.4% to 9% develop strictures or urethral obstruction as a delayed presentation.[53–55]

During the acute phase, cystoscopy reveals edema, erythema, and increased vascularity, which can be associated with a mild decrease in bladder capacity. Later, the bladder is pale, and telangiectasia is present. Focal areas of hyperemia and bullous edema may be present. Often, there is no focal area of bleeding. With extensive damage, necrosis and calcification can occur. Biopsy findings are dose- and time-dependent. In the first 24 hours, there is erythema due to hyperemia. This develops into a diffuse inflammatory response with hyperemia, edema, lymphocytic infiltration, and degeneration of the urothelium with atypia.[43,44,56] Shallow ulcers are occasionally seen but usually occur as a late response. This response lasts up to 4 months after therapy.[57] Later, sclerosing endarteritis, fibrosis, and atrophy occur. There may be edema and an inflammatory infiltrate. There can be ulceration, and healing is poor.[52,57,58] Treatment is symptomatic.

ANTIBIOTICS

Although most cystitis seen in the setting of oncologic care is related to antineoplastic agents, penicillins used in the treatment of chemotherapy-related infections represent another source. Methicillin, nafcillin, ticarcillin, piperacillin, carbenicillin, and penicillin G have all been implicated. The incidence of cystitis associated with the use of these agents is small, occurring in 4% to 8% of patients.[59] Symptoms are typical of cystitis. Laboratory investigation reveals eosinophilia, pyuria, hematuria, proteinuria, and negative urine cultures. The submucosal deposition of C3, IgG and IgM, and dimethoxyphenylpenicilloyl, a methicillin antigen, supports a hypersensitivity cause.[59–61] A diffuse hemorrhagic cystitis is seen at cystoscopy.[60] Biopsy specimens show an intense inflammatory reaction with erosion.[62] With repeated use, the time to development of symptoms shortens. Symptoms usually resolve promptly on cessation of the drug or substitution with an unrelated drug.[60,61]

REFERENCES

1. Stillwell TJ, Benson RC Jr, DeRemee RA, McDonald TJ, Weiland LH. Cyclophosphamide-induced bladder toxicity in Wegener's granulomatosis. Arthritis Rheum 1988;31:465–470.
2. Stillwell TJ, Benson RC Jr, Burgert EO Jr. Cyclophosphamide-induced hemorrhagic cystitis in Ewing's sarcoma. J Clin Oncol 1988;6:76–82.
3. Lawrence HJ, Simone J, Aur RJ. Cyclophosphamide-induced hemorrhagic cystitis in children with leukemia. Cancer 1975;36:1572–1576.
4. Fairchild WV, Spence CR, Solomon HD, Gangai MP. The incidence of bladder cancer after cyclophosphamide therapy. J Urol 1979;122:163–164.
5. Shaw IC, Graham MI. Mesna: A short review. Cancer Treat Rev 1987;14:67–86.
6. Cox PJ. Cyclophosphamide cystitis: Identification of acrolein as the causative agent. Biochem Pharmacol 1979;28:2045–2049.
7. Schoenike SE, Dana WJ. Ifosfamide and mesna. Clin Pharm 1990;9:179–191.
8. Chaviano AH, Gill WB, Ruggiero KJ, Vermeulen CW. Experimental Cytoxan cystitis and prevention by acetylcysteine. J Urol 1985;134:598–600.
9. Brock N, Pohl J, Stekar J. Detoxification of urotoxic oxazaphosphorines by sulfhydryl compounds. J Cancer Res Clin Oncol 1981;100:311–320.
10. Philips FS, Sternberg SS, Cronin AP, Vidal PM. Cyclophosphamide and urinary bladder toxicity. Cancer Res 1961;21:1577–1589.
11. Koss LG. A light and electron microscopic study of the effects of a single dose of cyclophosphamide on various organs in the rat. I. The urinary bladder. Lab Invest 1967;16:44–65.
12. Host H, Nissen-Meyer R. A preliminary clinical study of cyclophosphamide. Cancer Chemother Rep 1960;9:47–50.
13. Johnson WW, Meadows DC. Urinary-bladder fibrosis and telangiectasia associated with long-term cyclophosphamide therapy. N Engl J Med 1971;284:290–294.
14. Brugieres L, Hartmann O, Travagli JP, et al. Hemorrhagic cystitis following high-dose chemotherapy and bone marrow transplantation in children with malignancies: Incidence, clinical course, and outcome. J Clin Oncol 1989;7:194–199.
15. Forni AM, Koss LG, Geller W. Cytological study of the effect of cyclophosphamide on the epithelium of the urinary bladder in man. Cancer 1964;17:1348–1355.
16. Liedberg CF, Rausing A, Langeland P. Cyclophosphamide hemorrhagic cystitis. Scand J Urol Nephrol 1970;4:183–190.
17. Fauci AS, Haynes BF, Katz P, Wolff SM. Wegener's granulomatosis: Prospective clinical and therapeutic experience with 85 patients for 21 years. Ann Intern Med 1983;98:76–85.
18. Green TP, Mirkin BL. Prevention of cyclophosphamide-induced antidiuresis by furosemide infusion. Clin Pharmacol Ther 1981;29:634–642.
19. Droller MJ, Saral R, Santos G. Prevention of cyclophosphamide-induced hemorrhagic cystitis. Urology 1982;20:256–258.
20. Blume KG, Beutler E, Bross KJ, et al. Bone-marrow ablation and allogeneic marrow transplantation in acute leukemia. N Engl J Med 1980;302:1041–1046.
21. Brock N, Stekar J, Pohl J, Niemeyer U, Scheffler G. Acrolein, the causative factor of urotoxic side-effects of cyclophosphamide, ifosfamide, trofosfamide and sufosfamide. Arzneimittelforschung 1979;29:659–661.

22. Petru E, Schmahl D. Anticancer drugs: Second malignancies—risk reduction. Cancer Treat Rev 1987;14:337–343.
23. Schumacher MM, Dowd AL, eds. Physician's desk reference: Cytoxan. Oradell, NJ: ER Barnhart, 1991;723–725.
24. Tolley DA. The effect of N-acetyl cysteine on cyclophosphamide cystitis. Br J Urol 1977;49:659–661.
25. Ormstad K, Ohno Y. N-acetylcysteine and sodium 2-mercaptoethane sulfonate as sources of urinary thiol groups in the rat. Cancer Res 1984;44:3797–3800.
26. Thomas AE, Patterson J, Prentice HG, et al. Haemorrhagic cystitis in bone marrow transplantation patients: Possible increased risk associated with prior busulfan therapy. Bone Marrow Transplant 1987;1:347–355.
27. Atkinson K, Biggs J, Noble G, Ashby M, Concannon A, Dodds A. Preparative regimens for marrow transplantation containing busulfan are associated with haemorrhagic cystitis and hepatic veno-occlusive disease but a short duration of leucopenia and little oropharyngeal mucositis. Bone Marrow Transplant 1987;2:385–394.
28. Nevill TJ, Barnett MJ, Klingemann HG, Reece DE, Shepherd JD, Phillips GL. Regimen-related toxicity of a busulfan-cyclophosphamide conditioning regimen in 70 patients undergoing allogeneic bone marrow transplantation. J Clin Oncol 1991;9:1224–1232.
29. Arthur RR, Shah KV, Baust SJ, Santos GW, Saral R. Association of BK viruria with hemorrhagic cystitis in recipients of bone marrow transplants. N Engl J Med 1986;315: 230–234.
30. Miyamura K, Takeyama K, Kojima S, et al. Hemorrhagic cystitis associated with urinary excretion of adenovirus type 11 following allogeneic bone marrow transplantation. Bone Marrow Transplant 1989;4:533–535.
31. Blacklock H, Ball L, Knight C, Schey S, Prentice G. Experience with mesna in patients receiving allogeneic bone marrow transplants for poor prognostic leukaemia. Cancer Treat Rev 1983;10:45–52.
32. Heney NM, Koontz WW, Barton B, et al. Intravesical thiotepa versus mitomycin C in patients with Ta, T1 and TIS transitional cell carcinoma of the bladder: A phase III prospective randomized study. J Urol 1988;140:1390–1393.
33. Lamm D. Intravesical therapy of superficial bladder cancer. AUA Update Series 1983;2: 2–7.
34. Herr H, Laudone VP. Intravesical therapy for superficial bladder cancer. AUA Update Series 1989;8:90–95.
35. Lamm DL, Stogdill VD, Stogdill BJ, Crispen RG. Complications of bacillus Calmette-Guerin immunotherapy in 1,278 patients with bladder cancer. J Urol 1986;135:272–274.
36. Cantwell BM, Harris AL, Patrick D, Hall RR. Hemorrhagic cystitis after IV bleomycin, vinblastine, cisplatin, and etoposide for testicular cancer. Cancer Treat Rep 1985;70: 548–549.
37. Creagan ET, Ahmann DL, Schutt AJ, Green SJ. Phase II study of the combination of vinblastine, bleomycin, and cisplatin in advanced malignant melanoma. Cancer Treat Rep 1982;66:567–569.
38. Pode D, Perlberg S, Steiner D. Busulfan-induced hemorrhagic cystitis. J Urol 1983;130: 347–348.
39. Millard RJ. Busulfan-induced hemorrhagic cystitis. Urology 1981;18:143–144.
40. Benson RC, Kinsey JH, Cortese DA, Farrow GM, Utz DC. Treatment of transitional cell carcinoma of the bladder with hematoporphyrin derivative phototherapy. J Urol 1983;130:1090–1095.
41. Prout GR, Lin CW, Benson R, et al. Photodynamic therapy with hematoporphyrin derivative in the treatment of superficial transitional cell carcinoma of the bladder. N Engl J Med 1987;317:1251–1255.
42. Jayalakshmamma B, Pinkel D. Urinary-bladder toxicity following pelvic irradiation and simultaneous cyclophosphamide therapy. Cancer 1976;38:701–707.
43. Fajardo LF, Berthrong M. Radiation injury in surgical pathology: Part I. Am J Surg Pathol 1978;2:159–199.
44. Oration JP. Complications following radiation therapy in carcinoma of the cervix and their treatment. Am J Obstet Gynecol 1964;88:854–866.
45. Dean RJ, Lytton B. Urologic complications of pelvic irradiation. J Urol 1978;119:64–67.
46. Kucera H, Vavra N, Weghaupt K. Benefit of external irradiation in pathologic stage I endometrial carcinoma: A prospective clinical trial of 605 patients who received postoperative vaginal irradiation and additional pelvic irradiation in the presence of unfavorable prognostic factors. Gynecol Oncol 1990;38:99–104.
47. Jampolis S, Martin P, Schroder P, Horiot JC. Treatment tolerance and early complications with extended field irradiation in gynecological cancer. Br J Radiol 1977;50:195–199.
48. Montana GS, Fowler WC. Carcinoma of the cervix: Analysis of bladder and rectal radiation dose and complications. Int J Radiat Oncol Biol Phys 1989;16:95–100.
49. Montana GS, Fowler WC, Varia MA, Walton LA, Mack Y. Analysis of results of radiation therapy for stage II carcinoma of the cervix. Cancer 1985;55:956–962.
50. Buchler DA, Kline JC, Peckham BM, Boone ML, Carr WF. Radiation reactions in cervical cancer therapy. Am J Obstet Gynecol 1971;111:745–750.
51. Shiels RA, Nissenbaum MM, Mark SR, Browde S. Late radiation cystitis after treatment for carcinoma of the bladder. S Afr Med J 1986;70:727–728.
52. Ram MD. Visceral complications of supervoltage radiotherapy for carcinoma of the bladder. Br J Surg 1970;57:409–412.
53. Ray GR, Cassady JR, Bagshaw MA. Definitive radiation therapy of carcinoma of the prostate: A report on 15 years of experience. Radiology 1973;106:407–418.
54. Taylor WJ, Richardson RG, Hafermann MD. Radiation therapy for localized prostate cancer. Cancer 1979;43:1123–1127.
55. Harisiadis L, Veenema RJ, Senyszyn JJ, et al. Carcinoma of the prostate: Treatment with external radiotherapy. Cancer 1978;41:2131–2142.
56. Warren S VII. Effects of radiation on the urinary system. Arch Pathol 1942;34:1079–1084.
57. Haemorrhagic cystitis after radiotherapy. Lancet [Editorial] 1987;1:304–306.
58. Gowing NF III. Pathological changes in the bladder following irradiation. Br J Radiol 1960;33:484–487.
59. Relling MV, Schunk JE. Drug-induced hemorrhagic cystitis. Clin Pharm [Clinical Conference] 1986;5:590–597.
60. Bracis R, Sanders CV, Gilbert DN. Methicillin hemorrhagic cystitis. Antimicrob Agents Chemother 1977;12:438–439.
61. Marx CM, Alpert SE. Ticarcillin-induced cystitis: Cross-reactivity with related penicillins. Am J Dis Child 1984;138:670–672.
62. Cook FV, Farrar WE Jr, Kreutner A. Hemorrhagic cystitis and ureteritis, and interstitial nephritis associated with administration of penicillin G. J Urol 1979;122:110–111.

SECTION **4**

DIANE E. STOVER

Pulmonary Toxicity

Pulmonary disease can be caused by a wide spectrum of pathogens in patients with cancer. These include a variety of infectious agents and neoplastic disorders as well as pulmonary hemorrhage, pulmonary edema (cardiogenic and noncardiogenic) and leukocyte agglutinin reactions. Pulmonary toxicity caused by antineoplastic agents is being recognized more frequently, and the number of drugs known or suspected to cause lung disease is steadily increasing. Because continuing the offending agent may cause death and because withholding the agent may result in resolution of the pulmonary toxicity, it is important to recognize radiation and drug-induced pulmonary disease. In this section, parenchymal lung disease caused by irradiation and chemotherapy is discussed. Mechanisms of lung injury, histopathologic findings, clinical and laboratory features, and diagnosis and treatment of the abnormality produced by these agents are reviewed.

RADIATION-INDUCED PULMONARY TOXICITY

MECHANISM OF LUNG INJURY

Radiation can affect dividing and nondividing cells and can cause genetic and nongenetic damage.[1,2] In the lung, a hypothetical reconstruction of radiation injury might be as follows. Therapeutic radiation may result in nongenetic damage that is apparent in all cells, but capillary endothelial and type I cells (epithelial lining cells) appear most susceptible.[3] Many of these cells, whether dividing or not, undergo early necrobiosis and slough. Over time, capillaries regenerate, and the alveolar epithelium is repopulated by type II cells (surfactant-producing cells) because type I pneumonocytes do not regenerate. Some of these type II cells redifferentiate into type I cells. If the injury is severe, damage to other nondividing materials of the lung, such as proteins and polysaccharides, takes place. This can impede reconstruction of tissue architecture and result in functional derangement and scar formation. Genetic damage to dividing cells, such as endothelial cells or type II pneumonocytes, can also occur. Depletion of these cells may result during successive mitoses, causing a loss of integrity of pulmonary capillaries and exudation of fluid into the alveoli. At the physiologic level, loss of compliance, abnormal gas exchange, and respiratory failure can occur due to leakage of plasma proteins onto the alveolar surface. This type of genetic damage also explains why pneumonitis can happen so late after radiation. One might speculate that some endothelial cells initially remain normal but that, in the course of the next four cell divisions, chromosomal aberrations prevent further reduplication, which leads to loss of integrity of the capillary.[1]

Certain factors are critical to the development of radiation pneumonitis. In general, damage to the lung increases as the volume of lung tissue irradiated increases. Also, the toxic effects of radiation as measured by symptoms and signs, radiographic changes, and physiologic tests are proportionate to the total amount delivered to the lung. Radiation pneumonitis seldom occurs with doses of less than 20 Gy but is highly likely when doses exceed 60 Gy.[4] Because local control of lung cancer is greater when higher doses are delivered to the tumor,[5] methods are being devised to give high doses to the target tissue while sparing normal surrounding lung. One such technique, called *three-dimensional treatment planning,* is being evaluated.[6,7] In addition, a cooperative, randomized trial is assessing the value of combined chemotherapy, which includes drugs that are toxic to the lungs and high-dose radiation therapy.[8] In the future, in situ isolated lung perfusion for the treatment of unresectable pulmonary tumors, preceded or followed by high-dose irradiation, may be clinically applicable as well.[9] Whether these treatment modalities will have a sparing effect on the lung or whether they will be associated with an increase in pulmonary toxicity is unknown.

Besides the total radiation dose, the number of fractions into which it is divided and, to a lesser extent, the time span over which it is delivered are important factors.[10] The greater the number of fractions in which the radiation is given, the lower is the damaging effect. Fractionation is different from dose rate, which refers to output of the machine during radiation therapy. Dose rate certainly has an effect on lung tolerance: radiation delivered as 5 cGy/minute is less damaging than radiation delivered at 30 cGy/minute, which in turn is less damaging than radiation delivered at 2 to 3 Gy/minute. In summary, the incidence and severity of radiation damage to the lungs are related principally to the volume of lung tissue irradiated, the total dose, the fractions into which the total dose is divided, and the quality of the radiation.

HISTOPATHOLOGY

The histopathologic changes of radiation-induced pulmonary toxicity can be divided into early, intermediate, and late stages based on the time, course, and intensity of the radiation injury.[11] Early radiation damage (0–2 months after radiation) is characterized by injury to small vessels and capillaries with the development of vascular congestion and increased capillary permeability.[12] At this stage, a fibrin-rich exudate is present in the alveolar spaces. Hyaline membranes form on the alveoli, probably from condensation of the intraalveolar fibrin. Abnormalities in the intermediate stage (2–9 months after radiation) are characterized by obstruction of pulmonary capillaries by platelets, fibrin, and collagen. Alveolar-lining cells (primarily type II pneumonocytes) become hyperplastic, and the alveolar walls become infiltrated with fibroblasts. If the radiation injury is mild, these changes may subside entirely; however, when the injury is severe, a chronic phase (9 months or more after radiation) ensues that may persist or progress for months or years. The histopathologic appearance then is dominated by dense fibrosis, thickening of the alveolar walls, vascular subintimal fibrosis, and luminal narrowing. In some instances, the lung may shrink to less than half its original size with a thickened adherent pleura and scarred hilar structures.

CLINICAL FEATURES

Signs and Symptoms

The clinical syndrome of radiation pneumonitis develops in 5% to 15% of all irradiated patients. Factors that can add to the development of radiation pneumonitis include concomitant chemotherapy, previous irradiation, and withdrawal of steroids. There is not a significant difference in the incidence of radiation pneumonitis between the young and elderly, but the pneumonitis is inclined to be more severe in the latter.[13] Underlying chronic obstructive pulmonary disease does not appear to potentiate radiation damage.

Symptoms of acute radiation pneumonitis usually become evident 2 to 3 months after the completion of therapy; rarely, they occur within the first month and occasionally as late as 6 months after irradiation. In general, the early onset of symptoms implies a more serious and more protracted clinical course. The cardinal symptom of radiation pneumonitis is dyspnea.[11] It may be self-limited or may progress to severe respiratory distress depending on the extent and intensity of the injury. Patients may also have a nonproductive cough or a cough productive of small amounts of pinkish sputum. Frank hemoptysis early in the clinical course is distinctly uncommon; however, massive hemoptysis has been reported as a late complication of therapeutic pulmonary irradiation.[14] Fever is unusual but can be high and spiking; in severe cases, other constitutional symptoms may occur. Chest pain, which is rarely a prominent feature, may be due to fractured ribs, pleural changes, or coughing. Symptoms of airway obstruction can occur in the first few days of radiation therapy and are usually associated with swelling of a central bronchogenic carcinoma. Severe respiratory distress can result and may be prevented by the administration of steroids the day before and several days after the initiation of radiation therapy.

On physical examination, signs of pulmonary involvement are minimal. Occasionally, moist rales, a pleural friction rub, or evidence of pleural fluid may be heard over the area of irradiation. In severe cases, tachypnea and cyanosis may be present, and occasionally evidence of acute cor pulmonale appears, usually predicting a fatal outcome. Finger clubbing due to radiation is distinctly unusual and, if present, is most likely due to the underlying malignancy. Skin changes corresponding to the ports of irradiation are often present but provide no clue as to the presence or severity of the pulmonary reaction beneath.

Although patients with acute pneumonitis may show complete resolution of signs and symptoms, most develop gradual progressive fibrosis. In some cases, patients present with radiation fibrosis without a previous history of acute pneumonitis. The permanent changes of fibrosis take 6 to 24 months to evolve but usually remain stable after 2 years. Patients with fibrosis can be asymptomatic or can have varying degrees of dyspnea. The major complications of radiation pneumonitis occur late in the disease and are secondary to persistent fibrosis of a large volume of lung. These include cor pulmonale and respiratory failure.

Diagnostic Imaging

Although radiographic abnormalities are invariably found at the time clinical radiation pneumonitis is present, these changes may be seen in asymptomatic patients as well. Early radiographic changes include a ground-glass opacification, diffuse haziness, or indistinctness of the normal pulmonary markings over the irradiated area.[15] Later, the chest radiograph may show alveolar infiltrates or dense consolidation with or without air bronchograms. As the pneumonitis progresses to fibrosis, the radiographic appearance changes to that of linear streaks radiating from the area of pneumonitis and of contraction toward the hilar, the perimediastinal, or the apical areas. Pleural effusions, if present, are usually small and always coincident with the pneumonitis.[16] They can persist for long periods but often disappear spontaneously and never increase over a period of stability unless secondary complications occur, such as radiation-induced pericarditis. Mediastinal or hilar adenopathy and cavitation are almost always due to causes other than radiation pneumonitis.[2] Pneumothorax is occasionally associated with radiation fibrosis but not with acute pneumonitis.

One of the most characteristic features of radiation pneumonitis and fibrosis is that the radiologic changes are confined to the outlines of the field of radiation. In a few cases, extensive changes outside the field, even in the contralateral lung, have been observed. Obstruction of lymphatic flow from mediastinal irradiation,[17] hypersensitivity in response to radiation,[18] and absorption of x-rays by regions outside the irradiated ports are possible but poorly documented explanations of this phenomenon.[19]

Some data suggest that computed tomographic (CT) scans of the chest and gallium-67 citrate imaging are more sensitive than chest radiography in the detection of radiation changes.[20,21] Correlation of abnormalities seen in these tests with the development of physiologic dysfunction and clinical toxicity need clarification.

Pulmonary Function Tests

No gross physiologic changes occur in the lung until 4 to 8 weeks after completion of irradiation, usually coincident with the period of clinical pneumonitis. Then, one sees a decrease in lung volumes, which can progress.[22–25] These changes persist indefinitely with little evidence of recovery.[24] Gas exchange abnormalities, which include a decrease in diffusion capacity and arterial hypoxemia, especially with exercise, occur about the same time but show some tendency toward recovery after 6 to 12 months.[23–25] A fall in compliance coincidence with the clinical pneumonitis is usually seen in most subjects.[23] Accordingly, the elastic work of breathing is increased, and dyspnea, resulting from the increased workload, ensues.[23] Air flow parameters remain close to normal in most studies.[22–25]

DIAGNOSIS

The diagnosis of radiation pneumonitis can sometimes be made clinically based on the timing of irradiation in relation to symptoms and the typical chest radiographic appearance (*i.e.*, infiltrates corresponding to the margins of the irradiated portal). Differentiation from recurrent malignancy or infection often poses a problem, and then lung biopsy is necessary. Although histopathologic changes are nonspecific for radiation pneumonitis, when elements of the acute stages of radiation pneumonia (fibrin exudate in the alveoli) are seen adjacent to the more chronic stages (alveolar fibrosis and subintimal sclerosis), this entity can be diagnosed with reasonable certainty.[26]

Biochemical markers that indicate radiation lung injury before the onset of clinical pathologic events would be valuable in the early diagnosis and management of patients with radiation toxicity. In irradiated animals, studies demonstrate that surfactant found in the serum may be a marker and predictor for later radiation pneumonitis.[27] Studies are needed in humans to identify the sensitivity and specificity of monitoring serum surfactant levels as an early means to diagnose clinical radiation toxicity. No standard tests are used to monitor patients for radiation pneumonitis because most methods are of no predictive value.

TREATMENT

Three modalities of therapy have been used prophylactically and therapeutically for radiation-induced pneumonitis: corticosteroids, antibiotics, and anticoagulants. Of these, corticosteroid therapy is the most important.

Corticosteroid administration during irradiation in mice markedly improved the physiologic abnormalities and decreased mortality, an effect that had been attributed to the stimulation of surfactant synthesis and secretion by type II alveolar epithelial cells.[28] Despite this study and other animal studies indicating that steroids reduce mortality from radiation pneumonitis,[29] no controlled clinical trials in humans are available on the efficacy of steroid therapy in radiation pneumonitis. Ruben and Casarett[2] collected data from eight studies on humans and categorized them according to whether corticosteroids were used prophylactically or therapeutically. Corticosteroids given prophylactically failed to prevent radiation pneumonitis, but when they were administered as clinical pneumonitis occurred, an objective response was seen. In other reports, steroid therapy failed to ameliorate severe pneumonitis. Nonetheless, it is our practice to begin prednisone 1 mg/kg as soon as the diagnosis is reasonably certain. The initial dose is maintained for several weeks and then reduced cautiously and slowly. It has been our experience that if steroids are tapered too rapidly, symptoms can be exacerbated, necessitating higher doses for longer periods of time. Similarly, if corticosteroids are part of a chemotherapeutic regimen, stopping them abruptly can precipitate clinically evident radiation pneumonitis in recently treated patients.

What parameters, if any, to follow during the tapering schedule are not known, and no studies are available. Generally, we follow symptoms. Most authors agree that corticosteroids have no place in the treatment of radiation fibrosis.

In experimental and clinical reports, antibiotic administration has no effect on the course or outcome of radiation pneumonitis.[2,30] Although there is some rationale for the use of anticoagulants in view of the effects of irradiation on the vascular system, neither heparin injections nor oral anticoagulants have been found to be beneficial.[30]

CHEMOTHERAPY-INDUCED PULMONARY TOXICITY

Nineteen chemotherapeutic agents have been reported to cause cytotoxic drug-induced lung disease (see Table 63–13). An overview of the potential mechanisms of lung damage, a summary of the pathologic findings, and common clinical features of pulmonary toxicity are discussed in this section. Characteristics of pulmonary disease caused by some of these drugs are presented.

MECHANISMS OF PULMONARY INJURY

Although details about the pathophysiology of specific chemotherapeutic agents are generally not known, several mechanisms of pulmonary toxicity mediated by these agents have been proposed. Certain cytotoxic drugs may induce pulmonary injury by triggering the formation of reactive oxygen metabolites, including the superoxide anion, hydrogen peroxide, and hydroxyl radicals. These substances can produce direct toxicity through participation in redox reactions and subsequent fatty acid oxidation, which leads to membrane instability.[31] Oxidants can cause other inflammatory reactions within the lung. For example, the oxidation of arachidonic acid is an initial step in the metabolic cascade that produces immunoreactive substances, including prostaglandins and leukotrienes.[32] Cytotoxic drugs may also effect the local immune system. Because the lung is exposed to so many substances that can activate its immune system, there appears to be a "pulmonary immune tolerance state" to avoid unnecessary over reactions.[33] This tolerance state in part may be a result of effector and suppressor cell balance. Cytotoxic drugs can alter the normal effector and suppressor balance, which may cause tissue damage.[34–36] Other balance systems within the lung can be affected as well, such as the balance between collagenesis and collagenolysis.[33] Through modulation of fibroblast proliferation, excessive collagen deposition may result in severe irreversible pulmonary fibrosis. Bleomycin is one cytotoxic agent that has this potential.[37,38] Imbalance between the protease and antiprotease system also has been implicated in a number of pulmonary disorders, including drug toxicities.[33] Bleomycin and cyclophosphamide produce substances that can inactivate the antiprotease system, enhancing the effects of proteolytic enzymes on the lung. Drugs may damage the lung through a variety of other mechanisms, and considerable investigation needs to be done to define and clarify the exact mechanism of lung injury for each chemotherapeutic drug.

TABLE 63–13. Chemotherapeutic Agents Associated With Pulmonary Parenchymal Disease

Alkylating Agents	**Antimetabolites**
Busulfan	Methotrexate
Cyclophosphamide	Azathioprine
Chlorambucil	Mercaptopurine
Melphalan	Cytosine arabinoside
Nitrosoureas	**Miscellaneous**
Carmustine (BCNU)	Procarbazine
Lomustine (CCNU)	Vinblastine
Semustine (methyl-CCNU)	Vindesine
Chlorozotocin (DCNU)	VM-26
Antibiotics	
Bleomycin	
Mitomycin	
Neocarzinostatin (zinostatin)	

HISTOPATHOLOGY

The histopathologic changes of drug-induced pulmonary toxicity show common features. Similar to radiation-induced damage, abnormalities are seen in endothelial and epithelial cells. The vascular damage is characterized by endothelial swelling with exudation of fluid into the interstitium and the intraalveolar spaces. There is destruction and desquamation of type I pneumonocytes with delamellation and proliferation of type II pneumonocytes. Mononuclear cell infiltration and fibroblast proliferation with fibrosis are common findings; the character of the inflammatory cellular infiltrate may be a feature that distinguishes the toxicity of one drug from another. Bronchoalveolar lavage studies in patients with methotrexate pulmonary toxicity have shown the presence of a T-lymphocytic alveolitis, while studies on some patients with bleomycin toxicity have revealed a polymorphonuclear alveolitis.[34,39] Eosinophil infiltration has been associated with drugs that cause apparent hypersensitivity reactions, such as methotrexate, procarbazine, and bleomycin.[33,34,40,41]

(text continues on page 2368)

TABLE 63–14. Factors Associated With Increased Risk of Drug-Induced Pneumonitis

Risk Factor	*Drugs*
Total dose	Bleomycin[42,43]; carmustine[42]
Age	Bleomycin[43]
Oxygen therapy	Bleomycin[44–46]; cyclophosphamide[45]; mitomycin[47]
Simultaneous or prior radiation therapy to lungs	Bleomycin[48,49]; busulfan[50]; mitomycin[51]
Increased toxicity when given with other drugs	Carmustine[52]; mitomycin[53]; cyclophosphamide[54,55]; bleomycin[55,56]; methotrexate[54]
Preexisting pulmonary disease	Carmustine[57]

TABLE 63–15. Clinical and Pathologic Features of Chemotherapy-Induced Toxicity

Drug	*Mechanism of Injury*	*Histopathology*	*Clinical Features*	*Chest Roentgenogram*	*Diagnosis*	*Treatment*
Alkylating Agents						
Busulfan (Myleran)[42,50,65,76–80]	No studies, but direct toxicity to epithelial lining cells is suggested	Pneumocyte dysplasia (degeneration of type I cells; atypical hyperplastic type II cells), atypical bronchial lining cells, mononuclear cell infiltration, fibrosis	4% incidence; no direct dose-dependent toxicity; may be threshold dose (>500 mg); radiation and other alkylating agents may enhance toxicity, insidious onset after 4 years (8 mo to 10 y). Dyspnea, cough, weight loss, weakness, fever; crepitant basilar rales, pigmentation. Prognosis is poor.	Most common bibasilar reticular pattern; rarely pleural effusion, pulmonary ossification, normal chest radiograph	Suggested by history and bizarre pneumocytes in sputum or lavage fluid. Definitive diagnosis by open lung biopsy	Withdrawal of the drug; anecdotal reports of improvement with high-dose steroids. Mean survival after diagnosis is 5 mo
Cyclophosphamide (Cytoxan)[42,45,74,81–84]	May be toxic through production of reactive oxygen species	Endothelial swelling, pneumocyte dysplasia, lymphocytic and histiocytic infiltration, fibrosis	Less than 1% incidence; does not appear dose-dependent, but synergy with oxygen and other agents possible. Subacute onset 3 w to 8 y after initiation of therapy, up to 8 y after stopping therapy. Cough, dyspnea, fever; basilar rales	Commonly, bibasilar reticular pattern; diffuse pulmonary edema pattern also reported	As above	Drug withdrawal; corticosteroids may hasten improvement but have no documented effect on mortality. Overall recovery about 65%
Chlorambucil[33,85]	Unknown	Similar to busulfan; fibrosis may predominate	Rare reports; subacute onset 6 mo to 3 y after therapy. Cough, dyspnea, anorexia; bibasilar rales	Bibasilar reticular pattern; rarely, normal radiograph; alveolar infiltrates not reported	As above	Half of reported patients died despite cessation of drug and administration of steroids. Anecdotal reports of response to steroids
Melphalan (Alkeran)[33,86,87]	Unknown	Similar to busulfan; pneumocyte dysplasia more common than fibrosis	Rare (five documented reports); appears 1 to 48 mo after therapy. Progressive dyspnea, productive cough, fever, malaise; bibasilar rales	Reticular and alveolar infiltrates	As above	Despite cessation of drug, 3 of 5 patients reported died of disease. In most cases, patients were receiving steroids for underlying disease
Antibiotics						
Bleomycin[33,37,38,69,70,88–95]	Several possible mechanisms: (a) direct toxicity through generation of reactive oxygen metabolites; (b) leukocyte influx and lung injury from release of proteases; (c) increased collagen synthesis and subsequent pulmonary fibrosis	Endothelial blebbing; interstitial edema, necrosis of type I cells and metaplastic type II cells; inflammation with polymorphonuclear cells; fibroblast proliferation and fibrosis; occasionally eosinophilic infiltration	Incidence 2–40%; age- and dose-related; synergy seen with oxygen therapy, radiation, and other agents. Occurs during and shortly after stopping therapy. Cough, dyspnea, fever; tachypnea, crepitant rales. Hypersensitivity pneumonitis variant	Bibasilar reticular pattern; multiple nodules similar to metastatic disease; acinar pattern, especially with hypersensitivity reaction; rarely, localized infiltrate and cavitary nodules	Bronchoalveolar lavage might suggest diagnosis (polymorphonuclear alveolitis). Transbronchial or open lung biopsy required for diagnosis, especially to rule out other causes.	Drug withdrawal. In bleomycin hypersensitivity reactions, definite role for steroids; in other forms of bleomycin toxicity, efficacy less clear. Mortality estimated at 50%.

Mitomycin[33,51,53,73,96]	No studies, but probably similar to the alkylating agents	Similar to bleomycin; in patients with microangiopathic hemolytic anemia, prominent vascular changes are present.	3–12% incidence; does not appear dose-related, but possible synergy with oxygen, radiotherapy, and other agents. Dry cough and dyspnea; fever not seen; bibasilar rales	Diffuse reticular pattern; pleural effusions seen	Lung biopsy for definitive diagnosis; no bronchoalveolar lavage studies reported.	Drug withdrawal; steroids may alter outcome. Mortality approaches 50%.
Nitrosoureas*						
Carmustine (BCNU)[52,57,97–99]	Few studies; direct injury through generation of toxic oxidant molecules possible	Similar to bleomycin; fibrosis predominates.	20–30% incidence; dose-related; increased risk with preexisting lung disease and tobacco use; possible synergism with other agents; can be seen up to 17 y after drug stopped. Dry cough, dyspnea, bibasilar rales	Bibasilar reticular pattern; may be normal	As above	Early recognition and withdrawal of the drug; steroids not beneficial since most patients are on the drug for intracranial processes when toxicity develops. Mortality reported between 24% and 90%.
Antimetabolites						
Methotrexate[33,34,42,54,63,66]	Direct toxic effect may play a role but mechanism not known; hypersensitivity suggested by occurrence of eosinophils and presence of increased T lymphocytes in lavage fluid	Interstitial and alveolar infiltration of lymphocytes, eosinophils, and plasma cells; occasionally poorly formed, noncaseating granuloma; fibrosis unusual	8% incidence; synergism with other agents possible; occurs 12 d to 18 y after beginning therapy. Fever, chills, malaise, headache–a prodrome for days and weeks; cough, dyspnea, rales common. Skin rash in 17% and blood eosinophilia in 40%	Early interstitial infiltrates; later, alveolar infiltrates; hilar and mediastinal adenopathy, pleural effusions described; chest radiograph can be normal.	Clinical history suggestive; bronchoaleveolar lavage might suggest diagnosis (increase T cells in fluid), but lung biopsy required for diagnosis.	Discontinue drug, but reports of reinstitution without recurrence of the abnormality. Dramatic responses to steroids reported. Mortality 1%; outlook favorable
Cystosine arabinoside[103,104]	Unknown	Pulmonary edema; proteinaceous exudate with extravasation of red blood cells, no inflammatory cells	If given within 30 days of death, high incidence of pulmonary edema. Abrupt onset of dyspnea; gastrointestinal toxicity coexists.	Diffuse interstitial and alveolar pattern	Clinical picture suggests diagnosis.	Supportive; no studies
Miscellaneous						
Procarbazine (Matulane)[40,67,105]	Hypersensitivity	Mononuclear cell infiltration and scattered foci of eosinophils; fibrosis in one case	Acute onset within hours to days of first dose. Nausea, fevers, chills, arthralgias, urticaria, dry cough, and dyspnea. Blood eosinophilia common.	Interstitial Infiltrates; pleural effusion	Clinical picture highly suggestive of diagnosis.	Rapid recovery following discontinuation of drug. Role of steroids not known.
Vinca alkaloids (vinblastine and vindesine)[53,73,106,107]	Unknown	Dysplasia of alveolar lining cells; interstitial and alveolar influx of inflammatory cells; fibrosis	Most common reports of pulmonary edema in association with mitomycin; some patients subsequently developed pulmonary fibrosis. Dyspnea and wheezing seen with vindesine.	Diffuse interstitial and alveolar infiltrates with combination drugs; normal chest radiograph with vinca alkaloid alone	Clinical history suggests diagnosis.	Drug withdrawal; steroids probably beneficial. Prognosis poor if pulmonary infiltrates develop.

* Pulmomary toxicity has been reported with all other nitrosoureas, including, lomustine (CCNU), semustine (methyl-CCNU), and chlorozotocin (DCNU).[100–102]

CLINICAL FEATURES

Table 63–14 lists predisposing factors associated with enhancement of drug-induced pneumonitis.[42–57] Because bleomycin toxicity is relatively common, it deserves special mention. Although toxicity drastically increases with doses in excess of 450 to 500 mg, it can occur with much lower doses, especially when other risk factors are present. These factors include age greater than 60 years; simultaneous or prior irradiation to the lungs; simultaneous or subsequent oxygen therapy, especially with inspired doses equal to or greater than 35%; and a decrease in creatinine clearance time during the period of administration of bleomycin. A recent study described 9 of 45 patients (20%) who developed lung toxicity when they received bleomycin after cisplatin infusion.[58] Renal damage after cisplatin administration, with subsequent accumulation of bleomycin, was a likely cause of the high pulmonary toxicity and mortality rate of 67%. Extreme caution is recommended in the administration of combined bleomycin and cisplatin chemotherapy, and if possible, bleomycin should precede cisplatin infusion to minimize the risk of lung toxicity. Some data suggest that continuous infusion of bleomycin may be associated with less pulmonary toxicity than bolus therapy[59]; however, these data are inconclusive, and further studies are warranted.

Long intervals between drug administration and onset of clinical toxicity have been described. Late-onset pulmonary fibrosis has been reported many years after discontinuing cyclophosphamide[60] and carmustine.[61]

Signs and Symptoms

The cardinal symptom of drug-induced pulmonary toxicity is dyspnea. Nonproductive cough, fatigue, and malaise are other commonly associated complaints. Although symptoms usually develop over a period of several weeks to months, hypersensitivity drug-induced lung disease can develop over hours. Fever may be a common finding with this type of toxicity. Chest pain has been reported during infusion of bleomycin[62] or immediately after therapy with methotrexate[63]; however, it is an unusual manifestation of toxicity. Because hemoptysis is an uncommon feature of drug-induced pulmonary toxicity, when it is present, other diagnoses should be considered. Physical examination of the lungs may be normal or may reveal end-inspiratory "Velcro rales." Finger clubbing is distinctly unusual, but it may be related to the underlying malignancy.

Diagnostic Imaging

The most common radiographic abnormality associated with drug-induced pulmonary toxicity is a reticulonodular pattern, which may be basilar or diffuse. Pleural effusions are uncommon but occasionally have been reported in association with mitomycin, busulfan, methotrexate, and procarbazine toxicity.[64–67] Hypersensitivity lung disease associated with methotrexate and procarbazine may present with bilateral acinar infiltrates that clear rapidly.[67] In some instances, the chest radiograph is normal, even in the presence of histologically proved pulmonary infiltration and fibrosis.[66,68] Most commonly, methotrexate and carmustine toxicity have been reported with normal chest radiograph findings. Hilar adenopathy is distinctly unusual and has been reported only with methotrexate toxicity.[66] Cavitating and noncavitating nodules, simulating metastatic disease, have been seen with bleomycin toxicity.[69,70]

Both high-resolution thin-section CT chest scans and gallium scintigraphy have been shown to be more sensitive techniques than chest radiography to detect pulmonary parenchymal changes in association with drug toxicity.[71] The full relation of these changes to the development of functional or physiologic impairment is unclear, and further studies are needed. Although magnetic resonance spectrometry of lung parenchyma is in the early stages of development, eventually it may be used clinically to noninvasively differentiate among fibrosis, edema, acute pneumonitis, and hemorrhage.[72]

Pulmonary Function Tests

The most common abnormalities associated with chemotherapy-induced pulmonary toxicity are a reduced diffusing capacity for carbon monoxide and a restrictive ventilatory defect.[33] Isolated gas transport abnormalities manifested by a decrease in the diffusing capacity and arterial hypoxemia, especially with exercise, have been seen.

Screening pulmonary function tests to predict which patients receiving chemotherapy are likely to develop toxicity would be helpful but have not been established.

DIAGNOSIS

Although one might have a high clinical suspicion of drug-induced pulmonary toxicity, lung biopsy is usually necessary for a definitive diagnosis. Because pathognomonic pathologic changes associated with drug-induced pneumonitis often are not present, a biopsy is necessary to eliminate other specific diagnoses, such as opportunistic infection and malignancy. Through the use of bronchoalveolar lavage, several studies reported the presence of a characteristic or predominant cell associated with particular drugs.[34,39] Although these data might be of value in understanding the pathogenesis of drug-induced lung disorders, their usefulness in diagnosing drug toxicity is limited.

TREATMENT

The most effective way to manage pulmonary toxicity associated with chemotherapeutic agents is to prevent it. If it occurs, withdrawal of the offending agent is the cornerstone of therapy. Although no control studies in humans have systematically examined the efficacy of corticosteroids, a trial of these agents is probably warranted in most cases. The optimal dose and duration of therapy are not known; however, 1 mg/kg is usually initiated with a slow and careful tapering schedule because clinical deterioration after tapering has been reported.[73,74] One report described the case of a 23-year-old male patient who underwent a single lung transplantation because of presumed drug-induced pulmonary fibrosis 12 years after undergoing chemotherapy for acute lymphocytic leukemia.[75] The use of lung transplantation in the treatment of drug-induced pulmonary fibrosis is exciting and needs further evaluation.

Table 63–15 lists the characteristics of pulmonary disease caused by the commonly used chemotherapeutic agents.

REFERENCES

1. Gross NJ. The pathogenesis of radiation-induced lung damage. Lung 1981;159:115.
2. Rubin P, Casarett GW. Clinical radiation pathology. Philadelphia: WB Saunders, 1968.
3. Adamson ILR, Bowden DH, Wyatt JP. A pathway to pulmonary fibrosis: An ultrastructural study of mouse and rat following radiation to the whole body and hemithorax. Am J Pathol 1970;58:481.
4. Jennings FL, Arden A. Development of radiation pneumonitis: Time and dose factors. Arch Pathol 1962;74:351.
5. Perez C, Stanley K, Grundy G, et al. Impact of irradiation technique and tumor extent in tumor control and survival of patients with unresectable non-oat cell carcinoma of the lung. Cancer 1982;50:1091.
6. Emami B, Purdy JA, Manolis J, et al. Three-dimensional treatment planning for lung cancer. Int J Radiat Oncol Biol Phys 1991;21:217.
7. Goitein M, Abrams M, Rowell D, et al. Multi-dimensional treatment planning. II. Beam's eye view back projection through CT sections. Int J Radiol Oncol Biol Phys 1983;9:789.
8. Arriagada R, Le Chevalier T, Quoix E, et al. Chemotherapy effect on locally advanced non-small cell lung carcinoma: A randomized study on 353 patients. Proceedings of the 32nd annual ASTRO meeting 1990. Int J Radiat Oncol Biol Phys 1990;19:195.
9. Minchin RF, Johnson MR, Schuller HM, et al. Pulmonary toxicity of doxorubicin administered by in situ siolated lung perfusion in dogs. Cancer 1988;61:1320.
10. Wara WM, Phillips TL, Margolis LW, et al. Radiation pneumonitis: A new approach to the deviation of time-dose factors. Cancer 1973;32:547.
11. Gross NJ. Pulmonary effects of radiation therapy. Ann Intern Med 1977;86:81.
12. Maisin JR. The ultrastructure of the lung of mice exposed to a supralethal dose of ionizing radiation on the thorax. Radiat Res 1970;44:545.
13. Koga K, Kusumoto S, Watanabe K, et al. Age factor relevant to the development of radiation pneumonitis in radiotherapy of lung cancer. Int J Radiat Oncol 1988;14:367.
14. Isaacs RD, Wallie WJ, Wells UE, et al. Massive hemoptysis as a late complication of pulmonary irradiation. Thorax 1987;42:77.
15. Bate D, Guttman RJ. Changes in lung and pleura following two-million-volt therapy for carcinoma of the breast. Radiology 1957;73:679.
16. Bachman AL, Macken K. Pleural effusions following supervoltage radiation for breast carcinoma. Radiology 1959;72:699.
17. Smith JC. Radiation pneumonitis: Case report of bilateral reaction after unilateral irradiation. Am Rev Respir Dis 1964;89:264.
18. Holt JAG. The acute radiation pneumonitis syndrome. J Coll Radiol Aust 1964;8:40.
19. Bennett DE, Million RR, Ackerman LV. Bilateral radiation pneumonitis, a complication of the radiotherapy of bronchogenic carcinoma. Cancer 1969;23:1001.
20. Ikezoe J, Takashima S, Morimoto S, et al. CT appearance of acute radiation-induced injury in the lung. Am J Roentgenol 1988;150:765.
21. Kataoka M. Gallium-67 imaging for the assessment of radiation pneumonitis. Ann Nucl Med 1989;3:73.
22. Brady LW, German PA, Cander L. The effects of radiation therapy on pulmonary function in carcinoma of the lung. Radiology 1965;85:130.
23. Emirgil C, Heinemann HO. Effects of radiation of the chest on pulmonary function in men. J Appl Physiol 1961;16:331.
24. Prato FS, Kurdyak R, Saibil EA, et al. Regional and total lung function in patients following pulmonary irradiation. Invest Radiol 1977;12:224.
25. Wohl MEB, Griscom NT, Traggis DG, et al. Effects of therapeutic irradiation delivered in early childhood upon subsequent lung function. Pediatrics 1975;55:507.
26. Warren S, Spencer J. Radiation reaction in the lung. AJR 1940;43:682.
27. Rubin P, McDonald S, Maasilta P, et al. Serum markers for prediction of pulmonary radiation syndromes. Int J Radiat Oncol Biol Phys 1989;17:553.
28. Gross NJ, Narine KR. Experimental radiation pneumonitis: Corticosteroids increase the replicative activity of avelolar type 2 cells. Radiat Res 1988;115:543.
29. Gross NJ, Narine KR, Wade R. Protective effect of corticosteroids on radiation pneumonitis. Radiat Res 1988;113:112.
30. Moss WT, Haddy FJ, Sweany SK. Some factors altering the severity of acute radiation pneumonitis: Variation with cortisone, heparin, and antibiotics. Radiology 1960;75:50.
31. Freeman BA, Crapo JD. Biology of disease: Free radicals and tissue injury. Lab Invest 1982;47:412.
32. Lewis RA, Austen KF. The biologically active leukotrienes: Biosynthesis, metabolism, receptors, functions and pharmacology. J Clin Invest 1984;73:889.
33. Cooper JAD, White DA, Matthay RA. Drug-induced pulmonary disease: Part I. Cytotoxic drugs. Am Rev Respir Dis 1986;133:321.
34. White DA, Rankin JR, Stover DE, et al. Methotrexate pneumonitis: Lavage findings suggest an immune mediated disorder. Am Rev Respir Dis 1989;139:18.
35. Askenase PW, Hayden BJ, Gershon RK. Augmentation of delayed-type hypersensitivity by doses of cyclophosphamide which do not affect antibody responses. J Exp Med 1974;141:697.
36. L'age-Stehr J, Diamanstein T. Induction of autoreactive T lymphocytes and their suppressor cells by cyclophosphamide. Nature 1978;27:1663.
37. Absher M, Hildebran J, Trombley L, et al. Characteristics of cultured lung fibroblasts from bleomycin-treated rats: Comparison with in vitro exposed normal fibroblasts. Am Rev Respir Dis 1984;129:125.
38. Clark JG, Kostal KM, Marino BA. Bleomycin induced pulmonary fibrosis in hamsters: An alveolar macrophage product increases fibroblast prostaglandin E2 and cyclic adenosine monophosphate and suppresses fibroblast proliferation and collagen production. J Clin Invest 1983;72:2082.
39. White DA, Kris MG, Stover DE. Bronchoalveolar lavage cell populations in bleomycin-induced pulmonary toxicity. Thorax 1987;42:551.
40. Jones Se, Moore M, Blank N, et al. Hypersensitivity to procarbazine (Matulane) manifested by fever and pleuropulmonary reaction. Cancer 1972;29:498.
41. Holoye PY, Luna MA, McKay B, et al. Bleomycin hypersensitivity pneumonitis. Ann Intern Med 1978;88:47.
42. Ginsberg SJ, Comis RL. The pulmonary toxicity of antineoplastic agents. Semin Oncol 1982;9:34.
43. Blum RH, Carter SK, Agre K. A clinical review of bleomycin: A new antineoplastic agent. Cancer 1973;31:903.
44. Goldiner PL, Carlon GC, Cvitkovic E, et al. Factors influencing postoperative morbidity and mortality in patients treated with bleomycin. Br Med J 1978;1:1664.
45. Hakkinen PJ, Whiteley JW, Witschi HR. Hyperoxia, but not thoracic x-irradiation, potentiates bleomycin and cyclophosphamide-induced lung damage in mice. Am Rev Respir Dis 1982;126:281.
46. Tryka AF, Godleski JJ, Brian JD. Differences in effects of immediate and delayed hyperoxia exposure on bleomycin-induced pulmonary injury. Cancer Treat Rep 1984;68:759.
47. Franklin R, Buroker TR, Vaishampayan W, et al. Combined therapies in esophageal squamous cell cancer. Proc Am Assoc Cancer Res [Abstract] 1979;20:223.
48. Einhorn L, Krause M, Hornback N, et al. Enhanced pulmonary toxicity with bleomycin and radiotherapy in oat cell cancer. Cancer 1976;37:2414.
49. Samuels ML, Johnson DE, Holoye PY, et al. Large-dose bleomycin therapy and pulmonary toxicity: A possible role of prior radiotherapy. JAMA 1976;235:1117.
50. Soble AR, Perry H. Fatal radiation pneumonia following subclinical busulfan injury. AJR 1977;128:15.
51. Buzdar AU, Legha SS, Luna MA, et al. Pulmonary toxicity of mitomycin. Cancer 1980;45:236.
52. Durant JR, Norgard MJ, Murad TM, et al. Pulmonary toxicity associated with bischloroethylnitrosourea (BCNU). Ann Intern Med 1979;90:191.
53. Luedke D, McLaughlin TT, Daughaday C, et al. Mitomycin C and vindesine associated pulmonary toxicity with variable clinical expression. Cancer 1985;55:542.
54. White DA, Orenstein M, Godwin TA, et al. Chemotherapy-associated pulmonary toxic reactions during treatment for beast cancer. Arch Intern Med 1984;144:953.
55. Skarin AT, Rosenthal DS, Maloney WC. The treatment of advanced non-Hodgkin's lymphoma (NHL) with bleomycin, Adriamycin, cyclophosphamide, vincristine and prednisone. Blood 1977;49:759.
56. Bauer KA, Skarin AT, Balikian JP, et al. Pulmonary complications associated with combination chemotherapy programs containing bleomycin. Am J Med 1983;74:557.
57. Aronin PA, Mahaley MS, Rudnick SA, et al. Prediction of BCNU pulmonary toxicity in patients with malignant gliomas: An assessment of risk factors. N Engl J Med 1980;303:1983.
58. Rabinowits M, Souhami L, Gil RA, et al. Increased pulmonary toxicity with bleomycin and cisplatin chemotherapy combinations. Am J Clin Oncol 1990;13:132.
59. Cooper KR, Hong WK. Prospective study of the pulmonary toxicity of continuously infused bleomycin. Cancer Treat Rep 1981;65:419.
60. Alvarado CS, Boat TF, Newman AJ. Late-onset pulmonary fibrosis and chest deformity in two children treated with cyclophosphamide. J Pediatr 1978;92:443.
61. O'Driscoll BR, Hasleton PS, Taylor PM. Active lung fibrosis up to 17 years after chemotherapy with carmustine (BCNU) in childhood. N Engl J Med 1990;323:378.
62. White DA, Schwartzberg L, Kris MG, et al. Acute chest pain during bleomycin infusions. Cancer 1987;59:1582.
63. Walden PAM, Mitchell-Heggs PF, Coppin C, et al. Pleurisy and methotrexate treatment. Br Med J 1977;2:867.
64. Orwoll ES, Kiessling P, Patterson R. Interstitial pneumonia from mitomycin. Ann Intern Med 1978;89:352.
65. Smalley RV, Wall RL. Two cases of busulfan toxicity. Ann Intern Med 1966;64:154.
66. Sostman HD, Matthay RA, Putnam CE. Methotrexate-induced pneumonitis. Medicine 1976;55:371.
67. Ecker MD, May B, Keohane MF. Procarbazine lung. AJR 1978;131:527.
68. Weiss RB, Poster DS, Penta JS. The nitrosoureas and pulmonary toxicity. Cancer Treat Rev 1981;8:111.
69. Glasier CM, Siegel MJ. Multiple pulmonary nodules: Unusual manifestations of bleomycin toxicity. AJR 1981;137:155.
70. Talcott JA, Garnick MB, Stomper PL, et al. Cavitary lung nodules associated with combination chemotherapy containing bleomycin. J Urol 1987;138:619.
71. Taylor CR. Diagnostic imaging techniques in the evaluation of drug-induced pulmonary disease. Clin Chest Med 1990;11:87.
72. Vinitski S, Pearson MG, Karlik ST, et al. Differentiation of parenchymal lung disorders with in vivo proton nuclear magnetic resonance. Magn Reson Med 1986;3:120.
73. Gunstream SR, Seidenfeld JJ, Sobonya RE, et al. Mitomycin-associated lung disease. Cancer Treat Rep 1983;67:301.
74. Spector JI, Zimbler H, Ross JS. Cyclophosphamide and interstitial pneumonitis. JAMA 1980;243:1133.
75. Grossman RF, Frost A, Zamel N, et al. Results of single lung transplantation for bilateral pulmonary fibrosis. N Engl J Med 1990;322:727.
76. Koss LG, Melamed MR, Mayer K. The effect of busulfan on human epithelia. Am J Clin Pathol 1965;44:385.
77. Stover DE, Zaman MB, Hajdu SI, et al. Bronchoalveolar lavage in the diagnosis of

diffuse pulmonary infiltrates in the immunosuppressed host. Ann Intern Med 1984;101: 1.

78. Kuplic JB, Higley CS, Niewoehner DE. Pulmonary ossification associated with long-term busulfan therapy in chronic myeloid leukemia. Am Rev Respir Dis 1972;106: 759.
79. Heard BE, Cooke RA. Busulfan lung. Thorax 1968;233:1987.
80. Burns WA, McFarland W, Matthews MJ. Busulfan-induced pulmonary disease: Report of a case and review of the literature. Am Rev Respir Dis 1970;101:408.
81. Collis CH. Lung damage from cytotoxic drugs. Cancer Chemother Pharmacol 1980;4: 17.
82. Mark GJ, Lehimgar-Zadeh A, Ragsdale BD. Cyclphosphamide pneumonitis. Thorax 1978;33:89.
83. Alvarado CS, Boat TF, Newman AJ. Late-onset pulmonary fibrosis and chest deformity in two children treated with cyclophosphamide. J Pediatr 1978;92:443.
84. Maxwell I. Reversible pulmonary edema following cyclophosphamide treatment. JAMA 1974;229:137.
85. Cole SR, Myers TJ, Klatsky AU. Pulmonary disease with chlorambucil therapy. Cancer 1978;41:455.
86. Taetle R, Dickman PS, Feldman PS. Pulmonary histopathologic changes associated with melphalan therapy. Cancer 1978;42:1239.
87. Goucher G, Rowland V, Hawkins J. Melphalan-induced pulmonary interstitial fibrosis. Chest 1980;77:805.
88. Berend N. Protective effect of hypoxia on bleomycin lung toxicity in the rat. Am Rev Respir Dis 1984;130:307.
89. Frank L. Protection from O_2 toxicity by pre-exposure to hypoxia: Lung antioxidant enzyme role. J Appl Physiol 1982;53:475.
90. Wesselius LJ, Catanzaro A, Wasserman SI. Neutrophil chemotactic activity generation by alveolar macrophages after bleomycin injury. Am Rev Respir Dis 1984;129:485.
91. Kelley J, Newman RA, Evans JN. Bleomycin-induced pulmonary fibrosis in the rat: Prevention with an inhibitor of collagen synthesis. J Lab Clin Med 1980;96:954.
92. White DA, Stover DE. Severe bleomycin-induced pneumonitis: Clinical features and response to corticosteroids. Chest 1984;86:723.
93. Luna MA, Bedrossian CWM, Lichtiger B, et al. Interstitial pneumonitis associated with bleomycin therapy. J Clin Pathol 1972;58:501.
94. DeLena M, Guzzon A, Monfardini S, et al. Clinical, radiologic and histopathologic studies on pulmonary toxicity induced by treatment with bleomycin (NSC-125066). Cancer Chemother Rep 1972;56:343.
95. Jules KJ, White DA. Bleomycin-induced pulmonary toxicity. Clin Chest Med 1990;11: 1.
96. Jolivet J, Giroux L, Laurin S, et al. Microangiopathic hemolytic anemia, renal failure, and noncardiogenic pulmonary edema: A chemotherapy-induced syndrome. Cancer Treat Rep 1983;67:429.
97. Nathan CF, Arrick BA, Murray HW, et al. Tumor cell antioxidant defenses: Inhibition of the glutathione redox cycle enhances macrophage-mediated cytolysis. J Exp Med 1981;153:766.
98. Reznil-Schuller HM, Smith AC, Thenot JP, et al. Pulmonary toxicity of the anticancer drug, bis-chloroethyl nitrosurea (BCNU) in rats. Toxicologist 1984;4:29.
99. Selker RG, Jacobs SA, Moore PB. BCNU (1,3-bis(2-chloroenthyl)-1-nitrosourea) introduced pulmonary fibrosis. Neurosurgery 1980;7:560.
100. Cordonnier C, Vernant J-P, Mital P, et al. Pulmonary fibrosis subsequent to high doses of CCNU for chronic leukemia. Cancer 1983;51:1814.
101. Lee W, Moore RP, Wampler GL. Interstitial pulmonary fibrosis as a complication of prolonged methyl-CCNU therapy. Cancer Treat Rep 1978;62:1355.
102. Sordillo EM, Sordillo PP, Stover DE, et al. Chlorozotocin (DCNU)-induced pulmonary toxicity. Cancer Clin Trials 1981;4:397.
103. Haupt HM, Hutchins GM, Moore GW. Ara-C lung: Noncardiogenic pulmonary edema complicating cytosine arabinoside therapy of leukemia. Am J Med 1981;70:256.
104. Hewlett RI, Wilson AF. Adult respiratory distress syndrome (ARDS) following aggressive management of extensive acute lymphoblastic leukemia. Cancer 1977;39:2422.
105. Lokich JJ, Moloney WC. Allergic reaction to procarbazine. Clin Pharmacol Ther 1972;13:573.
106. Kris MG, Pablo D, Gralla RJ, et al. Dyspnea following vinblastine or vindesine administration in patients receiving mitomycin plus vinca alkaloid combination therapy. Cancer Treat Rep 1984;68:1029.
107. Konits PH, Aisner J, Sutherland J, et al. Possible pulmonary toxicity secondary to vinblastine. Cancer 1982;50:2771.

SECTION **5**

LAUREL J. STEINHERZ
JOACHIM YAHALOM

Cardiac Complications of Cancer Therapy

The treatment of cancer has been improved by the expansion of chemotherapeutic agents and the refinement of radiation therapy over the past three decades. However, many of the most effective antineoplastic agents and mediastinal irradiation produce toxic effects on the heart. This section describes some of these problems and discusses attempts at prevention and management.

CHEMOTHERAPY

ANTHRACYCLINES

The anthracyclines have been associated with cardiomyopathy since their introduction in the late 1960s. Early reports included isolated cases of unexplained cardiac failure in patients undergoing treatment with daunorubicin[1–4] and, in the early 1970s, with doxorubicin.[5–10] In 1983, Lefrak and colleagues[11] reported a series of 399 patients treated with doxorubicin. He found a 30% incidence of cardiac failure in the patients who received more than 550 mg/m^2 of doxorubicin and a lower incidence in those who received less. This introduced the concept of increasing cardiotoxicity with cumulative doses above a "safe threshold" cumulative dose. In 1974, Halazen and associates[12] reported a series of children with acute lymphoblastic leukemia in remission who were treated with two different maintenance protocols, one including and one excluding daunorubicin. There was a 10% incidence of cardiac failure in the children treated with daunorubicin and none in the other group. This report clearly demonstrated the relation of anthracycline treatment to the incidence of cardiac failure, and it excluded the influence of active malignancy or the stress of induction therapy as contributory factors. Von Hoff and colleagues demonstrated, in 5613 patients treated with daunorubicin[13] and in 4018 patients treated with doxorubicin,[14] a continuous exponential increase of incidence of cardiac failure with increasing cumulative dose. Subsequently, Bristow and colleagues[15,16] used endomyocardial biopsy to show that pathologic lesions progressively worsened in a linear relation to the increase in total cumulative dose, in contrast to the exponential increase in myocardial dysfunction. This contrast suggested a threshold of tolerable myocardial damage beyond which the administration of additional drug would result in clinical symptomatology. Both clinical and pathologic abnormalities increased at any dose level in patients who received mediastinal radiation therapy.[17]

Clinical Presentation

Anthracycline cardiomyopathy has been described as having three clinical presentations: acute, subacute, and late. The acute toxicity[18] presents as a myopericarditis and probably results from the combination of acute myocyte damage from drug exposure and the effects of the catecholamine and histamine[19,20] surge provoked by the administration of anthracyclines. This occurs within days of dose administration and includes transient arrhythmia,[21,22] pericardial effusion, and myocardial dysfunction, sometimes leading to transient cardiac failure and occasionally death.[15,18] Histologically, acute myocyte disruption and sometimes infiltration of the myocardium by granulocytes, lymphocytes, and histiocytes[23] are seen.

The classic subacute presentation has a more insidious onset and can appear immediately after the last dose or up to 30 months later,[24] with a peak onset of symptoms at 3 months from the last dose.[13] This insidious onset was duplicated by Jaenke[25] in rabbits treated with repeated sublethal doses of doxorubicin and then sacrificed at varying lengths of time after cessation of treatment. Rabbits treated with higher doses exhibited myocardial necrosis and lethal cardiac failure immediately after therapy, but the rabbits treated with low doses showed almost no myocardial damage when sacrificed immediately after treatment but showed increasing myocardial damage when sacrificed at increasingly later periods, even though no drug persisted in the blood or myocardium. The clinical picture presents with increasing tachycardia and fatigue, progressing in some to tachypnea, dyspnea, and finally pulmonary edema, right-sided congestive signs, and low cardiac output. The mortality of patients actually manifesting congestive heart failure in these early series ranged up to 60%, although some patients could be stabilized with intensive cardiac treatment,[26,27] and many showed remarkable improvement of cardiac function over the first few years after chemotherapy.[27–30] Evaluation of hemodynamics with exercise, however, has revealed significant underlying abnormalities even in asymptomatic patients with normal resting parameters.[31] The pathology noted on endomyocardial biopsy and autopsy within the first 2 years after completion of anthracyclines includes mitochondrial swelling, disruption and loss of myofibrils, and particularly swelling and distortion of the sarcoplasmic reticulum, producing intramyocyte vacuolization.[17,32,33] With mild toxicity, such damage is patchy; with higher doses and toxicity, it is found more extensively throughout the heart, with progression to myocyte necrosis and loss. Pathologic examination 41 to 47 months after chemotherapy reveals hypertrophy of the remaining myocytes without fibrosis and diminution of vacuolization, suggesting healing and compensation.[34]

The late presentation of anthracycline cardiomyopathy occurs 5 or more years after completion of anthracycline therapy (Table 63–16). It involves late clinical decompensation of patients who had recovered from subacute cardiac symptoms[35–37,39,40] (Fig 63–1) or the occurrence of de novo cardiac failure in patients with no previous symptoms 6 to 20 years after anthracycline therapy.[35–39,41] It has also been demonstrated subclinically as abnormal systolic cardiac function in 23%,[35–37] abnormal myocardial mass in 52%,[40,42] and abnormal diastolic function and exercise response in 80%[43,44] of patients. As with subacute toxicity, an increased incidence

TABLE 63–16. Late Cardiac Toxicity of Anthracyclines

Investigations	No. of Patients	*Anthracycline (mg/m²)* Range	Mean	Radiation Therapy	*Follow-up (years)* Range	Mean	No. of Abnormal Patients (%)	Methods of Evaluation	Types of Abnormalities Found
Steinherz et al, 1991[36,37]	201	200–1275	450	56	4–20	7	47 (23%)	ECHO, STI, Cath biopsy RNCA, 24 h ECG	47/201 ↓ FS, 9 ABN Biopsy 14 ABN 24 h ECG, 3 SD
Lipshultz et al, 1991[40]	115	45–550	334	No	1–15	6.4	66 (57%)	ECHO, FS, ESWS/VCF Exercise 24 h ECG	60/115 ↑ ESWS/ ↓ LV PW 32/115 ↓ FS 23/89 ABN 24 h ECG, 4VT
Hausdorf et al, 1988[42]	55	31–656	273	No	2–10	NS	NS	ECHO, carotid pulse Systolic/diastolic function ESWS, angiotensin II response	ABN diastolic function ↑ ESWS
Santoro et al, 1987[273]	26	NS	245	Yes	5–8	7	0	STI, ECHO, Rest RNCA	None
LaMonte et al, 1986[272]	19	83–229	176	Yes	1.3–5.9	3.25	5 (26%)	ECG, ECHO RNCA Rest and stress	2 ABN ECG 3 ABN EF rest 2 ABN EF stress
Weesner et al, 1991[43]	10	90–498	291	NS	4–13	7	NS	ECHO, Doppler, exercise, versus controls	Poor ↑ with stress of FS, aortic flow, and cardiac index
Larsen et al, 1992[45]	133	NS	219	51	NS	NS	≥110 (~90%)	ECG 24 h ECG	40 ABN ECG 110 ABN 24 h ECG 6 VPB pairs 4 VT
Jakacki et al, 1991[44]	57	≤350	263	16	2.1–20.7	5.4	≥40 (≥70%)	ECHO, ECG 24 h ECG RNCA Exercise	5 ABN FS, 18 ABN ECG ≥40 ABN 24 h ECG 9 ABN RNCA 25 ABN exercise

ABN, abnormal; Cath, cardiac catheterization; ECHO, echocardiogram; ECG, electrocardiogram; EF, ejection fraction; ESWS, end-systolic wall stress; FS, fractional shortening; LV, left ventricular; NS, not stated; PW, posterior wall thickening; RNCA, radionuclide cardiac angiography, SD, sudden death; STI, systolic time interval; VCF, velocity of circumferential fiber shortening; VPB, ventricular premature beats; VT, ventricular tachycardia.

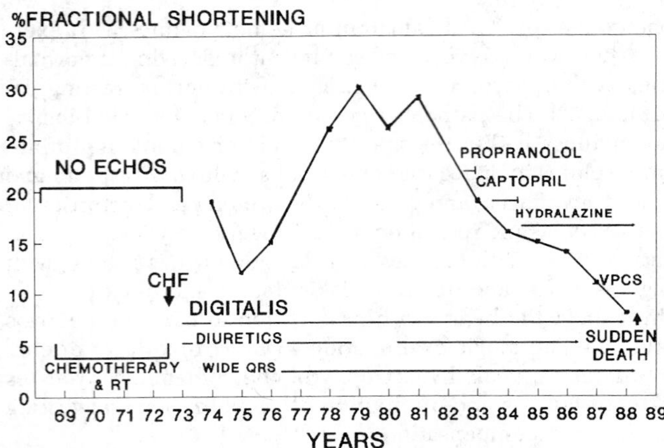

FIGURE 63–1. The clinical course of a patient after subclinical anthracycline cardiotoxicity. The initial increase and then progressive decrease of her fractional shortening (FS) on echocardiogram and increasing requirements for therapeutic support of cardiac function, can be seen. Despite an early FS of 11%, the patient gradually improved over the first 6 years. She discontinued diuretics, achieved modest exercise tolerance, and completed high school. The patient's FS on echocardiogram reached 30% 6 years after therapy. Eight years after doxorubicin therapy, however, she required increasing amounts of diuretics for recurrent edema. Ten years after chemotherapy, the patient had progressive deterioration of exercise tolerance and FS despite increasingly intensive medical management. During the last 2 years, she was found to have moderately frequent premature ventricular contractions but no syncope or runs of ectopic ventricular beats. She was deemed unsuitable for cardiac transplantation. Finally, 20 years after initial diagnosis and 17 years after her last anthracycline dose, the patient developed a tachy-brady arrhythmia that led to sudden syncope and cardiac arrest. CHF, congestive heart failure; VPCS, ventricular premature contractions; RT, radiotherapy.

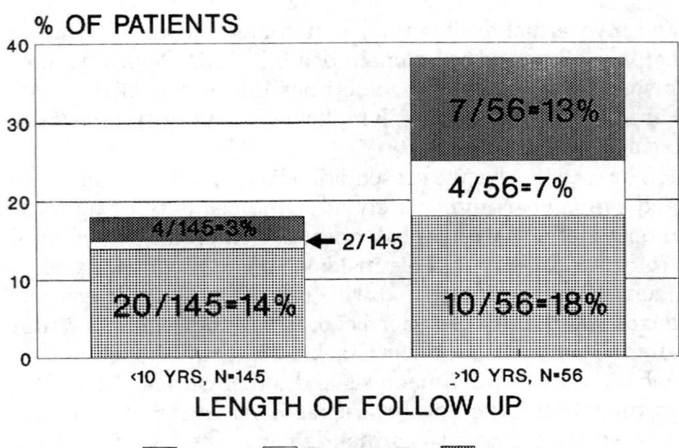

FIGURE 63–2. Percentage of patients found to have abnormal echocardiograms on long-term follow-up. Despite a similar cumulative anthracycline dose (495 versus 420 mg/m^2), 38% of those followed for 10 years or longer had decreased fractional shortening (FS), compared with 18% of those followed for less than 10 years ($p < 0.004$). More than half of abnormalities (11/21) seen in the group followed for 10 or more years were moderate (FS = 21–24%), or severe (FS $\leq$ 20%), while the degree of abnormality was mild (FS = 25–28%) in 77% (20/26) of the abnormal patients followed for less than 10 years.

of late abnormality correlates with increasing cumulative dose of anthracycline, and mediastinal irradiation is an additive risk factor.[36,37,40] Late abnormalities of resting echocardiograms, however, were found in patients treated with as little as 75 mg/m^2 of doxorubicin,[40] and late abnormalities of exercise response were seen in 55% of patients treated with low cumulative doses (median, 263 mg/m^2).[44] Abnormalities of myocardial mass are said to be more pronounced in patients treated in early childhood, implying a negative effect on myocardial growth.[40] Abnormalities of systolic function do not correlate with age during chemotherapy.[36] Measurements of systolic function[36,37] and myocardial wall thickness[40] deteriorate progressively with time after anthracyclines (Fig 63–2). Serious arrhythmias have been identified in symptomatic and asymptomatic patients at late cardiac follow-up, including ventricular tachycardia and fibrillation and second-degree heart block.[36,37,40,44,45] Several young patients with late cardiomyopathy have died suddenly up to 15 years after chemotherapy.[36,37] The pathology found on biopsy and autopsy of patients with late cardiotoxicity is predominantly fibrosis and hypertrophy of remaining myocytes, with little remaining vacuolization.[36,37,41] Thus, even asymptomatic patients who have been treated with anthracyclines need long-term cardiac follow-up, and new symptoms suggestive of arrhythmia and especially syncope need vigorous investigation. Cardiac status on noninvasive testing during the year after completion of therapy predicts the likelihood of late abnormality (Fig. 63–3) and indicates the advisable frequency of follow-up.[36,37]

Mechanisms of Pathogenesis

An understanding of the mechanisms of cardiotoxicity is vital to attempts at prevention. There are many mechanisms proposed, and several may interact to cause the multiple sites of intracellular injury seen histologically. Doxorubicin is found to bind to cardiolipin in the inner mitochondrial membrane,[46,47] with two deleterious results. The electron transfer in the respiratory chain, which is dependent on the binding of cardiolipin to cytochrome *c* for its interaction with cyto-

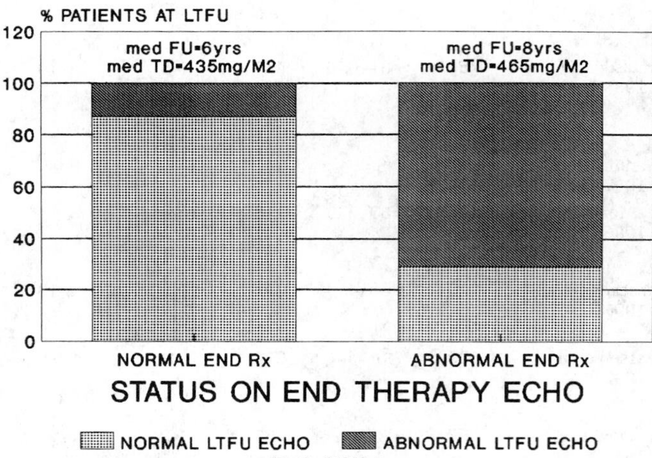

FIGURE 63–3. An echocardiogram taken after completion of anthracycline therapy has prognostic implications for cardiac function on late follow-up. Eighty-seven percent of patients who had normal fractional shortening on echocardiogram during the year after therapy remained normal at late follow-up, whereas only 29% of patients who were even mildly abnormal on end therapy echocardiogram were normal at late follow-up ($p < 0.0001$). ECHO, echocardiogram; LTFU, late follow-up.

chrome oxidase, and the activation by cardiolipin of the NADH-cytochrome *c* oxidoreductase complex (complex I–III), for the synthesis of adenosine triphosphate (ATP), are disrupted. This leads to depletion of ATP and phosphocreatine concentrations and depression of contractility.[48] In addition, the doxorubicin-cardiolipin complex promotes transfer of electrons through doxorubicin, forming a doxorubicin free radical that can reduce molecular oxygen, producing O_2^-.[46] This induces the generation of free hydroxyl radicals and H_2O_2, leading to mitochondrial membrane damage, further disruption of enzymatic respiration, and more extensive lipid peroxidation.[46,47] Oxidative damage is worsened by the concomitant decrease, during chemotherapy, of glutathione peroxidase, which normally serves as a free radical scavenger. Glutathione is especially important in myocytes, which lack catalase, which serves as a scavenger in other tissues. Free radical lipid peroxidation was identified[50] as an important mechanism of myocyte damage and has been found to depend, in the heart, on an iron-doxorubicin complex.[47,51,52] The resultant disruption of the sarcoplasmic reticulum and direct effects of the metabolite doxorubicinol have been shown to cause disturbances of Ca^{2+} transport,[47,53,54] which is critical to regulation of cardiac action potentials, contraction, and relaxation.[55] Chronically, there is alteration of contractile proteins and their enzymes with a shift in the ratio of prevalent isomyocin types and decreased production of α-myosin heavy chains, perhaps as an adaptation to chronic low-energy states.[56]

Prevention

MONITORING. Attempts at prevention of cardiomyopathy initially involved limitation of total cumulative dose below 450 to 550 mg/m^2. This limit was chosen to avoid the rapid increase in prevalence of clinical cardiac dysfunction in excess of 30%, which occurs above that dose range. Arbitrary dose limitation was inadequate because of variability of individual tolerance. Therefore, therapy has been modified according to serial monitoring of cardiac status, by various means, to identify increasing risk of unacceptable toxicity. Monitoring of systolic time intervals and of electrocardiograms (ECGs) for QRS voltage loss[57] or ST-T changes was too nonspecific or showed changes too late to direct prevention. Serial echocardiography has been helpful in identifying changes in systolic and diastolic function, especially in children, where echo images are clear and more easily measurable.[58–61] The fractional shortening is the most frequent parameter followed, although some recent groups follow end systolic wall stress and the relation between wall stress and velocity of circumferential fiber shortening.[61] Radionuclide cardiac angiography has been used by many investigators to follow systolic[62–65] and diastolic function,[66] and specific guidelines for modification of chemotherapy on the basis of radionuclide ejection fraction in adults, proposed by Schwartz and colleagues,[62] has gained wide acceptance. Adherence to these guidelines reduced the incidence of cardiac failure from 21% to 3% in this study. The addition of measurements of contractility during exercise for comparison with those at rest adds sensitivity according to some authors[63–65] but is less helpful according to others.[67] Recommendations for monitoring, including radionuclide studies and quantitation of pathologic damage by endomyocardial biopsy, have been offered by investigators from Stanford University Medical Center.[65] These recommendations, however, do not suggest monitoring until a cumulative dose of 450 mg/m^2 is reached, unless the baseline study is abnormal or unless the patient is over 70 years of age, has hypertension, has other cardiac disease, or was receiving mediastinal irradiation. Monitoring that follows these recommendations does not identify early sensitivity in patients without those particular risk factors. Another format for monitoring, using a combination of echocardiography and radionuclide studies, was formulated by the multiinstitutional Cardiology Discipline Committee of the Childrens Cancer Group.[58] These recommendations include cardiac evaluation before anthracycline administration and further monitoring before every other course until a cumulative dose of 300 mg/m^2 is reached and then for every course beyond this. Endomyocardial biopsy is suggested for abnormal or equivocal results. Although not yet included in routine monitoring, we hope that newer modalities, such as magnetic resonance imaging and indium-111-antimyosin scintigraphy,[68,69] will add to the efficacy of monitoring in the future.

SCHEDULE MODIFICATION. Other attempts to prevent cardiomyopathy involve decreasing the peak dose of anthracycline delivered to the heart by modification of schedules of delivery.[70–72] Legha and colleagues[70] demonstrated that patients receiving continuous infusions of doxorubicin developed lower peak plasma levels the longer the length of time of the infusion. Thus, levels with a 48-hour infusion were lower than with a 24-hour infusion, and a 96-hour infusion of the same dose per course produced still lower levels. Comparison of endomyocardial biopsy scores in patients receiving doxorubicin showed that patients receiving their dose by 48- or 96-hour infusion had significantly lower biopsy scores, indicating less cardiomyopathy than patients receiving the dose by 20-minute bolus. In addition, patients receiving 96-hour infusions had lower biopsy scores than those receiving 24-hour infusions. Infusions were administered through an indwelling intravenous line using a battery-powered, portable pump. Continuous infusion chemotherapy is usually given through a surgically implanted central venous catheter. A recent study by Shapira and colleagues[72] using radionuclide cardiac angiography to evaluate cardiotoxicity demonstrated a decline in left ventricular ejection fraction (LVEF) of only 6% after a total cumulative dose of 400 mg/m^2 administered by only 6-hour continuous infusion, compared with a drop of 21% in patients who received the same range of total doxorubicin dose by 20-minute bolus. More recently, Casper and colleagues[71] confirmed the cardioprotective effects of 72-hour infusion in a prospective randomized trial of 82 patients with soft tissue sarcoma. Schedules dividing the planned monthly doxorubicin dose into smaller weekly doses also decrease pathologic and physiologic abnormalities, allowing administration of higher cumulative doses.[73,74]

CARDIOPROTECTIVE AGENTS. Free radical scavengers, such as vitamin E,[75] *N*-acetylcysteine,[76] and other scavengers[77,78] have shown promise in animals but no clear benefit in patients. Similarly, trials of concomitant administration of coenzyme Q, verapamil,[79] prenylamine,[80,81] and other calcium-channel blockers; β-adrenergic and histamine blockers[82–84] to prevent the effects of excessive vasoactive agents; antiinflammatory agents, carnitine, digoxin,[85] and amrinone[86]; as well as encapsulation of the anthracycline in liposomes and binding to agarose[87] have not proved definitively useful in patients. The liposomes used during the patient trials of the last decade were highly unstable, and it is hoped that the new phase II trials with a more stable complex will show significant protection.[88] Attempts to exploit the importance of the iron-doxorubicin complex appear to be more successful. (+−)-1,2-bis(3,5-dioxopiperazinyl-1-yl)propane, known as ICRF-187 or ADR-529, is an iron chelator that has been shown to exhibit significant protection against anthracycline cardiotoxicity in various animal studies,[89,90] in a pilot study of 12 patients with various solid tumors,[91] and in a randomized therapeutic trial in women with breast cancer.[92,93] Patients were evaluated both by radionuclide ejection fraction and myocardial biopsy. Incidence of clinical toxicity, degree of decrease of ejection fraction, and biopsy score were significantly less in the ICRF arm of the studies. These results are being confirmed in a multicenter patient trial with similar monitoring. Recent animal studies have shown that there is no mediation of ICRF protection by changes of myocardial antioxidants[94] and that there is not merely a delay of appearance of the injury.[95] Examination of rabbits 3 months after discontinuation of therapy shows healing of lesions in those treated with ICRF.

NEW ANALOGS. Analogs of daunorubicin and doxorubicin have been studied in clinical trials. Many agents that appear to have decreased cardiotoxicity in animal studies and even in early clinical trials eventually have been found to have similar toxicity to the parent compound. Patients treated with zorubicin experienced cardiotoxicity, which was additive to prior anthracycline toxicity, and some developed cardiac failure.[96,97] 4′Epi-doxorubicin is another analog with cardiotoxicity similar to or possibly less than doxorubicin.[98–100] Incidents of atrioventricular block, ventricular fibrillation, decreased ejection fraction,[101] and decreased velocity of circumferential fiber shortening[102] have been reported in phase I and II trials with another analog, Aclarubicin. Demethoxy daunorubicin (idarubicin) has shown activity in patients whose malignancy has become resistant to daunorubicin, but it is also cardiotoxic.[103–105] The myelotoxicity of idarubicin is about four times that of daunorubicin. When given in amounts of equivalent myelotoxicity, the cardiotoxicity is also similar.[104,106] Thus, careful monitoring of this agent is warranted above a cumulative dose of 75 mg/m^2. Cardiac failure and subclinical decrease in ejection fraction occurred in patients treated with the analog esorubicin (DXDX). A 5% drop in mean LVEF was noted at 240 mg/m^2 and a 10% drop at 480 mg/m^2 of this agent.[107] Animal studies of 4′-deoxy-4′-iodo-doxorubicinol (I-DXR) indicate acute and chronic cardiotoxicity but possibly less than daunorubicin.[108] The ideal anthracycline has not been found.

Management

Clinical anthracycline cardiomyopathy needs to be managed with inotropic support and afterload reduction,[23] often initially by the intravenous route. Most patients can be stabilized and show clinical improvement. Patients who were refractory to treatment, had repeated bouts of pulmonary edema or increasing pulmonary resistance, and were free of malignancy benefited from cardiac transplantation.[109–111]

MITOXANTRONE

Mitoxantrone hydrochloride is an anthracenedione that is similar in structure to doxorubicin. Animal studies revealed conflicting findings in different species, including ECG abnormalities in treated monkeys, dose-related impairment of contractility in the rabbit heart,[112] and no ECG changes or progressive anthracycline-like lesions on endomyocardial biopsy specimens of beagle hearts.[113] Cases of cardiac failure and arrhythmia (mainly supraventricular) were reported from the early phase I and II trials of the National Cancer Institute.[114,115] The incidence of myocardial dysfunction and cardiac failure increased with increasing cumulative dose, as with doxorubicin.[114,116] Significant decrease in ejection fraction occurred in these trials around 110 mg/m^2,[114] and a rapid increase in incidence of cardiac failure was noted at 160 mg/m^2.[116] Recent studies have continued to detect cardiomyopathy and cardiac failure in patients with[117] and without[118] prior anthracycline therapy; and conduction delay, with prolongation of PR, QRS, and QT intervals on ECG was also reported.[119] A British patient trial reported a 46% incidence of abnormal LVEF using radionuclide angiography during rest and cold pressor stress in patients who received a wide range of doses.[120] An Italian trial reported ECG abnormalities in 41%, echocardiographic abnormalities in 66%, and a 15% or more decrease in radionuclide LVEF in almost 25% of patients receiving a cumulative dose of 28 to 84 mg/m^2.[121] The overall incidence, reported by Lederle Laboratories, of subclinical moderate to serious decrement in LVEF was 13%; and the incidence of cardiac failure, up to a cumulative dose of 140 mg/m^2, was 2.6%.[122]

AMSACRINE

Amsacrine (AMSA) is an acridine derivative used mainly in patients with nonlymphoblastic leukemia. It has been associated with myocardial infarction[123] and ventricular arrhythmias, including fatal ventricular fibrillation.[124–126] These arrhythmias often have been attributed to coexisting electrolyte abnormalities, particularly hypokalemia. Recently, AMSA has been safely administered even to patients with preexisting atrial[127] and ventricular[128] arrhythmias. Noninvasive monitoring of cardiac function during a prospective study of AMSA revealed reversible abnormalities on serial echocardiograms in 18 of 27 patients and cardiac failure in 7 of 27 patients.[129,130] Echocardiographic abnormalities generally appeared within 1 week of AMSA therapy and resolved in most cases once therapy was discontinued. Four patients died with persistent cardiac failure. The incidence of echocardiographic abnormalities was related to total dose of AMSA, rate of AMSA administration, and total dose of anthracyclines previously received. No patient who received less than 200 mg/m^2 of AMSA in 48 hours, after having previously received less than 400 mg/m^2 of anthracyclines, had echocardiographic abnormalities. In contrast, all patients who received 200 mg/m^2 or more of AMSA within 48 hours after having previously received more than 400 mg/m^2 of anthracyclines exhibited echocardiographic abnormalities.[129] Arlin and colleagues[131] treated 24 patients with preexisting myocardial dysfunction with more than 200 mg/m^2 of AMSA over 48 hours and reported no occurrences of cardiac failure in this group. Nine of the patients had radionuclide ejection fractions determined after AMSA treatment and 2 of these patients showed a further decrease of ejection fraction by more than 10%. It was not stated how soon after treatment the radionuclide angiograms were obtained. Therefore, it is possible that there were additional transient deficits that were not detected in this study. The absence, however, of any clinical cardiac failure in these heavily treated patients is significant.

CYCLOPHOSPHAMIDE

Investigators disagree about whether cyclophosphamide in doses under 100 mg/kg/week contribute to cardiomyopathy.[15,28,73,132] In our experience, it does not. Higher doses used for cytoreduction and immunosuppression before bone marrow transplantation can cause an acute hemorrhagic pancarditis. This was initially described in case reports,[133–135] animal studies,[136] and autopsy series[137,138] as involving a serosanguineous pericardial effusion, mural thickening with edema, and endocardial, myocardial, and epicardial hemorrhage. This results from endothelial capillary damage that allows extravasation of fluid and red cells into cardiac and pulmonary tissues. Reports of patient series[139–142] described the acute course, with an onset during the first week after treatment, peak toxicity at 7 to 9 days, and improvement over the next 3 weeks. Abnormal findings of diastolic dysfunction, small to moderate pericardial effusion, restrictive cardiomyopathy (sometimes mimicking pericardial tamponade), and later systolic dysfunction were found described in more than half of patients.[140–142] Most patients remained asymptomatic; some had mild symptoms of fluid retention, edema, and tachypnea; and a few had an extremely fulminant course of cardiac failure and shock that was resistant to intensive treatment and resulted in death. Previous anthracycline therapy and previous abnormal cardiac function were identified as risk factors, and the importance of dose and rate of delivery was stressed.[140] A weekly dose of 170 mg/kg over 4 days without anthracyclines and 120 mg/kg over 2 days after anthracyclines predicted risk for at least subclinical changes. More rapid delivery of 120 mg/kg over 24 hours produced fulminant cardiomyopathy in 1 patient.[135,137] Mildly symptomatic patients responded to diuretics and, if necessary, transient digitalization or intravenous inotropic agents. Those with the more fulminant course required prolonged intravenous inotropic support, respiratory assistance, and hemofiltration.[142] Pericardial drainage has not been helpful, and the effusion can be managed conservatively and improves with time.[143] To avoid this clinical cardiotoxicity, patients have been screened during the past decade with echocardiography or radionuclide studies to identify abnormal cardiac function. The pretransplantation regimen can then be adjusted for higher risk patients by administering the cyclophosphamide over additional days or by using a preparatory regimen without cyclophosphamide. A pretreatment radionuclide LVEF of less than 50% has been correlated with increased risk of cardiotoxicity.[144,145] Recent studies suggested that giving the cyclophosphamide in smaller doses twice a day decreased the incidence of systolic dysfunction, although changes in myocardial mass still occurred.[145] Children treated with anthracyclines for malignancy before transplantation who were evaluated during exercise at least 1 year after transplantation showed significant hemodynamic abnormalities. A small group of children with aplastic anemia who had not received anthracyclines, evaluated similarly, were normal.[146]

IFOSFAMIDE

Ifosfamide, an alkylating oxazaphosphorine related to cyclophosphamide, has been associated with atrial ectopy (including atrial fibrillation) and, less commonly, ST-T wave changes and bradycardia. These abnormalities were noted in patients who had received doses as high as 6.25 to 10 g/m^2 over 3 to 5 days.[147] ECG abnormalities, negative inotropic effects, and pathologic myocardial damage were also found in animals that received high doses of ifosfamide.[148,149]

RETINOIC ACID

Transretinoic acid is an agent that has proved effective for the treatment of acute promyelocytic leukemia. Its use is associated with RA syndrome in up to 25% of cases, characterized by fever, dyspnea, pleural and pericardial effusion, pulmonary infiltrates, peripheral edema, and transient myocardial dysfunction.[150] This is especially prevalent during the first 2 weeks of therapy and has responded to dexamethasone.

TAXOL

Taxol is a new antimicrotubule assembly inhibitor. It has activity against melanoma, refractory ovarian carcinoma, and non-small cell carcinoma of the lung through its induction of tubulin polymerization. Cases of significant disturbances of cardiac rhythm and conduction have been reported during phase I and II trials of this agent.[151] Significant sinus bradycardia (30–50 beats/minute) occurred in up to 29% of patients in the phase II trial for ovarian cancer.[152] Several patients exhibited progressive atrioventricular conduction delay from first-degree heart block, to complete heart block, to asystole[152] on continuous ECG monitoring during Taxol infusion as a single agent. The conduction delay reverted to normal with cessation of the infusion. Associated presyncope and syncope have been reported.[151] One patient required a demand pacemaker for further infusions. Episodes of sustained and nonsustained ventricular tachycardia have been reported with the combination of Taxol and cisplatin[153] during the Taxol infusion. Chest pain occurred in several patients receiving the combination, and a myocardial infarction, coincident with complete heart block, was documented in one man with coronary heart disease. It is not certain if the adverse effects on cardiac conduction relate to the Taxol itself or to its Cremophor EL vehicle. Preliminary experience with the synthetic analog Taxatere suggests a lesser potential for dysrhythmia. It has been recommended that continuous ECG monitoring accompany the use of these agents.[151]

HOMOHARRINGTONINE

Homoharringtonine is an alkaloid from the Chinese *cephalotaxus*. It is another drug that causes reversible atrioventricular block,[154] ventricular ectopy,[155] supraventricular tachycardia, and ST-T wave changes in animals[156] and patients.[154] It has also produced cardiac failure and hypotension, with vacuolar degeneration of the myocardium on pathologic examination.[154,156]

VINCRISTINE AND VINBLASTINE

Vincristine has been associated with cardiac autonomic dysfunction. One study demonstrated a loss of cyclic respiratory phase-related heart rate variation in 9 children during vincristine treatment.[157]

Vincristine[158] and vinblastine[159] have also been associated with myocardial infarction. Angina pectoris was reported in up to 38% of patients during treatment with vinblastine combined with cisplatin and bleomycin.[160] Another study of the same combination reported angina with infarct-like ECG changes and apical akinesia occurring repeatedly, during multiple courses, in a 47-year-old patient with normal coronary angiography.[161] This seemed to clearly implicate the chemotherapy as the cause.

MITOMYCIN C

Mitomycin C has been reported to increase the incidence of anthracycline cardiotoxicity when these agents are combined[162] due to enhancement of formation of superoxide and hydrogen peroxide.[163] It also has been described as a cause of acute congestive heart failure in a woman who received a cumulative dose of 225 mg/m^2 of mitomycin as a single agent[164] and in another patient when 30 mg/m^2 of mitomycin was added to treatment with 150 mg/m^2 doxorubicin.[165] The overall incidence of cardiotoxicity is said to be under 10% and limited to patients receiving a cumulative dose of at least 30 mg/m^2.[165,166]

5-FLUOROURACIL

The cardiotoxicity of 5-FU was first identified by Dent and McColl in 1975.[167] A survey of 1083 patients in 1982 reported cardiotoxicity in 1.1% of all patients and in 4.6% of patients with prior evidence of heart disease.[168] Since then, more frequent use of continuous-infusion 5-FU, increased awareness of the problem, and more sophisticated monitoring have increased the reported incidence. By 1990, there were more than 67 clinical cases described,[169] and an incidence ranging up to 68% of silent ischemic ECG changes was identified in patients monitored by continuous 24-hour ambulatory ECG during 5-FU infusion.[170] The clinical features of the cardiotoxicity included the following:

1. Precordial pain (both nonspecific and anginal)[169]
2. ECG ST-T wave changes (nonspecific and ischemic)[169,170]
3. Acute myocardial infarction (rare)[171,172]
4. Atrial arrhythmia (including atrial fibrillation) and, less frequently, ventricular ectopy (including refractory ventricular tachycardia and fibrillation)[170–173]
5. Ventricular dysfunction (usually global, less frequently segmental)
6. Cardiac failure, pulmonary edema, and cardiogenic shock (with and without ischemic symptoms)[172,174–177]
7. Sudden death[172,173]

In most cases, the arrhythmia was treatable and the ischemia-like symptoms and ECG changes disappeared (if the infusion was discontinued) or responded to nitrates, allowing the infusion to continue. The abnormalities of segmental and global ventricular function reverted to normal within days to weeks of cessation of infusion. Some patients needed intravenous inotropic and vasodilator support during the initial period.[174,175,177,178] In most cases with chest pain, with or without ECG changes, the CPK-MB fraction remained normal.[169,172,174,176] Most frequently, patients developed cardiac toxicity during the second or later course of treatment, but some experienced problems during the first course.[169] Those who developed cardiac toxicity and recovered usually had symptoms again when rechallenged with another infusion.[169,172] Some investigators reported success in preventing cardiotoxicity with calcium blockers such as nifedipine and diltiazem,[179] while others had less success.[176,180] There was no influence of age or sex on incidence.[169] Symptoms were reported in a 38-year-old man[177] and in several women in their 40s[169,174,175] with no prior cardiac history. Cardiac findings have occurred when 5-FU was given by infusion or bolus, as a single agent or with cisplatin and other drugs.[169] Although some felt that cardiac irradiation[181] and preexisting heart disease[168,170] were risk factors, others did not.[169,182] Several investigators documented normal coronary arteries in patients with severe symptoms.[172,175] One investigator excluded increased proclivity for coronary vasospasm by challenging a patient, who had previous angina, during 5-FU infusion with ergonovine during a posttreatment coronary study.[172] Findings on autopsy and endomyocardial biopsy have shown diffuse, interstitial edema, intracytoplasmic vacuolization of myocytes, and no inflammatory infiltrate.[183] Acute infarcts have been demonstrated pathologically in some, but not all, patients with clinical infarction.[169]

The ischemic-like pain and ECG findings, lack of CPK-MB fraction changes, and frequent response to nitrates and at times to calcium-channel blockers in the setting of anatomically normal coronary angiograms plus reversible contractility deficits suggest coronary vasospasm as a mechanism for 5-FU cardiotoxicity. The global dysfunction, however, possibly due to "stunned" myocardium, and the lack of universal response to coronary vasodilators leaves some questions about this hypothesis. Some investigators postulate a myocarditis or myocardiopathy pathogenesis.[184–186]

Although the mechanism is still uncertain, careful observation for cardiac symptoms and arrhythmia is warranted during drug infusion, especially in patients who were symptomatic in prior courses.

CISPLATIN

Cisplatin has been associated with arrhythmias such as atrial fibrillation[187] and with angina and ST-T wave changes on ECG.[188–191] These may be caused or exacerbated by electrolyte imbalances from the excessive hydration and forced diuresis required for the drug's administration.

INTERFERON

Cardiotoxicity has been identified in 44 of 432 patients from 15 phase I clinical trials of α-, α_2-, β-, and γ-interferon.[192] Significant abnormalities of cardiac rhythm and conduction,[192–195] ischemia and infarction,[192,196–198] and cardiomyopathy[192,199,200] were observed. These problems were identified with all types of interferon used except β-interferon, which was used in only a small subset of the patients.[192] No correlation with patient age, individual dose, or cumulative dose was identified, although some patients had less toxicity when retreated at doses lower than the dose that produced toxicity.[192,199] Cardiomyopathy was seen in patients after more prolonged treatment,[199] but the other forms of toxicity were seen frequently during the first 5 weeks of treatment, even within 1 to 7 days of initiation of therapy.[192] The occurrence of ischemia and infarction was definitely related to a prior history of ischemic heart disease and might have been related to increased myocardial oxygen demand, from the fever and stress of the influenza-like syndrome accompanying treatment, or to peripheral and coronary arterial constriction.[192] The arrhythmias were less clearly related to prior heart disease but might have been exacerbated by the features of this influenza-like syndrome as well. Arrhythmias and ischemic ECG changes were identified in mice treated with α-interferon with no myocardial lesions on necropsy, suggesting mediation by peripheral effects.[195] Arrhythmias have been seen in up to 20% of patients in clinical trials.[194] The arrhythmias observed include fatal[201] and reversible[202] ventricular fibrillation, ventricular tachycardia[193,194] atrial flutter and fibrillation, atrioventricular block, and less severe atrial and ventricular ectopy.[192] Sudden death occurred in 2 patients.[192] Cardiomyopathy, presenting as cardiac failure, with severe decrease in radionuclide ejection fraction to a range of 10% to 33%, was seen in 7 patients during prolonged administration of α- or α_2-interferon.[199,200,203,204] The cardiomyopathy was reversible in 4 of these patients after cessation of interferon, with and without inotropic, diuretic, and afterload reduction therapy. Congestive symptoms disappeared, and ejection fractions improved to a range of 29% to 46%. Two patients were retreated with lower doses of interferon without return of failure. Three of the patients with reversible cardiomyopathy had acquired immunodeficiency syndrome (AIDS) with Kaposi's sarcoma.[199] There is an AIDS-associated cardiomyopathy; however, this is not reversible. Two other patients had chronic myelogenous leukemia[203] and hairy cell leukemia,[200] and 2 more patients had other types of cancer.[204] Myocardial biopsy in 1 patient revealed only mild focal intramyocyte vacuolization.[199] The etiologic mechanism is unknown. In vitro studies have been conflicting. One study in isolated rat cardiac myocytes, incubated with interferon, showed inhibition of contractility and depletion of ATP,[205] while another similar study did not.[206] Some postulate an interaction between interferon and noradrenaline.[192,207] Cautious observation for cardiac symptoms and monitoring of rhythm appear to be warranted for these agents, with reduction in dose for significant abnormalities.

OTHER BIOLOGIC AGENTS

Interleukin-2 (IL-2) and tumor necrosis factor produced no reduction in ATP or decrease in contractility when incubated with isolated rat cardiac myocytes for 24 to 48 hours.[206] However, a major reduction in ventricular stroke work index was found in patients with a variety of solid tumors, who were monitored with indwelling arterial and pulmonary catheters during IL-2 treatment.[208] This resulted from a poor increase in cardiac index in comparison to the decrease in peripheral resistance. All patients developed a capillary leak syndrome requiring dopamine and crystaloid support. Deleterious effects on blood pressure, systemic resistance, and stroke work appeared to peak about 4 hours after individual doses and to worsen with subsequent doses.[208] In addition, there has been a significant (4–30% in various trials) incidence of apparent myocardial infarction with this agent.[208–213] One patient with elevated CPK-MB fraction, focal injury pattern on ECG, and segmental wall motion abnormality on radionuclide angiography underwent coronary angiography, which revealed normal coronary arteries.[214] This suggested a pathogenesis involving coronary vasospasm or focal myocarditis.

A new biologic agent, OK432, derived from *Streptococcus* sp was suspected of inducing an autoimmune cardiomyopathy; however, it was shown not to provoke the formation of antiheart antibody or ECG changes in rabbits or patients.[215] Continued evidence of lack of cardiotoxicity should remove an obstacle to the development of OK432 as an active anticancer agent.

OTHER AGENTS

Case reports have attributed cardiotoxicity to several other agents. Melphalan,[216] bis(helenalinyl)malonate,[217] mithramycin,[218] bis[1,2-bis(diphenylphosphino)ethane]gold(I) chloride (a cytotoxic antineoplastic drug containing gold),[219] teniposide (VM26),[220] etoposide,[221] and busulfan[222] have been implicated in this respect.

RADIATION-INDUCED HEART DISEASE

Cardiac complications resulting from mediastinal irradiation were considered rare and insignificant for a long period in the history of radiation therapy.[223,224] Since the mid-1960s, when follow-up information on a large number of patients who had been cured of Hodgkin's disease with higher dose of radiation became available, the heart has no longer been considered radioresistant.[225] Radiation-induced heart disease (RIHD) has now been characterized[226,227] and investigated in experimental animals,[228–231] and the pathologic features of RIHD damage have been described with regard to the coronary arteries and all three layers of the heart.[232–235]

Pericarditis and pericardial effusion have been regarded as the most common side effects of cardiac irradiation.[226] Modern techniques of irradiation, dose fractionation, and reduction of the heart volume irradiated in most malignancies, however, have substantially reduced the frequency of this complication during the last decade.[236] At the same time, accumulated evidence suggests that ischemic heart disease resulting from radiation-induced coronary artery disease (CAD) is the most formidable potential long-term risk of cardiac irradiation.

The clinical spectrum of RIHD involves most structures of the heart and is summarized in Table 63–17. Although the

TABLE 63–17. Clinical Spectrum of Radiation-Induced Heart Disease

Pericardial disease
Acute pericarditis during irradiation
Delayed acute pericarditis
Pericardial effusion
Constrictive pericarditis
Myocardial dysfunction
Valvular heart disease
Electrical conduction abnormalities
Coronary artery disease

pathologic and clinical manifestations of RIHD may overlap in many patients, they are discussed separately in the following paragraphs.

PERICARDIAL DISEASE

Incidence

The risk of radiation-induced pericardial disease depends on both the dose given and on the volume of the heart irradiated.[226,237,238] Even when a large volume of the heart (60% or more) is irradiated at or below 4000 cGy, the risk for mild pericarditis is below 5%, and severe pericarditis is rare.[236] Smaller heart volumes (20–30%) may tolerate up to 6000 cGy, with an expected 2% risk of mild pericarditis. The importance of both volume and dose in the production of radiation pericarditis in Hodgkin's disease was demonstrated in an analysis of mantle field radiation therapy practices at Stanford.[239] In instances in which the whole pericardium was irradiated, the pericarditis incidence was 20%, but when most of the left ventricle was excluded, it was reduced to 7%. When an additional block was implemented to shield most of the heart after 3000 cGy, the incidence was reduced to only 2.5%. All series that showed a high risk for pericarditis[240–242] were of patients treated with a radiation technique, energy, and fractionation schedules that are no longer considered to be an acceptable standard of care in most centers.[238] With current radiation therapy techniques for Hodgkin's disease and breast cancer, pericarditis is an infrequent event.[238,243,244]

Pathology

Clinical and pathologic changes involving the pericardium are the most common abnormalities described after cardiac irradiation. The macroscopic abnormalities consist of pericardial thickening and effusion.[226] The parietal pericardium is more frequently and severely involved.[226] Collagen replaces the normal adipose tissue, fibrinous exudate is present on the surface and interstitially, and proliferation of small blood vessels can be observed microscopically.[226] The pericardial fluid is protein-rich and may contain strands of fibrin. The fluid ranges in appearance from serous to grossly sanguineous.[227] Over time, the fibrinous exudate may organize with the fibrotic pericardium and epicardium to develop into constrictive pericarditis. The mechanism for pericardial fibrosis and effusion is not clear. It may result from increased capillary permeability and inhibition of the local fibrinolytic mechanism.[226,245] Radiation-induced hypothyroidism should also be considered as a cause of pericardial effusion after mediastinal irradiation.[246]

Acute Pericarditis During Radiation

Acute pericarditis during the course of radiation therapy is rare. It is almost always associated with massive mediastinal tumors adjacent to the heart. The signs and symptoms are of acute nonspecific pericarditis. It does not lead to a significant risk of late pericardial damage and is not an indication for interrupting the radiation course.[226]

Delayed Pericarditis

Radiation-induced pericarditis typically occurs within the first year after mediastinal irradiation. The common range is between 4 months to several years after treatment.[226,242,247–249] Pericardial disease presents either as an acute pericarditis, as a chronic pericardial effusion that may be asymptomatic, or as a combination of both. The symptoms of delayed acute pericarditis are indistinguishable from those of other types of pericarditis and usually consist of fever, pleuritic chest pain, pericardial friction rub, ST-T segment changes, and a decrease of the QRS voltage in the ECG.[226,227,242]

The differential diagnosis of pericardial effusion after radiation includes recurrent malignancy, idiopathic pericarditis, myxedema, and pericardial abscess.[227,250,251] It is estimated that 10% to 30% of patients with radiation-related pericardial effusion develop tamponade requiring pericardiocentesis.[241,252,253] Most cases of radiation-induced pericarditis and pericardial effusion resolve spontaneously, usually within 16 months.[253] About 20% of patients with delayed pericarditis progress within 5 to 10 years to develop symptomatic constriction requiring pericardiectomy.[254]

Treatment

Careful cardiac evaluation and monitoring with echocardiography and radionuclide ventriculography should be performed whenever RIHD is suspected.[247] Patients with mild symptoms and no hemodynamic compromise may be followed without treatment or receive symptomatic therapy with salicylates or other nonsteroidal antiinflammatory agents.[226,227] There are reports of a few patients who have received steroids with apparent improvement[255]; however, relapse of symptoms or unmasking of latent radiation injury after rapid withdrawal of steroid therapy has been reported.[256,257] Symptomatic pericardial effusion or clinical evidence for hemodynamic compromise warrants a drainage procedure. Pericardiocentesis with or without percutaneous placement of an indwelling catheter is successful in most patients.[251,258] Failure to relieve tamponade with pericardiocentesis, recurrence of effusion, or the presence of symptomatic constrictive pericarditis requires pericardiectomy.[229,242,259] The mortality of this procedure in patients with postirradiation pericarditis is high. Cameron and colleagues[260] reported a postoperative mortality of 21%, and a review by Ni and associates[261] showed an early mortality of 22% in patients operated for radiation-induced pericarditis and a late mortality (after more than 30 days) of 35%. The high rate of complication in previously irradiated patients is attributed to the existence of additional radiation injury to other cardiac and thoracic structures. Occult constrictive pericarditis requires no surgical intervention and usually has a good prognosis.[227]

MYOCARDIAL DYSFUNCTION

When myocardial dysfunction is detected after standard-dose mediastinal irradiation, it is typically mild or subclinical.[227,262,263] Impaired exercise capacity in asymptomatic patients after irradiation has been reported.[264,265] Noninvasive studies using echocardiography and radionuclide angiogram detected subtle left ventricular dysfunction in Hodgkin's disease patients evaluated a few years after mediastinal irradiation.[247,265,266] Most patients with abnormal ventricular function findings, however, do not have clinical heart failure.[263]

The magnitude of the potential contribution of cardiac irradiation to the risk of doxorubicin-induced cardiomyopathy is not well established, but some data suggest potentiation of anthracycline-induced cardiotoxicity when combined with radiation therapy.[13,17,26,267–269] The histopathologies of radiation heart disease and anthracycline heart disease are different,[270] and the combined effects are probably additive rather than synergistic.[226,270,271] Reducing the doxorubicin dose to 300 to 350 mg/m^2 in the setting of cardiac irradiation has been recommended.[13] In programs of combined modality therapy for Hodgkin's disease that included relatively low doses of doxorubicin (up to 250 mg/m^2) and mediastinal irradiation of 2000 to 4000 cGy, no significant clinical myocardial dysfunction was detected.[272–274] Longer follow-up is required, however, to fully appreciate the potential risk of combined-modality cardiac toxicity.[36]

Symptomatic myocardial dysfunction after a radiation dose that does not exceed 6000 cGy is rare.[226] The few patients described with intractable heart failure had myocardial fibrosis as part of pancarditis, a generalized process with damage to all three layers of the heart. The hemodynamic pattern is usually of restrictive cardiomyopathy and is difficult to distinguish from constrictive pericarditis.[226,227,245] Its coexistence with pericarditis explains the poor outcome of pericardiectomy when attempted under these circumstances.[226,261]

VALVULAR DISEASE

Clinically significant valvular heart disease resulting from mediastinal irradiation is rare.[226,227,275] In a review of radiation-associated valvular disease, only 10 patients with symptomatic postirradiation valvular disease could be found.[275] When echocardiographic studies were performed in asymptomatic Hodgkin's disease patients more than 7 years after mediastinal irradiation, however, valvular abnormalities were detected in a third of the patients.[263,276] Most of the changes were found in the mitral or aortic valves and consisted of thickening or regurgitation.[263,275–277] In one series,[264] mild pulmonary stenosis was detected in 3 patients 6 to 12 years after radiation therapy. Surgical intervention for postirradiation valvular disease had been performed in 5 patients but was successful in only 3 of them.[275] Fibrous thickening of the valvular endocardium was found in 13 of 16 necropsies of young patients who received over 3500 cGy to the heart, but none had apparent valvular dysfunction.[232] The mean interval from irradiation to detection of valvular disease in 32 asymptomatic patients was 11.5 years.[275] In symptomatic patients, the interval was 16.5 years.[275] With longer follow-up, more patients may manifest symptoms related to radiation-induced valvular damage.[232,275]

ELECTRICAL ABNORMALITIES

Many ECG abnormalities were recorded years after mediastinal irradiation, the most common clinically significant abnormality being complete atrioventricular block.[247,264,278–284] Slama and associates[282] reported that radiation-related atrioventricular block was typically infranodal and occurred at long intervals (mean, 12 years), after radiation doses above 4000 cGy, most frequently in patients with abnormal conduction on ECG before the advent of complete block, and most frequently in patients who had other radiation-related cardiac abnormalities. At postmortem examination, fibrosis of the conduction system has been reported.[279,282]

CORONARY ARTERY DISEASE

Experiments in laboratory animals,[228–231,285–287] analysis of pathologic specimens,[232] clinical observations,[240,288–290] and long-term risk analyses in large series of patients treated for Hodgkin's disease[291–294] all indicate that mediastinal irradiation may facilitate the development of CAD.

Studies in rabbits on an atherogenic diet and exposed to radiation showed extensive atherosclerotic coronary damage to a degree that was disproportionately higher than what might have been expected from the summation of the changes induced by radiation alone and by high-cholesterol diet alone.[286] Similar observations have also been made in other experimental animals.[287,288]

An autopsy study in 16 young (aged 15 to 33 years) patients who received over 3500 cGy to the heart showed that 16 of 64 (25%) major coronary arteries had significant stenosis (more than 76% obstruction) compared with only one of 40 (2.5%) obstructed coronary arteries in a group of age- and sex-matched controls.[232] In this study, the proximal portion of the arteries had significantly more narrowing than the distal parts. McEniery and colleagues[290] described coronary angiograms of 15 patients with CAD after chest irradiation. Eight of these 15 had significant narrowing (more than 50% in diameter) of the left main coronary artery, and 4 had severe ostial stenosis of the right coronary artery. Stenosis at the origin of the coronary arteries appears to be a common finding for radiation-associated CAD.[295,296] After mediastinal irradiation, there is a greater likelihood for right coronary, left main, or left anterior descending coronary artery lesions as opposed to circumflex lesions, which may be due to the fact that the former vessels, particularly at their origin, receive more radiation.[297] Coronary spasm after radiation therapy has also been documented in patients who developed acute myocardial infarction with patent coronary arteries.[290,298]

Reports of CAD in young patients who received mediastinal irradiation for Hodgkin's disease have long implicated that radiation is a facilitating factor in this multifactorial disease process.[227,232,288–290,297] Only recently, however, analyses of large data bases of patients with Hodgkin's disease demonstrated a significantly increased risk of mortality from myo-

TABLE 63–18. Relative Risk of Mortality From Myocardial Infarction After Mediastinal Irradiation for Hodgkin's Disease

Investigations	*Center*	*No. of Patients*	*No. of Lethal MI Events*	*Relative Risk*	*95% Confidence Interval*
Boivin et al, 1992[291]	Multiple	4665	68	2.6	1.1–5.9
Hancock et al, 1992[293]	Stanford	2060	45	3.2	1.5–5.8
Henry-Amar et al, 1991[292]	EORTC	1449	17	8.8	5.1–14.1
Tarbell et al, 1990[243]	JCRT	590	8	6.7	2.9–13.3

MI, myocardial infarction; EORTC, European Organization for Treatment and Research on Cancer; JCRT, Joint Center for Radiation Therapy (Boston).

cardial infarction after mediastinal irradiation. These studies are summarized in Table 63–18. Although only about 1% to 2% of Hodgkin's disease patients in these series died of myocardial infarction, the observed risk in all four series was still higher than expected.[243,291–293] Boivin and colleagues[291] analyzed the risk of mortality from CAD in 4665 patients treated for Hodgkin's disease and followed for an average period of 7 years. The age-adjusted relative risk of death with myocardial infarction after mediastinal irradiation was 2.6 and was even higher (relative risk, 4) when myocardial infarction was considered a direct cause of death. In this study, the onset of increased risk was rapid, occurring within the first 5 years of observation. None of the risk factors for CAD significantly altered the relative risk estimates.

Mantle radiation therapy techniques, better fractionation schemes, and modern equipment deliver smaller doses of radiation to the coronary arteries and may have a lower risk of promoting CAD.[238] In Boivin's study,[291] the relative risk for acute myocardial infarction was reduced from 6.33 for patients treated during the years 1940 to 1966 to 1.97 (with no significant difference from unity) for patients irradiated from 1967 to 1985. Alternatively, data from Stanford[293] showed no decrease in the risk of mortality from myocardial infarction for patients treated after 1972, compared with patients treated during earlier years.

Long-term mortality data from three trials that randomized breast cancer patients to receive postmastectomy radiation therapy as opposed to no additional treatment demonstrated a higher incidence of cardiac death in the irradiated group.[299–301] The excess in mortality did not appear until more than 10 years after treatment.[300,301] In one study, the increase in mortality risk was significant only in women who were irradiated for tumors in the left breast.[301] It was also increased in patients treated with orthovoltage irradiation as opposed to those treated with more modern supervoltage equipment.[301]

These data demonstrate the risk associated with coronary artery irradiation. The old breast irradiation techniques used in these particular studies delivered high doses of radiation to the heart.[238,302] These techniques are no longer in use in most centers. Long-term follow-up of patients in similar randomized trials who were treated with heart-sparing techniques did not show increased cardiovascular morbidity.[303,304] Prophylactic irradiation of the internal mammary nodes using a single anterior photon beam ("hockey stick" technique), which may deliver a high dose to the heart, is not indicated in most patients irradiated for breast conservation or after mastectomy.[305] Breast cancer patients irradiated with modern techniques, energies, and fractionation schedules are unlikely to receive a significant dose of radiation to the coronary arteries.[302]

The radiation threshold for an increased risk of CAD has not been determined. Lederman and associates[306] reported that patients with seminoma who received a relatively low dose of mediastinal irradiation (median, 2400 cGy) had more ischemic heart disease than a similar group of patients whose mediastinum was not irradiated. The observed cardiac risk in the irradiated group, however, did not differ significantly from the expected risk of a comparable normal population.

Monitoring and reduction of other contributing CAD factors in patients who receive mediastinal irradiation should be part of the follow-up of patients who undergo mediastinal irradiation. Early detection of CAD should be encouraged because angioplastic or surgical intervention may be indicated in special anatomic or clinical situations. Successful treatment of radiation-induced CAD with bypass surgery and with angioplasty has been reported.[290] In some cases, surgery may be technically difficult because of mediastinal and pericardial fibrosis.[290]

CONCLUSION

We look forward to the development of new chemotherapeutic agents that are active against malignant cells but free of cardiotoxicity. We also hope that future modifications in techniques of radiation therapy will further decrease cardiotoxicity from this mode of therapy. In the meantime, increased awareness and knowledge about the potential cardiotoxicity of these therapeutic modalities should enable physicians to adequately monitor patients and modify therapy to minimize serious acute and chronic cardiac sequelae. The increasing information about late cardiac effects should facilitate early diagnosis and therapeutic intervention for the benefit of previously treated patients.

REFERENCES

1. Tan CT, Tasaka H, Yu KP, et al. Daunomycin an antitumor antibiotic in the treatment of neoplastic disease. Cancer 1967;20:333–353.
2. Malpas JS, Scott RB. Rubidomycin in acute leukaemia in adults. Br Med J 1968;3: 227–229.

3. Bonadonna G, Monfardini S. Cardiac toxicity of daunorubicin. Lancet 1969;1:837.
4. Marmont AM, Damasio E, Rossi F. Cardiac toxicity of daunorubicin. Lancet 1969;1: 837–838.
5. Bonadonna G, Monfardini S, De Lena M, et al. Phase I and preliminary phase II evaluation of adriamycin. Cancer Res 1970;30:2572–2582.
6. Tan C, Etcubanas E, Wollner N, et al. Adriamycin in children with acute leukemia and other neoplastic diseases. In: Carter SK, DiMarco A, Ghione M, Krakoff IH, Mathe G, eds. International symposium on Adriamycin. V. Clinical activity and side effects. Berlin, NY: Springer-Verlag, 1972:204–212.
7. Tan C, Etcubans E, Wollner N, et al. Adriamycin: an antitumor antibiotic in the treatment of neoplastic disease. Cancer 1973;32:9–17.
8. O'Bryan RM, Luce JK, Tally RW, et al. Phase II evaluation of adriamycin in human neoplasia. Cancer 1973;32:1–8.
9. Blum RH, Carter SK. Adriamycin: A new anticancer drug with significant clinical activity. Ann Intern Med 1974;80:249–259.
10. Gilladoga AC, Manuel C, Tan CT, et al. Cardiotoxicity of adriamycin in children. Cancer Chemother Rep 1975;6:75–80.
11. Lefrak EA, Pitha J, Rosenheim S, et al. A clinicopathologic analysis of Adriamycin cardiotoxicity. Cancer 1973;32:302–314.
12. Halazun JF, Wagner HR, Gaeta JF, et al. Daunorubicin cardiac toxicity in children with acute lymphocytic leukemia. Cancer 1974;33:545–554.
13. Von Hoff DD, Layard M, Basa P. Risk factors for doxorubicin induced congestive heart failure. Ann Intern Med 1979;91:701–717.
14. Von Hoff DD, Rozencweig M, Layard M, et al. Daunomycin-induced cardiotoxicity in children and adults. Am J Med 1977;62:200–208.
15. Bristow MR, Billingham ME, Mason JW, et al. Clinical spectrum of anthracycline cardiotoxicity. Cancer Treat Rep 1978;62:873–879.
16. Bristow MR. Pathophysiologic basis for cardiac monitoring in patients receiving anthracyclines. In: Crooke ST, Reich SD, eds. Anthracyclines: Current status and new developments. New York: Academic Press, 1988:255–270.
17. Billingham ME, Bristow MR, Glastein E, et al. Adriamycin cardiotoxicity: Endomyocardial biopsy evidence of enhancement by irradiation. Am J Surg Pathol 1977;1:17–23.
18. Bristow MR, Thompson PD, Martin RP, et al. Early anthracycline cardiotoxicity. Am J Med 1978;65:823–832.
19. Bristow MR, Minobe WA, Billingham ME, et al. Anthracycline-associated cardiac and renal damage in rabbits: Evidence for mediation by vasoactive substances. Lab Invest 1981;45:157–68.
20. Bristow MR, Billingham ME, Daniels JR. Histamine and catecholamines mediate Adriamycin cardiotoxicity. Proc Am Assoc Cancer Res 1979;20:118.
21. Wortman JE, Lucas VS, Schuster E, et al. Sudden death during doxorubicin administration. Cancer 1979;44:1588–1591.
22. Dindogru A, Barcos M, Henderson ES, et al. Electrocardiographic changes following Adriamycin treatment. Med Pediatr Oncol 1978;5:65–71.
23. Porembka DT, Lowder JN, Orlowski JP, Bastulli J, Lockrem J. Etiology and management of doxorubicin cardiotoxicity. Crit Care Med 1989;17:569–572.
24. Gottlieb SL, Edmiston WA, Haywood LJ. Late, late doxorubicin cardiotoxicity. Chest 1980;78:880–882.
25. Jaenke RS. Delayed and progressive myocardial lesions after Adriamycin administration in the rabbit. Cancer Res 1976;36:2958–2966.
26. Gilladoga AC, Manuel C, Tan CTC, et al. The cardiotoxicity of Adriamycin and Daunomycin in children. Cancer 1976;37:1070–1078.
27. Goorin AM, Borow KM, Goldman A, et al. Congestive heart failure due to Adriamycin cardiotoxicity: Its natural history in children. Cancer 1981;47:2810–2816.
28. Alexander J, Dainiak N, Berger HJ, et al. Serial assessment of doxorubicin cardiotoxicity with quantitative radionuclide angiocardiography. N Engl J Med 1979;300:278–283.
29. Cohen M, Kronzon I, Lebowitz A. Reversible doxorubicin-induced congestive heart failure. Arch Intern Med 1982;142:1570–1571.
30. Saini J, Rich MW, Lyss AP. Reversibility of severe left ventricular dysfunction due to doxorubicin cardiotoxicity. Ann Intern Med 1987;106:814–816.
31. Yeung ST, Yoong C, Spink J, Galbraith A, Smith PJ. Functional myocardial impairment in children treated with anthracyclines for cancer. Lancet 1991;337:816–818.
32. Bristow MR, Mason JW, Billingham ME, Daniels JR. Doxorubicin cardiomyopathy: Evaluation by phonocardiography, endomyocardial biopsy, and cardiac catheterization. Ann Intern Med 1978;88:168–175.
33. Billingham ME, Mason JW, Bristow MR, et al. Anthracycline cardiomyopathy monitored by morphologic changes. Cancer Treat Rep 1978;62:865.
34. Koh E, Imashuku S, Kiyosawa N, Sawada T. Anthracycline- induced congestive heart failure in two pediatric leukemia cases and long term follow-up. Pediatr Hematol Oncol 1988;5:245–251.
35. Steinherz L, Murphy ML, Steinherz P, et al. Long-term cardiac follow up 4–13 years post anthracycline therapy. In: Doyle E, Engle MA, Gersony W, Rashkin W, Talner N, eds. Pediatric cardiology. New York: Springer Verlag, 1986:1058–1061.
36. Steinherz LJ, Steinherz PG, Tan CTC, Heller G, Murphy ML. Cardiotoxicity 4–20 years after completing anthracycline therapy. JAMA 1991;266:1672–1677.
37. Steinherz LJ, Steinherz PG. Delayed anthracyclines cardiac toxicity. In: DeVita VT, Hellman S, Rosenberg SA, eds. Cancer: Principles and practice of oncology, PPO updates, 1991;5:1–15.
38. Steinherz L, Steinherz P. Cardiac failure more than six years post anthracyclines. Am J Cardiol 1988;62:505.
39. Steinherz L, Steinherz P. Delayed cardiac toxicity from anthracycline therapy. Pediatrician 1991;18:49–52.
40. Lipshultz SE, Colan SD, Gelber RD, Perez-Atayde AR, Sallan SE, Sanders SP. Late cardiac effects of doxorubicin therapy for acute lymphoblastic leukemia in childhood. N Engl J Med 1991;324:808–815.
41. Goorin, AM, Chauvenet AR, Perez-Atayde AR, et al. Initial congestive heart failure, six to ten years after doxorubicin chemotherapy for childhood cancer. J Pediatr 1990;116:144–147.
42. Hausdorf G, Morf G, Beron G, et al. Long-term doxorubicin cardiotoxicity in childhood: Non-invasive evaluation of the contractile state and diastolic filling. Br Heart J 1988;60: 309–315.
43. Weesner KM, Bledsoe M, Chauvenet A, Wofford M. Exercise echocardiography in the detection of anthracycline cardiotoxicity. Cancer 1991;68:435–438.
44. Jakacki R, Silber J, Larsen R, Barber G, Goldwein J, Meadows A. Cardiac dysfunction following "Low risk" cardiotoxic treatment for childhood malignancy. Pediatr Res 1991;29:143A.
45. Larsen RL, Jakacki R, Vetter VL, Meadows AT, Silber J, Barber G. Electrocardiographic changes and arrythmias after cancer therapy in children and young adults. Am J Card 1992;70:73–77.
46. Goormaghtigh E, Huart P, Praet M, Brasseur R, Ruysschaert JM. Structure of the Adriamycin-Cardiolipin complex role in mitochondrial toxicity. Biophys Chem 1990;35: 247–257.
47. Fu LX, Waagstein F, Hjalmarson A. A new insight into Adriamycin-induced cardiotoxicity. Int J Cardiol 1990;29:15–20.
48. Kapelko VI, Saks VA, Novikova NA, Golikov MA, Kupriyanov VV, Popovich MI. Adaptation of cardiac contractile functions to conditions of chronic energy deficiency. J Mol Cell Cardiol 1989;21:79–83.
49. Myers CE, McGuire WP, Liss RH, Ifrim I, Grotzinger K, Young RC. Adriamycin: The role of lipid peroxidation in cardiac toxicity and tumor response. Science 1977;197: 165–167.
50. Rajagopalan S, Politi PM, Sinha BK, Myers CE. Adriamycin-induced free radical formation in the perfused rat heart: Implications for cardiotoxicity. Cancer Res 1988;48: 4766–4769.
51. Myers CE, Gianna L, Simone CB, Klecker R, Greene R. Oxidative destruction of erythrocyte ghost membranes catalyzed by the doxorubicin-iron complex. Biochemistry 1982;21:1707–1712.
52. Gutteridge JM. Lipid peroxidation and possible hydroxyl radical formation stimulated by the self-reduction of a doxorubicin-iron (III) complex. Biochem Pharmacol 1984;33: 1725–1728.
53. Olson RD, Mushlin PS, Brenner DE, et al. Doxorubicin cardiotoxicity may be caused by its metabolite doxorubicinol. Proc Natl Acad Sci USA 1988;85:3585–3589.
54. Pessah IN, Durie EL, Schiedt MJ, Zimanyi I. Anthraquinone-sensitized $Ca2+$ release channel from rat cardiac sarcoplasmic reticulum: Possible receptor-mediated mechanism of doxorubicin cardiomyopathy. Mol Pharmacol 1990;37:503–514.
55. Shenasa H, Calderone A, Vermeulen M, et al. Chronic doxorubicin induced cardiomyopathy in rabbits: Mechanical, intracellular action potential, and beta adrenergic characteristics of the falling myocardium. Cardiovasc Res 1990;24:591–604.
56. Cappelli V, Moggio R, Monti E, Paracchini L, Piccinini F, Reggiani C. Reduction of myofibrillar ATPase activity and isomyosin shift in delayed doxorubicin cardiotoxicity. J Mol Cell Cardiol 1989;21:93–101.
57. Minow RA, Benjamin RS, Lee ET, et al. QRS voltage change with Adriamycin administration. Cancer Treat Rep 1978;62:931–934.
58. Steinherz LJ, Graham T, Hurwitz R, et al. Guidelines for cardiac monitoring of children during and after anthracycline therapy: Report of the Cardiology Committee of the Childrens Cancer Study Group. Pediatrics 1992;89:942–949.
59. Bloom K, Bini R, Williams C, et al. Echocardiography in Adriamycin cardiotoxicity. 1978;Cancer 41:1265–1269.
60. Biancaniello T, Meyer RA, Wong KY, et al. Doxorubicin cardiotoxicity in children. J Pediatr 1980;97:45–50.
61. Borow K, Henderson I, Neuman A, et al. Assessment of left ventricular contractility in patients receiving doxorubicin. Ann Intern Med 1983;99:750–756.
62. Schwartz RG, McKenzie WB, Alexander J, et al. Congestive heart failure and left ventricular dysfunction complicating doxorubicin therapy: A seven year experience using serial radionuclide angiocardiography. Am J Med 1987;82:1109–1118.
63. Gottdiener JS, Mathisen DJ, Borer JS, et al. Doxorubicin cardiotoxicity: Assessment of late left ventricular dysfunction by radionuclide cineangiography. Ann Intern Med 1981;94:430–435.
64. Palmeri ST, Bonow RO, Myers CE, et al. Prospective evaluation of doxorubicin cardiotoxicity by rest and exercise radionuclide angiography. Am J Cardiol 1986;58:607–613.
65. McKillop JH, Bristow MR, Goris ML, et al. Sensitivity and specificity of radionuclide ejection fractions in doxorubicin cardiotoxicity. Am Heart J 1983;106:1048–56.
66. Lee BH, Goodenday LS, Muswick GJ, Yasnoff WA, Leighton RF, Skeel RT. Alterations in left ventricular diastolic function with doxorubicin therapy. J Am Coll Cardiol 1987;9: 184–188.
67. Bae JH, Schwaiger M, Mandelkern M, Lin A, Schelbert HR. Doxorubicin cardiotoxicity: Response of left ventricular ejection fraction to exercise and incidence of regional wall motion abnormalities. Int J Card Imaging 1989;3:193–201.
68. Estorch M, Carrio I, Berna L, et al. Indium-111-antimyosin scintigraphy after doxorubicin therapy in patients with advanced breast cancer. J Nucl Med 1990;31:1965–1969.
69. Jain D, Zaret BL. Antimyosin cardiac imaging: Will it play a role in the detection of doxorubicin cardiotoxicity? J Nucl Med 1990;31:1970–1974.
70. Legha SS, Benjamin RS, Mackay B, et al. Reduction of doxorubicin cardiotoxicity by prolonged continuous intravenous infusion. Ann Intern Med 1982;96:133–138.
71. Casper ES, Gaynor JJ, Hajdu SI, et al. A prospective randomized trial of adjuvant

chemotherapy with bolus versus continuous infusion of doxorubicin in patients with high-grade extremity soft tissue sarcoma and an analysis of prognostic factors. Cancer 1991;68:1221–1229.

72. Shapira J, Gotfried M, Lishner M, Ravid M. Reduced cardiotoxicity of doxorubicin by a 6-hour infusion regimen. Cancer 1990;65:870–873.
73. Torti FM, Bristow MR, Howes AE, et al. Reduced cardiotoxicity of doxorubicin delivered on a weekly schedule: Assessment by endomyocardial biopsy. Ann Intern Med 1983;99: 745–749.
74. Weiss AT, Manthel RW. Experience with the use of Adriamycin in combination with other anti-cancer agents using a weekly schedule with particular reference to lack of cardiac toxicity. Cancer 1977;40:2046–2052.
75. Sonneveid P. Effect of α-tocopherol on the cardiotoxicity of Adriamycin in the rat. Cancer Treat Rep 1978;62:1033–1036.
76. Villani F, Galimberti M, Monti E, et al. Effect of glutathione and N-acetylcysteine on in vitro and in vivo cardiac toxicity of doxorubicin. Free Radic Res Commun 1990;11: 145–151.
77. Perletti G, Monti E, Paracchini L, Piccinini F. Effect of trimetazidine on early and delayed doxorubicin myocardial toxicity. Arch Int Pharmacodyn Ther 1989;302:280–289.
78. Buc-Calderon P, Praet M, Ruysschaert JM, Roberfroid M. Increasing therapeutic effect and reducing toxicity of doxorubicin by N-acyl dehydroalanines. Eur J Cancer Clin Oncol 1989;25:679–685.
79. Kraft J, Grille W, Appelt M, et al. Effects of verapamil on anthracycline-induced cardiomyopathy: Preliminary results of a prospective multicenter trial. Hamatol Bluttransfus 1990;33:566–570.
80. Milei J, Marantz A, Ale J, Vazquez A, Buceta JE. Prevention of Adriamycin-induced cardiotoxicity by prenylamine: A pilot double blind study. Cancer Drug Deliv 1987;4: 129–136.
81. Milei J, Vazquez A, Boveris A, et al. The role of prenylamine in the prevention of Adriamycin-induced cardiotoxicity: A review of experimental and clinical findings. J Int Med Res 1988;16:19–30.
82. Bartoli KF, Decorti G, Candussio L, et al. Effect of ketotifen on Adriamycin toxicity: Role of histamine. Cancer Lett 1988;39:145–152.
83. Harman GS, Craig JB, Kuhn JG, et al. Phase I and clinical pharmacology trial of crisnatol (BWA770u mesylate) using a monthly single-dose schedule. Cancer Res 1988;48:4706–4710.
84. Klugmann FB, Decorti G, Candussio L, et al. Amelioration of 4'epidoxorubicin-induced cardiotoxicity by sodium cromoglycate. Eur J Cancer Clin Oncol 1989;25:361–368.
85. Reeves WC, Griffith JW, Wood MA, Whitesell L. Exacerbation of doxorubicin cardiotoxicity by digoxin administration in an experimental rabbit model. Int J Cancer 1990;45: 731–736.
86. Villani F, Manzotti C, Mella M, Monti E, Savi G, Zunino F. Effect of amrinone on anthracycline-induced lethal and cardiac toxicity in mice and rats. Med Oncol Tumor Pharmacother 1990;7:227–232.
87. Hacker MP, Lazo JS, Pritsos CA, Tritton TR. Immobilized Adriamycin: Toxic potential in vivo and in vitro. Sel Cancer Ther 1989;5:67–72.
88. Rahman A, Treat J, Roh JK, et al. A phase I clinical trial and pharmacokinetic evaluation of liposome-encapsulated doxorubicin. J Clin Oncol 1990;8:1093–1100.
89. Herman EH, Ferrans VJ. Reduction of chronic doxorubicin cardiotoxicity in dogs by pretreatment with (+) -1,2-bis(3,5-dioxopiperazinyl-l-yl) propane (ICRF-187). Cancer Res 1981;41:3436–3440.
90. Herman EH, Ferrans VJ, Jordan W, Ardalan B. Reduction of chronic daunorubicin cardiotoxicity by ICRF-187 in rabbits. Res Commun Chem Pathol Pharmacol 1981;31: 85–97.
91. Belt RJ. Prevention of Adriamycin-induced cardiotoxicity by ICRF-187 (NSC-169780). Proc Am Soc Clin Oncol 1984;3:27.
92. Speyer JL, Green MD, Kramer E, et al. Protective effect of the bispiperazinedione ICRF-187 against doxorubicin-induced cardiac toxicity in women with advanced breast cancer. N Engl J Med 1988;319:745–752.
93. Speyer JL, Green MD, Sanger J, et al. A prospective randomized trial of ICRF-187 for prevention of cumulative doxorubicin-induced cardiac toxicity in women with breast cancer. Cancer Treat Rev 1990;17:161–163.
94. Alderto P, Gross J, Green MD. Role of (±)-1,2-bis(3,5-dioxopiperazinyl-1-yl) propane (ICRF-187) in modulating free radical scavenging enzymes in doxorubicin-induced cardiomyopathy. Cancer Res 1990;50:5136–5142.
95. Herman EH, Ferrans VJ. Examination of the potential long-lasting protective effect of ICRF-187 against anthracycline-induced chronic cardiomyopathy. Cancer Treat Rev 1990;17:155–160.
96. Tan C, Mitta SK, Steinherz L, Miller DR. Phase I trial of Rubidazone (NSC-164011) in children with cancer. Med Pediatr Oncol 1981;9:347–353.
97. Benjamin RS, Mason JW, Billingham ME. Cardiac toxicity of Adriamycin-DNA complex and Rubidazone: Evaluation by electrocardiogram and endomyocardial biopsy. Cancer Treat Rep 1978;62:935–939.
98. Tan CTC, Hancock C, Steinherz LJ. Preliminary results of epirubicin in children with acute leukemia. In: Bonadonna G, ed. Advances in anthracycline chemotherapy: Epirubicin. Milan: Masson Italia Editori 1984:129–132.
99. Nielsen D, Jensen JB, Dombernowsky P, et al. Epirubicin cardiotoxicity: A study of 135 patients with advanced breast cancer. J Clin Oncol 1990;8:1806–1810.
100. Neri B, Cini-Neri G, Bandinelli M, Pacini P, Bartalucci S, Ciapini A. Doxorubicin and epirubicin cardiotoxicity: Experimental and clinical aspects. Int J Clin Pharmacol Ther Toxicol 1989;27:217–221.
101. Mortensen SA. Aclarubicin: Preclinical and clinical data suggesting less chronic cardiotoxicity compared with conventional anthracyclines. Eur J Haematol 1987;47(Suppl): 21–31.
102. Wojnar J, Mandecki M, Wnuk-Wojnar AM, Holowiecki J. Clinical studies on aclacinomycin A cardiotoxicity in adult patients with acute non lymphoblastic leukemia. Folia Haematol (Leipz) 1989;116:297–303.
103. Carella AM, Berman E, Maraone MP, Ganzina F. Idarubicin in the treatment of acute leukemias: An overview of preclinical and clinical studies. Haematologica 1990;75: 159–169.
104. Tan CT, Hancock C, Steinherz P, et al. Phase I and clinical pharmacological study of 4-demethoxydaunorubicin (Idarubicin) in children with advanced cancer. Cancer Res 1987;47:2990–2995.
105. Villani F, Galimberti M, Comazzi R, Crippa F. Evaluation of cardiac toxicity of idarubicin (4-demethoxydaunorubicin). Eur J Cancer Clin Oncol 1989;25:13–18.
106. Feig SA, Krailo MD, Harris RE, et al. Determination of the maximum tolerated dose of idarubicin when used in a combination chemotherapy program of reinduction of childhood ALL at first marrow relapse and a preliminary assessment of toxicity compared to that of daunorubicin: A report from the Children's Cancer Study Group. Med Pediatr Oncol 1992;20:124–129.
107. Ringenberg QS, Propert KJ, Muss HB, et al. Clinical cardiotoxicity of esorubicin (4'-deoxydoxorubicin,DxDx): Prospective studies with serial gated heart scans and reports of selected cases. A cancer and leukemia group B report. Invest New Drugs 1990;8: 221–226.
108. Danesi R, Marchetti A, Bernardini N, La Rocca RV, Bevilacqua G, Del Tacca M. Cardiac toxicity and antitumor activity of 4'-deoxy-4'-iodo-doxorubicinol. Cancer Chemother Phamacol 1990;26:403–408.
109. Aldouri MA, Lopes ME, Yacoub M, et al. Cardiac transplantation for doxorubicin-induced cardiomyopathy in acute myeloid leukemia. Br J Haematol 1990;74:541.
110. Arico M, Nespoli L, Pedroni E, Bonetti F, Vigano M, Burgio GR. Heart transplantation in a child with doxorubicin-induced cardiomyopathy. N Engl J Med 1988;65:1353.
111. Edwards BS, Hunt SA, Fowler MB, Valantine HA, Stinson EB, Schroeder JS. Cardiac transplantation in patients with preexisting neoplastic diseases. Am J Cardiol 1990;65: 501–504.
112. Tumminello FM, Leto G, Gebbia N, Gebbia V, Russo A, Rausa L. Acute myocardial effects of mitoxantrone in the rabbit. Cancer Treat Rep 1987;71:529–531.
113. Sparano BM, Gordon G, Hall C, Iatropoulos MJ, Noble FJ. Safety assessment of a new anticancer compound, mitoxantrone, in beagle dogs: Comparison with doxorubicin. II. Histologic and ultrastructural pathology. Cancer Treat Rep 1982;66:1145–1158.
114. Saletan S. Mitoxantrone: An active, new antitumor agent with an improved therapeutic index. Cancer Treat Rev 1987;14:297–303.
115. Shenkenberg TD, Von Hoff DD. Mitoxantrone: A new anticancer drug with significant clinical activity. Ann Intern Med 1986;105:67–81.
116. Posner LE, Dukart G, Goldberg J, Bernstein T, Cartwright K. Mitroxantrone: An overview of safety and toxicity. Invest New Drugs 1985;3:123–132.
117. Janmohammed R, Milligan DW. Mitoxantrone induced congestive heart failure in patients previously treated with anthracyclines. Br J Haematol 1989;71:292–293.
118. Pai GR, Reed NS, Ruddell WS. A case of mitozantrone-associated cardiomyopathy without prior anthracycline therapy. Br J Radiol 1987;60:1125–1126.
119. Ewer MS, Ali MK, Abraham K, et al. Electrocardiographic (ECG) changes in patients receiving mitoxantrone previously treated with Adriamycin. Proc Am Soc Clin Oncol 1990;9:81.
120. Cassidy J, Merrick MV, Smyth JF, Leonard RC. Cardiotoxicity of mitozantrone assessed by stress and resting nuclear ventriculography. Eur J Cancer Clin Oncol 1988;24:935–938.
121. Villani F, Galimberti M, Crippa F. Evaluation of ventricular function by echocardiography and radionuclide angiography in patients treated with mitoxantrone. Drugs Exp Clin Res 1989;15:501–506.
122. Duffy M, ed. Physicians Desk Reference. 45th ed. Montvale, NJ, 1991;1195.
123. Lindpaintner K, Lindpaintner LS, Wentworth M, et al. Acute myocardial necrosis during administration of amsacrine. Cancer 1986;57:1284–1286.
124. Legha SS, Latreille J, McCredie KB, et al. Neurologic and cardiac rhythm abnormalities associated with 4'-(9-acridinylamino) methanesulfon-m-anisidide (AMSA) therapy. Cancer Treat Rep 1979;63:2001–2003.
125. Von Hoff DD, Elson D, Polk G, et al. Acute ventricular fibrillation and death during infusion of 4'-(9-acridinylamino)methanesulfon-m-anisidide (AMSA). Cancer Treat Rep [Letter] 1980;64:356–357.
126. Falkson G. Multiple ventricular extrasystoles following administration of 4'-(9-acridinylamino)methanesulfon-m-anisidide (AMSA). Cancer Treat Rep 1980;64:358.
127. Arlin Z, Mehta R, Feldman E, Sullivan P, Pucillo A. Amsacrine treatment of patients with supraventricular arrhythmias and acute leukemia. Cancer Chemother Pharmacol 1987;19:163–164.
128. Puccio CA, Feldman EJ, Arlin ZA. Amsacrine is safe in patients with ventricular ectopy. Am J Hematol 1988;28:197–198.
129. Steinherz LJ, Steinherz PG, Mangiacasale D, Tan C, Miller DR. Cardiac abnormalities after AMSA administration. Cancer Treat Rep 1982;66:483–488.
130. Tan CTC, Hancock C, Steinherz PG, et al. Phase II study of 4'-(9-Acridinylamino)methanesulfon-*m*-anisidide (NSC 249992) in children with acute leukemia and lymphoma. Cancer Res 1982;42:1579–1581.
131. Arlin ZA, Feldman EJ, Mittelman A, et al. Amsacrine is safe and effective therapy for patients with myocardial dysfunction and acute leukemia. Cancer 1991;68:1198–1200.
132. Praga C, Beretta G, Vigo PL, et al. Adriamycin cardiotoxicity: A survey of 1273 patients. Cancer Treat Rep 1979;63:827–834.
133. Santos GW, Sensenbrenner LL, Burke PJ, et al. Marrow transplants in man utilizing cyclophosphamide: Summary of Baltimore experience. Exp Hematol 1970;20:78–81.

134. Buckner CD, Rudolph RH, Fefer A, et al. High-dose cyclophosphamide therapy for malignant disease: Toxicity, tumor, response, and the effects of stored autologous marrow. Cancer 1972;29:357–365.
135. Mullins GM, Anderson PN, Santo GW. High dose cyclophosphamide therapy in solid tumors: Therapeutic, toxic and immunosuppressive effects. Cancer 1975;36:1950–1958.
136. Storb R, Buckner CS, Dillingham LA, et al. Cyclophosphamide regimens in rhesus monkeys with and without marrow infusion. Cancer Res 1970;30:2195–2202.
137. Slavin RE, Millan JC, Mullins GM. Pathology of high dose intermittent cyclophosphamide therapy. Hum Pathol 1975;6:693–709.
138. Buja LM, Ferrans VJ, Graw RG. Cardiac pathologic findings in patients treated with bone marrow transplantation. Hum Pathol 1976;7:17–44.
139. Applebaum FR, Strauchen JA, Graw RG, et al. Acute lethal carditis caused by high dose combination chemotherapy: A unique clinical and pathological entity. Lancet 1976;1:58–62.
140. Steinherz L, Steinherz P, Mangiacasale D, et al. Cardiac changes with cyclophosphamide. Med Pediatr Oncol 1981;9:417–422.
141. Gottdiener JS, Applebaum FR, Ferrans VJ, et al. Cardiotoxicity associated with high-dose cyclophosphamide therapy. Arch Intern Med 1981;141:758–763.
142. Steinherz LJ, Steinherz PG. Cyclophosphamide cardiotoxicity. Cancer Bull 1985;37: 231–234.
143. Veys PA, McAvinchey R, Rothman MT, Mair GHM, Newland AC. Pericardial effusion following conditioning for bone marrow transplantation in acute leukemia. Bone Marrow Transplant 1987;2:213–216.
144. Bearman SI, Petersen FB, Schor RA, et al. Radionuclide ejection fractions in the evaluation of patients being considered for bone marrow transplantation: Risk for cardiac toxicity. Bone Marrow Transplant 1990;5:173–177.
145. Braverman AC, Antin JH, Plappert MT, Cook EF, Lee RT. Cyclophosphamide cardiotoxicity in bone marrow transplantation: A prospective evaluation of new dosing regimens. J Clin Oncol 1991;9:1215–1223.
146. Larsen RL, Barber G, Heise CT, August CS. Exercise assessment of cardiac function in children and young adults before and after bone marrow transplantation. Pediatrics 1992;89:722–729.
147. Kandylis K, Vassilomanolakis M, Tsoussis S, Efremidis AP. Ifosfamide cardiotoxicity in humans. Cancer Chemother Pharmacol 1989;24:395–396.
148. Herman EM, Mhatre RM, Warardekar VS, Lee IP. Comparison of the cardiovascular actions of NSC-109, 7824 (ifosfamide) and cyclophosphamide. Toxicol Appl Pharmacol 1972;23:178.
149. O'Connel TX, Berenbaum MC 1974 Cardiac and pulmonary effects of high doses of cyclophosphamide and isophosphamide. Cancer Res 1974;34:1586.
150. Frankel S, Weiss M, Warrell RP Jr. A "retinoic acid syndrome" in acute promyelocytic leukemia: Reversal by corticosteroids. Blood 1991;78:380a.
151. Rowinsky EK, McGuire WP, Guarnieri T, Fisherman JS, Christian MC, Donehower RC. Cardiac disturbances during the administration of Taxol. J Clin Oncol 1991;9: 1704–1712.
152. McGuire WP, Rowinsky EK, Rosenshein NB, et al. Taxol: A unique antineoplastic agent with significant activity in advanced ovarian epithelial neoplasms. Ann Intern Med 1989;111:273–279.
153. Rowinsky EK, Gilbert MR, McGuire WP, et al. Sequences of Taxol and cisplatin: A phase 1 and pharmacologic study. J Clin Oncol 1991;9:1692–1703.
154. Tan CTC, Luks E, Bacha DM, Steinherz P, Steinherz L, Mondora A. Phase I trial of homoharringtonine (NSC 141633) in children with refractory leukemia. Cancer Treat Rep 1987;71:1245–1248.
155. Ajani JA, Dimery I, Chawla SP, et al. Phase II studies of homoharringtonine in patients with advanced malignant melanoma: Sarcoma and head and neck, breast and colorectal carcinomas. Cancer Treat Rep 1986;70:375–379.
156. Jongii L, Hui Y, Xueying L, et al. Experimental studies on the toxicity of harringtonine and homoharringtonine. Chin Med J 1979;92:175–180.
157. Hirvonen HE, Salmi TT, Heinonen E, Antila KJ, Valimaki IA. Vincristine treatment of acute lymphoblastic leukemia induces transient autonomic cardioneuropathy. Cancer 1989;64:801–805.
158. Mandel EM, Lewinski U, Djaldetti M. Vincristine-induced myocardial infarction. Cancer 1975;36:1979–1982.
159. Lejonc JL, Vernant JP, Macquin I, et al. Myocardial infarction following vinblastine treatment. Lancet 1980;2:692.
160. Stefenelli T, Kuzmits R, Ulrich W, Glogar D. Acute vascular toxicity after combination chemotherapy with cisplatin, vinblastine, and bleomycin for testicular cancer. Eur Heart J 1988;9:552–556.
161. Zeymer U, Neuhaus KL. Infarct-typical changes in the electrocardiogram following chemotherapy with vinblastine. Dtsch Med Wochenschr 1989;114:589–92.
162. Buzdar AR, Leghe SS, Tashimal CK, et al. Adriamycin and mitomycin C: Possible synergistic toxicity. Cancer Treat Rep 1978;62:1005–1008.
163. Doroshow JH. Mitomycin-C enhanced superoxide and hydrogen peroxide in the rat heart. J Pharmacol Exp Ther 1981;218:206–211.
164. Sivanesaratnam V. FRCOG Mitomycin-C cardiotoxicity. Med J Aust 1989;151:300.
165. Verweij J, Funke-Kupper AJ, Teule GJJ, Pinedo HM. A prospective study on the dose dependency of cardiotoxicity induced by mitomycin C. Med Oncol Tumor Pharmacother 1988;5:159–163.
166. Verweij J, Van Der Burg ME, Pinedo HM. Mitomycin C-induced hemolytic uremic syndrome: Six case reports and review of the literature on renal, pulmonary and cardiac side effects of the drug. Radiother Oncol 1987;8:33–41.
167. Dent R, McColl I. 5-Fluorouracil and angina. Lancet 1975;1:347–348.
168. Labianca R, Beretta G, Clerici M, Fraschini P, Luporini G. Cardiac toxicity of 5-fluorouracil: A study of 1083 patients. Tumori 1982;68:505–510.
169. Lomeo AM, Avolio C, Iacobellis G, Manzione L. 5-Fluorouracil cardiotoxicity. Eur J Gynaec Oncol 1990;3:237–241.
170. Rezkalla S, Kloner RA, Ensley J, et al. Continuous ambulatory ECG monitoring during fluorouracil therapy: A prospective Study. J Clin Oncol 1989;7:509–514.
171. Collins C, Weiden PL. Cardiotoxicity of 5-fluorouracil. Cancer Treat Rep 1987;71: 733–736.
172. Freeman NJ, Costanza ME. 5-Fluorouracil-associated cardiotoxicity. Cancer 1988;61: 36–45.
173. Eskilsson J, Albertsson M, Mercke C. Adverse cardiac effects during induction chemotherapy treatment with cis-platin and 5-fluorouracil. Radiother Oncol 1988;13:41–46.
174. Jakubowski AA, Kemeny N. Hypotension as a manifestation of cardiotoxicity in three patients receiving cisplatin and 5-fluorouracil. Cancer 1988;62:266–269.
175. McKendall GR, Shurman A, Anamur M, Most AS. Toxic cardiogenic shock associated with infusion of 5-fluorouracil. Am Heart J 1989;118:184–186.
176. Patel B, Kloner RA, Ensley J, Al-Sarraf M, Kish J, Wynne J. 5-Fluorouracil cardiotoxicity: Left ventricular dysfunction and effect of coronary vasodilators. Am J Med Sci 1987;294: 238–243.
177. Misset B, Escudier B, Leclercq B, Rivara D, Rougier P, Nitenberg G. Acute myocardiotoxicity during 5-fluorouracil therapy. Intensive Care Med 1990;16:210–211.
178. Coronel B, Madonna O, Mercatello A, Caillette A, Moskovtchenko JF. Myocardiotoxicity of 5 fluorouracil. Intensive Care Med 1988;14:429–430.
179. Kleiman NS, Lehane DE, Geyer CE Jr, Pratt CM, Young JB. Prinzmetal's angina during 5-fluorouracil chemotherapy. Am J Med 1987;82:566–568.
180. Burger AJ, Mannino S. 5-Fluorouracil-induced coronary vasospasm. Am Heart J 1987;114:433–436.
181. Pottage A, Holt S, Ludgate S, Langlands A. Fluorouracil cardiotoxicity. Br Med J 1978;1: 547.
182. Jeremic B, Jevremovic S, Djuric L, Mijatovic L. Cardiotoxicity during chemotherapy treatment with 5-fluorouracil and cisplatin. J Chemother 1990;2:264–267.
183. Martin M, Diaz-Rubio E, Furio V, Blazquez J, Almenarez J, Farina J. Lethal cardiac toxicity after cisplatin and 5-fluorouracil chemotherapy: Report of a case with necropsy study. Am J Clin Oncol 1989;12:229–234.
184. Liss RH, Chadwick M. Correlation of 5-fluorouracil distribution in rodents with toxicity and chemotherapy in man. Cancer Chemother Rep 1974;58:777–786.
185. Suzuki T, Nakanishi H, Hayashi A, Nakahata N, Takano S, Ito G. Cardiac toxicity of 5-fluorouracil in rabbits. Jpn J Pharmacol 1972;27(Suppl):137.
186. Matsubara I, Kamiya J, Imai S. Cardiotoxicity effects of 5-fluorouracil in the guinea pig. Jpn J Pharmacol 1980;30:871–879.
187. Menard O, Martinet Y, Lamy P. Cisplatin-induced atrial fibrillation. J Clin Oncol 1991;9: 192–193.
188. Fassio T, Canobbio L, Gasparini G, Villani F. Paroxymal supraventricular tachycardia during treatment with cisplatin and etoposide combination. Oncology 1986;43:219–220.
189. Talley RW, O'Bryan RM, Gutterman JU, Brownlee RW, McCredie KB. Clinical evaluation of toxic effects of cis-diammine dichloroplatinum (NSC-119875). Phase I clinical study. Cancer Chemother Rep 1973;57:465–471.
190. Tomirotti M, Riundi R, Pulici S, et al. Ischemic cardiopathy from cis-diamminedichloroplatinum (CDDP). Tumori 1984;70:235–236.
191. Doll DC, List AF, Greco A, Hainsworth JD, Hande KR, Johnson DH. Acute vascular ischemic events after cisplatin-based combination chemotherapy for germ-cell tumors of the testis. Ann Intern Med 1986;105:48–51.
192. Sonnenblick M, Rosin A. Cardiotoxicity of interferon: A review of 44 cases. Chest 1991;99:557–561.
193. Friess GG, Brown TD, Wrenn RC. Cardiovascular rhythm effects of gamma recombinant DNA interferon. Invest New Drugs 1989;7:275–280.
194. Martino S, Ratanatharathorn V, Karanes C, Samal BA, Sohn YH, Rudnick SA. Reversible arrhythmias observed in patients treated with recombinant alpha 2 interferon. J Cancer Res Clin Oncol 1987;113:376–378.
195. Zbinden G. Effects of recombinant human alpha-interferon in a rodent cardiotoxicity model. Toxicol Lett 1990;50:25–35.
196. Dickson D. Death halts interferon trials in France. Science 1982;218:772.
197. Foon KA, Sherwin SA, Abrams PG, et al. Treatment of advanced non-Hodgkin's lymphoma with recombinant leukocyte A interferon. N Engl J Med 1984;311:1148–1152.
198. Brown TD, Koeller J, Beougher K, et al. A phase I clinical trial of recombinant DNA gamma interferon. J Clin Oncol 1987;5:790–798.
199. Deyton LR, Walker RE, Kovacs JA, et al. Reversible cardiac dysfunction associated with interferon alfa therapy in AIDS patients with Kaposi's sarcoma. N Engl J Med 1989;321:1246–1249.
200. Sonnenblick M, Rosenmann D, Rosin A. Reversible cardiomyopathy induced by interferon. Br Med J 1990;300:1174–1175.
201. Budd GT, Bukowski RM, Miketo L, Yen-Lieberman B, Proffitt MR. Phase I trial of ultrapure human leukocyte interferon in human malignancy. Cancer Chemother Pharmacol 1984;12:39–42.
202. Grunberg SM, Kempf RA, Itri LM, Venturi CL, Boswell WD, Mitchell MS. Phase II study of recombinant alpha interferon in the treatment of advanced non-small cell lung carcinoma. Cancer Treat Rep 1985;69:1031–1032.
203. Cohen MC, Huberman MS, Nesto RW. Recombinant alpha-2 interferon related cardiomyopathy. Am J Med 1988;85:549–550.
204. Sherwin SA. The interferons. Ann Intern Med 1987;106:425–426.

205. Lampidis TJ, Brouty-Boye D. Interferon inhibits cardiac cell function in vitro (41043). Proc Soc Exp Biol Med 1981;166:181–185.
206. Dorr Rt, Shipp NG. Effect of interferon, interleukin-2 and tumor necrosis factor on myocardial cell viability and doxorubicin cardiotoxicity in vitro. Immunopharmacology 1989;18:31–38.
207. Bialock JE, Stanton JD. Common pathways of interferon and hormonal action. Nature 1980;283:406–408.
208. Nora R, Abrams JS, Tait NS, Hiponia DJ, Silverman HJ. Myocardial toxic effects during recombinant interleukin-2 therapy. J Natl Cancer Inst 1989;81:59–63.
209. Rosenberg SA, Lotze MT, Muul LM, et al. A progress report on the treatment of 157 patients with advanced cancer using lymphokine-activated killer cell and interleukin-2 or high dose interleukin alone. N Engl J Med 1987;316:889–897.
210. Nora R, Belani C, Silverman H, et al. Immunotherapy of advanced cancer. N Engl J Med [Letter] 1987;316:275.
211. Nora R, Abrams J, Silverman HJ. Myocardial infarction (MI) in patients receiving high dose recombinant interleukin-2 (rIL-2). Proc Am Soc Clin Oncol 1987;6:245.
212. Fisher RI, Coltman CA, Doroshow JH, et al. Phase II clinical trial of interleukin-2 plus lymphokine-activated killer cells (IL2/LAK) in metastatic renal cell. Proc Am Soc Clin Oncol 1987;6:244.
213. Dutcher JP, Creekmore S, Weiss GR, et al. Phase II study of high dose interleukin-2 (IL-2) and lymphokine-activated killer (LAK) cells in patients (pts) with melanoma. Proc Am Soc Clin Oncol 1987;6:246.
214. Osanto S, Cluitmans FGM, Franks CR, et al. Myocardial injury after interleukin-2 therapy. Lancet 1988;2:48–49.
215. Torisu M, Goya T, Hayashi Y, Tanaka J, Sugisaki T, Yoshida T. Electrocardiogram studies on cancer patients treated with OK-432, a streptococcal preparation with potent biological response modifier activities. J Biol Response Mod 1989;8:665–75.
216. Sanz Manrique N, Valcarce Perez J, Broto Escapa P, et al. Enhancing factors in the cardiotoxicity of anthracyclines. An Esp Pediatr 1990;32:11–14.
217. Hall IH, Grippo AA, Holbrook DJ, et al. Renal, hepatic, cardiac and thymic acute toxicity afforded by bis(helenalinyl)malonate in BDF1 mice. Toxicity 1990;64:205–216.
218. Bashir Y, Tomson CR. Cardiac arrest associated with hypokalaemia in a patient receiving mithramycin. Postgrad Med J 1988;64:228–229.
219. Hoke GD, Macia RA, Meunier PC, et al. In vivo and in vitro cardiotoxicity of a gold-containing antineoplastic drug candidate in the rabbit. Toxicol Appl Pharmacol 1989;100:293–306.
220. Gebbia N, Flandina C, Leto G, et al. The role of histamine in doxorubicin and teniposide-induced cardiotoxicity in dog and mouse. Tumori 1987;73:279–287.
221. Schecter JP, Jones SE. Myocardial infarction in a 27 year old woman: Possible complication of treatment with VP-16–213 (NSC-141540), mediastinal irradiation or both. Cancer Chemother Rep 1975;59:887–888.
222. Winberger A, Pinkhas J, Sandbank U, et al. Endocardial fibrosis following busulfan treatment. JAMA 1975;231:495.
223. Desjardins AU. Action of roentgen rays and radium on the heart and lungs. AJR 1932;27: 153–176, 303–335, 447–495.
224. Leach JEL. Effect of roentgen therapy on the heart: Clinical study. Arch Intern Med 1943;72:715–745.
225. Cohn KE, Stewart JR, Fajardo LF, et al. Heart disease following radiation. Medicine (Baltimore) 1967;46:281–298.
226. Stewart JR, Fajardo LF. Radiation-induced heart disease: An update. Prog Cardiovasc Dis 1984;27:3:173–194.
227. Arsenian MA. Cardiovascular sequelae of therapeutic thoracic radiation. Prog Cardiovasc Dis 1991;33:5:299–312.
228. Stewart JR, Fajardo LF, Cohn KE. Experimental radiation-induced heart disease in rabbits. Radiology 1968;91:814–817.
229. Fajardo LF, Stewart JR. Experimental radiation-induced heart disease. I. Light mircoscopic studies. Am J Pathol 1970;59:299–316.
230. Lauk S, Kiszel Z, Buschmann J, et al. Radiation-induced heart disease in rats. Int J Radiat Oncol Biol Phys 1985;II:801–808.
231. Gillette EL, McChesney SL, Hoopes PJ. Isoeffect curves for radiation-induced cardiomyopathy in the dog. Int J Radiat Oncol Phys 1985;II:2091–2097.
232. Brosius FC, Waller BF, Robert WG. Radiation heart disease: Analysis of 16 young (aged 15 to 33 years) necropsy patients who received over 3,500 rads to the heart. Am J Med 1981;70:519–530.
233. Fajardo LF, Stewart JR, Cohn KE. Morphology of radiation-induced heart disease. Arch Pathol 1968;86:512–519.
234. Fajardo LF, Stewart JR. Pathogenesis of radiation-induced myocardial fibrosis. Lab Invest 1973;29:244–257.
235. Fajardo LF. Radiation-induced heart disease. In: Sternberg S, ed. Pathology of radiation injury. New York: Masson Publishing USA, 1982.
236. Stewart JR. Normal tissue tolerance irradiation of the cardiovascular system. In: Vaeth JM, Meyer JL, eds. Radiation tolerance of normal tissues. Front Radiat Ther Oncol 1989;23:302–309.
237. Stewart JR, Fajardo LF. Dose response in human and experimental radiation-induced heart disease: Application of the nominal standard dose (NSD) concept. Radiology 1971;99:403–408.
238. Corn BW, Trock BJ, Goodman RL. Irradiation-related ischemic heart disease. J Clin Oncol 1990;8:741–750.
239. Carmel RJ, Kaplan HS. Mantle irradiation in Hodgkin's disease. Cancer 1976;37: 2813–2815.
240. Appelfeld MM, Slawson RG, Spicer KM, et al. Long term cardiovascular evaluation of patients treated by thoracic mantle radiation therapy. Cancer Treat Rep 1982;66: 1003–1013.
241. Appelfeld MM, Wiernik PH. Cardiac disease after radiation therapy for Hodgin's disease: Analysis of 48 patients. Am Heart J 1983;51:1679–1681.
242. Ruckdeschel JC, Chang P, Martin RG, et al. Radiation-related pericardial effusions in patients with Hodgkin's disease. Medicine 1975;54:245–259.
243. Tarbell NJ, Thompson L, Mauch P. Thoracic irradiation in Hodgkin's disease: Disease control and long-term complications. Int J Radiat Oncol Biol Phys 1990;18:275–281.
244. Harris JR, Recht A. Conservative surgery and radiotherapy. In: Harris JR, Hellman S, Henderson IC, Kinne DW, eds. Breast diseases. 2nd ed. Philadelphia: JB Lippincott, 1991:406.
245. Fleming WH, Szakacs TE, King ER. The effects of gamma radiation on the fibrinolytic system of the dog lung and its modification by certain drugs: Relationship to radiation pneumonitis and hyaline membrane formation in the lung. J Nucl Med 1962;3:34–351.
246. Blayney DW, Longo D. Radiation-induced pericarditis. N Engl J Med 1982;306:550–551.
247. Gottdeiner JS, Katin MJ, Borer JS, et al. Late cardiac effects of therapeutic mediastinal irradiation: Assessment by echocardiography and radionuclide angiography. N Engl J Med 1983;308:569–572.
248. Totterman KJ, Personen E, Siltanen P. Radiation-related chronic heart disease. Chest 1983;83:875–878.
249. Gomm SA, Stretton TB. Chronic pericardial effusion after mediastinal radiotherapy. Thorax 1981;36:149–150.
250. Posner MR, Cohen GI, Skarin AT. Pericardial disease in patients with cancer. Am J Med 1981;71:407–413.
251. Carey RW, Sawicka JM, Choi NC. Cytologically negative pericardial effusion complicating combined modality therapy for localized small-cell carcinoma of the lung. J Clin Oncol 1987;5:818–824.
252. Stewart JR, Fajardo LF. Radiation-induced heart disease. Radiol Clin North Am 1971;3: 511–531.
253. Martin RG, Ruckdeschel JC, Chang P, et al. Radiation-related pericarditis. Am J Cardiol 1975;35:216–220.
254. Fajardo LF, Stewart JR. Radiation-induced heart disease. Human and experimental observations. In: Bristow MR, ed. Drug-induced heart disease. Amsterdam: Elsevier, North-Holland Biomedical Press, 1980:241–260.
255. Keelan MH, Rudders RA. Successful treatment of radiation pericarditis with corticosteroids. Arch Intern Med 1974;134:145–147.
256. Castellino RA, Glatstein E, Turbow MM, et al. Latent radiation injury of lungs or heart activated by steroid withdrawl. Ann Intern Med 1974;80:593–599.
257. Biran S. Corticosteroids in radiation-induced pericarditis. Chest 1978;74:96–98.
258. Krikorian JG, Hancock EW. Pericardiocentesis. Am J Med 1978;65:808–814.
259. Morton DL, Glancy L, Joseph WL, et al. Management of patients with radiation-induced pericarditis with effusion: A note on the development of aortic regurgitation in two of them. Chest 1973;64:291–297.
260. Cameron J, Osterle SN, Baldwin JC, et al. The etiologic spectrum of constrictive pericarditis. Am Heart J 1987;113:354–360.
261. Ni Y, von Segesser LK, Turina M. Futility of pericardiectomy for postirradiation constrictive pericarditis? Ann Thorac Surg 1990;49:445–448.
262. Savage DE, Constine LS, Schwartz RG, Rubin P. Radiation effects of left ventricular function and myocaridial perfusion in long-term survivors of Hodgkin's disease. Int J Radiat Oncol Biol Phys 1990;19:721–727.
263. Perrault DJ, Levy M, Herman JD, et al. Echocardiographic abnormalities following cardiac radiation. J Clin Oncol 1985;3:546–551.
264. Pohjola-Sintonen S, Totterman KJ, Salmo M, et al. Late cardiac effects of mediastinal radiotherapy in patients with Hodgkin's disease. Cancer 1987;60:31–37.
265. Burns RJ, Bar-Shlomo B, Druck MN, et al. Detection of radiation cardiomyopathy by gated radionuclide angiography. Am J Med 1983;74:297–302.
266. Gomez GA, Park JJ, Panahon AM, et al. Heart size and function after radiation therapy to the mediastinum in patients with Hodgkin's disease. Cancer Treat Rep 1983;67: 1099–1103.
267. Merrill J, Greco FA, Zimbler H, et al. Adriamycin and radiation: Synergistic cardiotoxicity. Ann Intern Med 1975;82:122.
268. Kinsella TJ, Ahmann DL, Giuliani ER, et al. Adriamycin cardiotoxibity in stage IV breast cancer: Possible enhancement with prior left chest radiation therapy. Int J Radiat Oncol Biol Phys 1979;5:1997–2002.
269. Mayer EG, Poulter CA, Aristizabal SA. Complications of irradiation related to apparent drug potentiation by Adriamycin. Int J Radiat Oncol Biol Phys 1976;1:1179–1188.
270. Eltringham JR, Fajardo LF, Stewart JR, et al. Investigation of cardiotoxicity in rabbits from Adriamycin and fractionated cardiac irradiation: Preliminary results. Front Radiat Ther Oncol 1979;13:21–35.
271. Petrovic D, Brown SM, Yatvin MB. Effects of Adriamycin and irradiation on beating of rat heart muscle cells in culture. Int J Radiat Oncol Biol Phys 1977;2:505–513.
272. LaMonte CS, Yeh SDJ, Straus DJ. Long-term follow-up of cardiac function in patients with Hodgkin's disease treated with mediastinal irradiation and combination chemotherapy including doxorubicin. Cancer Treat Rep 1986;70:439–444.
273. Santoro A, Bonadonna G, Valagusso P, et al. Long-term results of combined chemotherapy-radiotherapy approach in Hodgkin's disease: Superiority of ABVD plus radiotherapy versus MOPP plus radiotherapy. J Clin Oncol 1987;5:27–37.
274. Brice P, Tredaniel J, Monsuez JJ, et al. Cardiopulmonary toxicity after three courses of ABVD and mediastinal irradiation in favorable Hodgkin's disease. Ann Oncol 1991;2: 73–76.
275. Carlson RG, Mayfield WR, Normann S, Alexander JA. Radiation-associated valvular disease. Chest 1991;99:538–545.

276. Kadota RP, Burgert EO Jr, Driscoll DJ, et al. Cardiopulmonary function in long-term survivors of childhood Hodgkin's lymphoma: A pilot study. Mayo Clin Proc 1988;63:362–367.

277. Warda M, Khan A, Massumi A, et al. Radiation-induced valvular dysfunction. J Am Coll Cardiol 1983;2:180–185.

278. Cohen SL, Bharati S, Glass J, et al. Radiotherapy as a cause of complete atrioventricular block in Hodgkin's disease. Arch Intern Med 1981;141:676–679.

279. Mary-Rabine L, Waleffe A, Kulbertius HE. Severe conduction disturbances and ventricular arrhythmias complicating mediastinal irradiation for Hodgkin's disease: A case report. PACE 1980;3:612–617.

280. Tzivoni D, Ratzkowski E, Biran S, et al. Complete heart block following therapeutic irradiation of the left side of the chest. Chest 1977;71:231–234.

281. Kereiakes DJ, Morady F, Ports TA. High degree atrioventricular block after radiation therapy. Am J Cardiol 1983;51:1233–1234.

282. Slama M-S, LeGuludec D, Sebag C, et al. Complete atrioventricular block following mediastinal irradiation: A report of six cases. PACE 1991;14:1112–1118.

283. Strender LE, Lindahl J, Larsson LE. Incidence of heart disease and functional significance of change in the electrocardiogram 10 years after radiotherapy for breast cancer. Cancer 1986;57:929–934.

284. Watchie J, Coleman CN, Raffin TA, et al. Minimal long-term cardiopulmonary dysfunction following treatment for Hodgkin's disease. Int J Radiat Oncol Biol Phys 1987;13:513–524.

285. Amronim GD, Solomon RD. Production of arteriosclerosis in the rabbit: A quantitative assessment. Arch Pathol 1965;75:219–227.

286. Gold H. Production of arteriosclerosis in the rat: Effect of x-ray and high-fat diet. Arch Pathol 1961;71:268–272.

287. Artom C, Lofton HB, Clarkson TB. Ionizing radiation atherosclerosis and lipid metabolism in pigeons. Radiat Res 1965;26:165–177.

288. Kopelson G, Herwig KJ. The etiologies of coronary artery disease in cancer patients. Int J Radiat Oncol Biol Phys 1978;4:895–906.

289. Yahalom J, Hasin Y, Fuks Z. Acute myocardial infarction with normal coronary arteriogram after mantle field radiation therapy for Hodgkin's disease. Cancer 1983;52:637–641.

290. McEniery PT, Dorosti K, Schiavone WA, et al. Clinical and angiographic features of coronary artery disease after chest irradiation. Am J Cardiol 1987;60:1020–1024.

291. Boivin JF, Hutchison GB, Lubin JH, Mauch P. Coronary artery disease mortality in patients treated for Hodgkin's disease. Cancer 1992;69:1241–1247.

292. Henry-Amar M, Hayat M, Meerwaldt JH. Causes of death after therapy for early stage Hodgkin's disease entered on EORTC protocols. Int J Radiat Oncol Biol Phys 1990;19:1155–1157.

293. Hancock SL, Cox RS, Rosenberg SA. Correction: Death after treatment of Hodgkin's disease. Ann Intern Med [Letter] 1992;114:810.

294. Cosset JM, Henry-Amar M, Meerwaldt JH. Long-term toxicity of early stages of Hodgkin's disease therapy: The EORTC experience. Am Oncol 1991;2:77–82.

295. Handler CE, Livesey S, Lawton PA. Coronary ostial stenosis after radiotherapy: Angioplasty or coronary artery surgery? Br Heart J 1989;61:208–211.

296. Grollier G, Commeau P, Mercier V, et al. Post-radiotherapeutic left main coronary ostial stenosis: Clinical and histiological study. Eur Heart J 1988;9:567–570.

297. Annest LS, Anderson RP, Li W, et al. Coronary artery disease following mediastinal radiation therapy. J Thorac Cardiovasc Surg 1983;85:257–263.

298. Miller DD, Waters DD, Dangoisse V, et al. Symptomatic coronary artery spasm following radiotherapy for Hodgkin's disease. Chest 1983;83:284–285.

299. Host H, Brennhoud IO, Loeb M. Post-operative radiotherapy in breast cancer: Long-term results from the Oslo study. Int J Radiat Oncol Biol Phys 1986;12:727–732.

300. Jones JM, Ribeiro GG. Mortality patterns over 34 years of breast cancer patients in a clinical trial of post-operative radiotherapy. Clin Radiol 1989;40:204–208.

301. Haybittle JL, Brinkley D, Houghton J, et al. Postoperative radiotherapy and late mortality: Evidence from the Cancer Research Campaign trial for early breast cancer. Br Med J 1989;298:1611–1614.

302. Levitt SH, Fletcher GH. Trials and tribulations: Do clinical trials prove that irradiation increases cardiac and secondary cancer mortality in the breast cancer patient? Int J Radiat Oncol Biol Phys 1991;20:523–527.

303. Wallgren A, Arner O, Bergstrom J, et al. Radiation therapy in operable breast cancer: Results from the Stockholm trial in adjuvant radiotherapy. Int J Radiat Oncol Biol Phys 1986;12:533–537.

304. Stender LE, Lindahl J, Larsson LE. Incidence of heart disease and functional significance of changes in the electrocardiogram 10 years after radiotherapy for breast cancer. Cancer 1986;57:929–934.

305. Harris JR, Hellman S. Put the "hockey stick" on ice. Int J Radiat Oncol Biol Phys 1988;15:497–499.

306. Lederman GS, Sheldon TA, Chaffey JT, et al. Cardiac disease after mediastinal irradiation for seminoma. Cancer 1987;60:772–776.

SECTION 6

STEPHEN T. SONIS

Oral Complications of Cancer Therapy

The mouth is often a significant site of complications in the patient receiving therapy for cancer. Not only are patients with malignancies of the head and neck susceptible to such problems, but also affected are patients receiving treatment for more distant disease. Virtually all patients who receive radiation therapy to the head and neck develop oral side effects of their treatment, and about 40% of patients who are treated with chemotherapy develop oral complications. It has been demonstrated that aggressive oral evaluation before cancer therapy, intervention to eliminate potential sources of infection or irritation, and preventive measures taken during therapy result in a precipitous drop in the frequency of oral problems.[1]

In addition to affecting adversely the patient's ability to eat, speak, and control saliva, cancer therapy may have even more significant ramifications, especially relative to sepsis. Because of the mouth's vast bacterial and fungal flora, it is an important potential portal for these organisms in the myelosuppressed host; the mouth is the most frequently identifiable source of sepsis in the granulocytopenic cancer patient. Nevertheless, many of the oral problems associated with cancer therapy can be prevented or minimized with adequate pretherapy care and with aggressive preventive techniques during treatment.

ORAL COMPLICATIONS OF RADIATION THERAPY

For the most part, oral problems due to radiation therapy are the result of local tissue changes from direct irradiation. For this reason, implants tend to produce more problems than does beam irradiation. Radiation results in mucosal atrophy due to decreased cell renewal; fibrosis of the salivary glands, muscles, ligaments, and blood vessels; and damage to taste buds.[2]

Mucositis is the result of atrophic changes in the epithelium due to decreased cell renewal and usually is noted at a dose level of about 2000 cGy when therapy is administered at a rate of 200 cGy/day. Patients complain of generalized discomfort and drying of the mucosa; erythema is present; and any traumatized area may ulcerate. Generally, nonkeratinized epithelium of the cheeks, lips, soft palate, and ventral surface of the tongue is affected. Mucositis is extremely uncomfortable for the patient and may limit oral intake. Although it is self-limiting and usually resolves in 2 to 3 weeks after the termination of radiation treatment, severe mucositis may necessitate a temporary cessation of therapy. Ice chips or Popsicles are soothing. Patients should be instructed to avoid spicy or acidic foods. Unusually sharp teeth should be smoothed or eliminated. Removable prostheses should be used sparingly. Oral hygiene should be stressed.

Historically, treatment of mucositis has been palliative and aimed at minimizing mucosal trauma. Rinses such as Xylocaine Viscous, dyclonine hydrochloride (Dyclone), or Kaopectate and Benadryl provide varying degrees of relief.[3] Localized lesions can be treated with topical therapy using benzocaine in Orabase or benzocaine in a hydroxypropylcellulose base (Oratect gel). The latter purportedly provides lesion coverage for up to 4 hours.[4,5]

The successful use of sucralfate for the treatment of gastric ulcers has led to studies of its efficacy as a palliative rinse for the treatment of mucositis, but data are conflicting.[6–8] A number of studies have suggested that benzydamine HCl, a topical nonsteroidal antiinflammatory agent, can successfully soothe radiation- and chemotherapy-induced mucositis.[9–11] This drug is available in Europe and Canada, but not in the United States.

Biologically active treatments are also being studied for their potential efficacy in preventing or treating mucositis. The role of PGE2 in the development of or therapy for mucositis has been evaluated with mixed results. Data from early studies suggested that, although increases in plasma-extracted prostaglandin correlated with increases in mucositis, administration of moderate doses of prostaglandin inhibitors failed to affect the severity of lesions.[12] A later investigation, however, demonstrated that indomethacin administered orally at a dose of 25 mg four times a day delayed the onset and reduced the severity of mucositis induced by radiation therapy, compared with a placebo control.[13] Paradoxically, the administration of PGE2 by other investigators appeared to be beneficial in the treatment of mucositis.[14,15]

Another approach to the control of mucositis has been advocated by Spijkervet and colleagues.[16,17] They hypothesized that the selective elimination of gram-negative bacilli might have a favorable effect on mucositis since a shift to the latter was noted in patients receiving treatment for malignancies of the head and neck. Administration of lozenges of polymyxin E, tobramycin 1.8 mg, and amphotericin B 10 mg resulted in a reduced frequency of severe mucositis in response to radiation therapy.

Xerostomia is one of the most frequent side effects of irradiation to the head and neck and is due to changes in the salivary glands.[18–20] Generally, there is a direct relation between the dose of irradiation to the salivary glands and the extent of glandular changes.[21] Under 6000 cGy, changes in the salivary glands induced by irradiation, including edema and inflammation, are reversible. Over 6000 cGy, changes may be permanent, with fibrosis and glandular degeneration. Clinically, xerostomia has been reported with as little as two to three doses of 200 to 225 cGy.[21]

Xerostomia predisposes to increases in the number of oral bacteria because saliva is no longer available to help clear bacteria from the mouth, or as a source of IgA. The patient's ability to taste is altered.

The most consistent consequence of xerostomia is the development of radiation caries, which characteristically appears in the cervical regions or incisal edges of teeth a few months after the start of radiation therapy.[28] Left untreated, caries and decalcification may become so severe that the integrity of the tooth is compromised and fracture occurs. The causes of radiation caries include loss of salivary buffering capacity, lowered salivary pH, elimination of mechanical flushing, and decreased salivary IgA.

Treatment of xerostomia has four goals:

1. Stimulation of existing salivary flow
2. Replacement of lost secretions
3. Protection of the dentition
4. Reduction of sucrose intake

Stimulation of the patient's remaining salivary apparatus may be accomplished with sucrose-free lemon drops. Sugar-free chewing gum may satisfy the same objective; mint- and cinnamon-flavored gum should be avoided because it may irritate the mucosa. Saliva substitutes such as Xero-Lube or Salivart may be used before meals and at bedtime.[23]

Recent investigations by Fox and associates[25] and Greenspan and Daniels[24] indicate that relatively low doses of systemically administered pilocarpine may have a role in reducing radiation-induced xerostomia.

Prevention of radiation-induced caries is best accomplished by the aggressive use of fluorides.[26] Customized trays should be fabricated for patients so that they may deliver home fluoride treatments on a daily basis; this may be supplemented with fluoride rinses. Generally, acidulated fluorides are the most effective, although neutral fluorides may become necessary in patients with mucositis. Fluorides should be continued until full salivary function has returned. An alternative to fluoride-containing trays is the daily use of fluoride gel as a tooth brushing agent. Stannous fluoride 0.4% gel appears to be more effective than sodium fluoride 1.1% since it reduces detectable levels of caries-causing *Streptococcus mutans*.[7] In addition, scrupulous oral hygiene and aggressive professional maintenance are critical to minimizing the development of caries. Finally, the patient should be encouraged to avoid sucrose.

Loss of taste is a common sequela of radiation therapy. It usually is noted with a cumulative dose of between 1000 and 2000 cGy.[28] Most often, loss of the ability to differentiate sweet and salty is reported as often leading to an avoidance of foods with such tastes. Bitterness is common. Taste sensation usually returns 6 to 12 months after the completion of therapy.

The most serious local sequela of head and neck radiation therapy is osteoradionecrosis (ORN), which occurs when there is fibrotic thickening of blood vessels, replacement of bone marrow with connective tissue, subsequent lack of new bone formation, and bone death.[29] The bone becomes susceptible to infection, and its ability to heal is retarded. Patients develop open, foul-smelling wounds with areas of denuded bone. It is thought that ORN represents a defect in wound healing rather than a true osteomyelitis.[29] The reported incidence of ORN ranges from 4% to 44%; the actual frequency is about 15%. Ninety percent of cases occur in the mandible, which differs in vascularity and density compared with the maxilla. About 30% of cases occur spontaneously; the remainder are thought to be related to trauma, the most frequent form of which is tooth extraction. Most spontaneous cases of ORN occur within the first 6 to 24 months after treatment. By contrast, trauma-related osteonecrosis has two peaks of activity: the first peak typically occurs 3 months after radiation therapy, and the second peak occurs 2 to 5 years after treatment.[30,31]

Four major risk factors predispose to the development of ORN: (1) the anatomic site of the tumor, (2) the dose of radiation, (3) the dental status of the patient,[10] and (4) the type and source of radiation. Patients receiving radiation therapy to tumors anatomically related to the mandible develop ORN at five times the rate of patients with tumors at other sites. The risk of ORN is increased significantly at doses of 6000 cGy or more; the risk of developing ORN is increased twofold for patients receiving greater than 8000 cGy compared with patients receiving 5000 to 6000 cGy, and it is almost five times greater than for patients receiving 4000 to 5000 cGy. Dentulous patients are more likely to develop ORN than are edentulous patients. Furthermore, patients with dental disease are at twice the risk of developing ORN than patients without dental disease.[32] Therefore, meticulous oral hygiene, elimination of diseased teeth, aggressive prophylaxis, and follow-up should be stressed. Oral hygiene techniques for the patient receiving radiation therapy may include standard brushing and flossing. Water-irrigating devices (*e.g.*, Water-Pik) may be helpful for removal of food particles or other debris but are ineffective for the elimination of tooth-borne bacteria. Patients should be cautioned to use them at low pressure. Similarly, sucrose intake should be minimized, and topical fluorides should be used regularly. Patients receiving external-beam sources of radiation are at least twice as likely to develop ORN as those receiving radiation from implanted sources. Patients receiving supervoltage radiation therapy of 1 MeV or more are at significantly higher risk for osteonecrosis than are patients receiving particulate neutron beam therapy.[32]

For patients receiving interstitial radiation, a lead device may offer protection to the mandible and minimize the risk of ORN.[33]

Patients with poorly fitting prostheses are also at risk for ORN because breaks in the epithelium and pressure on supporting bone may cause infection and necrosis.

The issue of if and when dental extractions should be performed is unresolved.[31–32,34,35] At times when low-energy radiation was used, the common protocol was to extract all teeth in the path of the primary beam before the start of therapy to eliminate sources of infection and ORN. Improvements in the type of radiation used, more selective fields of radiation, increased concern for patient function and aesthetics, and the success of preventive dental protocols have modified this approach. An approach has evolved aimed at the elimination of actively infected teeth, with aggressive dental preventive techniques for the remaining dentition. It is important to note that sites of extractions performed before radiation therapy are also at increased risk for the development of ORN, although not at the same frequency as extraction sites created after the start of radiation therapy. Therefore, teeth demonstrating periapical pathology or active periodontal infection should be extracted as long as possible before the start of radiation therapy and at a minimum of 3 weeks before therapy. Nonrestorable teeth or teeth with deep caries and a significant risk of developing infection also should be eliminated. Teeth at marginal risk that are unlikely to become infected should be retained. When possible, extractions should be postponed until 1 year after the termination of radiation. Antibiotic prophylaxis is recommended. Endodontic therapy can be used as a temporary measure to "buy time" if a problem occurs during radiation therapy, although endodontics does not appear to have permanent efficacy in this group.[36]

Management of ORN depends on its severity. Most cases resolve spontaneously after about 6 months of conservative therapy consisting of local debridement and oral antibiotics. Hyperbaric oxygen therapy has been advocated for nonresolving cases.[37] In instances of intractable pain, severe trismus, orocutaneous fistulas, or persistent exposure of bone, surgical resection may be the only curative therapy available.

ORAL COMPLICATIONS OF CANCER CHEMOTHERAPY

Of all patients receiving chemotherapy, about 40% develop oral problems during each exposure to drug.[38] Although the spectrum of problems is wide, essentially all oral complications of chemotherapy occur through one of two major mechanisms: they are either a direct effect of the drug on the oral mucosa (direct stomatotoxicity) or an indirect result of myelosuppression (indirect stomatotoxicity; Fig. 63–4).

Not all patients are at equal risk of developing oral problems associated with their specific chemotherapy. Factors that influence the frequency and severity of these complications may be grouped into those that are related to the patient and those that are related to the drug. Patient-related factors include the types of malignancy, patient age, and the level of oral health before and during therapy.

Patients with hematologic malignancies (*e.g.*, leukemia, lymphoma) develop oral problems at two or three times the rate of patients with solid tumors.[39–41] This is probably because these patients are functionally myelosuppressed as a consequence of the malignancies.[42] Young patients tend to develop oral problems more frequently than older patients. Whereas 90% of patients between the ages of 1 and 20 years develop oral problems after chemotherapy, only 18% of patients over age 60 develop problems.[38] Part of the reason for this finding is attributable to the high incidence of hematologic malignancies in the younger age group. When oral problems are evaluated in patients with the same malignancy and the same chemotherapeutic regimen, however, this finding holds up. An explanation for this may be that cell renewal is decreased in older patients.[43] Additionally, the number of mitoses in the basal epithelium of younger patients is greater than in older patients. Patients in poor oral health, especially those with preexisting periodontal or pulpal disease, have a higher risk of developing oral infection in the face of chemotherapy-induced myelosuppression.[44–46] Similarly, patients with irritating prostheses or sharp or broken teeth are at increased risk for developing ulceration and mucositis. Patients in whom preexisting periodontal and dental disease is eliminated before therapy and who receive aggressive mouth care during treatment have a significant decrease in the frequency of oral problems associated with chemotherapy.[47–51]

Therapy-related variables also influence the frequency and severity with which patients develop problems. Probably the single most important factor in this area is choice of drug.[39,52–54] Although stomatotoxicity is a common side effect of many forms of chemotherapy, drugs differ significantly in the extent of the stomatotoxicity they cause. In many instances, stomatotoxicity is dose-related. This effect can be reduced by delivering an agent in divided doses rather than as a bolus.[53] Finally, concomitant therapy such as radiation increases the frequency and severity with which patients develop oral problems in response to chemotherapy.

DIRECT STOMATOTOXICITY

Direct stomatotoxicity is the consequence of the nonspecific effect of a drug on cells undergoing mitosis. Cells of the mouth undergo rapid renewal over a 7- to 14-day cycle. Chemotherapy causes a reduction in the renewal rate of the basal epi-

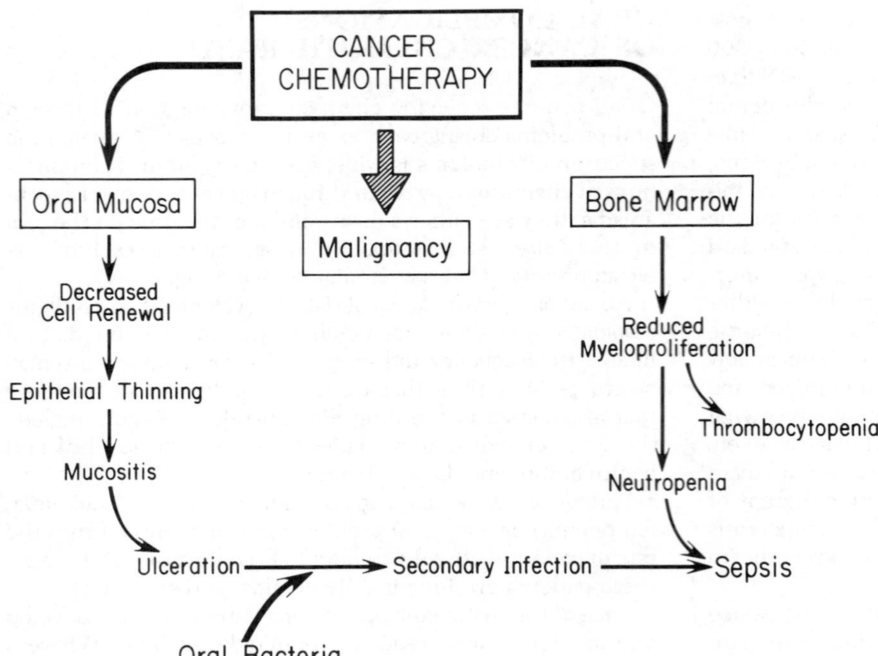

FIGURE 63–4. Effects of cancer chemotherapy on both the oral basal epithelial cells and the bone marrow stem cells.

thelium, which results in mucosal atrophy.[55,56] Diminished nutritional intake secondary to mucositis[57] may compound the problem because there is an overall decrease in cell migration and renewal after starvation or protein deprivation. Clinically, patients experience pain from mucositis and ulceration. Lesions are generally discrete initially but often progress to produce confluent areas of ulceration (Fig. 63–5). Nonkeratinized mucosa is most often affected. The buccal, labial, and soft palatal mucosa, along with the ventral surface of the tongue and the floor of the mouth, are the most common sites. Lesions do not progress outside the mouth (Fig. 63–6). Direct stomatotoxicity is usually observed 5 to 7 days after the administration of the drug. Left untreated, lesions generally heal without scarring within 2 to 3 weeks in the nonmyelosuppressed patient. A wide variety of agents may produce direct stomatotoxicity (Table 63–19).

The major clinical problem associated with direct stomatotoxicity is pain, with a consequent loss of function, especially ability to eat. Patients are miserable and are often unable to sleep because of oral pain. Treatment of direct stomatotoxicity is palliative (Table 63–20). A variety of agents are available, including Xylocaine viscous and Dyclone. A rinse of frequent benefit may be prepared by mixing equal proportions of elixir of Benadryl and Kaopectate. The use of milk of magnesia as

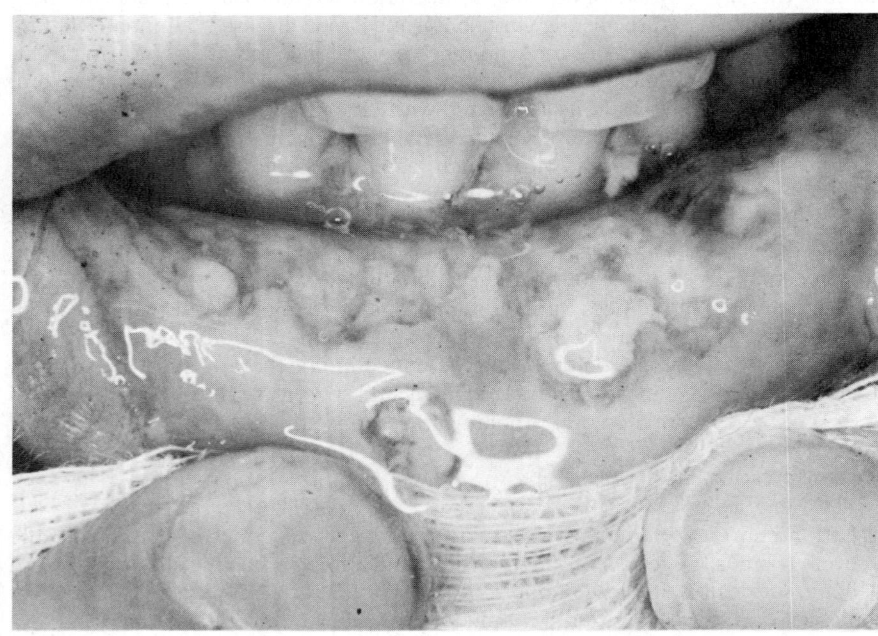

FIGURE 63–5. Mucositis of the labial mucosa due to stomatotoxicity secondary to methotrexate. Notice the severe disruption of epithelial integrity. (Sonis S, Fazio R, Fang L. Principles and practice of oral medicine. Philadelphia: WB Saunders, 1984)

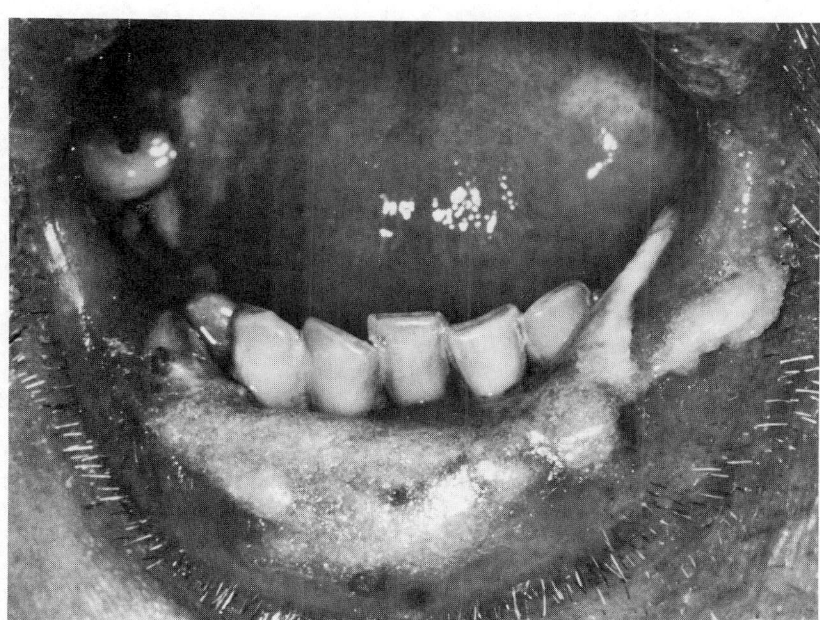

FIGURE 63–6. Severe breakdown of the labial mucosa as a result of direct stomatotoxicity. Notice the lack of involvement of nonmucosal surfaces. (Sonis S, Fazio R, Fang L. Principles and practice of oral medicine. Philadelphia: WB Saunders, 1984)

a vehicle for the delivery of palliative agents is to be avoided because of its desiccating effect on the mucosa. In severe cases, 2.5% to 5% cocaine rinses or spray may be used. The latter is recommended only in supervised inpatient settings because of the potential for neurotoxicity. In the case of discrete ulceration, ointments, such as benzocaine in Orabase, may be applied to the affected area after it is dried with a sponge. The use of systemic pain medication is often of value. Patients often find cold soothing; ice chips, Popsicles, and cold beverages may be helpful. Other approaches to the treatment of mucositis are discussed elsewhere in this section.

Cryotherapy reportedly has been helpful in marginally reducing the severity of chemotherapy-induced mucositis.[58] Additional controlled studies are required to confirm this observation.

The use of allopurinol, an inhibitor of orotidine-5′-phosphate decarboxylase, to prevent mucositis induced by 5-FU is unclear. Although two pilot studies suggested its efficacy, a larger, controlled investigation failed to substantiate its usefulness.[59–61] The vitamin A derivative, beta-carotene, may be beneficial in reducing the stomatotoxic effects of radiation therapy and chemotherapy, although large, well-controlled investigations are pending.[62]

TABLE 63–19. Cancer Chemotherapeutic Drugs That Produce Direct Stomatotoxicity

Alkylating Agents	**Natural Products**
Mechlorethamine	Bleomycin
	Dactinomycin
Antimetabolites	Daunorubicin
Cytarabine hydrochloride	Doxorubicin
Floxuridine	Mithramycin
Fluorouracil	Mitomycin
Mercaptopurine	Vinblastine sulfate
Methotrexate	Vincristine sulfate
Thioguanine	
	Other Synthetic Agents
	Hydroxyurea
	Procarbazine hydrochloride

Preliminary and anecdotal data suggest that some growth factors may have been positive modifiers of mucositis induced in myelosuppressed cancer patients.[63,64] Patients receiving human recombinant granulocyte colony-stimulating factor in conjunction with a stomatotoxic drug regimen for the treatment of transitional carcinoma of the bladder had an apparent reduction in mucositis. The effects of other growth factors on the development and course of mucositis is under investigation.[65]

Xerostomia is a common side effect of some forms of chemotherapy and accelerates the development of mucositis.[13] Management of xerostomia is discussed elsewhere in this section.

Plant alkaloids, particularly vincristine, may cause neurotoxicity that manifests as acute-onset dental pain, most frequently in the mandibular molar area, in the absence of odontogenic pathology.[66] The discomfort resolves after the drug is discontinued.

INDIRECT STOMATOTOXICITY

Indirect stomatotoxicity is the result of the effects of chemotherapy on a cell pool other than of the oral mucosa. The most significant target cells in this case are those of the bone marrow. Changes in the mouth that are associated with this action usually are noted at the patient's nadir and most often occur 12 to 14 days after drug administration.[20] The two most common forms of indirect stomatotoxicity are infection and hemorrhage.

The mouth is the most frequently identifiable source of sepsis in the granulocytopenic cancer patient.[64] Most often, oral infection is caused by bacteria, although fungal and viral infections also are relatively common. The degree and duration

TABLE 63–20. Formulary of Topical Medications for Specific Oral Problems

Problem	*Medication*	*Use*
General infection control	Chlorhexidine gluconate 0.12% oral rinse	Rinse twice daily after breakfast and at bedtime for 30 sec. Do not swallow.
	Povidone iodine rinse 0.5%	Rinse twice daily. Do not swallow.
Localized secondary topical lip infection	Neosporin	Apply to perioral lesions 2–5 times daily, depending on severity of lesion
Prevention of caries secondary to xerostomia	Acidulated fluoride rinse	Rinse daily for 1 min with 5 to 10 ml. Do not swallow. Switch to neutral fluoride if mucositis is present.*†
	Neutral fluoride rinse	Rinse daily for 1 min with 5 ml. Do not swallow. Switch back to acidulated fluoride rinse when mucositis resolves.
	Stannous fluoride gel 0.4%	Brush daily for 1 min, then hold in mouth and rinse for 30 sec. Do not swallow.†
	Sodium fluoride gel 1.1%	Brush daily at bedtime. Swish for 30 sec. Spit out and rinse.
Antifungal Agents		
Prevention and treatment of oral candidiasis	Nystatin oral suspension	Rinse and swallow 300,000 units 3–4 times daily. If intolerance to swallowing, rinse only.
	Clotrimazole troche 10 mg	Dissolve 1 tablet 5 times daily. The prophylactic use of clotrimazole for the prevention of candidiasis has not been adequately studied.
Treatment of candidiasis under dentures or at corners of mouth	Mycolog ointment	Apply to affected area 2 to 3 times daily or place under denture surface.
Palliation of mucositis (generalized)	Xylocaine viscous 2% solution	Swish 15 ml for 30 sec maximum every 3 h. Expectorate.
	Dyclonine hydrochloride 0.5% or 1% solution	Swish 15 ml for 30 sec every 2 to 3 h. Expectorate.
	Benadryl and Kaopectate mix solution of 50% each.	Swish 15 ml for 30 sec every 2 to 3 h. Expectorate.
Palliation of mucositis (localized)	Benzocaine in Orabase ointment	Apply to affected dried area every 2 to 3 h. Not to be used in presence of infection.
	Benzocaine 15% in Oratect gel.	Apply up to 4 times daily after drying mucosa.
Control of Local Bleeding		
Gingival	Topical thrombin solution	Apply to affected area with gauze sponge and hold in place with pressure for 30 min. Do not remove formed clots.
Mucosal surface bleeding	Microfibrillar collagen	Apply to dried site with dry sponge for 1 to 5 min. Do not use in closure of mucosal incisions.
Xerostomia		
Saliva substitutes	Salivart synthetic saliva spray	Spray as needed for xerostomia.
	Xerolube	Rinse as needed for xerostomia.
	Biotene chewing gum.	Use as needed.

* Fluoride gels in custom trays are preferred.
† Acidulated fluorides are contraindicated in patients with porcelain prostheses.

of granulocytopenia often determine the incidence and severity of infection. Although the normal flora is responsible for most infections, during myelosuppression, the oral flora changes to become primarily gram-negative (common isolated organisms include *Klebsiella, Serratia, Enterobacter, Escherichia coli, Pseudomonas,* and *Proteus*).[68] Most fungal infections are caused by *Candida albicans*.[69]

Bacterial infections may affect three sites in the mouth: the gingiva, the mucosa, and the teeth. Because the normal signs of inflammation and therefore infection are absent in the myelosuppressed patient, diagnosis is based on the presence of oral lesions in conjunction with fever and pain. Demonstration of a culturable local isolate in conjunction with a positive blood culture result confirms the diagnosis, although exotoxins and endotoxins from oral bacteria may produce fever in the absence of a positive blood culture.

Gingivae are a common site of infection, especially in the patient with preexisting periodontal disease.[70,71] Infection of this area presents as a necrotizing gingivitis that clinically resembles acute necrotizing ulcerative gingivitis (Vincent's disease). Patients develop painful necrosis of the marginal and papillary gingivae, usually beginning around one or two teeth and then spreading laterally. Fever and lymphadenopathy are present. The normal papillary architecture is eliminated, and a white, necrotic pseudomembrane is present. Treatment of necrotic gingivitis consists of parenteral antibiotics. Because spirochetes and fusiform organisms must be included in the spectrum of causative agents, coverage should include a penicillin as well as an agent specific for gram-negative organisms. The teeth should be gently debrided with cotton pellets soaked with 3% hydrogen peroxide. Frequent rinsing may be helpful.

Mucosal infection is usually due to secondary infection of ulcerations produced by direct stomatotoxicity or trauma (Fig. 63–7). Patients complain of pain and are febrile. Clinically, one observes ulceration, often deep, with a yellow-white necrotic center. The borders are often slightly raised and indurated. An erythematous border, usually associated with aphthous lesions, is conspicuously absent. Lesions are of variable size; the size of the lesion does not always relate directly to its potential to cause sepsis. The organisms causing these infections usually are mixed; therefore, isolation of organisms from the blood of septic patients is an important corroborating procedure in patients suspected of having an oral source.

It is often difficult to determine which mucosal lesions require antibiotic coverage. Patients with fever, neutropenia (fewer than 1000 leukocytes/mm^3), and an oral lesion must be presumed to have an oral source and should be appropriately treated until the leukocyte count recovers, the patient is afebrile, and the lesions begin to resolve.

Odontogenic infections in the myelosuppressed patient often present with confusing signs and symptoms because of the patient's inability to mount an inflammatory response.[52,72] Tooth pain and fever may be the only signs of odontogenic infection. Thorough dental examination, including radiographs, is often necessary to make a definitive diagnosis. Because many subacute odontogenic infections become symptomatic when the patient becomes myelosuppressed, the ideal treatment is elimination of questionable teeth before the initiation of chemotherapy. If this is not possible, and the patient develops a definite odontogenic infection, extraction to eliminate the source is the treatment of choice. This requires antibiotic and often platelet coverage. Extractions should be performed with as little trauma as possible, and block anesthesia should be avoided. Hemostatic gels should not be used because these may act as foci for bacterial infection. Primary closure of the wound with sutures is desirable.[73,74] Antibiotics should be continued for at least 1 week after extraction regardless of the patient's leukocyte count. Alternatively, if the patient is medically unstable, the necrotic pulp may be endodontically extricated and the tooth closed.

Oral fungal infections are common in the myelosuppressed cancer patient. Generally, these tend to be superficial infections of the oral mucosa caused by *C. albicans,* an organism present in about half of the normal population. Oral infection with *C. albicans* produces surface necrosis, which has a wide variety of clinical manifestations. Most frequently, lesions appear as raised, white curdy areas and can affect any of the oral soft tissues (Fig. 63–8). Angular cheilitis may also occur. Patients who wear removable prostheses may develop infections beneath their dentures that are broad, sensitive, erythematous macules. The major clinical significance of oral moniliasis is its potential regional or systemic spread. Patients are rarely febrile when *C. albicans* infections are limited to the mouth. Diagnosis is based on clinical appearance, the ability to scrape off the necrotic surface, and demonstration of the organism with potassium hydroxide smears.

The value of prophylactic antifungal medication is controversial.[74–78] One study concluded that patients whose leukocyte counts drop to 200 cells/mm^3 develop candidiasis despite topical medication. However, it appears that prophylactic use of topical antifungal agents begun simultaneously with chemo-

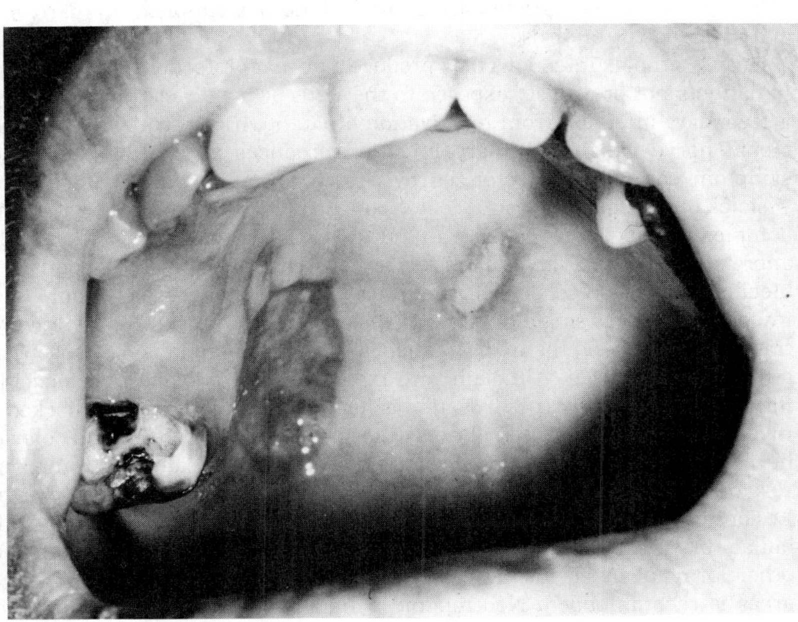

FIGURE 63–7. An unusual case of localized ulcerations of the hard palate in a patient hospitalized with fever of unknown origin. At the time of admission, the larger ulcer demonstrated evidence of infection. (Lockhart PB. Dental management of patients receiving chemotherapy. In: Peterson D, Sonis S, eds. Oral complications of cancer chemotherapy. Boston: Martinus Nijhoff, 1983)

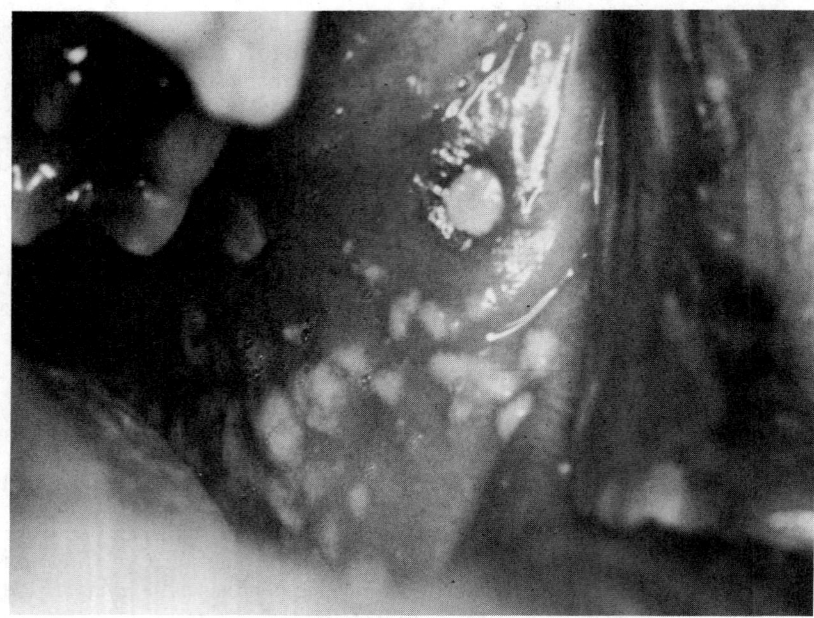

FIGURE 63–8. Candidiasis of buccal mucosa in a 49-year-old woman with acute myelogenous leukemia. Notice raised, white croppy areas of fungae. A small ulcer is also present.

therapy reduces both the frequency and severity of infection. The polyene antibiotics (nystatin) are probably the most often used, usually as a suspension that is rinsed and swallowed. Popsicles made of nystatin diluted in water are often soothing and provide prolonged contact with the mucosa. Alternatively, the imidazole agents in trouche form may be preferred. It appears that their efficacy is comparable to nystatin.[79] Patients complaining of esophageal pain or dysphagia should be evaluated for spread of infection (see Chap. 64),[80] which should be treated early and aggressively with a systemic antifungal agent (*e.g.*, amphotericin B).

Other deep fungal infections may occur in the myelosuppressed patient. Fortunately, however, these are relatively rare.

The two most common viral infections affecting the mouths of myelosuppressed patients are caused by herpes simplex and varicella zoster viruses.

Herpes simplex infections may produce a primary infection in patients not previously exposed to the virus or may cause a secondary infection from reactivation of latent virus in regional nerve ganglia. Primary infection produces an oral symptom complex characterized by acute-onset gingivitis, vesicles of the mucosa, and a coated tongue. This symptom complex usually is preceded by a viral prodrome of malaise, anorexia, and fever. The mouth is extremely tender. Gingival bleeding may be noted as well as fetor oris. Secondary herpes infection produces single or crops of vesicles, most often extraoral, at or beyond the mucocutaneous junction. Infections tend to be recurrent. Although rare in the normal person, intraoral secondary herpes infection is not uncommon in the myelosuppressed patient. Patients who are seropositive to herpes simplex virus because of prior exposure are at greater risk of infection compared with seronegative patients.[80–82] Lesions may have a variety of appearances, including vesicles, bullae, or small or large ulcers. Since the latter resembles other forms of mucositis, aggressive culturing of suspicious areas is recommended. Neutropenic patients experiencing herpes infections should be treated with acyclovir.[81–84] Extraoral lesions may become infected secondarily with bacteria. Healing often is helped by the presence of a lubricating ointment such as Neosporin.

The frequency of herpes simplex virus infections in patients receiving chemotherapy is not well resolved; the reported incidence ranges from about 11% to 48%. The differences in reported frequency are largely dependent on the method of diagnosis. In interpreting results, it must be remembered that herpes simplex virus is not an uncommon member of the normal oral flora and, in the absence of clinically detectable lesions, may not be of pathologic consequence.[85]

Chlorhexidine gluconate 0.12% may be efficacious in reducing the frequency and severity of mucositis and infection associated with chemotherapy and radiation therapy for bone marrow transplantations. The drug is used twice daily as a rinse. Side effects are minimal and include occasional burning, which may be reduced by dilution with water, and brown superficial tooth staining, which can be easily polished off.[86]

Thrombocytopenia predisposes to oral bleeding.[87,88] Bleeding may occur anywhere in the mouth but usually is provoked by trauma or preexisting periodontal disease. Minor mucosal trauma may result in hematoma formation or frank bleeding. Generally, hematoma formation is unusual with platelet counts greater than 25,000 cells/mm^3.[87] When patients are more profoundly thrombocytopenic, oral hematomas form relatively easily and are of clinical significance for two major reasons: (1) hematomas can act as sites of secondary infection, especially when there are breaks in the mucosa; and (2) unchecked submucosal bleeding in the sublingual area may result in elevation of the tongue and consequent respiratory compromise.

Spontaneous gingival bleeding is unusual with platelet counts greater than 10,000 cells/mm^3. Patients with preexisting periodontal disease are more likely to demonstrate gingival hemorrhage than are patients in good gingival health. Therefore, dental prophylaxis and good oral hygiene are of significant benefit in reducing the likelihood of this problem. If gingival bleeding does occur, topical thrombin-soaked gauze held under pressure is often helpful. For open mucosal oozing, microcrystalline collagen may produce hemostasis. When local measures fail, patients may require platelet transfusion. The use of stints or surgical gingival packs should be avoided because the pressure of these often causes necrosis. Furthermore, these appliances harbor bacteria and are irritating to the gingiva.

REFERENCES

1. Sonis ST, Woods PD, White BA. Pretreatment oral assessment. J Natl Cancer Inst 1990;9:29–32.
2. Reynolds WR, Hickey AJ, Feldman MI. Dental management of the cancer patient receiving radiation therapy. Clin Prevent Dent 1980;2:5–9.
3. Miaskowski C. Management of mucositis during therapy. NCI Monograph 1990;9:95–98.
4. Rodu B, Russell CM, Ray KL. Treatment of oral ulcers with hydroxyprophycellulose film. Compend Contin Educ Dent 1988;9:420–422.
5. Rodu B, Russell CM. Performance of a hydroxyprophycellulose film former in normal and ulcerated mucosa. Oral Surg 1988;65:699–703.
6. Preiffer P, Madsen EL, Hansen O, et al. Effect of prophylactic sucralfate suspension on stomatitis induced by cancer chemotherapy. Acta Oncol 1990;29:171–173.
7. Shenep JL, Kalwinsky DK, Hutson PR, et al. Efficacy of oral sucralfate suspension in prevention and treatment of chemotherapy-induced mucositis. J Pediatr 1988;113:758–763.
8. Scherlacher A, Beaufort-Spontin F. Radiotherapy of head-neck neoplasms: Prevention of inflammation of the mucosa by sucralfate treatment. HNO 1990;38:24–28.
9. Samaranayake LP, Robertson AG, MacFarlane TW, et al. The effect of chlorhexidine and benzydamine mouthwashes on mucositis induced by therapeutic irradiation. Clin Radiol 1988;39:291–294.
10. Lever SA, Dupuis LL, Chan SL. Comparative evaluation of benzydamine oral rinse in children with antineoplastic-induced stomatitis. Drug Intell Clin Pharm 1987;21:359–361.
11. Epstein JB, Stevenson-Moore P, Jackson S, et al. Prevention of oral mucositis in radiation therapy: A controlled study with benzydamine hydrochloride rinse. Int J Oncol Biol Phys 1989;16:1571–1575.
12. Tanner NS, Stanford IF, Bennett A. Plasma prostaglandins in mucositis due to radiotherapy and chemotherapy for head and neck cancer. Br J Cancer 1981;43:767–771.
13. Pillsbury HC, Webster WP, Rosenman J. Prostaglandin inhibitor and radiotherapy in advanced head and neck cancer. Arch Otolaryngol Head Neck Surg 1986;112:552–553.
14. Portender H, Rausch E, Kment G, et al. Local prostaglandin E2 in patients with oral malignancies undergoing chemo- and radiotherapy. J Craniomaxillofac Surg 1988;16:371–374.
15. Matejka M, Nell A, Kment G, et al. Local benefit of prostaglandin E2 in radiochemotherapy-induced oral mucositis. J Craniomaxillofac Surg 1990;28:89–91.
16. Spijkervet FK, Van Saere HK, Van Saene JJ, et al. Effect of selective elimination of the oral flora on mucositis in irradiated head and neck cancer patients. J Surg Oncol 1991;46:167–173.
17. Spijkervet FK, Van Saere HK, Van Saene JJ, et al. Mucositis prevention by selective elimination of the oral flora in irradiated head and neck cancer patients. J Oral Pathol Med 1990;19:486–489.
18. Shannon IL, Starche EN, Wescott WB. Effect of radiotherapy on whole saliva flow. J Dent Res 1977;56:693.
19. Baker DG. The radiobiological basis for tissue reactions in the oral cavity following therapeutic x-irradiation. Arch Otolaryngol 1982;108:21–24.
20. Engelmeier RL, King GE. Complications of head and neck radiation therapy and their management. J Prosthet Dent 1983;49:514–522.
21. Eneroth Cm, Henrikson CO, Jakobson PA. Effects of fractionated radiotherapy on salivary gland function. Cancer 1972;30:1147–1153.
22. Karmiol M, Walsh RF. Dental caries after radiotherapy of the oral regions. J Am Dent Assoc 1975;91:838–845.
23. Shannon IL, Tordahl JN, Starcke EN. Remineralization of enamel by saliva substitute designed for use by irradiated patients. Cancer 1978;41:1746–1750.
24. Greenspan D, Daniels TE. Effectiveness of pilocarpine in postradiation xerostomia. Cancer 1987;59:1123–1125.
25. Fox PC, Vander Ven PF, Baum BJ, et al. Pilocarpine for the treatment of xerostomia associated with salivary gland dysfunction. Oral Surg Oral Med Oral Pathol 1986;61:243–248.
26. Keys HM, McCasland JP. Techniques and results of a comprehensive dental care program in head and neck cancer patients. Int J Radiat Oncol Biol Phys 1976;1:859–865.
27. Keene HJ, Fleming TJ. Prevalence of caries-associated microflora after radiotherapy in patients with cancer of the head and neck. Oral Surg 1987;64:421–426.
28. MacCarthy-Leventhal EM. Postradiation mouth-blindness. Lancet 1959;2:1138–1139.
29. Epstein JB, Wong FL, Stevenson-Moore P. Osteoradionecrosis: Clinical experience and a proposal for classification. J Oral Maxillofac Surg 1987;45:104–110.
30. Murray CG, Herson J, Daly TE, et al. Radiation necrosis of the mandible: A 10-year study. Part 1. Factors influencing the onset of necrosis. Int J Radiat Oncol Biol Phys 1980;6:543–548.
31. Marx RE, Johnson RP. Studies in the radiobiology of osteoradionecrosis and their clinical significance. Oral Surg 1987;64:379–390.
32. Murray CG, Daly TE, Zimmerman SO. The relationship between dental disease and radiation necrosis of the mandible. Oral Surg 1980;49:99–104.
33. Levendag PC, Visch LL, Driver N. A simple device to protect against osteoradionecrosis induced by interstitial irradiation. J Prosthet Dent 1990;63:665–670.
34. Murray CG, Herson J, Daly TE, et al. Radiation necrosis of the mandible: A 10-year study. Part II. Dental factors: Onset, duration and management of necrosis. Int J Radiat Oncol Biol Phys 1980;6:549–553.
35. Marciani RD, Plezia RA. Management of teeth in the irradiated patient. J Am Dent Assoc 1974;88:1021–1024.
36. Markitziu A, Heling I. Endodontic treatment of patients who have undergone irradiation of the head and neck. Oral Surg 1981;52:294–297.
37. Mansfield MJ, Saunders DW, Heimbadi RD, et al. Hyperbaric oxygen as an adjunct in the treatment of osteoradionecrosis of the mandible. J Oral Surg 1981;39:585–589.
38. Sonis ST, Sonis AL, Lieberman A. Oral complications in patients receiving treatment for malignancies other than of the head and neck. J Am Dent Assoc 1978;97:468–472.
39. Sonis AL, Sonis ST. Oral complications of cancer chemotherapy in pediatric patients. J Pedodontics 1979;3:122–128.
40. Dreizen S, McCredie KB, Bodey GPN, et al. Quantitative analysis of the oral complications of antileukemic chemotherapy. Oral Surg 1986;62:650–653.
41. Bodey GP. Oral manifestations of myeloproliferative diseases. Postgrad Med 1971;49:115–121.
42. Lockhart PB, Sonis ST. Relationship of oral complications to peripheral blood leukocyte and platelet counts in patients receiving cancer chemotherapy. Oral Surg 1979;48:21–28.
43. Baraket NJ, Toto PD, Choukas NC. Aging and cell renewal of oral epithelium. J Periodontol 1969;40:599–602.
44. Peterson DW, Overholser CD. Increased morbidity associated with oral infection in patients with acute leukemia. Oral Surg 1982;53:32–36.
45. Greenberg MS, Cohen SG, McKifrick JC, et al. The oral flora as a source of septicemia in patients with acute leukemia. Oral Surg 1982;53:32–36.
46. Overholser CD, Peterson DE, William SL, et al. Periodontal infection in patients with acute nonlymphocytic leukemia: Prevalence of acute exacerbations. Arch Intern Med 1982;14:551–554.
47. Beck S. Impact of a systemic oral care protocol on stomatitis after chemotherapy. Cancer News 1979;2:185–199.
48. Epstein JB. Infection prevention in bone marrow transplantation and radiation patients. NCI Monograph 1990;9:73–85.
49. Hickey AJ, Toth BB, Lindquist SB. Effect of intravenous hyperalimentation and oral care on the development of oral stomatitis during cancer chemotherapy. J Prosthet Dent 1982;47:188–193.
50. Dreizen S, Bodey GP, Rodriquez V. Oral complications of cancer chemotherapy. Postgrad Med 1975;58:95.
51. Sonis S, Kunz A. Impact of improved dental services on the frequency of oral complications for patients with non-head and neck malignancies. Oral Surg Oral Med Oral Pathol 1988;65:19–21.
52. Dreizen S. Stomatotoxic manifestations of cancer chemotherapy. J Prosthet Dent 1978;40:650–655.
53. Volger W, Huguley C, Kerr W. Toxicity and antitumor effect of divided doses of methotrexate. Arch Intern Med 1965;115:285–293.
54. Woo SB, Sonis ST, Sonis AL. Oral herpes simplex virus infection in bone marrow transplant recipients. Cancer 1990;66:2375–2379.
55. Guggenheimer J, Verbin RS, Appel BN, et al. Clinicopathologic effects of cancer chemotherapeutic agents on human buccal mucosa. Oral Surg 1977;44:58–63.
56. Lockhart PB, Sonis ST. Alterations in the oral mucosa caused by chemotherapeutic agents. J Dermatol Surg Oncol 1981;7:1019–1025.
57. Aker SN. Oral findings in the cancer patient. Cancer 1979;43:2102–2107.
58. Mahood D, Dose AM, Loprinzi C, et al. Inhibition of fluorouracil-induced stomatitis by oral cryotherapy. J Clin Oncol 1991;9:449–452.
60. Clark PI, Slevin ML. Allopurinol mouthwash and 5-fluorouracil induced oral toxicity. Eur J Surg Oncol 1985;11:267–268.
61. Tsavaris N, Caragiauris P, Kosmidis P. Reduction of oral toxicity of 5-fluorouracil by allopurinol mouthwashes. Eur J Surg Oncol 1988;14:405–406.
62. Mills EE. The modifying effect of beta-carotene on radiation and chemotherapy induced oral mucositis. Br J Cancer 1988;57:416–417.
63. Bonilla MA, Gillio AP, Ruggeiro M, et al. Effects of recombinant human granulocyte colony-stimulating factor on neutropenia in patients with congenital agranulocytosis. N Engl J Med 1989;320:1574–1580.
64. Gabrilove JL, Jakubowski A, Scher H, et al. Effect of granulocyte colony-stimulating factor on neutropenia and associated morbidity due to chemotherapy for transitional-cell carcinoma of the urothelium. N Engl J Med 1988;318:1414–1422.
65. Sonis ST. Personal communication, 1992.
66. Rosenthal S, Kaufman S. Vincristine neurotoxicity. Ann Intern Med 1974;80:733–734.
67. EORTC International Antimicrobial Therapy Project Group. Three antibiotic regimens in the treatment of infection in febrile granulocytopenic patients with cancer. J Infect Dis 1978;137:14–29.
68. Dreizen S, Brown LR. Oral microbial changes and infections during cancer chemotherapy. In: Peterson DE, Sonis ST, eds. Oral complications of cancer chemotherapy. Boston: Martinus-Nijhoff, 1983:41–47.
69. Bodey GP. Fungal infections complicating acute leukemia. J Chronic Dis 1966;19:667–687.

70. Peterson DE: Bacterial infections: Periodontal and dental disease. In: Peterson DE, Sonis ST, eds. Oral complications of cancer chemotherapy. Boston: Martinus-Nijhoff, 1983:113–149.
71. Peterson DE, Minah GE, Overholser CD, et al. Microbiology of acute periodontal infection in myelosuppressed cancer patients. Clin Oncol 1987;5:1461–1468.
72. Lockhart PB. Dental management of patients receiving chemotherapy. In: Peterson DE, Sonis ST, eds. Oral complications of cancer chemotherapy. Boston: Martinus-Nijhoff, 1983:113–149.
73. Overholser CD, Peterson DE, Bergman SA. Dental extractions in patients with leukemia. J Oral Surg 1982;40:296–298.
74. Williford SK, Salisbury PL, Peacock JE, et al. The safety of dental extractions in patients with hematologic malignancies. J Clin Oncol 1989;7:798–802.
75. Epstein JB, Pearsall NN, Truelove EL. Oral candidiasis: Effects of antifungal therapy upon clinical signs and symptoms, salivary antibody and mucosal adherence of Candida albicans. Oral Surg 1981;51:32–36.
76. Taschdjian CL, Kosinn PH, Toni EF. Opportunistic yeast infections with special reference to candidiasis. Ann NY Acad Sci 1970;174:606–622.
77. Pizzuto J, Conte G, Aviles A, et al. Nystatin prophylaxis in leukemia and lymphoma. N Engl J Med 1978;299:661–662.
78. Carpentieri U, Haggard ME, Lockhart LH, et al. Clinical experience in preventions of candidiasis by nystatin in children with acute leukemia. J Pediatr 1978;92:593–595.
79. Gombert ME, duBouchet L, Aulicino TM, et al. A comparative trial of clotrimazole troches and oral nystatin suspension in recipients of renal transplants: Use in prophylaxis of oropharyngeal candidiasis. JAMA 1987;258:2553–2555.
80. Jones JM. Necrotizing Candida esophagitis: Failure of symptoms and roentgenographic findings to reflect severity. JAMA 1980;244:2190–2191.
81. Saral R, Burns WH, Laskin OL, et al. Acyclovir prophylaxis of herpes simplex virus infections. N Engl J Med 1981;305:63–67.
82. Wade JC, Newton B, McLaren C, et al. Intravenous acyclovir to treat mucocutaneous herpes simplex virus infection after marrow transplantation: A double blind trial. Ann Intern Med 1982;96:265–269.
83. Wade JC, Day LM, Crowley JJ, et al. Recurrent infection with herpes simplex virus after marrow transplantation: Role of specific immune response and acyclovir treatment. J Infect Dis 1984;149:750–756.
84. Saral R, Burns WH, Prentice HG:.Herpes virus infections. Clinical manifestations and therapeutic strategies in immunocompromised patients. Clin Haematol 1984;13:645–660.
85. Montgomery MT, Redding SW, LeMaistre CF. The incidence of oral herpes simplex virus infection in patients undergoing cancer chemotherapy. Oral Surg 1986;61:238–242.
86. Ferretti GA, Ash RC, Brown AT, et al. Chlorhexidine in prophylaxis against oral infections and associated complications in patients receiving bone marrow transplantation. J Am Dent Assoc 1987;114:292–294.
87. Stafford R, Lockhart P, Sonis ST, et al. Hemotologic parameters as predictors of oral involvement in the presentation of acute leukemia. J Oral Med 1982;37:38–41.
88. Lynch MA, Ship II. Initial oral manifestations of leukemia. J Am Dent Assoc 1977;75:932–940.

SECTION 7

CLAUDIA A. SEIPP

Hair Loss

Alopecia is a psychologically distressing yet common side effect of many chemotherapeutic agents and radiation therapy. As patients embark on new therapies, hair loss can induce a negative body image, alter interpersonal relationships, and arouse enough anxiety to cause some patients to reject potentially curative treatment.

Frank discussion of the problem by clinicians and oncology nurses with recognition of the patient's stress is helpful in preparing the patient to confront this loss.[1] Although methods for the prevention of total-scalp hair loss and the use of wigs after hair loss are not entirely satisfactory for all patients, caregivers can offer psychological support and some practical suggestions. Often, the presence of a spouse, family member, or friend during this discussion helps the patient to place the problem in perspective.

The hair loss caused by scalp irradiation is unpredictable. Epilation can begin at doses of 500 cGy and generally progresses with spotty areas of baldness as the course of treatment continues. The prospects for hair regrowth diminish with increasing doses.[2] Radiation ports on extremities have been noted to be hair-free 10 years after radiation therapy and may never have hair regrowth. In lower-dose ranges, regrowth begins 8 to 9 weeks after cessation of therapy. Patients should be cautioned that the new hair may be different in character from the pretreatment hair.[3]

The extent of body hair loss by patients in any chemotherapeutic program is both drug- and dose-dependent and is related to the frequency of cycle repetition. Often, it is caused by more than one drug used in combination (Table 63–21).[4] Long-term therapy may result in loss of pubic, axillary, and facial hair in addition to scalp hair. It should be emphasized to patients that alopecia from chemotherapy is reversible, with hair regeneration beginning 1 to 2 months after therapy is discontinued. Alteration in color and texture of hair may occur; hair may be a lighter or darker shade and is often curlier as it regrows.[5] Hair loss may begin 1 to 2 weeks after a single chemotherapeutic dose and reaches maximal loss within 2 months in most drug sequences. Doxorubicin and cyclophosphamide are common cytologic agents known to cause epilation after two cycles at doses of doxorubicin above 50 mg/m^2 and cyclophosphamide above 500 mg/m^2. Although agents differ in degree to which they cause hair loss, alopecia may be expected with other single-agent antibiotics, alkylating agents, nitrosoureas, and especially their combinations.[6]

HEAD COVERINGS

Most patients choose to cover their heads during periods of hair loss. Nurses and clinicians can suggest wigs or other head coverings such as stylish scarves, turbans, or hats. Wigs should be selected before hair loss begins so that the patient is prepared when alopecia occurs and so that hair color and style can be matched. Hairpieces are tax-deductable medical expenses and are covered by some medical insurance policies. Several small private businesses have been developed by former patients who distribute or sell head coverings of various designs. An American Cancer Society rehabilitation program called "Look Good, Feel Better" was developed specifically to assist women in compensating for hair loss and skin changes during cancer treatment.[7] Volunteer beauticians and cosmetologists help women look and feel more comfortable with changes in their appearance, such as dry, discolored, or blotching skin; discolored nails; and alopecia. Information is available through an American Cancer Society hotline (telephone number, 1-800-395-LOOK).

PREVENTION OF ALOPECIA

Since 1966, interventions have been proposed to prevent scalp hair loss from chemotherapy. The rationale for these procedures is to prevent drug circulation to the hair follicles by causing temporary vasoconstriction with either an occlusive

TABLE 63–21. Single Agents With Potential to Induce Reversible Alopecia*

Amsacrine	5-Fluorouracil
Bleomycin	Hydroxyurea
Cyclophosphamide	Ifosfamide
Dactinomycin	Methotrexate
Daunorubicin	Mitomycin
Doxorubicin	Melphalan
Epirubicin	Taxol
Etoposide	Vinblastine
Vincristine	

* The degree or onset of alopecia is dependent on dose, schedule of sequences, rate of delivery, route of delivery, and various combinations of agents.[4]

scalp tourniquet or localized hypothermia. The pharmacokinetics of the drugs to be used must be understood before either of these methods is considered. Occlusion of the superficial scalp veins must begin before the drugs are given and, to be effective, must be extended beyond the time of the peak plasma drug levels.[8–10]

Various types of scalp icing devices have been manufactured by several different U.S. companies. Although the Food and Drug Administration (FDA) had initially approved the marketing of cooling caps intended to cause localized scalp hypothermia, the FDA reviewed these applications early in 1990 and became concerned that the safety and efficacy of these devices had not been substantiated by adequate clinical data.[4,11–14] Regulatory action was initiated to address the following concerns:

1. The potential for scalp metastasis posed by the use of these devices
2. The potential for reducing drug circulation to other anatomic sites beyond the scalp, such as the skull and possibly the brain
3. The effectiveness of these devices in preventing hair loss and how specific cytologic doses and other variables affected the results achieved

The FDA halted the commercial distribution of these devices, and a year after their withdrawal, no company had come forward with supporting clinical evidence of reasonable safety and effectiveness.[15]

The safety limitations and inconclusive and conflicting reports of the usefulness of scalp hypothermia should be discussed with patients seeking information about these devices and hair preservation techniques.[16]

REFERENCES

1. Wagner L, Bye MG. Body image and patients experiencing alopecia as a result of cancer chemotherapy. Cancer Nurs 1979;2(5):365–369.
2. Moss WT, Brand WN, Battiford H. Radiation oncology: Rationale, techniques, results. 5th ed. St. Louis: CV Mosby, 1979:57–58.
3. Nordstrom RE, Holsti LR. Hair transplantation in alopecia due to radiation. Plast Reconstr Surg 1983;72:454–458.
4. Keller JF, Blausey LA. Nursing issues and management in chemotherapy-induced alopecia. Oncol Nurs Forum 1988;15:5, 603–607.
5. Cancer, cancer therapy, and hair. Lancet [Editorial] 1983;2:1177–1178.
6. Cline BW. Prevention of chemotherapy-induced alopecia: A review of the literature. Cancer Nurs 1984;7:221–228.
7. American Cancer Society Hotline. Personal communication, telephone 1-800-395-LOOK.
8. Dean JC, Salmon SE, Griffith KS. Prevention of doxorubicin-induced hair loss with scalp hypothermia. N Engl J Med 1979;302:1427–1429.
9. Satterwaite B, Zimm S. The use of scalp hypothermia in the prevention of doxorubicin-induced hair loss. Cancer 1984;54:34–37.
10. Robinson MH, Jones AC, Durant KD. Effectiveness of scalp cooling in reducing scalp alopecia caused by epirubicin treatment in breast cancer. Cancer Treat Rep 1987;71:913–914.
11. Middleton J, Franks D, Buchanan RB, et al. Failure of scalp hypothermia to prevent hair loss when cyclophosphamide is added to doxorubicin and vincristine. Cancer Treat Rep 1985;69:373–375.
12. Wheelock JB, Myers MB, Krebs HB, et al. Ineffectiveness of scalp hypothermia in the prevention of alopecia in patients treated with doxorubicin and cis-platin combinations. Cancer Treat Rep 1984;68:1387–1388.
13. Seipp CA. Scalp hypothermia: Indicators for precaution. Oncol Nurs Forum [Letter] 1983;10:12.
14. Whitman G, Cadman E, Chen M. Misuse of scalp hypothermia. Cancer Treat Rep 1981;65:507–508.
15. Harson C. Personal communication. November 1991.
16. Camp-Sorrell D. Scalp hypothermia devices: Current status. ONS News 1991;7:1.

SECTION 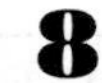

RICHARD J. SHERINS

Gonadal Dysfunction

Accompanying the success of cytotoxic chemotherapy in the treatment of cancer and nonmalignant disorders are new concerns for the long-term toxic effects of these therapies on normal host tissues. Although many of the acute and chronic toxicities of antineoplastic drugs have been well defined, comparatively little attention has been paid to gonadal dysfunction resulting from antitumor therapy. In part, this lack of attention has stemmed from the absence of any immediate or life-threatening symptoms resulting from gonadal injury; and, until recently, it has reflected the absence of a group of long-term cancer survivors who are concerned about their reproductive potential.

Neoplastic disease and its treatment can potentially interfere with any of the cellular, anatomic, physiologic, behavioral, or social processes that contribute to normal sexual and reproductive function. The tumor may directly involve the gonad, and cancer surgery itself may require incidental gonadectomy. For the male, genital mutilation or retroperitoneal lymph node dissection can result in failure of emission, retrograde ejaculation, loss of orgasm, and impotence (Table 63–22). Many drugs used in the treatment of cancer have profound and lasting effects on gonadal function. Both germ cell production and endocrine function may be affected. The magnitude of the effect varies with the drug class, the total dose administered, and the age and pubertal status of the patient at the time of therapy. Radiation therapy can also result in germ cell depletion and clinical hypogonadism, and, as with chemotherapeutic drugs, can induce mutagenic effects in the germ cell and teratogenic effects in the fetus. Recent evidence from rodent studies suggests that direct drug effects on sperm, as well as seminal transmission to the female of drugs administered to the male, may have adverse effects on the developing fetus and embryo without affecting male fer-

TABLE 63–22. Reproductive Consequences of Cancer and Cancer Therapy

Tumor	Direct gonadal involvement
	Hypothalamic and pituitary involvement
Surgery	Removal of gonad
	Neurogenic dysfunction
	Failure of emission
	Retrograde ejaculation
	Loss of orgasm
	Impotence
	Genital mutilation
Therapy	Germ cell depletion
	Clinical hypogonadism
	Mutagenic changes in germ cell
	Teratogenic effects on fetus
	Seminal transmission of drug

tility.[1,2] The reproductive consequences of cancer chemotherapy are drug-specific, dose-dependent, age-related, sex-dependent, and species-specific.

A separate category of effects concerns social and behavioral responses to the disruptions of cancer and its therapy. The nature of the patient's illness, the extent of necessary surgery, chemotherapy, or radiation therapy, and the patient's relationship with spouse and family all may play an important role in reestablishing normal sexual interest and function after treatment for cancer. Detailed reviews of the reproductive consequences of cancer and cancer therapy are available.[3–8]

CHEMOTHERAPY EFFECTS IN ADULT MEN

CLINICAL PATHOPHYSIOLOGY

Testicular function in adult men is particularly susceptible to injury by many chemotherapeutic agents. The primary histopathologic lesion produced by the drugs is one of progressive, dose-related depletion of the germinal epithelium lining the seminiferous tubule.[9–15] Frequently, the germinal tissue disappears completely, and only the supporting Sertoli cells remain lining the tubular lumen, a state described as *germinal aplasia.* The Leydig cells remain morphologically intact, although they may be functionally abnormal.

The clinical manifestations of germinal depletion (Table 63–23) are a marked reduction in testicular volume (atrophy), reduction in sperm count (oligospermia or azoospermia), and infertility. Because the gonad regulates pituitary gonadotropin secretion, serum follicle-stimulating hormone (FSH) and luteinizing hormone (LH) levels reflect the state of the seminiferous epithelium (Fig. 63–9). Germinal aplasia results in a fivefold increase in serum FSH levels (Fig. 63–10); and partial germinal depletion results in a lesser increase in FSH concentration.[16] By contrast, serum LH and testosterone levels tend to remain within normal limits in the presence of germinal depletion. The serum FSH level serves as a convenient marker for testicular germ cell loss. The changes in FSH are attributed to loss of inhibin, a peptide released from the Sertoli cells lining the seminiferous tubules of the testis, which normally inhibits FSH release from the pituitary.[7] Administration of hypothalamic gonadotropin-releasing hormone to patients with germinal aplasia results in an exaggerated LH response, however, suggestive of subtle Leydig's cell failure.[17] Furthermore, men with germinal aplasia, who maintain normal plasma LH and total testosterone concentrations, have been shown to have a 50% reduction in the amount of testosterone produced and in the level of circulating free testosterone[18] (see Table 63–23). This decrease in Leydig's cell function may account for the "selective" increase in plasma FSH level since, in steroid-replaced castrated male rats, it has been shown that high FSH levels accompanied by normal LH levels can be induced when testosterone is replaced at subphysiologic levels in association with high estradiol administration.[19]

SINGLE AGENTS

The anticancer agents most commonly associated with testicular germ cell depletion are listed in Table 63–24. Studies

TABLE 63–23. Evaluation of Gonadal Function in Men After Cancer Therapy

A. Sexual History
1. Pretreatment fertility history of both partners
2. Developmental: age of testicular descent, pubertal age, congenital anomalies of urinary tract or central nervous system
3. Surgical: orchiopexy, pelvic or retroperitoneal surgery, injury to genitals, spinal cord injury
4. Medical: venereal disease, mumps, renal disease, diabetes, epididymitis, tuberculosis, or other chronic illnesses
5. Drugs: many drugs interfere with spermatogenesis, erection, and ejaculation

B. Clinical and Laboratory Features of Germinal Aplasia

	Testis Size			*Hormone Profile*				
	Length × Width (cm)	*Volume (cc)*	*Sperm Count (million/ml)*	*FSH (mIU/ml)*	*LH (mIU/ml)*	*Testosterone (ng/100 ml)*	*Testosterone Production Rate (mg/d)*	*Free Testosterone (ng/100 ml)*
Normal men	5.0 × 3.0	16–30	20–100	4–25	4–20	250–1200	7.5	15.3
Germinal aplasia	3.7 × 2.3	8–15	0	25–90	8–25	200–700	3.5	8.6

FSH, follicle-stimulating hormone; LH, luteinizing hormone.

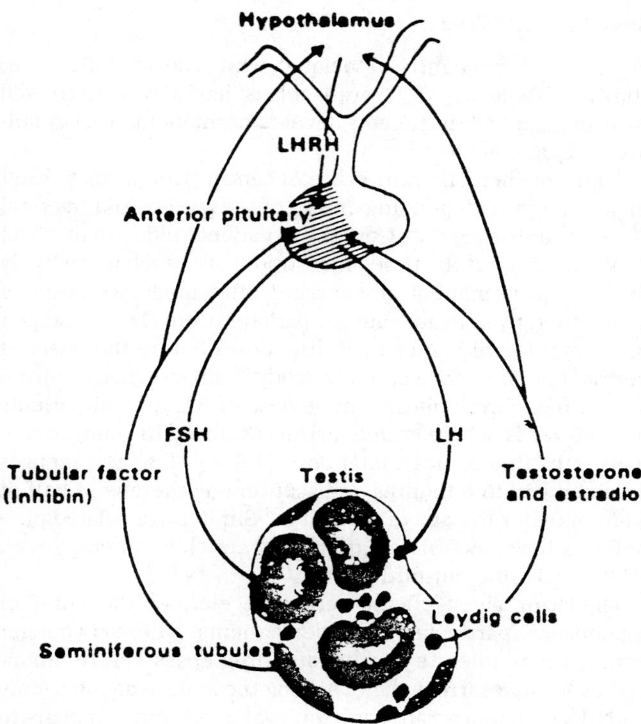

FIGURE 63–9. Hypothalamic-pituitary-testicular interrelations. Notice that leutinizing hormone (LH) acts primarily on Leydig's cells, whereas follicle-stimulating hormone (FSH) primarily affects the seminiferous tubules. LHRH, leutinizing hormone releasing hormone. (Sherins RJ, Winters SJ. Management of disorders of the testis. In: Melmon K, Morelli HP, eds. Clinical pharmacology: Basic principles and therapeutics. 2nd ed. New York: Macmillan, 1978:582)

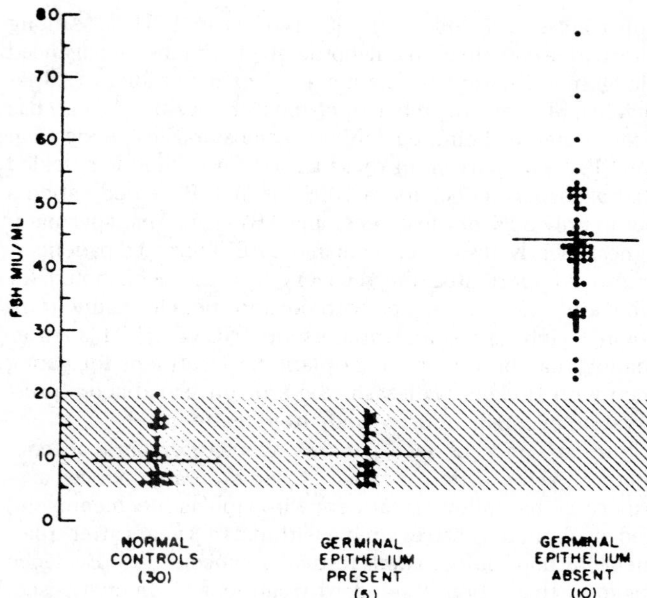

FIGURE 63–10. Serum follicle-stimulating hormone (FSH) levels in normal men and in men with germinal aplasia. (Van Thiel DH, Sherins RJ, Myers GH, et al. Evidence for a specific seminiferous tubular factor affecting follicle-stimulating hormone secretion in man. J Clin Invest 1972;51:1009–1019)

of men receiving single alkylating agents for lymphoma have been a major source of information about drug-related infertility. During alkylating agent therapy, the seminiferous epithelium is depleted in a dose-related fashion. Progressive but reversible oligospermia occurs in men receiving up to 400 mg of chlorambucil, whereas azoospermia and germinal aplasia occur in those patients treated with cumulative doses in excess of 400 mg.[12] Similarly, germinal aplasia is uncommon in patients receiving less than 6 to 10 g of cyclophosphamide.[9–15] Vinblastine, doxorubicin, procarbazine, and cisplatin have all been implicated as being toxic to the germinal epithelium in both animals and humans[13,20–23] although specific dose-toxicity relations have not been established for these drugs. Prospective evaluation of the effects of these and other single agents on testicular function is required to establish reliable data concerning the threshold drug dose above which seminiferous tubular damage becomes irreversible.

COMBINATION CHEMOTHERAPY

Combination drug regimens have a profound impact on spermatogenesis. The effects of nitrogen mustard, vincristine, procarbazine, and prednisone (MOPP) have been most carefully investigated, and it is clear that more than 80% of men receiving this regimen develop testicular atrophy, azoospermia, and elevated serum FSH levels resulting from germinal aplasia.[24–31] Procarbazine leads to particularly long-lasting testicular damage. Indeed, this drug alone induces germinal aplasia in adult male monkeys.[21]

Whereas the combination of MOPP and cyclophosphamide, vincristine, procarbazine, and prednisone (COPP)[32] produces irreversible germinal aplasia in most patients, this may not be true of other multimodal regimens in use.[33–36] Cyclophosphamide and doxorubicin, when used as adjuvant chemotherapy for soft tissue sarcoma, appear to produce irreversible testicular damage only in men over 40 years of age or in men receiving concomitant irradiation proximal to the gonads. Similar drug doses administered to younger patients produce

TABLE 63–24. Antitumor Agents Associated With Testicular Germ Cell Depletion

Degree of Risk	*Drug*
Definite	Chlorambucil
	Cyclophosphamide
	Nitrogen mustard
	Busulfan
	Procarbazine
	Nitrosoureas
Probable	Doxorubicin
	Vinblastine
	Cytosine arabinoside
	Cisplatin
Unlikely	Methotrexate
	5-Fluorouracil
	6-Mercaptopurine
	Vincristine
Unknown	Bleomycin

only transient, reversible elevations of serum FSH.[33,36] Among alternative combination chemotherapy regimens for advanced Hodgkin's disease, the combination of doxorubicin (Adriamycin), bleomycin, vinblastine, and dacarbazine (ABVD) has been touted as being equally efficacious and less toxic than MOPP. A comparison of these treatment regimens revealed that azoospermia occurs in 100% of MOPP-treated patients but in only 35% of those receiving ABVD and that spermatogenesis nearly always recovers in the ABVD-treated patients.[37] Improved spermatogenic recovery has also been noted for Hodgkin's patients treated with novantrone, vincristine (Oncovin), vinblastine, and prednisone (NOVP).[38] This information may be important in planning treatment for young men with Hodgkin's disease who are concerned about preservation of fertility during and after treatment.

Similar concerns face patients about to embark on chemotherapy for testicular cancer. Chemotherapy-induced azoospermia that follows treatment with vinblastine, bleomycin, and cisplatin may be reversible within 2 to 3 years after treatment for nonseminomatous testicular cancer.[23,39–44] Evidence suggests that when a standard treatment regimen is used, sperm count and semen quality recover 2 to 3 years after treatment in about half of patients, and these patients are capable of impregnating their partners. Importantly, about 75% of men with nonseminomatous testicular cancer have severely impaired sperm count and semen quality before chemotherapy is instituted[39–44]; and in about 40% of subjects, emission, ejaculation, and sexual function are compromised after retroperitoneal lymph node dissection.[45–47] These observations complicate interpretation of fertility status after therapy. In addition, some men with testicular cancer have been cryptorchid, which predisposes to infertility even when testicular nondescent is unilateral.[7]

CHEMOTHERAPY EFFECTS IN ADULT WOMEN

An assessment of the impact of cancer chemotherapy on ovarian function has been hampered by the relative inaccessibility of the ovary to biopsy and the resultant inability to obtain reliable estimates of the size of the germ cell population. Therefore, one must rely primarily on menstrual and reproductive history and on determinations of serum hormone levels to assess the functional status of the ovary.

CLINICAL PATHOPHYSIOLOGY

Examination of the ovaries of women who have developed chemotherapy-related ovarian failure frequently reveals arrest of follicular maturation or frank destruction of ova and follicles.[48–50] Clinically, these patients become amenorrheic and may complain of menopausal symptoms of estrogen deficiency such as "hot flashes," vaginal dryness, and dyspareunia. Abnormally low circulating estrogen levels result in marked elevation of serum FSH and LH, a manifestation of the loss of feedback inhibition of gonadotropin secretion consequent to drug-induced primary ovarian failure.

SINGLE AGENTS

Drugs most frequently associated with ovarian failure are shown in Table 63–25. Overall, at least half of women treated with single alkylating agents develop permanent ovarian failure and amenorrhea.[48–55]

Adjuvant chemotherapy in breast cancer patients may result in amenorrhea, depending on age of the patient and the total dose administered.[56,57] Generally, patients older than 35 to 40 years of age at the time of treatment are much more likely to develop permanent amenorrhea after moderate doses of chemotherapy than are younger patients. Conversely, younger patients tolerate higher total drug doses before the onset of permanent amenorrhea. In one study,[58] amenorrhea occurred after a mean cyclophosphamide dose of 5.2 g in all patients over 40 years, whereas amenorrhea occurred in younger subjects only after a mean total dose of 9.3 g. Further, menses resumed within 6 months of discontinuing therapy in half of women under the age of 40 years.[58] Similar age-related phenomena have been noted after adjuvant chemotherapy with L-phenylalanine mustard.[59]

Alkylating agent chemotherapy accelerates the onset of menopause, particularly in older patients, whereas younger patients may tolerate higher total drug doses before amenorrhea becomes irreversible. Among the antimetabolites, only high-dose methotrexate has been evaluated, and it appears to have no immediate ovarian toxicity.[60]

COMBINATION CHEMOTHERAPY

Most available information concerning the effects of combination chemotherapy regimens on ovarian function has come from the study of women receiving MOPP for Hodgkin's disease. Unlike the profound effects of this regimen on testicular function, MOPP produces ovarian dysfunction and amenorrhea in only 40% to 50% of treated women.[61–67] The frequency of ovarian injury is related to the age of the patient at the time of treatment, with persistent amenorrhea occurring much more commonly in subjects older than 35 to 40 years of age. Ovarian dysfunction in younger patients appears to be

TABLE 63–25. Antitumor Agents Associated With Ovarian Dysfunction

Degree of Risk	*Drug*
Definite	Cyclophosphamide
	L-Phenylalanine mustard
	Busulfan
	Nitrogen mustard
Unlikely	Methotrexate
	5-Fluorouracil
	6-Mercaptopurine
Unknown	Doxorubicin
	Bleomycin
	Vinca alkaloids
	Cisplatin
	Nitrosoureas
	Cytosine arabinoside

related to the total chemotherapy dose administered because permanent amenorrhea occurs in women receiving the highest cumulative drug doses. Although it is impossible to predict the effect of MOPP chemotherapy on ovarian function for any individual patient, it appears unlikely that those patients treated under age 25 will experience any significant therapy-related ovarian dysfunction during the initial 5 to 10 years after completion of treatment.[64-67] Continued long-term follow-up of women who maintain normal menses after chemotherapy will be necessary to determine whether these patients are still at risk for the development of premature ovarian failure and early menopause. Clinically, the current view is that changes in number of oocytes have little effect on the age of menopause until significant oocyte destruction is reached, and the rate of oocyte atresia is important.[68,68a]

CHEMOTHERAPY EFFECTS IN CHILDREN

Evaluation of the effects of chemotherapy on gonadal function in children is particularly complex because of the variables introduced by the continuum of sexual development present in this patient population. Knowledge of the pubertal status of the patient at the time of therapy and at the time of evaluation, along with recognition of the need to compare the results of hormonal evaluation with appropriate age-matched normal children, is required before definitive conclusions concerning drug effects can be drawn.

BOYS

Before the onset of puberty, the testicular germinal epithelium appears to be more resistant to moderate doses of alkylating agents than is the adult testis. Cyclophosphamide, in cumulative doses up to 20 g, produces only minor alterations in the testicular histology of prepubertal boys and no abnormalities in serum gonadotropin or testosterone levels.[69-71] At cumulative doses greater than 20 g, however, germinal aplasia has been documented.[72-74] Little information is available concerning the effects of other drugs on the immature testis, although recent data suggest that cytosine arabinoside and nitrosourea may be damaging to the germinal epithelium.[75,76]

Combination chemotherapeutic regimens have variable effects on reproductive function in boys. A commonly used antileukemic regimen, prednisone, 6-mercaptopurine, methotrexate, and vincristine, does not appear to cause damage to the testis in patients at any pubertal stage.[77] By contrast, MOPP administered to male patients during puberty appears to have profound effects on both germ cell production and endocrine function. After MOPP, gynecomastia, accompanied by elevation of both serum FSH and LH levels and by low normal serum testosterone levels, has been noted in many patients.[78,79] Testicular biopsy confirmed the occurrence of germinal aplasia in these patients. In contrast to prepubertal boys, some chemotherapy regimens administered during puberty may result in injury to Leydig's cells and the seminiferous epithelium, with gynecomastia being the clinical manifestation of this endocrine dysfunction. The reasons for the increased sensitivity to cytotoxic chemotherapy during puberty require further study.

GIRLS

Little information is available on the effects of cytotoxic drugs on the prepubertal and pubertal ovary. Postmortem studies of ovarian histology of girls treated with chemotherapy have revealed a spectrum of results ranging from normal histology to arrest of follicular maturation and frank ovarian destruction.[79-81] Most girls display impaired follicular maturation, although the total number of follicles is not reduced.[81] From clinical studies, delay in menarche or interruption of menses in girls treated with single-agent cyclophosphamide is uncommon.[70,74,82,83] Studies of girls with acute lymphocytic leukemia treated with vincristine, methotrexate, and 6-mercaptopurine have revealed normal ovarian function in more than 80% of patients.[84] It appears that the immature ovary is relatively insensitive to cytotoxic chemotherapy; however, follow-up of these patients will be required for many years to determine accurately the long-term effects of this therapy on reproductive potential.

RADIATION THERAPY

Radiation therapy plays a major role in the management of lymphoma, sarcoma, and other malignant diseases. Sometimes it is the only therapy, but varying strategies incorporating chemotherapeutic regimens are common. In considering the potential gonadal toxicity of radiation therapy, one must differentiate the consequences of radiation exposure from those that accrue from the chemotherapeutic agents administered. In contrast to the growing literature describing adverse effects of chemotherapy, there is a paucity of data concerning the effects of irradiation on gonadal function in humans. Furthermore, there are few data about the effects of age, gender, adjunctive chemotherapy, and fractionation of the radiation dose to gonadal toxicity.

MEN

The testis is highly radiosensitive, most likely because of rapid cell division of the germinal epithelium. There is limited discussion in the early literature of the effects of irradiation on testicular function of men receiving radiation therapy.[85,86] Until recently, there were few useful guides to the threshold dose for radiation damage to the human testis.[87-95] Studies of single-dose radiation exposure to normal volunteer men demonstrate a dose-dependent depletion and recovery of the germinal epithelium.[87,88] A marked but transient suppression of sperm production is evident with dosages as low as 15 cGy; transient aspermia is reported with doses of about 50 cGy, and more prolonged periods of aspermia are reported with higher doses. At 200 to 300 cGy, full recovery of sperm production requires 3 years; at 400 to 600 cGy, the interval is about 5 years; and above 600 cGy, sterility appears to be permanent. A recent assessment of the effects of conventionally fractionated irradiation on testicular function of men with Hodgkin's disease indicates that gonadal function is compromised at doses as low as 50 cGy, and that at 200 cGy, cumulative dose testicular dysfunction persists at least to 3 years.[94]

Unfortunately, there are no substantive studies of the effect of low-dose irradiation on testicular function in boys. In the few reports that appear, it is not possible to distinguish between the gonadal toxicity from chemotherapy and that caused by radiation therapy. In several recent studies, however, high doses of radiation (2400 cGy) delivered directly to the testes of boys with gonadal relapse from acute lymphoblastic leukemia produced marked testicular atrophy, with Leydig's cell impairment, androgen deficiency, and clinical hypogonadism.[96–98]

WOMEN

The medical literature is not adequate to counsel women precisely regarding the risks of ovarian dysfunction follow irradiation. There are only broad guidelines regarding the ovarian threshold. In comparison with men, gonadal exposure in women is complicated by the fact that the ovaries lie within the pelvis, often within the direct radiation beam, or considerably closer to major nodal areas where radiation scatter and beam leakage become critical. Although successful pregnancies have been reported after estimated fractionated ovarian doses of about 650 cGy, cessation of ovarian function is progressively more common with gonadal exposure above 150 cGy, and at 500 to 600 cGy, most women remain persistently amenorrheic.[99] Age is a significant factor in that women younger than age 20 have about a 70% chance of retaining regular cyclic menses after total nodal irradiation; whereas by age 30, only 20% of treated women retain normal ovarian function. Older women are virtually all sterile.[100,101] Existing data suggest that chemotherapy plus total nodal irradiation in women with Hodgkin's disease produces additive ovarian toxicity at any age.[100,101]

Further studies of the radiation dose received by the gonads during primary therapy to other sites are needed to determine the contribution to ovarian dysfunction and to define the circumstances under which repositioning or shielding of the ovary is necessary.

TECHNIQUES TO PROTECT FERTILITY

With the recognition that cytotoxic chemotherapy, radiation therapy, and surgery may destroy fertility has come increasing interest to protect the gonads from these adverse effects and to provide methods to store the germ cells for future use.

SUPPRESSION OF PITUITARY GONADOTROPIN

The subject of suppression of germ cell proliferation to prevent gonadal toxicity associated with cancer treatment is well discussed by Redman and Bajorunas.[102] Approaches to the suppression of gonadal function have included administration of testosterone in men,[103] oral contraceptives in women,[104] and hypothalamic gonadotropin-releasing hormone analogs in both men and women.[105] Unfortunately, none of these approaches has been proved effective despite encouraging preliminary results in experimental animals and humans.[106–111] Among the numerous possible factors contributing to these discrepancies is the fact that, in the human, there is usually inadequate time to suppress the germinal epithelium before instituting cancer therapy because of the urgency to treat the tumor as quickly as possible. Interspecies differences in response to pharmacologic manipulations are also well recognized.

TESTICULAR SHIELDING

Techniques to shield the testes from the direct radiation beam are employed during pelvic irradiation when the chance of gonadal injury may be high, but there have been few studies that accurately assess the dose received by the gonad when the treatment beam is directed to anatomically remote sites. Radiation scatter and leakage radiation can be important contributors to gonadal toxicity. For the testes, a threshold as low as 50 cGy, which is less than 1% of a typical treatment dose, means that use of a gonadal shield is required if the distance between the testes and the radiation field edge is less than 30 cm.[112] A simple and practical testicular shield has been developed for use near megavoltage radiation fields. This shield reduces testicular exposure to less than 10% of the patient's prescription dose; this effectively provides a threefold to tenfold reduction in testicular dose, depending on the distance from the field edge to the gonads.[113,114]

OOPHOROPEXY

For women, appropriate gonadal shielding is difficult because of the pelvic position of the ovary. Oophoropexy, a procedure by which the ovaries are surgically placed in the midline behind the uterus, appears to reduce ovarian exposure in about half women receiving pelvic irradiation.[99,115]

SPERM CRYOPRESERVATION

Pretreatment sperm banking is a reasonable approach to preservation of reproductive potential in some men undergoing sterilizing cancer therapy.[116–123] Unlike normal fertile donors whose semen is selected carefully for its subsequent excellent postthaw quality, pretreatment semen from cancer patients often shows both reduced sperm count (less than 20 million/ml) and poor motion characteristics (less than 50% motility). Analysis of semen in men with lymphoma or testicular cancer has shown that about half of patients have suboptimal semen quality before onset of treatment, which precludes cryobanking.[43,119–128]

Contributing factors that can impair semen quality include fever, stress, and the effects of systemic illness on pituitary gonadotropin release. In men with testicular cancer, there is often human chorionic gonadotropin secretion from the tumor, which stimulates increased estrogen production, which can also adversely affect the contralateral testis. Studies of pretreatment testicular function in patients with other malignancies are not yet available to determine if such adverse effects on semen quality are commonly seen with most cancers.

Cryobanking is feasible for men whose pretreatment semen has adequate numbers of reasonably motile cells; generally, more than 20 million/ml with at least 40% progressive motility is required to provide a postthaw specimen of adequate quality for subsequent insemination. For patients with a very low sperm count before cancer therapy, pooling of multiple specimens after freezing is frequently attempted but generally unsuccessful because quality of the postthaw specimen is actually more important than the total number of sperm. Freezing and thawing semen damages sperm and reduces semen quality below that present in the prebanked specimen.[129]

ASSISTED REPRODUCTIVE TECHNIQUES

For men, despite severe oligospermia after cancer treatment, fertility is often preserved and pregnancy achieved by coitus alone; such data are anecdotal. The key issue with return of a low count is retention of high-quality sperm.[130] Physicians can enhance fertility potential by artificial insemination of husband's sperm at the wife's midcycle LH surge. The technique of insemination is important as intrauterine placement of washed sperm appears to give a higher pregnancy rate than intracervical or intravaginal placement.[131] When there are a limited number of frozen specimens or the sperm count is severely reduced, the physician should consider using the sperm specimen for in vitro fertilization (IVF).[132] At IVF, insemination of eggs is usually performed with only 100,000 to 200,000 sperm and can be done with considerably fewer sperm under special conditions. Since multiple eggs are obtained during each IVF cycle, a single cryopreserved sperm specimen has many more eggs to fertilize than would be available if the specimen were used for an intrauterine insemination. In contrast to the egg, embryos can be frozen and subsequently thawed successfully for transfer at a later time.[133,134] IVF offers an important opportunity for both increased egg exposure and cryopreservation of supplemental embryos for a given limited sperm resource.

Assisted reproductive techniques can also be used in cancer patients before treatment is instituted with chemotherapy or radiation therapy. When time permits, IVF can be performed and resulting embryos cryopreserved. If increased estrogen exposure is contraindicated, such as in women undergoing treatment for breast cancer, an attempt can be made to wash out embryos from the uterus during several months of natural coitus and then to cryopreserve the embryos.[135,136] This approach is less efficient, however, because of a high rate of embryo loss in natural conception.[136]

MODIFIED NERVE-SPARING SURGERY

Retroperitoneal lymph node dissection commonly produces severe neurologic dysfunction in men, resulting in failure of emission, retrograde ejaculation, impotence, loss of orgasm, and infertility. Deliberate or inadvertent ligation of the hypogastric arteries may also result in vasculogenic impotence. These factors have stimulated renewed interest in modifying surgical procedures to reduce the adverse reproductive consequences of cancer surgery without diminishing its efficacy. Sexual function can now be preserved in 70% of men undergoing radical prostatectomy for localized prostate cancer[137,138] and in 83% of men undergoing radical cystoprostatectomy for invasive bladder cancer[139] by placing the incision in the lateral pelvic fascia more anteriorly above the neurovascular bundle supplying the penile corpora cavernosa.

Neural injury occurs in most men undergoing standard bilateral retroperitoneal lymph node dissection[45–47] for the staging and treatment of nonseminomatous germ cell tumors because of injury to the sympathetic innervation of the pelvic viscera. If the area surrounding the aortic bifurcation and sacral prominence is not disturbed, the final common pathways of the sympathetic innervation remain intact, and no neurologic deficit results. A modified bilateral node dissection sparing the final common sympathetic pathway is feasible without missing sites of potential nodal metastases[47] and allows about half of men to preserve ejaculatory function.[46,47] A modified unilateral retroperitoneal lymph node dissection preserves ejaculation in about 70% of men.[140–142]

ELECTROEJACULATION

The technique of electroejaculation, adopted from vast experience in veterinary practice, has been employed successfully to produce semen in neurologically impaired men.[143] From men with paraplegia[143,144] and in those with ejaculatory failure after retroperitoneal lymph node dissection,[145] it has been possible to collect semen of sufficient high quality to obtain pregnancies by insemination or IVF. Advances in sperm cryopreservation enhance the feasibility of using electroejaculation to obtain semen from such patients for subsequent use.

Retrograde ejaculation resulting from retroperitoneal lymph node dissection, however, can occasionally be treated successfully by administering adrenergic or anticholinergic drugs for several days to close the bladder neck.[7] Such treatment before a wife's midcycle ovulation can facilitate pregnancy by coitus. Additionally, sperm can be retrieved from a postejaculatory urine, washed, and then used as an inseminate.[7] If these simple approaches fail, then electroejaculation under anesthesia is a reasonable alternative.

GENETIC CONCERNS

The agents used to treat cancer are specifically designed to interfere with DNA, cellular metabolism, and cell division; hence, there is good reason to suspect that they may cause mutation and genetic disease in humans.[146]

Standard assays in the mouse at the Oak Ridge National Laboratory[147] show a linear dose-response curve for ionizing radiation as a cause of germ cell genetic damage at several loci. The Oak Ridge Laboratory has generated the experimental results used to set guidelines for radiation protection, specifically for germ cell effects in human populations. The data are based on just a few loci in a laboratory species that may not reflect directly the sensitivity of the human organism. For example, species may differ in their capacities to repair damage to germ cell DNA after environmental exposures.

Cancer treatments certainly cause genetic damage to somatic cells in humans. After all, some modern treatments cause cancer themselves and, at the level of the cell, cancer is a genetic disease. Also, cytogenic abnormalities are commonly seen after intensive cancer therapy. Despite considerable information about somatic effects in experimental systems, some data about germ cell effects in experimental animals, and much information about somatic cell mutation in humans, little is known about the sensitivity of the human gonad to mutagens. Dose-dependent abnormalities have been shown in meiotic chromosomes of the human testis after experimental irradiation, but no environmental agent has been causally linked to human germ cell mutation. Yet, in genetic counseling, in the area of mutagenicity of the human gonad, the ultimate measure of concern is human hereditary disease. Does cancer treatment cause hereditary damage in humans? Does it cause actual disease in the offspring, or mutational events without clinical significance? In theory, the effects of mutation may be neutral or even beneficial, as an essential element of biologic evolution.

Atomic bomb survivors in Japan have been extensively studied for possible genetic damage to their offspring.[148,149] The data are limited but are compatible with the interpretation that human germ cells may be much more tolerant of ionizing radiation than the standard laboratory mouse.[95,148–150] A recent evaluation of the same data suggests that the dose required to double the spontaneous mutation rate in humans is five times greater than the dose in the mouse.[148–150]

PREGNANCY OUTCOMES

The actual outcomes of pregnancies in survivors of cancer are published as case reports, small series, and some 14 retrospective case series (Table 63–26).[151–164] These are patients who all had cancer as a child or young adult, mostly finished cancer treatment, and then began a pregnancy. More than 844 cancer patients or survivors, nearly four fifths of them women, initiated a total of 1761 recognized pregnancies. Of 1389 liveborn outcomes, only 53 (about 4%) had a birth defect, a figure that resembles the rate of major malformations in the general population. The range of defects in the 14 studies included common malformations, such as congenital hip dysplasia, that may, in fact, represent deformity or the nongenetic extrinsic molding of fetal features. Only three of the disorders were purely genetic diseases, that is, mendelian traits or cytogenic defects, as were also, perhaps, the two instances of multiple congenital anomalies. Pendred's syndrome (goiter and deafness) is an autosomal recessive disease. Both parents had to have contributed a mutant gene; hence, one cannot be sure that therapy caused the mutation. The other two disorders, the possible trisomy 18 syndrome and Marfan's syndrome, may represent new mutants, but one cannot be sure. Of course, all these studies were hardly comparable and had such relatively small numbers of patients (given the rarity of genetic disease in the general population) that, even in the aggregate, they have low statistical power. With only two instances of possible mutants seen in some 1400 offspring, experience is obviously limited.

A National Cancer Institute study addressed late effects in some 2300 survivors of childhood and adolescent cancer, using siblings as controls. Only 22% had received any chemotherapy, and one third had received radiation therapy. Overall, fertility was slightly depressed in males, to about 85% of the rate in male controls.[165] Fertility was only slightly depressed in women. When fertility was examined as a function of the type of treatment received in the first year after diagnosis, patients (both men and women) who had been treated with alkylating agent chemotherapy and radiation therapy below the diaphragm were most severely affected.

Although fertility rates differed by tumor type and therapy, each case survivor had an average of about one child who had reached a mean age of about 11 years at the time of interview. Seven cancers were reported in the survivors' offspring (5 histologically confirmed), compared with 11 in the offspring of sibling controls (8 histologically confirmed).[166] This represents a slight but not statistically significant excess of cancer in the offspring of case survivors. In the first 5 years of age, the children of cancer survivors had three times the number of cancers expected based on rates from the Connecticut Tumor Registry; children of sibling controls had about half the expected number of cancers. After 5 years of age, there was no statistically significant difference. The excess seemed attributable to some hereditary cancers (retinoblastoma, Siple's syndrome, and Wilms' tumor) and to some known syndromes of familial cancer.

In short, there does not appear to be an overall excess risk of cancer in offspring.[167–170] What excess risk there was in the offspring appeared to be confined to the first 5 years of life, and could usually be attributable to a known hereditary or familial cancer and not to the cumulative dose of mutagenic agent.[170] There were few person-years of observation in the older adolescent age range, the ages when most of the case survivors were first diagnosed with cancer.

Cancer could be one indication of germ cell mutation. In a preliminary analysis, *genetic disease* was defined as a cytogenic syndrome, a single gene defect, or one of 15 simple malformations tracked for incidence by the Centers for Disease Control, such as neural tube defects, patent ductus arteriosus, and the like.[167] *Potentially mutagenic therapy* was defined as radiation therapy below the diaphragm or above the knee or chemotherapy with an alkylating agent. Finally, *sporadic* indicated that the offspring had no relative with a similar genetic disease; *familial* meant that there was a relative with a similar genetic disease or that the trait in the offspring was a recessive trait. The overall rate of genetic disease was 3.4% and was not different among the offspring of case survivors compared with sibling controls. Some possible differences in the rates of simple defects in the study groups, compared with population rates, probably arose from artifactual differences in defining the defects and differences in the length of follow-up. The case survivors whose offspring had sporadic genetic disease received potentially mutagenic therapies no more often than did those whose offspring were normal.

The study of genetic disease in offspring of cancer survivors had an 87% power for detecting a twofold excess and did not detect this excess, although the power is misleading because it mostly originates from the high background rate of simple birth defects, such as ventricular septal defect or cleft lip. One cannot be sure that such sporadic defects represent new mutations because they also might be due to the polygenic or multifactorial traits that arise from parental genes interacting with environmental factors.

Apart from genetic effects, female survivors may face problems carrying a pregnancy to term. Excess rates of premature delivery and low birth weight have been documented in several studies[158,159,163] but may be confined to women who had abdominal irradiation and were incapable of maintaining a full-term, normal-weight pregnancy, perhaps because of uterine fibrosis or vascular compromise.

TABLE 63–26. Large Series of Pregnancies in and by Survivors of Cancer

Investigations, Years Encompassed	*Exposed Parents*		*Completed Pregnancies*					
						Live Births		
	Total	*Females (%)*	*Total*	*Fetal Loss**	*Elective Abortions*	Normal	With Defect	Types of Defect
Li and Jaffe,[151] ?–1973	45	63	107	15	3	90	2	Hirschsprung's disease, asymptomatic heart murmur‡
Ross,[152] 1956–1973	58†	100	96	18	?	75	3	Pendred's syndrome, tetralogy of Fallot, hemangiomas, eczema and strabismus (1 stillborn with aplasia of the anterior abdominal wall)
Holmes and Holmes,[153] 1944–1975	48	60	93	12	3	77	6	Amblyopia, autism, scleroderma, rectal stenosis, absent fallopian tube and small uterus, slow learner and foot defect
Li et al,[154] ?–1978	146	58	286	45	10	236	8	Possible trisomy 18 syndrome; Marfan's syndrome; deafness, pyloric stenosis; Hirschsprung's disease (same as above); cardiac, brain, and multiple malformations
Blatt et al,[155] ?–1980	30	77	40	12	10	27	1	Congenital hip dysplasia
Horning et al,[156] 1968–1979	20	100	28	5	5	24	0	
Marradi et al,[157] ?–1982	14	57	23	?	?	21	2	Multiple congenital anomalies with mental and growth retardation, panhypopituitarism and cerebral atrophy, gatroschisis
Bundey and Evans,[158] ?–1973	24	83	48	3	0	44	1	Pyloric stenosis
Andrieu et al,[159] 1972–1976	22	100	30	9	4	21	1	Congenital hip dysplasia
Rustin et al,[160] 1958–1980	216†	100	374	90	36	267	8	Spina bifida, tetralogy of Fallot, talipes equinovarus, collapsed lung, umbilical hernia, desquamative fibrosing alveolitis (2 sibs), neonatal tachycardia (plus 2 anencephalic stillbirths and 1 sudden infant death)
Goldstein et al,[161] 1965–1983	?†	100	222	58	6	159	5	Not specified
Mulvihill et al,[162] 1957–1977	66	100	87	22	12	53	6	Neurosensory deafness‡, scoliosis and slow learner‡, hydrocephalus‡, cleft lip and palate‡, tracheomalacia
Li et al,[164] 1931–1979	181	65	246	53	32	190	5	Congenital hip dislocation (2), heart murmur, hypospadias, internal tibial torsion
Total	844	79	1761	373	132	1389	53	(4%)

* Fetal loss is defined as elective abortion, ectopic pregnancy, spontaneous abortion (miscarriage), or stillbirth.
† All gestational trophoblastic neoplasia.
‡ Exposed to cancer treatment during gestation.
(Modified with permission from Mulvihill JJ, Byrne J. Offspring of long-time survivors of childhood cancers. Clin Oncol 1985;4:333–343)

COUNSELING

Infertility must be viewed as an unfortunate complication of cancer chemotherapy and radiation therapy. An additional area of concern is the reproductive dysfunction that can result from cancer and cancer surgery. Not only can tumors directly involve the gonads and the genitalia, but also en bloc dissection of a tumor field may require removal of ovaries or testes. The psychosexual impact of mutilating surgery is not trivial.[171]

Counseling patients facing the high probability of therapy-induced sterility is important.[171–174] Several points should be considered. In cancer patients, there appears to be a high incidence of reduced sexual frequency, low sexual desire, erectile dysfunction, and difficulty reaching orgasm, not to mention infertility.[172–174] There is also the risk of seminal transmission of the mutagenic cancer drugs to the spouse through coitus.[1] Although most of men become infertile after cancer chemotherapy, it is impossible to predict for many drugs if or when spermatogenesis may resume, and standard contraceptive practices should therefore not be abandoned for couples not desiring pregnancy. Factors such as total drug dose administered, duration of time off therapy, and the type of drug or combination administered may be important determinants of reversibility. Recent evidence suggests that the use of procarbazine in combination chemotherapy regimens may be associated with more long-lasting testicular damage than that seen with alkylating agents alone. Certain drug regimens, such as vinblastine, bleomycin, and cisplatin, appear to be associated with a high probability of reversibility. Return of spermatogenesis is uncommon before 1 or 2 years off chemotherapy but may be expected to occur within 4 years off therapy, if at all. Individual patients should be followed carefully, with serial measurements of testicular volume, serum FSH, and sperm count taken as a matter of course.

Pretreatment sperm banking may be valuable to some patients interested in having children after the completion of chemotherapy or radiation therapy. Although the technology of freezing, preserving, and thawing human sperm has advanced considerably, ultimate conception rates using cryopreserved semen remain only 50% to 60% because of loss of semen quality after thawing. Unfortunately, many cancer patients have decreased sperm counts or sperm motility before receiving therapy, which mitigates against successful semen preservation. For example, at least half of patients with Hodgkin's disease and testicular cancer are oligospermic or azoospermic before receiving any therapy. Indeed, it appears that only 10% to 20% of newly diagnosed cancer patients produce semen of sufficient quality to consider cryopreservation. Nevertheless, sperm banking can be offered to patients if they are properly informed of the cost/benefit ratio of the procedure.

Although women older than 40 years of age frequently develop permanent chemotherapy-induced amenorrhea, many younger women maintain normal cyclic menses throughout the treatment period or resume them shortly after therapy is discontinued. Therapeutic guidelines for managing patients with cancer during pregnancy has been well reviewed.[3]

For couples with preserved fertility, genetic counseling should be offered, as outlined in Table 63–27.

TABLE 63–27. Guidelines for Genetic Counseling of Couples Seeking Pregnancy After Cancer Diagnosis

1. Inquire about family history of cancer.
2. Pregnancy is contraindicated during cancer treatment; birth control should be considered.
3. Discuss risk of infertility after cancer treatment, the option of sperm banking, and the possibility of healthy children if fertility is preserved.
4. Discuss theoretical concerns about mutational damage; data for humans are limited.
5. Pregnancy probably should be monitored with ultrasound; amniocentesis should be offered for usual reasons, not just because of cancer history.
6. Existing data on pregnancy outcome do not indicate an excessive risk of congenital or genetic problems above the 4% risk of any pregnancy resulting in a baby with a major malformation.

REFERENCES

1. Trasler JM, Hales BF, Robaire B. Paternal cyclophosphamide treatment of rats causes fetal loss and malformations without affecting male fertility. Nature 1985;316:144–146.
2. Hales BF, Smith S, Robaire B. Cyclophosphamide in the seminal fluid of treated males: Transmission to females by mating and effect on pregnancy outcome. Toxicol Appl Pharm 1986;84:423–430.
3. Allen HH, Nisker JA. Cancer in pregnancy: Therapeutic guidelines. New York: Futura, 1986.
4. American Cancer Society. Proceedings of the Workshop on Psychosexual and Reproductive Issues Affecting Patients with Cancer— 1987. Chicago: American Cancer Society Publ. No. 87-5M-4515, 1987.
5. Fox BW, Fox M. Biochemical aspects of the actions of drugs on spermatogenesis. Pharmacol Rev 1967;19:21–57.
6. Schilsky RL, Lewis BJ, Sherins RJ, et al. Gonadal dysfunction in patients receiving chemotherapy for cancer. Ann Intern Med 1980;93:109–114.
7. Sherins RJ, Howards SS. Male infertility. In: Harrison JH, ed. Campbell's urology. 4th ed. Philadelphia: WB Saunders, 1978:715–766.
8. Sieber SM, Adamson RH. Toxicity of antineoplastic agents in man: Chromosomal aberrations, antifertility effects, congenital malformations, and carcinogenic potential. Adv Cancer Res 1975;22:57–155.
9. Fairley KF, Berrie JU, Johnson W. Sterility and testicular atrophy related to cyclophosphamide therapy. Lancet 1972;1:568–569.
10. Kumar R, Biggart JD, McEvoy J, et al. Cyclophosphamide and reproductive function. Lancet 1972;1:1212–1213.
11. Miller DG. Alkylating agents and human spermatogenesis. JAMA 1971;217:1662–1665.
12. Richter P, Calamera JC, Morgenfeld MD, et al. Effect of chlorambucil on spermatogenesis in the human with malignant lymphoma. Cancer 1970;25:1026–1030.
13. Meistrich ML, Finch M, da Cunha MF, et al. Damaging effects of fourteen chemotherapeutic drugs on mouse testis cells. Cancer Res 1982;42:122–131.
14. Cheviakoff J, Calamera JC, Morgenfeld M, et al. Recovery of spermatogenesis in patients with lymphoma after treatment with chlorambucil. J Reprod Fertil 1973;33:155–157.
15. Quershi MJA, Goldsmith HJ, Pennington HJ, et al. Cyclophosphamide therapy and sterility. Lancet 1972;2:1290–1291.
16. Van Thiel DH, Sherins RJ, Myers GH, et al. Evidence for a specific seminiferous tubular factor affecting follicle-stimulating hormone secretion in man. J Clin Invest 1972;51:1009–1019.
17. Mecklenberg RS, Sherins RJ. Gonadotropin response to luteinizing hormone releasing hormone in men with germinal aplasia. J Clin Endocrinol Metab 1974;38:1005–1009.
18. Booth JD, Merriam GR, Clark RV, et al. Evidence for Leydig cell dysfunction in infertile men with a selective increase in plasma follicle stimulating hormone. J Clin Endocrinol Metab 1987;64:1194–1198.
19. Sherins RJ, Patterson AP, Brightwell D, et al. Alteration in the plasma testosterone/estradiol ratio: An alternative to the inhibin hypothesis. In: Bardin CW, Sherins RJ, eds. The cell biology of the testis. Ann NY Acad Sci 1982;383:295–306.
20. da Cunha MF, Meistrich ML, Reid HL, et al. Effect of chemotherapy on human sperm production. Proc Am Assoc Cancer Res 1979;20:100.
21. Sieber SM, Correa P, Dalgard DW, et al. Carcinogenic and other adverse effects of procarbazine in nonhuman primates. Cancer Res 1978;38:2125–2134.
22. Vilar O. Effect of cytostatic drugs on human testicular function. In: Mancini RE, Martini L, eds. Male fertility and sterility. New York: Academic Press, 1974:423–440.
23. Drasga RE, Einhorn LH, Williams SD, et al. Fertility after chemotherapy for testicular cancer. J Clin Oncol 1983;1:179–183.
24. Sherins RJ, DeVita VT. Effects of drug treatment of lymphoma on male reproductive capacity. Ann Intern Med 1973;79:216–220.
25. Asbjornsen G, Molne K, Kleep O, et al. Testicular function after combination chemotherapy for Hodgkin's disease. Scand J Haematol 1976;16:66–69.
26. Roeser HP, Stochs AE, Smith AJ. Testicular damage due to cytotoxic drugs and recovery after cessation of therapy. Aust NZ J Med 1978;8:250–254.
27. Chapman R, Sutcliffe SB, Rees L, et al. Prospective study: The effects of Hodgkin's disease and nitrogen mustard, vincristine, procarbazine and prednisolone on male gonadal function. Proc Am Soc Clin Oncol 1979;20:321.
28. Chapman RM, Sutcliffe SB, Rees LH, et al. Cyclical combination chemotherapy and gonadal function. Lancet 1979;1:285–289.
29. Chapman RM, Sutcliffe SB, Malpas JS. Male gonadal dysfunction in Hodgkin's disease. JAMA 1981;245:1323–1328.
30. Waxman JHX, Terry YA, Wrigley PFM, et al. Gonadal function in Hodgkin's disease: Long-term followup of chemotherapy. Br Med J 1982;285:1612–1613.
31. Whitehead E, Shalet SM, Blackledge G, et al. The effects of Hodgkin's disease and

combination chemotherapy on gonadal function in the adult male. Cancer 1982;49: 418–422.

32. Kreuser ED, Xiros N, Hetzel WD, et al. Reproductive and endocrine gonadal capacity in patients treated with COPP chemotherapy for Hodgkin's disease. J Cancer Res Clin Oncol 1987;113:260–266.
33. Evenson DP, Arlin Z, Welt S, et al. Male reproductive capacity may recover following drug treatment with the L-10 protocol for acute lymphocytic leukemia. Cancer 1984;53: 30–36.
34. Shamberger RC, Sherins RJ, Rosenberg SA. The effects of post-operative adjuvant chemotherapy and radiotherapy on testicular function in men undergoing treatment for soft tissue sarcoma. Cancer 1981;47:2368–2374.
35. Kreuser ED, Hetzel WD, Heit W, et al. Reproductive and endocrine gonadal functions in adults following multidrug chemotherapy for acute lymphoblastic or undifferentiated leukemia. J Clin Oncol 1988;6:588–595.
36. Meistrich ML, Chawla SP, da Cunha MF, et al. Recovery of sperm production after chemotherapy for osteosarcoma. Cancer, 1989;63:2115–2123.
37. Vivani S, Santoro A, Ragri G, et al. Gonadal toxicity after combination chemotherapy for Hodgkin's disease: Comparative results of MOPP vs ABVD. Eur J Cancer Clin Oncol 1985;21:601–605.
38. Hagemeister FB, Cabanillas FF, Valesquez WS, et al. NOVP: A novel chemotherapeutic regimen with minimal toxicity for treatment of Hodgkin's disease. Semin Oncol 1990;17:34–40.
39. Einhorn LH, Donahue J. Cis-diammine-dichloroplatinum, vinblastine and bleomycin combination chemotherapy in disseminated testicular cancer. Ann Intern Med 1977;87: 293–298.
40. Berthelsen JG, Skakkebaek NE. Gonadal function in men with testicular cancer. Fertil Steril 1983;39:68–73.
41. Berthelsen JG. Andrological aspects of testicular cancer. Int J Androl 1984;7:451–483.
42. Nijman JM, Schraffordt-Koops H, Kremer J, et al. Gonadal function after surgery and chemotherapy in men with stage II and III nonseminomatous testicular tumors. J Clin Oncol 1987;5:651–656.
43. Carroll PR, Whitmore WF Jr, Herr HW, et al. Endocrine and exocrine profiles of men with testicular tumors before orchiectomy. J Urol 1987;137:420–423.
44. Fossa SD, Theodorsen L, Norman N, et al. Recovery of impaired pretreatment spermatogenesis in testicular cancer. Fertil Steril 1990;54:493–496.
45. Kedia KR, Markland C, Fraley EE. Sexual function following retroperitoneal lymphadenectomy. J Urol 1975;114:237–239.
46. Narayan P, Lange PH, Fraley EE. Ejaculation and fertility after extended retroperitoneal lymph node dissection for testicular cancer. J Urol 1982;127:685–688.
47. Lange PH, Narayan P, Fraley EE. Fertility issues following therapy for testicular cancer. Semin Urol II 1984;4:264–274.
48. Belohorsky B, Siracky J, Sandor L, et al. Comments on the development of amenorrhea caused by myleran in cases of chronic myelosis. Neoplasm 1960;4:397–402.
49. Miller JJ, Williams GF, Leissring JC. Multiple late complications of therapy with cyclophosphamide including ovarian destruction. Am J Med 1971;50:530–535.
50. Sobrinho LG, Levine RA, DeConti RC. Amenorrhea in patients with Hodgkin's disease treated with antineoplastic agents. Am J Obstet Gynecol 1971;109:135–139.
51. Louis J, Limarzi LR, Best WR. Treatment of chronic granulocytic leukemia with myleran. Arch Intern Med 1956;97:299–308.
52. Galton DAG, Till M, Wiltshaw E. Busulfan: Summary of clinical results. Ann NY Acad Sci 1958;68:967–973.
53. Fosdick WM, Parsons JL, Hill DF. Long term cyclophosphamide therapy in rheumatoid arthritis. Arthritis Rheum 1968;11:151–161.
54. Uldall PR, Kerr DNS, Tacchi D. Sterility and cyclophosphamide. Lancet 1972;1:693–694.
55. Warne GL, Fairley KF, Hobbs JB, et al. Cyclophosphamide-induced ovarian failure. N Engl J Med 1973;289:1159–1162.
56. Dnistrian AM, Schwartz MK, Fracchia AA, et al. Endocrine consequences of CMF adjuvant therapy in premenopausal and postmenopausal breast cancer patients. Cancer 1983;51:803–807.
57. Samaan NA, DeAsis DN, Buzdar AU, et al. Pituitary-ovarian function in breast cancer patients on adjuvant chemoimmunotherapy. Cancer 1978;41:2084–2087.
58. Koyama H, Wada T, Nishizawa Y, et al. Cyclophosphamide-induced ovarian failure and its therapeutic significance in patients with breast cancer. Cancer 1977;39:1403–1409.
59. Fisher B, Sherman B, Rockette H, et al. L-phenylalanine mustard in the management of premenopausal patients with primary breast cancer. Cancer 1979;44:847–857.
60. Shamberger RC, Rosenberg SA, Seipp CA, et al. Effects of high-dose methotrexate and vincristine on ovarian and testicular function in patients undergoing postoperative adjuvant treatment of osteosarcoma. Cancer Treat Rep 1981;65:739–746.
61. Morgenfeld MC, Goldberg V, Parisier H, et al. Ovarian lesions due to cytostatic agents during the treatment of Hodgkin's disease. Surg Gynecol Obstet 1972;134:826–828.
62. Sherins R, Winokur S, DeVita VT, et al. Surprisingly high risk of functional castration in women receiving chemotherapy for lymphoma. Clin Res 1975;23:343.
63. Chapman RM, Sutcliffe SB, Malpas JS. Cytotoxic-induced ovarian failure in women with Hodgkin's disease: I. Hormone function. JAMA 1979;242:1877–1881.
64. Horning SJ, Hoppe RT, Kaplan HS, et al. Female reproductive potential after treatment of Hodgkin's disease. N Engl J Med 1981;304:1378–1382.
65. Schilsky RL, Sherins RJ, Hubbard SM, et al. Long-term followup of ovarian function in women treated with MOPP chemotherapy for Hodgkin's disease. Am J Med 1981;71: 552–556.
66. Whitehead E, Shalet SM, Blackledge G, et al. The effect of combination chemotherapy on ovarian function in women treated for Hodgkin's disease. Cancer 1983;52:988–993.
67. Specht L, Hansen MM, Geisler C. Ovarian function in young women in long-term remission after treatment for Hodgkin's disease stage II or III. Scand J Haematol 1984;32:265–270.
68. Thomford PJ, Jelovsek FR, Mattison DR. Effect of oocyte number and rate of atresia on the age of menopause. Reprod Toxicol 1987;1:41–51.
68a. Faddy MJ, Gosden RG, Gougeon A, et al. Accelerated disappearance of ovarian follicles in mid-life: Implications for forecasting menopause. Hum Reprod 1992;7:1342–1346.
69. Arneil GC. Cyclophosphamide and the prepubertal testis. Lancet 1972;2:1259–1260.
70. Pennisi AJ, Grushkin CM, Lieberman E. Gonadal function in children with nephrosis treated with cyclophosphamide. Am J Dis Child 1975;129:315–318.
71. Kirkland RT, Bongiovanni AM, Cornfeld D, et al. Gonadotropin responses to luteinizing hormone releasing factor in boys treated with cyclophosphamide for nephrotic syndrome. J Pediatr 1976;89:941–944.
72. Rapola J, Koskimies O, Huttanen NP, et al. Cyclophosphamide and the pubertal testis. Lancet 1973;1:98–99.
73. Etteldorf JN, West CD, Pitcock JA, et al. Gonadal function, testicular histology and meiosis following cyclophosphamide therapy in patients with nephrotic syndrome. J Pediatr 1976;88:206–212.
74. Lentz RD, Bergstein J, Steffes MW, et al. Post-pubertal evaluation of gonadal function following cyclophosphamide therapy before and during puberty. J Pediatr 1977;91: 385–394.
75. Lendon M, Hann IM, Palmer MK, et al. Testicular histology after combination chemotherapy in childhood for acute lymphoblastic leukemia. Lancet 1978;2:439–441.
76. Ahmed SR, Shalet SM, Campbell RHA, et al. Primary gonadal damage following treatment of brain tumors in childhood. J Pediatr 1983;103:562–565.
77. Blatt J, Poplack DG, Sherins RJ. Testicular function in boys after chemotherapy for acute lymphoblastic leukemia. N Engl J Med 1981;304:1121–1124.
78. Sherins RJ, Olweny CLM, Ziegler JL. Gynecomastia and gonadal dysfunction in adolescent boys treated with combination chemotherapy for Hodgkin's disease. N Engl J Med 1978;299:12–16.
79. Whitehead E, Shalet SM, Morris-Jones PH, et al. Gonadal function after combination chemotherapy for Hodgkin's disease in childhood. Arch Dis Child 1981;47:287–291.
80. Himelstein-Braw R, Peters H, Faber M. Morphologic study of the ovaries of leukemic children. Br J Cancer 1978;38:82–87.
81. Nicosia SV, Matus-Ridley M, Meadows AT. Gonadal effects of cancer therapy in girls. Cancer 1985;55:2364–2372.
82. Chiu J, Drummond KN. Long-term followup of cyclophosphamide therapy in frequent relapsing minimal lesion nephrotic syndrome. J Pediatr 1974;84:825–830.
83. DeGroot GW, Faiman C, Winter JSD. Cyclophosphamide and the prepubertal gonad: A negative report. J Pediatr 1974;84:123–125.
84. Siris EJ, Leventhal BG, Vaitukaitis JL. Effects of childhood leukemia and chemotherapy on puberty and reproductive function in girls. N Engl J Med 1976;294:1143–1146.
85. Bateman JL, Bond VP. The effects of radiations of different LET on early response in the mammal. Ann NY Acad Sci 1964;114:32–47.
86. Sanderman RF. The effects of irradiation on male human fertility. Br J Radiol 1966;39: 901–907.
87. Paulsen CA. The study of radiation effects on the human testis: Including histologic, chromosomal and hormonal aspects. Final Progress Report, AEC Contract AT (45-I)-225, Task Agreement 6, RLO–2225–2, 1973.
88. Rowley MJ, Leach DR, Warner GA, et al. Effect of graded doses of ionizing radiation on the human testis. Radiat Res 1974;59:665–677.
89. Ash P. The influence of radiation on fertility in man. Br J Radiol 1980;53:271–278.
90. Hahn EW, Feingold SM, Simpson L, et al. Recovery from aspermia induced by low-dose radiation in seminoma patients. Cancer 1982;50:337-340.
91. Nader S, Schultz PN, Cundiff JH, et al. Endocrine profiles of patients with testicular tumors treated with radiotherapy. Int J Radiat Oncol Biol Phys 1983;9:1723–1726.
92. Tomic R, Bergman B, Damber JE, et al. Effects of external radiation therapy for cancer of the prostate on the serum concentrations of testosterone, follicle stimulating hormone, luteinizing hormone and prolactin. J Urol 1983;130:287–289.
93. Clifton DK, Bremner WJ. The effect of testicular x-irradiation on spermatogenesis in man: A comparison with the mouse. J Androl 1983;4:387–492.
94. Shapiro E, Kinsella TJ, Makoch RW, et al. Effects of fractionated irradiation on endocrine aspects of testicular function. J Clin Oncol 1985;3:1232–1239.
95. Meistrich ML, von Beek MEAB. Radiation sensitivity of the human testis. Adv Radiat Biol 1990;14:227–268.
96. Brauner R, Czernichow P, Cramer P, et al. Leydig cell function in children after direct testicular irradiation for acute lymphoblastic leukemia. N Engl J Med 1983;309: 25–28.
97. Leiper AD, Grant DB, Chessells JM. The effect of testicular irradiation on Leydig cell function in prepubertal boys with acute lymphoblastic leukemia. Arch Dis Child 1983;58:906–910.
98. Blatt J, Sherins RJ, Niebrugge D, et al. Leydig cell function in boys following testicular relapse of acute lymphoblastic leukemia. J Clin Oncol 1985;3:1227–1231.
99. Thomas PRM, Winstantly D, Peckham MJ, et al. Reproductive and endocrine function in patients with Hodgkin's disease: Effects of oophoropexy and irradiation. Br J Cancer 1976;33:226–231.
100. Horning SJ, Hoppe RT, Kaplan HS, et al. Female reproductive potential after treatment for Hodgkin's disease. N Engl J Med 1981;304:1377–1382.
101. Fisher B, Cheung AYC. Delayed effect of radiation therapy with or without chemotherapy on ovarian function in women with Hodgkin's disease. Acta Radiol Oncol 1984;23:43–48.
102. Redman JR, Bajorunas DR. Suppression of germ cell proliferation to prevent gonadal

toxicity associated with cancer treatment. In: Proceedings of the Workshop on Psychosexual and Reproductive Issues Affecting Patients with Cancer. Chicago: American Cancer Society Publ. No. 87-5M-4515, 1987:90–94.

103. Redman J, Davis R, Evenson D, et al. Prospective, randomized trial of testosterone cypionate to prevent sterility in men treated with chemotherapy for Hodgkin's disease: Preliminary results. In: Proceedings of the 14th International Cancer Congress, Budapest. Basel: S Karger, 1986:440.
104. Chapman RM, Sutcliffe SB. Protection of ovarian function by oral contraceptives in women receiving chemotherapy for Hodgkin's disease. Blood 1981;58:849–851.
105. Johnson DH, Linde R, Hainsworth JD, et al. Effect of luteinizing hormone-releasing hormone agonist given during combination chemotherapy on post-therapy fertility in male patients with lymphoma: Preliminary observations. Blood 1985;65:832–836.
106. Glode LM, Robinson J, Gould SF, et al. Protection of spermatogenesis during chemotherapy. Drugs Exp Clin Res 1982;8:367–378.
107. Lewis RN, Dowling KJ, Schally AV. D-Tryptophan-6 analog of luteinizing hormone-releasing hormone as a protective agent against testicular damage caused by cyclophosphamide in baboons. Proc Natl Acad Sci USA 1985;82:2975–2979.
108. Delic JI, Bush C, Peckham MJ. Protection from procarbazine-included damage of spermatogenesis in the rat by androgen. Cancer Res 1986;46:1909–1914.
109. da Cunha MF, Meistrich ML, Nader S. Absence of testicular protection by a gonadotropin-releasing hormone analogue against cyclophosphamide induced testicular cytoxicity in the mouse. Cancer Res 1987;47:1093–1097.
110. Karashima T, Zalatnai A, Schally AV. Protective effects of analogs of luteinizing hormone releasing hormone agonist chemotherapy induced testicular damage in rats. Proc Natl Acad Sci USA 1988;85:2329–2333.
111. Jegou B, Velez de la Calle JF, Bauche F. Protective effect of medroxyprogesterone acetate plus testosterone against radiation-induced damage to the reproductive function of male rats and their offspring. Proc Natl Acad Sci USA 1991;88:8710–8714.
112. Fraas BA, Kinsella TJ, Harrington FS, et al. Peripheral dose to the testis: The design and use of a practical and effective gonadal shield. Int J Radiat Oncol Biol Phys 1985;11:609–615.
113. Kinsella TJ, Fraas BA, Glatstein E. Late effects of radiation therapy in the treatment of Hodgkin's disease. Cancer Treat Rep 1982;66:991–1001.
114. Pedrick TJ, Hoppe RT. Recovery of spermatogenesis following pelvic irradiation for Hodgkin's disease. Int J Radiat Oncol Biol Phys 1986;12:117–121.
115. Ray GR, Trueblood HW, Enright LP, et al. Oophoropexy: A means of preserving ovarian function following pelvic megavoltage radiotherapy for Hodgkin's disease. Radiology 1970;96:175–180.
116. Sherman JK. Synopsis of the use of frozen human semen since 1964: State-of-the-art of human semen banking. Fertil Steril 1973;24:397–412.
117. Ansbacher R. Artificial insemination with frozen spermatozoa. Fertil Steril 1978;29:375–379.
118. Curie-Cohen M, Luttrell L, Shapiro J. Current practice of artificial insemination by donor in the United States. N Engl J Med 1979;300:585–590.
119. Bracken RB, Smith KD. Is semen cryopreservation helpful in testicular cancer? Urology 1980;15:581–583.
120. Sanger WG, Armitage JO, Schmidt MA. Feasibility of semen cryopreservation in patients with malignant disease. JAMA 1980;244:789–790.
121. Scammell GD, Stedronske J, Edmonds DK, et al. Cryopreservation of semen in men with testicular tumor or Hodgkin's disease: Results of artificial insemination of their partners. Lancet 1985;2:31–32.
122. Rhodes EA, Hoffman DJ, Kaempfer SH. Ten years of experience with semen cryopreservation by cancer patients: Follow-up and clinical considerations. Fertil Steril 1985;44:512–516.
123. Reed E, Sanger WG, Armitage JO. Results of semen cryopresentation in young men with testicular carcinoma and lymphoma. J Clin Oncol 1986;4:537–539.
124. Thacil JV, Jewett MAS, Rider WD. The effects of cancer and cancer therapy on male fertility. J Urol 1981;126:141–145.
125. Chapman RM, Sutcliffe SB, Malpas JS. Male gonadal dysfunction in Hodgkin's disease: A prospective study. JAMA 1981;245:1323–1328.
126. Chlebowski RT, Heber D. Hypogonadism in male patients with metastatic cancer prior to chemotherapy. Cancer Res 1982;42:2495–2498.
127. Vigersky RA, Chapman RM, Berenberg J, et al. Testicular dysfunction in untreated Hodgkin's disease. Am J Med 1982;73:482–486.
128. Marmor D, Elefant E, Dauchez C, et al. Semen analysis in Hodgkin's disease before onset of treatment. Cancer 1986;57:1986–1987.
129. Cross NL, Hanks SE. Effects of cryopreservation on human sperm acrosomes. Hum Reprod 1991;6:1279–1283.
130. Burris AS, Clark RV, Vantman DJ, et al. A low sperm concentration does not preclude fertility in men with isolated hypogonadotropic hypogonadism after gonadotropin therapy. Fertil Steril 1988;50:343–347.
131. Free D, Stutts L, Merryman D, et al. A comparison of donor semen processing techniques for use in intrauterine inseminations and their corresponding pregnancy rates. Abstract #35. Orlando, FL: American Fertility Society, November 1991.
132. Schulman JD, Dorfmann A, Jones S, et al. Outpatient in vitro fertilization using transvaginal oocyte retrieval. N Engl J Med 1985;312:1639.
133. Fugger EF, Bustillo M, Katz LP. Embryonic development and pregnancy from fresh and cryopreserved sibling pronucleate human zygotes. Fertil Steril 1988;50:273–278.
134. Fugger EF, Bustillo M, Dorfmann AD, et al. Human preimplantation embryo cryopreservation: Selected aspects. Hum Reprod 1991;6:131–135.
135. Bustillo, M, Buster JE, Cohen SW, et al. Nonsurgical ovum transfer as a treatment in infertile women: Preliminary experience. JAMA 1984;251:1171–1173.
136. Buster JE, Bustillo M, Rodi IA, et al. Biology and morphology of donated human ova recovered by nonsurgical uterine lavage. Am J Obstet Gynecol 1985;153:211–217.
137. Walsh PC, Lepor H, Eggleson JC. Radical prostatectomy with preservation of sexual function: Anatomical and pathological considerations. Prostate 1983;4:473–485.
138. Quinlan DM, Epstein JI, Carter BS, et al. Sexual function following radical prostatectomy: Influence of preservation of neurovascular bundles. J Urol 1991;145:998–1002.
139. Walsh PC, Mostwin JL. Radical prostatectomy and cystoprostatectomy with preservation of potency: Results using a new nerve sparing technique. Br J Urol 1984;56:694–697.
140. Garnick MB, Richie JP. Toward more rational management for stage I testis cancer: Watch out for "watch and wait." J Clin Oncol 1986;4:1021–1023.
141. Pizzocaro G, Salvioni R, Zononi F. Unilateral lymphadenectomy in intraoperative stage I nonseminomatous germinal testis cancer. J Urol 1985;134:485–489.
142. Jewett MAS, Young-Soo PK, Goldberg SD, et al. Retroperitoneal lymphadenectomy for testis tumor with nerve sparing for ejaculation. J Urol 1988;13:1220–1226.
143. Thomas RJS, McLeisch G. McDonald IA. Electroejaculation of the paraplegic male followed by pregnancy. Med J Aust 1975;2:798.
144. Bennett CJ, Ayers JWT, Randolph JF, et al. Electroejaculation of paraplegic males followed by pregnancies. Fertil Steril 1987;48:1070–1072.
145. Bennett CJ, Seager SWJ, McGuire EJ. Electroejaculation for recovery of semen after retroperitoneal lymph node dissection. J Urol 1987;137:513.
146. Schull WJ. Reproductive problems: Fertility, teratogenesis and mutagenesis. Arch Envir Health 1984;39:207–212.
147. US Congress Office of Technology Assessment. Technologies for detecting heritable mutations in human beings. Washington, DC: US Government Printing Office, 1986.
148. Schull WJ, Otake M, Neel JV. Genetic effects of atomic bombs: A reappraisal. Science 1981;213:1220–1227.
149. Neel JV. Genetic effects of atomic bombs. Science 1981;213:1205.
150. Neel JV, Lewis SE. The comparative radiation genetics of humans and mice. Annu Rev Genet 1990;24:327–62.
151. Li FP, Jaffe H. Progeny of childhood-cancer survivors. Lancet 1974;2:707–709.
152. Ross GT. Congenital anomalies among children born of mothers receiving chemotherapy for gestational trophoblastic neoplasms. Cancer 1976;37:1043–1047.
153. Holmes GE, Holmes FF. Pregnancy outcome of patients treated for Hodgkin's disease: A controlled study. Cancer 1978;41:1317–1322.
154. Li FP, Fine W, Jaffe H, et al. Offspring of patients treated for cancer in childhood. J Natl Cancer Inst 1979;62:1193–1197.
155. Blatt J, Mulvihill JJ, Ziegler JL, et al. Pregnancy outcome following cancer chemotherapy. Am J Med 1980;69:828–832.
156. Horning SJ, Hippe RT, Kaplan HS, et al. Female reproductive potential after treatment for Hodgkin's disease. N Engl J Med 1981;304:1377–1382.
157. Marradi P, Schaison F, Alby N, et al. Les enfants nes de parents leucemiques. Nouv Rev Fr Hematol 1982;24:75–80.
158. Bundey S, Evans K. Survivors of neuroblastoma and ganglioneuroma and their families. J Med Genet 1982;19:16–21.
159. Andrieu JM, Ochoa-Molina ME. Menstrual cycle, pregnancies and offspring before and after MOPP therapy for Hodgkin's disease. Cancer 1983;52:435–438.
160. Rustin GJS, Booth M, Dent J, et al. Pregnancy after cytotoxic chemotherapy for gestational trophoblastic tumors. Br Med J 1984;288:103–106.
161. Goldstein DP, Berkowitz RS, Bernstein MR. Reproductive performance after molar pregnancy and gestational trophoblastic tumors. Clin Obstet Gynecol 1984;27:221–227.
162. Mulvihill JJ, Byrne J. Offspring of long-time survivors of childhood cancer. Clin Oncol 1985;4:333–343.
163. Mulvihill JJ, McKeen EA, Rosner F, et al. Pregnancy outcome in cancer patients: Experience in a large cooperative group. Cancer 1987;60:1143–1150.
164. Li FP, Gimbrere K, Gelber RD, et al. Outcome of pregnancy in survivors of Wilms' tumor. JAMA 1987;257:216–219.
165. Byrne J, Mulvihill JJ, Myers MH, et al. Effects of treatment on fertility in long-term survivors of childhood and adolescent cancer. N Engl J Med 1987;317:1315–1321.
166. Mulvihill JJ, Myers MH, Connelly RR, et al. Cancer in offspring of long-term survivors of childhood and adolescent cancer. Lancet 1987;2:813–817.
167. Mulvihill JJ, Byrne J, Steinhorn SA, et al. Genetic disease in offspring of survivors of cancer in the young. Am J Hum Genet 1986;39:A72.
168. Byrne J, Mulvihill JJ, Myers MH, et al. Reproductive problems and birth defects in survivors of Wilms' tumor and their relatives. Med Pediatr Oncol 1980;16:233–240.
169. Mulvihill JJ, Byrne J. Genetic counseling for the cancer survivor: Possible germ cell effects of cancer therapy. In: Proceedings of the Workshop on Psychosexual and Reproductive Issues Affecting Patients with Cancer. American Cancer Society Publ. No. #87-5M-4515, 1987:100–104.
170. Green DM, Zevon MA, Lowrie G, et al. Congenital anomalies in children of patients who received chemotherapy for cancer in childhood and adolescence. N Engl J Med 1991;325:141–146.
171. American Cancer Society. Proceedings of the Workshop on Psychosexual and Reproductive Issues Affecting Patients with cancer. American Cancer Society Publ. No. 87-5M-4515, 1987.
172. Schover LR, von Eschenbach AC. Sexual and marital relationships after treatment for nonseminomatous testicular cancer. Urology 1985;25:251–255.
173. Andersen BL. Sexual functioning morbidity among cancer survivors: Current status and future research directions. Cancer 1985;55:1835–1842.
174. Schover LR, Gonzales M, von Eschenbach AC. Sexual and marital relationships after radiotherapy for seminoma. Urology 1986;27:117–123.

SECTION **9**

MARGARET A. TUCKER

Secondary Cancers

As the success of modern cancer therapy has increased the duration of survival and curability of many patients, recognition of long-term complications of therapy also has increased. The successful treatment of first cancers involves radiation therapy and multiagent chemotherapy, each of which is used either as primary therapy or as an adjunct to therapy of the primary tumor, which often includes surgery. The increased use of adjuvant chemotherapy has placed a large number of patients at potential risk for developing a treatment-related malignancy.

In the past, discussion of secondary malignancies emphasized the treatments administered and the potential risk for appearance of a second tumor in relation to a specific agent. Whereas the initial reports considered single cases or small series of patients, there are now large populations of patients, such as those with Hodgkin's disease, pediatric cancers, or breast cancer, from which more accurate assessments of risks can be determined. Proper epidemiologic and statistical methods must be employed to avoid overestimating or underestimating the risks, especially in older populations in whom cancer is a more common occurrence.

More recently, it has become apparent that predisposing factors beyond the treatment itself may have a major impact on the risk for developing a second tumor. Alterations in the retinoblastoma locus, germline mutations in p53, and congenital or acquired immunodeficiency states are examples of some of the host factors that may increase the risk of developing a second tumor.

This chapter covers the important principles related to all these areas, emphasizing data available within the last few years. Some topics, such as the relation between the specific therapeutic agents and secondary cancers, were well reviewed by Li in a previous edition of this book[1] and by others.[2,3] A discussion of late effects and secondary malignancies is possible only if the primary treatment is successful. As more is learned about long-term toxicities, treatments can be altered to decrease these complications without compromising the success of treatments.

METHODS OF STUDYING SECONDARY MALIGNANCIES

Several methods have been used to study secondary cancers. Reports of individual cases or series have been important in establishing the occurrence of secondary cancers but have been of limited use in quantifying risks. The more useful epidemiologic methods for studying secondary cancer risk have included both cohort and case-control studies. In cohort studies, specific groups of patients are identified and observed for a number of years to determine the incidence of specific malignancies. Study groups providing large numbers of patients who may constitute a cohort include population-based tumor registries, multicenter clinical trials, and hospital-based patient groups. The groups to be followed may be defined by a first cancer of interest, such as ovarian cancer or Hodgkin's disease, or by an exposure of interest, such as single-agent cyclophosphamide or interstitial radiation therapy. The person-years of observation are accrued from the start of observation to the date of last follow-up, death, or diagnosis of the second tumor, whichever occurs first.[4] Tumor incidence rates from the general population specific for age, sex, race, and calendar year are multiplied by the accumulated person-years to derive the number of expected tumors. The observed number is then divided by the expected number to estimate the relative risk of a second tumor. When the 95% confidence interval does not include 1.0, the excess risk is statistically significant at the $p < 0.05$ level. This method yields a risk in the cohort that is compared with the general population.

The use of population-based tumor registries has some advantages, including relatively large numbers of patients, which allows the detection of even small risks (*e.g.*, the international cervical cancer study mentioned later[5]). In addition, the actual (observed) and the expected numbers of cancer cases come from the same reference population. Population-based registries have some disadvantages, however, including differential reporting of cancers to the registries by physicians and hospitals, variable follow-up, different autopsy rates, limited treatment data, and different diagnostic criteria for secondary cancers. Many registries record only initial therapy, and patients may be incompletely classified if they receive additional treatment. Finally, comparisons of rates of secondary cancers in cancer patients with rates in the general population are criticized because some types of cancer may have an intrinsically increased risk for specific secondary cancers, such as the retinoblastoma-osteosarcoma association.[6–8] Despite these limitations, these studies are informative and often produce the best data available. They tend, however, to give minimal estimates of risk because of the relatively incomplete follow-up. This source of error is less in the population-based tumor registries that are linked to national health care records.

Clinical trials are valuable sources of information on risks for secondary cancers. In clinical studies, initial evaluation of the patients and follow-up in the comparison arms of the trials are equivalent and usually as complete as possible. Patients within each arm have received comparable treatment, and the risks for secondary tumors may be directly compared between treatment arms. This controls for any intrinsic risk for a secondary cancer associated with the first cancer and also allows the comparison of risks from specific drug therapies or radiation exposure. Complete treatment information, including that administered for relapse, is usually available, so the risk of misclassification of exposure is minimized. The major disadvantage of most of the clinical trials is the relatively small number of study subjects involved. Examples of this type of analysis are the National Surgical Adjuvant Breast Project study of risks of adjuvant chemotherapy for breast cancers,[9] the study of ovarian cancer that combined data from several clinical trials,[10] and the Stanford and Milan Hodgkin's disease studies.[11,12]

Another type of analysis that is useful in the cohort studies is the actuarial or life-table risk.[13] This analysis gives the cumulative risk for a particular event, such as leukemia, expressed in a percentage at a particular time period—for example, 6.2% at 10 years. To calculate this life-table probability, person-years of follow-up, similar to those required for the estimation of relative risk compared with the general population, are necessary. The actuarial risk of a secondary cancer occurring can be compared between treatment arms using methods similar to those employed for the comparison of survival or disease-free survival (Fig. 63–11).[14] The limitation of this method is that it does not account for the baseline tumor rates in the general population. An example is the comparison of acute leukemia by age category in the Stanford population of Hodgkin's disease patients.[15] Within each chemotherapy category, the risk of leukemia is significantly higher among people treated after age 50 years than in those treated at a younger age. When the relative risks are examined, which take into account the higher risk for acute leukemia in the general population over age 50 years, the relative risk for all age groups is essentially the same.[11]

The other major approach is the case-control study, in which exposure to chemotherapy or radiation therapy is compared between patients who develop secondary cancers (cases) and those who do not (controls). The selection of appropriate controls is critical; they should be representative of the entire group from which both the cases and controls are derived. Bias in the selection of the control group can lead to spurious associations or can obscure a true association. Ideally, all therapy given to every person treated in the group from which the cases and controls were selected would be reviewed, and the cases compared with the rest of the subjects. In practice, this is not usually feasible since often hundreds or thousands of patients are involved and few develop secondary cancers. In this circumstance, it is much more cost-effective to collect the information on the cases and controls, the latter being representative of the patients who do not develop secondary cancers. The conclusions from such a study are only as valid as the control group selected.

INDIVIDUAL TREATMENT MODALITIES

RADIATION THERAPY

The carcinogenic effects of ionizing irradiation have been quantified in several groups, including occupational cohorts, people exposed to residential radon, atomic bomb survivors,

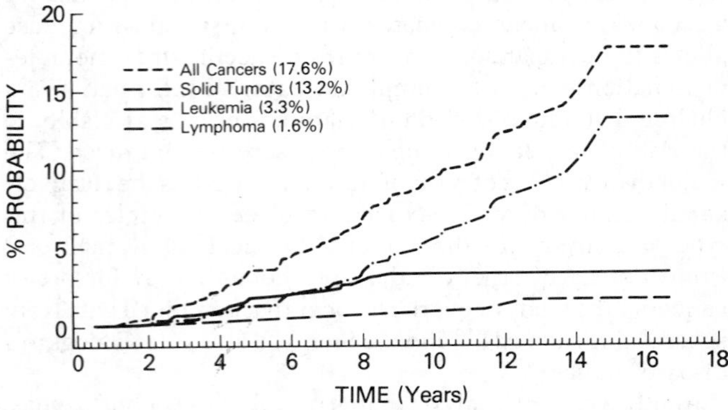

FIGURE 63–11. Actuarial risk of development of secondary malignancy after Hodgkin's disease for 1507 patients treated at Stanford University Medical Center. (Tucker MA, Coleman CN, Cox RS, et al. Risk of second malignancies following Hodgkin's disease after 15 years. N Engl J Med 1988;318:76–81)

and patients who undergo diagnostic and therapeutic procedures. This summary focuses on recent results in atomic bomb survivors and in patients treated with therapeutic irradiation. Many tumor types have been associated, at least in case reports, with irradiation to the tissue in which the malignancy developed; that is, there is no one radiation-induced tumor. With the exception of exposure associated with therapeutic irradiation, the doses have often been low. Extrapolation of radiation effects from low- to high-radiation-dose ranges cannot be done with certainty.[16] In the lower-dose ranges, the risk of a cancer developing increases with dose. Much of the recent effort in radiation epidemiology has focused on the shape (linear versus nonlinear) of the dose-response curves for different tumors. It is thought, however, that at the higher-dose ranges used therapeutically, the risk per centigray decreases, a phenomenon that has been attributed to cell killing at the higher doses.[16] Therapeutic irradiation doses usually fall within a relatively small range, making it difficult to establish a dose-response curve between irradiation doses and risk of a secondary cancer. Therefore, for a patient treated for cancer, the risk per centigray for the development of a secondary tumor cannot necessarily be determined with certainty.[2]

The largest population studies on the carcinogenicity of ionizing irradiation come from survivors of atomic bomb explosions. These people received one whole-body dose that ranged from 0 to 5 Gy. The radiation-related cancers included leukemia, multiple myeloma, and cancers of the lung, female breast, stomach, colon, esophagus, and urinary tract.[17] The relative risk for developing leukemia decreased with time (10.7% per year) after peaking at 5 to 10 years. Although the relative risk for the development of all cancers except leukemia increased with time, the rate of increase was small (4.9% per year).

Recent studies have sought to refine the risk estimates associated with irradiation of these cancers and to evaluate interactions with other known risk factors.[18] Previous evaluations of the cohorts have shown that the risk for breast cancer was greatest in those irradiated as children or adolescents and was lowest in those irradiated when over age 40 years. There was a clear dose response, with risk rising with increased radiation dose to the breast tissue. Parallel analyses of the Life Span Study (LSS) cohort and medically irradiated women in the United States demonstrated that for similar radiation dose levels, ages at exposure, and length of follow-up, similar excess rates of breast cancer were observed. This is remarkable since the age-specific rates of breast cancer are threefold to fivefold higher in the United States than in Japan. To evaluate the potential interaction of radiation with other breast cancer risk factors, Land and colleagues conducted a case-control study.[19,20] Age at first full-term pregnancy (relative risk, 1.08; 95% confidence interval, 1.03–1.13), number of live births (relative risk, 0.81; 95% confidence interval, 0.73–0.90), and cumulative months of lactation (relative risk, 0.98; 95% confidence interval, 0.97–0.99) were strongly associated with both premenopausal and postmenopausal breast cancer risk in the LSS women. Treatment of dysmenorrhea was a risk factor for postmenopausal breast cancer (relative risk, 3.01; p = 0.07). The relation between radiation and these risk factors is not simple. The increased risks associated with age at first pregnancy and treatment of dysmenorrhea were even higher in the women who received higher radiation doses, while the protective effects of number of children and cumulative months of lactation were more pronounced in the women who received higher doses. The interaction of radiation with the reproductive factors was not additive but appeared to be more than multiplicative. There was no clear evidence for an additive or multiplicative model for the treatment of dysmenorrhea. Therefore, even in the presence of radiation, the risk may be modulated by other risk factors for a specific tumor.

The risk of lung cancer also rises with increasing irradiation dose to the lungs. In a recent comparison of the histology of lung cancer in the LSS cohort with the lung cancers in uranium miners, 62% of the miners had small cell lung cancer, compared with 13% of the LSS cohort.[21] The percentages of squamous cell cancer were similar (29% in the miners versus 34% in the LSS population) and were related to smoking, but the percentage of adenocarcinomas was different (9% in the miners versus 43% of the LSS population). When the radiation dose was evaluated, there was a tendency for the proportion of small cell lung cancer to increase with radiation dose, while the proportion of adenocarcinomas decreased with increasing dose. The difference in the radiation dose seemed sufficient to explain the differences in the cell types of the lung cancer seen in the two groups.

No one specific type of cancer is seen after therapeutic irradiation. The secondary cancers can occur after any initial cancer when the survival is long enough. Radiation-induced leukemias frequently occur at about 5 years. Solid cancers typically occur more than 10 years after treatment but may occur earlier in particularly susceptible hosts.[9–12] Excess leukemia and cancers of the lung, breast, thyroid, stomach, bone, and connective tissues have been shown after radiation therapy for diverse tumors as described later. When it was evaluated, the risk of secondary solid cancers rose with increasing radiation dose to the site and with increasing time since treatment at least as long as 20 years. Even in the studies in which actual doses to the site were not estimated, the risk was usually highest in the field, lower at the border of the field, and much lower farther away. The excess risk is seen after both external-beam irradiation and interstitial radiation therapy.

The risk for cancer developing after diagnostic irradiation is much lower predominantly because the doses are so much lower. After diagnostic iodine-131 radiation therapy, no increased risk of cancer overall was found, but small increases were noted for endocrine tumors other than thyroid tumors, lymphomas, and leukemias.[22] An increased risk for breast cancer was found after repeated fluoroscopies in tuberculosis patients, particularly those exposed as adolescents[23]; these patients usually received a few gray. In contrast, Linos and associates[24] did not find that the risk of developing leukemia increased after radiation doses of 0 to 3 Gy when these amounts were delivered over long periods of time as part of routine medical care. Evans and colleagues[25] concluded that only about 1% of all cases of leukemia and less than 1% of all cases of breast cancer result from diagnostic radiation therapy.

CHEMOTHERAPY

The predominant secondary cancer associated with chemotherapy is acute nonlymphocytic leukemia (ANLL). Only selected publications of the large number of studies noting this association are mentioned here. Most ANLLs have occurred after treatment with alkylating agents or nitrosoureas for diseases that have prolonged survival. The findings are similar for Hodgkin's disease, pediatric cancers, ovarian cancer, multiple myeloma, polycythemia vera, gastrointestinal cancers, small cell lung cancer, and breast cancer.[9–12,26–33] The risk for leukemia rises with increasing cumulative dose of alkylating agents and nitrosoureas. The relative leukemogenicity of various drugs has not been fully established, but the risk appears to be different with different drugs. Greene and colleagues[10] found that single-agent cyclophosphamide was significantly less leukemogenic than melphalan in women treated for ovarian cancer. All the women who developed leukemia received high cumulative doses of cyclophosphamide or melphalan. This finding was confirmed and extended by Kaldor and colleagues.[34] In a study of 99,113 survivors of ovarian cancer, they found that the risk of leukemia was highest after chlorambucil or melphalan, followed by thiotepa, then cyclophosphamide and Treosulfan. For each drug evaluated, there was clear evidence of increased risk at higher doses. On the basis of small numbers, an elevated risk of leukemia was found after treatment with cisplatin and doxorubicin. In this study, the risk of developing leukemia after combined modality therapy with both radiation therapy and chemotherapy was no higher than the risk after chemotherapy alone.

It has been difficult to disentangle the effects of cumulative dose and duration of treatment, but when these attempts were made, total dose appeared to be more important than duration of treatment.[33–35] The time between cessation of drug treatment and the development of leukemia has also been explored; the risk for leukemia appears to be highest within a few years of completing treatment.[10,33,36] This, too, is difficult to evaluate since treatment of alkylating agents is stopped when people become pancytopenic, which may be a symptom of preleukemia. The observation needs to be evaluated further. The leukemias that occur after alkylating agent or nitrosourea chemotherapy have distinctive characteristics. The cell types are acute myeloblastic, including FAB M6, erythroleukemia. The leukemias typically occur between 2 and 10 years after therapy, with the peak time interval around 5 years. There is usually an antecedent period of pancytopenia, and the leukemia may manifest as part of the spectrum of myelodysplastic syndromes.[37] The leukemias are notoriously refractory to treatment, although there have been some reports of short-term success.[38,39] Clonal alterations in chromosomes 5 and 7 (translocations or deletions) are frequent (occurring in up to about 90% of patients).[40] This has led to the speculation that these chromosomes contain critical genes that are involved in the pathogenesis of the alkylating-agent-induced leukemias. The variance in host susceptibility to develop these leukemias has not been evaluated well but may relate to interindividual variation in drug metabolism.

A few reports were made of ANLL that followed combination chemotherapy including teniposide or etoposide.[41,42] The leukemias differ from those that follow alkylating agents in that they occur sooner (starting at around 15 months after treatment), there is no period of pancytopenia, the leukemias are frequently M4 or M5, and the most frequent chromosomal abnormalities involve chromosome 11q23.[43,44] The specific chromosomal abnormality has been used as corroboration of the importance of the epipodophyllotoxins in the leukemia risk since some in vitro studies indicated that DNA damage induced by these drugs is not random but is particularly frequent in the chromosome 11q regions. Among reported epipodophyllotoxin-related leukemias, however, only 40% to 80% have an abnormality on chromosome 11q.[43] Also, it is not clear that the translocations that have been associated with leukemia occurring after epipodophyllotoxins are due to that exposure since translocations involving chromosome 11q23—specifically, t(4;11)(q21;q23)—are common in acute lymphocytic leukemia (ALL) (the most frequent initial cancer) and since the translocation t(9;11)(p21;q23) is relatively specific for M5 leukemia of any cause. Several potential candidate genes in that region have been identified, including the protooncogene *ETS*1, *THY*1 surface antigen, *CD*3 surface antigen of T lymphocytes, *NCAM*, and a gene for ataxia-telangiectasia.[43]

The higher risks (cumulative risk of 12%) have been reported by Pui and associates[41] in children receiving relatively high doses of teniposide and other drugs, with or without radiation therapy, for ALL. Several of the children developed ANLL during active treatment of ALL. The data are difficult to evaluate because the children also received multiple other drugs, including cyclophosphamide, or radiation therapy. Radiation in much lower doses to equivalent areas in children treated for tinea capitis has caused an excess of leukemia. Potential interactions with radiation therapy and known or suspected leukemogenic drugs were not evaluated. Another unusual aspect of the relation was that the highest risk of leukemia occurred in the arm of the trial in which only 60% of the patients received 90% of the drugs. In the two other arms, with more patients with identical drugs (except for schedule), 84% of the patients received 90% of the drugs, and the risk of subsequent leukemia was much lower. The authors interpret these data as evidence that schedule is more important than dose.[41]

Others reported much lower cumulative risks (about 4% at 5 years) after treatment with etoposide in combination with other drugs.[42] Again, the potential interaction with alkylating or intercalating agents has not been adequately evaluated. Despite the limitations of these data, there is a suggestion that some of the chemotherapy combinations that include epipodophyllotoxins may confer some risk of leukemia. This is an important issue to resolve as soon as possible because of the widespread use of epipodophyllotoxins in curable diseases. Studies are underway to try to quantify the leukemia risk and to start to evaluate interactions with other drugs or radiation therapy.

Few solid tumors have been linked to treatment with chemotherapy. Bladder cancer has been associated with treatment with cyclophosphamide.[45–47] After daily oral cyclophosphamide at 100 mg/m² for 2 to 4 years, the cumulative risk of bladder cancer was 3.5% at 8 years and 10.7% at 12 years. The relative risk of developing bladder cancer was 6.8 (95% confidence interval, 3.2–14.3).[45] Bone sarcomas have also followed treatment with alkylating agents (discussed later).[48] In general, the risk for solid tumors after chemotherapy alone has been difficult to evaluate because the solid tumors occur later than the leukemias and because not enough people survive long enough after treatment by chemotherapy alone to detect substantial risks for solid tumors.

SECONDARY TUMORS IN PEDIATRIC, HODGKIN'S DISEASE, AND BREAST CANCER POPULATIONS

The two patient populations from which most of the secondary malignancy data have been derived are patients treated for pediatric malignancies and those treated for Hodgkin's disease. The spectrum of pediatric malignancies includes a number of diseases that have been correlated with specific genetic abnormalities, such as retinoblastoma,[8,49,50] Wilms' tumor,[51,52] and some soft tissue sarcomas.[53] The Hodgkin's disease populations treated in the modern era have received radiation therapy or chemotherapy or both; this is similar in the major series. Specific aspects of the treatment regimens can be studied for their carcinogenicity. Immunity, however, often is impaired in Hodgkin's disease patients, even long after treatment has been completed.[3] Despite the potential confounding factors, the excellent cure rates among these relatively young patients, coupled with the long-term follow-up of relatively large patient populations, have provided important data on the risk of developing secondary neoplasms. With the widespread use of adjuvant chemotherapy and primary radiation therapy for breast cancer, a third large patient population is available for study of treatment-related malignancy.

PEDIATRIC MALIGNANCIES

After treatment of childhood malignancies, there is a distinctive pattern of secondary cancers that has been well described.[54] The most common secondary cancer is bone sarcomas, followed by soft tissue sarcomas, leukemias, and cancers of the brain, thyroid, and breast. The most frequent initial cancer is retinoblastoma, followed by Hodgkin's disease, soft tissue sarcomas, Wilms' tumor, and brain cancers. This is not the usual distribution of childhood cancers; it reflects both the genetic predisposition to develop multiple tumors of heritable retinoblastoma and soft tissue sarcoma associated with Li-Fraumeni syndrome, the treatment associated with the specific cancers, and perhaps the immune dysfunction associated with Hodgkin's disease. Among 9170 patients treated for childhood cancers by members of the Late Effects Study Group (LESG) who survived 2 or more years, the risk of a secondary bone sarcoma was 133-fold increased (95% confidence interval, 98–176).[48] The relative risks by initial diagnosis were 999 for retinoblastoma, 649 for Ewing's sarcoma, 297 for rhabdomyosarcoma, 127 for Wilms' tumor, and 106 for Hodgkin's disease. The cumulative probability of developing secondary bone sarcoma at 20 years was 2.8% for the whole cohort and 14.1% for patients with retinoblastoma.[48]

To evaluate the relation between radiation dose and the risk of bone sarcoma, individual radiation dosimetry at the site of the development of the bone sarcoma was done for each case and its matched controls. The dosimetry accounted for the absorption characteristics of bone for different types of radiation. When the doses in cases and controls were compared, the risk for bone sarcoma rose dramatically to a 38-fold increase after radiation doses up to 60 Gy.[48] There was concern that the effect was due to an extremely high risk in the retinoblastoma patients, so the retinoblastoma patients were separated from all other patients, and the doses were compared. In each category of dose up to 40 Gy or more, the risks were equivalent in the retinoblastoma patients and all other patients. Although the cumulative risks for developing bone sarcoma are much higher after retinoblastoma than after other cancers, the relative risks, dose for dose, are similar. This is explained by the case-control matching on bilaterality of the retinoblastomas, which controlled for the genetic factors. Patients with heritable retinoblastomas have a higher baseline risk for secondary bone sarcoma, but their response to radiation is similar to patients with other childhood cancers.

In addition to the radiation dose, the exposure to chemotherapy was also evaluated (Table 63–28). There was an independent effect of exposure to alkylating agents in the risk for bone cancer (relative risk, 4.7; 95% confidence interval, 1.0–22).[48] The risk rose with increasing total dose of alkylating agents, suggesting a dose response. The effect of alkylating agents was much smaller than that of the radiation. In the presence of radiation to the site of the bone sarcoma, the alkylating agents added little to the risk. Other drugs did not appear to be associated with the risk of developing bone sarcoma. Although an increased risk for bone sarcoma associated with alkylating agents had not been previously reported, an increased risk for bone sarcoma after cyclophosphamide had been suggested after Ewing's sarcoma by Strong and colleagues[55] and after retinoblastoma by Draper and colleagues.[6] The findings of this study were consistent with previous observations.

Although the smaller number of secondary soft tissue sarcomas in the LESG cohort prohibited as extensive analyses as the bone sarcomas, the patterns of risk were similar. The risk for soft tissue sarcoma also increased with radiation dose to the site of the sarcoma, and there was a suggestion of a small effect of alkylating agent chemotherapy.[55a]

The risk for leukemia was also quantified in this cohort of 9170 survivors of pediatric cancer. Overall, the relative risk of developing leukemia was increased 14-fold (95% confidence interval, 9–22) and was highest (89-fold) after treatment of Hodgkin's disease.[33] The risk was associated with treatment with alkylating-agent chemotherapy, and it increased with the total dose of alkylating agents. Radiation dosimetry was done to estimate the radiation dose to the active bone marrow. In this study, no effect of radiation dose to the bone marrow was found, but the comparison group for the radiation-exposed cases and controls included patients who had received alkylating agents. There was no additional effect of the radiation that could be detected. This group did not include patients who had been treated with epipodophyllotoxins.

TABLE 63–28. Risk of Bone Sarcoma by Radiation Dose and Alkylator Score in LESG Study

	Alkylator Score		
Radiation Dose	*0*	*1 or 2*	*≥3*
None			
Relative risk	1.0*	4.8	8.5†
No of cases:controls	6:44	1:4	3:3
<1000 cGy			
Relative risk	1.3	0.4	1.3
No. of cases:controls	5:43	1:13	3:14
≥1000 cGy			
Relative risk	37.4‡	14.2‡	59.2‡
No. of cases:controls	21:45	11:26	13:12

LESG, Late Effects Study Group.
* Referent category.
† Trend in alkylator score in subjects not exposed to radiation; $p = 0.05$.
‡ $p < 0.05$.
(Tucker MA, D'Angio GJ, Boice JD, et al. Bone sarcoma linked to radiotherapy and chemotherapy in children. N Engl J Med 1987;317: 588–593)

Thyroid cancer risk after treatment of childhood cancer is increased 53-fold compared with general population rates.[56] The risk is highest after treatment of neuroblastoma (relative risk, 350); Wilms' tumor (relative risk, 132); non-Hodgkin's lymphoma (relative risk, 81); and Hodgkin's disease (relative risk, 67). Although there have been many quantifications of risk for thyroid cancer after radiation, most of the studies have evaluated much lower doses. This study evaluated therapeutic range radiation doses. Radiation dosimetry was done for the cases and controls to calculate the total dose to the thyroid. Doses to the thyroid of 2 Gy or more were associated with a 13-fold increased risk of thyroid cancer (95% confidence interval, 1.7–104). In this study, the comparison group received less than 2 Gy because all the case patients had received some irradiation to the thyroid. In other studies, patients receiving similar doses have been shown to have about a 10-fold increased risk of thyroid cancer compared with those receiving no radiation therapy. Therefore, the 13-fold increase shown in comparison with patients receiving less than 2 Gy may be about 130-fold increased compared with nonirradiated patients. The risk for thyroid cancer rose with increasing dose ($p < 0.001$), but this was derived almost entirely from the increase from less than 2 Gy to 2 Gy or more. The risk did not decrease, however, at radiation doses as high as 60 Gy related to the total dose of radiation to the thyroid. There was no increased risk of thyroid cancer associated with alkylating-agent chemotherapy. One of the a priori hypotheses to be tested by the study was whether or not dactinomycin protects against radiation-induced solid tumors, as had been previously suggested.[57] There was no diminution of risk associated with dactinomycin in conjunction with radiation therapy.[56]

The Children's Cancer Study Group also evaluated the risk for secondary cancers after ALL and found a sevenfold increased risk of developing a secondary cancer.[58] Most of this risk was due to the 22-fold risk of brain cancer. There was also a fourfold increased risk for lymphoma (n = 8) and leukemia, but the authors did not split the two cases of ANLL from the lymphomas. It is unlikely that the risk for ANLL would have been significantly increased. The brain cancers occurred in patients who were diagnosed before age 5 years and who received cranial or whole-body irradiation.

HODGKIN'S DISEASE

One of the most widely reported secondary cancers is leukemia after Hodgkin's disease. Virtually every group with an interest in Hodgkin's disease has reported their experience with treatment-related leukemias. These reports, however, are limited by the relatively small number of leukemias reported by any one center. Although the treatment-induced leukemias are a well-recognized phenomenon, several areas

TABLE 63–29. Relative Risk of Acute or Nonlymphocytic Leukemia According to Radiation Dose to Bone Marrow and Dose of Mechlorethamine-Procarbazine Chemotherapy

No. of Cycles	*Radiation Dose (Gy)*			
	0	*<10*	*10–20*	*>20*
0		1.0	1.6 (0.3–10)	8.2 (1.7–39)
≤6	9.1 (1.6–53)	8.6 (1.9–39)	22 (5.1–99)	9.4 (2–45)
>6	50 (8.1–310)	26 (4.4–150)	63 (9.6–410)	22 (3.7–130)

(Adapted from Kaldor JM, Day NE, Clarke EA, et al. Leukemia following Hodgkin's disease. N Engl J Med 1990;322:7–13)

of controversy persist. It is clear that the leukemias are related to alkylating-agent chemotherapy, but a major area of controversy is whether combined modality therapy confers a higher risk of leukemia than chemotherapy alone. Other areas of discussion are whether splenectomy contributes to risk of leukemia and whether age at treatment is important. One recent study had sufficient numbers of Hodgkin's disease patients and cases of leukemia to address these issues.[35] One hundred and sixty-three leukemias occurred among 29,552 patients with Hodgkin's disease. There was no difference in the relative risk of leukemia after chemotherapy alone (relative risk, 9; 95% confidence interval, 4.1–20) and after combined-modality therapy (relative risk, 7.7; 95% confidence interval, 3.9–15). The highest risk was after mechlorethamine-procarbazine, cyclophosphamide-procarbazine, or chlorambucil. Kaldor was able to evaluate risks associated with radiation and mechlorethamine-procarbazine therapy (Table 63–29).[35] A small risk for leukemia was seen after radiation therapy alone, and this risk rose with increasing radiation dose. The risk did not significantly or consistently vary across radiation doses for either number of chemotherapy cycles, but increased consistently with more cycles of chemotherapy in each radiation dose range. These investigators also found a twofold increased risk of leukemia in the patients who had undergone splenectomy, even when the dose of chemotherapy was taken into account.[35]

Although many studies have found an increased actuarial risk of leukemia in patients over age 50 years, Tucker and colleagues[11] found equivalent relative risks of acute nonlymphocytic leukemia in those treated over and under age 50 years (116 and 114, respectively). Kaldor and associates[35] reported that the relative risk for leukemia in patients treated under 38 years of age was higher than the relative risk in patients over 38 years old. The apparent discrepancy in the actuarial and relative risks is due to the higher rate of ANLL at older ages in the general population. When the age-specific rates are used, as in the relative risks, the risk for leukemia is equivalent in the different age groups. The risks for solid cancers at 15 years after treatment of Hodgkin's disease have also been quantified (Table 63–30).[11] Significantly elevated risks were found for lung cancer, non-Hodgkin's lymphoma, melanoma, stomach cancer, and bone and connective tissue sarcomas. This pattern of secondary cancers is distinctive and is similar to the distribution of cancers seen in immunosuppressed populations, such as renal transplantation patients or patients with non-Hodgkin's lymphoma. All cancers of the stomach, bone, and connective tissue (as well as a leiomyosarcoma of the small bowel) occurred within areas previously treated with radiation therapy. All those who developed lung cancer received radiation therapy and smoked. The relative risks for solid tumors increased with time, consistent with a radiation effect. The melanomas occurred without association with a specific treatment in patients who had dysplastic nevi.[59] Similar to patients with renal transplantation who develop melanoma, there is minimal lymphocytic host response at the base of the melanomas, which is an important prognostic factor.

Although an excess of thyroid cancer and breast cancer was anticipated at the 15 year follow-up (mean follow-up, 6.2 years), significant excesses were not seen.[11] Hancock and colleagues[60] subsequently found a 16-fold excess of thyroid cancer (mean follow-up, 9.9 years). The actuarial risk of developing thyroid cancer was 1.7% at 20 years. An insignificantly elevated breast cancer risk of 1.7 was seen after 15 years.[11] When the data were examined by age at radiation, because of the findings seen with tuberculosis fluoroscopy pa-

TABLE 63–30. Relative Risk of Second Cancers After Hodgkin's Disease

Site	*Observed Cases*	*Expected Cases*	*Observed/Expected Cases (95% Confidence Interval)*
All cancers	83	15.9	5.2 (4.2–6.5)
Acute nonlymphocytic leukemia	27	0.2	115 (76–167)
Solid tumors	46	14.5	3.2 (2.3–4.3)
Lung	14	1.8	7.7 (4.2–12.9)
Non-Hodgkin's lymphoma	9	0.5	18 (8.1–33.5)
Stomach	4	0.4	10 (2.8–26.4)
Melanoma	4	0.4	8.9 (2.4–22.8)
Bone	2	0.1	31 (3.5–111.8)
Connective tissue	2	0.1	15 (1.6–52.7)
Breast	3	1.8	1.7 (0.3–4.9)

(Adapted from Tucker MA, Coleman CN, Cox RS, et al. Risk of second malignancies following Hodgkin's disease after 15 years. N Engl J Med 1988;318:76–81)

tients and atomic bomb survivors, a 12-fold increased risk was seen in women who were treated before age 30. Hancock and colleagues[61] reevaluated this risk after more prolonged follow-up, and found a significantly elevated (fourfold) risk for breast cancer. Again, the highest risk was in women radiated before age 30.

The actuarial risks for leukemia, non-Hodgkin's lymphoma, and solid tumors at 15 years is demonstrated in Figure 63–11.[11] The risk for any secondary cancer (excluding nonmelanoma skin and simultaneous cancers) was 17.6% (±3.1%) compared with 2.6% (±1%) in the general population. The major component of the risk was due to the solid tumors, which, after a steep rise after 10 years, was 13.2% at 15 years. The risk for leukemia was 3.6%, with no new cases appearing after 9 years; the 1.6% risk for lymphoma rose slowly throughout the study period.[11] The 20-year cumulative risks have not yet been published. The risk for leukemia is unchanged, but the risks for non-Hodgkin's lymphoma and solid tumors have continued to increase, as anticipated.

The same pattern of second solid tumors has been confirmed in many subsequent studies, with some variations. Groups that did not use the spade field of irradiation as commonly did not report an excess of stomach cancer. The largest analysis of combined data sets was done by the International Database on Hodgkin's Disease.[62] The risks for secondary cancers were quantified 1 or more years after start of treatment of the Hodgkin's disease in 12,411 patients who accrued 82,850 person-years. Three hundred and sixty-seven solid secondary cancers, including basal cell carcinomas, occurred. The risk for solid tumors increased with time since treatment. The most common second solid tumor was lung cancer in both men and women. An excess of breast cancer was not seen until 15 to 19 years after treatment. Similar to the Stanford data, the risk for non-Hodgkin's lymphoma continued to increase over time and was not related to any treatment group.

Hodgkin's disease is one of the few tumors that occurs in both children and adults, and it is treated in similar manners in the two age groups. Age-at-treatment effects on the risk for secondary cancers can thus be evaluated (Table 63–31).[11,63] The risks for leukemia were similar. The risks for bone, connective tissue, and thyroid cancers, however, varied by age at treatment. In the Stanford data, the two patients who developed bone cancer were irradiated during their teenage years. Bone sarcomas, therefore, appear to be a consequence of irradiating growing bone rather than adult bone. In a similar manner, the risk for connective tissue sarcoma appears to be somewhat lower in adults. The risk for thyroid cancer also is much greater in those irradiated at an early age, which is consistent with data from atomic bomb survivors and from most groups developing radiation-induced thyroid cancer. The patients treated in the pediatric cohort have not yet attained the age when the "adult" cancers would likely manifest, so that the risks for lung, breast, and stomach cancers and melanoma cannot easily be compared.

In summary, the occurrence of a secondary leukemia after treatment of Hodgkin's disease is related to the cumulative dose of alkylating agents and, to a lesser extent, radiation. The radiation effect is only detectable in the patients who have not received alkylating agents. Secondary solid tumors and lymphomas occur with equal frequency in all treatment schemes, indicating that it is the disease itself or radiation therapy, or both, that is the etiologic agent. Given the increasing risk of the development of solid tumors and lymphomas, careful lifelong surveillance is indicated for Hodgkin's disease patients, with special attention given to new clinical signs or symptoms. Patients must be taught the necessity of not smoking, and for females, the importance of monthly breast self-examination. Mammography should be considered starting at 15 years after treatment. Patients with dysplastic nevi must be taught the necessity of monthly skin self-examinations, avoidance of sunburn, and routine professional skin examinations. With the knowledge of the substantial risks of secondary cancers, clinical trials are seeking to decrease this risk by attempting to decrease the exposure to both radiation therapy and alkylating agents without compromising the excellent therapeutic results.

BREAST CANCER

With the recommendations for the widespread use of adjuvant treatment of even low-stage disease, a large number of women are being exposed to cytotoxic therapy and can be expected to live for a long time.[64] Only relatively limited data are available to address the risk for secondary cancers. The follow-up

TABLE 63–31. Relative Risk of Specific Second Cancers After Treatment for Hodgkin's Disease in Two Age Groups

Site	*LESG Study (n = 1036; average follow-up = 5.1 y; average age = 12 y)*	*Stanford Study (n = 1507; average follow-up = 6.2 y; average age = 29 y)*
All cancers	16	7.4
Leukemia	89	66
Bone	106	31
Connective tissue	39	15
Thyroid	68	16*

* Risk of 16 from 1787 patients reported by Hancock and colleagues.[60]
(Adapted from Tucker MA, Coleman CN, Cox RS, et al. Risk of second malignancies following Hodgkin's disease after 15 years. N Engl J Med 1988;318:76–81; and Tucker MA, Meadows AT, Boice JD Jr, et al. Cancer risk following treatment of childhood cancer. In: Radiation carcinogenesis: Epidemiology and biological significance. New York: Raven 1984:211–224)

period in most groups is too short to adequately evaluate solid tumors, but several studies have examined the risk for leukemia associated with treatment of breast cancer.

Fisher and associates[9] reported the risk for leukemia in the National Surgical Adjuvant Breast Project clinical trials. The 10-year cumulative risk for leukemia after surgery alone was 0.06% (±0.05%) and was 1.37% (±0.74%) in the surgery plus locoregional radiation therapy group. Of note, two of the six cases of leukemia that occurred in the surgery plus radiation group were chronic lymphocytic leukemia, which is not a radiation-related cancer. The risk for leukemia plus myelodysplastic syndrome was 1.54% (±0.36%) after surgery plus chemotherapy that included melphalan. This risk was significantly higher than the risk with surgery alone. In contrast, Valagussa and associates[65] found no leukemia in 666 women treated with adjuvant cyclophosphamide, methotrexate, and fluorouracil.[65] These findings were extended by Curtis and associates[66] in a study of 82,700 women treated for breast cancer. The risk for leukemia after regional radiation alone was increased twofold, with an average dose of 7.5 Gy to active bone marrow. The risk associated with treatment with alkylating agents, without radiation, was increased tenfold; and with both radiation and alkylating agents, it was increased 17-fold. These radiation doses and chemotherapy doses are much higher than those used with adjuvant treatment or primary radiation therapy after lumpectomy. Women receiving melphalan were ten times more likely to develop leukemia than those receiving cyclophosphamide (relative risk, 31.4 versus 3.1). All the leukemias that developed after cyclophosphamide occurred in women who had received over 20,000 mg of cyclophosphamide.[66] The difference in the total dose of cyclophosphamide may explain the varying leukemia risks in these populations. Based on the risks found in their study, Curtis and associates[66] estimated that only about 5 in 10,000 patients treated with 6 months of a cyclophosphamide-based adjuvant regimen would be expected to develop a treatment-induced leukemia within about 10 years of breast cancer diagnosis.

Boice and colleagues[67] reported the risk of breast cancer in the contralateral breast of women who received radiation therapy for breast cancer between 1935 and 1982 in Connecticut. There was a small increase in risk associated with an average dose of about 3 Gy to the contralateral breast. Although the treatment varied substantially from recent practices, the total dose was within the range of what is delivered to the contralateral breast with current techniques. Fewer than 3% of all second breast cancers in the study could be attributed to previous radiation treatment. Consistent with the studies discussed previously, the risk was highest in women treated at a young age (under 45 years old). There was no increased risk in the women treated over age 45 years.

In summary, leukemia risk after breast cancer is due to treatment with alkylating agents, particularly melphalan. Risk is related to total dose of drug and is low in the dose range of cyclophosphamide currently used in the adjuvant setting. The risk for leukemia after older techniques of regional radiation therapy (chest wall and nodes) also appears to be minimally increased but is unknown after breast-conserving radiation therapy. The most common solid second primary cancer that occurs after breast cancer is contralateral breast cancer, but fewer than 3% of these tumors could be attributed to radiation. The effect of adjuvant tamoxifen and its increased use[64] on this radiation consequence is also unknown. Breast cancer patients are an important group to follow over time because, although the risks are much lower than those after treatment of Hodgkin's disease, breast cancer is a common tumor, and even a substantially decreased risk for secondary cancers compared with Hodgkin's disease could translate into a larger number of affected patients.

HOST FACTORS

Although the risks for second tumors after specific drugs and radiation doses are now being quantified, many questions remain. Several host characteristics have been identified that have a substantial effect on the level of risk associated with treatment. One of these is age at exposure. It is clear from multiple populations, including atomic bomb survivors, tuberculosis fluoroscopy patients, Hodgkin's disease patients, and breast cancer patients, that age at irradiation to the breast is a major determinant of risk for breast cancer. Women exposed over age 30 to 45 years, depending on the study, do not appear to be at increased risk for breast cancer, while those exposed at younger ages, particularly in adolescence, have an extremely high risk. From atomic bomb survivors, there is evidence that, in addition to the radiation, other host factors, such as age at first pregnancy, remain important in those who received relatively low doses to the breast. The effects of age and dose have not been fully explored, particularly at the therapeutic ranges, but it appears that in Hodgkin's disease patients, even doses in the therapeutic range confer high risk in young patients.

The risk for radiation-induced thyroid cancer is also modulated by the age at exposure to radiation. From several populations, including atomic bomb survivors, Marshall Islanders, tinea capitis patients, and Hodgkin's disease patients, the risk is higher after early childhood exposure. From the LESG study, the markedly increased risk is also seen not only at the lower doses previously reported, but also after therapeutic range doses up to 60 Gy or more. The data for an age effect in the development of bone sarcomas and perhaps connective tissue sarcomas are less compelling. The much smaller risks of bone, and to a lesser extent connective tissue sarcomas, after treatment of Hodgkin's disease in adults indicates an age effect. The difference in risk for bone sarcoma after treatment of childhood cancer in general versus adult cancers (such as cervical cancer[5]) again suggests that growing bone (and perhaps connective tissue) is more susceptible to treatment-induced sarcomas.

Age does not appear to have the same type of effect in alkylating-agent-induced leukemia. The relative risks by age groups are remarkably similar. The significantly increased actuarial risk of ANLL after Hodgkin's disease that is routinely seen in older patients (over 50 years) in most clinical series is due to the increased rate of ANLL in the general population at that age. The rates in children treated for Hodgkin's disease appear comparable to those in adults.

Immunosuppression also appears to have an effect on the risk for secondary cancers. The similarity in patterns of tumors after Hodgkin's disease, non-Hodgkin's lymphoma,[68] renal transplantation, and congenital or acquired immunodeficiency syndromes suggests that specific tumors are particularly affected by the immune status of the host. Non-Hodgkin's lymphoma, sarcomas, melanoma, and to a lesser extent lung cancer and stomach cancer, appear to be modulated by the immune system.

Probably the most important host factor is the patient's genetic susceptibility to developing cancer. The prototype of this is heritable retinoblastoma, in which patients with germline alterations in the RB locus have an excess of both radiation-induced and spontaneous osteosarcomas, with similar RB changes. As more tumor-suppressor genes, oncogenes, protooncogenes, and other important control genes are discovered and characterized, the individual susceptibility to specific agents may be clarified. The role of interindividual variation in the metabolism of specific drugs is only starting to be explored and may be a potent predictor of patients at risk for alkylating-agent-induced cancers. As the mechanisms of carcinogenesis are clarified, chemotherapy drugs may be able to be chemically modified to reduce risk without sacrificing efficacy.

CONCLUSION

Secondary, treatment-related cancers are seen because the initial treatment is successful. Attempts should be made to reduce this complication. Indeed, most investigators studying pediatric and Hodgkin's disease populations are developing treatment strategies to minimize late complications. Changes in therapy to minimize secondary cancers are best made in the context of a carefully designed study that includes the codification of treatment and follow-up procedures. It is through such careful studies that current treatments can be made less toxic while their efficacy is maintained or improved. Practicing oncologists are encouraged to participate in such studies so that this evolutionary process can proceed as expeditiously as possible.

REFERENCES

1. Li FP. Secondary cancers. In: DeVita VT Jr, Hellman S, Rosenberg SA, eds. Cancer: Principles and practice of oncology. 2nd ed. Philadelphia: JB Lippincott, 1985:2040–2049.
2. Coleman CN. Adverse effects of cancer therapy: Risk of secondary neoplasms. Am J Pediatr Hematol Oncol 1982;4:103–111.
3. Coleman CN. Secondary neoplasms in patients treated for cancer: Etiology and perspective. Radiat Res 1982;92:188–200.
4. Monson RR. Analysis of relative survival and proportional mortality. Comput Biomed Res 1974;7:325–332.
5. Boice JD Jr, Day NE, Anderson A, et al. Second cancer following radiation treatment for cervical cancer: An international collaboration among cancer registries. J Natl Cancer Inst 1985;74:955–975.
6. Draper GJ, Sanders BM, Kingston JE. Second primary neoplasms in patients with retinoblastoma. Br J Cancer 1986;53:661–671.
7. Abramson DH, Ellsworth RM, Kitchi FD, et al. Second nonocular tumors in retinoblastoma survivors: Are they radiation-induced? Ophthalmology 1984;91:1351–1355.
8. Hansen FM, Koufson A, Gallie BL, et al. Osteosarcoma and retinoblastoma: A shared chromosomal mechanism revealing recessive predisposition. Proc Natl Acad Sci USA 1986;82:6216–6220.
9. Fisher B, Rockette H, Fisher ER, et al. Leukemia in breast cancer patients following adjuvant chemotherapy or postoperative radiation: The NSABP experience. J Clin Oncol 1985;3:1640–1658.
10. Greene MH, Harris EL, Gershenson DM, et al. Melphalan may be a more potent leukemogen than cyclophosphamide. Ann Intern Med 1986;105:360–367.
11. Tucker MA, Coleman NC, Cox RS, et al. Risk of secondary malignancies following Hodgkin's disease after 15 years. N Engl J Med 1988;318:76–81.
12. Valagussa P, Santoro A, Bellani-Fossati F, et al. Second acute leukemia and other malignancies following treatment for Hodgkin's disease. J Clin Oncol 1986;4:830–837.
13. Kaplan EL, Meier P. Nonparametric estimation from incomplete observation. J Am Stat Assoc 1958;53:457–481.
14. Gehan EA. A generalized Wilcoxon test for comparing arbitrarily singly censored samples. Biometrika 1965;52:203–223.
15. Coleman CN, Kaplan HS, Cox R, et al. Leukemias, non-Hodgkin's lymphomas and solid tumours in patients treated for Hodgkin's disease. Cancer Surv 1982;1:733–744.
16. National Research Council, Committee on the Biologic Effects of Ionizing Radiations. Health effects of exposure to low levels of ionizing radiation. Washington, DC: National Academy of Science, 1990.
17. Preston DL, Kato H, Kopecky KJ, et al. Studies of the mortality of A-bomb survivors. Radiat Res 1987;111:151–178.
18. Land CE. A nested case-control approach to interactions between radiation dose and other factors as causes of cancer. RERF Commentary and Review Series CR 1-90. Hiroshima: Radiation Effects Research Foundation, 1990.
19. Land CE, Hayakawa N, Machado S, et al. A case-control interview study of breast cancer among Japanese A-bomb survivors. I. Main effects. RERF Technical Report (in press).
20. Land CE, Hayakawa N, Machado S, et al. A case-control interview study of breast cancer among Japanese A-bomb survivors. II. Interactions between epidemiologic factors and radiation dose. RERF Technical Report (in press).
21. Land CE. Histological types of lung cancer in Japanese A-bomb survivors and Colorado plateau uranium miners. Proceedings of the International Conference on Radiation Effects and Protection. Mito, Japan, 1992.
22. Holm LE, Wiklund KE, Lundell GE, et al. Cancer risk in population examined with diagnostic doses of ^{131}I. J Natl Cancer Inst 1989;81:302–306.
23. Hrubec Z, Boice JD Jr, Monson RR, Rosenstein M. Breast cancer after multiple chest fluoroscopies: Second follow-up of Massachusetts women with tuberculosis. Cancer Res 1989;49:229–234.
24. Linos A, Gray JE, Orvis AL, et al. Low-dose radiation and leukemia. N Engl J Med 1980;302:1101–1105.
25. Evans JS, Wennberg JE, McNeil BJ. The influence of diagnostic radiography on the incidence of breast cancer and leukemia. N Engl J Med 1986;315:810–815.
26. Reimer RR, Hoover RN, Fraumeni JF Jr, et al. Acute leukemia after alkylating-agent therapy for ovarian cancer. N Engl J Med 1982;307:1416–1421.
27. Greene MH, Boice JD Jr, Greer BE, et al. Acute nonlymphocytic leukemia after therapy with alkylating agents for ovarian cancer. N Engl J Med 1982;307:1416–1421.
28. Boice JD Jr, Greene MH, Killen JY, et al. Leukemia after chemotherapy with semustine (methyl-CCNU): Evidence of a dose-response effect. N Engl J Med [Letter] 1986;314:119–120.
29. Bergsagel DE, Bailey AJ, Langley GR, et al. The chemotherapy for plasma-cell myeloma and the incidence of acute leukemia. N Engl J Med 1979;301:743–748.
30. Berk PD, Goldberg JD, Silverstein MN, et al. Increased risk of acute leukemia in polycythemia vera associated with chlorambucil therapy. N Engl J Med 1981;304:441–447.
31. Boice JD Jr, Greene MH, Killen, et al. Leukemia and preleukemia after adjuvant treatment of gastrointestinal cancer with semustine (methyl-CCNU). N Engl J Med 1983;309:1079–1084.
32. Chak LY, Sikic BI, Tucker MA, et al. Increased incidence of acute nonlymphocytic leukemia following therapy in patients with small cell carcinoma of the lung. J Clin Oncol 1984;2:385–390.
33. Tucker MA, Meadows AT, Boice JD Jr, et al. Leukemia after therapy with alkylating agents for childhood cancer. J Natl Cancer Inst 1987;78:459–464.
34. Kaldor JM, Day NE, Pettersson F, et al. Leukemia following chemotherapy for ovarian cancer. N Engl J Med 1990;322:1–6.
35. Kaldor JM, Day NE, Clarke A, et al. Leukemia following Hodgkin's disease. N Engl J Med 1990;322:7–13.
36. Cuzik J, Erskine S, Edelman D, et al. A comparison of the incidence of the myelodysplastic syndrome and acute myeloid leukemia following melphalan and cyclophosphamide treatment for myelomatosis. Br J Cancer 1987;55:523–529.
37. Greene MH. Epidemiologic studies of chemotherapy-related acute leukemia. In: Cascinelli A, ed. Epidemiology and quantitation of environmental risk in humans from radiation and other agents. New York: Plenum, 1985:499–514.
38. Preisler HD, Early AP, Raza A, et al. Therapy of secondary nonlymphocytic leukemia with cytarabine. N Engl J Med 1983;308:21–23.
39. Vaughan WP, Karp JE, Burke PJ. Effective chemotherapy of acute myelocytic leukemia occurring after alkylating agent or radiation therapy for prior malignancy. J Clin Oncol 1983;1:204–207.
40. Le Beau MM, Albain KS, Larson RA, et al. Clinical and cytogenetic correlations in 63 patients with therapy-related myelodysplastic syndromes and acute nonlymphocytic leukemia: Further evidence for characteristic abnormalities of chromosomes no. 5 and 7. J Clin Oncol 1986;4:325–345.
41. Pui CH, Ribeiro RC, Hancock ML, et al. Acute myeloid leukemia in children treated with epipodophyllotoxins for acute lymphoblastic leukemia. N Engl J Med 1991;325:1682–1687.
42. Pedersen-Bjergaard J, Daugaard G, Hansen SW, et al. Increased risk of myelodysplasia and leukaemia after etoposide, cisplatin, and bleomycin for germ-cell tumours. Lancet 1991;338:359–363.
43. Whitlock JA, Greer JP, Lukens JN. Epipodophyllotoxin-related leukemia: Identification of a new subset of secondary leukemia. Cancer 1991;68:600–604.
44. Pedersen-Bjergaard J, Philip P, Larsen SO, et al. Chromosome aberrations and prognostic factors in therapy-related myelodysplasia and acute nonlymphocytic leukemia. Blood 1990;76:1083–1091.
45. Pedersen-Bjergaard J, Ersboll J, Hansen VL, et al. Carcinoma of the urinary bladder

after treatment with cyclophosphamide for non-Hodgkin's lymphoma. N Engl J Med 1988;318:1028–1032.

46. Wall RL, Clausen K. Carcinoma of the urinary bladder in patients receiving cyclophosphamide. N Engl J Med 1975;293:271–273.
47. Travis LB, Curtis RE, Boice JD Jr, Fraumeni JF Jr. Bladder cancer after chemotherapy for non-Hodgkin's lymphoma. N Engl J Med 1989;321:544–545.
48. Tucker MA, D'Angio GJ, Boice JD Jr, et al. Bone sarcomas linked to radiotherapy and chemotherapy in children. N Engl J Med 1987;317:588–593.
49. Cavenee WK, Murphee AL, Shull, et al. Prediction of familial predisposition to retinoblastoma. N Engl J Med 1986;314:1201–1207.
50. Lee WH, Bookstein R, Hong F, et al. Human retinoblastoma susceptibility gene: Cloning, identification, and sequence. Science 1987;235:1394–1399.
51. Arthur DC. Genetics and cytogenetics of pediatric cancers. Cancer 1986;58:534–540.
52. Koufos A, Hansen MF, Lampkin BC, et al. Loss of alleles at loci on human chromosome 11 during the genesis of WIlms' tumor. Nature 1984;309:170–172.
53. Malkin D, Li FP, Strong LC, et al. Germ line p53 mutations in a familial syndrome of breast cancer, sarcomas, and other neoplasms. Science 1990;250:1233–1238.
54. Meadows AT. Risk factors for second malignant neoplasms: Report from the Late Effects Study Group. Bull Cancer (Paris) 1988;75:125–130.
55. Strong LC, Herson J, Osborne BM, et al. Risk of radiation-related subsequent malignant tumors in survivors of Ewing's sarcoma. J Natl Cancer Inst 1979;62:1401–1406.

55a. Tucker MA, unpublished data. National Cancer Institute, 1992.

56. Tucker MA, Morris Jones PH, Boice JD Jr, et al. Therapeutic radiation at a young age is linked to secondary thyroid cancer. Cancer Res 1991;51:2885–2888.
57. D'Angio GJ, Meadows AT, Mike V, et al. Decreased risk of radiation-associated second malignant neoplasms in actinomycin-D treated patients. Cancer 1976;37:1177–1185.
58. Neglia JP, Meadows AT, Robison LL, et al. Second neoplasms after acute lymphoblastic leukemia in childhood. N Engl J Med 1991;325:1330–1336.
59. Tucker MA, Misfeldt D, Coleman CN, et al. Cutaneous malignant melanoma after Hodgkin's disease. Ann Intern Med 1985;102:37–41.
60. Hancock SL, Cox RS, McDougall IR. Thyroid diseases after treatment of Hodgkin's disease. N Engl J Med 1991;325:599–605.
61. Hancock SL, Tucker MA, Hoppe RT. Breast cancer after treatment for Hodgkin's disease. J Natl Cancer Inst (in press).
62. Kaldor JM, Lasset C. Second malignancies following Hodgkin's disease. In: Somers R, Henry-Amar M, Meerwaldt JH, et al, eds. Treatment strategy in hodgkin's disease. Colloque INSERM/John Libbey Eurotext 1990;196:139–150.
63. Tucker MA, Meadows AT, Boice JD Jr, et al. Cancer risk following treatment for childhood cancer. In: Boice JD Jr, Fraumeni JF Jr, eds. Radiation carcinogenesis: Epidemiology and biological significance. New York: Raven, 1984:211–224.
64. Early Breast Cancer Trialists' Collaborative Group. Systemic treatment of early breast cancer by hormonal, cytotoxic, or immune therapy. Lancet 1992;339:1–15, 71–85.
65. Valagussa P, Tancini G, Bonadonna G. Second malignancies after CMF for resectable breast cancer. J Clin Oncol 1987;5:1138–1142.
66. Curtis RE, Boice JD Jr, Stovall M, et al. Dose-dependent leukemia risk after drug and radiation treatment for breast cancer. N Engl J Med 1992;326:1745–1751.
67. Boice JD Jr, Harvey EB, Blettner M, et al. Cancer in the contralateral breast after radiotherapy for breast cancer. N Engl J Med 1992;326:781–785.
68. Travis LB, Curtis RE, Boice JD Jr, et al. Second cancers following non-Hodgkin's lymphoma. Cancer 1991;67:2002–2009.

Cancer: Principles & Practice of Oncology, Fourth Edition,
edited by Vincent T. DeVita, Jr., Samuel Hellman, Steven A. Rosenberg.
J.B. Lippincott Co., Philadelphia © 1993.

CHAPTER 64

Supportive Care and the Quality of Life of the Cancer Patient

SECTION 1

KATHLEEN M. FOLEY

Management of Cancer Pain

Pain is one of the most common symptoms leading to medical evaluation of the cancer patient. Numerous national and international surveys have demonstrated that 30% to 50% of patients in active therapy and as many as 60% to 90% of patients with advanced disease have pain.[1–6] Several studies that have focused on both patient and physician attitudes toward cancer pain suggest that cancer pain is perceived as the most feared consequence of cancer.[7,8] Sixty-nine percent of patients interviewed reported that they would consider suicide if their cancer pain became intolerable. For the clinician, pain represents a difficult diagnostic and therapeutic medical problem.[9,10]

Advances in the diagnosis and treatment of cancer, coupled with recent advances in our understanding of the anatomy, physiology, pharmacology, and psychology of pain perception, have led to improved care of the patient with pain of malignant origin. Specialized methods of cancer diagnosis and treatment provide the most direct approach to treating cancer pain by treating the cause of the pain. However, before the introduction of successful antitumor therapy, when treatment of the cause of the pain has failed, or when injury to bone, soft tissue, or nerve has occurred as a result of therapy, appropriate pain management is essential. Patients with cancer are managed most effectively by a multidisciplinary approach, using the expertise of a wide range of medical personnel.[2,11,12] The goal of pain therapy for patients receiving active treatment is to provide them with sufficient relief to tolerate the diagnostic and therapeutic approaches required to treat their cancer. For patients with advanced disease, pain control should be sufficient to allow them to function at a level that they choose and to die relatively free of pain. Critical to the management of cancer pain is the establishment of trust between the patient and physician; the physician must respect the pain complaint as serious, assess its nature and severity, and implement pain relief therapy.

BARRIERS TO CANCER PAIN RELIEF

Several barriers interfere with the appropriate management of patients with pain and cancer. Although pain can be controlled in most patients, an analysis of 11 published reports of cancer pain treatment covering nearly 2000 patients in nonhospice settings estimated that 50% to 80% did not have adequate control.[2] Several reports have focused on the observation that cancer pain is often improperly treated.[2,6–8,13–15] Various reasons have been cited for inadequate cancer pain management, including fear of addiction, lack of knowledge of analgesic drug therapy, assignment of low priority to pain management, lack of understanding of the pathophysiology of cancer pain, and overconcern about tolerance to analgesic medications. Patient-physician communication about pain symptoms is reported to be poor, and patients often underreport the amount of pain they experience or fail to report inadequate relief. Patients may also resist taking narcotic analgesics because of the stigma attached, and only take them when their pain is severe. Limited availability and lack of use of alternatives to systemic analgesics (*i.e.*, nerve blocks, palliative neurosurgery, and behavioral treatments) have also been reported to prevent adequate treatment.[4]

Finally, the attitudes of health-care providers toward pain and its impact on the patient influence the priority they and their patients place on pain therapy. Cleeland and colleagues have assessed the factors influencing the pain management practices of clinicians caring for cancer patients.[8] The authors studied clinicians' knowledge and attitudes toward cancer pain and its treatment in 91 physicians who participated in a statewide study. Of the participating physicians, 69% had managed the care of over 100 cancer patients in their current practice setting, and they represented the major medical and surgical subspecialties. Two groups of respondents were identified: one represented younger physicians with more specialized oncology training who had a liberal attitude toward pain management, while the larger group had a more conservative approach, placing a lower priority on pain management.

To further study these issues, Van Roenn and associates assessed physicians' knowledge and attitudes about cancer pain through a survey of the Eastern Cooperative Oncology group.[9] The 1177 oncologists who responded ranked the barriers as detailed in Table 64–1. This study clarified the current status of cancer pain treatment in the United States. Eighty-five percent of the respondents agreed that most patients with pain are undermedicated. Only half reported that pain control in their practice setting was either good or very good. Poor pain assessment was identified as the most important barrier to adequate pain management by 76% of physicians surveyed. In response to a case scenario, adjuvant medications were underused, and physicians failed to include a potent opioid in their most aggressive analgesic regimen 14% of the time. Concern about side effects by 65% of the physicians was cited as the reason for their reluctance to prescribe maximum analgesic therapy.

These data confirm the results of previous studies that have focused on the problems of inadequate pain control and serve as a useful outline for education to improve health-care professionals' and patients' knowledge about cancer pain and its treatment.

TABLE 64–1. ECOG Survey of Barriers to Adequate Cancer Pain Management

Characteristic	*Percent*
Inadequate assessment of pain and pain relief	76
Patient reluctance to report pain	48
Patient reluctance to take opiates	48
Medical staff reluctance to prescribe opiates	46
Lack of equipment skills	39
Nursing staff reluctance to administer opiates	28
Excessive state regulation of prescribing analgesics	12
Lack of psychological support services	8
Lack of available neurodestructive procedures	4
Lack of access to a wide range of analgesics	2
Lack of access to professionals who practice specialized methods	2

This table lists the percentage of 1177 oncologists' responses to a questionnaire survey describing their knowledge and attitudes about cancer pain management.
(Van Roenn JH, Cleeland CS, Gonin R, Hatfield A, Pandya KJ. Physicians' attitudes towards cancer pain management [in press])

EPIDEMIOLOGY

Although large-scale national epidemiologic studies on the incidence and severity of cancer pain are lacking, existing studies suggest that moderate to severe pain is experienced by one third of cancer patients receiving active therapy and by 60% to 90% of patients with advanced cancer. These data have been generated from several surveys of small groups of patients in specific medical-care settings.

Patients with cancer often have multiple causes of pain. In one survey 81% of patients reported two or more distinct pain complaints; 34% reported three pains.[3] More recent studies have focused on the factors that influence the prevalence of cancer pain.[5,10,13–18] Primary tumor type is one factor.[18] Patients with bone tumors and breast and prostate cancer have a much higher incidence of pain (60% to 80%) as compared with patients with lymphoma or leukemia.[1] The stage of disease is also a contributing factor. For example, only 15% of patients with nonmetastatic disease report pain. Certain types of tumors, because of their tendency for bony involvement or their occurrence in sites with proximity to neural structures, have a greater incidence of pain. Moreover, patient variables, such as anxiety and depression, markedly influence the patient's report and experience of pain.[17]

The data are very consistent in cross-cultural studies. Data from India, Thailand, Vietnam, and the Philippines report a similar prevalence of cancer pain in patients in active therapy and advanced disease.[4,20,21]

Studies have also focused not only on the prevalence of pain, but on its intensity, the degree of pain relief, and the impact of pain on quality of life. In one prospective study of pain prevalence and characteristics, 91 ambulatory patients with lung or colon cancer were interviewed.[22] They had reported persistent or frequent pain during the previous 2 weeks. One third of patients had more than one pain. The median pain duration was 4 weeks and the average pain intensity was moderate. Ninety percent experienced pain more than 25% of the time and 50% reported that pain interfered moderately or more with their general activity or work. A similar percentage reported moderate or greater pain interference with sleep, mood, and enjoyment of life. These data support the theory that pain is prevalent among well-functioning ambulatory patients and substantially compromises function in about half the patients who experience it.

In a study of patients with far-advanced disease cared for in a palliative care program, pain was the most common physical symptom associated with patients' perception of not feeling well. This symptom was significantly improved with analgesic therapies, but several other prominent symptoms, including weakness, anxiety, anorexia, nausea and vomiting, and confusion, were less readily treated. Several studies, including this one, have focused on the important observation that pain symptoms often represent only the "tip of the iceberg," and there is an enormous need to evaluate, rank, and treat all symptoms in dying patients to improve their quality of life.[24–27]

DEFINITION AND TYPES OF CANCER PAIN

DEFINITION OF PAIN

The definition of pain proposed by the International Association for the Study of Pain is "an unpleasant sensory and emotional experience associated with actual or potential tissue damage or described in terms of such damage."[28] Because pain is a subjective complaint, there is no definitive way to distinguish pain occurring in the absence of tissue damage from pain resulting from such damage. Pain as a somatic delusion or a masked depression is rare in cancer patients, and the presence of pain usually implies a pathologic process.

ANATOMY AND PHYSIOLOGY OF PAIN

Extensive investigations over the last 25 years have expanded our knowledge of ascending and descending central nervous system pathways that process and modulate nociceptive information. These advances provide a scientific rationale for the use of new and improved methods of cancer pain treatment.[29] A brief review of the neuroanatomy and physiology and pharmacology of pain provides a background for the later discussions of specific drug, anesthetic, and neurosurgical approaches.

Detailed information now supports the theory that activation of peripheral receptors in both superficial and deep structures as well as viscera by mechanical and chemical stimuli excites afferent discharges in two types of nerve fibers: thinly myelinated A-delta fibers and unmyelinated C fibers. These primary sensory afferents have their cell bodies in the dorsal root ganglion, and their axons enter the spinal cord via the dorsal root.

They ascend or descend from one or two segments in Lissauer's tract and synapse in specific lamina in the dorsal horn. There, they give rise to an extensive, highly branched terminal field. The small-diameter afferents that enter the cord in the lateral division of the dorsal root project densely to lamina I and lamina II in the dorsal horn. This projection includes both the unmyelinated and myelinated nociceptors, as well as some afferents that respond to innocuous thermal stimuli. Evidence suggests that myelinated nociceptors project to lamina I and V, unmyelinated nociceptors project to lamina II and possibly lamina I, and nonnociceptive myelinated afferents project to only deep lamina. Anatomic localization of nociceptive pathways within the dorsal horn reflects a very distinct relation between different lamina and their role in pain modulation.

The dorsal horn is an important site for modulating sensory input. Several ascending pathways arise from second-order neurons and decussate in the central gray of the spinal cord to become the neospinothalamic and paleospinothalamic tracts. These tracts project to discrete regions of the thalamus and cortex. The neospinothalamic pathways subserve pain intensity and localization, whereas the phylogenetically older paleospinothalamic pathway subserves the arousal and emotional component of pain. Descending pathways, the most important of which originate from the periaqueductal gray nuclei of the midbrain, synapse in the raphae magnus nucleus of the medulla. From this nucleus, a medial pathway, the dorsal longitudinal fasciculus, projects to the dorsal horn to modulate pain transmission. This pathway represents an important descending inhibitory pathway. A more laterally placed descending pathway from the locus ceruleus to the dorsal horn also plays a role in pain modulation at the spinal cord level.[30]

Neurotransmitters play a significant role in this modulatory system.[31] At the level of the nociceptive primary afferent, the neurotransmitters that appear to play an important role include substance P and the excitatory neurotransmitters glutamate, aspartate, and adenosine diphosphate. Dopamine, serotonin, norepinephrine, and the endogenous opioids enkephalin, β-endorphin, and dynorphin modulate pain at both the spinal and supraspinal sites. Attempts to enhance and mimic the role of these neurotransmitters in pain modulation have led to a series of clinical analgesic studies of, for example, amitriptyline.[32] Amitriptyline has analgesic properties independent of its antidepressant effects.[33,34] It appears to work by enhancing serotonin activity centrally by presynaptic inhibition of its reuptake and by activation of the descending inhibitory pain system. Recent studies with an NMDA antagonist suggest that pain can be inhibited at the level of the primary afferent by the use of these compounds, which alter the activity of the excitatory amino acid glutamate.[31]

Opiate receptors, stereospecific binding sites on the end of free nerve endings that bind endogenous and exogenous opioids, are localized in the ascending and descending pain pathways.[35] These receptors mediate the multiple pharmacologic effects of the opioid analgesics. Subpopulations of opioid receptors, including high-affinity and low-affinity μ receptors and δ, κ, and σ receptors, are localized to specific areas of the brain and spinal cord.

The identification of these subclasses of receptors that mediate different pharmacologic effects and that are located in specific cerebral and spinal sites offers the possibility of developing new analgesics targeted for specific receptors. For example, mu receptors modulate predominantly supraspinal analgesia, whereas delta receptors are the important receptors in modulating analgesia of the spinal cord level. The periaqueductal gray (PAG) region in the midbrain and the dorsal horn in the spinal cord are rich in these opioid receptors and are the supraspinal and spinal sites that mediate opioid analgesia.[36] These areas were identified as selective sites of analgesia after studies in animals and humans showed that electrical stimulation of the PAG region produces total body analgesia without motor or sensory changes. Administration of opioids directly into the PAG region inhibits pain transmission at the level of the spinal cord by activating this medial descending inhibitory pathway. The use of brain stem stimulation and the administration of the opioid analgesics directly into the cerebrospinal fluid bathing these selective sites in animals and cancer patients with pain are procedures based on this research. Pain transmission at the spinal cord level can be inhibited by the direct application of morphine, and these studies have led to the use of spinal opioid analgesia in clinical pain states.[37,38]

These advances in our understanding of pain modulatory systems and their neuroanatomic and neuropharmacologic correlates have had a major impact on the management of patients with pain. As our understanding of the neurobiology of pain expands, future studies will investigate therapeutic approaches directed at the primary afferent to prevent release of neurotransmitters as well as to modulate neurotransmitters within the central nervous system to enhance inhibitory pain systems.

TYPES OF PAIN

Three types of pain have been described based on the neuroanatomy and the neurophysiology of pain pathways: somatic, visceral, and neuropathic pain.[39] Each type results from either activation and sensitization of nociceptors and mechanoreceptors in the periphery (tumor compression or infiltration) by chemical (epinephrine, serotonin, bradykinin, prostaglandin, histamine) stimuli.

When nociceptors are activated in cutaneous or deep tissues, somatic pain results, typically characterized by a dull or aching but well-localized pain. Metastatic bone pain, postsurgical incisional pain, and myofascial and musculoskeletal pain are common examples of somatic pain.

Visceral pain results from activation of nociceptors from infiltration, compression, extension, or stretching of the thoracic, abdominal, or pelvic viscera. This typically occurs in patients with intraperitoneal metastases and is common with pancreatic cancer. This type of pain is poorly localized, is often described as deep, squeezing, and pressure-like, and when acute is often associated with significant autonomic dysfunction, including nausea, vomiting, and diaphoresis. Visceral pain is often referred to cutaneous sites that may be remote from the site of the lesion (*e.g.*, shoulder pain with diaphragmatic irritation). It may be associated with tenderness in the referred cutaneous site.

Neuropathic pain results from injury to the peripheral or central nervous system as a consequence of tumor compression or infiltration of peripheral nerves or the spinal cord, or from chemical injury to the peripheral nerve or spinal cord caused by surgery, irradiation, or chemotherapy. Examples of neuropathic pain include both metastatic and radiation-induced brachial and lumbosacral plexopathies, chemotherapy-induced peripheral neuropathies, paraneoplastic peripheral neuropathies, and phantom limb pain. Pain from nerve injury is often severe and is described as burning or dysesthetic, with a viselike quality. The pain is typically most common in the site of sensory loss and may be associated with hypersensitivity to nonnoxious and noxious stimuli. Intermittently, patients complain of paroxysms or burning or electric shock-like sensations.

These three types of pain may occur in the same patient, who may have pure somatic or visceral pain, or mixed somatic and neuropathic pain. These different types of pain account for different responses to drug and nondrug approaches. For instance, the nonsteroidal antiinflammatory drugs reduce chemical activation of nociceptors peripherally (*e.g.*, bone pain), whereas anesthetic approaches suppress the pain transmission in peripheral nerves. Management of both somatic and visceral pain suggests that these types of pain respond to a wide variety of approaches. The management of neuropathic pain is more complicated: changes in the peripheral nervous system and the central nervous system make this type of pain less responsive to a wide variety of pharmacologic, anesthetic, and neurosurgical approaches.

Evidence suggests that most cancer patients have both somatic and visceral pain, with neuropathic pain representing 15% to 20% of the significant pain problems in this population.[11,12,24,25] Certain adjuvant drugs appear to be more appropriate in the management of neuropathic pain; these issues are discussed in a later section.

TEMPORAL ASPECTS OF PAIN

Acute pain is characterized by a well-defined temporal pattern of pain onset, generally associated with subjective and objective physical signs and with hyperactivity of the autonomic nervous system. These signs provide the physician with objective evidence that substantiates the patient's complaint of pain. Acute pain is usually self-limited and responds to treatment with analgesic drug therapy and to treatment of its precipitating cause.

Acute pain can be further subdivided into subacute and episodic. Subacute pain comes on over several days, often with increasing intensity, and represents a pattern of progressive pain symptomatology. Episodic or intermittent pain occurs during confined periods of time on a regular or irregular basis. All of the pains in this category of acute pain have associated autonomic hyperactivity.

Chronic pain is the persistence of pain for more than 3 months, with a less well-defined temporal onset. The autonomic nervous system adapts, so chronic pain patients lack the objective signs common to those with acute pain. Chronic pain leads to significant changes in personality, lifestyle, and functional ability. For these patients, the management approach must include both the treatment of the cause of the pain and the treatment of the complications affecting their functional status, social interactions, and personalities.[40] This group of patients is a challenge to physicians in pain management, and this group also colors physicians' attitudes toward the management of acute pain problems. Treatment of chronic pain in the cancer patient is especially challenging because it requires a careful assessment of not only the intensity of the pain but its broad multidimensional aspects. Evidence suggests that the persistence of pain plays a major negative role in the quality of life of patients with pain and cancer.

Recently investigators have identified a series of specific pains in cancer patients with both acute and chronic pain states. Baseline pain is the average pain intensity experienced for 12 or more hours during a 24-hour period. Breakthrough pain is a transient increase in pain to greater than moderate intensity occurring on a baseline pain of moderate intensity or less. In a study of 70 adult inpatient cancer patients, 65% reported breakthrough pain.[41] The median number of reported pains was four, with a wide range. Most pains had a rapid onset and a brief duration. Breakthrough pain has a diversity of characteristics. In some patients, it marks the onset or worsening of pain at the end of the dosing interval or the regularly scheduled analgesic. In other patients, it is caused by an action of the patient, referred to as incident pain; sometimes the incident pain has a nonvolitional precipitant, such as flatulence. Most breakthrough pains are thought to be associated with a known malignant cause from direct tumor infiltration.

INTENSITY OF PAIN

Pain may also be defined on the basis of intensity, but there are limitations to a concept of pain based solely on its intensity.

In a study by Tearnan and associates, 451 cancer patients were asked to describe their pain in their own words.[42] A total of 129 distinct words were used by the patients; each patient used an average of 1.8 words. Ten words accounted for 67% of the total words used. Patients with specific pain etiologies could not be differentiated using word descriptors; in fact, the nature of the word did not define either the nature of the pain syndrome or its affective component.

Specific categorical scales of pain intensity have been used in which patients are asked to describe their pain as mild, moderate, severe, or excruciating.[43] Visual analogue scales have also been used.[19] These are often a 10-cm line anchored on either end by two points—no pain or worst possible pain—and the patient is asked to mark on the line the intensity of the pain. Numerical scales are commonly used, asking patients to rate their pain between "1=no pain" and "10=worst possible pain."

These scales have their limitations, but they are part of a series of validated instruments that include a measure of pain intensity as one of the components of the pain experience to be defined. In a study of physicians' and nurses' understanding of the language to describe pain, there was a close correlation among them of the level of intensity meant by the terms "ache," "hurt," or "pain."[44] Although health-care professionals may understand the common language of pain, there is an enormous discrepancy between their assessment and the patient's report of pain, particularly when the patient reports pain as moderate or severe. Peteet and colleagues interviewed cancer patients and physicians to obtain complete and direct information about pain treatment and the reasons for inadequate pain relief in individual cases.[10] They compared the ratings of pain severity by patients with those by physicians and found that patients tended to rate their pain as more intense than do physicians. In a study by Grossman and associates, the cancer patients' report of pain and the physicians' concurrent observation had a close correlation when patients reported mild pain.[45] However, when patients reported moderate to severe pain, the correlation of the nurse, house officer, and oncology fellow differed significantly from that of the patient: the concordance dropped from 78% for patients with mild pain to 20% for those with moderate to severe pain.

MEASUREMENT OF PAIN

These problems in communication about pain intensity strongly support the argument that multiple dimensions of the pain experience should be used to assess it adequately. Several validated instruments for pain measurement attempt to look at it in a multidimensional nature. The use of such methods can provide rapid evaluation in clinical settings of the major aspects of the pain experienced by cancer patients. Growing evidence suggests that they should be integrated into clinical trials and should be available for use on a routine basis to better define the pain symptomatology and to study the impact on pain by various treatment approaches.

Brief Pain Inventory

The Wisconsin Brief Pain Questionnaire is a self-administered, easily understood, brief method to assess pain.[46] It addresses the relevant aspects of pain (history, intensity, location, and quality) and the pain's ability to interfere with the patient's activities, and helps to provide an understanding of its cause. The history of pain and its relation to the patient's disease is assessed initially. If the patient admits to pain in the last month, he or she answers questions about current manifestations of pain. If the patient has no pain, he or she skips to the end of the questionnaire to complete demographic information. For patients with pain, a human figure drawing is provided for the patient to shade the area corresponding to the pain. Patients are asked to rate their pain at its worst, usual pain, and pain now. The pain scales consist of numbers from zero to ten; zero is labeled "no pain" and ten is labeled "pain as bad as you can imagine." Patients are asked to report the medications or treatments they receive for pain, the percent relief that these medications or treatment provide, and their belief about the cause of their pain. Finally, they are asked to rate how much the pain interferes with their mood, relations with other people, and functional ability (walking, sleeping, working, enjoying life). All patients, including those without pain, are asked for basic demographic information about marital status, education, occupation, spouse's occupation, and months since diagnosis.

This inventory has been translated into several languages and has been used to assess pain in cancer patients in such diverse settings as Vietnam, Mexico, the Philippines, and the University of Wisconsin Cancer Center.[20,21] Data from these studies suggest that cancer pain patients from widely different cultural and linguistic backgrounds respond in a similar fashion to rating the severity of their cancer-related pain and the interference caused by the pain.

McGill Pain Questionnaire

The McGill Pain Questionnaire (MPQ) is an extensively used pain assessment instrument that produces scores on four empirically derived dimensions, as well as several summary scores.[47] The instrument consists of 78 adjectives that cluster in 20 categories. Within each category, the adjectives are arranged in order of intensity from low to high. The categories are divided into four dimensions: sensory, affective, evaluative, and miscellaneous. The patient is asked to choose one adjective from each applicable category that describes an aspect of his or her current pain, and the score for each dimension is obtained by adding the rank values of the selected adjectives. A total summary score is derived by adding the scores across the four dimensions, and a total word count is also obtained. Finally, a rating of present pain intensity is made on a five-point scale.

Studies with this instrument have demonstrated that the factors derived reflect specific sensory qualities and combined emotional and sensory dimensions. This tool has also been used to assess distinct score profiles according to the nature of pain. For instance, patients with acute pain tend to use more sensory words, but patients with chronic pain tend to use more affective and reaction word subgroups.

Graham and associates obtained detailed findings for both single and multiple administrations of the MPQ with subject samples each composed of 18 cancer outpatients with pain.[47] The results were compared with similar but less extensive data from cancer patients reported by Melzack, and the data were remarkably similar.[48] Patients in both the Melzack and

Graham studies had a high consistency of pain descriptor subclass choice, ranging from 66% to 80% over four administrations.

The MPQ offers a methodologic approach to assess the sensory, affective, and evaluative components of pain, but it may be more difficult and cumbersome for patients to understand and complete and may be limited by its language constraints.

Memorial Pain Assessment Card

The Memorial Pain Assessment Card (MPAC) (Fig. 64–1) was initially developed by the Analgesic Studies Section of Memorial Sloan-Kettering Cancer Center to assess the relative potency of new and standard analgesic drugs. In that context, this method was found repeatedly to be a valid, reliable, efficient, and sensitive measure.[49]

The MPAC consists of three visual analog scales (VAS) that measure pain intensity, pain relief, and mood, and a set of pain severity descriptors adapted from the Tursky rating scale.[50] The card is 8.5″ by 11″ and is folded in the middle so that the four sides can be quickly presented to the patient. Three sides are imprinted with the 100-mm-long VAS scale; the fourth side is the set of Tursky adjectives. The pain intensity VAS is anchored by the terms "least possible pain" and "worst possible pain." The patient is asked to place a mark along the line to indicate his or her subjective judgment of pain intensity. The score on this and the other VAS is obtained by measuring in millimeters the distance between the left end of the line and the patient's mark. The Tursky pain adjective scale is a categorical measure of pain intensity. Eight intensity descriptors, ranging from "no pain" to "excruciating," are printed in a random arrangement and the patient is asked to circle the adjective that describes his or her subjective experience of pain severity. Side 3 of the MPAC is a pain relief VAS. Patients are asked to indicate with a mark the degree of pain reduction they experience after the most recent intervention, which is usually the administration of an analgesic drug. On side 4 the VAS measures the subjective experience of mood; on this side patients are asked to rate their current feeling, from "worst" to "best." The instructions for administration of these scales are simple and readily understood, and an experienced patient can complete the four ratings in less than 20 seconds.

The MPAC has been compared to the MPQ, the Profile of Mood States Questionnaire (a standardized self-report instrument that measures six dimensions of mood, reflecting degree and type of psychological distress), the Hamilton Rating Scale for Depression (an interviewer-rated scale evaluating the presence and severity of 17 symptoms typical of clinical depression), and the Zung Anxiety Scale (a standardized self-report scale that reports the presence and severity of various symptoms of anxiety).[49,51–53] The MPAC and the MPQ both provide reasonably equivalent assessments of the intensity dimension of pain. However, the evaluative scales of the MPQ did not correlate significantly with any of the measures of the MPAC, suggesting that the cognitive judgmental dimension of pain may be independent of the experiences of intensity, relief, and mood. None of the MPQ subscales correlated significantly with the VAS ratings of mood and pain relief.

These observations have led to the conclusion that the VAS mood scale on the MPAC represents a much more global assessment of general psychological distress rather than a spe-

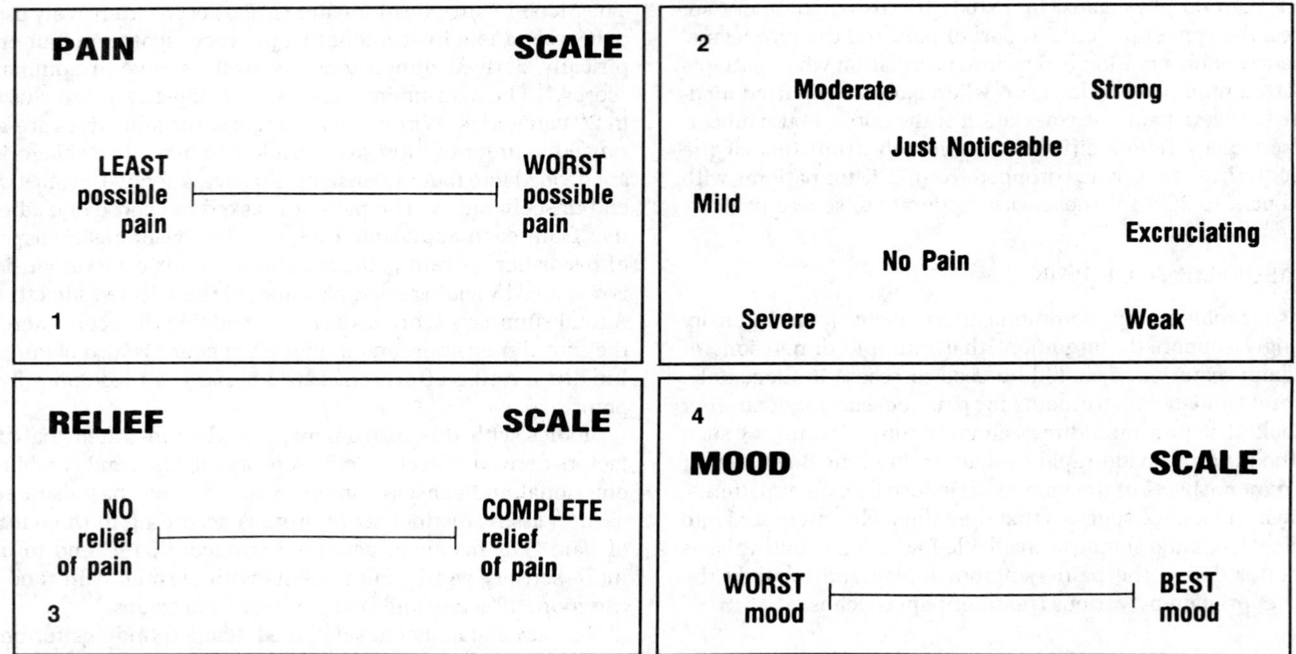

FIGURE 64–1. Memorial Pain Assessment Card, front **(1** and **4)** and back **(2** and **3)** sides. The card is folded along the broken line, and each measure is presented to the patient separately, in the numbered order. **(1)** Visual Analog Scale (VAS) Pain Intensity. **(2)** Modified Tursky Pain Descriptors Scale. **(3)** VAS Pain Relief. **(4)** VAS Mood. (Fishman B, Pasternak S, Wallenstein SL, Houde R, Holland JC, Foley KM. The Memorial Pain Assessment Card: A valid instrument for the evaluation of cancer pain. Cancer 1987;60:1151)

cific pain-related affect. This would suggest that the MPAC provides a broader assessment of the patient by its use of the mood scale, whereas the MPQ has a more narrow focus of simply representing pain-related emotional distress. What was particularly impressive was that in the use of any of the available scales, patients could differentiate pain and mood when they were explicitly asked. The perceptions of pain intensity and pain relief have different weights as components of psychological distress. The existence of such distinctions has important clinical and theoretical significance. Although the perception of pain intensity was found to contribute significantly to subjective distress, the perception of inadequate pain relief was a more important factor.

The MPAC provides valid, multidimensional information for the evaluation of pain and distress in cancer patients. It can distinguish pain intensity from pain relief and from global suffering, and it can be used to study the subtle interactions of these factors. With repeated administration it has now been demonstrated to be valid, reliable, easy to use, and nondisruptive. The MPAC and the BPI are the tools recommended for use in the clinical evaluation of individual patients and as an outcome measure in clinical trials.

CLASSIFICATION OF PATIENTS WITH CANCER PAIN

Five types of cancer pain patients can be identified, exemplifying the distinctions between acute and chronic pain (Table 64–2).[55] Although these categories are artificial, they serve as a useful preamble for discussion of the specific therapeutic approaches to the management of this group of patients.

Group I: Acute Cancer-Related Pain

Group I, patients with acute cancer-related pain, can be subdivided further according to etiology.

GROUP IA: TUMOR-ASSOCIATED PAIN. For Group IA patients, those with tumor-associated pain, pain is the major symptom prompting medical consultation and the diagnosis of cancer. In addition, pain has a special significance as the harbinger of their illness. Recurrent pain during the course of the illness or after successful therapy has the immediate implication of recurrent disease. Defining the cause of the pain may present a diagnostic problem, but effective treatment of its cause (*e.g.*, radiation therapy to bone metastases) usually is associated with dramatic pain relief in most patients.[56]

GROUP IB: PAIN ASSOCIATED WITH CANCER THERAPY. Group IB patients have postoperative pain, pain secondary to oral ulceration from chemotherapy, or myalgias secondary to steroid withdrawal. The cause of the pain is readily identifiable, and its course is predictable and self-limiting. These patients do not represent difficult diagnostic problems. Pain treatment directed at the cause of the pain is used to manage the transient symptoms. These patients endure significant pain for the promise of a successful outcome.

Group II: Chronic Cancer-Related Pain

Group II patients, those with chronic cancer-related pain, represent difficult diagnostic and therapeutic problems, in contrast to patients with acute cancer-related pain. They can be divided for discussion purposes into two groups: those with chronic pain from tumor progression, and those with chronic pain related to cancer treatment. Both groups share the characteristic of a pain symptom that has persisted for more than 3 months.

GROUP IIA: CHRONIC PAIN FROM TUMOR PROGRESSION. In patients with chronic pain associated with progression of disease (*e.g.*, patients with carcinoma of the pancreas, metastatic melanoma to bone, or Pancoast's syndrome), the pain escalates in intensity secondary to tumor infiltration of adjacent bone, nerve, or soft tissue.[58,59] Combinations of antitumor therapy, analgesic drug therapy, anesthetic blocks, and behavioral approaches to pain control are all applied with varying degrees of success. Psychological factors play a significant role in this group of patients, in whom palliative cancer therapy may be of little value and is physically debilitating.[60] The sense of hopelessness and fear of impending death may further add to and exaggerate the pain complaint; pain then becomes an aspect of the global "suffering" component.[61] Identifying both the pain and the "suffering" component is essential to the development of adequate therapy for these patients. The chronicity of the pain is associated with a series of psychological symptoms and signs, including sleep disturbances, reduced appetite, impaired concentration, or irritability, mimicking a depressive disorder. Management must be directed at controlling the pain, recognizing that antitumor therapy has failed. Analgesic therapy combined with a wide range of alternative approaches is necessary to provide adequate analgesia. Such patients are candidates for palliative care programs that address not only pain symptoms but the broader aspects of symptom management and psychological support.[23–25,62]

GROUP IIB: CHRONIC PAIN ASSOCIATED WITH CANCER THERAPY. Group IIB includes patients with chronic pain associated with cancer therapy, such as patients who develop pain after mastectomy, limb amputation (phantom limb), or thoracotomy. The nature of pain in these patients is secondary to nerve injury with the development of a traumatic neuroma. Treatment of the pain for these patients is

TABLE 64–2. Types of Patients With Pain From Cancer

I. Patients With Acute Cancer-Related Pain
   a. Associated with the diagnosis of cancer
   b. Associated with cancer therapy (surgery, chemotherapy, or radiation)
II. Patients With Chronic Cancer-Related Pain
   a. Associated with cancer progression
   b. Associated with cancer therapy (surgery, chemotherapy, or radiation)
III. Patients With Preexisting Chronic Pain and Cancer-Related Pain
IV. Patients With a History of Drug Addiction and Cancer-Related Pain
   a. Actively involved in illicit drug use
   b. In methadone maintenance program
   c. With a history of drug abuse
V. Dying Patients With Cancer-Related Pain

limited by the lack of available methods to remove the cause of the pain. Again, treatment is directed at the symptoms, not the cause. These patients closely parallel those in the general population with chronic intractable pain syndromes. Psychological factors play a significant role in how these patients adapt to and function with chronic pain. Defining this group is imperative: identifying the cause of the pain as not directly related to tumor markedly alters the patient's therapy, prognosis, and psychological state. Each of the primary modalities of cancer therapy is associated with a series of specific chronic pain syndromes with characteristic pain patterns and clinical presentations (Table 64–3). Although it is consoling to both the patient and the physician to realize that the pain does not represent recurrent or progressive disease, the persistence of the pain is a constant reminder of the previous diagnosis of cancer.

In these patients, all approaches aimed at maintaining the patient's functional status should be used. Alternative methods of therapy, in contrast to drug therapy, represent the major management approach. This group of patients is increasing in number and accounts for 25% of patients referred to a medical pain clinic.

Group III: Preexisting Chronic Pain and Cancer-Related Pain

Group III includes patients with a history of chronic nonmalignant pain who develop cancer and pain. Psychological factors play a significant role in this group of patients, whose psychological and functional status is already compromised by their chronic nonmalignant pain state.[28] These patients are at high risk of developing further functional incapacity and escalating chronic pain symptoms. However, their history should not be used in a punitive way to minimize or deny their complaints. Identifying this group of patients as a high-risk group helps to improve their psychological assessment and intervention.

TABLE 64–3. Pain Syndromes in Patients With Cancer

	References
Pain Syndromes Associated With Direct Tumor Involvement	1, 67
Tumor Infiltration of Bone	
Metastases to the cranial vault	68
Metastases to the base of skull	69
Jugular foramen syndrome	
Clivus metastases	
Sphenoid sinus metastases	
Vertebral body syndromes	70, 71
Fracture of the odontoid	72
C7–T1 metastases	59
L1 metastases	73
Sacral syndrome	74
Tumor Infiltration of Nerve	
Peripheral nerve	67
Peripheral neuropathy	
Intercostal neuropathy	67
Plexus	75, 76
Brachial plexopathy	
Lumbosacral plexopathy	73, 77
Celiac plexopathy	58
Root	70
Radiculopathy	
Leptomeningeal metastases	78, 79
Spinal cord	70, 71
Epidural spinal cord compression	
Intramedullary metastases	71
Brain	68
Intracranial metastases	
Tumor Infiltration of Viscera	
Infiltration of pleura	80
Small and large bowel obstruction	81
Infiltration of pelvis and bladder wall	74
Pain Syndromes Associated With Cancer Therapy	
Postsurgical Pain Syndromes	
Acute	67, 82
Postoperative pain	
Chronic	
Postthoracotomy syndrome	
Postmastectomy syndrome	67, 83
Postradical neck syndrome	67, 84, 85
Phantom limb syndrome	53
Postchemotherapy Pain Syndromes	
Acute	57, 87
Oral mucositis	
Bladder spasms	88
Jaw pain	89
Diffuse bone pain	90
Headache	90
Chronic	89
Peripheral neuropathy	
Aseptic necrosis fo the femoral head	91
Steroid pseudorheumatism	92
Postherpetic neuralgia	33, 34, 93
Postradiation Pain Syndromes	26
Acute	57
Oral mucositis, esophagitis	
Skin burns	26
Chronic	75, 94
Radiation fibrosis of brachial and lumbar plexus	
Radiation myelopathy	95
Radiation-induced second primary tumor	96, 97
Radiation fibrosis of bone	98
Infection-Induced Pain Syndromes	
Infected fistula in genitourinary and gynecologic cancers	74
Infected head and neck sites in head and neck cancer	99

Group IV: Patients With a History of Drug Addiction and Pain

Group IV includes patients with a history of drug addiction who have cancer-related pain. Three subgroups can be identified: patients actively involved in illicit drug use and drug-seeking behavior, those receiving methadone in a maintenance program, and those who have not used drugs for several years. Undertreatment with analgesic drugs occurs most commonly in this group of patients. Assessment of reported pain by physicians and nurses is colored by the fact that the pain symptoms are confused with drug-seeking behavior. Attention to the medical and psychological needs of these patients requires individualized assessment and consultation with experts in drug-related problems. The first subgroup represents a major management problem, straining the most tolerant of medical care systems.[63,64] Pain in the other two subgroups is readily managed, with the recognition that the psychological stresses consequent to the pain and cancer may place the patient at a high risk for recidivism.

Group V: Dying Patients With Pain

In dying patients in pain, diagnostic and therapeutic considerations are directed at maintaining the patient's comfort. This group is identified separately from Group II patients because the psychological factors further compound adequate pain management. The issues of hopelessness, death, and dying become more prominent, and the suffering component must be addressed.

Inadequate control of pain in the dying patient exacerbates the suffering component and demoralizes the family and the caregivers, who feel that they have failed in treating the patient's pain at a time when adequate treatment may matter the most. Rapid escalation of analgesic drug therapy, usually by the intravenous route, and attempts to ameliorate psychological symptoms should be used.

The risk-to-benefit ratios in analgesic approaches become less of an issue when the goal of pain therapy is the patient's comfort. In these patients, the physician must understand the temporal setting of pain in assessing the indications for and usefulness of the pain management approaches.

COMMON PAIN SYNDROMES

The common pain syndromes associated with cancer or cancer therapy are listed in Table 64–3. Numerous studies have demonstrated that pain in the cancer patient may have multiple causes. Several investigators have demonstrated that pain associated with direct tumor involvement is the most common cause; 78% of patients in an inpatient cancer pain population and 65% in an outpatient pain clinic were in this category.[11,65,66] Pain in bone is the most common site. Tumor infiltration of nerve and hollow viscus are the second and third most common painful sites.

A second category includes pain syndromes associated with cancer therapy. About 19% of patients in an inpatient population and 25% of those in an outpatient population were in this group.[1,12,66] The group includes patients in whom pain occurred during the course of therapy, during a therapeutic procedure, or as a result of chemotherapy, surgery, or radiation therapy. Each of these primary therapeutic modalities is associated with a series of specific pain syndromes with characteristic pain patterns and clinical presentations that have been well described in the literature.

The third major category of pain syndromes includes those unrelated to the cancer and the cancer therapy. About 3% of inpatients have pain unrelated to their cancer or cancer therapy; this figure increases to 10% in an outpatient cancer population.[1,12,65,66] Common syndromes seen in this population include osteoarthritis, lumbar disc disease, osteoporosis with a collapsed vertebral body, and peripheral neuropathy.

CLINICAL ASSESSMENT OF PAIN

Certain general principles should be followed in evaluating cancer patients who complain of pain. Lack of attention to these general principles is the major cause for misdiagnosis of a specific pain syndrome. As discussed above, multiple barriers exist in the assessment of pain, including the multidimensional nature of the subjective complaint of pain, the lack of a clearly defined language of pain, and poor communication between the patient and physician about pain (*e.g.*, underreporting by the patient and underassessing by the physician or nurse).[8] Sufficient information is now available on the scope of the problem of pain in cancer patients, and there are various assessment tools to refine and define the sensory and affective components of pain in this population; they should be integrated into clinical practice.

Adequate assessment is a critical component for defining the appropriate therapeutic strategy for each patient. The general principles are:

Believe the patient's complaint of pain.
Take a careful history of the patient's pain complaint.
Evaluate the patient's psychological state.
Perform a careful medical and neurologic examination.
Order and personally review the appropriate diagnostic studies.
Treat the pain to facilitate the appropriate workup.
Reassess the patient's response to therapy.
Individualize the diagnostic and therapeutic approaches.
Discuss advance directives with the patient and family.

Believe the Patient's Complaint of Pain

Critical to the management of the patient with cancer pain is the establishment of a trusting relationship with the physician. The complaint of pain is a symptom, not a diagnosis. Pain perception is not simply a function of the amount of physical injury sustained by the patient, but is a complex state determined by multiple factors. The diagnosis of a specific pain syndrome and a complete understanding of the patient's psychological state is not always made during the initial evaluation. In fact, it may take several weeks to define its nature because of the lack of radiologic or pathologic verification. It may take a similar period to fully comprehend each patient's psychological makeup. Numerous examples in the assessment of patients with pain and cancer highlight the limitation of the diagnostic process. It is not uncommon for patients with tumor infiltration of the brachial plexus from either lung or breast cancer to have pain for several weeks or months before the onset of objective radiologic and neurologic findings.[59,67]

A comprehensive evaluation involves taking a careful history, performing a detailed medical, neurologic, and psychological evaluation, developing a series of diagnosis-related hypotheses, and ordering the appropriate diagnostic studies.

Take a Careful History of the Patient's Pain Complaint

This should include the patient's description of:

Site of pain
Quality of pain
Exacerbating and relieving factors
Temporal pattern
Exact onset
Associated symptoms and signs
Interference with activities of daily living
Impact on the patient's psychological state
Response to previous and current analgesic therapies.

Multiple pain complaints are common in patients with advanced disease and must be ranked and classified.[3]

Evaluate the Patient's Psychological State

The patient's current level of anxiety and depression must be clarified and his or her past history of such symptoms must be defined. Knowledge of the patient's previous psychiatric history and need for past hospitalization for psychiatric care helps to clarify the patient's potential psychological risk.[60] Information on how the patient has handled previous painful events may provide insight into whether the patient has demonstrated chronic illness behavior or has a past history of a chronic pain syndrome.[40] It is important to know about a personal or family history of alcohol or drug dependence, to understand why the patient may be fearful or refuse to take opioid drugs.

Because each patient has his or her own understanding of the meaning of pain, it is useful to have the patient elaborate this meaning. Does he or she think it represents recurrent tumor, or is he or she convinced it is simply arthritis? Evidence suggests that when patients have a clear understanding of the meaning of their pain as representing recurrent tumor, they have increased psychological distress.

The importance of defining the psychological makeup of the patient with pain is supported by a variety of studies that have focused on the impact of suffering in patients with pain. Psychological factors play a significant role in accounting for the differences in pain experiences in cancer patients. A series of psychiatric syndromes have been described for cancer patients, with depression occurring in as many as 25% of patients.[60] The depression presents either as an acute stress response or as a major depression. Awareness of the common psychiatric syndromes when evaluating the pain complaint expands the physician's understanding of such a complaint.[60]

Although it is critical to know as much as possible about each patient with pain, some information may not be readily available in the first interview; in some instances it may never be available because of the lack of intellectual competence on the patient's part to define clearly the various components of the pain complaint. It is often necessary to verify the history from a family member who may provide information that the patient is unable or unwilling to provide. The family may be more objective in assessing a disability of a patient who underreports his or her symptoms. Similarly, in a patient who is a poor historian, the family member may be able to provide essential information that may alter the diagnostic approach. All attempts should be made to compile a careful history and define the medical, neurologic, and psychological profile of the pain complaint.

As patients become more active in defining advance directives and as they focus on the quality of life, it is critical to ask patients to define what they would do if the pain were intractable or intolerable. Do they have suicidal thoughts or a pact with a family member?[100] Do they have a family history of suicide? Do they have a family member who died a painful death? From our experience, patients who have had such an experience are particularly fearful of their own death.[16] Does the patient have drugs in reserve or a gun in the house that he or she might use in desperation? Such questions allow patients to discuss openly their fears of death and their need to take matters into their own hands rather than trust the health-care professional. Such open discussions can allow the physician to better define for the patient the options for care and to reassure the patient of the physician's commitment to care.[16] Because patients rarely offer this information unless requested, it is critical to develop specific questions that can be readily integrated into the initial history taken by the physician.

Perform a Careful Medical and Neurologic Examination

A medical and neurologic examination helps provide the necessary data to substantiate the history. Knowledge of the referral patterns of pain and the common cancer pain syndromes can direct the examination.[101] The characteristics of pain in breast-cancer patients with brachial plexopathy are so specific that they can help define the diagnosis of tumor infiltration of the brachial plexus from radiation fibrosis of the brachial plexus.[67,70] Similarly, the commonly described pain syndromes in cancer patients associated with a postmastectomy pain syndrome can readily be defined as separate from tumor infiltration of the brachial plexus.[71]

The physical and neurologic examination allows the physician to visually inspect and palpate the site of pain and to look for the associated physical and neurologic signs that might help to better define the nature of the pain symptom. Defining the degree of motor or sensory changes can help define the specific site in the nervous system that may be involved. Similarly, in patients with sensory loss, the presence of allodynia and hyperesthesia can further define the nature of the sensory problem. Moreover, the degree of muscle spasm, gait instability, and impaired coordination can only be fully assessed by such an evaluation.

Order and Personally Review the Appropriate Diagnostic Studies

Diagnostic studies confirm the diagnosis and define in patients with metastatic disease the site and extent of tumor infiltration. Computed transaxial tomography and MRI are the most useful diagnostic procedures in evaluating cancer patients with pain. The bone scan is a useful screening device and is more sensitive for demonstrating abnormalities in bone before changes appear on plain radiographs. However, a negative bone scan does not rule out bony metastatic disease, nor does a positive bone scan confirm the diagnosis of metastatic tumor. The physician should review the results personally with the radiologist to correlate any pathologic change with the site of pain.

Evaluation of the extent of metastatic disease may help to discover the relation of the pain complaint to possible recurrent disease. The use of tumor markers such as CEA, CA125, CA153, and PSA can be very useful in a patient in whom recurrent tumor is suspected. In certain pain syndromes the presence of recurrent disease is closely associated with the onset of pain (*e.g.*, in the appearance of late postthoracotomy pain syndrome in a patient after initial resolution of the postoperative pain).[72]

Treat the Pain to Facilitate the Appropriate Workup

No patient should be evaluated inadequately because of a significant pain problem. Early management of the pain while investigating the source will markedly improve the patient's ability to participate in the necessary diagnostic procedures. During the initial evaluation of the pain complaint, early consideration of the use of alternative methods of pain control, including anesthetic and neurosurgical approaches, should be considered (*e.g.*, the temporary use of a local anesthetic via an epidural catheter to manage sacral pain or the use of a percutaneous cordotomy in the patient with unilateral pain below the waist from a lumbosacral plexopathy). These approaches should not be considered for use only when all else fails, but should be an integral part of the assessment of the patient with pain.

Reassess the Patient's Response to Therapy

Continual reassessment of the response of the patient's pain complaint to the prescribed therapy provides the best method to validate the initial diagnosis as correct. If relief is less than predicted or if the pain worsens, reassessment of the treatment approach or a search for a new cause of the pain should be considered. A common example is the patient with epidural cord compression who develops a second block proximal to the one being radiated, with neurologic signs mimicking the original one.

Individualize the Diagnostic and Therapeutic Approach

Evaluation of the patient must be closely linked to the patient's level of function, ability to participate in the diagnostic workup, and willingness to undergo the necessary diagnostic approaches; objective evidence that treatment approaches may be beneficial; and life expectancy. Careful judgment is required to select diagnostic approaches that will have a direct impact on the choice of the therapeutic strategy or will answer a specific question. The random use of diagnostic procedures in these patients, particularly those with advanced cancer and significant pain, is inappropriate because it may have an adverse effect on their quality of life. Open discussion with the patient about the need for assessment as well as the therapeutic options is critical to allow the patient to be part of the decision-making process. In some patients, diagnostic procedures such as myelography or MRI are inappropriate because they will simply confirm the existence of a disease for which no treatment is available, or for which the treatment would be a major surgical procedure (*e.g.*, vertebral body resection) that would be inappropriate for a dying patient. Patient refusal of evaluation or treatment must be respected when the physician has fully explained the options and is convinced that the patient has an accurate understanding of the implications of no further workup or treatment.[16,103,104]

Discuss Advance Directives With the Patient and Family

When developing approaches for treatment, there must be an open discussion about advance directives so that the physician has a clear understanding of the patient's goal for therapy or his or her ambivalence in developing a therapeutic strategy. The physician must have unconditional positive regard for the patient, placing the control of symptoms of pain and treatment of psychological distress in the highest regard. Knowledge of the patient's decisions about resuscitation, living wills, and symptom management should he or she become incompetent improves the physician's ability to appropriately and humanely care for the dying patient with advanced disease.[73,74]

IMPACT OF A COMPREHENSIVE EXAMINATION ON THE MANAGEMENT OF CANCER PAIN

Although a comprehensive medical and neurologic evaluation is needed in cancer pain treatment, the full impact of such approaches are currently under study. The following information comes from a study of pain service consultations in a retrospective review of 226 consecutive consultations in a total of 190 patients and in 50 consecutive consultations evaluated prospectively in 46 patients.[66] Based on the history, examination, and results of imaging procedures, a pain diagnosis was derived and included the delineation of a somatic, visceral, or neuropathic lesion. Sixty percent of the consultations were requested in patients with known metastatic disease; in 64% of retrospectively studied consult patients and 64% of consultations evaluated prospectively a lesion was newly identified through the pain evaluation performed by the consultant. More than 50% of diagnoses were neurologic; the most common diagnosis was epidural spinal cord compression. The pain service evaluation resulted in a change of treatment and provided an opportunity for primary antineoplastic therapies to be considered. Radiation therapy was offered to 19% of the retrospective group and to 12% of the prospective study patients. Two percent of patients from both studies received chemotherapy, and 1% of retrospective study patients and 4% of prospective study patients were referred to surgery on the basis of the pain evaluation.

The prospective survey also tabulated specific neurologic diagnoses both related and unrelated to the pain complaint. Thirty-four percent (17 patients) had a neurologic diagnosis before evaluation by the pain consultant. Nine of the 17 diagnoses were confirmed, and the consultation led to a new neurologic diagnosis in an additional 18 patients. Thus, neurologic evaluation by the pain consultant confirmed neurologic diagnoses in 54% of patients; the most prevalent of these were epidural spinal cord compression in 9 and lumbosacral plexopathy in 9. Eight more cases of malignant lumbosacral plexopathy were identified by the pain consultant, far more than any other neurologic condition in this group of patients.

This study supports the observation that new pathology is commonly identified through a comprehensive assessment of pain in cancer patients. Equally important, many of these lesions were amenable to primary therapy, which may have direct analgesic consequences. About one fifth of the patients received primary antineoplastic therapy based on the pain evaluation, and another 6% received antibiotics.

Although the high prevalence of neurologic diagnoses may represent a bias in this Memorial study, it is critical to recognize that neurologic lesions make up a substantial portion of painful lesions in the cancer population. In a prospective study of the neurologic symptoms, neurologic diagnoses, and primary tumors in all patients with a history of systemic cancer referred to the Memorial Hospital's Neurology Consultation Service, the three most common symptoms in 851 patients were back pain (18.2%), altered mental status (17.1%), and headache (15.4%).[75] The most common neurologic diagnoses was brain metastases (15.9%), followed by metabolic encephalopathy (10.2%), pain associated with bone metastases only (9.9%), and epidural extension or metastases of tumor (8.4%). Physicians evaluating patients with cancer pain must have sufficient knowledge of these neurologic complications of cancer to appropriately evaluate and treat these patients.

MANAGEMENT OF CANCER PAIN

Recent advances in pain research provide the scientific rationale for using new, improved methods of treatment, including better and more effective use of standard drug therapy (nonnarcotic, narcotic, and adjuvant analgesic drugs), the development of new drugs, the use of novel methods and routes of drug administration, and the use of selective anesthetic and neurosurgical approaches to control pain. A variety of medical and surgical approaches to the management of cancer pain are currently available. The use of such techniques often depends on the clinical expertise in a particular center. Approaches such as drug therapy and some of the behavioral methods should be within the armamentarium of any physician or nurse who cares for patients with pain and cancer. Other approaches, such as specific anesthetic and neurosurgical techniques, require trained medical personnel who have clinical experience in managing cancer pain.

DRUG THERAPY

Analgesic drugs can be divided into three groups: nonnarcotic analgesics, such as aspirin and acetaminophen, and the nonsteroidal antiinflammatory drugs (NSAIDs), which act on the peripheral mechanisms of pain; narcotic agonist and antagonist drugs, which activate opiate receptors in the central and peripheral nervous system and mediate analgesia; and adjuvant analgesic drugs that produce analgesia in certain pain states (*e.g.*, amitriptyline in postherpetic neuralgia) or potentiate the opioid analgesics (Table 64–4).

Nonopioid Analgesics

Nonopioid analgesics are the drugs of choice for mild to moderate pain. The mechanism of action of their analgesic effect is controversial, but it is thought that they reduce or prevent sensitization of pain receptors to nociceptive stimuli by preventing prostaglandin synthesis through inhibition of cyclooxygenase activity. Their mechanism of action also includes nonprostaglandin inhibitory effects.[106] This class of drugs consists of a heterogenous group of substances that differ in chemical structure and pharmacologic action. Many of these drugs have analgesic, antiinflammatory, and antipyretic properties. All of the drugs in this class have an analgesic potency similar to or greater than that of aspirin. However, the analgesic effects of these drugs have a ceiling; that is, escalating the dose beyond a certain level does not produce additive analgesia. Experimental evidence suggests that these drugs may play a special role in the pain management of patients with bone metastases because of the documented role of prostaglandins in bone resorption in metastatic bone disease. Aspirin has been shown to have an antitumor effect in an animal bone tumor model.[107]

TABLE 64–4. Guidelines for the Rational Use of Analgesics in the Management of Cancer Pain

Start with a specific drug for a specific type of pain
Know the pharmacology of the drug prescribed
  Know the relative potency of the drug
  Know the duration of the analgesic effect
  Know the pharmacokinetics of the drug
  Know the equianalgesic doses for the drug and its route of administration
Administer analgesic on a regular basis
Gear the route of administration to the patient's needs

Oral	Sublingual
Buccal	Transmucosal
Rectal	Transdermal
Subcutaneous	Intravenous
Intrathecal	Intraventricular

Use a combination of drugs to provide additive analgesia
  Narcotic plus nonnarcotic (aspirin, acetaminophen, NSAIDs)
  Narcotic plus adjuvants
Anticipate and treat side effects
  Sedation
  Respiratory depression
  Nausea and vomiting
  Constipation
  Multifocal myoclonus and seizures
Management of the tolerant patient
  Use combinations of nonopioid and opioid drugs
  Use combinations of drug therapy, anesthetic and neurosurgical procedures
  Switch to an alternative opioid analgesic starting with half the equianalgesic dose
  Use epidural local anesthetics
  Reassess the nature of the pain
Prevent and treat acute withdrawal
  Taper drugs slowly
Anticipate complications
  Overdose
  Psychological dependence

In clinical practice, this class of drugs represents the first-line approach to the management of cancer pain with analgesics, but the choice and use of the nonnarcotic must be individualized. Each patient should be given an adequate trial of one nonnarcotic analgesic before switching to an alternative one. Such a trial should include administration of the drug to maximal levels at regular intervals. The gastrointestinal and hematologic side effects often limit their long-term use. There is controversy over the use of prophylactic antiulcer agents in cancer patients receiving these drugs. Histamine H_2 antagonist drugs reduce the incidence of gastroscopically diagnosed NSAID-induced duodenal ulcers.[108] It is unclear whether such an effect is associated with a decreased rate of perforation or bleeding. The duration of treatment with antiulcer agents concurrent with the use of these drugs is also under study. In cancer patients, the concurrent use of steroids should be avoided to limit the gastric effects of these two combinations.

For the patient with moderate pain, adding a narcotic to the nonnarcotic provides additive analgesia. Combinations with codeine, oxycodone, and propoxyphene are available, but these combinations often contain less than the full dose of 650 mg aspirin or acetaminophen. Prescribing each drug separately provides for a better method of individualizing pain control. This is particularly important when the patient requires escalation of the combination to provide analgesia, in which case the additional dosage of the NSAID may become excessive.

Several NSAIDs have been approved by the Food and Drug Administration for use as analgesics for mild to moderate pain and are listed in Table 64–5.

Guidelines for the use of NSAIDs in patients with cancer pain are largely empiric and drawn from clinical experience. If antiinflammatory effects are not essential and analgesia is the only goal, acetaminophen is probably safer than other NSAIDs, although it clearly has the potential for renal toxicity. Appropriate first-line drugs in patients with a bleeding diathesis or peptic ulcer disease should include acetaminophen and two of the salicylates—choline magnesium trisalicylate and salicylate. These are reported to have lower ulcer potential than other NSAIDs and at usual clinical doses do not impair platelet aggregation.

Because there is great variability among patients in their responses to different drugs, patients may require trials with several NSAIDs before finding an effective drug and dose regimen. Some authors have suggested that several weeks are necessary to judge the efficacy of the dose in the treatment of rheumatologic disorders. However, as an analgesic, pain relief should be obtained once steady-state levels are achieved (these depend on the drug's half-life and occur within three to five half-lives). If pain relief is not obtained, an alternative drug trial should be considered.

Opioid Agonists and Antagonists

The opioid analgesics, of which morphine is the prototype, vary in potency, efficacy, and adverse effects. These drugs produce their analgesic effects by binding to discrete opiate receptors in the peripheral and central nervous system. This group also includes a series of heterogenous substances with varying chemical structures. In contrast to the nonopioid analgesics, opioid analgesics do not appear to have a ceiling effect; that is, as the dose is escalated on a log scale, the increment in analgesia is linear to the point of loss of consciousness. Effective use of the opioid analgesics requires the balancing of the most desirable effects of pain relief to the undesirable effects of nausea, vomiting, mental clouding, sedation, constipation, tolerance, and physical dependence. These undesirable effects impose a practical limit on the dose useful for a particular patient.

Much of the difficulty encountered in the clinical use of these drugs arises from individual variation and differences of response of specific patients to the same drug dose. This difficulty is compounded by the lack of pharmacologic and pharmacokinetic data on many of the narcotic analgesics. This lack of information on the clinical pharmacology of these drugs and a series of uncontrolled survey-type studies have led to several controversies in the drug management of cancer pain. These include the type of pain that is responsive to opioid analgesics, the choice of the opioid drug, the appropriate route and method of administration, the extent to which tolerance limits the usefulness of opioid analgesics chronically, and concern about the risk of psychological dependence and substance abuse.[15,110,111] These controversies continue to affect the rational use of opioid analgesics in clinical practice.

Table 64–6 summarizes the most commonly used agents.

Principles of Opioid Drug Therapy

Start With a Specific Drug for a Specific Type of Pain. The WHO Cancer Pain Relief Program has advocated the use of an analgesic ladder (Fig. 64–2).[4] This approach advocates the use of nonopioid, opioid, and adjuvant analgesics alone or in combinations titrated to the needs of each patient.

Nonopioid drugs are the first-line approach for the patient with mild to moderate pain.[112] If pain is not relieved or if the side effects of the nonopioid are intolerable, opioid analgesics should be used.

Codeine, propoxyphene, and oxycodone (5 mg) make up the second step of the WHO analgesic ladder. These drugs have a higher analgesic potential than the nonopioids and are most often used in fixed oradose mixtures, limiting their use in increasing doses.

For moderate to severe pain—the third step of the ladder—morphine-hydromorphone, oxycodone, levorphanol, methadone, and oxymorphone are the drugs most commonly used. Chronic administration of meperidine produces central nervous system irritability and is not recommended for chronic cancer pain management.[113] Heroin is unavailable in the United States but has been demonstrated to be comparable to morphine in its analgesic, mood, and side effects.[114] Heroin does not bind to the opiate receptor and represents a pro-drug that must be metabolized to morphine and 6-acetylmorphine to produce it analgesic effects.[115]

WHO has recommended morphine as the drug of choice for cancer pain by the oral route based on its position on the Essential Drug List and has requested that it be made available worldwide. Alternatives to morphine include hydromorphone and levorphanol, both congeners of morphine. Hydromorphone has poor oral bioavailability with a short half-life. It is highly soluble and available in high-potency form (10 mg/ml). It is a useful alternative to morphine and to levorphanol. Levorphanol has good bioavailability but a long plasma half-life (12 to 16 hours). It must be used cautiously because with

TABLE 64–5. Nonopioid and Adjuvant Analgesic Drugs in the Management of Cancer Pain

Class/Drug	*Indications*	*Starting Oral Dose (mg) and Range/24 h)*	*Comments*
NSAIDs			
Aspirin	Soft-tissue and metastatic bone pain	650 650–1000	Used together with opioids, GI and hematologic effects; avoid combination with steroids
Acetaminophen	Like aspirin	650 650–1000	Fewer GI effects, no effects on platelet function, no significant antiinflammatory effects
Ibuprofen		400 200–800	Higher analgesic potential than aspirin, fewer GI and hematologic effects than aspirin
Choline magnesium trisalicylate	Like aspirin	1500 1000–4000	Antiinflammatory and analgesic effects, similar to aspirin without hematologic effects
Fenoprofen	Like aspirin	200 200–400	Like ibuprofen
Diflunisal	Like aspirin	500 500–1000	Longer duration of action than ibuprofen, higher analgesic potential than aspirin
Naproxen	Like aspirin	250 250–500	Like diflunisal
Anticonvulsants			
Phenytoin	Neuropathic pain acute lancinating type (tic)	100 100–300	Start with low dose, titrate slowly
Carbamazepine	Neuropathic pain acute lancinating type (tic)	100 200–800	Useful in paroxysmal nerve pain
Antidepressants			
Amitriptyline Imipramine	Neuropathic pain (*e.g.*, postherpetic neuralgia)	10 10–150	Start at low dose and titrate slowly; has analgesic properties
Antihistamines			
Hydroxyzine	Somatic and visceral pain	25 25–100	Additive analgesia in combination with opioids; antiemetic, antianxiety properties
Phenothiazines			
Methotrimeprazine	Somatic and visceral pain; useful in opioid-tolerant patients with GI obstruction and pain	5–15 IM	Anxiolytic and antiemetic effects; available only in IM preparation
Steroids			
Prednisone	Somatic and neuropathic pain (*e.g.*, inflammatory bone pain)	5 5–60	Antiinflammatory, antiemetic, analgesic effects
Dexamethasone	Reflex sympathetic dystrophy; brachial, lumbar plexopathy	0.5–16	
Neurostimulants			
Dextroamphetamine	Somatic and visceral pain (*e.g.*, postoperative pain)	2.5 2.5–10	Additive analgesia in combination with opioids; reduces sedative effects
Methylphenidate	Opioid-induced sedation	5 5–15	Additive analgesia in combination with opioids; reduces sedative effects
Caffeine		300 300–600	Additive analgesia in combination with opioids; reduces sedative effects

TABLE 64–6. Opioid Analgesics for Management of Cancer Pain

Drug and Equianalgesic Dose Relative Potency	*mg IM/PO*	*Plasma Half-Life (h)*	*Starting* Oral Dose (mg)*	*Available Commercial Preparations*
Morphine	10 IM 60 PO	3–4	30–60	Oral: tablet, liquid, slow-release tab Rectal: 5 mg–30 mg Injectable: SC, IM, I.V., epidural, intrathecal
Hydromorphone	1.5 IM 7.5 PO	2–3	2–48	Oral: tablets: 1, 2, 4, mg Injectable: SC, IM, I.V. 2 mg/ml & HP 10 mg/ml
Methadone	10 IM 20 PO	12–24	5–10	Oral: tablets, liquid Injectable: SC, IM, I.V.
Levorphanol	2 IM 4 PO	12–16	2–4	Oral: tablets Injectable: SC, IM, I.V.
Oxymorphone	1	2–3	NA	Rectal: 10 mg Injectable: SC, IM, I.V.
Heroin	5 IM 60 PO	3–4	NA	NA
Meperidine	75 IM 300 PO	3–4 (normeperidine, 12–16)	75	Oral: tablets Injectable: SC, IM, I.V.
Codeine	130 200	3–4	60	Oral: tablets and combination with ASA, acetaminophen, liquid
Oxycodone	15 30	—	5	Oral: tablets, liquid, oral formulation in combination with acetaminophen (tab and liquid) and aspirin (tab)

For these equianalgesic IM doses, the time of peak analgesia in nontolerant patients ranges from 30 minutes to 1 hour and the duration from 4 to 6 hours. The peak analgesic effect is delayed and the duration prolonged after oral administration.
* These doses are recommended starting IM doses from which the optimal dose for each patient is determined by titration and the maximal dose limited by adverse effects.

repeated administration accumulation will occur. Oxymorphone is only available in parenteral and suppository forms, limiting its wide use.

The role of methadone in cancer pain remains the most controversial.[109,116,117] Its bioavailability is 85%, and in single-dose studies its oral-to-parenteral potency ratio is 1:2. Its plasma half-life averages 24 hours but may range from 13 to 50 hours; its duration of analgesia is often only 4 to 8 hours. Repetitive analgesic doses of methadone lead to drug accumulation because of the discrepancy between its plasma half-life and the duration of analgesia. Sedation, confusion, and even death can occur when patients are not carefully monitored. The clinical use of methadone requires greater sophistication, and it should be considered as a second-line drug most useful in the patient with some prior opioid experience and a degree of tolerance. In the opioid-naive patient, initial doses should be titrated carefully.

The roles of the narcotic partial agonists such as buprenorphine and the mixed agonist-antagonists such as pentazocine, butorphanol, and nalbuphine are limited in cancer pain management.[118] Buprenorphine is available in the United States in a parenteral form only but is available worldwide in sublingual form. It is a useful first-line drug before the use of full agonist drugs because its analgesic efficacy is reduced in patients receiving narcotic-agonist drugs. Pentazocine is the only mixed agonist-antagonist available orally, but in the United States it is available only in combination with naloxone, aspirin, or acetaminophen. Escalation of the dose of pentazocine produces psychotomimetic effects, limiting its usefulness in chronic cancer pain management.

In short, the choice of the opioid analgesic depends on the patient's prior opioid experience and physical and neurologic status. Individualization is the rule.

Know the Equianalgesic Dose of the Drug and Its Route of Administration. Knowing the equianalgesic dose can ensure more appropriate drug use. Lack of attention to these differences in drug dose is the most common cause of undermedication of pain patients.[8] These doses have been derived from assessment of the relative analgesic potency of a drug.[119] Relative potency is the ratio of the doses of two analgesics required to produce the same effect. Estimates of relative potency allow calculation of the equianalgesic dose, which provides the basis for selecting the appropriate dose when switching drugs or the route of administration of the same drug. The values in Table 64–6 are based on studies in which 10 mg morphine was the standard dose. The equianalgesic dose is the recommended starting dose, with the optimal dose for each patient determined by dose adjustment.

Table 64–6 can be useful, but its limitations also need to be understood. One important controversy is the reported difference in relative potency for morphine. On the basis of a

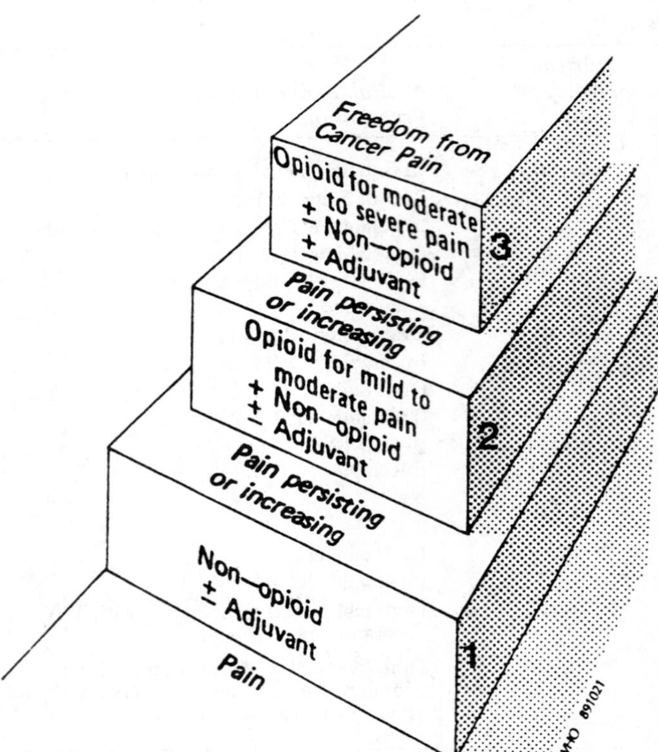

FIGURE 64–2. The World Health Organization's three-step ladder approach to analgesic drug therapy. (World Health Organization. Cancer pain relief. Geneva: World Health Organization, 1986)

series of survey studies, Twycross has suggested that the relative potency of morphine with repeated administration is 1:2 or 1:3.[120] As judged by single-dose studies in patients with both acute and chronic pain, the relative potency of intramuscular to oral morphine is 1:6.[119] The reason for this discrepancy relates to the fact that relative potency may differ in single-dose and repeated-dose studies. In practice, the 1:6 relative analgesic potency ratio should be used for patients with acute pain, the 1:2 or 1:3 ratio in patients treated with repeated doses on a chronic basis. Because of this discrepancy, patients are often undermedicated with morphine during the initial titration when a 1:3 ratio is used. Recent evidence suggests that morphine has an active metabolite, morphine-6-glucuronide, that may account for this difference.[121–123]

Administer Analgesics Regularly After Initial Titration. Medication should be given regularly, even if it means awakening the patient. The pharmacologic rationale of this approach is to maintain the plasma level of the drug above the minimum effective concentration for pain relief. In the initial titration patients should be advised to take their medication as needed to determine their total 24-hour requirements. This is also the timeframe for reaching the steady-state level of drug, which depends on the drug's half-life. For morphine, steady state can be reached in 24 hours; with methadone it may take up to 5 to 7 days to reach steady state. Therefore, full assessment of the analgesic efficacy of a drug regimen may take several days.

In patients on a fixed schedule, rescue medications equivalent to one half-life of the standing dose should be available to patients for breakthrough pain. This allows the physician to start with a safe dose and to use the total dose of rescue medication added to the fixed dose as the dose necessary on a 24-hour basis. Continuous intravenous and subcutaneous opioid infusions to manage both acute and chronic cancer pain are commonly used with a patient-controlled analgesic pump. The pump can be programmed to the patient's needs with a set "lock-out time" to prevent overdosing. This method of drug administration is very useful to manage patients with breakthrough pain. It is a significant advance in facilitating adequate titration of analgesics in chronic cancer patients, allowing discharge to home and hospice settings.[125]

Gear the Route of Administration to the Patient's Needs. Various methods of drug delivery of opioids have been developed in an attempt to maximize pharmacologic effects and minimize side effects. A recent review of the patterns of drug use in cancer pain patients throughout their illness demonstrates that from the onset of pain until death, most patients needed at least two routes of drug administration; 20% needed up to four approaches.[24] These data emphasize the need for these alternative routes and the development of guidelines for chronic drug management.

The oral route is preferable and easy. In general, orally administered drugs have a slower onset of action, delayed peak time, and longer duration of effect; drugs given parenterally have a rapid onset of action but a shorter duration of effect. Sustained-release preparations of morphine allow more convenient dosing of cancer pain patients every 8 to 12 hours. These preparations have found wide acceptance in clinical practice.[127,128]

For cancer therapy by the sublingual route, sublingual buprenorphine is used as part of the second step of the WHO analgesic ladder. The tablet is rapidly absorbed in 3 to 5 minutes with a 55% bioavailability.[118] In contrast, morphine is poorly absorbed by this route but reported anecdotally to be effective, probably secondary to swallowing the drug. Both fentanyl and methadone are well absorbed sublingually, but no commercial preparations exist.[129]

The buccal route has been studied with morphine, and absorption occurs if the tablet remains in contact with the gum for 1 to 2 hours.[130] This approach is impractical.

The transmucosal route has more advantages than the buccal route. Oral transmucosal fentanyl citrate (OTFC) is a new formulation of fentanyl incorporated into a palatable form for dissolution and absorption through the oral mucosa.[131] It produces rapid onset of analgesia, anxiolysis, and sedation in pediatric preoperative patients and in a pilot study in cancer pain has been used to provide rapid onset of analgesia in breakthrough pain.

For the rectal route, oxymorphone, hydromorphone, and morphine are available in suppositories. Oxymorphone suppositories (10 mg) produce analgesia equivalent to 10 mg of parenteral morphine.[132] Morphine pharmacokinetics after rectal absorption are controversial, and there are not enough data to clarify whether this route, like the oral route, undergoes presystemic elimination via the liver. Several studies support the use of sustained-release preparations of morphine that provide comparable analgesia via rectal absorption. The route similarly is practical for patients who require parenteral drug administration.

The transdermal route is a convenient way to deliver a potent, short-acting opioid on a continuous basis.[133] The drug is released through skin patches at a nearly constant amount per unit time with a concentration gradient from patch to skin. Serum fentanyl concentrations increase and steady-state levels are approached at 12 to 24 hours. After patch placement, the drug persists on the skin, with falling blood levels over 24 hours. In calculating the equianalgesic dose, a 1:20 to 1:30 ratio of fentanyl to parenteral morphine is being used in patients not tolerant to opioids.[133]

Parenteral routes include intermittent and continuous subcutaneous, intravenous, epidural, intraventricular, or intrathecal infusions.

The use of intermittent and continuous subcutaneous infusions avoids presystemic clearance by the liver and is most useful in patients who cannot tolerate oral analgesics because of gastrointestinal obstruction or intractable nausea and vomiting. It is the approach of choice for the patient with gastrointestinal obstruction and pain. Numerous series have reported the usefulness of this technique using morphine, heroin, hydromorphone, methadone, and levorphanol.[125,134,135] Pumps designed to infuse continuously but with options for bolus administration are connected to a 27-gauge butterfly needle that the patient can insert into a new subcutaneous site every third to sixth day. Focal erythematous swelling at the site of injection has been reported to occur for both morphine and methadone, appearing several months after the start of therapy.[135] Limited pharmacokinetic studies have demonstrated that systemic absorption of the drug from subcutaneous sites at steady state has a 70% to 100% bioavailability with hydromorphone.[136]

Intermittent and continuous intravenous infusions are used if intravenous access is available and the patient is hospitalized. This route allows for rapid titration of a patient in acute pain. Specific guidelines for the use of continuous infusions in patients with chronic pain have been developed.[137] This approach, as well as continuous subcutaneous infusion, is used to manage the dying cancer pain patient. The goal of therapy must be clearly delineated for patients, families, and staff to alleviate any concern that such an approach is a form of euthanasia. The intent is to provide patients with continuous relief of pain and suffering.[16]

Intermittent and continuous epidural and intrathecal opioid infusions are based on the demonstration of opiate receptors in the dorsal horn of the spinal cord and the ability of opioid drugs to suppress noxious stimuli at the spinal cord level.[35,36] Localized selective analgesia is produced without motor or sensory blockade. This approach has been developed to minimize the distribution of drugs to receptors in the brain stem and cerebral hemispheres, thereby avoiding the problematic side effects of systemic administration of opiates (sedation, drowsiness, and respiratory depression). The use of an intermittent bolus of opioid via an epidural catheter has been compared with continuous opioid administration, and both approaches provide effective analgesia.[138] The pharmacokinetics of epidural opioid administration demonstrate that there is significant systemic uptake after epidural injection, comparable to an intramuscular injection of the same drug and dose.[138] However, distribution of the drug directly into the cerebrospinal fluid is 10 to 100 times greater. Continuous epidural and intrathecal infusions have also been used with implanted pumps. Intrathecal administration has limited systemic uptake, making this theoretically a more useful approach. However, after both epidural and intrathecal administration there is significant rostral redistribution of drug in the cerebrospinal fluid, and rapid development of tolerance has been reported.

The clinical dilemmas are at what point should this approach be considered in the management of cancer patients with pain, and what are the risk-to-benefit ratios in the individual patient. Significant cross-tolerance is induced by systemic opiates, confounding the indications for this approach. Controlled analgesic studies of this approach in the long-term management of cancer patients are needed. Existing studies demonstrate that 10% of cancer patients need this approach to maximize analgesia. It is particularly useful when combined with local anesthetics in patients with neuropathic pain.[37,38,138–140]

For intermittent and continuous intraventricular opioid infusion, the major indication is pain in the cervical and craniofacial region from tumor infiltration. Doses between 1 and 7.5 mg/24 hours have been used, and patients have reported 70% excellent results, 25% good results, and 5% poor results.[141–143] The indications for this procedure, the type of pain, and the prior opioid exposure of the patients have not been fully delineated, making this a rarely used approach.

Use a Combination of Drugs. The use of a combination of drugs enables the physician to increase analgesic effects without escalating the narcotic dose. Combinations that produce additive analgesic effects include a narcotic plus a nonnarcotic (aspirin, acetaminophen, ibuprofen, choline magnesium trisalicylate), a narcotic plus an antihistamine (100 mg intramuscular hydroxyzine), and a narcotic plus an amphetamine (10 mg intramuscular dextroamphetamine).[144,145] Studies demonstrating the efficacy of these combinations were single-dose studies. Hydroxyzine in 25-mg doses has been used regularly, with anecdotal observations that it is an effective combination. Certain combinations do not provide additive analgesia; these include a narcotic plus a benzodiazepine or a narcotic plus a phenothiazine.

Anticipate and Treat Side Effects. The side effects of the narcotic analgesics often limit their effective use. The most common side effects are sedation, respiratory depression, nausea, vomiting, constipation, and multifocal myoclonus and seizures.

Sedation and drowsiness vary with the drug and dose and may occur after both single and repeated administration. They are mediated through activation of opiate receptors in the reticular formation and diffusely throughout the cortex. Management of these effects includes reducing the individual drug dose but prescribing the drug more frequently, or switching to an analgesic with a shorter plasma half-life. Amphetamines, methylphenidate, and caffeine can be used to counteract these sedative effects.[145–147] It is important to discontinue all other drugs that might exacerbate the sedative effects of the narcotic analgesic, including a wide variety of medications such as cimetidine, barbiturates, and other anxiolytic medications.

Respiratory depression is the most serious adverse effect of the opioid drugs. It occurs most commonly after short-term administration of the narcotic and is usually associated with other signs of central nervous system depression, including sedation and drowsiness. The narcotic-agonist drugs act on brain stem respiratory centers to produce, as a function of dose, increasing respiratory depression to the point of apnea. Tolerance to this effect develops rapidly with repeated drug administration, thereby allowing prolonged use without significant risk of respiratory depression.

Respiratory depression can be reversed by giving the short-acting narcotic antagonist naloxone (suggested dose, 0.4 mg/ml). Repeated administration, including an intravenous drip, may be necessary to prevent respiratory arrest in such patients. In patients receiving narcotics for prolonged periods who develop respiratory depression, diluted doses of naloxone (0.4 mg in 10-ml saline) should be titrated carefully to prevent the precipitation of severe withdrawal symptoms while reversing the respiratory depression. A useful dosing normogram for continuous intravenous infusion of naloxone has been developed in which two thirds of the initial bolus is started on an hourly basis and titrated against the patient's symptoms.[148]

In some patients the use of naloxone to reverse drug-induced respiratory depression can be dangerous. An endotracheal tube should be placed in the comatose patient before giving naloxone to prevent aspiration from excessive salivation and bronchial spasm induced by naloxone administration. In patients receiving meperidine over a longer period, naloxone may precipitate seizures by lowering the seizure threshold and by allowing the convulsant activity of the active metabolite normeperidine to become evident. In this instance, special attention must be given to the potential seizure effect of naloxone. If naloxone is used, diluted doses, slow titration, and appropriate seizure precautions are advised. There is insufficient clinical evidence to make more specific recommendations. If respiratory support can be effected by other means (that is, continuous stimulation to maintain the patient's wakefulness), such an approach may place the patient at less risk and clearly in less discomfort.

The narcotic analgesics produce nausea and vomiting by an action limited to the medullary chemoreceptor trigger zone. The incidence of nausea and vomiting is markedly increased in ambulatory patients. Tolerance develops to these side effects with repeated administration. Nausea with one drug does not mean that all drugs will produce it. Switching to alternative narcotic analgesics or using an antiemetic together with the narcotic analgesics is the way to obviate this effect.

Constipation results from the action of these drugs at multiple sites in the gastrointestinal tract and in the spinal cord to produce a decrease in intestinal secretions and peristalsis, resulting in a dry stool and constipation. When narcotic analgesics are started, a regular bowel regimen, including cathartics and stool softeners, should also be instituted. Several bowel regimens have been suggested because of their specific ability to counteract the effects of the narcotic drugs, but none has been studied in a controlled way.[149] Anecdotal surveys suggest that doses far above those used for routine bowel management are needed, and that careful attention to dietary factors along with the use of a bowel regimen can reduce patient complaints dramatically. Tolerance to this effect develops over time, but relatively slowly.

Multifocal myoclonus may occur with high doses of all of the opioid drugs. Multifocal myoclonus and seizures have been reported in patients receiving multiple doses of meperidine (250 mg or more per day), although signs and symptoms of central nervous system hyperirritability may occur with toxic doses of all the narcotic analgesics. In a series of cancer patients receiving meperidine, accumulation of the active metabolite normeperidine was associated with these neurologic signs and symptoms.[69] However, in a similar group of cancer patients with pain, subtle mood effects were noted after meperidine administration, which suggests a spectrum of central nervous system effects. Management of this hyperirritability includes discontinuing the meperidine, using intravenous diazepam if seizures occur, and substituting morphine to control the persistent pain. Because the half-life of normeperidine is 16 hours, it may take 2 or 3 days for the signs of central nervous system hyperirritability to clear completely. Meperidine is contraindicated in patients with chronic renal disease, but these complications noted in cancer pain occurred in patients with normal renal function.[113] In dying patients with myoclonus, the use of benzodiazepines or barbiturates has been reported anecdotally to suppress this sign, improving the patient's comfort.

Manage Tolerance. The earliest sign of the development of tolerance is the patient's complaint that the duration of effective analgesia has decreased. For reasons not yet understood, the rate of development of tolerance varies greatly among cancer patients.[111] Some demonstrate tolerance within days of initiating narcotic therapy; others remain controlled for many months on the same dose. Studies in an outpatient clinic population, a hospitalized population, and a homecare population revealed three patterns of drug use: those who rapidly increase their opioid requirements, those who stabilize at one dose for several weeks or months, and those who decrease or eliminate opioids.[24,65,137] Increased opioid requirements are most commonly associated with disease progression rather than tolerance alone. With the development of tolerance, increases in the frequency or the dose of the opioid are required to provide continued pain relief. Because the analgesic effect is a logarithmic function of the dose of opioid, a doubling of the dose may be needed to restore full analgesia. There appears to be no limit to the development of tolerance, and with appropriate dose adjustments patients can continue to obtain pain relief. Cross-tolerance among the opioid analgesics is not complete; therefore, it is advantageous to change to an alternate opioid, selecting half the predicted equianalgesic dose as the starting dose.

The use of analgesic combinations can reduce the amount of opioid required. Similarly, the use of bolus or continuous epidural local anesthesia in patients with perineal pain can dramatically reduce the need for systemic opioids and reverse tolerance.

Taper Drugs Slowly. The long-term administration of narcotic analgesics is associated with the development of physical dependence, a state in which the sudden cessation of the narcotic analgesic will produce signs and symptoms of withdrawal: agitation, tremors, insomnia, fear, marked autonomic nervous system hyperexcitability, and exacerbation of pain. Slowly tapering the dose of the narcotic analgesic will prevent such symptoms. The appearance of abstinence symptoms from the time of drug withdrawal is related to the elimination half-life for the particular drug. The type of abstinence syndrome similarly varies with the drug. For example, with morphine, withdrawal symptoms occur within 6 to 12 hours after drug cessation. Reinstituting the drug in doses of about 25% of the previous daily dose suppresses these symptoms.

Anticipate Complications. Overdose with narcotic analgesics occurs either intentionally, when a patient takes an excessive amount of drug in a suicide attempt, or unintentionally, when the recommended dosage accidentally produces excessive sedation and respiratory depression. In both instances, the complication can be treated effectively with naloxone. Intentional overdose in cancer patients occurs rarely, and concern for this is overemphasized. Overdose in patients previously stabilized on a narcotic regimen for cancer pain rarely is caused by drug intake alone. More commonly, it is the medical deterioration of the patient with a superimposed metabolic encephalopathy. Reducing the narcotic drug dosage and carefully assessing the patient's metabolic status usually provide the differential diagnosis. Patients who have taken an unintentional drug overdose should be scrutinized carefully to rule out other causes of excessive sedation, confusion, or respiratory depression. In such cases a reversal of these effects with naloxone is more therapeutic than diagnostic.

Psychological dependence or addiction is characterized by a concomitant behavioral pattern of drug abuse characterized by craving a drug for other than pain relief and overwhelming involvement in the use and procurement of the drug. This is a state distinct from tolerance and physical dependence, which are responses to the pharmacologic effects of long-term narcotic administration. The profound fear of causing psychological dependence plays a major role in a physician's reluctance to prescribe narcotic analgesics, particularly in cancer patients in the early phase of their disease.[8,9] Patients may share this fear, consistently taking less analgesic drug than is effective to control their pain. Increasing evidence suggests that cancer patients with pain can take narcotic analgesics for prolonged periods but can discontinue such drugs when adequate pain relief is achieved from other approaches. In almost all instances, dramatic escalation of drug intake is associated with progression of disease and subsequent death.[24,65,137] Very few patients with cancer and pain become psychologically dependent on the drugs and participate in drug-seeking and illicit drug use. Careful evaluation of patients who might be at risk for this complication is necessary, but such concern should not be punitive to the patient with severe cancer pain.

Adjuvant Analgesic Drugs

These drugs have a unique place in the management of cancer pain, but knowledge about their use is empirical. This group includes several heterogenous substances used to increase the analgesic effects of the opioid analgesics, to counteract their side effects, or to act as analgesics themselves. Any discussion of the use of these adjuvants must be prefaced with caveats:

1. These drugs have been developed and released for clinical indications other than analgesia, including nausea, vomiting, anxiety, mania, depression, and delirium.
2. These drugs are not as effective in relieving pain as are the narcotic analgesics, except for methotrimeprazine (Levoprome).
3. There are no efficacy studies for their co-analgesic properties in cancer patients.
4. The choice of these drugs should be individualized, using the simplest but most potent combination of drugs.

ANTICONVULSANTS. Phenytoin and carbamazepine are anticonvulsant drugs that suppress spontaneous neuronal firing and are the drugs of choice for treating trigeminal neuralgia and other neuropathic pains.[150] In cancer pain, carbamazepine has been useful in managing the acute shocklike neuralgic pain in the cranial and cervical distribution caused by either tumor infiltration or surgical nerve injury. It also has been effective in patients with stump pain secondary to traumatic neuroma and in patients with lumbosacral plexopathy. The starting dose is 100 mg slowly titrated to 400 to 800 mg/day, depending on the patient's needs.

Several studies have reported the use of clonazepam and valproate in patients with acute lancinating pain.[151,152] Clonazepam has been reported to be effective in patients with both trigeminal and posttraumatic neuralgia. Valproate has also been reported to be effective in both trigeminal and postherpetic neuralgia in a series of uncontrolled surveys.

In cancer patients, the use of carbamazepine is limited by the fact that the drug can cause both leukopenia and thrombocytopenia in about 2% of patients. Because cancer patients commonly have a compromised hematologic reserve, this effect may limit the use of carbamazepine. A trial of clonazepam or valproate may be indicated in patients who cannot tolerate carbamazepine.

PHENOTHIAZINES. Of the phenothiazine drugs, methotrimeprazine has definitive analgesic properties. In single-dose studies in patients with postoperative pain and chronic cancer pain, 15 mg intramuscular methotrimeprazine is equivalent to 15 mg intramuscular morphine.[153] This drug is useful in special circumstances. In the patient who is tolerant, it provides a temporary approach to produce analgesia by a nonopiate receptor mechanism. In the patient with bowel obstruction and pain, it avoids the constipating effects of the narcotics. In patients whose respiration is compromised, it avoids the respiratory-depressant effects of the narcotics, although it can produce significant sedative effects. In patients with pain and narcotic-induced nausea and vomiting, it acts as both an analgesic and an antiemetic.

Long-term administration of this drug in patients with cancer pain has not been fully assessed. The usual starting dose is 5 to 10 mg parenterally. Patients should be carefully observed for orthostatic hypotension and sedation.

BUTYROPHENONES. Haloperidol is the first-line drug in the management of the cancer patient with acute psychosis and delirium, but its role in pain management is less clear.[60] In animals it potentiates morphine analgesia. Several authors have reported its clinical usefulness in cancer patients with pain, suggesting that it works as a co-analgesic and thus allows reduction of the narcotic dose.[154] The doses suggested to produce co-analgesic effects are lower than those used to manage psychiatric symptoms; 0.5 to 1 mg orally two to three times daily is the suggested starting dose.

ANTIDEPRESSANTS. The tricyclic antidepressants may be the most useful group of psychotropic drugs used in pain management. Their analgesic effects are mediated by enhancement of serotonin activity. Animal studies demonstrate the direct analgesic effects of amitriptyline as well as its ability to enhance morphine analgesia. Amitriptyline has been reported to be useful in the management of patients with migraine, postherpetic neuralgia, diabetic neuropathy, and a series of chronic pain states.[33,34] No controlled studies in cancer patients with neuropathic pain have been done, but strong anecdotal information suggests a role for these drugs in the management of such patients and in the management of pain-related sleep disturbances.

The doses used for analgesia are far below those needed to produce an antidepressant effect, and the analgesic properties of these drugs appear to occur independently of their mood-altering effects. Patients should be started on low doses of 10 to 25 mg, then titrated up to achieve adequate analgesia in a 2- to 4-week trial. Blood levels should be measured to determine both patient compliance and drug absorption, because there are wide individual variations.

Recent studies suggest that both continuous dysesthesias as well as lancinating pains may respond to the use of these drugs. Most studies support the analgesic efficacy for amitriptyline, imipramine, and doxepin, with less impressive data for nortriptyline and desipramine. Side effects such as cardiotoxicity, sedation, dry mouth, constipation, and urinary retention may occur and affect the choice of drug.

In the management of the cancer patient with pain, these drugs are the first-line therapeutic approach to the management of patients with postherpetic neuralgia, posttraumatic nerve injury, peripheral neuropathy, and central pain states.

STEROIDS. A series of controlled and uncontrolled surveys suggest that the use of chronic steroid therapy improves the quality of life and reduces pain in patients with breast and prostate cancer. In a controlled study of corticosteroid use in patients with far-advanced disease, transient improvement in appetite, analgesia, and mood were noted, but they were not sustained after the initial effect.[155] Corticosteroids have been reported to have both specific and nonspecific benefits in managing acute and chronic pain. Their ability to produce euphoria, increased appetite, and weight gain contributes greatly to the sense of well-being in the cancer patient with pain.[156] Steroids reportedly reduce bone pain of metastatic origin and are used as oncolytic agents with certain types of tumors. Several studies demonstrate prolonged survival time and reduced narcotic doses to control pain in terminal cancer patients receiving steroids.[157] In certain cancer pain syndromes such as epidural cord compression, 85% of patients receiving 100 mg of dexamethasone as part of a radiation therapy protocol reported significant pain relief associated with marked reduction in analgesic requirements.[46] In patients with tumor infiltration of the brachial and lumbosacral plexus, steroids provide additive analgesic effects. In patients with leptomeningeal metastases or headache from increased intracranial pressure from tumor or superior sagittal sinus occlusion, steroids play a major role in controlling head pain or neck and back pain.

ANTIHISTAMINES. Hydroxyzine is the drug most widely studied as an analgesic in the management of patients with pain and cancer. A dose of 100 mg parenterally provides analgesia that is additive to morphine.[93] No data support the analgesic effectiveness of oral doses of 10 or 25 mg of hydroxyzine, although good evidence supports the observation that these doses are associated with anxiolytic and mild antiemetic effects. Hydroxyzine is indicated to provide additive analgesia in a cancer patient requiring additive anxiolysis or an antiemetic effect.

NEUROSTIMULANTS. Evidence supports the analgesic effects of dextroamphetamine, methylphenidate, and caffeine.[145–147] These drugs are most commonly used in patients with excessive sedation from opioids. In a controlled repeated-dose trial of oral methylphenidate in patients with advanced cancer, opioid-induced sedation was reversed and supplemental analgesia was concurrently provided.[146] In a follow-up survey of 50 advanced cancer patients receiving 15 mg of methylphenidate in divided doses, beneficial effects were noted in more than 90% of patients, but evidence suggested the need for escalating doses to maintain a comparable effect in some patients. Because cocaine was commonly used in the Brompton cocktail, it was evaluated for both its analgesic and mood-altering effects. In a well-controlled single-dose analgesic assay, cocaine 10 mg orally influenced mood but had no impact on analgesic efficacy or reversal of sedation.[158]

In clinical practice, dextroamphetamine in doses of 2.5 to 5 mg twice daily, methylphenidate in doses of 15 mg twice daily, and caffeine in doses of 300 mg twice daily are commonly used to reverse opioid-induced sedation. This is particularly useful in patients who are receiving effective analgesia but whose functional status is compromised by drowsiness.

DIPHOSPHONATES. This novel group of drugs, also named biphosphonates, includes four main groups.[159] These drugs act by inhibiting the bone-resorption effects of osteoclasts and have been found particularly useful in conditions characterized by osteoclastic hyperactivity, such as Paget's disease and malignant hypercalcemia.

Osteoclasts have been associated with pain due to bone metastases, and several authors have studied the effects of diphosphonates on cancer bone pain.[159,160] Three small uncontrolled studies in 8, 12, and 17 patients have suggested the presence of diphosphonate-induced analgesia.[161,163]

In a randomized study of 131 patients with metastatic bone cancer, diphosphonate APD 15 mg twice a day orally was studied against a control group.[164] Patients continued to receive antineoplastic therapy, and the authors reported a significant decrease in the incidence of fractures, hypercalcemia, bone pain, and the need for radiation therapy in patients receiving APD as compared with controls. The main limitations of this study were its unblinded nature and the fact that no stratification was made according to the prognostically relevant tumor variables.

In a randomized study of 57 patients with painful bone metastases from prostate cancer, Smith evaluated four protocols: 7.5 mg/kg intravenous etidronate followed by 200 mg of etidronate twice a day orally; 7.5 mg/kg intravenous etidronate plus placebo only; intravenous placebo plus 200 mg twice a day orally; or intravenous placebo plus placebo orally.[165] This randomized double-blind study assessed pain and analgesic consumption for 1 month. Smith reported no significant analgesic effects. The limitation of this study is its limited statistical power: only 14 patients received only drug and 14 patients received only placebo.

Bruera and associates studied 23 consecutive patients with cancer-related bone pain who participated in a double-blind crossover trial of intravenous clodronate 600 mg versus placebo; after 1 week the patients received the alternative therapy.[166] Pain intensity, analgesic consumption, and the investigators' blinded choice favored clodronate. No significant clinical or laboratory side effects were noted.

The utility of these compounds in the management of patients with bone pain remains to be clarified. They may provide interesting mechanisms that might be associated with additive analgesia.

MISCELLANEOUS ADJUVANT DRUGS. The use of local anesthetics and barbiturates is discussed below in the section on anesthetic approaches.

PSYCHOLOGICAL APPROACHES

Psychological approaches should be an integral part of the care of the cancer patient with pain. New disciplines in psychooncology and psychosocial oncology have developed that focus on the psychological and psychosocial complications of cancer.[60] A series of psychological variables contribute to the cancer pain experience and suffering, such as perception of control, the meaning of pain, fear of death, depressed mood, and hopelessness. The level of psychological distress experienced by each patient varies depending on personality, coping ability, social support, and medical factors. Pain has a profound impact on levels of emotional distress, and psychological factors such as depression and anxiety intensify the pain experience. Measures of emotional disturbance have been reported to be predictors of pain in advancing latter stages of cancer.

Cancer patients with lower levels of neuroticism, anxiety, and depression are less likely to report pain. From a study by the Psychosocial Collaborative Oncology Group, an increased frequency of psychiatric disorders was found in cancer patients with pain, in particular anxiety and depression. Of the patients studied by this group who received a psychiatric diagnosis, 39% had significant pain.[60]

The incidence of pain, depression, and delirium increases with high levels of physical debilitation in advanced disease. About 25% of all cancer patients experience severe depressive symptoms, with the prevalence increasing to 77% in those with advanced illness. Uncontrolled pain is a major factor in cancer suicide.[68] While relatively few cancer patients commit suicide, studies suggest that they are at increased risk.

Various psychological interventions have been advocated for patients with cancer pain. Optimal treatment is multimodal and requires pharmacologic, psychotherapeutic, and cognitive-behavioral approaches. The roles of the psychiatrist, psychologist, and social worker in cancer pain management are well described in the literature.[68,167]

The goals of short-term psychotherapy are to provide emotional support, continuity, and information and to assist patients in adapting to the crisis. Communication skills are of paramount importance for patient and family, particularly about pain and analgesic issues. The needs of the patient and family must be addressed. Psychotherapy in the cancer pain setting is primarily nonanalytic and focuses on current issues and exploration of reactions to cancer, which often provide insight into other life issues. Group interventions may also be helpful.

A specialized approach called cognitive-behavioral therapy has been used to treat pain disorders, including cancer pain.[167] This approach uses short-term therapeutic interventions based on theoretically and empirically derived principles that can be adapted to each patient's problems and needs. It includes a set of systematic mental and behavioral techniques designed to modify specific emotional, behavioral, and social problems as well as the global experiences of pain and distress. Its major goal is to enhance the sense of personal control or self-efficacy. In a multidisciplinary approach to cancer pain, not every patient needs referral for this therapy, but it is useful if all members of the pain team follow a cognitive-behavioral model. Because cognitive-behavioral therapy is a commonsense psychological approach consisting of specific techniques, it can be learned and practiced by any interested clinician, nurse, or social worker who can gain practical training in the use of these techniques and apply them effectively.

Various intervention methods have been developed and are arbitrarily divided into behavioral and cognitive methods for discussion purposes. These approaches must be targeted to each patient's needs.

Behavioral techniques include ways to modify physiologic pain reactions and pain behaviors. Relaxation training can be used by all caregivers who manage patients with pain and cancer. Its mechanism of action includes the reduction of muscle tension and it can provide the patient with a sense of improved self-control and a calming diversion of attention, breaking the associated pain/anxiety/tension cycle. Techniques include simple deep-breathing exercises to more specialized methods of biofeedback and hypnosis. Contingency management is another behavioral approach designed to modify dysfunctional pain behaviors and replace them with "well" behaviors.

Cognitive techniques are designed to modify dysfunctional mental processes or to teach adaptive coping strategies. Cognitive coping and cognitive modification are approaches in which distraction, focusing, and perception and interpretation of the meaning of pain are assessed.

ANESTHETIC AND NEUROSURGICAL APPROACHES

Anesthetic and neurosurgical approaches are most effective in treating patients with well-defined localized pain. Tables 64–7 and 64–8 outline the indications for their use. About 10% to 20% of cancer pain patients need these approaches together with pharmacologic approaches to provide adequate analgesia.

In a prospective study, Ventafridda and colleagues evaluated

TABLE 64–7. Types of Anesthetic Procedures Commonly Used in Cancer Pain

Type of Procedure	*Most Common Indications*
Inhalation therapy with nitrous oxide	Breakthrough pain, incident pain in patients with diffuse poorly controlled pain
Intravenous barbiturates (sodium pentobarbital)	Diffuse body pain and suffering inadequately controlled by systemic opioids
Local anesthetic by intravenous, subcutaneous, or transdermal application	Neuropathic pain in any site with local application to the area of hyperesthesia or allodynia
Trigger-point injections	Focal muscle pain
Nerve block:	
Peripheral	Pain in discrete dermatomes in chest and abdomen or in distal extremities
Epidural	Unilateral lumbar or sacral pain
	Midline perineal pain
	Bilateral lumbosacral pain
Intrathecal	Mildine perineal pain
	Bilateral lumbosacral pain
Autonomic	
Stellate ganglion	Reflex sympathetic dystrophy
Lumbar sympathetic	Reflex sympathetic dystrophy of the lower extremity
	Lumbosacral plexopathy
	Vascular insufficiency of the lower extremity
Celiac plexus	Midabdominal pain from tumor infiltration
Intermittent or continuous epidural infusion with local anesthetics	Unilateral and bilateral lumbosacral pain
	Midline perineal pain
	Neuropathic pain from the midthoracic region down
Intermittent or continuous epidural or intrathecal with local opioid analgesics	Unilateral and bilateral pain below the midthoracic region; often combined with local anesthetics
Intermittent or continuous intraventrical infusions with opioid analgesics	Head and neck pain and upper chest
Chemical hypophysectomy	Diffuse bone pain

two groups of patients for 3 months who presented with intractable cancer pain not responsive to specific anticancer therapies.[11] One group was treated with sequential pharmacologic approaches using the analgesic ladder. The second group was treated with a multimodal approach of analgesic therapy followed by the use of neurolytic blocks or chronic spinal opioid administration. Patients treated with neurolytic procedures combined with pharmacologic therapy showed a statistically significant degree of greater pain relief than those treated with drugs alone by the third week of therapy. However, by 6 weeks there was no statistical difference between the two groups. Complete pain relief without the need for analgesic drug therapy persisted up to 3 months in 29% of the patients who received spinal opiates, 25% treated with celiac ganglion neurolytic block, 24% with percutaneous cordotomy, 12% with chemical rhizotomy, and 7% with gasserian thermorhizotomy. This study demonstrated that although analgesic therapy is the mainstay of treatment, anesthetic and neurosurgical procedures provide an important but limited contribution to adequate analgesia.

In a study comparing a multimodal pain treatment approach combined with a home-based supportive care program, the same authors noted markedly improved analgesia and quality of life in the patients who were followed in a supportive care program compared with those who received pain therapy alone.[23] Again, these data support the construct that treating cancer pain requires a multidisciplinary approach that includes not only pain therapy but also symptom management and treatment of psychological distress.

Several factors are important in selecting the appropriate procedure for each patient. Because diffuse pain problems are common in cancer patients and most of the procedures are useful for well-defined localized pain, the role of these approaches is limited at best. Further complicating their use is the limited number of professionals who have expertise in these procedures. As patients become more cognizant of their disease and treatment options, they are often hesitant to undergo neurodestructive procedures. Patients often consider their pain to be an important marker for their disease and are frightened of the potential, although unlikely, complications of these procedures. As a result, these procedures are often performed late in the illness, and full evaluation of their effectiveness and duration of action is limited by the patient's overriding medical problems.

These procedures are often not very effective in managing neuropathic pain, except for the use of local anesthetics, and are most helpful in managing most types of somatic and visceral pain. However, cancer patients often have a mixed somatic, visceral, and neuropathic pain syndrome. We advocate early consideration for the use of some of these anesthetic and neurosurgical procedures in patients to improve their quality of life through adequate pain management.

ANESTHETIC APPROACHES

Nitrous Oxide

Nitrous oxide has analgesic properties and has been used in the management of patients with far-advanced disease to provide added analgesia. It is administered with oxygen through a nonrebreathing face mask in concentrations from 25% to 75%. Its use in combination with systemic narcotic analgesics is associated with improvement of symptoms of pain and anxiety and a demonstrable improvement in alertness.[168] Although long-term nitrous oxide use has been associated with the development of pancytopenia, its short-term use is relatively safe. This anesthetic approach should be considered in patients with breakthrough pain or incident pain to provide adequate analgesia to facilitate their care. The method offers a simple means to treat transient pain if excessive side effects occur from increasing opioid doses.

Intravenous Barbiturates

This approach has been advocated to manage dying patients who have inadequate analgesia or uncontrolled symptoms,

TABLE 64–8. Neuroablative and Neurostimulatory Procedures for Relief of Pain From Cancer

Site	*Procedure*	*Indications*
Neuroablative Procedures		
Nerve root	Rhizotomy	Useful in somatic and neuropathic pain from tumor infiltration of the cranial and rarely intercostal nerves
Spinal cord	Dorsal root entry zone lesion (DREZ)	Useful in unilateral neuropathic pain from brachial, intercostal, and lumbosacral plexopathy and postherpetic neuralgia
	Cordotomy	Useful in unilateral pain below the waist. Often combined with local neurolytic blocks in perineal and bilateral lumbosacral plexopathy; may be performed bilaterally
	Myelotomy	Useful in midline pain below the waist but rarely used because it involves extensive surgery
Brain stem	Mesencephalic tractomy	Useful in pain in the nasopharynx and trigeminal region
Thalamus	Thalamotomy	Useful in unilateral neuropathic pain in the chest and lower extremity
Cortex	Cingulotomy	Useful through a stereotactic approach for diffuse pain
Pituitary	Transsphenoidal hypophysectomy	Useful in pain control of bone metastases in endocrine-dependent tumors, breast, and prostate
Neurostimulatory Procedures		
Peripheral nerve	Transcutaneous and percutaneous electrical nerve stimulation	Useful in reducing painful dysesthesias from tumor infiltration of nerve or trauma (*e.g.*, neuroma)
Spinal cord	Dorsal column stimulation	Of limited use in neuropathic pain in the chest, midline, and lower extremities
Thalamus	Thalamic stimulation	Of rare use in neuropathic pain in the chest, midline, or lower extremity

who ask to be maintained in a sedated state. Intravenous thiopental titrated to a level of sedation was the approach advocated in a series of 17 terminally ill patients.[169] The authors suggested that the value of this approach is based on the use of one agent to treat both physical and psychological symptoms. This approach may be seen as a more generalized one to palliative care and should be considered only if the standard approaches with opioid analgesics and adjuvant drugs fail to provide adequate analgesia with minimal side effects. However, because it is the physician's responsibility to manage not only pain but also suffering, this may be a reasonable approach, particularly in the dying patient with profound dyspnea, myoclonus, or agitation. Further studies are needed to clarify the usefulness of this approach. In the published study, 13 of 17 patients developed somnolence and died; the somnolence lasted from 2 hours to 4 days, with an average of 23 hours. Four patients died without being somnolent.

The doses of thiopental varied. A standard solution consisted of 500 mg of thiopental in 250 ml of 5% dextrose and water. The drug was delivered at 20 to 80 mg/hour, titrated to the patient's need for sedation; the average dose was 107 mg/hour. In patients receiving ventilatory assistance the standard dose of thiopental was a 100- to 150-mg bolus followed by a continuous infusion of 150 mg/hour. The doses used in these studies were below those used in patients receiving respiratory assistance.

Several problematic symptoms often arise in the management of the dying patient, including intractable vomiting, profound dyspnea, extreme agitation and anxiety, and uncontrolled pain. Several authors have reported that most cancer patients have crescendo symptoms before death, requiring somnolence.[24,25,170] This approach offers one method to manage these difficult patients. Tachyphylaxis to thiopental has been described, but both the advantages and disadvantages of this approach must be further debated to define its place in the management of patients with advanced disease.

Local Anesthetics

Anecdotal reports and several controlled studies support the use of intravenous, subcutaneous, transdermal, intrapleural, and epidural local anesthetics in the management of patients with somatic, visceral, and neuropathic pain.[171–175]

Intravenous lidocaine should be considered as both a diagnostic and therapeutic approach in patients with neuropathic pain. If such patients obtain an analgesic response, a trial of oral mexiletine or the use of continuous subcutaneous lidocaine should be considered to determine whether prolonged relief may be possible. Although no studies have confirmed that the response to lidocaine predicts a response to mexiletine for pain, a comparable predictive value exists in the cardiac literature, where intravenous lidocaine's effectiveness in controlling ventricular arrhythmias predicts the usefulness of mexiletine for this same disorder.[171]

Cousins and colleagues reported the use of continuous subcutaneous infusions in two patients with cancer-related neuropathic pain, advocating this approach as an alternative one in patients who do not respond to standard opioid and adjuvant treatments as well as anesthetic approaches for neuropathic pain.[172]

The transdermal application of lidocaine using a 2%, 5%, or 10% ointment has been reported to be useful in patients with superficial hyperesthesia, dysesthesias, and significant allodynia. Spreading the ointment on the painful site can often provide transient pain relief. This has been best demonstrated in patients with postherpetic neuralgia. The advantage of such an approach is the limited degree of systemic uptake of the drug and the ability to reduce pain at its peripheral site of origin. This approach has been used in patients with peripheral skin lesions and open draining sores with associated inflammatory changes. Topical ointments used in and around the rectal area or oral solutions can provide pain relief in patients with superficial rectal/anal pain or oral mucositis or esophagitis.

Intrapleural local anesthetics have been used for acute pain in the chest wall and have been adapted for the management of chronic cancer pain.[174] A subcutaneously tunneled intrapleural catheter offered long-term relief of right upper quadrant pain from hepatic metastases in a patient with significant pain from tumor infiltration of the liver. This approach was successful for 6 weeks. The patient used 0.5% preservative-free bupivacaine given every 8 hours. This novel method offers an alternative approach for patients with local regional pain in the pleural and abdominal regions.

Epidural local anesthetics are used to manage patients with localized pain syndromes, usually below the waist. Intermittent and continuous epidural infusions of local anesthetics have been used to manage the difficult chronic pain associated with metastatic disease below the waist, often involving the sacrum and lumbosacral plexus.[140,175,176] This method consists of infusing a local anesthetic into a subcutaneous infusion pump or Ommaya reservoir that is connected to a catheter temporarily or permanently placed in the epidural space. If the amount and concentration of the anesthetic are varied, effective pain relief can be achieved without interrupting significant motor or autonomic function. The risk of infection is minimized because local anesthetics have antimicrobial effects. The use of continuous low-dose infusions of local anesthetics is associated with minimal systemic side effects. Further studies on the use of this technique in comparison with standard therapies are needed to define its place in the management of the cancer patient. Its major advantages are that the resultant analgesia is not cross-tolerant with the analgesic produced by the opioid analgesic, and that temporary use of this technique allows for reduction in the amount of systemic opiate drugs, therefore partially reversing tolerance. This has been a useful preliminary approach in patients for whom the use of spinal opiate analgesia is considered but who have developed tolerance from large doses of systemic opiates. Because tolerance develops to these analgesic effects, this approach is temporary (days to weeks) rather than long term. This approach is most useful in patients who experience an acute pain crisis, such as the patient with a pathologic hip fracture who is not a surgical candidate; this approach would allow the patient to move about in bed.

Peripheral Nerve Blocks

Peripheral nerve blocks are used both diagnostically to localize the nerve distribution and therapeutically to interrupt pain transmission within a determined nerve distribution.[140] This technique is limited to areas of the body in which the interruption of both motor and sensory function will not interfere with the patient's functional status. This approach is most commonly used with patients who have pain in the head, chest, or abdomen. This technique is also limited by the fact that each peripheral nerve subserves sensory function over many levels, and usually several nerves must be blocked to provide adequate analgesia. These techniques are most useful in patients with somatic pain; neuropathic pain is rarely controlled by peripheral nerve blocks alone. Examples of successful blocks include gasserian ganglion block for craniofacial pain, intercostal blocks for chest wall infiltration from tumor, and paravertebral blocks for radicular pain.[140,176]

In patients with somatic pain who respond to a local anesthetic block, neurolytic blockade with either alcohol or phenol may provide more prolonged relief. A block produced by phenol tends to be less profound and of shorter duration than that produced by alcohol. Phenol has local anesthetic as well as neurolytic effects. This is an advantage because it is painless to inject and provides a clear indication of the area affected by neurolysis. Some authors report that phenol has a more marked effect on blood vessels than does alcohol. It was originally believed that phenol's action as a neurolytic agent was based on its differential sparing of large myelinated fibers while destroying the small unmyelinated C fibers. However, this differential effect is not clinically significant, and a wealth of experimental evidence demonstrates these facts.[140]

Whatever the agent used, the most common peripheral neurolytic block is a paravertebral block for localized intercostal pain. From our experience in treating patients with chest wall pain, we advise that this procedure be done under fluoroscopic control or CT localization to accurately interrupt the individual intercostal nerve.

Epidural and intrathecal neurolytic blocks have been used primarily to manage patients with far-advanced disease whose pain is either unilateral in the chest or abdomen or midline in the perineum.[177] These approaches are less useful in managing upper and lower limb pain associated with brachial and lumbosacral plexopathy because of the high risk of motor weakness associated with effective neurolytic blockade by this route. Epidural phenol blocks are useful in chest wall pain over several dermatomes. Such an approach obviates the need for multiple paravertebral injections. Phenol is injected in small increments (1 to 2 ml per segment) over 2 or 3 days by an epidural catheter, and preliminary data demonstrate 80% pain relief in patients with documented somatic pain. Epidural and intrathecal phenol blocks have been used to manage perineal pain, but no studies have delineated the superiority of one approach to the other.

For an intrathecal block, a phenol-glycerine solution, which is viscous and hyperbaric, can be directed to the site by gravity. An 18-gauge spinal needle is used to introduce the phenol intrathecally, and the substance is injected in small increments (0.4 ml) to a total of 1 to 1.5 ml. With the use of alcohol, to produce a precise block of profound intensity and adequate duration, the patient must be carefully positioned so that the maximum concentration of the hypobaric alcohol solution reaches the posterior nerve roots. This means that the patient is placed in a lateral oblique position with the painful side uppermost. For bilateral pain, to produce a saddle or perineal block, the patient must be placed in a prone position with the affected segment uppermost over the break in the operating table. The injected alcohol will then spread over both posterior roots. Alternatively, each side may be blocked on separate occasions, 2 to 3 days apart, when the effect of the initial injection can be assessed before the second procedure is attempted.

A review of a large number of alcohol subarachnoid blocks reports an average of 60% good relief, 21% fair relief, and 18% poor relief.[140,176–178] Because the duration of pain relief has seldom been documented with careful follow-up studies, the overall estimate for relief of pain with both subarachnoid alcohol and phenol blocks suggests a mean duration of pain relief of between 2 weeks and 3 months.

Complications are of two kinds. With intrathecal injection a self-limiting spinal headache may occur. Complications that result from the action of neurolytic substances on nerve fibers include motor paresis, loss of sphincter function, impairment of touch and proprioception, and troublesome dysesthesias. Injection in the thoracic region has a low complication rate. In our experience, many cancer patients already have both motor and autonomic dysfunction before the use of neurolytic blockade; these often remain the same or may worsen. Patients should be informed of the risk of these procedures, with particular attention to the fact that they may develop motor paresis and bladder dysfunction, specifically incontinence, after the blockade.

The selection of patients for management with epidural or intrathecal neurolytic agents should be based on the following criteria: exhaustion of appropriate antitumor approaches; clear clinical and radiologic definition of the pain; poor candidacy for percutaneous cordotomy; failure of nonopioid, opioid, and adjuvant analgesics to produce adequate analgesia without significant side effects; a favorable response to diagnostic or epidural or intrathecal blocks, producing at least 75% pain relief; and myelography done before the procedure to rule out tumor infiltration of the subarachnoid space.

Autonomic Nerve Block

Sympathetic block is effective in conditions with vasomotor or visceromotor hyperactivity. This hyperactivity accompanies many of the cancer-related pain syndromes such as visceral pain or plexopathies. The most commonly used sympathetic block is that of the celiac ganglion for pain due to abdominal malignancy, including cancer of the pancreas, stomach, duodenum, liver, gallbladder, adrenal gland, and colon. Nociceptive fibers of the splanchnic, sympathetic, vagal, phrenic, and somatic nerves converge on the celiac ganglion, which is amenable to a regional block that is successful in from 70% to 85% of patients treated.[138,179,180]

Standardized approaches for the use of this technique have been described using CT monitoring or fluoroscopic control. After placement of the needle, 25 ml of absolute alcohol mixed with local anesthetic and contrast is injected. Bilateral needle placement has been reported to provide the best results, but anecdotal reports suggest that unilateral needle placement on the right provides comparable analgesia. The major side effect of the procedure is transient hypotension, and patients must be well hydrated and monitored carefully during the procedure and for 4 to 6 hours afterward. Significant neurologic complications occur in less than 1% of patients if proper technique is used. Complications include paraparesis, postural hypotension, and urinary difficulties.

Although there has been recent debate about the usefulness of this procedure in patients with pancreatic cancer, it should be considered as one of the approaches, together with pharmacologic approaches, in managing these patients.

Lumbar sympathetic block may provide significant relief of intractable urogenital pain or pain due to carcinomatous invasion of local nerves and plexus in the perineum and lower extremity.[181] This ganglion conveys visceral nociceptive afferents from the pelvic viscera. Pain caused by cancer of the sigmoid colon or rectum may be relieved by bilateral lumbar sympathetic block if the disease is confined to those viscera. Pain caused by cancer of the seminal vesicles or prostate may sometimes be relieved by bilateral lumbar sympathetic block. Similarly, pain caused by uterine cancer may be relieved if the disease is confined to the body of the uterus. In many instances, however, the block must be extended to the T12 ganglion. Good evidence suggests that lumbar sympathetic block alone is not useful in patients with lumbosacral plexopathy; therefore, the role of this procedure is limited to specific anatomic sites of pain.

Stellate ganglion block may sometimes be useful for pain in the face, upper neck, ear, and hemicranium. However, the potential complications of stellate ganglion block limit the use of this technique with neurolytic solution, as there is a high risk of spillage of the neurolytic material into the brachial plexus, with secondary nerve injury and focal pain.

Neuroadenolysis of the Pituitary

Chemical hypophysectomy is a special use of a neurolytic method. Several studies suggest that 35% to 95% of patients undergoing this approach report pain relief, with a median duration of 6 to 7 weeks and a maximum duration of 20 weeks.[182–184] The mechanism by which analgesia is produced may result from alcohol tracking up the pituitary stalk into the hypothalamus, with consequent disruption of the hypothalamic-thalamic endorphinergic pain pathways. Side effects include diabetic insipidus, cranial nerve palsies, cerebrospinal fluid leakage, and rarely meningitis. The lack of detailed clinical data limits critical assessment of these studies. This technique is rarely if ever used in patients with diffuse pain.

Trigger Point Injections

The use of trigger point injections is within the scope of the practicing physician.[185] Patients with significant musculoskeletal pain often describe specific, tender trigger point areas that, when injected with either saline or local anesthetic, are associated with significant pain relief. Effective relief of pain from trigger point injections, however, is not diagnostic of musculoskeletal pain alone, and an evaluation of the cause of the pain is still necessary to rule out the specific etiology.

NEUROSURGICAL APPROACHES

Neurosurgical approaches for cancer pain can be divided into two major categories—antitumor and antinociceptive.[186,187] These approaches are often used alone or in combination by neurosurgeons to provide improved pain relief.

Antitumor Approaches

Antitumor approaches are often more acceptable to patients because they focus on cancer treatment, offering the hope of prolonged survival. The major procedures are listed in Table 64–8 and include tumor removal from the spine, epidural space, or adjacent plexi; stabilization procedures for spinal fracture, instability, and subluxation; and implantation of regional delivery devices for epidural, intrathecal, and intraventricular opioid drugs.

Tumor removal through resection of spinal metastases is associated with dramatic improvement in pain in 70% to 90% of patients.[188,189] With the use of improved methods of internal fixation with methyl methacrylate and improved stabilizing procedures, the use of this approach has increased in patients with intractable continuous or incidental back and neck pain. Patients may also have an associated segmental instability associated with a pathologic fracture of the vertebral body or subluxation, syndromes that place patients at significant risk for neurologic dysfunction. Careful radiologic workup is necessary to define the specific anatomic basis for the spinal pain, but aggressive surgical approaches have improved the quality of life for many patients bedridden by uncontrolled back pain. In patients with epidural cord compression, the indications for surgery include uncontrolled pain in a patient with a pathologic fracture or a solitary relapse in the epidural space or vertebral body from a radioresistant tumor. In patients with radiosensitive tumors who relapse after radiation therapy, spinal surgery should be considered as a reasonable approach and is specifically indicated in the patient with an acute neurologic deterioration during radiation therapy. When percutaneous or open vertebral body biopsy is impossible, surgical resection should be strongly considered to define the primary tumor type in patients with undiagnosed lesions; this serves as both a diagnostic and therapeutic procedure.

In patients with paraspinal tumor or tumor infiltration of the plexus, en bloc resection of tumor has successfully provided pain relief and has served as a debulking antitumor procedure. In patients with Pancoast's syndrome, invasion of the spine or epidural extension is present in 20% at initial presentation and is associated with significant morbidity in up to 50% of patients when local treatment is ineffective. In the good-risk patient with plexopathy and spinal invasion, Sundaresan recommends surgery in which tumor is removed from the lower plexus, C8-T1, and the vertebral body is resected, with brachytherapy to provide further tumor control.[189]

In patients with tumor invasion of the paraspinal area (specifically the psoas and iliacus), radical resection of these tumor masses concurrent with spinal surgery, followed by brachytherapy, combines antitumor and antinociceptive therapies.

When considering the use of these neurosurgical procedures to provide palliative surgery with an antinociceptive component, the patient's extent of disease, performance score, prognosis, and ability to tolerate the surgery must all be weighed.

Antinociceptive Procedures

Antinociceptive procedures include neuroablative, neurostimulatory, and neuropharmacologic approaches.

Neuroablative procedures involve the production of a surgical or radiofrequency lesion along the nociceptive neural pathway. Sectioning of the posterior roots (rhizotomy), lesioning the lateral dorsal horn (dorsal root entry zone lesion), and interrupting the ascending neospinothalamic pathway (cordotomy) or the crossing interneuronal fibers (myelotomy) in the spinal cord are examples of neuroablative procedures performed for pain relief.

Cordotomy, either percutaneous or open, is the most common neuroablative procedure used to manage cancer pain.[187,190–192] It is the neurosurgical procedure of choice for patients with unilateral pain below the waist with a relatively short life expectancy. Cordotomy is usually effective for 1 to 3 years, with dysesthesias substituting for analgesia in patients living longer than 3 years. Pain in the chest wall or upper extremity may be successfully treated initially with cordotomy, but extensive data demonstrate that, with time, the level of analgesia drops, limiting the effectiveness of this approach. Somatic pain appears to be most responsive to cordotomy; visceral and neuropathic pain are less responsive for reasons that are not fully understood.

Percutaneous cordotomy is performed in a supine, awake patient through a lateral C1-2 approach.[187,190] A needle is advanced under fluoroscopic control until cerebrospinal fluid is obtained. A mini-myelogram is done to identify the dentate ligament. A cordotomy electrode is passed through the spinal needle and the spinal cord is punctured with the aid of impedance monitoring. Electrophysiologic stimulation is done to identify the spinothalamic tract and then a radiofrequency lesion is made in the appropriate painful site. Such a lesion interrupts pain and temperature on the contralateral side of the lesioned site. Patients typically report spontaneous relief of pain in this lesioned area.

The anatomic area at the lesion site includes fibers mediating respiration and autonomic function. These fibers are adjacent to the anterior horn and the cervical spinothalamic fibers. Near the lumbar spinothalamic tract are the fibers governing the intercostal muscles. This quadrant of the spinal cord also contains the sacral fibers to and from the bladder, which are closer to the spinothalamic fibers. These anatomic relations explain some of the complications associated with cordotomy: bladder dysfunction, respiratory compromise, and ipsilateral motor weakness.

From the literature that does not provide comparative studies in cancer patients with pain, pain relief can be obtained in 60% to 80% of patients immediately after cordotomy; results at 6 to 12 months are 40% to 50%.[187–190] In a retrospective survey of 40 percutaneous cordotomies in patients with predominant unilateral pain below the waist, 70% of patients obtained complete relief with continued use of some supplemental analgesics, 16% had moderate relief, and 13% did not benefit from the procedure.[186] In another study, Arbit reported that 16% of patients referred for percutaneous cordotomy could not undergo the procedure because of difficulty in positioning or with participating in the procedure, even with the use of increased analgesic drug doses and anesthetic assistance.[187] Careful patient selection is necessary for this procedure.

Open cordotomy is usually done below the cervicothoracic junction through a hemilaminectomy or full laminectomy. Open cordotomy should be reserved for the patient who cannot tolerate a percutaneous approach or for the patient with limited motor or sensory dysfunction from tumor infiltration below the waist in whom bilateral cordotomy is to be done for bilateral or midline pain.

The complications of cordotomy vary with the type of procedure (percutaneous or open) and are also strongly influenced by the patient's premorbid neurologic condition. Many patients have borderline bladder function and mild paresis from tumor infiltration that is transiently or permanently exacerbated by these procedures. In our series at Memorial Sloan-Kettering Cancer Center, 45% of patients had transient or permanent urinary retention.[192] After cordotomy there is often an unmasking of pain ipsilateral to the cordotomy site. This pain was reported in 22% of patients in our series.[187] In some patients it was difficult to clarify if this nerve pain was caused by unidentified tumor and really represented mirror pain, or was caused by the unmasking of tumor-related pain. In 60% of patients in the Arbit series, unmasking of pain on the contralateral side occurred because many patients had bilateral lumbosacral plexopathy. Dysesthesias characterized by burning pain in the area of sensory loss are reported in 1% to 2% of patients after a delay of several months to 2 years after the procedure. Ipsilateral motor weakness results from an inadvertent anterior extension of the lesion to involve the corticospinal tract. In our series, 7% of patients had transient paresis and 22% had permanent paresis. Most series report motor paresis in 10% to 20% of patients.

Respiratory complications occur in patients with a dysfunctional lung contralateral to the site of cordotomy. This is a predictable risk when patients undergo cordotomy on the same side as their only functioning lung: interruption of the reticulospinal fibers controlling the intercostal muscles and of the phrenic nerve may occur because of their proximity to the lateral spinothalamic tract in this spinal cord quadrant.

Several other complications, including headache, fever, and meningismus, are associated with the percutaneous procedure, as well as a Horner's syndrome because of interruption of the sympathetic tract.

In our series, 30% of patients demonstrated a profound depressive syndrome associated with significant pain relief.[192] Patients should be warned about this complication, but the factors contributing to its development have not been fully clarified. Rapid reduction in opioids, realization that with pain relief they must face their terminal illness, and other factors, including exhaustion, depression, and preexisting psychopathology, may all play a role in the appearance of this problematic complication. Psychological intervention and the use of tricyclic antidepressants have been effective in managing these patients.

Dorsal rhizotomy is the next most common neuroablative procedure used for cancer pain. It is performed by sectioning the posterior sensory rootlets, and a specific localized dermatomal pain level can be identified. It can be performed by an operative section of the nerve or as previously discussed by a neurolytic block. In patients with chest wall pain from tumor invasion, improved analgesia in 50% to 80% has been reported with dorsal rhizotomy.[193] Arbit has adapted this procedure to manage patients with significant chest wall pain.[194]

Rhizotomies of the trigeminal nerve, nervus intermedius, glossopharyngeal nerve, and portions of the vagus nerve are effective in controlling pain from head and neck tumors that invade the base of the skull.[195] Bilateral sacral rhizotomy has been reported to treat sacral or perineal pain involving the sacral plexus at the S2 and S3 levels. However, these patients have often had extensive radiation therapy, and wound closure in the irradiated skin over the sacrum may complicate recovery and increase the risk-to-benefit ratio. A neurolytic, epidural, or subarachnoid block is usually considered before surgical sacral rhizotomy.

The use of a dorsal root entry zone lesion is based on the recognition that nociceptive fibers enter lamina I and lamina II at the dorsal horn; interruption of this anterior lateral site has been associated with reduction in neuropathic pain in experimental animals. This approach has been used most commonly in avulsion of the brachial plexus, postherpetic neuralgia, and postradiation plexopathy. Because this approach has not been widely used in cancer pain, its usefulness for brachial and lumbosacral plexopathy is not established, but it is an interesting approach for such patients.[196] The procedure requires a several-level laminectomy to provide an adequate approach to this anatomic site, and this may be too extensive a procedure for the cancer patient with advanced disease. Further studies are necessary to determine its usefulness.

The midline commissural myelotomy approach has been used in patients with midline perineal or coccygeal pain or bilateral pain in the lower extremities. Using a limited midline myelotomy, Gildenberg and Hirschberg reported satisfactory pain relief in 10 of 14 patients with midline pain below the waist from cancer.[197] This procedure is based on the fact that nociceptive fibers cross in the anterior commissure from the dorsal horn to the contralateral spinothalamic pathway. This approach is used rarely if ever in patients with bilateral pain.

Cingulotomy has recently received attention in the treatment of some patients with cancer pain, using a stereotactic procedure with MRI to permit a radiofrequency lesion. Four patients with pain from widely metastatic, diffuse bone disease who were receiving opioid analgesics reported immediate pain relief with bilateral cingulate lesions.[198] The pain relief persisted until death in 2 to 6 weeks. This procedure was previously used to treat psychiatric illness and has a long history of use in severe chronic pain from a variety of neuropathic syndromes. The literature suggests that up to 50% of cancer patients have had moderate, marked, or complete relief for 3 months after the procedure. The extent to which the development of this improved method will alter the use of this technique needs to be clarified.

Neurostimulatory procedures involving the peripheral nerve and spinal cord are generally based on the gate theory of pain.[199] The original theory suggests that there is a neurophysiologic gating mechanism in the spinal cord, probably within the substantia gelatinosa. Noxious sensation is conducted via small-diameter peripheral nerve fibers and nonnoxious sensation via large-diameter fibers, and both send collaterals to the substantia gelatinosa and up the spinal dorsal columns. Stimulation of the small fibers tends to promote pain or "open the gate," whereas stimulation of the large fibers tends to inhibit pain or "close the gate." Because the large nerve fibers ascend in a compact bundle through the dorsal columns, they are accessible to selected electric stimulation. Retrograde firing of the large fibers ensues and pain sensation is inhibited at multiple levels of the spinal cord below that being stimulated.

Based on reports that high-frequency (50 to 100 Hz) percutaneous electrical nerve stimulation relieved chronic neurogenic pain, the use of transcutaneous electrical nerve stimulation (TENS) was reported effective in treating neuropathic pain. Although control studies are lacking, numerous clinical surveys suggest that this approach is useful for nociceptive and neuropathic pain. With the advent of sophisticated electronic devices, various patterns of electric stimulation are currently in use transcutaneously, including pulsed (burst), modulation (ramped), random, and complex wave forms, all designed to improve efficacy. Patients are instructed in proper electrode placement in a dermatomal pattern and are instructed to try both intermittent and continuous stimulation. By trial and error, analgesic effects should be observed either immediately or, in some cases, after the stimulation is discontinued.

TENS is used for a wide variety of pains and serves as a safe, noninvasive approach. Clinical experience suggests its usefulness in some patients with peripheral nerve pain. Several investigators have reported that it is useful in cancer pain for a wide variety of tumor-related and neuropathic pain syndromes.[200,201] Further studies are necessary to define the usefulness of TENS in the cancer patient with pain.

The dorsal column-stimulating technique involves the introduction of an electrode into the epidural or intrathecal space and advancing it to the appropriate level overlying the dorsal columns. This is done under local anesthesia and biplane fluoroscopy. Once in place, the electrode is implanted subcutaneously and an external transmitting electrode is placed over the receiving electrode and connected to a transmitter. A trial is then done to assess the efficacy of the electrode, check its position, and determine the patient's stimulatory parameters (frequency, amplitude, and duration of stimulatory cycles). The electrode that we have found most suitable is the quadripolar lead, a multielectrode lead that permits the physician to choose the pair of electrodes that produces the best response.[202,203]

The main indications for placement of a dorsal column stimulator are intractable dysesthetic or deafferentation pain of the limbs or trunk, such as radiation-induced brachial or lumbosacral plexopathy. This procedure is effective in 43% to 75% of patients and carries a low morbidity rate. The most common complication is failure of the device itself, which occurs in about 10% of patients annually. Other complications include infection, cerebrospinal fluid fistula, allergic or rejection response to the device material, and changes in stimulation over time, which may be related to cellular changes around the electrode or shifts in its position.

Thalamic stimulation involves the placement of electrodes in the medial thalamus and has been reported to be most useful for managing neuropathic pain from lesions in the central and peripheral nervous system. There are a series of reports on the usefulness of this technique in patients with head and neck cancer and prominent cranial neuropathic pain, but the limited use of this technique in these patients makes it difficult to define its specific role.[204]

Acupuncture has been used to treat both acute and chronic pain and is based on a sophisticated, elaborate system of diagnosis. The selected acupuncture points are manually or electrically stimulated with a needle until the patient feels the sensation. A wide variety of acupuncture techniques are available, ranging from a traditional Chinese approach to a Western adaptation. Laser acupuncture with external laser probes has also been used. The studies in cancer patients with pain represent large, uncontrolled, retrospective surveys. Minimal stimulation in manual acupuncture was used in all cases, and three acupuncture treatments represented an adequate trial. Fifty-two percent and 56% of patients reported some pain improvement for at least 7 days; an additional 30% and 22% had pain relief for 2 days or less or reported increased mobility alone.[205] A lack of detailed pain assessment in specific acupuncture techniques or a critical review of the patient population make it difficult to interpret these observations. Based on its current empirical use, this approach is relatively safe and may have some benefit in cancer patients with pain, but further studies are necessary to define its role.

PHYSIATRIC APPROACHES

Rehabilitation medicine plays an important role in the multidisciplinary approach to the patient with cancer pain. Physiatrists are concerned with a patient's physical functioning and provide expertise in assessing how impairment in a patient's physical capacity affects his or her ability to function. A wide variety of interventions are available, including TENS, diathermy (heating pads, ultrasound, hydrotherapy), and cryotherapy (ice and vapo-coolants). Assistive devices and braces, as well as therapeutic exercise and massage, are important. Trigger point injections and acupuncture have also been used. These interventions are commonly used in combination with other pain-therapy approaches, particularly behavioral and pharmacologic approaches.

A large body of data supports the use of rehabilitative interventions in acute and chronic nonmalignant pain, but similar studies have not addressed the rehabilitation needs of the cancer pain patient.[206] From our experience, neurologic dysfunction is one of the common components in patients with cancer pain, and aggressive neurorehabilitation is necessary to ambulate these patients and provide them with functional independence.

ALGORITHM FOR CANCER PAIN MANAGEMENT

An algorithm has been developed that integrates all of these management approaches for cancer pain. It attempts to integrate assessment techniques, drug therapy, behavioral approaches, and anesthetic and neurosurgical approaches and stresses continuity of care. Treatment begins with a diagnostic evaluation that addresses the medical, psychological, and social components of pain. A plan is developed to treat the cancer and the pain. If the anticancer treatment is effective, pain relief usually occurs and the drugs used for analgesia can be discontinued without difficulty. Pain treatment begins with the use of analgesic drugs as described in the analgesic ladder (see Fig. 64–2), starting with nonopioid drugs alone or in combination. If they are successful, no further therapy is necessary. If severe persistent pain does not respond to analgesic drugs or if the side effects of the drugs are not tolerated, the physician should consider switching analgesics (*e.g.*, from oral morphine to methadone), changing the route of administration (*e.g.*, from oral to subcutaneous), or performing a cordotomy for localized pain. A trial of an adjuvant drug together with the opioid and nonopioid drug would also be appropriate. In patients with excessive sedation or confusion, the use of a neurostimulant or haloperidol provides adequate treatment of the side effects of the opioid drugs and maintains the patient's analgesia while markedly reducing concurrent side effects. Alternatively, epidural or intrathecal opioids may be considered if systemic analgesics produce excessive side effects such as confusion or sedation. If the pain is localized (*e.g.*, intercostal pain from tumor infiltration of the chest wall), neurolytic blocks are indicated. If the pain is unilateral and below the waist, cordotomy should be considered. For diffuse pain, nitrous oxide inhalation may be tried. Cognitive-behavioral approaches must be integrated from the onset of treatment and should be used along with the medical and surgical approaches.

Whatever pain management techniques are used, the physician is responsible for providing continuing care, constantly reassessing both the diagnosis and the treatment to achieve optimum relief of pain and suffering for both patient and family.

The care of patients with cancer and chronic pain strains the resources of a single physician, especially after the patient's discharge from the hospital. Various supportive care and continuing care programs have been developed to manage dying patients, both in the hospital and at home. In these patients the focus of treatment shifts to symptom control and palliative comfort care. Palliative care services, home- and hospital-based palliative care teams, home- and hospital-based hospices, and high-technology home care programs are some of the approaches to care for patients with terminal illness.

A model of continuity of care for cancer centers has been developed at Memorial Sloan-Kettering Cancer Center.[207] This program centers on the patient and family and is coordinated by a nurse, using the expertise of the nurse, physician, and social worker. The nurse is responsible for day-to-day management of the patient's pain and works with the patient, family, and community physicians and nurses in symptom control and supportive care. Community health professionals work with the patient at home, and the team is available to the patient, family, and community health workers on a 24-hour-a-day basis.

To achieve continuity of care, the nurse-clinician, together with the social worker and the patient's primary physician, provides the essential link between the primary treating hospital (the cancer center), the patient, and the community. With the use of sophisticated cancer pain management, patients can die at home with adequate pain management.

FUTURE DIRECTIONS

The study of pain in cancer patients offers a unique opportunity to use clinical observations to advance our biologic knowledge. There is a critical need to expand both the research and educational efforts in cancer pain to improve the control of pain in these patients. Information on the basic mechanisms of pain modulation can be culled only from a careful study of these clinical pain problems. These patients can teach us the physiologic and psychological differences between acute and chronic pain problems, the importance of the evolution of psychological factors, the difference between pain and suffering, the clinical pharmacology of analgesic drugs, and the behavioral mechanisms humans use to suppress pain. The use of innovative approaches based on sound scientific principles and advances in research technology offer the opportunity to understand the complex phenomenon of pain.

REFERENCES

1. Foley KM. Pain syndromes in patients with cancer. In: Bonica JJ, Ventafridda V, eds. Advances in pain research and therapy. New York: Raven Press, 1979:59–75.
2. Bonica JJ. Cancer pain. In: Bonica JJ, ed. The management of pain. Philadelphia: Lea & Febiger, 1990:400.
3. Twycross RG, Fairfield S. Pain in far-advanced cancer. Pain 1982;14:303–310.
4. World Health Organization. Cancer pain relief. Geneva: World Health Organization, 1986.
5. Daut RL, Cleeland CS. The prevalence and severity of pain in cancer. Cancer 1982;50: 1913–1918.
6. Levin D, Cleeland CS, Dar R. Public attitudes toward cancer pain. Cancer 1985;56: 2337–2339.
7. Cleeland CS. Pain control: Public and physicians' attitudes. In: Hill CS, Fields WS, eds. Advances in pain research and therapy. New York: Raven Press, 1989:81–89.
8. Cleeland CS, Cleeland LM, Dar R, Rinehardt LC. Factors influencing physician management of cancer pain. Cancer 1986;58:796–800.
9. Van Roenn JH, Cleeland CS, Gonin R, Hatfield A, Pandya KJ. Physicians' attitudes towards cancer pain management: Results of the Eastern Cooperative Oncology Group Survey. Ann Intern Med (in press).
10. Peteet J, Tay V, Cohen G, MacIntyre J. Pain characteristics and treatment in an outpatient cancer population. Cancer 1986;57:1259–1265.
11. Ventafridda V, Tamburini M, DeConno F. Comprehensive treatment of cancer pain. In: Fields HL, Dubner R, Cervero F, eds. Advances in pain research and therapy. New York: Raven Press, 1985:617–628.
12. Moulin DE, Foley KM. A review of a hospital-based pain service. In: Foley KM, Bonica JJ, Ventafridda V, eds. Advances in pain research and therapy. New York: Raven Press, 1990:413–428.
13. Vainio A. Treatment of terminal cancer in Finland: A questionnaire survey. Acta Anesth Scand 1988;32:260–265.
14. Dorrepaal KL, Aaronson NK, van Dam F. Pain experience and pain management among hospital cancer patients. Cancer 1989;63:593–598.
15. Foley KM. The decriminalization of cancer pain. In: Hill CS, Fields WS, eds. Advances in pain research and therapy. New York: Raven Press, 1989:5–18.
16. Foley KM. The relationship of pain and symptom management to patient requests for physician-assisted suicide. J Pain Sympt Manag 1991;6:289–297.
17. Ahles TA, Blanchard EB, Ruckdeschel JC. The multidimensional nature of cancer-related pain. Pain 1983;17:277–289.
18. Ahles TA, Ruckdeschel JC, Blanchard EB. Cancer-related pain I. Prevalence in an outpatient setting as a function of stage of disease and type of cancer. J Psychosom Res 1984;28:115–119.
19. Ahles TA, Ruckdeschel JC, Blanchard EB. Cancer-related pain II. Assessment with visual analogue scales. J Psychosom Res 1984;28:121–124.
20. Cleeland CS, Ladinsky JL, Serlin RC, Thuy NC. Multidimensional measurement of cancer pain: Comparisons of US and Vietnamese patients. J Pain Symptom Manag 1988;3:23–27.
21. Cleeland CS. Assessment of pain in cancer: Measurement issues. In: Foley KM, Bonica JJ, Ventafridda V, eds. Advances in pain research and therapy. New York: Raven Press, 1990:47–56.
22. Portenoy RK, Miransky J, Thaler HT, et al. Pain in ambulatory patients with lung or colon cancer: Prevalence, characteristics and impact. Cancer 1992;70:1616–1624.
23. Ventafridda V, DeConno F, Ripamonti C, Gamba A, Tamburini M. Quality-of-life assessment during a palliative care programme. Ann Oncol 1990;1:415–420.
24. Coyle N, Adelhardt J, Foley KM, Portenoy RK. Character of terminal illness in the advanced cancer patient: Pain and other symptoms during the last 4 weeks of life. J Pain Sympt Manag 1990;5:83–93.
25. Ventafridda V, Ripamonti C, DeConno F, Tamburini M. Symptom prevalence and control during cancer patients' last days of life. J Palliat Care 1990;6:7–11.
26. Twycross R, Lack SA. Symptom control in far-advanced cancer. In: Pain Relief. London: Pitman Books, 1984.
27. Walsh TD, West TS. Controlling symptoms in advanced cancer. Br Med J 1988;296: 477–481.
28. IASP Subcommittee on Taxonomy. Pain terms: A list with definitions and notes on usage. Pain 1980;8:249–252.
29. Payne R. Pathophysiology of cancer pain. In: Foley KM, Bonica JJ, Ventafridda V, eds. Advances in pain research and therapy. New York: Raven Press, 1990:13–16.

30. Basbaum AI, Fields HL. Endogenous pain control mechanisms: Review and hypothesis. Ann Neurol 1978;451–462.
31. Wilcox GL. Excitatory neurotransmitters and pain. In: Bond MR, Charlton JE, Woolf CJ, eds. Pain research and clinical management. New York: Elsevier, 1991:97–118.
32. Spiegel K, Kalb R, Pasternak GW. Analgesic activity of tricyclic antidepressants. Ann Neurol 1983;13:462–465.
33. Watson CP, Evan RJ, Reed K, et al. Amitriptyline versus placebo in post-herpetic neuralgia. Neurology 1982;32:671–673.
34. Max MB, Culnane M, Shafer SC, et al. Amitriptyline relieves diabetic neuropathy pain in patients with normal or depressed mood. Neurology 1987;37:589–593.
35. Pasternak GW. Multiple opiate receptors. JAMA 1988;2599:1362–1367.
36. Yaksh TL. Spinal opiate analgesia: Characteristics and principles of action. Pain 1981;11: 293–346.
37. Max MB, Inturrisi CE, Kaiko RF, Grabinski PY, Li CH, Foley KM. Epidural and intrathecal opiates: Distribution in CSF and plasma and analgesic effects in patients with cancer. Clin Pharm Ther 1985;38:631–641.
38. Onofrio BM, Yaksh TL. Long-term pain relief: Intrathecal morphine infusion in 53 patients. J Neurosurg 1990;72:200–209.
39. Besson JM, Chrouch A. Peripheral and spinal mechanisms of nociception. Physiol Rev 1987;67:67–186.
40. Sternbach RA. Pain patients: Traits and treatment. New York: Academic Press, 1974.
41. Portenoy RK, Hagen N. Management of breakthrough pain. Prim Care Cancer 1991;11: 24–27.
42. Tearnan J, Blake H, Cleeland CS. Unaided use of pain descriptors by patients with cancer pain. J Pain Sympt Manag 1990;5:228–232.
43. Wallenstein SL. Measurement of pain and analgesia in cancer patients. Cancer 1984;53: 2217–2234.
44. McGrath PJ, Beyer J, Cleeland CS, Eland J, McGrath PA, Portenoy RK. Report of a subcommittee on assessment and methodologic issues in the management of childhood cancer. Pediatrics 1990;86:813–834.
45. Grossman SA, Sheidler VR, Swedeen K, Mucenski J, Pianladosi S. Correlation of patient and caregiver ratings of cancer pain. J Pain Sympt Manag 1991;6:53–57.
46. Daut RL, Cleeland CS, Flanery RC. The development of the Wisconsin Brief Pain Questionnaire to assess pain in cancer and other diseases. Pain 1983;17:197–210.
47. Graham C, Bond SS, Gertrovitch MM, Cook MR. Use of the McGill Pain Questionnaire in the management of cancer pain—replicability and consistency. Pain 1980;8:377–387.
48. Dubuison D, Melzack R. Classification of clinical pain descriptions by multiple group discriminant analysis. Exp Neurol 1976;51:480–487.
49. Fishman B, Pasternak S, Wallerstein SL, et al. The Memorial Pain Assessment Card: A valid instrument for the assessment of cancer pain. Cancer 1986;60:1151–1157.
50. Tursky B. The development of a pain perception profile: A psychophysical approach. In: Weisenberg M, Tursky B, eds. Pain: New perspectives in therapy and research. New York: Plenum Press, 1976:171–194.
51. Pollack V, Cho D, Reker D, Volavka J. Profile of mood states. The factors and their psychological correlates. J Nerv Ment Dis 1979;167:612–614.
52. Hamilton M. A rating scale for depression. J Neurol Neurosurg Psychiatry 1960;23: 56–62.
53. Zung W. The measurement of affects: Depression and anxiety. Mod Probl Pharmacopsych 1974;7:170–188.
54. Fishman B, Pasternak S, Wallenstein SL, et al. The Memorial Pain Assessment Card: A valid instrument for the assessment of cancer pain. Cancer 1986;60:1151–1157.
55. Foley KM. The treatment of cancer pain. N Engl J Med 1985;313:84–95.
56. Hellman S. The role of radiation therapy in the management of cancer. In: Foley KM, Bonica JJ, Ventafridda V, eds. Advances in pain research and therapy. New York: Raven Press, 1990:41–46.
57. Chapman CR, Hill HF. Prolonged morphine self-administration and addiction liability: Evaluation of two theories in a bone marrow transplant unit. Cancer 1989;63:1636–1655.
58. Saltzburg D, Foley KM. The management of pancreatic cancer pain. In: Reber H, ed. Surgical clinics of North America. Philadelphia: WB Saunders, 1989:629–650.
59. Kanner RM, Martini N, Foley KM. Incidence of pain and other clinical manifestations of superior pulmonary sulcus tumor (Pancoast's tumors). In: Bonica JJ, Ventafridda V, eds. Advances in pain research and therapy. New York: Raven Press, 1982:27–38.
60. Holland J, Rowland JH, eds. Handbook of psycho-oncology: Psychological care of the patient with cancer. New York: Oxford Press, 1989:369–382.
61. Cassell EJ. The nature of suffering and the goals of medicine. N Engl J Med 1982;306: 639–45.
62. Bruera E, Brenneis C, Michaud M, MacDonald RN. Influence of the pain and symptom control team on the patterns of treatment of pain and other symptoms in a cancer center. J Pain Sympt Manag 1989;4:112–116.
63. Macaluso C, Weinberg D, Foley KM. Opioid abuse and misuse in a cancer pain population. J Pain Sympt Manag 1988;3:S54.
64. Portenoy RK, Payne R. Acute and chronic pain. In: Lowinson JH, Ruiz P, Millman RB, eds. Comprehensive textbook of substance abuse. Baltimore: Williams & Wilkins, 1992.
65. Kanner RM, Foley KM. Patterns of narcotic drug use in a cancer pain clinic. Ann NY Acad Sci 1981;362:161–172.
66. Gonzales GR, Elliott KJ, Portenoy RK, Foley KM. Impact of a comprehensive evaluation in the management of cancer pain. Pain 1991;47:141–144.
67. Elliott K, Foley KM. Neurologic pain syndromes in patients with cancer. Neurol Clin North Am 1989;7:333–360.
68. Patchell R, Posner JB. Neurologic complications of systemic cancer. Neurol Clin North Am 1985;3:729–750.
69. Greenberg HS, Deck MD, Vikram B, et al. Metastasis to the base of the skull: Clinical findings in 43 patients. Neurology 1981;31:530–537.
70. Portenoy RK, Lipton RB, Foley KM. Back pain in the cancer patient: An algorithm for evaluation and management. Neurology 1986;37:134–138.
71. Posner JB. Back pain and epidural spinal cord compression. Med Clin North Am 1987;71: 185–205.
72. Sundaresan N, Galicich JH, Lane J. Treatment of odontoid fractures in cancer patients. J Neurosurg 1981;54:468–472.
73. Jaeckle KA, Young DF, Foley KM. The natural history of lumbosacral plexopathy in cancer. Neurology 1985;35:8–15.
74. Stillman M. Perineal pain: Diagnosis and management, with particular attention to perineal pain of cancer. In: Foley KM, Bonica JJ, Ventafridda V, eds. Advances in pain research and therapy. New York: Raven Press, 1990:359–378.
75. Kori S, Foley KM, Posner JB. Brachial plexus lesions in patients with cancer: Clinical findings in 100 cases. Neurology 1981;31:45–50.
76. Foley KM. Brachial plexopathy in patients with breast cancer. In: Harris JR, Hellman S, Henderson IC, Kinne D, eds. Breast diseases. Philadelphia: JB Lippincott, 1991: 722–729.
77. Evans RJ, Watson CPN. Lumbosacral plexopathy in cancer patients. Neurology 1985;35: 1392–1393.
78. Glass PJ, Foley KM. Carcinomatous meningitis. In: Harris JR, Hellman S, Henderson IC, Kinne D (eds). Breast diseases. Philadelphia: JB Lippincott, 1991:700–719.
79. Wasserstrom WR, Glass JP, Posner JB. Diagnosis and treatment of leptomeningeal metastases for solid tumors. Experience with 90 patients. Cancer 1982;49:759–768.
80. Macaluso C, Foley KM. Managing pain in patients with lung cancer. J Resp Dis 1988;9: 59–80.
81. Baines M, Oliver DJ, Carter RL. Medical management of intestinal obstruction in patients with advanced malignant disease: A clinical and pathological study. Lancet 1985;2:990–993.
82. Kanner RM, Martini N, Foley KM. Nature and incidence of post-thoracotomy pain. Proc ASCO 1982;1:152.
83. Granek I, Ashikari R, Foley KM. Postmastectomy pain syndrome: Clinical and anatomical correlates. Proc ASCO 1983;3:122.
84. Swift TR, Nichols FT. The droopy shoulder syndrome. Neurology 1984;34:212–215.
85. MacDonald DR, Strong E, Nielson S, et al. Syncope from head and neck cancer. J Neuro-oncol 1983;1:257–267.
86. Sherman RA, Sherman CJ, Parker L. Chronic phantom and stump pain among American veterans. Pain 1984;18:83–95.
87. Aker SN. Oral findings in the cancer patient. Cancer 1979;43:2103–2107.
88. Fair WR. Urologic emergencies. In: DeVita VT, Hellman S, Rosenberg SA, eds. Principles & Practice of Oncology. Philadelphia: JB Lippincott, 1985:1894–1906.
89. Lequesne PM. Neuropathy due to drugs. In: Dyck PJ, Thomas PK, Lambert EH, et al., eds. Peripheral neuropathy. 2d ed. Philadelphia: WB Saunders, 1983:2126–2179.
90. Huang ME, Ye YC, Chen SR, et al. Use of transretinoic acid in the treatment of acute promyelocytic leukemia. Blood 1988;72:567–572.
91. Ihde DC, DeVita VT. Osteonecrosis of the femoral head in patients with lymphoma treated with intermittent combination chemotherapy (including corticosteroids). Cancer 1975;36:1585–1588.
92. Rotstein J, Good RA. Steroid pseudorheumatism. Arch Intern Med 1957;99:545–555.
93. Portenoy RK, Duma C, Foley KM. Acute herpetic and postherpetic neuralgia: Review of clinical features and current therapy. Ann Neurol 1987;20:651–664.
94. Thomas JE, Cascino TE, Earle JD. Differential diagnosis between radiation and tumor plexopathy of the pelvis. Neurology 1985;35:1–7.
95. Jellinger K, Sturm KW. Delayed radiation myelopathy in man. J Neurol Sci 1971;14: 389–408.
96. Foley KM, Woodruff JM, Ellis F, et al. Radiation-induced malignant and atypical peripheral nerve sheath tumors. Ann Neurol 1980;7:311–318.
97. Payne R, Foley KM. Exploration of the brachial plexus in patients with cancer. Neurology 1986;36:329.
98. Harrington KD. Orthopaedic management of metastatic bone disease. Washington: CV Mosby, 1988.
99. Bruera E, MacDonald N. Intractable pain in patients with advanced head and neck tumors: A possible role for infection. Cancer Treat Rep 1986;70:691–692.
100. Breitbart WS, Holland J. Psychiatric aspects of cancer pain. In: Foley KM, Bonica JJ, Ventafridda V, eds. Advances in pain research and therapy. New York: Raven Press, 1990:73–88.
101. Kellgren JH. On the distribution of pain arising from deep somatic structures with charts of segmental pain areas. Clin Sci 1939–1942;4:35–46.
102. Journal of Pain and Symptom Management, Special Issue on Medical Ethics: Physician-Assisted Suicide and Euthanasia, 1991.
103. Emanuel LL, Emanuel EJ. The medical directive: A new comprehensive advance care document. JAMA 1989;261:3288–3293.
104. Annas G. The health care proxy and the living will. N Engl J Med 1991;324:1210–1213.
105. Clouston P, DeAngelis L, Posner JB. The spectrum of neurologic disease in patients with systemic cancer. Ann Neurol 1992;31:268–273.
106. Brooks PM, Day RO. Drug therapy: Nonsteroidal antiinflammatory drugs. N Engl J Med 1991;324:1718–1725.
107. Galasko CSB. Mechanisms of bone destruction in the development of skeletal metastases. Nature 1976;263:507–510.
108. Langman MJS. Treating ulcers in patients receiving anti-arthritic drugs. Q J Med 1989;73:1089–1091.
109. Foley KM. Controversies in cancer pain—medical perspective. Cancer 1989;63:2257–2266.
110. Portenoy RK, Foley KM, Inturrisi CE. The nature of opioid responsiveness and its implications for neuropathic pain: New hypotheses derived from studies of opioid infusions. Pain 1990;43:273–286.

111. Foley KM. Clinical tolerance to opioids. In: Basbaum AI, Besson JM, eds. Towards a new pharmacotherapy of pain. Chichester: John Wiley & Sons, 1991:181–204.
112. Ventafridda V, DeConno F, Panerai AE, Maresca V, Monza GC, Ripamonti C. Non-steroidal antiinflammatory drugs as the first step in cancer pain therapy: Double-blind, within-patient study comparing nine drugs. J Intl Med Res 1990;18:21–29.
113. Kaiko RF, Foley KM, Grabinski PY, et al. Central nervous system excitatory effects of meperidine in cancer patients. Ann Neurol 1983;13:180–185.
114. Kaiko RF, Wallenstein SL, Rogers AG, et al. Analgesic and mood effects of heroin and morphine in cancer patients with postoperative pain. N Engl J Med 1981;304:1501–1505.
115. Inturrisi CE, Max M, Foley KM, Chen J, Schultz M, Houde R. The pharmacokinetics of heroin in patients with chronic pain. N Engl J Med 1984;310:1213–1217.
116. Ventafridda V, Ripamonti C, Bianchi M, Sbanotto A, DeConno E. A randomized study on oral administration of morphine and methadone in the treatment of cancer pain. J Pain Sympt Manag 1986;1:203–207.
117. Sawe J, Hansen J, Ginsman C, et al. Patient-controlled dose regimen for methadone for chronic cancer pain. Br Med J 1981;282:771–773.
118. Ventafridda V, DeConno F, Guarise G, et al. Chronic analgesic study on buprenorphine action in cancer pain—comparison with pentazocine. Drug Res 1983;33:587–590.
119. Houde RW. Methods for measuring clinical pain in humans. Acta Anaesthesiol Scand (Suppl) 1982;74:25–29.
120. Twycross RG. Clinical experience with diamorphine in advanced malignant disease. Int J Clin Pharmacol Therap Toxicol 1974;9:184–198.
121. Paul D, Standifier KM, Inturrisi CE, Pasternak GW. Pharmacological characterization of morphine-6-glucuronide, a very potent morphine metabolite. J Pharmacol Exp Ther 1989;251:477–483.
122. Portenoy RK, Thaler HT, Inturrisi CE, Friedlander-Klar H, Foley KM. The metabolite, morphine-6-glucuronide, contributes to the analgesia produced by morphine infusion in pain patients with normal renal function. Clin Pharmacol Therap 1992;51:422–431.
123. Portenoy RK, Foley KM, Stulman J, et al. Plasma morphine and morphine-6-glucuronide during chronic morphine therapy for cancer pain: Plasma profiles, steady-state concentrations and the consequences of renal failure. Pain 1991;47:13–19.
124. Hagen N, Foley KM, Cebrone DJ, Portenoy RK, Inturrisi CE. Chronic nausea and morphine-6-glucuronide. J Pain Sympt Manag 1991;6:125–128.
125. Citron ML, Johnston-Early A, Boyer M, Brasnow SH, Hood M, Cohne MH. Patient-controlled analgesia for severe cancer pain. Arch Int Med 1986;146:734–736.
126. Coyle N, Adelhardt J, Foley KM, Portenoy RK. character of terminal illness in the advanced cancer patient: Pain and other symptoms during the last 4 weeks of life. J Pain Sympt Manag 1990;5:83–93.
127. Kaiko RF. Controlled-release oral morphine for cancer-related pain: The European and North American experiences. In: Foley KM, Bonica JJ, Ventafridda V, eds. Advances in pain research and therapy. New York: Raven Press, 1990:171–190.
128. Shepard K. Review of controlled-release morphine preparation Roxanol SR. In: Foley KM, Bonica JJ, Ventafridda V, eds. Advances in pain research and therapy. New York: Raven Press, 1990:191–202.
129. Weinberg DS, Inturrisi CE, Reidenberg B, et al. Sublingual absorption of selected opioid analgesics. Clin Pharm Therap 1988;44:335–342.
130. Bell MDD, Mishra P, Weldon P, et al. Buccal morphine—a new route of analgesia. Lancet 1985;1:71–73.
131. Fine PG, Marcus M, DeBaer AJ, Van der Oord B. An open-label study of oral transmucosal fentanyl titrate for the treatment of breakthrough cancer pain. Pain 1991;45:149–155.
132. Beaver WT, Feise GA. A comparison of the analgesic effects of oxymorphones by rectal suppository and intramuscular injection in patients with postoperative pain. J Clin Pharmacol 1977;17:276–291.
133. Portenoy RK, Southam MA, Gupta SK, et al. Transdermal fentanyl for cancer pain: Repeated dose pharmacokinetics. Anesthesiology 1992 (in press).
134. Coyle N, Mauskop A, Maggard J, et al. Continuous subcutaneous infusions of opiates in cancer patients with pain. Oncol Nurs Forum 1986;13:53–57.
135. Bruera E, Fainsinger R, Moore M, Thibault R, Spoldi E, Ventafridda V. Local toxicity with subcutaneous methadone. Pain 1991;45:141–145.
136. Moulin DE, Kreeft JH, Murray-Parsons N, Bouquillon AI. Comparison of continuous subcutaneous and intravenous hydromorphone infusions for management of cancer pain. Lancet 1991;337:465–468.
137. Portenoy RK, Moulin DE, Rogers A, Inturrisi CE, Foley KM. Intravenous infusion of opioids in cancer pain: Clinical review and guidelines for use. Cancer Treat Rep 1985;70: 575–581.
138. Gourlay GK, Plummer JL, Cherry DA, et al. Comparison of intermittent bolus with continuous infusions of epidural morphine in the treatment of severe cancer pain. Pain 1991;47:135–140.
139. Vainio A, Tigerstedt I. Opioid treatment for radiating cancer pain: Oral administration versus epidural techniques. Acta Anaesthesiol Scand 1988;32:179–185.
140. Cousins MJ, Bridenbaugh PO, eds. Neural blockade in clinical anesthesia and management of pain. 2d ed. Philadelphia: JB Lippincott, 1988.
141. Leavens ME, Hill CS, Cech DA, et al. Intrathecal and intraventricular morphine for pain in cancer patients: Initial study. J Neurosurg 1982;56:241–243.
142. Lobato RD, Madrid JL, Fatela LV, et al. Intraventricular morphine for control of pain in terminal cancer patients. J Neurosurg 1983;59:627–633.
143. Dennis CG, DeWitty RL. Long-term intraventricular infusion of morphine for intractable pain in cancer of the head and neck. Neurosurgery 1990;26:404–408.
144. Beaver WT. Comparison of analgesic effects of morphine sulfate, hydroxyzine and other combination in patients with postoperative pain. In: Bonica JJ, Ventafridda V, eds. Advances in pain research and therapy. New York: Raven Press, 1976:553–557.
145. Forrest WH, Brown B, Brown C, et al. Dextroamphetamine with morphine for the treatment of postoperative pain. N Engl J Med 1977;296:712–715.
146. Bruera E, Chadwich S, Brenneis C, et al. Methylphenidate associated with narcotics for the treatment of cancer pain. Cancer Treat Rep 1987;71:67–71.
147. Laska EM, Sunshine A, Mueller F, et al. Caffeine as an analgesic adjuvant. JAMA 1984;251:1711–1714.
148. Goldfrank L, Weisman RS, Errick JK, Lo MW. A normogram for continuous intravenous naloxone. Ann Emerg Med 1986;15:566–570.
149. Portenoy RK. Constipation in the cancer patient: Causes and management. In: Payne R, Foley KM, eds. Medical Clinics of North America: Cancer pain. New York: Raven Press, 1987:303–310.
150. Swerdlow M. Anticonvulsant drugs and chronic pain. Clin Neuropharmacol 1984;7: 51–82.
151. Caccia MR. Clonazepam in facial neuralgia and cluster headache: Clinical and electrophysiological study. Eur Neurol 1975;13:560–566.
152. Peris JB, Perera GLS, Devendra SV, et al. Sodium valproate in trigeminal neuralgia. Med J Aust 1980;2:278–281.
153. Beaver WT, Wallenstein SL, Houde RW, Rogers AG. A comparison of the analgesic effect of methotrimeprazine and morphine in patients with cancer. Clin Pharmacol Ther 1983;7:436–446.
154. Brevik H, Rennemo F. Clinical evaluation of combined treatment with methadone and psychotropic drugs in cancer patients. Acta Anesthesiol Scand (Suppl) 1982;74:135–140.
155. Bruera E, Roca E, Cedaro L, Carraro S, Chacon R. Action of oral methylprednisolone in terminal cancer patients: A prospective randomized double-blind study. Cancer Treat Rep 1985;69:751–756.
156. Weissman DE. Glucocorticoid treatment for brain metastases and epidural spinal cord compression—a review. J Clin Oncol 1988;6:543–551.
157. Tannock I, Gospodarowicz M, Meakin W, Panzarella T, Stewart L, Rider W. Treatment of metastatic prostate cancer with low-dose prednisone—evaluation of pain and quality of life as prognostic indices of response. J Clin Oncol 1989;7:590.
158. Kaiko RF, Kanner R, Foley KM, et al. Cocaine and morphine in cancer patients with chronic pain. Pain (Suppl 2) 1984;S203.
159. Fleisch H. Bisphosphonate: Mechanism of action. In: Burckhardt P, ed. Disodium pamidronate in the treatment of malignancy-related disorders. Bern: Hans Huber, 1989: 21–35.
160. Bisvoet OLM. Pamidronate in cancer therapy—the pharmacological background. In: The management of bone metastases and hypercalcemia by osteoclast inhibition. Switzerland: Hogrefe & Huber, 1990:9–11.
161. Schnur V. Etidronate for the relief of metastatic bone pain. J Urol 1984;131:404–407.
162. Hayward ML, Howell DA, O'Donnell JF, et al. Hypercalcemia complicating small-cell carcinoma. Cancer 1981;48:1643–1646.
163. Adami S, Salvago G, Guarrera G, et al. Dichloromethylene-diphosphonate in patients with prostatic carcinoma metastatic to the skeleton. J Urol 1985;134:1152–1154.
164. Van Holten A, Bijvoet ALM, Cleton FJ. Reduced morbidity from skeletal metastases in breast cancer patients during long-term biphosphonate treatment. Lancet 1987;2: 983–985.
165. Smith JA. Palliation of painful bone metastases from prostate cancer using sodium etidronate: Results of a randomized prospective, double-blind, placebo-controlled study. J Urol 1989;141:85–87.
166. Ernst DS, MacDonald RN, Paterson AHG, Jasen J, Bruera E. A double-blind, crossover trial of I.V. clodronate in metastatic bone pain. J Pain Sympt Manag 1992;7:4–11.
167. Loscalzo M, Amendola J. Psychosocial and behavioral management of cancer pain: The social work contribution. In: Foley KM, Bonica JJ, Ventafridda V, eds. Advances in pain research and therapy. New York: Raven Press, 1990:429–442.
168. Fosburg MT, Crone RK. Nitrous oxide analgesia for refractory pain in the terminally ill. JAMA 1983;250:511–513.
169. Green WR, David WH. Titrated intravenous barbiturates in the control of symptoms in patients with terminal cancer. South Med J 1991;84:332–337.
170. Roy D. Need they sleep before they die. J Palliat Care 1990;6:3–4.
171. Edwards WT, Habib F, Burney RG, Begin G. Intravenous lidocaine in the management of various chronic pain states. Reg Anesth 1985;10:1–6.
172. Brose WG, Cousins MJ. Subcutaneous lidocaine for treatment of neuropathic cancer pain. Pain 1991;45:141–148.
173. Rowbotham MC, Fields HL. Post-herpetic neuralgia: The relation of pain complaint, sensory disturbance, and skin temperature. Pain 1989;39:129–144.
174. Waldman SD, Cronen MC. Thoracic epidural morphine in the palliation of chest wall pain secondary to relapsing polychondritis. J Pain Sympt Manag 1989;4:38–40.
175. Jacobsen L, Chabal C, Brody MC, Mariano AJ, Chaney EF. A comparison of the effects of intrathecal fentanyl and lidocaine on established post-amputation stump pain. Pain 1990;40:137–142.
176. Ferrer-Brechner T. Anesthetic management of cancer pain. Semin Oncol 1985;12: 431–437.
177. Kuzucu EY, Derrick WS, Wilber SA. Control of intractable pain with subarachnoid alcohol block. JAMA 1966;195:541–548.
178. Swerdlow M. Complications of neurolytic blockade. In: Cousins MJ, Bridenbaugh PO, eds. Neural blockade in clinical anesthesia and management of pain. Philadelphia: JB Lippincott, 1980.
179. Ischia S, Luzzani A, Ischia A, et al. A new approach to the neurolytic block of the caeliac plexus: The transaortic technique. Pain 1983;16:333–341.
180. Brown DL, Bulley CK, Quiel EL. Neurolytic caelic plexus block for pancreatic cancer pain. Anesth Analg 1987;66:869–873.
181. Lofstrom B, Cousins MJ. Sympathetic neural blockade. In: Cousins MJ, Bridenbaugh PO, eds. Neural blockade in clinical anesthesia and management of pain. Philadelphia: JB Lippincott, 1980.

182. Gianasi G. Neuroadenolysis of the pituitary: An overview of development, mechanisms, technique and results. In: Benedetti C, Chapman CR, Moricca G, et al., eds. Advances in pain research and therapy. New York: Raven Press, 1984:647–678.
183. Katz J, Levin AB. Treatment of diffuse metastatic cancer pain by installation of alcohol into the sella turcica. Anesthesiology 1977;46:115.
184. Moricca G. Pituitary neuroadenolysis in the treatment of intractable pain from cancer. In: Lipton S, ed. Persistent pain: Modern methods of treatment. New York: Grune & Stratton, 1977.
185. Travell JG, Simons DG. Myofascial pain and dysfunction: The trigger-point manual. Baltimore: Williams & Wilkins, 1983.
186. Sundaresan N, DiGiacinto GV, Hughes EO. Neurosurgery in the treatment of cancer pain. Cancer 1989;63:2365–2377.
187. Arbit E. Neurosurgical management of cancer pain. In: Foley KM, Bonica JJ, Ventafridda V, eds. Advances in pain research and therapy. New York: Raven Press, 1990:289–300.
188. Sundaresan N, Galicich JH, Lane JM, Scher H. Stabilization of the spine involved by cancer. In: Dunsker DB, Schmidek HH, eds. The unstable spine. Orlando: Grune & Stratton, 1986:249–274.
189. Sundaresan N, Hilaris BS, Martini N. The combined neurosurgical-thoracic management of superior sulcus tumors. J Clin Oncol 1987;5:1739–1745.
190. Lahuerta T, Lipton SA, Wells JD. Percutaneous cervical cordotomy: Results and complications in a recent series of 100 patients. Ann Royal Col Surg Exp 1985;67:41–47.
191. Ischia S, Luzzani A, Ischia A, et al. Subarachnoid neurolytic block (L5, S1) and unilateral percutaneous cervical cordotomy for the treatment of neoplastic vertebral pain. Pain 1984;19:123.
192. Macaluso C, Arbit E, Foley KM. Cordotomy for lumbosacral, pelvic, and lower extremity pain of malignant origin: Safety and efficacy. Neurology 1988;38:110.
193. Barrash JM, Milan EL. Dorsal rhizotomy for the relief of pain of malignant tumor origin. J Neurosurg 1973;38:755–757.
194. Arbit E, Galicich JH, Burt M, et al. Modified open thoracic rhizotomy for treatment of intractable chest wall pain of malignant etiology. Ann Thoracic Surg 1989;48:820–823.
195. Giorgi C, Broggi G. Surgical treatment of glossopharyngeal neuralgia and pain from cancer of the nasopharynx. J Neurosurg 1984;61:952–955.
196. Nashold BS, Ostdahl RH. Dorsal root entry zone lesions for pain relief. J Neurosurg 1979;51:59–69.
197. Gildenberg PL, Hirschberg RM. Limited myelotomy for the treatment of intractable cancer pain. J Neurol Neurosurg Psychiatry 1984;47:94–96.
198. Hassenbusch SJ, Pillay PK, Barnett GH. Radiofrequency cingulotomy for intractable cancer pain using stereotaxis guided by magnetic resonance imaging. Neurosurgery 1990;27:220–223.
199. Melzack R, Wall PD. Pain mechanisms: A new theory. Science 1965;150:971–979.
200. Ventafridda V. Transcutaneous nerve stimulation in cancer pain. In: Bonica JJ, Ventafridda V, eds. Advances in pain research and therapy. New York: Raven Press, 1979: 509–515.
201. Thompson JW, Filshie J. Transcutaneous electrical nerve stimulation and acupuncture in palliative care medicine. In: Doyle D, Hanks G, MacDonald N, eds. Oxford University Press, 1992 (in press).
202. Hosobuchi Y. Subcortical electrical stimulation for control of intractable pain: Report of 122 cases. J Neurosurg 1986;64:543–553.
203. Levy RM, Lamb S, Adams JE. Treatment of chronic pain by deep brain stimulation: Long-term followup and review of the literature. Neurosurgery 1987;21:885–893.
204. Young RF, Brechner T. Electrical stimulation of the brain for relief of intractable pain due to cancer. Cancer 1986;57:1266–1272.
205. Filshie J. Acupuncture and malignant pain problems. Acupuncture in Medicine 1990;8: 38–39.
206. King JC, Kellcher MJ. The chronic pain syndrome: The interdisciplinary rehabilitative behavioral modification approach. Physical Medicine: State of the Art Reviews 1991;5: 165–186.
207. Coyle N, Monzillo E, Loscalzo M, et al. A model of continuity of care for cancer patients with pain and neuro-oncologic complications. Cancer Nurs 1985;8:111–119.

SECTION **2**

MARGUERITE S. LEDERBERG
MARY JANE MASSIE

Psychosocial and Ethical Issues in the Care of Cancer Patients

PSYCHOSOCIAL ISSUES: HISTORICAL BACKGROUND

The word cancer refers to a group of diseases that has struck fear in people's hearts for centuries. In the past, its fatal outcome, absence of known cause or cure, and association with pain and disfigurement made it particularly frightening. Physicians regarded the diagnosis as too painful to reveal to the patient and conspired, often unsuccessfully, with the family to create the illusion of a lesser illness. The same fear prevented the word from appearing in the press; patients and their families kept the diagnosis a secret from all but the closest acquaintances. A person who even suspected that he or she had cancer would often refuse to go to the doctor out of fatalistic resignation. Cancer was widely used as a metaphor for an insidious, destructive force in society. Fear, secrecy, and mythologic elaboration compounded the emotional burden and social stigma borne by patients and families.

In 1913, the American Cancer Society was founded to counter the public's fears and teach that early diagnosis and surgical treatment could be curative. However, negative attitudes have persisted. Only in the past 4 decades has a real, albeit still incomplete, change occurred in attitudes toward cancer in the United States. There is greater openness in public discussion and more candor in revealing the diagnosis to patients. Except for Scandinavia, few other countries have moved as far as the United States, but similar trends are under way throughout Western Europe.[1]

Several factors contributed to the change in attitudes in the United States:

1. Physicians and patients became more optimistic as radiation therapy and chemotherapy began to cure several common neoplasms of children and young adults.
2. Clinicians who spoke more openly with their patients found that such candor was unexpectedly well tolerated. A better understanding of the rationale for treatment helped patients handle side effects better, and truthful communication enhanced trust in the physician. During the 1950s, psychological studies showed that patients given accurate information adapted better to radical surgery.
3. Terminal care practices were reexamined. Following the lead of the European hospice movement and the pioneering work of Elizabeth Kubler-Ross, it became more widely understood that terminally ill patients benefited from an opportunity to discuss not only their illness but also their feelings and fears about death.
4. In the 1970s, advocacy of patients' rights became increasingly vocal. Physicians were required to discuss all diagnostic and treatment options to enable patients to participate in decisions. Informed consent for research patients became mandated by federal guidelines. In routine clinical care, the patient autonomy issue overlapped with and reinforced a growing demand for greater attention to quality of life during treatment. This problem was particularly acute in oncology, where the often severe side effects of treatment made special demands on patient trust. As physicians came to depend more on laboratory data and spent less time at the bedside, patients complained increasingly about the diminished

closeness to their new, more technology-oriented doctors.

Another impetus to exploring psychosocial issues in cancer was the recognition that psychological factors and their resulting behaviors are critical to the prevention and early detection of cancer. Much of the research effort in cancer prevention today, particularly that of smoking cessation, depends on the social sciences to develop ways of understanding and altering behavior.[2,3] Most recently, studies of the possible role of personality factors in altering not only risk but also survival, through neuroendocrine and neuroimmune mechanisms, has generated enormous public interest, far beyond what the scientific evidence can currently support. It has also stimulated extensive research that will, we hope, resolve the controversies during the next decades.[4,5] This issue is discussed later in this chapter.

The subspecialty of psychooncology developed in the wake of these developments. Since the mid-1970s, it has established a large body of information based on systematic clinical observations and scientific investigations, addressing two broad areas[6]:

1. The impact of cancer and its treatment on the psychological and social functioning of patients, their families, and the treating staff
2. The role of psychosocial factors and behaviors in cancer risk and survival.

PSYCHOLOGICAL IMPACT OF CANCER

Acute psychological distress is to be expected as a patient confronts the implications of cancer: possible death, pain, dependence on others, disability, disfiguring changes in the body, and loss of function, all of which endanger his or her relationships to others. The initial crisis is just the first of many, each requiring resiliency and rapid adaptation. Most patients cope adequately, keeping distress in a manageable range; some do not. To treat and prevent pathologic reactions, it is important to understand their causes, which are of three kinds: societal, biomedical, and patient-related (personal and interpersonal).

SOCIETAL FACTORS

Social factors play an immediate and important role in a patient's psychological adaptation to cancer but are seldom obvious to the patient.

In the past, patients came to the physician with a sense of doom at the mention of cancer, along with a deep sense of shame and the associated desire for secrecy. At the same time, they were more ready to trust their physician and accept his or her recommendations without question. Today—paradoxically in the face of far better outcomes—patients may come with less simple hope, more fear of treatment, and more mistrust of the doctor and the medical establishment.

The financial side of medical care is affecting physicians and patients more and more acutely. The issue of national health insurance is thought to have caused a major upset in the 1991 Pennsylvania senatorial election, making it clear how deeply the public fears medical pauperization. Patients and families may become easily angered when they perceive their physician as careless about this aspect of care. The same physician is also under enormous pressure to contain costs from both public and private sectors and may have to restrict length of stay or certain procedures in ways that also draw patient and family resentment. These sources of friction between physician and patient are less acute in countries with socialized medicine.

In the United States there is a large uninsured population whose health-care problems are well known. But even among the initially insured, identified cancer patients often become uninsurable. The policyholder becomes locked into a given job so as not to lose insurance benefits, causing a downward social drift that has yet to be fully documented.

Recent studies have shown a major effect of social class on cancer incidence and outcomes (see further discussion later in the chapter).[7,8] While this is mediated through many routes, psychological factors figure prominently among them. Socially disadvantaged patients are often more fatalistic and hopeless in their outlook and hence delay and seek less treatment. They also have many of the psychological risk factors outlined below.

Social rejection and job discrimination remain problems for cancer patients, although there has been a marked change in the handling of cancer in the media, and many famous personalities have come forward to speak about their own experience in ways that can be very meaningful to patients.

Alternative cancer therapies enjoy enduring popularity.[9] But there are now many naturalistic therapies that, while not scientifically proven, may increase a patient's sense of control and well-being and thus improve quality of life, as long as they are not used instead of proven treatments. They are becoming increasingly visible and popular, in direct proportion to the disillusionment with or mistrust of traditional medicine. (The possible scientific basis for claims of improved survival are discussed later in this chapter.)

These trends are affecting the practice of oncology in many ways. The growth of bioethics and the patients' rights movement have resulted in many changes of law and custom, including:

1. Many states require that a woman with stage I or II breast cancer be given the choice between breast-conserving treatment and mastectomy.
2. New York State gives the patient or family the ultimate authority in demanding resuscitation.
3. The Federal Patient Self-Determination Act requires all hospitals and nursing homes to advise patients at the time of admission of their right to refuse treatment.

The most dramatic intrusion of social policy into the practice of medicine is the debate over the legalization of euthanasia, which is discussed in the section below on ethical issues.

While these developments have brought difficult transition periods, the overall movement toward enabling patients to participate as fully and as early as possible in planning for their own care is a welcome one. One of the very positive outcomes of increased consumerism has been the emphasis on quality-of-life issues in evaluating cancer treatment. Today, an increasing number of treatment protocols that aim for prolonged survival rather than cure are factoring quality-of-life measures into the final outcomes.[10,11]

MEDICAL FACTORS

Once a patient receives a diagnosis of cancer, the vicissitudes of the disease and the treatment assume a central role in the patient's existence and emotional state.

Transition Points

Adaptational needs and distress are greatest at certain crises or transition points such as diagnosis, the start of primary treatment, the end of primary treatment (when concerns about possible recurrence increase), a change in treatment modalities, relapse, the transition from curative to supportive treatment, and during advanced and terminal disease.[12] The oncologist must be especially attuned to psychological distress at these points. For example, patients terminating an intensive course of treatment should be given an early follow-up appointment, reassured of the physician's ongoing availability, and warned that they may go through an unexpected period of increased anxiety.

Fear of Treatment

Today's patient is often very aware of the paradoxical toxicity of most cancer treatments and of the many unpleasant side effects they may have observed in friends or family members. Patient compliance and psychological adaptation improve if the oncologist is aware of these anxieties and allows the patient to discuss them.

Symbolically Meaningful Symptoms and Losses

Each patient brings his or her own history to bear on the illness. Construction workers value their stamina, computer operators their manual dexterity. Each will react with special intensity to a loss in their area of special functioning and may need special support.

Two related areas are of special significance to almost all patients: altered physical appearance and altered sexual functioning.[13–16] The first is easier to address; the second is often ignored out of patient and doctor embarrassment. Patients are deeply relieved and grateful when the doctor broaches these sensitive topics in an open, matter-of-fact manner.

Communication Problems

Physicians are often baffled when patients claim ignorance about matters they have clearly been told. Because anxiety interferes with information-processing, it is predictable that patients will need repeated statements to absorb complex and unwelcome news. This is particularly problematic when patients use an unusual amount of denial and systematically screen out the "bad" parts of the news. It becomes the oncologist's difficult task to gently confront denial when it interferes with important decision-making or necessary life adaptations.

Denial is a ubiquitous psychological defense mechanism that can range from very adaptive to very destructive. *Instrumental denial* prevents the patient from being active on his or her own behalf and must be confronted. *Affective denial* allows the patient to maintain an upbeat, hopeful stance even while making decisions that flow from a realistic assessment of his or her situation. This form of denial can be encouraged and is associated with better compliance and better quality of life.

Terminal Illness

In the past, terminal patients were often kept in the dark about their condition because protective families and physicians felt this was the most humane thing to do. This approach has been made obsolete by society's attention to patient's rights to participate in decisions about instituting and foregoing life-sustaining measures, especially cardiopulmonary resuscitation. The 1991 Federal Patient Self-Determination Act requires that all patients be asked on admission about their wishes concerning resuscitation. While both physicians and families may wish to avoid frank discussions with the fatally ill patient, almost all patients, even disturbed ones, are better off having frank discussions. Concern for how the patient may react, guilt for having failed the patient, and self-consciousness about how to present the issue cause many physicians to delay and avoid the discussion. This improves with encouragement, role-modeling, and practice. (The ethical problems associated with the terminal care period are discussed below.)

PATIENT-RELATED FACTORS

The patient's contribution to adaptation to illness is derived from several sources. Patients with a stable personality, no current psychiatric disorder, and no history of significant prior psychological problems can be expected to adapt well to cancer. These patients confront the facts, seek available information, and actively pursue treatment. They respond to the disease as a challenge, while poorer copers often try to avoid the implications of the illness and delay the decisions required for optimal care. The best predictor of good patient adjustment is good adaptation to prior life crises. However, some prior crises can make the diagnosis of cancer much more upsetting even in psychologically healthy patients. These include cancer in a close relative or friend, especially when it involves the same site as the patient's disease, and the coincidence of cancer with other crises such as grief, divorce, job loss, or another illness. Without the support of close, caring people, many patients unravel under the stress of cancer. Social supports have even been found to influence mortality rates and measures of immune function.[17,18]

Normal Psychological Responses to Cancer

The expected range of psychological responses to cancer must be defined to recognize when a patient requires further evaluation and support. The observed response to a diagnosis of cancer is similar to that of other life-threatening illnesses or major life changes. Initially, the person is often disbelieving. "I feel numb," "as if I am watching someone else," are common expressions used by patients at this time. This is a constructive attempt at keeping awareness within tolerable levels. The next stage is one of mixed anxious and depressed feelings, preoccupation with the implications of the illness, foreboding thoughts about the future, and a sense of helplessness. Attention and concentration are impaired; sleeping and eating patterns are disrupted. These acute symptoms dissipate over a few weeks as a treatment plan is agreed on and undertaken. During this critical time, the psychological distress and associated physiologic arousal make it difficult for the patient to fully absorb the diagnosis and treatment recommendations. Therefore, the physician should plan to repeat information several times and should not be surprised when patients appear to have poor comprehension and even poorer recall.

Although the acute response is limited to a few weeks, the overall adaptation lasts much longer. Weisman and Worden described the first 100 days after diagnosis as one of continuing "existential plight," and of course some level of concern remains indefinitely.[19] Psychologically healthy patients use ways of coping that have worked well in the past, obtaining and processing information about the treatment as well as help and advice from experienced others.

Psychosocial and Medical Factors Associated With Poor Adjustment

The vulnerability factors that identify patients at increased risk of poor adjustment and psychiatric problems fall into three major categories: psychological, social, and medical factors (Table 64–9). Prior psychiatric problems, alcohol or drug abuse, depression, and chronic anxiety are strong predictors for poor adjustment and for exacerbation of previous psychiatric difficulties. Evidence of unusually high initial distress that persists usually long with high levels of anxiety and depression, especially when coupled with behavioral evidence of poor coping, is also reason for concern. A negative attitude toward physicians and treatment and low expectations for the future do not bode well. Medical factors suggesting high vulnerability are advanced disease and poorly controlled symptoms, particularly pain and insomnia.[20] Several social factors are associated with poor adjustment: low socioeconomic status, chronic marital or family problems, perceived or actual poor support from others, and absence of affiliation with a meaningful social group, especially a religious one.

Abnormal Psychological Responses to Cancer

It is important for the oncologist to recognize when a patient's response is normal and self-limited and when it has become pathologic. The diagnosis of psychiatric disorders in cancer patients has been clouded by assumptions that severe depression is "normal" in cancer patients. In fact, when the level and severity of physical illness are controlled for, cancer patients have the same frequency of depression as other medically ill patients.[21]

TABLE 64–9. Psychological Problems of Cancer Survivors

Fears of termination of treatment
Preoccupation with minor physical problems
Adjustment to physical losses and handicaps
Difficulty with reentry into normal life (the Lazarus syndrome)
Perceived loss of job mobility
Awareness of insurance discrimination
Persistent sense of vulnerability to illness and death (the Damocles syndrome)
Persistent guilt (the survivor syndrome)

The incidence of psychiatric disorders in cancer patients has been determined by assessing ambulatory and hospitalized patients in three cancer centers using standard diagnostic criteria (Fig. 64–3).[22] Fifty-three percent of patients interviewed, although showing signs of stress, were coping adequately. The remaining 47% had a diagnosable psychiatric disorder. The most common by far was adjustment disorder with anxious and depressive symptoms, seen in two thirds of those with psychiatric disorders and one third of all patients interviewed. Depression was next, seen in 13% of those with a psychiatric diagnosis. Central nervous system complications resulting in organic mental disorders were present in 4%; prior psychiatric problems accounted for only 4% of cases.

Among hospitalized and more seriously ill patients, the frequency of major depression rises to 20%.[21] Organic mental disorders, primarily delirium, increase with worsening illness to a frequency of 20% in hospitalized cancer patients and 80% in the terminally ill.[20,23]

Six psychiatric disorders occur frequently enough in cancer patients to warrant a description of their clinical picture. Three represent a direct reaction to the illness: adjustment disorders (reactive anxiety and depression), major depression, and delirium. The others (primary anxiety disorders, personality disorders, and major mental illness) are preexisting conditions often exacerbated by illness.

ADJUSTMENT DISORDER WITH DEPRESSED, ANXIOUS, OR MIXED FEATURES (REACTIVE ANXIETY AND DEPRESSION). These common disorders are an exaggeration of the mixed anxiety and depression seen in self-limited stress responses. The key features are unusual persistence and undue interference with functioning.

Interventions are aimed at helping the patient resume successful coping by use of several modalities. Individual psychotherapy focuses on clarifying the medical situation and the meaning of illness and on reinforcing the patient's positive coping strategies. It is often desirable to include a spouse or family member to enhance support at home. Group therapy, with a focus on illness, is often helpful, as are behavioral methods such as relaxation and hypnosis. Couple and family therapy may be helpful when interpersonal issues are prominent. The decision to prescribe a psychotropic drug requires a high level of distress and the inability to carry out daily activities. Low doses of alprazolam, lorazepam, or oxazepam control symptoms and need not cause undue daytime sedation or risk withdrawal or dependence in these psychologically healthy patients. Alprazolam, because of its rapid onset and combined anxiolytic and antidepressant action, is particularly effective starting at doses of 0.25 mg one to three times per day. Bedtime sedation with a benzodiazepine (triazolam or temazepam) or a sedating antidepressant (amitriptyline) is effective and may improve daytime symptoms as well.

MAJOR DEPRESSION. All depression in cancer has a strong reactive component. However, major depressive episodes also occur and are responsive to treatment. Unfortunately, because it is often assumed that the patient is "appropriately" depressed, major depression is often undiagnosed and untreated.

Because of the associated medical illness, diagnosis cannot depend on vegetative signs such as fatigue, insomnia, weight

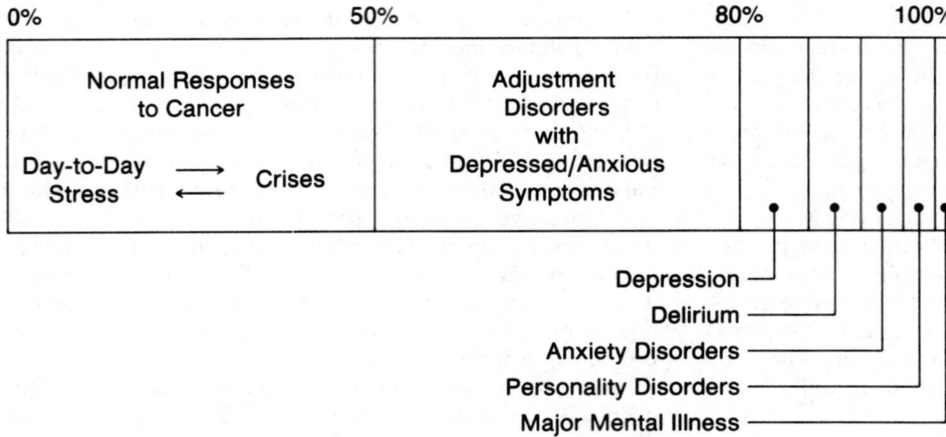

FIGURE 64–3. Incidence of psychiatric disorders in cancer patients. (Derogatis LB, Morrow GR, Fetting J, et al. The prevalence of psychiatric disorders among cancer patients. JAMA 1983;249:751)

loss, and anorexia, but rests on a constellation of psychological symptoms: dysphoric or sad mood, feelings of helplessness and hopelessness, loss of self-esteem and feelings of worthlessness or guilt, and a wish to die. Patients at high risk for major depression are those with a history of prior depression, inadequately controlled pain, an advanced stage of illness, and disease at certain sites such as the pancreas.[24] Some of the endocrine and ectopic hormone-secreting tumors also produce depression. Several drugs can produce severe depression as part of their central nervous system toxicity, both singly and additively; among chemotherapy agents, these include interferon, steroids, BCNU, vincristine, tamoxifen, and L-asparaginase.[25] Other commonly used drugs are antihypertensives, benzodiazepines, antiparkinsonian agents, and beta-blockers.

The presence of suicidal ideation requires careful assessment to determine if it reflects depressive illness or expresses a wish to have ultimate control over intolerable symptoms. Thoughtful clinical judgment is required to make this differentiation, especially in the patient with advanced disease. Breitbart has outlined factors that place a cancer patient at a high risk for suicide: poor prognosis and advanced illness, depression and hopelessness, uncontrolled pain, delirium, prior psychiatric history, history of previous suicide attempts or family history of suicide, history of recent death of friends or spouse, history of alcohol abuse, and few social supports.[26] At Memorial Sloan-Kettering Cancer Center, patients who have attempted suicide have been characterized by poorly controlled pain, mild encephalopathy, disinhibition secondary to medications, and hopelessness combined with distress about being unable to communicate discomfort to caregivers. If a patient is suicidal, a 24-hour companion is provided to establish constant observation, monitor the suicidal risk, and reassure the patient.

Depressed patients are usually treated with a combination of supportive psychotherapy and antidepressants. There are several reports of the efficacy of antidepressants in depressed patients with cancer.[27–30] The antidepressant agents that can be considered for use in cancer patients are the tricyclic antidepressants (TCAs), heterocyclic antidepressants, atypical antidepressants, monoamine oxidase inhibitors (MAOIs), psychostimulants, lithium carbonate, and benzodiazepines.[31] Table 64–10 shows the starting dose and range of therapeutic daily doses for drugs in these classes.

The antidepressants best documented in the oncology setting are the tricyclic antidepressants. They are started at a low dose (10 to 25 mg at bedtime), especially in debilitated patients, and the dose is increased by 25 mg every 1 to 2 days until a beneficial effect is achieved. For reasons that are unclear, depressed cancer patients often show a therapeutic response to a TCA at much lower doses (75 to 125 mg daily) than are usually required in physically healthy, depressed patients (150 to 300 mg daily). Patients are usually maintained on a TCA for 4 to 6 months after symptoms improve, after which time the dose is gradually lowered and discontinued.

The choice of TCA depends on the nature of the depressive symptoms, medical problems present, and side effects of the TCA. The depressed patient who is agitated and has insomnia will benefit from the use of a TCA with sedating effects, such as amitriptyline or doxepin. Patients with psychomotor slowing will benefit from use of the compounds with the least sedating effects, such as protriptyline or desipramine. The patient who has stomatitis secondary to chemotherapy or radiation therapy or who has slow intestinal motility or urinary retention should receive a TCA with the least anticholinergic effects, such as desipramine or nortriptyline.

Patients who cannot swallow pills may be able to take an antidepressant in an elixir (amitriptyline, nortriptyline, or doxepin) or in an intramuscular form (amitriptyline or imipramine). Intramuscular administration causes discomfort because of the volume of the vehicle; hence, 50 mg is usually the maximum dosage that can be delivered per intramuscular injection. Although TCAs have not yet been approved for intravenous use in the United States, several studies from Europe indicate their efficacy and safety by this route.[31] Hospital pharmacies can prepare some TCAs in rectal suppository form, but absorption by this route has not been studied in cancer patients.

Imipramine, doxepin, amitriptyline, desipramine, and nortriptyline are often used in the management of neuropathic pain in cancer patients. Dosing is similar to the treatment of depression, and analgesic efficacy, if it occurs, is usually observed at a dose of 50 to 150 mg daily; higher doses are needed occasionally. While the initial assumption

TABLE 64–10. Antidepressant Medications Used in Cancer Patients

Drug Name	*Starting Daily Dosage mg (PO)*	*Therapeutic Daily Dosage mg (PO)*
Tricyclic Antidepressants		
Amitriptyline	25	75–100
Doxepin	25	75–100
Imipramine	25	75–100
Desipramine	25	75–100
Nortriptyline	25	50–100
Heterocyclic Antidepressants		
Maprotiline	25	50–75
Amoxapine	25	100–150
Atypical Antidepressants		
Buproprion	15	200–450
Fluoxetine	20	20–60
Trazodone	50	150–200
Monoamine Oxidase Inhibitors		
Isocarboxazid	10	20–40
Phenelzine	15	30–60
Tranylcypromine	10	20–40
Lithium Carbonate	300	600–1200
Psychostimulants		
Dextroamphetamine	2.5 at 8 A.M. and noon	5–30
Methylphenidate	2.5 at 8 A.M. and noon	5–30
Pemoline	18.75 in A.M. and noon	37.5–150
Benzodiazepines		
Alprazolam	0.25–1.00	0.75–6.00

(Massie MJ, Holland JC. The cancer patient with pain: Psychological complications and their management. J Symptom Pain Manage [in press])

was that the analgesic effect resulted indirectly from the effect on depression, it is now clear that these tricyclics have a separate, specific analgesic action, probably mediated through several neurotransmitters, most prominently norepinephrine and serotonin.[32]

If a patient does not respond therapeutically to adequate blood levels of a TCA or cannot tolerate its side effects, a heterocyclic (maprotiline or amoxapine) or a second-generation (bupropion, trazodone, fluoxetine, sertraline) antidepressant can be used. The heterocyclic antidepressants have side-effect profiles similar to the TCAs. Maprotiline should be avoided in patients who are at high risk for seizures, because the incidence of seizures can be increased with this medication. Amoxapine has strong dopamine-blocking activity, so patients taking other dopamine blockers (*e.g.*, antiemetics) have an increased risk of developing extrapyramidal symptoms and dyskinesias.

The atypical antidepressants are generally considered to be less cardiotoxic than the TCAs and are increasingly being used. Bupropion is a relatively new drug in the United States, and there is little experience with its use in the medically ill. At present, it is not the first drug of choice for depressed patients with cancer, but it should be considered if a patient has a poor response to other antidepressants. Bupropion may be somewhat activating in medically ill patients. Because of its seizure potential it should be avoided in patients with seizure disorders and brain tumors and those who are malnourished.

Trazodone is strongly sedating and in low doses (50–100 mg at bedtime) is helpful in the treatment of the depressed cancer patient with insomnia. Effective antidepressant doses are often greater than 300 mg per day. Trazodone has been associated with priapism and should therefore be used with caution in male patients.

Fluoxetine, a selective inhibitor of neuronal serotonin uptake, has fewer sedative and autonomic effects than the TCAs. The most common side effects are mild nausea and a brief period of increased anxiety; hyponatremia is an uncommon adverse effect.[33] Fluoxetine can cause appetite suppression, which usually lasts for several weeks. Some cancer patients experience transient weight loss, but weight usually returns to baseline level and the anorectic properties of this drug have not been a limiting factor in this population. Fluoxetine may be particularly useful in depressed cancer patients who are additionally distressed from weight gain resulting from chemotherapy. Overall, the side-effect profile of fluoxetine suggests that it may be a relatively favorable treatment for depressed cancer patients; a multicenter study of its efficacy is currently under way. Sertraline, a recently approved serotonergic agent, has a shorter duration of action than fluoxetine, and possibly a more benign side effect profile. It is increasingly being used, starting with 25 mg per day, in the medically ill.

Patients who were taking lithium carbonate before cancer should be maintained on it throughout cancer treatment, although close monitoring is necessary when the intake of fluids and electrolytes is restricted, such as during preoperative and postoperative periods. The maintenance dose of lithium may need to be reduced in seriously ill patients. Lithium should be prescribed with caution in patients receiving cisplatin due to the potential nephrotoxicity of both drugs. Although several authors have reported that the leukocytosis produced by lithium could be beneficial in neutropenic cancer patients, the functional capabilities of these leukocytes have not been determined.[34] The bone-marrow stimulation appears to be transient; no mood changes have been noted in these patients.

If a patient has responded well to an MAOI for depression before treatment for cancer, its continued use is warranted. However, most psychiatrists are reluctant to start depressed cancer patients on MAOIs because the need for dietary restriction is poorly received by patients who already have dietary limitations and nutritional deficiencies secondary to cancer illness and treatment.

In cancer patients, low doses of the psychostimulants (dextroamphetamine, methylphenidate, and pemoline) promote a sense of well-being, decrease fatigue, and stimulate appetite.[35,36] An advantage of these drugs is their rapid onset of antidepressant action, compared with that of the TCAs. Psychostimulants can potentiate the analgesic effects of narcotic analgesics and are commonly used to counteract opioid-induced sedation. Occasionally they can produce nightmares, insomnia, and even psychosis.

Treatment with dextroamphetamine and methylphenidate is usually started at a dose of 2.5 mg at 8 A.M. and noon. Typically patients are maintained for 1 to 2 months, after which time about two thirds can be withdrawn without a recurrence of depressive symptoms. Those who develop recurrence of depressive symptoms can be maintained for up to 1 year. Tolerance may develop, and adjustment of the dose may be necessary.

Pemoline, a less potent and longer-acting psychostimulant, comes in a chewable tablet so patients who have difficulty swallowing can absorb the drug through the buccal mucosa.[36] We have begun to use pemoline frequently in a population of cancer patients with depressive symptoms, and it appears to be as effective as methylphenidate or dextroamphetamine. Pemoline should be used with caution in patients with renal impairment; liver function tests should be monitored periodically with long-term treatment.

The triazolobenzodiazepine alprazolam has been shown to be an effective antidepressant as well as an anxiolytic.[37] Alprazolam is particularly useful in cancer patients who have mixed symptoms of anxiety and depression.[38] Treatment is initiated with doses of 0.25 mg three or four times a day and titrated up to effective antidepressant doses, usually 4 to 6 mg per day.

Benzodiazepines are usually readily discontinued by cancer patients when the symptoms of anxiety abate. Concerns about addiction should not interfere with their use in the cancer setting. In fact, cancer patients often must be encouraged to take enough medication to provide relief from anxiety. Benzodiazepines should be tapered to avoid withdrawal.

DELIRIUM FROM CNS COMPLICATIONS. Delirium, the second most common psychiatric diagnosis among cancer patients, is due both to the direct effects of cancer on the CNS and the indirect CNS complications of the disease and treatment. Posner reported that 15% to 20% of hospitalized cancer patients have abnormalities of cognitive function that are not related to structural disease.[39] About one fifth of all consultation requests made to a psychooncology service were requests for assistance in the management of symptoms of delirium. Early symptoms are often unrecognized or misdiagnosed by medical and nursing staff as symptoms of depression or "poor coping." Early recognition is important: the underlying cause may be a treatable complication of cancer.

Any patient who shows the acute onset of agitation, impaired cognitive function, altered attention span, or a fluctuating level of consciousness should be suspected of having delirium. It is usually due to one or more of these causes: medications, electrolyte imbalance, failure of a vital organ or system, nutritional state, infections, vascular complications, or hormone-producing tumors. In a study of terminally ill cancer patients, over three fourths developed delirium with a multifactorial etiology.[23]

Many drugs can cause acute confusional states. Confusion is a common adverse effect of opioids. Among the more than 280 chemotherapeutic agents now available for cancer, delirium has been associated with methotrexate (with intrathecal or intravenous administration), 5-fluorouracil (5-FU), vincristine, vinblastine, bleomycin, BCNU, cisplatin, asparaginase, procarbazine, cytosine arabinoside, ifosfamide, and corticosteroids.[40,41] Other medications commonly prescribed to cancer patients that can cause confusional states are interleukin-2, amphotericin, and acyclovir.

All steroid compounds can cause symptoms ranging from minor mood disturbance to frank psychosis.[42] Disturbances may include affective changes (emotional lability, euphoria, depressed mood, anxiety), fears, paranoid interpretation of events and suspiciousness of others, with illusions, delusions, and hallucinations. Symptoms often develop 4 to 5 days after high-dose steroids are begun or when the dose is rapidly tapered, but they can also develop while patients are on maintenance dosages. It may be necessary to continue steroids despite psychiatric symptoms, in which case neuroleptics such as haloperidol can be used for symptom control. A steroid psychosis during one course of treatment does not necessarily predict recurrence with subsequent courses of steroids. No relation has been shown between the development of steroid psychosis and premorbid personality or psychiatric history.

Whole-brain irradiation, especially when combined with intrathecal chemotherapy, strongly predisposes patients to the development of later cognitive deficits. These are more severe in the very young and the very old, and result in IQ drops of as much as 20 to 25 points. Learning disabilities have been found even in the absence of documented IQ losses. Thus, despite some controversy, the preponderance of studies shows some residual deficits, leading to a search for new regimens to minimize them.[43,44]

Haloperidol is the most effective drug for prompt control of delirium and agitated or disruptive behavior. Intramuscular or intravenous injection of 0.5 to 2.0 mg reduces agitation without causing sedation or hypotension. It can be given intravenously at 1 mg/minute, if necessary, and repeated at 60-minute intervals, titrated against behavior. The patient should be changed to an oral dose of three-fourths the parenteral dose as soon as possible. For milder symptoms, 1 to 2 mg of trifluoperazine or 10 to 25 mg of thioridazine may be given orally twice a day.

ANXIETY DISORDERS: PREEXISTING PHOBIAS, PANIC ATTACKS, AND GENERALIZED ANXIETY. Persistent and incapacitating anxiety symptoms in cancer patients usually represent worsening of preexisting problems. Phobias, the most common form of abnormal fears, often revolve around physical illness, death, pain, needles, claustrophobia, or fear of solitude. Panic attacks may be precipitated, and chronic generalized anxiety syndromes are severely exacerbated. Long scanning procedures are intolerable to many patients, who require special handling and medication.[45] Agoraphobic patients may be unable to tolerate the night before surgery alone in the hospital and require relaxation of rules to allow the presence of a relative. They also need longer and higher levels of preoperative sedation, with coordination between the psychiatrist and the anesthesiologist. Specific fears of needles, pain, or the sight of blood require acknowledgment and individualized management, including medication, distraction, and desensitization.[46] Given this special care, patients are generally cooperative, grateful, and able to proceed with treatment.

Benzodiazepines are the drugs of choice for both acute and

chronic anxiety states. The most common side effects—sedation and confusion—occur more frequently in older patients and in those with impaired liver function. Short-acting benzodiazepines such as alprazolam, lorazepam, and oxazepam are often prescribed. Oxazepam and lorazepam are metabolized by conjugation and excreted by the kidney; hence, they are better tolerated by patients with impaired hepatic function and by those taking other medications with sedative effects (*e.g.*, analgesics). Lorazepam reduces vomiting in cancer patients receiving emetogenic cancer chemotherapies.

Clonazepam has been found useful in patients with organic mental disorders or seizure disorders who develop symptoms of depersonalization or anxiety. This longer-acting benzodiazepine is particularly useful for patients who have end-of-dose failure with recurrence of anxiety symptoms. It is effective in patients with organic mood disorders with symptoms of mania and as an adjuvant analgesic in patients with neuropathic pain.

PERSONALITY DISORDERS. Patients or families with "difficult" personalities frustrate and anger those who treat them. The stress of cancer exaggerates their normally maladaptive coping strategies and they become even more difficult than usual. The disorders can be recognized by the exaggeration of common characteristics: the paranoid person who is suspicious and constantly threatens litigation; the obsessive person whose excessive attention to details of care is accompanied by repeated criticism; the dependent person who demands care far beyond objective needs and who may be dependent on alcohol or drugs; the patient with borderline disorder who cannot conform to rules and who manipulates, divides, and may disturb other patients as well as staff; and the histrionic person who overdramatizes symptoms and distress.

Because personality disorders are not seen by patients as a problem, management usually depends on helping staff to understand the pattern and to contain their behavior. Many of these patients benefit from consistent limit-setting, applied in a quiet, kindly manner.

MAJOR MENTAL ILLNESS. Schizophrenia and bipolar (manic-depressive) illness are rare in the general population and hence uncommon in cancer patients. Careful management is needed to ensure the patient's cooperation with treatment and to prevent escalation of symptoms under stress. Previously prescribed neuroleptics should be continued, and management must be coordinated with the anesthesiologist when surgery is required because of potential paradoxical blood pressure reactions. Lithium should also be continued but may need to be stopped briefly during periods of fluid loss or restriction.

Indications for Psychiatric Evaluation

Many mild to moderately severe psychiatric disorders are managed successfully by the oncologist and a sensitive staff. However, as the above discussion makes clear, cancer patients experience several psychiatric disorders requiring accurate diagnosis for precise, effective treatment. Once treatment is outlined, management may often be done by the physician with help of social workers or other mental-health professionals. The more severe psychiatric problems require close collaboration between the oncologist and psychiatrist.

Table 64–11 outlines the indications for psychiatric consultation. Disorders directly related to illness, preexisting psychiatric disorders exacerbated by illness, and major mental disorders have been described, but four additional indications warrant discussion.

CAPACITY TO CONSENT TO OR REFUSE TREATMENT. A psychiatric consultation may be needed when a patient refuses a procedure critical to survival or when the capacity to give informed consent is in question. Rarely is legal advice or a judge's decision necessary for emergency treatment. However, when elective treatment is planned for a mentally impaired patient with no family, court direction may be needed. An increasingly common concern is the patient who refuses a clearly life-sustaining treatment, such as dialysis, as part of a decision to forego all further treatment. Physicians and nurses often are uncertain whether the patient is truly capable of assessing all the options. The presence of acute depression, which dulls mental processes and strongly biases decisions, poses a difficult and sometimes urgent reason for psychiatric consultation.

LEAVING AGAINST MEDICAL ADVICE. Requests to leave the hospital against advice are most commonly due to the presence of a confusional state secondary to illness or medication and as such often represent an acute danger to self, allowing for brief restraint and treatment after psychiatric evaluation. An acutely psychotic state or an exacerbated prior psychiatric disorder may also result in poor judgment. The cause of the behavior must be determined and a decision made as to whether the patient can be managed safely at home or whether he or she must remain in the hospital with a relative or companion. Often the severity of the patient's illness prevents safe transfer to a medical-psychiatric unit, but improvement occurs rapidly under the care of familiar medical staff, with one-to-one observation and low doses of a neuroleptic drug such as haloperidol.

SEXUAL DYSFUNCTION. Infertility and sexual dysfunction are often unavoidable consequences of irradiation, surgery, and chemotherapy. In men, the opportunity for sperm banking before treatment can both arouse and assuage con-

TABLE 64–11. Indications for Psychiatric Evaluation

Disorders directly related to illness
Adjustment disorders (reactive anxiety and depression)
Major depression and suicidal risk
Delirium from CNS complications
Preexisting disorders exacerbated by illness
Anxiety disorders
Personality disorders
Major mental disorders
Schizophrenia
Unipolar and bipolar mood disorder
Capacity to consent or to refuse treatment
Leaving against medical advice
Sexual dysfunction
Significant distress from conflict with family or staff

cerns about infertility. In women, psychological preparation for the premature menopause and sterility associated with chemotherapy or the altered sexual function that results from gynecologic surgery is very useful in diminishing the inevitable adverse reactions. Soon after completion of treatment, patients are reluctant to bring up sexual problems, and physicians and staff are equally reluctant to ask about them. In later follow-up visits, the burden is on the oncologist to inquire into the sexual problems common with several tumor sites: breast, testicular, and gynecologic neoplasms; prostate, bladder, and head and neck tumors; and Hodgkin's disease. An increasingly sophisticated literature on diagnosis and treatment is developing in this area.[15,16]

SIGNIFICANT DISTRESS FROM CONFLICT WITH FAMILY OR STAFF. Sometimes a case becomes imbued with persistent conflict. This may stem from the patient's personality but often involves the family's problems or, more rarely, the staff's inadvertent mishandling. A psychiatric consultation can provide an objective assessment that identifies and confronts the sources of the problematic behavior. Family meetings, possibly with the patient and selected staff members present, often help to ease family distress; similarly, staff conferences encourage a more concerted and effective approach to the family and patient.

Therapeutic Interventions in Cancer

The problems outlined above are amenable to three main types of therapeutic intervention: psychopharmacologic, psychological, and behavioral. Psychopharmacologic treatment has been described. The primary indications for all three modalities are reviewed in Table 64–12. An aggressive and eclectic approach combining several modalities is most useful.

The cornerstone is psychological support, which can take many forms, some carried out by many nonpsychiatric staff. Individual sessions for both patients and families offer counseling, advice, and information about illness, treatment, and expectation of side effects. Spiritual counseling is meaningful for many patients as they turn to their religion during the existential crisis created by cancer. The chaplain can offer not only spiritual solace but also the concrete support and services of others of the same faith. Psychotherapy usually consists of brief, crisis-oriented sessions to help patients regroup their defenses and cope successfully with the problems of illness. The one-to-one visit of a veteran patient who has successfully negotiated the same experience is often very helpful.

Group interventions have also proved to be useful for cancer patients in several ways. The first is an educational function: orientation and learning what is needed to adapt to a treatment or its consequences (*e.g.*, radiation, laryngectomy, ostomy). Second, groups encourage emotional learning and relieve anxiety by allowing patients to see how others are coping with the same problems and by encouraging the expression of feelings without fear of being ridiculed. Third, the advocacy provided by cancer groups often becomes a voice for more social awareness and change, while at the same time giving participants a valuable sense of strength and empowerment. These consumer groups can be effective whether led by a professional or self-directed, such as CanSurmount and I Can Cope. A recent and provocative use of groups is suggested by two studies in which immune function was improved and survival time increased by a group intervention; see below for further discussion.[47,48]

TABLE 64–12. Primary Indications for Each Therapeutic Approach

Intervention	*Treatment Modality*
Psychological	
Professional crisis intervention at points of maximal stress	
At time of diagnosis	Individual and group counseling
Before a new treatment	Crisis intervention
At relapse	Psychotherapy
At treatment failure	Counseling by clergy
Ongoing psychotherapy for patients with preexisting psychiatric disorders	
Nonprofessional (self-help)	
Provision of "practical" advice at times of crisis	Veteran and fellow patient counseling
Ongoing support	Self-help groups
Empowerment during chronic and survival phases	
Psychopharmacologic	
Some adjustment disorders	Antianxiety agents
Anxiety disorders	Antidepressants
Major depression	Analgesics
Delirium/dementia	Antipsychotics
Schizophrenia	
Manic-depressive illness	
Pain	
Nausea and vomiting	
Insomnia	
Behaviorial Interventions	
Anxiety and discomfort with procedures (bone-marrow aspiration, lumbar puncture)	Relaxation
	Biofeedback
Pain (adjunct to analgesics)	Systematic desensitization
Nausea and vomiting (anticipatory treatment-related)	Suggestion/imagery/ hypnosis
Eating disorders	Distraction
Some anxiety disorders	

Behavioral interventions such as relaxation, posthypnotic suggestion, autohypnosis, desensitization, and distraction are the newest additions to patient management and are particularly useful for the acute anxiety surrounding painful procedures or feared surgery, and for the conditioned nausea, vomiting, food aversions, and possible immune suppression found in patients receiving chemotherapy.[49–53]

An important role for the oncologist is to ensure that the patient and family have optimal access to the full range of financial, social, religious, psychological, and community resources available to them. In a large center social workers are trained to perform this function, but in more decentralized settings the oncologist should become familiar with a few key local resources and should use them systematically. The resulting improvements in coping benefit the patient and ease case management.

LONG-TERM SURVIVORS

Advances in cancer treatment have resulted in a rapidly growing population of over 5 million long-term survivors, many of them children and young adults. Early psychological studies using crude measures such as marriage and level of education showed few psychological effects, but recent investigators, using more refined measures, have shown more symptoms.[54–56] Figure 64–4 illustrates the magnitude of the effect in male leukemia survivors, who are about one standard deviation above the mean in their level of distress. The results for female survivors are comparable.

Much attention has been paid to the late medical effects of cancer. The ones with the most far-ranging psychological consequences include cognitive dysfunction secondary to brain radiation, which is most marked in the very young and very old; growth retardation in children; problems with sexual response and fertility (these are often submerged at the time of treatment but reemerge acutely later); chronic organ failure at all ages; and most poignantly the occurrence of a second malignancy.

The psychological issues outlined in Table 64–9 occur at many levels. There is a documented but paradoxical increase in distress when treatment is successfully terminated, because of the loss of the emotionally protective effect of the ongoing treatment. Psychiatric intervention is useful at this time. Memorial Sloan-Kettering Cancer Center has established a post-treatment resource program to address this and other issues important to survivors. Survivors forever remain aware of their vulnerability to disease, and remain more frightened of minor physical discomforts. Some manifest the guilt of the survivor syndrome, others rejoice in a sense of special worthiness and good fortune. Reentry into normal life can be very difficult for a patient with strong dependency traits or a patient whose family is very much out of tune with the patient's needs and capabilities. At work, survivors must cope with altered co-worker attitudes and with pervasive insurance discrimination, which in turn may lead to a loss of a career mobility; the dimensions of this need to be fully explored. Yearly checkups with the oncologist remain a recurrent frightening experience even after years pass. However, they are also an excellent opportunity for the physician to assess the survivor's overall adjustment and to institute appropriate supportive measures in psychological as well as physical areas.

Peer support has been found especially valuable for survivors, who provide each other with unique understanding and advocacy. Many patients can be referred to the National Coalition of Cancer Survivorship, and the American Cancer Society can direct patients to many other special survivor organizations, such as those for laryngectomy, ostomy, and mastectomy patients.

THE "WORRIED WELL": PSYCHOLOGICAL PROBLEMS IN HIGH-RISK GROUPS

The current explosion of information about the genetic contribution to the development of cancer has produced a new population: people whose family history is such that they are clearly at high risk for certain cancers. Table 64–13 lists cancers already known to be occasionally associated with recessive chromosomal abnormalities. With new DNA technologies, these numbers are increasing rapidly, creating psychological, social, legal, and ethical problems.

Psychologically, it is useful to differentiate between people who are afraid they *might* be at risk and people who are afraid because they know they *are* at risk. The first group can benefit from careful education about their increased risk, if any. Some will remain excessively anxious even in the absence of objective reason and may be said to suffer from cancerophobia; they benefit from psychological support and regular checkups with a trusted oncologist to prevent them from squandering

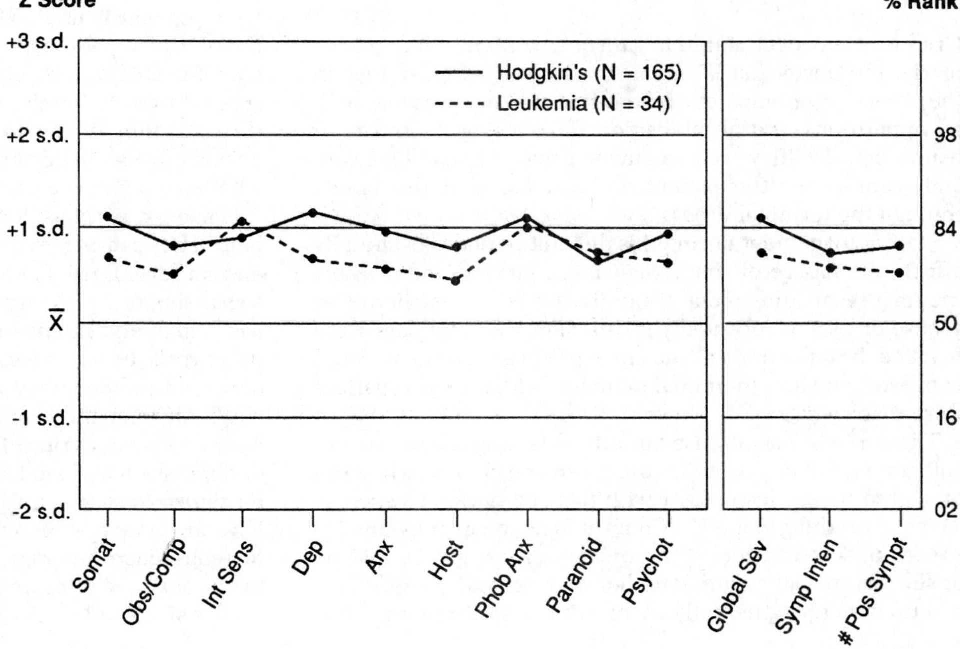

FIGURE 64–4. Comparison of psychological distress of male Hodgkin's disease and leukemia survivors in relation to normals: brief symptom inventory. (Lesko LM, Ostroff J, Smith K. Life after cancer: Survival and beyond. In: Current concepts in psycho-oncology. Memorial Sloan-Kettering Cancer Center, 1991, and Korn-blith AB, et al. Quality of life assessment of Hodgkin's disease survivors: A model for cooperative clinical trials. Oncology 1990; 4:93)

TABLE 64–13. Human Cancers Associated With Recessive Chromosomal Abnormalities

Cancer	*Chromosome or Region*
Bilaterial acoustic neuroma	22q
Bladder cancer	11p
Breast cancer	13q, 17p, 17q
Colorectal cancer	5q, 17p, 18, 22
Familial renal cell carcinoma	3p
Gastric carcinoma	13q
Multiple endocrine neoplasia (type 2A)	10
Neuroblastoma	1p32
Ovarian cancer	6q
Small cell lung cancer	3q13-p24, 13q, 17p
Uveal melanoma	2
Wilms' tumor	11p13

(Bodmer WF. Cancer genetics and the human genome. Hosp Prac 1991;29:73–85)

time and resources on numerous physicians.[58] The second group benefits from the same education but may need detailed genetic and psychological counseling to help them make difficult decisions regarding marriage, child-bearing, prenatal testing, and further personal testing or medical interventions such as prophylactic mastectomy.

Breast cancer is the most common cancer known to have a possible genetic component (in up to 30% of cases), and high-risk surveillance programs have been developed that have medical, surgical, educational, and psychological components.[59,60] Support groups have proven very helpful and have enabled many women who were too frightened to practice breast self-examination to begin to do it regularly.[60]

MANAGEMENT OF GRIEF

Grief is often encountered in cancer treatment. More particularly, the oncologist is intensely involved with families in the throes of anticipatory bereavement. This presents both an opportunity and an obligation for oncologists and their teams, because they are in a unique position to combine care and comfort for the patient with guidance of the family through the terminal illness.

Staff management during this difficult period substantially affects the nature of the bereavement process and possibly the long-term adjustment of family survivors. The bereaved spouse or parent repeatedly recalls how the final days were handled, how the news of the grave prognosis and death were conveyed, and how their final moments with the dying patient were managed.

The survivor has intense but mixed feelings about the oncologist. Gratitude about the care given and closeness because of shared memories coexist with nagging questions such as "Was everything done?" "Could it have been prevented?" "Were mistakes made?" The oncologist recognizes that he or she has special meaning to the survivors and accepts their reactions nonjudgmentally. A meeting 1 to 2 months after the death serves as an important setting in which troubling questions can be discussed. Autopsy findings, if available, provide a good opportunity to clarify concerns and relieve guilt. The meeting can also be used to monitor the course of grieving. The hallmarks of normal and abnormal grief are outlined below.[61,62]

Even when a death is clearly anticipated, the reaction of a relative to the actual event is often one of temporary disbelief. Despite visible deterioration in a dying spouse, the surviving partner may be unable to tolerate any real emotional awareness of the death and of what life will be like without the person. Available information suggests, however, that grief is tolerated better when the loss is expected and there has been some psychological preparation.

Once death has occurred, grieving has acute and chronic components. Acute waves of an overwhelming sense of loss, associated with crying and agitation, and usually precipitated by a reminder of the deceased, are superimposed on a chronic background of social withdrawal, preoccupation with the deceased, diminished concentration and attention, restlessness, depressed mood, anxiety, insomnia, and anorexia. The intense distress of the first few months looks like depression and may be clinically indistinguishable from it.

Over several months, the acute symptoms diminish in intensity and frequency. Reorganization of activities with resurgence of interest is seen. Preoccupation with the deceased is replaced by recall of memories associated with both pleasure and sadness. Satisfactory resolution of grief is marked by the readiness to invest deeply in new relationships and is assumed to be usually achieved by 1 year. However, the duration of normal grieving is quite variable and often extends well beyond a year. Parents, for example, are never the same again after the death of a child, and some never really recover. Older spouses from a long union often grieve acutely for 2 to 4 years, and some much longer.

The morbidity and mortality related to grief have been actively explored in the past decade. The symptoms were described above. Bereaved people often become more dependent on cigarettes, alcohol, and drugs to reduce distress, if these were previously used. They visit physicians more often than nonbereaved patients, with various physical complaints. Yet outcome studies indicate that most people recover with the support of only family, friends, and clergy. Peer counseling through the Widow-to-Widow programs, Compassionate Friends, or Candlelighters offers excellent support from others who have suffered a similar loss.

However, perhaps 20% of family survivors require special help. They can be identified early in bereavement by the presence of several risk factors, including perceived or actual poor social support, prior psychiatric history (especially alcoholism), high and intense initial distress, unanticipated death, concurrent life stresses or losses, prior high level of dependency on the deceased for primary support, and death of a child. Any one of these risk factors is sufficient reason to recommend psychiatric referral, particularly when high levels of depression and anxiety are sustained and there is little or no return to social functioning. Bereavement counseling allows the person to recount the details of the death and his or her subsequent feelings, to explore new ways of coping, and to try out new roles and experiences. An antidepressant to ensure sleep and reduce high levels of distress permits better daily functioning and often facilitates the exploration of painful feelings.

STRESSES ON ONCOLOGISTS

While recent studies have painted an increasingly clear picture of the emotional reaction of patients and their relatives, few studies have addressed the stresses on oncologists and their staffs, and the effect of these stresses on their personal and professional life.[63–65] These issues are important both for the well-being of medical professionals and for their impact on patient care. Studies consistently show that despite recurrent criticism that medicine has become uncaring and commercial, patients accept arduous treatment regimens largely because of their personal trust in their physician, and still expect to obtain their primary psychological support from him or her.[66] The harried, stressed oncologist cannot give sufficient attention to this aspect of medicine.

Physicians generally tolerate work stresses well. They have a strong intellectual and emotional commitment to their work and a well-tested capacity for hard work and discipline. However, they also have characteristics that predispose them to chronic stress. Many work long hours and seek little recreation, straining marital relations and upsetting children. Socializing becomes minimal except with colleagues. Strains in marriage and family life compound stresses at work. Conflicts with close colleagues endanger job performance and satisfaction and are especially difficult because resolution may be impossible. The need to care for patients while pursuing research and teaching activities adds special strains in the academic setting. Physical illness and frequent sleep loss are transient additional stressors; chronic fatigue is more insidious.

The practice of oncology brings special strains: the uncertainty inherent in treatment decisions; the unique toxicity inherent in treatments, especially those known to predispose to life-threatening complications such as bone-marrow transplants; and the repeated impact of patient deaths, especially patients to whom the oncologist has become attached. Some personal distress is inherent in confronting decisions about withholding or stopping life-sustaining measures and in discussing these decisions with the patient and family. The impact of patients' unrealistic expectations and the strain associated with the care of "problem" patients are additional sources of stress.[65] Caring for a colleague with cancer, while a compliment, is a double burden when treatments fail, and the loss is felt as a personal and a medical failure. Malpractice threats and suits increase, as do paperwork and outside intrusions on the ability to give the desired quality of care. Finally, it is poignantly clear that conscientious medical staff are not immune to irrational guilt, much less to ordinary sorrow. The wonder is not that symptoms of stress are observed, but rather how well physicians continue to cope.

The actual incidence of serious psychiatric problems in physicians is probably underreported. Depression, suicide, and alcohol and drug abuse are the most common psychiatric disorders seen. The rate of suicide among physicians is 100 physicians per year, or the equivalent of one medical-school class. When combined with the significant number who become dependent on drugs or alcohol, the reasons for concern become apparent; alcoholism is estimated to occur in 7% to 10% and drug abuse in 2% to 3% of physicians.

While neither of these have been examined in oncologists per se, the constant and continuing care of cancer patients, when combined with personality traits or personal problems, may provide a matrix for depression and psychological burnout. At the extreme it may lead to the need for peer review of professional competence. New legislation places increasing attention on physician competence and encourages doctors to identify their dysfunctional colleagues at an earlier and more treatable stage. Depressed physicians who continue to work cannot provide solid emotional support and therefore deprive their patients of a vital source of empathy.

What are the symptoms of emotional fatigue and burnout? The physician notices less zest and enthusiasm for work, with a sense of having to "drag in" to work. This may be coupled with feeling chronically tense, easily frustrated, and easily angered; depressed "down" moods frequently ensue. The need for a "few drinks after work" or experimentation with psychotropic drugs to "relax" are ominous signs, because the habits usually escalate. Insomnia is common, with either difficulty falling asleep, frequent awakening, or early-morning awakening. Appetite change may lead to weight gain or loss. Feeling exhausted or "tired all the time," headaches, and aches and pains are other indicators of distress.

Physicians tend to ignore these symptoms. At this point, the physician may "tune out" and feel detached from patients and unable to empathize. This is an early sign of stress in house staff, who say they feel less able to care and are cynical and pessimistic about the meaning of their work. They may begin working longer hours with a sense that "nobody can do it right but me" and "nobody works around here but me," when in fact they are less effective and efficient.

Physicians often delay seeking help for physical symptoms; unfortunately, they delay even longer in admitting to psychiatric problems and seeking help for them. To avoid becoming identified as a psychiatric patient, physicians hide their symptoms from family and colleagues, fearing the impact on their job and practice if it should become known. The warning signs of depression, the taking of secret drinks, and surreptitious use of pills are ignored. Family, colleagues, and even patients often collude in pretending nothing is wrong. The result is a paradoxical delay in identification and treatment of the physician.

Monitoring oneself for symptoms of emotional fatigue and acknowledging one's stress is very important in oncology. Survival tactics include recognizing one's limitations, not taking oneself too seriously, accepting the inadequacies of medicine, using gallows humor to lighten the meaning of painful events, working a "normal" work day for a few weeks, stopping when others do, taking a long weekend at recurrent intervals, maintaining a regular exercise program, and bringing to these measures the same care and consistency given to other responsibilities. When symptoms do not remit, psychiatric consultation should be sought.

Some training programs in oncology encourage awareness of personal reactions and provide regular meetings in which difficult patients and management of personal stresses are reviewed. They have proven useful and have been well described with oncology fellows.[65] Hospitals with liaison psychiatrists also have a built-in mechanism for attending to staff problems, especially among nurses and house staff. However, few resources exist for practicing oncologists after leaving training, and it is at this time when stresses may be greatest and the physician the most vulnerable. Actively seeking a supportive peer group is important.

More willingness to confront colleagues and to encourage them to seek treatment is necessary when significant symptoms are noted, especially because the professional arena is usually the *last* to be impaired, after personal and family functioning is already damaged. The motivation for intervention is human concern for a friend, together with the demands of optimal patient care, which require physicians to be strong enough to provide support and understanding to their patients. The severely distressed physician cannot meet this important requirement and endures much unnecessary personal suffering at the same time.

With the increasing complexity of therapeutic regimens, oncologists are working more and more as leaders or coleaders of treatment teams. Such leaders play a critical role in maintaining group morale, thereby diminishing staff stress and improving patient care. The main principles of good leadership are:

1. Modeling and expecting the delivery of high-quality patient care while also acknowledging realistic human limitations
2. Exercising authority clearly and consistently where appropriate, while supporting teamwork where appropriate
3. Encouraging and respecting in others the self-monitoring described above
4. Educating oneself about sources of help for one's staff, making them known, and using them.

Staff support groups are reportedly very effective in decreasing staff stress.[65,67] Oncologists may participate directly in such groups, but even if they choose not to, their well-publicized and genuine support for such groups is a key element of success.

PSYCHOSOCIAL AND BEHAVIORAL FACTORS IN CANCER RISK AND SURVIVAL

Psychosocial and behavioral factors affect both the risk of developing cancer and the length of survival once cancer has developed. Patients ask many questions about these issues as they attempt to understand why they got cancer and how they can positively affect the treatment outcome. Oncologists must be familiar with the present state of research to respond accurately and usefully.

Holland has reviewed the psychosocial and behavioral factors that may alter cancer risk and survival and has divided them into five areas: lifestyle and behaviors, social environments, personality and coping style, life events and emotional states, and behavioral and lifestyle interventions.[4,5]

LIFESTYLE AND BEHAVIORS

The effect of individual behaviors on altering exposure to carcinogens and the incidence of many cancers is well known. Cancer-prevention programs depend heavily on insights and techniques derived from psychology, psychiatry, and the social sciences for help in reducing smoking and alcohol intake and altering dietary practices and sexual behavior.[2,3] In addition, much of the improvement in survival for common cancers, such as breast and colon cancer, depends on early detection; psychiatry and the social sciences are needed to understand the complex factors that make people delay seeking consultation long after they have suspicious symptoms.

SOCIAL ENVIRONMENT

Socioeconomic status has been shown to be a key variable in the incidence and survival rates for many cancers, even under standardized treatment conditions.[6–8,68] This includes factors such as premorbid state of health and access to care, and also the other psychosocial factors described in this section. The absence of social ties also has been shown to prejudice cancer incidence and mortality, and in one study had an impact on natural killer-cell activity in women with breast cancer.[18]

PERSONALITY AND COPING STYLE

Although this area is of great interest to patients and to the lay press, data still do not strongly support the theory that a particular personality style predisposes to cancer. Early studies on type C personality have not been replicated.[69] Type A personality was shown to have at a most a 1.5 risk.[70] Greer's early work on the protective effect of the "fighting spirit" has been contradicted by three later studies.[71–74]

LIFE EVENTS AND EMOTIONAL STATES

The contribution of grief and depression to mortality from cancer does not appear to be as great as was previously assumed. Early studies showing some effects have been contradicted by later, better-designed ones.[75–79] While immune functions are perturbed after bereavement and in some other stressed states, the effects are probably too small to have clinical significance.[80]

BEHAVIORAL AND LIFESTYLE INTERVENTIONS

The impact of "mind on body" has been given impetus by two small but well-designed studies of group interventions that showed a positive effect on survival of breast-cancer patients and a positive effect on immune function in stage I and II melanoma patients.[47,48] However, three studies have shown no effects on mortality of intensive holistic supportive behavioral programs.[81–83] Follow-up and duplication attempts of the positive studies are currently under way.

Despite the sobering research trends described above, the wish, often translated into a magical belief, that one can cure the body with the power of the mind remains compelling. Its implied promises have spawned a growth industry of clinics and healers who encourage patients to use their mental powers to fight their cancer, with or without the help of traditional treatments. The accompanying emphasis on a healthy lifestyle and careful attention to nutrition is commendable. However, confusion is rampant between risk and survival factors. The well-known and powerful risk factors are conflated with ambiguous and weak survival factors, while the role of personality factors is inflated far beyond the existing evidence. The intense, cultlike aspect of many alternative programs encourages extreme hopes and beliefs and leads to equally extreme disappointments.

By placing the locus of power over cancer in the patient's mind, "healers" play into patients' (and families') universal tendency to feel they are to blame for their illness. It is only too common to see a nauseated, anorectic patient being badgered to eat by family members who demand that he or she demonstrate a "positive attitude." Worst of all, healers let patients bear personal responsibility for failure, or blame it on their having sought traditional treatment. The hapless patient has no choice but to join the universal chorus by blaming himself or "the cancer establishment."

Yet some of these programs have a core of constructiveness. Patients who feel energized and empowered to act on their own behalf, who maintain a healthful lifestyle, and who have a better subjective sense of hope and well-being will pursue and tolerate treatment more effectively and will have a better ongoing quality of life. If survival is improved, so much the better. The best traditional medical treatment has aimed for these results, but not often and not vigorously enough, as the demands of technology have elbowed aside the time- and labor-intensive demands of psychosocial interventions. It is to be hoped that the future will see a reconciliation between traditional cancer care and the more constructive aspects of alternative care.

COMMON ETHICAL DILEMMAS CONFRONTING THE CAREGIVER IN CANCER

The practice of medicine has been greatly affected by the development of the discipline of applied bioethics. Clinicians can no longer follow only their personal sense of what is right; they must now answer to a more informed and demanding public, as well as ethics committees and legal precedents. Oncology is at the heart of many controversial areas. Today's oncologists must have an understanding of the basic issues and the basic arguments.[84,85] We will present a brief review of the contemporary code of medical ethics and a description of the main areas likely to affect clinical oncologists.

MEDICAL CODE OF ETHICS

The medical code of ethics goes back to the Hippocratic oath and was restated by the American Medical Association in 1980. In the past two decades it has come under searching criticism and redefinition by bioethicists, who have criticized the profession as too paternalistic and monopolistic.

Beauchamp and Childress reviewed four basic principles that should guide the contemporary physician[85]:

1. *Respect for the patient's autonomy* implies honoring the patient's right to self-governance, privacy, and individual choice.
2. *Nonmaleficence* implies the obligation to do no harm.
3. *Beneficence* implies the obligation to help others to further their own best interests.
4. *Justice* is the hardest to define without many qualifiers, but in the context of clinical practice can be said to imply the duty to apply the first three principles to one's patients fairly and consistently.

From these principles are derived four sets of rules of conduct that should characterize the physician-patient relationship:

1. *Rules of veracity* bear directly on truth-telling and informed consent.
2. *Rules of privacy* stipulate that the physician must honor conditions of limited access to the patient. These two sets of rules have figured prominently in past statements of the profession.
3. *Rules of confidentiality* have long figured in medical codes of ethics, but are in fact profoundly eroded by economic, political, and legal developments, as well as purely technologic ones.
4. *Rules of fidelity* address the contractual nature of the physician-patient relationship in the legal arena, but also a broader concept of "promise-keeping" in the moral arena.

TRUTH-TELLING

A diagnosis of cancer can immediately present caregivers with an ethical dilemma, depending on the area in which they practice. In countries where the principle of autonomy is valued above all others, the physician is expected to tell the patient the diagnosis without any evasion. However, in many more countries, the principle of autonomy is much less valued than the principle of beneficence, or more exactly the principle of nonmaleficence. Thus, physicians are expected to shield the patient and to enter into a conspiracy with the patient's family. Practitioners who do not follow the locally accepted mode are surrounded by controversy.

INFORMED CONSENT FOR TREATMENT

Patients cannot give informed consent for treatment if they have not been given adequate information about their condition. Because there is an increasing pressure to require informed consent before treatment, truth-telling will probably become more widespread, especially because many cancer treatments are toxic. Public awareness of the toxicity of cancer treatment has risen steadily and has caused fear and anxiety. Improvements in outcomes in the last decade have been measured more by small but steady increments than by any major breakthroughs. Statistical analyses that point toward improved outcomes have been criticized.[86] Hence, the general public is even less likely to trust caregivers blindly.

Bone-marrow transplantation is an exception to the incremental improvement model because it offers a chance of cure to patients who would otherwise die. Unfortunately, the mortality rate from the procedure has remained around 15% to 20%, and the best results are obtained by selecting the healthiest patients, preferably those in remission. In a democratic society, it would appear difficult, or at the very least inconsistent, to justify putting a patient into such a high-risk/high-gain situation without obtaining consent from a fully informed patient. Nevertheless, this is still accepted practice in some countries. For the practice to be acceptable in these countries, the moral and professional caliber of the caregivers must be very high, and societal approval of the practice must run very deep.

INVESTIGATIONAL TREATMENTS

The special issues that surround investigational treatment are not unique to cancer. Being a clinical investigator puts the physician into a possibly irreducible conflict between concerns for research and his or her duty to the individual patient. Major abuses in previous decades have led to the development of mandatory institutional review boards (or ethics committees, as they are more often called in Western Europe).[87] A well-constituted, well-functioning institutional review board is the first and most important safeguard of the individual patient's welfare in a protocol (and the physician's, as well). But how can patients be protected from a caregiver's earnest zeal to accrue subjects who might not wish to participate in a given protocol? The best safeguard is a well-informed patient, aware of his or her right to refuse and able to give fully informed consent.

A second major controversy arises at the very core of the investigational process: Are randomized trials, by their very nature, unethical? This question was most recently highlighted by two articles in the May 30, 1991, issue of the *New England Journal of Medicine*. Hellman and Hellman invoked several arguments against the ethical validity of clinical trials[88]:

1. There is an irreducible conflict between the physician's duty to his or her patient and the researcher's responsibility to randomize.
2. Although patients may waive their rights to individual treatment, it is inconsistent with the physician's role to ask that they do so.
3. Terminally ill patients, said to have least to lose and most to gain, may also be least able to give informed consent that is truly voluntary.

The authors made a plea for pursuing research methods that avoid randomization.

In rebuttal, Passamani described the conditions for an ethical clinical trial[89]:

1. A fully informed patient
2. A condition of clinical equipoise where no treatment branch is clearly preferable to any other
3. A trial designed as a critical test of the alternatives
4. A data-monitoring committee prepared to stop the trial if that state of equipoise no longer exists.

He pointed out that many randomized trials have answered questions with counterintuitive results that might not have been established any other way.

TERMINAL CARE ISSUES

Although good medical care has resulted in the curing of many patients and has changed cancer from a rapidly fatal to a chronic disease, terminal care issues continue to present themselves regularly.

Truth-telling often recurs as an issue because many caregivers find it difficult to bring the patient or family to confront the grim reality. Sometimes the family will demand that the patient not be told, and may even remove the patient from a given physician's care when they fear he or she would be too frank. The ethics of surrogate decision-making are particularly important when family members must make decisions for newly incompetent patients. Currently, ethical and legal expectations are that the family, knowing the patient best, will act in a way that most closely approximates what the patient's wishes would have been. In reality, however, families often follow their own wishes. Furthermore, there are no guidelines to establish the competence of family surrogates. Many terminal care situations become quite chaotic when a very disturbed spouse or parent becomes the main decision-maker.

Medical technology has also brought about the need to make decisions for which our social, political, legal, ethical, and spiritual history has not prepared us: namely, decisions regarding the maintenance of life. These can be roughly divided into three categories: stopping the fight against death and winding down from active treatment to palliative care; accepting the arrival of death (namely, overcoming the magical expectations of cardiopulmonary resuscitation and allowing the dead to stay dead); and hastening the coming of death, which includes forms of passive and active euthanasia and assisted suicide.

In the United States these three areas have been the focus of intense public debate and changing policy. The first occurred during the 1970s, when increasing consumer disillusionment with the outcome of "high-tech" medicine led to more readiness on the part of physicians and patients to forego aggressive treatments. The second phase evolved during the 1980s, when there was a confrontation between the increasingly automatic practice of resuscitation and consumers' growing dread of "prolonged dying." This resulted in the development of "do not resuscitate" (DNR) regulations and the use of living wills and advance directives, by which patients can make their own wishes known while they are still competent. The last phase has only begun and is being discussed on many political and social fronts. It addresses the growing demand for the legalization of physician-assisted suicide and possibly euthanasia. Medical and legal organizations and many professional ethicists have opposed these measures, but grassroots support runs deep. A legal initiative to allow physician-assisted suicide was narrowly defeated in the state of Washington in November 1991, but further initiatives are expected in several western states.

THE PREGNANT CANCER PATIENT

The pregnant cancer patient is thrust into the furious crossfire of the right-to-life versus pro-choice debate, and such a patient almost always creates acute management controversies. Most recently, the Stoner case created a possible precedent. Mrs. Stoner had been forced to undergo a cesarean section against her will in a desperate effort to save her 23-week fetus while she was dying of advanced cancer. When both mother and infant died within a few days, the Stoner family sued the hospital. The case was settled out of court and the hospital published a set of guidelines designed to prevent future violation of the rights of pregnant patients. This is a welcome development in an era in which Curran has noted a rise in involuntary cesarean sections.[90] Nevertheless, the often competing interests of the mother and fetus make all treatment decisions momentous and conflict-ridden.

THE RIGHTS OF TRANSPLANT DONORS

The rights of transplant donors have also been a subject of controversy as increasingly bold recipients or their family members pursue potential donors. One patient sued his hospital to release the name of matched but unrelated and unwilling donors, and lost on the grounds of protecting the donor's right to privacy. This begged the issue of how much pressure could be brought to bear on a known donor. This was most recently addressed by the case of two half-siblings whose absent father sued to force their mother to permit them to provide a bone-marrow transplant for his older son from another union. The courts upheld the mother's refusal in a thoughtful opinion that, although it will not generalize automatically to other cases, will provide a useful guide to help caregivers analyze similar troubling situations.[90]

THE RIGHTS OF MINORS AS DECISION-MAKERS

Considering the rights of children and adolescents as decision-makers can profoundly complicate the practice of pediatric oncology due to potential conflicts between parents and children, especially adolescents. For every overt conflict, there are probably many that never become apparent to the caregivers. In keeping with the current trend toward empowering the recipient of medical care, King and Cross[91] and Leikin[92] offered guidelines for assessing and enhancing children's decision-making potential and for dealing with issues of death and dying.

THE RIGHTS OF GENETICALLY AT-RISK PATIENTS

As the ability to identify genetic markers for cancer has improved, the potential problems this may create for identified patients have become clearer. Lack of confidentiality leading to job discrimination, loss of insurability, and even loss of procreative freedom have already been reported. These and other related problems are being addressed by the Committee on Ethical, Legal, and Social Issues of the Human Genome Project and have been the focus of an Office of Technology Assessment Task Force.[93,94] Their publication on genetic monitoring in the workplace contains a current review of the legal and regulatory situation.[95]

REFERENCES

1. Holland JC, Marchini A, Tross S. An international survey of physician attitudes and practice in regard to revealing the diagnosis of cancer. Cancer Invest 1987;5:151–154.
2. Lerman C, Rimer BK, Engstrom PF. Reducing avoidable cancer mortality through prevention and early detection. Cancer Res 1989;49:4955–4962.
3. Ockene JK, Lindsay E, Berger L, Hymowitz N. Health-care providers as key change agents in the Community Intervention Trial for Smoking Cessation (COMMIT). Int Q Commun Health Educ 1990-1991;11:223–237.
4. Holland JC. Psychosocial variables: Are they factors in cancer risk or survival? In: Holland JC, Lesko LM, Massie MJ, eds. Current concepts in psycho-oncology. New York: Memorial Sloan-Kettering Cancer Center, 1991.
5. Levenson JC, Bemis C. The role of psychological factors in cancer onset and progression. Psychosomatics 1991;32:125–132.
6. Holland JC, Rowland J, eds. Handbook of psycho-oncology: Psychological care of the patient with cancer. New York: Oxford University Press, 1989.
7. Baquet CR, Horm JW, Gibbs T, Greenwald P. Socioeconomic factors and cancer incidence among blacks and whites. JNCI 1991;83:551–557.
8. Freeman H. Race, poverty and cancer. JNCI 1991;83:526–527, 1991.
9. Cassileth BR, Lusk EJ, Strouse TB, Bodenheimer BJ. Contemporary unorthodox treatments in cancer medicine: A study of patients, treatments and practitioners. Ann Intern Med 1984;101:105–12.
10. Aaronson NK. Methodologic issues in assessing the quality of life of cancer patients. Cancer 1991;67:844–850.
11. Hillner BE, Smith TJ. Efficacy and cost effectiveness of adjuvant chemotherapy in women with node-negative breast cancer. N Engl J Med 1991;324:160–168.
12. Holland JC. Clinical course of cancer. In: Holland JC, Rowland J, eds. Handbook of psycho-oncology. New York: Oxford University Press, 1989:134–145.
13. Bronheim H, Strain JJ, Biller JH. Four aspects of head and neck surgery, Part I: New surgical techniques and psychiatric consequences. Gen Hosp Psychiatry 1991;13:165–176.
14. Bronheim H, Strain JJ, Biller JH. Four aspects of head and neck surgery, Part II: Body image and interventions. Gen Hosp Psychiatry 1991;13:225–232.
15. Auchincloss S. Sexual problems in cancer patients; evaluation and management issues. In: Holland JC, Rowland JH, eds. Psycho-oncology: The psychological care of the patient with cancer. New York: Oxford University Press, 1989:383–413.
16. Schover LR, Jensen SB. Sexuality and chronic illness: A comprehensive approach. New York: Guilford Press, 1988.
17. House JS, Landis KR, Umberson D. Social relationship and health. Science 1988;240: 540–545.
18. Levy SM, Herberman RB, Whiteside T, et al. Perceived social support and tumor estrogen/progesterone receptor status as predictors of natural killer cell activity in breast cancer patients. Psychosom Med 1990;52:73–85.
19. Weisman AD, Worden JW. The existential plight in cancer: Significance of the first 100 days. Int J Psychiatry Med 1976;7:1–17.
20. Massie MJ, Holland JC. The cancer patient with pain: Psychiatric complications and their management. J Sympt Pain Manage 1992;7:99–109.
21. Bukberg J, Penman D, Holland JC. Depression in hospitalized cancer patients. Psychosom Med 1984;46:199–212.
22. Derogatis LB, Morrow GR, Fetting J, et al. The prevalence of psychiatric disorders among cancer patients. JAMA 1983;249:751–757.
23. Massie MJ, Holland JC, Glass E. Delirium in terminally ill cancer patients. Am J Psychiatry 1983;140:1048–1050.
24. Holland JC, Korzun AH, Tross S, et al. Comparative psychological disturbance in patients with pancreatic and gastric cancer. Am J Psychiatry 1986;143:982–986.
25. Lederberg MS, Holland JC. Psycho-oncology. In: Kaplan HI, Sadock BJ, eds. Comprehensive textbook of psychiatry. Baltimore: Williams & Wilkins, 1989:1249–1264.
26. Breitbart W. Suicide in cancer patients. In: Holland JC, Rowland JH, eds. Handbook of psycho-oncology: Psychological care of the patient with cancer. New York: Oxford University Press, 1989:291–299.
27. Rifkin A, Reardon G, Siris S, et al. Trimipramine in physical illness with depression. J Clin Psychiatry 1985;46:4–8.
28. Popkin MK, Callies AI, MacKenzie TB. The outcome of antidepressant use in the medically ill. Arch Gen Psychiatry 1985;42:1160–1163.
29. Costa D, Mogos I, Toma T. Efficacy and safety of mianserin in the treatment of depression of women with cancer. Acta Psychiatr Scand 1985;72(suppl 320):85–92.
30. Massie MJ, Lesko L. Psychopharmacological management. In: Holland JC, Rowland JH, eds. Handbook of psycho-oncology: Psychological care of the patient with cancer. New York: Oxford University Press, 1989:470–491.
31. Mucha H, Lange E, Bonitz G. Amitriptyline in der psychiatrischen therapie. Psychiatr Neurol Med Psychol [Leipz] 1970;22:116–120.
32. France RD. The future for antidepressants: Treatment of pain. Psychopathology 1987;20: 99–113.
33. Vishwanath BM, Navalgund AA, Cusano W, Navalgund KA. Fluoxetine as a cause of SIADH. Am J Psychiatry 1991;148:542–543.
34. Lyman GH, Williams CC, Preston D. The use of lithium carbonate to reduce infection and leukopenia during systemic chemotherapy. N Engl J Med 1980;302:257–260.
35. Fernandez F, Adams F, Holmes VF, et al. Methylphenidate for depressive disorders in cancer patients. Psychosomatics 1987;28:455–461.
36. Chiarello RJ, Cole JO. The use of psychostimulants in general psychiatry: A reconsideration. Arch Gen Psychiatry 1987;44:286–295.
37. Rickels K, Feighner JP, Smith WT. Alprazolam, amitriptyline, doxepin, and placebo in the treatment of depression. Arch Gen Psychiatry 1985;42:134–141.
38. Holland JC, Morrow GR, Schmale A, et al. A randomized clinical trial of alprazolam versus progressive muscle relaxation in cancer patients with anxiety and depressive symptoms. J Clin Oncol 1991;9:1004–1011.
39. Posner JB. Neurologic complications of systemic cancer. 1978;2:7–60.
40. Young DF. Neurological complications of cancer chemotherapy. In: Silverstein A, ed. Neurological complications of therapy: Selected topics. New York: Futura. 1982:47–113.
41. Drugs of choice for cancer chemotherapy. Medical Letter 1991;33:21–28.
42. Stiefel FC, Breitbart WS, Holland JC. Corticosteroids in cancer: Neuropsychiatric complications. Cancer Invest 1989;7:479–491.
43. Fletcher JM, Copeland DR. Neurobehavioral effects of central nervous system prophylactic treatment of cancer in children. J Clin Exp Neurol 1988;10:495–538.
44. Cousens P, Waters B, Said J, Stevens M. Cognitive effects of cranial irradiation in leukemia: A survey and meta-analysis. J Child Psychol Pyschiatr 1988;29:839–852.
45. Brennan SC, Redd WH, Jacobsen PB, et al. Anxiety and panic during magnetic resonance scans. Lancet 1988;2:512.
46. Jacobsen PB. Treating a man with needle phobia who requires daily injections of medication. Hosp Comm Psychiatry 1991;42:877–878.
47. Spiegel D, Bloom J Kraemer HC, et al. Effects of psychosocial treatment on survival of patients with metastatic breast cancer. Lancet 1989;2:888–891.
48. Fawzy FI, Kemeny ME, Fawzy NW, et al. A structured psychiatric intervention for cancer patients: II. Changes over time in immunologic measures. Arch Gen Psych 1990;47:729–735.
49. Loscalzo M, Jacobsen PB. Practical behavioral approaches to the effective management of pain and distress. J Psychosocial Oncol 1991;8:139–169.

50. Jacobsen PB, Redd WH. The development and management of chemotherapy-related anticipatory nausea and vomiting. Cancer Invest 1988;6:329–336.
51. Andrykowski MA, Otis JL. Development of learned food aversions in humans: Investigation in a natural laboratory of cancer chemotherapy. Appetite 1990;14:145–158.
52. Bovbjerg DH, Redd WH, Maier LA, et al. Anticipatory immune suppression and nausea in women receiving cyclic chemotherapy for ovarian cancer. J Consult Clin Psych 1990;58:153–157.
53. Manne SL, Redd WH, Jacobsen PB, Gorfinkle K, Schorr O, Rapkin S. Behavioral intervention to reduce child and parent distress during venipuncture. J Consult Clin Psych 1990;58:565–572.
54. Welch-McCaffrey D, Hoffman B, Leigh LA, et al. Surviving adult cancers, Part 2: Psychosocial implications. Ann Intern Med 1989;111:517–524.
55. Smith K, Ostroff J, Tan C, Lesko LM. Alterations in self-perceptions among adolescent cancer survivors. Cancer Invest 1991;9:581–588.
56. Mumma GH, Mashberg D, Lesko LM. Long-term psychosexual impact of marrow transplantation versus conventional chemotherapy. Gen Hosp Psychiatry 1992;14:43–55.
57. Loescher L, Welch-McCaffrey D, Leigh SA, et al. Surviving adult cancers, Part 1: Physiological effects. Ann Intern Med 1989;111:411–432.
58. Holland JC. Fears and abnormal reactions to cancer in physically healthy individuals. In: Holland J, Rowland JR, eds. Handbook of psycho-oncology: Psychological care of the patient with cancer. New York: Oxford University Press, 1989:13–21.
59. Scalfani L. Management of the high-risk patient. Sem Sup Oncol 1991;7:261–266.
60. Kash KM, Holland JC, Halper MS, Miller DG. Psychological distress and surveillance behaviors of women with a family history of breast cancer. JNCI 1992;84:24–30.
61. Osterweis M, Solomon F, Green M, eds. Bereavement: Reactions, consequences and care. Washington DC: National Academy Press, 1984.
62. Chochinov H, Holland JC. Bereavement: A special issue in oncology. In: Holland J, Rowland JR, eds. Handbook of psycho-oncology: Psychological care of the patient with cancer. New York: Oxford University Press, 1989:612–627.
63. Mount BM. Dealing with our losses. J Clin Oncol 1986;4:1127–1134.
64. Kash K, Holland JC. Special problems of physicians and house staff. In: Holland J, Rowland JR, eds. Handbook of psycho-oncology: Psychological care of the patient with cancer. New York: Oxford University Press, 1989.
65. Lederberg MS. Psychological problems of staff and their management. In: Holland J, Rowland JR, eds. Handbook of psycho-oncology: Psychological care of the patient with cancer. New York: Oxford University Press, 1989.
66. Penman D, Holland Jc, Bahna G, et al. Informed consent for investigational chemotherapy: Patients' and physicians' perceptions. J Clin Oncol 1984;2:849–855.
67. Lederberg MS. Group support for medical staff in high-stress settings. In: Alonzo A, Swiller HI, eds. Group psychotherapy in clinical practice. APA Press, 1992.
68. Cella DF, Orav J, Kornblith AB, Holland JC, et al. Socioeconomic status and cancer survival. J Clin Oncology 1991;9:1500–1509.
69. Temoshok L, Heller BW, Sageviel RW, et al. The relationship of psychological factors of prognostic indicators in cutaneous malignant melanoma J Psychosom Res 1985;29: 139–153.
70. Fox BH, Ragland DR, Brand RJ, Rosenman RH. Type A behavior and cancer mortality. Ann NY Acad Sci 1987;496:620–627.
71. Greer S, Morris T, Pettingale KW. Psychological response to breast cancer: Effect on outcome. Lancet 1979;2:785–787.
72. Cassileth BR, Lusk EJ, Miller DJ, et al. Psychological correlates of survival in advanced malignant disease? N Engl J Med 1985;312:1551–1555.
73. Holland JC, Korzun AH, Tross S, Cella DF, et al. Psychosocial factors and disease-free survival in Stage II breast cancer. Proc Am Soc Clin Oncol [Abstract] 1986;5:237.
74. Jamison RN, Burish TG, Wallston KA. Psychogenic factors in predicting survival of breast cancer patients. J Clin Oncol 1987;5:768–772.
75. Helsing KJ, Szklo M. Mortality after bereavement. Am J Epidemiol 1981;1124:41–52.
76. Bieliauskas LA, Garron DC. Psychological depression and cancer. Gen Hosp Psychiatry 1982;4:187–195.
77. Hahn RC, Petitti DB. Minnesota Multiphasic Personality Inventory-rated depression and the incidence of breast cancer. Cancer 1988;61:845–848.
78. Kaplan GA, Reynolds P. Depression and cancer mortality and morbidity: Prospective evidence from the Alameda County study. J Behav Med 1988;11:1–13.
79. Zonderman AB, Costa PT, Jr, McCrae RR. Depression as a risk for cancer morbidity and mortality in a nationally representative sample. JAMA 1989;262:1191–1195.
80. Stein M, Miller AH, Trestman RL. Depression of the immune system and health and illness. Arch Gen Psych 1991;48:171–177.
81. Bagenal FS, Easton DF, Harris E, et al. Survival of patients with breast cancer attending Bristol Cancer Help Centre. Lancet 1990;336:606–610.
82. Cassileth BR, Lusk EJ, Guerry D, et al. Survival and quality of life among patients receiving unproven as compared with conventional cancer therapy. N Engl J Med 1991;324:1180–1185.
83. Morganstein H, Gellert GH, Walter SD, et al. The impact of a psychosocial support program on survival with breast cancer; the importance of selection bias in program evaluation. J Chron Dis 1984;37:273–282.
84. Jonsen AR, Siegler M, Winslade WJ. Clinical ethics: A practical approach to ethical decisions in clinical medicine. New York: Macmillan, 1982.
85. Beauchamp TL, Childress JF. Principles of biomedical ethics. New York: Oxford University Press, 1989.
86. Bailar JC, Smith, EM. Progress against cancer? N Engl J Med 1986;314:1226–1232.
87. Beecher HK. Ethics and clinical research. N Engl J Med 1966;274:1354–1360.
88. Hellman S, Hellman DS. Of mice but not men: Problems of the randomized clinical trial. N Engl J Med 1991;324:1585–1589.
89. Passamani E. Clinical trials: Are they ethical? N Engl J Med 1991;324:1589–1592.
90. Curran WJ. Beyond the best interests of a child: Bone marrow transplantation among half-siblings. N Engl J Med 1991;324:1818–1819.
91. King NMP, Cross AW. Children as decision makers: Guidelines for pediatricians. J Pediatr 1989;115:10–16.
92. Leikin S. A proposal concerning decisions to forgo life-sustaining treatment for young people. J Pediatr 1989;115:17–22.
93. Wexler NS. Genetic jeopardy and the new clairvoyance. Prog Med Genet 1985;6:1.
94. Nelkin D, Tancredi L. Dangerous diagnostics: The social power of biological information. New York: Basic Books, 1989.

LESLIE R. SCHOVER
DROGO K. MONTAGUE
WENDY S. SCHAIN

SECTION 3

Sexual Problems

Sexual rehabilitation is an important aspect of restoring the quality of life to men and women who survive cancer treatment. Despite the attention to sexuality in our society, most cancer patients remain poorly informed about the impact of their disease and its treatment on sexual function, and about options available to them to overcome sexual problems related to cancer therapy. In the last 20 years we have seen important advances in our knowledge of the mechanisms of sexual function and how it may be impaired by cancer treatment. We also have evaluated treatment strategies in both the medical and psychological realms. However, this broader research base has had only a minimal impact on the counseling of cancer patients in clinical settings. The challenge of the 1990s is to implement sexual rehabilitation programs that are practical, economical, and effective.

The concept of sexual rehabilitation used in this chapter is not restricted to restoring firmer erections or overcoming dyspareunia, although these are common goals of treatment after cancer therapy. We also define sexual rehabilitation as remediation of the emotional impact of cancer diagnosis and treatment on body image, relationship satisfaction, and reproductive capacity.

Cancer treatments may damage one or more phases of the sexual response by affecting attitudes and emotions, central or peripheral components of the nervous system, the pelvic vascular system, and the hypothalamic-pituitary-gonadal axis. Sexual dysfunctions can be classified according to the phases of the sexual response cycle: desire, arousal, and orgasm.[1] It is very rarely a malignancy itself that interferes with sexual function, but rather the therapy needed to eradicate cancer that is the culprit. Not only does each treatment have its own peculiar impact on the various substrates of sexual function, but given that most types of cancer occur more often with age, many patients have a previous history of medical factors that could interfere with arousal or orgasm.

Clinicians need a clear idea of the types of problems to expect after specific cancer therapies. It is of limited value to study or make generalizations about groups of patients with the same diagnosis but different treatments (*i.e.*, gynecologic cancer survivors, or men with prostate cancer).[2] Thus, we will review the known impact of a variety of cancer treatments on sexual function.

PSYCHOLOGICAL IMPACT OF CANCER ON SEXUAL FUNCTION

In examining the impact of cancer treatment on sexual function, one must be aware of the general psychological effect of receiving a diagnosis of cancer as well as the more specific physiologic impairments related to certain types of cancer therapy. The diagnosis of cancer has traditionally been a source of terror and stigmatization. Cancer patients were viewed as unclean and marked for death. Although a very large change in these attitudes has occurred in the United States in this century, some men and women still regard cancer as a disease that renders them untouchable. Occasionally the spouse is the one who has these beliefs. A cessation of sexual activity because of a phobia about venereal contagion of cancer is seen more often in patients who are less educated and come from a rural or traditional ethnic background. Another common belief is that because sex is sinful and unclean, staying sexually active would interfere with cancer treatment. Some patients believe that the cancer is a punishment for some past sex-related behavior, such as having had an affair, sex with a prostitute, or an abortion. Obviously those who feel a high degree of sexual guilt are more likely to become celibate after a cancer diagnosis.

Cancer can also change a person's concept of his or her sexual attractiveness. Sometimes a very visible change results from treatment, such as loss of a nose or facial scarring from basal cell carcinoma. Other changes, such as a mastectomy or urostomy, are invisible to a casual observer but will be seen by the sexual partner. This creates dilemmas not only for married couples about whether to be open about nudity or try to conceal the change, but for single people about when to disclose the history of cancer treatment to a potential mate.[3] During chemotherapy, alopecia, pallor, skin changes, and weight changes are visible. Afterwards the patient may regain a physical appearance almost identical to that before the cancer treatment, but the experience of stigmatization lingers and can interfere with feeling sexually attractive. For example, about a quarter of long-term survivors of testicular cancer in one survey felt less attractive than before their illness.[4]

Affective disorders are increased in prevalence in cancer patients, although the prevalence depends on the type of assessment used.[5–7] In a study of sexual rehabilitation cases in a cancer center, low sexual desire was more common in men and women who were depressed and coping poorly with their cancer.[8] Several studies suggest that younger men and women who go through cancer treatment are more apt to be psychologically distressed, probably because they suffer more disruption of daily life goals, such as establishing a committed relationship, child-bearing, parenting, and advancing in their careers.[7,8] Clinical experience suggests that younger patients are also more apt to express distress over sexual dysfunction related to cancer treatment.

Cancer treatment does not result in an increased rate of divorce for adult patients.[9] Several studies suggest that the diagnosis does not produce marital distress in happy couples but may exacerbate conflict in couples already having problems. Sexual dysfunction and marital unhappiness tend to occur in tandem.[10–13] Some problems are related to disruption of traditional gender roles. For example, expression of nonsexual affection decreases more in couples in which the woman is the cancer patient.[8] This may be viewed as a result of the roles that society assigns to men and women. Women are socialized to be nurturant, and thus may feel quite competent to deal with an ill spouse. Men often feel helpless when faced with the disease, however, because there is little they can do to alleviate the wife's physical pain or fear, and they are often not skilled in providing emotional support. For both men and women, having a spouse go through cancer surgery produces significant psychological distress.[8,14] When a man has cancer, loss of sexual function and earning power are two events he often sees as a symbolic loss of masculinity.[15]

For younger, childless men, infertility after chemotherapy or radiation therapy also can cause long-term distress.[16] Unfortunately, many of these men do not take advantage of opportunities for sperm banking because they refuse to believe that their cancer treatment can really damage their fertility.[17] In young women survivors, not only is infertility a problem, but many fear that pregnancy could promote a cancer recurrence, especially those who had a hormone-sensitive breast cancer.[18] Current evidence suggests, however, that pregnancy at diagnosis of early-stage breast cancer or after successful local treatment does not affect disease-free survival in node-negative women.[19–21]

A problem that has both psychological and physiologic elements is loss of sexual desire during the debilitation of cancer treatment. Often chronic fatigue, nausea, or specific pain interfere with well-being. For most men and women, the energy level improves and pain decreases after cancer therapy is over. It is often at that time that they request help for a sexual problem that has become more salient as other areas of life are brought under control.

PHYSIOLOGIC IMPACT OF SYSTEMIC THERAPIES

Little research has been done on the impact of various systemic cancer therapies on sexual function. This section reviews what is known about sexual side effects of hormonal, chemotherapeutic, and biologic response modifiers.

HORMONAL THERAPY IN MEN

Men with metastatic prostate cancer typically receive hormonal regimens designed to reduce their amount of circulating serum testosterone. With the advent of luteinizing hormone-releasing hormone (LHRH) agonists such as buserelin or goserelin, the use of estrogenic compounds has decreased. The LHRH-agonist drugs do not have the estrogenic side effects of gynecomastia or cardiovascular toxicity.[22] Some men still prefer surgical orchiectomy, however, to avoid the expense or inconvenience of taking medication.[23] Although one might hypothesize that bilateral orchiectomy would impair sexual function because of a poor body image, one small case series found no difference in sexual function in men treated with surgery versus medication.[24] No evidence exists to suggest the superiority of one particular hormonal modality in preserving sexual function. All have the effect of reducing serum testosterone to prepubertal levels.

The typical dysfunctions related to hormonal therapy include a severe reduction in spontaneous desire for sex, difficulty getting subjectively aroused, difficulty achieving and maintaining rigid erections, and difficulty achieving orgasm. Men who can reach orgasm typically note reduced semen volume and sometimes decreased intensity of orgasmic pleasure.[25] It is also clear, however, that perhaps 15% to 20% of men can function quite normally after hormonal therapy has reduced serum testosterone levels to near zero.[22] This is true even in men treated with either orchiectomy or an LHRH-agonist plus the anti-androgen flutamide.[24] From clinical experience, men who maintain good sexual function are almost always under age 65. Some men cannot achieve good erections but have sufficient desire and arousability that they wish to have treatment to promote erectile rigidity.

The physician should avoid the word *castration* in educating patients about hormonal therapy, and should encourage positive expectations about maintaining sexual activity if desired.

HORMONAL THERAPY IN WOMEN

Women with breast cancer, and to a lesser extent those with endometrial cancer, face two issues related to hormonal therapy. The first is that they have traditionally been told not to risk using estrogens for postmenopausal hormonal replacement. The second is that many women with estrogen-receptor-positive disease are offered antiestrogen therapy, usually with tamoxifen.

Data increasingly demonstrate that women who take postmenopausal estrogen replacement live longer.[26,27] One factor is reduced risk of cardiovascular disease because of the beneficial effect of estrogen on lipid levels. Women who take estrogens also are less likely to have osteoporosis, with its increased risk of fatalities from complications of hip fractures. Without estrogen replacement, postmenopausal women may develop dyspareunia related to vaginal atrophy. Changes include decreased vaginal blood supply, less elasticity of the vaginal walls, decreased lubrication, and thinning of the mucosa. Although there have been conflicting epidemiologic studies, a recent review suggests that conjugated estrogens taken in a daily dose of 0.625 mg or less do not increase a woman's relative risk of breast cancer.[27] In another recent, large prospective study, women who used estrogen replacement therapy actually had reduced mortality from breast cancer compared with women who took no hormones.[26] Because of the known benefits of postmenopausal estrogen replacement, the American College of Obstetricians and Gynecologists recently stated that some clinicians may consider postmenopausal estrogen replacement for breast-cancer survivors who appear free of disease. The decision must be made on the basis of individual risks and benefits, the woman's informed consent must be elicited, and her oncologist must be informed.[28]

Tamoxifen has both estrogenic and antiestrogenic effects on different tissues.[29,30] While it can inhibit the growth of estrogen-receptor-positive breast-cancer cells, tamoxifen may actually produce estrogenic changes in the vaginal mucosa of postmenopausal women.[29,30] The impact of tamoxifen in exacerbating or alleviating symptomatic vaginal atrophy is unknown. Some women report increased hot flashes while on the drug.[30] Tamoxifen seems to prevent bone loss and lowers total serum cholesterol in women, making it a possible alternative to estrogens in breast-cancer survivors for long-term prevention of cardiovascular disease and osteoporosis.

CHEMOTHERAPY IN MEN

Although the toxic effects of chemotherapy on spermatogenesis are well known, recent evidence suggests that many men also develop dysfunction in the testicular Leydig's cells that produce testosterone.[31] Elevations in luteinizing hormone (LH) and decreases in total and free serum testosterone, as well as excessive rises in LH after LHRH stimulation, have been observed. It is unclear how often this translates into sexual dysfunction, but hypogonadal states are not uncommon in young men who survive treatment with combination chemotherapy.[31–33] In men with testicular cancer, low testosterone levels may also reflect congenital abnormalities in the remaining testicle.[34] Treatment with long-acting injectable forms of replacement testosterone can often alleviate loss of sexual desire or erectile dysfunction in these patients. In a pilot study of 46 men who had survived bone-marrow transplants for hematologic malignancies, both endocrine and autonomic nervous system abnormalities were predictive of sexual dysfunction.[33] Patients' psychological adjustment and the presence of graft versus host disease were also related to sexual variables.

Some chemotherapy drugs cause autonomic or sensory neuropathies, another possible mechanism for sexual dysfunction. No data are available on the association of autonomic neuropathy with erectile dysfunction after chemotherapy, but failure of the initial, emission phase of the male orgasm after chemotherapy has been observed.[34,35] Emission is mediated by short adrenergic neurons and involves contractions of the prostate and seminal vesicles, with simultaneous closure of the bladder neck. These men have dry orgasms, with pleasurable sensation and the striated muscle contractions of ejaculation, the second phase of orgasm, but no semen.

It is difficult to find case series detailing the sexual function of men treated with chemotherapy alone. The data available include men who also received radiation therapy or in some cases surgery. Nevertheless, it is helpful to look at the prevalence of sexual problems in men surviving treatment for hematologic, lymphatic, or testicular malignancies. In 60 men treated for Hodgkin's disease, sexual function was significantly worse than in a group of matched, healthy controls.[36] Eighteen percent of men reported a distinct worsening of sexual function after cancer therapy. In a group of men who had bone-marrow transplants, reports of sexual problems increased from 22% of the sample to 48% after cancer treatment.[33] The most common dysfunctions were low sexual desire, erectile dysfunction, and dry orgasm. In men treated for testicular cancer, including both studies of men with seminoma and nonseminomatous tumors, rates of low sexual desire ranged from 4% to 12%, erectile dysfunction from 9% to 15%, and difficulty reaching orgasm from 6% to 10%. About 20% of men reported engaging in sexual activity very infrequently or not at all. Diminished pleasure with orgasm is also a common complaint. Across studies, sexual dysfunction has been associated with more emotional distress and marital unhappiness, although causal relations could not be addressed in cross-sectional designs.[4,11–13,35]

Information is sparse on sexual function in patients given biologic response modifiers. There is one report that men treated with interferon-α for hairy cell leukemia had no unusual sexual problems.[37]

CHEMOTHERAPY IN WOMEN

Even less is known about the prevalence of sexual dysfunction in women after chemotherapy. Clinicians are increasingly concerned about measuring quality-of-life issues, hoping to determine the cost-benefit ratio for giving adjuvant chemotherapy, for example, in node-negative women with breast cancer.[38] As in men, alkylating agents seem to be the most damaging to the female gonads.[31] In premenopausal women receiving combination chemotherapy, those who are over age 30 are more apt to cease menstruating and less apt to resume menses after treatment. Even in younger women who recover menstrual cycles, permanent menopause tends to occur prematurely.[31,39,40] Because androgens are the hormones that promote sexual desire in women, it would be helpful to know what happens to ovarian androgen production after chemotherapy.[41,42] This issue has not been addressed. Loss of sexual desire is quite common clinically during extended chemotherapy treatment and afterwards.[26–28] It is unknown whether this represents psychological distress, impaired body image, or actual hormonal changes.

In addition to the typical symptoms of premature menopause, including severe vaginal dryness and loss of elasticity and vulnerability to urinary tract infections, women receiving drugs that cause stomatitis often report periodic vaginal irritation during courses of chemotherapy.[39,40] This exacerbates problems of dyspareunia. Monilial infections are also common, perhaps because of changes in vaginal pH related to premature menopause. Women who have viral sexually transmitted diseases, such as genital herpes or human papillomavirus, may have florid recurrences because of being immunosuppressed.

PHYSIOLOGIC IMPACT OF LOCAL THERAPIES

RADIATION THERAPY IN MEN

Radiation therapy can impair sexual function if treatment fields include the pelvis, or when gonadal or genital tissue receives radiation scatter from an adjacent field. In rare cases, the testes may receive enough radiation to damage Leydig's cell function, for example when testicular relapse of acute lymphocytic leukemia in pubertal boys was treated with a 2400-rad dose directly to the testes.[31] Circulating testosterone values have also been observed to decline temporarily after external-beam irradiation for prostate cancer, with full recovery to normal levels by 6-month follow-up.[43] During this period, men may experience a loss of sexual desire or have difficulty achieving erection, but such problems should be transient.

More controversy exists about the prevalence of permanent loss of erectile capacity after definitive external-beam irradiation to the pelvis for prostate cancer. Reported rates of erectile dysfunction have varied from 22% to 84%.[44] Unfortunately, most case series have been studied retrospectively. Because men with prostate cancer are typically elderly and have complex medical histories, many already have erectile dysfunction unrelated to their cancer diagnosis.[45,46] Goldstein has theorized that the fibrotic process taking place after radiation therapy accelerates existing pelvic arteriosclerosis or causes new stenoses in the arterial system necessary for erection.[44] In a retrospective case series, he and his colleagues found evidence of reduced arterial flow to the penis after pelvic irradiation for prostate cancer. One small prospective case series has not confirmed their findings, however.[47] Furthermore, the measure they used of vascular integrity has since been largely discredited.[48] One repeated finding is that men with excellent health and sexual function have a low rate of new erectile dysfunction after radiation therapy for prostate cancer, whereas those with barely adequate sexual function and risk factors for cardiovascular disease are more likely to develop severe impairments.[44,45] In one prospective study of 85 men, at 8 to 12 months after radiation therapy only 27% of those with unequivocally normal pretreatment sexual function had developed erection problems, versus 54% of the men who reported only "borderline" erectile rigidity and coital frequency before prostate cancer.[49] It would be helpful to have longer-term follow-up, however, because the vascular effects of posttreatment fibrosis may manifest themselves gradually, beginning at 6 to 12 months after treatment.

Other elements of sexual function may also be affected by external-beam irradiation for prostate cancer. Toward the end of the course of treatment, men often experience dysuria and gastrointestinal complications. Not only do these problems temporarily interfere with sexual desire, but urethral irritation can cause pain at ejaculation. These are usually transient symptoms, but the destruction of the prostate and seminal vesicles also leads to a permanent decline in semen volume at ejaculation. Many men notice only a few drops of semen or have completely dry orgasms.

Similar side effects on sexual function may be seen after radiation therapy for testicular cancer, but are less prevalent. The dose of radiation to the pelvic area is lower, but three retrospective surveys of testicular cancer patients suggest that men who received radiation therapy to the pelvis and retroperitoneum had increased rates of erectile dysfunction.[12,13,35] Men whose only cancer treatment was radiation therapy for seminoma also often reported decreases in semen volume.[13]

In the case of noninvasive penile cancer, interstitial irradiation can sometimes be used as definitive treatment, with preservation of the penis. The incidence of long-term side effects, such as radiation ulcers or fibrosis, that could interfere with functional erections is unknown.[50]

RADIATION THERAPY IN WOMEN

Pelvic irradiation in women produces sexual dysfunction through two mechanisms. One is the destruction of ovarian function, producing premature menopause in younger women. The prevalence of amenorrhea increases with doses over 150 rad. Although attempts have been made to shield the ovaries in women with Hodgkin's disease by moving them to the pelvic midline behind the uterus, results have been mixed.[31] As with chemotherapy, women under age 30 have more chance of regaining menses or perhaps having a successful pregnancy than do women over 30 treated with pelvic radiation therapy. In young adult women, a dose of 600 to 1000 rad to the ovaries will permanently destroy their function.[40] As with chemotherapy, researchers have not addressed the question of whether ovaries damaged by irradiation still produce androgens.

In addition to the effects of estrogen deprivation on the vagina and vulva, irradiation permanently damages the basal layer of vaginal epithelium, the endothelium of small vessels in the genital area, and the fibroblasts of the connective tissues in the subepithelium.[51] The net result is a gradual process of fibrosis that may continue for several years after treatment. After definitive external-beam plus intracavitary irradiation for cervical cancer, most women have some stenosis of the upper vagina.[51] In some women, fibrosis of the vaginal walls is severe enough to cause dyspareunia. Other common changes include pallor and thinning of the vaginal mucosa. Less lubrication is produced and intercourse may cause small lacerations, experienced as postcoital bleeding and irritation. A few women develop vaginal ulcers that can take months to heal. For the first several months after radiation therapy, the irritated vagina is in danger of agglutination or of developing tight, fibrous bands of scar tissue unless the woman continues to have sexual activity or uses a vaginal dilator to stretch the tissue several times a week.[52] Although estrogen replacement therapy has less effect on the irradiated vagina, it can relieve dyspareunia in some women.[53]

Few case series are available of women treated with irradiation alone.[51] Most gynecologic cancer patients studied have had a combination of surgery and irradiation, making it difficult to isolate the impact of one specific treatment on sexual function.[2,52] One study of women with early-stage cervical cancer randomized subjects to receive either definitive irradiation or radical hysterectomy.[54] Comparable and mild levels of sexual dysfunction were found in both groups at 6-month follow-up. A more recent case series compared 26 women treated with radical hysterectomy alone to 23 who underwent radiation therapy.[10] Sexual function in the two groups was equivalent when they were interviewed before treatment and at 6 months posttreatment. By 1-year follow-up however, women who had undergone radiation therapy had decreased sexual desire (27% versus 22% for the hysterectomy group), more arousal phase problems (29% versus 6%), and more dyspareunia (22% versus 0%). Their reports of painful intercourse correlated with gynecologists' ratings of the vaginal mucosa, vaginal size, and pain during pelvic examination. Despite conventional wisdom that women need a vaginal lubricant to have comfortable intercourse after pelvic irradiation, only about a quarter of the women reported a need for a lubricant by the 1-year mark. Compliance in using vaginal dilators was quite poor, despite sexual counseling given to each woman.

RADICAL PELVIC SURGERY IN MEN

Men have dreaded the possibility of radical pelvic cancer surgery because of the high rate of resultant erectile dysfunction. In recent years the work of Walsh and colleagues has elucidated the mechanism of erectile failure. The autonomic nerves of the prostatic plexus had been damaged by the removal of organs centrally located in the pelvis (the prostate, seminal vesicles, bladder, or rectum).[55] A method of sparing the prostatic nerve plexus was devised and applied to radical prostatectomy, radical cystectomy, and abdominoperineal resection.

When radical prostatectomy (removal of the prostate and seminal vesicles) was performed in the traditional manner, only about 10% of men recovered erections with normal rigidity. Using nerve-sparing procedures, Walsh reported a recovery rate of 74% when both neurovascular bundles are preserved and 69% with higher-stage tumors when only one bundle is left intact.[55] Recovery of erectile rigidity is gradual, taking a year or more for many men. The most recent and extensive case series from Johns Hopkins confirms earlier findings that men under age 50, those in whom both neurovascular bundles can be spared, and those with lower-stage tumors are more likely to recover functional erections.[56] Controversy remains, however. Other surgeons have not reported these success rates, although nerve-sparing certainly represents an advantage over conventional techniques.[57] Although two large case series suggested that nerve-sparing did not compromise surgical margins, a recent report questioned the efficacy of nerve-sparing prostatectomy either in preserving erectile capacity or in achieving good surgical margins in men with bulky clinical stage B2 tumors.[55,57,58] In a sample of 77 men, only 32% had clear margins and preserved potency.

Another troublesome issue is the definition used of potency. All of these studies use the criterion that the erection is firm enough to allow vaginal penetration and orgasm. Unfortunately, most men who ask for help for erectile dysfunction fit this definition. Most men do have partial erections after radical cancer surgery, and these can be sufficient for penetration with some difficulty and thrusting to the point of orgasm.[56,59] Nevertheless, the erection may not be fully rigid, so the ability to use different coital positions and produce pleasure for the woman are still unsatisfactory. When Walsh and colleagues assessed the quality of erections in finer detail in a group of men with preservation of only one neurovascular bundle, 69% met their usual criteria for potency, but only 32% described erections of normal rigidity.[60] This point is important, because men with nonrigid erections may wish further sexual rehabilitation, ending up in very much the same category as men with partial erections after traditional radical prostatectomy.

The surgeon often focuses exclusively on erectile function in discussing sexuality with a patient undergoing radical prostatectomy. It is important to inform men that desire for sex should not be impaired by surgery, because hormonal production is not altered. Sensation on the genital skin also remains normal, because the sensory nerves that innervate the genitals course along the pelvic sidewalls, where they are protected by fascia and are not in the surgical field. Because these same nerves control the striated muscle contractions of ejaculation and afferent impulses to the brain during orgasm, men can reach orgasm after radical prostatectomy, although without any ejaculation of semen, given the absence of the prostate and seminal vesicles. Many men have no idea that orgasm is possible without a firm erection and without semen. Thus, they make no attempt to resume sexual activity after radical prostatectomy, even though pleasure and orgasm from manual or oral stimulation are still options.

A few men (6% in one recent series) also suffer urinary incontinence after radical prostatectomy.[61] Seepage of urine during sexual activity may be embarrassing, although use of a condom can help.

Radical cystectomy includes not only removal of the prostate and seminal vesicles, but also the urinary bladder. In most cases only the prostatic urethra is removed, but complete urethrectomy is done if there is a risk of tumor extension to the urethral mucosa. As with radical prostatectomy, a pelvic lymphadenectomy is also part of the standard procedure. Urinary diversion may be done with an ileal conduit or more recently with alternate procedures to create a continent urinary reservoir.[62,63] Quality of life, including resumption of sexual activity, has been reported to be superior with a continent urinary diversion.[62] It is difficult to compare patient groups, however, because those who choose the longer surgery and risk of complications to have a continent diversion are often younger and more active than those who choose an ileal conduit.

Before the advent of the nerve-sparing procedure, 73 consecutive men were assessed before and at least 6 months after radical cystectomy with ileal conduit diversion.[59] Before surgery, 20% of the men were sexually inactive and 35% had at least mild erection problems. After surgery these rates increased to 50% and 91%, respectively. Men were more likely to have achieved orgasm after surgery if they had tried sexual activity more often and had recovered fuller erections. About half of the men who were orgasmic reported a reduction in the intensity of their pleasure. Treatment with preoperative pelvic irradiation or with complete urethrectomy did not have measurable additional impact on sexual function. Some reports suggest, however, that complete urethrectomy may further damage the autonomic nerves that control blood flow to the penis.[64] Two European studies also found some evidence that penile blood flow may be reduced after radical cystectomy because of intraoperative arterial ligation.[65,66]

Walsh and colleagues reported an 83% recovery of erections in men who had nerve-sparing radical cystectomy, dropping to 40% in men who had a subsequent complete urethrectomy.[55] Subsequently they reported a 71% rate of potency after cystectomy with ileocolic bladder reconstruction. They noted, however, that their patients were younger than most men undergoing radical cystectomy.[63] Although Walsh's group found that nerve-sparing did not compromise surgical margins, others warn that a nerve-sparing cystectomy may leave behind lymph nodes that are often the first site of metastatic disease in bladder cancer, compromising the completeness of surgery.[63,67]

Walsh has also suggested that nerve-sparing techniques should be applied to abdominoperineal resection.[55] He suggests that injury to nerves may be avoided with better recognition of the anatomy, not only of the prostatic plexus, but of the sacral nerve roots, the pelvic plexus, the neurovascular bundles in the perineum, and the hypogastric nerves in the retroperitoneum that mediate the emission phase of male orgasm. Sparing the prostatic nerve plexus may be most applicable to smaller, lower-stage tumors, however.[68]

After standard abdominoperineal resection, rates of erectile dysfunction have been reported from 15% to 80% in various case series.[68–76] Tumor stage does not predict recovery of erections, but as with other radical pelvic operations, younger men are more likely to recover fully.[68,70,72,73] Poor specification of the severity of erection problems in these studies makes it difficult to compare findings from different centers. Patients who underwent low anterior resection had a lower incidence of postoperative erectile dysfunction than those who had abdominoperineal resection.[69,71,77] For example, La Monica and colleagues reported a 55% rate of erection problems after abdominoperineal resection, compared with 20% after low anterior resection.[71] In another case series the respective rates were 67% and 30%.[74] Procedures that merely preserve the anal sphincter are not as successful in preventing erectile dysfunction, perhaps because the prostatic nerve plexus is often injured during surgery at that level.[72] Very low anterior resection may also damage the prostatic plexus.[68]

Impaired emission is also common after abdominoperineal resection because of dissection in the presacral area or between the seminal vesicles and rectum.[68,75] The prevalence of dry orgasm after surgery is unclear, because most published case series confuse failure of emission with inability to reach orgasm at all, or omit assessment of orgasm phase dysfunctions completely, focusing only on erectile capacity. Sympathetic nerve plexi involved in emission also are damaged during node dissections for tumors of the sigmoid colon. The incidence of dry orgasm increases with the extent of the dissection.[78] Although men who have dry orgasm still experience intense pleasure and have ejaculatory contractions of the bulbocavernosus muscles, they will need infertility treatment to have any hope of fathering a child.[79,80] Men in their reproductive years should consider sperm-banking before surgery.

Another surgical procedure that impairs the neurologic control of emission is retroperitoneal lymphadenectomy (RLND), performed to diagnose metastases from nonseminomatous testicular tumors. The standard bilateral node dissection usually damages sympathetic ganglia that send input to the short adrenergic neurons stimulating contractions of the prostate and seminal vesicles during emission.[12,81] This adrenergic system also mediates closure of the bladder neck at emission, so that dry orgasm after RLND sometimes is caused by simple retrograde ejaculation related to failure of the internal sphincter, and sometimes represents a more profound failure of the smooth muscle contractions of emission. The simplest way to differentiate the two patterns is to test for fructose and spermatozoa in urine voided after orgasm.[82]

Only two case series report detailed information on sexual function in a large sample of survivors of RLND who did not have additional chemotherapy or radiation therapy.[12,82] In one group of 47 men, only 38% consistently had dry orgasm.[12] In the other sample of 63 men, 85% had dry orgasm.[82] This discrepancy may represent different surgical technique, a shorter follow-up time in the second case series, or a different way of asking about the problem. RLND does not increase the prevalence of erectile dysfunction (seen in 6% of one and 2% of the other sample). Difficulty reaching orgasm was also rare (2% of men), but 24% of the men reported that their orgasms were less intense than before RLND.[12]

To preserve fertility and avoid dry orgasm, RLND has been

modified to spare some of the crucial sympathetic ganglia.[81,83] A recent review of nerve-sparing RLND in 75 patients found all were free of disease at 2 years postdiagnosis and none had dry orgasm.[81] The advent of highly successful combination chemotherapy for nonseminomatous testicular cancer has also led to surveillance programs for men with stage I tumors, avoiding RLND altogether.[84,85] These programs work best with highly motivated men who can travel to a regional center regularly for diagnostic tests, however, and relapse rates remain controversial.[81] Men who undergo RLND and have impaired emission can be treated by sympathomimetic agents to induce antegrade ejaculation of semen.[82,86] Another treatment that has value for some men is electrical stimulation of ejaculation.[87]

Only anecdotal accounts are available of sexual function after less common radical operations, including total pelvic exenteration, partial penectomy, and total penectomy.[25] Total pelvic exenteration is performed occasionally in men with large, localized tumors (for example, prostatic sarcomas). Given the extent of surgery, sparing the prostatic plexus is rarely possible. As with other radical pelvic procedures, however, sexual desire, penile sensation, and the ability to reach orgasm with striated muscle contractions are not impaired. Because most patients are relatively young, they often are interested in options to restore erectile function.

Penectomy is necessary when invasive, localized malignancies are found in the urethra or penis. Most are squamous cell carcinomas. There is growing evidence that cancer of the penis, like squamous cell carcinomas of the cervix, vulva, and anus, is promoted by the human papillomavirus.[88] Partners of men with penile cancer should be screened for evidence of human papillomavirus infection, although the efficacy of treatment of either partner in preventing cervical dysplasia is debatable.[89] Partial penectomy is usually chosen when the penile stump is long enough to allow a man to direct his urinary stream away from his body. After partial penectomy, most men have sufficient penile length and rigidity with erection to penetrate for intercourse. With thrusting, men report reaching a satisfying orgasm, even without the sensitive glans penis. For more proximal tumors, total penectomy is performed, including the creation of a perineal urethrostomy behind the scrotum. Because the internal sphincter is intact, men can control urination. Some men learn to reach orgasm after total penectomy, either through erotic dreams or fantasies, or from caressing the remaining erotically responsive areas.[25,90] Ejaculation of semen occurs through the perineal urethrostomy.

RADICAL PELVIC SURGERY IN WOMEN

As with men, there are several common misconceptions about the destructive impact of radical pelvic cancer surgery on a woman's sexual function. It is also difficult to find case series that assess sexual function in women who have had surgery alone, rather than combined treatment programs including chemotherapy or pelvic irradiation. Enough information exists to give a fairly complete picture, however.

Even having an abnormal Pap smear or experiencing the early symptoms of gynecologic cancer can disrupt sexual function.[91,92] Thus, estimates of changes in sexual function after cancer treatment should be based on recall of sexual function before gynecologic symptoms began to interfere.

Radical hysterectomy is a standard treatment for invasive early-stage cancer of the cervix. It includes removal of the uterus and surrounding ligaments, a pelvic node dissection, and resection of the cervix and upper one third to one half of the vagina. In women under age 40, at least one ovary is usually spared to avoid premature menopause. Some sex researchers have theorized that the cervix and uterus are essential for a woman's ability to have satisfying orgasms during intercourse, although empiric evidence from physiologic studies does not support this view.[93–95] If this were true, women after radical hysterectomy should experience a reduction in the frequency of coital orgasm and the intensity of orgasmic pleasure. One prospective study of women who had cervical conization found no impairment of sexual desire, frequency of activity, or ability to reach orgasm.[96] The percentage of women experiencing impaired sexual function after radical hysterectomy has ranged in several case series from 6% to 42%.[10]

To make sense of these variable results, one needs a large sample of women, studied prospectively and at adequate follow-up intervals using assessment techniques that examine sexual dysfunction in detail.[2,10] Only one case series meets these criteria and reports data for women treated with surgery alone.[10] Twenty-six women were interviewed and filled out questionnaires before radical hysterectomy and at 6 months and 1 year after surgery. No significant changes were observed in women's ability to reach orgasm from masturbation, partner noncoital stimulation, or intercourse. Only one woman felt that her orgasms had become less intense. Women also reported that sexual desire, arousal, and overall satisfaction were maintained at pre-illness levels. Dyspareunia occurred only 10% of the time for women evaluated at 1 year follow-up.

Vaginal sensory thresholds were studied in 26 women treated for cervical cancer.[51] There was some sensory loss at 6 and 12 months after surgery, compared with initial levels or with healthy control women. A good deal of recovery was seen by 2 years, however. Half of the women had also received radiation therapy, so that the impact of surgery alone cannot be assessed.

Only two studies of women treated for endometrial cancer are available, and both include women who had a combination of abdominal hysterectomy and pelvic radiation therapy.[97,98] Women experienced high rates of dyspareunia and decreased vaginal lubrication, as well as impairment in sexual frequency and satisfaction.

In women with invasive bladder cancer, radical cystectomy includes not only removal of the bladder and urethra, but also the uterus, adjacent ligaments, cervix, ovaries, and most of the anterior vaginal wall. The vagina is reconstructed, using the posterior wall to form either a shallower or narrowed vaginal barrel, depending on the approach taken.

Women with bladder cancer tend to be an elderly group, and many are no longer sexually active. Out of 39 consecutive women having radical cystectomy at one institution, only 9 were sexually active at the time of cancer diagnosis.[99] Interviews before and after surgery revealed that all women had severe dyspareunia on first attempting to resume coitus. By at least 6-month follow-up, however, 6 women were having regular sexual intercourse with at most mild pain. All of these women had been orgasmic with intercourse at least 50% of the time before the bladder cancer diagnosis, and continued to be orgasmic at least as often after surgery. No changes occurred in the type of stimulation needed to reach orgasm, and indeed 2 women became more easily orgasmic than in the past. Although 6 women also had pelvic radiation therapy, no additional impact of this treatment was evident in this very small sample.

The use of continent urinary diversions and modifications in surgical technique to spare more of the anterior vaginal wall are current trends that should improve women's sexual recovery after radical cystectomy.

Abdominoperineal resection for rectal cancer sometimes also includes removal of the uterus, cervix, uterine ligaments, ovaries, and posterior vaginal wall. The extent of surgery depends on tumor size and location, as well as the surgeon's preference. Little information has been published on women's sexual function after abdominoperineal resection. In one recent series of 18 women who were all sexually functional by self-report before cancer diagnosis, 78% had loss of sexual desire after surgery, 44% reported decreased overall satisfaction with sex, 34% had dyspareunia, and 6% (1 woman) could no longer achieve coital orgasm.[76] These rates of sexual dysfunction are about as expected. The loss of cushioning of the posterior vagina, as well as pelvic adhesions after surgery are common causes of dyspareunia. As with other pelvic cancer operations, loss of orgasmic capacity would not be expected. The colostomy may also affect a woman's body image and sexual desire.

Total pelvic exenteration is the most radical surgery performed for gynecologic cancer, most commonly locally recurrent cervical cancer. The uterus, tubes, ovaries, cervix, vagina, urethra, bladder, and rectum are excised. Both urinary and bowel diversions are needed. The vulva is usually left intact. The most common method currently of vaginal reconstruction is to use myocutaneous gracilis flaps from the thighs.[100] Although creating a neovagina extends the duration of surgery, it fills the defect created, helping the healing process. A neovagina created with myocutaneous flaps has the advantage of creating cushioned walls, but the vaginal lining consists of normal skin, rather than a mucosa that becomes self-lubricating as occurs with a split-thickness skin graft.[101] Women need to douche regularly to prevent odor from the neovagina, and also need a water-based lubricant for comfortable intercourse. It is unknown how many women learn to experience the sensation of thrusting during intercourse as erotic, but a few have complained that they perceive stimulation of the vaginal walls as coming from the inner thighs instead. When the clitoris is still present, many women continue to have orgasms from noncoital stimulation after total pelvic exenteration.[102,103] Many women do not resume sexual activity after exenteration, even if a vaginal reconstruction is performed.[104–106]

Radical vulvectomy not only removes the most erotically sensitive tissue of a woman's genital area, but often leads to dyspareunia because the vaginal introitus is narrowed by scar tissue and the exposed urethra is vulnerable to irritation. The pelvic lymph node dissection usually done as part of the procedure also usually produces severe lymphedema in the legs, which is both unsightly and uncomfortable. In women with in situ disease, use of wide local excision is superior to radical vulvectomy in preserving sexual function.[107,108] After radical vulvectomy, many women discontinue sexual activity, especially if they are older, or if the woman and her partner receive no sexual counseling.[109,110] Common sexual problems include loss of desire, loss of pleasurable genital sensations, dyspareunia, and difficulty reaching orgasm.[109,111]

The loss of the clitoris is not the major determining factor in whether women continue to be orgasmic after various surgical procedures to treat vulvar cancer, however.[112] A careful prospective study of 10 women undergoing radical vulvar surgery revealed that 50% regained the ability to reach orgasm, although there were elevations in genital sensory thresholds and increases in unpleasant sensations during sex that endured up to 2 years after treatment.[111] The most striking observation was that women's sexual satisfaction and level of activity recovered to pretreatment levels and seemed to depend more on the psychological intimacy of the marital relationship than on physiologic sexual function.

LOCAL TREATMENT FOR BREAST CANCER

A recent finding from two large studies is that women with early-stage breast cancer do not differ from healthy women of similar demographic background in terms of psychiatric disorders, sexual problems, or marital happiness.[113,114] This contradicts the conventional wisdom that the diagnosis of breast cancer and treatment by mastectomy is a permanent disruption of most women's sexual and marital relationships.

With the advent of breast-conservation surgery plus radiation therapy as an effective alternative to mastectomy for stage I or II disease, researchers have compared psychological and sexual adjustment after the two procedures. A recent review of 12 such studies, including four with randomized patient assignment to cancer treatment, reveals that the only consistent difference between treatment groups is a better body image for women with breast conservation.[9] This seemed to be true no matter how body image was measured, whether by standardized scales or by questions about feeling attractive sexually or feeling comfortable with nudity. Breast conservation has no clear advantage in terms of marital satisfaction, frequency of sex, sexual dysfunction, or sexual practices. Studies of breast reconstruction had similar results. One caveat, however, is that most researchers have not assessed the more subtle aspects of sexuality that might differ in women with a conserved or reconstructed breast compared to mastectomized women. These include duration of foreplay, use of breast caressing, erotic pleasure from breast caressing, and partner sexual satisfaction.

TREATMENT FOR PEDIATRIC CANCER

Little information is available about the impact of treatment for pediatric cancer on adult sexual function. Two large series of young adult survivors of childhood cancer reveal that rates of marriage are lower than in the general population.[115,116] In a study of over 2000 cancer survivors and sibling controls, there was no excess divorce rate among the cancer survivors.[116]

Only one research group has studied sexual issues. Twenty-eight young men who survived treatment for leukemia were compared to 25 men who survived other childhood cancers.[117] Overall, the men lagged behind developmental norms in terms of sexual attitudes, interest, and experience. The leukemia survivors were the most impaired, however. Only 32% of the leukemia group, compared with 64% of other survivors, were age-appropriate in their psychosexual development. Eighty-four percent of the mixed survivor group but only 57% of the leukemia group had experienced adolescent masturbation.

As more patients survive to adulthood, we need much better knowledge about the impact of pediatric cancer on sexual function.

ASSESSING SEXUAL FUNCTION IN CANCER PATIENTS

As this chapter illustrates, we now have a good knowledge of the impact of cancer on sexual function. In our work as clinicians and educators, however, it is painfully obvious to us that most men and women treated for cancer are never asked about sexual issues by their medical team. The most common reason clinicians give for not assessing sexuality is time pressure. Not only physicians but medical social workers and oncology nurses often are overwhelmed by the demands of a busy clinic. Complaints about time often mask other common concerns, however. Clinicians fear that discussing sexuality will be awkward or that they will not have remedies to offer for the patient's sexual problems.

We hope that this chapter helps clinicians feel more informed about sexual function and rehabilitation after cancer treatment, and more aware of the importance of these issues to patients. We urge the health-care professional to include one generic question about sex in an initial history or follow-up visit. The question can be prefaced by a statement emphasizing the normalcy of providing sexual health care: "I always ask patients about sexuality as part of a history," or "One aspect of every person's health is sexual health." The actual question should be open-ended, to elicit maximal information. For example, "What impact has your cancer diagnosis had on your sex life?" or "How concerned are you about the sexual side effects of your cancer treatment?" or "How well are you functioning now in your sex life?"

When cancer treatment is likely to cause sexual problems, options for rehabilitation should be mentioned at least briefly at the time of treatment disposition. Many clinicians think that this would be disruptive, and that discussing sex should wait until a follow-up visit. In our experience, however, knowing what to expect and what can be done to treat iatrogenic dysfunctions reduces the patient's anxiety.

It may be practical in a multispecialty setting to designate one trained physician, nurse, psychologist, or social worker as the sexual rehabilitation expert. If the primary physician is willing to invest a few minutes of extra time, however, we estimate that 80% to 90% of patients can benefit from brief sexual advice and information without a specialty consult.

A few patients need more intensive help. The patients at high risk to have significant sexual concerns are often younger and unmarried and may not have finished having children. Other common risk factors are being in a newer relationship or in a marriage that is troubled, with poor communication. Men who have many extramarital affairs often seek help for sexual problems after cancer treatment. The clinician should also be alert for the patient who has a history before the cancer diagnosis of poor psychological coping, sexual or physical abuse as a child, chemical dependency, or sexual dysfunction. High-risk patients should be identified and offered more intensive assessment and counseling.

ASSESSMENT BY INTERVIEW

The interview is the heart of a sexual assessment.[95] In a hospital setting it is important that interviews take place in a private setting, and that the patient can be assured that details of sexual behavior will not be documented in the medical chart. If the patient has a committed relationship, whether heterosexual, homosexual, marital, or cohabiting, we prefer to include both partners in the session. Not only do both partners have a chance to express their perspectives and hear information given by the clinician, but their behavior during the session provides insight into their relationship. If time permits, a few minutes alone with each partner can be added to assess sensitive issues such as masturbation or affairs. The clinician must hold such information in confidence, however.

Assessing General Issues

It is helpful to gain rapport by beginning the interview reviewing nonsexual issues, including the patient's demographic background, reaction to the cancer diagnosis and treatment plan, symptoms of major depression or anxiety, use of alcohol and street drugs, compliance with medical instructions, the quality of the patient's social support, shared leisure activities for the couple, expressions of caring and anger in the relationship, and communication of emotions each partner has about the cancer.

Some useful questions include the following:

1. "How has the illness affected your private time with your partner?" Especially for young couples with children, cancer treatment disrupts the family schedule so that spouses have no time just to sit together and talk, let alone have sex.
2. "Has there been a change in the amount of physical affection you show to each other?" A decrease in sexual activity is often paralleled by declining expressions of love and caring, especially in couples with marital conflict or when the wife is the cancer patient.[8] Even for the terminally ill, touching and intimacy continue to be important.[118]
3. "Every couple disagrees sometimes. If the two of you get angry with each other, how do you each express it?" The stress of cancer can accentuate marital conflict.
4. "Has the cancer diagnosis caused disagreements in the extended family?"
5. "Are you under serious financial stress?" Financial problems related to the illness can contribute to marital and sexual conflict.

Discussion of these issues leads naturally into an assessment of sexuality, as one more facet of the relationship.

Assessing Sexual Function

Questions about sexual function should be detailed and specific. The clinician's comfort in discussing sex will help ease the patient's embarrassment. It is helpful to begin with more general topics, such as:

1. How often does lovemaking occur?
2. Who is the initiator?
3. Does activity include manual or oral genital caresses? Can each partner reach orgasm through noncoital caressing, or only during intercourse? Patients who have tried having orgasms from manual or oral stimulation are more likely to resume sex if cancer treatment impairs erections.[59]
4. Do the partners communicate preferences for touch either verbally or nonverbally during sex? Cancer treatment can interfere with a long-term sexual routine, necessitating more sexual communication and negotiation than usual.
5. How has sex changed since the cancer diagnosis in terms of frequency, variety, and function?

The interviewer can ask about each phase of the response cycle:

1. How often does the patient feel a desire for sex?
2. Can a man get and keep firm erections? If he loses erections, at what point in the lovemaking does this occur?
3. Can a woman produce enough vaginal lubrication for comfort during sexual caressing?
4. Is there pain during sex? Describe the location and quality of the pain.
5. What kinds of stimulation help each partner to reach orgasm?
6. Has the quality of orgasmic pleasure changed?
7. Does the male partner have premature ejaculation?

When a dysfunction is identified, further questions should be asked about whether the onset was sudden or gradual and about the timing of onset in relation to cancer diagnosis and treatment. Other life stresses or medical problems that could have led to sexual dysfunction should not be overlooked. Does the problem occur with all types of sexual stimulation? With all partners? On every occasion? What about response to erotic materials? Does alcohol or drug use (including prescription medications) have an impact on the problem?

Some cancer patients are seropositive for the human immunodeficiency virus (HIV) and thus are at risk for transmitting it to a sexual partner. Others may be of unknown serologic status but have engaged in high-risk behaviors. Currently, any adult who is not in a monogamous relationship with a person known to be seronegative or at very low risk for HIV should be counseled about safer sex practices.[119]

ASSESSMENT BY QUESTIONNAIRE

Asking patients to fill out questionnaires can save valuable clinician time, especially in screening large numbers of patients to identify those with high levels of psychological, marital, or sexual distress. Such patients can then be targeted for more detailed interview assessment. If a screening program is set up, the inventories should be presented to the patient by a member of the health-care team with a rationale, a discussion of confidentiality, and an opportunity for the patient to ask questions or refuse to participate. Table 64–14 lists some questionnaires that we have found particularly useful.

The Sexual History Form is a multiple-choice inventory designed to be used on an item-by-item basis to arrive at a diagnosis of sexual dysfunction.[95] Some researchers who are comparing treatment groups or diagnostic groups prefer inventories with items that cluster into a numeric scale. Such questionnaires have been devised to study sexual function in female cancer patients and in male patients.[2,46]

MEDICAL ASSESSMENT OF MALE DYSFUNCTIONS

Medical assessment of men's sexual problems has focused on identifying the causes of erectile dysfunction. Several specialized examinations are available to evaluate the complex hormonal, vascular, and neurologic impacts of cancer treatment.

History

The evaluation begins with a clear definition of the sexual problem, as discussed above. The interviewer obtains a complete review of systems; past and current medication; surgeries; major injuries; radiation therapy, chemotherapy, angioplasty, or other medical treatments; illicit drug use; and a quantitative estimate of alcohol and tobacco consumption.

Physical Examination

The examiner notes the presence or absence of secondary sex characteristics and gynecomastia. After an abdominal examination, the femoral pulses are palpated. The external genitalia are carefully examined, including palpating the penis to identify plaques or fibrosis. During a rectal examination, anal sphincter tone, bulbocavernosus reflex, and the prostate are checked. The patient's gait is observed. Motor strength, sensation, and deep tendon reflexes in the lower extremities are also assessed.

Laboratory Studies

A complete blood count and screening profile check for occult systemic disorders such as hepatic or renal disease are done.

TABLE 64–14. Questionnaires for Cancer Patients With Sexual Problems

Area of Assessment	*Questionnaire*
Sexual function	Sexual History Form[95]
Marital satisfaction	Dyadic Adjustment Inventory[120]
Psychological distress	Brief Symptom Inventory[121]
Illness-related distress	Psychosocial Adjustment to Illness Scale[122]
Adjustment to cancer	Cancer Rehabilitation Evaluation System[123]

Serum testosterone and prolactin levels are also determined.[124] Some groups of cancer patients are at risk for hormonal abnormalities.[32–34] Because diabetes mellitus is a common cause of male erectile and ejaculatory disorders, a glucose tolerance test should be ordered when there is no other obvious cause for the sexual dysfunction.[125] Thyroid function can be assessed by determining serum thyroxine and thyroid stimulating hormone levels.

Nocturnal Penile Tumescence

Men normally have several erections each night during rapid-eye-movement sleep. When these erections are normal in number, duration, and rigidity, significant vascular, neurologic, or hormonal impairment is rarely a cause for erectile dysfunction during waking sexual activity. If nocturnal erections are impaired, an organic cause of the dysfunction is likely.[126,127] A cost-effective and accurate way to monitor erections during sleep is a Rigiscan home monitor.[128] This is one of the most helpful tests in planning treatment, because a normal study suggests that sexual counseling can be of benefit and obviates the need for further expensive, specialized examinations. An abnormal study, however, is not as definitive, because nocturnal erections can be impaired by sleep disorders, depression, low sexual desire, or the impact of normal aging in men who are still sexually functional.[127,129,130] Indeed, lower norms for rigidity should be used in men over age 60.

Vascular Assessment

Erection is initiated with neurotransmitter changes within the spongy tissue of the corpora cavernosa. Usually, the sinusoidal spaces within the corpora are small because of contraction of cavernosal smooth muscle, mediated by tonic α-adrenergic activation.[131] As an erection begins, neurotransmitter release, mediated by parasympathetic nerves, results in cavernosal smooth muscle relaxation. The sinusoidal spaces enlarge and blood flow into the corpora increases greatly. At the same time, small veins that normally drain the corpora are compressed between the expanding soft tissue and the tunica albuginea, resulting in decreased outflow of blood. At first the penis grows in length and circumference, but as the pressure continues to build within the corpora, the shaft becomes rigid.

Assessment of the arterial and venous hemodynamics of erection has been revolutionized by the discovery that erections can be induced by the injection of vasoactive substances directly into the corpora cavernosa.[48,132] A test penile injection of drugs such as papaverine, phentolamine, prostaglandin E_1, or combinations thereof will produce a firm erection in many men who do not have disease processes in the arterial or venous systems. However, anxiety can override the drugs, producing a false-positive test result in men with psychogenic erectile dysfunction.[133,134]

A further refinement of injection testing is dynamic infusion cavernosometry, in which a test injection is given while a needle with a pressure transducer is placed in the opposite corpus cavernosum. If full erection does not result after 10 to 20 minutes, saline is pumped into the penis briefly to attempt to obtain rigidity. Both the rate of infusion needed to maintain full erection and the intracavernous pressure 30 seconds after the infusion pump is stopped are noted. This evaluation attempts to measure the adequacy of the mechanism of venous occlusion during erection.[134,135] Although using Doppler technology to obtain penile blood pressures in the flaccid penis is no longer considered an adequate diagnostic test, pressures in the cavernosal arteries can be assessed successfully during these dynamic studies. When the cavernosometry is abnormal, the study can be repeated using contrast medium so that venous outflow can be radiographically assessed. Unfortunately, the dynamic cavernosometry procedure is also subject to interference by anxiety. Healthy young men who describe situational erection problems and have very normal Rigiscan studies may appear to have severe venous occlusive dysfunction on cavernosometry.[134]

Another important diagnostic study performed first before and then after intracavernous injection is the duplex ultrasound scan.[48] Changes in arterial circumference and rate of blood flow are an index of the adequacy of arterial supply to the penis.

The utility of these vascular evaluations may be limited in cancer patients. A simple test injection can help determine whether a man is a good candidate for using penile injections at home to obtain erections for sexual activity, although results in the office are often not as good as those in a sexual situation at home. Infusion cavernosometry and duplex ultrasound provide valuable information if vascular surgery is a treatment option, but that is rare in posttreatment cancer patients.

Neurologic Assessment

Unfortunately we still do not have a direct means to assess autonomic nervous system dysfunction that contributes to erectile problems.[136] Tests such as sacral evoked response or dorsal nerve somatosensory evoked potential testing assess only somatic nerve function and are rarely helpful with routine problems. Such tests could perhaps be useful in evaluating sexual function after treatment for tumors of the brain or spinal cord, especially in research studies. Penile sensory thresholds can be measured through either vibratory or electric stimulation tests.[137] Such testing can help assess complaints of loss of erotic penile sensation after cancer treatment.

MEDICAL ASSESSMENT OF FEMALE SEXUAL DYSFUNCTIONS

Methods available to the clinician who wants to determine the cause of a woman's sexual problem are far less sophisticated than the array of tests available for male dysfunctions. The pelvic examination continues to be the mainstay of the evaluation for female sexual problems. In women who are experiencing ovarian failure, indices of vaginal atrophy such as skin elasticity, thickness of pubic hair, fullness of the labia, caliber of the vaginal introitus, color and rugation of the vaginal mucosa, and vaginal depth are important.[138] The physician can use a speculum or fingers to attempt to reproduce pelvic pain that a patient experiences during intercourse.[139] The cause of the pain then becomes more evident.

Clinicians who examine women during systemic chemotherapy should look for an irritated vaginal mucosa. Immunosuppression also leaves a woman vulnerable to florid recurrences of genital herpes or human papillomavirus. The effects of pelvic and vaginal irradiation can include reduced vascularization of the mucosa, vaginal ulcers or stenosis, or more diffuse fibrous changes in the vaginal walls or adnexae.[52] A recently described syndrome of superficial pain and dyspareunia at the vaginal introitus, vulvar vestibulitis, can easily be missed during a routine pelvic examination.[140] Erythematous lesions in the vestibule produce exquisite pain when a cotton swab is touched to the local area. Ulcerations can often be seen on colposcopy. In our experience, vulvar vestibulitis is often triggered after gynecologic procedures such as topical chemotherapy or laser treatment for human papillomavirus.[141]

Researchers have attempted to measure vaginal blood flow, analogous to noninvasive examinations of penile vascular integrity. Unfortunately, such measurements in women must occur during sexual arousal and involve placing an instrument in the vagina. Many women are uncomfortable undergoing erotic stimulation under laboratory conditions. The instruments used also have limited reliability.[94] Neurologic measures of genital reflex arcs in women have also proven unreliable and have no clear correlation with sexual symptoms.[142,143] Sensory thresholds in women can be measured with electric stimulation, however, providing useful information on changes in sensitivity after cancer treatment.[51] Radioimmunoassays to measure serum levels of estradiol, prolactin, thyroid hormones, and follicle-stimulating hormone during amenorrhea or in the first 5 days of a menstrual cycle can help in deciding whether to prescribe replacement hormones for women showing signs of premature menopause after chemotherapy for cancers that are not hormone-sensitive (*e.g.*, leukemia or Hodgkin's disease).[40]

TREATING SEXUAL PROBLEMS IN CANCER PATIENTS

Our biggest challenge is to ensure that cancer patients benefit from the techniques of sexual rehabilitation now available. There is a dearth of outcome research on the effectiveness of such programs. Even in major cancer centers, it is rare to have a specialist in sexual health care on staff. When such a program does exist, our experience is that few physicians refer patients consistently to get help. The first step is to make sexual assessment routine in the clinic and hospital. A clinician within the primary treatment setting should be available to provide brief sexual counseling. The most effective way to present sexual rehabilitation to patients is as part of a more comprehensive program of psychosocial support. Sexuality is just one of the emotional issues facing men and women treated for cancer. It is increasingly obvious that psychological adjustment and supportive relationships are more important determinants of sexual satisfaction than is physiologic functioning.[51,95]

BRIEF SEXUAL COUNSELING

Brief counseling, the backbone of sexual rehabilitation, involves at least a few minutes and more often takes an hour or two. Of patients referred for sexual consultation in a cancer center, 73% were seen once or twice; 16% had three to five sessions.[8] Only a few of the patients who have brief counseling will need medical consultation by a urologist, gynecologist, or specialist in sexual medicine. Such experts should be linked in a referral network, however. Because sexual problems after cancer treatment are usually complex, a combined program of both counseling and medical or surgical intervention is often optimal. Thus, the clinician doing sexual counseling must have good communication and collaboration with the other specialists. They, in turn, should be well versed in treating sexual problems and in the iatrogenic effects of cancer treatment.

Table 64–15 lists the components of brief sexual counseling for cancer patients. Brief counseling has been described in more detail in a previous publication.[95] The American Cancer Society has developed guidebooks for men and women on sexuality and cancer.[144,145] They include diagrams, explanations of the sexual side effects of cancer treatments, and advice on sexual rehabilitation.

INTENSIVE SEX THERAPY

Perhaps 10% to 20% of cancer patients have severe sexual dysfunctions that call for the specialty skills of a trained sex therapist.[95] Indicators for referral to sex therapy include a sexual problem that preceded the cancer and remains a source of distress, sexual issues related to severe marital conflict, a dysfunction that has not responded to brief sexual counseling, or a sexual problem that is just one feature of poor psychological coping. Some patients endure cancer treatments that are so mutilating, such as total pelvic exenteration, total penectomy, radical vulvectomy, or facial disfigurement, that consultation with a mental-health professional trained in sex therapy should be routine during recovery, unless the patient declines.

Formal sex therapy is a short-term, symptom-focused treatment that ideally includes both partners.[146] Patients are assigned tasks between sessions that include sensate focus exercises and learning other sexual techniques found effective in reversing specific dysfunctions. Work on marital communication and individual psychological well-being are often part of treatment. Sex therapy can also enhance the results of medical or surgical rehabilitation, such as breast reconstruction or treatment of organic erectile dysfunction.

TREATING ORGANIC ERECTILE DYSFUNCTION

Most men with erectile dysfunction related to cancer treatment are candidates for one of three treatments: intracavernous injection therapy, a vacuum erection device, or a penile prosthesis. Surgery to improve arterial flow to the penis or to ligate penile veins is rarely appropriate in these patients.[147]

Intracavernous injection of vasoactive drugs to obtain an erection has become a popular method of treatment in recent years.[148] Men are taught how to inject themselves safely with a proper dose of medication just before beginning sexual activity at home. Men with neurologic damage from radical pelvic surgery often can obtain erections with quite low doses of medication.[149] Those with mild to moderate vascular impairment of erection may need larger doses or may be unable to use injections successfully. To be a good candidate for this treatment, a man should have the cognitive ability to learn the injection technique and the manual dexterity to perform the procedure. A committed spouse can also learn to give the injection. The patient should be compliant enough to follow

TABLE 64–15. Elements of Brief Sexual Counseling

Education	Attitude Change
Illustrate genital and pelvic anatomy using models or pictures	Debunk myths on cancer and sex:
Explain the normal sexual response cycle	Venereal contagion of cancer
Explain the impact of specific treatments on sexual function	Cancer as punishment for sins
Give advice on options for sexual rehabilitation:	Resuming sex is unhealthy
Sex therapy	Accept noncoital sex when coitus not possible
Vaginal dilators	Sex cannot always be spontaneous
Hormone replacement	Sex is not just for the young and healthy
Water-based lubricants	**Advice on Resuming Sex**
Vacuum erection device	Either partner can initiate sex
Home penile injections	Increase expression of nonsexual affection
Penile prostheses	Start slowly using sensate focus format[146]
Changes in medication	Discuss how to deal with physical attractiveness (mastectomy, ostomy, and so forth): desensitize to reality vs camouflage
Minimizing Physical Handicaps	**Resolving Couple Conflict**
Time sex to avoid pain and fatigue	Make private time for each other
Learn to cope with ostomy appliance, limb prosthesis, laryngectomy, and so forth	Discuss fears and sadness
Find comfortable positions	Negotiate illness-related changes in marital roles (wage-earner, childcare, budgeting, and so forth)
Female dyspareunia can benefit from lubricants and dilators	Act as team in dealing with conflict in extended family
Erectile dysfunction can be treated appropriately	
Use open sexual communication, verbal and nonverbal	

instructions precisely and to come in for reversal if priapism occurs.

Although priapism is rare at recommended doses, penile fibrosis becomes progressively more frequent with prolonged use of papaverine and phentolamine, the most popular drug combination.[150] In severe cases, fibrosis can cause pain and curvature of erection. Although prostaglandin E_1 has been recommended as a superior drug, a significant minority of men experience prolonged penile pain after using it.[151] In our program, a smaller but still significant rate of fibrosis is also seen with long-term use of prostaglandin E_1.[152] Thus, periodic follow-up examinations are crucial in treating men on intracavernous injection programs. This form of treatment is not ideal for a young man with a long life expectancy, but is often a good alternative to a penile prosthesis in an older patient who does not wish to have elective surgery.

The vacuum erection device (VED), shown in Figure 64–5, has also gained increasing popularity.[153,154] The VED works on a negative pressure principle. Either before starting sexual activity or preferably after obtaining some partial tumescence with foreplay, the man places the VED over his penis and uses a hand pump to create a vacuum around his penis. The vacuum leads to congestion of the spongy tissue of the corpora cavernosa and increased arterial inflow.[154] A constriction band is then transferred from the base of the pump to encircle the base of the erect penis, and the cylindrical pump is removed.

The resulting erection may be larger in circumference than a natural one, but unfortunately is often not firm proximal to the constriction band, so that the penis pivots. This can interfere with thrusting during intercourse. The band is also tight enough to constrict the urethra, resulting in retention of semen and occasional discomfort at orgasm for at least half the men who use the device. Most men can obtain usable erections, however. Over the first few months of use, dropout rates have been reported to be only about 20%.[153,154]

Complications of the VED are minimal. Some men experience bruising or discomfort with the device. It should be used with caution in men with low platelet counts or those on

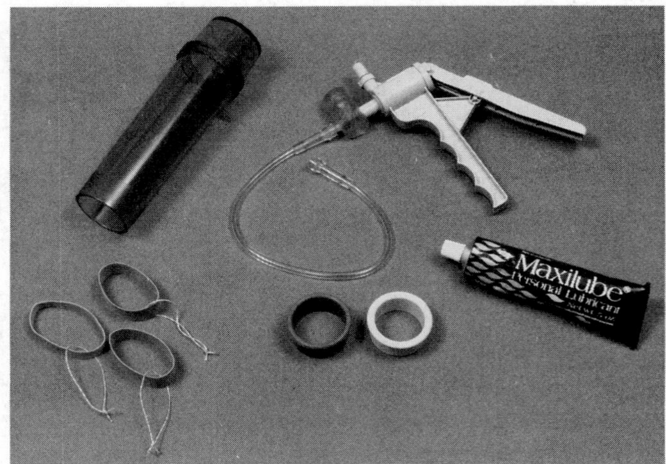

FIGURE 64–5. Vacuum erection device.

anticoagulants. The constriction band should not be used for more than 30 minutes, because penile ischemia can occur with the device.[155] Skin necrosis has been reported in one man with genital hypesthesia.[156] Men who obtain partial tumescence with sexual stimulation tend to have better erections with a VED than do men who no longer have any erectile changes at all.

Implantation of a penile prosthesis has the disadvantage of being potentially irreversible. If the prosthesis malfunctions or is removed, the capacity to have a normal erection may not return. On the other hand, with the improved reliability of prosthetic devices, surgery represents a permanent solution to erectile dysfunction for the vast majority of men who choose it.[157] A penile prosthesis may be the optimal treatment for irreversible erectile dysfunction in a patient with a long life expectancy.

Penile prosthesis surgery is successful in over 95% of cases. Infection around the prosthesis occurs in about 2% to 5% of cases and invariably requires removal of the prosthesis.[158] Later complications are usually mechanical device failures that require surgical revision. Late hematogenous infections of penile prostheses are rare.[159] No data are available on prosthetic complications related to the immunosuppression of cancer treatment, but the experience with organ transplant recipients suggests that the prosthesis is a safe treatment option.[160]

Although prosthesis implantation at the time of pelvic cancer surgery has been advocated, this practice has not gained widespread acceptance.[161] Surgeons are reluctant to prolong the cancer operation or to incur a risk of periprosthetic infection. Because many patients also recover erectile rigidity gradually after nerve-sparing surgery, an optimal time for prosthesis implantation appears to be at least 6 months after cancer surgery.

Prosthesis implantation is often done through a single 2- to 4-cm incision, without removing tissue and with minimal blood loss. Transfusions are rarely necessary. Some surgeons implant prostheses under local anesthesia on an outpatient basis, but more commonly the procedure is done under general or spinal anesthesia with a 1- to 2-day hospital stay.[162]

Three major types of penile prosthesis are most commonly used today: the rod prosthesis, the single-component hydraulic, and the multicomponent inflatable. Device failures are least likely to occur with simple rod prostheses but increase in frequency with increasing device complexity. A malleable prosthesis is one of the most simple, but even when the penis is bent for concealment, it does not look or feel flaccid. The erection obtained is shorter and narrower than a full, natural erection. The single-component hydraulic prosthesis (Fig. 64–6) also produces an erection similar to that with a malleable model, but the flaccid penis appears more natural for concealment.[163] In cancer patients who have had either pelvic irradiation or pelvic surgery, a malleable or single-component hydraulic prosthesis may be optimal, because no abdominal reservoir needs to be placed. The hydraulic type may be superior when repeated cystoscopies will be necessary.

Some men, however, desire the full penile girth and complete concealment of a multicomponent inflatable prosthesis (Fig. 64–7). The newest inflatable prosthesis also allows some elongation of the corpora cavernosa, so that the erect penis is more normal in length.[164] The fluid reservoir of a multicomponent prosthesis is usually implanted in the retropubic space via the penoscrotal incision, using special insertion tools. If the patient has had pelvic surgery or irradiation, however, the surgeon can avoid the risk of bowel injury by placing the reservoir extraperitoneally behind a rectus muscle.[165] A multicomponent inflatable prosthesis can also compensate for some of the loss of penile girth after urethrectomy.

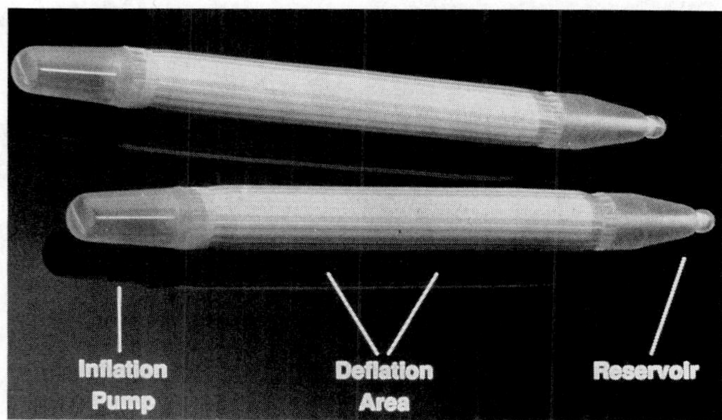

FIGURE 64–6. Single-component hydraulic penile prosthesis.

None of these treatments for erectile dysfunction can directly improve sexual desire, penile sensation, or the ability to reach orgasm, but often the renewed ability to have erections has a positive impact on a man's self-esteem and interest in initiating sex. If intercourse was a man's preferred aspect of sexual activity, the ability to engage in coitus again can improve sexual pleasure and facilitate reaching orgasm. None of these treatments is a cure for premature ejaculation, but that is the one sexual problem that does not increase in prevalence with cancer treatment.[8]

MEDICAL OR SURGICAL INTERVENTIONS FOR WOMEN

In contrast to the specific treatments for men's sexual problems, interventions for women are more closely linked to specific cancer therapies. Breast reconstruction can be considered a type of sexual rehabilitation, although enhancing sexual pleasure is not the primary motivation of most women who choose this surgery. Vaginal reconstructive surgery more

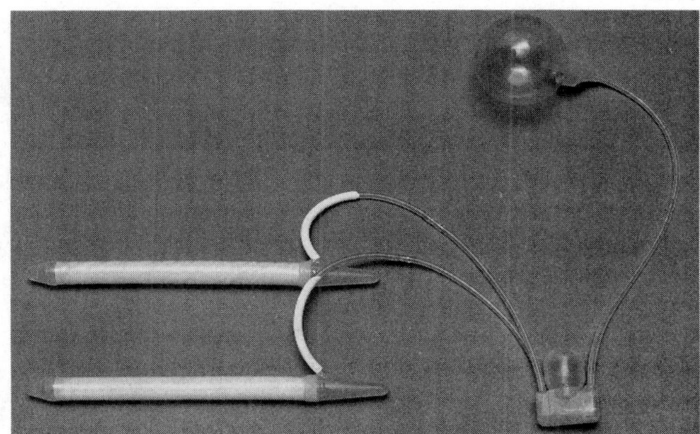

FIGURE 64–7. Multicomponent inflatable penile prosthesis.

closely parallels the penile prosthesis in that it restores the functional capacity for intercourse. After radical vulvectomy, some women need split-thickness skin grafts to repair stenosis of the vaginal introitus. Myocutaneous flap technology has also been used to perform reconstruction of the labia, both for cosmetic appearance and to provide cushioning for the urethra and vaginal entrance.[166]

Women who undergo premature menopause after cancer treatment need medical intervention. Those who do not have hormone-sensitive tumors should definitely be considered for hormonal replacement, given the benefits in preventing cardiovascular disease and osteoporosis, as well as the favorable impact on vaginal lubrication and elasticity.[26] As discussed above, even some women who are long-term survivors of node-negative breast cancer may decide that the benefits of estrogen replacement outweigh the risks.[28]

Women who have dyspareunia after cancer treatment can often benefit from learning exercises to relax the muscles that surround the vaginal entrance.[139] When a woman feels she can contract or relax these muscles at will, she may want to use a series of vaginal dilators of graduated size (Fig. 64–8). The goal of dilation is not usually to stretch the vagina physically, but to give the woman a sense that she can relax the vaginal entrance and accommodate penile penetration without pain. Steps in dilation include inserting the dilator and removing it, inserting it and holding it in the vagina for a few minutes, and being able to move the dilator without pain. Dilator size varies from about the length and thickness of a finger to that of an erect penis. When the woman can use the largest dilator without pain, she can approach penile penetration by gradually tolerating first one and then two fingers in her vagina during lovemaking, and then slowly guiding her partner's penis into her vagina while she stays relaxed in the female-superior position.

Water-based nonprescription lubricants are very helpful, not only in preventing pain with the use of dilators, but also in sexual activity for the woman with chronic vaginal dryness. Gel lubricants include Astroglide and Today Personal Lubricant. Suppositories can be used before sexual activity (Lubrin or Condommate). A vaginal moisturizer, Replens, can be used three times a week to provide more consistent hydration of the vaginal mucosa. Women with persistent superficial dyspareunia should be examined for vulvar vestibulitis, because combined surgery and counseling can often alleviate the pain.[141]

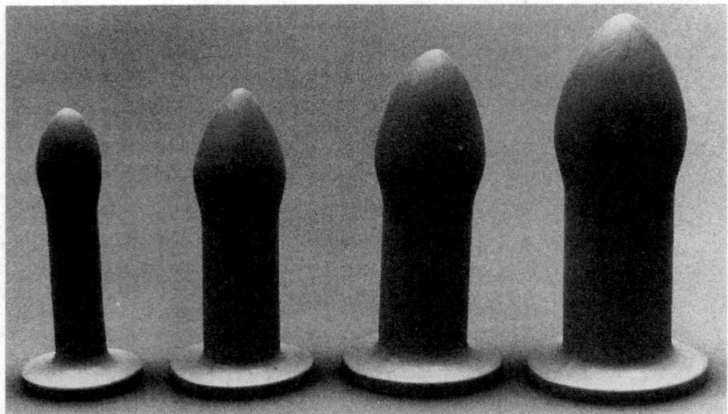

FIGURE 64–8. Graduated sizes of vaginal dilators.

REFERENCES

1. Schover LR, Friedman J, Weiler S, et al. The multiaxial problem-oriented system for sexual dysfunctions. Arch Gen Psychiatry 1982;39:614–619.
2. Andersen BL, Anderson B, deProsse C. Controlled prospective longitudinal study of women with cancer: I. Sexual functioning outcomes. J Consult Clin Psychol 1989;57:683–691.
3. Dackman L. Up front: Sex and the post-mastectomy woman. New York: Penguin Books, 1990.
4. Gritz ER, Wellisch DK, Wang H, et al. Long-term effects of testicular cancer on sexual functioning in married couples. Cancer 1989; 64:1560–1567.
5. Derogatis LR, Morrow GR, Fetting J, et al. The prevalence of psychiatric disorders among cancer patients. JAMA 1983;249:751–757.
6. Bukberg J, Penman D, Holland JC. Depression in hospitalized cancer patients. Psychosom Med 1984;46:199–212.
7. Kathol RG, Mutgi A, Williams J, Clamon G, Noyes R. Diagnosis of major depression in cancer patients according to four sets of criteria. Am J Psychiatry 1990;147:1021–1024.
8. Schover LR, Evans RB, von Eschenbach AC. Sexual rehabilitation in a cancer center: Diagnosis and outcome in 384 consultations. Arch Sex Behav 1987;16:445–461.
9. Schover, LR. The impact of breast cancer on sexuality, body image, and intimate relationships. CA 1991;41:112–120.
10. Schover LR, Fife M, Gershenson DM. Sexual dysfunction and treatment for early stage cervical cancer. Cancer 1989;63:204–212.
11. Rieker PP, Edbril SD, Garnick MB. Curative testis cancer therapy: Psychosocial sequelae. J Clin Oncol 1985;3:1117–1126.
12. Schover LR, von Eschenbach AC. Sexual and marital relationships after treatment for nonseminomatous testicular cancer. Urology 1985;25:251–255.
13. Schover LR, Gonzales M, von Eschenbach AC. Sexual and marital relationships after radiotherapy for seminoma. Urology 1986;27:117–123.
14. Keitel MA, Zevon MA, Rounds JB, Petrelli NJ, Karakousis C. Spouse adjustment to cancer surgery: Distress and coping responses. J Surg Oncol 1990;43:148–153.
15. Liss-Levinson WS. Clinical observations on the emotional responses of males to cancer. Psychother Theory Res Pract 1982;19:325–330.
16. Rieker PP, Fitzgerald EM, Kalish LA. Adaptive behavioral responses to potential infertility among survivors of testis cancer. J Clin Oncol 1990;8:347–355.
17. Cella DF, Najavits L. Letter to the editor: Denial of infertility in patients with Hodgkin's disease. Psychosomatics 1986;27:71.
18. Nugent P, O'Connell TX. Breast cancer and pregnancy. Arch Surg 1985;120:122–124.
19. Knob P. Physical and psychological distress associated with adjuvant chemotherapy in women with breast cancer. J Clin Oncol 1986;4:678–684.
20. Querleu D, Laurent JC, Verhaeghe M. Pregnancy following surgery for cancer of the breast. J Gynecol Obstet Biol Reprod 1986;15:633–639.
21. Riberio G, Jones DA, Jones M. Carcinoma of the breast associated with pregnancy. Br J Surg 1986;73:607–609.
22. Peeling WB. Phase III studies to compare goserelin (Zoladex) with orchiectomy and with diethylstilbestrol in treatment of prostatic carcinoma. Urology (Suppl) 1989;33:45–52.
23. Cassileth BR, Soloway MS, Vogelzang NJ, et al. Patients' choice of treatment in stage D prostate cancer. Urology (Suppl) 1989;33:57–62.
24. Rousseau L, Dupont A, Labrie F, Couture M. Sexuality changes in prostate cancer patients receiving antihormonal therapy combining the antiandrogen flutamide with medical (LHRH agonist) or surgical castration. Arch Sex Beh 1988;17:87–98.
25. Schover LR. Sexuality and fertility in urologic cancer patients. Cancer 1987;60(Suppl):553–558.
26. Henderson BE, Paganini-Hill A, Ross RK. Decreased mortality in users of estrogen replacement therapy. Arch Intern Med 1991;151:75–78.
27. Dupont WD, Page DL. Menopausal estrogen replacement therapy and breast cancer. Arch Intern Med 1991;151:67–72.
28. American College of Obstetricians and Gynecologists. Technical Bulletin 158: Carcinoma of the breast. Washington DC, 1991.
29. Jordan VC. Long-term adjuvant tamoxifen therapy for breast cancer: The prelude to prevention. Cancer Treatment Rev 1990;17:15–36.
30. Love RR. Antiestrogen chemoprevention of breast cancer: Critical issues and research. Prev Med 1991;20:64–78.
31. Gradishar WJ, Schilsky RL. Effects of cancer treatment on the reproductive system. Crit Rev Oncol Hematol 1988;8:153–171.
32. Vigersky RA, Chapman RM, Berenberg J, et al. Testicular dysfunction in untreated Hodgkin's disease. Am J Med 1982;73:482–486.
33. Baruch J, Benjamin S, Treleaven J, et al. Male sexual function following bone marrow transplantation for haematological cancer. Tenth World Congress for Sexology, Amsterdam, 1991.
34. Fossa SD, Klepp O, Molne K, et al. Testicular function after unilateral orchiectomy for cancer and before further treatment. Int J Androl 1982;5:179–184.
35. Nijman JM. Some aspects of sexual and gonadal function in patients with nonseminomatous germ-cell tumor of the testis (dissertation). Groningen, The Netherlands: Drukkerij Van Denderen BV, 1987.
36. Cella DF, Tross S. Psychological adjustment to survival from Hodgkin's disease. J Consult Clin Psychol 1986;54:616–622.
37. Schilsky RL, Davidson HS, Magid D, et al. Gonadal and sexual function in male patients with hairy cell leukemia: Lack of adverse effects of recombinant alpha-2-interferon. Cancer Treat Rep 1987;71:179–181.

38. Gelber RD, Goldhirsch A, Cavalli F, et al. Quality-of-life-adjusted evaluation of adjuvant therapies for operable breast cancer. Ann Int Med 1991;114:621–628.
39. Suttcliffe SB. Clinical problems and their management: Clinical problems in females with lymphoma. In: Proceedings of Workshop on Psychosexual and Reproductive Issues of Cancer Patients. Chicago: American Cancer Society, 1987.
40. Chapman RM. Effect of cytotoxic therapy on sexuality and gonadal function. Semin Oncol 1982;9:84–94.
41. Davidson JM, Myers LS. Endocrine factors in sexual psychophysiology. In: Rosen RC, Beck JG, eds. Patterns of sexual arousal: Psychophysiological processes and clinical applications. New York: Guilford Press, 1988:189–211.
42. Sherwin BB. A comparative analysis of the role of androgen in human male and female sexual behavior: Behavioral specificity, critical thresholds, and sensitivity. Psychobiology 1988;16:416–425.
43. Tomic R, Bergman B, Damber JE, Littbrand B, Lofroth PO. Effects of external radiation therapy for cancer of the prostate on the serum concentrations of testosterone, follicle-stimulating hormone, luteinizing hormone and prolactin. J Urol 1983;130:287–289.
44. Goldstein I, Feldman MI, Deckers PJ, et al. Radiation-associated impotence: A clinical study of its mechanism. JAMA 1984;251:903–910.
45. van Heeringen C, De Schryver A, Verbeek E. Sexual function disorders after local radiotherapy for carcinoma of the prostate. Radiother Oncol 1988;13:47–52.
46. Zinreich ES, Derogatis LR, Herpst J, et al. Pre- and posttreatment evaluation of sexual function in patients with adenocarcinoma of the prostate. Int J Radiat Oncol Biol Phys 1990;19:729–732.
47. Mittal B. A study of penile circulation before and after radiation in patients with prostate cancer and its effect on impotence. Int J Radiat Oncol Biol Phys 1985;11:1121–1125.
48. Lue TF, Abber JC. Penodynamics: Diagnostic studies of vasculogenic impotence. In: Montague DK, ed. Disorders of male sexual function. Chicago: Year Book Medical Publishers, 1988:95–104.
49. Banker FL. The preservation of potency after external beam irradiation for prostate cancer. Int J Radiat Oncol Biol Phys 1988;15:219–220.
50. Schover LR, von Eschenbach AC. Letter to the editor: Sexual rehabilitation of urologic cancer patients. CA 1985;35:319–320
51. Weijmar Schultz WCM, van de Weil HBM. Sexual functioning after gynaecological cancer treatment (dissertation). Groningen, The Netherlands: Drukkerij Van Denderen BV, 1991.
52. Abitbol MM, Davenport JH. The irradiated vagina. Obstet Gynecol 1974;44:249–256.
53. Pitkin RM, van Voorhis LW. Postirradiation vaginitis: An evaluation of prophylaxis with topical estrogen. Ther Radiol 1971;99:417–421.
54. Vincent CE, Vincent B, Griess FC, et al. Some marital-sexual concomitants of carcinoma of the cervix. South Med J 1975;68:552–558.
55. Walsh PC, Schlegel PN. Radical pelvic surgery with preservation of sexual function. Ann Surg 1988;208:391–400.
56. Quinlan DM, Epstein JI, Carter BS, Walsh PC. Sexual function following radical prostatectomy: Influence of preservation of neurovascular bundle. J Urol 1991;145:998–1002.
57. Catalona WJ, Dresner SM. Nerve-sparing radical prostatectomy: Extraprostatic tumor extension and preservation of erectile function. J Urol 1985;134:1149–1151.
58. Bigg SW, Kavoussi LR, Catalona WJ. Role of nerve-sparing radical prostatectomy for clinical stage B2 prostate cancer. J Urol 1990;144:1420–1424.
59. Schover LR, Evans RB, von Eschenbach AC. Sexual rehabilitation and male radical cystectomy. J Urol 1986;136:1015–1017.
60. Walsh PC, Epstein JI, Lowe FC. Potency following radical prostatectomy with wide unilateral excision of the neurovascular bundle. J Urol 1987;138:823–827.
61. Middleton RG, Smith JA, Melzer RB, et al. Patient survival and local recurrence rate following radical prostatectomy for prostatic carcinoma. J Urol 1986;136:422–424.
62. Boyd SD, Feinberg SM, Skinner DG, et al. Quality of life survey of urinary diversion patients: Comparison of ileal conduits versus continent Kock ileal reservoirs. J Urol 1987;138:1386–1389.
63. Marshall FF, Mostwin JL, Radebaugh LC, Walsh PC, Brendler CB. Ileocolic neobladder post-cystectomy: Continence and potency. J Urol 1991;145:502–504.
64. Kitamura T, Moriyama N, Shibamoto K, et al. Urethrectomy is harmful for preserving potency after radical cystectomy. Urol Int 1987;42:375–379.
65. Bergman B, Sivertsson S, Suurkala M. Penile blood pressure in erectile impotence following cystectomy. Scand J Urol Nephrol 1982;16:81–84.
66. Tizzani A, Casetta G, Carone R, et al. Defective erection in patients subjected to radical cystectomy: Diagnosis by Doppler test and stimulated sacral reflex. Minerva Urol Nephrol 1985;37:335–339.
67. Pritchett TR, Schiff WM, Klatt E, Lieskovsky G, Skinner DG. The potency-sparing radical cystectomy: Does it compromise the completeness of the cancer resection? J Urol 1988;140:1400–1403.
68. Santangelo ML, Romano G, Sassaroli C. Sexual function after resection for rectal cancer. Am J Surg 1987;154:502–504.
69. Balslev I, Harling H. Sexual dysfunction following operation of carcinoma of the rectum. Dis Colon Rectum 1983;26:785–788.
70. Danzi M, Ferulano GP, Abate S, et al. Male sexual function after abdominoperineal resection for rectal cancer. Dis Colon Rectum 1983;26:665–668.
71. La Monica G, Audisio RA, Tamburini M, et al. Incidence of sexual dysfunction in male patients treated surgically for rectal malignancy. Dis Colon Rectum 1985;28:937–940.
72. Neal D. The effects on pelvic visceral function of anal-sphincter-ablating and anal-sphincter-preserving operations for cancer of the lower part of the rectum and for benign colorectal disease. Ann R Coll Surg Engl 1984;66:7–13.
73. Kinn C, Ohman V. Bladder and sexual function after surgery for rectal cancer. Dis Colon Rectum 1986;29:43–48.
74. Williams NS, Johnston D. The quality of life after rectal excision for low rectal cancer. Br J Surg 1983;70:460–462.
75. Yeager ES, Van Heerden JA. Sexual dysfunction following proctocolectomy and abdominoperineal resection. Ann Surg 1980;191:169–170.
76. Cirino E, Pepe G, Pepe F, et al. Sexual complications after abdominoperineal resection. Ital J Surg Sci 1987;17:315–318.
77. Hjortrup A, Kirkegaard P, Friis J, et al. Sexual dysfunction after low anterior resection for midrectal cancer. Acta Chir Scand 1984;150:687–688.
78. Tomoda H, Furosawa M. Sexual and urinary dysfunction following surgery for sigmoid colon cancer. Jpn J Surg 1985;15:355–360.
79. Bergman B, Nilsson S, Petersen I. The effect on erection and orgasm of cystectomy, prostatectomy and vesiculectomy for cancer of the bladder: A clinical and electromyographic study. Brit J Urol 1982;51:114–120.
80. Biester RJ, Howards SS. Failure of seminal emission and retrograde ejaculation. In: Tanagho EA, Lue TF, McClure RD, eds. Contemporary management of impotence and infertility. Baltimore: Williams & Wilkins, 1988:285–290.
81. Donohue JP, Foster RS, Rowland RG, et al. Nerve-sparing retroperitoneal lymphadenectomy with preservation of ejaculation. J Urol 1990;144:287–292.
82. Nijman JM. Some aspects of sexual and gonadal function in patients with nonseminomatous germ-cell tumor of the testis (dissertation). Groningen, The Netherlands: Drukkerij Van Denderen BV, 1987.
83. Jewett MAS, Kong YP, Goldberg SD, et al. Retroperitoneal lymphadenectomy for testis tumor with nerve sparing for ejaculation. J Urol 1988;139:1220–1224.
84. Freedman LS, Parkinson MC, Jones WG, et al. Histopathology in the prediction of relapse of patients with stage I testicular teratoma treated by orchidectomy alone. Lancet 1987;2:294–298.
85. Herr HW, Whitmore WF, Sogani PC. Selection of testicular tumor patients for omission of retroperitoneal lymph node dissection. J Urol 1986;135:500–503.
86. Lange PH, Narayan P, Fraley EE. Fertility issues following therapy for testicular cancer. Semin Urol 1984;11:264–274.
87. Ohl DA, Denil J, Bennett CJ, et al. Electroejaculation following retroperitoneal lymphadenectomy. J Urol 1991;145:980–983.
88. Barrasso R, De Brux J, Croissant O, Orth G. High prevalence of papillomavirus-associated penile intraepithelial neoplasia in sexual partners of women with cervical intraepithelial neoplasia. N Engl J Med 1987;317:916–923.
89. Krebs HB, Helmkamp BF. Does the treatment of genital condylomata in men decrease the treatment failure rate of cervical dysplasia in the female sexual partner? Obstet Gynecol 1990;76:660–663.
90. Witkin MH, Kaplan HS. Sex therapy and penectomy. J Sex Marital Ther 1982;8:209–221.
91. Andersen BL, Lachenbruch PA, Anderson B, DeProsse C. Sexual dysfunction and signs of gynecologic cancer. Cancer 1986;57:1880–1886.
92. Campion MJ, Brown JR, McCance DJ, et al. Psychosexual trauma of an abnormal cervical smear. Br J Obstet Gynaecol 1988;95:175–181.
93. Ladas AK, Whipple B, Perry JD. The G spot. New York: Holt, Rinehart & Winston, 1982.
94. Rosen RC, Beck JG. Patterns of sexual arousal: Psychophysiological processes and clinical applications. New York: Guilford Press, 1988.
95. Schover LR, Jensen SB. Sexuality and chronic illness: A comprehensive approach. New York: Guilford Press, 1988.
96. Kilkku P, Gronroos M, Punnonen R. Sexual function after conization of the uterine cervix. Gynecol Oncol 1982;14:209–212.
97. Cochran SD, Hacker NF, Wellisch DK, Berek JS. Sexual functioning after treatment for endometrial cancer. J Psychosoc Oncol 1987;5:57–63.
98. Jenkins B. Patients' reports of sexual changes after treatment for gynecological cancer. Oncol Nursing Forum 1988;15:349–354.
99. Schover LR, von Eschenbach AC. Sexual function and female radical cystectomy: A case series. J Urol 1985;134:465–468.
100. Edwards CL, Loeffler M, Rutledge FN. Vaginal reconstruction. In: von Eschenbach AC, Rodriguez DB, eds. Sexual rehabilitation of the urologic cancer patient. Boston: GK Hall, 1981:251–264.
101. Masters WJ, Johnson VE. Human sexual response. Boston: Little, Brown, 1966.
102. Lamont JA, De Petrillo AD, Sargeant EJ. Psychosexual rehabilitation and exenterative surgery. Gynecol Oncol 1978;6:236–242.
103. Dempsey GM, Buchsbaum HJ, Morrison J. Psychosocial adjustment to pelvic exenteration. Gynecol Oncol 1975;3:325–334.
104. Morley GW, Lindenauer SM, Youngs D. Vaginal reconstruction following pelvic exenteration: Surgical and psychological considerations. Am J Obstet Gynecol 1973;116:996–1002.
105. Vera MI. Quality of life following pelvic exenteration. Gynecol Oncol 1981;12:355–366.
106. Andersen BL, Hacker NF. Psychosexual adjustment following pelvic exenteration. Obstet Gynecol 1983;61:331–338.
107. Disaia PJ, Creasman WT, Rich WM. An alternative approach to early cancer of the vulva. Am J Obstet Gynecol 1979;133:825–832.
108. Andersen BL, Turnquist D, LaPolla J, Turner D. Sexual functioning after treatment of in situ vulvar cancer: Preliminary report. Obstet Gynecol 1988;71:15–19.
109. Andreasson B, Moth J, Jensen SB, Bock JE. Sexual function and somatopsychic reactions in vulvectomy-operated women and their partners. Acta Obstet Gynecol Scand 1986;65:7–10.
110. Stellman RE, Goodwin JM, Robinson J, Dansak D, Hilgers RD. Psychological effects of vulvectomy. Psychosomatics 1984;25:779–783.
111. Weijmar Schultz WCM, van de Wiel HBM, Bouma J, Janssens J, Littlewood J. Psy-

chosexual functioning after the treatment of cancer of the vulva. Cancer 1990;66: 402–407.
112. Andersen BL, Hacker NF. Psychosexual adjustment after vulvar surgery. Obstet Gynecol 1983;62:457–462.
113. Psychological Aspects of Breast Cancer Study Group. Psychological response to mastectomy: A prospective comparison study. Cancer 1987;59:189–196.
114. Vinokur AD, Threatt BA, Caplan RD, Zimmerman BL. Physical and psychosocial functioning and adjustment to breast cancer: Long-term follow-up of a screening population. Cancer 1989;63:394–405.
115. Green DM, Zevon MA, Hall B. Achievement of life goals by adult survivors of modern treatment for childhood cancer. Cancer 1991;67:206–213.
116. Byrne J, Fears TR, Steinhorn SC, et al. Marriage and divorce after childhood and adolescent cancer. JAMA 1989;262:2693–2699.
117. Ropponen P, Aalberg V, Rautonen J, Kalmari H, Siimes MA. Psychosexual development of adolescent males after malignancies in childhood. Act Psychiatr Scand 1990;82: 213–218.
118. Lieber L, Plumb MM, Gerstenzang ML, et al. The communication of affection between cancer patients and their spouses. Psychosom Med 1976;38:379–389.
119. Goedert JJ. What is safe sex? Suggested standards linked to testing for human immunodeficiency virus. N Engl J Med 1987;316:1339–1341.
120. Spanier GB. Measuring dyadic adjustment: New scales for assessing the quality of marriage and similar dyads. J Marriage Fam 1976;38:15–28.
121. Derogatis LR, Melisaratos N. The Brief Symptom Inventory: An introductory report. Psychol Med 1983;13:595–605.
122. Derogatis LR. Psychosocial Adjustment to Illness Scale (PAIS and PAIS-SR): Scoring procedures and administration manual. Baltimore: Clinical Psychometric Research, 1983.
123. Ganz PA, Schag CAC, Cheng HL. Assessing the quality of life: A study in newly diagnosed breast cancer patients. J Clin Epidemiol 1990;43:75–86.
124. Maatman TJ, Montague DK, Martin LM. Cost-effective evaluation of impotence. Urology 1986;27:132–135.
125. Maatman TJ, Montague DK, Martin LM. Erectile dysfunction in men with diabetes mellitus. Urology 1987;29:589–592.
126. Meisler AW, Carey MP. A critical reevaluation of nocturnal penile tumescence monitoring in the diagnosis of erectile dysfunction. J Nerv Mental Dis 1990;178:78–89.
127. Schiavi RC. Nocturnal penile tumescence in the evaluation of erectile disorders: A critical review. J Sex Mar Ther 1988;14:83–97.
128. Kaneko S, Bradley WE. Evaluation of erectile dysfunction with continuous monitoring of rigidity. J Urol 1986;136:1026–1029.
129. Thase ME, Reynolds CF, Jennings JR, et al. Diagnostic performance of nocturnal penile tumescence studies in healthy, dysfunctional (impotent), and depressed men. Psychiatry Res 1988;26:79–87.
130. Schiavi RC, Schreiner-Engel P. Nocturnal penile tumescence in healthy aging men. J Geront 1988;43:146–150.
131. Lue TF, Tanagho EA. Functional anatomy and mechanism of penile erection. In: Tanagho EA, Lue TF, McClure RD, eds. Contemporary management of impotence and infertility. Baltimore: Williams & Wilkins, 1988:39–50.
132. Abber JC, Lue TF, Orvis BR, et al. Diagnostic tests for impotence: A comparison of papaverine injection with the penile-brachial index and nocturnal penile tumescence monitoring. J Urol 1986;135:923–925.
133. Buvat J, Buvat-Herbaut M, Dehaene JL, et al. Is intravascular injection of papaverine a reliable screening test for vascular impotence? J Urol 1986;135:476–478.
134. Montague DK, Lakin MM, Medendorp SV, Tesar LJ. Infusion pharmacocavernosometry and nocturnal penile tumescence findings in men with erectile dysfunction. J Urol 1991;145:768–771.
135. Lue TF. Functional study of penile veins. In: Tanagho EA, Lue TF, McClure RD, eds. Contemporary management of impotence and infertility. Baltimore, Williams & Wilkins, 1988:65–69.
136. Padma-Nathan H, Goldstein I. Neurologic assessment of the impotent patient. In: Montague DK, ed. Disorders of male sexual function. Chicago: Year Book Publishers, 1988:86–94.
137. Rowland DL, Greenleaf W, Mas M, Myers L, Davidson JM. Penile and finger sensory thresholds in young, aging, and diabetic males. Arch Sex Beh 1989;18:1–12.
138. Leiblum SR, Bachmann G, Kemmann E, et al. Vaginal atrophy in the postmenopausal woman: The importance of sexual activity and hormones. JAMA 1983;249:2195–2198.
139. Fordney DS. Dyspareunia and vaginismus. Clin Obstet Gynecol 1978;21:205–221.
140. Friedrich EG. Vulvar vestibulitis syndrome. J Reprod Med 1987;32:110–114.
141. Schover LR, Youngs DD, Cannata R. Psychosexual aspects of the evaluation and management of vulvar vestibulitis. Am J Obstet Gynecol 1992;167:630–636.
142. Blaivas JG, Zayed AAH, Labib KB. The bulbocavernosus reflex in urology: A prospective study of 299 patients. J Urol 1981;126:197–199.
143. Haldeman S, Bradley WE, Bhatia WN, et al. Pudendal evoked responses. Arch Neurol 1982;39:280–283.
144. Schover LR, Randers-Pehrson M. Sexuality and cancer: For the woman who has cancer, and her partner. Atlanta: American Cancer Society, 1991.
145. Schover LR, Randers-Pehrson M. Sexuality and cancer: For the man who has cancer, and his partner. Atlanta: American Cancer Society, 1991.
146. Wincze JP, Carey MP. Sexual dysfunction: A guide for assessment and treatment. New York: Guilford Press, 1991.
147. Lue TF, Carroll PR, Moore C. Treatment of impotence in cancer patients. Import Adv Oncol 1989;1:193–203.
148. Virag R, Shoukry K, Floresco J, Nollet F, Greco E. Intracavernous self-injection of vasoactive drugs in the treatment of impotence: 8-year experience with 615 cases. J Urol 1991;145:287–293.
149. Dennis RL, McDougal WS. Pharmacological treatment of erectile dysfunction after radical prostatectomy. J Urol 1988;139:775–776.
150. Lakin MM, Montague DK, Medendorp SV, Tesar L, Schover LR. Intracavernous injection therapy: Analysis of results and complications. J Urol 1990;143:1138–1141.
151. Stackl W, Hasun R, Marberger M. Intracavernous injection of prostaglandin E1 in impotent men. J Urol 1988;140:66–68.
152. Lakin MM, Montague DK, Schover LR, Chen RN, Ignaut CA. Fibrosis with intracavernous injection therapy utilizing prostaglandin E1 (PGE-1). [Abstract] Presented at the Annual Meeting of the American Urological Association, Washington, DC, May 1992.
153. Sidi AA, Becher EF, Zhang G, Lewis JH. Patient acceptance of and satisfaction with an external negative pressure device for impotence. J Urol 1990;144:1154–1156.
154. Turner LA, Althof SE, Levine SB, et al. Treating erectile dysfunction with external vacuum devices: Impact upon sexual, psychological and marital functioning. J Urol 1990;144:79–82.
155. Katz PG, Haden HT, Mulligan T, Zasler ND. The effect of vacuum devices on penile hemodynamics. J Urol 1990;143:55–56.
156. Meinhardt W, Kropman RF, Lycklama AAB, Nijeholt A, Zwartendijk J. Skin necrosis caused by use of negative pressure device for erectile impotence. J Urol 1990;144: 983.
157. Montague DK. Penile prostheses: An overview. Urol Clin N Amer 1989;16:7–12.
158. Montague DK. Periprosthetic infections. J Urol 1987;138:68–69.
159. Carson CC, Robertson CN. Late hematogenous infection of penile prostheses. J Urol 1988;139:50–52.
160. Kabalin JN, Kessler R. Successful implantation of penile prostheses in organ transplant patients. Urology 1989;33:282–284.
161. Bennett AH. Placement of penile prosthesis during surgery for malignancies. Urology 1987;20:276–277.
162. Kaufman JJ. Penile prosthetic surgery under local anesthesia. J Urol 1982;128:1190–1191.
163. Mulcahy JJ. The Hydroflex penile prosthesis. Urol Clin N Amer 1989;16:33–38.
164. Montague DK, Lakin MM. Early experience with the controlled girth- and length-expanding cylinder of the AMS Ultrex penile prosthesis. J Urol 1992;148:1444–1446.
165. Scott FB, Light JK, Fishman IJ. Treatment of impotency caused by cancer therapy: The inflatable penile prosthesis. Cancer Bull 1982;34:33–39.
166. Spauwen PHM, Bouma J, Burger MPM. Vulval reconstruction after cancer excision. Tenth World Congress of Sexology, Amsterdam, 1991.

SECTION 4

JOHN M. DALY
MICHAEL H. TOROSIAN

Nutritional Support

Proper preparation of cancer patients for major surgery, chemotherapy, and radiation treatment requires both physiologic and psychological intervention and support. The goal of therapy during the perioperative period in surgical patients is to prepare the patient to withstand the stress of major surgery and to minimize postoperative complications. The appropriate duration of the preoperative support period depends on the relative urgency of the surgical procedure compared with the operative risk and the natural history of the disease. A multitude of factors such as the patient's chronologic and physiologic age, the degree of metabolic derangements and nutritional deficits, the presence of organ dysfunction, the extent of obesity, and the stage of the primary disease should be considered relative to the timing and magnitude of the surgical procedure.

Protein-calorie malnutrition is a common problem in hospitalized medical and surgical cancer patients and occurs in most patients undergoing major upper-abdominal surgery. Among hospitalized patients, those with cancer have the highest incidence of protein-calorie malnutrition. Thus, evaluation of nutritional deficits is critical to determining operative risk and can influence the timing and extent of surgery.

Protein-calorie malnutrition results from decreased oral intake, increased enteral losses secondary to malabsorption or intestinal fistula, various forms of antineoplastic therapy, and tumor-induced alterations in host metabolism. In the absence of adequate exogenous nutrients, the body uses endogenous substrates to satisfy the ongoing requirements of both the host and the tumor for energy and protein. In patients with malignant obstruction of the gastrointestinal tract, the tumor itself may cause diminished nutrient intake. Multimodal therapy for malignant disease including surgery, chemotherapy, and radiation therapy exacerbates these metabolic derangements, further increasing the risk of significant postoperative morbidity and mortality.

Malnutrition associated with malignancy has major prognostic significance, and the association between weight loss and increased mortality in cancer patients has been known for several decades. The use of enteral and total parenteral nutrition allows clinicians to have an impact on the malnutrition associated with cancer. However, controversy remains as to whether nutritional intervention benefits the host and the tumor, and to what extent nutritional intervention affects clinical endpoints such as morbidity, mortality, and response to therapy.

CANCER CACHEXIA

Cancer cachexia is a group of symptoms and signs that includes inanition, anorexia, weakness, tissue wasting, and organ dysfunction. Common in patients with advanced metastatic disease, cachexia also occurs in patients with localized disease (Table 64–16). DeWys and associates noted substantial weight loss in some patients with breast cancer and most patients with gastric or pancreatic carcinoma.[1] The relation of cachexia to tumor burden, stage of disease, and tumor histology is inconsistent, and no single theory satisfactorily explains the cachectic state. Recent results suggest that cytokines and peptides secreted by the host in response to the tumor play a major role in the development of cachexia (Fig. 64–9). These mediators, such as cachectin/tumor necrosis factor and interferon-γ, exert profound effects on the host's intermediary metabolism. In the short term, these effects promote an acute-phase response by rerouting nutrients from the periphery to the liver. However, over the long term, these cytokines result in anorexia and abnormalities in carbohydrate, protein, and lipid metabolism.

TABLE 64–16. Potential Etiologies of Cancer Cachexia

Tumor	*Antineoplastic Therapy*
Dysphagia	Reduced intake in preparation for diagnostic and therapeutic intervention
Early satiety	Ileus
Bowel obstruction	Malabsorption
Malabsorption	Increased energy requirements
Competition for substrate	Anorexia
Alteration of host metabolism	Anosmia
Anorexia	Nausea and vomiting
Alteration of taste	GI mucosal damage
	Mastication and swallowing dysfunction
	Xerostomia
	Oropharyngeal ulcerations/ infections

DIMINISHED NUTRIENT INTAKE

Anorexia accompanies most neoplasms to some extent and is a major contributing factor to the development of the cachectic state. Often, loss of appetite is an important symptom of an underlying tumor. Several physiologic derangements have been cited as possible reasons for anorexia. Abnormalities in taste perception, such as reduced thresholds for sweet, sour, and salty flavors, have been shown. DeWys and Walters noted that a reduced taste sensitivity for sucrose and urea is associated with reduced caloric intake; reduced oral threshold for urea correlates with an aversion for red meat.[2] Deficiencies in zinc and other trace elements may contribute to altered taste sensation. Patients with hepatic metastases accompanied by hepatic insufficiency may develop anorexia and nausea from reduced clearance of lactate produced by anaerobic tumor metabolism of glucose.

The specific metabolic processes that affect nutrient intake in cancer patients are unclear. Lucke and colleagues noted the presence of a humoral factor that reproduces the metabolic characteristics of the tumor-bearing state in non-tumor-bearing animals.[3] DeWys and coworkers suggested that tumor peptides acting through neuroendocrine cells and neuroreceptors alter metabolic pathways.[1] Nakahara described a "toxohormone" capable of mimicking the cachectic state when injected into normal animals.[4] Antibodies to interferon-γ partially reversed the cachexia in animals with end-stage tumors.[5] Endogenously produced tumor necrosis factor/cachectin may also be a mediator in the development of cachexia in the tumor-bearing host. Krause and associates noted that abnormalities in the central nervous system metabolism of serotonin may be responsible for the anorexia associated with the tumor-bearing state.[6]

The local effect of the tumor may also lead to reduced food intake, particularly when the tumor obstructs the upper alimentary tract. Patients with cancer of the oral cavity, pharynx, or esophagus may have reduced nutrient intake because of dysphagia or odynophagia due to partial or complete obstruction. Patients with gastric cancer often have reduced gastric capacity or partial gastric outlet obstruction, leading to nausea, vomiting, and early satiety. Intestinal tumors and abdominal carcinomatosis can cause partial obstruction or blind-loop syndrome to interfere with nutrient absorption. Pancreatic carcinomas often cause exocrine enzyme deficiencies and malabsorption syndromes. Finally, psychological factors such as depression, grief, or anxiety resulting from the disease or its treatment may lead to poor appetite, abnormal eating behavior, and learned food aversions and thus to a diminished or unbalanced dietary intake.

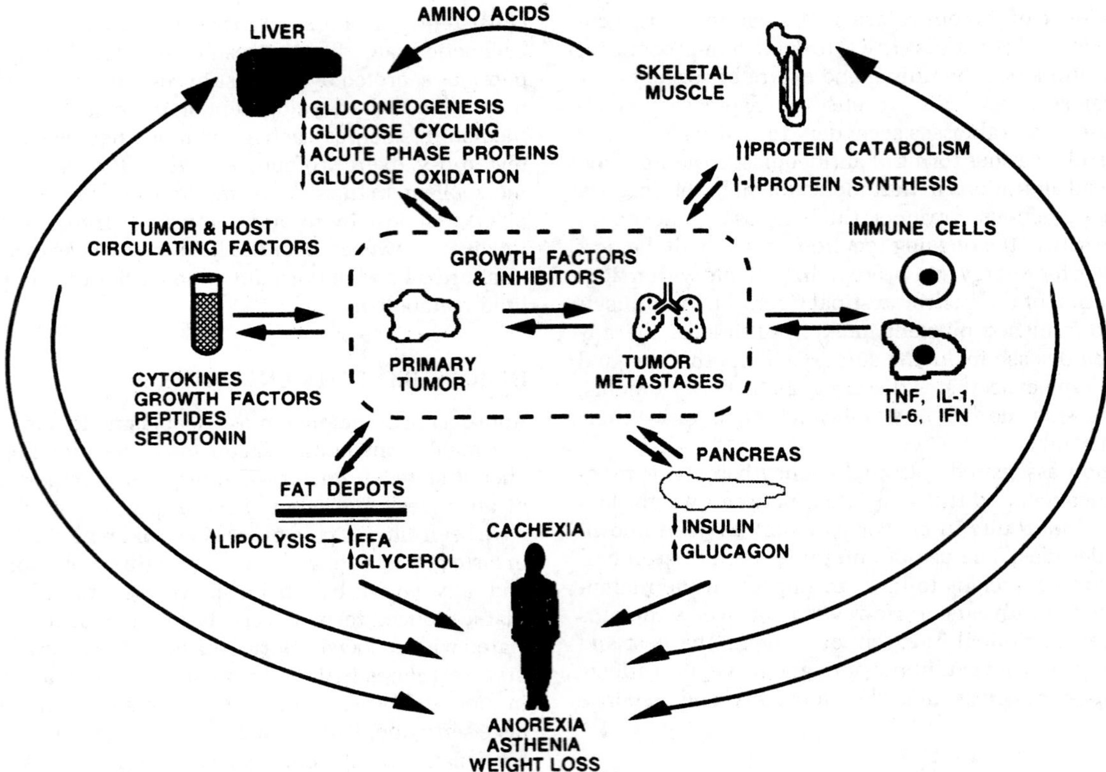

FIGURE 64–9. Mechanisms of metabolic abnormalities in tumor-bearing hosts.

ABNORMALITIES OF SUBSTRATE METABOLISM

Extensive changes in energy, carbohydrate, lipid, and protein metabolism have been demonstrated in patients with malignant disease.[7–9] Increased energy expenditure and inefficient energy use are frequently cited causes of malnutrition in tumor-bearing hosts.[10] The normal response to diminished food intake is a reduction in the basal metabolic rate (BMR); the BMR or resting energy expenditure consists of all the energy-requiring processes of vegetative function and accounts for 75% of total energy expenditure in normal people. The lack of a decreased response of BMR to semistarvation likens cancer cachexia to the septic state.

Energy requirements of cancer patients have been studied prospectively. Young could not conclude that resting metabolism was consistently elevated in cancer patients, although increased resting energy expenditure was found in leukemia and lymphoma patients.[10] Increases in resting metabolic rate paralleled advancing disease and reduced nutrient intake. Other investigators have shown an elevation in resting energy expenditure in patients with lymphomas, lung cancer, and head and neck cancers.[11] Shike and colleagues demonstrated in a group of patients with small cell lung carcinoma that basal energy expenditure was elevated compared with controls.[12] Responders to chemotherapy had a significant decrease in basal energy expenditure, while nonresponders exhibited no change. In 1983 Knox and coworkers measured energy expenditure in 200 malnourished cancer patients by indirect calorimetry.[13] Only 41% had a normal resting energy expenditure, while decreased and increased resting energy expenditure was observed in 33% and 26%, respectively. Similarly, Heber and associates found no clear evidence of hypermetabolism in noncachectic lung-cancer patients.[14] They argued that because malnourished patients normally have a decreased BMR as an adaptation to starvation, even predicted metabolic rates are inappropriately elevated in malnourished cancer patients.

Shaw and colleagues concluded that the alteration in metabolic rate depends on the type of tumor.[15] They demonstrated an elevated rate of energy expenditure in sarcoma-bearing patients associated with increased Cori cycle activity and glucose turnover, reduced glucose oxidation, and increased protein catabolism. Buzby and colleagues noted a reduction in metabolic rate associated with pancreatic cancer.[16] Patients with lower gastrointestinal neoplasms tended to be metabolically similar to normal volunteers, but patients with upper gastrointestinal tumors had an elevated metabolic rate.

Inefficient energy use by the tumor-bearing host was studied by Holroyde and Reichard, who reported increased Cori cycle activity in patients with malignancy.[9] This futile cycle, in which glucose is converted to lactic acid and subsequently reconverted to glucose by hepatocytes, wastes energy. The highest level of Cori cycle activity was seen in patients with the greatest energy expenditure and weight loss. Young suggested that increased rates of protein turnover also result in significant energy losses due to the failure of normal adaptation to starvation.[10] During the first 2 days of fasting, endogenous glycogen stores of muscle and the liver are depleted. Glucose use by the brain, leukocytes, and other tissues continues, resulting in the breakdown of protein for gluconeogenesis. In noncancer patients, muscle protein breakdown is gradually replaced by fat fuel metabolism, in which fatty acids are converted to ketone bodies. These are used for energy by peripheral tissues and eventually for up to 95% of energy use by the brain; this results in decreased glucose use, with sparing of muscle protein. In cancer patients, these adaptive mechanisms occur less commonly, resulting in increased glucose production and protein catabolism.

Although cancer patients have normal levels of circulating insulin and glucose, they have impaired insulin sensitivity (Table 64–17). Glucose intolerance is documented by hyperglycemia and delayed clearance of blood glucose in cancer patients after oral or intravenous glucose administration.[9,14,17] Glucose intolerance is due in part to decreased peripheral tissue sensitivity to insulin, but may also involve an attenuated islet cell secretory response to glucose.[17] Cancer patients also exhibit increased hepatic gluconeogenesis from alanine and lactate. Using carbon 14-labeled alanine, Waterhouse and coworkers found that the apparent increase in gluconeogenesis from alanine reflected a very rapid glucose turnover.[18] Feedback control of glucose production may be impaired because gluconeogenesis and Cori cycle activity are not inhibited by glucose administration in the cancer patient. Moley and associates[19] and Peacock and Norton[20] studied sarcoma-bearing rats and found that supplemental insulin administration preserves host lean body mass and even influences the duration of survival.

Shaw and Wolfe recently noted that patients with gastrointestinal tumors had elevated rates of basal hepatic glucose production.[21] They found a direct relation between tumor burden and the increased rate of gluconeogenesis. Furthermore, patients with the largest tumor burdens failed to suppress their own endogenous glucose production during glucose infusions.

Alterations in lipid metabolism in cancer patients include decreased fat stores and increased lipid mobilization.[22,23] Decreases in total body fat are common in these patients and are most likely related to insulin resistance. Increased oxidation of fatty acids also occurs. Glycerol and fatty acids, the byproducts of lipolysis, serve as substrates for gluconeogenesis and energy production, respectively, during periods of nutrient deprivation. Waterhouse found that fatty acids are the major substrates used in patients with progressive malignant disease.[24] Increased plasma clearance of endogenous fat stores and exogenously administered fat emulsions occurs in cancer patients in both fasting and fed states. Patients with malignancy fail to suppress lipolysis after glucose administration and continue to oxidize fatty acids.[25]

TABLE 64–17. Metabolic Changes in the Cancer Patient

Carbohydrate Metabolism
Insulin resistance
Glucose intolerance
Increased gluconeogenesis
Increased Cori cycle activity
Increased glucose turnover
Increased serum lactate

Fat Metabolism
Increased fatty acid mobilization
Increased fatty acid turnover
Increased glycerol turnover
Hyperlipidemia
Decreased lipoprotein lipase

Protein Metabolism
Increased whole body protein turnover
Increased skeletal muscle catabolism
Decreased skeletal muscle anabolism
Impaired keto-adaptation

Because loss of body fat occurs often in patients with cancer cachexia, Wilson and colleagues measured changes in intravenous fat clearance and the effects on such clearance by operation and total parenteral nutrition (TPN) in patients with colorectal cancer.[26] Fifteen out of 21 patients had increased rates of fat clearance. Fat clearance rates were reduced to nearly normal in the 14 patients who were retested 12 weeks after curative resection. In 7 malnourished patients who received intravenous nutrition, fat clearance was also reduced.

Several abnormalities of protein metabolism occur in cancer patients, including nitrogen depletion, decreased muscle protein synthesis, and abnormal plasma aminograms.[8] Nitrogen balance is negative in most patients with progressive malignancy. Amino acid trapping by tumor cells has been demonstrated clinically and experimentally. Norton and coworkers found that sarcoma-bearing limbs released less than 50% of the amount of amino acids released from tumor-free limbs.[27] Evidence obtained with whole-body protein studies using nitrogen 15-labeled glycine indicates that cancer patients have increased whole-body protein turnover, which contributes to increased energy expenditure.[27]

Muscle wasting and decreases in serum protein levels are common in patients with malignant disease. Eventually, severe wasting of host muscle mass occurs along with depletion of visceral and circulating proteins, due primarily to increased protein breakdown. Kien and Carmitta noted a close association of accelerated rates of whole-body protein turnover and energy expenditure in children with acute lymphocytic leukemia.[28] Fearon and associates demonstrated no correlation between increased turnover and increased resting energy expenditure in adults.[29]

While tumor-induced increases in muscle and visceral protein breakdown contribute to host cachexia, evidence is emerging that tumor tissues may regulate their own protein degradation. Recent work by Tayek and colleagues compared the rate of host muscle protein synthesis and tumor protein synthesis and degradation in rats bearing either syngeneic sarcoma or hepatoma.[30] Eighteen days after tumor implantation, synthesis of rat muscle protein was decreased, but liver protein synthesis increased, with a net decrease in total protein synthesis. The metabolic cost to the host of increased protein flux may be substantial and may contribute to the development of cachexia.

Changes in body composition occur in cachexia, such as increased extracellular fluid and total body sodium and decreased intracellular fluid and total body potassium. Cohn and coworkers, using prompt γ-neutron activation to evaluate total body nitrogen and a whole-body counter to measure potassium 40, found that total body potassium was diminished out of proportion to total body nitrogen.[31] On the basis of this finding, they concluded that endogenous nutrient losses in cancer patients were predominantly in the skeletal muscle compartment, because muscle makes up 45% of total body nitrogen and 85% of total body potassium. In normal volunteers, body cell mass (BCM) tended to decrease with increasing age as an absolute value and as a percentage of total body weight. In anorexia nervosa patients, there was a significant depletion of BCM but relative sparing of the BCM when expressed as a percentage of body weight. This reflects the normal adaptation to starvation, where fat use predominates and endogenous protein is spared. In cancer patients, there was a significant degree of weight loss accompanied by a proportional decline in BCM, indicating that protein is depleted to the same extent as fat stores.

A variety of micronutrient abnormalities (vitamin and trace metals) may occur in cancer patients. Because vitamin A plays a role in the histology of certain types of epithelia, it has been suggested that cancer patients may have abnormally low total carotenoid levels. However, no difference in total carotenoids and pro-vitamin A precursors have been noted between well-nourished normal volunteers and cancer patients.

ETIOLOGY OF CANCER CACHEXIA

The etiology of cancer cachexia remains controversial but is undoubtedly multifactoral. Cachexia is not simply a local effect of the tumor but is caused by systemic factors induced by the tumor (*i.e.,* a type of paraneoplastic syndrome). Most current theories hypothesize that tumors do not directly produce the mediators of cachexia but induce host tissues to secrete circulating factors that cause cachexia. Two classes of cachexia mediators believed to be important in the development of cancer cachexia are cytokines and regulatory hormones (Table 64–18).

Cytokines are soluble proteins secreted by host tissues in response to various stimuli, including cancer, sepsis, inflammation, starvation, and other pathophysiologic insults. Cytokines exert their effects on host tissues by autocrine, paracrine, or circulating/systemic mechanisms. Tumor necrosis factor/cachectin, interleukin-1, and interleukin-6 are specific cytokines implicated in the development of cancer cachexia by recent experimental evidence.

Tumor necrosis factor (TNF) or cachectin is a 17-kilodalton molecular weight protein secreted by macrophages in response to endotoxin or malignancy. When given to animals, TNF can reproduce many, but not all, of the changes seen in cancer cachexia. Anorexia, weight loss, depletion of fat stores, loss of protein mass, hypoproteinemia, and increased total body water have been documented in TNF-treated animals. Some of these effects can be prevented by inducing tolerance to TNF or can be reversed with anti-TNF antibodies. Thus, TNF may cause some of the adverse host effects of cancer cachexia, but it is certainly not the sole mediator. Furthermore, it has been difficult to detect circulating levels of TNF in cancer patients even with severe degrees of cachexia.

Interleukin-1 (IL-1) is a cytokine secreted by macrophages in response to endotoxin. This inflammatory cytokine causes anorexia, pyrexia, hypotension, decreased systemic vascular resistance, and increased cardiac output. Gene amplification of the IL-1 locus has been found in one cachectic, tumor-bearing animal model, and both IL-1 and TNF produce alterations in hepatic protein synthesis similar to the tumor-bearing state.

Interleukin-6 (IL-6) is secreted by macrophages stimulated by endotoxin and by fibroblasts in response to TNF or IL-1. This cytokine, also called β_2-interferon, hepatocyte-stimulating factor, and hybridoma growth factor, has many activities similar to TNF and IL-1. Elevated levels of IL-6 have been found in tumor-bearing animals and correlate with the hepatic acute-phase response to cancer.

Abnormalities in anabolic regulatory hormones may also play an important role in the development of cancer cachexia. Cancer is associated with numerous aberrations of intermediary metabolism, including glucose intolerance, increased glucose cycling, impaired glucose oxidation, and increased lipolysis. Hormonal changes may be integral to these metabolic alterations, and cachexia from cancer and other catabolic states has been associated with decreased insulin and increased glucagon levels. The resulting insulin:glucagon ratio, an anabolic hormone index, is significantly reduced and is asso-

TABLE 64–18. Circulating Host Factors That May Cause Cancer Cachexia

Factor	*Food Intake*	*Body Weight*	*Lipid Mass*	*Protein Mass*	*Measured in Circulation*	*Antibody Studies*
Cachectin/tumor necrosis factor	Decrease	Decrease	Decrease	Decrease	Animal studies correlate with cachexia (with stimulation). Human did not correlate with cachexia.	AB to TNF reversed anorexia and body composition changes in tumor-bearing mice
Interleukin-1	Decrease	Decrease	NA	NA	Undetectable levels in cancer cachexia	NA
Interleukin-6	NA	NA	NA	NA	Levels increased with increasing tumor burden	NA
Interferon-γ	Decrease	Decrease	NA	NA	NA	AB reversed cachexia and prolonged survival of tumor-bearing rat

NA, data not available; AB, antibody; TNF, tumor necrosis factor.
(Langstein H, Norton JA. Mechansisms of cancer cachexia. Hematol Oncol Clin North Am [February] 1991)

ciated with weight loss and continued catabolism. Although insulin alone is inadequate to reverse these metabolic abnormalities, the combined administration of the anabolic hormones insulin, growth hormone, and somatostatin can effectively treat some of the adverse host changes seen in cancer cachexia.[32]

Additional clinical and basic research is required to further elucidate the role of cytokines, hormones, and other circulating factors in the development of cancer cachexia and to devise effective therapeutic strategies to treat the cancer patient.

EFFECTS OF ANTITUMOR THERAPY ON NUTRITION

Antineoplastic therapy invariably affects the host, either by mechanical or physiologic alterations due to surgery, or at the cellular level with chemotherapy or radiation therapy.[33] The effects of therapy may add to the cachexia of malignancy and exacerbate the severe nutritional deficiency of cancer patients.

Surgery is the primary treatment modality of most solid cancers, particularly those of the gastrointestinal tract. The immediate metabolic response to major surgery in patients with cancer is similar to that of patients who have surgery for benign disease: increased nitrogen losses and energy requirements.[34] However, because cancer patients may have significant weight loss before surgery, their ability to cope with stress is impaired, resulting in increased morbidity and mortality. The physical insult, the associated pain, and the emotional and physiologic response to surgery cause an integrated endocrine and metabolic reaction designed to maintain homeostasis. There is an increased output of catecholamines, glucagon, and cortisol that results in hypermetabolism, weight loss, negative nitrogen balance, and retention of sodium and water. In addition to this general response to injury, operations on the oropharynx and gastrointestinal tract have specific nutritional sequelae, depending on the site of surgery.

Cancer chemotherapy may profoundly alter the host's nutritional state. The effects may be direct (by interfering with host cell metabolism or DNA synthesis and cellular replication) or indirect (by producing nausea, vomiting, changes in taste sensation, and learned food aversions). Most agents have the ability to stimulate the chemoreceptor trigger zone, resulting in nausea and vomiting. The rapid cell turnover in the alimentary tract mucosa makes it especially vulnerable to chemotherapy, resulting in stomatitis, ulceration, and decreased absorptive capacity. These effects result, in turn, in decreased intake and absorption of nutrients and further predispose the cancer patient to malnutrition. The bone marrow is another organ with a high cell turnover; toxicity is manifested by anemia, leukopenia, and thrombocytopenia. Neutropenia is, in turn, associated with an increased risk of sepsis.

Radiation therapy may also affect the host's nutritional state by its effects on the gastrointestinal tract. The severity of radiation injury is related to the dose of radiation and the volume of tissue treated. The adverse effects of radiation therapy are classified as early or late. Early effects are transient and are manifested by diarrhea, xerostomia, alterations in taste, and food aversions. Late radiation effects include intestinal strictures, fistulae, and malabsorption.

CONSEQUENCES OF MALNUTRITION IN THE CANCER PATIENT

The clinical relevance of severe malnutrition has been demonstrated by increased morbidity and mortality and poor treatment tolerance in malnourished tumor-bearing patients.[35,36] In 1932 Warren noted that malnutrition was a major factor contributing to mortality in cancer patients.[37] The protein-calorie malnutrition produced by the cancer-bearing state leads not only to obvious weight loss, but also to visceral and somatic protein depletion that compromises enzymatic, structural, and mechanical body functions. Impaired immunocompetence and increased susceptibility to infection often result, and these changes may be exacerbated by chemotherapy. Moreover, poor wound healing, increased wound infections, prolonged postoperative ileus, and longer hospital stays have all been linked to poor nutritional status in cancer patients. In patients undergoing colorectal cancer operations, the return to adequate oral food intake was significantly delayed in those patients classified as malnourished based on preoperative assessment.[38] Morbidity and mortality in malnourished patients was 52% and 12% respectively, compared with 31% and 6% in well-nourished patients.

In animal studies, severe protein restriction depressed both humoral and cellular immune responses. Daly and colleagues demonstrated that only 30% of tumor-bearing rats had a delayed hypersensitivity response to intradermal purified protein derivative after 2 weeks on an oral protein-free diet.[39] Protein repletion with 7 days of TPN or oral ad libitum feeding restored the response in 91% and 78% of rats, respectively. Only 17% of animals who remained on protein-free diets for 7 or more days showed a delayed hypersensitivity response. Law and associates found reduced titers of antibodies, reduced IgM-producing cells, reduced lymphocyte response to mitogens, and decreased delayed hypersensitivity in rats after 6 weeks on protein-free nutrition.[40]

In human studies, there is evidence for increased morbidity and mortality with depressed immunocompetence. In addition, it has been documented that nutritional therapy reverses anergy. Harvey and coworkers reported on 161 cancer patients undergoing nutritional support.[41] Of these, 32 were anergic before therapy. In 27 of these patients anergy was reversed, and three of this group died. Of the 5 patients who remained anergic, all died. Daly and associates documented that 51% of anergic patients undergoing cancer treatment had restoration of skin-test reactivity in response to TPN.[42]

The effect of malnutrition on host immune function is to depress host immune competence, particularly cell-mediated immunity. McEntee and coworkers further delineated the effects of malnutrition and nutrient administration in malnourished patients undergoing major surgery.[43] Acutely malnourished patients had significant reductions in absolute lymphocyte counts but no significant alterations in the proportion of T cells or T-cell helper and suppressor subsets. There was a marked impairment of the delayed cutaneous hypersensitivity response: 20 of 29 patients failed to respond to any of the seven antigens. Twenty patients responded positively to nutritional support with significant improvement in serum protein levels, absolute lymphocyte count, and delayed cutaneous hypersensitivity response, with a mean duration of 15 days of nutritional support. Other factors such as sepsis, trauma, steroids, and medications influence host immune function, but nutritional support is an important therapeutic intervention that can improve immunocompetence.

NUTRITIONAL ASSESSMENT

General indications of the need for nutritional assessment and therapeutic intervention with enteral or parenteral nutritional support include the patient's inability to eat or unwillingness to eat enough, and specific nutritional requirements due to cardiac, hepatic, or renal dysfunction. Using data from the patient's history, physical examination, and laboratory tests, together with knowledge of the anticipated method of treatment, the degree and duration of nutritional disability can be estimated and a nutritional management plan formulated.

The ability to ingest adequate quantities of nutrients orally is evaluated by dietary history and the extent of recent weight loss. A history of a recent (within 3 months) loss of 10% or more of body weight signifies substantial protein-calorie malnutrition. In our society, this determination is more important than measurement of the percentage of ideal body weight, because obesity is prevalent and the rapidity of weight loss indicates the severity of illness. Patient history includes questions regarding usual body weight; recent weight changes; special diets; problems with taste, chewing, or swallowing; food allergies and medications; alcohol ingestion; and bowel habits related to dietary intake. Physical examination may reveal evidence of undernutrition such as dry, scaly, and atrophic skin; muscle wasting; pitting, presacral, or pretibial edema; loss of muscle strength; and depletion of fat stores.

A thorough history and physical examination by an experienced physician is the simplest and one of the best methods of nutritional assessment. An excellent correlation has been demonstrated between the clinical diagnosis of malnutrition and nutritional status as determined by a battery of anthropometric and laboratory tests as well as analyses of total body potassium and total body nitrogen (Table 64–19). Thus, although laboratory tests and research tools such as total body potassium and nitrogen measurements allow quantification of nutritional status for comparative purposes, the diagnosis of malnutrition can be made by experienced medical personnel.

Several sophisticated tests have been devised to detect milder forms of malnutrition and to objectively quantify the patient's response to nutritional therapy. Anthropometric measurements quantify body habitus and body compartments and relate them to measurements of an age- and sex-matched normal population. The creatinine-height index, defined as the patient's 24-hour creatinine excretion divided by the expected 24-hour excretion of creatinine by a normal adult of the same height, provides another estimate of skeletal muscle mass in a patient with normal renal function. Substantial protein-calorie malnutrition is a level 75% or less of standard. A method for estimating body cell mass has also been developed by determining the ratio of exchangeable sodium to exchangeable potassium using isotope dilution techniques. This ratio increases with chronic malnutrition to a value greater than 1.22. Use of a whole-body counter allows determination of ^{40}K, a naturally occurring radioisotope, within the skeletal muscle mass. From this measurement total body potassium can be calculated, allowing an estimate of lean body mass. Measurement of total body nitrogen by γ-neutron activation is the gold standard for determining total body protein. These last three tests are not available for routine use in hospital centers, but they have been useful research tools in the assessment of body composition changes.

The degree of visceral protein depletion can be estimated by determining concentrations of serum proteins such as retinal-binding protein, prealbumin, transferrin, and albumin. The correlation of serum protein levels with protein-calorie malnutrition is directly related to the metabolic half-life of the individual serum proteins and the patient's hydrational state. Prealbumin and retinal-binding protein have the shortest half-lives and are depressed first, followed by serum transferrin and albumin levels. The half-lives of these proteins are 0.5, 2, 8, and 20 days, respectively. Thus, changes in prealbumin and retinal-binding protein reflect recent dietary changes, whereas transferrin and albumin are more closely related to nutritional status. A decrease in the serum concentration of these proteins may also be related to changes in the patient's salt and water balance. For example, serum albumin concentrations commonly decline after starting a malnourished patient on TPN. This depression in serum albumin concentration results from hydrational effects and does not reflect a worsening malnourished state (Fig. 64–10). With effective nutritional support, significant increases in serum transferrin

TABLE 64–19. Nutritional Assessment Using Clinical Evaluation and Objective Tests

Clinical Assessment	*Normal*	*Malnutrition* *Mild*	*Severe*
% Ideal body weight	112 ± 3	105 ± 5	81 ± 3
Albumin (g/dl)	39 ± 0.1	3.6 ± 0.3	3.1 ± 0.1
Transferrin (mg/dl)	208 ± 16	175 ± 27	147 ± 16
Total body nitrogen	1.80 ± 0.10	1.77 ± 0.20	1.40 ± 0.11
Total body potassium	0.108 ± 0.007	0.121 ± 0.011	0.077 ± 0.006
% Positive skin test	80	53	50

Mean ± SEM.
(Adapted from Baker JP, et al. N Engl J Med 1982;306:969–972)

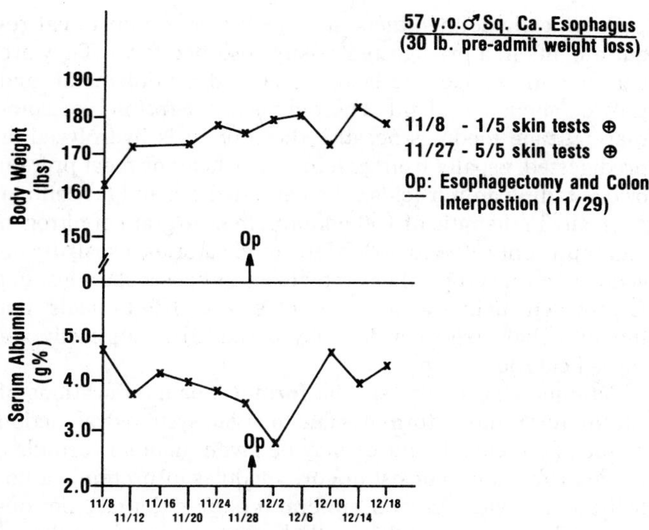

FIGURE 64–10. Body weight increases while serum albumin levels decrease during parenteral nutrition (IVH) before and after operation for a 57-year-old man with esophageal carcinoma.

and albumin levels typically occur after 7 to 10 days and 4 weeks of therapy, respectively.

The degree of visceral protein depletion has also been evaluated by determining the status of cell-mediated immunity as manifested by recall antigen skin testing and by the total blood lymphocyte count. Loss of immunocompetence is *not* a sensitive indicator of visceral protein depletion because weight loss usually exceeds 10% of the body weight before anergy develops secondary to malnutrition. Therefore, anergy associated with malnutrition signifies a significant deficiency of visceral protein and portends increased morbidity and mortality in hospitalized patients. Several factors result in anergy to recall skin testing, including age, presence of malignant disease, immunosuppression due to exogenous medications such as steroids, radiation therapy, stress, or sepsis. In the absence of these factors, nutritional repletion of the malnourished patient can result in reversal of skin-test anergy, and this reversal is associated with improved treatment outcome. Usually, however, improvement in other measurements of nutritional status such as body weight occur much in advance of improvement in delayed cutaneous hypersensitivity.

Complete nutritional assessment provides an estimate of body composition (fat, skeletal muscle protein, and visceral protein) to help identify and quantify the magnitude of clinical or subclinical malnutrition. A nutritional status scale can be used for classifying patients into nutritional categories of normal status, mild malnutrition, or severe malnutrition. The nutritional assessment should help to determine whether the goal of anabolic nutritional therapy should be repletion of nutritional deficits or maintenance of existing status. All of these measurements have proved accurate in population surveys, but they have varying sensitivity and lack specificity in individual patients. Thus, their major value lies in supporting the clinical diagnosis of malnutrition made by an experienced observer. Finally, blood analysis documents specific deficiencies that require correction.

Objective data can thus define the nebulous term nutritional status and allow both initial assessment of the patient and repeated evaluation of the efficacy of nutritional therapy. A prognostic nutritional index (PNI) to quantify the extent of malnutrition can be calculated as follows:

$$\text{PNI}(\%) = 158 - 16.6\,(\text{Alb}) - 0.78\,(\text{TSF}) - 0.20\,(\text{TPN}) - 5.8\,(\text{DH})$$

where Alb is albumin in g/dl, TSF is triceps skin fold in mm, TFN is transferrin in mg/dl, and DH is delayed hypersensitivity (0=negative, 1=less than 5 mm reactivity, and 2=5 or more mm reactivity).[16] In a large retrospective series of surgical patients, a PNI of below 30 (low risk) was associated with an 11.7% complication rate and 2% mortality. A PNI of 60 or above (high risk) was associated with an 81% complication rate and 59% mortality.

Studies such as these have helped to establish the relative importance of nutritional indices as predictive factors for postoperative morbidity and mortality in surgical patients. Almost all nutritional support teams have devised nutritional status scoring systems that allow repeated estimates of nutritional status during diagnostic and therapeutic management of the patient. A simple, practical definition of malnutrition that can be readily applied clinically includes an unintentional or unexplained loss of 10% or more of body weight, a serum transferrin level less than 150 mg/dl, and a serum albumin level less than 3.4 g/dl. Any two of these three criteria is an indication for nutritional support or therapy.

PREOPERATIVE NUTRITIONAL SUPPORT

After the need for preoperative nutritional support has been established, the most appropriate feeding regimen and the duration of nutritional support are determined (Fig. 64–11). The optimum duration of preoperative nutritional support varies with each patient. Generally, patients with severe malnutrition should receive at least 7 days of nutritional therapy during their workup and preparation for a major elective procedure. They should continue to receive postoperative nutritional support until oral intake is adequate. Obviously, the urgency of the operation determines the length of time available to correct existing nutritional deficiencies.

NASOENTERAL TUBE FEEDING

Nasoenteral tube feeding is the preferred method for providing short-term nutrition when the gastrointestinal tract is intact and sufficiently functional to tolerate and absorb adequate nutrients. When an elective operation is delayed and allows for longer preoperative preparation, nasointestinal or a surgical, endoscopic, or laparoscopic-placed tube feeding is preferred. Examples include patients with head and neck, esophageal, and gastric malignancies who are receiving preoperative chemotherapy or radiation therapy.

Solutions

The solution used should be nutritionally adequate, well tolerated, easy to prepare, and economical. Four types of enteral

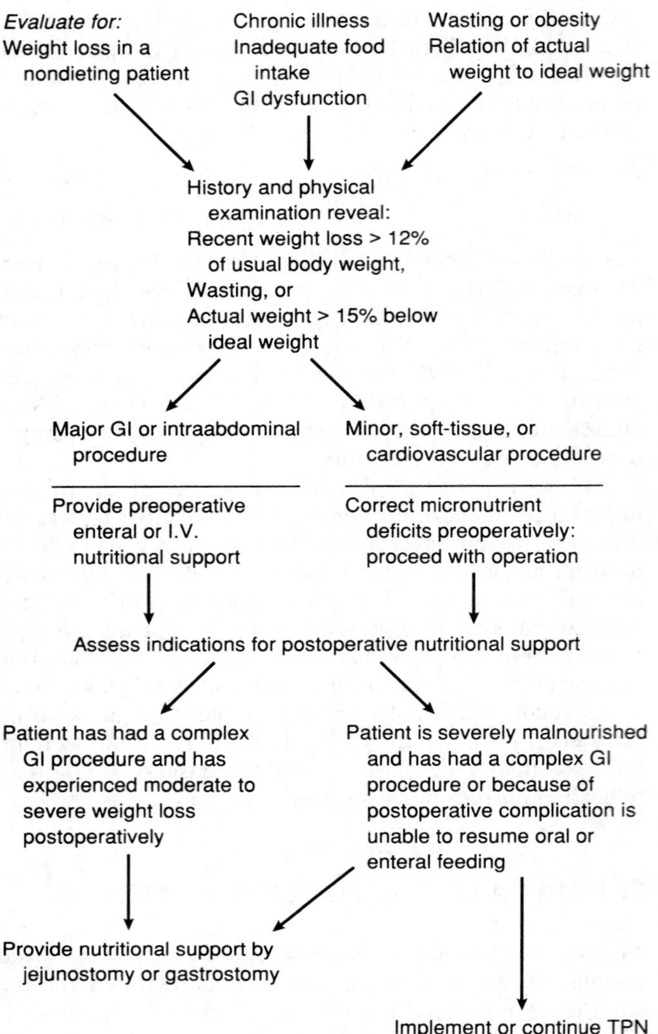

FIGURE 64–11. Nutritional management schema for cancer patients undergoing surgery.

formulas are available: blenderized tube-feeding formulas, nutritionally complete commercial formulas, chemically defined liquid diets, and modular formulas.

Blenderized tube feedings may be composed of any food that can be blenderized such as meat, whole or skim milk, vegetables, fruit, and cereal. Soy, safflower, sunflower, and corn oil are often used to increase caloric density and to supply a source of essential fatty acids. Other additives such as corn syrup or modular formulas can also be used to increase caloric density. Additional protein can be provided using dry milk powder, strained meats, or egg. Caloric concentrations of these formulas vary from 0.6 to 1.3 kcal/ml. These feedings are the least expensive but require both a larger-bore tube (14 Fr) and longer preparation time.

Nutritionally complete commercial formulas vary in protein, carbohydrate, and fat composition and are low to moderate in residue content. Most are lactose-free and contain about 1 to 1.5 kcal/ml. These formulas are the regimens of choice because they are relatively inexpensive and easily prepared and provide adequate nutrients.

Chemically defined diets provide complete nutritional requirements in a predigested, easily absorbed form. They are very low in residue, are lactose free and hyperosmolar, and provide about 1 kcal/ml. These diets differ from other commercial tube feedings because the protein is hydrolyzed or predigested, usually from casein, soy, wheat, or meat protein or crystalline amino acids. The carbohydrate and fat content is usually in the ratio of 150 nonprotein kcal/gram of nitrogen and represents 60% to 90% of the total calories, usually from sucrose, corn syrup solids, and glucose oligosaccharides. Fat is provided mainly as a source of essential fatty acids, but medium-chain triglycerides may be added as an easily absorbed caloric source.

Patients who require special formulas or modifications of commercial enteral formulas due to organ system dysfunction or specific metabolic needs may be given modular formulas. Modular formulas consist of core modules of protein, carbohydrate, fat, vitamin, and mineral mixtures that are not nutritionally complete individually but can be compounded to provide a complete diet specific to a patient's needs.

Tube Selection and Placement

Small-bore (8 to 10 Fr) flexible nasoenteral tubes of polyurethane and silicone elastomer have reduced major patient discomfort caused by large-bore rubber tubes. Nasogastric feeding uses a 91-cm-long tube, while the 109-cm tube with tungsten weight is used for spontaneous or directed passage of the tip through the pylorus into the distal duodenum or upper jejunum. Longer nasojejunal tubes should be used to reduce the risk of pulmonary aspiration. Placement of the weighted tube tip through the pylorus is facilitated by fluoroscopy and an inner stylet that stiffens the catheter. The exact position of the catheter tip must be documented by fluoroscopy or x-rays before starting feeding.

The bore size of the tube is determined by the viscosity and osmolality of the formula to be used. Isotonic formula flows well through a #8 French tube, while a high calorie-density (2 kcal/ml) formula requires at least a #10 French tube for proper infusion. As a general rule, the smallest bore tube that allows the formula to flow without clogging should be used for greater patient acceptance.

If preoperative enteral nutritional support is indicated for more than 6 weeks, the nutrient solution may be infused through a gastrostomy or jejunostomy tube. A gastrostomy tube has the advantage of being easy to care for because it is readily available and visible to the patient. Gastrostomy feedings are well tolerated because of the stomach's storage and dilutional functions, but the risk of aspiration is higher than with jejunostomy feedings. The tube may be placed using a percutaneous endoscopic technique, laparoscopic technique, or a minor surgical procedure under local, regional, or general anesthesia. Percutaneous endoscopic and laparoscopic gastrostomy have become quite popular as cost-effective and less morbid methods of permanent gastric intubation.

Tube feedings should be administered by continuous gravity drip or with pump infusion. Bolus feedings have been used in patients with nasogastric tubes, but this method is unsuitable for use with chemically defined hyperosmolar diets because of gastrointestinal complications. Clinical tolerance of the enteral nutrient solution is determined by the osmolality of the solution as well as the rate of infusion. The most common method is to begin infusion with a full-strength solution at 30 ml/hour and increase the rate every 12 to 24 hours over 2 to 4 days in increments of 10 ml/hour. Preoperative enteral feeding can be supplemented with peripheral parenteral nutrition to provide adequate caloric intake more quickly and safely. Nutritional/metabolic patient monitoring is performed as in patients receiving TPN. In addition, gastrointestinal complications such as nausea, vomiting, bloating, cramping, and diarrhea are common, and thus close monitoring is indicated (Table 64–20).

TOTAL PARENTERAL NUTRITION

Patients with severe malnutrition (weight loss greater than 12% of their usual body weight, serum albumin 2.5 g/dl or less, and serum transferrin 150 mg/dl or less) usually require intravenous nutritional support in the preoperative period. TPN is also indicated when nausea, vomiting, gastrointestinal tract obstruction, fistulae, or malabsorption make the gastrointestinal tract unavailable for nutrient administration and when rapid nutritional repletion becomes necessary to maximize the safety of operative intervention.

The hypertonic nutrient solution most commonly used for TPN consists of 15% to 25% dextrose, 4% to 5% crystalline amino acids, 10% fat emulsion, electrolytes, and vitamins. Each unit of base solution provides about 5.25 to 6.0 g nitrogen and 900 to 1000 calories in 1000 to 1100 ml of water. Specific water, electrolyte, calorie, and nitrogen requirements are individualized to avoid metabolic complications. Fluid requirements for normal maintenance can be estimated from either body weight (30 ml/kg) or body surface area (1400 ml/m^2) and adjusted for existing deficits and ongoing excessive losses. In febrile patients, insensible water losses can be appreciable. Knowledge of fluid and electrolyte losses occurring from the gastrointestinal tract are critical to proper intravenous replacement.

In patients who are at or above ideal body weight and have lost less than 12% of their usual body weight, protein is provided at 1.0 to 1.5 g per kg of current body weight for maintenance of body protein status (Table 64–21). If these patients exhibit a serum albumin level less than 3 g/dl or a serum transferrin concentration less than 150 mg/dl or if weight loss has exceeded 12%, then 1.5 to 2.0 g of protein per kg of current body weight is provided. In obese patients whose current body weight exceeds 120% ideal body weight, 1.0 to 1.5 g of protein per kg *ideal* body weight is given.

Daily caloric requirements for each patient are most precisely defined by measuring resting energy expenditure using indirect calorimetry. However, the costs involved prohibit the routine use of this approach outside the research setting. Caloric requirements can also be calculated on the basis of the Harris-Benedict formula:

Male: Basal Energy Expenditure (kcal) = 66 + 13.7 × weight (kg) + 5 × height (cm) − 6.8 age (y)

Female: Basal Energy Expenditure (kcal) = 655 + 9.6 × weight (g) + 1.7 × height (cm) − 4.7 × age (y)

Daily caloric requirements are met by providing 1000 kcal above the patient's basal energy expenditure or by giving 150% of the calculated or measured resting energy expenditure. An alternate method for determining caloric requirements is to calculate 35 kcal/kg/day for maintenance and 45 kcal/kg/day for anabolism. Dietary nitrogen requirements per day should be provided in a ratio of 1 g nitrogen to 125 to 150 calories. In obese patients whose body weight exceeds 120% ideal body weight, a caloric goal of 90% to 100% resting energy expenditure should be given to allow the use of excess endogenous fat tissue for calories.

The maximal rate of glucose oxidation in the adult is 7 g/kg/day. Patients with extremely high caloric requirements or severe glucose intolerance should have calories in excess of this amount supplied by lipid. Insulin should be given as needed to maintain serum glucose levels between 130 and 250 mg/dl. In intensive care unit patients who have fluctuating needs, insulin can be given as a separate intravenous infusion using a pump under close supervision. Glucose that is not oxidized is stored as either glycogen or lipids. Fatty infiltration of the liver and increased carbon dioxide production are clinical complications of excess glucose administration.

Lipid as a 10% solution is isotonic and can therefore be administered via either central or peripheral vein. This allows administration of more calories in the form of free fatty acids, which are a major source of energy for most peripheral tissues. Most patients can tolerate up to 2 g fat/kg/day, limiting the caloric supply of fat to 18 kcal/kg/day, or 1260 kcal/day for a 70-kg person. The daily dosage should not exceed 4 g fat/kg/day. Fat emulsions, supplied as either 10% or 20% solutions, can be infused over 6 to 8 hours. The more common practice is to have all nutrients (fat, glucose, and amino acids) admixed in a 3-L bag for administration. Serum triglyceride levels should be monitored to ensure that the patient can metabolize this amount of lipid. Energy requirements are best met by using a mixed fuel system supplying 30% of the nonprotein calories as lipids. If a predominantly glucose-based system is used, at least 1000 ml of a 10% lipid emulsion per week or 4% of calories per day should be given to prevent essential fatty acid deficiency.

In addition to calories and protein, electrolytes, vitamins, and trace elements are required nutrients. Daily requirements of electrolytes are as follows: sodium, 60 to 120 mEq; potassium, 60 to 100 mEq; chloride, 60 to 120 mEq; magnesium, 8 to 10 mEq; calcium, 200 to 400 mg; and phosphorus, 300 to 400 mg. These electrolyte maintenance requirements must be met daily. In selecting the proper nutrient formula, preexisting deficits, ongoing urine and gastrointestinal losses, and organ dysfunction (cardiac, hepatic, and renal) must be considered. Vitamin and trace metal preparations are commercially available to provide daily parenteral requirements. The latter formulation contains zinc, copper, chromium, and manganese. In some centers, 1000 units of heparin are added to each liter to reduce the risk of central venous catheter occlusion and subclavian vein thrombosis.

Administration of TPN and Patient Monitoring

The safest and most effective infusion route for administering hypertonic TPN solutions in adults has been the infraclavicular, percutaneous subclavian venous catheters. Tunneling of the catheters subcutaneously and use of the Seldinger method may reduce catheter-related infections. Double- and triple-

TABLE 64–20. Potential Complications of Enteral Nutritional Support

Problem	*Diagnosis*	*Therapy*	*Prevention*
Gastrointestinal Complications			
Offensive smell/taste	c/o smell, nausea, vomiting	Add flavorings	Use polymeric formulas
Gastric retention	Gastric residual >100 ml 4 h after a bolus, or >115% of vol/h, nausea and vomiting	Dilute formula, reduce bolus volume	Dilute formula and gradually increase toxicity and volume
Rapid infusion	Nausea and vomiting	Decrease rate, advance 25 ml/h q 12–24 h	Start gastr. feedings at 40–50 ml/h, jej. & duo feedings at 20–25 ml/h, advance 25 ml/h q 12–24 h
Lactose intolerance	Review of history, diarrhea, nausea, vomiting, lactose intolerance test	Switch to nonlactose formula	Use formulas with low lactose content
Excessive fat in diet	Review of history, nausea, vomiting	Switch to low-fat diet	Provide <30–40% of calories by fat
Fat malabsorption	Review of history, 72-h fecal fat assessment	Pancreatic enzyme supplements	Use low-fat formulas
Hyperosmolar solution	Osmolality > 300 mOsm, diarrhea, increased stool water content	Dilute to isotonicity, stop for 12 h, resume at slow rate, use Kaopectate, Lomotil	Use isotonic solutions, start at slow rate (40–50 ml/h), increase in 12–24 h increments
Cold feedings	Tubing cold to touch, diarrhea	Discontinue feedings until formula is warm	Start recently refrigerated formulas at 40 ml/h
Protein malnutrition	Albumin < 3 g/dl, diarrhea	Dilute solutions to isotonicity, use antidiarrheal	Start at slow rate (20–25 ml/h), increase in 12–24 h increments
Malabsorption	Diarrhea	Decrease flow rate to 25–50 ml/h or discontinue, use parenteral feeding	Start at slow rate (20–25 ml/h), increase gradually
Dehydration	Orthostatic hypotension, dry mucous membranes, constipation	Supplemental fluids	Monitor intake and output
Impaction	Rectal examination, constipation	Digital disimpaction	Monitor intake and output
Obstruction	Nausea, vomiting, constipation, obstructive series	Surgery	
Mechanical Complications			
Nasopharyngeal discomfort	Mouth breathing, sore throat, hoarseness	Sugarless gum, gargling with warm water and mouthwash, anesthetic lozenges, viscous or spray topical anesthetics	Use soft small-bore tubes or surgically inserted tubes for long-term nutrition
Nasal erosions	Erosions of nasal ala	Tape tube without pressure on nasal ala	Use soft small-bore tubes
Abscess of nasal septum	Pain, fever, chills	Remove tube, drainage, antibiotics	Use soft small-bore tubes, proper taping
Acute sinusitis	Pain, nasal congestion, fever, malodorous breath	Remove tube, hot compresses, analgesics	Use soft small-bore tubes
Acute otitis media	Severe throbbing ear pain, fever, chills, dizziness	Change tube to other nostril, antibiotics	
Rupture of esophageal varices	Hematemesis, melena, radiographic studies	Sedation, rest of esophagus	Use soft small-bore tube
Esophagitis	Heartburn, substernal & epigastric burning	Remove tube	Keep head of bed at 45°, keep gastric pH > 7 with H_2-blockers or antacids
Esophageal ulceration	Dysphagia, radiologic studies	Remove tube, esophagoscopy, and dilation	Use soft small-bore tube; with persistent vomiting, consider a jej. tube
TE fistula	Fistula present	Symptomatic	Use soft small-bore tube, gastric or jej. tube
Knotting of tube	Unable to remove tube	Cut tube and allow to pass per rectum; use McGill forceps to bring tube out mouth to cut tube	None

(continued)

TABLE 64–20. *(Continued)*

Problem	*Causes*	*Therapy*	*Prevention*
Metabolic Complications			
Hypokalemia	Insulin administration, diarrhea, severe malnutrition	K^+ supplements	Check electrolytes
Hypophosphatemia	Insulin administration, severe malnutrition	Phosphate supplements	
Hyponatremia	Over hydration	Water restriction	
Hypomagnesemia	Decreased carrier protein, inadequate delivery	Magnesium supplements	
Elevated transaminase	Activation of hepatic enzymes, excess caloric load	Reduce carbohydrates	
Vitamin K deficiency	Inadequate delivery	Vitamin K replacement	
Essential fatty acid deficiency	Low linoleic acid	Parenteral fat, 5 ml safflower oil qd	

lumen catheters are often used, with one port for TPN and other ports for blood-drawing, antibiotic administration, or chemotherapy administration. These functions must be carefully performed and monitored to preserve catheter sterility.

Meticulous care and maintenance of the catheter are critical to ensure long-term success with TPN. At any sign of unexplained fever or sepsis, the catheter should be changed over a guidewire using aseptic technique. Blood should be removed from the catheter for culture and the catheter tip cultured after its removal over the guidewire. A new catheter can be inserted using the Seldinger guidewire technique to reduce catheter-insertion complications until catheter sterility can be determined. If catheter infection is confirmed, a new catheter should be inserted at a distant site.

Parenteral nutrition is usually initiated by administering 1000 ml of the hypertonic solution at a constant rate using a pump over 24 hours. Once the patient can metabolize dextrose and amino acids in 1000 ml of the hypertonic solution during the 24-hour period, the flow rate can be increased to 2000 ml every 24 hours. Within 2 to 3 days of nutritional repletion, average adults should be able to tolerate their caloric and protein requirements intravenously. Close monitoring and the use of a nutrition support team can dramatically reduce the incidence of TPN-associated complications (Table 64–22).

TABLE 64–21. Solutions Used for Parenteral Nutrition

Solution	*Unit Volume (ml)*	*Amino Acids (g)*	*Dextrose (g)*	*Total Calories (kcal)*
Standard	1000	50	250	850
High-calorie	1000	50	350	1200
Low nitrogen	750	25	250	850
Low nitrogen/ high-calorie	750	25	350	1250
Peripheral	1000	29	50	170
Fat emulsion 10%	500	—	—	550
Fat emulsion 20%	500	—	—	1100

NUTRITION IN THE PERIOPERATIVE PERIOD

Planning for the operative procedure should take into account all aspects of treatment and monitoring and should meld nutritional support into the operative approach and postoperative management. Patients undergoing complex upper-gastrointestinal procedures such as esophagogastrectomy, total gastrectomy, and pancreaticoduodenectomy who have experienced moderate to severe weight loss preoperatively should have a feeding jejunostomy placed for postoperative nutritional support. Standard methods use a #8, #10, or #12 French catheter placed into the proximal jejunum using a Witzel technique and suturing the bowel to the anterolateral abdominal wall. A needle-catheter jejunostomy can also be used by inserting a small-diameter catheter for 15 cm into the proximal jejunum. Because small-bowel function returns within 6 hours of the operation, D_5W can be infused at a constant rate of 25 ml/hour in the recovery room. On the first postoperative day, a full-strength feeding formula is begun at a rate of 25 ml/hour. Usually the rate of infusion is increased in increments of 10 ml/hour every 12 to 24 hours until adequate caloric and protein goals are achieved. It is important to clinically assess the patient *frequently* to ensure that the infusion rate can be increased safely. Early postoperative enteral feeding may also be indicated in cancer patients requiring adjuvant chemotherapy or radiation therapy shortly after surgery.

In the malnourished patient undergoing a major, complex intraabdominal procedure, TPN is indicated when enteral feeding cannot be accomplished by jejunostomy. Use of TPN is also indicated in the patient who develops a major postoperative complication that does not allow resumption of adequate enteral or oral feeding. However, the metabolic profile of the malnourished preoperative patient differs from that of the stressed, complicated postoperative patient. In the absence of sepsis, resting energy expenditure postoperatively may be similar or slightly increased over preoperative levels. However, the altered hormonal milieu in the septic postoperative patient results in increased protein catabolism, gluconeogenesis, and glucose intolerance. Protein should be given at 1.5

TABLE 64–22. Potential Complications Associated With Total Parenteral Nutrition

Complications	*Diagnosis*	*Treatment*	*Prevention*
Mechanical			
Pneumothorax	Dyspnea, CXR	Tube thoracostomy, observation	Avoid emergency procedures, use Trendelenburg
Hemothorax	Dyspnea, CXR	Remove catheter, observation	
Venous thrombosis	Inability to cannulate	Remove catheter, heparin therapy	Use silicone catheters; add heparin to solution
Air embolism	Dyspnea, cyanosis, hypotension, tachycardia, precordial murmur	Trendelenburg; left lateral decubitus; attempt aspiration through line	Trendelenburg, Valsalva maneuver; tape intravenous connections
Catheter embolism	Sheared catheter	Fluoroscopic retrieval	Never withdraw catheter through needle
Arrhythmias	Catheter tip in right atrium	Withdraw catheter to SVC	Fluoroscopy, CXR
Subclavian artery injury	Pulsatile red blood	Remove needle, apply pressure, CXR	Review anatomy
Catheter tip misplacement	CXR	Redirect with a guidewire	Direct bevel of needle caudally
Metabolic			
Hyperglycemic, hyperosmolar, nonketotic coma	Dehydration with osmotic diuresis, disorientation, lethargy, stupor, convulsions, coma, glu 1000 mg/dl, osm 350 mOsm/L	Discontinue TPN, D1/2NS at 250 ml/h, insulin 10–20 u/h, bicarbonate, monitor glu, K, pH	Monitor glucose
Hypoglycemia	Headache, sweating, thirst, convulsion, disorientation, paresthesias	$D_{50}W$ I.V.	Taper TPN by 1/2 for 12 h then 12 h of $D_{50}W$ at 100 ml/h
CO_2 retention	Ventilator dependence, high RQ	Reduce glucose load	Provide 30–40% of calories with fat
Azotemia	Dehydration, elevated BUN	Reduce protein load, increase nonprotein calories, increase fluid	Monitor fluid balance
Hyperammonemia	Lethargy, malaise, coma, seizures	Discontinue amino acid infusions, infuse arginine	Avoid casein or fibrin hydrolysate
Essential fatty acid deficiency	Xerosis, hepatomegaly, impaired healing, bone changes	Fat administration	Provide 25–500 mg/kg/day of essential fatty acids
Hypophosphatemia	Lethargy, anorexia, weakness, arrhythmias	Supplemental phosphate	Treat causative factors: alkalosis, gram neg, sepsis, vomiting, malabsorption, provide 20 mEq/1000 cal
Abnormal liver function tests	Fatty infiltrate	Rule out other etiologies (*e.g.*, sepsis)	Provide balanced TPN solution
Hypomagnesemia	Weakness, nausea, vomiting, tremors, depression, hyporeflexia	Infuse 10% $MgSO_4$	Supply 0.35–0.45 mEq/kg/day
Hypermagnesemia	Drowsiness, nausea, vomiting, coma, arrhythmia	Dialysis, infuse calcium gluconate	Monitor serum levels

CXR, chest x-ray; RQ, respiratory quotient; BUN, blood urea nitrogen; SVC, superior vena cava; TPN, total parenteral nutrition.

g/kg/day. Lipid emulsions are used to provide at least 30% to 40% of calculated resting energy expenditure caloric requirements to reduce the occurrence of hyperglycemia, glycosuria, and abnormal fluid and electrolyte losses.

NUTRITION AND HOST METABOLISM

Despite the demonstration of metabolic abnormalities in cancer patients, it is unclear how efficacious enteral or parenteral nutrient administration can be in reversing derangements of substrate use. Jeevanandam and colleagues evaluated changes in whole-body protein kinetics before and after administration of TPN in malnourished cancer patients using a primed-continuous infusion of ^{15}N glycine.[44] After 10 days of TPN, whole-body protein breakdown decreased by 50% and 59% in cancer and noncancer patients respectively, whereas protein synthesis decreased by 21% and 33%. The mechanism of improved nitrogen balance during intravenous repletion is probably due to a significant reduction in protein breakdown. During oral or enteral nutritional repletion, improvement in nitrogen balance may be due to stimulation of protein synthesis.

To further define the alteration in protein kinetics that occur in patients with malignancy, Shaw and Wolfe performed a series of studies to determine rates of whole-body protein synthesis and metabolism in normal volunteers and in patients with either early or advanced gastrointestinal cancer.[45] This study demonstrated that gastrointestinal cancer patients and normal volunteers had similar basal rates of whole-body protein catabolism, but cancer patients had an increased rate of net protein loss. In patients with advanced disease and marked weight loss, a state of net protein synthesis could not be achieved, although whole-body protein synthesis became nearly equivalent to whole-body protein catabolism.

The effects of nutritional support in cancer patients are often complicated by the adverse effects of antineoplastic therapy. Drott and coworkers randomized 23 patients with metastatic testicular carcinoma to receive either TPN or spontaneous oral intake during their hospital stay coincident with multidrug chemotherapy.[46] Energy and nitrogen intakes were profoundly decreased in the spontaneous oral intake group, whereas intake decreased in the TPN group only at home while patients relied on oral intake alone. Despite the cytotoxic drugs, the TPN group remained in nitrogen balance when undergoing TPN. However, they lost substantial body weight and nitrogen over 10 weeks, which was a result of the prolonged anorexia all patients had after termination of chemotherapy. Thus, intermittent periods of adequate intravenous nutrition had only a marginal long-term impact. The clinical significance of improved nitrogen balance during chemotherapy administration remains controversial.

Several animal models have suggested that dietary nutritional depletion decreases tumor growth but results in marked wasting of the host (Fig. 64–12). Controversy exists as to whether nutritional repletion stimulates tumor growth out of proportion to enhancement of host nutritional status (Table 64–23). Numerous studies have demonstrated accelerated tumor growth in animals receiving nutrition support. Torosian and associates reported significant increases in the S, or DNA synthetic, phase of tumor cell cycle kinetics with potentiation of chemotherapy efficacy during parenteral nutrient administration.[47] Karpeh and colleagues reported that nutritional repletion resulted in significantly smaller tumors in the moderately immunogenic C1300 neuroblastoma and larger tumors in the nonimmunogenic TBJ neuroblastoma.[48] These results suggest that the influence of nutritional repletion on the tumor-bearing host varies specifically with the presence of an antitumor immune response.

Other studies in tumor-bearing animal models have demonstrated effects of specific nutrient alterations on tumor growth. Skeef and coworkers noted that zinc deficiency had a stimulatory effect on cAMP synthesis that was selective for hepatoma cells in an animal tumor model.[49] Both zinc deficiency and zinc excess resulted in a tendency toward decreased tumor growth in their hepatoma model. The effect of a protein-free diet or restricted intake and subsequent host repletion with TPN was examined by Grossie and associates.[50] Host body weight was significantly reduced both by the administration of a protein-free diet and restriction of standard diets

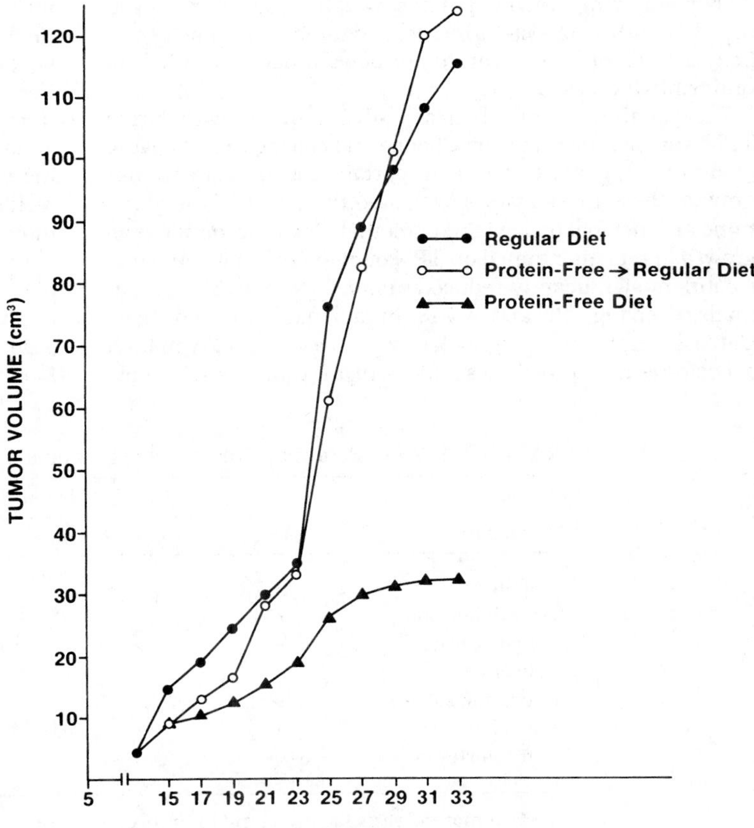

FIGURE 64–12. Tumor volume plateaus in animals on a protein-free diet. Animals switched from a protein-free to a regular diet on day 15 show a rapid increase in tumor volume to become similar to the regular diet group.

TABLE 64–23. Effects of Nutrition Supplementation on Tumor Growth

Animal/Tumor System	*Nutrition*	*Results*
W rats/AC-33	I.V. AA ± dextrose	↑ Tumor growth, no change tumor/host weight
	I.V. AA or TPN	↑ Tumor protein synthesis
	TPN	↑ Tumor weight, no change tumor/host weight
	TPN	↑ % S-phase tumor cells
F344/rats/MCA sarcoma	TPN	↑ Tumor weight proportional to TPN infused; tumor/host weight
SD rats/W256	Oral prot/carb diet	↑ Tumor volume
	Oral prot/carb diet or TPN	↑ Tumor volume, no change tumor/host weight
	TPN	↑ Tumor growth ↑ Tumor mitotic acitivty ↑ Tumor/host weight
Buff rats/Morris hepatoma	TPN	↑ H^3-thymidine labeling index of tumors
W rats/W-256	TPN	No significant ↑ tumor weight
ACI-N rats/Morris hepatoma	TPN	No change in tumor weight, protein content, or DNA synthesis

TPN, total parenteral nutrition; AA, amino acids; MCA, methylcholanthrene; SD, Sprague-Dawley; W, Walker.
(Adapted from Torosian M, Daly JM. Nutritional support in the cancer-bearing host. Cancer 1986;58: 1915–1929)

with diminished tumor growth. Subsequent host repletion with TPN resulted in a rebound of host weight and tumor growth, together with a consistent increase in tumor ornithine decarboxylase activity. However, tumor polyamine levels were not uniformly increased.

Further efforts to metabolically affect tumor growth during TPN were demonstrated by Chance and colleagues.[51] Because glutamine appears to be an important substrate for tumor growth, these investigators evaluated the effect of the glutamine antimetabolite acivicin on methylcholanthrene sarcoma growth in rats maintained on TPN or given rat chow. Acivicin treatment significantly reduced tumor growth by 67% in animals receiving TPN and by 71% in rats maintained on chow. Carcass weights were significantly increased by TPN in both acivicin-treated and saline-solution-treated tumor-bearing rats.

Thus, interest continues in methods to manipulate specific nutrients to selectively promote host anabolism while "starving" the tumor (Table 64–24). Unfortunately, this desired endpoint may be complicated by host metabolic requirements. For example, glutamine is an energy substrate of the intestinal tract. Recently, Grant and Snyder evaluated the use of L-glutamine in TPN in an animal model.[52] They noted that adding either 1% or 2% L-glutamine to TPN solutions did not result in any toxic clinical effects. Glutamine preserved the intestinal nitrogen content of the stomach and the colon compared with standard TPN and increased the nitrogen content of the small bowel greater than that seen in chow-fed animals. Adding 1% and 2% glutamine increased mucosal disaccharidase activity and protected the liver from fatty infiltration found with administration of standard TPN. Use of glutamine-

TABLE 64–24. Potential Treatments of Cancer Cachexia

	Metabolic Abnormalities				
Therapy	*Anorexia*	*Carbohydrate*	*Protein*	*Fat*	*Host Weight*
Insulin	+	++	+	+	+
Growth hormone	+	+	++		+
Somatostatin	+	+	+		
Acivicin		+	+		+
Hydrazine sulfate	+	++	+		+
Anti-TNF	+			+++	+
Anti-interferon-γ	++	+		+++	+

TNF, tumor necrosis factor. +, mild improvement; ++, moderate improvement; +++, marked improvement.

supplemented TPN may substantially reduce the adverse side effects of chemotherapy such as mucositis and enterocolitis.

Enterocolitis induced by radiation therapy and chemotherapy is a significant problem and often is the sole limiting side effect from the administration of antineoplastic therapy. Previous work in our laboratory noted that administration of an elemental diet to rats given methotrexate resulted in 100% mortality from severe enterocolitis (Fig. 64–13). Enteral feeding with polypeptides protected completely (100% survival) against methotrexate-induced enterocolitis.[53] Administration of glutamine with the elemental diet also resulted in increased survival (30%).[54] Thus, administration of a peptide-based diet or an elemental diet supplemented with glutamine, either enterally or parenterally, can protect against intestinal injury when either liquid elemental diets or TPN are used. Further studies in humans are clearly indicated to confirm these experimental results.

NUTRITION AND IMMUNITY

Immunosuppression is a common finding in the cancer patient. Malignancy, malnutrition, surgery, anesthesia, blood transfusions, chemotherapy, and radiation treatment have all been found to depress the immune system. Patients with cancer show depression of both cellular and humoral immune functions. Classically, T-cell proliferative responses to both mitogen and alloantigen are reduced with increasing tumor burden. Patients with advanced disease often lack a delayed-type hypersensitivity reaction to skin-recall antigens (anergy). Anergy is clearly predictive of increased sepsis and mortality in patients undergoing major surgery.[55]

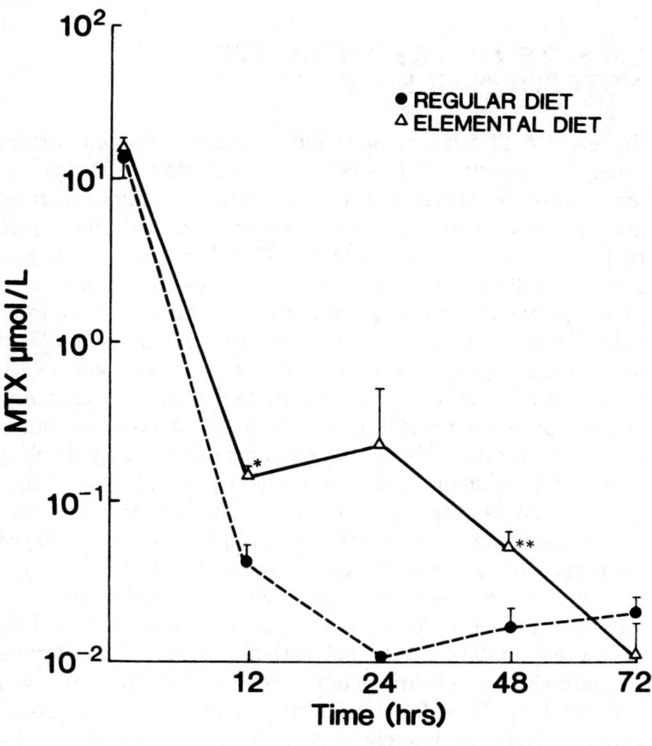

FIGURE 64–13. Plasma clearance of methotrexate (MTX) was significantly slower in animals given an elemental diet compared with a regular diet. Significantly greater toxicity (enterocolitis) was noted in the former group after receiving 20 mg/kg MTX.

In analyzing anergy, defects in T-cell activation have been found to be the primary abnormality in the delayed hypersensitivity response.[56] When removed from the "anergic environment" and cultured in vitro with recall antigen, however, T cells proliferate normally. These activated T cells then can elicit the delayed-type hypersensitivity response when reinjected into the patient. Cytotoxic T lymphocytes isolated from patients with breast, lung, and colon carcinomas as well as from sarcomas demonstrate decreased cytotoxicity to autologous tumor.[57] Natural killer cells, the body's putative first line against cancer, are also less active when isolated from tumor-bearing animals and patients.

In addition to the immunosuppression that occurs in the presence of malignancy, operative therapy intended to eradicate tumor may promote metastatic tumor growth. Patients undergoing diverting colostomy followed by colectomy for cancer have been shown to do less well than those treated by one operation.[58] Controlled experiments in animal models corroborate enhancement of tumor growth, but mechanisms remain obscure.[59] Functionally, T cells show depressed responses to mitogen or alloantigen. Although blood transfusions are often unavoidable in oncologic surgery, they may adversely affect outcome in the cancer patient. Perioperative blood transfusion has been associated with significantly poorer prognosis in patients with breast carcinoma, colon cancer, non-small cell lung cancer, and sarcoma.[60–63] The mechanisms involved are complex and multifactoral, but multiple blood transfusions depress the immune response manifested in vitro by poor T-cell proliferative indices and decreased effector-cell response to various lymphokines.

Certain nutrient substrates may have a major role in the nutritional support of the cancer patient. Specific amino acids, RNA, ω-3 fatty acids, and trace metals such as zinc have all been shown to affect host immune function.

Arginine is a semi-essential dibasic amino acid that is a component of the urea cycle (Fig. 64–14). It is converted by the enzyme arginase into ornithine and urea. Arginine has potent secretagogue effects on several endocrine and neuroendocrine glands.[64,65] Administration of arginine induces the secretion of growth hormone, prolactin, insulin, glucagon, insulin-like growth factor-1, pancreatic polypeptide, somatostatin, and catecholamines. In laboratory studies, arginine supplementation has thymotropic properties and enhances the responsiveness of thymic lymphocytes to mitogens in normal and traumatized animals.[66,67] Arginine enhances cellular immunity, as evidenced by improved skin allograft rejection in normal mice and improved delayed-type hypersensitivity responses and improved bacterial containment and survival in animal burn models. Arginine has also been demonstrated to have antitumor effects in both chemically and virally induced and transplanted solid tumor models. Studies from our laboratory have demonstrated beneficial effects of supplemental arginine in the tumor-bearing host by noting increased concanavalin A (con-A) mitogenic responses and IL-2 production by host splenocytes and increased host reactivity against tumor antigens in the tumor-bearing group.[68] Supplemental arginine significantly retarded the growth of C1300 neuroblastoma in protein-depleted mice and prolonged

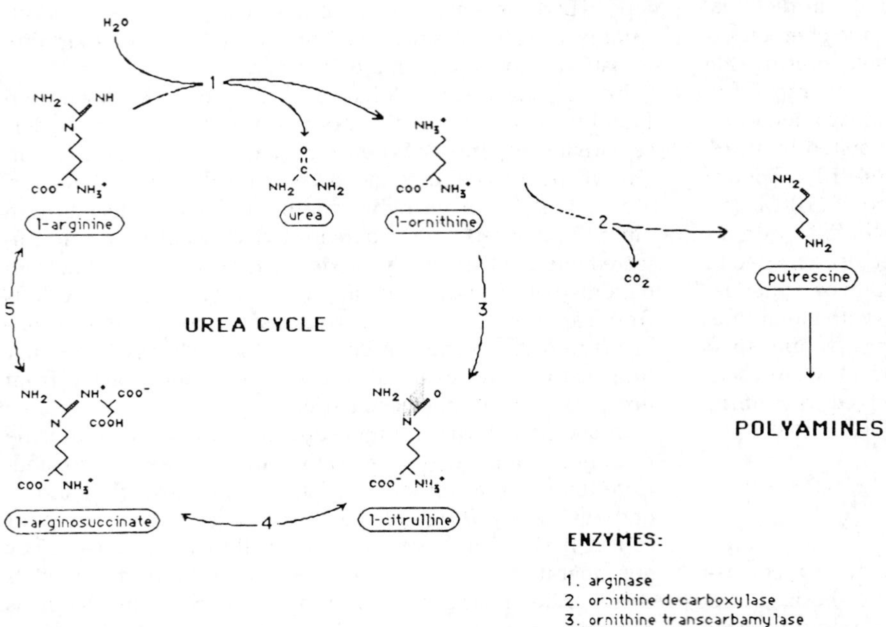

FIGURE 64–14. Arginine is a semi-essential amino acid within the urea cycle.

median host survival.[69] These effects were dependent on tumor antigenicity.

Few clinical studies have examined the role of oral or intravenous supplemental arginine in humans. In healthy volunteers, supplemental dietary arginine increased peripheral blood lymphocyte mitogenic response to con-A and phytohemagglutinin (PHA).[70] Our group investigated the effects of supplemental arginine in cancer patients undergoing major surgery.[71] Thirty patients were randomized to receive either supplemental arginine (25 g/day) or isonitrogenous L-glycine (43 g/day) as part of the graduated enteral diet for 7 days after surgery (Fig. 64–15). Supplemental arginine significantly increased mean mitogenic responses to con-A and PHA on postoperative days four and seven compared to postoperative day one (Fig. 64–16). No differences were found in the glycine-treated group. Mean CD4 phenotype levels on postoperative day seven were also significantly increased compared to the glycine group. Mean plasma levels of somatomedin-C were also significantly increased on day seven in the arginine group compared with the glycine group.

RNA has been demonstrated to be essential for the continued maturation of T cells in animal models. Absence of RNA from the diet results in depressed cell-mediated immune function, decreased survival after *Staphylococcus aureus* injection, and diminished rejection of allografts.[72] Fatty acids in the diet affect levels of arachidonic and eicosapentaenoic acid, resulting in changes in prostaglandin synthesis. Increased intake of ω-3 fatty acids has been reported to improve immunologic function by decreasing prostaglandin E_2 production after major injury. Animal studies by Alexander and coworkers have demonstrated improved response to infectious challenges in animals supplemented with ω-3 fatty acids.[73] Recent studies in cancer patients undergoing major upper gastrointestinal surgery demonstrated a significant reduction in postoperative infections, wound complications, and hospital length of stay in patients receiving arginine, RNA, and ω-3 fatty acids compared with patients receiving a standard diet (Fig. 64–17).[74]

EFFECTS OF PREOPERATIVE NUTRITIONAL SUPPORT

Since 1967, TPN has gained wide acceptance as an important route of nutrient administration. Recognition of the prevalence and consequences of malnutrition in the tumor-bearing host has promoted the use of TPN in these patients. More recently, however, routine use of TPN has been the subject of critical debate. Controversy exists regarding the role of preoperative TPN to significantly reduce perioperative morbidity, duration of hospital stay, and health-care costs. Most investigators agree that preoperative TPN is not indicated in well-nourished or mildly malnourished patients. Certainly, urgent operative procedures should not be delayed for nutritional intervention. The debate centers around the moderately to severely malnourished patient undergoing a high-risk procedure such as esophagectomy, total gastrectomy, and pancreaticoduodenectomy. Should elective procedures be delayed for nutritional repletion in these circumstances?

Numerous retrospective and prospective studies have examined the role of preoperative TPN (Table 64–25). Retrospective studies in surgical patients have generally demonstrated improved clinical outcome in patients who received perioperative TPN. In an analysis of 244 esophageal cancer patients, Daly and associates demonstrated a significant decrease in major complications in patients who received 5 or more days of TPN preoperatively compared with both concurrent and historical controls who did not receive TPN.[75] In other studies, preoperative TPN significantly reduced com-

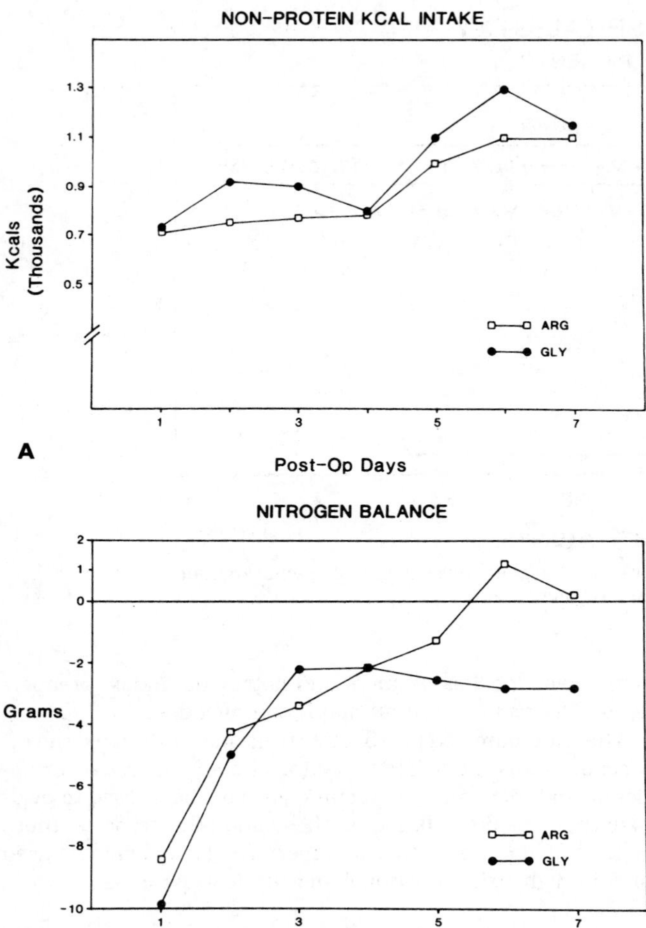

FIGURE 64–15. Postoperative patients were randomized to receive arginine (25 g/day) or glycine (43 g/day) in addition to standard enteral feeding by jejunostomy. Although caloric intake was similar, nitrogen balance was slightly improved in the arginine group.

lated to the patient and the planned operation. It also allows use of postoperative enteral feeding, which may be significantly more cost-effective.

In 1979 Heatley and associates studied 74 gastric cancer patients who either received preoperative TPN for 7 to 10 days or served as controls.[76] TPN patients had fewer wound infections and lost less body weight perioperatively than corresponding control patients. Muller and colleagues studied 125 patients with gastrointestinal cancer who were randomized to receive 10 days of preoperative TPN or standard diet.[77] Postoperative major morbidity and mortality were significantly lower in the TPN group. Muller and coworkers reported an extension of their work that included three groups: control, TPN (amino acids/glucose), and TPN-L (amino acids/glucose/lipid emulsion) patients.[78] Significant differences were seen in body-weight change, protein and immune parameters, and major complications and mortality comparing the TPN (amino acid/glucose) and control groups. The trial was changed before completion by stopping the TPN-L (amino acids/glucose/lipid emulsion) group due to greater complications in this group.

Studies by Starker[79] and Bellantone[80] and their colleagues included patients with benign and malignant disease. In the former study, 59 malnourished patients were divided into three groups based on initial response to TPN. Patients received TPN for 5 days to 6 weeks. The authors noted a high morbidity and mortality in patients who remained hypoalbuminemic after 1 week of TPN, suggesting the importance of administering preoperative TPN until nutritional deficits have been corrected.

Foschi and coworkers studied 64 patients who underwent preoperative transhepatic catheter biliary diversion for obstructive jaundice with or without preoperative TPN.[81] The nutritionally repleted group had significantly fewer major complications (18% versus 47%) and mortality (3.5% versus 12.5%) compared with control patients.

A multiinstitutional prospective randomized trial evaluated plications in patients deemed to be at high risk by their prognostic nutritional index.

Thus, clinical trials of perioperative TPN have demonstrated improved nutritional status as reflected by gain in body weight, improvement in serum protein levels, restoration of immune function, and improved nitrogen balance. Effects on clinical outcome remain less well defined. Preoperative TPN probably results in a significant reduction in postoperative complications and reduced mortality in the *severely malnourished, high-risk* group when given for an *adequate* length of time. Failure to demonstrate improved outcome with TPN in other trials may accurately reflect the limited value of TPN in well-nourished or moderately malnourished patients or in patients undergoing low-risk procedures. It is also possible that in these patients, the complications associated with TPN and the increased risk of nosocomial infections due to prolonged hospitalization negate any benefit and may result in net harm.

A useful approach to the nutritional management of elective surgical patients is shown in Figure 64–10. This approach uses a clinical assessment of nutritional and medical risk re-

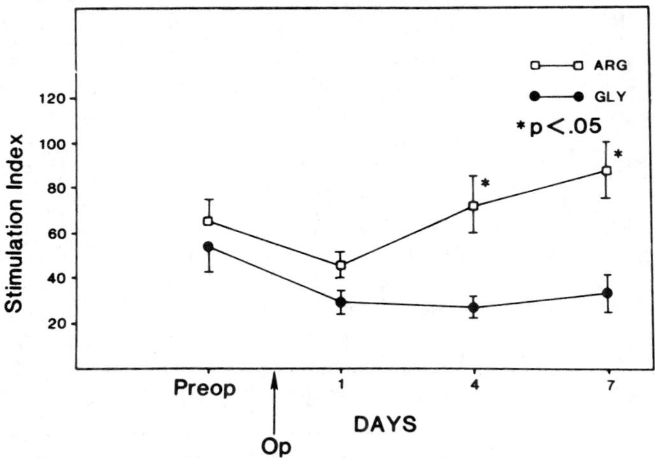

FIGURE 64–16. Peripheral blood T lymphocyte activation to ConA was significantly improved on postoperative days 4 and 7 in the arginine group compared with the glycine group.

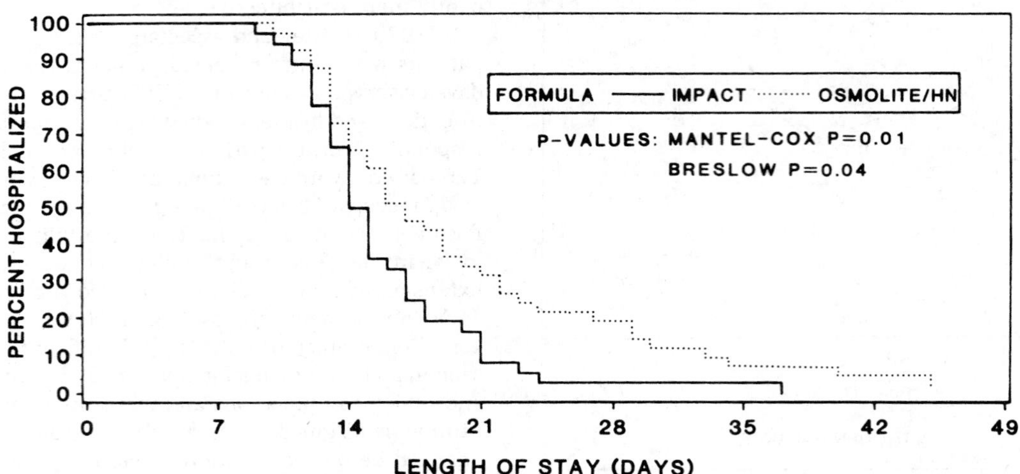

FIGURE 64–17. Length of hospital stay was significantly less in the group receiving supplemental arginine, RNA, and omega-3 fatty acids compared with a standard enteral diet.

TPN in surgical patients.[82] Two hundred and thirty-one TPN and 228 control patients were studied at ten Veterans Administration Medical Centers across the United States. Mortality rates and major postoperative complications were similar for both groups. A higher incidence of infectious complications was noted in the TPN group, while a higher noninfectious complication rate occurred in controls. In the subgroup of patients with severe malnutrition, measured by subjective global assessment and nutritional index, preoperative TPN reduced overall major complications.

These randomized prospective trials have evaluated the effects of preoperative TPN on clinical outcome in cancer patients, and meta-analysis techniques have been used to evaluate their results.[83] Based on these and other reports, there is general agreement that perioperative TPN should be used only in high-risk (nutritional and surgical) patients.

TABLE 64–25. Prospective Randomized Trials of Preoperative TPN in Surgical Patients

Investigations	*No. of Patients*	*Preoperative TPN Duration (days)*	*Complication Rate (%)* TPN vs Control	*Mortality Rate (%)* TPN vs Control
Holter, 1977	56	3	13 vs 19	7 vs 8
Heatley, 1979[76]	74	7–10	28 vs 25	15 vs 22
Holter, 1976	26	2	16 vs 18	ND
Moghissi, 1977	15	5–7	30 vs 50	ND
Preshaw, 1979	47	1	33 vs 17	ND
Simms, 1980	40	7–10	ND	0 vs 10
Lim, 1981	19	21–28	30 vs 50	10 vs 20
Schildt, 1981	15	14	38 vs 57	0 vs 0
Thompson, 1981	41	5–14	17 vs 11 vs 10	0 vs 0 vs 0
Sako, 1981	69	8–32	50 vs 56	50 vs 25
Mueller, 1982	125	10	11 vs 19	3 vs 11
Burt, 1982	18	14	ND	ND
Jenson, 1982	20	2	Sig in TPN group	ND
Starker, 1986[79]	59	5–42	12.5 vs 45	0 vs 10
Foschi, 1986[81]	64	20	18 vs 47	3.5 vs 12.5
Bellantone, 1988[80]	100	7	5.3 vs 22	5.3 vs 6.6

ND, not determined; TPN, total parenteral nutrition.
(Modified from Redmond HP, Daly JM. Preoperative nutritional therapy in cancer patients is beneficial. In: Simmons R, ed. Debates in clinical surgery. Chicago: Mosby-Year Book, 1991)

NUTRITIONAL SUPPORT WITH CHEMOTHERAPY AND RADIATION THERAPY

The use of nutritional support in the cancer patient receiving chemotherapy and radiation therapy remains controversial because of the lack of appropriate prospective randomized clinical trials to evaluate the effect of nutritional support on host survival and morbidity in these patients. Major flaws exist in most published clinical studies, including inadequate numbers of patients, inadequate duration/amount of nutritional support, heterogenous patient populations, and inappropriate study populations. Many clinical trials do not even stratify patients into malnourished versus well-nourished groups.

Numerous clinical reviews have correlated malnutrition with decreased survival in patients with advanced cancer receiving chemotherapy. Despite retrospective studies suggesting improved tolerance to chemotherapy in patients receiving nutritional support, prospective randomized trials have provided limited support for this concept. The primary toxicities evaluated in these trials include gastrointestinal (nausea, vomiting, stomatitis, and diarrhea), hematologic (leukopenia, anemia, and thrombocytopenia), and septic complications. The results are summarized in Table 64–26. In six trials that studied gastrointestinal toxicity, reduced toxicity was demonstrated in only one study and increased toxicity (stomatitis) was found in two studies; no difference in toxicity was found comparing TPN and control groups in three studies. Only two of eleven trials documented less hematologic toxicity in patients receiving TPN; in one trial of patients with advanced colorectal cancer, increased hematologic toxicity was observed. Finally, two of five clinical trials observed an increased incidence of septic complications in patients receiving TPN compared with the control group. A review of tumor response and length of survival in these clinical trials demonstrated similar outcome between patients receiving parenteral nutrition and control groups.

Weisdorf and associates in 1987 performed a prospective study of 137 bone-marrow transplant patients. In this large clinical trial, patients receiving TPN demonstrated improved overall survival, improved disease-free survival, and decreased incidence of relapse compared with control patients. This large prospective study demonstrates the possibility of using TPN to support patients through extremely aggressive chemotherapy treatment regimens.

Radiation therapy increases the potential for the development of severe nutritional deficits, and toxicity is related to degree of preexisting malnutrition, radiation site, and dose of radiation given. Published clinical trials of the efficacy of nutritional support in patients receiving radiation therapy suffer from the same defects as studies in chemotherapy patients. Most clinical radiation therapy studies have been conducted in patients with head and neck, esophageal, and abdominal/pelvic cancer (Table 64–27). An almost universal finding in studies of patients with advanced malignancy receiving radiation therapy is that TPN significantly increases weight gain. The significance of this weight gain is limited, however, as reduced toxicity and improved survival are difficult to demonstrate. Improved survival was found in one prospective study of 40 cancer patients receiving abdominal/pelvic radiation therapy, and fewer interruptions in radiation therapy treatments were seen in a similar patient population. However, insufficient numbers of patients have been evaluated to establish or refute the efficacy of nutritional support in patients receiving radiation therapy.

In summary, the efficacy of nutritional support in patients receiving adjuvant chemotherapy and radiation therapy remains to be determined. Few conclusions can be made from the limited information provided by existing prospective randomized trials. Nutritional support may play a more important role as adjuvant therapy regimens become more intense, such as bone-marrow transplantation. Furthermore, specific nutrients such as glutamine, arginine, and ω-3 fatty acids may play either a nutritive or pharmacologic role to prevent organ-

TABLE 64–26. Effect of Parenteral Nutrition on Chemotherapy Toxicity

Tumor Type	*No. of Patients*	*Gastrointestinal*	*Hematologic*	*Infections*
Lymphoma	41	—	ND	—
Colorectal	45	ND	↓	—
Testicular	30	ND	↑	↓
Metastatic sarcoma	27	—	ND	ND
Childhood metastatic	19	—	—	↓
Acute leukemia	23	—	ND	—
Lung, small cell	39	ND	ND	—
Lung, small cell	39	↓	ND	ND
Lung, small cell	31	—	ND	—
Lung, adenocarcinoma	43	↓	ND	ND
Lung, non-small cell	27	—	ND	—
Lung, squamous cell		↑	↑	—

↑, TPN group had reduced toxicity vs control group; ↓, TPN group had increased toxicity vs control group; —, information not provided; ND, no difference.
(Adapted from Koretz RL. J Clin Oncol 1984;2:535)

TABLE 64–27. TPN and Radiation Therapy

Cancer	*No. of Patients*	*Weight*	*Toxicity*	*% XRT Given*		*Survival*	
				TPN	*Control*		
Pelvic	32	↑TPN	ND	—	—	—	—
Abdominal/pelvic	20	↑TPN	ND	92	100	—	ND
Abdominal/pelvic	40	↑TPN	—	—	—	↑	—
Ovarian	81	—	—	—	—	ND	—
Abdominal/pelvic	25	—	ND	100	100	—	ND
Abdominal/pelvic	29	↑TPN	ND	91	82	ND	—

TPN, total parenteral nutrition; ND, no difference; XRT, radiation therapy.

specific toxicity. Once the mechanism of cancer cachexia and cellular mechanisms of adjuvant therapy toxicity have been elucidated, more specific nutrient regimens may be designed to prevent the development of cancer cachexia and reduce host toxicity associated with antineoplastic therapy.

REFERENCES

1. DeWys WE, Begg C, Lavin PT, et al. Prognostic effect of weight loss prior to chemotherapy in cancer patients. Am J Med 1980;69:491–497.
2. DeWys WD, Walters K. Abnormalities of taste sensation in cancer patients. Cancer 1975;36:1888–1896.
3. Lucke B, Borwick M, Zeckwer I. Liver catalase activity in parabiotic rats with one partner tumor bearing. J Natl Cancer Inst 1952;13:681–686.
4. Nakahara W. A chemical basis for tumor host relations. J Natl Cancer Inst 1960;24: 77–86.
5. Langstein H, Fraker D, Norton JA. Reversal of cancer cachexia by antibodies to interferon-gamma but not cachectin/tumor necrosis factor. Surg Forum 1989;40:408–410.
6. Krause R, Humphreys C, von Meyenfeldt M. A central mechanism for anorexia in cancer: A hypothesis. Cancer Treat Rep 1981;65(suppl):15–21.
7. Brennan MF. Uncomplicated starvation versus cancer cachexia. Cancer Res 1977;37: 2359–2364.
8. Brennan MF, Burt ME. Nitrogen metabolism in cancer patients. Cancer Treat Rep 1981;65(suppl):67–78.
9. Holroyde CP, Reichard A. Carbohydrate metabolism in cancer cachexia. Cancer Treat Rep 1981;65(suppl):55–59.
10. Young VR. Energy metabolism and requirements in the cancer patient. Cancer Res 1977;37:2336–2347.
11. Warnold I, Lundholm K, Schersten T. Energy balance and body composition in cancer. Cancer Res 1978;38:1801–1807.
12. Shike M, Russell D, Detsky A, et al. Changes in body composition in patients with small cell lung cancer: The effect of TPN as an adjunct to chemotherapy. Ann Intern Med 1984;101:303–309.
13. Knox LS, Crosby LO, Feurer ID, et al. Energy expenditure in malnourished cancer patients. Ann Surg 1983;197:152–162.
14. Heber D, Chlebowski RT, Ishibashi DE, et al. Abnormalities in glucose and protein metabolism in non-cachectic lung cancer patients. Cancer Res 1982;42:4815–4819.
15. Shaw JM, Humberstone DM, Wolfe RR. Energy and protein metabolism in sarcoma patients. Ann Surg 1988;207:283–289.
16. Buzby GP, Mullen JL, Matthews DC, et al. Prognostic nutritional index in gastrointestinal surgery. Am J Surg 1980;139:160–167.
17. Schein PS, Kesner D, Haller D, et al. Cachexia of malignancy: Potential role of insulin in nutritional management. Cancer 1979;43:2070–2076.
18. Waterhouse C, Jeanpretre N, Keilson J. Gluconeogenesis from alanine in patients with progressive malignant disease. Cancer Res 1979;39:1968–1972.
19. Moley JF, Morrison SD, Gornschboty DM, Norton JA. Body composition changes in rats with experimental cancer cachexia: Improvement with exogenous insulin. Cancer Res 1988;48:2784–2787.
20. Peacock JL, Norton JA. Impact of insulin on survival of cachectic tumor-bearing rats. J Parenter Enteral Nutr 1988;12:260–264.
21. Shaw JHF, Wolfe RR. Whole-body protein kinetics in patients with early and advanced gastrointestinal cancer—the response to glucose infusion and total parenteral nutrition. Surgery 1977;103:148–155.
22. Lundholm K, Edstron S, Edman L, et al. Metabolism in peripheral tissues in cancer patients. Cancer Treat Rep 1981;65(suppl):79–83.
23. Brennan MF. Cancer cachexia and rate of whole-body lipolysis. Metabolism 1986;35: 304–310.
24. Waterhouse C. Nutritional disorders in neoplastic diseases. J Chron Dis 1963;16:637–644.
25. Waterhouse C, Kemperman JH. Carbohydrate metabolism in subjects with cancer. Cancer Res 1971;31:1273–1278.
26. Wilson AW, Kirk CJC, Goode AW. The effect of weight loss, operation and parenteral nutrition on fat clearance in patients with colorectal cancer. Clin Sci 1987;73:489–495.
27. Norton JA, Stein TP, Brennan MF. Whole-body protein synthesis and turnover in normal and malnourished patients with and without known cancer. Ann Surg 1981;194:123–128.
28. Kien CL, Carmitta BN. Close association of accelerated rats of whole-body protein turnover (synthesis and breakdown) and energy expenditure in children with newly diagnosed acute lymphocytic leukemia. J Parenter Enteral Nutr 1987;11:129–134.
29. Fearon KCH, Hansell DT, Preston T, et al. Influence of whole-body protein turnover rate on resting energy expenditure in patients with cancer. Cancer Res 1988;48:2590–2595.
30. Tayek JA, Blackburn GL, Bistrian BR. Alterations in whole-body, muscle, liver and tumor tissue protein synthesis and degradation in Novikoff hepatoma and Yoshida sarcoma tumor growth studied in vivo. Cancer Res 1988;48:1554–1558.
31. Cohn SH, Gartenhaus W, Sawitsky A, et al. Compartmental body composition of cancer patients by measurement of total body nitrogen, potassium, and water. Metabolism 1981;30:222–229.
32. Bartlett DL, Torosian MH. Specific metabolic therapy of cancer cachexia. Arch Surg (in press).
33. McAnena OJ, Daly JM. Impact of antitumor therapy on nutrition. Surg Clin N Am 1986;66:1213–1228.
34. Stein JP, Buzby GP. Protein metabolism in surgical patients. Surg Clin N Am 1981;61: 519–527.
35. Copeland EM, Daly JM, Dudrick SJ. Nutrition as an adjunct to cancer treatment in the adult. Cancer Res 1977;37:2451–2456.
36. Nixon DW, Heymsfield SB, Cohen AE. Protein-calorie malnutrition in hospitalized cancer patients. Am J Med 1980;68:683–690.
37. Warren S. The immediate cause of death in cancer. Am J Med Sci 1932;184:610–615.
38. Meguid M, Mughal MM, Debonis D, et al. Influence of nutritional status on the resumption of adequate food intake in patients recovering from colorectal cancer operations. Surg Clin N Am 1986;66:1167–1176.
39. Daly JM, Copeland EM, Dudrick SJ. Effect of intravenous nutrition on tumor growth and host immunocompetence in malnourished animals. Surgery 1978;84:655–658.
40. Law DK, Dudrick SJ, Abdou NI. The effects of protein-calorie malnutrition on immunocompetence of the surgical patient. Surg Gynecol Obstet 1974;139:257–266.
41. Harvey KB, Bath A, Jr, Blackburn GL. Nutritional assessment and patient outcome during oncological therapy. Cancer 1979;43(suppl):2065–2069.
42. Daly JM, Dudrick SJ, Copeland EM. Intravenous hyperalimentation: Effect on delayed cutaneous hypersensitivity in cancer patients. Ann Surg 1980;192:587–592.
43. McEntee GP, Forster S, Duignan JP, O'Malley E. The effect of parenteral nutritional support on cell-mediated immunity. Int Ther Clin Monit 1988;8:138–143.
44. Jeevanandam M, Legaspi A, Lowry SF, Horowitz GD, Brennan MF. Effect of total parenteral nutrition on whole-body protein kinetics in cachectic patients with benign or malignant disease. J Parenter Enteral Nutr 1988;12:229–236.
45. Shaw JHF, Wolfe RR. Whole-body protein kinetics in patients with early and advanced gastrointestinal cancer—the response to glucose infusion and total parenteral nutrition. Surgery 1977;103:148–155.
46. Drott C, Unsgaard B, Schersten T, Lundholm K. Total parenteral nutrition as an adjuvant to patients undergoing chemotherapy for testicular carcinoma: Protection of body composition—a randomized, prospective study. Surgery 1977;103:499–506.
47. Torosian MH, Tsou KC, Daly JM, et al. Alteration of tumor cell kinetics by total parenteral nutrition: Potential therapeutic implications. Cancer 1984;53:1409–1415.
48. Karpeh MS, Kehne JA, Choi SH, et al. Tumor immunogenicity, nutritional repletion and cancer. Surgery 1987;102:283–290.
49. Skeef NS, Duncan Jr. A possible relation between dietary zinc and cAMP in the regulation of tumor cell proliferation in the rat. Br J Nutr 1988;59:437–442.
50. Grossie VB Jr, Ota DM, Ajani JA, Chang THE, Pateniz D, Nishioka K. Influence of total parenteral nutrition on tumor growth and polyamine biosynthesis of fibrosarcoma-bearing rats after induced-cachexia. J Parenter Enteral Nutr 1988;12:441–444.

51. Chance WT, Cao L, Nelson JL, Foley-Nelson T, Fischer JE. Acivicin reduces tumor growth during total parenteral nutrition. Surgery 1987;102:386–394.
52. Grant JP, Snyder PJ. Use of L-glutamine in total parenteral nutrition. J Surg Res 1988;33:506–513.
53. McAnena OJ, Harvey LP, Bonau RA, Daly JM. Alteration of methotrexate toxicity in rats by manipulation of dietary components. Gastroenterology 1987;92:354–360.
54. Fox AD, Kripke SA, DePaula J, Berman JM, Settle RG, Rombeau JL. Effect of a glutamine-supplemented enteral diet on methotrexate-induced enterocolitis. J Parenter Enteral Nutr 1988;12:325–331.
55. Meakins JL. Pietsch JB, Bubenik O, et al. Delayed hypersensitivity indicator of acquired failure of host defenses in sepsis and trauma. Ann Surg 1977;186:241–246.
56. Rode HN, Christou NV, Bubenik O, et al. Lymphocyte function in anergic patients. Clin Exp Immunol 1982;47:156–161.
57. Tartter PI, Martinelli G, Steinberg B, et al. Changes in peripheral T-cell subsets and natural killer cytotoxicity in relation to colorectal cancer surgery. Cancer Detect Prev 1987;9:359–364.
58. Lundy J, Lovett EJ, Hamilton S, et al. Immune impairment and metastatic tumor growth. Cancer 1979;43:945–951.
59. Weese JL, Ottery FD, Emoto SE. Does operation facilitate tumor growth? An experimental model in rats. Surgery 1986;100:273–277.
60. Tartter PI, Burrows L, Papatesta AE, et al. Perioperative blood transfusion has prognostic significance for breast cancer. Surgery 1985;97:225–230.
61. Burrows L, Tartter P. Effects of blood transfusions on colonic malignancy recurrence rate. Lancet 1982;2:662–664.
62. Blumberg N. Agarwal MM, Chuang C. Relation between recurrence of cancer of the colon and blood transfusion. Br Med J 1985;290:1037–1039.
63. Rosenberg SA, Siepp CA, White DE, et al. Perioperative blood transfusions are associated with increased rates of recurrence and decreased survival in patients with high-grade soft-tissue sarcoma of the extremities. J Clin Oncol 1985;3:698–709.
64. Merimee TJ, Lillicrap DA, Rabinowitz D. Effect of arginine on serum levels of human growth hormone. Lancet 1965;2:668–670.
65. Rakoff JS, Siver TM, Sinha YM, et al. Prolactin and growth hormone release in response to sequential stimulation by arginine and TRF. J Clin Endocrin Metab 1973;37:641–644.
66. Barbul A, Wasserkrug HL, Sisto DA, et al. Thymic and immune stimulatory actions of arginine. J Parenter Enteral Nutr 1980;4:446–449.
67. Barbul A, Wasserkrug HL, Seifter E, et al. Immunostimulatory effects of arginine in normal and injured rats. J Surg Res 1980;29:228–235.
68. Reynolds JV, Zhang SM, Thom AK, et al. Arginine as an immunomodulator. Surg Forum 1988;38:415.
69. Reynolds JV, Thom AK, Ziegler M, et al. Arginine, protein calorie malnutrition and cancer. J Surg Res 1987;45:513.
70. Barbul A, Sisto DA, Wasserkrug HL, et al. Arginine stimulates lymphocyte immune response in healthy humans. Surgery 1981;90:244.
71. Daly JM, Reynolds JV, Thom AK, et al. Immune and metabolic effects of arginine in surgical patients. Ann Surg 1988;208:512.
72. Rudolph RF, Kulkami AD, Schandle VB, et al. Involvement of dietary nucleotides in T-lymphocyte function. Adv Exp Med 1984;165:175–178.
73. Alexander JW, Saito H, Oglle C, Trocki O. The importance of lipid type in the diet after burn injury. Ann Surgery 1986;204:1–8.
74. Daly JM, Lieberman MD, Goldfine J, et al. Enteral nutrition with supplemental arginine, RNA and omega-3 fatty acids in postoperative patients: Immunologic, metabolic and clinical outcome. Surgery 1992;112:56–67.
75. Daly JM, Massar E. Giacco G, et al. Parenteral nutrition in esophageal cancer patients. Ann Surg 1982;196:203–208.
76. Heatley RV, Williams RHP, Lewis MH. Preoperative intravenous feeding: A controlled trial. Postgrad Med J 1979;35:541–45.
77. Muller JM, Dienst C, Brenner U, Pichlmaier H. Preoperative parenteral feeding in patients with gastrointestinal carcinoma. Lancet 1982;1:68–71.
78. Muller JM, Keller HW, Brenner U, Walter M. Holzmuller W. Indications and effects of preoperative parenteral nutrition. World J Surg 1986;10:53–63.
79. Starker PM, LaSala PA, Askanazi J, et al. The influence of preoperative total parenteral nutrition upon morbidity and mortality. Surg Gyn Obstet 1986;162:569–574.
80. Bellantone R. Doglietto G, Bossola M, et al. Preoperative parenteral nutrition of malnourished surgical patients. Acta Chir Scand 1988;22:249–251.
81. Foschi D, Cavagna G, Callioni F, et al. Hyperalimentation of jaundiced patients on percutaneous transhepatic biliary drainage. Br J Surg 1986;73:716–719.
82. Buzby GP, The Veterans Affairs TPN Cooperative Study Group. Perioperative TPN in surgical patients. N Engl J Med 1991;325:525–543.
83. Klein S, Simes J, Blackburn G. Total parenteral nutrition and cancer clinical trials. Cancer 1986;58:1378–1386.

SECTION **5**

FRANK J. BRESCIA

Specialized Care of the Terminally Ill

The modern concepts of palliative medicine were firmly established because of frustration with physicians and the health-care system to deliver effective, compassionate treatment to the dying.[1–3] In the roots of our past agricultural society, death at home was expected and familiar. However, by 1950, nearly half of the population in the United States died in the hospital. Today, at least 75% of Americans die in institutions.[4] Because medicine's primary objective became focused on curative intervention, the basic needs of terminally ill patients were often neglected. Unfortunately, prolonged and extensive diagnostic investigation was considered necessary by some physicians before the bothersome symptoms of dying patients were relieved. Often no treatment of symptoms was offered because the patient was considered terminal, or misdirected therapy was given to patients for every complaint without searching for an appropriate cause and remedy.

In 1974 America's first hospice opened in New Haven, Connecticut, starting with a home-care program and progressing to a 44-bed inpatient facility. Nearly 2000 American hospice programs and over 200 Canadian hospices flourished within 15 years. Of the patients they served, 92% had advanced malignancy.

In 1978 a hospice task force was started by the Department of Health, Education, and Welfare to examine the federal government's role in the care of the terminally ill.[5] Two years later, the Health Care Finance Administration funded 26 demonstration hospice programs to study the quality and utilization of hospice care by these organizations.

The terminally ill were reported to use 22% of all Medicare reimbursement expenses.[6] Because of an expected cost savings to the Medicare system of $30 million to $150 million, there was momentum to pass reimbursement legislation, which also had enormous political appeal.[7] Therefore, effective November 1, 1983, hospice services became part of the Medicare benefits program, featuring the following major components:

1. Physician-certified patient prognosis of 6 months or less
2. Annual reimbursement cap per patient to any individual hospice (initially this cap was $6,500)
3. Maximum of 210 days of hospice reimbursement
4. To encourage home-care usage, a 20% reimbursement cap on inpatient hospice days
5. Mandated home care and inpatient care, and spiritual, bereavement, and volunteer services.

PHILOSOPHY OF CARE

Despite the enormous advances in understanding and treating malignant illness, half of patients diagnosed will die of their disease.[8] The success in managing diverse, multiple, and difficult symptoms, which is important for all patients at all stages of disease, becomes the overriding imperative for those facing incurable cancer. The oncology literature began to aggressively examine measures to relieve pain and other symptoms in advanced disease as well as the unacceptable side effects of beneficial anticancer therapies.[9] With the initial promise of possible cure, the magnitude of side effects in cancer therapy seem unimportant to many patients.[10,11] However, when the reality of tumor recurrence and incurability must be faced, the patient is exceptionally wounded and vulnerable, sometimes more so than at the initial diagnosis.

Principles of good palliative medicine are no different from those of other medical care: clinical competency, experienced technical skills, and a compassionate bedside manner. However, at some point in the overall management of failing cancer therapy, the health-care team must recognize that the dying process has started. It is not death, but the indignity of the dying process, that terrifies most terminal patients.[12]

It has always been difficult to define the point that signals the beginning of the dying process. The decision that no further treatment should be directed against the tumor may create conflict between the patient and family. If the physician demands a trial of more conventional or experimental treatment in a patient who accepts his or her dying, this can create confusion, tension, and anger. The timing and acceptance among those involved with care decisions are crucial for preparing for the patient's imminent death.

Who are the known dying, the terminal (Table 64–28)? All patients known to be dying of advanced cancer are time-bound, but the terminal phase may be quite immediate, long-term, or indeterminate. Lynn considers the use of categorical terms such as terminal to be cumbersome, inadequate, and pejorative.[13] Unfortunately, these terms are used commonly for hospice admission criteria, court decisions, insurance claims, and public policy decisions.

The ability to effectively relieve the wide spectrum of difficult clinical problems begins with an understanding of tumor behavior and malignant pathophysiology. Ideally, if the tumor burden is diminished, the patient will experience subjective improvement of symptoms. A knowledge of both the natural history and tempo of progression for a specific malignancy allows the clinician to anticipate and therefore manage the changing signs and symptoms. The primary origin of the neoplasm, histology, grade, extent of disease (stage), and metastatic behavior must be evaluated early in the course of disease when the initial plan of care is formulated. The tumor's tempo of progression may vary among patients, even among those having the same primary site, histology, and stage. The patient's age, disease-free interval, tumor markers, hormone receptors, performance status, and previous response to adequate clinical trials all help to clarify the potential outcome.

TABLE 64–28. Terminal Illness Syndrome

- Causal illness with a progressive evolution
- Survival defined in days to weeks
- Karnofsky score < 40%
- Single or multiple organ failure
- Failure of conventional or proven treatment measures
- Absence of any other potential proven or experimental therapy
- Irreversible progressive complications

(Apilanez RV, Gonzalez de Langarica LR, Arribas EG. Terminal illness syndrome. Fourth European Conference on Clinical Oncology and Cancer Nursing. Madrid: Federation of European Cancer Societies, 1987:193)

The following are important considerations and questions when deciding the clinical options for patients with extensive disease:

1. Establish with certainty that the disease is beyond curative intervention.
2. What are the etiology, severity, and relation of the patient's tumor to the patient's present symptoms?
3. Are the symptoms compatible with the natural history of the specific cancer under treatment?
4. What potential limitations of function do the disease, diagnostic intervention, or treatment impose?
5. Where is the patient on the disease trajectory?
6. What issues need to be communicated with members of the treatment team, family, and patient?
7. What is a realistic therapeutic goal? Should the patient be treated at all?
8. Should systemic treatment be initiated for the overall illness, or should local therapy (*e.g.*, radiation therapy) be given for the specific complaint (*e.g.*, bone pain)?
9. Is the patient a reasonable candidate for experimental therapy?
10. Are there any other possible options, if the patient refuses the clinician's recommendations?[14,15]

The appropriateness of antineoplastic treatment in the asymptomatic patient with widespread disease may be questionable, because complete remissions are seldom noted and survival is not prolonged in most common advanced solid tumors.[16–18] Good clinical trials should be initiated if there is any degree of uncertainty for any possible useful outcome. Most importantly, patients with treatable cancer should never be referred to hospice settings.[19] Physicians, supported by their knowledge, training, and experience, must base their decisions not on what they would like to happen for their patients, but on the clinical reality, and must accept what most likely will occur. Decisions may be different when factors such as the patient's age, functional status, mental status, and concurrent illness are considered. Finally, the clinician's goal for the dying patient is quite simple: to relieve only by reducing the intensity of the distressful symptoms, canceling certain forms of treatment without avoiding the person as a patient. This is the ultimate meaning of patient nonabandonment.

SYMPTOM CONTROL

Traditionally, patients with end-stage cancer have not been the focus of major research interest. Yet these incurable patients may spend weeks to years suffering the poorly understood symptoms that normally accompany progressive malignancy. The emotional, social, and spiritual influences on a person's perception of any symptom, including pain, are personal and complex and become especially evident when the disease process is progressive, the tumor is advanced, the patient's lifestyle is limited, and the patient is expected to die.

For patients, persistent, unattended, and unrelieved pain may be linked to disturbing questions of suffering, abandonment, and perhaps for some even spiritual atonement. Furthermore, stressed and overwhelmed families may feel guilty and helpless, as well as angry at the caregivers for allowing unrelieved symptoms to continue until death.

The great variability of pain intensity and opioid usage as patients approach death underscores the need for careful ongoing assessment of distressing symptoms throughout the disease process.[20,21] A pain-free state may be an unrealistic goal in patients with advanced cancer.

The ability to control and manage physical complaints other than pain is extraordinarily difficult in patients who exhibit complicated multisystem signs and symptoms.[22–25] The clinician's dilemma is worsened by the patient's inability to undergo extensive or definitive diagnostic studies. Many distressing complaints may themselves be related to ongoing symptom-control therapy (*e.g.,* opioid-induced nausea, constipation, sedation; steroid-induced myopathy, insomnia, confusion).[26–38] Some symptoms are more easily corrected than others as the patient approaches death; others may be perceived as difficult or unacceptable by the family but are unnoticed by the patient (*e.g.,* moaning, grimacing, death rattles). Although the pathophysiology and treatment of cancer pain have been widely reviewed, there are no clear recommendations to manage every complex malignant symptom as patients approach death. (The reader is referred to a more comprehensive discussion of cancer pain by Dr. Kathleen Foley earlier in this chapter.) Common symptoms of advanced cancer are summarized in Table 64–29.

Unrelieved intolerable symptoms that accompany progressive malignancy are influenced by a variety of factors.[10,11] Similar tumor pathology will produce variable symptoms in different patients. Cancer patients may note distress of normal bodily sensations or minor symptoms may become exaggerated if recurrence of the cancer is feared. Thoughtful discussions of the true nature of a patient's complaints may help palliate the intensity of these somatic symptoms.

The difficulty of witnessing distressing symptoms in the dying patient may lead family members to seek hospitalization. Comfort measures directed toward these symptoms become the most important aspect of care once the patient enters the dying process. The clinician should have less concern about the potential negative consequences of the chosen symptom-control therapy (*e.g.,* steroid-induced bleeding, immunosuppression, narcotic masking pain).[39] In the last few days it may be appropriate and less distressing to eliminate much of the patient's medication for nonproblematic concurrent diseases (*e.g.,* hypertension, diabetes, thyroid).

TERMINAL EVENTS

There is little change in the quality of life of patients until 4 to 6 months before death, but the last weeks of life are especially dramatic, with increased dependency, weakness, confusion, and inability to manage simple functional and personal tasks such as bathing, walking, and continence. Coyle reviewed the prevalence and change of symptoms volunteered by 90 patients during the last 4 weeks of their terminal disease (Table 64–30).[32] Nearly 75% had three or more separate complaints near death, while some had as many as nine distinct symptoms. Less than 5% of these dying patients reported hallucinations, diarrhea, nightmares, hiccups, itch, or panic attacks.

The final phase of the dying process can be frightening for both patient and family, and sometimes is managed by clinicians with confusion, inadequacy, negligence, and apathy. Escalating symptoms during the last 48 to 72 hours usually foreshadow death. A prospective study of 120 terminal patients demonstrated that 63 had uncontrollable symptoms that appeared an average of 48 hours before death. Dyspnea appeared to be the most common uncontrollable problem, especially as death approached.[40] National Hospice Study data indicated that dyspnea occurred in 70.2% of dying patients during the last 6 weeks of life, and was usually associated with lung or pleural disease.[41] Other studies had a much lower incidence of this symptom.[35,42] It is rare, however, for symptoms to be

TABLE 64–29. Relation of Cancer Diagnosis and Symptoms Present at Time of Admission (n = 1103)

	Symptoms					
	Severe Pain (%)	*Confusion (%)*	*Anorexia (%)*	*Dyspnea (%)*	*Dysphagia (%)*	*Nausea (%)*
Total Patients	38	33	31	27	22	19
Primary Diagnosis						
Lung	31	43	35	51	21	16
Breast	39	38	30	30	22	13
Colon	36	25	34	17	12	30
Rectum and sigmoid	49	32	28	17	15	15
Prostate	57	32	18	28	22	8
Pancreas	44	21	54	21	13	35
Head and neck	42	11	22	11	62	2
Cervix	68	27	27	21	22	39
Ovary	32	38	35	21	17	56
Stomach	23	17	40	10	15	47

(Brescia FJ, Adler D, Gray G, et al. Hospitalized advanced cancer patients: A profile. J Pain Symptom Manage 1990;5:221–227)

TABLE 64–30. Prevalence of Symptoms 4 Weeks and 1 Week Before Death

Symptom	*4 Weeks Before Death (%)*	*1 Week Before Death (%)*
Fatigue	58	52
Pain	54	34
Generalized weakness	43	49
Mental haziness/confusion	24	28
Anxiety	21	18
Cough	6	7

(Modified from Coyle N, Adelhardt J, Foley KM, et al. Character of terminal illness in the advanced cancer patient: Pain and other symptoms during the last 4 weeks of life. J Pain Symptom Manage 1990;5: 83–93)

TABLE 64–31. Diagnoses and Survival (Diagnosis to Death) (n = 1107)

	Duration of Illness (%)			
	6 Mo or Less	*7–12 Mo*	*1–2 Y*	*2 Y or More*
Total Patients	24	18	21	37
Leading Diagnoses				
Lung	39	26	21	15
Breast	5	5	18	72
Colon	15	12	24	49
Rectum and sigmoid	16	16	24	45
Prostate	4	6	20	71
Pancreas	54	30	9	6
Head and neck	17	29	31	24
Cervix	8	11	38	43
Ovary	19	16	16	48
Stomach	50	28	11	11

(Calvary Hospital Clinical Database, 1989 [unpublished data])

so unmanageable near death that total sedation is required to ease the patient's suffering.

PREDICTING SURVIVAL

The ability to predict the life expectancy of an advanced cancer patient has been poor, even among experienced clinicians.[43–45] The life expectancy of 108 hospice patients was overly optimistic by an average of 3.4 weeks.[46] The patient's functional status (Karnofsky score) appears to be the most important variable in estimating survival. One study showed that half the patients whose Karnofsky scores were 10% to 20% died within 53 days if no symptoms were present, compared with 50% within 16 days if dry mouth, dyspnea, anorexia, dysphagia, and weight loss were present.[47]

Terminal cancer patients, despite the setting (home, hospital, or nursing home), appear to share a common three-step decline in the last weeks of life (15 weeks, 2 months, and 2 weeks before death), with the greatest functional dependency, obviously, close to death.[48,49] The interval from the initial cancer diagnosis to death was examined in 1107 patients admitted to a palliative care setting (Table 64–31). Of these patients, 63% were diagnosed with cancer and subsequently died within 2 years. Survival was inversely related to age: patients under 74 years were more likely to survive longer than older patients.[50] These data are important because they show that physicians have difficulty with the Medicare requirement to certify a 6-month prognosis and eligibility for hospice benefits.

CHALLENGES AND QUESTIONS

Numerous challenges face palliative medicine, and there are many barriers to appropriate terminal care, such as inadequate physician education regarding symptom control; government regulations hindering the prescribing of narcotics; retail pharmacy restrictions; reimbursement limits because of Medicare hospital regulations (*e.g.*, 6-month prognosis); and the fear of opioid addiction or tolerance by the physician, nurses, family, and patient.[19,51–53] Some important issues that must be further explored in the care of the dying are discussed below.

SITE OF DEATH

Despite the difficulties in keeping patients at home, most patients prefer to die at home.[54–57] The ability to allow patients to die at home in home-care hospice programs (55% to 72% of patients) may reflect the attitudes of staff and communication of the hospice philosophy rather than specific patient characteristics.[58] Wilkes found that only 3% of relatives of patients who died at home would have preferred the hospital setting.[59] The site of death was the consistent issue on which hospice-treated families demonstrated greater satisfaction over those families who received conventional care. However, in urban environments, dying at home may be difficult if not impossible, for example in the case of an elderly patient who lives alone, a patient with severe agitation, a patient who cannot get narcotics in pharmacies, or if such services are not covered by insurance.

A retrospective analysis of a home-care hospice program showed that pain was the single most important symptom that made hospitalization necessary, but this study could not determine whether the patients, despite the pain, could have remained at home.[60] The National Hospice Study reported that patients followed in hospital-based hospice programs were less likely to report having persistent pain, but this finding needs further analysis because a randomized trial of hospice care found no difference in pain-control outcomes between hospice and conventional care.[61] Another hospice program affiliated with a university hospital had 47% of their patients die at home, while 38% of patients had their care managed entirely without hospitalization.[62] In this study 71% of hospitalized patients received an average daily morphine dose of 75 mg; 53% of patients in the home had an average daily dose of 25 mg.

Dying at home is not always superior to the hospital setting. Families who strongly advocate death at home may not appreciate the enormous burden of 24-hour care of the sickest of patients and may eventually feel abandoned by their physicians and the health-care system. Unfortunately, many communities do not have the resources and trained professionals to meet the complex needs of terminal patients. The specific features of the patient, family, physician, program, or disease that impel hospitalization remain poorly defined.

LEGAL AND ETHICAL QUESTIONS IN HOSPICE CARE

There is always a rational place for therapy that comforts. In recent years, a medical consensus has emerged that patients have the right to refuse a treatment that no longer can remedy illness but only extends the agony of the dying process.[63–71] On whose authority are decisions of care finally made? Patients as people have the right to decide their own destiny; this premise is grounded in both common and constitutional law in the United States.[13,72] Thus, when competency exists, the patient's moral and legal right defines the soundness of the clinical action. However, situations may become quite complex for the physician. The patient may be competent and may understand the clinical issue at hand and the potential consequences of therapy, but because of his or her advanced state of illness, the symptoms endured, or the intensity, duration, and type of toxicity to past treatments, the patient's decisions may differ from those the physician anticipated.[73] The clinician may have moral conflicts if the patient talks of despair, harm to himself or herself, or avoidance of some treatment thought to be beneficial.[74,75]

Family members have the right to speak for their incompetent loved ones, but they often assume decision-making power for patients who are dying and frail but still competent. When patients lose the capacity to make decisions for themselves, family members usually render a substitute judgment of the patient's past wishes, not their own.

In some clinical situations there is an obligation *not* to provide some form of medical intervention to a dying patient. For example, both hunger and thirst are rarely recognized as problems in terminal patients by experienced clinicians.[76] Forcing fluid and food to patients is not warranted and is perhaps harmful with the onset of pulmonary congestion and edema and the need for a urinary catheter to manage increased urine output. Dehydration may result in some benefit to the dying person by enhancing sedation if hemoconcentration, hyperosmolality, azotemia, and hypercalcemia occur.

Trials of therapy should always be given when there is a clinical uncertainty of the outcome, but bad outcomes do not always mean the medical decisions of care were incorrect. For example, it is wrong to believe that therapy once begun cannot be stopped, because clinicians may omit clinical trials to patients who may benefit. Withdrawing treatment often appears to be more damaging and serious to the caregivers than if nothing had been initiated in the first place. What is indicated should be tried, and what is a failure should be stopped. Due to this misunderstood distinction and the fear of liability among good physicians, patients have suffered because clinicians have failed to give an adequate therapeutic trial or have kept patients on some form of futile intervention for long, exhausting, and costly periods of time.[77]

Major issues of conflict for clinicians in palliative settings include the futility of resuscitation, and inappropriate demands for resuscitation by the patient or family; the withholding of treatments such as chemotherapy, blood products, or antibiotics; and the withdrawal of some form of intervention, such as total parenteral nutrition, food, or hydration.[75,78–80] Physician-assisted suicide and active euthanasia are dilemmas that will soon confront physicians as attempts are made in our society to morally justify these actions as part of medical practice.[81–86]

Physicians must not have ill-conceived plans of medical care based on what they believe the patient's quality of life should be.[87] The urgency and challenge to promote adequate, acceptable patient comfort escalate as the patient enters the final days and hours. The anguish of any difficult manner of dying must be diminished, even if death is hastened—if not directly caused—by such therapy. These therapeutic decisions should be made with the patient's comfort as the objective, but should not be based on any public policy to seek death. The experience of most physicians who care for the dying is that there are few "unmanageable" patients, too few to change traditional medical practices and promote euthanasia and risk all the possible future abuses. However, as cost-containment controls are enacted, the criteria for limiting some treatments for certain patients must be publicly discussed and closely monitored.[88]

PERSONNEL ISSUES

Personnel remains the largest expenditure in hospice care and has the biggest impact on quality. It is difficult to attract and keep emotionally mature, competent, compassionate physicians to care for the dying.[89,90] Those involved in this work know both the gratification and the stress of dealing with the incurably ill. Witnessing dying and communicating tragic news to patients and their families produces an enormous strain on physicians.[91] The clinician is responsible for the timing and manner of discussing worsening clinical states. Attempting to offer realistic hope as well as helping the patient and family face the awful reality is no easy task, especially if the physician has previously avoided communication or is uncertain about treatment and outcome options. Other physicians, as well as family members, may feel that symptoms during the terminal phase are caused by the toxicity of some cancer treatment, and not by the obvious progressive cancer, and may blame the oncologist.

RESOURCE MANAGEMENT

Should those expected to die soon, despite therapy, use the scarce resources of well-trained clinicians and institutions?[92] Should oncologic treatment against the tumor continue because of demands by the patient or family, despite cost concerns? Because palliative care demands the skills of different disciplines, it remains costly.[93] Filling empty beds or meeting reimbursement needs should not be reasons for institutions to consider caring for the dying. Studies document that home-care hospice programs may save 10% to 20% of the total health care costs in the last year of life over inpatient medical care.[6,94–96] Savings of hospice care are more dramatic during the last 1 or 2 months of a patient's life, when diagnostic intervention and high-tech procedures are usually performed. Hospice care at home before the last 2 months of life appears more costly because of the need for expensive home services not usually seen in the conventional setting.[97] On average, conventional care of the cancer patient is more costly during the last year of a patient's life. There is an estimated annual savings of $4,000 if the patient is in a home-care hospice program and $1,300 if in a hospital-based hospice. If the patient remains in the hospice longer than 4 months, however, the costs are higher than conventional care.[98]

A study from western Australia found that the costs of providing 24-hour comprehensive medical and nursing care at home were comparable to those in acute hospitals during the last 3 months of life.[99] Vinciguerra reported a cost benefit of $256 per day for terminal patients receiving comprehensive multidisciplinary services for home treatment versus hospital care.[100] Despite the cost differences during the last 2 months of life, no negative effects were found in the National Hospice Study of patients who received hospice care.[95]

QUALITY ASSURANCE

How do we monitor the quality of medicine when the morbidity and mortality of advanced cancer is anticipated?[101] The problem is compounded because real alternatives of therapy and viable clinical options are severely limited in this population. Quality studies of patient care mandate the use of defined indicators of clinical care.[102–104] Mechanisms to monitor palliative care objectives, documentation of treatment outcomes, and evaluation of staff performance all must be included in these ongoing reviews of quality assurance.[19,75,105–112] Because these patients are so close to death, the review process must identify any inappropriate treatment or intervention. For example, an examination of the use of blood products in the terminally ill revealed that patients in conventional medical settings were five times more likely to get blood than in a hospital-based hospice and ten times more likely than those patients in home-care hospices.[113] Because satisfaction and comfort outcome measures appear similar in all three groups, this specific issue would suggest monitoring the use of blood products in this population.

Because the experience of terminal disease is interwoven with issues involving quality of life, psychosocial status, and suffering, as well as the devastating physical problems, outcome measurements can be cumbersome, complex, and almost impossible to interpret. The National Hospice Study examined 1754 patients to determine whether hospice care (home- or hospital-based) improved physical and overall quality of life outcomes compared to conventional medical care.[58] Home-care hospice patients did no worse than those in conventional care, with considerably lower cost. In general, studies showed that hospice care may offer equal or more satisfaction to patients and their families than conventional settings.[114]

RESEARCH

Although clinical studies are important in all medicine, advanced cancer patients are vulnerable and must be protected. Some clinical protocols may be inappropriate for this population. Therefore, the value and safety of the research project must be established beyond doubt. Symptom-control studies are ideal, if patients understand what is required and if possible adverse effects for patients are minimal.[19]

SUFFERING

Physicians should reflect on the concept of suffering in their daily work, especially if they are treating the dying. The objectives of medical care must emphasize patients' general well-being.[115] For example, patients may have distress beyond the severity of their pain, encompassing their psychosocial, spiritual, and cultural existence. Cassell addressed the need for medicine to recognize the patient as a person and to omit the traditional assignment of the body to medicine, and of the person to the category only of the mind.[116,117] If we accept this dichotomy, we depersonalize the patient and become the source of further suffering. This is especially evident as we examine the technological imperative of present-day medicine: doing something for patients because we *can* do it before asking whether we *ought* to do it.

Dying patients may reflect on and sometimes come to know the reasons for their own suffering because they have anguish that no other person can truly understand.[118] Suffering attacks a person's integrity and wholeness and dominates the patient's consciousness, causing sustained interior agony.[119] The diseased body becomes objectified, bound to time, place, and physical insult, and feels pain. When this perception of pain or physical insult can no longer be tolerated, the person assumes the role of a patient and seeks the advice of a physician.

It is the personal quest of the human spirit to search for meaning that enhances human dignity. The search for purpose is important and necessary because only the patient can give meaning to his or her life. Rosenthal, in an account of his own impending death, repeats that it is not death people are afraid of, but the incompleteness of their lives.[120] Indeed, each life and death have their own tempo and character. Somehow, the patient must touch the moment of discontinuity between life and death and at the same time discover that it was meaningful and worth something to have lived.

CONCLUSION

Uniting the humanity of the physician and those needing care requires an appreciation of our human drama.[121] The social ethic of medicine requires shared goals that allow patients a safe, comforting passage to a compassionate end. It is the unique ability of good clinicians to be concerned yet detached that allows a clear, logical awareness of what needs to be done for the sickest of human beings. Physicians must share the distress yet keep some distance, or they will become wounded and vulnerable themselves. These difficult cases call for attention to details that weaken the destructiveness of illness and aim to comfort.

Death is the only true democratic event. Although we must all die alone, our dependence on one another makes each death intensely shared. Illness radically tears apart the normal harmony of this interconnection of human lives, and the experience of patients dying with advanced cancer raises powerful, emotional, and sometimes conflicting issues for the physician. It is the compassionate and competent manner in which care is delivered at the end of life that helps these sickest of humans to transcend their suffering.

REFERENCES

1. Stoddard S. The hospice movement. Briarcliff Manor: Stein & Day, 1978.
2. Feifel H, ed. The meaning of death. New York: McGraw-Hill, 1959.
3. Kubler-Ross E. On death and dying. New York: Macmillan, 1969.
4. President's Commission for the Study of Ethical Problems in Medicine & Biomedical & Behavioral Research. Deciding to forego life-sustaining treatment. Washington DC, 1983:17.
5. Evolution of hospice. In: Mor V, ed. Hospice care systems. New York: Springer, 1987: 2.
6. Wachtel TJ, Mor V. Physicians' use of health resources for terminal cancer patients: Clinical setting versus physician specialty. South Med J 1987;80:1120–1124.
7. Bayer R, Feldman E. Hospice under the Medicare wing. Hastings Cent Rep 1982;12: 5–6.
8. Boring CC, Squires TS, Tong T. Cancer statistics, 1991. CA 1991;41:19–36.
9. Symposium on clinical pharmacology of symptom control. Med Clin North Am 1982;66.
10. Barsky AJ. Palliation and symptomatic relief. Arch Intern Med 1986;146:905–909.
11. Kane RL, Klein SJ, Bernstein L, et al. Hospice role in alleviating the emotional stress of terminal patients and their families. Med Care 1985;23:189–197.
12. Brescia FJ. An overview of pain and symptom management in advanced cancer. J Pain Symptom Manage 1987;2(Suppl):S7–S11.
13. Lynn J. Legal and ethical issues in palliative health care. Semin Oncol 1985;12:476–481.
14. Richter MP, Coia LR. Palliative radiation therapy. Semin Oncol 1985;12:375–383.
15. Abrams RA, Hansen RM. Radiotherapy, chemotherapy and hormonal therapy in the management of cancer pain. In: Abram SE, ed. Cancer pain: Current management of pain. Boston: Kluwer Academic, 1989:49–66.
16. Stoll BA. Quality of life as an objective in cancer treatment. In: Stoll BA, ed. Cancer treatment: Endpoint evaluation. New horizons in oncology. New York: John Wiley, 1983:113–138.
17. Braverman AS. Medical oncology in the 1990s. Lancet 1991;337:901–902.
18. Cellerino R, Tummarello D, Guidi F, et al. A randomized trial of alternating chemotherapy versus best supportive care in advanced non-small cell lung cancer. J Clin Oncol 1991;9:1453–1461.
19. Potter JF. A challenge for the hospice movement. N Engl J Med 1980;302:53–55.
20. Portenoy RK, Coyle N. Controversies in the long-term management of analgesic therapy in patients with advanced cancer. J Pain Symptom Manage 1990;5:307–319.
21. Brescia FJ, Portenoy RK, Ryan M, et al. Pain, opioid use and survival in hospitalized patients with advanced cancer. J Clin Oncol 1992;10:149–155.
22. Levy MH, Catalano RB. Control of common physical symptoms other than pain in patients with terminal disease. Semin Oncol 1985;12:411–429.
23. DeWys W. Management of cancer cachexia. Semin Oncol 1985;12:452–460.
24. Twycross RG, Lack SA. Symptom control in far-advanced cancer. London: Pitman Books, 1983.
25. Osoba D, ed. Effect of cancer on quality of life. Boston: CRC Press, 1991.
26. Kris MG, Gralla RJ. Management of vomiting caused by anticancer drugs. In: Foley KM, Bonica JJ, Ventafridda V, eds. Second International Congress on Cancer Pain: Advances in pain research and therapy, Vol. 16. New York: Raven Press, 1990:337–344.
27. Twycross RG. Management of constipation in the cancer patient with pain. In: Foley KM, Bonica JJ, Ventafridda V, eds. Second International Congress on Cancer Pain: Advances in pain research and therapy, Vol. 16. New York: Raven Press, 1990:317–326.
28. Baines MJ. Management of malignant intestinal obstruction in patients with advanced cancer. In: Foley KM, Bonica JJ, Ventafridda V, eds. Second International Congress on Cancer Pain: Advances in pain research and therapy, Vol. 16. New York: Raven Press, 1990:327–335.
29. Baines M. Nausea and vomiting in the patient with advanced cancer. J Pain Symptom Manage 1988;3:81–85.
30. Bruera E, MacDonald RN. Asthenia in patients with advanced cancer. J Pain Symptom Manage 1988;3:9–14.
31. Cowcher K, Hanks GW. Long-term management of respiratory symptoms in advanced cancer. J Pain Symptom Manage 1990;5:320–330.
32. Coyle N, Adelhardt J, Foley KM, et al. Character of terminal illness in the advanced cancer patient: Pain and other symptoms during the last 4 weeks of life. J Pain Symptom Manage 1990;5:83–93.
33. DeConno F, Ventafridda V, Saita L. Skin problems in advanced and terminal cancer patients. J Pain Symptom Manage 1991;6:247–256.
34. Hagen NA. An approach to cough in cancer patients. J Pain Symptom Manage 1991;6: 257–262.
35. Higginson I, McCarthy M. Measuring symptoms in terminal cancer: Are pain and dyspnoea controlled? J Royal Soc Med 1989;82:264–267.
36. Kolodzik PW, Eilers MA. Hiccups (singultus): Review and approach to management. Ann Emerg Med 1991;20:565–573.
37. Madden EJ. Itch. J Pain Symptom Manage 1986;1:97–99.
38. Collaud T, Rapin CH. Dehydration in dying patients: Study with physicians in French-speaking Switzerland. J Pain Symptom Manage 1991;6:230–240.
39. Levy MH. Integration of pain management into comprehensive cancer care. Cancer 1989;63:2328–2335.
40. Ventafridda V, Ripamonti C, DeConno F, et al. Symptom prevalence and control during cancer patients' last days of life. J Palliat Care 1990;6:7–11.
41. Reuben DB, Mor V. Dyspnea in terminally ill cancer patients. Chest 1986;89:234–236.
42. Fishbein D, Kearon C, Killian KJ. An approach to dyspnea in cancer patients. J Pain Symptom Manage 1989;4:76–81.
43. Pearlman RA. Inaccurate predictions of life expectancy: Dilemmas and opportunities. Arch Intern Med 1988;148:2537–2538.
44. Addington-Hall JM, MacDonald LD, Anderson HR. Can the Spitzer Quality of Life Index help to reduce prognostic uncertainty in terminal care? Br J Cancer 1990;62: 695–699.
45. Schonwetter RS, Teasdale TA, Storey P, et al. Estimation of survival time in terminal cancer patients: An impedance to hospice admissions? Hosp J 1991;6:65–79.
46. Forster LE, Lynn J. Predicting life span for applicants to inpatient hospice. Arch Intern Med 1988;148:2540–2543.
47. Reuben DB, Mor V, Hiris J. Clinical symptoms and length of survival in patients with terminal cancer. Arch Intern Med 1988;148:1586–1591.
48. Morris JN, Sherwood S. Quality of life of cancer patients at different stages in the disease trajectory. J Chronic Dis 1987;40:545–553.
49. Morris JN, Suissa S, Sherwood S, et al. Last days: A study of the quality of life of terminally ill cancer patients. J Chronic Dis 1986;39:47–62.
50. Brescia FJ, Adler D, Gray G, et al. Hospitalized advanced cancer patients: A profile. J Pain Symptom Manage 1990;5:221–227.
51. Adams AB. Dilemmas of hospice: A critical look at its problems. CA 1984;34:183–190.
52. Hyman RB, Bulkin W. Physician-reported incentives and disincentives for referring patients to hospice. Hosp J 1991;6:39–64.
53. Problems in the care of the dying patient. In Zimmerman JM, ed. Hospice: Complete care for the terminally ill. Baltimore: Urban & Schwarzenberg, 1981:1–12.
54. Parkes CM. Terminal care: Home, hospital, or hospice? Lancet 1985;1:155–157.
55. Ventafridda V, DeConno F, Vigano A, et al. Comparison of home and hospital care of advanced cancer patients. Tumori 1989;75:619–625.
56. Townsend J, Frank AO, Fermont D, et al. Terminal cancer care and patients' preference for place of death: A prospective study. Br Med J 1990;301:415–417.
57. McCusker J. The use of home care in terminal cancer. Am J Prev Med 1985;1:42–52.
58. Quality of life outcomes. In: Mor V, ed. Hospice care systems. New York: Springer, 1987:125–176.
59. Wilkes E. Dying now. Lancet 1984;1:950–952.
60. Brescia FJ, Sadof M, Barstow J. Retrospective analysis of a home care hospice program. Omega 1984;15:37–44.
61. Kane RL, Bernstein L, Wales J, et al. Hospice effectiveness in controlling pain. JAMA 1985;253:2683–2686.
62. Vinciguerra V, Degnan TJ, Sciortino A, et al. A comparative assessment of home versus hospital comprehensive treatment for advanced cancer patients. J Clin Oncol 1986;4: 1521–1528.
63. Smith DH, Granbois JA. The American way of hospice. Hastings Cent Rep 1982;12: 8–10.
64. Scham M, Scham A. Hospices: Medical and legal considerations. Leg Med 1985;297–322.
65. Veatch RM. Cross-cultural perspectives in medical ethics. Boston: Jones & Bartlett, 1989.
66. Wanzer SH, Federman DD, Adelstein SJ, et al. The physician's responsibility toward hopelessly ill patients: A second look. N Engl J Med 1989;320:844–849.
67. Tobias JS, Tattersall MH. Doing the best for the cancer patient. Lancet 1985;1:35–37.
68. Lo B, Jonsen AR. Ethical decisions in the care of a patient terminally ill with metastatic cancer. Ann Intern Med 1980;92:107–111.
69. Novack DH, Plumer R, Smith RL, et al. Changes in physicians' attitudes toward telling the cancer patient. JAMA 1979;241:897–900.
70. Roy DJ. Ethical issues in the treatment of cancer patients. J Palliat Care 1989;5:56–60.
71. Goetzler RM, Moskowitz MA. Changes in physician attitudes toward limiting care of critically ill patients. Arch Intern Med 1991;151:1537–1540.
72. Meisel A. Legal myths about terminating life support. Arch Intern Med 1991;151: 1497–1502.
73. Brock DW, Wartman SA. When competent patients make irrational choices. N Engl J Med 1990;322:1595–1599.
74. Brescia FJ. A philosophy of care: Notes of a death watcher. J Pain Symptom Manage 1988;3:212–214.
75. Brescia FJ. The goals and challenges of palliative care: Thoughts of a death watcher. J Pain Symptom Manage 1990;5:382–384.
76. Lynn J, ed. By no extraordinary means. Bloomington: Indiana University Press, 1986.
77. Brescia FJ. Killing the known dying: Notes of a death watcher. J Pain Symptom Manage 1991;6:337–339.
78. Cimino JE. Medical ethics and the decision to feed or not to feed: A physician speaks. Top Clin Nutr 1991;6:72–75.
79. Tomlinson T, Brody H. Futility and the ethics of resuscitation. JAMA 1990;264:1276–1280.
80. Emanuel EJ. A review of the ethical and legal aspects of terminating medical care. Am J Med 1988;84:291–301.
81. Battin MP. Euthanasia: The way we do it, the way they do it. J Pain Symptom Manage 1991;6:298–305.
82. Clouser KD. The challenge for future debate on euthanasia. J Pain Symptom Manage 1991;6:306–311.
83. Klagsbrun SC. Physician-assisted suicide: A double dilemma. J Pain Symptom Manage 1991;6:325–328.
84. Lachs J. Active euthanasia. J Clin Ethics 1990;1:113–115.
85. Goodwin JS. Mercy killing: Mercy for whom? JAMA 1991;265:326.
86. Singer PA, Siegler M. Euthanasia—a critique. N Engl J Med 1990;322:1881–1883.

87. Magno JB. The role of the physician when cure is no longer possible. Linacre Q 1991;58: 79–88.
88. Bayer R, Callahan D, Fletcher J, et al. The care of the terminally ill: Morality and economics. N Engl J Med 1983;309:1490–1494.
89. Cimino JE. Global trends of hospice care (unpublished data).
90. Ajemian I, Mount BM, eds. The R.V.H. manual on palliative/hospice care. Salem, N.H.: Ayer, 1980.
91. Whippen DA, Canellos GP. Burnout syndrome in the practice of oncology: Results of a random survey of 1000 oncologists. J Clin Oncol 1991;9:1916–1920.
92. Mor V, Kidder D. Cost savings in hospice: Final results of the National Hospice Study. Health Serv Res 1985;20:407–422.
93. Brody H, Lynn J. The physician's responsibility under the new Medicare reimbursement for hospice care. N Engl J Med 1984;310:920–922.
94. Hazzard WR. Geriatric medicine: Life in the crucible of the struggle to contain health-care costs. In: McCue JD, ed. The medical cost-containment crisis. Ann Arbor: Health Administration Press, 1989:266.
95. The cost of hospice. In: Mor V, ed. Hospice care systems. New York: Springer, 1987: 177–212.
96. Warren BH, Bell PL, Isikoff S, et al. Cost-containment and quality of life: An experiment in compassion for physicians. Arch Intern Med 1991;151:741–744.
97. Kidder D. The impact of hospices on the health-care costs of terminal cancer patients. In: Mor V, Greer DS, Kastenbaum R, eds. The hospice experiment. Baltimore: Johns Hopkins University Press, 1988:48–68.
98. Kidder D. Hospice services and cost savings in the last weeks of life. In: Mor V, Greer DS, Kastenbaum R, eds. The hospice experiment. Baltimore: Johns Hopkins University Press, 1988:69–87.
99. Gray D, MacAdam D, Boldy D. A comparative cost analysis of terminal cancer care in home hospice patients and controls. J Chronic Dis 1987;40:801–810.
100. Vinciguerra V, Degnan TJ, Budman DR, et al. Comparative cost analysis of home and hospital treatment. In: Mortenson LE, Engstrom PF, Anderson PN, eds. Advances in cancer control: Health care financing and research. New York: Alan R. Liss, 1986: 155–164.
101. Bulkin W, Lukashok H. Rx for dying: The case for hospice. N Engl J Med 1988;318: 376–378.
102. Donovan K, Sanson-Fisher RW, Redman S. Measuring quality of life in cancer patients. J Clin Oncol 1989;7:959–968.
103. Zweibel NR. Measuring quality of life near the end of life. JAMA 1988;260:839–840.
104. Latimer E. Auditing the hospital care of dying patients. J Palliat Care 1991;7:12–17.
105. Mor V, Masterson-Allen S. A comparison of hospice versus conventional care of the terminally ill cancer patient. Oncology 1990;4:85–91.
106. Rhymes J. Hospice care in America. JAMA 1990;264:369–372.
107. Krakoff IH. The case for active treatment in patients with advanced cancer: Not everyone needs a hospice. CA 1991;29:108–111.
108. McCann BA, Enck RE. Standards for hospice care: A JCAH hospice project overview. In: Engstrom PF, Anderson PN, Mortenson LE, eds. Advances in cancer control: Epidemiology and research. New York: Alan R. Liss, 1984:431–440.
109. Rees WD. Role of the hospice in the care of the dying. Br Med J 1982;285:1766–1768.
110. Powers JS, Burger MC. Terminal care preferences: Hospice placement and severity of disease. Public Health Rep 1987;102:444–449.
111. Wallston KA, Burger C, Smith RA, et al. Comparing the quality of death for hospice and nonhospice cancer patients. Med Care 1988;26:177–182.
112. Cimino JE. Concerns for hospice. N Y Med Q 1980;2:46.
113. Wachtel TJ, Mor V. The use of transfusions in terminal cancer patients: Hospice versus conventional care setting. Transfusion 1985;25:278–279.
114. Mor V, Greer DS, Kastenbaum R, eds. The hospice experiment. Baltimore: Johns Hopkins University Press, 1988.
115. Portenoy RK. Pain and quality of life: Theoretical aspects. In: Osoba D, ed. Effect of cancer on quality of life. Boston: CRC Press, 1991:279–292.
116. Cassell EJ. Recognizing suffering. Hastings Cent Rep 1991;21:24–31.
117. Cassell EJ. The nature of suffering and the goals of medicine. New York: Oxford University Press, 1991.
118. Frankl VE. Man's search for meaning. New York: Pocket Books, 1984.
119. Gunderman RB. Medicine and the question of suffering. Second Opin 1990;14:15–25.
120. Rosenthal T. How could I not be among you? New York: George Braziller, 1973.
121. Bennahum DA. Intimations of mortality reconsidered: Terminal care. Am J Med 1980;69: 488–490.

SECTION **6**

DONNA SAMMARINO

Dealing With the Dying Patient

Despite all our advances in health care, life can only be prolonged; death cannot be eradicated. As such, we must find ways of providing optimal care to people at all stages in their lives. This seemingly fundamental notion has become a complicated challenge in our increasingly technologic arena of health care. This chapter is intended to:

1. Identify and help one understand institutional obstacles that impede the provision of optimal care to the dying in hospitals
2. Provide insight into the issues and personal difficulties that arise for caregivers when dealing with the dying
3. Identify some of the specific care needs of the terminally ill
4. Formulate practical suggestions to maximize our effectiveness when dealing with the dying.

INSTITUTIONAL OBSTACLES

Acute-care hospitals remain the most common setting for death in our society due to the large concentration of caregivers and resources within these institutions.[1] Throughout life, until the dying process begins, a person's understanding of a hospital's mission to treat health-care needs is aligned with the hospital's ability to do so. However, the care of the dying is not necessarily within the hospital's repertoire of subspecialties.

Dealing with the dying can be a positive challenge and a rewarding experience, depending largely on what caregivers bring to the situation. We must gain a clearer understanding of the needs of the dying and also must appreciate the obstacles within our health-care system that can impede even the most well-intentioned of us from providing quality care to the dying.

Balfour Mount elucidated the differences between the needs of the terminally ill and the goals of an acute-care hospital.[2] He saw the mission of a general hospital to be fourfold: "to investigate, to diagnose, to cure, and to prolong life." For the terminally ill, the only appropriate goal is improvement of the quality of life through palliative care. The problem arises when we introduce into the acute-care environment patients who challenge the expertise of the health-care team. In the management of the dying, the skills of investigating and diagnosing are important, but with a view toward palliation and symptom management rather than cure and prolongation of life. What results is a misalignment between what the patient needs and what the staff can offer. The perception exists in this acute-care setting that "nothing can be done" for the dying patient. Therefore, the health-care team may feel frustrated and incompetent and may become angry or apathetic. What may appear on the surface as indifference may actually be a manifestation of guilt, anxiety, and insecurity. Often the staff distance themselves from patients and families, aggravating the problem.

Mount's study of attitudes toward the dying at the Royal Victoria Hospital in Montreal confirmed that there were deficiencies in the care of the dying. The medical, emotional, and spiritual needs of these patients and their families were often neglected. The staff felt inadequately prepared to meet their needs. Nurses did not welcome being assigned to dying patients. Physician visits decreased in frequency as the patients' length of stay increased. Nursing care decreased as death approached, despite the fact that patients' needs increased. For example, it took longer to answer the call bells of dying patients than those of patients with a better prognosis. Lack of communication and deficiencies in care led to patient isolation and to feelings of suspicion and mistrust among patients, family members, nurses, and physicians. Physicians and nurses felt poorly prepared to communicate openly and honestly with patients and families and as a result spent less time with the dying. Moreover, the staff felt that the efficient execution of their regular routines was disrupted by the dying patients.[2]

Hospital routines are designed to promote efficiency and to satisfy the needs of the staff in acute-care units.[2] Such routines can serve as obstacles as death approaches and the total emphasis is on diminution of suffering. Similarly, the physical environment of an acute-care hospital is not optimal for dying patients. Often, even if staff have the skills to render palliative care, the constraints of an acute-care environment can impede the implementation of such interventions. Visiting hours and policies are restrictive. Private rooms are reserved for isolation cases, not for the terminally ill. There is little room or time to deal with families. There is little training for staff to communicate appropriately with families, let alone include them as a unit of care.[3]

Terminally ill patients should always have the option of having loved ones present and available to them throughout this final phase of their illness. Most acute-care hospitals will make this provision only when the patient is deemed to be at the point of death. Even when loved ones are permitted, there is limited space; the room is crowded with sophisticated equipment of little value in the care of the terminally ill, and it is often difficult to remove. Acute-care hospitals also must comply with building codes, governmental regulations, and accreditation standards that make the creation of a more homelike environment for the terminally ill very difficult.[1]

There are real concerns about where to put the dying in an acute-care hospital. The impact of the death on the living, both bereaved family members and other patients, must be considered. Postmortem care and the transport of the body to the morgue are visible on the unit, despite institutional efforts to conceal them. Grieving families are entitled to time with the newly dead as part of the bereavement process. This is often impractical in an acute-care hospital: either another patient is waiting for the bed of the deceased, or the roommate needs treatment and support.

In their study of the hospitalized dying, Glaser and Strauss pointed out that as these patients are trying to exert some control over their remaining lives, they must expend a large amount of energy trying to learn how to be acceptable patients while in the hospital.[4] This type of energy expenditure is inappropriate and unfair: these patients are already struggling to enhance the quality of their remaining lives. Continued and inevitable loss of physical control is demoralizing, and the terminally ill have the ever-present awareness that they will soon cease to have any influence over anything.

PERSONAL OBSTACLES

It is not uncommon for dying patients to be perceived as socially dead even before their physical death occurs. The irony is that this occurs at the time of a person's greatest need.[5] Dying patients thus become victims of our inability to deal with them. Such distancing thwarts the patients' and families' attempts to process and integrate all that is happening. Rather, patients are left to analyze the reason for our abandonment and remain with a sense of shame for being terminal. There is a pervasive tendency to equate the inability to cure the incurable with failure. Dying patients are very sensitive to this notion, as it is often communicated to them by physicians.

Caring for and dealing with dying patients can be unsettling for caregivers, as it forces each of us to confront our mortality and arouses our preconceptions about dying. Ultimately we must gain some understanding, both as humans and collectively as a profession, of what it is that makes us uncomfortable around dying patients.[6] Only by acknowledging our personal limitations, as well as those of our health-care system in a death-denying society, can we even begin to help those at the most vulnerable, frightening part of their lives.

Part of understanding the plight of the dying is to question why we have been allowed to be remiss in this area of health care for so long, and why the deficiencies in terminal care are not more widely recognized. Mount offered two explanations.[2] First, health-care providers prefer to see themselves as sensitive and responsive to the needs of others. Second, patients are loath to criticize their physicians. Mount found that staff members were more likely to identify inadequacies in care on the parts of their colleagues than they were to acknowledge their own deficiencies. The staff attributed to their colleagues greater avoidance of discussions with patients about dying than they recognized in themselves.

A final possible explanation is that both the bereaved and the caregiver are likely to repress recollections of the dying experience of a loved one or patient. This decreases the chance that the caregiver's wisdom and expertise in this area will grow. It also makes it less likely that caregivers will be motivated—from without or within—to improve their delivery of terminal care.

THE DYING PROCESS

As with any other stage of life, there are tasks and needs unique to those living through the final stage. As with all developmental phases of life, there is pain and change, which ideally results in adaption. But how does one adapt to dying? There is a vast difference between having the cognitive awareness that death is universal and we each will someday die, and being the person confronted with the terminal illness. The crisis of dying calls into question our previous coping mechanisms of denial and repression of death.

People who are dying must reorient themselves by adjusting to all present and impending losses. The dying person experiences loss and death on various levels. There is social death, in which the dying person must learn to separate from the living. The phenomenon of losing our status and who we are is known as phenomenologic death. Psychological death involves the loss of the personality, the essence of a person. Psychological death occurs as the patient acknowledges that he or she will no longer exist. Simultaneously, a biologic death is occurring, and physical deterioration is an ever-present reminder that at the end of this experience, all that will be left are a person's remains.[7]

Our goal as caregivers is to make this overwhelming process

of dying more manageable for patients, families, and ourselves.

MEDICAL AND NURSING NEEDS OF THE TERMINALLY ILL

The care of the dying is both a science and an art. We must help patients cope with the high-tech medical environment that commonly surrounds them at the point of death. The concept of a "good death" should mean more than simply withholding aggressive measures. It also demands that we create an environment that allows for a peaceful, comfortable death. Doing so requires familiarity with the unique care needs of the terminally ill.

Inadequate or inappropriate management of pain and other symptoms is a major source of distress for dying patients. The pain of a terminal illness is not just physical pain. By the time a person has reached the terminal stage of disease, he or she suffers from many other types of pain, including mental, financial, interpersonal, and spiritual. Caregivers must pay attention to the whole person if they expect to affect this type of pain. However, a common error is to focus solely on the psychological and emotional needs of the dying; physical comfort comes first. Counseling a dying patient who is lying in a wet bed is ineffective.

Although the basic goals of pain management are somewhat similar in both cure-oriented and palliative contexts, the distinctive aspects of the situation of dying patients demand distinctive responses.

Acute pain can be significant but is usually of short duration. It can be classified as mild, moderate, or severe in intensity. Acute pain is associated with resolvable or reversible problems. For acute pain, treatment on a prn or as-needed basis is usually adequate. The patient's expectation is that the pain will be of finite duration, which is correct.

Unlike acute pain, chronic pain cannot be easily classified according to severity. Chronic pain can be seen as a "circular continuum of aching to agony."[8] The difference between tolerable chronic aching and intolerable chronic agony sometimes depends on the nature of the physical cause (*e.g.*, tumor involvement in bone or nerve plexus). However, equally important are the psychoemotional and social factors that inevitably exacerbate the pain. Unlike acute pain, chronic pain is not associated with recovery. It does not resolve rapidly, which in and of itself generates more anxiety and depression, which then lead to feelings of isolation and hostility.[8] Acute pain warns of a malfunction; chronic pain often dominates the patient's life to the exclusion of all else.

The terminally ill patient must receive whatever is necessary to control pain. Despite the recent advances in care of the dying, many practitioners still struggle with this concept. They continue to fear the legal repercussions of liberal narcotic use, which may depress respirations and blood pressure. They are also in a dilemma about the implications of assisted suicide or euthanasia. These fears are certainly well founded in an age of defensive medicine. The outcome, however, is a pervasive fear among patients, families, and the public at large that inadequate pain control will result in needless suffering. Fear of dying in pain is a common concern expressed by patients and families, and these fears are often valid.

A recent article in the *New England Journal of Medicine* took a strong stand on minimizing pain and suffering in a patient whose dying process is irreversible, even if this means potentially hastening death.[9] Wanzer and associates wrote that it is morally correct to use whatever narcotics are needed, in whatever doses and by whatever routes, even if this may decrease blood pressure or respirations or cause a loss of consciousness. Fears of addiction have no place in terminal care, and physicians, patients, and families alike must be reminded of this. Reassurance from the physician to patients and families that pain will be controlled should begin at the outset, when a fatal disease is diagnosed.

Other common physical symptoms experienced by the terminally ill that require skilled management are anorexia, nausea and vomiting, dry mouth, dyspnea, cough, hiccups, anxiety, confusion, depression, insomnia, constipation, incontinence, diarrhea, itch, and mental distress.[10] Narcotic and nonnarcotic medications are needed for the management of these and other symptoms. Benzodiazepines, metaclopramide, antihistamines, tricyclic antidepressants, phenothiazines, and other major and minor tranquilizers are used frequently.

The care needs of the terminally ill usually increase as death approaches. The patient becomes increasingly debilitated and dependent on staff for performing activities of daily living. Things that are usually taken for granted, such as mobility and personal hygiene, must now be performed by one human for another. Controlling all the symptoms requires tremendous time, patience, and compassion on the part of the caregivers. As Wanzer and associates wrote, "Dying patients may require palliative care of an intensity that challenges even that of curative efforts. . . [P]rofessionals . . . are still called upon to use intensive measures—extreme responsibility, extraordinary sensitivity and heroic compassion."[9]

PSYCHOEMOTIONAL NEEDS OF THE TERMINALLY ILL

The implications of a cancer diagnosis are vast. The emotional responses range from the expectation of cure, to hope for chronicity, to expectation of a terminal illness. For cancer patients, it is often difficult to determine when the dying process begins. Kastenbaum wrote that dying usually begins as a psychosocial event.[11] The optimal course of events is initiated by the physician's recognition that effective treatment options are no longer available. This should then be communicated to the patient. Ideally, the patient accepts the fact that nothing more can be done medically to preserve life. Once an acutely ill cancer patient becomes terminally ill, a grief response begins for all present, past, and future losses.

Merely contemplating one's own mortality causes some degree of anxiety. For terminally ill people, forced to confront their own imminent death, immense anxiety composed of specific fears is a major emotional response. There are fears of the unknown, loneliness, loss of self-control, loss of all loved ones, and loss of bodily functions. There are fears of pain and suffering, sorrow, regression, mutilation, decomposition, and premature burial.[7] Caregivers and family must help the dying to break down their anxiety into its components to make it manageable.

Depression, anger, guilt, and shame are common responses of the dying. Acceptance, withdrawal, detachment, and hope are also central issues. The nature and quality of hope change as the patient progresses through the stages of terminal illness. It is no longer hope of cure, but hope for a certain quality of remaining life. It is a day-to-day hope that enables the person to keep some control, dignity, and sense of worth.[7]

Caregivers also have an emotional response to cancer and to death and dying. With acute-care patients, although the prognosis is uncertain, caregivers can rely on experience to predict the direction things will take. In terminal care, the prognosis is known but what lies beyond is unknown to all.

To enable the dying to perform the last tasks of their lives with some degree of dignity and self-determination, caregivers must create a maximally supportive environment for those with limited energy. To do this, we are asked to put aside our professional and personal egos for a time and become active listeners. This requires a role reversal of sorts, which is often uncomfortable for physicians and nurses to perform. It means allowing the dying patients and their families to be our teachers and to communicate to us their real needs and concerns. This is not only the beginning, but the essence of what it takes to deal with dying patients.

WHAT CAN BE DONE?

Those who work closely with the terminally ill would like to maximize their effectiveness, despite institutional obstacles and individual limitations. A recent survey at a comprehensive cancer center revealed the following notable trends among the medical attending and nursing staff at the study institution.[12] The staff confirmed the existence of a patient population identified as terminally ill who required a significant amount of time and resources. They recognized the unique care needs of the terminally ill and acknowledged that certain institutional obstacles led to deficiencies in the care of this group in deference to the more acutely ill. For example, the staff recognized a tendency to respond first to the acutely ill patient if both types of patients required attention at the same time; they also admitted to some discomfort with this choice. They perceived that the continuity of care was inadequate in the present system, and the staff strongly preferred to follow their primary patients from the point of diagnosis through their final stages of life. They expressed an interest in finding solutions to more effectively deal with dying patients, and there was overwhelming support for the development of a formal program devoted to this end.

Irrespective of the setting of death, certain ways of relating to the dying person are essential. Thanatologic conversation is a unique type of communication between caregiver and patient. It is not ordinary conversation that occurs among friends, it is not the hierarchical conversation typical of the physician-patient relationship, and it is not the professional conversation of psychotherapy. It is an interaction between two humans, both acknowledging their common fate. It is a flexible communication that takes place in the present, with the awareness of the inevitable downhill course to follow. It requires a tremendous amount of empathy on the caregiver's part, with no place for sympathy or pity. It acknowledges the entire ambience of the dying process and thereby extends to family members and friends as well. The goals of such an interaction are to support and comfort patients and to help them find value in their remaining days.

For any interaction with the dying person to be effective, the caregiver must not fear the patient. A certain amount of death anxiety is normal when seeing a human who is dying or dead. However, caregivers must distinguish this general anxiety from more specific fears of the particular dying patient to whom they are attending. Caregivers commonly express fears that, although irrational, are important to recognize and deal with. Death and the process of dying are not contagious. Avoiding the dying patient does not confer immortality. Practitioners should not view their patients who become terminally ill as failures. This perception is self-serving and egocentric and creates additional anxiety for caregivers and patients. No patient wants to be seen as a failure, and it is equally uncomfortable for a practitioner to cast himself or herself as a failure.

Death has been viewed as the great equalizer among us, and this notion can help allay our fears of being with a dying patient. As Ajeman and Mount wrote, "The doctor, being himself a mortal man, should be diligent and tender in relieving his suffering patients inasmuch as he himself must one day be a like sufferer."[13]

Our efforts will be continually thwarted if we try to have every patient die a peaceful death with total acceptance and freedom from denial. This is rarely the case. We do ourselves and our patients an injustice by setting unrealistic goals. It is a myth to think we can help a person accept death. We cannot make the unknown familiar and eradicate all associated fears. We cannot render good and pretty that which is often bad and ugly. We as caregivers should repress this societally enforced tendency of avoiding unpleasantness when dealing with the dying.

To varying degrees throughout our lives, we all use the defense mechanism of denial with regard to death. Death is something we hold in abeyance somewhere out there in the distant future. Therefore, it is unrealistic for us as caregivers to believe that we can completely break down this protective mechanism, which has been nurtured for a lifetime. It is also unfair to our patients. At best, what usually occurs is that patients acknowledge the inevitable outcome: they will cease to be. As caregivers, we should strive to help the patients cope with the ramifications of this recognition.

It is equally important to acknowledge other limitations as clinical practitioners. Sometimes it is impossible to effectively manage all the symptoms of dying patients. This is particularly true when patients, along with other physically distressing problems, present with an altered mental state or mental distress of questionable etiology. These symptoms are often resistant to treatment, and we tend to throw up our hands in dismay due to our frustration and feelings of helplessness.

In these extraordinarily difficult cases, the desirable patient outcome of a peaceful, comfortable death will not be achieved. This can raise doubts for even the most caring and tenacious oncology practitioners as to our purpose: if we cannot even help a person die comfortably, what is the point? The main goal in this situation is not to turn away from the patient and family. Honest disclosure of the difficulty in controlling such symptoms can allay anxieties and offer reassurance that the symptom is not being ignored. We should also avoid focusing on the refractory symptoms to the exclusion of others. One is not seen as an inadequate physician or nurse because of the inability to manage *all* the distressing symptoms of the dying.

We caregivers must direct our energy toward what we can do for the dying. In many ways, it is the simplest offering of all. Yet perhaps because of its fundamental nature, we fail to recognize its importance and instead focus on our feelings of inadequacy or impotence. The most important thing we can offer our patients is our presence. We can easily relieve patients' fears that we will abandon and reject them because they are dying. We bring our skills and expertise in management and control of the symptoms of dying, but to be most effective we need to do more, and in this case, the more is less. We must learn to just be there: to listen, look, and try to understand what is happening for the particular person at this point in time. This concept is foreign to us and represents the total antithesis of our medical training. We need to relinquish control and take our cues from the patient. We should refrain from our tendency to stereotype and assume we know the needs of the dying. They will tell us if we just give them the time to do so.

From clinical experience, the willingness and ability to *listen* is the single most important characteristic a caregiver can bring to a dying patient. I have seen a sincerely concerned housekeeper, having daily contact and conversation with a dying patient, be more effective than the physician who was rushing in and out of the patient's room each morning reciting the plan for the day. In such circumstances, the greatest effectiveness comes from eliciting information from the patient about what he or she considers important and valuable. Not all dying patients want their hands held or their families maintaining a vigil at the bedside. We may assume this is how it should be because it makes us feel better, but we should not write the scripts for the dying.

The only way to overcome our trained tendency "to do" is to occupy our time by being with the patient and listening. This need not take endless hours that health-care professionals seldom have to spare. Rather, it is our sincerity and the quality of the time we give the person when we are present that is important. Certainly it is the dying patient who is most acutely aware of the passage of time.

Asking questions of the patient is encouraged. Certain questions may facilitate conversation, such as are you comfortable, do you feel like talking, what's on your mind, are you frightened. Then wait for the answer. Do not start something you cannot finish; if you are pressed for time, say so. Reassuring patients of your routine and thereby explaining your absences goes a long way toward allaying their fears of abandonment. Often is is us, not our dying patients, who impose unrealistic expectations on caregivers.

The dying often are acutely aware of and gain a sense of peace from the notion that life goes on. This brings a certain sense of familiarity and comfort in knowing that although life will cease to be for them, it goes on for others. This is why it is common for those of us who routinely talk with the dying to find ourselves discussing a multitude of topics totally unrelated to death. This, too, can be therapeutic and consoling; it should not be viewed as wasted time.

Entering into a relationship with a dying person involves some of the same dynamics as any other human interaction. Trust must be built through mutual understanding. The difference is that time is of the essence, so it behooves us to get it right the first time for the sake of the patient. Maintaining reasonable expectations of ourselves and our dying patients will allow a mutually fulfilling experience to occur. Caregivers need not underestimate the contribution their presence and genuine expressions of concern bring to a dying person. One of the few tangible guarantees we can give our patients is that we will not abandon or reject them, however threatened we are by their dying.

We must view the dying person from several different perspectives: in relation to the illness and the physical symptoms, in light of his or her psychological response to impending death, and in relation to others. There may come a time of pulling back on the patient's part. Usually this state of self-involvement comes after a period of enhanced emotional connection with and affirmation of feelings for those around him or her, both family and caregivers. At this time, it is helpful for us to shift our focus to the family and reassure them that their efforts have not been in vain. We should remember this advice for ourselves too at this time. This again requires our unselfish understanding, to step back and give the dying patient space and permission to begin to disconnect from all that he or she will soon lose totally.

There are few rules in thanatologic communication, but some pointers can enrich the experience. Throughout the dying process, honest communication must be maintained. To lie to or withhold information from the dying is cruel. Depriving them of such information could deny them crucial control over their remaining time. However, such disclosures should be handled sensitively, with the patient guiding the pace. Let the patient's level of comfort and understanding determine the pace, not your own. Ask questions and wait for answers. Of course, the ultimate question of "why" is completely unanswerable. As we discussed above, through all of this, hope is never totally taken away, but its nature changes. It is no longer hope for cure, but a hope to get through the next day with a sense of purpose and worth.

In being with people who are dying, try not to be afraid of them. Touch them, look at them, maintain eye contact, be aware of your body language. Pull up a chair so you are looking at them equally and not standing up and looking down at them in their beds. Listen and accept what you hear. Elicit their fears and concerns. Take action where you can and accept things over which you have no control. You cannot prevent death, but you can do your best to ensure that the dying guide their course to the extent possible.

It is really quite simple. Running away and leaving the matters of the dying to the clergy alone does not yield immortality or even professional fulfillment. The plight of the dying cannot be reversed, but it can be made easier if all members of the health-care team remember that the dying are still among the living; they are not yet dead. They should be treated with respect and sensitivity.

Greater effectiveness in dealing with the dying can really only be taught from doing so and being there. It is hoped that this chapter might make each of us more willing and able to learn.

REFERENCES

1. Grinslades S, Reko R. Hospital-based inpatient hospice units: Planning considerations. In: Corr CA, Corr DM, eds. Hospice care—principles and practice. New York: Springer, 1983:294–307.
2. Mount BM. The problem of caring for the dying in a general hospital: The palliative care unit as a possible solution. Can Med Assoc J 1976;115:119–121.
3. McNulty EB, Holdershy RA. Hospice, a caring challenge. Chicago: Charles L. Thomas, 1983.

4. Glaser BG, Strauss AL. Time for dying. Chicago: Aldine, 1968.
5. Cox JJ. Caring for the dying: Reflections of a medical student. Can Med Assoc J 1987;136: 577–579.
6. Bulkin W, Lukashok H. Rx for dying: The case for hospice. N Engl J Med 1988;318: 376–378.
7. Rando T. Grief, dying and death. Chicago: Research Press, 1984.
8. Lipman AG. Drug therapy of chronic pain. In: Corr CA, Corr DM, eds. Hospice care—principles and practice. New York: Springer, 1983:73–87.
9. Wanzer SH, Federman DD, Adelstein SJ, et al. The physician's responsibility toward hopelessly ill patients. N Engl J Med 1989;320:844–849.
10. Barnes M. Drug control of common symptoms. In: Corr CA, Corr DM, eds. Hospice care—principles and practice. New York: Springer, 1983:89–97.
11. Kastenbaum RJ. Death, society and human experience. St. Louis: CV Mosby, 1981.
12. Sammarino D. Caring for the terminally ill cancer patient within an acute-care cancer center: Analysis and alternatives. Unpublished master's thesis, Department of Health and Nutrition Science, Brooklyn College, 1990.
13. Ajeman I, Mount BM, eds. The R.V.H. manual on palliative hospice care. Salem, NH: Ayer, 1982.

GRACE H. CHRIST
ROSEMARY T. MOYNIHAN
MATTHEW LOSCALZO
LOIS L. WEINSTEIN

SECTION **7**

Providing Community Resources for Cancer Patients

A patient diagnosed with cancer may require a range of services over the course of the illness. As a consequence of the disease, treatment, and rehabilitation, the patient may need concrete services such as personal care, household assistance, medical equipment, child care, financial assistance, transportation, and information and counseling. These needs also may arise as a result of the demands of the health-care system, bureaucratic complications, financial limitations, and the emotional problems that patients and families often experience during a major illness. If these needs are unmet, patients may be unable to comply with intensive treatment regimens, may experience low morale that affects treatment-related decisions, may fail to resume active functioning after acute episodes of illness, and may experience an overall reduction in functioning and quality of life.

Resources to meet patients' concrete and emotional needs have never been more essential to treatment and recovery than in the contemporary medical climate. In recent years, the trend in the United States toward "dehospitalization" has affected oncology as well as other fields. Extended outpatient care, ambulatory surgical and radiation treatment centers, day treatment hospitals, and home administration of complex chemotherapies and associated treatments testify to the move away from the hospital as the locus of care. At the same time, cancer has become a chronic rather than an acute illness for increasing numbers of patients. The net effect of these trends is that greater demands are placed on informal and formal support systems in the family and community.

Demands for practical assistance in the home arise from patients' inability to meet daily living and treatment-related tasks. These tasks increase as the disease progresses and are complicated by the toxic side effects of treatment. Many of these needs, formerly handled in the hospital, must now be met by family members and other informal caregivers. Studies have documented, however, that this assistance often is inadequate.[1–3] In response to these changed conditions, studies on the prevalence of such needs identified barriers to service delivery and led to the development of new methods of delivery, new models of provision of care, different types of community services, and more comprehensive systems of care.

The services that cancer patients need can be divided into six categories:

1. *Cancer information, education, and counseling:* Individual or family counseling, support groups, veteran patient programs, marital counseling, sexual counseling, and spiritual counseling[4]
2. *Home care:* Personal care, including injections, care of catheters, stoma management, nasogastric tube feeding, pain management, occupational therapy, and so on; household assistance such as housecleaning, meal preparation, laundry, and shopping[5–7]
3. *Alternatives to home care:* Nursing homes, hospices, and so forth
4. *Equipment:* Wheelchairs, walkers, bath benches, hospital beds, intravenous poles and pumps, stoma bags, and the like[6,7]
5. *Financial assistance:* Income maintenance and help with the cost of treatment
6. *Transportation:* Ambulances, ambulettes, taxis, car services, and so on.[8]

This chapter presents the findings of recent research on the prevalence of these needs, defines the range of community resources available to meet them, describes new intervention models, and identifies evolving problems in the provision of community services. It also presents the range of resources available, reviews the indicators of need for such services, and describes ways of finding services in the community.

PREVALENCE OF NEEDS

Several recent studies have attempted to estimate the prevalence of cancer patients' needs for concrete assistance. Although earlier studies documented the importance of these needs and the fact that needs increased with progression of the disease and with age, their use of different definitions and measures of need and heterogenous samples of patients made it difficult to compare results.[3,9,10] In the more recent studies, careful definition of needs, better methods of data collection, and use of specific populations of patients at different stages of disease and treatment allowed comparisons of results.

In a randomized survey of 629 cancer patients selected from the Pennsylvania Cancer Registry and 397 support persons, Houts and colleagues found that 59% of the patients had at least one unmet psychosocial need during the first year after diagnosis.[2] The unmet need cited most often was for emotional support (25% of the patients cited this need). In a second study conducted with a stratified random sample of 433 significant others of patients who had recently died, Houts and colleagues found that 72% of the patients had had at least one unmet need during their final month of life.[11] The unmet needs reported most often were help with activities of daily living (42%), emotional support (21%), physical assistance (21%), communication problems with medical staff (20%), insurance (19%), and financial support (15%).

Mor and associates surveyed the unmet needs for concrete services of 217 patients with advanced cancer and family members who were already receiving agency services in New York City and found that age, duration of disease, education, income, gender, marital status, living arrangements, and pain were related to the degree of need.[3] More than half of the patients (51%) reported at least one unmet need, and most indicated unmet instrumental needs such as meal preparation, housekeeping, shopping, and home health care.

In a subsequent study, Guadagnoli and Mor interviewed 412 patients, 70% of whom received care in a private oncology practice in Rhode Island.[12] Ninety percent of these patients needed help with an activity of daily living. The unmet needs cited most often were help with heavy housework, shopping, and completing forms and other paperwork. Fewer than a third (26.7%) received help with at least one activity of daily living from a formal source. The vast majority (84%) received help with at least one daily living activity from informal sources (usually a family member). The level of unmet need (26%) in the second study was lower than expected, possibly because the patients lived in rural areas and fewer than two thirds of them (62%) had advanced disease.

The differences in these results were attributable to the fact that Houts assessed the need for emotional support, which accounted for 25% of the prevalence rate, but Mor did not. In the latter studies, the level of unmet need varied as a function of the level of confidence in the ability of others to provide help and the number of helpers available, as well as physical functioning and age.

Siegel and colleagues conducted in-depth interviews with 200 outpatients with advanced disease who were receiving chemotherapy at Memorial Sloan-Kettering Cancer Center and found that 62% reported at least one unmet need within the previous month; 39% reported two or more.[13,14] The mean number of unmet needs was about 1.7. Furthermore, the patients exhibited a marked lack of knowledge about the services available in their community. The estimation of prevalence of needs was based on a cross-sectional design and included patients who had been in treatment for different periods of time. If the sample had been followed longitudinally, the proportion of patients with one or more unmet needs at any point in the course of treatment would have been significantly greater.

Finally, in a survey of caregiver burden and unmet patient needs among 483 patients and their informal caregivers that did not include an assessment of the need for psychological counseling, only 18.9% of the patients reported an unmet need.[15] Because a more restricted definition of unmet need was used in this study, the prevalence rate was lower. In addition, patients with early- and late-stage cancer were included. Significant predictors of unmet needs were:

1. The patient's illness and treatment resulted in restricted ability to perform tasks of daily life.
2. The patient's financial resources were so limited that he or she was forced to apply for Medicaid or welfare.
3. The spouse was not the patient's caregiver.
4. The care provided was associated with a high level of burden.

Table 64–32 summarizes the results of these studies. The varying percentages of unmet needs were the result of dif-

TABLE 64–32. Recent Studies on the Prevalence of Cancer Patients' Unmet Psychosocial Needs

Source	Study Population	Prevalence
Included the Need for Emotional Counseling		
Houts et al[2]	Randomized survey of 629 patients and 397 support persons	59% reported at least one unmet need; 25% needed emotional support
Houts et al[11]	Randomized survey of 433 significant others of patients who had died	72% reported at least one unmet need during the final month of life
Did Not Include the Need for Emotional Counseling		
Mor et al[3]	217 patients and family members already receiving help from a cancer service agency	51% reported at least one unmet service need; the longer the duration of the disease, the higher the prevalence rate
Christ and Siegel[14]	200 outpatients with advanced disease	62% reported at least one unmet need; 39% reported two or more.
Used a Restricted Definition of Concrete Needs and Did Not Include the Need for Emotional Counseling		
Guadagnoli and Mor[12]	410 outpatients with early and late-stage disease	25% reported at least one unmet need
Siegel et al[24]	483 patients with early and late-stage disease and their informal caregivers	19% reported at least one unmet need

ferent stages of disease, inclusion or exclusion of the need for emotional support, and varying definitions of unmet need.

BARRIERS TO THE USE OF COMMUNITY RESOURCES

Several recent studies suggest that the primary reasons that patients have unmet needs is their lack of awareness that services exist and their inability to negotiate complex bureaucracies to obtain them in a timely manner.[6,8,13,16,17] In Siegel's study, for instance, in response to the question, "If the areas we have been talking about became a problem for you, would you know where to go to obtain help from an agency or a service?," 68% of the patients answered no. In addition to finding that patients and families were unaware of community resources, Parsons found that many lacked the mobility or strength to search for them, cope with the arduous process of establishing eligibility, and follow through on an application.[7]

Many authors have stressed the importance of informing patients and their families about available resources and providing guidance on how to use them to maximize comfort and functioning at home and to avoid unnecessary hospitalization. Dwyer and Held, who focused on the chronic phase of cancer and periodic changes in needs, wrote that patients and families should be told in advance about home-care services so they will know where to turn when they need help.[18] Lurie suggested a case advocacy approach that would ensure that programs are accessible to appropriate patients.[19]

Bennet pointed out that because of anxiety, physically ill patients have difficulty comprehending and integrating information.[20] After distributing written material on concrete services to 80 patients, she found, during a follow-up interview, that only 12 patients had read the material and that none of the patients believed it would be helpful. Thus, she concluded that written material should be distributed to patients in conjunction with individualized contact.

Grobe and associates recommended the use of a glossary of available services in the context of an extensive educational program that would enhance patients' awareness of potential needs and available resources.[7] Edstrom and Miller used a three-session course on home care to teach patients about aspects of physical care and how to find community resources to meet concrete needs.[16]

All of these studies, together with clinical experience, reveal several attitudinal and psychological barriers that prevent patients from learning about and using community resources. First, because they want to be independent, they would rather not ask for help and therefore usually do so only in a medical emergency. They are especially reticent about reporting nonmedical needs; however, if asked, they can specify which nonmedical needs are not being met and often want to know about the services available. Furthermore, asking patients if they need certain kinds of help implies that other patients have the same needs, which makes it easier for them to acknowledge their unmet needs. For these reasons, a system of universal outreach is essential.

Second, because patients are understandably focused primarily on their illness and treatment, they have difficulty assimilating information about services that are not relevant to their current needs. Some patients are threatened by information that forces them to acknowledge a probable deterioration in their functional status. Therefore, the timing of information should be individualized and patient-specific. Guadagnoli and coworkers postulated that intervention strategies are more effective when they are matched to a patient's readiness—that is, patients should be classified according to the following stages[21]:

1. The *precontemplation* stage, in which the patient needs help with a daily living activity but would not consider using formal services
2. The *contemplation* stage, in which the patient reports a need and is willing to receive help from a formal service, but has not yet received it
3. The *action* stage, in which the patient is trying to obtain formal services
4. The *maintenance* stage, in which the patient has used formal services in the past and would be willing to do so again.

Third, because their needs change over time, patients may need to be followed up. However, the growing number of patients treated on an outpatient basis and the limited staff available to serve them means that social work, nursing, or discharge planning staff cannot regularly follow up all outpatients. Hence, patients often are left to recognize their own unmet needs and to make those needs known.

NEW INTERVENTIONS

Using the findings from these prevalence studies, new interventions have been proposed and developed to address the problems that typically arise in obtaining community resources and to monitor patients' care:

1. A case-management training program for patients and families
2. A case-management patient and family monitoring program
3. A computer-automated telephone outreach system
4. New community resource manuals for patients and families and information hotlines
5. A training program for health professionals to heighten their awareness of the psychosocial needs of cancer patients and available resources.

All these programs aim to be cost-effective and focus primarily on outpatient care. Except for the case-management training program for patients and families, they focus on intervention over a longer period of time than earlier rehabilitation programs, which tended to focus on inpatients, were expensive, and covered a relatively brief period.

CASE-MANAGEMENT TRAINING PROGRAM

On the basis of Mor's survey,[3] Wool and colleagues[22] developed a 12-week training program for high-risk patients and their families to improve their problem-solving skills. The program combined an educational and counseling approach in which the case manager assessed patients' needs, provided information about existing resources, and guided patients in gaining access to these resources. The goal was to increase the family's autonomy and mastery, reduce their unmet needs, and counteract the common feeling of helplessness associated with serious illness. Thus, training patients to recognize problems as they arose was an important aspect of the program. To accomplish these goals, the case manager had regular meetings, both in person and on the telephone, with patients and caregivers to teach them problem-solving skills and impart information about current and anticipated needs. The case manager acted as a direct intermediary only when necessary. This training model is currently being tested in a randomized trial.

CASE-MANAGEMENT MONITORING PROGRAM

Polinsky and associates developed a 12-month case-management program for patients with stage I or stage II breast cancer that began 3 to 5 weeks after surgery and extended for 1 year.[23] This intervention included an initial assessment followed by periodic reassessments conducted primarily by telephone as well as in person if indicated, at least once every 6 weeks. During the initial in-depth assessment, patients received information about a broad range of resources. Throughout the 12 months that followed, the case manager provided new information about support-group meetings, presentations, and recent research findings, either by telephone or mail.

Although the program was not designed to include direct provision of counseling, case managers often provided counseling in the form of reassurance. Over the year, their time was accounted for by reassurance (58%), information (38%), and referrals (4%). They also served as advocates when a patient's efforts seemed ineffective (*e.g.*, correcting hospital billing errors). The average time of each case-management contact was 15.3 minutes. One case manager spent 374 hours during the year on the program with 69 newly diagnosed patients. The average case-management time spent on each patient per year was 5.4 hours. The efficacy of this program in improving patients' functional status, mood, and quality of life is now being studied in a randomized trial.

TABLE 64–33. Survey Questions Used in the Automated Telephone Outreach System to Assess Patients' Concrete Needs

Now, here is the first question, which is about the cost of your transportation to the hospital, including the cost of public transportation, other fares, parking, tolls, and gas. During the past month, when you came to the hospital, could you have used any help with these costs?

The second question is about the kind of transportation you usually take to the hospital. During the past month, would another kind of transportation have made the trip to the hospital easier?

The third question is about your medical prescriptions. During the past month, could you have used any help either paying for your prescriptions or getting them filled?

The fourth question is about the time you spend alone at home. During the past month, was there any time when you were alone in the house and felt too sick or weak to be alone?

The fifth question is about how you are managing bathing. During the past month, was there any time when you needed more help than you had when you were showering or bathing?

The sixth question is about how you are managing food shopping. During the past month, was there any time when you needed more help than you had to shop for food?

The seventh question is about how you are managing meal preparation. During the past month, was there any time when you needed more help than you had to prepare a meal?

The eighth question is about how you are managing light housekeeping like dusting, washing dishes, or making beds. During the past month, was there any time when you needed more help than you had to do light housework?

The ninth question is about how you are managing heavy housekeeping like mopping, vacuuming, doing the laundry, or cleaning the bathroom. During the past month, was there any time when you needed more help than you had to do heavy housework?

The tenth question is about how you are managing medical bills. Do you currently need help either understanding or paying your medical bills?

The eleventh question is about how you are managing to get medical information. Do you currently need help getting more information about your illness and its treatment?

Is there any other problem connected with your illness which you would like to discuss with a social worker?

TELEPHONE OUTREACH

In the second phase of their study, Siegel and associates attempted to reduce the prevalence of unmet needs by developing an intervention that would permit cost-effective, universal assessment of outpatients' needs as well as periodic reassessments to identify changing or emerging needs in a timely manner.[24] A computerized system telephoned patients periodically to conduct a brief needs assessment. This fully automated outreach system consisted of a specifically configured computer and custom-designed software that accepted a virtually unlimited number of patients and did not require a human operator.

In their earlier cross-sectional study, Christ and Siegel extracted a set of only 12 questions that allowed them to identify about 93% of the patients who reported one or more unmet concrete needs in response to the extensive list of concrete services covered during personal interviews with patients (see Appendix).[14] These 12 questions (Table 64–33) were then adapted for use in the telephone survey with the expectation that they would capture a similarly high proportion of patients who had one or more unmet needs. The questions specifically addressed needs related to the cost and mode of transportation to and from the hospital, medical prescriptions, supervision at home, personal care, food shopping, meal preparation, light and heavy housekeeping, medical bills, and medical information. If a patient said yes to any of the questions, a social worker called the patient within a week to discuss ways of solving the problem. In this way, the intervention coupled computer automation with professional service delivery.

The ability of the intervention to reduce the prevalence of unmet needs was then evaluated in an experimental trial. Patients were preassigned to the experimental or control group before accrual. The experimental group was entered onto the computer system to begin a series of three automated telephone surveys scheduled about 6 weeks apart. The results showed that the prevalence of unmet needs in the control group was higher than in the experimental group for 15 of the 21 specific needs; for eight of these needs, the difference exceeded 10%. Furthermore, in every domain of need, the proportion of patients who reported unmet needs for assistance with any task was lower among the patients in the experimental group than in the control group. Significant findings and trends in the data supported the conclusion that patients in the experimental group were less likely to experience unmet needs than were patients in the control group.

This automated outreach system appeared to be an especially cost-effective way of addressing the changing needs of the large number of patients who move in and out of outpatient care. It did not incur the considerable expense associated with other strategies used to screen patients needs. The expensive professional time was used for problem-solving in the return call. Because the problem was already identified, social workers found that the average length of a call was only 18 minutes.

In summary, the automated telephone screening survey holds promise as an effective strategy for early identification of patients with unmet needs. These patients can then be contacted by professionals who can further explore the nature and severity of their needs and their receptivity to and eligibility for available services in a timely way. The vast majority of patients with unmet needs may not otherwise come to professional attention, given the shortage of staff. In Siegel's cross-sectional study, only 11% of the patients had contact with a social worker in the 6 months before the intervention.

NEW RESOURCE AND EDUCATIONAL MATERIALS

Several new resource manuals and materials have been developed to inform patients about the community services available to them. Of particular note is the book *Facing Forward*, developed by the National Cancer Institute. This useful resource manual for cancer survivors can be obtained along with other materials by calling the Cancer Information Service (1-800-4-CANCER).

Another excellent resource manual for cancer patients and families is *Helping People Cope: A Guide for Families Facing Cancer*, which was developed by the Cancer Control Plan of the Pennsylvania Department of Health. This manual not only provides information about a broad range of community resource needs but also contains clear directions about how to obtain these services. It can be obtained by calling 1-800-537-4063.

These two sources of information take into account the changing health-care environment and data from recent studies of patients' needs, and are more comprehensive and practical than previous publications on the subject. Additional written materials for patients can be obtained from agencies listed in the appendix.

TRAINING PROGRAM FOR PROFESSIONALS

In response to Houts' survey, Barg and colleagues conducted a statewide 3-day continuing education program for health professionals in oncology in Pennsylvania.[25] The goals of the program were to:

1. Enhance the participants' knowledge regarding psychosocial support services
2. Develop consumer guides to community resources to improve and expand the use of existing support services
3. Increase the participants' knowledge about pain and symptom control to meet patients' physical and psychological needs
4. Increase the effectiveness of communication among patients, families, and caregivers.

When the program ended, the 409 participants were assessed to determine whether their attitudes and beliefs had changed as a result of the program. Later, the participants were assessed again to determine whether the program had led to new psychosocial initiatives within their institutions. The changes in both domains were significant and subsequently led to the development of a network for health providers who were interested in the psychosocial aspects of cancer. One recommendation from the program was to computerize regional resources for patients as a more timely, accurate, and cost-effective way to organize this information than the development of multiple directories. This led to a toll-free number that patients could call to obtain information about any cancer-related resource in the state. The information is updated every 6 months.

SERVICES FOR EVOLVING NEEDS

The fact that cancer has become a chronic illness in many instances has resulted in growing numbers of survivors who need rehabilitation. At the same time, the constant search for ways to reduce health-care costs is affecting the kinds of services available and how those services are delivered. Patients with prolonged chronic illness must deal with gradual debilitation, progression of disease, and fear of losing control over the disease. These stresses are heightened by the cost of medical care and surveillance, which can exhaust medical insurance and the family's resources.

Finally, chronically ill patients, although their numbers are increasing, have few positive models to emulate. Society's models tend to be either cured patients who can fill their roles in the community with no apparent impediments, or those who die heroically. Thus, cancer patients, as well as other chronically ill people, need new role models who illustrate the courage it takes to live day by day in this society with a chronic, sometimes terminal illness.

Cured patients must reenter a culture that values people who emerge unscathed from a crisis, yet they need ongoing social and psychological rehabilitation. They may have lost their hair or a breast, limb, or other organ; they may have gained or lost weight or suffered other effects of the disease or treatment, including infertility. They must live with the fear that the cancer will recur or that a new cancer will develop, possibly because of the treatment for the original cancer. Finally, they may confront discrimination from employers and medical insurance carriers.

Although most survivors adjust well to their illness, they are frustrated by the common notion that they can pick up where they left off. To most patients whose treatment has been successful, the illness represents a major discontinuity that brings about lasting changes in how they perceive themselves and their future. New resources are now being developed in the community to help survivors deal with these obstacles to developing meaningful and productive lives.[26]

Reducing the cost of health care is the dominant issue in

health-care policy for the 1990s. All purchasers of health care—governments, businesses, and people—experience the burden of mushrooming costs of medical care and the efforts to control them. These financial pressures are affecting patients in the following ways:

1. Their insurance premiums have increased but fewer costs are covered.
2. The number who lack insurance or have only limited coverage has increased dramatically.[27]
3. The kinds of treatment covered for a given diagnosis, the places where treatment can be provided, and coverage for outpatient care are increasingly restricted. The result is high turnover among staff of community agencies and changes in the way services are delivered and who is billed for them.

All these conditions have created an atmosphere in which patients are uncertain whether they will be able to obtain or afford the treatments that will prolong their lives. In other words, the cost of a particular treatment is becoming a major factor in a patient's decision about which course of treatment to pursue. Patients can no longer assume, as they have in the past, that the insurance company, the government, or the hospital will make it possible for them to receive recommended treatments. Furthermore, because of regulatory changes, a patient's financial liability may change during the course of treatment. For example, a new Medicare regulation asserts that hospitals must refer patients to selected outside vendors for equipment, absorb the cost of billing, and pay the vendors themselves if such services are not covered by Medicare. In the past, to avoid unfair restriction of trade, hospitals often avoided referring patients to specific vendors; this gave patients more choices of service providers.

Because less money is available for community resources at a time when those resources are increasingly necessary, it is even more urgent that professionals find cost-effective ways of facilitating patients' timely access to resources and thus reduce the risk of costly, uncomfortable medical crises that occur at home.

LIMITATIONS OF DISCHARGE-PLANNING SERVICES

In recent years, the emphasis on discharge planning has heightened the awareness of health professionals about the importance of careful coordination of posthospital care for cancer patients. Such coordination is crucial to ensure an uninterrupted flow of health services that will maximize patients' chances of recovering their normal functional status to the degree possible and will minimize the cost of care.[28] When the prospective payment system began to be phased into the health-care system in 1983, the length of stay for inpatients began to decline and the demand for outpatient services increased proportionately. Clearly, helping patients return home and remain there have become national priorities, and identifying supportive resources in the community and developing new services are necessary to achieve this end.

Until recently, most of the literature on the community resources available for cancer patients focused either on planning for the discharge of patients after an acute episode of illness or on patient care (at home or in a hospice) during the terminal phase of illness.[8,29–35] Little was written about patients' needs in the chronic phase, when progression of the disease and intensified treatment make the patient more and more debilitated but not yet in need of hospitalization or hospice care.[6,16,18]

Chronically ill patients may experience not only symptoms of the disease but also the sequelae of chemotherapy and radiation therapy, such as nausea and vomiting, anorexia, weight loss, aplastic anemia, and weakness.[16] As a result of improved methods of medical management, patients have greater tolerance for highly cytotoxic chemotherapeutic agents and can be treated on an outpatient basis.[18] However, because of variations in the course of the disease and the unpredictability of the side effects of treatment, medical crises may develop abruptly and cause concomitant changes in the types of home care a patient needs.[18] Discharge plans that appear to be satisfactory immediately after hospitalization cannot always anticipate a patient's future needs as the disease progresses. Thus, when further deterioration occurs months later, the patient is an outpatient and thus not as easily identified as requiring services because fewer screening mechanisms are available to determine his or her needs.[36]

NEED FOR A COMMUNITY RESOURCES NETWORK

To direct patients in a timely manner to the broad range of services available, practitioners must be aware of agencies and community services that address patients' needs. By so doing, they will be able to match individual patients with the appropriate community resources.[37] Most hospitals, clinics, and private physicians have developed resource manuals or computerized lists of cancer-specific resources available in their area. Ideally these manuals and lists are developed after needs assessments are conducted based on the diagnoses, treatments, and other characteristics of the patients treated and after the cost, quality, and appropriateness of the services provided by agencies have been reviewed.[37]

Private practitioners may have to give one person the responsibility for making referrals, maintaining relationships with vendors, reviewing the quality and performance of vendors periodically, and updating the list of resources. Auditing, surveying, or interviewing patients who have been referred to such services is necessary to evaluate the service providers. Generally, the most practical way to monitor the quality of the service is through ongoing communication with the vendors of these services. Establishing ongoing relationships with vendors and institutions ensures that the needs of all are presented and that changes are effectively made and maintained.

NEED FOR FINANCIAL ASSISTANCE

Medical Insurance

Medical insurance coverage is usually obtained through an employer or the federally and state-funded programs of Medicaid and Medicare. Because an employer may discontinue an employee's health insurance if the employee goes on leave without pay for an extended period and because individual policies are expensive and difficult to obtain, patients should make every effort to pay for their work-related group policy rather than allow it to lapse. Unfortunately, even people who have been free of disease for many years may have difficulty obtaining new or additional coverage. The state insurance representative and religious, fraternal, or advocacy organizations such as the American Association of Retired Persons and the National Coalition of Cancer Survivors may be helpful in finding individual policies for patients who have lost their insurance coverage.

Those who cannot obtain group insurance through an employer may be able to purchase direct-payment insurance. For example, Blue Cross/Blue Shield offers open enrollment in 12 states and high-risk pools have been set up in 22 states. To find out about Blue Cross/Blue Shield enrollment, call the organization's Washington office (202-626-4827). In states that do not have open enrollment, information about high-risk insurance can be obtained by calling (612) 854-9005 in Minneapolis.

Medicaid is funded by both federal and state governments and pays the medical expenses of people receiving welfare and those who fall within the Social Security Administration's definition of disability. In most states, people who are disabled but whose income exceeds the financial eligibility standards for Supplemental Security Income (SSI) are still eligible for Medicaid benefits, especially if they owe large medical bills not covered by other insurance. In some hospitals, applications for Medicaid can be made through the hospital billing department; otherwise, the patient must apply at a local welfare or social services office.

Medicare is a federal health-insurance program for people 65 or older. Medicare insurance is also extended to people who have received Social Security disability benefits for 2 years. Patients with disabilities such as kidney failure are eligible for Medicare without a 2-year wait. Specific instructions for obtaining these benefits can be obtained from the local Social Security office or by calling 1-800-234-5772.

Because Medicare does not cover medical bills completely, recipients may want to buy a Medicare supplementary insurance policy (Medigap). If the patient is older than 65, the American Association of Retired Persons and Blue Cross/Blue Shield have several policies for people diagnosed with cancer. People younger than 65 should call their state insurance department and ask for the names of the companies that sell Medicare supplementary policies to people under 65 on Medicare.

The American Cancer Society (ACS), the Leukemia Society of America, and other local religious and philanthropic agencies provide financial assistance for equipment, home care, transportation, certain pharmacy costs, and prostheses. The Crippled Children's Fund, managed by state health departments and funded by the federal government, also pays for some costs such as hospitalization, surgery, and appliances for patients younger than 21. (For sources of medical insurance, see the Appendix.)

Income Support

Because an ongoing source of income is a major concern for patients once paid-leave benefits from an employer are exhausted, Social Security disability benefits should be applied for early, because processing of claims can be time-consuming. Patients are eligible if they have accumulated sufficient quarters of Social Security coverage in the recent past. Children also are eligible for Social Security insurance on the basis of diagnosis and family income. The telephone number for children is 1-800-342-3009. Although the availability of other assets is not considered in the determination of eligibility for this benefit, the disease must have existed for 6 months and must be expected to last for at least 1 year. Also, the patient must be unable to work. (The requirement that the disease has existed for 6 months is often met while the application is being processed.) Application forms and detailed information can be obtained from the local Social Security office.

Patients can apply for SSI at the same time they apply for Social Security disability benefits. SSI provides income to elderly and disabled patients with extremely limited income and few assets and thus involves a means test. The amount of income or assets allowable varies from state to state. The SSI program may provide patients with income while they wait for disability benefits, then may be terminated once disability benefits are obtained and their income exceeds the limit. Children who have cancer may be eligible for this benefit if their parents' income meets the eligibility requirement.

State-administered public assistance programs provide financial assistance of various kinds, but the assistance varies greatly from state to state and within different jurisdictions. Generally, however, a patient's income must be extremely limited to qualify for these programs (*i.e.*, the patient must be receiving Aid to Dependent Children, food stamps, or general emergency relief funds). Additional pension funds and income support may be available from the Veterans Administration and from religious and fraternal organizations with which the patient is affiliated.

NEED FOR HOME HEALTH-CARE SERVICES

Home care for cancer patients consists of a wide range of health and personal services and equipment to support optimum recovery, restore functioning, and enhance patients' and families' quality of life throughout the course of care. The basic components of home care include personal care, medical care, skilled nursing, supportive counseling, case management, physical therapy, occupational therapy, nutritional counseling, and homemaking services.

Because of the variety of personnel who provide home care to patients and the fact that the titles used to denote these personnel vary according to geographic region, professionals and patients alike are often confused about the functions performed by home health-care personnel. In general, home-care personnel can be categorized as nonprofessionals or professionals according to their level of skill and training. Nonprofessional home-care personnel will be categorized here as companions, housekeepers, homemakers, and home health aides. Professional personnel include registered nurses, licensed practical nurses, social workers, physical therapists, and occupational therapists.

A companion may have little or no specific training and may stay with a patient to either supervise or ensure the patient's safety because he or she is confused or demented, weak, or extremely anxious. A housekeeper is responsible only for maintaining the household by performing such tasks as grocery shopping, cooking, and cleaning. A homemaker usually takes care of children in addition to maintaining the household. A home health aide has some training in the essentials of patient care and helps patients with bathing, dressing, toileting, and mobility; reminds them to take medications; gets their prescriptions filled; accompanies them to medical appointments; and performs light, minimal housekeeping tasks directly related to patient care (*e.g.*, changes the bed).

Registered nurses and practical nurses are responsible for monitoring the patient, making ongoing assessments of the patient's medical status, communicating this information to the physician, giving medications, supervising nonprofessional home health-care personnel, and teaching the patient and family how to manage special medical equipment or devices such as oxygen tanks and Broviac catheters and how to care for wounds or stomas. The social worker visits the patient and family at home and provides psychosocial counseling about adjusting to cancer, the stress of caring for the patient, and the family's fears or anticipation of the patient's death. In addition, the worker often assists with case management of entitlements and home-care services provided or funded by various agencies with the care rendered by the referring physician or hospital; more than one agency is often involved.

Medical Indicators of Need

The medical indicators of the type and intensity of home health-care services that a patient needs vary considerably and should be determined by evaluating several factors simultaneously:

1. The symptoms of the disease as defined by type, site, and stage of cancer
2. The type of treatment required (surgery, radiation therapy, chemotherapy)
3. Whether the treatment will be given on an inpatient or outpatient basis
4. The patient's insurance and personal and family resources.

Differences in need can be assessed most clearly at the time of the initial treatment, during treatment for recurrent or metastatic disease, and during palliative treatment for terminal illness.

Recently diagnosed patients tend to be less symptomatic and more functional and therefore usually require short-term (if any) home health care focused on their recovery from the initial treatment. Because surgery and radiation therapy, unlike chemotherapy, are discrete and time-limited, the patients' functioning is either compromised to a limited degree or affected significantly only for the immediate period of recuperation. Thus, there is a realistic expectation of increased functioning as each day passes. However, although the physical functioning of these patients usually improves quickly, the psychological impact of permanent or altered body functioning can create major impediments to adjustment at most stages of illness. Counseling to help the patient cope with bodily changes such as sexual functioning, the ability to communicate, appearance, and ambulation can significantly facilitate adjustment at home. Furthermore, any procedure that is done in the hospital reduces the need for home care because the patient receives complete care in the hospital and thus recuperates to a great extent before returning home. As a result, home care consists of teaching the patient to care for a surgical wound or ostomy or to manage a prosthesis, helping maintain the household while the patient regains strength and stamina, and providing physical or occupational therapy or special equipment during the recuperation period.

Because patients with recurrent or metastatic disease are often more symptomatic, their treatment is often long-term or chronic rather than acute. Consequently, many of these patients need some form of home care, usually for an indefinite period. Patients receiving systemic chemotherapy, which can be debilitating, are especially in need of this type of care. Furthermore, chemotherapy is often given on an outpatient basis, which taxes the patient's already limited energy by requiring frequent trips to the hospital or oncologist's office and increased interactions with a complex medical system. These patients (and those who receive similarly fatiguing radiation therapy on an outpatient basis, especially if it requires many daily treatments) usually need home health care to manage the side effects of treatment and the activities of daily living.

For patients with metastatic disease who are in the terminal stage of disease and require palliative treatment, home health care is a primary issue. Can the patient be managed at home rather than in an inpatient setting, given the nearly total care he or she requires? Because arranging appropriate home care for terminally ill patients involves acknowledging and preparing for their death both practically and psychologically, it is emotionally stressful. At this stage of the illness, most patients require home care from outside agencies because of their poor functional status and the exhaustion of family members who have cared for them during earlier stages of disease.

The home health-care team for terminally ill patients usually includes—in addition to traditional professional and nonprofessional home health-care personnel—clergy, volunteers, and a physician or a specially trained nurse or nurse practitioner who makes house calls. Hospice programs, which often help families to maintain their dying members safely and comfortably at home, attempt to provide such comprehensive services. For these reasons, the planning of appropriate home care for terminally ill patients is a complex process in which the patient's and family's medical, practical, and psychosocial needs must be addressed.

Social and Behavioral Indicators of Need

Several social and behavioral characteristics can be important indicators of the need for home health care. One indicator is the family's or friends' commitment and ability to care for the patient. The home-care needs of most patients are met by family members; patients who live alone are more likely to require help from outside agencies. Even if a patient lives with his or her family or has relatives nearby, however, the degree of the relatives' involvement can vary greatly. The family members' availability and willingness to help usually is demonstrated by their presence or absence at medical visits and the degree to which they take an active role in discussing treatment, the symptoms and progress of the disease, medications, and the general care of the patient. A family's ability to provide care also depends on its economic status, especially on the type of employment, work schedules, and other family illnesses and responsibilities.

A second behavioral indicator is the patient's Karnofsky status and general appearance at medical appointments.[38]

Does the patient appear relatively well-groomed? Does the patient's personal hygiene seem adequate? Are wounds or special medical devices being properly cared for? Are there any signs of decubitus ulcers or other symptoms that indicate the patient may not be well cared for? Is the patient's nutritional status adequate? Because of emotional stress, a patient may not recognize the degree of need and thus may not mention a need for home-care services until the situation becomes severe. Thus, problems observed by the physician may be an earlier indication of need for such services.

A third, often subtle, indicator is a noticeable change in the patient's or family's communication with the treatment team. For example, an increased number of telephone calls about the patient's condition—especially if they occur after normal office hours—from a patient or family member who typically calls infrequently and during office hours is often a sign that the patient requires more help at home than is available. Similarly, reduced contact with the medical system, manifest by missed or canceled medical appointments, also may indicate that the patient feels too ill to make the visits without additional help or that family members can no longer help as much as before. Finally, patients who make an increased number of emergency visits, either at the hospital emergency room or in unscheduled office visits, may well be signaling that they are uncomfortable with the existing home-care plan. In this situation, the family members also may be indicating that they feel overwhelmed by the responsibility of managing the patient's medical and emotional needs at home. These changes can alert the physician to the possibility that the patient or family is indirectly requesting additional help.

Resources

Patients receiving in- or outpatient care from a hospital can ask the hospital's social work or discharge planning department for information about home-care services and referrals. These hospital-based professionals have special expertise in assessing and enhancing the problem-solving abilities of patients and families concerning the medical plan and can link patients and families with entitlements and health resources in the community that will provide the needed services.

Patients who are not being treated by a hospital system can turn to a community agency, a local unit of the ACS, the departments of social work or discharge planning at a local hospital, or the local Visiting Nurse Association office. The type of care that patients need and their ability to pay for it are two major factors in exploring home-care resources. Three basic types of agencies provide home-care services: nonprofit (voluntary) home-care agencies, proprietary (for-profit) home-care agencies, and government-based services.

The services of nonprofit agencies are reimbursed by Medicare, Medicaid, and insurance carriers. These agencies, which include the Visiting Nurse Association, often have a sliding scale of fees based on the patient's ability to pay. These agencies regulate their own eligibility criteria and referral procedures. For example, a patient referred to the Visiting Nurse Association must demonstrate the need for skilled nursing to activate other services such as a home health aide. Because these agencies differ geographically in the hours of service per week they will provide, a patient who needs a great deal of care may require a plan that coordinates the services of several different agencies, including a visiting nurse for skilled nursing care, Meals on Wheels for nutrition, and a home health aide for general care. Other services can be coordinated through hospital-based home-care agencies or a community-based hospice in many areas.

Proprietary home-care agencies are privately owned businesses that recruit, train, and supervise a full range of home health-care workers who are assigned to clients under their supervision. Some are local; others have a nationwide network of offices. These agencies are listed in the Yellow Pages under "Home Health Agencies." Although the agencies provide comprehensive services and equipment at home 24 hours a day, 7 days a week, they are expensive and thus accessible only to patients who have strong financial support or excellent insurance coverage for home care for chronic diseases. Only proprietary agencies that are certified by Medicare will be reimbursed (80%) by Medicare. To be eligible for this type of home care under Medicare, patients must meet the following criteria:

1. A physician must certify the need for services and develop a specified plan of treatment.
2. The patient needs skilled care from a nurse or other therapist (skilled nursing services are strictly defined and interpreted by governmental and insurance company guidelines).
3. The patient cannot leave the house without help from another person, special transportation, or the aid of equipment such as a cane or wheelchair.

NEED FOR ALTERNATIVES TO HOME CARE

Patients who need care in an extended-stay facility after acute care in the hospital usually have preterminal or terminal disease. The most common social reasons for long-term institutional care are the lack of available family members or the need for home services 24 hours a day but an inability to pay. The usual medical indications for extended care are the progressive nature of the disease, coupled with a regimen of care that the family cannot manage at home. The decision to use this form of care must be made jointly by the patient, the family, and the treatment team to ensure that family relationships and the integrity of the family unit are maintained.

Many communities have institutions that provide extended care for patients with chronic illnesses; in some instances, a floor or wing of a building may be designated for patients who need long-term care. Most extended-care institutions accept cancer patients, and a few are devoted exclusively to them. The institutions can be nonprofit, proprietary, or under public auspices. Proprietary nursing homes accommodate the largest number of patients in extended-care institutions. Institutions that seek reimbursement from Medicare must meet Social Security Administration standards.

Terminal or preterminal cancer patients, in particular, tend to exceed Medicare's limit of 100 days of extended care. If a patient's stay is likely to exceed 100 days, the family must be prepared to assume the continuing financial responsibility. To avoid interrupting a patient's care, many institutions, including some proprietary ones, make financial arrangements with families of limited means, such as helping them file an application for Medicaid.

NEED FOR TRANSPORTATION SERVICES

In areas where services are accessible, transportation is available to patients with certain degrees of need and the financial resources to pay for it. Because the first step in obtaining such services is an awareness of their existence and the ability to apply for them, a social worker or discharge planner should arrange for transportation. Researchers have found that disadvantaged patients are more likely to keep medical appointments if transportation is arranged for them.[39] Because transportation services vary greatly in quality, they must be monitored constantly to protect patients. Certainly, patients should be surveyed concerning the quality of services; however, the most effective way to provide safe, reliable, and comfortable transportation is through ongoing communication with vendors to sensitize them to cancer patients' specific needs and concerns.

Ambulances

An ambulance is indicated when the patient's physical or mental condition is so serious that transport is impossible by any other means; in other words, if patients cannot sit, if they experience intense pain when they move, or if they have other conditions that require rapid transport to a hospital in optimal comfort in a vehicle containing life-saving equipment such as intravenous poles and tubes, oxygen tanks, cardiac monitors, and suction devices.

Transport by ambulance is expensive and seldom is completely covered by insurance. Medicare usually pays up to 80% of the customary charges of a one-way trip. The cost of transferring patients to their home, a nursing home, or another hospital (if that hospital provides treatment that is unavailable at the first hospital) also is reimbursed. In all these cases, however, a hospital or physician must provide documentation of the need for the service. Medicaid usually pays the entire cost of transport by ambulance for situations similar to those partially covered by Medicare. Because the reimbursement policies of private and commercial insurance carriers vary greatly, reviewing the specific policy is essential. Social workers and discharge planners often can negotiate with the ambulance and insurance companies to arrange the best accommodations for all involved.

Social work departments in medical centers maintain lists of ambulance services and the names of people to contact to arrange them. Although the Yellow Pages also lists ambulances, determining the quality and reliability of these services is impossible. In an emergency, a local police emergency unit can be called; in New York City, the police transport emergency cases to the emergency room of the nearest municipal hospital free of charge.

Ambulettes

An ambulette is the transportation of choice for patients who cannot walk or climb stairs without assistance but who can sit in a wheelchair and do not require acute care while in transit. The most common medical and physical reasons for using an ambulette are physical or mental senility, orthopedic impairments, neuromuscular disorders, severe cardiac disease, and acute side effects from treatments.

Ambulette service usually costs about 25% less than an ambulance. Medicare does not cover this service. In most states, Medicaid does cover it, but the hospital or physician must document the need. Private and commercial carriers sometimes pay for this service. Although insurance carriers initially may refuse to pay for the service, social workers often can negotiate with them by pointing out the higher cost of an ambulance.

Van, Car, and Taxi Services

Van, car, and taxi services are indicated for patients who are visually, physically, or cognitively impaired; weakened by illness or treatment; or otherwise unable to use public transportation. These services tend to be much less expensive than ambulances and ambulettes, and they are more convenient than mass transportation because they provide door-to-door service. Medicare and private and commercial insurance carries do not pay for these services; Medicaid usually does. Because vans usually pick up several patients during the same trip, patients often are forced to wait and may become uncomfortable.

These services can be obtained through social work departments in medical centers, which maintain lists and sometimes have special relationships with vendors to ensure quality and provide reduced rates to patients who need financial help.

Rail Services

Some wheelchair-bound patients who must travel long distances prefer to go by train. Carriers must be notified 48 hours in advance to make appropriate arrangements. (A slide board is useful for transferring the patient easily to a regular seat.) The patient should have a reservation, which should be confirmed before the patient arrives at the station. Trains lack facilities for stretcher patients.

The cost of transporting a wheelchair-bound patient by train is the same as for ordinary passengers. Medicare and private and commercial insurance carriers usually do not pay for train travel; however, some Medicaid programs do under certain circumstances. Travel arrangements are usually made simply by calling the railroad's reservation desk.

Airlines

For wheelchair-bound, stretcher-bound, or acutely ill patients who must travel long distances, air travel is often the best solution. Although each airline has different regulations, most require a letter from a physician describing the patient's condition and stating that the patient can tolerate the trip. If the patient must spend the entire trip on a stretcher, most airlines must be notified 48 hours in advance.

Medicare and private and commercial insurance companies usually do not pay for air travel. In many states, however, Medicaid does if the circumstances are unusual. A wheelchair-bound patient who can be moved to a regular seat pays the same fare as any other passenger. Stretcher-bound patients, on the other hand, must pay for a first-class seat (which must be physically removed) plus a second- or third-class seat if they are accompanied by a nurse or by equipment such as an intravenous pole and pump.

To make appropriate arrangements, notify the airline in advance. In addition, contact the airline before the flight to ensure that the flight will leave at the scheduled time and that the airline has all the necessary information about the patient. The necessary documentation should remain with the patient at all times, and a member of the health-care team should be available by telephone until the plane actually departs.

Volunteer Services

Volunteer transportation services are often underused because people do not know how to find them. Ground transportation is obtained most easily, but its availability, degree of comfort, predictability, and reliability vary greatly, depending on the volunteers' resources and commitment. Free air travel also is available under certain circumstances.

To locate services, contacting the local chapter of the ACS is a good first step. Other sources of information include the Red Cross, volunteer police and fire departments, religious groups, local men's and women's groups, visiting or public health nurses, and hospital social work departments. In addition, many commercial vendors who serve hospitals will provide free services for specific patients when asked. Obtaining free services is often limited only by one's imagination and by gaining access to the people who control the services. To save time when seeking free service, always try to contact the person at the top of the system.

The Corporate Angel Network (914-328-1313) offers free air travel by corporate jets, primarily for cancer patients who can sit up and do not need life-sustaining equipment. The network also will transport as many as three additional people (*e.g.,* a family member, a bone-marrow donor, and so on), depending on the size of the aircraft. The patient's physician must provide clearance for the patient in writing. Similar service is offered by an air transportation network in Toronto and Missouri, in cooperation with the Canadian Cancer Society (416-924-9333). Patients, family members, or social workers can contact these services directly. Using them requires advance notice and flexibility.

NEED FOR COUNSELING SERVICES

Counseling can be provided by self-help groups and by professional counselors, either individually or in groups. Counseling can range in duration from a single session to long-term traditional psychotherapy.

Many patients are reluctant to request professional counseling or even a self-help group, despite overwhelming reactions to a cancer diagnosis. Some are psychologically immobilized and cannot exert the emotional energy needed to get help. Others view a request for support as reflecting an inability to cope, a loss of autonomy, or a sign of mental illness. Many are unaware that counseling can help assuage the existential terror evoked by a cancer diagnosis or can alleviate grief over the loss of body function or appearance. Ironically, these same patients may later resent not having received enough emotional support. Such patients are more likely to use counseling services if those services are presented as an acceptable adjunct to the medical treatment plan, are universally prescribed, and are easily available.[40]

Because of increased coverage in the lay press, however, counseling has become more acceptable to patients. Consequently, increasing numbers of them are requesting professional counseling or self-help groups to solve the psychological, social, and practical problems created by their disease and treatment. Spiegel and colleagues suggested that group support that enhances mental health also may slow progression of the disease.[41]

Self-Help Groups

The number of self-help groups for people with a chronic illness such as cancer has grown astronomically. A self-help group now exists for every major disease listed by the World Health Organization.[42] All these groups share the philosophy that people who have experienced a crisis can make a unique contribution to others who are undergoing the same experience.

Several mechanisms have been suggested to explain the appeal of self-help groups. First, because they have been through the same crisis (*i.e.,* they have "experiential knowledge"), "veterans" can provide new members with insight and understanding.[43] As Katz and associates said, sharing a central problem is what defines members of a self-help group.[44]

A second mechanism through which group members experience benefits is the destigmatization and normalization of conditions and problems. A third mechanism is the helper-therapy principle, which suggests that "helpers" may benefit more than recipients of help because their role as adviser increases their sense of interpersonal competence, they learn from those they help, they receive social approval for helping others, and their own success in coping is reinforced.[45] Because members of self-help groups are both givers and receivers of care, all can benefit. Another benefit of self-help groups is the modeling of successful recovery—a role that veteran patients, such as Reach to Recovery volunteers, consciously adopt to encourage members' successful adaptation.

Contacts with veteran patients are reported to be helpful to almost all patients in highlighting the normal and universal nature of their reactions and reducing their sense of isolation. Patients learn from other patients about different coping strategies that can be used to deal with the myriad stresses associated with the disease and its treatment.

Some groups are organized and run by mental-health professionals; others are organized and controlled by patients. Some sponsor intense, short-term sessions for several months and then disband. Others have ongoing programs that involve the same members and are closed to newcomers. Still others are always open to new members. In all cases, the underlying group mechanisms are the same: members help one another by sharing their problems, being role models of successful recovery, and destigmatizing the illness.

Self-help groups in a specific geographic area can be found by contacting the local office of the ACS or the Cancer Information Service (1-800-4-CANCER), the National Self-Help Clearinghouse (1-800-422-6237), the social work or nursing department at the local hospital, or community organizations such as family service agencies or private counseling groups.

Professional Counseling

Although patients rarely report adverse reactions to self-help groups, they may feel that such groups are insufficient to meet their need for emotional support. Therefore, when patients are emotionally overwhelmed by their disease and treatment, are in an acute psychological crisis, have specific individual problems, or need to deal with preexisting personal and interpersonal problems that have been exacerbated by disease, professional counseling is recommended.

In addition to the traditional individual and group counseling, some medical centers now offer specialized counseling for patients and families. Specialized counseling has been developed in response to research findings that have documented the prevalence of particular concerns among cancer patients:

1. Marital counseling for couples whose relationship has been damaged by the stresses of diagnosis and treatment
2. Sexual counseling, especially for people with tumors directly related to areas of the body associated with sexuality
3. Drug or alcohol abuse counseling for patients or family members who have problems with substance abuse that either existed before the cancer diagnosis or have been exacerbated by the diagnosis and treatment.

Patients who need professional counseling represent a continuum ranging from those who are seriously mentally ill to those who are psychosocially vulnerable to those who, although resilient and well supported, can benefit from some counseling. Indeed, some *must* receive counseling to maintain their functioning and prevent their social and emotional breakdown.

Cancer patients with a history of mental illness or psychiatric treatment generally have an ongoing relationship with several supportive services in the community that may need information about their medical condition. Such patients should be urged to contact their therapists or mental health counselors about their medical condition or to ask a social worker or other mental health professional to transmit information about their medical status and arrange for continued psychological treatment and care. Because a cancer diagnosis can exacerbate mental illness or seriously affect day-to-day functioning, early psychosocial intervention may prevent a breakdown of functioning that would have lasting negative effects on the quality of a mentally ill patient's life, such as loss of a job or alienation of friends and relatives. Therefore, a referral for counseling is essential for these patients.

A much larger group of patients are not mentally ill but have social and psychological characteristics that place them at risk of emotional and social breakdown when confronted with a cancer diagnosis. Such reactions may interfere with their daily functioning and compliance with treatment. These patients are likely to have one or more of the following characteristics:

1. They live alone and have few friends or relatives to help them.
2. They are older than 75.
3. They have dependent children.
4. They are financially stressed (lack medical insurance or have only limited insurance).
5. They are undergoing multiple stresses or have experienced severe stress in the past.
6. They are experiencing other life crises such as loss of a job or a divorce.
7. Their family has a history of violence or sexual abuse or drug and alcohol abuse.
8. They have multiple cancers or other diseases.
9. They have another family member who also is ill.
10. They have a history of cancer in the family.

Although such patients may be more difficult to identify, they will benefit by obtaining emotional support services.

Finally, patients who are resilient and psychologically strong and have numerous personal, social, practical, and financial resources tend to express their needs specifically and are grateful when help is provided. Unfortunately, however, professionals often overlook their psychological and support needs and view them as coping well. These patients usually make rapid and highly effective use of emotional support services to better meet their high standards for functioning and often resent not having access to counseling services. As one patient said, "I knew I could cope well with a cancer diagnosis and I did, but I might have coped better with some help and would have liked to have known about counseling that could have been available to me."

In hospitals, counseling services are typically provided by social workers, nurses, psychiatrists, psychologists, and chaplains. Some hospitals refer patients directly for counseling; others offer counseling as part of routine psychosocial assessments. Mental health professionals in private practice provide these therapies, as do many special agencies for cancer patients, such as some local chapters of the ACS, religious organizations, and other mental health and family service agencies. Counseling services also can be found by contacting the social work or psychiatric department in the local hospital or cancer center or by calling the local ACS office or another cancer or community agency.

APPENDIX

Resources and Services

FINANCIAL ASSISTANCE FOR INCOME SUPPORT

Social Security Administration. Social Security Disability Insurance (SSDI) makes monthly payments to patients who cannot work because of disease or treatment. Eligibility does not depend on assets or income. Supplemental Security Income (SSI) makes monthly payments to disabled people with extremely limited income and assets.

State Departments of Social Services. Aid for Dependent Children provides monthly support for children of disabled parents. General Relief provides cash assistance in short-term emergencies. Food Stamps provides coupons to purchase food.

Veterans Administration. The State Disability Benefits Office provides payments through employers.

FINANCIAL ASSISTANCE FOR TREATMENT

Insurance. State departments of insurance can provide information about private insurance carriers. Medicaid pays the expenses of disabled patients. Eligibility requirements include limited assets and income. Medicare pays the medical expenses of patients older than 64 and those who have received SSDI for 2 years. Coverage for outpatient treatment and care is limited.

Philanthropic Agencies. The ACS pays some of the costs of transportation, treatment, home care, and dressings. The Crippled Children's Program pays for approved hospitalizations, operations, and appliances. The Leukemia Society of America pays some of the costs for leukemia patients such as transportation, drugs, and radiation therapy in specific instances.

HOME HEALTH CARE

Hospital-based home-care programs provide home-care personnel, and hospital departments of social work and discharge planning provide information about local home-care resources.

The Visiting Nurse Association and public health nurses provide home-care personnel and information about local proprietary agencies and other resources. Their services are covered by most insurance carriers.

Private home-care agencies provide personnel and usually require private pay or major medical insurance to cover the services of registered nurses only. These agencies are listed in the Yellow Pages or are recommended by hospital departments of social work and discharge planning or local visiting nurse services.

The ACS pays some home health-care fees, and the Leukemia Society of America selectively provides home-care services.

Hospices provide coordinated home care for terminally ill patients by using visiting nurse services and volunteers. Insurance coverage for these services varies.

Meals on Wheels, which delivers meals to patients' homes, is administered by a range of local social service and religious agencies.

EQUIPMENT

Hospital-based home-care programs, surgical supply companies, and pharmacies provide medical equipment for the home.

ALTERNATIVES TO HOME CARE

Terminal care and cancer-specific chronic care facilities provide inpatient care for terminally ill patients. Nursing homes provide chronic and terminal care of patients who cannot be cared for at home. Veterans Administration hospitals provide residential placement for veterans.

TRANSPORTATION

Private transportation companies provide ambulance, ambulette, taxi, van, or car transportation. See listings in the Yellow Pages.

The ACS provides transportation or money for transportation to the treatment center.

The American Red Cross provides free transportation to and from treatment centers when volunteers are available.

The Corporate Angel Network provides free air transport on corporate aircraft from home to the treatment center when flights are available. These flights are for ambulatory patients only.

Hospital transportation services arrange transportation to and from the hospital and, in some situations, provide funding for transportation.

The Leukemia Society of America provides some money for transportation to the treatment center.

Local religious organizations provide a range of vans and car services for members of their religious community.

Local volunteer ambulance and fire departments often provide free transportation to and from treatment centers when volunteers are available.

EMOTIONAL SUPPORT AND PLANNING SERVICES

The ACS sponsors the following self-help groups:

- Candlelighters: emotional support and information for parents of children with cancer
- CanSurmount: emotional support and information for patients with various cancer diagnoses
- International Association of Laryngectomees: emotional support and information to patients having their larynx removed
- Reach to Recovery: emotional support, exercises, and temporary prostheses for women undergoing mastectomy
- United Ostomy Association: emotional support, information, and advice to ostomy patients

Family service agencies provide information, practical help, emotional support, and psychological and behavioral therapies.

Hospital social work, psychiatric, nursing, and pastoral staff provide information, emotional support, and psychological and behavioral therapies.

Make Today Count provides group and individual emotional support and problem-solving for cancer patients with all diagnoses.

The National Coalition of Cancer Survivors is a clearinghouse for publications, self-help organizations of cancer survivors, and a resource for political advocacy.

The National Self-Help Clearinghouse provides information about self-help groups throughout the country.

Pastoral care and religious agencies provide emotional support and spiritual guidance.

Private practitioners provide emotional support and psychological and behavioral therapies.

EDUCATION AND INFORMATION

The ACS is a source of information about prevention, treatment, services, and rehabilitation.

The Breast Cancer Advisory Center provides medical advice to newly diagnosed breast cancer patients, makes referrals, and disseminates information.

The National Cancer Institute sponsors two services: the Cancer Information Service, a free nationwide telephone information service, and the National Cancer Information Clearinghouse, a source of indexes, abstracts, information, and free searches of resources.

AGENCIES AND ORGANIZATIONS

American Cancer Society. A voluntary organization that offers programs of cancer research and education and patient services and rehabilitation. Address: National Headquarters, 3340 Peachtree Road NE, Atlanta, GA 30326; (404) 329-7625

American Red Cross. Provides free transportation when volunteers are available. Address: National Headquarters, Washington, DC 20006; (202) 737-8300

Breast Cancer Advisory Center. Provides medical advice to breast cancer patients, makes referrals, disseminates information, gives lectures, and maintains a library of materials on breast cancer. Address: 11426 Rockville Pike, Suite 406, Rockville, MD 20859; (301) 984-1020

Cancer Information Service. A free, confidential, nationwide telephone information service sponsored by the National Cancer Institute that provides current, reliable information on research about cancer, local sources of cancer care, and free publications on a variety of subjects. The toll-free number 1-800-4-CANCER automatically connects callers to the Cancer Information Service serving their area. New York business number for professionals: (212) 794-7984

Candlelighters. An international organization that provides emotional support to parents of children with cancer. Address: National Headquarters, 2025 I (Eye) Street NW, Suite 1011, Washington, DC 20006; (202) 659-5136

Compassionate Friends, Inc. A self-help group that offers friendship and understanding to bereaved parents. Its primary goals are to aid parents in the positive resolution of grief experienced after a child's death and to foster the physical and emotional health of bereaved parents and siblings. Address: P.O. Box 1347, Oak Brook, IL 60521; (312) 323-5010

Concern for Dying. A nonprofit educational council dedicated to the belief in each person's right to participate in treatment decisions made during terminal illness. It offers counseling and information on death, dying, and burial, and provides copies of the living will. Address: 250 West 57th Street, New York, NY 10019; (212) 246-6962

Corporate Angels Network. Provides free air transportation on corporate planes *from* home *to* the treatment center when flights are available. Address: Westchester County Airport Building, White Plains, NY 10604; (914) 328-1313

Crippled Children's Program. Listed under Bureau of Handicapped Children in the telephone directory.

Hodgkin's Disease and Lymphoma Organization. Provides information and emotional support for patients with Hodgkin's disease and their families. Address: 518 Wingate Drive, East Meadow, NY 11154; (516) 999-6813

International Association for Enterostomal Therapy. Organizes enterostomal therapy nurses to promote education of patients, nurses, physicians, and other allied health professionals for rehabilitation of patients with abdominal stomas, fistulas, draining wounds, incontinence, and pressure sores. Address: 505 A Tustan Avenue, Suite 282, Santa Ana, CA 92705; (714) 972-1725

International Association of Laryngectomees. A voluntary organization of 286 member clubs that coordinates the activities of local laryngectomee clubs, which provide mutual support and encourage total rehabilitation. Address: 777 Third Avenue, New York, NY 10017; (212) 371-2900

Leukemia Society of America, Inc. A national voluntary health agency, supported primarily by donations from the public, that seeks to control and eradicate leukemia, Hodgkin's disease, and lymphomas. It supports a three-pronged program of research, patient aid, and public and professional education. Address: National Headquarters, 800 Second Avenue, New York, NY 10017; (212) 573-8584

Make-a-Wish Foundation of America. Grants the special wishes of seriously or terminally ill children, and consists of a network of 50 chapters. Located in Phoenix, AZ; (602) 234-0960

National Cancer Information Clearinghouse. Facilitates the exchange of information on public and patient educational materials; indexes, abstracts, and stores information received from people and organizations; and provides free searches of resources. Address: Office of Cancer Communication, National Cancer Institute, 9000 Rockville Pike, Bethesda, MD 20205; (800) 422-6237

National Home Caring Council. Provides a quick reference to all homemaker/home health aide services across the United States, including those it accredits. Address: 235 Park Avenue South, New York, NY 10003; (202) 547-6586

National Hospice Organization. A nonprofit, privately funded association of health professionals that promotes better, more appropriate care for terminally ill patients and ensures hospice care at the highest level. Publishes a quarterly newsletter, locator directory, and several reports. Address: 1909 North Fort Myer Drive, Suite 307, Arlington, VA 22209; (703) 243-5900

National League for Nursing. Provides a list of visiting nurse organizations in local areas. Address: American Public Health Association, 10 Columbus Circle, New York, NY 10019; (212) 582-1022

National Self-Help Clearinghouse. Provides information about self-help groups in specific communities and places patients in contact with one of 27 regional clearinghouses, which may be available to provide help in organizing self-help groups. Address: Graduate School and University Center, City University of New York, 33 West 43 Street, New York, NY 10036

Starlight Foundation. Grants the special wishes of terminally, chronically, and critically ill children. Address: 9021 Melrose Avenue, Suite 204, Los Angeles, CA 90069; (213) 205-0631

United Ostomy Association, Inc. A nonprofit service agency organized and run by ostomates that helps ostomy patients return to normal living through mutual aid and moral support by educating patients and the public about ostomy, contributing to improvement of ostomy equipment and supplies, and publishing the *Ostomy Quarterly* and educational literature for patients, the public, and professionals. At present, more than 500 local chapters exist through the United States and Canada. Address: 2001 W. Beverly Blvd., Los Angeles, CA 90057; (213) 481-2811

REFERENCES

1. Grobe ME, Ahmann DL, Ilstrup DM, et al. Assessment of the needs of cancer patients undergoing active anticancer therapy and the needs of their family members. Am Soc Clin Oncol 1983;2:61.
2. Houts PS, Yasko JM, Kahn B, et al. Unmet psychological, social and economic needs of persons with cancer in Pennsylvania. Cancer 1986;58:2355–2361.
3. Mor V, Guadagnoli E, Wool M. An examination of the concrete service needs of advanced cancer patients. J Psychosoc Oncol 1987;5:1–17.
4. Hermann, JF, Wojkowiak SL, Houts PS, Kahn SB. Helping people cope: A guide for families facing cancer. Harrisburg: Pennsylvania Department of Health, 1988.
5. Googe MC, Varricchio CG. A pilot investigation of home health-care needs of cancer patients and their families. Oncol Nurs Forum 1981;8:24–28.
6. Parsons J. A descriptive study of intermediate stage terminally ill cancer patients at home. Nurs Dig 1977;5:1–26.
7. Grobe ME, Ahmann DL, Alstrup DM. Needs assessment for cancer patients and their families. Oncol Nurs Forum 1982;9:26–30.
8. Putnam ST, McDonald MM, Miller MM, et al. Home as a place to die. Am J Nurs 1980;80:1451–1453.
9. Gold M. Life support: Families speak about hospital, hospice, and home care for the fatally ill. Mount Vernon, NY: Consumers Union Foundation, Institute for Consumer Policy Research, 1983.
10. Greer DS, Mor V, Morris JN, et al. An alternative in terminal care: Results of the National Hospice Study. J Chron Dis 1985;39:9–26.
11. Houts PS, Yasko JM, Harvey HA, et al. Unmet needs of persons with cancer in Pennsylvania during the period of terminal care. Cancer 1988;62:627–634.
12. Guadagnoli E, Mor V. Daily living needs of cancer outpatients. J Commun Health 1991;16: 37–47.
13. Siegel K. Continuing care of cancer patients—concrete needs: Progress report. New York: Memorial Sloan-Kettering Cancer Center, 1987.
14. Christ GH, Siegel K. Monitoring the quality-of-life needs of cancer patients. Cancer 1990;65:760–765.
15. Siegel K, Raveis VH, Houts P, et al. Caregiver burden and unmet patient needs. Cancer 1991;68:1131–1140.
16. Edstrom S, Miller MW. Preparing the family to care for the cancer patient at home: A home-care course. Cancer Nurs 1981;4:53.
17. Rose MA. Problems families face in home care. Am J Nurs 1976;76:416–418.
18. Dwyer JE, Held DM. Home management of the adult patient with leukemia. Nurs Clin North Am 1982;17:666–675.
19. Lurie A. The social work advocacy role in discharge planning. Soc Work Health Care 1982;8:75–85.
20. Bennet C. Testing the value of written information from patients and families in discharge planning. Soc Work Health Care 1984;9:95–100.
21. Guadagnoli E, Rice C, Mor V. Cancer patients' knowledge of and willingness to use agency-based services: Toward application of a model of behavioral change. J Psychosoc Oncol 1991;9(3):1–21.
22. Wool MS, Guadagnoli E, Thomas M, et al. Negotiating concrete needs: Short-term training for high-risk cancer patients. Health Soc Work 1989;14:184–195.
23. Polinsky ML, Fred C, Ganz PA. Quantitative and qualitative assessment of a case management program for cancer patients. Health Soc Work 1991;16:176–183.
24. Siegel K, Mesagno FP, Karus DG, et al. Reducing the prevalence of unmet needs for concrete services of patients with cancer. Cancer 1992;69:1813–1883.
25. Barg FK, McCorkle R, Jepson R, et al. A statewide plan to address unmet psychosocial needs of patients with cancer. J Psychosoc Oncol 1991;10(3).
26. Siegel K, Christ GH. Psychosocial consequences of long-term survivorship. In: Redman J, Lacher M, eds. Hodgkin's disease: Consequences of survival. Philadelphia: Lea & Febiger, 1989.
27. Vincenzino JV. Trends in medical care costs. Statistical Bulletin 1990;28–35.
28. Jessee WF, Doyle BJ. Discharge planning: Using audit to identify areas that need improvement. Quality Rev Bull 1979;5:25–29.
29. Hunter G, Johnson SH. Physical support systems for the homebound oncology patient. Oncol Nurs Forum 1980;7:21–23.
30. Shragen J, Halman M, Myers D, et al. Impediments to the cause and effectiveness of discharge planning. Soc Work Health Care 1978;4:65–80.
31. Wellisch DK, Fawzy FI, Landsverk J, et al. Evaluation of psychosocial problems of the homebound cancer patient: The relationship of disease and the sociodemographic variables of patients to family problems. J Psychosoc Oncol 1983;1(3):1–15.

32. Amado A, Cronk BA, Mileo R. Cost of terminal care: Home hospice versus hospital. Nurs Outlook 1979;27:522–526.
33. Cassileth BR, Donovan JA. History and implications of the new legislation. J Psychosoc Oncol 1983;1(1):59–69.
34. Marker WM, Simon VG. The hospice concept. Cancer 1978;28:225–237.
35. Rosenbaum EH, Rosenbaum DR. Principles of home care for the patient with advanced cancer. JAMA 1980;244:1484–1489.
36. Lindenberg RE, Coulton C. Planning for post-hospital care: A follow-up study. Health Soc Work 1980;5:45–50.
37. Polinsky ML, Ganz PA, Rofessart-O'Berry J, et al. Developing a comprehensive network of rehabilitation resources for referral of cancer patients. J Psychosoc Oncol 1987;5: 1–10.
38. Mor V, Laliberte L, Morris JN, et al. The Karnofsky Performance Status Scale: An examination of its reliability and validity in a research setting. Cancer 1984;53:2002–2007.
39. Bryan JL, Greger HA, Miller ME, et al. An evaluation of the transportation needs of disadvantaged cancer patients. J Psychosoc Oncol 1991;9(3):23–36.
40. Christ GH, Bowles ME, Kleban R, et al. Educational and support programs for breast-cancer patients and their families. In: Harris JR, Hellman S, Henderson C, eds. Breast diseases, 2d ed. Philadelphia: JB Lippincott, 1991:866–871.
41. Spiegel D, Kramer H, Bloom JR, et al. Effect of psychosocial treatment on survival of patients with metastatic breast cancer. Lancet 1989;2:888–891.
42. Gussow Z, Tracey GS. The role of self-help clubs in adaptation to chronic illness and disability. Soc Sci Med 1978;10:407.
43. Borkman T. A cross-national comparison of stutterers' self-help organizations. Speech Ther J 1974;29:6.
44. Katz S, Hedrick S, Henderson N. The measurement of long-term needs and impact. Health Med Care Serv Rev 1979;2:2–21.
45. Riessman F. The helper therapy principle. Soc Work 1965;10:27.

Cancer: Principles & Practice of Oncology, Fourth Edition,
edited by Vincent T. DeVita, Jr., Samuel Hellman, Steven A. Rosenberg.
J.B. Lippincott Co., Philadelphia © 1993.

John J. Mulvihill

CHAPTER **65**

Genetic Counseling of the Cancer Patient

Genetic counseling is a communication process that deals with the human problems associated with the occurrence or the risk of occurrence of a genetic disorder in a family. This process involves an attempt by one or more appropriately trained persons to help the individual or family: (1) comprehend the medical facts, including the diagnosis, the probable course of the disorder, and the available management; (2) appreciate the way heredity contributes to the disorder and the risk of recurrence in specified relatives; (3) understand the options for dealing with the risk of recurrence; (4) choose the course of action that seems appropriate to them in view of their risk and their family goals and act in accordance with that decision; and, (5) make the best possible adjustment to the disorder in an affected family member or to the risk of recurrence of that disorder.[1]

At the level of the cell, cancer is a genetic disorder, and it is appropriate that the total care of every patient with cancer includes attention to all five elements of genetic counseling. The definition emphasizes that genetic counseling is not a one-time event but rather an ongoing process of communication with the patient and his or her family. Such communication is a task for all clinicians and not exclusively for geneticists. One practical result of genetic counseling is addressing an inevitable question that most patients have but that some clinicians may not have time to consider in the midst of making a diagnosis and devising optimal therapy: "Why me?" This point was made in the ground-breaking book by cancer patient and advocate, Rose Kushner.[2] The answer is often unknown, but sometimes a patient's erroneous notions can be corrected with current evidence. In any case, it seems useful to offer the patient and relatives an opportunity to explore the known or perceived causes of his or her cancer; sometimes they are conspicuously genetic.

In practice, the need for formal genetic counseling of cancer patients may arise in three settings: at the time of diagnosis, to address questions of etiology; at the time of therapy, to address issues of reproduction and possible teratogenicity; and after survival has been achieved, to address the possibility of recurrence, risk in family members, and reproductive issues.

COUNSELING ABOUT GENETIC CAUSES OF CANCER

Genetics plays a role in the development of most human cancers. Four questions about the cancer patient may be posed to screen for the likelihood of genetic origins of the cancer:

1. Did the patient have a prior cancer, tumor, or growth?
2. Are there birth defects, dysmorphic features, or precursor lesions found on examination or by history?
3. Is there any clue in the pathology or description of the primary tumor that may suggest genetic origins?
4. Does any family member have cancer or a preneoplastic syndrome?

There are many features that suggest a person has a cancer of genetic origins and should be considered for more formal genetic counseling than usual (Table 65–1).[3–5] Some factors are suggested only by case series, and some are rigorously proved by analytic epidemiologic and prospective studies.

The criteria may identify persons or relatives at high risk for cancer because of genetic, congenital, or familial factors. The explanation may lie in a cytogenetic defect, a mendelian

TABLE 65–1. Identifying Patients and Families for Possible Genetic Counseling

Criterion	*Example*
Patients With a Cancer That Has One of These Features	
Bilateral, as separate primary neoplasms	Both kidneys, both breasts
Multifocal, within one organ	Multicentric colorectal cancers
An additional primary malignancy	Endometrial after colon cancer
At an atypical age	Breast cancer before 40 years
At an atypical site	Osteosarcoma of the mid-humerus
In the sex not usually affected	Breast cancer in a male
Associated with birth defects	Wilms' tumor with aniridia
Associated with a mendelian trait	Sarcoma in neurofibromatosis 1
Associated with a precursor lesion	Melanoma in dysplastic nevus syndrome
Associated with a rare disease	Lymphoma in immunodeficiency
A rare or unusual tumor type	Pheochromocytoma, sarcoma
Families With	
One first-degree relative* with a cancer with any of the above features	Siblings and children of a person with pheochromocytoma or melanoma arising in a dysplastic nevus.
Two first-degree relatives* with *any* cancer	Parents and siblings of a boy with sarcoma and his sister with brain tumor

* Brother, sister, parent, or child.
(Parry DM, Berg K, Mulvihill JJ, et al. Strategies for controlling cancer through genetics: Report of a workshop. Am J Hum Genet 1987;41:63–69; Parry DM, Mulvihill JJ, Miller RW, et al. Strategies for controlling cancer through genetics. Cancer Res 1987;47:1814–1817; Mulvihill JJ. Prospects for cancer control and prevention through genetics. Clin Genet 1989;36:313–319)

single-gene trait, in multifactorial inheritance or familial clustering, or even in environmental catalysts.

CHROMOSOMES AND SINGLE-GENE TRAITS

Every cancer probably has abnormal chromosomes, but they are usually acquired and doe not occur in every body cell.

Cancer can be a complication of a recognized syndrome of multiple malformations that has underlying constitutional chromosomal defects.[6] Such cytogenetic syndromes include Down's syndrome (trisomy 21) with various acute leukemias and perhaps testicular cancer; Klinefelter's syndrome (47,XXY) with nongonadal germ cell tumors and breast cancer; gonadal dysgenesis, including the full Turner's syndrome (if some Y chromosome material is present), with gonadoblastoma; trisomy 8 with preleukemia; the Miller syndrome of aniridia with Wilms' tumor and a deletion of 11q13; retinoblastoma with or without birth defects and a deletion of 13q14; and the fragile X syndrome with unusual cancers, including testicular cancer.[7]

Rare familial aggregations of specific cancers have been explained by constitutional translocations: t(3;8) in one family with renal cell carcinoma, an insertion of 11p13 into chromosome 2q32 with familial Wilms' tumor, an insertion of 13q14 into 3p12 with familial retinoblastoma, and a t(14;22) with familial meningioma.[8–11] Recognition of these rare families provides excellent opportunities for clinicians to make presymptomatic or prenatal diagnoses by vigorous identification and screening of persons at high risk. These families also present research opportunities for cancer biologists.

The ninth edition of *Mendelian Inheritance in Man* enumerates 2636 definite single-gene traits and 2281 others with suggestive but inconclusive evidence of mendelian inheritance behavior.[12] Of the 4917 traits, 338 conditions (in addition to 56 protooncogenes) have neoplasia as the sole feature, a frequent concomitant, or a rare complication.[13] The inference can be drawn that some 9% of known human genes influence the expression or suppression of neoplasia. Because these disorders have known or likely patterns of mendelian inheritance (*i.e.*, autosomal dominant, autosomal recessive, or X-linked inheritance), it is a simple matter to quote recurrence risks and offer counseling to a patient with a cancer that arose because of one of these mutant genes.

FAMILIAL AGGREGATION

As suggested in Table 65–1, no firm definition of a cancer family is available, and only empiric guidelines can be offered. Because 1 of every 4 Americans develops cancer, most persons have some relatives with cancer, and some, by chance, have many. In two clinical surveys, 6% of persons with cancer said they had three or more first-degree relatives with cancer.[14,15] Half of the cancer patients said they had no first-degree relative with cancer, about 30% said one, and 12% said two. The accuracy of a patient's report of cancer among relatives has been independently validated with medical records. The primary site of cancer was correct in 83% of first-degree, 67% of second-degree, and 60% of third-degree relatives.[16]

A working definition of familial cancer depends on the type and site of cancer, the age at diagnosis, the sex, the number of tumors, and the absolute numbers of affected relatives. It may be chance when 2 of 8 elderly sisters have breast cancer.

It would be unusual if both sisters were premenopausal or had bilateral disease. If brothers of any age had breast cancer, intuition recognizes a significant familial aggregation.

There are many reports of familial recurrences of exactly the same cancer, such as cancer of the breast, colorectum, ovary, or lung. Occasionally, closely related tumor types aggregate in relatives, such as squamous carcinomas of the lung and larynx or adenocarcinomas of the breast and ovary. The same pair of tumor types that cluster to excess in families also tend to occur as multiple primary neoplasms in one person. Of course, family members share many environmental factors, and there are clear instances of familial cancer due to environmental exposures, such as familial lung cancer and mesothelioma due to exposure to asbestos brought into the home on work clothes.[17]

At least two distinct patterns occur repeatedly enough to have gained the label of "cancer family syndrome." Many other patterns of familial cancer probably await delineation. One is the *cancer family syndrome of Lynch,* which is characterized by two or more generations with cancer of the colon and endometrium (and sometimes ovaries and breast) with diagnosis at an early age and with an excess of persons with multiple primary cancers.[18] Alternate names for the disorder are Lynch syndrome 2 or hereditary nonpolypotic colonic cancer, type 2; Lynch syndrome 1 is the term reserved for familial aggregation of colon cancers without polyposis or other cancers (*i.e.*, site-specific familial colon cancer). It is not clear that either Lynch syndrome is inherited as a simple single-gene trait.

The second distinct pattern is the *Li-Fraumeni cancer family syndrome* or *SBLA syndrome,* an acronym for the tumor types seen to excess: *s*arcomas; *b*reast, *b*one, and *b*rain tumors; *l*ung cancer, *l*aryngeal cancer, and *l*eukemia; and *a*drenal cortical neoplasia.[19] Constitutional mutations of the gene *p53* on chromosome 17p have been documented, and the predisposition to the syndrome is clearly a mendelian dominant trait with high penetrance.[20]

CLINICAL RECOMMENDATIONS

Identifying persons at high risk of cancer because of cytogenetic, mendelian, or familial determinants can lead to effective cancer screening and prevention through proper genetic counseling (see Table 65–1).[3–5] It is a persistent misperception that nothing can be done to manage genetic disease; in fact, the routes to prevention are numerous. Those at high risk for cancer may be enrolled in screening programs. Prenatal diagnosis can be offered for certain cytogenetic and mendelian predispositions to cancers. Patients with one cancer can be specifically screened for possible additional neoplasms. Prophylactic surgery may remove the target organ and prevent an inevitable cancer.[21] For example, prophylactic colectomy is done for patients with a polyposis syndrome or those at risk for familial colon cancer; gonadectomy is performed for cryptorchism, familial ovarian cancer, or gonadal dysgenesis; mastectomy is performed for familial breast cancer; and thyroidectomy is done for persons with the multiple mucosal neuroma syndrome. Interrupting gene-environmental interactions may prevent cancer by limiting environmental exposures in especially susceptible persons (*e.g.*, use of sunscreen, sun avoidance, chemoprevention in patients with xeroderma pigmentosum or albinism).

To offer genetic counseling to a person with or at high risk of developing cancer, the physician or counselor must first collect and interpret the family and personal medical histories, recognize any preneoplastic syndromes, assess the risk, begin counseling, and follow through with medical surveillance and perhaps prophylactic surgery.

Strategies for cancer prevention or for cancer genetics clinics, modeled after the practice of clinical genetics, have been advanced.[3–5,22–29] Disease-specific registries have expedited research and advanced preventive management (*e.g.*, syndromes of colorectal polyposis reported to the Immunodeficiency–Cancer Registry, NCI's research efforts on the Li-Fraumeni cancer family and dysplastic nevus syndromes).[19,30–33] Population-based registries of cancer families are underway in Iceland, Israel, and Utah, but only the latter seems to provide active prevention, probably because so many clinical studies are being conducted.[34–36] An innovative approach to identifying potential cancer families has been demonstrated in Utah and Texas.[37] In required health education classes, high school students complete a systematic medical family history. From 1980 through 1986, 24,332 family trees were collected at an estimated direct cost of $8.30 each; 1.7% were considered cancer-prone families.

The published experience indicates that the cancer prevention clinic serves mostly self-referred women who are concerned about a family history of breast cancer. Intake is done by a nurse or genetic counselor and usually includes family and medical histories for the consultant to complete. Medical records are sought to confirm reported diagnoses. In the University of Wisconsin model, a 3-hour clinic session is held in three parts: preview and general cancer prevention counseling (including a 16-minute videotape) by a social worker; instruction on disease-specific prevention and early detection by a health educator; and a review of family history and other risk factors leading to a specific age-adjusted risk assessment.[24] The Creighton University model (Fig. 65–1) emphasizes the research opportunities and the need for long-term follow-up with families.[23]

In the ideal situation, the genetic counseling of a person with an unusual personal or family history of cancer should include the following:

1. Review of the patient's family history for evidence of a preneoplastic syndrome or constellation of cancers that is considered to have a genetic etiology;
2. Review of the patient's environmental history for evidence of any unusual occupational, demographic, or medical exposures that may lead to cancer in a genetically susceptible person;
3. Review of the patient's medical history for evidence of a genetic condition predisposing to malignancy;
4. Clinical examination searching for dysmorphic features, congenital anomalies, abnormal cutaneous manifestations, or other abnormal findings that could form the basis for a syndromic diagnosis; and
5. Studies (*e.g.*, radiographs, peripheral blood karyotype) to confirm or rule out specific diagnoses.

If a single-gene disorder or chromosomal syndrome predisposing to cancer is diagnosed, the clinician can provide

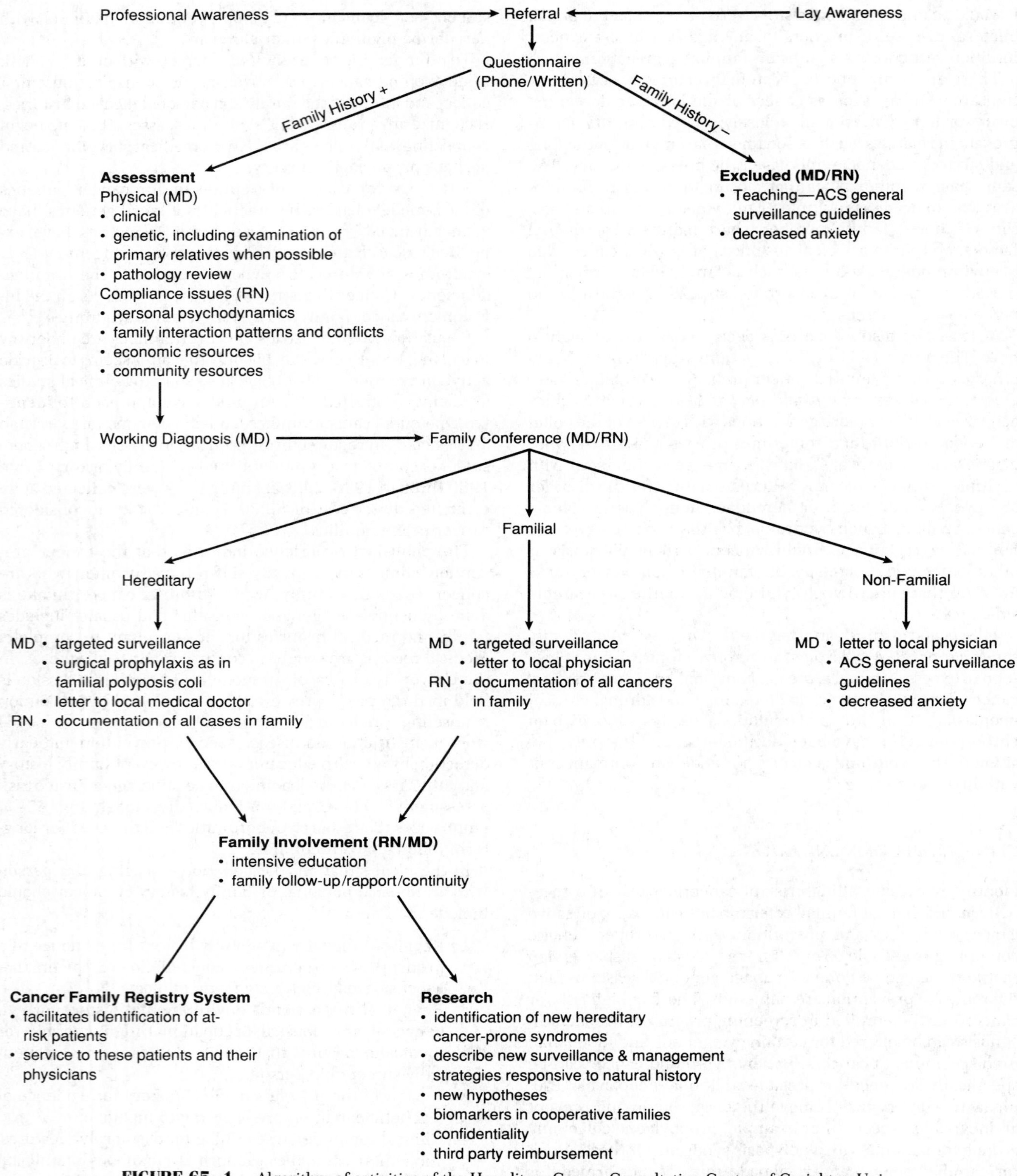

FIGURE 65–1. Algorithm of activities of the Hereditary Cancer Consultation Center of Creighton University. (Lynch HT, Fitzsimmons ML, Lynch J, et al. A hereditary cancer consultation clinic. Nebraska Med J 1989;74:351–359)

information on prognosis, offer appropriate genetic counseling, and recommend medical surveillance for the patient and at-risk family members with the intention of detecting early any further complications of the underlying condition, including cancer. For an increasing number of genetic disorders with neoplastic manifestations, it is becoming possible to identify affected fetuses or asymptomatic gene carriers in the family through the use of DNA tests (*e.g.*, for retinoblastoma, neurofibromatosis 1, Fanconi's anemia).

EMPIRIC RISK COUNSELING

For most patients, it is not possible to diagnose a specific cytogenetic or mendelian disorder. A counselor experienced in evaluating cancer families can sometimes offer empiric-risk estimates for future disease. In general, if a person develops a cancer, first-degree relatives (*i.e.*, parents, children, brothers, sisters) have a threefold risk of developing the same type of cancer. Until specific genes are found for common adult cancers, efforts are beginning to refine gross risk estimates by modifying them with information on other risk factors, calculating individual probabilities of disease, and discussing management options.

Breast Cancer Risk Counseling

One attempt to combine information on risk factors for breast cancer used age at menarche, age at first full-term livebirth, number of previous biopsies, and number of first-degree relatives with breast cancer.[38] A model of relative risks for various combinations of these factors was developed from case-control data from the Breast Cancer Detection Demonstration Project (Table 65–2). The baseline age-specific hazard rate (*i.e.*, rate for a patient without identified risk factors) was computed as the product of the observed age-specific composite hazard rate times the quantity 1 minus the attributable risk. The individualized breast cancer probabilities were calculated from information on relative risks and the baseline hazard rate. The resulting percentages, best applied to women undergoing regular mammography, are point estimates of the absolute probability of a woman's developing breast cancer in 10, 20, or 30 years after counseling (Table 65–3). This approach to individualizing the probability of developing breast cancer is used in the clinical research trial of tamoxifen as a way to prevent new clinical breast cancers.[39]

Another strategy for individualizing breast cancer risks assumes a genetic model of breast cancer predisposition that involves a rare dominant gene.[26,40] The counselor can offer calculated probabilities based on that model and on the specific pattern of affected relatives and their ages at diagnosis. This strategy has the disadvantage of ignoring other individual risk factors and assuming a genetic model for every familial case. (Familial does not always mean genetic.) Regardless of the method used to estimate risk, it is hoped that hearing a quantitative estimate of risk in a clinical setting may motivate women at high risk to undertake scrupulous surveillance. Some women have undergone prophylactic mastectomy, a controversial procedure that may be indicated for some women especially fearful of developing breast cancer.[41] If considered at all, proper counseling should precede a decision to operate.[42–44]

TABLE 65–2. Relative Risks for Selected Risk Factors

Risk Factor		*Relative Risk*
Age at menarche (y)		
≥14		1.00
12–13		1.10
<12		1.21
Number of breast biopsies		
Age <50 y		
0		1.00
1		1.70
≥2		2.88
Age ≥ 50 y		
0		1.00
1		1.27
≥2		1.62
Age at first term livebirth (y)	Number of first-degree relatives with breast cancer	
<20	0	1.00
	1	2.61
	≥2	6.80
20–24	0	1.24
	1	2.68
	≥2	5.78
25–29 or nulliparous	0	1.55
	1	2.76
	≥2	4.91
≥30	0	1.93
	1	2.83
	≥2	4.17

(Gail MH, Brinton LA, Byar DP, et al. Projecting individualized probabilities of developing breast cancer for white females who are being examined annually. JNCI 1989;81:1879–1886)

Follow-up studies of women counseled about their high risk of cancer revealed a low percentage who complied with the complete recommendation for surveillance.[41,45] One study showed only 40% performed monthly breast self-examination, and 69% went for clinic examinations; a surprising 94% had regular mammography.[45] The behavior seemed to reflect psychological distress from high anxiety. A small study found participation in a cancer prevention clinic correlated with prior involvement in cancer prevention activities, interest in cancer-specific information, and perceived risk level.[46]

Other Cancers

Table 65–4 summarizes familial recurrence risk estimates for several common sites of cancers. These common cancers are infrequently due to a single-gene trait inherited as a dominant or recessive trait, but more often, they have a low risk of recurrence. For the many people with no identifiable genetic determinants, the genetic counselor may reassure the patient that, based on current knowledge, the development of cancer was most likely a chance event, and that the risk of developing additional cancers in the patient or relatives is

TABLE 65–3. Projected Probability of Developing Breast Cancer Within 30 Years of Follow-up

Initial Age (y)	*Later Relative Risk**	*Initial Relative Risk (%)**					
		1	*2*	*5*	*10*	*20*	*30*
20		1.7	3.4	8.3	15.9	29.3	40.5
30	1	3.2	4.8	9.5	16.9	29.9	40.8
	2	4.7	6.3	10.9	18.2	30.9	41.7
	5	8.9	10.4	14.9	21.8	34.0	44.3
	10	15.6	17.1	21.2	27.6	38.8	48.3
	20	27.6	28.8	32.3	37.8	47.4	55.5
	30	37.7	38.7	41.8	46.4	54.7	61.7
40	1	4.4	5.6	9.1	14.6	24.6	33.5
	2	7.4	8.6	11.9	17.3	27.0	35.6
	5	15.9	17.0	20.0	24.9	33.7	41.5
	10	28.3	29.2	31.8	35.9	43.4	50.0
	20	47.5	48.1	50.0	53.1	58.5	63.4
	30	61.2	61.6	63.1	65.3	69.3	72.8
50		4.4	8.5	19.9	35.5	57.8	71.7

* The initial relative risk corresponds to the initial age at consultation. If the age is under 50 and the 30-year projection exceeds 50, a later relative risk at age 50 should be specified, because risk due to the number of biopsies varies with age (see Table 65–2).
(Gail MH, Brinton LA, Byar DP, et al. Projecting individualized probabilities of developing breast cancer for white females who are being examined annually. JNCI 1989;81:1879–1886)

TABLE 65–4. Empiric Familial Recurrence Risks for Selected Common Cancers

Cancer	*Mendelian Risk*	*Empiric Recurrence Risk**
Skin (Basal cell or squamous cell)		
General		1% (Depending on skin exposure)
Nevoid basal cell carcinoma syndrome	AD	
Xeroderma pigmentosum	AR	
Lung		
General		Relative risk of 3.0
Interstitial pulmonary fibrosis	AD	
P450-susceptible	AD	
Colorectal		
General		3–5%
Many polyposis syndromes	AD	
Turcot polyposis syndrome	AR	
Adenoma-carcinoma syndrome	AD	
Pancreas		
General		<1%
Hereditary pancreatitis	AD	
Breast		
General		See Tables 65–2 and 65–3
Cowden's disease	AD	
Certain families, especially with ovarian, linked to chromosome 17q	AD	
Ovarian carcinoma		
General		3–5%
Certain rare families	AD	
Prostate		
General		3%
Rare families	AD	

AD, autosomal dominant; AR, autosomal recessive.
* For first-degree relative (brother, sister, parent, child) with the same cancer.
(Mulvihill JJ. McKusick's mendelian inheritance in man: Oncology. Baltimore: Johns Hopkins University Press, 1993)

no greater than that of the population at large. The caveat should be added that future developments in the patient's or family's medical history may alter the patient's risk and that such developments should be brought to the counselor's attention.

GENETIC COUNSELING AT THE BEGINNING OF THERAPY

RISKS TO THE PATIENT

It is important to counsel the new cancer patient about the potential for decreased fertility caused by the cancer and its treatment. Cancer may affect the reproductive organs directly, or cancer surgery may impair reproduction. More likely, the use of alkylating agents, especially combined with radiotherapy below the diaphragm, predictably diminish reproductive potential. Alternate regimens that maintain excellent survival rates but decrease reproductive toxicity may be considered. Women have been offered oophoropexy to position ovaries outside radiotherapy fields to try to preserve fertility. Men may consider sperm banking before the therapy starts if they are interested in improving their potential for having natural children after the completion of cancer treatment, although the systemic effects of the cancer may have already impaired or reduced sperm production to below levels that can be effectively cryopreserved.

TERATOGENICITY

A rare but extremely unfortunate situation is the simultaneous diagnosis of cancer and pregnancy.[47] Pregnancy is contraindicated during cancer therapy because most cancer therapies are teratogens that are toxic to the fetus. Part of the advice at the onset of cancer therapy of a woman of reproductive age is to recommend birth control or at least to alert the woman of the potential for teratogenicity.

In human beings, largely based on experience of pregnant women exposed to the atomic bombs in Japan, as few as 10 cGy to the developing fetus between 8 and 15 weeks of gestational age is thought to result in some loss on IQ performance.[48,49] Microcephaly and short stature are the results of fetal exposure to higher doses of ionizing radiation. Each 100 cGy of fetal dose is calculated to lower IQ by 30 points. The older fetus is quite radioresistant. We documented normal findings in a 52-year-old man who, as a 30-week fetus, had been exposed to 180 to 300 cGy of radiation to the brain, given in the course of treating his mother's cervical cancer.[50]

If therapy has been inadvertently given to a woman with cancer who is later recognized to be pregnant or if life-saving therapy for a pregnant woman with cancer must begin, it may be possible to modify therapy to agents that are less likely to be teratogenic than others. For this purpose of genetic counseling, a registry of pregnancies exposed to cancer therapy was established at the NCI and is maintained at the University of Pittsburgh.[51] Because cancer treatment during pregnancy is a rare and sometimes accidental event, the exact teratogenicity of various chemotherapeutic agents will never be the subject of rigorous analytic epidemiologic study. It seems best to register the rare human experience as it accrues. The registry is available to answer immediate questions, for example, about the published and unpublished experience of vincristine given to women who are 5- to 6-weeks pregnant. Contrary to expectations, even substantial chemotherapy in the first trimester is not inevitably teratogenic. If a pregnancy exposed to cancer treatment is much wanted, there is some room for reassurance that gross malformations are not inevitable. However, given the experience with other human teratogens (*e.g.*, fetal alcohol syndrome), the least apparent manifestation of toxicity to the developing fetus is often a loss of higher brain function (*i.e.*, behavioral traits, IQ). It is better to expose no embryo or fetus to chemotherapy or radiotherapy.

GENETIC COUNSELING AFTER THERAPY ENDS

Former cancer patients should be told that there are major theoretical concerns about possible somatic and germ cell mutations. Cancer treatments are specifically designed to interfere with DNA, cellular metabolism, and cell division. There is good reason to suspect a priori that cancer treatments can cause mutation and genetic disease in human beings. They do so in mice and in somatic cells of human beings (*e.g.*, sustained chromosomal breakage or second cancers after cancer treatment). However, no environmental agent has been causally linked to human germ cell mutation, contrary to expectations. Despite intensive study of various parameters, genetic damage has not been seen in the offspring of the survivors of the atomic bombs in Japan.[52] Indicators of possible genetic damage have been birth defects, newborn survival, chromosomal abnormalities, a change in protein structure or function, and growth or development of malignancies.

In several large retrospective case series (Table 65–5), there was some room for reassurance that, despite expectations, no excess of birth defects or genetic diseases has been seen in the offspring of cancer survivors who maintain fertility enough to bear or father children. In 3687 liveborns from 15 cases series in the literature, the summary rate of birth defects and genetic disease is 4%, a rate comparable to that in the general population. The studies were not all directly comparable in how cancer survivors were identified and pregnancy outcomes were defined. In the single largest study, the NCI Five Center Study, family controls and population expected numbers were used, and no excess of genetic disease was seen.[66] That study alone had a 94% power to detect a 50% increase and did not find it.

Based on just two offspring with interventricular septal defects of the heart, the question was raised of possible adverse effects on pregnancies of women who had received dactinomycin.[67] Special analysis of the Five Center Study data could not confirm the association.[68]

Among 4256 offspring of survivors of childhood and adolescent cancer followed for over 32,000 person-years, 33 offspring had cancer; 25 of them had retinoblastoma, as did a parent of each.[69,70] Except for known hereditary or familial cancer syndromes, the offspring of survivors of cancer seem to have no excess of cancer.

TABLE 65–5. Large Series of Pregnancies Among Survivors of Cancer

	Exposed Parents		Completed Pregnancies					
						Liveborns		
Investigations	*Total*	*Females (%)*	*Total*	*Fetal Loss**	*Elective Abortions*	*Total*	*With Defects*	*Type of Defects*
Li and Jaffe, ?–1973[53]	45	63	107	15	3	90	2	Hirschsprung's disease, asymptomatic heart murmur‡
Ross, 1956–1973[54]	58†	100	96	18	?	75	3	Penred's syndrome, tetralogy of Fallot, hemangiomata, eczema and strabismus (1 stillborn with aplasia of the anterior abdominal wall)
Holmes and Holmes[55]	48	60	93	12	3	77	6	Amblyopia, autism, scleroderma, rectal stenosis, absent fallopian tube and small uterus, slow learner and foot defect
Li et al[56]	146	58	286	45	10	236	8	Possible trisomy 18 syndrome, Marfan's syndrome, deafness, pyloric stenosis, Hirschsprung's disease (same as above), cardiac, brain, and multiple malformations
Blatt et al, ?–1980[57]	30	77	40	12	10	27	1	Congenital hip dysplasia
Horning et al, 1968–1979[58]	29	100	28	5	5	24	0	
Marradi et al, ?–1982[59]	14	57	23	?	?	21	2	Multiple congenital anomalies with mental and growth retardation, panhypopituitarism and cerebral atrophy, gastroschisis
Bundey and Evans, ?–1973[60]	24	83	48	3	0	44	1	Pyloric stenosis
Andrieu and Ochoa-Molina, 1972–1976[61]	22	100	30	9	4	21	1	Congenital hip dysplasia
Rustin et al, 1958–1980[62]	216†	100	374	90	36	267	8	Spina bifida, tetralogy of Fallot, talipes eqinovares, collapsed lung, umbilical hernia, desquamative fibrosing alveolitis (2 sibs), neonatal tachycardia (plus 2 anencephalic stillbirths and 1 sudden infant death)
Goldstein et al, 1965–1983[63]	?†	100	222	58	6	159	5	Not specified
Mulvihill et al, 1959–1977[64]	66	100	87	22	12	53	6	Neurosensory deafness‡, scoliosis and slow learner‡, hydrocephalus‡, cleft lip and palate‡, hydrocephalus, tracheomalacia
Li et al, 1931–1979[65]	181	65	246	53	32	190	5	Congenital hip dislocation (2), heart murmur, hypospadias, internal tibial torsion
Mulvihill et al, 1945–1975[66]	2308	~50	?	?	?	2198	75	(Rate no different than control)
Green et al, 1960–1984[67]	60	58	?	?	?	100	8	Ventricular septal defect, tetralogy of Fallot, hydrocele, birth marks (2), skin tags, epidermal nevus
Total	3212	58	>4059	>373	132	3687	136	

* Fetal loss is defined as elective abortion, ectopic pregnancy, spontaneous abortion (miscarriage), or stillbirth; ?, uncertain.
† All gestational trophoblastic neoplasia.
‡ Exposed to cancer treatment during gestation.
(Modified from Mulvihill JJ, Byrne J. Offspring of long-time survivors of childhood cancers. Clin Oncol 1985;4:333–343)

CONCLUSION

Many questions remain about the proper care and counseling of survivors of cancer. Because no center and few nations will in the near future have much experience with pregnancies in or by cancer patients, it is hoped that collaborative international studies will prove feasible and gain wide support from clinicians. Currently, the ideal situation is that genetic and reproductive counseling should take place as soon as cancer is diagnosed (before therapy starts) and again when pregnancy is contemplated.

REFERENCES

1. Fraser FC. Genetic counseling. Am J Hum Genet 1974;26:636–659.
2. Kushner R. Why me? New York: Holt, Rinehart, and Winston, 1982.
3. Parry DM, Berg K, Mulvihill JJ, et al. Strategies for controlling cancer through genetics: Report of a workshop. Am J Hum Genet 1987;41:63–69.
4. Parry DM, Mulvihill JJ, Miller RW, et al. Strategies for controlling cancer through genetics. Cancer Res 1987;47:6814–1817.
5. Mulvihill JJ. Prospects for cancer control and prevention through genetics. Clin Genet 1989;36:313–319.
6. Mulvihill JJ. Childhood cancer, the environment, and heredity. In: Pizzo PA, Poplack DG, eds. Principles and practice of pediatric oncology, 2nd ed. Philadelphia: JB Lippincott, 1993.
7. Phelan MC, Stevenson RE, Collins JL, et al. Fragile X syndrome and neoplasia. Am J Med Genet 1988;30:77–82.
8. Cohen AJ, Li FP, Berg S, et al. Hereditary renal cell carcinoma associated with a chromosomal translocation. N Engl J Med 1979;301:592–595.
9. Yunis JJ, Ramsay NKC. Familial occurrence of the aniridia-Wilms' tumor syndrome with deletion 11p13–14.1. J Pediatr 1980;96:1027–1030.
10. Strong LC, Riccardi VM, Ferrell RE, et al. Familial retinoblastoma and chromosome 13 deletion transmitted via an insertional translocation. Science 1981;213:1501–1503.
11. Bolger GB, Stamberg J, Kirsch IR, et al. Chromosome translocation t(14;22) and oncogene (c-*sis*) variant in a pedigree with familial meningioma. N Engl J Med 1985;312:564–567.
12. McKusick VA. Mendelian inheritance in man. 9th ed. Baltimore: Johns Hopkins, 1990.
13. Mulvihill JJ. McKusick's mendelian inheritance in man: Oncology. Baltimore: Johns Hopkins University Press. 1993.
14. Müller HJ. Familial cancer in Basel: Some aspects. In: Müller HJ, Weber W, eds. Familial cancer. Basel: Karger, 1985:1–5.
15. Albano WA, Lynch HT, Recabaren JA, et al. Family cancer in an oncology clinic. Cancer 1981;47:2113–2118.
16. Love RR, Evans AM, Josten DM. The accuracy of patient reports of a family history of cancer. J Chron Dis 1985;38:289–293.
17. Li FP, Lokich J, Lapey J, Neptune WB, Wilkins EW Jr: Familial mesothelioma after intense asbestos exposure at home. JAMA 1978;240:467.
18. Lynch HT, Lynch JF, Cristofaro G. Genetic epidemiology of colon cancer. In: Lynch HT, Hirayama T, eds. Genetic epidemiology of cancer. Boca Raton: CRC Press, 1989: 251–277.
19. Li FP, Fraumeni JF Jr, Mulvihill JJ, et al. A cancer family syndrome in twenty-four kindreds. Cancer Res 1988;48:5358–5362.
20. Malkin D, Li FP, Strong LC, Fraumeni JF Jr, et al. Germ line *p53* mutations in a familial syndrome of breast cancer, sarcomas, and other neoplasms. Science 1990;250:1233–1238.
21. Weber W, Dürig M, eds. Hereditary cancer and preventive surgery. Basel: Karger, 1990: 118.
22. Blattner WA. The interdisciplinary approach to cancer families. In: Mulvihill JJ, Miller RN, Fraumeni JF Jr, eds. Genetics of human cancer. New York: Raven Press, 1972.
23. Lynch HT, Fitzsimmons ML, Lynch J, et al. A hereditary cancer consultation clinic. Nebraska Med J 1989;74:351–359.
24. Josten DM, Evans AM, Love RR. The cancer prevention clinic: A service program for cancer-prone families. J Psychosoc Oncol 1986;3:5–20.
25. Ponder BAJ. Familial cancer: Opportunities for clinical practice and research. Eur J Surg Oncol 1987;13:463–473.
26. Kelly PT. Risk counseling for relatives of cancer patients: New information, new approaches. J Psychosoc Oncol 1987;5:65–79.
27. LeMarec B, LeGail E, Journel H, et al. Le conseil génétique en cancérologie. Presse Med 1986;15:1369–1371.
28. Williams CJ. Managing families genetically predisposed to cancer: The "cancer-family syndrome" as a model. In: Chaganti RSK, German J, eds. Genetics in clinical oncology. New York: Oxford University Press, 1985:222–240.
29. Philippe P. Les familles à cancer. Paris: Éditions Maloine, 1985:181–191.
30. Bussey HJF. Familial polyposis coli. Baltimore: Johns Hopkins, 1975:104.
31. Burt RW, Bishop DT, Lynch HT, et al. Risk and surveillance of individuals with heritable factors for colorectal cancer. Bull World Health Org 1990;68:655–665.
32. Kersey JH, Shapiro RS, Filipovich AH. Relationship of immunodeficiency to lymphoid malignancy. Pediatr Infect Dis J 1988;7:S10–S12.
33. Goldstein AM, Dracopoli NC, Ho EC, et al. Further evidence for a locus for cutaneous malignant melanoma-dysplastic nevus (CMM/DN) on chromosome 1p and evidence for genetic heterogeneity. Am J Hum Genet (in press).
34. Tulinius H. Familial cancer registration in Iceland. In: Müller HJ, Weber W, eds. Familial cancer. Basel: Karger, 1985:263–267.
35. Steinitz R, Costin C, Ben-Hur M, et al. Clusters of families in a population-based cancer registry: Methodological problems. In: Müller HJ, Weber W, eds. Familial cancer. Basel: Karger, 1985:272–274.
36. Skolnick M. The Utah genealogical data base: A resource for genetic epidemiology. In: Cairns J, Lyon JL, Skolnick M, eds. Banbury report 4. Cold Spring Harbor, NY: Cold Spring Harbor Laboratory, 1980:285–297.
37. Williams RR, Hunt SC, Barlow GK, et al. Health family trees: A tool for finding and helping young family members of coronary and cancer prone pedigrees in Texas and Utah. Am J Public Health 1988;78:1283–1286.
38. Gail MH, Brinton LA, Byar DP, et al. Projecting individualized probabilities of developing breast cancer for white females who are being examined annually. JNCI 1989;81:1879–1886.
39. Fisher B, Redmond C. New perspective on cancer of the contralateral breast: A marker for assessing tamoxifen as a preventive agent. JNCI 1991;464:1278–1280.
40. Claus EB, Risch N, Thompson WD. Autosomal dominant inheritance of early onset breast cancer: Implications for risk prediction. Cancer (in press).
41. Mulvihill JJ, Safyer AW, Bening JK. Prevention in familial breast cancer: Counseling and prophylactic mastectomy. Prev Med 1982;11:500–511.
42. Lynch HT, Lynch JF, Fusaro RM. Clinical importance of familial cancer. In: Müller HJ, Weber W, eds. Familial cancer. Basel: Karger, 1985:6–12.
43. Lerman C, Rimer B, Engstrom P. Cancer risk notification: Psychosocial and ethical implications. J Clin Oncol 1991;9:1275–1282.
44. Wapnir IL, Rabinowitz B, Greco R. A reappraisal of prophylactic mastectomy. Surg 1990;171:171–184.
45. Kash KM, Holland JC, Helper MS, Miller DG. Psychological distress and surveillance behaviors of women with a family history of breast cancer. JNCI 1992;84:24–30.
46. Evans AM, Love RR, Meyerowitz BE, et al. Factors associated with active participation in a cancer prevention clinic. Prev Med 1985;14:358–371.
47. Allen HH, Nisker JA, eds. Cancer in pregnancy: Therapeutic guidelines. Mt. Kisco, NY: Futura Publishing, 1986.
48. United Nations Environment Programme. Radiation: Doses, effects, risks. Oxford, Blackwell, 1991:89.
49. Miller RW, Mulvihill JJ. Small head size after atomic irradiation. Teratology 1976;14: 355–357.
50. Mulvihill JJ, Harvey EB, Boice JD Jr, et al. Normal findings 52 years after in utero radiation exposure. Lancet 1991;338:1202–1203.
51. Mulvihill JJ, Stewart KR. A registry of pregnancies exposed to chemotherapeutic agents. Teratology 1986;33:80C.
52. Neel JV, Satoh C, Goriki K, et al. Search for mutations altering protein charge and/or function in children of atomic bomb survivors: Final report. Am J Hum Genet 1988;42: 663–676.
53. Li FP, Jaffe H. Progeny of childhood-cancer survivors. Lancet 1974;2:707–709.
54. Ross GT. Congenital anomalies among children born of mothers receiving chemotherapy for gestational trophoblastic neoplasms. Cancer 1976;37:1043–1047.
55. Holmes GE, Holmes FF. Pregnancy outcome of patients treated for Hodgkin's disease: A controlled study. Cancer 1978;41:1317–1322.
56. Li FP, Fine W, Jaffe H, et al. Offspring of patients treated for cancer in childhood. JNCI 1979;62:1193–1197.
57. Blatt J, Mulvihill JJ, Ziegler JL, et al. Pregnancy outcome following cancer chemotherapy. Am J Med 1980;69:828–832.
58. Horning SJ, Hippe RT, Kaplan HS, et al. Female reproductive potential after treatment for Hodgkin's disease. N Engl J Med 1981;304:1377–1382.
59. Marradi P, Schaison F, Alby N, et al. Les enfants nés de parents leucémiques. Nouv Rev Fr Hematol 1982;24:75–80.
60. Bundey S, Evans K. Survivors of neuroblastoma and ganglioneuroma and their families. J Med Genet 1982;19:16–21.
61. Andrieu JM, Ochoa-Molina ME. Menstrual cycle, pregnancies and offspring before and after MOPP therapy for Hodgkin's disease. Cancer 1983;52:435–438.
62. Rustin GJS, Booth M, Dent J, et al. Pregnancy after cytotoxic chemotherapy for gestational trophoblastic tumours. Br Med J 1984;288:103–106.
63. Goldstein DP, Berkowitz RS, Bernstein MR. Reproductive performance after molar pregnancy and gestational trophoblastic tumors. Clin Obstet Gynecol 1983;27:221–227.
64. Mulvihill JJ, McKeen EA, Rosner F, et al. Pregnancy outcome in cancer patients: Experience in a large cooperative group. Cancer 1987;60:1143–1150.
65. Li FP, Gimbrere K, Gelber RD, et al. Outcome of pregnancy in survivors of Wilms' tumor. JAMA 1987;257:216–219.
66. Mulvihill JJ, Byrne J, Steinhorn SA, et al. Genetic disease in offspring of survivors of cancer in the young. Am J Hum Genet 1986;39:A72.
67. Green DM, Zevon MA, Lowrie G, et al. Congenital anomalies in children of patients who received chemotherapy for cancer in childhood and adolescence. N Engl J Med 1991;325:141–146.
68. Byrne J, Nicholson HS, Mulvihill JJ. Absence of birth defects in offspring of women treated with dactinomycin. N Engl J Med 1992;326:137.
69. Mulvihill JJ, Myers MH, Connelly RR, et al. Cancer in offspring of long-term survivors of childhood and adolescent cancer. Lancet 1987;2:813–817.
70. Hawkins MM, Draper GJ, Smith RA. Cancer among 1,348 offspring of survivors of childhood cancer. Int J Cancer 1989;43:975–978.

Cancer: Principles & Practice of Oncology, Fourth Edition,
edited by Vincent T. DeVita, Jr., Samuel Hellman, Steven A. Rosenberg.
J.B. Lippincott Co., Philadelphia © 1993.

Lynn H. Gerber
Stephen Levinson
Jeanne E. Hicks
Patrice Gallelli
Jessie Whitehurst
Donna Scheib
Barbara C. Sonies

CHAPTER **66**

Evaluation and Management of Disability: Rehabilitation Aspects of Cancer

The oncologist or oncologic surgeon may be most concerned with the ablation of tumor and with the ultimate survival of the patient, and the patient may be just as concerned with issues of function, quality of life, and with independence in life routines. Factors predicting whether a patient will have a good functional outcome after cancer treatment include the site, stage, type, and rate of growth of tumor, but other factors may be as influential. These typically include coexisting medical conditions, concomitant use of medications, age or life stage, and psychosocial variables such as motivation, depression, or optimism. The impact of cancer treatments on function, much of which is not appreciated until well after primary treatment has been completed, is often significant. Key examples of this are the long-term effects of irradiation on the brachial plexus or the central nervous system (CNS).

Often, as a result of the underlying disease process or of its treatment, patients are forced to accept a degree of physical dependence on others. Long-term disability, however, is a treatable and often preventable complication of cancer and cancer therapy. Early intervention by the cancer rehabilitation team can significantly reduce the morbidity associated with malignant disorders.

Disability in a significant portion of patients undergoing treatment for cancer has been well documented.[1] The causes of disability are varied and often difficult to predict from the tumor type alone. Most obvious are the direct effects of primary and metastatic lesions. Invasion of soft tissues can cause pain and, if skeletal structures are involved, loss of bony integrity.[2] Invasion of the digestive tract or liver can lead to generalized wasting, and invasion of the lungs or pleura can lead to respiratory compromise.

CNS involvement can result in cognitive impairment, or if the spinal column is involved, in quadriplegia or paraplegia. This can affect mobility and gross physical function, and it may interfere with essential body functions such as respiration and waste elimination. Bulbar involvement may impede autonomic or motor control, and it may lead to dysfunctional speech and swallowing. Peripheral nerves may be compromised by the direct effects of a tumor or its metastases, resulting in the loss of critical sensory or motor functions.

Venous compression may result in edema or in deep venous thrombosis that can lead to life-threatening pulmonary embolus. Edema can result from lymphatic obstruction. Left untreated, the swollen extremity can become a major burden to the patient, impeding mobility, causing pain and discomfort, and leading to the development of permanent changes in skin consistency. The edematous extremity can become infected or necrotic, with tissue breakdown leading to severe morbidity and mortality.

A tumor may result in disability through its systemic effects. Paraneoplastic syndromes resulting in myopathy, neuropathy, and cerebellar dysfunction are well documented.[3,4] Perhaps the most significant causes of disability are related to cancer treatment. Chemotherapy-related neuropathies are commonly related to agents such as vincristine, cisplatin, DDC, and DDI. Radiation treatment often results in neuropathies, plexopathies, and myelopathies in lymphedema and in tissue fibrosis. Irradiation effects are often not evident until months or years after the completion of all treatment. Surgery can lead to the loss of a limb or of important functional elements. Prolonged bed rest can lead to severe deconditioning and significant psychological morbidity.

New treatment strategies may be associated with disability and with new challenges to the rehabilitation specialist. Limb-salvage procedures may preserve anatomy and body image, although occasionally at the expense of function. Early involvement of the cancer rehabilitation team can help to predict the degree of disability and to help the patient make an informed decision about a variety of treatment options. Strategies to help adapt to the loss of critical musculoskeletal elements can often be devised before treatment actually begins.

The patient undergoing immunotherapy with agents such as interleukin-2 (IL-2) presents another set of challenges, including phenomenal fluid shifts.[5] Intraoperative irradiation can result in a more concentrated delivery of radiation to the tumor bed, but it has been our experience that severe delayed peripheral neuropathy and pain are frequent sequelae. Rehabilitation can play a role in the evaluation, treatment and prevention of disability.

THE ROLE OF REHABILITATION

Rehabilitation is a phased process, which should begin soon after diagnosis if a disability is anticipated. It should continue until the patient has reached maximal functional benefit.

THE PRETREATMENT EVALUATION

A complete functional assessment should be made at the time of staging, with particular attention to the home environment, the patient's occupation, and his or her valued roles. This assessment focuses attention on strategies that can preserve the aspects of function that are most important to the patient. Potential problem areas can be identified and possible solutions explored.

If multiple treatment options exist, discussion should center on the functional impact of each potential treatment program and the rehabilitation strategies that are required to maintain or restore full function. When surgery is planned, the rehabilitation team can make preparations in advance, such as the provision of adaptive equipment and gait aids to promote independence. Prosthetic and orthotic devices can be planned before surgery, and initial prosthetic fitting can even take place in the operating room. When radiation therapy is planned, the patient can be trained in an exercise program designed to minimize the effects of radiation fibrosis.

REHABILITATION DURING THE TREATMENT PHASE

Treatment should begin with mobility to prevent the complications of prolonged bed rest. Pain management using heat, cold transcutaneous electrical nerve stimulation (TENS) can help prevent a patient becoming a chronic pain patient. Gait and functional retraining can the proceed even as the patient receives chemotherapy or radiation therapy. Other problems such as peripheral neuropathies, myopathies, myelopathies, and pathologic fractures can be addressed as rapidly as they arise.

REHABILITATION OF THE CANCER SURVIVOR

After treatment has been completed, the cancer patient may need continued treatment to maintain strength and range of motion (ROM), control pain, and return to normal activity. There may be residual effects of the disease or its treatment, and the patient may suffer from nutritional deficits and from a loss of physical capacity. Psychosocial issues may be a critical factor.[6] The survivor often has an impaired body image, and patients always perceive themselves as being different from the rest of the world. The fear of recurrence is a real one, but cancer survivors often deny obvious signs of recurrent tumor.[7]

Vocational counseling and retraining are important aspects of returning the cancer patient to the community. Adaptive strategies are often needed to facilitate the return to work. Job discrimination is a real problem that may interfere with the rehabilitative process and that must be overcome.[8,9] The clinical oncology and cancer rehabilitation teams often must serve in an advocacy role.

Sexual rehabilitation is an important aspect of cancer survivorship that is often ignored.[10,11] Pain during intercourse is a common problem that can often be overcome using modified sexual practices. Infertility may be a secondary issue during the acute phase of cancer treatment, only to emerge as a primary concern in the survivor.[12] Teratogenesis and the complications of pregnancy may be concerns.[13]

The child with cancer presents a special set of circumstances.[14–16] The rehabilitation team often must treat the entire family. Siblings may feel particularly vulnerable, or they may feel resentment about the attention received by the patient. Parents may feel guilt that they may have inadvertently caused the illness, and parents may sometimes place blame on each other. Classmates may have difficulty understanding what the patient has been through, and they may, out of their own fear, treat the patient as if cancer were a communicable disease. Growth and development are frequently impaired. Although the survivor of childhood cancer usually regains much of the development that was lost or delayed after treatment has been completed, residual short stature, uneven growth, and cognitive impairment are frequent long-term sequelae of treatment.[17–20]

Late neurologic complications of cancer include plexopathies, peripheral neuropathies, and myelopathies, all of which can be the result of late radiation effects or of tumor recurrence. Abnormal brain development or cognitive impairment can result from intrathecal chemotherapy or from brain irradiation, although late deterioration should always lead to the suspicion of recurrent metastatic disease. Paraneoplastic syndromes, including cerebellar degeneration, encephalomyelitis, subacute necrotizing myelopathy, peripheral neuropathies, myopathies, and myasthenic syndrome, are uncommon but documented late complications that may not resolve with resolution of the malignancy.[3,21] Chronic pain related to radiation fibrosis, radiation neuritis, or tumor recurrence may result in the need for late rehabilitative interventions.

A swollen extremity in the cancer survivor always warrants further investigation. Swelling may be the result of deep venous thrombosis, lymphatic tumor invasion, or venous obstruction by tumor. Lymphedema, often related to radiation fibrosis or previous surgery, should be a diagnosis of exclusion. Rehabilitation management may require the use of compressive garments or pumps, exercise, and the use of moisturizing creams. The use of a compression pump in the face of recurrent lymphatic involvement may increase the likelihood of further tumor spread. Radiation fibrosis may require the use of exercise, splinting, orthotic appliances, moisturizing creams, or surgery.

REHABILITATION OF THE TERMINAL PATIENT

Even in the patient in whom there is no chance of survival, rehabilitation can play a critical role in the prevention of unnecessary morbidity. Pain control is of utmost importance. Prevention of skin ulcers, contractures, and generalized wasting can improve the quality of life. Maintaining mobility through the use of exercises and adaptive devices can maximize patient independence and minimize the burden to others.

THE CANCER REHABILITATION TEAM

Rehabilitation is a complex discipline that involves the interaction of numerous treatment providers, each with a particular area of training. The rehabilitation team is usually composed of physiatrists, occupational and physical therapists, speech and language pathologists, vocational counsellors, and a variety of other professionals as determined by the particular needs of the individual patient.

Although any rehabilitation specialist can serve as the team leader, we feel that, if possible, the rehabilitation team should be led by a medical rehabilitation specialist. A *physiatrist* is a physician who has specialty training in the field of physical medicine and rehabilitation. This training includes a core of information about the causes and effects of functional disability, the basic biomechanics of human motion, methods of functional assessment, and adaptive strategies. This physician is usually well equipped to prescribe and train patients in the use of orthotics, prosthetics, and adaptive equipment.

The *physical therapist* is an allied health specialist well informed in the basic mechanics of human motion and exercise. Physical therapists often institute and supervise an exercise program to improve mobility, strength, and stamina. If involved early in the course of treatment, they can instruct the patient and the family in a basic exercise program to prevent muscle atrophy or contractures and maintain fitness. Typically, physical therapists provide assessments of ROM, manual muscle testing, and gait. They use orthotics and other adaptive devices to correct specific neuromuscular impairments, such as a foot drop, and they may treat edema using exercise, compressive pumps, and elastic stockings. They are particularly adept at the use of superficial and deep heating modalities, traction, hydrotherapy, and electrical stimulation in the management of open wounds, contractures, and pain. Working with occupational therapists, they may address issues such as bed mobility and the use of wheel chairs or custom seating.

Occupational therapists are specialists who evaluate and treat dysfunction in daily living activities, including self-care, work, and leisure-related activities, placing emphasis on those roles and activities that the patient most values. They often help to develop alternative strategies for performing basic self-care activities and other valued roles, making use of adaptive equipment where indicated. Bathroom safety is an issue of particular importance to the cancer patient, and occupational therapists frequently recommend or provide devices such as a raised toilet seat or bedside commode, a tub or shower transfer bench or chair, a hand-held shower hose, and grab bars.

Occupational therapists are often involved with the evaluation of wheelchairs and custom seating for assisted mobility. They play a major role in the assessment and management of hand dysfunction and often make use of therapeutic hand exercises, splints, and braces to restore function. Vocational issues are often the responsibility of the occupational therapist, although in some institutions, a separate *vocational counselor* is a part of the rehabilitation team. In some cases, the occupational therapist performs a home visit to evaluate the home environment and physical changes that are needed for the patient to be safe and independent.

The *social worker* provides important input into the rehabilitation process for the cancer patient, evaluating the complete home environment and determining the availability, willingness, and strengths of family members who can assist with care and support of the patient. The social worker may help the family evaluate its financial resources and provide information on available support services.

Speech pathologists evaluate communication skills and the mechanics of speech and swallowing. In many institutions, they perform cognitive assessments and training in basic memory skills. They may provide vocal retraining and instruction in alaryngeal speech, and they may provide equipment for alternative methods of communication such as with an alphabet board or a computer. They assess functional integrity and compensatory ability of structures and mechanisms needed to achieve adequate communication, deglutition, nutrition, hydration, and cognition. They are often involved with the evaluation and treatment of dysphagia and work with *maxillofacial prosthetists* in the restoration of facial appearance and oral function.

Audiologists assess the integrity of the peripheral and central auditory mechanism in relation to presurgical and postsurgical, intraoperative, and ototoxic effects on hearing. They provide advice for preserving or restoring hearing using augmentative devices.

A *psychologist* can play a crucial role as a member of the cancer rehabilitation team. Virtually all cancer patients must address issues of death and dying and many need the support of someone trained in this area. Patients may have difficulty dealing with changes in their body image, particularly with the loss of a limb. *Clinical neuropsychologists* may be involved with the evaluation of cognitive impairment.

The *rehabilitation nurse* is a nurse who has specialty training in rehabilitative aspects of nursing care. Particular emphasis is placed on bowel and bladder management in the patient with neurogenic disorders of waste elimination and on wound management. The rehabilitation nurse may be involved with ostomy care and with the training of the patient or family in the management of catheters, ostomy equipment, and surgical dressings.

The *prosthetist-orthotist* is involved with the fitting and fabrication of braces and artificial limbs. In oncology, the prosthetists often provide valuable input about appropriate prosthetic or orthotic components that may be used. In cases of limb-sparing procedures, the orthotist often needs to fabricate devices that substitute for weak muscle groups or unstable joints.

A variety of other practitioners may be involved as part of the rehabilitation team. These may include the chaplains, recreational therapists, nutritional services, psychiatrists, and pain management specialists. By assembling an optimal mix of specialists, it is possible to minimize the disability that results from malignancy and its treatment.

FUNCTIONAL EVALUATION

It is necessary for rehabilitation specialists to evaluate the impact of cancer diagnoses on complex behaviors and activities and its impact on anatomic structures and physiologic processes. These evaluations, often called global or functional assessments, are multidimensional and combine objective measures and subjective reports.

Typically, the evaluations include joint ROM data, strength measures and measurements of stamina and often measures of pain intensity. Some evaluations include measures of the psychological impact of cancer on patients and their adjustment to it.[22] Most functional assessments include indices that reflect independence in self-care, mobility, bowel or bladder functioning, and cognitive performance if indicated.

These measurement tools are useful as long as they are reliable, sensitive to the magnitude of change expected, easy to use, and standardized for the cancer population.[23]

COMMON FUNCTIONAL IMPAIRMENTS IN ONCOLOGY

The common functional impairments caused by cancer therapy are summarized in Table 66–1.

IMMOBILITY AND ITS IMPACT

Bed rest in cancer patients is associated with numerous metabolic and physiologic changes that may impair the patient's medical and functional recovery.[24] Bone loss is well documented and, in extreme cases, may lead to hypercalcemia.[25–27] In patients who are already osteoporotic or who have metastatic involvement of the skeletal system, this may predispose to pathologic fractures and further disability. The use of agents to minimize bone loss is somewhat controversial.[28,29] Muscle atrophy can be quite rapid, often leading to an inability to walk in as short a time as a week. Changes in muscle physiology and fiber type have been documented as well.[30,31] As muscle mass becomes reduced, the amount of soft tissue covering bony prominences can become marginal, predisposing to the development of pressure ulcers (decubiti). Prolonged pressure over the nerves and particularly over the peroneal nerve as it crosses the fibular head may lead to a mononeuropathy and foot drop. Lack of motion about the joints may result in contractures and changes in muscle and joint physiology.[32,33] Lack of mobility can lead to the development of deep venous thrombosis and pulmonary embolus.[34] All of these factors can significantly reduce mobility and independence.

Generalized Deconditioning

As a rule of thumb, each week of immobility requires as much as a month of rehabilitation to regain functional mobility.

TABLE 66–1. Functional Impairments Caused by Cancer Therapy

Musculoskeletal Problem	*Primary Cancer Therapy*			
	Surgery	*Chemotherapy*	*Irradiation*	*Immunotherapy*
Atrophy/weakness	×	×	×	×
Contracture	×		×	
Decubiti/wound complications	×	×	×	×
Edema	×	×	×	×
Gait deficits	×	×	×	
Joint instability	×		×	
Neuropathy (sensory and motor)	×	×	×	
Pain	×		×	
Generalized deconditioning (cardiotoxicity)		×	×	×
CNS involvement (UMN/LMN)	×	×	×	
Cosmetic deficits	×		×	

UMN/LMN, upper motor neuron/lower motor neuron.
(Modified from Gerber LH, McGarvey CL. Musculoskeletal deficits and rehabilitation intervention in the cancer patient. In: Wittes RE, ed. Manual of oncologic therapeutics. Philadelphia: JB Lippincott, 1991:417)

Complications such as pathologic fractures and pressure ulcers can further prolong the hospital stay. Although it is sometimes impossible to fully mobilize a patient receiving chemotherapy or major surgery, some degree of mobilization under a physical therapist's supervision may significantly reduce morbidity. For the patient who is mildly restricted by disease or treatment, active ambulation at least once or twice daily should be strongly encouraged. If this is not possible, an exercise program in bed may be started, using resistance against gravity or against an elastic band. A tilt table may be used to maintain or restore cardiovascular conditioning in the patient who is unable to stand. This helps to minimize heel cord contractures. In patients with severe dependent edema, compressive garments may help to maintain the vascular volume and to reduce the degree of the edema while facilitating ambulation. Exercises, by increasing muscular tone and facilitating venous compression, can help to maintain cardiovascular volume.

Skin Care

Prevention of skin breakdown should be of utmost importance in the bed-bound patient. Above all else, the patient must not be allowed to remain in a single position for more than 2 hours. If the patient is unable to position himself or herself in bed, repositioning should be done with pillows or cushions, taking care not to encourage the development of contractures by, for example, persistently flexing the neck, hips, or knees. Air-cushioned beds can help to reduce the incidence of pressure injuries, but they do not substitute for proper nursing care. Sequential air chamber mattresses seem to be as effective as older designs, provided that an intervening cushion such as an egg-crate or sheepskin mattress is not used. Shear forces and direct pressure may be important in the development of decubiti. Care should therefore be taken to avoid leaving the patient slouched in a chair or in bed with the head elevated, because these positions can predispose to ischial and sacral pressure wounds, respectively.

If skin becomes dry, aqueous remoisturizing creams should be applied. Greasy agents can predispose to maceration and breakdown. Irradiated skin is of particular concern, due to the loss of normal resilience and healing capacity. Moisturizing agents may be required for the remainder of the patient's lifetime. Careful attention to hygiene is important with irradiated skin, and all open cuts and abrasions should receive scrutiny, because these can easily become infected.

When complications arise, they should be treated promptly. Areas of skin redness that do not blanch should be considered to be early pressure ulcers (stage I) and treated by removing pressure over the affected area. Most tissue damage in pressure ulcers occurs in the deep layers of the dermis and underlying tissues, such that the visible portion of the ulcer may represent only a fraction of the total extent. If actual skin breakdown occurs, care should be taken to keep the wound clean and to avoid the accumulation of purulent exudates. Packing should be used to prevent loculation of fluid, and frequent dressing changes should be used to keep the wound clean. All necrotic tissue should be debrided daily, if necessary. In many instances, hydrotherapy (whirlpool) can aid in the process of debridement and cleansing.

Packing the wound with an antiseptic solution such as Dakin's or povidone-iodine should be done only if the wound is known to be clinically infected, because such solutions can actually retard the healing process. In the case of noninfected small lesions, absorptive hydrocolloid occlusive dressings can be effective in promoting healing, provided they are used in accordance with the manufacturer's recommendations. The use of occlusive dressings with larger wounds is controversial. Although we have seen many cases of complete resolution with the use of absorptive granules and occlusive dressings in deeper wounds, the potential exists for developing a superinfection. Occlusive dressings cannot be used as a substitute for adequate nursing care.

With proper management, virtually any pressure ulcer can heal in a healthy well-nourished patient. Unfortunately, most cancer patients do not have the luxury of a healthy intact immune system with which to lay down new connective tissue. For this reason, it is often necessary to maintain care to an open pressure or surgical wound until well after all chemotherapy has been completed. In any case, good nutrition should never be ignored as a factor in would healing. Dietary supplementation with ascorbic acid, B complex vitamins, and minerals, particularly zinc, should always be considered in cases of delayed wound healing. In some cases, it may be necessary to use a skin graft or myocutaneous transfer (flap) procedure to close a wound. This is particularly true over irradiated tissues, in which the capacity for healing may be permanently impaired.

Contractures

In cases of prolonged disuse, collagen fibers within muscles, tendons, and ligaments shorten, resulting in a loss of joint motion and the development of a contracture. This problem is particularly evident at the shoulder, where the joint capsule is fairly redundant, but also occurs in all major joints of the body. Heel cords are prone to severe shortening, with hamstring and hip flexor contractures contributing to impaired mobility.

ROM exercises should be done actively by the debilitated patient or passively by nursing or by the family at least two to three times each day, moving all major joints through their full ROM in all directions. In the case of the shoulder, this includes external and internal rotation full abduction, and flexion. If flexion and abduction need to be limited (*e.g.*, in the patient after mastectomy or axillary lymph node dissection), internal and external rotation should be done to stretch the joint capsule.[35] Splinting may be used to maintain functional hand and foot position. An example of each is presented in Figures 66–1 and 66–2.

Radiation fibrosis may potentiate the development of contractures, and its continuing long-term effects may make recovery of ROM especially difficult. The rehabilitation team should instruct the patient in a home stretching program at the earliest possible time, impressing the need to continue this faithfully. A long-term stretching program may be required because of the tendency for irradiated tissues to develop persistent fibrosis. Compliance with the exercise recommendations is essential.

If contractures do occur, they may require months of therapy to regain full motion. Stretching exercises should be done at least once or twice daily under the guidance of a physical therapist. This may be supplemented by the use of superficial

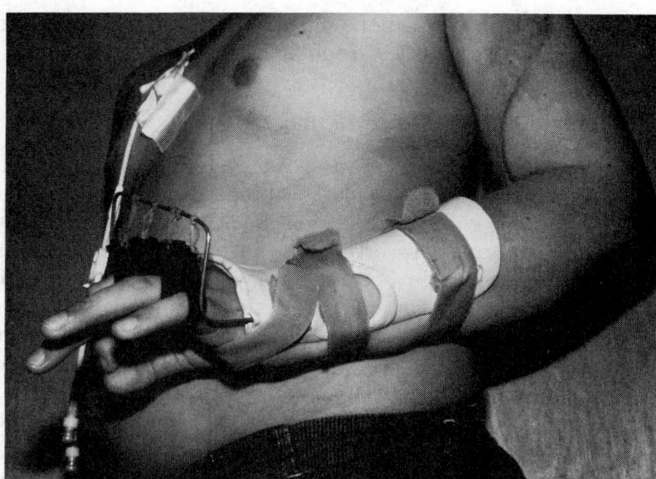

FIGURE 66–1. Functional, dynamic hand splint used to compensate for weak extensors.

or deep heating modalities, particularly ultrasound, which can help to increase the pliability of collagen, facilitating stretching. However, ultrasound may increase the tendency for metastasis, and caution should be used if it is thought that malignant cells may be present in the insonofied area.[36] This problem is of minimal concern in systemic malignancies. In extreme conditions, surgical release or manipulation under anesthesia may be considered.

METABOLIC PROBLEMS

Metabolic problems can result from tumor involving the endocrine organs, metastasis to these organs, the secretion of ectopic hormones by tumors, or cancer treatments.[37,38]

Rehabilitation professionals should be aware of the metabolic changes produced by malignancy and cancer treatments. The chemical alterations, symptoms, and physical findings produced by these entities can influence rehabilitation goal and treatment planning for patients. The metabolic changes often include electrolyte disturbances as hyponatremia, hypercalcemia, hypoglycemia, hyperuricemia, hyperkalemia; lactic acidosis; and hormonal overactivity syndromes such as hypercortisolism, hyperthyroidism, and hyperparathyroidism. Signs and symptoms related to these metabolic disturbances include anorexia, nausea, vomiting, myalgias, altered mental states, seizures, psychosis, cardiac arrhythmias, muscle weakness, lethargy, fatigue, and hyperpnea. These problems limit the delivery of rehabilitation programs.

Exercise may produce lactic acidosis and hypoglycemia, and it should be avoided in these patients. Patients with hyperkalemia or hypokalemia may be more susceptible to arrhythmia. Patients have problems following directions and have poor carryover with altered mental states due to metabolic problems. In this instance, rehabilitation programs may have to be put on hold.

When symptoms or findings that may suggest metabolic problems are observed, staff should notify the primary care physician. In treating patients with cancer, it is good to review the patient chart before each treatment session to see if any new metabolic problems that may alter the rehabilitation program have occurred.

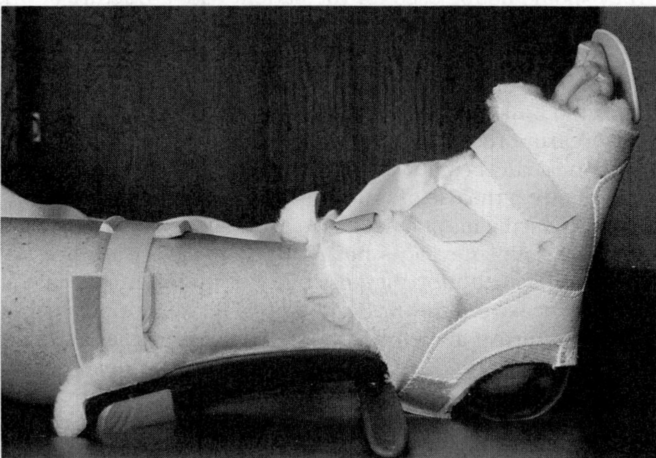

FIGURE 66–2. Multipodus splint to maintain foot and ankle in functional (neutral) position.

MYOPATHY

Tumor-associated myopathy may result in mobility and activities-of-daily-living (ADL) deficits. The myopathy may be a result of direct tumor invasion of muscle and other soft tissues, paraneoplastic syndrome, carcinomatous myopathy, steroid myopathy, or carcinomatous neuromyopathy.

Direct Tumor Invasion

Tumors that invade muscle include soft tissue sarcomas, rhabdomyosarcoma, lymphoma, osteogenic sarcoma, and metastatic tumor. The invasion of muscle by tumor is usually nonreversible and the resultant myopathy remains. Rhabdomyosarcoma and lymphoma may respond to chemotherapy and irradiation with shrinkage of the tumor and improvement in muscle strength. Soft tissue tumors are often excised with surrounding muscle and other soft tissue. Metastatic tumors may be irradiated or removed. After tumor and muscle resection, exercise to increase or preserve joint motion and to strengthen remaining muscles is essential to ensure optimal functioning of the limb. Re-education of surgically transposed muscles may need to be done. Radiation causes soft tissue changes that may produce muscle shortening and joint contracture. A stretching program should be prescribed and supervised for the duration of the radiation course.

Paraneoplastic Syndrome

Nonmetastatic paraneoplastic syndromes of malignancy have been recognized with polymyositis and dermatomyositis. Malignancy primarily occurs in association with dermatomyositis rather than with polymyositis.[39] The incidence is thought to be higher in men over 50 years of age.[40] The literature between 1975 and 1983 reports an incidence of malignancy of 7% to 8%.[41] A study by Lakhanpal mentions a 25% incidence of malignancy in a polymyositis and dermatomyositis group and a 17% incidence in the control group.[42] The most commonly associated malignancies with polymyositis and dermatomyositis are breast (18%) and lung (16%).[43]

Patients with this syndrome have decreased endurance, muscle weakness, pain, decreased joint motion, and problems with ambulation, self-care, sexual performance, and work related activity. Treatment to increase joint motion with stretching exercise, to increase muscle strength with isometric exercise, to improve mobility with gait aides and bracing, and to improve ADL with assistive devices are all appropriate. The patient should be instructed in energy conservation, joint protection, and sexual and vocational counseling.[44,45]

Carcinomatous Myopathy

Carcinomatous myopathy may be seen with metastatic malignant disease. Histologically, there is widespread muscle necrosis and minimal or no inflammatory response. Clinically, there is proximal muscle weakness in this type of myopathy.[46]

Because of the necrosis of muscle, it is thought that these patients would probably not respond well to an exercise program, but function should be maintained if possible. They should be given appropriate pain relieving modalities and assistive and mobility devices to help with ADL and safe ambulation. The environment should be altered to help ensure safety and easy access.

Carcinomatous Neuropathy and Myopathy

This entity occurs with metastatic disease and affects peripheral nerve and muscle due to toxic or immunopathologic effects of the tumor. Diminished reflexes and sensation occur.[46]

The rehabilitation treatment is similar to that recommended in the management of carcinomatous myopathy. However, distal weakness occurs in addition to the proximal weakness, and appropriate bracing to improve ankle dorsiflexion may be needed. If weakness is severe, an electric scooter may be needed. Several assistive devices to help with hand function are useful.

Steroid Myopathy

Steroid muscle weakness is really a selective atrophy of type II fibers in proximal muscles. It tends not to affect neck flexor muscles. It may be superimposed on the weakness of carcinomatous myopathy or polymyositis and dermatomyositis associated myopathy and exacerbate it. It is caused by catabolic and anabolic effects of steroid on muscle. Amino acids leak into the circulation, and there is decreased incorporation of protein into muscle. The condition may be diminished by providing exercise to enhance protein metabolism by muscle.[47] Isometric exercise can be used to accomplish this goal. It may take up to 1 year after cessation of steroids for steroid-induced muscle weakness to return to normal.[48]

BONE DESTRUCTION

For several types of cancer, many patients develop metastases to bone during the course of the disease.[28,49,50] Most metastatic lesions result from carcinoma of the breast, lung, kidney, and colon, and prostate, bladder, ovaries, and uterus are frequent sites of primary lesions.[51] Leukemias, lymphomas, and myelomas may invade the bone marrow. The axial skeleton and the proximal extremities are most often affected.

Evaluation of Skeletal Involvement

The most frequent symptom associated with bony involvement is pain, usually localized, dull, aching, and more severe at night. Patients with multiple sites of involvement frequently describe pain as sharp or burning in nature. If this pain is brought on by weight bearing it may indicate a pathologic fracture. Bone involvement may result in neuropathic or radicular pain through entrapment or compression of nerves or nerve roots. Any cancer patient with new localized pain symptoms or cancer survivor with atypical pain should be evaluated for skeletal metastases. A bone scan provides the simplest means of screening for bony lesions. The plain x-ray film provides the best method for characterizing the local extent of lesions. A computed tomography (CT) scan may be needed to further evaluate the extent of cortical involvement. Magnetic resonance imaging (MRI) does not provide good visualization of bone and is not suitable for this purpose.

Prevention and Management of Pathologic Fractures

Pathologic fractures can limit mobility in a marginally functioning patient and, in some cases, lead to significant morbidity and mortality. Hip fractures are particularly debilitating and often difficult to stabilize, and they may lead to a significant hemorrhage. Prevention of pathologic fracture is important. Fracture should be considered imminent if the size of a lytic lesion exceeds 60% of the total bone width, if cortical involvement exceeds 50%, or if the axial extent of cortical destruction exceeds 13 mm in the femoral neck and 30 mm elsewhere.[52] Pain with weight bearing suggests a need to reduce load on the affected structure.

A cane used in the hand opposite the affected extremity can theoretically remove about 50% of body weight from that extremity. Attachments, such as a quadruped base (quad-cane) or a forearm support (forearm or Lofstrand crutch), may help to stabilize the cane, but they cannot overcome the simple physics of gravitation loading. Canes or single crutches can be used for the patient who has pain with weight bearing, but they should not be used for the patient with a fracture or one that is imminent.

Bilateral support is essential for the patient in whom no weight bearing is required. For the more debilitated patient, a simple walker suffices. For the more active patient, axillary or forearm crutches may be used. Toe touch of the affected leg can usually be allowed, but in the patient who has difficulty coordinating the use of crutches or walker, total avoidance of weight bearing may be needed to avoid sudden weight bearing if the assistive device is not properly placed. Care must be taken to evaluate for the possibility of metastatic disease in the upper extremities. It is quite possible to develop a pathologic fracture of an involved humerus if it is used as a weight-bearing structure. The patient should be cautioned against torquing the affected extremity, because this can often lead to fracture, even without weight bearing.

After an affected extremity has been unweighted, options for stabilization can be considered. Radiation often can be used to treat lesions of the long bones. Irradiation does not directly repair damaged bone, and irradiated bone heals much more slowly than normal bone. For small lesions, irradiation with the use of a cane may be all that is required. For larger lesions, surgical stabilization should be considered if possible. Intramedullary rods or methylmethacrylate can be used to increase strength of the invaded bone or, if used prophylactically, to stabilize a painful lesion and prevent fractures.[53] This gives the patient a more functional limb and allows increased mobility.

Destruction of the femoral head or acetabulum may be treated with hip joint arthroplasty, making ambulation a possibility while providing excellent palliation of pain. Fractures of the ischium may be painful during sitting and should be treated with cushions to reduce weight bearing over the fracture. Fractures of a single portion of the pelvic ring are generally not a problem. Multiple fractures, however, can interfere with ambulation and should be addressed appropriately. Fractures of the iliac wing may be painful during active hip flexion and abduction, due to the attachments of the iliacus and gluteal abductors, respectively. Assistive devices used to avoid activation of these muscles during ambulation can provide significant relief of pain.

Ribs are a common site of bony involvement and fracture. Generally, only a rib belt is required. Pathologic fractures of nonweight-bearing bones can be managed with splinting or sling immobilization while irradiation is delivered. ROM or isometric exercises may be appropriate to maintain function. If a dominant upper extremity is involved, assistive devices and training in one-handed strategies by an occupational therapist can significantly improve function. Devices such as reachers and dressing aids can help the patient to avoid torquing the spine or hips if the risk of fracture is high.

SPINAL COLUMN INVOLVEMENT

The emergency management of tumor-related spinal cord compression is discussed elsewhere. The rehabilitation team can assist in the prediction, prevention, and rehabilitation of vertebral column and spinal cord dysfunction resulting from malignant invasion or as a side effect of treatment. Prevention of disabling vertebral collapse requires a high index of suspicion for any patient with known or suspected malignancy, past or present, that frequently metastasizes to bone, such as tumors of breast, lung, and prostate.

Evaluation of Suspected Spine Involvement

One of the earliest indicators of spine involvement is pain.[54] The diagnosis of mechanical back pain should be one of exclusion in this population. Particular features that should alert the clinician are pain that is unrelated to activities or position, pain that is worse at night or when lying down, and pain associated with neurologic symptoms such as sciatica, muscle weakness, sensory loss, and particularly loss of bowel or bladder control. Hyperreflexia may be masked by peripheral neuropathy or plexopathy related to chemotherapy or irradiation, and patients with extensive metastatic involvement of the vertebral column may have little or no pain.

In the patient who presents with neurologic deficits, the physician must always rule out spinal cord compression by tumor. Other causes of paraparesis in the cancer patient include peripheral neuropathy, lumbosacral plexitis, radiation myelitis, and pseudotumor, often from radiation fibrosis. Radiation-related paraparesis may not occur for some time after the completion of all treatment. We have seen patients with radiation myelitis presenting as long as 7 years after having been declared free of disease.

Screening of suspected spinal involvement with a bone scan can be helpful, although this technique may not image epidural or intramedullary tumors. Myelography, previously the method of choice for detection of epidural involvement in cases of neurologic symptoms, has largely been supplanted by the use of magnetic resonance imaging (MRI).[55–58] Intramedullary tumors are particularly difficult to detect by any imaging modality, and they may mimic radiation myelitis.[59] Suspicion is often based on clinical grounds alone.

Issues of Stability

The prevention of serious spinal cord injury should be the primary initial goal of the cancer rehabilitation team in treating the patient with known vertebral destruction by primary or metastatic disease. Although radiation treatment may be used to control tumor growth and to relieve spinal cord compression, this does not address the issue of spinal stability.

Although no good models of vertebral collapse from tumor exist, it has been assumed that spinal stability in the cancer patient can be addressed in much the same way that it is in the patient with a traumatic injury of the spine.[60] The most widely accepted method of stability evaluation involves the concept of three columns.[61,62] This method considers the spine to be made up of three supporting columns, consisting of the anterior, middle, and posterior structures of the vertebrae, roughly divided into equal thirds. Any two of these supporting columns must be intact for the spine to be stable. For example, complete destruction of a vertebral body is usually unstable, because the posterior structures (facet joints) can easily sublux. A simple compression fracture, however, is usually stable because the posterior and middle columns are relatively intact. Of particular concern are lesions at the atlantoaxial and thoracolumbar junctions, due to the significant bending and torquing moments generated at these interfaces.

Whenever possible, an unstable lesion of the bony spine should be stabilized surgically, because virtually no brace can be completely effective in preventing subluxation. Irradiated bone heals slowly and often incompletely, and continued malignant destruction may sometimes occur. It is desirable from the rehabilitation standpoint to mobilize the patient as quickly as possible to prevent the complications associated with immobility. Even if there is extensive vertebral destruction, surgical stabilization can usually be accomplished by means of rods, strut grafts, and cement.[63,64] Occasionally, extensive multilevel involvement may make it impossible to find adequate healthy bone to which stabilizing hardware can be attached, or the patient's health may preclude any surgical option. In such cases, bracing may provide the only means of protecting the spinal canal.

Although a variety of spinal orthotics is available, some commonly used neck and back braces have no place in the management of the unstable spine. The soft cervical collar, for example, may provide comfort to the patient with neck pain, but it provides virtually no significant limitation in cervical motion. Beyond a doubt, the only cervical orthotic that provides virtually complete immobilization of all but the lowest cervical segments is the halo brace.[65] This device is attached directly to the skull using bone pins and to the chest using a plastic vest or plaster cast. Unfortunately, many cancer patients cannot tolerate the degree of chest immobilization resulting from this type of brace.

If it becomes necessary to use a more "practical" cervical stabilization orthotic, selection should be based on the level of potential instability and the directions of motion that might lead to instability.[66] The Philadelphia collar, consisting of a foam collar with rigid supports, provides moderately successful stabilization of higher segments in flexion and extension but inadequate stabilization at lower levels and inadequate stabilization for side bending and rotation, and it is of limited usefulness as a spinal stabilization brace.

Two alternatives that provide excellent stabilization of lower segments in flexion and extension are the two-poster and sternal occipital mandibular immobilization (SOMI) braces. The SOMI is particularly useful in managing debilitated patients, due to its open design and the ease with which it can be applied, because all components are attached from the front. It can be used with a light-weight chest piece as supplied, or it can be bolted onto a lower spinal orthotic, as shown in Figure 66–3, making it useful in cases of multilevel instability. An alternative cervical thoracic orthosis is the Yale brace, which essentially consists of a Philadelphia collar attached to a thoracic extension. With any of these orthotics, the patient must be informed that the brace is a compromise solution, and that care is indicated, particularly with motions not well supported by the particular brace.

Stabilization of the thoracolumbar regions is generally done using two basic types of bracing. Metal braces such as the Jewitt or the Taylor-Knight orthoses can be fit to the patient rapidly, providing optimal limitation of flexion and extension (Fig. 66–4). The custom-molded plastic thoracolumbosacral orthotic, or body jacket, additionally provides limitation in rotation as well. Body jackets can be padded to enhance comfort, and they can be perforated to reduce heat build-up, which is a frequent problem. They can be fabricated using a one-piece anterior opening design that can be applied independently by the patient, although a two-piece "clam shell" design is preferred in the unstable spine, because it can be donned and doffed with assistance by "log-rolling" the patient to apply first the back half and then the front half. Unfortunately, these braces are frequently poorly tolerated in the debilitated patient with atrophic skin. Elastic back braces and corsets, often used in the management of mechanical low back pain, do not provide adequate limitations in motion to be used for spinal stabilization, although rigid corsets may be worthy of consideration in the patient who absolutely cannot tolerate anything else.

High thoracic lesions and cases of extensive vertebral involvement may require the use of a combination orthotic. A cervical extension or SOMI brace can, for example, be attached to a body jacket, providing restricted mobility of the entire spine, as shown in Figure 66–5. These braces should be worn whenever the patient is upright or travels in a motor vehicle. When the patient lies in bed without the brace, the head of the bed should not be elevated by more than 30°. Patients should be cautioned against twisting or torquing their backs, because this may potentiate the injury. Cervical orthoses should be worn even when the patient is recumbent and removed only in a supervised setting.

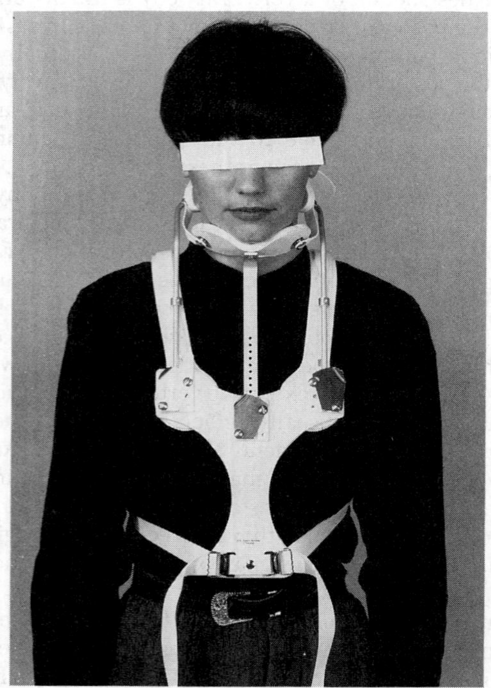

FIGURE 66–3. Sternal occipital mandibular immobilization brace (SOMI).

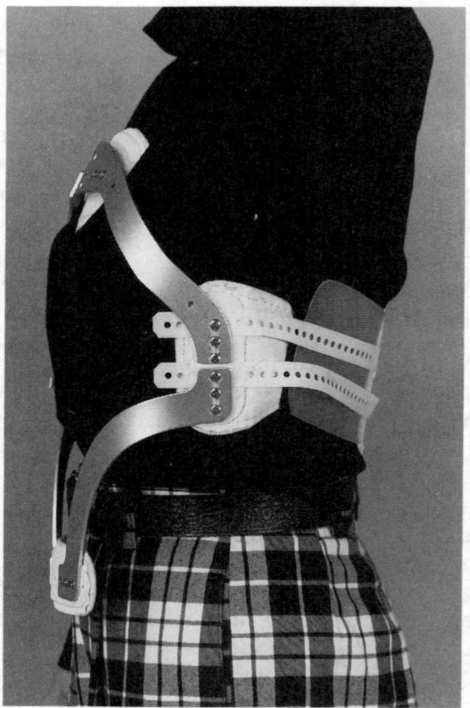

FIGURE 66–4. Taylor-Knight orthosis.

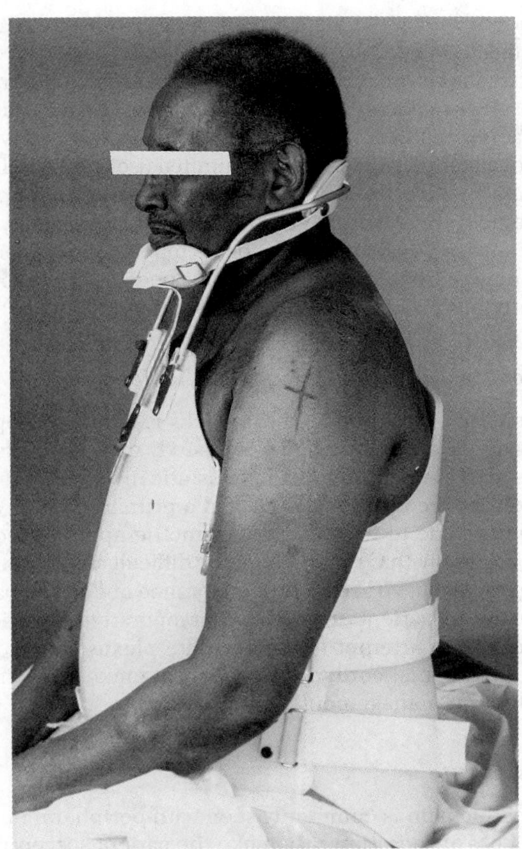

FIGURE 66–5. SOMI brace attached to a body jacket.

Spinal Cord Injury Syndromes

Spinal cord disorders in cancer patients may result from malignant invasion, bony compression or trauma, syrinx or hematoma formation, radiation myelitis, or vascular events. Radiation myelitis is directly related to radiation dose and often does not develop until years after the completion of therapy.[67] Spinal cord dysfunction has been associated with high-dose intrathecal chemotherapy.[68,69]

The degree of functional impairment in a spinal cord disorder is related to the level of the lesion and to its degree of completeness. The level of a lesion is by American convention the last fully functional spinal root level. For example, a C5 (cervical root 5) quadriplegic has intact function of the biceps brachii (innervated primarily by C5 and C6), with intact sensation over the shoulders and lateral aspects of the arms. A C5 quadriplegic is able to bring the hand to the mouth but requires assistance for most self-care. A level of C4 is required for unassisted breathing. C6 quadriplegics have intact wrist extension, allowing some light grasp through the tenodesis effect. C7 quadriplegics are able to extend the elbows, making it possible for them to lift themselves, performing their own weight shifts. C8 and T1 are required for intact hand function.

The remaining thoracic segments are of significance primarily in the motor control of trunk stability. In the lower spine, the degree of functional use of the legs is more vague due to the extensive overlap of motor segments. Generally, hip and knee extensor strength of sufficient magnitude to overcome gravity (3/5) are essential for safe ambulation. Although long leg braces can be used for paraplegic ambulation, the level of energy required is usually beyond the capability of many healthy persons, let alone the patient debilitated by cancer. Short leg braces or ankle-foot orthoses (AFOs) can be used effectively to compensate for the loss of ankle dorsiflexors and plantarflexors. In selected patients with intact hip musculature, AFOs that limit dorsiflexion can be used to create an extension moment at the knee, substituting for quadriceps function during the stance phase of gait.

Damage of the central portion of the spinal cord may occur with the outer portions being spared. This may occur with intramedullary tumors, with syrinx formation, or in certain vascular events. The central cord syndrome is characterized by loss of upper extremity function, with relative sparing of function in the legs. If only one side of the spinal cord is involved, the Brown-Sequard syndrome results, in which motor function is affected on the ipsilateral side while most sensory function is affected on the contralateral side.

Rehabilitation in Spinal Cord Impairment

Because of the complexities involved with spinal cord dysfunction, rehabilitation should be provided by those familiar with management of spinal cord injury. Assisted mobility using manual or motorized wheel chairs or crutches or canes with braces are usually required. Adaptive equipment and strategies for self-care may be needed in the cancer patient with spinal cord involvement.

Bowel and bladder dysfunction in this patient population is virtually universal, requiring particular attention. Even in the patient with apparent normal voiding, silent bladder, and sphincter spasticity may lead to infection, bladder reflux, and significant morbidity. We have seen cases of hydronephrosis with almost complete destruction of the kidneys in asymptomatic persons. Foley catheters may be used for short-term management if there are other medical indications. Otherwise, intermittent catheterization done frequently enough to keep the bladder volume less than 500 ml is the method of choice during the acute phase. A urologist should be consulted after the patient has stabilized. Regular use of laxatives as part of a bowel training program are frequently required.

Autonomic dysreflexia or hyperreflexia is a true emergency in the spinal cord impaired patient. When the spinal cord level is T6 or above, uncontrolled vasoconstriction and severe hypertension may result. Paradoxically, the heart rate is often slowed due to the intact vagus nerve. The first objective should be to lower the blood pressure as quickly as possible. Sitting the patient upright helps to reduce intracerebral pressure. A fast-acting agent such as sublingual nifedipine may be used initially, followed by a longer-acting agent such as nitroprusside, if needed. After the blood pressure has been stabilized, the cause, usually a noxious stimulus, should be isolated and corrected. The most common cause is an overdistended bladder, and distended bowel and skin trauma are other possible explanations.

NEUROPATHIES AND PLEXOPATHIES

Peripheral nerve involvement is a common diagnostic dilemma in the cancer patient. Dysfunction of peripheral nerves usually results from the use of cisplatin or vincristine and irradiation.[20,70–74] Peripheral neuropathies and plexopathies can be the result of direct tumor invasion or a paraneoplastic syndrome.

Chemotherapy-Induced Neuropathies

Generally chemotherapy-related neuropathies tend to be distal and symmetric. Occasionally, initial symptoms are unilateral, mimicking a mononeuritis or invasive lesion. Vincristine and cisplatin are documented causes of autonomic neuropathies.[75,76] In some instances, this has been severe enough to mimic spinal cord involvement.[77] Cytarabine (ara-C) has caused brachial plexus neuropathy.[78] Suramin, largely an experimental drug, has caused a profound polyneuropathy mimicking Guillain-Barré syndrome. Agents that are lipid soluble or that have metabolites with a prolonged half-life may lead to a progressive neuropathy, even after discontinuance of the drug.[79]

Vincristine seems to induce distal axonal degeneration similar to that of other toxic neuropathies.[20] Because of this, the duration of the neuropathy tends to be prolonged because of the time needed for nerve fiber regeneration. Many patients receiving this agent develop sensory complaints of numbness and paresthesias. Some patients develop severe neuropathic pain. Often the degree of motor neuropathy is significant, sometimes resulting in a virtual quadriparesis. Although it may take months after cessation of chemotherapy to recover function, recovery is usually complete. Neurotoxicity is one of the most common reasons for limiting the dosage of vincristine chemotherapy.

Neuropathies due to cisplatin generally tend to be less frequent and often milder. Unfortunately, we have treated several patients who have developed a severe permanent neuropathy from the use of cisplatin. There does not seem to be any common factor that can be used to predict the development of lasting neuropathy. Rarely is an adjustment in cisplatin dosage indicated.[70]

Brachial Plexopathies

Radiation-induced brachial plexopathy is an uncommon problem in the conservative management of breast cancer if supraclavicular and axillary lymph nodes are irradiated. It may be seen as a late effect of mantle irradiation for Hodgkin's disease. Onset of symptoms is usually delayed. In one study, onset of symptoms occurred with a median time of 4.5 months after the cessation of radiation treatment, and full recovery was usually observed.[74] In another study, symptoms began more than 1 year after therapy, and the overall prognosis for recovery was poor.[72]

Differentiation of radiation from neoplastic plexitis is essential. Severe pain has been documented in 80% of patients with infiltrating tumor, but only 19% of patients with radiation injury described this finding.[80] Horner's syndrome is more common in cases of tumor involvement, and lymphedema is a much more common concomitant finding in radiation injury. The distribution of involvement of the brachial plexus is an important diagnostic criterion, with 72% of patients with invasive tumor having involvement of the lower trunk and 78% of patients with radiation injury having involvement of the upper trunk.

Electrodiagnostically, myokymic discharges are virtually diagnostic of radiation plexitis, occurring in 63% of patients.[81] Other abnormalities are common in both types of injury, with nerve conduction studies being of limited usefulness.[82] Tumor detection by MRI provides definitive evidence of neoplastic involvement. Even without visible tumor during surgery, neoplastic disease has sometimes been found microscopically, and it may not be possible to rule out neoplastic plexopathy for many months after the onset of symptoms.[73,83]

Lumbosacral Plexopathy and Radiculopathy

Involvement of the lumbosacral plexus is common in pelvic tumors due to direct invasion.[84] In a study of 11 patients with lumbosacral plexopathy, 6 had metastatic involvement, 2 had radiation-induced plexopathy, 1 had a primary tumor, and 2 had neuritis due to intraarterial chemotherapy.[85] Direct imaging of tumor with CT or MRI may be difficult after irradiation or surgery. We have seen a preponderance of delayed painful plexopathy in patients receiving intraoperative radiation. It is important to attempt to differentiate plexus lesions from those of the spinal cord, due to the difference in treatment, rehabilitation management, and prognosis.

Management

Neuropathic pain is commonly seen with peripheral neuropathies. Loss of sensation may make the patient susceptible to skin injury. The patient with insensate skin should be cautioned about the avoidance of potential injuries from burns and sharp objects and about the need for daily skin inspection to avoid the development of infection. Loss of proprioceptive feedback, particularly in the patient with impaired vision, may interfere with simple fine motor tasks and with ambulation. A cane can provide proprioceptive feedback to the upper extremities in the patient with impaired proprioception in the lower extremities. Motor impairment is treated similarly to other neurologic disorders, with bracing and adaptive devices as needed.

REHABILITATION ASPECTS OF PAIN CONTROL

In addition to the use of narcotic agents, which has become the mainstay of palliative treatment in the cancer patient, the physical modalities of pain control may significantly help to alleviate suffering. More aggressive approaches, including nerve blocks and rhizotomies, have been used with limited success. Sympathetic nerve blocks and sympathectomies may be effective in patients with the reflex sympathetic dystrophy syndrome. Trigger point injections are sometimes helpful in musculoskeletal pain disorders.

The use of physical modalities can be particularly effective adjunct in the management of pain in the cancer patient. Heat modalities, including superficial heat, shortwave diathermy and ultrasound may provide relief in musculoskeletal pain syndromes, but ultrasound may help to spread lymphatic disease. Other heat modalities increase circulation to the affected area, questionably increasing the potential for metastatic spread. Therapeutic cold can sometimes help to reduce pain.

Electrical stimulation has met with increasing criticism in the literature, but we have found electrical stimulation to be effective in reducing narcotics usage in a variety of cancer patients with a variety of pain syndromes. It seems to be particularly effective in the management of phantom limb pain and in treating radiculopathy and incisional pain. If effective, the patient can be provided with a pocket-sized TENS unit, which can be used as needed. Electrodes should be placed at the site of maximum pain or, in the case of referred pain, at the site of the lesion. A conventional high-frequency setting is usually most effective. Many TENS units are available at modest cost.

LYMPHEDEMA AND DEEP VENOUS THROMBOSIS

The swollen extremity is often a diagnostic dilemma in the patient with a history of cancer. Because of the possibility of malignant compression or invasion of lymphatics or venous drainage, and because of the possibility of deep venous thrombosis, a swollen extremity should always be fully evaluated in the cancer patient or cancer survivor. Idiopathic lymphedema, rather than edema secondarily caused by infection or tumor, should be a diagnosis of exclusion. Tumor can usually be excluded by imaging studies such as CT, MRI, or bone scan, or in extreme instances, by lymphangiogram.

Deep venous thrombosis can usually be ruled out using impedance plethysmography or ultrasound.[86,87] If certainty is required, a venogram can be done. Suspected pulmonary embolism can be evaluated with a ventilation-perfusion scan or more definitively by pulmonary angiography. The greatest risk of embolization is from proximal thromboses.[88]

Lymphedema in the cancer patient is frequent with lymph node involvement or after lymph node dissection. Late edema is usually related to radiation therapy and the gradual development of fibrous tissue. Edema in a nonirradiated extremity should always be thoroughly evaluated, and remediable causes, such as infection or cardiovascular causes, should be treated.

The simplest means of minimizing edema is to keep the affected extremity elevated as often as possible. Legs should be placed on an elevated foot support, preferably keeping the feet above the level of the heart. Arms should be rested on a high table surface. A sling may be of short-term benefit. Isometric exercises, by increasing muscle tone, may help to minimize edema.

The mainstay of lymphedema management is the compressive garment. Compressive stockings in the legs and elastic sleeves in the arms can significantly reduce swelling. These are designed with a pressure gradient such that the pressure exerted by the garment distally is greater than that proximally. This is to ensure fluid flow in a proximal direction. Compressive garments should always be used over the entire extent of the edema. A stocking that only reaches the knee tends to develop tightness and occlude lymphatic and venous return if there is significant edema in the thigh. Ready-made garments are available in a variety of sizes. These should not be confused with the thin elastic support hose frequently used on hospital wards that are ineffective in edema management.

Patients with long-standing lymphedema should usually be fitted for custom-made compressive garments, which provide an optimized pressure gradient. Care should be taken with the use of compressive garments in insensate patients and in those with open wounds due to the potential for impaired circulation and local ischemia. The one major drawback of elastic garments is that they are extremely difficult to don and doff. A newer nonelastic compressive orthotic, which consists of a series of adjustable straps, is much easier to apply, but it is rather unsightly.[89]

In some patients, the use of compressive garments alone is not sufficient to manage severe lymphedema. For these patients, compressive pumps may provide the answer. These pumps consist of an inflatable garment that is cyclically filled with air, pressing fluid out of the affected extremity. There are two types of pumps: single-chamber devices and sequential multichamber devices. Single-chamber pumps are relatively inexpensive and can easily be used by the patient at home. Sequential devices can be extremely effective, although at a higher cost.[90] Sequential pumping can be so effective as to put the patient with cardiovascular compromise into cardiovascular overload. It is often preferable to start use of this device in an inpatient setting. In some cases, it may be necessary to use the sequential pump at home on a nightly basis, wearing compressive stockings during the day. Caution when using compressive pumps and other techniques should be taken if there is a potential for residual tumor to be mobilized into venous or lymphatic channels.

BOWEL AND BLADDER DISORDERS

Oncologic patients develop bowel and bladder difficulties for a variety of reasons. Bowel obstruction or urethral or ureteral compromise is usually the result of malignant invasion or compression. Constipation and urinary hesitancy are frequently related to the use of medication, particularly narcotics and drugs with anticholinergic properties. Input from the rehabilitation team is most often needed if there is neurologic dysfunction or in ostomy care.

Management of Bowel Dysfunction

Disorders of fecal elimination are frequently the most significant complaint of the cancer patient. Constipation is extremely common and is best treated using dietary modifications and medication. Often, a high-fiber diet with copious fluid intake is all that is required to ensure regularity. If fiber supplements are used, the patient should be cautioned about the absolute need for fluid intake, because bulk in the absence of fluid can lead to impaction. If necessary, stool softeners such as docusate (*e.g.*, docusate sodium, 50–200 mg/day) can be added to reduce straining. A stimulant medication such as metoclopramide (metoclopramide hydrochloride, 10 mg 30 minutes before meals and at bedtime) can be used for delayed gastric emptying.

When spontaneous defecation does not occur, a stimulant agent may be required. A mild preparation with a well-controlled transit time, such as an over-the-counter senna preparation, is preferred. A standard dose of senna (*e.g.*, Senokot, 2 tablets) at bedtime usually results in controlled defecation in the morning. Stronger agents such as bisacodyl (5–15 mg) or magnesium hydroxide (milk of magnesia, 30 ml) may be used in more recalcitrant cases, although it should be kept in mind that magnesium is mildly nephrotoxic. Cathartics such as magnesium citrate should be used as a last resort and only if there is no suspicion of obstruction or impaction.

In the patient with neurogenic bowel dysfunction, stimulation from below may be required. Digital stimulation, or if needed, use of a glycerin or bisacodyl (10 mg) suppository, should usually be sufficient to initiate evacuation. Rarely, an enema may be required. By instituting a regular bowel training program in which full evacuation is achieved on a daily or every-other-day basis through the use of medications and rectal stimulation, it is usually possible to achieve continence.

Diarrhea in the cancer patient is usually the result of chemotherapy. Standard antidiarrheal preparations, narcotics, and anticholingergics may be used. If occurring in the face of antibiotics, pseudomembranous colitis resulting from infection with *Clostridium difficile* should always be ruled out. Other bacterial or parasitic diarrheas should be treated with appropriate antibiotics, as determined by stool culture or smear. Narcotic antidiarrheals should be avoided in this case due to the potential for developing toxic megacolon. Viral diarrhea should be allowed to run its course.

Management of the Neurogenic Bladder

Proper evaluation and management of bladder dysfunction in cancer patients with neurologic abnormalities is essential to the prevention of significant morbidity. Although bladder dysfunction is often arbitrarily divided into disorders of incontinence or reduced bladder capacity and disorders of retention, this model is overly simplistic. Patients with spinal cord or brain stem involvement should always undergo formal evaluation of bladder function.

There may be various combinations of a spastic or flaccid bladder and a spastic or flaccid urinary sphincter.[91] The combination of a spastic bladder and sphincter is the most dangerous, because this can lead to reflux, causing hydronephrosis or upper tract infection, or to autonomic hyperreflexia. Medications such as oxybutynin (oxybutynin chloride, 5 mg 2–4 times daily) can be used to reduce bladder spasticity, but mechanical means of drainage may be needed.[92] Urinary tract infections are frequent in the patient with neurogenic bladder, and proper evaluation and treatment is mandatory.

In the acute phase of management, an indwelling catheter is usually sufficient if there are appropriate medical indications. Catheters should be removed as soon as the patient is stable, so as to minimize the risk of infection. In the patient who appears to be voiding normally, evaluation for possible retention should still be done. Postvoid residual urine volumes as determined by catheterization or by ultrasound should be less than 50 ml. If the patient does exhibit retention, intermittent catheterization should be instituted, taking care to catheterize frequently enough to keep bladder volumes less than 500 ml. In the incontinent patient without retention, condom (Texas) catheters may be used for men. Collection devices for women are often less than satisfactory.

Management of the Ostomy Patient

Cancer patients may have ostomies for a variety of reasons. Ureteral stints are often used in patients with ureteral obstruction, occasionally in combination with a temporary ostomy for kidney drainage. Patients with bladder carcinoma may have a ureteral diversion to an ileal loop, which is drained through an ostomy. Patients with bowel carcinoma or other types of bowel obstruction may need a temporary or permanent ostomy for fecal elimination. This may be required at any level of the small bowel or colon. Ileostomies, involving diversion of the terminal small bowel, are sometimes problematic because of the volume of fluid present in the fecal contents before entry into the colon. An ileal pouch is sometimes created surgically as a reservoir for urine or ileal fluid as a means of providing continence.

In cases of neck tumors or if there is impaired swallowing, a gastrostomy may be required for supplemental nutrition. This can often be placed by percutaneous endoscopic gastrostomy (PEG), eliminating the need for major surgery. Tracheostomies are often used in cases of head or neck tumors or if there is a need for prolonged access to the airway, as in the patient with severe cognitive impairment and uncontrolled tracheal secretions. Gastrostomies and tracheostomies are discussed in more detail in the section on head and neck cancer.

Ostomy training should be a regular part of the cancer patient's rehabilitation process.[93] Proper clean technique avoids the likelihood of infection. Proper attention to skin care should avoid maceration and breakdown. Occasionally, a bowel training program can be instituted for colostomy patients, regularizing emptying and sometimes eliminating the need for an ostomy bag. A variety of ostomy collections systems are available, including one-piece collection bags that are applied directly to the skin using an adhesive and two-piece collection bags involving an occlusive seal that is applied to the skin and a separate detachable bag.[94] Collection bags may be closed and disposed of with each use or open, allowing for drainage and reuse. One- and two-piece barriers may be used to help patients maintain continence. Support groups for ostomy patients are available in most areas, and a variety of patient information materials are available.[95–100]

PSYCHOSOCIAL ASPECTS OF CANCER REHABILITATION

The rehabilitation team has an opportunity to help plan, supervise, and reinforce behaviors that may ameliorate symptoms of distress. These should be directed toward reducing stress and anxiety, improving fitness and performance, enhancing coping, and maintaining optimism.

Management of Stress

Cancer staging and treatment planning often require patients to go through multiple steps, during or after which choices have to be made. This is a particularly stressful time for patients and their families. Relaxation training using relaxation tapes and a low-level aerobic program is effective in reducing anxiety and depression. The rehabilitation process requires a commitment to participate in therapies on the part of the patient. This therapeutic alliance, oriented toward patient valued outcomes often addresses some aspects of the uncertainty that lies ahead and permits patients to be proactive in their own care.

Management of Depression

Cancer patients are psychologically vulnerable for several reasons. Often these include facing a serious illness with concerns about life expectancy and disability. Some cancer patients worry that the treatments and their results may cause family and friends to spurn them. The rehabilitation team can provide support and can suggest exercise at an appropriate level that may confer a sense of mastery, control, and offer the antidepressant benefits associated with exercise.

REHABILITATION AND MANAGEMENT OF SPECIFIC TUMORS

BREAST CARCINOMA

Rehabilitation interventions for patients undergoing modified or radical mastectomy, lumpectomy, and axillary dissection have usually included treatment for painful or immobile shoulders or swollen upper extremities or to restore functional activity. Because treatments for control of breast cancer vary widely, the rehabilitation interventions must be customized. Clinical experience has taught that a three-level axillary dissection is associated with more lymphedema than a less complete dissection. The patient with the more extensive surgery needs closer monitoring of upper extremity edema. The patient receiving chest irradiation is likely to experience chest wall tenderness and possible rib fractures and should be informed and monitored for the occurrence of these problems.

The prognosis of breast cancer is good and because its expression may occur in any decade of life after the first, early rehabilitation may play an important role in preserving function and returning the patient to her previous level of activity. A direct relation between physical therapy and good shoulder motion is established.[101] The converse has been demonstrated. Delaying physical therapy as little as 7 to 10 days postoperatively results in moderately severe limitation of shoulder abduction.[102] Some caution must be exercised in introducing shoulder motion immediately postoperatively, because this may result in increased axillary drainage and delayed wound healing.[35,102]

Most of the studies cited were performed in women receiving radical or modified radical mastectomy. However, one prospective study compared radical mastectomy with lumpectomy patients with respect to arm motion and found the latter group had better motion at 3 months.[103] None of the women received axillary dissection. Another study demonstrated no difference between a group receiving modified radical mastectomy or lumpectomy and axillary dissection at 1 or 2 years after definitive therapy.[104]

Typically, arm mobilization begins on postoperative day 1 or 2, with joint rotation to tolerance but restricted abduction and flexion to 40°. By day 4, flexion is gradually advanced to 45° and increased by 10° to 15° per day if tolerated. Abduction is held at 45° until the drains are removed and then advanced to tolerance.[35]

The incidence of lymphedema is not precisely known. This is in part a result of lack of uniform measurement techniques to assess it and few prospective, long-term studies to evaluate it. There are several types of upper extremity lymphedema, each of which may be characterized by its time of onset after treatment and associated clinical findings. The first is acute, transient, and mild, occurring within a few days of surgery, and is a result of cutting of lymphatic channels. It usually responds within a week of onset after arm elevation and hand pumping (*i.e.*, making a fist and releasing it). The second is acute, painful, and occurs 4 to 6 weeks postoperatively as a result of acute lymphangitis or phlebitis. This type can successfully be treated with arm elevation and use of antiinflammatory medication. The third type is an acute erysipeloid form, often occurring after an insect bite or minor injury or burn. It may be superimposed on a chronic edematous limb. This form of edema often requires arm elevation and antibiotics. Compression pumping or wrapping is contraindicated if there is infection. The fourth and most common form of lymphedema is usually insidious and painless and not associated with erythema. This form is most frequently apparent 18 to 24 months after surgery. If it develops much later than that, the physician should suspect recurrent tumor in the axilla or chest wall. This form of edema is thought to be due to lymphatic ablation and resultant increased interstitial pressure causing impedance of lymph flow. Successful treatment of this form of edema usually requires the use of compression pumps, single channel or multichannel systems, plus a compression garment. Careful attention to arm positioning so that gravity is eliminated and protection from sun, insect bites, and trauma are important therapeutic interventions.

Although arm motion and lymphedema are two of the most common findings seen in the breast cancer patient, a variety of other sequelae are common to this population (Table 66–2).

The patient undergoing mastectomy is usually provided with a temporary prosthesis that is Dacron filled. This may be used

TABLE 66–2. Clinical Problems After Mastectomy or Axillary Dissection Often Requiring Rehabilitation

Problem	*When Likely to Occur*
Pain	
Incisional	0–2 wk
Dysesthesiae	0–2 wk
Muscle spasm	0–2 wk
Chest wall	3 mo–2 y (usually with radiation)
Edema	
Transient (arm)	0–2 mo
Persistent (arm)	>1 y
Breast	0–2 mo
Weakness	
Serratus anterior	0–3 mo
Loss of motion	
Shoulder	0–3 mo

even if the patient is not comfortable wearing a bra and is simply pinned to an undergarment. After the incision is well healed, a definitive breast prosthesis can be fitted. This is usually done at 3 to 6 weeks postoperatively. There are a variety of types available.[105] Patients who elect breast reconstruction often have a tissue expander placed initially in anticipation of a definitive reconstruction. These patients may benefit from a temporary prosthesis until they are reconstructed.

HEAD AND NECK CANCER

There are approximately 42,000 new cases of oral, pharyngeal, and laryngeal cancers every year.[106] Despite constituting only about 5% of all malignancies, they present with profound deficits and cosmetic deformities. Because these cancers involve body parts that are highly visible, structurally complex, and crucial to survival, optimal interactions between medical treatment and rehabilitative care are necessary to assure adequate physiologic function, socially acceptable cosmesis, and quality psychosocial status.

Approximately 50% of these patients are expected to be disease free after a 5-year period.[106] Survivorship presents major challenges to patients, their families, and their acquaintances. To maintain medical and therapeutic compliance and disease-free status, long-standing habits of tobacco and alcohol abuse must be addressed. Vocational adaptations or changes may be required if return to work is necessary. Alternations of self-concept and body image may lead to seclusion and avoidance of activities such as eating in restaurants or attendance at social and religious activities. Due to isolation and pain, many patients become depressed and fail to thrive. We cannot measure survival in this population just by looking at morbidity or mortality statistics.

The goals of the rehabilitation team in the management of head and neck cancer are to provide counseling and therapeutic intervention aimed at maximizing functional capabilities, compensating for lost function, and preventing secondary complications that may result from disuse and cancer treatment. If we view head and neck cancer as a chronic disease, we must address these goals throughout the course of the disease and provide timely and appropriate interventions in the pretreatment, treatment, posttreatment (survivorship), and terminal stages of the illness.

The functional deficits (items 1 through 7) and needs (items 8 and 9) common to head and neck patients are as follows:

1. Psychosocial deficits
2. Communication or speech deficits
3. Mastication, deglutition, and nutrition deficits
4. Sensory deficits of taste, smell, or vision
5. Auditory and vestibular dysfunction
6. Neck and shoulder dysfunction
7. Disfigurement
8. Tracheostomy management
9. Oral hygiene management

The patient undergoing partial glossectomy or removal of small tumors of the tonsil or palate may experience mild deficits in speech and swallowing that can easily be addressed by therapeutic exercises and prosthetic management. A partial laryngectomy could result in severe swallowing difficulties, including aspiration, but only mild problems with speech and voice. A total laryngectomy requires extensive speech therapy training to use augmentative communication systems or to learn new voice production techniques. In some cases, secondary surgical procedures such as tracheoesophageal fistula (TEF) or tracheoesophageal puncture (TEP) for voice restoration are suggested. The patient undergoing total glossectomy and laryngectomy may require alternative communication systems, or synthetic speech devices, and text telephone (TT) for the communicatively impaired (formerly called telecommunication devices for the deaf [TDD]) and computers for communication.

Tumors of the Aerodigestive System

Tumor sites are from the nose and nasopharynx to the lower border of the cricoid cartilage, including the accessory sinuses and glands. Primary locations of head and neck cancers include:

Oral cavity: tongue, floor of mouth, buccal mucosa, retromolar region, gingivae, lips, roof of mouth, cheeks
Oropharynx: tongue base, pharyngeal walls, soft palate, tonsils, faucial pillars
Nasopharynx
Hypopharynx: pyriform sinuses, postcricoid
Larynx: glottic, supraglottic, subglottic
Salivary glands: parotid, submandibular glands
Cervical nodes

A summary of assessment and treatment components for head and neck cancer patients is given in Table 66–3.

Pretreatment Evaluation

Most head and neck cancers are squamous cell carcinomas arising from the epithelial lining of the aerodigestive tract.[107] Most grow and present as malignant ulcerations of the surface mucosa, sores that do not heal, or areas of leukoplakia and erythema. The most common sites for head and neck cancers are in the oral cavity (including the lips), pharynx, larynx, and salivary glands.[107] Signs and symptoms depend on the tumor location and may include dysphagia, vocal changes, sensory and motor deficits, or pain. In-depth medical evaluation to asses the extent of the tumor begins with diagnostic staging procedures, including a biopsy.

Thorough dental and maxillofacial prosthetic evaluations are needed to examine the structure and function of the oral cavity before medical intervention. Evaluation includes radiographs, impressions and casts, and recording of baseline data. The prosthetist consults with the oncologist and surgeon about the therapy plan, design, and fabrications of the initial surgical prosthesis, implants, and obturators (Fig. 66–6). For patients receiving irradiation and chemotherapy, a plan is developed for dental and oral care before or early in the medical intervention program to control oral infections, stomatitis, and conditions that may lead to later problems. Some patients require dental extractions before irradiation.[108]

Pretreatment evaluation by the clinical social worker, vocational rehabilitation counselor, and an occupational therapist can help to alleviate emotional distress by anticipating

TABLE 66–3. Assessment and Treatment Components for Head and Neck Cancer Patients

Components	*Pretreatment*	*Treatment*	*Survivorship*
Oral sensorimotor examination	×	×	
Clinical examination of oropharyngeal swallow	×	×	
Hearing and balance assessment	×	×	
Speech and voice assessment	×	×	
Dental examination and treatment	×	×	×
Nutrition assessment	×	×	
Instrumental swallowing assessment		×	
Speech and voice therapy		×	
Augmentative/alternative communication		×	×
Dysphagia therapy		×	×
Prosthetic management		×	×
Feeding and dietary management		×	×
Physical therapy		×	
Medical/surgical management	×	×	×
Nursing education	×	×	
Intubation, tracheostomy, stoma management		×	×
Cognitive and memory assessment	×	×	
Communication, language, reading, writing, assessment	×	×	
Lifestyle counseling	×	×	×
Family counseling	×	×	×
Vocational rehabilitation		×	
Community support groups		×	×

changes in vocational and family roles and financial resources.[109]

Before surgery, chemotherapy, or irradiation, a series of baseline diagnostic procedures should be performed to assess premorbid levels of speech and swallowing function that can be used after treatment for assessment of progress. It is important to establish whether any changes are due to treatment or were preexisting. The sensory motor function of the oropharynx, including the tongue, jaw, velum, teeth, oral mucosa, face, and neck areas must be assessed clinically. This examination should include an oral motor examination of the sensation and motion of the structures innervated by cranial nerves V, VII, VIII, IX, X, and XII, which are essential to speech, swallowing, hearing, oral sensation, taste, smell, and saliva-

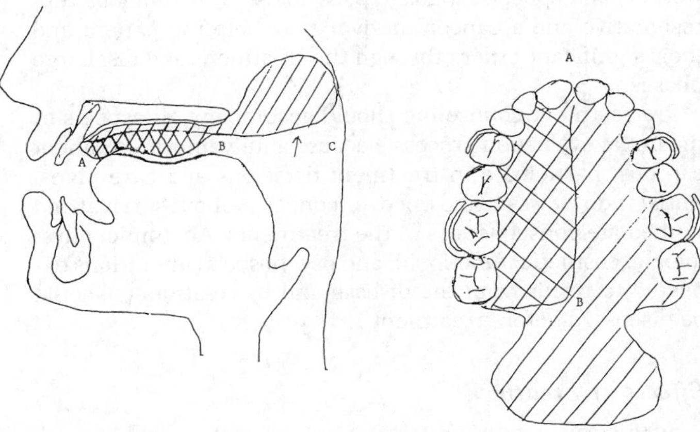

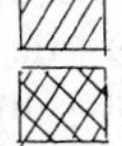

FIGURE 66–6. Palatal augmentation obturator: Speech prosthesis for a hemiglossectomy with soft palate resection. (Courtesy of Jack Light, DDS)

tion.[110] In a complete workup of preoperative function the aerodigestive system should be examined radiographically for masses, lesions, and structural deviations. Speech should be assessed and recorded to determine whether articulation, vocal quality, pitch, resonance, frequency, or prosody has changed subsequent to disease progression. Long-standing patterns of deviant speech or misarticulations should be described, because old errors can contribute to the success of speech therapy.

Because many tumors and medications can affect the VIII (auditory) nerve and its pathway to the cortex and cause hearing impairment, hearing levels, emission, balance, and vestibular functioning should be assessed by an audiologist or an otolaryngologist before surgery.[111] Impaired auditory acuity can reduce ability of the patient to monitor his or her speech production, and the patient may not demonstrate maximal progress during speech rehabilitation.

Before starting cancer treatment, it is important to evaluate the nutritional status and food preferences of each patient.[112,113] A pretreatment screening assessment should examine mastication, jaw alignment, dental status and deviations, oral hygiene, periodontal condition, and salivary flow. The examiner should question whether there are any complaints of difficulty swallowing pills, painful swallowing, choking, reflux or heartburn, or avoidance of certain food textures or prolonged duration of eating. Patients at risk of aspiration should be advised that they may require a temporary or permanent feeding tube.

Screening for existence of cognitive dysfunction (*e.g.*, memory, reasoning, problem-solving ability) and personality or affective disorders is important to determine potential areas of noncompliance. Language usage and comprehension, reading, written expressions, and fine motor coordination should be assessed informally or through interviews, especially for patients who have CNS involvement.

Pretreatment Counseling

Rehabilitation begins at the time of diagnosis and often requires a support team of medical and lay specialists, including the oncologist, dentist, prosthodontist, surgeon, nurse, social worker, and speech-language pathologist.[114] A religious representative and a cancer survivor may help the patient and their significant others through the treatment and discharge phases.

Pretreatment counseling should accompany all aspects of the initial evaluation process, because a fully informed patient can best participate in treatment decisions and care plans. Initial interviews should uncover concerns about survival and immediate consequences of the treatments. Anatomic, physiologic, cosmetic, functional, and psychosocial alterations expected to result from the disease and its treatments should be discussed before treatment.

Effects of Treatment

SENSORY ALTERATIONS. Head and neck cancer patients may experience temporary or permanent auditory or vestibular deficits related to ototoxic medications. Surgical or radiation treatments may affect the functions of the ear or eustachian tubes and diminish auditory acuity. Before treatment, auditory and vestibular testing procedures should be explained, and the need for follow-up monitoring should be mentioned during early counseling sessions. Because these patients are likely to experience alterations in taste and smell as a consequence of the disease and its treatments, counseling should increase awareness of hazards from smoke, spoiled foods, and oral hygiene and include the compensatory use of other senses.[115–117]

SWALLOWING AND NUTRITION. Nutritional status before and during cancer treatment influences recovery.[118] Previous lifestyles and food preferences, combined with the effects of the disease, may cause compromised nutritional status and weight loss. Swallowing abilities may be impaired due to muscular, structural, and sensory changes. Patients need to be informed that they can experience added structural and functional changes from irradiation, chemotherapy, or surgery that can further alter eating and swallowing.[119,120] They should know that there are therapeutic interventions that can restore those functions and reduce the risk of aspiration. Occasionally, swallowing techniques and compensations may be taught and practiced during these pretreatment sessions. The major reason for pretreatment counseling about potential difficulties in swallowing is to prepare the patient for the possibility of therapy and to facilitate compliance and success.

COMMUNICATION ISSUES AND ALTERNATIVES. Because alterations of speech and voice occur after treatment for head and neck cancer, discussion of possible communication changes is important. Counseling allows for exploration of current communication abilities, styles, and needs and the introduction to alternative and augmentative communication methods. It is imperative that the patient be provided with options for communication of basic needs immediately after surgery.[121] A variety of alternatives should be offered, such as use of a buzzer or a bell for general alerting, writing (*i.e.*, pad and pencil, magic slate), or an alphanumeric and picture board communication system. Several types of electrolarynx (*e.g.*, neck and intraoral instruments) should be demonstrated before medical or surgical treatment. Voice and telephone amplifiers can enhance whispered or dysphonic speech. Patients should be assured that a variety of communication options and voice restoration procedures are available later in their course of treatment. This can be accomplished with visits from cancer survivors who have undergone successful speech rehabilitation or with films and literature from the American Cancer Society.

DENTAL PROSTHETIC AND ORAL HYGIENE ISSUES. Counseling, education, and dental evaluation should begin in the pretreatment phase of the disease to effect positive treatment outcomes. Consultation from a maxillofacial prosthetist should be sought for patients who undergo ablative surgery.[122,123] Dental damage and infections may be prevented if patients are seen before or early in their treatment. Regular oral hygiene, attention to dental health, and prophylactic use of fluorides and other soft tissue treatment may be necessary for the remainder of the patient's life.[124] Prophylactic extraction of viable teeth within the field of radiation exposure is often recommended to prevent subsequent jaw necrosis secondary to dental decay.[108]

LIFESTYLE ISSUES. The association between tobacco and oral cancer has been well established, and multiple studies confirm an independent and synergistic relation between head and neck cancer and consumption of alcohol and tobacco.[125] Successful rehabilitation and subsequent survival can be greatly compromised if habits are not changed. Counseling efforts, strategies, and support groups must be introduced early to facilitate modifications in lifestyles that allow the best recovery and prevent mortality from intercurrent and recurrent disease.

Presurgical nursing, self-care counseling, and education may be needed to educate the patient and family to manage tracheostomy or laryngectomy tubes, stoma and secretions, tube feedings, and associated equipment and supplies and to introduce suctioning, oral hygiene, and irrigation techniques.

PAIN. Because pain occurs in most head and neck cancers, pain control issues, including pharmacologic intervention, should be discussed early and throughout the course of care. Tolerances, past experiences, and coping styles need exploration. Whenever possible, objective scales and subjective descriptions of pain should be used.[126,127]

Rehabilitation Issues

CANCER TREATMENT INVENTIONS. Rehabilitation that includes preservation of function and acceptable appearance is a prime consideration for surgical planning. Many surgical reconstructive approaches for voice and cosmetic rehabilitation have been developed during the last 40 years; some are performed as part of the primary surgery, and others are secondary procedures.[128] The surgeon and maxillofacial prosthodontist must evaluate and consult preoperatively, sharing information about the dynamics and limitations of various prosthetics in relation to surgical reconstruction and clinical conditions. If voice restoration surgery (*i.e.*, TEF) is considered as a primary procedure, consultation with and evaluation by a trained speech-language pathologist can provide information that is critical to successful vocal rehabilitation.[129,130]

Neurophysiologic intraoperative monitoring by trained audiologists neurologists, anesthetists, and other physicians is becoming an accepted standard of care in many hospital settings.[131,132] The application of evoked potential measurements and techniques to surgical monitoring may help to avoid or reduce the risk of injury to the auditory and facial nerve pathways.[133]

POSTOPERATIVE SWALLOWING, SPEECH, AND COMMUNICATION EVALUATIONS. On referral of the physician, depending on patient tolerance, the speech-language pathologist reassesses the structure and function of the orolaryngopharyngeal mechanisms for speech and swallowing capabilities postoperatively. In most instances, postsurgical nutrition is provided nonorally (*e.g.*, PEG, nasogastric tube, Keo feed tube). Before resumption of oral intake, the speech-language pathologist conducts a clinical evaluation of oropharyngeal swallow (bedside swallowing evaluation). Careful clinical evaluation of the anatomy and physiology, including range, rate, and coordination of movement, tone and reflexes during a variety of tasks that may include manipulation of material in the mouth, and sensory and speech observations, can reveal much about the oral stages of swallowing, including mastication, bolus preparation and transport.[110,134] However, only instrumental approaches, such as the modified barium swallow, provide objective information about the neuromuscular events of the pharyngeal phase to reveal dangers such as pooling, reflux, reduced peristalsis and aspiration.[134–137] Endoscopy, ultrasound, and scintigraphy provide critical objective information about pharyngeal and laryngeal events, tongue and hyoid movements, and the presence and amount of aspiration.[138] After clinicians gain a thorough understanding of the swallow, they can introduce and objectively judge the efficacy of a variety of management techniques during the radiographic studies.

Dynamic radiographic evaluation by videofluoroscopy and ultrasound can provide useful feedback in evaluation of speech.[139] Some medical centers assess vocal and resonance parameters with instrumentation such as videostroboscopy, nasometry, acoustic spectrographic analysis, palatometers, and glossometers.[140] The severity of speech disorders in this population is a direct result of site and size of the tumor and the variety of reconstructive surgical procedures and prosthetic applications. Reduction of speech intelligibility is due to deviations in articulation, oral and nasal resonance patterns, voice production and quality characteristics, changes of speaking rate and prosody, and preexisting speech impairment. Tests of articulation in a variety of contexts, voice and resonance ratings, measures of diadochokinesis, speaking rate, speech and breathing efficiency, and judgments of overall intelligibility are administered postoperatively. Video and audio tape recordings are useful for patient feedback and documenting progress. A clinical tool called Performance Status Scales assesses the specific areas of dysfunction unique to this population, which is understandability of speech, normalcy of diet, and eating in public.[141] This scale can be administered by untrained professionals, is reliable, and can discriminate across the broad range of head and neck cancers. The scale can be a useful tool to screen patients who deviate from the expected course of recovery and who are in need of further rehabilitation.

As soon as the patient is medically or surgically stable, oral-motor exercises should be initiated to aid maximal return of the sensorimotor functions requisite for speech and swallowing. These exercises are designed to facilitate, maintain, and increase the ROM, strength, speed, flexibility, and sensation of the oral muscles and structures. Exercises are especially important to reduce mandibular fixation and increase range of jaw motion in patients who have had jaw reconstruction.[142] Lingual, labial, and velar exercises are important in retraining speech articulation and often involve teaching compensatory movement patterns or using sensory and reflex stimulation to enhance perception and execution of motion.[143–145] Fibrosis or contractions of facial and neck muscles can often be prevented by early and ongoing application of sensory stimulation and massage coupled with specific exercises to increase ROM.[146]

Irradiation and chemotherapy cause a variety of symptoms, including significant diminution of salivary flow and oral dryness (xerostomia); thick, sticky oral secretions; mucositis of the oropharyngeal mucosa; esophagitis; oral pain; dental caries; and taste changes, appetite loss, and nausea.[147–149] Use of various tastes, spices, textures, or olfactory input may be used to stimulate salivary flow in postirradiation patients and for swallowing treatment. Artificial saliva and spray have limited or temporary benefits.[149] Pilocarpine appears to have some potential for increasing salivary flow in selected patients.[149] Careful continual dietary planning and modification are necessary to ensure proper nutrition and to encourage eating when it is so unpleasant. Foods may need to be modified to make them taste better or to be less spicy. The addition of sauces, gravy, margarine, or butter may compensate for oral dryness. Moist, soft, or smooth foods such as buttered noodles, puddings, yogurt, ices, hot or cold soups, juice, purees, liquids, and dietary supplements (*e.g.,* Ensure or Sustacal) are moist and are easier to swallow if there is mouth pain or dryness. Papain dissolves thick oral secretions and can be swabbed in the mouth before eating.[150,151] If pain is more severe, topical anesthetics can be applied orally before a meal.[124] The use of fluoride trays can help to manage dental caries.[152] Dental monitoring and good oral hygiene are essential throughout treatment.

Because most head and neck patients have excisions of the structures needed for swallowing and bolus transport, swallowing retraining is an essential component of rehabilitation.[150,151,153–156] Although some patients may benefit from prosthetic swallowing devices or obturators, most can be retrained to swallow by therapeutic techniques. Modification of head, trunk, or body position may be crucial in swallowing retraining to improve bolus flow and reduce pooling in the hypopharynx that may lead to aspiration after swallowing. For many patients, a safe swallow procedure combines airway protection and head positioning to reduce the threat of aspiration or bolus penetration into the laryngeal vestibule.[155] This technique is especially important because aspiration is a major complication of head and neck cancer and a major cause of respiratory complications.[157]

Swallowing treatment is done by the speech-language pathologist or swallowing therapist and involves indirect and direct strategies for feeding and deglutition.[155] Indirect swallowing treatment does not involve the use of food, but direct treatment strategies involve modifications of temperature, bolus size, and texture of the food and in feeding positions. Indirect treatment strategies to retrain patterns needed for bolus manipulation and transport can be used while the patient is taking nothing orally and intubated. Because many head and neck cancer patients can not handle thin liquids or tough, sinuous foods after surgery, thickeners are often added to foods. Many patients benefit from preparing all foods to pureed consistency. A variety of special spoons, syringes, and adapted eating devices may be necessary to transport food from the oral cavity to the pharynx in patients who have had glossectomies or other oral surgical procedures.[119,158] Because the effects of irradiation or chemotherapy treatment are not immediately apparent, the patient may have progressive changes in dental status, smell, taste, and salivary flow that should be monitored. If the patient is found to have hoarseness or a gurgling voice that persists after eating, aspiration into the laryngeal area may occur. Elevated temperature can indicate aspiration pneumonia that should be monitored by periodic chest radiographs.

TRACHEOSTOMY CARE AND PRECAUTIONS. Head and neck surgery often involves creation of a temporary or permanent tracheostomy. The nursing staff can teach self-care and hygiene techniques and stress the importance of keeping the airway open and free of foreign substances. Patients should be encouraged to cough deeply to aerate the lungs and bring secretions to the tube opening. In the early postsurgical period, suctioning may be needed to remove thick secretions from the airway. Patients usually require continuous humidity in the inspired air just after surgery and may continue to need humidification to reduce mucosal crusting from dried secretions. The stoma must be protected from dust, aerosol sprays, powders, and other foreign substances by wearing a crocheted bib or other coverings. A protective stoma cover must be worn during showering to prevent water from entering the airway. Special stoma equipment (Keith-White tracheostomy Snorkel, Gauthier Medical Inc., Rochester, MN or Larkel Snorkel, Seidel Medicine, West Germany) is available for those who wish to resume swimming and water sports. Neck breathers should be instructed to wear medical alert bracelets (American Cancer Society), carry medical data cards, and place emergency instructions in their cars and homes so that special procedures such as mouth-to-neck breathing are clearly visible when needed.

EARLY COMMUNICATION OPTIONS. After head and neck surgery, especially if the laryngopharyngeal area has been changed, verbal communication may be sufficiently altered or compromised so that written communication becomes the primary mode of expression. Premorbid spelling, grammar, legibility, condition of the hands, and composition abilities dictate the ease of using writing to substitute for speaking. In most cases, the written conversational interchanges should be short phrase-length units, rather than long narratives. The patients and their families often need instruction on how to use key ideas and telegraphic writing to facilitate written interactions.

In the early stages of treatment and recovery, an artificial speaking device is widely recommended by head and neck surgeons and speech-language pathologists. These instruments are relatively inexpensive ($200–$600) and are reimbursable through most insurance policies. They are easy to operate and often can be used successfully after a few training sessions. The most commonly used instruments are the neck and intraoral electrolarynx devices. They are battery powered tone generators that convey sound through tissue of the neck or directly into the mouth by catheter to be articulated into speech. However, inability to obtain a good neck seal with the instrument or soreness and pain due to surgery or irradiation may preclude the early use of this type of speech aid. Despite adjustment for loudness and pitch levels, these instruments produce a monotonous, robot-like sound. The third type of electrolarynx, the Pneumatic External Reed larynx, diverts air from the tracheostomy site past a vibrating membrane into the mouth by rubber tubing and is not commonly used in this country.

Speech synthesizers and other communication aids with digital displays and paper printouts are available. One inexpensive device allows the user to request basic needs, spell words, generate simple questions and statements, and to phone the police, fire department or medical help in an emergency (Vocaid, Texas Instruments). A variety of more sophisticated synthetic speech systems have been developed for the severely speech and motor handicapped person. These devices can be used successfully by the laryngectomized glossectomy patient who is unable to use an electrolarynx. The use of the TT and fax machines may be helpful for electronic communication needs in the work setting.

REHABILITATION OF IMPAIRED SPEECH PRODUCTION. Speech production requires precise coordination of respiration, phonation, resonation, articulation, and cognition. If these are impaired by head and neck cancer, speech therapy can restore function and is essential for rehabilitation.

For laryngectomized patients, speech rehabilitation may consist of several techniques; esophageal speech, voice restoration through TEP or TEF, and voice prosthesis.[159–161] The electrolarynx was discussed in the previous section.

Esophageal Speech. To produce esophageal speech, air is injected or inhaled and trapped in an esophageal reservoir and then released with volitional control through the pharyngoesophageal (PE) segment and articulated in a normal manner. The PE segment is formed by the inferior pharyngeal constrictor, cricopharyngeal, and upper esophageal sphincter muscles. These serve as the substitute vibratory source for the production of voice.[160,161] Attainment of esophageal speech is successful in only 26% to 46% of patients because of several limiting factors. Among these are scarring of the tissues, nerve damage, poor relaxation or tension of the sphincter, impaired intellectual ability, hearing loss, and unavailability of trained instructors.[162–166] The combination of pharyngectomy and esophagectomy along with laryngectomy make learning esophageal speech impossible. Partial glossectomy or base of the tongue resection also compromises ability to learn esophageal speech.

TEP and TEF Prostheses. Singer and Blom described a procedure for voice restoration that creates a fistula or puncture between the tracheal stoma and the esophagus.[167] The puncture is stented with a catheter, and after maturation of the fistula (approximately 2–10 days), a one-way valved silicone voice prosthesis is sized and inserted into the fistula (Figs. 66–7 and 66–8).[130,168] The TEP prosthesis protects the airway during swallowing. If the tracheostomy is occluded with a finger or a tracheostomy valve, the prosthesis opens to shunt air from the lungs into the area of the PE segment.[159]

Speech restoration treatment for TEP requires collaboration of the speech-language pathologist and the surgeon. Patients are selected preoperatively using results of the air insufflation test, radiographic studies, and pharyngeal plexus blockade to rule out pharyngeal spasm.[164,169,170] The procedure may be unsuccessful if the patient has pharyngoesophageal spasm, myopharyngeal strictures, or hypotonia of the PE segment.[171] To alleviate failure, several procedures can be used: presurgical selective myotomy of the pharyngeal constrictor muscles, lysis of scar tissue that prevents vibration of the PE segment, constriction bands or digital pressure to increase tension of the PE segment, or dilation of the esophageal sphincter.[168,171] TEP surgery has been found to be successful for patients with reconstruction flaps and gastric pull-up procedures, advanced tumors and those who have had large doses of radiation.[171]

The speech-language pathologist and otolaryngologist fit the patient with the appropriate speaking valve after the surgery. Patients are then trained on insertion, care, and management of the TEP and valve. Patients must learn to coordinate the timing of the occlusion of the stoma with exhalation to achieve optimal speech production. A tape on voice reconstruction after total laryngectomy is available to train patients and professionals (Blom, Singer, Cine-med, Woodbury, CT). Functional communication is often achieved after a few therapy sessions. Perceptual and acoustic studies and subjective speech rating suggest near-normal speech characteristics and excellent intelligibility.[162,167,172] Self sufficiency in care and self-insertion may take longer in patients with impaired visual acuity, manual dexterity or cognitive capacity.

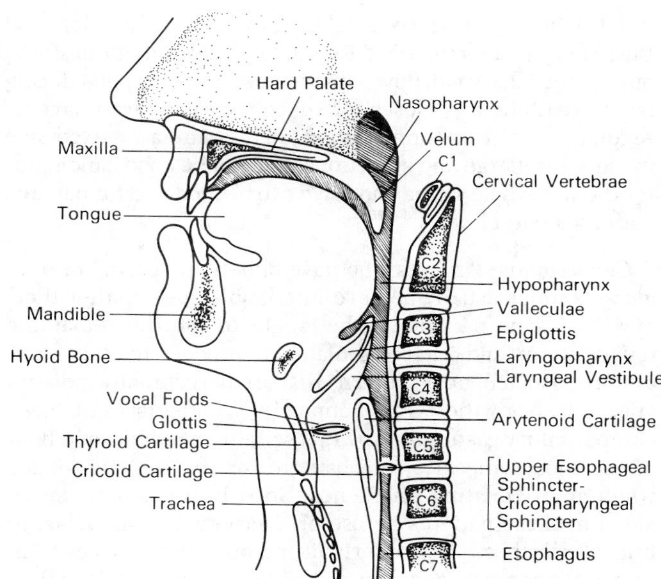

FIGURE 66–7. Sagittal view of oropharyngeal structures.

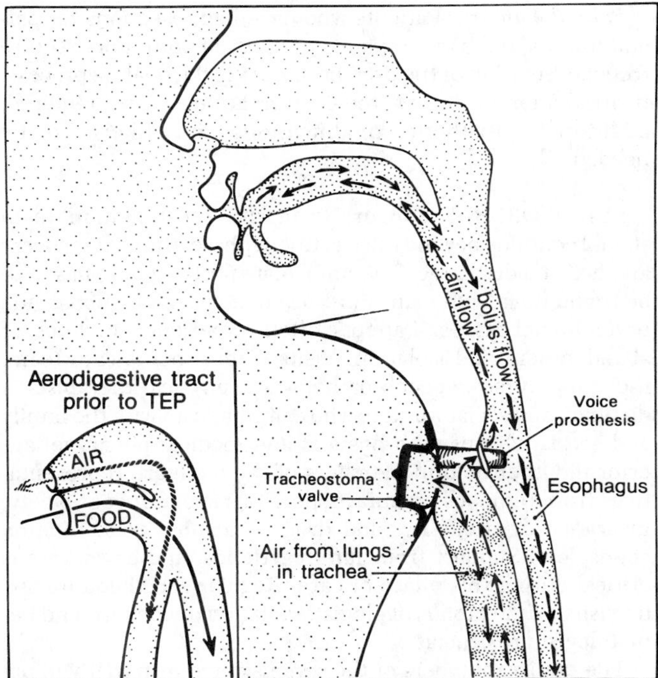

FIGURE 66–8. Sagittal view of oropharyngeal structures after tracheoesophageal puncture, with voice prosthesis and breathing valve in place.

A tracheostomy valve developed by Baxter, Mueller, and Bivona eliminates the need for digital occlusion of the stoma during speech. An airflow sensitive diaphragm opens during quiet breathing and closes for speech. Patients who have irregularities of the configuration of the stoma or excessive mucous discharge and secretions may not be good candidates for the valve. The stoma and valve can be modified for patients with these problems.[173–175]

Glossectomy. Patients who have undergone partial or total glossectomies usually achieve intelligible speech after therapy.[143–145] The patient can be taught to use the remaining tongue stump and other articulators to produce modifications of normal articulatory patterns that are perceptually indistinguishable from the target sound.[144,176] Patients must learn compensatory gestures of the lips, velum, mandible, and floor of the mouth muscles to substitute for the missing tongue when approximating phonemes. Speech production can be aided in these patients by use of a variety of oral, velar, or lingual prostheses. A properly fitting oral prosthesis can improve appearance and can simulate tongue-palate contact needed to produce speech sounds and achieve correct oral resonance.[177,178] Fitting prosthetic appliances and dentures in some irradiated patients may have to wait for several years after treatment.[108] Speech therapy may continue to be needed for 3 to 12 months beyond the surgical treatments, depending on the extent and type of tumor and treatments, cognitive factors, and the complexity of new speech, voice, and communication systems.

Composite Resections. Patients who have had composite resections that involve the tongue, jaw, and neck usually experience the greatest difficulty with speech and swallowing rehabilitation. Major problems after surgery can be caused by surgical ankyloglossia and absence of buccal gingival sulci.

Palatal Tumors. Patients who have had resections for palatal tumors and have implants or surgical obturators require frequent revision of the prosthesis during the healing process. If irradiation or other medical treatments are required, additional prosthetic modifications are likely to be needed.[108,123,179,180]

SURVIVORSHIP. Support from the rehabilitation team should continue beyond the treatment phase, through recovery and hospital discharge. The immediate posthospital phase can be frightening, with many unresolved medical, functional, and psychosocial issues. Patients often experience feelings of abandonment and isolation. Visits from a home-care team, including nurses, speech pathologists, physical therapists, a dietitian, and social workers who communicate with the family and act as liaisons with hospital and medical personnel are critical. Other helpful members of the team are representatives from religious organizations, American Cancer Society, insurance or disability, and drug or alcohol rehabilitation counselors. Support from family, friends, and coworkers is critical during this phase of care. Regular scheduled follow-up visits by the otolaryngologist, radiation oncologist, and hematologist are crucial.

The family members of the seriously and terminally ill patient need counseling about their feelings and fears. Social workers, psychologists, hospice workers, and clergy are best prepared to deal with the issues of death and feelings of anxiety. The speech pathologist, although not specifically trained, is often involved in assisting the patient to develop methods for expression of feelings and may be the person who initiates referral for counseling.[163]

SUPPORT GROUPS. The interactions and support of the various community and lay groups for cancer patients under the auspices of the American Cancer Society can be a crucial factor in adjustment to the disease and in maintenance of a healthy life style. These groups can provide educational materials, counseling, recreational activities, equipment, transportation, and financial and vocational assistance for cancer survivors. The International Association of Laryngectomies is one group that provides cancer patients with specific activities for speech and swallowing retraining, purchase of an electrolarynx, and hospital visitation and provides family members with counseling and other assistance. Groups to reduce smoking and alcohol abuse can often provide a positive milieu and enhance the quality of life of these patients.

TUMORS OF THE CENTRAL NERVOUS SYSTEM

CNS tumors may be primary or metastatic. In the case of metastatic lesions, the prognosis is related to the particular type of primary malignancy, but the neurologic deficits observed are related to the location of the metastatic lesions.[181] Chemotherapy and irradiation may cause CNS deficits in the absence of an intracranial lesion.[182] Primary malignant neoplasms of the CNS are most commonly gliomas, most frequently glioblastoma multiforme.[183,184] Lymphomas, relatively rare among CNS neoplasms, are relatively common in patients with the acquired immunodeficiency syndrome (AIDS).[185–187] Additional CNS neoplasms are angiosarcoma and germinomas.[188–191]

Although the long-term prognosis of glioblastomas is poor, many patients live for several years, during which time rehabilitation can play a significant role in minimizing disability and improving the quality of life. In children, advances have resulted in significant improvements in survival.[192,193] Long-term sequelae in survivors of childhood cancer may result in residual cognitive deficits that may require ongoing measures.[17,194]

The type, location, and depth of the CNS tumor dictate the severity and form of deficits in speech, language, cognition, memory, and personality. Different symptoms result from lesions of the right or left hemisphere, from frontal, temporal, parietal, and occipital tumors, and from surface versus deep tumors. Primary tumors can cause a wide variety of deficits in the areas of cognition, language, memory, perception, reading, writing, behavior, and affect. Whenever possible, it is important to have some premorbid, pretreatment assessment or estimate of these functions for comparison and for use in later family counseling sessions.

Changes in cognitive function may resemble those usually associated with patients who have had strokes if the lesions are specific to a specific lobe or hemisphere. If the lesions are spotty throughout the CNS, cognitive behavior may resemble that of the dementias. Subcortical lesions, especially to the left ventral tract of the thalamus, most often mimic cortical lesions to the language areas. Sensory and motor deficits are related to the area of involvement, with unilateral cortical lesions often presenting a picture virtually identical to that of stroke.

Rehabilitation treatments should include intellectual and communicative assessment as soon as possible after diagnosis of a tumor. The speech-language pathologist or neuropsychologist uses standardized test batteries of the various modalities, including speech, language, writing, auditory and visual perception, attention, reading, memory, gesture, comprehension, and verbal and nonverbal problem solving in their assessment of patient status. The results of these tests are used to formulate an individualized treatment plan and to evaluate progress of disease or progress in treatment. For some patients with severe disability, a variety of augmentative and alternative communication systems may be used to substitute for verbalization. Specialized switches and adaptations to other equipment and environmental control systems, assistive technology, and computer use may be useful avenues for rehabilitation.

Because swallowing abnormalities are common in CNS tumors, a high index of suspicion is necessary. The swallowing evaluation should include an oral motor examination and a modified barium swallow using video fluoroscopy. Swallowing and dietary modifications or tube feedings may be needed by some patients.

Difficulties with mobility and self-care should be handled similarly to that of other neurologic impairment syndromes. Orthotics and assistive devices may be used to substitute for lost motor function. In some cases, a wheel chair may be needed. Particular attention should be given to the avoidance of shoulder, hand and heel cord contractures in the hemiplegic patient, using splinting and ROM exercises as appropriate. Additional adaptive equipment, such as reachers, dressing aids, and bathroom equipment, may be used as needed. Treatment should involve counseling about the modification of expectations of work ability, life style, and roles. The spouse and family should be included in counseling before, during, and after treatment.

SARCOMAS OF THE EXTREMITIES

The three most commonly seen extremity sarcomas requiring rehabilitation are soft tissue sarcomas, osteosarcoma, and Ewing's sarcoma. Management of these usually is surgical, often amputation. Early detection and treatment has made limb-sparing surgeries possible without compromising outcome.[195–197] Sixty percent of all soft tissue sarcomas occur in the extremities with a 3:1 ratio of lower extremity (45%) to upper extremity (15%) involvement.[197] Approximately 75% of lower extremity sarcomas originate at or above the knee. Osteosarcomas are the most common primary bone malignancy of children and adolescents.[198] This type of tumor is most frequently located in the metaphyseal ends of long bones. Seventy-five percent of all osteosarcomas occur in the extremities, with most occurring in the femur (40%).[199] The axial skeleton, clavicle, and scapula are rarely involved.[198] Ewing's sarcoma is second only to osteosarcoma as the most common malignant bone tumor of children and adolescents.[200] As with soft tissue sarcomas and osteosarcomas, Ewing's most frequently affects the extremities. Approximately 60% of these sarcomas originate in the extremities (*i.e.*, femur, 21%; tibia or fibula, 23%; foot, 2%; humerus, 11%; hand or forearm, 2%), and approximately 40% appear in the flat bones (*e.g.*, pelvis, vertebral body, scapula).[200,201]

Pretreatment Phase

During the pretreatment phase, the rehabilitation staff should be familiar with the medical history, perform a thorough musculoskeletal evaluation and a functional assessment, and educate the patient and family about the expected course of treatment. An effort should be made to ascertain the patient's prognosis and his or her understanding of the disease and treatment options available. Knowledge of the patient's support system, vocational and avocational interests is useful in planning the optimal treatment program.

After the history is obtained, a complete musculoskeletal evaluation should be performed. This should include a general observation of the patient and close inspection of the affected area. Particular attention should be paid to the overall ROM, strength, sensation, pain intensity, edema, deep tendon reflexes, pulses, and joint alignment. The functional assessment to determine the patient's level of independence for bed mobility, transfers, ambulation, and self-care should be added at this time. The team must evaluate endurance levels for basic activities, such as walking on level surfaces, inclines and stairs, and use of gait assistance.

A crucial aspect of the pretreatment evaluation is the education of the patient and family. Patients who have a good understanding of what they may face and with whom they may need to interact postoperatively often progress faster, are more satisfied with their levels of progress, and cooperate more with their specialists than those who are unaware of their treatment. Patients need information about what their functional capabilities will be after surgery. For example, a patient who is to receive an above-knee amputation should be shown a prosthesis that would be appropriate for him or her or be introduced to another above-knee amputee of similar age, size, and medical history. A patient receiving a forearm excision may be shown a splint or brace appropriate for this type of surgery or view photographs of patients who have received a similar procedure. The pretreatment phase is an ideal time to instruct patients on the use of assistive devices such as crutches, cane, or walker that may be necessary for use after surgery. It is an appropriate time for demonstrating exercises that may be beneficial after surgery.

Surgery Phase

Before the early 1970s, amputation was the standard treatment for soft tissue sarcomas and osteosarcomas of the extremities. Despite this radical surgical approach, the 5-year survival rate for these patients was less than 50%.[202,203] However, advances in diagnosis and treatment have dramatically improved 5-year survival rates for patients with extremity soft tissue sarcomas to 70% to 80% and for osteosarcoma to 50% to 60%, and they have improved functional use of the extremity.[204] Surgical advances in limb-salvage procedures and the use of neoadjuvant and adjuvant chemotherapy and radiation therapy have promoted limb-sparing procedures as an alternative to more ablative procedures such as amputation.[205]

These procedures seem to preserve function, although they may prolong rehabilitation postoperatively.

AMPUTATIONS. Despite advances in treatment, there are cases in which amputation is indicated as the primary surgical option. Figure 66–9 shows various amputation levels. If the tumor is located in such a position that its removal would not ensure resection of all gross disease or if resection would sacrifice major nerves, blood vessels, or muscle, resulting in a poorly functioning limb, amputation is the treatment of choice. Other considerations that may favor amputation are pathologic fracture and skeletal immaturity. However, advances in endoprosthetic replacement have resulted in the increased ability to perform limb-salvage surgeries despite these factors and are discussed elsewhere in this chapter.[206] This chapter does not discuss basic amputee management because there are many other resources for this topic.[207] It is more important to discuss the problems unique to the oncologic amputee. The rehabilitation of patients with high-level amputations, including shoulder disarticulation, forequarter amputation, hip disarticulation, and hemipelvectomy, is the primary focus of this section.

Amputation of a limb, for any reason, has many psychological, social, and physical impacts. Amputations due to trauma, although devastating in their abrupt nature, are usually not life threatening. In contrast, the oncologic amputee often confronts a life-threatening diagnosis in which anxiety about the extent of involvement and choices about how to treat it are anxiety inducing. Treatments and their side effects (*e.g.*, alopecia, nausea, vomiting, fatigue) may produce fear, pain, altered body image, and change in customary roles. All these factors must be addressed for successful rehabilitation of this patient population, who tends to be younger and may have more significant problems with acceptance of their loss than vascular patients. The oncologic amputee often has greater rehabilitation potential.

Oncologic amputations are usually at higher levels than those due to other medical problems. The use of prosthetic devices in such cases requires higher energy expenditure and may result in the patient having limited physical capacity.[208] In the extreme case, some older patients may not be able to use a prosthetic limb because of the amount of energy required. Prostheses for above the knee amputees with very short residual limbs, hip disarticulations, or hemipelvectomy (and prostheses for the shoulder disarticulation or forequarter amputee) are difficult to fit, because there is less area to anchor

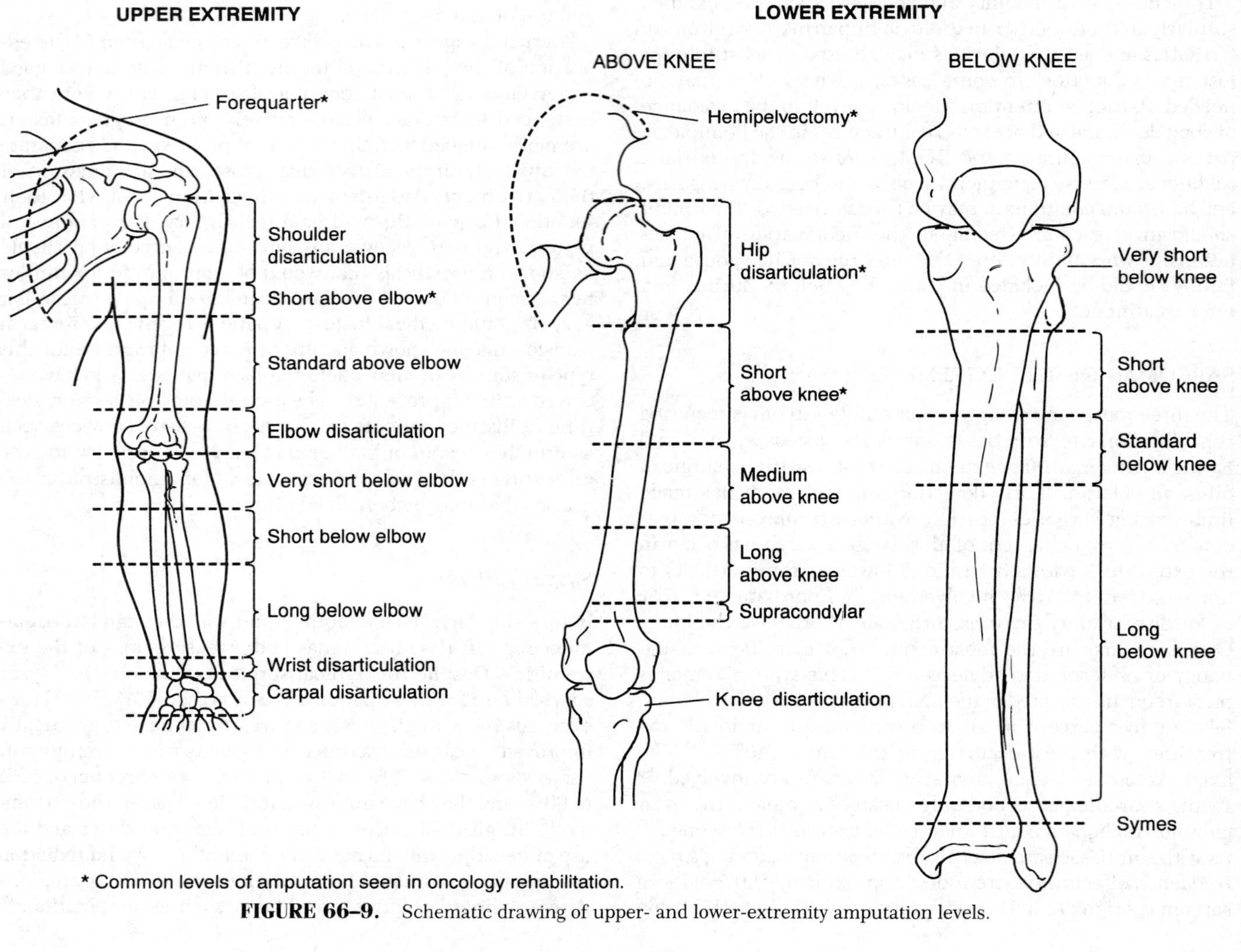

FIGURE 66–9. Schematic drawing of upper- and lower-extremity amputation levels.

or suspend the prosthesis. The weight of the prosthesis is often considerable, and the problem of adequately distributing pressure to minimize discomfort becomes a major aspect of prosthetic fitting. Interim inspections are essential so that modifications can be made to alleviate high-pressure areas before fabrication of the final prosthesis.

The oncologic amputee may undergo additional treatments, such as chemotherapy and radiation therapy, that may delay healing of the incision or produce stump volume fluctuations secondary to chemotherapy side effects. A rigid dressing applied in the operating room may aid in reducing edema and promoting healing. After a prosthetic socket is fabricated, maintaining a proper fit is always challenging in this patient population. Volume changes and muscle atrophy occur, and weight maintenance is difficult due to the chemotherapy-induced nausea, vomiting, and loss of appetite. If the period of chemotherapy lasts for only a few months, prosthetic fitting should be delayed until completion of chemotherapy and weight stabilization. However, the obvious psychological and physical disadvantages of delaying prosthetic fitting must be kept in mind and considered in the rehabilitation team's decisions. In general, it is advisable to obtain a prosthesis as soon as the incision is healed. Socket fit can be adapted by changing stump sock thickness, using a temporary flexible socket with adjustable closures, using a series of flexible sockets in a rigid frame, or modifying a permanent socket by filling it entirely or by padding specific areas.[199]

During this treatment time, prosthetic training may be hampered by decreased stamina, fatigue, and anemia. Daily fluctuations may require alterations in rehabilitation treatments. Occasionally, an amputated limb may receive irradiation that may interfere with prosthetic fitting by causing pain and skin breakdown in the irradiated area. Extra padding and vigorous stump management can aid in coping with the resulting problems.

Shoulder Disarticulation or Forequarter Amputation. The rehabilitation of high-level upper extremity amputations should concentrate on training the patient in one-handed activities, training the uninvolved hand in fine motor activities such as writing skills if the amputated limb was the dominant one, strengthening of the remaining extremity, and addressing postural and cosmetic issues (Figs. 66–10 and 66–11). The patient may tend to lean toward the affected side due to the weight imbalance, resulting in neck and back problems. This can be avoided with ROM exercises of the neck and trunk and postural training exercises using a mirror for visual feedback. A functional prosthesis is rarely recommended and is often rejected by patients because of its weight, lack of coordinated multiarticular movement, psychological unacceptability, and ready adaptation to one-handed activities.[209] The patient who desires a functional prosthesis is usually the exception and requires extensive training to coordinate shoulder and elbow movement with hook opening and closing. Despite the ineffectiveness of a functional prosthesis for most patients, all patients should be fitted with a cosmetic shoulder cap to provide symmetry and a shelf for clothing. A purely cosmetic, light-weight full arm and hand may be used to assist with psychological adjustment.[209] Rehabilitation team members can provide ideas for clothing modification and instruction in the use of assistive devices, as needed.

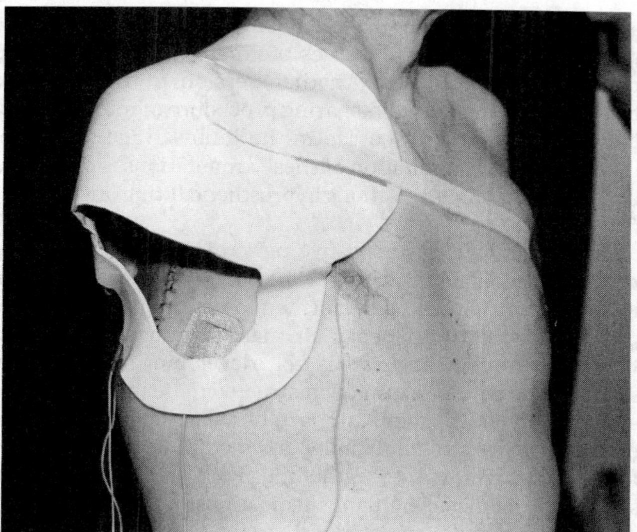

FIGURE 66–10. Custom-molded plastic shoulder cap for a forequarter amputee.

Hip Disarticulation and Hemipelvectomy. Malignant, bony lesions of the middle and distal femur and soft tissue tumors of the middle and lower thigh that are not amenable to limb salvage usually require hip disarticulation. This surgical procedure involves disarticulation of the hip joint, with complete removal of the femur and most muscles of the lower extremity. Hemipelvectomy, removal of the entire lower extremity and hemipelvis with disarticulation of the sacroiliac joint and pubic symphysis, is most often used for lesions of the proximal thigh

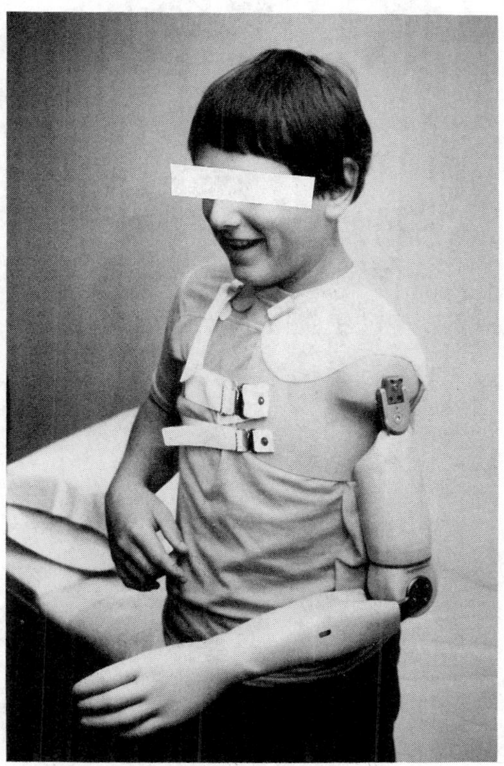

FIGURE 66–11. Forequarter prosthesis.

and buttocks. Similar to the standard hemipelvectomy is a modified version that preserves the iliac wing and improves patient rehabilitation.[210] Another version of the standard hemipelvectomy is a limb-sparing procedure of internal hemipelvectomy that is discussed in the limb-salvage section of this chapter. Rehabilitation of these amputations is quite similar, with only slight variations in prosthetic fitting and training (Fig. 66–12).

The immediate postoperative period is usually one of bed rest for 3 to 5 days. During this period, exercises on the uninvolved limb should be performed to maintain strength and promote circulation. Special air mattresses are usually provided to prevent pressure areas from developing in the surgical site, and the patient is usually instructed to lie predominantly on the uninvolved side. A trapeze bar should be placed over the patient's bed to allow independence in bed mobility and for upper extremity strengthening. Pain and phantom sensation are managed by pain medications, but TENS can be used if TENS pads are not placed on the flap area. Placement of pads to the translumbar area has given some relief of phantom pain. Compression wrapping with elastic bandages or the use of a commercial girdle with the involved side sewn closed aids in reducing pain and controlling postoperative edema.

After the period of bed rest, increased mobility should be encouraged. Initially, the patient may start on the tilt table to accommodate to the upright position. However, sitting on or at the bedside for several short periods may aid in adjusting

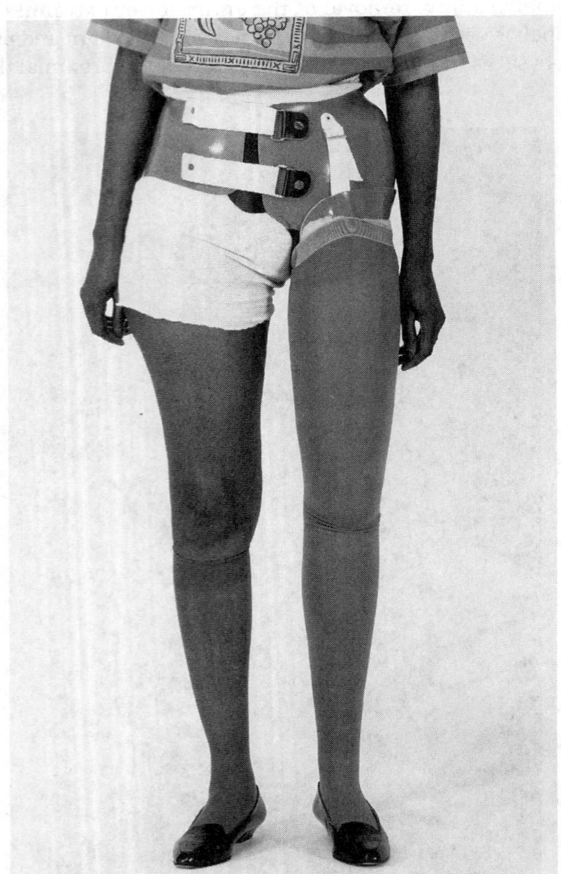

FIGURE 66–12. Hemipelvectomy prosthesis.

to this position. Re-educating the patient to become ambulatory involves a series of steps. Parallel bars are used initially, with the patient advancing to a walker and finally crutches as he or she develops increased strength, balance, and coordination. Activities that promote improved sitting and standing balance include sitting at the edge of a mat and reaching, catching, or kicking a foam or rubber ball with and without upper extremity support. Catching and throwing activities within the parallel bars challenge and improve standing balance. During sitting activities, a wedge or air (*e.g.*, Roho) cushion should be provided to enable equal weight distribution. This is particularly important for the hemipelvectomy patient who lacks a bony weight-bearing surface on the amputated side. After good balance and independent ambulation on level surfaces have been achieved, the patient may be advanced to more difficult activities such as stair climbing, getting up and down from the floor, opening doors, and riding on escalators.

Fitting for a prosthesis should occur after the suture line is well healed, surgical swelling has subsided, and the residual limb appears firm and nontender. Before obtaining a prosthesis, all patients should be informed of the potential benefits and the limitations of prosthetic use at this level. After such discussion with the rehabilitation team, the patient should be fitted if he or she so desires and prosthetic wearing is thought appropriate. The prosthetic socket is usually a plastic laminate that contours the remaining pelvis or abdomen and extends around the intact pelvis for additional pressure distribution. An endoskeletal unit with a foam covering is usually prescribed because it weighs less than a wooden exoskeletal type, but the exoskeletal type may be prescribed for the very active child or adult. The knee unit most often prescribed is a constant friction single axis knee, but occasionally, a safety knee may be prescribed. The safety knee allows increased stability in stance phase from a weight activated breaking system. A SACH (single axis, cushioned heel) foot is adequate at this level, but some patients are fitted with energy-storing feet, such as the Seattle foot or the Carbon Copy II, that simulate more natural foot mechanics.

Interim examinations are essential in this population. Modifications can be made to the socket, length, and alignment. The stability of the prosthesis depends on proper alignment of the hip, knee, and ankle joints and is crucial for successful ambulation. The prosthesis should be 1 to 2 cm shorter than the sound limb to aid in foot clearance. Other specific items to be checked are well documented elsewhere.[207]

After completion of the prosthesis, prosthetic training should begin. Instruction in an exaggerated pelvic tilt is necessary for bending of the prosthetic knee. This movement is more easily accomplished by those patients who have had hip disarticulations or modified hemipelvectomy because they have retained their entire pelvis or their iliac crest on the amputated side. Other gait deviations include vaulting and hip hiking to aid in advancement of the prosthetic limb. Vaulting is done to clear the prosthetic foot and to use up time needed for the prosthesis to take a step. It is sometimes impossible to eliminate vaulting, particularly in the younger amputee who needs and wants to walk fast. Vaulting is contraindicated only if there are leg or foot problems on the sound side.[207]

Patients with hip disarticulation may ambulate without any assistive devices, but most require at least a cane. Almost all patients with hemipelvectomy require a cane or pair of crutches for ambulation. Because these levels require increased energy expenditure for prosthetic use, some patients abandon the prosthesis and use crutches. It has been the experience of these authors that patients older than 50 and those younger than 18 prefer to use crutches, despite adequate prosthetic training. Few patients require the use of wheelchairs. Back pain and scoliosis should be monitored, especially in the growing child. If prosthetic use is impractical or not desired, a custom-made sitting jacket may be prescribed to stabilize the remaining pelvis and equalize the sitting surface.

Patients undergoing lower extremity amputation should be referred to occupational therapy to assess their safety in bathroom activity, need for adaptive devices for dressing and to review vocational and avocational interests. Adaptation of the environment may be useful to this population in preserving independence and conserving energy.

LIMB SALVAGE. Limb-sparing surgery implies removal of a soft tissue or bone sarcoma while preserving the extremity with a satisfactory functional and cosmetic result. Reconstruction should provide limb function that is equal or superior to the function of a prosthetic device. Sarcomas may arise in any part of the extremity. The functional outcome is determined in most part by the extent of soft tissue and bony structures resected. Knowledge of the anatomy and function of the musculoskeletal and nervous systems is fundamental in the treatment of these patients. With this knowledge, the rehabilitation team can better predict the outcome of the intended treatments and plan for the appropriate rehabilitation interventions.

Buttockectomy is an en bloc resection of the gluteus maximus muscle. Hip ROM and stretching exercises are recommended postoperatively. Gait deviations are usually absent, except for minor difficulty in stair climbing. A prosthetic buttock contour can be fabricated out of thermoplastic material or cloth covered foam and attached to the patient's underwear to provide a cosmetic appearance.

Internal hemipelvectomy is a procedure in which a portion of the hemipelvis and proximal femur are resected while leaving the extremity intact. A prolonged period of bed rest with skeletal traction is required postoperatively to allow fusion of the femur with the remaining pelvis. Strengthening and ROM exercises of the uninvolved extremities would be appropriate during this time. After the period of bed rest, a hip spica cast is most often indicated until further stabilization occurs, but ambulation with partial weight bearing can be performed while in the cast. Leg-length discrepancies are common and should be corrected with shoe lifts. Partial weight-bearing restrictions are usually maintained until total union occurs.[199] Most patients are independent ambulators with bilateral Lofstrand crutches, but depending on the extent of surgical resection, some may only require a cane. Common gait deviations include Trendelenburg and lateral trunk bending due to hip weakness and leg-length discrepancies. Rehabilitation efforts should be directed at minimizing these deficits.

Adductor group excisions typically result in significant postoperative drainage. Bed rest is recommended until drainage has decreased or drainage tubes are removed. Lower extremity edema and mild tightness are common after this procedure. Leg elevation, compression garments, active ROM exercises, and stretching are recommended to manage these problems. Gait deviations are rare, as is the need for assistive devices after this procedure.

Rehabilitation after quadriceps excision requires a period of bed rest with the extremity in a knee immobilizer for proper positioning and healing of the surgical site. Exercises on the uninvolved extremity should be encouraged and ankle exercises and hip isometrics on the operated limb. After drainage has decreased, ambulation may begin with partial weight bearing. An AFO should initially be prescribed that blocks dorsiflexion and allows 5° of plantarflexion. This creates an extension moment at the knee to provide knee stability during stance phase. With training, it has been shown through biomechanical analysis that some patients can learn to substitute hip extensors and plantarflexors adequately to control the knee joint. In such cases, ambulation can occur without an orthosis.

Management of patients after hamstring group excisions should include strengthening exercises for the quadriceps, knee ROM program, and stretching exercises to prevent knee flexion contractures. Little functional loss is attributed to this surgery if the sciatic nerve is not sacrificed. If the nerve is resected, motor and sensory loss below the knee occurs. The patient should be placed in an ankle splint in the neutral position postoperatively to prevent ankle contractures. Instruction in proper foot care including shoe wear is necessary to prevent skin ulcerations. A dorsiflexion-assist AFO is needed to provide foot clearance.[199]

Gastrocnemius muscle excision interferes with the patient's ability to properly push off at the end of stance phase. A rocker bottom on the sole of the patient's shoe aids in this motion. Active heel cord stretching should be performed to prevent heel cord tightening.[199]

Tumors involving the distal femur or proximal tibia can, in selected patients, be treated by limb-salvage surgery. Surgical treatment options include en bloc resection of the involved bone and soft tissue with autogenous grafting or allografting and arthrodesis of the knee, replacement with an endoskeletal prosthesis, or rotationplasty.[206,211] An expandable endoprosthesis has been developed that allows this procedure to be performed on a growing child.[206]

Rehabilitation after arthrodesis or arthroplasty is generally prolonged. Postoperative bed rest is recommended for 1 to 2 weeks with the leg elevated and immobilized in a posterior knee splint. If no wound healing problems are encountered, active exercises may begin after the period of bed rest. Quadriceps setting, gluteal setting, ankle pumps, and assisted straight-leg raising are encouraged. Weight-bearing limitations are determined on an individual basis, but most patients are progressed initially from no weight bearing to partial weight bearing to full weight bearing. Active ROM of the knee for those receiving arthroplasty usually begins 3 weeks postoperatively.[212]

Arthrodesis has the advantage of providing a stable limb that can withstand greater physical demands than arthroplasty, but the functional and cosmetic deficit of a fused knee must be considered. Successful arthroplasty has its advantages over arthrodesis in that it provides improved mobility of the reconstructed limb. However, complications of the endoprosthesis are common and can interfere with full functional restoration.[211]

Rotationplasty is a procedure that is performed instead of above-knee amputation. In this procedure, the distal femur is resected, and the distal portion of the limb is rotated 180°. The ankle is in a reversed position, and acts as the knee joint. The plantarflexors of the ankle act to extend the knee, and the dorsiflexors act to flex the knee. The functional result is that of a below-knee amputation and is superior to the function of an above-knee amputation. Vigorous rehabilitation should be instituted to achieve 90° of plantar flexion and to restore strength in the ankle musculature for the ankle to adequately perform as a knee joint. Prosthetic fitting includes weight-bearing surfaces to be distributed to the ischium and heel pad and has been described elsewhere.[206,213]

Soft tissue sarcomas adjacent to the scapula may require partial or total scapulectomy. A partial scapulectomy removes any extent of the scapula while preserving the glenohumeral joint, but the glenohumeral joint is sacrificed in a total scapulectomy. Near-total shoulder function with mild limitations in ROM can be expected after partial scapulectomy. However, after total scapulectomy, active motion at the shoulder is severely limited, and strength at the shoulder girdle is lost.[214] Preservation of function at the elbow and hand make this procedure superior to forequarter amputation.

Sarcomas deep to the scapula or involving the proximal humerus that do not involve the brachial plexus or axillary vessels can be treated with a Tikhoff-Lindberg resection. This procedure involves resection of the distal clavicle, upper humerus, and part or all of the scapula.[210] Partial shoulder and elbow function is maintained by muscle transfers and skeletal reconstruction. A custom prosthesis is used to maintain the length of the humerus. All patients should be fitted with a cosmetic shoulder mold similar to that for the forequarter amputee. If the cosmetic deficit is not as great, an off-the-shelf shoulder pad can be used instead of the shoulder mold.

Postoperatively, the arm should be maintained in an arm sling to restrict abduction and prevent distal traction on the reconstructed shoulder. Arm edema should be controlled with elastic stockinet. Active hand exercises aid in preventing and controlling edema. After drain removal and incisional healing, active exercises at the elbow can begin within the sling. At approximately 3 weeks postoperatively, passive ROM at the shoulder and forearm can begin. Progressive ROM and strengthening exercises should be encouraged after the arm is out of the sling. Excesses of 9 kg (20 lb) should not be lifted with the reconstructed arm.[199] Although shoulder function is limited, elbow, wrist, and hand function is usually preserved, making the functional outcome of this procedure more desirable than the alternative of forequarter amputation.

Other surgical resections in the upper extremity, including deltoid and triceps excisions, result in the obvious limitations. Due to the proximity of the major neurovascular structures in the upper extremity, many resections involve the median, radial, or ulnar nerves. After such resections, static and dynamic splinting must be employed to preserve functional use of the involved areas.

This information about rehabilitation progression constitutes general guidelines. Each surgical procedure must be individualized. Most limb-sparing surgeries are combined with other modalities, such as chemotherapy and radiation therapy. The effects of these treatments on the functional outcomes of the surgical procedures must be considered and are discussed in subsequent sections.

Effects of Chemotherapy

Extremity sarcoma patients receiving chemotherapy may experience complications that warrant rehabilitation intervention. Common musculoskeletal sequelae associated with chemotherapy that may affect mobility include nausea, vomiting, edema, peripheral neuropathy, cardiopulmonary toxicity, CNS dysfunction, immunosuppression, and delayed wound healing. Early rehabilitation intervention can lessen the degree of functional deficits that may result from the above sequelae. The rehabilitation varies in accordance with the medical status changes of the patient during or proceeding the chemotherapy course. Bouts of nausea and vomiting require careful monitoring and adjustment of treatment goals.

Fluctuations in fluid volume of the involved extremity should be treated using compression garments, active exercise, and, if appropriate, compression pumping or manual lymph drainage. Heat, cold, vibration, or compression can decrease the tingling or sharp pain associated with chemotherapy-induced neuropathies. If partial or complete loss of muscle function has occurred (*e.g.*, foot drop), ROM exercises and stretching of the affected joint can prevent contractures. Similarly, if muscle function has been disrupted, appropriate bracing can improve ambulation or basic daily living skills.

Cardiopulmonary toxicity can limit a patient's stamina and overall activity level. A carefully prescribed, closely monitored walking program is an excellent choice of exercise for increasing endurance in a patient with a compromised cardiovascular system. The goal of this form of endurance training is to progress the patient from a level of low exercise tolerance to a functionally and physiologically improved level.

CNS dysfunction resulting from chemotherapy treatment can manifest itself in motor and sensory losses. Motor dysfunction can range from subjective weakness with no objective findings to objective weakness with impaired function or even paralysis. Sensory loss can vary from mild paresthesia to severe objective sensory loss that significantly limits function. Rehabilitation can intervene by providing appropriate exercise and functional training, adaptive devices for assistance with impaired daily living activities, and assistive devices to aid in gait abnormalities resulting from weakness or sensory loss.

Immunosuppression may limit a patient's activity level, possibly confining them to bed rest. An exercise program that may be performed at bedside can be designed to decrease the unwanted effects of bed rest. Exercises can include active-assistive ROM, active ROM, isometrics, or resistive exercises. An immunosuppressed patient's blood counts should be closely monitored, and progression on therapy should follow medical status improvement (see Table 66–1).[215] Chemotherapy treatment can often delay wound healing. Delayed or inadequate wound healing should be treated immediately and can be managed by whirlpool or protection of the involved extremity by splinting or bracing.

Effects of Irradiation

Extremity sarcoma patients frequently receive radiation therapy preoperatively to reduce size and deep fixation of a tumor or postoperatively to eliminate or reduce residual tumor.[216] Radiation may produce pain, edema, delayed wound healing, leg-length discrepancy, or significant tissue fibrosis with possible contracture of the affected joint, any of which may occur early or remote from treatment. The goal of rehabilitation is to lessen the degree of functional deficit that may subsequently occur.

Pain control is often achieved with a TENS unit used on a high-frequency conventional setting. Modalities such as heat and cold can be used after the course of irradiation but should be avoided during treatment due to skin sensitivity or radioenhancement. Edema resulting from fibrosis of lymphatic channels can often be controlled with proper extremity positioning, compression garments or, if necessary, intermittent compression pumping. The use of whirlpool, debridement, or splinting or bracing of the involved area may be indicated for facilitation of wound healing.

Irradiation of growing bones, as in the case of adjuvant treatment of Ewing's sarcoma, may result in epiphyseal closure and leg-length discrepancy. Rehabilitation can supply shoe lifts, reducing future risk of scoliosis or muscle or joint imbalances. Fibrosis of joint tissues secondary to radiation treatment is a challenging problem for the rehabilitation specialist. Tissue fibrosis may continue 6 to 12 months after treatment. Patients must be encouraged to stretch and perform ROM exercises during and for 1 year after radiation treatment.

LUNG CANCER

Lung cancer may be one of four types: squamous cell, large cell, small cell, and adenocarcinoma. These four types are further classified as non-small cell lung cancer (NSCLC) and small cell lung cancer (SCLC). SCLC often has extensive local disease when diagnosed and is associated with early widespread metastasis. It carries the worst prognosis and has the lowest long-term 5-year survival rate. All types of lung cancer can metastasize to brain, liver, and bone.[217]

The treatment for lung cancer depends on the type and stage of the disease. Surgery is indicated for primary resectable lesions without distant metastasis. The primary tumor may be resected with a solitary brain metastasis, in which case, there is a 25% 5-year survival rate.[218] Surgical resection varies in extent and may include a pneumonectomy, lobectomy, or wedge segmental resection. At times, resection of the chest wall with reconstruction and insertion of plastic mesh may be needed.

Radiotherapy may be used as a preoperative adjunctive treatment to shrink the tumor, allowing surgery to be done. In this instance, it is associated with increased survival.[219] Radiotherapy as a primary treatment for unresectable tumor has a 5% 5-year survival rate.[220] Radiotherapy may be used in low doses for palliative treatment of superior vena cava syndrome secondary to tumor compression. High-dose radiation therapy is associated with lung tissue radiation effects.

Rehabilitation of the patient with lung cancer is generally divided into a preoperative or pretreatment phase and a postoperative phase. The pretreatment phase consists of a medical review of the chart to ascertain the stage and type of the tumor and whether metastasis is present. The physician should review the planned medical treatment. In addition to assessment of current medical status in regard to cardiopulmonary function, tests should be done for hemoglobin, hematocrit, and electrolytes. The current vocational status and family support situation should be assessed. A preoperative physical examination with particular attention to chest wall expansion, musculoskeletal status, and cardiopulmonary status is requisite. The patient is generally educated in proper coughing and breathing techniques (*i.e.*, diaphragmatic, segmental). It should be explained to the patient that these exercises help air to enter the lungs better, increase the efficiency of the respiratory muscles, increase chest mobility, and decrease risk of pneumonia.[221] Lower extremity exercises after surgery to prevent thrombophlebitis are explained.

During the postoperative stage, the patient's pulmonary function and chest excursion are again assessed.[221] Specific breathing exercises are started after the patient is extubated. Posture and lower extremity exercises are addressed. Chest wall pain is often relieved by use of a TENS unit. After pain is controlled and the patient is allowed to ambulate, some assessment of endurance should be made. Endurance exercises should be gradually introduced into the rehabilitation program.

In patients with metastatic disease of the brain, speech and language deficits should be included in a cognitive, language, and swallowing evaluation. Depending on the location of the metastasis, there may be focal motor and sensory deficits. Ambulatory aids, bracing or splinting, and occupational therapy intervention for assistive devices and safety equipment may be needed. Bone metastasis may need unweighting with crutches or a walker and spinal bracing and pain management.

Depending on the prognosis of the patient, there should be discussions with him or her and the family about adjustment to whatever disabilities there may be. Careful assessment of whether the person can continue working should be made.

HEMATOPOIETIC TUMORS

Leukemias

Leukemia is the uncontrolled proliferation and incomplete maturation of leukocyte and lymphocyte precursors appearing in bone marrow and peripheral blood. The type of leukemia depends on the cell line affected—myeloid, monocyte, or lymphocyte. Leukemia may occur in acute or chronic forms.

The acute leukemias include acute myelogenous leukemia (AML) and acute lymphoblastic leukemia (ALL). They are more common in childhood. Both leukemias are associated with anemia, fatigue, fever, bleeding gums, gastrointestinal tract or urinary tract symptoms, easy bruising, and pallor. Headache, mental changes, and cranial nerve palsy are common in ALL with CNS involvement. Joint pain is often seen with ALL but rarely in AML. The prognosis for AML even with treatment is poor.[222] ALL responds much better to treatment, and complete remissions are often seen. Treatment of AML consists of cytosine ara-C, daunorubicin, and m-amsacrine. The mainstay treatment in ALL consists of vincristine and prednisone.

Chronic myelogenous leukemia (CML) is not usually seen before 20 years of age, and chronic lymphocytic leukemia (CLL) is generally seen after 50 years of age. Both present with abdominal discomfort, organ enlargement, malaise, and fatigue. Anemia, low platelet count, bruising, and cutaneous bleeding are seen with CML. Chemotherapeutic agents may suppress the disease, but only bone marrow transplantation is curative.[223]

The rehabilitation team must address the effects of the leukemia itself and the side effects of medications and irradiation.

A leukemia that doesn't respond completely to treatment has a course of remissions and exacerbations that seriously affects the ability to attend school or continue working. Long periods of rest may be needed during treatment or during times of low platelets. Generalized deconditioning and decreased muscle strength occur. Steroids contribute to decreased strength when they cause a myopathy. They may be associated with osteoporosis, compression fractures, and painful aseptic necrosis of bone. CNS leukemia is associated with altered cognition, cranial nerve abnormalities, and other neurologic deficits. Vincristine causes peripheral neuropathy. Hair loss occurs with some chemotherapeutic agents. Bone marrow transplantation requires a 6-week hospital stay, usually with confinement in a bone marrow hospital unit because of the necessary immunosuppression (*e.g.,* leukocyte count $<1000/mm^3$).

Management of muscle weakness, decreased endurance, focal neurologic deficits, joint pain, cosmesis, and psychosocial and vocational problems are a challenge to rehabilitation specialists in this group of patients. The type and intensity of exercises allowable depends mainly on the platelet count and hemoglobin level. Exercise should be nonresistive when the platelet count is less than $50,000/mm^3$. No exercise is performed with counts below $20,000/mm^3$.[224] Aerobic or endurance exercise is limited when hemoglobin is less than 8 to 10 g/dl.[225] Whenever exercise and activity is possible, it should be encouraged. Patients undergoing bone marrow transplantation are always placed on an exercise program to increase strength and endurance. They are on high-dose steroid therapy and particularly susceptible to steroid myopathy, osteoporosis, and aseptic necrosis. Their exercise program includes weight-bearing activities, upper extremity ROM, an isometric program, and back extension exercises. An aerobic program is introduced when platelet and hemoglobin levels permit.[224,225]

Bracing and splinting are needed for neurologic deficits. Assessment of activity of daily living and issuance of safety equipment and assistive devices may be needed. Energy-conservation education is important. Assisting the patient and family with coping with acute and chronic problems is essential. A wig should be available during hair loss due to chemotherapy. Children should be tutored while they are unable to attend school.

Lymphomas

Lymphomas represent a malignant group of tumors that arise principally from lymph node cellular structures, other reticuloendothelial organs, and bone marrow. These tumors are classified as Hodgkin's disease and non-Hodgkin's lymphomas. The type of cells and their growth pattern help to differentiate the types of lymphomas. Knowledge of the stage of the disease is important because medical and rehabilitation treatment regimens are oriented to the stage-specific problems and prognosis.

Hodgkin's disease arises in lymph nodes and commonly involves bone marrow, liver, lung, and bone. There is a bimodal distribution of incidence, with peaks between 15 and 35 years of age and above age 50. Significant progress has been made in the medical management of this disease, and 75% of patients are cured.[226] Stage IV disease carries a less favorable prognosis, as does disease occurring after age 50. Relapses may occur anytime during the life of the patient.

Treatment consists of combination chemotherapy and radiation therapy. Many multidrug regimens exist. Choice of an appropriate drug regimen depends on the stage of the disease. Most of the regimens include prednisone, and side effects of osteoporosis, compression fracture, myopathy, and aseptic necrosis may be seen in 10%.[227] Other drugs with potential side effects that need to be addressed by rehabilitation include doxorubicin (Adriamycin), which produces decreased cardiac ejection fraction, and vincristine, which causes peripheral neuropathy. Combination regimens may result in hair loss, aspermia, and early menopause. Prolonged bed rest results in muscle weakness and decreased endurance. Treatment with radiotherapy can result in skin tightness, restricted joint motion, and aspermia.

The disease itself can be asymptomatic subtype (A) or symptomatic subtype (B). Systemic symptoms of fever, night sweats, weight loss, and decreased endurance are present with stage I through IVB disease.

Non-Hodgkin's lymphoma (NHL) is three times as common as Hodgkin's disease. The peak incidence occurs between the ages of 50 and 59.[228] These lymphomas are tumors of B and T cells and can originate in any lymphatic organ. Staging is similar to Hodgkin's disease (stage I–IVA or B). An international classification of NHL is based on the grade of the tumor (*i.e.,* low, intermediate, high). For purposes of prognosis, NHL can be classified according to its biologic behavior into indolent (favorable) lymphomas and aggressive (unfavorable) lymphomas. Indolent lymphomas are low grade and progress over many years. They are not currently curable by medical treatment. The aggressive lymphomas are fatal in a short time if not treated. Long-term disease-free survival occurs for 50% of patients. Aggressive high-grade lymphomas, such as Burkitt's, have a high propensity for metastasis to the CNS (*i.e.,* meningeal carcinomatosis), causing symptoms of headache, diplopia, cranial nerve palsy, and weakness. Spinal cord compression can occur if lymphoma involves the epidural space. CNS and spinal cord involvement can occur with NHL and Hodgkin's disease.

Other problems that arise with lymphomas include increased susceptibility to infection, pleural and pericardial effusion, and superior vena cava syndrome due to compression of the superior vena cava by enlarged lymph nodes.

Chemotherapy and irradiation regimens for NHL are chosen according to the grade and type of tumor. Vincristine, prednisone, and cyclophosphamide are commonly used in these regimens. Side effects are similar to those described under Hodgkin's disease.

As for patients with any type of cancer, it is important to know the type and stage of lymphoma, the treatment indicated, side effects, and the general prognosis when planning a rehabilitation regimen. In general, patients have to cope with disease-related problems and the effects of complex chemotherapeutic and radiotherapy regimens. Some patients may have an early complete cure and be left with no residual problems. Others may have had more advanced or more malignant disease with incomplete remissions or recurrences and disease- and treatment-related morbidity. In this latter group, vocational and school status should be assessed. All members of the rehabilitation team are involved in the management of these patients.

Neurologic involvement may require bracing, mobility aides, assistive devices, and speech and language evaluation.

Unweighting lower extremity joints involved with aseptic necrosis is appropriate. Muscle weakness and deconditioning should be addressed with appropriate strengthening and endurance exercises. The same precautions about platelet and hemoglobin levels hold true for lymphomas and leukemias.

Particular attention should be paid to unweighting bony lower extremity lesions if there is more than 50% cortical involvement. Appropriate spinal bracing for vertebral involvement should be addressed. Unstable lesions should be evaluated surgically. If the patient has advanced disease and surgery cannot be done, choice of a body jacket for thoracic and lumbar lesions and a four-poster brace for cervical lesions may need to be used to help prevent spinal cord compression. When treating patients in rehabilitation, any early signs of spinal cord compression such as new weakness, sensory deficits, or reflex changes should be reported to the primary physician, because radiation therapy may be effective in reducing the size of spinal metastasis and relieving spinal compression. Likewise, any signs of superior vena cava syndrome such as increased dyspnea, facial edema, and dilated chest wall veins should be reported, because irradiation may palliate these symptoms.

REFERENCES

1. Lehmann JF, DeLisa JA, Warren CG, deLateur BJ, Bryant PLS, Nicholson CG. Cancer rehabilitation: Assessment of need, development and evaluation of a model of care. Arch Phys Med Rehabil 1976;59:410.
2. Habermann ET, Lopez RA. Metastatic disease of bone and treatment of pathological fractures. Orthop Clin North Am 989;20:469.
3. Palma G. Paraneoplastic syndromes of the nervous system. West J Med 1985;142: 787.
4. Bateman DE, Weller RO, Kennedy P. Stiffman syndrome: A rare paraneoplastic disorder? J Neurol Neurosurg Psychiatry 1990;53:659–696.
5. Van Healst-Pisani CM, Pisani RJ, Kovach JS. Cancer immunotherapy: Current status of treatment with interleukin 2 and lymphokine-activated killer cells. Mayo Clin Proc 1989;64:451.
6. Welch-McCaffrey D, Hoffman B, Leigh SA, Loescher LJ. Surving adult cancers. Part 2: Psychosocial implications. Ann Intern Med 1989;111:517.
7. Hoffman B. Current issues of cancer survivorship. Oncology 1989;3:85.
8. Hoffman B. Cancer survivors at work: Job problems and illegal discrimination. Oncol Nurs Forum 1989;16:39.
9. Tebbi CK, Bromberg C, Piedmonte M. Long-term vocational adjustment of cancer patients diagnosed during adolescence. Cancer 1989;63:213.
10. Schover LR, Schain WS, Montague DK. Sexual problems of patients with cancer. In: De Vita VT Jr, Hellman S, Rosenberg SA, eds. Cancer: Principles and practice of oncology. Philadelphia: JB Lippincott, 1989:2206.
11. Smith DB. Sexual rehabilitation of the cancer patient. Cancer Nurs 1989;12:10.
12. Levy MJ, Stillman RJ. Reproductive potential in survivors of childhood malignancy. Pediatrician 1991;18:61.
13. Green DM, Zevon MA, Lowrie G, Seigelstein N, Hall B. Congenital anolmalies in children of patients who received chemotherapy for cancer in childhood and adolescence. N Engl J Med 1991;325:141.
14. Kazak AE. Psychological issues in childhood cancer survivors. J Assoc Pediatr Oncol Nurses 1989;6:15.
15. Chang PN. Psychosocial needs of long-term childhood cancer survivors: A review of literature. Pediatrician 1991;18:20.
16. List MA, Ritter-Sterr C, Lansky SB. Cancer during adolescence. Pediatrician 1991;18: 32.
17. Glauser TA, Packer RJ. Cognitive deficits in long-term survivors of childhood brain tumors. Childs Nerv Syst 1991;7:2.
18. Goldwein JW. Effects of radiation therapy on skeletal growth in childhood. Clin Orthop Rel Res 1991;262:101.
19. Maguire A, Murray JJ, Craft AW, Kernahan J, Welbury RR. Radiological features of the long-term effects from treatment of malignant disease in childhood. Br Dental J 1987;162:99.
20. Ryan JR, Emami A. Vincristine neurotoxicity with residual equinocavus deformity in children with acute leukemia. Cancer 1983;51:423.
21. Hammack JE, Kimmel DW, O Neill BP, Lennon VA. Paraneoplastic cerebellar degeneration: A clinical comparison of patients with and without Purkinje cell cytoplasmic antibodies. Mayo Clin Proc 1990;65:1423.
22. Derogatis L, Abeloff M, Melisaratos N. Psychological coping mechanisms and survival time in metastatic breast cancer. JAMA 1979;242:1504.
23. Bergner M, Bobbitt R, Carter W, Gilson B. The sickness impact Profile: Development and final revision of a health status measure. Med Care 1981;19:787.
24. Wilmore DW. Catabolic illness: Strategies for enhancing recovery. N Engl J Med 1991;325:695.
25. Gross M, Roberts JG, Foster J, Shankardass K. Calcaneal bone density reduction in patients with restricted mobility. Arch Phys Med Rehabil 1987;68:158.
26. Stewart AF, Adler M, Byers CM, Segre GV, Broadus AE. Calcium homeostasis in immobilization: An example of resorptive hypercalcemia. N Engl J Med 1982;306:1136.
27. Claus-Walker J, Halstead LS, Rodrigues GP, Henry YK. Spinal cord injury hypercalcemia: Therapeutic profile. Arch Phys Med Rehabil 1982;63:108.
28. Scher HI, Yagoda A. Bone metastases: Pathogenesis, treatment, and rationale for use of resorption inhibitors. Am J Med 1987;82:6.
29. Vico L, Chappard D, Alexandre C, et al. Effects of a 120 day period of bedrest on bone mass and bone cell activities in man: Attempts at countermeasure. Bone Miner 1987;2: 383.
30. Booth FW. Physiologic and biochemical effects of immobilization on muscle. Clin Orthop Rel Res 1987;219:15.
31. Häggmark T, Eriksson E, Jansson E. Muscle fiber type changes in human skeletal muscle after injuries and immobilization. Orthopedics 1986;9:181.
32. Akeson WH, Amiel D, Abel MF, Garfin SR, Woo SL-Y. Effects of immobilization on joints. Clin Orthop Rel Res 1987;219:28.
33. Woo SL-Y, Gomez MA, Sites TJ, Newton PO, Orlando CA, Akeson WH. The biomechanical and morphological changes in the medial collateral ligament of the rabbit after immobilization and remobilization. J Bone Joint Surg 1987;69-A:1200.
34. Mohr DN, Ryu JH, Litin SC, III ECR. Recent advances in the management of venous thromboembolism. Mayo Clin Proc 1988;63:281.
35. Lotze MT, Duncan MA, Gerber LH, Woltering EA, Rosenberg SA. Early versus delayed shoulder motion following axillary dissection. Ann Surg 1981;193:288.
36. Lehmann JF, De Lateur BJ. Diathermy and superficial heat, laser and cold therapy. In: Kottke FJ, Lehmann JF, eds. Krusen's handbook of physical medicine and rehabilitation. Philadelphia: WB Saunders, 1990:283.
37. Glover D. Metabolic emergencies. New York: JB Lippincott, 1991:7.
38. Glover D. Paraneoplastic syndrome: Endocrine effects. Philadelphia: JB Lippincott, 1991.
39. Dalakas M. Polymyositis dermatomyositis, and inclusion body myositis. N Engl J Med 1991;325:1487.
40. Cairncross GJ. Effects of cancer on the nervous system. In: Wiites R, ed. Manual of oncological therapeutics. New York: JB Lippincott, 1991.
41. Manchul LA, Jina-Prichard KI, Tenenbaum J, et al. The frequency of malignant neoplasms in patients with polymyositis-dematomyositis. Arch Intern Med 1985;145:1835.
42. Lakhanpal S, Bunch TW, Strup IL, et al. Polymyositis-dermatomyositis and malignant lesions: Does an association exist? Mayo Clin Proc 1986;61:645.
43. Bohm A. Clinical presentation and diagnosis of polymyositis and dermatomyositis. In: Dalakas M, ed. Polymyositis and dermatomyositis. London: Butterworths, 1987:28.
44. Hicks JE. Comprehensive rehabilitation management of patients with polymyositis and dermatomyositis. In: Dalakas M, ed. Polymyositis and dermatomyositis. London: Butterworths, 1987:293.
45. Hicks JE, Miller F, Plotz P, et al. Strength improvement without CPK elevation in a polymyositis patient on isometric exercise program. Arthitis Rheum 1988;31:559.
46. Rosenberg N, Carry M, Rengel S. Association of inflammatory myopathies with other connective tissue disorders and malignancies. In: Dalakas M, ed. Polymyositis and dermatomyositis. London: Butterworths, 1987.
47. Dalakas M. Treatment of polymyositis and dermatomyositis with corticosteroids. In: Dalakas M, ed. Polymyositis and dermatomyositis. London: Butterworths, 1987.
48. David DS, Greico H, Cushman P. Adrenal glucocorticoids after twenty years: A review of their clinically relevant consequences. J Chron Dis 1970;22:637.
49. Paterson AHG. Bone metastases in breast cancer, prostate cancer and myeloma. Bone 1987;1(suppl 1):S17.
50. Nielsen OS, Munro AJ, Tannock IF. Bone mestatases: Pathophysiology and management policy. J Clin Oncol 1991;9:509.
51. Bocchi L, Lazzeroni L, Maggi M. The Surgical treatment of metastases in long bones. Ital J Orthop Traumatol 1988;14:167.
52. Menck H, Schulze S, Larsen E. Metastasis size in pathologic femoral fractures. Acta Orthop Scand 1988;59:151.
53. Galasko CSB. Skeletal metastases. Clin Orthop Rel Res 1986;210:18.
54. Rodichok LD, Harper GR, Ruckdeschel JC, et al. Early diagnosis of spinal epidural metastases. Am J Med 1981;70:1181.
55. Rodichok LD, Ruckdeschel JC, Harper GR, et al. Early detection and treatment of spinal epidural metastases: The role of myelography. Ann Neurol 1986;20:696.
56. Beltran J, Noto AM, Chakeres DW, Christofordis AJ. Tumors of the osseous spine: Staging with MR imaging versus CT. Radiology 1987;162:565.
57. Godersky JC, Smoker WRK, Knutzon R. Use of magnetic resonance imaging in the evaluation of metastatic spinal Disease. Neurosurgery 1987;21:676.
58. Smoker WRK, Godersky JC, Knutzon RK, Keyes WD, Normal D, Bergman W. The role of MR imaging in evaluating metastatic spinal disease. Am J Neuroradiol 1987;8: 901.
59. Winkelman MD, Adelstein DJ, Karlins NL. Intramedullary spinal cord metastasis. Arch Neurol 1987;44:526.
60. Errico TJ, Kostuik JP. Diagnosis and treatment of metastatic disease of the spinal column: A review. Contemp Orthop 1986;13:15.
61. Denis F. Spinal Instability as defined by the three-column spine concept in acute spinal trauma. Clin Orthop Rel Res 1984;189:65.
62. Pal GP, Sherk HH. The vertical stability of the cervical spine. Spine 1988;13:447.
63. Onimus M, Schraub S, Bertin D, Bosset JF, Guidet M. Surgical treatment of vertebral metastasis. Spine 1986;11:883.
64. Galasko CSB. Spinal instability secondary to metastatic cancer. J Bone Joint Surg [Br] 1991;73:104.

65. Cooper PR, Marvilla DR, Sklar FH, Moody SF, Clark K. Halo immobilization of cervical spine Fractures. Indications and results. J Neurosurg 1979;50:603.
66. Johnson RM, Owen JR, Hart DL, Callahan RA. Cervical orthoses. A guide to their selection and use. Clin Orthop Rel Res 1981;154:34.
67. Sutherland IA, Myers SJ. Radiation myelopathy. Arch Phys Med Rehabil 1976;57:81.
68. Hahn AF, Feasby TE, Gilbert JJ. Paraparesis following intrathecal chemotherapy. Neurology 1983;33:1032.
69. Werner RA. Paraplegia and quadriplegia after intrathecal chemotherapy. Arch Phys Med Rehabil 1988;69:1054.
70. Loehrer PJ, Einhorn LH. Drugs five years later. Cisplatin. Ann Intern Med 1984;100: 704.
71. Reinstein L, Ostrow SS, Wiernik PH. Peripheral neuropathy after cis-platinum (II) (DDP) therapy. Arch Phys Med Rehabil 1980;61:280.
72. Basso-Ricci S, della Costa C, Viganotti G, Ventafridda V. Report on 42 cases of post-irradiation lesions of the brachial plexus and their treatment. Tumori 1980;66:117.
73. Barr LC, Kissin MW. Radiation-induced brachial plexus neuropathy following breast conservation and radical radiotherapy. Br J Surg 1987;74:855.
74. Salner AL, Botnick LE, Herzog AG, et al. Reversible brachial plexopathy following primary radiation therapy for breast cancer. Cancer Treat Rep 1981;65:797.
75. Wheeler JS Jr, Siroky MB, Bell R, Babayan RK. Vincristine-induced bladder neuropathy. J Urol 1982;130:342.
76. Rosenfeld CS, Broder LE. Cisplatin-induced autonomic neuropathy. Cancer Treat Rep 1984;68:659.
77. Raphaelson MI, Stevens JC, Newman RP. Vincristine neuropathy with bowel and bladder atony. Mimicking spinal cord compression. Cancer Treat Rep [Letter] 1983;67:604.
78. Scherokman B, Filing-Katz MR, Tell D. Brachial plexus neuropathy following high-dose cytarabine in acute monoblastic leukemia. Cancer Treat Rep 1985;69:1005.
79. La Rocca RV, Meer J, Gilliatt RW, et al. Suramin-induced polyneuropathy. Neurology 1990;40:954.
80. Kori SH, Foley KM, Posner JB. Brachial plexus lesions in patients with cancer: 100 cases. Neurology 1981;31:45.
81. Harper CM Jr, Thomas JE, Cascino TL, Litchy WJ. Distinction between neoplastic and radiation-induced brachial plexopathy, with emphasis on the role of EMG. Neurology 1989;39:502.
82. Mondrup K, Olsen NK, Pfeiffer P, Rose C. Clinical and electrodiagnostic findings in breast cancer patients with radiation-induced brachial plexus neuropathy. Acta Neurol Scand 1990;81:153.
83. Hoang P, Ford DJ, Burke FD. Post-mastectomy pain after brachial plexus palsey: Metastases or radiation neuritis. J Hand Surg 1986;11B:441.
84. Jaeckle KA, Young DF, Foley KM. The natural history of lumbosacral plexopathy in cancer. Neurology 1985;35:8.
85. Pettigrew LC, Glass JP, Maor M, Zornoza J. Diagnosis and treatment of lumbosacral plexopathies in patients with cancer. Arch Neurol 1984;41:1282.
86. Ricci MA. Deep venous thrombosis in orthopedic patients. Current techniques in precise diagnosis. Orthop Rev 1984;13:185.
87. Dauzat MM, Laroche J-P, Charras C, et al. Real-time B-mode ultrasonography for better specificity in the noninvasive diagnosis of deep venous thrombosis. J Ultrasound Med 1986;5:625.
88. Moser KM, LeMoine JR. Is embolic risk conditioned by location of deep venous thrombosis. Ann Intern Med 1981;94:439.
89. Vernick SH, Shapiro D, Shaw FD. Legging orthosis of venous and lymphatic insufficiency. Arch Phys Med Rehabil 1987;68:459.
90. Klein MJ, Alexander MA, Wright JM, Redmond CK, LeGasse AA. Treatment of adult lower extremity lymphedema with the Wright linear pump: Statistical analysis of a clinical trial. Arch Phys Med Rehabil 1988;69:202.
91. Madersbacher H. The various types of neurogenic bladder dysfunction: An update of current therapeutic concepts. Paraplegia 1990;28:217.
92. Wyndaele JJ. Pharmacotherapy for urinary bladder dysfunction in spinal cord injury patients. Paraplegia 1990;28:146.
93. Broadwell DC, Jackson BS. Principles of ostomy care. St. Louis: CV Mosby, 1982.
94. ConvaTec. A professionals guide for counseling ostomy patients. Princeton, NJ: Squibb and Sons, 1989.
95. Broadwell DC, Sorrells SL. Ileostomy care. Plainfield, NJ: Patient Education Press, 1988:21.
96. Broadwell DC, Broadhurst BB. Colostomy care. Plainfield, NJ: Patient Education Press, 1989:26.
97. Broadwell DC, Broadhurst BB. Urinary diversion. Plainfield, NJ: Patient Education Press, 1989:24.
98. ConvaTec. An ostomy is for living. Princeton, NJ: Squibb & Sons, 1983.
99. ConvaTec. For a better way of living with a colostomy . . . everyday. Princeton, NJ: Squibb & Sons, 1985.
100. ConvaTec. For a better way of living with an ileostomy . . . everyday. Princeton, NJ: Squibb & Sons, 1985.
101. Pollard K, Callum K, Altman D. Shoulder movement following mastectomy. Clin Oncol 1976;2:343.
102. Flew TJ. Wound drainage following radical mastectomy: The effect of restriction of shoulder movement. Br J Surg 1966;66:302.
103. Atkins H, Hayward JL, Klugman DJ. Treatment of early breast cancer: A report after 10 years of a clinical trial. Br Med J 1972;2:423.
104. Gerber L, Lampert M, Wood C. Comparison of pain, motion and edema after modified radical mastectomy or local excision with axillary dissection and radiation. Breast Cancer Res Treat 1992;21:139.
105. After mastectomy: Finding the right prosthesis. Consumer Reports 1975;105:652.
106. Mathog RH. Rehabilitation of head and neck cancer patients: Consensus on recommendations from the International Conference on Rehabilitation of the Head and Neck Cancer Patient. Head Neck 1991;Jan/Feb:1–2.
107. Zagar G, Norante J. Head and neck tumors. 6th ed. Atlanta: American Cancer Society, 1983.
108. Silverman S. Radiation effects. 3rd ed. Atlanta: American Cancer Society, 1990:9.
109. Dudgeon B, DeLisa L, Miller R. Head and neck cancer: A rehabilitation approach. Am J Occup Ther 1980;34:243.
110. Sonies BC, Weiffenbach J, Atkinson J, Brahim J, Macynski A, Fox P. Clinical examination of motor and sensory function of the adult oral cavity. 1987;1:178.
111. Blakley BW, Black O, Meyers SF, Rintelmann WF, Schweitzer V, Schwan SA. Ototoxicity. Head Neck 1991;Jan/Feb:2–3.
112. Aker S, Tilmont G, Harrison V. A guide to good nutrition during and after chemotherapy and radiation. Health Sciences Learning Research Center. Fred Hutchinson Cancer Research Center, 1976.
113. Bradford K. A practical application of nutrition for the patient with head and neck cancer. Cancer Bull 1977;29:35.
114. Argerakis GP. Psychosocial considerations of head and neck cancer patients. Dent Clin North Am 1990;34:285.
115. DeWys WD, Walters K. Abnormalities of taste sensation in cancer patients. CA 1975;36: 1888.
116. Kelly D. Speech rehabilitation of the laryngectomized patient. Cancer Bull 1977;29: 39.
117. Marunick MT, Kapur K, Beumer J, McGregor IA, Urken M. Mastication. Head Neck 1991;Jan/Feb:6–7.
118. Donaldson S. Nutrititional consequences of radiotherapy. Cancer Res 1977;37:2407.
119. Fleming S, Hamlet S, Nelson R, Muz J. Deglutition. Head Neck 1991;Jan/Feb:4–5.
120. Hamlet S, Jones L, Patterson R, Michou G, Cislo C. Swallowing recovery following anterior tongue and floor of mouth surgery. Head Neck 1991;13:334.
121. McKenna JP, Fornataro-Clerici LM, Menamin PGM, Leonard RJ. Laryngeal cancer: diagnosis, treatment and speech rehabilitation. Am Fam Physician 1991;44:123.
122. Urken ML, Buchbinder D, Weinberg H, et al. Functional evaluation following microvascular oromandibular reconstruction of the oral cancer patient: A comparative study of reconstructed and nonreconstructed patients. Laryngoscope 1991;101:935.
123. Burgess EM. Surgery as related to prosthetics and orthotics. Bull Prosthet Res 1974;Fall: 15–21.
124. Wright WE, Haller JM, Harlow SA, Pizzo PA. An oral disease prevention program for patients receiving radiation and chemotherapy. J Am Dent Assoc 1985;110:43.
125. Silverman S, Shillitoe E. Etiology and predisposing factors. 3rd ed. Atlanta: American Cancer Society, 1990:32.
126. Ingall JRF, Saper JR, Kish J, Kuch K, Evans R. Pain. Head Neck 1991;Jan/Feb:9–10.
127. McCaffery M, Beebe A. Pain: Clinical manual for nursing practice. St Louis: CV Mosby, 1989.
128. Siddoway JR, Gursel E, Sullivan W, Hayden R. Cosmetic rehabilitation of the head and neck cancer patient. Head Neck 1991;Jan/Feb:3.
129. Hamaker RC, Singer MI, Blom ED. Primary voice restoration of laryngectomy. Arch Otolaryngol 1985;111:182.
130. Singer MI. Tracheoesophageal speech: Vocal rehabilitation after total laryngectomy. Laryngoscope 1983;93:1454.
131. Instrumental guidelines for diagnosis of dysphagia. American Speech and Hearing Association, 1992;34(Suppl):7.
132. Miller A, Miller B. Does intraoperative monitoring of auditory evoked potentials reduce incidence of hearing loss as a complication of microvascular decompression of the cranial nerves? Neurosurgery 1989;Feb.
133. Hammerschlag PE, Cohen NL. Introperative monitoring of facial nerve function in cerebellopontine angle surgery. Otolaryngol Head Neck Surg 1990;Nov.
134. Logemann JA. Manuel for the videofluorographic study of swallowing. San Diego: College-Hill Press, 1986.
135. Staple TW, Ogura JH. Cineradiography of the swallowing mechanism following supraglottic subtotal laryngectomy. Radiology 1966;87:226.
136. Muz J, Mathog RH, Hamlet SL, Kling LPDA. Objective assessment of swallowing function in head and neck cancer patients. Head Neck 1991;13:33.
137. Litton WB, Leonard JR. Aspiration after partial laryngectomy: Cineradiographic studies. Laryngoscope 1969;79:887.
138. Sonies BC. Instrumental procedures for dysphagia diagnosis. New York: Thieme Medical Publishers, 1991:13.
139. Sonies BC. Ultrasound imaging and swallowing. New York: Springer-Verlag, 1991:10.
140. Fletcher SG, Jacobs RF, Kelly D. Speech Production. Head Neck 1991;Jan/Feb:8–9.
141. List MA, Ritter-Sterr C, Lansky SB. A performance status scale for head and neck cancer patients. CA 1990;66:564.
142. Beumer J, Zlotolow I, Curtis T. Rehabilitation. 3rd ed. Atlanta: American Cancer Society, 1990:21.
143. Skelly M, Spector DJ, Donaldson RC. Compensatory physiologic phonetics for the glossectomee. J Speech Hear Disord 1971;36:101.
144. Skelly M, Donaldson RC, Fust RS. Changes in phonatory aspects of glossectomee intelligibility through vocal parameter manipulation. J Speech Hear Disord 1972;37: 379.
145. Skelly M, Donaldson R, Schinsky I. Substitution consistency as a factor in glossectomy intelligibility. J Missouri Hear Assoc 1972;5:21.
146. Stockmeyer S. An interpretation of the approach of Rood to the treatment of neuromuscular dysfunction. Am J Phys Med 1967;46:1.
147. Mendenhall WM, Parsons JT, Stringer SP. The role of radiation therapy in laryngeal cancer. CA 1990;40:3.

148. Moore GK, Getchell T, Mistretta C, Mozell M, Kern R. Taste/smell. Head Neck 1991;Jan/Feb:7–8.
149. Nelson R, Fox P, Marks J. Salivation. Head Neck 1991;Jan/Feb.
150. Larsen G. Guidelines for head and neck rehabilitation. Fred Hutchinson Cancer Research Center, 1979.
151. Larsen G. Rehabilitating dysphagia mechanica, paralytica, pseudobulbar. J Neurosurg Nurs 1976;8:14.
152. Keyes HM, McCasland JP. Techniques and results of a comprehensive dental care program in head and neck cancer patients. Int J Radiat Oncol Biol Phys 1976;1:859.
153. Doberneck RC, Antoine JE. Deglutition after resection of oral, laryngeal, and pharyngeal cancers. Surgery 1974;75:87.
154. Trible WM. The rehabilitation of deglutition following head and neck surgery. Laryngoscope 1967;77:518.
155. Logemann JA. Swallowing and communication rehabilitation. Semin Oncol Nurs 1989;5: 205.
156. Desjardins RP, Laney WR. Prosthetics rehabilitation after cancer resection in the head and neck. Surg Clin North Am 1977;57:809.
157. Fine R, Krell W, Ranella K, Sessions D, Williams M. Respiratory problems and rehabilitation in the head and neck cancer patient. Head Neck 1991;Jan/Feb.
158. Fleming S. Treatment of mechanical swallowing disorders. Boston: Butterworths, 1984: 157.
159. Westmore SJ, Johns ME, Baker SR. The Singer-Blom voice restoration procedure. Arch Otolaryngol 1981;107:674.
160. Schaefer SD, Johns DF. Attaining functional esophageal speech. Arch Otolaryngol 1982;108:647.
161. Miller S. The role of the speech-language pathologist in voice restoration after total laryngectomy. CA 1990;40(3).
162. Robbins J, Fisher HB, Blom EC, Singer MI. A comparative acoustic study of normal esophageal and tracheoesophageal speech production. J Speech Hear Disord 1984;49: 202.
163. Keith RL, Darley FL. Laryngectomee rehabilitation. Houston: College-Hill Press, 1979.
164. Singer MI, Blom ED. Medical techniques for voice restoration after total laryngectomy. CA 1990;40(3).
165. Jacobs JR, Pearson BW, Singer M, Hamaker R, Blom E, Tucker H. Rehabilitation of the patient following total laryngectomy. Biol Assoc Med 1989;8(11):455–457.
166. Lehmann W, Krebs H. Interdisciplinary rehabilitation of the laryngectomees. Recent Results Cancer Res 1991;121:442.
167. Singer MI, Blom ED. An endoscopic technique for restoration of voice after laryngectomy. Ann Otol Rhinol Laryngol 1980;89:529.
168. Singer MI, Blom ED, Hamaker RC. Further experience with voice restoration after total laryngectomy. Ann Otol Rhinol Laryngol 1981;90:498.
169. Blom ED, Singer MI, Hamaker RC. An improved esophageal insufflation test. Arch Otolaryngol 1985;111:211.
170. Juarbe C. Overview of results with trachea esophageal puncture after total laryngectomy. Bol Assoc Med Puerto Rico 1989;8:455.
171. Baugh RF, Lewin JS, Baker SR. Vocal rehabilitation of tracheoesophageal speech failures. Head Neck 1990;Jan/Feb:69–73.
172. Baggs T, Pine S. Acoustic characteristics: Tracheo-esophageal speech. J. Commun Disord 1983;16:299.
173. Doyle P, Grantmyre A, Myers C. Clinical modification of the tracheostoma breathing valve for voice restoration. J Speech Hear Disord 1989;54:189.
174. Cantu E, Shagets FW, Fifer RC. Customized valve housing. Laryngoscope 1986;96: 1065.
175. Barton D, DeSanto L, Pearson BW, Keith R. Anendostomal tracheostomy tube for leakproof retention of the Blom-Singer stomal valve. Otolaryngol Head Neck Surg 1988;999:38.
176. Heller KS, Levy J, Sciubba JJ. Speech patterns following partial glossectomy for small tumors of the tongue. Head Neck 1991;13:340.
177. Aramy MA, Down JA, Berry QC. Prosthodontic rehabilitation for glossectomy patients. J. Prosthet Dent 1982;48:78.
178. Davis JW, Lazarus C, Hurst PS. Effects of a maxillary glossectomy prosthesis on articulation and swallowing. J Prosthet Dent 1987;57:715.
179. Drane J. Role of maxillofacial prosthetics. Cancer Bull 1977;29:41.
180. Panje WR. Mandibular reconstruction with the trapezius osteomusculocutaneous flap. Arch Otolaryngol 1985;111:223.
181. Zochodne DW, Cairncross JG. Metastasis to the central nervous system. Cancer Growth Prog 1989;8:32.
182. Pluss JL, DiBella NJ. Reversible central nervous system dysfunction due to tamoxifen in a patient with breast cancer. Ann Intern Med 1984;101:652.
183. Paoletti P, Spanu G. Surgical therapy of malignant gliomas. J Neurosurg Sci 1990;34: 289.
184. Brandes A, Soesan M, Fiorentino MV. Medical treatment of high grade malignant gliomas in adults: An overview. Anticancer Res 1991;11:719.
185. O Neill BP, Illig JJ. Primary central nervous system lymphoma. Mayo Clin Proc 1989;64: 1005.
186. Grote TH, Grosh WW, List AF, Wiley R, Cousar JB, Johnson DH. Primary lymphoma of the central nervous system. A report of 20 cases and a review of the literature. Am J Clin Oncol 1989;12:93.
187. Remick SC, Diamond C, Migliozzi JA, et al. Primary central nervous system lymphoma in patients with and without the acquired immune deficiency syndrome. A retrospective analysis and review of the literature. Medicine (Baltimore) 1990;69:345.
188. Mena H, Ribas JL, Enzinger FM, Parisi JE. Primary Angiosarcoma of the central nervous system. Study of eight cases and review of the literature. J Neurosurg 1991;75: 73.
189. Horowitz MB, Hall WA. Central nervous system germinomas. A review. Arch Neurol 1991;48:652.
190. Black PM. Brain tumors. (II.) N Engl J Med 1991;324:1555.
191. Black PM. Brain tumors. (I.) N Engl J Med 1991;324:1471.
192. Friedman HS, Horowitz M, Oakes WJ. Tumors of the central nervous system. Improvement in outcome through a multimodality approach. Pediatr Clin North Am 1991;38:381.
193. Harwood-Nash DC. Primary neoplasms of the central nervous system in children. Cancer 1991;67(suppl 4):1223.
194. Gamis AS, Nesbit ME. Neuropsychologic (cognitive) disabilities in long-term survivors of childhood cancer. Pediatrician 1991;18:11.
195. Eilber R, Huth J, Mina J. Progress in the recognition and treatment of soft tissue sarcomas. Cancer 1990;65:660.
196. Quill G, Gitelis S, Morton T. Complications associated with limb salvage for extremity sarcomas and their management. Clin Orthop Rel Res 1990;260:242.
197. Sondak V, Economow J, Eilber F. Soft tissue sarcoma of the extremity and retroperitoneum: Advances in management. Adv Surg 1991;24:333.
198. Meyer W, Malawer M. Osteosarcoma. Ped Clin North Am 1991;38:317.
199. Lampert M, Gahagen C. Rehabilitation of the sarcoma patient. In: McGarvey CL, ed. Physical therapy for the cancer patient. New York: Churchill-Livingstone, 1990:123.
200. Horowitz M. Ewing's sarcoma: Current status of diagnosis and treatment. Oncology 1989;3:101.
201. Delephine N, Delephine G, Desbois J. Present trends in the treatment of Ewing's sarcoma. Biomed Pharmacother 1990;44:249.
202. Kraybill W, Emani B, Lyss A. Management of soft tissue sarcomas of the extremities. 1991;109:233.
203. Eilber F, Eckhardt J, Morton D. Advances in the treatment of sarcomas of the extremity: Current status of limb salvage. 1984;54:2695.
204. Yang JC, Rosenberg SA. Surgery for patients with soft tissue sarcomas. Semin Oncol 1989;16(4):289–296.
205. Elias AE. Advances in the diagnosis and management of sarcomas. 1990;2:474.
206. Finn HA, Simon MA. Limb salvage surgery in the treatment of osteosarcoma in skeletally immature individuals. 1991;262:108.
207. Lower limb prosthetics. New York: New York University Medical Center, 1987.
208. Nowroozi F, Salvanelli M, Gerber L. Energy expenditure in hip disarticulation and hemipelvectomy amputees. Arch Phys Med Rehabil 1983;64:300.
209. Griffith E. Rehabilitation of children with bone and soft tissue sarcomas: A physiatrist's viewpoint. NCI Monogr 1981;56:137.
210. Sugarbaker P, Nicholson T. Atlas of extremity sarcoma surgery. Philadelphia: JB Lippincott, 1984.
211. Harris I, Leff A, Gitelis S. Function after amputation, arthrodesis or arthroplasty for tumors about the knee. 1990;72A:1477.
212. Rao B, Champion J, Gore D. Limb salvage procedures for children with osteosarcoma: An alternative to amputation. 1983;18:901.
213. Murray M, Jacobs P, Gore D. Functional performance after tibial rotationplasty. 1985;67A:392.
214. Ward B, McGarvey C, M. L. Excellent shoulder function is obtainable after partial or total scapulectomy. Arch Surg 1990;125:537.
215. Pfalzer C. Aerobic exercise for patients with disseminated cancer. Clin Management 1988;8:28.
216. Shiu M, Hadju S. Management of soft tissue sarcoma of the extremity. Semin Oncol 1981;8:172.
217. Shank B, Sher H. Controversies of treatment of small cell carcinoma of the lung. Cancer Invest 1985;3:367.
218. Magilligan DJ. Surgical approach to lung cancer with solitary cerebral metastasis: Twenty five years' experience. Ann Thorac Surg 1986;42:360.
219. Warren J. Preoperative irradiation of cancer of the lung: Final report of a therapeutic trial: A collaborative study. Cancer 1975;36:914.
220. Perez CA, Stanley K, Grundy G, et al. Impact of irradiation technique and tumor extent in tumor control and survival of patients with un resectable oal cell carcinoma of the lung. Report by the Radiation Therapy Oncology Group. Cancer 1982;50:1091.
221. Shea B, Vlad G. Rehabilitation of the lung cancer patient. In: McGarvey CL, ed. Clinics in physical therapy: Physical therapy for the cancer patient. New York: Churchill-Livingstone, 1990:29.
222. Robinson LL, Nesbit ME. Treatment of acute leukemia in childhood. In: Wierner PH, ed. Contemporary issues in clinical oncology: Leukemia and lymphomas. New York: Churchill-Livingstone, 1985:1.
223. Marmont AM. Allogenic bone marrow transplantation for chronic granulocytic leukemia: Progress and controversies. Acta Haematol (Basel) 1987;78(suppl 1):181.
224. Holtzman L, Chesney K. Rehabilitation of the leukemia/lymphoma patient. New York: Churchill-Livingstone, 1990:85.
225. Hicks JE. Exercise for cancer patients. In: Basmajian JV, Wolf S, eds. Therapeutic exercise. Baltimore: Williams & Wilkins, 1990:351.
226. Fisher RI. Hodgkins disease. New York: JB Lippincott, 1991:268.
227. Proswitz LR, Lawson JP, Firedlander GE, et al. Avascular necrosis of bone in Hodgkin's disease patients treated with combined modality therapy. Cancer 1981;47:2793.
228. Fisher RI. Non-Hodgkin's lymphoma. New York: JB Lippincott, 1991.

Cancer: Principles & Practice of Oncology, Fourth Edition,
edited by Vincent T. DeVita, Jr., Samuel Hellman, Steven A. Rosenberg.
J.B. Lippincott Co., Philadelphia © 1993.

Ellen J. Gallina

CHAPTER **67**

Practical Guide to Chemotherapy Administration for Physicians and Oncology Nurses

Chemotherapy administration in an office, hospital, or home should be performed only by specially trained personnel. Physicians and oncology nurses must be knowledgeable about cytotoxic agents, proficient in drug administration, skilled in venipuncture, and familiar with recommendations for safe handling and disposal of chemotherapeutic agents to provide safe treatment, protect themselves, and conserve the environment.

Although certain aspects of all drug administration, such as verification of correct drug, dose, and route of administration, are similar, chemotherapeutic agents differ because their lethal potential is greater if errors in dosing or administration occur. It is essential to patient safety that the persons preparing and administering these drugs have in-depth knowledge about each cytotoxic agent, its classification, mechanism of action, routes of administration, coinciding normal dosage ranges, common side effects and toxicities, special precautions, and management of symptoms.[3–6,8–10,17,24]

Before initiating treatment, a baseline assessment of the patient, including current height and weight, should be obtained and recorded. Throughout the course of treatment, monitoring for toxicity and adverse side effects should continue.[1,4,5,15]

This data provides the basis for decisions about the current treatment. The importance of asking the patient specific questions cannot be overemphasized. Patients often respond by saying that things are "okay," but when queried about specific points, they provide details that may alter the treatment plan. For instance, a patient being treated with vincristine may not advise the clinician about having difficulty buttoning shirts or opening pill containers, because the patient may be unaware of the association between the symptom and the drug.

At the beginning of each cycle of therapy, weight should be rechecked. For patients who have excess weight from ascites, edema, or overeating, consideration should be given to adjusting dosing for "ideal" body weight. Patients should be weighed without prostheses.

Chemotherapy is generally ordered in units of mg/m^2. Because errors in calculating body surface areas (BSA) can easily occur, it is prudent to recalculate the BSA and dosage before preparing the drug.[5,20] Doses should be compared against standard practice or against a protocol, if appropriate, and with dispensed drug before actual drug administration. Accuracy in dosing is crucial to patient safety.

Pertinent laboratory data and clinical assessment should be monitored before each treatment. Education of the patient and family regarding the treatment regimen, side effects of each agent, and how to manage them and a discussion about the risks associated with treatment must be initiated before the first treatment and reviewed periodically. Patients must understand what measures they can take to alleviate symptoms and which symptoms and problems require prompt reporting. Instructions should include appropriate phone numbers to call.[1,8–11,15,20] The information should be given verbally and in writing for later reference. Having information in writing allows the patient to refresh his or her memory and provide a family member with pertinent information. Educational information designed for patients about chemotherapy in general, specific drugs, clinical trials, and eating hints are available through the National Cancer Institute (NCI) and other agencies. Many institutions have preprinted materials for patient education that can be purchased.

DRUG ADMINISTRATION

After reverifying the drug, dose, and route of administration and checking the labels on the dispensed drug, confirm the patient's identification. This is particularly important in busy outpatient settings where patients do not wear identification bands. Verify before treatment that informed consent has been obtained from patients participating in clinical trials. Additional questions about the protocol and research trial should be addressed at this time.

When you choose an intravenous site for drug administration, begin by carefully inspecting both arms for the best vein.[1,4,5,9,20] Choose a distal site first, feeling and palpating for soft, pliable veins, large enough to handle the needle. Avoid veins that are hard, sclerosed, or fragile. Using arms with compromised or impaired circulation, such those on the side of a mastectomy, lymph node dissection, invading neoplasm, or with active phlebitis or extravasation, is not recommended. Upper extremities should not be used in patients with superior vena cava syndrome. Lower extremities should be generally avoided and never be used to administer vesicant agents. (Specific information regarding vesicant administration is discussed later in the chapter.) The distal veins of the hand and arms should be used first. Avoid areas over wrists and antecubital fossae if possible. Measures such as using warm packs or holding the patient's arm under warm water may assist in obtaining access.

In choosing a catheter for venipuncture, clinicians should use the one with which they are most comfortable. Needle gauge and size are determined by the size of the vein, the chemotherapy, and the fluid needed for drug administration.[5,6,17,20] Choose the smallest-gauge needle to meet these criteria. For patients with difficult access, seek assistance of a colleague if more than two venipunctures are attempted.

If access continues to be problematic, alternate means of vascular access should be discussed with the patient. The clinician should consider several questions when recommending alternate access devices for the patient. Will more than one intravenous line frequently be needed for blood, blood products, and therapy? Will continuous infusions of vesicants be part of the long-term treatment plan? In these situations, external Silastic catheters are more appropriate for patient care and safety. If an implantable venous port is planned, placement should be on the side of the nondominant arm whenever possible. This decreases the chances of needle dislodgement or coring of the port septum during continuous infusions resulting from increased movement of the dominant arm.

After a suitable line is placed, it should be secured, allowing visualization of the insertion site, particularly if irritants or vesicants are to be administered. Never use the chemotherapeutic agent to test the line. Venous integrity can be assessed using a running line of normal saline or dextrose and water. Observe the site for swelling or pain. Assess blood return by gently drawing back with a syringe, being careful not to exert undue pressure, particularly if vesicants are to be administered. Gently palpate the tip of the needle as fluid runs through for a "buzz" or "bruit" sensation. Observe the flow rate of the intravenous fluid. Consideration should be given to securing the venous line with an arm board if increased mobility could disrupt the line integrity. These steps to monitor venous patency should be taken throughout the treatment.

The control of chemotherapy-induced nausea and vomiting is integral to quality patient care, fostering patient compliance, and maximizing quality of life.[1-10] Antiemetics should be administered before chemotherapy and prophylactically at predetermined intervals based on the emetogenic characteristics of the drugs, the patients's age and gender, and the patients's response to prior antiemetics. In the outpatient setting, caution should be used with agents that have a sedative effect especially if patients are traveling alone or driving.

Chemotherapy should be administered sequentially, as ordered, especially if the patient is being treated on a clinical trial. If multiple drugs are being administered, flush the line with 5 to 10 ml of a compatible solution between agents and again at the end of the infusion to prevent the drug from leaking as the line is discontinued.

Monitor the patient throughout treatment for adverse or allergic reactions. Be prepared to intervene promptly. For patients who are at increased risk for sensitivity or anaphylactic reactions to chemotherapy, attempts to block the histamine receptors before retreatment have been successful in some circumstances. One regimen used at Memorial Sloan-Kettering Cancer Center includes diphenhydramine (50 mg every 6 hours), around-the-clock (ATC) with cimetidine (300 mg every 6 hours), ATC or ranitidine (150 mg every 6 hours), and ATC beginning the evening before chemotherapy. Dexamethasone (20 mg) is administered intravenously immediately before initiating the therapy.

For patients on continuous infusions of chemotherapy, inspection and assessment of the intravenous site for signs and symptoms of infiltration should be performed every 4 hours. Patients should be advised of the signs and symptoms to report. Care should be taken to ensure compatibility of chemotherapy with maintenance intravenous fluids, additives, and antiemetics to prevent precipitation or other adverse drug interactions. Flush the line before and after any drug of unknown compatibility is administered. If compatibility of a concomitant infusion cannot be ascertained, use separate intravenous lines. Instruct all staff involved in caring for these patients to follow these principles. Continuous infusions of chemotherapy should be placed on a rate controller device to avoid inadvertent bolus of the drug and to maintain consistent blood levels.

Administration of chemotherapy through central access lines has become increasingly common, particularly in patients with difficult venous access and those who require intensive or long-term therapy. Verify the location of the catheter tip before the line is used. If treatment may be given in a variety of settings or by various persons, a standardized policy outlining specific procedures should be in place to verify the purpose, location, and patency of the device. Implantable ports used for purposes other than venous access may be surgically placed in locations on the body where venous ports are usually placed. Ports used for epidural drug administration may be found in the upper chest area; venous ports may be placed below the nipple line, where a peritoneal port or a hepatic artery port may be located. Even the most experienced clinician would have difficulty making a determination based on physical assessment in these cases. Making an assumption about the purpose of these devices is risky.

As alternate uses for implantable ports increase, it becomes the challenge and the responsibility of the care givers to maintain detailed records of placement, removal, type, and anatomic locations of these devices.[14] Although the burden of this should not be on the patient, educating the patient about the specific purpose of the port can help to decrease problems. Advising patients to alert or remind health care personnel about the device in place and what it is or is not to be used for can help, especially if the patient may require care outside of the usual setting. Written documentation about the device, carried by the patient, minimizes the risk of inappropriate port use. Telling a patient that the port is for "chemotherapy" is inadequate and could lead to delivery of medications or intravenous fluids into an inappropriate region such as the peritoneal cavity or epidural space. This clearly opens a new area in risk management.

Before administering therapy through an intravenous implantable port, assess catheter integrity for presence of blood return and for signs and symptoms of infection, prior infiltration, or port erosion through the skin.[13,14] Use only a noncoring, nonsiliconized needle long enough to pass through the skin and touch the back of the port without being easily dislodged. Ports located deeply in tissue or ones placed in overweight patients require the longest needles. Needle gauge depends on type and volume of the fluid and drug to be administered. Larger-gauge needles are better suited for administration of high volumes of fluids and blood products, and smaller-gauge needles are better for continuous infusions.

Access the port after it is cleansed with a bactericidal agent. Spread the skin taut over the port using the thumb and forefinger to anchor it while the already fluid-primed needle is inserted with the other hand at a 90° angle directly into the center of the port. The back of the port can be felt by gently pressing on the needle at the bend of the angle or at the hub if a straight noncoring needle is used. Patients can be taught easily to reconfirm needle placement using this technique. The angled needle can be supported with a 2-in × 2-in gauze before covering it with a clear occlusive dressing. For patients who experience pain during port access, the skin over the port can be numbed with an ice pack before needle insertion. It is not uncommon for a patient to be admitted to have a port placed and to have treatment initiated immediately after. Ask the surgical team to access the device and leave the noncoring needle in place at the completion of the surgical procedure. The postoperative pain and swelling over the port insertion site are severe enough in many cases that accessing the port after the patient has returned from surgery becomes impossible. Postoperative swelling makes it more difficult to ascertain if fluid is infiltrating around the needle exit site.

Venous access ports may not have a blood return after just a few uses. This can result from a positional line, a fibrin sheath at the end of the catheter, an intraluminal clot, or venous thrombosis.[2,5] Assessment is necessary to ascertain the cause of any lack of blood return. Verify that the needle is in the port septum by pressing on the needle until it comes in contact with the base of the port. Attempt to withdraw blood again. If there is still no blood return, reaccess the port, making sure that the needle is directly in the center of the septum, and retest for blood return. Sometimes this simple measure corrects the problem. In other cases, the catheter tip may have temporarily adhered to the vein wall resulting in lack of blood return. Use a 3- to 5-ml syringe to flush, and gently pull back on the line. Have the patient change position from side to side, raise hands above his or her head, sit forward and cough, or bear down with a Valsalva maneuver while opening his or her mouth. Attempt to withdraw blood again.

If none of these measures is effective, a fibrin sheath may cover the tip of the catheter. Initiate an infusion of normal saline or 5% dextrose and water, and run the line wide open. Observe the intravenous flow rate. Inspect the port site for symmetry and signs of swelling or leakage around the needle entry site. Have the patient slowly turn his or her head from side to side, and observe for changes in the fluid flow. If none of these symptoms exist, it is probably safe to use the port without a blood return. However, if swelling occurs or if the intravenous flow rate changes as the patient changes position, the catheter may be kinked or partially occluded. Reconfirmation of the location and of overall catheter integrity using a contrast agent is recommended before proceeding with chemotherapy, especially if vesicants are to be administered. Communicate the specific problem to the radiology department or service personnel so that they may thoroughly evaluate the problem. The catheter may be kinking when the patient turns his or her head, causing back pressure in the line. The radiologic examination should include such an assessment.

After line placement and catheter integrity are radiologically confirmed, consider using an antiembolic agent, such as urokinase, to attempt to dissolve an intraluminal clot. Catheter occlusion may also be the result of venous thrombosis. Clinicians should be mindful of the signs and symptoms associated with thrombosis when assessing for these complications.

REGIONAL DRUG ADMINISTRATION

Chemotherapy can be administered directly into a particular cavity or region. These regions may have temporary or semipermanent lines in place through which drugs are delivered. The physician or oncology nurse must understand the general principles of chemotherapy and its administration and the unique aspects of regional therapy.

Therapy can be delivered into the peritoneal cavity by a percutaneous catheter or an implantable port. Before initiating treatment, fluid distribution within the cavity is assessed radiologically using contrast material. This provides information about cavity perfusion and patient tolerance to the amount of fluid administered during the flow study, which can be useful in predicting treatment problems.

Further assessment of the patient includes inspection of the abdominal area for symmetry, infection, and existing ascites. Ascites may need to be drained before treatment for comfort and to allow adequate drug distribution. Access the catheter to assess patency and to determine if drainage is possible. These catheters frequently have a one-way valve effect that interferes with fluid drainage. Drug delivery fluid volume may need to be altered or therapy may need to be postponed until the peritoneal cavity can be drained. Perform these assessments before drug preparation to avoid drug waste and increased cost.[2,18]

Patients should have information about the rationale for intraperitoneal therapy and about the specific agents so that they may fully participate in the treatment and report problems promptly.[17] Therapy should begin after the patient has emptied his or her bladder to facilitate comfort. Although the goal is to deliver the treatment in approximately 20 minutes, factors such as pain, bloating, increased pressure on the diaphragm, and restricted fluid flow frequently alter delivery time. Narcotic analgesia may be required during treatment particularly with vesicant drugs. Close supervision of the patient and needle entry site is necessary to avoid extravasation of a vesicant. Patients should remain in bed, with the head of the bed slightly elevated for comfort. After the treatment, instruct the patient to change position (*e.g.*, side to side, flat and upright) to enhance fluid distribution throughout the peritoneal cavity. Because approximately 1 L of fluid is absorbed in 24 hours, patients should understand that some of the uncomfortable side effects, like bloating, will decrease over 24 hours but not subside until after the last dose of the cycle. Some patients find it painful to have their ports accessed; using ice to chill the skin covering the port sometimes decreases the discomfort associated with needle insertion. For patients receiving treatment every 12 hours, consider leaving the noncoring needle in place. Flush the catheter with normal saline, and cover the site with a dry sterile dressing. Reconfirm needle placement in the septum before initiating each treatment.

Implantable pumps and ports can be placed into the hepatic artery. Implantable pumps deliver drugs as a continuous infusion over a maximum of 14 days, followed by a 2-week rest period.[2,17,19] The pump is emptied of remaining drugs and refilled with 10,000 U of heparin and enough saline to make a 50-ml solution. Fifty milliliters of 50% glycerol may be used in the main chamber to maintain pump function after treatment. The glycerol lasts 5 to 6 weeks. Boluses of a drug may be delivered through the side port of the pump. Depending on the patient's anatomy, there may be one or two side ports.

For patients with two side ports, the total dose of the drug is divided and delivered into each port. As with other implanted devices, an initial flow study using radiopaque dye is performed to assess the degree of perfusion. The study is repeated periodically for therapeutic assessment and to evaluate mechanical problems. Experience and technical expertise are particularly important because the septa of the pump and side ports are smaller than other venous access devices. Familiarity with normal pressure and resistance when using this device is essential for early identification of problems and intervention. Assess pump and catheter integrity promptly whenever a question arises. Assessment, recording, and monitoring of the amount of residual fluid remaining in the pump is important to determine pump functioning and therapeutic management.

Education is integral for this population of patients. Patients should not fly in airplanes or have significant changes in altitude without notifying their physician or oncology nurse. Changes in altitude can alter the pump's rate of flow, as can changes in body temperature from fever or hot baths, possibly increasing the toxicity from accelerated drug infusion. Premature emptying of the pump could result in the pump's clotting off. Patient education literature about the pump is available from the manufacturer of the device.

The drugs most frequently administered through the pump are FUDR with or without leucovorin and Decadron. Mitomycin or BCNU are most frequently administered through the side ports. Drug infusion through the side port requires a pump to deliver the drug against the arterial pressure.

Implantable access devices placed into the hepatic artery are used in patients who are not candidates for the implantable pump but who would benefit from drug delivery directly into the region. Assessment of catheter integrity, tip location, and degrees of pressure and resistance when the line is flushed are essential for ports placed in the hepatic artery. The port is accessed as is any other vascular access device; however, do not attempt to aspirate for blood return to minimize the risk of clotting. The line is flushed with normal saline after the port is accessed with a fluid-primed noncoring, nonsiliconized needle to evaluate patency. In some patients, a pulsing of the saline in the line can be observed. The catheter patency is maintained on a weekly basis and after discontinuance of treatment with 300 to 1000 U of heparin, depending on physician preference.

Patients must be instructed to keep the area around the catheter clean, because the port is often located in the upper pubic region. Frequent inspection for signs and symptoms of infections must be emphasized in practice and in patient education. Bolus therapy or continuous infusions are administered through the port. Carefully selected patients can manage effectively at home with an ambulatory infusion pump connected to the port. Flushing the port at home by the patient or family member is frequently taught.

Chemotherapy can be administered intrapleurally though chest tubes immediately postoperatively for therapeutic management or after chest tube placement for the management of pleural effusions. Experience in determining air leaks and the side effects of agents is essential. Patients require narcotic analgesics when drugs such as mitomycin are infused, despite incomplete recovery from anesthesia. Resealable chest tubing is required to prevent leakage of the chemotherapy from the tubing and prevent exposure to these agents by the staff caring for the patient. Chest drainage is treated as chemotherapy waste.

Drug administration though the Ommaya reservoir requires extreme caution, meticulous technique, and verification of the drug dose, volume, and route of administration.[6] Drug errors can be fatal in this situation.

CUTANEOUS REACTIONS ASSOCIATED WITH CHEMOTHERAPY ADMINISTRATION

Chemotherapy agents are described as irritants, nonirritants, and vesicants. Irritants are capable of producing venous pain at the injection site or along the vein, with or without an inflammatory reaction.[12,20] The symptoms do not usually last for long periods and present themselves as complaints of local discomfort and burning. The symptoms can be reduced by decreasing the flow rate of the chemotherapy and increasing the simultaneous intravenous hydration. Other measures to minimize the venous discomfort include applying ice to numb the area or heat, which is thought to dilate the veins and decrease discomfort.[1] The application of topical hydrocortisone cream (1%) has been effective in some patients. Drugs more commonly associated with irritation include dacarbazine, carmustine, and plicamycin. Doxorubicin, a potent vesicant, can be irritating without causing underlying tissue damage. The clinician must respond promptly to any patient complaint of pain or burning. Differentiating the irritating effects of these agents from the signs and symptoms of extravasation is crucial and a challenge even for the most experienced clinician. Continuous monitoring of venous patency throughout treatment with attention to any changes is essential for determining the situation. If either problem occurs, promptly stop administration of the drug and allow the maintenance intravenous line to flow freely. Patients usually feel relief from the irritant effects within 10 to 15 minutes. If there are no signs of infiltration of the drug and the discomfort has been altered by stopping the drug, slowly restart it. The rate of the drug should be adjusted in accordance with the patient's tolerance.

VESICANT DRUG ADMINISTRATION

A vesicant is an agent capable of producing severe tissue damage and necrosis if the drug is extravasated into the surrounding tissue.[12] Drugs capable of causing extravasation include dactinomycin, daunorubicin, doxorubicin, idarubicin, mitomycin, mechlorethamine, vinblastine, and vincristine.

The best management of a vesicant extravasation continues to be prevention. It cannot be emphasized enough that the person administering a vesicant must be highly skilled in techniques of intravenous line placement and well versed in the risks, signs, symptoms, and interventions of extravasation. He or she must be sensitive to subtle changes in venous patency during drug delivery and attentive to all patient complaints and comments during treatment.

Good lighting, a relaxed approach, and application of heat to the arm facilitate selection of a site for vesicant administration. The clinician must critically assess the veins of both upper extremities, with attention to overall venous integrity, visibility, evidence of compromised circulation, location, and time of previous venipunctures above the site of potential access. Veins above a recent site of access or attempted access should not be used for 24 or more hours. Veins chosen should be resilient and large; however, smaller veins may be used if the needle can be easily threaded. Veins over joints, wrists, and the antecubital area should be avoided. Lower extremities should never be used for vesicants, because extravasation in these areas can result in greater injury and have a more negative effect on quality of life. The forearm often offers the best choices of veins because there is more soft tissue and fewer nerves and tendons. Distal veins of the forearm should be chosen first. The overall guiding principle should be to choose a vein that, if the drug did infiltrate, would have the least debilitating effects on the extremity.

It is recommended that the physician or oncology nurse responsible for the vesicant administration should be the person to place the line. This allows the care giver to understand the type of vein being used and the amount of trauma associated with needle insertion. Clinicians must be willing to recommend a short delay in treatment if choices of access are impaired by recent venipunctures or if access is poor enough to recommend an alternate means of access. In the hospital setting, it is a good idea to coordinate routine blood sampling with the phlebotomy team to avoid delays in treatment resulting from limited venous choice because of phlebotomy in the antecubital area.

For patients receiving mechlorethamine, which can cause immediate vomiting, or for those who may have difficulty keeping the extremity still, an arm board or some other method of gentle restraint should be used to minimize the risk of needle dislodgement and infiltration from the sudden movement. Patients are usually amenable to this precaution if they comprehend the risks associated with the administration of vesicants.

After suitable access is obtained using a needle or catheter, the line should be gently secured with tape, leaving the insertion site exposed. Using the degree of ease of needle or catheter insertion as a baseline, the physician or oncology nurse can begin to monitor the site for any signs or symptoms of impaired venous integrity by running a maintenance intravenous line with normal saline. Initial baseline assessment also includes evaluation for swelling or inflammation around the insertion site, changes in rate of flow of the maintenance intravenous solution, a blood return, a "buzz" or "bruit" when the needle or catheter tip is gently palpated with the forefinger, and complaints of pain or burning by the patient.

These criteria must be continuously assessed throughout treatment. Before injecting the vesicant, gently flush the line using a syringe with 5 to 10 ml of saline. Never test venous integrity with the vesicant. Inject the vesicant at a rate of 1 to 2 ml at a time, pausing to allow additional maintenance fluid to infuse. Continue to recheck patency and to ask the patient for feedback.

Respond to complaints promptly by stopping the drug immediately and assessing the situation to determine if this is an extravasation, an irritation, or an flare reaction, which is described later. There may not be a disruption in blood return if there is a tiny leak or if an underlying part of the vein was punctured. Apply a tourniquet above the intravenous site; if the vein is intact, the intravenous flow rate should slow down. If there is any doubt, discontinue the infusion and administer the therapy in an alternate site. With vesicants, it is better to err on the side of safety. After vesicant administration, allow additional maintenance intravenous fluid to infuse. The severity of the extravasation depends on the drug, its concentration, and the amount of drug infiltrated, and the use of additional intravenous fluid further dilutes the drug.

Continuous infusions of vesicants used in the treatment of leukemias, lymphomas, and sarcomas present additional challenges. Vesicants prescribed for this route of administration should only be initiated though a central venous line resting in the superior vena cava. The intensive monitoring required for these infusions precludes peripheral administration. Extreme caution must be exercised with these infusions because of the risk of vesicant infiltration into the chest or neck area. Before initiating therapy, catheter tip location and catheter integrity must be confirmed. Questionable lines should be verified radiologically using contrast medium. Standardized orders for monitoring infusions and specific interventions for suspected infiltrations should be initiated at the time of therapy and reviewed with the personnel who will be caring for the patient (Fig. 67–1). This is particularly important if the drug is being infused through an implanted venous port. Needle dislodgement can occur at any time but especially when the patient is asleep or sedated. Because of this increased risk, the use of venous access ports for home infusions of vesicants is strongly discouraged.

In rare instances, such as the patient with superior vena cava syndrome, a catheter may be placed in the inferior vena cava for the delivery of a vesicant. To minimize the risk of extravasation and avert the significant damage resulting from such an extravasation, the line should be placed immediately before the initiation of therapy. The patient must remain on bed rest. Interventions to reduce chances of catheter kinking or breakage from increased flexion of the leg must be taken. The patient needs to understand thoroughly the risks associated with the use of ports and inferior vena cava catheters for this drug therapy. Documentation of the patient's consent and understanding should be placed in the medical record.

PHYSICIAN'S ORDERS

Chemotherapy: Continuous Infusion of a Vesicant

DATE AND TIME OF ORDER: ____________________

START DATE: ____________ STOP DATE: ____________

________________ is receiving a continuous infusion of a
(patient name)

vesicant, ________________ for ________ days.
(name of drug(s))

1. Infuse chemotherapy via **CENTRAL ACCESS ONLY**. Do not administer the vesicant peripherally.
2. Check the catheter insertion site and needle entry site every 2 hours for signs and symptoms of infiltration.
   If there are signs of redness, swelling or leakage at the needle or catheter insertion site OR if there is any question regarding the integrity of the infusion, take the following steps:
   A. STOP the chemotherapy infusion **IMMEDIATELY.**
   B. STOP other fluids infusing through the line.
   C. Flush the line with normal saline and the appropriate amount of heparin, specific to the device.
   D. Notify the following persons **IMMEDIATELY:**
   Attending Physician: ________________ M.D.
   Medical Oncology Fellow: ________________ M.D.
   BEEPER #: ____________
   House Officer
   Plastic Surgery Service
   Chemotherapy Nursing/Pharmacy
   E. After medical consultation, discontinue all IV's infusing through the affected site.
   F. Save chemotherapy and tubing in a plastic bag for chemotherapy to pick up.
   G. Apply ____________ compresses for 24 hours.
   H. Medications to be administered IN THE EVENT OF A VESICANT INFILTRATION: (VERIFY orders with attending physician/fellow prior to administration.)
   ____
   ____

Physician Name: ________________ Date: ____________

Physician Signature: ________________________ M.D.

FIGURE 67–1. Physician's orders for chemotherapy.

EXTRAVASATIONS

The management of extravasations resulting from chemotherapy continues to be controversial. Studies in humans are limited because of incidence and ethical issues. Many studies in animals have been inconclusive.[12,17,20]

Despite the best efforts, extravasations do occur and can present in a delayed fashion, because they are undetected at the time of drug administration. After extravasation is suspected, prompt intervention is essential. Stop the drug immediately. Attempt to withdraw any remaining drug from the line. Administer an antidote in accordance with institutional guidelines and policies through the infiltrated line or subcutaneously around the site of infiltration. Apply heat or cold as indicated.[12] Table 67–1 lists antidotes recommended by the Oncology Nursing Society. In many institutions, a plastic surgery consultation is immediately initiated, especially if the clinician is sure that the drug did infiltrate.

A standardized plan for systematic follow-up of the patient should be in place and initiated with each suspected or actual extravasation. It should include the following data: patient demographics, name of the vesicant infiltrated, dose, amount suspected to have infiltrated, specific location of infiltration, presenting signs and symptoms (*e.g.*, redness, swelling, pain, blisters, necrosis), and range of motion at time of presentation. Management of extravasation, interventions, and plans for follow-up must be included. Patients should receive written information about the home care of the infiltration and be advised of the appropriate persons to contact with questions or problems. Because a delay in intervention can adversely affect the outcome and because patients can be reluctant to call if they are uncertain if it is appropriate, the care giver should follow-up at specified intervals by phone or office visit (Fig. 67–2). For monitoring purposes, baseline and periodic photographs are recommended. These serve as a visual record of the efficacy of treatments and interventions and as an educational tool for colleagues.

FLARE REACTION

A flare reaction can occur with the administration of anthracyclines, particularly doxorubicin. This reaction occurs within minutes of initiating treatment and is evidenced by erythematous streaking around the injection site and along the vein. Pruritus, urticaria, and patchy erythema may be present. Pain and burning at the site occur infrequently and aid in differentiating a flare reaction from an infiltration. The reaction is transient, often subsiding within 30 to 45 minutes of onset. It may recur with future doses of doxorubicin.

Prompt intervention is essential to determine whether the reaction is a flare phenomenon or an infiltration. Stop the drug immediately and allow the intravenous solution to infuse freely. Reassess catheter patency and assess for signs and symptoms of extravasation. After extravasation has been ruled out, hydrocortisone cream (1%) may be applied to the areas of inflammation. Restart the drug administration at a slower rate. These measures may alleviate the symptoms.

The occurrence of a flare reaction does not preclude future

(text continues on page 2579)

TABLE 67–1. Antidotes for Vesicant or Irritant Drugs

Drug Classification	Specific Agent	Local Antidote	Positive Effect: Animal Studies	Positive Effect: Clinical Case Reports	Antidote Preparation	Method of Administration	Comments
Alkylating agents	Mechlorethiamine (nitrogen mustard)	Isotonic sodium thiosulfate 1 g/10 ml (manufacturer's recommendations)	None	Yes[1]	Mix 4 ml of 10% Na thiosulfate with 6 ml sterile water for injection (1/6 molar solution results)	1. Inject 5–6 ml (0.2–0.24 g) I.V. through the existing line and SQ into the extravasated site with multiple injections. 2. Repeat dosing SQ over the next several hours. 3. Apply cold compresses. 4. No total dose established.	1. ACTION: chemical neutralization 2. Initiate treatment immediately and liberally.
	Mitomycin C (Mutamycin)	Topical DMSO (RIMSO)	Yes[2]	None	1–2 ml of 1 mmol DMSO 50–100%	1. Apply topically one time to the site.	1. Probably not effective for distal or delayed ulcers 2. Initiate treatment immediately. 3. ACTION: carrier solvent or oxygen radical scavenger
Plant alkaloids	Vinblastine (Velban) Vincristine (Oncovin)	Hyaluronidase (Wydase) 150 U/ml (manufacturer's recommendations)	Yes[3]	None	Add 1 ml USP sodium chloride (150 U/ml results)	1. Inject 1–6 ml (150–900 U) SQ into the extravasated site with multiple injections. 2. Repeat dosing SQ over the next several hours. 3. Apply *warm* compresses. 4. No total dose established.	1. ACTION: enhances absorption and dispersion of the extravasated drug 2. Corticosteroids and topical cooling appear to worsen toxicity 3. Warm compresses increase systemic absorption of the drug.
	Vindesine (Eldisine)	Hyaluronidase (Wydase)	Yes[4]	None			

	Teniposide (VM-26) Etopiside (VP-16-213 VePesid)	150 U/ML					
Anthracycline antibiotics	Doxorubicin (Adriamycin) Daunomycin (Cerubidine)	Topical DMSO	Yes[5–9]	Yes[10–11]	1–2 ml of 1 mmol DMSO 50–100%	1. Apply topically one time to the site. 2. Apply cold compresses.	1. Probably best to initiate treatment immediately 2. ACTION: carrier solvent or oxygen free radical 3. Cold compresses block cytotoxicity of doxorubicin.
	Bisanirene	Sodium bicarbonate 1 mEq/1 ml (premixed)	Yes[12]	Yes[12]	Mix equal parts of 1 mEq/ml sodium bicarbonate with sterile normal saline (1:1 solution). Resulting solution is 0.5 mEq/ml	1. Inject 2–6 ml (1.0–3.0 mEq) I.V. through the existing line and SQ into the extravasated site with multiple injections 2. Appy cold compresses. 3. Total dose not to exceed 10 ml of 0.5 mEq/ml solution (5.0 mEq).	1. ACTION: chemical activation 2. Dilute bicarbonate chemically degrades the drug.

1. Owen O, Dellatorre DL, Scott EJ, Cohen MR. Accidental intramuscular injection of mechlorethamine. Cancer 1980;45:2225–2226.
2. Dorr R, Soble MJ, Liddil JD, Keller JH. Mitomycin C skin toxicity studies in mice: Reduced ulceration and altered pharmokinetics with topical dimethyl sulfoxide. J Clin Oncol 1986;4:1399–1404.
3. Dorr RT, Alberta DS, Woods MW. Vinca alkaloid ulceration: Experimental mouse model and effects of local antidotes. Proc Am Assoc Cancer Res 1982;23:109.
4. Dorr RT, Alberts DS. Skin ulceration potential without therapeutic anticancer activity for epipodophyllotoxin commercial diluents. Invest New Drugs 1983;1:151–159.
5. Desai MH, Teres D. Prevention of doxorubicin-induced skin ulcers in the rat and pig with dimethyl sulfoxide (DMSO). Cancer Treat Rep 1982;66:1371–1374.
6. Svingen BA, Powis G, Appel PL, Scott M. Protection against Adriamycin-induced skin necrosis in the rat with dimethyl sulfoxide and alpha tocopherol. Cancer 1981;41:3395–3399.
7. Dorr RT, Alberta DS. Failure of DMSO and vitamin E to prevent doxorubicin skin ulceration in the mouse. Cancer Treat Rep 1983;67:499–501.
8. Nobbs P, Barr RD. Soft tissue injury caused by antineoplastic drugs is inhibited by topical dimethyl sulphoxide and alpha tocopherol. Br J Cancer 1983;48:873–876.
9. Soble M, Dorr R, Plezia P, Breckenridge S. Dose dependent skin ulcers in mice treated with DNA binding antitumor antibiotics. Cancer Chemother Pharmacol 1987.
10. Olver IN. Use of dimethyl sulfoxide in limiting tissue damage caused by extravasation of doxorubicin. Cancer Treat Rep 1983;67:407–408.
11. Lawrence HJ, Goodnight SH. Dimethyl sulfoxide and extravasation of anthracylcine agents. [Letter] Ann Intern Med 1983;98:1025.
12. Dorr RT, Peng YM, Alberts DS. Bisantrene solubility and skin toxicity studies: Efficacy of sodium bicarbonate as a local antidote. Invest New Drug 1984;2:351–357.

(With permission from the ONS Cancer Chemotherapy Guidelines—Module V. Recommendations for the management of extravasations and anaphylaxis. Oncology Nursing Society, 1988:8–9)

CHEMOTHERAPY NURSING

Extravasation Flow Sheet

Pt. Name ______________________ M.R. # ______________________

Date ______________________ Date Extravasation Occurred ______________________

Name and Volume of Drug Extravasated ______________________

Attending Physician ______________________ Physician Notified ______________________

Patient Telephone # ______________________ Preferred Calling Time ______________________

Appearance of Extravasation Site
Exact Location (*describe and doc. on diagram*)

____

____

Dimensions ______________________

Appearance of Skin at Site ______________________

____

____

Nursing Interventions (* *indicates requires M.D. order*)

________ Antidote Administered* ______________________ ________ Hydrocortisone cream applied

________ Cold Compresses ________ Warm Compresses

________ Dermatology Consult* ________ Plastic Surgery Consult*

________ Initiated Wound Care (*describe*) ______________________

________ Patient Education Card Reviewed ________ Plan for Follow-up Reviewed

________ Baseline Photograph Obtained

Follow Up Flow Sheet

	Day 1	Day 3	Day 5	Day 7	Day 14	Day 21	Day 28	Day 35**	Day 42**
Pain									
Edema									
Skin Changes									
Change Mobility									
Color of area									
Fever									
Date									
R.N. Initial									
Tel. Call. Visit									

**** may omit if patient without positive signs of extravasation**

FIGURE 67–2. Flow sheet for managing extravasations.

treatment. The flare may recur at the next treatment, but it is usually milder than the first reaction. The literature suggests pretreatment with antihistamines or corticosteroids. Documentation of the event should be included in the medical record.

HANDLING AND DISPOSAL OF CHEMOTHERAPY

Because chemotherapy is currently administered in many settings, health care personnel and support personnel (*e.g.*, maintenance, sanitation) continue to be at increased risk of exposure to antineoplastic drugs. Many are rightfully concerned. Because the risks from prolonged exposure are unknown and no safe level of exposure has been identified, meticulous attention must be given to handling and disposal of these agents.[1,3–11,33]

The goal must be to protect health care personnel, support persons, and the environment from the potential hazards of these agents. The Office of Safety and Health Administration has issued guidelines for safe handling and disposal, which focus on minimizing exposure through absorption and inhalation.[28]

All personnel having contact with cytotoxic agents must become aware of the possible risks and how to effectively minimize them before they handle the chemotherapy drugs.[29–32] Antineoplastic drug preparation requires specific training and attention to manufacturer guidelines.[36–38]

All drugs should be prepared aseptically in a class II biologic safety cabinet, which is cleaned, serviced, and maintained at specified intervals. The environment should be clean and free of interruptions; no food, drinks, or cosmetics should be present.

Personnel preparing chemotherapy should wear disposable surgical gowns, which tie in the back and have cuffs. Unpowdered latex gloves should be worn at all times when preparing chemotherapy.[28,36,37] Gloves should be changed hourly or more frequently if needed. A thermoplastic face shield or goggles and an air purifying respirator should be worn when drugs are prepared outside of a biologic safety cabinet. Measures to avoid exposure to drug leakage or aerosolization should be taken, no matter where the drug is prepared. Care should be taken to ensure that intravenous tubing is secured in the infusion container and all lines are clamped and capped to avoid inadvertent drug spills. Drugs should be transported to the patient in a sealed, zip-closed plastic bag.

Proper administration techniques provide optimal protection from exposure. Physicians and nurses must be well versed in proper handling and disposal of chemotherapy.[30–32] Many clinicians wear lab coats as a barrier, rather than gowns, but drug can be readily absorbed into a lab coat, and it does not provide maximal protection. If the coat is to have any barrier benefit, it should be worn closed, with the sleeves down, and changed frequently.

To reduce further potential exposure, intravenous tubing should be primed in the biologic safety cabinet. If this is not feasible, the clinician can back-prime the secondary tubing that is connected to the chemotherapy by piggybacking it into the side arm of a compatible intravenous solution. This technique maintains a closed system. An alternative method is to wrap a sterile gauze around the tip of the needle and slowly prime the chemotherapy tubing into a zip-closed bag. Care must be taken to protect the sterility of the infusion line. Syringes containing chemotherapy can be primed in a similar fashion. After chemotherapy is discontinued, gauze should be held at the disconnection site to catch any droplets of the drug. All waste should be disposed of in the zip-closed bag and discarded as hazardous waste.

All chemotherapy should be disposed of in accordance with applicable state, local, and federal regulations for handling hazardous waste. Written guidelines should be placed in all areas where chemotherapy is dispensed, administered, or handled.[34,35,38]

All waste associated with chemotherapy—gloves, gowns, gauze, tubings, and syringes—should be treated as hazardous waste. Drugs containing solutions to be wasted should first be transferred to resealable containers. Needles and syringes should be disposed of intact into a leak-proof, puncture-proof container to avoid aerosolization leaks or spills. Gloves should be worn by all persons handling bodily waste of a patient who has received chemotherapy within the last 48 hours.

Patients receiving therapy at home must also be educated in proper handling and disposal of chemotherapy waste.[38] The Environmental Protection Agency has made available patient fact cards, entitled "Disposal Tips For Home Health Care," which explain how to handle needles and syringes. Patients should be urged to contact their state or community environmental programs or local sanitation departments for specific details in their areas.

In cases of accidental exposure to the drug, contaminated clothing should be removed promptly and the affected skin washed thoroughly with soap and water. If the eye is involved, immediately flood the eye for 5 minutes with water or isotonic eye wash. Prompt medical follow-up is recommended after all exposures. Document exposure of personnel according to institutional policy.[28,34–38]

A spill kit should be maintained in all dispensing and treatment areas in the event of an accidental drug spill. These kits can be purchased or assembled. They should contain two pairs of disposable gloves, disposable protective garments including shoe covers, safety goggles, respirator, absorbent plastic-backed pads, disposable towels, two resealable hazardous waste bags, a scoop for picking up glass, and a container for disposal of glass fragments.

Spills should be cleaned promptly. Traffic through the area should be restricted until clean-up is completed. Windows and doors should remain closed to minimize aerosolization. After the waste is cleaned and disposed of, the area should be washed three times with detergent and then flushed with water.

Smaller spills of less than 5 ml of unconcentrated drug should be promptly cleaned using absorbent toweling. Wash the affected area three times with soap and water. Reusable items can be washed by specially trained personnel wearing a double pair of unpowdered latex gloves.

Physicians and oncology nurses have a responsibility to protect themselves and the environment from the potential hazards of chemotherapeutic agents through safe practice techniques. An ongoing review of the current literature regarding practice issues and changes should be basic to all clinical practice settings using this treatment modality.

CONCLUSION

Successful treatment and management of chemotherapy requires in-depth knowledge and skill by the physician and oncology nurse. Clinicians must maintain competency and clinical expertise to deliver continued quality of care in a complex, changing climate.

REFERENCES

1. Perry MC. The chemotherapy source book. Baltimore: Williams & Wilkins, 1992:780–882.
2. Lokich JJ. Cancer chemotherapy by infusion. Chicago: Precept Press, 1987:3–113, 502–524.
3. Carter S, Bakowski M, Hellman K. Chemotherapy of cancer. 3rd ed. New York: Wiley Medical, 1987:325–340.
4. Baird SB, McCorkle R, Grant M. Cancer nursing. Philadelphia: WB Saunders, 1991: 291–321.
5. Otto SE. Oncology nursing. St. Louis: Mosby, 1991:253–317.
6. Chabner BA, Collins JM. Cancer chemotherapy principles and practice. Philadelphia: Lippincott, 1990:449–464.
7. Groenwald SL, Frogge MH, Goodman M, Yarbro CH. Cancer nursing principles and practice. Boston: Jones and Bartlett, 1990:230–284.
8. Cancer chemotherapy guidelines. Recommendations for cancer chemotherapy. Pittsburgh: Oncology Nursing Society, 1988.
9. Cancer chemotherapy guidelines. Recommendations for nursing practice in the acute care setting. Pittsburgh: Oncology Nursing Society, 1988.
10. Cancer chemotherapy guidelines. Recommendations for nursing practice in the outpatient setting. Pittsburgh: Oncology Nursing Society, 1988.
11. Cancer chemotherapy guidelines. Recommendations for nursing practice in the home care setting. Pittsburgh: Oncology Nursing Society, 1988.
12. Cancer chemotherapy guidelines. Recommendations for the management of extravasation and anaphylaxis. Pittsburgh: Oncology Nursing Society, 1988.
13. Access device guidelines. Recommendations for nursing education and practice. Modules 1–3. Pittsburgh: Oncology Nursing Society, 1989.
14. Wickman R. Advances in venous access devices and nursing management strategies. Nurs Clin North Am 1990;25:345–364, 1990.
15. Brown MH, Kiss ME, Outlaw E, Viamontes C. Standards for oncology nursing practice. Somerset, NJ: Wiley and Sons, 1986:59–101, 595–610.
16. Brager BL, Yasko JM. Care of the client receiving chemotherapy. Reston, VA: Reston Publishing, 1984:53–89.
17. DeVita VT, Hellman S, Rosenberg SA. Cancer: Principles and practice of oncology. 3rd ed. Philadelphia: Lippincott, 1989:2369–2402.
18. Swenson KK, Erikkson JH. Nursing management of intraperitoneal chemotherapy. Oncol Nurs Forum 1986;13:33–39.
19. Roemeling R, MacDonald M, Langevin T, et al. Chemotherapy via implanted infusion pump: New perspectives for delivery of long-term continuous treatment. Oncol Nurs Forum 1986;13:17–24.
20. Fischer DS, Tish Knobf M. The cancer chemotherapy handbook. 3rd ed. Chicago: Year Book Medical, 1989:199–233, 557–558.
21. Ziegfeld CR. Core curriculum for oncology nursing. Philadelphia: WB Saunders, 1987: 225–234.
22. Ashwanden P, Belcher A, Hubbard Mattson EA, et al. Oncology nursing advances, treatments and trends into the twenty-first century. Rockville, MD: Aspen, 1990:53–57, 303–309.
23. Lynch M, Yanes L. Flowsheet documentation of chemotherapy administration. Oncol Nurs Forum 1991;18:777–782.
24. Dorr RT, Fritz WL. Cancer chemotherapy handbook. New York: Elsevier, 1980:75–93, 101–137.
25. Alberts DS, Dorr RT. Case report: Topical DMSO for mitomycin-C-induced skin ulcerations. Oncol Nurs Forum 1991;18: 693–695.
26. Rudolf R, Larson DL. Etiology and treatment of chemotherapeutic agent injuries: A review. J Clin Oncol 1987;5:1116–1126.
27. Reed WP, Newman KA, Applefeld MM, Sutton FJ. Drug extravasation as a complication of venous access ports. Ann Intern Med 1985;102:788–790.
28. U.S. Department of Labor, Office of Occupational Medicine, Occupational Safety and Health Administration. Work practice guidelines for personnel dealing with cytotoxic (antineoplastic) drugs, No 8-1.1, Washington, DC: U.S. Government Printing Office, 1986.
29. Venitt S, Crofton-Sleigh C, Hunt J, et al. Monitoring exposure of nursing and pharmacy personnel to cytotoxic drugs: Urinary mutation assays and urinary platinum as markers of absorption. Lancet 1984;1:74–76.
30. Miller S. Issues in cytotoxic drug handling safety. Semin Oncol Nurs 1987;3:133–141.
31. Valanes M, Shortridge L. Self-protective practices of nurses handling antineoplastic drugs. Oncol Nurs Forum 1987;14:23–27.
32. Cloak M, Connor T, Stevens K, et al. Occupational exposure of nursing personnel to antineoplastic agents. Oncol Nurs Forum 1985;12:33–39.
33. Stellman JM, Zoloth R. Cancer chemotherapeutic agents as occupational hazards: A literature review. Cancer Invest 1986;4:127–135.
34. Gullo SM. Safe handling of antineoplastic drugs: Translating the recommendations into practice. Oncol Nurs Forum 1988;15:595–601.
35. Barhammand BA. Difficulties encountered in implementing guidelines for handling antineoplastics in the physician's office. Cancer Nurs 1986;9:138–143.
36. Power LA, Anderson RW, Cortopassi R, Gera JR, Lewis RM. Update on safe handling of hazardous drugs: The advice of experts. Am J Hosp Pharm 1990;47:1050–1060.
37. ASHP technical assistance bulletin on handling cytotoxic and hazardous drugs. Am J Hosp Pharm 1990;48:1033–1049.
38. Stevens KR. Safe handling of cytotoxic drugs in home chemotherapy. Semin Oncol Nurs 1989;5:15–20.

Cancer: Principles & Practice of Oncology, Fourth Edition,
edited by Vincent T. DeVita, Jr., Samuel Hellman, Steven A. Rosenberg.
J.B. Lippincott Co., Philadelphia © 1993.

CHAPTER 68

Information Systems in Oncology

SECTION 1

SUSAN MOLLOY HUBBARD

Information Retrieval Systems

Ready access to current information on effective and promising new investigational therapies is crucial if patients with cancer are to receive state-of-the-art treatment. This is particularly important given the explosive growth of knowledge and the pace of research advances in the field of medicine. Results of a survey of 432 primary care practitioners and 88 of their opinion leaders indicated that two of three physicians claimed that the volume of medical literature was unmanageable.[1] More than 78% reported that they had problems sorting out irrelevant material when examining the medical literature. Fifty-four percent were unaware of recently proven clinical advances regarding the use of digitalis preparations in the elderly, and knowledge deficiencies were documented for five other medical advances that were used as marker studies. Survey data indicated that these physicians felt that critical, "validated" reviews were the most useful means of meeting their information needs. Experts in continuing medical education and information science have been attempting to develop innovative systems that assist physicians to manage what promises to be an ongoing information explosion.[2–10]

Automated systems for improving access to medical knowledge and accelerating the pace of technology transfer have been developed by the National Cancer Institute (NCI). These computerized resources provide ready access to bibliographic citations of the published cancer research literature (*i.e.*, CANCERLIT database) and validated, peer-reviewed syntheses of current information on the prognosis and treatment of all major cancers (*i.e.*, PDQ database). Both of these computerized information systems are designed to facilitate research and patient care by assisting health professionals to maximize use of current medical knowledge. This chapter summarizes the information systems that are currently available from the NCI, existing mechanisms for distributing these resources, enhancements that are under development, and ongoing efforts to electronically link patient records, clinical and laboratory information, and decision support to our automated information systems.

HISTORICAL PERSPECTIVE

Index Medicus, inaugurated in 1879, was the first systematic classification of the medical literature. The first year's volume contained 17,000 citations from 700 periodicals. In 1992, a single month of *Index Medicus* averaged more than 31,000 citations and annual coverage exceeded 373,000 articles.[11,12] The rapid growth of the medical literature manual preparation of *Index Medicus* a logistic nightmare by the early 1950s, prompting the staff of the National Library of Medicine (NLM) to develop a computer-based medical literature analysis and retrieval system (MEDLARS). MEDLARS automated the process of organizing, indexing, publishing, and searching *Index Medicus.* This pioneering use of early computing technology led to the introduction of MEDLINE in 1971, an on-line version of the *Cumulated Index Medicus.* Rapid acceptance of MEDLINE by the medical and scientific community stimulated the growth of nationwide access systems by commercial telecommunication networks and the development of a variety of additional scientific and medical databases for distribution over the MEDLARS system. By the end of 1991, MEDLINE alone contained over 7 million medical references.

In 1971, the National Cancer Act mandated the creation of an international databank to foster rapid and effective exchange of cancer data throughout the world.[13] Faced with responsibility for organizing, updating, and disseminating a rapidly growing collection of knowledge, staff at the NCI decided to establish a computerized information program to complement its peer-reviewed scientific journals. NCI staff immediately began to develop cancer databases for distribution on MEDLARS and a series of database-derived publications designed to meet the information needs of those who without access to on-line systems.[14]

The first on-line information system to be made available was a bibliographic database called CANCERLIT, created in 1974.[5,6] Each literature citation was formatted in a unit record structure similar to the records in MEDLINE to enable NCI to distribute CANCERLIT on the NLM's computer system. Because NCI staff anticipated that users would want access to summary data from each article, abstracts were created and included in each citation. CANCERLIT is a comprehensive resource of the published cancer literature containing over 900,000 citations screened, indexed, abstracted, and keyed from over 3000 biomedical journals, books, monographs, government-sponsored reports, and proceedings.

Other than presenting abstracts of ongoing research from conference proceedings, the CANCERLIT database does not provide information on clinical research in progress. To fill this need, in 1974, NCI staff developed CLINPROT, a computerized database that summarized the investigational treatment protocols sponsored by the Institute. Each protocol record was created using the full clinical research protocol as the source document and indexed with special terms that allowed users to retrieve protocols by tumor type and treatment. As with CANCERLIT, each unit record was formatted to allow distribution and on-line searching on the NLM computer system. However, the CLINPROT database did not provide information on state-of-the-art treatment. Moreover, summaries were not indexed by stage, histologic type, participating investigators, or institutions. This made it difficult for physicians to identify clinical trials appropriate for cancer patients that were being conducted in a particular location. CLINPROT did not lend itself to use in clinical care or decision making, but it instead served as an on-line catalog of clinical research that provided physicians designing treatment protocols with information on research performed by others. Moreover, as with all MEDLARS databases, effective information retrieval required knowledge of the NLM's specialized searching language. A trained search intermediary, usually a medical librarian, was required to search the cancer databases effectively.

The growing power of personal computers in the 1980s and the introduction of powerful operating systems permitted greater speed and flexibility in telecommunications among computers and an enormous increase in the capacity to store and manipulate large quantities of data. New software technologies quickly emerged to support the development and distribution of large factual databases. Recognizing the power of this computer technology, the director of the NCI conceived PDQ, an on-line database containing up-to-date information on state-of-the-art cancer treatment to speed the diffusion of information about advances in cancer treatment and to facilitate the integration of new medical knowledge and research advances into clinical practice.[15]

THE PDQ SYSTEM

The PDQ information system is a computerized resource that provides three general types of information: up-to-date guidelines cancer treatment that are synthesized, peer reviewed, and continually updated by cancer experts; summaries of clinical trials that are open to patient accrual; and a directory of physicians and organizations that provide cancer care. The information in PDQ enables users to identify the full range of treatment alternatives that are state-of-the-art therapy for all major cancers; locate clinical trials for patients who are candidates for treatment research; and identify physicians and treatment facilities for consultation and referral. The PDQ information retrieval system that is distributed on NLM's MEDLARS system is designed with a user-friendly, menu-driven interface that internally links diverse types of information and allows users to search and display information without learning a specialized search language (Fig. 68–1).[16]

PDQ's cancer information file contains treatment recommendations that summarize current state-of-the-art therapy for all major cancers. Treatment information is presented in two formats: a peer-reviewed file of "state-of-the-art statements" that are written to meet the information needs of clinicians and a corresponding file of overviews written in simpler language for patients, their families, and the general public. The state-of-the-art statements provide current information that can assist clinicians in deciding whether a standard or investigational therapy is appropriate for their cancer patient. Each state-of-the-art statement provides up-to-date data on prognosis, relevant staging and histologic classifications, therapies that constitute current standards of cancer care, and references to seminal literature. Abstracts have been incorporated into the system, allowing users to retrieve them for review if so desired. Each patient information summary contains references to patient education materials that are readily available through NCI and other sources.

PDQ's cancer information file is being enhanced with information on the cause and management of untoward sequelae of cancer or its treatment. PDQ contains 20 "supportive care" summaries on the management of patient care issues, such as pain, nutrition, sleep disorders, radiation enteritis, nausea, vomiting, and oral complications. The file is being expanded to peer-reviewed information on innovative approaches to cancer prevention and promising investigational drugs. Prognostic and treatment information for rare tumors is also under development.

The cancer information file contains a *news file* that contains items of interest, including summaries of the most recent changes to the state-of-the-art statements; NCI's clinical alerts; NIH Consensus Development Conferences dealing with cancer; information on NCI's group C drugs and its treatment referral center; current database vendors, including foreign MEDLARS centers; and NCI's high-priority clinical trials.

The prognostic and treatment information in the cancer information file was developed and is maintained by an Editorial Board of cancer specialists with input from experts

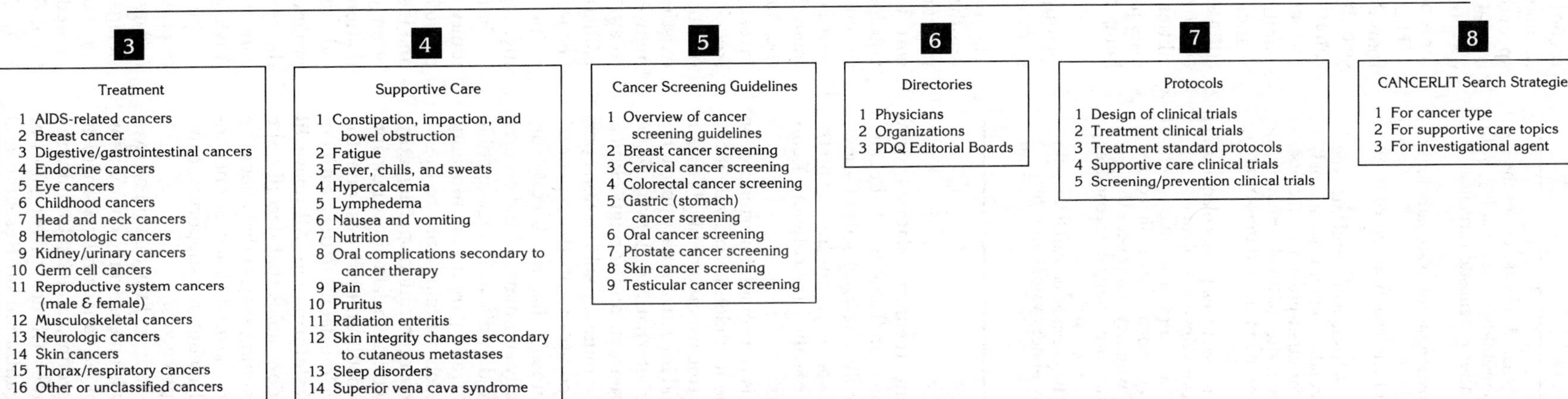

PDQ Menu
The following information is available in PDQ.
1 Information about PDQ
2 PDQ News
3 Treatment
4 Supportive Care
5 Screening
6 Directories
7 Protocols
8 CANCERLIT Search Strategies
9 Exit PDQ
3
Treatment
1 AIDS-related cancers
2 Breast cancer
3 Digestive/gastrointestinal cancers
4 Endocrine cancers
5 Eye cancers
6 Childhood cancers
7 Head and neck cancers
8 Hemotologic cancers
9 Kidney/urinary cancers
10 Germ cell cancers
11 Reproductive system cancers (male & female)
12 Musculoskeletal cancers
13 Neurologic cancers
14 Skin cancers
15 Thorax/respiratory cancers
16 Other or unclassified cancers
4
Supportive Care
1 Constipation, impaction, and bowel obstruction
2 Fatigue
3 Fever, chills, and sweats
4 Hypercalcemia
5 Lymphedema
6 Nausea and vomiting
7 Nutrition
8 Oral complications secondary to cancer therapy
9 Pain
10 Pruritus
11 Radiation enteritis
12 Skin integrity changes secondary to cutaneous metastases
13 Sleep disorders
14 Superior vena cava syndrome
5
Cancer Screening Guidelines
1 Overview of cancer screening guidelines
2 Breast cancer screening
3 Cervical cancer screening
4 Colorectal cancer screening
5 Gastric (stomach) cancer screening
6 Oral cancer screening
7 Prostate cancer screening
8 Skin cancer screening
9 Testicular cancer screening
6
Directories
1 Physicians
2 Organizations
3 PDQ Editorial Boards
7
Protocols
1 Design of clinical trials
2 Treatment clinical trials
3 Treatment standard protocols
4 Supportive care clinical trials
5 Screening/prevention clinical trials
8
CANCERLIT Search Strategies
1 For cancer type
2 For supportive care topics
3 For investigational agent

FIGURE 68–1. The PDQ file structure. This diagram from the PDQ User Guide depicts the menu hierarchy from the "main PDQ menu," shown at the top of the diagram. PDQ's user interface uses menu selections to prompt users to select the information desired. Each item of the main PDQ menu has a series of submenus that are arranged in hierarchical order. User commands provide shortcuts for moving through the hierarchy of menus.

TABLE 68–1. Guidelines for the Development of Treatment Statements

1. Open with a prognostic statement that clearly describes the success of treatment in terms of curability (or treatability) with current modalities and states whether prognostic variables influence treatment outcome.
2. Provide clinically relevant information on the histopathologic classification of the malignant cells.
3. Describe the most clinically useful and widely accepted staging classification.
4. Provide current survival data for each stage or histologic type.
5. Provide treatment information (standard and investigational) options by stage of dissemination or other prognostic factors such as histology (*e.g.*, lung cancer), sites of involvement (*e.g.*, rhabdomyosarcoma), or location of the primary tumor (*e.g.*, brain neoplasms).
6. Indicate whether the therapeutic alternatives produce equivalent results and whether there are reasons for selecting one treatment over another in a particular clinical setting.
7. List only therapies with superior and documented efficacy as potential therapeutic alternatives with key references that document treatment efficacy if cure or prolonged disease-free survival is achievable.
8. Clearly state that patients should be considered candidates for investigational therapies currently under evaluation if no effective treatment exists.

around the country. Treatment recommendations were drafted using the guidelines shown on Table 68–1. Because PDQ provides a current and critically analyzed body of knowledge that encompasses an entire specialty, on-line use on the NLM implementation has been certified for category I continuing medical education credits.

Because a major goal of PDQ is to provide information on therapeutic research, the treatment guidelines provide information on ongoing studies, directing users to clinical trials if effective therapies do not exist and investigational approaches represent important therapeutic alternatives. A *protocol file* containing over 1500 active American and foreign clinical trials, 30% to 35% of which are voluntary submissions performed without federal support, complements the cancer information file. All treatment protocols that are directly supported by the NCI are automatically summarized and entered into PDQ. Each protocol is indexed by disease, stage-specific eligibility criteria, phase of investigation, treatment modality, drugs, and drug regimens, and each contains links to the directory records of physicians and organizations participating in the trial so that users can easily retrieve data on participants by geographic location. Each protocol summary describes the study objectives, eligibility criteria, the details of the treatment program, and dose and schedule information. All phase III protocols contain dose-modification tables that describe the dose and schedule adjustments (sliding scales) that should be used when significant toxicity to normal tissue is encountered.[17] The PDQ protocol file also contains supportive care, early detection, and prevention protocols.

A *physician directory* contains address information on over 19,000 physicians. This directory is an electronic compilation of the membership directories of 17 cancer-related medical societies, NCI's clinical trials groups, and its Community Clinical Oncology Program grantees. Clinical investigators of the NCI and the European Organization on Research and Treatment of Cancer (EORTC) are also listed. Each person's record includes the physician's full name, address, telephone number, medical specialties, information on oncologic subspecialty board certification, and organizational affiliations. The PDQ implementation that distributed on the NLM system uses interfile linkages to automatically retrieve all protocols for a physician if requested by the user.

The *organization directory* includes information on more than 2500 organizations at which NCI supports clinical research and hospitals with cancer programs certified by the American College of Surgeons' Commission on Cancer. Information on organizations is retrievable by name, city, state, country, or postal code. Each organization record includes the name, address, and telephone number of a person at the institution who has agreed to answer questions from PDQ users about the organization's cancer treatment programs and facilities. As in the physician directory, PDQ on the NLM system uses interfile linkages to automatically retrieve all protocols being conducted at an organization if requested by the user.

CURRENCY OF THE TREATMENT RECOMMENDATIONS

The major rationale for developing PDQ as an on-line database was the ability to use computer technology to rapidly and easily maintain the currency of the information. A multidisciplinary core Editorial Board of 30 cancer specialists (including an oncology nurse) and an 80-member Advisory Board maintains the currency of the treatment information. Each month, core board members receive a printout of the state-of-the-art statements that fall within their purview and relevant articles from the current literature that report cure with an established or investigational treatment program; improvement in disease-free or overall survival that is equivalent to or better than that produced by regimens cited as "standard" treatment in the existing statement; significantly less acute or long-term treatment-induced toxicity with equivalent results to standard treatments cited in the existing statement; and significant palliation for cancers for which no effective therapies exist. Separate Editorial Boards have been established to develop, refine, and update the state-of-the-art information on screening, early detection, cancer prevention, and supportive care.

Monthly meetings of the Board afford members the opportunity to discuss data from the current treatment literature, propose modifications and refinements to PDQ statements, and identify the need for new state-of-the-art statements and other file enhancements. Modifications to the cancer information file are based on Board discussions. Articles that provide data suggesting improved results with investigational programs are also reviewed and highlighted or referenced in the text if the data merit. On average, 20% to 25% of the cancer information statements are modified each month. The Advisory Board provides input and peer review by mail.

The PDQ protocol file is maintained by a monthly mailing to protocol coordinators at medical centers nationwide who update the status and update the matrix of participating physicians and organizations to ensure that the protocols remain accurate. Twice each year, the protocol summaries are reviewed by the principal investigators to ensure that the protocol details remain accurate. Each month, approximately 35% of the active protocols in PDQ undergo a change of description, status, or investigators. On average, 60 new protocols are abstracted, indexed, and entered into PDQ each month and about 50 are closed and transferred to the closed protocol file.

Each physician and organization in PDQ is sent a printout of the directory record annually and must validate the accuracy of the listing by return mail. Update requests are mailed to one twelfth of the PDQ directory each month. Physicians and organizations are encouraged to submit changes whenever they occur. More than 93% of the directory records have been revalidated or corrected by return mail every year, making the file one of the most accurate directories in existence.

In September of 1992, the PDQ Screening and Prevention file was introduced on-line. It includes *Guidelines* for screening for cancers of the breast, cervix, colon and rectum, stomach, oral cavity, prostate, skin, and testes. For each site, in addition to the actual screening *Guideline*, there is background information describing studies of the efficacy of screening as a means of accomplishing the early detection of cancer in asymptomatic individuals and reducing mortality.

The Screening and Prevention Editorial Board reviews the published literature and discusses the clinical data at a bimonthly meeting. The data are analyzed with regard to whether the specific technique detects cancers earlier and whether there is evidence that earlier detection results in improved treatment outcome. The editorial board determines whether the narrative should be changed to accommodate the new literature and whether new evidence is sufficient to change actual guidelines. Board members discuss the quality of the data and the gaps in knowledge as the basis for their decisions about establishing or revising screening guidelines. Critical parameters considered for a specific technique include sensitivity, specificity, and predictive value. Four measures of improved outcome are considered: (1) a decrease in cause-specific mortality; (2) a reduction in the incidence of advanced stage cancers; (3) an increase in survival; and (4) a shift in stage distribution. Evidence of improved outcome is categorized into five levels in decreasing order of strength:

1. Evidence obtained from at least one properly randomized well-designed and well-conducted trial
2. Evidence obtained from well-designed and well-conducted trials without randomization
3. Evidence obtained from well-designed cohort or case-control analytic studies, preferably from more than one center or research group
4. Evidence obtained from multiple time series with or without the intervention
5. Opinions of respected authorities based on clinical experience, descriptive studies, or reports of expert committees

The levels of evidence supporting improved outcome are specified in the narrative and taken into account by the editorial board in arriving at screening guidelines. Statements are sent yearly to an external advisory board for review and comment.

SYSTEM IMPLEMENTATION

As implemented on the NLM's MEDLARS system, PDQ is completely menu driven. The main menu (see Fig. 68–1) prompts users to select a number to select information about PDQ (*i.e.*, a description of the database and instructions on database searching); a list of the members of the various PDQ Editorial Boards; the news file; cancer information; directories of physicians and organizations; protocols, or information on preformulated CANCERLIT searches. Throughout a PDQ search, users may return to previous menus and change files by entering a simple command, restart from the main menu, or exit from PDQ at any time during a search.

Prognostic and treatment information contained in the cancer information file are selectable options from a menu that is dynamically generated when the user selects a cancer diagnosis. Treatment information for each cancer diagnosis is provided in two formats: state-of-the-art information and information for patients (Fig. 68–2). Because, for many users, the cancer information file is the entry point into the PDQ files, each description of stage-specific treatment options on the NLM implementation indicates the number of clinical trials that may be found in the protocol file for that subset of patients. PDQ also offers users the opportunity to review the abstracts of any of the literature that is cited in the state-of-the-art statements. A series of preformulated search statements that enable the user to search the CANCERLIT database

CANCER INFORMATION MENU

Breast Cancer

Information for Patients	State-of-the-Art Information
1 Description	**4** Prognosis
2 Stage Explanations	**5** Cellular Classification
3 General Treatment Options	**6** Stage Information
	7 Treatment by Cell Type/Stage

8 Display all information

9 Continuation options for citation abstracts, **CANCERLIT** searches and protocols.

*** Enter desired number and press CR**

FIGURE 68–2. The cancer treatment information menu. Once a specific clinical diagnosis is selected this menu is displayed for that diagnosis. By making *selections 1 → 3,* the user can display information written for patients based on the state-of-the-art recommendations made for physicians. These summaries are written in lay language with references to printed materials written for cancer patients. By making *selections 4 → 7,* the user can display the state-of-the-art statements that are written to meet the technical information needs of clinicians caring for cancer patients. Key references from the medical literature, abstracts, and the number of active trials for each type and stage are available for review. *Selection 8* allows the user to display all of the information. *Selection 9* contains the continuation options that are available for the selected diagnosis. If the user has selected treatment information about a particular stage, the diagnosis and stage are used for continuing searches.

for additional literature on treatment questions are available as a menu selection (see Figs. 68–1 and 68–2).

Users may select protocols for a particular cancer diagnosis and stage by choosing the continuation option on the cancer information menu (see Fig. 68–2). This option automatically retrieves all trials that are open to the last type or stage of cancer defined by the user from the protocol file without reformulation of the search criteria. Users may also select protocols as the primary retrieval option from the main menu or by typing a simple command (*i.e.*, prot) at most prompts. Users can retrieve protocols from PDQ by diagnosis, stage, therapeutic agent, treatment modality, phase of clinical investigation, title word, patient age, geographic region, cancer center, cooperative group, ID number, and any combination of these parameters (see lower part of Fig. 68–1). In 1992, PDQ began to provide users with the capability of narrowing their protocol retrievals by patient-related criteria, such as menopausal status, and protocol-specific eligibility criteria, such as prior chemotherapy. Dose and schedule modifications for normal tissue toxicity are provided for all phase III and standard therapy protocols and most adjuvant trials. Detailed summaries describing the administration of treatment regimens considered to be state-of-the-art (*e.g.*, CMF, MOPP, ABVD) are provided as *standard therapy protocols.*

After a protocol set is defined, PDQ informs the user how many protocols met the search criteria. At this point, the user may redefine the criteria or decide to display or print information in a range of formats by selecting one of PDQ's print options. A customized print format can be created from a menu containing all protocol data elements. Users can select and order the items as desired and can maintain the customized format for the entire session or redefine it any time. In 1991, NCI incorporated a large portion of its CLINPROT database into PDQ. Users who wish to retrieve information on over 7000 closed and completed protocols may now do so.

Users can retrieve information about physicians by entering a name, medical specialty, a particular geographic location, or a combination of these parameters. After a data set is defined, PDQ offers a variety of print and display options that enable the user to review physician profiles in varying degrees of detail. Protocols for which a physician is a principal investigator or those that are being conducted at an organization can also be displayed using interfile linkages. The directory of organizations can be searched in a similar fashion.

AVAILABILITY

More than 35,000 domestic and 4000 foreign centers have access to the cancer databases on the MEDLARS system. Over 3500 student codes are also in effect. There are currently 16 principal foreign MEDLARS centers that offer database access to foreign medical institutions and physicians. Sixteen, including the Pan American Health Organization, offer access to CANCERLIT, and 12 offer access to PDQ. An on-line service, called EuroCODE, operated by the EORTC makes PDQ available to its participating organizations.[18] Once logged into the EORTC's EuroCODE computer system, physicians can register, randomize, and enter patients on EROTC clinical trials, search PDQ, or exchange electronic mail with colleagues.[19] NCI staff plan to make PDQ and CANCERLIT widely available to Latin American and Caribbean countries on the academic network, BITNIS, with an easy to use front end that will permit users to formulate their search query before logging onto the on-line system. Any hardware that can emulate an 80-character ASCII terminal can be used to search PDQ by a 300, 1200, or 2400 baud modem. Transmission of PDQ data over commercial telecommunication networks allows users to access PDQ without incurring long-distance charges. PDQ is also licensed to commercial vendors and academic and nonprofit health care organizations with computerized medical information systems.

A wide range of implementations exist for access by PDQ users. Some have been developed by the NCI and others by private vendors. Implementations fall into two general categories: on-line time-sharing systems with dial-up access and "local" implementations that reside on a single computer or a local area network for use by groups of individuals. Local access to PDQ is currently available from NCI as MUMPS or C language versions. PDQ is also offered as a local system on CD-ROM by two commercial sources. Subscriptions to the CD-ROM products are sold on an annual basis. They can be purchased to run on a DOS-based personal computer or a local area network. PDQ is provided alone on CD-ROM and as a component of products that also contain oncologic textbooks and other bibliographic databases. At least one vendor plans to release a CD-ROM product for the Macintosh computer family. The availability of NCI databases on CD-ROM should serve to markedly increase the awareness and usage of PDQ and CANCERLIT throughout the world, particularly in regions where access to on-line systems is difficult and cost is a consideration.

As part of an initiative to increase information dissemination to underserved populations, NCI is providing subscriptions to a commercial CD-ROM product containing PDQ and CANCERLIT to over 40 demonstration sites in selected domestic and foreign underserved areas for a 3-year demonstration period. These sites will serve as cancer information distribution centers, enabling the NCI to disseminate up-to-date information on cancer research findings and current standards of patient care to new and hitherto largely unreachable audiences.

NCI's Cancer Information Service (CIS) network uses CD-ROM technology to handle PDQ inquiries from the public. NCI plans to augment the CIS system with a new 800 number that will handle inquiries from physicians and other health professionals. The new service will be introduced in early 1993 and provide rapid and easy access to PDQ to those who do not have ready access to PDQ in other ways, especially disadvantaged and underserved health care professionals.

USER DOCUMENTATION AND PDQ ACCESS

Enhancements are continually being incorporated into PDQ to increase its clinical and educational value and ease of use. User documentation consists of a User Guide for the version that is distributed over the NLM system, which provides an overview of the system, explicit instructions for the inexperienced user on how to search each file, and advanced searching techniques for the expert searcher.[20] The guide is sold through the National Technical Information Service and subscribers automatically receive updates as they are printed. There is also a Quick Reference Guide that summarizes frequently used system functions and commands and a publication on the terminology in PDQ that explains how PDQ is indexed, the associations among indexed terms, and an index of drug synonyms. These resources are available free of charge through the NCI.

PDQ ACCESS is a telecommunications program that totally automates the dial up and log-on procedures to the NLM's MEDLARS system. The PDQ ACCESS software is provided free of charge to everyone who subscribers to the PDQ User Guide. Two versions of the PDQ ACCESS program are available: one for IBM-compatible computers and the other for the Macintosh family of computers.[21]

The PDQ ACCESS program automatically captures each search session to disk, enabling users to print the search after the on-line session is over. The PDQ ACCESS program also automates a link from PDQ to CANCERLIT. After a preformulated literature search in PDQ is selected, the PDQ ACCESS program connects the user to CANCERLIT and automatically executes the search and captures the results to a disk file. When the CANCERLIT search is complete, the PDQ ACCESS program returns the user to the PDQ search session. NLM's telecommunications package, GRATEFUL MED, also provides access to CANCERLIT, PDQ, and all of the preformulated CANCERLIT searches in PDQ.

CANCERFAX

Recent advances in technology allow facsimile (fax) boards to be placed inside personal computers so that the computer can act as a fax machine, sending and receiving documents simultaneously. When coupled with digital voice technology and software that interprets user selections from a touch-tone telephone, information from a database like PDQ can be delivered to a caller without human intervention. In 1991, NCI staff began distributing the treatment guidelines from PDQ using fax technology.[22] The service, CancerFax, allows users to dial into one of NCI's computers (301-402-5874) from the handset on their fax machine and retrieve a faxed image of any of PDQ's state-of-the-art, patient information statements or news articles. The service is available 24 hours each day, and there is no cost to the user other than the telephone call. In addition to the prognostic and treatment information contained in PDQ's cancer information file, CancerFax provides the current information on databases vendors, NCI's scientific journals, its database-derived publications, and its patient education materials. At the end of 1992, the CancerFax service had handled over 29,000 calls approximately 2400 queries per month.

Advances in computer technology have led to the development of natural language processing systems that have programs for speech recognition, language understanding, and language generation.[23] A text processing translation system has been used to facilitate the translation of text from PDQ's cancer information file into Spanish for distribution on CancerFax. The machine translator processes the source language text, producing a literal translation. This draft is reviewed, edited, and finalized by Spanish-speaking health professionals and oncologists and distributed on CancerFax.

In July 1992, NCI also introduced CancerNet, an electronic service that enables computer users to obtain free access to the treatment guidelines in PDQ 24 hours a day, 7 days a week on INTERNET's electronic bulletin board. INTERNET, a web of computer networks that reaches all over the world, trades information over high-speed datalines. This new service is another example of the NCI's efforts to make effective and efficient use of technology to facilitate its information dissemination initiatives. In the first 6 months, CancerNet was accessed over 8000 times (1400 times/month); one third of the users were from foreign countries. The technology is expected to play an increasingly important role in the dissemination of ICIC services and products as high-speed networks become more widely used.

NEW INITIATIVES

As part of its challenge to develop novel communication technologies, NCI is identifying emerging communication technologies that can facilitate the dissemination of information on cancer through the federal government's small business innovation research (SBIR) program. Areas of research include improving telecommunication access; optimizing the user interface; the ongoing refinement of touch-tone interfaces to facsimile (CancerFax); the development of other advanced personal computing technologies such as portable digital storage devices; and voice-recognition interfaces for information dissemination applications.[24]

Future plans include the development of links in PDQ that will make it easy for users to move between protocol summaries and published abstracts or articles on the trial that are cited in the CANCERLIT database. A drug file that would provide information on indication, does, mechanism of action, pharmacology and phase of development of investigational agents listed in the PDQ protocol file is under development. This enhancement will enable users to move easily between a protocol summary or state-of-the-art statement in the cancer information file to a relevant summary in the drug file or citations in the CANCERLIT database. Advances in fiberoptic communication technology offer the potential for future integration of images into PDQ as new developments in computer and communication technologies make it feasible.

CLINICAL INFORMATION SYSTEMS FOR DECISION SUPPORT

Hospital-based information systems have been developed to automate the collection, retrieval, and analysis of information for rapid and flexible access in clinical settings. Most systems process clinical, laboratory, and administrative data to support inpatient care, clinical research, and hospital operations. Some also use computer-based logic to support clinical decision making without additional data entry requirements.[25,26] The logic incorporated in these systems generates medical alerts that provide physicians with interpretations of physiologic data and medical advice (*e.g.*, drug interaction warnings, recommendations for additional tests) and guide them in the efficient management of patients in light of their past medical history and current problem list. Information systems also have been designed to deal specifically with diagnostic problems.[5,6,10,27,28]

Protocol-derived clinical algorithms have been developed to specify data-collection requirements (*e.g.*, frequency of radiologic studies, laboratory tests), to flag abnormal values, and to help oncologists to administer treatments as prescribed in a written protocol. Many of the oncology systems developed during the last decade also provided clinical databanks for statistical analysis, often with special displays or prompts to help remind physicians about protocol details.[29-32] Advice provided through algorithms implemented on a computer have been shown by investigators to improve oncology protocol compliance significantly for the cooperative group with which they worked.[33] However, this system was unable to analyze complex, ambiguous, or unusual clinical situations, involved data entry and program management centrally at the university rather than at the cooperating oncologist's office, and required considerable central effort to prepare the appropriate algorithm for each clinic visit. These limitations precluded the system's use in routine practice.

There is ongoing interest in the development of decision-support systems that formulate advice by following lines of reasoning similar to those used by human experts. Systems such as these capture and analyze patient data, apply medical knowledge, and interact with the physician to provide patient-specific recommendations on a course of action.[6,9,10] ONCOCIN is a decision-support system that integrates a clinical data management environment with an expert system provides customized treatment advice for cancer patients and clinical trial data management.[34] It presents, on a picture-quality display screen, a flow sheet that duplicates the traditional paper version. The graphic flow sheet is divided into sections, similar to those that separate classes of data on the paper flow sheet, and the physician can open sections for review or data entry by selecting them with a mouse device. ONCOCIN has several features that facilitate clinical trials data management:

1. *Registers and menus for data entry.* When physicians wish to enter data such as the current white blood cell count, they select the corresponding box on the flow sheet. An appropriate register containing values appears on the screen. They can use a mouse to indicate the proper value, which appears in the appropriate box on the flow sheet.
2. *Graphic data entry.* A paper flow sheet traditionally includes drawings of the human torso and chest x-ray views on which a physician is able to indicate areas of disease involvement. ONCOCIN also permits data to be entered and retrieved with a mouse.
3. *Guidance during data entry.* ONCOCIN uses current and past data on the patient to guide its assessment of the appropriate protocol-directed treatment for the current visit. The program indicates what information is needed to make an informed recommendation by displaying question marks in the appropriate boxes on the flow sheet. As clinical data are entered on the graphic flow sheet, they are passed to a "reasoner" that uses them plus knowledge about the protocol or treatment program to consider whether therapy should be administered and, if so, whether dosage adjustments are indicated. This decision-support program then displays its recommendations in the appropriate column on the flow sheet. If physicians wish to administer different dosages or to delay therapy, they indicate their changes in treatment by entering the new doses.

In addition to knowing the rules for chemotherapy administration in specific clinical trials, ONCOCIN keeps track of the data required by the protocol and provides reminders to the physician when laboratory studies or radiologic examinations are indicated. ONCOCIN can generate order forms, which can be printed and used to arrange tests on subsequent appointments. At the end of each clinic visit, ONCOCIN produces a hard copy of the flow sheets that can be placed in the patient's chart for backup and review. Although it has been documented that the data management and clinical consultation provided by this system can exert a significant influence on physician behavior, the overall impact of this and other systems on medical practice has been limited to selected settings.[35] However, there is increasing interest in using computer technology to meet the practicing physician's need for up-to-date medical information and expert medical advice.[6,10,11,36,37] Interest is due in part to the availability of increasingly powerful and sophisticated microcomputers, greatly improved graphical interfaces, and affordable, easily used, software tools, coupled with the growing concern about the increase in medical knowledge, medicolegal accountability, and cost-effective practice.[38,39] A key requirement for physician acceptance of automated information and decision support systems appears to be the smooth integration of the computer programs into the routine patient-care environment. Narrowly defined systems that serve a single purpose and require users to make special or duplicate efforts to access them have met with limited success, even though the information they provide has been shown in some cases to be accurate and valuable for patient care.[40,41]

Several recent developments may accelerate the pace at which the logistic problems are addressed. In an initiative to address technologic solutions to the current health care crisis, the Institute of Medicine (IOM) commissioned an 18-month study to examine the status of patient records and computer-based approaches to their management.[42] The study recommended the development of information systems to address the deficiencies in the paper-based medical record and help physicians to access and manage clinical information effectively.[43] Acknowledging that such systems must provide a critical mass of capabilities to achieve widespread and routine use, the IOM has recommended the establishment of a public and private computer-based patient record institute to develop and implement standards to ensure intersystem compatibility and data sharing.

Research in medical informatics is focusing on intersystem compatibility. Physician workstations are being designed with an "open systems architecture" that allows new applications to be added easily.[44] This permits the development of cost-effective systems that can integrate innovations in user interface and database technology as well as data from computer-based hospital information systems and decision support tools.[45] Designers of such systems have begun to systematically study the work patterns of physicians and analyze clinical practices to identify information needs in the context of patient care.[46] Future systems should help physicians find pertinent information and provide innovative ways to assist them in determining how the data apply to a specific clinical question.[47]

Several academic centers have developed and successfully implemented strategically placed computer workstations developed under grants from the NLM. These networked workstations are designed to instill query habits in the daily clinical activities of young physicians in training.[48–50] They facilitate one-stop, integrated information shopping.

One of these systems allows users to maintain patient records, check findings with two diagnostic decision support systems (*i.e.,* RECONSIDER and DXplain), look up drugs on various databases, and search PDQ by a licensed, local implementation and search the medical literature.[48]

In radiation therapy, two groups have reported their experiences with the development and use of workstation-based expert systems designed to serve as consulting resources to the practicing radiotherapist and as a teaching aid to residents in training.[51,52] Both groups reported satisfaction with the power, capability, and utility of the workstations and expressed enthusiasm about the development and integration of anatomic atlases, treatment planning guides, dosimetric calculations, tutorials, and decision-support tools like ONCOCIN for protocol management.

DEVELOPMENT OF AN INTEGRATED ONCOLOGY WORKSTATION

NCI is currently supporting efforts to enhance computerized support for clinical decision-making through the development of an *integrated oncology workstation* (IOW). This workstation integrates an electronic patient record; automated clinical and laboratory systems; access to information resources such as PDQ, CANCERLIT, the full text of this and other oncologic textbooks (through OncoDisc); and access to decision-support software such as ONCOCIN, which is currently undergoing refinement. A prototype for this workstation has been designed as an advanced, yet affordable, desk-top personal computer or technical workstation. Extensive integration of this data-management function with laboratory, financial, and office-management systems is under development to enhance the utility of the IOW.

Users on networked workstations will be able to retrieve and manipulate patient records, integrate laboratory and diagnostic test results into the medical record and the flow sheet, obtain decision support, manage clinical trials data, and easily obtain context-specific (*i.e.,* patient- or problem-specific) information from integrated electronic databases and textbooks. Commercial development of the workstation is being conducted as a collaborative project with the medical informatics group at Stanford University and private industry under the auspices of the Federal Technology Transfer Act (FTTA).[53] The FTTA authorizes the NCI to enter into a Cooperative Research and Development Agreement (CRADA). The CRADA is a mechanism for facilitating commercial development that permits private sector partners to obtain exclusive license rights in exchange for participation in product development and marketing.

Another development that may hasten the integration of computer technology into medical practice is the introduction of a fully electronic medical journal, the *Online Journal of Clinical Trials.*[54,55] Subscribers must have a personal computer with a 286 or higher-level processor, two megabytes of memory, a VGA monitor, a modem, and Microsoft's Windows software. Subscribers will be notified of new articles by fax and can have instant access to them, complete with tables and figures, on their video terminals. The software also allows readers to browse through previously published articles. The concept is innovative but not without its critics. Concern has been expressed about the fate of traditional customs of review, authorship, and attribution. However, the introduction of an online journal reflects a growing recognition that the current process by which clinical research is reviewed, edited, and published requires substantial streamlining to expedite the rapid dissemination of important clinical advances—the principal goal of PDQ, CancerFax, CancerNet, and NCI's clinical alert mechanism.[56–58]

As the biologic revolution continues, it has become clear that computer and communication technology has a major role to play in information management and decision support. Future systems should assist physicians not only to find pertinent information but also to determine how the data apply to specific clinical situations. An improved understanding of the nature of medical knowledge, the way it should be used for optimal decision-making, and the logistical issues that serve as barriers to widespread use, pose continued challenges for system developers.

REFERENCES

1. Williamson JW, German PS, Weiss R, Skinner EA, Bowes F. Health science information management and continuing education of physicians. A survey of U.S. primary care practitioners and their opinion leaders. Ann Intern Med 1989;110:151–160.
2. Association of Medical Colleges. Physicians of the twenty-first century: Report of the panel on the general education of the physician and college preparation for medicine. J Med Educ 1984;59:1–208.
3. Covell DG, Uman GC, Manning PR. Information needs in office practice: Are they being met? Ann Intern Med 1985;103:596–599.
4. Medical education in the information age. Proceedings of the Symposium on Medical informatics. Washington, DC: Association of Medical Colleges, 1986.
5. Bankowitz RA, Mc Neill MA, Challinor SM, Parker RC, Kapoor WN, Miller RA. A computer-assisted medical diagnostic consultation service. Ann Intern Med 1989;110: 824–832.
6. Greenes RA, Shortliffe EH. Medical informatics: An emerging academic discipline and institutional priority. JAMA 1990;263:1114–1120.
7. Connelly DP, Rich EC, Curley SP, Kelly JT. Knowledge resource preferences of family physicians. J Fam Pract 1990;3:353–359.
8. Osheroff JA, Forsythe DE, Buchanan BG, Bankowitz RA, Blumenfeld BH, Miller RA. Physicians' information needs: Analysis of questions posed during clinical teaching. Ann of Intern Med 1991;114:576–581.
9. Wyatt J. Uses and sources of medical knowledge. Lancet 1991;338:1368–1373.
10. Wyatt J. Computer-based knowledge systems. Lancet 1991;338:1431–1436.
11. Lindberg DAB, Schoolman HM. The National Library of Medicine and medical informatics. West J Med 1986;145:786–790.
12. Lindberg DAB. Information systems to support medical practice and scientific discovery. Method Inform Med 1989;28:202–206.
13. 92nd Congress. National Cancer Act of 1971. Public Law 92–218, Sec. 1828, Dec. 23, 1971.
14. Masys DR, Hubbard SM. Technical information progress of the National Cancer Institute. J Am Soc Info Sci 1987;38:60–64.
15. Hubbard SM, Henney JE, DeVita VT. A computer database for information on cancer treatment. N Engl J Med 1987;316:315–318.
16. Hubbard SM, DeVita VT. PDQ: An innovation in information dissemination linking cancer research and clinical practice. In: DeVita VT, Hellman S, Rosenberg SA, eds. Important advances in oncology: 1987. Philadelphia: JB Lippincott, 1987:263–277.
17. Perry, DJ, Hubbard, SM, Masys, DR, Tingley, DE. Dose modification for PDQ. In: Stead WW, ed. Symposium on Computer Applications in Medical Care. 11th ed. Los Angeles: Computer Society Press, 1987:739–742.
18. Perry DJ, Hubbard SM, Young RC. PDQ: A new source of information on cancer therapy. Eur J Cancer Clin Oncol 1989;25:1907–1908.
19. EuroCODE. A new approach to collaborative research in clinical oncology. Eur J Cancer Clin Oncol 1989;25:1905–1906.
20. Van Camp AJ. PDQ search aids. Database Searcher 1990;6:24–28.
21. Perry DJ, Sloane EM, Hubbard SM, Tingley DE, DeVita VT. Keeping up with the cancer literature—PDQ and CANCERLIT. J Clin Oncol 1988;6:1649–1652.
22. Hubbard SM. Getting the "fax" on cancer treatments. Oncology Times [Editorial] 1991;13: 2.
23. Joshi AK. Natural language processing. Science 1991;254:1242–1249.
24. Gomez E, Demetriades JE, Babcock D, Peterson J. The Department of Veteran's Affairs optical patient card workstation. In: Clayton PD, ed. Assessing the value of medical informatics. New York: McGraw Hill, 1992:378–380.

25. Warner HR. Computer-assisted medical decision-making. New York: Academic Press, 1979.
26. McDonald CJ, Hui SL, Smith DM, et al. Reminders to physicians from an introspective computer medical record. Ann Intern Med 1984;100:130–138.
27. Barnett GO, Cimino JJ, Hupp JA, et al. DXplain: An evolving diagnostic decision-support system. JAMA 1987;258:67–74.
28. Miller RA, Pople HE, Myers JD. Internist-1: An experimental computer-based diagnostic consultant for general internal medicine. N Engl J Med 1982;307:468–476.
29. Friedman RH, Frank AD. Use of a conditional rule structure to automate clinical decision support: A comparison of artificial intelligence and deterministic programming techniques. Comput Biomed Res 16:378–394.
30. Friedman RB, Entine SM, Carbone PP. Experience with an automated cancer protocol surveillance system. Am J Clin Oncol 1983;6:583–592.
31. Wirtschafter DD, Scalise M, Henke C, et al. Do information systems improve the quality of clinical research? Results of a randomized trial in a cooperative multi-institutional cancer group. Comput Biomed Res 1981;14:78–90.
32. Lenhard RE, Blum BI, Sunderland JM. The Johns Hopkins oncology clinical information system. J Med Syst 1983;7:147–174.
33. Wirtschafter DD, Carpenter JT, Mesel E. A consultant-extender system for breast cancer adjuvant chemotherapy. Ann Intern Med 1979;90:396–401.
34. Hickam DH, Shortliffe EH, Bischoff MB, et al. The treatment advice of a computer-based chemotherapy protocol advisor. Ann Intern Med 1985;103:928–936.
35. Kent DL, Shortliffe EH, Carlson RW, et al. Improvements in data collection through physician use of a computer-based chemotherapy treatment consultant. J Clin Oncol 1985;3:409–417.
36. Schwartz WB, Patil RS, Szolovits P. Artificial intelligence in medicine: Where do we stand? N Engl J Med 1987;316:685–688.
37. Perry CA. Knowledge bases in medicine: A review. Bull Med Libr Assoc 1990;78:271–282.
38. Shortliffe EH. Computer programs to support clinical decision making. JAMA 1987;258:67–74.
39. Shortliffe EH, Wulfman CE, Rindfleisch TC, Carlson RW. An integrated oncology workstation. Bethesda: National Cancer Institute, 1990.
40. Kent DL, Shortliffe EH, Carlson RW, et al. Improvements in data collection through physician use of a computer-based chemotherapy treatment consultant. J Clin Oncol 1985;3:409–417.
41. Hickam DH, Shortliffe EH, Bischoff MB, et al. The treatment advice of a computer-based chemotherapy protocol advisor. Ann Intern Med 1985;103:928–936.
42. Institute of Medicine. Committee on Improving the Patient Record. The computer-based patient record: An essential technology for health care. Washington, DC: National Academy Press, 1991.
43. Shortliffe EH, Tang PC, Detmer DE. Patient records and computers. Ann Intern Med 1991;115:979–981.
44. Young CY, Tang PC, Annevelink J. An open systems architecture for development of a physicians workstation. In: Clayton PD, ed. Assessing the value of medical informatics. New York: McGraw Hill, 1992:491–495.
45. Annevelink J, Young CY, Tang, PC. Heterogenous database integration in a physician's workstation. In: Clayton PD, ed. Assessing the value of medical informatics. New York: McGraw Hill, 1992:368–372.
46. Fafchamps D, Young CY, Tang PC. Modelling work practices: Input to the design of a physician's workstation. In: Clayton PD, ed. Assessing the value of medical informatics. New York: McGraw Hill, 1992:788–792.
47. Rennels GD, Shortliffe EH, Miller PM, et al. A computational model of reasoning from the clinical literature. Comput Method Prog Biomed 1987;24:139–149.
48. Broering N. The MAClinical workstation project at Georgetown University. Bull Med Libr Assoc 1991;79:276–281.
49. Clayton PD, Anderson RK, Hill C, McCormack M. An initial assessment of the cost and utilization of the integrated academic information system (IAIMS) at Columbia Presbyterian Medical Center. In: Clayton PD, ed. Assessing the value of medical informatics. New York: McGraw Hill, 1992:109–113.
50. Clark AS, Shea S. Free text database in an integrated academic information system (IAIMS) at Columbia Presbyterian Medical Center. In: In: Clayton PD, ed. Assessing the value of medical informatics. New York: McGraw Hill, 1992:333–337.
51. Laramore GE, Altschular MD, Banks G, et al. Applications of databases and AI/expert systems in radiation therapy. Am J Clin Oncol 1988;11:387–393.
52. Zusag TW, McDonald S, Miller BA, Purdy JA, Rubin P. Radiation oncology resident's computer workstations. Int J Radiat Oncol Biol Phys 1991;22:147–157.
53. Esterhay R, Hubbard S. The integrated oncology workstation (IOW): A collaborative project under the Federal Technology Transfer Act (FTTA). Proc ASCO (in press).
54. Palca J. New journal will publish without paper. Science 1991;253:1480, 1991
55. Kassirer JP. Journals in bits and bytes. N Engl J Med 1992;326:195–196.
56. DeVita VT, Hubbard SM. NCI's breast cancer clinical alert: Rationale and results. Resident Staff Physician 1989;35:49–55.
57. Huth EJ. Prepublication release of scientific data and the right of the public to know: Adapting to our times. J Infect Dis 1989;159:407–411.
58. Steinbrook R. Informing physicians about promising new treatments for severe illness. JAMA 1990;263:2078–2082.

SECTION 2

COLIN B. BEGG

Research Data Management

Every prospective clinical research study is constructed with the goal of addressing specific scientific objectives, and each is completed, if successful, with an interpretive analysis of the results. However, to progress from the initial idea to the results, the researcher must have a system for conducting the study and collecting the data. Research data management is the discipline devoted to the collection, storage, retrieval, and quality control of the data required for evaluating the scientific objectives of the study. It plays a crucial role in determining the success or failure of the study. This role is especially important in cancer studies because of the relative complexity of the clinical interventions in this field and the fact that the endpoints are frequently multifaceted, subjectively interpreted, and involve follow-up over a significant period.

There are two motivating factors for paying careful attention to data management in the development phase of a research study. The first is that medical records are rarely maintained with the kind of detail that is necessary to answer the scientific objectives of research studies, and any data assembled retrospectively from the medical record is likely to be incomplete and of poor quality. Second, the data collection methods should be uniform for all patients and should be developed in close conformity with the methodologic principles of good study design. This can only be ensured with careful attention to these principles during the design and development of the study. If not, there is the possibility that unforeseen biases may compromise a study that appears to be methodologically sound. For example, in a randomized trial involving long-term follow-up, it is important that the schedules for evaluating patients over time are similar for the treatments under comparison, or reporting biases may influence one of the treatment groups disproportionately. In studies with multiple endpoints, such as phase I and II studies of new agents in which a variety of adverse reactions are possible, absence of careful data collection tools may lead to underreporting of toxicities.

There are four key components to research data management: protocol development, data collection, computing, and quality control. The protocol should contain, in addition to the scientific background and the goals of the study, detailed information on all important logistical aspects of the study, including the data collection forms and a schedule for their completion. After the protocol is open to patient accrual, it is important that there is a system for checking patient eligibility and for prospective registration and randomization of all patients entered in the study. Collection and abstraction of the data is often complex because the medical intervention is often delivered over a period of weeks or months, may have to be adjusted over time in the individual patient due to adverse reactions, and may be multimodal. The outcomes, such as graded toxicities, may have to be derived from secondary data collected over time (*e.g.,* blood counts) or subjectively interpreted. Because of the volume of data collected and the requirements of the statistical analysis, computerization of the data is invariably required. A system of quality control is necessary to protect the integrity of the database, because errors can occur in a variety of ways and are especially likely in complex studies.

In addition to being crucial to the success of the study, the process of data management spans a number of disciplines. Forms development and data abstraction can be performed by data managers, people who have knowledge of biology, medical terminology, and the medical record. This role is often played by nurses, who can also apply their expertise in protocol development to check that details of the intervention under study are factually correct, consistent, and feasible. However, the active involvement of the principal investigator and a statistician is also extremely important to ensure that the appropriate data are being targeted, that the data are being coded in a manner amenable to statistical analysis, and that the logistics of data collection are structured in such a way as to validate the scientific principles embedded in the study design. A team approach of this nature is essential for a successful study with high-quality data.

PRINCIPLES OF STUDY DESIGN

There are many methodologic principles and related techniques that are relevant to the design of clinical research studies, far too many to discuss in a comprehensive way in this chapter. This section instead addresses a few general principles and the relevance of data management planning to ensuring their observance. These principles are concerned with the composition of the source population of patients, the integrity of the sampling procedure (*e.g.*, the patients selected for the trial), the degree to which the intervention under study is prescribed, and the accuracy and completeness of the endpoints. In practice, the role of the statistician or epidemiologist is to make sure that the appropriate design is selected to address the targeted hypotheses of the study.

Typically, the composition of the source population is defined by a set of eligibility criteria in the study protocol. The study may target a broad or a focussed group of patients, depending on the extensiveness of these criteria, and there has been considerable debate on the relative merits of broad or strict criteria.[3] In any event, the results of the trial will be interpreted in the context of the population under study, and the clear characterization of the source population is important from a reporting standpoint. From the data management perspective, the primary goal is to ensure that the patients recruited to the study belong to the source population by fulfilling the eligibility criteria.

In reporting the results of therapeutic trials, the principle of "intent to treat" is frequently invoked, especially in randomized trials.[41] The data analyst includes all patients randomized in the analysis, even though some patients may never have received the allocated treatment for one reason or another. In this way, any bias that may be caused by conscious or inadvertent exclusion of patients with an unrepresentative prognostic profile is avoided, at the cost of reporting aggregate results for groups of patients, not all of whom received the intervention under study. This principle is equally important in uncontrolled or nonrandomized studies. To ensure that the analyst has at least the opportunity to assess the outcome of the study in the total sample of patients selected for inclusion in the study, it is essential to have a system for prospective registration of patients, with the registration taking place after completion of the informed consent but before initiation of the intervention. A registration system of this nature, using an independent office, is in place in all of the cooperative groups and many of the cancer centers. In the absence of a formal system of registration, it is important that all patients recruited to the study be cataloged, so that there is full information on all the patients for whom there was intent to treat.

If the study is randomized, the legitimacy of the process of randomization is crucial to the integrity of the study. The treating physician must play no role in or be able to predict the selection of treatment. Many organizations have an independent office to control the randomization process, but if the study is conducted locally, the logistics of the randomization process must be constructed to ensure the blinding of the allocation procedure.[2] Organizational issues are crucial in studies in which the treatment selection remains unknown to the physician and the patient during the study (*i.e.*, double-blind studies).

A clinical research study invariably involves one or more prescribed interventions on the patients. These could be medical, surgical, radiotherapeutic, diagnostic, or a combination of modalities. The prescribed nature of the intervention distinguishes the experimental nature of a clinical trial from an observational study, in which the extent of the intervention is determined on a patient by patient basis by the physician. This distinction is extremely important with regard to the credibility of the study in that, in an observational study, it is likely that the aggressiveness of the intervention is influenced by the prognosis of the patient, with the result that any apparent treatment difference observed may be spurious (*i.e.*, due to systematic differences in the prognostic composition of the groups of patients being compared, rather than due to the intervention).[4] Because the major methodologic advantage of a study is the fact that the intervention strategies are prescribed rather than elective, it is important that the interventions actually be delivered as prescribed. Such protocol compliance is necessary to validate the results of the research, and monitoring its success is an important data management objective.

The quality of the study depends on the accuracy and completeness of the data. Of paramount importance are the primary endpoints, which must be carefully defined to ensure that the necessary supportive data are collected. For example, if reduction in tumor volume (*i.e.*, tumor response) is the endpoint, measurements at predefined times are required; if survival is the endpoint, regular follow-up of surviving patients is necessary to validate the statistical analysis; and graded toxicities require regular monitoring of the patient and scheduling of laboratory tests. If the outcomes must be assessed subjectively, carefully defined assessment scales are essential to reduce interobserver and intraobserver variability, and the logistical circumstances of the assessment must be constructed to minimize observer biases. For example, in studies of diagnostic technologies, it is sometimes necessary to "blind" test raters from information from other tests conducted on the patient. Care in developing study forms, coding conventions, documentation of codes, and precise data collection schedules is necessary to ensure that the special methodologic requirements of the study are protected.

In structuring the data management system to satisfy important methodologic goals, the data collected must conform to the specific objectives of the study. The required data and the tools for their collection are different from those that are necessary for regular clinical support. The research database is different from a clinical database, even though there may be a lot of overlap in practice. For example, in diagnostic imaging studies, information on the suspected presence of disease usually are carefully coded by site in a manner that permits precise anatomic correlations between the tests and the surgical and pathologic evaluations to a far greater level of precision than is necessary in everyday clinical care. An important conceptual error that is frequently made is the belief that clinical databases, if complete, are adequate resources for clinical research. In fact, only by constructing research databases prospectively, in a manner designed to address the preceding methodologic concerns, can an appropriate resource for clinical research be developed.[5]

RESEARCH DATA MANAGEMENT METHODOLOGY

In the following sections, the major components of a system for research data management are discussed. In each case, the most important tasks are identified and cataloged, tools for facilitating the tasks are described, and the expertise necessary at each stage of the process is discussed. Most of the concepts are sufficiently general that they apply to all kinds of clinical research studies, even though the examples presented are primarily derived from medical oncology trials.

PROTOCOL DEVELOPMENT

The research protocol is the guiding document for the study, and it should specify in detail all important logistical components of the plans for data collection and analysis. Although the format of protocols may vary considerably across modalities, every protocol should address a number of key issues, as indicated in Table 68–2. Care in protocol development is vital to a successful study, and a major data management role is to ensure that the study plan as embodied in the protocol is feasible, consistent, and unambiguous and that the necessary tools for conducting the protocol are in place before the study commences.

TABLE 68–2. Skeleton of Protocol

Study objectives
Definition of the patient population
Registration and randomization of patients
Description of the interventions
Definitions of endpoints
Data collection
Biostatistics
Informed consent procedures

The study population is usually defined in terms of a list of eligibility criteria. Ideally, this list is short, and the exclusion factors are designed only to exclude patients inappropriate to the hypothesis under study, those for whom the intervention is inappropriate on medical grounds, or those for whom evaluation of the endpoints is likely to be compromised. Experienced data managers and nurses can play a useful role in ensuring that the appropriate tests for determining eligibility are planned and that the relevant data are recorded on the data collection forms.

The prospective registration of all patients entered on the study is important for ensuring the scientific integrity of the results. This process is usually accomplished together with randomization if the study is randomized. At a minimum, the protocol must contain enough information about the registration and randomization procedures to enable study participants to enter patients into the trial in an efficient manner and to convince scientific reviewers of the validity of the treatment assignment processes and treatment blinding procedures, if appropriate.

The interventions under study should be entirely prescribed. In practice, the treatment of cancer patients is sufficiently complex and dynamic that modifications are frequently necessary during the progress of the study. Guidelines for protocol modifications should be specified in the protocol to the maximal extent possible to minimize the likelihood of elective treatment modifications and to preserve the experimental nature of the study.

Careful, objective definitions of the primary endpoints are essential. Their absence can introduce "noise" into the results and inhibit the meaningful comparison of the results with those of similar studies. Wherever possible, accepted reporting standards should be used, such as the National Cancer Institute's (NCI) common toxicity criteria.[6] It is important that the endpoints correspond to the written study objectives in the protocol and that, if there are multiple objectives, precisely quantified endpoints be defined for each of them.

The protocol should contain a summary of the data collection schedules and a list of data collection forms to ensure that all personnel contributing to the conduct of the study are familiar with the plans. It is wise to have these materials in place before the study is activated, because it is often impossible to retrieve data retrospectively.

There are several biostatistical issues that are essential to successful protocol development. The design of the study must be justified in logical and quantitative statistical terms, and the latter must address a projected sample size. This usually involves calculations specifying the power of the study to detect statistically significant effects or the precision to which the targeted endpoints can be estimated. Formal calculations of this nature are neither relevant nor meaningful for small exploratory (*i.e.*, pilot) studies. The feasibility of the study should be addressed by projecting the accrual rate and the time required to complete the study.

Protocol development should be a team effort, with all relevant parties contributing to and understanding all aspects of the protocol. From the biostatistical and data management perspective, the major task is to ensure that the study design is capable of addressing the stated scientific hypotheses and that the logistical plans for managing the conduct of the study and collecting the data can produce a database that contains high-quality, complete data that are free from methodologic biases.

DATA COLLECTION

The process of data collection is greatly facilitated if attention is given to the creation of protocol-specific data management tools. These tools include data collection forms and various checklists to guide the study participant in the conduct of the study.

The design of the data collection forms is central to the conduct of the study, and this task requires the active involvement of the principal investigators in addition to the data manager. The forms embody the database for the study; it is in their design that the investigators come to grips with the nuts and bolts of how the scientific objectives are going to be reflected in the data with regard to the coding of endpoints and the demarcation of subsets of patients.

It is advisable to create forms that are self-coding to the maximal extent possible; text responses are minimized and as many items as possible are translated into single or multiple digit codes. This facilitates the eventual computer data entry and retrieval, and it ensures that the appropriate data summarization takes place at the optimal time with regard to access to secondary data, minimizing the risk of interpretive errors in data abstraction.[7] Another important consideration is the layout of the paper forms. They should be designed so that data items collected at approximately the same time are contiguous. The values to be entered on the computer should be positioned to maximize efficiency and ease of data entry (*e.g.*, all codes on the left-hand margin of the form, with explanatory text to the right of the code). Using boxes to collect the codes can help to enforce proper form completion, because the boxes dictate maximal field length.

Another ideal attribute of data forms is that they should be parsimonious. Investigators are inclined to want to record every datum imaginable to prevent items from being missed that eventually turn out to be important. However, the volume of data collected is inversely associated with quality.[8] The scientific credibility of any observed association is qualitatively greater if the hypothesis is targeted in the design of the study, and the collection of excessive data is likely to lead to unscientific data dredging. For all of these reasons, a tightly-organized, defined, parsimonious dataset is ideal.

If a variety of studies are being conducted on an ongoing basis, the form design and the coding conventions should reflect the continuity of the research effort. Coding conventions for outcomes, pathology, staging, and other relevant variables should be consistent across studies if feasible. This reduces the risk of transcription errors because data managers and other persons are less likely to be confused by conflicting conventions, and it facilitates the aggregation of data across studies for general statistical analyses. Consistency of coding also simplifies the task of computer database management.

Timing of data collection is usually important in cancer studies, and the precise schedule for completing the forms deserves attention. In medical oncology studies, flow sheets are often used in the clinic to record supplementary data and as a primary source for toxicity data. The flow sheets are unusual in that they represent an amalgamation of the goals of collecting data for research and providing data for clinical support.

Data collection can take place in a variety of settings, depending on the type of study. If the study investigators or nurses complete the data forms, the role of the data manager may be focussed on entering data into the computer and retrieving data for reports of the study results. In studies in which the data collection is performed by data managers and abstraction of results from the medical record or from flow sheets is involved, the data managers generally require significant knowledge of medical terminology, anatomy, and biology and expertise in specific aspects of the protocol, such as formulas for evaluating the correctness of drug dosages and similar technical issues.

It can be helpful for the data manager to create additional tools to assist in the conduct of the study and to improve protocol compliance. An eligibility checklist is useful to guard against the registration of ineligible patients. If the study is in any way complex, a patient calendar can be a useful resource to remind the physicians and nurses of the required tests and treatments throughout the course of the study. Table 68–3 displays part of such a calendar from a study of E-MVAC chemotherapy and recombinant human granulocyte colony-stimulating factor in the treatment of urothelial tract tumors. The calendar serves as a daily reminder and is designed to maximize protocol compliance. It can be amended if unscheduled delays in protocol treatment occur.

COMPUTING

Computing has become an essential feature of research data management for all but the smallest studies. A computer database allows easy and flexible access to the data for quality control and reporting purposes. Statistical analyses invariably involve the use of a computer, and many modern statistical methods are impossible to use without a computer.

What are the attributes of a good computer system for storing a clinical research study? First, it must be structured in such a way that retrieval and analysis of the data are relatively simple. An important ingredient of this is the user friendliness of the software; fortunately, the computer industry has made enormous strides in this respect in recent years. Second, the system should be designed to minimize the number of errors in the data. Many coding errors can be detected at data entry if built-in checks ensure that coded values are in the admissible range for the data item. Other logical checks can be built into any system to ensure that logically related items are consistent with each other. For example, a date of relapse should not occur later than a date of remission. Double entry of data is a technique that can virtually eliminate coding errors, at the expense of doubling the time required to enter the data. However, the quality of the computer support is only of limited usefulness without a carefully organized data management system, as outlined in the preceding sections.

The creation of a research database to encompass multiple studies presents a far greater database management challenge. It is necessary to consider the overlapping features of the individual studies, and in addition to the preceding attributes, there are many other desirable characteristics. The first concerns the consistency of a number of database features across studies. Data items that are common to different studies should

TABLE 68–3. Patient Calendar for Study of Urothelial Tumors

Day 0	Methotrexate (34 mg/m^2)
Day 1	PE & KPS
	CBC & Differential counts
	LAP
	SMA-12
	Creatinine
	Vinblastine (3.4 mg/m^2)
	Adriamycin (45 mg/m^2)
	Cisplatin (70 mg/m^2)
Day 2	Differential count
Day 3	PE
	Differential count
	Creatinine
Day 4	rh-G-CSF (5 μg/kg/day SQ)
Day 5	rh-G-CSF (5 μg/kg/day SQ)
Day 6	rh-G-CSF (5 μg/kg/day SQ)
Day 7	PE & KPS
	CBC & differential count
	LAP
	SMA-12
	Creatinine
	rh-G-CSF (5 μg/kg/day SQ)
Day 8	rh-G-CSF (5 μg/kg/day SQ)
Day 9	rh-G-CSF (5 μg/kg/day SQ)
Day 10	CBC & differential counts
	Bone marrow (selected patients)
	rh-G-CSF (5 μg/kg/day SQ)
Day 11	rh-G-CSF (5 μg/kg/day SQ)
Day 12	rh-G-CSF (5 μg/kg/day SQ)
Day 14	PE & KPS
	CBC & differential counts
	LAP
	SMA-12
	Creatinine
	Bone marrow (selected patients)
	Methotrexate (34 mg/m^2)
	Vinblastine (3.4 mg/m^2)
(Note: Dose modification schedules should be examined)	
Day 15	rh-G-CSF (5 μg/kg/day SQ)
Day 16	rh-G-CSF (5 μg/kg/day SQ)
Day 17	rh-G-CSF (5 μg/kg/day SQ)
Day 18	rh-G-CSF (5 μg/kg/day SQ)
Day 19	rh-G-CSF (5 μg/kg/day SQ)
Day 21	Methotrexate (34 mg/m^2)

PE, physical examination; KPS, Karnovsky performance status; CBC, complete blood counts; LAP, leukocyte alkaline phosphatase; SMA-12, standard chemistry screen; rh-G-CSF, recombinant granulocyte colony-stimulating factor; SQ, subcutaneous.

be coded in a consistent manner, if feasible. Important common variables include stage, pathologic classifications, and tumor response criteria. Most items collected in cancer studies are applicable to a variety of sites and types of studies. Consistency of this nature facilitates aggregate analyses of multiple studies, in addition to expediting data transfer, education of new personnel, and the maintenance of quality control. A second type of consistency involves the naming of data items, and this has benefits similar to consistent coding. A third area concerns the user interface for data entry and retrieval. For example, if data entry screens are constructed with a consistent layout, data entry efficiency is improved when data entry operators or data managers are involved in a variety of studies.

A second general goal that becomes increasingly important as the number of studies and data items increase is the performance of the system. Most modern database management systems are relational, and the performance (*i.e.*, speed of operation) is determined by the manner in which the database architecture is constructed and maintained in an on-going manner by performance tuning.[9] These activities require the input of an experienced database administrator. The integration of multiple studies and investigators necessitates an effective and flexible security system to ensure that access to individual studies is limited to designated persons. As a general rule, it is advisable that data entry privileges for an individual study be severely restricted, ideally to a single person, but that access for retrieval of data be more broadly available.

There are many commercial software packages to aid in the construction of the database. Typically, database management packages provide a convenient structure and a language of commands to achieve this goal. For all but the simplest databases, it is necessary to use the package to construct the database system in the required format, and the extent of the developmental effort increases with the complexity of the database. Because the market is changing rapidly and there are many products available, it is not worthwhile to discuss the merits of individual products. However, there are two general characteristics of a product that have an important bearing on its usefulness, depending to some extent on the size and complexity of the database. The first issue is hardware independence. Many products available are designed specifically for the host computer and its operating system. However, there are nonproprietary packages that have been designed to work on a variety of hardware platforms. This capability increases the opportunity to develop a distributed database, in which parts of the database can reside on different computers, and it increases the options for changing the hardware in the future with minimal disruption. Therefore, hardware independence is an insurance against future unforeseen changes in hardware requirements. Second, many packages can now communicate with each other. This greatly facilitates data transfer. Of special importance is the link between the database and the statistical packages that are to be employed. For some products, direct links of this nature are available, permitting interactive statistical analysis and data retrieval without the user having to log in and log out of each product.

Computing is an essential component of research data

management. Modern technology offers the potential for efficient storage, retrieval, and analysis of the data, in addition to providing a valuable tool for enhancing quality control of the data. However, the construction of the database is a complex task for all but the simplest studies and requires significant expertise in computer science.

QUALITY CONTROL

There are several areas in which the quality and reliability of a research study can be compromised. We can group these into three broad categories, each of which requires an entirely different approach to quality control: accuracy of the computer record, compliance with the protocol, and accurate reporting of the results of the study.

Accuracy of the Computer Record

In transcribing results from their source (*e.g.*, point of collection, medical records, data forms) to the computer, it is desirable to minimize the number of random errors. This is an objective issue, and quality control can be influenced in an algorithmic manner. Because most computer errors are due to transcription errors by the data manager on abstracting the data (*e.g.*, from the chart) or typing errors during data entry, some of the errors are potentially identifiable by computer logical checks. For example, if a keyed value of a coded item is outside the admissible range, it can be flagged at data entry. More complex checking is also possible. For example, stage can be logically mapped to disease extent, such that inconsistencies can be identified when either item is keyed. These logical associations can apply to key dates, such as date of registration and date of response or date of death. There are many potential logical inconsistencies in a typical research database that can be used to advantage in flagging errors.

An alternative approach that can dramatically reduce typing errors is to enter all data twice, to allow the computer to match each item with itself. This technique is guaranteed to virtually eliminate all simple typing errors, at the cost of doubling the time for data entry. Although it may be advisable in some situations, it is not always necessary or practical to implement double data entry. For example, if an experienced data entry operator is keying the data, the error rate may be so low that double data entry is not cost effective. In a busy clinic environment where a nurse or data manager is keying the data, it may be unrealistic to consider this technique.

Protocol Compliance

A good research protocol clarifies in detail all aspects of the research study. Of particular importance are the definition of the source population of patients, the description of the prescribed interventions, and the definitions and schedules for evaluating endpoints. To ensure that the results of a study are reliable, it is important that the study be conducted in compliance with these protocol guidelines. Quality control in this context involves techniques for monitoring and enhancing protocol compliance.

One way to promote protocol compliance for an individual study is to carefully prepare data management tools to facilitate the conduct of the study, as outlined previously. Realistically, long-term success in this area also requires on-going evaluations of individual investigators with regard to patient management and endpoint assessment and feed-back of the results to improve performance. A useful approach is to perform random, retrospective audits for individual patients. Typically, this is not a simple thing to do because it can involve a detailed examination of the medical record for information regarding eligibility, work-up, protocol modifications, and endpoint evaluation. Medical judgments are an important ingredient of this process, and audits of this nature usually involve a team of data managers, clinicians, and possibly nurses, depending on the nature of the study. Routine audits have become a standard requirement for most of the cooperative group cancer trials in recent years.[10] Audits can be beneficial in identifying problems with the accuracy of the data recorded on forms. By comparing the study forms with the medical record, it may be possible to identify relevant events that were not reported on the forms, such as laboratory values missing from a flow sheet.

Accurate Reporting of Results

An institutional or global concern is the accuracy of the study results that are eventually disseminated through journals, conference presentations, and other media. It is vital for the process of science that the published findings be an accurate reflection of the results of the study as conducted, or the study will not be reproducible and may be misleading. For example, if the study involves 50 patients, but the investigators report the results as if only 40 had been studied without at least documenting the number of exclusions and reasons for exclusion and if the chosen 40 are selected (even unconsciously) on the basis of favorable outcomes, the implications of the reported results will be misleading and overoptimistic. It is important that the results of clinical research studies be reported factually and completely.

Quality control of research reporting is not an issue that is commonly addressed, although it is an extremely important aspect of the research process. The induced biases are probably more profound in this area than in the areas discussed in the previous sections.[11] Moreover, recent incidents of false reporting of scientific research have led to tremendously adverse publicity for the host institutions and for the field of research in general. Practical problems in setting up a system of review include the fact that individual protocols may spawn many publications, perhaps only involving subgroups of patients, but other publications may involve aggregation of data from many protocols. The sampling frame for selecting studies for auditing purposes is not obvious. This is an issue that requires development in the future.

MULTIINSTITUTIONAL STUDIES

A considerable proportion of clinical research studies undertaken are multiinstitutional studies. The multiinstitutional approach was developed in response to the need for studies with relatively large numbers of patients, especially large randomized clinical trials and studies of rare diseases. Although individual multiinstitutional studies are occasionally organized to tackle a specific high-priority objective, most of the multiinstitutional studies in cancer are conducted by one of the numerous cooperative groups of institutions, each of which conducts many studies in an ongoing basis.

The conduct of multiinstitutional studies compared with single-institution studies, presents a special organizational challenge to data management. The challenge is to ensure protocol compliance, standardization of data, and timely data collection from a large group of contributing investigators scattered geographically. The role of the coordinating center is crucial to the development and conduct of these studies. The coordinating center orchestrates all logistical aspects of the study, including registration and randomization of patients, protocol development, forms development, creation of the computer database, quality control of submitted data, and statistical analysis.

The coordinating center is responsible for consistently conducting the study at each of the contributing institutions, and it must ensure that the data are submitted in a timely fashion. To accomplish this as effectively as possible, a system of reminders is necessary to trigger the submission of relevant data forms at each stage of the protocol. Special data management tools are necessary over and above those described earlier for local studies. The coordinating center is also responsible for quality control, and much of its data processing function is geared toward monitoring the quality of the data submitted to identify inconsistencies and missing data. This can be accomplished by computer logical checks and by manual examination of the submitted data by experienced data managers. To evaluate protocol compliance, eligibility and accuracy of the data occasional audits of individual institutions are useful. This is now mandated by the NCI for the cooperative groups.[12]

Recent advances in computer technology have offered the opportunity for many of the manual aspects of this process to be bypassed by allowing remote data entry at the participating institutions, including on-line registration and randomization. In this setting, the task of the coordinating center is to create a computing environment that preserves the quality control capabilities of a central office and database, while allowing the local institutions to take advantage of the new technology. The challenge is to create a software environment that allows, for example, registration and randomization on a local workstation in a manner that preserves the scientific integrity of the registration process.

Another role of the coordinating center is the sequential monitoring of the data. The statistical monitoring of the primary endpoints may or may not involve a formal plan for terminating the study, and in this respect, the monitoring is similar to a single-institution study.[13] An additional data management role is to detect the occurrence of unforeseen adverse side effects while the trial is in progress, because individual reactions may not cause concern locally.

The general principles of data management outlined earlier are applicable to multiinstitutional studies. The multiinstitutional setting merely creates some additional logistical complexities. Multiinstitutional studies are necessary for the conduct of many types of trials due to sample size limitations at individual institutions.

CONCLUSIONS

Planning the data management of a clinical research study is a task that is crucial to its success. Failure to determine the precise data requirements for achieving the scientific objectives of the study and a suitable schedule for the data collection can seriously compromise the validity of the study, because use of medical records to obtain outcome data retrospectively is frequently problematic. Data management plans should be initiated in the earliest stages of planning the study and should address all aspects of the study, encompassing protocol development, forms development, patient registration, data collection procedures, computing, and quality control. This resource-intensive approach to data management is only worthwhile if the study objectives are of sufficient scientific importance. As Medawar pointed out, "An experiment not worth doing is not worth doing well."[14]

The conduct of the study is enhanced by the development and use of specially developed data management tools. These include carefully prepared data collection forms, eligibility checklists, patient-specific calendars to prompt scheduled interventions and tests, and other reminders and supportive documentation. The precise coding of the data and the schedule for their collection are especially important for standardizing the results.

The conclusions of the study are limited in their validity by the quality of the data, and quality control is therefore an important aspect of the process. It should involve methods to limit the number of transcription errors in abstracting and keying the data and efforts to evaluate protocol compliance, patient eligibility, and the correctness of outcomes involving judgment, such as the determination of tumor response. A frequently ignored aspect of quality control concerns the veracity of the results eventually reported in publications. Of particular concern is the completeness of the census of patients registered in the study, because the selective reporting of subgroups of patients has an important bearing on the credibility of the results.

Computing plays an increasingly important role in the conduct of clinical research. The computer is essential for data storage and statistical analysis, but it can also be used to provide tools for enhancing the conduct of the study and for improving quality control. The construction of a computer research database is not a simple task when many different kinds of studies are involved, and this aspect of clinical research is assuming an increasing share of the budget for conducting studies. For example, the conversion of the Southwest Oncology Group from a hierarchical to a relational system took 5 programmers 4 years to complete.[15] Other groups have had similar experiences.

The successful implementation of a data management system for supporting clinical research requires the input of several disciplines. The active involvement of the principal investigator and a statistician is essential to ensure that the appropriate data are recorded in a manner capable of addressing the scientific objectives of the study but free from analytic biases. Computer science personnel are usually necessary to develop and maintain an efficient database management system, except for relatively simple, individual studies. A team approach is essential for the successful conduct of clinical research.

REFERENCES

1. Peto R, Pike MC, Armitage P, et al. Design and analysis of randomized clinical trials requiring prolonged observation of each patient: I. Introduction and design. Br J Cancer 1976;34:585–612.
2. Zelen M. The randomization and stratification of patients to clinical trials. J Chron Dis 1974;27:365–375.
3. Begg CB. Selection of patients for clinical trials. Semin Oncol 1988;15:434–440.
4. Silverman WA. Human experimentation: A guided step into the unknown. New York: Oxford University Press, 1985.
5. Byar DP. The use of data bases and historical controls in treatment comparisons. Recent Results Cancer Res 1988;111:95–98.
6. Wittes RE. Manual of oncologic therapeutics. Philadelphia: JB Lippincott, 1989:627–632.
7. Van der Patten E, van der Valden JW, Siers A, Hamersma EAM. A pilot study on the quality of data management in a cancer clinical trial. Controlled Clin Trials 1987;8:96–100.
8. Knatterud GL. Methods of quality control and of continuous audit procedures for controlled clinical trials. Controlled Clin Trials 1981;1:327–332.
9. Sandberg G. A primer on relational data base concepts. IBM Syst J 1981;20:23–40.
10. Wolter JM. Quality assurance in a cooperative group. Cancer Treat Rep 1985;69:1189–1193.
11. Begg CB: Publication bias and the dissemination of clinical research. JNCI 1989;81:107–115.
12. Mauer JK, Hoth DF, Macfarlane DK, et al. Site visit monitoring program of the clinical cooperative groups: Results of the first 3 years. Cancer Treat Rep 1985;69:1177–1187.
13. O'Brien PC, Fleming TR. A multiple testing procedure for clinical trials. Biometrics 1979;35:549–556.
14. Medawar PW. The threat and the glory. New York: Harper Collins, 1990.
15. Blumenstein BA. The relational database model and multiple multicenter clinical trials. Controlled Clin Trials 1989;10:386–406.

Cancer: Principles & Practice of Oncology, Fourth Edition,
edited by Vincent T. DeVita, Jr., Samuel Hellman, Steven A. Rosenberg.
J.B. Lippincott Co., Philadelphia © 1993.

CHAPTER 69

Newer Approaches to Cancer Treatment

SECTION 1

STEVEN A. ROSENBERG

Gene Therapy of Cancer

Gene therapy can be defined as a therapeutic technique in which a functioning gene is inserted into the cells of a patient to correct an inborn genetic error or to provide a new function to the cell. Increased understanding of gene regulation in eukaryotic cells and the development of improved techniques for inserting and expressing foreign genes into mammalian cells have opened new possibilities for cancer therapy based on these gene transfer techniques. In May 1989, the first successful transfer of foreign genes into a human was performed in a patient with advanced melanoma.[1] This early trial using a bacterial "marker" gene led to the first gene therapy approaches with advanced cancer that began in January 1991. This chapter reviews the current status and potential future applications of gene therapy in the treatment of patients with cancer.

INTRODUCTION OF FOREIGN GENES INTO MAMMALIAN CELLS

A variety of techniques are available for the introduction of DNA into eukaryotic cells (Table 69–1), including coprecipitation with calcium phosphate, the use of polycations or lipids complexed with DNA, encapsulation of DNA in lipid vesicles or erythrocyte ghosts, or the exposure of cells to rapid pulses of high voltage electric current (*i.e.*, electroporation).[2] DNA has also been introduced into cells by direct microinjection or by the use of high-velocity tungsten microprojectiles. These techniques are capable of integrating multiple copies of DNA into the genome although the efficiency of the integration varies widely with the technique, different genes, and different cell types. The efficiency of most of these physical transfection techniques is less than 1 in 10,000 and can be lower than 1 in 1 million.

Recently techniques have been developed using viral vectors to introduce DNA into mammalian cells.[2–12] These techniques have the potential for infecting all cells exposed to the virus. In developing techniques for the use of viral vectors, it was necessary to develop vectors that stably incorporated into the target cell without damaging it. Early work used transforming DNA viruses such as papovaviruses, simian virus 40, polyomavirus, or adenoviruses. More recently, murine and avian retroviruses have been used for DNA transduction and have proven practical and safe. These retroviral vectors can infect multiple cell types, although cell replication is necessary for integration into the genome using this approach.

Retroviruses are viruses in which the viral genes are encoded in RNA rather than DNA. After infection of the cell the viral RNA is converted to DNA by the action of reverse transcriptase. The DNA then enters the nucleus and integrates randomly into the genome. This integrated provirus is indistinguishable from other cellular genes and replicates with the cell during mitosis. The integration of the provirus into the cell genome and the subsequent formation of progeny virus may have no effect on the viability of the infected cell.

Because practical applications of gene therapy involve in-

TABLE 69–1. Methods for Inserting Genes Into Mammalian Cells

Coprecipitation with calcium phosphate
Polycations complexed with DNA
Lipids complexed with DNA
Encapsulation of DNA in lipid vesicles
Exposure of cells to pulses of high-voltage electric current (electroporation)
Microinjection
High-velocity tungsten microprojectiles
Retroviruses
DNA viruses (*e.g.*, adenoviruses, vaccinia, herpes simplex)

troduction of the foreign gene by the retrovirus without actual replication of new retroviral particles in the host, special techniques using packaging cell lines have been developed.[2–12] Retroviral vectors can be produced with the deletion of the viral protein coding sequences and introduction of the exogenous gene. These modified retroviruses retain the encapsulation sequences required for production of RNA transcripts into virions and the necessary sequences for integration and expression of the vector in the host cell genome.

To obtain these replication defective vector preparations, special "packaging cell lines" were produced that contain the helper virus genome but lack the encapsulation or psi sequence. The packaging cell line cannot produce active virions that contain viral RNA. Introduction of the retroviral vector provides the necessary encapsulation sequence that in conjunction with the viral coding sequences in the packaging cell line produces virions containing the vector RNA. The most popular packaging cell lines have been derived from NIH 3T3 cells.[2–12] The possibility exists however that replication competent virus may be produced by recombination of the vector encapsulation sequences with the viral coding sequences present in the packaging cell line. A variety of workers, have engineered modifications of the packaging cell lines and the retroviral vectors to minimize the possibility of helper virus generation including deletions if specific sequences in the 5′ and 3′ long terminal repeats (LTR), thereby requiring at least two recombinations to produce replication competent virus. The particular retroviral vector that we have used, designated LNL6 derived from the N2 vector, was engineered to contain a stop codon at the site of the *GAG* start codon, further reducing the possibility that any competent virus would be produced.[6,7]

The development of improved retroviral vectors for introduction of genes into eukaryotic cells is an active area of current investigation. The need exists for the consistent production of high-titer virus capable of efficient transduction into a broad array of target cell lines. The need for cell replication and DNA synthesis required for provirus integration limits the usefulness of these retroviruses to the introduction of DNA into rapidly dividing cells. Although integration of the retroviral genome is often stable, in some cases, there is substantial instability of the inserted genes, and loss of inserted genetic material with cell replication can occur. The random integration of the retrovirally derived DNA into the cell genome can lead to insertional mutagenesis through disruption of essential cellular genes or by activating otherwise quiescent cellular genes. A major area of current interest involves the development of retroviral vectors with appropriate internal promoters that can express multiple genes in the same retroviral construct. In retroviral vectors in which one gene is promoted by the retroviral LTR and another from internal promoters the interactions between these promoters can lead to marked inhibition of expression of one of the inserted genes.

Despite these problems, retroviral vectors represent the most efficient means of stably integrating DNA into large numbers of target cells by coincubation of the packaging cell line or the retroviral vector preparation with the target cell. Future developments are aimed at the development of retroviral vectors that can be introduced systemically into an intact animal and targeted specifically to selected cells. Although techniques for accomplishing this are not currently feasible, this represents an area of active investigation.

Viruses other than the murine and avian retroviruses are being explored for possible use as expression vectors (reviewed elsewhere[13]). Human adeno-associated viruses can be achieved in high concentrations and appear to be nonpathogenic, however difficulties in producing these preparations in the absence of contaminating helper viruses and concern about the long-term consequences of integration of these adenoviruses into cells have limited their usefulness. Vaccinia viruses, herpesviruses, bovine viruses, and papillomaviruses and others are being explored for their usefulness in gene transduction into human cells.

CANCER THERAPY USING GENE-MODIFIED TUMOR-INFILTRATING LYMPHOCYTES

STUDIES OF TUMOR-INFILTRATING LYMPHOCYTES

Tumor-infiltrating lymphocytes (TIL) are lymphocytes that infiltrate into growing tumors and can be grown by culturing single-cell suspensions obtained from tumors in interleukin-2 (IL-2).[14–21] TIL cultures can be readily established from most murine and human tumors. To prepare TIL, a single-cell suspension is made from a freshly resected tumor, generally by enzymatic digestion, and is incubated in complete medium containing IL-2. Although lymphocytes comprise a minor subpopulation of the enzymatic digest, some lymphocytes contain IL-2 receptors, presumably because of their interaction with antigens in the tumor cell surface. These lymphocytes begin to grow under the influence of IL-2 in the culture medium. Although tumor cells also grow, the lymphocytes outgrow the tumor cultures, and when these lymphocytes have specific lytic activity or lymphokine-activated killer (LAK) activity, tumor cells are destroyed. By 2 to 3 weeks after initiating the culture, pure populations of lymphocytes without contaminating tumor cells can be obtained.

Extensive studies of murine TIL have been conducted in vitro and in vivo. In vitro, murine TIL are $CD8^+$ and often have specific cytolytic function directed against the tumor from which they were derived.[22] TIL can specifically secrete cytokines when cocultured with their specific tumor.[23,24] Extensive in vivo studies have demonstrated the effective therapeutic impact of the administration of TIL into mice with established cancer.[14,15,23,25]

The administration of TIL plus IL-2 is from 50 to 100 times more effective than LAK cells and IL-2 in treating established 3-day lung micrometastases.[14,15] Although TIL can be specifically lytic, it appears that specific secretion of cytokines such as interferon-γ and tumor necrosis factor (TNF) are the best correlates of the in vivo antitumor effectiveness of TIL.[23] Although most specifically lytic TIL are therapeutically effective in vivo, nonlytic TIL that specifically secrete interferon-γ can also effectively eliminate established lung micrometastases. These studies of transplantable mouse tumors led to the study and application of TIL derived from human cancers.

TIL can be grown from approximately 80% of human cancers of various histologies, including melanoma, renal cell cancer, colon cancer, breast cancer, and bladder cancer.[16–21] From approximately 33% of patients with melanoma, TIL can be derived that have specific cytolytic activity for fresh cancer cells and not normal cells from the same patient, including lymphocytes, fibroblasts, or Epstein-Barr virus (EBV)-transformed B cells.[16,17,21] It is difficult, however, to generate specifically cytolytic TIL from tumors other than melanoma, and we have been unsuccessful in finding TIL with specific lysis with patients with colon cancer and breast cancer. Rare cultures from patients with renal cancer can exhibit specific cytolytic activity.[26] TIL derived from human tumors are mainly $CD3^+$ and can be $CD8^+$ or $CD4^+$ or mixtures of both. Some cultures contain $CD56^+$ non-MHC-restricted killer cells.

The specific lysis of autologous tumor by TIL is MHC restricted. Specific lysis of TIL can be inhibited by antibodies to CD3 or MHC class I molecules.[21] When specific TIL are tested against a panel of HLA-typed allogeneic melanomas, the cross-reactivity of lysis follows a pattern of HLA specificities.[27] HLA-A2 appears to be a common restriction element for the recognition of melanoma antigens on allogeneic melanomas. We transfected the gene for HLA-A2 into allogeneic non HLA-A2 melanomas and showed that HLA-A2-restricted TIL could lyse allogeneic melanomas expressing the transfected HLA-A2 gene in 6 of 6 patients.

The recognition of specific antigens by TIL has led to studies attempting to define the nature of these antigens. By repeated immunoselection using TIL with specific lysis tumor lines can be isolated that are resistant to lysis by autologous TIL.[28] These immunoselected tumors can then be used to identify multiple tumor antigens present on a single tumor.

In seeking other assays for detecting tumor specific antigens, we determined that specific cytokine release by TIL cocultured with the autologous human tumor is an indicator of specific immune recognition of tumor antigens.[24] The specific secretion of cytokines, such as granulocyte-macrophage colony-stimulating factor (GM-CSF), TNF, and interferon-γ after incubation with autologous tumor have shown patterns similar to that seen with the use of lytic TIL. Using this cytokine release assay, specific reactivity has been identified in TIL from patients with breast cancer and melanoma. We are currently exploring the use of this assay to identify tumor-specific antigens in other tumors.

In pilot trials, the treatment of patients with advanced melanoma using TIL plus IL-2 has resulted in objective responses in 38% of 50 patients.[29] This is approximately twice the level of response seen with IL-2 alone or LAK cells plus IL-2. Prior nonresponsiveness to therapy with IL-2-based regimens does not compromise the ability to respond to TIL plus IL-2 therapy. In vitro lysis of autologous tumor by TIL has a weak but significant correlation with clinical response, and we are currently testing whether specific cytokine release correlates with clinical response.[30]

Studies have been conducted in patients with metastatic melanoma treated with TIL labeled with indium 111 to test whether administered TIL localized to tumor deposits.[31–32] Clear tumor localizations of TIL were seen on 13 of 18 nuclear scan series. Similarly, paired biopsies of tumor and normal skin showed a substantial concentration of ^{111}In-labeled TIL in tumor compared with normal skin. It appears that TIL can concentrate in tumor deposits. Approximately 0.015% of the injectate accumulates per gram of tumor. The accumulation of TIL in tumor has played an important role in the development of gene therapies using TIL transduced with cytokine genes.

GENE TRANSFERS INTO HUMANS USING TUMOR-INFILTRATING LYMPHOCYTES

Attempts to follow the in vivo distribution and survival of human TIL after systemic administration to humans were limited by the problems associated with using radioactive ^{111}In as a label for the cells. ^{111}In has a half-life of 2.8 days, and the combination of the natural decay of the isotope and the spontaneous release of ^{111}In from the cell limited the time we could use these cells for study to 1 to 2 weeks. The autoirradiation of the TIL by the ^{111}In led to potential damage of the TIL, which could alter their function. Information was needed about how long infused TIL persisted in vivo, where they were located in the body, and whether the in vivo accumulation of TIL at the tumor site, draining lymph nodes, or in the circulation correlated with clinical antitumor effect. The opportunity to reisolate administered TIL from the tumor site would also provide information about the functional characteristics of TIL that traffic to tumor sites and whether any of these properties correlated with in vivo antitumor effects.

The introduction of new genes into TIL provided a possibility for genetically marking the cell to answer many of these questions. An introduced gene has many potential advantages as a cell marker that no other exogenous label can provide. The label becomes part of the permanent genome of the cell and does not leach away from the original cell, as would a radioactive label. The label is not diluted as the cells proliferate, and every daughter cell is labeled. The label is lost as soon as the cell dies and does not become sequestered or reused in other cells. The vital function of the cells is not changed by the marker label. A new functional property, such as the use of a selectable marker gene, can be introduced into the cell that would permit the specific recovery of the marked cells. Depending on the gene inserted, sensitive detection methods are available, such as the polymerase chain reaction (PCR), which enable the identification of as few as one marked cell in one million unmarked cells.

A clinical protocol was conducted using retroviral mediated gene transfer to introduce the gene coding for neomycin phosphotransferase, a bacterial protein capable of rendering the cell resistant to G418, a neomycin analog otherwise lethal to all eukaryotic cells.[1] Because gene transfer studies had never been approved in humans, the potential risks and benefits of this proposed technology were carefully analyzed by a variety of review groups, including the Clinical Research Committees of the National Cancer Institute; the National Heart, Lung and Blood Institute; the National Institutes of Health (NIH) Biosafety Committee; the Gene Therapy Subcommittee of the Recombinant DNA Advisory Committee (RAC), the full RAC, and the Food and Drug Administration. Final approval was required from the Director of the NIH, who gave his approval to proceed in January 1989. A variety of factors were considered by these review groups. It was necessary to demonstrate that marker genes could insert and express in human TIL, that the marked TIL were not significantly altered, that the marked cells could be detected in animal models, and that there was low risk to the patient and no risk to the public in using this new technology.

In initial studies, TIL obtained from cancer patients were grown in culture and transduced with the retroviral vector N2 from the PA317 packaging cell line.[6] N2 was a derivative of the Moloney murine leukemia virus in which the *GAG, POL,* and *ENV* genes were removed or truncated and the bacterial NeoR gene inserted. To further decrease the development of replication, competent virus the LNL6 vector was derived from the N2 vector.[7] This vector contained a stop codon at the site of the gag start codon. Substitution of the 5′ Moloney leukemia virus sequences with those of the Moloney sarcoma virus sequences minimized the homology between the vector and helper virus genome, which decreased the potential frequency of recombination. The PA317/LNL6-C8 cell line was used to produce the transduction vector used in these clinical studies and provided high-titer retroviral vector without helper virus contamination.

A variety of preclinical studies preceded the clinical administration of gene transduced TIL into humans.[33–34] These studies were conducted with the N2 and the LNL6 vectors.

The gene coding for neomycin phosphotransferase could be readily introduced into human TIL using these vectors.[1,33,34] An example of the growth of the nontransduced and transduced TIL in IL-2 is shown in Figures 69–1 and 69–2. Examples of the ability of the transduced cells to resist exposure to the neomycin analog G418 are also shown in these figures. Only the transduced and not the nontransduced cells could grow in G418 concentrations of 0.4 mg/ml or higher.

The proviral sequences in transduced TIL populations were demonstrated on Southern blots by hybridization of *Sac*1-digested DNA with ^{32}P-labeled NeoR probes (Fig. 69–3). A single copy of the expected 3.2-kb NeoR-hybridizing fragment was present without rearrangement or deletion in the transduced TIL populations but was not detectable in nontransduced cells. The integration and expression of the transduced TIL

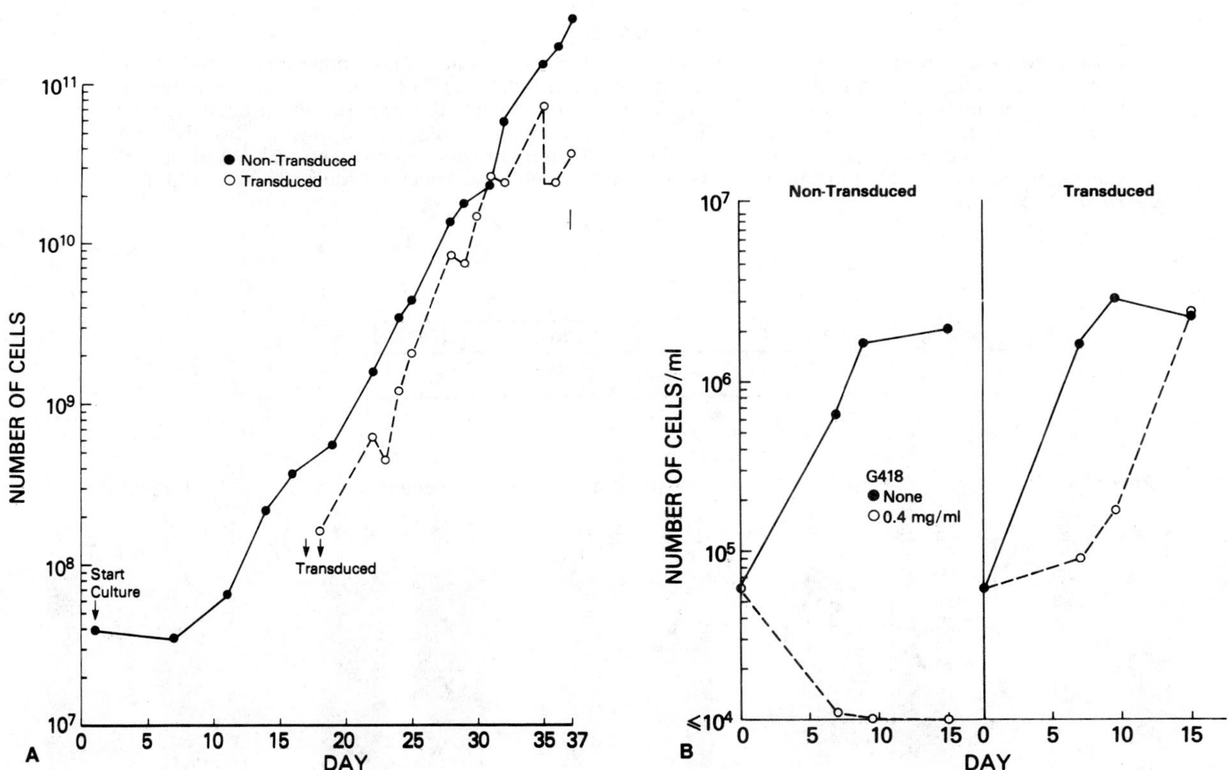

FIGURE 69–1. Growth of nontransduced and transduced human tumor-infiltrating lymphocytes (TIL) in culture. When TIL reach approximately 3×10^8 cells, an aliquot is transduced, and the transduced and nontransduced cells are grown in parallel. **(A)** Growth rates for the two populations appear to be similar. **(B)** The effect of 0.4 mg/ml of G418 on nontransduced and transduced TIL. The nontransduced TIL die in the presence of G418. The transduced TIL show a short lag after exposure to G418 and then begin to grow at a rate equivalent to that of the nontransduced cells. (Kasid A, Morecki S, Aebersold P, et al. Human gene transfer: Characterization of human tumor-infiltrating lymphocytes as vehicles for retroviral-mediated gene transfer in man. Proc Natl Acad Sci USA 1990;87:473–477)

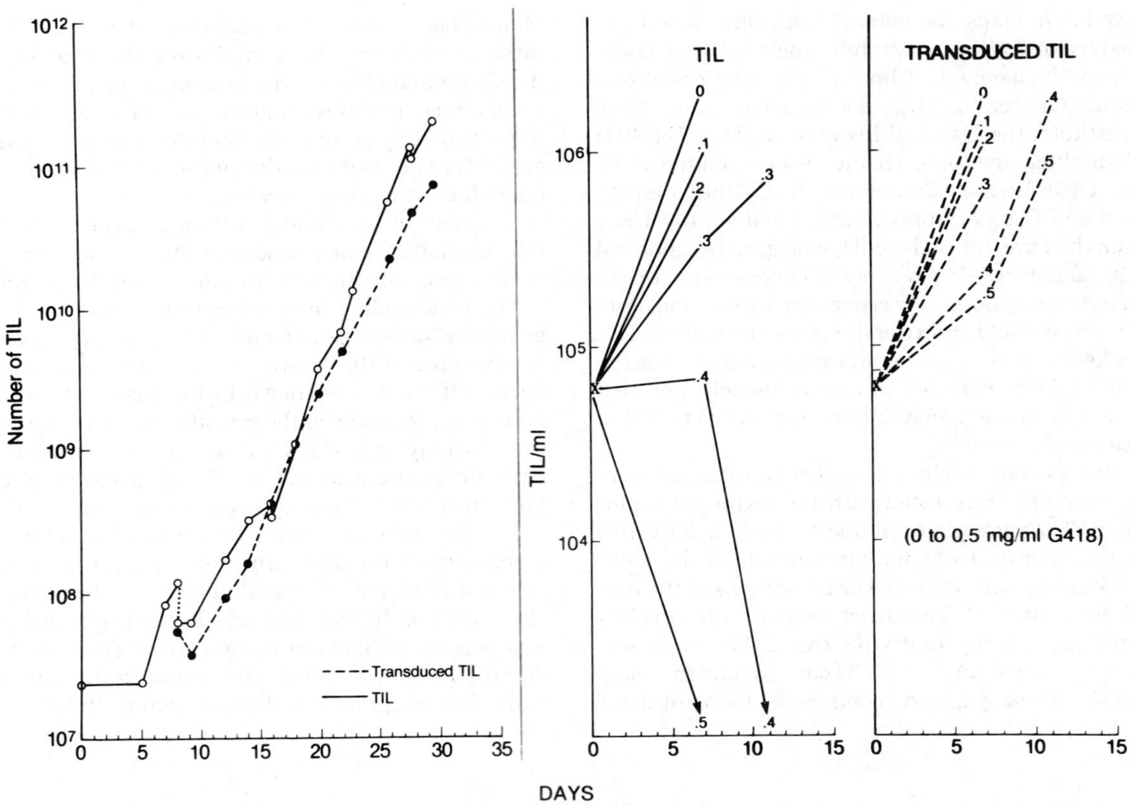

FIGURE 69–2. Growth of transduced and nontransduced human tumor-infiltrating lymphocytes (TIL) in culture (*left*). Growth of nontransduced TIL in varying concentration of G418 (*middle*). At concentrations of 0.4 and 0.5 mg/ml G418, nontransduced TIL die. Growth of transduced TIL in various concentrations of G418 (*right*). Transduced TIL grow successfully in G418 concentrations as high as 0.5 mg/ml. (Rosenberg SA, Aebersold P, Cornetta K, et al. Gene transfer into humans—Immunotherapy of patients with advanced melanoma, using tumor-infiltrating lymphocytes modified by retroviral gene transduction. N Engl J Med 1990;323:570–578)

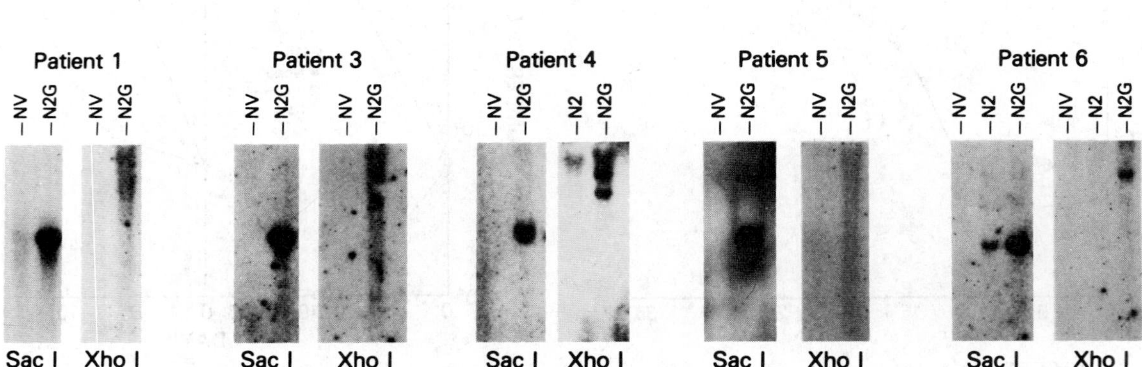

FIGURE 69–3. Detection and integration of vector DNA in human tumor infiltrating lymphocytes (TIL) transduced with the *NeoR* gene. The *Sca*1-digested DNA shows the expected 3.2 kilobase *NeoR* hybridizing fragment in the transduced but not in the nontransduced cells. The *Sca*1-digested DNA revealed multiple clones of transduced TIL containing proviral DNA integrated into different sites of the host chromosome. (Kasid A, Morecki S, Aebersold P, et al. Human gene transfer: Characterization of human tumor-infiltrating lymphocytes as vehicles for retroviral-mediated gene transfer in man. Proc Natl Acad Sci USA 1990;87:473–477)

appeared stable during extended cell cultures even in the absence of G418. Restriction digest with *Sca,* which did not cut within the provirus, revealed multiple clones of transduced TILs containing proviral DNA integrated into different sites of the chromosome. Neomycin phosphotransferase activity could also be demonstrated in the transduced cells.

Extensive tests were performed on the transduced and nontransduced populations to test whether the transduction procedure altered the phenotypic and functional characteristics of the TIL.[1,33] Because the antigenic specificity of the TIL depended on the presence of T-cell receptors, we used human genomic and cDNA probes specific for β and γ T-cell receptors to study the pattern of gene rearrangement in the TIL.[33] As illustrated in Figure 69–4, T-cell receptor-β gene rearrangements appeared similar in the nontransduced and transduced selected populations. The study of Northern blots for cytokine mRNA expression revealed similar patterns between the transduced and the nontransduced TIL; TIL expressed mRNA for TNF-α and TNF-β but not for IL-6, GM-CSF, IL-1β or interferon-γ.[33] Similarly, studies of the phenotype and cytotoxicity of transduced and nontransduced cells appeared to reveal substantial similarity unaffected by cell transduction. It appeared from these studies that the gene for *NeoR* could be inserted and expressed in human TIL and that the marked TIL were not significantly altered.

Before initiating clinical trials, studies were performed to see if marked cells could be detected in animals.[34] Despite extensive efforts, it has not been possible to introduce genes into short-term murine lymphocyte cultures by any available technique. Extensive efforts have been made using retroviral vectors, calcium phosphate precipitation, and electroporation to stably insert genes into short-term murine cultures without success. It has, however, been possible to insert genes into selected long-term mouse lymphocyte lines, and these long-term cultures were used to test the detection and recovery of marked cells in animal models. Culver and coworkers inserted the *NeoR* gene into long-term cultures of sperm whale myoglobin specific murine helper T cells (clone 14.1), which were maintained by repeated cycles of stimulation in vitro with myoglobin in the presence of antigen presenting cells.[34] These murine helper T cells were transduced with the N2 vector and the retroviral SAX vector, which expressed *NeoR* and human adenosine deaminase genes. After selection of these cells in G418, they were injected into nude mice to test the persistence of the cells in vivo. In these studies, G418-resistant cells were readily recovered from the spleens of recipient animals several months after injection. These cells could be grown in vitro and shown to express neomycin phosphotransferase activity. Animal experiments suggested that marked cells could survive and could be recovered in animal models, although it should be emphasized that these studies were not performed with murine TIL.

Safety considerations were paramount in our preclinical evaluation of the use of retroviral vectors for transduction of human cells.[1,35] Sterility tests and tests for replication competent virus capable of detecting one viral particle per milliliter of solution were performed on the viral supernatants and on the gene modified cells after expansion in culture. In no case did we ever find evidence of replication competent viruses in cells administered to patients.

After presentation of much of this information to the appropriate regulatory committees, permission was received to treat as many as 10 patients with advanced melanoma having life expectancies of 90 days or less. In these trials patients

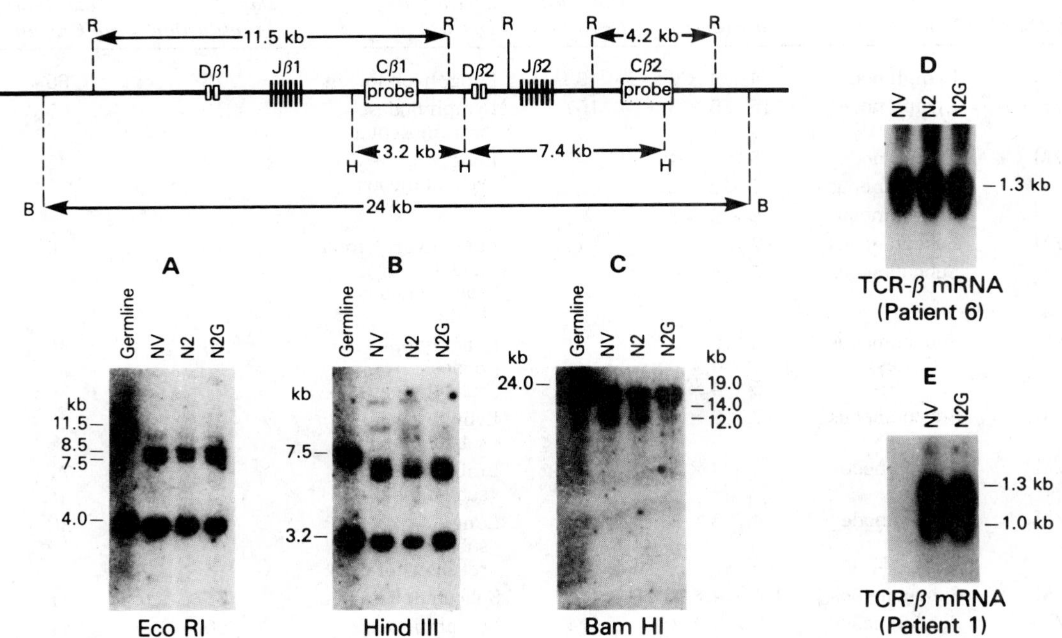

FIGURE 69–4. T-cell receptor-β gene rearrangements in nontransduced and transduced tumor-infiltrating lymphocytes. Similar patterns of gene rearrangements were seen in the transduced and nontransduced populations. (Kasid A, Morecki S, Aebersold P, et al. Human gene transfer: Characterization of human tumor-infiltrating lymphocytes as vehicles for retroviral-mediated gene transfer in man. Proc Natl Acad Sci USA 1990;87:473–477)

received an aliquot of gene modified cells with nonmodified cells as part of their standard TIL treatment for advanced melanoma.[1,29] Ten patients with advanced melanoma were treated using *NeoR* gene-modified cells. The results in the first 5 patients have been published.[1] The characteristics of the 10 patients are presented in Table 69–2. They vary in age from 26 to 52, and all had extensive melanoma with multiple lesions, including lesions in brain, lung, liver, subcutaneous tissue, adrenal gland, and other sites. Characteristics of the infused gene transduced and nontransduced TIL administered to the first 5 patients are also presented in Table 69–3.

Lymphocytes grew to a maximum of 63,400-fold over a 65-day period. Estimates of the percent of transduced cells by semiquantitative PCR analysis revealed that from 1% to 11% of the cells were transduced. Semiquantitative Southern blot analysis estimated that 4% to 18% of cells were transduced. In each patient, evidence for the insertion of the *NeoR* gene was demonstrated using Southern blots. Expression of the neomycin phosphotransferase was detected in all of the transduced cell populations and none of the nontransduced cells. The expression of the *NeoR* gene was demonstrated by successfully culturing TIL from 4 of the 5 initial patients in the neomycin analog G418.

A primary goal of our studies was the detection of these gene-marked cells in blood and tumor samples. Samples of peripheral blood and tumor samples were taken from all patients before and at various times after the infusion. Because of the pattern of tumor spread, multiple tumor biopsies could not be obtained from all patients. PCR analyses were performed in a blinded fashion by at least two investigators, and the results on all positive samples were confirmed in a second independent assay. The results of these assays on the first 5 patients is presented in Figure 69–5. Circulating peripheral blood mononuclear cells containing the *NeoR* gene were consistently present in the first 19 to 22 days after cell infusion. Cells were detected in the peripheral blood on day 51 in 1 patient and on day 60 on another patient. One of the patients underwent resection of a lesion 64 days after the infusion of gene modified cells. TIL in this specimen contained the *NeoR* gene, and TIL were reinfused on day 94. In this patient, gene-modified cells were detected in the circulation on day 121 and day 189 after the initial infusion.

An attempt was made to estimate the number of gene-modified cells in the circulation using semiquantitative PCR analysis.[1] In patient 1 the incidence of transduced TIL in peripheral blood was approximately 1 in 5000 mononuclear cells on day 1, 1 in 8000 on day 2, and 1 in 16,000 on day 4 after cell infusion. Another patient had 1 transduced cell in 300 on day 3, 1 in 1500 on day 6, 1 in 3000 on day 14, and 1 in 10,000 on day 19. TIL grown from the tumor in one of the patients grew successfully in G418, indicating that the *NeoR* gene was present and was expressed in these cells. Multiple

TABLE 69–2. Characteristics of Patients Receiving Tumor-Infiltrating Lymphocytes Transduced With the NeoR Gene

		Tumor Harvest				*Infused Cells*		
Patient	*Age/Sex*	*Site*	*Size (cm)*	*Total No. of Cells Obtained* ($\times 10^{-7}$)	*Sites of Evaluable Disease*	*Day of Transduction*	*Total Days of Growth*	*Fold Expansion**
1	52/M	Lymph node	4 × 4 × 2	33	Lung, liver spleen	13	60	16,100
2	46/F	Lymph node	5 × 5 × 3	157	Lymph nodes, intramuscular	19	65	5,000
3	42/M	Lymph node Subcutaneous Subcutaneous	6 × 5 × 4 2 × 2 × 2 2 × 2 × 2	205	Lung, subcutaneous	12	48	35,100
4	41/M	Subcutaneous Subcutaneous	2 × 1 × 1 5 × 4 × 4	41	Lung, liver, lymph nodes, subcutaneous brain	16	36	9,500
5	26/F	Subcutaneous (6 sites)	2 × 2 × 2 to 5 × 4 × 2	71	Lung, lymph nodes, subcutaneous	8	30	5,300
6	38/M	Subcutaneous	17 × 9 × 6	150	Lymph nodes, subcutaneous	21	36	12,818,000
7	43/M	Lymph node	5 × 4 × 3	100	Brain, subcutaneous	21	71	4,000
8	53/M	Lymph node	4 × 3 × 3	22	Lung, subcutaneous, retroperitoneum,	20	36	79,400
9	30/M	Subcutaneous	6 × 4 × 3	100	Subcutaneous	31	41	2,300
10	30/M	Subcutaneous	5 × 5 × 3	14	Lymph nodes, intraperitoneal	20	41	10,000

* Calculated fold expansion of cells administered. Not all cultured cells were given; some cells were diverted for experimental studies or lost to contamination.

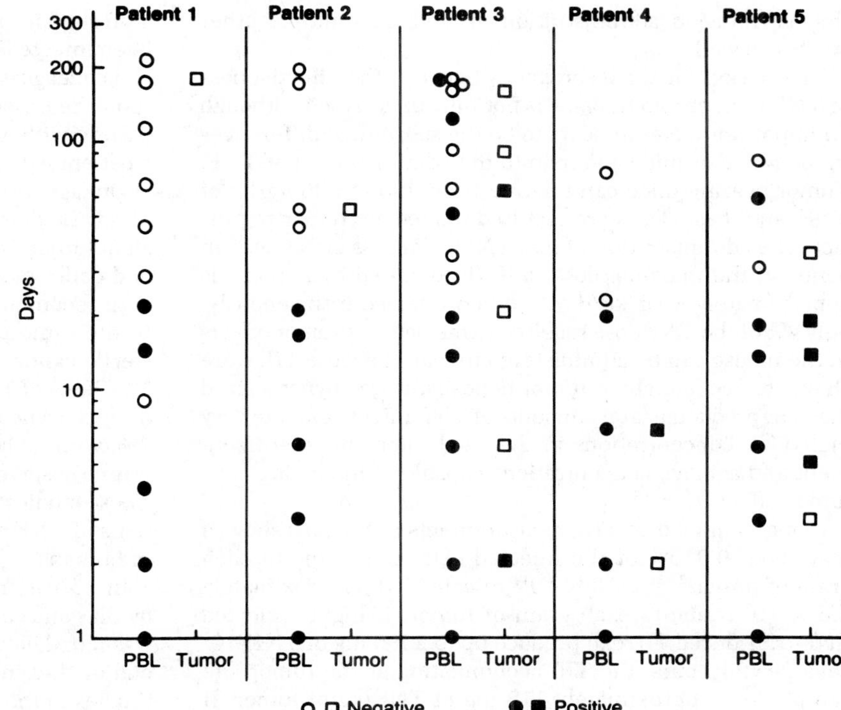

FIGURE 69–5. Results of polymerase chain reaction assays on peripheral blood mononuclear cells and tumor biopsy of 5 patients receiving *NeoR* gene-modified tumor-infiltrating lymphocytes (TIL). Gene-modified cells were consistently seen in the circulation for approximately 21 days after infusion. *NeoR* gene-modified TIL were found in tumor biopsies up to 64 days after TIL infusion. (Rosenberg SA, Aebersold P, Cornetta K, et al. Gene transfer into humans—Immunotherapy of patients with advanced melanoma, using tumor-infiltrating lymphocytes modified by retroviral gene transduction. N Engl J Med 1990;323:570–578)

specimens taken at autopsy performed on 3 patients who received gene-modified cells about 6 months earlier revealed no PCR-positive cells, with the exception of one specimen in a single renal cortex biopsy that was thought to be a false positive; the opposite renal cortex was negative.

Two of the 10 patients had an objective regression of cancer, including 1 patient who had complete regression of multiple lung lesions, subcutaneous deposits, and oral mucosal deposits, which has persisted for more than 2 years. The antitumor effects were due to the TIL and IL-2 treatment and not to any direct function of the modified gene.

All of the safety studies in the patients have been negative. All viral supernatants used for gene transduction and all infused TIL were sterile for bacteria, fungi, and mycoplasma and negative on S^+L^- assays for ecotropic, xenotropic, and amphotropic infectious viruses and on NIH 3T3 amplification tests. PCR analysis for the presence of the amphotropic helper virus 4070A envelope genes and reverse transcriptase assays of all TIL were negative. All infused TIL stopped growing shortly after IL-2 was withdrawn from the culture medium. Western Blot assays of the patient's serum to antibodies to 4070A viral P30 GAG protein and S^+L^- assays for virus performed at various times up to 180 days after cell infusion were negative.[1]

These studies demonstrated that it was possible to use retroviral mediated gene transfer to introduce foreign genes into cells that could be readministered safely to humans.[1] These studies also showed that small numbers of lymphocytes could persist for long periods in the circulation and at tissue sites and suggested that TIL might be suitable vehicles for the introduction of other genes that might improve the therapeutic efficacy of these cells or be suitable for the introduction of genes to correct inherited genetic defects, such as severe combined immunodeficiency disease based on adenosine deaminase deficiency.

THERAPY USING TUMOR-INFILTRATING LYMPHOCYTES TRANSDUCED WITH THE GENE FOR TUMOR NECROSIS FACTOR

Initial studies using TIL transduced with the *NeoR* gene provided the basis for attempts of the gene therapy of cancer using TIL transduced with genes that would increase their therapeutic efficacy. The first gene selected for these studies was the gene coding for production and secretion of the cytokine TNF.

A variety of considerations led to the hypothesis that TIL secreting large amounts of TNF would increase the therapeutic efficacy of the TIL. Extensive animal research in the Surgery Branch, NCI, and in many other groups demonstrated that the injection of recombinant TNF could mediate the necrosis and regression of a variety of established experimental murine cancers.[36–38] The combined administration of TNF and IL-2 mediated far greater antitumor effects against subcutaneous and liver tumors than either cytokine alone.[39] The exact mechanisms of the antitumor effects of TNF are not clearly understood, although it appears that TNF has a significant effect on the vascular supply of tumors.[38] Membrane-bound TNF may be involved in direct tumor lysis as well.[40]

The animal experiments led to extensive tests of recombinant human TNF administered to humans with advanced cancer.[41–45] In the Surgery Branch, NCI, 38 patients with advanced cancer were treated using escalating doses of recombinant TNF administered in conjunction with IL-2.[41] No antitumor effects of TNF administration were seen in these studies nor were antitumor responses seen after bolus or continuous infusion administration of TNF in multiple other studies as well.

The reason for the discrepancy between the effectiveness of TNF in mice and humans is not fully understood, although an important factor appears to be the substantial differences in tolerance of mice and man to the administration of TNF. Tumor-bearing mice can tolerate from 400 to 500 μg/kg of TNF, and these doses are required to mediate tumor regression; the administration of less TNF is far less effective.[38] In contrast, the maximal dose of TNF tolerated by humans is approximately 8 μg/kg/day.[41] When injected intravenously, only 2% of the TNF dose required to mediate antitumor effects in the mouse can be administered to man. Because TIL were shown to accumulate at tumor deposits, it was hypothesized that TIL producing large amounts of TNF might generate very high TNF concentrations in the local tumor microenvironment and achieve concentrations capable of mediating antitumor effects.

Using ^{111}In-labeled TIL, measurements in humans showed that about 0.015% of the injected cells can traffic to each gram of tumor.[31,32] Of 3×10^{11} injected TIL, approximately 4.5×10^{7} traffic to each gram of tumor. If highly selected TNF-transduced TIL can produce up to 2500 mg of TNF/10^6 cells per 24 hours, the TIL accumulating at the tumor site can produce approximately 112 mg of TNF/kg of tumor. If we estimate that only a small percentage of the tumor is the interstitial fluid volume, the equivalent TNF concentration in the interstitial fluid should exceed the 400 ug/kg that murine models predict is necessary to mediate tumor destruction. These concentrations at the tumor site are approximately 100 times the concentration that can be achieved at the tumor in humans by the intravenous injection of TNF.

An indirect estimate of the impact of high local concentrations of TNF at the tumor site may be achieved by introducing the gene for TNF into murine tumors and studying the effects of this TNF secretion on the growth of these tumor cells when injected in vivo. These studies using cytokine genes transduced into tumors are considered in more detail in a subsequent section of this chapter. Transduction of tumors with the TNF gene can result in the production of from 10 to 12 ng of TNF/10^6 cells/24 hours.[46] Nontransduced tumor cells do not produce TNF. When the murine tumors producing TNF are injected into syngeneic mice, they grow to about 5 mm and then often spontaneously regress, leading to the cure of mice. Nontransduced tumors or tumors transduced with *NeoR* gene alone grow and kill the mice.

In similar studies, the TNF gene was introduced into human melanoma cells and injected into nude mice. These tumor cells grow and then often regress while nontransduced human tumors grow and kill the nude mice. Local production of TNF by human tumors can also lead to their destruction. We have not detected TNF in the serum of animals bearing TNF-transduced tumors. When transduced tumors have been removed from animals and placed back into culture, assays of culture supernatants have shown that these cells are continuing to make TNF.

These studies have shown that high local concentrations of TNF in the tumor microenvironment can lead to tumor regression and hold promise that TIL accumulating at tumor sites producing large amounts of TNF might lead to tumor regression in humans.

In support of this hypothesis are studies in which TNF has been injected directly into tumor nodules in humans. Bartsch and colleagues injected TNF directly into tumors and observed tumor regression in 1 of 3 melanoma patients.[47] An additional patient with a squamous cell cancer of the oral pharynx and a patient with malignant histiocytoma also showed significant shrinkage after TNF was injected into the tumor. A double blind, randomized, placebo-controlled study of the intralesional injection of recombinant TNF was reported by Kahn and colleagues.[48] One Kaposi's sarcoma lesion was injected with recombinant TNF and another Kaposi's sarcoma lesion in the same patient was injected with the same volume of sterile saline. The TNF reduced the cross-sectional area of 12 (92%) of 13 of the injected lesions and caused a complete disappearance of two lesions. The placebo response rate was 7%, with no complete response observed ($p < 0.01$). There was no observed disease progression in any TNF treated lesion. These studies suggested that achieving high local concentrations of TNF at the tumor site could lead to tumor regression in humans.

In 25 patients with metastatic renal cell cancer reported by Blay and colleagues using LAK cells and IL-2, a correlation was found between serum levels of TNF at 48 hours after the end of IL-2 infusion and response to this immunotherapy.[49] Studies in the Surgery Branch using TIL in animals also suggested that those TIL that specifically secreted cytokines, including TNF, were the TIL with the most potent antitumor activities, and this cytokine secretion correlated far better than direct tumor lysis with the antitumor efficacy of TIL against established metastases.[23] These studies suggested that secretion of TNF by lymphocytes might play a role in the response to immunotherapy and increased production of TNF might increase therapeutic effects. Clinical trials were begun with humans using the systemic administration of TIL transduced with the gene for TNF.

The TNF retroviral vector used in these studies was generated by inserting the native full-length human TNF-cDNA gene containing the native signal peptide sequence into the retroviral vector LXSN developed by Miller and colleagues.[10–12] A schematic representation of the TNF retroviral vector is shown in Figure 69–6. The human TNF gene is promoted by the retroviral LTR and the *NeoR* gene by the SV40 early promoter. Both the promoters are placed in the same orientation. To prevent synthesis of viral proteins from the vector, alterations have been made in the basic vector backbone, including insertion of a stop codon in place of the *GAG* start codon. Similarly, part of the vector has been replaced with the homologous region from the Moloney murine sarcoma virus which is very similar to the Moloney murine leukemia virus but does not make a glycosylated protein. The TNF vector producing cell lines were generated by transfection of the PA317 packaging cell line as discussed earlier in this review.

Although this retroviral vector readily transduced murine and human tumor cells with *TNF* and *NeoR* genes, it was more difficult to get consistent transduction and expression of the *TNF* gene in human TIL. Despite multiple attempts to optimize the transduction procedure, transduction efficiencies in the range of 0.1% to 10% have been common. Some patients' TIL appear to be more readily transduced than others, and the reasons underlying this difference are unclear. Using se-

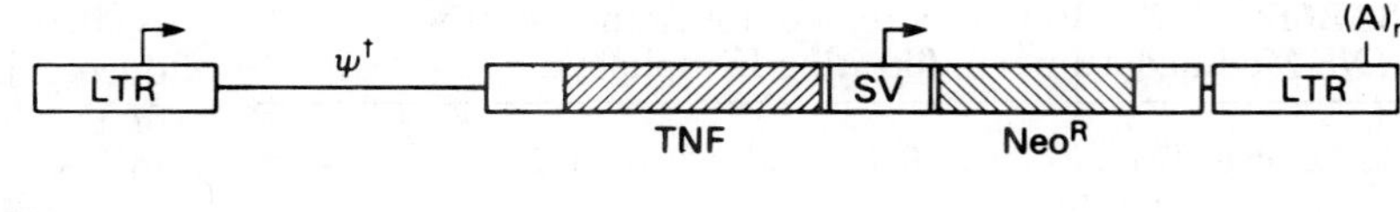

FIGURE 69–6. Schematic diagram of the tumor necrosis factor (TNF) *NeoR* retroviral construct. The TNF gene is promoted by the retroviral long terminal repeat (LTR) and the *NeoR* gene promoted by the SV40 early promoter.

lection in G418, it was possible in one study to increase the percent of transduced cells from 3.2 ± 1.0% to 57.8 ± 7.5% (Table 69–3). The increased secretion of TNF was stable over time (Table 69–4). It has been possible to achieve TNF production by transduced TIL in selected patients in excess of 100 pg/10^6 cells/24 hours, and in selected cells, TNF levels in excess of 500 pg/10^6 cells/24 hours have been achieved in some patients. TIL producing TNF grow well in culture and retain their growth dependence on IL-2.

After extensive review, the protocol for the use of these TNF gene-modified TIL was approved and treatment of patients with TNF-modified TIL begun on January 29, 1991. A schema of the approved protocol is shown in Table 69–5. In this protocol, escalating numbers of TNF transduced TIL are administered to patients in the absence of IL-2 administration. This cautious escalation of the use of TNF-transduced TIL was instituted because of the potential toxic side effects that could be induced in patients due to the TNF secretion. As of April, 1992, 6 patients have been entered into this protocol, and it is too early to determine whether TIL producing TNF will be more effective than unmodified TIL (Table 69–6). These studies represent a prototype for the use of TIL potentially modified by other genes for use in the gene therapy of cancer.

OTHER POTENTIAL MODIFICATIONS OF TUMOR-INFILTRATING LYMPHOCYTES FOR CANCER THERAPY

In addition to the introduction of the *TNF* gene into TIL, several other genetic modifications of TIL may improve their therapeutic efficacy. A list of some of these possibilities is shown in Table 69–7.

TABLE 69–3. Transduction of Human Tumor-Infiltrating Lymphocytes With the Genes for Tumor Necrosis Factor and Neomycin Phosphotransferase

Concentration of G418 Used for Selection (mg/ml)	*No. of Patients*	*Percentage of Transduced Cells (Mean ± SEM)**
0	10	3.2 ± 1.0
0.1	4	9.0 ± 2.0
0.3	12	40.9 ± 6.5
0.5	9	57.8 ± 7.5

* Estimated on semiquantitative Southern blots after 5 days of selection in G418.
(Hwu, et al. J Immunol [in press])

The increased local secretion of interferon-α or interferon-γ by TIL may have antitumor effects for several reasons. Interferon-α has a direct antiproliferative effect against some tumor cell types, and high local concentrations at the tumor site may impede tumor growth. In addition, interferon-α and interferon-γ can upregulate major histocompatibility antigens and other molecules on the cell surface, such as tumor antigens or adhesion molecules and increase the immunogenicity of these tumor cells. The introduction of other cytokine genes that may be involved in antitumor activity such those for as IL-6, IL-1α, IL-7, and RANTES, may also have antitumor effects because of their ability to modulate the immune response at the tumor site.

Modifications of tumor cells that do not affect secretory functions but could alter a different functional aspect of the cell might be useful. TIL do not bear Fc receptors and therefore cannot mediate antibody-dependent cellular cytotoxicity. However, because TIL target to tumor sites and have cytolytic capacity, the transduction of TIL with the gene for Fc receptors may induce the ability to mediate antibody-dependent cellular cytotoxicity and be a potent therapeutic tool in conjunction with the administration of monoclonal antibodies.

TIL depend on IL-2 for their continued survival, and the high doses of IL-2 required to cause TIL proliferation in vivo can be associated with substantial toxicity when administered to patients. Transduction of the gene for IL-2 receptors into TIL may increase the sensitivity of TIL to administered IL-2 and lessen the need for the high doses currently required.

TABLE 69–4. Tumor Necrosis Factor Production in Transduced Tumor-Infiltrating Lymphocytes

Patient Number	*Days After Transduction*	*TNF (pg/ml/10⁶ cells/24 h)*	
		No Vector	*Transduced**
1142.9†	34	5	380
	45	10	119
	52	8	554
1143.A†	24	55	245
	31	62	216
	49	53	228
888 MEL‡	18	0	28,280
	97	0	31,170

* Transduced TIL selected in 0.3–0.5 mg/ml G418 for 5 days. Transduced tumor (888 MEL) selected continuously in 0.6 mg/ml G418. The increased secretion of TNF was stable over time.
† Representative patient TIL cultures.
‡ Melanoma cell line.

TABLE 69–5. Revised Protocol for Administering *TNF*-Modified Tumor-Infiltrating Lymphocytes

1. Escalate *TNF*-modified TIL *twice weekly;* no IL-2.
   10^8 cells
   3×10^8
   10^9
   3×10^9
   10^{10}
   3×10^{10}
   10^{11}
   3×10^{11}
2. Reduce cell dose to *one tenth* of maximal tolerated dose. Escalate as in (1) every *3 weeks* with 180,000 IU of IL-2 per 1 kg body weight.
3. After treating 3 patients, discuss with the FDA (possibly start at a higher cell dose with IL-2).

Eshhar and his coworkers provided an intriguing possibility for extending the use of TIL to tumors for which reactive monoclonal antibodies exist.[50] These workers made chimeric T-cell receptors by combining the genes coding for the constant region of the T-cell receptor with the variable region of monoclonal antibodies. When these genes are transfected into hybridoma cells, they confer the reactivity of the monoclonal antibody to the hybridoma. These chimeric T-cell receptors can result in triggering lysis or cytokine release from the appropriate hybridoma line. An example of this phenomenon is shown in Table 69–8. We are currently attempting to produce chimeric T-cell receptors by using the constant region of the human T-cell receptor with the variable region of monoclonal antibodies that recognize human gastrointestinal or ovarian tumors. The transduction of these chimeric T-cell receptor genes into TIL may induce the TIL to exhibit the non MHC restricted reactivity of the monoclonal antibody.

GENE THERAPY OF CANCER USING TUMOR TRANSDUCED WITH CYTOKINE GENES TO INCREASE IMMUNOGENICITY

The introduction of genes coding for cytokines into tumor cells can increase the immunogenicity of tumor cells and decrease tumor growth.[46,51–58] The potential use of these gene-modified tumor cells for active immunization against cancer or for the generation of lymphocytes to be used in adoptive immunotherapy represents an attractive approach to the gene therapy of cancer. The introduction of cytokine genes into tumor cells can also provide a sensitive assay for identifying cytokines with antitumor activity and elucidate the types of tumor cells susceptible to this type of cytokine gene therapy. A summary of studies introducing cytokine genes into murine tumors is shown in Table 69–9.

Tepper and colleagues introduced the gene for interleukin-4 (IL-4) into the J558L BALB/c plasmacytoma and the K485

TABLE 69–6. Gene Therapy With Tumor-Infiltrating Lymphocytes Transduced With the Gene for Tumor Necrosis Factor

Patient Number	*Age*	*Sex*	*Sites of Metastatic Disease*	*Cell Doses Administered*
1	30	F	Brain, subcutaneous, adrenal	1.1×10^8
				3.0×10^8
				1.0×10^9
				3.0×10^9
				5.4×10^9
2	44	M	Lymph nodes, subcutaneous, intramuscular	1.0×10^8
				3.1×10^8
				1.1×10^9
				3.0×10^9
3	53	F	Liver, subcutaneous, retroperitoneum	1.0×10^8
				3.0×10^8
				9.6×10^8
				3.0×10^9
				1.0×10^{10}
				2.4×10^{10}
				1.0×10^{11}
				1.0×10^{10} + IL-2
				2.8×10^{10} + IL-2
				9.0×10^{10} + IL-2
4	25	M	Brain, lung, subcutaneous, mediastinum	1.0×10^9
				1.0×10^{10}
				4.2×10^{10}
5	30	M	Lymph nodes, subcutaneous	8.5×10^9 + IL-2
				1.1×10^{11} + IL-2
6	48	M	Lung, lymph nodes	3.0×10^{10} + IL-2
				4.9×10^{10} + IL-2

TABLE 69–7. Genetic Modification of Tumor-Infiltrating Lymphocytes for Use in the Gene Therapy of Cancer

Gene Insertion	*Rationale*
Tumor necrosis factor	Interfere with the blood supply of tumors
Interferon-α or -γ	Upregulate major histocompatibility antigens on tumors and increase susceptibility to T-cell killing
Cytokines, (*e.g.*, IL-1 α, IL-6, IL-7, RANTES)	Modulate immune response to tumors
Fc receptor	Enable TIL to mediate antibody dependent cellular cytotoxicity
Chimeric T-cell receptor (constant region of T-cell receptor and variable region of monoclonal antibody)	Broaden the specificity of TIL recognition of tumors
IL-2 receptor	Increase the sensitivity of TIL to administered IL-2

mammary cancer.[51] IL-4 was studied because of its ability to activate MHC-restricted and MHC-unrestricted cytotoxic lymphocytes and macrophages. Tumor cells expressing the IL-4 gene showed reduced tumor growth that was related to the secretion of IL-4. The mixture of nontransfected with transfected tumor cells resulted in growth inhibition, indicating that the local production of IL-4 could lead to antitumor effects against parental tumor cells at the same site although no effect was seen on tumor cells at distant sites. The rejection of the IL-4-producing tumors was associated with a dense macrophage and eosinophil infiltrate at the tumor site.

Many workers, including Fearon and coworkers,[52] Gansbacher and colleagues,[53] and Ley and associates,[54] introduced the *IL2* gene into tumor cells using calcium phosphate transfection or retroviral mediated gene transduction. These workers used different tumors including colon cancer, melanoma, sarcomas, and mastocytomas, and all showed that introduction and expression of the *IL2* gene could lead to inhibition of growth of the tumor. This activity could be blocked by anti-CD8 or anti-MHC class I antibodies. $CD8^+$ cells were required in vivo to mediate these effects. Fearon and colleagues hypothesized that the failure of the immune response to the parental tumor was due in part to the failure of T-cell help that could be overcome by the local production of cytokines such as IL-2.[52]

Asher and coworkers conducted extensive studies of the retroviral mediated transduction of the *TNF* gene into mouse sarcomas, and these studies are used here as an example of the results obtained by other workers using the *TNF* gene and genes coding for other cytokines.[46] The introduction of *TNF* genes into a murine sarcoma and subsequent cloning of the tumor cells revealed that different clonal tumor populations had widely varying but stable expression of TNF secretion. An example of the variation of TNF secretion in clonal tumor lines is shown in Figure 69–7. TNF can exist in a secreted or membrane-bound form and both types of TNF were found in these tumor cells.

Cells secreting high levels of TNF would grow to a size of several millimeters and then often spontaneously regressed. In contrast, cells producing low or no levels of TNF grew progressively and killed the animals (Fig. 69–8). The growth inhibition could be inhibited by the administration of anti-TNF antibodies, as shown in Figure 69–9. The mechanism of tumor rejection was related to an immune effect in the host; lymphocyte depletion in the mouse using antibodies to $CD4^+$ or $CD8^+$ T-cell subpopulations could result in abrogation of tumor inhibition. It appeared that both cell subpopulations were necessary to mediate antitumor effects. As was shown by other investigators using other cytokine genes, the mixture of cytokine-producing cells and noncytokine-producing parental cells resulted in the inhibition of the mixture. Studies by Blankenstein and associates[55] and Teng and colleagues[56] using a BALB/c plasmacytoma and a UV-induced skin tumor, respectively, showed tumor growth inhibition that could be blocked by anti-TNF antibody and *TNF* gene-modified tumor cells.

Other cytokines are being studied for their potential to reduce tumor growth when introduced into tumor cells. No effect

TABLE 69–8. Transfecting Chimeric T-Cell Receptor Genes That Alter the Specificity of MD.45 Hybridoma Line

*Transfected Chimeric Genes**	*Stimulator Cells*					
	EL-4†	*A20‡*	*TNP A20*	*TNP Mouse Spleen*	*TNP Human Lymphocyte*	*TNP KLH*
	(IL-2 production, U/ml)					
	17	0	0	0	0	0
$V_L\ C_\beta$	50	0	0	1	1	0
$V_H\ C_\beta$	15	0	23	5	2	6
$V_H\ C_\beta + V_L\ C_\alpha$	72	0	108	10	20	150

* Variable region from anti-TNP antibody plus constant region of T cell receptor
† MD.45: Murine hybridoma that lyses H-2^b target cells (EL-4)
‡ A20: B cell lymphoma from BALB/c mice (H-2^d)
(Gross G, Waks T, Eshhar Z. Expression of immunoglobulin T-cell receptor chimeric molecules as functional receptors with antibody-type specificity. Proc Natl Acad Sci USA 1989;86:10024–10028)

TABLE 69–9. Introduction of Cytokine Genes Into Murine Tumors

Gene Inserted	*Investigations*	*Tumor*	*Method*	*Comments*
IL-4	Tepper et al[51]	J558L BALB/c plasmacytoma K485 mammary cancer	Electroporation or calcium phosphate	Tumor growth reduced or eliminated; related to IL-4 secretion; nontransfected cells at same site inhibited; dense macrophage and eosinophil infiltrate
IL-2	Fearon et al[52]	CT26 BALB/c colon cancer B16 C57BL/6 melanoma	Calcium phosphate	Mediated generation of CTL; activity blocked by anti-CD8 and anti-MHC class I antibodies; tumor growth inhibited; CD8+ cells required in vivo
	Gansbacher et al[53]	CMS-5 BALB/c sarcoma	Retroviral transduction	Tumor growth inhibited; correlated with IL-2 secretion; CTL activity induced; nontransduced cells at same site
	Ley et al[54]	P815 DBA/2 mastocytoma	Not stated	Growth inhibited
TNF	Asher et al[46]	MCA-205 C57BL/6 sarcoma	Retroviral transduction	Tumor growth inhibited; correlated with TNF secretion; blocked by anti-TNF antibody; membrane-associated TNF detected; nontransduced cells at same site inhibited
	Blankenstein et al[55]	J558L BALB/c plasmacytoma	Retroviral transduction	Tumor growth inhibited; blocked by anti-TNF antibody and anti-TNF antibody and anti-CR3 antibody; dense macrophage infiltrate (IL-6 transfected tumor showed no growth inhibition)
	Teng et al[56]	1591 UV induced skin tumor	Liopfection or calcium phosphate	Tumor growth inhibited; mediated generation of CTL; increased membrane class I expression
Interferon-γ	Gansbacher et al[57]	CMS-5 BALB/c sarcoma	Retroviral transduction	Tumor growth inhibited; mediated generation of CTL; increased membrane class I expression
G-CSF	Colombo et al[58]	C-26 BALB/c colon cancer	Retroviral transduction	Tumor growth inhibited; blocked by anti-G-CSF antibody; tumor growth inhibited in nude mice

IL, interleukin; TNF, tumor necrosis factor; G-CSF, granulocyte colony-stimulating factor.

was seen by Blankenstein and coworkers after introducing the *IL6* gene into tumors.[55] Gansbacher and associates saw tumor growth inhibition after introducing the gene for interferon-γ into the CMS-5 BALB/c sarcoma.[57] This growth inhibition was associated with an increased expression of membrane class I antigens. Colombo and colleagues introduced the gene for granulocyte colony stimulating factor (G-CSF) into the C26 BALB/c colon cancer and showed growth inhibition that could be blocked by anti-G-CSF antibody.[58]

Golumbek and colleagues demonstrated that active immunization with *IL4* gene-modified tumor cells could reduce the growth of established tumor deposits at distant sites in mice.[59] It is possible that the use of other cytokines or cytokines in combination may provide a more potent immune stimulus sufficient to reduce growth or cause regression of distant tumors.

Alternatively, the use of gene-modified tumor cells could be used to generate immune lymphocytes for use in the adoptive immunotherapy of cancer. Fearon and coworkers[52] and Gansbacher and colleagues[53] showed that IL-2-modified tumor cells could induce the generation of specific cytotoxic T lymphocytes that could not be raised to the original parental tumor. Experiments are underway to use these cytolytic cells for the adoptive therapy of established tumor deposits.

Based on these considerations, a clinical protocol has been developed to use tumor cells modified by transduction with the *IL2* and *TNF* genes for the treatment of patients with advanced cancer. A schema of the protocol is shown in Table 69–10.

OTHER APPROACHES TO GENE THERAPY

Many innovative techniques are being proposed to apply the technology of gene manipulation to cancer treatment. Several of these current approaches are summarized in Table 69–11.

In contrast to gene modification of lymphocytes and tumor cells ex vivo as discussed previously, several groups have ex-

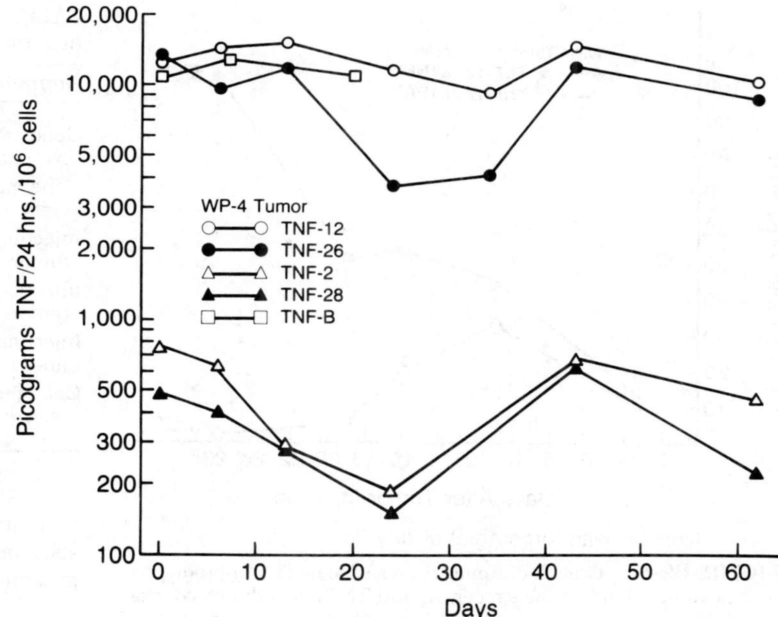

FIGURE 69–7. Secretion of tumor necrosis factor (TNF) by transduced murine tumor cell lines. Some clones produced higher levels of TNF than other clones and this production was consistent over 2 months of growth in culture. (Asher AL, Mulé JJ, Reichert CM, et al. Studies of the anti-tumor efficacy of systemically administered recombinant tumor necrosis factor against several murine tumors in vivo. J Immunol 1987;138:963–974)

plored approaches to the direct injection of genes into tumors in situ. Nabel and colleagues have proposed using DNA in liposomes for direct injection of the gene coding for the HLA-B7 alloantigen into tumors.[60] Murine studies have suggested that these liposomes are taken up by cancer cells and the DNA is incorporated into the cell genome. The expressed foreign alloantigen is then designed to trigger an immune response that stimulates immune reactions against bystander nonmodified tumor cells. Roth and colleagues have proposed injecting, directly into tumors, antisense genes intended to block the effects of the *K-RAS* gene that is involved in cell proliferation.[61,62] Alternate approaches to inject *P53* suppressor genes directly into cancers in an attempt to suppress cell growth are also being explored.

Several groups are attempting to use "suicide" genes in cancer treatment. Culver and colleagues have developed an approach to the treatment of experimental brain tumors using the direct injection into brain cancers of a cell line producing retroviral particles carrying the herpes thymidine kinase (*TK*) gene.[63] The incorporation of the *TK* gene into tumor cells will make them sensitive to the drug gancyclovir. In this approach it is hoped that the death of cells containing the *TK* gene will cause a "bystander effect," which will result in the death of adjacent cancer cells as well. Attempts to use this approach in patients with brain cancer have begun at the National Institutes of Health. Freeman and colleagues have proposed using the *TK* gene inserted into ovarian cancer cells that will then be injected into the tumor-bearing host. Treatment with

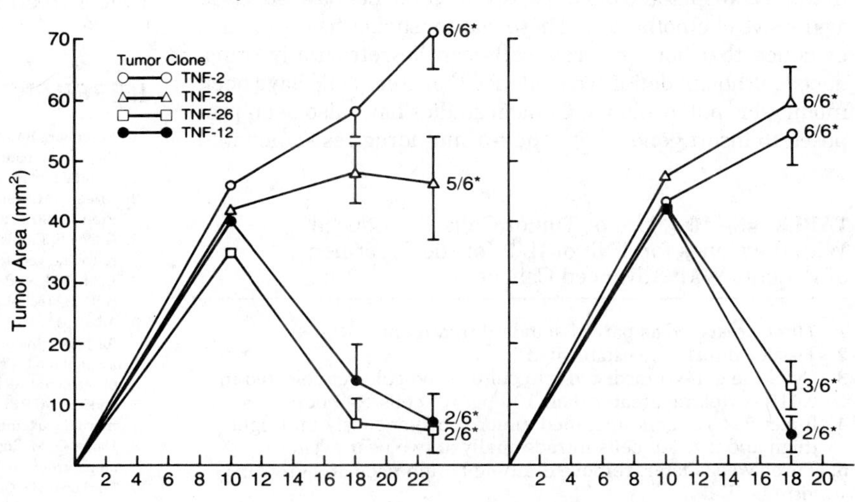

FIGURE 69–8. Growth of tumor necrosis factor (TNF)-producing murine tumor clones after injection into mice. High-producing TNF clones grew for about 10 days and then regressed, but low-producing clones grew progressively and resulted in death of the mice. (Asher AL, Mulé JJ, Reichert CM, et al. Studies of the anti-tumor efficacy of systemically administered recombinant tumor necrosis factor against several murine tumors in vivo. J Immunol 1987;138:963–974)

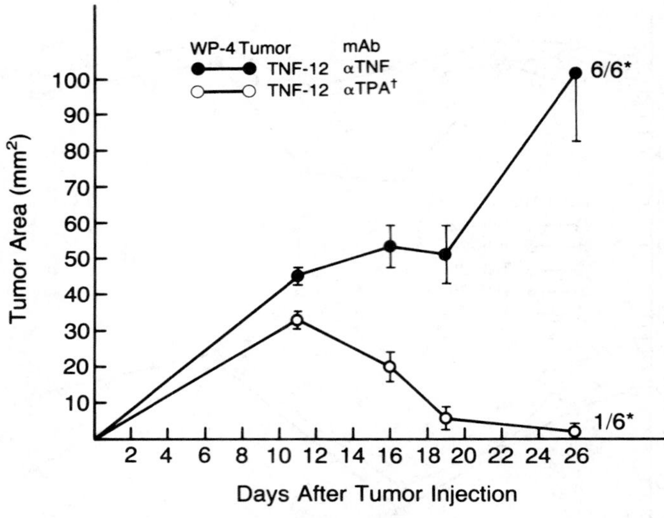

FIGURE 69–9. Growth of tumor necrosis factor (TNF)-producing murine tumor clones in mice receiving anti-TNF antibody or a control anti-TPA antibody. In animals receiving control antibody, the tumor grew for approximately 11 days and then regressed. Progressive tumor growth was seen after anti-TNF antibody was administered, indicating that TNF production is involved in the regression of these TNF gene-modified tumors. (Asher AL, Mulé JJ, Reichert CM, et al. Studies of the anti-tumor efficacy of systemically administered recombinant tumor necrosis factor against several murine tumors in vivo. J Immunol 1987;138:963–974)

gancyclovir results in the destruction of these cells and possible lysis of adjacent tumor cells as well. This approach is being directed toward the treatment of patients with diffuse intraperitoneal ovarian cancer.

Approaches to introduce foreign genes into bone marrow cells have also been proposed in patients with cancer. Brenner and colleagues at St. Jude Children's Research Hospital have inserted marker genes into the bone marrow cells of children with acute myeloid leukemia or neuroblastoma. These studies are designed to determine whether recurrence after autologous bone marrow transplantation is caused by cancer cells in the retransplanted bone marrow or cells that have survived aggressive chemotherapy. These marker studies have provided evidence that bone marrow cells can be retrovirally transduced, although definitive evidence that stem cells have been modified is not available. Clinical studies have also been proposed to insert genes that code for multidrug resistance into bone marrow cells to attempt to protect the marrow against subsequent aggressive chemotherapy treatment. This approach may allow larger doses of chemotherapy to be used.

TABLE 69–10. Use of Tumor Cells Transduced With the Genes for TNF or IL-2 for the Treatment of Patients With Advanced Cancer

1. Tumor resected as part of standard treatment
2. Tissue culture line established
3. Cytokine gene transduced into culture and cultures selected in G418 (cytokine greater than 100 pg/10^6 cells/24 hours)
4. Inject 2×10^8 gene-modified tumor subcutaneously into right thigh and 2×10^7 cells intradermally at two nearby sites.
5. Three weeks later, remove draining lymph node and grow in vitro in IL-2.
6. Adoptive immunotherapy using these cells plus IL-2

TABLE 69–11. Current Approaches to the Gene Therapy of Cancer in Humans

Approach	*Aim*
Gene modification of lymphocytes	Increase antitumor activity
Gene modification of tumor cells	Increase tumor immunogenicity
Injection of class I genes into tumors	Increase tumor immunogenicity
Injection of antisense genes into tumors	Block expression of oncogenes
Injection of retroviral producer lines into tumors	Introduce "suicide" genes into cancer cells
Gene modification of bone marrow cells	Increase resistance to chemotherapeutic drugs

CONCLUSIONS

Ongoing studies are using gene transfer technology for the development of new approaches to cancer treatment. Initial studies using TIL modified by transduction with the *NeoR* gene showed that retroviral mediated gene transfer can be safely and practically used for the introduction of genes into humans. Attempts are underway to use this technology to introduce the genes for TNF into TIL to attempt to improve the therapeutic efficacy of these cells. Other approaches to the gene therapy of cancer involve attempts to modify tumor cells to increase their immunogenicity for use in active immunization against cancer or to raise immune lymphocytes for use in adoptive transfer. Some researchers are attempting to clone the gene that codes for tumor antigens in animal and human systems. The identification of these genes could potentially result in their incorporation into viruses for use in active immunization against cancer that may have applications for cancer treatment and prevention.

REFERENCES

1. Rosenberg SA, Aebersold P, Cornetta K, et al. Gene transfer into humans—Immunotherapy of patients with advanced melanoma, using tumor-infiltrating lymphocytes modified by retroviral gene transduction. N Engl J Med 1990;323:570–578.
2. Kriegler M. Gene transfer and expression. A laboratory manual. New York: Stockton Press, 1990:1–242.
3. Gilboa E, Eglitis MA, Kantoff PW, et al. Transfer and expression of cloned genes using retroviral vectors. Biotechniques 1986;4:504–512.
4. Eglitis MA, Anderson WF. Retroviral vectors for introduction of genes into mammalian cells. Biotechniques 1988;6:608–614.
5. Adam MA, Miller AD. Identification of a signal in a murine retrovirus that is sufficient for packaging of nonretroviral RNA into virions. J Virol 1988;62:3802–3806.
6. Armentano D, Yu SF, Kantoff PW, et al. Effect of internal viral sequences on the utility of retroviral vectors. J Virol 1987;61:1647–1650.
7. Bender MA, Palmer TD, Gelinas RE, et al. Evidence that the packaging signal of Moloney murine leukemia virus extends into the *gag* region. J Virol 1987;61:1639–1646.
8. Danos O, Mulligan RC. Safe and efficient generation of recombinant retroviruses with amphotropic and ecotropic host ranges. Proc Natl Acad Sci USA 1988;85:6460–6464.
9. Markowitz D, Goff S, Bank A. Construction and use of a safe and efficient amphotropic packaging cell line. Virol 1989;167:400–406.
10. Miller AD, Buttimore C. Redesign of retrovirus packaging cell lines to avoid recombination leading to helper virus production. Mol Cell Biol 1986;6:2895–2902.

11. Miller AD, Trauber DR, Buttimore C. Factors involved in the production of helper virus-free retrovirus vectors. Somatic Cell Mol Genet 1986;12:175–183.
12. Miller AD, Rosman GJ. Improved retroviral vectors for gene transfer and expression. Biotechniques 1989;7:980–986.
13. Friedmann T. Progress toward human gene therapy. Science 1989;244:1275–1281.
14. Rosenberg SA, Spiess P, Lafreniere R. A new approach to the adoptive immunotherapy of cancer with tumor-infiltrating lymphocytes. Science 1986;223:1318–1321.
15. Spiess PJ, Yang JC, Rosenberg SA. In vivo antitumor activity of tumor-infiltrating lymphocytes expanded in recombinant interleukin-2. JNCI 1987;79:1067–1075.
16. Muul LM, Spiess PJ, Director EP, et al. Identification of specific cytolytic immune responses against autologous tumor in humans bearing malignant melanoma. J Immunol 1986;138:989–995.
17. Itoh K, Tilden AB, Balch CM. Interleukin 2 activation of cytotoxic T-lymphocytes infiltrating into human metastatic melanomas. Cancer Res 1986;46:3011–3017.
18. Kurnick JT, Kradin RL, Blumberg R, et al. Functional characterization of T lymphocytes propagated from human lung carcinomas. Clin Immunol Immunopathol 1986;38:367–380.
19. Rabinowich H, Cohen R, Bruderman I. Functional analysis of mononuclear cells infiltrating into tumors: Lysis of autologous human tumor cells by cultured infiltrating lymphocytes. Cancer Res 1987;47:173–177.
20. Miescher S, Whiteside TL, Moretta L, et al. Clonal and frequency analyses of tumor-infiltrating T lymphocytes from human solid tumors. J Immunol 1987;138:4004–4011.
21. Topalian SL, Solomon D, Rosenberg SA. Tumor-specific cytolysis by lymphocytes infiltrating human melanomas. J Immunol 1989;142:3714–3725.
22. Barth RJ, Bock SN, Mulé JJ, et al. Unique murine tumor-associated antigens identified by tumor infiltrating lymphocytes. J Immunol 1990;144:1531–1537.
23. Barth RJ, Mulé JJ, Spiess PJ. Interferon gamma and tumor necrosis factor have a role in tumor regressions mediated by murine $CD8^+$ tumor-infiltrating lymphocytes. J Exp Med 1991;173:647–658.
24. Schwartzentruber DJ, Topalian SL, Mancini M, et al. Specific release of granulocyte-macrophage colony-stimulating factor, tumor necrosis factor-α, and IFN-γ by human tumor-infiltrating lymphocytes after autologous tumor stimulation. J Immunol 1991;146:3674–3681.
25. Yang JC, Perry-Lalley D, Rosenberg SA. An improved method for growing murine TIL with in vivo antitumor activity. J Biol Response Modif 1990;9:149–159.
26. Belldegrun A, Muul LM, Rosenberg SA. Interleukin 2 expanded tumor-infiltrating lymphocytes in human renal cell cancer: Isolation, characterization, and antitumor activity. Cancer Res 1988;48:206–214.
27. Hom SS, Topalian SL, Simoni ST, et al. Common expression of melanoma tumor-associated antigens recognized by human tumor-infiltrating lymphocytes: Analysis by HLA restriction. J Immunother 1991;10:153–164.
28. Topalian SL, Kasid AL, Rosenberg SA. Immunoselection of a human melanoma resistant to specific lysis by autologous tumor infiltrating lymphocytes: Possible mechanism for immunotherapeutic failures. J Immunol 1990;144:4487–4495.
29. Rosenberg SA, Packard BS, Aebersold PM, et al. Use of tumor-infiltrating lymphocytes and interleukin-2 in the immunotherapy of patients with metastatic melanoma. A preliminary report. N Engl J Med 1988;319:1676–1680.
30. Aebersold P, Hyatt C, Johnson S, et al. Lysis of autologous melanoma cells by tumor infiltrating lymphocytes: Association with clinical response. JNCI 1991;83:932–937.
31. Fisher B, Packard BS, Read EJ, et al. Tumor localization of adoptively transferred indium-111 labeled tumor infiltrating lymphocytes in patients with metastatic melanoma. J Clin Oncol 1989;7:250–261.
32. Griffith KD, Read EJ, Carrasquillo JA, et al. In vivo distribution of adoptively transferred indium-111 labeled tumor infilrating lymphocytes and peripheral blood lymphocytes in patients with metastatic melanoma. JNCI 1989;81:1709–1717.
33. Kasid A, Morecki S, Aebersold P, et al. Human gene transfer: Characterization of human tumor-infiltrating lymphocytes as vehicles for retroviral-mediated gene transfer in man. Proc Natl Acad Sci USA 1990;87:473–477.
34. Culver K, Cornetta K, Morgan R, et al. Lymphocytes as cellular vehicles for gene therapy in mouse and man. Proc Natl Acad Sci USA 1991;88:3155–3159.
35. Cornetta K, Morgan RA, Anderson WF. Safety issues related to retroviral-mediated gene transfer in humans. Human Gene Ther 1991;2:5–14.
36. Carswell EA, Old LJ, Kassel RC, et al. An endotoxin-induced serum factor that causes necrosis of tumors. Proc Natl Acad Sci USA 1975;72:3666–3670.
37. Wang AM, Creasy AA, Ladner MB, et al. Molecular cloning of the complementary DNA for human tumor necrosis factor. Science 228:149–154.
38. Asher AL, Mulé JJ, Reichert CM, et al. Studies of the anti-tumor efficacy of systemically administered recombinant tumor necrosis factor against several murine tumors in vivo. J Immunol 1987;138:963–974.
39. McIntosh JE, Mulé JJ, Merino MJ, et al. Synergistic antitumor effects of immunotherapy with recombinant interleukin-2 and recombinant tumor necrosis factor-alpha. Cancer Res 1988;48:4011–4017.
40. Kriegler M, Perez C, DeFay K, et al. A novel form of TNF/cachectin is a cell surface cytotoxic transmembrane protein: Ramifications for the complex physiology of TNF. Cell 1988;53:45–53.
41. Rosenberg SA, Lotze MT, Yang JC, et al. Experience with the use of high-dose interleukin-2 in the treatment of 652 cancer patients. Ann Surg 1989;210:474–485.
42. Spriggs Dr, Sherman ML, Michie H, et al. Recombinant human tumor necrosis factor administered as a 24-hour intravenous infusion. A phase I and pharmacologic study. JNCI 1988;80:1039–1044.
43. Sherman ML, Spriggs DR, Arthur KA, et al. Recombinant human tumor necrosis factor administered as a five-day continuous infusion in cancer patients: Phase I toxicity and effects on lipid metabolism. J Clin Oncol 1988;6:344–350.
44. Feinberg B, Kurzrock R, Talpaz M, et al. A phase I trial of intravenously-administered recombinant tumor necrosis factor-alpha in cancer patients. J Clin Oncol 1988;6:1328–1334.
45. Moritz T, Niederle N, Baumann J, et al. Phase I study of recombinant human tumor necrosis factor alpha in advanced malignant disease. Cancer Immunol Immunother 1989;29:144–150.
46. Asher AL, Mulé JJ, Kasid A, et al. Murine tumor cells transduced with the gene for tumor necrosis factor-α. Evidence for paracrine immune effects of tumor necrosis factor against tumors. J Immunol 1991;146:3227–3234.
47. Bartsch HH, Pfizemaier K, Schroeder M, et al. Intralesional application of recombinant human TNF factor alpha induces local tumor regression in patients with advanced malignancies. Eur J Cancer Clin Oncol 1989;25:285–291.
48. Kahn J, Kaplan J, Zeigler P, et al. Phase II trial of intralesional recombinant tumor necrosis factor alpha (rTNF) for aids associated Kaposi's sarcoma (KS). Proc Am Soc Clin Oncol 1989;8:4.
49. Blay JY, Favrot MC, Negrier S, et al. Correlation between clinical response to interleukin-2 therapy and sustained production of tumor necrosis factor. Cancer Res 1990;50:2371–2374.
50. Gross G, Waks T, Eshhar Z. Expression of immunoglobulin T-cell receptor chimeric molecules as functional receptors with antibody-tupe specificity. Proc Natl Acad Sci USA 1989;86:10024–10028.
51. Tepper RI, Pattengale PK, Leder P. Murine interleukin-4 displays potent anti-tumor activity in vivo. Cell 1989;57:503–512.
52. Fearon ER, Pardoll DM, Itaya T, et al. Interleukin-2 production by tumor cells bypasses T helper function in the generation of an antitumor response. Cell 1990;60:397–403.
53. Gansbacher B, Zier K, Daniels B, et al. Interleukin 2 gene transfer into tumor cells abrogates tumorigenicity and induces protective immunity. J Exp Med 1990;172:1217–1224.
54. Ley V, Roth C, Langlade-Demoyen P, et al. A novel approach to the induction of specific cytolytic T cells in vivo. Res Immunol 1990;141:855–863.
55. Blankenstein T, Qin Z, Uberla K, et al. Tumor suppression after tumor cell-targeted tumor necrosis factor α gene transfer. J Exp Med 1991;173:1047–1052.
56. Teng MN, Park BH, Koeppen HKW, et al. Long-term inhibition of tumor growth by tumor necrosis factor in the absence of cachexia or T-cell immunity. Proc Natl Acad Sci USA 1991;88:3535–3539.
57. Gansbacher B, Bannerji R, Daniels B, et al. Retroviral vector-mediated γ-interferon gene transfer into tumor cells generates potent and long lasting antitumor immunity. Cancer Res 1990;50:7820–7825.
58. Colombo MP, Gerrari G, Stoppacciaro A, et al. Granulocyte colony-stimulating factor gene transfer suppresses tumorigenicity of a murine adenocarcinoma in vivo. J Exp Med 1991;173:889–897.
59. Golumbek PT, Lazen by AJ, Levitsky, HI, et al. Treatment of established renal cancer by tumor cells engineered to secrete interleukin-4. Science 1991;254:713–716.
60. Stewart MJ, Plautz GE, Del Buono L, et al. Gene transfer in vivo with DNA-liposome complexes: Safety and acute toxicity in mice. Hum Gene Ther 1992;3:267–275.
61. Roth JA, Mukhopadhyay T, Tainsky MA, et al. Molecular approaches to prevention and therapy of aerodigestive tract cancers. Review article. Monogr Natl Cancer Inst 1992;13:15–21.
62. Mukhopadhyay T, Tainsky M, Cavender AC, Roth JA. Specific inhibition of K-ras expression and tumorigenicity of lung cancer cells by antisense RNA. Cancer Res 1991;51:1744–1748.
63. Culver KW, Ram Z, Wallbridge S, et al. In vivo gene transfer with retroviral vector-producer cells for treatment of experimental brain tumors (see comments). Cellular Immunology Section, National Cancer Institute, National Institutes of Health, Bethesda, MD. Science 1992;256:1550–1552.

ZVI Y. FUKS
SAMUEL HELLMAN

SECTION **2**

Three-Dimensional Conformal Radiotherapy

Three-dimensional conformal radiation therapy (3D-CRT) is a mode of high precision radiotherapy. It is based on treatment designs which shape the isosurface of a given radiation dose to accurately conform the anatomic boundaries of the tumor in its entire three-dimensional configuration. Dynamic modes or multiple static coplanar and noncoplanar field arrangements are used to build the tumor dose while concomitantly minimizing the dose to the surrounding normal tissues. This approach permits increased tumor doses beyond those feasible with current conventional two-dimensional (2D) radiotherapy without increasing the risk of normal tissue complications. The improved tumor coverage and the increased tumor dose are likely to improve tumor control, although the benefit from 3D-CRT still must be demonstrated. 3D-CRT has been implemented using photon beams, protons, or heavy charged particles. In this chapter, we limit the discussion to 3D conformal photon-beam radiotherapy only.

Until several years ago, photon-beam 3D therapy was not considered practical, because its planning and implementation require the use of powerful computers not readily available at the time. The emergence of new computer technologies in the last decade enabled an accelerated development of several of the systems essential for full-scale 3D-CRT programs. New 3D treatment planning systems, powerful workstations capable of fast computations of elaborate mathematical functions, specialized computer-driven radiation producing machines, multileaf collimators, and on-line imaging devices that monitor automated treatments and assure their quality, have recently been introduced for patient use in several centers. The current clinical experience, although based on only a few hundred patients treated so far, indicates that this approach has an enormous potential and should become available for routine clinical use in the foreseeable future.

BIOLOGIC BASIS OF THREE-DIMENSIONAL CONFORMAL RADIOTHERAPY

The specific goal of 3D conformal radiotherapy is to improve the likelihood of local tumor control. Efforts to develop 3D-CRT in this context can be justified only if improved local control can be shown to have a significant impact on the overall therapeutic outcome. Because of the inability to define the boundaries between tumor and normal tissues, radiation target volumes have classically included a "safety" margin of surrounding normal tissue. Treatments have been frequently constrained by normal tissue tolerance rather than by specific tumor parameters. When attempts were made to increase tumor doses, reductions in the normal tissue safety margins were required, frequently leading to inadvertent tumor misses and subsequent marginal recurrences.[1–4] Although the introduction of computed tomography (CT)-assisted treatment planning has significantly improved the ability to define tumor target volumes for radiation beams, the problem of geographic misses has not been completely eliminated because of the limited use of CT information in conventional 2D treatment planning.[5,6] Only one or a few CT slices are used, mostly at the level of the central axis, and treatment planning at off-center levels is not based on detailed CT anatomic information.

The new techniques of 3D treatment planning provide complete anatomic and dose information for the entire tumor volume, and recent studies using 3D systems have indeed documented significant improvements in target coverage as compared with CT-assisted 2D treatment planning.[7,8] However, improved tumor coverage in itself is apparently not sufficient to produce maximal local tumor control. Local failure after radiotherapy is related to the degree of inherent radioresistance of the tumor clonogenic stem cells and to a variety of epigenetic and microenvironmental factors.[9–13] Because some of these parameters vary significantly even within the same tumor, it leads to clonal heterogeneity in terms of the sensitivity to the effects of radiation.[14] This apparently contributes to the observed phenomenon that in many human tumors the relation of tumor control probability to dose is substantially shallower than would be expected from the Poisson distribution that describes the randomness of cell killing by ionizing radiation.[15] There have been concerns that in many human tumors a significant dose escalation will be required before an effect on local control is detected.[15] However, underdosed regions within the tumor or marginal misses may contribute to "flattening" of dose-response curves. Besides causing local failures, such geometric and dosimetric inaccuracies would flatten the population average of dose-response curves and obscure the beneficial effects of dose increases in achieving improved local control. The use of 3D-CRT is likely to eliminate or minimize these sources of uncertainty and should maximize the likelihood of observing dose effects on the probability of local control.

Another major concern has been that efforts to improve survival by enhancement of local control alone may be offset by the subsequent appearance of metastatic disease, arising from micrometastases already present at the time of initial diagnosis.[16,17] However, clinical and experimental studies on patterns of failure after curative locoregional therapy (*i.e.*, surgery, radiotherapy) show that the incidence of metastatic disease significantly increases when initial treatment fails to control the primary tumor.[1,4,18] A recent study of 679 surgically staged B-C/NO prostatic cancer patients treated at Memorial Sloan-Kettering Cancer Center with interstitial ^{125}I source implantations showed that the actuarial 15-year distant metastasis-free survival for 351 locally controlled patients was 77%, compared with 24% in 328 patients who relapsed locally ($p > 0.001$).[18] The association of the local failure and the development of metastatic disease was uniformly observed across the spectrum of biologic variants, from the less aggressive stage B1N0–grade I to the highly malignant stage CN0–grade III tumors.[18] Similar associations between local failure and metastatic disease have been reported in carcinoma of the breast, lung, rectum, prostate, uterine cervix, endometrium and vagina, tumors of the head and neck, and in soft tissue sarcoma (Table 69–12).[18–37] These data suggest that

TABLE 69–12. Impact of Local Control on the Incidence of Distant Metastases in Human Tumors

Investigations	*Site*	*Stage*	*No. of Patients*	*Distant Metastases (%)* LC	LF
Chauvet[20]	Breast	T1–2/N0–1	202	9	20
Perez[51]	Lung	III	365	46	58
Chung[52]	Lung	T1–2/N0–2	118	39	89
		N0	51	24	90
		N1–2	67	52	59
Merino[49]	Head and neck	I–IV	5019	8	17
Leibel[48]	Head and neck	I–IV	2860	17	40
Lee[50]	Nasopharynx	I	196	3	20
Fuks[47]	Prostate	B–C/N0	679	24	77
Perez[58]	Prostate	B–C	317	22	58
Kuban[59]	Prostate	A2–C	286	18	61
Paunier[53]	Cervix	I–IV	1705	6	30
Anderson[54]	Cervix	IIB–IV	122	30	90
Perez[55]	Cervix	I–IV	1054	18	66
Stokes[56]	Endometrium	I	304	4	50
Perez[57]	Vagina	I–IV	149	20	54
Schild[60]	Rectum	B2–C3	139	28	90
Vigliotti[61]	Rectosigmoid	B1–C3	103	32	93
Markhede[62]	Soft tissue sarcoma	All	97	41	71
Suit[63]	Soft tissue sarcoma	All	204	25	61
Gustafson[36]	Soft tissue sarcoma	All	375	25	56

LC, local control; LF, local failure.

local failure exerts a dominant effect on the probability of spread to remote sites even in tumors with an inherent propensity for early and frequent metastatic dissemination (*e.g.*, breast, lung).

The association of local relapse and metastatic spread has led to the postulate that improving the local control can decrease the incidence of metastatic failure.[1,4,18] This hypothesis is consistent with recent investigations on the mutagenic origin of metastatic tumor cells. There is compelling evidence that cancer arises by a pleiotropic and multistage process. Mutagenic alterations in positive and negative regulatory genes seem equally prevalent among human cancers, because genetic instability and growth requirements grant selective advantages to to specific tumor clonogens.[37–40] The acquisition of metastatogenic properties seems to represent the ultimate outcome of tumor progression in this selective process.[37–42] It has been postulated that multiple mutational events in several recessive suppressor and dominant regulatory genes are involved in the transformation of nonmetastatic clonogens into cells with metastatic potential.[1,4,37–43] Mutagenic deactivation of recessive suppressor genes, such as *RB1, NM23,* and *p53* were shown to be associated with the metastatic conversion, and the function of several normal genes has been shown to be suppressed, ectopically expressed, or upregulated in metastatic tumor cells.[41–46] Suppressed expression of the major histocompatibility complex (MHC), increased expression of several oncogene and regulatory protooncogene products, and ectopic expression of enzymes involved in the metastatic cascade (collagenase type IV, heparanase, and cathepsin proteases) were found to be upregulated in metastatic versus nonmetastatic cells, and their demonstration has been considered evidence for the metastatic phenotypes.[43,46–50]

The realization that this multistep mutational process exists may elucidate the mechanism by which local failure enhances the rate of metastatic disease. It is likely that tumor cell clonogens remaining in residual tumors after failure to eradicate the primary lesion are primed with at least some of the initial events required for completion of the metastatic conversion. The enhanced mitotic activity that is typical for the early phases of the regrowth of locally failing primary residual lesions provides an opportunity for a rapid progression of the mutations required for completion of the metastatic conversion, facilitating subsequent events of metastatic spread and the increase in metastatic disease (Fig. 69–10).[51–53]

If a reasonably similar growth rate is assumed for the locally relapsing tumor and for the distant metastases in a given patient, the hypothesis previously described suggests that the relapsing tumor would become clinically detectable first and the distant metastases only later on. Clinical studies on the temporal relation between local relapse and distant metastases in prostatic cancer patients are consistent with this assumption.[18] Figure 69–11 shows that the median for local relapse-free survival after ^{125}I implantation in patients with stage B-C/N0 prostate cancer was 51 months, compared with 71

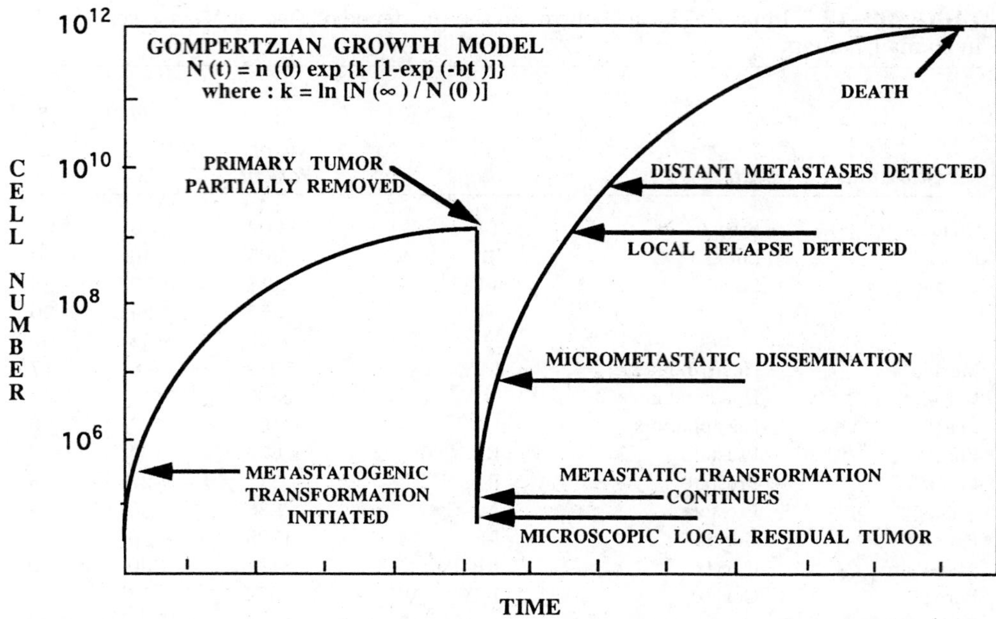

FIGURE 69–10. A hypothetical model that describes the effect of local failure on the development of metastatic disease. The growth pattern of the tumor is modeled according to Gompertzian growth kinetics. In this case, an assumption is made that the multistep process of mutations responsible for the metastatic conversion is initiated in stem cell clonogens of the primary lesion early in its subclinical growth phase, when the mitotic frequency is high. Another hypothetical assumption made is that the metastatic conversion is not completed when the primary lesion is clinically detected and only partially removed. The growth kinetic of the residual microscopic primary lesion is significantly accelerated according to the Gompertzian model. This provides an opportunity for an accelerated completion of the mutational metastatic transformation within residual tumor stem cell clonogens. According to this model, the clinical detection of the primary tumor lesion should precede the detection of metastatic disease.

months for the distant metastases-free survival in the same group of patients ($p < 0.001$). The same line of logic suggests that distant metastases in patients with local control, apparently already existing as micrometastases before treatment, would be detected earlier than metastases resulting from local relapse. Figure 69–12 shows that the median time to distant

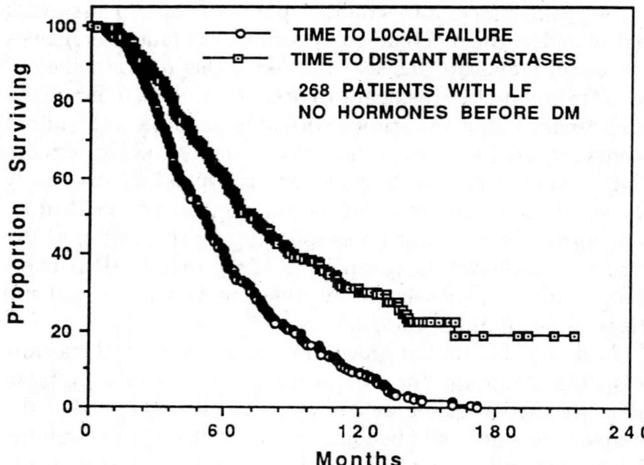

FIGURE 69–11. Kaplan-Meier time-adjusted analysis comparing local relapse-free survival (LRFS) and distant metastases-free survival (DMFS) in 268 patients with stage B-C/N0 carcinoma of the prostate who developed local failures after retropubic ^{125}I implantations. The criteria for inclusion in this analysis required that patients did not receive hormonal therapy before distant metastases were detected.

metastases in patients with stage B-C/N0 carcinoma of the prostate in local control after ^{125}I implantation was 36 months, compared with 54 months in patients with local relapse ($p > 0.001$). The hypothetical impact of local failure on the metastatic outcome highlights the need for a complete eradication of the primary tumor lesion during the initial attempt at curative therapy, and the concept serves as a basis for recent protocols designed to test the effect of improved local control by 3D-CRT on the metastatic outcome.[1,4]

THREE-DIMENSIONAL SIMULATION PROCEDURES

Essentially all imaging methods are suitable sources for acquisition of the detailed anatomic information required for 3D treatment planning, but dose calculation formalisms require that the anatomic information be presented in terms of electron density ratios, which can be obtained only from CT images.[54] Although magnetic resonance imaging (MRI), PET scanning, ultrasound, and monoclonal imaging are useful in providing complementary anatomic information on the target volume and the adjacent normal organs, the simulation process for 3D treatment planning is essentially based on CT. Conventional simulators are still used in 3D treatment planning, mainly to determine the positioning of the patient, fit the patient immobilization devices (*e.g.,* facial or body thermoplastic masks, alpha cradle body molds, head and feet rests), define the isocenter, and produce localization marks

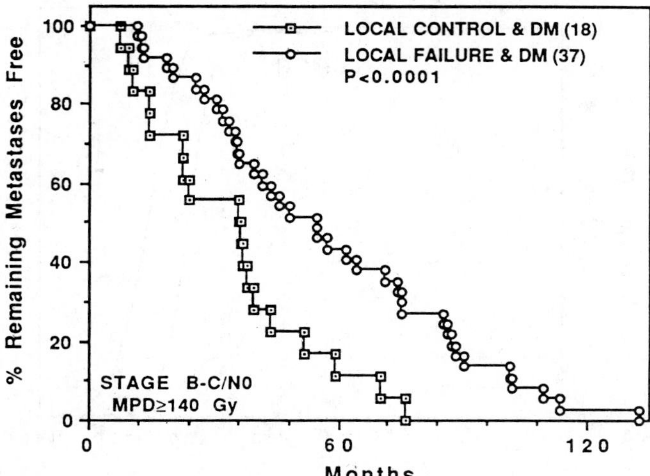

FIGURE 69–12. Time-dependent probability of remaining distant metastases free for 37 patients who developed local and distant relapses and for 18 locally controlled patients who developed distant metastases. Times to distant failure were calculated from ^{125}I implantation. Inclusion in this analysis required that patients received a mean peripheral implant dose (MPD) to the prostate of 140 Gy or more (to decrease the likelihood of occult local relapse), developed distant metastases regardless of whether they developed local recurrences, and did not receive hormonal therapy before distant metastases were detected.

on the patient's skin. The patient is then scanned on a flat table top in the treatment position, with opaque catheters placed over the predetermined simulation skin marks, so that the isocenter location can be visualized on the CT scans. The number of CT slices obtained and the spacing between slices depends on the size, shape, and location of the region of interest and the treatment technique. To produce the best 3D reconstruction, the interslice spacing should be 3 to 5 mm, and the slice thickness should be chosen to avoid overlaps or gaps between images.

BIOLOGIC TARGET VOLUME AND CRITICAL ORGANS

The biologic target volume (BTV) for treatment is defined as the volume of tissue that includes the tumor and the regions considered to be at risk for microscopic tumor extensions.[55] Usually, 5- to 10-mm margins are added to the BTV as visualized on CT to compensate for treatment set-up errors and other uncertainties. The contours of the BTV and the surrounding normal tissues are delineated manually on every CT slice with the aid of a track ball, digitizer pad, or light pen. The degree of effort required for manual extraction of anatomic features from the large number of CT slices and the lack of accuracy associated with the extraction of low contrast structures represent two of the challenging problems of current 3D treatment planning systems. Artificial intelligence and new image processing technologies are being explored for their potential to facilitate the anatomic extraction process.

A 3D structural reconstruction of the BTV and its surrounding normal organs is then performed using the beam's eye view (BEV) technique, in which the anatomic structures are displayed as if the viewer is positioned at the beam's source, observing the structures that are in the path of the beam from every spatial angle possible around the isocenter.[56,57] This mode of display facilitates the selection of beam shapes and directions that minimize radiation to the normal tissues while simultaneously conforming to the accurate shape of the tumor. Real time display of solid surfaces has recently been introduced to enhance the imaging involved in this process.[58]

SELECTION OF BEAMS AND CALCULATION OF DOSE DISTRIBUTIONS

Most current 3D-CRT plans are based on a multidirectional coplanar and noncoplanar static field arrangements. After beam directions and shapes are defined with the BEV technique, dose calculations are performed and dose distributions are displayed to evaluate the adequacy of the treatment plan. Dose computations are performed for the entire 3D space, and because of their enormous complexity, they require the use of powerful computers. Modern methods of 3D dose calculations are based on parameters of radiation transport through the entire geometry of the tissues and its pleiotropic interactions with absorbing media and account for variations in tissue composition and density.[59]

The techniques most commonly used are the radiologic path length method, the scatter integration technique, and the more advanced delta-volume method, differential pencil beam dosimetry, and the Fourier convolution methods.[59–65] The pencil beam method, for example, divides the beams into many narrow beams (*i.e.*, pencils), and the dose is computed by summation of the contributions from the individual pencil beams. The method accounts for the transport of radiation in the full three dimensions to include contributions from the primary photons, scattered photons, and secondary electrons, and it improves the accuracy of the computed dose distributions for curved patient surfaces and inhomogenous internal structures.[66]

After the field arrangement and dose calculations are completed, the selected beam shapes are used to produce treatment blocks. The digital information of the computer-stored images can be used to produce reconstructed beam films that serve as templates for block fabrication.[66] The digital data can be used for automated block fabrication by numerically controlled milling machines or to guide individual leaf positioning in computer controlled multileaf collimators.[66]

QUANTITATIVE EVALUATION OF TREATMENT PLANS

The traditional method for evaluation of dose distributions, in which isodose curves are superimposed onto 2D CT displays of body sections, is inadequate for 3D treatment plan evaluation. New methods for graphic presentation of spatial 3D dose distributions superimposed or covering 3D anatomic configurations of the tumor and normal organ structures have been described.[67,68] To differentiate anatomy from dose information, different surface rendering techniques must be used. For example, the anatomy may be shown as a stack of contours and the dose as a mesh of points or as a solid transparent surface. Volumetric displays of the 3D CT data with dose can be implemented, in which the entire volume of CT pixel data can be shown in a semitransparent manner, much like a radiograph from arbitrary angles. Graphic presentations of spatial dose distributions are highly useful for rapid qualitative evaluations of treatment plans and for the identification of "hot" or "cold" spots within a given plan. However, such methods are by themselves insufficient for the final selection of the most appropriate plan, and complementary information must be obtained from quantitative numeric evaluation methods.

Integral dose-volume histograms (DVH) represent the current most useful numeric evaluation method.[69,70] In this approach, the volume (or the percentage of the total organ volume) receiving at least the dose D is presented as a function of D (Fig. 69–13). DVHs are convenient condensations of the dose distribution data. One DVH is generated for the tumor and one for each organ involved in the treatment plan. The compilation of the curves is used for evaluating or comparing treatment plans in a convenient and rapid manner. However, there are limitations to the use of DVHs. If the dose-volume histograms do not cross one another, the curve that is found furthest to the left in the case of normal organ DVHs or furthest to the right in the case of tumor DVHs (see Fig. 69–13A) is regarded as the best plan. Frequently, the ranking of the DVHs in rival plans is more ambiguous, because the histograms often cross one another (see Fig. 69–13B), and it is not evident which plan is better. If there are several rival plans and many organs, DVH comparisons can become quite complex and demanding. DVHs do not provide spatial information, and the positions of hot or cold regions cannot be obtained directly from the DVH; spatial dose distributions must be used. DVHs do not incorporate the complex trade-offs between tumor control and normal tissue toxicities. Although dose-volume histograms represent an advancement over spatial dose distribution displays, numeric scoring functions that correlate with biologic endpoints have been suggested to improve the selection process of the best plan.

The most popular numeric scoring functions are the normal tissue complications probabilities (NTCP) and tumor control probabilities (TCP), which employ a further condensation of dose distribution data to yield a single number for each structure.[71–74] Normal tissue tolerance doses required for NTCP calculations are derived from clinical data and are fit to a function that has a sigmoid shape. Complication probability data for normal tissues, even for uniform whole organ irradiation, are scarce, and the accuracy of the available data is unknown. A recent compilation of organ tolerance doses has been developed by Emami and coworkers.[71] The aim was to obtain tolerance doses for 5% and 50% complication probabilities for uniform whole organ and for two-thirds and one-third partial organ irradiation. Whenever possible, the data were obtained from the literature, and otherwise, the dose was based on the best judgment of the participating investigators, but the consistency and accuracy of the input data were not adequately tested. Although the absolute value of the calculations based on these data may have large uncertainties, their relative values may still prove useful in evaluating rival plans (Fig. 69–14), because certain systematic errors are likely to cancel out in ranking treatment plans.

The model currently used to calculate TCP is based on the work of Goitein.[75] TCP is given by the product of the TCPs for small subvolumes of the tumor in which the dose is uniform. The tumor control for each subvolume is obtained from the estimated control for the whole tumor using binomial statistics. This model, although similar to one developed by Brahme, includes the effect of population heterogeneity on TCP.[76] The input data for these calculations are the target dose-volume histogram, TCP at the prescribed dose, and the normalized slope of the dose-response function at the 50% tumor control level. Because of microscopic disease there can be a nonzero TCP at zero dose, and an additional parameter, the probability of no tumor, is included.

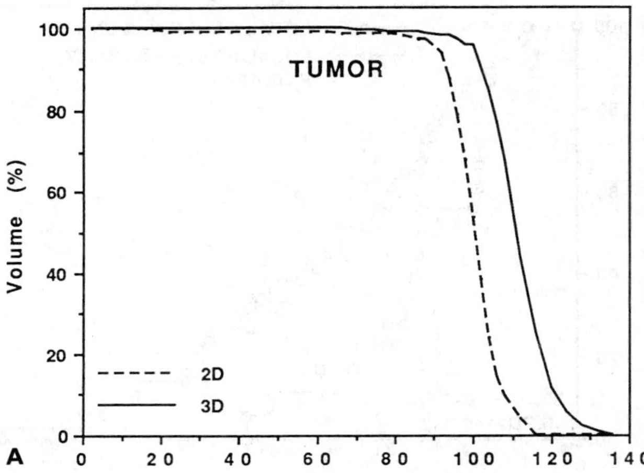

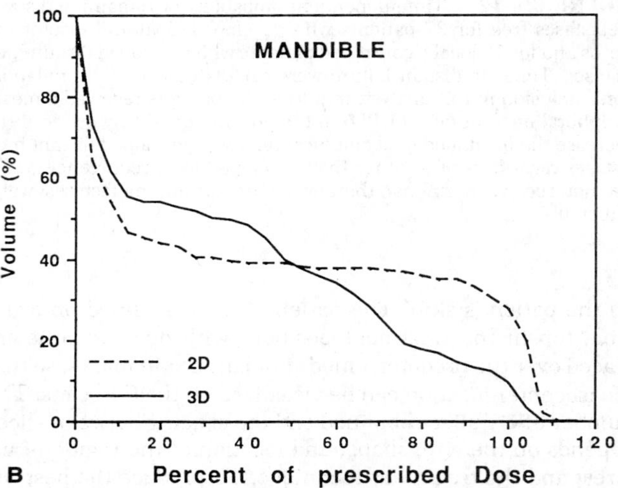

FIGURE 69–13. Dose-volume histograms (DVH) derived from a conventional 2D and a conformal 3D treatment plan for a patient with carcinoma of the nasopharynx. The doses were normalized to the prescribed minimum tumor dose, and the volumes are presented as the percentage of the total target volume. **(A)** This graph demonstrates the tumor DVH. Both plans cover the total target volume with at least 80% of the prescribed dose, but the 2D treatment plan shows a steep falloff beginning at approximately 80% of the prescribed dose, and the 3D plan carries the total tumor volume to 100%, with portions of the tumor receiving up to 120% of the prescribed dose. **(B)** DVHs for the mandible in the same patient. At the low dose levels, the 2D plan seems to offer less mandibular dose. However, the two DVHs cross each other at approximately 50% of the prescribed dose, and 40% of the mandible is carried to significantly higher doses with the 2D plan than the 3D plan.

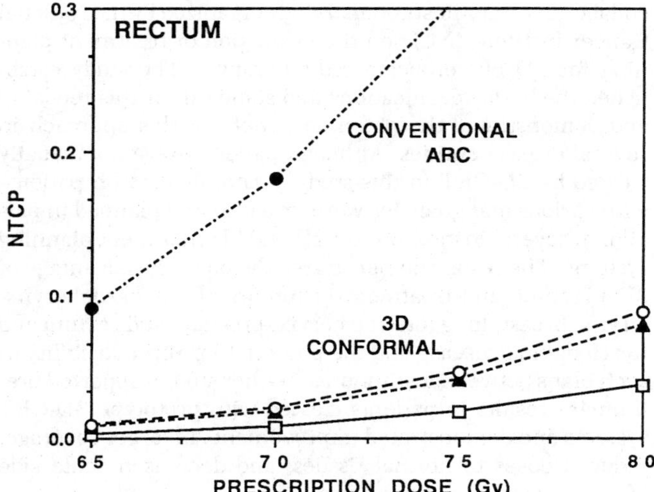

FIGURE 69–14. Calculated rectal normal tissue complication probabilities (NTCP) as a function of dose in a patient with carcinoma of the prostate. Treatment was planned with a conventional 2D, bilateral, 120° arc approach (●) or with three different 3D conformal plans involving four fields (□), six fields (▲), or eight fields (○). Rectal NTCP for each plan was calculated for a range of prescribed doses of between 65 and 80 Gy. Calculations were made assuming a strong volume effect for rectal NTCP. A potential for tumor dose escalation is demonstrated with the 3D plans because the calculated risks of toxicity to the rectum remained at acceptably low levels with all 3D planned doses.

The primary utility from calculating NTCP and TCP is that they can be used to rank treatment plans. Even though the absolute value of the calculations may be uncertain, it is their relative values that are needed for numeric evaluations. Together with DVHs and spatial dose distributions, these parameters yield a fairly complete representation of a treatment plan as required for its evaluation.

COMPUTER-AIDED OPTIMIZATION OF TREATMENT PLANNING

The process of 3D treatment planning described so far indicates that the amounts of data that need to be managed and analyzed in each plan is so voluminous that decisions regarding the selection of the most adequate plan may become an intellectually demanding task. Because there are no restrictions for the use of coplanar and noncoplanar field combinations, the number of evaluations and decision making processes involved in the planning of a single case may easily exceed practical constraints in terms of manpower and time factors involved.

There has been great interest in the development of expert systems for computer-aided optimization of 3D treatment planning.[6,74,77] Because there is virtually an infinite number of combinations possible, the specifications for this approach in terms of input of beam arrangements, weights, intensity, distributions, NTCP, TCP, and machine parameters to yield the highest possible therapeutic ratio need to be restricted to make computer-aided optimization a practical tool. However, the probability of finding a better solution increases as the domain of search for the optimal solution increases. Because a larger number of beams can improve the ratio of tumor dose to normal tissue dose, optimized 3D conformal plans, in general, contain a larger number of beams than a conventional 3D plan. The maximal benefit from computer-aided optimization is associated with the availability of new treatment machines that are capable of rapidly delivering large numbers of arbitrarily shaped fields under automated computer control.

THREE-DIMENSIONAL CONFORMAL THERAPY DELIVERY SYSTEMS

The application of 3D-CRT requires new performance standards of treatment delivery systems and the formulation of new specifications for their function. Most commercial linear accelerators have been reconfigured to allow automated computer controlled movements of the gantry and the treatment couch, as required for the delivery of successive multisegment or dynamic treatments within a reasonable treatment time. Another major development has been the introduction of new beam shaping devices. Three-dimensional plans frequently entail 10 or more fields, with all fields delivered every day. The introduction of multileaf collimators (MLC) provides an ideal solution for this need. The multileaf collimator is a secondary collimator system, which consists of independently movable high-Z material rods or leaves. Each leaf is operated by an individual motor, and the function of all motors is coordinated under computer control. The leaves on both sides can be automatically positioned to shape the treatment beam according to a preprogrammed plan. Successive multisegment therapy can be employed, in which each segment's aperture conforms to the specific shape of the tumor from that angle. A photograph of a recently developed MLC is shown in Figure 69–15. This MLC can be retrofitted onto existing linear accelerators, and other types of MLCs are currently designed as built-in components. The spatial resolution with currently available MLCs is approximately the projected leaf width in the patient plane (usually 1 cm), although narrower leaf widths may be available in the future for treatment of small target volumes. Integration of automated collimator beam shaping with other automated motions of the machine is being developed to produce the full range of static and dynamic conformal therapy.

Other modes of beam modulation within the aperture or the open part of the field are frequently needed. This has been classically accomplished by custom-made compensators manually attached to the head of the treatment machine. For multifield conformal therapy, however, automated systems are preferred, and such capabilities have been provided by techniques of beam scanning within the radiation field. For example, the Scanditronix MM50 racetrack microtron is capable of scanning photon and electron beams under computer control. The elementary electron fields used in this scanning process can be as narrow as 1.4 cm for 50-MeV electrons. Although the elementary field widths for scanning photon beams are considerably larger, they can still be used to obtain field shaping where less resolution is acceptable, or they can be used in conjunction with MLC if finer resolution is required.

Another useful system recently introduced is the on-line treatment imaging system that permits fluoroscopy-like reviews of the actual treatment fields as given daily to the patient. Although the component structure of these devices differs

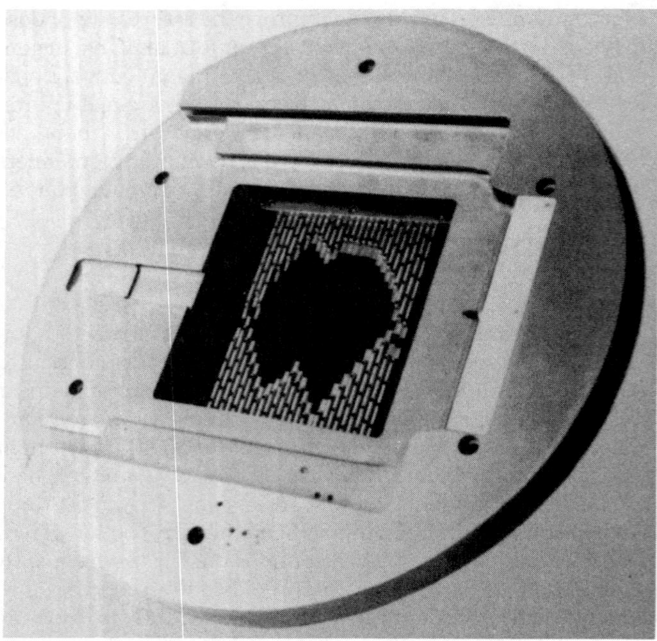

FIGURE 69–15. A computer-controlled multileaf collimator for photon beam shaping. This particular multileaf collimator features 52 leaves, each driven by a dedicated motor, and the function of all motors is coordinated by a computer. The resolution of each leaf is 10 mm at the 100-cm isocenter. The leaves can be driven under the computer control to shape the beam according to preplanned specifications. (Courtesy of Varian Associates)

between manufacturers, they all have in common an imaging detector attached to the machine gantry, methods of digitizing and analyzing image data with a computer, and a video display system. The images can be contrast enhanced or modified in other ways to highlight and enhance details that are difficult to observe with conventional screen film systems. The major potential of these systems for conformal therapy is the speed with which each field can be verified. It should be possible in the near future to use these systems in a feedback mode to compensate for set-up errors or patient movements. For example, before daily treatment begins, two orthogonal images can be obtained, the output can be compared with a preplanned configuration by the computer, and deviations that exceed tolerance limits can be adjusted automatically by computer controlled movements of the gantry, couch, and the MLC setting positions. On-line imaging devices will play a crucial role in the verification of conformal 3D treatments and probably contribute to improving the accuracy of all radiation treatments.

PRELIMINARY CLINICAL EXPERIENCE

The clinical application of 3D conformal radiotherapy is still in its developmental phase. Because 3D treatment planning systems are only beginning to emerge and treatment delivery systems are still in a testing mode, the number of published reports on clinical experiences with 3D conformal therapy is small. A major development has been the completion of a collaborative multiinstitutional study organized by the National Cancer Institute (NCI) on the evaluation of treatment planning for 3D photon-beam radiotherapy.[78] The study established the basic specifications and standard for this modality and demonstrated the potential benefit of this approach in several disease entities. Although patients were not actually treated by 3D-CRT in this study, anatomic data on patients with various malignancies were provided and planned in parallel in several institutions on 2D and 3D treatment planning systems. The results demonstrated the potential advantage of 3D planning and treatment in tumors of the nasopharynx, larynx, breast, lung, uterine cervix, prostate, and rectum and for Hodgkin's disease and the potential for reproducibility of such plans between institutions.[78] Other studies reported preliminary results in patients treated with prototype 3D-CRT systems and demonstrated improvements in target coverage, reduced doses to normal tissues, and decreased acute side effects in several tumors types.

NASOPHARYNX

Leibel and colleagues studied at Memorial Sloan-Kettering Cancer Center (MSKCC) the advantages of 3D-CRT in patients with carcinoma of the nasopharynx.[8] The study entailed 10 previously untreated patients and 5 patients treated for locally recurrent disease. The previously untreated patients received initially 5040 cGy with conventional two lateral opposed fields to the primary tumor and the cervical lymph nodes, and the 3D-CRT component was limited to a boost of 1980 cGy given to the region of the primary tumor. The patients with locally recurrent disease received the entire treatment (1620–2160 cGy; median, 1960 cGy) by 3D-CRT. All patients were planned independently by two teams. One team performed a conventional 2D plan employing bilateral opposed fields, and the other performed a 3D plan using the BEV technique to select the most optimal field configurations and BEV-derived tumor-conforming blocks for delivery of treatment. Comparisons of dose distributions, DVHs, TCPs, and NTCPs for the 2D and 3D plans were performed for the target volume and for each normal organ in each patient. Overall, the 3D plans consistently showed improved tumor coverage and reduced underdosed tumor volumes. Despite the fact that there was no intentional effort to increase the dose beyond prescription dose, the mean dose with the 3D plan was found to be higher in all cases tested (Fig. 69–16), resulting in an overall mean increase of 13%. This was achieved mainly from the improved ability to avoid tumor underdosage. The 3D plans also resulted in a significant reduction of normal tissue doses, with the traditional 2D plans involving almost twice as much normal tissue volumes carried to high-dose levels as compared with the 3D plans. An analysis of the uncomplicated tumor control probability demonstrated that with the 3D approach there was with an overall mean increase of 15% in the predicted uncomplicated control (Fig. 69–17). This translates roughly to an expected advantage from an increment of approximately 1000 cGy in effective tumor dose. Whether further escalation of the tumor volume dose is possible without exceeding normal tissue tolerance in this disease is currently being investigated in a phase I dose escalation study.

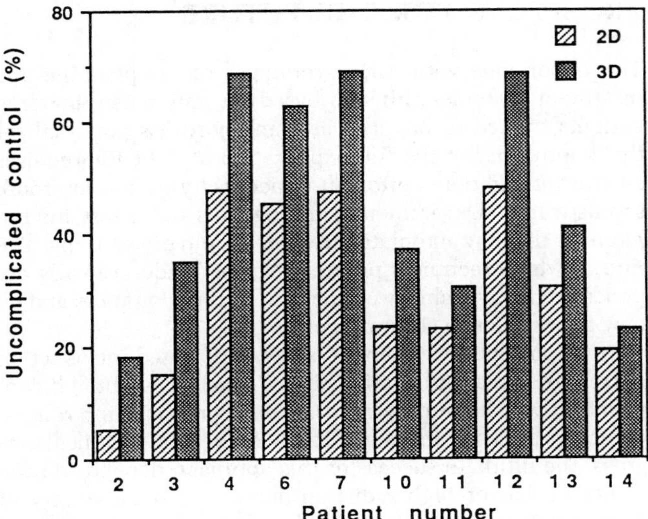

FIGURE 69–16. The probability of uncomplicated control in patients with carcinoma of the nasopharynx. The treatment was prescribed to deliver 50 Gy through conventional two lateral opposed fields to the nasopharynx and the cervical lymph node-bearing areas. Subsequently, a 19.6-Gy boost dose was planned by traditional 2D or a 3D conformal approach. The score in each case was calculated from the normal tissue complication probabilities and tumor control probabilities for the entire prescribed course of 70 Gy. Because the complication probability for the parotid gland is near unity, this organ was excluded from the calculations.

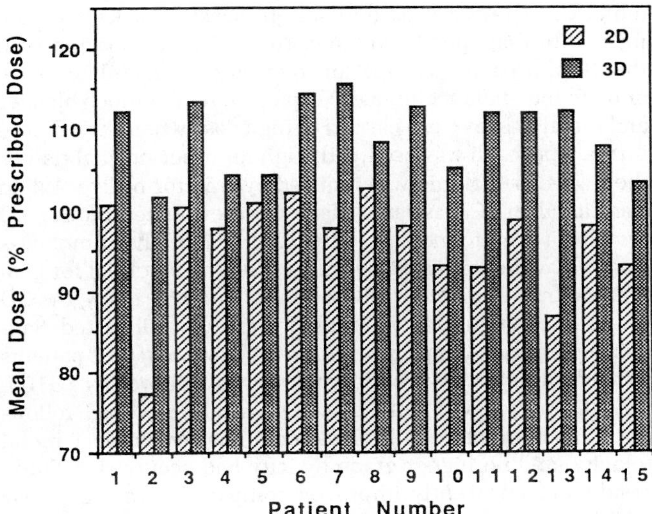

FIGURE 69–17. Comparison of the mean tumor dose in patients with carcinoma of the nasopharynx planned with a conventional 2D or a conformal 3D treatment plan. The mean dose is expressed in terms of the percentage of the prescribed minimum tumor dose.

BRAIN

The University of Michigan conducted a series of studies on 3D-CRT of brain tumors.[79–81] To demonstrate that 3D planning is practical and applicable to the treatment of high-grade astrocytomas, 50 patients were treated with cerebral irradiation delivered in a focussed, nonaxial techniques employing from two to five beams.[79] Patients were immobilized with a mask-marker immobilization system, using a commercially available thermoplastic mesh indexed and mounted to a rigid frame attached to the therapy couch. Studies employing weekly simulation indicate that patient treatment position movement can be restricted by this immobilization system to 2 mm over the course of treatment.[80] The tumor plus a 3.0-cm margin was treated to 4500 cGy and the tumor plus a 1.5-cm margin were then boosted to 5940 cGy using beam orientations that maximally spared normal parenchyma. DVH curves demonstrate dosimetric advantages to nonaxial techniques over conventional parallel-opposed orientations. Assessment of the nonaxial techniques in selected cases indicated that uniform target volume coverage could be maintained with a typical reduction of 30% in the total amount of brain tissue treated to the 95% isodose line.[79] DVH analysis demonstrated an approximation of brachytherapy dose confinement through the use of multiple nonaxial noncoplanar beam orientations. Of 12 patients with recurrent astrocytoma treated with this technique to a dose of 3060 cGy, 7 showed improvement in Karnofsky status or decrease in steroid dependence and the average survival exceeded 9 months, demonstrating the potential of this approach.[81]

LUNG

Armstrong and colleagues compared 3D conformal treatment planning with the traditional 2D approach for 10 patients with non-small cell lung cancer.[82] Patients were simulated in custom Alpha-cradle molds and scanned with CT using 1.0-cm slice thicknesses from below the larynx to the upper abdomen and 0.5-cm thickness through the levels containing visible nodal and primary disease. The objective was to deliver 5040 cGy to elective nodal volumes and 7020 cGy to all visible disease. Significant underdosing occurred in 2% of the gross target volume with the 3D approach, compared with 15% with 2D. Three-dimensional treatment reduced significantly the dose to normal tissues outside of the target volume. In some patients, as much as 30% of the uninvolved lung received 2000 cGy or more with the 2D plan, although no portion of the contralateral lung received over 2000 cGy with the 3D plan. Esophageal NTCPs were reduced from 33% with 2D to 22% with 3D. Using the doses generally delivered to normal tissues with traditional 2D planning methods as constraints, the data suggest that with the 3D approach the dose to the primary tumor can be escalated by at least 20% to 30% in appropriate cases.

PROSTATE

The University of Michigan carried out several studies on 3D-CRT for prostate cancer. Ten Haken and colleagues compared 3D treatment plans with conventional 2D plans in 17 patients with stage C carcinoma of the prostate.[7] CT scans and BEV displays were used to generate a six-field 3D treatment plan consisting of a two parallel lateral opposed fields and two sets of oblique fields directed at ±45° with respect to the lateral fields. For each field, an interactive BEV display was produced showing the target in its correct 3D perspective, and an autoblock program was used to design focused blocks that conformed to that specific volume. Normal tissue sparing with the 3D approach was superior to traditional 2D bilateral arc or open four-field techniques. Typically, half as much bladder and rectal tissues were carried to high dose when the 3D conformal approach was used, although for other normal tissues the high-dose volume was reduced by a factor of five. When traditional 2D CT-assisted plans were evaluated on the 3D system, it was found that only 72 ± 7% of the tumor was covered by the 95% isodose, suggesting the potential for geographic misses in 20% to 35% of the patients. Using the 3D six-field technique, a dose escalation study was initiated. Sandler reported preliminary results in the first 15 stage C patients treated with 4500 cGy to the whole pelvis, followed by a 3100-cGy 3D-guided boost to the prostate. Within an average follow-up of 16.5 months, only 2 patients showed grade I rectal toxicity, and no higher grade toxicity had occurred.[83] These results are apparently improved compared with the 2-year 60% moderate to severe rectal complications reported in a recent study of patients treated with conventional techniques to 7500 cGy or higher, but longer follow-up is required to confirm this observation.[84]

Soffen and colleagues from the Fox Chase Institute in Philadelphia compared a four-field 3D conformal static technique with conventional 2D techniques to determine the advantages of the 3D approach in treating patients with B1 (Gleason Score 2–5) disease.[85,86] A DVH analysis demonstrated that an average of 14% of the bladder, and the rectal dose was eliminated using the 3D approach. Grade 2 or higher acute toxicity occurred in 60% of the 2D treated patients, compared with 31% in the 3D treated patients ($p > 0.05$). The researchers emphasized the need for careful patient immobilization so that the margins of normal tissue surrounding the prostate in the high-dose radiation volume can be reduced without compromising the precision of treatment.

At MSKCC, Leibel and colleagues treated 73 patients with stages A2 through C disease in a phase I dose escalation study to explore the highest feasible tumor doses and their effect on the outcome.[87] The entire prostate, seminal vesicles, and the pelvic organs were reconstructed in their full 3D configuration from consecutive 5 to 10 mm CT slices obtained throughout the pelvis. The BEV planning technique was used to select the most optimal field configurations for the individual patient, and BEV-derived tumor-conforming blocks were used for individualized treatment in each case. Thirty-six patients received 6480 cGy, 25 received 7020 cGy, and 12 received 7560 cGy. Complete tumor regressions in all patients were confirmed by digital rectal examinations. Sixty-seven patients have been followed for more than 6 months (median, 12 months, with 36 followed for at least 1 year and 10 for >2 years), regarded as sufficient to analyze acute toxicity and response to treatment. Serum PSA normalized within a median of 3 months after treatment (range, 1–9 months) in 80% of the patients. Eleven of the 14 patients with abnormal posttreatment PSA have developed bone metastases, although the prostates remained normal to rectal digital examination. Acute toxicities were mild. Grade 1 or acute gastrointestinal toxicity developed in 49% and grade 1 or 2 acute genitourinary toxicity in 76% of the patients, but severe acute toxicities were not observed. There have been no late complications within a median follow-up of 12 months (range, 6–36).

PROSPECTS FOR THE FUTURE

The experience with early prototypes of 3D planning and treatment systems, although based on only a few hundred patients treated so far, indicates an enormous potential for this approach, but the full exploitation of 3D-CRT requires significant additional effort. It is necessary to develop more sophisticated 3D treatment planning tools and to test and implement the new automated treatment delivery systems. The rate at which technical progress can be made critically depends on the availability of new and faster computers and on new approaches to software design.

An important development is the anticipated introduction of treatment planning optimization, which is essential if conformal 3D radiotherapy is to become practical for routine clinical use at the community level. But beyond technical progress, the ultimate success of this approach depends on the ability to deliver high radiation doses to a large variety of tumors without significantly increasing the toxicity to transited normal tissues. If higher radiation doses are indeed feasible without adverse effects on the surrounding normal tissues, the ultimate limitation to 3D-CRT could be due to dose directly applied to the tumor bed. As with all irradiated tissue, the maximal tolerable dose within the tumor bed is a function of volume. Large volumes are expected to have a lower tolerance than smaller volumes, for which primary integrity may rely on migration of important stromal elements from adjacent less irradiated normal tissues. More should be done to understand the limitations on dose due to the target volume, rather than the transited normal tissues. Current 3D-CRT systems are adequate to support phase I or II dose escalation and toxicity studies, and several institutions have already initiated such studies.

The efficacy of the treatment depends on the tumor being reasonably well defined by the imaging procedures, so that a relatively small margin can be added with the expectation that a target volume has been appropriately identified and covered. If this is not the case and tumor extends beyond the target volume, conformal therapy offers no better opportunity for control; in fact, it may offers less likelihood of tumor control, because simpler techniques would more likely include unidentified tumor. There are no imaging techniques that can provide information about the existence of microscopic deposits of tumor cells. The current resolutions of magnetic resonance and radiolabeled monoclonal antibody imaging are not sufficient to provide such information, although there is potential for such developments in the future, especially with magnetic resonance spectroscopy. Anther exciting prospect of magnetic resonance spectroscopy is its potential to add biologic information to 3D conformal radiotherapy, such as the state of tumor oxygenation, cell cycle parameters, and other biologic variables that can be used to determine appropriate time-dose relations. As chemotherapy becomes more effective in controlling occult micrometastatic disease, as evidenced by the current success of adjuvant treatment, combined-modality approaches for improving local control increase in their importance. Three-dimensional conformal radiotherapy will afford opportunities for improved local control, and it will reduce the dose to transited normal tissues and decrease toxicities associated with combinations of radiation and chemotherapy.

The extraordinary increase in the complexity of treatment that results from the application of conformal radiotherapy should be recognized. This invites possibilities for errors and requires extraordinary attention to assurances that the treatment is being given in accordance with the treatment plan. With conventional radiotherapy, quality control depends on static portal images made at periodic intervals through treatment. For 3D-CRT to be regarded as safe, much more sophisticated on-line verifications are required, which should allow feedback and control loops to provide automated mechanisms for error corrections during treatment. All of this suggests that treatment will be quite expensive and extremely time consuming, raising issues of cost-benefit evaluations and cost containment. The true clinical advantages of 3D conformal therapy and the justification for its high cost will not be known until future phase III studies are conducted to test whether improved local control can be achieved and whether it affects the outcome in several human cancers.

REFERENCES

1. Fuks Z, Leibel SA, Kutcher GE, Mohan R, Ling CC. Three dimensional conformal treatment: A new frontier in radiation therapy. In: DeVita VT Jr, Hellman S, Rosenberg SA, eds. Important advances in oncology. Philadelphia: JB Lippincott, 1991:151–172.
2. Suit H, Urie M. Proton beams in radiation therapy. JNCI 1992;84:155–164.
3. Castro JR, Chen GT, Blakley EA. Current considerations in heavy charged particle radiotherapy. Radiat Res 1985;8:227S–234S.
4. Leibel SA, Ling CC, Kutcher GJ, Mohan R, Cordon-Cardo C, Fuks Z. The biological basis of conformal three-dimensional radiation therapy. Int J Radiat Oncol Biol Phys 1991;21:805–811.
5. Munzenrider JE, Pilepich M, Rene-Ferrero JB, Tchakarova I, Carter BL. Use of body scanner in radiotherapy treatment planning. Cancer 1979;40:170–179.
6. Goitein M. The utility of computed tomography in radiation therapy: An estimate of outcome. Int J Radiat Oncol Biol Phys 1979;5:1799–1807.
7. Ten Haken RK, Perez-Tamayo C, Tesser RJ, McShan DL, Fraass BA, Lichter AS. Boost treatment of the prostate using shaped fixed beams. Int J Radiat Oncol Biol Phys 1989;16:193–200.
8. Leibel SA, Kutcher GJ, Harrison LB, et al. Improved dose distributions for 3D conformal boost treatments in carcinoma of the nasopharynx. Int J Radiat Oncol Biol Phys 1991;20: 823–833.
9. Deacon JM, Peckham MJ, Steel GG. The radioresponsiveness of human tumours and the initial slope of the cell survival curve. Radiat Oncol 1984;2:317–323.
10. Fertil B, Malaise EP. Intrinsic radiosensitivity of human cell lines is correlated with radioresponsiveness of human tumors analysis of 101 published survival curves. Int J Radiat Oncol Biol Phys 1985;11:1699–1707.
11. Steel GG, McMillan TJ, Peacock JH. The picture has changed in the 1980s. Int J Radiat Biol 1989;56:525–537.
12. Suit HD, Baumann M, Skates S, Convery K. Clinical interest in determinations of cellular radiation sensitivity. Int J Radiat Biol 1989;56:725–737.
13. Weichselbaum RR, Rotmensch J, Swan SA, Beckett MA. Radiobiological characterization of 53 human tumor cell lines. Int J Radiat Biol 1989;56:553–560.
14. Peters LJ, Withers HR, Thames HD, Fletcher GH. Keynote address. The problem: Tumor radioresistance in clinical radiotherapy. Int J Radiat Oncol Biol Phys 1981;8: 101–108.
15. Thames HD, Schulthheiss TE, Hendy JH, Tucker SL, Dubry BM, Brock WA. Can modest escalations of dose be detected as increased tumor control? Int J Radiat Oncol Biol Phys 1991;22:241–246.
16. DeVita VT, Lippman M, Hubbard SA, Idhe DC, Rosenberg SA. The effect of combined modality therapy on local control and survival. Int J Radiat Oncol Biol Phys 1986;12: 487–501.
17. Suit HD. Potential for improving survival rates for the cancer patient by increasing the efficacy of treatment of the primary lesion. Cancer 1982;50:1227–1234.
18. Fuks Z, Leibel SA, Wallner KE, et al. The effect of local control on metastatic dissemination in carcinoma of the prostate: Long term results in patients treated with ^{125}I implantation. Int J Radiat Oncol Biol Phys 1991;21:549–566.
19. Fisher B, Anderson S, Fisher ER, et al. Significance of ipsilateral breast tumour recurrence after lumpectomy. Lancet 1991;338:327–331.
20. Chauvet B, Reynaud-Bougnoux A, Calais G, et al. Prognostic significance of breast relapse after conservative treatment in node-negative early breast cancer. Int J Radiat Oncol Biol Phys 1990;9:1125–1230.
21. Perez CA, Pajak TF, Rubin P, et al. Long term observations of the pattern of failure in patients with unresectable non-oat cell carcinoma of the lung treated with definitive radiotherapy. Report by the Radiation Therapy Oncology Group. Cancer 1987;59:1874–1881.
22. Chung CK, Stryker JA, O'Neill M, DeMuth WE. Evaluation of adjuvant postoperative radiotherapy for lung cancer. Int J Radiat Oncol Biol Phys 1982;8:1877–1880.
23. Merino OR, Lindberg RD, Fletcher GH. An analysis of distant metastases from squamous cell carcinoma of the upper respiratory and digestive tracts. Cancer 1977;40:145–151.
24. Leibel SA, Kutcher GJ, Harrison LB, et al. Improved dose distributions for 3D conformal boost treatments in carcinoma of the nasopharynx. Int J Radiat Oncol Biol Phys 1991;20: 823–833.
25. Lee AW, Sham JS, Poon YF, Ho JH. Treatment of stage I nasopharyngeal carcinoma: Analysis of the patterns of relapse and the results of withholding elective neck irradiation. Int J Radiat Oncol Biol Phys 1989;17:1183–1190.
26. Kuban DH, El-Mahdi AM, Schellhammer PF. Effect of local tumor control on distant metastasis and survival in prostatic adenocarcinoma. Urology 1987;30:420–426.
27. Perez CA, Pilepich MV, Zivnuska F. Tumor control in definitive irradiation of localized carcinoma of the prostate. Int J Radiat Oncol Biol Phys 1986;12:523–531.
28. Paunier JP, Delclos L, Fletcher GH. Cause, time of death, and sites of failure in squamous cell carcinoma of the uterine cervix on intact uterus. Radiology 1967;88:552–562.
29. Anderson P, Dische S. Local tumor control and subsequent incidence of distant metastatic disease. Int J Radiat Oncol Biol Phys 1981;7:1645–1648.
30. Perez CA, Kuske RR, Camel HM, et al. Analysis of pelvic tumor control and impact on survival in carcinoma of the uterine cervix treated with radiation therapy alone. Int J Radiat Oncol Biol Phys 1988;14:613–621.
31. Stokes S, Bedwinek J, Kao MS, Camel HM, Perez CA. Treatment of stage I adenocarcinoma of the endometrium by hysterectomy and adjuvant irradiation: A retrospective analysis of 304 patients. Int J Radiat Oncol Biol Phys 1986;12:339–344.
32. Perez CA, Camel HM, Galakatos AE, et al. Definitive irradiation in carcinoma of the vagina: Long-term evaluation of results. Int J Radiat Oncol Biol Phys 1988;15:1283–1290.
33. Schild SE, Martenson JA Jr, Gunderson LL, et al. Postoperative adjuvant therapy of rectal cancer: An analysis of disease control, survival and prognostic factors. Int J Radiat Oncol Biol Phys 1989;17:55–62.
34. Vigliotti A, Rich TA, Romsdahl MM, Withers HR, Oswald MJ. Postoperative adjuvant radiotherapy for adenocarcinoma of the rectum and rectosigmoid. Int J Radiat Oncol Biol Phys 1987;13:999–1006.
35. Markhede G, Angervall L, Stener B. A multivariate analysis of the prognosis after surgical treatment of soft tissue tumors. Cancer 1982;49:1721–1733.

35a. Suit HD, Mankin HJ, Wood WC, et al. Treatment of the patient with stage MO soft tissue sarcoma. J Clin Oncol 1988;6:854–862.

36. Gustafson P, Rooser B, Rydholm A. Is local recurrence of minor importance for metastases in soft tissue sarcoma? Cancer 1991;67:2083–2086.
37. Vogelstein B, Fearon ER, Kern SE, et al. Allelotype of colorectal carcinomas. Science 1989;244:207–211.
38. Fearon ER, Vogelstein B. A genetic model for colorectal tumorigenesis. Cell 1990;61: 759–767.
39. Hollstein M, Sidransky D, Vogelstein B, Harris CC. Mutations in human cancers. Science 1991;253:49–53.
40. Bishop M. Molecular themes in oncogenesis. Cell 1991;64:235–249.
41. Kerbel RS. Towards an understanding of the molecular basis of the metastatic phenotype. Invasion Metastasis 1989;9:329–337.
42. Sobel ME. Metastasis suppressor genes. JNCI 1990;82:267–276.
43. Liotta LA, Steeg PS, Stettler-Stevenson WG. Cancer metastasis and angiogenesis: An imbalance of positive and negative regulation. Cell 1991;64:327–336.
44. Steeg PS, Bevilacqua G, Kopper L, et al. Evidence for a novel gene associated with low tumor metastatic potential. JNCI 1988;89:200–203.
45. Cance WG, Brennan MF, Dudas ME, Cordon-Cardo C. Altered expression of the retinoblastoma gene product in human sarcomas. N Engl J Med 1990;323:1457–1462.
46. Cordon-Cordo C, Fuks Z, Eisenbach L, Feldman M. Expression of HLA-A,B,C antigens on primary and metastatic tumor cell populations of human carcinomas. Cancer Res 1991;51:6327–6380.
47. Greenberg AH, Egan SE, Wright JA. Oncogenes and metastatic progression. Invasion Metastasis 1989;9:360–378.
48. Muschel R, Liotta RA. Role of oncogenes in metastasis. Carcinogenesis 1988;9:705–710.
49. Vlodavsky I, Michaeli RI, Bar-Ner M, et al. Involvement of heparanase in tumor metastasis and angiogenesis. Isr J Med Sci 1988;24:464–470.
50. Sloane BF, Dunn TR, Honn KV. Lysosomal cathepsin B. Correlation with metastatic potential. Science 1981;212:1151–1153.
51. Steel GG, McMillan TJ, Peacock JH. The picture has changed in the 1980s. Int J Radiat Biol 1989;56:525–537.
52. Tubiana M. Repopulation in human tumors. Acta Oncol 1988;27:83–88.
53. Withers HR, Taylor JMG, Maciejewski B. The hazards of accelerated tumor clonogens repopulation during radiotherapy. Acta Oncol 1988;27:131–146.
54. Mohan R. Three-dimensional radiation treatment planning. Aust Phys Eng Sci Med 1989;12:73–91.
55. Urie MM, Goitein M, Doppke K, et al. The role of uncertainty analysis in treatment planning. Int J Radiat Oncol Biol Phys 1991;21:91–107.
56. McShan DL, Silverman A, Lanza DM, Reinstein LE, Glicksman AS. A computerized three-dimensional treatment planning system utilizing interactive colour graphics. Br J Radiol 1979;52:478–481.
57. Goitein M, Abrams M, Rowell D, Pollari H, Wiles J. Multi-dimensional treatment planning: II. Beam's eye-view, back projection, and projection through CT sections. Int J Rad Oncol Biol Phys 1983;9:789–797.
58. Three-dimensional displays in planning radiation therapy: A clinical perspective. Photon

Treatment Planning Collaborative Working Group. Int J Radiat Oncol Biol Phys 1991;21: 79–89.
59. Three-dimensional dose calculations for radiation treatment planning. Photon Treatment Planning Collaborative Working Group. Int J Radiat Oncol Biol Phys 1991;21:25–36.
60. Cunningham JR. Scatter-air Ratios. Phys Med Biol 1972;17:42–51.
61. Larson KB, Prasad SC. Absorbed-dose computations for inhomogeneous media in radiation treatment planning using differential scatter-air ratios IEEE. Proceedings of the Second Annual Symposium on Computer Application in Medical Care, 1978:93–99.
62. Wong JW, Slessinger ED, Hermes RE, Offutt CJ, Roy T, Vannier MW. Portal dose images. I. Quantitative treatment plan verification. Int J Radiat Oncol Biol Phys 1990;18: 1455–1463.
63. Chui CS, Mohan RM. Extraction of pencil beam kernels by the deconvolution method. Med Phys 1988;15:138–144.
64. Mohan R, Chui CS. Use of Fourier transforms in calculating dose distribotions for irregularly shaped fields for three dimensional treatment planning. Med Phys 1987;14: 70–77.
65. Boyer AL, Mok EC. Fourier convolution incorporating inhomogeneities. Med Phys 1985;12:507.
66. Mohan R, Chui C, Lidofsky L. Differential pencil beam dose computation model for photons. Med Phys 1986;13:64–73.
67. Photon Treatment Planning Collaborative Working Group. State of the art of external photon beam radiation treatment planning. Int J Radiat Oncol Biol Phys 1991;21:9–23.
68. Photon Treatment Planning Collaborative Working Group. Three-dimensional displays in planning radiation therapy: A clinical perspective. Int J Radiat Oncol Biol Phys 1991;21:79–89.
69. Shipley WU, Tepper JE, Prout GR, et al. Proton radiation as boost therapy for localized prostatic carcinoma. JAMA 1979;241:1912–1915.
70. Drzymala RE, Mohan R, Brewster L, et al. Dose-volume histograms. Int J Radiat Oncol Biol Phys 1991;21:71–78.
71. Emami B, Lyman J, Brown A, et al. Tolerance of normal tissue to therapeutic irradiation. Int J Radiat Oncol Biol Phys 1991;21:109–122.
72. Burman C, Kutcher GJ, Emami B, Goitein M. Fitting of normal tissue tolerance data to an analytic function. Int J Radiat Oncol Biol Phys 1991;21:123–135.
73. Kutcher GJ, Burman C, Brewster L, Goitein M, Mohan R. Histogram reduction method for calculating complication probabilities for three-dimensional treatment planning evaluations. Int J Radiat Oncol Biol Phys 1991;21:137–146.
74. Munzenrider JE, Brown AP, Chu JC, et al. Numerical scoring of treatment plans. Int J Radiat Oncol Biol Phys 1991;21:147–163.
75. Goitein M. The probability of controlling an inhomogeneously irradiated tumor. In: Evaluation of treatment planning for particle beam radiotherapy. Bethesda: National Cancer Institute, 1987:5.8.1–5.8.17.
76. Brahme A. Dosimetric precision requirements in radiation therapy. Acta Radiol Oncol 1984;23:379–391.
77. Mohan R, Mageras GS, Baldwin MS, et al. Clinically relevant optimization of 3D conformal treatments. Med Phys 1992;19:933–943.
78. Three-dimensional photon treatment planning: Report of the Collaborative Working Group on the evaluation of treatment planning for external beam radiotherapy. Int J Radiat Oncol Biol Phys 1991;21:1–206.
79. Thornton AF, Hegarty TJ, Ten-Haken RK, et al. Three-dimensional treatment planning of astrocytomas: A dosimetric study of cerebral irradiation. Int J Radiat Oncol Biol Phys 1991;20, 1309–1315.
80. Thornton AF, Ten-Haken RK, Gerhardsson A, Correll M. Three-dimensional motion analysis of an improved head immobilization system for simulation, CT, MRI, and PET imaging. Radiother Oncol 1991;20:224–228.
81. Thornton AF, Sandler HM Jr, Ten-Haken RK, Greenberg HS. Retreatment of recurrent high grade astrocytoma using three-dimensional external beam treatment planning. [Abstract] Proceedings of the 9th Annual Meeting of the Europeen Society for Therapeutic Radiology and Oncology (ESTRO), Notectini, Italy, 1990:274.
82. Armstrong JG, Burman C, Leibel SA, et al. Conformal three dimensional treatment planning may improve the therapeutic ratio of high dose radiation therapy for lung cancer. Int J Radiat Oncol Biol Phys 1991;21(suppl 1):146.
83. Sandler HM Jr, Perez-Tamayo C, Licter A. Dose escalation in the treatment of stage C (T3) prostate cancer: Report on the rectal toxicity observed in a prospective series using a conformational external beam technique. [Abstract] Proceedings of the 9th Annual Meeting of the Europeen Society for Therapeutic Radiology and Oncology (ESTRO), Notectini, Italy, 1990:329.
84. Smit WGJM, Helle PA, van Putten WLJ, Wijnmaalen AJ, Seldenrath JJ, van der Werf-Messing BHP. Late radiation damage in prostate cancer patients treated by high dose external radiotherapy in relation to rectal dose. Int J Radiat Oncol Biol Phys 1990;18: 23–29.
85. Soffen EM, Hanks GE, Hwang CC, Chu JHC. Conformal static field therapy for low volume low grade prostate cancer with rigid immobilization. Int J Radiat Oncol Biol Phys 1991;20:141–146.
86. Soffen EM, Epstein BE, Hunt MA, Hanks GE. Decreased acure morbidity with conformal static field radiation therapy treatment of early prostate cancer as compared to non-conformal techniques. Int J Radiat Oncol Biol Phys 1991;21(suppl 1):152.
87. Leibel S. Personal communication.

ELLEN S. VITETTA
JONATHAN W. UHR
PHILIP E. THORPE

SECTION 3

Immunotoxin Therapy

GENERAL PRINCIPLES

Chemotherapy and radiotherapy have been used successfully to treat a variety of malignancies. They act by killing rapidly dividing or metabolizing cells whether malignant or normal. For this reason, there have been increasing efforts to develop new approaches that offer better selectivity for malignant cells. One emerging modality is immunotoxin therapy.

The concept of immunotoxin therapy is appealing. An antibody or other cell-binding ligand with specificity for tumor cells is biochemically or genetically linked to a potent toxin. When injected into a patient with cancer, the ligand carries the toxin to the tumor cells. Once bound to the cells, the toxin is internalized and kills the cell. Even though monoclonal antibodies and other ligands are rarely tumor specific, they often react with a limited array of normal tissues that are not life sustaining.

Despite its conceptual simplicity, the development of immunotoxins for clinical use has been challenging. Immunotoxins are large, complex molecules in which each component, including the cell-binding moiety, the crosslinker, and the toxin, plays a critical role in the effectiveness of the agent.

COMPONENTS OF AN IMMUNOTOXIN

LIGAND PORTION

Antibodies and Antibody Fragments

Monoclonal antibodies directed against molecules on tumor cells have been most frequently used as the ligand portion of immunotoxins. Such antibodies are seldom tumor specific and often recognize differentiation antigens present on the non-neoplastic cell at the time it became malignant. Immunotoxins directed against tumor-associated antigens often kill the tumor cells and certain nonneoplastic cells of the same lineage. Antibodies can crossreact with molecules on normal cells in a spurious and unpredictable fashion. When the nonmalignant cells are not life sustaining, this damage may be acceptable. In contrast, cross-reactions with life-sustaining tissue, even if minor, may be life threatening when these reagents are administered in vivo.[1] These cross-reactions are often difficult to detect by screening monoclonal antibodies on cell lines and normal tissues. For example, if the density of the cross-reacting antigen is low, it may not be possible to visualize cross-reactions by standard techniques of immunofluorescence or immunoperoxidase. Thus, even antigens of low density may be effective targets for immunotoxins.[2,3] Nonhuman primates can be useful for determining toxicities for the rare instances where a monoclonal antibody crossreacts with epitopes expressed on the cells.

A second consideration in the use of monoclonal antibodies as targeting agents is their immunogenicity. Because most monoclonal antibodies are of murine origin, they induce antibody responses in patients, unless they are immunosuppressed because of their disease or prior therapy. The development of chimeric antibodies having human constant (C_H and C_L) domains and murine variable (V_H and V_L) domains and of humanized murine antibodies having mouse hypervariable regions grafted onto human framework regions have reduced the immunogenicity of murine monoclonal antibodies.[4–7] However, even if this approach is successful in reducing the immunogenicity of the antibody portion of an immunotoxin, the toxin will probably induce an immune response. This has led to the practical consideration of treating persons who are immunosuppressed because of their disease or using various immunosuppressive regimens in conjunction with immunotoxin therapy.[8–10] However, the use of immunosuppressive agents may not be desirable if an intact immune system is needed to suppress regrowth of tumors.

Antibodies can be used as intact IgG molecules or as their $F(ab')_2$, Fab', or Fab fragments.[11,12] Fv fragments have also been used to generate fusion proteins.[13,14] IgG and $F(ab')_2$ molecules are divalent and bind to target cells more avidly than Fab or Fab' fragments. They generally have superior cytotoxic activity as immunotoxins.[15] Although $F(ab')_2$ molecules are less immunogenic and do not bind to Fc receptors, they are often partially inactivated by coupling to toxins.[12] Because they lack an Fc portion, they have a shorter half-life in vivo.[16] Univalent fragments have little antigenicity but often have lower potencies as immunotoxins and rapid clearance in vivo both of which reduce their antitumor activity relative to their IgG and $F(ab')_2$ counterparts.[12,15–18]

Although not often appreciated, only 5% to 25% of specific monoclonal antibodies make potent immunotoxins. For an immunotoxin to be effective, it must bind avidly to cells, be rapidly internalized, and be routed to intracellular compartments where toxins can translocate into the cytosol.[19–22] Many antibodies must be screened to select the ones which make effective immunotoxins.[23] Screening involves an indirect immunotoxin assay in which appropriate target cells are first treated with the test antibody and then with a Fab' immunotoxin directed against the immunoglobulin portion of the immunotoxin.[23,24] If effective killing is obtained, the test antibody invariably makes a potent immunotoxin when directly conjugated to the same toxin or ribosome-inactivating protein (RIP).

Even when an effective immunotoxin is used, the heterogeneity of tumor cells undoubtedly leads to the escape of antigen-negative mutants, necessitating the use of combinations (*i.e.*, "cocktails") of effective immunotoxins directed against different target cell antigens.[25,26]

Growth Factors

Growth factors can sometimes be used as carriers for toxins, and these constructs are called oncotoxins. Although growth factors bind to normal cells, tumor cells frequently express elevated levels of growth factor receptors.[27–30] If the normal cells are not life sustaining, it may be possible to devise dose-regimens that provide an acceptable therapeutic index. Fibroblast growth factor (FGF), melanocyte-stimulating hormone-α (MSH-α), epidermal growth factor (EGF), transforming growth factor-α (TGF-α), insulin-like growth factor (IGF), and interleukin-2, -4, and -6 have been coupled to toxins to create oncotoxins (Table 69–13). Advantages of using growth factors as ligands include their lack of immunogenicity, generally high affinity for their receptors, and the availability of cloned genes for generating growth factor-toxin fusion proteins.[31–38] However, many growth factors are rapidly cleared in vivo and may require continuous administration for long periods.[39] Another potential problem is that growth of some tumor cells may be stimulated by a few molecules of bound oncotoxins, insufficient to kill the cells.[40,41] Circulating levels of these ligands or their soluble receptors can be elevated in animals and patients with malignant disease resulting in competition for the oncotoxin and inhibition of its target cell cytotoxicity.[42,43] Despite these considerations, the use of oncotoxins has enormous potential and is currently being explored in animal studies and in phase I clinical trials.

TOXIN PORTION

The toxins that have been used to form immunotoxins are derived from bacteria and plants and are inhibitors of protein synthesis.[44] They are the most powerful cell poisons known, and when effectively targeted, fewer than 10 molecules in the cytosol of the target cell can be lethal.[45,46] Because toxins inhibit protein synthesis, they kill resting cells and, hence,

TABLE 69–13. Growth Factor–Toxin Fusion Proteins

Growth Factor	*Toxin*	*Type of Cancer*	*References*
IL-2	PE40	T-cell leukemia	14
	DAB486	Hodgkin's lymphoma	63, 137
		non-Hodgkin's lymphoma, T-cell leukemia	138
IL-4	DAB389	Non-Hodgkin's lymphoma	139
	PE40	Sarcoma, colon adenocarcinoma	140
IL-6	PE40	Myeloma, hepatoma	141
			142
TGF-α	PE40	Epidermoid carcinoma, prostate carcinoma, ovarian carcinoma, liver carcinoma, breast carcinoma	143 144
EGF	PE40	Epidermoid carcinoma	144
IGF	PE40	Breast carcinoma, hepatoma	145
FGF	Saporin		146
	PE40	Hepatoma, colon carcinoma, ovarian carcinoma, breast carcinoma	147
MSH-α	DT	Melanoma	148

IL, interleukin; TGF, tumor growth factor; EGF, epidermal growth factor; IGF, insulin-like growth factor; MSH, melanocyte-stimulating hormone.

have the potential of killing tumor cells that are not in cycle at the time of the treatment and that are spared by conventional chemotherapy. Toxins that have been used for the construction of immunotoxins are described in Table 69–14.[47] They share several features. All are synthesized as single chain peptides and are processed posttranslationally or in the target cell to which they are delivered into two-chain molecules with interchain disulfide bonds.[44,48,49] All have subunits or domains devoted to binding to cells, to translocation across membranes, and to the destruction of the protein synthetic machinery of the cell.[36]

The most frequently used plant toxins are ricin and abrin, both of which are synthesized as single chain polypeptides and then processed posttranslationally into mature toxins consisting of disulfide bonded A and B subunits.[44] The B-chain is a galactose-specific lectin that binds to glycoproteins and glycolipids on the surface of all cell types in higher animals and the A-chain is an N-glycosidase that translocates across the membrane of an intracellular vesicle and inhibits protein synthesis by removing an adenine residue from the 28S RNA (60S ribosomal subunit) that is needed for the binding of elongation factor-2 (EF-2).[44,50,51] The B-chain, and probably the A-chain, contain translocation domains that enable the A-chain to traverse cell membranes and enter the cytosol.[52]

RIPs analogous to the A-subunit of ricin (RTA) or abrin have been found in many plants and several of these have been used to form immunotoxins, such as bryodin, momordin, saporin, gelonin, trichosanthin, and pokeweed antiviral protein (PAP).[53–61] These single-chain RIPs are evolutionarily related to RTA and inactivate ribosomes in an identical fashion. However, because they lack the equivalent of the B-chain, they can only enter cells after being targeted by an appropriate ligand. Their main advantage over the toxin A-chains is that rigorous purification to eliminate B-chain or toxin is not required.

The bacterial toxins, like the plant toxins, are also synthesized as single polypeptide chains and have domains devoted to binding, translocation, and inhibition of protein synthesis.[36] The most frequently used bacterial toxins are *Pseudomonas* exotoxin A (PE) and diphtheria toxin (DT). DT is processed by the bacterium into the mature form consisting of two disulfide bonded chains analogous to the A- and B-chains of ricin and abrin.[48,49] PE is processed in the target cell to which it is delivered into a disulfide-bonded two-chain molecule.[36] The enzymatic domain of these toxins kills cells by catalyzing a modification of EF-2 that prevents its participation in protein synthesis.[62] The bacterial toxins have been successfully cloned, expressed and truncated into versions containing the active A-chain and the translocation domain without the nonspecific cell-binding domain.[63,64] These have been coupled to a variety of ligands (see Table 69–13) and the resulting oncotoxins are highly potent to target cells.

CROSSLINKER

For their use in in vivo therapy, the ligand and the toxin portions of the immunotoxins must be coupled in such a way as to remain stable in the blood and tissues and yet be labile within the target cell so the toxin subunit can enter the cytosol. A variety of crosslinkers that generate linkages that meet these requirements have been developed. The choice of a crosslinker depends on whether an intact toxin, A-chain, or RIP is used.

Holotoxin Immunotoxins

Linkers used to couple holotoxins usually introduce a free thiol group into the antibody or ligand and an alkylating function into the toxin.[65,66] The two derivatized proteins are then reacted to produce a conjugate containing a thioether linkage. This linkage is stable to reduction and precludes dissociation of the toxin from the antibody. Holotoxin-immunotoxins retain the natural disulfide bond between the A- and B-chain that is necessary for the release of the A-chain inside the cell. For in vivo use, the lectin site on the B-chain must be blocked to prevent the immunotoxin from binding to and killing cells nonspecifically. The blockade can be accomplished sterically by attaching the ligand by a short crosslinker to the toxin or by using galactose-based affinity labels that bind covalently to the lectin site of the toxin.[67–70]

A-Chain Immunotoxins

Unlike holotoxin-containing immunotoxins, those containing toxin A-chains must have a disulfide bond introduced between the ligand and the A-chain, because bonds that cannot be reduced (*e.g.,* thioethers) generate ineffective immunotoxins.[15] The linker used to couple the A-chain to the ligand is usually a heterobifunctional crosslinker that introduces an activated thiol group into the ligand. The derivatized ligand is then mixed with reduced A-chain and the free thiol group in the A-chain displaces the leaving group from the activated thiol group of the ligand to form a disulfide linkage. The resulting immunotoxin is then purified to remove free A-chain and free antibody. These constructs retain full antigen-binding activity but the disulfide bond is usually not as stable as that generated with a thioether linkage.[17,71,72] A-chain can be released in vivo in the circulation or in the tissues. This is probably due to reduction by glutathione, albumin or other thiol-containing molecules. Immunotoxins prepared with hindered crosslinkers (*e.g.* SMPT) are much more stable and may have fewer side effects probably because less A chain is released in vivo.[72]

Fab and Fab′ fragments of antibodies are coupled to A-chain by forming a disulfide bridge between the free cysteine residue near the hinge region and the free cysteine residue of the A-chain.[73] The thiol group in the antibody fragment is generally activated with Ellman's reagent and the derivative is mixed with reduced A-chain. Coupling then occurs by a thiol-disulfide exchange reaction. Because the thiol group of the antibody fragment is distant from the antigen combining site, the A chain does not interfere with the antigen-binding activity of the Fab′/Fab fragment.[73]

Ribosome-Inactivating Protein Immunotoxins

Immunotoxins containing RIPs are formed by linking the antibody and the RIP by a disulfide bond. However, unlike toxin A-chains, RIPs do not contain a free thiol group, and one must be introduced by treating the RIP with a thiolylating reagent.[47,74,75] The coupling reaction between the thiolylated RIP and the antibody is then performed in the same manner as for the A-chain immunotoxins.

TABLE 69–14. Structure and Function of Toxins and Ribosome-Inactivating Proteins Used for Immunotoxin Therapy

Toxin	*Structure of Mature Form*	*Receptor*	*A-Chain Action*
DT	Binding site; A —SS— B	Heparin-binding EGF-like growth factor precursor[149]	ADP-ribosylation of EF-2
DT(CRM-45)	A —SS— B	None	ADP-ribosylation of EF-2
PE	B — — A (I II III)	α_2-macroglobulin receptor-LDL receptor-related protein[150]	ADP-ribosylation of EF-2
PE40	— A (II III)	None	ADP-ribosylation of EF-2
Ricin, abrin	A —SS— B	Galactose-containing oligosaccharide	N-glycosidase for 28S ribosomal RNA
Blocked ricin, abrin	A —SS— B (X, X)	None	N-glycosidase for 28S ribosomal RNA
RTA	A —SH	None	N-glycosidase for 28S ribosomal RNA
RIP (gelonin, saporin)	A	None	N-glycosidase for 28S ribosomal RNA

▩, translocation domain; A, cytotoxic domain; B, binding domain; DT, diphtheria toxin; PE, *Pseudomonas* endotoxin A; EF-2, elongation, factor-2.

Recombinant Immunotoxins

Recombinant oncotoxins have been prepared with truncated PE or DT (see Table 69–13). This has been accomplished by cloning the genes for the toxins and mutagenizing them to delete segments encoding the cell-binding domain. The truncated forms of PE are PE40 and PE40lys, and the truncated forms of DT are CRM45, DAB486, and DAB389. The genes for the modified toxins are spliced to the gene encoding the ligand, and the entire oncotoxin is synthesized as a fusion protein in *E. coli*. Oncotoxins retain the activities of the ligand and the toxin, and they are highly stable in vivo because they contain a nonreducible peptide bond.[76]

PRECLINICAL EVALUATION

CYTOTOXIC POTENCY

The potency of an immunotoxin depends on the affinity of the antibody, the cell surface molecule that the antibody recognizes, and the capacity of that cell surface molecule to enter an intracellular compartment that is effective for A-chain translocation.[12,20,77,78] In the case of DT-containing immunotoxins, A-chain translocation occurs in an acidic compartment, such as late endosomes.[79,80] In the case of ricin and RIP immunotoxins, translocation occurs in a nonacidic compartment, possibly the trans-Golgi network.[81] The epitope on the surface molecule that the antibody recognizes may also play a critical role in intracellular routing and subsequent potency of the immunotoxin.[20,22,82] Those epitopes lying closer to the membrane appear to provide better targets possibly because they position the toxin closer to the lipid bilayer through which the toxin must ultimately pass to kill the cell.[82]

Immunotoxins containing blocked holotoxin or genetically engineered bacterial toxins are usually more potent that those containing A-chains or RIPs, although there are exceptions.[37,69,78,83,84] In the case of blocked abrin and ricin immunotoxins, their superior potency is probably attributable to the fact that the immunotoxin is partially degraded inside the target cell, and the unblocked toxin or toxin fragments that are released then kill the cell.[85] In the case of the oncotoxins, translocation domains in the toxin may form pores in the membrane that enable the A-chain-like domain to enter the cytosol and kill the cell. Immunotoxins prepared with A-chains and RIPs often have greatly enhanced toxicity in the presence of lysosomotropic amines and carboxylic ionophores.[86–88] These agents work by slowing the fusion of endosomes with lysosomes (where A-chains are enzymatically destroyed), or by delaying the transit of the immunotoxin through a compartment favorable for A-chain translocation (such as the trans-Golgi). B chains and B-chain immunotoxins also enhance the toxicity of some A-chain immunotoxins presumably by facilitating intracellular events involved in translocation.[89–91] Carboxylic ionophores have also been used successfully to potentiate the activity of immunotoxins in vivo by administering them in emulsions or coupled to albumin.[92,93]

HEPATOTOXICITY AND LIVER CLEARANCE

Immunotoxins prepared with blocked ricin, RTA, abrin A-chain, DT, PE, and certain RIPs (*e.g.* saporin) cause hepatotoxicity in rodents of a severity that varies from moderate to dose limiting.[64,94–99] However, the mechanisms by which these immunotoxins cause liver damage are not the same. In the case of RTA, mannose and fucose-containing oligosaccharides are recognized by avid receptors on parenchymal and nonparenchymal cells of the liver and by other cells of the RES.[100,101] This results in rapid clearance, modest hepatic damage, and reduction in antitumor activity.[25,72,94,99] This problem has been circumvented by using chemically or enzymatically deglycosylated RTA or by using recombinant RTA expressed in a nonglycosylating cell.[102,103] In the case of blocked ricin-immunotoxins, the natural oligosaccharides on the A- and B-chains and those used to block the B-chain's lectin sites result in liver homing and marked liver damage.[100–102,104] Deglycosylation of the B-chain reduces its ability to potentiate the toxicity of A-chain immunotoxins and is therefore predicted to reduce their potency.[105] In the case of immunotoxins containing DT, PE, saporin, or abrin A-chain, the mechanisms underlying hepatotoxicity have not been elucidated. However, hepatotoxicity is not mediated through recognition of oligosaccharides on the toxin because none of these toxins is glycosylated. Conceivably, liver cells express a receptor for some portion of the toxin molecule. Alternatively, these toxins, like RTA, may bind to serum proteins for which liver cells have avid receptors.[106]

ANTITUMOR EFFECTS

A variety of animal tumor models have been used to evaluate immunotoxin therapy. In these models, immunotoxins are usually administered shortly after animals are injected with tumor cells to ascertain their effectiveness in treating minimal disease. In other studies, they have been administered to animals with large, established tumors. Although immunotoxins are generally more efficacious in the setting of minimal disease, some immunotoxins have had major antitumor effects on established tumors.[3,18,25,61,107–112] Chemotherapy or radiotherapy given in conjunction with immunotoxin therapy markedly improves their antitumor effects, as do β-adrenergic blockers and emulsified monensin.[92,113–118]

Cocktails of immunotoxins directed against different determinants on tumor cells have antitumor activity that is superior to that of single immunotoxins because the cocktail diminishes the probability that antigen-deficient variants or mutants will escape killing.[25,26] Taken together, these results indicate that immunotoxins will have their greatest impact in the clinic when used as a cocktail in conjunction with other debulking therapies. The ideal scenario is probably to administer an immunotoxin cocktail at a time when patients have minimal residual disease. It is encouraging that combined modalities have in certain experimental tumors reduced the tumor burden to a level where the immune system of the host can suppress the growth of remaining tumor cells.[3,115] If the immune system is functional, it may not be necessary to kill every tumor cell to induce a prolonged remission.

IMMUNOTOXIN-RESISTANT MUTANTS

Subpopulations of tumor cells that are resistant to immunotoxins pose the same problem for immunotoxin therapy as it does for chemotherapy. In several rodent tumor models, the inability of immunotoxin therapy to cure the animals is due to the survival and subsequent outgrowth of immunotoxin-resistant tumor cells.[25,26] Various types of mutants have been identified. The most common are antigen-loss mutants that lack the target antigen entirely or express it at levels too low for immunotoxin-mediated killing.[25,26] This type of mutant can be eradicated with cocktails of two or more immunotoxins recognizing different target antigens. Rarely, the mutants express the target antigen but have some deficiency in their intracellular transport system.[25,26] This type of mutant should also succumb to an immunotoxin cocktail provided that the deficiency in entry is not common to both antigen-entry pathways. Mutants having toxin-resistant ribosomes have not been observed despite deliberate attempts to raise them. Mutations in ribosomes that confer A-chain resistance may be lethal. Alternatively, there may be multiple copies of genes encoding ribosomal components that make simultaneous mutations in all copies highly improbable.

CLINICAL TRIALS

SOLID TUMORS

The first clinical trials with RTA and PE-based immunotoxins were carried out in patients with solid tumors, including melanoma, breast cancer, and colon cancer. For several reasons, these tumors are among the least likely to respond to immunotoxin therapy. Tumor cells in solid epithelial tumors are not very accessible to immunotoxins. Compression of draining lymphatics and elevation of interstitial pressure within the tumor reduce the amount of an antibody that enters the tumor to approximately 0.001% of the injected dose per gram of tumor.[120,121] The immunotoxin that enters the tumor is absorbed by tumor cells adjacent to the vasculature and often fails to reach tumor cells deeper in the tumor mass.[122] Patients with solid tumors are usually not intrinsically immunosuppressed and frequently develop neutralizing antibodies against the immunotoxin that preclude further courses of immunotoxin therapy.[123,124] Antibodies raised against antigens on solid epithelial tumors frequently crossreact with life-sustaining normal tissues.[1,125]

Few phase I–II clinical trials involving systemic therapy with immunotoxins in solid tumors are ongoing. The results of several trials are presented in the next sections, and their major features are summarized in Table 69–15.

Melanoma

The first phase I immunotoxin trial was carried out in patients with metastatic melanoma.[126] The antibody portion of the immunotoxin was directed against a high molecular weight antigen on melanoma cells and the toxin was native RTA. The two components were linked by a disulfide bond generated with the SPDP-crosslinker. Twenty-two patients were treated in the phase I trial. Toxicities included hypoalbuminemia in 20 patients, weight gain and edema in 6 patients, and low voltage electrocardiograms in 16 patients. These toxicities are characteristic of vascular leak syndrome (VLS). The maximal tolerated dose (MTD) was greater than 3 mg/kg, and 17 of the patients made antibody against the immunotoxin. One patient had a complete remission, and 9 had mixed responses or stabilized disease. Pharmacokinetic data are not available, but immunoperoxidase staining indicated the presence of RTA and mouse immunoglobulin in the metastatic lesions of 5 patients after 24 hours of therapy. In the ensuing phase II trial, 43 patients were treated, and 3 had partial responses, 1 had a mixed response, and 9 had stabilization of their disease.[127] Toxicities were similar to those described in the phase I trial. In another phase II trial, the immunotoxin was administered in conjunction with cyclophosphamide to decrease the antibody response against the immunotoxin.[123] In this trial, 1 patient developed seizures, neutropenia, and anemia, but this may have been attributable to cyclophosphamide rather than the immunotoxin. Four of the 20 patients treated had partial responses. Thirteen patients evaluated for an immune response made antibodies against the immunotoxin. Cyclophosphamide did not reduce the immunogenicity of the immunotoxin, and it is unclear if it contributed to the clinical responses.

Colon Carcinoma

A phase I study of an immunotoxin containing native RTA and a monoclonal antibody that recognizes glycoprotein, gp72, on the surface of colon carcinoma cells was conducted in 17 patients with metastatic colorectal carcinoma.[124] Toxicities included fever, hypoalbuminemia, flu-like symptoms, proteinuria, and mental status changes (*e.g.*, fatigue, slurred speech, irritability, expressive aphasia), all of which reversed when treatment was discontinued. The MTD was greater than 1 mg/kg. Five of the 16 patients had mixed tumor regressions, including 2 with a reduction of hepatic metastases, 3 with a reduction in subcuticular metastases, and 1 with a decrease in pulmonary metastases. Virtually all patients made antibodies against the RTA (HARA) and the mouse Ig (HAMA) of the IgM and IgG classes.

Breast Carcinoma

Nine patients with metastatic breast carcinoma were treated with recombinant RTA coupled to an antibody (260F9) that reacts with an antigen expressed on approximately 50% of breast cancer cells. The immunotoxin was administered by bolus injection (4 patients) or continuous infusion (5 patients).[1,128] The patients receiving the bolus infusion developed symptoms of VLS, even at the lower doses. Continuous infusion of the immunotoxin in 5 patients resulted in less severe VLS, but severe neurologic toxicity occurred in 3 patients, commencing with plexopathies at the site of previous chest wall irradiation and progressing to sensor motor neuropathies in all extremities. Neuropathies worsened over a period of 2 to 3 months. During the following 6 months, the patients recovered motor function but had persistent paresthesias. A nerve biopsy of 1 patient at the time of maximal symptoms revealed axonal loss and segmental demyelination consistent with toxic injury to the Schwann cells. It was found that the 260F9 antibody intensely stained the nerve sheath, suggesting that the antibody recognized an epitope present on Schwann cells or myelin.

The major dose-limiting toxicity of this immunotoxin was due to targeting of the RTA to normal neural tissue, rather

TABLE 69–15. Summary of Clinical Trials

Disease	*Phase*	*Immunotoxin*	*Maximal Tolerated Dose (Total)*	*Toxicity*	*Antibody Response*	$T_{1/2}$ *(h)*	*Clinical Response*	*Reference*
Metastatic melanoma	I	Xomazyme-Mel	>3 mg/kg	VLS, myalgia	17/21 (81%)	ND	1/22 CR 9/22 mixed or stabilized	126
	II	Xomazyme-Mel		VLS	ND	ND	3/43 PR 1/43 MR′ 9/43 stabilization	127
	II	Xomazyme-Mel plus cyclophosphamide		VLS	13/13 (100%)	ND	4/20 PR	123
Colorectal carcinoma	I	Anti-gp72-RTA	>1 mg/kg	VLs, aphasia	15/16 HARA (94%) 16/17 HAMA (94%)	ND	5/16 mixed tumor regressions	124
Metastatic breast carcinoma	I	260F9-rRTA (bolus)	>50 μg/kg	VLS, myalgia paresthesia	4/4 (100%)	8.3	1/4 resolution of lung nodules	128
	I	260F9-rRTA (continuous infusion)	0.4 mg/kg	VLS, myalgia, neuropathies	4/5 HARA (80%) 3/5 HAMA (60%)	4–6	0/5	1
Ovarian carcinoma	I	Anti-OVB3-PE		SGOT/SGPT elevations, abdominal pain, encephalopathy			0/23	125
Non-Hodgkin's lymphoma	I/II	Anti-CD19-blocked ricin (bolus)	0.25 mg/kg	SGOT/SGPT elevations thrombocytopenia	12/15 (78%)	ND	1/25 CR 2/25 PR 10/25 mixed or transient	129
	I	Anti-CD19-blocked ricin (continuous infusion)	0.35 mg/kg	SGOT, SGPT elevations thrombocytopenia edema	26/43 (60%)	ND	2/43 CR 5/43 PR 11/43 transient	130
	I	Fab′ anti-CD22-dgA	75 mg/m² (1.8 mg/kg)	VLS, myalgia, pulmonary edema rhabdomyolysis	4/14 HARA (29%) 1/14 HAMA (7%)	1.4	5/13 PR	131
	I	IgG anti-CD22-dgA	30 mg/m² (0.7 mg/kg)	VLS, myalgia, pulmonary edema, rhabdomyolysis	8/24 HARA (33%) 7/24 HAMA (29%)	7.8	6/24 PR 1/24 CR	Amlot et al (submitted)
B-cell chronic leukemia	I	Anti-CD5 (T101)-RTA	ND	Fever	1/4 HARA (25%) 0/4 HARA	ND	4/5 transient rapid fall in circulating leukemic cells	132
T-cell lymphoma	I	Anti-CD5 (H65)-RTA	3.3 mg/kg	VLS, dyspnea	10/12 (86%)	1.2–2.9	4/14 PR	133
NHL, Hodgkin's disease	I	IL-2-DAB486		Hepatic transaminase elevations, hypoalbuminemia, hypersensitivity, creatine elevations, thrombocytopenias	(60%)	0.08	3/47 CR	134 (J. Nichols, personal communication)
Steroid-resistant GVHD	II	Anti-CD5 (H65)-RTA		VLS, myalgia; hematuria, tremors	6/23 HAMA (26%) 6/23 HARA (26%)	1.5–3.9	9/32 CR 7/32 PR 6/32 MR	135

ND, not determined; VLS, vascular leak syndrome; CR, complete response; PR, partial response.

than nonspecific effects common to all RTA-immunotoxins. In the bolus infusion protocol, the MTD was approximately 50 μg/kg, and in the continuous infusion protocol, the MTD was 400 μg/kg. After bolus administration, the peak serum concentrations of immunotoxin were between 200 and 850 μg/ml, the $T_{½}$ was 1.8 hours, and the $T_{½}\beta$ was 8.3 hours. Using the continuous infusion protocol the $T_{½}$ was 4-6 hours. One of 4 patients who received bolus administration showed resolution of a lung nodule, which was the sole site of disease. All 4 patients made antibody against the immunotoxin. None of 5 patients who received the continuous infusion of immunotoxin showed clinical responses, and 4 patients made HARA and 3 made HAMA. Because of the cross-reactivity of this immunotoxin with normal neural tissue, trials with this immunotoxin were discontinued.

Ovarian Carcinoma

OVB3 antibody linked to PE was administered intraperitoneally to 23 patients with advanced ovarian carcinoma.[125] Therapeutic levels of immunotoxin were achieved in peritoneal fluid at all doses of the immunotoxin. At higher doses, therapeutic levels were also achieved in the serum. Side effects included transient elevations of liver enzymes, fever and abdominal pain that was sufficiently severe to require treatment. The dose-limiting toxicity was neurologic. Two patients developed encephalopathy (*e.g.,* confusion and aphasia) after two doses of the immunotoxin and took several months to recover. A third patient developed severe encephalopathy after three doses resulting in seizures, coma, and ultimately death. It was found that the OVB3 antibody was weakly reactive with cells in the cerebellum. No objective responses were achieved.

HEMATOLOGIC MALIGNANCIES

Several clinical trials have been conducted in which immunotoxins have been used to treat lymphomas and leukemias. Hematologic tumors are particularly likely to respond to immunotoxin therapy for several reasons. It is possible to treat such diseases with immunotoxins directed against normal lymphocyte and myeloid cell markers, because the normal cells that are killed with the tumor cells are rapidly replenished from progenitor cells in the marrow. Many antibodies that react with tumor cells but not with life-sustaining tissues are available. The tumor cells in large solid lymphomas may be more accessible than those in epithelial tumors, which frequently contain dense connective tissue. Patients with lymphoid malignancies are often immunosuppressed by their disease and by prior therapy. Not all patients make antiimmunotoxin antibodies so that immunotoxin therapy can be given in multiple courses.

Four types of immunotoxin constructs have been used to treat lymphomas and leukemias, as described in the next few sections.

Blocked-Ricin Immunotoxins

In two phase I trials, an anti-CD19-blocked ricin immunotoxin was administered to patients with refractory lymphomas and leukemias.[129,130] This immunotoxin was highly potent and specific in vitro. CD19 is present on virtually all B-cells and tumor cells from non-Hodgkin's lymphoma (NHL), chronic lymphocytic leukemia (CLL), and some types of non-T-cell acute lymphocytic leukemia (ALL). In the first phase I trial, daily bolus injections of the immunotoxin were administered to 23 patients with NHL, 1 with non-T-ALL, and 1 with CLL. All patients had relapsed after prior chemotherapy or bone marrow transplantation. Toxicities included transient elevation of hepatic transaminase, transient thrombocytopenia, low-grade fevers, and hypoalbuminemia without edema. Of the 25 patients treated, 1 had a complete response after 3 courses of therapy, 2 had partial responses, and 10 had transient or mixed responses. The two partial responses occurred in patients where bone marrow was the only site of tumor. The MTD was 250 μg/kg. Twelve of the 15 patients made antibodies against the immunotoxin. Blood levels of the immunotoxin were approximately 200 nM but were maintained only transiently. In a subsequent trial, anti-CD19-blocked ricin immunotoxin was administered by a 7-day continuous infusion protocol. Forty-three patients were treated, including 33 with NHL, 5 with CLL, and 5 with non-T-ALL. Toxicities that defined MTD included elevations of SGOT and SGPT that lasted from 1 to 2 weeks and thrombocytopenia. In addition, 23 patients developed transient hypoalbuminemia, 11 developed peripheral edema, and 30 developed fever. Twenty-six of the 43 patients made HAMA or HARA. Of the 43 patients treated, there were 2 complete responses, 5 partial responses, and 11 transient responses. Almost 50% of the patients with low- and intermediate-grade NHL or CLL had significant responses; less frequent responses were seen in patients with high-grade NHL and non-T-ALL.

Deglycosylated-RTA Immunotoxins

Two phase I trials have been carried out with immunotoxins consisting of anti-CD22 antibody coupled to chemically deglycosylated RTA.[131] The patient population was similar to that treated with the CD19-blocked ricin immunotoxin. CD22 is a normal B-lymphocyte antigen that is expressed on cells from 60% to 70% of patients with B-cell lymphomas. A total of 41 patients with $CD22^+$ tumor cells were entered into the two trials. An average of 50% of the tumor cells in the patients expressed CD22. The remaining tumor cells lacked the antigen or expressed it at levels too low to be detected by indirect immunofluorescence analyses. One immunotoxin consisted of an intact IgG antibody (RFB4) coupled by a stable cross-linker (SMPT) to chemically deglycosylated ricin A-chain. The other immunotoxin was an Fab′ fragment of the same antibody coupled by a cystine bond to deglycosylated ricin A-chain. The RTA was deglycosylated to prevent the immunotoxins from homing to and damaging cells in the liver and RES that have receptors for the mannose and fucose residues on native RTA. The IgG immunotoxin had an IC_{50} on Daudi cells in vitro of 10^{-12} M, and the Fab′ immunotoxin had an IC_{50} of 10^{-11} M. Both constructs were more than 100,000 times more toxic to cells expressing CD22 than they were to cells lacking CD22. Fifteen patients were treated with the Fab′ immunotoxin and 26 with the IgG immunotoxin.

In both cases, dose-related toxicities included VLS and myalgia, and dose-limiting toxicities included aphasia, pulmonary edema, and rhabdomyolysis. In the earlier phases of the trial, the presence of pulmonary parenchymal lymphoma predisposed patients to rapidly appearing and severe pulmonary edema during treatment; therefore, patients with pulmonary lymphoma were later excluded from entry.

The MTD for the Fab′ immunotoxin was 75 mg/m^2 (1.8 mg/kg) and the MTD for the IgG immunotoxin was 30 mg/m^2 (0.7 mg/kg). The $T_{½}$ of the Fab′ immunotoxin averaged 1.3 hours, but that of the IgG immunotoxin averaged 7.8 hours. Only a single phase of clearance was visible in the recipients of the Fab′ immunotoxin, but in 9 patients receiving IgG-IgA, distinct α and β phases of clearance were observed, with a $T_{½}\beta$ that ranged from 6 to 17 hours. The highest serum levels obtained were 15.8 μg/ml for the Fab′ immunotoxin and 11.3 μg/ml for the IgG immunotoxin. In 2 patients treated with the IgG immunotoxin, serum was taken 24 hours after administration of the IgG immunotoxin and the concentration and cytotoxic activity of this circulating immunotoxin were determined. The immunotoxin was fully active, indicating that it was highly stable in vivo. Overall, 28% of the patients treated with the Fab′ immunotoxin and 37% treated with the IgG immunotoxin made antibodies against the RTA, the mouse immunoglobulin, or both, but the Fab′ portion of the immunotoxin was less immunogenic than the IgG portion. After one course of treatment, the clinical responses for the Fab′ and the IgG immunotoxin were very similar. At 1 month, 6 of 24 evaluable patients who had received the IgG immunotoxin had partial responses, and an additional patient had a complete response. Five of 12 patients who received the Fab′ immunotoxin had partial responses. In all cases, responses were transient and lasted between 1 and 4 months.

It can be concluded that the Fab′ construct was less immunogenic than the IgG construct. The Fab′ construct was shorter lived but similar in efficacy. VLS and myalgias were observed in patients treated with both constructs. Because these side effects were the same as those observed in patients treated with immunotoxins containing other antibodies and recombinant or native RTA, they cannot be attributed to the specificity of the antibody, the Fc portion of the antibody, or the carbohydrate portion of the A-chain.

Native RTA Immunotoxins

Five patients with refractory CLL were treated with 24 mg/m^2 of anti-CD5-RTA prepared with the T101 antibody.[132] Toxicities included VLS and fever. No objective responses were achieved although 4 of 5 patients had a rapid and transient decreases in circulating leukemic cells. One of the 4 patients made HARA, and none made HAMA. The lack of efficacy may be due to the fact that CLL cells internalize the immunotoxins poorly.

In another trial, an anti-CD5 -RTA prepared with the H65 antibody was administered to 14 patients with cutaneous T-cell lymphoma in a dose escalation protocol.[133] VLS was observed in virtually all patients and the dose-limiting toxicity was dyspnea. The MTD was 3.3 mg/kg and the $T_{½}$ ranged from 1.2 to 2.9 hours. Ten of 12 patients evaluated made HAMA/HARA, and in 7 of 11 cases, this antibody blocked immunotoxin-mediated killing. All patients but 1 had a decrease in circulating CD3$^+$/CD5$^+$ lymphocytes, and 4 of 14 patients had partial responses lasting from 3-5 months. Palliation of disease was observed in all patients.

Diphtheria Toxin Oncotoxins

Human IL-2 fused to DT-AB486 has been used to treat a variety of malignancies of lymphoid, epidermoid, or sarcomatoid types.[134] The fusion protein was administered to 72 patients with IL-2R$^+$ malignancies, and 47 were evaluable for a response. Side effects at MTD included transient hepatic transaminase elevations, hypoalbuminemia, hypersensitivity-like syndromes, and occasional transient creatine elevations and thrombocytopenias. Antibodies against DT were present in approximately 30% of the patients before treatment and in 60% after one or two courses of therapy. Preliminary studies indicated that the response rates in patients with circulating antibodies were similar to those without antibodies. However, the $T_{½}$ of this oncotoxin was so short (5–10 minutes) that the presence of antibodies may have been irrelevant. Of 47 patients treated with different dose schedules ranging from bolus injection to 6-hour infusions, complete responses were seen in 3 patients and these responses lasted from 9 to 24 months. Although the IL-2 oncotoxin is directed against the tumor cells, it also has the potential of killing activated IL-2R$^+$ T cells in these patients. Elimination of T cells may be directly or indirectly involved in tumor regressions. This possibility remains to be explored.

GRAFT-VERSUS-HOST DISEASE

Although not a malignant disease, we include a description of the efficacy of an immunotoxin in treating GVHD, because it makes the important point that immunotoxins are extremely effective therapeutic agents in settings where the target cells are readily accessible to the blood and where it is not necessary to kill all the target cells for benefit to be obtained.

Thirty-two patients were treated with anti-CD5(H65)-RTA.[135] The CD5 antigen is expressed on most T cells and a minority of B cells. Most of the patients had visceral and skin involvement. The immunotoxin was administered in 7 to 14 doses, and the $T_{½}$ ranged from 1.5 to 3.9 hours. Toxicities included VLS, hematuria, and tremors. Nine of the 32 patients had a complete response, 7 had a partial response, and 6 had mixed responses. In 26 patients with evaluable skin disease, 11 had complete resolution of their disease, and 8 showed improvement. Resolution of disease was seen in 6 of the 22 patients with gastrointestinal involvement, and 3 of 22 patients with liver involvement. The success of these trials demonstrates that clinical responses could be induced at safe doses of the immunotoxin and that the side effects were tolerable. There was marked reduction in mononuclear cells staining with anti-CD5 and anti-CD3 antibodies in all 7 patients studied, demonstrating that the target cells were eliminated. It is not clear whether the responses are attributable to elimination of the CD5$^+$ T cells, the CD5$^+$ B cells, or both.

CONCLUSIONS

Several important lessons have been learned from the phase I–II clinical trials. The side effects of immunotoxin therapy are different from those of conventional chemotherapy. In particular, the damage to rapidly regenerating normal tissues observed with conventional chemotherapy is absent with immunotoxin therapy, with the exception of anti-CD19-blocked ricin immunotoxins and IL2-DAB486 that, for obscure reasons, cause thrombocytopenia. Liver toxicity is a consistent side effect in recipients of DT- and PE-containing immunotoxins. Blocked ricin immunotoxins cause liver toxicity, VLS, and myalgias. Immunotoxins containing native RTA cause VLS and myalgias but little liver toxicity, and those containing recombinant or deglycosylated RTA cause VLS and myalgias but no liver toxicity.

Because the side effects of immunotoxin therapy and chemotherapy differ, it is important to test these modalities in combination. In vitro and animal studies indicate that these two forms of therapy are markedly synergistic.

VLS observed with immunotoxins containing ricin or RTA rapidly reverses after treatment is discontinued or corticosteroids are given. The mechanism underlying VLS is not known. Possibilities include a direct effect of the RTA on vascular endothelium (for which we have some preliminary experimental evidence) or RTA-induced release of cytokines (*e.g.* TNF, IFN-, IL-2) that cause increased vascular permeability. Myalgias and muscle weakness may be caused by VLS-induced extravasation of immunotoxins into skeletal muscle. A generalized reduction in cardiac voltage, as determined by electrocardiogram, is usually observed after administration of RTA immunotoxins. The cause is unknown, but it could be a result of fluid accumulation in the chest wall. Electrocardiographic changes have not been associated with any other abnormalities, including abnormalities in echocardiograms, elevations in cardiac enzymes in sera, or clinical evidence of cardiac dysfunction.

There are circumstances in which VLS or myalgia become dose limiting, including rhabdomyolysis, pulmonary edema (particularly if there is a concomitant pulmonary neoplasia or infection), and psychoneurologic alterations. The latter are usually manifested by mental confusion and aphasia and are transient. The mechanisms involved in neurologic changes are not known, but they could be related to VLS. No permanent sequelae have resulted.

The severe neurotoxicity observed in two trials for breast and ovarian carcinoma emphasizes the importance of carefully screening antibodies for unexpected cross-reactivities with life-sustaining tissues and, if possible, for selecting antibodies that are cross-reactive with their homologs in nonhuman primates.

Optimal regimens for administration of the immunotoxins have not yet been devised so that the $T_{½}$s are generally shorter than would be predicted to induce an optimal therapeutic response. The short $T_{½}$s are due to a combination of factors. Immunotoxins prepared from antibodies that lack an Fc portion are not resorbed into the blood after filtration in the glomerulus, and they have inherently short serum half-lives. Immunotoxins prepared from glycosylated toxins (*e.g.* ricin) are cleared by cells with carbohydrate receptors in the liver and the RES. The crosslinkers used to form the immunotoxins that were used in some of the first clinical trials were unstable, and this instability has been shown in animal tumor models to diminish antitumor activity. Because of the short $T_{½}$, it is probably advisable to consider continuous infusion protocols. It should be noted, however, that sustaining the blood levels of immunotoxins over days or weeks could lead to additional toxicities from cross-reactions with cells in less accessible tissues.

Antibody responses against the antibody portion and the toxin portion of the immunotoxins have been observed. It is not known to what extent these antibodies can prevent repeated courses of therapy. A high and sustained level of serum antibody will probably inhibit further therapy by increasing the rate of clearance from the blood or neutralizing the toxin. However, little is known about the persistence of these antibody responses, the generation of memory cells, and what proportion of the antibodies are neutralizing. HAMA can probably be partially overcome by humanizing the antibodies, but it is unlikely that humanization will significantly reduce antibody responses against the toxins. The latter will probably require the prior or simultaneous administration of immunosuppressive agents or the derivatization of immunotoxins with agents that render them nonimmunogenic. In patients who are immunosuppressed because of their disease, immune responses are less frequent, but even in these patients, immune responsiveness depends on the immunogenicity of the construct. Blocked ricin-immunotoxins are considerably more immunogenic than RTA-immunotoxins in a similar population of patients.

Clinical responses in phase I and II patients are encouraging considering that most patients had bulky disease and that the targeted antigen may not have been expressed on all tumor cells. This is particularly true in lymphoma and leukemia. In one trial, as few as 15% of the tumor cells in some patients were positive for the targeted antigen.[131] This situation may also be true for some of the other targeted antigens, although it has not been reported. In future trials, it will be important to determine the phenotype of residual tumor cells to establish whether their escape is due to deficiency of the target antigen, to other resistance mechanisms, or to inaccessibility to the immunotoxin. If the first possibility is true, survival of the residual cells might be prevented by the use of immunotoxin cocktails directed against two or more target antigens. It will also be important to correlate response rates in phase II trials with the percentage of antigen-positive cells in tumor samples and with the size, location, and grade of the tumors. The response rate may also correlate with the incidence of VLS, because a moderate degree of VLS may promote access of the immunotoxin to the tumor. If clinical responses were not achieved in phase I trials but unacceptable toxicities were absent, it is possible that clinical responses may be achieved in the setting of minimal disease.

Although not specifically addressed in the clinical trials carried out to date, a general problem in targeting immunotoxins is the identification and phenotype of the malignant progenitor cell. In the case of NHL, it appears that the renewal cell bears surface immunoglobulin and has the phenotype of a mature B cell. This can be deduced from the complete remissions induced by treatment with antibody to the tumor immunoglobulin idiotype in some patients with NHL.[136] In contrast, the bulk of tumor cells in CLL are mature, nondividing lymphocytes, and the phenotype of their progenitor cell has not yet been determined. It is important to develop in vitro assays for progenitor cells to verify that candidate immunotoxins have cytotoxic activity against the malignant stem cells in the neoplastic disease to be treated.

The immunotoxin field has undergone an impressive evolution since its inception one decade ago. Although drug development is a lengthy and complex process (and no less so for the immunotoxins), it is extremely encouraging that one immunotoxin (*i.e.*, anti-CD5-A-RTA) has received approval to be marketed for the treatment of GVHD. The speed with which this occurred is due in no small part to the impact of immunology, pharmacology, and molecular and cell biology on the rational design of these reagents. Optimization of immunotoxins for cancer therapy will be more complex, but there is every reason to believe that success for treating some tumors will be achieved.

REFERENCES

1. Gould BJ, Borowitz MJ, Groves ES, et al. Phase I study of an anti-breast cancer immunotoxin by continuous infusion: Report of a targeted toxic effect not predicted by animal studies. JNCI 1989;81:775–781.
2. Fulton RJ, Uhr JW, Vitetta ES. In vivo therapy of the BCL1 tumor: Effect of immunotoxin valency and deglycosylation of the ricin A chain. Cancer Res 1988;48:2626–2631.
3. Krolick KA, Uhr JW, Slavin S, Vitetta ES. In vivo therapy of a murine B cell tumor (BCL1) using antibody-ricin A chain immunotoxins. J Exp Med 1982;155:1797–1809.
4. Morrison SL, Johnson MJ, Herzenberg LA, Oi VT. Chimeric human antibody molecules: Mouse antigen-binding domains with human constant region domains. Proc Natl Acad Sci USA 1984;81:6851–6855.
5. Shaw DR, Khazaeli MB, Lobuglio AF. Biological activity of mouse/human chimeric antibodies of the four human IgG subclasses with specificity for a tumor-associated antigen. Proc Am Assoc Cancer Res 1988;29:421.
6. Jones PT, Dear PH, Foote J, Neuberger MS, Winter G. Replacing the complementarity-determining regions in a human antibody with those from a mouse. Nature 1986;321:522–525.
7. Shaw DR, Khazaeli MB, Sun LK, et al. Characterization of a mouse/human chimeric monoclonal antibody (17-1A) to a colon cancer tumor-associated antigen. J Immunol 1987;138:4534–4538.
8. Lederman JA, Begent RHJ, Bagshawe KD, et al. Repeated anti-tumor antibody therapy in man with suppression of the host response by cyclosporin A. Br J Cancer 1988;58:654–657.
9. Lobuglio AF, Khazaeli MB, Lee J, et al. Pharmacokinetics and immune response to Xomazyme-Mel in melanoma patients. In: Antibody Immunoconj Radiopharm 1988;1:305–310.
10. Pai LH, FitzGerald DJ, Tepper M, Schacter B, Spitalny G, Pastan I. Inhibition of antibody response to *Pseudomonas* exotoxin and an immunotoxin containing *Pseudomonas* exotoxin by 15-deoxyspergualin in mice. Cancer Res 1990;50:7750–7753.
11. Raso V, Griffin T. Specific cytotoxicity of a human immunoglobulin directed Fab′-ricin A conjugate. J Immunol 1980;125:2610–2616.
12. Ghetie M-A, May RD, Till M, et al. Evaluation of ricin A chain-containing immunotoxins directed against CD19 and CD22 antigens on normal and malignant human B-cells as potential reagents for in vivo therapy. Cancer Res 1988;48:2610–2617.
13. Batra JK, FitzGerald DJ, Chaudhary VK, Pastan I. Single-chain immunotoxins directed at human transferrin receptor containing *Pseudomonas* exotoxin A or diphtheria toxin: Anti-TFR (Fv)-PE40 and DT388-anti-TFR (Fv). Mol Cell Biol 1991;11:2200–2205.
14. Chaudhary VK, Gallo MG, FitzGerald DJ, Pastan I. A recombinant single-chain immunotoxin composed of anti-tac variable regions and a truncated diphtheria toxin. Proc Natl Acad Sci USA 1990;87:9491–9494.
15. Masuho Y, Kishida K, Saito M, Umeto N, Hara T. Importance of the antigen-binding valency and the nature of cross-linking bond in ricin A chain conjugates with antibody. J Biochem 1982;91:1583–1591.
16. Holton OD, III, Black CDV, Parker RJ, et al. Biodistribution of monoclonal IgG1, F(ab′)2 and Fab′ in mice after intravenous injection. Comparison between anti-B cell (anti-LyB8. 2) and irrelevant (MOPC21) antibodies. J Immunol 1987;139:3041.
17. Fulton RJ, Tucker TF, Vitetta ES, Uhr JW. Pharmacokinetics of tumor-reactive immunotoxins in tumor-bearing mice: Effect of antibody valency and deglycosylation of the ricin A chain on clearance and tumor localization. Cancer Res 1988;48:2618–2625.
18. Engert A, Martin G, Pfreundschuh M, et al. Anti-tumor effects of ricin A chain immunotoxins prepared from intact antibodies and Fab′ fragments on solid human Hodgkin's disease tumors in mice. Cancer Res 1990;50:2929–2935.
19. Bjorn MJ, Ring D, Frankel A. Evaluation of monoclonal antibodies for the development of breast cancer immunotoxins. Cancer Res 1985;45:1214–1221.
20. Engert A, Burrows F, Jung WE, et al. Evaluation of ricin A chain-containing immunotoxins directed against CD30 as potential reagents for the treatment of Hodgkin's disease. Cancer Res 1989;50:84–88.
21. Goldmacher VS, Scott CF, Lambert JM, et al. Cytotoxicity of gelonin and its conjugates with antibodies is determined by the extent of their endocytosis. J Cell Physiol 1989;141:222–234.
22. Press OW, Martin P, Thorpe PE, Vitetta ES. Ricin A-chain containing immunotoxins directed against different epitopes on the CD2 molecule differ in their ability to kill normal and malignant T cells. J Immunol 1988;141:4410–4417.
23. Till M, May RD, Uhr JW, Thorpe PE, Vitetta ES. An assay that predicts the ability of monoclonal antibodies to form potent ricin A chain-containing immunotoxins. Cancer Res 1988;48:1119–1123.
24. Weltman JK, Pedroso P, Johnson S-A, Davignon D, Fast LD, Leone LA. Rapid screening with indirect immunotoxin for monoclonal antibodies against human small cell lung cancer. Cancer Res 1987;47:5552–5556.
25. Thorpe PE, Wallace PM, Knowles PP, et al. Improved anti-tumor effects of immunotoxins prepared with deglycosylated ricin A chain and hindered disulfide linkages. Cancer Res 1988;48:6396–6403.
26. Thorpe PE, Blakey DC, Brown AN, et al. Comparison of two anti-Thy 1.1-abrin A-chain immunotoxins prepared with different cross-linking agents: Antitumor effects, in vivo fate, and tumor cell mutants. JNCI 1987;79:1101–1112.
27. Libermann TA, Nusbaum HR, Razon N, Kris R, Lax I, Soreq H. Amplification, enhanced expression and possible rearrangement of EGF receptor gene in primary brain tumors of glial origin. Nature 1985;313:144–147.
28. Leonard WJ, Depper JM, Robb RJ, Waldmann TA, Greene WC. Characterization of the human receptor for T cell growth factor. Proc Natl Acad Sci USA 1983;80:6957–6961.
29. Hendler FJ, Ozanne BW. Human squamous cell lung cancers express increased epidermal growth factor receptors. J Clin Invest 1984;74:647–651.
30. Kronke M, Depper JM, Leonard WJ, Vitetta ES, Waldmann TA, Greene WC. Adult T cell leukemia: A potential target for ricin A chain immunotoxins. Blood 1985;65:1416–1421.
31. FitzGerald D, Pastan I. Targeted toxin therapy for the treatment of cancer. JNCI [Review] 1989;81:1455–1463.
32. FitzGerald D, Pastan I. Redirecting *Pseudomonas* exotoxin. Semin Cell Biol 1991;2:31–38.
33. Greenfield L, Bjorn MJ, Horn G, et al. Nucleotide sequence of the structural gene for diphtheria toxin carried by corynebacteriophage beta. Proc Natl Acad Sci USA 1983;80:6853–6857.
34. Gray GL, Smith DH, Baldridge JS, et al. Cloning, nucleotide sequence, and expression in Escherichia coli of the exotoxin A structural gene of *Pseudomonas aeruginosa*. Proc Natl Acad Sci USA 1984;81:2645–2649.
35. Leong D, Coleman KD, Murphy JR. Cloned fragment A of diphtheria toxin is expressed and secreted into the periplasmic space of *Escherichia coli* K12. Science 1983;220:515–517.
36. Ogata M, Chaudhary VK, Pastan I, FitzGerald DJ. Processing of *Pseudomonas* exotoxin by a cellular protease results in the generation of a 37,000 Da toxin fragment that is translocated to the cytosol. J Biol Chem 1990;256:20678–20685.
37. Kondo T, FitzGerald D, Chaudhary VK, Adhya S, Pastan I. Activity of immunotoxins constructed with modified *Pseudomonas* exotoxin A lacking the cell recognition domain. J Biol Chem 1988;263:9470–9475.
38. Johnson VG, Wilson D, Greenfield L, Youle RJ. The role of the diphtheria toxin receptor in cytosol translocation. J Biol Chem 1988;263:1295–1300.
39. Bacha P, Forte S, Kassam N, et al. Pharmacokinetics of the recombinant fusion protein DAB486IL-2 in animal models. Cancer Chemother Pharmacol 1990;26:409–414.
40. Walz G, Zanker B, Murphy JR, Strom TB. A kinetic analysis of the effects of interleukin-2 diphtheria toxin fusion protein upon activated T cells. Transplantation 1990;49:198–201.
41. Walz G, Zanker B, Brand K, Waters C, Genbauffe F, Zeldis JB, Murphy JR, Strom TB. Sequential effects of interleukin-2/diphtheria toxin fusion protein of T-cell activation. Proc Natl Acad Sci USA 1989;86:9485–9488.
42. Balkwill F, Osborne R, Burke F, Naylor S, Talbot D, Durbin H, Tavernier J, Fiers W. Evidence for tumor necrosis factor/cachectin production in cancer. Lancet 1987;2:1229–1232.
43. Kay NE, Burton J, Wagner D, Nelson DL. The malignant B-cells from B-chronic lymphocytic leukemia patients release TAC-soluble interleukin-2 receptors. Blood 1988;72:447–450.
44. Olsnes S, Pihl A. Toxic lectins and related proteins. In: Cohen P, van Heyningen S, eds. Molecular action of toxins and viruses. New York: Elsevier, 1982:51–105.
45. Eiklid K, Olsnes S, Pihl A. Entry of lethal doses of abrin, ricin and modeccin into the cytosol of HeLa cells. Exp Cell Res 1980;126:321–326.
46. Yamaizumi M, Mekada E, Uchida T, Okada Y. One molecule of diphtheria toxin fragment A introduced into a cell can kill the cell. Cell 1978;15:245–250.
47. Thorpe PE, Ross WC. The preparation and cytotoxic properties of antibody-toxin conjugates. Immunol Rev 1982;62:119–158.
48. Gill DM, Dinius LL. Observations on the structure of diphtheria toxin. J Biol Chem 1971;246:1485–1491.
49. Collier RJ. Diphtheria toxin: Mode of action and structure. Bacteriol Rev 1975;39:54–85.
50. Endo Y, Tsurugi K. RNA *N*-glycosidase activity of ricin A-chain. Mechanism of action of the toxic lectin ricin on eukaryotic ribosomes. J Biol Chem 1987;262:8128–8130.
51. Endo Y, Mitsui K, Motizuki M, Tsurugi K. The mechanism of action of ricin and related toxic lectins on eukaryotic ribosomes. The site and the characteristics of the modification in 28S ribosomal RNA caused by the toxins. J Biol Chem 1987;262:5908–5912.
52. Neville DM Jr, Hudson TH. Transmembrane transport of diphtheria toxin, related toxins, and colicins. Annu Rev Biochem 1986;55:195–224.
53. Casellas P, Dussossoy D, Falasca AI, et al. Trichokirin, a ribosome-inactivating protein from the seeds of *Trichosanthes kirilowii* Maximowicz. Purification, partial characterization and use for preparation of immunotoxins. Eur J Biochem 1988;176:581–588.
54. Stirpe F, Wawrzynczak EJ, Brown ANF, et al. Selective cytotoxic activity of immunotoxins composed of a monoclonal anti-Thy 1.1 antibody and the ribosome-inactivating proteins, bryodin and momordin. Br J Cancer 1988;58:558–561.

55. Wang QC, Ying WB, Xie H, Zhang Z, Yang Z, Ling L. Trichosanthin-monoclonal antibody conjugate specifically cytotoxic to human hepatoma cells in vitro. Cancer Res 1991;51:3353–3355.
56. Ramakrishnan S, Houston LL. Prevention of growth of leukemia cells in mice by monoclonal antibodies directed against Thy 1.1 antigen disulfide linked to two ribosomal inhibitors: Pokeweed antiviral protein or ricin A chain. Cancer Res 1984;44:1398–1404.
57. Uckun FM, Ramakrishnan S, Houston LL. Increased efficiency in selective elimination of leukemia cells by a combination of a stable derivative of cyclophosphamide and a human B-cell-specific immunotoxin containing pokeweed antiviral protein. Cancer Res 1985;45:69–75.
58. Stirpe F, Barbieri L. Ribosome-inactivating proteins up to date. FEBS Lett 1986;195:1–8.
59. Thorpe PE, Brown AN, Ross WC, et al. Cytotoxicity acquired by conjugation of an anti-Thy1.1 monoclonal antibody and the ribosome-inactivating protein, gelonin. Eur J Biochem 1981;116:447–454.
60. Stirpe F, Gasperi-Campani A, Barbieri L, Falasca A, Abbondanza A, Stevens WA. Ribosome-inactivating proteins from the seeds of *Saponaria officinalis* L. (soapwort), of *Agrostemma githago* L. (corn cockle) and of *Asparagus officinalis* L. (asparagus), and from the latex of *Hura crepitans* L. (sandbox tree). Biochem J 1983;216:617–625.
61. Thorpe PE, Brown AN, Bremner JA Jr, Foxwell BM, Stirpe F. An immunotoxin composed of monoclonal anti-Thy 1.1 antibody and a ribosome-inactivating protein from *Saponaria officinalis*: Potent antitumor effects in vitro and in vivo. JNCI 1985;75:151–159.
62. Vasil ML, Kabat D, Iglewski BH. Structure-activity relationships of an exotoxin of *Pseudomonas aeruginosa*. Infect Immunol 1977;16:353–361.
63. Williams DP, Parker K, Bacha P, et al. Diphtheria toxin binding domain substitution with interleukin-2: Genetic construction and properties of a diphtheria toxin-related interleukin-2 fusion protein. Protein Eng 1987;1:493–498.
64. Jinno Y, Chaudhary VK, Kondo T, Adhya S, FitzGerald DJ, Pastan I. Mutational analysis of domain I of *Pseudomonas* exotoxin. Mutations in domain I of *Pseudomonas* exotoxin which reduce cell binding and animal toxicity. J Biol Chem 1988;263:13203–13207.
65. Houston LL, Nowinski RC. Cell-specific cytotoxicity expressed by a conjugate of ricin and murine monoclonal antibody directed against thy 1.1 antigen. Cancer Res 1981;41:3913–3917.
66. Youle RJ, Neville DM Jr. Anti-Thy 1.2 monoclonal antibody linked to ricin is a potent cell-type-specific toxin. Proc Natl Acad Sci USA 1980;77:5483–5486.
67. Thorpe PE, Ross WC, Brown AN, et al. Blockade of the galactose-binding sites of ricin by its linkage to antibody. Specific cytotoxic effects of the conjugates. Eur J Biochem 1984;140:63–71.
68. Houston LL. Inactivation of ricin using 4-azidophenyl-β-D-galactopyranoside and 4-diazophenyl-β-D-galactopyranoside. J Biol Chem 1983;258:7208–7212.
69. Breitmeyer J, Nadler L, Coral F, Eliseo L, Blattler WA, Schlossman S. Blocked ricin immunotoxin therapy of malignant lymphoma. Proceedings of Monoclonal Antibody Immunoconjugates in Cancer Therapy, Chicago, September, 1989:28–29.
70. Moroney SE, Dalarcao LJ, Goldmacher VS, Lambert JM, Blattler WA. Modification of the binding site(s) of lectins by an affinity column carrying an activated galactose-terminated ligand. Biochemistry 1987;26:8390–8398.
71. Blakey DC, Watson GJ, Knowles PP, Thorpe PE. Effect of chemical deglycosylation of ricin A chain on the in vivo fate and cytotoxic activity of an immunotoxin composed of ricin A chain and anti-Thy 1.1 antibody. Cancer Res 1987;47:947–952.
72. Thorpe PE, Wallace PM, Knowles PP, et al. New coupling agents for the synthesis of immunotoxins containing a hindered disulfide bond with improved stability in vivo. Cancer Res 1987;47:5924–5931.
73. Stanworth DR, Turner MW. Immunochemical analysis of immunoglobulins and their sub-units. In: Weir DM, ed. Handbook of experimental immunology. Oxford: Blackwell Scientific Publications, 1978:1–102.
74. Wawrzynczak EJ, Thorpe PE. Methods for preparing immunotoxins: Effects of the linkage on activity and stability. In: Vogel CW, ed. Immunoconjugates: Antibody conjugates in radioimaging and therapy of cancer. New York: Oxford University Press, 1987:28–55.
75. Lambert JM, Senter PD, Yau-Young A, Blattler WA, Goldmacher VS. Purified immunotoxins that are reactive with human lymphoid cells. J Biol Chem 1985;260:12035–12041.
76. Murphy JR, Bisha W, Williams D, et al. Genetic assembly and selective toxicity of diphtheria-toxin-related polypeptide hormone fusion proteins. Biochem Soc Symp 1987;53:9–23.
77. Ramakrishnan S, Houston LL. Comparison of the selective cytotoxic effects of immunotoxins containing ricin A chain or pokeweed antiviral protein and anti-Thy 1.1 monoclonal antibodies. Cancer Res 1984;44:201–208.
78. Shen G-L, Li J-L, Ghetie M-A, et al. Evaluation of four CD22 antibodies as ricin A chain-containing immunotoxins for the in vivo therapy of human B-cell leukemias and lymphomas. Int J Cancer 1988;42:792–797.
79. Guillemot JC, Sundan A, Olsnes S, Sandvig K. Entry of diphtheria toxin linked to concanavalin A into primate and murine cells. J Cell Physiol 1985;122:193–199.
80. Bacha P, Williams DP, Waters C, Williams JM, Murphy JR, Strom TB. Interleukin 2 receptor-targeted cytotoxicity. Interleukin 2 receptor-mediated action of a diphtheria toxin-related interleukin 2 fusion protein. J Exp Med 1988;167:612–622.
81. Van Deurs B, Tnnessen TI, Petersen OW, Sandvig K, Olsnes S. Routing of internalized ricin and ricin conjugates to the Golgi complex. J Cell Biol 1986;102:37–47.
82. Press OW, Vitetta ES, Farr AG, Hansen JA, Martin PJ. Evaluation of ricin A-chain immunotoxins directed against human T cells. Cell Immunol 1986;102:10–20.
83. Thorpe PE, Mason DW, Brown AN, et al. Selective killing of malignant cells in a leukaemic rat bone marrow using an antibody-ricin conjugate. Nature 1982;297:594–596.
84. Bacha P, Murphy JR, Reichlin S. Thyrotropin-releasing hormone-diphtheria toxin-related polypeptide conjugates. J Biol Chem 1983;258:1565.
85. Wawrzynczak EJ, Watson GJ, Cumber AJ, et al. Blocked and non-blocked ricin immunotoxins against the CD4 antigen exhibit higher cytotoxic potency than a ricin A-chain immunotoxin potentiated with ricin B-chain or with a ricin B-chain immunotoxin. Cancer Immunol Immunother 1991;32:289–295.
86. Casellas P, Bourrie BJP, Gros P, Jansen F. Kinetics of cytotoxicity induced by immunotoxins. Enhancement by lysosomotropic amines and carboxylic ionophores. J Biol Chem 1984;259:9359–9364.
87. Ramakrishnan S, Houston LL. Inhibition of human acute lymphoblastic leukemia cells by immunotoxins: Potentiation by chloroquine. Science 1984;223:58–61.
88. Raso V, Lawrence J. Carboxylic ionophores enhance the cytotoxic potency of ligand- and antibody-delivered ricin A chain. J Exp Med 1984;160:1234–1240.
89. McIntosh DP, Edwards DC, Cumber AJ, et al. Ricin B chain converts a non-cytotoxic antibody-ricin A chain conjugate into a potent and specific cytotoxic agent. FEBS Lett 1983;164:17–20.
90. Vitetta ES, Cushley W, Uhr JW. Synergy of ricin A chain-containing immunotoxins and ricin B chain-containing immunotoxins in in vitro killing of neoplastic human B cells. Proc Natl Acad Sci USA 1983;80:6332–6335.
91. Vitetta ES, Fulton RJ, Uhr JW. Cytotoxicity of a cell-reactive immunotoxin containing ricin A chain is potentiated by an anti-immunotoxin containing ricin B chain. J Exp Med 1984;160:341–346.
92. Ramakrishnan S, Bjorn MJ, Houston LL. Recombinant ricin A chain conjugated to monoclonal antibodies: Improved tumor cell inhibition in the presence of lysosomotropic compounds. Cancer Res 1989;49:613–617.
93. Casellas P, Jansen FK. Immunotoxin enhancers. In: Frankel AE, ed. Immunotoxins. Norwell, MA: Kluwer Academic Publishers, 1988;351–371.
94. Harkonen S, Stoudemire J, Mischak R, Spitler LE, Lopez H, Scannon P. Toxicity and immunogenicity of monoclonal anti-melanoma antibody-ricin A chain immunotoxin in rats. Cancer Res 1987;47:1377–1382.
95. Stirpe F, Derenzini M, Barbieri L, et al. Hepatotoxicity of immunotoxins made from saporin, a ribosome-inactivating protein from *Saponaria officinalis*. Virchows Arch [B] 1987;53:259–271.
96. Blakey DC, Skilleter DN, Price RJ, et al. Comparison of the pharmacokinetics and hepatotoxic effects of saporin and ricin A-chain immunotoxins on murine liver parenchymal cells. Cancer Res 1988;48:7072–7078.
97. Kanellos J, MacKenzie IF, Pietersz GA. In vivo studies of whole ricin monoclonal antibody immunoconjugates for the treatment of murine tumours. Immunol Cell Biol 1988;66:403–415.
98. Zaleberg JR, Pietersz G, Toohey B, Zimet A, Hennessy O, McKenzie IFC. Phase I–II study of a ricin monoclonal antibody conjugate in colon cancer. In: Monoclonal antibody immunoconjugates for cancer. San Diego, CA: Abstract from 4th International Conference, 1989.
99. Jansen FK, Blythman HE, Carriere D, et al. Immunotoxins: Hybrid molecules combining high specificity and potent cytotoxicity. Immunol Rev 1982;62:185–216.
100. Blakey DC, Skilleter DN, Price RJ, Thorpe PE. Uptake of native and deglycosylated ricin A-chain immunotoxins by mouse liver parenchymal and non-parenchymal cells in vitro and in vivo. Biochim Biophys Acta 1988;968:172–178.
101. Skilleter DN, Paine AJ, Stirpe F. A comparison of the accumulation of ricin by hepatic parenchymal and non-parenchymal cells and its inhibition of protein synthesis. Biochim Biophys Acta 1981;677:495–500.
102. Thorpe PE, Detre SI, Foxwell BMJ, et al. Modification of the carbohydrate in ricin with metaperiodate-cyanoborohydride mixtures. Effects on toxicity and in vivo distribution. Eur J Biochem 1985;147:197–206.
103. O'Hare M, Roberts LM, Thorpe PE, Watson GJ, Prior B, Lord JM. Expression of ricin A chain in Escherichia coli. FEBS Lett 1987;216:73–78.
104. Skilleter DN, Price RJ, Thorpe PE. Modification of the carbohydrate in ricin with metaperiodate and cyanoborohydride mixtures: Effect on binding, uptake and toxicity to parenchymal and non-parenchymal cells of rat liver. Biochim Biophys Acta 1985;842:12–21.
105. Vitetta ES, Thorpe PE. Immunotoxins containing ricin A or B chains with modified carbohydrate residues act synergistically in killing neoplastic B cells in vitro. Cancer Drug Deliv 1985;2:191–198.
106. Ghetie MA, Uhr JW, Vitetta ES. Covalent binding of human 2-macroglobulin to deglycosylated ricin A chain and its immunotoxins. Cancer Res 1991;51:1482–1487.
107. Jansen FK, Blythman HE, Carriere D, et al. High specific cytotoxicity of antibody-toxin hybrid molecules (immunotoxins) for target cells. Immunol Lett 1980;2:97–102.
108. FitzGerald DJ, Willingham MC, Pastan I. Antitumor effects of an immunotoxin made with *Pseudomonas* exotoxin in a nude mouse model of human ovarian cancer. Proc Natl Acad Sci USA 1986;83:6627–6630.
109. Manske JM, Buchsbaum DJ, Hanna DE, Vallera DA. Cytotoxic effects of anti-CD5 radioimmunotoxins on human tumors in vitro and in a nude mouse model. Cancer Res 1988;48:7107–7114.
110. Hara H, Luo Y, Haruta Y, Seon BK. Efficient transplantation of human non-T-leukemia cells into nude mice and induction of complete regression of the transplanted distinct tumors by ricin A-chain conjugates of monoclonal antibodies SN5 and SN6. Cancer Res 1988;48:4673–4680.
111. Bernhard MI, Foon KA, Oeltmann TN, et al. Guinea pig line 10 hepatocarcinoma model: Characterization of monoclonal antibody and in vivo effect of unconjugated antibody and antibody conjugated to diphtheria toxin A chain. Cancer Res 1983;43:4420–4428.

112. Hwang KM, Foon KA, Cheung PH, Pearson JW, Oldham RK. Selective antitumor effect on L10 hepatocarcinoma cells of a potent immunoconjugate composed of the A chain of abrin and a monoclonal antibody to a hepatoma-associated antigen. Cancer Res 1984;44:4578–4586.
113. Weil-Hillman G, Uckun FM, Manske JM, Vallera DA. Combined immunochemotherapy of human solid tumors in nude mice. Cancer Res 1987;47:579–585.
114. Pearson JW, Sivam G, Manger R, Wiltrout RH, Morgan AC Jr, Longo DL. Enhanced therapeutic efficacy of an immunotoxin in combination with chemotherapy against an intraperitoneal human tumor xenograft in athymic mice. Cancer Res 1989;49:4990–4995.
115. Sironi M, Canegrati MA, Romano M, Vecchi A, Spreafico F. Chemotherapy-increased antineoplastic effects of antibody-toxin conjugates. Cancer Treat Rep 1984;68:643–645.
116. Pirker R, FitzGerald DJP, Raschack M, Frank Z, Willingham MC, Pastan I. Enhancement of the activity of immunotoxins by analogues of verapamil. Cancer Res 1989;49:4791–4795.
117. Yokota S, Hara H, Luo Y, Seon BK. Synergistic potentiation of in vivo anti-tumor activity of anti-human T-leukemia immunotoxins by recombinant interferon and daunorubicin. Cancer Res 1990;50:32–37.
118. Pearson JW, FitzGerald DJP, Willingham MC, Wiltrout RH, Pastan I, Longo DL. Chemoimmunotoxin therapy against a human colon tumor (HT-29) xenografted into nude mice. Cancer Res 1989;49:3562–3567.
119. Smyth MJ, Pietersz GA, McKenzie IF. Use of vasoactive agents to increase tumor perfusion and the antitumor efficacy of drug-monoclonal antibody conjugates. JNCI 1987;79:1367–1373.
120. Jain RK, Baxter LT. Mechanisms of heterogeneous distribution of monoclonal antibodies and other macromolecules in tumors: Significance of elevated interstitial pressure. Cancer Res 1988;48:7022–7032.
121. Sands H. Radioimmunoconjugates: An overview of problems and promises. Antibody Immunoconjugates Radiopharm 1988;1:213–226.
122. Osdol WV, Fujimori K, Weinstein JN. An analysis of monoclonal antibody distribution in microscopic tumor nodules: Consequences of a "binding site barrier." Cancer Res 1991;51:4776–4784.
123. Oratz R, Speyer JL, Wernz JC, et al. Anti-melanoma monoclonal antibody-ricin A chain immunoconjugate (XMMME-001–RTA) plus cyclophosphamide in the treatment of metastatic malignant melanoma: Results of a phase II trial. J Biol Response Modif 1990;9:345–354.
124. Byers VS, Rodvien R, Grant K, et al. Phase I study of monoclonal antibody-ricin A chain immunotoxin XomaZyme-791 in patients with metastatic colon cancer. Cancer Res 1989;49:6153–6160.
125. Pai LH, Bookman MA, Ozols RJ, et al. Clinical evaluation of intraperitoneal *Pseudomonas* exotoxin immunoconjugate OVBB-PE in patients with ovarian cancer. J Clin Oncol 1991;9(12):2095–2103.
126. Spitler LE, del Rio M, Khentigan A, et al. Therapy of patients with malignant melanoma using a monoclonal anti-melanoma antibody-ricin A chain immunotoxin. Cancer Res 1987;47:1717–1723.
127. Spitler LE. Clinical studies: Solid tumors. In: Frankel AE, ed. Immunotoxins. Norwell, MA: Kluwer Academic Publishers, 1988;493–515.
128. Weiner LM, O'Dwyer J, Kitson J, et al. Phase I evaluation of an anti-breast carcinoma monoclonal antibody 260F9-recombinant ricin A chain immunoconjugate. Cancer Res 1989;49:4062–4067.
129. Grossbard ML, Freedman AS, Kinsella JM, Epstein CL, Blattler WA, Nadler LM. Immunotherapy with anti-B4-blocked ricin (Anti-B4–BR): Phase 1 trials of continuous infusion in patients with B-cell neoplasms. Am Soc Hematol [Abstract] 1991;.
130. Grossbard ML, Freedman AS, Ritz J, et al. Serotherapy of B-cell neoplasms with anti-B4-blocked ricin: A phase 1 trial of daily bolus infusion. Blood 1992;79:576–585.
131. Vitetta ES, Stone M, Amlot P, et al. A phase I immunotoxin trial in patients with B cell lymphoma. Cancer Res 1991;15:4052–4058.
132. Hertler AA, Schlossman DM, Borowitz MJ, Blythman HE, Casellas P, Frankel AE. An anti-CD5 immunotoxin for chronic lymphocytic leukemia: Enhancement of cytotoxicity with human serum albumin-monensin. Int J Cancer 1989;43:215–219.
133. Le Maistre CF, Rosen S, Frankel A, et al. Phase I trial of H65-RTA immunoconjugate in patients with cutaneous T-cell lymphoma. Blood 1991;78:1173–1182.
134. Le Maistre F, Rosenblum M, Reuben J, et al. Phase I study of genetically engineered DAB486IL-2 in IL-2-receptor expressing malignancies. Blood 1990;76:360a.
135. Byers VS, Henslee PJ, Kernan NA, et al. Use of an anti-pan T-lymphocyte ricin A chain immunotoxin in steroid-resistant acute graft-versus-host disease. Blood 1990;75:1426–1432.
136. Miller RA, Maloney DG, Warnke R, Levy R. Treatment of B-cell lymphoma with monoclonal anti-idiotypic antibody. N Engl J Med 1982;306:516–522.
137. Waters CA, Schimke PA, Snider CE, et al. Interleukin 2 receptor-targeted cytotoxicity. Receptor binding requirements for entry of a diphtheria toxin-related interleukin 2 fusion protein into cells. Eur J Immunol 1990;20:785–792.
138. Kiyokawa T, Shirono K, Hattori T, et al. Cytotoxicity of interleukin 2-toxin toward lymphocytes from patients with adult T cell leukemia. Cancer Res 1989;49:4042–4046.
139. Lakkis F, Steele A, Pacheco-Silva A, Rubin-Kelly V, Strom TB, Murphy JR. Interleukin 4 receptor targeted cytotoxicity: Genetic construction and in vivo immunosuppressive activity of a diphtheria toxin-related murine interleukin 4 fusion protein. Eur J Immunol [Abstract] 1991;21:2253–2258.
140. Puri RK, Ogata M, Leland P, Feldman GM, FitzGerald D, Pastan I. Expression of high-affinity interleukin 4 receptors on murine sarcoma cells and receptor-mediated cytotoxicity of tumor cells to chimeric protein between interleukin 4 and *Pseudomonas* exotoxin. Cancer Res 1991;51:3011–3017.
141. Siegall CB, Chaudhary VK, FitzGerald DJ, Pastan I. Cytotoxicity of an interleukin 6–*Pseudomonas* exotoxin fusion protein on human myeloma cells. Proc Natl Acad Sci USA 1988;85:9738–9742.
142. Siegall CB, Kreitman RJ, FitzGerald DJ, Pastan I. Antitumor effects of interleukin 6–*Pseudomonas* exotoxin chimeric molecules against the human hepatocellular carcinoma, PLC/PCF/5 in mice. Cancer Res 1991;51:2831–2836.
143. Pai LH, Gallo MG, FitzGerald DJ, Pastan I. Antitumor activity of a transforming growth factor a-*Pseudomonas* exotoxin fusion protein (TGF-a-PE40). Cancer Res 1991;51:2808–2812.
144. Siegall CB, FitzGerald DJ, Pastan I. Selective killing of tumor cells using EGF or TGFa-*Pseudomonas* exotoxin chimeric molecules. Cancer Biology 1990;1:345–350.
145. Prior TI, Helman LJ, FitzGerald DJ, Pastan I. Cytotoxic activity of a recombinant fusion protein between insulin-like growth factor I and *Pseudomonas* exotoxin. Cancer Res 1991;51:174–180.
146. Lappi DA, Maher PA, Martineau D, Baird A. The basic fibroblast growth factor-saporin mitotoxin acts through the basic fibroblast growth factor receptor. J Cell Physiol 1991;147:17–26.
147. Siegall CB, Epstein S, Spein E, et al. Cytotoxic activity of chimeric proteins composed of acidic fibroblast growth factor and *Pseudomonas* exotoxins on a variety of cell types. FASEB J 1991;5:2843–2849.
148. Murphy JR, Bishai W, Borowski M, Miyanohara A, Boyd J, Nagle S. Genetic construction, expression, and melanoma-selective cytotoxicity of a diphtheria toxin-related melanocyte-stimulating hormone fusion protein. Proc Natl Acad Sci USA 1986;83:8258–8262.
149. Naglich JG, Methereal JE, Russel DW, Erdels L. Expression cloning of a diphtheria toxin receptor: Identity with a heparin-binding EGF-like growth factor precursor. Cell 69:1051–1061.
150. Kounnas MZ, Morris RE, Thompson MR, FitzGerald DJ, Strickland DK, Saelinger CB. The α_2-macroglobulin receptor/low density lipoprotein receptor-related protein binds and internalizes *Pseudomonas* exotoxin A*. J Biol Chem 1992;267:12420–12423.

SECTION 4

CHARLES W. YOUNG
RAYMOND P. WARRELL, JR

Differentiating Agents

Cancer can be perceived as an inappropriate accumulation of cells that are capable of varying degrees of differentiation. This concept is inherent in the familiar diagnostic adjectives, which range from "well differentiated" through "poorly differentiated" to "anaplastic." In the usual course of disease progression, there is an inverse relation between the degree of cytologic differentiation and the clinical aggressiveness of the neoplastic condition. It is now clear that the neoplastic change is not immutable; some cancer cells can be induced to undergo phenotypic changes, characterized by morphologic maturation along the expected pattern for the tissue of origin and by the loss of replicative capacity. This process is referred to as "terminal" differentiation, and drugs that predictably induce these changes are considered to be differentiating agents.

For several decades it had been recognized that a residual mass comprised solely of differentiated cells may be observed after aggressive therapy of certain tumors, particularly neuroblastoma and germ cell neoplasms. Whether this phenomenon resulted from treatment-induced cytodifferentiation or selective destruction of less differentiated tumor cell population was not established. In the past 2 decades, interest in differentiation therapy of cancer as a planned therapeutic approach was aroused by reports that cytodifferentiation of cancer cell lines could be produced in vitro by treatment with a wide variety of physiologic and xenobiotic molecules.[1–4] Although the theoretic interest of these cell culture observations has been widely accepted, their clinical relevance was considered to be questionable. However, clinical applications of this approach have been convincingly established in at least one disorder, acute promyelocytic leukemia.[5–9]

Cancer is associated with genetic abnormalities that range in extent from translocations, such as t(9;22) in chronic myelogenous leukemia (CML) and t(15;17) in acute promyelocytic leukemia, to the extensive multichromosomal defects that characterize colorectal cancer and breast cancer.[10–14] In colorectal cancer, anatomic and physiologic correlations exist between the progressive loss of genetic integrity and sequential changes from an apparently normal mucosa to one that shows hyperproliferation and then dysplasia, adenoma, locally invasive carcinoma, and eventually metastatic carcinoma. Similarly, in CML progression from the chronic to the accelerated and blastic phases is accompanied by further chromosomal loss, particularly at the p53 locus.[15–17] Simplistically, the genetic abnormalities in cancer cells result in a physiologic block at a stage of differentiation that retains proliferative capacity; moreover, the neoplastic cells no longer respond to controls that normally govern growth and differentiation. Differentiation therapy reasserts certain critical aspects of normal control that eventually leads to loss of proliferative capacity. Because these controls are presumably physiologic, differentiation therapy should be considerably less toxic than conventional cytotoxic therapies.

A wide variety of drugs or physical conditions induce cytodifferentiation (Table 69–16). Not all cancer cells or cancer cell lines are responsive to inducing agents in vitro; frequently, those that do respond differentiate under the influence of several different agents. These observations suggest that, although responding cells may have a rather "localized" block to differentiation, they retain sufficient intact genetic information to fully respond after the localized block has been circumvented. Conceivably, nonresponding lines have undergone more extensive genetic injury or may have multiple blocks that not relieved by a single agent. Extending this concept, dysplastic or precancerous cells that have undergone minimal genetic change may have only a partial block to differentiation and be quite responsive to induced maturation. Accordingly, the early stages of preneoplastic transition may also be an appropriate place for the use of differentiating agents. This idea is supported by the considerable overlap between agents that produce differentiation and those that have chemopreventive activity in model systems.

This chapter summarizes relevant clinical and laboratory information related to differentiation agents currently undergoing extensive clinical testing. Because mechanisms of drug-induced differentiation are largely unknown, clinical trials have usually been empirically based on activity observed for a given drug in model systems. Hematologic disorders, largely leukemia and myelodysplastic syndromes, have received particular attention because phenotypic stages of normal differentiation in blood cells are well characterized. Furthermore, because the neoplastic cell population in these patients can be conveniently and repeatedly sampled during the course of treatment, there is an opportunity to delineate whether cytotoxicity or cytodifferentiation is occurring in responding patients.

TABLE 69–16. Cytodifferentiation Agents in Cell Culture

Class	*Example*
Retinoids	All-*trans*-retinoic acid
	13-*cis*-retinoic acid
Vitamins	1,25-Dihydroxyvitamin D_3
Fatty acids	Butyrate
Interferons	
Phorbol esters	
Planar/polar compounds	Dimethyl sulfoxide (DMSO)
	Hexamethylene bisacetamide (HMBA)
	Dimethylformamide (DMF)
Cytotoxics	Cytosine arabinoside (ara-C)
	Tiazofurin
	5-Bromodeoxyuridine
	Antifolates
	Aclacinomycin
Cyclic-AMP Modulators	Cholera toxin
	Forskolin
	Isobutylmethylxanthine
Analogs	8-Cl/Br-cyclic-AMP
	Dibutyryl-cyclic AMP

RETINOIDS

BACKGROUND

The term retinoids includes the naturally occurring and synthetic analogues of vitamin A (retinol) a fat-soluble dietary substance essential for growth, normal embryologic development, and vision.[18,19] The physiologic morphogen, all-*trans*-retinoic acid (tretinoin) is synthesized in vivo from retinol; when supplied exogenously, tretinoin can replace retinol in all biologic functions except that of supporting vision. Retinoids produce biologic effects by interaction with a series of nuclear receptors that are analogous to the receptors of steroids and thyroid hormone.[20–23] At least three RA-receptor (RAR) subtypes—α, β, and γ—have been identified, along with a second receptor family, termed RXR.[23] Tretinoin and its naturally occurring isomer 13-*cis*-retinoic acid (isotretinoin) induce cytodifferentiation of a wide variety of tissues and cells in culture.[2,3,24,25] RARA is expressed in hematopoietic cells and has been shown to mediate RA-induced differentiation in certain myeloid cells.[26]

ALL-*TRANS*-RETINOIC ACID IN ACUTE PROMYELOCYTIC LEUKEMIA

Clinical evaluation of tretinoin (all-*trans*-retinoic acid; RA) in acute promyelocytic leukemia (APL) was undertaken because of numerous reports that documented retinoic acid-induced differentiation of APL cells in vitro.[3,24,27] Studies of normal human bone marrow progenitor cells treated with RA in vitro suggest that normal granulopoiesis is stimulated, possibly by increasing responsiveness to cytokines and growth factors.[28] Leukemic blasts freshly obtained from patients with acute myeloid leukemia (AML) show variable responsiveness to RA exhibiting stimulation and inhibition of colony formation.[29]

REMISSION INCIDENCE

Since the original report by Huang and colleagues in 1988, studies from China, France, and the United States have conclusively documented the activity of all-*trans*-RA in (APL).[5] Table 69–17 summarizes the clinical activity of the drug in APL from reported studies in 207 of these cases.[5–9,30] The treatment groups are not homogenous because previously treated and newly diagnosed patients were included in these series. Moreover, with the recent advances using molecular genetic techniques for the diagnosis of APL, a number of patients were included in these series who had a morphologic diagnosis of APL but who did not have the disease as it can now be molecularly defined. These issues notwithstanding, the initial response to all-*trans*-RA in a patient with APL documented by cytogenetics or molecular studies is very high (95–100% if patients who died before being fully evaluated are excluded).

REMISSION DURATION

The actual number of patients maintained solely on all-*trans*-RA in continuous complete remission (CR) is quite small; nonetheless, it is clear that CRs induced by all-*trans*-RA tend to be brief. The median duration of CR in the New York series was 4 months, ranging from 1 to 10 months for 13 patients.[8] CR durations in other series are similar although a few patients in China are reported to have had CR durations exceeding 1 year.[5,6,9] Three groups have indicated that induction treatment with all-*trans*-RA, followed by "consolidation" or "maintenance" with standard chemotherapy, yields a CR duration that seems to be at least equivalent to results achieved with conventional chemotherapy, albeit with considerably shorter follow-up.[7–9] There appears to be no benefit (and there may be some disadvantage) to continuous treatment with all-*trans*-RA during complete remission.

RETINOID RESISTANCE

Patients who relapse while taking all-*trans*-RA usually cannot be reinduced into CR by further treatment with all-*trans*-RA, although there seems to be no increased resistance to reinduction with conventional chemotherapy.[5–9] One report from China suggested that occasional patients who were induced with RA and then taken off could be successfully retreated at relapse.[9] In the New York series, CR could not be recaptured in any patient who relapsed during all-*trans*-RA treatment despite a twofold escalation of the daily drug dosage.[8,31] The reasons for relapse and acquired resistance to retinoid therapy are subjects of intense research interest. Potential mechanisms include accelerated drug clearance from plasma, further acquired mutations in retinoid receptors, or sequestration by cellular retinoic acid binding proteins in normal tissues.

CLINICAL PHARMACOLOGY

Retinoic acid is normally found in the body and circulates in plasma at concentrations of approximately 1 to 2 ng/ml. Physiologic amounts of RA are likely derived by oxidation of vitamin A (retinol) that has been absorbed from the gastrointestinal tract.[18,19] An isomerase reaction may convert some of the material to 13-*cis*-RA. Pharmacologic amounts of all-*trans*-RA are highly protein bound, probably nonspecifically to albumin.[32] A membrane transport mechanism has not been identified and the drug appears to enter cells by simple diffusion where it is bound to several cellular retinoic acid-binding proteins (CRABP). RA bound to CRABP is transferred to the cell nucleus and then binds to various retinoic acid receptors. Signaling events after receptor binding of RA are poorly characterized, although a number of RA-responsive genes have been identified.

After a single oral all-*trans*-RA dose of 45 mg/m^2, peak plasma drug concentrations of approximately 300 ng/ml (10^{-6} M) are achieved within 1 to 2 hours.[31,32] The drug rapidly disappears from plasma with a half-life of approximately 40 minutes. The plasma half-life of 13-*cis*-RA is 12–14 hours.[33] Only trace amounts of RA metabolites (<1% of the administered dose) are excreted in urine. The drug does not penetrate the cerebrospinal fluid and thus the agent is not effective treatment for CNS leukemia.[32]

Continuous daily treatment with all-*trans*-RA is associated with a marked decrease in plasma drug concentrations,[31,32] an effect not observed with other retinoids.[34,35] The reduction in plasma levels has been correlated with clinical relapse in patients with APL.[31] Conceivably, relapse from remissions induced by all-*trans*-RA may be due to an inability to sustain effective "cytodifferentiating" concentrations in vivo during prolonged administration.

TABLE 69–17. Clinical Trials Using All-*trans*-Retinoic Acid as Remission Induction Treatment for Acute Promyelocytic Leukemia

Site	*No. of Patients*	*No. in Complete Remission*	*Complete Responses (%)*	*References*
Shanghai	100	85	85	5, 6
Suzhou	50	47	94	9
Paris	22	14	64	8
New York	35	27	77	8*

* And R. P. Warrell, Jr, unpublished data.

PREDICTING RESPONSE TO RETINOIC ACID WITH CELL CULTURE, CYTOGENETIC, AND MOLECULAR STUDIES

Short-term (7-day) cultures of freshly aspirated blasts from patients with APL can be cultured in the presence of RA at various concentrations (usually 10^{-6} or 10^{-7} M). The Chinese and French groups have reported that the in vitro response to all-*trans*-RA predicts for clinical effectiveness.[5,7,9] However, the interpretation of differentiation in vitro is somewhat more qualitative than quantitative, and clinical exigencies often dictate the choice of treatment before obtaining such results. Relapsing patients may retain in vitro sensitivity to the drug yet remain clinically resistant.[31]

APL is associated with a specific cytogenetic abnormality, t(15;17), that results in the fusion of the *RARA* gene on chromosome 17 with a previously unknown gene, initially named *MYL,* and now renamed *PML* (for promyelocytic leukemia).[36–38]

It appears that the initial clinical response to all-*trans*-RA is most closely correlated with presence of the t(15;17) translocation as assessed by conventional cytogenetics or by molecular detection of the rearranged RARA receptor.[39,40] Molecular testing is usually performed using probes for *RARA* and Northern blot analysis or by reverse transcriptase-polymerase chain reaction (RT/PCR) using specific primers.[41] Each of these tests varies in its sensitivity and specificity, and proper interpretation of the laboratory result is critical. A cytogenetic result that indicates the presence of the t(15;17) is pathognomonic for APL, is associated with molecular rearrangement of the RARA receptor, and is positively correlated with clinical response to all-*trans*-RA. A "negative" result—indicating a normal karyotype or technical failure—is problematic. Some patients with typical or equivocal evidence of APL by light microscopy and with reportedly normal karyotypes have shown the typical rearrangement of RAR-α by molecular testing, and each of these patients subsequently responded to all-*trans*-RA. All patients tested who have had a negative RT/PCR test for the *RARA* mutation also failed to exhibit t(15;17) by cytogenetic analysis, and none of these patients responded clinically.[41] This result is not surprising, because relatively few metaphases are evaluated by cytogenetics, but only minute amounts of rearranged *RARA*-encoded mRNA are necessary to detect the mutation.

ADVERSE CLINICAL EFFECTS

Compared with most anticancer drugs used in oncologic practice, all-*trans*-RA must be considered highly safe with few serious adverse reactions. The drug shares adverse reactions common to other retinoids and its principal side effects are listed in Table 69–18.

Headache occurring several hours after drug ingestion is the most common side effect of all-*trans*-RA. Mild analgesics generally suffice for control and the patient usually develops a tolerance to the effect. Pseudotumor cerebri, a known consequence of vitamin A toxicity, has been documented in several patients. These persons have required serial lumbar punctures, high-dose corticosteroids, and narcotic analgesics. Children have proven markedly more sensitive than adults to the CNS effects of all-*trans*-RA, and this effect is dose limiting in children.

TABLE 69–18. Adverse Effects of All-*Trans*-Retinoic Acid

Skin or Mucous Membranes
Skin dryness, itching, peeling
Genital excoriations
Angular cheilitis, lip cracking

Central Nervous System
Headache
Intracranial hypertension ("pseudotumor cerebri")

Metabolic Effects
Hypertriglyceridemia
Hypercholesterolemia

Hematologic Effects
Marked leukocytosis

Gastrointestinal Effects
Hepatic toxicity (increased SGOT, alkaline phosphatase, bilirubin)

Cardiovascular Effects
Congestive heart failure
Fluid overload
Lower extremity edema
Episodic hypotension
Decreased left ventricular ejection fraction
Pericardial effusion

Pulmonary Effects
Respiratory distress
Pleural effusion
Radiographic infiltrates

Dry skin, itching, flaking, nasal stuffiness, xerostomia, and cheilitis are relatively common although these reactions rarely disabling. Skin and mucous membrane effects can be managed with topical lubricants. Occasional scrotal and penile ulcerations have been observed. Bone pain occurs in 10% to 20% of patients. This effect tends to occur early during remission induction and usually remits despite continued therapy. The pain may transiently become quite intense and narcotics can be required for adequate analgesia.

Hypertriglyceridemia, a known side effect of other retinoids, has been observed with all-*trans*-RA. Hypercholesterolemia occurs to a less striking degree. Adverse consequences specifically related to hyperlipidemia have not been described. Retinoids are fat soluble and restrictions on dietary fat may decrease bioavailability of the drug. Hepatic toxicity is a well-known side effect of retinoids. Transient increases in serum transaminases, alkaline phosphatase, and bilirubin have been observed during RA treatment, and these effects may persist for several weeks after the drug is stopped. Permanent liver damage (even in posttransplant patients) has not been reported. As a group, the retinoids are exceptionally potent teratogens. All-*trans*-RA should not be administered to women who are pregnant, and a pregnancy test should be performed before therapeutic use in women of child-bearing age.

Leukocytosis (increase in peripheral leukocytes to $\geq$20,000 cells/mm^3) may occur in as many as 40% of APL patients treated with all-*trans*-RA. Although the development of leukocytosis was originally equated with an unfavorable outcome, additional experience suggests that an elevated leukocyte count, unaccompanied by the "retinoic acid syndrome," actually represents a positive biologic response to the drug and requires no specific treatment in the absence of other signs of leukostasis.[7] The peripheral blood leukocytes comprise a spectrum of myeloid cells including myeloblasts, promyelocytes, "intermediate cells", and granulocytes. Disseminated intravascular coagulopathy is usually not exacerbated by the leukocytosis.

Approximately 10% to 20% of patients with APL treated with all-*trans*-RA have experienced a syndrome characterized by high fever, respiratory distress, radiographic pulmonary infiltrates, and pleural or pericardial effusions.[42] This syndrome has occasionally been accompanied by impaired myocardial contractility and episodic hypotension. Although originally attributed to pneumonia or congestive heart failure, this reaction is now seen as a characteristic feature of all-*trans*-RA treatment in APL and represents by far the most serious reaction encountered with the use of this agent. Autopsy has revealed extensive infiltration of myeloid cells into lungs, skin, kidney, liver, and lymph nodes. Although leukocytosis is frequently observed with this syndrome, onset of the reaction may occur with a relatively normal leukocyte count in up to one third of cases.[42]

After reports of benefit in the "capillary leak syndrome" associated with interleukin-2 treatment, short courses of corticosteroids (*e.g.*, dexamethasone, 10 mg intravenously every 12 hours for 3 or more days) have been used and clinical symptoms have reversed in some patients.[42,43] Early recognition of the syndrome (especially unexplained fever and dyspnea) is critical, and the appearance of these signs should prompt immediate steroid treatment.

RETINOIC ACID-INDUCED DIFFERENTIATION

Although differentiation as a practical method of cancer treatment has been difficult to document conclusively, several lines of suggest that differentiation is a principal effect of all-*trans*-RA. This evidence includes changes in morphology, increased proliferative activity demonstrated by RNA/DNA flow cytometry, emergence of mature antigens on the surface of leukemic cells by immunophenotype studies, and persistence of the 15;17 translocation in morphologically mature cells documented by fluorescence in situ hybridization. One of the most distinctive aspects of all-*trans*-RA treatment is the appearance of cells derived from the leukemic clone visibly undergoing maturation. This process is obvious in the bone marrow and in the peripheral blood where cells can be found that are intermediate in maturation between promyelocytes and neutrophils.[8] Typically, these cells form indented vacuolated nuclei and lose their hypergranular appearance. Occasionally, one or more Auer rods can be found in the peripheral blood in cells that otherwise appear as mature polymorphonuclear neutrophils.

Using DNA/RNA flow cytometry, the S-phase component generally remains unchanged or increases during treatment with all-*trans*-RA.[44,45] This effect is clearly distinct from cytotoxic therapy (including low-dose cytosine arabinoside) wherein the proportion of cells in S-phase decreases markedly. Consistent with the phenomenon of leukocytosis described above, this effect probably indicates that cells treated with all-*trans*-RA in vivo undergo one or more cycles of mitosis before maturing to a cell incapable of further division. In studies of APL patients, cell surface immunophenotyping of the neoplastic cells showed progression from a pattern of immature marker expression at presentation toward the appearance of mature granulocytic markers during remission; however, midway during remission induction, morphologically maturing cells were observed in the peripheral blood that simultaneously expressed mature and immature markers on the same cell (Fig. 69–18).[8] Using fluorescence in situ hybridization (FISH), the karyotypes of maturing cells in peripheral blood have been examined for the presence of clonal abnormalities by using a molecular probe for chromosome 17.[46] The PCC/FISH studies showed that approximately one third of these mature cells contained the chromosome 17 translocation while patients were undergoing induction treatment. After achieving complete remission, however, no mature cells containing the chromosome 17 translocation could be found.

Although this evidence is important, none of these data conclusively document that differentiation is the only mechanism whereby all-*trans*-RA exerts a therapeutic effect. To the extent that leukemic cells suppress normal hematopoiesis, all-*trans*-RA may cause a modest antiproliferative effect on the leukemic clone that could still be sufficient to eventually permit regrowth of normal cells. There is also no evidence that an abundance of mature cells derived from the leukemic

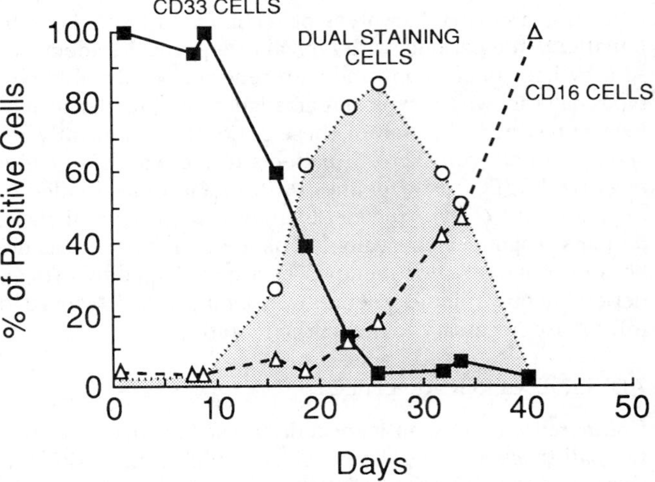

FIGURE 69–18. Cell immunophenotyping studies of peripheral blood leukocytes taken from a patient with acute promyelocytic leukemia undergoing treatment with all-*trans*-retinoic acid. Surface marker studies were performed to show the presence of cells that expressed only immature (CD33; *closed squares, solid line*) or mature (CD16; *open diamonds, dashed line*) myeloid surace antigens. A unique population of "intermediate" cells transiently appeared between days 15 and 33 of treatment (*open circles, dotted line*) that simultaneously disappeared as the patient entered complete remission (day 40), when only mature cell surface antigens were expressed. (Data provided by D. A. Scheinberg and reprinted with permission from Warrell RP Jr, Frankel SR, Miller WH Jr, et al. Differentiation therapy of acute promyelocytic leukemia with tretinoin [all-*trans*-retinoic acid]. N Engl J Med 1991;324:1385–1393)

clone persist during complete remission. However, the tests used to evaluate ongoing differentiation during remission (*e.g.*, immunophenotyping, PCC/FISH) are relatively insensitive. Studies using detection of restriction fragment length polymorphisms are clearly desirable to further explore this proposed mechanism.[47]

13-*CIS*-RETINOIC ACID

Due to its widespread availability, 13-*cis*-retinoic acid (isotretinoin) has been broadly evaluated as a method of cancer treatment and cancer prevention; the field has been extensively reviewed.[48,49] Because of the established relation between retinoic acid and the physiologic maturation of squamous epithelium, particular emphasis has been placed on the study of isotretinoin in preneoplastic and fully cancerous lesions of that tissue.

Effects in Squamous Neoplasms

Hong and colleagues demonstrated isotretinoin to be effective in reversing oral leukoplakia, a known precursor to squamous cancer.[50] The principal toxic effects of cheilitis, facial erythema, and dryness and peeling of the skin were acceptable in most patients. They were able to maintain remission of leukoplakia by a low-dose regimen of isotretinoin.[51] In a follow-up study, Hong and colleagues demonstrated that 12 months of therapy with high oral doses of isotretinoin significantly reduced the incidence of second primary cancers in patients who were free of disease from a previously treated squamous cell carcinoma of the head and neck.[52] The isotretinoin therapy had no evident effect on the rate or timing of recurrence of the original primary cancer. The isotretinoin dosage used in the study produced significant side effects; one third of the isotretinoin patients did not complete the planned 12-month course because of toxicity or noncompliance. Less toxic regimens are being sought.

Meyskens and Lippman observed objective antitumor effects of isotretinoin in advanced squamous cell carcinoma of the skin; however, the major response rates with the drug as a single agent were low.[53,54] Lippman and coworkers subsequently evaluated the combination of isotretinoin and interferon-α-2a in patients with advanced squamous cell cancer of the skin or cervix.[55,56] The preclinical basis for this combination was that interferon, a known differentiating agent, was synergistic with retinoic acid in differentiation induction of HL-60 and neuroblastoma and in growth inhibition in four additional human cell lines.[4,57–59] The drug dosages were identical in the skin and cervix cancer trials (isotretinoin, 1 mg/kg/day orally; interferon α-2a, 3 million units daily by subcutaneous injection).

In 32 patients with advanced cutaneous squamous cell carcinoma of the skin, 19 of 28 evaluable patients had a major response; the response was complete in 7 patients (25%).[55] Major response was observed in 13 of 14 patients with advanced local disease, 4 of 6 with regional disease, and 2 of 8 with distant metastases. The median duration of response was greater than 5 months. In the trial in patients with squamous cervix cancer, the isotretinoin plus interferon combination produced a major response in 13 of 26 patients; at the time of assessment, 9 of the 13 "nonresponders" had stable disease, and only 4 patients demonstrated frank progression.[56] Although it cannot be stated that these antitumor responses are the result of drug-induced differentiation rather than immune modulation or some other mechanism, the two drugs produce synergistic differentiating effects in at least two cell model systems. Moreover, cytotoxic side effects in normal organ systems were limited to granulocytopenia in a small proportion of the treatment population.

Effects in Hematopoietic Neoplasms and Embryonal Tumors

Because of the differentiation induction of retinoic acid in leukemic and embryonal tumor models isotretinoin has also been evaluated in myeloproliferative disorders and germ cell neoplasms. It is not clear whether 13-*cis*-retinoic acid has significant activity APL. There are scattered reports of responses and failures in this disorder; however, a detailed assessment has not been undertaken.[27,60–63]

Isotretinoin has produced transient responses in patients with mycosis fungoides, but it did not produce useful effects in an extended evaluation in patients with myelodysplastic syndromes.[64,65,66–68] It was also inactive in a phase II assessment in patients with nonseminomatous germ cell tumors.[69]

1,25-DIHYDROXYVITAMIN D_3

1α,25-dihydroxyvitamin D_3 ($1,25(OH)_2D_3$), the active form of the hormone, contributes to physiologic differentiation in a variety of cell types.[70] The biologic effects of $1,25(OH)_2D_3$ are mediated through interaction with nuclear receptors analogous to thyroid, steroid, and retinoic acid receptors.[71] These receptors have been identified in a variety of cells, including normal and neoplastic cells of hematopoietic, colonic, and breast epithelial lineages.[72–74] Epidemiologic data suggest that an adequate dietary vitamin D intake reduces the incidence of colorectal cancer, and calcium or vitamin D supplementation protects against induction of colon cancer in some rodent models.[75–77] $1,25(OH)_2D_3$ is growth inhibitory to breast, colonic, and melanoma cancer cell lines, but does not induce differentiation;[78–81] However, it greatly enhances butyrate-induced differentiation in colon cancer cell lines.[79,80]

$1,25(OH)_2D_3$ induces differentiation of HL-60 cells along the monocyte-macrophage pathway.[82–84] Koeffler and colleagues demonstrated that a high concentration of $1,25(OH)_2D_3$ (10^{-6} M) induced in vitro differentiation of blast cells from patients with acute myeloblastic leukemia as assessed by morphology, phagocytosis, and superoxide production.[85] At a lower concentration (10^{-9} M), there was no effect. Based on these results, this group treated 18 patients with myelodysplastic syndrome with 2 μg/day of $1,25(OH)_2D_3$; 8 patients had partial or minor peripheral blood responses during the period of drug administration. However, no patient showed significant improvement of peripheral blood or bone marrow findings, and 9 patients developed hypercalcemia that precluded further study.[85] New analogs of vitamin D_3 have been synthesized that retain the differentiating activity while minimizing effects on calcium mobilization.[86–88] Several of these agents have been proposed for clinical investigation.

LOW-DOSE CYTOSINE ARABINOSIDE

In low concentrations, cytosine arabinoside (ara-C) induces terminal cytodifferentiation in HL-60 and K562 leukemia cells.[89–92] At higher concentrations, ara-C produces cytotoxic effects by inhibition of DNA synthesis and by incorporation into DNA and RNA. The mechanism by which ara-C and other inhibitors of DNA synthesis produce cellular differentiation in culture is not established. In HL-60 and K562 cells it is postulated that a low but predictable rate of terminal differentiation occurs in the absence of added inducers. At "subcytotoxic" concentrations, ara-C may slow the rate of DNA synthesis and prolong the S phase, causing a shift in the cellular balance from proliferation toward differentiation.

Low-dose ara-C has been extensively evaluated in patients with myelodysplastic syndromes and in elderly persons with AML.[93–97] A variety of dosages and schedules have been examined. Although complete remissions have been induced in some patients, it remains unclear whether low-dose ara-C merits an established place in the management of these diseases. It is also uncertain to what extent these regimens produce their effects by cytodifferentiation, rather than by cytotoxicity.

In a review of the published results on 751 patients treated with low-dose ara-C up to 1986, Cheson and coworkers projected the following CR rates for the 507 evaluable patients: 32% for patients with primary AML; 16% for AML secondary to prior chemotherapy; and 16% for patients with myelodysplastic syndromes (MDS).[98] The median survival of these three groupings was 9 months, 3 months, and 15 months, respectively.[98] The status of low-dose ara-C has also been reviewed for MDS.[99,100] In a randomized prospective comparison study of low-dose ara-C versus supportive therapy, the CR rate from low-dose ara-C was only 8%.[101] Despite a longer progression-free survival in ara-C treated patients, total survival was similar in the two groups (8.7 versus 6.9 months with ara-C and supportive care). Although response rates may be higher in some subgroups of the myelodysplastic syndromes, low-dose ara-C does not have an established role in management of MDS.

Although some contribution of differentiation induction to the therapeutic effects produced by low-dose ara-C can not be excluded, the available data suggest that the principal mechanism was cytotoxicity. Myelosuppression was evident in 88% of patients.[98] In patients for whom bone marrow hypoplasia was not observed, concerns have been raised about the frequency of observation. Although examples of mature cells with the malignant genotype have been reported in patients undergoing low-dose ara-C therapy, the heterogeneity of the entities under treatment and the paucity of observations do not permit definitive conclusions.

TIAZOFURIN

Tiazofurin is one of a numerous inhibitors of purine synthesis developed as candidate anticancer agents. Their synthesis was stimulated by observations that cancer cells commonly have upregulated the guanylate biosynthetic pathway by increased expression of inosine 5′-monophosphate (IMP) dehydrogenase, the rate-limiting step in guanylate biosynthesis.[102] Recent studies demonstrate that two isoenzymes of IMP dehydrogenase exist in human cells.[103] Neoplastic cells display a selective increase in mRNA for the type II isoenzyme, while the rate of expression of type I IMP dehydrogenase mRNA remains relatively constant.[103–105]

Tiazofurin (2-β-D-ribofuranosylthiazole-4-carboxamide), is metabolized to tiazofurin adenine dinucleotide, a highly selective inhibitor of IMP dehydrogenase.[106,107] The drug has displayed cytotoxic and cytodifferentiating effects in cell culture systems, with a clear correlation between these effects and a decrease in cellular levels of GTP.[108–111] Consistent with this proposed relation, tiazofurin-induced differentiation in cell culture can be reproduced by mycophenolic acid, another inhibitor of IMP dehydrogenase, and abrogated by the addition of guanosine to the culture medium.[107–111]

Tricot and colleagues have treated patients with refractory acute myeloblastic leukemia and blast crisis of chronic myelocytic leukemia with a protocol combining tiazofurin and allopurinol.[112,113] The concept of the protocol is to lower cellular GTP pools by the combined effects of inhibition of IMP dehydrogenase (through tiazofurin) and inhibition of guanine salvage (guanine plus hypoxanthine/guanine phosphoribosyl transferase plus PRPP with or without guanylate plus ribose-1-phosphate) by elevating plasma hypoxanthine levels through the use of allopurinol. Hypoxanthine and guanine are competitive substrates for the purine salvage pathway but hypoxanthine would enter the guanylate pools only through the action of IMP dehydrogenase.

The regimen appears to have produced the greatest therapeutic effect in patients with blast crisis of CML; 9 of 11 patients returned to the chronic phase of the disorder.[113] One patient with AML in first relapse achieved a complete remission of 10 months duration.[112] Although the response in AML was considered to be due to the drug's cytotoxic effects, the absence of marrow hypoplasia and the consistent presence of chromosomal abnormalities in the responding CML patients suggested differentiation induction as a contributing mechanism.[112] Although of considerable theoretic interest, this program is not readily extended to wide usage as it required frequent specialized biochemical observations and tiazofurin dose adjustments. Adverse effects included drowsiness, nausea, vomiting, pleuropericarditis, headache, skin rash, myalgia and hypertension.

PLANAR-POLAR INDUCERS

Hexamethylene bisacetamide (HMBA) entered clinical trials largely because of its capacity to induce terminal differentiation in murine erythroleukemia cells (MELC). The studies with HMBA extended the original observations of Friend and colleagues with dimethyl sulfoxide (DMSO).[114] HMBA and related planar-polar compounds induce differentiation in numerous other neoplastic cell lines.[115] This field has been the subject of several recent reviews.[1,116,117] Numerous biochemical events have been associated with HMBA-induced differentiation; recent data indicate that the drug produces an activation of the β isozyme of protein kinase C.[118,119] The effects of HMBA mimic those of transforming growth factor-β (TGF-β) in a number of systems. The two agents are synergistic in MELC.[120] However, in the HT29 colon cancer cell line, the effects of HMBA appear to result from its capacity to induce the synthesis of TGF-β1.[121,122]

The initial clinical evaluations of HMBA have been based on drug concentrations and durations of exposure derived from the extensive studies in the MELC system. In all cell culture models, prolonged exposure to HMBA has been required to induce cellular commitment to differentiation. In MELC, 1 mM was the minimal effective concentration in 5-day cultures; 5 mM was optimal, producing erythroid differentiation in over 95% of cells, and 10 mM was cytotoxic. Most clinical studies of HMBA have employed continuous intravenous infusions given for 5 or 10 days. The 5-day regimens used steady-state HMBA levels between 1 and 2 mM.[123,124] In the 10-day regimens, the $[HMBA]_{ss}$ has been 1 mM.[125] Renal and central nervous system toxicity precluded the use of steady state concentrations $\geq$2 mM.[123,124] The limiting side effect of prolonged infusions has been thrombocytopenia. Because HMBA is rapidly cleared from plasma, and the drug is only moderately soluble, intravenous treatment programs have required administration of large fluid volumes.[123–126] Although extended studies of the intravenous drug have been limited, these impediments may be obviated by the development of an oral formulation and the documentation that oral HMBA is fully bioavailable.[127]

There have been no major clinical responses to HMBA given by the 5-day schedule in the phase I studies or in a subsequent phase II assessment in patients with myelodysplastic syndromes (MDS).[123,124,128] With the 10-day schedule, one sustained complete response has been observed in a patient with lung cancer.[125] Although 5-day courses of HMBA produced no apparent remissions in MDS, Andreeff and coworkers observed 2 CRs and 6 PRs in 22 evaluable patients with MDS or acute myeloid leukemia treated on a 10-day schedule.[128,129] In 1 patient with monosomy 7 who entered CR, HMBA administration produced an increase in granulocytes with the monosomy 7 marker, as demonstrated by direct FISH.

The extensive excretion of HMBA and active metabolites in the urine, coupled with the availability of an oral formulation of HMBA, make it a potentially useful chemotherapeutic or chemopreventive agent in patients with recurrent superficial bladder tumors.[126,130,131] Russo and colleagues have demonstrated that HMBA has growth-inhibitory effects on bladder cancer cells in studies with short-term culture of shed cells and with an established cell line.[132]

Future studies of planar-polar compounds may also involve assessment of newer analogs, several of which are approximately 100-fold more active than HMBA in differentiation induction in the MELC system.[133] One of these compounds demonstrates a 33-fold increase in growth-inhibitory potency against the HT-29 human colon cancer line.

CYCLIC AMP MODULATION

Increase cytodifferentiation is observed in a broad range of cell culture systems with the combined use of "triggering agents" (*e.g.*, retinoic acid, HMBA, interferons) and substances that increase intracellular levels of 3′,5′-cyclic adenosine monophosphate (cAMP) by inducing an increase in its synthesis (*e.g.*, cholera toxin, PGE_1, forskolin, isoproterenol) or a decrease in its degradation by phosphodiesterase (*e.g.*, isobutylmethylxanthine).[134–137] Analogs of cAMP (*e.g.*, dibutyryl-cAMP, 8-Br-cAMP) are also effective for this purpose.[138,139] cAMP modulation is only a weak inducer of cytodifferentiation in the absence of the triggering agents. Although widely examined in the preclinical systems, differentiation regimens including a cAMP modulatory component have not yet received a meaningful clinical assessment.

CONCLUSIONS

With the striking exception of the major therapeutic activity of all-*trans*-retinoic acid in treating APL, the use of single agents to induce differentiation and eventual regression of advanced cancer has been clinically disappointing. Success of differentiation therapy may be increased by the use of combination regimens. Except for the combination of isotretinoin and interferon-α, combination regimens have not received extended clinical evaluation. Nevertheless combination regimens of differentiating agents themselves are possible and justified by preclinical data. Many of the triggering agents (*e.g.*, retinoic acid, DMSO, HMBA, $1,25(OH)_2D_3$, interferons) have nonoverlapping toxicities but produce enhanced differentiation effects in combination.[140] It is reasonable to explore the combined use of inducers with pharmacologic modulators needed to maintain adequate plasma concentrations of the active agent, or inducers with enhancing agents (*e.g.*, cAMP-elevating regimens).

Differentiation therapy was initially conceived as altering the phenotypic behavior of neoplastic cells, rather than eliminating that population. Theoretically, this could result in a pseudochimeric state in which a morphologically normal mixture of genetically normal and abnormal cells would be present on a continuing basis. In APL patients in complete remission after therapy with all-*trans*-retinoic acid, the *RARA/PML* gene fusion is frequently detectable by PCR techniques; however, the numbers of genetically abnormal cells are dramatically decreased, implying a therapy-induced adjustment of the proliferative balance between the normal and neoplastic cell populations.

What is the proper dosage schedule and duration for new candidate differentiation regimens? In the successful treatment of APL and the encouraging regimens for squamous cancers of skin and cervix the drugs are given daily for weeks or months. Because drug-induced differentiation does not kill cells acutely, even differentiated cells may survive for prolonged periods, and some tumor cells may resume proliferation when therapy is interrupted. Chronic therapy of some weeks' duration may be more likely to show a clinical effect than a more intense course that can only be given a few days each month.

It is reasonable to explore possible interface between cytotoxic and differentiation regimens. Currently, differentiation therapy appears to work best when the target cells have a low number of genetic mutations. When this concept is extended to precancerous lesions, differentiation therapy merges with chemoprevention. The use of isotretinoin in delaying the development of new primary head and neck cancer provides a paradigm for differentiation therapy after initial ablative therapy of cancer. In ongoing APL studies, the sequence is reversed. Tretinoin is used to induce remission with good patient tolerance; however, because resistance to continuous retinoid therapy is expected in most patients, responding patients are shifted to cytotoxic regimens while still in remission; the utility of this approach will be assessable over the next several years.

REFERENCES

1. Reuben RC, Khanna PL, Gazitt Y, et al. Inducers of erythroleukemic differentiation. Relationship of structure to activity among planar-polar compounds. J Biol Chem 1978;253:4214–4218.
2. Strickland S, Mahdavi V. The induction of differentiation in teratocarcinoma stem cells by retinoic acid. Cell 1978;15:393–403.
3. Breitman TR, Selonick SE, Collins SJ. Induction of differentiation of the human promyelocytic leukemia cell line (HL-60) by retinoic acid. Proc Natl Acad Sci USA 1980;77:2936–2940.
4. Rossi GB. Interferons and cell differentiation. In: Gresser I, ed. Interferon. London: Academic Press, 1985:31–68.
5. Huang ME, Ye YC, Chen JR, et al. Use of all-*trans* retinoic acid in the treatment of acute promyelocytic leukemia. Blood 1988;72:567–572.
6. Wang ZY, Sun GL, Lu JX, et al. Treatment of acute promyelocytic leukemia with all-*trans* retinoic acid in China. Nouv Rev Fr Hematol 1990;32:34–36.
7. Castaigne S, Chomienne C, Daniel MT, et al. All-*trans* retinoic acid as a differentiation therapy for acute promyelocytic leukemia: I. Clinical results. Blood 1990;76:1704–1709.
8. Warrell RP Jr, Frankel SR, Miller WH Jr, et al. Differentiation therapy of acute promyelocytic leukemia with tretinoin (all-*trans*-retinoic acid). N Engl J Med 1991;324:1385–1393.
9. Zi-Xing C, Yong-Quan X, Ri Z, et al. A clinical and experimental study of all-*trans* retinoic acid-treated acute promyelocytic leukemia patients. Blood 1991;78:1413–1419.
10. Vogelstein B, Fearon ER, Hamilton SR, et al. Genetic alterations during colorectal-tumor development. N Engl J Med 1988;319:525–532.
11. Fearon ER, Cho KR, Nigro JM, et al. Identification of a chromosome 18q gene that is altered in colorectal cancers. Science 1990;247:49–56.
12. Baker SJ, Preisinger AC, Jessup JM, et al. *P53* gene mutations occur in combination with 17p allelic deletions as late events in colorectal tumorigenesis. Cancer Res 1990;50:7712–7722.
13. Miyaki M, Seki M, Okamoto M, et al. Genetic changes and histopathological types in colorectal tumors from patients with familial adenomatous polyposis. Cancer Res 1990;50:7166–7173.
14. Sato T, Akiyama F, Sakamoto G, et al. Accumulation of genetic alterations and progression of primary breast cancer. Cancer Res 1991;51:5794–5799.
15. Kelman Z, Prokocimer M, Peller S, et al. Rearrangements in the *p53* gene in Philadelphia chromosome positive chronic myelogenous leukemia. Blood 1989;74:2318–2324.
16. Mashal R, Shtalrid M, Talpaz, et al. Rearrangement and expression of *p53* in the chronic phase and blast crisis of chronic myelogenous leukemia. Blood 1991;75:180–189.
17. Feinstein E, Cimino G, Gale RP, et al. *P53* in chronic myelogenous leukemia in acute phase. Proc Natl Acad Sci USA 1991;88:6293–6297.
18. Blomhoff R, Green MH, Green JB, et al. Vitamin A metabolism: New perspectives on absorption, transport, and storage. Physiol Rev 1991;71:951–990.
19. De Luca LM. Retinoids and their receptors in differentiation, embryogenesis, and neoplasia. FASEB J 1991;5:2924–2933.
20. Evans RM. The steroid and thyroid hormone superfamily. Science 1992;240:889–895.
21. Petkovich M, Brand NJ, Krust A, et al. A human retinoic acid receptor which belongs to the family of nuclear receptors. Nature 1987;330:444–450.
22. Giguere V, Ong ES, Segui P, et al. Identification of a receptor for the morphogen retinoic acid. Nature 1987;330:624–629.
23. Mangelsdorf DJ, Ong ES, Dyck JA, et al. Nuclear receptor that identifies a novel retinoic acid response pathway. Nature 1990;345:224–229.
24. Breitman TR, Collins SJ, Keene BR. Terminal differentiation of human promyelocytic leukemic cells in primary culture in response to retinoic acid. Blood 1981;57:1000–1004.
25. Sidell N, Altman A, Haussler M, et al. Effects of retinoic acid on the growth and phenotypic expression of several human neuroblastoma cell lines. Exp Cell Res 1983;148:21–30.
26. Collins SJ, Robertson KA, Mueller LM. Retinoic acid-induced granulocytic differentiation of HL-60 myeloid leukemia cells is mediated directly through the retinoic acid receptor (RAR-alpha). Mol Cell Biol 1990;10:2154–2163.
27. Flynn PJ, Miller WJ, Weisdorf DJ, et al. Retinoic acid treatment of acute promyelocytic leukemia: In vitro and in vivo observations. Blood 1983;62:1211–1217.
28. Douer D, Koeffler PH. Retinoic acid enhances colony stimulating factor induced growth of normal human myeloid progenitor cells in vitro. Exp Cell Res 1982;138:193–198.
29. Lawrence HJ, Conner K, Kelly MA, et al. *Cis*-retinoic acid stimulates the clonal growth of some myeloid leukemia cells in vitro. Blood 1987;69:302–307.
30. Chen Z, Sun G-L, Chen S-S, et al. All-*trans*-retinoic acid and acute promyelocytic leukemia in China: From clinic to molecular biology. Conference Proceedings for Retinoids: New Trends in Research and Clinical Application, Palermo, 1991:102.
31. Muindi J, Frankel SR, Miller WH Jr, et al. Continuous treatment with all-*trans* retinoic acid causes a progressive reduction in plasma drug concentrations: Implications for relapse and retinoid "resistance" in patients with acute promyelocytic leukemia. Blood 1992;79:299–303.
32. Muindi J, Frankel SR, Huselton, C, et al. Clinical pharmacology of oral all-*trans* retinoic acid in patients with acute promyelocytic leukemia. Cancer Res 1992;52:2138–2142.
33. Goodman GE, Einspahr JG, Alberts DS, et al. Pharmacokinetics of 13-*cis*-retinoic acid in patients with advanced cancer. Cancer Res 1982;42:2087–2091.
34. Brazzell RK, Colburn WA. Pharmacokinetics of the retinoids isotretinoin and etretinate: A comparative review. J Am Acad Dermatol 1982;6:643–651.
35. Brazell RK, Vane FM, Ehmann CW, et al. Pharmacology of isotretinoin during repetitive dosing to patients. Eur J Clin Pharmacol 1983;24:695–702.
36. Larson RA, Kondo K, Vardiman JW, et al. Evidence for a 15;17 translocation in every patient with acute promyelocytic leukemia. Am J Med 1984;76:827–841.
37. de The H, Chomienne C, Lanotte M, et al. The t(15;17) translocation of acute promyelocytic leukaemia fuses the retinoic acid receptor gene to a novel transcribed locus. Nature 1990;347:558–561.
38. Kakizuka A, Miller WH Jr, Umesono K, et al. Chromosomal translocation t(15;17) in human acute promyelocytic leukemia fuses the RAR-alpha receptor with a novel putative transcription factor PML. Cell 1991;66:663–674.
39. Biondi A, Rambaldi A, Alcalay M, et al. *RAR-α* gene rearrangements as a genetic marker for diagnosis and monitoring in acute promyelocytic leukemia. Blood 1991;77:1418–1422.
40. Miller WH Jr, Warrell RP Jr, Frankel S, et al. Novel retinoic acid receptor-α transcripts in acute promyelocytic leukemia responsive to all-*trans*-retinoic acid. JNCI 1990;82:1932–1933.
41. Miller WH, Kakizuka A, Frankel SR, et al. Reverse transcriptase/polymerase chain reaction amplification for *PML/RAR-alpha* clarifies diagnosis and detects minimal residual disease in acute promyelocytic leukemia. Proc Natl Acad Sci USA 1992;89:2694–2698.
42. Frankel SR, Weiss M, Warrell RP. A "retinoic acid syndrome" in acute promyelocytic leukemia: Reversal by corticosteroids. Blood 1991;78:380a.
43. Vetto JT, Papa MZ, Lotze MT, et al. Reduction of toxicity of Interleukin-2 and lymphokine-activated killer cells in humans by the administration of corticosteroids. J Clin Oncol 1987;5:496–503.
44. Andreeff M, Darzynkiewicz, Sharpless TK, et al. Discrimination of human leukemia subtypes by flow cytometric analysis of cellular DNA and RNA. Blood 1980;55:282–293.
45. Frankel SR, Scheinberg DA, Miller WH Jr, et al. Differentiation therapy of acute promyelocytic leukemia with all-trans retinoic acid. Proc Am Soc Clin Oncol 1991;10, 225.
46. Pinkel D, Strauma T, Gray JW. Cytogenetic analysis using quantitative, high sensitivity, fluorescence hybridization. Proc Natl Acad Sci USA 1986;83:2934–2938.
47. Fearon ER, Burke PJ, Schiffer CA, et al. Differentiation of leukemia cells to polymorphonuclear leukocytes in patients with acute nonlymphoblastic leukemia. N Engl J Med 1986;315:15–24.
48. Lippman SM, Kessler JF, Meyskens FL Jr. Retinoids as preventive and therapeutic anticancer agents (Part I). Cancer Treat Rep 1987;71:391–405.
49. Lippman SM, Kessler JF, Meyskens FL Jr. Retinoids as preventive and therapeutic anticancer agents (Part II). Cancer Treat Rep 1987;71:493–515.
50. Hong WK, Endicott J, Itri LM, et al. 13-*Cis*-retinoic acid in the treatment of oral leukoplakia. N Engl J Med 1986;315:1501–1505.
51. Lippman SM, Toth BB, Batsakis JG, et al. Low-dose 13-cis-retinoic acid maintains remission in oral premalignancy: More effective than β-carotene in randomized trial. Proc Am Soc Clin Oncol 1990;9:59.
52. Hong WK, Lippman SM, Itri LM, et al. Prevention of second primary tumors with isotretinoin in squamous cell carcinoma of the head and neck. N Engl J Med 1990;323:795–801.
53. Meyskens FL Jr, Gilmartin E, Alberts DS, et al. Activity of isotretinoin against squamous cell cancers and preneoplastic lesions. Cancer Treat Rep 1982;66:1315–1319.
54. Lippman SM, Meyskens FL Jr. Treatment of advanced squamous cell carcinoma of the skin with isotretinoin. Ann Intern Med 1987;107:499–501.
55. Lippman SM, Parkinson DR, Itri LM, et al. 13-*Cis*-retinoic acid and interferon α-2a: Effective combination therapy for advanced squamous cell carcinoma of the skin. JNCI 1992;84:235–241.
56. Lippman SM, Kavanagh JJ, Paredes-Espinoza M, et al. 13-*Cis*-retinoic acid plus interferon α-2a: Highly active systemic therapy for squamous cell carcinoma of the cervix. JNCI 1992;84:241–245.
57. Hemmi H, Breitman TR. Combinations of recombinant human interferons and retinoic acid synergistically induce differentiation of the human promyelocytic leukemia cell line HL-60. Blood 1987;69:501–507.
58. Higuchi T, Hannigan GE, Malkin D, et al. Enhancement by retinoic acid and dibutyryl cyclic adenosine 3′,5′-monophosphate of the differentiation and gene expression of human neuroblastoma cells induced by interferon. Cancer Res 1991;51:3958–3964.
59. Frey JR, Peck R, Bollag W. Antiproliferative activity of retinoids, interferon α and their combination in five human transformed cell lines. Cancer Lett 1991;57:223–227.
60. Nilsson B. Probable in vivo induction of differentiation by retinoic acid of promyelocytes in acute promyelocytic leukemia. Br J Haematol 1984;57:365–371.
61. Daenen S, Vellenga E, van Dobbenburgh OA, et al. Retinoic acid as antileukemic therapy in a patient with acute promyelocytic leukemia and *Aspergillus* pneumonia. Blood 1986;67:559–561.
62. Fontana JA, Rogers JS, Durham JP. The role of 13 *cis*-retinoic acid in the remission induction of a patient with acute promyelocytic leukemia. Cancer 1989;57:209–217.
63. Wijermans PW, Rebel VI, Ossenkoppele GJ, et al. Combined procoagulant activity

and proteolytic activity of acute promyelocytic leukemic cells: Reversal of the bleeding disorder by cell differentiation. Blood 1989;73:800–805.

64. Kessler JF, Meyskens FL Jr, Levine N, et al. Treatment of cutaneous T-cell lymphoma (mycosis fungoides) with 13-*cis*-retinoic acid. Lancet 1983;1:1345–1347.
65. Warrell RP Jr, Coonley CJ, Kempin SJ, et al. Isotretinoin in cutaneous T-cell lymphoma. Lancet 1983;1:629.
66. Greenberg BR, Durie BGM, Barnett TC, et al. Phase I–II study of 13-*cis*-retinoic acid in myelodysplastic syndrome. Cancer Treat Rep 1985;69:1369–1374.
67. Picozzi VJ, Swanson GF, Morgan R, et al. 13-*Cis* retinoic acid treatment for myelodysplastic syndromes. J Clin Oncol 1986;4:589–595.
68. Koeffler HP, Heitjan D, Mertelsmann R, et al. Randomized study of 13-*cis* retinoic acid *vs* placebo in the myelodysplastic disorders. Blood 1988;71:703–708.
69. Gold EJ, Bosl GJ, Itri LM. Phase II trial of 13-*cis* retinoic acid in patients with advanced nonseminomatous germ cell tumors. Cancer Treat Rep 1984;68:1287–1288.
70. Suda T, Shinki T, Takahashi N. The role of vitamin D in bone and intestinal cell differentiation. Annu Rev Nutr 1990;10:195–211.
71. Fuller PJ. The steroid receptor superfamily: Mechanisms of diversity. FASEB J 1991;5: 3092–3099.
72. Kizaki M, Norman AW, Bishop JE, et al. 1,25-dihydroxyvitamin D_3 receptor RNA. Expression in hematopoietic cells. Blood 1991;77:1238–1247.
73. Meggouh F, Lointier P, Saez S. Sex steroid and 1,25-dihydroxyvitamin D_3 receptors in human colorectal adenocarcinoma and normal mucosa. Cancer Res 1991;51:1227–1233.
74. Eisman JA, Suva LJ, Sher E, et al. Frequency of 1,25-dihydroxyvitamin D_3 receptor in human breast cancer. Cancer Res 1981;41:5121–5124.
75. Garland C, Shekelle RB, Barrett-Connor E, et al. Dietary vitamin D and calcium and risk of colorectal cancer: A 19 year prospective study in men. Lancet 1985;1:307–309.
76. Pence BC, Buddingh F. Inhibition of dietary fat-promoted colon carcinogenesis in rats by supplemental calcium or vitamin D. Carcinogenesis 1988;9:187–190.
77. Sitrin MD, Halline AG, Abrahams C, et al. Dietary calcium and vitamin D modulate 1,2-dimethylhydrazine-induced colonic carcinogenesis in the rat. Cancer Res 1991;51: 5608–5613.
78. Frampton RJ, Omond SA, Eisman JA. Inhibition of human cancer cell growth by 1,25-dihydroxyvitamin D_3 metabolites. Cancer Res 1983;43:4443–4447.
79. Tanaka Y, Bush KK, Klauck TM, et al. Enhancement of butyrate-induced differentiation of HT-29 human colon carcinoma cells by 1,25-dihydroxyvitamin D_3. Biochem Pharmacol 1989;38:3859–3865.
80. Tanaka Y, Bush KK, Eguchi T, et al. Effects of 1,25-dihydroxyvitamin D_3 and its analogs on butyrate-induced differentiation of HT-29 human colonic carcinoma cells and on the reversal of the differentiated phenotype. Arch Biochem Biophys 1990;276:415–423.
81. Colston K, Colston MJ, Feldman D. 1,25-Dihydroxyvitamin D_3 and malignant melanoma: The presence of receptors and inhibition of cell growth in culture. Endocrinology 1981;108:1083–1086.
82. McCarthy DM, San Miguel JF, Freake HC, et al. 1,25-Dihydroxyvitamin D_3 inhibits proliferation of human promyelocytic leukemia (HL60) cells and induces monocyte-macrophage differentiation in HL60 and normal human bone marrow cells. Leuk Res 1983;7:51–55.
83. Tanaka H, Abe E, Miyaura C, et al. 1,25-Dihydroxyvitamin D_3 induces differentiation of human promyelocytic leukemia cells (HL-60) into monocyte-macrophages, but not into granulocytes. Biochem Biophys Res Comm 1983;117:86–92.
84. Manglesdorf DJ, Koeffler HP, Donaldson CA, et al. 1,25-Dihydroxyvitamin-D_3-induced differentiation in a human promyelocytic leukemia cell (HL-60): Receptor-mediated maturation to macrophage-like cells. J Cell Biol 1984;98:391–398.
85. Koeffler HP, Hirji K, Itri L, et al. 1,25-Dihydroxyvitamin D_3: In vivo and in vitro effects on human preleukemic and leukemic cells. Cancer Treat Rep 1985;69:1399–1407.
86. Zhou J-Y, Norman AW, Lubbert ED, et al. Novel vitamin D analogues that modulate leukemic cell growth and differentiation with little effect on either intestinal calcium absorption or bone calcium mobilization. Blood 1989;74:82–93.
87. Perlman K, Kutner A, Prahl J, et al. 24-Homologated 1,25-dihydroxyvitamin D_3 compounds: Separation of calcium and cell differentiation activities. Biochemistry 1990;29: 190–196.
88. Norman AW, Jhou JY, Henry HL, et al. Structure-function studies on analogues of 1α,25-dihydroxyvitamin D_3: Differential effects on leukemic cell growth, differentiation, and intestinal calcium absorption. Cancer Res 1990;50:6857–6864.
89. Lotem J, Sachs L. Different blocks in the differentiation of myeloid leukemic cells. Proc Natl Acad Sci USA 1974;71:3507–3511.
90. Sachs L. The differentiation of myeloid leukaemic cells: New possibilities for therapy. Br J Haematol 1978;40:509–517.
91. Griffin J, Munroe D, Major P, et al. Induction of differentiation of human myeloid leukemia cells by inhibitors of DNA synthesis. Exp Hematol 1982;10:774–781.
92. Luisi-DeLuca C, Mitchell T, Spriggs D, et al. Induction of terminal differentiation in human K562 erythroleukemia cells by arabinofuranosylcytosine. J Clin Invest 1984;74: 821–827.
93. Baccarani M, Tura S. Differentiation of myeloid leukemia cells: New possibilities for therapy. Br J Haematol 1979;42:485–487.
94. Castaigne S, Daniel MT, Tilly H, et al. Does treatment with ara-C in low dosage cause differentiation of leukemic cells? Blood 1983;62:85–86.
95. Wisch JS, Griffin JD, Kufe DW. Response of preleukemic syndromes to continuous infusion of low-dose cytarabine. N Engl J Med 1983;309:1599–1602.
96. Ishikura H, Sawada H, Okazaki T, et al. The effect of low dose ARA-C in acute non-lymphoblastic leukaemias and atypical leukaemia. Br J Haematol 1984;58:9–18.
97. Degos L, Castaigne S, Tilly H, et al. Treatment of leukemia with low-dose ara-C. A study of 160 cases. Semin Oncol 1985;12(suppl 3):196–199.
98. Cheson BD, Jasperse DM, Simon R, et al. A critical appraisal of low-dose cytosine arabinoside in patients with acute non-lymphocytic leukemia and myelodysplastic syndromes. J Clin Oncol 1986;4:1857–1864.
99. Cheson BD. The myelodysplastic syndromes: Current approaches to therapy. Ann Intern Med 1990;112:932–941.
100. List AF, Garewal HS, Sandberg AA. The myelodysplastic syndromes: Biology and implications for management. J Clin Oncol 1990;8:1424–1441.
101. Miller KB, Kim K, Morrison FS, et al. Evaluation of low dose ara-C versus supportive care in the treatment of myelodysplastic syndromes: An intergroup study by the Eastern Cooperative Oncology Group and the Southwest Oncology Group. Blood 72(suppl 1): 215A.
102. Weber G. Biochemical strategy of cancer cells and the design of chemotherapy: G.H.A. Clowes Memorial Lecture. Cancer Res 1983;43:3466–3492.
103. Natsumeda Y, Ohno S, Kawasaki H, et al. Two distinctive cDNAs for human IMP dehydrogenase. J Biol Chem 1990;265:5292–5295.
104. Konno Y, Natsumeda Y, Nagai M, et al. Expression of human IMP dehydrogenase types I and II in Escherichia coli and distribution in human normal lymphocytes and leukemic cell lines. J Biol Chem 1991;266:506–509.
105. Nagai M, Natsumeda Y, Konno Y, et al. Selective up-regulation of type II inosine 5′-monophosphate dehydrogenase messenger RNA expression in human leukemias. Cancer Res 1991;51:3886–3890.
106. Cooney DA, Jayaram HN, Gebeyehu G, et al. The conversion of 2-β-D-ribofuranosylthiazole-4-carboxamide to an analogue of NAD with potent IMP dehydrogenase inhibitory properties. Biochem Pharmacol 1982;31:2133–2136.
107. Jayaram HN, Dion RL, Glazer RI, et al. Initial studies on the mechanism of action of a new oncolytic thiazole nucleoside, 2-β-D-ribofuranosylthizole-4-carboxamide (NSC 286193). Biochem Pharmacol 1982;31:2371–2380.
108. Olah E, Natsumeda Y, Ikegami T, et al. Induction of erythroid differentiation and modulation of gene expression by tiazofurin in K562 leukemic cells. Proc Natl Acad Sci USA 1988;85:6533–6537.
109. Kharbanda SM, Sherman ML, Spriggs DR, et al. Effects of tiazofurin on protooncogene expression during HL-60 cell differentiation. Cancer Res 1988;48:5965–5968.
110. Yamaji Y, Natsumeda Y, Yamada S, et al. Synergistic action of tiazofurin and retinoic acid on differentiation and colony formation of HL-60 leukemia cells. Life Sci 1990;46: 435–442.
111. Kiguchi K, Collart FR, Henning-Chubb C, et al. Induction of cell differentiation in melanoma cells by inhibitors of IMP dehydrogenase: Altered patterns of IMP dehydrogenase expression and activity. Cell Growth Diff 1990;1:259–270.
112. Tricot GJ, Jayaram HN, Lapis E, et al. Biochemically directed therapy of leukemia with tiazofurin, a selective blocker of inosine 5′-phosphate dehydrogenase activity. Cancer Res 1989;49:3696–3701.
113. Tricot G, Jayaram HN, Zhen W, et al. Biochemically directed therapy with tiazofurin of refractory leukemia and myeloid blast crisis of chronic granulocytic leukemia. Proc Am Assoc Cancer Res 1991;32:184.
114. Friend C, Scher W, Holland JG, et al. Hemoglobin synthesis in murine erythroleukemia cells in vitro: Stimulation of erythroid differentiation by dimethylsulfoxide. Proc Natl Acad Sci USA 1971;68:378–382.
115. Sekiya S, Kimura H, Yamazawa K, et al. Induction of human embryonal carcinoma cell differentiation using *N,N*′-hexamethylene bisacetamide in vitro. Gynecol Oncol 1990;36:69–78.
116. Reuben RC, Rifkind RA, Marks PA. Chemically induced murine erythroleukemic differentiation. Biochim Biophys Acta 1980;605:325–346.
117. Marks PA, Sheffery M, Rifkind RA. Induction of transformed cells to terminal differentiation and the modulation of gene expression. Cancer Res 1987;47:659–666.
118. Melloni E, Pontremoli S, Michetti M, et al. Protein kinase C activity and hexamethylenebisacetamide-induced erythroleukemia cell differentiation. Proc Natl Acad Sci USA 1987;84:5282–5286.
119. Melloni E, Pontremoli S, Sparatore B, et al. Introduction of the β-isoenzyme of protein kinase C accelerates induced differentiation of murine erythroleukemia cells. Proc Natl Acad Sci USA 1990;87:4417–4420.
120. Yamashita T, Eto Y, Shibai H, et al. Synergistic action of activin A and hexamethylene bisacetamide in differentiation of murine erythroleukemia cells. Cancer Res 1990;50: 3182–3185.
121. Schroy P, Rifkin J, Coffey RJ, et al. Role of transforming growth factor β_1 in induction of colon carcinoma differentiation by hexamethylene bisacetamide. Cancer Res 1990;50: 261–265.
122. Hafez MM, Infante D, Winawer S, et al. Transforming growth factor β_1 acts as an autocrine-negative growth regulator in colon enterocytic differentiation but not in goblet cell maturation. Cell Growth Different 1990;1:617–626.
123. Egorin MJ, Sigman LM, Van Echo DA, et al. Phase I clinical and pharmacokinetic study of hexamethylene bisacetamide (NSC 95580) administered as a five-day continuous infusion. Cancer Res 1987;47:617–523.
124. Rowinsky EK, Ettinger DS, Grochow LB, et al. Phase I and pharmacologic study of hexamethylene bisacetamide in patients with advanced cancer. J Clin Oncol 1986;4: 1835–1844.
125. Young CW, Fanucchi MP, Walsh TD, et al. Phase I trial and clinical pharmacological evaluation of hexamethylene bisacetamide administration by ten-day continuous intravenous infusion at twenty-eight-day intervals. Cancer Res 1988;48:7304–7309.
126. Egorin MJ, Zuhowski EG, Cohen AS, et al. Plasma pharmacokinetics and urinary excretion of hexamethylene bisacetamide metabolites. Cancer Res 1987;47:6142–6146.
127. Ward FT, Kelley JA, Roth JS, et al. A phase I bioavailability and pharmacokinetic

study of hexamethylene bisacetamide (NSC 95580) administered via nasogastric tube. Cancer Res 1991;51:1803–1810.

128. Rowinsky EK, Conley BA, Jones RJ, et al. Efficacy of hexamethylene bisacetamide in myelodysplastic syndromes: 5-Day exposure to maximal levels. Proc Am Assoc Cancer Res 1990;31:190.
129. Andreeff M, Stone R, Young C, et al. Treatment of myelodysplastic syndromes and acute myeloid leukemia with hexamethylene bisacetamide. Blood 1990;76(suppl 1): 251a.
130. Snyder SW, Egorin MJ, Geelhaar LA, et al. Induction of differentiation of human promyelocytic leukemia cells (HL60) by metabolites of hexamethylene bisacetamide. Cancer Res 1988;48:3613–3616.
131. Subramanyam B, Callery PS, Egorin MJ, et al. An active, aldehydic metabolite of the cell-differentiating agent hexamethylene bisacetamide. Drug Metab Dis 1989;17:398–401.
132. Russo P, Sheinfeld J, Cordon-Cardo C, et al. Changes in phenotype and growth induced by hexamethylene bisacetamide and *cis*-retinoic acid in human urothelial carcinoma cells obtained from bladder washings. Surg Forum 1990;38:685–688.
133. Breslow R, Jursic B, Yan ZF, et al. Potent cytodifferentiating agents related to hexamethylenebisacetamide. Proc Natl Acad Sci USA 1991;88:5542–5546.
134. Olsson IL, Breitman TR. Induction of differentiation of the human histiocytic lymphoma cell line U-937 by retinoic acid and cyclic adenosine 3',5'-monophosphate-inducing agents. Cancer Res 1982;42:3924–3927.
135. Fontana J, Munoz M, Durham J. Potentiation between intracellular cyclic-AMP-elevating agents and inducers of leukemic cell differentiation. Leuk Res 1985;9:1127–1132.
136. Strickland S, Smith KK, Marotti KR. Hormonal induction of differentiation in teratocarcinoma stem cells: Generation of parietal endoderm by retinoic acid and dibutyryl cAMP. Cell 1980;21:347–355.
137. Lando M, Abemayor E, Verity MA, et al. Modulation of intracellular cyclic adenosine monophosphate levels and the differentiation response of human neuroblastoma cells. Cancer Res 1990;50:722–727.
138. Cho-Chung YS. Role of cyclic AMP receptor proteins in growth, differentiation, and suppression of malignancy: New approaches to therapy. Cancer Res 1990;50:7093–7100.
139. Tagliaferri P, Katsaros D, Clair T, et al. Synergistic inhibition of growth of breast and colon human cancer cell lines by site-selective cyclic AMP analogues. Cancer Res 1988;48:1642–1650.
140. Breitman TR, He R. Combinations of retinoic acid with either sodium butyrate, dimethyl sulfoxide, or hexamethylene bisacetamide synergistically induce differentiation of the human myeloid leukemia cell line HL60. Cancer Res 1990;50:6268–6273.

SECTION 5

C.A. STEIN

Antisense Inhibition of Gene Expression

HISTORICAL BACKGROUND

Antisense oligodeoxynucleotides are short fragments of DNA, usually 15 nucleotide bases or longer. The term "antisense" refers to the fact that these molecules are complementary to the "sense" strand of mRNA. Due to Watson-Crick base pairing, antisense oligodeoxynucleotides form DNA-mRNA duplexes in an antiparallel fashion. In theory, this process can inhibit the function of the mRNA, which normally is translated into protein in the cytoplasm by the ribosome. If the protein in question is vital for cellular or viral growth and reproduction, inhibition of its synthesis by antisense oligodeoxynucleotides could lead to a diminution in cellular or viral viability. The use of oligodeoxynucleotides as antisense inhibitors of gene expression holds forth the promise of a specific, genetically based therapeutic approach.

There are two other antisense approaches to inhibition of gene expression that are being actively investigated. The first is antisense RNA. For example, a plasmid expressing the *MYC* gene cloned in the antisense orientation produces *MYC*-encoded mRNA, also with the antisense orientation.[1] The RNA-RNA hybrids formed may result by several different mechanisms in inhibition of *MYC* mRNA translation into protein. However, because this method is not currently at a stage of therapeutic consideration, it is not covered in this chapter. An additional antisense approach is provided by the ribozyme, an oligoribonucleotide that catalyzes the specific scission of a complementary mRNA strand.[2–4] Their development as therapeutic agents, while of potentially great interest, is behind that of oligodeoxynucleotides.

Since the commercialization of the oligomer synthetic process in the mid-1980s, the relative ease of availability of these materials has led to wide variety of antisense experiments in various test systems, many successful, others not. There are also many reviews on the subject.[5–18]

CLASSES OF OLIGODEOXYNUCLEOTIDES

In the quest for nuclease-resistant oligomers, many modifications to the structure of normal or phosphodiester (PO) DNA (Fig. 69-19) have been made. Some of these are briefly described in the following sections.

METHYLPHOSPHONATE OLIGOMERS

The biochemistry and biologic effects of these materials have been reviewed by Miller and colleagues.[19] As shown in Figure 69–19, they possess four different substituents at each phosphorus atom, a property known as chirality; lack ionizable groups; and are uncharged. This can lead to solubility problems at long chain length that may be overcome by including, for example, a single PO residue at the 5' end. Methylphosphonate oligomers have significant antiviral activity, especially against

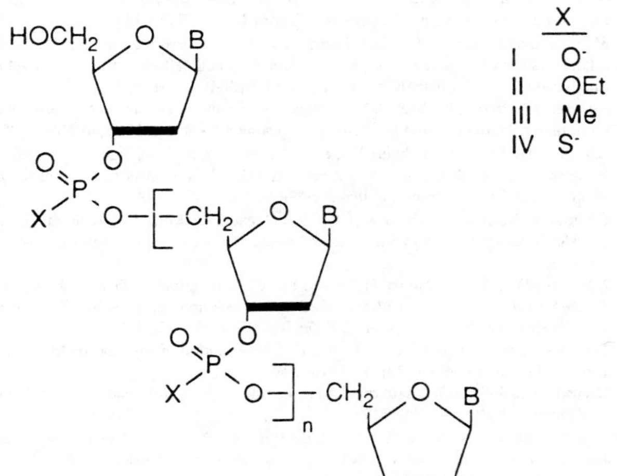

	X
I	O⁻
II	OEt
III	Me
IV	S⁻

$HOCH_2$ O B; O P O; X O—[— CH_2 O B; O P O; X O—]$_n$— CH_2 O B; HO

FIGURE 69–19. The structure of an oligodeoxynucleotide. B represents the nucleotide bases adenine, cytosine, guanine, or thymine. When X = O, the structure is that of a phosphodiester (PO) or normal oligodeoxynucleotide. When X = methyl (Me), methylphosphonate; X = S, phosphorothioate (PS) oligodeoxynucleotide. (Stein CA, Cohen J. Oligodeoxynucleotides as inhibitors of gene expression: A review. Cancer Res 1988;48:2659–2668)

vesicular stomatitis virus and human immunodeficiency virus-1 (HIV-1), but they do not elicit RNase H activity.[20,21]

PHOSPHOROTHIOATE OLIGOMERS

The subject of phosphorothioate oligomers has been reviewed elsewhere.[22,23] The compounds (see Fig. 69–19) were first synthesized by Stec and coworkers.[24] The charge and solubility are retained, but hybridizability with complementary mRNA is poorer than that of the PO oligomers. Phosphorothioate (PS) oligomers are nuclease resistant and have been shown to be sequence-specific inhibitors of HIV-1 and herpes simplex virus (HSV) replication.[25–28] However, they also have several nonsequence specific effects on HIV-1 replication, including competitive inhibition of the viral reverse transcriptase with respect to template primer binding and binding to cell surface CD4 and interference with the binding of the HIV-1 envelope glycoprotein gp120, a ligand for CD4.[29,30] These compounds are also chiral.

INTERACTIONS OF OLIGONUCLEOTIDES WITH CELLS

Many classes of oligonucleotides are polyanions. Because of their charge, it had been supposed that they could not readily pass through cell membranes. However, the existence of cell-surface DNA has been recognized for several years. Bennett and associates discovered a 30-kd protein on the surface of peripheral blood lymphocytes that binds double stranded DNA.[31] Lymphocytes that bear this membrane protein can cap the bound DNA over a period of 30 to 45 minutes, with internalization occurring within 2 hours.[31,32] The DNA receptor protein, however, does not seem to bind oligodeoxynucleotides. Loke and colleagues demonstrated that cellular association of oligomer could be inhibited by other phosphodiester homopolymers and phosphorothioate oligomers, but not by heparin, ribose-5-phosphate, or uncharged thymidine methylphosphonate oligomers.[33] They isolated an 80-kd cell-surface protein that appeared to be responsible for specific oligomer binding to HL60 cells. Yakubov and coworkers found two cell-surface oligomer binding proteins (79 kd and 90 kd).[34] Gasparro and associates identified three high-affinity double-stranded DNA-binding proteins on the surface of human peripheral blood lymphocytes.[35] These included a 28-kd species, a 79-kd species, and a protein of approximately 59 kd. The researchers did not comment on the role that any of these proteins might have with respect to internalization of cell-surface DNA.

Stein and colleagues demonstrated by flow cytometric analysis in HL60 cells that the Michaelis Constant (K_m) of a 5′-fluorescein (F)-labeled phosphodiester 15-mer homopolymer of thymidine from the cell surface is 22 nM.[36] It has also been shown in HL60 cells that there is only one unique site on the cell surface that binds oligonucleotides. A phosphorothioate 28-mer homopolymer of cytidine, known as SdC28, is a competitor of oligomer binding, and has a $K_c \sim 3$ nM. Cell membrane-bound fluorescence can be seen to cluster on the cell surface and the specific binding of oligomers to HL60 cells is calcium dependent. Cell surface-bound oligonucleotide appears to be nuclease resistant.[37] However, most oligomer internalization appears to be consequent to pinocytosis or fluid-phase endocytosis. This is a process in which the cell entraps and internalizes external liquid that contains dissolved solute (*e.g.*, oligonucleotide). It is mechanically similar to the process of receptor mediated endocytosis, although no specific receptors are present. It is likely that a smaller percentage of oligomer internalization may be accounted for by adsorptive endocytosis. In HL60 cells, we have shown that the pinocytosis rate is under the control of protein kinase C, a major signal transduction protein.

Several strategies, mostly relying on 5′ modification, have been employed to increase the cellular internalization of oligonucleotides. Investigators have linked poly-L-lysine (which is internalized by pinocytosis) to the 5′ terminus of an oligomer complementary to vesicular stomatitis virus or HIV mRNA sequences. Enhanced antiviral activity was observed.[38–41] Oligomers modified with a 5′ cholesteryl or lipid residue increase intracellular internalization, and the cholesteryl modification renders homopolymeric PS oligomers more potent HIV inhibitors than the unmodified parent. These effects may relate to the ability of 5′-cholesteryl oligomers to bind to low-density lipoprotein (LDL) and to be at least partially internalized by the LDL receptor.[42–46] However, the detergent properties of these molecules may contribute to nonspecific cellular cytotoxicity. A phosphorothioate oligomer complementary to an *MYC*-encoded mRNA sequence has been liposome encapsulated and shown to reduce levels of MYC protein in HL60 cells after fusion.[47]

After a phosphodiester oligonucleotide is internalized in a cell, it is vulnerable to nuclease digestion by cellular DNAses. For example, in microinjected *Xenopus* oocytes, an unmodified 17-mer was degraded with a half-life of only about 10 minutes.[48] In *Xenopus* embryos and in human plasma ($T_{\frac{1}{2}}$ = 7.7 minutes), this process occurred primarily because of 3′ exonuclease activity, and is vitiated by heat inactivation.[49–51] Some label originating from intracellularly digested oligomer (as nucleotide 5′ triphosphate) may be incorporated into the de novo synthesis of genomic DNA, but relatively long oligomers may be expelled from the cell by the process of exocytosis.[52] On the other hand, oligonucleotides that have been microinjected into cells seem to be quickly translocated to the nucleus.[53,54] This is unlike the behavior observed when fluorescent oligomers are allowed to "passively diffuse" into cells. In this case, a perinuclear pattern of fluorescence with nuclear sparing has been observed.[36] Little is known about the intracellular organellar distribution of oligonucleotides.

PHARMACOLOGY OF OLIGODEOXYNUCLEOTIDES

Relatively little information exists about the pharmacology of oligodeoxynucleotides because of the difficulties and cost involved in large-scale oligonucleotide synthesis. Preliminary studies with a methylphosphonate oligomer (8-mer) targeted to the splice acceptor junction of the HSV-1 immediate early mRNA 4 and 5 have shown efficacy in preventing the development of herpetic lesions when applied to the ear skin of a mouse.[9] The oligomer was distributed to all tissues except the brain, although other investigators, using ^{14}C-labeled methylphosphonates complementary to rat insulin mRNA, found accumulation preferentially in the brain, followed by kidney, lung, heart, and muscle.[55] Organ accumulation was sequence independent. As much as 99% of a 12-mer methylphosphonate oligomer may be eliminated in the urine within one hour.[56]

Iverson and coworkers studied the pharmacokinetics of a single injection of phosphorothioates of different lengths in rats.[57] Included was a 27-mer complementary to the HIV-1 rev sequence used by Matsukura and associates.[27,28] The plasma concentration of oligomer versus time could be fitted to a two-compartment model. Peak plasma levels were achieved in 10 to 20 minutes after intravenous injection and at 90 minutes after intraperitoneal injection. Little of the compound was associated with formed blood elements. The initial distribution half-time, representing distribution out of the plasma ($t_{1/2}\alpha$, intravenous administration) was 23 ± 3 minutes, and the actual half-time, representing total body elimination ($t_{1/2}\beta$) was 33.9 hours. Similar values were determined for an intraperitoneal injection approach. The plasma clearance of oligomer was not affected by length (*e.g.*, 21-, 27-, and 40-mer) or base composition. The researchers suggest that the long elimination half-time can lead to infrequent repetitive dosing to maintain therapeutically effective tissue concentrations.

Oligomer, within 3 hours, was found to appear in liver, fat, and muscle. Within 12 hours, the liver contained over 40% of the administered dose. About 5% of the dose accumulated in the kidney. After 12 hours, less than 1% of the injected dose remained circulating in the plasma, compared with the 58% that was tissue associated. Approximately one third of a 100 μg-dose of oligomer was recovered in the urine within 24 hours of injection and virtually all of it, as the parent compound, within 3 days. Fecal excretion was minimal. Toxicity included a twofold to sixfold rise in lactate dehydrogenase, peaking at 24 hours and normalizing within 3 days. Smaller increases in serum glutamic oxalacetic transaminase (SGOT) and serum glutamic pyruvic transaminase (SGPT) were seen.

MECHANISM OF THE ANTISENSE EFFECT

After internalization, and presumably after liberation from an endosomal compartment, sequence-specific oligomers can bind to their complement, forming an RNA-DNA hybrid. RNAse H is a virtually ubiquitous cytoplasmic enzyme that cleaves the RNA strand of an RNA-DNA duplex, and it is this activity, rather than translation inhibition, that may account for most antisense effects.[58] RNAse H activity can be elicited when the DNA strand is phosphodiester. This activity is also present when the DNA strand is phosphorothioate, but it is absent with methylphosphonate oligomers.[25,59] If a sample of the cell-free reticulocyte lysate translation system, which is poor in RNAse H activity, is doped with exogenously added RNAse H, translation into protein of an added mRNA proceeds poorly in the presence of a complementary 17-mer oligomer.[60] Antisense activity is also diminished in reticulocyte lysate if a competitive inhibitor of RNAse H activity (poly(rA)-oligo dT) is added.[61] Because the cleavage of mRNA by RNAse H is irreversible and should lead to dissociation of the oligomer from its target, the process of RNase H cleavage of mRNA is catalytic with respect to oligomer. After enzymatic cleavage, the mRNA appears to be rapidly degraded and usually cannot support translation. In one report of a cell-free translation system, incubation of rabbit globin mRNA with oligomers complementary to β-globin led to loss of the intact message and the appearance of RNA fragments.[62,63] The size of these mRNA pieces corresponded to cleavage occurring at binding sites complementary to the oligomer. However, in intact cell systems, mRNA fragments are rarely observed. Successful sequence specific antisense experiments have been performed with nuclease-resistant methylphosphonate oligomers, which are not substrates for RNAse H activity. Translation arrest in this case must occur through another, yet unknown mechanism.

The location of the best targets for antisense oligonucleotides has been discussed by several researchers.[14,64] In a cell free translation system, the best inhibition results from targeting of the 5′ cap or the initiation codon (AUG) regions of the globin message molecule. In contrast, in HL60 cells, the 5′ cap region of the *MYC* message, which is thought to occur as a stem and bulge region, was a significantly better target than the initiation codon region.[65] The first splice junction site was about as effective a target as the initiation codon region. Effectiveness was dependent on oligomer length, with an 18-mer complementary to the initiation codon region being twice as effective as a 15-mer and a 12-mer only 25% as effective. Daaka and colleagues targeted the 5′ cap region of the *HRAS* message, as expressed in NIH3T3 fibroblasts.[37] Other regions targeted included a region upstream of the initiation codon, and the initiation codon region. Cells were treated with 25 or 50 μM oligomer, and dose-dependent decreases in the amount of p21 HRAS protein were observed. All three oligomers were effective, but the most effective oligomer was the one targeted to the 5′ cap region. Other workers constructed PO oligomers complementary to regions on the HIV-1 mRNA.[66] Greatest efficacy, as assessed by ability to inhibit HIV-1 induced syncytia formation and to diminish viral p24 GAG protein production, was found for an oligomer complementary to the polyadenylation signal region (*i.e.*, 5′ to the mRNA poly A tail). This was followed by oligomers targeted to the 5′ cap and untranslated regions. The internal *TAT* splice acceptor site and the splice acceptor site upstream of the *ENV* initiator were also good targets. On the basis of currently available information, it is clear that there is no general rule about the preferred target site.

SEQUENCE-SPECIFIC ANTISENSE INHIBITION OF GENETIC EXPRESSION

HEMATOPOIETIC CELL LINES

MYC

The initial work with antisense *MYC* constructs was performed in peripheral blood lymphocytes by Heikkila and coworkers.[67] The oligomer was a 15-mer complementary to the first five codons of the human *MYC*-encoded mRNA and included the initiation codon. A single addition of the oligomer (30 μM) blocked the increase in MYC protein production after mitogen (*e.g.*, phytohemagglutinin) stimulation. The effect persisted for 24 hours, and treatment with noncomplementary oligomers was ineffective. The treatment with antisense oligomer and concomitant decrease in MYC protein levels led to cell cycle blockade at the G_1/S interface, but did not block cell cycle traversal from G_0 to G_1. Treatment was associated with a dramatic decrease in the mitotic index. Similar results, including blockade of entry into S phase, were found in human T lymphocytes, in which an anti-MYC phosphodiester oligomer blocked the proliferative response to interleukin-2 (IL-2).[68] The identical 15-mer was used by Wickstrom and associates in HL60 cells to inhibit MYC translation.[69] In this cell line, the *MYC* gene is amplified as much as 30-fold and is expressed in large quantities. A significant reduction in MYC protein levels at a concentration of 10 μM was observed. The antisense oligomer decreased proliferation by 50% at 4 μM.

Holt and colleagues, using HL60 cells, employed oligomers complementary to the 5′ initiation codon region, but the sequences were different than those cited previously.[70] Evidence was found for the formation of an RNA-DNA duplex that was S1 nuclease resistant, and the antisense oligomer could inhibit MYC translation by 50% to 90% at 4 μM. The growth rate of the cells was decreased by 50% over the 5-day experiment, and some of the cells underwent myeloid differentiation. No accumulation of cells in any one phase of the cell cycle was observed.

Other experiments with HL60 cells have produced very different results. Loke and coworkers found that a 50 μM concentration of antisense oligomer was required to decrease intracellular MYC protein to 30% of control; this decrease took place over a 24-hour period.[47] An identical phosphorothioate oligomer was ineffective at reducing intracellular MYC protein levels. However, the PO and PS antisense, but not sense oligomers, when encapsulated in liposomes, could inhibit MYC protein expression within several hours after fusion, but the effect was transient. Other experiments using HL60 cells revealed little inhibition after incubation with an antisense MYC oligomer, even if it was dosed daily.[71] There was, however, a decrease in ability to form colonies in soft agar, and an increase in nitroblue tetrazolium and sudan black staining, indicating at least partial, intermediate granulocytic differentiation.

When the 15-mer anti MYC oligomer was linked to poly-L-lysine and complexed with heparin, 50% inhibition of the growth of L929 cells was achieved at 1 μM.[72] This was associated with a decrease in MYC protein expression and in MYC mRNA levels, although no degraded RNA products could be detected. A 21-mer oligomer, targeted to the aberrantly transcribed first intron of *MYC*, inhibited growth of several Burkitt's lymphoma cell lines in culture.[73] Such transcripts are not found in normal cells nor in the Burkitt's cell line KK124, in which the oligomer had no effect. Levels of MYC protein were decreased after 48 hours. Experiments of this type demonstrate the attractive therapeutic potential of oligodeoxynucleotides, because, theoretically, translation of the normal MYC transcripts were unaffected.

In an in vitro system, transcription of *MYC* could be suppressed by a 27-mer targeting 115 base pairs upstream from

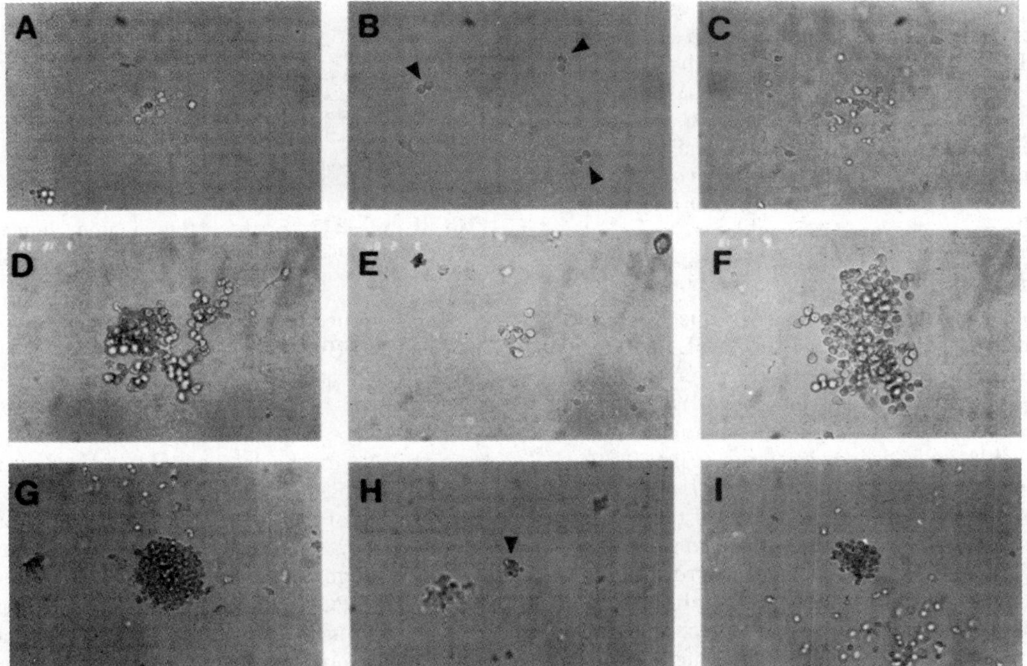

FIGURE 69–20. Development of human hematopoietic colonies cloned in plasma clot culture from normal bone marrow cells in the presence of oligonucleotides. **(A–F)** CFU-GM-derived colonies; **(G–I)** CFU-E-derived colonies. GM colony development after 4 days of exposure to c-*MYB* sense, C-*MYB* antisense, or myeloperoxidase antisense PO oligonucleotides is depicted in **A**, **B**, and **C**, respectively. Arrows in **B** point to cell doublets. GM colony development after 12 days of exposure to c-*MYB* sense, c-*MYB* antisense, or myeloperoxidase antisense PO oligomers is shown in **D**, **E**, and **F**, respectively. Erythroid colony development after 7 days of exposure to c-*MYB* sense, c-*MYB* antisense, or coagulation factor V antisense PO oligomers is shown in **G**, **H** (*arrow*), and **I**, respectively. (Gewirtz A, Calabretta B. A c-*myb* antisense oligodeoxynucleotide inhibits normal human hematopoiesis in vitro. Science 1988;242:1303–1306)

the transcription origination site.[74] This is presumably due to the formation of a DNA triple helix. The oligomer can insert itself into the major groove of a Watson-Crick double helix. Binding of the oligomer to the double helix is a consequence of so-called Hoogsteen base pairing and is stable, in the presence of divalent cations, for CG . . . C and TA . . . T triplets. It is unclear to what extent triple helix formation is a process that can occur in vivo.

MYB

The protein product of this protooncogene appears to play a role in the maintenance of the dedifferentiated phenotype in hematopoietic cells. The 18-mer PO oligomers targeted to the 5′ regions of the *MYB*-encoded mRNA were effective at suppressing the growth of HL60 cells after 5 days in culture.[75] An oligomer with a two-base mismatch was only slightly effective. Measurement of DNA content revealed that most cells were in the G_1 phase of the cell cycle. This finding is similar to that after antisense inhibition of *MYC*. However, no phenotypic differentiation was observed after treatment. In peripheral blood T lymphocytes, incubation with the 18-mer led to decreased proliferation after phytohemagglutinin stimulation.[76] Intranuclear expression of MYB protein decreased with the 18 mer PO oligomer, and with a 15-mer and the 18-mer, cells were also blocked at the G_1/S interface.[77] *MYB*-encoded mRNA detected by the polymerase chain reaction (PCR) was markedly diminished after 12 hours of treatment with antisense oligomer.[78] Antisense inhibition of *MYB* translation was also accompanied by decreases in cellular levels of DNA polymerase-α and PCNA mRNAs, both of whose protein products play a role in de novo DNA synthesis.[79]

One problem with the eventual use of an anti-MYB oligomer in clinical practice in, for example, the extracorporeal purging of autologous bone marrow, is that the normal function of *MYB* is compromised. For example, in cultures of normal human bone marrow, incubation with the 18-mer antisense PO oligomer caused a mean decrease in granulocyte-macrophage colony-forming units (CFU-GM) of 68% (Fig. 69-20), in CFU-E of 67% (Fig. 69-21), and in CFU-Meg of 76%.[80] The number of cells per colony was also dramatically reduced. CFU-CM colonies, even in the presence of GM-CSF or IL-3, and CFU-G colonies, even in the presence of G-CSF, were reduced in number of cells per colony after antisense *MYB* treatment. Levels of *MYB*-encoded mRNA were also dramatically reduced after treatment with the antisense oligomer (Fig. 69-22).

It has been demonstrated that normal and leukemic cells exhibit differential sensitivity to the effects of the antisense oligomer.[81] In mixed cultures of blast cells from patients with acute myelogenous leukemia and normal marrow elements, only the normal elements could be detected after antisense treatment. If this treatment is generally applicable to the leukemic marrow, and can be shown to effect a high cell kill, it may become therapeutically attractive.

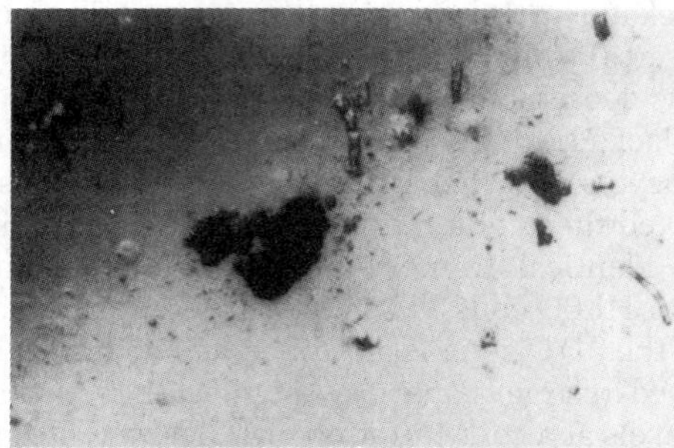

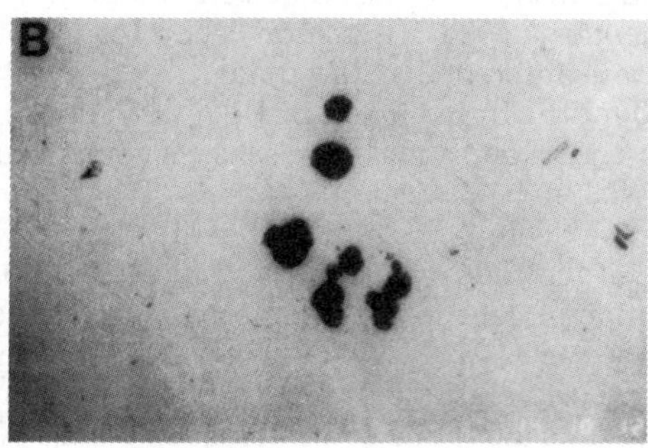

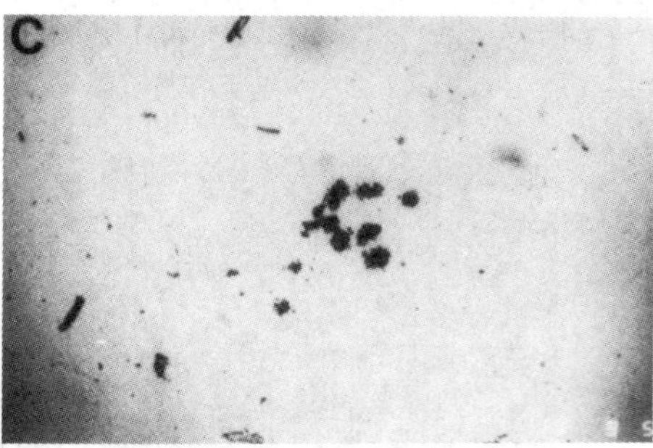

FIGURE 69–21. Erythroid bursts from human bone marrow MY10$^+$ mononuclear cells. **(A)** Control. **(B)** Colonies after treatment with a c-*MYB* sense PO oligomer. **(C)** Colonies after treatment with a c-*MYB* antisense PO oligomer. (Caracciolo D, Venturelli D, Valtieri M, et al. Stage-related proliferative activity determines c-*myb* functional requirements during normal hematopoiesis. J Clin Invest 1990;85:55–61)

BCL2

The *BCL2* gene plays a role in the survival and growth of normal lymphoid cells. It is also implicated in the t(14:18) translocation that is found in most cases of follicular lymphoma, in which high levels of *BCL2*-encoded mRNA is found. In 65% to 75% of these cases, a novel BCL2/immunoglobulin fusion mRNA can be detected.[82] Reed and associates used 20-mer PO and PS oligomers complementary to the initiation codon region of the human BCL2 mRNA.[83] Both inhibited the growth of 697 leukemia cells in a dose dependent fashion, but the PS oligomer was more potent (Fig. 69-23). However, although the PO oligomer inhibited proliferation after 2 to 3 days, the PS oligomer required 3 to 6 days for maximal effect. A concentration-dependent decrease in BCL2 protein expression (Fig. 69-24) was also observed (75–95%, PO oligo, 150 μM, 4 days: 70% PS oligomer, 25 μM). Cellular viabilities rapidly declined after 3 days of treatment (PO and PS oligomers), which was attributed to the role of *BCL2* in promoting lymphoid survival. These results highlight some of the similarities and differences between PO and PS oligomers with respect to their biologic interactions. However, the *BCL2* gene appears to be an excellent target for the purging of autologous bone marrow in patients with follicular lymphoma.

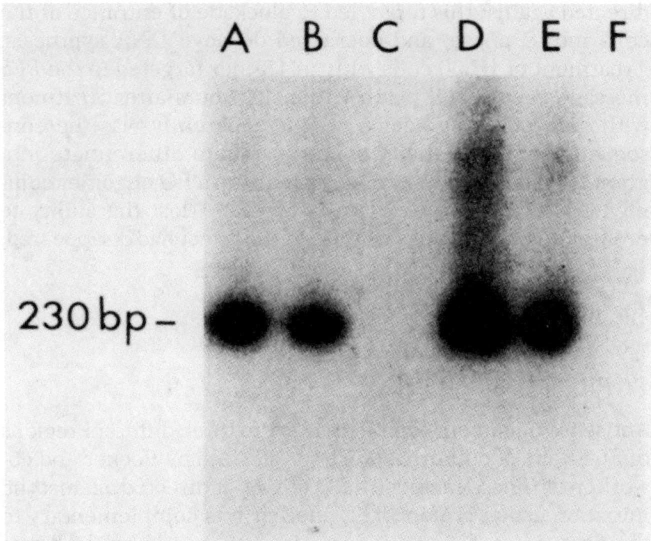

FIGURE 69–22. Expression of c-*MYB* mRNA in bone marrow progenitors cultured in the presence of c-myb oligomers. MY10^{+} mononuclear cells are shown in lanes A–C. Mononuclear cells depleted of adherent phagocytic cells and T lymphocytes are shown in lanes D–F. Control lanes (no oligomer) are A and D. mRNA from cells incubated with c-*MYB* sense is in lanes B and E. mRNA from cells incubated with c-*MYB* antisense is in lanes C and F. C-*MYB* mRNA was amplified by the polymerase chain reaction and detected by a radiolabeled 50-mer spanning the nucleotide region 2351 to 2400. (Caracciolo D, Venturelli D, Valtieri M, et al. Stage-related proliferative activity determines c-*myb* functional requirements during normal hematopoiesis. J Clin Invest 1990;85:55–61)

CSF1R and CSF1

Differentiation of HL60 cells into macrophages, induced by phorbol esters or 1,25-dihydroxy vitamin D_3, is associated with increased transcription of the *CSF1R* (formerly called FMS) message, which codes for the CSF1 receptor.[84,85] Treatment with an antisense PO oligomer complementary to the *CSF1R*-encoded mRNA inhibited macrophage formation induced by phorbol ester, but not by 1,25-dihydroxy vitamin D_3. Granulocytic differentiation induced by DMSO was not affected. Similar results were obtained using oligomers targeted against the mRNA of CSF1. Synergistic inhibition of macrophage formation was suggested by combination of the two oligomers. In a murine cell line, a 15-mer PO oligomer targeted to the initiation codon region of the CSF1 mRNA (5 μM) reduced cell proliferation by 63% at 24 hours, and decreased membrane levels of CSF1 protein over a 3-hour period.[86] Inhibition of proliferation could be increased to 95% if an anti-CSF1 monoclonal antibody was added to the cell cultures.

Myeloblastin

This is a serine protease, initially described by Bories and colleagues in HL60 cells.[87] It is down regulated during differentiation of myeloblasts with DMSO or 1,25-dihydroxy vitamin D_3. Specific diminution of myeloblastin mRNA translation was accomplished by an 18-mer PO oligomer complementary to a sequence beginning at position 95 downstream of the initiation codon. Oligomer was added to the growing cells every 8 hours, and by 7 days, cells began to assume a differentiated phenotype. After 10 days, myeloblastin protein had also markedly decreased. By day 12, 80% of the cells exhibited the typical morphologic characteristics of monocytic differentiation, and few cells remained in S phase. The changes are virtually identical to what was seen after treatment of HL60 cells with phorbol esters, which are known to induce monocytic differentiation. Use of the antisense oligomer, in this case, has allowed the function of the myeloblastin protein to be ascertained, a task that otherwise would have been possible only with difficulty.

BCR-ABL

This fusion gene results from the translocation of the *ABL* protooncogene from chromosome 9 to the *BCR* (breakpoint cluster region) of chromosome 22.[88] Transcripts of this hybrid gene are found only in patients with hematologic neoplasms, predominately chronic myelogenous leukemia. After determination of the base sequence of the *BCR-ABL* junction region, a complementary 18-mer PO oligomer was constructed and added to cells derived from a patient with CML.[88] The number of colonies formed in soft agar in 10 days declined from 60% to 90%. An oligomer with a two-base mismatch was ineffective. The antisense oligomer did not affect clonogenic growth

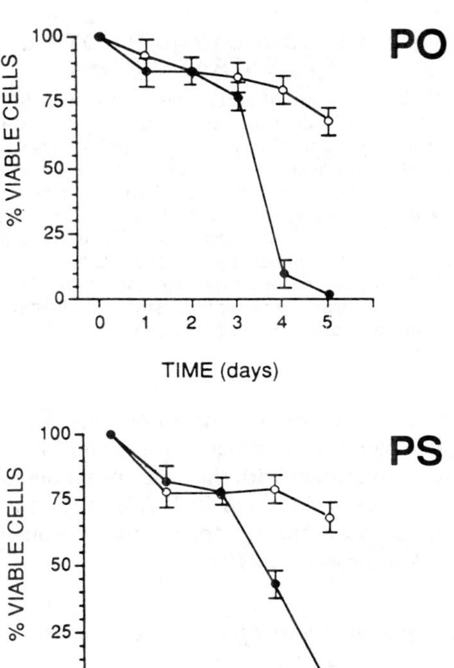

FIGURE 69–23. Influence of *BCL2* antisense oligonucleotides on the viability of 697 leukemia cells. The leukemia cells were cultured with PO and PS oligomers. The percentage of viable cells was determined by trypan blue dye exclusion. Open circles indicate sense oligomers, and closed circles indicate antisense oligomers. (Reed JC, Stein CA, Subasinghe C, et al. Antisense-mediated inhibition of BCL2 protooncogene expression and leukemic cell growth and survival: Comparisons of phosphodiester and phosphothioate oligodeoxynucleotides. Cancer Res 1990;50:6565–6570)

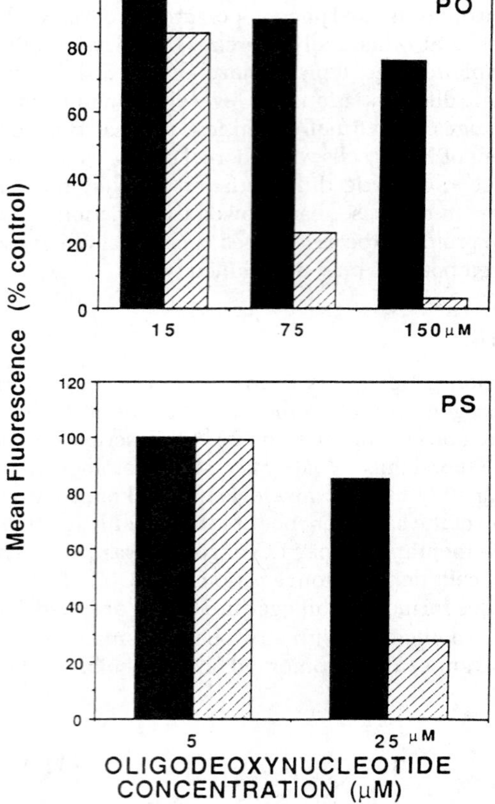

FIGURE 69–24. Immunofluorescence analysis of *BCL2*-encoded protein levels after oligodeoxynucleotide treatment of 697 leukemia cells. Cells were treated for 2 days with PO and 4 days with PS oligomers. Black columns are sense oligomers, hatched columns are antisense oligomers. Cells were then labeled with anti-*BCL2* antiserum and analyzed by fluorescence-activated cell sorting. Data are expressed as percent of mean fluorescence relative to cells not treated with oligomer. (Reed JC, Stein CA, Subasinghe C, et al. Antisense-mediated inhibition of *BCL2* protooncogene expression and leukemic cell growth and survival: Comparisons of phosphodiester and phosphothioate oligodeoxynucleotides. Cancer Res 1990;50:6565–6570)

from normal hematopoietic progenitor cells. Similar results were found in patients' cells that carried different breakpoints. Furthermore, treatment with the antisense molecule led to a dramatic decrease in levels of BCR-ABL mRNA as detected by RT-PCR. However, no attempt was made to quantitate levels of BCR-ABL protein (p210).

Other Targets in Hematopoietic Cells

PO antisense oligomers have been used to inhibit the α and β genes of the T-cell receptor, and treatment results in failure of lymphokine production after exposure to specific antigen.[89] Anti-IL2 and anti-IL4 PO oligomers reduced cellular proliferation and levels of lymphokine message in two different T-cell lines, and a PO oligomer targeted to the growth hormone mRNA reduced secreted immunoreactive growth hormone levels and the cellular proliferation of rat lymphocytes.[90,91] The gene *CDC2*, which codes for a p34 serine-threonine protein kinase, increases in expression as cells traverse the cell cycle after G_1.[92] Treatment of T cells with a PO oligomer directed against this target led to blockade of entrance of the cells into S phase, and decreased de novo DNA synthesis. Treatment of HL60 cells with an 18-mer targeted to the *FES* message caused cell death within 24 hours after treatment with differentiating agents.[77] This apparently was the consequence of the inability of these cells to differentiate into granulocytes. Myeloma cells treated with a PO oligomer complementary to the prothymosin-α mRNA lost the ability to proliferate for 24 hours.[93] By day 2, the effect had disappeared.

GROWTH REGULATORY TARGETS IN NONHEMATOPOIETIC CELLS

FGFB

Antisense oligomers complementary to three different regions of *FGFB*-encoded mRNA were synthesized by Becker and coworkers.[56] These included a PO oligomer directed against the initiation codon region (#1); another was complementary to the first splice donor-acceptor site (#2), and the third was complementary to the second splice donor-acceptor site at condons 94–95 (#3). WM75 cells, derived from a human melanoma in the vertical growth phase, when treated with a single dose (50 μM) of oligomer #2, were growth inhibited by 60% at day 8. When the metastatic melanoma line WM 983-B was treated with oligomer #3, similar growth inhibition was observed. The sense and five-base mismatched oligomers had no effect on proliferation. Competition experiments performed with sense oligomer in the presence of antisense oligomer revealed that the inhibition of growth was reversible within 48 hours. Treatment with the antisense oligomers reduced the ability of the melanoma cells to clone in soft agar.

Another source of FGFB is in neural tissue, particularly the brain. It has been suggested that this fibroblast growth factor may directly promote glial cell tumor growth directly or indirectly secondary to stimulation of angiogenesis.[94] PO 15-mer oligomers were synthesized and targeted, as previously described, to the initiation codon (#1) and first splice donor-acceptor regions (#2) of the FGFB mRNA. Incubation with oligomer #2 markedly reduced the growth rate of SNB-19 human glioma cells (25 μM). The effect was dose dependent and plateaued at higher concentrations. The sense strand had no effect on growth, and the antiproliferative effect was vitiated by addition of exogenous FGFB. Similar results were obtained after incubation with oligomer #1. This correlated with a 67% reduction in FGFB protein content and a 55% reduction in cell number, implying that the diminution in cell number was directly related to the inhibitory effects on FGFB mRNA translation by the oligomer. The proliferation of nontransformed astrocytes, prepared from temporal lobe biopsies, was not inhibited by either antisense oligomer. These results suggest the possibility of a local therapeutic strategy for high-grade human glioma, a uniformly fatal disease.

HRAS

The protein product of the *HRAS* gene is involved in signal transduction across cell membranes, and p21, the protein product of the *HRAS* oncogene, binds guanosine nucleotide phosphates, and possesses GTPase activity. Yu found that the most common pathway of *RAS* activation in human cancer involves a point mutation in the 12th or 61st amino acid codon of *HRAS*.[95] This mutation is found in a variety of radiation-induced and chemically induced tumors.

Brown and associates inserted the murine RAS p21 coding region into an RNA expression vector.[96] A methylphosphonate oligonucleotide was targeted to the first 11 nucleotides of the initiation codon region. When the in vitro run off mRNA transcripts were translated in cell-free systems in the presence of the antisense oligomer, a 59% inhibition of translation was observed at 25 μM. The effect was dose dependent and was maximal (virtually 100%) above 100 μM. Lower levels of inhibition were observed for oligomers with one- and two-base mismatches. Because methylphosphonate oligomers do not elicit RNAse H activity, it was proposed that the mechanism of the antisense effect depended on blocking the ribosome from interacting with the translation initiation site.[97] At no point was the morphology of the cells affected.

Yu and colleagues targeted methylphosphonate oligomers (8-mers) to the twelfth amino acid codon of a wild type and a mutant *HRAS*-encoded mRNA transcript.[95] The oligomers effectively inhibited translation in cell-free systems, and the translation inhibition was diminished in the presence of oligomers with one- or two-base mismatches. The exquisite sequence specificity was further demonstrated when the mutant HRAS transcript was used in the cell-free translation system. There was a single nucleotide change, from guanine to thymine, in the twelfth amino acid codon. At 200 μM, inhibition was most pronounced (84%) with the oligomer containing the single-base mismatch and somewhat less so (65%) with the oligomer complementary to the wild type gene. At 50 μM, only the exact complement of the mutated HRAS message produced any inhibition whatsoever in the cell-free translation system. Experiments of this type suggest an important role for antisense oligomers in which the transcripts from normal and mutant alleles must be discriminated and highlights novel potential therapies if these results can be applied in cellular or tissue systems.

MYCN

The 15-mer PO oligomers were synthesized as targets to the initiation codon of the *MYCN*-encoded mRNA in the CHP 100 neuroepithelial cell line.[98] CHP 100 cells contain only one copy of the *MYCN* gene. Diminished cellular staining for MYCN protein was observed after 16 hours of exposure to 100 μM oligomer. The sense oligomer was ineffective at reducing cellular MYCN protein levels, and no effects on *MYC* expression were seen. Cellular proliferation and DNA synthesis were also reduced by the antisense oligomer. Morphologically, there was a decrease in cellular heterogeneity, with an increase in the number of flat, epithelial-like cells (*i.e.*, S cells), which are contact inhibited, do not clone in soft agar, and are not tumorigenic in nude mice. The researchers suggested using implantable microinfusion pumps to study the effects of antisense oligomers when infused at a constant rate into nude mice.

Other Targets In Nonhematopoietic Cells

Cope and coworkers treated the malignant keratinocyte line SCC-25 with 15-mer PO oligomers complementary to the cellular retinol-binding protein 1 (cRBP) and to the human nuclear retinoic acid receptor-α (hnRARA).[99] At a concentration of 30 μM antisense cRBP, a 90% loss of retinol binding in the cytoplasm was observed over 16 hours. This oligomer had no effect on the binding of retinoic acid to hnRAR. When the cells were treated with the antisense hnRARA construct, nuclear binding of retinoic acid was blocked to a similar extent. These decreases in binding were shown to directly correlate with decreases in levels of the respective retinoid binding proteins. In cells treated with either oligomer, the typical retinol-dependent induction of alkaline phosphatase activity did not occur. Cells treated with the cRBP antisense construct rounded up, lost cell-cell attachments, and exhibited decreased adherence to the substratum. Sense oligomers had few if any biologic effects.

The colonic adenocarcinoma line, LoVo, and its doxorubicin-resistant subline, LoVo/Dx, overexpress the *MYB* oncogene.[100] The researchers treated the cells with 18-mer PO oligomers complementary to codons 2–7 of the MYB mRNA. The proliferative rate was markedly decreased, as was *MYB* expression.

Proliferating cell nuclear antigen (PCNA) is a nuclear protein that is a cofactor of DNA polymerase-δ. Jaskulski and colleagues prepared 18 mer PO oligomers extending from nucleotides 4–21 and 22–39 of the mouse PCNA mRNA.[101] The mitotic index of the cells treated with the antisense oligomer was decreased, and by 16 hours, no cells undergoing mitosis could be detected. These effects were even more striking when the oligomers were used individually and could be correlated with a decrease in levels of PCNA protein. After determination of the amount of DNA per cell, it was concluded that the cell cycle block must have occurred at the G_1/S boundary or early in the S phase.

The use of antisense oligomer to reverse the pleiotropic drug-resistant phenotype has been considered. Rivoltini and coworkers, using the LoVo cell line and its resistant sublines LoVo/H and LoVo/Dx, treated these cells with 15-mer PO oligomers complementary to the initiation codon region of the p170 mRNA (160 μM on day 1 and 80 μM on day 2).[102] After 3 days, cell-surface p170 was down-modulated, and in the LoVo/Dx cells, the MDR phenotype was reverted, with the cells becoming almost as sensitive to doxorubicin as after treatment with verapamil. Studies further investigating these intriguing observations should appear shortly.

Although the potential of specific genetic therapy is huge and theoretically within reach, in reality, daunting problems remain. Technically, foremost among these are the problems of scale and cost. Although it is soon likely that several grams of an antisense oligomer can be relatively easily synthesized, it is not clear that technology exists to cost effectively synthesize the at least 1 kg of material required for adequate phase I testing in humans. This problem is reflected in the relative paucity of pharmacokinetic and pharmacodynamic data referable to oligonucleotides. Nevertheless, the breathtaking progress in this field over a very short span of years and the ever increasing number of targets known to be susceptible to antisense inhibition of gene expression must be taken as an excellent harbinger of the eventual development of a novel, specific, antineoplastic therapy, which is in its earliest stages.

REFERENCES

1. Griep A, Westphal H. Antisense myc sequences induce differentiation of F9 cells. Proc Natl Acad Sci USA 1988;85:6806–6810
2. Cech T, Bass B. Biological catalysis of RNA. Ann Rev Biochem 1986;55:599–629.
3. Haseloff J, Gerlach W. Simple RNA enzymes with new and highly specific endoribonuclease activities. Nature 1988;334:585–591.
4. Sarver N, Cantin E, Chang P, et al. Ribozymes as potential anti-HIV-1 therapeutic agents. Science 1990;247:1222–1225.
5. Stein CA, Cohen J. Oligodeoxynucleotides as inhibitors of gene expression: A review. Cancer Res 1988;48:2659–2668.
6. Zon G. Oligonucleotide analogues as potential chemotherapeutic agents. Pharm Res 1988;5:539–549.
7. van der Krol AR, Mol JN, Stuije AR. Modulation of eukaryotic gene expression by complementary RNA or DNA sequences. Biotechniques 1988;6:958–976.
8. Marcus-Sekura C. Techniques for using antisense oligodeoxyribonucleotides to study gene expression. Analyt Biochem 1988;172:289–295.
9. Miller PS, Ts'o POP. A new approach to chemotherapy based on molecular biology and nucleic acid chemistry: Matagen (masking tape for gene expression). Anticancer Drug Des 1987;2:117–128.
10. Paoletti C. Anti-sense oligonucleotides as potential antitumour agents: Prospective views and preliminary results. Anticancer Drug Des 1988;2:325–331.
11. Goodchild J. Conjugates of oligonucleotides and modified oligonucleotides: A review of their synthesis and properties. Bioconjugate Chem 1990;1:165–183.
12. Tidd D. A potential role for antisense oligonucleotide analogues in the development of oncogene targeted cancer chemotherapy. Anticancer Res 1990;10:1169–1182.
13. Dolnick B. Antisense agents in pharmacology. Biochem Pharmacol 1990;40:671–675.
14. Helene C, Toulme JJ. Specific regulation of gene expression by antisense, sense and antigene nucleic acids. Biochim Biophys Acta 1990;1049:99–125.
15. Knorre D, Vlassov V. Antisense oligonucleotide derivatives as gene-targeted drugs. Biomed Sci (USSR) 1990;1:334–343.
16. Uhlmann E, Peyman A. Antisense oligonucleotides: A new therapeutic principle. Chem Rev 1990;90:543–584.
17. Calabretta B. Inhibition of protooncogene expression by antisense oligodeoxynucleotides: Biological and therapeutic implications. Cancer Res 1991;51:4505–4510.
18. Cohen J, ed. Oligodeoxynucleotides: Antisense inhibitors of gene expression. London: Macmillan, 1989.
19. Miller P. Non-ionic antisense oligonucleotides. In Cohen J, ed. Oligodeoxynucleotides: Antisense inhibitors of gene expression. London: Macmillan, 1989:79–95.
20. Agris C, Blake D, Miller P, et al. Inhibition of vesicular stomatitis virus protein synthesis and infection by sequence-specific oligodeoxyribonucleoside methylphosphonates. Biochemistry 1986;25:6268–6275.
21. Sarin P, Agrawal S, Civeira M, et al. Inhibition of acquired immunodeficiency syndrome virus by oligodeoxynucleoside methylphosphonates. Proc Natl Acad Sci USA 1988;85: 7448–7451.
22. Stein C, Cohen J. Phosphorothioate oligodeoxynucleotide analogues. In Cohen J, ed. Oligodeoxynucleotides: Antisense inhibitors of gene expression. London: Macmillan, 1989:97–117.
23. Stein C, Tonkinson J, Yakubov, L. Phosphorothioate oligodeoxynucleotides. Pharmacol Ther 1991;52:365–384.
24. Stec W, Zon G, Egan V. Automated solid-phase synthesis, separation and stereochemistry of phosphorothioate analoges of oligodeoxyribonucleotides. J Am Chem Soc 1984;106: 6077–6079.
25. Stein C, Subasinghe C, Morgan N, et al. Physicochemical properties of phosphorothioate oligodeoxynucleotides. Nucleic Acids Res 1988;16:3209–3221.
26. Matsukura M, Zon G, Shinozuka K, et al. Phosphorothioate oligodeoxynucleotides as inhibitors of the replication of HIV. Gene 1988;72:343–347.
27. Matsukura M, Zon G, Shinozuka K, et al. Regulation of viral expression of HIV in vitro by an antisense phosphorothioate oligodeoxynucleotide against rev in chronically infected cells. Proc Natl Acad Sci USA 1989;86:6244–6248.
28. Gao W, Hanes R, Vazquez-Padua M, et al. Inhibition of herpesvirus type 2 growth by phosphorothioate oligodeoxynucleotides. Antimicrob Agents Chemother 1990;34:808–821.
29. Majumdar C, Stein C, Cohen J, et al. HIV reverse transcriptase stepwise mechanism: Phosphorothioate oligodeoxynucleotide as primer. Biochemistry 1989;28:1340–1346.
30. Stein C, Pal R, Hoke G, et al. Phosphorothioate oligodeoxynucleotide interferes with binding of CD4 to gp 120. J Acquir Immune Defic Syndr 1991;4:686–693.
31. Bennett R, Gabor GT, Merritt M. DNA binding to human leukocytes: Evidence for a receptor-mediated association, internalization, and degradation of DNA. J Clin Invest 1985;76:2182–2190.
32. Rogers J, Kerstiens J. Capping of DNA on phytohemagglutinin-stimulated human lymphoblasts. J Immunol 1981;126:703–705.
33. Loke SL, Stein, CA, Zhang XH, et al. Characterization of oligonucleotide transport into living cells. Proc Natl Acad Sci USA 1989;86:3474–3478.
34. Yakubov LA, Deeva EA, Zarytova VF, et al. Mechanism of oligonucleotide uptake by cells: Involvement of specific receptors? Proc Natl Acad Sci USA 1989;86:6454–6458.
35. Gasparro FP, Dall'Amico R, O'Malley M, et al. Cell membrane DNA. A new target for psoralen photoadduct formation. Photochem Photobiol 1990;52:315–321.
36. Stein CA, Tonkinson J, Zhang LM, et al. Unpublished observations.
37. Daaka Y, Wickstrom E. Target dependence of antisense oligodeoxynucleotide inhibition of c-Ha-*ras* p21 expression and focus formation in T24-transformed NIH3T3 cells. Oncogene Res 1990;5:267–275.
38. Leonetti JP, Degols G, LeBleu B. Biological activity of oligonucleotide-poly(L-lysine) conjugates: Mechanism of cell uptake. Bioconjugate Chem 1990;1:149–153.
39. Lemaitre M, Bayard B, Lebleu B. Specific antiviral activity of a poly(L-lysine)-conjugated oligodeoxyribonucleotide sequence complementary to vesaicular stomatitis virus N protein mRNA initiation site. Proc Natl Acad Sci USA 1989;84:648–652.
40. LeMaitre M, Bayard B, Lebleu B. Specific antiviral activity of a poly(L-lysine)-conjugated oligodeoxyribonucleotide sequence complementary to vesicular stomatitis virus N protein mRNA initiation site. Proc Natl Acad Sci USA 1987;84:648–682.
41. Stevenson M, Iversen P. Inhibition of human immunodeficiency virus type 1-mediated cytopathic effects of poly(L-lysine)-conjugated synthetic antisense oligodeoxyribonucleotides. J Gen Virol 1989;70:2673–2682.
42. Boutourin A, Gus'kova E, Ivanova E, et al. Synthesis of alkylating oligonucleotide derivatives containing cholesterol or phenazinium residues at their 3′ terminus and their interaction with DNA within mammalian cells. FEBS Lett 1989;254:129–132.
43. Shea R, Marsters J, Bischofberger N. Synthesis hybridization properties and antiviral activity of lipid-oligodeoxynuycleotide conjugates. Nucleic Acids Res 1990;18:3777–3783.
44. Letsinger R, Zhang G, Sun D, et al. Cholesteryl-conjugated oligonucleotides: Synthesis, properties, and activity as inhibitors of replication of human immunodeficiency virus in cell culture. Proc Natl Acad Sci USA 1989;86:6553–6556.
45. Stein CA, Pal R, DeVico A, et al. Mode of action of 5′-linked cholesteryl phosphorothioate oligodeoxynucleotides in inhibiting syncytia formation and infection by HIV-1 and HIV-2 in vitro. Biochemistry 1991;30:2439–2444.
46. Stein CA, Tonkinson J, Yakubov L, et al. unpublished observations
47. Loke SL, Stein CA, Zhang XH, et al. Delivery of c-myc antisense phosphorothioate oligodeoxynucleotides to hematopoietic cells in culture by liposome fusion: Specific reduction in c-myc protein expression correlates with inhibition of cell growth and DNA synthesis. Curr Top Microbiol Immunol 1988;141:282–289.
48. Cazenave C, Chevrier M, Thuong N, et al. Rate of degradation of [α]- and [β]-oligodeoxynucleotides in *Xenopus* oocytes. Implications for anti-messenger strategies. Nucleic Acids Res 1987;15:10507–10521.
49. Dagle J, Walder J, Weeks D. Targeted degradation of mRNA in *Xenopus* oocytes and embryos directed by modified oligonucleotides: Studies of An2 and cyclin in embryogenesis. Nucleic Acids Res 1990;18:4751–4757.
50. Dagle J, Weeks D, Walder J. Pathwasys of degradation and mechanism of action of antisense oligonucleotides in *Xenopus laevis* embryos. Antisense Res Devel 1991;1: 11–20.
51. Eder P, DeVine R, Dagle J, Walder J. Substrate specificity and kinetics of degradation of antisense oligonucleotides by a 3′-exonuclease in plasma. Antisense Res Devel 1991;1: 141–151.
52. Zon G. Pharmaceutical considerations. In Cohen J, ed. Oligodeoxynucleotides: Antisense inhibitors of gene expression. London: Macmillan, 1989:243–248.
53. Chin DJ, Green GA, Zon G, et al. Rapid nuclear accumulation of injected oligodeoxyribonucleotides. New Biologist 1990;12:1091–1100.
54. Leonetti JP, Mechti N, Degols G, et al. Intracellular distribution of microinjected antisense oligonucleotides. Proc Natl Acad Sci USA 1991;88:2702–2706.
55. Maguire DK, Han H. Synthesis and metabolism of oligonucleoside methylphosphonates. Proc Austral Biochem Soc 1988;20:26.
56. Becker D, Meier C, Herlyn M. Proliferation of human malignant melanomas is inhibited by antisense oligodeoxynucleotides targeted against basic fibroblast growth factor. EMBO J 1989;8:3685–3691.
57. Iverson P, Mata J, Zon G. The single injection pharmacokinetics of an antisense phosphorothioate oligodeoxynucleotide against rev (art/trs) for the human immunodeficiency virus (HIV) in the adult male rat. Personal communication.
58. Wintersberger U. Ribonucleases H of retroviral and cellular origin. Pharmacol Ther 1990;48:259–280.
59. Cazenave C, Stein CA, Loreau N, et al. Comparative inhibition of rabbit globin mRNA translation by modified antisense oligodeoxynucleotides. Nucleic Acids Res 1989;17: 4255–4273.
60. Minshull J, Hunt T. The use of single-stranded DNA and RNase H to promote quantitive hybrid arrest of translation of mRNA/DNA hybrids in reticulocyte lysate cell-free translation. Nucleic Acids Res 1986;14:6433–6451.
61. Walder R, Walder J. Role of RNase H in hybrid-arrested translation by antisense oligonucleotides. Proc Natl Acad Sci USA 1988;85:5011–5015.
62. Dash P, Lotan I, Knapp, M, et al. Selective elimination of mRNAs in vivo: Complementary oligodeoxynucleotides promote RNA degradation by an RNase H-like activity. Proc Natl Acad Sci USA 1987;84:7896–7900.
63. Cazenave C, Loreau N, Thuong N, et al. Enzymatic amplification of translation inhibition of rabbit β-globin mRNA mediated by anti-messgnger oligodeoxynucleotides covalently linked to intercalating agents. Nucleic Acids Res 1987;15:4717–4736.
64. Goodchild J. Inhibition of gene expression by oligonucleotides. In Cohen J, ed. Oligodeoxynucleotides, antisense inhibitors of gene expression. London: Macmillan, 1989: 53–77.
65. Bacon T, Wickstrom E. Walking along human c-myc mRNA with antisense oligodeoxynucleotides: Maximum efficacy at the 5′ cap region. Oncogene Res 1991;6:13–19.
66. Goodchild J, Agrawal S, Civeira M, et al. Inhibition of human immunodeficiency virus replication by antisense oligodeoxynucleotides. Proc Natl Acad Sci USA 1988;85:5507–5511.
67. Heikkila R, Schwab G, Wickstrom E, et al. A c-*myc* antisense oligodeoxynucleotide inhibits entry into S phase but not progress from G_0 to G_1. Nature 1987;328:445–449.
68. Harel-Bellan A, Ferris D, Vinocour M, et al. Specific inhibition of c-myc protein biosynthesis using an antisense synthetic deoxyolignucleotide in human T lymphocytes. J Immunol 1988;140:2431–2435.
69. Wickstrom EL, Bacon T, Gonzalez A, et al. Human promyelocytic leukemia HL-60 cell proliferation and c-myc protein expression are inhibited by an antisense penta-

decadeoxynucleotide targeted against c-myc mRNA. Proc Natal Acad Sci USA 1988;85: 1028–1032.

70. Holt J, Redner R, Nienhuis A. An oligomer complementary to c-myc mRNA inhibits proliferation of HL-60 promyelocytic cells and induces differentiation. Mol Cell Biol 1988;8:963–973.
71. Bacon T, Wickstrom E. Daily addition of an anti-c-*myc* DNA oligomer induces granulocytic differentiation of human promyelocytic leukemia HL-60 cells in both serum-containing and serum-free media. Oncogene Res 1991;6:21–32.
72. Degols G, Lenoetti JP, Mechti N, et al. Antiproliferative effects of antisense oligonucleotides directed to the RNA of c-*myc* oncogene. Nucleic Acids Res 1991;19:945–948.
73. McManaway ME, Neckers LM, Loke SL, et al. Tumour-specific inhibition of lymphoma growth by an antisense oligodeoxynucleotide. Lancet 1990;335:808–811.
74. Cooney M, Czernuszewicz G, Postel E, et al. Site-specific oligonucleotide binding represses transcription of the human c-*myc* gene in vitro. Science 1988;241:456–459.
75. Anfossi G, Gewirtz A, Calabretta B. An oligomer complementary to c-*myb*-encoded mRNA inhibits proliferation of human myeloid leukemia cell lines. Proc Natl Acad Sci USA 1989;86:3379–3383.
76. Gewirtz A, Anfossi G, Venturelli D, et al. G_1/S transition in normal human T-lymphocytes requires the nuclear protein encoded by c-*myb*. Science 1989;245:180–183.
77. Ferrari S, Donelli A, Manfredini R, et al. Differential effects of c-*myb* and c-*fes* antisense oligodeoxynucleotides on granulocytic differentiation of human myeloid leukemia HL60 cells. Cell Growth Differ 1990;1:543–548.
78. Churilla A, Braciale T, Braciale V. Regulation of T lymphocyte proliferation: Interleukin 2-mediated induction of c-*myb* gene expression is dependent of T lymphocyte activation state. J Exp Med 1989;170:105–121.
79. Venturelli D, Travale S, Calabretta B. Inhibition of T-cell proliferation by a MYB antisense oligomer is accompanied by selective down-regulation of DNA polymerase α expression. Proc Natl Acad Sci USA 1990;87:5963–5967.
80. Gewirtz A, Calabretta B. A c-*myb* antisense oligodeoxynucleotide inhibits normal human hematopoiesis in vitro. Science 1988;242:1303–1306.
81. Calabretta B, Sims R, Valtieri M, et al. Normal and leukemic hematopoietic cells manifest differential sensitivity to inhibitory effects of c-*myb* antisense oligodeoxynucleotides: An in vitro study relevant to bone marrow purging. Proc Natl Acad Sci USA 1991;88:2351–2355.
82. Weiss L, Warnke R, Sklar J, et al. Molecular analysis of the t(14;18) chromosomal translocation in malignant lymphoma. N Engl J Med 1987;317:1185–1189.
83. Reed JC, Stein CA, Subasinghe C, et al. Antisense-mediated inhibition of *BCL2* protooncogene expression and leukemic cell growth and survival: Comparisons of phosphodiester and phosphothioate oligodeoxynucleotides. Cancer Res 1990;50:6565–6570.
84. Wu J, Zhu JQ, Han KK, et al. The role of the c-*fms* oncogene in the regulation of HL-60 cell differentiation. Oncogene 1990;5:873–877.
85. Sherr C, Rettenmier C, Sacca R, et al. The c-*fms* proto-oncogene product is related to the receptor for the mononuclear phagocyte growth factor, CSF-1. Cell 1985;41:665–676.
86. Birchenall-Roberts M, Ferrer C, Ferris D, et al. Inhibition of murine monocyte proliferation by a colony-stimulating factor-1 antisense oligodeoxynucleotide. J Immunol 1990;145:3290–3296.
87. Bories D, Raynal MC, Solomon DH, et al. Down-regulation of a serine protease, myeloblastin, causes growth arrest and differentiation of promyelocytic leukemia cells. Cell 1989;59:959–968.
88. Szczylik C, Skorski T, Nicolaides N, et al. Selective inhibition of leukemia cell proliferation by *BCR-ABL* antisense oligodeoxynucleotides. Science 1991;253:562–565.
89. Zheng H, Sahai B, Kilgannon P, et al. Specific inhibition of cell-surface T-cell receptor expression by antisense oligodeoxynucleotides and its effect on the production of an antigen-specific regulatory T-cell factor. Proc Natl Acad Sci USA 1989;86:3758–3762.
90. Harel-Bellan A, Durum S, Muegge K, et al. Specific inhibition of lymphokine biosynthesis and autocrine growth using antisense oligonucleotides in Th1 and Th2 helper T cell clones. J Exp Med 1988;168:2309–2318.
91. Weigent D, Blalock J, LeBoeuf R. An antisense oligodeoxynucleotide to growth hormone messenger ribonucleic acid inhibits lymphocyte proliferation. Endocrinology 1991;128: 2053–2057.
92. Furukawa Y, Piwnica-Worms H, Ernst T, et al. *CDC2* gene expression at the G_1 to S transition in human T lymphocytes. Science 1990;250:805–808.
93. Sburlati A, Manrow R, Berger S. Prothymosin α antisense oligomers inhibit myeloma cell division. Proc Natl Acad Sci USA 1991;88:253–257.
94. Morrison R. Suppression of basic fibroblast growth factor expression by antisense oligodeoxynucleotides inhibits the growth of transformed human astrocytes. J Biol Chem 1991;266:728–734.
95. Yu A, Chen D, Black R, et al. Sequence specific inhibition of in vitro translation of mutated or normal *ras* p21. J Exp Pathol 1989;4:97–108.
96. Brown D, Yu A, Miller P, et al. Modulation of *ras* expression by anti-sense, nonionic deoxyoligonucleotide analogs. Oncogene Res 1989;4:243–254.
97. Miller P, McParland K, Jayaraman K, et al. Biochemical and biological effects of nonionic nucleic acid methylphosphonates Biochemistry 1981;20:1874–1880.
98. Rosolen A, Whitesell L, Ikegaki N, et al. Antisense inhibition of single copy N-*myc* expression results in decreased cell growth without reduction of c-*myc* protein in a neuroepithelioma cell line. Cancer Res 1990;50:6316–6322.
99. Cope F, Wille J. Retinoid receptor antisense DNAs inhibit alkaline phosphatase induction and clonogenicity in malignant keratinocytes. Proc Natl Acad Sci USA 1989;86:5590–5594.
100. Melani E, Rivoltini L, Parmiani G, et al. Inhibition of proliferation by c-*myb* antisense oligodeoxynucleotides in colon adenocarcinoma cell lines that express c-*myb*. Cancer Res 1991;51:2897–2901.
101. Jaslkulski D, DeRiel J, Mercer W, et al. Inhibition of cellular proliferation by antisense oligodeoxynucleotides to PCNA cyclin. Science 1988;240:1544–1546.
102. Rivoltini L, Colombo M, Supino R, et al. Modulation of multidrug resistance by verapamil or *mdr1* anti-sense oligodeoxynucleotide does not change the high susceptibility to lymphokine-activated killers in *mdr*-resistant human carcinoma (LoVo) line. Int J Cancer 1990;46:727–732.
103. Caracciolo D, Venturelli D, Valtieri M, et al. Stage-related proliferative activity determines c-*myb* functional requirements during normal hematopoiesis. J Clin Invest 1990;85:55–61.

SECTION 6

WILLIAM S. DALTON

Overcoming the Multidrug-Resistant Phenotype

The problem of clinical drug resistance is well known to those involved in the care of cancer patients. Despite improvements in the treatment of many cancers, including hematologic and solid tumors, most patients will relapse and die of their disease. Modern chemotherapeutic regimens are capable of inducing remissions in many newly diagnosed patients, but treatment of relapsed disease is usually less rewarding. The drug resistance that eventually develops in the patients with recurrent disease is one of "acquired" resistance. Drugs that were initially effective in reducing tumor burden become ineffective by selecting for drug-resistant cells over time. Hematologic tumors such as acute leukemia and malignant lymphoma are good examples of diseases that manifest acquired resistance. Unlike acquired drug resistance, tumors that are relatively insensitive to chemotherapeutic drugs from the onset of disease, such as non-small cell lung cancer and colon cancer, are described as having "intrinsic" drug resistance.

Failure of chemotherapy to induce a response may be due to several different factors. These factors may be considered at the level of the entire organism or at the level of individual cells. At the level of the entire organism, physiologic factors play a major role in the successful outcome of therapy. The physiologic disposition of drugs considers absorption, distribution, metabolism, and elimination as key principles in successful cancer chemotherapy. These factors determine whether the drug actually reaches the tumor and can be manipulated by changing route of administration, drug dosage, and scheduling. Because these factors may be more readily addressed they have been given the term "temporary resistance."[1]

A more permanent form of drug resistance occurs at the genetic level. Compared with normal cells, malignant cells are genetically more unstable.[2] Genetic changes such as mutations, deletions, translocations, and gene amplification can lead to an inheritable form of drug resistance that is passed from one generation of cells to another. These genetic changes can lead to altered protein products that may be directly involved in the development of drug resistance. Chemotherapy becomes a selection factor, eradicating drug-sensitive cells and leaving behind a smaller population of drug-resistant cells. The resistant cells eventually proliferate, resulting in recurrent disease that is drug resistant.

Individual mechanisms of cellular drug resistance vary according to tumor type and the family of drugs used in the treatment of disease. One form of cellular drug resistance is the overexpression of an integral plasma membrane protein given the name P-glycoprotein or P-170.[3,4] This resistance may be acquired or intrinsic and is usually associated with natural product drugs such as the anthracyclines and vinca alkaloids. P-glycoprotein acts as a drug efflux pump that actively extrudes drugs from tumor cells, preventing a cytotoxic drug from reaching the cellular site of action. Although there are other important mechanisms of cellular drug resistance, this section focuses on multidrug resistance due to the overproduction of P-glycoprotein. Overcoming or preventing this form of drug resistance may represent a new approach to cancer treatment and improve treatment outcomes.

Multidrug resistance (MDR) is a term that describes the phenomenon by which a cancer becomes resistant to multiple drugs that have little similarity in their chemical structure and mechanism of action.[3,4] The drugs involved in MDR are primarily natural products and include antibiotics such as doxorubicin and mitomycin C and plant products, including the vinca alkaloids and podophyllotoxins. However, even certain antimetabolites such as trimetrexate and synthetic compounds such as mitoxantrone may be involved in the MDR mechanism.[5,6] Table 69–19 lists some of the drugs that have been associated with MDR.

STRUCTURE AND FUNCTION OF P-GLYCOPROTEIN

P-glycoprotein (P-gp) consists of 1280 amino acids that are arranged in such a way that the protein appears to have two similar halves.[4] The amino acid sequence predicts that each half consists of six separate segments that span the entire width of the cell membrane. The sequence information also reveals two segments of the protein that are likely to bind the energy-containing molecule ATP. Only a small portion of the protein extends to the outside of the cell, and it is this portion of the protein that is glycosylated. Most of the protein resides inside the cell and consists of two homologous domains that bear the ATP-binding sites. These ATP-binding sites on the P-gp molecule suggest that the protein is involved in an energy-requiring function, such as the transport of molecules from inside the cell to the outside.

The structural similarities between P-gp and other known membrane transport proteins support the contention that P-gp is involved in drug transport.[7,8] Presumably, chemotherapeutic drugs enter the cell and, before they reach their critical target, are bound to P-gp and actively pumped out of the cell, reducing the overall intracellular accumulation of drug (Fig. 69–25). How drugs actually bind to the P-gp and are extruded from the cell is unknown. An alternative explanation likens the mammalian P-gp to the bacterial transport protein, hemolysin-B, which transports the toxin α-hemolysin.[9] In this setting, drugs bind a carrier protein and the drug protein complex is actively transported from the cell (Fig. 69–26). No candidate for a carrier protein has been identified. In either case, P-gp must be in high concentrations in the plasma membrane if it is involved in the transport of drugs out of the cell.

TABLE 69–19. Chemotherapeutic Drugs Exhibiting Cross-Resistance in Multidrug Resistance

Doxorubicin	Taxol
Daunorubicin	Trimetrexate
Vincristine	Mitomycin C
Vinblastine	Dactinomycin
Etoposide	Mitoxantrone

Although P-gp is involved in the transport of drugs out of neoplastic cells, its normal function is unknown. Analyzing for the presence of P-gp in normal tissue may give us clues to the normal function of this molecule. Fojo and colleagues were the first to report on a large survey of *MDR1* expression in normal human tissues.[10] Using a technique to detect MDR1 mRNA, they found a high degree of expression in normal adrenal gland and kidney. Intermediate levels were detected in the lung, liver, and colon. Tumors derived from those tissues that express a higher intermediate level of MDR1 RNA (*e.g.*, renal cell carcinoma) may explain the intrinsic drug resistance observed in these tumors.

Using flow cytometry, Chaudhary and Roninson examined *MDR1* expression in human bone marrow.[11] These investigators found that early hematopoietic precursor cells, defined as high expressors of CD34 antigen and capable of self-renewal in tissue culture, produce high levels of P-gp. Functional analysis demonstrated that these cells could exclude the dye rhodamine 123 (a substrate for P-gp) and that this exclusion could be attenuated by inhibitors of P-gp (*e.g.*, verapamil). Using the polymerase chain reaction (PCR), it was shown that the lymphoid region of the bone marrow—where most of early progenitor cells are thought to reside—express MDR1 RNA. P-gp expression has been associated with the

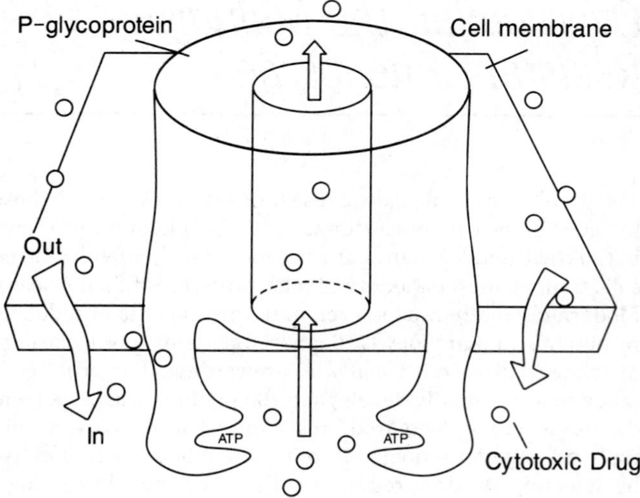

FIGURE 69–25. Model of P-glycoprotein as an energy-dependent drug efflux pump. In this model, cytotoxic drugs bind directly to P-glycoprotein and are transported from the intracellular to the extracellular space.

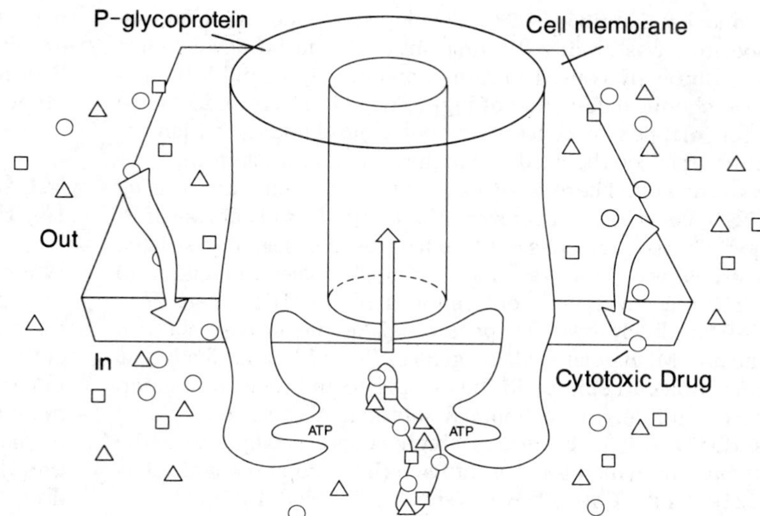

FIGURE 69–26. In this model, P-glycoprotein transports an intracellular protein that serves as a carrier for cytotoxic drugs. This model is analogous to other transport molecules known to transport proteins to the extracellular space.

CD34 phenotype in myelodysplastic syndrome and acute myeloid leukemia.[12] These hematopoietic stem cell malignancies are notoriously resistant to drugs.

With the development of monoclonal antibodies against P-gp, the cellular location of P-gp can be determined. Using the monoclonal antibody MRK-16, Thiebaut and coworkers found that P-gp was distributed in a highly site-specific fashion.[13] Immunohistochemical staining with the MRK-16 antibody demonstrated that P-gp was distributed along the apical surface of epithelial cells of the proximal tubules of the kidney, superficial columnar epithelial cells of the colon in jejunum, and limited to hepatocytes lining the biliary canaliculi of the liver. These results suggested that P-gp served a function in the normal excretion of compounds and possibly drugs into the urine, gastrointestinal tract, and bile. Immunohistochemical studies using monoclonal antibodies HYB-241 and HYB-612 have shown that endothelial cells of human capillary blood vessels in the brain and testes express high levels of P-gp.[14] This finding suggests a physiologic role for P-gp in reducing the amount of drugs in critical anatomic sites that have been known to be sanctuaries for malignant cells.

METHODS OF DETECTION OF MULTIDRUG RESISTANCE

General methods of detecting MDR in tissues are shown in Table 69–20. These approaches include assessing DNA amplification, measuring messenger mRNA, and quantitating the amount of protein. Although the amplification of the *MDR1* gene has been observed in tumor cell lines, gene amplification is an uncommon event in the clinical setting, and overexpression of the *MDR1* gene is usually not associated with gene amplification.[15] Most investigators have turned to measuring the *MDR1* message or actual detection of the gene product, P-gp. To evaluate the role of P-gp in clinical drug resistance, it is important to develop assays that are specific for the *MDR1* gene but sensitive enough to detect minute concentrations that may be present in small tissue specimens.[16] An added confounding factor in the clinical setting is the fact that P-gp is expressed in certain normal tissues. Assays must be specific and sensitive and be able to discriminate between normal and neoplastic tissue.

Initial studies analyzing the role of *MDR1* in human tumor specimens used biochemical analyses of bulk tumor tissue. Bell and colleagues first reported the presence of P-gp in ovarian cancer by detecting the protein in bulk tumor specimens using an immunoblot analysis.[17] Gerlach and associates, using a similar immunoblot technique, detected P-gp in a series of sarcoma patients.[18] Fojo and colleagues[10] and later Goldstein and colleagues[19] were successful in measuring MDR1 RNA in various human tumors by extracting total RNA from bulk tissue and detecting the *MDR1* message with gene-specific probes. Although these initial analyses were considered to be specific for *MDR1*, they were relatively insensitive and did not differentiate between normal and neoplastic tissue.

Methods to differentiate expression of *MDR* in normal and tumor cells have been developed. In situ hybridization with nucleic acid probes on tissue sections allows the detection of MDR mRNA in tumor cells.[20] This technique, however, is very laborious and can be difficult to interpret. Because of the difficulties in performing mRNA in situ hybridization, attention has been directed to the use of monoclonal antibodies in immunohistochemical detection.

Several antibodies are available for detection of P-gp. The

TABLE 69–20. Methods of Detecting Multidrug Resistance

1. DNA analysis for amplification (Southern blot)
2. Analysis of RNA
   - Northern blot
   - Slot-blot
   - RNase protection assay
   - In situ hybridization
   - Polymerase chain reaction analysis
3. Analysis for protein
   - Western blot
   - Immunohistochemistry
   - Flow cytometry

monoclonal antibody C219, developed by Victor Ling and associates, was among the first antibodies to be developed.[21] This antibody is used in immunoblot analysis and immunohistochemical detection of P-gp. The epitopes for C219 have been mapped to conserve cytoplasmic domains, which requires that cells be fixed so that the antibody may gain entrance into the cell. There is also a problem of specificity in using C219, because it recognizes *MDR1* and *MDR3* isoforms of P-gp.[22] Cross-reactivities of C219 have been observed in striated musculature.[23] Several monoclonal antibodies in addition to C219 react with different epitopes of the MDR1 P-gp. The C494 antibody is MDR1 specific and does not cross-react with the non-MDR-related *MDR3* gene of P-gp.[22] This antibody also recognizes an epitope in the cytoplasm and requires fixation before immunohistochemical staining. A third monoclonal antibody, JSB-1, recognizes a highly conserved epitope in the cytoplasm, which is different from the epitope recognized by C219.[24] Like C494, JSB-1 is specific for MDR1 P-gp.[25]

Tsuruo and colleagues developed a monoclonal antibody, MRK-16, that has a high affinity for MDR1.[26] Unlike the antibodies mentioned previously, MRK-16 recognizes an external epitope on the outer surface of the plasma membrane of living cells. The use of MRK-16 does not require prior fixation to detect P-gp. This particular characteristic allows the use of flow cytometry in detecting P-gp in living cells. Two new monoclonal antibodies, HYB-241 and HYB-612, have been developed by Hybritech (San Diego, CA) in collaboration with Biedler and associates at Memorial Sloan-Kettering Cancer Center in New York.[14] These two antibodies recognize external epitopes of MDR1 but recognition is restricted to a 180-kd P-gp, and they do not recognize the 170-kd form of P-gp. Whether this limits the usefulness of these antibodies in P-gp detection in clinical samples is unknown.

Immunohistochemical detection of P-gp in clinical samples holds particular promise, because it is a practical, readily performed procedure.[16,27] The primary advantages of immunohistochemistry in the clinical setting include the ability to detect P-gp a single cell, allowing for small sample size, and the ability to discriminate P-gp expression in normal cells from that found in tumor cells. This latter feature is especially important considering the heterogenous nature of clinical specimens. The sensitivity and specificity of immunohistochemical detection of P-gp have been improved, and this method holds considerable promise for practical application in the clinical setting.[23–30]

The advent of the PCR provided probably the most sensitive and reliable means of detecting MDR1 RNA. Using this approach, it is possible to analyze the most minute of clinical specimens.[31] PCR is so sensitive, however, that it raises the question of what threshold level of *MDR1* expression is necessary to confer multidrug resistance. Levels detected below a theoretical threshold level may actually cause a tumor to be called drug resistant although it is still sensitive to drugs. This problem illustrates the need for proper controls, usually in the form of drug-sensitive and drug-resistant cell lines for a particular tumor type, when performing assays for MDR detection. Several PCR methods have been developed to quantitate MDR1 RNA in tumor specimens.[32–34]

The multitude of assays and techniques used in clinical studies may produce various results for a given tumor type, and investigators must be aware of the strengths and weaknesses of each assay. In the clinical situation, a combination of complementary assays such as immunohistochemistry and PCR may provide the best information about the presence of MDR in human tumors.

MULTIDRUG RESISTANCE IN HEMATOLOGIC TUMORS

When first diagnosed, hematologic tumors are sensitive to most chemotherapeutic agents used. However, after relapse, the response rate is less and usually of shorter duration. The anthracyclines, vinca alkaloids, and epipodophyllotoxins are integral components of treatment regimens used in the treatment of leukemias, malignant lymphomas, and multiple myeloma. Complete remissions are common with initial induction therapy, but if relapse occurs, patients usually acquire drug resistance and frequently die of their disease.

ACUTE LYMPHOCYTIC LEUKEMIA

Complete hematologic remissions are achieved in 70% to 90% of patients with newly diagnosed adult or childhood acute lymphoblastic leukemia (ALL).[35] Sustained remissions are more common in childhood than adult ALL. Expression of P-gp in ALL blast cells is detected infrequently at initial diagnosis (Table 69–21). Goldstein and coworkers[19] and Rothenberg and colleagues[36] found overexpression of the *MDR1* gene in fewer than 15% of patients with childhood ALL at presentation or at relapse. Acquisition of the MDR phenotype, however, may be more frequent in adult ALL. As shown in Table 69–21, Musto and associates[37] and others[38–40] have found expression of the MDR phenotype in 50% or more of cases of re-

TABLE 69–21. Multidrug Resistance in Acute Leukemias

	Pretreatment		*Relapsed*	
Malignancy/ Investigations	*No. of Patients*	*MDR+ (%)*	*No. of Patients*	*MDR+ (%)*
Acute Lymphocytic Leukemia (ALL)				
Childhood ALL				
Goldstein et al[19]	9	1 (11)	20	3 (15)
Rothenberg et al[36]	9	1 (11)	19	3 (16)
Adult ALL				
Goldstein et al[19]	15	2 (13)		
Musto et al[37]	20	2 (10)	12	7 (58)
Herweijer et al[38]	8	4 (50)	1	1
Adult T-cell Leukemia-Lymphoma (ATL)				
Kuwazuru et al[41]	20	8 (40)	6	6 (100)
Acute Non-Lymphocytic Leukemia (ANLL)				
Goldstein et al[19]	24	3 (13)	5	4 (80)
Herweijer et al[38]	7	1 (14)	10	8 (80)
Holmes et al[45]	8	2 (25)	8	5 (62)
Ito et al[46]	10	1 (10)	14	2 (15)
Musto et al[37]	12	1 (8)	8	6 (75)
Nooter et al[47]	6	1 (17)	10	6 (60)
Sato et al[44]	36	9 (25)	17	9 (53)

lapsing adult ALL. These observations are consistent with the lower rate of successful reinduction in relapsed adult ALL.

Patients with adult T-cell leukemia-lymphoma (ATL) syndrome appear to have a high prevalence of P-gp overexpression. Remissions are usually of short duration and are associated with the emergence of acquired drug resistance despite the use of intensive chemotherapy induction regimens. In a study by Kuwazuru and colleagues, 25 patients with the ATL syndrome were studied for the presence of P-gp using immunoblot analyses.[41] At initial presentation, 8 of 20 patients were positive for P-gp. Of 6 patients who had relapsed and were refractory to chemotherapy, all were positive for P-gp. Similarly, Herweijer and coworkers found a higher frequency of *MDR1* expression in T-cell-lineage ALL, implying that lymphoblast lineage may relate to *MDR* overexpression.[38]

ACUTE NONLYMPHOCYTIC LEUKEMIA

Like ALL, patients with acute nonlymphocytic leukemia (ANLL) have a high probability of going into a complete remission; however, if relapse occurs, they are unlikely to be cured due to the emergence of drug resistance.[42] The anthracycline daunorubicin is one of the most active agents used in the treatment of ANLL. Studies have shown that the intracellular concentration of daunorubicin in leukemic cells is an important determinant of response to therapy.[43] The presence of P-gp on cells could lower the intracellular concentration of daunorubicin, thereby decreasing efficacy.

Table 69–21 shows the incidence of P-gp in newly diagnosed and relapsed ANLL patients from several studies using different methods of detection for *MDR1*. Between 10% and 20% of cases of newly diagnosed ANLL appear to express the *MDR1* message or its P-gp product. Although few patients have been studied serially, P-gp or its message occurs in more than 50% of patients with relapsed ANLL. In a study by Sato and colleagues, 88% of patients who had P-gp-negative disease obtained a complete remission, compared with 58% of patients whose leukemic cells contained moderate of high levels of *MDR1* message.[44] The number of patients requiring two courses of induction therapy to obtain a complete remission was substantially higher among patients with high *MDR* expression. Moreover, the median duration of response for patients with low levels of *MDR* expression was twice as long as that observed for patients with high levels of *MDR* expression, indicating that *MDR* expression affects overall outcome in patients receiving conventional cytarabine-daunorubicin induction and consolidation treatment.

The prevalence of P-gp in myelodysplastic syndromes has been investigated. Holmes and associates found elevated levels of MDR1 RNA in 7 of 19 cases of myelodysplastic syndrome (MDS).[45] List and colleagues, using immunocytochemical staining and flow cytometry to detect P-gp, found increased expression in 7 of 32 patients (22%).[12] P-gp detection was limited to blast cells and leukemic monocytes and was otherwise absent from terminally differentiated blood cells. Among patients who developed ANLL that was preceded by a myelodysplastic syndrome, the incidence of P-gp increased to 75%. Among patients with secondary leukemia related to prior treatment for hematologic disorders including Hodgkin's disease, 9 (82%) of 11 patients had overexpression of P-gp on their leukemic cells.

Patients with acute leukemias preceded by myelodysplastic syndrome or patients with secondary leukemias related to treatment of other hematologic disorders usually have a poor response to conventional induction therapy. The high incidence of *MDR1* expression in these patient populations may explain the poor treatment outcome.

CHRONIC LEUKEMIAS

The expression of P-gp has also been examined in chronic lymphocytic and chronic myelocytic leukemias. Chronic lymphocytic leukemia (CLL) is characterized by the progressive increase in malignant lymphocytes in the peripheral blood, bone marrow, and lymphoid tissues. Chemotherapy is able to control proliferation of these abnormal lymphocytes; however, cure is generally not possible. In a study by Holmes and coworkers measuring *MDR1* expression, moderate levels of MDR1 RNA were found in 4 of 7 untreated CLL patients and 14 of 27 previously treated patients.[48] In a study by Herweijer and colleagues using a sensitive RNAse protection assay, 17 of 17 patients expressed at least some MDR1 mRNA in their cells.[38] These same investigators found detectable message for the *MDR3* gene in all CLL patients. No correlation was observed between *MDR1* expression and prior treatment. However, the *MDR3* expression was generally higher in treated patients than in untreated patients. The investigators speculated that a particular splice variant of *MDR3* may be functional in conferring drug resistance in CLL.

The importance of the type of method used in detecting MDR in CLL was reported by Cumber and colleagues.[49] These investigators used the monoclonal antibody MRK-16, which recognizes an external epitope of P-gp on the external surface of cells. Initial studies using this antibody showed only 12% of the lymphocyte samples from CLL patients had increased P-gp on their cells. Treatment of the leukemic cells with neuraminidase to remove sialic acid residues increased the proportion of patients expressing P-gp on their cells from 12% to 52%. The investigators think that abnormal sialalation patterns on the surface of cells masked the epitope recognized by MRK-16, creating false-negative results.

In chronic myelocytic leukemia, *MDR1* expression generally has been limited to blast cells seen in the terminal phase of the disease. Goldstein and associates analyzed the RNA of 9 patients with chronic myelogenous leukemia.[19] Three patients were in the chronic phase of their CML, and 6 patients were in the blast phase. All 3 patients who were in chronic phase showed no *MDR1* expression in their leukemic cells. In contrast, 5 of 6 patients in the blast phase of their disease showed overexpression of *MDR1*. Similarly, two different studies using immunocytochemistry or RNA analysis found that 50% of patients in the blast phase of their CML expressed *MDR1*.[50,51] This increased expression may partially explain the poor results of treatment for the blast phase of CML.

LYMPHOMA

The clinical course of patients with malignant lymphoma closely parallels the laboratory animal models of acquired drug resistance. Most patients with newly diagnosed non-Hodgkin's lymphomas and advanced Hodgkin's disease respond to initial chemotherapy. Responses to treatment are observed with a wide variety of single agents or combinations of drugs. However, most patients relapse and eventually develop drug-resistant disease.

The parallel to animal models of multidrug resistance is even more striking when the frequency of P-gp expression is considered. Newly diagnosed and untreated patients rarely express the P-gp in detectable amounts, but patients with recurrent and drug-refractory disease frequently have detectable levels of P-gp. In a consecutive series of 42 patients with newly diagnosed malignant lymphomas, Miller and colleagues using immunocytochemistry found detectable levels of P-gp in only 1 patient.[52] Goldstein and coworkers, using RNA slot blot methods, found P-gp in 4 of 18 previously untreated patients.[19] These findings contrast with the high frequency of P-gp expressed in previously treated patients with recurrent and clinically drug-resistant disease. Miller and colleagues[52] found P-gp in 7 (64%) of 11 patients, and Goldstein and associates[19] found it in 3 (60%) of 5 patients. These studies suggest that incidence of detectable levels of P-gp closely parallels the clinical response to chemotherapy.

MULTIPLE MYELOMA

Multiple myeloma is a malignancy of the plasma cell, the most mature cell in the B-cell series. Advances in the treatment of multiple myeloma have been made over the last 3 decades and are manifest both in prolongation of survival from less than 1 year to almost 3 years and in a better quality of life.[53,54] These improvements are attributed to the development of more effective chemotherapy, which includes the natural products vincristine and doxorubicin. Despite initial responses seen in most patients, all patients develop drug resistance and eventually die of their disease.

At the University of Arizona, over 100 patients with multiple myeloma have been studied for the expression of P-gp.[55] In newly diagnosed patients, fewer than 5% of patients have P-gp on their cells. When treated with alkylating agents alone (*e.g.*, melphalan), the incidence of P-gp remains basically unchanged. As patients receive more treatment, including vincristine and doxorubicin, the incidence of P-gp increases. When patients become refractory to vincristine and doxorubicin (Adriamycin), as used in the VAD regimen of continuous infusion of vincristine and doxorubicin given over 4 days, more than 75% of patients express P-gp on their tumor cells. Epstein and colleagues, using the C219 monoclonal antibody and flow cytometry, found that most patients who failed VAD treatment had P-gp-positive myeloma cells.[56] In multiple myeloma, the development of MDR appears to be acquired and related to the type of chemotherapy received.

MULTIDRUG RESISTANCE IN SOLID TUMORS

The incidence of MDR in human tumors was first shown in a series of five ovarian cancer patients who had undergone chemotherapy before surgery. In the study, Bell and coworkers found two tumors exhibiting overproduction of P-gp as revealed by Western blot analysis using the monoclonal antibody C219.[17] Since this first paper appeared in 1985, several studies have been performed using various methods of detection to determine the incidence of MDR in solid tumors. The largest study performed was reported by Goldstein and colleagues.[19] These investigators studied over 400 human cancers and were able to group tumors into four groups based on their level of expression of MDR1 RNA (Table 69–22). Not surprisingly, tumors that had a high level of *MDR1* message tended to originate from normal cells that were also known to express high levels. These tumors included most untreated colon cancers, renal carcinomas, hepatoma, adrenal cortical carcinoma, pheochromocytoma, islet cell tumors of the pancreas, and carcinoid tumors. Tumors that occasionally expressed *MDR1* were neuroblastoma, breast cancer, and bladder cancer. Those untreated cancers that rarely if ever expressed *MDR1* were esophageal carcinoma, gastric carcinoma, head and neck cancer, Wilms' tumor, and ovarian cancer. The investigators found that posttreatment relapsed breast cancers, pheochromocytoma, and neuroblastoma had increased levels of *MDR1* expression.

Perhaps the most impressive studies demonstrating the value of P-gp as a prognostic factor comes from the retrospective studies of Chan and associates.[57] These investigators studied 30 cases of rhabdomyosarcoma and undifferentiated sarcoma from children. P-gp was detected in 9 patients, 4 at diagnosis and 5 at subsequent biopsy. All 9 patients who had P-gp-positive tumors relapsed after chemotherapy. Of the 20 patients who had P-gp-negative tumors and responded to chemotherapy, only 1 relapsed. The overall probability of survival was significantly different in these two groups of patients with childhood soft tissue sarcoma.

TABLE 69–22. Expression of *MDR1* in Untreated Solid Tumors

Tumor	*No. of Samples*	*Percent Positive*
Tumors With Moderate to High Expression		
Colon	41	85
Renal	50	80
Hepatoma	12	100
Adrenocortical	9	77
Pheochromocytoma	20	75
Islet cell	4	50
Carcinoid	9	77
Tumors With Low Expression		
Breast	57	15
Bladder	6	16
Esophageal	14	0
Gastric	2	0
Head and Neck	14	0
Melanoma	3	0
Ovarian	16	0
Prostate	3	0
Thyroid	4	0
Wilms' Tumor	20	0

(Modified from Goldstein LJ, Galski H, Fojo A, et al. Expression of a multidrug resistance gene in human cancers. JNCI 1989;81:116–124)

Similar results have been reported in children with neuroblastoma.[58] Tumors positive for P-gp as detected by immunocytochemistry predicted for poor response to chemotherapy compared with P-gp negative tumors. Relapse-free survival and overall survival were also worse in patients whose tumors were positive for P-gp. Although these studies were retrospective, they provide strong preliminary evidence that P-gp is an important prognostic factor in these childhood solid tumors.

Studies to detect P-gp in breast cancer have produced interesting results regarding level of expression and stage of disease. Several studies using various methods, including immunodetection or measurement of RNA, have shown that the level of expression in breast cancer is relatively low.[59,60] However, two studies, both involving locally advanced breast cancer, have shown that most patients express P-gp on their tumors. Using the C219 monoclonal antibody, Ro and colleagues observed frequent expression of P-gp in tumors after preoperative chemotherapy.[61] This expression was significantly associated with a poor response to chemotherapy. In a second study by Verrelle and coworkers,[62] the expression of P-gp in locally advanced breast cancer was analyzed using immunohistochemical staining with the monoclonal antibody C494, which is considered specific for the MDR1 protein.[22] This study of 20 previously untreated patients found a surprisingly high incidence of P-gp expression in tumor cells from patients with primary, locally advanced breast cancer. Eighty-five percent of the patients expressed P-gp in at least some of their tumor cells. Seven patients who had a high degree of staining in most tumor cells had a worse prognosis, with fewer patients responding to therapy and with shorter durations of response.

These studies demonstrate that, as a tumor grows, there may be a higher likelihood of expressing P-gp. The numbers of patients in these studies were small, and confirmatory studies are necessary.

Cordon-Cardo and colleagues studied 22 patients with non-small cell lung cancers using an immunohistochemical stain.[63] Only two of the 22 lung cancers showed any positive staining cells in the tumor. A similar study by Lai and associates found very low levels of MDR1 RNA in small cell and non-small cell lung cancers.[64] It would appear that *MDR1* expression plays an insignificant role in drug resistance in lung cancer.

REVERSING MULTIDRUG RESISTANCE

Efforts to overcome drug resistance that can be attributed to overexpression of *MDR1* include several possibilities: the use of high-dose chemotherapy to increase intracellular concentrations; the use of noncross-resistant regimens as proposed by the Goldie-Coldman hypothesis; targeting P-gp-positive cells with monoclonal antibodies or conjugates; and the use of chemosensitizing agents or agents that are able to inhibit the function of P-gp. This last approach has received much attention in the laboratory and in the clinic. Tsuruo and colleagues observed that the calcium channel blocker verapamil was able to overcome resistance in vivo and in vitro to vincristine and doxorubicin.[65] Since the initial observation of Tsuruo and coworkers, a great deal of effort has been devoted to identifying other chemosensitizing agents capable of reversing MDR.[66,67]

All of these agents have been identified empirically, and several them are listed in Table 69–23. These agents share the property of inhibiting anticancer drug binding to P-gp, blocking enhanced drug efflux and allowing increased intracellular concentrations of the anticancer drug (Fig. 69–27).[7,8,9] Exactly how these chemosensitizing agents inhibit P-gp function is unknown, but it has been shown that the chemosensitizers themselves bind to P-gp.[68,69] What is not clear is the nature of the P-gp binding sites. It is unknown whether the chemosensitizers share binding sites with anticancer drugs or whether these agents inhibit P-gp function through allosteric changes. Because some of these agents can modulate calcium metabolism (*e.g.*, verapamil, trifluoperazine), it is possible that the MDR reversal effect is mediated by indirect means, through modulation of calcium-dependent P-gp phosphorylation.[70]

The effect of chemosensitizers such as verapamil and cyclosporine on cytotoxic drug accumulation has been investigated in tumor cells from patients with drug-resistant disease.[36,71,72] In these studies of patients with hematologic neoplasms, verapamil increased the accumulation of vincristine or daunorubicin. In studies of patients with myeloma or acute lymphocytic leukemia, verapamil increased drug accumulation in cells shown to express P-gp.[36,71] In a study by Nooter and colleagues, cyclosporin A was more effective than verapamil in increasing daunorubicin intracellular accumulation in leukemic cells from patients with acute nonlymphocytic leukemia.[72] The degree of cyclosporin-A-induced increase in daunorubicin accumulation correlated with the levels of overexpression of the *MDR1* gene in these leukemic cells. This in vitro analysis of human leukemic cells obtained from patients with drug-resistant, P-gp-positive disease demonstrated that drug accumulation can be increased by chemosensitizers such as verapamil and cyclosporin A. What remains to be demonstrated, however, is an increase in cellular drug accumulation when chemosensitizers are given in the clinical situation.

With the evidence that P-gp overexpression occurs in patients with drug-resistant diseases, pilot studies have been conducted to determine if verapamil is capable of overcoming

TABLE 69–23. Chemosensitizers Known to Modulate P-glycoprotein Function

Chemical Class	*Example*
Calcium channel blockers	Verapamil
Calmodulin inhibitors	Trifluoperazine
Indole alkaloids	Reserpine
Quinolines	Quinine
Lysosomotropic agents	Chloroquine
Steroids	Progesterone
Triparanol analogs	Tamoxifen
Detergents	Cremophor EL
Cyclic peptide antibiotics	Cyclosporines

(Citations for individual agents can be found in Beck WT. Modulators of P-glycoprotein associated multidrug resistance. In: Ozols RF, ed. Drug resistance, vol. II. Norwell, MA: Kluwer Academic Publishers, 1991)

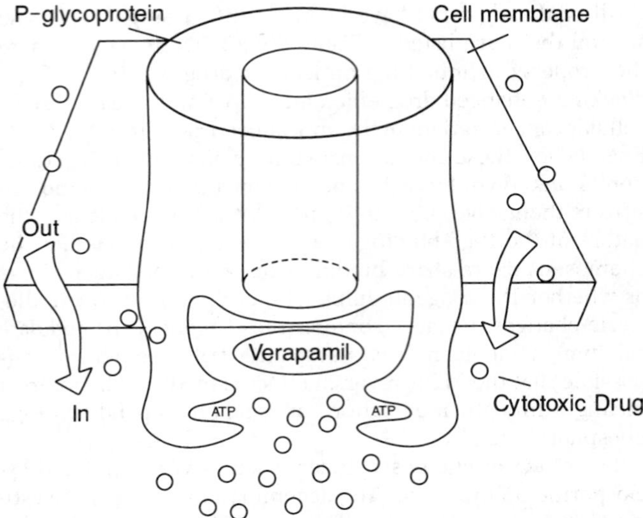

FIGURE 69–27. Chemosensitizers, such as verapamil, may block the enhanced efflux of cytotoxic drugs by directly binding to P-glycoprotein and inhibiting its function.

clinical drug resistance.[71,73–78] Benson and associates reported preliminary findings of a phase I study investigating the combination of vinblastine and verapamil in 17 patients with solid tumors.[73] Both verapamil and vinblastine were given as continuous infusion for 5 days. Cardiac toxicity was dose limiting, and there was no augmentation of vinblastine toxicity. In a similar study, Ozols and colleagues examined the combination of intravenous verapamil with doxorubicin in 8 patients who had drug-resistant ovarian cancer.[75] No patients benefitted from this treatment, and cardiac toxicity was dose limiting.

In a study of multiple myeloma patients with drug-resistant disease by Dalton and coworkers, 5 of 7 patients overexpressed P-gp on their tumor cells as determined by immunohistochemical staining and RNA analysis.[71] All patients had developed progressive disease while receiving a regimen containing vincristine and daunorubicin (VAD). At the time of progressive disease, continuous infusion verapamil was added to the VAD regimen. Two of the 7 patients who were refractory to VAD alone responded after verapamil was added to the regimen. Both patients who responded had P-gp-positive tumors. In two patients whose tumors overexpressed P-gp, verapamil increased the intracellular accumulation of vincristine or doxorubicin in vitro. This study has been expanded to 22 patients, with 5 patients showing a partial response.[76] Durations of response have been short, with a median response duration of 5.4 months. Two other studies using verapamil as a chemosensitizing agent have been reported in preliminary form in patients with drug-resistant myeloma.[77,78]

In a report by Gore and colleagues, 7 patients who were resistant to 4-day continuous infusion vincristine and doxorubicin were administered a low dose of verapamil by continuous infusion.[77] Four of 7 patients had a further reduction in paraprotein levels of greater than 25%. Two patients had a greater than 50% response with the addition of verapamil to the chemotherapeutic regimen. A second preliminary report by Trumper and associates studied 10 patients who had developed drug-resistant myeloma.[78] Only 1 of 10 patients responded after verapamil was added to the VAD regimen. Based on these pilot studies, prospective, randomized, controlled studies are indicated. A prospective randomized study is being conducted by the Southwest Oncology Group to determine the value of adding verapamil to the VAD chemotherapy regimen.

A similar pilot study was conducted in patients with drug-resistant non-Hodgkin's lymphoma.[52] Verapamil was administered as a continuous 5-day infusion at escalating doses until dose-limiting cardiotoxicity intervened. The verapamil was combined with cyclophosphamide and a 4-day infusion of vincristine and doxorubicin and oral dexamethasone. Patients were carefully selected for drug resistance based on disease progression while receiving combination chemotherapy or a relapse within 3 months of receiving doxorubicin and vincristine-containing chemotherapy regimen. Clinical drug resistance was confirmed by a high incidence of *MDR1* expression. Five complete remissions (28%) and eight partial remissions (44%) were observed among 18 patients studied. Cardiovascular side effects observed most frequently included first-degree heart block, hypotension, sinus bradycardia, and junctional rhythms.[79] Effects on mean arterial pressure, heart rate, and PR interval were time- and dose-related. Severe, symptomatic congestive heart failure was rarely observed. The most common noncardiovascular side effects were constipation, peripheral edema, and weight gain.

From these studies it can be concluded that the cardiovascular side effects associated with continuous, high-dose intravenous verapamil therapy are significant and dose limiting. Further research is clearly needed to develop less toxic and more efficacious chemosensitizers to be used clinically.

Clinical studies using other chemosensitizers listed in Table 69–23 have been reported. Miller and colleagues reported that the calmodulin inhibitor, trifluoperazine, was capable of causing a second response to doxorubicin in patients who had received this drug in prior regimens.[80] Drug-limiting toxicity was due to extrapyramidal site effects commonly seen with trifluoperazine. Trump and coworkers reported a phase I clinical trial of high-dose oral tamoxifen administered in conjunction with 5-day continuous infusion vinblastine.[81] Neurotoxicity was dose limiting and resolved rapidly when tamoxifen was discontinued. There was no indication that tamoxifen enhanced the expected toxicity of vinblastine. Like verapamil, the dose-limiting toxicities of these potential chemosensitizers have been attributed to the inherent toxicity of the chemosensitizer and not due to enhanced chemotherapy toxicity.

Theoretically, chemosensitizers may alter or enhance the toxicity of chemotherapeutic drugs by inhibiting the function of P-gp in normal tissues, including the kidney, liver, colon, and capillary endothelial cells of the brain. Preliminary studies using high doses of cyclosporin A as a chemosensitizer found hyperbilirubinemia as a side effect.[82–84] This toxic effect may be related to cyclosporin A inhibiting the normal function of P-gp in hepatic biliary canaliculi.[23] A phase II study of epidoxorubicin plus cyclosporin A in patients with colorectal cancer observed a greater than expected frequency of severe neutropenia.[85] P-gp occurs in normal hematopoietic (CD34 positive) precursor cells.[11] High doses of cyclosporin A may have increased intracellular concentrations of epidoxorubicin in this hematopoietic compartment, resulting in severe neutropenia. A second explanation for this enhanced toxicity may be changes in clearance of the cytotoxic drug by cyclosporin A. Studies of cyclosporin A plus etoposide have reported a prolonged clearance of etoposide when cyclosporin A was added.[82] These studies illustrate the importance of measuring pharmacokinetics of chemosensitizers and cytotoxic drugs in clinical trials so that therapeutic and toxicity results may be interpreted correctly.

Strategies for developing new chemosensitizing agents are outlined in Table 69–24. Currently, compounds are screened for activity on an empiric basis using in vitro cytotoxicity assays. Promising agents are then evaluated in in vivo models to determine the therapeutic index and efficacy. Studies of structure-activity relations of chemosensitizers performed by Beck and colleagues have demonstrated that modulators of P-gp are usually lipid soluble at physiologic pH and possess a basic nitrogen atom and at least one planar aromatic ring.[86,87] Notable exceptions to these generalities exist (*e.g.*, cyclosporin A). Rationale drug design by molecular modeling as proposed by Beck and colleagues should ultimately provide more effective and less toxic chemosensitizers, but more basic information about P-gp binding sites and exactly how P-gp exports anticancer drugs is needed.[86]

One approach to reducing toxicity is to develop stereoisomers of effective chemosensitizers that have fewer side effects. Both the R and S optical isomers of verapamil are equally effective in reversing MDR, but the R isomer is 10 times less cardiotoxic than the S isomer.[88] Clinical studies are using R-verapamil as a chemosensitizer. The optical isomers quinine and quinidine also appear to have equal activity in reversing resistance. Quinine is less toxic than quinidine, and the therapeutic index for quinine may be superior in the clinical setting.[89]

A transgenic mouse was developed for testing agents as potential chemosensitizers in reversing drug resistance. In this model developed by Mickisch and associates, transgenic mice express the multidrug resistance gene in their bone marrow cells and are resistant to leukopenia induced by natural products such as anthracyclines.[90] This drug resistance can be circumvented in a dose-dependent manner by simultaneous administration of agents such as verapamil and quinine. This *MDR1*-transgenic mouse model may serve as a reliable system for evaluating the bioactivity of potential chemosensitizing agents.

TABLE 69–24. Strategies for Developing Chemosensitizers to Overcome Multidrug Resistance

1. Drug screening of candidate drugs
   A. Evaluate efficacy using in vitro cytotoxicity assays with drug-resistant cell lines and short-term cultures of fresh tumor specimens
   B. Determine therapeutic index by analyzing in vivo activity in murine tumors, xenografts, or transgenic mouse models
2. Develop analogs of known chemosensitizers for
   A. Molecular modeling
   B. Structural activity relations
3. Identify P-glycoprotein binding sites by
   A. Biochemical methods—competitive photoaffinity labeling experiments
   B. Molecular methods—effect of P-glycoprotein site-directed metagenesis on drug binding

TABLE 69–25. Clinical Evaluation of Chemosensitizing Agents to Overcome Multidrug Resistance

1. Select promising agents from preclinical screening (see Table 69-23)
2. Phase I trials of chemosensitizing (CS) agent plus chemotherapy
   A. Determine maximal tolerated dose of CS for phase II trials
   B. Evaluate pharmacokinetics of CS (serum levels of CS agent should approximate levels known to be active in vitro)
3. Phase II trials of CS agent plus chemotherapy
   A. Choose tumor types known to be associated with MDR
   B. Monitor P-glycoprotein before and after therapy
   C. Monitor pharmacokinetic levels of both CS and chemotherapy
4. Phase III trials of CS agent plus chemotherapy in MDR-positive tumors
   A. Patients randomized to chemotherapy alone versus chemotherapy plus CS. Consider cross-over design for patients receiving chemotherapy alone to chemotherapy plus CS at time of progressive disease
   B. Monitor P-glycoprotein levels before and after therapy

After a promising potential chemosensitizing agent has been identified by a preclinical means, it is important to design clinical trials so that meaningful data may be obtained regarding potential activity of chemosensitizing agents (Table 69–25). In phase I trials, it is important to perform pharmacokinetic analyses of the chemosensitizers to ensure that levels required for activity in vitro can be obtained clinically. If toxicity of the chemosensitizer plus chemotherapy is acceptable and adequate concentrations of the chemosensitizer are obtained, phase II testing may be performed. Cancers known to be associated with MDR and P-gp should be treated in phase II trials, and analysis for P-gp in individual patients enrolled in study should be attempted. Pharmacokinetic analysis of anticancer drugs would be helpful in determining if chemosensitizers alter the physiologic disposition of anticancer drugs. Ultimately, phase III testing of the chemosensitizer and chemotherapy will be required to determine if treatment outcome is improved in specific diseases by the use of chemosensitizers.

Tumors that are considered drug-sensitive at diagnosis but acquire an MDR phenotype at relapse pose an interesting problem for protocol design. It is unclear how these initially drug-sensitive tumors become P-gp positive at relapse, but tumor heterogeneity and cell selection by cytotoxic drugs presumably play a role. At diagnosis, only a minority of tumor cells may express P-gp and treatment with chemotherapy provides a selection advantage for the few cells that are P-gp positive early in the course of disease. An alternative explanation is that natural-product-derived chemotherapy actually induces the expression of *MDR1,* leading to P-pg-positive tumors at relapse. A possible therapeutic approach to tumors that acquire MDR is outlined in Table 69–26. Using chemosensitizers early in the course of disease may prevent the emergence of MDR by eliminating the few cells that are P-gp positive at the beginning. In vitro studies have shown that selection of drug-resistant cells by combining verapamil and doxorubicin does prevent the emergence of P-gp, but that an alternative drug resistance mechanism develops, which is secondary to altered topoisomerase II function.[91]

Reasons for possible failure of chemosensitizers to reverse

TABLE 69–26. Possible Approaches to Overcoming Clinical Multidrug Resistance in Tumors With Acquired Drug Resistance

1. Use chemosensitizers plus natural product agents (*e.g.*, anthracyclines, vinca alkaloids) as initial treatment to prevent *MDR* overexpression.
2. Follow with noncross-resistant drugs, such as antimetabolites and alkylating agents.
3. Consider high-dose chemotherapy as a form of consolidation therapy.
4. Use biologics or differentiating agents as maintenance therapy.

clinical MDR as shown in Table 69–27. Other mechanisms of natural product resistance may emerge after treatment with cytotoxic drugs and chemosensitizers. One such non-P-gp mechanism is due to altered topoisomerase II function that may confer resistance to anthracycline and epipodophyllotoxins.[92] A second mechanism of MDR that involved enhanced drug efflux but is non-P-gp mediated has also been described.[93,94] This mechanism of drug resistance due to enhanced drug efflux is unaffected by verapamil or other commonly known chemosensitizers. The clinical relevance of these alternative drug resistance mechanisms remains to be determined.

CONCLUSIONS

There are many ways by which a cancer may develop drug resistance at the cellular level. Clinical studies suggest that a common form of multidrug resistance in human cancers results from the expression of the *MDR1* gene that encodes for P-gp. This glycoprotein functions as a plasma membrane, energy-dependent, multidrug efflux pump that reduces the intracellular concentration of cytotoxic drugs. This mechanism of resistance may account for de novo resistance in common tumors, such as colon cancer and renal cancer, and for acquired resistance, as observed in common hematologic tumors such as acute nonlymphocytic leukemia and malignant lymphomas. Although this type of drug resistance may be common, it is by no means the only mechanism by which cells become drug resistant.

With the understanding that P-gp is a common mechanism of drug resistance in certain tumors, it is reasonable to try to prevent or circumvent this form of resistance. Pilot studies using chemosensitizers indicate that these agents may reverse resistance in a subset of patients. These same preliminary studies also indicate that drug resistance is multifactoral, because not all drug-resistant patients have P-gp-positive tumor cells and only a few patients appear to benefit from the use of chemosensitizers. The development of more efficacious and less toxic agents may improve the therapeutic outcome when they are added to cytotoxic drugs.

To define the role of chemosensitizers in reversing multidrug resistance in the clinic, it will be important to perform randomized, prospective, controlled clinical trials. Factors that should be considered in designing these trials include the type of tumor studied, which should have a high expression of P-gp, de novo or acquired; the presence or absence of P-gp on patients' tumor cells at the time of administering chemosensitizers; and the type and dose of chemosensitizer used. Only after demonstrating efficacy in well-designed clinical trials can the use of chemosensitizers be integrated into the everyday practice of clinical oncology.

TABLE 69–27. Possible Reasons for Failure of Chemosensitizers to Reverse Clinical Multidrug Resistance

1. Levels of the chemosensitizing agents are inadequate at the tumor site.
2. Levels of P-glycoprotein increase as the tumor progresses.
3. The *MDR*1 gene mutates, resulting in decreased binding of the chemosensitizing agent to P-glycoprotein.
4. Alternative non-P-glycoprotein mechanisms of resistance emerge during treatment that are unaffected by chemosensitizers.

REFERENCES

1. DeVita VT. The problem of resistance. PPO Updates 1990;4:11.
2. Goldie JH, Coldman AJ. Genetic instability in the development of drug resistance. JNCI 1989;81:116–124.
3. Pastan I, Gottesman M. Multiple-drug resistance in human cancer. N Engl J Med 1987;316:1388–1393.
4. Bradley G, Guranka PF, Ling V. Mechanisms of multidrug resistance. Biochem Biophys Acta 1988;948:87–128.
5. Assaraf YG, Molina A, Schimke RT. Sequential amplification of dihydrofolate reductase and multidrug resistance genes in Chinese hamster ovary cells selected for stepwise resistance to the lipid-soluble antifolate trimetrexate. J Biol Chem 1989;264:18324–18326.
6. Dalton WS, Durie BGM, Alberts DS, Gerlach JH, Cress AE. Characterization of a new drug resistant human myeloma cell line which expresses P-glycoprotein. Cancer Res 1986;46:5125–5130.
7. Higgins CF, Hiles ID, Salmond PC, et al. A family of related ATP-binding submits coupled to many distinct biological processes in bacteria. Nature 1986;323:448–450.
8. Gros P, Croop J, Housman D. Mammalian multidrug resistance gene: Complete cDNA sequence indicates strong homology to bacterial transport proteins. Cell 1986;47:371–380.
9. Gerlach JH, Endicott JA, Juranka PF, et al. Homology between P-glycoprotein and a bacterial hemolysin transport protein suggests a model for multidrug resistance. Nature 1986;316:820.
10. Fojo AT, Ueda K, Slamon DJ, et al. Expression of a multidrug resistance gene in human tumors and tissues. Proc Natl Acad Sci USA 1987;84:265–269.
11. Chaudhary PM, Roninson IB. Expression and activity of P-glycoprotein, a multidrug efflux pump, in human hematopoietic stem cells. Cell 1991;66:85–94.
12. List AF, Spier CM, Cline A, et al. Expression of the multidrug resistance gene product (P-glycoprotein) in myelodysplasia is associated with a stem cell phenotype. Br J Haematol 1991;78:28–34.
13. Thiebaut F, Tsuruo T, Hamada H, et al. Cellular localization of the multidrug-resistance gene product P-glycoprotein in normal human tissues. Proc Natl Acad Sci USA 1987;84:7735–7738.
14. Cordon-Cardo C, O'Brien JP, Casals D, et al. Multidrug-resistance gene (P-glycoprotein) is expressed by endothelial cells at blood-brain barrier sites. Proc Natl Acad Sci 1989;86:695–698.
15. Fuqua SAW, Moretti-Rojas IM, Schneider SL, et al. P-glycoprotein expression in human breast cancer cells. Cancer Res 1987;47:2103–2106.
16. Dalton WS, Grogan TM. Does P-glycoprotein predict response to chemotherapy, and if so, is there a reliable way to detect it? JNCI 1991;83:80–81.
17. Bell DR, Gerlach JH, Kartner N, et al. P-glycoprotein expression in ovarian cancer: Evidence for multidrug resistance. J Clin Oncol 1985;3:311–315.
18. Gerlach JH, Bell DR, Karakousis C, et al. P-glycoprotein in human sarcoma: Evidence for multidrug resistance. J Clin Oncol 1987;5:1452–1460.
19. Goldstein LJ, Galski H, Fojo A, et al. Expression of a multidrug resistance gene in human cancers. JNCI 1989;81:116–124.
20. Chabner BA, Fojo A. Multidrug resistance: P-glycoprotein and its allies—the elusive foes. JNCI 1989;81:910–913.
21. Kartner N, Evernden-Porelle D, Bradley G, et al. Detection of P-glycoprotein in multidrug-resistant cell lines by monoclonal antibodies. Nature 1985;316:820–823.
22. Georges E, Bradley G, Gariepy J, et al. Detection of P-glycoprotein isoforms by gene-specific monoclonal antibodies. Proc Natl Acad Sci USA 1990;87:152–156.
23. Thiebaut F, Tsuruo T, Hamada H, et al. Immunohistochenical localization in normal

tissues of different epitopes in a multidrug transport protein P170: Evidence for localization in brain capillaries and crossreactivity of one antibody with a muscle protein. J Histochem Cytochem 1989;37:159–164.

24. Scheper RJ, Bulte JWM, Brakke JGP, et al. Monoclonal antibody JSB-1 detects a highly conserved epitope on the P-glycorptoein associated with multi-drug-resistance. Int J Cancer 1988;42:389–394.
25. Schinkel AH, Roelofs MEM, Borst P. Characterization of the human MDR3 P-glycoprotein and its recognition by PGP-specific monoclonal antibodies. Cancer Res 1991;51:2628–2635.
26. Hamada H, Tsuruo T. Functional role for the 170- to 180-kDa glycoprotein specific to drug-resistant tumor cells revealed by monoclonal antibodies. Proc Natl Acad Sci USA 1986;83:7785–7789.
27. Weinstein RS, Kuszak JR, Kluskens LF, Coon JS. P-glycoproteins in pathology: The multidrug resistance gene family in humans. Human Pathol 1990;21:34–48.
28. Chan HSL, Bradley G, Thorner P, et al. A sensitive method for immunocytochemical detection of P-glycoprotein in multidrug-resistant human ovarian carcinoma cell lines. Lab Invest 1988;59:870–875.
29. Dalton WS, Grogan TM, Rybski JA, et al. Immunohistochemical detection and quantitation of P-glycoprotein in multiple drug-resistant human myeloma cells: Association with level of drug resistance and drug accumulation. Blood 1989;73:747–752.
30. Grogan TN, Dalton WS, Rybski J, et al. Optimization of immunocytochemical P-glycoprotein assessment in multidrug resistant plasma cell myeloma using 3 antibodies. Lab Invest 1991;63:815–824.
31. Saiki RK, Scharf S, Faloona F, et al. Enzymatic amplification of β-globin genomic sequences and restriction site analysis for diagnosis of sickle cell anemia. Science 1985;230: 1350–1354.
32. Noonan KE, Beck C, Holzmayer TA, et al. Quantitative analysis of MDR1 (multidrug resistance) gene expression in human tumors by polymerase chain reaction. Proc Natl Acad Sci USA 1990;87:7160–7164.
33. Murphy LD, Herzog CE, Rudick JB, Tito Fojo A, Bates SE. Use of the polymerase chain reaction in the quantitation of the *mdr1* gene expression. Biochemistry 1990;29:10351–10356.
34. Futscher BW, Blake LL, Grogan TM, Dalton WS. Quantitative PCR analysis of *mdr1* expression in clinical specimens. Anal Biochem 1993 (in press).
35. Champlin R, Gale RP. Acute lymphoblastic leukemia in recent advances in biology and therapy. Blood 1989;73:2051–2066.
36. Rothenberg ML, Mickley LA, Cole DE, et al. Expression of the *mdr1*/P-170 gene in patients with acute lymphoblastic leukemia. Blood 1989;74:1388–1395.
37. Musto P, Melillo L, Lombardi G, Matera R, Di Giorgio G, Carotenuto M. High risk of early resistant relapse for leukemic patients with presence of multidrug resistance associated P-glycoprotein positive cells in complete remission. Br J Haematol 1991;77: 50–53.
38. Herweijer H, Sonneveld P, Baas F, Nooter K. Expression of mdr1 and mdr3 multidrug-resistance genes in human acute and chronic leukemias and association with stimulation of drug accumulation by cyclosporine. JNCI 1990;82:1133–1140.
39. Kato S, Ideguchi H, Muta K, Nishimura J, Nawata H. Mechanisms involved in the development of Adriamycin resistance in human leukemias. Leuk Res 1990;14:567–573.
40. Mattern J, Efferth T, Back M, Ho AD, Volm M. Detection of P-glycoprotein in human leukemias using monoclonal antibodies. Blut 1989;58:215–217.
41. Kuwazuru Y, Hanada S, Furukawa T, et al. Expression of P-glycoprotein in adult T-cell leukemia cells. Blood 1990;76:2065–2071.
42. Champlin R, Gale RP. Acute myelogenous leukemia: Recent advances in therapy. Blood 1987;69:1551–1562.
43. Kokenberg E, Sonneveld P, Delwel R, Sizoo W, Hagenbeek A, Lowenberg B. In vivo uptake of daunorubicin by acute myeloid leukemia (AML) cells measured by flow cytometry. Leukemia 1988;2:511–517.
44. Sato H, Preisler H, Day R, et al. Mdr1 transcript levels as an indication of resistant disease in acute myelogenous leukemia. Br J Haematol 1990;75:340–345.
45. Holmes J, Jacobs A, Carter G, Janowska-Wieczorek A, Padua RA. Multidrug resistance in haemapoietic cell lines, myelodysplastic syndromes and acute myeloblastic leukemia. Br J Haematol 1989;72:40–44.
46. Ito Y, Tanimoto M, Kumazawa T, et al. Increased P-glycoprotein expression and multidrug-resistant gene (mdr1) amplification are infrequently found in fresh acute leukemia cells: Sequential analysis of 15 cases at initial presentation in relapse stage. Cancer 1989;63:1534–1538.
47. Nooter K, Sonneveld P, Oostrum R, Herweijer H, Hagenbeek T, Valerio D. Overexpression of the mdr1 gene in blast cells from patients with acute myelocytic leuekmia is associated with decreased anthracycline accumulation that can be restored by cyclosporine. Int J Cancer 1990;45:263–268.
48. Holmes JA, Jacobs A, Carter G, et al. Is the *mdr1* gene relevant in chronic lymphocytic leukemia? Leukemia 1990;4:216–218.
49. Cumber PM, Jacobs A, Hay T, Fisher J, Whittaker JA, Tsuruo T. Expression of the MDR gene (*mdr1*) and epitope masking in chronic lymphatic leukemia. Br J Haematol 1990;76:226–230.
50. Tsuruo T, Sugimoto Y, Hamada H, et al. Detection of multidrug resistance markers, P-glycoprotein and *mdr1* mRNA, in human leukemia cells. Jpn J Cancer Res 1987;78: 1415–1419.
51. Carulli G, Petrini M, Marini A, et al. P-glycorptoein in acute nonlymphoblastic leukemia and in the blastic crisis of myeloid leukemia. N Engl J Med 1988;319:797–798.
52. Miller TP, Grogan TM, Dalton WS, Spier CM, Scheper RJ, Salmon SE. P-glycoprotein expression in malignant lymphoma and reversal of clinical drug resistance with chemotherapy plus high dose verapamil. J Clin Oncol 1991;9:17–24.
53. Kyle RA. Diagnosis and management of multiple myeloma and related disorders. Prog Hematol 1986;14:257–282.
54. Buzaid AC, Durie BGM. Management of refractory myeloma: A review. J Clin Oncol 1988;6:889–905.
55. Grogan TM, Spier CM, Salmon SE, et al. P-glycoprotein expression in human plasma cell myeloma: An acquired trait related to prior chemotherapy. Blood 1993 (in press).
56. Epstein J, Xiao H, Oba BK. P-glycoprotein expression in plasma-cell myeloma is associated with resistance to VAD. Blood 1989;74:913–917.
57. Chan HSL, Thorner PS, Haddad G, Ling V. Immunohistochemical detection of P-glycoprotein: Prognostic correlation is soft tissue sarcoma of childhood. J Clin Oncol 1990;8:689–704.
58. Chan HSL, Haddad G, Thorner PS, et al. P-glycoprotein expression as a predictor of the outcome of therapy for neuroblastoma. N Engl J Med 1991;325:1608–1614.
59. Merkel DE, Fuqua SAW, Tandon AK, et al. Electrophoretic analysis of 248 clinical breast cancer specimens for P-glycoprotein overexpression or gene amplification. J Clin Oncol 1989;7:1129–1136.
60. Schneider J, Bak M, Efferth TH, et al. P-glycoprotein expression in treated and untreated human breast cancer. Br J Cancer 1989;60:815–818.
61. Ro J, Sahin A, Ro JY, et al. Immunohistochemical analysis of P-glycoprotein expression correlated with chemotherapy resistance in locally advanced breast cancer. Hum Pathol 1990;21:787–791.
62. Verrelle P, Meissonnier F, Fonck Y, et al. Clinical relevance of immunohistochemical detection of multidrug resistance P-glycoprotein in breast carcinoma. JNCI 1991;83: 111–116.
63. Cordon-Cardo C, O'Brien JP, Boccia J, Casals D, Bertino JR, Melamed MR. Expression of the multidrug resistance gene product (P-glycoprotein) in human normal and tumor tissues. J Histochem Cytochem 1990;38:1277–1287.
64. Lai S-L, Goldstein LJ, Gottesman MM, et al. *MDR1* gene expression in lung cancer. JNCI 1989;81:1144–1150.
65. Tsuruo T, Iida H, Tsukagoshi S, et al. Overcoming of vincristine resistance in P388 leukemia in vivo and in vitro through enhanced cytotoxicity of vincristine and vinblastine by verapamil. Cancer Res 1981;41:1967–1972.
66. Kessel D, Wilberding C. Anthracycline resistance in P388 murine leukemia and its circumvention by calcium antagonists. Cancer Res 1985;45:1687–1691.
67. Ramu A, Spanier R, Rahaminoff H, et al. Restoration of doxorubicin responsiveness in doxorubicin-resistant P388 murine leukemia cells. Br J Cancer 1984;50:501–507.
68. Yang CPH, Mellado W, Horwitz SB. Azidopine labeling of multidrug resistance-associated glycoproteins. Biochem Pharmacol 1988;37:1417–1421.
69. Safa AR. Photoaffinity labeling of the multidrug resistance-related P-glycoprotein with photoactive analogs of verapamil. Proc Natl Acad Sci USA 1988;85:7187–7191.
70. Hamada H, Hagiwara KI, Nakajima T, et al. Phosphorylation of the 170,000 to 180,000 glycoprotein specific to multidrug-resistant tumor cells: Effects of verapamil, trifluoperazine, and phorbol esters. Cancer Res 1987;47:2860–2865.
71. Dalton WS, Grogan TM, Meltzer PS, et al. Drug-resistance in multiple myeloma and non-Hodgkin's lymphoma: Detection of P-glycoprotein and potential circumvention by addition of verapamil to chemotherapy. J Clin Oncol 1989;7:415–424.
72. Nooter K, Sonneveld P, Oostrum R, Herweijer H, Hagenbeek T, Valerio D. Overexpression of the *mdr1* gene in blast cells from patients with acute myelocytic leukemia is associated with decreased anthracycline accumulation that can be restored by cyclosporin-A. Int J Cancer 1990;45:263–268.
73. Benson AB, Trump DL, Koeller JM, et al. Phase I study of vinblastine and verapamil given by concurrent IV infusion. Cancer Treat Rep 1985;69:795–799.
74. Presant CA, Kennedy PS, Wiseman C, et al. Verapamil reversal of clinical doxorubicin resistance in human cancer. Am J Clin Oncol 1986;9:355–357.
75. Ozols RF, Cunnion RE, Klecker RW, et al. Verapamil and Adriamycin in the treatment of drug-resistant ovarian cancer patients. J Clin Oncol 1987;5:641–647.
76. Salmon SE, Dalton WS, Grogan TM, et al. Multidrug-resistant myeloma: Laboratory and clinical effects of chemosensitizers. Blood 1991;78:44–50.
77. Gore ME, Selby PJ, Millar B, et al. The use of verapamil to overcome drug resistance in myeloma. Proc Am Soc Clin Oncol 1988;7:228.
78. Trumper LH, Ho AD, Wulf G, et al. Addition of verapamil to overcome drug resistance in multiple myeloma. Preliminary clinical observations in 10 patients. J Clin Oncol 1989;7:1578–1579.
79. Pennock GD, Dalton WS, Roeske WR, et al. Systemic toxic effects associated with high dose verapamil infusion and chemotherapy administration. JNCI 1991;83:105–110.
80. Miller RL, Bukowski RM, Budd GT, et al. Clinical modulation of doxorubicin resistance by the calmodulin inhibitor trifluoperazine: A phase I trial. J Clin Oncol 1988;6:880–888.
81. Trump D, Rogers M, Fine R, et al. Phase I trial of high dose Tamoxifen and 5 day infusion of vinblastine as an approach to reverse multidrug resistance. Proc Am Assoc Cancer Res [Abstract] 1990;31:205.
82. Yahanda AM, Adler KM, Hardy R, Brophy NA, Halsey J, Sikic B. A phase I trial of etoposide with cyclosporine as a modulator of multidrug resistance. Proc Am Soc Clin Oncol [Abstract] 1991;10:102.
83. Samuels B, Ratain M, Mick R, et al. Phase I trial of multidrug resistance modulation with cyclosporin-A. Proc Am Assoc Cancer Res [Abstract] 1991;32:195.
84. List AF, Spier C, Greer J, Azar C, Hutter J, Wolff S, Salmon S, Futscher B, Dalton W. Biochemical modulation of anthracycline resistance (MDR) in acute leukemia with cyclosporin-A [Abstract]. Proc Am Soc Clin Oncol [Abstract] 1992;11:264.
85. Verweij J, Herweijer H, Oosterom R, et al. A phase II study of epidoxorubicin in colorectal cancer and the use of cyclosporin-A in an attempt to reverse multidrug resistance. Br J Cancer 1991;64:361–364.

86. Beck WT. Modulators of P-glycoprotein associated multidrug resistance. In: Ozols RF, ed. Drug resistance, vol II. Norwell, MA: Kluwer Academic Publishers, 1991.
87. Zamora JM, Pearce HL, Beck WT. Physical-chemical properties shared by compounds that modulate multidrug resistance in human leukemia cells. Mol Pharmacol 1988;33:454–462.
88. Keilhauer C, Emling F, Raschack M, et al. The use of R-verapamil (R-VPM) is superior to racemic VPM in breaking multidrug resistance (MDR) of malignant cells. Proc Am Assoc Cancer Res 1989;30:503.
89. Lehnert M, Dalton WS, Roe D, Emerson S, Salmon SE. Synergistic inhibition by verapamil and quinine of P-glycoprotein-mediated multidrug resistance in a human myeloma cell line model. Blood 1991;77:348–354.
90. Mickisch GH, Merlino GT, Galski H, Gottesman MM, Pastan I. Transgenic mice that express the human multidrug-resistance gene in bone marrow enable a rapid identification of agents that reverse drug resistance. Proc Natl Acad Sci USA 1991;88:547–551.
91. Dalton WS. Reversing multidrug resistance in the laboratory and clinic. Proc Am Assoc Cancer Res 1990;31:520.
92. Danks MK, Yalowich JC, Beck WT. Atypical multiple drug resistance in a human leukemic cell line selected for resistance to teniposide (VM-26). Cancer Res 1987;47:1297.
93. Dalton WS, Cress AE, Alberts DS, Trent JM. Cytogenetic and phenotypic analysis of a human colon carcinoma cell line resistant to mitoxantrone. Cancer Res 1988;48:1882.
94. Taylor CW, Dalton WS, Parrish PR, et al. Different mechanisms of decreased drug accumulation in doxorubicin and mitoxantrone resistance variants of the MCF7 human breast cancer cell line. Br J Cancer 1991;63:923–929.

SECTION 7

WILLIAM J.M. HRUSHESKY
GEORG A. BJARNASON

The Application of Circadian Chronobiology to Cancer Chemotherapy

Most clinicians give little thought to the time of day at which a drug is given. In general, patients receive drugs at times that are convenient for the staff administering them. A growing body of data suggests that therapeutic effect may be maximized and toxicity may be minimized if drugs are administered at carefully selected times of the day.[1] This potential for a marked improvement in therapeutic index is especially critical for therapies with narrow ratios of efficacy to toxicity, like most anticancer treatment regimens.[2]

The toxicities of at least 20 chemotherapeutic agents depend on the time of day in murine systems. The anticancer efficacy of many of these agents, given singly or in combinations, depends on circadian factors.[3] Clinical data show that the dosing time of 5-fluorouracil (5-FU), floxuridine, 4′-O-tetrahydropyranyl-doxorubicin, and oxaliplatin markedly affect their toxicities, safely achievable dose intensity, and perhaps their therapeutic efficacy.[4–9] The toxicity and therapeutic efficacy of combination chemotherapy with cisplatin and doxorubicin were found to depend on the time of day that they were administered.[10–12]

This reproducible temporal variability in antitumor effect and normal tissue toxicity can be explained in part by two important observations. First, experimental and clinical studies have documented that the pharmacokinetics of many anticancer drugs (and most other drugs studied) show consistent and reproducible circadian temporal variation, depending on the time of their administration.[1,13–16] Second, most normal tissues are reproducibly rhythmically more or less sensitive to the effects of drugs at specific times of day.[17] Some tumors also exhibit similar rhythmic susceptibility patterns during the circadian cycle.[18,19] These circadian rhythmic variations in drug pharmacokinetics and tissue susceptibility may be exploited to select a time for treatment that results in an increased tumor cell killing and reduced toxicity.

The availability of portable infusion pumps capable of delivering a single or multiple drugs, each with their optimal circadian scheduling, has made the clinical application and testing of these principles possible.

CHRONOBIOLOGY

Chronobiology is the quantitative study of the temporal relations of biologic phenomena. Even the most superficial quantitative study of biodynamics demonstrates that biophysical and biochemical processes vary with respect to time in a regular and predictable periodic manner across several rhythmic frequencies.[20,21] De Mairan's early 18th century observations that the leaves of the mimosa plant open during the day and close at night and that this pattern continues faithfully in constant darkness constitutes an important partial proof of the endogenicity of circadian time structure.[22] Richter further generalized these findings to mammals, documenting the persistence of diurnal activity rhythms in rats housed in constant darkness.[23] In a landmark study, Johnson found that the activity rhythm of animals under constant darkness fit a period different from 24 hours and postulated an internal physiologic rhythm that was not directly dependent on the daily fluctuations of environmental conditions.[24]

Endogenous biologic rhythms have been demonstrated at all biologic levels, from yeasts and nucleated unicells to man, and at all levels of biologic organization, including the entire organism, organ system, organ tissue, cell, and subcellular unit.[20,21,25] Each patient's hospital record demonstrates tight coordination of all vital signs. Figure 69–28 demonstrates the circadian rhythms of activity, pulse, temperature, and systolic, diastolic, and mean blood pressure in a typical person.

The existence of a molecular time-keeping mechanism, "clock-gene," was first inferred for *Drosophila melanogaster* by Konopka and Benzer.[26] Subsequently, molecular biologists used several mutant strains to identify an important "clock gene" that has been named *per* (for period). In several other species (*e.g., Neurospora, Chlamydomonas*), single-gene mutations have been shown to alter such basic clock properties as period length, light entrainability, and temperature compensation.[27,28] A mammalian clock gene mutation was found that dramatically alters the period of the circadian locomotor rhythm of golden hamsters.[29]

There is considerable evidence to suggest that the suprachiasmatic nucleus (SCN) of the hypothalamus is a site of critically important circadian pacemaker cells in mammals. Meijer and Rietveld reviewed this subject.[30] The most definitive experimental evidence for primacy of the SCN in circadian organismic time keeping demonstrates that circadian rhythmicity can be restored to SCN-lesioned arrhythmic hamsters by implantation of fetal brain tissue containing SCN cells.[31–34] Ralph and colleagues demonstrated that small neural grafts from the SCN of normal hamsters and τ-mutant ham-

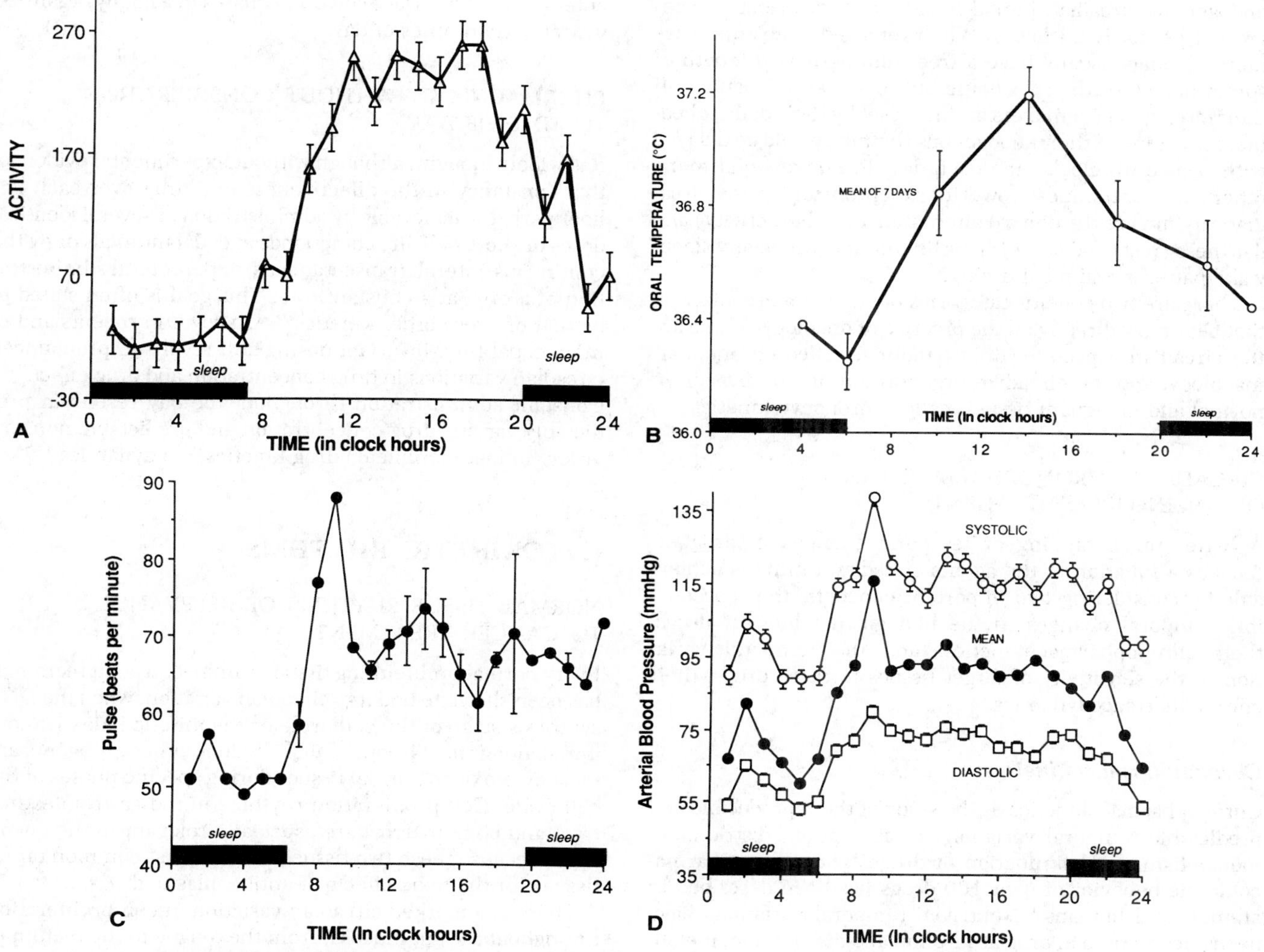

FIGURE 69–28. All physiologic functions are temporally organized within circadian time. **(A)** Hourly averages of continuously monitored activity. **(B)** Intermittent oral temperature obtained every 4 hours for 7 consecutive days. **(C)** Hourly averages of continuously monitored pulse. **(D)** Hourly averages of continuously monitored systolic, diastolic, and mean arterial blood pressure. The activity pattern documents the sleep onset, wakefulness onset, and amount of activity throughout the day. The temperature pattern documents the daily rise of temperature, which anticipates daily arising, peaks in the afternoon, and falls throughout each night. Pulse and blood pressure behave similarly throughout the day, dropping substantially during sleep and rising sharply after morning arousal. This rapid morning rise in circadian hemodynamic variables has been prominently associated with a high frequency of heart attacks and strokes at this time of day.

sters restored circadian rhythms to arrhythmic animals whose own nucleus had been ablated.[35] The restored rhythms always exhibited the period of the donor genotype.

Genetic time-keeping mechanisms most likely evolved in response to regular variations in physical demands of the environment. The two motive forces for this temporal evolution would be biologic economy and systematic stability. It could be thermodynamically wasteful if not lethal for cellular and organismic tasks to be unordered in time or too easily affected by environmental cycles. The multifrequency resonance structure of living organisms helps to keep the life processes within acceptable homeostatic limits by reinforcing temporal order. Biologic processes are sequential, ordered, and depend on the completion of one event to initiate the next.

At least three major biologic rhythms have been defined that correspond to obvious periodic changes in the environment: the circadian rhythm (20–28 hours, the solar day); the circatrigintan rhythm (30 ± 7 days, the lunar month); and the circannual rhythm (12 ± 2 months, the year). These three rhythms weave the temporal fabric from which each earth-born organism is tailored, and they have left an indelible imprint on every biologic process. Of each of the biofrequency domains, the circadian rhythm has been most thoroughly investigated. Moore-Ede and coworkers reviewed its potential importance in health and disease.[36,37] The basic properties of biologic rhythms are similar in plants and animals; they are endogenous and genetic in origin, persist without time cues, and are regularly influenced by cyclic variations of certain environmental factors called synchronizers.[20]

When precisely measured under constant conditions, the

endogenous circadian period lengths of the various species are not precisely 24 hours. When removed from time cues human beings usually have a free-running period length of somewhat more than 24 hours but less than 25 hours.[38] If their circadian pacemakers are not reset by their daily schedule, the timing of their endogenous rhythms would be delayed with respect to clock time each day. In humans and many other species, the most powerful synchronizers of the circadian rhythm are the diurnal alternation of light (activity) and darkness (rest) and our 24-hour life routine, especially sleep-wake patterns and meal timing.

There are two general categories of circadian organization that bear most directly on the practice of oncology. These are the circadian aspects of drug handling, called chronopharmacology, and the circadian organization of cell division in normal and malignant tissues, called chronocytokinetics.

CIRCADIAN CHRONOPHARMACOLOGY OF ANTINEOPLASTIC AGENTS

A better understanding of temporal changes in drug effects as a function of the agents circadian timing is achievable by considering two important concepts: the reproducible temporal changes in the biologic handling of drugs, their chronopharmacokinetics, and the temporal variation in the sensitivity of target tissues to these drugs, their chronopharmacodynamics.

Chronopharmacokinetics

Chronopharmacokinetics, is the study of the reproducible and predictable temporal variations in absorption, distribution, metabolism, and elimination of drugs. The chronopharmacokinetic behavior of over 100 drugs has been described in animals and humans.[1] Nontrivial temporal variations have been documented in drug absorption and distribution, metabolism, and excretion.[39–42] This has been well documented in vivo for many drugs metabolized through the P-450 system. This may be due to temporal variation in the microsomal concentration of the various P-450 isoenzymes. Reproducible circadian variation has been documented in the activity of at least 13 major hepatic drug metabolizing enzyme systems, including those responsible for hepatic glucuronidation and sulfation and for glutathione conjugation.[43,44]

Chronopharmacodynamics

Rhythmic changes in the susceptibility of a biosystem is well documented for many cytotoxic agents, in vivo and in vitro, for cells removed at specific circadian phases. Sometimes the susceptibility can be explained and quantified in terms of bioperiodic changes in the concentration of receptors of a given system for a given drug. Circadian rhythms in cellular defense mechanisms such as oxygen free radical defense mechanisms, such as glutathione and the concentration of other nonprotein-bound sulfhydryl compounds can also be responsible for time-of-day dependence of drug effect.[45–51]

For cytotoxic anticancer drugs, rhythmic changes in specific normal tissue functions, such as cell division, can also help explain the temporal variation in sensitivity of rapidly proliferating tissues. The cells of every tissue appropriately studied enter or exit the various cell cycle phases in a highly organized way at certain times of day.[52]

PHARMACOLOGY WITHOUT CONSIDERATION TO TIME OF DAY

It is widely thought, although without experimental evidence, that constancy in the effectiveness of a drug over each 24-hour period is achievable by administration of several identical doses of short-half-life compounds at equal intervals or by the continuous enteral, transcutaneous, or parenteral administration of a drug at a constant rate. This goal is often stated to be that of "zero-order kinetics." As shown in rodents and in man, equal time-invariant dosing still results in pronounced circadian variations in drug concentration and drug effect.[25,53] Constant administration throughout the day results in predictably varying drug concentration and predictable nonzero order (in fact, nonlinear) drug kinetics and dynamics.[14,54]

CYTOKINETIC RHYTHMS

NORMAL TISSUE RHYTHMS OF RELEVANCE TO CANCER TREATMENT

Every normal proliferating tissue examined in adult mammals has been shown to undergo circadian variation, when the DNA synthesis stage of the cell cycle or the mitotic index is monitored along the 24-hour scale.[55,56] Chemotherapy agents are most cytotoxic to normal tissues during specific phases of the cell cycle. Cell proliferation rhythms in the gastrointestinal tract and bone marrow are especially relevant to the oncologist, because these two tissues are the most common target tissues for the toxic effects of antineoplastic drugs.

There is a marked circadian variation in cell proliferation throughout the gut mucosa, from the tongue to the rectum in mice and rats.[52,57] There are major variations seen in the amplitude of the rhythms in the various regions, but the phasing in the different regions of the gut is remarkably similar. Similar rhythms have been thoroughly documented in the gastrointestinal tract in humans, with the highest DNA synthetic activity each day between 5 to 9 A.M. each morning (Fig. 69–29A).[58]

The bone marrow is the most common tissue to limit dose intensity of common anticancer treatment. The production of all types of blood cells undergoes strong regular temporal variations, and circadian and seasonal rhythms in blood cell production have been described.[59] The relative number of bone marrow stem cells and progenitor cells, such as CFU-S, CFU-GM and CFU-E, have significant, predictable circadian variation in rodents. These findings have been confirmed in normal humans.[60–64] The marrow activity rhythms are reflected by circadian rhythms in the cellular components of the peripheral blood.[65,66] The studies of Smaaland of a group of 16 normal controls unequivocally confirmed the earlier findings of Mauer and Killman.[62–64] The percentage of cells in DNA synthesis measured by flow cytometry demonstrated a large variation along the circadian time scale for each 24-hour profile, with a range of variation from 29% to 339% from the lowest to highest value. The mean value of the lowest DNA synthesis for each 24-hour period was 8.7% ± 0.6% (8

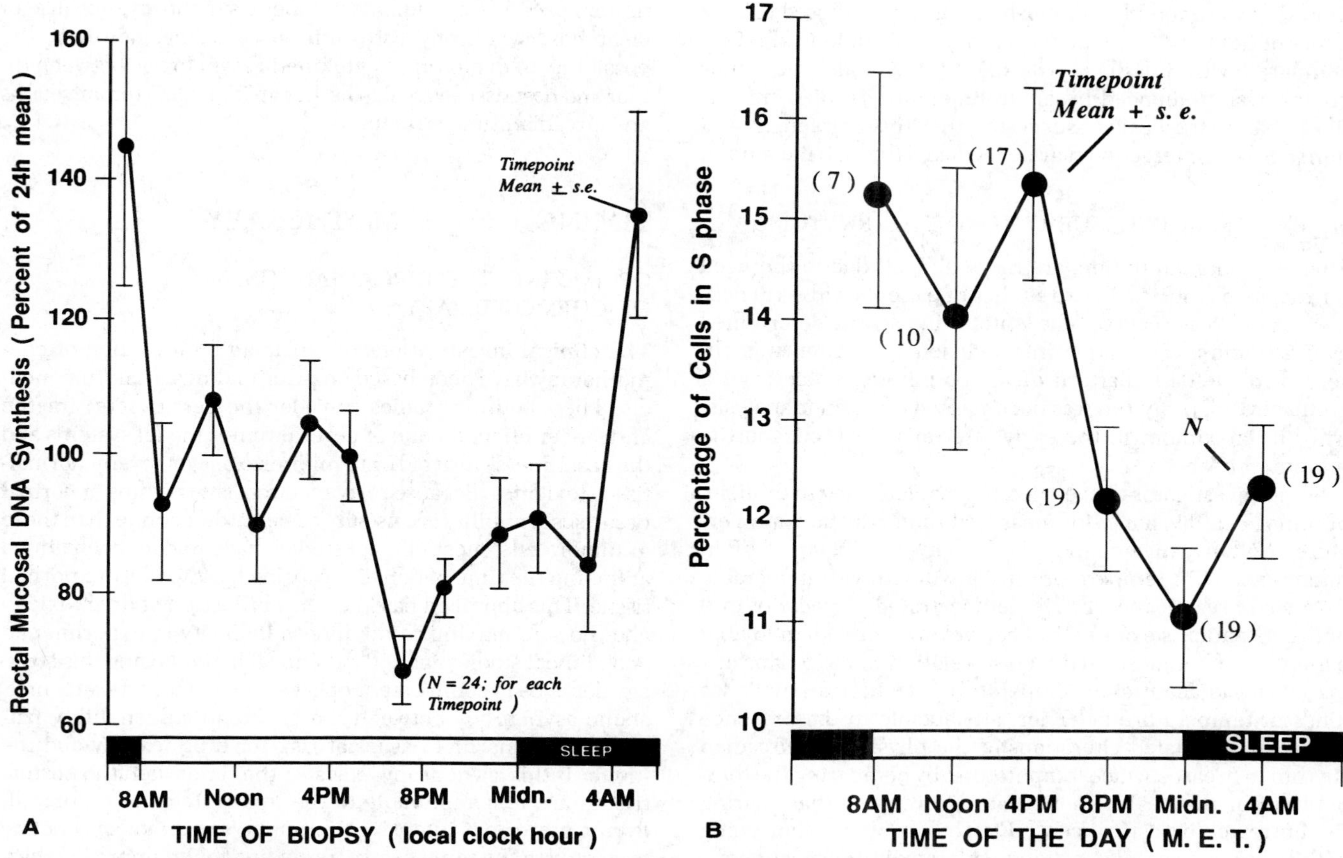

FIGURE 69–29. **(A)** The pattern of tritiated thymidine uptake by samples of human colorectal mucosa as a function of the time of day the samples were obtained. The data are presented as averages for 24 persons, each expressed relative to that person's 24-hour mean DNA synthetic capacity. Flexible colonoscopy was performed every 2 hours, round the clock, in each of 24 normal persons. Three mucosal tissue samples were obtained at each time of day from each subject, and one of these samples was immediately incubated with labeled thymidine. After appropriate washing and processing, the amount of radioactively labeled thymidine incorporated into DNA was measured. This histogram demonstrates that DNA synthetic capacity is highest in the early morning, before usual daily awakening (4 A.M. and 6 A.M. samples). DNA synthetic capacity is lowest in the evening hours, before daily sleep onset (8 P.M. and 10 P.M. samples). This tight circadian organization ($p < 0.001$) is similar in phasing and amplitude in fed and fasted states (data not shown). (Buchi KN, Moore JG, Hrushesky WJM, Sothern RB, Rubin NH. Circadian rhythm of cellular proliferation in the human rectal mucosa. Gastroenterology 1991;101:410–415). **(B)** The cytofluorometrically determined average percentage of cells in S phase actively synthesizing DNA. Bone marrow punctures were performed on as many as 19 healthy persons at up to six times of day. Samples were stained appropriately and then evaluated by flow cytometry. Samples obtained between 6 A.M. and 2 P.M. had the greatest average proportion of cells undergoing DNA synthesis. Samples obtained around midnight averaged much lower DNA synthesis activity ($p < 0.001$). (Smaaland R, Laerum OD, Lote K, Sletvold O, Sothern RB, Bjerknes R. DNA synthesis in human bone marrow is circadian stage dependent. Blood 1991;77:2603–2611). Concurrent inspection of these two panels reveals that the morning hours are associated with the greatest DNA synthetic activity for both chemotherapy-sensitive tissues. The evening hours are associated with far less DNA synthetic capacity in the bone marrow and the gut.

P.M. to 4 A.M.), and the mean value of the highest was 17.6% ± 0.6% (8 A.M. to 4 P.M.), which was a twofold difference, with the highest DNA synthetic activity between 7 A.M. and 4 P.M. (see Fig. 69–29B). This has now been confirmed in cancer patients.[66a]

MURINE TUMOR TISSUE CYTOKINETIC RHYTHMS

Another focus of interest has been the investigation of whether tumor cells proliferate rhythmically within the circadian reference frame and how their circadian pattern of cell division relates to those of nonmalignant host target tissues. Earlier-stage better-differentiated hepatomas seem more tightly tied to host circadian time structure than are later-stage more-undifferentiated malignancies.[18] Similar circadian variations in DNA synthesis have been demonstrated in Lewis lung carcinoma cells after implantation into mice.[19,67]

In an attempt to determine whether tumor tissue communicates with circadian control mechanisms, Waldorp investigated whether the length of the daily photoperiod altered tumor growth rate in a mouse colon adenocarcinoma cell line.[68] Significantly greater tumor size, weight, and group mortality were found in tumor-bearing mice exposed to a 12 hours of light and 12 hours of darkness schedule (12L:12D) compared with 6L:18D or 18L:6D. In this model the tumor growth was influenced by environmental circadian milieu. Blask[69] and Hrushesky[70] suggested that this day length and tumor growth interaction may be mediated through melatonin.

HUMAN TUMOR TISSUE CYTOKINETIC RHYTHMS

Studies on human tumors are more difficult due to the need for repeated biopsies. In two studies of patients with skin nodules from breast cancer, the mitotic index was determined over 24 hours.[71,72] A large interindividual variation was observed in the daily pattern of tumor mitotic indices, but a group circadian rhythm was documented by cosinor analysis, with the maximum in the early afternoon (3 P.M.) and the minimum near 3 A.M.[73]

Some investigators have tried to correlate the rhythmicity of tumor cell division with measured tumor surface temperature. Stoll investigated the relation between uptake of ^{32}P in tumors and skin temperature in 19 women with inoperable advanced breast cancer.[74] He demonstrated periodicity in 9 of the 19 patients examined. The cycle was circadian in all 9 patients and demonstrated a close relation to circadian fluctuation in adjacent skin temperature. Gautherie found two kinds of temperature behavior, attributable to the presence of cancer associated alterations of the physiologic circadian rhythm in breast surface temperature, by comparing the temperature of the healthy contralateral breast to that bearing the untreated breast cancer.[75] First, there was a shortening of the circadian period in patients with rapidly growing tumors. These cancers subsequently proved to be poorly differentiated. Second, he found the persistence of a normal 24-hour rhythm in the slow-growing tumors, but with a decreased amplitude and a 6-hour phase advance, compared with the temperature pattern of the contralateral normal breast. The maximal mitotic index and maximal surface temperature coincided in circadian time.

Klevecz looked at cell proliferation in the ascites fluid from 30 patients with ovarian cancer.[76] A highly significant circadian rhythm in tumor cell DNA synthesis was found. Its peak (*i.e.*, mid to late morning) was found to be almost 12 hours out of phase with the proliferation in benign mesothelial cells from the same patients.

Smaaland has documented coordinated circadian patterns of DNA synthesis in the malignant lymph nodes of 24 patients with non-Hodgkin's lymphoma. Fine-needle aspirates were obtained from each patient every 4 hours for at least 24 hours. Flow cytometry was used to determine the proportion of cells in each sample that were actively synthesizing DNA (S-phase). DNA synthesis of these lymphomas was coordinated within the day, peaking during early sleep, out of phase with normal bone marrow, which peaks in the first half or middle of each day.[77] Both raw data and best fitting cosine curves can be used to demonstrate this phase relation of DNA synthesis in normal bone marrow and malignant lymph node tissue involved with non-Hodgkin's lymphoma. S-phase active bone marrow toxins may therefore be less toxic and more effective in the treatment of malignant lymphoma.

In summary, there is some evidence to suggest that human tumors preserve circadian cytokinetic synchrony. Because of clear host synchrony with different phasing, however, the possibility of exploiting a cytokinetic asynchrony between tumor and host tissue is real, whether an individual tumor retains any circadian time structure.

TIMING OF CHEMOTHERAPY

OPTIMIZING THE CIRCADIAN TIMING OF CHEMOTHERAPY

The clinical investigations of circadian optimization of chemotherapy have been based on prior findings in murine models. These murine studies consider the best time(s) for the anticancer effect on one or several tumor model systems and the best time(s) to avoid or to minimize one or several normal-tissue toxicities. Because relevant circadian rhythms of normal tissue susceptibility are usually easier to determine than those of tumor cells, most clinical studies have to date been aimed at finding the time of delivery causing least toxicity to normal tissue. This approach has allowed a reduction of drug toxicity and the safe maximization of dose intensity in experimental and clinical studies.[3,6,8,10,78,81] Clinical benefit using this strategy depends to some extent on a certain cytokinetic and metabolic asynchrony between the circadian susceptibility patterns of the normal tissues at risk for drug toxicity and the tumor. If this asynchrony exists, at the time when the normal tissues are less vulnerable to the toxic effects of a drug, allowing more dose intensive treatment, the tumor may not be protected to the same extent, providing for an improved therapeutic index.

Some researchers have given chemotherapy treatment to tumor-bearing animals at a time when a high percentage of the malignant cell population in the tumor is occupying a more drug-sensitive cell-cycle phase. In mice bearing methylcholanthrene-induced sarcoma, cyclophosphamide was given during the time of day associated with the highest G_2-phase distribution of sampled tumor cells. This strategy achieved 44% growth inhibition and 13% tumor cures.[79] Based on the finding that cyclophosphamide could synchronize tumor cells in M phase, tumor cure rate was improved to 53%, if vinblastine was given 12 hours after cyclophosphamide during the M phase of synchronized tumor cells.[80] Similar results have been reported for cyclophosphamide treatment in Lewis lung carcinoma-bearing mice.[67]

In a clinical trial based on these murine findings, 63 cancer patients with various tumors were randomized to receive the same 40-hour sequential chemotherapy regimen (*i.e.*, methotrexate or 5-FU, followed by vinblastine and cyclophosphamide). In the group receiving the treatment, at times taking into account the circadian rhythm of tumor proliferation, the antitumor effectiveness appeared better with respect to response rate (85% versus 58%), duration of response, and survival.[82] Braly and Klevecs are currently conducting a clinical trial in ovarian cancer patients in which intraperitoneal tumor cell samples are obtained every 1 to 4 hours for as long as 72 hours before treatment. Treatment timing is assigned to that time of day at which the predictably highest tumor cell S-phase fraction occurs.

METHODOLOGY FOR DETERMINING OPTIMAL CIRCADIAN DRUG TIMING

The clinical study design that ensures discovery of the optimal time of day for a given anticancer agent requires at least six arms; randomization to treatment at one of six equispaced times of day. This is unfortunately difficult because of the number of patients required. Therefore, surrogate information, such as DNA synthesis rhythms in target tissues and circadian pharmacokinetic changes, is combined with information obtained in large groups of mice or rats treated at each of six equispaced circadian stages. Preclinical experiments are usually performed in rats or mice of the same strain, sex, and age with free access to food and water. Like human beings with cancer who are living on a regular schedule of nocturnal sleep and diurnal activity, these animals have been synchronized for 2 weeks or longer in a lighting regimen usually consisting of 12 hours of light and 12 hours of darkness (LD 12: 12) or an other specified LD-time regimen. As a time reference in these studies, the hours after light onset (HALO) in the animal cage is universally accepted. This circadian reference point corresponds approximately to the time humans go to sleep, and it has proven helpful in extrapolating rhythm data from nocturnally active rodents to humans.[83] Sleep or rest onset is a particularly stable reference point, because many endocrinologic rhythms are fixed and reinforced by light regimen and sleep onset secondarily.[83]

Data Analysis

Biodynamics are described by time series analyses that resolve rhythmic patterns and trends in biologic variability. Time series record the values of the variable(s) in question over at least one full period, for circadian rhythms at least 24 hours, and depict these values as a function of sampling time. Several excellent specialized methods are available to analyze rhythmic time series data objectively.[84,85] A method commonly used to complement Chi squared standard ANOVA and life table analysis is the cosinor method. This method was originally described by Halberg and colleagues.[86] This method is a simple regression technique that uses the least squares fit of the raw data or data as percentage of daily mean to the best fitting cosine function.

Marker Rhythms for Cancer Chronochemotherapy

In assigning a time of day to administer chemotherapeutic agents, certain assumptions about interindividual circadian synchrony are made. This can easily be checked by establishing internal timing markers, which can be used as reference points independently of and complementary to clock hour.[87] Hrushesky and associates studied this in patients with small and large tumor burdens.[88] Biologic measurements were done every 2 hours during wakefulness and once during midsleep over three circadian cycles. At this sampling frequency and duration, oral temperature, heart rate, and blood pressure were poor choices as reference rhythms. Urinary volume and sodium excretion rhythms were affected by tumor burden. The rhythm characteristics of urinary potassium excretion were not different in patients with large or small tumor burden. The daily time peak of potassium excretion was near its usual afternoon timing. Urinary cortisol excretion was highly rhythmic in all patients studied. The daily peak was quite normal in patients with good performance status and moderate tumor burden. In bedridden patients with large tumor burdens, the peak occurred somewhat later in the day, with a higher circadian amplitude and mean cortisol excretion, indicating that circadian treatment studies should be limited to persons with good performance status. When markers of circadian time structure are obtained densely over several cycles (5–7 days), it has been discovered that circadian coordination with the environment is maintained up until very shortly before death from widespread cancer. Ultimately, marker rhythms may be used to tailor the timing of chemotherapy to each patient. Currently, we may realistically aim to give chemotherapy in the correct sixth to quarter of the day (*i.e.*, the best predicted timing ±2–3 hours).

CHRONOBIOLOGIC DATA FOR CHEMOTHERAPY AGENTS

Preclinical chronotoxicologic studies have investigated whether mice or rats tolerate the same dose of an anticancer agent differently depending on when in their circadian cycle it is given.[89] Table 69–28 summarizes data for 20 antineoplastic agents given to normal mice or rats by bolus or continuous infusion, intravenously, or intraperitoneally, evaluating a range of toxicities from lethal toxicity to organ specific toxicities. Table 69–29 summarizes 10 studies involving seven antineoplastic agents in seven different transplantable tumor systems in mice and rats. In these experimental systems, giving chemotherapy at the optimal time with regard to reduced toxicity improved the effectiveness of the treatment. In these nocturnally active animals, hours after light onset (HALO) correspond to hours after humans go to sleep.

FLUOROPYRIMIDINES

FUDR Animal Data

Animal studies have shown FUDR bolus and continuous infusion to be highly circadian stage dependent with regard to toxicity and antitumor activity.[90,130] Single boluses of FUDR in doses from 1000 mg/kg to 2000 mg/kg were given at one of six equally distributed circadian stages to more than 300 CD_2F_1 mice. Survival varied reproducibly by more than 50%, depending on the circadian stage of injection, with the best drug tolerance in the daily late activity span (18–20 HALO). The animals died with severe gut and bone marrow damage.[90]

Because of its short half-life, FUDR is usually given by prolonged infusion. Therefore, circadian patterned infusion studies were performed. FUDR (1000 mg/kg) was given by continuous intravenous infusion over 48 hours to female 344 Fisher rats. Drug was delivered by constant rate infusion or by variable rate infusion, with peak drug delivery during one of six different times of day. FUDR lethal toxicity, which was secondary to gut damage, was lowest 4 to 6 hours later (22-04 HALO) than the best time for bolus FUDR. This was also the best time with regard to tumor response in animals with

TABLE 69–28. Chronotoxicity of Anticancer Agents in Murine Models

Agent and Route	*Least Toxic Time in Rodents, HALO* (no. of tested times)†*	*Least Toxic Time for Humans‡ Resting 22-06*	*Measure of Toxicity§*
Antimetabolites			
FUDR I.V. bolus[90]	18–20 (6)	16–18	Lethal toxicity
FUDR I.V. infusion[91]	22–04 (6)	20–02	Lethal toxicity
FUDR IP[92]	02 (6)	24	Lethal toxicity
5-FU IP[93]	19 (11)	17	Gastrointestinal
5-FU IP[94]	02 > 12 (2)	24 > 10	Marrow
5-FU I.V.[95]	20 > 14 (2)	18 > 12	Marrow
5-FU IP[96]	05–07 (6)	03–05	Lethal toxicity
5-FU IP[97]	05 > 17 (2)	03 > 15	Lethal toxicity
5-FU IP[92]	10 (6)	08	Lethal toxicity
Methotrexate I.V.[98,99]	17.5 (4)	15.5	Lethal, marrow, renal, liver
Methotrexate IP[100]	14 (4)	12	Weight loss
Ara-C IP[101]	03–12 (8)	01–10	Lethal toxicity
Antitumor Antibiotics			
Doxorubicin IP[102,103]	08–10 (6)	06–08	Lethal—early, marrow
Doxorubicin I.V.[102,103]	15 (6)	13	Lethal—late, cardiac
Daunorubicin IP[104]	10 (6)	8	Lethal toxicity
Epirubicine IP[105]	02–06 (6)	24–04	Lethal toxicity
THP-doxorubicin I.V.[106]	07–10 (6)	05–08	Lethal, marrow
Mitoxantrone IP[107]	16 (4)	14	Lethal toxicity
Platinum Analogs			
Cisplatin IP, I.V.[108,109]	17–19 (6)	16–18¶	Lethal, renal, marrow
Oxaliplatin I.V.[110]	16 (6)	14	Lethal, marrow, jejunal
Caboplatin I.V.[111]	16 (6)	14	Lethal, marrow, jejunal
Vinca Alkaloids			
Vinblastine I.V.[112]	18–19 (6)	16–17	Lethal
Vincristine IP[113]	13 (6)	11	Lethal
Etoposide I.V.[114,115] ‖	07–11 (6)	05–09	Lethal
Alkylating Agents			
Cyclophosphamide IP[116]	07, 19 (6)	05, 17	Bladder
Cyclophosphamide IP[117,118]	12–13 (6, 5)	10–11	Lethal
Ifosfamide IP[119]	22–23 (6)	20–21	Lethal
Peptichemio I.V.[120]	15 (6)	13	Lethal, marrow, intestinal
Mitomycin C I.V.[121,122]	17–20 (6)	15–18	Lethal
Melphalan IP[123]	10 (6)	08	Marrow

* HALO, Hours after light on in animal cage; least toxic time refers to the time when treatment results produce least toxicity to the target tissue or the whole animal. Toxicity was not always tested at the same times for the same agents.
† Number of circadian times tested in the given experiment. If only a few times tested, 2 > 15 indicates that treatment was less toxic if given at 2 than if given at 15 HALO.
‡ Extrapolated from animal data for humans sleeping from 10 P.M. to 6 A.M. Human time = (HALO + 22) − 24.
§ Usually lethal toxicity. If autopsy was performed to determine tissue sustaining most toxcity, this is mentioned.
‖ The vehicle is more toxic to moce than VP-16 plus the vehicle; therefore, these data may reflect vehicle toxicity and are suspect.
¶ L:D–8:16 schedule used. May transfer later.

TABLE 69–29. Effectiveness of Anticancer Agents in Murine Tumor Systems When Each Agent is Given at Its Least Toxic Circadian Time

Agent	*Tumor*	*HALO**	*Index†*	*Effectiveness (%)*	
				Control‡	*Circadian Timed*
CY (+ Ara-C)	L1210 leukemia	8	Cure rate	44	94[124]
Doxorub (+CY)	L1210 leukemia	13	Cure rate	0–8	56–68[125]
Ara-C	L1210 leukemia	8	Cure rate	11	23[126]
L-PAM + D	Breast-adeno ca	10	PR	12.5	50[127]
Cisplatin (+D)	Immunocytoma	18	CR	24	60[128]
FUDR infusion	Breast-adeno ca	22–04	PR	0	25[91]
5-FU	Colon-adeno ca	2	PR	§[94]	
CY	T9 + T10 sarcoma	2	Cure rate	14% improvement[79]	
CY	L1210 leukemia	12	Cure rate	27% improvement[118]	
CY	Ehrlich's ascites	4	Cure rate	13% improvement[129]	

CY, cyclophosphamide; D, doxorubicin.
* If more than one agent was given, HALO (hours after light onset) refers to the timing of the agent outside the brackets.
† Index of effectiveness as measured by cure rate; PR, partial response; CR, complete response.
‡ Effectiveness of treatment if not given at the best circadian time.
§ Tumor growth delay was significantly better with treatment at 2 HALO than at 12 HALO.

a transplanted 13762-adenocarcinoma given 700 mg/kg of FUDR as a 48-hour intravenous infusion. Because some of the circadian shaped infusions studied were toxicologically and therapeutically inferior to constant rate infusion, the circadian pattern and not the quasi-intermittency of circadian FUDR administration was primarily responsible for these circadian pharmacodynamic differences.[90,91]

FUDR Clinical Data

In a series of clinical studies, von Roemeling and Hrushesky used a 14-day continuous infusion of FUDR. To achieve a variable rate infusion pattern, the daily drug dose was divided into four portions of 68%, 15%, 2%, and 15%. Each portion was infused over a 6-hour span. This type of infusion with its peak drug delivery between 3 P.M. and 9 P.M. was found to give substantially less toxicity than a constant infusion of the same dose.[6] In a crossover study and a second randomized study, patients with metastatic malignancies treated with equal dose intensities experienced less frequent and less severe diarrhea, nausea, and vomiting after the variable-rate infusion described previously compared with a flat-rate infusion. In a third study, the dose intensity of variable rate infusion was escalated stepwise to determine the maximal tolerated dose. Patients receiving the time-modified FUDR infusion tolerated an average of 1.45-fold more drug per unit time while experiencing minimal toxicity. Valvassori confirmed in 111 cancer patients that FUDR is well tolerated when given by this circadian schedule.[131]

This FUDR schedule was found to be active in 63 consecutive evaluable patients with metastatic renal cell cancer, with five complete responses and ten partial responses to give a 24 ± 5.1% (95% confidence limits) objective response rate.[5] Other researchers have confirmed this. Huben similarly treated a group of good performance status patients without prior therapy and found a 60% objective response rate.[132] Damaschelli also found the regimen to be active.[133] More recently, Venook treated 29 patients and also found a 21% objective response rate. Dexeus and colleagues, using a somewhat different circadian schedule of FUDR in 42 patients with metastatic renal cell cancer, reported a partial response in 4 patients (10%; 95% confidence limits 3–24%). Another 4 patients (10%) had partial responses at metastatic sites but no response in the primary kidney tumor.[134] Hrushesky and colleagues are conducting a prospective randomized multicenter trial comparing a 14 day circadian infusion of FUDR with a 14 day flat FUDR infusion in patients with metastatic renal cell cancer.

Continuous FUDR intravenous infusion for 14 out of 21 to 28 days is the most consistently active and useful chemotherapy for metastatic RCC. FUDR toxicity and safely achievable dose intensity are each favorably modified by circadian infusion, giving most of each day's dose in the evening hours. An NCI-sponsored multicenter international study is currently determining the effect of circadian optimization on response frequency and quality and patient survival.

In 50 patients with liver metastases from colorectal cancer receiving FUDR as intrahepatic infusion, toxicity in the form of cholestasis and jaundice was several-fold less frequent, less severe, and occurred later when circadian infusion was employed compared with a flat infusion. Patients receiving the circadian modified infusion tolerated a 70% higher average dose intensity. Response rates in the two groups were similar.[7]

Focan and colleagues have reported preliminary data from a randomized study of intravenous 5-FU and intrahepatic FUDR in 38 previously untreated patients with liver metastases from colorectal cancer.[133a] Patients in arm A received a flat infusion, and patients in arm B received a circadian infusion with peaks for 5-FU at 4 A.M. and for FUDR at 4 P.M. Stomatitis was dose limiting. No hepatic toxicity was noted. After the third course, toxicity (alopecia, neutropenia, and skin) became lower in arm B despite a higher dose intensity. More courses could be delivered in arm B. The response rate was similar in both arms (50–60%). The median survival was superior in arm B (40+ months versus 19.6 months in arm A).

More recent animal studies indicate that the optimal systemic FUDR infusion should most likely peak 4 to 6 hours later than was originally extrapolated from the bolus studies.[91] Even more benefit may be expected in future clinical studies using FUDR infusion if this is taken into account.

5-Fluorouracil Animal Data

Popovic found that the best tolerance to 5-FU, with 30% mortality, was in middle to late rest phase (5–7 HALO), but 100% mortality was observed in animals treated in the late activity phase (20–22 HALO).[96] Burns randomized mice to receive 5-FU treatment at 5 or 17 HALO. The single intraperitoneal bolus dose of 5-FU killing 50% of the animals (LD_{50}) was significantly higher in early rest (5 HALO) than in midactivity (17 HALO) phase.[97] Gonzales and coworkers concurrently tested the lethal toxicity of a single intraperitoneal 5-FU and FUDR bolus injections at one of six different time points in Balb/c mice.[92] 5-FU was least toxic in late rest (10 HALO), and FUDR was least toxic in early rest (2 HALO). Gardner found that the impairment of water absorption by small intestine in vitro and the incidence of diarrhea in vivo differed as a function of treatment time when 5-FU was given to rats.[93] The intestinal toxicity was minimal after treatment in late activity (19 HALO) when the maximum of small intestine mucosa cells were in the postmitotic resting phase (G_1) and less susceptible to the effects from 5-FU. Peters and colleagues tested the antitumor and bone marrow toxicity of 5-FU in transplantable mouse colon cancer-bearing mice. Better antitumor activity and less marrow toxicity was found in the early rest phase compared with treatment given in the early activity phase.[94] Minshull has confirmed these data with regard to bone marrow toxicity in Wistar rats.[95] Overall, these preclinical data indicate that this drug, like FUDR, is probably best given in the first half of the daily sleep span.

5-Fluorouracil Clinical Data

Murine data from investigating 5-FU-induced lethal toxicity and human pharmacology data for 5-FU were the basis for subsequent clinical trials, giving the highest dose of 5-FU centered in the second half of the daily sleep span at 4 A.M.[14,96,97] Lévi and associates used a 5-day circadian continuous infusion of 5-FU every 3 weeks in 30 patients with metastatic colorectal cancer. The delivery rate varied in a circadian manner and was highest at 4 A.M. and null from 6 to 10 P.M. An intrapatient dose escalation by 1 g/m^2/course was planned from 5 g/m^2/course (usual schedule) to 9 g/m^2/course according to toxicity criteria. The mean highest tolerated dose was 7.5 g/m^2/course, considerably higher than that recommended for a constant infusion of 5-FU.[4,9]

The clinical data available indicate that the combination of 5-FU and leucovorin (LV) is more effective in shrinking tumors than 5-FU alone in patients with metastatic colorectal cancer.[135] In a phase II trial using patients with metastatic colorectal cancer, 5-FU, LV, and oxaliplatin were infused continuously for 5 days every 3 weeks.[9] Oxaliplatin (25 mg/m^2/day) was infused for 12 hours, with peak delivery at 4 P.M., and 5-FU (700 mg/m^2/day) and LV (300 mg/m^2/day) were infused concurrently for 12 hours with peak delivery at 4 A.M. Fifty-four of the 93 patients had an objective response (58%; 95% confidence limits, 48% to 68%) regardless of previous chemotherapy. In a subsequent phase II study, this circadian schedule was used in 37 patients with fluoropyrimidine-resistant colorectal cancer. After a mean number of eight courses, a partial response rate was achieved in 16 of 37 patients (43%).[135a] The timing of oxaliplatin was based on previous experimental and clinical studies.[78,110] These findings await confirmation in a ongoing randomized study comparing a flat infusion of these agents with the schedule described here.

A phase I trial was conducted to identify the optimal dose rate of delivery for admixtures of 5-FU and LV given for 14 days as a flat continuous infusions.[136] The optimal dose rate for 5-FU and LV was found to be 200 mg/m^2/day and 5 mg/m^2/day, respectively. In a phase I study of a 14-day circadian infusion of 5-FU and LV, with the infusion peaking at 4 A.M., Bjarnason and colleagues determined the maximum tolerated dose (MTD) for 5-FU and LV, given as a continuous circadian infusion over 14 days, with 64% of the daily dose given over 7 hours around 3 to 4 A.M.[137] LV was first escalated by 5 mg/m^2/day to 20 mg/m^2/day, followed by escalation of 5-FU by 50 mg/m^2/day. Patients who developed ≥grade II toxicity had the peak of the infusion shifted from 3 to 4 A.M. to 9 to 10 P.M., to determine if this reduced toxicity. This timing corresponds to the time of least toxicity from 5-FU in more recent murine studies, testing nonlethal doses.[93–95] Recent clinical studies of 5-FU pharmacokinetics, 5-FU metabolism, and gut cytokinetics also suggest that an evening infusion peak may be less toxic than an infusion peaking at 3 to 4 A.M.[54,58,146] The MTD for an infusion peaking at 3 to 4 A.M. was reached at dose level 5 (5-FU 250 mg/m^2/day-LV 20 mg/m^2/day). In 6 patients developing ≥grade II toxicity, the peak of the infusion was shifted to 9 to 10 P.M. Toxicity was reduced in all 6 patients and further dose escalation was possible in 3 patients. The MTD for an infusion peaking at 9–10 P.M. was reached at dose level 6 (5-FU 300 mg/m^2/day-LV 20 mg/m^2/day). Stomatitis and hand-foot syndrome was dose limiting. There was no bone marrow toxicity. The recommended dose for phase II studies using this schedule is 5-FU 250 mg/m^2/day and LV 20 mg/m^2/day with the infusion peak at 9 to 10 P.M. This is a 300% and 25% higher dose for LV and 5-FU, respectively, than was suggested to be safe for a flat infusion. A phase II study is ongoing in metastatic colorectal cancer. The addition of leucovorin may alter the circadian time-dependent toxicity of 5-FU by diverting its mechanism of action more toward the inhibition of thymidylate synthetase and away from incorporation into RNA. Preliminary animal studies of 5-FU and LV pharmacodynamics indicate that the addition of LV may change the circadian optimum for 5-FU from the second half toward the first half of the daily sleep span.[138]

Mechanisms of Fluropyrimidine Circadian Pharmacodynamics

Several studies have shown that plasma drug levels vary significantly during continuous infusion of 5-FU.[139–141] Two studies demonstrated a circadian rhythm in the plasma concentration of 5-FU in patients receiving this drug as a continuous venous infusion at a constant rate for 5 to 14 days.[14,54]

Harris found the peak value for plasma 5-FU at 11 A.M. and the trough value at 11 P.M. The ratio of the maximal concentration of 5-FU to the minimal concentration observed was almost fivefold higher.[54] Petit found the peak value for plasma 5-FU at 1 A.M. and the trough value at 1 P.M., 10 hours earlier than Harris.[14] The difference may be related to the fact that the patients in the second study received cisplatin at a fixed time of day before each 5-day 5-FU infusion (450–966 mg/m^2/day), but the patients in the first study received only 5-FU in a lower dose (300 mg/m^2/day) and for a longer time span. Pharmacokinetic interactions between cisplatin and 5-FU have been documented, with a single dose of cisplatin increasing subsequent plasma levels of 5-FU given by continuous infusion.[142]

More than 80% of an administered dose of 5-FU is rapidly catabolized in the liver and extrahepatic sites.[143] Catabolism largely determines the availability of 5-FU for anabolism to its active nucleotide analogs. The activity of dihydropyrimidine dehydrogenase (DPD), the rate-limiting enzyme for fluoropyrimidine catabolism, is highly circadian stage dependent ($p < 0.0001$) in the rat liver, with a peak in late rest (10 HALO).[144] Harris showed that this leads to a circadian variation of 5-FU catabolism in the isolated perfused rat liver with the peak and trough elimination rates of 5-FU in late activity (19 HALO) and midrest (7 HALO) respectively. There was a reciprocal relation between the elimination rates of 5-FU and 5-FU catabolites.[145]

Tuchman [146] and Harris[54] independently demonstrated a circadian variation of DPD activity in human mononuclear cells with peak values occurring at 10 P.M. to 2 A.M. and at 1 A.M., respectively (*i.e.*, early rest period). A inverse relation between DPD activity in peripheral blood mononuclear cells and plasma 5-FU concentration was demonstrated by Harris in his study of cancer patients receiving a protracted continuous infusion if 5-FU.[54] The timing of peak values for DPD activity in humans (*i.e.*, early rest) differs somewhat from the time of peak values of DPD activity determined in rats (*i.e.*, late rest). The reason for this discrepancy is not clear, but it emphasizes the variability that may exist between species. The activity of the initial enzyme in fluoropyrimidine anabolism, thymidine kinase, recently has been shown to be rhythmic in the rat spleen, with a pattern opposite to that of DPD.[146a]

The activities of other enzymes of importance in fluoropyrimidine activation; dihydrouracil dehydrogenase, uridine phosphorylase, and thymidine phosphorylase have each been shown to be circadian rhythmic in the mouse liver.[147] Daher did not find a circadian variation in the activity of thymidine phosphorylase in the rat liver.[148] Thymidine phosphorylase is the major enzyme responsible for the phosphorolysis of FUDR to 5-FU.

Reproducible circadian patterns in the activities of catabolic and anabolic enzymes relevant to the biochemical pharmacology of fluoropyrimidines are responsible, at least in part, for the marked circadian pharmacodynamics of 5-FU and FUDR.

ANTHRACYCLINES

Animal Toxicity Studies

Early chronotoxicity studies of intraperitoneal doxorubicin in hybrid mice and F344 rats demonstrated its profound circadian pharmacodynamics.[149] When doxorubicin was given in early activity (14 HALO), it was much better tolerated than when given in early rest (2 HALO). These results were confirmed by Sothern in a more detailed study, in which the toxicity of doxorubicin given intravenously and intraperitoneally was investigated.[103] The timing of best tolerance for doxorubicin was found to be to some extent dependent on the route of administration.[102,103] Early mortality (*i.e.*, day 5–20) from doxorubicin was only seen after intraperitoneal administration, with late rest (8 HALO) being the time of least toxicity. Late mortality, starting on day 40, was found to be similar for intraperitoneal and intravenous administration, with early activity (15 HALO) the time of least toxicity for both routes. Sothern has demonstrated that circadian stage, not time of day, characterizes doxorubicin susceptibility rhythms of mice in continuous light.[83] The time of least toxicity coincided with the low point of the rectal temperature rhythm in animals in constant light and in animals on a schedule of alternating light and darkness. Intraperitoneal daunorubicin, compared with doxorubicin, had an earlier time of least toxicity (10 HALO versus 14 HALO).[104] Experimental data are also available for the time of epirubicin and 4′-O-tetrahydropyranyl doxorubicin.[105,106]

Mitoxantrone was tested at four circadian times in $B_6D_2F_1$ mice, and found to be most toxic in early rest (3–7 HALO). Pharmacokinetic monitoring showed that this coincided with the time for the longest half-life and the largest area under the curve (AUC) for mitoxantrone compared with treatment at the three other time points.[107] The least toxic time was at 16 HALO, about 8 hours later than for doxorubicin.

The time of day associated with lowest doxorubicin toxicity to bone marrow, gut, and heart tissue, as well as its best antitumor activity occurs just before usual daily awakening, when normal tissue oxidative defense systems are most robust.

Animal Tumor Response Studies

In LOU rats bearing an immunocytoma, a single injection of doxorubicin induced a faster tumor regression, but a faster regrowth of tumor, when doxorubicin was given near the time of best tolerance, just before daily awakening (06 HALO).[150]

Several studies have used doxorubicin in combination with other chemotherapy agents. Halberg and coworkers gave sequential chemotherapy with doxorubicin and melphalan to female Fisher rats that were previously inoculated with 13762 mammary adenocarcinoma.[127] The best responses to treatment, as measured by tumor size, complete remissions, and duration of remission, were observed when the drugs were given just before usual awakening (10 HALO), near the time of best normal tissue tolerance in rodents.

Studies of intraperitoneal doxorubicin and cisplatin in immunocytoma-bearing LOU rats documented a striking circadian stage dependence of tumor response and toxicity. The maximal tumor response and least toxicity was observed when cisplatin was administered in the middle to latter part of the daily activity span, and doxorubicin was administered near the end of the daily resting span.[128]

Scheving studied the response rate to intraperitoneal doxorubicin and cyclophosphamide in mice bearing advanced L1210 leukemia.[125] The variation in cure rate ranged from 8% to 68% in male animals and 0% to 56% in female animals, depending on the time of treatment. The maximal cure rate was recorded when the two drugs were administered 3 hours apart during the early activity cycle, corresponding to the time of best tolerance for doxorubicin.

Clinical Studies

Several clinical studies have used the combination of doxorubicin and cisplatin. In the first randomized-crossover study, which accrued 23 patients between 1979 and 1982, patients with metastatic ovarian cancer (11) and bladder cancer (12) alternated between treatments with doxorubicin (60 mg/m^2) at 0600 or 1800 with cisplatin (60 mg/m^2) given 12 hours later.[151] Nadir blood counts were moderate, and recovery was complete within 21 days, using morning doxorubicin and evening cisplatin. Evening doxorubicin and morning cisplatin produced statistically significantly lower nadirs with less than full recovery by day 28. Nephrotoxicity from the first course of treatment was entirely avoided by the use of the favorable circadian schedule, but treatment with morning cisplatin and evening doxorubicin resulted in an average creatinine clearance fall of 30 ml/minute after the first course of treatment. Cisplatin urinary pharmacokinetics were concurrently studied and contrasted in patients receiving morning or evening cisplatin. These studies were performed in a general clinical research center, where vigorous comparability of all oral and intravenous fluid and calorie delivery were maintained. It was found that peak urinary cisplatin concentration and the AUC of cisplatin concentration were each much higher for the patients receiving cisplatin in the morning. There was a good correlation between the peak urinary concentration and degree of subsequent permanent kidney damage.[13,151] These data are consistent with the animal data described previously.[128]

In a study conducted between 1982 and 1986, 37 patients with ovarian cancer were accrued and randomized to receive doxorubicin (60 mg/m^2) at 0600 (schedule A) or 1800 (schedule B), with cisplatin (60 mg/m^2) given 12 hours later, monthly for 9 months.[10,151] Evaluation of bone marrow toxicity in patients who received at least 8 of 9 planned treatments revealed more cumulative marrow toxicity in patients treated on schedule B. Most patients on this schedule had to have greater than 33% doxorubicin dose reductions and some treatment delays because of marrow toxicity. Patients on schedule A had fewer dose reductions, treatment delays, and fewer episodes of infection, bleeding, and transfusions (Fig. 69–30). This study confirmed all the preliminary toxicity results uncovered in the initial crossover study. Average achievable dose intensity, expressed in mg/kg/week or as percentage of planned dose intensity, was lower for schedule B than schedule A. This prospectively randomized study hinted at a survival advantage for patients treated on schedule A. At 5 years, 44% of patients treated on schedule A were alive, but 11% of those treated using schedule B survived 5 years.

The same two-drug combination of doxorubicin and cisplatin was given to 43 patients with advanced transitional cell carcinoma of the bladder. Patients were randomized to receive schedule A or schedule B. Overall, 57% had an objective response, and 23% had a complete response (35 evaluable patients). The numbers of patients per treatment group did not allow interpretation of schedule-dependent differences in response, but toxicity evaluation confirmed that schedule A was superior, with lower toxicity despite higher dose intensity.[12]

Similar schedule dependency with regard to toxicity was observed by Lévi using 4′tetrahydropyranyl doxorubicin (THP) and cisplatin in patients with advanced ovarian cancer.[8] Thirty-one patients were randomized to chemotherapy according to one of two schedules (*i.e.,* schedule A or schedule B). Patients on schedule A received their chemotherapy at times predicted to be least toxic by animal experiments: THP (50 mg/m^2) by intravenous bolus at 6 A.M. and cisplatin (100 mg/m^2) by a 4-hour infusion from 4 to 8 P.M. Patients on schedule B received THP at 6 P.M. and cisplatin infusion from 4 to 8 A.M. The overall response rate was 64%, 73% on schedule A and 57% on schedule B. Schedule A was associated with two to three times less hematologic and renal toxicity than schedule B ($p < 0.01$). Three of 4 patients withdrawn from this protocol because of severe toxicity were on schedule B. Full planned doses of these drugs could be given for three or more courses to fourfold as many patients on schedule A compared with schedule B. A randomized trial is ongoing.

The Gynecology Oncology Group has reported a phase II study of patients with advanced or recurrent endometrial cancer.[152] Doxorubicin (60 mg/m^2) was given over 30 minutes at 6 A.M., followed by cisplatin (60 mg/m^2) given over 30 minutes at 6 P.M. every 28 days. The number of treatment courses ranged from two to eight, with a median of six. A preliminary review of 25 evaluable patients shows 4 (16%) of 25 complete responses, 9 (36%) of 25 partial responses, and 8 (32%) of 25 with stable disease. This 52% objective response rate was three times the predicted response rate and is currently being followed-up with additional clinical trials.

Lévi is studying chronotherapy with doxorubicin in patients with metastatic breast cancer, comparing a flat infusion with a sinusoid infusion, giving the highest dose of doxorubicin from 3 to 7 A.M.[153] Stomatitis was the main dose limiting factor on both schedules, but hematologic toxicity was more pronounced on the flat infusion schedule. In another study Lévi found better hematologic tolerance to 4′-O-tetrahydropyranyl doxorubicin if this agent was given at 0600 compared with 1800 in patients with metastatic cancer.[154]

Each of several circadian clinical trials of doxorubicin or its analogs with cisplatin or its analogs demonstrate substantial advantage to timing the anthracycline early at, or just before, usual awakening and platinum compounds late in the afternoon or in the early evening.

Mechanism

Circadian variation of plasma concentration of doxorubicin was noticed in mice.[155] In humans receiving bolus or infusional therapy with doxorubicin, similar circadian changes in doxorubicin pharmacokinetics were found with higher levels late in the day.[156]

Some of the bone marrow toxicity and all of the cardiac toxicity of doxorubicin may be related to the NADPH-dependent doxorubicin semiquinone-mediated generation of free radicals, such as hydroxyl and superoxide anions, that can be detoxified by several pathways, primarily the glutathione cycle.[157] A circadian rhythm in the level of total glutathione and reduced glutathione (GSH) in cardiac tissue has been documented in mice and rats, with highest levels in the early activity span, corresponding to the time of lowest lethal toxicity of intravenous doxorubicin in these animals.[50,158] He-

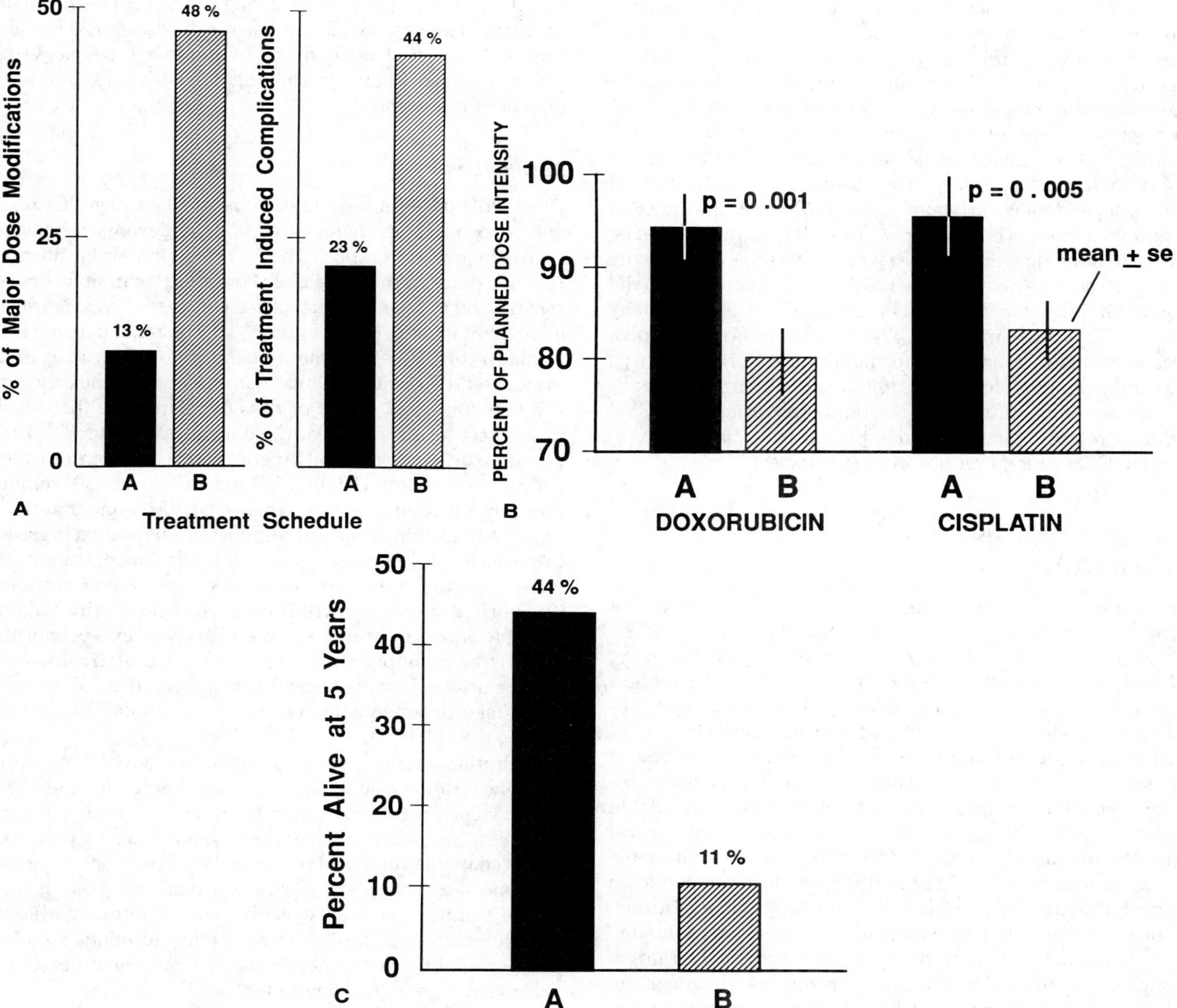

FIGURE 69–30. **(A)** The frequency of dose modifications and treatment delays forced by therapy on each circadian schedule and the frequency of treatment-associated complications. Each of 37 patients were randomized to receive monthly treatment courses of doxorubicin and cisplatin at one of two times of the day. Patients randomized to receive morning doxorubicin and evening cisplatin (A, *solid bars*) had to have only about 1 in 10 of their treatment courses modified (13%), but treatment with doxorubicin in the evening and cisplatin in the morning (B, *hatched bars*) forced major dose or schedule modifications in almost one of every two treatment courses (48%) ($p < 0.001$). On the right of the first panel, it can be seen that patients treated on schedule A had serious complications in almost one of every five treatment courses (23%); patients treated on schedule B had complications in more than three of every five courses (44%) ($p < 0.001$), even though this group of patients received less drug less frequently. **(B)** The average achievable dose intensity of each drug for patients treated on schedule A (*solid*) or schedule B (*hatched*) for doxorubicin and cisplatin. Toxicity forced reduction of doxorubicin dose if schedule A (*solid bars*) was used to 95% of the planned dose. When schedule B (*hatched bars*) was employed, only 80% of planned dose could safely be given ($p < 0.001$). Moreover, 96% of scheduled cisplatin could be given if schedule A (*solid bars*) was employed, but only 83% of the planned dose could be administered if schedule B (*hatched bars*) was used ($p < 0.005$). **(C)** This panel contrasts the relative probability that patients treated with schedule A (*solid bar*) are alive 5 years after study entry (44%) with the relative probability of survival for patients treated on schedule B (*hatched bar*), which was 11%.

patic GSH concentration in rodents exhibits a similar circadian rhythmicity, and similar rhythmicity in GSH occurs in other tissues in the rat, differing in amplitude and frequency from the hepatic cycle.[159,160] Substantial circadian differences in the nonprotein-bound sulfhydryl concentration (>90% GSH) in nucleated cells of human bone marrow has been documented.[49] More than fivefold higher levels were present at 8 A.M. than at 8 P.M. in 5 healthy volunteers. Smaaland found a time-dependent covariation between GSH content and DNA synthesis in human bone marrow from 10 healthy volunteers, when 70 bone marrow samples were collected every 4 hours over a 24-hour period.[51] These results are in keeping with the human findings that doxorubicin produced less myelotoxicity when given in the morning. The toxicity of other antineoplastic agents that cause the formation of free radicals (*e.g.*, alkylating agents, bleomycin, mitomycin C, antitumor antibiotics) could be affected by the temporal variation in GSH levels. Cyclophosphamide and ara-C toxicities have been related to GSH concentrations in target tissues.[48]

PLATINUM ANALOGS

Animal Studies

Cis-diamminedichloroplatinum (CDDP) represents the parent compound in this group. There is a circadian rhythm in the lethal toxicity of CDDP (11 mg/kg given intraperitoneally) when studied in female 344 Fisher rats.[108,161] The highest tolerance for cisplatin occurred in middle to late activity 17–19 HALO). The nephrotoxicity of a lower nontoxic dose of CDDP (5 mg/kg intraperitoneally) was found to be least at the same circadian time.[162] This was further confirmed in a study giving CDDP intravenously to male $B_6D_2F_1$ mice.[163] In both species, the drug was best tolerated if given near or just after the middle of the activity span, regardless of the route of administration. CDDP induced renal failure was the main cause of drug-related mortality. Two nonnephrotoxic platinum analogs, carboplatin and oxaliplatin, are also best tolerated near the middle of the activity span, even though their target organs of toxicity are mainly bone marrow and the intestine, rather than the kidney for CDDP.[110,111] A new cisplatin analog, B-85-0040, is likewise best tolerated near the middle activity span.[164]

Cisplatin and each of its analogs, which have been studied, are least toxic and most effective when given in the second half of the daily activity span.

Clinical Studies

Modern cancer treatment is polypharmaceutical, and most clinical studies with CDDP have been done with combination chemotherapy. Combinations with doxorubicin have been discussed previously and have confirmed the time of least toxicity in humans to be in the evening.

Caussanel has reported a randomized phase I trial of a 5-day flat continuous venous infusion of oxaliplatin compared with a circadian-modulated infusion with its peak at 1600.[78] Toxicity was assessed for 94 courses in 23 patients. There was far less neutropenia ($p < 0.05$) and less frequent and less severe distal paresthesias ($p < 0.001$) and a trend to less emesis ($p = 0.15$) in patients receiving the circadian-modulated infusion. With dose escalation, the mean dose was 33% higher in the circadian-modulated arm by the fourth course. Oxaliplatin has been studied in combination with 5-FU and LV as discussed previously.[9]

Mechanism

Cisplatin's dose-limiting toxicity is renal damage. Cisplatin and other platinum analogs are eliminated from the body primarily by renal excretion. The fact that glomerular filtration rate increases in the middle of the activity span in laboratory rodents and in humans could play a part in the circadian stage-dependent toxicity of platinum.[165,166] The renal damage from cisplatin correlates with the concentration of free drug in the urine, and the greatest tubular damage occurs when the drug is given during the phase of the circadian cycle that results in highest urinary cisplatin concentration.[108,162,167] Free-platinum urinary excretion kinetics were studied in 11 cancer patients receiving CDDP (60 mg/m^2) over 30 minutes monthly.[13] Patients received their CDDP treatment at 6 A.M. or at 6 P.M. Evening cisplatin administration resulted in greater urine output, lower peak urinary platinum concentration, and lower areas under the curve of urinary cisplatin concentration. The normal circadian rhythm, characteristic of urine volume, 1 month after the treatment was disrupted by the morning CDDP treatment but not by the evening CDDP treatment.[168] Plasma protein binding of cisplatin has been found to be circadian stage dependent in humans, with its daily maximum around 4 P.M.[169]

Hydration reduces cisplatin nephrotoxicity.[170] An intraperitoneal saline load was given or withheld in female Fisher rats concurrently with cisplatin at six separate circadian times.[109] A marked rhythm in the amount of kidney protection achieved by the fluid load was observed. Hydration improved outcome most when given with platinum at its optimal circadian timing. Diethyldithiocarbamate or tetraethylthiocarbamate, which act through nucleophile excretion, protected from cisplatin induced nephrotoxicity only at times of day associated with high cisplatin toxicity.[171]

Cisplatin and its analogs are not cell cycle specific, but circadian rhythms have been well documented for renal cytokinetics.[172,173] Other cellular defenses of importance may be tied to cell cycle; for example, the urinary activity of many metabolically important renal tubular enzymes has a circadian rhythm in animals and healthy human volunteers.[162,174–176] A specific index of proximal tubular damage is an increase in the urinary excretion of (β-N-acetylglucosaminidase (β-NAG), a lysosomal enzyme released into the urine by normal proximal tubular cells.[177] Lévi documented in rats that β-NAG was released into the urine in proportion to the degree of histologically confirmed renal dysfunction induced by cisplatin.[162] This enzyme was present in the urine of normal animals, and its base line concentration was found to display a high-amplitude circadian rhythm. When cisplatin was given at its most toxic time, the circadian rhythm of urinary β-NAG was maintained, but the mean and peak levels increased fivefold in direct proportion to the subsequent rise in BUN. When cisplatin was given at a favorable circadian stage, these groups demonstrated a smaller β-NAG rise and had little histologic renal damage with only a small rise in BUN. Other thiol-rich proteins or amino acids such as GSH may play a role in the mechanism of circadian renal toxicity from platinum.[178]

Boughattas has looked at tissue concentration of cisplatin and carboplatin in spleen, kidney, and colon of mice given eight weekly courses of these drugs at one of three dosing times.[179] There was half the tissue accumulation of platinum when these drugs were given at their least toxic circadian times.

ALKYLATING AGENTS

Melphalan, peptichemio, cyclophosphamide, ifosfamide, and threosulfan toxicities are all characterized by circadian rhythms in murine tolerance.[117–120,123,180,181] These drugs have different times for best tolerance (see Table 69–28), perhaps because some of them must be metabolized to become active by different metabolic processes.

Three studies looked at the time-dependent anticancer activity of alkylating agents. Badran gave a single intraperitoneal dose of cyclophosphamide to female mice bearing transplantable mammary carcinoma at one of six circadian stages. Animals treated in the resting span (2, 6, and 10 HALO) developed significantly smaller tumors.[182] Focan treated sarcoma bearing mice with cyclophosphamide. Best antitumor effect was found if the drug was given early rest (02 HALO), coinciding with the G_2 phase of the sarcoma cells.[79] Cardoso observed maximal cure rate and least toxicity in leukemic mice when cyclophosphamide was given at the end of the rest period (12 HALO).[118] Anticancer activity was usually superior when the cytoxan was given in the second half of the daily sleep span, or just before or just after usual daily awakening.

Bladder toxicity from cyclophosphamide in male CD1-mice was minimal after dosing in midrest (7 HALO) or midactivity (19 HALO).[116] Most mucosal damage was induced with dosing in late rest (11 HALO) or late activity (23 HALO). These results suggest a 12-hour cycle in the sensitivity of the bladder to cyclophosphamide.

Mitomycin C can produce prolonged myelosuppression among other toxicities.[121,122] This drug was least toxic when given to mice in mid to late activity (17–20 HALO). Histologic evaluation of all target organs revealed that the lethal toxicity so profoundly modified by drug timing may well be related to the vexing clinical problem of mitomycin C induced microangiopathic disease.[122] No clinical work has been done to investigate this possibility.

Although the circadian timing of each alkylating agent studied markedly affects its toxicity, their optimal times are quite different. Clinical trials are needed to follow-up on the murine data.

CYTOSINE ARABINOSIDE

A single fixed dose of cytosine arabinoside (ara-C) administered daily for 6 days to mice was found to be least toxic when given in the rest span (2,5–7 HALO). The same dose of ara-C killed 15% of the animals if given in the rest span compared with 75% if given in the activity span.[183,184] Haus applied this finding to the treatment of leukemic mice.[126] Each animal received eight intraperitoneal injections of ara-C at 3-hour intervals over 24 hours. This was given on days 1, 6, 10, and 14. In one group of animals, the doses at the various injection times varied in amount according to a sinusoidal pattern, ranging from 7.5 mg/kg given at the predicted time of lowest resistance to 67.5 mg/kg given at the predicted time of highest resistance. Another group of animals received the same total doses in eight equal doses over each 24-hour period. A doubling of survival was observed in the sinusoidally treated group (23%) compared with the group given constant doses (11%).

In an attempt to unequivocally demonstrate rhythmic variation in tolerance to ara-C, studies were carried out by two different laboratories using the same experimental design as described previously, but on nontumor-bearing mice.[101] Eight differently timed circadian-shaped treatment schedules and one constant-dose schedule were used. The most favorable survival was achieved in the sinusoidal treatment arms in which the highest dose was given in the rest period (from 3.5–12.5 HALO). The homeostatic treatment achieved only 12.5% survival; 25% to 38% of the animals given treatment on "unfavorable" sinusoidal schedules survived, and the "favorable" sinusoidal treatments produced survival rates of 73% to 80%.

Hromas used flow cytometry to look at the effect of ara-C on the chronobiology of the bone marrow DNA synthesis in mice.[185] At all times, ara-C flattened the rhythm of bone marrow DNA synthesis; however, it had it's greatest effect if given when there were relatively more cells moving into S phase (18 HALO) or in S phase (0 HALO) than if few cells were in S phase (12 HALO) or cells were leaving S phase (6 HALO).

Scheving treated L1210 leukemic mice with a combination of intraperitoneal ara-C and cyclophosphamide at one of six circadian stages.[124] Best results with regard to cure rate and survival were observed when cyclophosphamide was given in late rest (8 HALO) and ara-C given by the sinusoidally shaped schedule found to be optimal in previous studies. In the animals receiving ara-C in the optimal fashion, the cure rate ranged from 44% to 94%, depending on the timing of the cyclophosphamide dose. Only 1.4% of these animals died from drug toxicity. When another group of animals was treated with the same drugs without chronobiologic consideration, 30% died from acute drug toxicity.

When vincristine was added to the best schedule of ara-C and cyclophosphamide described previously, best results (52% cure rate) were achieved when vincristine was given in late activity (23 HALO). When methylprednisolone was added to this three-drug scheme, best results were obtained when prednisolone was given in early activity (11 HALO or 14 HALO).[186] Attempts were made to improve the response rate further by adding cisplatin to this schedule.[187] The least toxic time for cisplatin was in late activity (20 HALO). With reduced drug dosage to decrease toxicity from this combination chemotherapy regimen, a 88% cure rate was obtained in these L1210 leukemic animals.

Rose confirmed the circadian variation in toxicity for ara-C and cyclophosphamide given as single agents.[188] The optimal therapeutic responses of leukemic mice treated in the least toxic way by ara-C or cyclophosphamide at maximal tolerated dose levels were no better than those achieved in leukemic mice receiving equitoxic, but results were achieved lower doses of these drugs by the conventional method and at other circadian stages. The design and analysis of this study have been criticized.[189]

Cytosine arabinoside alone or in combination with other cytotoxic agents was much more effective and much less toxic when given during the usual daily sleep span.

METHOTREXATE

Intravenous methotrexate was found to be most toxic in rats in late activity (23.5 HALO), with least toxicity in terms of marrow, renal, and liver toxicity in midactivity (17.5 HALO).[98] The pharmacokinetics of methotrexate were found to be circadian stage dependent, with the longest half-life after treatment at the most toxic time. The time of day of maximal toxicity coincided with the nadir for plasma corticosterone concentration. In subsequent studies by the same researchers, high plasma levels of exogenously administered corticosterone protected against methotrexate toxicity, but suppressed levels markedly increased toxicity unrelated to time.[99] Giving oral melatonin daily for 6 weeks before methotrexate treatment increased its toxicity at all time points.[190]

Labat found intraperitoneal methotrexate to be most toxic to male Swiss mice when given in early rest (2 HALO), as estimated by the relative weight loss after therapy.[100] The highest AUC values in this study were found after treatment in early rest. This observation is consistent with the work of English and with his earlier data, showing that the inhibition by methotrexate of the activity of renal dihydrofolate reductase (DHFR), the target enzyme for methotrexate, is maximal in the early rest period.[191] These results indicate clearly that methotrexate is least toxic when given in the middle of the daily activity span.

In a very limited two times of day study, Robinson did not find circadian variation in the pharmacokinetics for methotrexate in six lymphoma patients receiving the drug as a part of the CHOP chemotherapy.[16] Methotrexate was given as a 30 minute continuous infusion starting at 0600 or 1800, with each patient serving as his own control. The timing of oral methotrexate may be important in children on maintenance therapy for acute lymphoblastic leukemia.[192]

Methotrexate is metabolized only to a minor extent in rodents and is excreted largely unchanged in roughly equal amounts in the urine and in the bile, but in humans, the major route is renal excretion.[193] Variation in plasma clearance rate in rodents may be caused by variations in renal filtration rate or biliary output.

6-MERCAPTOPURINE

The course of 118 children with ALL, who had achieved complete remission with a standard induction protocol and had received meningeal prophylaxis with intrathecal methotrexate and cranial irradiation, was reviewed.[192] Maintenance therapy consisted of daily 6-mercaptopurine (6-MP), weekly methotrexate (MTX), and monthly vincristine and prednisone. For compliance reasons, 82 children took their 6-MP and MTX in the morning, and 36 children took these medications in the evening. Regression analysis showed that, for those children surviving free of disease for longer than 78 weeks, the risk of relapsing was 4.6 times greater for the morning schedule than for the evening schedule ($p = 0.006$).

Studies of orally administered 6-MP and MTX have shown a poor correlation between the given dose and peak serum levels.[194] Absorption of MTX and 6-MP is better if the drugs are taken in a fasting state.[195,196] The bioavailability of 6-MP can be very low and unpredictable, and in some patients, the drug is undetectable in blood.[197] Evans and colleagues have shown that relapsing children have significantly faster clearance rates of MTX and therefore are exposed to substantially lower serum concentrations of the drug.[198] Peeters and associates reported that relapsing patients receive significantly less methotrexate during the first and second years of therapy.[199]

Balis and colleagues could not demonstrate any difference in the pharmacokinetics of MTX and 6-MP between morning and evening dosing in 17 children with ALL.[200] Koren and colleagues have studied the pharmacokinetics of intravenous MTX at 10 A.M. and 9 P.M. in 6 children with ALL.[200a] There was a significant fall in MTX plasma clearance at night ($p < 0.05$). Langevin and coworkers studied the pharmacokinetics of 6-MP in 6 children on this treatment for ALL.[201] After evening dosing, the AUC was significantly larger, and 6-MP had a longer half-life compared with morning dosing. Koren and colleagues compared the disposition pharmacokinetics of 6-MP administered in the morning or in the evening in 13 children with ALL.[202] The elimination half-life was longer, and the AUC, especially the AUC of the postdistributive phase, was significantly larger after evening dosing of the drug. In the same study, 12 children receiving the 6-MP in the morning were switched to an evening dose. Within 2 weeks there was a sharp fall in peripheral leukocyte counts in all patients. The leukocyte count during maintenance therapy was found to be significantly related to risk of relapse, giving patients with higher cell counts the poorer outcome.[203] The antileukemic effect of 6-MP is related to the incorporation of 6-MP derived neucleotides (6-TGN) into DNA. The erythrocyte concentration of 6-TGN achieved after a standard dose of 6-MP varied widely and was not correlated with the dose of 6-MP but was predictive of outcome in children on maintenance therapy (6-MP given in the morning after overnight fasting) for ALL.[204] Giving a constant dose of MTX and 6-MP, without modification with regard to achieved serum concentrations or induced toxicity, may expose these children to very different amounts of drugs over time and can affect their ultimate prognosis.

The anticancer pharmacodynamics of these antimetabolites, as reflected by the survival of children with ALL, is superior if the drugs are given in the evening. The time of day also affects the pharmacokinetics of each of these agents.

PLANT ALKALOIDS

The time for least toxicity in mice varies considerably for plant alkaloids. Vincristine is least toxic in early activity (13 HALO), and vinblastine is least toxic in midactivity (18 HALO).[112,113] Etoposide is best tolerated in late rest (7–11 HALO).[115] The solvent for VP-16 was more toxic to rodents than the combination of solvent and VP-16, and therefore these data may not truly reflect the circadian pharmacodynamics of VP-16.[114] The toxic response to the VP-16 plus solvent and solvent alone were time dependent, and the lethality patterns were about 180° out of phase with one another.

Focan demonstrated a circadian variation in vindesine serum concentration in 9 patients receiving this drug as a 48-hour continuous constant-rate infusion, with peak at about midday.[15] In a study of 34 patients receiving cisplatin (given at 6 P.M. daily for 3 days) and etoposide (given at 7 A.M. or 7 P.M., daily for 3 days), less hematologic toxicity was found in the group receiving etoposide at 7 A.M.[205] Focan reported a randomized trial using 124 patients with previously untreated advanced lung cancer.[206] Etoposide (100 mg/m^2) was given on days 1, 2, and 3 at 6 A.M. (group A) or at 6 P.M. (group B). Cisplatin (100 mg/m^2) was given on day 4 at 6 P.M. Animal studies have predicted that the 6 A.M. etoposide dose (group A) would be less toxic. Interim analysis of 76 patients and 126 courses confirmed lesser hematologic toxicity in group A, but cisplatin was better tolerated in group B. No differences could be established in the overall dose intensities of drugs or in the frequency of tumor response. The most commonly used plant alkaloids, vincristine and vinblastine, may be less toxic if given during the first half of the daily activity span.

ADRENAL CORTICOSTEROIDS

Adrenal corticosteroids are widely used as antiemetic agents in patients receiving chemotherapy and as an integral part of the chemotherapy protocol in some hematologic malignancies. The activity of several hepatic drug-metabolizing enzymes are influenced by corticosterone in mice.[44] It is not surprising that these agents can modulate the efficacy and toxicity of some chemotherapy agents. English and colleagues documented that the time of maximal toxicity for methotrexate is in the late activity period.[98] This coincides with the time of the lowest level of serum corticosterone. In another study, these researchers gave dexamethasone or corticosterone to the animals for 10 days before a dose of methotrexate.[99] The dexamethasone suppressed the corticosterone level and abolished its normal circadian rhythm, but the corticosterone resulted in high corticosterone plasma levels throughout the day. The dexamethasone-treated animals all died from the methotrexate treatment within 5 days, regardless of the time of administration. Less toxicity was observed in the animals receiving the corticosterone than in those receiving either dexamethasone or placebo steroids before treatment. In the control group, the late activity span was again found to be the time of worst methotrexate toxicity. In vitro work with L1210 murine leukemia cells has indicated that cortisol and methylprednisolone can inhibit uptake of methotrexate by these lymphoblastoid cells.[207] Prednisolone has improved the therapeutic index of several alkylating agents in nonsteroid-responsive cancer cell lines, but exogenous corticosteroids decreased the antitumor effect of cyclophosphamide in Erlich ascites carcinoma-bearing female mice.[129,208] Giving ACTH 24 hours before doxorubicin raised GSH levels to their circadian maxima in a variety of murine tissues and protected against toxicity from intravenous doxorubicin in mice.[102] Children with ALL had better survival rates when maintenance chemotherapy consisting of daily 6 mercaptopurine and weekly methotrexate was given in the evening rather than in the morning.[192] This time coincides with the lowest level of plasma cortisol.

ACTH, corticosteroids, and melatonin are agents that demonstrate the potential for manipulating some circadian toxicity patterns.[190] Giving oral melatonin daily for 6 weeks before methotrexate treatment increased the toxicity at all time points in rats, but especially at time points for which melatonin was artificially high.[190] Extending the period during which melatonin is high is theoretically equal to extending the dark phase in photoperiodic species.[209] This chronobiotic approach to making each time of day predictably the optimal time requires much more preclinical and clinical work to make it practical. There is every reason to believe, for example, that the optimal chronobiotic for one cytotoxic agent may differ from that for another. The effective use of a chronobiotic depends intimately on when it is given—when in circadian terms and when relative to the drugs whose toxic to therapeutic ratios are to be modulated.

BIOLOGIC RESPONSE MODIFIERS AND GROWTH FACTORS

Biologic response modifiers are a new important class of weapon in the armamentarium against cancer. We are at a very early stage in our understanding of these agents and their potential therapeutic applications. Early data indicate that these agents may be even more circadian stage dependent with regard to toxicity and therapeutic efficacy than the traditional chemotherapeutics. This is logical because the xenobiotics, reactive chemicals, and antimetabolites that have served as the mainstay for systemic cancer therapy usually have multiple metabolites and many subcellular targets, unlike the receptor-mediated and highly specific activity of peptides.

In humans, erythropoietin, which stimulates bone marrow erythroid precursors to produce new erythrocytes, peaks at around 8 P.M., and reticulocyte numbers peak some 5 hours later.[210,211] Wood gave recombinant human erythropoietin (rhEPO) to female CD_2F_1 mice at one of six circadian stages. The reticulocyte response to rhEPO varied almost sevenfold as a function of its circadian timing, with the greatest response occurring when rhEPO was given before usual awakening compared with later in the day.[212] Vysula and colleagues have looked at the time-dependent activity of G-CSF in rodents.[216a] In two separate studies, 89 female C3HeB/FeJ mice were given either G-CSF or sterile normal saline. In the first study, G-CSF was given in a dose of 5 μg/kg for 5 consecutive days at one of six equispaced times of day. Leukocytes were measured at baseline and daily for 13 days after G-CSF administration. In the second study, mammary adenocarcinoma was inoculated and a single 25 μg/kg dose of G-CSF was given 7 days later when tumor was palpable. Tumor volume was measured daily for 9 days after the G-CSF administration. The rise in leukocytes after G-CSF was found to be circadian-stage dependent, with the maximum rise in total leukocyte count after dosing in the mid-activity phase. Unexpectedly, G-CSF was found to have antitumor activity, with the maximum tumor reduction at the time of best leukocyte count response.

Interleukin-2 (IL-2) has profound circadian-dependent effects on DNA synthesis in many organs of CD2F1 mice.[213,214] Feuers studied the circadian-dependent effect of IL-2 on enzymes of lipid, amino acid, and carbohydrate metabolism in male CD2F1 mice.[215] IL-2 had no significant effect if given during the light span. When treatment was given in the dark span, IL-2 produced statistically significant increases in enzymes of glycolysis and lipid synthesis, but amino acid metabolism was decreased. Von Roemeling gave recombinant IL-2 to mice at one of six circadian stages.[216] Significant circadian rhythmicity (>50% of daily mean) affected spleen weight of control mice, as well as the proportion of suppressor T cells in spleen and bone marrow, and Lyt-5.2$^+$ cells in bone marrow. IL-2 increased the number of spleen cells by 16% overall, but up to threefold more when it was given during the activity span of the animals ($p < 0.02$). Toxicity as gauged by wet-dry lung weight was minimal but clearly circadian stage dependent. Daily administration of IL-2 to mice bearing Meth A sarcoma had opposite effects on the balance between host and cancer, depending on the time of administration. IL-2 given just before usual daily awakening halved tumor growth compared with diluent-treated mice. IL-2 given in the middle of daily activity more than doubled tumor growth rate compared with concurrent diluent treatment or to IL-2 treatment just before awakening.[70]

The toxicity of tumor necrosis factor (TNF) in mice is highly circadian stage dependent, with 90% mortality in late rest (10 HALO) and only 10% mortality in midactivity (18 HALO) after a 750 to 1000 μg/kg dose was given intravenously.[217]

Clinical experience with toxicity and some physiologic observations indicate that the best time to give interferon may be in the evening.[218–220] Under physiologic conditions, interferon plasma levels are negligible in the morning, but they tend to increase in the late afternoon.[221] There is a circadian variation of several lymphocyte subsets, including monocytes, with the lowest level in the morning and highest levels at night.[211] These are one type of the effector cells for interferon. Interferon causes a marked but transient rise in the plasma 11-hydroxycorticosteroids, with a peak about 8 hours after injection. Evening administration did not interfere with the normal rhythm of corticosteroids, with a peak in the morning.[220] However, a peak in plasma steroids in the evening, induced by morning interferon, may hinder the normal rise in circulating lymphocytes in the evening. Gatti looked at circadian changes in the enhancement of the natural killer (NK) cell activity after exposure to interferon-γ of peripheral blood mononuclear cells obtained from 7 healthy volunteers over 24 hours.[222] Maximal enhancement of NK activity was attained in blood removed in the second part of the night or in the early morning, in phase with the peak of the spontaneous NK activity in these volunteers. A phase I clinical trial of a 21-day circadian infusion of interferon-α has been reported.[223] The investigators gave interferon-α2 as a continuous circadian modulated infusion to 10 patients with metastatic melanoma or renal cell cancer for 21 days with a treatment-free interval of 10 days between courses. The largest proportion of the 24-hour dose was given from 6 P.M. to 10 P.M. The starting dose was 15 MU/m^2/day. Doses were escalated as high as 20 MU/m^2/day. Dose-limiting toxicity was fatigue in 9 of the 10 patients. All patients experienced a grade I flu-like syndrome limited to the first 4 to 5 days of each treatment course. A mild dose-dependent somnolence was noted in 2 patients. Grade III–IV neutropenia was observed in 25% of all courses in 5 patients.

PRACTICAL IMPLICATIONS OF CIRCADIAN EFFECTS

Each cytotoxic or biologic agent that has been tested at different circadian stages in rodents shows a significant circadian stage dependency for toxicity. In most cases of tumor-bearing animals given chemotherapy, the time of least toxicity has coincided with or was close to the time of best antitumor activity. There are compelling experimental data suggesting that the therapeutic index of commonly applied anticancer agents can be improved by the optimal circadian timing of treatment. Clinical trials have confirmed the decreased toxicity and demonstrated that maximal safe dose intensity is dependent on the time of drug therapy. Additional prospective, randomized studies are required to demonstrate if a better response rate or survival can be achieved in patients given chemotherapy based on these principles.

These data have significant implications for new anticancer drug discovery and development. Usually, drugs leave murine toxicology, done at the beginning to middle of the daily rest span in the mice and rats, and are immediately tested in humans at a similar clock hour, in the first half or middle of the patient's daily activity span (*i.e.*, the opposite circadian time). It is not common practice to optimize or fix the circadian stage of drug administration in phase I–II trials. This process of anticancer drug selection introduces a clear selection bias for agents that are safe and active in the rest span and may explain in part why many drugs reaching phase I–II studies are ultimately abandoned because of toxicity or lack of activity at achievable doses. Phase III studies, comparing a "standard treatment" to a new treatment, may be comparing apples and oranges if all agents in all arms are not given at their optimal times. These concepts apply even more urgently to research using the various new biologic response modifiers and growth factors. Early data indicate that these agents are even more profoundly circadian stage dependent with regard to response and toxicity than the classic cytotoxic agents.

Toxicity is an important endpoint in itself in patients receiving chemotherapy. Chemotherapy-induced toxicity affects the quality of life for these patients and increases costs of health care. Even if we observe similar response rates but less toxicity by using chronochemotherapy, something important has been gained. Toxicity becomes an important issue with regard to adjuvant treatment. A large proportion of patients receiving adjuvant treatment are not destined to have recurrence of their cancer, but receive adjuvant chemotherapy as an insurance policy against future relapse. It is important to be able to offer patients in this situation safe and effective chemotherapy.

Evidence from studies with chronochemotherapy in animals and humans confirm that this scheduling method reduces bone marrow toxicity but also reduces other types of toxicity such as gastrointestinal and renal toxicity. This scheduling method therefore offers the possibility of giving more dose-intensive chemotherapy without more toxicity and could work well in conjunction with other strategies for high-dose chemotherapy. Dose intensity is in itself a time-dependent variable, because the pharmacokinetics and pharmacodynamics of the major anticancer agents depend on the time of delivery. This fact complicates even further the practice of dose-intensity calculation.

We are still at an early stage in understanding the mechanisms responsible for the circadian dependency of toxicity and efficacy. Interindividual variation in the best timing for certain drugs is a potential problem. Ideally, the best treatment time should be determined for each person according to measurable internal marker rhythms.[88] More work is needed in this area to optimize the benefits of chronochemotherapy for each patient. Clinical trials have, however, documented that we can gain substantially by delivering many drugs at or near the optimal time of day for that drug.

REFERENCES

1. Reinberg A, Smolensky MH. Circadian changes of drug disposition in man. Clin Pharmacokinet 1982;7:401–420.
2. Hrushesky WJ. Chemotherapy timing: An important variable in toxicity and response. In: Perry MC, Yarbro JM, eds. Toxicity of chemotherapy. Orlando: Grune & Stratton, 1984:449–477.
3. Lévi F, Boughattas NA, Blazsek I. Comparative murine chronotoxicity of anticancer agents and related mechanisms. In: Reinberg A, Smolensky M, Labrecque G, eds. Annual review of chronopharmacology, vol 4. Oxford: Pergamon Press, 1987:283–331.
4. Lévi F, Soussan A, Adam R, Caussanel J, Metzger G, Misset JL. Programmable-in time pumps for chronotherapy of patients with colorectal cancer with 5-day circadian-modulated venous infusion of 5-fluorouracil. Proc Am Soc Clin Oncol [Abstract] 1989;8: A429.
5. Hrushesky WJM, von Roemeling R, Lanning RM, Rabatin JT. Circadian-shaped infusion of floxuridine for progressive metastatic renal cell carcinoma. J Clin Oncol 1990;8:1504–1513.
6. von Roemeling R, Hrushesky WJM. Circadian patterning of continuous floxuridine infusion reduces toxicity and allows higher dose intensity in patients with widespread cancer. J Clin Oncol 1989;7:1710–1719.
7. Wesen C, Hrushesky WJM, Roemeling R, Lanning R, Rabatin J, Grage T. Circadian modification of intra-arterial 5-fluoro-2′-deoxyuridine infusion rate reduces its toxicity and permits higher dose intensity. J Infus Chemother 1992;2(2):69–75.
8. Lévi F, Benavides M, Chevelle C, et al. Chemotherapy of advanced ovarian cancer with 4′-O-tetrahydropyranyl doxorubicin and cisplatin: A randomized phase II trial with an evaluation of circadian timing and dose-intensity. J Clin Oncol 1990;8:705–714.
9. Lévi F, Misset JL, Brienza S, et al. A chronopharmacologic phase-II clinical trial with 5-fluorouracil, folinic acid, and oxaliplatin using an ambulatory multichannel programmable pump. Cancer 1992;69:893–900.
10. Hrushesky WJM. Circadian timing of cancer chemotherapy. Science 1985;228:73–75.
11. Hrushesky JM. Circadian scheduling of chemotherapy increases ovarian patient survival and cancer responses significantly. Proc Annu Meet Am Soc Clin Oncol [Abstract] 1987;6:A473.
12. Hrushesky WJM, Roemeling RV, Wood PA, Langevin TR, Lange P, Farley E. High-dose intensity systemic therapy of metastatic bladder cancer. J Clin Oncol 1987;5: 450–455.
13. Hrushesky WJM, Borch R, Levi F. Circadian time dependence of cisplatin urinary kinetics. Clin Pharmacol Ther 1982;32:330–339.
14. Petit E, Milano G, Levi F, Thyss A, Bailleul F, Schneider M. Circadian rhythm-varying plasma concentration of 5-fluorouracil during a five day continuous infusion at a constant rate in cancer patients. Cancer Res 1988;48:1676–1679.
15. Focan C, Mazy JM, Zhou J, Rahmani R, Cano JP. Circadian variation of vindesine serum concentrations during continuous infusion. In: Reinberg A, Smolensky M, Labreque G, eds. Annual review of chronopharmacology, vol 5. Oxford: ergamon Press, 1988:411–414.
16. Robinson BA, Begg EJ, Colls BM, Jefferey GM, Sharman JR. Circadian pharmacokinetics of methotrexate. Cancer Chemother Pharmacol 1989;24:397–399.
17. Scheving LE. Chronobiology of cell proliferation in mammals: Implications for basic research and cancer chemotherapy. In: Edmunds LN, ed. Cell cycle clocks. New York: Marcel Dekker, 1984:455–499.
18. Nash RE, Echave Llanos JM. Circadian variation in DNA synthesis of fast-growing and slow-growing hepatoma: DNA synthesis rhythm in hepatoma. JNCI 1971;47: 1007–1012.
19. Burns ER, Scheving LE, Tsai TH. Circadian rhythms in DNA synthesis and mitosis in normal mice and in mice bearing the Lewis lung carcinoma. Eur J Cancer 1979;15: 233–242.
20. Aschoff J. Comparative physiologyıurnal rhythms. Ann Rev Physiol 1963;25:581.
21. Bünning E. Die physiologische Uhr. Berlin: Springer Verlag, 1963.
22. De Mairan J. Observation botanique. Hist Acad R Sci Paris 1729;:35–36.
23. Richter CPA. A behavioristic study of the activity of the rat. Comp Physiol Monogr 1922;1.
24. Johnson MS. Activity and distribution of certain wild mice in relation to biotic communities. J Mammal 1926;7:245–277.
25. Reinberg A. Clinical chronopharmacology, an experimental basis for chronotherapy. Drug Res 1978;28:1861.
26. Konopka RJ, Benzer S. Clock mutants of drosophila melanogaster. Proc Nat Acad Sci USA 1971;68:2112–2116.
27. Hall JC, Rosbash M. Mutations and molecules influencing biological rhythms. Ann Rev Neurosci 1988;11:373–393.
28. Dunlap JC. Closely watched clocks: Molecular analysis of circadian rhythms in *Neurospora* and *Drosophila*. Trends Genet 1990;6(5).
29. Ralph MR, Menaker M. A mutation of the circadian system in golden hamsters. Science 1988;241:1225–1227.
30. Meijer JH, Reitveld WJ. Neurophysiology of the suprachiasmatic circadian pacemaker in rodents. Physiol Rev 1989;69:671–707.
31. Sawaki Y, Nihonmatsu I, Kawamura H. Transplantation of the neonatal suprachiasmatic nuclei into rats with complete bilateral suprachiasmatic lesions. Neurosci Res 1984;1: 67–72.
32. Drucker-Colin R, Aguilar-Roblero F, Garcia-Hernandez F, Fernandez-Cancinoa F, Rattoni FB. Fetal suprachiasmatic nucleus transplants: Diurnal rhythm recovery of lesioned rats. Brain Res 1984;311:353–357.
33. DeCoursey PJ, Buggy J. Restoration of locomotor rhythmicity in SCN-lesioned golden hamsters by transplantation of fetal SCN. Neurosci Abstr 1986;12:210.
34. Lehman MN, Silver R, Gladstone WR, Kahn RM, Gibson M, Bittman EL. Circadian rhythmicity restored by neural transplant. Immunocytochemical characterization of the graft and its integration with the host brain. J Neurosci 1987;7:1626–1638.
35. Ralph MR, Foster RG, Davis FC, Menaker M. Transplanted suprachiasmatic nucleus determines circadian period. Science 1990;247:975–978.
36. Moore-Ede MC, Czeisler CA, Richardson GS. Circadian timekeeping in health and disease. Part 1. Basic properties of circadian pacemakers. N Engl J Med 1983;309: 469–476.
37. Moore-Ede MC, Czeisler CA, Richardson GS. Circadian timekeeping in health and disease. Part 2. Clinical implications of circadian rhythmicity. N Engl J Med 1983;309: 530–536.
38. Aschoff J. On the perception of time during prolonged temporal isolation. Hum Neurobiol 1985;4:41–52.
39. Bruguerolle B. Temporal aspects of drug absorption and drug distribution. In: Lemmer B, ed. Chronopharmacology: Cellular and biochemical interactions. New York: Markel Dekker, 1989:3–13.
40. Belanger MP, Labreque G. Temporal aspects of drug metabolism. In: Lemmer B, ed. Chronopharmacology: Cellular and biochemical interactions. New York: Markel Dekker, 1989:15–34.
41. Waterhouse JM, Minors DS. Temporal aspects of renal drug elimination. In: Lemmer B, ed. Chronopharmacology: Cellular and biochemical interactions. New York: Markel Dekker, 1989:35–50.
42. Koopman MG, Krediet RT, Arisz L. Circadian rhythms and the kidney. Neth J Med 1985;28:416–423.
43. North C, Feuers RJ, Scheving LE, Pauli JE, Tsai TH, Casciano DA. Circadian organization of thirteen liver and six brain enzymes of the mouse. Am J Anat 1981;162: 184–199.
44. Radzialowski FM, Bousquet WF. Daily rhythmic variation in hepatic drug metabolism in rat and mouse. J Pharmacol Exp Ther 1968;163:229–238.
45. Hughes A, Jacabon HI, Wagner RK, Jungblut PW. Ovarian independent fluctuations of estradiol receptor levels in mammalian tissues. Mol Cell Endocrinol 1976;5:379–388.
46. Wirz-Justice A. Neurophsychopharmacology and biological rhythms. In: Mendlewics J, ed. Biological rhythms and behavior. Basel: Karger, 1982.
47. Wirz-Justice A, Wehr TA, Goodwin FK, et al. Antidepressant drugs slow circadian rhythm in behaviour and brain neurotransmitter receptors. Psychopharmacol Bull 1980;16:45.
48. Adams J, Carmichael J, Wolf CR. Altered mouse bone marrow glutathione transferase levels in response to cytotoxins. Cancer Res 1985;45:1669–1673.
49. Bellamy WT, Alberts DS, Dorr RT. Daily variation in non-protein sulfhydryl levels of human bone marrow. Eur J Cancer Clin Oncol 1988;24:1759–62.
50. Hrushesky WJM, Dell I, Eaton J, Halberg F. Circadian-stage-dependent effect of doxorubicin upon reduced glutathione in the murine heart. Proc Annu Meet Am Assoc Cancer Res [Abstract] 1982;23:12.
51. Smaaland R, Svardal AM, Lote K, Ueland PM, Laerum OD. Glutathione content in human bone marrow and circadian stage relation to DNA synthesis. JNCI 1991;83: 1092–1098.
52. Scheving LE, Tsai TS, Feuers RJ, Scheving LA. Cellular mechanisms involved in the action of anticancer drugs. In: Lemmer B, ed. Chronopharmacology: Cellular and biochemical interactions. New York and Basel: Markel Dekker, 1989:317–369.
53. Haus E, Halberg F, Kuhl JFW, Lakatua DJ. Chronopharmacology in animals. Chronobiologia 1974;1(suppl 1):122.
54. Harris BE, Song R, Soong SJ, Diasio RB. Relationship between dihydropyrimidine dehydrogenase activity and plasma 5-fluorouracil levels with evidence for circadian variation of enzyme activity and plasma drug levels in cancer patients receiving 5-fluorouracil by protracted continuous infusion. Cancer Res 1990;50:197–201.
55. Scheving LE. Circadian rhythms in cell proliferation: Their importance when investigating the basic mechanism of normal versus abnormal growth. In: von Mayersbach H, Scheving LE, Pauli JE, eds. 11th International Congress of Anatomy, part C: Biological rhythms in structure and function. New York: Alan R Liss, 1981:39–79.
56. Hrushesky WJM, Merdink J, Abdel-Monem M. Circadian rhythmicity characterizes monoacetyl polyamine urinary excretion. Cancer Res 1983;43:3944–3947.
57. Scheving LE, Burns ER, Pauli JE, Tsai TH. Circadian variation and cell division of

the mouse alimentary tract, bone marrow and corneal epithelium. Anat Rec 1978;191: 479–486.
58. Buchi KN, Moore JG, Hrushesky WJM, Sothern RB, Rubin NH. Circadian rhythm of cellular proliferation in the human rectal mucosa. Gastroenterology 1991;101:410–15.
59. Sletvold O, Smaaland R, Laerum OD. Cytometry and time-dependent variations in peripheral blood and bone marrow cells: A literature review and relevance to the chronotherapy of cancer. Chronobiol Int 1991;8:235–250.
60. Stoney PJ, Halberg F, Simpson HW. Circadian variation in colony-forming ability of presumable intact murine bone marrow cells. Chronobiologia 1975;2:319–324.
61. Bartlett P, Haus E, Tuason T, Sacket-Lundeen L, Lakatua D. Circadian rhythm in number of erythroid and granulocytic colony forming units in culture (ECFU-C and GCFU-C) in bone marrow of BDF1 male mice. In: Haus E, Kabat HF, eds. Proceeding of the 15th International Conference on Chronobiology. Basel: S Krager, 1984:160–164.
62. Killman SA, Cronkite EP, Fliedner TM, Bond VP. Mitotic indices of human bone marrow cells. I. Number and cytologic distribution of mitosis. Blood 1962;19:743–750.
63. Mauer AM. Diurnal variation of proliferative activity in the human bone marrow. Blood 1965;26:1–7.
64. Smaaland R, Laerum OD, Lote K, Sletvold O, Sothern RB, Bjerknes R. DNA synthesis in human bone marrow is circadian stage dependent. Blood 1991;77:2603–2611.
65. Morley AA. A neutrophil cycle in healthy individuals. Lancet 1966;ii:1220.
66. Ponassi A, Morran L, Bonanni F, et al. Normal range of blood colony forming cells (CFU-C) in humans. Blut 1979;39:257.
66a. Smaaland R, Abrahamsen JF, Svardal AM, Lote K, Ueland PM. DNA cell cycle distribution and glutathione (GSH) content according to circadian stage in bone marrow of cancer patients. Br J Cancer 1992;66:39–45.
67. Flentje M, Akokan G, Reinecke D, Klein HO. Diurnal variations of tumor growth and its influence on cytostatic treatment. Blut 1981;43:85–88.
68. Waldrop RD, Saydjari R, Rubin NH, Rayford PL, Townsend CM, Thompson JC. Photoperiod influences the growth of colon cancer in mice. Life Sci 1989;45:737–744.
69. Blask DE, Pelletier DB, Hill SM, et al. Pineal melatonin inhibition of tumor promotion in the *N*-nitroso-*N*-methylurea model of mammary carcinogenesis: Potential involvement of antiestrogenic mechanisms in vivo. J Cancer Res Clin Oncol 1991;117:1–7.
70. Hrushesky WJM, Sánchez P, Wood PA, et al. Heterogeneity of interleukin-2 therapeutic activity. Proc Am Assoc Cancer Res [Abstract] 1992;33:A1791.
71. Voutilainen A. Über die 24-stunden-rhythmik der mitozfrequenz in malignen tumoren. Acta Pathol Microb Scan 1953;99(Suppl):1–104.
72. Tähti E. Studies of the effect of x-irradiation on 24 hour variations in the mitotic activity in human malignant tumours. Acta Pathol Microbiol Scand 1956;117:1–61.
73. Garcia-Sainz M, Halberg F. Mitotic rhythms in human cancer reevaluated by electronic computer programs. Evidence for chronopathology. JNCI 1966;37:279–292.
74. Stoll BA, Burch WM. Surface detection of circadian rhythm in ^{32}P content of cancer of the breast. Cancer 1968;21:193–196.
75. Gautherie M, Gros C. Circadian rhythm alteration of skin temperature in breast cancer. Chronobiologia 1974;4:1–17.
76. Klevecz RR, Shymko RM, Blumenfeld D, Braly PS. Circadian gating of S phase human ovarian cancer. Cancer Res 1987;47:6267–6271.
77. Smaaland R, Lote K, Sothern RB, Laerum OD. Circadian and circannual variation in DNA synthesis in non-Hodgkin's lymphoma. Biological rhythms and medications: The Fifth International Conference of Chronopharmacology, Amelia Island, FL [Abstract] 1992;:AIV-12.
78. Caussanel JP, Lévi F, Brienza S, et al. Phase I trial of 5-day continuous venous infusion of oxaliplatin at circadian rhythm-modulated rate compared with constant rate. JNCI 1990;82:1046–1050.
79. Focan C, Barbason H, Betz EH. Influence du rythme nycthéméral des division cellulaires sur l'efficacité de la cyclophosphamide contre des sarcomes induits par le méthylcholanthréne. C R Acad Sci (Paris) 1973;276:136–137.
80. Focan C, Schyns-Mosen J, Barbason H, Betz EH. Kinetically scheduled sequential chemotherapy with cyclophosphamide and vinblastine in methylcholanthrene-induced sarcoma of mice. In: Reinberg A, Smolensky M, Labrecque G, eds. Annual review of chronopharmacology, vol 3. Oxford: Pergamon Press, 1986:191–194.
81. Bjarnason GA, Hrushesky WJM. Circadian cancer chemotherapy: Clinical trials. J Infus Chemother 1992;2(2):79–88.
82. Focan C. Sequential chemotherapy and circadian rhythm in human solid tumors. Cancer Chemother Pharmacol 1979;3:197–202.
83. Sothern RB, Halberg F, Hrushesky WJM. Circadian stage not time of day characterizes doxorubicin susceptibility rhythm of mice in continuous light. In: Reinberg A, Smolensky M, Labrecque G, eds. Annual review of chronopharmacology, vol 5. Oxford: Pergamon Press, 1988:385–388.
84. Scheving LE. Chronobiology, a new perspective for chronobiology in medicine. In: Saletu E, ed. Proceedings of the 11th International Neuro-psycho-pharmacologium Congress. Oxford: Pergamon Press, 1978:629–646.
85. Benton LA, Berry SJ, Yates FE. Ultradian rhythmic models of blood pressure variation in normal human daily life. Chronobiologia 1990;17:95–116.
86. Halberg F, Johnson EA, Nelson W, Runge W, Sothern E. Autorhythmometry procedures for physiological self measurement and their analysis. Physiol Tech 1972;1:1–11.
87. Haus E, Nicolau GY, Lakatua D, Sackett-Lundeen L. Reference values for Chronopharmacology. In: Reinberg A, Smolensky M, Labrecque G, eds. Annual review of chronopharmacology, vol 4. Oxford: Pergamon Press, 1987:333–424.
88. Hrushesky WJM, Haus E, Lakatua DJ, Halberg F, Langevin T, Kennedy BJ. Marker rhythms for cancer chrono-chemotherapy. In: Haus E, Kabat HF, eds. Chronobiology 1982–1983. New York: Krager, 1985:493–499.
89. Mormont C, Boughattas N, Lévi F. Mechanisms of circadian rhythms in the toxicity and efficacy of anticancer drugs: Relevance for the development of new analogs. In: Lemmer B, ed. Chronopharmacology: Cellular and biochemical interactions. New York and Basel: Markel Dekker, 1989:395–437.
90. Roemeling Rv, Hrushesky WJM. Circadian pattern of continuous FUDR infusion reduces toxicity. In: Pauli JE, Scheving LE, eds. Advances in chronobiology, Part B. New York: Alan R Liss, 1987:357–373.
91. von Roemeling R, Hrushesky WJM. Determination of the therapeutic index of floxuridine by its circadian infusion pattern. JNCI 1990;82:386–393.
92. Gonzalez RB, Sothern RB, Thatcher G, Nguyen N, Hrushesky WJM. Substantial difference in timing of murine circadian susceptibility to 5-fluorouracil and FUDR. Proc Annu Meet Am Assoc Cancer Res [Abstract] 1989;30:A2452.
93. Gardner MLG, Plumb JA. Diurnal variation in the intestinal toxicity of 5-fluorouracil in the rat. Clin Sci 1981;61:717–722.
94. Peters GJ, Van Dijk J, Nadal JC, Van Groeningen CJ, Lankelman J, Pinedo HM. Diurnal variation in the therapeutic efficacy of 5-fluorouracil against murine colon cancer. In Vivo 1987;1:113–118.
95. Minshull M, Gardner MLG. The effect of time of administration of 5-fluorouracil on leukopenia in the rat. Eur J Cancer Clin Oncol 1984;20:857–858.
96. Popovic P, Popovic V, Baughman J. Circadian rhythm and 5-fluorouracil toxicity in C_3H mice. Biomed Thermol 1982;25:185–187.
97. Burns RE, Beland SS. Effect of biological time on the determination of the LD_{50} of 5-fluorouracil in mice. Pharmacology 1984;28:296–300.
98. English J, Aherne GW, Marks V. The effect of timing of a single injection on the toxicity of methotrexate in the rat. Cancer Chemother Pharmacol 1982;9:114–117.
99. English J, Aherne GW, Marks V. The effect of abolition of the endogenous corticosteroid rhythm on the circadian variation in methotrexate toxicity in the rat. Cancer Chemother Pharmacol 1987;19:287–290.
100. Labat C, Mansour K, Malmary MF, Terrissol M, Oustrin J. Chronotoxicity of methotrexate in mice after intraperitoneal administration. Chronobiologia 1987;14:267–75.
101. Scheving LE, Haus E, Kuhl JFW, Pauly JE, Halberg F, Cardoso SS. Different laboratories closely reproduce characteristics of circadian rhythm in tolerance of mice for arabinofuranosylcytosine. Cancer Res. 1976;36:113–1137.
102. Lévi F, Halberg F, Haus E, et al. Synthetic adrenocorticotropin for optimizing murine circadian chronotolerance for Adriamycin. Chronobiologia 1980;7:227–244.
103. Sothern RB, Nelson WL, Halberg F. A circadian rhythm in susceptibility of mice to the anti-tumor drug Adriamycin. In: Proceedings of the 12th International Conference of the International Society for Chronobiology. Milano: Il Ponte, 1977:433–438.
104. Sothern RB, Halberg F, Good R, Simpson H, Grage T. Differing characteristics of circadian rhythms in murine tolerance to chemically related antibiotics: Adriamycin and daunomycin. In: Walker CA, Soliman K, Winget C, eds. Chronopharmacology. Gainesville, FL: University Presses of Florida, 1981.
105. Mormont MC, Roemeling RV, Sothern RB, et al. Circadian and seasonal dependence in the toxicological response of mice to epirubicin. Invest New Drugs 1988;6:273–284.
106. Lévi F, Mechkouri M, Roulon A, et al. Circadian rhythm in tolerance of mice for the new anthracycline analog 4′-tetrahydropyranyl Adriamycin (THP). Eur J Cancer Clin Oncol 1985;121:1245–1251.
107. Metzger G, Bizi E, Mechkouri M, Halleck M, Lévi F. A pharmacokinetic mechanism for the circadian rhythm in mitoxantrone toxicity in mice. Proc Am Ass Cancer Res [Abstract] 1990;31:A2375.
108. Hrushesky WJM, Lévi F, Halberg F, Kennedy BJ. Circadian stage dependence of cisdiamminedichloroplatinum lethal toxicity in rats. Cancer Res 1982;42:945–949.
109. Lévi F, Hrushesky WJM, Halberg F, Langevin TR, Haus E, Kennedy BJ. Lethal nephrotoxicity and hematologic toxicity of *cis*-diamminedichloroplatinum ameliorated by optimal circadian timing and hydration. Eur J Cancer Clin Oncol 1982;18:471–477.
110. Boughattas N, Lévi F, Fournier C, et al. Circadian rhythm in toxicities and tissue uptake of 1,2-diamminocyclohexane (*trans*-1)oxalatoplatinum(II) in mice. Cancer Res 1989;49:3362–3368.
111. Boughattas N, Lévi F, Hecquet B, et al. Circadian time dependence of murine tolerance for carboplatin. Toxicol Appl Pharmacol 1988;96:233–247.
112. Mormont MC, Berestka J, Mushiya T, et al. Circadian dependence of vinblastine toxicity. In: Reinberg A, Smolensky M, Labrecque G, eds. Annual review of chronopharmacology, vol 3. Oxford: Pergamon Press, 1986:187–190.
113. Halberg F, Gupta B, Haus E, et al. Steps toward a chronopolychemotherapy. Proceedings of the 14th International Congress of Therapeutics. Paris: L'Expansion Scientifique Francaise, 1977:151–196.
114. Tsai TH, Scheving LE. Murine circadian variation in susceptibility to epipodophillotoxin (VP16) as well as to the solvent alone in which it was suspended. In: Reinberg A, Smolensky M, Labrecque G, eds. Annual review of chronopharmacology, vol 3. Oxford: Pergamon Press, 1984:389–392.
115. Lévi F, Mechkouri M, Roulon A, et al. Circadian rhythm in tolerance of mice for etoposide. Cancer Treat Rep 1985;69:1443–1445.
116. Hacker MP, Ershler WB, Newman RA, Fagan MA. Chronobiologic fluctuation of cyclophosphamide induced urinary bladder damage. Chronobiologia 1983;10:301–306.
117. Haus E, Fernandes G, Kuhl JFW, Yunis EJ, Lee JP, Halberg F. Murine circadian susceptibility rhythm to cyclophosphamide. Chronobiologia 1974;1:270–277.
118. Cardoso SS, Avery T, Venditti JM, Goldin A. Circadian dependence of host and tumor response to cyclophosphamide in mice. Eur J Cancer 1978;14:949–954.

119. Snyder NK, Smolensky M, Hsi BP. Circadian variation in the susceptibility of male Balb/c mice to iphosphamide. Chronobiologia 1981;8:33–44.
120. Lévi F, Horvath C, Mechkouri M, et al. Circadian-time dependence of murine tolerance for the alkylating agent peptichemio. Eur J Cancer Clin Oncol 1987;23:487–497.
121. Klein F, Danober L, Roulon A, Lemaigre G, Mechouri M, Lévi F. Circadian rhythm in murine tolerance for the anticancer agent mitomycin C. In: Reinberg A, Smolensky M, Labrecque G, eds. Annual review of chronopharmacology, vol 5. Oxford: Pergamon Press, 1988:367–370.
122. Sothern RB, Haus R, Langevin TR, et al. Profound circadian stage dependence of mitomycin-C toxicity. In: Reinberg A, Smolensky M, Labrecque G, eds. Annual review of chronopharmacology, vol 5. Oxford: Pergamon Press, 1988:389–392.
123. Simpson HW, Stoney PJ. Circadian variation of melphalan (L-phenylalanine nitrogen mustard) toxicity to murine bone marrow: Relevance to cancer treatment protocols. Br J Haematol 1977;35:459–464.
124. Scheving LE, Burns R, Pauly JE, Halberg F, Haus E. Survival and cure of leukemic mice after circadian optimization of treatment with cyclophosphamide and 1-β-D-arabinofuranosylcytosine. Cancer Res 1977;37:3648–3655.
125. Scheving LE, Burns ER, Pauly JE, Halberg F. Circadian bioperiodic response of mice bearing advanced L1210 leukemia to combination therapy with Adriamycin and cyclophosphamide. Cancer Res 1980;40:1511–1515.
126. Haus E, Halberg F, Scheving L, et al. Increased tolerance of mice to arabinosylcytosine given on schedule adjusted to circadian system. Science 1972;177:80–82.
127. Halberg F, Nelson W, Lévi F, Culley D, Bogden A, Taylor DJ. Chronotherapy of mammary cancer in rats. Int J Chronobiol 1980;7:85–99.
128. Sothern RB, Levi F, Haus E, Halberg F, Hrushesky WJ. Control of a murine plasmacytoma with doxorubicin-cisplatin: Dependence on circadian stage of treatment. JNCI 1989;81:135–145.
129. Kodama M, Kodama T. Influence of corticosteroid hormones on the therapeutic efficacy of cyclophosphamide. Gann 1982;73:661–666.
130. Roemeling R, Mormont MC, Walker K, Olshefski R. Cancer control depends upon the circadian shape of continuous FUDR infusion. Proc Annu Meet Am Assoc Cancer Res [Abstract] 1987;28:A1293.
131. Valvassori L, Bellegotti L, Marchiano A, et al. Continuous circadian-shaped infusion FUDR effectively reduces toxicity. Proc Am Soc Clin Oncol [Abstract] 1989;8:A427.
132. Huben RP, Dragone N, Perrapato SD. Continuous infusion FUDR chemotherapy in the treatment of metastatic renal cell carcinoma. Am Urol Assoc [Abstract] 1990;: A413.
133. Damascelli B, Marchiano A, Spreafico C, et al. Circadian continuous chemotherapy of renal cell carcinoma with an implantable, programmable infusion pump. Cancer 1990;66:237–241.
133a. Focan C, Lévi F, Couturier SL, et al. Chronotherapy of hepatic metastases from colorectal cancer by local and general infusion. Proc Annu Meet Am Soc Clin Oncol [Abstract] 1992;11:A542.
134. Drexus FH, Logothetis CJ, Sella A, et al. Circadian infusion of floxuridine in patients with metastatic renal cell carcinoma. J Urol 1991;146:709–713.
135. Arbuck SG. Overview of clinical trials using 5-fluorouracil and leucovorin for the treatment of colorectal cancer. Cancer 1989;63(suppl 6):1036–1044.
135a. Lévi F, Brienza JL, Misset R, et al. Circumvention of clinical resistance of metastatic colorectal cancer to 5-fluourouracil (5-FU) with circadian rhythm modulated chemotherapy. Proc Am Soc Clin Oncol [Abstract] 1992;11:A500.
136. Anderson N, Lokich J, Bern M, Wallach S, Moore C, Williams D. A phase I clinical trial of combined fluoropyrimidines with leucovorin in a 14-day infusion. Demonstration of biochemical modulation. Cancer 1989;63:233–237.
137. Bjarnason GA, Kerr I, Doyle N, MacDonald M, Sone M. Phase I study of 5-fluorouracil (5-FU) and leucovorin (LV) by 14 day continuous infusion chronotherapy in patients with metastatic adenocarcinoma. Eur J Cancer [Abstract] 1991;2:A528.
138. Markiewicz M, Martynowicz M, Sanchez S, Wood P, Hrushesky WJM. Reversal of circadian 5-fluorouracil lethality pattern by leucovorin in mouse. 20th international conference on chronobiology. Israel [Abstract] 1991;.
139. Erlichman C, Fine S, Elhakim T. Plasma pharmacokinetics of 5-FU given by continuous infusion with allopurinol. Cancer Treat Rep 1986;70:903–904.
140. Poplin E, Chabot G, Rutkowski K, Baker L. Continuous infusion (CI), low-dose 5-fluorouracil (FUra): Plasma concentrations. Proc Am Assoc Cancer Res [Abstract] 1988;29:A753.
141. Gudauskas G, Goldie JH. The pharmacokinetics of high-dose continuous 5-fluorouracil infusion. Proc Am Assoc Cancer Res and Am Soc Clin Oncol [Abstract] 1978;18:C-230.
142. Bastian G, Demarcq C, Leteutre F, et al. Pharmacokinetics of 5 fluorouracil: Effect of association with cisplatinum during long term infusion. Proc Am Soc Clin Oncol [Abstract] 1986;5:A213.
143. Mayers CE. The pharmacology of fluoropyrimidines. Pharmacol Rev 1981;33:1–15.
144. Harris BE, Song R, HE Y, Diasio RB. Circadian rhythm of rat liver dihydropyrimidine dehydrogenase. Biochem Pharmacol 1988;37:4759–4762.
145. Harris BE, Song R, Soong S, Diasio RB. Circadian variation of 5-fluorouracil catabolism in isolated perfused rat liver. Cancer Res 1989;49:6610–6614.
146. Tuchman M, Roemeling R, Lanning R. Source of variability of dehydropyrimidine dehydrogenase (DPD) activity in human blood mononuclear cells. In: Reinberg A, Smolensky M, Labrecque G, eds. Annual review of chronopharmacology, vol 5. Oxford: Pergamon, 1988:399–402.
146a. Zhang R, Liu T, Soong SJ, Diasio RB. Circadian rhythm of rat spleen cytoplasmic thymidine kinase: Possible relevance to 5-fluorodeoxyuridine chemotherapy. Biological rhythms and medications: The Fifth International Conference of Chronopharmacology, Amelia Island, FL [Abstract] 1992;:AIV-12.
147. el Kouni MH, Naguib FMN, Cha S. Circadian rhythm of dihydrouracil dehydrogenase (DHUDase), uridine phosphorylase (UrdPase), and thymidine phosphorylase (dThdase) in mouse liver. FASEB J 1989;3:A397.
148. Daher G, Zhang R, Soong SJ, Diasio RB. Circadian variation of fluoropyrimidine catabolic enzymes in rat liver: Possible relevance to 5-fluorodeoxyuridine chemotherapy. Drug Metab Dispos 1991;19:285–287.
149. Kuhl JFW, Grage F, Halberg F, Rosene G, Scheving LE, Haus E. Ellen-effect: Tolerance of Adriamycin by mice and rats depend on circadian timing of injection. Int J Chronobiol 1973;1:335–336.
150. Good RA, Sothern RB, Stoney PJ, Simpson E, Halberg E, Halberg F. Circadian stage dependence of Adriamycin-induced tumor regression and recurrence rates in immunocytoma bearing LOU rats. Chronobiologia 1974;4:177–183.
151. Hrushesky WJM, von Roemeling R, Sothern B. Circadian chronotherapy: From animal experiments to human cancer chemotherapy. In: Lemmer B, ed. Chronopharmacology: Cellular and biochemical interactions. New York: Marcel Dekker, 1989:439–473.
152. Barrett R, Blessing J, Webster K, Twiggs L. Circadian-timed combination doxorubicin-cisplatin chemotherapy for advanced endometrial carcinoma. Gynecol Oncol 1990;36: 285–297.
153. Bailleul F, Lévi F, Metzger G, Regensberg C, Reinberg A, Mathé G. Chronotherapy of advanced breast cancer with continuous doxorubicin infusion via an inplantable programmable device. Proc Annu Meet Am Assoc Cancer Res [Abstract] 1987;28: A771.
154. Lévi F, Bailleul F, Misset JL, et al. Clinical chronopharmacologic optimization of hematologic tolerance for the anticancer agent 4'-O-tetrahydropyranyl Adriamycin. Preliminary results. In: Reinberg A, Smolensky M, Labrecque G, eds. Annual review of chronopharmacology, vol 3. Oxford: Pergamon Press, 1986:199–202.
155. Sqalli A. Chronopharmacociétique clinique et expérimentale de la doxorubicine. Thésis Doctorat Es-Sciences. Toulouse, France: Université Paul Sabatier, 1988.
156. Sqalli A, Oustrin J, Houin G, Bugat R, Carton M. Clinical chronopharmacokinetics of doxorubicin. In: Reinberg A, Smolensky M, Labreque G, eds. Annual review of chronopharmacology, vol 5. Oxford: Pergamon Press, 1988:393–396.
157. Bachur NR, Gordon SL, Gee MW. A general mechanism for microsomal activation of quinone anticancer agents to free radicals. Cancer Res 1978;38:1745–1750.
158. Boor PJ. Cardiac glutathione: Diurnal rhythm and variation in drug-induced cardiomyopathy. Res Commun Chem Pathol Pharmacol 1979;24:27–36.
159. Jakoby WB, Habig WH. Glutathione transferases. In: Enzymatic basis of detoxification, vol 2. New York: Academic Press, 1980.
160. Farooqui MYH, Ahmed AE. Circadian periodicity in tissue glutathione and its relationship with lipid peroxidation in rats. Life Sci 1984;34:2413–2418.
161. Halberg E, Halberg F, Venner KJ, et al. Twenty-four hour synchronized chronotolerance of cisdiamminedichloroplatinum (II) by rats on 8-h and 12-h photofraction gauged by acrophase and paraphase of rectal temperature. In: Reinberg A, Halberg F, eds. Chronopharmacology. New York: Pergamon Press, 1979:377.
162. Lévi FA, Hrushesky WJM, Blomquist CH, et al. Reduction of cis-diamminedichloroplatinum nephrotoxicity in rats by optimal circadian drug timing. Cancer Res 1982;42: 950–955.
163. Boughattas AN, Levi F, Roulon A, et al. Similar circadian rhythm in murine host tolerance for two platinum analogs: Carboplatin (cbdca) and oxaliplatin (i-ohp). Proc Annu Meet Am Assoc Cancer Res [Abstract] 1987;28:451.
164. von Roemeling R, Portuese E, Salzer M, et al. Improved therapeutic index of cisplatin analogue: B-85-0040 by circadian timing. Prog Clin Biol Res 1990;341B:11–20.
165. Cal JC, Dorian C, Cambar J. Circadian and circannual changes in nephrotoxic effects of heavy metals and antibiotics. In: Reinberg A, Smolensky M, Labrecque G, eds. Annual review of chronopharmacology, vol 3. Oxford: Pergamon Press, 1986:143–176.
166. Wesson LG. Diurnal circadian rhythms of renal function and electrolytes excretion in heart failure. Int J Chronobiol 1979;6:109–117.
167. Guarino AM, Moller DS, Arnold ST, et al. Platinate toxicity: Past, present, and prospects. Cancer Treat Rep 1979;63:1475–1483.
168. Kanabrocki EL, Scheving LE, Halberg F, Brewer RL, Bird TJ. Circadian variations in presumably healthy men under conditions of peace time army reserve unit training. Space Life Sci 1973;4:258–270.
169. Hecquet B, Maynadier J, Bonneterre J, Adenis L, Demaille A. Time dependency in plasmatic protein binding of cisplatin. Cancer Treat Rep 1985;69:79–83.
170. Ozols RF, Corden BF, Jacob J. High-dose cisplatin in hypertonic saline. Ann Intern Med 1984;100:19–24.
171. Roemeling RV, Olshefski R, Langevin T, et al. Cisplatin Chronotherapy and disulfiram rescue reduce toxicity without interfering with anticancer activity: Animal findings and preliminary clinical experiences. Chronobiol Intern 1986;3:55–64.
172. Ivanova LN. Diurnal rhythm of the mitotic activity of the various regions of the mouse nephron. Bull Exp Biol Med 1967;64:88–89.
173. Farutina LM, Bogatova RI. Circadian rhythm of mitotic division of kidney cells in rats of different sexes. Bull Exp Biol Med 1969;67:78–80.
174. Lindahl PE, Surowiak J. The circadian fluctuation of the amount of free phosphate and the activity of acid phosphatase in the kidneys of mice and the effect of UV radiation upon this rhythm. Acta Physiol Scand 1970;80:254–268.
175. Margolis R. The effect of continuous illumination (LL) and continuous darkness (DD) on the daily rhythms of membrane-bound and microsomal enzymes in the adrenal gland and kidney of the rat. Am J Anat 1977;149:469–476.
176. Maruhn D, Stozyk K, Gielow L, Bock KD. Diurnal variations of urinary enzyme excretion. Clin Chim Acta 1977;75:427–433.
177. Robinson D, Price RG, Dance N. Rat urine glycosidases and kidney damage. Biochem J 1967;102:533–538.

178. Nakano S, Gemba M. Potentiation of cisplatin-induced lipid peroxidation in kidney cortical slices by glutathione depletion. Jpn J Pharmacol 1989;50:87–92.

179. Boughattas NA, Lévi F, Fournier C, et al. Stable circadian mechanism of toxicity of two platinum analogs (cisplatin and carboplatin) despite repeated dosage in mice. J Pharmacol Exp Ther 1990;256:672–679.

180. Sothern RB, Rosene G, Nelson W, Jovonovich JA, Wurcher T, Halberg F. Circadian rhythm in tolerance of melphalan by mice. In: Proceedings of the 12th International Conference of the International Society for Chronobiology. Milano: Il Ponte, 1977: 443–450.

181. Anagnou J, Mayer D, von Mayersbach H. Circadian toxicity of cytostatic drugs. Chronobiologia 1979;6:73.

182. Badran AF, Echave-Llanos JM. Persistence of mitotic circadian rhythm of a transplantable mammary carcinoma after 35 generations: Its bearing on the success of treatment with endoxan. JNCI 1965;35:285–290.

183. Cardoso SS, Scheving LE, Halberg F. Mortality of mice as influenced by the hour of the day of drug (ara-C) administration. Pharmacologist 1970;12:302.

184. Scheving LE, Cardoso SS, Pauly JE, Halberg F, Haus E. Variation in susceptibility of mice to the carcinostatic agent arabinosylcytosine. In: Scheving LE, Pauly JE, eds. Chronobiology. Tokyo: Igaku-Shoin, 1974:213–217.

185. Hromas RA, Hutchinson JT, Markel DE, Scholes VE. Flow cytometric analysis of the effect of ara-C on the chronobiology of bone marrow DNA synthesis. Chronobiologia 1981;8:369–373.

186. Burns ER, Scheving LE. Circadian optimization of the treatment of L 1210 leukemia with 1-β-D-arabinofuranasylcytosine, cyclophosphamide, vincristine and methylprednisolone. Chronobiologia 1980;7:41–51.

187. Scheving LE, Burns ER, Halberg F, Pauly JE. Combined chronotherapy of L1210 leukemic mice using 1-β-D-arabinofuranasylcytosine, cyclophosphamide, vincristine, methylprednisolone and cisdiamminedichloroplatinum. Chronobiologia 1980;7:33–40.

188. Rose WC, Trader MW, Laster WR, Schabel FM. Chronochemotherapy of 11210 leukemic mice with cytosine arabinoside or cyclophosphamide. Cancer Treat Rep 1978;62: 1337–1349.

189. Halberg F, Haus E, Scheving LE, Good RA. On methods for testing and achieving cancer chronotherapy. Cancer Treat Rep 1979;63:1428–1430.

190. English J, Aherne GW, Arend J. Effect of corticosteroids and melatonin on the circadian rhythm of methotrexate toxicity in the rat. In: Reinberg A, Smolensky M, Labrecque G, eds. Annual review of chronopharmacology, vol 1. Oxford: Pergamon Press, 1984: 145–148.

191. Malmary-Nebot MF, Labat C, Casanovas AM, Oustrin J. Aspect chronobiologique de l'action du méthotrexate sur la dihydrofolate réductase. Ann Pharm Fr 1985;43:337–343.

192. Rivard GE, Infante-Rivard C, Hoyoux C, Champagne J. Maintenance chemotherapy for childhood acute lymphoblastic leukemia: Better in the evening. Lancet 1985;2: 1264–1266.

193. Henderson ES, Adamson RH, Denham C, Oliverio VT. The metabolic fate of tritiated methotrexate. 1. Absorption, excretion and distribution in mice, rats, dogs and monkeys. Cancer Res 1965;25:1008.

194. Poplack DG, Balis FM, Zimm S. The pharmacology of orally administered chemotherapy. A reappraisal. Cancer 1986;58(suppl 2):473–480.

195. Pinkerton CR, Welshman SG, Glasgow JFT, Bridges JM. Can food influence the absorption of methotrexate in children with acute lymphoblastic leukemia? Lancet 1980;2: 944–945.

196. Riccardo R, Balis FM, Ferrara P, Lasorella A, Poplack DG, Mastrangelo R. Influence of food intake on bioavailability of oral 6-mercaptopurine in children with acute lymphoblastic leukemia. Pediatr Hematol Oncol 1986;3:319–324.

197. Zimm S, Collins J, Roccardi R, et al. Variable bioavailability of oral mercaptopurine: Is maintenance chemotherapy in acute lymphoblastic leukemia being optimally delivered. N Engl J Med 1983;308:1005–1009.

198. Evans WE, Crom WR, Abromowitch M, et al. Clinical pharmacodynamics of high dose methotrexate in acute lymphocytic leukemia: Identification of a relation between concentration and effect. N Engl J Med 1986;314:471–477.

199. Peeters M, Koren G, Jakubovicz D, Zipursky A. Physician compliance and relapse rates of acute lymphoblastic leukemia in children. Clin Pharmacol Ther 1988;43: 228–232.

200. Balis FM, Jeffries SL, Lange B, et al. Chronopharmacokinetics of oral methotrexate and 6-mercaptopurine: Is there diurnal variation in the disposition of antileukemic therapy? Am J Pediatr Hematol Oncol 1989;11:324–326.

200a. Koren G, Ferrazzini G, Sohl H, Robieux I, Johnson D, Giesbrecht E. Chronopharmacology of methotrexate pharmacokinetics in childhood leukemia. Chronobiol Intern 1992;9(6):424–438.

201. Langevin AM, Koren G, Soldin S, Greenberg M. Pharmacokinetic case for giving 6-mercaptopurine maintenance doses at night. Lancet [Letter] 1987;2:505–506.

202. Koren G, Langevin AM, Olivieri N, Giesbrecht E, Zipursky A, Greenberg M. Diurnal variation in the pharmacokinetics and myelotoxicity of mercaptopurine in children with acute lymphocytic leukemia. Am J Dis Child 1990;144:1135–1137.

203. Schmiegelow K, Pulczynska MK, Seip M. White cell count during maintenance chemotherapy for standard-risk childhood acute lymphoblastic leukemia: Relation to relapse rate. Pediatr Hematol Oncol 1988;5:259–267.

204. Lennard L, Lilleyman JS. Variable mercaptopurine metabolism and treatment outcome in childhood lymphoblastic leukemia. J Clin Oncol 1989;7(12):1876–1823.

205. Krakowski I, Levi F, Mechkouri M, et al. Dose intensity of etoposide (VP16)-cisplatin (CDDP) depends upon dosing time. Proc Annu Meet Am Assoc Cancer Res [Abstract] 1988;29:A776.

206. Focan C. Chronotherapy in lung and ovarian cancer. J Cancer Res Clin Oncol [Abstract] 1990;116:*16.20.04*.

207. Zagar RF, Frisby SA, Oliverio VT. Cellular transport and antitumor activity of methotrexate in combination with clinically useful drugs. Proc Am Assoc Cancer Res [Abstract] 1972;13:33.

208. Shepherd R, Harrap KR. Modulation of the toxicity and antitumor activity of alkylating drugs by steroids. Br J Cancer 1982;45:413.

209. Carter DS, Goldman BD. Antigonadal effects of timed melatonin infusion in pinealectomised male Djungarian hamsters (*Phodopus sungorus sungorus*): Duration is the critical parameter. Endocrinology 1983;113:1267–1267.

210. Wide L, Bengtsson C, Birgegard G. Circadian rhythm of erythropoetin in human serum. Br J Haematol 1989;72:85–90.

211. Haus E, Lakatua DJ, Swoyer J, Sackett LL. Chronobiology in hematology and immunology. Am J Anat 1983;168:467–517.

212. Wood PA, Sanchez de la Peña S, Hrushesky WJM. Evidence for circadian dependency of recombinant human erythropoietin (rhEPO) response in the mouse. In: Reinberg A, Smolensky M, Labreque G, eds. Annual review of chronopharmacology. Oxford: Pergamon Press, 1990;7:173–176.

213. Scheving LA, Tsai TH, Feuers RJ, Smolensky MH, Young JD, Scheving LE. Differential effect of interleukin-2 on [^{3}H]TdR incorporation into DNA in the thymus, spleen and bone marrow of CD2F1 male mice. In: Reinberg A, Smolensky M, Labrecque G, ed. Annual review of chronopharmacology, vol 5. Oxford: Pergamon Press, 1988;381–382.

214. Tsai TH, Scheving LA, Feuers RJ, Young JD, Scheving LE. Circadian influence of IL-2 in stimulating DNA synthesis in the lung, liver and pancreas of CD2F1 male mice. In: Reinberg A, Smolensky M, Labreque G, eds. Annual review of chronopharmacology, vol 5. Oxford: Pergamon Press, 1988:397–398.

215. Feuers RJ, Scheving LA, Tsai TH, Young JD, Scheving LE. A preliminary report of circadian effects of interleukin-2 (IL-2) on the activity of enzymes of intermediary metabolism of mice. Prog Clin Biol Res 1990;341B:473–482.

216. von Roemeling R, DeMaria L, Salzer M, et al. Circadian stage dependent response to IL-2 in mouse spleen and bone marrow. In: Reinberg A, Smolensky M, Labreque G, eds. Annual review of chronopharmacology. Oxford: Pergamon Press, 1990:7:211–214.

216a. Vyzula R, Whighton T, Traynor K, et al. Comparative circadian organization of the myelopoetic and unexpected oncomodulary effects of granulocyte colony stimulating factor. Third Meeting of the Society for Research on Biological Rhythms, Amelia Island, FL [Abstract] 1992;:A139.

217. Langevin T, Young J, Walker K, Roemeling R, Nygaard S, Hrushesky WJM. The toxicity of tumor necrosis factor (TNF) is reproducibly different at specific times of the day. Proc Annu Meet Am Assoc Cancer Res [Abstract] 1987;28:A1580.

218. Bocci V. Administration of interferon at night may increase its therapeutic index. Cancer Drug Deliv 1985;2:313–318.

219. Abrams PG, McClamrock E, Foon KA. Evening administration of alpha interferon. N Engl J Med [Letter] 1985;312:443–4445.

220. Morgano A, Puppo F, Criscuolo D, Lotti G, Indiveri F. Evening administration of alpha interferon: Relationship with the circadian rhythm of cortisol. Med Sci Res 1987;15: 615–616.

221. Bocci V. The physiological interferon response. Immunol today 1985;6:7–9.

222. Gatti G, Masera R, Cavallo R, et al. Circadian variation of interferon-induced enhancement of human natural killer (NK) cell activity. Cancer Detect Prevent 1988;12: 431–438.

223. Deprés-Brummer P, Lévi F, DiPalma M, et al. A phase I trial of 21-day continuous venous infusion of α-interferon at circadian rhythm modulated rate in cancer patients. J Immunol 1991;10:440–447.

SECTION 8

HARVEY I. PASS
THOMAS F. DELANEY

Photodynamic Therapy

It is only recently that photodynamic therapy (PDT) has been investigated on a large scale, although the concept of a light-activated sensitizer resulting in specific or nonspecific cell death is not new. PDT was first used in 1900, when acridine and light were combined to kill paramecia, and the first oncologic use of PDT was in 1903, when eosin and light were employed in the treatment of skin cancer.[1,2] In the following years, many chemicals were used to promote photochemically induced cytotoxicity.[3]

Since Hauseman's initial experiments in 1911 with hematoporphyrin (HP), there has been a continued interest in porphyrin-based photosensitizers.[3] During the late 1940s, a key development was made. HP (probably a fairly impure preparation) was found to selectively concentrate or to be preferentially retained in malignant tissues.[4,5] Lipson improved the tumor-localizing properties of HP by synthesizing a complex porphyrin mixture called hematoporphyrin derivative (HPD).[6–9] Gregorie extended Lipson's observations by demonstrating that HPD is retained in a large percentage of squamous and adenocarcinomas.[10] Lipson's work on tumor detection resulted in a single attempt to manage a large, recurrent breast cancer by multiple injections of HPD and light treatments. The tumorous lesion was not cured, but there was objective evidence of photodynamically induced cytotoxic effect.[11] Several years later, Kelly reported results with intravenous HPD followed by light delivered through a fiberoptic device to treat a patient with recurrent bladder cancer. Shortly afterward, Dougherty described his first of a sustained series of studies throughout the 1970s and 1980s exploring the mechanism and applications of HPD-based PDT for the treatment of diverse human malignancies.[12–17] It was through Dougherty's continued efforts that PDT evolved to the level it is practiced today.

MECHANISM OF PHOTODYNAMIC THERAPY

Photodynamic therapy requires three simultaneously present components for cytotoxicity: a sensitizer, light, and oxygen. PDT is an oxygen-dependent photochemical oxidative process that should not be confused with laser techniques, including carbon dioxide or neodymium-yttrium-aluminum-garnet lasers. The laser techniques, used at much longer wavelengths (10,600 and 1064 nm, respectively), are associated with heat production to produce a desiccating-cutting action. Moreover, the wavelength of the sensitizers used dictates the proper light spectrum and the depth of treatment effect with photodynamic therapy. PDT may have more promise as a primary cancer modality than the laser techniques, primarily because PDT offers some tumor selectivity due to selective sensitizer retention compared with sensitizer concentrations in normal tissue. This differential cytotoxicity separates PDT from other chemically based forms of cancer treatment.

COMPONENTS OF PHOTODYNAMIC THERAPY

PHOTOSENSITIZERS

The most widely used sensitizers in clinical studies have been hematoporphyrin derivative (HPD; Photofrin I) or a further purified mixture of HPD known as dihematoporphyrin ether (DHE; Photofrin II). HPD localizes in tumors and has photodynamic properties that, when activated by 630-nm light, lead to cytotoxicity. The absorption at longer wavelengths, although small in comparison with its major absorptive peak, allows greater tissue penetration and obviates the problems associated with light absorbance by naturally present biologic chromophores such as hemoglobin.[18] The relative impurity of HPD has been improved by the availability of Photofrin II (PII) that, although more homogenous, also contains hematoporphyrin, hydroxyethylvinyl deuteroporphyrin, and protoporphyrin.

The distribution of different porphyrins is determined by the individual chemical properties, including lipophilicity or hydrophilicity, polarity, pH, anionic or cationic change, and aggregate size.[19] HPD is predominantly associated with the lipoproteins LDL and VLDL, and the components not associated with tumor localization (*i.e.*, HP, HVD, protoporphyrin) are associated with albumin.[20] LDL is the main early carrier, but it later becomes almost exclusively associated with HDL. PII accumulates in and is retained by vascular endothelium by endocytosis, but its selectivity to tumor as a result of abnormal tumor vascular endothelium remains to be elucidated.[21–23] Intracellular accumulation of the drug is most certainly affected by the concentration of soluble and structural protein such as collagen and may be influenced by diminished local lymphatic drainage in tumors. Although the serum half-life is relatively short in humans (20–30 hours for a 5-mg bolus), the photosensitizing component remains in the skin or at least at low levels (2–5%) in the serum for at least 4 to 6 weeks.[18]

SELECTIVE TUMOR RETENTION

One of the attributes of porphyrin-based photodynamic therapy is the ability of tumor tissue to retain substantial levels of sensitizer for a longer period than normal tissue. Why DHE is retained to a greater extent in tumors than in normal tissues is unknown. In vitro studies to determine if tumor cells are more photosensitive or selectively retain HPD fail to show a difference between normal and cancerous cells. NIH3T3 cells transformed by the *RAS* oncogene have identical PDT survival curves compared with the parent NIH3T3 line, and Perry found no differences in sensitivity to PDT or in vitro survival curves of thoracic oncologic lines compared with a normal lung fibroblast.[24,25] Differences in in vivo retention of sensitizer between tumor and normal tissues have been demonstrated by numerous methods, including using fluorescent and radioactively labeled sensitizer. In examining and kinetics of PII delivery in flank tumors of animals in vivo, sensitizer levels fall significantly in tumor only after 48 hours and are significantly greater than those seen in the muscle and the skin.[24] Route of delivery and the type of tumor play a role in the kinetics of delivery. Maximal tumor to tissue ratios shortly after HPD administration were demonstrated by Tochner after intraperitoneal injection of HPD in an ovarian cancer ascites model.[26] Because the drug was directly injected into the ascites fluid containing the tumor cells, drug availability was greater because there was no dependence on vascular delivery.

The difference between in vivo tumor and normal cell sensitizer uptake and retention probably depends on several environmental factors. Leaky tumor neovascular effects, retention within the tumor vascular endothelial cells with subsequent disruption of tumor oxygen and nutrient delivery, poorly developed tumor lymphatics, lower tumor pH, binding to lipoproteins, and subsequent receptor mediated endocytosis may all contribute to the selective retention. The trapping of porphyrin aggregates by macrophages may be favored in tumor-associated monocytes, which could contribute to a host of immunologic circumstances.

LIGHT

Any source of light having the appropriate spectral characteristics can be used for photodynamic therapy. Lasers, specifically argon pump-dye lasers, are used, exciting Kiton red or rhodamine B to produce up to 5 watts of red light, which corresponds to one of the minor spectral peaks of Photofrin II. The laser can be coupled to one or more fiberoptic cables to propagate the light with minimal energy loss to the tip, cleaved (for forward light projection), bulbous (for isotropic spherical distribution), or coated with cylindrical scattering material to yield light perpendicular to the midpoint of the fiber axis. The amount of energy delivered depends on the dose rate of light from the fiber and the duration of light delivery. The light distribution can be calibrated with a power meter at the tip before treatment, and the rate of light delivery is always gauged to prevent hyperthermic effects.

OXYGEN

PDT cytotoxicity probably occurs through photooxidative reactions. When oxygen is absent from the system or present at levels less than 2%, cells are resistant to photodynamic therapy cytotoxicity.[27,28] The light-excited sensitizer loses or accepts an electron with oxygenation of secondary radicals or transfer of energy to oxygen to yield singlet oxygen with resultant hydroperoxyl products.[29] Such products, although short lived, lead to cell death at various targets.

The most striking and immediate cellular response observed after PDT is damage to membranes, particularly the plasma membrane.[30,31] Shortly after light treatment, cells withstand trypsin removal from plastic surfaces. Such early changes imply that membrane proteins have cross-linked with residual double bonds of the plastic. Within hours of treatment, visible damage is seen by cessation of normal cellular movement and the formation of multiple membrane blebs.[32] The blebs, which are often as large as the cell itself, develop as balloon-like structures protruding from the cell membrane and indicate severe membrane damage.[33,34] After cell blebbing, there is no longer cell division, and cell lysis follows. Other experimental indications of membrane distortion after PDT are constituent leakage from intact cells or isotope from red blood cell ghosts.[35,36] Other cellular membranes may be at risk, including the nucleus, mitochondria, lysosome, Golgi apparatus, and endoplasmic reticulum. Membranes, by virtue of the HPD or DHE water-lipid partition coefficient, are good targets for PDT damage. Mitochondrial damage after PDT has been demonstrated by specific inhibition of oxidative phosphorylation and electron transport enzymes and reduction in cellular ATP levels.[37,38]

Although production of DNA strand breaks has been observed after PDT, such lesions may not be responsible for cellular death.[39,40] Incorporation of bromodeoxyuridine into cellular DNA has been shown to sensitize cells to ionizing radiation and chemotherapy drugs but not to PDT.[41,42] PDT is not mutagenic in in vitro systems.[43,44] These last two facts indicate that DNA is not a primary target for PDT-induced cytotoxicity. The HPD or DHE uptake studies clearly define initial binding within the plasma membrane followed, in time, by migration to internal cellular regions.[45]

MECHANISMS OF PHOTODYNAMIC THERAPY

SENSITIZER DOSE

Cells exposed to increasing amounts of sensitizer exhibit an increase in light-induced cytotoxicity, and drug uptake depends on drug concentration, length of incubation (*i.e.*, the longer the incubation with PII, the greater the PDT cytotoxicity), and protein concentration of the media environment (*i.e.*, the higher the protein concentrations, the less the PDT cytotoxicity).[46] As the volume of cells increase, there is a linear increase in HPD uptake, and larger cells may have greater susceptibility to PDT than smaller cells treated under identical conditions.[47]

DOSE RATE EFFECTS

The degree of PDT cytotoxicity depends on the rate at which the dose of energy is given. The greater the dose rate delivery to the tumor cells at a given energy, the greater the PDT cytotoxicity.[48] The ability of the cells to escape PDT cytotoxicity at low dose rates, but equal energies, may be related to their ability to repair sublethal damage or remove toxic oxidative products. These potential repair capabilities may have significant clinical implications, because light dose delivery to the tumor falls off exponentially as a function of the distance from the light point of entry. With low levels of light at low dose rates, tumor tissue may escape treatment and may locally recur.

INHERENT PHOTODYNAMIC THERAPY SENSITIVITY OF CELL LINES

Despite various histologies of malignancies at a given anatomic site, no real differences in the parameters that influence survival after similar doses of PDT has been elucidated. Corrections of sensitizer uptake with regard to total cellular protein, volume, and cell size make no difference, and the survival characteristics in vitro of adenocarcinoma, squamous cell carcinoma, large cell carcinoma, small cell carcinoma, and mesothelioma are quite similar.[25] The modest difference in cell survival after PDT may be partially explained by the cells inherent ability to form colonies (*i.e.*, its plating efficiency).

IMMUNE MECHANISMS AND PHOTODYNAMIC THERAPY

One of the more interesting aspects of PDT that is being pursued is the relation between immune mechanisms and PDT. An immunosuppressive element of PDT was recognized in the 1980s. Elmets and Bauer reported a 50% suppression of contact hypersensitivity after PDT treatment, and this was a sustained phenomenon for a period of at least 2 weeks.[49] Moreover, the immunosuppressive characteristics could be adoptively transferred. A direct effect on effector cells and evidence that PDT could cause release of vasoactive peptides, priming factors, or substances that influence immune status as a secondary messenger has been demonstrated. Ortner illuminated murine peritoneal mast cells previously incubated with protoporphyrin and documented progressive inhibition of histamine secretion at low fluences, while histamine was released at high dose rates.[50] Henderson and Donovan have reported release of proctoglandins from peritoneal murine macrophages after PII-based PDT.[51] This release was associated with cellular membrane disruption. Lynch was able to demonstrate that the macrophage was the cell that mediates the adoptively transferred suppression of contact hypersensitivity after PDT.[52]

Tumor necrosis factor is released in a dose-dependent fashion from PDT stimulated peritoneal murine macrophages, and it is possible to potentiate this TNF release with pretreatment with interferon.[53] Such an effect could have implications for indirect mechanism of tumor killing by PDT though cytokine stimulation or effect of the cytokine on tumor vascular to cause hemorrhagic necrosis due to endothelial cell destruction.

A great interest in the use of immune mechanisms for increasing specificity of PDT has developed. Levy conjugated hematoporphyrin to monoclonal antibody and selectively eliminated a suppressor subset of T lymphocytes.[54] Elimination resulted in tumor regression by the HP-monoclonal antibody becoming an immunotoxin that selectively destroys the suppressor T cell alone so other cytotoxic T lymphocytes can destroy the cancer. A more direct use of monoclonal antibody-sensitizer conjugates has been reported by Pogrebniak; greater specificity, less normal tissue destruction, and greater long-term cures were described for a in vivo murine model.[55]

Whether these immune mechanisms are truly active in vivo in humans requires further verification. Nevertheless, Shumaker[56] described an increase in T-cell lymphocytes and plasma cells in bladders of patients undergoing bladder PDT, and Nseyo[57] documented cytokine production in the urine of patients receiving bladder PDT. Clinically, psoralen photosensitization has been used as a light-activated therapy with extracoporeal photophoresis to treat cutaneous T-cell lymphoma.[58] Patients who respond have a selective destruction of the malignant T-cell clone.

TISSUE EFFECTS IN VIVO

The response to PDT in vivo is rapid, with no palpable tumor present within 1 to 2 days after treatment. Where there is regrowth of tumor, it usually occurs after 1 to 2 weeks at the edges of the wound.[18] The original injury to the tumor is a marked coagulation necrosis, and regrowth could be due to inherent tumor cell resistance, hypoxia, inadequate drug uptake, or inadequate drug-light dose concentration. Vascular damage is probably one of the primary targets of in vivo PDT, and tumor blood flow studies confirm a marked decrease in blood flow with PDT. Such vascular damage results in tumor hypoxia and cytotoxicity. This PDT induced vascular damage can be amplified with use of hypoxic cell sensitizers just before or within 30 minutes of the PDT treatment. Misonidazole selectivity binds hypoxic cells and once within the tumor helps amplify the PDT effect.[59]

PHOTODYNAMIC THERAPY FOR MALIGNANCIES

CLINICAL STUDIES

Initial efforts with HPD photodynamic therapy were in patients with cutaneous and subcutaneous malignancies. Since that time, several thousand patients have been treated with PDT for a wide variety of malignancies involving various organ systems. For most patients, conventional treatment had failed or it had been refused. The first trials were designed to develop techniques to treat particular anatomic sites and to gather dose, toxicity, and response information. As additional experience with this modality has accumulated, there has been increasing emphasis on the development of controlled clinical studies to help define the role of modality in the current management of patients with cancer.

CUTANEOUS AND SUBCUTANEOUS TUMORS

Malignancies involving the skin that have been treated with PDT include basal and squamous cell carcinomas, malignant melanomas, mycosis fungoides, recurrent metastatic breast carcinoma, and Kaposi's sarcomas (Table 69–30).[60] Patients received sensitizer by intravenous injection and were treated with red light 72 to 96 hours after injection of HPD. Both external surface illumination and interstitial implantation have been used for some larger lesions. Most patients in the early reports had disease that had not been controlled by prior surgery, chemotherapy, and ionizing radiation. Although investigators used different criteria to judge response, it is clear that responses have been obtained even after extensive prior treatment, and differential responses are seen between tumor and adjacent normal tissue within the light field.

Treatment is effective to a depth of 5 to 10 mm, depending on the drug and light doses and the mode of light delivery. The discovery of photobleaching (photodestruction) of porphyrins during illumination has been an important development in the treatment of skin lesions.[61] By reducing the injected dose of photosensitizer, the drug concentration in the normal skin surrounding tumors may be low enough that any residual drug is photobleached and destroyed during light delivery. This permits large increases in light delivery to the tumors (which still contain active photosensitizer) with much less risk of injury of normal skin. For primary lesions involving skin, investigators report high complete response rates that are often durable. Complete responses have been achieved, lasting up to 4 years.[60]

Bandieramonte and coworkers treated 43 basal cell carcinomas and 18 metastatic breast cancer lesions. Using light

TABLE 69–30. Results of Photodynamic Therapy for Cutaneous or Subcutaneous Tumors

Investigations	*Tumor Type*	*Patients/Sites*	*Light Dose (J/cm²)*	*Response Rate (%)*			*Comments*
				CR	*PR*	*NR*	
Kennedy[65]	Basal cell	3/38	90	100	0	0	None recur at 35 mo
Bandieramonte[62]	Basal/breast	7/61	60–100	50	31	19	Follow-up 4–16 mo
Waldow[64]	Basal/SCCa	6/9	8–60	100	0	0	Follow-up 8–24 mo
Pennington[66]	Basal/SCCa	6/53	30	68	NA	NA	Most recur at 6 mo
Wilson[67]	Basal/SCCa	37/151	56–216	88	12	0	61% PR retreated to CR
Santoro[63]	Basal cell	50/292	120–150	93.5	6.5	0	Topical porphyrin
Schuh[73]	Breast	14/NA	26–288	15	69	15	Palliative, longest CR was 6 mo

J, joules; CR, complete response, eradication of tumor; PR, partial response, greater than 50% reduction in tumor size; NR, no response; SCCa, squamous cell carcinoma; NA, not available.

doses of 60 to 120 J/cm², clinically complete responses were seen in 26 (43%) of 61, and 16 (26%) of 61 had partial responses.[62] Side effects included cutaneous photosensitivity and discomfort during and after treatment. Pain appeared to be related to tumor necrosis and was more severe with larger and more deeply infiltrating lesions. This group reported using a topically applied porphyrin, tetraphenylporphinesulfonate, for the treatment of 50 patients with 292 basal cell carcinomas less than 2 mm thick.[63] Complete responses were seen with 273 lesions (93.5%). Recurrences were observed in 29 (10.6%). The advantage of the topically applied photosensitizer is that the patient is spared cutaneous photosensitivity. Because of limited depth of penetration by the topical photosensitizer preparation, this approach is only suitable for patients with superficial lesions (<2 mm thick).

Waldow and associates reported treatment of six basal cell lesions and three cases of Bowen's disease or squamous cell carcinomas.[64] All lesions had clinically complete responses, with follow-up times of 8 to 24 months. Kennedy reported durable, complete responses for 38 primary basal cell carcinomas in 3 patients.[65] Pennington and coworkers, however, reported a less favorable experience for 53 primary basal cell or squamous cell skin tumors.[66] Using HPD 5 mg/kg and 30 J/cm², complete responses were achieved in 52% of the basal cell lesions and 81% of the squamous cell lesions. However, over half of the squamous lesions and most of the basal cell lesions recurred at the time of the 6 month follow-up visit. No attempts were made to determine whether alterations of the drug or light dose would affect the response duration.

The group at Roswell Park reported 133 complete and 18 partial responses in 151 basal cell lesions in 37 patients with acceptable normal tissue response and excellent cosmesis.[67] They delivered light doses of 180 to 133 J/cm² 48 to 72 hours after injection of 1 mg/kg of DHE. With 12 months minimum follow-up, recurrences were seen in 13 of 133 complete responders. Most patients who had recurrences had morpheoform basal cell epitheliomas, which the researchers suggested might be more effectively treated with higher light doses or intralesional fiber optic implantation. Eleven of the 18 partial responders were given a repeat course of photoradiation therapy. All had complete responses and remained free of disease at 1 year after treatment.

Excellent treatment results have been reported for managing multiple basal cell carcinomas in patients with nevoid basal cell carcinoma syndrome, with an 82.5% pathologic complete response rate.[68] A higher complete response rate was seen for power densities above 40 mW/cm² and total light doses greater than 70 J/cm². Multiple lesions of Bowen's disease have been treated with excellent response, although complete eradication of tumors required more than one course of treatment.[69]

Of particular interest is the finding by Kennedy that ALA (5-aminolevulinic acid), a precursor of protoporphryin IX in the biosynthetic pathway for heme, can be applied *topically* to photosensitize skin tumors.[70] Because ALA in aqueous solution passes readily through abnormal keratin but not through normal keratin, topical application induces photosensitization that is restricted primarily to abnormal epithelium. This permits photodynamic therapy to these lesions without causing systemic photosensitivity. The response rate for basal cell carcinomas after a single treatment has been 90% complete response and 7.5% partial response for the first 80 lesions treated.

Dose-seeking studies to determine the optimal treatment schedule for skin lesions are in progress. Gilson and colleagues found more complete responses with 1.5 or 2.0 mg/kg of DHE than with 1.0 mg/kg, although this was accompanied by higher frequency of skin necrosis (which healed in all cases). The relation between the drug and light dose necessary to control tumor is complex and nonlinear.[71] Lower drug doses (*e.g.*, 1.0 mg/kg of DHE) offer the advantage of greater normal tissue sparing and superior depth of treatment effect because of photobleaching of photosensitizer. However, drug dose reductions are accompanied by dramatic increases in the light dose necessary to control tumor, which may be a practical problem for large lesions.

Pigmented melanomas are almost completely unresponsive to PDT because of extremely efficient light absorption by melanin. Nonpigmented lesions, however, can be effectively controlled by PDT. Control of Kaposi's sarcomas as large as 3 cm in diameter has been reported.[60]

Photoradiation has been evaluated for treatment of recurrent breast cancer on the chest wall. Such patients have disease that is difficult to control on the chest wall despite multiple local therapies. Chest wall recurrence of breast cancer is frequently associated with the development of distant metastases. Although focal tumor nodules on the chest wall can be controlled with PDT, new lesions often appear outside of the treatment field. Attempts at treatment of the entire ipsilateral chest wall in patients with diffuse or multifocal involvement have only produced transient responses.[72–74]

HEAD AND NECK TUMORS

Photodynamic therapy should prove to be a useful addition to head and neck oncology because of the accessibility of this area to endoscopy and laser light and because these patients tend to develop multiple primary malignancies. Photodynamic therapy can be repeated when necessary and can be used in sites that have been previously irradiated. Treatment appears to be more effective in early-stage lesions, but relative indications for its use with respect to radiation or surgery need to be defined. Although PDT was initially attempted for patients with lesions that had not been controlled with surgery or irradiation, it appears to be most effective in patients with *early* tumors of the head and neck.[75,76] These patients often have curative surgical or irradiation options; PDT must establish itself as highly reliable and effective before it can be deemed "standard treatment" for such patients. It may have an important role in patients with field cancerization with large areas of superficial premalignant and malignant change for which PDT may be able to produce complete responses with normal tissue preservation.[76]

Wile and coworkers reported on 21 patients with head and neck tumors recurrent in the primary site who were treated with HPD and red light (Table 69–31).[77] Most had squamous cell carcinomas refractory to conventional therapy. Complete responses were seen in 6 patients (29%), and partial responses were seen in 11 patients (52%). The complete responses were durable in 4 of the 6 patients at follow-up times from 8 to 18 months. These occurred in patients with tongue, soft palate, and nasopharyngeal lesions. In 10 patients with regional head and neck cancer recurrences in soft tissues, results were less favorable: 2 complete responses and 3 partial responses. In these patients, tumor rapidly recurred at the margins of the treated field, and the overall disease process did not appear substantially altered by treatment.

Schuller and colleagues documented short response durations in patients with recurrent or metastatic tumors in the head and neck region.[78] Takata found significant necrosis of tumors of the larynx, oropharynx, and tongue by PDT, but pathologic examination of biopsy and surgical specimens revealed nests of viable tumor below the mucosa, suggesting inadequate light delivery and dose inhomogeneity.[79] Grossweiner described 10 patients with early-stage squamous cell carcinoma of the head and neck region who had refused or could not tolerate conventional therapy or with advanced or recurrent disease after conventional therapy who were treated with photodynamic therapy by superficial or interstitial illumination. With follow-up of 6 to 18 months, eight complete responses and one partial response were seen. One patient failed to respond to treatment.[80] Gluckman found encouraging results with photodynamic therapy for earlier-stage squamous carcinomas of the oropharynx and larynx, with control of tumor of up to 2 years.[76] Twenty-five of 41 patients with superficial, less advanced tumors were treated (13 with oral cavity and oropharynx, 6 with recurrent laryngeal lesions after radiation therapy, 6 with tumors at miscellaneous sites). Eleven of the 13 with oropharyngeal lesions obtained complete responses, but less success was seen with the laryngeal and miscellaneous lesions.

Durable control of carcinoma in situ with PDT was reported by Schweitzer.[81] Freche and De Corbiere reported treatment of 32 patients with severe dysplasia, carcinoma in situ, or microinvasive carcinoma of the true vocal cord without anterior commissure involvement.[82] Twenty five patients (72%) had eradication of their disease, with follow-up times as long as 4.5 years. Seven patients had tumors that failed to respond to treatment, probably due to inadequate light delivery. All patients developed a local laryngeal reaction of a laryngitis type with edema and petechiae. Dysphonia persisted for 1 to 2 months, but normal voice returned in all cases.

Photodynamic therapy has been effective in eradicating papillomas caused by papillomavirus in animals and is being evaluated clinically for the eradication of laryngeal papillomatosis.[83]

TABLE 69–31. Results of Photodynamic Therapy for Head and Neck Tumors

Investigations	*Tumor Type*	*No. of Patients*	*Light Dose (J/cm^2)*	*Response Rate (%)*			*Comments*
				CR	*PR*	*NR*	
Takata[79]	Squamous	6	34–390	0	100	0	Primary site
Wile[77]	Squamous	21	17–91	29	52	19	Primary site
Wile[77]	Squamous	10	17–91	20	30	50	Regional soft tissue
Grossweiner[80]	Squamous	10	60–100	80	10	10	9 of 10 have early cancer
Freche[82]	Squamous	23	~270 J	72	0	28	Early cancer
Gluckman[76]	Squamous	25	50–100	56	24	20	Early cancer
Gluckman[76]	Squamous	8	50–100	87.5	12.5	0	Carcinoma in situ
Gluckman[76]	Squamous	8	50–100	0	0	100	Advanced cancers

J, joules; CR, complete response, eradication of tumor; PR, partial response, greater than 50% reduction in tumor size; NR, no response; NA, not available.

CENTRAL NERVOUS SYSTEM MALIGNANCIES

Because of the grim prognosis with high-grade gliomas, there has been interest in PDT for these tumors (Table 69–32). Diamond and coworkers reported the inactivation of glioma cells in tissue culture with hematoporphyrin and light and significant destruction of gliomas transplanted subcutaneously and intracranially in rats.[84–87]

Perria and associates first reported the use of PDT as part of a treatment program for malignant brain tumors, with intraoperative PDT using a low power helium-neon laser to a modest dose of 9 J/cm^2 to the tumor bed after resection.[88] Survival ranged from 6 to 44 weeks, and no significant complications of treatment were seen.

Laws and coworkers from the Mayo Clinic reported a phase I feasibility study with PDT for the treatment of malignant brain tumors.[89] All patients were thought to be surgically incurable and had gross recurrent tumor after conventional therapy at the time of treatment. Two of the patients showed a transient decrease in the size of the mass or resultant mass effect on computed tomography (CT) scans after the procedure. In a subsequent report, Laws described a total of 23 patients with brain tumors treated with PDT, most of whom were treated after tumor resection.[90] Two patients developed transient worsening of neurologic function, and 2 had wound infections after PDT. The longest survivor in this series lived 37 months after PDT.

McCulloch described the use of intraoperative PDT delivered by external illumination to the resection cavity in patients with primary gliomas or recurrent metastatic lesions.[91] The patients with glioblastoma all underwent radical resection with PDT and received radiation therapy. Three patients were alive 17 to 42 months after treatment. Energy densities of 100 to 150 J/cm^2 and total energies of 2000 to 2500 J were employed. In their experience, cerebral edema was encountered after PDT but was manageable with steroids and osmotic agents.

Kostron reported intraoperative intratumoral injection and intraarterial injection of hematoporphyrin derivative in a modification of the usual intravenous photosensitization for PDT. Their approach was well tolerated, although the intratumoral injection required a second operation 3 days later for light delivery. Histologic examination immediately after intravenous and intraarterial injection demonstrated a predominantly vascular effect, but the direct injection resulted in a direct cellular effect with few vascular changes.[92]

Two series by Kaye[93] and Muller[94] demonstrated that high-dose adjuvant photoradiation therapy can be delivered at the time of resection of cerebral gliomas with an acceptable level of risk, although increased intracranial pressure and cerebral edema may be seen in some patients. Higher light doses appear to be more effective than lower light doses. Investigators in this area are exploring the use of a light diffusing lipid solution or a lipid-filled balloon to homogenously illuminate the resection cavity to high dose. However, the limited depth of photodynamic effects, ranging from 0.5 to 1.0 cm, which has been seen after illumination of the resection cavity highlights the need for the development of photosensitizers and techniques to adequately treat deep-seated tumors and infiltrating gliomas cells beyond the limits of grossly evident tumor, possibly using multiple interstitial fibers.

LUNG NEOPLASMS

The primary use of PDT in patients with lung cancer or endobronchial metastases has been to palliate endobronchial obstruction in patients with intrinsic lesions of the bronchus causing partial or complete obstruction. The patient receives 2 mg/kg of PII intravenously 48 to 72 hours before endobronchial illumination and is then removed from direct contact with sunlight but may be exposed to incandescent or fluorescent lighting for up to 12 hours each day. After the elapsed time, the patient is then exposed to 630-nm light usually from an argon pump-dye laser. Two methods are used to accomplish tumor illumination, both of which require quartz fibers linked to the laser for light transmission. The tumor can be directly implanted with the fiber for a length 0.5 to 2.0 cm, which shields the normal bronchus to the greatest extent and results in more uniform tumor illumination. For this interstitial treatment, a cylindrical fiber illuminator provides uniform illumination in all planes perpendicular to the fiber. Alternatively, an "end-cleaved" fiber can be used for surface illumination of the tumor. In both techniques, the light dose can be calibrated before treatment using a light power meter. The length of time that the tumor is exposed to the light dictates the total amount of energy (J) that constitutes the treatment. The amount of energy used for endobronchial tumor illumination has been loosely standardized but depends on the site and method of treatment and ranges from 5 to 900 J/cm^2.

TABLE 69–32. Results of Photodynamic Therapy for Brain Tumors

Investigations	*Tumor Type*	*No. of Patients*	*Light Dose (J/cm^2)*	*Response Rate (%)*			*Comments*
				CR	*PR*	*NR*	
Laws[89]	Glioma/Met	5	810 J	NA	NA	NA	No toxicity; phase I
McCulloch[91]	Glioma/Met	16	1260–2520 J	NA	NA	NA	Cerebral edema after PDT
Kaye[93]	Glioma/Met	23	70–230	NA	NA	NA	No toxicity; phase I–II
Kostron[92]	Glioma	14	15/120	NA	NA	NA	Well tolerated
Muller[94]	Glioma	32	8–68	19	13	68	25% cerebral edema
Perria[88]	Glioma	8	720–2400 J	NA	NA	NA	PDT after resection

J, joules; CR, complete response, eradication of tumor; PR, partial response, greater than 50% reduction in tumor size; NR, no response; Met, tumors metastatic to the brain; PDT, photodynamic therapy.

PDT has no immediate effect on hemostasis; after the patient is treated with light, no attempt is made to remove the obstruction until 72 hours later at a "clean-up" bronchoscopy. During this second bronchoscopy, multiple biopsies are performed without hemorrhage, which enables to bronchus to be opened to the bronchial wall. After hemorrhage is encountered, the endoscopist is beyond the phototherapy effect, and the session is terminated after ensuring airway hemostasis.

The relative advantages of PDT for endobronchial obstruction relief include its nonthermal nature and selective retentive properties that make it more akin to a specific cytotoxic modality. There is no real chance for airway ignition due to high inspired oxygen tensions, and the treatment takes relatively little time to perform (*i.e.,* 10–12 minutes to deliver 250 J/cm^2). The superficial nature of the treatment is a mixed blessing because, unlike Nd:YAG laser, there is no chance for extra-airway perforation of vessels. The delay in relieving the airway obstruction to allow the avascular necrosis to occur and a second bronchoscopy are obvious disadvantages of this technique, along with the inability to have an impact on acute hemostasis that can be performed with the Nd:YAG laser. Because PII is the only sensitizer approved in the United States for human use, and even that use is confined to experimental investigations, the obligatory 4 to 6 week avoidance of sunlight can severely limit the patient's independence. An ongoing prospective, randomized trial is attempting to define efficacy and toxicity comparisons between endobronchial PDT and Nd:YAG therapy for bronchial obstruction. Until definitive advantages are illustrated, it is the endoscopist's choice as to which method of airway relief is used, depending on training and equipment constraints.

The ability to compare results of PDT for management of malignant endobronchial lesions has been limited by the lack of standardization of protocols regarding the timing of laser treatment after sensitizer injection, sensitizer dose, treatment energy, and method of treatment (*i.e.,* tumor insertion or surface treatment). Moreover, the definition of a response has not been uniform, with some investigators defining a complete response as an anatomical improvement in the endobronchial component, while others call no evidence of tumor histologically, cytologically, or endoscopically a complete response. In a series of 10 patients treated uniformly with regard to dose rate (400 mW/cm^2, and energy (200–250 J/cm^2 with 2 mg/kg of sensitizer 72 hours before light), 80% of the patients were objectively improved, and there was a 20% histologically complete response rate. A summary of the published results is given in Table 69–33.[95–107]

The complications of endobronchial PDT can be immediate or late, depending on previous treatments, technique, or patient compliance. Hemorrhage can occur in previously irradiated patients. Pneumothorax after PDT and reversible pulmonary infiltrates may represent sensitized lung with injury.[95] Skin sensitization is the most common complication and can be minimized by limiting patient sun exposure for at least 4 weeks.

Photodynamic techniques have been investigated in the diagnosis of early lung cancer in an attempt to detect the small carcinoma (in situ lesions) or superficial lung tumors that cover a large endobronchial area. The method involves intravenous injection of hematoporphyrin D (HpD) or PII.[98–101] All of the current systems function by using the selective retention properties of malignant tissue in a temporal fashion after the sensitizer is delivered to the patients. With the use of an imaging intensifying, wavelength detecting device, wavelengths of approximately 405 nm (blue-violet) are used to selectively produce characteristic reddish fluorescence from tissue containing significant amounts of the sensitizer. As described by Lam, due to the preferential retention of the PII by the tumor, tumor fluorescence is higher than surrounding normal tissues.[108] The endoscopist can image the areas of red fluorescence distinct from the green autofluorescence, or a ratio for different areas of red to green fluorescence can be calculated, with the areas of highest ratios indicating the likely sites of tumor.

The most striking disadvantage of this technique is the requirement that patients receiving the sensitizer avoid sunlight for 4 to 6 weeks to avoid severe skin burn. Lam reported the use of low dose (0.25 mg/kg) PII instead of the usual 2 to 3 mg/kg dose in conjunction with a ratioing fluorometer probe.[108] The red-green ratios of known normal areas was 0.9

TABLE 69–33. Results of Photodynamic Therapy for Bronchial Obstruction

Investigations	*No. of Patients*	*Response Rates (%)* Complete	*Partial*	*Minimal*
Kato et al[96]	13	77	22	0
Kato et al[97]	60	0	48	52
Edell and Cortese[98]	30	70	30	0
Doiron and Balchum[99]	38	34	66	0
Balchum et al[100]	22	91	9	0
Balchum et al[100]	236	100	0	0
Vincent et al[101]	21	12	83	5
Forbes et al[103]	17	22	30	48
Lam et al[104]	7	89	11	0
Hugh-Jones and Gardner[105]	15	80	20	0
Pass et al[95]	10	20	60	20
Li and Zhao[106]	74	14	78	8
Benov et al[107]	25		76	24

to 1.8, and the red-green ratio in biopsy-proven tumor areas was 4.8 (3.0–9.5). Increasing the dose of PII by 700% (to 2 mg/kg) increased the ratio in the tumor area by only 64% (to 7.9). Moreover, skin photosensitivity testing after the 0.25 mg/km PII but before the additional 1.75 mg/g revealed no skin reaction to as high a dose as 30 J/cm^2, a light dose commonly used to eradicate recurrent skin malignancies (after giving the patient the usual 2 mg/kg dose of sensitizer).

Success in detecting these occult neoplasms has been reported from all centers involved in their development. Nevertheless, the systems still lack specificity because areas of cellular atypia or moderate or marked digress concentrate sensitizer and have low levels of fluorescence. Moreover, false positives have been reported with metaplasia. Ongoing efforts must concentrate on the miniaturization of the system, simultaneous digital computerized video imaging of the airway, fluorescence ratios, and methods to decrease the chance for nonspecific skin toxicity that may involve alternate routes of sensitizer delivery or use of differences in autofluoresence between normal and tumor tissue without sensitizer use.

It would seem logical that, if these areas of early or occult lung cancer could be localized by standard bronchoscopic methods or by the fluorescence activation principles as covered above, these superficial lesions would be most amenable to possible complete eradication by endobronchial photodynamic therapy. The Japanese were among the first to recognize this potential route of treatment and reported a series of 8 patients who had "early-stage central type" lung cancer (*i.e.,* x-ray and endoscopic findings suggesting the absence of lymph node involvement, and disease confined to the bronchial wall) who did not undergo resection due to patient refusal or medical contraindication, who were treated with photodynamic therapy.[109] Complete tumor remission as defined by no evidence of endoscopic, cytologic, or histologic tumor was obtained in all cases. Variable sensitizer doses, from 2.5 to 5 mg/kg were used, with a wide range of energies (90–600 J/cm^2).[104] Of these 8 patients, 1 was described in a follow-up report as the first 5-year disease-free survivor treated only by photodynamic therapy.[110] This pioneering group has subsequently updated their results in early-stage lung cancer in 40 cytology-positive only patients, of which 26 were treated without surgical resection. An impressive 100% initial complete remission rate has been reported, with 3 (12%) late recurrences, although autopsy confirmation in 10 deaths supposedly unrelated to cancer was not 100%.[111] The 16 surviving patients are free of disease 21 to 112 months post PDT at the time of the report (July 1990). More sobering results were recorded for 14 patients who, due to uncertainty of the PDT effect, had surgical resection of 15 PDT-treated lesions, of which 67% showed residual carcinoma.

In smaller but similar series of 13 patients with 14 carcinomas who had a complete endobronchial response to PDT, 11 of 13 had no local recurrence 3 to 53 months after treatment.[98] Most of these squamous carcinomas were less than 1 cm^2 in surface area. This surface area corresponds to the most recent recommendations from Hayatas group for best PDT results in early lung cancer.

The concept of endobronchial PDT for occult or early-stage lung cancer will be the subject of numerous reports in the future; currently, the best therapy for the patient with no medical contraindication to resection is surgical removal of the cancer. Moreover, thoracic surgeons and pulmonary physicians must keep in mind that if an "early" lung cancer is visible endoscopically, there is a 25% chance that the regional lymph nodes are involved with metastatic cancer. With the current sensitizers, the nodal basins will not be affected by endobronchial PDT. Moreover, the major problem with early-stage or occult lung cancers is the development of a second primary malignancy, often in the airway. Unless this disease is thought to be occult multicentric disease and all visible airways are illuminated, this late cause of death will be unaffected.

The number of patients for whom this therapy would be relevant must be mentioned. Because only 1% of patients on initial screening were found to have early lung cancer (which raises doubts about the cost effectiveness of such screening), few patients will then fall into the favorable cytologically positive, roentgenographically and endoscopically negative group with lesions smaller than 1 cm^2. Perhaps more patients can be defined in the future as high-risk patients on the basis of more sophisticated sputum analysis with monoclonal antibody markers and be followed for the development of in situ cancer amenable to PDT.

We need to refine the sensitizers to circumvent the 6-week avoidance of light. Newer sensitizers, conjugation of sensitizers to monoclonal antibody, or perhaps aerosol delivery of sensitizer topically to the airway will affect these problems.

The use of PDT for treatment of large pleural surfaces contaminated by malignancy, such as stage IIIB lung cancer, isolated pleural metastases, or mesothelioma, has been addressed at the National Cancer Institute, with the groundwork beginning in 1986. A series of in vitro, in vivo, small and large animal, and phantom modeling experiments were designed as a prelude to human investigations. A feasibility and phase I trial of intrapleural PDT for the treatment of pleural malignancies, including stage IIIB lung cancer isolated pleural metastases to the hemithorax, and mesothelioma has been ongoing since November of 1989 to define the maximal tolerated dose of photodynamic therapy that can be delivered to the chest cavity after maximal cytoreductive surgery. Light delivery to the thorax is accomplished after pleurectomy or modified extrapleural pneumonectomy to debulk the disease to 5 mm thickness maximum using dilute intralipid for light dispersion.[112] Seven photodiodes are strategically placed in the chest to record ongoing cumulative and real time light dose. After the maximal tolerated dose of PDT has been defined, a phase II trial of efficacy in the treatment of uniform histologic types (*e.g.,* mesothelioma) is planned. In such patients, whose curative options are close to zero with standard treatment, the advent of an intraoperative adjuvant that may obtain at least local control could be the first step toward improving survival.

OCULAR TUMORS

PDT has been attempted for control of choroidal malignant melanoma, a tumor managed traditionally by enucleation, but in recent years, there has been interest in local or external particle beam irradiation in addition to laser photocoagulation or transscleral diathermy (Table 69–34).[113–115] Complete responses have been seen in patients with small or medium lesions, with the final appearance of the tumor that of a large

TABLE 69–34. Results of Photodynamic Therapy for Ocular Tumors

Investigations	*Tumor Type*	*Patients/Eyes*	*Light Dose (J/cm²)*	*Response Rate (%)*			*Comments*
				CR	*PR*	*NR*	
Murphree[116]	Melanoma	9/9	50–400	22	66	12	CRs nonpigmented
Bruce[113]	Melanoma	24/24	300–3000	41	6	53	CRs in small tumors
Murphree[116]	Retinoblastoma	6/9	50–400	11	78	11	All recur later

J, joules; CR, complete response, eradication of tumor; PR, partial response, greater than 50% reduction in tumor size; NR, no response.

chorioretinal scar. Posttreatment complications include transient chemosis, iritis, and lid swelling in all patients, managed with cycloplegics and corticosteroid drops. Exudative retinal detachment worsened or developed in most patients.

Most investigators have used high energy densities for treatment, and there are no comments about the pigmentation in the lesions treated. Melanin is an efficient absorber of red light, and high energy densities must be used if sufficient light is to reach the deepest portions of pigmented lesions. Thermal effects may have been present at the power densities (dose rates) employed and increased the risk of damage to uninvolved normal tissue. Murphree and Gomer achieved no complete responses in patients with pigmented choroidal melanomas.[116]

Photodynamic destruction of retinoblastoma cells in vitro has been reported, but generally the response to PDT in humans has been disappointing.[117]

ESOPHAGEAL MALIGNANCIES

PDT has been attempted for cure and palliation of esophageal malignancies (Table 69–35). In the United States, where patients most often present with bulky tumor and adjacent nodal involvement indicative of advanced-stage disease, investigators have reported palliation of esophageal obstruction using PDT. In Japan and China, where mass screening clinics have been able to detect early esophageal carcinomas, PDT has been attempted with curative intent.

McCaughan and coworkers reported the treatment of 40 patients with esophageal tumors (19 adenocarcinomas, 19 squamous carcinomas, and 2 melanomas) in whom conventional treatments were unsuccessful.[118] Patients received HpD or DHE, followed by the delivery of red light by an optical fiber passed through a flexible endoscope. Four patients with stage I tumors had a complete response. One with squamous cancer subsequently died of recurrent disease at 18 months, but 2 with adenocarcinoma were alive and free of disease at 11 and 23 months after treatment. A third patient with melanoma died of another cancer 31 months after treatment. Of the 35 patients who could be evaluated 1 month after PDT, the average improvement in food intake was from a liquid to a soft diet. Of the 28 patients assessable one month after PDT, the average minimal esophageal diameter opening increased from 6 to 9 mm. Nine patients with complete obstruction were treated; of the 7 survivors at 1 month, all were able to tolerate oral intake of food. Side effects of treatment included six pleural effusions, of which five resolved without treatment; six strictures requiring dilation, and three tracheoesophageal fistulas (one in a patient with tracheal invasion and one in a patient who had had prior laryngeal surgery). Because of the advanced nature of most of their cases, overall survival was poor, averaging 7.7 months for patients with adenocarcinoma and 5.8 months for patients with squamous carcinomas.

Thomas and colleagues treated 14 patients with locally advanced esophageal cancer using high-dose photodynamic

TABLE 69–35. Results of Photodynamic Therapy for Esophageal and Gastric Tumors

Investigations	*Tumor Type*	*No. of Patients*	*Light Dose (J/cm²)*	*Response Rate (%)*			*Comments*
				CR	*PR*	*NR*	
McCaughan[118]	Esophagus	40	300–600 J/c	10	NA	NA	Most improve swallowing
Thomas[119]	Esophagus	14	60–337	14	86	0	All improve swallowing
Aida[120]	Esophagus	4	270–360	50	50	0	Early stage; CR's NED at 1, 2 y
Aida[120]	Esophagus	5	270–360	0	100	0	Advanced stage
Hayata[121]	Gastric	4	34–960	100	0	0	3/4 recur by 27 mo.
Hayata[121]	Gastric	12	34–960				Resected after PDT; 5 of 12 had no tumor in specimen

J, joules; J/c: joules per centimeter; CR, complete response, eradication of tumor; PR, partial response, greater than 50% reduction in tumor size; NR, no response; NED, no evidence of disease.

therapy.[119] All patients achieved a measurable improvement in the severity of dysphagia persisting from 1 to 28 weeks. Two patients had complete eradication of tumor proven by histologic examination of the subsequently resected esophagus. The complication rate was 16% and included mediastinitis and bronchoesophageal fistula.

Aida and Hirashima treated 4 patients with superficial carcinomas of the esophagus.[120] Two had endoscopically complete responses and remained disease-free at one and two years after treatment. The other two patients went on to surgical resection and were found to have residual tumor cells in portions of the tumor thought to have been inadequately illuminated. Their advanced cases showed partial responses.

UPPER GASTROINTESTINAL MALIGNANCIES

PDT may have some applicability in early-stage gastric cancer for patients who cannot undergo curative surgery. The shape of the stomach and deep rugae complicate the delivery of light. The technical aspects of light delivery must be addressed if adequate PDT is to be given. Because of the difficulty in diagnosing early-stage cases and the propensity of gastric carcinomas to metastasize to adjacent lymph nodes, PDT for most gastric cancers in the United States will probably be limited to palliation of medically inoperable cases.

The practice of screening for gastric cancers in Japan has detected some early gastric cancers that have been treated by PDT in patients who refused or were not eligible for surgery. Hayata and coworkers in Japan treated 16 patients with early-stage gastric carcinoma (see Table 69–35).[121] Four were treated by PDT alone because of medical inoperability or refusal of surgery, while the other 12 patients had resection after PDT. Complete disappearance by endoscopic visualization was obtained in all 4 patients treated with PDT alone. One patient remained disease free at 30 months, 1 had a recurrence at 27 months and was retreated, and 2 patients died with recurrent disease at 5 and 13 months. Of the 12 patients who had resection after PDT, there was no evidence of tumor in the operative specimen in 5. Okuda reported endoscopic PDT treatment of 5 patients with early and 1 patient with advanced gastric cancer.[122]

LOWER GASTROINTESTINAL MALIGNANCIES

Fluorescence assays of human and murine colorectal cancers that had received intravenous HpD demonstrate preferential localization of HpD in adenocarcinomas and tubular adenomas, with the mean HpD concentration twofold to sixfold higher in tumor compared with surrounding normal mucosa.[123–125] It has been possible to destroy experimental colon cancers without producing any damage to adjacent normal colon exposed to similar light doses.[126] For experimental tumors undergoing necrosis caused by PDT slough, the defect heals by regeneration of the normal colon, and photosensitization does not reduce the mechanical strength of the colonic wall.[127] Barr treated 10 patients with colorectal cancers unsuitable for operation because of metastatic disease or underlying medical debility.[128] Light was delivered with an optical fiber passed through the colonoscope and into from 1 to 4 points within the lesion. Intraluminal ultrasound measurements showed a reduction in mean tumor depth from 18.8 to 12.6 mm with four patients reporting some degree of symptomatic improvement. PDT was suitable for treatment of small tumors or for small areas of persistent tumor where the bulk of tumor could be removed by alternative techniques.

GENITOURINARY MALIGNANCIES

The first reported human use of PDT was for a patient with transitional cell carcinoma of the bladder. Kelly and Snell observed destruction of tumor in the subsequent cystectomy specimen only in sites that had been illuminated.[12] This has been one of the most active areas of interest in PDT (Table 69–36). Emphasis has been on treatment of superficial transitional cell cancers not involving the muscularis of the bladder (*e.g.*, Tis, Ta, T1 tumors).

TABLE 69–36. Results of Photodynamic Therapy for Urinary Bladder Tumors

Investigations	*Tumor Type*	*Patients/Sites*	*Light Dose (J/cm^2)*	*Response Rate (%)*			*Comments*
				CR	*PR*	*NR*	
Hisazumi[133]	TCCa	9/36	F 50–300	50	19	31	Ta, T1 tumors; all CR ≤2 cm
Tsuchiya[132]	TCCa	8/NA	F 120–360	100	0	0	Ta-T2; two recur at 6–18 mo
Benson[134]	TCCa	4/NA	F 150	100	0	0	CIS; recur elsewhere in bladder
Benson[136]	TCCa	10/NA	WB 25–45	60	20	20	CIS or CIS and T2 tumors
Prout[135]	TCCa	19/50	F 100–200	24	50	26	Ta, T1, CIS tumors
Nseyo[138]	TCCa	19/NA	WB 5–60	37	53	10	Ta, T1, CIS tumors
Harty[140]	TCCa	7/NA	WB 25+F	78	0	22	4/7 develop contracted bladder
Dugan[143]	TCCa	12/NA	WB 15				PDT prophylaxis reduces recurrences, 33% vs 83%

J, joules; CR, complete response, eradication of tumor; PR, partial response, greater than 50% reduction in tumor size; NR, no response; TCCa, transitional cell carcinoma; F, focal; WB, whole bladder; CIS, carcinoma in situ; Ta, papillary tumor confined to mucosa; T1, tumor invading lamina propria; T2, tumor invading muscle superficially; PDT, photodynamic therapy.

Sensitizer is selectively retained by murine bladder tumors and tumor destruction can be achieved with the appropriated combination of photosensitizer and light.[129,130] Benson demonstrated localization of sensitizer in transitional cell carcinoma in situ and severely dysplastic epithelium in the urinary bladder after intravenous administration and subsequent illumination of the bladder with violet light.[131] Their observations were confirmed at histologic examination of the bladders after cystectomy with the only false-positive findings at sites of regenerative mucosal activity around healing biopsy areas. Other groups have found preferential fluorescence in tumors compared with normal bladder mucosa.[132,133]

Light dose and light delivery technique have been important for tumor control and complications of treatment. High-dose (100–200 J/cm^2) focal light treatment has been used to control papillary lesions. However, much lower doses (~15 J/cm^2) have been used for the whole-bladder treatment, which has been used to control carcinoma in situ or microscopic disease after resection of papillary lesions. The Mayo Clinic group initially reported biopsy-proven complete tumor responses in 4 patients with recurrent, previously treated transitional cell carcinomas of the bladder that were focally illuminated using optical fibers introduced through the cystoscope after intravenous HpD injection.[134] A collaborative group of American and Chinese urologists treated 50 papillary tumors and three areas of carcinoma in situ in 20 patients with focal PDT to the involved sites.[135] The carcinomas in situ were all eliminated, and 74% of the papillary lesions had complete responses to treatment. The complete response rate was only 33% for lesions larger than 1.5 cm. Two groups from Japan reported that the highest complete remission rate was seen for lesions smaller than 1 cm.[132,133]

Because of the tendency of tumors to later recur at other sites in the bladder that had not been illuminated and because of the interest in treating diffuse, multifocal carcinoma in situ, several groups switched to using a modified optical fiber with a spherical diffusing bulb to illuminate the entire bladder.[136,137] In 10 patients with carcinoma in situ alone, biopsy and urinary cytology at follow-up examination 3 months after treatment showed complete disappearance of tumor.[136] Two patients with both carcinoma in situ and papillary, noninvasive lesions were found to have disappearance of the former but persistence of the latter. Of these 12 patients, 3 subsequently developed focal recurrent disease at 6 to 9 months after treatment. Hisazumi treated 2 other patients with carcinoma in situ, both of whom had a complete response to treatment. Both developed acute posttreatment inflammatory symptoms for 2 to 3 weeks and a transient reduction in bladder capacity that resolved by 3 months.[137]

Nseyo and colleagues treated 19 patients with resistant superficial transitional cell carcinoma of the bladder.[138,139] Seven patients (37%) had complete responses to treatment, and 10 (53%) had partial responses. All patients had irritative urinary tract symptoms after treatment; 4 patients developed bladder shrinkage that did not resolve. Among 4 patients treated with muscle invading disease (≥T2), control of gross hematuria was the only benefit seen. Harty and associates described the development of a contracted bladder with hydroureteronephrosis and vesicoureteral reflux in 4 of 7 patients treated with 25 J/cm^2 to the whole bladder, with or without additional focal treatment.[140] Deep bladder biopsies showed replacement of smooth muscle by fibrous tissue. Careful attention to light dose and treatment technique and photosensitizer localization in tumor compared with normal bladder is important if this is to be a safe and effective treatment for superficial bladder cancer.[141,142]

In a controlled trial, the toxicity of the therapy appears acceptable. Dugan and associates reported the preliminary results of a randomized trial of observation versus PDT after transurethral resection for patients with high-grade or recurrent low-grade papillary superficial bladder cancer.[143] PDT patients received 2 mg/kg of DHE followed 40 to 50 hours later by 15 J/cm^2 with 630-nm red light to the whole bladder. With median follow-up of 1 year, there were 10 recurrences (83%) of 12 in the observation group, compared with 4 (33%) of 12 in the PDT group ($p = 0.0014$); 91% of the PDT patients experienced acute irritative symptoms after treatment, but these were self-limited. Bladder capacity over time was equivalent in both groups. The final report from this trial will be an important factor in determining the efficacy and safety of bladder PDT. In another ongoing trial, patients with refractory or recurrent superficial transitional cell carcinoma in situ in the bladder are being treated with PDT as an alternative to cystectomy.

GYNECOLOGIC MALIGNANCIES AND INTRAABDOMINAL PHOTODYNAMIC THERAPY

An early report on the use of PDT for gynecologic malignancies described treatment of 5 patients with recurrent tumors involving the vaginal vault.[144] Two complete responses were seen, one in a patient with recurrent ovarian cancer and the other in a patient with melanoma. These were durable at 10 and 12 months. The only toxicity observed was cutaneous phototoxicity.

Multiple other reports subsequently appeared, primarily describing cases of gynecologic cancer recurring in the vagina or skin after conventional treatment (Table 69–37).[145–150]

PDT is being investigated as an adjuvant therapy to be delivered to patients with ovarian cancer at the time of second-look laparotomy. Tochner and coworkers were able to control an experimental murine ovarian ascites tumor in 17 of 20 animals using intraperitoneally administered HpD and four intraperitoneal light treatments.[26] On the basis of these experimental findings, a phase I study was initiated in which PDT was administered to the peritoneal surface of patients with minimal thickness intraperitoneal tumor at the time of surgical resection.[152–154] The study was completed with the determination of a maximal tolerated dose of photodynamic therapy that could be delivered to the peritoneal cavity after major cytoreductive surgery. Of the 54 patients with refractory ovarian cancer, sarcoma, colon cancer, or mucinous adenocarcinoma diffusely involving the peritoneal cavity, 39 were able to undergo adequate surgical cytoreduction to receive intraoperative photodynamic therapy. With median follow-up of 22 months, 9 of 39 patients remained free of disease. Phase II studies at the maximal tolerated dose are planned.

CONCLUSIONS

PDT represents another modality for the treatment of human malignancy. Light-activated photosensitizers have definite antitumor activity in in vitro and in vivo experimental systems.

TABLE 69–37. Results of Photodynamic Therapy for Gynecologic Tumors

Investigations	*Tumor Type*	*Patients/Sites*	*Light Dose (J/cm²)*	*Response Rate (%)*			*Comments*
				CR	*PR*	*NR*	
Ward[144]	Vagina	5/5	NA	40	60	0	CRs durable at 10, 12 mo
Soma[145]	Vagina	1/NA	NA	100	0	0	NED at 1 y
Dahlman[146]	Vulva	2/2	NA	50	0	50	CR in carcinoma in situ
Rettenmaier[147]	Vagina/perineum	6/9	20–40	22	45	33	Treatment well tolerated
McCaughan[148]	Vulva/vagina	5/5	Variable	80	20	0	Follow-up 5–15 mo
Lobraico[151]	Vulva/vagina	7/45	Variable	76	18	6	Edema, erythema after PDT
Corti[149]	Vagina	15/15	60–240	53	40	7	Duration of CR 2.5–25 mo
Lele[150]	Skin	7/NA	Variable	100	0	0	PDT with palliative intent
Lele[150]	Vagina/cervix	11/NA	Variable	18	18	64	CRs durable at 28, 36 mo

J, joules; CR, complete response, eradication of tumor; PR, partial response, greater than 50% reduction in tumor size; NR, no response; NED, no evidence of disease; PDT, photodynamic therapy; NA, not available.

Much of the early clinical work involved treatment of patients with advanced, recurrent disease who had not responded to conventional therapy. Because good responses with acceptable toxicity have been obtained in these patients, active investigation continues and is aimed at defining the most appropriate sites and applications for the technique. Because of the limited depth of light penetration in tissue, the most promising sites may be those where there is limited thickness of tumor, such as in superficial skin lesions or early-stage carcinomas involving the aerodigestive tract, bronchial tree, or the genitourinary tract. Other potential uses include those where PDT could be combined with surgical or chemotherapeutic debulking, such as pleural mesothelioma or advanced stage ovarian cancer. Whether PDT can be of benefit in surgical cases for which the margins of resection are close is an interesting question.

The hematoporphyrin derivative, dihematoporphyrin ethers, and benzoporphyrin monoacid ring A are currently only approved for use as investigational compounds in clinical studies. If ongoing trials of PDT in superficial bladder cancer, obstructing esophageal cancer, and non-small cell lung cancer show encouraging results, application to the Food and Drug Administration for approval of DHE as a photosensitizer for general clinical use for these indications is planned. Laboratory work to better understand mechanism of photosensitizer localization and cytotoxicity continues, as do investigations into alternative photosensitizers with improved tumor localization, less cutaneous photosensitivity, and absorption peaks at deeper penetrating wavelengths of light. Attempts at measurement of singlet oxygen, if successful, will permit the development of more meaningful dosimetry to correlate response with actual tissue levels of the purported cytotoxic agent. Hopefully, these and other developments in the field of PDT will improve the treatment for patients with cancer.

REFERENCES

1. Raab O. Uber die Wirkung Fluoreszierenden Stoffen. Infusoria Z Biol 1900;39:524.
2. Jesionek A, Tappeiner VH. Zur Behandlung der hautcarcinomit mit fluorescierenden stoffen. Muench Med Wochenshr 1903;47:2042.
3. Hausman W. Die sensibilisierende Wirkung des hematoporphyrins. Biochem Z 1911;30:276.
4. Auber H, Banger G. Unter suchungen uber die rolle der porphyrine bei geschwulstkranken menschen und tieren. Z Krebsforsch 1942;53:65.
5. Figge FHJ, Weiland GS, Manganiello LOJ. Cancer detection and therapy. Affinity of neoplastic embryonic and traumatized tissue for porphyrins and metalloporphyrins. Proc Soc Exp Biol Med 1948;68:640.
6. Lipson RL, Baldes EJ. The photodynamic properties of a particular hematoporphyrin derivative. Arch Dermatol 1960;82:508.
7. Lipson RL, Blades EJ. The use of a derivative of hematoporphyrin in tumor detection. JNCI 1961;26:1.
8. Lipson RL, Baldes EJ. Hematoporphyrin derivative: A new aid for endoscopic detection of malignant disease. J Thorac Cardiovasc Surg 1961;42:623.
9. Grey M, Lipson RL, Mack JVS, et al. Use of hematoporphyrin derivative in detection and management of cervical cancer. Am J Obstet Gynecol 1967;9:766.
10. Gregorie HG, Horger EO, Ward JL, et al. Hematoporphyrin derivative for detection and management of cancer. Ann Surg 1968;167:82.
11. Lipson RL, Gray MJ, Baldes EJ. Hematoporphyrin derivative for detection and management of cancer. Proceedings of the 9th International Cancer Congress, Tokyo, 1966:393.
12. Kelly JF, Snell NE, Berenbaum MC. Photodynamic destruction of human bladder carcinoma. J Urol 1976;115:150.
13. Dougherty RJ. Activated dyes vs anti-tumor agents. JNCI 1974;51:1333.
14. Dougherty TJ, Crindley GE, Fiel R, et al. Photoradiation therapy II. Cure of animal tumors with hematoporphyrin and light. JNCI 1975;55:115.
15. Dougherty TJ, Kaufman JE, Goldfarb A, et al. Photoradiation therapy for the treatment of malignant tumors. Cancer Res 1978;38:2628.
16. Dougherty TJ. Photoradiation therapy. Urology 1984;23:61.
17. Dougherty TJ. Photosensitizers: Therapy and detection of malignant tumors. Photochem Photobiol 1987;45:874.
18. Pass HI Photodynamic therapy for lung cancer. Chest Surg Clin North Am 1991;1:135–151.
19. Lin C-W. Selective localization of photosensitizers in tumors: A review of the phenomenon and possible mechanisms. In: Kessel D, ed. Photodynamic therapy of neoplastic disease. Boston: CRC Press, 1990:79–101.
20. Barel A, Jori G, Perin A, Romandini P, Pagnan A, Biffanti S. Role of high-, low-, and very low-density lipoproteins in the transport and tumor-delivery of hematoporphyrin, in vivo. Cancer Lett 1986;32:145.
21. Bugelski PJ, Porter CW, Dougherty TJ. Autoradiographic distribution of hematoporphyrin derivative in normal and tumor tissue of the mouse. Cancer Res 1981;41:4606.
22. Selman SH, Kreimer-Birnbaum M, Klaunig JE, Goldblatt PJ, Keck RW, Britton SL. Blood flow in transplantable bladder tumors treated with hematoporphyrin derivative and light. Cancer Res 1984;44:1924.
23. Star WM, Marijnissen HPA, van den Berg-Blok AE, Versteeg JAC, Franken KA, Reinhold HS. Destruction of rat mammary tumor and normal tissue microcirculation by hematoporphyrin derivative photoradiation observed in vivo in sandwich observation chambers. Cancer Res 1986;46:2532.
24. Pass HI, Evans S, Matthews WA, et al. Photodynamic therapy of oncogene-transformed cells. J Thorac Cardiovasc Surg 1991;101:795–799.
25. Perry RR, Matthews W, Pass HI, et al. Sensitivity of different human lung cancer histologies to photodynamic therapy. Cancer Res 1990;50:4272–4276.
26. Tochner Z, Mitchell JB, Smith P, et al. Photodynamic therapy of ascites tumours within the peritoneal cavity. Br J Cancer 1986;53:733.
27. Mitchell JB McPherson S, DeGraff W, et al. Oxygen dependence of hematoporphyrin derivative-induced photoinactivation of Chinese hamster cells. Cancer Res 1985;45:2008.
28. Lee See K, Forbes IJ, Betts WH. Oxygen dependency of phototoxicity with maematoporphyrin derivative. Photochem Photobiol 1984;39:631.

29. Foote CS. Mechanisms of photooxygenation. In: Doiron DR, Gomer CJ, eds. Porphyrin localization and treatment of tumors. New York: Alan R Liss, 1984:3.
30. Christensen T, Moan J, Smedshammer L, et al. Influence of hematoporphyrin derivative (HPD) and light on the attachment of cells to the substratum. Photochem Photobiophys 1985;10:53.
31. Denstaman SC, Dillehay LE, Williams JR. Enhanced susceptibility of HPD-sensitized phototoxicity and correlated resistance to trypsin detachment in SV40 transformed IMR-90 cell. Photochem Photobiophys 1985;10:53.
32. Volden G, Christensen T, Moan J. Photodynamic membrane damage of hematoporphyrin derivative-treated NHIK 3025 cells in vitro. Photochem Photobiophys 1981;3:105.
33. Jewell SA, Bellomo G, Thor H, et al. Bleb formation in hepatocytes during drug metabolism is caused by disturbances in thiol and calcium ion homeostatis. Science 217: 1257.
34. Borrelli MJ, Wong RSL, Dewey WC. A direct correlation between hyperthermia-induced blebbing and survival in synchronous G_1 CHO cells. J Cell Physiol 1986;126:181.
35. Tom M, Dubhelman AR, Prinsze C, et al. Photodynamic therapy membrane and enzyme photobiology. In: Henderson B, Dougherty T, eds. Photodynamic therapy. New York: Marcel Dekker, 1992.
36. Sonoda M, Murali-Krishna C, Riesz P. The role of singlet oxygen in the photochemolysis of red blood cells sensitized by phthalocyanine sulfonates. Photochem Photobiol 1987;46: 635.
37. Hilf R, Murant RS, Narayanan U, Gibson SL. Hematoporphyrin derivative-induced photosensitivity of mitochondrial succinate dehydrogenase and selected cytosolic enzymes of R3230AC mammary adenocarcinomas of rats. Cancer Res 1984;44:1483.
38. Hilf R, Murant RS, Narayanan U, Gibson SL. Relationship of mitochondrial function and cellular adenosine triphosphate levels to hematoporphyrin derivative-induced photosensitization in R3230AC mammary tumors. Cancer Res 1986;46:211.
39. Gomer CJ. DNA damage and repair in CHO cells following hematoporphyrin photoradiation. Cancer Lett 1980;11:161.
40. Moan J, Waksvik H, Christensen T. DNA single-stand breaks and sister chromatid exchanges induced by treatment with hematoporphyrin and light or by x-rays in human NHIK 3025 cells. Cancer Res 1980;40:2915.
41. Mitchell JB Russo A, Kinsella TJ, Glatstein E. The use of non-hypoxic cell sensitizers in radiobiology and radiotherapy. Int J Radiat Oncol Biol Phys 1986;12:1513.
42. Russo A, DeGraff W, Kinsella TJ, et al. Potentiation of chemotherapy cytotoxicity following iododeoxyuridine incorporation in Chinese hamster cells. Int J Radiat Oncol Biol Phys 1986;12:1418.
43. Gomer CJ, Rucker N, Banerjee A, Benedict WF. Comparison of mutagenicity and induction of sister chromatid exchange in Chinese hamster cells exposed to hematoporphyrin derivative, ionizing radiation, or ultraviolet radiation. Cancer Res 1983;43: 2662.
44. Ben-Hur E, Fujihara T, Suzuki F, Elkind MM. Genetic toxicology of the photosensitization of Chinese hamster cells by phthalocyanines. Photochem Photobiol 1987;45: 227.
45. Kessel D. Sites of photosensitization by derivatives of hematoporphyrin. Photochem Photobiol 1986;44:489.
46. Rizzoni WE, Matthews W, Pass HI, et al. In vitro photodynamic therapy of human lung cancer. Influence of dose rate, hematoporphryn concentration and incubation, and cellular targets. Surg Forum 1987;38:452–455.
47. Bohmer RM, Morstyn G. Uptake of hematoporphyrin derivative by normal and malignant cells: Effect of serum, pH, temperature, and cell size. Cancer Res 1985;45:5328–5334.
48. Matthews W, Cook J, Pass HI. In vitro photodynamic therapy of human lung cancer: Investigation of dose-rate effects. Cancer Res 1989;49:1718–1721.
49. Elmets CA, Bowen KD. Immunological suppression in mice treated with hematoporphyrin derivative photoradiation. Cancer Res 1986;46:1608–1611.
50. Ortner MJ, Abhold RH, Chignell CF. The effect of protoporphyrin on histamine secretion by rat peritoneal mast cells: A dual phototoxic reaction. Photochem Photobiol 1981;33: 355–360.
51. Henderson BW, Donovan JM. Cellular prostaglandin E release after photodynamic therapy. Lasers Med Sci 1988;3:103.
52. Lynch DH, Haddad S, King VJ, Ott MJ, Straight RC, Jolles CJ. Systemic immunosuppression induced by photodynamic therapy (PDT) is adoptively transferred by macrophages. Photochem Photobiol 1989;49:453–458.
53. Evans S, Matthews W, Perry R, Fraker D, Norton J, Pass HI. Effect of photodynamic therapy on tumor necrosis factor production by murine macrophages. JNCI 1990;82: 34–39.
54. Jiang FN, Liu D.J Neyndorff H, et al. Photodynamic killing of human squamous cell carcinoma cells using a monoclonal antibody-photosensitizer conjugate. JNCI 1991;83: 1218–1225.
55. Pogrebniak HW, Matthews W, Black C, et al. Targeted phototherapy with sensitizer-monoclonal antibody and light. Surg Forum 1991;42.447–449.
56. Shumaker BP, Hetzel FW. Clinical laser photodynamic therapy in the treatment of bladder carcinoma. Photochem Photobiol 1987;46:899–901.
57. Nseyo UO, Whalen RK, Duncan MR, Berman B, Lundahl SL. Urinary cytokines following photodynamic therapy for bladder cancer. Urology 1990;36:167–171.
58. Heald PW, Perez MI, McKiernan G, Christensen I, Edelson RL. Extracorporeal photochemotherapy for CTCL. Prog Clin Biol Res 1990;337:443–447.
59. Gonzalez S, Arnfield MR, Meeker BE, et al. Treatment of Dunning R3327-AT rat prostate tumors with photodynamic therapy in combination with misonidazole. Cancer Res 1986;46:2858–2862.
60. Dougherty TJ. Photosensitization of malignant tumors. Semin Surg Oncol 1986;2:24.
61. Mang TS, Dougherty TJ, Potter WR, et al. Photobleaching of porphyrins used in photodynamic therapy and implications for therapy. Photochem Photobiol 1987;45:501.
62. Bandieramonte C, Marchesini R, Melloni E, et al. Laser phototherapy following HpD administration in superficial neoplastic lesions. Tumori 1984;70:327.
63. Santoro O, Bandieramonte G, Melloni E, et al. Photodynamic therapy by topical mesotetraphenylporphinesulfonate tetrasodium salt administration in superficial basal cell carcinomas. Cancer Res 1990;50:4501.
64. Waldow SM, Lobraico RV, Kohler IK, et al. Photodynamic therapy for treatment of malignant cutaneous lesions. Lasers Surg Med 1987;7:451.
65. Kennedy J. Photoradiation therapy for cancer at Kingston and Hamilton. In: Kessel D, Dougherty TJ, eds. Pophyrin photosensitization. New York: Plenum Press, 1983: 53.
66. Pennington DG, Waner M, Knox A. Photodynamic therapy for multiple skin cancers. Plast Reconst Surg 1987;82:1067.
67. Wilson BW, Mang TS, Cooper MC, et al. Use of photodynamic therapy for the treatment of extensive basal cell carcinomas. Facial Plastic Surgery 1990;6:185.
68. Tse DT, Kerstein RC, Anderson RL. Hematoporphyrin derivative photoradiation therapy in managing nevoid basal-cell carcinoma syndrome: A preliminary report. Arch Opthalmol 1984;102:990.
69. Robinson PJ, Carruth JAS, Fiarris GM. Photodynamic therapy: A better treatment for widespread Bowen's disease. Br J Dermatol 1988;119:59.
70. Kennedy JC, Pottier RH, Pross DC. Photodynamic therapy with endogenous protoporphyrin IX. Basic principles and present clinical experience. J Photochem Photobiol B 1990;6:143.
71. Potter WR, Mang TS, Dougherty TJ. The theory of photodynamic therapy dosimetry: Consequences of photodestruction of sensitizers. Photochem Photobiol 1987;46:97.
72. Aberizk WJ, Silver B, Henderson IC, et al. The use of radiotherapy for treatment of isolated locoregional recurrence of breast carcinoma after mastectomy. Cancer 1986;58: 1214.
73. Schuh M, Nseyo UO, Potter WR, et al. Photodynamic therapy for palliation of locally recurrent breast carcinoma. J Clin Oncol 1987;5:1766.
74. Sperduto PW, DeLaney TF, Thomas G, et al. Photodynamic therapy for chest wall recurrence in breast cancer. Int J Radiat Oncol Biol Phys 1991;21:441.
75. Gluckman JL, Waner M, Shumrick K, et al. Photodynamic therapy. A viable alternative to conventional therapy for early lesions of the upper aerodigestive tract. Arch Otolaryngol Head Neck Surg 1986;112:949.
76. Gluckman JL. Hematoporphyrin photodynamic therapy. Is there truly a future in head and neck oncology? Laryngoscope 1991;191:36.
77. Wile AG, Novotny J, Mason GR, et al. Photoradiation therapy of head and neck cancer. Am J Clin Oncol 1984;6:39.
78. Schuller DE, McCaughan JS Jr, Rock RP. Photodynamic therapy in head and neck cancer. Arch Otolargyngol 1985;111:351.
79. Takata C, Imakiire M. Cancer of the ear, nose, and throat. In: Hayata Y, Dougherty TJ, eds. Lasers and hematoporphyrin derivative in cancer. New York: Igaku-Shoin, 1983:70.
80. Grossweiner LI, Hill JH, Lobraico RV. Photodynamic therapy of head and neck squamous cell carcinoma: Optical dosimetry and clinical trial. Photochem Photobiol 1987;46: 911.
81. Schweitzer VG. Photodynamic therapy for treatment of head and neck cancer. Otolarygol Head Neck Surg 1990;102:225.
82. Freche C, De Corbiere S. Use of photodynamic therapy in the treatment of vocal cord carcinoma. J Photochem Photobiol 1990;B6:291.
83. Shikowitz MJ, Steinberg BM, Abramson A.L. Hematoporphyrin derivative therapy of papillomas: Experimental study. Arch Otolaryngol Head Neck Surg 1986;112:42.
84. Diamond I, Granelli SG, McDonough AF, et al. Photodynamic therapy of malignant tumours. Lancet 1972;2:1175.
85. Boggan JE, Walter R, Edwards MSB, et al. Distribution of hematoporphyrin derivative in the rat 9L gliosarcoma brain tumour analyzed by digital videofluorescence microscopy. J Neurosurg 1984;61:1113.
86. Little FM, Gomer CJ, Hyman S, et al. Observations in studies of quantitative kinetics of tritium labelled hematoporphyrin derivatives (HpDI and HpDII) in the normal and neoplastic rat brain model. J Neurooncol 1984;2:361.
87. Berenbaum MC, Hall GW, Hoyes AD. Cerebral photosensitization by hematoporphyrin derivative. Evidence for an endothelial site of action. Br J Cancer 1986;53:81.
88. Perria C, Carai M, Balzoi A, et al. Photodynamic therapy of malignant brain tumors: Clinical results of difficulties, with questions about and future prospects for the neurosurgical applications. Neurosurgery 1988;23:557.
89. Laws ER Jr, Cortese DA, Kinsey JH, et al. Photoradiation therapy in the treatment of malignant brain tumors: A phase I (feasibility) study. Neurosurgery 1981;9:672.
90. Laws ER Jr, Wharen RE, Anderson RE. Photoradiation therapy of malignant gliomas. In: Wilkens RH, Rengachary SS, eds. Neurosurgery Update, 1990:260.
91. McCulloch GAJ, Forbes IJ, See KL, et al. Phototherapy in malignant brain tumors. In: Doiron DR, Gomer CJ, eds. Porphyrin localization and treatment of tumors. New York: Alan R Liss, 1984:709.
92. Kostron H, Weiser G, Fritsch E, et al. Photodynamic therapy of malignant brain tumors: Clinical and neuropathological results. Photochem Photobiol 1987;46:937.
93. Kaye AH, Morstyn G, Brownbill D. Adjuvant high-dose photoradiation therapy in the treatment of cerebral glioma: A phase 1–2 study. J Neurosurg 1987;67:500.
94. Muller PJ, Wilson BC. Photodynamic therapy of malignant primary brain tumors: Clinical effects, post-operative ICP, and light penetration of the brain. Photochem Photobiol 1987;46:929.
95. Pass HI, Delaney T, Smith PD, et al. Bronchoscopic phototherapy at comparable dose rates: Early results. Ann Thorac Surg 1989;47:693–699.
96. Kato H. Lung cancer. In: Hayata Y, Dougherty TJ, eds. Lasers and hematoporphyrin derivative in cancer. Tokyo: Kgaka-Shion, 1983:39.
97. Kato H, Aizawa K, Ono J, et al. Clinical measurement of tumor fluorescence using a

new diagnostic system with hematoporphyrin derivative, laser photoradiation, in a spectroscope. Lasers Surg Med 1984;4:49–58.
98. Edell ES, Cortese DA. Detection and phototherapy of lung cancer. In: Morstyn G, Kaye A, eds. Phototherapy of cancer. London: Harwood Academic Publishers, 1990:185.
99. Doiron DR, Balchum OJ. Hematoporphyrin derivative photoradiation therapy of endobronchial lung cancer. In: Andreoni A, Bucedda R, eds. Porphyrin in tumor phototherapy. New York: Plenum Press, 1984:195.
100. Balchum OJ, Doiron DR, Huth GC. Photodynamic therapy of obstructing lung cancer. In: Doiron DR, Gomer CJ, eds. Porphyrin localization and treatment of tumors. New York: Alan R Liss, 1984:721.
101. Balchum OJ. Photodynamic therapy of endobronchial lung tumors. [Abstract] Clayton Foundation Conference, 1987.
102. Vincent RG, Dougherty TJ, Rao U. Photoradiation therapy in the treatment of advanced carcinoma of the trachea and bronchus. In: Doiron DR, Gomer CJ, eds. Porphyrin localization and treatment of tumors. New York: Alan R Liss, 1984:759.
103. Forbes IJ, Ward AD, Jacka FJ, et al. Multidisciplinary approach to phototherapy in tumors. In: Doiron DR, Gomer CJ, eds. Porphyrin localization and treatment of tumors. New York: Alan R. Liss, 1984:693.
104. Lam S, Kostashuk EC, Coy P, et al. A randomized comparative study of the safety and efficacy of photodynamic therapy using Photofrin II combined with palliative radiotherapy alone in patients with inoperable non-small cell bronchogenic carcinoma: A preliminary redport. Photochem Photobiol 1987;5:893–898.
105. Hugh-Jones P, Gardner WN. Laser photodynamic therapy for inoperable bronchogenic carcinoma. J Med 1987;243:565–581.
106. Li JH, Zhao HZ. Photodynamic therapy of bronchogenic carcinoma. Proceedings of the Third Biennial Meeting of the International Photodynamic Association [Abstract] 1990:8:5–10.
107. Benov E, Kostadinov D, Vlasov V. Photoradiation therapy of bronchial cancer. Proceedings of the Third Biennial Meeting of the International Photodynamic Association [Abstract] 1990;8:3–31.
108. Lam S, Palcic B, McLean D, et al. Detection of early lung cancer using low dose Photofrin II. Chest [Abstract] 1990;97:333–337.
109. Hayata Y, Kato H, Konaka C, et al. Photoradiation therapy with hematoporphrin derivative in early and stage 1 lung cancer. Chest 1984;86:169–177.
110. Kato H, Konaka C, Kawate N, et al. Five-year disease-free survival of a lung cancer patient treated only by photodynamic therapy. Chest 1986;90:768–770.
111. Kato H, Konaka C, Yamamoto H, et al. Photodynamic therapy in early stage lung cancer. Proceedings of the Third Biennial Meeting of the International Photodynamic Association [Abstract] 1990;8:4–31.
112. Pass HI, Tochner Z, Delaney T, et al. Intraoperative photodynamic therapy for malignant mesothelioma. [Abstract] Ann Thorac Surg 1990;50:687–688.
113. Bruce RA Jr, McCaughan JS. Lasers in uveal melanoma. Ophthamol Clin North Am 1989;2:597.
114. Tse DT, Dutton JJ, Weingeist TA, et al. Hematoporphyrin photoradiation therapy for intraocular and orbital malignant melanoma. Arch Opthalmol 1984;102:833.
115. Sery TW, Shield JA, Augsburger JJ, et al. Photodynamic therapy of human ocular cancer. Ophthal Surg 1987;18:413.
116. Murphree AL, Cote M, Gomer CJ. The evolution of photodynamic therapy techniques in the treatment of intraocular tumors. Photochem Photobiol 1987;46:919.
117. Sery TW. Photodynamic killing of retinoblastoma cells with hematoporphyrin and light. Cancer Res 1979;39:96.
118. McCaughan JS Jr, Nims TA, Guy JT, et al. Photodynamic therapy for esophageal tumors. Arch Surg 1989;124:74.
119. Thomas RJ, Abbott M, Bhathal PS, et al. High-dose photoradiation of esophageal cancer. Ann Surg 1987;206:193.
120. Aida M, Hirashima T. Cancer of the esophagus. In: Hayata Y, Dougherty TJ, eds. Lasers and hematoporphyrin derivative in cancer. New York: Igaku-Shoin, 1983:57.
121. Hayata T, Kato H, Okitsu H, et al. Photodynamic therapy with hematoporphyrin derivative in cancer of the upper gastrointestinal tract. Semin Surg Oncol 1985;1:1.
122. Okuda S, Mimura S, Otani T, et al. Experimental and clinical studies on HpD-photoradiation therapy for upper gastrointestinal cancer. In: Andreoni A, Cubeddu R, eds. Porphyrins in tumor phototherapy. New York: Plenum Press, 1984:413.
123. Agrez MV, Wharen RE, Anderson RE, et al. Hematoporphyrin derivative: Quantitative derivative: Quantitative uptake in demethylhydrazine-induced murine colorectal carcinoma. J Surg Oncol 1983;24:173.
124. Wooten RS, Ahlquist DA, Anderson RE, et al. Localization of hematoporphyrin derivative to human colrectal cancer. Cancer 1989;64:1569–1576.
125. Dal Fanter M, Bottiroli G, Spinelli P. Behavior of hematoporphyrin derivative in adenomas and adenocarcinomas of the colon: A microfluorometric study. Lasers Med Sci 1988;3:165.
126. Barr H, Tralau CJ, Lewin M, et al. Selective destruction of experimental colon cancer using photodynamic therapy. Br J Surg 1988;75:611.
127. Barr H, Tralau CJ, MacRobert AJ, et al. Photodynamic therapy in the normal rat colon with phthalocyanine sensitisation. Br J Cancer 1987;56:111.
128. Barr H, Krasner N, Boulos PB., et al. Photodynamic therapy for colorectal cancer: A quantitative pilot study. Br J Surg 1990;77:93.
129. Shulok JR, Klaunig JE, Selman SH, et al. Cellular effects of hematoporphyrin derivative photodynamic therapy on normal and neoplastic rat bladder cells. Am J Pathol 1986;122: 277.
130. Jocham D, Staehler G, Chaussy C, et al. Laserbehandlung von blasentumoren nach photosensibilisierung mit hämatoporphyrin-derivat. Urologe 1981;20:340.
131. Benson RC Jr, Farrow GM, Kinwey JH, et al. Detection and localization of in situ carcinoma of the bladder with hematoporphyrin derivative. Mayo Clin Proc 1982;57: 548.
132. Tsuchiya A, Obara N, Miwa M, et al. Hematoporphyrin derivative and laser photoradiation in the diagnosis and treatment of bladder cancer. J Urol 1983;130:79.
133. Hisazumi H, Misaki T, Miyoshi N. Photoradiation therapy of bladder tumors. J Urology 1983;130:685.
134. Benson RC Jr. Laser photodynamic therapy for bladder cancer. Mayo Clin Proc 1986;61: 859.
135. Prout GR Jr, Lin C, Benson R Jr, et al. Photodynamic therapy with hematoporphyrin derivative in the treatment of superficial transitional-cell carcinoma of the bladder. N Engl J Med 1987;317:1251.
136. Benson RC Jr. Treatment of diffuse transitional cell carcinoma in situ by whole bladder hematoporphyrin derivative photodynamic therapy. J Urology 1985;134:675.
137. Hisazumi H, Miyoshi N, Naito K, et al. Whole bladder wall photoradiation therapy for carcinoma in situ of the bladder: A preliminary report. J Urology 1984;131:884.
138. Nseyo UO, Dougherty TH, Sullivan L. Photodynamic therapy in the management of resistant lower urinary tract carcinoma. Cancer 1987;60:3113.
139. Nseyo UO, Whalen TK, Duncan MR, et al. Urinary cytokines following photodynamic therapy for bladder cancer: A preliminary report. Urology 1990;36:167.
140. Harty JI, Amin M, Wieman TJ, et al. Complications of whole bladder dihematoporphyrin ether photodynamic therapy. J Urol 1989;141:1341.
141. Nseyo UO, Dougherty TJ, Boyle DG, et al. Study of factors mediating effect of photodynamic therapy of bladder in canine bladder model. Urology 1988;32:41.
142. Star W, Marijnissen HPA, Jansen H, et al. Light dosimetry for photodynamic therapy by whole bladder wall irradiation. Photochem Photobiol 1987;46:619.
143. Dugan M, Crawford E, Nseyo U, et al. A randomized trial of observation (obs) vs photodynamic therapy after transurethral resection (TUR) or superficial papillary bladder carcinoma. Proc Am Soc Clin Oncol [Abstract] 1991;10:173.
144. Ward BG, Forbes IJ, Cowled PA, et al. The treatment of vaginal recurrences of gynecologic malignancy with phototherapy following hematoporphyrin derivative pretreatment. Am J Obstet Gynecol 1982;142:356.
145. Soma H, Akiya K, Nutahara S, et al. Treatment of vaginal carcinoma with laser photoirradiation following administration of haematoporphyrin derivative. Ann Chir Gynaecol 1982;71:133.
146. Dahlman A, Wile AG, Burns RG, et al. Laser photoradiation therapy of cancer. Cancer Res 1983;43:430.
147. Rettenmaier MA, Berman ML, Disaia PJ, et al. Gynecologic uses of photoradiation therapy. In: Doiron DT, Gomer CJ, eds. Porphyrin localization and treatment of tumors. New York: Alan R Liss, 1984:767.
148. McCaughan JS Jr, Schellhas HF, Lomano J, et al. Photodynamic therapy of gynecologic neoplasms after presensitization with hematoporphyrin derivative. Lasers Surg Med 1985;5:491.
149. Corti L, Tomio L, Maluta S, et al. Photodynamic therapy in gynecological cancer. Lasers Med Sci 1989;4:155.
150. Lele SB, Piver MS, Mang TS, et al. Photodynamic therapy in gynecologic malignancies. Gynecol Oncol 1989;34:350.
151. Lobraico RV, Waldow SM, Harris DM, et al. Photodynamic therapy for cancer of the lower female genital tract. Colops Gynecol Laser Surg 1986;2:185.
152. DeLaney TF, Sindelar W, Smith P, et al. Initial experience with photodynamic therapy for intraperitoneal carcinomatosis. In: Sharp F, Mason WP, Leake RE, eds. Ovarian cancer: Biological and therapeutic challenges. London: Chapman and Hall Medical, 1990:371.
153. Sindelar WF, DeLaney TF, Tochner Z, et al. Technique of photodynamic therapy for disseminated intraperitoneal malignancies: Phase I study. Arch Surg 1991;126:318.
154. DeLaney TF, Sindelar WG, Tochner Z, et al. Phase 1 study of debulking surgery and photodynamic therapy for disseminated intraperitoneal tumors. Int J Radiat Oncol Biol Phys [Abstract] 1991;21:183.

CLAIR J. BEARD
C. NORMAN COLEMAN
TIMOTHY J. KINSELLA

SECTION **9**

Radiation Sensitizers

The cause of the failure of irradiation to locally control solid tumors is multifactorial but may be divided into three broad categories: an excessive number of clonogenic cells, intrinsic cellular characteristics, and environmental factors. Intrinsic cellular characteristics include cell kinetics of a tumor and the capacity to repair radiation damage.[1,2] Intratumoral cellular and environmental heterogeneity makes it likely that multiple factors are operative.[3–7]

A cell that might be sensitive to irradiation under normal physiologic conditions may become resistant due to its microenvironment within the tumor.[8] The nutritional status, pH, and degree of oxygenation contribute to treatment resistance.[9–11] Although each factor is likely to be important, clinical and laboratory research has focused on tumor hypoxia as a potentially important factor limiting local control after treatment with radiation therapy.[12–16] This chapter emphasizes two major areas of radiation sensitization under investigation: the hypoxic cell sensitizers and the halopyrimidines. Although a substantial effort in the development of radiation sensitizers has focused on the oxygen effect and the halopyrimidines, there are numerous potential factors causing radiation failure, and even an effective hypoxic cell or halopyrimidine sensitizer is not a panacea for local tumor persistence.[9,17–20]

THERAPEUTIC STRATEGIES FOR HYPOXIC CELLS

Hypoxic cell sensitizers fall within the broader category of chemical modifiers of cancer treatment.[8,9,21–23] Chemical modifiers are usually not cytotoxic by themselves but modify or enhance the tissue response to standard radiation therapy. The ultimate utility of a radiotherapy or chemotherapy modifier depends on its ability to alter the therapeutic index, which is the ratio of toxicity to efficacy. For a modifier to be beneficial, it must enhance curability more than toxicity; tumor cells must be more affected than normal tissues. Conceptual knowledge of the mechanism of radiation cell killing, the competition model, and the physiology of hypoxia are briefly reviewed to facilitate the understanding of the current therapeutic approaches.

MECHANISMS OF RADIATION CELL KILLING AND THE COMPETITION MODEL

Radiation causes cell death by damaging a critical target within the cell. Evidence for chromosomal DNA as the principle target is circumstantial but overwhelming; nuclear membrane damage may also be important.[24] Ionizing radiation interacts with molecules inside the cell to produce free radicals directly within the DNA (direct effect) or in molecules able to diffuse to and damage the DNA (indirect effect). Cell death probably occurs after a sufficient number of double-stranded DNA breaks are produced by ionization of the DNA or during the enzymatic repair process.[25]

Although the precise mechanism of radiation damage is not fully understood, the competition model is useful for visualizing the potential roles of hypoxic sensitizers and protectors. Figure 69–31 illustrates the competition model. DNA· represents ionized (damaged) DNA; its fate is determined by two competing processes, protection and sensitization.

In theory, an oxygen mimetic hypoxic cell sensitizer can replace oxygen leading to the stable lesion, DNA-sensitizer; the precise chemistry of this interaction is unknown.[26] The processes in which DNA radicals are stabilized by oxygen or an oxygen-mimetic sensitizer is called sensitization. Two of the primary clinical approaches to irradiation and chemotherapy modification are hypoxic-cell sensitization and thiol modulation. Before reviewing the currently available literature, it may be helpful to review the physiology and clinical importance of tumor hypoxia.

THE OXYGEN EFFECT

Awareness of the importance of oxygen in tissue response to irradiation can be traced back to 1921, when Holthusen found

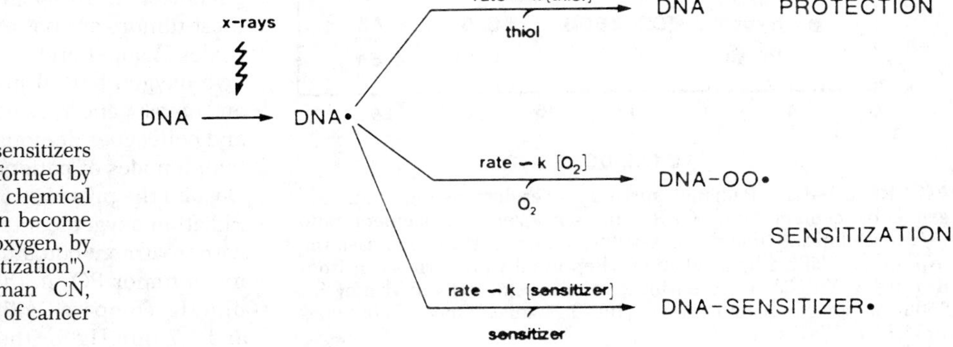

FIGURE 69–31. Competition between sensitizers and protectors. The DNA radical (DNA·) formed by the ionizing radiation may rapidly undergo chemical restitution ("protection"), or the lesion can become stabilized by oxygen or, in the absence of oxygen, by an oxygen-mimetic radiosensitizer ("sensitization"). (Reprinted with permission from Coleman CN, Bump EA, Kramer RA. Chemical modifiers of cancer therapy. J Clin Oncol 1988;6:709–733)

that larger doses of radiation were needed to inactivate sea urchin eggs rendered hypoxic by liquid nitrogen.[15] Since that time, it has been repetitively demonstrated in vitro that to achieve the same proportion of cell killing, about three times the radiation dose is required for hypoxic cells compared with that for well oxygenated cells.[27] The ratio of dose required for a given level of cell killing under hypoxic conditions compared with the dose needed in air is called the oxygen enhancement ratio (OER) (Fig. 69–32).[24] It is estimated that even a 2% or 3% proportion of hypoxic cells within a tumor may double the radiation dose needed for permanent local control.[14,27] For relatively large single doses of radiation, the OER is in the range of 3, and for clinically relevant smaller doses of radiation (200 cGy per fraction) the OER is approximately 2.[28,29] Oxygen has the ability to sensitize cells to ionizing radiation even at clinically relevant radiation doses.

Hypoxic cells are relatively radioresistant, but how important is hypoxia in clinical radiotherapy? Although the answer to this question remains unknown, this is an area of intense laboratory and clinical research and much information suggests that hypoxia may be important in certain situations.

TYPES OF HYPOXIA

The classic model of chronic hypoxia was developed by Thomlinson and Gray who found the pathologic appearance in lung cancer specimens of small necrotic volumes at set distances from capillaries.[30] They calculated that hypoxic but viable cells could be present at a radial distance of up to 130 to 150 μm from the nearest capillary, because oxygen is metabolized and consumed by the cells closest to the vessel. In this model, it is assumed that the nutrient vessel remains patent and that the hypoxic cells are confined to the area surrounding the necrosis (Fig. 69–33). These chronically hypoxic cells have diffusion limited hypoxia.

A second kind of hypoxia can be demonstrated in animal tumors. Due to the dysfunctional opening and closing of tumor vessels, transient or intermittent hypoxia occurs.[31,32] In the intermittent hypoxia model, cells irradiated when blood flow is present behave radiobiologically as oxygenated cells. When blood flow transiently stops, existing oxygen and other nutrients are rapidly exhausted, leaving cells that were perfused by that vessel in a temporarily ischemic state. If irradiation is given when these cells are not perfused, these cells will behave radiobiologically as hypoxic cells. These intermittently hypoxic cells can be conceived as having perfusion-limited hypoxia. Experiments in murine systems indicate that, in general, the percentage of hypoxic cells within a tumor remains relatively stable during a course of fractionated irradiation rather than increasing, as might be expected with the selective killing of aerobic cells.[16,33,34] A process called reoxygenation occurs between radiation fractions and may explain the success of fractionated radiotherapy in curing relatively large size tumors.[33] The mechanism of reoxygenation is unknown, and the degree to which it occurs during radiation therapy in the clinic awaits the further development of methods to identify and quantitate hypoxic cells.

Although the dominant form of tissue hypoxia in human tumors is unknown, the potential existence of two types of hypoxia has important implications for attempts to overcome hypoxic radioresistance. A radiosensitizer that diffuses well through tissue without being rapidly metabolized should reach the inner core of chronically hypoxic cells as well as the well-perfused intermittently hypoxic cells.

IDENTIFYING HYPOXIC CELLS

Clinical assays able to identify and quantitate hypoxic cells in a simple and reproducible manner would have great utility in the evaluation of tumor hypoxia. Ideally, these assays would identify areas of chronic and intermittent hypoxia. Although indirect evidence of tumor hypoxia exists, attention has recently been turned to direct measurement of hypoxia in tumors. Oxygen electrodes can be introduced directly into tumors with visual or under computed tomography (CT) guidance.[35–38] Although these techniques are complicated and most tumors are not accessible for implantation of the electrodes, Vaupel and colleagues were able to measure the in vivo oxygen partial pressure values of normal breast tissue and breast cancer, as demonstrated by Figure 69–34. Gatenby and colleagues demonstrated the presence of hypoxia in the lymph nodes of patients with head and neck malignancies.[38] Despite the presence of intratumoral heterogeneity, the preradiation oxygen content in the lymph nodes correlated well with treatment outcome. For tumors of 4 cm in diameter, the mean tumor PO_2 in the complete remission group was 20.6 mm Hg, compared with 8.8 mm Hg for the partial responders and 4.7 mm Hg for the nonresponders.

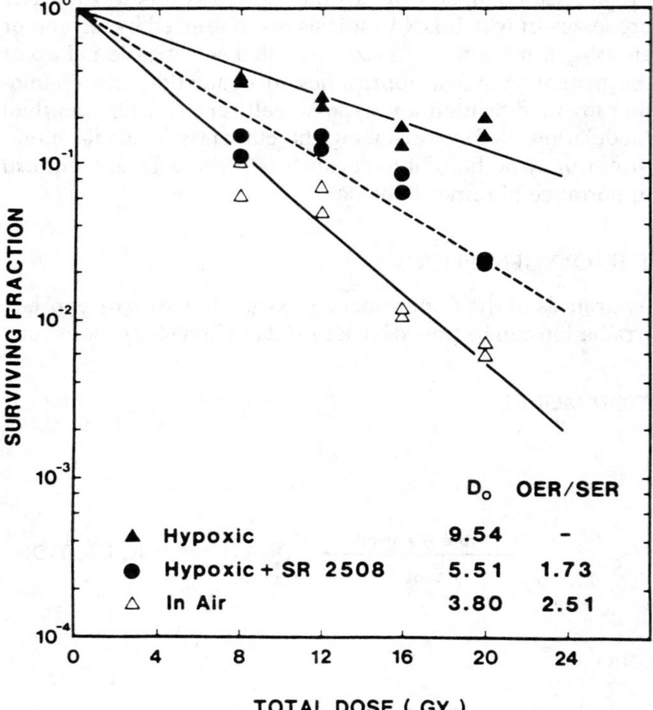

FIGURE 69–32. Radiation survival curves demonstrating the oxygen enhancement ratio (OER) and sensitizer enhancement ratio (SER) at clinically relevant doses. Oxygen or sensitizer increase the hypoxic cell killing by irradiation. (Reprinted with permission from Brown JM, Yu NY. Radiosensitization of hypoxic cells in vivo by SR 2508 at low radiation doses. Int J Radiat Oncol Biol Phys 1984;10:1207–1212)

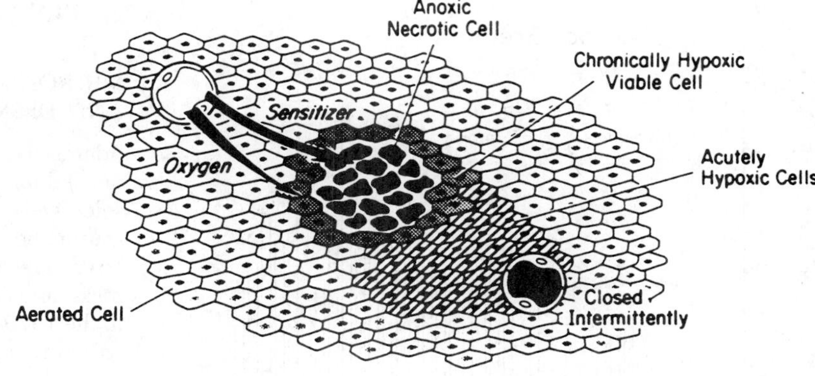

Approaches to Chronic Hypoxia

- Increase Oxygen Delivery
  - Transfusion
  - Hyperbaric Oxygen
  - Perfluorochemical
  - Altered Hgb Affinity for O_2
- Hypoxic Cell Sensitizers
  - ± Thiol modification
- Bioreductive Agents
  - Mitomycin-C
  - Nitroimidazoles
- ? Hyperthermia

Approaches to Acute Hypoxia

- Altered Oxygen Delivery
  - Likely to have minimal impact
- Hypoxic Cell Sensitizers
  - ± Thiol modification
- Bioreductive Agents
  - Would need rapid action under hypoxia
- ? Hyperthermia
- ? Chemotherapy

FIGURE 69–33. Chronic and intermittent hypoxia. Chronically hypoxic cells (*left side*) are diffusion limited. Intermittently hypoxic cells (*right side*) are perfusion limited in that they are hypoxic only if blood flow stops in their nutrient vessel. Possible methods of overcoming acute and chronic hypoxia are suggested. (Reprinted with permission from Coleman CN. Chemical modification of radiation and chemotherapy. In: Cancer: Principles and practice of oncology. Philadelphia: JB Lippincott, 1989:2435–2449)

^{31}P magnetic resonance spectroscopy (MRS) can be used to examine intact tissue and has the advantage of being non-invasive and easily repeated. ^{31}P techniques measure intratumoral phosphorus metabolites and assess tumor metabolism. Metabolism is affected by several physiologic factors including blood flow and oxygen tension. Several investigators have attempted to correlate MRS readings with hypoxia but the heterogeneity of MRS spectral parameters, interfering signals from surrounding tissues, and the presence of hypoxic but metabolically active tumor cells have limited its usefulness.[36,39–42] A similar technique that may be useful is positron emission tomography (PET) scanning for measuring anaerobic glycolysis (indirectly representing hypoxia).[43]

Hypoxic cells preferentially reduce and bind misonidazole at a rate that is three times faster that oxygenated cells.[44] Radiolabeled misonidazole can then be used to indicate the presence of tumor hypoxia.[45–48] Tumor selective retention of fluorinated nitroimidazoles has been demonstrated in vivo by Maxwell and coworkers using magnetic resonance spectroscopy.[49] ^{3}H-misonidazole has been used to identify hypoxic cells in solid animal tumors, multicellular spheroids, and human tumors labeled in vivo.[50–57] Unfortunately, the large doses of ^{3}H required limit the use of this technique in the clinic.

A histologic technique allowing direct visualization of chronic and intermittently hypoxic cells in mice involves sequential intravenous injection of two fluorescent stains, Hoechst 33342, a DNA-binding dye, and DiOC7, a carbocyanine dye.[3,58] Each dye defines cells near blood vessels that were open for the few minutes after administration of the stains. The presence of cells containing one dye and not the other indicates that their perfusion was intermittent.[59]

Ideally, it should be possible to assess the hypoxic state of the cell using intrinsic markers of properties of the cells. Chronic or severe hypoxia can induce metabolic and phenotypic changes in the tumor. Sutherland and colleagues have observed the increased production of a group of proteins, oxygen regulated proteins (ORPs), and reduction of intracellular glutathione content. The induction of ORPs is a general phenomenon that has been observed in a variety of human and rodent cell lines.[60] Although the kinetics vary for the different ORPs, in general synthesis peaks by about 12 hours into hypoxic incubation and declines to aerobic levels after 12 hours of reoxygenation.[61] Whether or not it will be possible to detect stress protein levels or other intrinsic markers in tumors remains to be determined.

A model being used to evaluate cellular phenotypic changes induced by ischemia and reperfusion described by Hlatky and coworkers has demonstrated metabolic (reductive enzyme induction) and phenotypic changes (differentiation) caused by the cellular environment.[62] Although the ideal technique to assess tissue hypoxia remains to be established, methods such as those described will be critical for the understanding of the cellular biology and may be ultimately useful for the tailoring of a treatment plan based on the pretreatment characteristics of the particular tumor.

APPROACHES TO HYPOXIA IN THE CLINIC

Clinicians have attempted to increase oxygen delivery to hypoxic tumors with the use of hyperbaric oxygen, erythrocyte transfusions, and perfluorocarbons.[63–70] The use of the hyperbaric oxygen chamber was the first widely explored approach. A total of nine prospective randomized trials were performed, but only three gave statistically significant positive results for the use of hyperbaric oxygen.[71] Because of the difficulty in hyperbaric oxygen administration, radiation therapy

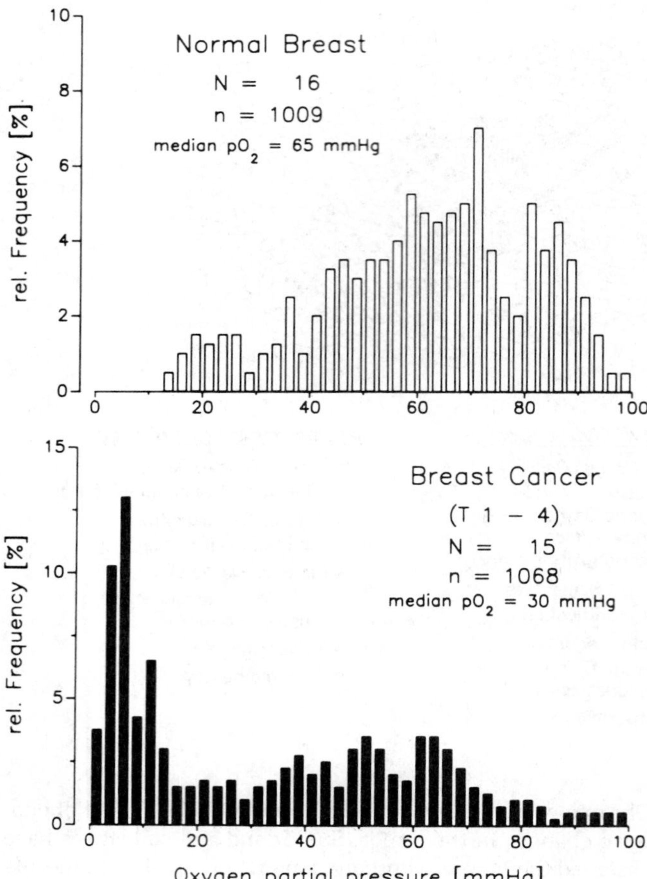

FIGURE 69–34. Frequency distributions of measured oxygen partial pressures (pO_2 histograms) for normal breast tissue (*top*) and for breast cancers (pooled data for pathologic stages T1–T4, *bottom*). (Reprinted with permission from Vaupel P, Schlenger K, Knoop C, Hockel M. Oxygenation of human tumors: Evaluation of tissue oxygen distribution in breast cancers by computerized O_2 tension measurements. Cancer Res 1991;51:3316–3332)

was often administered in few high-dose fractions that did not take full advantage of reoxygenation and that might have led to increased normal tissue injury.[69,71] Nevertheless, the results were of biologic interest.

A second approach toward increased oxygen delivery involved the use of erythrocyte transfusions. Retrospective studies looking at the effect of low initial hemoglobin on local tumor control or overall survival yielded indirect evidence that radiotherapy is less effective in the presence of anemia.[67–70] These findings should be interpreted with caution, because it can be difficult to correct for other important prognosticators such as stage and size of tumors in a retrospective setting.[72] However, a prospective, randomized trial using erythrocyte transfusion did improve the results of treatment of cervical cancer.[68] A phase I–II study of the perfluorochemical oxygen-carrying emulsion Fluosol-DA and 100% O_2 as adjunct to radiotherapy in the treatment of advanced malignancies of the head and neck was sufficiently promising to proceed to a phase III trial (now in progress).[72–74] Although these data are not conclusive, they are sufficiently encouraging to lead to efforts to develop other methods of overcoming hypoxia.

HYPOXIC CELL SENSITIZERS

METRONIDAZOLE, MISONIDAZOLE, AND DESMETHYMISONIDAZOLE

Adams and colleagues described the properties that would be needed for a hypoxic cell sensitizer.[75] The compound should selectively sensitize hypoxic cells at a clinically safe concentration, be chemically stable with slow metabolic breakdown, be capable of diffusing a considerable distance through a tumor mass, and be effective at clinically relevant radiation doses.[33] In the 1970s, researchers began to study drugs with a chemical structure associated with increased electron affinity. The nitroimidazole compounds have been the most interesting and most tested class of drugs meeting these criteria.

The effectiveness of a sensitizer is generally expressed as the sensitizer enhancement ratio (SER). The SER (like the OER) is the dose of radiation required to produce a defined level of killing without sensitizer divided by the dose of radiation required for the same level of cell killing with the sensitizer. Because oxygen is the best "oxygen-like" sensitizer, the SER should, at best, equal the OER, unless the sensitizer has inherent cytotoxic properties or provides sensitization by mechanisms beyond the oxygen effect.[76]

The first compound tested was the 5-nitroimidazole, metronidazole. Marketed as Flagyl and already approved for use in humans as an antitrichimonal agent, metronidazole had an SER of 1.3 to 1.6, depending on the dose of drug used.[27] In the classic randomized trial by Urtasun and colleagues, patients with glioblastoma multiforme were treated with 330 cGy three times a week for 3 weeks with metronidazole plus irradiation or irradiation alone.[77] The median survival of the sensitizer group, 7 months, was superior to the 3 month median survival of the controls ($p = 0.02$). However, almost all the patients died by 1 year, and the results of the sensitizer group were not superior to historical controls given standard radiation therapy. This study indicated that an oxygen-mimetic sensitizer could demonstrate clinical activity, but that it should be added to the most effective irradiation schema.

Misonidazole was the first in a series of 2-nitroimidazole compounds to be used in the clinic. Because the 2-nitroimidazole compounds are more electron affinic than metronidazole, they are more efficient as hypoxic cell sensitizers (*i.e.*, they produce a greater amount of sensitization for a given dose). Oral misonidazole was evaluated in clinical trials for a wide range of tumor sites. Unfortunately, the maximal tolerated single dose that could be administered was limited by nausea and vomiting and the total dose that could be administered was limited by neuropathy.[78,79] Because of the toxicities associated with misonidazole, it was necessary to use a modest drug dose with only a few radiation fractions, yielding a low SER and leaving most of the radiation fractions unsensitized. In retrospect, it would have been surprising if misonidazole produced a major therapeutic benefit in the clinic.[8]

When Dische reviewed the results of 33 clinical trials with misonidazole, only five showed some possible benefit to the use of this drug.[80] Four of these five positive trials were from twelve head and neck cancer studies. A large randomized trial in Denmark (1979–1985) suggested that misonidazole was of benefit for male patients with pharyngeal cancer, with an overall disease-free survival rate of 46% for the misonidazole group, compared with 26% for controls. The misonidazole group had a superior 3-year survival rate, 59% compared with 39% for controls (*p* value not stated).[81] This finding was not confirmed in a retrospective analysis of the RTOG trial, in which patients with stage III and IV head and neck malignancies experienced no benefit with the addition of misonidazole to standard radiotherapy in terms of local or regional control, disease-free survival, or overall survival.[82]

ETANIDAZOLE

Using pharmacokinetic principles, Brown, Lee, Workman, and coworkers developed a series of misonidazole analogs designed to be as potent as misonidazole but less toxic.[83–88] These drugs were designed to be less lipid soluble to decrease their ability to permeate nervous system tissue and to facilitate metabolic clearance. Because the critical element in oxygen mimetic sensitization is the concentration of drug only at the time of irradiation, rapid elimination is desirable because drug remaining after irradiation would produce toxicity without benefit. The two compounds judged to be of greatest interest were etanidazole (SR 2508) and pimonidazole (Ro-03- 8799).[83–89]

Etanidazole produces significantly less neurotoxicity than misonidazole and doses of up to 36 to 40 g/m^2 can be given over 4 to 6 weeks.[90,91] In the RTOG phase I trial, 30% of patients experienced a peripheral neuropathy when receiving a total of 34 to 36 g/m^2.[90,91] A retrospective evaluation of the phase I data indicated that the risk of neuropathy in any given patient could be predicted from their individual pharmacokinetic profile (Fig. 69–35).[91] A series of plasma levels obtained at several specific time points after administration of etanidazole are used to generate the area under the concentration versus time curves (AUC) that remains constant throughout a course of treatment.[91,92] For a single dose of 2 g/m^2, a typical single-dose AUC is approximately 2.2 mM.hour but can be more than 5 mM.hour. Multiplying the single dose AUC by the number of drug administrations yields the total AUC, a measure of drug exposure. The risk of neurotoxicity increases with increasing AUC with slightly more drug being tolerated as the overall treatment course lengthened.

As part of a phase II trial for patients with locally advanced adenocarcinoma of the prostate, this model was tested prospectively. The ability to predict, and subsequently prevent, peripheral neuropathy was investigated.[93] Single-dose and total-dose AUCs were calculated for all patients (Fig. 69–36). Group I patients received "standard" etanidazole, 2 g/m^2, three times per week for a total of 17 doses or 34 g/m^2 without schedule modification. Group II patients underwent a schedule modification for an individual AUC more than 2.2 mM.hour (predicted cumulative AUC 36 mM.hour). Group III patients were scheduled to receive 1.8 g/m^2 for 19 doses, but their individual dose size was adjusted to limit their cumulative AUC to approximately 40 mM.hour. The baseline incidence of neurotoxicity in the group I patients was decreased from 65% to 55% with simple dose or schedule modification (group II). However, using pharmacokinetically derived dose individualization, group III patients received 19 treatments as scheduled, but the incidence of neuropathy was decreased to 1 in 19 patients (see Fig. 69–36). By eliminating the high single-dose AUC, the patients in schedule III actually received a higher total dose of drug. Future trials will incorporate the principle of pharmacokinetic monitoring and dose individualization in an attempt to minimize the incidence of peripheral neuropathy and optimize the total amount of sensitizer administered.

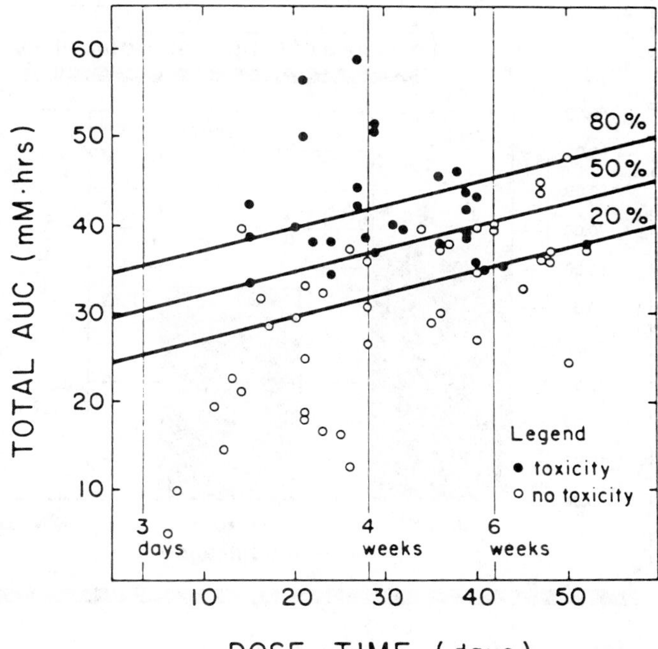

FIGURE 69–35. Risk of developing peripheral neuropathy by drug exposure and duration of treatment course. The total area under the curve (AUC) (mM·h) is derived from the single-dose AUC times the number of doses given. Circles indicate patients without neuropathy (*open circle*) and those with neuropathy (*closed circle*). The three curves indicate the 20%, 50%, and 80% risk of developing peripheral neuropathy. (Reprinted with permission from Coleman CN, Halsey J, Cox RS, et al. Prediction of the neurotoxicity of the hypoxic cell radiosensitizer SR 2508 from the pharmacokinetic profile. Cancer Res 1987;47:319–322)

Efficacy data for etanidazole are not yet available. Randomized clinical trials for head and neck cancer are ongoing under the auspices of the RTOG and in a multicenter European trial.[94,95] Because etanidazole is excreted in the urine, high concentrations have been found in bladder tumors.[96,97] This has generated interest in the use of etanidazole in bladder and prostate cancer. For esophageal tumors, combined-modality treatment with cisplatin, 5-fluorouracil and irradiation plus etanidazole (on the nonchemotherapy weeks) is being evaluated. Because of the relatively high likelihood of distant disease for many of these patients with esophageal cancer, a major improvement in local control rate, possibly with the avoidance of surgery, would affect the quality of life more than survival. The data using combined-modality therapy for esophageal cancer is encouraging in this regard.[98]

Although etanidazole does not appear to penetrate the normal blood-brain barrier (BBB), the BBB integrity may be lost in the presence of a brain tumor.[99–101] As part of a phase I continuous infusion etanidazole plus brachytherapy protocol, the ability of etanidazole to penetrate into malignant gliomas was investigated.[102] In this study, all of the 22 brain tumor patients studied had various concentrations of etanidazole in their brain tumor tissue, confirming the results of Newman

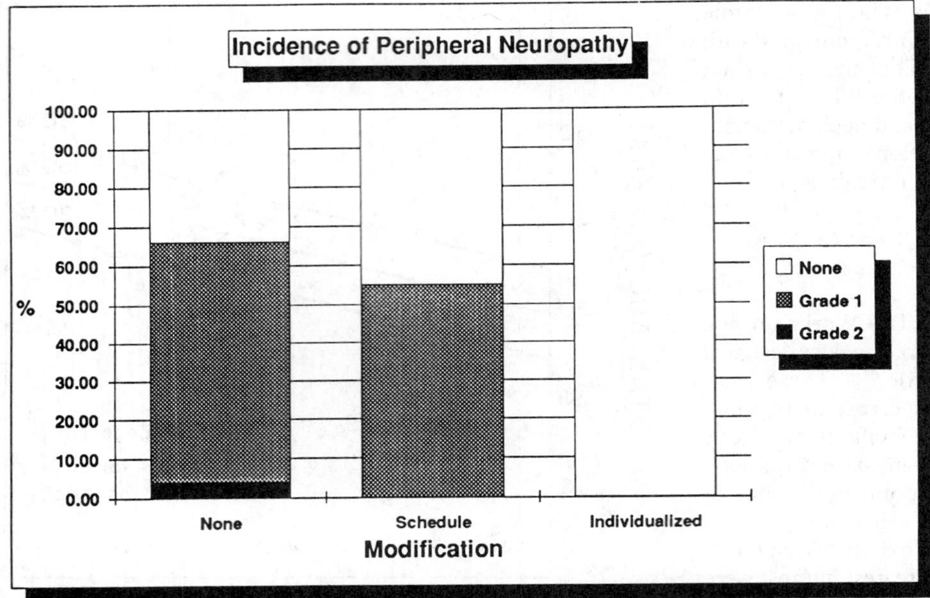

FIGURE 69–36. Risk of developing peripheral neuropathy by modification of etanidazole exposure during treatment using single and total AUC measurements. (Reprinted with permission from Coleman NC, Buswell L, Noll L, et al. The efficacy of pharmacokinetic monitoring and dose modification of etanidazole in the incidence of neurotoxicity: Results from a phase II trial in locally advanced prostate cancer. Radiother Oncol 1991)

and coworkers[103] Etanidazole is currently being evaluated as part of a phase I study of accelerated fraction external-beam irradiation with or without a sensitized implant for patients with newly diagnosed high-grade glioma.

Etanidazole has been evaluated as a continuous infusion accompanying brachytherapy based on laboratory data indicating that a continuous exposure of etanidazole may produce an SER that could exceed the OER.[27,76,104] The precise mechanism of this additional enhancement is unknown but involves metabolic reduction of the drug under hypoxic conditions. Seventy-seven patients were treated on a phase I protocol using continuous infusion etanidazole of 48 or 96 hours' duration while undergoing brachytherapy for locally advanced tumors.[105] A previously unreported toxicity called the cramping arthralgia syndrome limited dose escalation to 20 to 21 g/m^2 over 48 hours and 23 to 24 g/m^2 for patients receiving 96-hour infusions. The cramping arthralgia syndrome consists of relatively severe muscle and joint aches that disappear within hours or days after discontinuing the etanidazole.[93,106] The more classic peripheral neuropathy was only seen in 2 patients. Phase II trials are now ongoing.

Pimonidazole is a basic, lipophilic drug that is concentrated in the acidic environment within tumors.[107,108] It is a more efficient hypoxic cell sensitizer than etanidazole on a molar basis due to its higher electron affinity.[109] A phase I trail using pimonidazole plus etanidazole was conducted in an attempt to increase hypoxic cell sensitization by combining two drugs with different dose-limiting toxicities.[110] For the 48 patients who received both drugs, there was some evidence for toxicity interaction with 40% of the patients not receiving the planned cumulative dose secondary to toxicity.[111] Similar results were reported by Newman and colleagues in their phase I trial and phase I–II trial in brain tumor patients.[112,113] In a recently completed phase III trial of external-beam irradiation (5000 cGy in 5 weeks) with or without pimonidazole, followed by intracavitary treatment, cervical cancer patients who were randomized to receive pimonidazole actually had a lower incidence of clinical complete regression, and statistically significantly lower local control, freedom from distant metastases, disease-free survival, and overall survival.[114] Known prognosticators seemed to be balanced between the two arms of the trial, and the reason for the poor outcome of the sensitizer patients is currently being investigated, although there is speculation that the pimonidazole may have decreased tumor perfusion. No additional clinical trials with pimonidazole are planned.

NIMORAZOLE

The Danish Head and Neck Cancer Group (DAHANCA) is evaluating a 5-nitroimidazole, nimorazole, in a randomized trial of 421 patients with squamous cell cancer of the larynx and pharynx.[115] Patients were randomized to nimorazole (1.2 g/m^2) or placebo with each of the 30 fractions of radiotherapy. Results to date demonstrate a statistically significant improvement in locoregional control (52% versus 33% at 4 years, $p = 0.013$). The dose-limiting toxicity of nimorazole was nausea and vomiting. Although not as electron affinic as the 2-nitroimidazole compounds, an advantage of nimorazole may be the ability to administer it with each radiation treatment. The final results of this study will be of great interest.

DUAL-FUNCTION HYPOXIC CELL SENSITIZERS

This group of compounds is preferentially activated to their toxic species in the presence of hypoxia. This series of 2-nitroimidazole compounds under development additionally has a dual action: oxygen-mimetic sensitization (from the 2-nitroimidazole ring) and an alkylating function (from the aziridine side chain). The prototype for this group is RSU-1069, a 2-nitroimidazole containing a monofunctional, alkylating aziridine ring. RSU-1069 induced a dose-dependent loss of up to 50% of the clonogenic KHT cells in the absence of radiation and greater hypoxic cell sensitization activity than misonidazole in experimental systems.[116–120] Phase I testing revealed severe nausea, limiting its use in the clinic at the present time.[121] However, less toxic analogs, such as RB 6145, are under preclinical development.[122]

BENZOTRIAZINE DIOXIDE

SR 4233 (3-amino-1,2,4-benzotriazine-1,4-dioxide) is a newly developed bioreductive agent developed by Zeman, Brown, and coworkers.[123] It is particularly cytotoxic to hypoxic cells in vitro with 25 to 100 times more drug required to produce a given level of cell killing in aerobic conditions compared with anaerobic ones.[123–125] The mechanism of action remains to be fully defined, but the drug appears to induce DNA strand scission resulting from an oxidative damage to pyrimidines.[126] The free radical 1-electron reduction product, formed rapidly under hypoxic conditions, is thought to be the toxic species.[124,127,128] Analysis of DNA and chromosomal breaks after hypoxic exposure to SR 4233 suggest that DNA double-strand breaks are the primary lesion causing cell death.[129]

Due at least in part to its hypoxic cell cytotoxicity, SR 4233 has been shown to markedly enhance radiation-induced tumor killing in vitro.[124,128,130] This enhancement is seen when SR 4233 is given before or after irradiation.[131] The theoretical benefit to the use of an effective bioreductive agent is indicated in Figure 69–37, which shows the surviving fraction of cells after radiation doses with sensitizers of different properties.[132] Brown mathematically simulated cell survival curves under hypothetical and varied scenarios of irradiation and tumor properties, demonstrating the theoretical benefit to the use of a hypoxic cell toxin.[132,133] In Figure 69–37, it is assumed that a tumor has 20% hypoxic cells and that complete reoxygenation occurs between 200-cGy fractions. Each time a treatment is given, the tumor has 20% hypoxic cells. The curves for SER 1.5 and 2.5 indicate the impact of a hypoxic cell radiosensitizer (*e.g.*, etanidazole) of various potentcies. Similarly, Hyp Cyt indicates the impact of a hypoxic cytotoxic agent that is given with each treatment of irradiation and that kills 50% or 90% of the hypoxic cells. A hypoxic cell sensitizer is less effective than a hypoxic cell cytotoxin if a sufficient number of doses of the hypoxic cell cytotoxin can be administered. Such laboratory and theoretical modeling results are intriguing, and SR 4233 is now in phase I clinical trials.

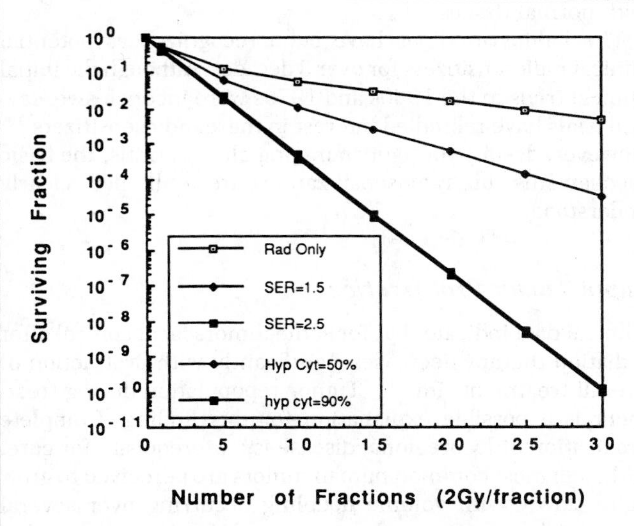

FIGURE 69–37. Surviving fraction of cells of a tumor with 20% hypoxic cells as a function of the number of 2-Gy fractions, assuming no reoxygenation between fractions and no tumor cell repopulation. The lines for SER = 1.5 or 2.5 and Hyp Cyt = 50% or 90% show the projected effect of adding to each radiation dose a hypoxic cell radiosensitizer or a hypoxic cell cytotoxin, each with two efficacies. The lines for SER = 2.5 and Hyp Cyt = 50% and 90% are superimposed. (Reprinted with permission from Brown JM. Therapeutic advantage of hypoxic cells in tumors: A theoretical study. JNCI 1991;83:1778–1784)

TREATMENT WITH RADIATION SENSITIZERS

ALTERATION OF BLOOD FLOW

As a consequence of the introduction of bioreductive agents, attention has been turned to agents that modify blood flow within the tumor and actually induce hypoxia so that the hypoxic cells may then be targeted with bioreductive-cytotoxic radiation sensitizers or hyperthermia.[134] The microcirculation of tumors has been studied extensively and is characterized by low pressure, intermittent stasis, spontaneous hemorrhage, bidirectional flow, and regions of hypoxia.[36,135–137] Tumor vessels are generally thin walled and fragile, lacking the muscular and neuronal components necessary for normal dilation and constriction in response to vasoactive stimuli.[138] Because tumors already have compromised blood flow, a minor change in blood pressure may increase their proportion of hypoxic cells. There is a major interest in the use of systemically administered agents, such as hydralazine, nicotinamide, or flunarazine to alter tumor blood flow and secondarily modulate hypoxia.

Studies have centered on hydralazine, primarily because of its use as an antihypertensive agent. In transplanted rodent and dog tumors, intravenously administered hydralazine has resulted in rather dramatic reductions in tumor blood flow as measured by flow cytometry, MRS, and laser Doppler flowmetry.[139–142] The reduced blood flow and resulting hypoxia seem to potentiate the activity of bioreductive drugs used alone or with irradiation or irradiation with hyperthermia.[128,139,140,143] Unfortunately, the dramatic decrease in blood flow seen in animal tumors has been difficult to recreate in transplanted human tumors xenografted into mice.[144,145] Additionally, Horsman and coworkers demonstrated that a 10% decrease in blood pressure actually resulted in a blood flow increase of approximately 30%.[146]

Another factor that may limit the use of blood flow reduction in the clinic includes the possibility that high doses of agents such as hydralazine could produce focal areas of hypoxia in critical normal tissues and increase the normal tissue toxicity of the bioreductive agents.[139,140] A second potential problem is the heterogeneity of blood vessels within a single tumor mass. Studies have shown that tumor vessels in different parts of the same tumor may respond differently to hydralazine with induction of complete vascular stasis in some areas with relatively normal perfusion in others. The reason for this is unclear but more work will be needed before it is known if this overall approach of blood flow modification is effective or safe in the clinic.

GLUTATHIONE MODIFICATION

Glutathione (GSH), a ubiquitous tripeptide thiol, has important functions in a wide range of cellular functions including metabolism, transport, and protection. GSH is involved in the free radical scavenging of radiation-induced lesions such as hydroxyl radicals, peroxy radicals, and organic radicals, and is a substrate for enzymatic reduction and detoxification of electrophiles such as alkylating agents by means of glutathione-S-transferase. It is the protective functions that are of interest in cancer therapy (see Fig. 69–33).[8] The discovery by Griffith and Meister that GSH synthesis could be manipulated by BSO (D,L-buthionine-S,R-sulfoximine) has generated great interest in glutathione manipulation as a method of sensitizing cells to the effects of irradiation.[147,148]

L-BSO

Glutathione is a tripeptide, gammaglutamyl-cysteinyl-glycine. The enzyme γ-glutamylcysteine synthetase acts to combine glutamate with cysteine to produce gammaglutamylcysteine. Glutathione synthetase then acts on this product plus glycine to produce glutathione. L-BSO inhibits the enzyme gammaglutamylcysteine synthetase and prevents the de novo synthesis of GSH. The kinetics of GSH depletion depend on the pharmacokinetics of L-BSO and on the rate of depletion and resynthesis of GSH. Although data from human studies are not yet available, Kramer and colleagues demonstrated that after a single-dose of L-BSO to mice, the time course for depletion and recovery of GSH concentration varies from tissue to tissue with liver, stomach, and lung recovering faster than kidney and heart.[149]

To understand and optimally use L-BSO, it is critical to be able to monitor GSH concentration within tumor and normal tissue. O'Dwyer and coworkers are measuring GSH concentration in circulating monocytes to monitor GSH depletion, but it is not clear that this correlates with thiol content of tumor or critical normal tissues.[150] Ongoing work with MRS to measure the cellular thiol reduction-oxidative state is encouraging but the technique has not yet been applied to solid tumors.[151] BSO is currently under investigation in the phase I setting as a chemomodifier of alkylating agents, and no toxicity has been demonstrated with doses of 1000 to 4800 mg/m^2/dose in the twenty patients entered.[150,152]

GSH Depletion and Radiation Therapy

The clinical utility of GSH depletion to decrease protection, as illustrated in Figure 69–33, depends greatly on the therapeutic ratio (*i.e.*, extent of depletion, loss of protection) in the target tissue compared with the effect of GSH depletion (*i.e.*, loss of protection and other functions) in normal tissues. Some researchers have found that GSH depletion alone sensitizes hypoxic cells to radiation without affecting the sensitivity of aerobic cells.[153–156] Under these circumstances, GSH depletion would produce a therapeutic advantage. Other investigators found various degrees of aerobic sensitization after GSH depletion, a discrepancy due to the much greater degree of GSH depletion in the latter experiments.[157–161] In any case, GSH depletion by itself is not likely to be a useful strategy to enhance the radiation effect.

Hodgkiss and colleagues demonstrated that GSH depletion can greatly enhance the efficacy of a single dose of misonidazole.[162] Similar results have been obtained with BSO and other hypoxic cell sensitizers such as etanidazole and pimonidazole.[162–167] The work by Kramer and coworkers revealed that BSO significantly enhanced the SER of etanidazole with fractionated radiotherapy in vitro from 1.2 to 1.4 in the relatively aerobic RIF tumor model and from 1.4 to 1.8 in the relatively hypoxic MCA tumor model.[149] Etanidazole toxicity, measured as the LD_{50} dose, was doubled in animals receiving BSO but only at doses of etanidazole that exceeded the optimal therapeutic dose.

The enhancement of hypoxic sensitization by L-BSO may be most important in cells that have a high endogenous concentration of GSH, a phenomena seen in several human tumor cell lines.[168–170] This hypothesis was tested by Degraff and coworkers who analyzed five nitroimidazole hypoxic cell sensitizers in A549 cells (high in GSH) and V79 cells (low in GSH).[184] They were able to demonstrate enhanced sensitization in the A549 cells after pretreatment with BSO, particularly with the sensitizer pimonidazole but also with etanidazole. Although the available data are limited, these results are interesting and it may be that L-BSO can be used to enhance the cytotoxicity and sensitizing effects of clinically available hypoxic cell sensitizers like etanidazole.

HALOPYRIMIDINE RADIOSENSITIZERS

Another strategy to improve the efficacy of radiation therapy is the use of the halogenated pyrimidine analogs (*e.g.*, IUDR, BUDR, FUDR, 5-FU). These drugs are taken up and metabolized only by cells actively synthesizing DNA.[194,195] Drug uptake by adjacent or dose-limiting normal tissues could limit the therapeutic gain for radiosensitization of tumor compared with normal tissues.

The halopyrimidines have been recognized as potential clinical radiosensitizers for over 3 decades. Although the initial clinical trials in the 1960s and 1970s were inconclusive, several trials have rekindled interest in these radiosensitizers.[196] However, despite these encouraging clinical trials, the basic mechanisms of radiosensitization are still not clearly understood.

Rapid Tumor Proliferation

Clinical data indicate that for some tumors local control after radiation therapy decreases significantly with protraction of overall treatment time.[171] Tumor repopulation during treatment is a possible explanation for this finding. Complete eradication of locoregional disease is a prerequisite for cure. Although most common human tumors are perceived to grow quite slowly with volume doubling occurring over several weeks or longer, it must be recognized that clinical or radiographic volume changes reflect a combination of tumor cell proliferation and tumor cell loss. Cell loss factors in human tumors have been estimated to be as high as 80% to 99%.[197] Tumor volume doublings over many weeks can disguise clonogenic doubling times that can be as rapid as 1 week or less. In a typical conventional fractionated radiotherapy course lasting 6 to 7 weeks, such potentially rapid tumor cell proliferation could significantly reduce tumor cell killing by up to 3 to 4 logs and result in a treatment failure.

With the use of in vivo BrdUrd/IdUrd labeling of S-phase DNA in human tumors followed by analysis with flow cytometry, there is limited but confirmatory data supporting the argument that a sizable proportion of human tumors are proliferating rapidly as measured by the potential doubling time (T_{pot}) as seen in Table 69–38.[171,184] T_{pot} is equal to the cell cycle time divided by the growth fraction (multiplied by log 2). T_{pot} measurements before treatment are thought to be of importance because they may be a reliable indicator of a human tumor's ability to proliferate during therapy.[198] The clinical relevance of pretreatment T_{pot} measurements in at least one common human tumor (head and neck) was highlighted recently.[172]

Metabolic Studies

IUDR, BUDR, and FUDR are a family of deoxyuridine analogs in which the halogen atom is substituted for the methyl group at the 5 position on the pyrimidine ring. FUDR is the deoxyribonucleoside derivative of 5-fluorouracil (5-FU). Structurally, IUDR and BUDR are analogs of thymidine (TDR) and are recognized by the same cellular enzymes that process thymidine to its triphosphate form (dTTF). Thymidine kinase (TK) is the rate-limiting enzyme in this salvage pathway. DNA polymerase then uses IdUTP or BUTP as a substrate for synthesis of DNA. The radiosensitizing effect of IUDR and BUDR are closely associated with DNA incorporation (*i.e.*, radiosensitization parallels the percentage of TDR replacement).[173,174]

The molecular mechanism of radiosensitization by IUDR and BUDR is thought to be induction of highly reactive free radicals (*e.g.*, uracilyl radical) within DNA.[196] Radiation damage as measured by clonogenic survival and induction of single- and double-strand DNA breaks may be increased twofold to threefold with prior incorporation of these analogs.[199,200] This effect on irradiation is most noticeable in the clinically relevant range of radiation dose as measured by changes in the shoulder, alpha component of the LQ formula, or survival at 200 cGy.[174–177]

Although the fluoropyrimidines (FUDR, 5-FU) share similar metabolic pathways as the TDR analogs, the mechanism of radiosensitization is less well understood and presumably does not involve DNA incorporation. Both FUDR and 5-FU inhibit thymidylate synthase (TS) after conversion to FdUMP using TK. This inhibition is believed to be the principle mechanism of cytotoxicity and possibly radiosensitization mediated through imbalances in the triphosphate pool and subsequent altered DNA damage repair.[178] Because 5-FU affects processing of nuclear RNA to ribosomal RNA, these RNA effects might be related to radiosensitization.

Although the interaction of fluoropyrimidines and irradiation has been recognized for over 30 years, there are surprisingly few in vitro data despite the renewed clinical interest.[179] In vitro radiosensitization by 5-FU appears to be schedule dependent, with maximal sensitization occurring only if cytotoxic doses of 5-FU are administrated after irradiation.[180,181] In vivo, the combination of 5-FU and irradiation has proved to be slightly greater than additive in cell killing, but the schedule dependency was weak.[182,183] Another laboratory has been evaluating the in vitro interaction of FUDR and irradiation in human colon cancer cells to further relate TS inhibition and radiosensitization.[184] FUDR was selected instead of 5-FU because FUDR is a more specific inhibitor of TS and has no RNA effects. These results suggest that FUDR radiosensitization occurs with preincubation and does not require extended drug exposure. It appears more related to the effect of extended TS inhibition on cell kinetic changes than to the actual time course of inhibition. Several questions persist regarding the in vitro and in vivo mechanisms of fluoropyrimidine radiosensitization that need further study.

TABLE 69–38. Summary of Potential Doubling Times in Some Common Human Tumors After S-phase Radiosensitizers Have Been Used

Tumor Site (no. of tumors)	*T_{pot} (median)*	*T_{pot} (range)*
Colorectal (100)	5.9 d	2–23 d
Esophageal and gastric (22)	9.8 d	6.8–14 d
Head and neck (102)	5.5 d	1.8–30 d
Malignant glioma (10)	8.4 d	2–13.5 d

(Modified from Miller EM, Kinsella TJ. Radiosensitization by fluorodeoxyuridine: Effects of thymidylate synthase inhibition and cell synchronization. Cancer Res 1992 [in press])

Clinical Results and Future Trial Design

Over the last decade, there has been a resurgence in clinical investigation of halogenated pyrimidines as radiosensitizers for several different tumor sites. As a result, there appears to be an improvement in locoregional tumor control and survival with acceptable normal tissue toxicities.[185–187,189–193] A better understanding of halogenated pyrimidine metabolism opens the possibility of using biochemical modulators of key enzymes (*e.g.*, leucovorin, 5-aminothymidine) to further improve clinical radiosensitization.

Most clinical trials with the TDR analogs (*e.g.*, BUDR, IUDR) have been phase I and II studies involving continuous prolonged (several days or longer) infusions in patients with poorly radioresponsive tumors such as high-grade gliomas and sarcomas, colorectal liver metastases.[185–187] Phase III trials are ongoing for these tumor types and others at the NCI and within RTOG. The optimal clinical approach for BUDR or IUDR has not been clearly defined. Theoretically, the clinical approach should result in adequate DNA replacement (probably only 3% to 10%) in all tumor cells.[188] Based on tumor cell kinetic and radiobiologic data, this most likely will require prolonged continuous relatively low-dose infusion.[188] The use of nontoxic modulators might improve the therapeutic gain, and clinical protocols are being designed to address this approach.

Clinical trial results with the fluoropyrimidine (principally 5-FU) are even more impressive. Several phase III studies have documented an improvement in local control and survival in cancers of the rectum, anus, esophagus, pancreas, and larynx.[189–193] In some trials, study design did not allow a direct comparison to irradiation alone.[192] 5-FU has been administered by bolus or continuous infusion alone or with other drugs (*e.g.*, mitomycin C, cisplatin) that cloud the issue of additive cytotoxicity compared with true sensitization of irradiation.[191,193]

Many ongoing trials have assumed that continuous infusion 5-FU (±leucovorin modulation) is superior as a radiosensitizer, although the preclinical data are confusing.[184,201] It is hoped that further experimental studies will help shape the next generation of clinical trials in fluoropyrimidine radiosensitization.

CONCLUSIONS

This chapter has only addressed two general approaches to radiosensitization. The lack of success to date has been due in part to the toxicities of these compounds at therapeutic doses (*e.g.*, misonidazole) and lack of knowledge of optimal drug timing and scheduling in conjunction with the radiotherapy. Nevertheless, these early efforts have yielded much important information, including identification and quantification of hypoxia in human tumors, newer aspects of assessing tumor cell kinetics, a better understanding of drug pharmacokinetics and toxicities, and interesting results in some of the clinical hypoxic radiosensitizer and halopyrimidine trials. Other radiation-modification approaches are being developed and include the use of altered irradiation schedules based on cell survival parameters or on tumor cell kinetics, and combinations of irradiation and systemic therapies such as chemotherapy, hormonal therapy, biologics, and radioprotectors. Entirely novel approaches, such as GSH depletion and hypoxic cytotoxic therapies, are undergoing evaluation in early clinical trials. Through incremental advances in cancer biology and drug development, there has been steady progress in the radiation modifier field. Combined with improved systemic therapies and surgical approaches, these have the possibility to improve local control, survival, and quality of life.

REFERENCES

1. Barker JL, Montague ED, Peters LJ. Clinical experience with irradiation of inflammatory carcinoma of the breast with and without elective chemotherapy. Cancer 1980;45: 625–629.
2. Norin T, Onyango J. Radiotherapy in Burkitt's lymphoma: Conventional or superfractionated regimen. Int J Radiat Oncol Biol Phys 1977;2:399–406.
3. Fertil B, Malaise EP. Intrinsic radiosensitivity of human cell lines is correlated with radioresponsiveness of human tumors: Analysis of 101 published survival curves. Int J Radiat Oncol Biol Phys 1985;11:1699–1707.
4. Courtenay VD. Radioresistant mutants of L5178Y cells. Radiat Res 1969;38:186–203.
5. Peters LJ, Withers HR, Thames HD, Fletcher GH. Keynote address: The problem: Tumor radioresistance in clinical radiotherapy. Int J Radiat Oncol Biol Phys 1982;8: 101–108.
6. Weichselbaum RR, Nove J, Little JB. Radiation Response of human tumor cells in vitro. In: Radiation biology in cancer research. New York: Raven Press, 1980:345–352.
7. Carmichael J, Hickson ID. Keynote address: Mechanisms of cellular resistance to cytotoxic drugs and x-irradiation. Int J Radiat Oncol Biol Phys 1991;20:197–202.
8. Coleman CN, Bump EA, Kramer RA. Chemical modifiers of cancer therapy. J Clin Oncol 1988;6:709–733.
9. Coleman CN. Hypoxia in tumors: A paradigm for the approach to biochemical and physiological heterogeneity. JNCI 1988;80:310–317.
10. Koch CJ, Meneses JJ, Harris JW. The effect of extreme hypoxia and glucose on the repair of potentially lethal and sublethal radiation damage by mammalian cells. Radiat Res 1977;70:542–551.
11. Varnes ME, Dethlefsen LA, Biaglow JA. The effect of Ph on potentially lethal damage recovery in A549 cells. Radiat Res 1986;108:80–90.
12. Dische S. Review of hypoxic cell sensitizers. Int J Radiat Oncol Biol Phys 1991;20: 147–152.
13. Gray LH, Conger AO, Ebert M, et al. The concentration of oxygen dissolved in tissues at the time of irradiation as a factor in radiotherapy. Br J Radiol 1953;26:638–648.
14. Hall EJ. Welcome and overview. Int J Radiat Oncol Biol Phys 1982;8:323–325.
15. Holthusen H. Beitrage zur biologie der Strahlenwirkung; untersuch ungen an ascarideneiern. Arch Ges Physiol 1921;187:1–24.
16. Howes AE. An estimation of the changes in the proportions and absolute numbers of hypoxic-cells after irradiation of transplanted C3H mouse mammary tumors. Br J Radiol 1969;42:441–447.
17. Adams GE. Hypoxia-mediated drugs for radiation and chemotherapy. Cancer 1980;48: 696–709.
18. Brown JM. Keynote address: Hypoxic cell radiosensitizers: Where next? Int J Radiat Oncol Biol Phys 1989;16:987–993.
19. Fowler JF. Chemical Modifiers of radiosensitivity-theory and reality: A review. Int J Radiat Oncol Biol Phys 1985;11:665–674.
20. Gonzalez DG. Hypoxia and local tumor control. Part I. Radiother Oncol 1991;20:5–7.
21. Coleman CN, Glover DJ, Turrisi AT. Radiation and chemotherapy sensitizers and protectors. Cancer chemotherapy: Principles and practice. Philadelphia: WB Saunders, 1989:225–252.
22. Coleman CN. Modification of radiotherapy by radiosensitizers and cancer chemotherapy agents. I. Radiosensitizers. Semin Oncol 1989;16:169–175.
23. Coleman CN. Hypoxic cell radiosensitizers: Expectations and progress in drug development. Int J Radiat Oncol Biol Phys 1985;11:323–329.
24. Hall EJ. Cell survival curves. In: Radiobiology for the radiologist. 3rd ed. Philadelphia: JB Lippincott, 1988:1–16.
25. Ward JF. Mechanisms of DNA repair and their potential modification for radiotherapy. Int J Radiat Oncol Biol Phys 1986;12:1027–1032.
26. Finklestein E, Glatstein E. Seduced by oxygen. Int J Radiat Oncol Biol Phys 1988;14: 205.
27. Hall EJ, Astor MA, Biaglow J, et al. The enhanced sensitivity of mammalian cells to killing by x-rays after prolonged exposure to several nitroimidazoles. Int J Radiat Oncol Biol Phys 1982;8:447–451.
28. Brown JM, Yu NY. Radiosensitization of hypoxic cells in vivo by SR 2508 at low radiation doses. Int J Radiat Oncol Biol Phys 1984;10:1207–1212.
29. Skarsgard LD, Harrison I, Durand RE, et al. Radiosensitization of hypoxic cells at low doses. Int J Radiat Oncol Biol Phys 1986;12:1075–1078.
30. Thomlinson RH, Gray LH. The histological structure of some human lung cancers and the possible implications for radiotherapy. Br J Cancer 1955;9:539–549.
31. Chaplin DJ, Durand RE, Olive PL. Acute hypoxia in tumors: Implications for modifiers of radiation effects. Int J Radiat Oncol Biol Phys 1986;12:1279–1282.
32. Chaplin DJ, Olive PL, Durand RE. Intermittent blood flow in a murine tumor: Radiobiological effects. Cancer Res 1987;47:597–601.
33. Hall EJ. The oxygen effect and reoxygenation. In: Radiobiology for the radiologist. 3rd ed. Philadelphia: JB Lippincott, 1988:137–160.
34. van Putten LM. Tumor reoxygenation during fractionated radiotherapy: Studies with a transplantable osteosarcoma. JNCI 1968;40:441–451.
35. Carter DB, Silver IA. Quantitative measurements of oxygenation in normal tissues and in the tumors of patients before and after radiotherapy. Acta Radiol 1960;53:233–256.
36. Vaupel P, Frinak S, O'Hara M. Direct measurement of reoxygenation in malignant mammary tumors after a single large dose of irradiation. Adv Expt Med Biol 1984;180: 773–782.
37. Vaupel P, Schlenger K, Knoop C, Hockel M. Oxygenation of human tumors: Evaluation of tissue oxygen distribution in breast cancers by computerized O_2 tension measurements. Cancer Res 1991;51:3316–3322.
38. Gatenby RA, Kessler HB, Rosenblum JS, et al. Oxygen distribution in squamous cell carcinoma metastases and its relationship to outcome of radiation therapy. Int J Radiat Oncol Biol Phys 1988;14:831–838.
39. Fu KK, Wendland MF, Iyer SB, et al. Correlations between in vivo 31P NMR spectroscopy measurements, tumor size, hypoxic fraction and cell survival after radiotherapy. Int J Radiat Oncol Biol Phys 1990;18:1341–1350.
40. Okunieff P, Kallinowski F, Vaupel R, Neuringer LJ. Effects of hydralazine-induced vasodilation on the energy metabolism of murine tumors studied by in vivo 31P-nuclear magnetic resonance spectroscopy. JNCI 1988;80:745–750.
41. Okunieff P, Ramsay J, Tokuhiro T, et al. Estimation of tumor oxygenation and metabolic rate using 31P MRS. correlation of longitudinal relaxation with tumor growth rate and DNA synthesis. Int J Radiat Oncol Biol Phys 1988;14:1185–1195.
42. Rofstad EK, DeMuth P, Fenton BM, et al. 31P NMR spectroscopy and HbO_2 cryospectrophotometry in prediction of tumor radioresistance caused by hypoxia. Int J Radiat Oncol Biol Phys 1989;16:919–924.
43. Frank JA, Alger JR, Bizzi A, et al. In vivo proton magnetic resonance spectroscopy (^{1}HMRS) of human gliomas. Annual Meeting of the American Society for Clinical Oncology, Bethesda, 1990:349.
44. Chapman JD, Franko AJ, Sharplin JA. A marker for hypoxic cells in tumors with potential clinical applicability. Br J Cancer 1981;43:546–550.
45. Biaglow JE. Cellular electron transfer and radical mechanisms for drug metabolism. Radiat Res 1981;86:212–242.
46. Ling L, Streffer C, Sutherland R. Decreased hypoxic toxicity and binding of misonidazole by low glucose concentration. Int J Radiat Oncol Biol Phys 1986;12:1231–1234.
47. Biaglow JE, Varnes ME, Roizin-Towle L, et al. Biochemistry of reduction of nitroheterocycles. Biochem Pharm 1986;35:77–90.
48. Raleigh JA, Franko AJ, Treiber EO, et al. Covalent binding of a fluorinated 2-nitroimidazole to EMT-6 tumors in Balb/C mice: Detection by F-19 nuclear magnetic resonance at 2.35 T. Int J Radiat Oncol Biol Phys 1988;12:1243–1246.
49. Maxwell RJ, Workman R, Griffiths JR. Demonstration of tumor-selective retention of

fluorinated nitroimidazole probes by ^{19}F magnetic resonance spectroscopy in vivo. Int J Radiat Oncol Biol Phys 1989;16:925–930.

50. Chapman JD. The detection and measurement of hypoxic cells in solid tumors. Cancer 1984;54:2441–2449.
51. Horowitz M, Blasberg R, Molnar P, et al. (^{14}C) Misonidazole binding to EMT-6 and V-79 spheroids. Cancer Res 1983;43:3800–3807.
52. Rasey JS, Koh W, Grierson JR, Grunbaum Z, Krohn KA. Radiolabeled fluoromisonidazole as an imaging agent for tumor hypoxia. Int J Radiat Oncol Biol Phys 1989;17:985–991.
53. Franko AJ, Chapman JD, Koch CJ. Binding of misonidazole to EMT-6 and V-79 spheroids. Int J Radiat Oncol Biol Phys 1982;8:737–739.
54. Hlatky L, Hong C, Sachs R. Patterns of misonidazole binding as observed in the sandwich system. Int J Radiat Oncol Biol Phys 1989;16:943–948.
55. Hlatky L, Ring CS, Sachs RK. Detection of an intrinsic marker in hypoxic cells. Cancer Res 1989;49:5162–5166.
56. Sutherland RM, Sordat B, Bamat J, et al. Oxygenation and differentiation in multicellular speroids of human colon carcinoma. Cancer Res 1986;46:5320–5329.
57. Urtasun RC, Chapman JD, Raleigh JA, et al. Binding of ^{3}H-misonidazole to solid human tumors as a measure of tumor hypoxia. Int J Radiat Oncol Biol Phys 1986;12:1263–1267.
58. Olive PL, Chaplin DJ, Durand RE. Pharmacokinetics, binding and distribution of Hoechst 33342 in spheroids and murine tumours. Br J Cancer 1985;52:739–746.
59. Trotter MJ, Chaplin DJ, Durand RE, Olive PL. The use of fluorescent probes to identify regions of transient perfusion in murine tumors. Int J Radiat Oncol Biol Phys 1989;16: 931–934.
60. Heacock CS, Sutherland RM. Induction characteristics of oxygen regulated proteins. Int J Radiat Oncol Biol Phys 1986;12:1287–1290.
61. Kwok TT, Sutherland RM. The relationship between radiation response of human squamous carcinoma cells and specific metabolic changes induced by chronic hypoxia. Int J Radiat Oncol Biol Phys 1989;16:1301–1305.
62. Hlatky L, Coleman CN. Modification of cell phenotype by ischemia/reperfusion. Seventh International Conference on Chemical Modifiers of Cancer Treatment. Clearwater, FL, 1991:27–28.
63. Brady LW, Plenk HP, Hanley JA, et al. Hyperbaric oxygen therapy for carcinoma of the cervix—stages IIb, IIIA, IIIB, and IVA. Results of a randomized study by the Radiation Therapy Oncology Group. Int J Radiat Oncol Biol Phys 1981;7:991–998.
64. Churchill-Davidson I, Sanger C. High pressure oxygen and radiotherapy. Lancet 1955;10: 1091–1095.
65. Dische S. Hyperbaric oxygen. The Medical Research Council's trials and their clinical significance. Br J Radiol 1978;51:888–894.
66. Rubin P, Hanley J, Keys HM, et al. Carbogen breathing during radiation therapy. The Radiation Therapy Oncology Group study. Int J Radiat Oncol Biol Phys 1979;5:1963–1970.
67. Bush RS. The significance of anemia in clinical radiation therapy. Int J Radiat Oncol Biol Phys 1986;12:2047–2050.
68. Dische S, Saunders MI, Wharburton MF. Hemoglobin, radiation, morbidity, and survival. Int J Radiat Oncol Biol Phys 1986;12:1335–1337.
69. Henk JM. Does hyperbaric oxygen have a future in radiation therapy? Int J Radiat Oncol Biol Phys 1981;7:1125–1131.
70. Hong A, Rojas A, Dische S. Normobaric oxygen as a radiosensitizer of hypoxic tumor cells. Int J Radiat Oncol Biol Phys 1989;16:1097–1100.
71. Dische S. Hypoxia and local tumor control. Part 2. Radiother Oncol 1991;20:9–11.
72. Dische S. Radiotherapy and anaemia: The clinical experience. Radiother Oncol 1991;20: 35–40.
73. Rose C, Lustig R, McIntosh N, et al. A clinical trial of Fluosol-DA 20% in advanced squamous cell carcinoma of the head and neck. Int J Radiat Oncol Biol Phys 1988;12: 1325–1327.
74. Lustig R, McIntosh LN, Rose C, et al. Phase I/II study of Fluosol DA and 100% oxygen as an adjuvant to radiation in the treatment of advanced tumors of the head and neck. Int J Radiat Oncol Biol Phys 1989;16:1587–1593.
75. Adams GE, Dische SE, Fowler JF, Thomlinson RH. Hypoxic cell sensitizers in radiotherapy. Lancet 1976;1:186–188.
76. Taylor YC, Brown JM. Radiosensitization in multifraction schedules, II. Greater sensitization by 2-nitroimidazoles than by oxygen. Radiat Res 1987;112:134–145.
77. Urtasun RC, Bond P, Chapman JD, et al. Radiation and high-dose metronidazole in supratentorial glioblastomas. N Engl J Med 1976;294:1364–1367.
78. Dische S, Saunders MI, Flockhart IR, et al. Misonidazole—A drug for trial in radiotherapy and oncology. Int J Radiat Oncol Biol Phys 1979;5:851–860.
79. Wasserman TH, Phillips TL, Johnson RJ, et al. Initial United States clinical and pharmacologic evaluation of misonidazole (Ro-07-0582), an hypoxic cell radiosensitizer. Int J Radiat Oncol Biol Phys 1979;5:775–786.
80. Dische SE. Chemical sensitizers for hypoxic cells: A decade of experience in clinical radiotherapy. Radiother Oncol 1985;3:97–115.
81. Overgaard J, Hansen HS, Anderson AP. Misonidazole combined with split course radiotherapy in the treatment of invasive carcinoma of the larynx and pharynx. Int J Radiat Oncol Biol Phys 1989;16:1065–1068.
82. Fazekas J, Pajak TF, Wasserman T, et al. Failure of misonidazole-sensitized radiotherapy to impact upon outcome among stage III–IV squamous cancers of the head and neck. Int J Radiat Oncol Biol Phys 1987;13:1155–1160.
83. Brown JM, Lee WW. Pharmacokinetic considerations in radiosensitizer development. In: Radiation sensitizers, their use in the clinical management of cancer. New York: Masson Publishing, 1980:2–13.
84. Brown JM, Yu NY. The optimum time for irradiation relative to tumor concentration of hypoxic cell sensitizers. Fr J Radiol 1980;53:915.
85. Brown JM, Yu NY, Brown DM, et al. SR-2508: A 2-nitroimidazole amide which should be superior to misonidazole as a radiosensitizer for clinical use. Int J Radiat Oncol Biol Phys 1981;7:695–701.
86. Brown JM. Clinical perspectives for the use of new hypoxic cell sensitizers. Int J Radiat Oncol Biol Phys 1982;8:1491–1497.
87. Dische S, Bennett MH, Orchard R, et al. The uptake of the radiosensitizing compound Ro 03-8799 (pimonidazole) in human tumors. Int J Radiat Oncol Biol Phys 1989;16: 1089–1092.
88. Hall EJ, Biaglow J. Ro-07-0582 as a radiosensitizer and cytotoxic agent. Int J Radiat Oncol Biol Phys 1977;7:521–530.
89. Maughan TS, Newman HFV, Bleehan NM, et al. Abnormal clinical pharmacokinetics of the developmental radiosensitizers pimonidazole (Ro 03-8799) and etanidazole (Sr 2508). Int J Radiat Oncol Biol Phys 1990;18:1151–1156.
90. Coleman CN, Wasserman TH, Urtasun RC, et al. Phase I trial of the hypoxic cell radiosensitizer SR-2508: The results of the five to six week drug schedule. Int J Radiat Oncol Biol Phys 1986;12:1105–1108.
91. Coleman CN, Halsey J, Cox RS, et al. Prediction of the neurotoxicity of the hypoxic cell radiosensitizer SR 2508 from the pharmacokinetic profile. Cancer Res 1987;47: 319–322.
92. Workman P, Ward R, Maughan TS, et al. Estimation of plasma area under the curve for etanidazole (SR 2508) in toxicity prediction and dose adjustment. Int J Radiat Oncol Biol Phys 1989;17:177–181.
93. Coleman CN, Buswell L, Noll L. The efficacy of pharmacokinetic monitoring and dose modification of etanidazole on the incidence of neurotoxicity: Results from a phase II trial in locally advanced prostate cancer. Int J Radiat Oncol Biol Phys1992;22(3):565–568.
94. Wasserman TH, Lee DJ, Cosmatos D, et al. Clinical trials with etanidazole (SR-2508) by the Radiation Therapy Oncology Group (RTOG). Radiother Oncol 1991;20:129–135.
95. Chassagne D, Sancho-Garnier H, Charreau I, et al. Progress report of a phase II and III trial with etanidazole (SR-2508): A multicentre European study. Radiother Oncol 1991;20:121–127.
96. Awwad HK, El Merzabani MM, El Badawy S, et al. Misonidazole in the preoperative and radical radiotherapy of bladder cancer. In: Radiation sensitizers, their use in the clinical management of cancer. New York: Masson Publishing, 1980:381–386.
97. Awwad H, el Badawy S, Zagloul M, et al. Pharmacokinetics of etanidazole (SR-2508) in bladder and cervical cancer: Evidence of diffusion from urine. Proceedings of the Chemical Modifiers of Cancer Treatment, Paris, 1988:3–13.
98. Whittington R, Coia LR, Haller DG, et al. Adenocarcinoma of the esophagus and esophago-gastric junction: The effects of single and combined modalities on the survival and patterns of failure following treatment. Int J Radiat Oncol Biol Phys 1990;19: 813–815.
99. Eifel PJ, Brown JM. Pharmacokinetics and toxicology of continuously infused nitroimidazoles. Int J Radiat Oncol Biol Phys 1983;10:1311–1314.
100. Pardridge WM. Recent advances in blood-brain barrier transport. Ann Rev Pharmacol Toxicol 1988;28:25–39.
101. Workman P. Controversy in drug delivery to tumors in the brain. In: Drug delivery in cancer treatment. European School of Oncology Monograph. Berlin: Springer Verlag, 1990:1–50.
102. Hurwitz SJ, Coleman CN, Riese N, et al. Distribution of etanidazole into human brain tumors: Implications for treating high grade gliomas. Int J Radiat Oncol Biol Phys 1992;22(3):573–576.
103. Newman HFV, Bleehan NM, Ward R, Workman P. Hypoxic cell radiosensitizers in the treatment of high grade gliomas: A new direction using combined Ro 03-8799 (pimonidazole) and SR 2508 (etanidazole). Int J Radiat Oncol Biol Phys 1988;15: 677–684.
104. Fu K, Hurst A, Brown JM. The effects of misonidazole and continuous low dose irradiation. In: Radiation sensitizers, their use in the clinical management of cancer. New York: Masson Publishing, 1980:167–175.
105. Coleman CN, Noll L, Howes AE, et al. Initial results of a phase I trial of continuous infusion SR 2508 (etanidazole): A Radiation Therapy Oncology Group study. Int J Radiat Oncol Biol Phys 1989;16:1085–1088.
106. Coleman CN, Noll L, Riese N, et al. Final report of the phase I trial of continuous infusion etanidazole (SR 2508): A Radiation Therapy Oncology Group study. Int J Radiat Oncol Biol Phys 1992;22(3):577–580.
107. Cobb LM, Nolan J, Butler SA. Distribution of pimonidazole and RSU 1069 in tumour and normal tissues. Br J Cancer 1990;62:314–318.
108. Lespinasse F, Thomas C, Bonnay M, et al. Ro 03–8799: Preferential relative uptake in human tumor xenografts compared to a murine tumor: Comparison with SR-2508. Int J Radiat Oncol Biol Phys 1989;16:1105–1109.
109. Bleehan NM, Maughan TS, Workman P, et al. The combination of multiple doses of etanidazole and pimonidazole in 48 patients: A toxicity and pharmacokinetic study. Radiother Oncol 1991;20:137–142.
110. Honess DJ, Wasserman TH, Workman P, et al. Additivity of radiosensitization by the combination of SR 2508 (etanidazole) and Ro 03-8799 (pimonidazole) in a murine tumor system. Int J Radiat Oncol Biol Phys 1988;15:671–675.
111. Bleehan NM, Newman HFV, Maughan TS, Workman P. A multiple dose study of the combined radiosensitizers Ro 03-8799 (pimonidazole) and SR 2508 (etanidazole). Int J Radiat Oncol Biol Phys 1989;16:1093–1096.
112. Newman H, Bleehan NM, Workman P. A phase I study of the combination of two hypoxic cell radiosensitizers, Ro-03-8799 and SR 2508: Toxicity and pharmacokinetics. Int J Radiat Oncol Biol Phys 1986;12:1113–1116.
113. Newman HFV, Ward R, Workman P, Bleehan NM. The multi-dose clinical tolerance

and pharmacokinetics of the combined radiosensitizers, Ro 03-8799 (pimonidazole) and SR 2508 (etanidazole). Int J Radiat Oncol Biol Phys 1988;15:1073–1084.

114. Dische S, Chassagne D, Machin D. Randomized controlled trial of the use of pimonidazole (Ro 03-8799) in the treatment of advanced carcinoma of the cervix. Seventh International Conference on Chemical Modifiers of Cancer Treatment. Clearwater, FL, 1991;7:172–173.
115. Overgaard J, Hansen HS, Lindelov B, et al. Nimorazole as a hypoxic radiosensitizer in the treatment of supraglottic larynx and pharynx carcinoma. First report from the Danish Head and Neck Cancer Study (DAHANCA) protocol 5-85. Radiother Oncol 1991;20:143–149.
116. Adams GE, Ahmed I, PWS, Stratford IJ. Radiation sensitization and chemopotentiation with RSU 1069, a compound more effective than misonidazole in vitro and in vivo. Br J Cancer 1984;49:571–578.
117. Ahmed I, Jenkins TC, Walling JM. Analogues of RSU-069: Radiosensitization and toxicity in vitro and in vivo. Int J Radiat Oncol Biol Phys 1986;12:1079–1081.
118. Chaplin DJ, Durand RE, Stratford IJ. The radiosensitizing and toxic effects of RSU-1069 on hypoxic cells in a murine tumor. Int J Radiat Oncol Biol Phys 1986;12:1091–1095.
119. Deacon JM, Holliday SB, Ahmed I, et al. Experimental pharmacokinetics of RSU-1069 and its analogs: High tumor/plasma ratios. Int J Radiat Oncol Biol Phys 1986;12:1087–1090.
120. Stratford IJ, O'Neill P, Sheldon PW, et al. RSU 1069, a nitroimidazole containing a aziridine group. Biochem Pharm 1986;35:105–109.
121. Horwich A, Holliday SB, Deacon JM, Peckham MJ. A toxicity and pharmacokinetic study in man of the hypoxic cell radiosensitizer RSU1069. Br J Radiol 1986;59:1238–1240.
122. Sebolt-Leopold JS, Vincent PW, Beningo KA, et al. Pharmacologic/pharmacokinetic evaluation of emesis induced by RSU 1069 and its control by antiemetic agents. Seventh International Conference on Chemical Modifiers of Cancer Treatment. Clearwater, FL, 1991:152–153.
123. Zeman EM, Brown JM, Lemmon MJ, et al. SR-4233: A new bioreductive agent with high selective toxicity for hypoxic mammalian cells. Int J Radiat Oncol Biol Phys 1986;12:1239–1242.
124. Zeman EM, Hirst VK, Lemmon MJ, et al. Enhancement of radiation-induced tumor cell killing by the hypoxic cell toxin SR 4233. Radiother Oncol 1988;12:209–218.
125. Baker MA, Zeman EM, Hirst VK, Brown JM. Metabolism of SR 4233 by Chinese hamster ovary cells: Basis of selective hypoxic cytotoxicity. Cancer Res 1988;48:5947–5953.
126. Edwards DI, Virk NS. Repair of DNA damage induced by SR 4233. Seventh International Conference on Chemical Modifiers of Cancer Treatment. Clearwater, FL, 1991:229–230.
127. Laderoute KR, Eryavec E, McClelland RA, et al. The production of strand breaks in DNA in the presence of the hydroxylamine of SR-2508 (1-[N-(2- hydroxylethyl)acetamido]-2-nitroimidazole at neutral pH. Int J Radiat Oncol Biol Phys 1986;12:1215–1218.
128. Brown JM, Lemmon MJ. Potentiation by the hypoxic cytotoxin SR 4233 of cell killing produced by fractionated irradiation of mouse tumors. Cancer Res 1990;50:7745–7749.
129. Biedermann KA, Wang J, Giaccia AI, et al. DNA and chromosomal damage and repair after hypoxic treatment of cells with SR 4233. Seventh International Conference on Chemical Modifiers of Cancer Treatment. Clearwater, FL, 1991:227–228.
130. Brown JM, Lemmon MJ. SR 4233: A tumor specific radiosensitizer active in fractionated radiation regimens. Radiother Oncol 1991;20:151–156.
131. Zeman EM, Brown JM. Pre- and post-irradiation radiosensitization by SR 4233. Int J Radiat Oncol Biol Phys 1989;16:967–971.
132. Brown JM. Therapeutic advantage of hypoxic cells in tumors: A theoretical study. JNCI 1991;83:178–184.
133. Brown J, Koong A, Lemmon MJ. A comparison of the relative efficacies of combining either a hypoxic cell radiosensitizer, increased tumor oxygenation or a hypoxic cytotoxin, with fractionated irradiation. Seventh International Conference on Chemical Modifiers of Cancer Treatment. Clearwater, FL, 1991:272–273.
134. Chaplin DJ, Horsman MR, Peters CE, et al. Tumour blood flow and its modulation: Implications for bioreductive drug activity in vivo. In: Selective activation of drugs by redox processes. New York: Plenum, (in press).
135. Warren BA. The vascular morphology of tumors. In: Tumor blood circulation. Boca Raton: CRC Press, 1978:1–47.
136. Eddy HA, Cassarett GW. Development of the vascular system in hampster malignant neurilemmoma. Microvasc Res 1973;6:63–82.
137. Dewhirst MW, Oliver R, Tso CY, et al. Heterogeneity in tumor microvasculature response to radiation. Int J Radiat Oncol Biol Phys 1990;18:559–568.
138. Denekamp J, Hill S. Angiogenic attack as a therapeutic strategy for cancer. Radiother Oncol 1991;20:103–112.
139. Chaplin DJ, Horsman MR.Changes in tumour blood flow induced by chemical modifiers of radiation response. Seventh International Conference on Chemical Modifiers of Cancer Treatment. Clearwater, FL, 1991:56–57.
140. Chaplin DJ, Peters CE, Horsman MR, Trotter M. Drug induced perturbations in tumor blood flow:therapeutic potential and possible limitations. Radiother Oncol 1991;20:93–101.
141. Horsman MR, Chaplin DJ, Brown JM. Radiosensitization by nicotinamide in vivo: A greater enhancement of tumor damage compared to that of normal tissue. Radiat Res 1987;109:479–489.
142. Okunieff P, Walsh CS, Vaupel P, et al. Effects of hydralazine on in vivo tumor energy metabolism, hematopoietic radiation sensitivity, and cardiovascular parameters. Int J Radiat Oncol Biol Phys 1989;16:1145–1148.
143. Horsman MR, Overgaard J, Chaplin DJ. The interaction between RSU 1069, hydralazine, and hyperthermia in a C3H mammary carcinoma as assessed by tumor growth delay. Acta Oncol 1988;27:861–862.
144. Cole S, Robbins L. Manipulation of oxygenation in a human tumor xenograft with BW12C or hydralazine: Effect of misonidazole or RSU 1069. Radiother Oncol 1989;16:235–243.
145. Guichard M, Lespinasse F, Trotter M, Chaplin D. The effect of hydralazine on blood flow and misonidazole toxicity in human tumor xenografts. Radiother Oncol 1991;20:117–123.
146. Horsman MR, Christensen KL, Overgaard J. Relationship between the hydralazine-induced changes in murine tumor blood supply and mouse blood pressure. Seventh International Conference of Chemical Modification of Cancer Treatment. Clearwater, FL, 1991:54–55.
147. Griffith OW, Meister A. Potent and specific inhibition of glutathione synthesis by buthionine sulfoximine (S-n-butylhomocysteine sulfoximine). J Biol Chem 1979;254:7558–7560.
148. Griffith OW. Mechanism of action, metabolism, and toxicity of buthionine sulfoximine and its higher homologs, potent inhibitors of glutathione synthesis. J Biol Chem 1982;254:13704–13712.
149. Kramer RA, Soble M, Howes AE, Montoya VP. The effect of glutathione (GSH) depletion in vivo by buthionine sulfoximine (BSO) in the radiosensitization of SR 2508. Int J Radiat Oncol Biol Phys 1989;16:1325–1329.
150. O'Dweyer PJ, Hamilton TC, Young RC, et al. Depletion of glutathione in normal and malignant tumor cells in vivo by buthionine sulfoximine: Clinical and biochemical results. Seventh International Conference of Chemical Modifiers of Cancer Treatment. Clearwater, FL, 1991:313–315.
151. Livesey JC, Golden RN, Shankland Z, et al. Magnetic resonance spectroscopic measurement of cellular thiol reduction-oxidation state. Seventh International Conference on Chemical Modifiers of Cancer Treatment. Clearwater, FL, 1991:307–308.
152. Bailey H, Spriggs D, Tutsch K, et al. Phase I trial of intravenous L-buthionine sulfoximine and melphalan: An attempt at modulation of glutathione chemoprotection. Seventh International Conference of Chemical Modifiers of Cancer Treatment. Clearwater, FL, 1991:319–320.
153. Brown JM. The mechanisms of cytotoxicity and chemosensitization by misonidazole and other nitroimidazoles. Int J Radiat Oncol Biol Phys 1982;8:675–682.
154. Bump EA, Yu NY, Brown JM. Radiosensitization of hypoxic tumor cells by depletion of intracellular glutathione. Science 1982;127:544–545.
155. Clark EP, Epp ER, Biaglow JE, Morse-Gaudio E. Glutathione depletion, radiosensitization, and misonidazole potentiation in hypoxic Chinese hamster ovary cells by buthionine sulfoximine. Radiat Res 1984;98:370–380.
156. Louie KG, Behrens BC, Kinsella TJ, et al. Radiation survival parameters of antineoplastic drug-sensitive and -resistant human ovarian cancer cell lines and their modification by buthionine sulfoximine. Cancer Res 1985;45:2110–2115.
157. Mitchell JB, Cook JA, DeGraff W, et al. Keynote address: Glutathione modulation in cancer treatment: Will it work? Int J Radiat Oncol Biol Phys 1989;16:1289–1295.
158. Biaglow JE, Varnes ME, Tuttle SW, et al. The effect of L-buthionine sulfoximine on the aerobic radiation response of A549 human lung carcinoma cells. Int J Radiat Oncol Biol Phys 1986;12:1139–1142.
159. Rice GC, Bump EA, Shrieve DC, et al. Quantitative analysis of cellular glutathione by flow cytometry utilizing monochlorobimane: Some applications to radiation and drug resistance in vitro and in vivo. Cancer Res 1986;46:6105–6110.
160. Russo A, Mitchell JB, Finkelstein E, et al. The effects of cellular glutathione elevation on the oxygen enhancement ratio. Radiat Res 1985;103:232–239.
161. Van der Schans GP, Vos O, Roos-Verheij WSD, et al. The influence of oxygen on the induction of radiation damage in DNA in mammalian cell after sensitization by intracellular glutathione depletion. Int J Radiat Biol 1986;50:453–465.
162. Hodgkiss RJ, Middleton RW. Enhancement of misonidazole radiosensitization by an inhibitor of glutathione biosynthesis. Int J Radiat Biol 1983;43:179–183.
163. Lespinasse F, Biscay P, Malaise EP, Guichard M. SR-2508 plus buthionine sulfoximine or SR-2508 alone: Effects on the response and the glutathione content of a human tumor xenograft. Radiat Res 1987;110:149–154.
164. Ling CG, Wong RSL, Basas RD. Glutathione depletion and cytotoxicity of buthionine sulphoximine and SR2508 in rodent and human cells. Int J Radiat Oncol Biol Phys 1990;16:325–330.
165. McNally NJ, Soranson JA. Radiosensitization by misonidazole during recovery of cellular thiols following depletion by BSO or DEM. Int J Radiat Oncol Biol Phys 1989;16:1331–1334.
166. Phillips TL, Mitchell JB, DeGraff WG, et al. Modification in SR 2508 sensitization in hypoxic V79 cells by manipulation of glutathione (GSH) levels. Int J Radiat Oncol Biol Phys 1989;16:1335–1340.
167. Yu NY, Brown JM. Depletion of glutathione in vivo as a method of improving the therapeutic ratio of misonidazole and SR 2508. Int J Radiat Oncol Biol Phys 1984;10:1265–1269.
168. DeGraff WG, Russo A, Gamson J, Mitchell JB. Evaluation of nitroimidazole hypoxic cell radiosensitizers in a human tumor cell line high in intracellular glutathione. Int J Radiat Oncol Biol Phys 1989;16:1021–1024.
169. Phillips TL, Mitchell JB, DeGraff W, et al. Variation in sensitizing efficiency for SR 2508 in human cells dependent on glutathione content. Int J Radiat Oncol Biol Phys 1986;12:1627–1635.
170. Stratford IJ, Hickson ID, Robson CN, Stephens M. Radiosensitizing and cytotoxic effects of nitroimidazoles in CHO cells expressing elevated levels of glutathione-s-transferase. Int J Radiat Oncol Biol Phys 1989;16:1307–1310.
171. Fowler JF, Lindstrom MJ. Loss of local control with prolongation of radiotherapy. Int J Radiat Oncol Biol Phys 1992;22(2):457–467.
172. Begg AC, Hofland I, Moonen L, et al. The predictive value of cell kinetic measurements in a European trial of accelerated fractionation in advanced head and neck tumors: An interim report. Int J Radiat Oncol Biol Phys 1990;19:1449–1453.

173. Kinsella TJ, Mitchell JB, Russo A, et al. The use of halogenated thymidine analogs as clinical radiosensitizers: Rationale, current status, and future prospects: Monhypoxic sensitizers. Int J Radiat Oncol Biol Phys 1984;10:1399–1406.
174. Kinsella TJ, Dobson PP, Mitchell JB, et al. Enhancement of x-ray induced DNA damage by pretreatment with halogenated pyrimidine analogs. Int J Radiat Oncol Biol Phys 1987;13:733–739.
175. Iliakis G, Kurtzman S, Pantelias G, et al. Mechanism of radiosensitization by halogenated pyrimidines: Effect of BrdU in radiation induction of DNA and chromosome damage and its correlation with cell killing. Radiat Res 1989;119:286–304.
176. Fornace AJ, Dobson PP, Pantelias G, et al. Enhancement of radiation damage of cellular DNA following unifilar substitution with iododeoxyuridine. Int J Radiat Oncol Biol Phys 1990;18:873–878.
177. Lawrence TS, Davis MA, Maybaum J, et al. The effect of single versus double stranded substitution on halogenated pyrimidine-induced radiosensitization and DNA strand breakage in human tumor cells. Radiat Res 1990;123:192–198.
178. Berger SH, Berger FG. Thymidylate synthase as a determinant of 5-fluoro-2'-deoxyuridine response in human colonic tumor cell lines. Mol Pharmacol 1988;34:474–479.
179. Heidelberger C, Griesbach L, Montag BJ, et al. Studies on fluorinated pyrimidines II. Effects on transplanted tumors. Cancer Res 1958;18:305–317.
180. Byfield JE, Calabro-Jones P, Klisak I, et al. Pharmacologic requirements for obtaining sensitization of human tumor cells in vitro to combined 5-fluorouracil and x-rays. Int J Radiat Oncol Biol Phys 1982;8:1923–1933.
181. Ishikawa T, Tanaka Y, Ishituska H, et al. Comparative antitumor activity of 5-fluorouracil and 5-deoxy-5-fluorouridine in combination with radiation therapy in mice bearing colon 26 adenocarcinoma. Jap J Cancer Res 1989;80:583–591.
182. Nakajima M, Miyamoto M, Tamabe T, et al. Enhancement of mammalian cell killing by 5-fluorouracil in combination with x-rays. Cancer Res 1979;39:3763–3767.
183. Weinberg MJ, Rauth AM. 5-Fluorouracil infusion and fractionated doses of radiation: Studies with a murine squamous cell carcinoma. Int J Radiat Oncol Biol Phys 1987;13: 1691–1699.
184. Miller EM, Kinsella TJ. Radiosensitization by fluorodeoxyuridine: Effects of thymidylate synthase inhibition and cell synchronization. Cancer Res 1992;52(7):1627–1684.
185. Tochner Z, Kinsella TJ, Rowland J, et al. Treatment of unresectable sarcomas of adults with hyperfractionated irradiation and iododeoxyuridine. Br J Radiol 1989;19:107–111.
186. Rodriguez R, Kinsella TJ. Halogenated pyrimidines as radiosensitizers for high grade glioma. Int J Radiat Oncol Biol Phys 1991;21:859–862.
187. Chang AE, Kinsella TJ, Rowland J, et al. A phase I study of intra-arterial iododeoxyuridine in patients with colorectal liver metastases. J Clin Oncol 1989;7:662–668.
188. Rodriquez R, Miller E, Fowler JF, et al. Continuous infusion of halogenated pyrimidines. Int J Radiat Oncol Biol Phys 1991;20:1380–1381.
189. Gastrointestinal Tumor Study Group. Prolongation of the disease-free interval in surgically treated rectal carcinoma. N Engl J Med 1985;312:1465–1472.
190. Gastrointestinal Tumor Study Group. Further evidence of effective adjuvant combined radiation and chemotherapy following curative resection of pancreatic cancer. Cancer 1987;59:2006–2010.
191. Krook JE, Moertel CG, Gunderson LL, et al. Effective surgical adjuvant therapy for high risk rectal carcinoma. N Engl J Med 1991;423:709–715.
192. The Department of Veterans Affairs Laryngeal Cancer Study Group. Induction chemotherapy plus radiation compared with surgery plus radiation in patients with advanced laryngeal cancer. N Engl J Med 1991;324:1685–1690.
193. Sischy B, Doggett RLS, Krall JM. Definitive irradiation and chemotherapy for radiosensitization in management of anal carcinoma: Interim report in Radiation Therapy Oncology Group No. 8314. JNCI 1989;81:850–856.
194. Goz B. The effects of incorporation of 5-halogenated deoxyuridines into the DNA of eukaryotic cells. Pharmacol Rev 1978;29:249–272.
195. Myers CE. The pharmacology of the fluoropyrimidines. Pharmacol Rev 1981;33:1–13.
196. Kinsella TJ, Mitchell JB, Russo A, et al. The use of halogenated thymidine analogs as clinical radiosensitizers: Rationale, current status, and future prospects: Nonhypoxic sensitizers. Int J Radiat Oncol Biol Phys 1984;10:1399–1406.
197. Steel G. Growth kinetics of tumors. Oxford: Clarendon Press, 1977.
198. Fornace AJ, Dobson PP, Pantelias G, et al. Enhancement of radiation damage of cellular DNA following unifilar substitution with iododeoxyuridine. Int J Radiat Oncol Biol Phys 1990;18:873–878.
199. Kinsella TJ, Dobson PP, Mitchell JB, et al. Enhancement of x-ray induced DNA damage by pretreatment with halogenated pyrimidine analogs. Int J Radiat Oncol Biol Phys 1987;13:733–739.
200. Fowler JF. Potential for increasing the differential response between tumors and normal tissues: Can proliferation rate be used? Int J Radiat Oncol Biol Phys 1986;12:641–645.
201. Lawrence TS. The effects of leucovorin and dipyridamole on fluoropyrimidine-induced radiosensitization. Int J Radiat Oncol Biol Phys 1991;20:377–381.

SECTION **10**

THOMAS W. GRIFFIN
MARY AUSTIN-SEYMOUR

Heavy Particle Beam Radiation Therapy

Advances in the field of radiation oncology have substantially improved the outlook for significant numbers of cancer patients, but failure to control locoregional disease is still a major problem. Heavy particle radiation therapy can address at least a part of this problem by offering a therapeutic gain over conventional photon and electron radiation therapy in several clinical situations.

Heavy particle beams in clinical use include fast neutrons, protons, helium ions, heavy ions (*e.g.* carbon, neon, argon), and negative pions.[1–3] Fast neutrons are used for their radiobiologic properties that potentially are superior to those of conventional photons and electrons. Protons and helium ions are used for their ability to achieve dose distributions that are potentially superior to those obtainable with conventional radiations. Heavy ions and pions have potential biologic and dose distribution advantages.

BIOLOGIC EFFECTS OF HEAVY PARTICLE BEAMS

The biologic effects of a radiation beam depend on the spatial distribution of the ionizing events produced in tissue. The rate at which charged particles deposit energy per unit distance is known as the linear energy transfer (LET), expressed in keV/μm. Protons, helium ions, electrons, and photons are sparsely ionizing, characterized by a low LET. Conversely, fast neutrons, heavy ions, and pions are densely ionizing and are referred to as high-LET radiations. Review of the possible causes of cancer treatment failure with conventional radiation therapy suggests that there are major areas in which neutrons and other high-LET radiations may offer a biologic advantage.

TUMOR CELL HYPOXIA

The oxygen enhancement ratio (OER) is defined as the ratio of the dose of radiation required to produce a specified biologic effect under anoxic conditions to the dose required to produce the same effect under well-oxygenated conditions. With photons, the oxygen enhancement ratio for most mammalian cells is 2.5 to 3.0. With neutrons, heavy charged particles, or pions, the oxygen enhancement ratio is significantly smaller (1.4 to 1.7), and the protection conferred on tumor cells by hypoxia is diminished. In practice, the clinical advantage of high-LET radiations may be less than suggested by the differences in oxygen enhancement ratios. Not all tumor cells are severely hypoxic, and reoxygenation may occur during intervals between dose fractions, diminishing the influence of hypoxic cells on tumor recurrence.[4]

RELATIVE BIOLOGIC EFFECTIVENESS

The relative biologic effectiveness (RBE) of an ionizing radiation is the ratio of the dose of that radiation compared with the dose of a reference radiation required to produce a specific endpoint in a specific tissue. A potential area of therapeutic gain from high-LET radiations exists if tumor cells are relatively radioresistant because of their increased capacity to accumulate sublethal radiation injury. This situation is reflected in a wide shoulder for the tumor-cell-survival curve. With neutrons and other high-LET radiations, most cell killing results from single lethal events, producing cell-survival curves that are almost exponential in the range of clinical relevance. Tumors characterized by a large capacity to accumulate and repair sublethal radiation injury should have a higher value of relative biologic effectiveness for high-LET radiations than for normal tissues.[5] However, Howlett and others have shown that RBE values of neutrons for different experimental tumors vary considerably, and no general statement about which types of tumors are best treated with high-LET radiations can be made.[6]

TUMOR CELL KINETICS

The cell-cycle-dependent variation of radiosensitivity is similar for neutrons and γ-rays, but the magnitude of the difference is smaller for neutrons and other high-LET particle beams.[7] Whether this properly constitutes a therapeutic advantage for high-LET radiations cannot always be predicted. Tumors in which cells are slowly cycling, tumors in which cells redistribute poorly between phases of their cell cycles, and tumors in which the cell cycle spectrum is dominated by cells in resistant phases are more effectively treated with high-LET radiations.

REPAIR OF POTENTIALLY LETHAL DAMAGE

Repair of potentially lethal damage occurs after low-LET irradiation, but it is observed less frequently after high-LET irradiation.[8] If, as has been suggested by Hall and Kraljevic, potentially lethal damage repair after low-LET irradiation occurs in nutritionally deprived tumor cells but not in normal tissue cells, the use of high-LET radiation beams would be therapeutically advantageous in tumors with these types of cell populations.[9]

PHYSICAL EFFECTS OF PARTICLE BEAMS

Fast neutron beams can be generated for radiation therapy by bombarding a target containing tritium (T) with accelerated deuterium (d) ions in a dT generator or by bombarding a suitable target, such as beryllium (Be) with protons (p) or deuterons (d) accelerated in a cyclotron or linear accelerator. The dT generator produces a monoenergetic 14-MeV neutron beam, and the proton-on-beryllium (p-Be) reactions produce neutron beams with a spectrum of energies. High-energy particle accelerators are required to produce medically useful beams of heavy charged particles.

Neutrons have no dose distribution advantages over photons, but protons, helium ions, heavy ions, and negative pions have significant dose distribution advantages over conventional photons and electrons. These charged particles preferentially deposit energy and more effectively destroy tumor cells near the end of their path. By appropriate determination of range (or path length) in tissue and by spreading the peak area, the high-effect region (*i.e.* the spread Bragg peak) can be made to correspond to the target volume.

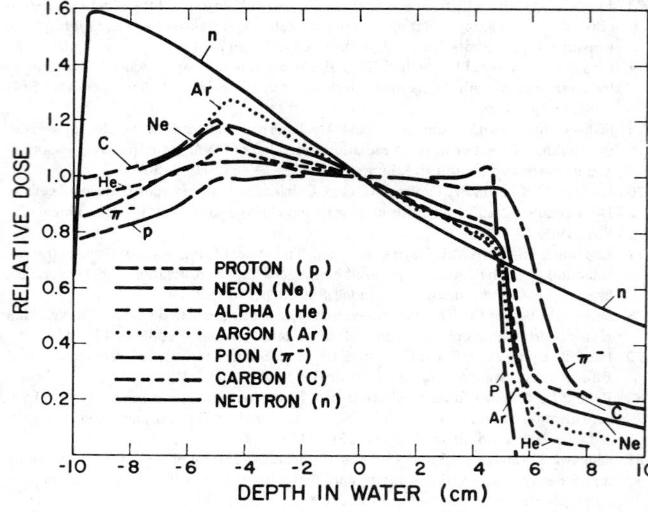

FIGURE 69–38. Comparison of depth dose (spread peak curves) for various charged particles of clinical interest.

The complex effects of heavy particles in tissues are a function of the energy, weight, velocity, and tract structure of the accelerated particle and the technique of beam delivery. Figure 69–38 compares the physical parameters of the clinically useful heavy particles. Table 69–39 illustrates the biologic and physical characteristics of these particles.

FAST NEUTRON CLINICAL STUDIES

Fast neutron radiation therapy was first used as a cancer treatment tool by Robert Stone at the Lawrence Berkeley Laboratory in 1938.[10] Using the Berkeley cyclotron, Dr. Stone treated a series of patients with advanced malignancies in various locations to high doses. Almost all of the long-term survivors from that clinical trial had severe radiation sequelae in their normal tissues. This result was initially thought to be due to an increased RBE of neutrons for late effects, and it deterred further clinical investigation of fast neutrons for approximately 20 years. Later experiments, however, showed that the daily treatment doses used in Stone's clinical work corresponded to a much higher equivalent photon dose than Stone had assumed.[11] An exhaustive review of Stone's work revealed that the early and late normal tissue effects observed in his patients could be accounted for by the equivalent photon doses received.[12] The influence of his fractionation scheme on tissue response, and the change of RBE with fraction size, caused his patients to be inadvertently treated to extremely high radiation doses.

Dr. Catterall reintroduced fast neutrons as a cancer treatment in the late 1960s on the basis of the new knowledge gained from the early neutron therapy experience. After several hundred patients were treated on the Hammersmith Hospital cyclotron, she concluded that fast neutron radiation therapy, using appropriate fractionation, was well tolerated

TABLE 69–39. Comparison of Relative Physical and Biologic Parameters of Particles in Clinical Use

High LET Advantage	*Protons*	*Helium*	*Pions*	*Neutrons*	*Heavy Ions*			
					C	*Ne*	*Si*	*Ar*
Physical depth dose	+++	+++	+++	No	+++	+++	++	+
RBE	No	+	+	++	++	++	+++	+++
OER	No	+	+	+++	+	++	+++	+++

+, slight advantage; ++, moderate advantage; +++, very significant advantage.

and that many advanced tumors responded amazingly well.[13] Based on her encouraging results, 38 cancer treatment centers in North America, Europe, Asia, and Africa began clinical treatments with fast neutron beams of various energies. Initially, clinical trials were confined to converted physics-laboratory-based particle accelerators that were poorly suited for patient treatment. In the mid-1980s, hospital-based neutron generators became available with treatment delivery systems comparable to those of modern, conventional linear accelerators. Approximately 15,000 patients have been treated with neutrons, resulting in a fairly extensive worldwide database.

SALIVARY GLAND CANCERS

The case for high-LET radiation therapy is strong for salivary gland tumors. Tumors with low growth fractions and long doubling times are predicted to be more sensitive to high-LET than to low-LET radiations. Reduced variation in radiosensitivity throughout the cell cycle predicts that slowly growing tumors with slowly cycling cells, such as salivary gland cancers, would be advantageously treated with high-LET radiations. Batterman and colleagues published pioneering work clinically defining the RBE of fast neutrons for various human malignancies.[14] One of the highest RBEs of neutrons was found in adenoid cystic carcinomas (8.0 with fractionated neutron therapy), which indicates an inherent radiosensitivity of this tumor to high-LET radiation. The RBE for adenoid cystic carcinomas is substantially higher than that for normal mesenchymal tissues. Treating an adenoid cystic carcinoma with 2000 neutron cGy would be approximately equivalent to 16,000 photon cGy in its tumor effect, but equivalent to only 6000 to 6600 photon cGy in its effect on normal tissues. This differential effect gives rise to a therapeutic gain factor of approximately 2.5 and is thought to be the underlying reason for the success of high-LET radiations in salivary gland malignancies. Clinical trials have confirmed these predictions.

In excess of 300 patients have been treated for locally advanced, unresectable salivary gland tumors with fast neutrons.[15] Patients have been treated with neutrons alone and mixed beam irradiation over short (4 weeks) and long (8 weeks) overall treatment times. The results are remarkably consistent and demonstrate long-term locoregional tumor control rates of approximately 67% compared with average long-term locoregional tumor control rates of approximately 26% for low-LET radiations (Tables 69–40 and 69–41).[15–37] The normal tissue complication rates have been marginally higher with low-energy, fixed-beam neutron generators, but they have been equivalent to megavoltage photons when high-energy or isocentric hospital-based neutron generators were employed.[24,30,31] Subsequently, the National Cancer Institute (NCI) and the Medical Research Council (MRC) of Great Britain jointly sponsored a prospective, randomized phase III clinical trial directly comparing fast neutron to megavoltage photon and electron radiation therapy for patients with locally advanced, unresectable salivary gland tumors using laboratory-based and hospital-based neutron generators.[24] This study demonstrated a long-term locoregional tumor control rate of 67% for neutrons compared with 17% for photons ($p < 0.005$) in this group of patients with advanced tumors (up to 16 cm. in maximum dimension) (Table 69–42). The normal tissue toxicities were not statistically significantly different between the two groups.

An analysis of patients treated on the national neutron registry in a phase IV fashion at the University of Washington was recently accomplished.[37] Grouping patients according to

TABLE 69–40. Local Control Rates for Malignant Salivary Gland Tumors Treated With Low LET Radiotherapy

*Investigations**	*Local Control (patients)*	*Local Control Rate (%)*
Borthne[16]	8/35	23
Fitzpatrick[17]	6/50	12
Fu[18]	6/19	32
Shidnia[19]	6/16	38
Elkon[20]	2/19	11
Rossman[21]	6/11	54
Rafla[22]	9/25	36
Dobrowsky[23]	7/17	41
Griffin[24]	2/12	17
Vikram[25]	5/49	10
Stewart[26]	9/19	47
Guillamondegui[27]	9/15	60
Ravasz[28]	3/12	25
Total	79/299	26

* Patients were treated with photon or electron-beam irradiation with or without radioactive implants. Patients treated de novo and for gross disease after a postsurgical recurrence are included but not patients who were treated postoperatively for microscopic residual disease.

TABLE 69–41. Local Control Rates for Malignant Salivary Gland Tumors Treated With Neutron Radiotherapy

*Investigations**	*Local Control (patients)*	*Local Control Rate (%)*
Saroja[29]	71/113	63
Catterall[30]	50/65	77
Duncan[31]	12/22	55
Ornitz[32]	3/8	38
Batterman[33]	21/32	66
Maor[34]	6/9	67
Eichhorn[35]	3/5	60
Skolyszewski[36]	2/3	67
Buchholz[37]	40/52	77
Total	208/309	67

* Patients treated de novo and for gross disease after a postsurgical recurrence are included but not patients who were treated postoperatively for microscopic residual disease.

treatment status, actuarial 5-year locoregional tumor control rates were 92% for patients treated definitively with fast neutrons (without a prior surgical procedure), 63% for patients treated postoperatively for gross (measurable by computed tomography) residual disease, and 51% for patients treated for recurrent disease after a surgical procedure. (Fig. 69–39) The p values associated with these differences were 0.12 and 0.01, respectively (two-sided log rank test). There were no cases of radiation-induced facial nerve damage. Figure 69–40 illustrates patient survival as a function of presentation. The difference between patients treated primarily and those treated for recurrent disease is significant at the $p = 0.03$ level. These results have been confirmed by other series.[30]

PROSTATE CANCER

Fast neutron radiation therapy has been predicted to be advantageous in this tumor system for many of the same reasons as it was for salivary gland tumors. Based on these same biologic considerations, an RTOG-sponsored phase III study was designed and conducted between 1977 and 1983 randomizing patients between photons and a mixture of neutrons and photons using physics-laboratory-based machines. The 10-year results are now available from this study. These results confirm the radiobiology-based predictions, and they demonstrate statistically significant advantages for neutrons in terms of locoregional tumor control, survival, and disease-specific survival.[38] Ten-year locoregional control rates on this study were 70% for mixed beams compared with 58% for photons ($p = 0.03$); 10-year survival rates were 46% for mixed beams compared with 29% for photons ($p = 0.04$); and 10-year disease-specific survival rates were 58% for mixed beams compared with 43% for photons ($p = 0.05$). No significant differences were found in complication rates. Although statistically significant advantages were seen with neutron therapy for all relevant endpoints at 10 years, this study has been criticized on the basis of photon locoregional tumor control and survival rates that appear to be inferior to other photon retrospective series published in the medical literature. Although these differences are probably due to patient selection factors, a confirmatory study was designed using state-of-the-art, hospital-based cyclotrons.

One hundred seventy-eight patients were randomized on this follow-up study comparing 2040 neutron cGy delivered in 12 fractions over 4 weeks against 7000 photon cGy delivered in 35 fractions over 7 weeks. The depth-dose properties and isocentric delivery capabilities of the hospital-based, high-energy neutron beams allowed treatment with neutrons alone to this deep-seated tumor, whereas the prior study using lower energy physics-laboratory-based equipment was limited to mixtures of photons and neutrons in the experimental treatment arm. After stratification for stage, Gleason grade, and the presence or absence of surgical nodal staging, 89 patients were randomized to each treatment arm. Patients with high grade, stage B2, stage C, or stage D1 tumors were eligible for the study. The two treatment arms were balanced for all known prognostic factors.

A preliminary analysis of this study is presented in Figures 69–41 and 69–42. The median follow-up time at the time of this analysis is only two years. Currently, locoregional tumor control rates favor neutrons with a 94% control rate for neutron-treated patients compared with an 86% control rate for photon-treated patients ($p = 0.04$). It is too early (with this slow growing tumor system) to expect any significant differences to show up in survival rates, and no significant differences have been seen. Survival rates are 85% for neutron-treated patients compared with 80% for photon-treated patients (p = not significant). Only two deaths can be attributed to prostate cancer (both on the photon treatment arm); the rest have been due to intercurrent disease or homicide. The preliminary results from this second generation randomized study confirm the results of the prior study showing an increased effectiveness for fast neutron beam irradiation over standard photon radiation therapy in the radiation field.

TABLE 69–42. Salivary Gland RTOG-MRC Randomized Study Results

Endpoint	*Treatment*	*Total Evaluable*	*One-Year Survival*	*Two-Year Survival*
Locoregional tumor control	Photons	12	17% (±11)	17% (±11)
	Neutrons	13	67% (±14)	67% (±14)
Survival	Photons	12	67% (±12)	25% (±14)
	Neutrons	13	77% (±12)	62% (±14)

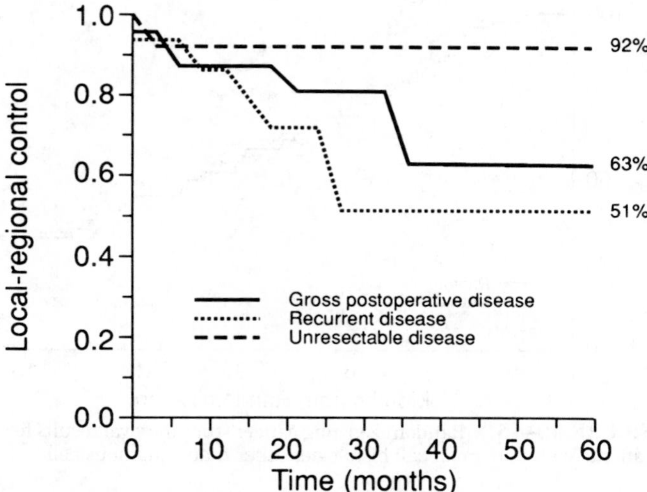

FIGURE 69–39. Actuarial locoregional control of salivary gland tumors for patients stratified according to their disease status at presentation. Curves are shown as a function of time from the start of neutron irradiation. The patients with unresectable disease are shown by the dashed curve, the patients with gross postoperative disease are shown by the solid curve, and patients with recurrent disease are shown by the dotted curve.

NON-SMALL CELL LUNG CANCER

Fast neutron radiation therapy was first systematically investigated for lung cancer by Einhorn and colleagues using a Russian cyclotron generating a neutron beam of 6.2 MeV mean energy.[39] Although no improvements were seen in survival rates, combinations of neutrons and photons demonstrated at autopsy an increased tumor sterilization with increasing neutron dose. The disease sterilization rates in the chest at autopsy were 33% (149 of 429) for photon-treated patients, 48% (45 of 93) for patients receiving 20% of their

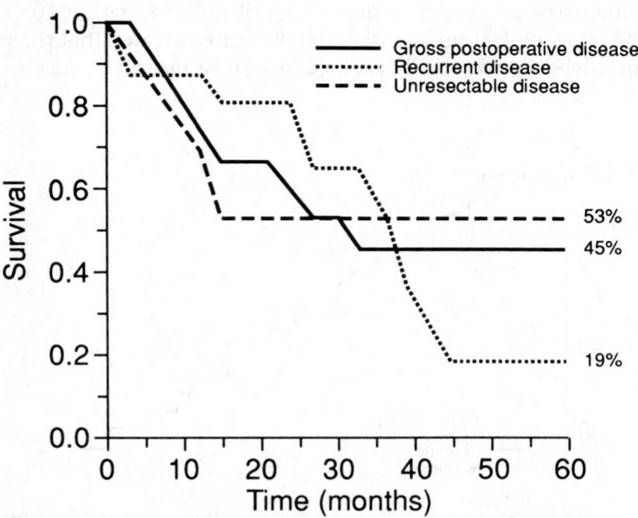

FIGURE 69–40. Actuarial survival for patients with salivary gland tumors stratified according to their disease status at presentation. Curves are shown as a function of time from the start of the neutron irradiation. The patients with unresectable disease are shown by the dashed curve, the patients with gross postoperative disease are shown by the solid curve, and patients with recurrent disease are shown by the dotted curve.

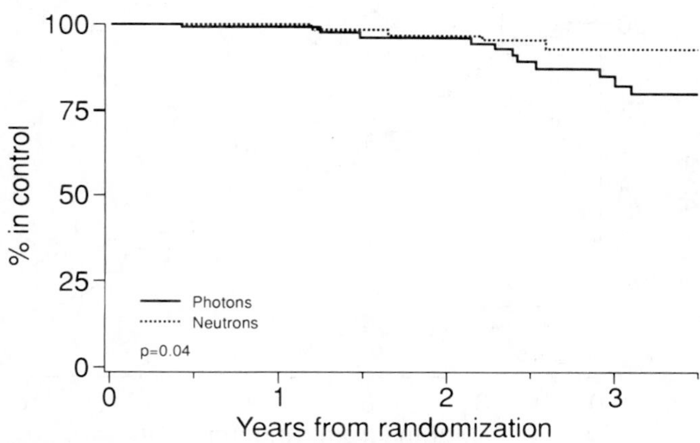

FIGURE 69–41. Locoregional tumor control rates from a randomized prostate cancer study comparing 20.4 neutron Gy with 70 photon Gy. The results are significant at the $p = 0.04$ level.

total dose with neutrons, and 57% (49 of 65) for patients receiving 37% of their total dose with neutrons. The University of Washington reported a 70% local control rate using high-energy neutrons, and M.D. Anderson reported a 91% high-energy neutron local control rate for patients with superior sulcus tumors.[40,41] Sawada, using the NIRS facility in Chiba, Japan, demonstrated improved survival rates for neutron radiation therapy over photon radiation therapy for patients in this same situation.[42] An RTOG-sponsored randomized trial comparing photons to neutrons to mixtures of photons and neutrons using low-energy equipment failed to demonstrate significant differences in median survival or local control, although local tumor control was difficult to evaluate due to obscuring pneumonitis in the low-energy neutron and mixed beam treatment fields. Early treatment failures tended to be dominated by distant metastases, and longer-term (3-year) survival rates favored the neutron-treated and mixed beam-treated patient groups over the photon-treated group (37% versus 25% versus 12%). The normal tissue severe complication rate was significantly higher in patients treated with low-energy neutrons than it was for patients treated with mixed beam or photons (30.9% versus 14.5% versus 5.4%).[43]

A definitive phase III clinical trial using hospital-based, state-of-the-art neutron equipment was subsequently designed for

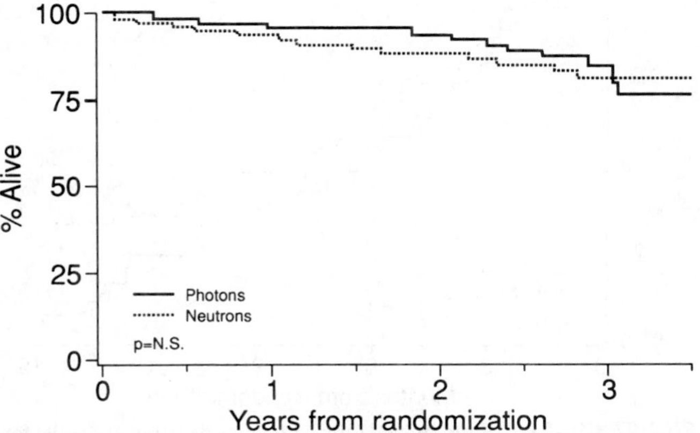

FIGURE 69–42. Survival rates from a randomized prostate cancer study comparing 20.4 neutron Gy with 70 photon Gy.

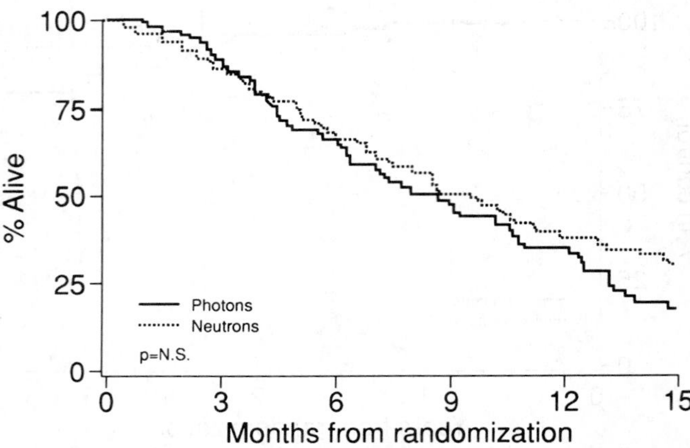

FIGURE 69–43. Results of overall survival from a randomized study comparing fast neutrons with photons for locally advanced non-small cell lung cancer. The differences in the survival curves fail to reach statistical significance.

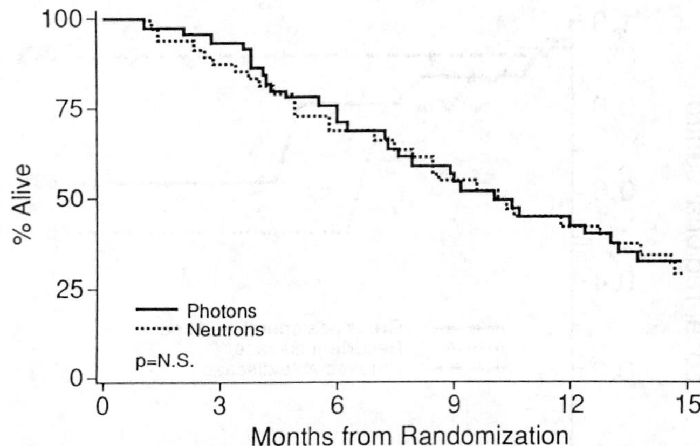

FIGURE 69–45. Randomized lung cancer study survival results for patients with non-small cell histologies other than squamous cell.

patients with inoperable non-small cell carcinomas of the lung. After stratification by prognostic factors and treating institution, patients were randomized to receive 6600 photon cGy delivered in 33 fractions over 7 weeks or 2040 neutron cGy delivered in 12 fractions over 4 weeks. Two hundred patients were entered on this study; 99 patients were randomized to photons, and 101 patients were randomized to neutrons. Tumors confined to the ipsilateral hemithorax and draining regional lymph nodes in patients with a Karnofsky performance score of 70 or better were eligible. The two treatment arms were balanced for all known prognostic factors.

Local tumor control was difficult to evaluate, as it is on all lung cancer studies, due to obscuring radiation pneumonitis in the treatment fields. Actuarial survival curves are depicted for the entire group, patients with squamous cell histologies, patients with non-squamous cell histologies, and patients with favorable prognostic factors in Figures 69–43 through 69–46. There is a trend favoring neutrons in the entire study population that is statistically significant in patients with squamous cell carcinomas ($p = 0.02$; Fig. 69–44). No differences are observed in patients with non-squamous cell histologies. The advantage for neutrons in the patient population with favorable prognostic factors (patients without pleural effusions, without weight loss greater than 5% of body weight, without T4 or N3 tumors) is significant at the $p = 0.03$ level (see Fig. 69–46). There were only four major treatment-related complications (grades 4 or 5) in this study population, with two complications observed in each treatment arm (p = not significant).

Locoregional treatments of non-small cell lung cancer can only show survival benefits in patients who do not have a high probability of harboring occult distant metastases at the time their disease presents itself. Patients with squamous cell cancers, superior sulcus tumors, and patients with favorable prognostic indicators fall into this category. Prior studies have demonstrated improved disease sterilization rates for treatments using fast neutrons, and have demonstrated that these improved locoregional results can lead to improved survival

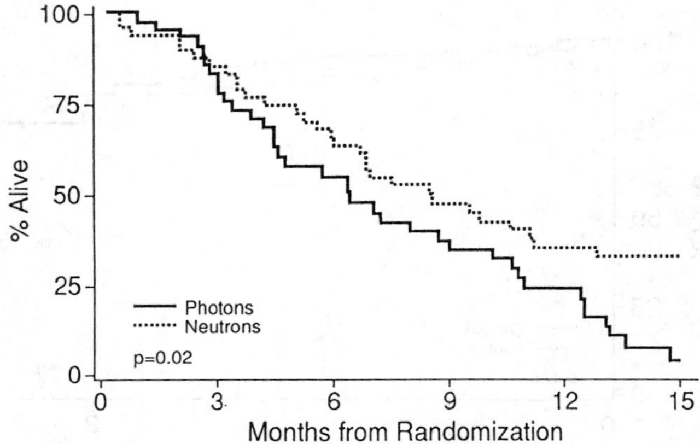

FIGURE 69–44. Randomized lung cancer study survival results for patients with squamous cell histologies. The differences are significant at the $p = 0.02$ level.

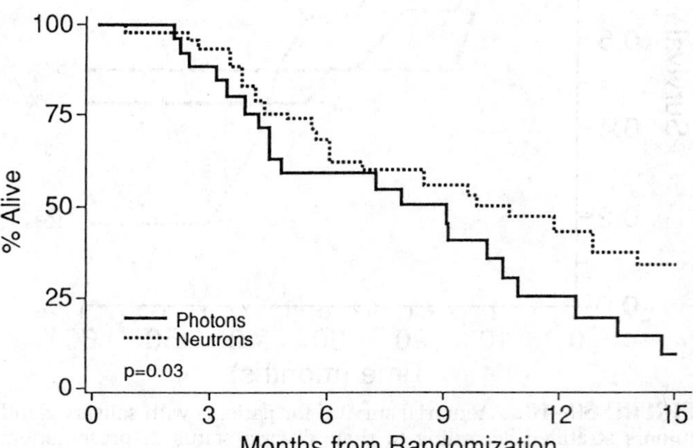

FIGURE 69–46. Randomized lung cancer study results for patients with non-small cell histologies and in good prognostic categories (excludes patients with T4, N3, pleural effusions, weight loss >5% of body weight). The difference is significant at the $p = 0.03$ level.

rates in patients where the risk of distant metastases is not overwhelming. The results of this study thus far appear to confirm these findings.

SQUAMOUS CELL HEAD AND NECK CANCERS

More patients have been treated for squamous cell carcinomas of the head and neck with neutrons than have been treated with neutrons for any other tumor system. Seven phase III randomized studies have been completed; six using low-energy or laboratory-based neutron generators of marginal capability, and a seventh using state-of-the-art equipment. Results from the six low-energy, laboratory-based studies were equivocal. Some reported dramatic improvement in complete response rates and locoregional tumor control with neutrons, and others reported no significant differences.[44–49] Direct comparisons of these trials are made difficult due to the diversity of treatment techniques and equipment, total radiation doses, and patient populations. A seventh prospective, randomized, phase III study using hospital-based cyclotrons was designed to definitively answer questions concerning the role of fast neutrons in treatment of squamous cell carcinomas of the head and neck.

One hundred and seventy-eight patients were entered on this study directly comparing state-of-the-art fast neutron radiation therapy with state-of-the-art photon and electron radiation therapy; 89 patients were randomized to each treatment arm. Patients with T3 or T4 tumors, or T2N+ tumors originating in the oral cavity, oropharynx, hypopharynx, supraglottic larynx, and glottic larynx received 7000 photon cGy in 35 fractions over 7 weeks or 2040 neutron cGy in 12 fractions over 4 weeks. The complete response rate in the neutron-treated group of patients is 70%, compared with 50% in the low-LET-treated group of patients ($p = 0.003$); with relatively short follow-up, this increased complete response rate has resulted in an improvement in locoregional tumor control (53% for neutrons compared with 35% for low-LET radiations). The survival rates are illustrated in Figure 69–47. There are no significant differences in major complication rates between the two groups.

Although fast neutron radiation therapy may ultimately demonstrate a statistically significant improvement in locoregional tumor control in this tumor system, it is unlikely, based on the shapes of the survival curves, that this improvement will result in an associated improvement in survival.

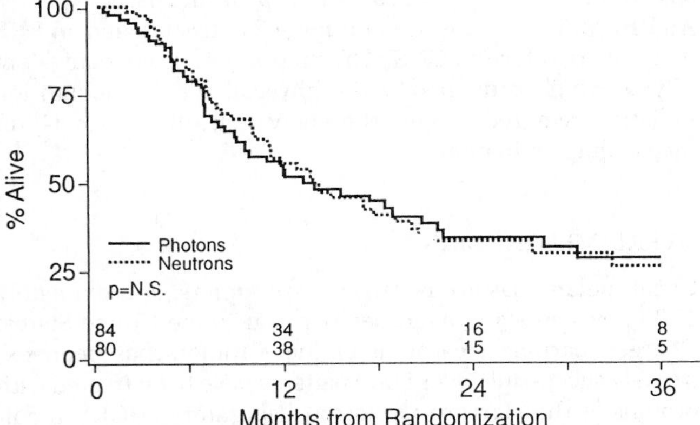

FIGURE 69–47. Survival results from a randomized study comparing 20.4 neutron Gy with 70 photon Gy for squamous cell carcinomas of the head and neck.

TABLE 69–43. Local Control Rates for Soft Tissue Sarcomas Treated Definitively With Radiotherapy

*Investigations**	*Local Control (patients)*	*Local Control Rate (%)*
Neutrons		
Hammersmith[49]	26/50	52
NIRS[50]	7/12	58
Fermi Laboratory[51]	13/26	50
MANTA[32]	4/10	40
TAMVEC[52]	18/29	62
Edinburgh[53]	5/12	42
Hamburg/Eppendorf[54]	27/45	60
Heidelberg/Essen[55]	31/60	52
Louvain[56]	4/19	21
Amsterdam[57]	8/13	61
Seattle[58]	15/21	71
Total	158/297	53
Photons or Electrons		
McNeer[59]	14/25	56
Windeyer[60]	13/22	59
Duncan[63]	5/25	20
Tepper[61]	17/51	33
Leibel[62]	0/5	0
Total	49/128	38

* Patients treated de novo or for gross disease after surgery are included but not patients treated postoperatively for microscopic residual disease or for limited macroscopic residual disease.

SARCOMAS

Although no phase III randomized studies have been completed investigating the role of fast neutrons in treatment of sarcomas of soft tissue, bone, or cartilage, a considerable experience has been amassed in non-randomized settings. Tables 69–43 through 69–45 compare neutron results with historical photon results reported in the literature for soft tissue sarcomas, osteogenic sarcomas, and chondrosarcomas, respectively.[49–69] The summed locoregional tumor control rates for inoperable, locally advanced soft tissue sarcomas are 53% for neutrons compared with 38% for low-LET photons and electrons. The locoregional results for locally advanced osteogenic sarcomas are 55% for neutrons compared with 21% for photons and electrons, and the results for locally advanced chondrosarcomas are 49% for neutrons compared with 33% for low-LET radiations. The results of fast neutron radiation therapy for these sarcomas are remarkably consistent and appear to demonstrate an improvement in locoregional tumor control rates over historical results. These results cannot be considered definitive until randomized studies are completed.

TABLE 69-44. Local Control Rates for Osteogenic Sarcomas Treated Definitively With Radiotherapy

*Investigations**	Local Control (patients)	Local Control Rate (%)
Neutrons		
MANTA[32]	1/1	100
TAMVEC[52]	0/1	0
Fermi Laboratory[51]	2/9	22
Amsterdam[57]	0/3	0†
Edinburgh[63]	1/5	20
NIRS[64]	33/41	80
Seattle[58]	3/13	23
Total	40/73	55
Photons		
DeMoor[65]	9/43	33
Beck[66]	1/21	5
Tudway[67]	5/9	56
Total	15/73	21

* Patients treated postoperatively for microscopic residual disease or for limited macroscopic residual disease are not included.
† Persistent mass and calcification treated as failure, and local control rates may be underestimated.

TABLE 69-45. Local Control Rates for Chondrosarcomas Treated Definitively With Radiotherapy

*Investigations**	*Local Control (patients)*	*Local Control Rate (%)*
Neutrons		
MANTA[32]	7/9	78
TAMVEC[52]	4/4	100
Fermi Laboratory[51]	9/16	56
Amsterdam[57]	0/6	0†
Edinburgh[63]	0/5	0†
NIRS[64]	1/2	50
Seattle[58]	4/9	44
Total	25/51	49
Photons		
McNanny[68]	3/10	30
Harwood[69]	7/20	35
Total	10/30	33

* Patients treated postoperatively for microscopic residual disease or for limited macroscopic residual disease are not included.
† Persistent mass and calcification treated as failure, and local control rates may be underestimated.

CHARGED PARTICLE CLINICAL STUDIES

As with neutrons (uncharged particles), charged particle radiation therapy was first suggested by physicists. However, despite 2 decades of small volume treatment for pituitary diseases, the investigation of large field charged particle cancer treatment did not begin until the mid 1970s. The first clinical cancer trials in the United States used protons (hydrogen nuclei) at the Harvard Cyclotron Laboratory (HCL), helium ions (α particles) at the University of California Lawrence Berkeley Laboratory (LBL), and pi mesons (subatomic particles) at the Los Alamos Meson Physics Facility. Heavier nuclei (*e.g.*, neon, carbon, silicon) were introduced at LBL later in that decade.

The initial accrual of clinical data to heavy charged particle studies was slow because of limitations on beam availability and the need to develop pioneering treatment techniques. In the United States almost 3600 cancer patients have been treated with protons and helium ions.[70] In other parts of the world, smaller numbers of patients have been treated at several proton facilities including the USSR, Switzerland, and Japan. Almost 230 patients were treated with pi mesons in the United States before that project was closed.[71] Subsequently over 700 patients have been treated with pi mesons in Switzerland and Canada. Heavy charged particle therapy has been used in over 400 patients. Virtually all patients receiving treatment with charged particles have been treated in laboratory-based treatment facilities located at some distance from their affiliated medical centers.

PROTONS AND HELIUM IONS

Protons and helium ions are charged particles that have a finite penetration in tissue. This unique characteristic results in dose distributions that are superior in many clinical situations to those obtainable with photons or electrons. The finite range and well-defined lateral edge allows smaller treatment volumes and lower doses to adjacent critical organs when compared with photons or electrons. Figure 69-48 shows a helium ion treatment plan for a chordoma at C2; in this plan the distal edge of the posterior field (with a cord block) is matched exactly to the lateral penumbra of the lateral fields.

Although the primary distinguishing characteristic of protons and helium ions compared with photons is their finite range in tissue, protons and helium ions differ slightly in relative biologic effectiveness (RBE) compared with megavoltage photons. The RBE for protons is 1.1.[72,73] Dose is expressed in the units of cobalt Gray equivalent (CGE) where CGE equals proton Gy $\times$ 1.1. The RBE for helium ions depends on fraction size, position in the spread out Bragg peak and tissue type.[74,75] An RBE value of 1.3 is used for non-CNS tissues, and an RBE of 1.6 is used for the CNS. The unit of dose is Gy-equivalent (GyE), which is defined as the physical dose of helium ion radiation required to give the equivalent effect of 1 Gy of megavoltage radiation.

UVEAL MELANOMAS

Uveal melanomas are relatively rare tumors; approximately 1200 new cases are diagnosed per year in the United States. Charged particle treatment of these tumors has been extremely successful. Over 2000 patients have been treated with protons at the Harvard Cyclotron Laboratory (HCL) in collaboration with Massachusetts General Hospital and Massachusetts Eye and Ear Infirmary or with helium ions at the Lawrence Berkeley Laboratory (LBL) in collaboration with the University of California-San Francisco.[70]

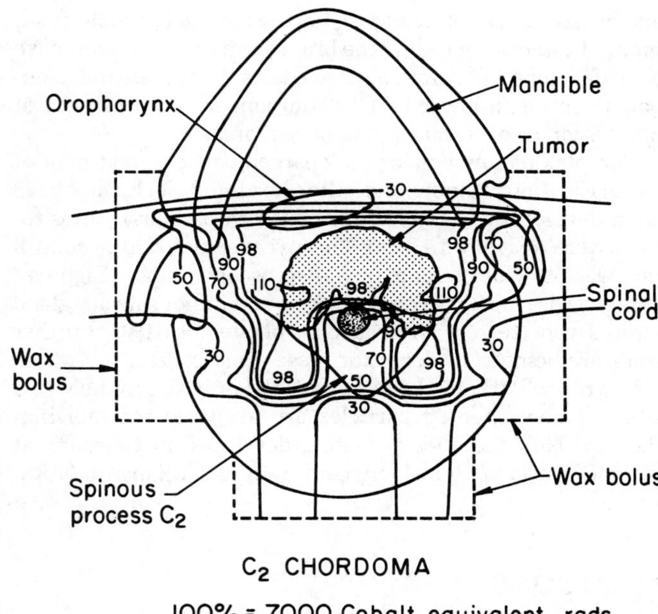

FIGURE 69–48. Composite treatment plan for precision high-dose helium irradiation of a chordoma of the upper cervical spine.

Charged particle treatment of uveal melanoma has employed high doses of radiation. Most patients have received the equivalent of 7000 cGy in five fractions over 8 to 9 days.[76,77] The treatment volume is small because the charged particles have minimal scatter and there is no radiation distal to the end of the particle range. Precise planning and delivery methods have been used for these treatments.[78]

The goal of charged particle treatment is to eradicate the melanoma while preserving a cosmetically intact eye and visual function. Local control rates after charged particle treatment have been very high (Table 69–46): the actuarial 5-year local control rate is 96.3% for the HCL patients and 96.8% for the LBL patients.[79,80] All but a small number of patients have maintained a cosmetically intact eye. In the HCL experience the 5-year actuarial eye retention rate is 89%, and in the LBL experience, the rate is 83%.[81,80] Vision of 20/200 or better has been maintained in 65% to 70% of the HCL patients.[82,83] At 5 years, 80% of the HCL patients and 76% of the LBL patients are without evidence of metastatic disease.[84] Survival rates for patients treated with protons have been compared using known prognostic factors with survival rates for patients undergoing enucleation.[80,85] The results show no differences in survival after the two different treatments.

SARCOMAS

The next largest group of cancer patients receiving proton or helium ion treatment are patients with sarcomas of the skull base and cervical spine. Charged particle radiation in the postoperative setting has achieved a significant clinical gain for patients with these uncommon tumors. Despite the rarity of these tumors, 320 patients with chordomas or chondrosarcomas in the skull base or cervical spine have been treated with protons or helium ions.[85,215] These tumors are locally aggressive and are located immediately adjacent to critical structures such as the brain stem, spinal cord, temporal lobes, and optic nerves and chiasm. Surgical resection is usually incomplete. Postoperative photon radiation achieves local control in approximately 35% to 40% of patients.[86] Proton and helium ion radiation can deliver a substantially higher dose than photons to the residual tumor. The 5-year actuarial local control rates are 60% to 77% for patients treated with helium ions or protons after surgery.[87,88] Survival rates at 5 years are 62% to 88%.

In the HCL proton experience, patients received a median dose of 68.5 CGE (range, 56.8–77.4 CGE) using 1.8 CGE fractions. Patients with chondrosarcomas have a better prognosis than patients with chordomas. The 5-year actuarial local control rate is 91% for chondrosarcomas (85 patients) and 65% for chordomas (130 patients).[70] Tumor volume is another prognostic factor with small volumes having higher local control rates.[89] Patients treated with helium ions at LBL have received a mean dose of 67 GyE (range, 36–80 GyE). The usual fractionation was 2.0 to 2.5 GyE four days per week. Patients with tumor volume less than 20 ml had a 5-year actuarial local control rate of 80% while patients with larger tumor volumes had a 33% local control rate.[87] Patients with recurrent disease had a poorer outcome than previously untreated patients.[90] A small number of patients with sacral chordomas have received helium ion treatment.[91]

The achievements of proton therapy discussed in this section have been accomplished using physics laboratory facilities with fixed, horizontal beams. The next generation of proton facilities in the United States will be hospital based machines with isocentric gantries. Such a facility has been built at Loma Linda University and plans for several other facilities are being developed.

TABLE 69–46. Results of Charged Particle Treatment for Uveal Melanoma

Results	*Protons**	*Helium Ions**
Local control	96.3%	96.8%
Eye retention	89%	83%
Survival without metastases	80%	76%

* Five-year actuarial rates.

HEAVY CHARGED PARTICLES

Heavy charged particle radiotherapy has been investigated at the University of California Lawrence Berkeley Laboratory in collaboration with the University of California-San Francisco Department of Radiation Oncology. Heavy charged particles have high-LET properties and improved dose localization properties compared with x-rays because of a defined depth of penetration in tissue. Most of the clinical work with heavy charged particles has been done with neon. A small number of patients have been treated with silicon and carbon.

Between 1979 and 1988, a total of 239 patients had received neon treatment with a neon dose of 1000 cGy or greater.[92] Neon doses were gradually escalated while acute and late toxicities were monitored until toxicity limits were reached. The preclinical in vitro and in vivo measurements of neon RBE relative to megavoltage x-rays were 2.0 to 3.5, depending on fraction size, beam energy, size of the extended Bragg peak, type of tissue irradiated and biologic endpoint chosen.[93–98] The clinical RBE for acute normal tissue reactions was consistent with the experimental data in the range of 2.0 to 3.5 (average 2.5). The RBE for the CNS is higher and the dose to the brain and spinal cord is limited to 1000 cGy whenever possible.[4,5] The neon dose is expressed as equivalent dose using the units of GyE (GyE=neon physical Gy × RBE).

Neon treatment of many different tumor sites has been explored and include prostate cancer, soft tissue and bone sarcomas, paranasal sinus cancers, salivary gland tumors, advanced head and neck cancer, malignant gliomas, lung cancer, esophageal cancer, gastric cancer, pancreatic cancer, biliary tract cancer, and melanoma. Promising results were seen in advanced prostate cancer, macroscopic soft tissue and bone sarcomas, paranasal sinus cancers, macroscopic salivary gland cancers, and biliary tract cancers (Table 69–47). Further studies including randomized trials are in progress or are being initiated for these disease sites.

Twenty-one patients with locally advanced prostate cancer received a neon boost after megavoltage treatment to the pelvis. The median total dose was 7500 cGy, and the median neon dose was 11 Gy. The 5-year actuarial local control rate is 89%, and the disease-specific survival (DSS) is 61%.[100] Disease-specific survival analysis reflects the events of death from disease or treatment complications. A phase III trial is in progress for patients with stage C and D1 disease; this trial compares neon and photon boosts to the prostate.

Twelve patients with soft tissue sarcomas were treated with a median total dose of 60 GyE and a median neon dose of 14 Gy. Nineteen patients with bone sarcomas were treated. The median total dose used in this group of patients was 69.6 GyE and the median neon dose was 16.8 Gy. The actuarial 5-year local control rate is 56% for patients with macroscopic soft tissue sarcoma and 59% for patients with macroscopic bone sarcoma.[92] The excellent dose localization properties of neon allow treatment in challenging tumor locations where high doses of x-rays or neutrons cannot be delivered safely. These tumor locations include soft tissue sarcomas of the retroperitoneum and trunk and bone sarcomas arising in the spine

TABLE 69–47. Results of Neon Treatment for Malignant Disease

Tumor	*No. of Patients*	*5-Year Local Control (%)*	*5-Year Disease-Specific Survival (%)**
Prostate	21	89	61
Soft tissue sarcoma	12	56	56
Bone sarcoma	19	59	45
Paranasal sinuses	12	69	69
Salivary gland	18	61	59
Biliary tract	8	44	29

* Disease-specific survival scores death from disease and treatment complications as events.

and clivus. Elegant techniques for the charged particle treatment of tumors encircling the brain stem or spinal cord have been developed.[100] A randomized trial is in progress that compares neon with lower-LET helium ions in the treatment of macroscopic soft tissue and bone sarcomas.

Complex techniques for the charged particle treatment of paranasal sinus tumors and other head and neck sites have been developed.[101] Twelve patients with paranasal sinus tumors were treated with neon. The 5-year actuarial local control rate was 69% for patients with macroscopic tumor. Eighteen patients with locally advanced major and minor salivary gland tumors were treated. The local control rate was 61%.[92] Further trials are being considered for these disease sites.

Lawrence Berkeley Laboratory is the only site in the world where heavy charged particles are available for radiation therapy. New facilities are being developed in Germany at G.S.I. Darmstadt-Heidelberg University and in Japan at NIRS, Chiba.

PI MESONS

Pi mesons (pions) were first investigated clinically at the Los Alamos Meson Physics Facility (LAMPF) between 1974 and 1981. Patient treatment with pions were later started at the TRI University Meson Facility (TRIUMF) in Vancouver, Canada, and the Paul Scherrer Institute (PSI) in Villigen, Switzerland. Clinical investigations are continuing at these facilities. Pions have improved depth dose characteristics and increased RBE compared with photons. The interaction of pions with tissue is characterized by the pion star that is formed as pions are captured by nuclei. Preclinical in vivo measurements of RBE indicated a pion RBE of 1.5 in the range of 2 to 3 Gy per fraction.[102–104] Phase I–II clinical experience at LAMPF is consistent with an RBE in the range of 1.4 to 1.6 for acute normal tissue reactions and late sequelae.[71] Phase III studies are planned for gliomas, sarcomas, and prostate. Encouraging phase I–II results for the treatment of unresectable soft tissue sarcomas have been reported.[105]

BORON NEUTRON-CAPTURE THERAPY

An isotope of boron, boron 10 has the capacity to capture neutrons and concentrate their cell killing effects in a small volume. When the nucleus of a boron atom captures a neutron, it undergoes a fission reaction producing lithium and helium nuclei that deposit approximately 2.35 million electron volts in energy over short distances comparable to cellular dimensions. If boron atoms are selectively concentrated in tumor cells, by attaching them to tumor-specific antibodies or through other means, this energy could be removed from an external neutron beam and concentrated in malignant cells. If a sufficient concentration differential of boron atoms is achieved between tumor and normal tissues, then the destruction of target tumor cells will be selectively enhanced relative to surrounding normal tissue structures, and the effectiveness of neutron radiotherapy would be greatly increased.

Shortly after the neutron was discovered by Chadwick in 1932, Locher proposed the use of boron neutron capture therapy (BNCT) as a possible treatment for human malignancies.[106] A few years later, Kruger[107] and Zahl[108] demonstrated the biologic effectiveness of the fission fragments produced by the interaction of slow neutrons with ^{10}B. The first clinical trials for human malignancies were carried out for malignant gliomas of the brain using a reactor beam at the Brookhaven National Laboratories with borax used as the ^{10}B carrier agent.[109,110] These and other subsequent trials carried out in the 1960s showed no therapeutic benefit for this form of treatment and moreover, showed considerable damage to the endothelial linings of the blood vessels. This was attributed to the high concentration of ^{10}B in the blood at the time of treatment and to the poorly penetrating characteristics of the collimated reactor beams used for treatment. The development of new ^{10}B-carrier agents has led to a resurgence of interest in BNCT on the part of the medical community.

Although most BNCT work has used thermal and epithermal nuclear reactor generated slow neutron beams, it is possible to enhance accelerator-produced fast neutron beams by BNCT. When a fast neutron beam penetrates tissue, a small "thermalized" neutron flux develops naturally due to neutron-nuclear interactions, and it is possible to use this thermalized component to specifically enhance the microdosimetric radiation dose to tumor cells via BNCT techniques.[111] The use of fast neutrons for BNCT avoids the problems of poor depth dose, poor skin sparing, poor collimation, and the radiation safety considerations associated with slow neutron beams generated from nuclear reactors. Typical fast neutron doses used in a course of radiotherapy are in the range of 18 to 20 neutron Gy.

Because only low-energy neutrons can be captured by boron atoms, the effective low-energy component of fast neutron beams has been measured by activation of Sodium in a $NaNO_3$ solution, and model calculations have been performed based on Monte Carlo simulations for cell survival. This model predicts that over a standard course of fast neutron radiotherapy, 30 μg/g concentrations of boron in the tumor cells would result in a tenfold to 100-fold increase in tumor cell kill. Using a Poisson model for tumor control, a tenfold improvement in

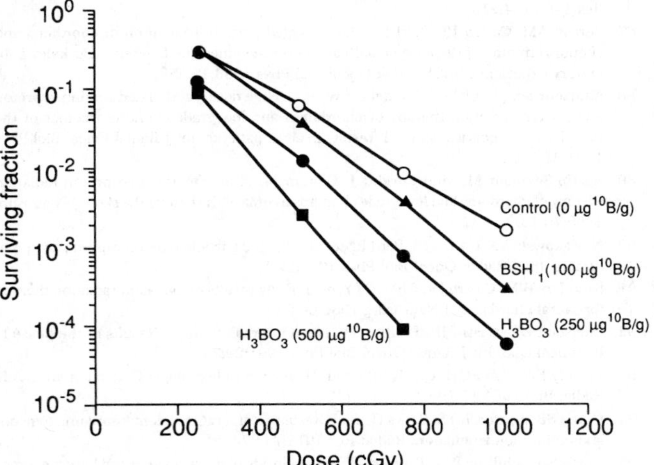

FIGURE 69–49. Survival of Chinese hamster ovary cells after fast-neutron-beam irradiation. Cells incubated with boron-containing compounds before irradiation show enhanced cell killing.

cell kill would increase a tumor control rate from 20% to 85%. Concentration differentials (tumor to normal tissue) of 30 to 50 μg/g have been achieved with modern boron carrier technology. These newer carriers include: sodium borocaptate, tumor specific antibodies, chlorpromazine, misonidazole, thiouracil, porphyrins, amino acids, nucleosides, and steroids.

Radiobiologic measurements made in vitro verify these model calculations (Fig. 69–49), and the size of these measured effects agree with the models.[112]

Boron neutron capture therapy, in a theory described by Lochner in 1936, should result in a dramatic improvement in the results of treatment for tumors that can concentrate quantities of boron in excess of 30 μg/g of tumor above surrounding normal tissue. With the development of new carrier agents for boron and with studies that now demonstrate that cyclotron-generated fast neutron beams can be enhanced by boron capture, BNCT has the potential to become a practical clinical reality.

REFERENCES

1. Griffin TW, Wambersie A, Laramore GE, et al. High LET heavy particle trials. Int J Radiat Oncol Biol Phys 1988;14:583.
2. Suit HD, Griffin TW, Castro JR, et al. Particle radiation therapy research plan. Am J Clin Oncol 1988;11:330.
3. Von Essen CF, Blattman H, Crawford JF, et al. The piotron: Initial experience, preparation and experience with pion therapy. Int J Radiat Oncol Biol Phys 1982;8:1499.
4. Gray LH, Conger AE, Ebert M, et al. Concentration of oxygen dissolved in tissues at time of irradiation as a factor in radiotherapy. Br J Radiol 1950;26:638.
5. Tenforde TJ, Azal SM, Parr, SS, et al. Cell survival in rat rhabdomyosarcoma tumors irradiated in vivo with extended peak silicon ions. Radiat Res 1982;92:208.
6. Howlett JF, Thomlinson RH, Alper T. A marked dependence on the conformative effective causes of neutrons on tumor line and its implications for clinical trials. Br J Radiol 1975;48:40.
7. Gragg RL, Humphrey RM, Thomas HT, et al. The response of Chinese hamster ovary cells to fast neutron radiotherapy beams. I. Variations in relative biologic effectiveness with position in the cell cycle. Radiat Res 1978;76:283.
8. Gragg RL, Humphrey RM, Meyn RE. The response of Chinese hamster ovary cells to fast neutron radiotherapy beams. II. Sublethal and potentially lethal damage recovery capabilities. Radiat Res 1977;71:461.
9. Hall EJ, Kraljevic J. Repair of potentially lethal radiation damage: Comparison of neutron and x-ray RBE and implications for radiation therapy. Radiology 1976;121:731.
10. Stone RS, Larkin JC. Treatment of cancer with fast neutrons. Radiology 1942;39:608.
11. Fowler JF, Morgan RL. Pre-therapeutic experiments with fast neutron beam from Medical Research Council's cyclotron. VIII: General review. Br J Radiol 1963;36:115.
12. Sheline GE, Phillips TL, Field SB, et al. Effects of fast neutrons on human skin. AJR 1971;111:31.
13. Catterall M. The treatment of advanced cancer by fast neutrons from the Medical Research Council's cyclotron at Hammersmith Hospital, London. Eur J Cancer 1974;10:343.
14. Batterman JJ, Breur K, Hart GAM, et al. Observations on pulmonary metastases in patients after single doses and multiple fractions of fast neutrons and cobalt-60 gamma rays. Eur J Cancer 1981;17:539.
15. Koh W, Laramore GE, Griffin TW, et al. Fast neutron radiation for inoperable and recurrent salivary gland cancers. Am J Clin Oncol 1989;12:316.
16. Borthne A, Kjellevold K, Kaalhus O, et al. Salivary gland malignant neoplasms: Treatment and prognosis. Int J Radiat Oncol Biol Phys 1986;12:747.
17. Fitzpatrick PJ, Theriault C. Malignant salivary gland tumors. Int J Radiat Oncol Biol Phys 1986;12:1743.
18. Fu KK, Leibel S, Levine M, et al. Carcinoma of the major and minor salivary glands: Analysis of treatment results and sites and causes of failures. Cancer 1977;40:2882.
19. Shidnia H, Hornback N, Hamaker R, et al. Carcinoma of major salivary glands. Cancer 1980;45:693.
20. Elkon D, Colman M, Hendrickson F. Radiation therapy in the treatment of malignant salivary gland tumors. Cancer 1978;41:502.
21. Rossman K. The role of radiation therapy in the treatment of parotid carcinomas. AJR 1975;123:492.
22. Rafla S. Malignant parotid tumors: Natural history and treatment. Cancer 1977;40:136.
23. Dobrowsky W, Schlappack O, Karcher KH, et al. Electron-beam therapy in treatment of parotid neoplasm. Radiother Oncol 1986;6:293.
24. Griffin TW, Pajak TF, Laramore GE, et al. Neutron vs. photon irradiation of inoperable salivary gland tumors: Results of an RTOG-MRC cooperative study. Int J Radiat Oncol Biol Phys 1988;15:1085.

25. Vikram B, Strong EW, Shah JP, et al. Radiation therapy in adenoid-cystic carcinomas. Int J Radiat Oncol Biol Phys 1984;10:221.
26. Stewart JG, Jackson A, Chew M. The role of radiation therapy in the management of malignant tumors of the salivary glands. AJR 1968;102:100.
27. Guillamondegui OM, Byers RM, Luna MA, et al. Aggressive surgery in the treatment for parotid cancer: The role of adjunctive postoperative radiotherapy. AJR 1975;123: 49.
28. Ravasz LA, Terhhard CHJ, Hordijk GJ. Radiotherapy in epithelial tumors of the parotid gland: Case presentation and literature review. Int J Radiat Oncol Biol Phys 1990;19: 55.
29. Saroja KR, Mansell J, Hendrickson R, et al. An update on malignant salivary gland tumors treated with neutrons at Fermilab. Int J Radiat Oncol Biol Phys 1987;13:1319.
30. Catterall M, Errington RD. The implications of improved treatment of malignant salivary gland tumors by fast neutron radiotherapy. Int J Radiat Oncol Biol Phys 1987;13:1313.
31. Duncan W, Orr JA, Arnott SJ, et al. Neutron therapy for malignant tumors of the salivary glands: A report of the Edinburgh experience. Radiother Oncol 1987;8:97.
32. Ornitz R, Herskovic A, Bradley E, et al. Clinical observations of early and late normal tissue injury and tumor control in patients receiving fast neutron irradiation. In: High LET radiations in clinical radiotherapy. Elmsford, NY: Pergamon Press, 1979.
33. Battermann JJ, Mijnheer BJ. The Amsterdam fast neutron therapy project: A final report. Int J Radiat Oncol Biol Phys 1986;12:2093.
34. Maor M, Hussey D, Fletcher GH, et al. Fast neutron radiotherapy for locally advanced head and neck tumors. Int J Radiat Oncol Biol Phys 1981;7:155.
35. Eichhorn HJ. Pilot study on the applicability of neutron radiotherapy. Radiobiol Radiother 1981;3:262.
36. Skolyszewski J, Byrski E, Chrzanowska A, et al. A preliminary report on the clinical application of fast neutrons in Krakow. Int J Radiat Oncol Biol Phys 1982;8:1781.
37. Buchholz TA, Laramore GE, Griffin BR, et al. The role of fast neutron radiotherapy in the management of advanced salivary gland malignancies. Cancer 1992:2779–2788.
38. Laramore GE, Krall JM, Thomas FJ, et al. Fast neutron radiotherapy for locally advanced prostate cancer: Final report of an RTOG randomized clinical trial. Am J Clin Oncol (in press).
39. Eichhorn HJ. Results of a pilot study on neutron therapy with 600 patients. Int J Radiat Oncol Biol Phys 1982;8:1561.
40. Livingston RB, Griffin BR, Higano C, et al. Combined treatment with chemotherapy and neutron irradiation for limited non-small cell lung cancer: A SWOG study. J Clin Oncol 1987;5:1756.
41. Komaki R, Mountain C, Holbert J, et al. Superior sulcus tumors: Treatment selection and results for 85 patients without metastases at presentation. Int J Radiat Oncol Biol Phys 1990;19:31.
42. Sawada K, Fukuma S, Seki Y, et al. Clinical experience in patients with Pancoast tumor treated by fast neutron radiotherapy. Gan No Rinsho 1983;A7:111.
43. Laramore GE, Bauer M, Griffin TW, et al. Fast neutron and mixed beam radiotherapy for inoperable non-small cell carcinoma of the lung. Am J Clin Oncol 1986;9:233.
44. Catterall M, Bewley D, Sutherland I. Second report on a randomized clinical trial of fast neutrons compared with x or gamma rays in treatment of advanced cancers of the head and neck. Br J Med 1977;1:1942.
45. Maor M, Schoenfeld DA, Hendrickson FR, et al. Evaluation of a neutron boost in head and neck cancer: Results of the randomized RTOG trial 78-08. Am J Clin Oncol 1986;9: 61.
46. Duncan W, Orr JA, Arnott SJ, et al. Fast neutron therapy for squamous cell carcinoma in the head and neck region: Results of a randomized trial. Int J Radiat Oncol Biol Phys 1987;13:171.
47. Griffin TW, Davis R, Hendrickson F, et al. Fast neutron radiation therapy for unresectable squamous cell carcinomas of the head and neck: The results of a randomized RTOG study. Int J Radiat Oncol Biol Phys 1984;10:2217.
48. Griffin TW, Pajak T, Maor M, et al. Mixed neutron/photon irradiation of unresectable squamous cell carcinomas of the head and neck: The final report of a randomized trial. Int J Radiat Oncol Biol Phys 1989;17:959.
49. Catterall M. The treatment of advanced cancer by fast neutrons from the Medical Research Council's cyclotron at Hammersmith Hospital, London. Eur J Cancer 1974;10: 343.
50. Tsunemoto H, Morita S, Arai T, et al. Results of clinical trial with 30 MeV d-Be neutrons at NIRS. In: Treatment of radioresistant cancers. Amsterdam, Elsevier-North Holland, 1974.
51. Cohen L, Hendrickson F, Mansell J, et al. Response of sarcomas of bone and soft tissue to neutron beam therapy. Int J Radiat Oncol Biol Phys 1984;10:821.
52. Salinas R, Hussey DH, Fletcher GH. Experience with fast neutron therapy for locally advanced sarcomas. Int J Radiat Oncol Biol Phys 1980;6:267.
53. Duncan W, Dewar JA. A retrospective study of the role of radiotherapy in the treatment of soft tissue sarcoma. Clin Radiol 1985;36:629.
54. Franke HD, Hess A, Brassow F, et al. Clinical results after irradiation of intracranial tumors, soft tissue sarcomas, and thyroid cancers with fast neutrons at Hamburg-Eppendorf. In: Progress in Radio-Oncology II. New York: Raven Press, 1982.
55. Schmitt G, Schnabel K, Sauerwein W, et al. Neutron and neutron-boost irradiation of soft tissue sarcomas: A 4.5 year analysis of 139 patients. Radiother Oncol 1983;1:23.
56. Wambersie A. The European experience in neutron therapy at the end of 1981. Int J Radiat Oncol Biol Phys 1982;8:2145.
57. Battermann JJ, Breur K. Fast neutron therapy for locally advanced sarcomas. Int J Radiat Oncol Biol Phys 1981;7:1051.
58. Laramore GE, Griffeth JT, Boespflug M, et al. Fast neutron radiotherapy for sarcomas of soft tissue, bone, and cartilage. Am J Clin Oncol 1989;12:320.
59. McNeer GP, Cantin J, Chu F, et al. Effectiveness of radiation therapy in the management of sarcoma of the soft somatic tissues. Cancer 1968;22:391.
60. Windeyer W, Dische S, Mansfield CF. The place of radiotherapy in the management of fibrosarcoma of the soft tissues. Clin Radiol 1966;17:32.
61. Tepper JE, Suit HD. Radiation therapy alone for sarcoma of soft tissue. Cancer 1985;56: 474.
62. Leibel SA, Tranbaugh RF, Wara WF, et al. Soft tissue sarcomas of the extremities: Survival and patterns of failure with conservative surgery with postoperative irradiation compared to surgery alone. Cancer 1985;56:475.
63. Duncan W, Arnott SJ, Jack WJL. The Edinburgh experience of treating sarcomas of soft tissue and bone with neutron irradiation. Clin Radiol 1986;37:317.
64. Hokada E, Maruyama K, Takada N, et al. Multimodality treatment, including fast neutron radiotherapy, for osteosarcoma. Cancer Bull 1979;31:216.
65. deMoor NG. Osteosarcoma: A review of 72 cases treated by megavoltage radiation therapy with or without surgery. S Afr J Surg 1975;13:137.
66. Beck JC, Wara WM, Bovill EG, et al. The role of radiation therapy in the treatment of osteosarcoma. Radiology 1976;120:163.
67. Tudway RC. Radiotherapy for osteogenic sarcoma. J Bone Joint Surg 1961;43:61.
68. McNaney D, Lindberg RD, Ayala AG, et al. Fifteen year radiotherapy experience with chondrosarcoma of bone. Int J Radiat Oncol Biol Phys 1982;8:187.
69. Harwood AR, Krajbich JI, Fornasier VL. Radiotherapy of chondrosarcoma of bone. Cancer 1980;45:2769.
70. Suit H, Urie M. Clinical gains to be realized from proton beams in radiation therapy (in press).
71. Schmitt G, von Essen CF, Greiner R, et al. Review of the SIN and Los Alamos pion trials. Radiat Res 1985;104:272.
72. Urano M, Goitein M, Verhey L, et al. Relative biological effectiveness of a high energy modulated proton beam using a spontaneous murine tumor in vivo. Int J Radiat Oncol Biol Phys 1980;6:1187.
73. Urano M, Verhey LJ, Goitein M, et al. Relative biological effectiveness of modulated proton beams in various murine tissues. Int J Radiat Oncol Biol Phys 1983;10:509.
74. Phillips TL, Fu KK, Curtis SB. Tumor biology of helium and heavy ions. Int J Radiat Oncol Biol Phys 1977;3:109.
75. Lyman JT. Computer modeling of heavy charged-particle beams. In: Pion and heavy ion radiodtherapy pre-clinical and clinical studies. New York: Elsevier Biomedical, 1979.
76. Gragoudas ES, Goitein M, Koehler A, et al. Proton irradiation of choroidal melanomas. Arch Ophthalmol 1978;96:1583.
77. Saunders WM, Char DH, Quivey JM, et al. Precision high dose radiotherapy: Helium ion treatment of uveal melanoma. Int J Radiat Oncol Biol Phys 1985;11:227.
78. Goitein M, Miller T. Planning proton therapy of the eye. Med Phys 1983;10:275.
79. Munzenrider JE, Verhey L, Gradoudas ES, et al. Conservative treatment of uveal melanoma: Local recurrence after proton beam therapy. Int J Radiat Oncol Biol Phys 1989;17:493.
80. Linstadt D, Castro J, Char D, et al. Long-term results of helium ion irradiation of uveal melanoma. Int J Radiat Oncol Biol Phys 1990;19:613.
81. Munzenrider JE, Gragoudas ES, Seddon JM, et al. Conservative treatment of uveal melanoma: Probability of eye retention after proton treatment. Int J Radiat Oncol Biol Phys 1988;15:553.
82. Seddon JM, Gragoudas ES, Polivogianis L, et al. Visual outcome after proton beam irradiation of uveal melanoma. Ophthalmology 1986;93:666.
83. Gragoudas ES, Seddon JM, Egan K, et al. Long-term results of proton beam irradiated uveal melanomas. Ophthalmology 1987;94:349.
84. Gragoudas ES, Seddon JM, Egan KM, et al. Metastasis from uveal melanoma after proton beam irradiation. Ophthalmology 1988;95:992.
85. Seddon JM, Gragoudas ES, Egan KM, et al. Relative survival rates after alternative therapies for uveal melanoma. Ophthalmology 1990;97:769.
86. Austin-Seymour M, Munzenrider JE, Goitein M, et al. Progress in low-LET heavy particle therapy: Intracranial and paracranial tumors and uveal melanomas. Radiat Res 1985;104:219.
87. Berson AM, Castro JR, Petti P, et al. Charged particle irradiation of chordoma and chondrosarcoma of the base of skull and cervical spine: The Lawrence Berkeley Laboratory experience. Int J Radiat Oncol Biol Phys 1988;15:559.
88. Munzenrider JE, Liebsch NJ, deBois W, et al. High dose fractionated combined proton and photon radiation therapy of chordomas and low-grade chondrosarcomas of the skull base and cervical spine. I. results in adult patients. Int J Radiat Oncol Biol Phys 1991;21:166.
89. Austin-Seymour M, Munzenrider J, Goitein M, et al. Fractionated proton radiation therapy of chordoma and low-grade chondrosarcoma of the base of the skull. J Neurosurg 1989;70:13.
90. Nowakowski VA, Castro JR, Petti PL, et al. Charged particle radiotherapy of paraspinal tumors. Int J Radiat Oncol Biol Phys 1991;22:1.
91. Saunders WM, Castro JR, Chen GTY, et al. Early results of ion beam radiation therapy for sacral chordoma. J Neurosurg 1986;64:243.
92. Lindstadt DE, Castro JR, Phillips TL. Neon ion radiotherapy: Results of the phase I/II clinical trial. Int J Radiat Oncol Biol Phys 1991;20:761.
93. Blakely EA, Ngo FQH, Curtis SB, et al. Heavy-ion radiobiology: Cellular studies. Adv Radiat Biol 1984;11:295.
94. Curtis SB, Tenforde TS, Parks D, et al. Response of a rat rhabdomyosarcoma to neon- and helium-ion irradiation. Radiat Res 1978;74:274.
95. Curtis SB, Schilling WA, Tenforde TS, et al. Survival of oxygenated and hypoxic tumor cells in the extended-peak regions of heavy charged-particle beams. Radiat Res 1982;90: 292.
96. Leith JT, Woodruff KH, Howard J, et al. Early and late effects of accelerated charged particles on normal tissues. Int J Radiat Oncol Biol Phys 1977;3:103.

97. Leith JT, Smith P, Ross-Riveros P, et al. Cellular response of a rat brain tumor to a therapeutic neon ion beam. Int J Radiat Biol 1977;32:401.
98. Tobias CA, Blakely EA, Alpen EL, et al. Molecular and cellular radiobiology of heavy ions. Int J Radiat Oncol Biol Phys 1982;8:2109.
99. Castro J. Personal communication.
100. Castro JR, Collier M, Petti PL, et al. Charged particle radiotherapy for lesions encircling the brain stem of spinal cord. Int J Radiat Oncol Biol Phys 1989;17:477.
101. Castro JR, Reimers MM. Charged particle radiotherapy of selected tumors in the head and neck. Int J Radiat Oncol Biol Phys 1988;14:711.
102. Raju MR, Carpenter S, Tokita N, et al. Effects of fractionated pions on normal tissues. I. Mouse skin. Int J Radiat Oncol Biol Phys 1980;6:2663.
103. Peters LJ, Withers HR, Mason KA, et al. Effects of fractionated pions on normal tissues. II. Mouse jejunum. Int J Radiat Oncol Biol Phys 1980;6:1667.
104. Chaplin DJ, Douglas BG, Saito T, et al. Preclincal evaluation of pions in vivo: Experience at TRIUMF. Radiother Oncol 1990;17:7.
105. Greiner RH, Blattmann JH, Thum P, et al. Dynamic pion irradiation of unresectable soft tissue sarcoma. Int J Radiat Oncol Biol Phys 1989;17:1077.
106. Locher GL. Biological effects and therapeutic possibilities of neutrons. Am J Roentgenol Radium Ther 1936;36:1.
107. Kruger PG. Some biological effects of nuclear disintegration products on neoplastic tissue. Proc Natl Acad Sci 1940;26:181.
108. Zahl PA, Cooper FS, Dunning JR. Some in vivo effects of localized nuclear disintegration products on a transplantable mouse sarcoma. Proc Natl Acad Sci 1940;26:589.
109. Farr LE, Sweet WH, Robertson JS, et al. Neutron capture therapy with boron in the treatment of glioblastoma multiforme. AJR 1954;71:279.
110. Godwin JT, Farr LE, Sweet WH, et al. Pathological study of eight patients with glioblastoma multiforme treated by neutron capture therapy using boron-10. Cancer 1955;8:601.
111. Waterman FM, Kuchnir FT, Skaggs LS, et al. The use of ^{10}B to enhance the tumour dose in fast-neutron therapy. Phys Med Biol 1978;23:592.
112. Laramore GE, Livesey J, Wootton P, et al. Boron neutron capture therapy: A means of increasing the effectiveness of fast neutron radiotherapy. In: Proceedings of the 9th International Congress of Radiation Research. Academic Press, San Diego (in press).

SECTION 11 Hyperthermia

JAMES R. OLESON

Temperature elevation to 42°C to 45°C for 10 to 60 minutes can lethally damage bacterial and mammalian cells. This fact, first observed in ancient times, was rediscovered in the 19th century when patients with malignant tumors who had fevers related to bacterial infections occasionally had regressions in tumor size. Coley deliberately induced fevers in cancer patients using pyrogenic bacterial toxins and observed some partial responses.[1]

The development of radiofrequency generators in the early 1900s and their application in diathermy allowed the testing of effects due to temperature rise localized to a tumor, rather than whole-body hyperthermia.[2,3] Although investigation of combined hyperthermia and irradiation soon followed, a series of reports by Crile in the 1960s probably stimulated the modern quantitative study of effects of hyperthermia on cancer.[4–6] Crile demonstrated thermal enhancement of radiation effect and cure of melanomas implanted on the feet of mice with water bath heating; no normal tissue damage was observed from exposures to 44°C for 30 minutes. Since the early 1960s, systematic laboratory investigation of hyperthermia has expanded, and these investigations continue to support use of hyperthermia in cancer therapy. Several reviews provide further information.[7–10]

BIOLOGIC BACKGROUND

EFFECTS OF HYPERTHERMIA ALONE

When the logarithm of the surviving fraction of cells is plotted as a function of time of exposure to given temperatures above 41°C, the resulting cell survival curve is similar to that resulting from radiation exposure (Fig. 69–50). An initial shoulder region for short exposure times is followed by a linear portion representing cell killing that is an exponential function of time.[11] At temperatures below 42.5°C, the rate of cell killing diminishes with exposure times longer than about 200 minutes, providing evidence of the development of thermotolerance, a fundamentally important and universal phenomenon.[12] For a given effect, such as the percentage of cell killing, the exposure time must be reduced by one half for each 1°C increase in temperature. For temperatures below 42.5°C in thermotolerant cells, the heating time must be reduced by about one half for each 0.5°C increase in temperature for an isoeffect.

Thermal sensitivity varies during the cell cycle. Chinese hamster ovary (CHO) cells exhibit the greatest thermal sensitivity during M and S phases, and mild thermal exposure of CHO causes a cell cycle delay in G_2 of about 6 hours.[13,13a,14] Relative thermal sensitivity varies with different cell lines and is not correlated with radiation sensitivity.[15] Earlier reports suggested erroneously that malignant cells were intrinsically more thermally sensitive than normal cells, but the

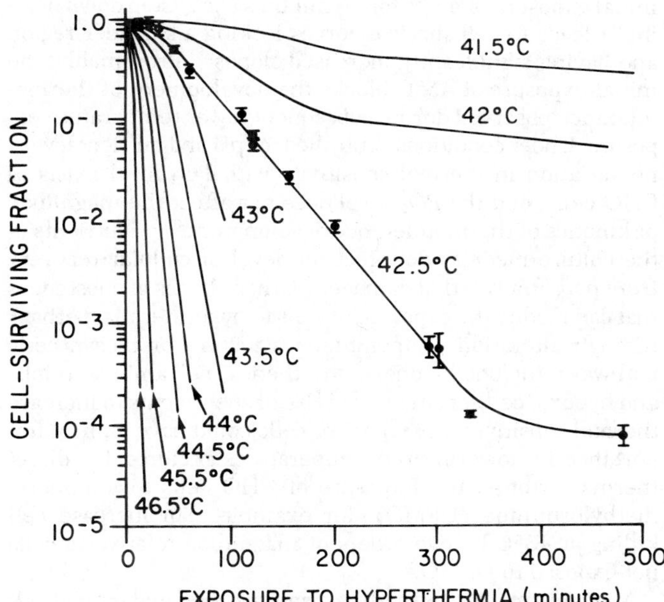

FIGURE 69–50. Survival curves for Chinese hamster ovary cells in vitro exposed to various temperatures for different periods. Similar to radiation survival curves, there is a shoulder and an exponential portion. Prolonged exposure to 42.5°C and below leads to flattening of the curves with minimal further cell killing, corresponding to thermotolerance induction. (Modified from Dewey W, Hopwood L, Sapareto S, et al. Cellular responses to combinations of hyperthermia and radiation. Radiology 1977;123:463–474)

altered physiologic milieu of malignant cells in vivo may lead to thermal sensitization relative to normal cells.[16,17] The shoulder of the survival curve of preheated cells is reproduced with a second exposure, implying recovery from sublethal damage produced with the first exposure. Part of this recovery is separate from thermotolerance induction.[18]

The ratio of slopes of survival curves for preheated and single heated cells, respectively, gives a thermotolerance ratio (TTR) that varies as a function of the fractionation interval. Exposure to temperatures above 42.5°C for more than 30 minutes induces a maximal TTR at 6 to 16 hours, after the first or priming exposure. This effect requires at least 24 hours for complete decay in L1A2 cells.[19] The magnitude and kinetics of thermotolerance vary with cell lines and may vary within subclonogenic lines.[20,21]

Acidic pH inhibits the magnitude and rate of expression of thermotolerance, although the pH effects in cells adapted to low pH are less marked.[22–24] Intracellular, not extracellular, pH determines the thermosensitivity of cells.[24a] Induction of thermotolerance is associated temporally with synthesis of proteins with molecular masses in the range of 20 to 100 kd, particularly 70 kd, which are called heat shock proteins (HSP).[25–27] If these proteins are induced by agents other than heat, cells can become thermotolerant. Whether the HSP are enzymes or structural proteins is unknown. HSP are highly conserved in prokaryotic and eukaryotic cells, suggesting an important role of the HSP in the cellular stress response.[27a] A possible function is that HSP may participate in "rescuing" denatured proteins.[28]

Other agents and conditions can modify the cellular effects of hyperthermia from those illustrated in Figure 69–50. Incubation of cells at temperatures from 40°C to 43°C after an initial exposure of 45°C for 20 minutes (*i.e.*, "step down heating") leads to cell survival curves lacking a shoulder region and having significantly increased slopes.[29] Presumably, the initial exposure at 45°C blocks the development of thermotolerance observed during subsequent lower temperature exposure. Under conditions controlled for pH and nutrient levels, no variation in thermal sensitivity with PO_2 level exists in CHO cells, and the PO_2 level does not affect the magnitude or kinetics of thermotolerance development.[30,31] Nutrients in the culture medium do affect the level of cellular recovery from potentially lethal damage.[32] Other classes of substances that can modify the exposure of cells to hyperthermia, perhaps through alteration of membrane structure or biosynthetic pathways, include alcohols, anesthetics, polyamines, thiols, and hypoxic cell sensitizers.[7,33] Use of such agents to increase thermal sensitivity of malignant cells could have clinical importance by lowering the temperatures required for direct thermal cytotoxicity. Exposure of CHO cells to α-difluoromethylornithine (DFMO), for example, can increase cell killing at 43°C by two orders of magnitude relative to cells not exposed to DFMO.[34]

Mechanisms of thermal damage are not understood, although effects on the cell membrane and nucleus are associated with heat exposure.[35–37a] An Arrhenius plot analysis gives the energy of activation of the assumed chemical reaction that is rate limiting for thermal cell killing to be about 140 to 150 kilocalories per mole, similar to that required for protein denaturation.[14] This implies that heat-induced aggregation of cellular proteins is involved in cell killing.

A rapid mode of interphase cell death can occur. At lower levels of heat, stressed cells become morphologically abnormal with multinucleation; these are nonclonogenic.[37b,37c] Thermotolerant cells have fewer heat-induced morphologic changes immediately after a second heat challenge, suggesting a protective role of thermotolerance in stabilizing cell structures. Other observations indicate that recovery from heat-induced changes is stimulated in the thermotolerant cell, suggesting induction or activation of repair enzymes by HSP.

EFFECTS OF COMBINED HYPERTHERMIA AND IRRADIATION

In 1963, Belli and Bonti demonstrated temperature dependence of the radiation response of mammalian cells in tissue culture, suggesting thermal lability of enzymes involved in repair of radiation damage.[38] Ben-Hur and colleagues showed that temperature elevation above 41°C increases the slope of the exponential portion of the radiation survival curve of CHO cells, confirming enhancement of lethal damage expression.[39] The effects of incubation at temperatures below 40.5°C after irradiation are principally on the shoulder of the survival curve, indicating a reduced capacity for sublethal damage repair. At 41°C, the shoulder of the survival curve is absent. Survival of CHO cells depends on the sequence of hyperthermia and irradiation, with sixfold lower survival resulting from simultaneous exposure to 42.5°C and irradiation compared with heat preceding or after the irradiation by more than 5 minutes.[40] Thermal radiosensitization is greater for S-phase cells than G_1 cells, complementary to the cell cycle dependence of survival from irradiation alone.[13] Survival also is lower for the very low dose rates typical of brachytherapy than for those used in teletherapy.[41,42] Cell survival with hyperthermia and irradiation depends on intracellular pH; this is of particular significance in vivo, because acid pH also reduces the rate of thermotolerance development at 42°C to 42.5°C.[24,43–46] The effect of thermotolerance on thermal cytotoxicity, radiosensitivity, and thermal radiosensitization is complex, but in general terms, thermotolerance does not modify radiation sensitivity of cells but does decrease direct thermal cytotoxicity and thermal radiosensitization.[47–51]

EFFECTS OF HYPERTHERMIA COMBINED WITH CHEMOTHERAPEUTIC AGENTS

Many chemotherapeutic agents (*e.g.*, doxorubicin, bleomycin, cisplatin, mitomycin C, nitrosoureas) have increased cytotoxicity in vivo with an increase in temperature.[7] When thermotolerance is induced, an associated tolerance for the effects of drugs occurs in some cases.[52,53] Wallner and Li illustrated the importance of the duration of exposure of cells to a drug and heat-drug sequencing.[54] Maximal potentiation with simultaneous exposure also occurs with cyclophosphamide and mitomycin. Although an increased number of DNA crosslinks in CHO cells exposed to cisplatin at 43°C compared with 37°C exists, the precise mechanisms of thermal potentiation of drug effects are not known. In vivo, pH, PO_2, and drug pharmacokinetics can lead to more complex sequencing effects.[54–55d]

Acquired resistance to some chemotherapeutic agents can be partially overcome by hyperthermia, suggesting a role for hyperthermia in treating drug-resistant disease.[55e] Hyperthermia can increase uptake and retention of monoclonal antibodies in solid tumors.[55f]

IN VIVO EFFECTS OF HYPERTHERMIA

Effects of hyperthermia alone or in combination with other agents in vivo have been studied in rodents, large animals, and humans. Many variables can influence the effects of hyperthermia in vivo.[56] Most importantly, blood circulation is a mechanism for transporting heat, affecting the temperatures produced in tissues with heating by any means.[57,58] The amount of blood flow and temperature dependence of flow itself influence the delivery of nutrients to the cells and the metabolic status and pH.[59] Tumor vessels resemble leaky capillaries and venous sinusoids without the vascular smooth muscle that allows normal vasoactivity, such as thermally induced vasodilation.[58] Stasis of blood flow and vascular destruction can occur in tumor microcirculation under conditions that produce only reversible reactive change in normal tissues, creating one of the most important rationales for advantageous differential effects of hyperthermia between tumors and normal tissues. Areas of low blood perfusion in tumors can reach preferentially higher temperatures than normal tissue, further enhancing the differential effects of heat.

Measurements of extracellular pH in animal and human tumors confirm that acidic pH conditions occur in some tumors, presumably from low PO_2 and nutrient levels producing anaerobic glycolysis and high lactic acid levels.[45] The pH shift does not correlate consistently with tumor size, histology, or other characteristics. Glucose infusions to lower tumor pH during hyperthermia may take advantage of increased thermal cytotoxicity, reduced thermotolerance, and reduced recovery from sublethal hyperthermic damage.[60,61]

Thermotolerance occurs in vivo.[62] A priming treatment of 43.5°C for 30 minutes in C3H mammary carcinoma tumors, for example, leads to maximal thermotolerance 16 hours later and a complete decay time of 120 hours.[63] Thermotolerance can also be induced in the tumor vessels.[59a] The implications of thermotolerance development for fractionation of hyperthermia and irradiation in treatment regimens are complex and significant.

The kinetics of repair of sublethal damage and thermotolerance induction and decay in vivo may vary between tumor and normal tissue. Simultaneous irradiation and heat results in equal sensitization of tumor and normal tissue under uniform temperature conditions, producing no therapeutic gain.[64,65] When an interval of at least 2 hours separates radiation and heat, with radiation administered before heat, there is consistently a ratio of enhancement of radiation effect in tumor compared with normal tissue (*i.e.*, therapeutic gain) of 1.2 to 1.5.

The expression of direct thermal injury in normal tissues follows that expected from interphase death of cells rather than postmitotic death as in the case of radiation injury.[37b] Studies involving scoring of development of rodent leg contracture, for instance, show peak damage between 2 and 15 days after hyperthermia, and radiation damage peaks at 20 to 25 days and then progresses for as long as 365 days.[66] This pattern of difference is found in intestinal crypts, testis, and kidney. In normal feline brain, the histologic appearance and time course of repair of thermal injury are similar to the acute necrosis produced by vascular infarction.[67] In murine jejunal tissue, hyperthermia accelerates the expression and increases the magnitude of late radiation fibrosis.[68]

The threshold for normal tissue injury is sharply marked as a function of time and temperature of exposure. A 20% increase in time of exposure or a 0.5°C increase in temperature in the range of 42.0°C to 45.5°C increases the likelihood of necrosis from 0% to 100% in rodent tissue.[69] Few clinical studies report severe normal tissue thermal injury or potentiation of radiation effects in superficial tissues if there has been careful monitoring of the temperatures achieved and the patients' perceptions. Normal tissue temperatures rarely exceed safe limits of 42°C to 43°C and usually reach highest levels corresponding to locations predictably receiving the greatest power deposition. Hyperthermia techniques causing temperature elevation in deep visceral sites infrequently cause serious injury; however, the potential location and magnitude of temperature elevation is more difficult to predict and is less well perceived by the patient. Little information exists on the toxic or therapeutic in vivo effects of combined hyperthermia and chemotherapeutic agents, although hyperthermia can alter drug pharmacology.[69a–72]

Relating the tissue effects of hyperthermia to a thermal dose is a desirable but elusive goal. From Arrhenius associations, formulas for combinations of time and temperature can be derived that give isoeffects in cultured cells and in animal tissues.[73] The formulas may be useful for comparing clinical treatments, but they do not predict absolute levels of effects, are difficult to apply to nonuniform temperature distributions, do not express effects of fractionated therapy, and may not express correctly the variation of thermal radiosensitization with pH.[74] The use of a thermal isoeffective dose is still investigational.

The prospective, randomized phase III study of Dewhirst and collaborators was one of the most important therapeutic trials in animals.[75] Treatment with combined hyperthermia and radiotherapy produced a statistically significant improvement in freedom from disease progression compared with radiotherapy or hyperthermia alone. The complete response rate and duration were inversely correlated with the tumor volume, but the relative improvement in response was greater for large tumors than small tumors. The average site-nonspecific minimal temperature was the thermal measure best correlating with response; the equivalent of 41.3°C for 30 minutes, plus radiation, nearly doubled the complete response rate from 35% to 65% compared with radiotherapy alone.

TECHNICAL ASPECTS

THERMOMETRY

Typical temperature distributions in tumors are nonuniform. Methods for measuring temperatures are limited in practice to invasive placement of probes at only a few sites, introducing the problem of inferring the overall temperature distribution from spatially limited samples.[76,77] Methods of calculating temperature distributions are being developed but cannot be applied routinely because the principal determinants of temperature rise, absorbed power density, and blood perfusion rate are not accurately known.[78] Proper choice, use, and calibration of thermometers to limit errors of measurement require many different considerations for each hyperthermia technique.[79] Standard practice includes the use of single sensors, multiple sensors, or periodically translated sensors within catheters placed into tumor sites.[80] The selection of the number of sensors and sites of measurement bears directly on the likelihood of sampling prognostically important temperatures or defining prospectively what temperature distributions are required for efficacious treatment. Adherence to quality assurance guidelines can help to systematize treatments.[81]

METHODS OF HEATING

Available heating methods include ultrasound or electromagnetic applicators. The principle of heat production is that energy is absorbed in tissue in doing work against the molecular viscosity or electrical resistance of tissue constituents.[82,83] These dissipative processes causing heat production do not involve ionization, unlike absorption mechanisms for diagnostic and therapeutic radiation. Local heat production results in a temperature rise that depends on the specific heat of the tissue and the heat transport processes of conduction and convection (*i.e.*, blood flow); chemical or metabolic heat production levels are themselves temperature dependent and may contribute to the local temperature rise.[57] Heating methods consist of noninvasive and invasive techniques of depositing power in localized volumes, regional vascular perfusion techniques, and whole-body hyperthermia techniques. Heating superficial tumors in a water bath is common for laboratory study of small rodent tumors, but this technique is inappropriate for bulky human tumors. Special techniques are required for achieving temperature uniformity even in small rodent tumors.[84] Many of these methods have been evaluated in a multiinstitutional effort.[84a]

NONINVASIVE TECHNIQUES

Ultrasound applicators with focused or unfocused stationary beams and with focused scanning beams are available for the frequency range of 0.5 to 10 MHz, for which the penetration depth in tissue varies from about 10 to 0.5 cm, respectively. Lack of ultrasound propagation across air spaces, marked absorption in bone, and reflections from tissue interfaces constitute fundamental problems with ultrasound. The depths of penetration and ability to focus, however, are advantages over electromagnetic techniques, especially for deep-seated tumors.[85,85a]

Electric currents in the frequency range of 0.2 to 13 MHz can be capacitively coupled into tissue to result in resistive heating by using two or more surface electrodes or plates.[82] The currents flow in divergent paths between the plates, and large plates must be used for significant power absorption in deep sites relative to superficial sites near the plates. The power absorption is not focused or localized in tumor, and excessive superficial fat heating is a problem for fat layers thicker than about 1.5 cm. At frequencies of 10 to 30 MHz, current carrying coils external to the body can create an intense magnetic field that in turn induces eddy current flow within the body.[86] The resulting power deposition generally diminishes with increasing depth, so these techniques are best suited for tumors at superficial and intermediate depths. Radiated electromagnetic fields in the frequency range of 60 to 2450 MHz penetrate to depths of about 15 to 1.5 cm, respectively. Single microwave applicators commonly are limited to heating superficial lesions, and multiapplicator arrays can achieve heating at depth in the body without excessive superficial normal tissue heating.[87]

Sharp focusing of the power is not possible with these techniques, and as with the other electromagnetic approaches, it is necessary to rely on blood perfusion in tumor lower than normal tissue for preferential temperature elevation in tumor.

INVASIVE TECHNIQUES

Interstitial Hyperthermia

Greater localization and control of power deposition within a tumor volume is possible using interstitial techniques that can be combined with conventional interstitial irradiation treatments.[88] Electric current at 0.5 MHz flowing between implanted metallic needles results in resistive heating of intervening tumor.[89] Alternatively, nonmetallic catheters can accommodate miniature microwave antennas operating at 433 to 2450 MHz that radiate power into surrounding tumor.[90] Interstitial ferromagnetic seeds can be heated inductively to produce conductive or "hot source" heating of the implanted tumor.[91]

Regional Vascular Perfusion

Isolation of the major artery and vein of an extremity from the systemic circulation and connection of these vessels to an extracorporeal heated perfusion circuit results in temperature elevation of an entire limb.[92] This approach has been used for treating extremity melanoma and sarcoma with chemotherapy-containing heated perfusates.

Whole-Body Hyperthermia Techniques

Currently used methods of inducing systemic temperature rise depend on limiting the heat loss from the body while inducing heat absorption through conduction across the skin surface from heated water or infrared power absorption.[93–95]

CLINICAL RESULTS

EFFICACY OF COMBINED HYPERTHERMIA AND RADIOTHERAPY

Several studies reported treatment to small superficial metastatic nodules by hyperthermia alone, radiotherapy alone, or combined radiotherapy and hyperthermia. A variety of heating techniques and radiation fractionation schemes was used, and temperature distributions were not always characterized. Despite these problems, there is surprising consistency in results as summarized by Overgaard and as updated in Table 69–48.[98] Complete response rates with hyperthermia alone are about 15%, about 35% with radiotherapy, and about 70% with combined radiotherapy and hyperthermia. The rate of toxicity, principally thermal burns and blisters, is usually about 10%

TABLE 69–48. Complete Response of Superficial Tumors to Treatment

Investigations	*Lesions*	*Total No. of Tumors*	*Radiotherapy Alone†*	*Radiotherapy and Hyperthermia†*	*Significance (p)*
Valdagni et al[132] *	Neck nodes	43	36.8%	82.3%	0.015
Arcangeli et al[99,133]	Neck nodes; melanoma mets.	81	42%	79%	<0.05
			14% (24 mo)	58% (24 mo)	<0.05
Steeves et al[134]	Superficial tumors	90	31%	65%	
Lindholm et al[120]	Superficial tumors, superficial	85	25%	46%	
	matched pairs only	56	25%	57%	0.0027
Van der Zee et al[121]	Breast cancer recurrences	113	55%	90%	<0.001
Kim et al[122,126]	Melanoma recurrences	97	45%	66%	
Li et al[123]	Superficial tumors	124	29%	53.8%	
	Superficial matched pairs only	62	29%	68%	
Scott et al[131]	Superficial tumors, matched pairs only	62	39%	87%	<0.01
Corry et al[125]	Superficial tumors	21	30%	62%	
Perez et al[101a]	Superficial tumors	218	28%	32%	
	Subset ≤3 cm dia. CR ≥12 mo	48	15%	80%	

* Prospective, randomized trials; *p* values shown when reported.
† Complete response rates.

to 15%. No evidence exists of enhanced late effects of radiotherapy in these studies. These trials have established safety and efficacy for combined treatment in superficial lesions, particularly if prior radiotherapy limits additional doses to suboptimal levels.

Other trials, summarized in Table 69–49, confirm that tumor volume, radiation dose, and measures of minimal tumor temperature are prognostic factors for response to hyperthermia and radiotherapy. Arcangeli and coworkers found a highly significant correlation of complete response rate with minimal thermal isoeffective dose.[99] Dunlop and colleagues found improvement in response rates from 35% to 86% with at least two hyperthermia treatments in which a tumor minimal isoeffective dose of 20 minutes at the equivalent of 43°C (Eq 43) was achieved.[100] Kapp and coworkers randomized prospectively treatment to small superficial lesions with radiotherapy plus two or six weekly fractions of hyperthermia and observed no differences in complete response rate or duration of response.[101] Perez and colleagues found no overall difference in complete response rates of tumors treated with radiotherapy or radiotherapy plus hyperthermia treatment and argued that poorly defined criteria for matching microwave applicators to tumor size resulted in inadequate treatment of tumors larger than 3 cm in diameter.[101a] These researchers proposed that quality assurance and control for hyperthermia treatments would be essential for obtaining good results.

For superficial tumors treated with radiotherapy plus one or two hyperthermia treatments per week, the complete response rate depended greatly on the cumulative time for which 90% of intratumoral temperatures exceeded 40.5°C.[101b]

These results imply that the number of hyperthermia treatments is less important for complete response than the cumulative duration and extent of temperature elevation.[101b–d] Radiation dose is important, and in specific diseases, many other prognostic factors may be important.[101e,101f] The use of frequency distribution of temperature parameters (*e.g.*, temperature exceeded by 10% or 50% of tumor temperatures) and cumulative time may provide the basis for a hyperthermia treatment dosimetry.[102]

TABLE 69–49. Prognostic Variables for Complete Response to Hyperthermia and Radiotherapy

Investigations	*Prognostic Variables*
Kim et al[122,126]	Volume, radiation dose/fx, T_{min}
Dewhirst and Sim[75]	Volume, T_{min} (not site specific)
Oleson et al[105]	Volume, radiation dose, T_{min} averaged over all treatments, HT technique
Sim et al[127]	Volume, radiation dose, HT technique, number of intratumoral sites ≥ 42.5°C
Arcangeli et al[99,133]	Volume, minimum equivalent time at 42.5°C
Luk et al[128]	Total radiation dose, recurrence status, minimum daily average temperature, volume
Van der Zee et al[130]	Mean minimum tumor temperature
Dunlop et al[100]	Number of HT treatments for which T_{min} ≥ 20 min equals 43
Scott et al[124,131]	T_{ave} ≥ 43°C, greatest tumor diameter, site and histology
Kapp et al[101,101e]	Histology, radiation dose, volume; mean T_{min} (borderline significance); no dependence on 2 vs 6 HT treatments
Leopold et al[101b]	Cumulative min for T_{90} ≥ 40.5°C, radiation dose, tumor depth

HT, hyperthermia treatment.

EVALUATION OF HYPERTHERMIA FOR DEEP TUMORS

The reported trials on superficial tumors define important biologic aspects of treatment with hyperthermia and radiotherapy. Control of bulky deep locoregional disease, however, limits the curability of many common human tumors.[103] Development and phase I equipment evaluation for inducing hyperthermia in deep sites, especially interstitial techniques, magnetic induction coils, and capacitively coupled plates, annular microwave phased arrays, and focused ultrasound, is the subject of extensive current investigation.[104] If deep sites can be implanted, interstitial hyperthermia techniques can provide higher average temperatures than noninvasive techniques.[105] Toxicity is similar to irradiation alone, except that in pelvic sites, tumor necrosis and slough can occur acutely, precipitating development of fistulas.

Trials using a commercially available magnetic induction coil (Magnetrode) that included extensive temperature measurements revealed that most intratumoral sites do not exceed 42°C to 43°C with this device, although marked temperature elevation in core regions of bulky tumors is possible, presumably because of low blood perfusion.[107,108] Japanese investigators reported clinical testing of capacitively coupled radiofrequency devices (13.6 MHz and 8 MHz), and a report of multipoint measurements in 60 deep-seated tumors revealed a maximal tumor center temperature of more than 43°C in 38% of tumors, a lowest intratumoral temperature of more than 42°C in 11%, and temperature variation greater than 2°C in 81%.[109,109a,110] Localized pain was the major power-limiting factor.[111] The capacitively coupled radiofrequency device can produce significant temperature rise in deep tumors at a variety of anatomic locations with limited toxicity and with significant nonuniformity of the temperature distribution.

Investigators at the University of Utah have extensively evaluated an annular microwave array (AA) for heating intraabdominal and pelvic malignancies.[108,112,112a] Measurement of temperature distributions across at least one tumor diameter was typical. In pelvic tumors, pain during the hyperthermia treatments occurred in most of 43 patients, and there were 8 patients with serious late complications. In 73% of 175 treatments for 43 patients, temperatures over 42°C were achieved. Applied electromagnetic power levels were limited by patient discomfort and safety considerations. Serious toxicity with these techniques has been infrequent. In deep sites, most of the tumor volume may not reach temperatures and durations of temperature elevation sufficient to result in direct thermal cytotoxicity, and enhancement of radiation effect by hyperthermia may be more limited than is evident in superficial tumors.[112b,112c] Determining the extent and distribution of temperature elevation and number of treatments needed for significant improvement in local control compared with radiation alone will require prospective studies.

Study of focused ultrasound for treatments of deep tumors has been limited. Lele used scanned focused ultrasound transducers to treat tumors at depths of 12 cm with volumes up to about 10 × 10 × 10 cm.[85] The incidence of pain from bone or periosteum heating and other toxic effects was negligible, and the desired temperature of 43°C were achieved in 43 of 44 tumors in 30 patients. Similar success has been demonstrated by others.[113]

Few reports exist using electromagnetically produced locoregional hyperthermia with chemotherapy. A trial of ifosfamide plus etoposide combined with hyperthermia for soft tissue sarcoma and bone sarcoma did show activity (complete responses in 6 of 38 patients) and temperature parameters such as T_{20mean}, T_{90mean}, and T_{50mean} (*i.e.*, mean temperature exceeded by 20%, 90%, 50% of monitored sites) correlated with outcome.[69b,69c]

Most reports of whole-body hyperthermia have been phase I trials that showed considerable toxicity. However, a radiant heating device has allowed routine heating of mildly sedated patients to 41.8°C for 2 hours with minimal toxicity.[94] This device promises to facilitate more systematic study of whole-body hyperthermia with chemotherapy and localized radiotherapy. Selection of a chemotherapeutic agent for which there is clear evidence of therapeutic gain with whole-body hyperthermia is difficult. Carboplatin with whole-body hyperthermia improved therapeutic gain in rat tumors.[69a] Altered pharmacokinetics of systemic agents, acid pH in tumors, and thermal modulation of macrophage activity are factors that can be exploited for therapeutic gain.[114,115]

TRENDS IN HYPERTHERMIA

There has been considerable progress in analyzing mechanisms of action of hyperthermia alone and in combination of chemotherapy and irradiation. Significant potentiation of some chemotherapeutic agents and radiation is possible, and efficacy of thermoradiotherapy has been demonstrated in small superficial tumors. Research supports a strong rationale for hyperthermia in cancer therapy.

It is pertinent to question why clinical testing of hyperthermia treatment has not led to more demonstrations of efficacy over the last 10 to 15 years and why most clinical trials of hyperthermia treatment are still phase I feasibility and toxicity studies. To demonstrate dose-effect relations (phase II), it is necessary to establish a dosimetry system. This has been difficult for temperature distributions that are typically highly nonuniform. Even the sophisticated technology for measuring temperatures at multiple intratumoral sites has been developed only with difficulty in recent years; in early trials, the temperature at only one site in a tumor may have been monitored, and this approach gives no indication whatsoever of spatial nonuniformity of tumor temperature. After a dosimetry system is established, there must be heating devices available that are capable of producing and controlling the desired temperature distribution. In general, electromagnetic heating systems do not produce highly focused power deposition in tumors, and applied power levels are limited by excessive normal tissue temperatures rather than tumor temperatures. The marked limitations of heating devices have been recognized slowly and in retrospect. Concepts of thermal dosimetry are being developed that may provide a basis for treatment prescription.[102]

Many of these problems can be addressed through adequate quality assurance programs, and the importance of such programs was recognized in a series of articles.[81,116–119] Lack of quality assurance guidelines in the past has contributed to the difficulty of performing meaningful single or multiple institutional trials.

There is little justification for phase III trials of hyperthermia until a dose-response relation has been demonstrated for the tumor studied and until there is demonstration that the desired thermal dose can be delivered routinely to the tumor site being studied.

REFERENCES

1. Coley-Nauts H, Swife W, Coley B. The treatment of malignant tumors by bacterial toxins as developed by the late William B. Coley, M.D., reviewed in light of modern research. Cancer Res 1946;6:205–216.
2. Susskind C. The "story" of nonionizing radiation research. Bull N Y Acad Med 1979;55: 1152–1163.
3. Westermark N. The effect of heat upon rat-tumors. Skandin Arch F Physiol 1927;52: 257–322.
4. Rohdenburg GL, Prime F. The effect of combined radiation and heat on neoplasms. Arch Surg 1921;2:116–129.
5. Selawry OS, Carlson JC, Moore GE. Tumor response to ionizing rays at elevated temperatures. AJR 1958;80:833–839.
6. Crile G Jr. The effects of heat and radiation on cancers implanted on the feet of mice. Cancer Res 1963;23:372–380.
7. Hahn GM. Hyperthermia in cancer. New York: Plenum Press, 1982.
8. Urano M, Douple EB, eds. Hyperthermia and oncology, vols 1 and 2. Zeist, Netherlands: VSP, 1988.
9. Hand JW, James JR, eds. Physical techniques in clinical hyperthermia. Letchworth, England: Research Studies Press, 1986.
10. Oleson JR, Calderwood SR, Coughlin CT, et al. Biological and clinical aspects of hyperthermia in cancer therapy. Am J Clin Oncol 1988;11:368–380.
11. Dewey WC, Hopwood LE, Sapareto SA, et al. Cellular responses to combinations of hyperthermia and radiation. Radiology 1977;123:463–474.
12. Gerner E, Schneider M. Induced thermal resistance in HeLa cells. Nature 1976;256: 500–502.
13. Westra A, Dewey WC. Variation in sensitivity to heat shock during the cell-cycle of Chinese hamster cells in vitro. Int J Radiat Biol 1971;19:467–477.

13a. Dewey WC, XiLian L, Wong RSL. Cell killing, chromosomal aberrations, and division delay as thermal sensitivity is modified during the cell cycle. Radiat Res 1990;122: 268–274.

14. Sapareto SA, Hopwood LE, Dewey WC, et al. Effects of hyperthermia on survival and progression of chinese hamster ovary cells. Cancer Res 1978;38:393–400.
15. Gerweck LE, Burlett P. The lack of correlation between heat and radiation sensitivity in mammalian cells. Int J Radiat Oncol Biol Phys 1978;4:283–285.
16. Giovanella BC, Stehlin JS Jr, Morgan AC. Selective lethal effect of supranormal temperatures on human neoplastic cells. Cancer Res 1976;36:3944–3950.
17. Overgaard J, Nielsen OS. The role of tissue environmental factors on the kinetics and morphology of tumor cells exposed to hyperthermia. Ann N Y Acad Sci 1980;335: 254–278.
18. Nielsen OS, Overgaard J. Effect of extracellular pH on thermotolerance and recovery of hyperthermic damage in vitro. Cancer Res 1979;39:2772–2778.
19. Nielsen OS, Overgaard J. Influence of time and temperature on the kinetics of thermotolerance in L1A2 cells in vitro. Cancer Res 1982;42:4190–4196.
20. Rofstad EK, Midthjell H, Brustad T. Heat sensitivity and thermotolerance in cells from five human melanoma xenografts. Cancer Res 1984;44:4347–4354.
21. Leith JT, Bliven SF, Glicksman AS. Similarity of thermotolerance characteristics in heterogeneous human colon tumor subpopulations after exposure to fractionated heat doses (44°C). Radiat Res 1985;104:128–139.
22. Gerweck LE. Modification of cell lethality at elevated temperatures: The pH effect. Radiat Res 1977;70:224–235.
23. Holahan PK, Dewey WC. Effect of pH and cell cycle progression on development and decay of thermotolerance. Radiat Res 1986;106:111–121.
24. Hahn GM, Shiu EC. Adaptation to low pH modifies thermal and thermochemical responses of mammalian cells. Int J Hyperthermia 1986;2:379–387.

24a. Chu GL, Wang Z, Hyun WC, et al. The role of intracellular pH and its variance in low pH sensitization of killing by hyperthermia. Radiat Res 1990;122:288–293.

25. Hahn GM, Li GC. Thermotolerance and heat shock proteins in mammalian cells. Radiat Res 1982;92:452–457.
26. Li GC. Elevated levels of 70,000 Dalton heat shock protein in transiently thermotolerant chinese hamster fibroblasts and in their stable heat resistant variants. Int J Radiat Oncol Biol Phys 1985;11:165–177.
27. Lindquist SL. The heat shock response. Ann Rev Biochem 1986;55:535–572.

27a. Carper SW, Duffy JJ, Gerner EW. Heat shock proteins in thermotolerance and other cellular processes. Cancer Res 1987;47:5249–5255.

28. Pelham HRB. Speculations on the function of the major heat shock proteins. Cell 1986;46:959–961.
29. Henle KJ. Sensitization to hyperthermia below 43°C induced in Chinese hamster ovary cells by step-down heating. JNCI 1980;64:1479–1483.
30. Gerweck LE, Richards B, Jennings M. The influence of variable oxygen concentration on the response of cells to heat or x-irradiation. Radiat Res 1981;85:314–320.
31. Gerweck LE, Bascomb F. Influence of hypoxia on the development of thermotolerance. Radiat Res 1982;90:356–361.
32. Li GC, Shiu EC, Hahn GM. Recovery of cells from heat-induced potentially lethal damage: Effects of pH and nutrient environment. Int J Radiat Oncol Biol Phys 1980;6: 577–582.
33. Stone HB, Dewey WC. Biologic basis and clinical potential of local-regional hyperthermia. In: Phillips T, Wara W, eds. Radiation oncology, vol 2. New York: Raven Press, 1987:1–41.
34. Fuller DJM, Gerner EW. Sensitization of chinese hamster ovary cells to heat shock by alpha-difluoromethylornithine. Cancer Res 1987;47:816–820.
35. Lepcock JR. Involvement of membranes in cellular responses to hyperthermia. Radiat Res 1982;92:433–438.
36. Konings AWT, Ruifrok ACC. Role of membrane lipids and membrane fluidity in thermosensitivity and thermotolerance of mammalian cells. Radiat Res 1985;102: 86–98.
37. Roti Roti JL, Uygur N, Higashikubo R. Nuclear protein following heat shock: Protein removal kinetics and cell cycle rearrangements. Radiat Res 1986;107:250–261.

37a. Dewey WC. Failla Memorial Lecture: The search for criticial cellular targets damaged by heat. Radiat Res 1989;120:191–204.

37b. Vidair CA, Dewey WC. Two distinct modes of hyperthermic cell death. Radiat Res 1988;116:157–171.

37c. Borrelli MJ, Thompson LL, Cain CA, Dewey WC. Time-temperature analysis of cell killing of BHK cells heated at temperatures in the range of 43.5°C to 57.0°C. Int J Radiat Oncol Biol Phys 1990;19:389–399.

38. Belli JA, Bonte FJ. Influence of temperature on the radiation response of mammalian cells in tissue culture. Radiat Res 1963;18:272–276.
39. Ben-Hur E, Elkind MM, Bronk BV. Thermally enhanced radioresponse of cultured chinese hamster cells: Inhibition of repair of sublethal damage and enhancement of lethal damage. Radiat Res 1974;58:38–51.
40. Sapareto S, Raaphorst G, Dewey WC. Cell killing and the sequencing of hyperthermia and radiation. Int J Radiat Oncol Biol Phys 1979;5:343–347.
41. Spiro IJ, McPherson S, Cook JA, et al. Sensitization of low-dose rate irradiation by nonlethal hyperthermia. Radiat Res 1991;127:111–114.
42. Jones EL, Lyons BE, Douple EB, Dain BJ. Thermal enhancement of low dose rate irradiation in a murine tumour system. Int J Hyperthermia 1989;5:509–523.
43. Gillette EL, Ensley BS. Effect of heat, radiation, and pH on mouse mammary tumor cells. Int J Radiat Oncol Biol Phys 1983;9:1521–1525.
44. Wike-Hooley JL, Haveman J, Reinhold HS. The relevance of tumour pH to the treatment of malignant disease. Radiother Oncol 1984;2:343–366.
45. Thistlethwaite AJ, Leeper DB, Moylan DJ III, et al. pH distribution in human tumors. Int J Radiat Oncol Biol Phys 1985;11:1647–1652.
46. Chu GL, Wang Z, Hyun WC, et al. The role of intracellular pH and its variance in low pH sensitization of killing by hyperthermia. Radiat Res 1990;122:288–293.
47. Haveman J. Influence of pH and thermotolerance on the enhancement of x-ray induced inactivation of cultured mammalian cells by hyperthermia. Int J Radiat Biol 1983;43: 281–289.
48. Holahan EV, Highfield DP, Holahan PK, et al. Hyperthermic killing and hyperthermic radiosensitization in Chinese hamster ovary cells: Effects of pH and thermal tolerance. Radiat Res 1984;97:108–131.
49. Holahan PK, Dewey WC. Effect of pH and cell cycle progression on development and decay of thermotolerance. Radiat Res 1986;106:111–121.
50. Haveman J, Luinenburg M, Wondergem J, et al. Effects of hyperthermia on the linear and quadratic parameters of the radiation survival curve of mammalian cells: Influence of thermotolerance. Int J Radiat Biol 1987;51:561–565.
51. Wynstra JH, Wright WD, Roti JL. Repair of radiation-induced DNA damage in thermotolernce and nonthermotolerant LeLa cells. Radiat Res 1990;124:85–89.
52. Morgan JE, Honess DJ, Bleehen NM. The interaction of thermal tolerance with drug cytotoxicity in vitro. Br J Cancer 1979;39:422–428.
53. Herman TS, Sweets CC, White DM, et al. Effect of heating on lethality due to hyperthermia and selected chemotherapeutic drugs. JNCI 1982;68:487–491.
54. Wallner KE, Li GC. Effect of drug exposure duration and sequencing on hyperthermic potentiation of mitomycin-C and cisplatin. Cancer Res 1987;47:493–495.
55. Meyn RE, Corry PM, Fletcher SE, et al. Thermal enhancement of DNA damage in mammalian cells treated with *cis*-diaminadichloroplatinum(II). Cancer Res 1980;40: 1136–1139.

55a. Douple EB, Jones EL, Kellogg KC, Van Buren T. Treatment sequence effects of combined cisplatin and hyperthermia in a murine tumor system. Hyperthermic oncology, 1988, vol 1, summary papers. London: Taylor & Francis, 1989:221–222.

55b. Herman TS, Teicher BA, Holden SA. Trimodality therapy (drug/hyperthermia/radiation) with BCNU or Mitomycin C. Int J Radiat Oncol Biol Phys 1990;18:375–382.

55c. Raaphorst GP, Feeley MM, Martin L. Enhancement of sensitivity to hyperthermia by lonidamine in human cancer cells. Int J Hypethermia 1991;7:763–772.

55d. Herman TS, Teicher BA, Collins LS. Effect of hypoxia and acidosis on the cytotoxicity of four platinum complexes at normal and hyperthemric temperatures. Cancer Res 1988;48:2342–2347.

55e. Laskowitz DT, Elion GB, Dewhirst MW, et al. Hyperthermia-induced ehancement of melphalan activity against a melphalan-resistant human rhabdomyosarcoma xenograft. Radiat Res 1992;129:218–223.

55f. Cope DA, Dewhirst MW, Friedman HS, et al. Enhanced delivery of a monoclonal antibody (Fab') 2 fragment to subcutaneous human glioma xenografts using local hyperthermia. Cancer Res 1990;50:1803–1809.

56. Urano M, Gerweck LE, Epstein R, et al. Response of a spontaneous murine tumor to hyperthermia: Factors which modify the thermal response in vivo. Radiat Res 1980;83:312–322.
57. Jain RK, Ward-Hartley K. Tumor blood flow—Characterization, modifications, and role in hyperthermia. IEEE Trans Sonics Ultrasonics 1984;SU-31:504–526.

58. Reinhold HS, Endrich B. Tumor microcirculation as a target for hyperthermia. Int J Hyperthermia 1986;2:111–137.
59. Streffer C. Metabolic changes during and after hyperthermia. Int J Hyperthermia 1985;1:305–319.
59a. Song CW, Chelstrom LM, Sung JH. Effects of a second heating on blood flow in tumors. Radiat Res 1990;122:66–71.
60. Ward-Hartley KA, Jain RK. Effect of glucose and galactose on microcirculatory flow in normal and neoplastic tissues in rabbits. Cancer Res 1987;47:371–377.
61. Thistlethwaite AJ, Alexander GA, Moylan DJ III, et al. Modification of human tumor pH by elevation of blood glucose. Int J Radiat Oncol Biol Phys 1987;13:603–610.
62. Urano M. Kinetics of thermotolerance in normal and tumor tissues: A review. Cancer Res 1986;46:474–482.
63. Nielsen OS, Overgaard J, Kamura T. Influence of thermotolerance on the interaction between hyperthermia and radiation in a solid tumor in vivo. Br J Radiol 1983;56: 267–273.
64. Dewey WC, Freeman ML, Raaphorst GP, et al. Cell biology of hyperthermia and radiation. In: Meyn RE, Withers HR, eds. Radiation biology in cancer research. New York: Raven Press, 1980:589–621.
65. Overgaard J. Simultaneous and sequential hyperthermia and radiation treatment of an experimental tumor and its surrounding normal tissue in vivo. Int J Radiat Oncol Biol Phys 1980;6:1507–1517.
66. Stone HB, Harding RP. Reversible injury after mild hyperthermia. Int J Radiat Oncol Biol Phys 1986;12:823–827.
67. Lyons BE, Obona WG, Borcich JK, et al. Chronic histological effects of ultrasonic hyperthermia on normal feline brain tissue. Radiat Res 1986;106:234–251.
68. Peck JW, Gibbs FA Jr. Assay of premorbid murine jejunal fibrosis based on mechanical changes after x-irradiation and hyperthermia. Radiat Res 1987;112:525–543.
69. Morris CC, Meyers R, Field SB. The response of the rat tail to hyperthermia. Br J Radiol 1977;50:576–580.
69a. Ohno S, Siddik ZH, Baba H, et al. Effect of carboplatin combined with whole body hyperthermia on normal tissue and tumor in rats. Cancer Res 1991;51:2994–3000.
69b. Issels RD, Wadepohl M, Tiling K, et al. Regional hyperthermia combined with systemic chemotherapy in advanced abdominal and pelvic tumors: First results of a pilot study employing an annular phased array applicator. Rec Res Cancer Res 1988;107:236–243.
69c. Issels RD, Prenninger SW, Nagele A, et al. Ifosfamide plus etoposide combined with regional hyperthermia in patients with loclly advanced sarcomas: A phase II study. J Clin Oncol 1990;8:1818–1829.
70. Marmor JB. Interactions of hyperthermia and chemotherapy in animals. Cancer Res 1979;39:2269–2276.
71. Zakris EL, Dewhirst MW, Riviere JE, et al. Pharmacokinetics and toxicity of intraperitoneal cisplatin combined with regional hyperthermia. J Clin Oncol 1987;5:1613–1620.
72. Page RL, Thrall DE, George SL, et al. Quantitative estimation of the thermal dose-modifying factor for cis-diamminedichloroplatinum (CDDP) in tumor-bearing dogs. Int J Hyperthermia 1992;8:761–769.
73. Field SB. Studies relevant to a means of quantifying the effects of hyperthermia. Int J Hyperthermia 1987;3:291–296.
74. Overgaard J. Some problems related to the clinical use of thermal isoeffect doses. Int J Hyperthermia 1987;3:329–336.
75. Dewhirst MW, Sim DA. The utility of thermal dose as a predictor of tumor and normal tissue responses to combined radiation and hyperthermia. Cancer Res 1984;44: 4772s-4780s.
76. Fessenden P, Lee ER, Samulski TV. Direct temperature measurement. Cancer Res 1984;44:4799s-4804s.
77. Divrik AM, Roemer RB, Cetas TC. Inference of complete temperature fields from a few measured temperatures: An unconstrained optimization method. IEEE Trans Biomed Eng 1984;31:150–160.
78. Strohbehn JW, Roemer RB. A survey of computer simulations of hyperthermia treatments. IEEE Trans Biomed Eng 1984;31:136–149.
79. Cetas TC. Thermometry. In: Lehmann JR, ed. Therapeutic heat and cold. 3rd ed. Baltimore: Williams & Wilkins, 1982:35–69.
80. Gibbs FA Jr. Thermal mapping in experimental cancer treatment with hyperthermia: Description and use of a semiautomatic system. Int J Radiat Oncol Biol Phys 1983;9: 1057–1063.
81. Dewhist MW, Phillips TL, Samulski TV, et al. RTOG quality assurance guidelines for clinical trials using hyperthermia. Int J Radiat Oncol Biol Phys 1990;18:1249–1259.
82. Guy AW. Biophysics of high frequency currents and electromagnetic radiation. In: Lehmann JF, ed. Therapeutic heat and cold. 3rd ed. Baltimore: Williams & Wilkins, 1982:199–277.
83. Frizzell LA, Dunn F. Biophysics of Ultrasound. In: Lehmann JF, ed. Therapeutic heat and cold. 3rd ed. Baltimore: Williams & Wilkins, 1982:353–385.
84. Gibbs FA Jr, Peck JW, Dethlefsen LA. The importance of temperature uniformity in the study of radiosensitizing effects of hyperthermia in vivo. Radiat Res 1981;87: 187–197.
84a. Final report on the NCI hyperthermia equipment evaluation contractors group, part 1. London: Taylor & Francis, In: J Hyperthermia [Special issue] 1988;4:1–132.
85. Lele PP. Physical aspects and clinical studies with ultrasonic hyperthermia. In: Storm FK, ed. Hyperthermia in cancer therapy. Boston: GK Hall Medical, 1983:333–365.
85a. Ebbini ES, Cain CA. A spherical-section ultrasound phased array applicator for deep localized hyperthermia. IEEE Trans Biomed Eng 1991;38:634–643.
86. Oleson JR. A review of magnetic induction methods for hyperthermia treatment of cancer. IEEE Trans Biomed Eng 1984;31:91–97.
87. Bach Andersen J. Regional electromagnetic heating. In: Hand JW, James JR, eds. Physical techniques in clinical hyperthermia. Letchworth, England: Research Studies Press, 1986:65–97.
88. Oleson JR. Interstitial hyperthermia. In: Withers HR, Peters LJ, eds. Innovations in Radiation Oncology Research. Berlin: Springer-Verlag, 1987:303–312.
89. Joseph C, Astrahan M, Lipsett J, et al. Interstitial hyperthermia and interstitial iridium-192 implantation: A technique and preliminary results. Int J Radiat Oncol Biol Phys 1981;7:827–833.
90. Lyons BE, Britt RH, Strohbehn JW. Localized hyperthermia in the treatment of malignant brain tumors using an interstitial microwave antenna array. IEEE Trans Biomed Eng 1984;31:53–62.
91. Stea B, Cetas TC, Cassady JR. Interstitial thermoradiotherapy of brain tumors: Preliminary results of a phase I clinical trial. Int J Radiat Oncol Biol Phys 1990;19:1463–1471.
92. Cavaliere R, Mondovi B, Moricca G, et al. Regional perfusion hyperthermia. In: Storm FK, ed. Hyperthermia in cancer therapy. Boston: GK Hall Medical, 1983:369–399.
93. Bull J, Lees D, Schuette W, et al. Whole body hyperthermia: A phase I trial of a potential adjuvant to chemotherapy. Ann Intern Med 1979;90:317–323.
94. Robins HI, Dennis WH, Neville AJ, et al. A nontoxic system for 41.8°C whole body hyperthermia. Results of a phase I study using a radiant heat device. Cancer Res 1985;45:3937–3944.
95. Parks L, Minaberry C, Smith D, et al. Treatment of far advanced bronchogenic carcinoma by extracorporeally induced systemic hyperthermia. J Thorac Cardiovasc Surg 1979;78:883–892.
98. Overgaard J. Rationale and problems in the design of clinical studies. In: Overgaard J, ed. Hyperthermic oncology 1984, vol 2. London: Taylor & Francis, 1985:325–338.
99. Arcangeli G, Benassi M, Cividalli A, et al. Radiotherapy and hyperthermia. Analysis of clinical results and identification of prognostic variables. Cancer 1987;60:950–956.
100. Dunlop PRC, Hand JW, Dickinson RJ, et al. An assessment of local hyperthermia in clinical practice. Int J Hyperthermia 1986;2:39–50.
101. Kapp DS, Petersen IVA, Cox RS. Two or six hyperthermia treatments as an adjunct to radiation therapy yield similar tumor responses: Results of a randomized trial. Int J Radiat Oncol Biol Phys 1990;19:1481–1495.
101a. Perez CA, Gillespie B, Pajak T, et al. Quality assurance problems in clinical hyperthermia and their impact on therapeutic outcome: A report by the Radiation Therapy Oncology Group. Int J Radiat Oncol Biol Phys 1989;16:551–558.
101b. Leopold KL, Dewhirst MW, Samulski TV, et al. Cumulative minutes with T_{90} greater than Temp index is predictive of response to hyperthermia and radiation. Int J Radiat Oncol Biol Phys 1993 (in press).
101c. Oleson JR, Dewhirst MW, Harrelson JM, et al. Tumor temperature distributions predict hyperthermia effect. Int J Radiat Oncol Biol Phys 1989;16:559–570.
101d. Leopold KA, Dewhirst M, Samulski T, et al. Relationship among tumor temperature, treatment time, and histopathological outcome using preoperative hyperthermia with radiation in soft tissue sarcoma. Int J Radiat Oncol Biol Phys 1992;27:989–998.
101e. Kapp DS, Barnett TA, Cox RS. Hyperthermia and radiation therapy of local-regional recurrent breast cancer: Prognostic factors for response and local control of diffuse or nodular tumors. Int J Radiat Oncol Biol Phys 1991;20:1147–1164.
101f. Valdagni R, Liu F-F, Kapp DS. Important prognostic factors influencing outcome of combined radiation and hyperthermia. Int J Radiat Oncol Biol Phys 1988;15:959–972.
102. Oleson JR, Samulski TV, Leopold KA, et al. Sensitivity of hyperthermia trial outcomes to temperature and time: Implications for thermal goals of treatment. Int J Radiat Oncol Biol Phys 1993 (in press).
103. Kapp DS. Site and disease selection for hyperthermia clinical trials. Int J Hyperthermia 1986;2:139–156.
104. Gibbs FA Jr. Regional hyperthermia: A clinical appraisal of noninvasive deep-heating methods. Cancer Res 1984;44:4765s-4770s.
105. Oleson JR, Sim DA, Manning MR. Analysis of prognostic variables in hyperthermia treatment of 161 patients. Int J Radiat Oncol Biol Phys 1984;10:2231–2239.
107. Oleson JR, Manning MR, Heusinkveld RS. Hyperthermia by magnetic induction: II. Clinical experience with concentric electrodes. Int J Radiat Oncol Biol Phys 1984;10: 2231–2239.
108. Sapozink MD, Gibbs FA Jr, Thomson JW, et al. A comparison of deep regional hyperthermia from an annular phased array and a concentric coil in the same patients. Int J Radiat Oncol Biol Phys 1985;11:179–190.
109. Abe M, Hiraoka M, Takahashi M, et al. Multi-institutional studies on hyperthermia using an 8-MHz radiofrequency capacitive heating device (Thermotron RF-8) in combination with radiation for cancer therapy. Cancer 1986;58:1589–1595.
109a. Kakehi M, Ueda K, Mukojima T, et al. Multi-institutional clinical studies on hyperthermia combined with radiotherapy or chemotherapy in advanced cancer of deep-seated organs. Int J Hyperthermia 1990;6:719–740.
110. Hiraoka M, Shiken J, Alzuta K, et al. Radiofrequency capacitive hyperthermia for deep-seated tumors. I. Studies on thermometry. Cancer 1987;60:121–127.
111. Hiraoka M, Shiken J, Akuta K, et al. Radiofrequency capacitive hyperthermia for deep-seated tumors. II. Effects of thermoradiotherapy. Cancer 1987;60:128–135.
112. Sapozink MD, Gibbs FA Jr, Egger MJ, et al. Regional hyperthermia for clinically advanced deep-seated pelvic malignancy. J Clin Oncol 1986;9:162–169.
112a. Sapozink MD, Joszef G, Astrahan MA, et al. Adjuvant pelvic hyperthermia in advanced cervical carcinoma. I. Feasibility, thermometry and device comparison. Int J Hyperthermia 1990;6:985–996.
112b. Feldman HJ, Molls M, Adler S, et al. Hyperthermia in eccentrically located pelvic tumors: Excessive heating of the perineal fat and normal tissue temperatures. Int J Radiat Oncol Biol Phys 1991;20:1017–1022.

112c. Petrovich Z, Langholz B, Gibbs FA. Regional hyperthermia for advanced tumors: A clinical study of 353 patients. Int J Radiat Oncol Biol Phys 1989;16:601–607.

113. Hynynen K, Shimm D, Anhalt D, et al. Temperature distributions during clinical scanned, focused ultrasound hypethermia treatments. Int J Hyperthermia 1990;6:891–908.

114. Riviere JE, Page RL, Dewhirst MW, et al. Effect of hyperthermia on cisplatin pharmacokinetics in normal dogs. Int J Hyperthermia 1986;2:351–358.

115. Klostergaard J, Barta M, Tomasovic SP. Hyperthermic modulation of tumor necrosis factor-dependent monocyte/macrophage tumor cytotoxicity in vitro. J Biol Response Modif 1989;8:262–277.

116. Shrivastava P, Luk K, Oleson J, et al. Hyperthermia quality assurance guidelines. Int J Radiat Oncol Biol Phys 1989;16:559–587.

117. Waterman FM, Dewhirst MW, Fessenden P, et al. RTOG quality assurance guidelines for clinical trials using hyperthermia administered by ultrasound. Int J Radiat Oncol Biol Phys 1991;20:1099–1107.

118. Sapozink MD, Corry PM, Kapp DS, et al. RTOG quality assurance guidelines for clinical trials using hyperthermia for deep-seated malignancy. Int J Radiat Oncol Biol Phys 1991;20:1109–1115.

119. Emami B, Stauffer P, Dewhirst MW. RTOG quality assurance guidelines for interstitial hyperthermia. Int J Radiat Oncol Biol Phys 1991;20:1117–1124.

120. Lindholm CE, Kjellen E, Nilsson P, et al. Microwave-induced hyperthermia and radiotherapy in human superficial tumors: Clinical results with a comparative study of combined treatment versus radiotherapy alone. Int J Hyperthermia 1987;3:393–411.

121. van der Zee J, van Rhoon GC, Wike-Hooley, et al. Thermal enhancement of radiotherapy in breast carcinoma. In: Overgaard J, ed. Hyperthermic oncology 1984, vol 1. London: Taylor & Francis, 1985:345–348.

122. Kim JH, Hahn EW, Ahmed SA, et al. Clinical study of the sequence of combined hyperthermia and radiation therapy of malignant melanoma. In: Overgaard J, ed. Hyperthermic oncology 1984, vol 1. London: Taylor & Francis, 1985:387–390.

123. Li R-Y, Zhang T-Z, Lin S-Y, et al. Effects of hyperthermia combined with radiation in the treatment of superficial malignant lesions in 90 patients. In: Overgaard J, ed. Hyperthermic oncology 1984, vol 1. London: Taylor & Francis, 1985:395–397.

124. Scott RS, Johnson RJR, Story KV, et al. Local hyperthermia in combination with definitive radiotherapy: Increased tumor clearance, reduced recurrence rate in extended follow-up. Int J Radiat Oncol Biol Phys 1984;10:2119–2123.

125. Corry PM, Spanos WJ, Tilchen EJ, et al. Combined ultrasound and radiation therapy treatment of human superficial tumors. Radiology 1982;145:165–169.

126. Kim JH, Hahn EW, Antich P. Radiofrequency hyperthermia for clinical cancer therapy. NCI Monogr 1982;61:339–342.

127. Sim DA, Oleson JR, Grochowski KJ. An update of the University of Arizona human clinical hyperthermia experience including estimates of therapeutic advantage. In: Overgaard J, ed. Hyperthermic oncology 1984, vol 1. London: Taylor & Francis, 1985:367–370.

128. Luk KH, Pajak TF, Perez CA, et al. Prognostic factors for tumor response after hyperthermia and radiation. In: Overgaard J, ed. Hyperthermic oncology 1984, vol 1. London: Taylor & Francis, 1985:353–358.

130. van der Zee J, van Putten WLJ, van den Berg AP, et al. Retrospective analysis of the response of tumors in patients treated with a combination of radiotherapy and hyperthermia. Int J Hyperthermia 1986;2:337–349.

131. Scott R, Gillespie B, Perez CA, et al. Hyperthermia in combination with definitive radiation therapy: Results of a phase I/II RTOG study. Int J Radiat Oncol Biol Phys 1988;15:711–716.

132. Valdagni R, Armichetti M, Pani G. Radical radiation alone versus radical radiation plus microwave hyperthermia for N3 (TNM-UICC) neck nodes: A prospective clinical trial. Int J Radiat Oncol Biol Phys 1988;115:13–24.

133. Arcangeli G, Arcangeli GC, Guerra A, et al. Tumor response to heat and radiation: Prognostic variables in the treatment of neck node metastases from head and neck cancer. Int J Hyperthermia 1985;1:207–217.

134. Steeves RA, Severson SB, Paliwal BR, et al. Matched-pair analysis of response to local hyperthermia and megavoltage electron therapy for superficial human tumors. Endocurietherapy/Hyperthermia Oncol 1986;2:163–170.

Cancer: Principles & Practice of Oncology, Fourth Edition,
edited by Vincent T. DeVita, Jr., Samuel Hellman, Steven A. Rosenberg.
J.B. Lippincott Co., Philadelphia © 1993.

Gregory A. Curt

CHAPTER **70**

Unsound Methods of Cancer Treatment

Things are seldom what they seem, skim milk masquerades as cream.

—Gilbert and Sullivan, "HMS Pinafore"

DEFINITION AND MAGNITUDE OF THE PROBLEM

In earlier editions of this text, this chapter was called "Unproven Methods of Cancer Treatment." However, the term *unproven* is nonjudgmental and at best is a euphemism for the unsound therapies described in this chapter. After all, many of the newer methods of cancer treatment described elsewhere in this edition are, in some sense, "unproven" in that their precise role in clinical treatment remains uncertain. The two distinguishing characteristics of *unsound* methods of cancer treatment (whether we want to label them unproven, unorthodox, nontraditional, complementary, or alternative therapies) are promotion without sufficient preclinical data to justify use in patients, and unmethodical treatment of patients that cannot detect either meaningful responses or therapy-related side effects.

A recent and somewhat surprising development has been the beginning of scientific and impartial evaluation of alternative cancer treatments. This healthy trend has been seen with the Bristol Cancer Help Centre (holistic care), the Livingston Wheeler Clinic (autogenous vaccines and diet), and the Burzynski Research Institute (antineoplaston therapy). These are discussed later in this chapter.

Not surprisingly, purveyors of unsound methods generally offer "nontoxic" or "natural" approaches to cancer treatment. These unorthodox practitioners are largely physicians who escape regulatory control by the Food and Drug Administration (FDA) and offer their particular treatment approach to well-educated patients with early-stage disease. At a time when 50% of the serious cancers diagnosed in the United States are curable with existing therapies, and access to scientifically sound experimental trials has been considerably simplified with the National Cancer Institute's Physician Data Query computerized information system, it seems inconsistent that unsound methods of cancer treatment should continue to be a significant public health problem. However, the problem remains enormous.

Until recently, it was difficult to accurately estimate the magnitude of the use of unsound cancer remedies. In 1984 the Subcommittee on Health and Long-Term Care of the U.S. House of Representatives concluded that Americans spent $10 billion on unsound and unscientific remedies, with some $4 billion to $5 billion being spent annually on useless cancer treatments.[1] The cost in human terms is impossible to estimate.

One survey found that 13% of inpatients treated at a large urban cancer center had used or were using an unorthodox treatment regimen in addition to therapy prescribed by their oncologists.[2] Although this represents a highly selected inpatient population at a university referral center, this estimate of the frequency of use of unsound treatments is supported by a more recent Harris telephone survey of over 6000 American households. The study, undertaken for the Division of Consumer Affairs of the Food and Drug Administration in 1986, reports that 15% of all cancer patients had used one or more questionable cancer treatments.[3] This sample estimate, applied to the 6 million Americans who are alive today with a previous diagnosis of cancer, would project that about one million Americans have used one or more unsound cancer treatments.

What factors contribute to the continuing appeal of "alternative" cancer treatments? An interesting and perhaps predictable component to cancer quackery has always been an element of faddism. Indeed, the popularity of different methods of unsound cancer treatment has often paralleled advances in orthodox clinical cancer medicine. In the 1940s and 1950s, when radiation therapy was beginning to improve control of locoregional disease, cancer quackery became device-oriented: cancer patients were treated with the oscilloclast (a device that supposedly "retuned" disharmonic electrons and restored health) and the orgone energy accumulator (purportedly capable of concentrating a visible and ubiquitous cosmic energy into depleted erythrocytes). During the 1960s and 1970s, when chemotherapy was beginning to become accepted as an effective treatment for patients with advanced cancer, useless drugs were offered by nonscientific practitioners. This era saw the use of krebiozen and laetrile in thousands of cancer patients, and "freedom of choice" became the banner under which cancer patients demanded access to organized quackery.

There have been two recent fundamental shifts in the practice of unsound cancer treatment. The first, and most predictable, is a new focus on treatments that might be called "biologic." Since the beginning of the 1980s, thousands of cancer patients have paid millions of dollars for treatment with antineoplastons (proteins derived from urine that are said to be capable of differentiating tumors) or with Dr. Lawrence Burton's immunoaugmentative therapy (falsely represented as being able to boost immune response). Differentiating agents and immunotherapy are among the most promising leads in mainstream cancer treatment, and the biologic trend in unsound cancer therapy in the 1980s continues the device orientation of the 1940s and 1950s and the drug orientation of the 1960s and 1970s. In each case, the unsound practitioners echo the most promising theories of the day in offering their own peculiar brand of optimism. This optimism is derived from the promise that, in addition to being scientifically avant-garde, the alternative therapy is safer, more natural, less toxic, yet uniquely effective.

The second recent shift in alternative medicine involves the perception of cancer and other diseases as symptoms of metabolic imbalance rather than illnesses in and of themselves. The lifestyle approach to cancer holds that the disease can be effectively prevented and treated by changes in diet, supplements of enzymes and vitamins, or avoidance of stress, pollutants, and impurities. This is the world of "metabolic therapy," where laetrile is no longer a drug, but instead is reborn as "vitamin B_{17}." In addition, because metabolic therapy holds that the cancer is merely a symptom of more fundamental underlying processes, tumor progression does not necessarily indicate treatment failure. Instead, the effectiveness of treatment can be monitored by subjective feelings, by blood assays available only to the practitioner, or through other irrelevant observations, such as iridology (anatomic diagnosis by examination of the iris).

The result of all of these unsound approaches is the same: patients spend time and money on useless therapies. The potential for greater harm is obvious. Cancer patients who seek and obtain unsound therapy may not receive treatments of proven efficacy or appropriate experimental treatment approaches based on sound science. In addition, some of the most popular unsound treatments are potentially harmful in themselves.

A list of unsound therapies is given in Table 70–1, and detailed statements on each approach are available from the American Cancer Society.

TREATMENT REGULATION

It is useful, from an historical perspective, to understand how quackery affected drug regulation in the United States before reviewing the evolution of past and present unsound cancer treatments. The FDA is responsible for regulating the avail-

TABLE 70–1. Unsound Methods of Cancer Treatment

Alivizatos therapy (Greek cancer cure)	Dimethyl sulfoxide (DMSO)	Koch antitoxins
Antineoplastons	Dotto electronic reactor	Krebiozen
Bamfolin	Ferguson plant products	Laetrile (amygdalin, vitamin B_{17})
Beard method	Fonti method	Low's method
Bonifacia anticancer goat serum	Francis diet	Macrobiotic diet
Cancer-lipid concentrate	Fresh cell therapy	Makari intradermal cancer test
Carcin and neo-carcin	Frost method	Metabolic therapy
Carzodelin	Gerson method	Mucorhicin
C.N.T.	Glover serum	Multiple enzyme therapy
CH-23	Grape diet	Orgone energy devices
Chase dietary method	Hill Hadley vaccine	Polonine
Collodaurim and bichloracetic acid	Hemacytology index	Psychic surgery
Chaparral tea	Hett cancer serum	Revici method
Clam extracts (mercenene)	Hoxsey method	Spears hygenic system
Contreras method	Immunoaugmentative therapy (IAT)	Ultraviolet blood irradiation
Cresson method	Iscador	
Crofton immunization	Issel's combination therapy	
Cytec lung cancer screening	KC-555	
Diamond carbon compound	Kanfer handwriting test	
	Kelly malignancy index	

ability of drugs, biologicals, and medical devices in the United States and has the ultimate authority to approve or disapprove new treatments in cancer and other diseases. Much of the FDA's current regulatory authority came from an obvious hoax in cancer therapy at the turn of the century—the so-called "golden age of quackery."[4]

The case involved Dr. O.A. Johnson of Kansas City, Missouri, and his "Mild Combination Treatment" for cancer. As shown in Figure 70–1, prospective patients were invited to send for Dr. Johnson's books, *Cancer and Its Cure* and *My 125-Page Testimonial Book*—titles that have a contemporary ring in today's world of unsound cancer treatments. Those who could not visit the doctor were asked to fill out a symptom sheet so that cures could be "effected at home." Recognizing that the Mild Combination Treatment was fraudulent, the Bureau of Chemistry (the forerunner of today's FDA) prosecuted Dr. Johnson under the Food and Drug Act of 1906. The case eventually reached the Supreme Court and was decided in favor of Dr. Johnson. Justice Oliver Wendell Holmes, writing the majority opinion, interpreted existing laws to pertain only to drug labeling and not therapeutic claims. As long as the treatment materials were properly labeled, Dr. Johnson could not be prosecuted for "mistaken praise" of the Mild Combination Treatment.[4]

President Taft and Congress responded by amending the Food and Drug Act, making "false and fraudulent" therapeutic claims a criminal offense. However, legal proof of fraudulence was often difficult in practice, and in 1938 Congress passed a new Food and Drug Act that required proof of safety before a drug could be marketed. The new law strengthened the FDA's ability to cope with fraudulent cancer therapists, and the subsequent years saw a series of successful criminal prosecutions. During this era the Koch therapy, Hoxsey's herbal tonic, and krebiozen became subjects of highly visible public trials that also resulted in seizures of drug supplies and injunctions against further drug distribution. By 1960, FDA Commissioner George Larrick could state, "The Food and Drug Administration has had considerable success in combatting quackery in the courts. There have been some heavy fines and some prison sentences. Such actions have had a strong deterrent effect."[5]

In 1962, however, the FDA's responsibilities and priorities changed with the passage of the Kefauver-Harris amendments to the 1938 Food and Drug Act. These amendments required evidence of drug efficacy and safety before marketing. As a result, the FDA increasingly turned its attention to the control of the pharmaceutical industry. Between 1962 and 1987, over 7000 previously available prescription drugs were removed from the U.S. market. During the same interval, the FDA's commitment to combatting quackery decreased proportionately; less than 0.001% of the FDA budget is currently committed to combatting health fraud.

THE ERA OF UNSOUND DEVICES

The period between 1940 and 1950 saw the use of several fraudulent devices in the treatment of cancer. One of the more interesting therapists was Dr. Wilhelm Reich, a Viennese colleague of Sigmund Freud. Reich's studies of character analysis and sexuality during the 1930s were considered seminal to the new discipline of psychoanalysis.

Between 1936 and 1939, Reich's research took him to Norway, where he claimed discovery of orgone, a visible and ubiquitous cosmic energy that he described as "the most powerful force in the universe." In 1940, Reich emigrated to the United States, where he purchased a 300-acre estate in Rangeley, Maine, which he named, appropriately enough, Organon. The estate eventually housed the Orgone Energy Ob-

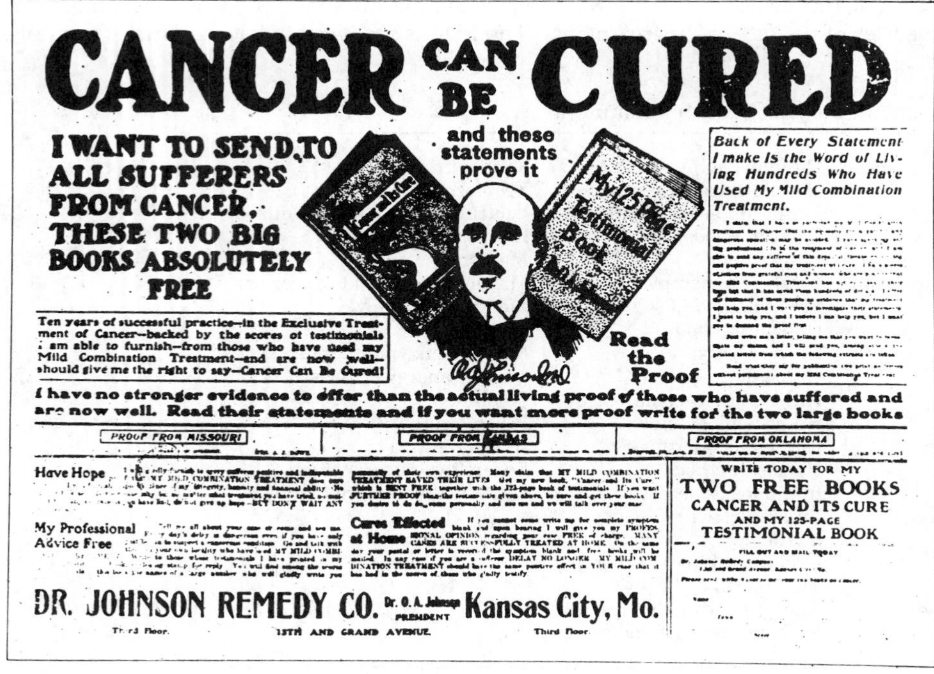

FIGURE 70–1. A 1908 advertisement of Dr. Johnson's Mild Combination Cancer Treatment. Litigation involving this reached the Supreme Court and resulted in important changes in U.S. drug regulation. (Courtesy of the U.S. Food and Drug Administration History Office)

servatory, the Wilhelm Reich Foundation, laboratories, and its own printing facilities.[6]

In Rangeley Reich designed and built "orgone energy accumulators," treatment devices resembling telephone booths constructed of metal, wood, and asbestos board. Specialized cone-shaped instruments were also designed to treat the head. Hundreds of these devices were leased throughout the United States at the then-remarkable cost of $250 per month. Treatment response was judged by blood tests performed in Reich's laboratories. Volume I of the 1942 edition of *The International Journal of Sexual Economy and Orgone Research* has a strangely contemporary tone in describing the four blood tests for cancer: a culture test, a biologic resistance test, a disintegration test, and a blue margin test. This battery of studies was purported to be capable of distinguishing between healthy and "cancerous" blood and was even purported to be able to detect cancer *before* the development of a tumor.

Reich had developed not only his own theories of cancer etiology (orgone depletion in erythrocytes) but also a completely self-contained system for diagnosis, treatment, and prevention of cancer.[7,8] It was an unimpeachable and self-fulfilling system that anticipated many common characteristics of unsound cancer therapies today.

However, this was an era of organized opposition to cancer quackery. The FDA consulted a group of independent clinicians and physicists who examined several orgone accumulators and concluded that orgone energy could be neither accumulated nor measured, and that Reich's principles had no scientific merit or clinical utility. In 1954 a federal injunction was issued against Reich and his foundation, demanding a recall of orgone accumulators and banning interstate advertisements in Reich's pamphlets and magazines.

Proponents of the orgone energy theories charged that the FDA investigation interfered with freedom of the press and was part of an organized government effort to prevent effective and nontoxic cancer treatments from being widely distributed.[9] Reich was held in criminal contempt of the FDA injunction when he continued to lease and distribute orgone accumulators, claiming that courts and juries had no jurisdiction in matters of "natural law."[4] Despite an appeal to the Supreme Court, Reich was sentenced to 2 years in prison, where he died in 1957.

Although orgone energy devices are not part of the contemporary scene of cancer quackery, several common themes remain all too familiar: a charismatic "scientist" with an appealing—albeit unsupportable—theory of cancer and its treatment; unverifiable measures of success; and faithful proponents who believe that orthodox medicine wants to suppress innovation.

At the same time on the west coast of the United States, Dr. Albert Abrams was pioneering other devices—equally unsound in principle and profitable in practice—for the diagnosis and treatment of cancer. Abrams' diagnostic technique involved analyzing patient blood specimens in a "radioscope"—a tuning apparatus capable of detecting radiofrequencies associated with disease. After a blood specimen was dried on filter paper and inserted into the machine, the patient had to hold metal plates connected to the radioscope while the operator completed an examination with a plastic wand. This examination was described as sufficiently sensitive to "inform the doctor whether or not the patient has cancer, or a tendency towards cancer, long before there has been any visible disturbance of tissue."[10] To treat what the radioscope diagnosed, Abrams developed the oscilloclast, a device said to be capable of restoring electronic vibrations in diseased tissue.

Eventually the fraud blossomed into a mail-order business sponsored by the Electronic Medical Foundation. Radioscopes were "perfected" to diagnose blood specimens mailed in on postcards by practitioners who rented an oscilloclast directly from Abrams. A diagnosis was promptly returned with recommended oscilloclast treatment settings. At the height of its popularity in 1950, oscilloclasts were rented to more than 3000 practitioners for a $250 deposit and $5 per month. As a result, Abrams was able to endow his Electronic Medical Foundation with some $3 million.[11]

However, a comprehensive investigation by the FDA demonstrated that the radioscope could not distinguish colored water from blood. The radioscope diagnosis of a specimen from an 11-week-old rooster was sinus infection and bad teeth.[12] In 1958, after a series of appeals, the Electronic Medical Foundation was prohibited from interstate shipment of the devices. In 1962 the Foundation was dissolved.

The story has an ironic twist: the officers of the Electronic Medical Foundation subsequently founded the National Health Federation, an organization established to represent, protect, and promote alternative medicine in the United States. During the ensuing years, the National Health Federation would become increasingly organized supporters of the Hoxsey therapy, krebiozen, and laetrile.

THE ERA OF UNSOUND DRUGS

The 1950s saw the first successful use of cancer chemotherapy but also was an era in which fraudulent drugs were promoted.

THE HOXSEY TREATMENT

One of the most popular health scams of the 1950s was the Hoxsey method of cancer treatment. In his 1956 book *You Don't Have to Die*, Harry Hoxsey described his approach as "essentially chemotherapy" for "the systemic treatment of cancer."[13] The Hoxsey method involved two medicines: the "pink medicine" (potassium iodide and pepsin) and the "black medicine" (cascara in an extract of licorice, red clover, burdock root, stillingia root, berberis root, poke root, and the bark of the buckthorn and prickly ash).[14] This complex of plant products was attributed to Hoxsey's great-grandfather, who observed that his horse was cured of cancer after grazing on these plants.

Hoxsey initially peddled his therapy from state to state and was convicted of practicing medicine without a license in Illinois and Iowa. He finally established clinics in Texas and Pennsylvania, where patients were examined, uniformly diagnosed as having cancer, and routinely offered treatment at a cost of $400. At the height of its popularity in the late 1950s, more than 10,000 "cancer" patients were receiving Hoxsey's medicines.[4]

Because of the treatment's popularity, there were many contemporary attempts to validate antitumor activity by independent review. In 1957, a site visit by the University of British Columbia to Hoxsey's Texas clinic concluded, "The medications are of no value in the treatment of cancer. We have found that the methods of diagnosis are inadequate, that treatments do not affect the progress of disease, that no serious attempt is made to evaluate results and that no significant research has been done."[15]

This was followed by a detailed FDA examination of 400 cases of cancer "cured" by Hoxsey's regimen. Patients were found to fall into one of three categories: those who never had a diagnosis of cancer, those who had been previously cured of cancer by conventional therapy, or those (the majority) who had cancer that had not responded to the regimen.[16] In short, no cures could be documented and no evidence of antitumor activity was found.

These reviews led to a series of highly public trials during which Hoxsey proponents countered the prosecution by lobbying Congress with a prayer campaign against the FDA. After ten years of litigation, the Hoxsey cancer treatment was finally banned from U.S. sales, although by that time over $50 million had been spent on the drugs.[17] This approach is still available in Mexico.

KREBIOZEN

The growing popularity of krebiozen in the late 1950s and early 1960s, after the invalidation of Hoxsey's herbal medicines, began a new era in unsound cancer treatments. Unlike Hoxsey's folksy midwestern tonics, krebiozen and subsequent popular unsound remedies had a pseudoscientific ring of authenticity and were increasingly promoted by more convincing, scientifically trained proponents with the support of an organized constituency.

Krebiozen was initially manufactured as an antihypertensive by Dr. Stevan Durovic, a Yugoslavian physician who claimed to produce the drug by extracting the serum of horses injected with sterile extracts of *Actinomyces bovis,* a pathogenic fungus that causes lumpy jaw disease in animals. The original 2 grams of krebiozen (an estimated 200,000 doses) were purportedly produced from 2000 horses in Argentina and brought into the United States in Durovic's suitcase in 1949.

In the United States, Durovic met Dr. Andrew Ivy, a professor emeritus at the University of Illinois. Ivy became convinced that krebiozen had antitumor activity after an experiment in which Durovic demonstrated disease "improvement" in seven of twelve animals treated with the drug.[18] These results were never reproduced. Instead, Ivy, a respected scientist, began treating a series of patients after deciding that the drug was nontoxic by administering it to himself.

In 1951, the results of krebiozen treatment in 22 cancer patients were announced at a press conference at the Drake Hotel in Chicago. The results of the trial were never submitted for publication; instead, pamphlets published by the newly organized Krebiozen Research Foundation were distributed to the press, claiming improvement in most patients treated. Although 8 patients had died during the course of the trial, death was said not to be due to progressive cancer, and the fact was omitted that 2 additional patients had died in the interval between publication of the pamphlet and the press conference.

After Ivy's announcement, small quantities of krebiozen were provided to several medical centers to allow them to reproduce the results of the initial clinical trial. During the subsequent 12 years, independent investigators could not confirm that krebiozen had any antitumor activity. However, this did not stop the Krebiozen Research Foundation from issuing reports and independently publishing monographs claiming impressive treatment responses in individual patients.

Between 1951 and 1963, krebiozen was distributed by the Krebiozen Research Foundation to thousands of general practitioners throughout the United States. Physicians could receive an injectable ampule of krebiozen for a "research donation" of $9 and use it in any way they saw fit. Business was brisk. The initial 200,000 doses were rapidly depleted, and in 1960 Durovic manufactured an additional 100,000 ampules from horse serum and horse meat. It was claimed that, like the original batch of krebiozen, the treatment material contained lipopolysaccharides consisting of galacturonic acid, glucosamine, arabinose, and xylose, combined with glycerol.

In 1962 the Kefauver-Harris amendments to the Food and Drug Act required sponsors of investigational drugs to submit plans for the rational clinical development of new agents. Although Durovic submitted such a plan for krebiozen to the FDA in June 1963, he withdrew the package without review a month afterward, making interstate shipment of krebiozen illegal. Several concurrent observations led to subsequent criminal proceedings. In 1963 FDA chemists analyzed samples of krebiozen submitted by Ivy and Durovic. The white power was found to be creatine, a simple organic acid widely distributed in muscle tissues and inactive as an antitumor agent. Analysis of pre-1960 ampules of krebiozen revealed nothing but mineral oil, while those vials manufactured after 1960 contained mineral oil and trace quantities of methylhydantoin, a soluble form of creatine.

Independent analysis of the clinical results of krebiozen treatment was equally revealing. In 1962 the Krebiozen Research Foundation selected its 504 best responses (from over 4000 patients on whom records were available) and sent them to the National Cancer Institute (NCI) for independent review and analysis. Because these cases were inadequately documented for careful review, FDA officials spent considerable effort confirming diagnoses and reconstructing treatment duration, dose, and response. This information was submitted to an independent 24-member panel of experts appointed by the NCI. In 1963 that committee reported that review of all 504 cases established that krebiozen had no antitumor activity. From the NCI's perspective, the case was closed and there was no justification to pursue clinical trials.[19]

The FDA undertook its own independent analysis of an additional 4307 cases submitted by the Krebiozen Research Foundation. Again, no convincing evidence for antitumor activity could be demonstrated.

In short, krebiozen had been promoted for the treatment of thousands of cancer patients at a cost of millions of dollars. The treatment materials were falsely labeled. Moreover, although indiscriminate prescription made retrospective review of the thousands of available records particularly time-consuming and expensive, there was no evidence of reproducible antitumor activity in any malignancy.

In 1964 Ivy, Durovic, and the Krebiozen Research Foundation were indicted on 49 counts of violation of the Food, Drug and Cosmetic Act, including mail fraud, mislabeling of drugs, and conspiracy to defraud the public. Although the defendants were found innocent after a highly public 9-month trial, the interstate distribution of krebiozen was stopped.[20]

This decision was followed by a series of demonstrations by krebiozen supporters, who argued that the government, industry, and organized medicine had worked in concert to deny the public an effective and nontoxic cancer treatment. Proponents blocked the FDA Commissioner's office and lobbied Congress to reverse the FDA decision. Eventually, 11 senators demanded an impartial trial of krebiozen. Durovic offered to sell the NCI bulk krebiozen for such a study for $170,000 per gram; the same quantity of pure creatine from chemical suppliers was available for 30 cents.

However, interest in krebiozen evaporated when Durovic unexpectedly left the United States for Switzerland after withdrawing substantial amounts of cash from Foundation bank accounts. At the time, he was under investigation by the Internal Revenue Service for nonpayment of taxes on $904,907 of unreported income. Ivy renamed krebiozen "carcalon"—Greek for a natural substance that slows down a cancerous process—and continued to prescribe the drug from his Chicago office.[21] At the request of the Illinois State Medical Society, the governor appointed the Illinois Krebiozen Committee to oversee continued "controlled scientific testing of krebiozen" by Ivy. The committee never gave a report, and at the time of Ivy's death in 1977 there was still no evidence that krebiozen was useful in the treatment of cancer.

LAETRILE

Laetrile is a generic term for a group of cyanogenic glucosides that can be isolated from several natural sources, including the pits of edible fruits such as apricots, cherries, pears, apples, and peaches.[22,23] The term was coined by E.T. Krebs, "because this apricot-kernel preparation was *lae*vorotary to polarized light and because amygdalin was chemically a maloni*trile*."[24] The principal constituent of laetrile is amygdalin, a compound first isolated in 1830 and chemically synthesized in 1924.[25,26] As early as 1935 it was found that the β-glycoside linkage in amygdalin could be hydrolyzed by emulsin (an enzyme found in almonds) or specific β-glucosidases to release one molecule of hydrogen cyanide and benzaldehyde and two molecules of glucose.

In the 1920s, Ernest Krebs Sr. was the first to use oral amygdalin in the treatment of cancer. The preparation proved toxic, however, and it was not until 1952 that Krebs' son, E.T. Krebs, reported the development of a "safe" parenteral formulation.

Laetrile's purported mechanism of action is shown below. It was hypothesized that β-glucosidases would activate amygdalin to glucose, benzaldehyde, and toxic hydrogen cyanide. Hydrogen cyanide could be itself detoxified by rhodanese (thiosulfurtransferase), which would convert the hydrogen cyanide to inactive thiocyanate.[27]

$$\text{Amygdalin} \xrightarrow{\text{glycosidases}} \begin{matrix}\text{HCN}\\ \text{benzaldehyde}\\ \text{glucose}\end{matrix} \xrightarrow{\text{rhodanese}} \text{thiocyanate}$$

To explain amygdalin's specific antitumor effects and lack of toxicity, proponents further postulated that cancer cells have high intracellular levels of β-glucosidase and low levels of rhodanese, while the opposite is true in normal tissues. There are several critical flaws in this theory. First, normal and malignant tissues appear to have comparable levels of rhodanese, and tumor tissues lack β-glucosidase activity.[28,29] Indeed, there appears to be little detectable in vivo β-glucosidase activity, so that virtually all of a parenteral amygdalin dose is excreted intact in the urine.[23] Moreover, laetrile itself is inactive in vitro and in vivo against murine and human tumors in several preclinical assays, even when β-glycosidase is administered concurrently.[30–34] Indeed, control animals in comparative studies showed improved survival, suggesting that amygdalin is toxic without being active against disease.

Because β-glycosidase is not found in mammalian tissues, up to 10 grams of amygdalin can be administered intravenously without toxicity. However, gut bacteria have glycosidase and can release cyanide from amygdalin. Cyanide toxicity can occur after the administration of oral laetrile, and death from cyanide poisoning has been reported after such treatment.[35] Moreover, although cyanide is proposed as the active component to laetrile, cyanide itself has been tested as a potential antitumor agent and appears to be more toxic to normal than malignant tissues.[36–38]

Thus, there is no evidence for selective activation of amygdalin by malignant tissues, preferential inactivation of hydrogen cyanide by normal tissues, or usefulness of hydrogen cyanide as a chemotherapeutic agent. The drug has proved inactive in every in vivo and in vitro system in which it was tested. So why did laetrile become the most popular and celebrated unsound cancer therapy of contemporary medicine?

As Wallace Jansen has noted, by the mid-1950s the laetrile business was controlled by Andrew McNaughton, an international entrepreneur with a flair for manipulating the press.[4] In 1961 McNaughton founded Bioenzymes International, Ltd., and began to manufacture laetrile in Mexico and Canada. In 1963 a strongly pro-laetrile paperback book, *Laetrile—Control for Cancer, The Authorized Story*, was published with an introduction by McNaughton.[39] Several of the chapters were reprinted in newspapers and magazines, and so began an intense public interest in and demand for the drug. However, with neither preclinical nor clinical evidence that laetrile was useful in the treatment of cancer, the FDA began a series of actions against Krebs and the McNaughton Foundation. The Canadian FDA followed by prohibiting distribution of laetrile in Canada. Manufacture and distribution continued in Mexico, where apricot pits were largely imported from the California fruit-packing industry.

In 1970 the McNaughton Foundation of Canada submitted an investigational new drug application (INDA) to the U.S. FDA. The INDA was granted, but the FDA withdrew its approval a month later. Dr. Charles Edwards, then FDA commissioner, cited "serious preclinical and clinical deficiencies" in the application.[40] For example, while chemical analysis of Canadian laetrile in the 1960s found amygdalin contents between 87% and 98%, Mexican production suffered from problems in quality control.[41] FDA analysis of laetrile from Mexican laboratories indicated that a 500-mg tablet might contain anywhere from 42 to 450 mg of amygdalin, while the parenteral product was 14% to 87% pure. Indeed, vials of injectable laetrile were found to be contaminated with bacteria, fungus, and isopropyl alcohol.[42]

However, the FDA's reversal only strengthened the public's conviction that the "establishment" was intent on keeping a useful product away from patients. An article in the *Harvard Political Review* ignored available evidence and concluded that "vested interests have prevented the use of an inexpensive and effective cancer cure."[43] At the same time, the legal prosecution of the ultraconservative physician Dr. John Richardson under a California law that made prescription of laetrile a felony galvanized the John Birch Society. Laetrile proponents established the International Association for Cancer Victims and Friends in 1963, and in 1972 Robert Bradford, a John Bircher, founded the Committee for Freedom of Choice in Cancer Therapy. Together with the National Health Foundation, these organizations mounted an effective campaign to "legalize" laetrile on the premise that the patient and physician should have ultimate authority in choosing treatment and that the government should not regulate medical practice. As Lerner notes in assessing the laetrile phenomenon, this was a time when antiestablishment groups and ultraconservatives united in the name of "freedom of choice."[44]

Their efforts at the state level were highly successful. In a 1977 *New England Journal of Medicine* editorial entitled "Laetrilomania," Dr. F.J. Ingelfinger summarized contemporary developments: "In Alaska, Laetrile may be prescribed by doctors, and an Oklahoma judge legalized importation of drug from Mexico. Indiana, if the physician-governor signs the bill passed by his legislature, would become the first state to approve the manufacture and sale of the substance as well as its use. Bills that prohibit interference with the sale or use of laetrile are well on their way in Arizona, Florida, Massachusetts, and Minnesota."[45]

During the next year, additional legislation to approve laetrile at the state level followed the celebrated case of Rutherford versus the United States. In this 1978 case, Glenn Rutherford enjoined the FDA from interfering with his constitutional right to obtain nontoxic therapy (laetrile) for his terminal malignancy. Both the U.S. District Court in Oklahoma and the Court of Appeals ignored the fact that Rutherford's "terminal" rectal polyp had been surgically cured. Instead, they ruled that safety and efficacy have no meaning in the treatment of terminally ill patients and that the designation of terminal illness could be made by any licensed physician. The FDA was directed to provide regulations for the distribution of laetrile to any terminal cancer patient who desired it.[46] Although this decision was eventually overturned by the Supreme Court, laetrile gained additional political credibility and 23 states moved to legalize laetrile therapy.

Despite widespread laetrile use, evidence that the drug was effective remained unconvincing. By 1978 it was estimated that more than 70,000 Americans had been treated with laetrile.[47] A small retrospective analysis of laetrile treatment response was undertaken by the California Cancer Commission in 1953; no antitumor activity was found in 44 patients with a variety of tumors.[48] By far the largest retrospective analysis of laetrile efficacy was undertaken by the NCI in 1978.[47] Case reports of patients who might have benefited from laetrile were solicited from 385,000 physicians, 70,000 health professionals, and pro-laetrile groups. Only 93 cases were submitted, of which 67 could be evaluated. Of these, 6 patients were felt to have had an objective treatment response (2 lymphoma, 2 adenocarcinoma, 1 carcinoid, 1 squamous cell lung cancer). The authors admitted that the design of the study made it impossible to rule out intentional or unintentional submission of inaccurate information, but concluded that if laetrile has antitumor activity, it must be vanishingly small. The proper denominator for the six responses is not the 67 cases selected for best response but the 70,000 patients known to have been treated with the drug.

The issue of laetrile's usefulness in cancer treatment remained unsettled. Some prominent physicians urged legalization as a way to "make forbidden fruit less tempting," while others urged prospective clinical trials.[45,49] In 1978 the NCI submitted its own INDA for a clinical trial of amygdalin to the FDA. The NCI ensured quality control in the production of the drug as well as prospective, well-designed, and well-implemented clinical trials. In a small phase I study, a single patient developed cyanide toxicity after eating almonds during laetrile treatment; almonds not only contain small quantities of amygdalin but also have β-glycosidase activity.[50] In the larger phase II trial, no responses were seen in 178 patients with a variety of cancers.[51] The resolution of laetrile's activity as an anticancer drug came 30 years and 70,000 patients too late.

UNSOUND CANCER TREATMENTS POPULAR TODAY

As discussed at the beginning of this chapter, there have been two fundamental developments in the contemporary practice of unsound cancer medicine. The first is a predictable shift towards treatments that might be considered biologic, while the second is the development of the concept that cancer is a symptom of underlying metabolic disturbances and can be prevented and treated by diet, vitamins, and avoiding stress.

IMMUNOAUGMENTATIVE THERAPY

Immunoaugmentative therapy (IAT) is a scientifically unsupportable treatment dispensed by the Immunology Researching Center in Freeport, Bahamas. The center was established in 1977 by Lawrence Burton, a PhD zoologist, after he failed to receive approval for clinical studies of IAT in the U.S. from the FDA.[52] The treatment is based on the theory that cancer develops because of "immunoincompetence," which Burton can measure and restore using a series of protein fractions derived from the blood of patients and healthy donors.

Patients receiving IAT first undergo a series of immunocompetence blood tests that are computer-analyzed to select each patient's treatment regimen. The treatment itself consists of four "immune serum protein fractions" called blocking protein, tumor antibody, tumor complement, and deblocking protein. Based on the computer analysis of the patient's immune profile, some or all of these fractions may be prescribed as daily subcutaneous injections. Stabilization of the immune system usually requires several weeks on the island, after which patients leave with a cache of sera and computer projections for further treatment.[53] The initial treatment costs about $10,000, and patients are required to make follow-up visits for immune system "tune-ups."[53] The clinic also provides patients with assistance in filing claims for third-party reimbursement.

In 1978, a year after the clinic was established, the Bahamian government requested a review of IAT by a committee of physician-scientists from the Pan-American Health Organization. This panel found neither a scientific rationale for IAT nor clinical evidence for its efficacy, and unanimously recommended that the center be closed.[54] Despite these findings, the clinic remained open (for the treatment of non-Bahamians only) and over 3000 patients, most of them Americans with cancer, have received IAT for cancer treatment or prevention.

Because of political pressure at the state level, IAT was approved for the treatment of cancer in Florida and Oklahoma in 1981.[55,56] In addition, there have been unsuccessful congressional proposals to exempt IAT from FDA control.[57] As with laetrile in the previous decade, an unsound cancer treatment was essentially legalized by individual states without regard to either therapeutic effectiveness or potential toxicity.

However, subsequent independent analysis of IAT treatment materials has shown them to be devoid of purported content or biologic activity. In each case, analysis of the IAT treatment reagents revealed diluted blood proteins, the major component of which was albumin.[58] Specific immunoglobulins, macroglobulins, and complement activity said to be essential to the activity of the regimen were undetectable. Treatment materials were found to be uniformly contaminated with bacteria and hepatitis, and an epidemic of nocardia abscess formation was reported at IAT injection sites.[59,60] Even more worrisome was Burton's use of IAT in the treatment of acquired immunodeficiency syndrome (AIDS), a disease that he ascribes to the immunodepressant effects of sexual lubricants.[61] Since the IAT laboratories pool blood specimens before processing them into treatment reagents, contamination of reagents with the human immunodeficiency virus (HIV) is possible. Indeed, of 72 vials of IAT treatment materials available to the NCI for analysis, 37 (51%) were positive for antibodies to HIV, and the Centers for Disease Control were subsequently reproducibly able to culture viable AIDS virus from Burton's treatment materials.[58,62]

Therefore, IAT is without scientific rationale or documented clinical activity; rather, patients are treated with a series of inert blood products capable of transmitting bacterial infection, hepatitis, and AIDS. Because of these findings, in July 1985 the Bahamian clinic was closed as a hazard to its laboratory workers. After 6 months of demonstrations in Freeport and Washington, the clinic reopened. By then, Burton had already moved to establish clinics in Mexico.

IAT is an unsound and potentially harmful approach to the treatment of cancer and AIDS. Unfortunately, as reported by the Congressional Office of Technology Assessment, which devoted considerable attention to IAT in its report on alternative cancer treatments, attempts to evaluate this approach impartially have not met with Burton's cooperation.[63]

ANTINEOPLASTONS

Antineoplaston treatment is an alternative biologic therapy offered by Dr. Stanislaw Burzynski at the Burzynski Research Institute in Houston. The treatment is based on the theory that medium-sized peptides normally present in urine are capable of controlling tumor growth and differentiating cancer cells in vivo. In the early 1970s Burzynski, then a faculty member at the Baylor College of Medicine, used gel filtration techniques to isolate peptides from normal urine that inhibited in vitro growth of several human cell lines.[64]

In 1977 Burzynski left Baylor to establish the Burzynski Research Institute. There, the initial peptide fraction, called antineoplaston A, was subfractionated into antineoplaston A_1, A_2, A_3, A_4, A_5, A_{10}, and AS2-1.[65] Each fraction is said to be composed of low-molecular-weight peptides in the 2000 to 5000 dalton range. The active component in each of these peptides has recently been identified as 3-[N-phenylacetylaminopiperidine]-2,5-dione, a substance that is not known to occur in urine.[65] In treating cancer patients, the dosage of each antineoplaston fraction is determined individually by first measuring pretreatment levels of antineoplastons in serum and urine. Burzynski claims that this ambient antineoplaston profile is a valuable aid in cancer diagnosis and also uses the assay to monitor response to antineoplaston therapy.[66]

The period of full-dose antineoplaston treatment may require from 6 weeks to more than a year.[67] Therapy is administered via Hickman catheter, although newly available capsules for oral administration "appear to produce better results in some forms of cancers."[67] The cost of each treatment (exclusive of monitoring and laboratory testing) is $45, regardless of dose, and the therapy is claimed to be nontoxic. The clinic accepts responsibility for billing third-party insurers, although a cash deposit of $5000 has been requested from patients at the beginning of therapy.[68]

In small phase I studies, clinical activity, including complete responses, is claimed in carcinoma of the lung, prostate, stomach, colon, breast, and bladder.[69–72] Independent confirmation of these results, however, has not yet occurred. A site visit to the Burzynski Research Institute by the Canadian Ministry of Health in 1982 found no evidence of therapeutic efficacy, and medical claims for antineoplaston treatments were subsequently disallowed in Canada.[73] In 1985 a follow-up of 36 antineoplaston-treated patients followed by 25 Canadian physicians found no evidence of partial or complete responses. Indeed, 34 of the 36 patients had died, and the only two survivors had had prior curative therapy.[74]

The NCI has always had a policy of investigating potential new treatments from alternative practitioners, so long as the methods could be evaluated and prioritized using the science criteria for development of other agents; that is, these unorthodox approaches should play on a level field with orthodox medicine. As part of an effort to uncover new leads from alternative medicine, NCI investigators from the Cancer Therapy Evaluation Program examined a series of best-case responses submitted by the Burzynski clinic.[75] Seven patients with primary brain tumors on no other therapy showed disease response on antineoplaston therapy. Based entirely on this clinical evidence, the NCI will sponsor a phase II trial of antineoplastons in high-grade glioma, low-grade glioma, anaplastic glioma, and pediatric brain tumors in 1993. The drug will be supplied by Burzynski, but the trials will be performed by NCI-supported investigators. We hope that well-implemented and impartial studies will determine, 15 years after broad clinical use, whether this approach has any merit.

METABOLIC THERAPIES

Current metabolic approaches to the treatment of cancer represent a wide spectrum of alternative interventions, including enzyme therapy, cellular therapy, dietary manipulation, vitamin treatment (including vitamin B_{17} [laetrile] and megavitamins), and detoxification with enzymes or hydrogen peroxide. In each case, cancer is viewed as a symptom of a more basic and underlying metabolic imbalance. Therefore, the metabolic therapist believes that cancer can be prevented and treated with metabolic interventions.

The idea is not new. In the early 1900s, Dr. William Koch prescribed a regimen of cancer treatment that was based on the theory that malignancies were nothing more than a protective response to toxic compounds generated within the body.[76] Cancer could be treated by oxidizing these toxic compounds with Koch's "antitoxin" preparation in combination with diet and enema therapy. Although Koch's antitoxin was, in essence, distilled water (Koch actually labeled the drug one part glyoxylide to one trillion parts water), the treatment was enormously popular and remains available today.[4]

There has been a renaissance of interest in the metabolic and holistic therapy of cancer. Treatments offered at these centers vary widely, depending on the philosophy of the program. For example, the International Health Institute was established by dentist William Kelley, who believes that cancer is caused by pancreatic enzyme deficiency. He developed the Kelley enzyme test or the "self-test for cancer." For a "donation" of $50, patients receive a nutritional lifestyle program and the procedure for the enzyme test. Patients are instructed to take six to eight pancreatic tablets after each meal for 4 weeks. The analysis then runs as follows:

> If at the end of this time:
> You feel worse, have a loss of appetite, nausea, headache, goopy, sick, toxic or in general listless: you can be assured there is a cancerous condition present in your body.
> You feel better, have more energy and a brighter, happier outlook: you can be assured there is a precancerous condition in your body.
> You feel no different: you can be reasonably assured there is not a cancerous condition present in your body.[77]

Overall, not very reassuring, although the institute's nutritional program explains "how to avoid cancer or how to proceed if you're a victim." The program might include a low-protein diet (buttermilk allowed), mineral supplements (for example, blackstrap molasses), yogurt enemas, and induced sweating.

Some of the clinics offer more "traditional" alternative treatments. For example, the Biomedical Center in Tijuana still uses herbal tonics based on Hoxsey's original methods. Most of the clinics have evolved with the times, however. Diet, an important component of many metabolic therapies, is especially emphasized by the East West Center for Macrobiotics and the Kushi Foundation. The emphasis here is on the traditional Oriental philosophy of yin and yang: cancers of "yin" organs (colon, stomach, bladder) are treated with "yang" foods (cooked vegetables, fruit, fish), and cancer of "yang" organs (lung, liver) are treated with "yin" food (raw vegetables, no fruit, no fish).[78–80] Kushi recommends that patients avoid meat, dairy products, sweets, processed foods, hot spices, and "toxic and unnatural" conventional cancer treatments.[81] Because the macrobiotic diet is deficient in calories, vitamins D and C, and iron, nutritional deficiencies have been reported in children and adults, and there is no evidence that this approach is useful as a cancer treatment.[82–88]

Others, most notably Dr. Linus Pauling, have espoused nutritional supplements as primary cancer treatment. Ewan Cameron, in the mid-1960s, hypothesized that vitamin C might inhibit tumor cell invasion and metastasis. The theory, also called the orthomolecular treatment of cancer, is predicated on the notion that vitamin C augments collagen production or stabilization and decreases tumor cell production of enzymes, such as hyaluridase, required for basement membrane invasion.[89,90] An initial clinical trial of high-dose vitamin C (10 g/day) appeared to improve survival, at least when compared with historical controls.[91] However, because of the problems inherent in this kind of retrospective analysis, the NCI supported two successive trials at the Mayo Clinic. The first, a standard phase II study, used vitamin C therapy in patients who had disease refractory to standard therapy; no evidence of tumor regression or subjective benefit was observed.[92] The second study was a randomized, double-blind, placebo-controlled trial of high-dose vitamin C in patients who had had no prior therapy; again, no evidence of tumor regression was observed.[93]

Interestingly, vitamin C can prevent development of carcinogen-induced malignancies in some animal models, and the NCI is supporting chemoprevention studies using vitamin C. However, available evidence now indicates that ascorbic acid has no role in primary cancer treatment.[94]

However, nutritional and megavitamin therapy for the treatment of cancer and other diseases has developed into a profitable health-fraud industry in the United States.[87,95] Here, practitioners can obtain degrees in "nutrition" by mail: $1000 for a bachelor's degree, $2000 for both bachelor's and master's degrees, and $4000 for bachelor's, master's, and PhD degrees.[96,97] Some diploma mills even provide a computer program that will prescribe specious nutritional supplements based on the patient's dietary history. In addition to high-dose vitamin C, these "health and wellness" clinics might prescribe:

Megadose vitamin A (3000 to 300,000 units/day) for "immune stimulation" and "epithelial integrity."[86] These doses of vitamin A are not known to have such effects and may, in fact, be associated with significant toxicity. Indeed, the ingestion of 5000 to 10,000 units of vitamin A for 30 days can cause increased intracranial pressure, fetal abnormalities, and hepatic and renal toxicity.[98,99]

Megadose vitamin E (up to 3200/IU/day) as an "antioxidant."[100] Vitamin E has no known use in cancer treatment. Although doses of 300 IU or less a day are considered nontoxic, increased triglycerides are seen at 600 IU/day, depression and fatigue at 900 IU/day, and nausea, diarrhea, headache, and blurred vision at 3200 IU/day.[101–103] Double-blind studies have shown no effect of vitamin E on work performance or libido, and high doses in experimental animals can cause teratogenesis, depressed bone calcification, and testicular atrophy.[101,104]

Vitamin B_{15} (also known as pangamic acid, 15, or pangamate). Vitamin B_{15} is not known to be a vitamin at all. Prescribed as a dietary supplement in health stores, analysis reveals that preparations consist of dimethylglycine hydrochloride (DMG) or diisopropylamine dichloroacetate (DIPA).[105] Both compounds are, indeed, known carcinogens of no nutritional value.[106,107] Although pangamic acid is illegal in the United States as either a drug or a vitamin, it remains freely available in health stores because the FDA cannot trace the thousands of vitamin B_{15} retailers.[88,108]

Most metabolic clinics offer a combined program of diet, vitamin therapy (sometimes including laetrile), and detoxification with wheatgrass therapy or coffee enemas. Again, the underlying principle for these approaches is the theory that reversing the metabolic imbalances that "actually caused" the malignancy will control or cure the disease. For example, the portal delivery of caffeine to the liver by a coffee enema is thought to increase bile production, alkalinize the intestine, and detoxify impurities.[109,110] Yet there are internal inconsistencies to the theory; for example, drinking coffee is prohibited during treatment.

The Centro Medico Del Mar in Mexico, established by Dr. Ernesto Contreras, also offers orthodox treatment in addition to its metabolic program of laetrile, cell therapy, interferon, and enzyme enemas. However, laboratory tests, chemotherapy, and surgery are not included in the cost of Contreras' 3-week program. Other practitioners, such as Hans Nieper of Germany, routinely include standard anticancer chemotherapy as part of a metabolic program that includes tumor vaccines, vitamin A, anavit (enzymes extracted from pineapple), squalene (shark-liver extract), carnivora (Venus flytrap extract), laetrile, and selenium and zinc (minerals that supposedly promote tissue healing). Should the tumor respond to effective drugs, practitioner and patient can ascribe the regression to the chemotherapy or any other aspect of the program.

IRIDOLOGY

Metabolic therapists may offer not only an unsound cancer treatment but also may compound the problem with unsound methods of cancer diagnosis. One such technique is iridology, the science of reading the iris to diagnose disease.[111,112] As shown in Figure 70–2, the iridologist studies a homunculus superimposed within the iris, and from the physiologic black stripes therein can make organ-specific diagnoses. Because the technique is purported to be more sensitive than standard diagnostic imaging techniques, the iridologist claims to be able to detect preclinical or subclinical disease. Of course, this can then be conveniently "cured" (*i.e.*, reversal of iris changes) with a medically useless intervention. Double-blind studies in which ophthalmologists and iridologists have examined photographs from patients and healthy controls have shown the technique to be without merit.[113,114] Still, iridology is a common technique for diagnosing disease and following therapeutic response in homeopathic and metabolic clinics.

INVESTIGATING ALTERNATIVE THERAPIES

There have been two recent attempts to investigate the clinical efficacy of alternative therapies. These studies are important because they were conducted with the approval of the unorthodox clinic by impartial investigators trained in science. Cassileth and coworkers studied 158 matched cohorts of patients with metastatic or recurrent colon cancer treated at either the Livingston-Wheeler Clinic in San Diego (autogenous immune-enhancing vaccine, bacillus Calmette-Guérin, vegetarian diet, and coffee enemas) or the University of Pennsylvania.[115] Although there was no difference in survival between these two groups, the quality of life was significantly and uniformly better in those patients receiving only conventional care. This study, then, does not support the assumption

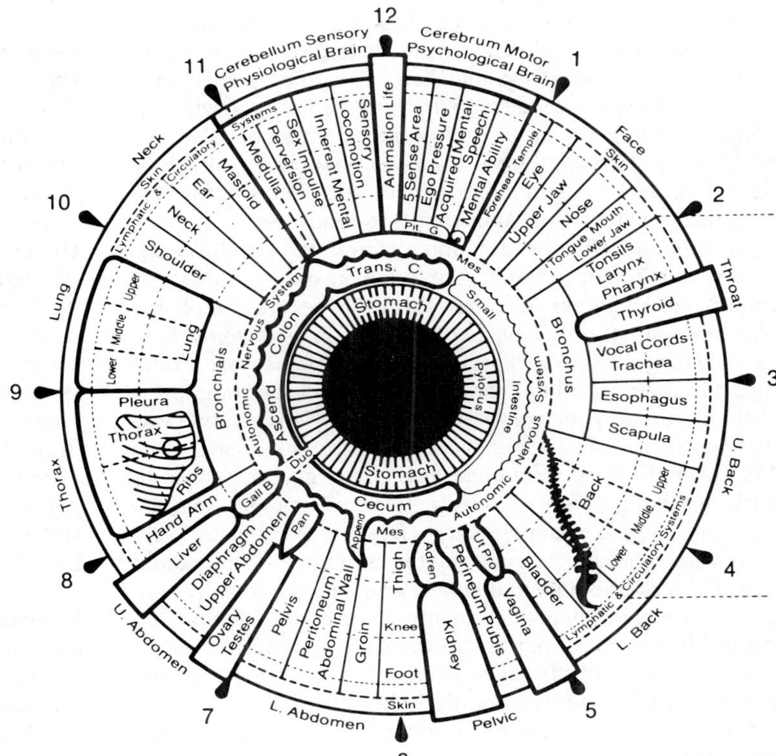

FIGURE 70–2. The iridology homunculus. Metabolic and holistic practitioners commonly use changes in the iris to diagnose organ-specific cancer and follow "disease response." Although inexpensive and noninvasive, iridology is also useless. (Adapted from Worrall RS. Iridology: Diagnosis or delusion. In: Stalker D, Glymour C, eds. Examining holistic medicine. Buffalo: Prometheus, 1985)

that alternative therapies (with emphasis on self-help and absence of the toxicity of conventional treatments) lead to a better quality of life.

The Bristol Cancer Help Centre (BCHC) was established in Great Britain in 1979 to offer a more holistic approach to cancer treatment, including a vegetarian diet, counseling, healing, and development of a more positive attitude. Patients also may continue conventional treatment. Bagenal and associates studied 334 women with breast cancer followed for 3 years at BCHC, comparing them with 461 consecutive breast-cancer patients seen at a single cancer center or two general hospitals over the same time period.[116] Overall, women seen at BCHC were about twice as likely to die from their disease and three times more likely to develop metastases as women receiving conventional care. These results must be interpreted with caution, however, since the BCHC cohort was significantly younger than the more general population. However, for the first time, alternative approaches are being evaluated scientifically, and preliminary evidence does not suggest any clinical advantage.

THE SIMONTON METHOD: AN UNPROVEN ADJUNCT TO CANCER TREATMENT

There is one unproven (as opposed to unsound) method that deserves mention in this chapter, if only because of its current popularity. The Simonton method of relaxation and imagery is basically a self-help program designed to be used in conjunction with standard medical treatment.[117] The program is described in detail in Dr. O. Simonton's best-selling book *Getting Well Again*.[118] The techniques, which are simple and largely easily self-taught, include a program of relaxation and mental imagery performed three times daily, drawing analysis, identification and reduction of stress, exercise, counseling or group therapy, and a "sensible diet." Since first published in 1978, the book has gone through over 20 editions. Stephanie Matthews-Simonton has recently written another popular text, *The Healing Family*, which describes now family members can participate in the Simonton method.[119] There is nothing here that is patently unsound, but is it of any use?

Dr. Simonton first became interested in the psychological factors that might influence treatment response during his training in radiation oncology. In 1975 he and Stephanie Matthews-Simonton published a study in *The Journal of Transpersonal Psychology* in which 152 patients were examined for their "attitude" profile at the time of completing radiation therapy for a variety of cancers. This attitude was then retrospectively correlated with treatment responses.[120] Not surprisingly, patients who had had a good response to radiation therapy were optimistic; those with progressive disease had a sense of hopelessness. Despite the obvious problems with this kind of analysis, the Simontons conjectured that stress, depression, and hopelessness might actually contribute directly (independent of other behavior such as smoking or alcohol consumption) to the development of cancer. For example, in *Getting Well Again* the Simontons note that several studies have temporally linked the development of cancer to severe psychological trauma, such as the loss of a loved one.[121–124]

In a leap of faith, the Simontons hypothesized that positive thinking and stress reduction might be useful as therapy and established the Cancer Counseling and Research Center (recently renamed the Simonton Cancer Center) in Fort Worth, Texas, to teach and administer their program. The center conducts regular counseling and training workshops for patients and professionals. A 10-day "phase I" program of group therapy, training in relaxation and imagery, and counseling, intended primarily for patients, is offered at the Simonton's Southern California clinic. In addition, more extensive "phase II" workshops are conducted to instruct professionals in the Simonton techniques; more than 4000 such counselors have been trained.[125] Finally, the Simontons have produced a series of audiotape cassettes describing the program that can be purchased by mail.[126]

In today's climate of "self-help" or "how-to" literature, the Simonton techniques have become enormously popular, and there are certain appealing facets to the program. It is relatively inexpensive and recommended only as an adjunct to proven therapy. An American Cancer Society review notes other potentially positive aspects to the method: it gives the patient a sense of control, promotes relaxation and well-being, and has no known deleterious effects.[127] R.M. Mack, a physician with metastatic lung cancer, detailed the usefulness of the Simonton techniques in a deeply personal note in *The New England Journal of Medicine,* and equal praise has appeared in other journals as well.[128–132]

However, the literature on mindset and cancer is much more confused than the Simontons would have us believe. For example, *Getting Well Again* limits its discussion to studies in which development of cancer has followed bereavement and asks the reader to accept that depression and carcinogenesis are causally linked. Alternative explanations are not discussed. For example, a patient under stress may be more likely to visit a doctor—behavior that might lead to early detection.[133] Moreover, as Wellisch and Yager discuss in their excellent review, "Is There a Cancer-Prone Personality?," the studies that link depression and disease use faulty personality measurements, have inherent selection bias, and are statistically imprecise.[134] Indeed, there is an equal body of evidence to suggest that no relationship between psychological attitude and cancer exists.[135–137] For example, a controlled study demonstrated no correlation between psychological attributes and development of breast cancer.[136] A 24-year follow-up comparison of a large number of World War II veterans discharged because of "psychoneurosis" showed no increase in cancer incidence compared with controls.[138] A carefully controlled 22-year study of 191 chronically depressed patients demonstrated an incidence of cancer equal to age-matched controls.[139] A recent, well-controlled, prospective study indicated that attitude appears to have no effect on time to recurrence or survival of patients with stage II breast cancer or high-risk melanoma.[140] Indeed, animal studies suggest that stress has a protective effect in carcinogenesis and can inhibit the growth of implanted experimental tumors.[141]

By ignoring this information, the Simontons fail to acknowledge that this is an area of controversy; indeed, although some of these studies have appeared since the first printing of *Getting Well Again*, the book has remained unrevised through more than 20 printings.[142] Friedlander has written a balanced review of the Simonton hypothesis and concludes, correctly, that the method is unproven.[143] Only well-designed negative studies can show if it is unsound.

PATIENT CHARACTERISTICS AND THE ROLE OF HEALTH PROVIDERS

Logic might suggest that patients who adopt unsound methods of cancer treatment might be unsophisticated consumers with diseases for which there is no effective standard therapy. However, analysis in this area once again defies logic. In one important review of the contemporary popularity of unsound cancer treatments, Cassileth and coworkers compared 304 cancer inpatients at the University of Pennsylvania Cancer Center with 356 cancer patients under the care of 138 alternative practitioners at 19 clinics.[2] In decreasing order of popularity, unsound or unproven cancer treatments included metabolic therapy (161 patients), diet (134 patients), megavitamins (92 patients), imagery (89 patients), spiritual healing (71 patients), and immunotherapy (57 patients). Practitioners of unsound therapies were likely to be physicians (60%) and 18% had subspecialty boards. Insurance covered some costs of treatment in a third of the patients being treated.

When compared with patients being treated with standard therapy, those adopting unsound or unproven (imagery) approaches were more likely to be white ($p>0.00001$) and better educated ($p>0.00001$). Of these, patients who selected imagery were the most educated, with 79% having some college education. This finding is also supported by the recent FDA telephone survey of 6000 American households in which higher levels of education were the single best predictor of likelihood to adopt an unsound treatment approach.[3]

Another surprising finding of the Cassileth study is that patients who opted for unsound therapy were more likely to be asymptomatic and have earlier (and perhaps more conventionally curable) stages of disease. Of the 325 patients concomitantly receiving both standard and unsound treatments, 40% discontinued standard therapy in favor of the unorthodox approach. One expected finding was that patients who opted for nontraditional care distrusted the medical establishment.

There are some important lessons for health professionals in this analysis. Patients who seek alternative or unsound cancer therapies are intelligent and inquisitive and unlikely to be persuaded that an approach is useless simply because the proponent lacks scientific credentials or has not published in peer-reviewed journals. Moreover, those who offer these useless approaches are generally convinced that they can help the patient. The clinician needs to understand and be able to discuss the seemingly attractive although useless treatments patients hear about through the media or from well-intentioned friends.

There are various sources of updated information on unsound remedies. The American Cancer Society and the American Society of Clinical Oncology maintain committees that critically review and publish the facts on questionable treatments. Other organizations, such as the National Council Against Health Fraud (Box 1276, Loma Linda, CA 92354), the Center for Medical Consumers and Health Care Information (237 Thompson Street, New York, NY 10012), the Consumer Product Safety Commission (Food & Drug Administration, Rockville, MD 20892), and the National Consumer League (1028 Connecticut Avenue, NW, Washington, DC 20036), have additional consumer-oriented information.

However, the most important protection against health fraud is the practitioner's willingness to discuss the disease and available treatments in an open and supportive fashion.[144,145] The NCI's Physician Data Query computer database on current state-of-the-art (phase III) and scientifically sound experimental (phase I and II) therapies is a useful resource in guiding patients to the best available care. In addition, a recent NCI booklet, *What Are Clinical Trials All About?*, is a helpful educational tool that explains how bona-fide clinical studies are performed and gives patients the information they need to know to learn if a trial is logical and well-run.[146] In today's world of alternative treatments, education has replaced legislation as the first defense against unsound cancer therapy.

REFERENCES

1. Quackery: A $10 billion scandal. Subcommittee on Health and Long-Term Care, of the Select Committee on Aging, House of Representatives, 98th Congress, 2d session, 1984 (Committee publication 98-435).
2. Cassileth BR, Lusk EJ, Strouse TB, Badenheimer BA. Contemporary unorthodox treatments in cancer medicine: A study of patients, treatments and practitioners. Ann Intern Med 1984;101:105–112.
3. Louis Harris Survey on the Use of Questionable Cancer Products. Food and Drug Administration, Division of Consumer Affairs, 1987.
4. Jansen WF. Cancer quackery, the past in the present. Semin Oncol 1976;6:526–536.
5. Why the FDA doesn't crack down. Consumer Reports, May 1985:282–284.
6. Reich W. The Orgone Energy Accumulator: Its scientific and medical use. Rangeley, Maine: Orgone Institute Press, 1951.
7. Reich W. Selected writings, an introduction to orgonomy. New York: Farrar, Strauss & Cudahy, 1960.
8. Reich W. Cosmic superimposition: Man's orgonotic roots in nature. Rangeley, Maine: Wilhelm Reich Foundation, 1951.
9. Orgone energy devices. In: Unproven methods of cancer management. New York: American Cancer Society, 1975:176.
10. Hart FJ, ed. Electronic Medical Digest. San Francisco: Electronic Medical Foundation, 1952.
11. Young J. The medical messiahs: A social history of health quackery in 20th-century America. Princeton, NJ: Princeton University Press, 1987.
12. Milstead JL, Davis JB, Dubiele M. Quackery in the medical device field. Proceedings of the Second National Congress on Medical Quackery, 1963:30–35.
13. Hoxsey HM. You don't have to die—The amazing story of the Hoxsey cancer treatment. New York: Milestone Books, 1956.
14. Food and Drug Administration. Report on the background of Harry M. Hoxsey and the Hoxsey Cancer Center, 1952.
15. Mather JM, et al. Report of a committee of faculty members of the University of British Columbia concerning the Hoxsey treatment for cancer. December 19, 1957.
16. FDA Notices of Judgment DD 5654, 5212 and 5202.
17. Press Release HEW-020, U.S. Department of Health, Education & Welfare, Food & Drug Administration, September 21, 1960.
18. Durovic S. Cancer and krebiozen: A new concept in cancer. Today Japan Orient West 1961;6:51–55.
19. Report of the Director, National Cancer Institute, to the Secretary, Department of Health, Education and Welfare, concerning decision of the Institute not to undertake clinical testing of krebiozen. Released October 16, 1963.
20. FDA Notices of Judgment No. 121, FDA Papers, June 1968, p. 43.
21. Hartwell W. Dr. Ivy: Life begins anew at 74. Chicago's American, April 2, 1967.
22. Vierhover A, Mach H. Biochemistry of amygdalin. Am J Pharm 1935;197:392–450.
23. Greenberg DM. The vitamin fraud in cancer quackery. West J Med 1975;122:345–348.
24. Beard HH. A new approach to the conquest of cancer, rheumatic and heart disease. New York: Pageant Press, 1958.
25. Robiquet B. Les amande ameres et l'iele volafle qu'elles focurscent. Ann Chim Phys 1830;14:352–382.
26. Van Meter CT, Gennaro AR. Natural products. In Remington's pharmaceutical sciences, 14th ed. Easton, Pa.: Merck, 1915:474–475.
27. Dorr RT, Paxinos J. The current status of laetrile. Ann Int Med 1978;89:389–397.
28. Gal EM, Fung FH, Greenberg DM. Studies on the biological action of malonitriles. II. Distribution of rhodanese (transulfurase) in tumor-bearing animals, and the effect of malonitriles thereon. Cancer Res 1952;12:574–579.
29. Conchie J, Findley J, Levvy GA. Mammalian glycosidases: Distribution in the body. Biochemistry 1959;71:318–325.
30. Koeffler PH, Lowe L, Golde DL. Amygdalin (laetrile): Effect of clonogenic cell from human myeloid leukemia cells and normal human marrow. Cancer Treat Rep 1980;64:105–110.
31. Stock CC, Martin DS, Suiguira K, et al. Antitumor tests of amygdalin in animal tumor system. Surg Oncol 1978;10:81–88.
32. Wodinsky I, Swiniarski J. Antitumor activity of amygdalin set on a spectrum of transplantable rodent tumors. Cancer Chemo Rep 1975;59:939–950.
33. Laster WR, Schabel FM. Experimental studies of the antitumor activity of amygdalin MF (NSC 15780) above and in combination with beta-glucosidase (NSC 128056). Cancer Chemo Rep 1975;59:957–965.
34. Toxicity of laetrile. FDA Drug Bull 1977;7:25.

35. Laetrile, not so harmless. Emerg Med 1978;10:155–156.
36. Bickis IJ, Quastel JH. Effects of metabolic inhibitors on energy metabolism of Ehrlich ascites carcinoma cells. Nature 1965;205:44–46.
37. Browne WE, Wood CD, Smith AW. Sodium cyanide as a cancer chemotherapeutic agent: Laboratory and clinical studies. Am J Obstet Gynecol 1960;80:907–915.
38. Perry IH. The effect of prolonged cyanide treatment on body and tumor growth in rats. Am J Cancer 1935;25:592–598.
39. Kittler GD. Laetrile: Control for cancer, the authorized story. New York: Paperback Library, 1963.
40. Edwards CC. Statement before the Subcommittee on Intergovernmental Relations of the Committee on Government Operations. June 9, 1970:21–22.
41. Levi L, French WW, Bickis IJ, Henderson WB. Laetrile: A study of its physiochemical and biochemical properties. Can Med Assoc J 1965;92:1057–1061.
42. Davignon P, Trissel LA, Kleinman LM. Pharmaceutical assessment of amygdalin (laetrile products). Cancer Treat Rep 1978;62:99–104.
43. Diamond GEB. Cancer research: Who profits? Harvard Political Review 1977;5(3): 17–21.
44. Lerner IJ. The whys of cancer quackery. Cancer 1984;53:815–819.
45. Ingelfinger FJ. Laetrilomania. N Engl J Med 1977;296:1167–1168.
46. Rutherford vs. United States, 524F 2d 1137 (10th Cir 1976).
47. Ellison NM, Byar DP, Newell GR. Results of the National Cancer Institute's retrospective laetrile analysis. N Engl J Med 1978;299:549–557.
48. California Medical Association, Cancer Commission: The treatment of cancer with "laetrile." Calif Med 1953;78:320–326.
49. Moertel CG. A trial of laetrile now. N Engl J Med 1977;298:218–219.
50. Moertel CG, Ames MM, Kovach JS, et al. A pharmacologic and toxicological study of amygdalin. JAMA 1978;255:591–594.
51. Moertel CG, Fleming TR, Rubins J, et al. A phase II trial of amygdalin (laetrile) in human cancer. N Engl J Med 1982;306:201–206.
52. Immunoaugmentative therapy. Food and Drug Administration publication T82-14. Rockville, MD: U.S. Department of Health and Human Services, 1982.
53. Immunoaugmentative therapy: Cancer research and treatment (IAT Information Center patient brochure). Freeport, Bahamas: Immunology Researching Center, 1984.
54. Report to the Ministry of Health of Bahamas on the site visit to the Immunology Researching Center, Ltd., Freeport, Grand Bahamas Island, Bahamas. Washington DC: Pan-American Health Organization, Regional Office of the World Health Organization, 1978:29–31.
55. The cancer therapeutic research act. Fla. Stat. 402.36, 1982.
56. The immunoaugmentative therapy act, Oklahoma House Bill 1633, 1982.
57. Page H. Easy "cures" for cancer still support. JAMA 1981;246:714–715.
58. Curt GA, Katterhagen G, Mahaney FX. Immunoaugmentative therapy: A primer on the perils of unproven treatment. JAMA 1986;255:505–507.
59. Curt GA. Warning on immunoaugmentative therapy. N Engl J Med 1984;311:859.
60. Cutaneous nocardiosis in cancer patients receiving immunotherapy—Bahamas. MMWR 1984;33:471–477.
61. Burton L. Immunoaugmentative therapy. Read before the Fourth Annual "Health by Choice" Conference, Atlanta, May 1983.
62. Isolation of human T-lymphotropic virus type III/lymphoadenopathy-associated virus from serum proteins given to cancer patients—Bahamas. MMWR 1985;34:489–490.
63. Congressional Office of Technology Assessment Report. U.S. Congress, Office of Technology Assessment, Unconventional Cancer Treatments, OTA-H-405. Washington, DC: U.S. Government Printing Office, September 1990.
64. Burzynski SR, Georgiades J. Effect of urinary peptides on DNA, RNA and protein synthesis in normal and neoplastic cells. Fed Proc 1973;32:766.
65. Burzynski SR. Antineoplastons: History of research. Drugs Exper Clin Res 1986;12: 1–9.
66. Liau MC, Szopa M, Burzynski B, Burzynski SR. Quantitative assay of plasma and urinary peptides as an aid for the evaluation of cancer patients undergoing antineoplaston therapy. Drugs Exper Clin Res 1986(Suppl 2);13:61–70.
67. Burzynski Research Institute, Houston, TX. Patient information brochure, undated.
68. Antineoplastons. CA 1983;33:57–59.
69. Burzynski SR, Kubove E. Toxicology studies on antineoplaston A_{10} injections in cancer patients. Drug Exper Clin Res 1987(Suppl 1);12:1–12.
70. Burzynski SR, Kubove E. Initial clinical study with antineoplaston A_2 injections in cancer patients with 5 years follow-up. Drug Exper Clin Res 1987(Suppl 1);12:1–12.
71. Burzynski SR, Kubove E, Burzynski B. Phase I clinical studies of antineoplaston A_3 injections. Drug Exper Clin Res 1987(Suppl 1);13:37–43.
72. Burzynski SR, Kubove E, Burzynski B. Phase I clinical studies of antineoplaston A_5 injections. Drug Exper Clin Res 1987(Suppl 1);13:37–43.
73. Blackstein and Sagal. The treatment of cancer patients with antineoplastons at the Burzynski Clinic in Houston, Tex. Report to the Ministry of Health, Province of Ontario, 1982.
74. Antineoplastons A2, AS2-1, A_3, A_5 and A_{10}. Memorandum from JD Sproul, Bureau of Prescription Drugs, to Dr. Ian Henderson, Director, Toronto, Ontario, Canada, March 15, 1985.
75. Mead JAR. Developmental Therapeutics Program, NCI: Letter to JD Sproul. Preclinical evaluation of antineoplastons by Southern Research Institute, December 1, 1983.
76. Koch WF. A new and successful treatment and diagnosis of cancer. Detroit Medical Journal, July 1979.
77. Kelley WD. One answer to cancer—An ecological approach to the successful management of malignancy. Grapevine, TX: The Kelley Research Foundation, 1969.
78. Kohler JC, Kohler MA. Healing miracles from macrobiotics: A diet for all diseases. New York: Parker, 1979.
79. Esko E. The cancer prevention diet. Brookline, MA: East West Foundation, 1981.
80. Enloe CH. Yin Yang and Mao. Nutrition Today 1974;9:24.
81. Kushi M. A dietary approach to cancer. In: Diet and Cancer. Brookline, MA: East West Foundation, 1981.
82. Sherlock P, Rothchild EO. Scurvy produced by a Zen macrobiotic diet. JAMA 1987;199: 794–798.
83. Roberts IF, West RJ, Ogilvie D, et al. Malnutrition in Infants receiving cult diets: A form of child abuse. Br Med J 1979;1:296–298.
84. Robson JRK, Konlande JE, Larkin FA, et al. Zen macrobiotic dieting problems in infancy. Pediatrics 1974;53:326–329.
85. Bowman BB, Kushner RF, Dawson SC, Levin B. Macrobiotic diets for cancer treatment and prevention. J Clin Oncol 1984;2:702–711.
86. Herbert V. Unproven (questionable) dietary and nutritional methods in cancer prevention and treatment. Cancer 1986;58:1930–1941.
87. Herbert V. Faddism and quackery in cancer nutrition. Nutr Cancer 1984;6:196–206.
88. Shils ME, Hermann MG. Unproved dietary claims in the treatment of patients with cancer. Bull NY Acad Med 1982;58:323–340.
89. Cameron E, Campbell A. The orthomolecular treatment of cancer. Clinical trial of high-dose ascorbic acid supplements in advanced human cancer. Chem Biol Interact 1974;9:285–315.
90. Cameron E. Hyaluronidase and cancer. New York: Pergamon Press, 1966.
91. Cameron E, Pauling L. Supplemental ascorbate in the supportive treatment of cancer: Prolongation of survival times in terminal human cancer. Proc Natl Acad Sci USA 1976;73:3685–3689.
92. Greagen ET, Moertel CG, O'Fallon JR, et al. Failure of high-dose vitamin C (ascorbic acid) therapy to benefit patients with advanced cancer. N Engl J Med 1979;301:687–690.
93. Moertel CG, Fleming TR, Creagen ET, et al. High-dose vitamin C versus placebo in the treatment of patients with advanced cancer who have had no prior therapy: A randomized double-blind comparison. N Engl J Med 1985;312:137–141.
94. Abdel-Galil AM. Preventive effect of vitamin C (L-ascorbic acid) on methylcholanthrene-induced soft tissue sarcomas in mice. Oncology 1986;43:335–337.
95. Herbert V, Barnet S. Vitamins and "health" foods: The great American hustle. Philadelphia: George F. Stickley, 1981.
96. Herbert V, Jarvis WT, Monaco GP. Commentary: Obstacles to nutrition education. Health Values 1983;7:38–41.
97. Herbert V. Will questionable nutrition overwhelm nutrition? Sci Am J Clin Nutr 1981;34: 2848–2853.
98. Yaffe SF, Filer LJ Jr. Use and abuse of vitamin A. In ADA Handbook of Clinical Dietetics. New Haven: Yale University Press, 1981:81–83.
99. Dubiele MA, Rucker RB. Dietary supplements and health foods. A critical evaluation—vitamins and minerals. J Nutr Ed 1983;2:47–53.
100. Jukes TH. Megavitamins and food fads. In: Hodes RE, ed. Human nutrition, Vol. 4. New York: Plenum Press, 1979:257–292.
101. Tsai AC, Kelley JJ, Peng B, Cook N. Study on the effect of megavitamin E supplementation in man. Am J Clin Nutr 1978;31:831–837.
102. DiPalma JR, Richie DM. Vitamin toxicity. Am Rev Pharm Toxicol 1977;17:133–148.
103. Anderson TW. Vitamin E in angina pectoris. Can Med Assoc J 1974;110:401–406.
104. Roberts HJ. Perspective on vitamin E as therapy. JAMA 1981;246:129–131.
105. Herbert V. Pangamic acid (vitamin B_{15}). Am J Clin Nutr 1979;32:1534–1540.
106. Colman N, Herbert V, Bardner A, Gelernt M. Mutagenicity of dimethylglycine when mixed with nitrite: Possible significance in human use of pangamates. Proc Soc Exp Biol Med 1980;164:9–12.
107. Gelernt MD, Herbert V. Mutagenicity of diisopropylamine dichloroacetate, the "active constituent" of vitamin B_{15} (pangamic acid). Nutr Cancer 1982;3:129–133.
108. McPherrin EW, Herbert V, Herbert R. Vitamin B_{15}: Anatomy of a health fraud. New York: American Council of Science and Health, 1981.
109. Manner HW, DiSanti SJ, Michalsen TL. The death of cancer. Chicago: Advanced Century Publishing Corporation, 1978.
110. Eisele JWS, Reay DT. Deaths related to coffee enemas. JAMA 1980;244:1608–1609.
111. Banner D. Applied iridology and herbology. Orem, UT: Bioworld Publishers, 1982.
112. Worrall RS. Iridology: Diagnosis or delusion? In: Stalker D, Glymour C, eds. Examining holistic medicine. Buffalo: Prometheus Books, 1985:167–179.
113. Simon A, Worthen DM, Mites JA. An evaluation of iridology. JAMA 1979;242:1385–1387.
114. Worrall RS. Pseudoscience—A critical look at iridology. J Am Optom Assoc 1984;55: 735–739.
115. Cassileth BR, Lusk EJ, Guerry D, et al. Survival and quality of life among patients receiving unproven compared with conventional cancer therapy. N Engl J Med 1991;324:1180–1185.
116. Bagenal FS, Eastor DF, Harris E, et al. Survival of patients with breast cancer attending Bristol Cancer Help Centre. Lancet 1990;336:606–610.
117. Simonton Cancer Counseling and Research Center brochure, undated.
118. Simonton OC, Matthews-Simonton S, Creighton JL. Getting well again. New York: Bantam, 1980.
119. Matthews-Simonton S. The healing family. New York: Bantam, 1984.
120. Simonton OC, Matthews-Simonton S. Belief systems and management of the emotional aspects of malignancy. J Transpersonal Psychology 1975;7:29–47.
121. Greene WA, Young LE, Swisher SW. Psychological factors and reticuloendothelial disease: Observations on a group of women with lymphomas and leukemias. Psychosom Med 1956;18:1252–303.
122. Greene WA. The psychosocial setting of the development of lymphoma and leukemia. Ann NY Acad Sci 1966;164:394–406.
123. Schamle AH, Iker HP. The effect of hopelessness in the development of cancer in women with atypical cytology. Psychosom Med 1964;26:634–635.
124. LeShan L, Worthington RE. Some recurrent life history patterns observed in patients with malignant disease. J Ment Dis 1954;124:460–465.

125. Kolata G. Texas counselors use psychology in cancer therapy. Smithsonian 1980:49–56.
126. Publications CCRC brochure, undated.
127. Simonton OC. Unproven methods of cancer management. CA 1982;32:58–61.
128. Mack RM. Lessons from living with cancer. N Engl J Med 1984;311:1640–1644.
129. Kennedy AM. Coping with cancer: New ways to deal with its physic devastation. Medical World News, Oct. 15, 1979:36–46.
130. Scarf M. Images that heal: A doubtful idea whose time has come. Psychology Today 1986;14:32–46.
131. Kirsch ML. The Simonton method of visualization: Nursing implications and a patient's perspective. Cancer Nursing 1980;3:295–300.
132. Wright ME. Book review of Getting Well Again. Contemporary Psychology 1979;24: 1019–1020.
133. Hanley CA. Illness behavior and psychosocial correlates of cancer. Soc Sci Med 1977;11: 223–225.
134. Wellisch DK, Yager J. Is there a cancer-prone personality? CA 1983;33:145–153.
135. Graham S, Snell LM, Graham JB, et al. Social trauma in the epidemiology of cancer of the cervix. J Chronic Dis 1971;24:711–725.
136. Green S, Maris T. Psychological attributes of women who develop breast cancer: A controlled study. J Psychosom Res 1975;19:147–153.
137. Muslin HL, Gyarfas K, Pieper WJ. Separation experience and cancer of the breast. Ann NY Acad Sci 1966;125:802–806.
138. Keehn RJ, Goldberg ID, Beebe GW. 24-Year follow-up of any veteran with disability separations for psychoneurosis in 1944. Psychosom Med 1978;26:27–46.
139. Niani T, Jasskleainen J. Cancer morbidity in depression persons. J Psychosom Res 1978;22:117–120.
140. Cassileth B, Lusk EJ, Miller DS, Brown LL, Miller C. Psychosocial correlates of survival in advanced malignant disease. N Engl J Med 1984;312:1551–1555.
141. Fox BH. Current theory of psychogenic effects on cancer incidence and prognosis. J Psychosoc Oncol 1983;1:17–31.
142. Fox BH. Premorbid psychological factors as related to cancer. J Behavioral Med 1978;1: 45–133.
143. Friedlander ER. Dream your cancer away: The Simontons. In: Stalker D, Glymour C, eds. Examining holistic medicine. Buffalo: Prometheus Books, 1985:273–285.
144. Monaco GP. The primary care physician: The first line of defense in the battle against health fraud. Medical Times 1986;114:43–48.
145. Jarvis W. Helping your patients deal with questionable cancer treatments. CA 1986;36: 293–301.
146. Nealon E. What are clinical trials all about? NIH Publication No. 86-2706, 1986.

Index

Page numbers followed by *f* indicate figures; those followed by *t* indicate tabular material; **CF** indicates color figures.

B

D

F

H

I

M

N

P

Q

R

S

T

U

ISBN 0-397-51323-2

DIVISION OF RADIATION ONCOLOGY
UNIVERSITY HOSPITALS
410 WEST 10TH AVENUE
COLUMBUS, OHIO

DIVISION OF RADIATION ONCOLOGY
UNIVERSITY HOSPITALS
410 WEST 10TH AVENUE
COLUMBUS, OHIO